TEXTBOOK
OF
ENDOCRINOLOGY

Sixth Edition

Edited by

ROBERT H. WILLIAMS, M.D.

Late Head of the Division of Endocrinology and Metabolism,
University Hospital; Professor of Medicine, School of
Medicine, University of Washington, Seattle

With Contributions by Forty-nine Authorities

W. B. SAUNDERS COMPANY

PHILADELPHIA • LONDON • TORONTO • MEXICO CITY • RIO DE JANEIRO • SYDNEY • TOKYO

W. B. Saunders Company: West Washington Square
Philadelphia, Pa. 19105

1 St. Anne's Road
Eastbourne, East Sussex BN21 3UN, England

1 Goldthorne Avenue
Toronto, Ontario M8Z 5T9, Canada

Apartado 26370 — Cedro 512
Mexico 4, D.F., Mexico

Rua Coronel Cabrita, 8
Sao Cristovao Caixa Postal 21176
Rio de Janeiro, Brazil

9 Waltham Street
Artarmon, N.S.W. 2064, Australia

Ichibancho, Central Bldg., 22-1 Ichibancho
Chiyoda-Ku, Tokyo 102, Japan

Library of Congress Cataloging in Publication Data

Williams, Robert Hardin.

Textbook of endocrinology.

1. Clinical endocrinology.   I. Title. [DNLM: 1. Endocrine
  diseases.   2. Endocrine glands. WK100 T355]

RC648.W55 1981   616.4   79–67306

ISBN 0–7216–9398–9

Listed here is the latest translated edition of this book together with
the language of the translation and the publisher.

Polish (*3rd Edition*) — Lekarskich, Warsaw, Poland

Spanish (*5th Edition*) — Salvat Editores, Barcelona, Spain

French (*4th Edition*) — Flammarion, Paris, France

Italian (*5th Edition*) — Piccin Editore, Padova, Italy

Japanese (*5th Edition*) — Hirokawa Publishing Company, Tokyo, Japan

Serbo-Croat (*4th Edition*) — Medicinska Knjiga, Belgrade, Yugoslavia

Textbook of Endocrinology

ISBN 0-7216-9398-9

Last digit is the print number: 9   8   7   6   5   4   3   2

CONTRIBUTORS

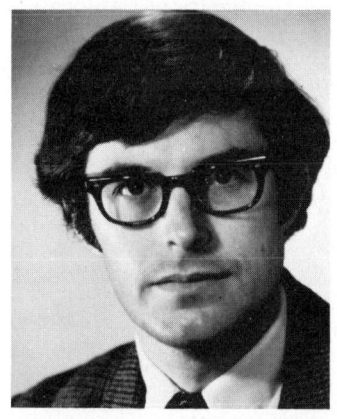

JOHN W. ADAMSON, M.D.
Professor of Medicine, University of Washington School of Medicine; Chief, Hematology Section, Veterans Administration Medical Center, Seattle.

Hormones and the Formed Elements of the Blood

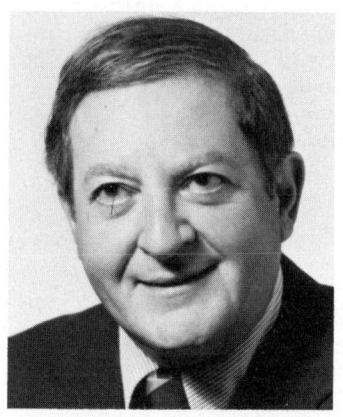

G. D. AURBACH, M.D.
Chief, Metabolic Diseases Branch, National Institutes of Health, Bethesda.

Parathyroid Hormone, Calcitonin, and the Calciferols

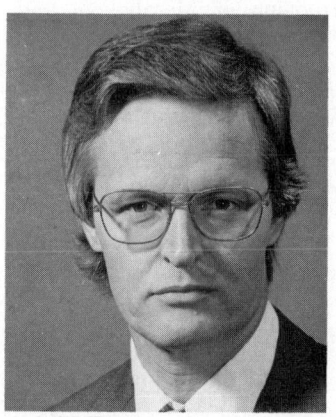

C. WAYNE BARDIN, M.D.
Director, Center for Biomedical Research, The Population Council, New York.

The Testes

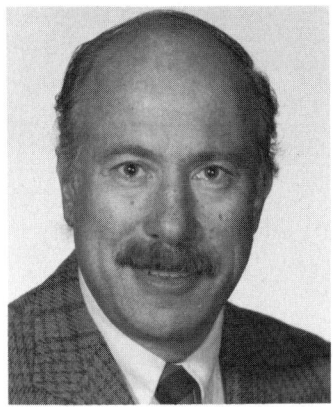

EDWIN L. BIERMAN, M.D.

Professor of Medicine, Head, Division of Metabolism and Endocrinology, University of Washington School of Medicine; Attending Physician, University of Washington Affiliated Hospitals, Seattle.
Disorders of Lipid Metabolism; Obesity; Aging and Hormones

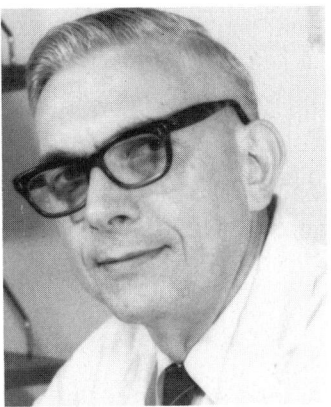

ROBERT M. BLIZZARD, M.D.

Professor and Chairperson, Department of Pediatrics, University of Virginia School of Medicine, Charlottesville.
Autoimmunity and Endocrine Disease

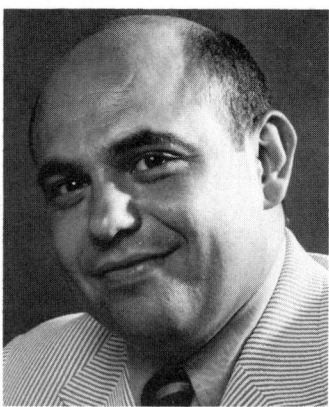

FELIX A. CONTE, M.D.

Associate Professor of Pediatrics, University of California, San Francisco.
Disorders of Sex Differentiation

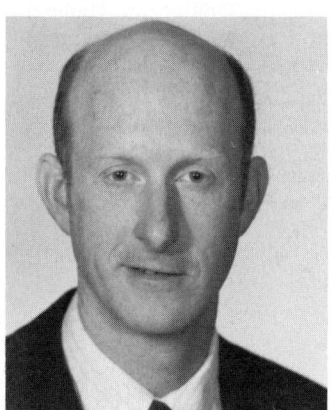

DAVID C. DALE, M.D.

Professor of Medicine, University of Washington School of Medicine; Attending Physician, University of Washington Hospital, Seattle.
Hormones and the Formed Elements of the Blood

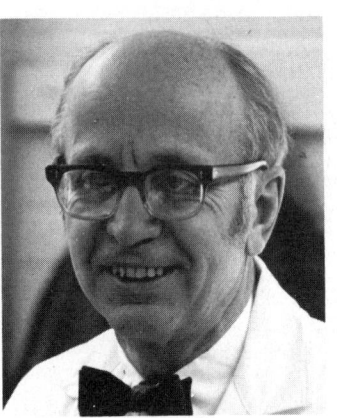

WILLIAM H. DAUGHADAY, M.D.

Professor of Medicine, Washington University School of Medicine; Physician, Barnes Hospital, St. Louis.
The Adenohypophysis

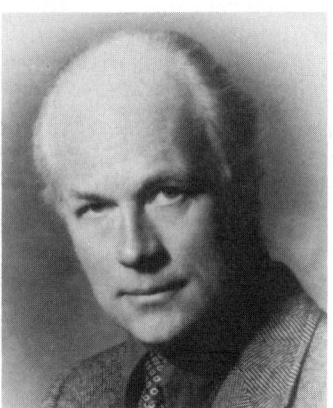

JOHN W. ENSINCK, M.D.

Professor of Medicine, University of Washington School of Medicine; Program Director, Clinical Research Center, University Hospital, Seattle.
Disorders Causing Hypoglycemia

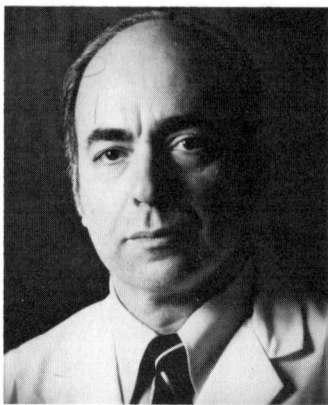

DANIEL D. FEDERMAN, M.D.

Professor of Medicine, Harvard Medical School; Physician, Affiliated Hospital Center, Beth Israel Hospital, and Massachusetts General Hospital, Boston.
General Principles of Endocrinology

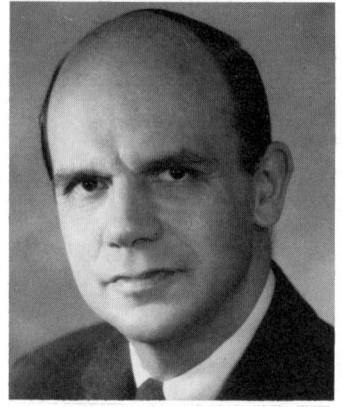

ANDREW G. FRANTZ, M.D.

Professor of Medicine and Chief, Division of Endocrinology, Columbia University College of Physicians and Surgeons; Attending Physician, Presbyterian Hospital, New York.
The Breasts

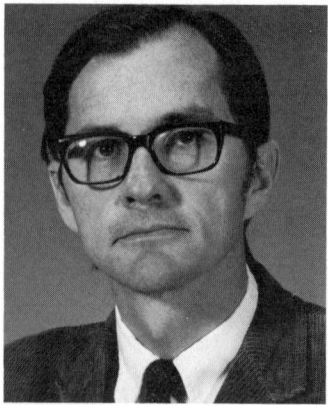

JOHN A. GLOMSET, M.D.

Investigator, Howard Hughes Medical Institute; Professor of Medicine, Adjunct Professor of Biochemistry, University of Washington School of Medicine, Seattle.
Disorders of Lipid Metabolism

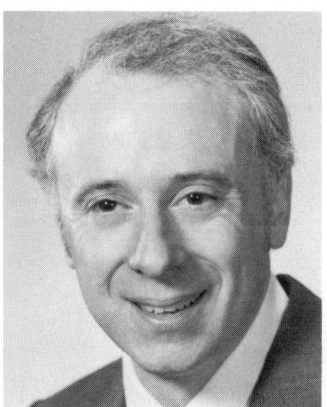

JOSEPH L. GOLDSTEIN, M.D.

Paul J. Thomas Professor of Medicine and Genetics, Chairman, Department of Molecular Genetics, University of Texas Health Science Center at Dallas; Senior Attending Physician, Parkland Memorial Hospital, Dallas.
Genetics and Endocrinology

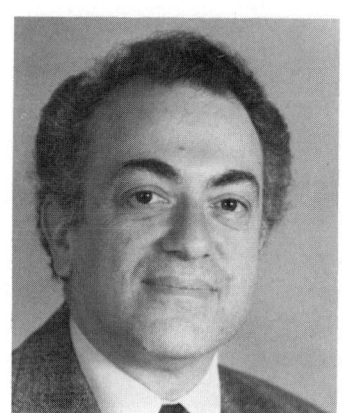

ROBERT I. GREGERMAN, M.D.

Chief of Endocrinology Section (Clinical Physiology Branch) of the National Institute on Aging, National Institutes of Health, Gerontology Research Center, Baltimore City Hospitals; Associate Professor of Medicine, Johns Hopkins University School of Medicine, Baltimore.
Aging and Hormones

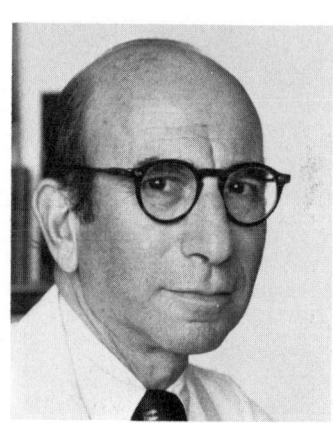

MELVIN M. GRUMBACH, M.D.

Professor of Pediatrics, Chairman, Department of Pediatrics, and Director of Pediatric Services, University of California, San Francisco.
Disorders of Sex Differentiation

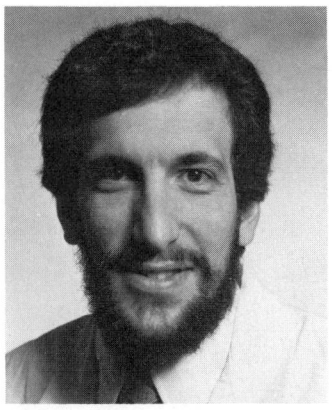

CARL GRUNFELD, M.D.
Assistant Professor of Medicine, University of California, San Francisco; Co-Director of Special Diagnostic Treatment Unit, Veterans Administration Medical Center, San Francisco.
Endocrine Systems: Mechanisms of Disease, Target Cells, and Receptors

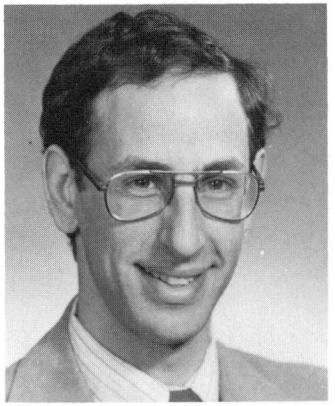

JEFFREY B. HALTER, M.D.
Associate Professor of Medicine, University of Washington School of Medicine; Associate Director of the Geriatric Research, Education and Clinical Center, Veterans Administration Medical Center, Seattle.
The Endocrine Pancreas and Diabetes Mellitus

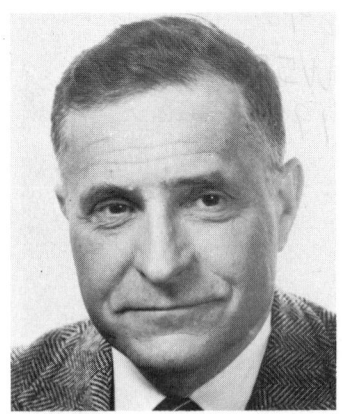

JULES HIRSCH, M.D.
Professor and Senior Physician, Rockefeller University and Hospital of the Rockefeller University, New York.
Obesity

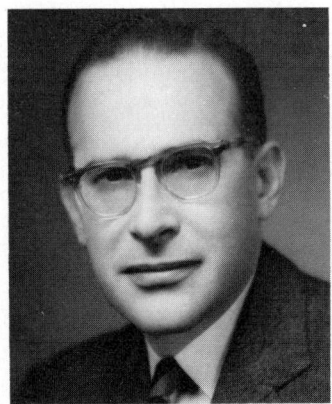

SIDNEY H. INGBAR, M.D.
William Bosworth Castle Professor of Medicine, Harvard Medical School; Director, Thorndike Laboratories; Chief, Endocrinology Division, Beth Israel Hospital, Boston.
The Thyroid Gland

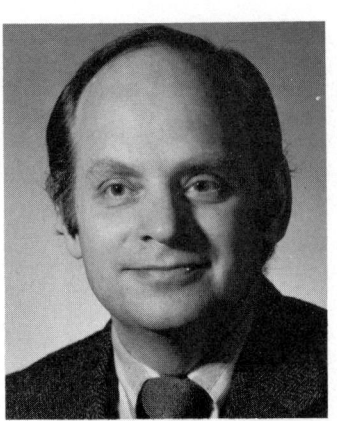

SEYMOUR J. KLEBANOFF, M.D., Ph.D.
Professor of Medicine, Chief, Division of Allergy and Infectious Diseases, University of Washington School of Medicine, Seattle.
Hormones and the Formed Elements of the Blood

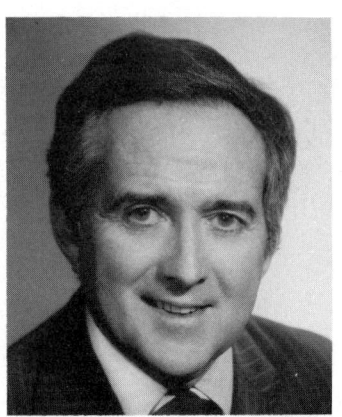

JOHN H. LARAGH, M.D.
Hilda Altshul Master Professor of Medicine, Director of Cardiovascular and Hypertension Center and Chief, Division of Cardiology, The New York Hospital-Cornell Medical Center, New York.
The Renin-Aldosterone Axis for Blood Pressure, Electrolyte Homeostasis, and Diagnosis of Blood Pressure

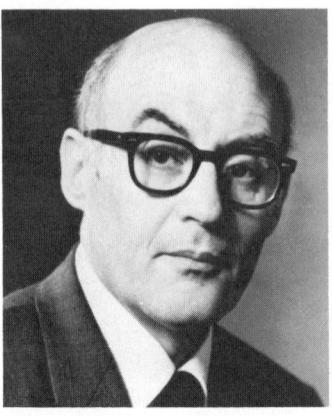

ALEXANDER LEAF, M.D.

Professor of Medicine, Harvard Medical School; Ridley Watts Professor of Preventive Medicine and Chairman, Department of Preventive Medicine and Clinical Epidemiology, Harvard Medical School; Physician, Medical Services, Massachusetts General Hospital, Boston.
Effect of Hormones on Water, Sodium, Chloride, and Potassium Metabolism

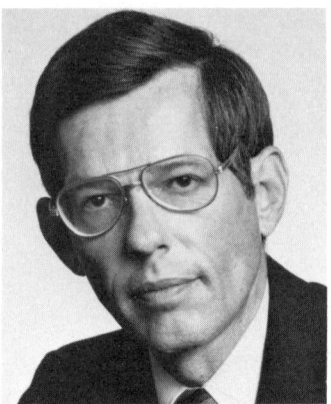

JAMES B. LEE, M.D.

Professor of Medicine, State University of New York at Buffalo; Attending Physician, Erie County Medical Center; Consultant, Veterans Administration Hospital, Buffalo.
The Prostaglandins

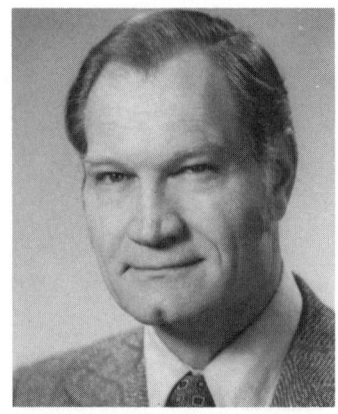

GRANT W. LIDDLE, M.D.

Professor and Chairman, Department of Medicine, Vanderbilt University School of Medicine; Physician-in-Chief, Vanderbilt University Hospital, Nashville.
The Adrenals

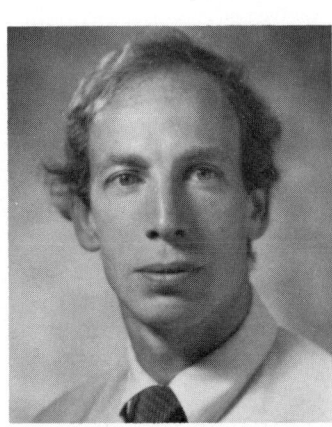

MARC E. LIPPMAN, M.D.

Head, Medical Breast Cancer Section, National Cancer Institute; Associate Professor of Medicine and Pharmacology, Uniformed Services University of the Health Sciences, Bethesda.
Endocrine Responsive Cancers of Man

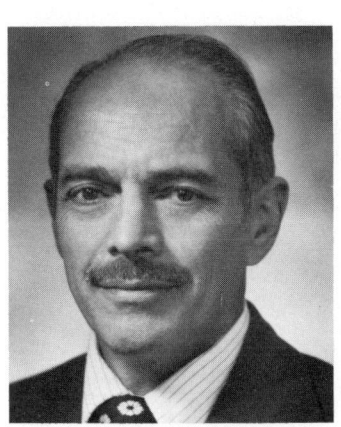

MORTIMER B. LIPSETT, M.D.

Professor of Medicine, Uniformed Services University of the Health Sciences; Director, Clinical Center, National Institutes of Health, Bethesda.
Endocrine Responsive Cancers of Man

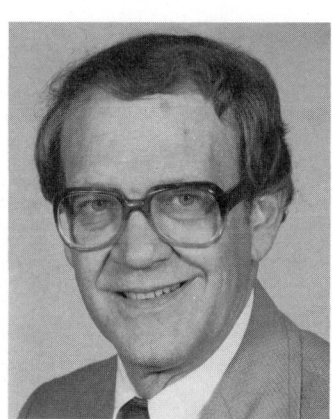

PAUL C. MACDONALD, M.D.

Director, Cecil H. and Ida Green Center for Reproductive Biology Sciences; Professor of Obstetrics and Gynecology and Biochemistry, The University of Texas Southwestern Medical School at Dallas.
The Endocrinology of Pregnancy

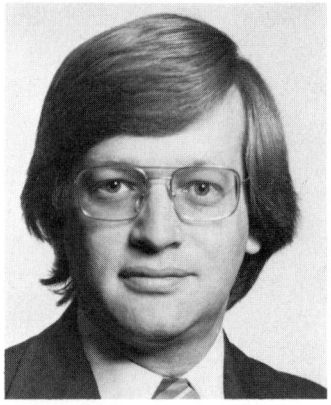

STEPHEN J. MARX, M.D.

Senior Investigator, Metabolic Disease Branch, National Institute of Arthritis, Metabolism and Digestive Diseases, Bethesda.
Parathyroid Hormone, Calcitonin, and the Calciferols

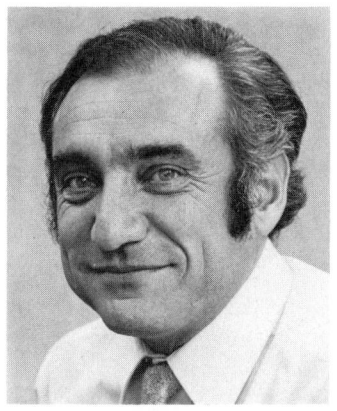

KENNETH L. MELMON, M.D.

Professor of Medicine and Pharmacology, Chairman, Department of Medicine, Stanford University School of Medicine; Physician-in-Chief, Stanford University Hospital, Stanford; Veterans Hospital, Palo Alto; Santa Clara Valley Medical Center, San Jose.
The Endocrinology Function of Selected Autacoids: Catecholamines, Acetylcholine, Serotonin, and Histamine

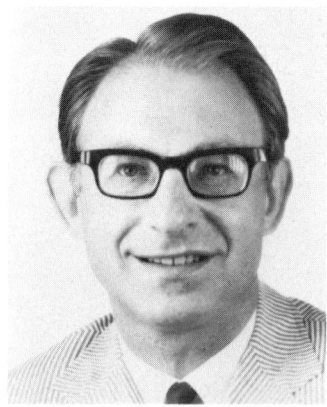

ARNO G. MOTULSKY, M.D.

Professor of Medicine and Genetics, University of Washington School of Medicine; Attending Physician, University Hospital, Seattle.
Genetics and Endocrinology

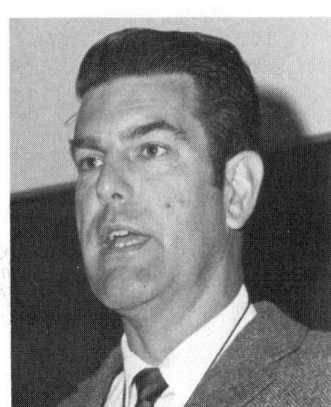

WILLIAM D. ODELL, M.D., Ph.D.

Chairman, Department of Medicine, Professor of Medicine and Physiology, University of Utah College of Medicine, Salt Lake City.
Humoral Manifestations of Cancer

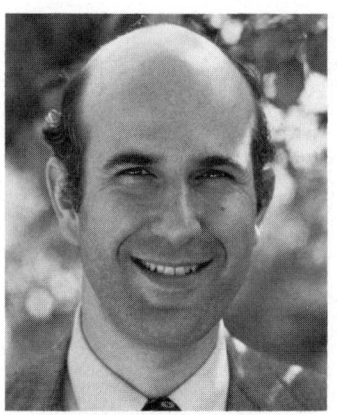

GILBERT S. OMENN, M.D., Ph.D.

Professor of Medicine (Medical Genetics), University of Washington School of Medicine; Attending Physician, University of Washington Hospital, Harborview Medical Center, Veterans Administration Hospital; Consulting Physician, Children's Orthopedic Hospital, Seattle.
Dysmentation from Metabolic Alterations

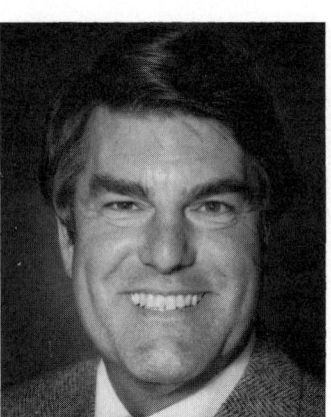

FRANK PARKER, M.D.

Professor and Chairman, Department of Dermatology, University of Oregon Medical Center; Attending Physician, Veterans Administration Hospital, Portland.
Skin and Hormones

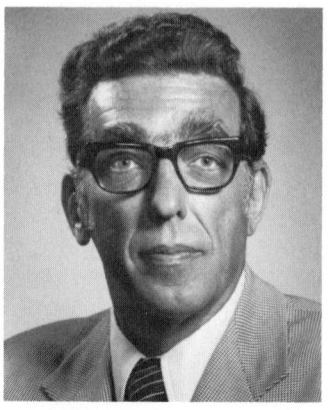

C. ALVIN PAULSEN, M.D.
Professor of Medicine, University of Washington School of Medicine, Seattle.
The Testes

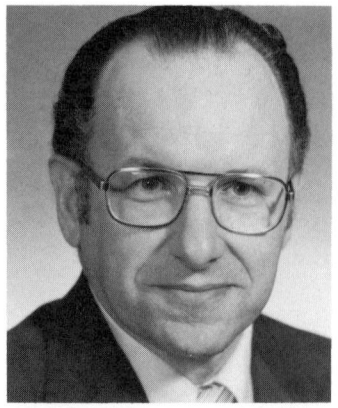

DANIEL PORTE, JR., M.D.
Professor of Medicine, Director, Diabetes Research Center, University of Washington School of Medicine; Associate Chief of Staff for Research and Development, Head, Division of Endocrinology and Metabolism, Veterans Administration Medical Center, Seattle.
The Endocrine Pancreas and Diabetes Mellitus

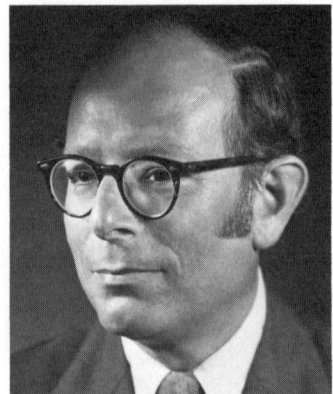

SEYMOUR REICHLIN, M.D., Ph.D.
Professor of Medicine, Tufts University School of Medicine; Senior Physician and Chief, Endocrine Division, New England Medical Center Hospital; Program Director, Clinical Study Unit, New England Medical Center Hospital, Boston.
Neuroendocrinology

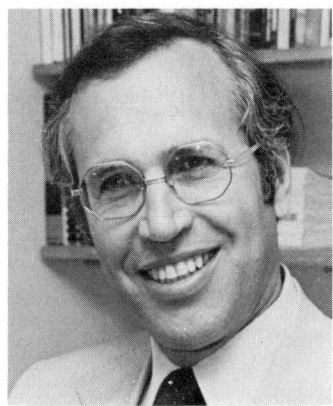

ROBERT M. ROSE, M.D.
Professor and Chairman, Department of Psychiatry and Behavioral Sciences, The University of Texas Medical Branch; Medical Staff, The University of Texas Medical Branch; Psychiatrist-in-Chief, John Sealy Hospital, Galveston.
Psychoendocrinology

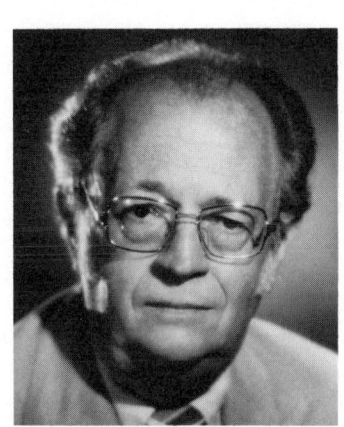

GRIFF T. ROSS, M.D., Ph.D.
Deputy Director, The Clinical Center, National Institutes of Health, Bethesda.
The Ovaries

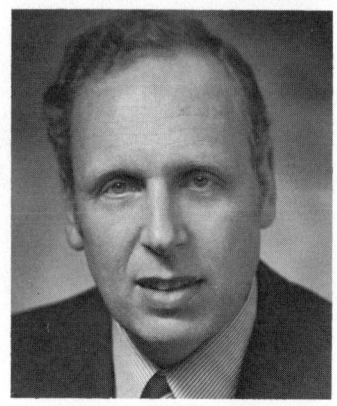

JESSE ROTH, M.D.
Chief, Diabetes Branch, National Institute of Arthritis, Diabetes and Digestive and Kidney Diseases, National Institutes of Health, Bethesda.
Endocrine Systems: Mechanisms of Disease, Target Cells, and Receptors

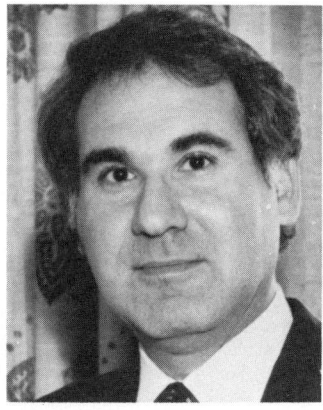

EDWARD J. SACHAR, M.D.

Lawrence C. Kolb Professor and Chairman, Department of Psychiatry, Columbia University College of Physicians and Surgeons; Director, New York State Psychiatric Institute; Attending Psychiatrist and Director, Psychiatry Service, Presbyterian Hospital, New York.
Psychoendocrinology

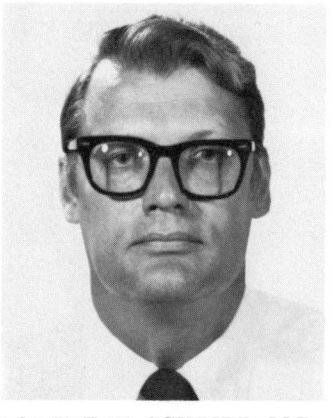

ROBERT W. SCHRIER, M.D.

Professor and Chairman, Department of Medicine, University of Colorado School of Medicine; Attending Physician, University Hospital, University of Colorado Health Sciences Center, Denver.
Effect of Hormones on Water, Sodium, Chloride, and Potassium Metabolism

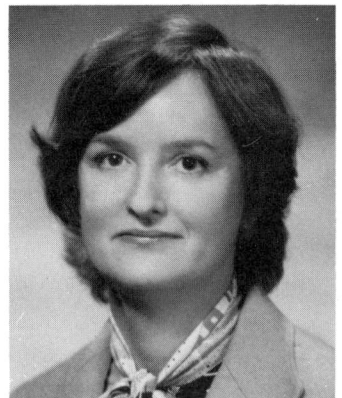

JEAN E. SEALEY, D.Sc.

Associate Professor of Physiology in Medicine, Cornell University Medical College, New York.
The Renin-Aldosterone Axis for Blood Pressure, Electrolyte Homeostasis, and Diagnosis of Blood Pressure

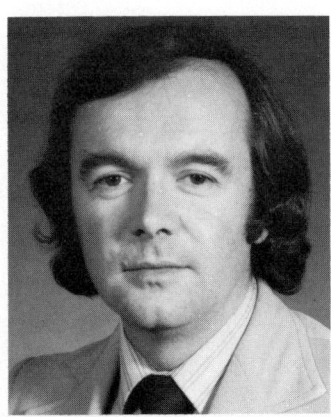

EVAN R. SIMPSON, B.Sc., Ph.D.

Associate Professor of Biochemistry and Obstetrics and Gynecology, University of Texas Health Science Center at Dallas.
Endocrinology of Pregnancy

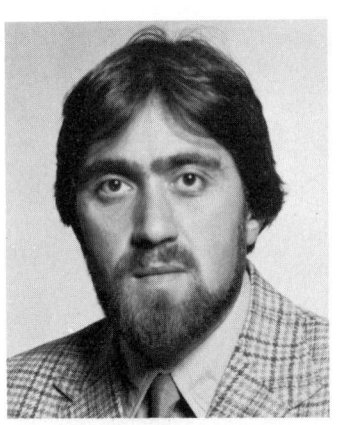

ALLEN M. SPIEGEL, M.D.

Senior Investigator, Metabolic Diseases Branch, National Institute of Arthritis, Diabetes, Digestive and Kidney Diseases, Bethesda.
Parathyroid Hormone, Calcitonin, and the Calciferols

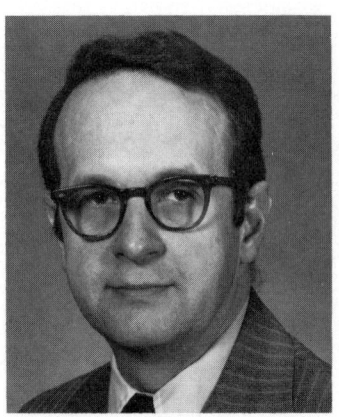

LOUIS E. UNDERWOOD, M.D.

Associate Professor of Pediatrics, University of North Carolina School of Medicine; Attending Pediatrician, North Carolina Memorial Hospital, Chapel Hill.
Hormones in Normal and Aberrant Growth

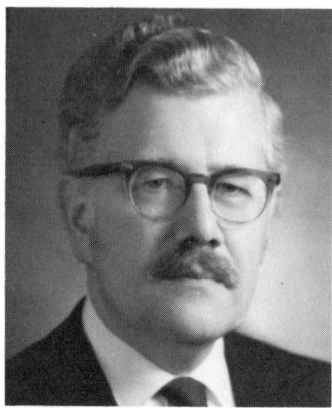

PAUL P. VAN ARSDEL,
JR., M.D.

Professor of Medicine and
Head, Section of Allergy, University of Washington School
of Medicine; Attending Physician, University Hospital,
Seattle.
*Allergy, Immunology, and
Hormones*

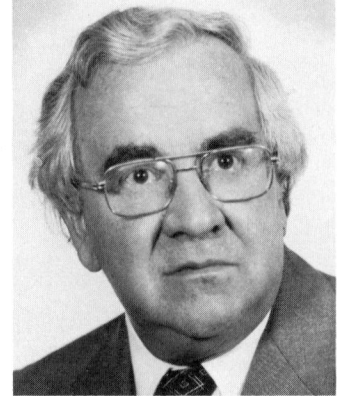

RAYMOND L. VANDE
WIELE, M.D.

Professor and Chairman, Department of Obstetrics and
Gynecology, Columbia University College of Physicians
and Surgeons; Director, International Institute for the
Study of Human Reproduction,
Columbia University; Director, Obstetrical and Gynecological Service, Presbyterian
Hospital, New York.
The Ovaries

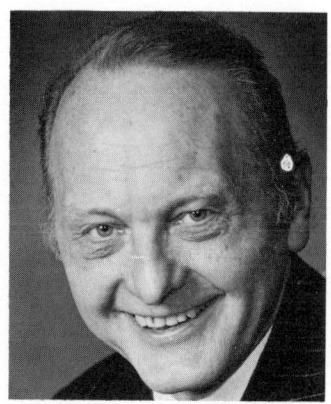

JUDSON J. VAN WYK,
M.D.

Kenan Professor of Pediatrics,
University of North Carolina
School of Medicine; Attending
Pediatrician, North Carolina
Memorial Hospital, Chapel
Hill.
*Hormones in Normal and
Aberrant Growth*

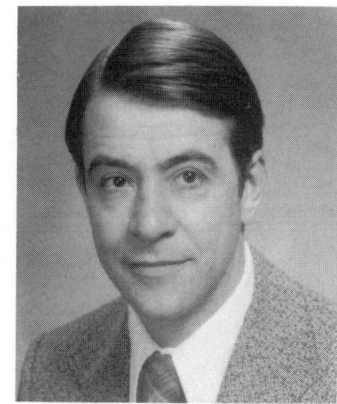

KENNETH A. WOEBER,
M.D.

Chief, Department of Medicine, Mt. Sinai Hospital; Professor of Medicine, University
of California, San Francisco.
The Thyroid Gland

PUBLISHER'S FOREWORD

The sudden death of Dr. Robert H. Williams in November 1979 interrupted his work on this edition in mid-course. There was a necessarily lengthy interval of reorganization and rededication to completion of the work by his former associates before his own chapters could be brought to final form.

Meanwhile some contributions had been reviewed by Dr. Williams and submitted for typesetting. Editorial and production work went ahead in the usual way on these chapters in preparation for 1980 publication. The chapters submitted earliest (Chapters 1, 3, 13, 18, 21, 24, 25, 26, 27, 30, and 31) are presented here as approved by Dr. Williams.

Inevitably delays and difficulties hampered preparation of a few chapters, and some were not delivered for printing until the spring of 1981. The complete table of contents and the list of contributors found in this edition follow Dr. Williams' plans.

W. B. Saunders Company

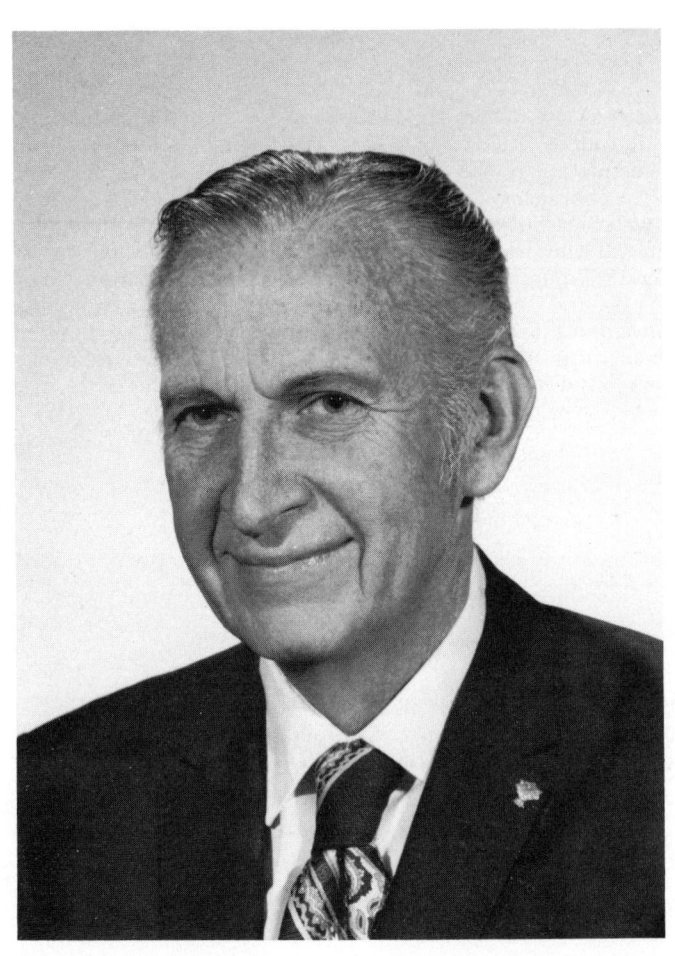

In Memoriam

This Sixth Edition of Williams' *Textbook of Endocrinology* is dedicated to Dr. Robert H. Williams, who died November 4th, 1979, while it was in preparation. Dr. Williams' contributions to medical research, teaching, and organization are legion; but he is best known throughout the world as an author and the editor of this *Textbook*.

The philosophy of the book was clearly stated in the Preface to the First Edition:

Tremendous progress has been made in the field of endocrinology in the past three decades. During this period many of the hormones have been made available in pure form and much has been learned of the manner in which they influence propagation, growth, maturation and general metabolic activities. With the accumulation of knowledge of the mechanisms by which the hormones influence bodily functions, there has been acquired a much better understanding of the clinical endocrinopathies. Moreover, attention has recently turned to the role of the endocrines in heart failure, hypertension, gerontology, immunology, hematology and in the therapy of neoplasms and neoplasms and collagen diseases.

The rapidity and extent of advances in endocrinology have made it increasingly difficult for the student and physician to take full advantage of information available for the understanding, diagnosis and treatment of clinical disorders. It is the realization of these difficulties that prompted the writing of this book. The main objective is to provide a condensed and authoritative discussion of the management of clinical endocrinopathies, based upon the application of fundamental information obtained from chemical and physiologic investigations.

The authors chosen to collaborate in writing this book are men who have maintained intimate contact with progress in both basic and clinical investigations and who have had great experience in the practical application of this information. Since they have also demonstrated excellent teaching ability, they are well qualified to present a clear and well-balanced discussion of their subject.

The *Textbook* soon received universal acceptance. It introduced generations of medical students and house officers to the field of endocrinology, and this exposure led many to select a career in research, teaching, or practice of endocrinology.

The *Textbook* became the standard reference book on endocrinology for both the general physician and the specialist. Its influence spread around the world, reaching physicians not only in English but also in French, Greek, Italian, Japanese, Polish, and Spanish editions. Many contributors have learned that their international reputation depended not so much on their own research contributions as on the fact that they authored chapters in Williams' *Textbook of Endocrinology*.

Dr. Williams defined his goals for the Sixth Edition in a letter to the contributors as follows:

There has accumulated such a vast amount of material dealing with different phases of endocrinology and metabolism that we must be highly selective in the phases for coverage and the extent of coverage. It is our objective to mention the most important components and to deal with them in a brief and clear manner. In areas of controversy it is important to mention that the points are controversial, but for the author to give his best judgment for the present.

The challenge has been to present the essence of a field which has continued to exhibit logarithmic growth within the confines of a book of roughly the same size. "Unless we make a great effort to restrict the length, we will end up with a heavy and expensive book that may either be left on the shelf unusually long or not be acquired in the first place."

It was the essence of Dr. Williams' genius as a teacher of endocrinology at the bedside, in the lecture hall, and through his textbook that he was not content to transmit simply the basic facts of endocrinology but also conveyed the excitement of endocrinology and its promise of the future.

Those of us who have worked to complete this work that he initiated hope that it measures up to the exalted standards he set. The world has lost a remarkable teacher and author.

WILLIAM H. DAUGHADAY, M.D.

CONTENTS

CHAPTER 1

General Principles of Endocrinology

By Daniel D. Federman

INTRODUCTION

The functions of the endocrine glands can be recognized in four principal areas. First is the maintenance of the *milieu intérieur,* a narrowly regulated mixture of substrates, cofactors, enzymes, and conditions that provide an optimum environment for the biochemic machinery of the body. A second challenge, imposed by more marked environmental changes, is the response to emergency demands, such as starvation, infection, trauma, and psychologic stress. Third, many hormones play roles in the smooth, sequential integration of growth and development. Finally, specialized endocrine tissue contributes to the processes of sexual reproduction, including gametogenesis, coitus, fertilization, and nourishment of the fetus and newborn.

This chapter focuses on the mechanisms that integrate the endocrine system. The other survival systems of the body have an anatomic continuity that is essential to their function. This continuity is found in the cardiovascular, respiratory, gastrointestinal, and urinary systems. In contrast, the endocrine glands are widely scattered about the body, with no interconnections other than with the vascular system and, in some instances, autonomic innervation. In the absence of anatomic linkage, it is necessary to look elsewhere for the principles that integrate the activities of the endocrine organs. To summarize, the meshing of endocrine physiology depends on functional interactions rather than on structural continuity.

FUNCTIONAL INTERACTIONS OF HORMONES

The interactions among hormones in regulating bodily processes can be summarized by recognizing that few processes under hormonal control are regulated by only one hormone and that few hormones have only one role.

One Function: Multiple Hormones

Although not all bodily processes are hormone-dependent, those that are dependent are rarely sensitive to only one hormone. For instance, the brain depends on a constant supply of oxygen and glucose. Just as cardiac and pulmonary functions have primary responsibility for the maintenance of cerebral oxygenation, so endocrine function is responsible for the maintenance of the cerebral glucose supply. To achieve a stable blood sugar, four processes are involved: carbohydrate ingestion, hepatic glycogenolysis, gluconeogenesis, and glucose sparing by use of other energy

1

Table 1–1. THE DEFENSE OF BLOOD SUGAR

Process	Hormones Involved
Glucose intake and absorption	Cortisol ← ACTH ← CRF Thyroxine ← TSH ← TRH
Glycogenolysis	Glucagon (between meals) Epinephrine (in emergencies) (Insulin suppression) Cortisol Thyroxine
Gluconeogenesis	Cortisol GH Glucagon (Insulin suppression) Epinephrine
Use of alternative energy sources	Epinephrine GH (Insulin suppression)

sources.[1] The hormonal bases of each of these processes may be reviewed in Table 1–1, above.

Food Ingestion

Cortisol is a dominant factor in appetite. The secretion of cortisol requires corticotropin (ACTH) from the pituitary, and that in turn is stimulated by a putative corticotropin-releasing factor (CRF). Similarly, both appetite and gastrointestinal absorption of glucose are influenced by thyroxine (T_4) and triiodothyronine (T_3), secretion of which is stimulated by thyrotropin (TSH) and thus by thyrotropin-releasing hormone (TRH). A falling blood sugar also stimulates hunger; the hormonal mediation, if any, is unclear.

Glycogenolysis

Excess carbohydrate is stored as glycogen in both muscle and liver. The breakdown of hepatic glycogen to glucose-6-phosphate (G-6-P) and thence to glucose is the second line of defense of the blood sugar. Within approximately 1 to 2 hours of the last meal, as the temporarily raised blood sugar is falling, hepatic glycogenolysis begins. This process is influenced by at least three hormones: A release of glucagon stimulates glycogenolysis, and the falling level of insulin removes a brake on the process that was present immediately after eating. Epinephrine may play a small role in stimulating glycogenolysis between meals, but it is quantitatively more important in stress.

Gluconeogenesis

Depending on the age, sex, weight, and preceding nutritional status of the individual, the breakdown of hepatic glycogen will defend the blood sugar during fasting for from 8 to 14 hours. At some time during this period, gluconeogenesis comes into play. The production of glucose from amino acids, glycerol, and lactate can sustain the blood sugar for weeks or months. Gluconeogenesis is stimulated by at least three hormones (cortisol, glucagon, and growth hormone [GH]) and is released from inhibition by insulin as that hormone falls to a low level. In addition, lipolysis releases glycerol, and thus hormones that stimulate lipolysis play a role in blood glucose preservation. These hormones include epinephrine, norepinephrine, GH, and several others. Similarly, the breakdown of protein to release alanine and glutamine is favored by cortisol and by the absence of insulin.

Glucose Sparing

The use of alternate fuels is an important additional means of defending the blood glucose; indeed, some consider it the principal mechanism. Fatty acids, a preferred substrate for both cardiac and skeletal muscle, are released from adipose tissue stores when insulin levels are low and the levels of other hormones, such as glucagon and GH, are high. The oxidation of fatty acids, which does not require insulin, and of ketone bodies inhibits glycolysis and allows the release of lactate and pyruvate, which are substrates for gluconeogenesis. Similarly, lipolysis releases glycerol, which is reconverted to glucose on returning to the liver. The resort to alternate fuels, akin to the triggering of gluconeogenesis, is initiated before hepatic glycogen stores are depleted. Thus the full range of intermediary metabolic processes is mobilized in a coordinate manner, for which the balance between insulin and opposing hormones is the prime regulator.

In summary, the maintenance of a single circulating metabolite, the blood glucose, involves at least 10 hormones and 6 endocrine glands. The relations among the hormones can be additive, cooperative, preparative, or opposing, and it is only by considering the whole system that the process is understood.

One Hormone: Multiple Actions

The obverse of multihormonal involvement in a single goal is the principle that few hormones have but a single effect. For example, in the regulation of the level of blood glucose, insulin works at multiple sites: It promotes glucose entry into muscle and adipose tissue; it affects both glycogenolysis and gluconeogenesis; it regulates lipolysis; and it favors the synthesis rather than the breakdown of muscle protein stores. Similarly, epinephrine promotes glycogenolysis and peripheral lipolysis and also inhibits insulin secretion by the pancreas — all steps that tend to raise the blood sugar. Parathyroid hormone (PTH) also illustrates the multiple effects of one hormone, for it stimulates release of calcium and phosphate from bone, promotes reabsorption of calcium by the renal tubule, and stimulates synthesis of the biologically active form of vitamin D. All of these actions contribute to raising the serum calcium.

NEUROENDOCRINE INTEGRATION

The nervous and endocrine systems are the principal mediators of physiologic adaptation to environmental stress. In general terms, neural reactions are faster and are therefore more important immediate responses, whereas hormonal effects serve to complete a homeostatic adaptation. It is not surprising, therefore, that neural influences play a major role in unifying the responses of endocrine glands. Three types of neuroendocrine interaction can be discerned: the hypothalamic regulation of pituitary function, the combination of neural and endocrine responses to stimuli, and the neural control of endocrine secretion.

Hypothalamus and Pituitary Gland

One of the major areas of recent advance is the elucidation of the regulation of anterior pituitary function by the central nervous system.[2, 3] It has long been known that the anterior pituitary gland, although housed within the cranium, is not a neural structure. Harris and others postulated that pituitary function is regulated by tropic and inhibitory factors secreted by certain hypothalamic neurons. These versatile cells are thus, at one end, proper citizens of the central nervous system, having electrical synapses with other hypothalamic neurons, the reticular formation and hippocampus, and many other parts of the brain. At their distal termini, however, the hypothalamic cells are secretory structures, producing small polypeptides that are released directly into the hypophyseal portal system for delivery via a secondary capillary plexus to the cells of the anterior pituitary.

Several anatomic features of the hypothalamus contribute to the functioning of the hypothalamus-pituitary unit. First, there is no blood-brain barrier at the hypothalamus; therefore, circulating messages such as the serum sodium or cortisol level have direct access to regulatory sites. Second, the hypothalamus contains centers for other crucial functions, including thirst, hunger, osmoregulation, blood pressure, and pulse rate. Third, the portal circulation allows substances of hypothalamic origin to reach the pituitary gland in concentrations that cannot be duplicated elsewhere in the body. Finally, investigation has revealed the linkage of pituitary secretion to sleep onset and depth as well as to vision, smell, and body mass.

Autonomic Nervous System

A second type of neuroendocrine interaction is exemplified by the autonomic nervous system and endocrine collaboration in the regulation of blood pressure. The major determinants of blood pressure are intravascular volume and vascular tone. In the control of intravascular volume, sodium and water balance are influenced by vasopressin, cortisol, angiotensin, and aldosterone, as well as by cardiorenal function. The sympathomimetic amines are critical in the regulation of vascular tone, but vascular sensitivity to catecholamines is influenced by both cortisol and T_4. This effect of thyroid hormone is associated with an increase in β-adrenergic receptors in vascular smooth muscle. β-adrenergic stimulation of renin is also important in the release of renin, and thus in the enlistment of the angiotensin-aldosterone response.

Neural Control of Endocrine Function

Neural regulation of endocrine cell function provides another means of cooperative response to challenge. Individual adipose tissue cells receive both α- and β-adrenergic nerve fibers, and lipolysis versus fat synthesis is partly determined by adrenergic impulses. In the hypothalamic-hypophyseal unit, α-adrenergic impulses release GH and inhibit prolactin (PRL), whereas β-adrenergic signals inhibit GH release. Similarly, the parathyroid gland has a rich autonomic innervation. *In vitro*, β-adrenergic agents raise cAMP levels in the parathyroid gland and also promote PTH release; it seems likely that β-adrenergic stimulation, perhaps via adenyl cyclase activation, mediates part of the hypocalcemic stimulation of PTH secretion.[4] A similar possibility is provided by the autonomic innervation of the pancreatic islets, in which α-adrenergic stimulation restrains insulin release. In certain circumstances, insulin release is inhibited even when glucose levels are rising; this phenomenon may be part of the explanation of stress hyperglycemia.

Examined temporally, peripheral neuroendocrine regulation is of immediate or short-range responsiveness and allows for adaptation to changes in posture and to acute stressful demands. Central neuroendocrine patterns, on the other hand, have longer time frames, ranging from the diurnal rhythm of ACTH to the monthly cycles of gonadotropins and even to the generation-long aspects of reproduction, such as with PRL.

REGULATION OF ENDOCRINE FUNCTION

There are three major classes of hormones: steroid, peptide, and amino acid. The steroid hormones are generally lipid-soluble and circulate in plasma bound to transport proteins such as cortisol-binding globulin or sex steroid–binding globulin. The half-lives of these hormones vary from 60 min for testosterone to 100 min for cortisol. In order to exert their biologic effect, steroids enter cells and bind to specific cytosol receptor proteins. The protein or polypeptide hormones are generally water-soluble and circulate unbound in plasma. Their half-lives vary from 5 to 60 min. The short peptide or amino acid hormones have some characteristics intermediate to those of the steroids and polypeptides. The diamino acid T_4 circulates attached to not one but three binding proteins and has a plasma half-life of a week. In contrast, epinephrine is not protein bound and has a plasma half-life of less than 1 min.

The effect of a hormone ultimately depends on its interaction with a receptor, and a major determinant of this step is the circulating level of the hormone. This section deals with the regulation of hormone level, and Chapter 2 discusses the hormone:receptor interaction and its consequences.

Basal Secretion

Curiously little is known about the basal secretion of endocrine glands *in situ* when no tropic stimulation or homeostatic challenge exists. *In vitro* studies of parathyroid tissue have shown that a basal level of PTH secretion persists however high the calcium level is raised in the medium. Basal secretion *in vivo* is difficult to study without catheterizing efferent veins. Mere measurement of the plasma levels of most hormones does not answer the question, since few assays can reliably distinguish absent levels from low levels of peptide hormones in the blood. When one adds the confusion produced by the heterogeneity of circulating peptide hormones, the significance of extremely low plasma levels is difficult to ascertain.

Neuroregulation is a principal determinant of basal secretion by the hypothalamus-pituitary unit.[5] ACTH is secreted in a diurnal rhythm that is presumed to reflect variable intensity of stimulation by the hypothalamus. Although CRF has not yet been isolated, the pituitary gland cultured *in vitro* has no rhythm of secretion, and its well-established diurnal pattern is thought to reflect a hypothalamic electrical pattern. Nyctohemeral secretion has been defined for a number of hormones. GH and PRL are both released in a sharp burst within 1 hour of the onset of deep sleep. A similar nocturnal surge of luteinizing hormone (LH) release is characteristic during puberty but is not seen in either the child or the adult. Finally, both follicle-stimulating hormone (FSH) and LH are secreted cyclically, provided the individual is a genetic female and there is appropriate secretion of estrogen and progesterone by the ovary. All of these rhythmic hormonal patterns are presumed to be secondary to central nervous system events mediated through hypothalamic releasing hormones.

Stimulated Secretion

The output of hormone from an endocrine gland can always be increased over the basal level. The principal stimuli to increased output are a change in the level of a circulating metabolite and an increase in the blood level of a tropic hormone.

Change in a Circulating Metabolite

PTH secretion is regulated principally by the plasma level of calcium and, to a lesser degree, by inorganic phosphate and magnesium. When the serum calcium level falls, PTH secretion is increased; the converse is true when the level of calcium rises (Fig. 1–1). The effects of altered calcium can be demonstrated *in vitro*, indicating that the calcium level has a direct influence on the synthesis and release of hormone. The mechanism of this influence is poorly understood, but, as cited earlier, a β-adrenergic receptor inhibited by a high ambient calcium may be involved.

The regulation of insulin secretion by the pancreatic beta cell reflects a higher order of complexity.[6] The dominant influence is the level of blood glucose; to stimulate insulin release, glucose must enter the beta cell and be metabolized. Amino acids such as arginine also release insulin, as do glucagon and certain enteric hormones (Fig. 1–2). The glucose-sensitive control is primary, however, for when the blood glucose level is low, neither amino acids nor glucagon or the glucagon-like enteric insulin secretagogues will release insulin. On the other hand, catecholamines with α effects depress insulin secretion, suggesting that the autonomic innervation of the pancreas also plays a role in insulin secretion. Finally, there may be local ("paracrine") factors as well: Glucagon increases and somatostatin decreases insulin release, but whether these islet cell products act locally is not yet certain. Thus, in the control of insulin secretion, the regulated substance (glucose) plays a dominant role, but other nutrients, hormones, neural input, and local factors are each important.

Increase in the Blood Level of a Tropic Hormone

The second general mechanism for increasing the output of an endocrine gland is the stimulating effect of a tropic hormone. Perhaps the simplest example of tropic hormone function is the stimulation of thyroid hormone secretion by pituitary TSH (Fig. 1–3). In this case, "simplest" refers to

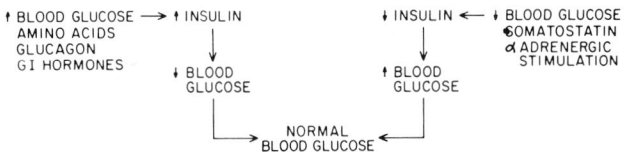

Figure 1–2. Although the regulated substance, glucose, plays a dominant role in the regulation of insulin release, additional factors are important.

the fact that one tropic hormone works on one gland to stimulate the secretion of one type of hormone: T_4 and T_3.[7] The thyroid follicle has one secretory site, the epithelial cell; there appears to be a single receptor for TSH; and throughout the life of the individual the tropic hormone controls the action of the thyroid.

In the next order of complexity, one tropic hormone elicits two different responses. In the adult, ACTH stimulates adrenal secretion of both cortisol and androgens. (ACTH also plays a small role in aldosterone synthesis, but the mechanism of this transient and low-level response is almost certainly different.) Cortisol is a C_{21} steroid, whereas the androgens are C_{19} steroids. Although the initial steps in the synthesis of both hormones are the same, the biosynthetic pathways diverge beyond 17-OH-progesterone; yet one tropic hormone, acting at a prior step, the conversion of cholesterol to pregnenolone, is able to stimulate both syntheses (Fig. 1–4).

A converse relationship, in which two tropins are required for one event, is illustrated by the role of gonadotropins in ovulation. FSH initiates maturation of a cohort of graafian follicles at the onset of a new menstrual cycle; FSH also stimulates synthesis of the LH receptor. After follicular maturation and the resulting rise in plasma estradiol, there is an abrupt surge in both FSH and LH and ovulation results (Fig. 1–5). Neither gonadotropin is sufficient alone to achieve release of the egg.

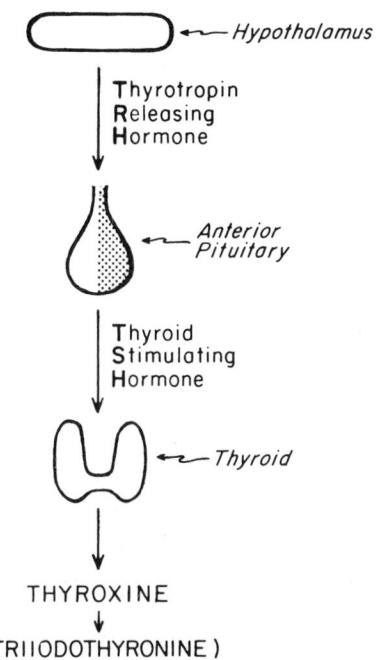

Figure 1–3. The simplest pattern of hypothalamic-hypophyseal interaction: one releasing hormone stimulates one pituitary tropic hormone, and it stimulates one hormonal pathway in the thyroid.

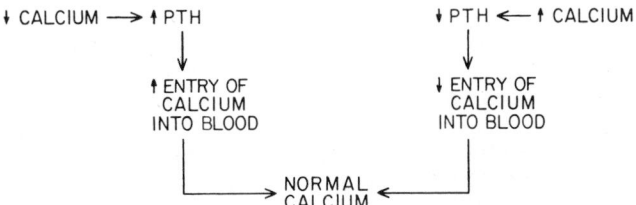

Figure 1–1. The dominant influence on parathyroid hormone (PTH) secretion is the level of serum calcium, i.e., the substance regulated. In turn, suppression or release of PTH is the principal control of the level of calcium in the blood. (For additional, but less important, influences see text.)

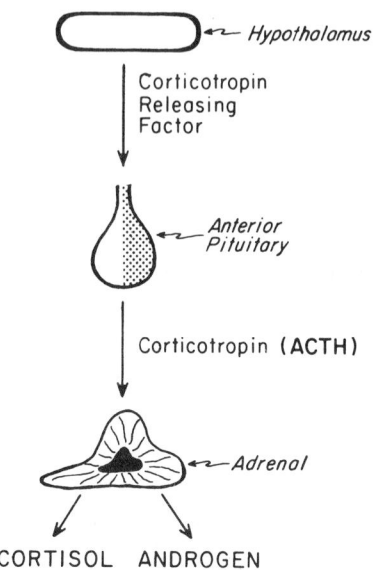

(I Releasing Hormone → I Tropin → 2 Hormones)

Figure 1–4. The pituitary control of adrenal secretion represents an increase in complexity over the thyroid (cf. Figure 1–3). One hypothalamic releasing hormone stimulates one pituitary tropin, but the latter elicits activity in two biosynthetic pathways of the adrenal.

Feedback Regulation

The inhibition of active secretion is another critical feature of normal endocrine function. The principal control is negative feedback acting either directly, secondary to change in a circulating metabolite, or indirectly, via a tropic hormone. An example of negative feedback by a metabolite is the suppressive effect of hypercalcemia on the secretion of

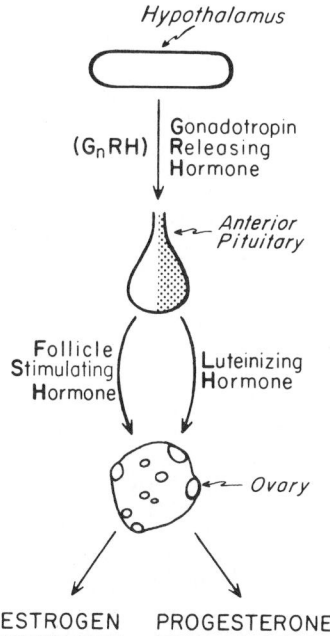

(I Releasing Hormone → 2 Tropins → 2 Hormones)

Figure 1–5. Gonadotropin regulation involves one releasing hormone that stimulates two pituitary tropins and, in turn, two target gland hormones.

PTH. The linear relationship between serum calcium and PTH secretion is shown in Fig. 1–6. The existence of such stoichiometry can be used in diagnosing hyperparathyroidism. If the serum immunoreactive PTH(iPTH), even though not absolutely high, is elevated for a given serum calcium value, the diagnosis of hyperparathyroidism is likely. In basing clinical decisions on this relationship, the clinician is paying tribute to the sensitivity of the normal gland to negative feedback.

Feedback regulation via a tropic hormone is widely represented in normal physiology. The circulating T_4 and T_3 levels condition the sensitivity with which the anterior pituitary gland responds to hypothalamic TRH. A protein synthesized in the pituitary suppresses the response to TRH. When the circulating T_4 is high, less of the protein is formed; when T_4 deficiency occurs, more of the intermediary control protein is produced. The sequence can be schematized as in Fig. 1–7. Similar negative feedback is exerted by cortisol on ACTH release, although this appears to affect the hypothalamus more than the anterior pituitary (Fig. 1–8).

The regulation of gonadotropin secretion in the male appears to add an additional level of complexity to the pattern seen in the thyroid and adrenal glands. After 40 years of speculation, there is now convincing evidence of a protein, inhibin, that is secreted by the Sertoli cells and that inhibits FSH release (Fig. 1–9). The role of testosterone, the principal product of the Leydig cells, is more controversial. Both in the testis and in the periphery, testosterone is aromatized to estradiol. Several areas of the brain — importantly, the hypothalamus — are capable of this transformation, and there are estradiol and testosterone receptors in brain tissue. Dynamic studies of the suppression of LH by testosterone and estradiol suggest that both steroids are required for the normal control of LH release.[8] The testosterone-to-estradiol conversion occurs in the tissue in which estradiol is the active agent; in other words, the tissue is producing from the "prohormone" (testosterone) the compound to which it is sensitive. The negative feedback regulation of gonadotropins thus involves (a) inhibition by inhibin of the pituitary FSH response to LH-releasing hormone (LRH), (b) inhibition of LRH and perhaps of its effect on the pituitary by testosterone and its metabolite estradiol, and (c) perhaps a cooperative role of estradiol in blunting the LRH stimulation of FSH.

Evidence for *positive* feedback regulation has been obtained much more recently, predominantly from studies of the menstrual cycle.[9] During the follicular phase, there is a rapid rise in plasma estradiol. At a critical level, the elevated estradiol produces both an enhanced release of LRH and an increased pituitary responsiveness to the releasing hormone. Similarly, the plasma progesterone, formerly thought to be the secretory evidence of the corpus luteum, begins to rise before ovulation and appears to exert a positive feedback role on FSH. The effect of the rising levels of estrogen and progesterone is the midcycle surge of LH and FSH that triggers ovulation (Fig. 1–10).

The consequences of basal secretion, tropic stimulation, and feedback inhibition are balanced in an equilibrium that can be interpreted by resorting to control theory. In their regulatory roles, most hormones must be adjusted to changes in exogenous or endogenous stimuli. We have seen that neural regulation allows prompt response and that endocrine regulation allows sustained adaptations to altered circumstances. In addition, the opposing influences of tropic stimulation and negative feedback allow rapid responses but prevent overshoot and its maladaptive consequences. Further insurance is provided by the counterpoise of agonist and antagonist for both specific steps and

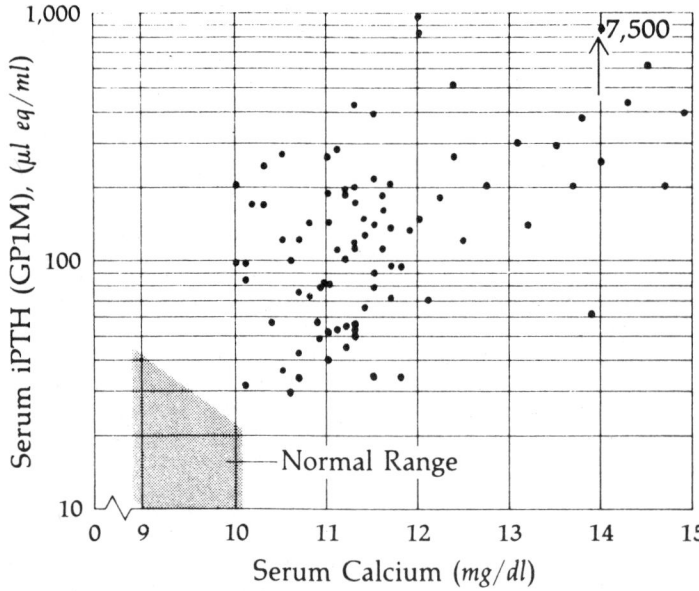

Figure 1–6. The relationship between serum calcium and iPTH. In normal individuals, the upper border of the shaded area reflects the negative feedback of serum calcium on PTH release. In contrast, patients with hyperparathyroidism show a positive correlation between calcium and iPTH. Some patients have iPTH levels that, although within the normal range, are elevated for their serum calcium.

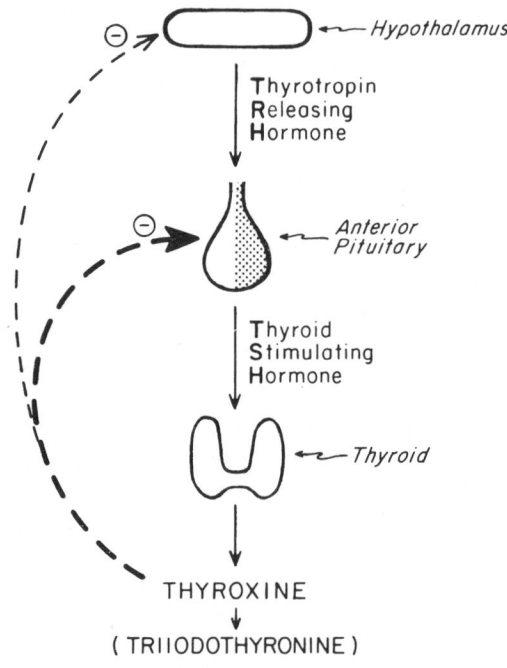

Figure 1–7. The feedback regulation of thyroid secretion. The thyroid hormone(s) acts predominantly at the pituitary by restraining the effect of TRH on TSH synthesis and release.

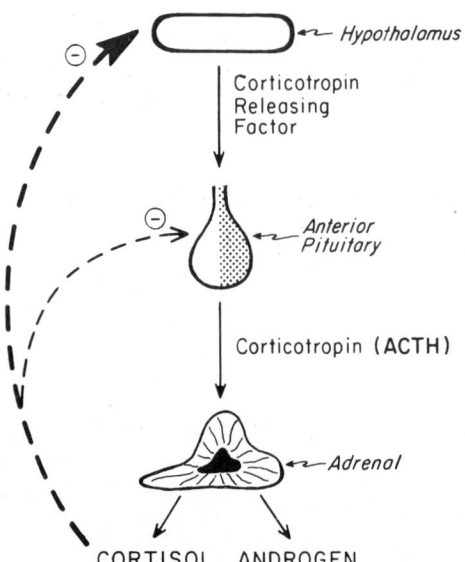

Figure 1–8. The feedback regulation of ACTH release is exerted by circulating cortisol, acting principally at the hypothalamus. Although the synthesis of adrenal androgens is thus controlled by cortisol dynamics, intrinsic adrenal factors modulate the androgenic response to ACTH.

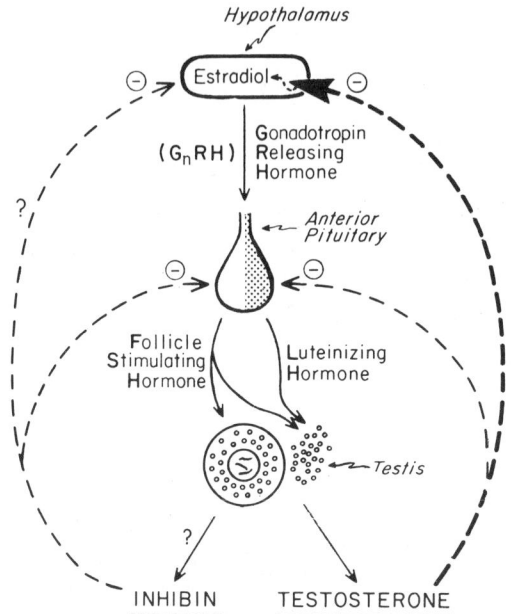

(I Releasing Hormone ⟶ 2 Tropins ⟶ I (?2) Hormone(s))

Figure 1–9. The feedback regulation of gonadotropin secretion in the male includes two features not seen before now. The inhibition of LH by testosterone is exerted by both testosterone and estradiol, the latter derived from testosterone by an aromatose within the hypothalamic cells. FSH regulation is less well understood, but one factor is a protein, inhibin. This substance is produced in the testicular tubules but not clearly under the direct influence of FSH.

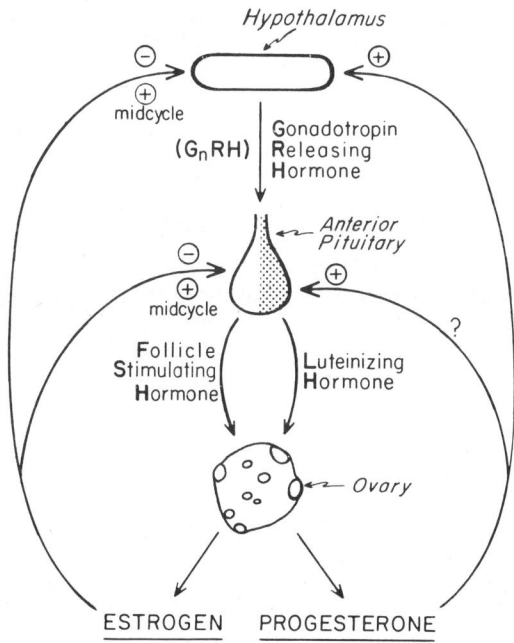

(I Releasing Hormone ⟶ 2 Tropins ⟶ 2 Hormones)

Figure 1–10. The most perplexing balance of feedback influences is that controlling gonadotropin in the female. Estrogen secreted by the ovarian follicles exerts a negative restraint on both FSH and LH release. Ordinarily, the FSH is an inverse reflection of the complement of follicles; but, at midcycle, estrogen and perhaps progesterone exert a positive feedback influence on both hypothalamus and pituitary, resulting in a surge of FSH and LH.

overall goals. Finally, there is adaptation at the target tissue: The regulation of hormone receptors further modulates the effect of sustained deficient or excess secretion. In sum, each excursion from the basal level of secretion entrains both biologic effects and corrective reactions. The result is an extraordinary combination of daily maintenance, emergency responsiveness, and long-range adaptation.

Metabolism of Hormones

The metabolic degradation of circulating hormones provides an additional means for regulating the exposure of tissue to active compounds. The possibilities include alteration of the molecule, consumption at the site of action, and hepatic and renal excretion. All these approaches are used, although to different degrees for different compounds.

Steroid Hormones

The metabolic degradation of cortisol can be used to illustrate the principles that have been cited. The fastest way to inactivate cortisol is by reduction of the double bond in ring A to produce dihydrocortisol (Fig. 1–11A). This step, which occurs in the liver, is sensitive to the state of hepatic function and is accelerated by T_4. T_4 also affects the metabolism of testosterone, and in addition to regulating the rate, influences the direction of testosterone metabolism. At a branched pathway leading to androsterone, a weak androgen, and etiocholanolone, an inactive steroid, thyroid hormones induce the 5-α reductase that produces androsterone (Fig. 1–11B). The level of a hormone is a balance between its production and its degradation.

Peptide Hormones

Less is known about the metabolism of the protein and peptide hormones, but a few points can be made. Their half-lives tend to be quite short, ranging from 5 to 6 min (ACTH) to 20 min (GH) to 60 min or more (gonadotropins). At least one peptide hormone, PTH, is cleaved in the circulation into two fragments, of which only one (the amino terminal portion) has significant biologic activity. There is recent evidence, contradicting what had previously been thought, that the peptide hormones enter cells with their receptors; this step could serve to bring the hormone to the lysosomes for intracellular degradation and inactivation.[10]

Hormone:Hormone Interactions

Hormones influence each other's synthesis, action, metabolism, and transport. These processes provide an additional source of integration of the endocrine system.

Synthesis

The synthesis of epinephrine in the adrenal medulla is completed when a methyl group is added to norepinephrine in a step catalyzed by phenylethanolamine-N-methyl transferase (PNMT). This enzyme is induced by cortisol, which is produced in the adrenal cortex and delivered to the medulla in concentrations that cannot be duplicated by systemic administration (Fig. 1–12). Control of synthesis of the principal medullary product, therefore, is exerted by a major product of the cortex. Another example of hormonal induc-

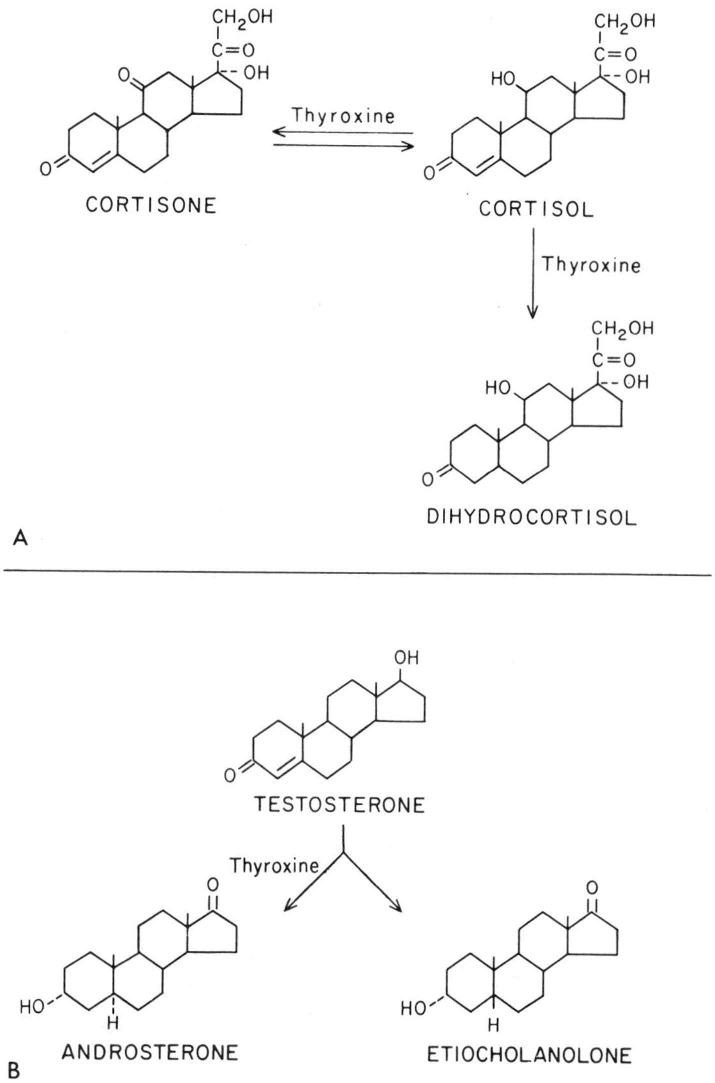

Figure 1–11. *A,* Thyroxine stimulates the conversion of cortisol to both cortisone and dihydrocortisol. The former reaction is reversible, but the ring A reduction yielding dihydrocortisol is an irretrievable step toward inactivation and excretion. *B,* Thyroxine favors the reduction of testosterone to androsterone, a weak androgen, over the pathway to etiocholanolone.

tion of hormone synthesis is the effect of PTH on vitamin D.

Preparatory Influences of Hormones

Certain hormones influence others by stimulation of the latters' receptors. Estrogen induces a progesterone-

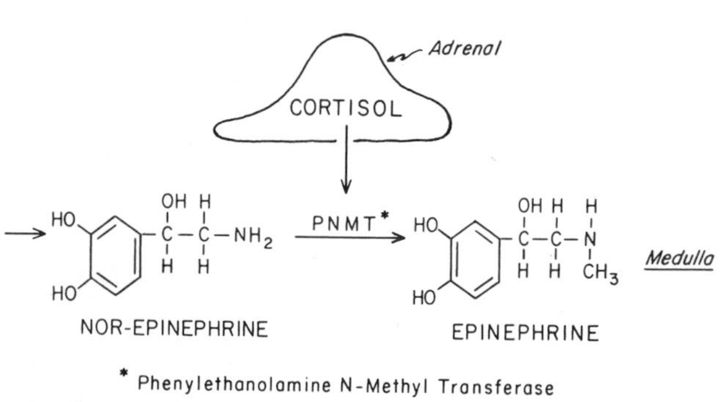

Figure 1–12. Cortisol, produced in the adrenal cortex, reaches the medulla via a local circulation. The resulting high concentration of cortisol induces the enzyme that catalyzes the completion of epinephrine synthesis.

binding protein in the uterine myometrium and endometrium. During the follicular phase of the menstrual cycle, therefore, one of the functions of estrogen is to prepare a receptor for the progesterone that will be produced after ovulation. A major clinical implication of this sequence is the progesterone–withdrawal bleeding test, which is used to evaluate patients with amenorrhea. If a patient has FSH (and therefore estrogen) of her own, the endometrium is proliferative and contains the progesterone-binding protein. Administered progestin presumably attaches to the endometrium; when the drug is discontinued, bleeding occurs.

FSH induces the formation of an androgen-binding protein in the Sertoli cells of the seminiferous tubules and in certain epithelial cells of the epididymis.[11] It also induces formation of the Leydig cell receptors for LH. The stage is then set for pituitary LH to attach to the Leydig cells and stimulate testosterone formation; the testosterone then binds to the testicular tubules and epididymis to exert its effect.

As mentioned previously, T_3 induces certain β-adrenergic receptors, thus partly accounting for the diminished effectiveness of catecholamines in myxedematous patients and the apparent hypersensitivity to the amines in hyperthyroid individuals.

Permissive Actions

The physiologic effect of a hormone depends in great measure on the other hormones present, that is, on the metabolic state of the individual. GH is considered the anabolic agent *par excellence*, but unless there is effective insulin present GH has a devastatingly catabolic effect. In 18 hours, it can precipitate ketoacidosis in a juvenile diabetic patient lacking insulin.

Transport and Metabolism of Hormones

Mention has been made previously of the effects of T_4 and T_3 on testosterone and cortisol metabolism. A subtler interaction between one hormone and the metabolism of another can be found in the influence of the sex steroids on hormone transport proteins. T_4 and cortisol, among other hormones, circulate bound to specific transport proteins, T_4-binding globulin (TBG) and cortisol-binding globulin (CBG). The level of each of these binding globulins is raised by estrogen. As the fraction of free hormone is diminished, a slight increase in production occurs and a new steady state is reached with a revised fractional disappearance rate that restores the expected net daily exposure of peripheral tissues to active hormones.

The case of the sex steroids is more intriguing. Testosterone and estradiol circulate bound to the same protein, sex steroid–binding globulin (SSBG or TEBG). As with the other hormone-binding globulins, testosterone lowers and estrogen raises the level of the binding protein, with consequent changes in the fractional amounts of the free hormones and, therefore, their metabolism. Testosterone is converted to estradiol in several tissues, however, and certain effects of these two hormones depend on the ratio between them. Thus, to interpret the influence of changes in sex steroid levels, one must take into account any resulting change in transport and metabolism.[12]

The role of nonendocrine tissues in hormone metabolism is being recognized increasingly as a source of endocrine regulation and occasionally as a cause of disease. One example of this phenomenon is the production of estrogen in the postmenopausal woman. The adrenal androgen androstenedione can be aromatized to the estrogen estrone in both the liver and the adipose tissue. The physiologic significance of this source of estrogen is unclear, but several pathologic implications have been suggested, including a role in endometrial or breast carcinoma, for the excessive production of estrone alleged to occur in obesity.[13]

The importance of diverse pathways and sites of hormone metabolism and interconversion can be illustrated by a consideration of some of the fates of testosterone (Fig. 1–13). Testosterone can be converted to a more potent androgen, to an estrogen, or to a weaker androgen. Some of these steps occur where testosterone is made (the testis) or where it acts (the brain, prostate, etc.), and some occur in the liver. Certain cells are capable of two of the transformations.

Both within such cells and in the organism as a whole, the relative use of alternate metabolic routes provides an added control well beyond the point of synthesis.

PATTERNS OF HORMONE BIOSYNTHESIS

Although more than 25 hormones of differing structure and function are known, certain common features of their biosynthesis and secretion provide recognizable patterns. The steroid hormones share a common pathway of synthesis; the dimeric glycoprotein hormones have one chain common to all and one unique chain that confers both biologic and immunologic specificity. The protein hormones, in common with other secretory proteins, are initially synthesized as prehormones; several have a pre-prohormone step as well.

Steroid Hormones

Steroid hormones are produced in the adrenal gland, ovaries, and testes; they regulate a wide range of physiologic functions. Cortisol controls the blood sugar and the balance of intermediary metabolism but is also involved in responses to stress. Aldosterone is the principal regulator of intravascular volume and therefore of the response to postural changes. Androgens and estrogens control reproductive function as well as provide an anabolic stimulus. In other words, the processes regulated by steroid hormones range from moment-to-moment reactions of the vascular tree to the generation-long concern of the species for reproduction.

A priori, one might anticipate that the production of hormones of such diverse roles would follow clearly separate pathways. Quite the contrary (as shown in Fig. 1–14), common pathways are used for the synthesis of these hormones by both the adrenal gland and the gonads. The immediate precursor of steroid synthesis is stored cholesterol, which is either synthesized intracellularly or incorporated attached to a carrier lipoprotein. For all steroids, the initial step is conversion of cholesterol to pregnenolone; ACTH, angiotensin, and the gonadotropins stimulate the side-chain cleavage enzyme that catalyzes this reaction. The adrenal cortex uses pregnenolone to produce C_{21} glucocorticoids, C_{19} androgens, and the mineralocorticoids. The gonads begin with the same precursors and the same initial pathways but then use later steps to produce the C_{19} androgens and the C_{18} estrogens. Small amounts of the sex steroids are also produced in the adrenal.

Important clinical consequences stem from these evolutionary choices. In congenital adrenal hyperplasia, impairment of cortisol biosynthesis leads to compensatory excessive ACTH, which results in androgen excess. In the genetic female, the result is virilization of the external genitalia. In the genetic male with untreated congenital adrenal hyperplasia, both sexual precocity and growth acceleration reflect the common pathways of biosynthesis used by both

Figure 1–13. The diverse fates of testosterone illustrate the critical role of hormone metabolism in determining hormone effects. Although a potent androgen in itself, testosterone also serves as a prohormone for the stronger androgen dihydrotestosterone (1) and for the estrogen estradiol (2). Certain tissues can make both transformations. In addition, testosterone is converted to a weak androgen (3) or excreted as the glucuronide (4). Finally, testosterone can be interconverted to androstenedione (5), which is also aromatized (to estrone).

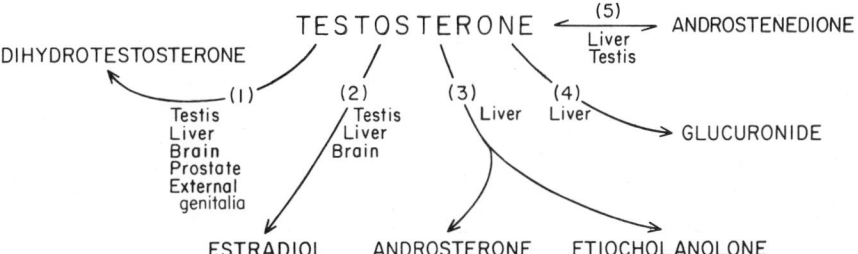

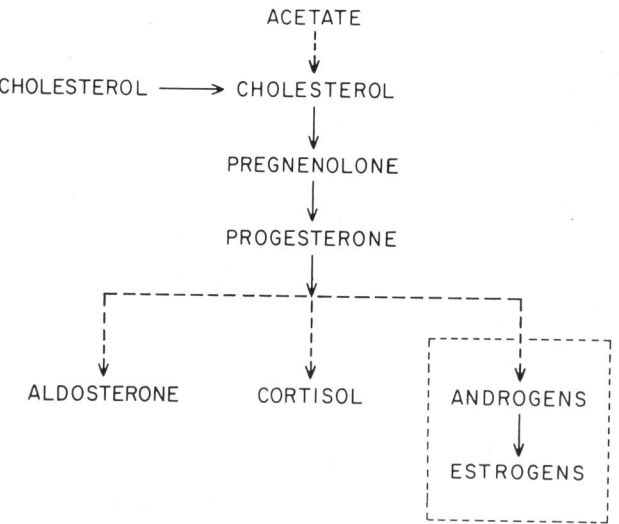

Figure 1–14. This schema of steroid hormone synthesis shows that hormones of diverse roles are produced from a common initial pathway that is present in both adrenal and gonad. The adrenal makes aldosterone, cortisol, and androgens; the gonad is specialized for the steps enclosed in the box.

adrenal gland and gonads. Indeed, gonadal tumors arising in such patients are so similar to adrenal cells in both biochemistry and histopathology that their classification as adrenal or gonadal tissue has defied consensus. An additional instance of clinical overlap is the syndrome produced by absence of a 17-hydroxylase that normally occurs in both adrenal and testis. In genetic males, 17-hydroxylase deficiency produces pseudohermaphroditism (a female phenotype) combined with hypertension and hypokalemia because of the hypersecretion of mineralocorticoids. Finally, occasional gonadal tumors contain an 11-hydroxylase and thus produce cortisol, and some adrenal tumors make excess androgen or estrogen or both. Thus many clinical disorders reflect the unifying role of the common pathways of steroid synthesis.

Glycoprotein Hormones

Four hormones include a carbohydrate moiety that plays a role in both the mechanism of action and the physiologic disposition of the compound. The two pituitary gonadotropins (FSH and LH), the placental gonadotropin (hCG), and thyrotropin (TSH) all differ in physiologic function, target glands, and secretory patterns. Nevertheless, their synthesis is ordered on a unique pattern that helps to account for both their physiologic roles and the derangements seen in disease.[14] Each of the glycoprotein hormones is composed of two chains (Fig. 1–15). The α chain is common to FSH, LH, and TSH; the α chain of hCG has minor amino acid differences from the others but is immunologically indistinguishable. In contrast, the β chain is unique in each of the four and confers both biologic and immunologic specificity on the hormone. The β chain, however, is not active by itself but

only when bridged to the α chain. Thus, when the α and β chains of the four hormones are separated and then randomly reannealed, the new combinations each have the biologic and immunologic characteristics of their β chain.

Peptide Hormones

The common features of the synthesis of peptide hormones derive not from their structure but from the steps in their synthesis. The circulating form of a peptide hormone is not usually the initial protein formed. Rather, a preprotein is formed, with an amino acid sequence at the N-terminal part. This preprotein ordinarily is short-lived; for PTH, it exists less than 1 min.[15] It is thought, however, to function as a signal protein[16] or as a leader sequence[15] that serves to move the protein from the rough endoplasmic reticulum, where it was synthesized, to the intracisternal space from which it will move to the Golgi apparatus. From there, the hormone is incorporated into secretory granules and then extruded from the cell as part of the excitation-secretion coupling that is activated by a fall in extracellular calcium. Removal of the signal segment leaves, in the case of PTH, insulin, and perhaps glucagon, a prohormone that is also longer than the active molecule. In the case of insulin, the prohormone serves to bring the α and β chains into positions that permit the disulfide bridges to form. The roles of other prohormones are not yet clear.

The details of peptide hormone synthesis have several points of relevance for the clinical endocrinologist. Insulinomas release proportionately larger amounts of proinsulin than the normal pancreas does; a plasma level of proinsulin of greater than 25% is strong evidence of a beta cell neoplasm. Release of proglucagon by alpha cell tumors has also been reported.[16] A similar circumstance may explain the paradox of clinical improvement despite maintained elevation of plasma GH in acromegalics treated with irradiation. The molecule being assayed as GH may be a cross-reacting but larger species. Here, as elsewhere that "big hormones" have been described, further study is needed to distinguish true prohormones from aggregations of smaller units in plasma, attachments of hormone molecules to nonhormone proteins, and other possibilities. Although unable to penetrate this thicket, the clinician needs to recall basic physiology when trying to interpret anomalous laboratory results.

A second implication of the secretory protein mechanism is the possibility that hypofunction may result from failure of the intraglandular cleavage of the preprotein or proprotein.[17] If this failure were to prevent export of the hormone, the gland could be rich in precursor while the body was poor of the product. If the prehormone was secreted *and* if an immunoassay detected it as the hormone, one would encounter hypofunction despite measurable hormone. Finally, the presence of hepatic or renal disease might lead to accumulation of hormone precursors in the circulation and thus to potentially confusing assay results.[18]

Another example of pathology arising from this mechanism of synthesis of secretory proteins is the production of hormones by nonendocrine malignant tumors. Far from being rare, ectopic secretion may be a routine aspect of malignancy.[18] The secreted compound is not always biologically active, however. Depending on the assay used, one may have measurable hormone without the corresponding endocrine syndrome, and conversely, clinical findings may exist without the presumed "responsible" hormone being found, that is, when another compound with similar biologic activity is produced. Correlation of immunoassay with a biologic assay, such as radioreceptor assay, is sometimes useful in illuminating these problems.

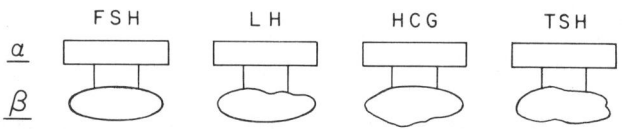

Figure 1–15. The glycoprotein hormones share a common α chain but have distinct β chains that confer biologic and immunologic specificity.

MECHANISMS OF HORMONE ACTION

The current understanding of hormone effector mechanisms is developed in the next chapter. For the purpose of this chapter it is necessary only to emphasize the integrating influence of the fact that, despite great variation in structure and physiologic function, most hormones work via one of two principal mechanisms.

Steroid hormones enter the cells of their target tissues and are bound to cytosol receptors of low affinity but high specificity.[19] The hormone-receptor complex is translocated into the nucleus, where it attaches to specific sites on the nuclear chromatin. Transcription of particular sequences of DNA is initiated, the resulting messenger RNA is exported, and ribosomal translation of the message leads to the synthesis of unique proteins that mediate the hormonal action. For most human target tissues, the nature of these proteins is not yet clear. By analogy with work done in other species, however, it appears that many organs may be the target of one hormone, that both receptor and chromatin binding are critical in making a particular organ a target, and that intracellular transformation of the hormone may be an additional control.

A similarly embracing generalization applies to most of the peptide hormones, but the steps are quite different. Until recently, peptide hormones were thought to stop at the cell surface and attach to specific protein receptors in the membrane.[20] The receptors are coupled to one of several species of adenylate cyclase. The bound hormone initiates adenylate cyclase activity, releasing cyclic adenosine monophosphate (cAMP) from adenosine triphosphate (ATP). The cAMP then initiates a cascade of phosphorylations and dephosphorylations of intracellular proteins. At the end of this sequence, the peptide hormone exerts its "biologic action." As with the steroid hormones, the molecule that is the immediate effector is, in most instances, not yet known.

The integrating theme is that multiple hormones, coming from different glands and having a wide range of actions, have their effects by one of two principal mechanisms. These two mechanisms account for most of the known hormones, but there are important exceptions that warrant mention. The thyroid hormones behave almost like steroid hormones, but they escape the requirement for a cytoplasmic receptor and instead attach directly to nuclear receptors.[21] Conversely, catecholamines appear to exert their β effects via adenyl cyclase activation at the cell membrane.

Finally, these generalizations should not hide the fact that the mechanisms of action of some of the principal hormones, including insulin, GH, and PRL, and the α effects of catecholamines have not been defined and may obey different principles.

GENETIC CONTROL OF ENDOCRINE FUNCTION

Many endocrine disorders are now recognized as hereditary, with mendelian pedigrees that reflect the action of a single gene. Such diseases affect the synthesis of hormones (congenital adrenal hyperplasia, goitrous cretinism) and hormone action (testicular feminization, pseudohypoparathyroidism). Genetic mechanisms are therefore operating from the biosynthesis of the hormone to its transport and intracellular binding and action. In addition, however, there are several disorders in which single genes control the differentiation and secretory function of multiple endocrine glands that otherwise have no obvious interconnection.

Table 1–2. SYNDROMES OF MULTIPLE ENDOCRINE ADENOMATOSIS

Multiple Endocrine Neoplasia I
Glands involved	Pituitary
	Parathyroid
	Pancreatic islets
Associated abnormalities	Peptic ulcer
	Lipomas
	Zollinger-Ellison syndrome
Genetics	Autosomal dominant
	Large number of new mutations

Multiple Endocrine Neoplasia IIA
Glands involved	Thyroid
	Adrenal
	Parathyroid
Associated abnormalities	Cushing's syndrome
	Diarrhea
Genetics	Autosomal dominant
	50% new mutations

Multiple Endocrine Neoplasia IIB
Glands involved	Thyroid
	Adrenal
Associated abnormalities	Neuromas
	Marfanoid habitus
	Heavy-lipped facies
Genetics	Autosomal dominant
	50% new mutations

Foremost of these syndromes are those of multiple endocrine adenomatosis (MEA) (Table 1–2) and polyglandular deficiency.

Multiple Endocrine Adenomatosis

Multiple Endocrine Neoplasia — Types I and II

Multiple endocrine neoplasia type I (MEN I) affects the parathyroid gland, pituitary gland, and pancreas. The pathology and pathophysiology are remarkably nonspecific, for the affected glands may contain adenomas, hyperplasia, or carcinoma. The cells may be inactive, normally active, or hyperfunctioning. Any abnormality in one of the glands can be combined with different lesions in the others and occasionally with disease of an entirely separate endocrine organ. Within one affected family there may be marked variations from one individual to another in the clinical findings. The features of MEN I suggest a mutant gene that can trigger simultaneous abnormality in three endocrine glands that are not directly interrelated. By inference, the wild-type allele must regulate both cell division and secretion in the pituitary, parathyroid, and pancreas. These glands therefore have a connection that is not otherwise apparent.

In MEN IIA, medullary carcinoma of the thyroid, pheochromocytoma, and parathyroid hyperplasia coexist. The medullary carcinomas tend to arise in zones of hyperplasia in the midportions of the thyroid lobes. They are typically multicentric and occur at younger ages than in individuals who have the sporadic, nonfamilial form of medullary cancer of the thyroid. The pheochromocytomas of MEN IIA show distinct features that contrast with those of sporadic pheochromocytomas: They occur at earlier ages, and they are more often bilateral and malignant. An additional feature of MEN IIA, seen in about 60% of cases, is parathyroid hyperplasia. Although there has been speculation that this hyperplasia might be secondary to calcitonin excess, the evidence to date suggests it is an independent consequence of the mutant gene.

MEN IIB (sometimes termed MEN III) is a similar abnormality in which medullary carcinoma and pheochromocytoma occur with a marfanoid habitus, mucosal neuromas, and a typical facies, but without coexisting parathyroid hyperplasia. Both of the MEN II disorders, as with MEN I, are inherited as autosomal dominant traits, with high penetrance but also with high *de novo* mutation rates: About 50% of cases occur without a positive family history.

The findings of the MEN syndromes, as well as some of the abnormalities of ectopic hormone secretion by malignant tumors, have suggested to Pearse and others that a number of endocrine glands may have a common embryologic origin.[22] The initial formulation suggested that the affected tissues shared the capacities to take up precursors of biogenic amines and to decarboxylate the intermediate products to produce active hormones. The sequence of *a*mine *p*recursor *u*ptake and *d*ecarboxylation was expressed in the acronym APUD to describe the cells or system involved. It was suggested that cells containing chromaffin and neural tissue had a common origin in the neuroectoderm of the embryo. From this origin, isolated cells could have migrated during early embryogenesis to sites as disparate as the thyroid gland, adrenal gland, hypothalamus, pancreas, and gut. Indeed, some recent studies have suggested that the cells of the anterior pituitary gland are also derived from the neuroectoderm. There seems little doubt that common origins for cells in widely dispersed tissues will be conclusively demonstrated and that this ontogeny provides an additional source of unity within the endocrine system.

Polyendocrine Deficiencies

Just as there are hereditary syndromes of hyperplasia and hyperfunction, there are several familial disorders in which hypofunction is seen in multiple endocrine tissues. Perhaps the most frequent disorder is one in which adrenal and parathyroid deficiencies occur in association with candidiasis in children. Some patients also have hypothyroidism and gonadal deficiency. Circulating antibodies against the endocrine tissues are common in these patients, and the histopathology of the destroyed tissues suggests a cytotoxic immune mechanism. The genetics of the polyendocrine deficiencies is not so well established as that of the MEN disorders. Nevertheless, the clustering in families suggests a gene that has something to do with an immunologic aspect of differentiation of the adrenal, thyroid, and parathyroid glands.

In summary, the syndromes of hyperfunction or hypofunction of unrelated endocrine glands reveal the presence of single genes controlling the differentiation, replication, function, and immunologic identity of these glands. Although the mechanisms are not well understood at this time, the inference is plain: Genetic integration of disparate endocrine glands is an additional source of unity within the system.

ENDOCRINE GLAND TOPOGRAPHY

The "ductless" glands are traditionally treated separately because their products, the hormones, reach their target tissues via the blood stream. But many hormones have local effects in addition to distant ones, and such effects seem to require the high concentration that a local vasculature can provide. Review of some examples helps to account for why the endocrine glands are located in their special niches.

The hypothalamus regulates pituitary function via small peptides that are secreted in the hypothalamus and then traverse the hypophyseal portal system to reach the anterior pituitary gland in high concentration. The secretory cells of the ovaries, specifically those in the follicle surrounding the oocyte, play a critical role in the nourishment and survival of the egg. A parallel phenomenon exists in the testes. Testosterone secreted by the Leydig cells reaches the seminiferous tubules in high concentration and stimulates spermatogenesis. As was mentioned earlier, cortisol reaches the adrenal medulla via a local circulation and induces the enzyme that completes the synthesis of epinephrine.

The pancreas provides another example of the physiologic importance of a portal circulation. Both insulin and glucagon are secreted into the portal vein and reach the liver before passing into the general circulation. This phenomenon has at least three significances. First, the liver is a principal site of action of insulin and may be the only target for glucagon; each hormone is thus delivered in high concentration. Second, both insulin and glucagon have a hepatotropic effect distinct from their influences on intermediary metabolism. Finally, since the liver is a principal site of metabolism for peptide hormones, insulin and glucagon can be partially metabolized after having acted on the liver. Indeed, there is a paradox in the metabolism of the two hormones by the liver: Approximately 50% of insulin, which has many peripheral actions, is extracted by the liver, whereas only 10–20% of glucagon is extracted, and yet this hormone has no proven extrahepatic actions.

In summary, the integrating theme of this section is a recognition of the fact that, although called "messengers," most hormones have a local effect at a site they reach in high concentration through local circulation.

SUMMARY OF MECHANISMS OF INTEGRATION

This chapter has stressed the thesis that the functioning of endocrine glands is cohesively integrated through numerous mechanisms. First, most hormone-dependent processes involve multiple hormones and most hormones have multiple effects. Second, there is a constant interplay of neural and endocrine forces, both in the basal state and in emergency responses. Third, there are several broadly defined classes of hormones that share pathways of biosynthesis, transport, and mechanisms of action. Finally, the hereditary endocrine disorders reveal interrelations among certain glands. In evaluating patients with suspected endocrine disease, the clinician should review the phyisologic pattern and the manifold layers and controls involved; he then will be in the best position to identify the pathologic alteration.

CLINICAL ENDOCRINOLOGY

Clinical endocrinology is a subspecialty of medicine, and the general principles of diagnosis and therapy are applicable within this subspecialty. Perhaps the most important caveat is to avoid the intellectual trap awaiting the consultant as he confronts a new patient — unconsciously asking, "Does this patient have one of my diseases or not?" The proper question is: "What is wrong with this patient, and do I know anything special that will contribute to a correct diagnosis?"

Certain features of endocrine disorders differentiate them from other diseases that the internist sees. Although these features are usually obvious, their explication may be a useful background for the discussion of laboratory tests that follows. All endocrine disorders are merely quantitative departures from the norm; that is, all normal persons have cortisol and parathyroid hormone and insulin, but a normal person does not have a little bit of pneumococcal pneumonia or cancer. These quantitative changes are superimposed on a wide variety of normal constitutions; for example, excess hirsutism is much more obvious in a blue-eyed, blond Scandinavian than in a swarthy person of Mediterranean background.

The changes due to endocrine disease occur against a changing background of normal findings, including diurnal variations, sleep-entrained rhythms, monthly cycles (menses), growth and development, and aging. Endocrine function must constantly be assessed against this changing background. Meningitis is abnormal whether the patient is 5, 25, or 65, but vaginal bleeding has an entirely different significance at each of those ages.

Endocrine changes tend to develop gradually and to be well tolerated by the patient as only fractional differences from his prior state. Thus, direct questioning may be unrevealing because the patient has adapted to the changes so gradually as not to realize they are symptoms. Indeed, patients often attribute the symptoms of endocrine disease to the normal passage of time or to aging.

A careful, sensitive, subtle, thorough history and physical examination provide the fundamental approach to the evaluation of a patient with suspected endocrine disease. The specific items to be emphasized are developed elsewhere in this text, but a useful general principle is to try to come away from the initial history-taking and physical with an estimate of the likelihood or unlikelihood of an endocrine disorder. The selection, pursuit, and interpretation of laboratory examinations are heavily influenced by the clinician's impression after the initial examination.

Generally speaking, there are too many endocrine laboratory tests, and it is easy to waste money in ordering them. One should therefore be aware of appropriate screening tests and of their reliability and should formulate sharply the questions one wants to answer with the help of the laboratory. Some examples may be useful.

The best test to exclude subtle hyperthyroidism in an ambulatory cardiac patient with new onset of atrial fibrillation but with no clinical features of hyperthyroidism would be different from the test ordered to confirm a clinically obvious case of Graves' disease. If the clinician believes a disease is *not* present, he is in general seeking a sensitive test that reveals abnormality early in the development of the disease. For hyperthyroidism, the most sensitive test in general use is the serum T_3; this test should be used to exclude the diagnosis of hyperthyroidism or to detect it in a borderline case. On the other hand, since the serum T_4 is elevated in better than 90–95% of patients with clinically definite Graves' disease, and since the T_4 is easier and more widely available than the T_3, it would be the proper test to *confirm* the diagnosis when it is strongly suspected.

There is seldom one endocrine test that is best for detecting all perturbations of function of a given gland: there is no "perfect" thyroid function test. The serum T_3 is extremely reliable in detecting mild hyperthyroidism but is insensitive and therefore often misleading as a test for hypothyroidism. In some series, as many as 50% of myxedematous patients have a normal serum T_3. On the contrary, the most sensitive test for detecting primary hypothyroidism is the serum TSH, which is typically elevated before the serum T_4 is measurably depressed. Yet, the TSH is a poor test by which to separate hyperthyroid patients from normal persons.

A second important need is to distinguish clearly between tests meant to establish the presence of altered endocrine function and tests addressed to localizing the probable pathology. For example, a morning plasma cortisol after the patient has taken 1.0 mg of dexamethasone the previous midnight will reliably exclude Cushing's syndrome better than 99% of the time for a total cost of $20.20 (two tablets of dexamethasone, 20¢; plasma cortisol, $20). But the detailed dynamic testing so useful in demonstrating whether Cushing's syndrome is of pituitary, adrenal, or ectopic origin may cost $1500.00 or more when one includes the charges for hospitalization, laboratory determinations, and professional fees. The author has seen numerous occasions when a frustrating and ultimately fruitless effort to pinpoint the pathology was launched before the existence of hypercortisolism had been established.

The clinician must decide whether the resting level of a hormone is an adequate measurement or whether the physiology must be perturbed in order to make the result meaningful. As an illustration, the plasma level of GH in normal individuals oscillates several times a day between values that, if sustained, would be consistent with acromegaly and, if the maximum achieved by the individual, would be diagnostic of hypopituitarism. In studying GH, therefore, it is advisable to set an appropriate physiologic challenge before determining the value. If one is trying to exclude acromegaly — perhaps in an alcoholic patient whose appearance suggests acromegaly — it is best to measure a GH value in an ambulatory, otherwise unstressed individual 1 hour after ingestion of 100 g of glucose. If the GH level after glucose is less than 3 ng/ml, the diagnosis of acromegaly has been excluded. Alternatively, if one wishes to test pituitary function in a child who appears abnormally short, a prior period of active exercise or administration of glucagon ½ hour before drawing the GH level would be more revealing than would a prior period of rest. If the GH level does not rise after such a challenge, definitive evaluation is appropriate.

A fourth caution is the need to be clear about the limitations of tests that are ordered. For example, peptide hormone assays in clinical laboratories are rarely able to distinguish reliably between low and low normal values, but they are excellent in distinguishing between low and high values. Specifically, few clinical laboratories can consistently distinguish a low normal level of LH from a low level of LH. Therefore, the screening test for male hypopituitarism, in which gonadotropin deficiency is often the first feature, should not be an LH but a serum testosterone. If the testosterone is low, the question one then asks the laboratory is: "Is the deficiency of testosterone due to pituitary disease or to gonadal disease?" If it is due to pituitary disease, the LH should be low. If the defect is primarily in the testes (and thus the negative feedback of testosterone has been withdrawn), then the pituitary LH should be increased. The laboratory is now being used to distinguish low from high, and this is done with great reliability. As a generalization, therefore, the detection of hypofunction of pituitary tropic hormones is first assessed by looking at the functioning of the target gland; once that is established, measurement of the tropic hormone is an effective approach to determining the site of pathology.

Finally, it is critical to recall the influence of drugs, hepatic and renal functions, and age and general body health on the results of laboratory tests. When care is taken, however, and when laboratory tests are ordered and interpreted within the context of alert and subtle clinical evaluation, the modern laboratory provides a precision and a sensitivity of diagnosis never previously possible in endocrine disease.

REFERENCES

1. Felig, P., and Koivisto, V.: Body fuel metabolism, In *The Year in Metabolism 1977.* Freinkel, N. (ed.), New York, Plenum Press, 1978.
2. Guillemin, R.: The expanding significance of hypothalamic peptides, or, Is endocrinology a branch of neuroendocrinology? *Recent Prog. Horm. Res. 33*:1, 1977.
3. Schally, A. V.: Aspects of hypothalamic regulation of the pituitary gland. Its implications for the control of reproductive processes. *Science 202*:18, 1978.
4. Abe, M., and Sherwood, L. M.: Regulation of parathyroid hormone secretion by adenyl cyclase. *Biochem. Biophys. Res. Commun. 48*:396, 1972.
5. Weitzman, E. D.: Circadian rhythms and episodic hormone secretion in man. *Ann. Rev. Med. 27*:225, 1976.
6. Unger, R. H., and Dobbs, R. E.: Insulin, glucagon, and somatostatin secretion in the regulation of metabolism. *Ann. Rev. Physiol. 40*:307, 1978.
7. Sterling, K., and Lazarus, J. H.: The thyroid and its control. *Ann. Rev. Physiol. 39*:349, 1977.
8. Santen, R. J.: Is aromatization of testosterone to estradiol required for inhibition of luteinizing hormone secretion in men? *J. Clin. Invest. 56*:1555, 1975.
9. Yen, S. S. C.: The human menstrual cycle (integrative function of the hypothalamic-pituitary-ovarian-endometrial axis), In *Reproductive Endocrinology.* Yen, S. S. C., and Jaffe, R. B. (eds.), Philadelphia, W. B. Saunders Company, 1978.
10. Kolata, G. B.: Polypeptide hormones: What are they doing in cells? *Science 201*:895, 1978.
11. Fritz, I. B., Rommerts, F. G., et al.: Regulation by FSH and dibutyryl cyclic AMP of the formation of androgen-binding protein in Sertoli cell–enriched cultures. *J. Reprod. Fertil. 46*:17, 1976.
12. Anderson, D. C.: Sex-hormone-binding globulin. *Clin. Endocrinol. 3*:69, 1974.
13. Siiteri, P. K., and MacDonald, P. C.: Role of extraglandular estrogens in human endocrinology, In *Handbook of Physiology,* Section 7: *Endocrinology,* Vol. II, Part I. American Physiological Society. Geiger, S. R., Astwood, E. B., and Greep, R. O. (eds.), Baltimore, Williams and Wilkins, 1973.
14. Odell, W., Wolfsen, A., et al.: Ectopic peptide synthesis: A universal concomitant of neoplasia. *Trans. Assoc. Am. Physicians xc*:204, 1977.
15. Habener, J. F., and Potts, J. T., Jr.: Biosynthesis of parathyroid hormones. *N. Engl. J. Med. 299*:580, 635, 1978.
16. Blobel, G., and Sabatini, D.: Ribosome-membrane interactions in eukaryotic cells. In *Biomembranes.* Vol. 2. Manson, L. A. (ed.), New York, Plenum Press, 1971.
17. Yalow, R. S.: Heterogeneity of peptide hormones: Its relevance in clinical radioimmunoassay. *Adv. Clin. Chem. 20*:1, 1978.
18. Blackman, M. R., Rosen, S. W., et al.: Ectopic hormones. *Adv. Intern. Med. 23*:85, 1978.
19. Chan, L., and O'Malley, B. W.: Steroid hormone action: Recent advances. *Ann. Intern. Med. 89*:694, 1978.
20. Catt, K. J., and Dufau, M. L.: Peptide hormone receptors. *Ann. Rev. Physiol. 39*:529, 1977.
21. Sterling, K.: Thyroid hormone action at the cell level. *N. Engl. J. Med. 300*:117, 173, 1979.
22. Pearse, A. G. E., and Takor, T. T.: Neuroendocrine embryology and the APUD concept. *Clin. Endocrinol. 5*(Suppl.):229s, 1976.

CHAPTER 2

Endocrine Systems: Mechanisms of Disease, Target Cells, and Receptors

By Jesse Roth
and Carl Grunfeld

AN INVITATION TO THE CLINICIAN

The authors have intended this chapter to cover a broad subject for a wide audience. Throughout, general principles are emphasized, and disease applications are included. For the medical student or young physician, whose basic science background is recent, the chapter is intended to provide a link between the science and his or her growing framework of knowledge of clinical endocrinology. The experienced physician, who knows endocrine diseases, will find that the science adds a new dimension and rationality to his or her clinical wisdom. In addition to emphasizing the "big picture," the authors have included some details to provide the reader with enough background to tackle easily other chapters in this book as well as reviews and original articles in the literature. This chapter might be used both as a quick introduction and as a reference for recurrent stimulation and integration. Because individual sections will be referred to more often than the whole chapter, some points have been covered more than once.

This chapter deals with the biochemical basis of endocrine disorders. An endocrine system represents an orderly sequence of biochemical events. The first step is the biochemical recognition of a biological need, which, in turn, leads to regulation (stimulation or inhibition) of hormone release. The final step is a biochemical event at the target cell that meets that biological need. From the first step to the last are a very large number of biochemical events, all of which must be intact for the system to work properly. Disruption of any of the steps results in an endocrine disorder. The aim of this chapter is to present in general principles the biochemical events by which endocrine systems operate so that the physician dealing with the patient who has an endocrine disorder can understand the mechanism of the disorder and utilize diagnostic tests and therapeutic interventions in a rational way. Equally important, an understanding of the overall biochemical framework will enable the physician to deal effectively with newly described diseases as well as new diagnostic and therapeutic modes. Fortunately for everyone who studies endocrinology, nature has chosen to use widely a very limited number of biochemical mechanisms. Therefore, despite the existence of more than 50 different hormones, only a relatively few principles are needed to characterize all of the hormones.

Outline of an Endocrine System

To organize the subsequent discussion, let us recount in outline the essential components of an endocrine system (Figs. 2–1 and 2–2). First there is the body of secretory cells. There must be a sufficient number of appropriately programed secretory cells that are capable of releasing, upon command, an adequate amount of biologically active hormone.

The secretory mechanism does not know when to release hormone or how much. Therefore the secretory cells have available to them information from sensing systems that are capable of appreciating conditions in the internal and external environment. Since a secretory cell is typically subject to multiple influences, the multiple (often conflicting) signals must be integrated within the secretory cell to yield a single signal that tells the secretory cell how much hormone to release for how long a time period. Traditionally, we have thought that hormone release was an active process whereas lack of release simply indicated lack of a release signal. It has become quite

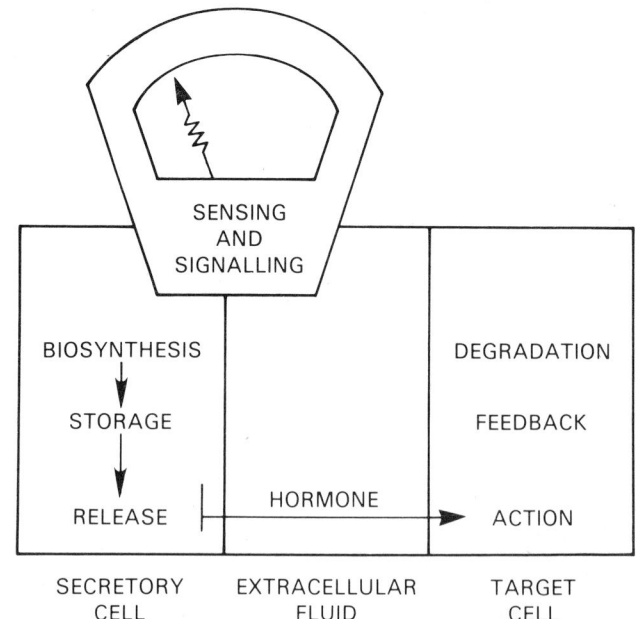

Figure 2–1. Essential elements of an endocrine system. The secretory cell typically is a unique cell type that can synthesize (store) and release the hormone. Associated with the secretory cell are sensing and signaling devices that regulate the magnitude and duration of hormone release (and biosynthesis). The blood or extracellular fluid carries the hormone to target cells throughout the body where it acts, generates feedback signals, and is degraded.

clear now that inhibition of release is also an active process that is actively signaled and regulated by means similar to the stimulatory signals. For example, insulin release is stimulated by glucose and glucagon and is inhibited by somatostatin, catecholamines, and prostaglandins. Thus the rate and duration of hormone release are governed by active inhibitory as well as stimulatory events.

With the release of an appropriate amount of biologically active hormone into the extracellular fluid, the next stage begins, namely the delivery of the hormone to target cells throughout the body. When the hormone arrives at the target cell, the next major series of events begins. How does the target cell recognize the hormone? The hormone molecule may represent only one of every 10^5 to 10^9 molecules to which the cell is exposed. Recognition of the active hormone is provided by the receptor. The receptor molecule specifically recognizes the bioactive hormone and manifests its recognition by binding it. In addition to recognition, the combination of hormone with receptor must initiate a series of biochemical events at the target cell that will result in the final biological effect(s). The nature of the biological effect that is produced depends heavily on the cell type that is being acted upon. Thus the hormone should be viewed as a signal molecule whose interaction with the cell leads to a modification of processes that already exist within the target cell, either accelerating or inhibiting processes that have been programed by differentiation into that specific cell type. For example, glucagon acts on fat cells to accelerate lipolysis, on liver cells to accelerate glycogenolysis and stimulate uptake of amino acids, and on β-cells to enhance the secretion of insulin.

Once the desired biological effect has been achieved by the target cells, two more processes must take place. First, the accomplishment of the desired biological goal must be recognized by the secretory cell (i.e., there must be feedback inhibition). Second, all of the biochemical

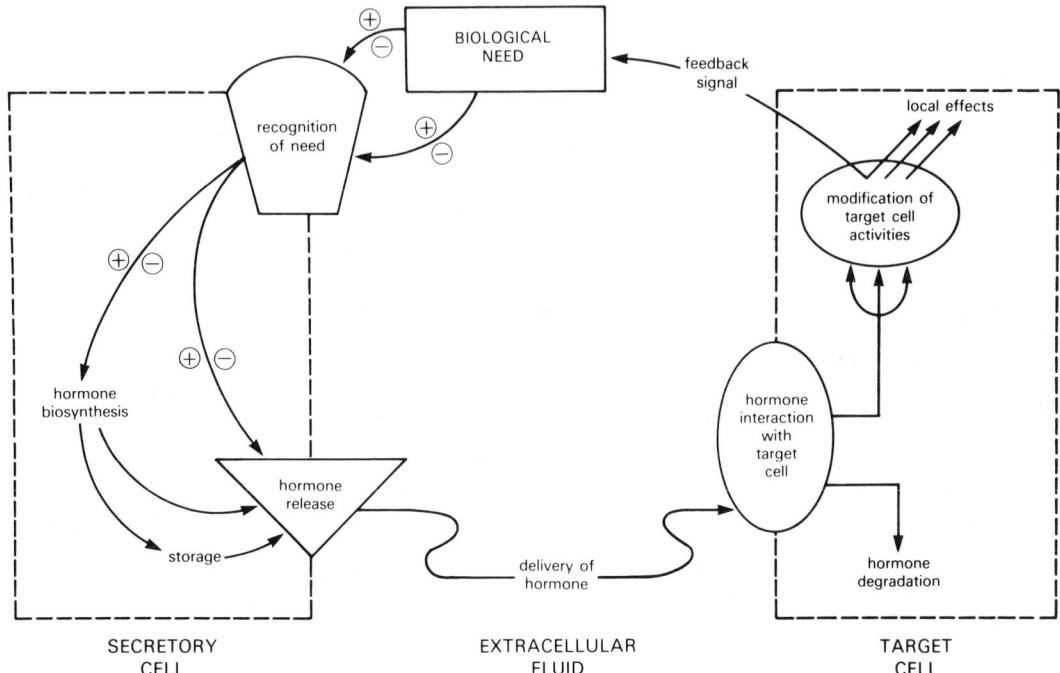

Figure 2–2. Overall scheme of an endocrine system. The keystone of an endocrine system is a biological need. Recognition of the need is carried out by a sensing or signaling system which often (though not always) is in the secretory cell itself. Often several needs are expressed through one type of endocrine secretory cell (e.g., plasma glucose, amino acids, fatty acids, and ketones regulate insulin secretion) and a single need may be expressed through multiple types of hormone-secreting cells (e.g., glucose regulates insulin, glucagon, GIP, and growth hormone). The sensing and signaling system, in recognizing the biological need, sends signals to stimulate or inhibit release of the hormone. Often there are several sensing systems and their multiple signals are integrated within the secretory cell. In addition, there may be independent signals to regulate hormone biosynthesis (and storage). Hormone, released into blood or extracellular fluid, is delivered to target cell and acts as the intercellular messenger from secretory cell to target cell. Hormone interaction with elements of the target cell leads to modification of cellular processes that are already present in the target cell. Most hormones produce a multiplicity of effects in any single target cell, only a minority of which are recognized outside the target cell (as feedback signals) to announce that the biological need has been met. Often hormone interaction with the target cell may lead to hormone degradation. Typically, defects on the left half of the figure are lumped together as defects in hormone secretion, and defects on the right are grouped as target cell defects.

messages that have been generated in the secretory cell, in the plasma, and at the target cell must decay at an appropriate speed so that fresh information can be appreciated and acted upon.

A General Approach to Endocrine Disorders

This scheme should provide the physician with a general approach to any suspected endocrine disorder. Is the biological abnormality that is observed in the patient under hormonal regulation? Which target cell(s) or hormone(s) is involved? Does the abnormality represent an excessive effect or an insufficient effect or some of both? (See Table 2–1.) Is an appropriate amount of biologically active hormone being delivered to the target cell? If yes, that focuses our attention on the target cell. Is there something wrong with the target cell itself? Alternatively, is the target cell being misled by an abnormal signal? For example, immunoglobulins from patients with Graves' disease can simulate the effects of TSH on the thyroid gland, or certain drugs can mimic the actions of estrogens on multiple target cells. A further discussion of target cell mechanisms will form a major portion of this chapter.

If the target cell is not receiving an adequate amount of

Table 2–1.   HORMONE DEFICIENCY STATES COMPLICATED BY SECONDARY HORMONE EXCESS

Condition	Hormone that Is Deficient	Hormone Present in Excess	Result of Hormone Excess
Defect in thyroid hormone biosynthesis	T_3, T_4	TSH	goiter
Defect in adrenal steroid biosynthesis	cortisol cortisol cortisol	ACTH androgen mineralocorticoid	skin darkening virilization hypertension
Menopause; ovariectomy	estrogen	pituitary or hypothalamic factor	hot flashes
Insulin-dependent (Type I) diabetes	insulin	glucagon	aggravation of hyperglycemia and ketogenesis
Hypopituitarism (due to destructive lesion)	one or more hormones of anterior pituitary	prolactin	amenorrhea, infertility, galactorrhea

Typically we categorize endocrine disorders as states in which either the hormone effect is deficient or the hormone effect is excessive. This table illustrates that a single disorder may manifest some features due to deficiency of one hormone and some features due to excess of another hormone.

biologically active hormone, the next question is to decide whether the delivery system is at fault; is the secretory cell releasing appropriately but the hormone cannot reach the target cell? For example, are there anti-hormone antibodies that are intercepting the hormone? Is hormone being inactivated excessively or otherwise being lost from the body at an inappropriately rapid rate?

After having considered the delivery system, we turn our attention to the secretory cells. Are the secretory cells releasing an inadequate amount of biologically active hormone? If so, is it because they are not producing the requisite hormone precursors (e.g., hypothyroidism due to a defect at an early step in thyroid hormone biosynthesis, which can be the result of an inborn deficit, excessive ingestion of iodide, or goitrogens in the food or water supply)? Is it because the secretory cells are incapable of converting precursors to the normal hormone, or unable to store hormone appropriately, or are there too few secretory cells, or is some other aspect of hormone production deranged?

For example, three inborn defects of the insulin molecule have been found; in two, there is a defect at a site on the proinsulin molecule where proinsulin is cleaved to produce insulin so that the conversion of precursor to hormone cannot be completed. In the third, there is an amino acid substituted in the biologically important region of insulin itself, which yields a molecule that has a reduced ability to bind to insulin receptors and is even more defective in its ability to stimulate a biological response. In all three examples, the measurements of plasma insulin by radioimmunoassay give an overestimate of the bioactivity of the circulating hormone.

Alternatively, is it the sensing or signaling system that regulates the secretory cell that is inadequate, either failing to recognize the appropriate signals or responding to inappropriate signals? Likewise, excessive (more properly "inappropriate") hormone production should be analyzed in a similar way. At what level is the excess generated? Excessive stimulation or inadequate inhibition? Is the messenger coming from its usual site of production or is it being produced ectopically? Is the stimulator a normal messenger in excess or an abnormal messenger? Are the normal negative feedback signals present? Are they recognized?

For example, insulin release from islet cell adenomas typically is subnormally responsive to glucose, excessively responsive to leucine or glucagon, and inadequately suppressed by hypoglycemia. Growth hormone release in patients with acromegaly is often excessively responsive to TRH and typically is inadequately suppressed by hyperglycemia. In a few cases of acromegaly, peripheral tumors have been found that contain material that is capable of stimulating growth hormone release from pituitaries *in vitro*. Although our understanding of most endocrine diseases is still insufficient to allow a complete formulation of this type, this overall scheme should be a permanent tool with which the physician can approach patient problems at the present time as well as provide a framework for integrating new information.

Historical Perspective on Endocrine Disorders

In learning any field, most people prefer to ignore the historical development. They want to know where we are today, not how we got here. Endocrinology and biochemistry are both young disciplines. Our understanding of endocrine systems is clearly still quite incomplete. The portions of the system that we do understand clearly relate to what we have been able to measure. The portions of the system that have been the most studied, about which we have the most information, and that have attracted the most workers in the field have been given the most importance. Like the blind men examining the elephant in the ancient Indian legend, we have examined only a small part of the whole from which we extrapolate to the entirety. While this analogy exaggerates the true state of endocrinology, it should serve as a warning to the contemporary physician and scientist.

As emphasized earlier, for an endocrine system to function properly, every step from the first to the last must be intact. Hormone biosynthesis, release, and delivery to the target cell have received the most attention, although they represent but a minority of the events in the pathway. As a result, the hormone has dominated the thoughts of endocrinologists, both the investigators and the physicians. Events at the target cell have been less well studied. The sensing and signaling systems that regulate the secretory cell and the mechanisms for signal decay are even less well understood. That the known dominates the unknown in the system should not mislead the reader. An endocrine disorder occurs whenever any of the myriad steps in the complex system fails. Statistically speaking, it is likely that defects will occur with approximately equal frequency at each step. However, because our understanding of the hormone has advanced much further than our understanding of the other components of the system, our interpretation of endocrine disorders has been excessively weighted at the level of the hormone.

As a first approximation, whenever the biological effect of a hormone was excessive or deficient we ascribed it to a quantitative excess or deficiency of that hormone. Only later and more slowly have we recognized that diseases can occur at other sites within the pathway (Table 2–2). Thus, vasopressin deficiency (diabetes insipidus) was recognized long before vasopressin resistance (nephrogenic diabetes insipidus), parathyroid hormone deficiency before parathyroid hormone resistance (pseudohypoparathyroidism), and growth hormone deficiency before growth hormone resistance (Laron-type dwarfism). Thus target cell defects were much more slowly recognized than secretory

Table 2–2. EXAMPLES OF BIOLOGICAL DEFECTS PRODUCED BY HORMONE DEFICIENCY OR TARGET CELL INSENSITIVITY

Biological Defect	Hormone-Deficient State	Target Cell Insensitivity
Inadequate water reabsorption by kidney tubules	diabetes insipidus	nephrogenic diabetes insipidus
Hypocalcemia	hypoparathyrodism	pseudohypoparathyroidism
Short stature	growth hormone deficiency	Laron-type dwarfism
Hyperglycemia	insulin-dependent (type I) diabetes mellitus	insulin-independent (type II) diabetes mellitus
Failure of virilization	androgen deficiency	testicular feminization

defects. Even at the level of target cell defects, complete refractoriness to the hormone was more readily recognized than partial defects, i.e., subnormal sensitivity but not total refractoriness. Again, total refractoriness was much easier to measure than subnormal sensitivity.

Disorders of glucose metabolism present such an example. With the isolation of insulin in 1921, hyperglycemic and hypoglycemic conditions were formulated simply in terms of insulin deficiency and insulin excess. Only 30 or 40 years later, with the development of methods to measure insulin accurately, did it become clear that this formulation was too simple; many of the patients, in fact the majority of hyperglycemic patients, have normal or supernormal amounts of biologically active insulin that is being delivered to the target cells and yet the target cells do not respond adequately. Thus we can conclude that these patients have defects at the level of the target cell. Some respond to insulin half as well or one third as well as normal persons while others respond substantially less well. None of them are totally refractory to insulin (possibly a lethal defect). Rather the defect is a quantitative one.

In some of these patients with target cell defects, defects have been detected at the level of the receptor or at later steps within the target cell. With new techniques introduced in the last decade, receptor defects have been characterized in some detail. On the other hand, our technology for studying other events at the target cell has been inadequate, and our recognition of defects at these sites has clearly lagged. Throughout the rest of this chapter, historical perspectives will be introduced not simply for "completeness" but rather as a constant warning that our current formulation of endocrinology and of endocrine disorders remains heavily biased by historical forces. While the past represents our sole supply of current information, it also serves as the major impediment to our progress toward future understanding.

TARGET CELLS

Breadth of Target Cells

Hormone-producing cells represent only a limited number of cell types. Thus 50 or so different hormones are produced by an even smaller number of cell types. On the other hand, essentially all cells of the body are target cells for one or more hormones. While a small number of hormones have been known to regulate nearly all cells of the body, e.g., thyroid hormones or glucocorticoids, the traditional view in endocrinology has been that each hormone had a limited number of cell types as targets. Classic examples of hormones with a limited range of target tissues include TSH, which stimulates thyroid acinar cells; ACTH, which stimulates cells in the adrenal cortex; and LH, which stimulates cells in the gonads.

It is now known that all three of these hormones are capable of stimulating lipolysis in fat cells (although their physiological role in fat metabolism is unclear). More important, it is clear that TSH acts to stimulate the stromal tissue of the thyroid gland. In fact, its effects on the stroma including blood vessels and connective tissue may be even greater than its effects on the acinar cells. ACTH is also known to have effects on a large number of cell types.

Glucagon traditionally was thought to act only on the liver to stimulate glycogen breakdown. Now it is clear that glucagon also stimulates lipolysis by fat cells, stimulates amino acid uptake by liver, and has a direct effect on the β-cells of the pancreas to increase insulin secretion. By studying the ability of glucagon to activate the enzyme adenylate cyclase and stimulate cyclic AMP production, we have been able to add a large number of other tissues to the list of glucagon-sensitive cells. Likewise, insulin had been though to act only on skeletal muscle and heart muscle. It was later found that fat and liver are also insulin-sensitive. With increasing study, it is now clear that fibroblasts, monocytes, and many other tissues are also insulin-sensitive.

Thus, as a general rule, most hormones affect a very wide range of tissues and, as our skill increases in measuring biochemical events within cells, the number of target cells known to be influenced by a given hormone is expanding continuously. As will be discussed later, the specific receptors for a given hormone have been found on many more types of cells than would have been predicted on the basis of our current understanding of their physiology.

Nature of the Target Cell Response

The biological response of a given cell type to a particular hormone depends largely on the differentiated nature of that cell. The hormone is a signal that causes the cell to do certain things. The program of responses to that particular hormone is built into the target cell by processes of differentiation. Thus insulin acts on the fat cells to stimulate glucose transport and lipid biosynthesis; in liver it stimulates amino acid transport and glycogen synthesis; it acts on the α-cells of the pancreatic islets to inhibit glucagon secretion; and when infused into the cerebrospinal fluid of experimental animals it causes a decrease in food intake and weight loss. Thus the target cell, by its differentiation, determines whether or not it will be responsive to a particular hormone and determines what the nature of the response shall be.

Breadth of Responses

When a hormone acts on a target cell, it typically does not activate a single process but rather regulates numerous biochemical events within the cell (Fig. 2–2). When thyrotropin acts on a thyroid cell, it not only stimulates iodide uptake and hormone biosynthesis and release, it also regulates glucose metabolism and phospholipid synthesis as well as the biosynthesis of all major classes of macromolecules. ACTH not only acts to stimulate hormone biosynthesis and release but also regulates a large number of other biological processes in the adrenal. In addition, it regulates more complex functions, such as blood flow, cell growth, differentiation, and regulatory mechanisms of all kinds.

When a hormone acts on a cell to produce a biological effect, the achievement of that biological effect may be recognized back at the level of the secretory cell. For example, hormone output by the thyroid or the adrenal is recognized by the hypothalamus and pituitary, which leads to a reduction in trophic hormone secretion by the pituitary. On the other hand, the vast majority of hormone-mediated events at the target cell are not recognized outside the target cell (Fig. 2–2). Thus the classic negative-feedback loop that we associate with endocrine systems should be recognized as only a very limited part of the target cell's response.

Table 2–3. COMPARISON OF TWO CLASSES OF HORMONES

		Peptides	Steroids and 1,25(OH)₂-Vitamin D
*Solubility**	— in aqueous (polar) solvents	excellent	limited
	— in nonaqueous (nonpolar) solvents	poor	excellent
Synthesis and Degradation	— biosynthetic pathway	single peptide; prohormones	multiple enzymes
	— extraglandular transformation of bioactivity	very rare	common
	— storage of preformed hormone	often substantial	minimal
	— degradation products	irreversibly inactive	sometimes retain or regain activity
In Plasma	— binding proteins	very rare	yes
	— half-life	short (minutes)	long (hours)
At the Target Cell	— initial binding site	cell surface receptor	cytoplasmic receptor
	— principal site of action	plasma membrane	nucleus
	— principal mechanism of action	stimulate production of soluble intracellular ("second") messenger	stimulate production of specific mRNA's

Catecholamines follow the patterns of the peptide hormones except that biosynthesis is via a multienzyme pathway like that for steroids and 1,25(OH)₂-vitamin D. Iodothyronines follow the pattern of the steroids except (1) a protein (thyroglobulin) acts as hormone precursor and as a large reservoir of stored hormone, as with peptide hormones; (2) half-lives in plasma are measured in days; and (3) receptors, i.e., major initial sites of interaction, are in the nucleus.

*For brevity, we designate the peptide hormones (and growth factors) as well as catecholamines as "water-soluble hormones" and the steroids, 1,25(OH)₂-vitamin D, and iodothyronines as "lipid-soluble hormones"; the latter term is convenient but somewhat inaccurate since these hormones are amphophilic, are very soluble in amphophilic solvents such as alcohols, and only variably soluble in pure aqueous or pure lipid solvents.

Target Cell Responsiveness

A fundamental concept in endocrinology is that hormone levels rise and fall, often rapidly, in response to changing body needs. We are much less comfortable with the idea that normally the target cell also fluctuates continuously and often widely in its responsiveness to hormone. The magnitude of each biological effect that results from the interaction of hormone with target cell will depend equally on the amount of hormone present and the

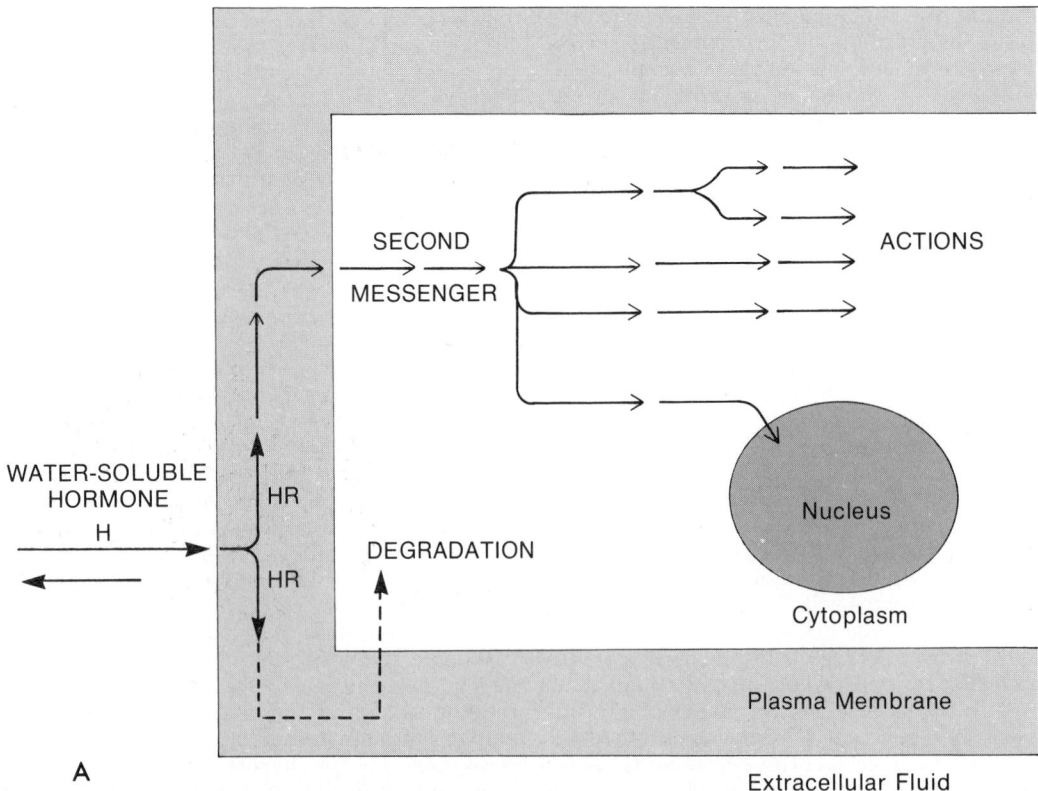

Figure 2–3. Two types of target cell interactions. *A*, The water-soluble hormones (peptides and catecholamines; abbreviated H) interact reversibly with receptors on the outer surface of the target cell. The hormone-receptor complex (HR) interacts with one or more membrane components which, in the absence of further participation of hormone, leads to stimulation of a common intracellular pathway (e.g., synthesis of cAMP and activation of protein kinase) which then activates multiple (branched) pathways within the cell. Hormone need not enter the cell for expression of hormone action; when it does enter, it is largely for purposes of degradation (broken line). Some effects of these hormones may be modifications of nuclear events, but these are not invariably present and represent only a minority of the events observed.

Illustration continued on opposite page

responsiveness of the target cell. Thus, a given concentration of hormone will have a large or small effect depending on the state of the target cell.

PEPTIDE HORMONES AND CATECHOLAMINES

Up to this point, our discussion has covered all hormones. To discuss further the mechanisms by which hormones interact with their target cells, it is useful to divide all the hormones into two major classes on the basis of their solubility. A comparison of these two classes is given in detail in Table 2–3 and Figure 2–3. Those hormones that are lipid-soluble (iodothyronines, steroids, and 1,25(OH)$_2$-vitamin D, a sterol) readily traverse the lipid-rich membrane of the target cell and first interact with intracellular components (Fig. 2–3B).* The specific receptors for the steroids and 1,25(OH)$_2$-vitamin D are soluble cytoplasmic components. The complexes of hormone with receptor, after one or more transformations, move to the

*Evidence is accumulating that entry of these agents into the cytoplasm of the target cells may be regulated by specific biological processes at the cell membrane.

nucleus where they regulate one or more aspects of gene expression (Fig. 2–3B). Similarly, thyroid hormones regulate gene expression but have their receptors in the nucleus; it is unclear what role, if any, is played by cytoplasmic components.

The vast majority of hormones are water-soluble. This class includes the peptide hormones as well as the catecholamines. They do not readily traverse the lipid barrier posed by the plasma membrane of the cell but interact directly with receptors located on the cell surface (Fig. 2–3A). As shown in Table 2–3, the chemical nature of the individual hormone determines many features of how that hormone operates biochemically, especially its interaction with its target cells.

The overall scheme by which peptide hormones and catecholamines activate target cells is shown in Figure 2–3A and Table 2–4. The hormone (extracellular messenger) carries the signal from the secretory site to the cell surface. On the outer surface of the cell on the plasma membrane is a receptor that recognizes the hormone and binds it. The combination of hormone with receptor initiates a transmembrane message which results for most hormones in the activation of the adenylate cyclase at the inner surface of the plasma membrane. Adenylate cyclase, an enzyme that is restricted to the cell membrane, converts

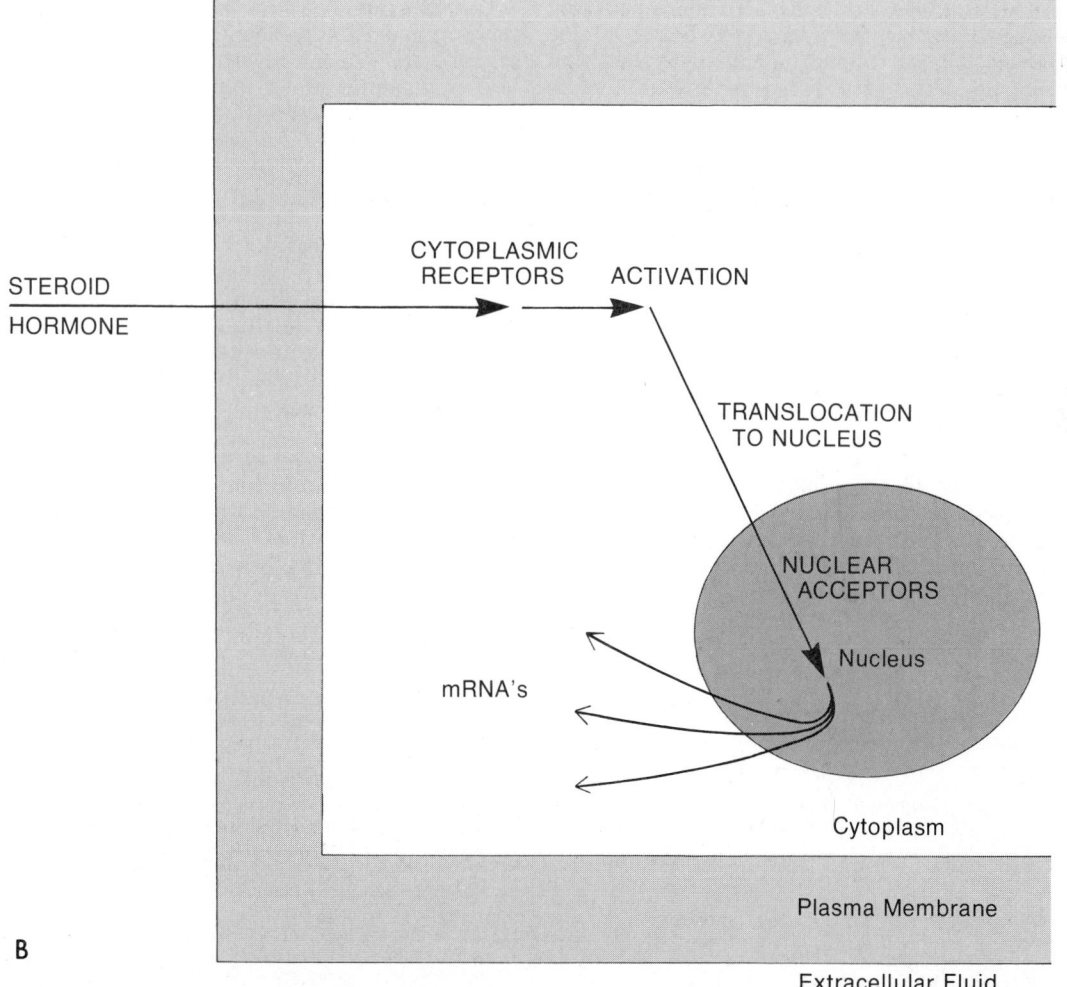

Figure 2–3 *Continued.* *B,* The lipid-soluble hormones (steroids and 1,25(OH)$_2$-vitamin D) readily enter the cell and bind to cytoplasmic receptors. Binding is followed by an activation process and translocation to the nucleus where the activated receptors bind to DNA and nuclear proteins ("nuclear acceptors") and thereby stimulate the production of specific mRNA's for a relatively small number of proteins. The iodothyronines are the same except that they appear to lack cytoplasmic receptors. The solid-headed arrows indicate steps in which the hormone molecule actually participates.

Table 2–4. EARLY STEPS IN THE ACTION OF MANY WATER-SOLUBLE HORMONES
AT THE TARGET CELL

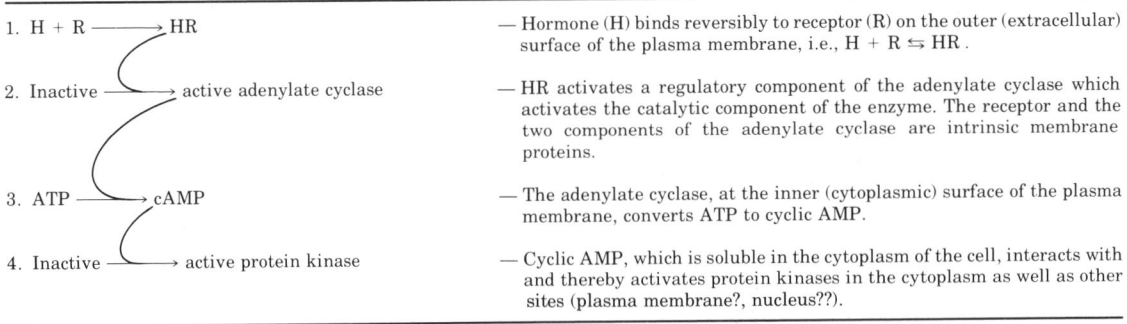

1. H + R ⟶ HR	— Hormone (H) binds reversibly to receptor (R) on the outer (extracellular) surface of the plasma membrane, i.e., H + R ⇌ HR.
2. Inactive ⟶ active adenylate cyclase	— HR activates a regulatory component of the adenylate cyclase which activates the catalytic component of the enzyme. The receptor and the two components of the adenylate cyclase are intrinsic membrane proteins.
3. ATP ⟶ cAMP	— The adenylate cyclase, at the inner (cytoplasmic) surface of the plasma membrane, converts ATP to cyclic AMP.
4. Inactive ⟶ active protein kinase	— Cyclic AMP, which is soluble in the cytoplasm of the cell, interacts with and thereby activates protein kinases in the cytoplasm as well as other sites (plasma membrane?, nucleus??).

ATP to cyclic AMP. The latter is a soluble "second messenger" which can diffuse widely through the cell, where it activates protein kinase, an enzyme that phosphorylates intracellular proteins, especially enzymes, and thereby regulates their activity. The steps from adenylate cyclase activation through cyclic AMP production to protein kinase activation represent a common intracellular pathway for all hormones that act through cAMP. As shown schematically in Figures 2–3A and 2–4A, the fact that the intracellular pathways branch accounts for the very large number of biological effects that are produced by a single target cell. For the minority of water-soluble hormones that do not act through adenylate cyclase and cAMP (insulin, prolactin, growth hormone, α-adrenergic catecholamines), other intracellular messengers with similar pathways are postulated.

In this scheme each step leads only to the next step. In Figure 2–4B, we have modified the scheme to show that each step is capable not only of initiating the next step but also of initiating feedback and feedforward regulatory events of both the negative and positive type.

Receptor Specificity

As a first approximation, all of the cells in the body are exposed to an equal concentration of each of the hormones (Fig. 2–5). What gives specificity to this system of communication? Receptors! The receptor recognizes the bioactive hormone from among all the other substances to which the cell is exposed. It binds the bioactive hormone and essentially ignores everything else in plasma. Often hormone may be present at 10^{-9} to 10^{-12} M whereas the total concentration of other proteins and peptides is about 10^{-3}

M. Thus the hormone recognized by the receptor represents one molecule in one million or even one in a billion.

The receptor manifests its recognition by binding the hormone. Binding of hormone to receptor is necessary but not sufficient. The combination of hormone with receptor must do something to begin the chain of biochemical events within the target cell that leads ultimately to the biological action(s) or effect(s) of that hormone acting on that target cell. These two processes (binding and activation) are quantified independently.

Let us examine these two processes with reference to the hormone. For hormone to bind to receptor, some region of the hormone molecule must have a structure that is complementary to a region of the receptor. The tightness of the fit between the hormone and its specific receptor is described or measured in terms of "affinity," abbreviated K (Table 2–5). For hormones and hormone derivatives (agonists as well as antagonists) that are active in that particular system, the affinity, K, is finite, i.e., K > 0, whereas K = 0 for substances that are not active through that particular receptor. Let us examine insulin as a specific example.

The receptor for insulin has a specificity (and affinity) that is quite well conserved throughout all of vertebrate evolution, whereas the insulins of different species do differ somewhat from one another in their affinity for receptor (Fig. 2–6). Among insulins, acting through the insulin receptor to produce the characteristic metabolic responses of insulin, chicken and turkey insulins have two or three times higher affinity for the receptor than beef, pork, and human insulins, which in turn have twofold greater affinity than fish insulin > proinsulin > guinea pig insulin > insulin-like growth factors and somatome-

---

STRAIGHT ARROW — STEP 1→ STEP 2→ -- → STEP n

H + R ⇌ HR ⟶ E₁, E₂, E₃

A

Common   Branched
Pathway   Pathway

MODULATION OF TARGET CELL — FEED BACK & FORWARD - POS. & NEG.

H + R ⇌ HR ⟶ E₁, E₂, E₃

B

Figure 2–4. Target cell pathways: direct and modulatory. *A,* A traditional scheme of how each step within the target cell leads directly to the next: hormone binds to receptor; HR complex activates a common intracellular pathway which, via branched pathways, ultimately leads to characteristic biological effects, designated E₁, E₂, E₃. In *B,* we have added schematically other arrows to indicate that hormone binding to receptor can also produce modulation, both negative and positive, proximally and distally, within the target cell itself. Though not illustrated here, later steps in the pathway, in addition to activating the next step, also participate in modulatory reactions. The arrows in *A* illustrate the intrinsic capacity or direct program for biological action by the target cell in response to the hormone; the additional arrows in *B* illustrate that the sensitivity of the target cell — the magnitude of the responses (E₁, E₂, E₃) to a signal of a given size — is highly regulated on a continuous basis. (From Roth, J.: Transductive coupling by cell surface receptor — I. In *Physical Chemical Aspects of Cell Surface Events in Cellular Regulation.* DeLisi, C., and Blumenthal, R. (eds.), New York, Elsevier/North-Holland, 1979.)

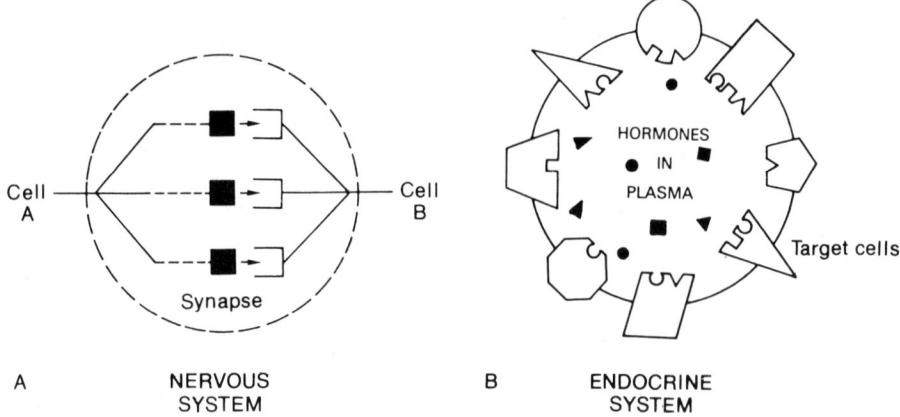

Figure 2–5. Chemical messengers: specificity and problems of recognition. *A*, Schematic representation of a synapse, showing that only a single species of transmitter (■) is being released from one cell to travel a microscopically short distance to interact with a single species of receptor (⊐–) on another cell, and the whole interaction occurs within the confines of an isolated private space. Thus the demands placed on the specificity and uniqueness of the recognition system are limited. This is in contrast to *B*, which is a schematic representation of the endocrine system. As a first approximation, all cells of the body are exposed to equal concentrations of all of the hormones. Specificity lies entirely in the ability of each specific receptor type to recognize its own hormone and to ignore all others to which it is exposed. Thus the demands on this system for specificity are very great. (From Roth, J., et al.: Hormone receptors, human disease, and disorders in receptor design. In *Hormones and Cell Culture,* Book A. Sato, G. H., and Ross, R. (eds.), Cold Spring Harbor Laboratory, 1979.)

dins (Fig. 2–6). These insulins and insulin-like molecules all have a finite affinity for the receptor and overall have structures that are quite similar to one another.* They all differ from one another to some extent in their structure; where they differ in affinity, we can safely assume that the region of the hormone responsible for binding to receptor is somewhat different. All other hormones and sub-

---

*In the case of the insulin family of peptides, the structures show obvious similarities. An extreme example where this is not the case is the opiate alkaloids from plants which are biologically very similar to opiate peptides that are native to nerve cells; both bind to a common set of receptors and compete with one another for binding. It is presumed that these alkaloids and peptides have molecular regions in common whose three-dimensional configurations are extremely similar, despite the obvious gross differences in overall chemical structures.

Table 2–5. HORMONE INTERACTION WITH RECEPTOR — QUANTITATIVE CONSIDERATIONS

(1) $H + R \rightleftarrows HR$

H = hormone
R = receptor
HR = hormone-receptor complex

(2) Affinity = $K = \dfrac{[HR]}{[H][R]}$

Free = Total − Bound
$[H] = [H_0] − [HR]$
$[R] = [R_0] − [HR]$

— We have expressed K, the affinity or equilibrium constant, as the association reaction, $H + R \rightleftarrows HR$
— Therefore K here is more precisely K_a, the association form
— $K_a = 1/K_d$ where K_d is the affinity expressed as a dissociation reaction, i.e., $HR \rightleftarrows H + R$

(3) $E = f([HR])$
Magnitude of bioeffect, E, is some function, f, of the size of the signal to the cell, [HR]

(4) $[HR] = K[H][R] \overset{*}{\simeq} K[H][R_0]$

(5) $E = f(K[H][R]) = f(K,[H],[R_0])$

(6) Conclusion: Concentration of hormone, concentration of receptor, and affinity of receptor for hormone are effectively coequal determinants in signaling the cell.

---

*$K[H][R] = \dfrac{K[H][R_0]}{1 + K[H]}$ but for $H < K^{-1}$ (which is typical), $K[H] < 1$, and $1 + K[H]$ is approximately 1 and always < 2. Therefore, under most physiological circumstances, $K[H][R]$ is very nearly $K[H][R_0]$.

stances have no affinity for this particular receptor (i.e., $K = 0$) and are inactive in this system. We should emphasize that it is the affinity, $K > 0$ or $K = 0$ as well as relative K among bioactive hormones, that defines specificity, and it is the precisely defined specificity that is the essence of a receptor.

The relative affinity of each different insulin for receptor correlates extremely well with its biological potency (Fig. 2–6). Thus the avian insulins are two to three times more potent than beef, pork, and human insulins, which are twofold more potent than fish insulin, and so on. Although there is a several hundred fold difference in affinity and biopotency between the most potent and least potent, all of the insulins and insulin-like factors, if present in high enough concentrations, are capable of eliciting the maximal biological response (Fig. 2–6). Thus a fish insulin molecule bound to a receptor is just as effective in generating the biological signal to the cell as a chicken insulin molecule bound to a receptor, but it requires four to six times more fish insulin molecules in the medium than chicken insulin molecules to produce the same number of insulin-receptor complexes, because the relative affinities differ by four to six times.

Intrinsic Activity

The ability of a hormone when bound to a receptor to elicit a biological response is measured in terms of the "intrinsic activity" of that hormone. All active hormones or hormone analogues (in addition to having affinity or $K > 0$) have intrinsic activity > 0, and are referred to as "agonists" (Table 2–6). If we arbitrarily assign 100% to the intrinsic activity of the native hormone, then agonists with intrinsic activity < 100% are "partial agonists"; > 100% are "super agonists"; = 100% are "full agonists." Substances that bind to receptor ($K > 0$) but do not activate (intrinsic activity = 0) are designated "antagonists" (Table 2–6).

Using synthetic variants of many hormones, scientists have been able to show that in general the region of the hormone that binds (determines affinity) is distinct from the region of the hormone that activates (determines intrinsic activity). Antagonists bind to the hormone-binding site on the receptor molecule and thereby prevent the

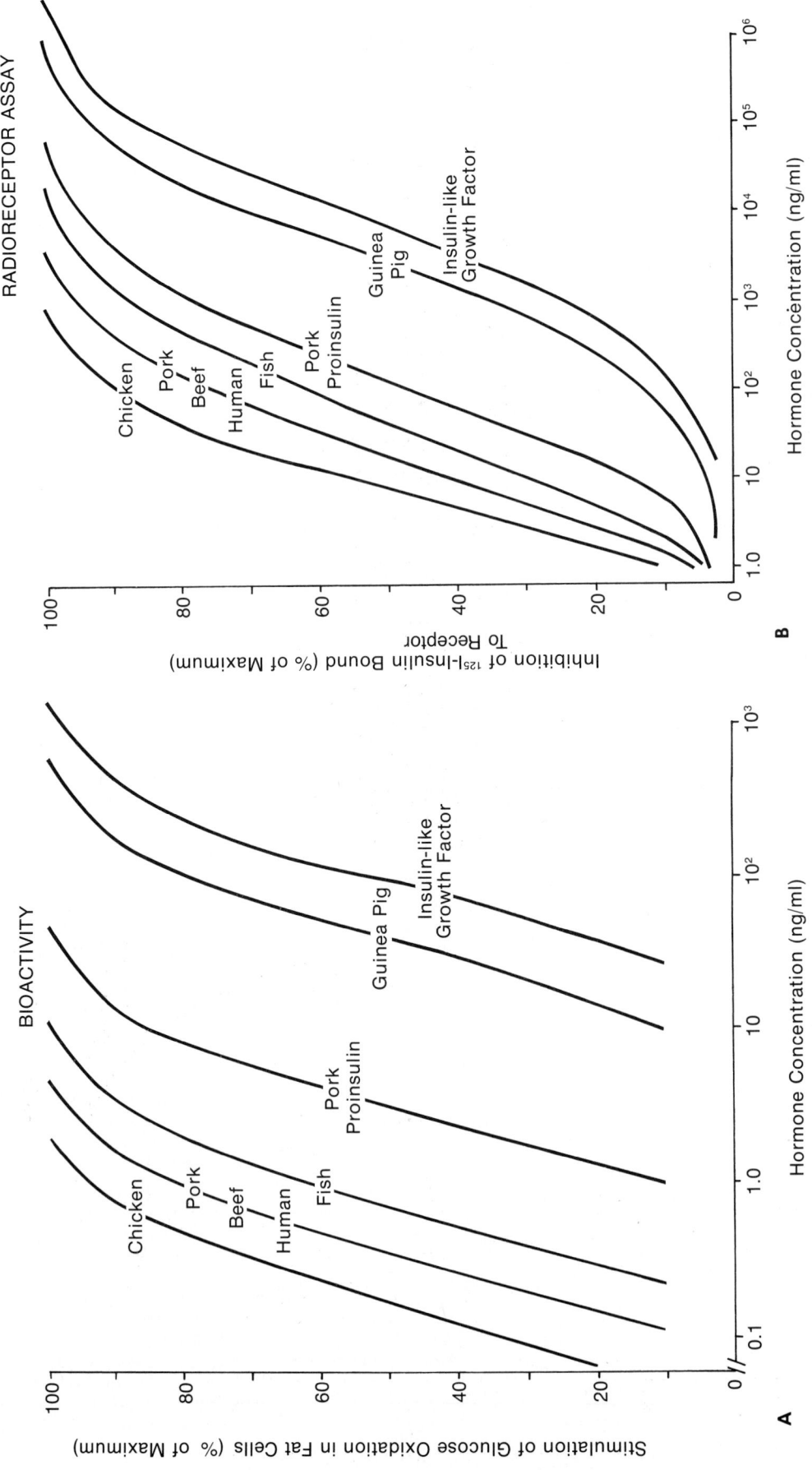

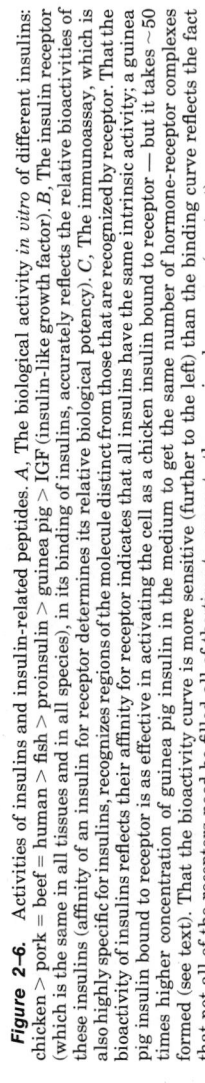

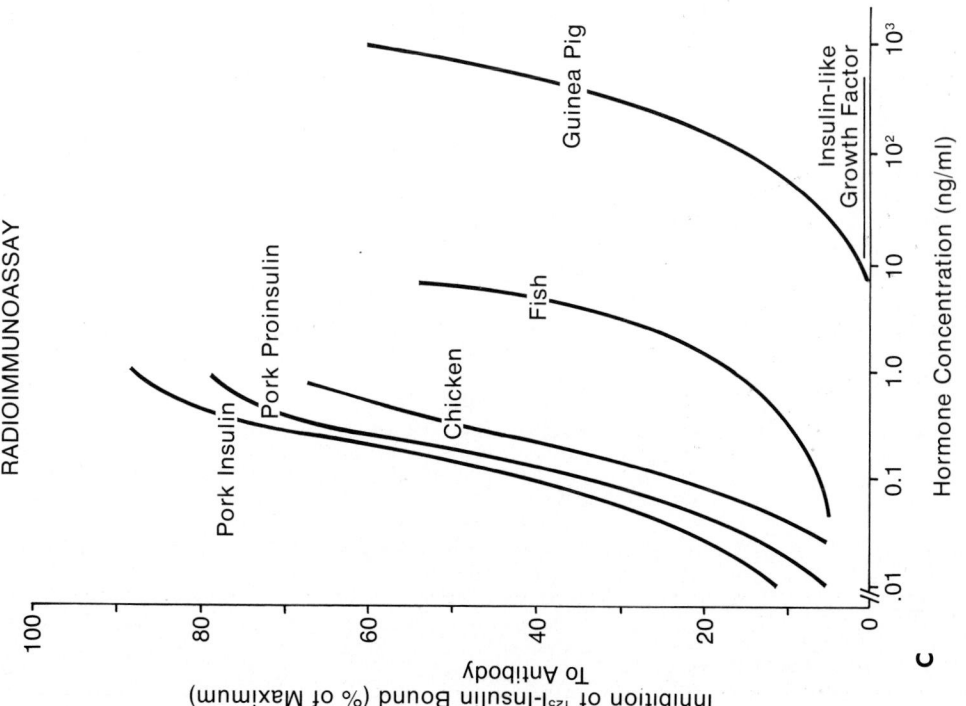

Figure 2–6. Activities of insulins and insulin-related peptides. *A,* The biological activity *in vitro* of different insulins: chicken > pork = beef = human > fish > proinsulin > guinea pig > IGF (insulin-like growth factor). *B,* The insulin receptor (which is the same in all tissues and in all species), in its binding of insulins, accurately reflects the relative bioactivities of these insulins (affinity of an insulin for receptor determines its relative biological potency). *C,* The immunoassay, which is also highly specific for insulins, recognizes regions of the molecule distinct from those that are recognized by receptor. That the bioactivity of insulins reflects their affinity for receptor indicates that all insulins have the same intrinsic activity; a guinea pig insulin bound to receptor is as effective in activating the cell as a chicken insulin bound to receptor — but it takes ~50 times higher concentration of guinea pig insulin in the medium to get the same number of hormone-receptor complexes formed (see text). That the bioactivity curve is more sensitive (further to the left) than the binding curve reflects the fact that not all of the receptors need be filled all of the time to generate the maximal response (see text).

RADIOIMMUNOASSAY

Inhibition of ^{125}I-Insulin Bound (% of Maximum) To Antibody

Hormone Concentration (ng/ml)

Pork Insulin

Pork Proinsulin

Chicken

Fish

Guinea Pig

Insulin-like Growth Factor

C

Table 2–6. DEFINITION OF AGONISTS AND ANTAGONISTS AT THE RECEPTOR

Classification	Affinity	Intrinsic Activity
Native hormone = agonist = full agonist	finite	= 100%
Antagonist = full antagonist	finite	= 0
Partial agonist (= partial antagonist)	finite	> 0, < 100
Superagonist	finite	> 100%
Inactive (with respect to this receptor)	zero	—

All agonists and antagonists that act at the level of receptor bind to receptor and therefore all have some finite affinity for receptor (affinity or $K > 0$). Inactive materials do not bind to receptor (affinity or $K = 0$). The intrinsic activity of the natural hormone is typically assigned a value of 100% and arbitrarily designated as a full agonist. Analogues with intrinsic activity > 100% are superagonists, while those with intrinsic activity < 100% are partial agonists or antagonists. Those whose intrinsic activity = 0 are (full) antagonists while those with intrinsic activity > 0 but < 100% are partial agonists (and also, by definition, partial antagonists.)

binding of bioactive hormone to the receptor, but the antagonist-receptor complex is unable to initiate the biological response. Administered alone, antagonists typically have no observed bioactivity. Their bioactivity relates to the fact that they reduce or block completely the activity of agonist present at the same time. Note that "partial agonists" (intrinsic activity < 100% but > 0) are in fact also "partial antagonists" because the effectiveness of native hormone is reduced in the presence of partial agonists. Here we use "antagonists" and "antagonism" in a narrow sense to refer to interactions at the receptor. These words are also used more broadly, to describe any situation in which one hormone reduces the biological effect of another, irrespective of whether the interaction is taking place at the receptor. In fact, most antagonisms are post-receptor.

In the previous example we pointed out that naturally occurring insulins vary widely in their biological potency (effectiveness per unit of hormone) owing to differences in their affinity for receptor. All have the same intrinsic activity: when bound to receptor they are equally effective in generating the biological signal and, at high enough concentrations, can stimulate the system maximally. Two exceptions may be the insulin of the hagfish and a mutant insulin found in one patient with diabetes, mentioned earlier, in which intrinsic activity is < 100%; thus these two insulins are partial agonists (or partial antagonists).

Many synthetic variants of hormones have intrinsic activity greater or less than 100% (superagonists: intrinsic activity > 100%, and pure antagonists: intrinsic activity = 0, are highly prized pharmacologically), but native hormones as a rule are all full agonists. Two exceptions to this rule are (1) progesterone, which may act as an antagonist for other steroid hormones at the level of receptor (see later); and (2) a low-affinity analogue of a native hormone that may have intrinsic activity that is moderately reduced. Oxytocin, when acting on the kidney as a low-affinity analogue of vasopressin to stimulate water reabsorption, may have intrinsic activity ~ 70% that of vasopressin.

Information Transfer

When the hormone binds to receptor, the complex acts to activate the target cell. While hormone cannot do anything without receptor and vice versa, it is useful to consider the problem of which has the information for cell activation. Hormone? Receptor? Both? (Table 2–7.) This question has been a difficult one to answer. (The nearly equal roles of egg and sperm in transfer of information to the offspring became known only at the turn of this century!) For some well known ligand-receptor systems (all outside of endocrinology), the key information is largely within the ligand. The receptor acts to concentrate, process, and/or direct the translocation of the ligand to an intracellular site where the ligand acts. However, if the ligand can get in without receptor, the effect will occur. For example, the cholera toxin molecule contains within it an enzyme that acts intracellularly; the enzyme actually performs the action of the toxin, while the surface receptor for the toxin acts to expedite and direct the intracellular movement and exposure of the toxin's enzyme.

Similarly, cholesterol that is contained within the low-density lipoprotein (LDL) carries important information to the cholesterol-synthesizing apparatus within the cell. The receptor for LDL concentrates, translocates, and directs the delivery of LDL to lysosomes where the cholesterol is released (from the LDL) and then performs its function as a signal. Experimentally, cholesterol introduced intracellularly without the ligand does the same.

Another example of where the essential information is largely within the ligand are viruses. If the infectious nucleic acid of the virus is introduced into the cell, infection ensues. The receptor for the virus acts to concentrate the virus and expedite delivery of the viral genome to the interior of the cell; the receptor is not directly involved in the infection.

By contrast, for the water-soluble hormones that have been studied, the receptor appears to contain the full program of information, and the ligand acts only to get that information expressed by the receptor (Table 2–7). One of the best studied examples is insulin. The evidence is derived largely from studies with antibodies directed against the receptor that are present in patients with the syndrome of extreme insulin resistance and autoimmunity. These antibodies bind directly to the receptor molecule. Antibody binding impairs insulin binding and vice versa. However, individual antibodies and the hormone both have a unique binding site on the receptor. Not only do the antibody molecules block insulin binding but they also mimic insulin

Table 2–7. INFORMATION TRANSFER

A. Hormone + Receptor $\leftrightarrows$ Hormone-Receptor Complex → Activation of Cell Process
B. Where is the message? H? R? or HR?
C. Classes
  1. Ligand has the message

    Receptor acts only to concentrate, process, and/or translocate the ligand to intracellular site. Experimentally, an element of ligand (in the absence of receptor) can activate the relevant biological event.

      1. toxins: cholera, diphtheria (enzyme)
      2. low-density lipoproteins (cholesterol)
      3. viruses (nucleic acid)

  2. Receptor has the message

    Receptor has the full program for activation of the cell and experimentally receptor in the absence of specific natural ligand can produce full effect. Ligand's function is to get the receptor to express its program.

      1. polypeptide hormones: insulin, TSH
      2. acetylcholine (nicotinic) receptors
      3. IgE receptors

  3. Receptor and ligand

    Both receptor and ligand together contribute information to cell activation.

      1. egg and sperm

Table 2–8. BIOLOGICAL EFFECTS OF INSULIN THAT ARE MIMICKED BY ANTI-RECEPTOR ANTIBODY*

A. Transport process at the cell surface
— hexoses
— amino acids
B. Intracellular disposition of substrates
— glucose oxidation to CO_2
— glucose incorporation into glycogen and lipids
— amino acid incorporation into protein
— inhibition of lipolysis
C. Effects on specific enzymes
— lipoprotein lipase
— glycogen synthase
— pyruvate dehydrogense
— acetyl CoA carboxylase
— inhibition of phosphorylase
D. Other
— simulate effects of insulin on phosphorylation of cellular proteins

*Anti-receptor antibody indicates autoantibodies directed against receptor for insulin which are found in serum of patients with Type B extreme insulin resistance. Except where indicated, the processes are accelerated or activated.

action (Table 2–8). They stimulate the transport of glucose and amino acids, which are processes at the cell membrane, and also stimulate more specific intracellular actions of insulin including activation of glycogen synthase, inactivation of phosphorylase, and increased synthesis of lipoprotein lipase. The latter is a slow delayed effect of insulin on enzyme synthesis. Thus an antibody binding to the receptor (even not at the insulin-binding site) is capable of getting the receptor to express its program of activation. Concanavalin A, a plant protein that also binds to the insulin receptor and alters insulin binding, can also promote insulin-like events at the target cells; this again suggests that the binding of ligand to the receptor causes the receptor to express its intrinsic biological capability. There is further evidence, to be presented in detail later, that shows that the receptor has the information; when two or more active ligands that are related in structure both bind to two or more receptor types, the nature of the biological effect produced is determined by which receptor is occupied and is independent of which ligand is bound (see later).

The ability of antibodies from patients with Graves' disease to alter TSH binding and to mimic multiple actions of TSH suggests that for this system, too, the receptor has all the essential information. Another example may be the steroid hormones and their cytoplasmic receptors, though more detailed information about these systems is needed. Two other examples of signaling systems in which the receptor rather than the ligand has the key information are the acetylcholine receptor which transmits the nerve impulse to skeletal muscle and the IgE receptor on the surface of basophils which can activate histamine and/or serotonin release in the absence of the ligand (IgE). (The classic example where both moieties provide nearly equal amounts of information is the interaction of egg with sperm.)

In summary, for some nonhormonal ligands information for biological activation of the target cell is within the ligand. The evidence for peptide hormones suggests that the receptor has the full program of information and that the hormone acts to cause the receptor to express its intrinsic program of information (see Table 2–7). The implications for therapy are clear. If all the information is within receptor, then strategies for hormone replacement need no longer be restricted to hormone analogues. Other molecules that bind to receptor, even at sites distant from the hormone-binding site, may be effective and useful agonists.

Definition of Receptor

Up to here we have described both functional and structural aspects of a bioactive hormone but have restricted our description of the receptor to its function: the receptor provides the target cell with a mechanism for recognizing the hormone; the hormone-receptor complex initiates activation of the target cell; and probably the hormone activates the cell surface receptor which in turn activates the cell. The purpose of this section is to add structural aspects of the receptor and thereby describe what investigators in the field of endocrinology mean when they use the term "receptor."

The chemical moiety on the target cell that provides recognition of the hormone is presumed to be the same as the binding site for the hormone and is the minimal unit referred to as "receptor." This binding site may be an integral part of a larger molecule, which in turn may be only one type of subunit within a larger complex. Currently, most writers do not distinguish the binding site from the whole molecule from the whole complex, and use "receptor" to refer to all of them.

Not only must the hormone be recognized but the combination of hormone with receptor must produce a biochemical event ("activation") that initiates the series of biochemical events that result ultimately in a biologically meaningful event. Thus the concept of "receptor" implies that the same molecule that has the binding or recognition site can participate normally in the initiating event in cell activation. This part of the molecule may be referred to as "effector." Thus, in all likelihood, one molecule contains both "recognition" and "activation" regions which may be separate, identical, or partially overlapping.

Everyone agrees that when the "recognition" and "activation" regions are present intact in a bona fide target cell, this constitutes a "receptor." The concept of receptor becomes less clear when the pathway is incomplete and the final biologically meaningful event cannot be achieved, e.g., when the ligand that binds is an antagonist, when the target cell has one or more later steps that are defective, or when the molecular complex or subunits that have the "recognition" and "activation" region have been freed from the rest of the cell or cell membrane.

The concept of the "receptor," and hence its definition, is in transition from a functional to a structural basis. As the molecular structures of the component parts become defined, the term will become more precise. In the ultimate, we expect that a "binding region" and "activation region" will be defined as entities within the receptor molecule; the receptor molecule, with other subunits that are closely associated with it, will constitute a receptor unit or complex. The definition will not require these molecules to have derived originally from fully active target cells, so long as they are accurate functional and structural replicas of the molecules that are present and functioning in legitimate target cells.

Receptor Status

In every case, the actual proximate biochemical event produced by a hormone-receptor complex is unknown, even for hormone-receptor systems that activate adenylate cyclase early in their action at the target cell. Is an enzymatic function activated? Is the receptor an ion channel or a transport protein? It is important to understand that the name "receptor" is actually a temporary designation and implies a major element of ignorance. Ultimately, when the receptor's function is defined in precise biochemical and

Table 2–9. RECEPTORS: PROGRESSION OF NAMES IN RELATION TO KNOWLEDGE

State of Knowledge	Designation (hemoglobin as example)
1. Binding property detected	1. Oxygen-*binding substance* of erythrocytes
2. Protein nature of the binding substance	2. Oxygen-*binding protein*
3. Recognition of the relationship of its binding properties (O_2, CO_2, CO) to physiological functions (respiration, oxidation)	3. Oxygen *receptor*
4. Purification of the material, analysis of its structure, and recognition of the physical and/or chemical processes it carries out	4. *Real name:* hemoglobin (or oxygen–carbon dioxide transport protein of erythrocytes)

This table indicates that the term "receptor" indicates an intermediate stage in our understanding of the material. Binding of ligand is necessary but not sufficient; to be designated a "receptor," the relationship of the binding process to a biological process is needed based on the specificity of the binding for a series of materials known to be biologically related. Thus implicit in "receptor" is a relationship to a set of biological events. When the receptor's structure and biochemical actions are determined, the term "receptor" is replaced by a unique, more precise name. The example of hemoglobin is not intended to be historically accurate but is an easily understood hypothetical example.

structural terms, "receptor" will be replaced by a specific biochemical designation.

A trivial (nonhistorical, hypothetical) illustration, with hemoglobin as an example, should help the reader to grasp this concept more clearly (Table 2–9). When red cells were found to have a substance that binds oxygen, we might have named it the "oxygen-binding substance" of erythrocytes. When its protein nature was discovered, we might have changed the designation to "oxygen-binding protein." When the oxygen-binding properties were found to conform identically to the specificity of a known biological process *in vivo* (respiration and oxidation) on the basis of its behavior with O_2, CO_2, CO, and oxidizing and reducing agents, we might have promoted it to the temporary rank of "oxygen receptor" of erythrocytes. When its structure was fully defined, we would have promoted it further and called it "hemoglobin."

In a similar fashion, an insulin-binding substance or protein is elevated to insulin receptor when the specificity for insulin and insulin-related molecules conforms to the specificity of the biological process (metabolic effects that are characteristic of insulin action). When the full nature of this molecule is defined, we will change its name to the insulin-dependent protease, oxygenase, Ca^{++} channel, or what have you, or even give it a single trivial but unique name.

In summary, "receptor" is a temporary designation which requires (1) that the material have the ability to bind hormone, (2) that the specificity of the binding conform precisely to the specificity of the recognition process for a particular biological process,* and (3) that the biochemical event initiated by the ligand-receptor complex be as yet undefined.

---

*In trying to define the receptor, the absolute affinity of the receptor for hormone is usually irrelevant, whereas the relative affinity of a series of hormone analogues for binding to receptor is crucial. Actually, it is typical for the "apparent" affinity ("K") based on the biological response to be much greater than the true affinity (K) of hormone for receptor; i.e., the concentration of hormone that produces the half-maximal biological effect is usually much lower than the hormone concentration that produces occupancy of 50% of the receptors. In fact, when several biological effects in the same cell are produced by a hormone acting through the single pool of receptors, the effects often differ in their apparent "K." These observations are related to the fact that typically the maximal capacity of the hormone-receptor complex to stimulate exceeds the maximal capacity of the target cell to respond (see under the heading Integration and Control).

Cell Surface Receptors

Receptor Structure

The cell surface receptors for hormones are all integral proteins of the cell membrane, and therefore insoluble in aqueous media except in the presence of detergents. They are much larger and more complex than the hormones. Most peptide hormones have a single peptide chain (only a few have two chains), and total molecular weights range from 300 to 50,000 daltons. The receptors that have been studied have several subunits, each of 30,000 daltons or more, with overall molecular weights of several hundred thousand up to one million or more. Several of the features of cell surface receptors have been contrasted with those of their hormone counterparts to indicate why progress with the hormones has been much faster than that with the receptors (Table 2–10). Although our knowledge about the structure of the receptor is limited, a great deal of information has been gathered about the specificity of the receptors, regulation of their number and affinity, their involvement in disease states, and their role in transmitting biological information.

Plasma Membrane

The plasma membrane, which covers the outer surface of the cell, is a key structure in the hormone–target cell interaction. All of the components of the target cell that are involved in the initial steps in the action of peptide hormones and catecholamines — receptor, transmembrane signals or coupling, and adenylate cyclase — are components of the plasma membrane. Furthermore, some of the important later events in hormone action involve components of the

Table 2–10. COMPARISON OF HORMONES AND CELL SURFACE RECEPTORS

	Hormone	Cell Surface Receptor
1. Highly concentrated in a localized site	yes	no
a. extirpation		
b. purification		
2. Soluble in simple solvents	yes	no
3. Simple structure	yes	no
4. Bioeffect when introduced *in vivo* or *in vitro*	yes	no
5. Present in blood	yes	no
6. Name of its own	yes	no

This table outlines the reasons why progress in our knowledge of the hormones has been much faster than progress in our knowledge of cell surface (and other) receptors. In fact, hormones or receptors that are exceptions to the rules act to emphasize the cogency of the rules. For example, (1) hormones that have secretory cells that are diffusely distributed have been difficult to study in terms of function because surgical extirpation of all of the cells is impossible. Hormones that are not present in high concentrations in a gland have been difficult to purify. On the other hand, acetylcholine receptors, which are very highly concentrated in the electric organs of marine organisms, have been among the first receptors to be purified. (2) The cytoplasmic receptors for steroids, which are water-soluble, have been better characterized earlier than receptors for peptide hormones which, when freed from the membrane, require the continuous presence of detergents in order to stay soluble. (3) The receptors for certain toxins are simple lipids; they were the first to have their structures determined. Most hormone receptors are large, complex proteins, typically with several subunits, and are more complex than even the largest of the hormones. (4) The hormones have an assay system intrinsic to their nature (the gland is extirpated and glandular extracts are injected into the hormone-deficient animal), whereas assays for receptors require more sophisticated forms of reagents. (5) Those receptors that are normally present on blood cells have been more accessible to study, especially in humans. (6) That nearly all receptors are known only by the name of their partners may represent a subtle but potent barrier to their early study.

Table 2–11. COMPONENTS OF THE PLASMA MEMBRANE

Lipids — 50% (few components repeated often)	phospholipids and cholesterol	1. Continuous lipid bilayer: impermeable to water 2. Partial asymmetry to bilayer, i.e., inside ≠ outside 3. Amphipathic components — hydrophilic and lipophilic regions to each molecule 4. Fluid in two dimensions, i.e., lateral mobility of components >>> "flip-flop" 5. Mechanisms for "flip-flop"
Proteins — 40% (great variety)	peripheral	1. Located most often on the inner surface of the membrane 2. Attached noncovalently to integral proteins 3. Extractable in high salt; soluble in aqueous solvents

	integral	1. Embedded in the lipid bilayer
		2. Soluble in detergents; insoluble in aqueous solvents
		3. Absolute asymmetry (i.e., sidedness is essential); three regions to the protein
		   (a) External — carbohydrate side chains, i.e., glycoprotein — hydrophilic
		   (b) Intramembranous — lipophilic (i.e., hydrophobic) amino acids
		   (c) Internal — water-soluble amino acids — often negatively charged
		4. Mobility = lateral only; speed = 1/100th speed of lipids

Carbohydrate — 10%	glycoproteins	1. Covalently linked to asparagine, serine, or threonine groups on the extracellular portion of (all) integral proteins 2. Similar to carbohydrates of plasma glycoproteins 3. Core carbohydrates (close to peptide backbone) are synthesized separately from the terminal branched carbohydrates that are inserted later during biosynthesis
	glycolipids	1. Includes cerebrosides and gangliosides 2. Carbohydrate groups are linked to sphingosine core

plasma membrane, e.g., transport systems for hexoses, amino acids, and ions; membrane proteins that are phosphorylated following addition of hormone; and morphological changes. (Similarly, hormone secretion is a process that is also closely related to cell membranes.) Thus an understanding of the key features of cell membranes is essential background for contemporary endocrinology.

Lipids. The structure and function of the plasma membrane are logically related. A prime essential function of the plasma membrane is to insulate the inside of the cells from the extracellular environment. This function is performed by the lipids of the cell membrane which form a continuous bilayer that is impervious to aqueous solvent. The major lipid components are phospholipids and cholesterol, each of which has a water-soluble (hydrophilic) region and a larger lipid-soluble (lipophilic or hydrophobic) region (Table 2–11). When mixed in an aqueous environment they naturally form the characteristic bilayer with the hydrophobic regions facing inward and the hydrophilic regions in contact with the aqueous solvent on both surfaces of the bilayer (Fig. 2–7). The bilayer itself is a two-dimensional liquid; lipid molecules in one half of the bilayer move laterally very rapidly within their plane of the membrane but only rarely cross over to the opposite plane ("flip-flop"). It is now clear that special biochemical mechanisms are used to promote "flip-flop," as opposed to formation of the bilayer and lateral mobility which are physical properties of these lipids in an aqueous environment.

A first impression is that the two faces of the bilayer are mirror images of one another. In fact, there is a definite polarity to natural membranes which is retained when membrane sheets form vesicles and vice versa. This asymmetry is reflected in a small but definite difference in lipid composition of the two halves of the membrane.

Proteins. The proteins constitute almost the same total mass as the lipids in the membrane but differ in many ways. For example, the lipids are represented by a small number of molecular species that are repeated, whereas the proteins present a very wide variety of species, some of which are represented by only a few molecules per cell. The lipid composition is similar from one cell type to another, whereas the types of proteins and their number per cell are unique to each cell type and, for a given cell, unique to its current state of function and differentiation. The lipids show a relative but not overwhelming asymmetry, whereas the proteins are totally asymmetric. The strict asymmetry is essential for their function; i.e., the proteins will not perform at all or their performance of function will not be biologically useful if their symmetry is reversed. The asymmetry is imposed initially during the biosynthetic process and is maintained by the lipid bilayer, which is a very effective barrier to flip-flop of the proteins. If a natural membrane is disrupted by detergent and then the detergent is removed to allow the membrane to form again, most proteins will be oriented randomly; i.e., only half of the molecules will be properly oriented.

Peripheral Versus Integral Proteins. The membrane proteins are divided into two groups based on their behavior in solvents. Peripheral proteins are usually found associated with the plasma membrane but can be removed by high salt (or other changes in the aqueous solvent) without destroying the membrane, and they remain soluble in an aqueous solvent after removal from the membrane. Presumably, in nature the peripheral proteins are linked noncovalently to integral proteins and are most commonly (or exclusively) on the cytoplasmic surface of the plasma membrane.

Integral proteins, which include the cell surface receptors, adenylate cyclase, and the transport systems for ions, glucose, and other small molecules, are embedded in the lipid bilayer. They can be removed from the membrane only by addition of detergents or other methods that disrupt the membrane, and they remain soluble only so long as detergent is present. The typical integral proteins studied thus far span the membrane (Fig. 2–7D), having three distinct regions: (1) A portion of the molecule which is in the extracellular fluid (which always has covalently linked carbohy-

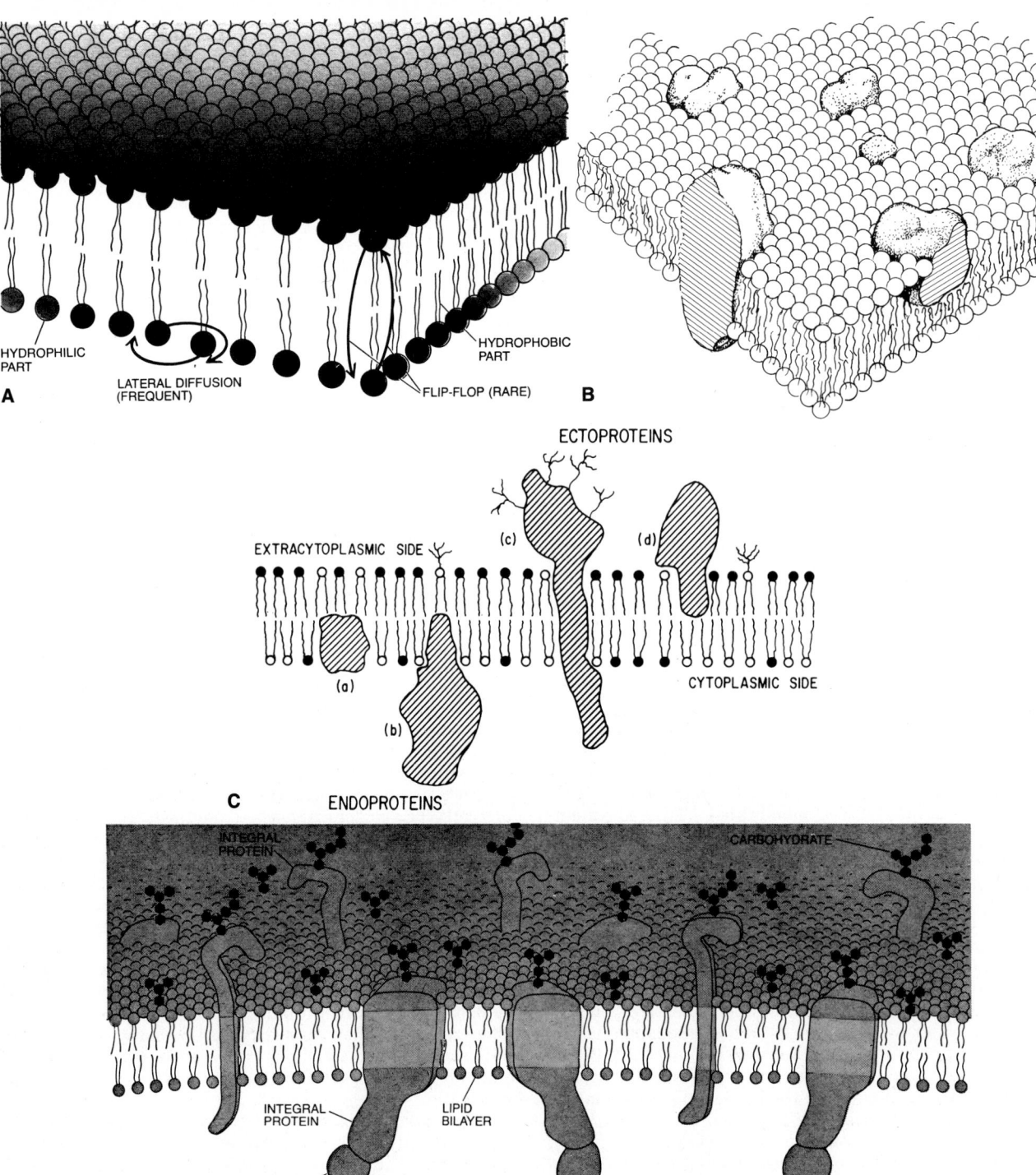

Figure 2-7. Organization of the plasma membrane. The figure has four schematic representations of the plasma membrane, each of which illustrates some of its features. *A*, Three-dimensional representation of the lipid bilayer devoid of any protein or carbohydrate. Note that the lipids form a continuous sheet. The hydrophilic region of each lipid molecule is represented by a globular figure; collectively they form the two surfaces of the bilayer. The hydrophobic (lipophilic) portion of each lipid molecule is represented by a pair of wavy lines to signify the long acyl (fatty acid) side chains. These constitute the interior of the bilayer. The figure also shows that lateral diffusion of the lipid molecules occurs frequently while exchange of lipids between the two surfaces ("flip-flop") is rare. *B*, Addition of integral proteins into the lipid bilayer. Note that the proteins, although they represent almost half of the membrane mass, constitute only a small minority of the surface. Each of the integral proteins has some portion embedded in the hydrophobic region of the bilayer. The protein may completely traverse the membrane and be exposed at both surfaces or may have exposure restricted to one surface or the other; each protein may have one or more subunits. Also, note the great diversity of proteins in contrast to the relative uniformity of the lipids. *C*, Two-dimensional sketch showing that the lipids of the bilayer, while they have an overall symmetry, do differ between the cytoplasmic (intracellular) and extracytoplasmic (extracellular) sides. Again, the integral membrane proteins are shown to be embedded in the lipophilic region of the lipid bilayer and exposed to one or both surfaces. The four proteins, labeled *(a)*, *(b)*, *(c)*, and *(d)*, are intended to display, in a hypothetical way, the possible diversity of structural arrangements of integral proteins. Carbohydrate groups, shown as branched lines, are restricted to the extracytoplasmic surface attached to proteins (glycoproteins) and lipids (glycolipids). *D*, A more complete picture of the proteins and carbohydrates. First, all of the integral proteins in this figure traverse the membrane and have exposure at both surfaces, which is the most common case. The portion of the protein that is embedded in the membrane is very rich in amino acid residues that are hydrophobic (have aromatic or long aliphatic side chains), shown by the shaded region. Note that the peripheral proteins of the membrane are restricted to the cytoplasmic side and are attached noncovalently to the integral proteins; the carbohydrate groups are restricted to the extracytoplasmic (extracellular) surface and are attached covalently to an integral protein or to the hydrophilic portion of a lipid molecule. Note that the proteins have a definite fixed orientation (inside ≠ outside) and move laterally in the plane of the bilayer but at much slower speeds than the lipids. (*A* and *D* from Lodish, H. S., and Rothman, J. E.: The assembly of cell membranes. *Sci. Am. 240*:48, Jan. 1979. Copyright © 1979 by Scientific American, Inc. All rights reserved. *C* from Rothman, J. E., and Lenard, J.: Membrane asymmetry. *Science 195*:743, Feb. 25, 1977. Copyright 1977 by the American Association for the Advancement of Science.)

drate chains). (2) A long segment composed of amino acids that are hydrophobic, i.e., have side chains that are richly aromatic (tyrosine, phenylalanine, and tryptophan) or aliphatic (leucine, valine, isoleucine). It is this piece that keeps the protein embedded in the membrane and gives it the characteristic solubility properties. (3) The cytoplasmic segment, which is water-soluble and is often rich in amino acids that have extra negative charges (glutamic and aspartic acids).

Carbohydrates. The carbohydrate groups of the integral proteins are restricted to the extracellular (N-terminal) region. The carbohydrates of the membrane proteins have not been explored in great detail but are thought to be similar to those on plasma glycoproteins. Core carbohydrates are attached to the side chains of the asparagine (via the γ-NH_2), serine (via $-OH$), and threonine (via $-OH$) moieties of the nascent peptide chains, before completion of the synthesis of the polypeptide chain. The complex branched carbohydrates are assembled separately and added later in large pieces. The role played by the carbohydrates is not yet well defined.

Biosynthesis of Receptors

Receptors, like other cell proteins, are continuously synthesized and degraded. If the concentration of receptor or other protein is unchanging, it simply indicates that the rates of synthesis and degradation are equal. The turnover of receptors is thought to be rapid. For example, in one type of cultured cells the insulin receptor has a half-life of about 6 hours. Changes in receptor concentration can be initiated in a few minutes.

The biochemical and cellular events in the synthesis of cell surface receptors and other integral proteins of the plasma membrane are not yet well understood but are thought to resemble in many ways the processes used for the synthesis of export proteins (e.g., digestive enzymes, peptide hormones, and plasma proteins). It is thought that their synthesis begins on ribosomes associated with the rough endoplasmic reticulum (ER), and processing of the nascent proteins continues in the cisternae of the rough endoplasmic reticulum and later in the Golgi or other organelles closely associated with rough ER. In addition to modification of the protein itself, other unsolved problems include the initial association of the protein with the membrane, addition of carbohydrate groups, association of receptor subunits, and final insertion and later removal of the receptor from the plasma membrane.

Intracellular Receptors for Peptide Hormones

Receptors for insulin, prolactin, and other polypeptide hormones are not restricted to the plasma membrane but have been detected in other membranous structures of the cell including the rough endoplasmic reticulum, Golgi, and the nuclear membrane. These receptors are very similar to the receptors on the plasma membrane, though some modest differences have been noted. The role of these receptors and their origins are unclear. Are they receptors in the process of synthesis and delivery to the plasma membrane? Have they been on the plasma membrane and then internalized as part of receptor or hormone degradation or processing? Or are they permanently in place on internal membranes? Do these receptors have any fundamental role in hormone action? These questions are unanswered at present. Although both hormone and receptors do get into cells (see later), it is widely agreed that the interaction of hormone in extra-cellular fluid with receptors at the outer surface of the plasma membrane is the essential first step.

Approaches to Receptors

Methods

The most widely used method for the direct study of the interaction of a hormone with receptor on the cell surface, introduced about 10 years ago for the study of ACTH and angiotensin, utilizes the interaction *in vitro* of receptor, labeled hormone, and unlabeled hormone, and is similar in principle to other competitive ligand assays. The hormone is labeled with radioactivity (typically ^{125}I) at high specific radioactivity under especially mild conditions so that the bioactivity is retained by the labeled hormone. To minimize side reactions, especially degradation of hormone and receptor, the receptor preparations are preferably whole intact cells or highly purified plasma membranes, and the reaction is usually carried out at a reduced temperature ($<< 37°$ C) for several hours. When equilibrium is reached, the receptor preparation is separated from the medium by sedimentation or filtration, and the radioactivity associated with the membranes or cells is counted ("total binding"). The portion of radioactivity in the membrane or cell pellet that is bound to specific receptors is designated "specific binding"; it represents the saturable component of binding and varies with the hormone concentration (Fig. 2–8). The remainder of the radioactivity that is associated with the membrane or cell pellet, designated "nonspecific binding," represents an unsaturable component; operationally it represents that portion of the total binding that is present even when there is an excess of unlabeled hormone (Fig. 2–8). At each hormone concentration, specific binding equals total binding minus nonspecific binding.

If the labeled hormone and unlabeled hormone react identically in the system, degradation is negligible or corrected for, and the reactants are at thermodynamic equilibrium, then the binding data can be analyzed by any of several methods to give the total receptor concentration and affinity of hormone for receptor (Figs. 2–8 and 2–9). Obviously the system can be used to measure and characterize either the receptor or the hormone.

Membrane-bound receptors can be solubilized in detergents and then studied as soluble proteins (in the continuous presence of detergent). The receptor protein can be labeled biosynthetically by growing the cells in the presence of amino acids or sugars that contain radioactive or heavy isotopes. The hormone can be tagged with fluorescent, radioactive, or electron-dense (e.g., iron or gold) moieties; in conjunction with ultrasensitive light detectors, or radioautography and electron microscopy, these hormone preparations can be used to track the hormone after it makes contact with the receptor on the cell. For most studies, the hormone is reacted with the receptor *in vitro* or in cell culture. However, tagged hormones can be injected *in vivo*, followed by study of the interaction with receptors *in vitro*. Recently, methods have been introduced to study the interaction of hormone with receptor in the whole animal *in vivo* (Fig. 2–10).

Studies in Humans

Receptors for hormones are present on many if not most tissues, and these receptors are extremely similar, if not identical, to the receptors on recognized target cells. Unlike experimental animals in which all tissues are accessible for study, the range of fresh human tissues available for study is quite limited.

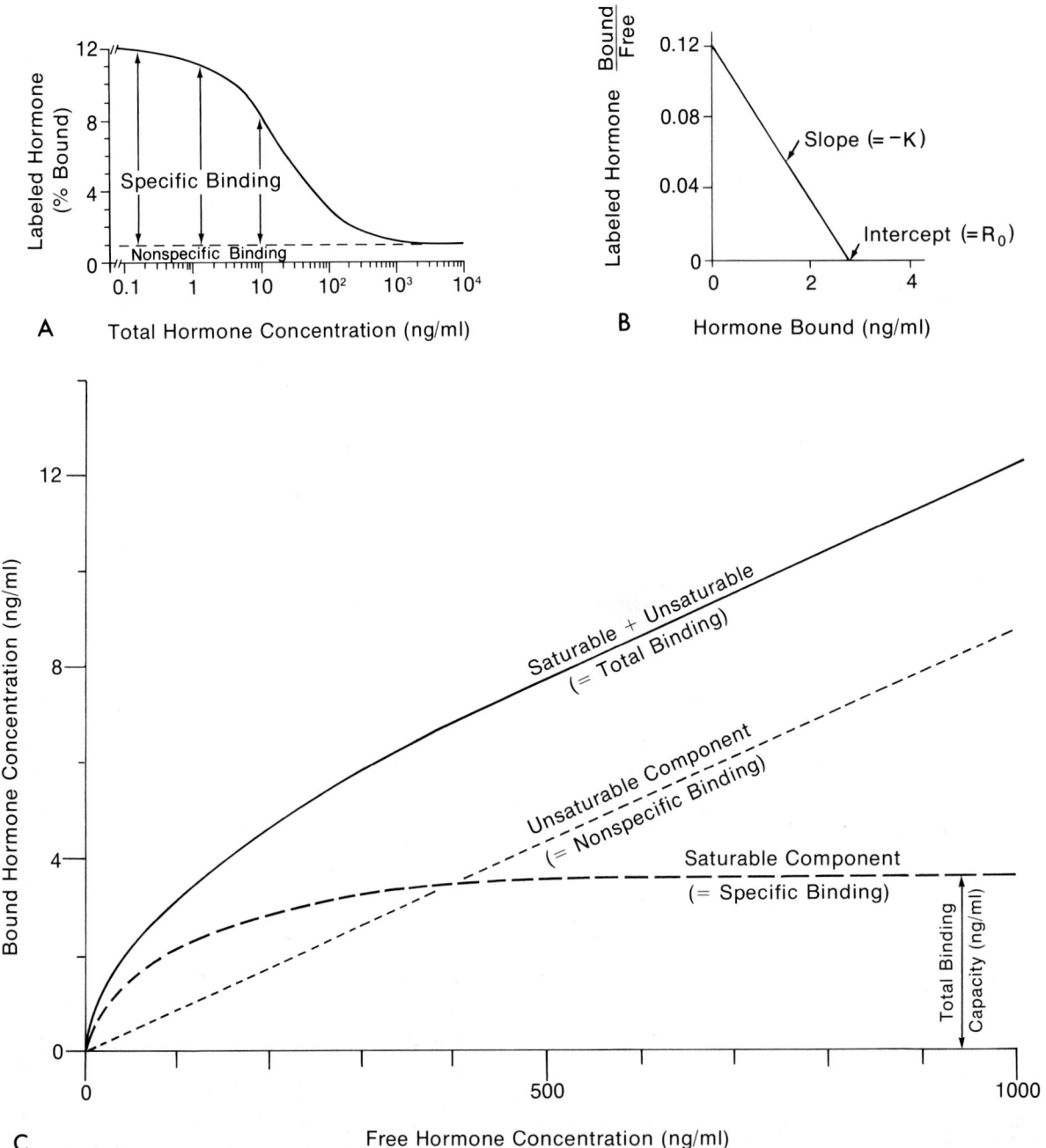

Figure 2–8. Graphic analysis of hormone binding to receptor. Hormone is bound to a single set of receptors that have a fixed uniform affinity. *A,* A competition curve, which most closely resembles the raw data; the percentage of labeled hormone bound to cells ("total binding") is plotted as a function of the total hormone concentration. Note that even at very high hormone concentrations, there is some binding of labeled hormone ("nonspecific binding"); at each hormone concentration, "specific binding" equals total binding minus nonspecific binding. *B* shows the same data but nonspecific binding has been subtracted, and the data are plotted as bound/free of labeled hormone as a function of the concentration of (specifically) bound hormone. The advantage of this graphical analysis (Scatchard plot) is that the slope of the line is proportional to $-K$, the equilibrium constant of the hormone-receptor interaction, and the intercept with the horizontal axis represents the total binding capacity or receptor concentration (R_0). *C,* The same data are plotted (solid line) as concentration of (total) bound hormone as a function of the concentration of free hormone. This represents the sum of the saturable (or specific) binding (heavy broken line) and unsaturable (or nonspecific) binding (light broken line). The tangent to the initial part of the saturable curve (not shown) has a slope proportional to K, and the limiting value of the saturable binding component represents the binding capacity.

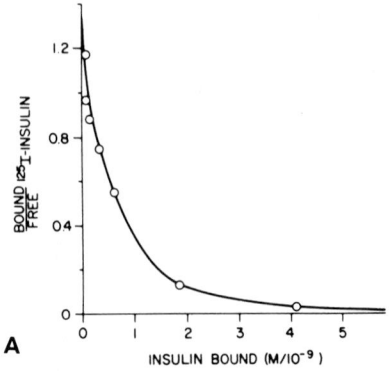

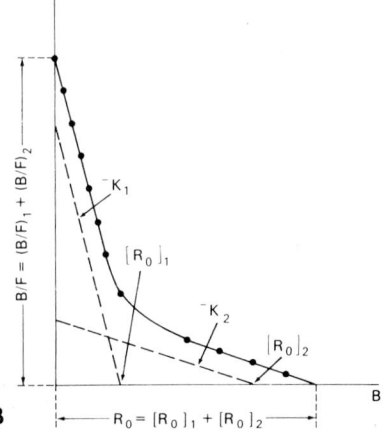

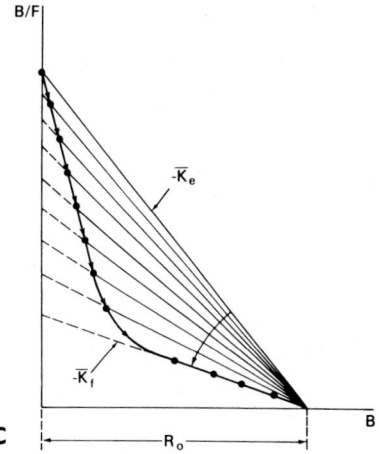

Figure 2–9.   Graphic analysis of insulin binding to insulin receptors. Insulin binding to its receptors is more complex than the binding shown in Figure 2–8. *A,* Scatchard plot of insulin binding to the insulin receptor. Note that it is curvilinear, in contrast to the previous example (Fig. 2–8*B*) which was linear. Two different interpretations of the curvilinear plot are presented (two sites versus negative cooperativity). *B,* The same curve is shown to be the sum of binding of insulin to two distinct independent receptor populations, one with higher affinity, K_1, and lower capacity, $[R_0]_1$, and another with lower affinity, K_2, and higher capacity, $[R_0]_2$. *C,* The same curve is presented as a single population of receptors with an affinity that is inversely related to receptor occupancy, i.e., negative cooperativity. At each level of occupancy, the line through the point has a slope that represents (the negative of) the average affinity, $\bar{K}$, which ranges from K_e, the limiting value for unoccupied receptors, to K_f, the limiting value for occupied receptors. (*A* from DeMeyts, P., Roth, J., et al.: Insulin interactions with its receptors: Experimental evidence for negative cooperativity. *Biochem. Biophys. Res. Commun. 55*:154, 1973. *B* and *C* from DeMeyts, P., and Roth, J.: Cooperativity in ligand binding: A new graphic analysis. *Biochem. Biophys. Res. Commun. 66*:1118, 1975.)

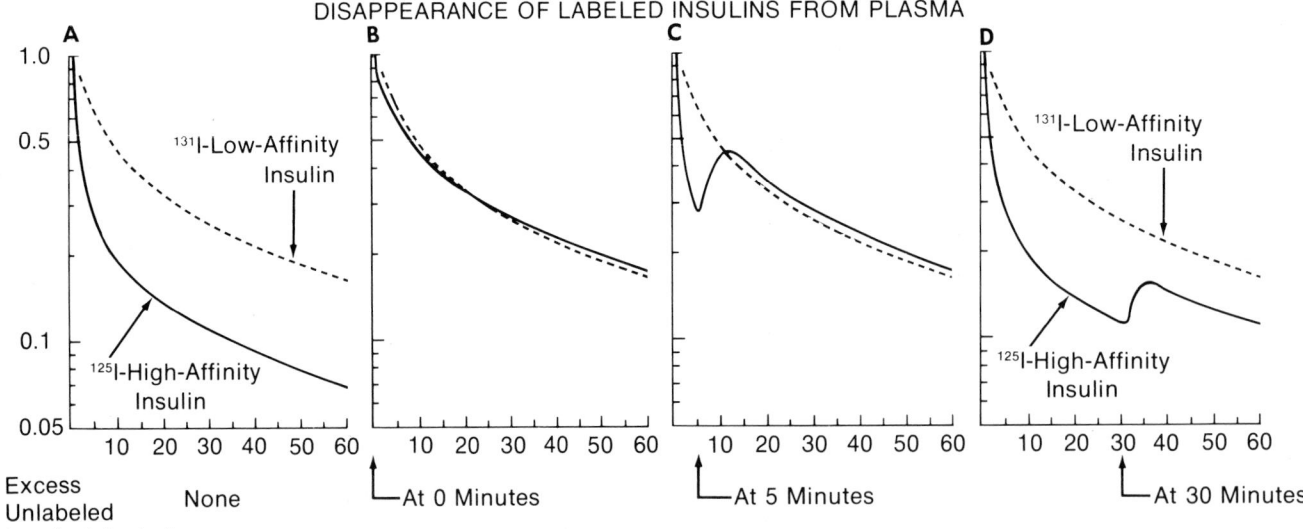

Figure 2–10. Insulin binding to insulin receptors in the whole animal *in vivo.* To demonstrate the insulin receptor *in vivo,* rabbits were injected intravenously with a mixture of two labeled insulins. Labeled insulin that has a low affinity for receptor (e.g., guinea pig insulin, broken line) quickly (first 5 minutes) distributed into the physical space characteristic of insulin and disappeared from plasma at a relatively slow rate (A through D). Labeled insulin that has high affinity for receptor (e.g., pork insulin, solid line) disappears from plasma more quickly because it distributed into the physical space and was also binding to receptors on cells (A). When unlabeled insulin (in an amount sufficient to saturate the insulin receptor) was injected at the same time as the labeled insulins (B), the disappearance from plasma of the high-affinity insulin was changed to match that of the low-affinity insulin. Intermediate-size doses of unlabeled insulin (which partially saturated receptors) yielded intermediate effects on the labeled high-affinity insulin (not shown). In C, the high dose of unlabeled insulin was injected 5 minutes after the labeled insulins; note that much of the high-affinity labeled insulin that had disappeared from plasma was returned to the plasma compartment. In D, when the injection of unlabeled insulin was delayed until 30 minutes after the injection of labeled insulins, there was still an effect, though less marked, on the high-affinity insulin. In other experiments (not shown), labeled proinsulin, which has low affinity for receptor, gave results like guinea pig insulin; chicken insulin, which has an affinity greater than that of pork insulin, showed an even larger effect due to receptor binding. Results similar to those shown here have been found in rats and humans by others.

To study the status of insulin receptors in patients, freshly obtained monocytes, granulocytes, erythrocytes, adipocytes, and placenta have been used successfully. Circulating blood cells including lymphocytes and platelets have also been used to study other receptors. In most of these studies, the accessible tissue is not regarded as a major target cell for the hormone. Rather, the receptor on the accessible tissue is being used to mirror events at other more relevant (but not easily accessible) sites. For example, the circulating monocyte, a favorite cell for studying insulin receptors, is used to reflect events in liver, muscle, and other important targets. That the monocyte does possess an insulin-sensitive pathway for hexose metabolism is unimportant to the argument. Investigators who use these tissues to study receptors must validate the extrapolation of the data from the accessible (irrelevant) cells to events at the inaccessible (but relevant) cells. Findings that are identical in two or more different tissues (e.g., erythrocytes and monocytes) strengthen the argument that the findings with blood cells reflect events at other sites.

While fresh cells can be used *in vitro* to determine the status of receptors *in vivo,* cultured cells are used to characterize the nature of the receptor free from *in vivo* influences, especially when genetic defects are suspected. Fibroblasts in culture have been most widely used. More recently B-lymphocyte cell lines have been established from individual patients to complement the fibroblast studies. Because the expression of receptors by cells in culture is influenced by many variables, the interpretation of results is easier when two or more types of cultured cells from the same patient give concordant results.

The two *in vitro* methods (fresh cells and cultured cells) measure receptors on only a single cell type and often this cell is not a major target for the hormone. Another method, which complements the two *in vitro* approaches, measures receptors in the whole organism *in vivo.* This method is illustrated in Figure 2–10 and described in the legend.

Receptor Regulation

Quantitative Aspects

The hormone (H) combines with receptor (R) to form hormone-receptor complexes (HR). The number or concentration of HR complexes, which determines the magnitude of the signal to the cell, depends equally on hormone concentration, [H]; receptor concentration, [R] or [R_0]; and the affinity, K, with which hormone and receptor interact (see Table 2–5). The implication is simple (though historically unanticipated): fluctuations in hormone concentration, an essential feature of endocrine systems, are no more important than changes in receptor affinity or changes in receptor concentration. All three have an equal influence on cell activation (see Table 2–5).

While the affinity of the native hormone in one species may differ from that in another species, the affinity of the hormone within an organism undergoes few or no significant changes. Thus the hormone affects the concentration of hormone-receptor complex ([HR]) largely or exclusively by one mechanism, changes in the concentration of hormone. On the other hand, *in vivo* the receptor affects [HR] by two mechanisms — regulation of both the concentration of the receptor and the affinity of receptor for hormone.

Changes in Receptor Concentrations and Affinity

We are accustomed to the notion that hormone concentrations fluctuate widely in response to changes within the organism. With the advent of methods to measure directly the binding of hormone to its receptors, it has become evident that the concentration and affinity of receptors also change rapidly, in response to signals from inside and outside the cell. Given that the receptors are at the crossroads between the interior and exterior of the cell, retrospectively it is not surprising that they are so responsive to the environment.

Whereas the effect produced by changing hormone concentrations is intuitive to most readers, the effect of changing receptor concentrations or receptor affinity may require more thought. Both receptor concentration and affinity regulate the effectiveness of a given concentration of hormone, i.e., are major determinants of cell responsiveness. An increase or decrease in receptor affinity shifts the dose-response curve (bioeffect versus hormone concentration) to the left or right, respectively, without any change in the shape of the curve or the maximal response observed at high concentrations of hormone. As will be elucidated later, changes in receptor concentration typically produce an almost identical left or right shift with little or no effect on the shape of the dose-response curve or the maximal response observed (see later).

The major differences in effect between a change in receptor concentration and receptor affinity are more subtle. The affinity, expressed as the equilibrium constant, K, not only represents the concentrations of the products divided by the reactants (see Table 2–5) but also is the quotient of the association and dissociation rate constants, $\overrightarrow{k}/\overleftarrow{k}$ (Table 2–12). Thus a change in affinity always brings with it a change in the kinetics of the system, which is typically but not exclusively expressed in the dissociation rate. While any increase in affinity typically slows the dissociation rate, a large increase in affinity may produce a dissociation rate that is intolerably slow from a physiological (regulatory) point of view. Changes in receptor concentration do not have comparable kinetic consequences.

Further, from our earlier discussion of specificity, it should be pointed out that essentially the same chemical bonds that link hormone to receptor provide recognition ("specificity") and determine the strength of the linkage ("affinity"). Thus extreme changes in affinity may not be truly independent of specificity. Probably for these two reasons (kinetics and specificity), receptor affinity *in vivo* fluctuates in a relatively much narrower range than receptor concentration; affinity is used for subtle changes and has kinetic consequences

Table 2–12. THE RELATIONSHIP OF AFFINITY OR EQUILIBRIUM CONSTANT TO KINETICS

(1) As shown in Table 2–5

$$H + R \rightleftharpoons HR$$

and

$$K = \frac{[HR]}{[H][R]}$$

H = free hormone
R = free receptor
HR = hormone receptor complexes
K = equilibrium constant

(2) At all times, the rate of formation

of HR $= \overrightarrow{k}$ [H][R] $\overrightarrow{k}$ = association rate constant

and

the rate of dissociation of HR $= \overleftarrow{k}$ [HR] $\overleftarrow{k}$ = dissociation rate constant

(3) At equilibrium, since [HR] remains constant, the rate of HR formation = the rate of HR dissociation

or

$$\overrightarrow{k} [H][R] = \overleftarrow{k} [HR]$$

(4) By transposition

$$\frac{\overrightarrow{k}}{\overleftarrow{k}} = \frac{[HR]}{[H][R]} = K$$

(5) Conclusion

$$\text{Equilibrium constant, } K = \frac{\overrightarrow{k}}{\overleftarrow{k}} = \frac{\text{association rate constant}}{\text{dissociation rate constant}}$$

Table 2–13. BIOLOGICALLY RELEVANT REGULATORS OF THE INSULIN RECEPTOR

Insulin	Exercise	Cell program
Other hormones	Diet	— differentiation; maturation
pH; other ions	— Calories, Composition	— growth; cell cycle
Ketone bodies	— Fiber	— tumor; transformation
Drugs	Eating	— viral infection

Receptor affinity and concentration are both affected by insulin (homologous effect). Insulin binding to receptors, by physicochemical mechanisms, acutely reduces the affinity of the receptor. To regulate receptor concentration, insulin must bind to its receptor as well as activate post-binding processes. The two other hormones that affect insulin receptors (heterologous effect) that have been widely studied are growth hormone, which affects largely receptor concentration, and glucocorticoids, which often affect receptor affinity, at least in experimental animals. The insulin receptor is very sensitive to pH, even within the range observed *in vivo*, and to a lesser extent to other common ions. Ketone bodies, especially β-OH-butyrate, have effects under some conditions. Both the sulfonylureas and biguanides have been reported to increase receptor concentration. Exercise, both acutely and chronically, increases insulin binding to receptors. Insulin binding is very sensitive to diet, with high calories, high carbohydrates, and high fat reducing receptor concentration. Dietary fiber, both soluble and insoluble, increases insulin binding to receptor. Eating causes a shift in the insulin-binding curve. There may be diurnal changes in insulin binding independent of eating and exercise. Any major change in cell program can alter insulin binding, typically by altering receptor concentration. In addition to effects on the receptor, some of these agents can also alter target cell sensitivity by regulating post-receptor events (which may be in the same direction as or the opposite direction from their effects on the receptor).

while changes in receptor concentration are used for small as well as very large changes in target cell sensitivity without kinetic consequences.

In our exposition here, general rules will be followed by specific examples, especially the receptor for insulin which has been studied in some detail (Table 2–13).

Physicochemical Factors

The structure and function of the receptor and the hormone, like those of all other proteins, are heavily influenced by the physicochemical environment which includes the solvent, the ionic composition (including pH), and temperature. For individual receptors, one or more of these influences may be especially strong. The binding of insulin to its receptor is unusually pH-dependent (Fig. 2–11A) and temperature-dependent. ACTH binding to its receptors has a strong inverse relation with the Ca^{++} concentration in the medium (Fig. 2–11B), and angiotensin binding to its receptor is related to the concentration of Na^+.

Membrane Lipids

In addition to its direct effects on the proteins (and their interaction with one another), the physicochemical environment can affect the lipid matrix of the plasma membrane and thereby affect the structure and function of the proteins of the membrane. For example, some of the effects of salts and of temperature on the receptors may be through effects on the lipids of the plasma membrane. The types and proportions of lipid components of the membrane (cholesterol content; saturation of the fatty acid side chains; the nature of the polar groups of the phospholipids) strongly influence the function of the receptor and other integral membrane proteins such as adenylate cyclase. The lipids of the membrane are potentially rapidly exchangeable with the lipids of the environment, so that changes in plasma lipids can result in changes in the membrane lipids, which in turn may affect the behavior of the membrane proteins.

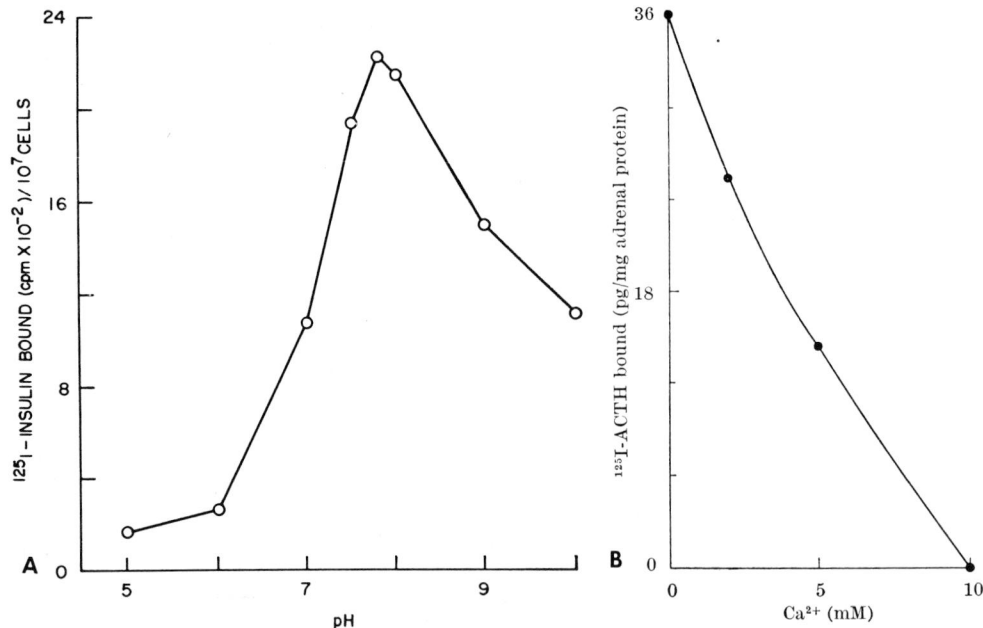

Figure 2–11. Effects of ions on hormone binding to receptor. Insulin binding to its receptor is exquisitely sensitive to pH, and ACTH binding to its receptor is very sensitive to [Ca^{++}]. Note that these changes occur even within the range of ion concentrations that occur *in vivo*, suggesting that they are physiologically relevant regulators. (*A* from Gavin, J. R., III, Gorden, P., et al.: Characteristics of the human lymphocyte insulin receptor. *J. Biol. Chem. 248*:2202, 1973. *B* reproduced by permission from Lefkowitz, R. J., Roth, J., and Pastan, I.: Effects of calcium on ACTH stimulation of the adrenal: Separation of hormone binding from adenyl cyclase activation. *Nature 228*:864, 1970. Copyright © 1970 Macmillan Journals Limited.)

Genetics, Growth, and Development

The type of receptors that a cell has and their number are highly dependent on the cell's genetic make-up and developmental program. Thus normal events such as differentiation and growth as well as pathological events such as viral infection or tumor transformation are often associated with major changes at the level of receptors. A corollary relates to interpretation of studies that show that some factor alters a particular receptor; is the influence of that factor narrow and direct or does the factor primarily act to change the whole program of the cell and only indirectly influence the receptor?

Homologous Hormone

It had been recognized for some time that exposure of a cell to a very high concentration of a stimulatory agent, especially a drug, could lead to diminished or total loss of responsiveness to that agent (desensitization or tachyphylaxis). More recently it has become clear that this represents the extreme of a more general and actually physiological process; the sensitivity of a target cell to stimulation by hormone is often related inversely to the chronic level of hormone to which the cell has been exposed, even over the range of endogenous hormone concentrations commonly encountered *in vivo*. Processes at the target cell that regulate its sensitivity often occur rapidly, and the receptor is one of the important and common sites where this regulation is exercised; the decrease in the concentration of receptor in response to the concentration of homologous hormone to which the cell is exposed is often referred to as "down regulation," while an increase in receptors is referred to as "up regulation."

In general, an increase in the chronic level of hormone produces a fall in the steady-state concentration of its receptor (one exception is prolactin, which in some tissues causes

an increase in its own receptors). This effect requires that the agent be an agonist (binding of ligand to receptor is necessary but not sufficient), and often post-receptor processes are also required. For example, regulation of the insulin receptor by insulin requires that the cell be metabolically intact and functioning. The cellular processes by which homologous hormone regulates its own receptors are not known in detail but appear to be multiple, including in some cases reversible inactivation at the cell surface, internalization of receptor with or without accelerated destruction, and possibly effects on receptor biosynthesis and insertion into the membrane.

Negative Cooperativity

A much less common mechanism by which a hormone may regulate the sensitivity of its target cell is by affecting receptor affinity. In the case of insulin, progressive saturation of receptors progressively lowers the affinity of all of the receptors for that hormone (Fig. 2–9 *C*), largely by an instantaneous increase in the rate of dissociation of hormone from receptor. This implies interaction among the receptor sites — "cooperativity"; because hormone binding lowers affinity, it is referred to as "negative cooperativity." This is the opposite of what occurs with hemoglobin, where binding of one oxygen enhances the affinity of both oxygen-binding sites and is referred to as "positive cooperativity."

The effect on affinity appears to be a physicochemical event concomitant with hormone binding to receptor, which occurs even when the cell has been broken or the receptor freed from the membrane by solubilization in detergent. In the case of insulin, the region of the hormone molecule responsible for inducing negative cooperativity has actually been mapped; the region on the hormone molecule as well as those on the receptor that mediate the cooperativity has been fully conserved throughout vertebrate evolution.

Heterologous Hormone

One hormone (A) can affect the workings of another hormone (B) by altering plasma levels of hormone B (most often by regulating its secretion rather than its degradation) or by altering the responsiveness of the target cells to hormone B. One of the sites on target cells that is often affected is the receptor; both the concentration and affinity of specific receptors for hormone B can be modulated by effects of hormone A, acting through hormone A receptors, either directly on the target cells for hormone B or indirectly on other cells that ultimately affect target cells for hormone B.

These heterologous effects (of one hormone on the receptors of another) appear to be very widespread and may be part of the phenomenon of "priming," where the action of one hormone (A) is a prerequisite for the development of sensitivity of the target cell to another hormone (B). The effect on one target cell type may differ from that on another, and the effect on a given target cell type may vary with particular conditions (age, metabolic status, and growth). At present, we are unable to provide the reader with any rules that are of predictive value except that the steroid and thyroid hormones seem to be especially active in this regard.

The following examples of heterologous effects have been selected because they may have important clinical consequences. Estrogens increase oxytocin binding to receptors of the uterus, possibly enhancing the sensitivity of that organ to oxytocin. FSH and estrogen (the action of FSH may actually be due to stimulation of estrogen production) increase the concentration of LH receptors in the ovary, thereby enhancing its sensitivity to LH. Both glucocorticoids and growth hormone regulate the insulin receptor, consistent with the effect of both of these hormones to reduce insulin sensitivity. Thyroid hormone increases the concentration of β-type catecholamine receptors, possibly accounting at least in part for an enhanced β-adrenergic effect in hyperthyroid patients.

Regulation of the Insulin Receptor

A brief review of the insulin receptor, the most widely studied from this point of view, will be presented to close this section (Table 2–13). The insulin receptor is highly responsive to the physical and chemical environment, especially to pH and temperature; growth and differentiation (e.g., premature versus term and older infants); circulating level of insulin itself; and effects of other hormones, especially glucocorticoids and growth hormone. In addition the receptor is regulated by intracellular concentrations of cAMP (part of the effects of growth may be mediated by cAMP), drugs (e.g., sulfonylureas), metabolites (e.g., B-OH-butyrate), diet (e.g., total calories, carbohydrate and fat content, type of fats, fiber), and exercise. In many cases changes in glucose tolerance, insulin sensitivity, and insulin secretion can be related to the receptor changes.

The Role of Cell Surface Receptors in Endocrine Disorders

To illustrate the breadth of involvement of receptors in disease states, the discussion will first focus on conditions in which events at the target cell appear to dominate the pathophysiology. Later, the discussion will turn to conditions in which circulating hormone (excess or deficient) clearly plays the dominant role to show that even in these

Table 2–14. INVOLVEMENT OF INSULIN RECEPTORS IN DISORDERS OF GLUCOSE TOLERANCE AND INSULIN SENSITIVITY

I. Target Cell Dominates (i.e., plasma hormone concentration discordant with clinical state)
  A. Insulin Resistance
    1. Moderate resistance
      (a) clinical
        (1) obesity
        (2) type II (insulin-independent) diabetes, obese and thin
        (3) acromegaly
      (b) experimental animals
        (1) glucocorticoid excess
        (2) growth hormone excess
        (3) uremia
    2. Extreme resistance
      (a) immunological (anti-receptor antibodies)
        (1) type B
        (2) ataxia-telangiectasia
        (3) IgA or IgE deficiency
        (4) NZO mouse
      (b) no autoimmunity (? role of genetics)
        (1) type A
        (2) leprechaunism
        (3) lipoatrophic diabetes
  B. Insulin Supersensitivity
      (1) anorexia nervosa
      (2) glucocorticoid deficiency (in experimental animals)
      (3) growth hormone deficiency
II. Hormone Dominates (i.e., plasma hormone concentration concordant with clinical state)
  A. Insulin Deficiency
    (a) clinical
      (1) type I (insulin-dependent) diabetes
      (2) pancreatic diabetes (e.g., chronic pancreatitis)
    (b) experimental animals
      (1) streptozotocin-induced hypoinsulinemia
      (2) hypoinsulinemic diabetic Chinese hamster
  B. Insulin Excess
    (1) insulinoma
    (2) infants of diabetic mothers
    (3) other hypoglycemias in the newborn
    (4) chronic insulin excess in experimental animals
  C. Disorders of Receptor Design (specificity spillover)
    (1) infants of diabetic mothers
    (2) non-islet cell tumors with hypoglycemia

conditions, events at the target cell, especially at the receptor, may play important roles in modifying the clinical course. Because they have been so widely studied, disorders of glucose metabolism will serve as the most frequent examples (Table 2–14) followed wherever possible by a broader range of disorders.

Moderate Insulin Resistance in Obesity

The insulin resistance of obesity is the most common of all target cell defects. In the majority of obese patients, irrespective of glucose tolerance, the plasma insulin concentrations are higher than normal and there is a reduced responsiveness to insulin that is largely or entirely ascribable to a reduced concentration of insulin receptors (Figs. 2–12 and 2–13). (In some animal models, post-receptor defects may also contribute to a moderate or substantial extent, as in ob/ob mouse and Zucker fatty rat, respectively.) The high correlation between hyperinsulinemia (measured in the basal state), insulin resistance, and reduction in insulin receptors not only is found in groups of patients but carries over to individual patients as well; for example, the obese patients with normal sensitivity to insulin have normal levels of insulin and of insulin receptors, and affected patients who are treated with calorie-restricted diets for a few weeks show an amelioration of all three defects. Since amelioration of the defects can occur even with patients

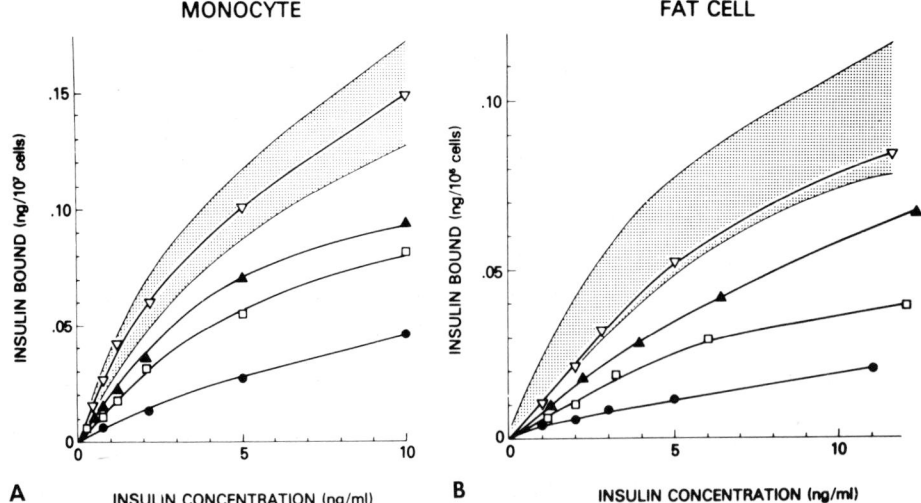

Figure 2–12. Insulin binding to receptors on cells of obese patients. *A,* Circulating monocytes. *B,* Adipocytes. For each graph four obese patients were selected to show the range of findings. The upper curve in each represents an obese patient who was indistinguishable from normal; these patients had normal receptors, normal levels of plasma insulin, and normal sensitivity to insulin. The two middle curves in each graph show a moderate decrease in receptor concentration which was associated with moderate hyperinsulinemia and insulin resistance. The lower curve in each graph shows a more severe deficiency of insulin receptors in a patient who had more severe hyperinsulinemia and insulin resistance. Dietary treatment (600 Kcal/day) for several weeks (not shown) is associated with restoration of receptor concentration to normal (or near-normal) levels.

who are still markedly overweight, the triad of defects is not due to the mass of fat tissue but is presumably related to the overeating that sustains the obesity.

Thin Diabetics

Many thin patients with insulin-independent (type II) diabetes have the same defects; again, correlation of the three defects is high in groups of patients as well as individual patients, before and after treatment with sulfonylureas. (While the sulfonylureas and the biguanides appear to have beneficial effects at the level of the receptor for insulin, the long-term safety and efficacy of the sulfonylurea drugs have

been seriously questioned, and the biguanides have been removed from the U.S. market.) Again, patients with normal sensitivity to insulin have normal levels of insulin and receptors for insulin.

Acromegaly and Other Conditions

In patients with acromegaly the patterns of glucose metabolism and insulin sensitivity are similar to those in obese patients. Again, the deficiency of insulin receptors is correlated with the elevation of plasma insulin; both correlate with the elevation of plasma growth hormone (Fig. 2–14). In contrast to patients with obesity or type II diabe-

RELATIONSHIPS BETWEEN FAT CELL INSULIN RECEPTORS AND INSULIN
SENSITIVITY *IN VITRO* AND *IN VIVO* IN OBESE SUBJECTS

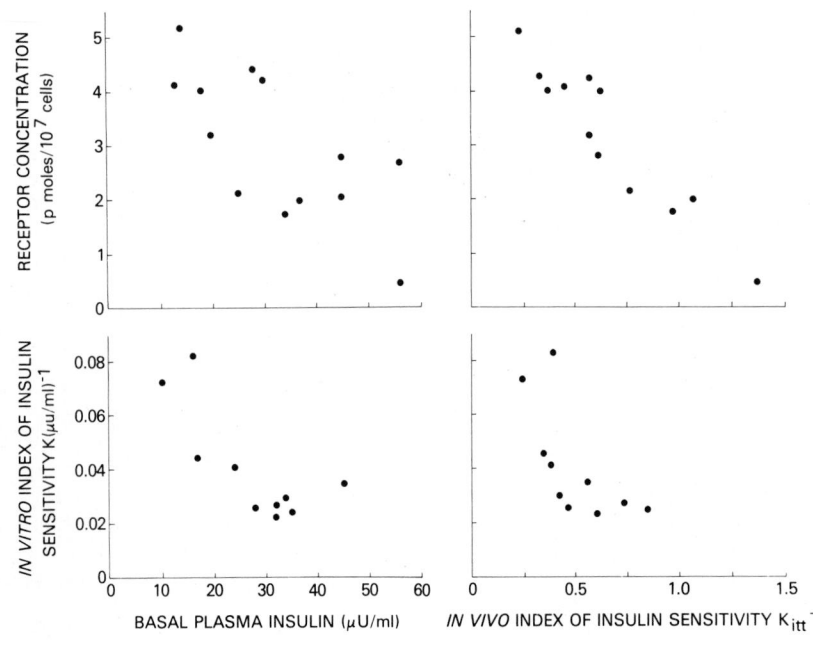

Figure 2–13. Correlations of variables in obese patients. *In vitro* measurements of insulin receptor concentration and insulin sensitivity in adipocytes were compared in individual patients with *in vivo* measurements of basal levels of plasma insulin and insulin sensitivity. Note that the basal plasma insulin, receptor concentration, and insulin sensitivity are closely related.

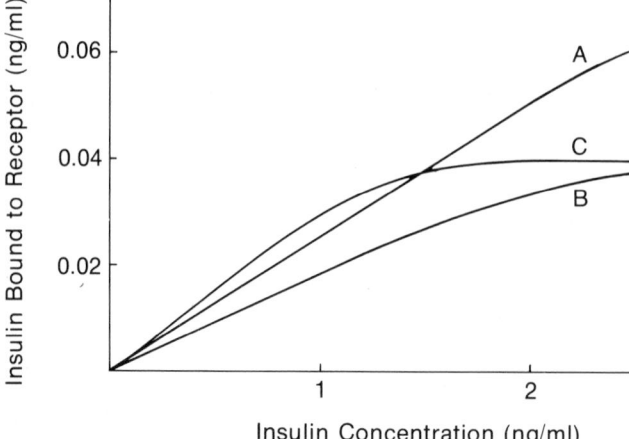

Figure 2–14. Insulin binding to receptors in acromegaly. These curves are schematic representations of insulin binding *in vitro* to circulating monocytes from three patients with acromegaly. The upper curve *(A)* shows binding indistinguishable from normal and represents a patient with a modest elevation in plasma growth hormone but normal plasma insulin levels and normal insulin sensitivity. The lower curve *(B)* shows only a decrease in receptor concentration in a patient with elevated plasma growth hormone, elevated levels of plasma insulin, and moderate insulin resistance. Note that insulin binding is reduced at every level of insulin to which the cells are being exposed. The middle curve *(C)* represents a patient who has the same decrease in receptor concentration as the patient in curve *B* but in whom receptor affinity is elevated above normal at low levels of insulin; the net result is a normal level of insulin binding at resting levels of insulin and reduced levels of insulin binding at stimulated levels of circulating insulin.

tes, there is in some patients with acromegaly an adjustment of the affinity of the receptor for insulin which partially offsets the effect of the decrease in receptor concentration; the increase in receptor affinity appears to help these patients maintain normal glucose tolerance despite the reduction in receptor concentration (Fig. 2–14C).

The blood glucose, plasma insulin, and insulin sensitivity with glucocorticoid excess or with uremia closely resemble the findings in obesity and acromegaly, but the changes in the insulin receptor in humans appear thus far to be more complex and dependent on more variables than in experimental animals.

Extreme Insulin Resistance

In contrast to the common forms of insulin resistance, which are typically moderate in degree, there are conditions associated with insulin resistance of a much more severe degree. The two major classes of these disorders to be discussed here are both associated with defects at the level of the target cell: those associated with autoantibodies directed at the receptor for insulin and another group of disorders that appear to be inborn. Both classes of patients have hyperinsulinemia (basal and stimulated) and impaired responsiveness to exogenous insulin that is much more marked than that observed in patients with obesity or other forms of moderate insulin resistance.

Autoantibodies to Insulin Receptors. Autoantibodies to the insulin receptor have been found in patients wtih an unusual form of diabetes associated with extreme insulin resistance (designated Type B extreme insulin resistance with acanthosis nigricans). These patients typically have other signs and symptoms of autoimmunity, although only a minority have a well defined autoimmune disorder such as lupus erythematosus or Sjögren's syndrome. They have extreme hyperinsulinemia and are typically very resistant (though not totally refractory) to both endogenous and exogenous insulin. ^{125}I-insulin binding to their circulating cells, studied *in vitro,* is markedly reduced (Fig. 2–15), and their plasma, or purified immunoglobulins from their plasma, can reproduce the binding defect when interacted with normal cells (Fig. 2–16). The defect in insulin binding can be reversed by removal of the antibody from the receptor.

These antibodies, which are specific for insulin receptors (Fig. 2–16), bind to the receptor, but their binding sites on the receptor are not identical with the site that binds insulin. The antibodies not only inhibit insulin binding but also mimic, at least acutely, all of the metabolic effects of insulin including rapid membrane effects (transport of glucose and amino acids), rapid activation of intracellular enzymes (glycogen synthase and pyruvate dehydrogenase), and slow processes such as stimulation of synthesis of lipoprotein lipase (see Table 2–8). While these antibodies are acutely insulinomimetic, they act chronically to desensitize the cells at post-receptor sites. Thus, clinically, most of the

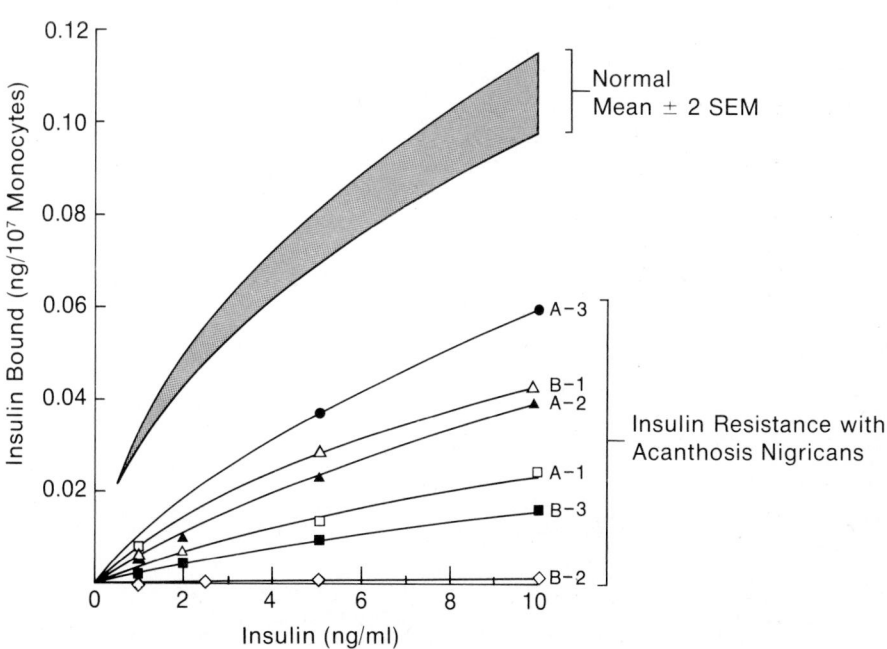

Figure 2–15. Insulin binding to receptors in patients with extreme insulin resistance. Insulin binding *in vitro* to monocytes from normal subjects (upper curve) and six patients with extreme insulin resistance. *B* indicates patients with Type B extreme insulin resistance, i.e., with anti-receptor antibodies. *A* indicates patients with Type A extreme insulin resistance, which probably represents an inborn defect in insulin receptors. For comparison (not shown), obese patients range from the lower part of the normal range to the upper range of patients with extreme insulin resistance shown here.

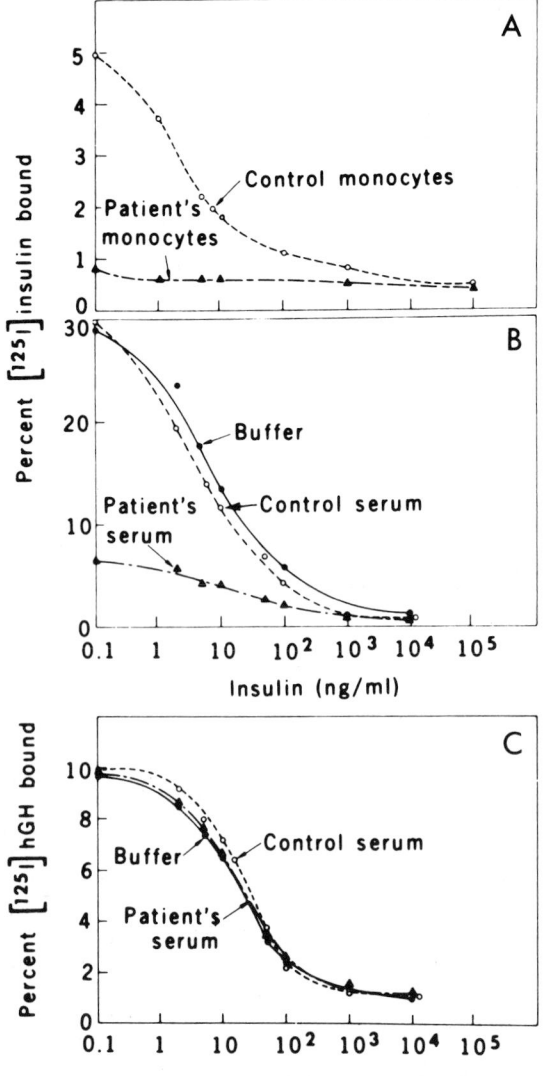

Figure 2–16. Effect of anti-receptor antibodies on insulin binding to its receptors. *A,* Insulin binding to receptors on fresh monocytes, expressed as a competition curve, from a normal subject and a patient with Type B extreme insulin resistance. *B,* Cultured cells with normal insulin receptors were exposed briefly to normal serum, buffer, or serum from the patient with anti-receptor antibodies. The cells were washed, and then the binding of ^{125}I-insulin was measured. Note that exposure of normal cells to anti-receptor antibody produced a defect in insulin binding similar to that found with the patient's own cells *(A).* *C,* The same study as in *B* except that the binding of ^{125}I-growth hormone was studied. This antibody, which interferes with insulin binding to its receptors, had no effect on growth hormone binding to its receptors.

time, the antibodies produce insulin-resistance by inhibiting insulin binding and by desensitizing at post-receptor sites. However, in several of the patients at some time in the course of their disease, the insulin-mimicking effect predominated, with hypoglycemia that in at least one case was severe and protracted.

In addition to patients with Type B syndrome, insulin-resistant diabetes has been associated with autoantibodies to the insulin receptor in some patients with other disorders of immune function (e.g., ataxia-telangiectasia; isolated IgA deficiency) and in the New Zealand Obese (NZO) mouse, which has an autoimmune background genetically (see Table 2–14).

Genetic Disorders. The earliest and best studied genetic disorders of a hormone receptor are those associated with the androgen-resistant states, which will be covered later under intracellular receptors. For hormones with cell surface receptors, those related to insulin have been most extensively studied, although the genetic or inherited nature of these disorders is not yet fully established. The disorders have been found in at least three groups of patients with extreme hyperinsulinemia and insulin resistance who differ from the type B patients in that they do not have anti-receptor antibodies or other signs of autoimmunity: (1) types A (and C) extreme insulin resistance with acanthosis nigricans (adolescent females); (2) leprechaunism (infants); and (3) lipoatrophic diabetes (all ages including adults). In some, insulin binding to receptors is markedly diminished when measured on freshly isolated blood cells (see Fig. 2–15), and a comparable defect has also been detected in cultured cell lines derived from the patients' fibroblasts or B-lymphocytes. In others, insulin binding is not diminished, either *in vivo* or in cultured cells, suggesting strongly that there is a defect at a step in insulin action, either in the receptors (beyond binding) or at a site beyond the receptor.

It seems safe to predict that genetic defects will be detected in receptors for most or all of the hormones and will account for some fraction of the congenital defects in hormone sensitivity (e.g., vasopressin-resistant diabetes insipidus, growth hormone–resistant dwarfism, and pseudohypoparathyroidism). It should be emphasized that the putative defect may or may not alter hormone binding to receptor, and that post-receptor defects may be clinically indistinguishable from receptor defects.

Supersensitivity to Insulin

Target cell defects at the opposite pole, which include anorexia nervosa, glucocorticoid deficiency, and growth

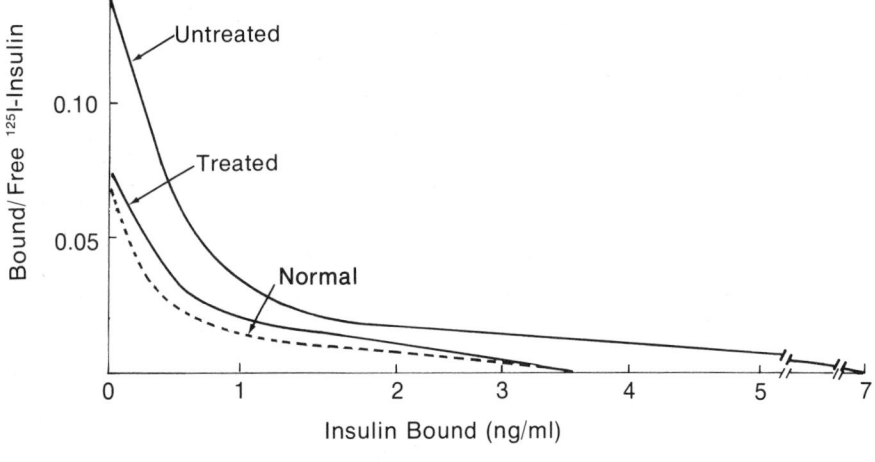

Figure 2–17. Insulin binding to receptors in anorexia nervosa. Scatchard plot (cf. Figs. 2–8 and 2–9). ^{125}I-insulin binding to fresh erythrocytes from patients with untreated anorexia nervosa (upper solid line) is compared to binding to receptors on cells from normal subjects (broken line) and patients with anorexia nervosa after a period of refeeding (lower solid line).

Table 2–15. ANTI-RECEPTOR ANTIBODIES

Condition	Receptor Against Which Antibody Is Directed	Major Effect In Vivo	Mechanism
Graves' disease	TSH	hyperthyroidism	mimics action of TSH
Myasthenia gravis	acetylcholine, nicotinic type	muscle weakness	reduces concentration of receptors by accelerating degradation of receptor
Type B extreme insulin resistance	insulin	insulin resistance	inhibits insulin binding; desensitizes cell at post-receptor level
		(rarely, hypoglycemia)	(mimics insulin; proliferation of low-affinity receptors)
Allergic disorders	adrenergic — β_2	decreased responsiveness to catecholamines; ? enhanced sensitivity to allergens	reduces binding of agonist

hormone deficiency, are characterized by low normal or subnormal levels of blood glucose associated with low normal or subnormal levels of circulating insulin and a heightened responsiveness to injected insulin. In patients with anorexia nervosa, the concentration of insulin receptors is elevated (Fig. 2–17) and may well contribute to the heightened sensitivity to insulin; refeeding restores insulin sensitivity, plasma insulin, and receptors to normal (Fig. 2–17).

Autoantibodies to Other Receptors

Autoantibodies directed against a cell surface receptor have been detected thus far in four conditions (Table 2–15), one presented earlier and three to follow. From studies of these autoantibodies as well as of antibodies generated against receptors in experimental animals, it is clear that antibodies to receptor can block or reduce hormone binding, mimic hormone action, and reduce the sensitivity of the target cell at the level of the receptor or at later steps (Table 2–15). Because of the breadth of possible effects of an anti-receptor antibody (or antibodies to other endocrine-related membrane components), such antibodies should be considered in the differential diagnosis of any endocrine-related disorder, especially (but not only) in patients in whom there are other suggestions of disturbed immune regulation.

TSH Receptors. A majority of patients with Graves' disease, the most common form of hyperthyroidism, have circulating antibodies that bind to the TSH receptors on the thyroid. Typically these antibodies, in binding to the TSH receptor, both inhibit the binding of TSH and mimic the effect of TSH; i.e., they stimulate the thyroid as does TSH (Table 2–15) but this stimulation is largely independent of feedback inhibition by T_3 and T_4 (Fig. 2–18). Presumably these antibodies represent LATS (long-acting thyroid stimulator), an activity found in plasma of patients with Graves' disease by investigators almost three decades ago.

Catecholamine Receptors. Autoantibodies directed against one of the β-type adrenergic receptors have been found in a substantial minority of patients with a wide range of atopic or allergic disorders. These patients manifest reduced sensitivity to stimulation by β-adrenergic agents, but the role of this antibody in their primary (allergic) disorder is not yet defined (Table 2–15).

Acetylcholine Receptors. Although not an endocrine disorder, myasthenia gravis is introduced here because it is associated with autoantibodies to a cell surface receptor, the nicotinic-type acetylcholine receptor found on motor end-plates of skeletal muscle. The antibody does not block ligand binding or mimic the action of the neurotransmitter. Rather, it appears now that antibody bound to receptor accelerates degradation of receptor, which results in a

chronic diminution in the number of receptors and thereby a reduced sensitivity to stimulation by ligand (Table 2–15).

Modulation of the Target Cell in Response to Hormone Deficiency

Insulin (see Table 2–14). In experimental animals, insulin deficiency (starvation; streptozotocin-induced destruction of β-cells; "spontaneous" in Chinese hamsters) is associated with an elevation in the concentration of insulin receptors. In humans, this process is less constant and less marked, so that insulin-deficient humans with type I diabetes may or may not have an increase in insulin binding, and the magnitude of the increase is less than that observed in animals. The milder degree of insulin deficiency associated with chronic pancreatitis is associated with an increase in receptors but again is less marked than in animals, and acute starvation in humans of normal weight produces a marked reduction in levels of circulating insulin but no change in the insulin receptor. In addition to effects on the receptor, insulin deficiency (with or without starvation) can result in many changes in the target cell at steps beyond insulin binding, especially in the levels of many enzymes that metabolize glucose and other related substrates. Thus the overall effect of insulin deficiency on the target cell is complex; it may vary among different cells (e.g., hepatocyte versus adipocyte), and the response to insulin may be reduced despite an elevation in insulin binding to receptors.

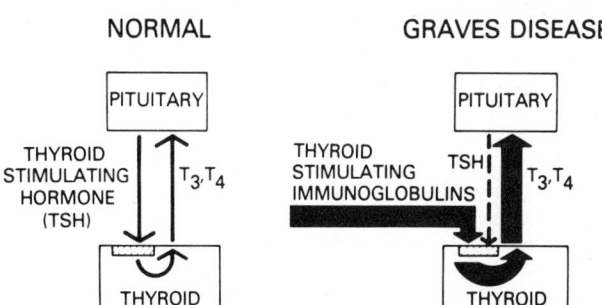

Figure 2–18. Thyroid stimulators in normal persons and in patients with Graves' disease. In normal people, the pituitary releases TSH which binds to its specific receptors on the surface of thyroid cells and stimulates intracellular events that lead to the release of T_3 and T_4. The thyroid hormones, among their many effects, act on the hypothalamus and pituitary to reduce TSH secretion ("negative feedback"). In patients with Graves' disease, autoantibodies (immunoglobulins) bind to the TSH receptor and stimulate the same intracellular pathways as TSH, resulting in the release of thyroid hormones (T_3, T_4) even in the absence of TSH. Typically, the elevated levels of thyroid hormones suppress TSH secretion but have no effect on the circulating levels of the thyroid-stimulating immunoglobulins. (From Kahn, C. R., et al.: Receptors for peptide hormones. New insights into the pathophysiology of disease states in man. *Ann. Intern. Med.* 86:205, 1977.)

While insulin deficiency itself sometimes elevates the receptor concentration, the ketosis and acidosis that supervene can both reduce insulin binding to receptor. A fall in the pH of the extracellular fluid acutely, on a physiochemical basis, reduces the affinity of the receptor for insulin (see Fig. 2–11A). In addition, over a period of hours acidosis *per se* leads to a decrease in the concentration of insulin receptors that can be marked. Thus what begins as a state of hormone deficiency may be complicated by severe defects at the level of the target cell, both at the receptor and at the post-receptor sites.

ACTH. A somewhat analogous condition may be the changes in the responsiveness of the adrenal to ACTH. In the first few hours following ACTH withdrawal (hypophysectomy), the adrenal cortex of the rat displays heightened sensitivity to ACTH, measured as activation of early steps (adenylate cyclase) or late steps (steroid release). With time, the sensitivity at early steps persists but the steroidogenic response to ACTH diminishes markedly. In humans with chronic ACTH deprivation, steroid hormone production by the adrenal cortex is subnormally responsive to ACTH, and the responsiveness can be restored to normal by continual ACTH replacement. In summary, hormone deficiency often results in changes in the target cell's capacity to respond. Some of these changes act to enhance sensitivity while others reduce sensitivity; with chronic deficiency, the latter may predominate.

Modulation of the Target Cell in Response to Hormone Excess

As pointed out earlier, chronic hormone excess can lead to desensitization of the target cell, both at the level of hormone binding to receptor and at post-receptor steps. Patients with choriocarcinomas, with extremely high plasma levels of biologically active hCG, are often refractory to the effects of the hormone, both endogenous and exogenous, presumably because of desensitization at the receptor and at (multiple) post-receptor sites. Destruction of the tumor and elimination of the hormone excess restores the sensitivity of the target cells to the hormone. (Does a similar scheme explain why patients with medullary carcinoma of the thyroid who have extremely elevated concentrations of thyrocalcitonin in plasma have no detectable disturbance in calcium metabolism?) Patients treated chronically with β-adrenergic drugs often show decreased catecholamine binding along with reduced sensitivity which can be reversed by withdrawal of the drug. Patients with insulinomas often have a reduction in insulin binding to receptors and are often much less responsive than normal subjects to high levels of circulating insulin.

It should be emphasized that excessive levels of circulating hormone, decreased binding of hormone to receptor, post-receptor defects, and reduced sensitivity of the target cell often coexist, irrespective of which defect is primary. Thus a single primary defect can lead secondarily to all the others and even aggravate itself. Therefore, studies done at steady state often fail to permit a unique decision about the initiating event. While in the four examples cited in the previous paragraph hormone excess obviously antedated the target cell defects, other conditions (e.g., those with moderate insulin resistance, cited earlier) are often less easy to decipher except by much more extensive study.

States of Insulin Excess. The target cell's response to hormone excess may not always be restricted to a simple pattern. To illustrate this point (see Table 2–14), several conditions in which insulin excess is a dominant feature are presented here. In experimental animals daily injections of insulin in progressively increasing doses produce, as expected, a decrease in receptor concentration and reduced sensitivity to insulin. As noted earlier, patients with insulinomas show a similar pattern, which may permit them to maintain (even in the fasting state) normal levels of blood glucose for surprisingly long periods in the face of very high circulating levels of biologically active insulin. Some of these patients also have an increase in receptor affinity (mechanism?), in addition to the decrease in receptor, analogous to the changes found in some patients with acromegaly. The increase in receptor affinity, which in acromegaly appears to be beneficial, in patients with insulinomas appears to be detrimental and may be an important determinant of the patient's course. Thus, for a given elevation of plasma insulin, there is typically a characteristic decrement in receptor concentration; but the increase in receptor affinity, which is very variable among individual patients, appears to account for differences in the ability of an individual patient to maintain a normal blood glucose in the face of a given level of circulating insulin.

Neonates with hypoglycemia due to insulin excess (because of nesidioblastosis, Beckwith's syndrome, or maternal diabetes) may represent another example in which secondary modulations at the target cell become major determinants of the clinical course. With normal maturation in late fetal and early postnatal life, there appears to be a progressive fall in the concentration of insulin receptors. Hyperinsulinemia at this stage of life is associated with a delay in the maturation of many biochemical systems (these babies are classically big and immature). These infants appear to have elevated concentrations of insulin receptors which we interpret as a manifestation of their biochemical immaturity. Thus, the hyperinsulinemia, which is a dominant factor in the disorder, instead of causing target cell desensitization as it often does in other conditions, appears to produce a heightened sensitivity to insulin by its effects on maturational events. The persistently elevated concentration of receptors may account, in part, for the observation that amelioration of the hyperinsulinemia in these babies does not uniformly do away with the hypoglycemia.

Other Considerations. Up to this point, in discussing the response of the target cell, we have not distinguished the maximal capacity to respond (biological effect per unit time when hormone is present in excess) from target cell sensitivity (the concentration of hormone needed to produce half, or some other fraction, of the maximal response). For our discussion of hormone effects on target cell responsiveness, ACTH effects on the adrenal provide a useful example. With ACTH deficiency, the adrenal gland atrophies. When suddenly exposed to a very high concentration of hormone, its maximal capacity to generate steroids is subnormal but it may well produce its steroidogenic response at low levels of hormone. (This is analogous to denervated muscle which responds to unusually low levels of stimulation but whose maximal capacity to work is reduced.) With chronic ACTH excess (as in bilateral adrenal hyperplasia) the adrenal glands are markedly hypertrophied and a high concentration of exogenous ACTH produces a massive output of steroids but the concentration of ACTH needed to stimulate steroidogenesis (threshold or half-maximal response) may be elevated above normal. The fairy-tale equivalents might be the nervous dwarf and the lethargic or hard-of-hearing giant; the former is easy to stimulate but his maximal performance is subnormal, while the latter requires strong stimuli to be aroused but his maximal performance is greater than normal. In analyzing target cell responsiveness, this distinction should be made whenever possible.

In summary, an excess or deficiency of circulating hormone can produce typical effects which are familiar and in addition modify the responsiveness of the target cell to itself (homologous effects) at the receptor as well as at post-receptor sites. Because in individual conditions and patients the magnitude and direction of the changes at each of the target cell sites may differ, the overall change in responsiveness can vary widely. While essential for diagnostic purposes, measurements of circulating hormone levels, even in conditions where they are the dominant force, provide only a partial understanding of the pathophysiology; measurements of receptor and post-receptor events, whenever possible, can add substantially. In addition, it should be recalled that one effect of a hormone can be to alter the physiology of another hormone at any level, including sensing, secretion, transport in plasma, degradation, and at multiple target cell sites. Finally, a hormone acting on its target cell can lead secondarily to major changes (e.g., food intake, body composition, or ionic environment) that profoundly affect many processes including multiple endocrine-modulated pathways.

Hormone Excess, Specificity Spillover, and Disorders of Receptor Design

In our presentation of the role of the target cell and its receptors in endocrine disorders, conditions dominated by the target cell were followed by a discussion of disorders in which hormone deficiency or excess was the dominant problem but the target cell played an important modifying role. In this section the discussion will continue with disorders of hormone excess but specifically situations in which one or more effects of the hormone excess are exerted through the receptor of another hormone. We designate these conditions as "disorders of receptor design" or "specificity spillover." As before, examination of the target cell and its receptors provides insights into pathophysiology and strategies for therapeutic intervention that were not apparent from measurements of plasma hormone alone.

Specificity Spillover. As noted earlier, essentially all cells in the body are exposed to essentially equal concentrations of each hormone (see Fig. 2–5B), and, ideally, to insure specificity, each hormone should have a single unique class of receptors (Fig. 2–19). In fact, one hormone may have strong affinity for its own receptor and in addition (Fig.

Table 2–16. PRIMARY INTERACTION OF HORMONE WITH TARGET (EFFECTOR) CELL

I. External Cell Surface (Plasma Membrane)
  A. Peptide hormones, divided into families*
    1. Glycoprotein hormones: TSH, FSH, LH, chorionic gonadotropin
    2. Growth hormone, prolactin, placental lactogen
    3. Insulin; insulin-like growth factors (IGF) including the somatomedins; relaxin; nerve growth factor (NGF)
    4. Gastrin; cholecystokinin-pancreozymin (CCK-PZ)
    5. Pancreatic glucagon; gut glucagon; secretin; vasoactive intestinal peptide (VIP); gastric inhibitory polypeptide (GIP)
    6. ACTH, α-MSH
    7. Enkephalins, endorphins, β-lipotropin
    8. Posterior pituitary nonapeptides: oxytocin, vasopressin, vasotocin
    9. Epidermal growth factor (EGF); urogastrone
    10. Calcium-regulating: parathyroid hormone, thyrocalcitonin
    11. Hypothalamic peptides: TRF, LHRH, somatostatin
  B. Catecholamines
  C. Nonhormones related to endocrinology
    1. Prostaglandins
    2. Neurotransmitters and bioactive amines: acetylcholine, serotonin, histamine
    3. Neurotensin; substance P
    4. Other: cholera toxin, low-density lipoproteins, hepatic receptor for glycoproteins
II. Intracellular
  A. Steroid-like hormones
    1. Adrenal: glucocorticoids, mineralocorticoids
    2. Sex: estrogens, androgens, progestins
    3. Sterols: 1,25(OH)$_2$-vitamin D
  B. Iodothyronines

*The division of the peptide hormones into families 1 through 9 is based on similarities in overall structure or in amino sequences and/or reactivity either at the receptor or with anti-hormone antibodies. Potential for spillover at the receptor (two or more ligands binding to two or more types of receptor within a family) is suggested for I:A1 through A8; B; C1 and C2, and II: A1 and A2. While the text stresses the pathological consequences of spillover at the receptor, possible physiological interplay and pharmacological mechanisms should be considered as well.

2–19) have some affinity for the receptor of another hormone ("specificity spillover"). The spillover or "cross-reactions" are not at all random; rather, they occur because of similarities in structure between the two hormones. The fifty or so different hormones belong to a much smaller number of families of hormones (Table 2–16); while each family may be unique, within a family (by definition) there are structural similarities.

A purely speculative teleological interpretation is that all of the hormones that exist today were derived evolution-

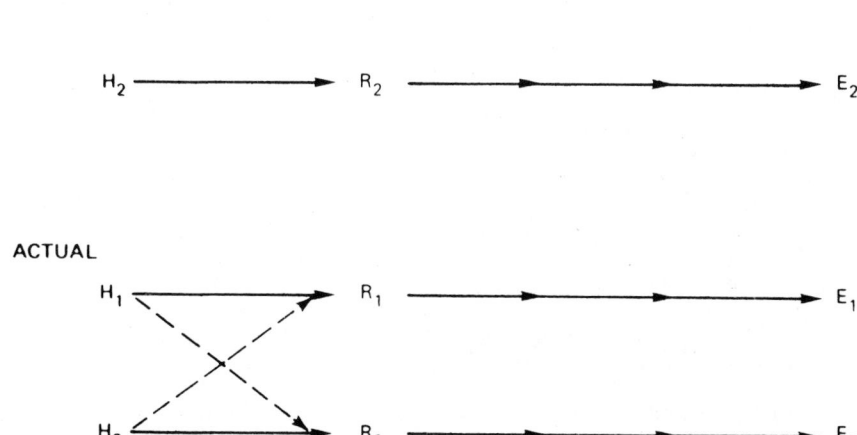

IDEAL

$H_1 \longrightarrow R_1 \longrightarrow E_1$

$H_2 \longrightarrow R_2 \longrightarrow E_2$

ACTUAL

$H_1 \longrightarrow R_1 \longrightarrow E_1$

$H_2 \longrightarrow R_2 \longrightarrow E_2$

Figure 2–19. Specificity spillover. Ideally, a hormone (H_1) should have a unique receptor (R_1) through which it produces its characteristic effects (E_1), and likewise a second hormone (H_2) should have its unique receptor (R_2) for its effects (E_2). Actually one hormone (H_1), in addition to high affinity for its own receptor (R_1), may have some affinity for the receptor (R_2) of another related hormone; likewise, H_2 may have some affinity for R_1.

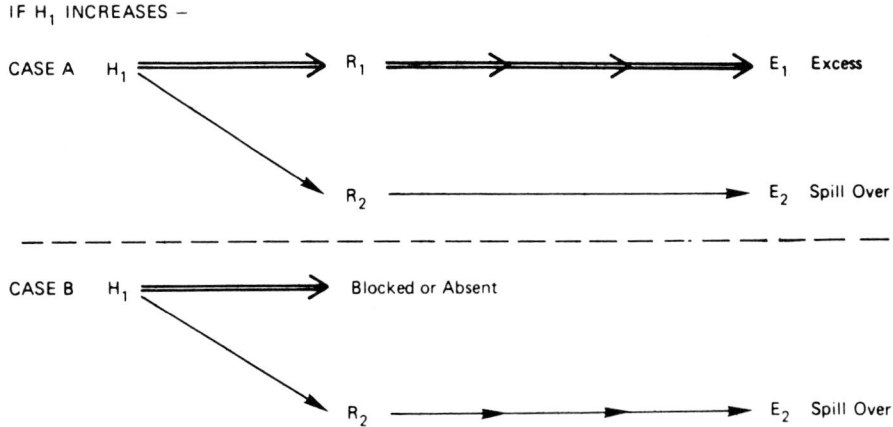

Figure 2–20. Disorders of receptor design. Hormone 1 (H_1) is present in excess. In *Case A*, H_1 binds to R_1 to produce an excess of E_1, the characteristic effect of H_1 binding to R_1. In addition, the concentration of H_1 is sufficiently great so that, despite its lower affinity, it binds to R_2, receptor of a related hormone, forming H_1R_2 complexes which produce E_2 (spillover), biological effects characteristically associated with H_2 binding to R_2. In *Case B*, the primary pathway is blocked or absent so that the only effect of H_1 is via the spillover pathway.

arily from a much smaller number of ancestral prototypes. To gain diversity, the genes responsible for the hormones and their receptors were duplicated one or more times and, by undergoing multiple mutations, achieved one or more signaling systems in addition to the original. While one hormone has high affinity for its own receptor, it may well retain some affinity for the receptor of its relative (Fig. 2–19). Thus evolutionarily, diversity was purchased at some cost in specificity, and there is some "degeneracy" in the specificity of the systems.

At physiological levels of hormones, the affinity of hormone 1 for receptor 2 is so low (relative to the concentrations of reactants) that the spillover is of negligible consequence. Now consider what may occur when hormone 1 is present in excess (Fig. 2–20). Clearly, hormone 1 through its own receptor (R_1) will produce an excess of its typical effect (E_1). In addition, because its concentration is so high, hormone 1 may now produce sufficient complexes with receptor 2 (R_2) to trigger that pathway which results in effects (E_2) characteristic of hormone 2, even in the absence of the latter hormone. Alternatively, its own target cell pathway may be absent or blocked, so that the only effects of excess hormone 1 may be those exercised through pathway 2. (Recall that the effects observed are not determined by which hormone is present but rather by the receptor that is activated; hormone 1 or 2 when it reacts with receptor 2 produces effects (E_2) characteristic of hormone 2. Likewise both hormones when reacted with receptor 1 produce effects (E_1) characteristic of receptor 1.)

In Table 2–17 we have listed some disease states in which one or more manifestations of hormone excess may be due to interaction of one hormone with the receptor for another. Several of these situations are described in detail in the text, involving insulin and the insulin-like growth factors, growth hormone and prolactin, adrenal steroids, and sex steroids.

Effects of Insulin in Infants of Diabetic Mothers. Insulin and the insulin-like growth factors are structurally quite similar but the latter do not react with antibodies to insulin and therefore are not detected by radioimmunoassay for insulin. Each reacts strongly with its own receptor and weakly with the receptor for the other (Fig. 2–21). Both can produce all the metabolic effects of insulin but insulin is more potent. Both can stimulate cell growth but in this action the growth factors are more potent. In infants of diabetic mothers, the high level of glucose, amino acids, or other substrates that cross the placenta from the mother to the fetus is thought to cause the hypersecretion of insulin by the infant's B-cells. These infants manifest metabolic symptoms typical of insulin excess (excess deposition of glycogen and fat as well as postnatal hypoglycemia), presumably effects of insulin through its own receptor. In addition they have signs of excessive growth (increased body length and macrosomia), due possibly, at least in part, to effects of insulin through growth factor receptors (Fig. 2–21). Interestingly, infusions of insulin into fetal baboons in utero re-create both the metabolic and growth abnormalities typical of infants of diabetic mothers.

Hypoglycemia with Non-Islet Cell Tumors. Another example of spillover in this family of hormones is in pa-

Table 2–17.   CANDIDATES FOR SPECIFICITY SPILLOVER

Clinical Condition	Hormone in Excess	Reacts with Receptor for	To Produce
Infants of diabetic mothers	insulin	insulin-like growth factors	excess skeletal growth, macrosomia (? retardation of biochemical maturation)
Non-islet cell tumors	IGF-II	insulin	hypoglycemia
Acromegaly	growth hormone	prolactin	galactorrhea; amenorrhea; infertility
Choriocarcinoma	hCG	TSH	hyperthyroidism
Untreated Addison's disease "Autonomous" overproduction of ACTH by pituitary or ectopic tissue	ACTH	α-MSH	skin darkening
Primary hypothyroidism in childhood	TSH	LH, FSH	precocious puberty
Glucocorticoid excess	hydrocortisone	aldosterone	hypertension
Androgen excess	testosterone	estrogen	estrogen-like effects

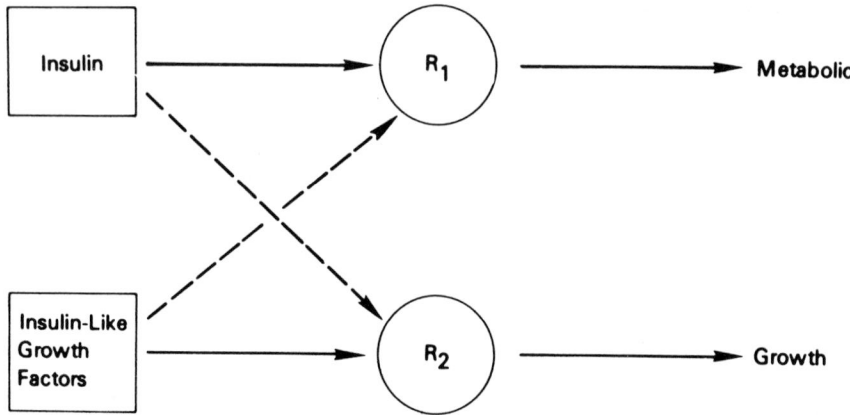

Figure 2–21.   Interaction of insulin and insulin-like growth factors at the target cell. Insulin binds with high affinity to its own receptors (R_1) to produce the metabolic effects we characteristically associate with insulin action. Insulin-like growth factors bind to their own receptors (R_2) to stimulate growth, as by cell division. Each ligand binds with lower affinity to the opposite receptor; the nature of the effect that is produced depends entirely on which receptor is occupied and is independent of which ligand is bound. (Experimentally, bivalent antibodies to R_1 mimic only the metabolic effects of insulin; monovalent antibodies to R_1 block the metabolic effects of both insulin and the growth factors but fail to affect the growth-promoting effects of either ligand.) In infants of diabetic mothers, insulin is present in excess, which through its own receptor (R_1) produces characteristic metabolic effects; we postulate that excess insulin, acting through growth factor receptors (R_2), causes excess skeletal growth and macrosomia and possibly slows the maturation of biochemical pathways. Some non-islet cell tumors produce an insulin-like growth factor, which binds to insulin receptors to produce insulin-like metabolic effects including hypoglycemia.

tients with tumor-associated hypoglycemia. While patients with β-cell tumors have hypoglycemia that is due to inappropriate secretion of insulin, patients with hypoglycemia associated with non-islet cell tumors do not have elevated levels of immunoassayable insulin. Instead, about a third to a half of these patients have in their circulation elevated levels of one of the insulin-like growth factors (IGF-II) that is not detected by radioimmunoassays for insulin but is measured by specific radioreceptor assays (and bioassays). Presumably the insulin-like growth factor at high levels in the circulation interacts with the insulin receptor to produce an excess of the metabolic effect typical of insulin action (Fig. 2–21). In fact, the available (free) IGF in the plasma of these patients has as much insulin-like bioactivity as the insulin in plasma of patients with insulinomas.

Galactorrhea with Acromegaly.   Prolactin excess of any etiology may lead to amenorrhea, infertility, and galactorrhea. In female patients with pituitary tumors (without acromegaly), plasma prolactin is often elevated; while a minority of these patients have galactorrhea, the latter is almost always associated with an elevated plasma prolactin. Among females with pituitary tumors associated with acromegaly, there is also an increased prevalence of elevated prolactins and galactorrhea (but not as frequently as in the former group). Remarkably, though, most of our acromegalic patients with galactorrhea did not have elevated prolactins.

Recall that growth hormone, in addition to its growth-promoting activity, is also a full prolactin agonist (Fig. 2–22). Thus the total prolactin-like activity is best repre-

sented as the sum of the prolactin plus growth hormone, each measured by its specific radioimmunoassay. Ordinarily, the contribution of GH to total prolactin is slight, but in patients with acromegaly, the elevated growth hormone can provide a substantial portion of the total prolactin bioactivity. In most of our acromegalic patients with galactorrhea who had normal prolactin levels by radioimmunoassay, the sum of GH + prolactin was pathologically elevated. We suggest that in these patients, growth hormone, which is present at high levels in plasma, is acting through the prolactin receptor (along with endogenous prolactin) to produce the excess of prolactin-like effects.

Spillover Among Steroid Hormones.   The potential for specificity spillover is not limited to peptide hormones (Table 2–16 footnote and Table 2–17). All naturally occurring glucocorticoids have some affinity for mineralocorticoid receptors and, at high concentrations, in addition to excess glucocorticoid effects, can produce effects of mineralocorticoid excess. Androgens at high concentrations can mimic all of the effects of estrogens. Several investigators have proposed that, in addition to the chemical conversion of androgens to estrogen ("aromatization"), natural androgens have an affinity for estrogen receptors which accounts (at least in part) for their estrogen-like effects.

Other Functions of Cell Surface Receptors

From the earlier discussion, the reader recognizes that the hormone-receptor interaction not only performs the fundamental functions of recognition and activation but also can regulate receptor concentration and affinity as well as

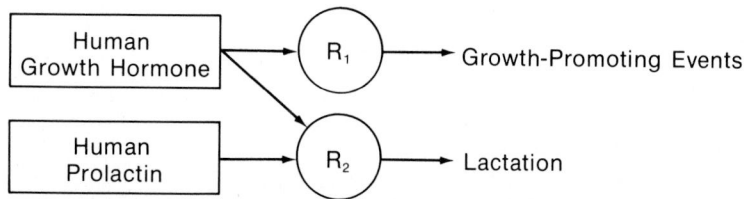

Figure 2–22.   Interaction of growth hormone and prolactin at the target cell in humans. Prolactin binds to its specific receptors (R_2) to produce characteristic prolactin-like effects including lactation (in appropriately primed breast tissue). Growth hormone binds to its own specific receptors (R_1) to stimulate growth-promoting events. In addition, growth hormone binds with about the same affinity as prolactin to prolactin receptors (R_2), where it produces prolactin-like effects. Thus, in human plasma the total concentration of effective prolactin-like activity is best represented as the sum of growth hormone and prolactin. While the contribution of growth hormone to the total prolactin activity is trivial under most conditions, in patients with acromegaly (or in newborns) the concentration of growth hormone may be sufficiently elevated to provide a substantial prolactin-like effect, including simulation of the syndrome of prolactin excess — amenorrhea, infertility, and galactorrhea.

Table 2–18. FUNCTIONS OF THE RECEPTOR-HORMONE INTERACTION*

A. Fundamental
1. Recognition
2. Activation
B. Additional
1. Reservoir for plasma hormone
2. Regulate degradation of hormone
3. Regulate degradation of receptor
4. Regulate receptor concentration and receptor affinity
5. Cross-link and translocate hormone-receptor complexes
6. Regulate post-receptor events

*From Roth, J.: Transductive coupling by cell surface receptor — I. In *Physical Chemical Aspects of Cell Surface Events in Cellular Regulation.* DeLisi, C., and Blumenthal, R. (eds.), New York, Elsevier/North-Holland, 1979.

post-receptor events. Table 2–18 lists the multiple functions performed by cell surface receptors. The discussion here will describe two — the role of specific receptors in hormone degradation and as a possible reservoir for plasma hormone.

Receptors as Reservoirs

The lipid-soluble hormones have intracellular receptors for hormone action and typically have a distinctly separate binding protein in blood that acts as a reservoir for plasma hormone. The water-soluble hormones have cell surface receptors and typically lack binding proteins in blood. We have found for insulin that the cell surface receptors may act as reservoirs for plasma hormone *in vivo.* Thus, hormone released into blood by the secretory cells is rapidly taken up by receptors throughout the body; the concentration of insulin receptors is so high, relative to hormone concentration and the affinity of the interaction, that most of the hormone is bound. As the concentration of hormone falls, hormone that dissociates from receptor helps to replenish the pool in plasma. Initially (up to 10 minutes) all or most of the bound insulin is dissociable and available to resupply the plasma, whereas at later times only part of the receptor-bound hormone is available (see Fig. 2–10). Thus the receptors throughout the body act as a reservoir (albeit a leaky one), with a net uptake of hormone when the hormone concentrations in plasma are rising and a return of hormone to plasma when plasma hormone concentrations are falling.

Hormone Degradation

Hormone binding to receptors, while initially reversible, often leads to irreversible association of the hormone with the cell, internalization, and degradation of the hormone, presumably in the lysosomes. Receptor-mediated degradation is probably the major pathway for the degradation of most peptide hormones *in vivo,* but other pathways are also present. In the case of insulin, we estimate that about 70% of the hormone is degraded via the receptor and the remainder by other (nonreceptor) mechanisms at the cellular level, which are poorly understood; little or none is degraded in plasma. A corollary is that in conditions associated with receptor deficiency, the lifetime of circulating insulin is prolonged, and elevated concentrations of receptor are associated with a shortened life span for the circulating hormone.

For some peptide hormones of low molecular weight (e.g., oxytocin, angiotensin), there may be significant degradation by proteases in plasma. Another mechanism for degradation of hormones *in vivo* is unique to the glycoprotein hormones (TSH, LH, FSH, and hCG). These hormones, like many other circulating glycoproteins, typically have a sialic acid at the peripheral end of their carbohydrate side chains. Removal of the sialic acid (mechanism unknown) results in the exposure of a free galactose which is specifically recognized and bound by a receptor present on the surface of hepatocytes, followed by internalization and destruction of the hormone. Thus asialo forms of the glycoprotein hormones (and other asialoglycoproteins) are rapidly removed from plasma and destroyed. This accounts for the observation that the asialo form of hCG is at least as active biologically as native hCG *in vitro* but has markedly reduced or absent effects *in vivo,* because of its accelerated destruction. The hepatic receptor for asialoglycoproteins and some of the other cell surface receptors of relevance to endocrinology are presented in Table 2–19.

Post-Receptor Events at the Target Cell

The post-receptor events for the water-soluble hormones were presented in outline earlier. We now will present them in depth with particular emphasis on applications to disease states. As a prelude, we will present the historical context in which this area developed to show the pivotal role it has played in casting present thoughts about mechanisms of hormone action.

Historical Perspective

As recently as a quarter of a century ago, mechanisms of hormone action at the target cell were only vaguely understood, and the formulation of relevant questions about them was rare. Endocrinologists were largely concerned with physiology. Their interest in chemistry was focused on bio-

Table 2–19. OTHER CELL SURFACE RECEPTORS RELATED TO ENDOCRINOLOGY

Ligand	Cell Surface Receptor	Relevant Biological Event
Asialoglycoproteins (including asialo forms of hCG, LH, TSH, and FSH)	Integral protein of hepatocyte; recognizes terminal free galactose, which is exposed following removal of terminal sialic acid	Accelerated clearance (and destruction) of asialo forms of plasma glycoproteins including the glycoprotein hormones
Low-density lipoproteins (LDL)	Specific integral protein present on many (most) types of cells	Cholesterol is the biosynthetic precursor of steroid hormones; LDL, which is rich in cholesterol, is a major source of intracellular cholesterol for hormone synthesis
Cholera toxin	GM_1 ganglioside (present on essentially all human cells)	Cholera toxin (ADP)-ribosylates one subunit of the adenylate cyclase, leading to "irreversible" activation
Plant lectins	Each lectin binds to one or a few types of simple sugars in the carbohydrate side chains of integral proteins; a single lectin typically binds to many different cell surface proteins	Mimic hormone action; modify receptors for hormones; other modifications of target cells

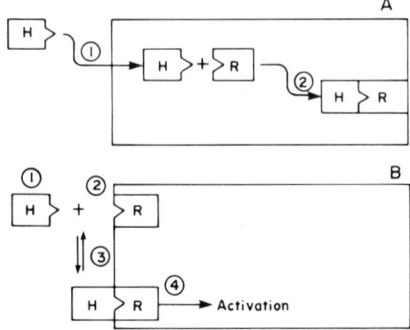

Figure 2–23. Historical development of concepts about interaction of hormones with target cells.

A, Early ideas: It was thought that most (all) hormones readily entered cells ①; the initial interaction of hormone *(H)* with a component of the cell occurred intracellularly ②; the process was irreversible ②; and that cellular component (to which the hormone bound) was directly involved in the final biologically relevant event. While we have designated that cellular component as *R* for receptor, receptors were rarely discussed by endocrinologists. Further, each hormone was considered to be unique.

B, Later ideas: The distinction was made between lipid-soluble hormones and water-soluble hormones ①. Within each class, generalizations were established for post-receptor events as well as initial events. Concepts about receptors emerged, and receptors for the water-soluble hormones were located on the cell surface ②. The initial interaction of hormone with its cell surface receptor was recognized as a reversible event ③; subsequent activation steps ④ involved membrane-bound as well as soluble intracellular moieties; and the biochemical distance between the first step and final step in the target cell widened markedly. (From Roth, J., et al.: Hormone receptors, human disease, and disorders in receptor design. In *Hormones and Cell Culture*, Book A. Sato, G. H., and Ross, R. (eds.), Cold Spring Harbor Laboratory, 1979.)

synthesis, isolation, purification, and characterization of hormone molecules; this interest was shared with the biochemists, who at that time were focused on soluble proteins.

The membranes of the cell and receptors for hormones were neglected, and theories of hormone action were rarely considered. It was thought that the hormone interacted directly with the components of the cell that produced the final biological effect and that hormones entered cells freely and bound (irreversibly) to the enzyme whose action they regulated (Fig. 2–23). A modification of that formulation was proposed for insulin and vasopressin; since the most prominent effect of these hormones is to promote the movement of small molecules (glucose and water, respectively) across cell membranes, it was thought that they interacted directly with membrane components linked closely to the transport systems and thereby promoted the translocation of the small molecules. Because these hormones (as well as oxytocin) have disulfide bridges in their structure (the structure of these hormones was elucidated in the early fifties), it was proposed further that these hormones bound covalently by disulfide interchange with cell components. Further, the mechanism of action of each hormone was considered to be unique for that hormone. Alternatively, the few unified general approaches to mechanism typically provided a single mechanism for all hormones with no distinction between water-soluble and lipid-soluble hormones.

Research over the next 25 years progressively increased the biochemical distance between the first step, contact of the hormone with target cell, and the final biologically relevant event. Simultaneously, the similarities among the hormones at a biochemical level progressively took hold over the obvious physiological differences among them. A major breakthrough was the discovery by Sutherland and co-workers that epinephrine (and many other hormones) acts on the liver (and other tissues) to stimulate the activity of a membrane-bound enzyme, adenylate cyclase, which catalyzes the conversion intracellularly of ATP to cyclic AMP. The latter is a soluble compound that can strikingly mimic the effects of specific hormones on their particular target cells. Sutherland and associates proposed the "second-messenger hypothesis" that the hormone or "first messenger" carried the message from the secretory cell to the target cell but the action of the hormone at the cellular level was carried out by cAMP, the "second messenger."

Subsequent progress occurred both distal and proximal to this enzyme and its product. It was established that the major (? sole) role of cAMP is to activate a protein kinase and that phosphorylation and dephosphorylation of cellular proteins (especially enzymes) by kinases and phosphatases play a major role in hormone action distal to cAMP.

At the same time it became clear that the initial interaction of peptide hormones with the cell takes place on the outer cell surface (or plasma membrane) rather than inside the cell (Fig. 2–23); that the interaction is rapid, reversible, and hormone-specific; that hormone binding is not tantamount to activation of adenylate cyclase; and that the receptor molecule is a molecular entity distinct from the cyclase that is regulated independently and participates on its own in physiological and pathological processes.

Meanwhile, intracellular sites for the binding of steroid hormones were defined (in concordance with old ideas) but the receptor proteins were not found to be enzymes. Rather, the further action of these hormones requires transfer to the nucleus where they regulate gene expression, processes that were just being explored in mammalian cells.

Now, the distance is great between the first step and the last in hormone action at the target cell, and a limited number of biochemical mechanisms apply widely. Progress has brought receptors into sharp focus, made clear the distinction between the water-soluble and lipid-soluble hormones, and also showed extraordinary similarity among hormones within either group. The lipid-soluble hormones, with their intracellular receptors, regulate cells by actions within the nucleus at the level of DNA, while the water-soluble hormones, with their cell surface receptors, act through cAMP or other soluble intracellular messengers on kinases and phosphatases that regulate cellular processes by phosphorylation and dephosphorylation mechanisms.

Hormone-Sensitive Adenylate Cyclase

Most peptide hormones, many biogenic amines, and some prostaglandins activate their target cells by stimulating the production of cAMP, the so-called second messenger of hormone action. This section deals with the steps by which hormone bound to its receptor leads to activation of adenylate cyclase and conversion of ATP to cyclic AMP (Fig. 2–24).

Physiologically, for extracellular messengers such as hormones to produce an increase in the intracellular concentration of cAMP, three proteins are required, all of which are intrinsic proteins of the plasma membrane: the specific receptor, the regulatory component of adenylate cyclase, which, as its name suggests, regulates the activity of the third protein, the catalytic component, which actually effects the conversion of ATP to cAMP (Table 2–20).

When assayed in membrane preparations *in vitro,* the enzyme typically displays some basal activity, which varies very widely. It is unclear whether this basal activity corresponds to the *in vivo* unperturbed state or is due to an artifactual stimulation during preparation for the assay. Hormones and other activators increase this activity; the magnitude of the stimulation and the sensitivity to low concentrations of hormone are greater in intact cells than in broken cell preparations.

In addition to hormone bound to receptor, three other agents are ubiquitous activators of the enzyme — GTP, fluo-

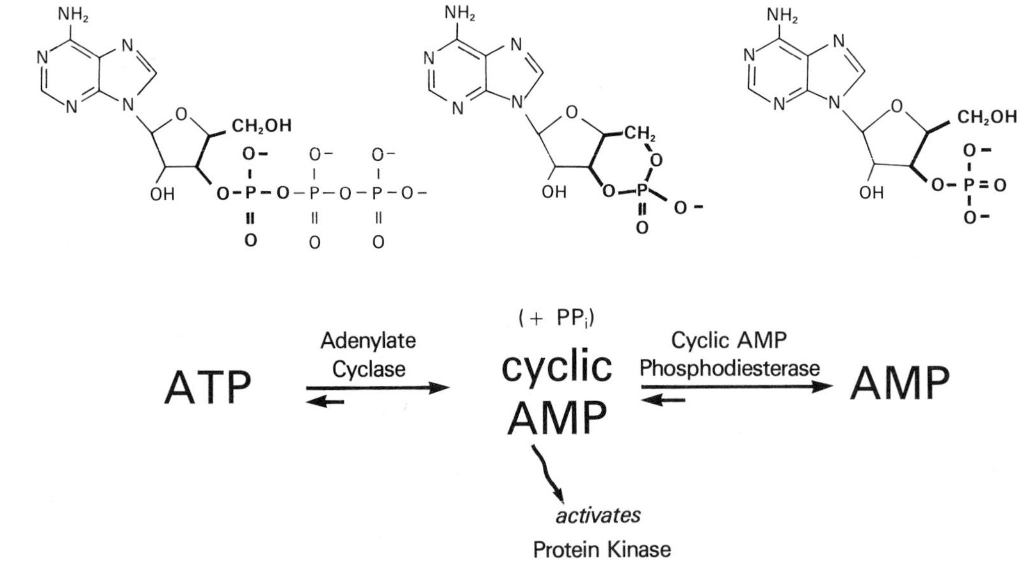

$$ATP \xrightleftharpoons[]{\text{Adenylate Cyclase}} \text{cyclic AMP} \xrightleftharpoons[]{\text{Cyclic AMP Phosphodiesterase}} AMP$$

(+ PP$_i$)

cyclic AMP *activates* Protein Kinase

Figure 2–24. Enzymatic formation and destruction of cyclic AMP. Cyclic AMP is synthesized enzymatically from ATP (more correctly, Mg^{++}• ATP) by removal of the pair of terminal phosphates (to yield pyrophosphate, PP$_i$) and formation of a cyclic link between the hydroxymethyl in the 5′ position and the remaining phosphate in the 3′ position — hence its proper name, adenosine 3′,5′ cyclic monophosphate. Cyclic AMP is destroyed enzymatically by hydrolysis of the new bond to yield AMP. Note that both reactions are thermodynamically reversible but the forward reactions are highly favored.

ride, and cholera toxin (Table 2–20, Fig. 2–25). All four classes of activators appear to act on the regulatory component which in turn activates the enzyme. Thus the regulatory protein is the sole proximal mediator of activation of the catalytic unit.

In the normal resting state, the hormone-binding site of the receptor is empty and has a high affinity for hormone (Fig. 2–25 *I*). The regulatory protein, which is free of nucleotides or, more likely, with a GDP bound to its nucleotide binding site, is inactive (Fig. 2–25 *II*). The catalytic unit is inactive, having a low affinity for its natural substrate, Mg^{++}·ATP, and can be recognized in this state by its preference for a pharmacological form of substrate, Mn^{++}·ATP.

Hormone bound to receptor leads to dissociation from the regulatory component of GDP and its replacement by GTP (Fig. 2– 25 *II*). The regulatory component with GTP bound activates the catalytic component (Fig. 2–25 *III*) and confers on it high affinity for its substrate, Mg^{++}·ATP, which is rapidly converted to cAMP.

Table 2–20. PROTEIN COMPONENTS OF HORMONE-SENSITIVE CYCLASE

I. Receptor for hormone or other extracellular messenger (abbreviated R)
  1. hormone binding site on extracellular face
  2. one or more different receptors per target cell, all of which interact with the same pool of regulatory and catalytic components
  3. each individual receptor may be composed of multiple subunits

II. Catalytic protein (abbreviated C)
  1. converts ATP to cAMP
  2. Mn^{++}·ATP much better substrate than Mg^{++}·ATP
  3. not stimulated by hormones, GTP, or toxins
  4. MW ~ 200,000
  5. labile relative to I and III

III. Guanine nucleotide-binding regulatory protein (abbreviated G/F)
  1. binds GTP and fluoride (F$^-$)
  2. modified (ribosylated) by toxin action
  3. confers upon catalytic protein the ability to use Mg^{++}·ATP
  4. mediates the activation of catalytic protein by hormone, GTP, F$^-$, and toxins
  5. GTPase, i.e., catalyzes GTP → GDP
  6. absent or defective in some conditions
  7. relatively more stable than II
  8. MW ~ 50,000

The binding of GTP to the regulatory component not only leads to activation of the catalytic component but also activates processes that favor turning off of the activation at two or possibly more sites; the receptor is converted to a lower-affinity form that favors dissociation of hormone from receptor (Fig. 2–25 *I*), and a GTPase that is intrinsic to the regulatory component hydrolyzes the bound GTP to GDP (Fig. 2–25 *II*). Since the regulatory component with GDP bound is inactive, continued activity appears to require continuous replenishment of free GTP for binding to the regulatory component. These two inactivation processes (decrease in affinity of receptor for hormone and hydrolysis of GTP), which are mediated by the regulatory component, are in addition to other potential inactivation processes which include irreversible binding of hormone to receptor and hormone-stimulated aggregation of receptor, followed by internalization of hormone and receptor with translocation to lysosomes. It remains to be determined what role GTP and the regulatory protein play in these processes and other mechanisms of desensitization at receptor and post-receptor sites.

Organization of the Components. The three components (receptor, regulatory component, and catalytic component) are modular, which means that components from different tissues or species can be combined within natural membranes to yield a fully functional unit. As a first approximation they float free in the membrane and are free to move laterally to permit interactions one with another. However, there is evidence that some cells may have mechanisms that restrict the distribution of the three components or limit the extent and nature of their movements. The regulatory component, since it exchanges information with the receptor, must bind to one or more components of the receptor, but it is not known which form of the regulatory component binds to which components of the receptor or the duration or frequency of such interactions. Likewise, since the regulatory component activates the catalytic component and regulates it, these two components must be physically in contact at some time, at least when the regulatory unit has GTP bound, but details about these interactions are not yet known.

When more than one type of receptor is present on a single

Figure 2–25.   Activation of adenylate cyclase by hormone.

I. Receptor

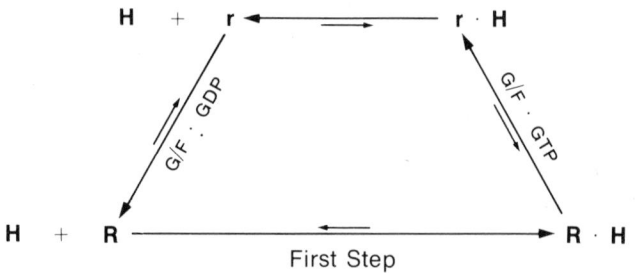

R = receptor in its high affinity, slowly dissociating state
r = receptor in its low affinity, rapidly dissociating state
H = hormone

The first step is binding of hormone to receptor; if the receptor-hormone complex (R·H) is effective in activating the regulatory component of the enzyme (G/F), i.e., conversion G/F·GDP → G/F·GTP, then the conversion of the receptor from its high-affinity to low-affinity state (R → r) will be favored, which favors dissociation of the hormone from receptor. The fall in affinity of receptor requires both an agonist ligand and intact regulatory protein. The mechanism for reestablishment of the high-affinity state of the receptor (r → R) is unclear, though we have suggested in the diagram that G/F·GDP (or possibly free G/F) may favor the reaction.

II. Regulatory
Component of
Adenylate
Cyclase

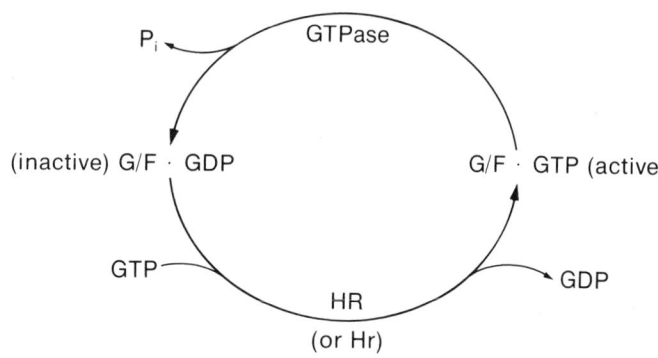

G/F = regulatory component which is sensitive to guanine nucleotides and fluoride
GTP = guanosine triphosphate
GDP = guanosine diphosphate

The regulatory component (G/F) with GDP bound (abbreviated G/F·GDP) is inactive. Hormone bound to receptor (HR or Hr) promotes the exchange of GDP for GTP, thereby converting G/F·GDP → G/F·GTP; the latter is the active form of the regulatory component which activates the catalytic component. The G/F protein has an intrinsic GTPase activity which rapidly inactivates the regulatory component by converting G/F·GTP → G/F·GDP. Cholera toxin, by covalently modifying G/F, inactivates the GTPase, allowing the accumulation of G/F·GTP that remains in the active GTP form.

III. Catalytic
Component of
Adenylate
Cyclase

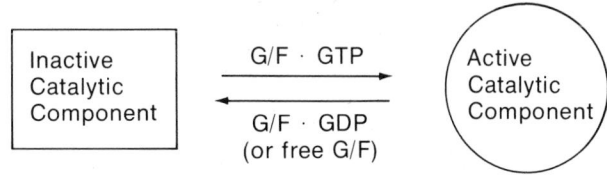

The inactive catalyst can be recognized by its (pharmacological) property of being much more active with Mn^{++}· ATP than with Mg^{++}· ATP, the physiological substrate. The active form of the regulatory component (G/F· GTP) confers on the enzyme the ability to react well with Mg^{++}· ATP.

IV. Substrate
and Product

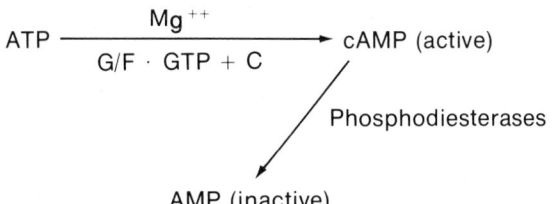

C = catalytic component of adenylate cyclase

In traditional biochemistry the nucleotides such as ATP contain high-energy phosphate bonds that are used to store the chemical energy produced by oxidative processes (oxidative phosphorylation). This energy in the ATP is then used to synthesize other chemical bonds such as glycogen synthesis and protein synthesis or for mechanical work (muscle contraction). In the reactions described here, the nucleotides are used as signals and as regulators rather than as energy suppliers. Thus the high-energy phosphate bond in cAMP, formed from ATP, is not used for energy transfer but as a signal; likewise for the GTP that activates the regulatory until of adenylate cyclase. In the case of phosphorylation of proteins (see later), the phosphate on the protein retains the high energy donated by ATP but that is dissipated during the hydrolysis that reconverts the protein to its dephospho- form.

cell, as is often the case, it appears that they compete for a single pool of regulatory and catalytic units, and their individual effects are combined at the level of the regulatory component. To emphasize the extent of modularity of the components, it appears that any receptor capable of activating adenylate cyclase in any cell can activate regulatory component from any source, and any catalytic component that is hormone-sensitive can be activated by regulatory component of any source.

Clinical Implications of Modularity.   That the three components of the hormone-sensitive cyclase system are modular has important physiologic and pathologic implications. It means that addition of any receptor to the plasma membrane of a cell that has the two components of the enzyme will confer on that cell responsiveness to the corresponding ligand. For example, the adenylate cyclase of the normal adrenal cortical cell is responsive specifically to ACTH (1) because it possesses functionally intact ACTH receptors *and*

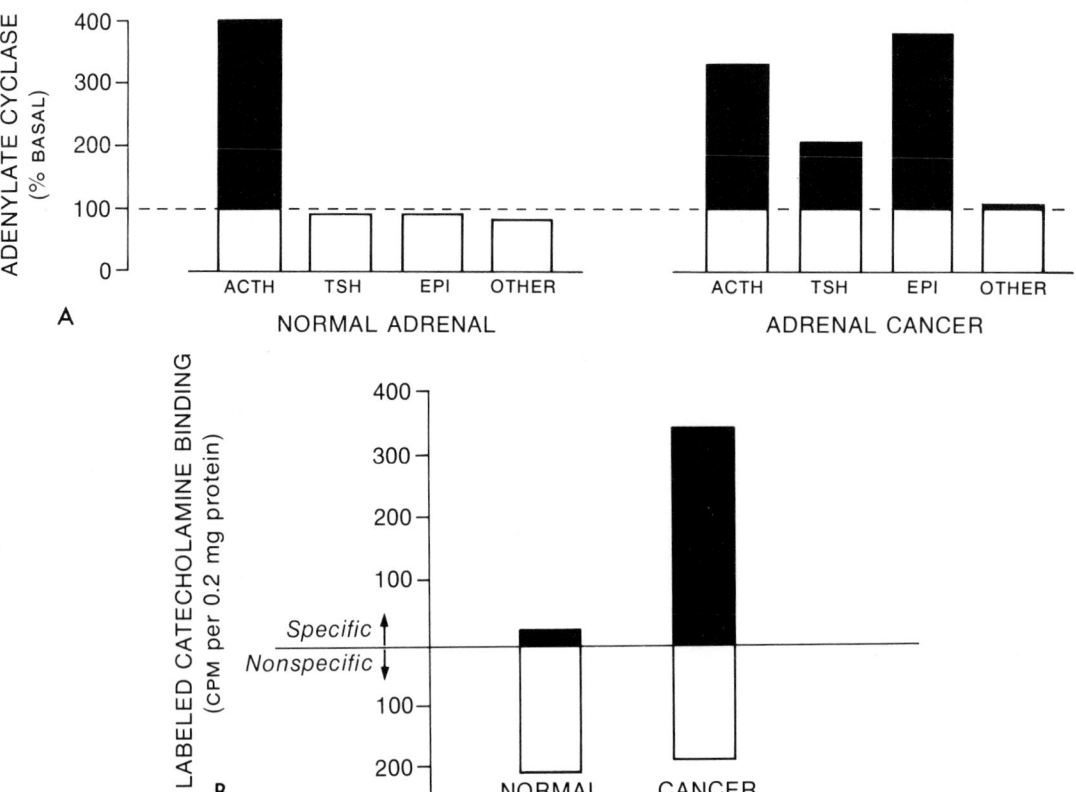

Figure 2–26. Ectopic receptors.

A, Left: In the normal rat adrenal, only ACTH stimulates adenylate cyclase. *Right*: In a corticosterone-producing adrenal cancer of the rat, ACTH as well as catecholamines and TSH stimulate the enzyme. (Adapted from Schorr, I., and Ney, R. L.: Abnormal hormone responses of an adrenocortical cancer adenyl cyclase. *J. Clin. Invest. 50*:1295–1300, 1971.)

B, The cancer, but not the normal adrenal, has high concentrations of receptors for β-adrenergic catecholamines. (Adapted from Williams, L. T., et al.: Ectopic β-adrenergic receptor binding sites: Possible molecular basis of aberrant catecholamine responsiveness of an adrenocortical tumor adenylate cyclase. *J. Clin. Invest. 59*:319–324, 1977.)

(2) because it lacks all other receptors that can link to adenylate cyclase. Insertion into the plasma membrane of adrenal cortical cells of β-adrenergic receptors or TSH receptors (ectopic receptors), which can link to the adenylate cyclase, confers on the cell responsiveness to epinephrine or TSH. An adrenal tumor with ectopic receptors is shown in Figure 2–26. There are many pathologic conditions in which a target cell responds to a hormonal signal to which it is normally unresponsive. The release of growth hormone by the normal pituitary is unaffected by TRH, but in many patients with acromegaly TRH stimulates growth hormone release. There are pheochromocytomas that are responsive to glucagon. The development by the cell of ectopic receptors provides the most likely interpretation.

To extend this concept, consider again conditions characterized by autonomous overproduction of hormone or, more generally, apparently unregulated hyperfunction of any target cell. In many cases, the apparent autonomy or unregulated function represents unexpected effects of a humoral stimulator; i.e., the target is marching to a different drummer.* Earlier we gave examples of abnormal stimulators acting on normal receptors, one of which was immunoglobulins in patients with Graves' disease that bind to TSH receptors on the thyroid. Probably a more frequent mechanism is stimulation of the target cell by normal levels of a normal ligand

*"If a man does not keep pace with his companions, perhaps it is because he hears a different drummer. Let him step to the music he hears. . . ." — Henry David Thoreau

acting through a normal form of receptor that has no business being there (an ectopic receptor). The therapeutic consequences are obvious; when we can determine which ligand-receptor system is responsible for the abnormal activation (as in the case of the adrenal tumor described earlier), we can aim specific therapy at the ligand or the receptor — treatment with T_3 to suppress TSH or with propranolol to block β-adrenergic receptors.

Coupling. The term "coupling" is used to characterize the efficiency with which a hormone or other extracellular messenger molecule that is bound to a receptor on the cell surface has its information converted into cAMP or other intracellular messenger. Some cells are uncoupled. Thus rat hepatoma (HTC) cells in culture have receptor and regulatory component but lack the catalytic component; they can bind hormone and produce the active form of the regulatory component but do not elevate their levels of cAMP in response to hormone. Likewise, cell lines exist that have a regulatory component that is defective or absent (S49 mouse lymphoma UNC and cyc⁻ variants, respectively) so that they are also unresponsive to hormone, despite the presence of receptor and catalytic components. These situations probably are similar to physiological or experimental conditions in which alterations in coupling have been detected. In addition to systems that are completely uncoupled, there are systems in which the coupling may be relatively efficient or inefficient, described as tightly or loosely coupled. Coupling depends not only on the number and structural integrity of the proteins themselves but also on the lipid and other

Table 2–21. ACTION OF CHOLERA TOXIN

1. Cholera toxin, which is an oligomer composed of one A (enzymatic) peptide and 4 to 6 B (receptor-binding) peptides, binds via the B peptide to receptor (GM_1 gangliosides) on the plasma membrane.

2. A major portion (A_1 peptide) of the A peptide molecule is released from the B peptides and is now enzymatically active.

3. $NAD + \underset{\text{(active GTPase)}}{G/F} \xrightarrow{A_1 \text{ peptide}} ADP \cdot ribose \cdot G/F + nicotinamide + H^+$
   $\phantom{3. NAD + G/F \xrightarrow{A_1 peptide} ADP \cdot ribose \cdot}\underset{\text{(inactive GTPase)}}{}$

components of the membrane as well as the physical-chemical milieu such as temperature, solvent, and ions.

Disease Applications. Since the production of cAMP in response to hormone requires at least three proteins that can interact properly, perturbations that change any of the proteins or their ability to interact will alter the sensitivity of the target cell to hormone. In addition to changes at the level of receptor, an increasing number of alterations in coupling are being reported and defined. In hypothyroid states, sensitivity of the adenylate cyclase to its hormonal stimuli is reduced, by both receptor and coupling mechanisms. In hyperthyroidism, sensitivity of adenylate cyclase to hormonal stimuli is enhanced by tighter coupling and possibly also at the level of receptor. The two best studied examples are cholera and pseudohypoparathyroidism.

Cholera. Toxins such as cholera toxin as well as related bacterial toxins, including one from *Escherichia coli,* contain an enzyme that covalently links an ADP-ribose to the regulatory component of the adenylate cyclase which irreversibly inactivates the GTPase activity of that component (Table 2–21). With its GTPase inactivated, a regulatory protein molecule that is activated by the binding of GTP will remain in its active form indefinitely and will continue to activate the catalytic component continuously, even in the absence of further extracellular stimuli. The severe diarrhea characteristic of cholera is thought to be due entirely to continuous activation of the adenylate cyclase of certain cells of the intestinal lining.

The toxin, in addition to the enzyme, has another protein subunit, which is recognized by cell surface receptors; the receptor is not a protein but a lipid component of the membrane, the GM_1 ganglioside. Absence of GM_1 in the membrane confers resistance to the toxin, and an increase in GM_1 heightens sensitivity to it.

Pseudohypoparathyroidism. This condition, the prototype of hormone resistance at the target cell, is a group of inherited disorders characterized by resistance to the effects of parathyroid hormone. In the face of an adequate or superabundant supply of endogenous hormone, patients with this disorder have hypocalcemia and hyperphosphatemia, which

are unaltered by exogenously administered hormone. In most of the patients (Type I), the administration of parathyroid hormone fails to elicit the typical rise in the level of cyclic AMP in urine, which suggests they have a defect at an early step in hormone action at the target cell (Table 2–22). The vast majority of these patients (designated in the table as Type Ia) have a reduced amount ($\sim 50\%$ of normal) of the regulatory component of adenylate cyclase, demonstrated in their erythrocytes and other cells. Interestingly, patients with pseudohypoparathyroidism have been reported to have subnormal responsiveness to several other hormones (TSH, TRH, glucagon, gonadotropins). The tentative conclusion is that most patients with this disorder suffer from a generalized deficiency of the regulatory component of adenylate cyclase which for unknown reasons has severe consequences for the action of parathyroid hormone but variable or less severe effects on other systems that require the regulatory component. In the small minority of patients with pseudohypoparathyroidism who have normal levels of regulatory protein, the pathway for parathyroid hormone action is presumed to be defective at other early (Type Ib) or late steps (Type II), as yet undefined (Table 2–22).

Action of Cyclic AMP

In the previous discussion we described the steps by which hormone binding to receptor leads to the conversion of ATP to cyclic AMP. In this section we will describe the action of cAMP and the pathway for its destruction. All of the actions of cAMP in mammalian and other eukaryotic cells are thought to be due to its ability to activate a single group of closely related enzymes known as cAMP-dependent protein kinases, which can be soluble or membrane-bound. In response to cyclic AMP, as will be described in detail later, these enzymes phosphorylate cellular proteins and thereby modify (activate or inactivate) their biological functions.

The cyclic AMP–dependent protein kinases have a regulatory subunit and a catalytic subunit (Fig. 2–27). In the absence of cAMP, the regulatory subunit is bound to the catalytic unit and the latter is inactive. Cyclic AMP, which is soluble and diffuses within the cell, can bind reversibly to specific sites on the regulatory subunit; with cAMP bound, the regulatory subunit dissociates from the catalytic unit, which is now active. Free cAMP, but not cAMP bound to the regulatory unit, is rapidly inactivated by hydrolysis (Fig. 2–28). A rise in the concentration of cAMP favors binding to the regulatory unit and activation of kinase. A fall in the concentration of the second messenger favors its dissociation from the regulatory unit, which reassociates with the catalytic unit, quenching its activity.

Table 2–22. PSEUDOHYPOPARATHYROIDISM

A. Clinical Definition	Circulating Hormone	Serum Ca^{++} and P	Response of Serum Ca^{++}/P to Exogenous Hormone
Normal	normal	normal	normal
Hypoparathyroidism	reduced	affected	normal
Pseudohypoparathyroidism	elevated	affected	defective

B. Localization of Target Cell Defect	Rise in Urinary cAMP Following Administration of Parathyroid Hormone	Erythrocyte Content of Regulatory Component
Normal or hypoparathyroidism	normal	normal
Pseudohypoparathyroidism Type Ia	defective	reduced
Type Ib	defective	normal
Type II	normal	normal

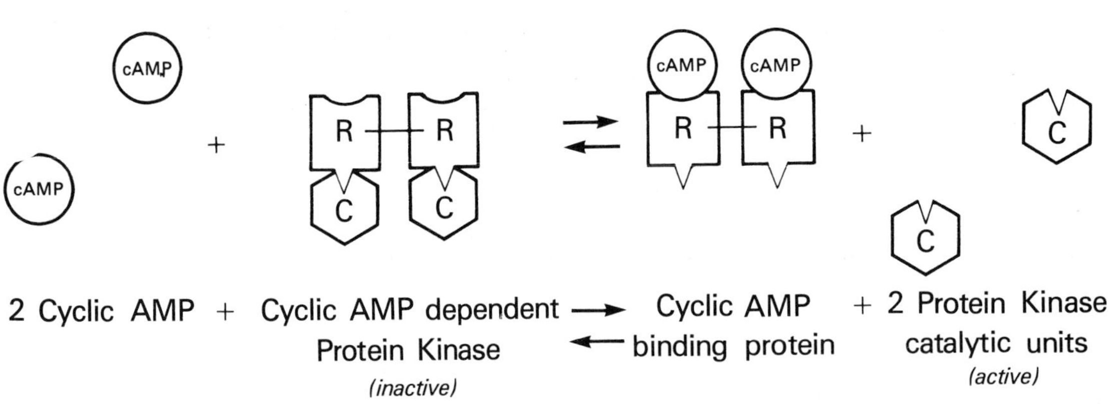

2 Cyclic AMP + Cyclic AMP dependent ⟶ Cyclic AMP + 2 Protein Kinase
Protein Kinase ⟵ binding protein catalytic units
(inactive) *(active)*

Figure 2–27. Effect of cAMP on protein kinase. The cyclic AMP–dependent protein kinases consist of four subunits, two catalytic subunits *(C)* and a dimeric regulatory subunit (R–R), which can bind two molecules of cyclic AMP. When cyclic AMP binds to the regulatory dimer of the holoenzyme, the two catalytic subunits are released and become fully active. With removal of cyclic AMP, the regulatory dimer reassociates with the catalytic subunits, inactivating the latter. Recent data indicate that a total of four cyclic AMP molecules bind to the regulatory dimer.

Note that R is widely used as an abbreviation for "receptor" as well for "regulatory" components, especially for the regulatory component of the cyclic AMP–dependent protein kinases. Also note that C is widely used as an abbreviation for the catalytic component of an enzyme, especially for the adenylate cyclase and the cAMP-dependent protein kinase.

Action of cAMP-Dependent Protein Kinases

A "kinase" is an enzyme that phosphorylates its substrate. Protein kinases constitute a subgroup of these enzymes that use proteins as their substrates; they transfer a phosphate from ATP to the hydroxyl group on a serine (or much less often, threonine or tyrosine) of the substrate (Fig. 2–29). Introduction of the covalently linked phosphate typically modifies the activity of that protein in a specific way, either activating or inactivating it (for examples, see Table 2–23). Only some of the protein kinases are regulated by cAMP; hence the distinction of cAMP-independent from cAMP-dependent enzymes. The effects of the cAMP-dependent protein kinases on their substrates are reversed by the action of a group of enzymes, phosphoprotein phosphatases, which remove the phosphate by hydrolysis and restore the original activity of the protein (Fig. 2–29).

The hormonal regulation of the enzymes that control glycogen metabolism presents an excellent example. Glucagon and catecholamines stimulate glycogen breakdown and also inhibit glycogen synthesis, while insulin has the opposite effect on both processes. The enzymes that promote glycogenolysis are active in their phospho- form and inactive in their dephospho- form while the reverse is true for glycogen synthase, the major enzyme in glycogen formation (Table 2–23).

More precisely, in the liver (Fig. 2–30), catecholamines, acting through β-type receptors, or glucagon, through its receptor, stimulate the synthesis of cAMP, which activates cyclic AMP–dependent protein kinase, which has a relatively broad spectrum of proteins as substrates. One of its substrates is another protein kinase, phosphorylase kinase, which is phosphorylated and thereby activated. Phosphory-

lase kinase, which has a narrower range of substrates, phosphorylates the enzyme phosphorylase, which initiates glycogen breakdown (Figs. 2–30 and 2–31). Phosphorylase kinase also phosphorylates glycogen synthase, thereby inactivating it, inhibiting further synthesis of glycogen (Fig. 2–31). Insulin, by mechanisms that are as yet unclear, promotes the removal of the phosphates on glycogen synthase and phosphorylase, thereby promoting glycogen synthesis and inhibiting its breakdown. A similar overall scheme is thought to integrate the effects of these hormones on the enzymes that regulate gluconeogenesis in liver and lipolysis in fat cells.

It should be emphasized that the individual kinases and phosphatases may have a broad or narrow range of substrates, and their access to substrates and their effects may be sharply modified by geographical constraints (cellular organization). Further, multiple sites on a single enzyme may be phosphorylated, and this can affect its activity directly as well as modify its susceptibility to further activation or inactivation. Finally, a single hormone, acting through one or more receptors, may ultimately act on a single enzyme via multiple pathways (Fig. 2–31).

Another enzyme that is under reciprocal control through phosphorylation and dephosphorylation is pyruvate dehydrogenase (Fig. 2–32). It is active in its original (dephospho-) form and inactive in its modified (phospho-) form (Table 2–23). Insulin, through specific phosphatases, promotes its activation. It is inactivated by a cAMP-independent kinase; the latter may be activated indirectly via the action of catecholamines. Discussion of this enzyme is introduced here to indicate that in addition to the hormones, a large number of intracellular substances including substrate, product, other metabolites, cofactors, and ions have impor-

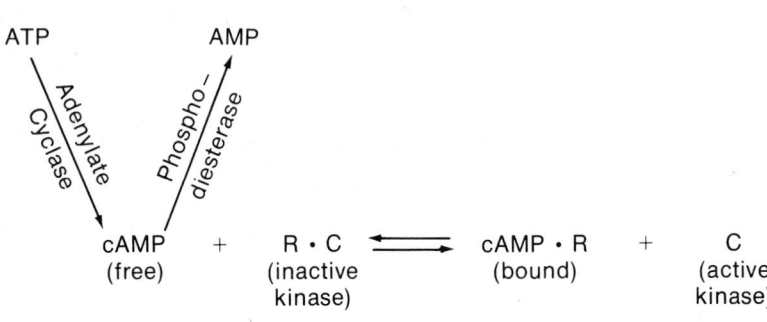

Figure 2–28. Life cycle of cyclic AMP. This figure combines information from Figure 2–24 and 2–27 to show that free cAMP is available for destruction by phosphoidiesterase or for binding to protein kinases. When bound to the protein kinase, cAMP molecules are protected from hydrolysis but following dissociation are again vulnerable.

Table 2–23. HORMONAL CONTROL OF ENZYMATIC ACTIVITY BY PHOSPHORYLATION AND DEPHOSPHORYLATION

Activator	Active Form	Enzyme	Inactivator	Inactive Form
Epinephrine	Phospho-	Phosphorylase kinase Phosphorylase Triglyceride lipase	Insulin	Dephospho-
Insulin	Dephospho-	Glycogen synthase Pyruvate dehydrogenase	Epinephrine	Phospho-

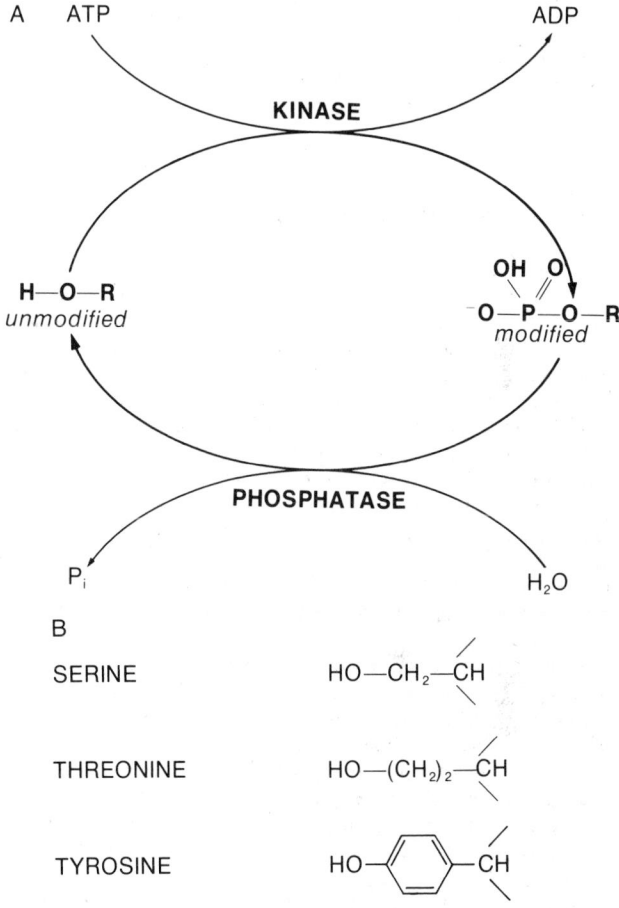

Figure 2–29. In the phosphorylation of ("unmodified") protein, a protein kinase causes ATP to donate a phosphate group to the hydroxyl group on the side chain of a serine; phosphoprotein phosphatase causes hydrolysis of the phosphate bond and return of the substrate to its dephospho- or unmodified form. The net result is converison of ATP $\longrightarrow$ ADP + P_i. Only specific serines in each protein are involved; specificity is conferred by the amino acid groups in the region of that serine. Threonine and tyrosine also have hydroxyl groups that can undergo these transformations, but are much less commonly involved.

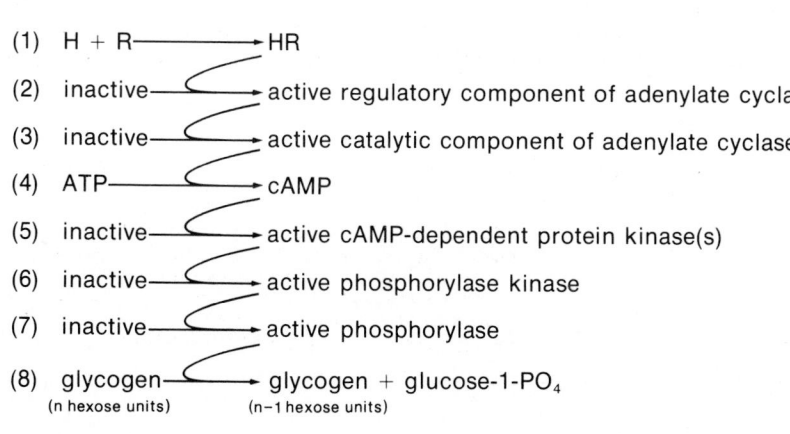

Figure 2–30. Outline of how hormones stimulate glycogenolysis. Hormones (glucagon and β-adrenergic amines) bind to specific receptors in liver which initiate a series of biochemical events that lead to hydrolysis of glycogen. Many steps require cofactors: GTP is needed for step 2, and Ca^{++} for step 6 and probably other steps. The details of these steps are provided later. In addition to stimulating glycogenolysis, these hormones also inhibit glycogen synthesis (see later). A similar scheme is thought to be involved in other cAMP-dependent processes, e.g., hormonal stimulation of lipolysis in adipocytes.

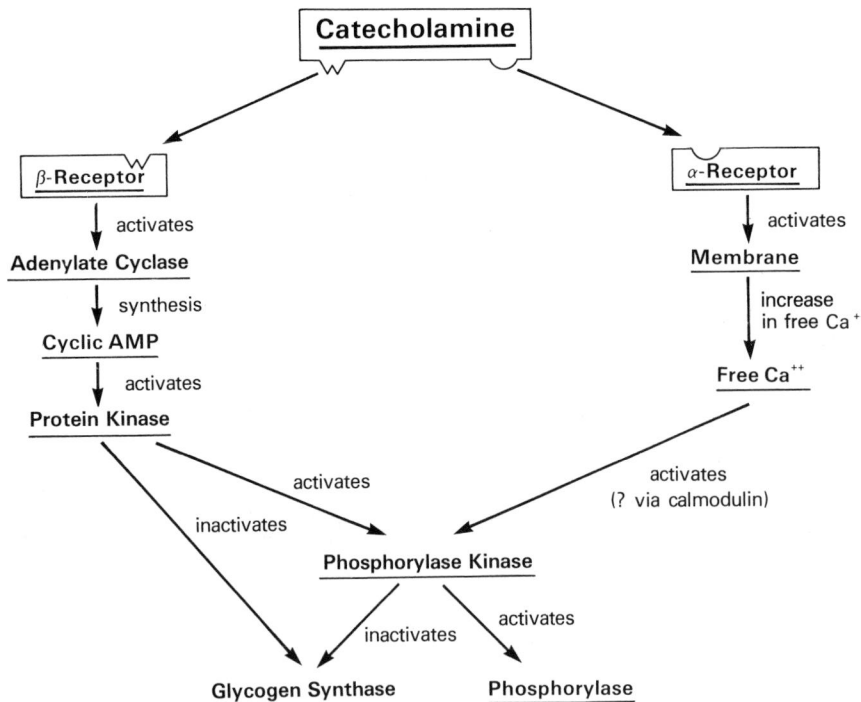

Figure 2–31. Two pathways for catecholamine effects on glycogen metabolism. A hormone can influence a distal pathway by more than one mechanism. Catecholamines increase glycogenolysis and decrease glycogen synthesis by activity at both α- and β-type adrenergic receptors, which are often on the same cells. The binding of catecholamines to the β-receptor stimulates the formation of cyclic AMP. Protein kinase mediates the action of cyclic AMP; it inactivates glycogen synthase and activates phosphorylase kinase which in turn activates phosphorylase. The binding of catecholamines to the α-receptor increases the intracellular concentration of free calcium which activates phosphorylase kinase via calmodulin (see later). Phosphorylase kinase not only activates phosphorylase but also inactivates glycogen synthase.

tant regulatory effects on the enzyme itself as well as on the enzymes that modify the activity of the enzyme (Fig. 2–32, inset). To develop this theme further, we shall return to the example of glycogen.

When the glycogen content of the cell is constant, it does not indicate that the cell and its enzymes are at rest. Rather, the rates of synthesis and degradation are equal; the enzymes responsible for its synthesis and degradation show a steady level of activity but only because the activation and inactivation (phosphorylation and dephosphorylation) processes, which are going on continuously, are in balance. The inputs to this system from endogenous intracellular signals are continuous and are the major influences on each of these pathways. The external signals in the form of hormones

change this balance directly by affecting the enzymes that modify the enzyme or less directly by changing the concentrations of the endogenous small molecules that regulate both the enzyme itself and its modifying enzymes.

At first glance it appears that the cell is simply wasting ATP by phosphorylating and dephosphorylating enzymes continuously, especially when it uses more than one cyclic cascade in series to regulate a single pathway. Actually, these cyclic cascades, regulated by enzymes and small molecules, provide regulation that is very sensitive to low concentrations of signal molecule, great amplification of the signal, rapid responses, and equally rapid return to the basal state. In fact each additional cascade cycle enhances the capacity for amplification and control.

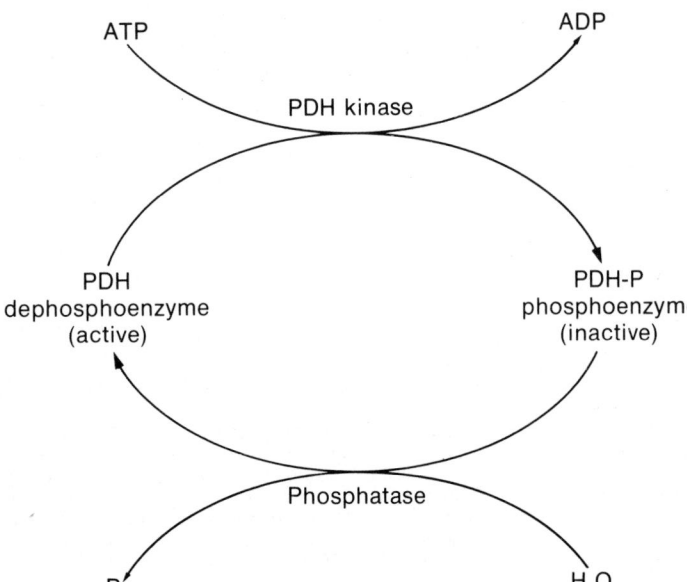

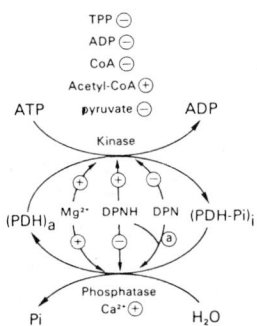

Figure 2–32. Regulation of pyruvate dehydrogenase. The main figure shows the phosphorylation (inactivation) of the enzyme pyruvate dehydrogenase (PDH) by a specific kinase and the dephosphorylation (activation) by a phosphatase. The inset shows some of the other biologically relevant regulators of the covalent interconversion of this enzyme. (a) indicates that DPN antagonizes the inhibition by DPNH; ⊕ and ⊖ indicate activation and inactivation, respectively. (Inset from Stadtman, E. R., and Chock, P. B.: Interconvertible enzyme cascades in metabolic regulation. In *Current Topics in Regulation.* Vol. 13. New York, Academic Press, 1978.)

Table 2–24. REGULATORS OF PHOSPHODIESTERASE ACTIVITY

Enhance
Calmodulin + Ca^{++}
Nucleotides
Hormones with cell surface receptors
— insulin, insulin-like factors
— catecholamines, ACTH
— prostaglandins
Hypothyroid state

Reduce
Nucleotides
Insulin-deficient diabetes
Hyperthyroidism
Hormones with intracellular receptors
— iodothyronines
— adrenal steroids
— sex steroids
Drugs
— methylxanthines
— sulfonylureas
— benzodiazepines
Catecholamines

Phosphodiesterase

Cyclic nucleotide phosphodiesterase is the name for the enzyme activity that inactivates cAMP by hydrolyzing it to AMP (see Figs. 2–24 and 2–28). The activity is found in essentially all cells, and multiple forms of the enzyme exist in individual cells. Most of the enzymes are soluble or easily freed from the membrane; that is, they are peripheral proteins of the membrane. They vary widely in their absolute and relative affinities for cyclic AMP and cyclic GMP. As can be seen in Table 2–24, hormones can act to enhance or reduce phosphodiesterase activity, thereby modifying the lifetime of cyclic AMP. Likewise, intracellular signals such as nucleotides and Ca^{++} as well as drugs can have effects (Table 2–24).

Second Messenger for Insulin

The long sought after soluble intracellular ("second") messenger for insulin action has recently been reported by several laboratories in several cell types including liver and fat. Though not yet characterized in detail, it appears to be a small ($\sim$ 1000-dalton) peptide which is thought to be generated not from insulin but from a protein of the plasma membrane of the target cell by the action of a membrane-bound protease. Among other effects, the soluble peptide activates an insulin-sensitive enzyme, pyruvate dehydrogenase, in mitochondria, apparently by activating a specific phosphatase which converts the enzyme from its phospho- (inactive) to its dephospho- (active) form (Fig. 2–32). Although this messenger has been detected in several different tissues, it is not yet known whether it is the sole mediator of all of the metabolic effects of insulin in all tissues.

Cyclic GMP

In addition to adenylate cyclase, cAMP and its dependent kinase system, most cells have guanylate cyclase, an enzyme that converts GTP to cyclic GMP, as well as protein kinases that are activated specifically by this cyclic nucleotide. Despite these similarities to cAMP, cGMP has not yet been implicated as the second messenger for any hormone, although it may play the role of second messenger for a neurotransmitter, acetylcholine.

Calcium

Calcium plays a key role in many cellular processes. It is ubiquitously present in its free form in extracellular fluids and in bound form within cells. Free Ca^{++} ion in cells, imported from the outside or liberated from intracellular storage sites, is thought to be the active intracellular form. As will be seen, in some situations Ca^{++} is acting as a soluble intracellular second messenger in the classic cAMP mode.

Calcium ion has a potent effect on many vital biologic processes, including cell division, cell movement, and muscle contraction. In endocrine systems, Ca^{++} is essential for the secretion of most hormones and for hormonal regulation of many metabolic pathways in target cells. Ca^{++} is thought to exert its effects by first binding to a calcium-binding protein. In effect, these proteins are the intracellular receptors for Ca^{++}. The calcium-binding proteins, which are active only when Ca^{++} is bound, then combine with enzymes or other effector proteins and thereby modify their activity — typically to activate a biochemical pathway that leads ultimately to a physiological response (Table 2–25).

The most widespread by far of the calcium-binding proteins is calmodulin. This protein is present in all nucleated cells, and its structure is very highly conserved phylogenetically. It has many structural similarities to troponin C and to parvalbumin, two other calcium-binding proteins found in striated muscle where they appear to be receptors and mediators of Ca^{++} action. Calmodulin has four binding sites for Ca^{++} with K_d for Ca^{++} in the low micromole range. About 30% of its amino acids have acidic side chains (aspartic and glutamic acids); the extra COO^- groups on these amino acids are clustered in such a way as to form the binding sites on the protein that bind the Ca^{++}.

The concentration of free Ca^{++} in the extracellular fluid is relatively high compared with its concentration inside cells, which is 10^{-8} to 10^{-7} M. In the resting state, the concentration of free Ca^{++} inside cells is kept low by the binding of free Ca^{++} to intracellular binding substances and by the action of pumps (ATPases) in the membrane (which are activated by Ca^{++}) that extrude it from the cell. Calmodulin, in the resting state, has few or no Ca^{++} ions bound and is inactive. Activation of the cell leads to a precipitous rise in the intracellular concentration of free Ca^{++} ($\sim 10^{-6}$M) derived from the extracellular fluid and/or intracellular storage sites. The increase in Ca^{++} concentration promotes its binding to calmodulin; binding of Ca^{++} to calmodulin alters the configuration of the protein and converts it into its active form (Table 2–25). It now binds to calcium-sensitive proteins and thereby alters their activity. It is thought that all Ca^{++}-sensitive cellular processes use calmodulin or another closely related calcium-binding protein as the mediator of Ca^{++} action. The rise in free Ca^{++}, by stimulating the Ca^{++} pumps to extrude Ca^{++}, also promotes restoration of the

Table 2–25. MECHANISM OF Ca^{++} ACTION

$$Ca^{++} + \underset{\text{(inactive)}}{\text{calmodulin}} \leftrightarrows \underset{\text{(active)}}{Ca^{++} \cdot \text{calmodulin}}$$

$$Ca^{++} \cdot \underset{\text{(inactive)}}{\text{calmodulin} + \text{enzyme}} \leftrightarrows Ca^{++} \cdot \underset{\text{(active)}}{\text{calmodulin} \cdot \text{enzyme}}$$

Under resting conditions, the intracellular concentration of free Ca^{++} is low, and most of the calmodulin (or other Ca^{++}-binding protein) is in its inactive (Ca^{++}-free) form. A rise in the concentration of intracellular free Ca^{++} (from extracellular fluid or intracellular storage sites) favors binding of Ca^{++} to calmodulin; the $Ca^{++} \cdot$ calmodulin complex can now bind efficiently to a calcium-sensitive enzyme, thereby converting it from its inactive to active form.

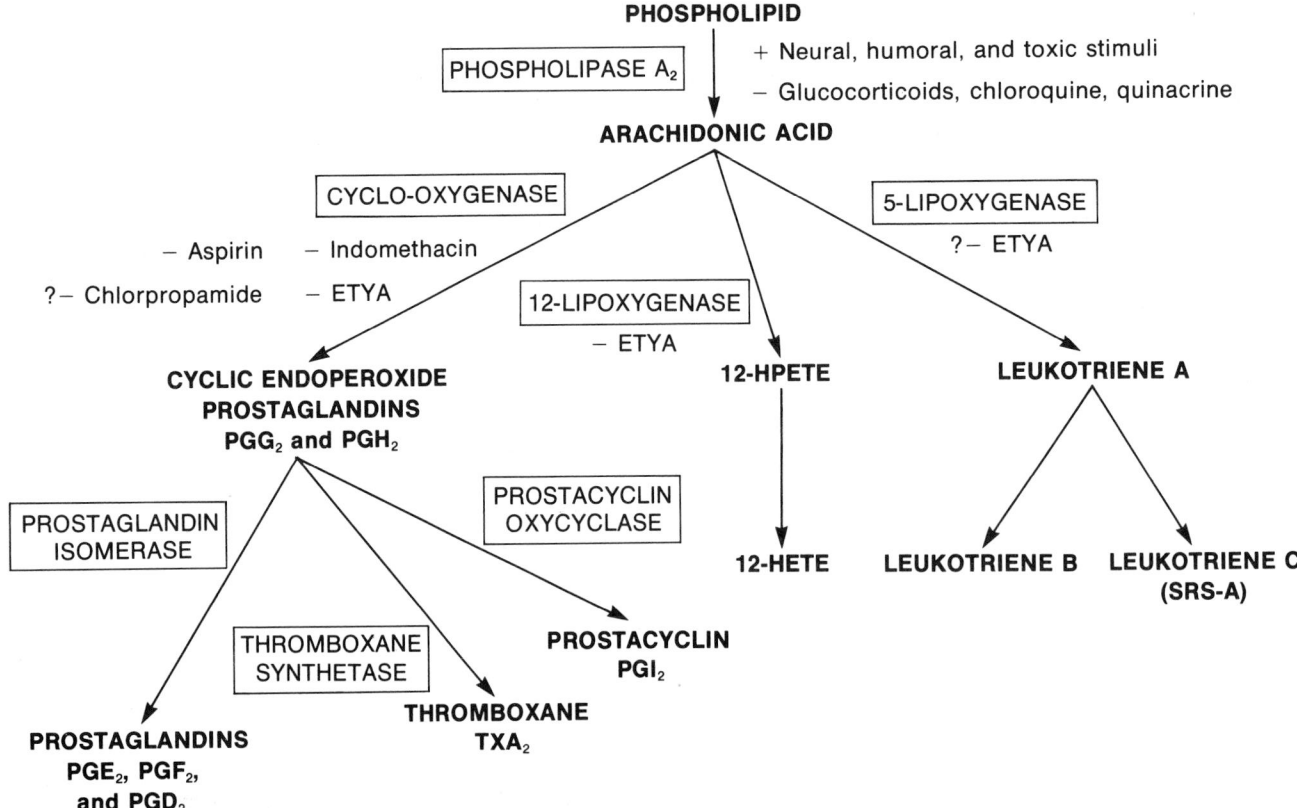

Figure 2–33. Synthesis of prostaglandins. Neural, hormonal, or toxic stimuli activate membrane-bound phospholipase A_2, which releases arachidonic acid from membrane phospholipid, usually phosphatidylcholine. Glucocorticoid hormones, chloroquine, and quinacrine inhibit the phospholipase. Free arachidonic acid is rapidly converted to the cyclic endoperoxide prostaglandins PGH_2 and PGG_2 by a cyclo-oxygenase. Aspirin, indomethacin, and other nonsteroidal anti-inflammatory agents as well as eicosatetraynoic acid (ETYA) inhibit the cyclo-oxygenase. The endoperoxide prostaglandins are substrates for three types of enzymes. Prostaglandin isomerase synthesizes the prostaglandins PGE_2, PGF_2, and PGD_2. Prostacyclin oxycyclase synthesizes the prostacyclin PGI_2, and thromboxane synthetase makes thromboxane. TXA_2. In addition, arachidonic acid is converted by lipoxygenases to other bioactive compounds such as 12-HETE and the leukotrienes, including leukotriene C, the slow-reacting substance of anaphylaxis (SRS-A). ETYA also inhibits the lipoxygenases.

resting state — fall in free Ca^{++}, dissociation of Ca^{++} from calmodulin, and a return of calmodulin to its inactive form.

The effects of cAMP and Ca^{++} as intracellular messengers are often intertwined and can be in the same or opposite directions. Effects of Ca^{++} are often very short-lived (milliseconds) while effects of the nucleotide are a bit longer (seconds or minutes), in contrast to hormones that have half-lives of minutes to hours.

Some forms of adenylate cyclase are Ca^{++}-sensitive. Many phosphodiesterases are also Ca^{++}-sensitive. Their activities are markedly enhanced by Ca^{++} · calmodulin. Phosphorylase kinase, which is activated by cAMP-dependent protein kinase, absolutely requires Ca^{++} for activity. In fact, this enzyme is composed of four subunits, one of which is calmodulin; that is, calmodulin is an intrinsic component of this enzyme.

Prostaglandins

The prostaglandins and their offspring, the prostacyclins and thromboxanes, are major modifiers of hormone action at the target cell. The peptide hormones, in addition to generating their own intracellular messengers, often stimulate the formation and release of prostaglandins and prostaglandin derivatives, which then act on the cell itself and its neighbors to amplify, broaden, or attenuate the effects of the hormone acutely and may also play a major role in regulating target cell sensitivity. Steroid hormone action may also involve effects on the prostaglandin system. In addition, the prostaglandin family is affected by numerous drugs, espe-cially anti-inflammatory agents such as aspirin, indomethacin, and glucocorticoids.

The immediate precursor of the prostaglandins is arachidonic acid. Man and many other mammals can convert linoleic acid, a long-chain (C_{18}) unsaturated fatty acid, to arachidonic acid. Either linoleic or arachidonic acid must be supplied in the diet; that linoleic acid is an essentially fatty acid is thought to relate solely to its role as a precursor of prostaglandins. Thus, it is similar to vitamin D and vitamin A in that an essential dietary (vitamin-like) constituent is the precursor of a hormonal (hormone-like) extracellular messenger.

Arachidonic acid is found as the free acid in plasma, as a cholesterol ester, in triglycerides, and in glyceride linkage in phospholipids of the plasma membrane; it is largely in the latter state that it acts as the immediate precursor of prostaglandins. Phospholipase A_2, an enzyme of the plasma membrane, hydrolyzes the phospholipid to yield free arachidonic acid, which is itself inactive. However, arachidonic acid is modified enzymatically and nonenzymatically to a series of prostaglandins as well as a series of other active molecules, the prostacyclins and thromboxanes (Fig. 2–33). The compounds resemble the cholesterol-derived hormones in that a widely available fat-soluble constituent of the cell is acted on by a series of enzymes to produce the active compounds; again, like the steroid hormones, one active form, formed early in the biosynthetic pathway, can be active itself as well as act as a precursor of one or more active forms of different specificity. These in turn can act as well as be precursors for others (cf. progesterone → androgen → estrogen).

In their mechanism of action, the prostaglandins and prostaglandin derivatives act like water-soluble (peptide and catecholamine) hormones in that their receptor binding sites are on the extracellular surface of the cell and they often activate adenylate cyclase (or guanylate cyclase).

The action of the prostaglandins secreted by the hormone's target cell is largely local on the target cell itself and on its neighbors; in addition, they can affect blood flow which is often an important adjunct of hormone action at the target cell. Prostaglandins also modulate secretion of hormones, especially in response to stimulation by hormones or by small molecules (e.g., insulin secretion in response to glucose or hormones, thyroid hormone secretion in response to TSH, progesterone synthesis in ovaries). Although the major effects of prostaglandins are largely local, one exception worthy of mention is the hypercalcemia associated with malignancy, which in some cases can be caused by prostaglandins produced by the tumor and carried in blood to bone where they stimulate Ca^{++} release.

In summary, the prostaglandin family of substances plays a major role in endocrinology, especially in regulating hormone secretion and hormone action at the target cell. Although they are not usually considered hormones (because of their very widespread production and their local action), their biosynthesis and modes of action share many features with the hormones. Given their number and complexity and the limited tools that we now have for their study, it is easy to imagine that the majority of their functions are as yet undiscovered.

Methylation of Membrane Phospholipids

In the preceding sections, it has become clear that the lipids of the plasma membrane, in addition to their fundamental role in providing a permeability barrier for the cell, have functions that are relevant to endocrinology, as in the function of membrane proteins such as receptors and adenylate cyclase and as precursors for the biosynthesis of prostaglandins and related messenger molecules. Recently, methylation of membrane lipids has been found to be affected by hormones and is an important modifier of hormone action at the target cell. For this discussion, let us recall that the lipid bilayer is roughly symmetrical but shows a definite asymmetry with regard to several components (see Fig. 2–7C). In particular, phosphatidylethanolamine (PE) is more abundant on the inner (cytoplasmic) face, and phosphatidylcholine (PC) is more abundant on the outer (extracellular) face (Fig. 2–34). Two enzymes (methyltransferases) are present in the plasma membrane which can add methyl

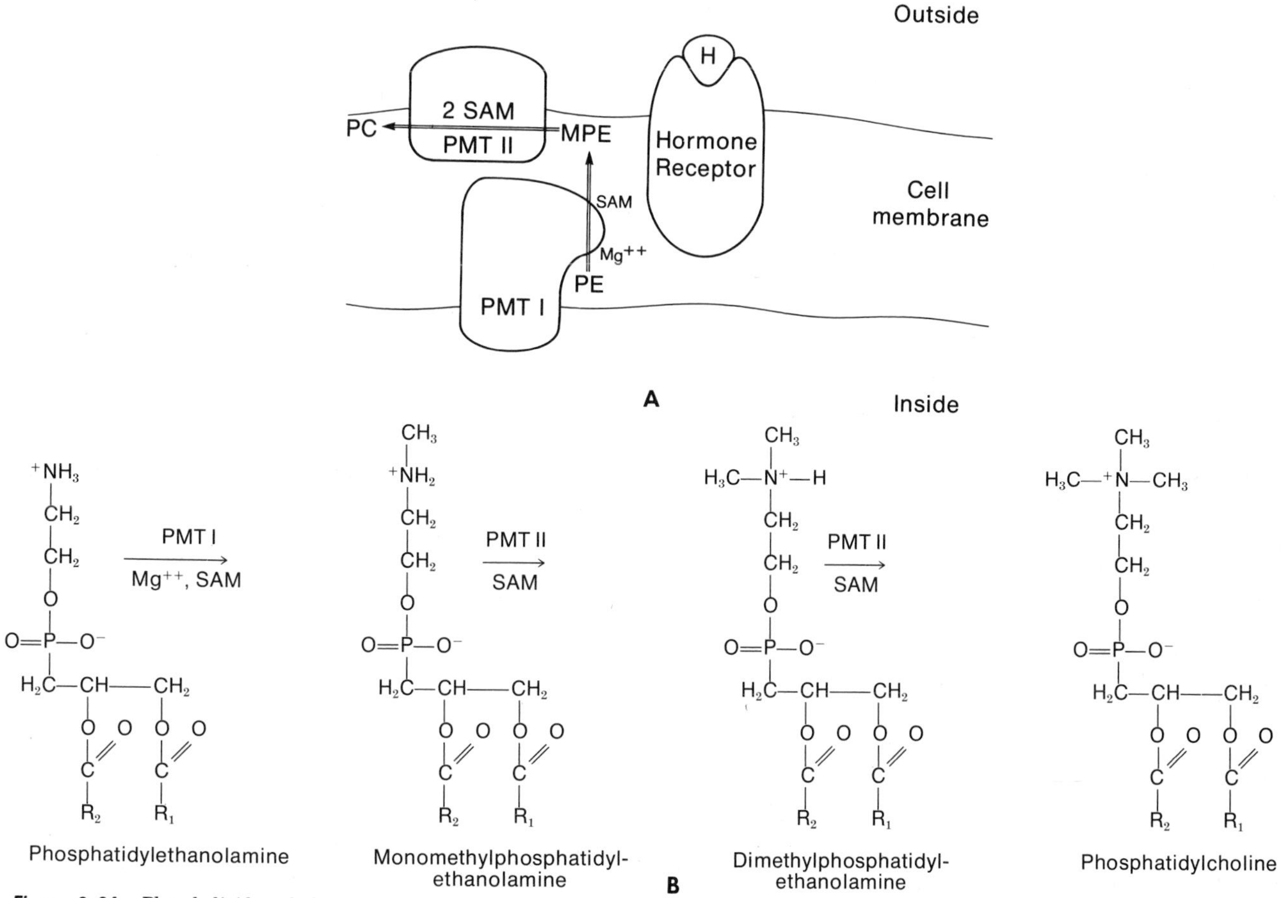

Figure 2–34. Phospholipid methylation in the cell membrane.

A, Phospholipid methyltransferase I (PMT I) on the inside of the plasma membrane catalzyes the methylation of phosphatidylethanolamine (PE) to form phosphatidyl-N-monomethylethanolamine (MPE). This reaction requires S-adenosyl-methionine (SAM), as the methyl donor, and magnesium. The net result is that the product (MPE) is translocated to the outer leaflet of the plasma membrane and is reoriented ("flip-flop"). The MPE is then methylated twice by phospholipid methyltransferase II (PMT II) on the outer surface, resulting in the synthesis of phosphatidylcholine (PC). The reaction catalyzed by PMT I increases the fluidity of the membrane. Catecholamine binding to the β-adrenergic receptor increases the activity of PMT I. An increase in the synthesis of PC by PMT II increases the exposure of β-receptors. Under appropriate conditions in certain cells, catecholamines, concanavalin A, IgE, and benzodiazepines may increase the activity of PMT I and II. The final product, phosphatidylcholine, is the substrate for phospholipase A_2, which generates arachidonic acid, the prostaglandin precursor.

B, The reactions catalyzed by PMT I and PMT II: Phospholipid methyltransferase I (PMT I) in the presence of magnesium transfers a methyl group from S-adenosyl methionine (SAM) to phosphatidylethanolamine (PE), forming monomethylphosphatidylethanolamine. Phospholipid methyltransferase II then sequentially transfers a methyl group first from SAM to monomethylphosphatidylethanolamine, forming dimethylphosphatidylethanolamine (DPE), and then transfers an additional methyl group from another SAM molecular to DPE, forming phosphatidylcholine.

groups to PE and thereby convert it to PC, associated with an increase in the fluidity of the membrane in that region (facilitating the lateral movement of proteins) and a flip-flop in the phospholipids so that a PE on the inner face is converted to a PC on the outer face of the lipid bilayer (Fig. 2–34).

Binding of a β-adrenergic agonist to its specific receptor, for example, stimulates methylation of the phospholipids. Increased methylation of the phospholipids *per se* enhances coupling — the efficiency with which hormone bound to receptor activates cAMP production. (In general, increased fluidity of the membrane enhances coupling while reduction in fluidity diminishes coupling between receptor and cyclase.) Since GTP but not cholera toxin or fluoride enhances agonist-induced stimulation of methylation, it is likely that the hormone-receptor complex, HR, is the proximal stimulator of the methylation, without involvement of cAMP or the catalytic unit of adenylate cyclase; the role, if any, of the regulatory unit of adenylate cyclase in activation of methylation is only secondary to its effects on occupied receptors (HR) analogous to those shown in Figure 2–25 *I*.

Increased methylation of membrane phospholipids causes an increase in the number of adrenergic receptors available for binding, probably by unmasking preexisting receptors. Inhibition of methylation reduces receptor number, presumably by masking receptors. The agonist appears to activate methylation in a localized region near the receptor; thus, one cell with two or more sets of receptors can produce methylation effects that are independent of each other.

Increased methylation of membrane phospholipids, in addition to increasing membrane fluidity and unmasking receptors, may have other important effects. Recall that phospholipase A_2, a Ca^{++}-requiring enzyme of the plasma membrane, cleaves membrane phospholipids to release arachidonic acid, a free fatty acid that is acted upon by enzymes in the plasma membrane to form prostaglandins and their derivatives. Inhibition of methylation inhibits both Ca^{++} uptake and arachidonic acid release. Increased methylation promotes Ca^{++} fluxes, which are part of many signaling systems, possibly including activation of phospholipase A_2.

Phospholipid methylation may also be a major mechanism of increasing the availability of arachidonic acid for release by phospholipase A_2; phosphatidylcholine, which has two fatty acids per molecule, is enriched in arachidonic acid, so that the flip-flop of the phospholipid, induced by methylation, may be a major mechanism to maintain or increase the supply of substrate to phospholipase A_2.

Phospholipase A_2 also appears to be important in agonist-induced desensitization of β-adrenergic receptors. Inhibition of the enzyme enhances sensitivity and prevents desensitization, while activation of phospholipase A_2 stimulates desensitization. Methylation of phospholipids, by effects on phospholipase A_2, may be an important regulator of desensitization of receptors.

A further point of interlocking effects should be mentioned. The action of phospholipase A_2 on phosphatidylcholine, in addition to releasing arachidonic acid, leaves behind in the membrane lysophosphatidylcholine, a form of the phospholipid that lacks one of the two fatty acids, which is detergent-like and promotes fusion of membranes. These effects may enhance activation of other processes.

In summary, methyltransferases in the membrane that can be activated by hormone binding to receptor can produce multiple effects on the target cell including possibly changes in the receptor, coupling processes, availability of Ca^{++}, and regulation of arachidonic acid metabolism.

LIPID-SOLUBLE HORMONES

This section covers the seven major classes of lipid-soluble hormones, with emphasis on the features they have in common and how, as a group, they differ from water-soluble hormones. Individual hormones will be introduced only to highlight principles or because a unique feature of that hormone has special biological or clinical importance. The first part of this section covers the traditional series of events at the target cell — interaction of hormones with receptors and subsequent biological effects. In later sections, we examine these hormones with respect to their biosynthesis (in the gland as well as at extraglandular sites, including target cells) and their transport in blood, especially where these processes are closely related to mechanisms of human disease.

Events at the Target Cell

Initial Interactions

As a first approximation, all of the lipid-soluble hormones freely traverse the lipid bilayer of the plasma membrane by a process best characterized as passive diffusion. These hormones have their receptors inside the cells, and the nucleus is the major site at which they act (see Fig. 2–3). While there is evidence that these hormones may also be soluble within the lipids of the plasma membrane, and elements of the membrane may modify their entry, the role of these processes is still poorly defined.

For the six cholesterol-derived hormones (the five steroids and the sterol, 1,25(OH)$_2$-vitamin D), the receptors are soluble cytoplasmic proteins, with molecular weights estimated to be in the range of 50,000 to 300,000 daltons. The binding of hormone to its receptor is followed by one or more events (as yet, not fully characterized) that result in activation of the complex and translocation to the nucleus (see Fig. 2–3). The activation process may change the size, shape, conformation, and chemical properties of the receptor protein.

Events in the Nucleus

The important unique feature of the activated hormone-receptor complex is its high affinity for binding to components of the nucleus; the unactivated receptor appears to be quite capable of entering the nucleus but its affinity for nuclear components is very low. Thus, entry of hormone into the target cell and binding to receptor lead quickly to a reduction in the number of cytosol receptors and their appearance in the nucleus in the form of hormone-receptor complexes bound to the nucleus. Binding is largely to the nuclear chromatin, which is a mixture of DNA and protein, including both histone and nonhistone proteins. The nuclear binding sites associated with chromatin are defined as nuclear acceptors. The nuclear acceptor sites are much more plentiful than cytosol receptors, so that even when the latter are saturated with hormone, the number of free nuclear acceptor sites is not reduced significantly.

The nature of the interaction between hormone-receptor complexes and chromatin is as yet poorly defined. It has not been possible to identify chemically any of the putative nuclear acceptors. Studies of the progesterone receptor suggest that the receptor has two protein subunits, both of which have progesterone bound; subunit A binds with little specificity to DNA, and subunit B binds to chromatin protein derived from target cells (Fig. 2–35). It is suggested that

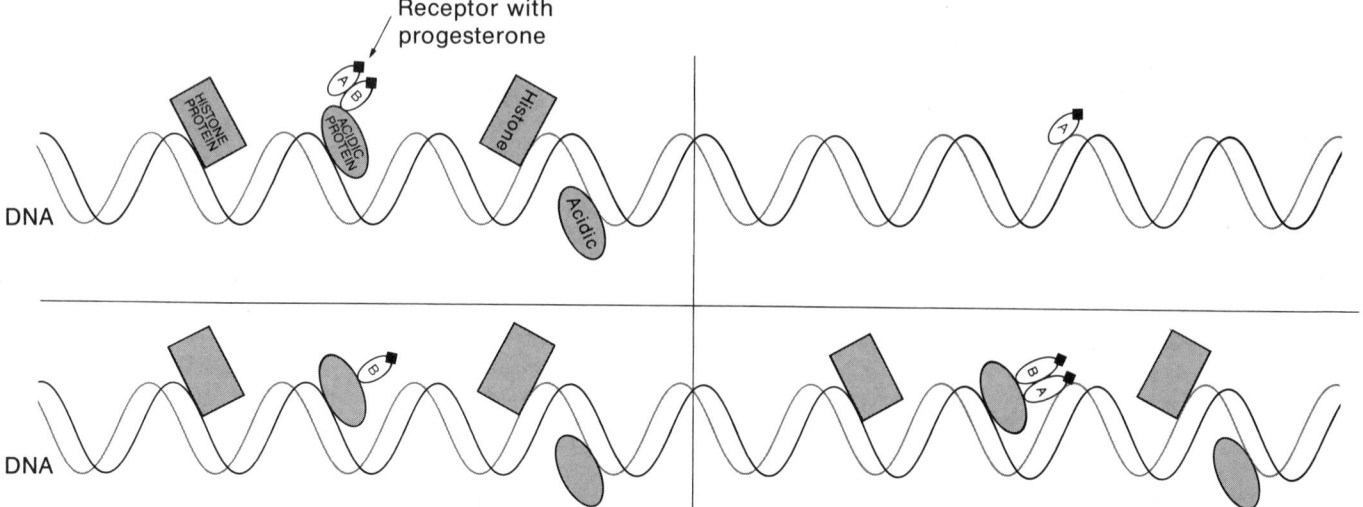

Figure 2–35. The progesterone receptor is a dimer composed of two different subunits designated A and B, each of which binds hormone. When progesterone is bound to the receptor subunits, the intact dimer is capable of binding (via the B subunit) to a nuclear acceptor protein in the acid (nonhistone) fraction of intact chromatin (upper left panel). With a progesterone attached, the isolated B subunit can also bind to the acidic chromatin (lower left panel). With a progesterone attached, the isolated A subunit can bind to naked (protein-free) DNA (upper right panel). It is speculated that with the intact receptor the interaction of the B subunit with the acidic chromatin acceptor protein directs the A subunit to the proper sites on the DNA of the target cell's nucleus. (lower right panel).

subunit B provides site specificity for the action of subunit A on DNA.

Biological Consequences

The major (if not sole) action of the lipid-soluble hormones is to increase the production of specific messenger RNAs, which leads to the increased production of new or existing proteins by the target cells. Under most conditions, the vast majority of the cell's DNA is prevented from being expressed, and each cell is making only a relatively small number (a thousand) of different proteins, which represents only a minute fraction of its total potential repertoire. The lipid-soluble hormones act to relieve these constraints at specific regions on the DNA, leading to synthesis of specific mRNA and protein. In general, steroid hormone action affects only about 1% of the proteins expressed by the cell; i.e., changes are limited and specific. In some cases, the specific proteins affected have been identified: sex steroids act on the hen oviduct to increase production of ovalbumin, avidin, and other egg proteins; glucocorticoids act to increase specific enzymes in liver; 1,25(OH)$_2$-vitamin D stimulates intestinal mucosa to produce a protein needed for Ca^{++} absorption. In some cases, an effect of the hormone may lead to effects on differentiation of the cell. Since differentiation represents a major change in the whole program of the cell, a very large number of proteins may be changed secondarily.

It is now clear that the primary complementary RNA transcript of DNA must be processed in several stages before it appears in the cytoplasm as a functional mRNA. This processing not only determines whether the transcript will ever get from the nucleus to the cytoplasm but also has effects on its lifetime in the cytoplasm and its efficiency as a template for protein synthesis. Although an increase in the synthesis of a specific protein may be affected by changes at any of these steps, it is thought that an increase in the rate of transcription of DNA is the major cause of the increase in number of the mRNA molecules, which is responsible for the increase in protein concentration.

It should also be emphasized that the ultimate expression of some hormone action may be inhibition of a biological event. Inhibition is more difficult to detect and may result from direct inhibition at the level of nuclear DNA or by an activation process that yields proteins that counter the effects of other proteins or inactivate them.

Decay of the activation process is associated with dissociation of the hormone from receptor and presumably return of the receptor to the cytoplasm, where it rejoins the pool of cytosol receptors available for binding hormone. The mechanisms governing these events are not well defined.

Do these hormones have extranuclear effects on mitochondrial DNA or on processes not involving DNA and protein synthesis? Further study is needed.

Distribution of Receptors

The breadth of distribution of receptors for each of the hormones appears to be related to the range of target cells. That glucocorticoid receptors are found in a very wide range of cell types is consistent with the idea that glucocorticoids act very widely. The other cholesterol-derived hormones appear to have receptors in a much narrower range of cells, consistent with a narrower spectrum of target cells on which they are known to act. However, methods for the detection of receptors can be quite insensitive. Therefore, the finding in any cell of a biological or biochemical effect that is hormone-sensitive and specific (on the basis of comparative effects of well characterized analogues) should be considered prima facie evidence for existence of a specific receptor, even if it is not yet demonstrable by direct binding methods.

Specificity of Receptors

The definition of these receptors, like those of the polypeptide and catecholamine hormones, is based on specificity of binding and its relationship to subsequent events, especially biological action. As a first approximation, each of the hormones has a unique receptor which is the same for all cells in which it is found. Several important modifications of this rule should be raised.

1. Androgen action is expressed through two sets of distinct receptors. One receptor, which binds testosterone strongly, is found in some tissues including testis, kidney, ovary, and uterus. The other type of androgen receptor, which binds dihydrotestosterone (DHT) with much higher affinity than testosterone, is found in other tissues (prostate, seminal vesicle, epididymis, and levator ani). Testosterone is the secreted form of the hormone. In liver and in some of the target cells such as prostate that have dihydrotestosterone-favoring receptors, there is an enzyme that reduces testosterone to its dihydro- form. In other target cells such as levator ani, which have the DHT-favoring receptors but lack the reductase, testosterone may be the active hormone, though it is a less effective hormone in this tissue.

2. Testosterone can have estrogen-like actions. Two mechanisms may account for it. Many tissues can convert ("aromatize") testosterone to an active estrogen, estradiol. Also there is evidence that testosterone has a low but finite affinity for estrogen receptors and when bound to estrogen receptors can produce all of the effects of an estrogen-estrogen receptor complex; it is a full estrogen agonist of low affinity. This would qualify as an example of specificity spillover (see earlier under peptide hormones).

3. All natural glucocorticoids and mineralocorticoids, in addition to a high affinity for their own receptors, have some affinity for the receptor of the other class of adrenal steroids. Thus, extreme endogenous overproduction of cortisol, a glucocorticoid, may also result clinically in mineralocorticoid excess (Na^+ retention, K^+ loss, hypertension) by specificity spillover. Conversely, does the persistence of normal mineralocorticoid production in patients with defects in glucocorticoid biosynthesis (e.g., patients with ACTH deficiency) produce some glucocorticoid effect which is absent in patients in whom both hormones are deficient, such as those with Addison's disease?

4. Progesterone, in addition to binding and acting through its own receptors, binds to glucocorticoid receptors, where it acts as an antagonist, and binds to androgen receptors, where it acts as a weak agonist.

Antagonists

Synthetic specific antagonists of steroid hormones may act in several ways. The simplest mechanism is competition at the level of receptor; the antagonist binds but does not activate (i.e., intrinsic activity is very low or absent). Such a mechanism accounts for the acute action of spironolactone, an inhibitor of aldosterone binding to mineralocorticoid receptors. However, with chronic administration of a constant dose of the drug, plasma aldosterone may rise to very high levels, yet without breakthrough of the aldosterone effect, which would be expected if the effect of the drug were simply competitive at the level of the receptor. Presumably, in addition, the drug desensitizes the tissue by additional mechanisms, such as depletion or inactivation of cytosol receptors or nuclear acceptors. Side effects of the drug (decreased menses; gynecomastia and impotence) are thought to be related to competition for androgen receptors and to effects on steroid biosynthetic pathways in adrenal and gonadal tissues.

Nafoxidine, an estrogen antagonist, clearly demonstrates the possibility of multiple mechanisms. Acute nafoxidine binds to estrogen receptors and translocates them to the nucleus; concomitantly there are estrogen effects, showing that nafoxidine is an agonist acutely. However, following treatment with nafoxidine, receptors with nafoxidine bound become inactivated, and the cytosol is therefore depleted of free receptor; this coincides with the antagonist stage of nafoxidine action.

Iodothyronines

The action of thyroid hormone and its receptor at the level of the nucleus is very similar to that described for the cholesterol-derived hormones — binding to chromatin, increased synthesis of specific mRNA's, and increased production of a limited number of proteins. The major difference is that the initial binding site of hormone is in the nucleus (in contrast to the cytosol receptors and nuclear acceptors). It has been suggested that mitochondria and the plasma membrane may be additional sites for direct action of thyroid hormones but as yet their physiological role is unsettled.

The active form of the hormone is T_3, which is usually produced in small amounts by the thyroid gland and in much larger amounts by deiodination of T_4 at multiple peripheral sites. While T_3 has high affinity for receptors, it is not certain whether T_4 has reduced or absent affinity for receptors, that is, whether all of T_4 action requires conversion to T_3 or whether T_4 can act directly as an agonist with reduced affinity.

Consistent with the wide range of target cells for the iodothyronines, receptors for them are found in a very wide range of cell types, as is the case with glucocorticoid receptors. Among the specific proteins whose production is stimulated by the action of thyroid hormones are adult hemoglobin in tadpole erythrocytes, growth hormone in rat pituitary cells (in culture), and the components of the Na^+-K^+ ATPase in plasma membrane of liver and other cells. The iodothyronine-stimulated increase in the number of ATPase units is thought to be important in the thermogenesis that is characteristic of this hormone.

Regulation

The receptors for the lipid-soluble hormone undergo substantial regulation. Differentiation that represents a major change in cell program is a major factor which accounts for the wide differences in receptor concentration between target and nontarget cells. The hormone itself can regulate its own receptors and those for other hormones. An effect of T_3 is to reduce the concentration of its own receptors. Progesterone reduces the concentration of both its own receptors and estrogen receptors. Estrogens increase the concentration of both its receptors and progesterone receptors. This is in addition to the widespread effect of the lipid-soluble hormones on receptors for water-soluble hormones (see earlier, regulation of receptors in the section on polypeptide hormones and catecholamines).

Specific Disease Implications

Cancer. Many breast cancers respond to hormonal therapy, which can be either ablation or estrogen administration. Why cancers that are hormone-sensitive respond to both addition and subtraction of hormones is unclear but receptor measurements have been found to be useful in determining which patients will respond. As a first step, a patient whose cancer has a low level of estrogen receptors is not likely to respond to hormone therapy and is best suited for chemotherapy. Of those with high levels of estrogen receptors, a significant portion will respond to hormone therapy. Since estrogen receptors are necessary but not sufficient, methods have been investigated to see if the estrogen receptor is coupled to an intact estrogen-response pathway. As noted earlier, one effect of estrogen is to increase the level of progesterone receptors. Studies show that patients with high levels of estrogen receptors who also have high levels of progesterone receptors are more likely to respond (than those with high levels of estrogen receptors but low or absent progesterone receptors) because it indicates the post-receptor pathway for estrogen action is intact.

Similar applications have been made to other cancers. Lymphocytes are typically very sensitive to glucocorticoids and can be killed by high doses of these steroids. Sensitivity and resistance of leukemic cells to killing by glucocorticoids is closely related to their content of glucocorticoid receptors. Similar approaches apply to other "hormone-sensitive" tumors such as endometrial and prostatic cancers.

Genetic Disorders. In addition to cancer, the other major area of study of receptors for the lipid-soluble hormones relates to states of hormone resistance, especially of genetic origin. While most of the lipid-soluble hormones have been studied to some extent, those associated with androgen resistance have been studied in exquisite detail; these should be the prototypes for the others, in addition to having been the pioneer area in the field.

Androgen resistance at the target cell level has been studied in detail using cultured fibroblasts of affected patients. Binding of hormone may be deficient owing to absence of receptors or owing to receptors that are reduced in number or affinity. In addition, binding may be normal in cells maintained at low (less than body) temperatures but reduced at higher temperatures; this suggests that the receptor may have a structural alteration away from the binding site that makes the receptor excessively susceptible to degradation. (Substitution of an abnormal amino acid in the bioactive region of a protein often disturbs function, whereas a substitution outside the bioactive region may leave the function normal but causes the molecule to be highly susceptible to degradation.) Alternatively, binding may be entirely normal but subsequent steps — e.g., activation or binding to nuclear acceptors — may be defective.

Transport of Lipid-Soluble Hormones

Binding Proteins in Plasma

In contrast to the polypeptide hormones, which as a rule circulate as the free form in plasma, all of the lipid-soluble hormones bind reversibly to one or more plasma proteins. The majority of each hormone is bound, ranging from 60% for aldosterone to more than 99% for T_4. In humans, transcortin (corticosteroid-binding globulin, CBG) has high affinity for both progesterone and cortisol. The level of CBG is increased by estrogens. Sex hormone–binding globulin (SHBG) binds dihydrotestosterone, testosterone, and estradiol with high affinity. Circulating levels of this protein are increased by estrogens and hyperthyroidism and reduced by androgens and hypothyroidism. Thyroid hormones (T_4 and to a lesser extent T_3) are bound to thyroid-binding globulin (TBG) and thyroid-binding prealbumin (TBPA). TBG levels are increased by estrogen action and reduced by testosterone and glucocorticoids. In addition, albumin and possibly other plasma proteins provide high-capacity, low-affinity sites for all of the lipid-soluble hormones.

Under *in vivo* conditions, binding to these proteins is rapidly reversible. Thus, as a first approximation, the binding proteins act simply as a reservoir for plasma hormone; only the minority of plasma hormone that is free is avail-able to enter target cells or subject to metabolic transformation, and the supply of free hormone is buffered by the large supply of bound hormone. Because the binding proteins typically bind more than one species of hormone, and because hormone levels are potent regulators of the concentration of binding protein, a change in concentration of one hormone can have multiple effects on the availability of another hormone, acutely by competition at the level of protein binding, or chronically by altering the concentration of binding protein. While it is widely accepted that only free hormone is active, there are sufficient data to the contrary (bound hormone is available for action and for metabolic transformation) to leave the issue unsettled. Probably free hormone is the major but not sole active form of the hormone. Clinically, considerations of the binding proteins are most important as they affect measurements of hormone levels in blood; typically we measure total hormone rather than free hormone concentration. Finally, the binding proteins are not biologically essential since extreme elevations or total absence has trivial consequences.

The binding proteins are clearly distinct from the target cell receptors, especially in their specificity for bioactive hormone. As an example, dexamethasone, a potent synthetic glucocorticoid agonist, has high affinity for cellular receptors but does not bind at all to transcortin (CBG), the major glucocorticoid-binding protein in blood.

Access to the Central Nervous System

The central nervous system has anatomical barriers ("blood-brain barrier") that limit the access of polypeptide hormones to most parts of the brain. These hormones, when present in blood, reach the brain only via a limited number of regions where this barrier is absent or reduced, as hypothalamus. The lipid-soluble hormones, like other lipid-soluble substances, have much easier and wider access to brain tissue, and effects of these hormones in the central nervous system are substantial. Thyroid hormones in blood have profound effects on neuronal development and organization in the young — the permanent deleterious effect of thyroid hormone deficiency in early life. Estrogens and androgens, blood-borne, early in life also affect neuronal development in a permanent way. In addition, these hormones have effects on the behavior of adults, at least in animals.

Hormone Biosynthesis

Implications for Ectopic Hormone Production

Since all of the machinery to produce peptides and proteins is present in essentially every cell, the introduction into the cytoplasm of a messenger RNA for a peptide hormone will result in production of the corresponding hormone. Clearly, first a portion of the DNA must be transcribed and the complementary RNA must be processed and exported from the nucleus, but fundamentally the process is easy. On the other hand, biosynthesis of the seven lipid-soluble hormones (from cholesterol or tyrosine) requires a very large number of gene products including complex organized enzymatic machinery that is present in only a limited number of differentiated cells; thus ectopic hormone production, in the classic sense, does not occur. The only tumors that synthesize lipid-soluble hormones are those derived from cell types that normally produce such hormones.

Localization of Synthesis, Peripheral Transformations, and Degradation

The peptide hormones are normally synthesized completely from simple precursors to the complete final active form within a single secretory cell of a unique type, and when degraded are fully inactivated irreversibly. The lipid-soluble hormones do not conform to this pattern. (1) Synthesis of the active form of the hormone molecule may require action of more than one cell, e.g., dihydrotestosterone, $1,25(OH)_2$-vitamin D, and most of the triiodothyronone. (2) Complete *de novo* synthesis of the active hormone from cholesterol is often carried out in more than one organ (androgen by adrenals and gonads, progesterone by ovary and placenta, estrogens by adrenals and gonads). (3) The synthetic pathway from cholesterol often has another active hormone as precursor (progesterone as precursor of androgens, androgens as precursor of estrogens). (4) Peripheral (extraglandular) sites can convert an inactive form to an active form or transform one active form into another (estrogen to 2-OH estrogen, which may have its own unique biological properties, or androgen to estrogen); postmenopausal women vary widely in their manifestation of estrogen deficiency such as osteoporosis and atrophy of vaginal mucosa possibly because of differences in their extraovarian production of estrogen. (5) The active forms of the hormone may be represented by more than one chemical form; both androgens and estrogens provide examples. (6) The active hormones and chemically related species are widespread in nature and some of these may not be destroyed in the digestive tract. For example, licorice ingestion can lead to a clinical state that resembles mineralocorticoid excess because of its content of a mineralocorticoid agonist. Many substances can lead to gynecomastia (e.g., marijuana and cardiac glycosides), probably by interacting with target cell receptors for sex steroids.

Implications of These Complexities

For a steroid hormone to act, not only must the hormone bind to receptor to form a complex but the complex must be activated, translocate and bind to nuclear acceptors, regulate DNA expression, and permit recycling of receptors. While affinity for receptor may be simple, what we call intrinsic activity is the product of a series of successive complex steps; both natural and synthetic hormones may differ in their ability, when combined to receptor, to carry out each of these steps. Second, although there are only eight receptor types for the seven hormones, each receptor recognizes multiple forms of active hormone. Further, an active form of hormone may interact with more than one receptor type. The supply of hormone available to the cell is modulated proximally by binding proteins which may bind more than one active hormone, and the effect of the binding protein is modulated physically and biologically by these and other hormones. The supply of hormone to the blood is regulated in a very complex way because each of the hormones is produced by actions of multiple enzymes in several glands as well as extraglandular organs. Finally, the existence of related substances in nature that can enter the body relatively intact and interact with target cells in biologically relevant fashion further complicates the possible mechanisms. Thus, the patient who appears to have excessive or deficient effects of a lipid-soluble hormone requires substantially more thought on the part of the physician to determine whether the primary problem is at the target cell or before the target cell. Further, measurements of hormone levels in blood must be interpreted so as to consider whether all of the active forms recognized by the receptor are being measured and whether all of the forms measured are active and available to the cell. Overproduction and underproduction can be generated at multiple sites including the target cell itself. Finally, the ability of a natural material to bind to receptor does not predict what its biological effect will be.

FINAL CONSIDERATIONS

In this section are three subjects: (1) target cell defects; (2) integration of the elements of an endocrine system including "spare receptors" and the relationship of receptors to the final biological events at the target cell; and (3) new (undiscovered) diseases. Much of the material is a direct extension of earlier sections, and logic might suggest that this material belongs earlier. However, because some of the concepts are subtle or summary in nature, we have chosen to postpone them to this point.

Target Cell Defects

We suspect that the primary defect is at the target cell when (1) clinically the patient is deficient in the bioeffect of a particular hormone; (2) plasma levels of the putative hormone are normal or (more often) elevated; and (3) administration of the exogenous hormone elicits no response or a response that is unexplainedly low. (The finding of decreased binding to receptors on fresh cells from the patient would heighten that suspicion and focus our attention on the target cell receptors.)

The first possibility to consider is whether the apparent elevation in plasma hormone levels may actually represent interference in the assay by anti-hormone antibodies or other hormone-binding substance in the patient's plasma. Thus, in some insulin radioimmunoassays, circulating anti-insulin antibodies (due to prior treatment with insulin or, rarely, autoantibodies) make it appear that the patient has elevated concentrations of plasma insulin. The next step is to be certain that the hormone assay is measuring the bioactive hormone, rather than a closely related material that is biologically less active or actually an antagonist, as in one patient with a genetically defective insulin, mentioned earlier. The third possibility is that the bioactive hormone does not have access to the target cell because anti-hormone antibodies or other hormone-binding proteins prevent access to receptors of target cells; for example, euthyroid patients with elevated levels of TBG have elevated levels of plasma thyroxine (but normal levels of free T_4 and T_3). A fourth possibility is that slowly developing extreme hormone excess (e.g., choriocarcinoma producing hCG or possibly medullary cell carcinoma producing thyrocalcitonin) may lead to a state of extreme resistance at the level of the target cell, involving receptor and post-receptor mechanisms.

Target cell defects may be mimicked by other disorders. As a trivial example, iodide-deficient patients have some findings that suggest resistance to TSH by the thyroid gland. Plasma levels of thyroid hormone are subnormal, circulating TSH is elevated, TSH receptors are probably reduced, and thyroid hormone release in response to TSH is subnormal. Typically, the thyroid gland is intact but simply lacks some element from the outside that is needed for expression of one of its biological responses to TSH. Likewise, patients with a deficiency of apoprotein B (abetalipoproteinemia) have findings that suggest subnormal sensitivity of the adrenal to ACTH. Plasma ACTH is elevated with normal levels of circulating glucocorticoids, and the steroid response to an infusion of ACTH is subnormal. Cholesterol, which is the precursor of all steroid hormones, in humans is largely derived from low-density lipoprotein (LDL), which is one of the cholesterol-containing substances that are absent from these patients; in the adrenal, high-density lipoprotein (HDL) and endogenous synthesis do not completely make up for the deficiency of LDL cholesterol needed for hormone synthesis. Again, the real problem is the shortage of an externally derived material needed for expression of the target cell's response.

Defects in Hormone Biosynthesis (or Delivery) Masquerading as Target Cell Insensitivity

With the lipid-soluble hormones, another confusing possibility has been encountered. Some patients thought to be testosterone-resistant (at the target cell) were actually found to lack the enzyme that converts testosterone to dihydrotestosterone (DHT); it was not realized that DHT was the major active substance for some target cells. Thus a defect in hormone biosynthesis masqueraded as a target cell defect. Similarly, some patients with vitamin D resistance lack the ability to convert precursors into the active form of the hormone, 1,25(OH)$_2$-vitamin D. They are resistant to the precursors but not to the active hormone. Again, a condition characterized by a defect in biosynthesis had appeared to be a target cell defect. With the lipid-soluble hormones (and the prostaglandin family), where biosynthesis of hormones includes a series of precursors of varying bioactivity with transformation occurring at multiple tissue sites, our ignorance of which moiety is actually acting at the target cell may be misleading.

As an extension of the previous discussion, we now raise a general question: Is the peripherally acting species identical with the species recognized at the level of feedback inhibition? Glucocorticoids seem to vary in their ability to act as glucocorticoids peripherally (prevent symptoms of glucocorticoid deficiency) and their ability to suppress ACTH output by the pituitary. Does this relate to the finding that patients with ACTH hypersecretion from the pituitary are less sensitive to circulating glucocorticoids than normal, and some patients suppress better with an apparently equal dose of one glucocorticoid than another? Estrogens may provide another example. It is thought that the same estrogenic moieties that produce peripheral effects act centrally (hypothalamus and pituitary). But estrogens can both stimulate and inhibit gonadotropin and prolactin secretion. For prolactin, it appears that the stimulatory moiety is estrogen itself while the inhibitory agent is 2-OH estrogen, a catechol estrogen formed locally. Again, hormone biosynthetic events may occur so closely to hormone action at the target cell that a defect in hormone biosynthesis or transformation may appear to be a defect in hormone action at the target cell. A related observation concerns LHRH. This hormone is normally secreted in a pulsatile pattern. The administration of the hormone in a pulsatile manner yields good responses, whereas the same dose of hormone as a continuous infusion produces resistance to the hormone at the level of the target cell.

Integration and Control

Early in this chapter, the endocrine system was discussed in broad general terms. Then individual components of the system were described. The purpose of this section is to return to a complete endocrine system and in simple semi-quantitative terms show how a whole system works. Rather than a general theoretical and rigorous analysis, simple examples will be used to show what mechanisms the body actually employs — especially to illustrate the flexibility, constraints, and levels of control. (While the discussion is quite broadly applicable to all hormones, we have based the discussion heavily on the hormones that work through cAMP because this is the largest group of hormones and the available data are extensive.)

As a first approximation, all target cells are exposed to the same concentration of hormone (Fig. 2–36a). Thus the hormone is providing a uniform signal to all cells. However, we find that some cell types are much more responsive than others (Fig. 2–36b and c); *low concentrations of insulin produce much greater effects on fat cells than on muscle cells.* Some cell types are responsive some of the time but not at other times (the liver of the young fetus is not responsive to insulin) while other cell types are uniformly unresponsive. This difference among cell types is provided by early steps at the target cell, either through the receptor or early postreceptor (coupling) processes. (It is easy to conceive of biological situations in which a cell that is normally responsive to a hormone may temporarily ignore external events, as during cell division or repair of injury.)

Moreover, within a single cell type, we find that individual processes that are sensitive to the same hormone through the same proximal pathway in the target cell may differ widely in their sensitivity to hormone (Fig. 2–37). Low concentrations of insulin at the fat cell are much more effective at inhibiting lipolysis than stimulating glucose oxidation or lipogenesis; in the liver, glycogen metabolism is much more sensitive to insulin than amino acid transport. Further, a particular pathway that is typically under hormonal control may become totally unresponsive while other pathways in the cell remain sensitive to hormone. Thus a uniform intracellular signal produces widely divergent effects distally in the target cell. These differences within a single target cell are presumably regulated distally beyond the major branch points described earlier. By analogy, we see central overall regulation by the hormone (cf. the national or federal government), control for the whole cell by the receptor and early coupling steps (cf. government at the state or provincial level), and distal regulation of individual pathways (cf. city or county government).

Let us now examine the variables and how they relate to one another. The hormone molecule provides potential for very wide changes quantitatively but very limited possibilities otherwise. The concentration of hormone can be varied rapidly over a very wide range by an increase in secretion and much more slowly by changes in degradation rate. But the affinity of the hormone (for receptor) and the intrinsic activity of the hormone are essentially invariant *in vivo*. In essence, hormone as a biological regulator is dependent solely on hormone secretion rates. The concentrations of

---

*We have ignored the existence of target tissues that are exposed to concentrations of hormone different from those in plasma; for example, the endocrine (and exocrine?) cells of the pancreas and the cells of the liver are exposed to much higher concentration of islet cell hormones (insulin, glucagon, somatostatin) than are peripheral tissues such as fat and muscle. It appears that these tissues accommodate to their situation by adjusting their responsiveness; resting levels of hormone, despite their absolute magnitude, elicit small responses, and elevations of hormone concentration above that level stimulate the cell.

In this discussion we are also ignoring the fact that within a target tissue there is a wide range of variation in sensitivity; for example, thyroid cells in small follicles are more responsive to TSH than those in large follicles, there is variability among follicles of the same size, and individual cells within a single follicle show variations. For this discussion we assume that all cells of a single type are homogeneous but differ from all cells of another type.

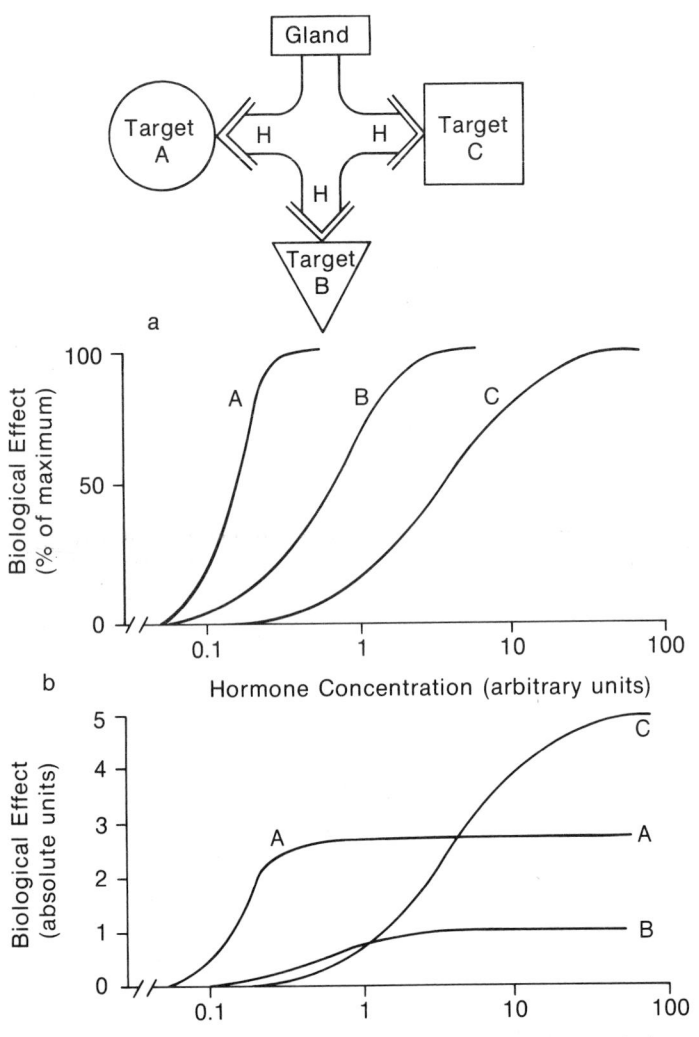

Figure 2–36. *a,* Again, as a general rule, the hormone provides a uniform signal to all target cells. *b* and *c* show, in a schematic way, that the responses of three different target tissues to a single hormone often differ widely even when they have in common the same receptor species with the same affinity for hormone.

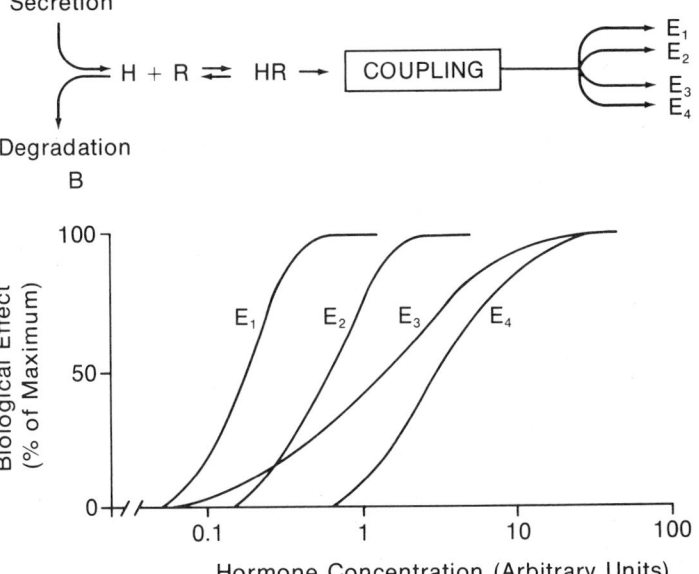

Figure 2–37. *A,* Recalling the simplified scheme in Figure 2–4*A,* hormone in the extracellular fluid, which is continuously modulated by secretion and degradation, interacts with receptors to form HR complexes that activate the cell. The subsequent steps that link the HR complexes to the individual distal pathways are grouped together as "coupling" events. E_1, E_2, E_3, and E_4 represent individual biological events.

B, Four separate biological events in a single target cell can have widely different dose-response relationships, even when they share the same receptors and intermediate steps.

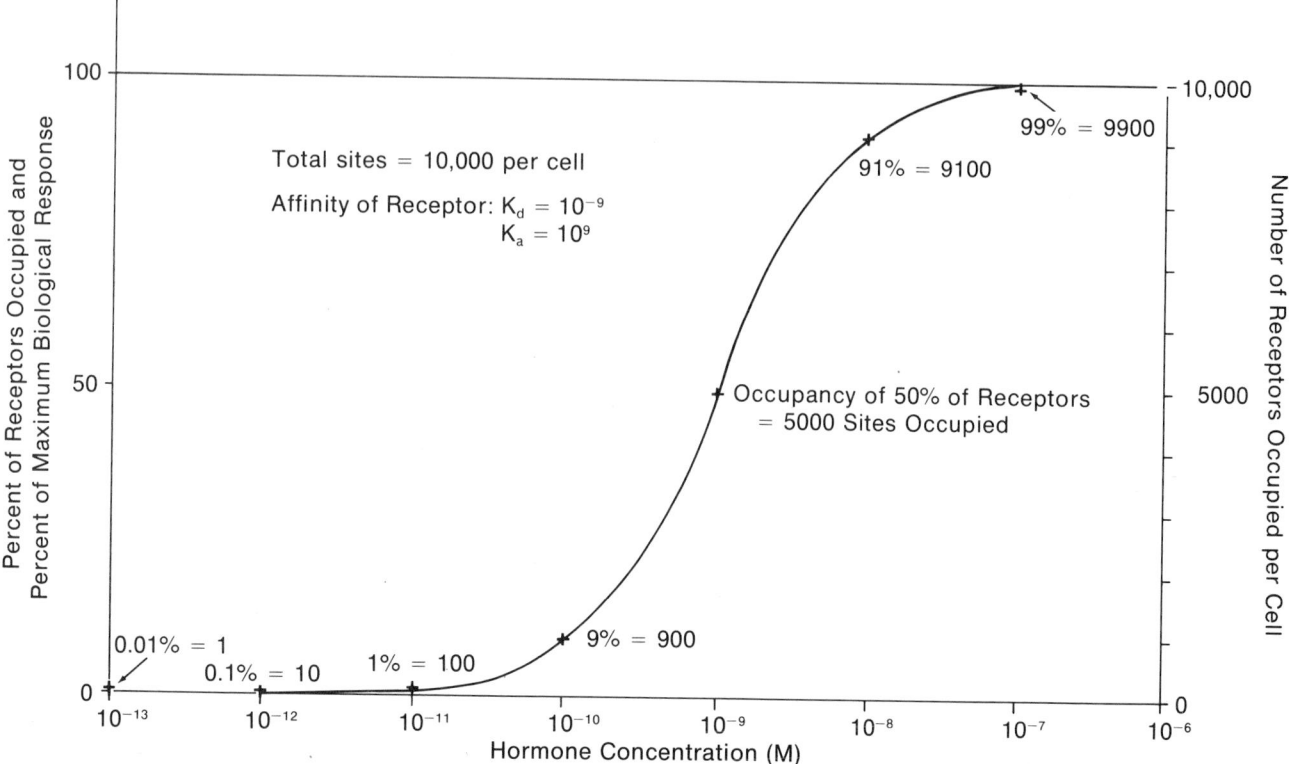

Figure 2–38. This figure illustrates a very simple relationship between hormone binding to receptor and the biological response (E): [HR] is directly proportional to the biological effect over the whole dose-response curve. The receptors are homogeneous with a fixed affinity, and $K_d = 10^{-9}$ or $K_a = 10^9$. At $[H] = 10^{-9} = K_d$, half of the receptors are occupied, and the biological response is half maximum. At $[H] = 10^{-10}$ M, only about 10% of the receptors are occupied. At $[H] < 10^{-10}$ M, the fraction of receptors occupied is small, but with 10,000 receptors per cell, the number of occupied receptors is finite. Note that even at $[H] = 10^{-13}$ (four orders of magnitude less than K_d), the number of receptors occupied is not 0, a fact that will be of importance in the later discussion. Also note that at $[H] < 10^{-10}$ M, a tenfold increase in [H] produces a tenfold increase in [HR], while at $[H] \geq 10^{-10}$ M, a tenfold increase in [H] produces less (often much less) than a tenfold increase in [HR].

hormone are very low compared with the affinity of the receptors; resting $[H] \ll K_d$ and stimulated $[H] < K_d$. Thus receptors are never saturated under physiological conditions — hormone concentration is essentially always limiting relative to receptors. Physiologically we are always dealing with a situation where a further increase in hormone concentration is appreciated at the level of the receptor — an increase in [H] always produces an increase in [HR].

To understand the consequences of this relationship between hormone and receptor, let us examine the quantitative relationship between hormone concentration and the concentration of hormone-receptor complexes on the cell (Fig. 2–38). If we simply look at the percentage of receptors occupied, then at low concentrations of hormone ($[H] \ll K_d$), it appears that receptor occupancy is trival; i.e., the curve approaches 0% occupancy of receptors. But if we assume that there are 10,000 receptors per cell (a reasonable number for most systems), then the absolute number of complexes formed is quite respectable even at low hormone concentrations. One advantage of this arrangement is that the system is more sensitive to relative changes in hormone concentration; notice that at receptor occupancy (occupied receptors/total receptors, or $[HR]/[R_o]$) below 10%, [HR] is linearly related to [H], whereas at occupancies of 10 to 90%, [HR] is linear with log [H] — a fold increase in H is more effective in generating HR at the lowest part of the curve than at the middle part. Other advantages will be shown later.

Now let us relate receptor occupancy to final biological effects. *In vivo*, as hormone concentration is increased, the maximal biological effect is normally achieved before all of the receptors are occupied! To understand how this is ac-

complished and its consequences, let us first examine a simple hypothetical system and then manipulate it stepwise until we reproduce the natural condition.

Let's start with a single set of homogeneous receptors that regulate a single final event (E) in a very simple relationship — when [HR] is 0, E is 0; each increase in [HR] produces a comparable increase in E, and when [HR] is maximal, E is maximal (Fig. 2–38). Notice that the curve that relates [H] to [HR] is superimposable on the curve that relates [H] to E. If we simply increase or decrease the affinity (K) of the receptor (for hormone), the two curves shift together left or right; the system is simply more sensitive or less sensitive to hormone (Fig. 2–39). Now let us restore the original affinity but reduce receptor concentration by 50% (Fig. 2–40). Now at every hormone concentration, E is reduced by 50% and, at very high concentrations of hormone, only half of the final effect can be achieved. With further reductions in receptor concentration, E is proportionally reduced. Note that under these conditions where the capacity to respond (distally) exceeds the capacity to stimulate (proximally), a portion of the cell's capability is not utilizable.

Now let us restore the original conditions but double receptor concentration to 20,000 (Fig. 2–41); 10,000 occupied receptors are still required to activate 10,000 units of E, but now with 20,000 total receptors per cell, 10,000 receptors are occupied at much lower levels of hormone. With further increases in receptor concentration (keeping everything else the same), the dose-response curve relating [H] to E shifts left and becomes steeper, more sensitive absolutely and relatively (Fig. 2–41). This in fact is the typical case; the maximal capacity of the receptor (and other steps) to stimulate far exceeds the maximal capacity

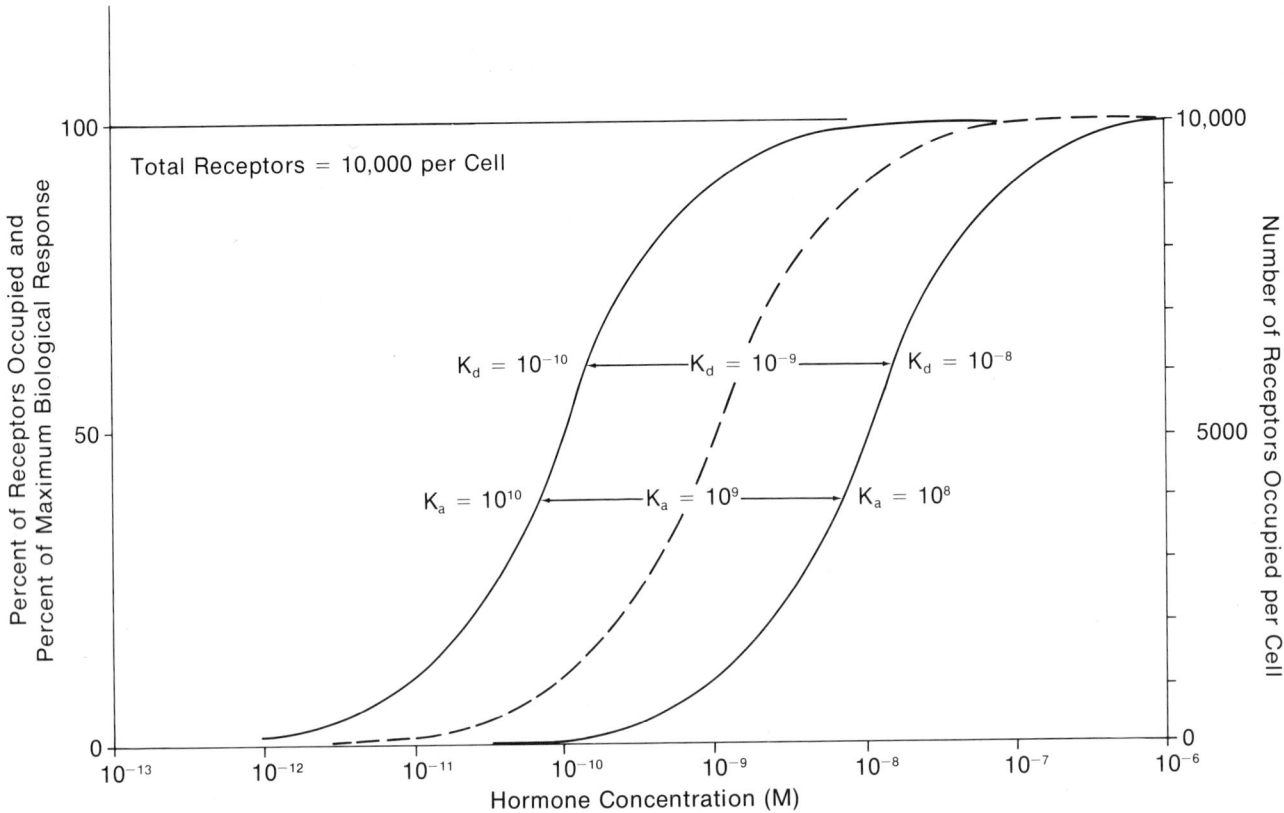

Figure 2–39. This figure illustrates that a change in affinity simply shifts (to the left or to the right) the binding curve along with the biological response curve. Remember, however, that such a change in affinity is often accompanied by a comparable change in the dissociation rate constant (of hormone from receptor).

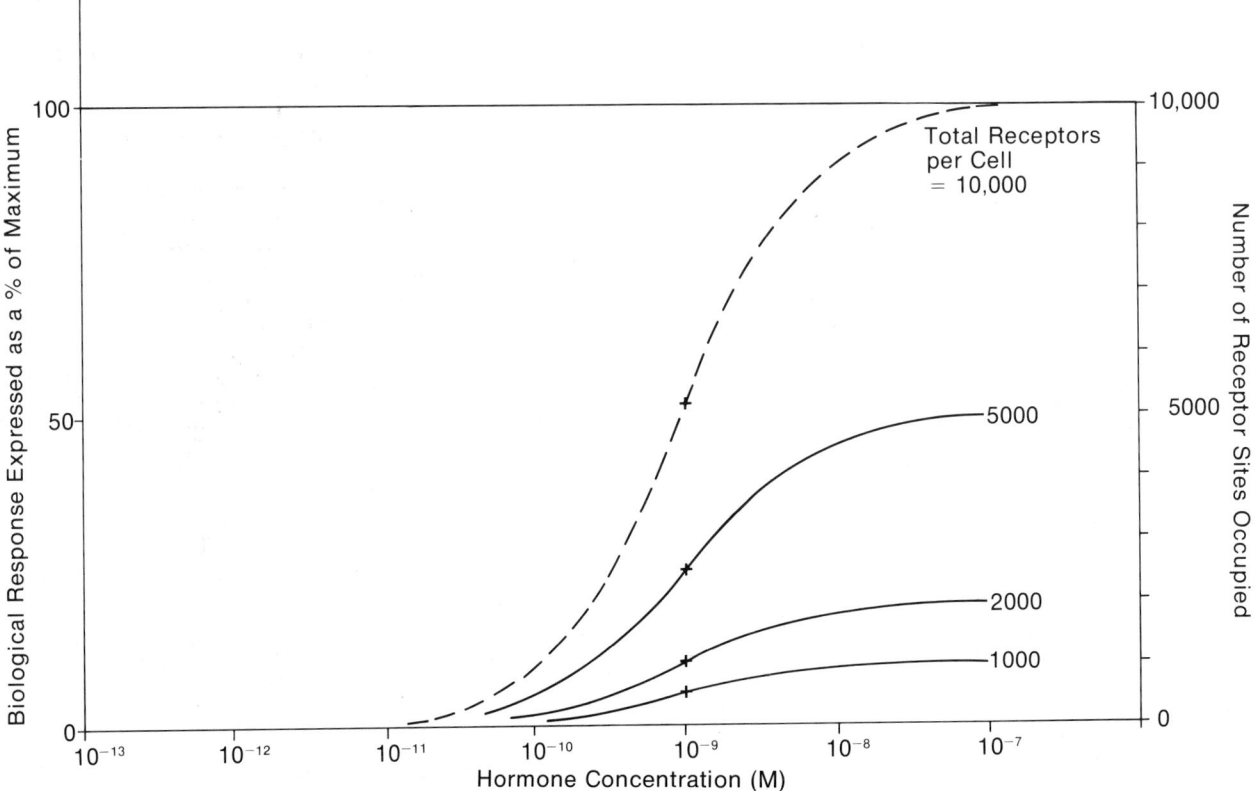

Figure 2–40. The original curve (----) represents the binding curve and biological response curve for $K_d = 10^{-9}$, total receptor sites = 10,000 per cell, and a capacity of the cell to respond to 10,000 occupied receptors. When only the number of receptor sites per cell is reduced, there is at each hormone concentration a proportionate reduction in [HR] and in biological response. Note that with [H] = 10^{-9}, the biological response is half of the maximal response that can be achieved with that number of receptors. Expressed differently, when the curves are normalized to their own maximum, the curves are all superimposable.

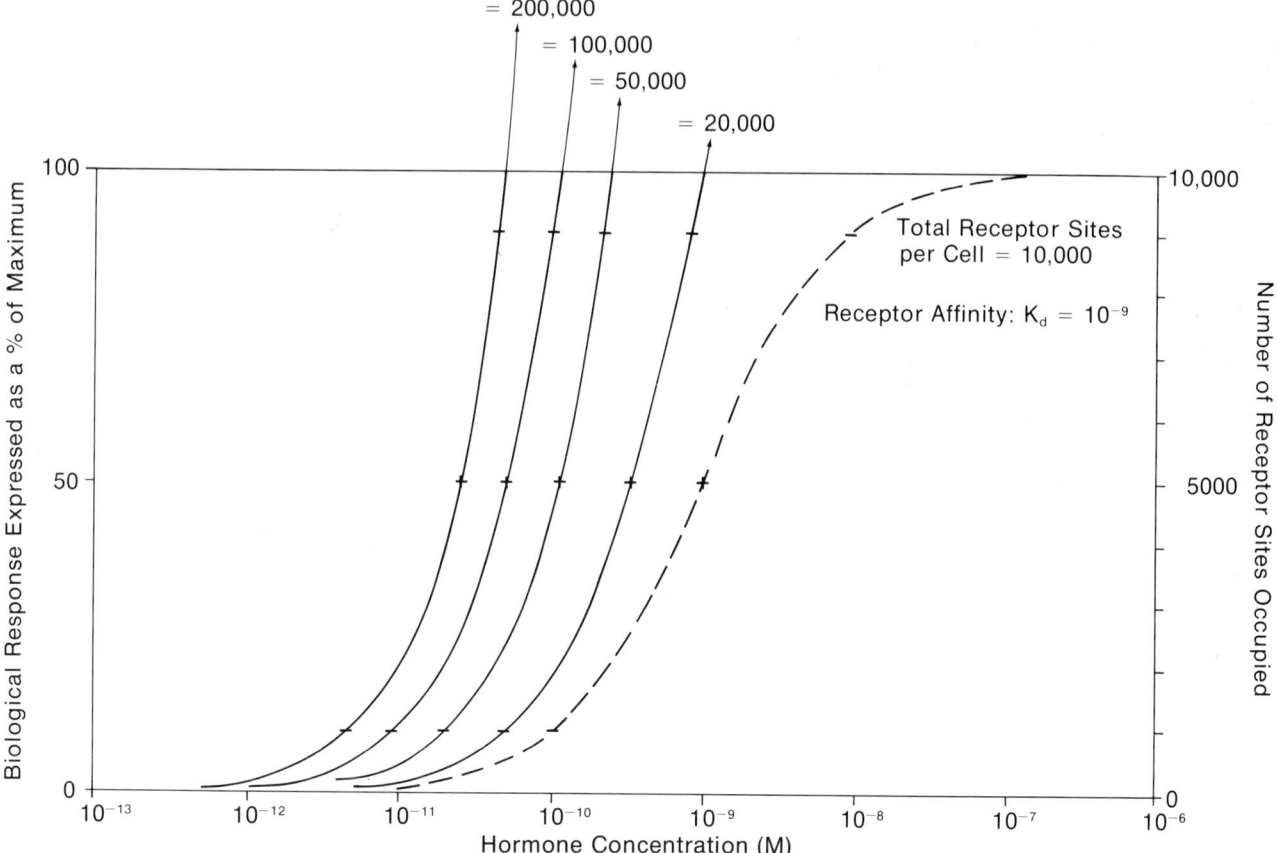

Figure 2-41. The original curve (----) is the same as before (10,000 receptors per cell, $K_d = 10^{-9}$, and the maximal response is achieved with 10,000 receptors occupied). When receptors are increased in number (all else unchanged), the biological response curve shifts to the left and is steeper. The maximal biological response is the same as before, and occurs when 10,000 receptor sites are occupied. However, the larger number of receptor sites permits 10,000 receptors to be occupied at lower concentrations of hormone.

Receptors/Cell	Capacity to Stimulate / Capacity to Respond	Degree of Spareness of Receptors	[H] Needed To Achieve 50% of Maximal Response
10,000	1	0	1.0×10^{-9}
20,000	2	50%	0.35×10^{-9}
50,000	5	80%	0.1×10^{-9}
100,000	10	90%	0.05×10^{-9}
200,000	20	95%	0.03×10^{-9}

Note the following: (1) All of the receptors are being used to achieve the heightened sensitivity; none are truly "spare." (2) The initial fivefold (and tenfold) increase in the number of receptors increases sensitivity tenfold (and twentyfold). (3) While the original dose-response curve (from 10% to 90% of the maximal effect, marked by small horizontal bars on each curve) covered two logs, the other curves cover one log or less. (4) The last three curves at the left are essentially parallel to one another, i.e., at this level of receptor number, a shift in receptor affinity and receptor number would be indistinguishable at steady state, but only the former would have kinetic consequences. (5) While the maximal capacity of the cell to stimulate may be uniform for all proximal (common) pathways, the maximal capacity of each distal (branched) pathway to respond may vary widely. Since the position of the biological response curve (relative to K_d of the receptor) will depend on the *ratio* of stimulatory-response capacity, each distal effect may have its own biological response curve.

of the distal steps to respond. Note that by simply increasing the receptor concentration, the biological response curve can be shifted indefinitely far to the left, and a hormone concentration of 10^{-12} M can be very effective despite an affinity that is quite low, e.g., $K_d = 10^{-9}$ ($K_a = 10^9$). Notice also that under these conditions changes in receptor concentration produce, at steady state, shifts in the curve that are indistinguishable from changes in affinity.

Where the curve sits (how far left) depends on the *ratio* of stimulatory capacity to response capacity. Since the position of a biological response curve depends on the ratio of stimulatory capacity to response capacity, the multiple effects in a given cell (E_1, E_2, E_3) can each have an individual curve although they share common sets of receptors and other proximal steps. Further note that all of the distal capacity is regulatable and usable.

Spare Receptors

The term spare receptors is used to denote the phenomenon that the maximal biological response is achieved at hormone concentrations where not all of the receptors are occupied. For example, we say there is 90% spareness if occupancy of 10% of the receptors produces the maximal biological effect. The term is misleading for several reasons. First, none of the receptors are spare — all are being used. When we say that 10% of the receptors are occupied, we really mean that all of the receptors are occupied 10% of the time. Second, the degree of spareness is not dependent on the absolute number or concentration of receptors but on the ratio of receptors to the capacity of the distal event to respond. In fact, the degree of spareness for a single cell varies from one response or effect to another. The advantages of this design (i.e., very high concentration of receptors relative to other elements of the system) are that it permits very wide shifts in the position of the biological response curve without changes in receptor affinity; it allows all of the distal capacity to be under hormonal regulation; it permits each of the multiple responses in a given cell to have its own dose-response curve; and it causes most of the secreted hormone to be receptor-bound even when the affinity (K) of the receptor is quite low.

Another advantage of this arrangement (receptor concentration > affinity > hormone concentration, and within the target cell having proximal capacity to stimulate, > distal capacity to respond) is that it adds a kinetic-time dimension to hormonal control over target cell responses. Keep in mind that the natural decay rates of all of the signal molecules (the hormone as well as the signal elements in the target cell) are very rapid. This is implicit in the finding that a given steady-state concentration of hormone produces a given steady-state effect, and changes in hormone concentration produce changes in effect; if the activated intermediates were very long-lived, any concentration of hormone sufficient to produce any finite [HR] would, in time, achieve the maximal effect.

To illustrate how spareness of receptors adds a kinetic-time dimension, let us observe the effect of short bursts of hormone secretion of fixed duration but of progressively increasing magnitude (Fig. 2–42). A small burst yields a small response of short duration; a greater burst of hormone yields greater responses but also of short duration, until we achieve a hormone level that produces the maximal response. Further increases in the magnitude of the hormone concentration produce further increases in [HR] but no further increases in the magnitude of the effect; but now, after hormone concentration falls to baseline levels, the response will continue for longer, because it will take longer for [HR] and other intermediates to decay to baseline levels. Thus, levels of [H] that achieve [HR] greater than those needed to produce the maximal effect (expressed per minute) do produce greater effects when measured as integrated effects. This was noted early during studies of *in vivo* action of ACTH. Small doses produce small increases in output of adrenal steroids per minute; larger doses produce a larger output per minute. Further increases in ACTH produce no further increases in output per minute but prolong the duration of the maximal effect. *In vivo*, when hormone concentrations vary widely and quickly, time (or duration of the elevation in hormone concentration) can be used to increase the net effect at the target cell. That the proximal events at the target cell can be stimulated further at a time when the distal response (per unit time) is maximal also

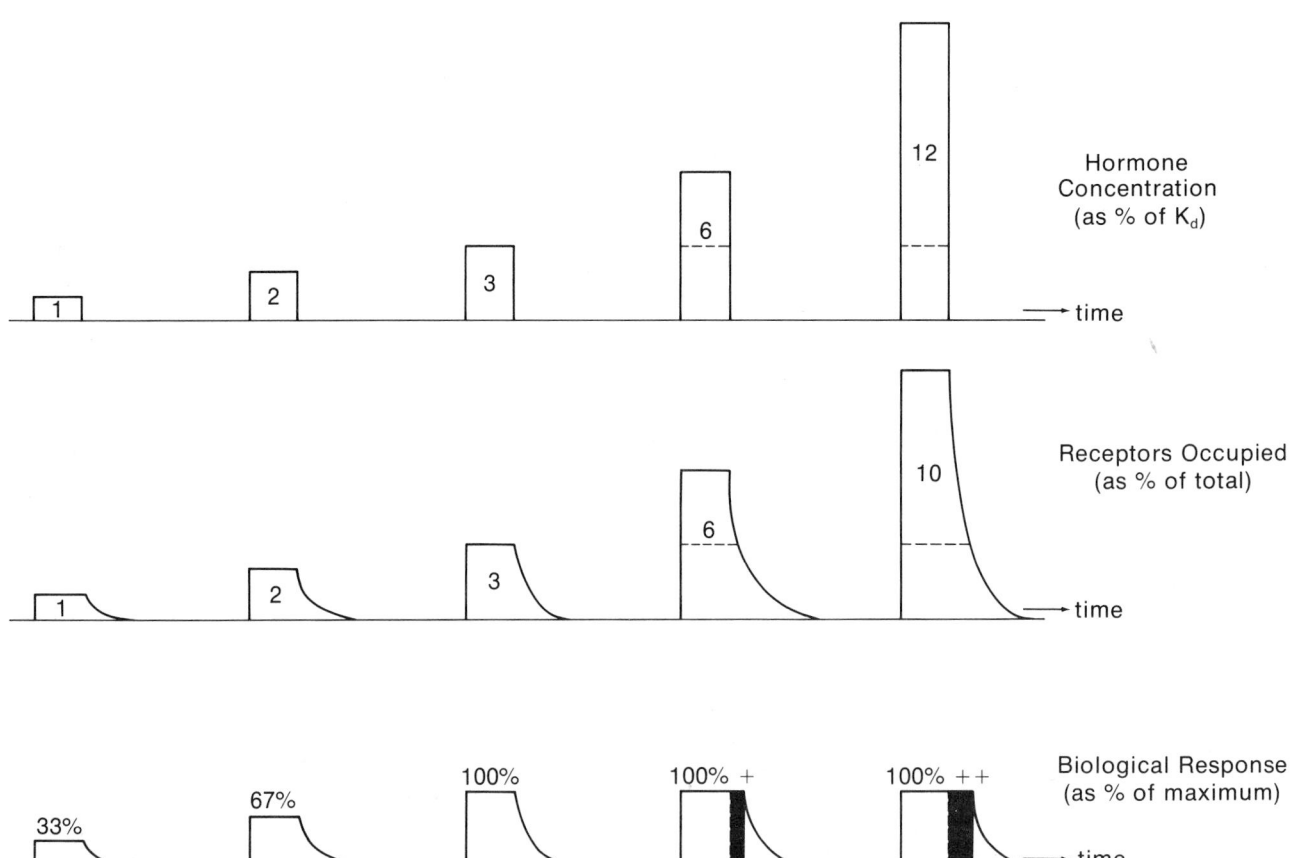

Figure 2–42. This figure shows the effect of spare receptors on the duration of the biological response. In this diagram, we relate hormone concentration, [H], to the concentration of occupied receptors, [HR], to the biological response as a function of time. In each case the target cell was exposed briefly to hormone. In this system, the biological response, expressed per unit time, is maximal when [H] = 3 units. Note that at [H] > 3 there is a further increase in receptor occupancy but no further increase in biological response per unit time, but the duration of the maximal response is prolonged (marked by the blackened area), and the integrated biological response is increased. In this exampler we selected the dissociation of hormone from receptor as the only element in the decay process that was slow enough to be measured. Since the hormone in the medium and post-receptor events in the target cell also have finite decay rates, the effect *in vivo* here would be even more marked than the effect we have schematically illustrated here.

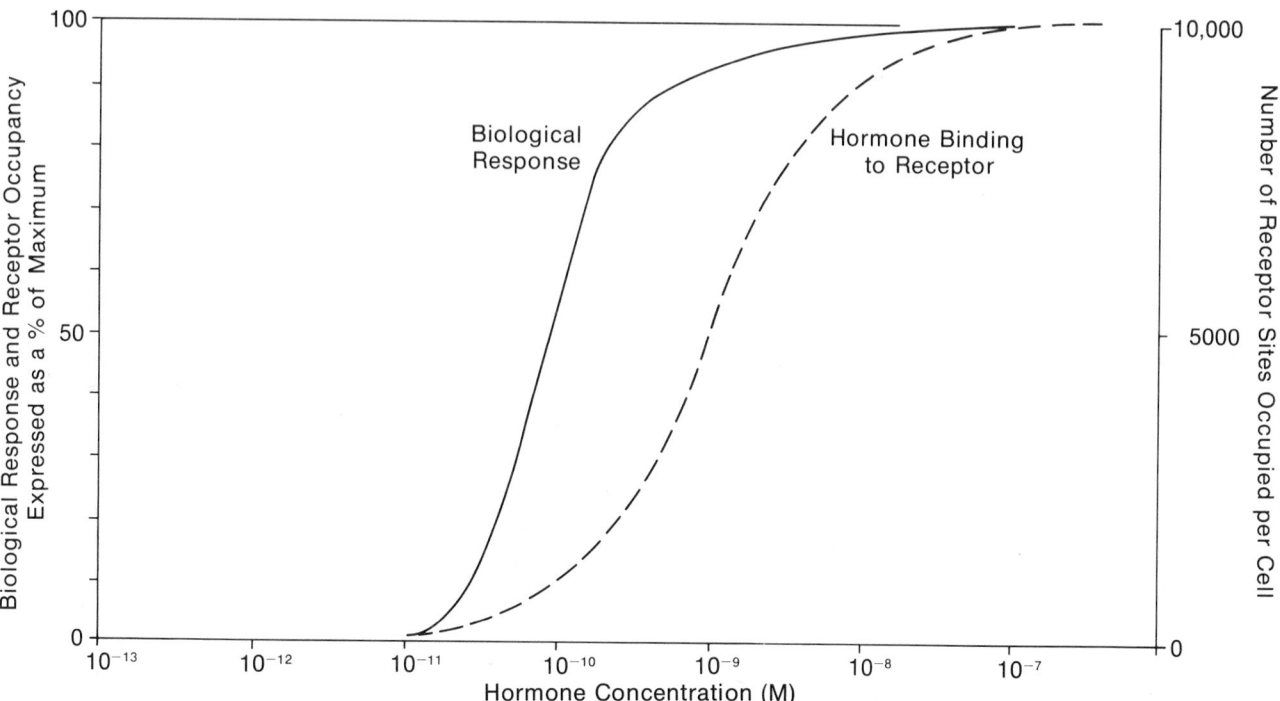

Figure 2–43. In this figure the curve representing the binding of hormone to receptor (----) is as before ($K_d = 10^{-9}$; 10,000 receptor sites per cell; all receptor sites need to be filled to achieve the maximal response — no spareness). However, in contrast to all of the previous figures in this group, where coupling was linear, coupling is more efficient, so that the biological response curve is more sensitive to small numbers of occupied receptors ("tight" coupling). Notice that an increase in coupling efficiency with no spareness of receptors produces an effect similar to that produced by simply increasing receptor number, i.e., "spare" receptors.

allows regulatory events — desensitization processes — to increase further as hormone concentration is increased further.

What is the relationship between [HR] and the early events in hormone action? For hormones that act through adenylate cyclase, multiple components are required: hormone receptors, G/F subunit, adenylate cyclase, cAMP-dependent kinases, and substrates. Different target organs vary in the amount of spareness at each of these steps. In virtually all systems maximal activation is achieved before the cAMP concentration reaches its limit. In general, the spareness between the first step (HR) and the final biological effect (E) is actually due to cumulative spareness generated at multiple steps between them.

In our analysis, we treated coupling as a constant and linearly related to [HR]. This need not be so (Fig. 2–43). In fact, the efficiency of coupling can be regulated and often is not linear; the coupling processes may be more effectively stimulated at low [HR] than at high [HR] or, less often, there may be a threshold effect — the response may be absent until a finite [HR] is achieved.

A Teleological Synthesis

To appreciate this design, let us consider what might happen when a new endocrine system evolves. First we need a pair of ligands (hormone and receptor) that have an affinity for one another. This happens because chemical groups in the two moieties can form enough noncovalent bonds to provide for binding. Most important, we need specificity; i.e., the match should be unique. This requires multiple binding sites in a precise three-dimensional arrangement. This matching to yield multiple bonds is the basis of both specificity and affinity. The fact that specificity, which

is so crucial, is linked to the absolute affinity of binding puts severe constraints on how much the affinity can be manipulated without altering specificity.

To convert a pair of matching ligands into an endocrine system requires that a unique cell type devote a major portion of its efforts to producing hormone so that it can make enough hormone to fill the extracellular fluid space with hormone at an effective concentration. To achieve meaningful concentrations of hormone in plasma, synthesis and secretion can be increased, or degradation minimized. However, rapid responsiveness of the system requires that the hormone concentration be rapidly changeable. That requires high rates of secretion (and synthesis) as well as rapid degradation. What are the relative limitations of [H] and [R]? Given the desirability of a rapid rate for hormone degradation, the limits on hormone concentration are then determined by how much of an endocrine cell's total metabolism can be diverted to hormone production (typically a very large fraction) and what fraction of the total cells of the body differentiate into cells that produce that hormone (typically a small fraction). On the other hand, receptors typically represent only a small minority ($\ll 1\%$) of the total protein of the cell and can be turned over much more slowly without loss of flexibility, so that receptor production is a much smaller burden on the target cell's activities than is hormone production for the hormone-producing cell. Under most conditions *in vivo*, the concentration of [HR] is the product of $K \times [H] \times [R]$. Given the limitations imposed on K, which is often low, and the limitations on [H], if rapid degradation is to be achieved, then the burden falls on [R]; it is increased to permit low [H] and low K to work.

Having a teleological rationalization for the relationship between [H], K, and [R], the reader may now find it easier, in reviewing the earlier discussion, to appreciate the relationship of [HR] to post-receptor events and in general of having the maximal capacity of each step exceed the maximal capacity of the step that follows. A more detailed and erudite discussion is provided by Stadtman and Chock.

Summary

The exquisite control by hormones of biological events depends on the quantitative relationship among the individual elements of the system. Some typical features include: (1) $[H] < K_d < [R]$; (2) the capacity of the proximal target cell elements to stimulate exceeds by far the capacity of the distal target cell elements to respond; (3) at the target cell, in general, the maximal capacity of one (proximal) step exceeds that of the next (distal) step; and (4) decay of the activated elements is rapid. For regulation, hormone concentration is varied widely, as is receptor concentration. Receptor affinity is regulated much more narrowly to regulate the rate of hormone dissociation and for more subtle adjustments, as are early coupling steps. Individual distal pathways can be regulated widely, independent of one another. Finally, it should be appreciated that investigators try to study the system at steady state but *in vivo* it is always dynamic, and kinetic considerations are of great importance.

AN INVITATION TO THE CLINICIAN

Endocrinology is a discipline in which biochemistry and physiology can be related closely to each other and to clinical medicine. In managing a patient with an endocrine-related disorder, the physician must continuously keep in mind this interplay of science and medicine. While obviously useful in dealing with known disorders, the principles presented here on biochemical mechanisms and endocrine disorders should be even more useful when the physician encounters in a patient a disorder that does not appear to match one of the known disease entities or when the observed pathophysiology fails to conform to known patterns. It is here that principles and patterns of biochemistry or pathophysiology derived elsewhere can lead to creative (and carefully considered) extrapolations to novel situations. The physician at the bedside should continuously be alert to the possibility that the observed disorder is as yet unmapped and should be prepared to enlist the aid of scientific colleagues to map these unexplored regions of clinical medicine. Good luck!

REFERENCES

Peptide Hormones and Catecholamines

CELL MEMBRANE STRUCTURE AND FUNCTION

1. Singer, S. J., and Nicolson, G. L.: The fluid mosaic model of the structure of cell membranes. *Science* 175:720–731, 1972.
2. Rothman, J. E., and Lenard, J.: Membrane asymmetry. *Science* 195: 743–753, 1977.
3. Shattil, S. J., and Cooper, R. A.: Role of membrane lipid composition, organization and fluidity in human platelet function. *Prog. Hemost. Thromb.* 4:59–86, 1978.
4. Cooper, R. A., and Shattil, S. J.: Membrane cholesterol — is enough too much? *New Engl. J. Med.* 302:42–51, 1980.
5. Lodish, H. F., and Rothman, J. E.: The assembly of cell membranes. *Sci. Am.* 240:48–63, 1979.

6. den Kamp, J. A. F. O.: Lipid asymmetry in membranes. *Ann. Rev. Biochem.* 48:47–71, 1979.

RECEPTORS, RECEPTOR REGULATION, AND DISEASES

7. Roth, J., Lesniak, M. A., Bar, R. S., Muggeo, M., Megyesi, K., Harrison, L. C., Flier, J. S., Wachslight-Rodbard, H., and Gordon, P.: An introduction to receptors and receptor disorders. *Proc. Soc. Exp. Biol. Med.* 162:3–12, 1979.
8. Roth, J.: Insulin binding to its receptor: Is the receptor more important than the hormone? *Diabetes Care* 4:27–32, 1981.
9. Catt, K. J., Harwood, J. P., Aquilera, G., and Dufau, M. L.: Hormonal regulation of peptide receptors and target cell responses. *Nature* 280:109–116, 1979.
10. Lefkowitz, R. J., Wessels, M. R., and Stadd, J. M.: Hormones, receptors and cyclic AMP: Their role in target cell refractoriness. *Curr. Top. Cell. Regul.* 17:205–230, 1980.
11. Gorden, P., Carpentier, J. L., Freychet, P., and Orci, L.: Internalization of polypeptide hormones: Mechanism, intracellular localization and significance. *Diabetologia* 18:263–274, 1980.
12. Dufau, M. L., and Catt, K. J.: Gonadotropin receptors and regulation of steroidogenesis in the testes and ovary. *Vitam. Horm.* 36:461–592, 1978.
13. Means, A. R., Dedman, J. R., Tash, J. S., Tindall, M. V. S., and Welsh, M. J.: Regulation of testis Sertoli cell by follicle stimulating hormone. *Ann. Rev. Physiol.* 42:59–70, 1980.
14. Goldstein, J. L., and Brown, M. S.: The low-density lipoprotein pathway and its relationship to atherosclerosis. *Ann. Rev. Biochem.* 46:897–930, 1977.
15. Brown, M. S., Kovanen, P. T., and Goldstein, J. L.: Receptor-mediated uptake of lipoprotein-cholesterol and its utilization for steroid synthesis in the adrenal cortex. *Recent Prog. Horm. Res.* 35:215–249, 1979.

ANTI-RECEPTOR ANTIBODIES

16. Flier, J. S., Kahn, C. R., and Roth, J.: Receptors, antireceptor antibodies and mechanisms of insulin resistance. *New Engl. J. Med. 300*: 413–419, 1979.
17. Kahn, C. R.: The role of insulin receptors and receptor antibodies in states of altered disease. *Proc. Soc. Exp. Biol. Med.* 162:13–21, 1979.
18. Harrison, L. C., Van Obberghen, E., Grunfeld, C., King, G. L., and Kahn, C. R.: Modulation of the insulin receptor by insulin receptor autoantibodies. *Prog. Clin. Biol. Res.* 42:109–126, 1980.
19. Venter, J. C., Fraser, C. M., and Harrison, L. C.: Autoantibodies to β_2 adrenergic receptors: A possible cause of adrenergic hyporesponsiveness in allergic rhinitis and asthma. *Science* 207:1361–1363, 1980.
20. Mehdi, S. Q., and Kriss, J. P.: Preparation of radiolabeled thyroid stimulation immunoglobulins (TSI) by recombining TSI heavy chains with ^{125}I-light chains: Direct evidence that product binds to membrane thyrotropin receptor and stimulates adenylate cyclase. *Endocrinology* 103:296–301, 1978.
21. McKenzie, J. M., Zakarija, M., and Sato, A.: Humoral immunity in Graves' disease. *Clin. Endocrinol. Metab.* 7:31–46, 1978.
22. Kidd, A., Okita, N., Row, V. V., and Volpé, R.: Immunologic aspects of Graves' and Hashimoto's diseases. *Metabolism* 29:80–99, 1980.
23. Drachman, D. B.: Myasthenia gravis. *New Engl. J. Med.* 298:136–142, 186–193, 1978.
24. Drachman, D. B.: Acetylcholine receptors and myasthenia gravis. *Proc. Soc. Exp. Biol. Med.* 162:22–30, 1979.

SPECIFICITY SPILLOVER AND ECTOPIC RECEPTORS

25. Higgins, H. P., and Hershman, J. M.: The hyperthyroidism due to trophoblastic hormone. *Clin. Endocrinol. Metab.* 7:167–175, 1978.
26. Roth, J., Lesniak, M. A., Megyesi, K., and Kahn, C. R.: Hormone receptors, human disease and disorders in receptor design. In: *Hormones and Cell Culture,* Book, A., Sato, G. H., and Ross, R. (eds.), Cold Spring Harbor Conferences on Cell Proliferation, Vol. 6, 1979, pp. 167–186.
27. Schorr, I., and Ney, R. L.: Abnormal hormone responses of an adrenocortical cancer adenyl cyclase. *J. Clin. Invest.* 50:1295–1300, 1971.
28. Matsukura, S., Kakita, T., Hirata, Y., Yoshimi, H., Fukase, M., Iwasaki, Y., Kato, Y., and Imura, H.: Adenylate cyclase of GH and ACTH producing tumors of human: Activation by non-specific hormones and other bioactive substances. *J. Clin. Endocrinol. Metab.* 44: 392–397, 1977.
29. Williams, L. T., Gore, T. B., and Lefkowitz, R. J.: Ectopic β-adrenergic receptor binding sites: Possible molecular basis of aberrant catecholamine responsiveness of an adrenocortical tumor adenylate cyclase. *J. Clin. Invest.* 59:319–324, 1977.

CYCLIC AMP AND PHOSPHORYLATION

30. Robison, G. A., Butcher, R. W., and Sutherland, E. W.: *Cyclic AMP.* New York, Academic Press, 1971.

31. Ross, E. M., and Gilman, A. G.: Biochemical properties of hormone-sensitive adenylate cyclase. *Ann. Rev. Biochem. 49*:533–565, 1980.
32. Abramowitz, J., Iyengar, R., and Birnbaumer, L.: Guanyl nucleotide regulation of hormonally responsive adenylate cyclase. *Mol. Cell. Endocrinol. 16*:129–146, 1979.
33. Rodbell, M.: The role of hormone receptors and GTP-regulatory proteins in membrane transduction. *Nature 284*:17–22, 1980.
34. Levitzki, A.: The β-adrenergic receptor and its mode of coupling to adenylate cyclase. *CRC Crit. Rev. Biochem. 10*:81–112, 1981.
35. Moss, J. M., and Vaughn, M.: Activation of adenylate cyclase by choleragen. *Ann. Rev. Biochem. 48*:581–600, 1979.
36. Chasin, M., and Harris, D. N.: Inhibitors and activators of cyclic nucleotide phosphodiesterase. *Adv. Cyclic Nucleotide Res. 7*:225–264, 1976.
37. Wells, J. N., and Hardman, J. G.: Cyclic nucleotide phosphodiesterases. *Adv. Cyclic Nucleotide Res. 8*:119–143, 1977.
38. Stadtman, E. R., and Chock, P. B.: Interconvertible enzyme cascades in metabolic regulation. *Curr. Top. Cell. Regul. 13*:53–97, 1978.
39. Steinberg, D.: Interconvertible enzymes in adipose tissue regulated by cyclic AMP-dependent protein kinase. *Adv. Cyclic Nucleotide Res. 7*:157–197, 1976.
40. Nimmo, H. A., and Cohen, P.: Hormonal control of protein phosphorylation. *Adv. Cyclic Nucleotide Res. 8*:145–266, 1977.
41. Rosen, O. M., Rangel-Aldao, R., and Erlichman, J.: Soluble cyclic AMP-dependent protein kinases: Review of the enzyme isolated from bovine cardiac muscle. *Curr. Top. Cell. Regul. 12*:39–74, 1977.
42. Roach, P. J., and Larner, J.: Covalent phosphorylation in the regulation of glycogen synthase activity. *Mol. Cell. Biochem. 15*:179–200, 1977.
43. Cohen, P.: The role of cyclic AMP-dependent protein kinase in the regulation of glycogen metabolism in mammalian skeletal muscle. *Curr. Top. Cell. Regul. 14*:118–196, 1978.
44. Soderling, T. R.: Regulatory functions of protein multisite phosphorylation. *Mol. Cell. Endocrinol. 16*:157–179, 1979.
45. Krebs, E. G., and Beavo, J. A.: Phosphorylation-dephosphorylation of enzymes. *Ann. Rev. Biochem. 48*:923–959, 1979.
46. Curnow, R. T., and Larner, J.: Hormonal and metabolic control of phosphoprotein phosphatase. In *Biochemical Actions of Hormones*. Vol. VI. Litwack, A. (ed.), New York, Academic Press, 1979, pp. 77–119.

OTHER INTRACELLULAR MESSENGERS

47. Rasmussen, H., and Goodman, D. B. P.: Relationships between calcium and cyclic nucleotides in cell activation. *Physiol. Rev. 57*:421–509, 1977.
48. Assimacopoulos-Jeannet, F. D., Blackmore, P. F., and Exton, J. H.: Studies on α-adrenergic activation of hepatic glucose output: Studies on the role of calcium in α-adrenergic activation of phosphorylase. *J. Biol. Chem. 252*:2662–2669, 1977.
49. Wang, J. H., and Wassman, D. M.: Calmodulin and its role in the second messenger system. *Curr. Top. Cell. Regul. 15*:47–108, 1979.
50. Means, A. R., and Dedman, J. R.: Calmodulin in endocrine cells and its multiple roles in hormone action. *Mol. Cell. Endocrinol. 19*:215–228, 1980.
51. Kretsinger, R. H.: Structure and evolution of calcium-modulated proteins. *CRC Crit. Rev. Biochem. 8*:119–174, 1980.
52. Cohen, P., Klee, C. B., Dicton, C., and Shenolikar, S.: Calcium control of muscle phosphorylase kinase through the combined action of calmodulin and troponin. *Ann. N.Y. Acad. Sci. 356*:151–161, 1980.
53. Cheung, W. Y.: Calmodulin plays a pivotal role in cellular regulation. *Science 207*:19–27, 1980.
54. Klee, C. B., Crouch, T. H., and Richman, P. G.: Calmodulin. *Ann. Rev. Biochem. 49*:489–516, 1980.
55. Goldberg, N. D., and Haddox, M. K.: Cyclic GMP metabolism and involvement in biological regulation. *Ann. Rev. Biochem. 46*:823–896, 1977.
56. Kuo, J. F., Shoji, M., and Kuo, W. N.: Molecular and physiopathologic aspects of mammalian cyclic GMP-dependent protein kinase. *Ann. Rev. Pharmacol. Toxicol. 18*:341–355, 1978.
57. Murad, F., Arnold, W. P., Mittal, C. F., and Braughler, J. M.: Properties and regulation of guanylate cyclase and some proposed functions for cyclic GMP. *Adv. Cyclic Nucleotide Res. 11*:175–204, 1979.
58. Jarrett, L., and Seals, J. R.: Pyruvate dehydrogenase activation in adipocyte mitochondria by an insulin-generated mediator from muscle. *Science 206*:1407–1408, 1979.
59. Larner, J., Galasko, G., Cheng, K., DePaoli-Roach, A. A., Huang, L., Daggy, P., and Kellogg, J.: Generation by insulin of a chemical mediator that controls protein phosphorylation and dephosphorylation. *Science 206*:1408–1410, 1979.
60. Czech, M. P.: Insulin action and the regulation of hexose transport. *Diabetes 29*:399–409, 1980.
61. Hirata, F., and Axelrod, J.: Phospholipid methylation and biological signal transmission. *Science 209*:1082–1090, 1980.
62. Monacada, S., and Vane, J. J.: Pharmacology and endogenous roles of prostaglandin endoperoxides, thromboxane A$_2$ and prostacyclin. *Pharmacol. Rev. 30*:293–331, 1978.
63. Samuelsson, B.: Prostaglandins and thromboxanes. *Recent Prog. Horm. Res. 34*:239–253, 1978.
64. Harris, R. H., Ramwell, P., and Gilmer, P. J.: Cellular mechanisms of prostaglandin action. *Ann. Rev. Physiol. 41*:653–668, 1979.
65. Lands, W. E. M.: The biosynthesis and metabolism of prostaglandins. *Ann. Rev. Physiol. 41*:633–652, 1979.

DISEASE APPLICATIONS

66. Kahn, C. R., Megyesi, K., Bar, R. S., and Flier, J. S.: Receptors for peptide hormones: New insights into the pathophysiology of disease states in man. *Ann. Intern. Med. 86*:205–219, 1977.
67. Olefsky, J. M.: Insulin resistance and insulin action: An *in vitro* and *in vivo* perspective. *Diabetes 30*:148–162, 1981.
68. Williams, L. T., Lefkowitz, R. J., Watanabe, A. M., Hathaway, D. R., and Besch, H. R., Jr.: Thyroid hormone regulation of β-adrenergic receptor number. *J. Biol. Chem. 252*:2787–2789, 1977.
69. Malbon, C. C., Moreno, F. J., Cabelli, R. J., and Fain, J. N.: Fat cell adenylate cyclase and β-adrenergic receptors in altered thyroid states. *J. Biol. Chem. 253*:671–678, 1978.
70. Levine, M. A., Downs, R. W., Jr., Singer, M., Marx, S. J., Aurbach, G. D., and Spiegel, A. M.: Deficient activity of guanine nucleotide regulatory protein in erythrocytes from patients with pseudohypoparathyroidism. *Biochem. Biophys. Res. Comm. 94*:1319–1324, 1980.
71. Farfel, Z., Brickman, A. S., Kaslow, H. R., Brothers, V. M., and Bourne, H. R.: Defect of receptor-cyclase coupling in pseudohypoparathyroidism. *New Engl. J. Med. 303*:237–242, 1980.

Steroid Hormones, Sterols, and Iodothyronines

GENE EXPRESSION

72. Watson, J. D.: *The Molecular Biology of the Gene*. 3rd ed., Menlo Park, CA, W. A. Benjamin, 1976.
73. Baxter, J. D., and Ivarie, R. D.: Regulation of gene expression by glucocorticoid hormones. In *Receptors and Hormone Action*. Vol. II. O'Malley, B. W. and Birnbaumer, L. (eds.), New York, Academic Press, 1978, pp. 251–296.
74. O'Malley, B. W., Roop, D. R., Lai, E. C., Nordstrum, J. L., Catterall, J. F., Swaneck, G. E., Colbert, D. A., Tsai, M. J., Dugalczyk, A., and Woo, S. L. C.: The ovalbumin gene: Organization, structure, transcription and regulation. *Recent Prog. Horm. Res. 35*:1–42, 1979.
75. Rosen, J. M., Matusik, R. J., Richards, D. A., Gupta, P., and Rodgers, J. R.: Multihormonal regulation of gene expression at the transcriptional and post transcriptional levels in the mammary gland. *Recent Prog. Horm. Res. 36*:157–187, 1980.
76. Leder, P., Konkel, D. A., Nishioka, N., Leder, A., Hamer, D. H., and Kaehler, M.: The organization and evolution of cloned globin genes. *Recent Prog. Horm. Res. 36*:241–257, 1980.

RECEPTORS AND MECHANISMS

77. O'Malley, B. W., and Schrader, W. T.: The receptors of steroid hormones. *Sci. Am. 234*:32–43, 1976.
78. Gorski, J., and Gannon, F.: Current models of steroid hormone action: A critical review. *Ann. Rev. Physiol. 38*:425–450, 1976.
79. Katzenellenbogen, B. S.: Dynamics of steroid hormone action. *Ann. Rev. Physiol. 42*:17–35, 1980.
80. Thompson, E. B., and Lippman, M. A.: Mechanism of action of glucocorticoids. *Metabolism 23*:159–202, 1974.
81. Baxter, J. D.: Glucorticoid hormone action. *Pharmacol. Ther. B 2*:605–659, 1976.
82. Munck, A., and Lering, K.: Glucocorticoid receptors and mechanisms of action. In *Receptors and Mechanisms of Action of Steroid Hormones*. Part 2. Pasqualine, J. R. (ed.), New York, Marcel Dekker, 1977, pp. 311–397.
83. Baxter, J. D., and Rousseau, G. G.: *Glucocorticoid Hormone Action*. Heidelberg, Springer-Verlag, 1978.
84. Feldman, D., Funder, J. W., and Edelman, I. S.: Subcellular mechanisms in the action of adrenal steroids. *Am. J. Med. 53*:545–560, 1972.
85. Chan, L., and O'Malley, B. W.: Mechanism of action of the sex steroids. *New Engl. J. Med. 294*:1322–1328, 1372–1381, 1976.
86. Mainwaring, W. I. P.: *The Mechanism of Action of Androgens*. Heidelberg, Springer-Verlag, 1977, pp. 1–172.
87. Clark, J. H., Markcaverich, B., Upchurch, S., Eriksson, H., Hardin, J. W., and Peck, E. J., Jr.: Heterogeneity of estrogen binding sites: Relationship to estrogen responses. *Recent Prog. Horm. Res. 36*:89–125, 1980.
88. Haussler, M. R., and McCain, T. A.: Basic and clinical aspects related to vitamin D metabolism and action. *New Engl. J. Med. 297*:974–983, 1041–1050, 1977.
89. Oppenheimer, J. H.: Thyroid hormone action at the cellular level. *Science 203*:971–979, 1979.

90. Baxter, J. D., Eberhardt, N. L., Apritelli, J. W., Johnson, L. K., Ivarie, R. D., Schachter, B. S., Morris, J. A., Seeburg, P. H., Goodman, H. M., Latham, K. R., Polansky, J. R., and Martial, J. A.: Thyroid hormone receptors and response. *Recent Prog. Horm. Res. 35*:97–146, 1979.

DISEASE APPLICATIONS

91. Lippman, M.: Steroid hormone receptors in human malignancy. *Life Sci. 15*:143–152, 1976.
92. Jensen, E. V., and De Sombre, E. R.: The diagnostic implications of steroid hormone binding in malignant tissues. *Adv. Clin. Chem. 19*:57–89, 1977.
93. McGuire, W. L.: Steroid hormone receptors and disease: Breast cancer. *Proc. Soc. Exp. Biol. Med. 162*:22–25, 1979.

94. McGuire, W. L.: Steroid hormone receptors in breast cancer treatment: Strategy. *Recent Prog. Horm. Res. 36*:135–146, 1980.
95. Bardin, C. W., Bullock, L. P., Sherins, R. J., Mowszowicz, I., and Blackburn, W. R.: Androgen metabolism and mechanism of action in male pseudohermaphroditism: A study of testicular feminization. *Recent Prog. Horm. Res. 29*:65–105, 1973.
96. Griffen, J. E., and Wilson, J. D.: The syndromes of androgen resistance. *New Engl. J. Med. 302*:198–209, 1980.
97. George, F. W., and Wilson, J. D.: Pathogenesis of the Henny feathering trait in the Sebright Bantam chicken. Increased conversion of androgen to estrogen in skin. *J. Clin. Invest. 66*:57–65, 1980.

CHAPTER 3

The Adenohypophysis

By William H. Daughaday

PITUITARY MORPHOLOGY

Anatomy

The pituitary gland is a complex structure lying in a bony walled cavity, the *sella turcica,* in the sphenoid bone at the base of the skull (Fig. 3–1). The sella turcica is separated superiorly from the cranial cavity by a tough reflection of the dura mater, the *diaphragma sellae,* through which the pituitary stalk and its attendant blood vessels reach the main body of the gland. The pituitary is a small organ with normal dimensions of about 10 mm × 13 mm × 6 mm and weighs about 0.5 g. The anterior lobe constitutes 75 % of the total weight of the gland. In women the gland increases in size during pregnancy and may approach 1 g in weight. The *pars intermedia,* which is present in the pituitary of most vertebrates, is virtually missing from the human pituitary. The terminology recommended by the International Commission on Anatomical Nomenclature is presented in Table 3–1.

The pituitary is formed early in embryonic life from the fusion of two ectodermal hollow processes of diverse origins. An evagination from the roof of the primitive oral region, Rathke's pouch, extends upward toward the base of the brain and is met by an outpouching of the floor of the third

ventricle, destined to become the neurohypophysis. Rathke's pouch undergoes much more extensive proliferation to form the anterior lobe. A pair of lateral buds arises from Rathke's pouch and extends superiorly to invest the neural stalk with cells that later become the *pars tuberalis.* In humans the pars tuberalis is a thin cloak of cells on the anterior surface of the stalk; in other species the pars tuberalis forms a complete collar about the neural stalk.

The lumen of Rathke's pouch is nearly obliterated by the proliferation of the anterior and posterior lobes of the hypophysis. It persists in adult human beings as small colloid-filled cysts and clefts at the juncture of the *pars distalis* and the neurohypophysis. The connection of Rathke's pouch with the oral cavity is separated by the developing sphenoid bone. Small remnants of tissue derived from Rathke's pouch, the so-called pharyngeal pituitary, may persist into adult life within or just below the sphenoid bone. These cells contain granules, and growth hormone (GH) and prolactin (PRL) have been detected by radioimmunoassay. It is speculated that the pharyngeal pituitary may be of secretory significance after removal of the main body of the pituitary gland.

Secretory granules appear in the fetal pituitary toward the end of the first trimester. At about the same time, several pituitary hormones can be detected by radioimmunoassay. The age at which hormonal secretion is initiated and main-

73

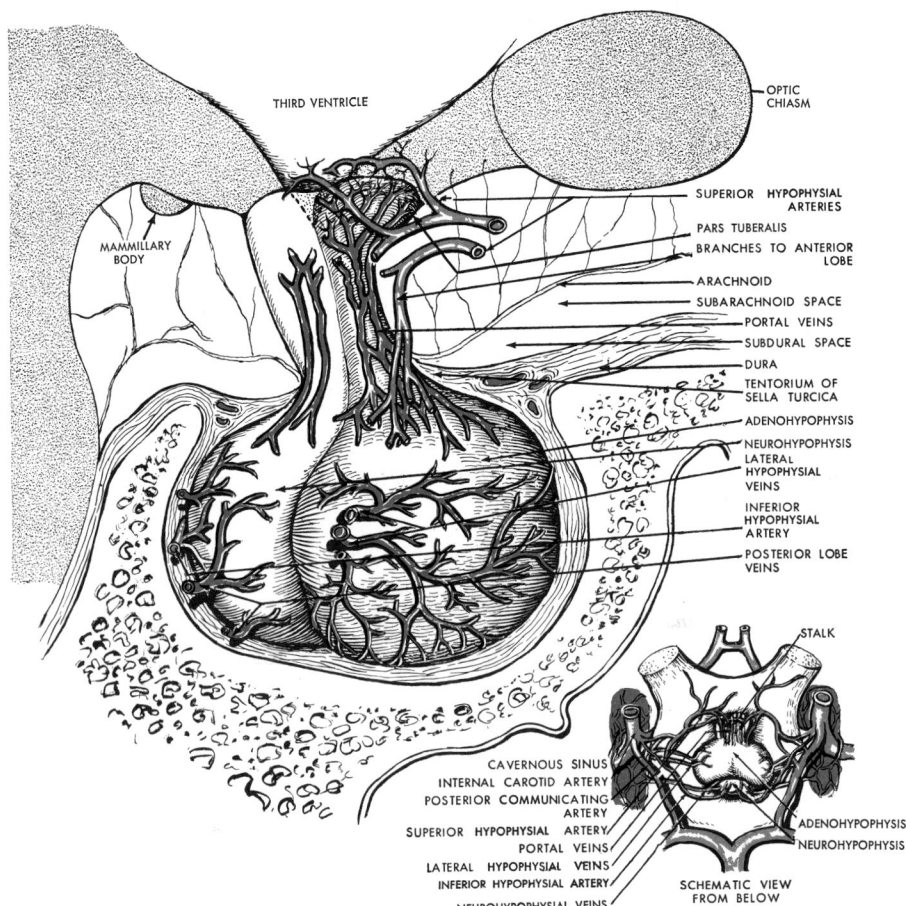

THIRD VENTRICLE

OPTIC CHIASM

SUPERIOR HYPOPHYSIAL ARTERIES
PARS TUBERALIS
BRANCHES TO ANTERIOR LOBE
ARACHNOID
SUBARACHNOID SPACE
PORTAL VEINS
SUBDURAL SPACE
DURA
TENTORIUM OF SELLA TURCICA
ADENOHYPOPHYSIS
NEUROHYPOPHYSIS
LATERAL HYPOPHYSIAL VEINS
INFERIOR HYPOPHYSIAL ARTERY
POSTERIOR LOBE VEINS

MAMMILLARY BODY

STALK

CAVERNOUS SINUS
INTERNAL CAROTID ARTERY
POSTERIOR COMMUNICATING ARTERY
SUPERIOR HYPOPHYSIAL ARTERY
PORTAL VEINS
LATERAL HYPOPHYSIAL VEINS
INFERIOR HYPOPHYSIAL ARTERY
NEUROHYPOPHYSIAL VEINS

ADENOHYPOPHYSIS
NEUROHYPOPHYSIS

SCHEMATIC VIEW FROM BELOW

Figure 3-1. Relationships of pituitary and its blood supply to neighboring structures. (Modified from drawing by Frank Netter. © Ciba Pharmaceutical Products.)

tained under feedback control has not been definitely established in man. In the case of corticotropin (ACTH), this control may be established by the 12th week. Evidence for this belief has been derived from an analysis of the genital lesions that occur in severe cases of the adrenogenital syndrome. The malformations of the labia and vagina result from excess ACTH stimulation of defective fetal adrenal secretion and excess androgenic steroid secretion at about the 12th week of gestation.

The pituitary receives its blood supply from two sources (Fig. 3–1). Arterial blood reaches it from branches of the superior hypophyseal artery, a branch of the internal carotid artery. Venous blood enters the pituitary by a physiologically important portal system that originates in specialized vascular structures of the median eminence, the gomitoli, which comprise short straight terminal arterioles with muscular walls surrounded by a dense capillary network. Blood from these capillaries is collected into long portal veins that course down the anterior surface of the pituitary stalk to drain into the sinusoidal capillaries of the anterior lobe. There are also short portal veins that originate in the neurohypophysis and terminate in the anterior lobe sinusoidal capillaries. Direct observation in the living animal has confirmed that the direction of blood flow in the portal veins is mainly from the median eminence to the pituitary. These vessels transport neurohumors from the hypothalamus to the adenohypophysis (see Chapter 11). Some studies suggest that there also may be retrograde flow from the adenohypophysis to the median eminence. If such flow exists, it could carry pituitary hormones that might influence hypothalamic function.

The detailed vascular organization within the pituitary gland has been clearly recognized only with the help of the electron microscope. The pituitary sinuses are lined with endothelium. Between the basement membrane of the sinusoidal endothelium and the parenchymal cells there exists a perisinusoidal space. Scattered cells with cytoplasmic projections, as well as extracellular granules believed to be extruded secretory granules from the pituitary parenchymal cells, are found in the perisinusoidal spaces.

Table 3–1. DIVISION OF PITUITARY GLAND*

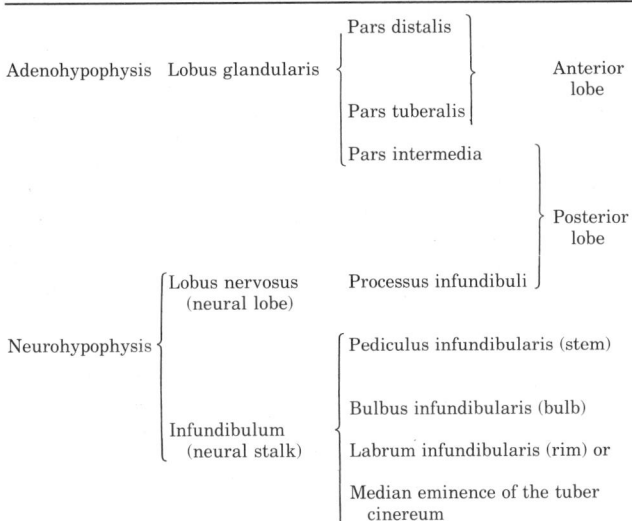

Adenohypophysis	Lobus glandularis	Pars distalis	Anterior lobe
		Pars tuberalis	
		Pars intermedia	
Neurohypophysis	Lobus nervosus (neural lobe)	Processus infundibuli	Posterior lobe
	Infundibulum (neural stalk)	Pediculus infundibularis (stem)	
		Bulbus infundibularis (bulb)	
		Labrum infundibularis (rim) or	
		Median eminence of the tuber cinereum	

*Terminology recommended by the International Commission on Anatomical Nomenclature.

The blood supply to the posterior lobe arises from the inferior hypophyseal arteries and is therefore largely separate from the blood supply to the anterior lobe. Venous blood from both pituitary lobes drains into the cavernous sinus by a number of veins.

The nerve supply of the anterior lobe is limited to fine nerves derived from the carotid plexus that accompany the arteriolar branches. These nerves appear to have a vasomotor function. A few neural fibers traversing from the posterior lobe to the anterior lobe have been described, but their significance in regulating adenohypophyseal function is denied by most authorities.

Cell Types

The human pituitary is a confederation of five largely independent functional units, each represented by a specific cell type synthesizing and, with one exception, releasing one or two pituitary hormones. The time-honored classification of pituitary cells into acidophil, basophil, and chromophobe types is clearly inadequate to explain the independent secretion of six major hormones and the secretion of other hormonal peptides whose physiologic significance remains to be established.

Despite the complexities of the cytologic classification of adenohypophyseal cell types, progress has been made by the application of histochemical, immunofluorescent, and electron microscopic techniques. The results of studies of a number of investigators have strengthened the concept that each major hormone is secreted by a distinct cell type, except that both gonadotropins are secreted by a single cell. It is logical to classify the pituitary cells on the basis of the hormone secreted. The following descriptions are derived primarily from the immunoelectron microscopic studies of Pelletier et al.[7]

Somatotroph Cells

The human somatotroph cells are easily recognized as numerous large, nearly round, membrane-bound secretory granules measuring 350 to 500 nm in diameter (Fig. 3–2). These cells are predominantly located in the lateral wings of the adenohypophysis.

Lactotroph Cells

Lactotroph cells can be distinguished from somatotroph cells by their affinity for erythrosin or carmosin stains. In the lateral wings of the human pituitary are a limited number of these cells, which react with immunofluorescent staining with antisera against PRL. The lactotroph cells contain secretory granules of about 275 to 350 nm in diameter that are generally round or slightly ovoid (Fig. 3–3).

The relative number of lactotroph cells is increased in fetal pituitaries and during pregnancy. This proliferation of lactotroph cells is the result of the very high concentration of circulating estrogens during human pregnancy.

Thyrotroph Cells

Positive identification of the human thyrotroph cells has been achieved by immunofluorescent staining. Thyrotroph cells, located predominantly in the central "mucoid" wedge of the adenohypophysis, are large and polyhedral. By electron microscopy the granules are small, 50 to 100 nm in diameter, and of inconstant electron density (Fig. 3–4).

In the thyroprivic state, striking changes occur in pituitary thyrotroph cells. The endoplasmic reticulum becomes greatly enlarged, forming cisternae that occupy most of the cytoplasm. Similar but less marked hypertrophy of the Golgi apparatus occurs. In addition, secretory granules virtually disappear from the cell, indicating that storage of

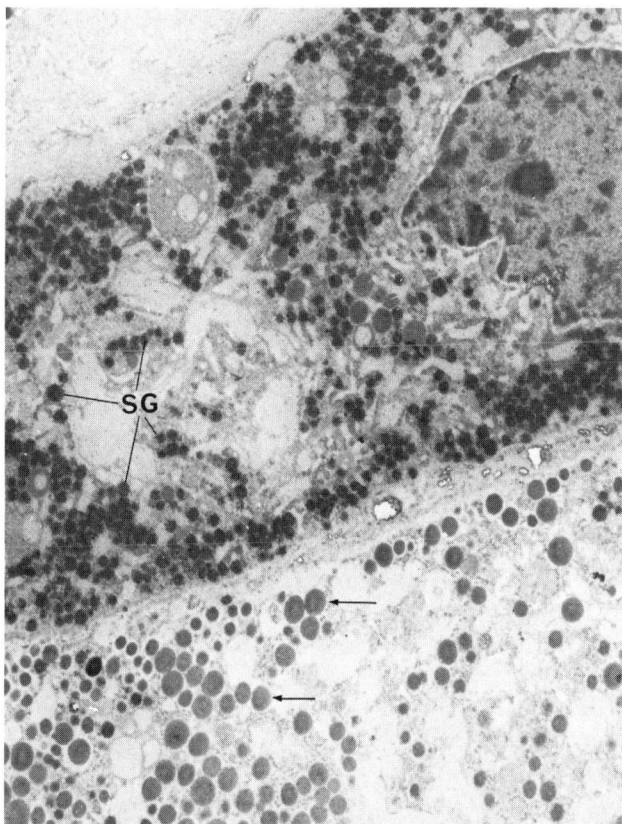

Figure 3–2. Immunohistochemical localization of GH in an ultrathin section from human pituitary. The accumulation of molecules of the peroxidase antiperoxidase complex indicating the presence of PRL can be observed on the secretory granules of a specific cell type. A weak diffuse reaction can also be seen in the cytoplasm. Magnification × 1600. (Reprinted by permission from G. Pelletier et al.: Identification of human anterior pituitary cells by immunoelectron microscopy. J. Clin. Endocrinol. *46*:534, 1978.)

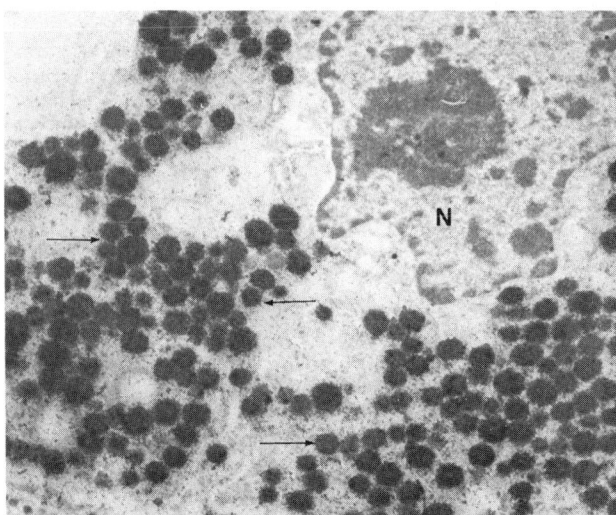

Figure 3–3. Localization of PRL. Reaction product is mainly concentrated in the secretory granules with some degree of diffusion in the cytoplasm. The nucleus (N) is completely free of reaction. The granules *(arrows)* of another cell type, probably a GH cell, are completely negative. Magnification × 11,000. (Reprinted by permission from G. Pelletier et al.: Identification of human anterior pituitary cells by immunoelectron microscopy. J. Clin. Endocrinol. *46*:534, 1978.)

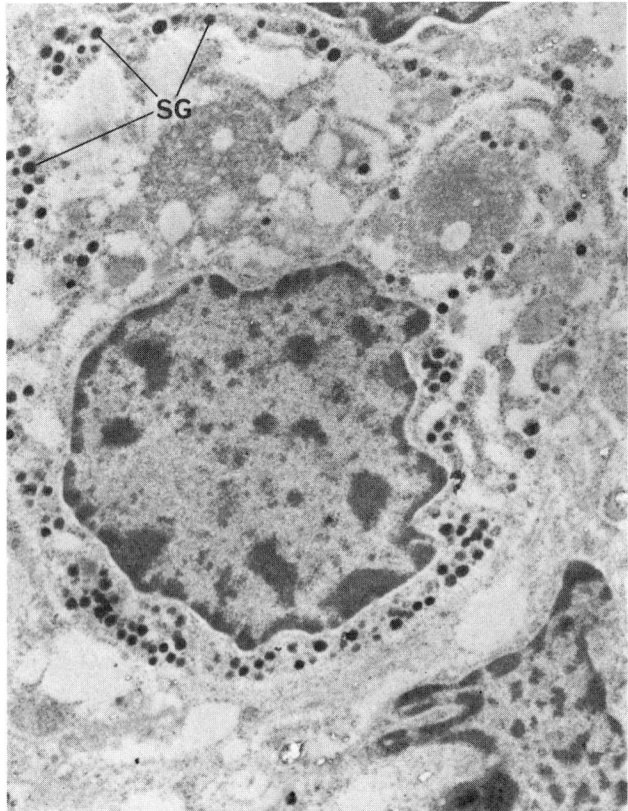

Figure 3–4. Localization of TSH-β in a cell characterized by small secretory granules. The positive reaction is restricted to the secretory granules (SG). Magnification × 15,000. (Reprinted by permission from G. Pelletier et al.: Identification of human anterior pituitary cells by immunoelectron microscopy. J. Clin. Endocrinol. 46:534, 1978.)

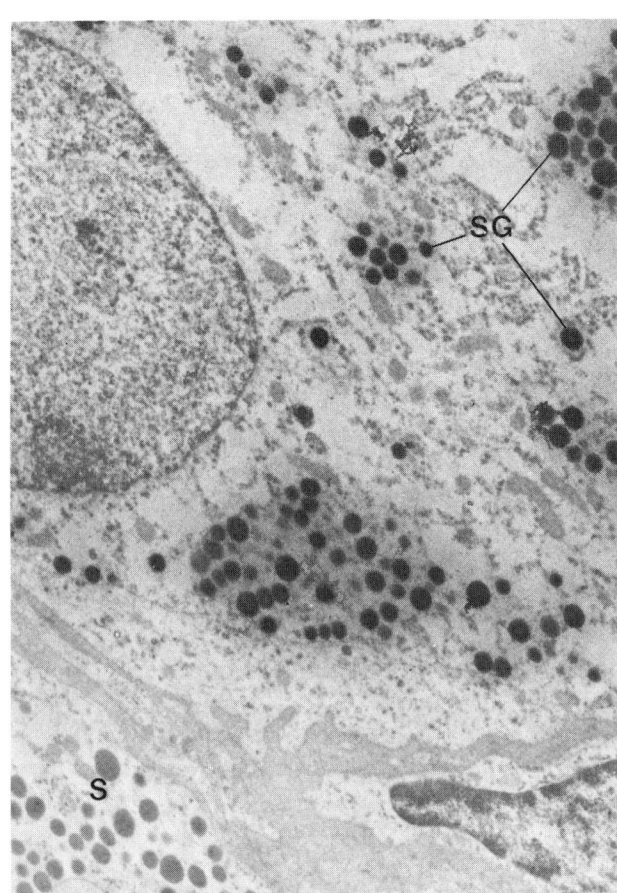

Figure 3–5. Localization of LH-β in a gonadotrophic cell. The secretory granules (SG) are immunostained. The same type was also shown to react with antibodies to FSH-β. Another cell type, probably a somatotroph (S), is completely negative. Magnification × 14,000. (Reprinted by permission from G. Pelletier et al.: Identification of human anterior pituitary cells by immunoelectron microscopy. J. Clin. Endocrinol. 46:534, 1978.)

hormone does not keep pace with secretion. The hypertrophied thyrotroph cells are easily recognized and are called "thyroidectomy cells."

Gonadotroph Cells

The human gonadotroph cell is most clearly recognized by immunofluorescent methods employing specific antisera raised against the β chain of LH or FSH. These cells are sparsely granulated, usually angular in shape, and distributed singly throughout the pituitary. By immunoelectron microscopy, the secretory granules range in diameter from 275 to 375 nm (Fig. 3–5). Nearly all cells react with both antisera, and it is concluded that a single gonadotroph cell secretes both LH and FSH.

Corticotroph-Lipotroph Cells

Identification of the cells of the human pituitary that secrete ACTH has been achieved by immunostaining. Immunoreactive cells are distributed throughout the pituitary. By immunoelectron microscopy, the secretory granules are large, 375 to 550 nm, and react with antibody more intensely at the periphery of the granules. These granules are the largest of any adenohypophyseal cell (Fig. 3–6).

ACTH is synthesized as a large precursor that contains not only ACTH but also β lipotropin, which contains the amino acid sequence of β MSH (see Fig. 3–7). This explains why antibodies directed against β MSH also stain corticotroph cells. Similar reactive cells are also present where the neuro-

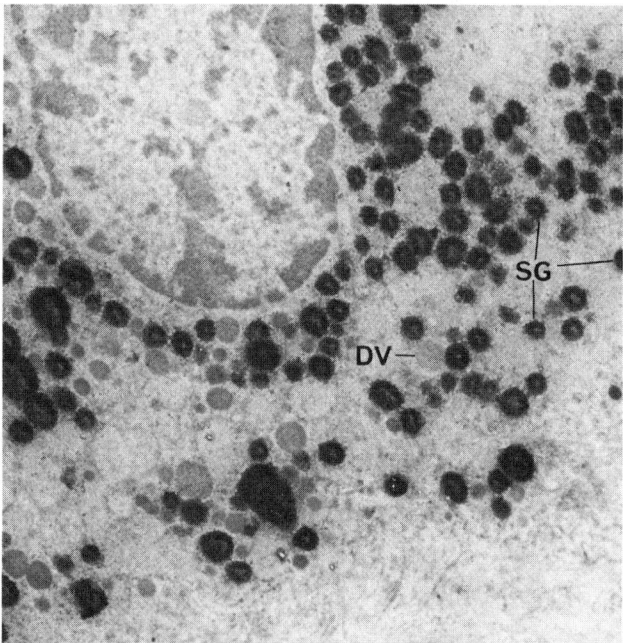

Figure 3–6. Pituitary cell that has been immunostained for ACTH. Many secretory granules (SG) are strongly labeled, the reaction being more intense at the periphery of the granules. Other dense vesicles (DV) are unstained. Magnification × 15,000. (Reprinted by permission from G. Pelletier et al.: Identification of human anterior pituitary cells by immunoelectron microscopy. J. Clin. Endocrinol. 46:534, 1978.)

hypophysis is in apposition to the adenohypophysis. These cells in the neurohypophysis may be the human counterpart to the pars intermedia. β endorphin has also been identified in corticotroph cells. Additional cells are also inconstantly present in the pars tuberalis.

The hyaline deposits that develop in corticotroph cells (Crooke's cells) in the presence of elevated plasma corticosteroid levels of any cause represent microtubular deposits and are not immunologically cross-reactive with ACTH antibodies.

Nonsecretory Cells

About one quarter of the pituitary cells do not stain with the usual histologic acid and basic stains and have been called chromophobe cells. When examined with an electron microscope, most of these cells contain a variable number of secretory granules. It is likely that most of these cells are degranulated secretory cells, many of them lactotroph cells.

Another cell of the human adenohypophysis is the follicular or stellate cell. These cells have long cell processes adjacent to perivascular spaces and other processes in contact with those from other stellate cells to form primitive pituitary follicles. In certain areas, microvilli and cilia may be present. There are few, if any, secretory granules seen by electron microscopy, and the function of stellate cells is still uncertain.

Pituitary Hormones

The human adenohypophysis contains six hormones of established functional significance. In addition, the pitu-

itary contains a number of smaller peptides of uncertain significance. These peptide and protein hormones as well as related hormones of the placenta can be assigned to three distinct families on the basis of molecular structure and biochemical evolution. Table 3-2 lists the members of the corticotropin, glycotropin, and somatotropin families and summarizes their basic chemical structure.

CORTICOTROPIN-RELATED PEPTIDE HORMONES

Structures

The corticotropin-related peptides compose a family of simple peptides that are synthesized as a single carbohydrate containing prohormone of about 31,000 daltons ("31 K" precursor) (Fig. 3-7). Within the large prohormone are the sequence of the 39 amino acids of ACTH and the 91 amino acids of β lipotropin (β LPH). This latter portion of the molecule is devoid of carbohydrate substituents. Conversion of the prohormone to ACTH and other biologically active peptides must require proteolytic cleavages of the prohormone molecule.

In many animal species, and probably also in the human fetus, ACTH is cleaved after the 13th amino acid to yield α MSH and a CLIP peptide representing amino acids 18–39 of the original ACTH molecule. Also, in nonhuman species, β LPH is cleaved to yield β MSH, which comprises amino acids 41–58 of the β LPH molecule. These cleavages occur predominantly in the intermediate lobe. This lobe is rudimentary in adult human beings and the formation of MSH in adult human beings does not occur to any significant extent.

β LPH is also subject to proteolytic cleavage to yield γ LPH

Table 3-2. HUMAN ADENOHYPOPHYSEAL AND RELATED PLACENTAL HORMONES

	Amino Acids	Carbohydrate	Molecular Weight
I. Corticotropin-related peptide hormones: Single small peptides derived from common precursor.			
1. α-Melanocyte-stimulating hormone (α MSH) (α Melanotropin*)	13 AA	O CHO	1,823
2. Corticotropin (ACTH)	39 AA	O CHO	4,507
3. γ Lipotropin (γ LPH)	58 AA	O CHO	5,810
4. β Lipotropin (β LPH‡)	91 AA	O CHO	9,500
II. Glycoprotein hormones: Composed of two dissimilar peptides. The α chain is similar in structure or identical. The β chain differs from each hormone and confers specificity.			
1. Follicle-stimulating hormone (FSH) (Follitropin*)	α 89 AA† β 115 AA	18% CHO 5% Sialic acid	32,000
2. Luteinizing hormone (LH) (Lutotropin*)	α 89 AA† β 115 AA	16% CHO 1% Sialic acid	32,000
3. Thyrotropin (TSH)	α 89 AA† β 112 AA	16% CHO 1% Sialic acid	32,000
4. Human chorionic gonadotropin (HCG) (Choriogonadotropin*)	α 92 AA β 144 AA	31% CHO 12% Sialic acid	46,000
III. Somatomammotropin hormones: Single peptide chains with 2 or 3 SS bonds. No carbohydrate.			
1. Prolactin (PRL)	198 AA	O CHO	23,510
2. Growth hormone (GH) or somatotropin	191 AA	O CHO	22,650
3. Chorionic somatomammotropin (CS) (Choriomammotropin*)	191 AA	O CHO	21,700

*IUPAC-IUB nomenclature not adopted in this book.

†The primary amino acid sequence of LH, FSH, and TSH is identical.

‡Precursor molecule of β MSH, the endorphins, and enkephalins; see Fig. 3-7. The hormonal status of these peptides in the pituitary has not been established.

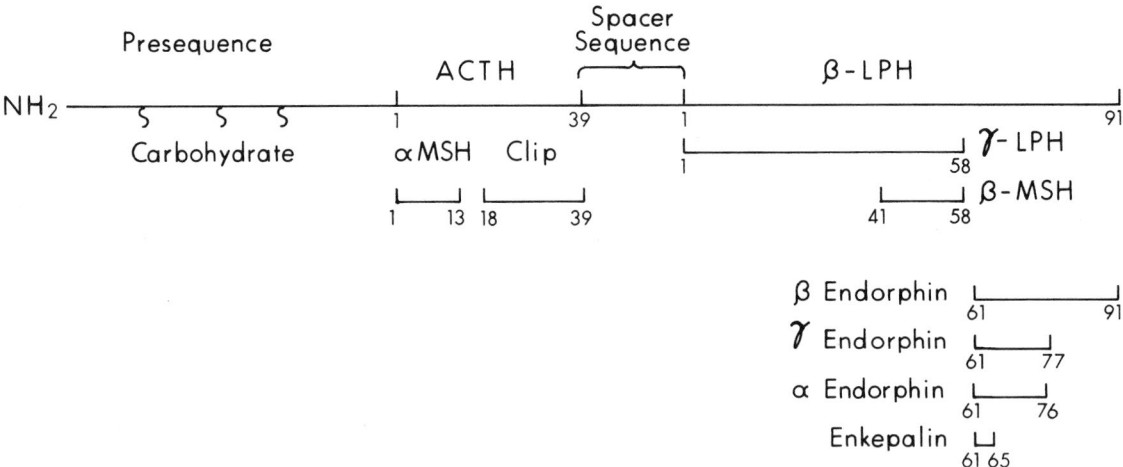

Figure 3–7. Diagrammatic representation of the proposed structure of the ACTH-LPH precursor molecule. (Modified from Roberts, J. L., and Herbert, E.: Characterization of a common precursor to corticotropin and beta-lipotropin: Identification of beta-lipotropin peptides and their arrangement relative to corticotropin in the precursor synthesized in a cell-free system. Proc. Natl. Acad. Sci. USA *74*:5300, 1977.)

(amino acids 1–58 of β LPH). These two substances constitute the major peptides of human serum reacting with the β MSH radioimmunoassay. Of great interest is the fact that the amino acids of β LPH contain the amino acid sequences of the opioid peptides, α endorphin (amino acids 61–76), γ endorphin (amino acids 61–77), and β endorphin (amino acids 61–91). These peptides are also formed in the brain by neurons composing a distinct peptidergic system related to pain perception (see Chapter 11). Although β endorphin is secreted in parallel with ACTH, the significance of pituitary secretion is as yet unestablished.

To summarize: Corticotropin-related peptides are synthesized as a single large molecular weight prohormone that is activated by proteolytic cleavage to yield ACTH, the LPH's, the MSH's, and the opioid peptides. The actual hormones secreted by individual cell types concerned with these hormones appear to be determined by post-translational proteolytic cleavage.

The amino acid sequences of human ACTH, α MSH, and simian β MSH are shown in Fig. 3–8. The homology between β MSH and ACTH suggests gene duplication. The minimum amino acid sequence required for melanocyte-stimulating activity is 4–10 of the ACTH molecule, which is present also as amino acids 7–13 of the β MSH molecule.

The minimum requirement for corticotropic action resides in the first 13 amino acids of ACTH, beginning with the N-terminal amino acid. The addition of amino acid residues 14 through 20 progressively increases biologic activity up to that of the native hormone. Synthetic ACTH peptide containing the first 24 amino acids is available for clinical use (cosyntropin). This peptide is fully active in stimulating corticosteroid secretion but does not react with most antibodies developed in rabbits against porcine ACTH. The most potent immunologic determinants reside in the carboxyl tail of the peptide chain representing amino acids 22–39.

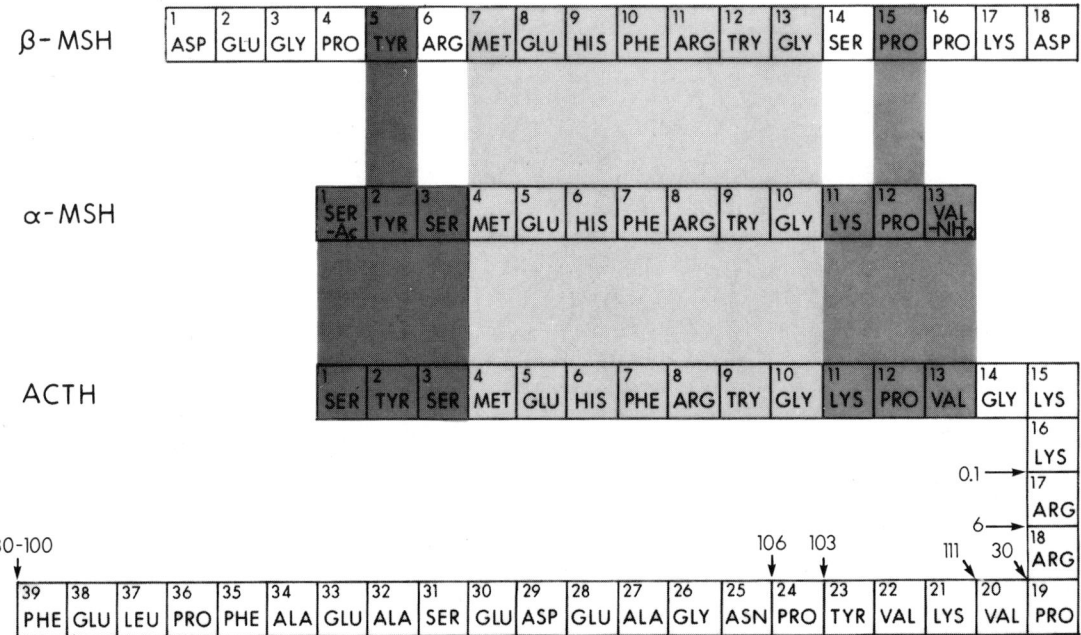

Figure 3–8. Structures of simian β MSH, α MSH, and human ACTH. The free amino end of each chain is residue No. 1. The figures are shaded to emphasize similar sequences of amino acids. The figures with arrows on the ACTH molecule indicate the biologic activity, according to Hofman, of the peptide beginning at the N terminal amino acid to the point indicated. The biologic activities are for porcine ACTH and may be presumed identical to human ACTH.

CORTICOTROPIN

Adrenal Actions

Corticotropin (ACTH) is bound by specific receptors on the surface of the adrenal cortical cell. The affinity of binding of these receptors for ACTH is high (association constant about 10^{12}), which permits concentration of ACTH from plasma. In the presence of calcium, the ACTH receptor complex activates adenyl cyclase, which in turn increases the concentration of cyclic AMP (cAMP) in the adrenal cell. The net result of increased intracellular cAMP is the phosphorylation of key enzymes and histones that leads to the biologic actions of the hormone. Increased steroidogenesis results from stimulation of the conversion of cholesterol to pregnenolone. The remaining enzymatic steps involved in formation of the 3-keto Δ 4–5 configuration in ring A and hydroxylations at 11 β, 21–OH, and 17 α-OH positions are not rate-limiting in the synthesis of cortisol. ACTH action also stimulates RNA synthesis and synthesis of new adrenal proteins. This increases the synthetic machinery of the adrenal cell and increases adrenal weight.

The marked depletion of adrenal ascorbic acid following ACTH administration remains largely unexplained despite the fact that this response provided the first practical end point for bioassay for ACTH. Ascorbic acid is not required for steroidogenesis, and the vitamin may actually inhibit steroidogenesis. Loss of ascorbic acid from the adrenal may facilitate hormonal synthesis.

Extra-Adrenal Actions

ACTH has a number of actions on isolated extra-adrenal tissues. It promotes lipolysis in fat cells and stimulates amino acid and glucose uptake in muscle. In addition, ACTH stimulates the pancreatic beta cell to secrete insulin and the somatotroph cells of the pituitary to secrete GH.

Although these varied extra-adrenal actions of ACTH attest to the versatility of the ACTH molecule, they are not evident at the plasma levels achieved during endogenous ACTH release. It is possible that the extreme hypersecretion of ACTH that occurs in certain pituitary tumors (see Nelson's syndrome) could be having extra-adrenal effects.

Pituitary Storage

The amount of ACTH stored in the adenohypophysis is small; the entire human gland contains only about 50 U or 0.25 mg, of the active peptide. The daily secretion only amounts to 1 to 5 U, but much larger amounts are secreted in conditions of stress.

Measurement

Although plasma ACTH was formerly measured by rat bioassays and radioreceptor assays, clinical measurement of plasma ACTH is now preformed by radioimmunoassay.

Plasma Concentration

As shown in Fig. 3–9, the plasma ACTH concentration of healthy adult subjects is usually less than 50 pg/ml. Hospitalized patients with the stress of nonendocrine illness may have plasma ACTH levels up to 600 pg/ml. Normally there

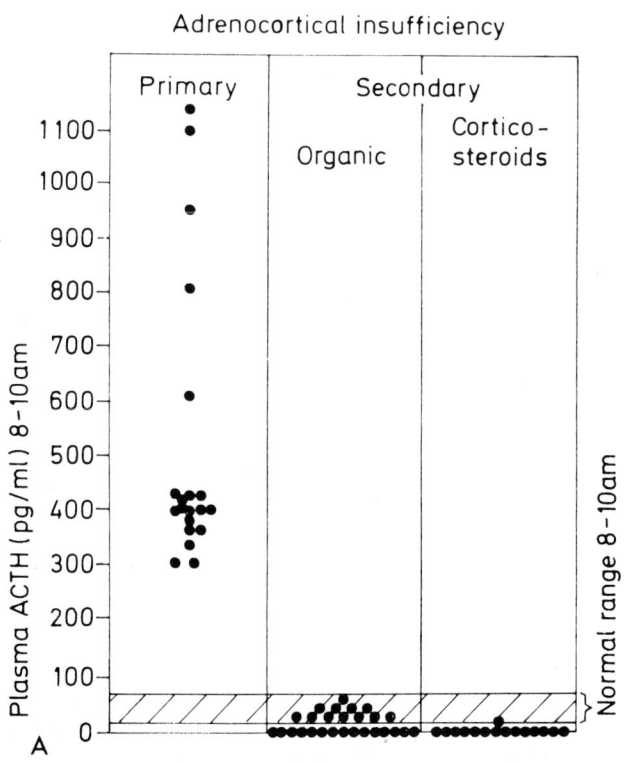

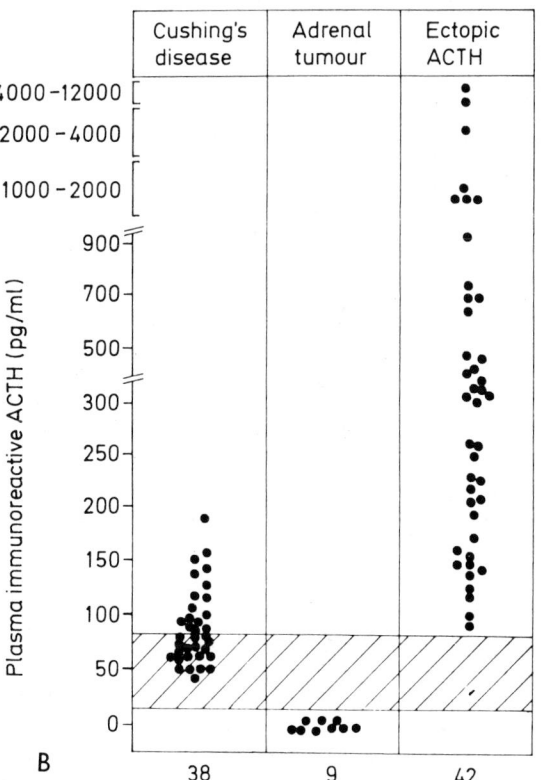

Figure 3–9. *A,* Measurements of plasma ACTH by radioimmunoassay in normal subjects (hatched area) and patients with adrenocortical insufficiency. *B,* Measurements in patients with different types of hyperadrenalcorticism. (*A* and *B* reproduced from Rees, L. H., Holdaway, I. M., et al.: ACTH secretion and clinical investigations. In *Some Aspects of Hypothalamic Regulation of Endocrine Functions.* Symposium, Vienna, June 3–6, 1973. F. K. Schattauer Verlag, Stuttgart, 1974, with permission.)

is a diurnal pattern of plasma ACTH, with the lowest levels reached between 6 PM and 11 PM. Plasma levels begin to rise in the early morning hours and reach a peak between 6 AM and 8 AM. The rise in plasma ACTH is closely followed by a rise in plasma cortisol. ACTH is secreted in a pulsatile manner. This renders the interpretation of individual plasma levels difficult.

In primary hypoadrenocorticism, plasma ACTH is often elevated to concentrations greater than 1000 pg/ml. Similar concentrations are encountered in plasma from patients with extrapituitary cancers producing ACTH and in patients with Cushing's disease after adrenalectomy.

Metabolism and Secretory Rate

ACTH leaves the plasma rapidly; the half-life is approximately 25 min. The adrenal cortex has an unusual affinity for ACTH, but the adrenal is not responsible for removing more than a relatively small fraction of ACTH from the plasma. The 24-hour secretion is only about 3 U.

Regulation

The secretion of ACTH by the adenohypophysis is under dual control. The first type of control is "long loop" feedback inhibition of ACTH secretion by circulating cortisol. After adrenalectomy, cortisol levels fall and ACTH secretion rises; the converse holds true after the administration of cortisol. Current evidence indicates that cortisol acts primarily on the pituitary corticotroph cells, but an additional site of feedback in the hypothalamus may well exist.

The second level of ACTH regulation is exerted by the hypothalamus through the secretion of corticotropin-releasing hormone (CRF). This mechanism is involved in a number of neurogenic stimuli for ACTH release (e.g., circadian rhythm, pulsatile secretion, response to pain, anxiety, pyrogen, hypoglycemia, and vasopressin).

The possibility of a "short loop" feedback of ACTH inhibition on its own secretion in certain restricted experimental conditions has been entertained, but there is no evidence that this effect is significant in man.

Melanocyte-Stimulating Hormones and Lipotropins

Action

The melanocyte-stimulating hormones (MSH) disperse pigment granules of melanocytes in certain fish and amphibians. The action permits animals to blend inconspicuously with their environments. In these species, MSH is localized predominantly in the pars intermedia, and the release of MSH is under neurohumoral control. As previously noted, the human intermediate lobe is vestigial and α and β MSH are not formed in significant amounts. β and γ LPH as well as ACTH have weak melanocyte-stimulating activity that contributes to the hyperpigmentation associated with increased ACTH secretion. Administration of α MSH to human beings had led to slight increases in pigmentation.

The lipotropins were originally recognized by their ability to mobilize lipid from adipose tissue in rabbits. This response is not demonstrable in many other species. There is no evidence that β or γ LPH have significant effects on fat metabolism of human beings.

Plasma Concentration

Plasma from patients with untreated Addison's disease and other conditions associated with ACTH hypersecretion contains increased melanocyte-stimulating activity when added to frog skin *in vitro*. α MSH has not been detected in human plasma by radioimmunoassay. "β MSH"-like activity has been detected in radioimmunoassays developed for human β MSH. The molecular size of the material detected is larger than β MSH and corresponds to β and γ LPH, however. The results of assays expressed in terms of weight of MSH for normal men and women are between 0 and 100 pg/ml. Greatly increased levels are noted in Addison's disease, corticotroph tumors of the pituitary, and ectopic ACTH-producing tumors. In most patients a close correlation exists between ACTH and "β MSH" concentration.

Pituitary Storage

Human pituitaries contain about 300–400 μg of "β MSH" immunoactivity per g of wet pituitary. Most of this immunoactivity is actually β-LPH.

Metabolism and Secretion

There is little information concerning the metabolism of lipotropins in man. One can presume that the half-life would be less than 20 min. Estimates of total daily secretion in man are not available.

The kidney is important in removing the LPH's from plasma. The elevated "MSH" concentrations in uremia may account for the hyperpigmentation that occurs. Estimates of total daily secretion in man are not available.

Regulation

The regulation of MSH secretion has been extensively studied in lower animals. The predominant hypothalamic control is exerted by a MSH-inhibiting factor. The existence of a MSH-releasing factor is suggested by some evidence.

GLYCOPROTEIN HORMONES

Structure of FSH, LH, TSH, and hCG

The glycoprotein hormones of the pituitary and placenta comprise a closely related family of hormones derived by biochemical evolution from a common primitive molecule. Included in this group of hormones are the thyrotropic hormone of the pituitary (TSH), the follicle-stimulating and luteinizing gonadotropins of the pituitary (FSH and LH), and the human chorionic gonadotropic hormone (hCG) of the placenta. All these hormone molecules have two peptide chains (α and β) each with carbohydrate substituent groups attached. The sugars that account for 15–31% of the molecular weight include fucose, mannose, galactose, glucosamine, and galactosamine. Sialic acid is inconstantly present. Even with homology of amino acid sequence, major differences in carbohydrate composition exist. Also, there is microheterogeneity of the carbohydrate components of a single hormone, which suggests that the addition of these components to the peptide chain is not under rigorous control.

The amino acid sequences of the α chain are identical or very similar for all these hormones. The isolated α chains lack biologic activity. Hormonal specificity in the complete molecule is conferred by the β chains, which have greater differences in amino acid sequences between the various hormones.

Proof that the hormonal specificity resides within the β chain has come from recombination experiments of the separate α and β chains. Isolated β chains may have slight intrinsic biologic activity, but total activity is regained after the α and β chains are recombined. Hybrids formed from the α chain of TSH and the β chain of LH possess LH activity. The converse recombination hybrid of α LH and β TSH results in a molecule with TSH activity.

The β chain of a glycoprotein hormone is responsible for the specificity of binding to cell receptors. The α chain may be more directly involved in activation of adenylate cyclase.

Gonadotropins

Actions

The pituitary gland contains two hormones whose primary action is on the gonads. FSH stimulates follicular development in the ovary and gametogenesis in the testes. LH, sometimes called the *interstitial cell–stimulating hormone* (ICSH), acts primarily in promoting luteinization of the ovary and in stimulating Leydig cell function of the testes.

The urine of postmenopausal women contains substantial amounts of gonadotropic substances of pituitary origin that have been isolated and partially characterized; this urinary gonadotropin qualitatively resembles FSH but has less than 1/25 the biologic potency of the pituitary hormone. Moreover, the dose response curve in bioassays has a different slope. These findings indicate that a change in the structure of the FSH molecule occurs either during its stay in the circulation or during its passage through the kidney.

The effects of gonadotropins are clearly recognized following administration to women with hypopituitarism. FSH, either isolated from human pituitaries or extracted from the urine of postmenopausal women, stimulates the development of one or more primordial follicles. After a period of 10–14 days of treatment with FSH, ovulation can be achieved by the addition of LH or hCG. Under physiologic conditions, LH contributes to follicular development by synergizing with FSH. During the period of follicular development and growth, thecal cells are active in the secretion of estrogens. When estrogen levels reach a certain critical level, they trigger a surge of FSH and LH secretion that results in ovulation. This midcycle peak is the result of a unique *positive* feedback that is to be contrasted with the *negative* feedback, which can also be demonstrated for gonadal hormones and is common for other tropic hormones with target glands. The function of the corpus luteum is maintained by LH. If pregnancy occurs, CG produced by trophoblastic cells maintains the corpus luteum of pregnancy. (This subject is discussed in detail in Chapter 7.)

The gonadotropic hormones can restore spermatogenesis and testosterone in men with hypopituitarism. FSH is primarily concerned with the restoration of spermatogenesis and must be administered with CG for 70–80 days, a time span much longer than that required for the development of the mature ovarian follicle in hypogonadotropic women.

Cellular Actions

The effects of LH and FSH on isolated ovaries, corpora lutea, and cultures of granulosa cells have been extensively studied.

In corpora lutea, LH (and hCG) promote steroidogenesis by stimulating the conversion of cholesterol to pregnenolone. The effects of LH on ovarian tissue can be reproduced by the addition of cAMP or dibutyryl cAMP.

The initial actions of LH on the Leydig cells of the testes are entirely comparable to those on the corpus luteum, but because of the enzymatic complement of the testes, the major product is testosterone rather than progesterone.

The actions of FSH are less well defined. It does stimulate testicular cAMP but is without effect on corpus luteum cAMP.

Pituitary Storage

The content of gonadotropins is low in the pituitaries of prepubertal children. In menstruating women, pituitary LH averages about 700 IU and the FSH about 200 IU by bioassay. Radioimmunoassay values are about 5 times greater. After menopause occurs, LH rises to about 1700 IU, with a comparable rise in FSH. The pituitary gonadotropin content of men is not greatly different from that of menstruating women.

Measurement

Formerly, urinary gonadotropins were measured by bioassay in rats and mice, but these methods have been replaced by radioimmunoassay. Most radioimmunoassays for LH also cross-react with CG, but specific radioimmunoassays have been developed with the β chains of LH and hCG that do not cross-react.

The radioimmunoassay of FSH is more difficult than that of LH. Many antisera raised in rabbits against partially purified human FSH cross-reacted extensively with LH and were unsuitable for use. When a sufficient number of rabbits are immunized, however, a few show the desired specificity for FSH. One such antibody is available in the United States from the National Pituitary Agency. A purified human FSH preparation is required for radiolabeling, but less highly purified pituitary extracts suffice for standards.

Different standards for radioimmunoassay have been used and the results expressed in several ways. The material currently being distributed by the National Pituitary Agency for standardization is a crude pituitary extract (LER 907) that has a biologic potency of 20 IU FSH and 48 IU LH per mg when expressed in terms of the Second International Reference Powder (IRP) (a preparation of urinary gonadotropins). When the radioimmunologic potency is compared directly with the Second IRP, LER 907 contains about 219 IU/mg of LH, or five times its apparent biologic activity, and 38 IU/mg of FSH. Other workers are using highly purified FSH and LH preparations for standardization and expressing results on a weight basis. Results are variously reported as mIU/ml or in terms of weight of LER 907. Assay results in Britain and in Europe are often expressed per liter.

Plasma and Urine Gonadotropins

Gonadotropins are present in plasma at all ages (Fig. 3–10). A twofold rise in gonadotropins occurs at the time of

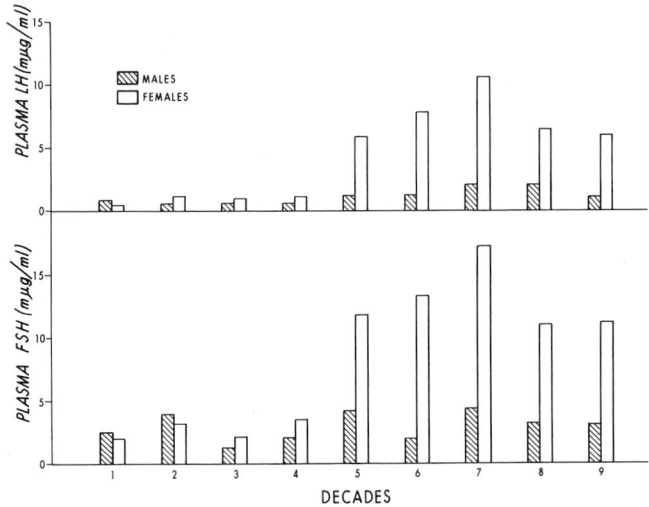

Figure 3–10. Plasma LH and FSH levels in normal males and females in relation to age. Each bar represents the mean value for 5–10 individuals. All women in the 5th decade were postmenopausal, and this group had significantly higher mean LH and FSH levels than premenopausal women. The mean LH (but not FSH) level in men during the 7th and 8th decades was also found to be significantly higher (p < 0.02) than the mean level during the 3rd and 4th decades. (Reproduced from Schalch, D. S.: Gonadotropin secretion in the human. In *The Neuroendocrinology of Human Reproduction.* Mack, H. C., and Sherman, A. I. (eds.), Springfield, Ill., Charles C Thomas, 1971, with permission.)

puberty. In ovulating women, there is a slight initial rise in FSH followed by a slow decline during the follicular phase of the cycle (Fig. 3–11). Preceding ovulation there is a sharp peak of excretion of both gonadotropins, with the greater rise in LH and a lesser rise in FSH. Except for the ovulatory spike, the concentrations of LH and FSH in men are not greatly different from those in women. There is no abrupt change in plasma gonadotropins in men as a function of age; increases in plasma LH occur in the seventh and eighth decades of life. In women, however, a marked increase in both FSH and LH occurs after the menopause, usually in the fifth decade.

Following gonadectomy of men and women, there is a marked rise in plasma FSH and LH.

In general, the urinary excretion of LH and FSH parallels plasma concentrations, with the important exception that little gonadotropic hormone is found prepubertally (Fig 3–12). After puberty, a tenfold rise in urinary LH occurs. Urinary measurements, either for 24 hours or for a designated period of time, are preferred by many pediatric endocrinologists. Gonadotropins, particularly in children, may be secreted in episodic bursts, especially at night. Urine collections provide a means of integrating the fluctuations of plasma content.

Radioimmunoassays have also been developed for the separate α and β chains of the gonadotropins. Free α chain exists in the pituitary and peripheral plasma when hormone secretion is stimulated. β chain is rarely present in plasma normally but has been detected in certain pathologic states.

Metabolism and Secretory Rate

FSH and LH disappear from the plasma in a complex manner, with a half-life of between 20 and 40 minutes for LH and about twice this figure for FSH. The urinary excretion of immunoassayable FSH may be as high as 36%, but that of LH is considerably smaller, less than 5%. Detailed

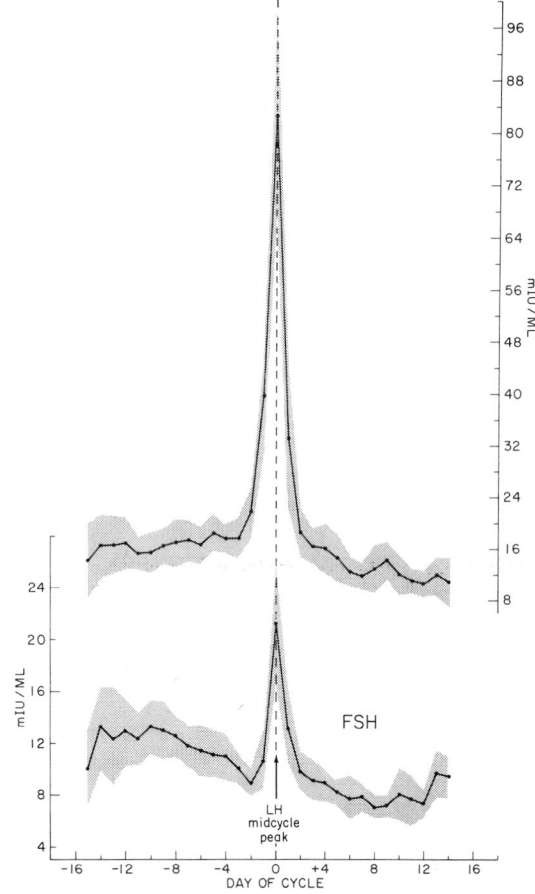

Figure 3–11. Changes in serum LH and FSH during the menstrual cycle. This represents the average value for 16 normal menstrual cycles. (Reproduced from Ross, G. T., Cargille, C. M., et al.: Pituitary and gonadal hormones in women during spontaneous and induced ovulatory cycles. *Recent Progr. Hormone Res.* 26:1, 1970, with permission.)

studies of clearance of LH from the plasma have been conducted on women with the constant infusion techniques. The metabolic clearance rate is about 25 ml/min, and it is not affected by the gonadal function of the individual. Daily production rates of LH in normal women during most of the menstrual cycle are about 500–1100 IU/day, with much higher levels occurring during the preovulatory period. In postmenopausal women, LH production is between 3000 and 4000 IU/day. When these production rates are compared to the scanty information concerning pituitary content of LH, it is evident that complete turnover of stored gonadotropin occurs every 12–24 hours, indicating that gonadotropin synthesis is an active process in the pituitary.

In contrast to the pituitary gonadotropins, the half-life of hCG in the plasma is about 8 hours by bioassay and considerably longer by radioimmunoassay. Renal clearance of hCG is about 1 ml/min, which is about seven times that of LH. The total daily production of hCG may reach as high as 30 mg during the first trimester of pregnancy.

The marked differences in plasma and renal clearances of hCG and LH occur despite the fact that the amino acid sequences of the two peptides are closely similar. Differences in the carbohydrate substituents of the molecule are important determinants of metabolism. CG differs from LH in its high sialic acid content (12% as compared to 0.1%). Enzymatic removal of the sialic acid greatly shortens plasma half-time and increases hepatic extraction without

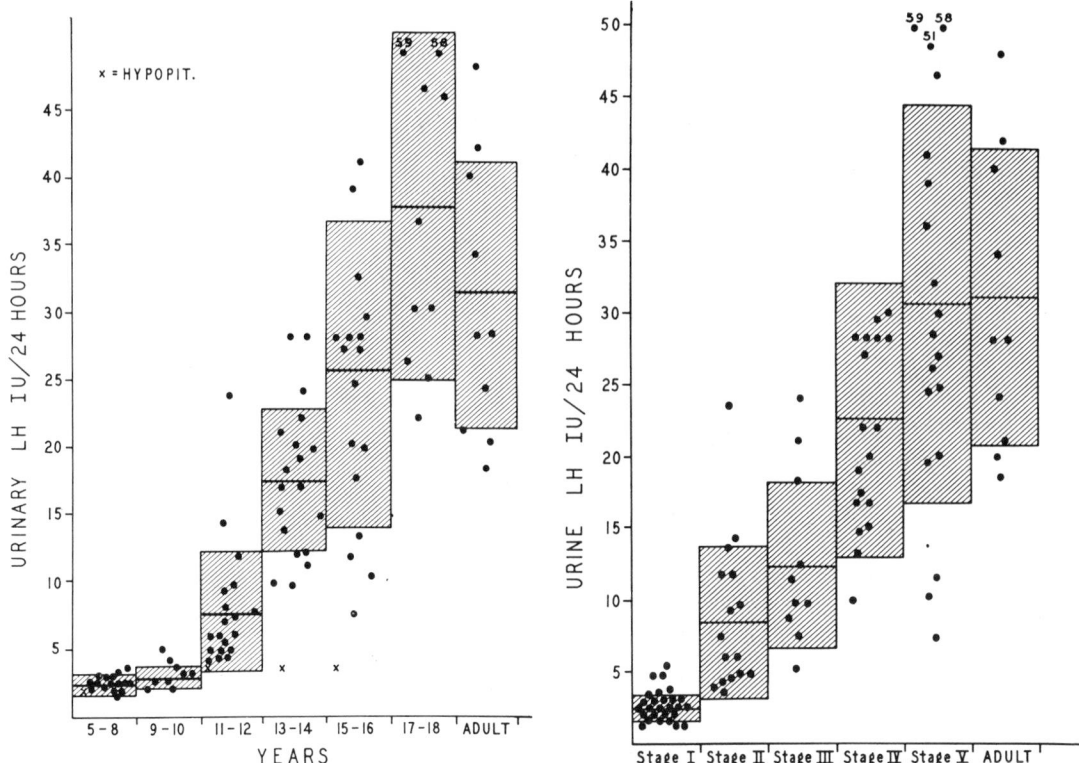

Figure 3–12. Urinary secretion of LH in normal boys and men. Changes in girls during puberty are similar but occur about 1 year earlier. Changes in urinary FSH show a less dramatic rise during puberty. (Reproduced from Baghdassarian, A., Guyda, H., et al.: Urinary excretion of radioimmunoassayable luteining hormone (LH) in normal male children and adults, according to age and stage of sexual development. *J. Clin. Endocrinol.* 31:428, 1970, with permission.)

affecting intrinsic biologic activity at the tissue level. The long half-life of hCG facilitates the rapid rise in plasma concentration early in pregnancy and may have teleologic significance.

Regulation

The secretion of FSH and LH is regulated by feedback inhibition by sex steroids. A single hypothalamic hormone, the LH releasing hormone (LRH), also stimulates the release of FSH. The possibility of an additional hypophysiotropic hormone acting solely on FSH release has not been completely eliminated.

After gonadectomy, plasma FSH and LH concentrations rise markedly because of the absence of "feedback" inhibition of sex steroids. Estrogens are potent inhibitors of LH and FSH release, but testosterone is less effective. The role of other testicular secretions in pituitary FSH suppression remains conjectural. It is likely that sex steroids act on both the pituitary and the hypothalamus to modify gonadotropin secretion.

The gonadotroph cell secretes both FSH and LH in response to stimulation by a single releasing factor (LRH). It is also clear that the ratio of FSH to LH is not constant but varies at different ages and at different times of the menstrual cycle. Sex steroids acting on the pituitary greatly influence the pattern of gonadotropins secreted in response to LRH. FSH secretion in the male may be suppressed by a peptide substance, inhibin, secreted by Sertoli cells of the testicular tubule. As is the case with other cells secreting peptide hormones, there appears to be a pool of gonadotropins that is promptly secreted by an infusion of LRH. Somewhat later, a reserve pool of stored and newly synthesized gonadotropin is mobilized.

Thyrotropin

Actions

Thyrotropin (TSH) is bound by receptors on the thyroid cell surface. A critical component of the receptor is a specific ganglioside. Of great interest is that cholera toxin also shares an affinity for this ganglioside. TSH exerts its effects on the thyroid cell by increasing the cellular content of cAMP. In Graves' disease there is a thyroid-stimulating immune globulin that can react with the thyrotropin receptor. In so doing, antibody activates adenylate cyclase and the resultant cellular consequences in a manner similar to TSH.

TSH exerts profound effects on many aspects of thyroid function. Increases in thyroid size and vascularity are easily recognized after the administration of the hormone to experimental animals. Microscopically, the height of the follicular epithelium is increased, and the amount of colloid is reduced. TSH increases iodide uptake, thyroglobulin synthesis, iodotyrosine and iodothyronine formation, thyroglobulin proteolysis, and thyroxine (T_4) and triiodothyronine (T_3) release from the thyroid gland. Other alterations in thyroid cell biochemistry not directly related to hormone production and release follow TSH administration. There is an increase in oxygen uptake, phospholipid synthesis, RNA synthesis, and glucose utilization. Administration of TSH to a number of animal species induces exophthalmos due to the deposition of mucopolysaccharide-rich edema fluid in the retro-orbital tissue. Separation of thyrotropic and exophthalmos-producing activities has been accomplished by chromatography of bovine pituitary extracts. Despite these experimental findings, it is unlikely that the pituitary is responsible for exophthalmos in humans. Current evidence would favor either an antibody-mediated or a cell-mediated autoimmune process.

Storage

There is little information concerning the concentrations of TSH in human pituitaries as a function of age and sex. Bioassay of a limited number of human pituitaries showed a content of about 4 IU. This low concentration made the isolation or characterization of human TSH difficult.

Measurement

TSH and the thyroid-stimulating immunoglobulin (TSI) have been measured by *in vivo* bioassay, radioreceptor assay, and histocytochemical assay. Although these methods have been used extensively in the past for research applications, they are seldom applied clinically at the present time. The radioimmunoassay of TSH is a useful, well-standardized procedure.

Plasma Concentration

By radioimmunoassay, normal human plasma contains less than 5 μU/ml. In about 10% of normal individuals, TSH is undetectable with current clinical radioimmunoassays (Fig. 3–13). In patients with primary hypothyroidism, plasma TSH concentrations are elevated to as much as 50 times normal (Fig. 3–14). With replacement treatment, TSH levels fall to normal; the rate of fall is dependent on the type and dosage of thyroid hormone administered. In most cases of hyperthyroidism, plasma TSH levels are low because of suppression by the elevated levels of circulating thyroid hormone.

Metabolism and Secretion

When ^{131}I-TSH is injected into normal adults, it is promptly distributed into a volume only slightly larger than the plasma volume. Over the next 2 hours, the disappearance is exponential with a mean half-life of about 50 min. On the basis of a mean plasma concentration of 2.7

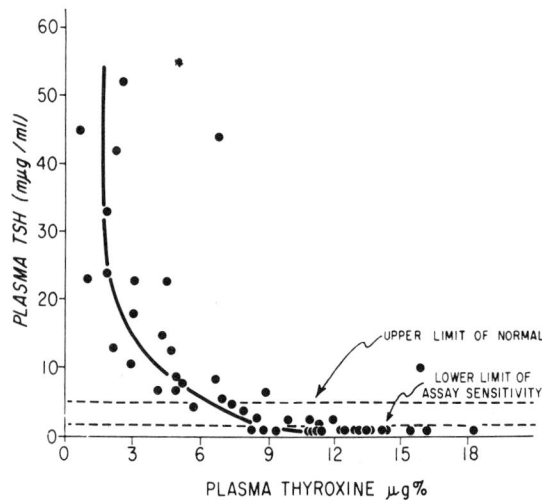

Figure 3–14. Relationship between plasma thyroxine and plasma TSH. (Reproduced from Reichlin, S., and Utiger, R. D.: Regulation of the pituitary-thyroid axis in man: relationship of TSH concentration to concentration of free and total thyroxine in plasma. *J. Clin. Endocrinol.* 27:251, 1967, with permission.)

μU/ml, Odell et al.[31] calculated pituitary secretion to be 165 mIU/day.

In hypothyroidism, disappearance of TSH from plasma is slow, but because of the high concentration of TSH in plasma, the total secretory rate ranges from 390–23,025 mIU/day.

Regulation

The secretion of TSH by the adenohypophysis is determined partially by the level of circulating thyroid hormone and partially by thyrotropin-releasing hormone (TRH). After sectioning of the pituitary stalk, thyroid activity is maintained at a higher level than after hypophysectomy, suggesting that at least minimal TSH secretion persists under such conditions. The negative feedback control of TSH secretion exercised by circulating thyroid hormone is exerted primarily at the pituitary level (see Chapter 11).

SOMATOMAMMOTROPIN HORMONES

Structures

Characterization

GH and PRL of the pituitary and chorionic somatomammotropin (CS) of the placenta have similar chemical structures and overlapping biologic actions. The amino acid structures of human GH and CS have been completely established. Both hormones contain 191 amino acids with two intramolecular S-S bonds in the same location (between half-cystines at positions 53 and 165 and between 182 and 189) (Fig. 3–15).

Examination of the amino acid sequences reveals that 161 of the 191 amino acids are identical in the two hormones. Of the remaining 30, 19 are highly compatible substitutions requiring only a simple base change in the DNA template, 4 are relatively compatible, and only 7 of the amino acid differences cannot be easily explained.

Prolactin (PRL) is a simple protein slightly larger than GH consisting of 198 amino acids in a single peptide chain. Two intramolecular S-S bridges occupy the same relative positions as those in GH and CS, and, in addition, there is a

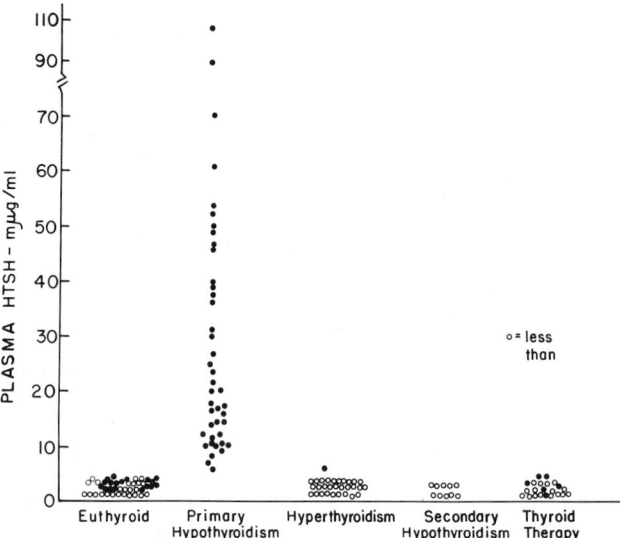

Figure 3–13. Plasma TSH measured by radioimmunoassay in hypothyroidism of several types and normal subjects. (Reproduced from Utiger, R. D. Immunoassay of human plasma TSH. In *Current Topics in Thyroid Research.* New York, Acadmic Press Inc., 1965, p. 513, with permission.)

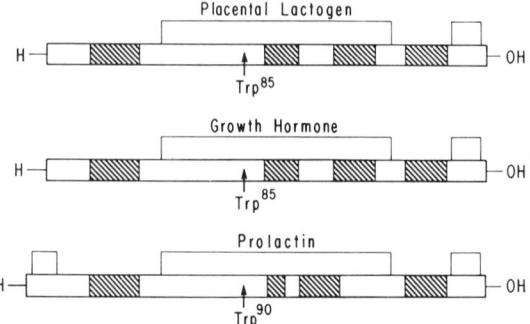

Figure 3–15. Diagram of basic structural properties of human chorionic somatomammotropin (HPL), human GH, and ovine PRL. The bars represent the peptide chains with the amino terminal to the left and the carboxyl terminal to the right. The shaded portions of each bar represent the recognizable areas, suggesting replicating sequences. The lines above the bars diagrammatically represent the position of disulfide bridges. (Reproduced from Niall, H. D., Hogan, M. L., et al.: *Proc. Nat. Acad. Sci.* USA 68:866, 1971, with permission.)

third disulfide bridge at the amino end of the molecule. There are six regions of the ovine PRL molecule comprising about 146 amino acids that appear to correspond closely to portions of the GH and human CS molecules (Fig. 3–15). Forty-nine of the amino acids in these sequences are identical, and an additional 68 are acceptable substitutions.

The structural homologies of these three hormones provide a strong indication that they evolved from a single progenitor hormone. GH and CS are so closely related in structure that one may assume the evolutionary divergence of these two peptides is comparatively recent. Niall et al. have identified an amino acid pattern that appears to repeat itself four times in each molecule (Fig. 3–15). From this they surmise that tandem duplication of the genetic information has occurred in the course of evolution of the primitive somatomammotropin.

Prolactin

Actions

PRL acts directly on tissues and does not regulate the function of a secondary endocrine gland. The initiation and maintenance of lactation is the only known function of PRL in human beings. PRL has little effect on the mammary gland without the presence of certain other hormones; full lactation requires preparation of the breast tissue by estrogens, progestins, corticosteroids, and insulin. When the gland has been primed, PRL brings about milk secretion. In many species, milk cannot be removed by suckling unless oxytocin (OT) stimulates contraction in the myoepithelial cells of the mammary alveoli and ductules to force the milk into the larger collecting ducts and cisterns. In women, however, OT is not required for successful nursing.

The action of PRL on the crop sac of pigeons and doves is a fascinating facet of comparative endocrinology. Following the hatching of the young, a nutritious material is formed by proliferation and desquamation of the crop epithelium. This crop "milk" is used for feeding the young. The action of PRL on the crop sac is direct because local proliferation will surround an area of the crop sac into which PRL is injected.

PRL has a luteotropic action on the ovary in rats. FSH and LH bring about follicular development, ovulation, and the initial development of the corpus luteum, but they are unable to sustain the secretory activity of the corpus luteum in the rat. PRL maintains luteal secretion but has no effect on ovarian follicles. By prolonging the secretory life of the corpus luteum, PRL plays an important role in early pregnancy. In other mammals, including ungulates, rabbits, guinea pigs, and probably humans, PRL does not have an important role in maintaining the secretory life of the corpus luteum.

PRL induces changes in maternal behavior in some animals that are important for the protection of the young. It promotes nesting behavior in some species of birds. Effects of PRL on reproductive behavior have also been demonstrated in cold-blooded animals.

PRL has general metabolic actions in the hypophysectomized animal that are unrelated to reproduction and are similar to those of somatotropin (STH). An increase in the weight of the liver and several other organs has been observed in PRL-treated pigeons.

Similar GH-like effects have been observed in humans by some but not all investigators after the administration of large doses of PRL. The possible significance of these various actions of PRL under physiologic conditions remains to be determined. As yet there is no known role of the hormone in the male sex.

Pituitary Storage

The normal human pituitary contains little PRL, about 100 μg. A significant increase in the content of PRL occurs during pregnancy.

Measurement

PRL is measured clinically by radioimmunoassay. In addition, PRL can be measured by radioreceptor assay employing membranes prepared from pregnant rabbit mammary glands and ^{125}I-labeled ovine PRL.

Plasma Concentration

The mean serum PRL of women is about 10 ng/ml with upper limits of normal about 20 ng/ml (Fig. 3–16). The mean plasma concentrations of men and prepubertal children is slightly lower. During the hours of sleep there is a moderate progressive rise in PRL concentration (Fig. 3–17). Some have reported a slight rise in PRL associated with the midcycle period in women.

Lactation

In pregnancy, plasma PRL begins to rise in the first trimester and increases progressively during pregnancy. At the time of delivery, the PRL concentration averages about 200 ng/ml (Fig. 3–16). The rise in plasma PRL almost exactly parallels the increase in placental somatomammotropin. Human pregnancy is unusual because comparable rises in PRL have not been found in pregnancy in other species, including the rhesus monkey. The rise in PRL during human pregnancy may be the result of the very high level of estrogens that are present in the human species. PRL is present in amniotic fluid in concentrations greater than fetal or maternal plasma during the second trimester. There is evidence that this PRL is synthesized by the amniotic epithelial lining.

During pregnancy, the combined effects of both pituitary and placental mammotropic hormones, estrogens, and progesterone develop the secretory apparatus of the breast for subsequent lactation. Actual lactation is suppressed in

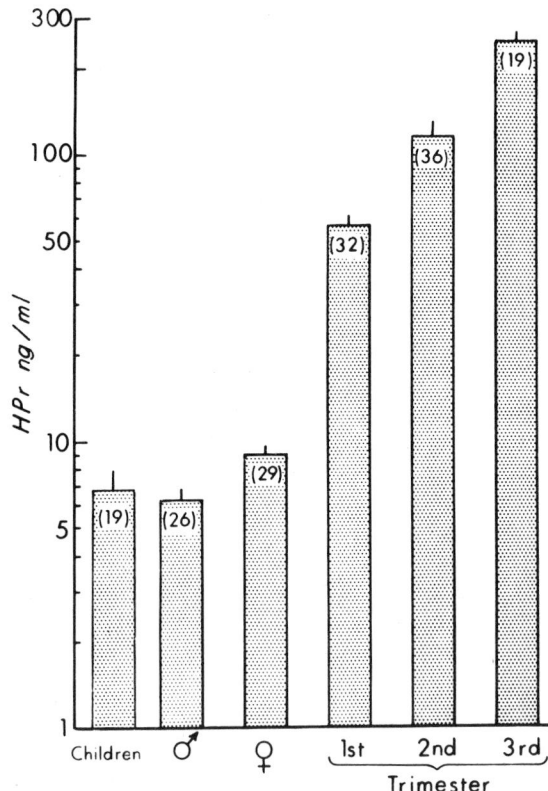

Figure 3–16. PRL levels in prepubertal children and adult men and women and in the three trimesters of pregnancy. (Reproduced from Jacobs, L. S., Mariz, I. K., et al.: A mixed heterologous radioimmunoassay for human prolactin. *J. Clin. Endocrinol. 34*:484, 1972, with permission.)

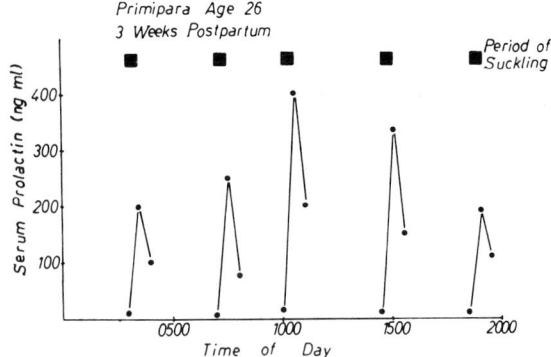

Figure 3–18. Changes in serum PRL immediately before and after nursing in a 26-year-old woman 3 weeks after delivery. (Reproduced from Hwang, P., Guyda, H., et al.: A radioimmunoassay for human prolactin. *Proc. Nat. Acad. Sci.* USA 68:1902, 1971, with permission.)

greatly elevated after the immediate postpartum period. The stimulation of the nipple by suckling initiates a neuroendocrine reflex that results in a surge of PRL secretion (Fig. 3–18). This period of PRL secretion primes the breast for the next episode of nursing. As nursing continues, the magnitude of PRL secretion promoted by suckling becomes attenuated. It is possible for lactation to continue more or less indefinitely as long as the repeated stimulus of nursing occurs. There are cases on record of the development of lactation in nonpuerperal women who allow infants to suckle repeatedly.

Metabolism and Secretion

PRL has a volume of distribution that approximates that of extracellular fluid. After exogenous administration or suppression of endogenous secretion, PRL disappears from plasma rapidly. The disappearance curve is complex, but the major portion of PRL has a plasma half-life of 20–30 min. As in the case of GH, both liver and kidneys are important sites of degradation.

Regulation

Mechanical stimulation of the female breast for as little as 5 min can lead to a secretion of PRL in some nonlactating adult women (Fig. 3–19). Similar stimulation of the male breast does not result in PRL secretion. Tactile stimulation of a nonmammary region of the same dermatome fails to stimulate PRL. It is known that the breast, particularly the nipple and areola, is richly endowed with specialized nerve endings. These sensory receptors initiate the impulses that eventually reach the area in the hypothalamus that regulates PRL secretion.

A number of drugs that affect dopaminergic mechanisms influence PRL secretion by altering hypothalamic secretion of a PRL inhibitory factor (PIF). Alpha methyldopa, an agent that inhibits dopamine synthesis, can induce nonpuerperal lactation and hyperprolactinemia. On the other hand, levodopa, which crosses the blood-brain barrier and increases dopamine concentrations in hypothalamic neurons, inhibits normal PRL secretion in normal women and also in many pathologic states associated with hyperprolactinemia (Fig. 3–20). Dopamine itself is secreted into the portal vessels and may be the PIF. Dopamine may also stimulate the secretion of a hypothalamic PRL-inhibiting peptide. In addition, L-dopa can be converted into dopamine

pregnancy by a direct inhibition of mammary secretory activity by the high levels of estrogen and progesterone. Following delivery, estrogen and progesterone levels fall rapidly, and the lactogenic action of PRL is unopposed. During lactation, basal levels of PRL in plasma are not

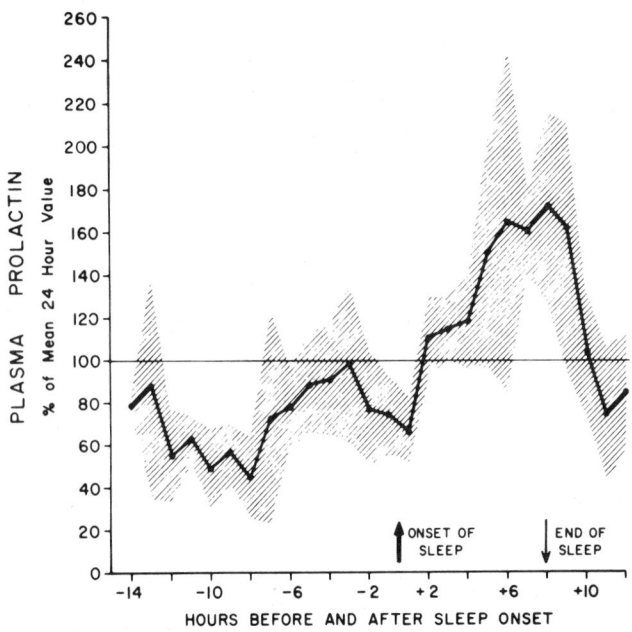

Figure 3–17. Serum PRL levels in six normal subjects to show the diurnal pattern. Note rise in serum PRL during the later hours of sleep. (Reproduced from Frantz, A. G.: Prolactin. New Engl. J. Med. 294:201, 1978.)

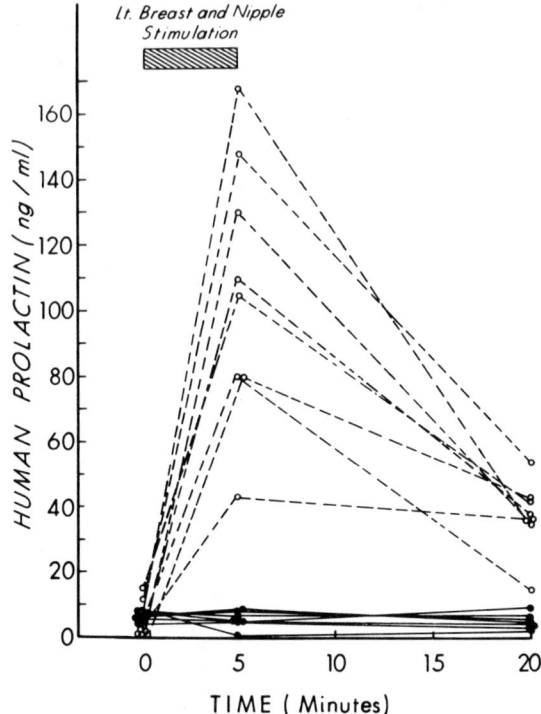

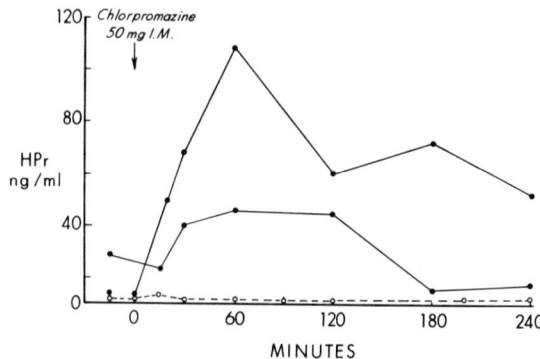

Figure 3–21. Changes in plasma PRL following IM injection of 50 mg. of chlorpromazine. Results in two normal women (●) and in a patient with panhypopituitarism (○).

obtained hourly for 3 hours. Examples of normal responses are shown in Fig. 3–21.

In addition to a PIF, the hypothalamus may also contain prolactin releasing factors (PRF). TRH is one such releasing substance. As shown in Fig. 3–22, TRH is a potent stimulus for PRL secretion in humans, but it is unlikely that TRH is an important releasing factor for PRL *in vivo*. The acute secretion of PRL in suckling is unattended by a parallel increase in TSH secretion. Other examples of the dissociation in the secretion of TSH and PRL could be cited.

A number of nonspecific stimuli result in PRL secretion, including surgical stress, uremia, and exercise. The physiologic significance of this PRL secretion is obscure.

Growth Hormone

Actions

The metabolic processes controlled by GH are multiple and complex. Despite intensive investigation for more than three decades, the molecular basis for most GH effects remains unknown. For detailed summaries of existing knowledge, the reader is referred to the Handbook of Physiology. In this section, the overall effects of GH on body composition and intermediary metabolism will first be considered. Next, the cellular actions of GH that are exerted directly will be contrasted with those that are the result of intermediary tissue growth factors in somatomedins.

Figure 3–19. Changes in plasma PRL before and at intervals after mechanical stimulation of breast and nipple in eight normal women (--○--) and eight normal men (–●–). This response in women is not demonstrable in many normal women. (Reproduced from Kolodny, R. C., Jacobs, L. S., et al.: Mammary stimulation causes prolactin secretion in non-lactating women. *Nature* [*London*] 238:284, 1972, with permission.)

within the adenohypophysis and inhibit PRL secretion directly.

Tranquilizing drugs, including the phenothiazines and reserpine, that interfere with dopaminergic transmission may induce nonpuerperal lactation and hyperprolactinemia in women. As a test of PRL secretory reserve, 25 or 50 mg of chlorpromazine is given intramuscularly and samples are

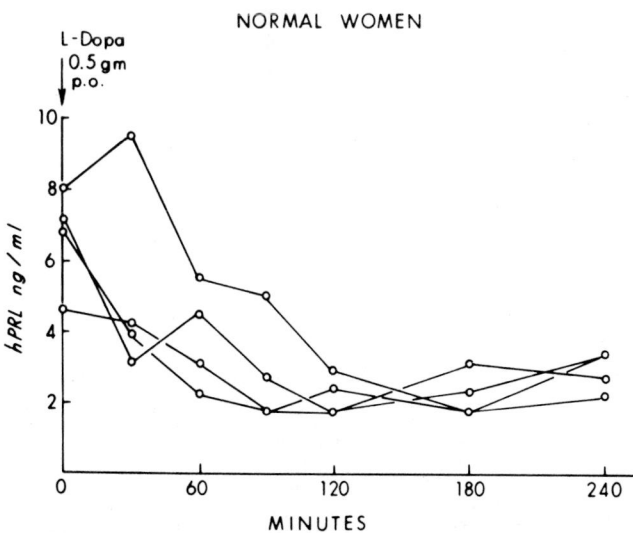

Figure 3–20. Changes in serum PRL following ingestion of 0.5 gm of L-dopa by four normal women. (Reproduced by permission from Jacobs, L. S., and Daughaday, W. H.: Physiologic regulation of prolactin secretion in man. In *Lactogenic Hormones, Fetal Nutrition and Lactation*. Josimovich, J. B., Reynolds, M., et al. (eds.), New York, John Wiley and Sons, 1974.)

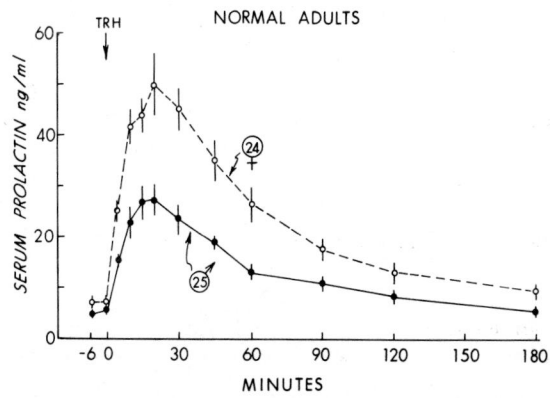

Figure 3–22. Serum PRL changes after injection of TRH (100 to 400 μg) into normal men (●) and women (○). (Reproduced from Jacobs, L. S., Snyder, R. D., et al.: Prolactin response to thyrotropin releasing hormone in normal subjects. *J. Clin. Endocrinol.* 36:1069, 1973, with permission.)

Body Composition

By comparing the body composition of subjects with hypopituitarism before and after GH treatment with that of normal subjects, certain differences are apparent. In hypopituitarism in children it is axiomatic that the skeletal growth is decreased. There is an even greater impairment of lean body mass. Muscle, the largest component of lean body mass, has been quantitated. The number of muscle nuclei, as well as protoplasmic mass, is decreased relative to height, and GH administration to hypopituitary children corrects these deficits of muscle. GH also has a viscerotropic effect on the heart, pancreas, liver, and kidneys.

In children with hypopituitarism the percentage of body fat is increased. This fat accumulation is recognized clinically as a characteristic pudginess and an increased skinfold thickness that rapidly disappear during the early months of treatment with GH.

GH has effects on the relative volume of body fluids. In acromegaly, the plasma volume, erythrocyte mass, and interstitial fluid volume are relatively increased. An opposite deviation probably occurs in hypopituitarism but has not been definitively studied.

Intermediary Metabolism

The administration of GH to GH-deficient animals and humans leads to changes in intermediary metabolism. There is an increased protein synthesis that results from a number of integrated processes, including enhanced amino acid transport, increased ribosomal number, increased mRNA, and the enzymatic apparatus for protein synthesis. The diversion of amino acids to protein synthesis and away from oxidative pathways leads to a decrease in urea formation and positive nitrogen balance.

Fat mobilization from depots to the liver is accelerated. Fatty acid oxidation is augmented relative to amino acid and carbohydrate oxidation. Ketogenesis is promoted.

Uptake of carbohydrate by muscle is inhibited by GH largely because of decreased responsiveness to insulin. This may be attributed partially to increased fatty acid utilization, the so-called glucose–fatty acid cycle, and partially to decreased insulin receptor affinity and number. Despite hyperinsulinism, glucose utilization is impeded and plasma glucose tends to rise. Islet hypertrophy occurs, which in some cases leads to islet exhaustion.

Actions in Humans

Knobil and Greep, in 1957, demonstrated that simian GH was potent in hypophysectomized monkeys, as compared to the ineffectiveness of nonprimate GH's. Soon thereafter, human GH was prepared and tested in humans. With daily doses of 1–10 mg/day, major metabolic changes are induced in patients with hypopituitarism and even in normal adult individuals. Nitrogen balance becomes strongly positive; plasma and urine urea values promptly fall. Although daily nitrogen retention decreases with continued GH treatment, it is still adequate to maintain a greatly increased growth rate in pituitary dwarfs. The retention of sodium, chloride, potassium, magnesium, and phosphorus is concomitant with the positive nitrogen balance (Fig. 3–23). Calcium is retained by the body despite hypercalciuria. This unexpected finding is explained by increased gastrointestinal absorption of calcium. Plasma phosphorus levels may rise after GH administration, but this has been inconstant. Alkaline phosphatase levels are little changed.

In view of the well-documented diabetogenic effects of GH in some experimental animals, carbohydrate metabolism has been carefully studied after GH administration in humans. When GH is administered to fasting normal and hypophysectomized subjects, little change occurs in plasma glucose and insulin concentrations. If glucose is administered 2 hours after GH, however, glucose disappearance from plasma is inhibited. More prolonged administration of GH does not produce diabetes unless very large doses are administered because of compensatory hyperinsulinism. The diabetogenic influence of GH is most easily demonstrated when it is administered to hypophysectomized diabetic patients. In these patients as little as 1 mg of human GH daily leads to exacerbation of diabetes. These observations attest to the diabetogenic action of human GH, which is masked in the presence of normal pancreatic reserve.

Direct Cellular Actions

Although the general effects of GH *in vivo* are well recognized, the molecular mechanisms by which GH exerts its effects on cells remain in doubt. GH acts directly on a number of cell types within the body. Table 3–3 lists some of the organ perfusion and isolated cell systems that are known to respond to GH. GH reacts with specific receptors on the cell wall that have been best studied in a line of

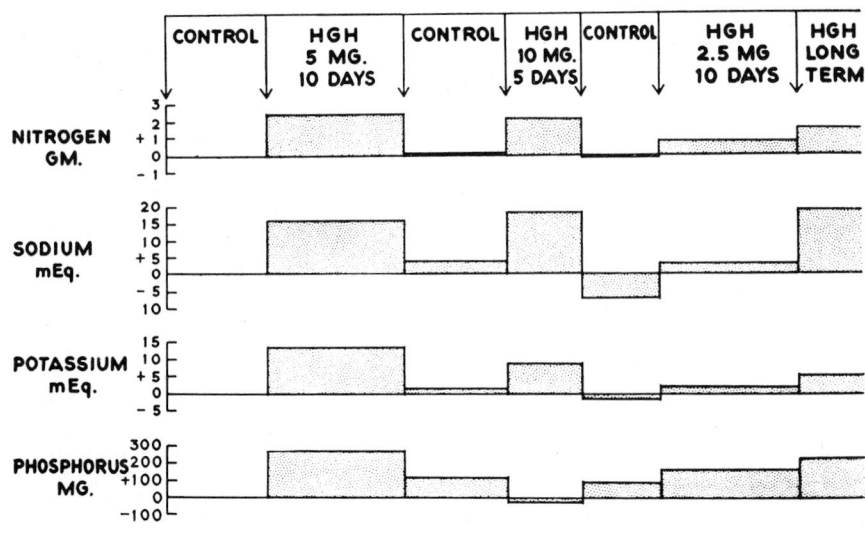

Figure 3–23. The effects of GH treatment of an 11½-year-old girl with pituitary dwarfism on the balances of nitrogen, sodium, potassium, and phosphorus. Changes above the initial control baseline represent retention of the substance and below the line, loss. (Reproduced from Hutchings, J. J., Escamilla, R. F., et al.: Metabolic changes produced by human growth hormone (Li) in a pituitary dwarf. *J. Clin. Endocrinol. 19*:759, 1959, with permission.)

Table 3–3. DIRECT ACTIONS OF GH ON ISOLATED TISSUES AND ORGANS

I. Liver
  Perfusion
    RNA synthesis[1]
    Plasma protein synthesis[2]
    Somatomedin release[3]
  Cell Culture
    Replication[4]

II. Muscle
  Diaphragm
    Amino acid transport and incorporation[5]
  Heart
    Amino acid transport and incorporation[6]
  Vascular smooth muscle cell culture
    Outgrowth[7]

III. Fat
  Amino acid incorporation[8]
  Lipolysis by dexamethasone-sensitized adipocytes[9]

IV. Hematopoietic tissue
  Thymocytes, mitosis[10]
  Malignant lymphoblasts
    ^{3}H-Thymidine incorporation
    ^{3}H-Uridine incorporation
    ^{3}H-Leucine incorporation[11]
  Bone marrow
    Number of erythroid colonies, potentiation of erythropoietin[12]

[1]Jefferson, L. S., and Korner, A.: *Biochem. J. 104*:826, 1967.
[2]Griffin, E. E., and Miller, L. L.: *J. Biol. Chem. 249*:5062, 1974.
[3]McConaghey, P., and Sledge, C. B.: *Nature 225*:1249, 1970.
[4]Moon, H. D., Jentoft, V. L., and Li, C. H.: *Endocrinology 70*:31, 1962.
[5]Kostyo, J. L., Hotchkiss, J., and Knobil, E.: *Science 130*:1653, 1959.
[6]Hjalmarson, A., Isaksson, O., and Ahren, K.: *Am. J. Physiol. 217*:1795, 1969.
[7]Ledet, T.: *Diabetes 25*:1011, 1976.
[8]Goodman, H. M.: *Endocrinology 83*:300, 1968.
[9]Fain, J. N., Kouacev, V. P., and Scow, R. O.: *J. Biol. Chem. 240*:3522, 1965.
[10]Whitfield, J. F., MacManus, J. P., and Rixon, R. H.: *Horm. Metab. Res. 3*:28, 1971.
[11]Desai, L. S., Lazarus, H., Li, C. H., and Foley, G. E.: *Exp. Cell Res. 81*:330, 1973.
[12]Golde, D. W., Bersch, N., and Li, C. H.: *Science 196*:1112, 1977.

cultured human lymphocytes. The second messenger for GH action remains unknown because the activated GH-receptor complex does not transmit its information by activating adenylate cyclase. There is also little evidence that guanylate cyclase is activated. Most GH effects are delayed and appear to require a period of protein synthesis.

Somatomedins

Some of the effects of GH are not exerted directly but are mediated indirectly by inducing the formation of a second hormonal messenger, the somatomedins or insulin-like growth factors (Fig. 3–24). The evidence for this hypothesis has been largely developed by studies of cartilage. The metabolic activity of this growth tissue *in vivo* is crucially dependent on GH secretion; nevertheless, direct addition of GH to cartilage *in vitro* is without effect. Cartilage from hypophysectomized rats is markedly stimulated by serum from normal individuals but not by serum of GH-deficient individuals. GH treatment restores somatomedin levels of subjects with hypopituitarism within 24–72 hours. The active components of the serum that are responsible for this action are several closely related peptides called somatomedins. Two somatomedin peptides with molecular weights of about 8000 have been isolated, and their amino acid sequences have been established. Because of the similarity of structure to proinsulin, these peptides have been named insulin-like growth factors (IGF) I and II. There is a high

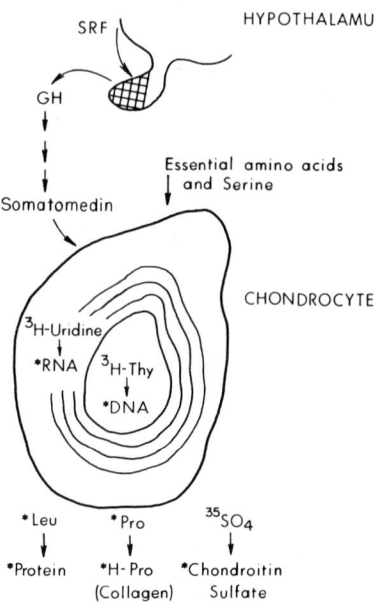

Figure 3–24. GH action on cartilage is mediated by somatomedin (sulfation factor). This peptide is produced by GH action on liver and possibly kidney. It acts directly on chondrocytes to stimulate many aspects of cartilage metabolism necessary for cartilage replication and matrix formation.

degree of homology of structure of IGF and proinsulin (Fig. 3–25). The connecting peptide of 12 amino acids is much abbreviated compared to that of proinsulin and does not contain any of the amino acid sequences of human C-peptide. This portion of the IGF I molecule is not cleaved prior to secretion.

The somatomedins circulate as a macromolecular complex consisting of the somatomedin peptide and a plasma-binding protein binder. The entire complex has a molecular size of about 120,000 daltons. The components are dissociated at high hydrogen ion concentrations. The somatomedin-binding protein complex is probably retained within the vascular space and is probably not biologically active. Dissociation is thought to occur to permit passage through capillary membranes and entrance into dense tissues such as cartilage.

Receptors for somatomedin exist on chondrocytes, hepatocytes, adipocytes, and muscle cells as well as other cell types. In most cases these receptors also bind insulin to some extent. This cross reactivity is not surprising in view of the similarity of the structures of insulin and IGF I and II.

The site or sites of somatomedin synthesis in the body are not established, although the liver seems to be an important source of somatomedins.

Somatomedin peptides are released by isolated hepatocytes and perfused rat liver. In the case of the perfused rat liver, the release and synthesis of somatomedin is stimulated by GH acting synergistically with T₃ and corticosteroids. In some experiments PRL and insulin also increase somatomedin release from the perfused rat liver.

Somatomedins exert a pleiotypic effect on cartilage (Fig. 3–24); many aspects of matrix formation, cell growth, and replication are stimulated. In most laboratory studies the stimulation of thymidine uptake into DNA or the uptake of sulfate into chondroitin sulfate (sulfation factor activity) have been measured. Somatomedins also have insulin-like effects on some tissues. They can inhibit lipolysis and increase glucose oxidation in adipocytes and stimulate glucose and amino acid uptake by diaphragm and heart muscle.

Although the *in vitro* effects of somatomedin-containing

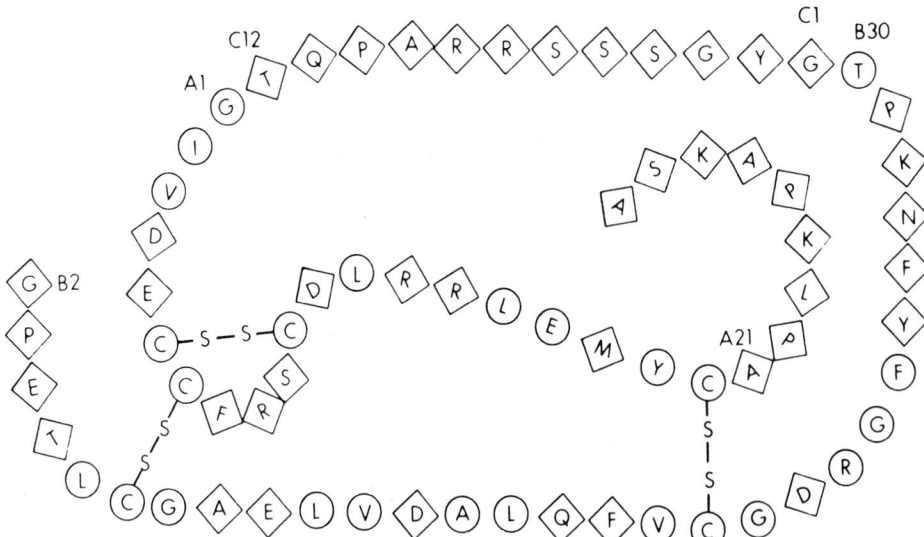

Figure 3–25. Primary structure of IGF I according to Rinderknecht and Humbel. The simplified single letter designation of amino acids is employed. Portions of the molecule homologous to residues 2–30 of the B chain of insulin and 1–21 of the A chain of insulin are designated. Amino acids in circles are identical in IGF I and insulin molecules. The two chains are joined by an abbreviated 12-amino acid sequence that contains no identical amino acids with the connecting peptide of proinsulin. IGF II has a structure with 76% identical residues but has only 67 amino acid residues rather than 70. (Structure according to Rinderknecht, E., and Humbel, R. E.: *J. Biol. Chem.* 253:2769, 1978.)

serum or isolated somatomedin peptides are readily observed, definite evidence of *in vivo* effects of purified somatomedins has been difficult to demonstrate because of the limited supplies. Recently, van Buul-Offers et al. administered a partially purified somatomedin devoid of insulin or GH contamination to mice with congenital hypopituitarism. This resulted in a stimulation of sulfate uptake by cartilage and an increase in body weight and length.

Somatomedin can be measured by *in vitro* bioassay, radioreceptor assay, and radioimmunoassay. The test systems for bioassay have included costal cartilage from hypophysectomized rats, normal pigs, and embryonic chicks. The end points for most assays have been sulfate uptake or thymidine incorporation. If preliminary gel filtration at low pH is conducted, somatomedin fractions can be assayed on isolated fat cells and chick fibroblasts. Radioreceptor assays for several of the somatomedin peptides have been developed with ^{125}I-labeled somatomedin peptide and membranes from human placenta or rat liver. A radioligand assay has been described employing the binding component of plasma.

The radioimmunoassay of somatomedin peptides has been developed in several laboratories and the somatomedin-C RIA is now available for clinical use.

Plasma concentrations are usually expressed in units (U). One U of somatomedin is the somatomedin activity of 1 ml of pooled normal adult human serum. Most results of IGF (NSILA-s) assays have been reported in terms of μU/ml of insulin equivalents, the insulin-like action of the IGF standard having been assayed in a fat cell assay. Normal serum appears to contain about 0.5 μg of somatomedin peptide per ml. As will be discussed later, levels of somatomedin are reduced in hypopituitarism and elevated in hypersomatotropism.

Although these assays have provided much information about the concentrations of somatomedin in health and disease, they have their limitations. The radioligand and radioimmunoassays do not react equally with all forms of somatomedin. The precision of bioassays is often unsatisfactory, and inhibitors of bioactivity exist in serum.

Pituitary Storage

Fortunately, the human pituitary is particularly rich in GH, and the somatotropic granule resists autolytic dissolution after death. Despite the fact that radioimmunoassays suggest a much higher content, the yield of somatotropin

with present extraction methods is between 8 and 16% of the dry weight of human pituitaries, equivalent to 4–8 mg of hormone per gland. No significant changes in GH content with age are evident.

Plasma Concentration

The level of circulating radioimmunoassayable GH in the well-rested adult prior to breakfast is less than 3 ng/ml. With moderate exercise, such as is incurred by ambulatory patients coming to the hospital, higher values may be observed. A rise in plasma GH occurs in many individuals 2–4 hours after ingestion of a meal and during fasting prolonged beyond one night.

The effects of age on plasma GH are of interest. In the first days of life, very high levels of GH occur, but there is great variability among infants. After 2 weeks of age, lower mean levels are found. In pubertal children, the basal plasma GH concentration is not greatly different from that reported for adults, but more peaks of GH may occur during the day with physical activity and at night. GH continues to be secreted after the period of skeletal growth has been completed. GH secretory responses to provocative stimuli are generally unimpaired even in elderly individuals.

The diurnal pattern of GH secretion has been characterized by obtaining blood samples every 20 or 30 min throughout the 24 hours under nonstressful conditions. During most of the day, plasma GH levels of normal adults are less than 3 ng/ml, with one or two sharp spikes 3–4 hours after meals. The most consistent period of GH secretion for both children and adults occurs about 1 hour after the onset of deep sleep (Fig. 3–26). Subsequent smaller peaks of plasma GH may be observed later during the sleep period. The initial surge of GH secretion is correlated with the onset of stage III or IV sleep and not with any recognized general metabolic clues. Delay in the onset of deep sleep will correspondingly delay the onset of the GH peak. Plasma levels of glucose, fatty acids, and insulin are not changed by the sudden secretion of GH, but after the peak, the individual is more resistant to administered insulin and glucose tolerance is slightly decreased. There is evidence that REM (rapid eye movement) sleep inhibits the GH peak and may be important in the termination of the sleep-related GH secretion. Despite the fact that a substantial fraction of total GH secretion occurs 1–2 hours after the onset of deep sleep, the significance of this pattern of GH secretion remains to be determined. It has been suggested

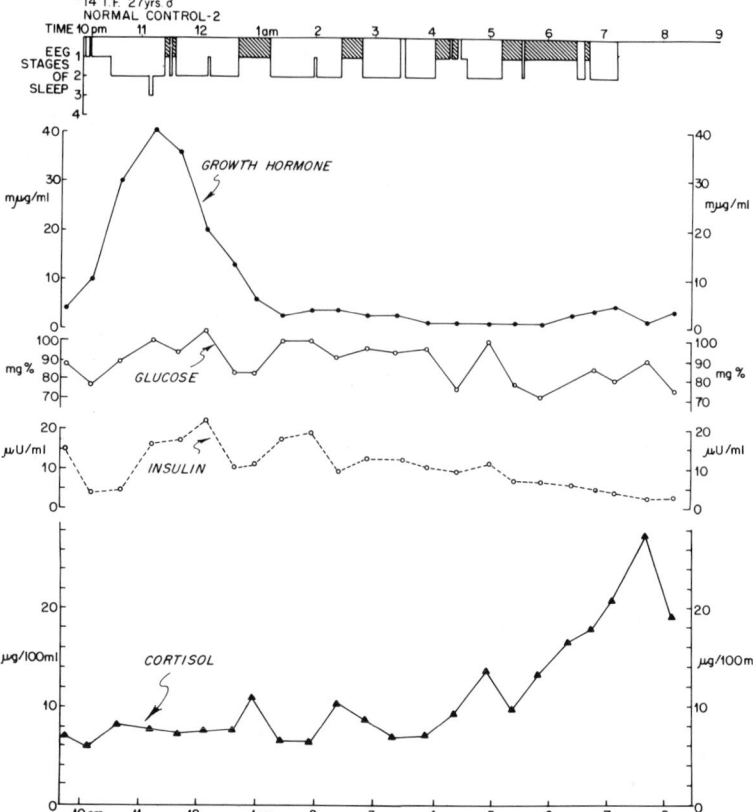

Figure 3–26. Changes in GH, glucose, insulin, and cortisol concentrations in plasma during the hours of sleep. The bars at the top of the graph indicate the stages of sleep. The shaded portions are periods of rapid eye movement sleep (REM). (Reproduced form Takahashi, Y., Kipnis, D. M., et al.: Growth hormone secretion during sleep. *J. Clin. Invest.* 47:2, 1968, with permission.)

that sleep-related GH secretion is important in anabolic and repair processes. Abnormalities of GH secretion during sleep could influence skeletal growth.

Metabolism and Secretory Rate

Administered hormone disappears from plasma with an initial half-life of about 20–25 min. A similar half-life in the disappearance of endogenous hormone has been reported following pituitary suppression with glucose or after hypophysectomy in patients with acromegaly. The clearance rate for human GH determined by the constant infusion method is between 100 and 150 ml/m^2 of body surface/min. No consistent changes with age or sex exist. GH clearance is normal in patients with acromegaly but is decreased in those with hyperthyroidism and in many persons with diabetes mellitus.

Attempts have been made to estimate GH secretory rates on the basis of the basal GH levels and the metabolic clearance of GH. This calculation disregards the marked fluctuation of plasma GM that may occur throughout the day and night. To obviate this difficulty, investigators have resorted to continuous or repetitive sampling to arrive at an integrated 24-hour GH concentration. This has been found to be 1.8 ± 1.0 (SD) ng/ml in men, somewhat higher in women, and 5.6 ± 3.6 ng/ml in preadolescent and adolescent boys.

Attempts to estimate GH secretion by measuring GH in a 24-hour urine collection have not been successful because of nonspecific interference with radioimmunoassays.

Regulation

In human beings, the secretion of GH is stimulated by a rapid fall in plasma sugar, but slowly developing hypoglycemia may not activate GH secretion.

The physiologic and pharmacologic factors that alter GH secretion are listed in Table 3–4.

To test the adequacy of the GH secretory response, 0.05 to 0.1 U of insulin per kg of body weight is given intravenously with careful observation of the patient. The rise in plasma GH follows the nadir of blood sugar and reaches a maximum by 45–60 min (Fig. 3–27). A rapid fall in blood sugar to less than 50% of the initial level or below 50 mg/100 ml represents an adequate stimulus for most subjects. A much smaller fall in blood sugar is adequate to stimulate GH release in many individuals. Administration of glucose with insulin prevents the rise in GH levels in the plasma that is observed with insulin alone. The importance of glucose utilization by the GH regulatory center is suggested by the observation that 2-deoxyglucose (which inhibits the utilization of glucose in the tissues) stimulates the secretion of GH.

Table 3–4. FACTORS INFLUENCING NORMAL GH SECRETION

	GH Secretion	
	Augmented	Inhibited
Neurogenic	1. Stages III and IV sleep 2. Stress (traumatic, surgical, infectious, psychogenic) 3. α Adrenergic agonists 4. β Adrenergic antagonists 5. L-Dopa	1. REM sleep 2. Emotional deprivation 3. β Adrenergic agonists 4. α Adrenergic antagonists
Metabolic	1. Hypoglycemia (fasting) 2. Falling fatty acid level 3. Amino acids 4. Uncontrolled diabetes 5. Uremia 6. Hepatic cirrhosis	1. Hyperglycemia 2. Rising fatty acid level 3. Obesity
Hormonal	1. Low somatomedin(?) 2. Estrogens 3. Glucagon 4. Vasopressin	1. Somatostatin 2. Hypothyroidism 3. Large doses of corticosteroids 4. Medroxyprogesterone

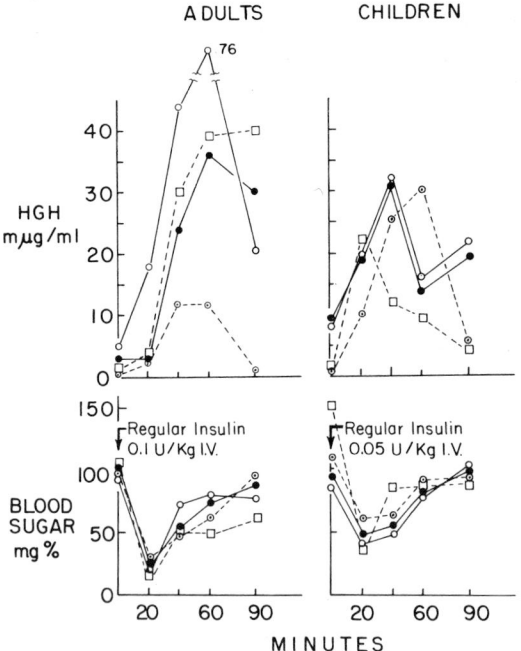

Figure 3–27. Plasma GH concentrations in normal adults and children after the induction of hypoglycemia with insulin. (Courtesy of M. L. Parker.)

It is of interest, but still unexplained, that obese patients do not respond to provocative stimuli with GH secretion as regularly as do individuals of normal weight.

Oral or intravenous administrations of amino acids stimulates GH secretion. Arginine is one of the most potent amino acids in causing GH release (Fig. 3–28). This amino acid also stimulates the release of insulin, which precedes the release of GH, but the release of the two hormones is unrelated. The reasonable suggestion has been made that the secretion of GH induced by amino acids is a mechanical for stimulating protein synthesis when precursors are available.

In clinical testing, arginine hydrochloride, 0.5 g/kg body weight, is given intravenously over a 30-min period. Blood samples for GH determination are obtained every 30 min for 2 hours. Peak values occur usually 60–90 min after the start of the infusion. A rise in serum GH greater than 7–10 ng/ml is considered normal.

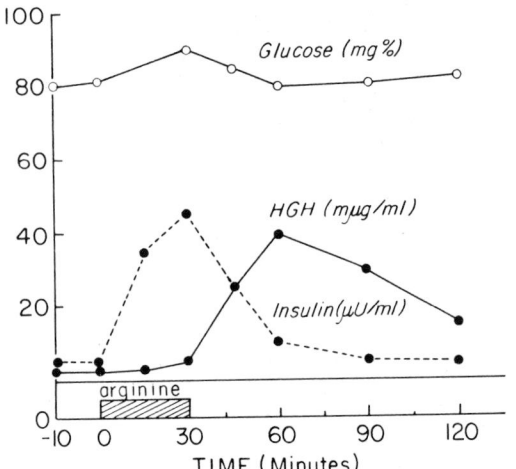

Figure 3–28. The typical effects of intravenous arginine (0.5 gm/kg body weight) on plasma glucose, human GH, and insulin. (From Hammod, Parker, and Daughaday, unpublished.)

As has already been mentioned, plasma GH levels are elevated after exercise and after certain types of excitement.

The secretion of GH is influenced by catecholamine agonists and antagonists. Normally the administration of 500 mg of L-Dopa by mouth leads to the secretion of GH between 90 min and 2 hours later. This response is inhibited by α blocking agents and not by the dopamine antagonist, halperidol. This suggests that L-Dopa is converted to norepinephrine in the hypothalamus, α Blockers such as phentolamine will decrease the GH response to hypoglycemia arginine but do not affect the GH secretion associated with sleep. The converse occurs with propranolol, a β blocker; the GH responses to a number of metabolic stimuli are augmented.

The effect of serotonergic pathways on GH secretion are controversial. Methysergide, a serotonin antagonist, decreases the GH response to hypoglycemia but increases the sleep-associated GH secretion. Cyproheptadine, on the other hand, is a serotonin antagonist that does not affect GH release during sleep.

The effects of other hormones on the secretion of GH have received considerable attention. Plasma GH levels are higher in many women after exercise, hypoglycemia, or arginine infusion than in men. This sex difference is due to estrogens, because relatively brief administration of potent estrogens will increase the GH response induced in men by arginine administration. Corticosteroid excess occurring in spontaneous hyperadrenocorticism and after high-dose corticosteroid administration impairs the plasma GH response to hypoglycemia and inhibits the sleep-related peak of GH secretion.

Hypothyroidism in the rat greatly reduces the GH content of the pituitary and the concentration of the hormone in plasma. In man, a similar but less profound change in GH secretion occurs. Although the basal plasma levels of GH are not depressed in clinical hypothyroidism, the rise in plasma GH in response to hypoglycemia is frequently subnormal in hypothyroid children.

HYPOPITUITARISM
Etiology

Primary hypopituitarism may result from surgical ablation, radiation, nonsecretory pituitary tumors (discussed later), metastatic tumors, infarction, and a number of infiltrative or granulomatous processes.

Pituitary infarction is most commonly associated with postpartum uterine hemorrhage, but it may occur from time to time in patients with evidence of diabetic microvascular disease and in patients with sickle cell anemia. Rare cases of hypopituitarism due to cavernous sinus thrombosis, temporal arteritis, carotid aneurysm, and trauma have been reported. Pituitary necrosis occurs frequently in catastrophic anoxic states. Usually the condition is observed at autopsy in patients who were on respirators for a long time. Except for diabetes insipidus, clinical manifestations are rarely recognized.

Sheehan's syndrome is the association of pituitary necrosis with hemorrhage or severe shock at the time of delivery. Pituitary hyperplasia takes place during pregnancy owing to estrogen stimulation of lactotropic cell proliferation. After delivery, the succulent gland normally undergoes involution. Postpartum hemorrhage, with its attendant shock and frequent coagulation abnormalities, is the precipitating cause of ischemic necrosis. There is a correlation between the severity and duration of hypotension and the extent of the adenohypophyseal lesion.

The exact pathogenesis of the pituitary vascular lesion is difficult to reconstruct. Sheehan postulated that severe arteriolar spasm develops in vessels supplying the critical hypothalamic areas from which hypothalamic-pituitary portal veins arise. This spasm leads to pituitary ischemia and cellular damage. When the circulation is restored, it is likely that severe edema occurs. This swelling, which occurs in a hyperplastic gland encased in the bony confines of the sella turcica, leads to further circulatory impairment and eventual cellular necrosis.

When circulation is re-established, pituitary hemorrhage develops. Disappearance of glandular elements after necrosis is so extensive that only small nests of recognizable pituitary cells may be found in condensed stroma lying in an otherwise empty sella turcica.

The neurohypophysis is generally spared because it is less dependent on the portal vessels for its nutrition; in unusual cases damage to the neurohypophysis is extensive and diabetes insipidus results.

In early life, infiltration with cholesterol-laden histiocytes (Hand-Schüller-Christian disease) may lead to adenohypophyseal and neurohypophyseal damage. Pituitary infiltration by hemosiderin-laden macrophages (hemochromatosis) or by sarcoid granuloma may involve the pituitary as well as the thyroid and adrenal glands. The resulting multiglandular syndrome presents difficult diagnostic problems. The pituitaries of certain patients examined at necropsy show only a diffuse fibrosis of uncertain origin.

Tuberculosis and syphilis, once significant causes of hypopituitarism, are now very rarely seen. Isolated instances have been reported in which mycoses, brucellosis, and other infections have led to hypopituitarism.

In disease processes producing destruction in the pituitary, clinical manifestations of hypopituitarism are usually absent until about 75% of the gland is destroyed. With more refined laboratory procedures, it is possible to detect lesser losses of functional reserve. As the extent of pituitary destruction increases, clinical evidence of hormonal deficiencies usually occurs in the following order: (1) gonadotropins, (2) GH (growth failure in children), (3) TSH, (4) corticotropin, (5) PRL. Clinical evidence of PRL deficiency is only recognized in postpartum necrosis of the pituitary. In other types of hypopituitarism, plasma PRL is often normal or increased because of interruption of normal portal transport of PIF. Exceptions to this sequence are frequent.

Pituitary hypofunction can result from disease processes attacking the hypothalamus that either destroy the ability to synthesize new hypophysiotropic hormones or impair the transport of these hormones to the pituitary. Disease processes that may produce hypothalamic hypopituitarism include suprasellar tumors (craniopharyngiomas, optic gliomas, etc.), trauma, infection, hydrocephalus, congenital malformations, and granulomas (histiocytosis and sarcoid). Although this mechanism of pituitary hypofunction has been suspected, it is only recently that evidence obtained by administration of TRH and LRH has definitely established the existence of secondary hypopituitarism. In most cases of secondary hypopituitarism involving more than one hormone, PRL secretion is increased rather than decreased.

Sheehan's Syndrome

The occurrence of pituitary necrosis after obstetric bleeding or shock formerly was a frequent endocrine condition. Fortunately, with the general availability of blood banks and improved obstetric care, this condition has become rare in countries with advanced medical care. Usually the clinical history is sufficient to make the diagnosis. Blood loss is profuse and shock prolonged. Postpartum enlargement of the breasts and lactation generally are not noted. Pubic hair shaved for delivery may never grow back and axillary hair may fail to grow. Asthenia and loss of vigor are usually severe. Later, signs of hypothyroidism develop, but frank myxedema may be delayed for years — even decades. Menses, if they return at all, are infrequent. Vaginal mucosal atrophy develops, and the uterus exhibits hyperinvolution.

Because the extent of pituitary necrosis in Sheehan's syndrome is highly variable, the clinical features may be few and involve only partial insufficiency of only one or two hormones. On the other hand, severe panhypopituitarism may be present.

Pathophysiology

Corticotropin Deficiency

The clinical features of complete ACTH deficiency in humans is most clearly defined after the discontinuation of replacement therapy following complete hypophysectomy. Clinical adrenal insufficiency is evident within 2 weeks by the appearance of nausea, vomiting, and eventual hypotensive collapse. Secondary adrenal insufficiency decreases glycogen reserve and fasting gluconeogenesis resulting in hypoglycemia. In most cases of spontaneous hypopituitarism, ACTH deficiency is partial and cortisol replacement may not be required to maintain life.

In women, the loss of axillary and pubic hair and a general decrease in body hair are the result of a decrease in adrenal androgen production (Fig. 3–29). Loss of libido may in part be due to adrenal androgen deficiency.

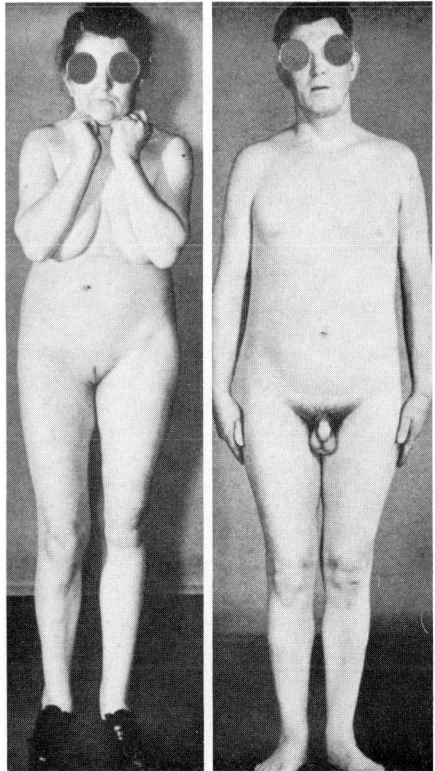

Figure 3–29. *Left,* hypopituitarism of 12 years' duration produced by postpartum necrosis of the adenohypophysis. Note good nutritional state, myxedematous facies, normal breasts, and absence of pubic hair. *Right,* hypopituitarism in a man produced by a chromophobe adenoma of the pituitary. Note the excellent nutritional state.

Salt and Water Metabolism

The hypophysectomized patient is able to conserve body sodium far better than the patient with Addison's disease. Hyponatremia, if it does occur, is more likely to be caused by excessive water retention than by sodium loss. Aldosterone secretion continues under the control of the renin angiotensin system and will rise after salt restriction. Nevertheless, ACTH deficiency limits maximum aldosterone secretion. Rarely, aldosterone deficiency as well as cortisol deficiency are present in patients with long-standing panhypopituitarism.

Anterior pituitary deficiency decreases urine volume in a patient with diabetes insipidus. Urine volumes are seldom more than 4–5 L a day, as compared to 6–12 L in individuals with diabetes insipidus whose adenohypophysis is intact. The apparent improvement of diabetes insipidus in hypopituitarism can be attributed to the low rate of glomerular filtration resulting from GH and adrenal steroid deficiencies and increased tubular reabsorption of water due to adrenal insufficiency. Conversely, treatment in patients with combined neural and adenohypophyseal deficiency with cortisol or other corticosteroids may increase the severity of diabetes insipidus.

Hypo-osmolality without hypovolemia can occur within the first week after surgical hypophysectomy or cryohypophysectomy. Excessive administration of water to such patients can lead to dangerous water intoxication. In most cases, the hypo-osmolality is the result of inappropriate secretion of vasopressin. Adrenal insufficiency further impairs water diuresis. This limitation of free water clearance is a manifestation of cortisol and not mineralocorticoid deficiency.

Melanocyte-Stimulating Peptides

Patients with hypopituitarism lose skin pigmentation and have impaired ability to acquire a suntan. This has been generally attributed to a loss of melanocyte-stimulating peptides, but it is now clear that the human pituitary does not secrete either α or β MSH in significant amounts. Therefore our understanding of pigmentary control in hypopituitarism is incomplete.

Thyrotropin Deficiency

The time of onset and severity of symptoms of hypothyroidism in spontaneous hypopituitarism is variable. In the complete absence of TSH the changes are predictable. Four to 8 weeks after the withdrawal of thyroid replacement from hypophysectomized patients, the clinical signs and symptoms of severe hypothyroidism appear: torpor, cold intolerance, dryness of skin, and myxedema. In the presence of a waxy pallor, fine wrinkles about the mouth suggest the diagnosis of hypopituitarism (Fig. 3–30). The serum T_4 reaches extremely low levels, 1–2 μg/100 ml, and the serum cholesterol level is usually elevated. Little radioiodine accumulates in the thyroid, and other deficiencies of iodine metabolism develop. The radioactive iodine uptake in the thyroid is restored to the normal range after 1–5 days of treatment with TSH. Other laboratory tests of thyroid hypofunction are also corrected by TSH.

Exceptional patients do not develop hypothyroidism after total hypophysectomy. Thyroid autonomy of a nodular goiter is the usual explanation. In a few cases, actual hyperthyroidism has been described. In several documented cases, this has been associated with plasma thyroid-

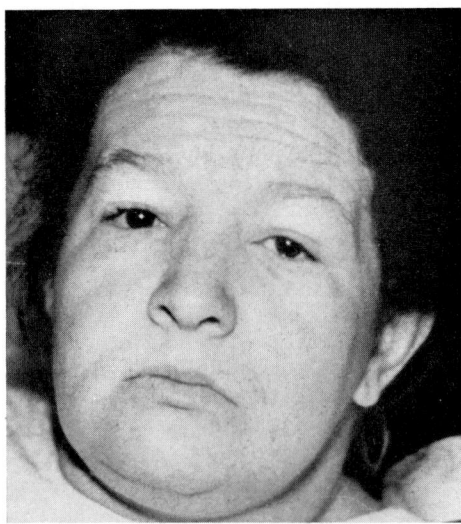

Figure 3–30. The facies of a patient with hypopituitarism. Note the myxedematous appearance and indolent expression.

stimulating immunoglobulin (TSI). This unusual situation provides evidence that TSI is not dependent on pituitary function.

Gonadotropin Deficiency

The loss of pituitary gonadotropins leads to profound gonadal atrophy. In men, the testes are atrophic, soft, and less tender than normal to pressure. Libido and potency decrease; sperm disappear from the semen. The loss of testosterone leads to decreased beard growth, loss of axillary and pubic hair, and a general decrease in body hair. In women, menstruation ceases; there is profound atrophy of the uterus and vagina; and libido decreases.

Prolactin Deficiency

The failure of lactation in patients with Sheehan's syndrome has already been discussed.

Growth Hormone Deficiency

Impaired skeletal growth is recognized in children with hypopituitarism and will be discussed later. In adults, GH deficiency is less easily recognized. It is likely that some of the loss of muscle strength and endurance may be the result of GH deficiency. GH deficiency may be responsible for the contraction of plasma and interstitial fluid volumes and may contribute to the impaired erythropoiesis that leads to the mild refractory anemia.

GH deficiency affects carbohydrate metabolism in several ways. GH and cortisol deficiencies are largely responsible for the increased insulin sensitivity of patients with hypopituitarism. Fasting hypoglycemia results partly from increased insulin sensitivity and decreased alanine and glutamine mobilization from muscle for gluconeogenesis. GH deficiency also is directly responsible for decreased insulin secretory capacity. This impairment may lead to hyperglycemia after an oral glucose challenge.

General Metabolism

The notion that hypopituitarism frequently leads to cachexia persists despite much evidence to the contrary. Actually the extreme malnutrition described in some of the initial case reports of hypopituitarism is rarely encountered (Fig. 3–29). This emaciation was probably the result of lower standards of medical care and social welfare. Patients with hypopituitarism have a normal distribution of body weight.

Differential Diagnosis

Panhypopituitarism must be distinguished from a number of conditions commonly exhibiting similar clinical manifestations (Table 3–5).

Anorexia Nervosa

Chronic malnutrition leads to decreased secretion of ACTH, TSH, and gonadotropins, but GH secretion may be increased. The term *anorexia nervosa* is applied to individuals whose malnutrition is attributable to a psychogenic disturbance in eating. The majority of cases of anorexia nervosa occur in unmarried women between the ages of 15 and 35 years. Anorexia nervosa is not a distinct psychiatric entity but a clinical feature found in a number of psychic illnesses, including psychoneurosis and schizophrenia. For some patients, food and the process of eating have assumed an unacceptable sexual significance. These patients rarely complain of their emaciated appearance but may experience bloating, constipation, and vomiting.

Amenorrhea is common in women whose body weight has fallen below 80% of ideal weight. There is evidence of estrogen deficiency with breast and vaginal atrophy. Gonadotropin levels are low and the response to LRH is subnormal. If nutritional adequacy is restored by psychotherapy or other means, the response to LRH is restored when body weight approaches normal and may actually be supranormal for a time. Dryness of the skin, tendency to hypothermia, and reduced oxygen consumption (low basal metabolic rate) all may suggest hypothyroidism. There may also be a slight lowering of plasma T_4 and TSH. The T_3 level is regularly much reduced and there is a reciprocal increase in rT_3 (3, 3'5'-triiodothyronine). Plasma cortisol in anorexia nervosa is usually considerably reduced because of decreased rate of metabolism of corticosteroids. In the rare male with anorexia nervosa, a decrease in serum testosterone is found. In women, sufficient adrenal androgen is secreted to maintain axillary and pubic hair, the presence of which provides an important bedside indication that chronic panhypopituitarism is not present. The diagnosis of anorexia nervosa is usually suspected on the basis of distorted attitudes about food and the inappropriate self-image expressed by the patient and the knowledge that hypopituitarism is rarely associated with major weight loss. The disease can be distinguished from true hypopituitarism in most cases by (1) the infrequency of marked wasting in hypopituitarism, (2) the preservation of axillary and pubic hair in anorexia nervosa, (3) the higher levels of urinary steroid excretion in anorexia nervosa, and (4) the normal or elevated concentration of plasma GH.

Table 3–5.   DIFFERENTIAL DIAGNOSIS OF PANHYPOPITUITARISM

1. Anorexia nervosa
2. Thyroidal hypothyroidism
3. Chronic liver disease
4. Hemochromatosis
5. Myotonia dystrophica

Thyroidal Hypothyroidism

Thyroidal hypothyroidism presents with many features in common with panhypopituitarism. The clinical features of hypothyroidism and even myxedema are common to both conditions. Both conditions may be associated with amenorrhea. The loss of axillary and pubic hair is less extreme in most women with thyroidal as compared to pituitary hypothyroidism. Urinary 17-OH corticosteroids are often very low but plasma cortisol is normal in thyroidal hypothyroidism. The two conditions are easily distinguished by measuring plasma TSH, which will be distinctly elevated in thyroidal hypothyroidism. Some hypopituitary patients will have levels of TSH by radioimmunoassay that are normal and occasionally slightly elevated. The TSH in these individuals is probably functionally impaired.

Chronic Liver Disease

The diagnosis of hypopituitarism is often suspected in men with alcoholic liver cirrhosis or hemochromatosis when testicular atrophy is combined with general debility. In most cases the underlying primary disease process can be recognized, and simple hypopituitarism ruled out, by laboratory procedures. Morphologic evidence of extensive pituitary destruction is rarely found at necropsy in these diseases.

Myotonia Dystrophica

Individuals with myotonia dystrophica complain of progressive muscular weakness, and the characteristic myotonia may not be recognized. They develop premature balding and cataracts. The facial features suggest accelerated aging. The possibility of hypopituitarism may arise because of the development of testicular atrophy in men. Panhypopituitarism is easily excluded by endocrine tests.

Establishing the Diagnosis

An unequivocal diagnosis of panhypopituitarism must be established before a patient is committed to a lifetime of replacement therapy. Two lines of evidence help establish the diagnosis of hypopituitarism in a patient with compatible symptoms and physical findings: (1) evidence of a possible cause of pituitary damage and (2) laboratory evidence of hormonal deficiencies.

The great majority of cases of pituitary insufficiency of the adult are the result of pituitary tumor or postpartum necrosis of the pituitary. Careful roentgenograms of the sella turcica and determination of visual fields will demonstrate tumors that lead to hypopituitarism. Historical evidence of catastrophic postpartum collapse can be obtained from most patients with Sheehan's syndrome, but 20 or more years may intervene from the accident of pregnancy before the diagnosis of hypopituitarism is suspected.

Laboratory procedures for demonstrating hormonal deficiencies are now highly developed. It is unnecessary to document all the hormonal biochemical abnormalities existing in hypopituitarism, but procedures of proven differential value should be selected. Elaborate studies of carbohydrate and insulin tolerance are nonspecific and dangerous. Direct radioimmunoassay measurements of pituitary hormones in blood have made these indirect indices obsolete.

When the corticosteroid levels are normal or borderline, evaluation of impaired ACTH secretory reserve is of some practical value. To do this it is important to document that the adrenal can respond to exogenous ACTH. If this is normal, the simplest procedure available to measure the pituitary response is the measurement of the plasma cortisol rise after insulin-induced hypoglycemia. Metyrapone can be administered to lower plasma cortisol by preventing 11-hydroxylation to provide a stimulus for ACTH secretion. Metyrapone is given for 1 or 2 days in doses of 750 mg by mouth every 4 hours to adults; children are given 15 mg/kg of body weight. Metyrapone tartrate, 30 mg/kg of body weight, can be given intravenously for 4 hours. A failure of the urinary 17-OH corticosteroids to double or the plasma 11-deoxycortisol to exceed 10 μg/dl is abnormal.

TSH secretion is easily evaluated by radioimmunoassay and is helpful in the presence of reduced plasma T_4. Administration of TSH is rarely employed in diagnosis at the present time. It is time-consuming and expensive.

The administration of 400 μg of TRH intravenously helps one to identify those patients with hypothalamic disease as a cause of hypothyroidism. A delayed rise in plasma TSH will occur. Unfortunately, some patients with primary pituitary disease also will have an abnormal TSH response.

PRL levels are not regularly depressed in patients with panhypopituitarism, and so a normal or moderately elevated serum PRL does not militate against the diagnosis of hypopituitarism. Presumably, small nests of lactotroph cells, which are isolated from normal portal flow, hypersecrete sufficiently to maintain normal plasma concentrations. PRL measurements are helpful in recognizing prolactinomas in patients with pituitary tumors presenting as hypopituitarism.

GH measurements are only helpful when performed after one of the provocative procedures (see Pituitary Dwarfism, p. 97, for details).

Radioimmunoassays of serum and urine LH and FSH are most helpful in the evaluation of hypopituitarism in women beyond the menopause. In this age group, gonadotropins are normally high. Gonadotropin measurements are less helpful in other patients because the results observed in patients with hypopituitarism and in hospitalized nonendocrine patients overlap. Measurements of LH and FSH after administration of LRH are not recommended for clinical diagnosis unless hypothalamic disease is suspected. If LRH is used, it may be administered for 3–4 days in adequate dosage, i.e., 100 μg tid im, to distinguish between hypothalamic and primary pituitary diseases.

Treatment

Replacement of pituitary hormones, although theoretically sound, has little practical use except in attempts to restore fertility. Fortunately, potent hormonal preparations are readily available to replace the secretions of the adrenals, thyroid, and gonads.

Experience dictates that a gradual restoration of T_4 should be instituted. An initial dose of 0.05 mg of L-T_4 is prudent with severe hypothyroidism. The dose of T_4 is increased gradually to a full maintenance dose (0.15–0.2 mg L-T_4/day).

Replacement treatment with corticosteroids is mandatory if pituitary destruction is complete and desirable if hypopituitarism is moderate. For simple maintenance therapy relatively small doses are required, 12.5–25 mg of cortisone acetate or its equivalent of the newer synthetic analogues. During fever, gastrointestinal upsets, or surgical procedures, larger doses are indicated. There is no need to prescribe mineralocorticoids routinely to patients with hypopituitarism if they salt their foods normally.

The administration of androgens to men with hypopituitarism improves general strength and vigor, as well as restoring libido and potency. Methyltestosterone, in doses of 20–30 mg daily by mouth, is sufficient. Some patients prefer to receive an intramuscular injection of a slowly absorbed preparation such as testosterone enanthate, 200 mg every 2–3 weeks. Estrogen replacement is desirable in young women to correct vaginal mucosal atrophy and to maintain breast development. Also, estrogen administration may minimize bone calcium losses. To induce ovulation in women with hypopituitarism, menotropin, a form of FSH isolated from the urine of postmenopausal women, is given under careful medical supervision. When the ovarian response is established after 2–3 weeks treatment by monitoring estrogen production, ovulation is achieved by the administration of CG. Although experience with this form of therapy in patients with panhypopituitarism is limited, the evidence would suggest that the ovary remains responsive to FSH even after many years of hypopituitarism. There is a real risk of multiple births with this type of treatment.

Treatment of male hypogonadism in patients with panhypopituitarism with gonadotropins requires three or four months. Fertility has been restored in a few cases treated with menotropin and CG for prolonged periods.

With replacement of all target gland hormonal deficiencies, the clinical response is gratifying to both patient and physician. The patient with severe hypopituitarism is transformed from a vegetating invalid to an active member of society. The signs of hypothyroidism disappear. Energy and strength increase nearly to normal. If provision is made for increased doses of corticosteroids during periods of metabolic stress, the prognosis for a long and useful life is excellent.

Isolated Deficiencies

The condition known as hypogonadotropic eunuchoidism has been well characterized (Chapter 6). The analogous syndrome in women of amenorrhea secondary to decreased gonadotropin secretion is also well defined. Male hypogonadotropic eunuchoidism associated with hyposmia (Kallman's syndrome) is a familial disorder, often with some members of the family sexually normal but hyposmic. Hypogonadotropic eunuchoidism is characterized by gonadal inactivity, little or no gonadotropins in urine and plasma, and responses of the gonad to exogenous gonadotropins. Although most cases of hypogonadotropic hypogonadism exhibit deficiencies of both gonadotropins, there are rare cases in which the secretion of only a single pituitary gonadotropin was impaired.

Isolated deficiency of ACTH secretion is a definite clinical entity. Symptoms of weakness, hypoglycemia, weight loss, and decreased female sex hair suggest the diagnosis. The plasma and urinary steroid levels are low and rise to normal after ACTH treatment. Following the administration of metyrapone, the expected rise in plasma 11-deoxycortisol or urinary tetrahydro-11-deoxycortisol does not occur. To make the diagnosis, clinical and laboratory evidence of other pituitary hormone deficiencies must be absent.

The diagnosis of isolated TSH deficiency is likely when clinical features of hypothyroidism exist, plasma TSH is not elevated, and there are no deficiencies of other pituitary hormones. In this condition the plasma TSH, as measured by radioimmunoassay, is not invariably lower than normal. Cases have been reported in which the plasma TSH has been normal or slightly elevated but still inappropriately low for the degree of hypothyroidism. There is some evidence that TSH secreted in these cases has decreased thyroid-stimulating activity. The administration of TRH will in most cases result in a rise in plasma TSH that is normal in magnitude but usually delayed in onset. This result indicates that the TSH deficiency is the result of a hypothalamic disorder. The diagnosis of TSH deficiency can also be established by noting a rise in plasma T_3 or radioiodine uptake after the administration of bovine TSH, 10 IU for 3 days.

The existence of isolated PRL deficiency has rarely been recognized in patients who fail to lactate after delivery. Basal PRL levels are low, and no response to phenothiazine challenge occurs.

Isolated GH deficiency has been established in many cases of dwarfism. This will be described at length in the next section.

PITUITARY DWARFISM

Definition

Impairment in GH secretion either due to abnormal function or destruction of somatotroph cells or due to a lack of hypothalamic stimulation in childhood leads to the impaired growth that is called pituitary dwarfism.

Etiology

The etiology of pituitary dwarfism is varied. In only a minority of the affected children is there evidence of pituitary destruction. Skull films will reveal evidence of craniopharyngioma or pituitary tumor in about one third of the cases. Most children with such tumors will grow normally for a period of years, with later failure of skeletal growth. In some patients, lytic lesions of bone in the skull, usually combined with diabetes insipidus, suggest histiocytosis.

Midline defects, such as cleft palate, absence of the septum pellucidum, optic nerve hypoplasia, and nystagmus, indicate involvement of the pituitary in a more general embryonic malformation. The basic defect in GH secretion may lie in the hypothalamic STH-regulating centers.

About 10% of the cases of pituitary dwarfism are familial. Analysis of a number of pedigrees of the familial form of hyposomatotropism indicates transmission as a recessive gene. Less commonly, a dominant pattern has been observed. The pituitary dysfunction is usually limited to the secretion of STH. A delayed but otherwise normal puberty occurs. Affected women can become pregnant and deliver normal-sized offspring. Lactation is normal. The diagnosis of GH deficiency in these patients has been unequivocally established by radioimmunoassay.

Most cases of pituitary dwarfism have no familial basis and are not the result of any recognizable disease process affecting the pituitary gland. The possibility of birth trauma is suggested by an increased frequency of breech and difficult deliveries. In about one third of the cases, isolated GH deficiency is present. In the remaining cases, other pituitary deficiencies exist.

Clinical Features

The size and appearance of the infants at birth are unremarkable except for the occasional presence of microphallus in male infants. Although growth failure may be recognized as early as 6 months, more frequently this is not recognized until the child is 1–3 years of age. Untreated, there is continued slow growth through childhood at about 50–60% normal velocity (Fig. 3–31). Body proportions and facial

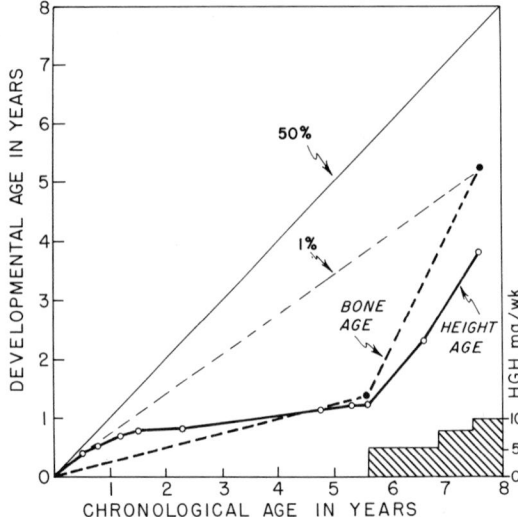

Figure 3–31. Extreme retardation of skeletal age and height age in a pituitary dwarf, plotted according to the convention of Lawson Wilkins. The rapid advancement of growth and bone maturation after treatment with human GH is also shown. (Reproduced from Daughaday, W. H., and Parker, M. L.: The pituitary in disorders of growth. *Disease-a-Month*, August, 1962, by permission of Year Book Medical Publishers, Inc.)

features remain immature. Many affected children are pudgy, with deposition of fat over the iliac crests and lower abdomen (Fig. 3–32). Primary teeth appear at the expected age, but the eruption of secondary teeth is delayed. In adult life, many pituitary dwarfs develop fine wrinkles about the mouth and eyes that give a paradoxical appearance of immaturity combined with presenility.

General health often remains surprisingly good, with normal response to illness and trauma. Only about 10% of the subjects suffer from symptomatic hypoglycemia. Low fasting blood sugars and impaired glucose tolerance are more common. The insulin response to glucose is usually subnormal.

Mental development usually keeps up with chronologic age, and, because of small stature, these children may seem unusually bright. At first, adverse emotional reactions to small stature may not be recognized, but psychologic adjustment becomes increasingly difficult with age.

Laboratory Evaluations

Determination of bone age by hand and other roentgenographs is an important procedure in evaluating growth problems. In pituitary dwarfism, epiphyseal maturation is usually retarded to the same extent as height. The sella turcica is abnormally small in about 10–20% of cases.

Although the clinical picture may suggest pituitary dwarfism, diagnosis can be accepted only when confirmed by radioimmunoassay. A single determination of plasma GH in the basal state is of limited usefulness because the basal plasma levels of most normal children are so low that they cannot be differentiated with confidence from those of hypopituitary dwarfs. For this reason, GH determinations should be carried out after provocative challenge. Many tests have been proposed. Hypoglycemia induced by insulin given intravenously in a dose of 0.05–0.1 U/kg body weight will stimulate GH secretion in most normal children if the plasma sugar falls below 50 mg/dl or 50% of the fasting level. Peak GH levels are usually reached at 45 or 60 min. Simultaneous measurement of serum cortisol will also provide information concerning the normality of the pituitary

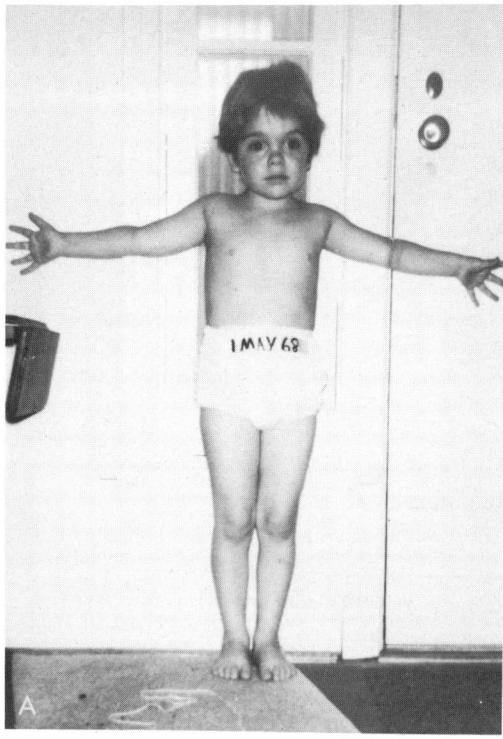
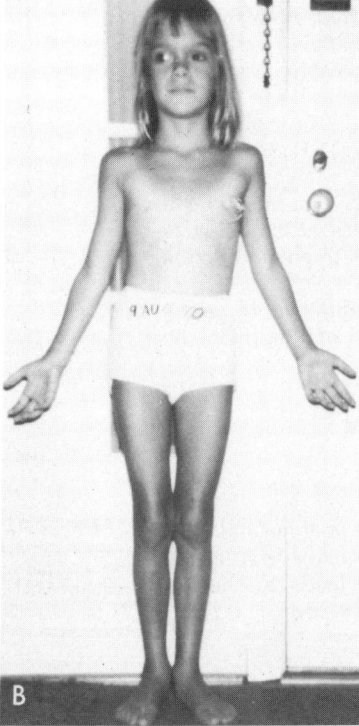

Figure 3–32. *A*, A 6-year-old girl with hyposomatotropic dwarfism secondary to a craniopharyngioma. Note infantile chubbiness and facial features. Height, 37 inches. *B*, Fifteen months later after she had been treated with 2.5 mg of HGH twice weekly, her height had increased to 48¼ inches. In addition to her gain in height, note her obvious loss of infantile fat and more mature facial features.

adrenal axis. Conducting this test may lead to serious hypoglycemic symptoms if the blood sugar falls excessively. For this reason, insertion of an inlying needle for glucose administration and careful professional observation during the test is mandatory. Alternatively, the drop in blood sugar may be insufficient to stimulate GH secretion.

Arginine infusion, 0.5 g/kg given intravenously over 30 min, and L-dopa (500 mg for children over 70 lbs, 250 mg for children 30–70 lbs, and 125 mg for children less than 30 lbs) provide alternative provocative stimuli, well adapted for diagnostic studies. It is advisable to allow the patient to rest horizontally in a quiet room during the L-dopa test to minimize possible syncope, nausea, and vomiting.

More potent stimuli of GH secretion result when L-dopa and arginine administration are combined or when propranolol is added. Stilbestrol, 3 mg/day, by mouth for 3 days has also been advocated as a method for increasing borderline responses.

In all these provocative tests, blood samples can be drawn with the patient fasting and at 20-min intervals for 80 min. A rise in plasma GH levels above 7–10 ng/ml is usually considered normal, although rigorous validation of these limits has not been provided. It is possible that patients with physiologically significant partial GH deficiency will not be recognized by the more vigorous testing procedures.

Differential Diagnosis

The number of conditions that lead to short stature are legion. A functional classification of some of these conditions is given in Table 3–6.

Decreased Skeletal Response

The great majority of children below the third percentile of stature prove to have normal levels of GH and somatomedin. The bone and height ages are usually retarded to some extent. Short members of the family are common, and delayed sexual maturation may have occurred in parents or siblings. These children are currently diagnosed as having idiopathic short stature or constitutional delay. Undoubtedly as techniques of investigation improve, this group of children will be resolved into subgroups due to a number of somatomedin receptor and postreceptor defects. The short stature of certain races, most evident in African pygmies, probably is also due to similar limited hormonal responsiveness.

Psychosocial Dwarfism

This is a form of reversible hypothalamic hyposomatotropism due to psychogenic inhibition. Affected children show

Table 3–6. CAUSES OF IMPAIRED GH SECRETION AND ACTION

I. Decreased GH secretion
    Hypothalamic: decreased secretion of GH-releasing hormone
    Isolated GH deficiency
    Combined GH and other pituitary hormones
    Functional GH deficiency—emotional deprivation
    Primary pituitary deficiencies or destruction

II. Defective GH action
    Defective GH receptor — Laron dwarfism
    Secretion of abnormal GH (?)
    Nutritional impairment of GH-induced somatomedin formation—
      kwashiorkor

III. Impaired skeletal response to somatomedin or (?) GH
    Constitutional short stature
    Gonadal dysgenesis
    Primary cartilaginous or bone disease
    Chronic renal disease
    Corticosteroid excess
    Chronic inflammatory disease

IV. Complex disorders
    Hypothyroidism
    Diabetes mellitus

---

marked growth impairment with little or no overt evidence of nutritional impairment. Characteristically the family environment is extremely bad and lacking in normal emotional support. In at least some cases the growth failure cannot be attributed to lack of available food because bizarre patterns of excessive eating and drinking have been reported. When first studied these children have been observed to have low somatomedin levels and impaired GH secretion. Characteristically, a rapid reversal of the hormone abnormalities and resumption of normal growth ensue after entering the neutral environment of the metabolic ward or convalescent center. It is postulated that the extreme emotional deprivation has inhibited GH secretion by neurogenic pathways.

Defective Growth Hormone Action

When dwarfism is associated with normal or increased secretion of GH by radioimmunoassay and low levels of somatomedin, a defect in GH action is suspected unless malnutrition is present. Patients with Laron dwarfism have severe proportionate growth retardation and a phenotypic appearance of pituitary dwarfism. Serum GH levels are moderately to greatly elevated and somatomedin levels are invariably low. After the administration of human GH, there is neither a rise in serum somatomedin (Fig. 3–33) nor a sustained stimulation of growth velocity. The disease is more common in Oriental Jews and Mediterranean populations but also has been reported in other racial groups. It is transmitted as a mendelian autosomal recessive gene. Although the molecular defect in this disease has not been established, a defect in the GH receptor is suspected.

Recently, patients have been described (Kowarski et al.) who had normal levels of GH associated with very low serum somatomedin concentrations. Unlike patients with Laron dwarfism, there was a normal rise of somatomedin after the administration of human GH. More prolonged hGH treatment restored normal growth velocities. It is suspected that these children secreted a biologically inactive GH.

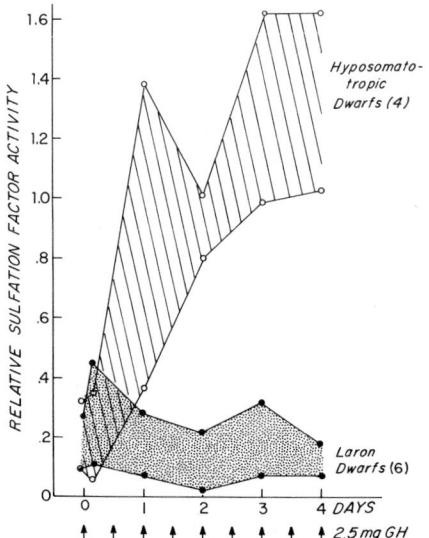

Figure 3–33. Comparison of somatomedin (sulfation factor) activity of hyposomatotropic and hypersomatotropic (Laron) dwarfs before and after twice-daily GH administration. (Reproduced from Daughaday, W. H., Laron, Z., et al.: Defective sulfation factor generation: a possible etiological link in dwarfism. *Trans. Assoc. Am. Physicians* 82:129, 1969, with permission.)

Hypothyroidism

Hypothyroidism is associated with a striking slowing of growth velocity and an even greater slowing of bone maturation. In experimental hypothyroidism of rats, there is a virtual cessation of GH synthesis. In humans an impairment in GH secretion and somatomedin release is inconstant. Provocative tests of GH secretion are often normal despite severe growth retardation, and somatomedin levels may be within normal limits. It would appear that the most significant impairment is in the ability of cartilage and other growth target tissues to respond to GH and somatomedin.

Gonadal Dysgenesis (Turner's Syndrome)

The short stature of patients with gonadal dysplasia is often confused with pituitary dwarfism. Growth retardation is only moderate, and bone maturation is little impaired. The diagnosis may be strongly suspected in short girls with primary amenorrhea and congenital anomalies, such as webbing of the neck, short metacarpal or metatarsal bones, increased carrying angle of the elbows, and coarctation of the aorta. Rarely, the short stature may be associated with gonadal dysplasia without external congenital anomalies. Cytologic examination of the buccal smear should be included in the diagnostic evaluation of all stunted girls. The absence of the normal female chromatin body will permit unequivocal recognition of 80% of individuals with gonadal dysplasia. In doubtful cases, complete characterization of the karyotype is desirable. Patients have been described with XO/XX or other X chromosomal mosaicism who present with short stature and few of the classic features of Turner's syndrome.

Diabetes Mellitus

Uncontrolled diabetes mellitus retards normal growth. In a few cases GH levels have been reported to be elevated and somatomedin levels low. It is likely that this pattern is the result of the disorder of intermediary metabolism with resultant secondary caloric and other nutritional deficits rather than of insulin deficiency directly.

Malnutrition

Growth failure is an invariant finding of serious malnutrition. The pattern of GH secretion is inconstant in various types of undernutrition. In marasmus, which results from a deficiency of total food intake, GH levels in plasma may be normal or slightly elevated. In kwashiorkor, protein intake is markedly deficient but caloric intake is relatively more adequate. In the florid forms of kwashiorkor that exist in Africa, serum GH levels are markedly elevated but serum levels of somatomedin are low. A hypothesis to explain this pattern is that hepatic synthesis of somatomedin is limiting and that the elevation of serum GH may be the result of decreased negative feedback of somatomedin on GH secretion. The hormonal disturbance is rapidly corrected by nutritional rehabilitation.

Systemic Inflammatory Disease

The possibility of an occult systemic inflammatory condition should be considered in children with growth failure.

Patients with juvenile rheumatoid arthritis, rheumatic fever, and inflammatory bowel disease may attract attention because of growth failure rather than because of the primary manifestations of these diseases. The true nature of the diagnosis generally becomes evident after a thorough clinical examination with appropriate laboratory procedures. The old-fashioned sedimentation rate test is a useful screening procedure.

Chronic Renal Disease

Patients with chronic azotemia or renal acidosis often present initially with short stature.

Primary Skeletal Disorders

There are a number of congenital and hereditary diseases of the skeleton, such as hypophosphatemic rickets, pseudohypoparathyroidism, achondroplasia, epiphyseal dysplasia, and neurofibromatosis, that occasionally have to be considered in the diagnosis of short stature. Usually these diseases cause disproportionate growth that is readily recognized. When presented with such cases, the physician should refer to texts dealing with congenital disorders of the skeleton.

Corticosteroid Excess

Impairment of skeletal growth is an extremely sensitive indicator of spontaneous or iatrogenic corticosteroid toxicity. Associated cushingoid obesity is common and if the corticosteroid excess persists for 1 year or more, radiologically recognizable osteopenia may be present. The familiar features of Cushing's syndrome may be present to a variable extent. Termination of corticosteroid excess leads to the resumption of normal growth velocities but "catch-up" growth may not occur. Although GH secretion can be inhibited by massive doses of corticosteroids, there usually is normal GH secretion in children with this type of GH impairment. In clinical cases also, measurements of serum somatomedin have given conflicting answers depending on the assay method used. It is likely that the most significant defect is at the level of skeletal tissue response to somatomedins.

Treatment

Administration of human GH to pituitary dwarfs leads to a marked acceleration of growth with doses as small as 2.5 IU twice a week (Fig. 3–29). There is no advantage of intermittent treatment. Increases in height of 10–15 cm are frequently achieved within the first year. Thereafter, more moderate growth rates are encountered and higher doses of hormone may be required to maintain accelerated growth. An occasional child will respond initially but subsequently prove refractory. High levels of antibody against human GH have been found in the plasma of a few such patients. In other cases, the refractoriness remains unexplained. Withholding the hormone for several months may restore the response to subsequent GH administration.

In the past, supplies of human GH in the United States have depended on a nationwide collection of cadaver pituitaries conducted by the National Pituitary Agency. The GH has been allocated for clinical investigation. Human GH is prepared commercially and is available in other countries at considerable expense. Additional supplies of the hormone are urgently needed. It is hoped that the microbial synthesis of GH achieved by recombinant gene technology will soon provide the GH required for therapy.

Other therapeutic agents are of limited value in treatment of hyposomatotropism. Thyroid deficiency should be corrected, but overtreatment will cause excessive advancement of bone maturation. Cortisone treatment should be avoided if possible but may be required if hypoglycemia or other symptoms of hypoadrenocorticism are a problem.

Androgenic steroids have a restricted use for patients who are refractory to human GH or for children over 12 years for whom GH is not available. If care is taken to prescribe a minimal dose of androgen, stimulation of growth without undue virilization or prohibitive advance in bone maturation can be achieved. GH treatment should be continued because synergism exists between the action of these two growth-promoting agents. Eventual height may be increased slightly and growth obtained at a time appropriate for psychologic development. In the past, excessive androgen doses have been used with the unfortunate result of premature closure of the epiphysis.

PITUITARY TUMORS

Pathology

Adenomas are classified as microadenomas if their diameter is less than 10 mm and as macroadenomas if they are larger (Fig. 3–34). Enclosed adenomas are entirely confined to the osteoaponeural sheath of the sella turcica; invasive adenomas extend beyond the confines of the sheath. Pituitary adenomas lack true capsules, and the margin between normal adenohypophysis and adenoma may be marked only by condensation of normal cells interspersed by adenomatous cells and a varying amount of condensed normal stroma. With growth of the adenoma there is at first localized, and later more generalized, pressure on the bony sella, leading to sellar expansion. It is now recognized that macroadenomas possess an impressive ability to invade neighboring bony and vascular structures. Inferiorly, the tumor can penetrate the thin sellar floor and enter the sphenoid sinus and even present within the nasopharynx. Lateral invasion will carry tumor cells into the carotid sheath and the structures of the cavernous sinus, effectively eliminating the possibility of surgical care. Superior extension of either the enclosed or the invasive adenoma may exert a pressure on the optic chiasm.

Further upward progression of a pituitary tumor into the hypothalamus may produce disturbed consciousness, hyperphagia, and abnormal temperature regulation. Obstruction of cerebrospinal fluid drainage with creation of hydrocephalus can occur with craniopharyngiomas but is rare with pituitary adenomas. Particularly invasive pituitary tumors may break into the middle and posterior fossae and produce brain stem manifestations. Rarely, distant metastases on the spinal meninges and even in the liver have been reported.

All pituitary tumors but particularly corticotroph and somatotroph adenomas undergo hemorrhagic infarction — "pituitary apoplexy."

Cell Types

Prolactinoma. Lactotroph cell tumors, commonly called prolactinomas, are the most common pituitary tumor. More than 60% of patients formerly believed to harbor nonsecretory tumors have shown elevations of serum PRL. About half of the tumors at the time of operation are microadenomas,

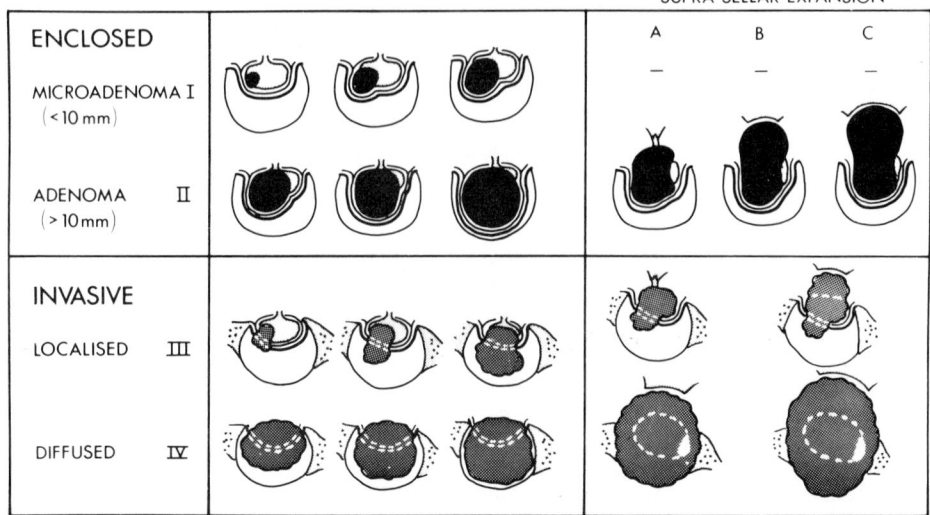

SUPRA SELLAR EXPANSION

Figure 3–34. A classification of pituitary tumors based on tumor size and evidence of tumor invasiveness. Shown are diagrammatic representations of coronal tomograms showing four classes with three degrees of severity within each class. Suprasellar extension is separately considered. (Reproduced with permission from Hardy, J.: *Transsphenoidal surgery of hypersecreting pituitary tumors.* In *Diagnosis and Treatment of Pituitary Tumors.* Kohler, P. O., and Ross, G. T., (eds.), New York, American Elsevier Publishing Co., 1973.)

which produce endocrine symptoms but with little tendency to enlarge. These tumors present as yellowish or pinkish growths; frequently there is a soft necrotic center.

Somatotroph Cell Adenoma. This tumor is almost invariably associated with gigantism or acromegaly. Macroadenomas are frequently locally invasive. As many as 20% of the tumors are mixed somatotroph and lactotroph cell tumors, as determined by immunostaining of the separate cell types. Less frequently the same cell has been shown to contain both hormones, indicating a derivation from a common stem cell.

Corticotroph Adenomas. These are present in nearly all cases of pituitary hyperadrenal corticism, i.e., Cushing's disease. Because they may be as small as 2 mm in diameter, many of these tumors were not considered functionally significant until recently. Despite their neoplastic nature, most corticotroph tumors are functionally partially suppressed by the high levels of cortisol that their secretions have provoked. If the patients undergo bilateral total adrenalectomy, ACTH secretion rises and 10% or more of the tumors show progressive growth. Clinically this is recognized by severe pigmentation and is called Nelson's syndrome. These tumors are characterized by their great invasiveness with a tendency to produce cranial nerve and vascular involvement.

Thyrotroph and Gonadotroph Cell Adenomas. These adenomas are distinctly unusual. In some cases the tumors have arisen after years of hypersecretion prompted by thyroid and gonadal failure respectively. There are only a few cases of thyrotroph adenomas that have induced hyperthyroidism.

Chromophobe or Nonsecretory Cell Tumors. These tumors of the pituitary were, until recently, considered to be the most common type of pituitary adenoma. Only about 15% of adenomas have recognized secretory granules by conventional staining techniques, but a much higher fraction of secretory granules are seen when examined by electronmicroscopy. More than half of the so-called "chromophobe" adenomas are associated with PRL secretion and others secrete GH and ACTH. Some tumors without elevations of serum gonadotropins secrete gonadotropins or their isolated α chains *in vitro*. The application of highly sensitive radioimmunoassay methods has therefore established that even in the absence of clear clinical manifestations most pituitary tumors are secreting at least small amounts of one or more pituitary hormones.

Topical Distribution of Pituitary Tumors (Fig. 3–35). The secretory cells of the adenohypophysis are not uniformly

distributed throughout the anterior pituitary. Somatotroph and lactotroph cells are more common in the lateral wings of the pituitary whereas the cells secreting glycoprotein hormones and corticotropins are concentrated within the central mucoid wedge of the gland. In Hardy's[72] experience the pituitary adenomas are similarly predominantly distributed. He notes a tendency for the prolactinomas to be deeper and more posterior in the lateral wing than somatotroph tumors. Not all neurosurgeons agree with these generalizations.

Nonpituitary Sellar and Parasellar Tumors

Craniopharyngiomas are the most important nonpituitary tumors arising in the vicinity of the sella turcica. They

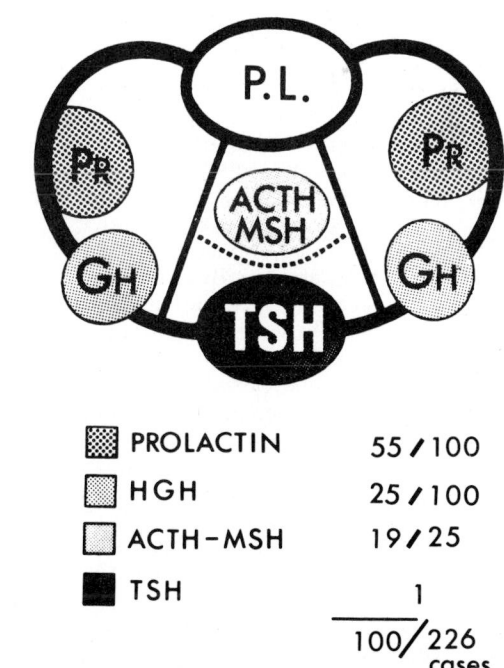

▦ PROLACTIN	55	100
▨ HGH	25	100
☐ ACTH-MSH	19	25
■ TSH		1
		100/226 cases

Figure 3–35. Diagrammatic representation of the most likely location of pituitary microadenomas. There is general acceptance of the usual lateral location of somatotroph adenomas and prolactinomas. Corticotroph adenomas may or may not have the localization shown. Only a few thyrotroph adenomas have been recognized. (Reproduced with permission from Hardy, J.: *Transsphenoidal approach to the pituitary.* In *Microneurosurgery,* Rand, R. W. (ed.), St. Louis, C. V. Mosby Co., 1978, pp. 105–130.)

arise from remnants of Rathke's pouch and vary greatly in structure from simple cysts containing dark oily fluid to solid tumors composed of columnar cells on a basement membrane in a pattern that resembles adamantinomas. Occasionally, squamous cells with masses of cornified tissue replace the columnar cells in areas of the tuumor. The frequent occurrence of areas of calcification is a helpful diagnostic characteristic for the radiologist, suggesting craniopharyngioma rather than some other type of pituitary neoplasm.

Meningiomas, chordomas, teratoid tumors, and metastatic tumors of varied origin may involve the sella turcica and mimic nonsecretory pituitary adenomas clinically.

Experimental Tumors

Pituitary tumors occur spontaneously or can be experimentally induced in a number of animal species, especially in rats and mice. In many cases, the tumor develops after the induction of a hypersecretory state. Thyroidectomy leads to the development of TSH-secreting tumors in mice, and gonadectomy has led to pituitary tumors that secrete gonadotropins and ACTH. Estrogen administration stimulates the pituitary lactotroph cells and has led to tumors that secrete PRL and GH. The development of pituitary tumors with these endocrine manipulations is increased by radiation. At present, experimental pituitary tumors have been characterized that secrete MSH, ACTH, TSH, GH, and PRL. Successful transplantation of some of these tumors requires a hormonally deficient recipient, indicating that tumor growth is not truly autonomous. Several types of experimental tumors have been successfully established as cloned cell lines in cell culture. The cell lines of GH- and PRL-secreting rat pituitary tumors have been used extensively in studies of a hormonal biosynthesis and its regulation.

Radiologic Diagnosis

Plain Films

The diagnosis of functioning pituitary microadenomas is based on clinical findings and radioimmunoassay measurements of hormone levels, often with appropriate stimulatory or inhibitory procedures. Because less than 5% of patients with Cushing's disease and less than 33% of patients with prolactinomas have abnormalities in their conventional sella x-rays, a negative examination has no value in excluding this diagnosis. In screening patients with hypopituitarism or field defects, coned-down views of the sella are clearly important in the diagnosis of macroadenomas and craniopharyngiomas (often recognized by the presence of intrasellar or suprasellar calcification).

Normally the sella turcica measures less than 12 × 15 mm in vertical and saggital dimensions or a lateral area measured by planimetry of less than 130 mm². Some radiologists prefer an estimate of sellar volume (lateral area × sellar lateral width as detected in the frontal projection). An increase in sellar volume suggests the possibility of a macroadenoma of the pituitary but also may occur in the physiologic hyperplasia of pregnancy, the hyperplasia of hypothyroidism, and the empty sella syndrome (see p. 000). In most cases of macroadenomas, the posterior clinoid processes are porotic and displaced posteriorly. An asymmetric pituitary adenoma can occasionally be recognized on the plain film as a clearly defined double floor of the sella turcica (Fig. 3–36).

Tomographic Sections

Tomographic sections of the sella at 2-mm intervals are sufficient in the radiologic demonstration of macroadenomas but 1-mm intervals should be employed for suspected microadenomas. Microadenomas may present as a localized scalloping, porosity, or focal cortical break in the sellar wall or as a discrete bulging or "blister" of the anterior or inferior sellar floor (Fig. 3–37). In anterior tomograms such tumors are often recognized by a slanting floor or a localized blister. These subtle abnormalities are not pathognomonic of pituitary tumors and can occur in a small percentage of patients otherwise considered normal. Since the diagnosis of microadenomas is often based on endocrine and not radiologic criteria, these radiologic changes are of help to the neurosurgeon in planning his operative procedurés.

Tomograms are also of use in detecting early invasive adenomas by showing the extent of bone destruction and sphenoid sinus invasion (Fig. 3–38).

Computerized Axial Tomography (CAT Scans)

This procedure, particularly after the injection of a radiologic contrast agent, provides a useful, relatively noninvasive examination of the suprasellar area that will detect most but not all superior extensions of pituitary tumors (Fig. 3–39). Some tumors, it should be noted, are isodense with cerebrospinal fluid and cannot be differentiated from the normal suprasellar cistern. A homogeneous intrasellar density less than that of brain tissue suggests either an empty sella syndrome or a pituitary cyst. The claim has been made that some microadenomas can be detected with larger doses of contrast agents and properly selected CAT scan sections. Most pituitary tumors show enhancement after intravenous injection of contrast material. If only a rim of enhancement occurs, a cystic lesion is to be suspected.

Carotid Angiograms

Carotid angiograms are useful in ruling out the possibility of an intrasellar carotid aneurysm or meningioma.

Because of the intrinsic risk of the procedure, particularly in patients with Cushing's disease, it is not usually performed in patients with intrasellar enclosed adenomas.

Intrathecal Air or Metrizamide Contrast Studies

These studies are still considered to be more reliable than simple CAT scans in providing detailed information about suprasellar extention. Metrizamide usually is associated with less stress and less severe headaches than is air and may be the procedure of choice. The physician should be aware of the stressful nature of these procedures, and when ACTH secretion is in doubt, corticosteroid coverage should be provided.

Parasellar Manifestations

Headaches

These are a troublesome complaint of more than three quarters of the patients with pituitary tumors. Traction on the diaphragma sellae or surrounding dural structures would appear to be the most common cause of headache.

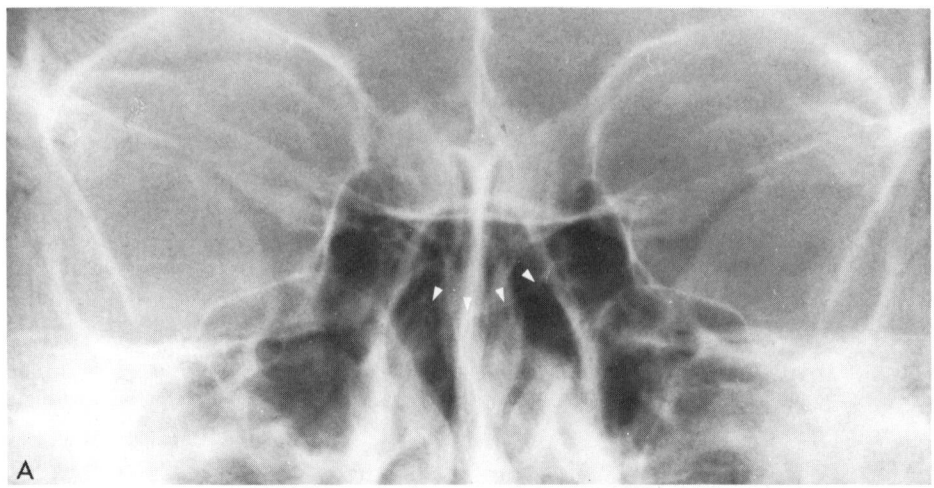

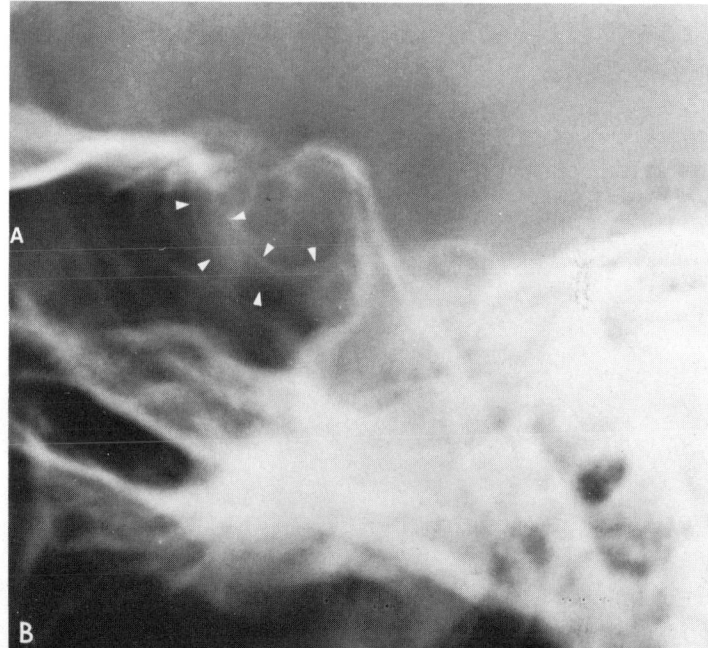

Figure 3–36. Plain skull radiographs. "Double floor" of the sella turcica. 18-year-old girl with a PRL-secreting adenoma. *A*, Coned-down frontal projection. The floor of the sella turcica (white arrowheads) slopes downward from left to right. *B*, Coned-down lateral projection (A = Anterior). The inclination of the sella floor appears as a "double floor" in lateral projection (white arrowheads). This usually indicates sellar erosion. (Courtesy of T. P. Naidich and C. J. Moran, Washington University School of Medicine.)

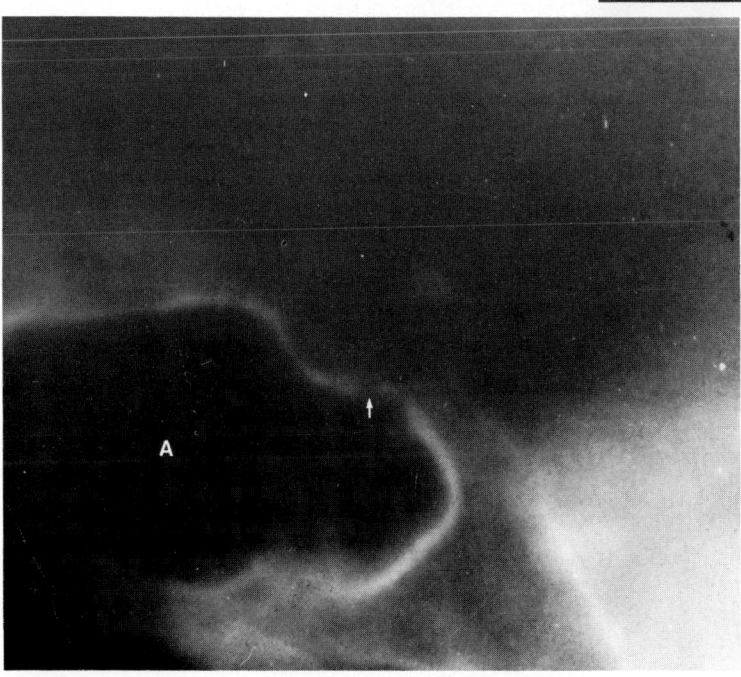

Figure 3–37. Polytomography of the sella turcica in lateral projection (A = Anterior). Thirty-five-year-old woman with a PRL-secreting microadenoma. There is focal erosion of the cortical margin of the sellar floor (white arrow). (Courtesy of T. P. Naidich and C. J. Moran, Washington University School of Medicine.)

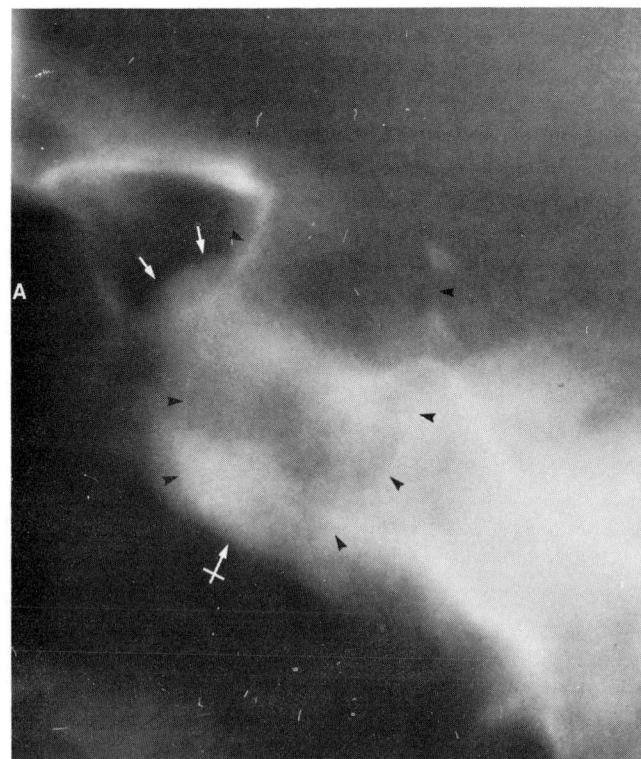

Figure 3–38. Polytomography of the sella turcica in lateral projection (A = Anterior). Fifty-year-old man with a nonsecreting adenoma. There is massive expansion of the sella turcica (black arrows) with marked extrasellar tumor extension through the sphenoid sinus (white arrows) into the roof of the nasopharynx (crossed white arrow). (Courtesy of T. P. Naidich and C. J. Moran, Washington University School of Medicine.)

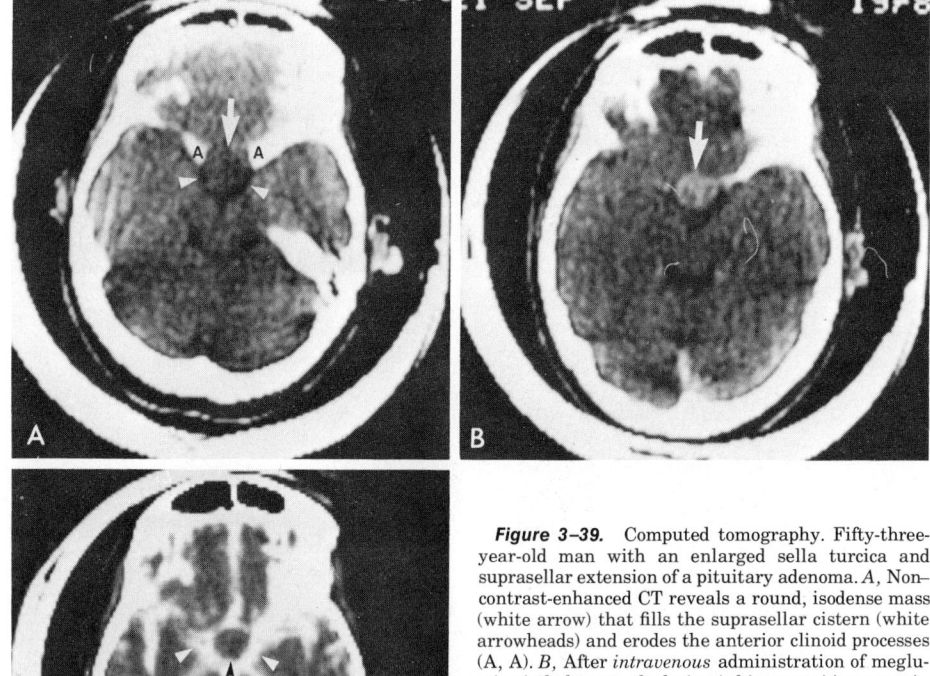

Figure 3–39. Computed tomography. Fifty-three-year-old man with an enlarged sella turcica and suprasellar extension of a pituitary adenoma. *A,* Non–contrast-enhanced CT reveals a round, isodense mass (white arrow) that fills the suprasellar cistern (white arrowheads) and erodes the anterior clinoid processes (A, A). *B,* After *intravenous* administration of meglumine iothalamate, the lesion (white arrow) increases in density (tumor contrast enhancement) and is more easily detected. *C,* After opacification of the CSF by *intrathecal* administration of metrizamide, CT demonstrates the lesion (black arrowhead) as a filling defect in the metrizamide-opacified suprasellar cistern (white arrowheads). The midbrain (M) is outlined by metrizamide in the perimesencephalic cistern. (Courtesy of T. P. Naidich and C. J. Moran, Washington University School of Medicine.)

The lining of the sphenoid sinus and the walls of large blood vessels in the region of the sella are also capable of giving rise to painful sensations. The location of the headache is inconstant: In one large series of patients with pituitary adenomas, 31% were frontal, 19% orbital, 16% temporal, 10% occipital, 7% vertical, and 2% generalized; in the remaining 15%, the headaches were insufficiently characterized for tabulation. Most commonly, the headaches are of moderate severity and are intermittent. Occasionally, headaches are accompanied by nausea and vomiting.

Visual Deficits

Loss of vision due to pressure on the optic nerves may be noted by patients with macroadenomas. Other patients are unaware of small or even advanced visual field defects. As a tumor presses upward from the bony confines of the sella turcica, the optic chiasm and optic nerves are at first displaced superiorly. Continued displacement is prevented by the anterior arterial arc of the circle of Willis (Fig 3–1), which overlies the optic nerves and serves as a nonyielding constricting band against which the optic nerves are compressed. Most tumors protrude between the two arms of the optic nerves and exert pressure on the inferior medial aspect of the nerves. With this type of impingement, the earliest losses of visual field are recognized in the superior temporal quadrant. Later a quadrantic loss of the visual field extends to hemianopia. Further damage to the optic nerve leads to scotomas, loss of vision in the nasal fields, and finally total blindness.

Extensive damage to the optic nerve leads to pallor of the optic disk. Papilledema is rare. Anisocoria occurs if the loss in vision in one eye greatly exceeds that in the other. Because of the vagaries of tumor growth and the anatomic variations in the location of the optic chiasm, other patterns of visual loss may occur. Repeated examinations of the visual fields are an essential part of the management of pituitary tumors. Accurate measurements are particularly urgent during periods of radiation therapy, when swelling of the tumor can result in sudden worsening of vision.

Cranial Nerves

Involvement of cranial nerves, other than the optic nerves, occurs infrequently (10–20% of patients with macroadenomas) despite the proximity of the third, fourth, and sixth cranial nerves to any sellar mass. Impairments of third nerve function are recognized more frequently than those of other cranial nerves. Occasionally the olfactory nerves or tracts are disrupted, with loss of the sense of smell.

Hypothalamus

Large pituitary tumors may compress or infiltrate the hypothalamus, producing a variety of manifestations, such as disturbances in appetite, sleep, and temperature regulation. Deficiencies of adenohypophyseal function occurring in suprasellar tumors can be the result of damage to the hypothalamic centers regulating adenohypophyseal function. Involvement of uncinate lobe can result in uncinate seizures.

Vascular Involvement

Pituitary tumors may invade the large vessels that ring the sella turcica, with subsequent thrombosis or hemor-

rhage. The blood supply of pituitary tumors is easily impaired, and infarctions of tumors followed by cystic degeneration are common. Hemorrhage into a tumor, "pituitary apoplexy," leads to severe headache, abrupt loss of vision or other cranial nerve deficits, mental obtundity, hypotension and hyperthermia. Prompt evacuation of the clots and control of bleeding may save life and vision.

Hormonal Deficiencies

The normal pituitary may be compressed to a shell about a tumor mass. The clinical evidences of hypopituitarism correlate roughly with the degree of destruction of normal tissue. Symptoms are usually not detected unless more than three quarters of the pituitary has been destroyed. Even with very large tumors, the signs of hormonal deficiency rarely equal in severity those that occur after hypophysectomy. Hypogonadism is usually the earliest sign of hypopituitarism, but this can be the result of PRL excess as well as due to loss of normal pituitary tissue. Symptoms of hypothyroidism are common with many poorly functioning macroadenomas. Adrenal insufficiency rarely is symptomatic except under conditions of severe stress, but ACTH reserve is commonly lost, as demonstrated by the failure of the urinary steroids to increase after the administration of metyrapone.

Disruption of the neurohypophyseal regulation of water metabolism leading to diabetes insipidus only occurs in about 10% of untreated cases of pituitary tumors. Patients with untreated somatotroph or corticotroph tumors almost never have diabetes insipidus. Minor disturbances of water regulation are easily overlooked unless careful measurements of the osmolality of urine and plasma are made in the hydropenic state. Following surgical treatment of pituitary tumors, transitory or permanent diabetes insipidus frequently develops.

Clinical Characteristics

Clinical syndromes of hypersecretion of PRL, GH, ACTH, and TSH are recognized in association with pituitary adenomas.

Prolactinomas

Incidence

Prolactinomas are the most common secretory tumor of the pituitary. In women, about half the tumors are microadenomas, whereas the remainder are macroadenomas at the time of diagnosis. The frequency of microprolactinomas in men is much lower. It remains unclear whether the rarity of microadenomas in men can be related to late recognition or whether the growth characteristics of prolactinoma are different in women. As previously mentioned, there is the possibility that estrogens, particularly as increased during pregnancy or as administered as contraceptive drugs, may have led to an increase in the frequency of this tumor.

Clinical Manifestations

Women with microadenomas usually present with amenorrhea with or without galactorrhea. Fully 20–33% of young women with amenorrhea of greater than six months duration have persistent hyperprolactinemia, but less than half of the patients with hyperprolactinemia experience galactorrhea. Galactorrhea usually consists of the discharge of a few drops of milk only with pressure. Some patients fail to note galactorrhea until the physician manually expresses the milk. Rarely, profuse galactorrhea will wet clothing and be a cause of annoyance and embarrassment to the patient. Galactorrhea associated with normal menses is usually unassociated with sustained hyperprolactinemia. Some of these patients may have increased PRL levels after mechanical breast stimulation and not at the time PRL measurements are made. In other patients this form of galactorrhea simply represents mammary hypersensitivity to normal concentrations of sex steroids and PRL.

The duration of symptoms prior to diagnosis of microadenomas may be very long. Years and even decades of increased menstrual irregularity may precede the onset of amenorrhea. Amenorrhea and galactorrhea may follow pregnancy (the Chiari-Frommel syndrome) or be unassociated with pregnancy (del Castillo's syndrome or Forbes-Albright syndrome). These eponyms have out-lived their usefulness and should be abandoned. Many patients with prolactinomas have been given birth control pills for various periods because of preceding menstrual disturbances. The persistence of hyperprolactinemia after stopping these pills is one cause of postpill amenorrhea.

Men with pituitary tumors may present to physicians because of visual impairment, headache, or other parasellar complaints. About two thirds of such men have noted loss of libido and potency. In the past, these symptoms have been attributed to compressive atrophy of normal adenohypophyseal tissue. The fact that bromocriptine treatment can, in at least some cases, restore serum testosterone levels and correct the impairment in libido and potency indicates that PRL suppression of hypothalamic release of LRF is involved.

Endocrine Diagnosis

Hyperprolactinemia is present when repeated measurements of plasma PRL are elevated. In most laboratories the upper limit of normal PRL is 20 ng/ml for healthy ambulatory subjects, although a wider range exists for hospitalized nonendocrine sick patients. Repeated measurements are necessary because secretion by prolactinomas is often variable. Patients with prolactinomas lose their nocturnal peak of secretion but this is not a useful diagnostic observation.

The diagnosis of a prolactinoma requires the exclusion of the large number of functional causes of hyperprolactinemia, some of which are also associated with amenorrhea and galactorrhea. Table 3–7 lists these conditions and medications that have been recognized as principal causes of functional hyperprolactinemia.

The diagnosis of prolactinoma is reasonably secure if there is radiologic evidence of a pituitary tumor with hyperprolactinemia.

When there is no radiologic evidence of a pituitary tumor, the diagnosis of prolactinoma presents more of a challenge. The following criteria have been proposed for the diagnosis of prolactinomas.

1. *Level of Plasma Prolactin.* Cases of amenorrhea and galactorrhea of functional causes rarely have serum PRL levels in excess of 100 ng/ml.

2. *TRH Responsiveness.* Most patients with prolactinomas do not have significant rise in serum PRL after the iv administration of 400 μg of TRH, whereas normal individuals have a reproducible rise. There is doubt about the

Table 3–7. CAUSES OF HYPERPROLACTINEMIA

I. Increased neurogenic afferent impulses
    Chest wall lesions
    Suckling and nipple stimulation
    Stress

II. Hypothalamic etiologies
    Diffuse hypothalamic disease (encephalitis, etc.)
    Granulomatous and infiltrative disease (sarcoid, histiocytosis)
    Tumors (craniopharyngiomas, meningiomas, etc.)
    Metabolic (uremia)
    Traumatic (stalk section)

II. Pituitary diseases
    Prolactinomas
    Mixed lactotroph and somatotroph adenomas
    Stem cell adenomas

IV. Endocrine
    Estrogens
      Pregnancy
      Contraceptive pills
    Hypothyroidism

V. Impaired dopaminergic transmission
    DA-blocking drugs
      Phenothiazines
      Butyrophanones
      Benzamides: (metoclopramide sulpiride)
    DA-depleting agents
      α Methyldopa
      Reserpine

specificity of this test because patients with drug-induced hyperprolactinemia also may fail to respond to TRH. This may mean that any lactotroph cell that is in a vigorous secretory phase may not be responsible to TRH and that the test is not specific for neoplastic lactotroph cells.

3. *Dopaminergic Inhibition.* Dopamine blocking agents such as chlorpromazine act primarily on the hypothalamus to block dopaminergic transmission of PRL inhibition. In normal subjects, chlorpromazine and related drugs stimulate PRL secretion, and most patients with prolactinomas fail to respond. Unfortunately, the frequency of false positive and false negative results has led investigators to seek more refined testing procedures. L-Dopa and bromocriptine, a dopaminergic drug, inhibit PRL secretion of normal subjects, patients with functional hyperprolactinemia as well as patients with prolactinoma. Dopamine infusions can also lower PRL levels in these conditions so that these responses do not assist in the diagnosis of prolactinoma. There is good experimental evidence that dopaminergic pathways in the hypothalamus suppress PRL secretion in normal individuals and that dopamine and dopaminergic drugs also act directly on the pituitary to inhibit normal lactotroph and prolactinoma secretion of PRL. Two pharmacologic tests have been proposed, but not yet generally accepted, to test the integrity of hypothalamic regulation of PRL secretion. In the first procedure, proposed by Fine and Frohman, the patient is pretreated with carbidopa before L-dopa administration. Carbidopa blocks pituitary formation of dopamine from L-dopa but does not block hypothalamic formation of L-dopa because it is excluded from the hypothalamus by the blood-brain barrier. When this test was applied to patients with prolactinomas, no fall in PRL occurred, whereas normal patients did show the expected fall (Fig. 3–38).

Another pharmacologic test that may be clinically useful is the administration of the experimental drug nomifensine. This drug's principal action is to inhibit axonic reuptake of dopamine; therefore, it is an indirect dopaminergic agent that inhibits normal PRL secretion by hypotha-

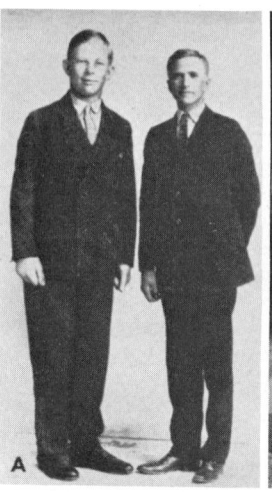
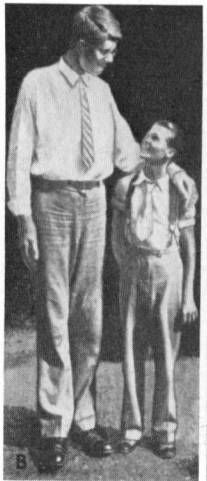
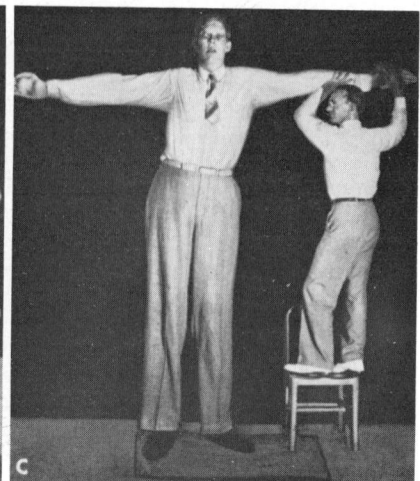

Figure 3–40. One of the most notable examples of GH excess in the human was Robert Wadlow, later known as the "Alton Giant." Although weighing only 9 pounds at birth, he soon commenced to grow excessively and by 6 months of age weighed 30 pounds. At 1 year of age he had reached a weight of 62 pounds. Growth continued throughout his life. Shortly after his death, which occurred at the age of 22 years from cellulitis of the feet, he was found to be 8 feet 11 inches in height and 475 pounds in weight by the careful measurements of Dr. C. M. Charles. (*A* and *B*, from Fadner, F.: *Biography of Robert Wadlow*, 1944. Courtesy of Bruce Humphries, Publishers. *C*, Courtesy of C. M. Charles and C. M. MacBryde.)

lamic action. Because the pituitary does not have dopaminergic axons, the drug is unable to act directly on prolactinomas to suppress secretion. Muller et al. have reported no inhibition of PRL secretion in a series of patients with prolactinoma.

From the previous discussion it is evident that the differentiation of functional from neoplastic PRL hypersecretion remains a problem, particularly in those patients with PRL levels below 100 ng/ml and normal radiographic examinations of the sella turcica. It is hoped that the second generation of pharmacologic tests will resolve this dilemma.

Medical Treatment of Prolactinomas

Although ablative therapy (see p. 00) is effective in many cases, there is a clear place for the medical treatment of prolactinomas. A great deal of experience has been accumulated in other parts of the world. Bromocriptine mesylate in doses of 5–10 mg/day has been highly effective in the reduction of PRL levels, control of galactorrhea, and restoration of menstrual cycles. Although this drug has been successful in restoring fertility in women and has been followed by pregnancy and delivery, its use in the United States is not authorized by the FDA. In about 10% of women who become pregnant while taking bromocriptine, there is evidence of increase in tumor size that in some cases impairs vision. The risk to fetus and mother has not been sufficiently evaluated to the satisfaction of the FDA, which limits approval of the medication for short-term treatment of amenorrhea and galactorrhea associated with hyperprolactinemia due to varied etiologies, excluding demonstrable pituitary tumors. The FDA recommends that contraception measures other than oral contraception be used in women receiving bromocriptine.

These recommendations seem unnecessarily restrictive in view of the extensive European experience. In particular, the drug has proved effective in women after failure of surgical or radiation therapy of known pituitary tumors. The drug may also prove to be effective in a number of cases of invasive prolactinomas by actually reducing tumor size. Isolated case reports have shown unequivocal shrinkage of tumor mass by CAT scans.

Undoubtedly this area of clinical research will remain very active, and the safety and therapeutic indications of the drug will be established.

Somatotroph Adenomas

Definition

Hypersomatotropism can be defined as an elevation of the mean GH level, usually greater than 10 ng/ml. Functional hypersomatotropism occurs in certain types of severe nutritional deficiencies, uncontrolled diabetes mellitus, chronic liver and renal disease, and rarely growth failure (Laron dwarfism). In the absence of these conditions, when associated with clinical features of overgrowth, nearly all cases are due to a somatotroph adenoma.

Incidence

Symptoms of GH excess can begin at any age but are most frequently recognized between the third and fifth decades of life. Rarely, the condition begins in childhood at a time when open epiphyses permit the exaggerated skeletal growth that leads to gigantism (Figs. 3–40 and 3–41). No clear sex or racial predisposition is recognized. Multiple cases in a family have been reported but most cases are sporadic. Acromegaly is a rare manifestation of the multiple endocrine adenomatosis syndrome (MEA I).

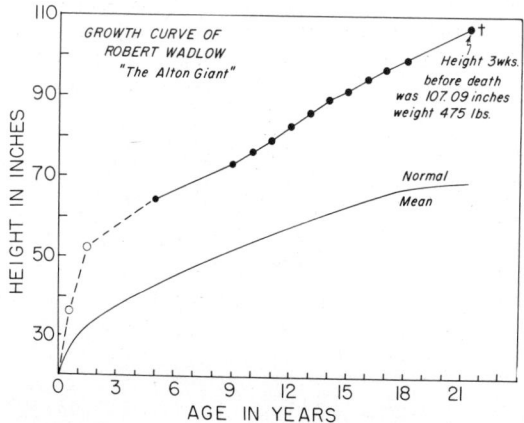

Figure 3–41. Growth curve of the Alton giant. The first two points (open circles) are estimates based on recorded weights and presumed normal body composition. (Reproduced from Daughaday, W. H., and Parker, M. L.: The pituitary in disorders of growth. *Disease-a-Month*, August, 1962, by permission of Year Book Medical Publishers, Inc.)

Clinical Manifestations (Table 3–8)

The earliest clinical feature of acromegaly is the coarsening of facial features and the soft-tissue swelling of the feet and hands (Figs. 3–42 and 3–43). This is recognized by the patient through a change in appearance and a need for larger rings, gloves, and shoes. These changes often occur so gradually that they are not recognized by the patient or by relatives until they are well advanced. A book of snapshots taken over the years may be more reliable than the patient's memory in charting the progression of the disease. The dermal changes are the result of connective tissue proliferation and the accumulation of intercellular matrix. The deposition of hyaluronates leads to interstitial edema that has been confirmed by measurement of interstitial fluid volume. After successful correction of hypersomatotropism this edema regresses in a few weeks. As the duration of acromegaly increases, collagenization of the dermis progresses, and regression after restoration of normal GH levels is less and less complete.

Other changes in the skin occur. There is increased coarse body hair. There is an increase in size and function of sebaceous and sweat glands. Most patients complain of excessive perspiration and of an offensive body odor. Moderate darkening of the skin is noted by many patients. Fibroma molluscum is recorded in 25% of patients.

Bony proliferation is seen on radiographs of the hands as cortical thickening and distal tufting (Fig. 3–44). The deformities of the skull are often striking. The mandible increases in length as well as in thickness. The resulting underbite is easily recognized. The calvarium may be thickened; bony ridges and muscle attachments are exaggerated. The frontal, mastoid, and ethmoid sinuses may enlarge to a remarkable degree.

The ribs continue to elongate because of proliferation at the cartilage–bone junction. These changes have been con-

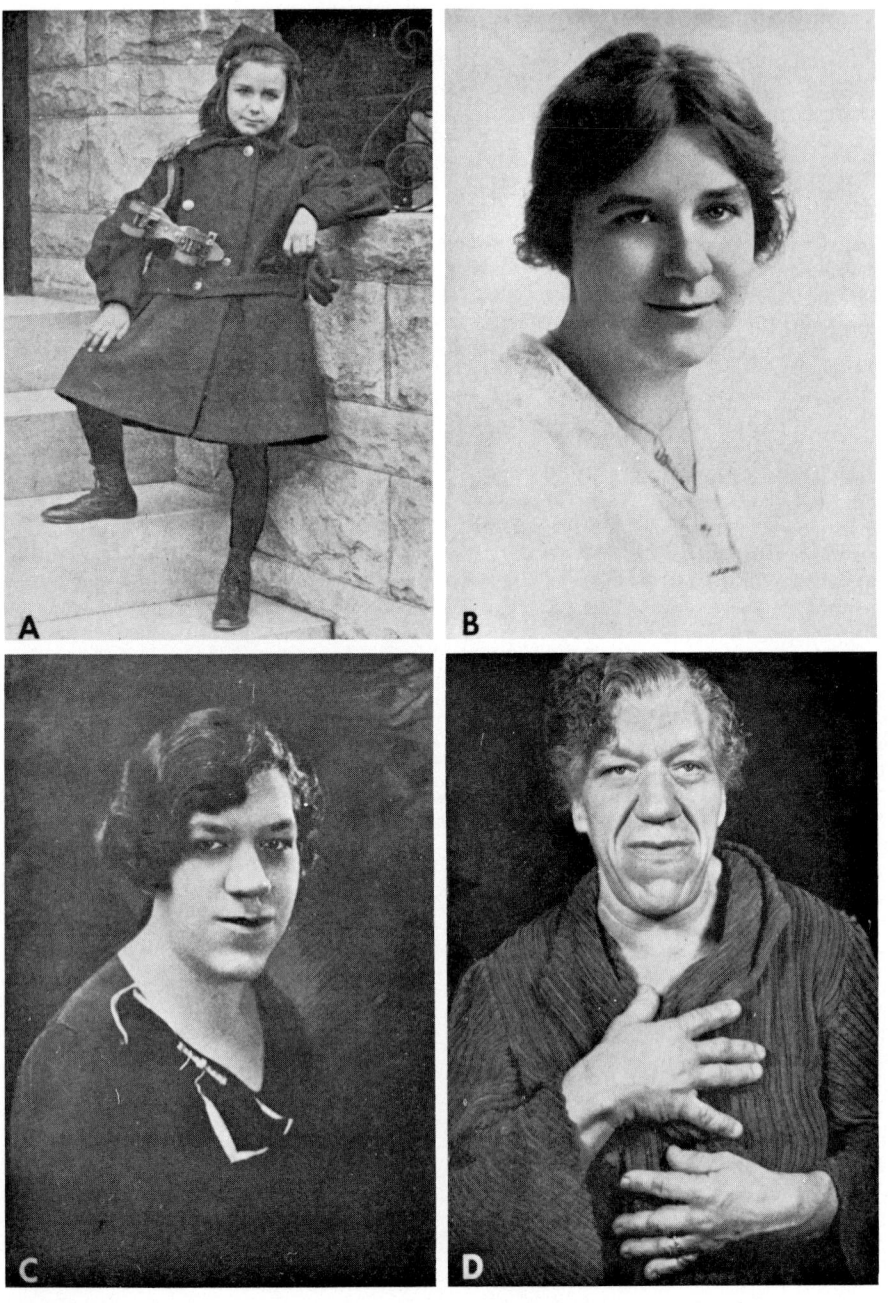

Figure 3–42. The progression of acromegaly is illustrated in these photographs. *A*, normal, age 9 years; *B*, age 16 years with possible early coarsening of features; *C*, age 33 years, well-established acromegaly; *D*, age 52 years, end stage acromegaly with gross disfigurement. (Reproduced from Mendeloff, A. I., and Smith, D. E. (eds.): Acromegaly, diabetes, hypermetabolism, proteinuria and heart failure. Clinical Pathological Conference. *Am. J. Med. 20*:133, 1956, with permission.)

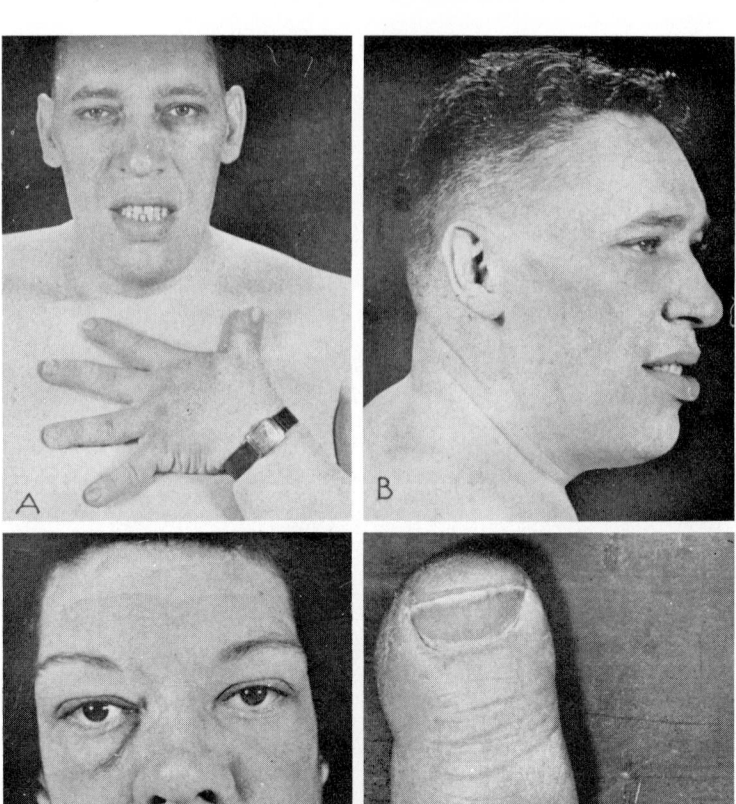

Figure 3–43. Acromegaly. A and B, Note the large and elongated head, large hand, nose, ears, and lips. There are also prognathism and slightly increased interdental spaces. C, Note the coarse features. D, Large blunt-pointed thumb.

Table 3–8. ACROMEGALY: FREQUENCY OF MANIFESTATIONS

	Per Cent
Parasellar Manifestations	
Enlarged sella	93 (80–93)
Headache	87 (75–87)
Visual impairment	62 (5–62)
Uncinate fits	7
Rhinorrhea	15
Pituitary apoplexy	(3)
Papilledema	3
GH Excess	
Weight gain	39
Hypermetabolism	70
Hyperhidrosis	60
Impaired glucose tolerance	25 (37)
Clinical diabetes mellitus	12 (13)
Acral growth	100
Prognathism	Common
Arthritic complaints	(64)
Osteoporosis	Common
Soft-tissue growth	100
Hypertrichosis	53
Pigmentation	40
Fibroma molluscum	27
Visceromegaly	Common
Goiter	25
Disturbances of Other Hormones	
Lactorrhea (?PRL excess)	4
Hyperadrenocorticism	Rare
Hyperthyroidism	Rare
Increased libido	38
Decreased libido, male	23

Most of the data for the preparation of this chart were obtained from Davidoff. When other sources were used, the figures are placed in parentheses.

firmed by biopsy. In long-established acromegaly, costal growth leads to a deep barrel chest. Periosteal growth of the vertebrae occurs, and osteophytic proliferation of the articular margins of joints are frequently recognized.

Cartilage proliferation of the larynx results in a deep husky voice. The tongue is often enlarged and furrowed, and the salivary glands are enlarged.

In long-standing acromegaly, joint symptoms are common. These may be limited to backache or arthralgias or may progress to crippling degenerative arthritis. The initial response to GH excess is articular cartilage proliferation, which sometimes can be recognized radiographically by a widening of the joint spaces (Fig. 3–45), but later as the disease progresses, the articular cartilage may undergo necrosis and erosion may develop.

Involvement of peripheral nerves is common. Acroparesthesias are noted in about 20% of the patients. In many cases, this complaint is due to entrapment of nerves by bony or soft tissue overgrowth. Compression of the median nerve in the carpal tunnel space leads to weakness and sensory changes in the hands. Peripheral neuropathy can also be due to perineural and endoneural fibrous proliferation. Peripheral nerves are often palpably enlarged. Peripheral neuropathy is particularly severe in untreated gigantism. Much of the debility that such patients experience is attributable to this cause. Foot drop, muscular atrophy, and even Charcot's joint have been reported.

In addition to muscular weakness due to neuropathy, there is electromyographic and biopsy evidence of a proximal muscle myopathy.

Enlargement of the heart is found almost universally in acromegalic patients at necropsy, even in the absence of any functional impairment. Clinicians are impressed by the

109

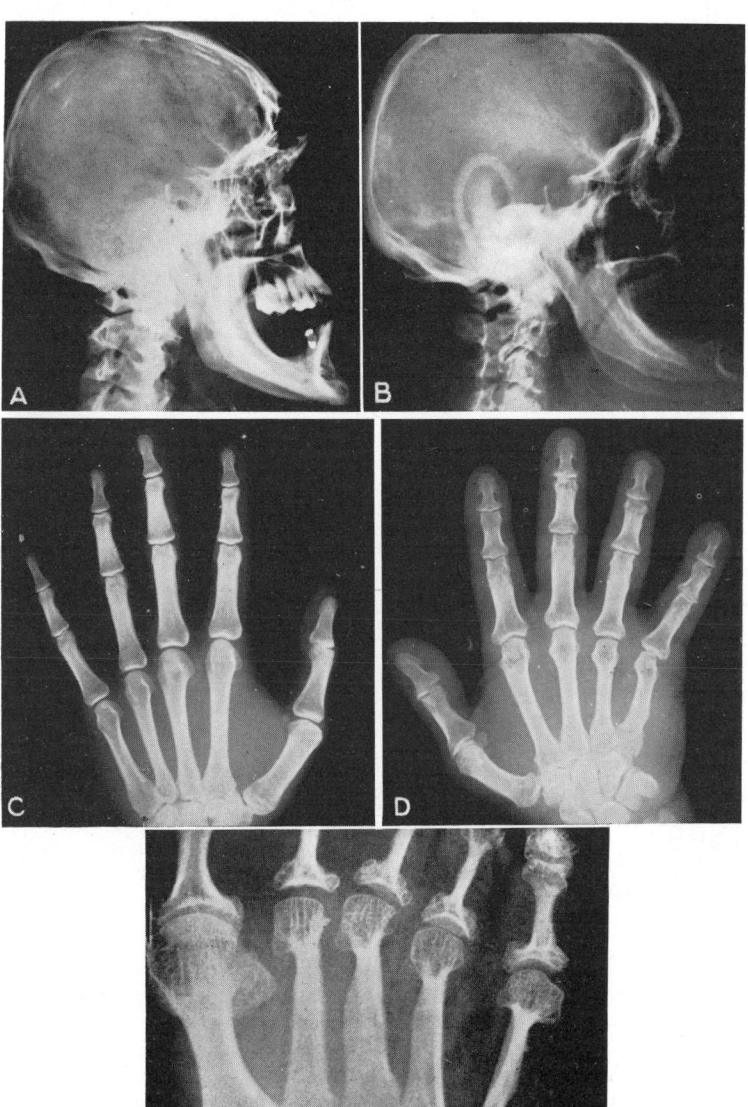

Figure 3–44. *A* and *B*, Enlarged sella turcica, large paranasal sinuses, and marked elongation of the mandible, *C*, The hand of a normal Norwegian-Swedish male who weighs 220 pounds and is 6 feet 4 inches in height. Though he is regarded as being "big-boned," or having a "big frame," there are many differences in the roentgenogram of his hand and that of the acromegalic hand *(D)*, which shows marked thickening of the soft tissues, widened bones, periosteal reaction, small osteophytes, tufting and mushrooming of the terminal phalanges, and spur formation. *E*, Note that the trabeculae in the bone ends are thickened and widely spaced, appearing porotic, while the shafts are narrow and dense; there is a sudden transition from a dense, narrow pipe-stem shaft to a squared and porotic bone end. (*E* is reproduced with modification from Kellgren, J. H., Ball, J., et al.: Articular and other limb changes in acromegaly; clinical and pathological study of 25 cases. *Q. J. Med. 21*:405, 1952, with permission.)

fact that acromegalic patients may develop unexplained progressive congestive heart failure in the fifth and sixth decades. At necropsy, the size of the myocardial fibers is increased, and the fibers are separated by interstitial fibrosis.

Hepatomegaly is often detected on physical examination

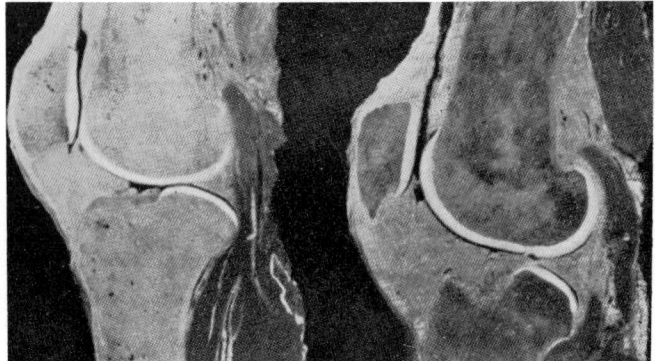

Figure 3–45. The knee on the left is normal, whereas the one on the right shows acromegalic arthropathy, with marked thickening of ligaments, meniscus, and fat pad. There is an enlarged femoral condyle with thickening of the articular cartilage. (Reproduced with modification from Kellgren, J. W., Ball, J., et al.: Articular and other limb changes in acromegaly; clinical and pathological study of 25 cases. *Q. J. Med. 21*:405, 1952, with permission.)

and is regularly observed at necropsy. The thyroid, parathyroid, spleen, and pancreas also are larger than normal.

A remarkable increase in the size of the kidneys can occur. The combined weight of the kidneys of one of our patients was 870 g, and there are reports in the literature of even larger kidneys. The glomeruli may be twice normal in diameter, and comparable increases in the size of the renal tubules occur. Remarkable changes in renal function have been described. In one patient the inulin clearance was 325 ml/min (normal for his size is 131 ml/min); the tubular reabsorption of glucose was 1068 mg/min (normal value is 385 mg/min); and the tubular secretion maximum for para-aminohippurate was 165 mg/min (normal value is 76 mg/min).

GH increases tubular reabsorption of phosphate and leads to the mild hyperphosphatemia.

Impaired glucose tolerance is present in nearly half the cases of acromegaly, but clinical diabetes mellitus occurs in only about 10% of patients. Even in those patients whose plasma glucose response to oral glucose is normal, the plasma insulin response is increased, indicating insulin resistance. The insulin response to tolbutamide is also exaggerated. It is widely suspected that diabetes develops only in those acromegalic patients who have a hereditary disposition to diabetes; in the remaining patients the insulin secretory reserve is believed to be sufficient to overcome insulin antagonism. Rarely, severe insulin resistance may be encountered in acromegalic individuals with diabetes. Pathologically the islets of Langerhans may be enlarged, and beta cells may be packed with granules even in the presence of diabetes.

The frequency of degenerative diabetic complications occurring in acromegalic diabetics has aroused much interest. Diabetic retinopathy is not unusual, but the pathologic changes of intercapillary glomerulosclerosis are infrequently observed.

Growth Hormone Secretion

Plasma GH may be very slightly elevated (5–20 ng/ml) or may reach massive concentrations (>1000 ng/ml). Many patients exhibit little fluctuation of plasma GH throughout a 24-hour period. In other patients, GH levels are strikingly inconstant, with abrupt rises occurring at short intervals (Fig. 3–46). In almost all cases the sleep-related peak of GH secretion is absent.

Peaks of GH secretion can be provoked in some acromegalic patients by mixed meals or arginine infusions. The influence of changes of blood sugar on GH secretion is of interest. Hypoglycemia can increase GH secretion in some patients, and glucose administration may provoke a paradoxical rise in plasma GH. The GH responses to these metabolic stimuli require hypothalamic participation. Persistence of these responses suggests that a disorder of hypothalamic regulation exists in certain patients with hypersomatotropism.

GH measurements are of great practical value in diagnosis and the monitoring of therapeutic responses. Plasma GH measurement makes possible unequivocal diagnosis before significant acromegalic disfigurement. Blood should be obtained from hospitalized patients in the basal state before breakfast. Transient functional elevations of plasma GH occur in ambulatory patients, particularly in young women, and must be distinguished from pathologic hypersecretion. Functional GH secretion can be suppressed by obtaining samples of blood 90 min after administration of 75 g of glucose by mouth. Under these conditions, plasma GH normally is less than 5 ng/ml. Levels between 5 and 10 ng/ml are indeterminant, and higher values support the diagnosis of hypersomatotropism. Most acromegalic patients have substantially higher values.

The apparent lack of correlation of plasma GH levels and the stigmata of the disease has led to misunderstandings.

Often clinicians have not considered the important influence of duration of hypersomatotropism. Clinical manifestations of pathologic growth are cumulative, so that severe hypersomatotropism of short duration can be present with less marked acromegaly than that with mild hypersomatotropism of long duration. There are also age-dependent differences in tissue responsiveness, younger patients being more responsive than older. In some patients, acromegalic changes represent the residual high tide mark of past GH secretion that has ebbed at the time of study. Although not common, spontaneous improvement in hypersomatotropism can occur because of hemorrhagic infarction of tumors. Also, from what has been said, it should be remembered that one or two random GH measurements may not accurately reflect total GH secretion. Despite these limitations, GH measurements provide a much more reliable guide to therapy than do minor fluctuations of symptoms and signs. Recently it has been reported that measurements of somatomedin provide a more sensitive index of persistent acromegaly. Elevations of somatomedin were definite, with only slight elevations of plasma GH.

Secretion of Other Hormones

Certain clinical features suggest the existence of hyperthyroidism in acromegalic patients. Goiter is found in about one quarter of the patients, and excess sweating is a common finding in the active disease. Although the basal metabolic rate is commonly moderately elevated, more specific measurements of thyroid function (serum T_4, radioiodine uptake) have characteristically been normal. A decreased concentration of thyroxine-binding globulin and an increased capacity of thyroxine-binding prealbumin occur in some patients with acromegaly. Measurements of plasma TSH have failed to show elevation of this hormone. At operation or necropsy, a multinodular goiter has generally been found without histologic evidence of hypersecretion. The hypermetabolism of acromegaly, therefore, seems to be a direct effect of GH excess. Hypothyroidism may develop late in the course of acromegaly after normal pituitary tissue has been compressed by the adenoma or destroyed by treatment.

Galactorrhea occurs in some young women with acromegaly and is usually associated with an elevation of plasma PRL, but it should be noted that more women have an elevated PRL than actually lactate. Also, lactation may occur with GH excess alone because human GH itself is a potent lactogenic hormone.

ACTH secretion is usually adequate to maintain basal cortisol secretion. Urinary 17-hydroxycorticosteroid excretion is usually normal, but a decrease in ACTH reserve may be uncovered with metyrapone administration. Failure of ACTH secretion may complicate the later stages of the disease. Rarely, cases have been observed in which clinical and laboratory evidence of hyperadrenocorticism has been found in acromegaly.

Decreased gonadotropin secretion is the usual consequence of somatotroph tumors. Sexual immaturity is common in giants. About one third of men with acromegaly develop impotence, and nearly all women note menstrual irregularities or amenorrhea during the course of their disease. Completion of normal pregnancy is unusual.

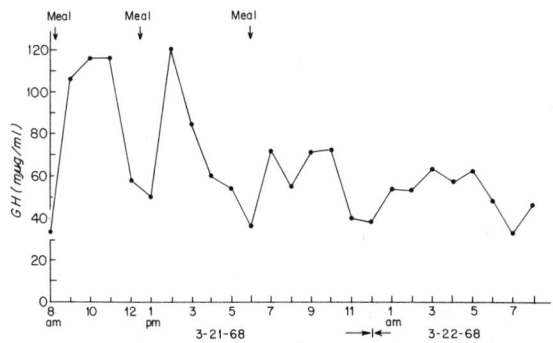

Figure 3–46. Serial GH measurements made during a 24-hour period in an acromegalic patient exhibiting marked instability of GH levels. Note rises of plasma GH occurring after meals and the absence of a defined sleep-related GH peak at night. (Reproduced from Cryer, P. E., and Daughaday, W. H.: Regulation of growth hormone secretion in acromegaly. *J. Clin. Endocrinol.* 29:386, 1969, with permission.)

Associated Neoplasia

A variety of tumors have developed in rats receiving GH injections for prolonged periods, but there is little solid clinical evidence linking high levels of circulating GH with an increased frequency of neoplasia. Pituitary adenomas are associated with adenomas of the parathyroid, islets of Langerhans, and adrenal cortex in the multiple endocrine adenomatosis syndrome. This possibility should be considered in evaluating patients with acromegaly.

Medical Treatment

Ablative therapy (see below) is preferable to presently known medical treatment. There are cases, however, in which surgical or radiation therapy, or both, have failed to control hypersomatotropism. European authors have reported that bromocriptine and certain other dopaminergic drugs have induced substantial lowering of GH levels and symptomatic improvement. This use of bromocriptine has not been approved in the U.S. by the FDA. The long-term benefit of such treatment remains to be determined.

Corticotroph Adenomas (Cushing's Disease)

Definition

In 1932, Harvey Cushing proposed that small basophilic pituitary tumors could produce the syndrome that now bears his name. At the present time, the term Cushing's disease is applied to this condition, whereas other forms of hyperadrenocorticism are referred to as Cushing's syndrome.

Association with Cushing's Disease

Cushing's proposal was not immediately accepted because some neurosurgeons and pathologists failed to find pituitary adenomas in patients with this condition. Moreover, the production of ACTH by nonpituitary tumors as a cause of Cushing's syndrome was not separated from Cushing's disease until recently. In untreated patients with Cushing's disease, radiologic evidence of a pituitary lesion is usually lacking.

Within the past five years, Cushing's hypothesis that corticotroph adenomas are responsible for most cases of the disease has received general acceptance. The most convincing evidence has been provided by the finding at transsphenoidal exploration of the sella of corticotroph microadenomas in nearly all cases and by the cure of the disease by adenomectomy.

The striking finding is that adenomas less than 2 mm in size can be the cause of a devastating systemic disease. In the past such adenomas were usually disregarded. The small size of the corticotroph tumors as compared to other pituitary tumors is probably the result of the earlier ascertainment rather than a difference in basic tumor biology. Only a moderate increase in ACTH secretion is required for marked alterations in appearance and well-being of a patient. It is likely that medical attention is sought much earlier than with other pituitary tumors.

Incidence

Corticotroph adenomas can occur at any age but are rare in childhood. The disease occurs two to three times more frequently in women than in men. Onset is generally in the third to fifth decade of life.

Corticotropin Measurements

The level of ACTH in untreated patients with Cushing's disease obtained under normal morning fasting conditions is only moderately elevated. In about one half of the cases the levels are within the normal range (Fig. 3–9B). Importantly, there is no diurnal rhythm of ACTH secretion, although pulsatile secretion may be maintained. The secretion of ACTH by corticotroph adenomas is regulated to a greater or lesser extent by corticosteroids. High levels of corticosteroids (dexamethasone 2 mg q 6 hrs) will inhibit corticotroph levels, and adrenalectomy leads to a substantial rise in plasma levels despite adequate replacement therapy.

Clinical and Laboratory Manifestations

Since these features are largely the results of hypersecretion of cortisol, they are described in Chapter 5.

Nelson's Syndrome

Progressive growth of corticotroph adenomas occurs in 10% of patients with Cushing's disease subjected to adrenalectomy. These tumors secrete large amounts of ACTH and lipotropin (LPH)-related peptides. It is not established whether ACTH itself or a peptide derived from β LPN is the effective melanocyte-stimulating substance causing intense pigmentation.

Rarely, patients who had intense pigmentation but no evidence of adrenal dysfunction have been described with pituitary tumors. Such tumors may secrete only melanocyte-stimulating peptides.

Gonadotroph and Thyrotroph Tumors

These unusual tumors have been described only in isolated case reports. Both types of tumor occasionally develop after long periods of hypersecretion secondary to target gland insufficiency (hypogonadism or hypothyroidism). In certain cases, tumor regression has simply followed target hormone replacement therapy, so that restraint is indicated before instituting ablative therapy. Occasionally, a pituitary tumor will secrete only α chain glycoprotein without intact hormone. Such cases can only be detected with specific radioimmunoassay.

There have been several cases of TSH-secreting pituitary tumors associated with hyperthyroidism.

Ablative Treatment

The goals of ablative treatment are to prevent parasellar extension and to correct hormonal hypersecretions without affecting secretion of other pituitary hormones. Unfortunately, these goals are difficult to achieve.

Surgical Adenomectomy

The treatment of pituitary microadenomas has been revolutionized by the widespread application of transsphenoidal microsurgery. This procedure, initially favored by Harvey Cushing in the second and third decade of this century, fell into disfavor because of the risk of infection. Its reintroduction by Guiot, Hardy, and others has been made safe by antibiotics and by video radiographic monitoring and selective by the operating microscope, which has permitted recognition of adenomatous tissue and its removal by special instruments. The surgical approach and visualization are shown in Fig. 3–47.

Transsphenoidal microsurgery has been reported to cure between 70 and 90% of small prolactinomas, somatotroph adenomas, and corticotroph adenomas. Although cryohypophysectomy, thermal hypophysectomy, and local implantation of radioactive material are definitely effective in many cases of pituitary tumor, their lack of visual control and selectivity has led most centers to abandon these therapies.

The surgical treatment of large or invasive adenomas is less satisfactory. Transsphenoidal adenomectomy fails to yield endocrine cures in over half of all endocrine-secreting tumors, but sellar mass and most of the suprasellar extension can be removed. The failure of endocrine cure may be due to failure to recognize small intrasellar remnants or the presence of parasellar invasion of bony and vascular structures.

When suprasellar extension is large, particularly when angulation occurs or visual loss is extensive, frontal hypophysectomy is usually preferable to the transsphenoidal approach. These operations may prevent or delay parasellar tumor manifestations but usually are unsuccessful in correction of hormone hypersecretion.

Radiation Treatment

Gamma radiation administered by supravoltage, or Cobalt 57, sources has been used extensively. Control of tumor size and prevention of parasellar complications can usually be achieved, but control of hormonal hypersecretion is often incomplete. The hormonal response to therapy is slow, and two years may be required to assess the full effect of treatment. The details of therapy are not germane to this discussion, but there is risk in exceeding 5500 R. The total dose of radiation should be given as a single course of treatment through multiple ports. With modern supravoltage equipment, reactions are rarely encountered, and late damage to cranial nerves and hypothalamic tissues is seldom recognized. Very rarely, sarcomas of the sellar region have developed many years after pituitary radiation.

Treatment with accelerated protons permits a greater dose of radiation to be focused on the pituitary with less damage to intervening and neighboring tissue. Doses equivalent to 10,000 R can be administered through multiple or rotational ports. Employment of the Bragg effect allows a greater delivery of radiation directly to the pituitary. The treatment carries a greater risk of cranial nerve and hypothalamic damage than was first claimed, but the overall responses to treatment appear quite satisfactory. A disadvantage of this form of treatment is the limited

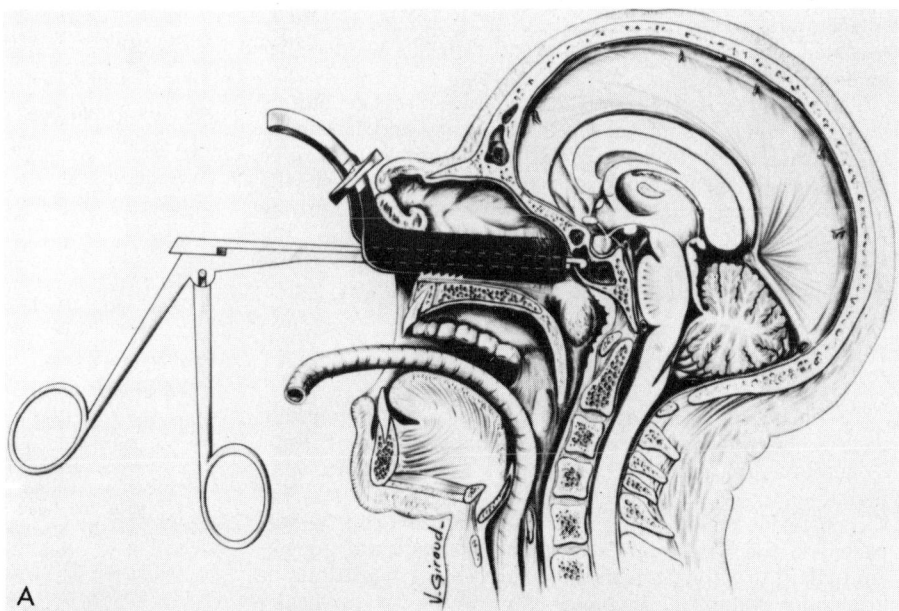

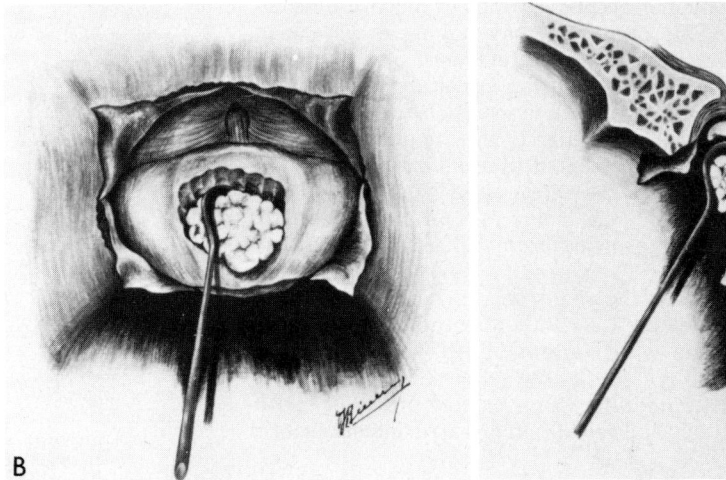

Figure 3–47. *A*, Transsphenoidal approach to the pituitary gland. (Reproduced with permission from Hardy, J.: In *Microneurosurgery*. Rand, R. W. (ed.), St. Louis, C. V. Mosby Co., 1978, pp. 105–130.) *B*, Selective adenomectomy leaving normal pituitary tissue undisturbed. (Reproduced with permission from Hardy, J.: Transsphenoidal microsurgery of the normal and pathological pituitary. In *Clinical Neurosurgery*. Vol. 16. Ojemann, R. G. (ed.). Congress of Neurological Surgeons. Baltimore, Williams and Wilkins, 1969, pp. 185–217.)

number of centers where it is available. Because radiation damage is cumulative, proton beam radiation is not recommended after conventional gamma radiation.

Local implantation of radioactive isotopes of yttrium, gold, and strontium is seldom done in this country because of the frequency of rhinorrhea and meningitis.

ECTOPIC PRODUCTION OF PITUITARY HORMONES

This subject is discussed at length in Chapter 31. It is only necessary to note that ACTH radioimmunoactivity is present in nearly all small cell carcinomas (oat cell) of the lung and less frequently in other carcinomas. It is evident that the secretion of biologically active ACTH and the development of hyperadrenocorticism secondary to ectopic ACTH production is less common. In nearly all cases ACTH production is directly correlated with production of LPH-related peptides.

Gonadotropin production by tumors is usually limted to α chain and CG. Such secretion is characteristic of choriocarcinoma and teratoid tumors but also has been noted with hepatic, gastric, and bronchial carcinomas.

TSH-like activity is produced by choriocarcinomas and may be the cause of hyperthyroidism. It is still unclear whether this is caused by CG or by a separate chorionic TSH.

GH and PRL secretion by bronchial tumors has been reported, but in each case the production has been rather modest.

There is a fascinating correlation between certain pulmonary and upper abdominal carcinoid tumors and acromegaly and gigantism. In some cases the tumors seemed to be secreting GH, but in other cases, despite an enlarged sella turcica, GH excess has been cured by removal of the primary tumor. At least in certain cases such tumors have not contained GH but a GH-releasing factor (GHRF). Further confirmation of this finding is needed.

EMPTY SELLA SYNDROME

This is a radiologic diagnosis applied to an enlarged sella with replacement of much of the adenohypophyseal tissue by cerebrospinal fluid. In the usual views of the sella, symmetric enlargement is evident with little displacement of the posterior clinoid processes. The diagnosis can be suspected if the CAT scan shows an homogeneous density equivalent to water but this is also present with pituitary or arachnoid cysts. The diagnosis can only be unequivocally established by pneumoencephalography or metrizamide encephalography. This procedure may not be necessary in some cases unless there is other evidence of a pituitary tumor. Patients with this condition are often obese women complaining of headache. This association may be one of ascertainment rather than direct causation because this population is highly represented in adult patients getting skull films. Very rarely, the empty sella syndrome is associated with visual field defects due to traction on the optic nerves and chiasm resulting from collapse of pituitary parenchyma.

The pathogenesis of the empty sella syndrome is varied. Most cases seem to be the result of incompetence of the diaphragma sellae, which allows direct transmission of cerebrospinal fluid pressure to the sellar contents. In other cases, a pituitary tumor may have existed previously with subsequent necrosis and resorption or extrusion of necrotic tissue.

Endocrine studies of patients with the empty sella syndrome have usually shown no impairment of pituitary hormone secretion despite extensive parenchymal loss. Some patients do exhibit inadequate secretion of one or more hormones. PRL secretion may be moderately elevated in some cases.

The presence of an empty sella is not incompatible with a microadenoma causing galactorrhea, acromegaly, or Cushing's disease.

The clinical importance of the empty sella is its recognition and the avoidance of unneeded surgical or radiation therapy.

REFERENCES

The following references have been selected to allow the interested student or physician to extend his or her knowledge. Many articles cited are reviews and not primary references. Obviously, this list of references neither is comprehensive nor reflects scientific priority.

General Reviews and Texts

1. Besser, G. M. (ed.): The hypothalamus and pituitary. *Clin. Endocrinol.* 6:1, 1977.
2. Greep, R. O., and Astwood, E. B. (eds.): The pituitary gland and its neuroendocrine control, In *Handbook of Physiology*, Section 7: Endocrinology. Vol. 4. American Physiological Society. Baltimore, Williams and Wilkins, 1974.
3. Harris, G. W., and Donovan, B. T.: *The Pituitary Gland.* Vols. 1–3. Berkeley, University of California Press, 1966.
4. Lock, W., and Schally, A. V.: *The Hypothalamus and Pituitary in Health and Disease.* Springfield, Ill., Charles C Thomas, 1972.
5. Rimoin, D. L., and Schimke, R. N.: *Genetic Disorders of the Endocrine Glands.* The C. V. Mosby Co., St. Louis, 1971.

Pituitary Morphology

ANATOMY

6. Bergland, R.M., Ray, B. S., et al.: Anatomical variations in the pituitary gland and adjacent structures in 225 human autopsy cases. *J. Neurosurg.* 28:93, 1968.
7. Pelletier, G., Robert, F., et al.: Identification of human anterior pituitary cells by immunoelectron microscopy. *J. Clin. Endocrinol. Metab.* 46:534, 1978.
8. Stanfield, J. P.: The blood supply of the human pituitary gland. *J. Anat.* 94:257, 1960.

Pituitary Hormones

CORTICOTROPIN

9. Bachelot, I., Wolfsen, A. R., et al.: Pituitary and plasma lipotropins: demonstration of the artifactual nature of β MSH. *J. Clin. Endocrinol. Metab.* 44:939, 1977.
10. Gilkes, J. J., Rees, L. H., et al.: Plasma immunoreactive corticotrophin and lipotrophin in Cushing's syndrome and Addison's disease. *Br. Med. J.* 1:996, 1977.
11. Gill, G. N.: Mechanism of ACTH action. *Metabolism* 21:571, 1972.
12. Guillemin, R., Vargo, T., et al.: β-Endorphin and adrenocorticotropin are secreted concomitantly by the pituitary gland. *Science* 197:1367, 1977.
13. Lefkowitz, R. J., Roth, J., et al.: ACTH receptors in the adrenal: specific binding of ACTH-125I and its relation to adenyl cyclase. *Proc. Nat. Acad. Sci. USA.* 65:745, 1970.
14. Liddle, G. W., Island, D., et al.: Normal and abnormal regulation of corticotropin secretion in man. *Recent Progr. Horm. Res.* 18:125, 1962.
15. Metcalf, M. G., and Beaven, D. W.: The metopirone test of pituitary corticotrophin release. Evaluation of 101 tests. *Am. J. Med.* 45:176, 1968.
16. Nicholson, W. E., Liddle, R. A., et al.: Adrenocorticotrophic hormone biotransformation, clearance, and catabolism. *Endocrinology* 103:1344, 1978.
17. Orth, D. N., and Nicholson, W. E.: High molecular weight forms of human ACTH are glycoproteins. *J. Clin. Endocrinol. Metab.* 44:214, 1977.
18. Rees, L. H., Holdaway, I. M., et al.: ACTH secretion and clinical investigations. In *Some Aspects of Hypothalamic Regulation of Endocrine Functions.* Symposium, Vienna, June 3–6, 1973. Stuttgart-New York, F. K. Schattauer Verlag, 1974.
19. Smith, A. G., Shuster, S., et al.: Plasma immunoreactive β-melanocyte-stimulating hormone and skin pigmentation in chronic renal failure. *Br. Med. J.* 1:658, 1975.

GONADOTROPINS

20. Forest, M. G., De Peretti, E., et al.: Hypothalamic–pituitary–gonadal relationships in man from birth to puberty. *Clin. Endocrinol.* (Oxf.) 5:551, 1976.
21. Ross, G. T., Cargille, C. M., et al.: Pituitary and gonadal hormones in women during spontaneous and induced ovulatory cycles. *Recent Progr. Horm. Res.* 26:1, 1970.
22. Sherman, B. M., Halmi, K. A., et al.: LH and FSH response to gonadotropin-releasing hormone in anorexia nervosa: effect of nutritional rehabilitation. *J. Clin. Endocrinol. Metab.* 41:135, 1975.
23. Vaitukaitis, J. L., Ross, G. T., et al.: Gonadotropins and their subunits: basic and clinical studies. *Recent Progr. Horm. Res.* 32:289, 1976.
24. Vande Wiele, R. L., Bogumil, J., et al.: Mechanisms relating the menstrual cycle in women. *Recent Progr. Horm. Res.* 26:63, 1970.
25. Wollensen, F., Swerdloff, R. S., et al.: LH and FSH responses to luteinizing-releasing hormone in normal human males. *Metabolism* 25:845, 1976.
26. Wollensen, F., Swerdloff, R. S., et al.: LH and FSH responses to luteinizing-releasing hormone in normal fertile women. *Metabolism* 25:1275, 1976.

THYROTROPIN

27. Hall, R., Ormston, B. J., et al.: The thyrotrophin-releasing hormone test in diseases of the pituitary and hypothalamus. *Lancet* 1:759, 1972.
28. Kourides, I. A., Weintraub, B. D., et al.: Pituitary secretion of free alpha and beta subunits of human thryotropin in patients with thyroid disease. *J. Clin. Endocrinol. Metab.* 40:872, 1975.
29. Mayberry, W. E., Gharib, H., et al.: Radioimmunoassay for human thyrotropin. Clinical value in patients with normal and abnormal thyroid function. *Ann. Intern. Med.* 74:471, 1971.
30. Mullin, B. R., Pacuszka, T., et al.: Thyroid gangliosides with high affinity for thyrotropin: potential role in thyroid regulation. *Science* 199:77, 1978.
31. Odell, W. D., Wilber, J. F., et al.: Studies of thyrotropin physiology by means of radioimmunoassay. *Recent Progr. Horm. Res.* 23:47, 1967.
32. Pierce, J. G.: Eli Lilly Lecture. The subunits of pituitary thyrotropin — their relationship to other glycoprotein hormones. *Endocrinology* 89:1331, 1971.

PROLACTIN

33. Bern, H. A., and Nicoll, C. S.: The comparative endocrinology of prolactin. *Recent Progr. Horm. Res.* 24:681, 1968.
34. Daughaday, W. H., and Jacobs, L. S.: Human prolactin, In *Reviews of Physiology, Biochemistry and Experimental Pharmacology.* Berlin, Springer-Verlag, 1972.
35. Frantz, A. G.: Prolactin. *N. Engl. J. Med.* 298:201, 1978.
36. Topper, Y. J.: Multiple hormone interactions in the development of mammary gland *in vitro. Recent Progr. Horm. Res.* 26:287, 1970.
37. Tyson, J. E., Hwang, P., et al.: Studies of prolactin secretion in human pregnancy. *Am. J. Obstet. Gynecol.* 113:14, 1972.

GH AND SOMATOMEDINS

38. Daughaday, W. H.: Hormonal regulation of growth by somatomedin and other tissue growth factors. *Clin. Endocrinol. Metab.* 6:117, 1977.
39. Furlanetto, R. W., Underwood, L., et al.: Estimation of somatomedin-C levels in normals and patients with pituitary disease by radioimmunoassay. *J. Clin. Invest.* 60:648, 1977.
40. Pecile, A., and Mueller, E. E. (eds.): Growth Hormone and Related Peptides. (International Congress Symposium). Elsevier-North Holland Pub. Co., New York, 1976.
41. Van Wyk, J. J., and Underwood, L. E.: The somatomedins and their actions. *Biochem. Actions Horm.* 5:101, 1978.

Hypopituitarism

IN ADULTS — ANOREXIA NERVOSA, EMPTY SELLA SYNDROME

42. Bell, J., Benveniste, R., et al.: Isolated deficiency of follicle stimulating hormone: further studies. *J. Clin. Endocrinol. Metab.* 40:790, 1975.
43. Beumont, P. J., George, G. C., et al.: Body weight and the pituitary response to hypothalamic releasing hormones in patients with anorexia nervosa. *J. Clin. Endocrinol. Metab.* 43:487, 1976.
44. Cleveland, W. W., Green, O. C., et al.: A case of proved adrenocorticotropin deficiency. *J. Pediatr.* 57:376, 1960.
45. Daughaday, W. H.: Sheehan's syndrome in endocrine causes of menstrual disorders, In *Endocrine Causes of Menstrual Disorders.* Givens, J. R. (ed.), Chicago, Year Book Medical Publishers, 1978.
46. Frankel, R. J., and Jenkins, J. S.: Hypothalamic-pituitary function in anorexia nervosa. *Acta Endocrinol.* 78:209, 1975.

47. Haddock, L., Vega, L. A., et al.: Adrenocortical, thyroidal and human growth hormone reserve in Sheehan's syndrome. *Johns Hopkins Med. J.* 131:80, 1972.
48. Jordan, R. M., Kendall, J. W., et al.: The primary empty sella syndrome, analysis of the clinical characteristics, radiographic features, pituitary function and cerebrospinal fluid adenohypophyseal hormone concentrations. *Am. J. Med.* 62:569, 1977.
49. Kovács, K., : Necrosis of anterior pituitary in humans. I. *Neuroendocrinology* 4:170, 1969.
50. Marshall, J. C., Harsoulis, P., et al.: Isolated pituitary gonadotrophin deficiency: gonadotrophin secretion after synthetic luteinizing hormone and follicle stimulating hormone-releasing hormone. *Br. Med. J.* 4:643, 1972.
51. Miyai, D. M., Azukizaqa, M., et al.: Familial isolated thyrotropin deficiency. *N. Engl. J. Med.* 287:972, 1972.
52. Neelon, F. A., Goree, J. A., et al.: The primary empty sella: clinical and radiographic characteristics and endocrine functions. *Medicine* 52:73, 1973.
53. Rabin, D., Spitz, I., et al.: Isolated deficiency of follicle-stimulating hormone, clinical and laboratory features. *N. Engl. J. Med.* 287:1313, 1972.
54. Schalch, D. S., and Burday, S. Z.: Antepartum pituitary insufficiency in diabetes mellitus. *Ann. Intern. Med.* 74:357, 1971.
55. Sheehan, H. L.: Post-partum necrosis of anterior pituitary. *J. Pathol. Bacteriol.* 45:189, 1937. Reprinted in *Am. J. Obstet. Gynecol.* 111:851, 1971.

IN CHILDREN — DWARFISM AND RELATED DISORDERS

56. Collu, R., Brun, G., et al.: Reevaluation of levodopa-propranolol as a test of growth hormone reserve in children. *Pediatrics* 61:242, 1978.
57. Daughaday, W. H., Laron, Z., et al.: Defective sulfation factor generation: a possible etiologic link in dwarfism. *Trans. Assoc. Am. Phys.* 82:129, 1969.
58. Goodman, H. G., Grumbach, M. M., et al.: Growth and growth hormone. II. Comparison of isolated growth-hormone deficiency and multiple pituitary hormone deficiencies in 35 patients with idiopathic hypopituitary dwarfism. *N. Engl. J. Med.* 278:57, 1968.
59. Hopwood, N. J., Forsman, P. J., et al.: Hypoglycemia in hypopituitary children. *Am. J. Dis. Child.* 129:918, 1975.
60. Howse, P. M., Rayner, P. H. W., et al.: Nyctohemeral secretion of growth hormone in normal children of short stature and in children with hypopituitarism and intrauterine growth retardation. *Clin. Endocrinol.* 6:347, 1977.
61. Hoyt, W. F., Kaplan, S. L., et al.: Septo-optic dysplasia and pituitary dwarfism. *Lancet* 1:893, 1970.
62. Joss, E. E.: Growth hormone deficiency in childhood. Evaluation of diagnostic procedures. *Monogr. Paediatr.* 5:1, 1975.
63. Kaplan, S. L., Grumbach, M. M., et al.: Thyrotropin-releasing factor (TRF) effect on secretion of human pituitary prolactin and thyrotropin in children and in idiopathic hypopituitary dwarfism: further evidence of hypophysiotropic hormone deficiencies. *J. Clin. Endocrinol. Metab.* 35:825, 1972.
64. Laron, Z.: Syndrome of familial dwarfism and high plasma immunoreactive growth hormone. *Isr. J. Med. Sci.* 10:1247, 1974.
65. Pimstone, B.: Endocrine function in protein-calorie malnutrition. *Clin. Endocrinol.* 5:79, 1976.
66. Powell, G. F., Brasel, J. A., et al.: Emotional deprivation and growth retardation stimulating idiopathic hypopituitarism. I. Clinical evaluation of the syndrome. *N. Engl. J. Med.* 276, 1271, 1967.
67. Powell, G. F., Brasel, J. A., et al.: Emotional deprivation and growth retardation stimulating idiopathic hypopituitarism. II. Endocrinological evaluation of the syndrome. *N. Engl. J. Med.* 276:1279, 1967.
68. Preece, M. A., Tanner, J. M., et al.: Dose dependence of growth response to human growth hormone in growth hormone deficiency. *J. Clin. Endocrinol. Metab.* 42:477, 1976.
69. Rona, R. J., and J. M. Tanner: Aetiology of idiopathic growth hormone deficiency in England and Wales. *Arch. Dis. Child.* 52:197, 1977.
70. Tanner, J. M., Whitehouse, R. H., et al.: The effect of human growth hormone treatment for 1 to 7 years on the growth of 100 children with growth hormone deficiency low birthweight, inherited smallness, Turner's syndrome, and other complaints. *Arch. Dis. Child.* 46:745, 1971.
71. Weldon, V. V., Gupta, S. K., et al.: Evaluation of growth hormone release in children using arginine and L-dopa in combination. *J. Pediatr.* 87:540, 1975.

Pituitary Tumors

GENERAL

72. Hardy, J.: Transsphenoidal microsurgery of the normal and pathological pituitary. *Clin. Neurosurg.* 16:185, 1969.
73. Hoff, J. T., and Patterson, R. H.: Craniopharyngiomas in children and adults. *J. Neurosurg.* 36:299, 1972.

74. Kohler, P. O.: Diagnosis and Treatment of Pituitary Tumors. The National Institute of Child Health & Human Development, and the National Cancer Institute, Bethesda, Md., 1973, American Elsevier Publishing Co., Inc., N.Y., 1973.
75. McCormick, W. F., and Halmi, N. S.: Absence of chromophobe adenomas from large series of pituitary tumors. *Arch. Pathol. 92*:233, 1971.
76. Naidich, T. P., Pinto, R. S., et al.: Evaluation of sellar and parasellar masses by computed tomography. *Radiology 120*:91, 1976.
77. Russfield, A. B.: Pituitary Tumors, In *Pathology Annual.* Vol. 2. Sommers, S. C. (ed.), New York, Appleton-Century-Crofts, 1967.
78. Shaffi, O. M., and Wrightson, P.: Dural invasion by pituitary tumours. *N. Z. Med. J. 81*:386, 1975.
79. Weisberg, L. A.: Pituitary apoplexy. Association of degenerative change in pituitary adenoma with radiotherapy and detection by cerebral computed tomography. *Am. J. Med. 63*:109, 1977.
80. Weisberg, L. A., Zimmerman, E. A., et al.: Diagnosis and evaluation of patients with an enlarged sella turcica. *Am. J. Med. 61*:590, 1976.

PROLACTINOMAS

81. Bergh, T., Nillius, S. J., et al.: Hyperprolactinaemia in amenorrhoea — incidence and clinical significance. *Acta Endocrinol. 86*:683, 1977.
82. Bergh, T., Nillius, S. J., et al.: Hyperprolactinaemic amenorrhoea — results of treatment with bromocriptine. *Acta Endocrinol. 88*:147, 1978.
83. Carter, J. N., Tyson, J. E., et al.: Prolactin secreting tumors and hypogonadism in 22 men. *N. Engl. J. Med. 299*:847, 1978.
84. Fine, S. A., and Frohman, L. A.: Loss of central nervous system component of dopaminergic inhibition of prolactin secretion in patients with prolactin-secreting pituitary tumors. *J. Clin. Invest. 1*:973, 1978.
85. Franks, S., Jacobs, H. S., et al.: Hyperprolactinaemia and impotence. *Clin. Endocrinol. 8*:277, 1978.
86. Franks, S., Murray, M. A. F., et al.: Incidence and significance of hyperprolactinaemia in women with amenorrhoea. *Clin. Endocrinol. 4*:597, 1975.
87. Franks, S., Nabarro, J. D., et al.: Prevalence and presentation of hyperprolactinaemia in patients with "functionless" pituitary tumors. *Lancet 1*:778, 1977.
88. Halmi, N. S., VanGilder, J., et al.: Pathogenesis of prolactin-secreting pituitary adenomas. *Lancet 2*:1019, 1978.
89. Thorner, M. O., and Besser, G. M.: Bromocriptine treatment of hyperprolactinaemic hypogonadism. *Acta Endocrinol. 88*:131, 1978.

SOMATOTROPH ADENOMAS

90. Belforte, L., Camanni, F., et al.: Long-term treatment with 2-Br-α-ergocriptine in acromegaly. *Acta Endocrinol. 85*:235, 1977.
91. Besser, G. M., Wass, J. A. H., et al.: Acromegaly — results of long-term treatment with bromocriptine. *Acta Endocrinol. 88*:187, 1978.
92. Cryer, P. E., and Daughaday, W. H.: Adrenergic modulation of growth hormone secretion in acromegaly: alpha- and beta-adrenergic blockade produce qualitatively normal responses but no effect on L-dopa suppression. *J. Clin. Endocrinol. Metab. 44*:997, 1977.
93. Daughaday, W. H.: Extreme gigantism. *N. Engl. J. Med. 297*:1267, 1977.
94. Kellgren, J. H., Ball, J., et al.: The articular and other limb changes in acromegaly. *Q. J. Med. 21*:405, 1952.
95. Lamberg, B. A., Kivikangas, V., et al.: Conventional pituitary irradiation in acromegaly. Effect on growth hormone and TSH secretion. *Acta Endocrinol. 82*:267, 1976.
96. Low, P. A., McCleod, J. G., et al.: Peripheral neuropathy in acromegaly. *Brain 97*:139, 1974.
97. Muggeo, M., Bar, R. S., et al.: The insulin resistance of acromegaly: evidence for two alterations in the insulin receptor on circulating monocytes. *J. Clin. Endocrinol. Metab. 48*:17, 1979.
98. Nagulesparen, M., Trickey, R., et al.: Muscle changes in acromegaly. *Br. Med. J. 2*:914, 1976.
99. Schwinn, G., Dirks, H., et al.: Metabolic and clinical studies on patients with acromegaly treated with bromocriptine over 22 months. *Eur. J. Clin. Invest. 7*:101, 1977.
100. Smallridge, R. C., Rajfer, S., et al.: Acromegaly and the heart. An echocardiographic study. *Am. J. Med. 66*:22, 1979.
101. Strauch, G., Lego, A., et al.: Reversible plasma and red blood cells volumes increases in acromegaly. *Acta Endocrinol. 85*:465, 1977.
102. Wright, A. D., Hill, D. M., et al.: Mortality in acromegaly. *Q. J. Med. 39*:1, 1970.

CORTICOTROPH ADENOMAS

103. Hopwood, N. J., Kenny, F. M., et al.: Incidence of Nelson's syndrome after adrenalectomy for Cushing's disease in children — results of a nationwide survey. *Am. J. Dis. Child. 131*:1353, 1977.
104. Moore, T. J., Dluhy, R. G., et al.: Nelson's syndrome: frequency, prognosis, and effect of prior pituitary irradiation. *Ann. Intern. Med. 85*:731, 1976.
105. Salassa, R. M., Kearns, T. P., et al.: Pituitary tumors in patients with Cushing's syndrome. *J. Clin. Endocrinol. 19*:1523, 1959.
106. Tyrrell, J. B., Brooks, R. M., et al.: Cushing's disease, selective transphenoidal resection of pituitary microadenomas. *N. Engl. J. Med. 298*:753, 1978.

GONADOTROPH AND THYROTROPH ADENOMAS

107. Baylis, P. H.: Case of hyperthyroidism due to a chromophobe adenoma. *Clin. Endocrinol. 5*:145, 1976.
108. Cunningham, G. R., and Huckins, C.: An FSH and prolactin-secreting pituitary tumor: pituitary dynamics and testicular histology. *J. Clin. Endocrinol. Metab. 44*:253, 1977.
109. Demura, R., Kubo, O., et al.: FSH and LH secreting pituitary adenoma. *J. Clin. Endocrinol. Metab. 45*:653, 1977.
110. Friend, J. N., Judge, D. M., et al.: FSH-secreting pituitary adenomas: stimulation and suppression studies in two patients. *J. Clin. Endocrinol. Metab. 43*:650, 1976.
111. Jawadi, M. H., Ballonoff, L. B., et al.: Primary hypothyroidism and pituitary enlargement — radiological evidence of pituitary regression. *Arch. Intern. Med. 138*:1555, 1978.
112. Kourides, I. A., Ridgway, E. C., et al.: Thyrotropin-induced hyperthyroidism: use of alpha and beta subunit levels to identify patients with pituitary tumors. *J. Clin. Endocrinol. Metab. 45*:534, 1977.
113. Vagenakis, A. G., Dole, K., et al.: Pituitary enlargement, pituitary failure, and primary hypothyroidism. *Ann. Intern. Med. 85*:195, 1976.

Ectopic Production of Adenohypophyseal Hormones

114. Bertagna, X. Y., Nicholson, et al.: Corticotropin, lipotropin, and beta-endorphin production by a human nonpituitary tumor in culture — evidence for a common precursor. *Proc. Nat. Acad. Sci. USA 75*:5160, 1978.
115. Bloomfield, G. A., Holdaway, I. M., et al.: Lung tumours and ACTH production. *Clin. Endocrinol. 6*:95, 1977.
116. Caplan, R. H., Koob, L., et al.: Cure of acromegaly by operative removal of an islet cell tumor of the pancreas. *Am. J. Med. 64*:874, 1978.
117. Odell, W., Wolfsen, A., et al.: Ectopic peptide synthesis: a universal concomitant of neoplasia. *Trans. Assoc. Am. Phys. 90*:204, 1977.
118. Saeed uz Zafar, M., Mellinger, R. C., et al.: Acromegaly associated with a bronchial carcinoid tumor: evidence for ectopic production of growth hormone-releasing activity. *J. Clin. Endocrinol. Metab. 48*:66, 1979.

CHAPTER 4

The Thyroid Gland

By Sidney H. Ingbar
and Kenneth A. Woeber

PHYLOGENY

In its phylogeny, its embryogenesis, and certain aspects of its function, the thyroid gland reveals its primitive relation to the gastrointestinal tract.

The ability of the thyroid to metabolize iodine and incorporate it into a variety of organic compounds is found widely throughout the animal and plant kingdoms. Monoiodotyrosine (3-monoiodo-L-tyrosine, MIT) and diiodotyrosine (3,5-diiodo-L-tyrosine, DIT) have been found in a variety of invertebrate fauna, including mollusks, crustaceans, coelenterates, annelids, and insects, as well as in certain marine algae. In these lower forms, however, no recognizable thyroid tissue is present. Clearly recognizable thyroid tissue is confined to the vertebrates and is present in all species thereof. A close link to the thyroid of higher vertebrates is evident in the ammocoete, the larval form of the lamprey. Here, the endostyle is also capable of carrying out iodinations, but prior to metamorphosis a protease appears in the endostyle that can hydrolyze the iodoprotein formed. Presumably, this permits the endostyle to lose its connection with the pharynx, as occurs during metamorphosis, and to assume its adult function as an endocrine organ which secretes iodothyronines, including 3,5,3',5'-tetraiodo-L-thyronine (thyroxine; T_4) and 3,5,3'-triiodo-L-thyronine (T_3). (See Figure 4–1 for the structural formulas of the thyroid hormones, their precursors, and certain of their metabolites.)

Except perhaps in some lower vertebrates, control of thyroid function is mediated by a pituitary thyrotropin (thyroid-stimulating hormone; TSH). In higher vertebrates, control of TSH secretion is, in turn, influenced by a TSH-releasing hormone (TRH) of hypothalamic origin. In many lower vertebrates, a functional response of the pituitary-thyroid axis to TRH cannot be elicited, though TRH is clearly present within the brain. (For a thorough review of comparative thyroidology with extensive references, see Gorbman, 1978.)

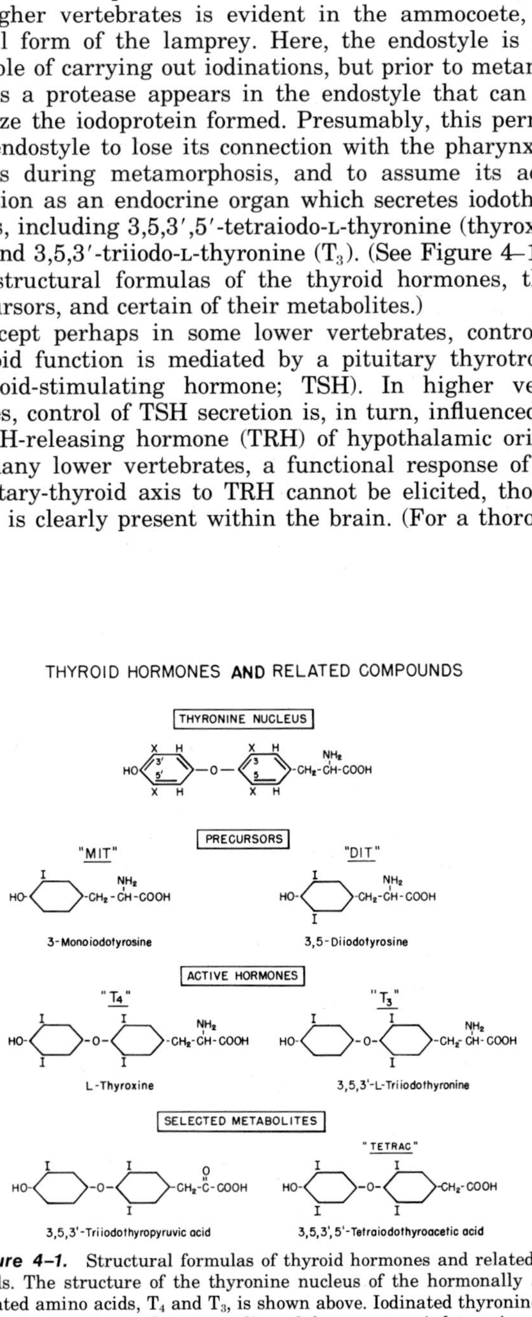

The phylogenetic association of the thyroid gland and the gastrointestinal (GI) tract is evident in several functional respects. Thus the salivary and gastric glands, like the thyroid, are capable of concentrating iodide in their secretions many times over, although iodide transport in these sites is not responsive to stimulation by thyrotropin (thyroid-stimulating hormone, TSH). In the rare form of goitrous hypothyroidism due to lack of the thyroid iodide transport mechanism, salivary transport of iodide is also defective (Stanbury, 1978). The salivary gland also contains enzymic mechanisms similar to those in the thyroid that are capable of iodinating tyrosine when provided with hydrogen peroxide. Although it is unlikely that the salivary gland forms significant quantities of iodoproteins under normal circumstances, when completely thyroidectomized rats are given large doses of iodide, specific stigmata of hypothyroidism are reversed and synthesis of DIT and T_4 occurs, probably within a protein matrix. Such iodoproteins may be formed in GI structures, pass into the lumen, and be digested, and the iodinated amino acids may well be absorbed. The similarity of function to that found in prevertebrates and in the ammocoete is thus apparent.

ANATOMIC AND FUNCTIONAL EMBRYOLOGY

The human thyroid anlage is first recognizable at about 1 month after conception when the embryo is approximately 3.5–4.0 mm in length. An extensive discussion of its subsequent development is available (Boyd, 1964). Briefly, the primordium begins as a thickening of epithelium in the pharyngeal floor which later forms a diverticulum. With continuing development, the median diverticulum undergoes relative caudal displacement, and the primitive stalk connecting the primordium with the pharyngeal floor undergoes elongation (thyroglossal duct). During its caudal displacement, the primordium assumes a more bilobate shape, coming into contact and fusing with the ventral aspect of the fourth pharyngeal pouch. Normally, the thyroglossal duct undergoes dissolution and fragmentation by about the second month after conception, leaving at its point of origin a small dimple at the junction of the middle and posterior third of the tongue, the foramen cecum. Cells of the lower portion of the duct differentiate to thyroid tissue, forming the pyramidal lobe of the gland. Concomitantly, histologic alterations occur. Complex interconnecting cordlike arrangements of cells interspersed with vascular connective tissue replace the solid epithelial mass. These transform to tubule-like structures at about the third month of fetal life, and shortly thereafter, follicular arrangements devoid of colloid appear, followed by colloid-filled follicles.

Numerous studies have been conducted on the functional development of the thyroid in laboratory animals of various species. Although some discordance in the findings has been noted, several general features have emerged. Thyroprotein resembling thyroglobulin appears just prior to or at the time that follicular structure is first apparent. Evidently, this antecedes by a short period the capacity to collect iodine, although results of some studies suggest that early iodine accumulation is virtually concurrent with the appearance of MIT, DIT, T_4, and T_3. Other results suggest that iodide transport, organic binding (binding of iodine to tyrosine), and iodotyrosine-coupling functions appear in sequence. The continued an-

THYROID HORMONES AND RELATED COMPOUNDS

Figure 4–1. Structural formulas of thyroid hormones and related compounds. The structure of the thyronine nucleus of the hormonally active iodinated amino acids, T_4 and T_3, is shown above. Iodinated thyronines are formed through the oxidative coupling of the precursor iodotyrosines, MIT and DIT, in varying combination. 3,5,3'-Triiodothyropyruvic acid is derived by oxidative deamination from T_3. "Tetrac" is derived from T_4 by oxidative deamination followed by decarboxylation.

atomic and functional development of the thyroid after these functions have begun, and perhaps even before, is dependent upon TSH. Its origin is necessarily fetal since the placenta is impermeable to maternal TSH.

Despite obvious difficulties in studying this problem, the ontogeny of thyroid function and its regulation in the human fetus is fairly well defined. (For extensive reviews of this topic, see Fisher, 1974, and Fisher and Dussault, 1975). The capacity of future follicular cells to form thyroglobulin is apparently established as early as the twenty-ninth day of gestation. Nonetheless, the ability to concentrate iodide and to synthesize T_4 is delayed until about the eleventh week. Significant accumulation of radioactive iodine given to the mother begins soon thereafter. Early growth and development of the thyroid do not seem to be TSH-dependent, since the capacity of the pituitary to synthesize and secrete TSH is not apparent until the tenth to twelfth week. Following this, rapid changes in pituitary and thyroid function take place. Probably as a consequence of hypothalamic maturation and increasing secretion of TRH, serum TSH concentration increases rapidly from about 18 to 26 weeks, following which it remains largely unchanged at levels higher than those found in the mother. Thyroxine-binding globulin (TBG), the major thyroid hormone–binding protein in plasma, is detectable in serum by the tenth gestational week, and increases in concentration progressively to term. This doubtless accounts in part for the progressive increase in serum T_4 concentration that occurs in the second and third trimesters, but increased secretion of T_4 must also play a role, since the concentration of unbound or free T_4 also rises.

The peripheral metabolism of T_4 in the human fetus differs markedly from that in the adult in both the quantitative and the qualitative senses. Overall, on the basis of unit body mass, rates of production and degradation of T_4 greatly exceed those found in the adult. In addition, in all species thus far studied, the specific enzymatic pathways by which T_4 is metabolized differ greatly from those in the adult, favoring the formation of 3,3′,5′-triiodo-L-thyronine (reverse T_3; rT_3) at the expense of T_3. These differences in T_4 metabolism during fetal and adult life are discussed more fully in a later section.

Several aspects of fetal thyroidology are especially worthy of note from the clinical standpoint. Rarely, thyroid tissue may develop from remnants of the thyroglossal duct near the base of the tongue. Such lingual thyroid tissue may be the sole functioning thyroid present; its surgical removal will then lead to hypothyroidism. More commonly, elements of the thyroglossal duct may persist and later give rise to thyroglossal cysts, or thyroid tissue progenitors may migrate with adjacent cardiovascular structures to occupy a place within the mediastinum. Functionally, the patterns of iodine metabolism in certain defects of hormone synthesis apparent after birth may represent or mimic a particular stage in the functional development of the fetal thyroid. Examples are evident in genetically determined goiters or in tumors of the mature gland that are not capable of carrying out organic iodinations or of synthesizing active hormones from precursor iodotyrosines. In addition, it is clear that the fetal pituitary-thyroid axis functions as a unit that is essentially independent of that of the mother. Transplacental passage of TSH from mother to fetus is negligible or nearly so, and the same is true of maternal T_4 and T_3, whether endogenous or exogenous in origin. Consequently, it is fruitless to administer thyroid hormones to the mother in an effort to forestall fetal hypothyroidism, whether spontaneous or induced by goitrogens given to the mother (e.g., for the treatment of maternal thyrotoxicosis). In addition, observation of neonates who lack thyroid function reveals that somatic development during fetal life is largely independent of thyroid hormones. Thyroid hormones almost certainly condition late-phase skeletal maturation, possibly influence late prenatal maturation of the lung, and clearly are required for normal development of the brain and intellectual function, either before birth or soon thereafter, but neonatal hypothyroidism is extremely difficult to detect by physical examination. Rather, this very common disease, which occurs at least once in every 4000–5000 newborns throughout the world, must be sought with measurements of the serum T_4 or TSH concentration.

ANATOMY AND HISTOLOGY

The thyroid is normally one of the largest of the endocrine organs, weighing approximately 20 g in North American adults. Moreover, the potential of the thyroid for growth is tremendous. Goiters weighing many hundred grams are not rare. The normal thyroid is made up of two lobes joined by a thin band of tissue, the isthmus. The latter is approximately 0.5 cm thick, 2 cm wide, and 2 cm high. The individual lobes normally display a rather pointed superior pole and a poorly defined blunt inferior pole merging medially with the isthmus. Each lobe is approximately 2.0 or 2.5 cm in both thickness and width at its largest diameter and is approximately 4.0 cm in length. Occasionally, especially when the remainder of the gland is goitrous, a pyramidal lobe is discernible as a finger-like projection directed upward from the isthmus, generally just lateral to the midline, usually on the left. The right lobe of the thyroid is normally more vascular than the left, is often the larger of the two, and tends to enlarge more in disorders associated with a diffuse increase in size.

The thyroid is closely affixed to the anterior and lateral aspects of the trachea by loose connective tissue. The upper margin of the isthmus generally lies just below the cricoid cartilage, which therefore provides a convenient landmark for locating the gland. The lobes themselves lie along the lower half of the lateral margins of the thyroid cartilage. Lying between the thyroid gland and the subcutaneous tissue are the thin infrahyoid muscles. Lateral to the gland are the carotid sheaths and sternocleidomastoid muscles, while the recurrent laryngeal nerves lie in the grooves between the lateral lobes and the trachea. Two pairs of parathyroid glands are normally situated on or beneath the posterior surface of the thyroid lobes.

Two main pairs of vessels constitute the major arterial blood supply. The superior thyroid arteries, arising from the external carotids, and the inferior thyroid arteries from the subclavians enter their respective poles. The thyroid gland is exceptionally well vascularized. Estimates of thyroid blood flow range from 4 to 6 ml/min/g, well in excess of the blood flow to the kidney (3 ml/min/g). In severe hyperplasia as in diffuse toxic goiter, blood flow rates greater than 1 liter/min may occur. Increased flow is evident clinically in the presence of a thrill or audible bruit over the gland or in its immediate vicinity. There is rich lymphatic drainage. Its function relative to the endocrine activity of the gland is uncertain, but reports suggest that the lymph contains a higher concentration of newly released radioiodine than does thyroid venous blood, probably in the form of iodoprotein.

The thyroid is innervated by both the adrenergic and cholinergic nervous systems, arising from the cervical ganglia and the vagus nerve, respectively. Afferent fibers pass through the laryngeal nerves and regulate an active vasomotor system. One function of neurogenic stimuli is to regulate blood flow to the thyroid. Although acute changes in blood flow do not appear to alter the rate of hormonal release, the rate of perfusion influences the delivery of TSH, iodide, and metabolic substrates and may eventually influence glandular function and growth.

In addition to vasomotor innervation, there exists a network of adrenergic fibers that terminates near the basement membrane of the follicular wall. Moreover, specific, saturable adrenergic receptors are present in thyroid plasma membranes. These findings, together with the ability of adrenergic (and other) amines to affect iodine and intermediary metabolism of the thyroid *in vitro* and *in vivo*, indicate that the adrenergic nervous system can influence thyroid function through a direct effect on the follicle cell, as well as by changing glandular blood flow. This is discussed more fully in a later section on Factors That Influence Thyroid Hormone Economy.

The thyroid is invested with a thin fibrous capsule that penetrates the gland, forming irregular pseudolobules. The gland itself is firm yet resilient. The cut surface of a normal gland has a spotted beefy red appearance. Minute vesicles (the follicles) from which the amber-colored, sticky colloid exudes are more or less evenly distributed throughout.

With light microscopy, the gland is seen to be composed of closely packed sacs, called acini or follicles, which are invested with a rich capillary network. The interior of the follicle is filled with the clear, proteinaceous colloid, which normally is the major constituent of the total thyroid mass. The diameter of the follicles varies considerably, even within a single gland, but averages about 200 μ. As might be expected, the iodine-accumulating function of the individual follicle varies with its surface area. The wall of the follicle is lined by a single layer of closely packed cuboidal cells, approximately 15 μ high. The cell height of the acinar epithelium varies with the degree of glandular stimulation, becoming columnar when active and flat when inactive. The epithelium rests upon a well-defined basement membrane that stains positively with reagents for mucopolysaccharides and separates the follicular cells from the surrounding capillaries. From 20 to 40 follicles are demarcated by connective tissue septa to form a lobule supplied by a single artery. The function of an individual lobule may vary from that of its neighbors.

With electron microscopy, the thyroid is seen to have many features in common with other secretory cells but some which are peculiar to the thyroid. From the apical aspect of the follicular cell, numerous microvilli extend into the colloid. It is at or near this surface of the cell that such crucial reactions as iodination and the initial phase of hormone secretion, namely colloid resorption, occur. The nucleus of the follicular cell has no distinctive features. The cytoplasm contains an extensive endoplasmic reticulum (ER) laden with microsomes. The ER is distinctive in being composed of a network of wide irregular tubules that contain the precursor of thyroglobulin. The carbohydrate component of thyroglobulin is probably added to this precursor in the Golgi apparatus which is located apically. Lysosomes and mitochondria are scattered throughout the cytoplasm. Upon stimulation by TSH, there occurs enlargement of the Golgi apparatus, formation of pseudopodia at the apical surface, and appearance in the apical portion of the cell of many droplets that contain colloid taken up from the follicular lumen. (For an extensive review of thyroid ultrastructure, see Fawcett et al., 1969).

In addition to the follicular cell, the thyroid contains a population of other cells, termed parafollicular or C cells, that are important because they are the source of the calcium-lowering hormone calcitonin. These cells arise during embryonic development from the last pair of pharyngeal pouches, but ultimately come to rest either among the cells of the follicular epithelium or in the thyroid interstitium. They differ from the cells of the follicular epithelium in never bordering upon the follicular lumen and in being rich in both mitochondria and α-glycerophosphate dehydrogenase. C cells undergo hyperplasia early in the syndrome of familial medullary carcinoma of the thyroid and give rise to this tumor in both its familial and sporadic forms.

IODINE METABOLISM: THE SYNTHESIS, SECRETION, AND METABOLISM OF THE THYROID HORMONES

In the most general sense, the function of the thyroid in higher forms, including man, is to secrete such quantities of hormone as are necessary to meet the demands of the peripheral tissue. This section will deal with the overall metabolism of one of the major components of the thyroid hormones, iodine; the reactions by which iodine is incorporated into them; the synthesis of the specific protein, thyroglobulin, which serves as a matrix in which the hormones are formed and stored; and the processes by which the hormones are released into the blood. Consideration will also be given to the peripheral transport of the hormones and the avenues along which they are excreted or degraded. A subsequent section will deal with the regulation of thyroid function.

Extrathyroid Metabolism of Iodide

Formation of normal quantities of thyroid hormone ultimately depends upon the availability of adequate quantities of exogenous iodine. Although efficient mechanisms exist to conserve iodine in the presence of iodine deficiency, they do not entirely entirely succeed in preventing depletion of iodine stores; ultimately, this may lead to insufficient hormone production. Normally, iodine balance is maintained from dietary sources, i.e., food and water, but increasingly, especially in more highly developed cultures, iodine may enter the body via medications, diagnostic agents, and dietary supplements and as a result of the use of iodine by the food-processing industry. Increases in available iodine modify both the metabolism of iodine and the clinical tests by which it is assessed; this will be discussed more fully in the section on laboratory tests.

It is difficult to assign normal limits to the daily dietary intake of iodine since this varies widely throughout the world, depending on the iodine content of soil and water and upon culturally established dietary preferences. Even in any single area, considerable variation in iodine intake can be expected among different individuals and in the same individual from day to day. In most areas of the United States, for example, dietary iodine intake is in the range of 500 μg daily, while in Japan, where large quantities of foods rich in iodine are characteristically consumed, intakes as high as several milligrams per day have been commonplace. In other areas of

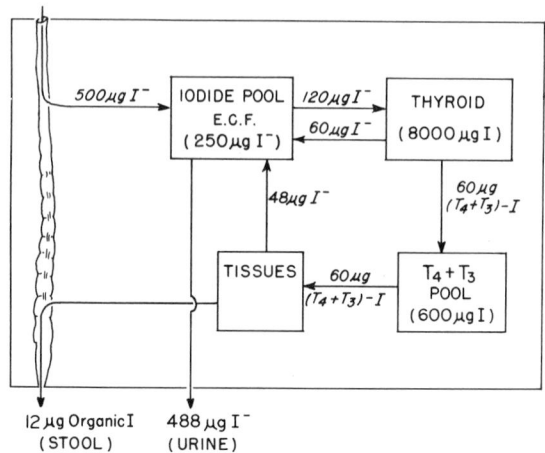

Figure 4–2. Diagram depicting normal pathways of iodine metabolism in a state of iodine balance. Note that most (approximately 90%) of body iodine store is present in the thyroid (chiefly in the organic form). Approximately 10% is present as iodide. Arrows indicate daily flux of iodine from one compartment to another. In this example, one-fifth of the iodide entering the iodide space (120/608) is accumulated by the thyroid. Peak thyroid uptake of I* should be 20%, and the rate of turnover of thyronine-iodine peripherally 10%/day.

the world, iodine intakes substantially less than those of the United States are apparently well tolerated without overt widespread thyroid dysfunction. As with pharmacologically induced alterations in iodine intake, such variations in the common dietary intake, when sustained, are reflected in differences in the kinetics of iodine metabolism and hence must be taken into account in assigning normal limits to tests designed to evaluate thyroid function. Figure 4–2 is a schema of the major pathways of overall iodine metabolism, summarizing the movement of iodine into, out of, and among the various compartments of body iodine. The numerical values presented are approximations to the normal means in the United States, but even here rather wide variations are encountered. Iodine used in the synthesis of thyroid hormone is drawn from the inorganic iodide of the extracellular fluid (ECF). This iodide is partly replenished both by iodide lost from the thyroid into the blood (iodide leak) and by iodide liberated through deiodination of thyroid hormones in peripheral tissues. Ultimately, however, the diet is the most important source of iodide. Iodine is ingested in both the inorganic and the organically bound form. The rapidity of absorption of organically bound iodine and the form in which it is absorbed are uncertain, but eventually the iodine is made available as inorganic iodide. Iodide itself is rapidly and efficiently absorbed from the GI tract, and little is lost in the stool.

In the body, iodide is largely confined to the ECF. It is also found, however, within the red blood cell and is concentrated in the intraluminal fluids of the GI tract, notably the saliva and gastric juice, from which it is ultimately reabsorbed and reenters the ECF. In addition, until bound to organic compounds (chiefly tyrosine), iodide brought into the thyroid by active transport is in essence a portion of the extracellular iodide, since, like iodide in the other two extensions of the extracellular iodide space, it is in rapid equilibrium with iodide in the main compartment. The concentration of iodide in the ECF is normally quite low, approximately 1.0–1.5 μg/100 ml and the content of the peripheral pool approximately 250 μg. Thus only a very small percentage of total body iodine is

present in the iodide compartment, and this is turned over, i.e., removed and replenished, several times daily.

There are two main avenues for the removal of iodide from the ECF. Small quantities of iodide are lost in expired air and through the skin, but the major clearance of iodide occurs via the thyroid and the kidneys. The processes by which thyroid clearance occurs and the subsequent fate of the iodide thereby removed will be considered in detail later. An appreciation of the renal mechanism for iodide clearance is important, since renal removal of iodide determines the availability of iodide to the thyroid (and vice versa). Although iodide is almost completely filterable at the glomerulus, the renal iodide clearance rate in adults normally approximates 30–40 ml/min. Thus filtered iodide is largely reabsorbed, but reabsorption is passive rather than active. In man, unlike other animals, the renal iodide clearance rate is unaffected by the excretion of chloride or other anions and is apparently independent of the plasma iodide concentration and hence the filtered load. Iodide clearance is minimally affected by the rate of urine flow per se and is uninfluenced by physiologic agents, such as TSH, or drugs that alter thyroidal iodide transport. As with other urinary components that are passively reabsorbed, the renal clearance of iodide varies with changes in glomerular filtration rate (GFR), the iodide clearance increasing or decreasing disproportionately when GFR is acutely increased or decreased, respectively. Thus, when intrinsic renal function is normal, the kidneys can be considered passive participants in iodide metabolism, not really sharing in the physiologic adjustments designed to maintain thyroidal homeostasis under abnormal circumstances.

Normally about 500 μg of iodine is cleared into the urine daily, almost entirely in the inorganic form. This quantity is only slightly less than the average daily dietary intake, reflecting the scant loss of iodine through other avenues. Among these, the GI tract is the most important, about 12 μg of iodine being lost in the stool daily, mainly in the organic form. Under abnormal circumstances, substantial losses of iodine may occur. In nephrosis or other proteinuric states, T_4 and T_3 are excreted in the urine in association with their transport proteins. Iodinated tyrosines are lost in the urine in the rare familial disorder in which the enzyme iodotyrosine dehalogenase is lacking from both the thyroid and peripheral tissues. Fecal loss of organic iodine may be excessive when GI absorption is impaired, as in chronic diarrheal states or under the influence of certain dietary constituents, such as soybean products. Finally, notable losses of iodine may occur through lactation.

The second major site of removal of iodide from the ECF is the thyroid. Iodide removed from the plasma by the thyroid is not irreversibly lost, however, since ultimately it will be secreted into the circulation as either iodinated thyronines, T_4 and T_3, or as inorganic iodide. The thyroid contains by far the largest pool of body iodine, under normal circumstances approximately 8000 μg, most of which is in the form of iodinated amino acids. Normally this pool of iodine turns over quite slowly (about 1%/day).

Synthesis and Secretion of the Thyroid Hormones

The structural formulas of the thyroid hormones, their precursors, and several related compounds are shown in Figure 4–1, and the major steps in the synthesis and se-

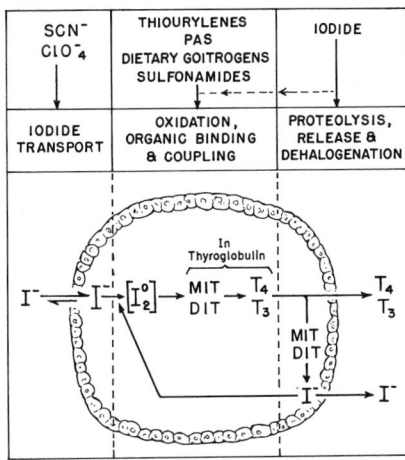

Figure 4–3. Diagram of the major steps in thyroid hormone biosynthesis. In this diagram, the follicular outline is intended merely to differentiate the intrathyroid from the interstitial compartment and should not be construed as indicating that the reactions shown necessarily occur in the follicular lumen. Note that the concentration of intrathyroid iodide maintained by the iodide transport mechanism is greater than that in the extracellular fluid. The processes of iodide oxidation, organic binding, and coupling of iodotyrosines are grouped together since they appear to be closely related oxidative reactions. The precise proportions of the iodide liberated from iodotyrosines by dehalogenation that are reused or released into the extracellular fluid are unknown. Shown above are the major inhibitors of the several steps in hormone biosynthesis. Large quantities of iodide inhibit organic binding and coupling (dashed lines), but this effect is usually transient. Although not shown, the lithium ion, like iodide, is an inhibitor of proteolysis and release.

cretion of the hormones are shown in Figure 4–3. It is convenient to consider the metabolism of iodine leading to the biosynthesis of thyroid hormones as occurring in three sequential stages: (1) active transport of iodide into the thyroid, (2) oxidation of iodide and iodination by the oxidized form of tyrosyl residues within thyroglobulin to yield the hormonally inactive iodotyrosines, and (3) coupling of iodotyrosines to form the hormonally active iodothyronines, notably T_4 and T_3. The hormones thus formed are held in peptide linkage within the specific thyroprotein, thyroglobulin, which is the major component of the intrafollicular colloid. Release of hormones, in addition, involves two additional groups of reactions: (1) hydrolysis of thyroglobulin by a thyroid protease and by peptidases, liberating free iodinated amino acids; (2) passage of iodothyronines into the blood, while the iodotyrosines undergo intrathyroid deiodination.

Iodide Transport

Except when the plasma concentration of inorganic iodide is greatly increased, synthesis of adequate quantities of hormone requires that iodide enter the thyroid more rapidly than would be possible by simple diffusion from the ECF. The thyroid, however, contains a transport mechanism (the iodide-concentrating, -transport, or -trapping mechanism) that subserves this end and provides sufficient iodide substrate for subsequent steps in hormone formation (comprehensively reviewed by Bastomsky, 1974). Iodide transported into the gland either is oxidized and organified or is free to diffuse back into the ECF. Under normal circumstances the rate of inward clearance of iodide exceeds the combined rates of organic

binding* and back diffusion, with the result that intrathyroid concentration gradients for iodide in excess of unity are maintained within the gland. Such gradients are often referred to as thyroid/plasma (T:P) or thyroid/serum (T:S) ratios. Although most of the inorganic iodide within the thyroid is located within the follicular lumen, the actual iodide-concentrating mechanism is located within the acinar cell itself. The interior of the cell maintains a negative electrical potential with respect to both the interstitium and the follicular lumen. Presumably, iodide is actively transported into the cell against this negative potential and then diffuses along the electrochemical gradient into the luminal area.

The exact biochemical mechanism of active iodide transport is unknown. However, like other active transport mechanisms, thyroid iodide transport is an energy-requiring process, highly dependent upon continued generation of phosphate bond energy. In addition, active iodide transport is closely related to the function of the sodium (Na^+)-, potassium (K^+)-dependent ATPase system. Although TSH increases the activity of both the iodide transport and ATPase systems, the two do not respond in parallel in other circumstances. Hence the precise nature of their relationship remains uncertain. ATPase, acting on ATP at the cell membrane, may make phosphate bond energy available for iodide transport. Alternatively, reversible exchange of iodide for phosphate in a specific carrier may take place. The nature of the iodide carrier is unknown, but lecithins capable of reversibly binding iodide have been extracted from thyroid tissue.

The activity of the iodide transport mechanism is influenced by a variety of physiologic factors, the most important of which is the level of TSH stimulation. Iodide transport activity is enhanced by TSH and decreased by hypophysectomy. The other major factor that influences iodide transport activity is an internal autoregulatory system through which the intrinsic activity of the iodide transport mechanism and its responsiveness to TSH stimulation are caused to vary inversely with the glandular content of organic iodine (reviewed by Ingbar, 1978). As a result of these influences, T:P ratios can be extremely high when the thyroid is depleted of organic iodine or is intensely stimulated by TSH. In animals, under appropriate conditions, ratios of several hundred have been observed, and high ratios are also found in most patients with thyroid hyperfunction, regardless of its cause. The ability of the thyroid to transport iodide and to maintain iodide concentration gradients vis-à-vis the ECF is not unlimited, however. Rather, there exists a maximal rate of inward iodide transport. Thus, progressive increases in the concentration of iodide in the ECF are associated with progressively decreasing values of the T:P ratio, while the concentration of iodide that has been actively transported into the gland rises progressively, ultimately reaching a maximum. Absolute values of both the T:P ratio and the iodide transport maximum vary with the functional state of the gland.

The thyroid mechanism for concentrating iodide is shared by other monovalent anions, including perchlorate and pertechnetate. These and other anions act as competitive inhibitors of iodide transport, a property that may relate to similarity of their partial specific molecular volumes. Thiocyanate, another monovalent anion that inhibits iodide transport, is not itself concentrated within the thyroid and may possibly act by uncoupling thyroid oxidative phosphory-

---

*For brevity, "organic binding," "organic iodine," "organified," and similar terms are often used. These expressions signify that iodide is bound to organic compounds, chiefly as iodotyrosine.

lation. The ability of perchlorate and thiocyanate to inhibit iodide transport is the basis for their use in the perchlorate- or thiocyanate-discharge tests for defects in the thyroid organic-binding mechanism, and concentration of the radio-active anion pertechnetate makes this a valuable agent for thyroid imaging (see later section on thyroid function tests).

The ability of the thyroid to concentrate iodide is shared by other tissues of endodermal origin, notably the salivary and gastric glands. The effect of metabolic inhibitors and inhibitory anions on iodide transport in these other tissues is similar to that on iodide transport in the thyroid. A rare disorder arises from the absence of an effective thyroid iodide transport mechanism. In patients with this disorder the salivary and gastric iodide concentration mechanisms are also lacking. Whether the result of disease or the action of pharmacologic agents, inadequate iodide transport results in goiter and hypothyroidism. Both can be overcome, however, by administering additional iodine. This increases the iodide concentration in plasma and permits sufficient iodine for hormone synthesis to enter the gland by simple diffusion.

In addition to iodide brought into the thyroid by active transport from the ECF, iodide is generated in the thyroid by the deiodination of iodotyrosines liberated during the hydrolysis of thyroglobulin. A portion of this iodide is reorganified, while the remainder is lost from the gland as the so-called "iodide leak."

Oxidation of Iodide and Organic Iodinations

After its transport into or regeneration within the thyroid, iodide enters into a series of reactions which ultimately lead to the synthesis of the active thyroid hormones. (For a review of the organic-binding and coupling mechanisms, see Taurog, 1974.) The first of these reactions involves oxidation of iodide and incorporation of the resulting intermediate into the hormonally inactive iodotyrosines, MIT and DIT. Iodide thus metabolized is removed from the iodide pool and can no longer be discharged by thiocyanate, perchlorate, or other inhibitors of iodide transport. In most species, oxidation of iodide is normally rapid. After administration of radioiodine ($I*$),* the isotope is almost immediately found in organic combination, mainly in soluble thyroprotein, principally thyroglobulin, and to a limited extent in subcellular particulate proteins, lipids, and nucleic acids. These iodinated products are probably the result of random rather than specifically directed iodinations.

The iodinations that lead to formation of iodotyrosines occur within a preformed thyroprotein molecule rather than in free amino acids that are then incorporated into protein. Oxidation of thyroid iodide is almost certainly mediated by a peroxidase. Enzymes with peroxidatic activity have been demonstrated in the thyroid of many species, including man, especially in particulate subcellular fractions. A peroxidase in hog thyroid has been substantially purified and appears to be a heme protein; this accounts for the requirement of organic iodinations for molecular oxygen and their ready inhibition by cyanide and azide. In vitro, thyroid peroxidase, when afforded a source of hydrogen peroxide, readily iodinates thyroglobulin as well as other proteins. The reaction catalyzed by peroxidase in vitro has many properties of the

---

The abbreviation I is employed to denote any of the radioactive isotopes of iodine, since they cannot be distinguished from one another physiologically or biochemically. When a specific isotope of iodine is referred to, it will be appropriately designated.

iodination reaction in vivo, including inhibition by antithyroid agents and by high concentrations of iodide (Wolff-Chiakoff effect). The evanescent product of the peroxidation of iodide, i.e., the active iodinating form, is uncertain, but may be the iodinium ion (I^+) or a free radical of iodine. Current evidence suggests that the hydrogen peroxide that serves as the oxidant of iodide is generated through the auto-oxidation of flavin enzymes acting as NADH- and particularly NADPH-oxidases. In this way, generation of hydrogen peroxide is linked to electron transfers consequent to substrate oxidations within the thyroid.

Radioautographic and histochemical evidence, as well as the demonstration that thyroid cell ghosts that are virtually devoid of intracellular contents are capable of carrying out organic iodination, suggests that iodinations occur at the cell-colloid interface. As judged from studies in vitro, soluble inhibitors of organic iodinations, principally ascorbic acid and reduced glutathione, exist in thyroid tissue. These may inhibit iodinations by reducing either the oxidized form of iodine or hydrogen peroxide itself. Thus mitochondrial systems may provide a source of hydrogen peroxide and cell membrane the iodide-peroxidase, while the cytoplasmic fraction may contain regulatory inhibitors of organic iodinations.

Organic iodinations are conditioned by the extent of thyroid stimulation by TSH. They are retarded in the hypophysectomized rat and are promptly increased by administration of TSH. Iodinations are susceptible to inhibition by a great number of pharmacologic agents, including the usual antithyroid drugs, most of which are inhibitors of peroxidase and also have intrinsic reducing activity. Iodinations are also inhibited by freezing, cooling, or storage of the thyroid tissue. Defects in the organic-binding mechanism of variable severity occur in humans and lead to the development of goitrous hypothyroidism or, if less severe, to goiter without hypothyroidism. In certain instances of this type, the thyroid is found to be lacking in peroxidase. In others, peroxidase is present, and the defect may reside in inadequate production of hydrogen peroxide or abnormalities in thyroglobulin that render it less readily iodinated.

Formation of Iodothyronines

Formation of MIT and DIT, via oxidation and organic binding of iodide, is followed by the synthesis of the hormonally active iodothyronines, T_4 and T_3. Since noniodinated thyronine cannot be demonstrated in thyroglobulin, it seems certain that T_4 and T_3 must arise from iodinated precursors. Synthesis of T_4 from DIT requires the fusion of two DIT molecules to yield a structure with two diiodinated rings linked by an ether bridge. Concomitantly, there occurs a net loss of the alanine side chain from the ring that ultimately contains the phenolic hydroxyl group (beta or outer ring). This reaction is commonly termed the coupling reaction. In aqueous media, this or analogous reactions take place when DIT or derivatives of DIT are allowed to stand under oxidative conditions. Nevertheless, the manner in which T_4 is synthesized in vivo remains uncertain. Two general hypotheses have received major consideration. (See Taurog, 1974.) The first is that T_4 and T_3 are formed by the interaction of a peptide-bound DIT with an oxidation product of DIT or MIT, respectively. In the case of DIT, the suggested product is 3,5-diiodo-4-hydroxy-phenylpyruvic acid (DIHPPA). In vitro, DIHPPA has been shown to be a product of oxidative systems that yield T_4 from DIT. Moreover, when DIHPPA is added to solutions of DIT, T_4 is formed, with pyruvic acid and ammonia as by-products. Additional studies in vitro have revealed formation of labeled T_4 when thyroglobulin is incubated with labeled DIHPPA. As small quantities of DIHPPA and its monoiodinated analogue, MIHPPA, the suggested precursor of T_3, have been found in thyroid tissue, this mechanism of synthesis of iodothyronines *in vivo* seems quite possible. It is attractive since it does not require the extensive structural alterations in the thyroglobulin molecule during iodothyronine synthesis required by the alternative hypothesis.

The most commonly held view concerning the synthesis of T_4 and T_3 differs from that described above in that it requires the coupling of two iodotyrosines, both of which are initially held in peptide bond within the thyroglobulin molecule. A free radical mechanism whereby two molecules of DIT yield T_4 via a quinol ether intermediate has been proposed, but it is apparent that, whatever the intermediates in the reaction, coupling of two peptide-bound iodotyrosines would require disruption of the peptide bonds holding the iodotyrosyl group that yields the beta ring of the thyronine nucleus. This would obviously require substantial changes in the structure of thyroglobulin as iodothyronines are formed. Such rearrangements are possible, however, since T_4 can be formed *in vitro* during iodination of thyroglobulin or even of proteins that are not normally iodinated, such as casein, insulin, or albumin. Moreover, both *in vivo* and *in vitro*, the enhanced synthesis of iodothyronines that accompanies increasing iodination of thyroglobulin is associated with an increase in both the sedimentation constant of the protein and its stability to conditions that induce dissociation. These changes are consistent with the occurrence of a major change in the structure of the protein consequent to the synthesis of T_4 and T_3.

Synthesis of iodothyronines requires oxidative conditions. There is increasing thought that the reaction is mediated by a peroxidase, perhaps the same peroxidase that mediates the initial oxidation of iodide, since there are interesting similarities between the two reactions. Virtually all agents that inhibit organic binding also inhibit coupling. In addition, cell-free particulate fractions can yield T_4 from free DIT when provided with a source of hydrogen peroxide. Moreover, synthesis of labeled iodothyronines from prelabeled iodotyrosines is demonstrable when prelabeled thyroglobulin is incubated with thyroid peroxidase and a source of hydrogen peroxide in the absence of free iodide. Despite this evidence that peroxidase may mediate both the organic-binding and the coupling mechanisms, there are certain physiologic differences between the two. The coupling reaction is much more sensitive to a variety of factors. Inhibition of coupling with continued generation of MIT and DIT occurs in response to small doses of antithyroid agents or during the acute response to large amounts of iodide. Iodine deficiency and lack of TSH impair the synthesis of iodothyronines relatively more than the synthesis of iodotyrosines. Finally, a failure of coupling, without a failure of organic binding, may be the cause of certain cases of goitrous hypothyroidism in man. Here, inadequate secretion of iodothyronines occurs, and although the thyroid contains ample iodotyrosines, little T_4 and T_3 are found. It is thus uncertain whether the organic-binding and coupling reactions are indeed separate or whether they are mediated by a similar mechanism. Perhaps they are the same but are differentially affected by other factors, possibly the inherent oxidative potential of the gland.

Storage and Release of Hormones

The thyroid is unique among the endocrine glands by virtue of the large store of hormone that it contains and the slow overall rate at which the hormone normally turns over. This aspect of thyroid hormone economy has homeostatic value in that the large hormone reservoir provides prolonged protection against depletion of circulating hormone should synthesis cease. In normal man, administration of completely blocking doses of antithyroid agents for as long as 2 weeks results in little lowering of the serum T_4 concentration, and plasma concentrations of TSH are not increased. Thus an important aspect of hormone economy is the storage function of the thyroid. Analyses reveal that the normal thyroid contains about 8000 μg of iodine, of which as much as 10% may be inorganic. Direct analyses of human thyroids performed when iodine intake was generally lower indicated that the organic iodine is constituted as follows: MIT, 17–28%; DIT, 24–42%; T_4, 35%; T_3, 5–8%. More recent analyses show that the T_4:T_3 ratio may be greater than 10:1 (Chopra et al., 1973).

Thyroglobulin is the storage form of the thyroid hormone. Although it had been thought that thyroglobulin is excluded completely from the peripheral blood, immunochemical analyses suggest that the protein may be present in the plasma of most normal individuals. Direct cannulation reveals that the lymphatics are the avenue through which thyroglobulin normally enters the blood. It is very unlikely, however, that peripheral hydrolysis of thyroglobulin contributes significantly to the T_4 and T_3 found in the blood. Rather, T_4 and T_3 enter the blood directly after their liberation from thyroglobulin by proteolytic cleavage within the follicular cell.

The mechanisms whereby this cleavage occurs have been extensively clarified by submicroscopic, histochemical, and biochemical studies. (See review by Greer and Haibach, 1974.). The sequence is best observed after stimulation of the resting thyroid by TSH. Within a few minutes after such stimulation, formation of pseudopodia is evident at the apical surface of the follicular cell, followed by endocytosis of colloid to yield multiple vesicles (colloid droplets). That these vesicles contain colloid is evident in that they are PAS-positive and contain ^{14}C-amino acids or radioiodine previously allowed to accumulate in the luminal contents. The process of endocytosis apparently involves destabilization of the apical membrane, since membrane stabilizers, such as chlorpromazine, inhibit this process. The process is not confined to thyroglobulin, since isolated thyroid cells are capable of accumulating latex particles, and this process is stimulated by factors that enhance the endocytosis of colloid. Concomitantly with endocytosis, there occurs a migration of dense bodies, rich in esterases and acid phosphatase and apparently identical with lysosomes, from the basal toward the apical end of the cell. Fusion of lysosomes with colloid droplets occurs. The resulting "phagolysosomes" have histochemical characteristics of both component particles and are likely the site of the physiologically active protease. The latter is an acid hydrolase similar in properties to cathepsin D. Hydrolysis of thyroglobulin is thought to occur in the phagolysosomes, which gradually regain the ultrastructural properties and basal location of lysosomes as hydrolysis is completed. Microtubular and microfilamentous structures, similar to those found in other organs, are present in the thyroid cell. They are apparently involved in the secretory process, since inhibitors of both the former (vincristine, vinblastine, colchicine) and the latter (cytochalasin B) inhibit the secretory process.

Studies *in vitro* with subcellular fractions of thyroid tissue containing phagolysosomes have shed light on the biochemical processes by which thyroglobulin is hydrolyzed. It appears that hydrolysis is facilitated by reduction of disulfide bonds in thyroglobulin, this being effected by a transhydrogenase that uses reduced glutathione (GSH). The availability of GSH, in turn, depends upon the activity of a second enzyme, glutathione reductase, that uses NADPH to reduce oxidized glutathione. If true, the proposed mechanism would link the secretory process to intermediary metabolism and biologic oxidations within the gland.

Although it had been thought that iodothyronines liberated by this process were entirely free to enter the blood, there being no mechanism within the gland to effect their degradation, it now appears that the thyroid is capable of deiodinating both T_4 and T_3 and generating the latter from the former. However, the contribution of this process to T_3 secretion under normal conditions is probably small. In the rat, for example, the T_3:T_4 ratio in the thyroid venous effluent is similar to that in the gland as a whole, and, as will be seen below, little T_3 is apparently secreted by the normal human thyroid. It is possible, however, that significant quantities of T_3 are generated from T_4 in circumstances in which secretion of T_3 relative to T_4 is disproportionately great.

Iodotyrosines liberated from thyroglobulin are subject to the action of a microsomal iodotyrosine dehalogenase, an NADPH-dependent enzyme found in the peripheral tissues as well as in the thyroid. This enzyme liberates iodide from MIT and DIT and normally prevents their entry into the blood in appreciable quantities. It is inactive against peptide-bound iodotyrosines or free iodothyronines, and hence differs from the mechanism for T_4 deiodination described above. Activity of the thyroid iodotyrosine deiodinase system is enhanced by TSH administration, possibly because of increased NADPH generation, rather than an increase in enzyme concentration. Iodide liberated from MIT and DIT is partly used for hormone synthesis and partly lost from the gland as "iodide leak."

There is much evidence that the thyroid does not behave as a single homogeneous functioning unit. Radioautographic studies reveal variations in function among different areas of the gland and in different follicles. In addition, it seems clear that the thyroid contains at least two pools of organic iodine which turn over at different rates. One pool, representing more newly iodinated materials, is smaller but turns over more rapidly than the other, larger pool of older hormone (last come — first served). This may result from the contiguity of the sites for iodination and colloid resorption. In truth, there may be many iodine pools in the thyroid turning over at different rates, just as there are many subtle differences in the thyroglobulin molecules within a single thyroid.

The storage function of the thyroid is not perfectly maintained, even under normal conditions. As noted above, some thyroglobulin can be detected by radioimmunoassay (RIA) in the blood of most normal individuals, and the frequency of detection is increased by pregnancy. Increased concentrations are present in the serum of patients with nontoxic goiter, in whom there is a correlation between the serum thyroglobulin and goiter size, and in patients with hyperthyroidism, in whom there is a correlation with the degree of hyperfunction. Serum thyroglobulin concentrations are often increased in patients with differentiated thyroid tumors, but do not distinguish benign from malignant forms. Serum thyroglobulin concentrations decline when the tumor is removed, and, in patients with thyroid cancer, later elevation is a useful indicator of metastatic recurrence. Large quantities of thyroglobulin are released into the blood during surgical manipulation of the thyroid and radiation thyroiditis, and probably in patients with subacute thyroiditis as well. In both forms of thyroiditis, serum T_4 and T_3 concentrations may be increased sufficiently to produce thyrotoxicosis.

Uncertainty exists concerning the extent to which iodotyrosines are normally released into the blood. Recently developed sensitive and highly specific RIA methods have revealed measurable, but low (approximately 6 ng/dl), concentrations of DIT in the serum of normal individuals. Values are decreased in untreated hypothyroidism, remain low during T_4 replacement therapy, and are increased in hyperthyroidism, suggesting strongly that the DIT is a product of thyroid secretion. Some contribution may be made, however, by the peripheral tissues, which are capable of cleaving the ether link of T_4 and T_3. Large quantities of iodotyrosines are lost from the thyroid in the inherited form of goitrous hypothyroidism that results from a lack of iodotyrosine dehalogenase in both the thyroid and peripheral tissues. Here. iodotyrosines both escape from the gland and escape deiodination in the periphery. As a consequence, they are excreted into the urine, either intact or as their keto-acid metabolites. The resulting losses of iodine produce a state of conditioned iodine deficiency; this is in large part responsible for the development of the goiter and can be overcome by dietary iodine supplementation (Stanbury, 1978). A similar syndrome can be produced in animals by administration of the inhibitors of iodotyrosine dehalogenase, mononitrotyrosine or dinitrotyrosine (Green, 1971). The extent to which mild forms of the disorder are responsible for sporadic nontoxic goiter in man is unknown.

The processes of proteolysis and release are inhibited by several agents. Most important among these is iodine. Inhibition of hormone release is responsible for the rapid improvement in thyrotoxicosis that iodine induces in the hyperthyroid patients. The full mechanism by which this effect is mediated is uncertain, but iodine inhibits the stimulation of thyroid adenylate cyclase produced by TSH and by the stimulatory immunoglobulins of Graves' disease. Increasing iodination of thyroglobulin also increases its resistance to hydrolysis by the thyroid acid protease. Lithium also inhibits thyroid hormone release, though its mechanism of action is poorly understood and may differ from that of iodine. It inhibits both the increase in adenylate cyclase activity produced by TSH and the stimulation of I* release from prelabeled thyroid produced by dibutyryl cyclic AMP. (See Emerson, et al., 1973, for references.)

Thyroid Iodoproteins

Thyroglobulin is the principal iodoprotein of the thyroid gland. It constitutes virtually all of the follicular colloid and is therefore the major component of the normal thyroid mass. It is furthermore the repository of virtually all the active hormones, T_4 and T_3, within the gland and of most of their immediate precursors, MIT and DIT. Retention within the gland of this large protein permits maintenance of the unique storage function of the thyroid. Because of its distinctive character and the relative ease with which it can be isolated in highly purified form, it has been a source of interest not only to thyroidologists but also to biochemists and immunochemists and, more recently, to molecular biologists. (For a detailed review of the chemistry and synthesis of thyroglobulin and other thyroid iodoproteins, see Ui, 1974.) Thyroglobulin is a glycoprotein containing approximately 10% by weight of carbohydrates, which include glucosamine, mannose, fucose, galactose, and sialic acid. Its molecular weight is approximately 660,000, and its sedimentation constant ($S^0_{20,w}$) approximately 19. Terminal amino acid analysis suggests that thyroglobulin is composed of four peptide chains. Individual chains may exist in the 6–7S (monomeric) or 12S (dimeric) form in saline extracts of the thyroid. However, iodoproteins with sedimentation constants of 27S and 32S are also found. The latter may represent more highly iodinated forms of the 19S molecule.

The thyroglobulin molecule contains approximately 120 tyrosyl residues, of which a varying but relatively small portion are naturally iodinated. During iodination *in vitro*, even when excess iodine is added, approximately 30% of the tyrosyl residues remain uniodinated, but these can be iodinated when the molecule is unfolded in 8 M urea. Small amounts of T_4 are formed *in vitro* during the iodination of thyroglobulin, especially if thyroid peroxidase is present, but not if the molecule has been subjected to enzymatic digestion, suggesting that peptide chain length is an important factor in T_4 formation. Although suggested by earlier work, it does not seem likely that iodinated amino acids exist as end groups in the thyroglobulin molecule. Results of some studies suggest that in natural thyroglobulin T_4 is commonly surrounded by particular amino acids, indicating that T_4 formation is favored by a unique amino acid sequence at the site of coupling. The I/N ratio in thyroglobulin is highly variable among different species and among animals of the same species. In addition, even within a single animal, thyroglobulin can be shown by chromatographic techniques to be heterogeneous in several respects, including iodine content. In general, newly iodinated thyroglobulin is lowest in iodine content, and is most susceptible to dissociation by dilution or exposure to alkaline pH.

The site and mode of synthesis of thyroglobulin have been studied both by radioautography and by biochemical analysis following administration of labeled amino acids and sugars. Pulse-chase experiments show that labeled amino acids are quickly incorporated into 3–8S and 12S proteins. Soon thereafter, 17–18S proteins are seen to be labeled, and a shift of activity from the 12S to the former zone progressively occurs. By contrast, the 3–8S fraction does not appear to be a source of labeled amino acid for the heavier fractions. The 17–18S "prethyroglobulin" is transformed to 19S "mature thyroglobulin" through iodination, and further iodination is thought to produce the 27S variety. Synthesis of the peptide skeleton of thyroglobulin occurs in the rough ER of the follicular cell, where a portion of the carbohydrate components may be added. The partly synthesized molecule then moves through the channels of the ER to the Golgi apparatus where glycosylation is completed. The protein then moves to the apex of the cell, where at least much of the iodination takes place at or near the cell-colloid interface. Much of the iodination takes place in newly synthesized thyroglobulin just before or just as it is extruded into the colloid by a process of exocytosis.

In recent years, great attention has been focused on the nonthyroglobulin proteins of normal and diseased glands, particularly the soluble protein(s) with a sedimentation coefficient of approximately 4 (4S or S-1 iodoprotein). Small quantities of this protein are found in normal thyroids of both man and other species, and larger quantities have been detected in a wide variety of thyroid disorders, particularly those associated with glandular hyperfunction, irrespective of the rate of T_4 and T_3 synthesis. Thus the protein is abnormally abundant in frankly dyshormonogenetic goiters with or without hypothyroidism, in some cases of simple nontoxic goiter, in the diffuse toxic goiter of Graves' disease, in endemic goiter, and in Hashimoto's disease. A similar protein is also found in some thyroid neoplasms. Very often in these conditions an abnormal iodoprotein of similar properties appears in the serum, producing an unusually large discrepancy between the protein-bound iodine (PBI) and T_4-iodine concentrations. The iodoprotein in both serum and thyroid has the electrophoretic mobility of serum albumin; hence, that form found in the thyroid has been designated thyralbumin. From studies in patients with nontoxic goiter, it appears that the secretion of the iodoprotein is under physiologic control, since its release from the thyroid is enhanced by TSH and decreased by suppressive doses of T_4. In rare cases, the thyroid and, less frequently, the plasma contain an iodoprotein similar or identical in properties to the T_4-binding prealbumin. (For references in this area, see Otten et al., 1971.)

Transport, Turnover, and Metabolism of the Thyroid Hormones

Hormone Transport

Considerations relative to the transport and metabolism of the thyroid hormones have come to occupy an increasingly important place in clinical and experimental thyroidology. At any level of thyroid function, the concentrations of thyroid hormones in the blood will be determined in large measure by their association with thyroid hormone–binding proteins. Consequently, in measuring such concentrations as an aid to diagnosis, one must take cognizance of the state of the hormone-protein binding interaction. Further, the metabolic transformations of thyroid hormones that take place in peripheral tissues influence their biologic potency and perhaps the nature of their biologic effect. Consequently an understanding of thyroid physiopathology in many clinical states demands considerable knowledge of thyroid hormone metabolism, interpreted in the broadest sense. This topic will be discussed, therefore, in substantial detail.

Hormones and Their Derivatives in Blood

It has recently become clear that there exists in the plasma a wide variety of iodothyronines and their metabolic derivatives. Of these, T_4 is highest in concentration and is the only one that arises solely by direct secretion from the thyroid gland. In normal man, T_3 is secreted to a slight extent from the thyroid, but most of the T_3 present in the plasma is derived from the peripheral tissues, where it is generated by the enzymatic removal of a single iodine atom (monodeiodination) from T_4. The remaining iodothyronines and their derivatives are all generated in the peripheral tissues from T_4 and T_3. Principal among them are rT_3 and 3,3'-diiodo-L-thyronine (3,3'-T_2), but also present are trace concentrations of other diiodothyronines, monoiodothyronines, and conjugates thereof with glucuronic or sulfuric acid. Deaminated derivatives of T_4 and T_3 which bear an acetic acid, rather than an alanine, side chain are also present in very low concentrations. (See Figures 4–1 and 4–4 for structural formulas.)

Although it is clear that these derivatives, including T_3, can enter the plasma from the peripheral tissues, it is uncertain to what extent a portion of them is degraded and whether they exert a metabolic action locally prior to their exit into the blood or their local degradation. What is known of these matters, and others related to their formation, transport, metabolism, and action, is discussed below. Emphasis will be placed on T_4, T_3, and rT_3, since these are the components of greatest clinical import at present.

Extracellular Binding Proteins. Upon entering the blood, the major secretory products of the normal thyroid gland, T_4 and T_3, as well as the products of peripheral T_4 and T_3 metabolism, are bound to particular proteins in a firm but reversible bond (see review by Woeber and Ingbar, 1974, for more extensive discussion and references). Much of what is known about the specific binding of the thyroid hormones, including its initial demonstration, has been derived from study of serum enriched with labeled hormone by the tech-

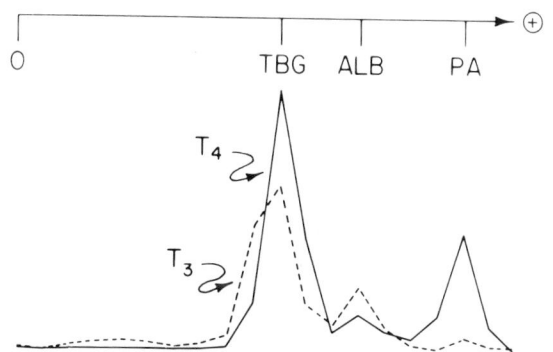

Figure 4–4. Pathways of the sequential monodeiodination of thyroxine (T_4) and its derivatives. Asterisk indicates which compounds would contain radioactive iodine if the original T_4 were labeled in its outer ring. Arrows pointing to left indicate 5'-monodeiodination, and arrows pointing to the right, 5-monodeiodination. Not shown is deiodination of 3'-T_1 and 3-T_1 to thyronine. (From Sakurada et al.: *J. Clin. Endocrinol. Metab.* 46: 916, 1978. ©1978 The Endocrine Society.)

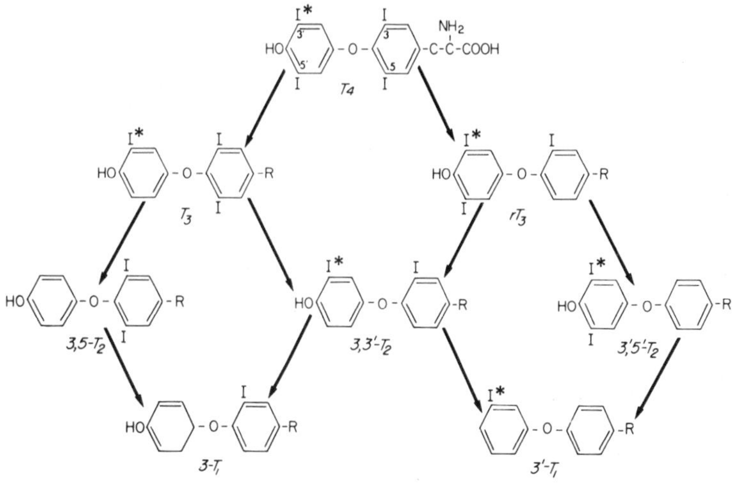

nique of zonal electrophoresis, particularly in filter paper, but also in starch, agar, or polyacrylamide gels. Although these electrophoretic techniques result in some distortions of the hormone-protein interactions, they are quantitative rather than qualitative. Electrophoretic studies have disclosed two plasma proteins with which T_4 is mainly associated, a T_4-binding inter-α globulin (TBG) and a T_4-binding prealbumin (TBPA). To a limited extent, T_4 is also bound to albumin; T_3, on the other hand, is bound mainly by TBG and, to a small extent, by albumin (Fig. 4–5). Despite some data suggesting that T_3 might be bound to a slight extent by TBPA, the bulk of evidence suggests that, for practical purposes, T_3 is not bound by TBPA at all. In view of the fact that TBG binds both T_4 and T_3, a more appropriate designation than the commonly employed T_4-binding globulin would be "thyronine-binding globulin," a term that would not necessitate altering the universally accepted abbreviation, TBG.

TBG has been isolated from human plasma by several groups. For a review of the properties of TBG and TBPA, see Nicoloff, 1978. From their studies, it appears that its molecular weight is approximately 60,000 and its concentration in normal plasma approximately 2 mg/100 ml. This quantity is capable of binding approximately 20 μg of T_4. TBG is a glycoprotein which contains about 9 moles of neuraminic acid per mole. Treatment of the protein with bacterial neuraminidase alters its electrophoretic mobility but does not

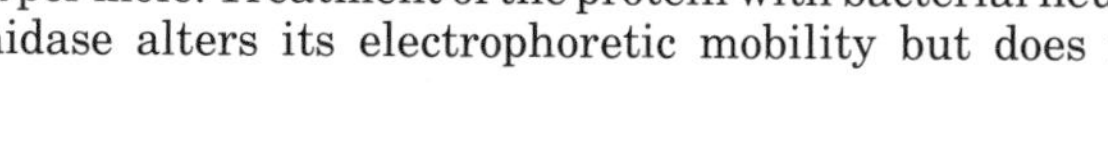

influence its ability to bind T_4. In normal man, its half-time in plasma is about 5 days and its metabolic clearance rate approximately 800 ml/day, so that its production rate is about 16 μg daily.

TBPA has also been isolated from human plasma, in which it exists in part as a complex with retinol (vitamin A)-binding protein. Its molecular weight is approximately 50,000 and its concentration in plasma approximately 25 mg/100 ml. This quantity of TBPA can bind about 200 μg of T_4. Binding of T_4 is independent of the association with retinol-binding protein. TBPA is poor in carbohydrate but rich in tryptophan. In normal man, its half-time in plasma is about 2 days, and its production rate about 1 g daily.

Although both TBG and TBPA are capable of binding T_4 avidly, their binding sites exhibit substantially different properties. The TBG molecule appears to have one thyronine binding site. Its affinity for T_3 is, however, less than that for T_4, the equilibrium constant for the latter reaction being about 10^{10} liters/mole. TBG is the main binding protein for rT_3, but its affinity for rT_3 is far lower still than that for T_3. TBG binds the dextro-isomer of T_4 apparently as well as it binds the naturally occurring levo-isomeric form. Deamination of the iodothyronine molecule greatly reduces the binding to TBG; the acetic and propionic acid analogues of T_4 and T_3 are bound by TBG little if at all. Binding by TBG is inhibited by a variety of organic compounds, including phenytoin, tetrachlorthyronine, salicylate, anilinonaphthalenesulfonic acid, and o, p'-DDD (dichlorodiphenyldichloroethane).

Like TBG, the TBPA molecule has but one major binding site, the equilibrium constant for the interaction with T_4 being about 10^8 liters/mole. D-Thyroxine is not bound appreciably by TBPA, and deamination of the alanine side chain yields products that interact much more strongly than do the parent compounds. Thus tetraiodothyroacetic acid (tetrac) and tetraiodothyropropionic acid are bound to TBPA more strongly than is T_4. Moreover, the triiodinated analogues, unlike T_3 itself, are bound by TBPA quite strongly. A variety of organic compounds are potent inhibitors of the T_4-TBPA interaction; these include barbital, salicylate and some of its congeners, 2,4-dinitrophenol, and penicillin.

Owing to the quantitatively variable results provided by different electrophoretic techniques, there has been considerable confusion as to the relative importance of TBG and TBPA in determining the overall intensity of T_4 binding in plasma. However, by means of refined electrophoretic techniques and of immunochemical removal of TBPA from serum by a specific antibody, it has been possible to demon-

Figure 4–5. Diagram depicting the electrophoretic migration of radioiodine-labeled T_4 and T_3 in normal human serum. TBG, thyronine-binding globulin; ALB, albumin; PA, prealbumin, also shown as T_4-binding prealbumin (TBPA). T_4 is bound predominantly by TBG, to a lesser extent by TBPA, and to a slight extent by albumin. T_3 is bound by TBG and by albumin, but little, if at all, by TBPA.

strate that TBG is normally responsible for the transport of most of the T_4 (about 77%) and, with the serum T_4 concentration, is by far the major determinant of the free T_4. TBPA plays a far lesser role, except when TBG is lacking, and even then, rather marked variations in TBPA influence the concentration and turnover of T_4 only slightly. Much effort has been directed toward the elucidation of the function of the T_4-binding proteins. Certain conclusions seem indisputable. Thus, as a result of their interaction with the transport proteins, the iodinated amino acids acquire macromolecular properties which profoundly alter their metabolism. The negligible normal urinary excretion of T_4 and T_3 is almost certainly due to their limited filterability at the glomerulus. Furthermore, as will be seen, values for the volume of distribution and rate of turnover of the hormones are also affected by their protein associations, so that they resemble more closely those of the plasma proteins than those of unbound amino acids.

In vitro, the interaction between the thyroid hormones and their binding proteins has been found to conform to a reversible binding equilibrium which can be expressed by conventional equilibrium equations. For those formulations which follow, T_4 is used as the hormone prototype, with the understanding that similar interactions apply in the case of T_3. In addition, TBG is used as the prototype binding protein, in view of the predominant role that it plays in hormone transport. The interaction between T_4 and TBG can be expressed as follows:

$$T_4 + TBG \underset{}{\overset{k}{\rightleftharpoons}} T_4 \cdot TBG$$

Here, TBG represents the unoccupied binding sites of the protein; k, the equilibrium constant for the interaction; and $T_4 \cdot TBG$, the binding sites on TBG occupied by T_4. This interaction can also be expressed by the mass-action relationship, wherein

$$\frac{(T_4 \cdot TBG)}{(T_4)(TBG)} = k$$

rearranging,

$$\frac{(T_4)}{(T_4 \cdot TBG)} = \frac{1}{(TBG)k}$$

and

$$(T_4) = \frac{(T_4 \cdot TBG)}{(TBG)k}$$

These expressions predict that T_4 will exist in the plasma in both the bound and free forms and this has been shown to be the case by direct analysis. Although the concentration of free T_4 in normal human serum cannot generally be measured directly, the proportion of hormone that is free can be measured by radioisotopic techniques, and the concentration can then be calculated as the product of the total hormone concentration and the fraction that is free. In normal serum, the free T_4 is approximately 0.03% of the total, and its absolute concentration is about 2 ng/100 ml.

It is also evident from the preceding formulas that the proportion of free hormone is inversely related to the concentration of unoccupied binding sites and their binding affinity for the hormone in question. For example, the lesser affinity of TBG for T_3 results in a proportion of free T_3 (0.30%) that is about ten times that of T_4. Further, the absolute concentration of free T_4 is seen to be a direct function of the ratio of the

concentrations of occupied and unoccupied binding sites on TBG.

Studies *in vitro* in which T_4 has been allowed to interact with both plasma and tissues have led to an expansion of the formulation as follows:

$$T_4 \quad \begin{array}{l} + TBG \overset{k_1}{\rightleftharpoons} T_4 \cdot TBG \\ + CBP \overset{k_2}{\rightleftharpoons} T_4 \cdot CBP \overset{k_3}{\rightarrow} \end{array}$$

Here, CBP represents the unoccupied binding sites on cellular binding proteins; k_2, their affinity for T_4; $T_4 \cdot CBP$, occupied binding sites on CBP; and k_3, the rate at which T_4 in the cell is irreversibly metabolized to other products, such as T_3, rT_3, tetrac, or conjugates.

This formulation indicates that it is the free hormone that is available to the tissues and that can, therefore, both induce metabolic effects and undergo degradation. The bound form of the hormone then acts merely as a metabolically inert reservoir. It also follows that it should be the concentration of the free hormone that acts as an important determinant of the metabolic state and that homeostatic mechanisms would seek to defend.

It is useful to examine the effects of hormone binding not only on the static concentration of free and bound hormone in the blood, but also on the dynamic aspects of hormone metabolism. Two factors influence the plasma concentration of T_4 (or any other hormone or metabolite), its rate of entry into the plasma, usually by secretion from the thyroid, and the efficiency of those processes that lead to its removal from plasma. A convenient means of expressing the latter is as a metabolic clearance rate, analogous to a renal clearance rate, which relates the quantity of T_4 removed from the plasma per unit time to the quantity available for removal, i.e., its plasma concentration. Thus

$$MCR = D/[P]$$

where MCR is the metabolic clearance rate (volume/time), D is the absolute disposal or removal rate (amount/time), and [P] is the plasma concentration (amount/volume). Transposing,

$$[P] = D/MCR$$

However, under steady-state conditions, the production rate of T_4 (PR) and disposal rate, D, are equal. Hence,

$$[P] = PR/MCR$$

This relationship simply indicates that for any level of T_4 production, be it increased, normal, or decreased, the total plasma T_4 concentration will vary inversely with its MCR. However, if only the free T_4 is readily able to leave the plasma and enter the cells, while the bound T_4 is largely confined to the intravascular space, then a change in the fraction of total T_4 that is free, by changing the fraction that is available to the tissues, will change the MCR in a parallel manner. This would explain why a primary increase in hormone binding, without any change in thyroid function, will increase the plasma total T_4 concentration, and why a decrease in hormone binding will have the converse effect. (See Figure 4–6.)

This formulation, which has come to be known as the "free thyroxine hypothesis," is better termed the "free thyroid

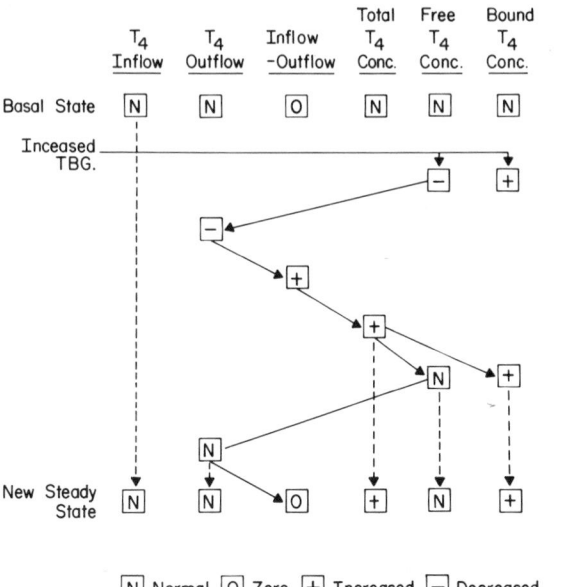

Schema of the Sequence Following an Increase in Plasma TBG Concentration

Figure 4-6. The sequence of events following an increase in TBG: its effects on the turnover of T_4 and on the serum concentration of total and free T_4. Converse consequences would follow a decrease in TBG.

hormone hypothesis," in view of the fact that it is equally applicable to other thyromimetic compounds, including T_3, whose predominant metabolic importance is unquestioned. Though supported by a wealth of correlative data linking changes in hormone binding to changes in hormone metabolism, the validity of the hypothesis has been questioned because of instances in which alterations in hormone turnover cannot be explained by changes in extracellular binding. Such criticism is itself invalid, however, since the hypothesis does not attribute to extracellular binding of hormone the sole regulatory role, merely an important regulatory role, in hormone metabolism. Indeed, a variety of other factors play upon hormone metabolism, causing it to vary, either from tissue to tissue or within a single tissue, in response to physiologic stimuli or pharmacologic agents. Among them are differences in: (1) the permeability of various vascular beds to the circulating protein-thyroid hormone complex; (2) the nature and concentration of intracellular binding sites for the hormones; (3) the nature and concentration of hormone-metabolizing enzymes; and (4) factors such as local blood flow, intracellular pH, and cofactor concentration that may influence any or all of the above. Such factors, acting independently of extracellular hormone binding, can influence the tissues in which circulating hormones predominantly accumulate, the rate at which they accumulate, the overall rate at which they are metabolized once within the cell, and the specific products that result. (For a review with references, see Nicoloff, 1978.)

Cellular Binding Proteins. The free thyroid hormone hypothesis implies the existence within the cell or on its surface of sites with which T_4 and T_3 engage in a reversible binding interaction. The existence of such sites has been clearly demonstrated, though their characterization is still incomplete. Proteins that bind T_4 and T_3 have been identified in the cytosol of many tissues of different species, including human liver. Some studies suggest that the cytosol binding proteins for T_4 and T_3 are distinct from one another, while others do not (see Hamada and Nishimoto, 1979, for references). In the earlier view, entry of hormone into the cell would be conditioned by a simple competitive binding equilibrium between intracellular and extracellular, extravascular binding proteins. It is now clear, however, that this conception is vastly oversimplified. Specific, saturable binding sites for T_3 and T_4 have been found in cell nuclei, mitochondria, and plasma membrane of diverse organs. These are thought to be related to hormone action, and will be discussed more fully in a later section. In addition, T_3 and probably T_4 are actively transported into the cell, at least into the isolated hepatocyte (Eckel et al., 1979; Krenning et al., 1979). How these various sites and processes interrelate in delivering T_4 and T_3 to their loci of action and of degradation in the cell or on the cell surface is at present quite unclear.

Pathways of Hormone Metabolism

Qualitative and Quantitative Aspects. The demonstration that athyreotic patients given a mixture of highly purified stable and radioiodine-labeled T_4 by mouth or vein display in their serum substantial concentrations of stable and labeled T_3 provided the first conclusive evidence that the peripheral tissues of man have the capacity to convert T_4 to the more active hormone, T_3 (Braverman et al., 1970), ending many years of uncertainty whether this was the case. There followed a vast number of studies of peripheral thyroid hormone metabolism in man and animals, and in tissue preparations *in vitro*, all made possible by sensitive RIA methods for measuring the concentrations of various iodothyronines and their derivatives and by physicochemical techniques for effectively separating them from one another. The result has been a prodigious expansion of knowledge in this area, and an appreciation that the deiodination of thyroid hormones is not a mere nonspecific process leading to hormone degradation and disposal, but rather comprises a group of specific, regulated processes that generate diverse metabolites of varying thyromimetic activity. The material that follows is a brief summarization of the salient features of current information in this area. (For reviews and references, see Ingbar and Braverman, 1975; Schimmel and Utiger, 1977; Cavalieri and Rapoport, 1977; and Burman, 1978.)

In normal man, approximately 80% of the metabolism of T_4 and the various products derived from it proceeds by enzymatic monodeiodination, i.e., removal of one iodine atom at a time. These reactions occur in sequence, so that a progression of less fully iodinated thyronines is generated. T_4 itself is acted upon by one or the other of two monodeiodinating enzymes. One, a 5'-monodeiodinase, removes an iodine atom from the outer ring of the molecule to yield T_3; the other, a 5-monodeiodinase, removes an iodine atom from the inner ring to yield rT_3. T_3 and rT_3 are themselves subject to the action of 5'- and 5-monodeiodinases that yield all of three possible forms of diiodo-L-thyronine (T_2), 3,5-T_2, 3'5'-T_2, and 3,3'-T_2, and these in turn are monodeiodinated to yield the two possible types of monoiodo-L-thyronine (T_1), 3'-T_1 and 3-T_1. Studies with ^{125}I-labeled precursors have also revealed serum conjugates of these partially deiodinated iodothyronines with glucuronic or sulfuric acid. Ultimately, monoiodothyronines lose their iodine, leaving for excretion in the urine the iodine-free thyronine ring and its metabolites. The deaminated and decarboxylated derivatives of T_4 and T_3, tetrac and triac, are also formed and, having entered the blood, are rapidly metabolized by deiodination and conjugation, followed by biliary excretion.

Table 4–1. APPROXIMATE VALUES OF THE PLASMA CONCENTRATION, CLEARANCE RATE, AND PRODUCTION RATE OF THYROID HORMONES AND SOME METABOLITES

Compound	Plasma Concentration (ng/dl)	Metabolic Clearance Rate (l/day)	Production Rate (μg/day)
T_4	8000	1	60
T_3	120	25	30
Reverse T_3 (rT_3)	25	120	30
3,3'-T_2	?	600	?

As judged from studies with radioiodine-labeled hormones, approximately 20% of outer-ring iodine in T_4 and T_3 is eliminated in organic form by fecal excretion, probably comprising a mixture of T_4, T_3, and their various derivatives in both the free and conjugated forms.

From kinetic studies, it has been estimated that approximately 35% of the T_4 secreted in normal man is deiodinated to yield T_3, and about 40% to yield rT_3. Hence, with a normal T_4 production rate of 90 μg daily, approximately 26 μg of T_3 and 30 μg of rT_3 would be produced by peripheral deiodinations. When these values are compared to estimated total daily production rates for T_3 and rT_3 (Table 4–1), the remarkable conclusion that emerges is that nearly all (at least 80%) of normal T_3 production and all of rT_3 production can be accounted for by peripheral generation from T_4, rather than direct thyroid secretion. The conclusion that the normal thyroid secretes little if any T_3 and essentially no rT_3 is consonant with the concentration of these iodothyronines relative to that of T_4 within the thyroid gland. Though it is clear that some of the T_3 and rT_3 produced from T_4 in the peripheral tissues can leave those tissues and enter the blood, it is uncertain to what extent T_3 and rT_3 are degraded locally before they can enter blood or whether they may be retained intact at their site of origin, sequestered in pools that exchange only slowly with the plasma compartment. Thus, the foregoing estimates of the rate of conversion of T_4 to T_3 and rT_3, having been made solely on the basis of measurements in blood, must be considered minimal estimates. Evidently, T_3 is metabolized mainly by 5-monodeiodination and rT_3 by 5'-monodeiodination; both processes yield 3,3'-T_2.

Tetrac is generated peripherally from T_4, but the proportion of T_4 metabolized by this pathway is uncertain. Estimates of tetrac production rate suggest that about 4 μg of tetrac are produced daily, accounting for approximately 5% of total T_4 disposal (Table 4–1).

Enzymology. Although some inferential evidence has been obtained from studies of T_4 metabolism in man or intact animals, most of what is known about the specific enzymes that mediate iodothyronine metabolism has come from *in vitro* studies of tissue slices, homogenates, or subcellular fractions. (See review by Visser, 1978.) Since it is generally the case that rT_3 is very rapidly degraded in such systems, far more is known of the mechanism for generating T_3 from T_4 (T_3-neogenesis) than is the case for rT_3. Nonetheless, contrary to early suggestions, it is clear that the 5'- and 5-monodeiodinations of T_4 that lead to the formation of T_3 and rT_3, respectively, are mediated by two separate enzymes that share some properties, but differ in others. Such differences permit the generation of T_3 and rT_3 to vary independently of one another, as they indeed do in various conditions. Neither enzyme has as yet been purified and characterized, but the 5'-monodeiodinase, at least, is mainly located in the microsomal fraction, though its specific activity in liver is greatest in the plasma membrane. Both enzymes require for maximal activity soluble cofactors, chief among them reduced glutathione (GSH). Both enzymes may act as transhydrogenases in a two-step process. In this formulation, hydrogen from a –SH group on the enzyme molecule is first substituted for an iodine at either the 5'- or the 5-position of the T_4 molecule, with the formation of a sulfenyl iodide group within the enzyme. The sulfenyl iodide is then reduced and the enzyme reactivated by GSH. Both enzymes in liver are inhibited uncompetitively by propylthiouracil (PTU), probably because this agent interacts with the sulfenyl iodide to yield a mixed disulfide. The enzymes have strikingly different pH optima, that of the 5'-monodeiodinase on the acid side, and that of the 5-monodeiodinase on the alkaline side, of neutrality. Thus, variations in intracellular pH may modify the proportionate relationship between T_3 and rT_3 formation.

The activity of the 5'-monodeiodinase in liver is influenced in a parallel fashion by conditions that alter cellular GSH concentration. However, its activity may depend not so much on the available –SH concentration as on the oxidation-reduction poise, since addition of oxidized glutathione (GSSG) is inhibitory. *In vitro*, T_3 neogenesis by liver preparations is decreased if donor animals are starved, are made diabetic or hypothyroid, or are given large doses of adrenal glucocorticoids, PTU (but not methimazole), or certain iodinated x-ray contrast dyes. Such decreases have been variously ascribed to decreased enzyme concentration, depletion of cofactor, or enzyme inhibition. Though far less is known of the regulation of the hepatic 5-monodeiodinase for T_4, its activity appears to be unaffected by starvation or glucocorticoids, though it is greatly decreased by hypothyroidism.

To a large extent, the sequential monodeiodinations of several forms of T_3, T_2, and T_1 shown in Figure 4–4 have also been shown to be enzyme-mediated. A central question is how many enzymes mediate these reactions. The preponderance of current evidence suggests that there may be only two enzymes involved, one mediating all 5'-monodeiodinations (arrows pointing to the reader's left in Figure 4–4), the other mediating all 5-monodeiodinations (arrows pointing to the reader's right).

A remarkable feature of these enzymes, at least in the rat, is the extent to which their individual activities vary from tissue to tissue, and the extent to which, in different tissues, they are differently affected by the same stimuli. Since these differences probably have important, and may even have profound, physiologic ramifications, a few examples will be cited. Thus, *in vitro* studies indicate that pituitary has an extremely active 5'-monodeiodinase and a relatively inactive 5-monodeiodinase, while brain displays the converse pattern, and liver and kidney have more nearly equal activities of the two enzymes. Further, hypothyroidism retards and hyperthyroidism accelerates T_3-neogenesis in liver and kidney, but they have opposite effects on T_3-neogenesis in pituitary. Starvation impairs T_3-neogenesis in liver, but leaves the activity of this process in kidney and pituitary unchanged. As a final example, PTU inhibits the 5'-monodeiodinase in liver, but not, apparently, in pituitary.

Physiologic Implications. (See Ingbar and Borges, 1979.) There is no question that in regard to all classical thyromimetic actions, T_3 is several times more active than T_4 is. Since approximately one-third of all T_4 gives rise to T_3 during the course of its metabolism, the question arises whether all the metabolic activity of T_4 can be ascribed to the T_3 that it gives rise to, i.e., whether T_4 is merely a prohormone for T_3, as thyroglobulin is for T_4. In a variety of systems, the metabolic effectiveness of T_4 is decreased by agents that inhibit T_3-neogenesis, indicating that much or most of the activity of T_4 stems from formation of T_3, but the question whether T_4 has some intrinsic biologic activity remains unresolved.

In classic tests for bioactivity, rT_3 appears to be extremely inactive. This, together with evidence that T_3-neogenesis and rT_3-neogenesis can vary independently of one another, has given rise to the concept that the choice between 5'-monodeiodination and 5-monodeiodination of T_4 is a choice between hormone activation and hormone inactivation. If T_4 must give rise to T_3 in order to exert most of its metabolic effect, then the initial monodeiodination of T_4 emerges as an important branch point for metabolic regulation, and further, the many conditions cited earlier in which T_3-neogenesis is impaired should be associated with a general deficit of active thyroid hormone at the tissue level, but this has not yet been shown to be the case.

In the older view of thyroid hormone economy, peripheral tissues depended for their supply of thyroid hormone solely on hormone secreted by the thyroid gland and delivered to them by the blood. In the light of the new knowledge of peripheral hormone metabolism, this concept must change. The supply of active hormone to a particular tissue must now be seen as a function of multiple variables: the rate of secretion of T_4 (and T_3) from the thyroid gland; the rate at which the tissue receives in the blood T_3 generated by other organs; and the rate at which the tissue itself can convert T_4 to T_3 for its own use. As indicated earlier, tissues vary in the rate at which they carry out T_3-neogenesis and vary, too, in the extent to which their rate of T_3-neogenesis is changed by factors that alter T_3-neogenesis elsewhere. Therefore, it is possible, indeed likely, that the extent to which there occurs a metabolic perturbation in response to some factor that alters peripheral T_4 metabolism will vary both with the nature of that factor and from tissue to tissue. In starvation, for example, the pituitary may perceive no deficit of thyroid hormone, because pituitary T_3-neogenesis is unaltered, though it is inhibited elsewhere. In view of evidence that T_3 generated locally within the pituitary from T_4 is an important determinant of TSH secretion (see Larsen and Silva, 1979), this would explain why in starved subjects there is no compensatory TSH secretion, despite an overall decrease in the rate of T_3-neogenesis and a striking decline in serum T_3 concentration.

Finally, consideration must be given to the possibility that those metabolites of T_4 that are now considered to be metabolically inactive (rT_3, the various monoiodothyronines and diiodothyronines, tetrac, and triac) are not truly lacking in thyromimetic activity. Traditionally, tests for the bioactivity of such compounds almost always involved their systemic administration, and were predicated on the assumption that they could be present in tissues only as a result of delivery from the bloodstream. Since the derivatives of T_4, without exception, are cleared from the blood and degraded more rapidly than T_4 is, some extremely so, their access to tissues may have been extremely limited in both amount and time, making them appear to be inactive. What is needed now are studies to determine whether the various physiologic derivatives of T_4 have particular metabolic actions in the very tissues within which they are being generated.

Hormone Turnover. The availability of radioiodine-labeled thyroid hormones and their derivatives has made possible studies of their overall metabolism in man and experimental animals *in vivo* that have provided useful information concerning this aspect of thyroid hormone economy in normal and disease states. (For a review of this topic with extensive references, see Nicoloff, 1978.) With few exceptions, studies in man have involved administration of compounds labeled with radioiodine in their 3'-position, either by a single intravenous injection or by continuous infusion, followed by serial measurements of the concentration of administered compound in the blood. When subjected to appropriate kinetic analysis, the data permit calculation of the metabolic clearance rate of the administered compound and often of its component functions, the volume of

distribution, and the fractional rate of turnover. Such studies can also provide quantitative evidence of the fate of the labeled iodine atoms, and occasionally have been used to provide qualitative information concerning pathways of hormone metabolism, but yield no evidence of the fate of the unlabeled compounds that remain when the radioiodine is removed. Nevertheless, in a state of physiologic equilibrium, the quantity of hormone degraded or excreted per unit time must equal the rate of hormone secretion, which can be measured indirectly in this manner. Furthermore, in a homeostatically regulated system, the rate of hormone disposal may well determine the requisite rate of hormone manufacture. Hence considerable interest is focused upon such measurements. As judged from such studies, T_4 in the normal adult has a volume of distribution of approximately 10 liters; that is, the extrathyroid amount of T_4 is equivalent to the quantity that would be contained in 10 liters of plasma. Since the normal concentration of T_4 in plasma approximates 8 $\mu g/100$ ml, the extrathyroid pool of T_4 is approximately 800 μg. In the young or middle-aged adult, the fractional rate of turnover of T_4 in the periphery is normally about 10%/day (half-time, 6.7 days). Thus about 1.1 liter of the peripheral T_4 distribution space is cleared of hormone daily, a volume that contains approximately 90 μg of T_4. The fractional rate of turnover and rate of clearance of T_4 are much smaller than those of other hormones. The slower turnover of T_4 is doubtless a reflection of the predominant extent to which T_4 is bound, leaving only a small fraction free for metabolic turnover. If only the free T_4, which is about 1/3000 of the total, is available for metabolic turnover, then the rate of clearance of free T_4 would be at least 3000 liters/day or more than 120 liters/hr.

The kinetics of T_3 metabolism differ greatly from those of T_4, owing in part to differences in the intensity of their binding to TBG. A single dose of T_3 is rapidly cleared from the plasma as a result of both widespread distribution and rapid cellular metabolism. Its volume of distribution in the normal adult is almost 40 liters and its fractional turnover rate about 60%/day. Hence, the MCR of T_3 is about 24 liters/day. At a mean normal serum T_3 concentration of 120 ng/dl, this would indicate a normal daily production rate for T_3 of approximately 30 ng. As indicated earlier, much of normal T_3 production in man occurs via the deiodination of T_4 in peripheral tissues, rather than by thyroid production and secretion.

The overall metabolism of several of the peripheral metabolites of T_4 has also been studied by related techniques. The distribution and metabolism of rT_3 is exceedingly rapid. Soon after the intravenous administration of labeled rT_3, most of the radioiodine present in serum is composed of various products of rT_3 metabolism, rather than rT_3 itself. An extremely large metabolic clearance fate of rT_3 (approximately 120 liters/day) and a very low concentration in plasma (about 25 ng/dl) combine to yield daily production rates for rT_3 of about 30 ng. The turnover and metabolism of $3,3'-T_2$ are even faster than those of rT_3. As judged from continuous infusion studies, $3,3'-T_2$ has a metabolic clearance rate of approximately 600 liters/day (Gavin et al., 1978). Its production rate in normal individuals is uncertain, owing to lack of agreement concerning its concentration in plasma.

Alterations in the Transport, Turnover, and Metabolism of the Thyroid Hormones

The free thyroid hormone hypothesis assigns to the concentration of free hormones a role as a major determinant of the quantity of hormone available to the cells and, hence, the absolute rate of hormone turnover and the metabolic state of the patient. It assigns to the proportion of free hormone a role as a major determinant of the proportionate distribution and metabolism of hormone. In addition, the hypothesis encompasses the operation of cellular factors that may influence the distribution, effectiveness, and metabolism of the hormone, independently of alterations in extracellular binding. These have been brought strongly into prominence by recent interest in specific pathways of thyroid hormone metabolism and the manner in which they are altered in various abnormal states.

Extracellular Abnormalities. Abnormalities in the interaction between the thyroid hormones and their binding proteins, predominantly TBG, are of two types: those that result primarily from a change in the number or affinity of available binding sites, and those that result primarily from a change in the concentration of the hormone. The static, kinetic, and physiologic consequences of these two types of change differ greatly from one another.

These differences can best be appreciated by considering the sequential perturbations that follow abnormalities of each type. Consider first the consequences that would follow from an increase in the concentration in plasma of TBG. (See Figure 4–6.) Initially, the number of unoccupied binding sites would increase, resulting initially in a shift of hormone from the free to the bound state, a decrease in its MCR, and initially a decrease in the quantity of hormone removed from the plasma. With a normal or perhaps increased influx of T_4 into the plasma, the total concentration of hormone would increase progressively until such time as the concentration of free hormone had been restored to normal. At this time, the total and bound concentrations of hormone, which are numerically almost equal, would be increased; hence, the proportion of free hormone and the MCR would remain decreased. The plasma concentration of T_4 would have risen sufficiently to counterbalance the decrease in the proportion of free T_4 and decrease in MCR, so that both the absolute concentration of free T_4 and its dependent variable, the rate of hormone disposal to the tissues, would be normal. The patient would remain euthyroid. This sequence is almost precisely that which has been observed for both T_4 and T_3 in a variety of states associated with an increased TBG in plasma. The converse consequences would be predicted and have been observed in states associated with decreased TBG (see Table 4–2 and section on laboratory tests for a description of the circumstances in which TBG is altered).

Thus it can be seen that, although primary alterations in TBG alter the total concentrations of hormone in plasma and the kinetics of T_4 metabolism, they do not ultimately influence the absolute quantity of hormone that enters the cell, acts, and is degraded in unit time. Therefore, they do not influence the total turnover of hormone or the metabolic state of the patient. These remain a function of the rate of hormone production or supply, and when homeostatic mechanisms are normal, hormone production and the metabolic state of the patient will be normal too.

Far different consequences follow a primary alteration in the rate of hormone supply. (See Figure 4–7.) For example, in hyperthyroid states, hypersecretion of hormone leads to an increase in total hormone concentration. As a result, the concentration of unoccupied binding sites on TBG decreases, and the concentrations of both free and bound hormone rise. As a consequence of the fixed quantity of TBG available, the mass action expression dictates that the concentration of free hormone would increase to a disproportionately great extent and that the proportion of free hormone would therefore rise. *In vivo*, these changes would be reflected in an increase in the MCR of T_4, an increase in the rate of hormone disposal to the tissues, and a hypermetabolic state. Converse consequences occur when the supply of hormone is decreased, as in hypothyroidism. Here, as in the case of primary alterations in hormone binding, the flux of hormone to the tissues and the metabolic state of the patient are again determined by the rate of hormone production. In the final analysis, therefore, barring metabolically wasteful loss of hormone, the metabolic state of the patient over any prolonged period is determined by the rate of hormone production. The effect of alterations in binding is merely to change the plasma concentration, partition, and clearance rate of the hormone for a given rate of hormone production.

Alterations in the extracellular binding of T_4 and T_3 can also occur because of the presence in blood of abnormal binding proteins. In some patients with thyroid disease, particularly those with chronic thyroiditis, immunoglobulins capable of specifically binding T_4, T_3, or both are demonstrable in serum by electrophoretic or protein-fractionation

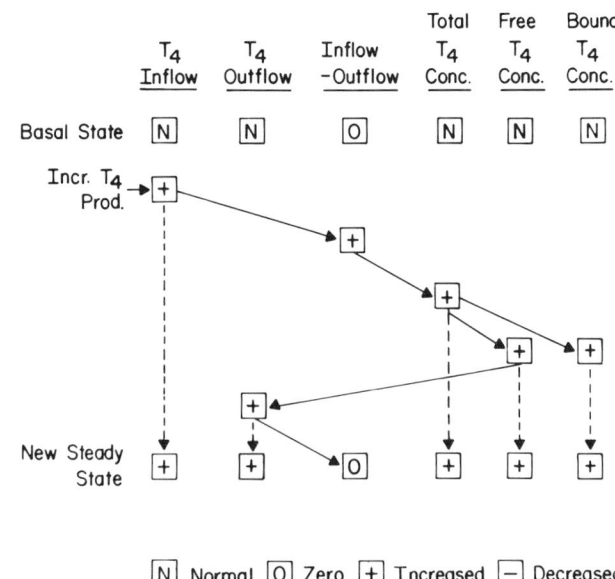

Schema of the Sequence Following an Increase in the Production or Supply of Thyroxine

Figure 4–7. The sequence of events following a sustained increase in T_4 secretion: its effects on the turnover of T_4 and on the serum concentration of total and free T_4. Converse consequences follow a decrease in T_4 secretion.

Table 4–2. CIRCUMSTANCES ASSOCIATED WITH ALTERATIONS IN THE CONCENTRATION OF TBG

1. *Increased Concentration of TBG*
   Pregnancy
   Neonatal state
   Estrogens and hyperestrogenemic states
   Oral contraceptives
   Acute intermittent porphyria
   Infectious and chronic active hepatitis
   Biliary cirrhosis
   Genetic determination
   Perphenazine (Trilafon)

2. *Decreased Concentration of TBG*
   Androgenic or anabolic steroids
   Large doses of glucocorticoids
   Active acromegaly
   Nephrotic syndrome
   Major systemic illness
   Genetic determination

techniques. Such antibodies affect the measured concentration of T_4 or T_3 by two mechanisms. First, they enhance the overall binding of their antigen in plasma, increasing its concentration in the blood and producing kinetic consequences similar to those associated with an increase in TBG. Second, the antibodies introduce artifacts into the RIA measurement of their specific antigen in blood. Depending on the type of RIA procedure employed, endogenous antibody against T_4 or T_3 can produce values for the serum T_4 or T_3 concentration that are spuriously high or low, suggesting the presence of hyperthyroidism or hypothyroidism.

Very recently, a new syndrome associated with abnormal binding of T_4 in serum has been described, and has come to be known as familial isolated hyperthyroxinemia. Evidently, the syndrome, which has an autosomal dominant mode of transmission, is not overly rare, as a substantial number of families with this disorder are being identified. Patients with this disorder are euthyroid. They display, however, an elevation of serum total T_4 concentration, though the free T_4 concentration is normal, owing to the presence in serum of abnormal protein that binds T_4 and that migrates electrophoretically with serum albumin. Because the protein does not bind T_3, serum T_3 concentration and in vitro T_3 uptake tests are normal. The abnormal protein has not been isolated or characterized. (For additional discussion of anti-T_4 and anti-T_3 antibodies, and of isolated hyperthyroxinemia, see later section on States Associated with Abnormal Hormone Concentrations in Blood.)

Cellular Abnormalities. As predicted by the free thyroid hormone hypothesis, factors intrinsic to the cell can, in certain circumstances, play a primary role in mediating alterations in the overall rate of hormone metabolism, with or without changes in the specific pathways by which hormone metabolism proceeds. This was first demonstrated in the case of phenobarbital, an agent known to induce hypertrophy of the smooth endoplasmic reticulum. In rats, phenobarbital produces an increase in the liver/plasma concentration ratio for T_4 but not for T_3. The peripheral clearance of the two hormones is increased, that for T_4 resulting from an increase in both fecal and deiodinative removal, and that for T_3 from an increase in the fecal component alone. Despite these losses of T_4, its concentration in plasma is maintained as a result of compensatory hyperfunction of the thyroid. These changes occur without a net change in extracellular hormone binding, indicating that they are cellular in origin. The foregoing response to phenobarbital typifies the effect of an increase in the cellular disposal of T_4 in which disposal is not associated with metabolic action and in which the pituitary and hypothalamus do not appear to be primarily affected.

Phenytoin, like phenobarbital, accelerates the peripheral metabolism of T_4, an effect that is demonstrable both in the rat and in man. Here, too, the effect cannot be ascribed to an alteration in the extracellular binding of hormone. Indeed, the concentrations of total and free T_4 are subnormal while the total T_1 secretion rate is unchanged. There is no uniformity of data concerning the effect of phenytoin on serum T_3 and TSH concentrations. Some data suggest, however, that phenytoin accelerates the peripheral conversion of T_4 to T_3, thereby maintaining serum T_3 concentration and obviating the need for increased TSH secretion, despite the subnormal serum concentrations of total and free T_4. If this is indeed the case, it would represent an example of diversion of the T_4 metabolism into pathways that enhance its metabolic effectiveness.

Alterations in thyroid status themselves induce changes in cellular mechanisms for T_4 disposal. In patients with thyrotoxicosis, the metabolic clearance rates of T_4 and T_3 are increased, and the converse is true in patients with hypothyroidism. These changes are partly due to alterations in extracellular binding of the hormones, but a variety of evidence suggests that cellular factors operate as well. In experimental thyrotoxicosis and hypothyroidism in the rat, overall degradation of T_4 in liver preparations in vitro is accelerated or retarded, respectively, both 5'- and 5-monodeiodinases varying in concentration with the metabolic state. Most interesting is the observation that in the pituitary, in contrast, the rate of 5'-monodeiodination of T_4 varies inversely with the metabolic state.

Greatest interest currently attaches, however, to the wide variety of circumstances in man and animals in which the conversion of T_4 to T_3 and the serum T_3 concentration are decreased owing, evidently, to an increase in the activity of the 5'-monodeiodinase for T_4, at least in certain tissues. These conditions have come to be known generically as the "low T_3 syndrome." To the extent that decreases in serum T_3 concentration, unassociated with decreased serum total and free T_4 concentrations, are indicative of a decrease in overall T_3 production rate, then the low T_3 syndrome in man is associated with acute or chronic caloric deprivation, especially deprivation of carbohydrate; uncontrolled diabetes; chronic liver disease; virtually any acute or chronic systemic illness; accidental or surgical trauma; and even anesthesia itself. In the case of starvation, chronic liver disease, and diabetes mellitus, the decrease in T_3 production is not merely inferred from a decrease in serum T_3 concentration, but has been directly demonstrated by kinetic studies. (See reviews by Schimmel and Utiger, 1977, and Cavalieri and Rapoport, 1977.) Moreover, in the case of starvation and diabetes, decreased T_3-neogenesis has been demonstrated in studies of rat liver in vitro. A variety of pharmacologic agents also impair peripheral conversion of T_4 to T_3, producing a low T_3 syndrome. Among them are PTU; large doses of glucocorticoids; propranolol; amiodarone, an agent used in the treatment of angina pectoris; and certain iodinated x-ray contrast dyes, such as iopanoic acid. In the case of PTU and propranolol, this effect may contribute to their beneficial action in the treatment of hyperthyroidism. For similar reasons, glucocorticoids and iodinated x-ray contrast media may also have utility under these circumstances.

In almost all varieties of the low T_3 syndrome, there occurs a reciprocal increase in the serum concentration of rT_3. As judged from studies in patients with cirrhosis, or those undergoing starvation, the increase in serum rT_3 concentration does not reflect a major increase in rT_3 production, but rather a decrease in its metabolic clearance rate. Studies in animal tissues indicate that this is due to a decrease in the major pathway of rT_3 metabolism, 5'-monodeiodination to yield $3,3'-T_2$. Thus, the decrease in T_3 production and in rT_3 degradation, reflected in reciprocal changes in their concentration in serum, stems from a coordinate decrease in the activity of the 5'-monodeiodinases for T_4 and rT_3 (see Fig. 4–4), possibly because they are, in fact, the same enzyme.

In the majority of patients with the low T_3 syndrome, serum TSH concentration is not appreciably increased, and gives no evidence, therefore, of responding to the lowered serum T_3 concentration. Why this should be is uncertain. Possibly, T_3 production from T_4 within the pituitary is unaffected, so that normal feedback inhibition of TSH secretion is maintained. It is also unclear why, if the T_3-generating pathway of T_4 metabolism is slowed in these patients and the rT_3-generating pathway largely unchanged, overall metabolism of T_4 is not slowed and serum T_4 concentration increased. Conceivably, some as yet undisclosed pathway of T_4 metabolism is activated under these circumstances.

The most important area of uncertainty in respect to the

low T_3 syndrome, particularly as it occurs during illness or after trauma, concerns the metabolic state of the patient. Current thinking would dictate that a lowering of T_3 production would lead to a state of peripheral thyroid hormone insufficiency, at least in some tissues. Whether this is indeed the case is unclear, largely owing to a lack of sensitive and specific tests for the degree of peripheral thyroid hormone action that can be carried out in a clinical setting. The problem is compounded by the possibility that individual tissues may respond differently to stimuli that decrease T_3-neogenesis, so that some tissues lack T_3 and others do not. Because of these complexities, the question is one that is unresolved, but it urgently requires resolution. Only then can the derivative question of central importance be addressed, whether the low T_3 syndrome represents a beneficial adaptation to illness or whether it contributes to the illness adversely and should be treated.

A remarkable finding is that peripheral iodothyronine metabolism in the fetus is grossly different from that in the mother or in other adults. In general, 5'-monodeiodination of T_4 is greatly retarded, so that the rate of T_3-neogenesis is low. Concomitantly, 5-monodeiodinations are accelerated so that both rT_3 formation and the degradation of any T_3 formed are increased. At about the time of delivery, iodothyronine metabolism switches to a more mature pattern, a change that is induced by glucocorticoids, at least in part. This general pattern of fetal iodothyronine metabolism appears to have fundamental biologic significance, since it has been observed in all of the several mammalian species thus far studied, including man, and in the chick embryo as well. (See Borges et al., 1980, for references.) T_3-neogenesis appears to be limited in both the dawning and twilight of life, since the decrease in serum T_3 concentration associated with senescence may reflect decreased generation from T_4.

REGULATION OF THYROID FUNCTION

In common with other endocrine organs, the function of the thyroid gland is closely regulated in order that constancy of the internal metabolic milieu be maintained. Regulation of the thyroid, however, seems more complex and more extensive than that of other endocrine organs. Figure 4–8 is a schema of regulatory mechanisms affecting the thyroid as currently conceived. Like the gonads and adrenal cortices, the thyroid participates with the hypothalamus and pituitary in a classic type of feedback control. In addition, intrinsic regulatory mechanisms exist within the thyroid that create an inverse relationship between glandular organic iodine and the activity of hormonogenetic mechanisms. Such autoregulatory mechanisms are apparently found in no other endocrine gland. Teleologically, they subserve an important purpose, for in the case of no other endocrine gland is the rate of hormone synthesis potentially so susceptible to acute fluctuations in the availability of a requisite substrate such as iodine. Furthermore, relative to other hormones with effects on metabolic processes (e.g., insulin, glucocorticoids, parathyroid hormone), the effects of thyroid hormones, although less dramatic, are much longer lasting. Hence, it is homeostatically important that fluctuation in hormone secretion be prevented, if possible, rather then merely compensated for after it has occurred. This is achieved in part by the storage function of the gland. A large intraglandular store of hormone that buffers the effect of acute increases or decreases in hormone synthesis can thus be maintained. Autoregulatory mechanisms within the gland, in turn, tend to maintain the constancy of the thyroid hormone pool. Finally, the classic feedback mechanism senses variations in the

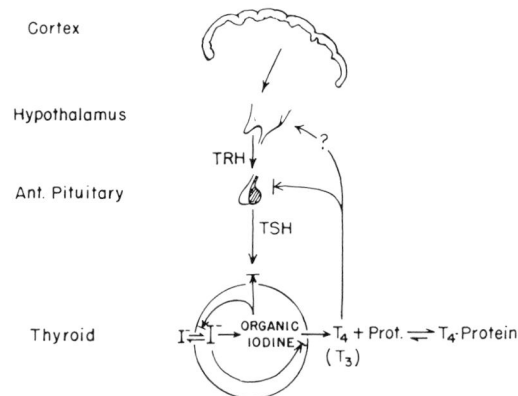

Figure 4–8. Diagram of the factors that regulate thyroid function. Thyroid hormones (T_4 and T_3) in the pituitary, as reflected by their unbound concentrations in blood, inhibit secretion of thyroid-stimulating hormone (TSH). The TSH-releasing hormone (TRH) sets the threshold in the pituitary at which this negative feedback occurs. Factors regulating the secretion of TRH are uncertain but may include influences from higher centers and a stimulatory effect of the thyroid hormones. Autoregulatory control of thyroid function is also shown. High concentrations of intrathyroid iodide decrease the rate of release of thyroid iodide. In addition, the magnitude of the organic iodine pool inversely influences the iodide transport mechanism and the response to TSH.

availability of thyroid hormones and their metabolic impact at the periphery; it is generally concerned, therefore, with correcting abnormalities in the effective concentration of thyroid hormones in the blood, however small, once they have occurred.

The Hypothalamic-Pituitary-Thyroid Complex

Abundant anatomic and functional evidence obtained in animals and man has long indicated a close functional relationship between the anterior pituitary gland and the thyroid gland. More recently, the classic concept of an independent pituitary-thyroid axis, to which these findings led, has been extended to accommodate evidence of a similar nature with respect to the hypothalamus, leading to the concept of a hypothalamic-pituitary-thyroid complex, whose function is modified by still higher centers in the brain. Thus, extensive data obtained from endocrine and neurophysiologic observation and experimentation provided inferential, and ultimately direct, evidence for secretion by the pituitary of a thyroid stimulator and secretion by the hypothalamus of a stimulator of the pituitary, the function of the entire complex being modified in a classic negative feedback manner by the availability of the thyroid hormones. (See Florsheim, 1974, and Reichlin, 1978, for extensive discussions and references.) These observations culminated in the isolation and characterization of the respective stimulators, thyroid-stimulating hormone (thyrotropin, TSH) and TSH-releasing hormone (TRH) (see Fig. 4–9). Subsequently developed radioimmunoassays for TSH and TRH, and chemical synthesis of the latter, have led to an extensive if not yet complete understanding of the mechanism by which secretion of TSH is regulated in man and animals, and have provided extremely valuable tools for use in the diagnosis of thyroid disease.

It is now clear that regulation of TSH secretion results from a complex interaction, mainly or entirely at the level of the pituitary thyrotroph, in which TRH acts to stimulate first the release and later the synthesis of TSH, while thy-

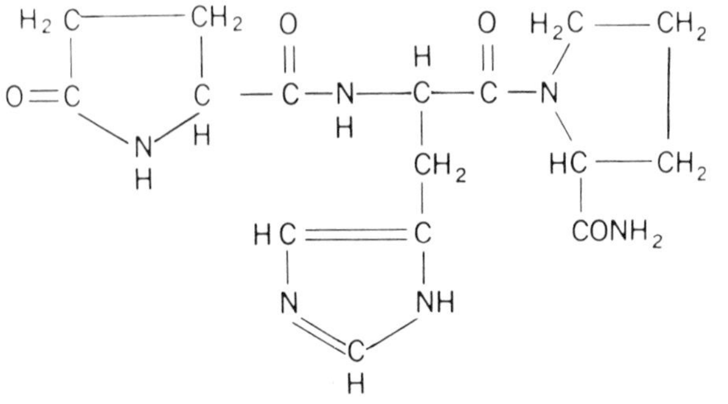

L-Pyroglutamyl-L-Histidyl-L-Proline amide

Figure 4–9. Formula of TRH: pyroglutamyl-histidyl-proline amide.

roid hormones act to inhibit these functions. These inhibitory effects are not merely a direct antagonism of the effects of TRH, since they can be observed when the hypothalamic source of TRH is destroyed or the pituitary gland is separated from it *in vivo* or *in vitro*. Moreover, the degree of thyroid hypofunction that results from destruction of the appropriate areas of the hypothalamus is less severe than that which follows hypophysectomy, and the degree of residual thyroid function in the former circumstance can be varied by raising or lowering the concentration of thyroid hormones in the blood. Thus it appears that the thyroid hormones mediate the feedback regulation of TSH secretion and TRH determines its set-point. Despite numerous experiments to the point, there is no convincing evidence that thyroid hormones directly modify the secretion of TRH. Indeed, all known properties of the interrelation between TRH and thyroid hormones in the regulation of TSH secretion can be explained adequately by what is known of their interaction at the level of the pituitary alone.

TRH, a modified tripeptide (pyroglutamyl-histidyl-proline amide), is synthesized by peptidergic neurons in the supraoptic and paraventricular nuclei of the hypothalamus, whence it is transported to and stored in the median eminence. From here, TRH enters the hypophyseal portal venous system, in which it traverses the pituitary stalk, and is carried to the cells of the anterior pituitary gland. Thyrotroph and lactotroph cells contain specific, saturable receptors to which TRH binds, eliciting a stimulation of adenylate cyclase. The resulting increase in cyclic AMP concentration is evidently responsible for the subsequent manifestations of TRH action, since these are mimicked by exposure of pituitary *in vitro* to stable derivatives of cyclic AMP. Under the influence of TRH, secretion of TSH is promptly stimulated; enhanced synthesis of TSH follows. The response to TRH requires extracellular Ca^{2+} and oxidative metabolism within the pituitary, but the prompt stimulation of TSH release does not depend upon new protein synthesis. The concentrations of TRH required to stimulate the secretion of TSH must be exceedingly minute, since amounts as small as a few micrograms can increase the serum TSH concentration in man, even after systemic administration.

The mechanism by which thyroid hormones inhibit the synthesis and secretion of TSH, and effectively antagonize the action of TRH, remains problematical. It is perfectly clear from circumstances in which hormone binding by TBG is abnormal that feedback regulation of TSH secretion is more closely related to the concentrations of free T_4 and free T_3 than the concentrations of their bound counterparts, presumably because it is the former and not the latter that

have access to the tissue. Considerable uncertainty exists, however, as to how feedback regulation is effected and which of the two hormones is more important in this regard. Observations in patients with mild thyroid failure or iodine deficiency reveal a closer correlation of the serum TSH concentration with the serum T_4 than the serum T_3 concentration. Nonetheless, T_3 delivered to the pituitary in the bloodstream is certainly capable of inhibiting secretion of TSH; this is, of course, the basis of the thyroid suppression test. A possible resolution of the question is provided by the demonstration that pituitary tissue actively converts T_4 to T_3, and that T_3 present in the pituitary from this source plays a major role, with T_3 from the plasma, in regulating TSH secretion. Acute enhancement of TSH secretion by minute doses of PTU and inhibition of the suppressive effect of T_4 on TSH secretion of iopanic acid support this conclusion, since both are agents that inhibit T_3-neogenesis. Thus, three factors, apart from TRH, may condition the level of TSH secretion: the rate of secretion of T_4 by the thyroid; the level of T_3 in the blood generated by peripheral conversion of T_4 to T_3; and the rate of conversion of T_4 to T_3 within the pituitary itself. An intriguing observation in this regard is the recent finding in the rat that T_3 administration acutely inhibits synthesis of the 5'-monodeiodinase that converts T_4 to T_3 within the pituitary. This action, which is the converse of the effect of T_3 on 5'-monodeiodination in liver and kidney, may serve to modulate the ability of T_4 within the pituitary to inhibit the secretion of TSH. Whether T_4 per se has a direct inhibitory action on TSH secretion, apart from its role as a precursor of T_3, is uncertain.

Pituitary tissue contains high-affinity, limited capacity nuclear receptors for T_3 that also bind T_4, but with lesser affinity. Feedback inhibition of TSH secretion is apparently mediated at the nuclear level, since pretreatment with inhibitors of protein synthesis prevents the inhibitory effect of thyroid hormones on TSH secretion. Evidently, thyroid hormones induce the synthesis of a protein that, in turn, somehow inhibits the secretion of TSH. This is consonant with the demonstrated effect of thyroid hormones to stimulate nucleic acid and protein synthesis in other tissues.

Some degree of regulation of TSH secretion may also occur at the level of the TRH receptor on the surface of the thyrotroph. Thyroid hormone may decrease receptor density, an effect which would lessen the response to TRH. Estrogens, in contrast, appear to enhance receptor density and increase the response to TRH.

One aspect of the regulatory control of TSH secretion in man that has important clinical implications is the extremely delicate poise of the pituitary feedback mechanism and its sensitivity to extremely small alterations in the availability of thyroid hormone. Small doses of thyroid hormones, sufficient only to produce very small alterations in their plasma concentrations, greatly diminish the response to exogenous TRH. Conversely, large doses of iodide, when administered to euthyroid subjects, inhibit hormone release and produce very slight decreases in serum T_4 and T_3 concentrations. Though all values remain well within the normal range, prospective studies have revealed that this is uniformly accompanied by distinct increases in basal serum TSH concentration and the response to TRH (see Fig. 4–10).

Although TRH and thyroid hormones are the major regulators of TSH secretion, other factors play a role as well. Somatostatin (growth hormone release–inhibiting factor) decreases the response to TRH *in vitro* and *in vivo*, and the infusion of antisomatostatin antiserum to rats enhances both basal serum TSH concentrations and the response to TRH. Chronic administration of L-dopa decreases basal

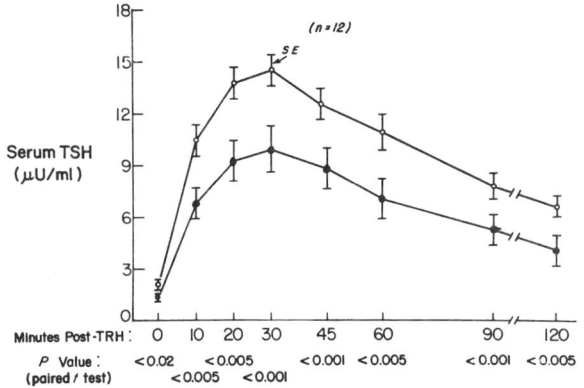

Figure 4–10. Increased response of the serum TSH concentration to the administration of TRH in euthyroid volunteers given iodide (190 mg daily for 10 days). During iodide administration, mean serum T_4 concentration decreased from 8.0 to 6.6 μg/dl and mean serum T_3 concentration from 128 to 110 ng/dl. (From Vagenakis, A. G., et al.: Hyperresponse to thyrotropin-releasing hormone accompanying small decreases in serum thyroid hormone concentrations. *J. Clin. Invest.* 54:913, 1974.)

serum TSH concentration in hypothyroid patients, and decreases the response to TRH. Similar effects follow dopamine infusion and the administration of bromocriptine, a stimulator of the dopamine receptor. Conversely, blockade of the dopamine receptor by metoclopramide increases basal serum TSH concentration in both euthyroid and hypothyroid patients, and increases the response to TRH. These findings leave little doubt that dopamine is a physiologic inhibitor of TSH secretion, but its mechanism of action is unknown. Pharmacologic doses of glucocorticoids inhibit the response of the serum TSH concentration to TRH, and may decrease secretion of TRH as well.

There are several other aspects of the physiology of TRH, apart from its role in TSH secretion, that are of importance and interest. Exogenous TRH elicits secretion of prolactin at threshold doses that are the same as those for stimulation of TSH secretion. As with TSH, the prolactin response to TRH is modified by the prevailing levels of thyroid hormones, though not to as marked an extent. The role of TRH as a physiologic modulator of prolactin secretion is uncertain, however. In humans, nursing increases the serum prolactin concentration, but the serum TSH concentration is unchanged. TRH may also subserve a role as a neurotransmitter. It is found in areas of brain apart from the hypothalamus, in spinal cord, in cerebrospinal fluid, and in portions of the GI tract. Application of TRH elicits a depressing effect in single-neuron preparations, and administration of TRH clearly produces a variety of behavioral effects in animals.

Exogenous TRH elicits the secretion of growth hormone in patients with renal failure and in some patients with acromegaly. The basis for these anomalous responses is unknown. (For a very comprehensive review of the mechanisms that regulate the secretion of TSH, with extensive references, see Scanlon et al., 1978).

Thyroid Autoregulation

The pronounced changes in thyroid iodine and intermediary metabolism, size, and histology that accompany variations in the secretion of TSH suggest that TSH is the major regulator of thyroid structure and function. There is ample evidence, however, that the thyroid is the seat of a group of intrinsic responses that modify several aspects of its own function, most importantly its responsiveness to TSH. In contrast to the classic feedback control effected via TSH, which seeks to defend the plasma or tissue concentrations of the thyroid hormones, these so-called autoregulatory mechanisms seek to maintain constancy of thyroid hormone stores. They are, therefore, most clearly evident in situations in which thyroid iodine content is varied by changes in iodine ingestion or by abnormalities in thyroid iodine utilization. The actual extent to which these autoregulatory responses are operative in diverse states of thyroid function is uncertain. Nevertheless, it appears likely that their participation as a first line of defense of thyroid homeostasis is extensive. In man, increases in iodine ingestion are not accompanied by either increased serum hormone or decreased TSH concentrations. Hence, the decreased efficiency of thyroid iodide extraction manifested in the lowered thyroid uptake of radioactive iodine (RAIU) that follows excessive iodine ingestion is doubtless mediated by autoregulatory inhibition of iodide transport. Conversely, acute iodide depletion is associated with an enhanced autoregulatory response. In the iodine-deficient rat, goiter development antecedes any demonstrable increase in serum TSH concentration. Similarly, in both sporadic nontoxic goiter and the goiter associated with moderate iodine deficiency, serum TSH concentration is usually normal. Such findings support the logical hypothesis that, by enhancing the morphologic and functional response to TSH, autoregulatory mechanisms are a major factor in the ability of the thyroid to overcome the influence of factors that impair hormone synthesis.

Operationally, autoregulatory responses are those that are demonstrable when the level of TSH is constant, i.e., when TSH either is totally lacking or is provided in standard quantities. Although a variety of intrathyroid processes are influenced by iodine (see section on the pharmacology of iodine), the classic type of autoregulatory response is that which affects the activity of the thyroid iodide transport mechanism, as judged from both thyroid/serum iodide concentration ratios and iodide transport maxima. In the hypophysectomized rat, regardless of whether standard doses of TSH are administered, variations in the dietary iodine intake are associated with inverse changes in iodide transport activity. However, the inhibition of iodide transport induced by supplemental iodine, whether given chronically or acutely, is abolished if administered iodide is prevented from binding to tyrosine by concomitant administration of propylthiouracil. This and other evidence indicates that it is organic rather than inorganic iodine that exerts an autoregulatory influence on iodide transport. Although an iodinated inhibitor of iodide transport has been postulated as the responsible agent, no such inhibitor has been specifically demonstrated.

The organic iodine content of the thyroid also influences glandular morphology. Thyroids of hypophysectomized rats subjected to prolonged iodine deficiency are larger than those of iodine-sufficient hypophysectomized controls. Moreover, in hypophysectomized rats, depletion of thyroid iodine greatly increases the growth response of the thyroid to standard doses of TSH.

Some or all of the foregoing effects of iodine may reflect an autoregulatory influence of iodine on certain aspects of thyroid intermediary metabolism. In the thyroid of hypophysectomized rats the stimulatory response of several metabolic functions to TSH varies inversely with glandular organic iodine content. These include the rate of glucose dissimilation and the rate of incorporation of glucose carbon into CO_2, lactate, lipid, and nucleic acid. These effects, in turn, may be a consequence of an inhibition by organic iodine of the adenylate cyclase response to TSH. Since iodine neither inhibits the enzyme directly nor reduces binding of TSH to its plasma membrane receptor, it is presumed to act on the mechanism by which binding of TSH is coupled to cyclase activation. (For references to this effect of iodine, see Uchimura et al., 1979. For a more extensive review of thyroid autoregulation, see Ingbar, 1978a.)

FACTORS THAT INFLUENCE THYROID HORMONE ECONOMY

The widespread metabolic role of the thyroid hormones, the diverse processes involved in the synthesis, secretion, and metabolism of the hormones, and the complex mode of regulation of thyroid function suggest that a great many factors could influence one or more aspects of thyroid hormone economy. This is indeed the case. In general, the factors can be considered in the following categories: endogenous variables, pharmacologic agents, environmental alterations, and dysfunction or diseases of other organ systems.

Thyrotropin (Thyroid-Stimulating Hormone, TSH)

In many respects, TSH can be considered the major regulator of the morphologic and functional state of the thyroid. Removal of TSH stimulation is followed by hypovascularity and atrophy of the gland, accompanied by decreased synthesis and secretion of hormone, whereas converse effects are produced by stimulatory doses of TSH. As indicated earlier, it is not certain that all adjustments in thyroid function in response to a variety of stimuli are mediated by changes in the rate of TSH secretion. Intrinsic autoregulatory mechanisms may be the first sensors of changes in the rate of hormone synthesis and may respond appropriately to alter thyroid sensitivity to constant degrees of TSH stimulation. If this response is inadequate to maintain continued secretion of requisite quantities of hormone, modification of the rate of TSH secretion follows.

TSH is a glycoprotein hormone secreted by a specific cell type, the thyrotroph, located principally in the anteromedial portion of the adenohypophysis. Highly purified preparations of TSH have been obtained from a variety of mammalian species as well as man, and the molecular weights are in the range of 28,000 to 30,000. In common with the other glycoprotein hormones, luteinizing hormone (LH), follicle-stimulating hormone (FSH), and chorionic gonadotropin (CG), TSH is composed of two different glycopeptide subunits, α and β, that are held together by noncovalent forces. Within any species, the α subunits of these glycoprotein hormones are virtually identical with respect to amino acid sequence, but differences do exist in their oligosaccharide components. Greater differences are evident in the composition of the specific β subunits of these hormones, though strong similarities nevertheless exist. The biologic activity of the isolated subunits is negligible, but activity can be restored by recombination of the corresponding specific subunits. Of even greater interest is the observation that recombination of α subunits of any of the hormones with a specific β subunit yields physiologic activity corresponding to that of the parent hormone of the β subunit. Immunologic specificity, like physiologic activity, appears to reside in the β subunits.

Pituitary extracts yield greater quantities of α subunits than β subunits, suggesting that the latter are limiting in the biosynthesis of the complete glycoprotein hormone. In addition, high molecular weight forms of TSH ("big" TSH) and of its β subunit ("big" TSH-β) have been identified in pituitary extracts and may account for the heterogeneity that has been noted with respect to electrophoretic and chromatographic behavior. The foregoing findings raise the possibility that certain disturbances of function may result from abnormalities in the synthesis or secretion of TSH or its constituent subunits. (See Pierce, 1978, for a review of the chemistry of TSH.)

The development of sensitive and highly specific radioimmunoassays for TSH, and more recently for TSH-β and the α subunit, has made possible their measurement in serum. The TSH in human serum normally ranges in concentration from 0.5 to 3 μU/ml and has a specific activity of approximately 5 μU/mg using an international human reference standard. Free α subunit is detectable in serum from normal subjects and is increased in serum from postmenopausal women and from patients with primary hypothyroidism. Free TSH-β is often undetectable normally, but is present in serum from hypothyroid patients. In normal subjects, the secretion rate of TSH is approximately 100 mU/day. This value is greatly increased in patients with primary hypothyroidism and reduced in patients with hyperthyroidism. (See Kourides et al., 1977b, for a discussion of TSH and subunit kinetics.)

Earlier work using insensitive radioimmunoassays yielded contradictory data as to whether the concentration of TSH in serum undergoes a circadian variation. This issue has now been resolved by the availability of assays with sensitivities of the order of 0.2 μU/ml, which have revealed that TSH in serum displays both briefly episodic and circadian variations (Parker et al., 1976). The former variation is characterized by fluctuations at 1- to 2-hour intervals, suggesting that TSH is secreted in a pulsatile manner. The circadian variation is characterized by a nocturnal surge that antecedes the onset of sleep and appears not to be determined by the cortisol rhythm or by fluctuations in the serum T_4 and T_3 concentration. When the onset of sleep is delayed, the nocturnal TSH surge is accentuated and prolonged, whereas early onset of sleep results in a surge of lesser magnitude and shorter duration. These observations suggest that secretion of TSH is subject to a fundamental circadian rhythm that is modulated by sleep-associated inhibitory influences. A qualitatively similar variation in serum TSH concentration has been reported to occur in patients with mild primary hypothyroidism. In patients with severe hypothyroidism, the circadian variation may disappear.

Although TSH is capable of inducing lipolysis *in vitro*, its major effects *in vivo* are on the structure and function of thyroid gland. The effect of TSH on intrathyroid iodine metabolism is to enhance essentially all processes leading to the synthesis and secretion of hormone. Abolition of TSH secretion by hypophysectomy or suppression is followed by decreased activity of the thyroid iodide transport mechanism. In addition, organic binding is inhibited, as indicated both by kinetic analysis and by an increase in the proportion of newly accumulated intrathyroid iodine present in the inorganic form. A decreased fraction of organified iodine is present as iodothyronines, indicating a decrease in the rate of coupling of iodotyrosines. In the intact animal, the fractional release of glandular I* is retarded, indicating a decrease in proteolysis of thyroglobulin. Following administration of TSH, iodide transport activity is increased, apparently owing to the induction of specific protein, possibly the iodide carrier. Organic-binding reactions are also enhanced, and a very prompt stimulation of the coupling reaction occurs. Proteolysis of thyroglobulin and release of glandular iodine are accelerated. Finally, the rate of iodotyrosine dehalogenation is increased, possibly because of increased availability of NADPH, rather than increase in concentration of the enzyme. Clinically, the effects of TSH on iodine metabolism are evident in an increased RAIU and thyroid iodide clearance rate, an increase in the rate of release of glandular I*, and an increase in serum T_4 and T_3 concentrations.

In view of suggestive evidence that the several stages in thyroid hormone synthesis may be closely linked to or dependent upon thyroid energy metabolism, considerable interest has centered upon the effects of TSH on glandular intermediary metabolism. In brief, TSH stimulates thyroid oxygen consumption, glucose assimilation, and glucose oxidation via the hexose monophosphate shunt and glycolytic and tricarboxylic acid cycles. As a consequence, production of carbon dioxide and lactate from exogenous glucose is increased. Oxygen consumption and carbon dioxide production are increased by TSH in the absence of exogenous glucose, indicating increased oxidation of endogenous substrate. TSH acutely increases the total thyroid content of NADP and also increases the $NADP^+/NADPH$ ratio. TSH also has a pronounced and rapid effect on phospholipid metabolism. Accelerated turnover of thyroid phospholipids is evident, particularly among the phosphomonoinositides, changes in phosphatidic acid and phosphatidyl serine being less prominent. Incorporation of glucose and glycerol carbon into thyroid phospholipids is also accelerated. The glandular concentration of inorganic phosphate is increased by TSH, reflecting hydrolysis of organic phosphates. This may serve as a stimulus to oxidative metabolism. TSH stimulates the synthesis of purine and pyrimidine precursors and their incorporation into nucleic acids. Uptake of α-aminoisobutyrate by thyroid cells is enhanced by TSH, and leucine incorporation is accelerated in the thyroid of rats given TSH. Thus TSH stimulates both catabolic and anabolic processes in the thyroid, the former presumably supplying energy requisite for the latter.

There is now compelling evidence that cyclic AMP is the intracellular mediator of many of the effects of TSH on the thyroid. Activation of adenylate cyclase by TSH requires binding of the hormone to a specific receptor on the plasma membrane of the thyroid cell and may involve membrane phospholipids as the coupling mechanism. The TSH receptor has been partly characterized and contains gangliosides

that may be important in the binding interaction. Recent work has indicated that prostaglandins can mimic many of the effects of TSH on the thyroid. However, indomethacin, an inhibitor of prostaglandin synthetase, does not block the effects of TSH, indicating that prostaglandins are not obligatory intermediates in TSH action. (See Field, 1978, for a comprehensive review of TSH action.)

Iodine

In addition to its role as a requisite substrate for thyroid hormone biosynthesis, iodine participates in a number of clinically important interactions with the thyroid. Elucidation of the nature and mechanism of these interactions has for some years constituted a fascinating avenue of clinical and physiologic exploration. (See Nagataki, 1974; and Ingbar, 1978a, for more extensive considerations of the various effects of iodine on the thyroid.)

Effects on Thyroid Hormone Synthesis

The effect of iodine on the rate of thyroid hormone synthesis depends on the amount and duration of iodine administration. When administered acutely, small to moderate amounts of stable iodine do not influence the percentage of thyroid uptake of concomitantly administered I.* In addition, direct analysis reveals little change in the fraction of accumulated iodine that has undergone organification or in the proportions of the several iodinated amino acids formed. Hence these small acute does result in an increased rate of thyroid hormone synthesis, at least for a time.

With progressively larger acute doses of iodide, more complex consequences result. The quantity of iodine that undergoes organification displays a biphasic response to increasing doses of iodide, at first increasing, then declining as a result of at least a relative blockade of organic binding. This decreasing yield of organic iodine from increasing doses of iodide is termed the acute Wolff-Chaikoff effect. The mechanism of the acute effect is uncertain, but it has been shown that this effect depends upon the establishment within the thyroid of a sufficiently high concentration of inorganic iodide. Under these conditions, the reactive form of iodine generated by oxidative mechanisms may complex with iodide to yield a form that is relatively inefficient in iodinating tyrosine. In common with other situations in which the proportionate rate of organic binding is decreased, as when propylthiouracil is administered, qualitative changes in hormone synthesis also occur. Of that iodine that is bound to organic compounds, little if any is incorporated into T_4 and T_3, a subnormal proportion appears as DIT, and MIT becomes the major product formed. It is unlikely that organic-iodinations are completely inhibited during the acute Wolff-Chaikoff effect, but from chromatographic evidence it appears that synthesis of the hormonally active iodothyronines is abolished. Thus the thyroid rejects both quantitatively and qualitatively the large quantity of iodide acutely administered, and the massive increase in thyroid hormone formation that would otherwise occur is prevented. (See Figure 4–11 for a schematic representation of the Wolff-Chaikoff effect.)

In man, induction of at least a partial blockade of organic binding by an acute dose of iodide is what is responsible for the iodide discharged from the thyroid during the iodide-perchlorate discharge test. In normal man, somewhat more than 2 mg of iodide must be given acutely in order to induce a Wolff-Chaikoff effect and hence to inhibit the uptake and

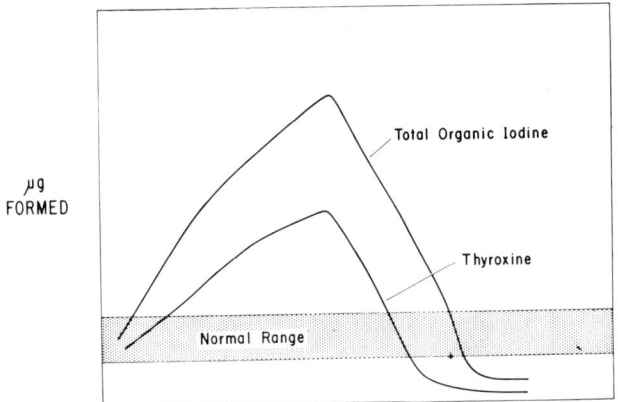

THE WOLFF — CHAIKOFF EFFECT

μg FORMED

Total Organic Iodine

Thyroxine

Normal Range

Figure 4–11. Schema of the Wolff-Chaikoff effect. Progressively increasing doses of iodide, given acutely, are associated with an increase and then a decrease in total organic iodinations and in T_4 synthesis. It is uncertain whether values really fall below the normal level in normal subjects.

organic binding of a concomitantly administered dose of I*. That is why substantially smaller doses of iodide are employed in the iodide-perchlorate discharge test. Abnormal sensitivity to the Wolff-Chaikoff effect in terms of the dose of iodide required for its elicitation is conditioned by one or both of two factors. Susceptibility is increased when the iodide transport mechanism is activated. Here the increase in intrathyroid iodide concentration produced by a given dose of iodide is enhanced. This may explain the enhanced susceptibility of some patients with Graves' disease or of normal individuals given TSH. Susceptibility is also increased when there is an underlying defect in the organic-binding mechanism. One or another of these factors, or both, likely accounts for the increased susceptibility seen in patients who have previously developed goiter during chronic iodide administration or for that seen in many patients with Hashimoto's disease or with Graves' disease previously treated with surgery, ^{131}I, or antithyroid drugs. Such patients are likely to develop goiter if given iodides chronically, and in them the defective organic-binding mechanism may be a forerunner of eventual thyroid failure.

When moderate or large doses of iodide are administered repeatedly, the relative inhibition of organic binding and inhibition of iodothyronine formation are at least partly relieved. This so-called "escape" or "adaptation" phenomenon occurs because, with continued iodine administration, iodide transport activity decreases, and the thyroid iodide concentration becomes insufficient to maintain a full Wolff-Chaikoff effect. This response is demonstrable in the hypophysectomized animal and hence is a manifestation of the thyroid autoregulatory inhibition of iodide transport discussed earlier. It allows synthesis of iodothyronines to resume, despite continued iodide administration, and thereby forestalls the development of goitrous hypothyroidism. The reduction in iodide transport which permits adaptation reduces the thyroid iodide clearance rate and hence the RAIU. Nonetheless, the quantity of iodine accumulated and organified is well in excess of normal, though the rate of secretion of T_4 is not enhanced. Hence it is evident that during chronic iodine administration the thyroid forms and releases noncalorigenic forms of iodine. Probably much of the iodine lost from the gland in this manner is iodide. In normal individuals the magnitude of this so-called "iodide leak" varies directly with the dietary iodine intake. In unusual circumstances, adaptation does not occur, and synthesis of hormone is chronically inhibited, leading to the development of goiter and hypothyroidism (iodide myxedema). This disorder, to which patients with Hashimoto's disease, certain patients with Graves' disease, patients who have undergone hemithyroidectomy, and patients with cystic fibrosis are prone, is discussed more fully in the section dealing with disorders that lead to hypothyroidism.

Effect on Thyroid Hormone Release

In the clinical setting, probably the most important effect of pharmacologic doses of iodine on the thyroid is their ability to induce a prompt inhibition of hormone release. When the thyroid iodine is labeled with I* and large doses of antithyroid agents are administered to prevent recycling of I* released from the gland, administration of iodine is followed soon thereafter by a decrease in the rate of disappearance of I* from the gland (Fig. 4–12). This effect is most clearly evident in hyperfunctioning thyroids but can also be demonstrated in the normal thyroid, though with some difficulty because of the relatively slow initial rate of ra-

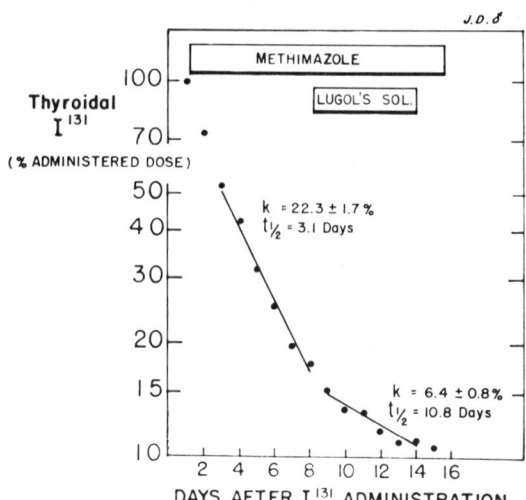

Figure 4–12. Effect of iodine on the thyroid turnover of ^{131}I in a patient with Graves' disease. The initial turnover rate of 22.3%/day is much faster than that observed in normal patients and is abruptly slowed by the administration of Lugol's iodine.

dioiodine turnover. Alternative methods of analysis have shown that iodine not only decreases the fractional turnover of thyroid radioiodine but also decreases the actual T_4 secretion rate.

This effect of iodine is doubtless the mechanism whereby iodine rapidly lowers the serum T_4 concentration and acutely alleviates thyrotoxicity in the patient with diffuse toxic goiter. The response to iodine in this disorder cannot be ascribed to the persistence of an acute Wolff-Chaikoff effect with inhibition of T_4 synthesis, since the ameliorative effect is much more rapid than that produced by even large doses of antithyroid agent. Neither can the response to iodine be ascribed to an effect on the peripheral metabolism or metabolic effectiveness of T_4, since none can be demonstrated. In most patients with otherwise untreated diffuse toxic goiter, the decrease in serum T_4 concentration during iodine administration does not continue into the hypothyroid range, but rather stabilizes at a normal or high normal value. The reason for this is uncertain, but in normal individuals the decline in serum T_4 and T_3 concentrations induced by iodine appears to elicit an increase in TSH secretion that counteracts the effect of iodine (Vagenakis et al., 1973). Whether normalization of the serum T_4 concentration by iodine in the thyrotoxic patient also elicits secretion of TSH has not been studied.

The mechanism by which iodine inhibits secretion of T_4 is unknown. Clearly the effect is mediated at the thyroid level rather than through an action on TSH, in view of its occurrence in Graves' disease. Moreover, the effect is demonstrable in the autonomously hyperfunctioning thyroid nodule, in which disorder the secretion of TSH is also lacking. The effect of iodine on the secretory mechanism is not confined to an effect on the release of T_4 itself but is likely an effect on the mechanism of proteolysis, since iodine acutely inhibits its "iodide leak."

Involution of Thyroid Hyperplasia

One of the most important and enigmatic effects of iodine on the thyroid is its ability to diminish the hypervascularity and hyperplasia that characterize the diffuse toxic goiter of Graves' disease. This effect, which greatly facilitates surgical therapy of this disorder, is not an obligatory action of iodide on the thyroid, since intense hyperplasia characterizes the thyroid gland of patients with iodide myxedema. In the latter disorder, pharmacologic quantities of iodide inhibit hormone synthesis, while in Graves' disease some binding of iodine to organic compounds doubtless occurs, even during treatment with antithyroid agents. The involuting effect of iodine may reflect an autoregulation of thyroid intermediary metabolism, since the rat thyroid which is rich in iodine uses glucose less efficiently and forms therefrom less carbon dioxide, lactate, and lipid than does the thyroid which is poor in iodine (unpublished observations of Nagataki). Decreased energy metabolism in the thyroid may retard anabolic processes necessary for maintenance of hyperplasia, while decreased production of acid metabolites may be responsible for the reduction in vascularity that iodine produces.

Adrenergic Nervous System and Bioactive Amines

The effects of the adrenergic nervous system and of catecholamines on various aspects of thyroid function have long been a subject of interest. Studies of varying design in varying species have yielded variable results. As a consequence, there has been considerable doubt whether the adrenergic nervous system has any significant influence on thyroid function. Considerable clarification, however, has come in recent years, principally from the studies of Melander and co-workers. These investigators have shown that the extent of adrenergic innervation of the thyroid varies from species to species and with the age of the animal, possibly explaining the variable results obtained by other investigators. In man and the mouse, abundant adrenergic fibers terminate in the thyroid in relation to both arterioles and follicle cells. Stimulation of the cervical sympathetic trunks in mice whose thyroid glands have been prelabeled with I* and then suppressed by exogenous T_4 induces formation of colloid droplets and an increase in blood I* concentration. Unilateral stimulation induces colloid droplet formation only within the distribution of the stimulated nerve. Moreover, a direct stimulatory effect of catecholamines on thyroid hormone secretion is indicated by the demonstration that exogenous norepinephrine, epinephrine, and dopamine induce release of I* from the prelabeled and T_4-suppressed thyroid of the mouse. Direct stimulatory effects of these catecholamines on iodine and intermediary metabolism have also been demonstrated. In common with TSH, the catecholamines exert their effects through activation of the adenylate cyclase–cyclic AMP system. In contrast to TSH, however, their stimulatory effects on adenylate cyclase activity and on thyroid hormone synthesis and secretion are inhibited by adrenergic antagonists. Evidence of a stimulatory effect of serotonin on thyroid hormone synthesis and secretion has also been obtained. Serotonin may have functional significance in the rat, a species in which the thyroid is particularly rich in serotonin-containing mast cells that degranulate in response to TSH. (See Melander et al., 1977, for pertinent references.)

There is also evidence that catecholamines are involved in the regulation of TSH secretion. Norepinephrine appears to have a stimulatory influence and dopamine an inhibitory influence on TSH secretion. In the rat, dopamine-β-hydroxylase inhibitors and α-adrenergic antagonists, but not β-adrenergic antagonists, decrease the serum TSH concentration and prevent the cold-induced surge in TSH secretion. Since the cold-induced surge of TSH is probably dependent on TRH, the modulating influence of catecholamines on TSH secretion is in all likelihood mediated by TRH.

As might be expected, the effects of catecholamines on thyroid hormone economy in man have been less well defined. Depending on the magnitude and timing of the dose, acute administration of epinephrine may either increase or decrease the RAIU, and thyroid function is normal in most patients with pheochromocytoma. No significant alterations in thyroid function or serum T_4 concentration are seen in patients given the usual pharmacologic doses of adrenergic blocking agents, though propranolol may impair, to a modest extent, the peripheral conversion of T_4 to T_3.

Evidence for a role of biogenic amines in the regulation of TSH secretion in man is beginning to emerge. In patients with hypothyroidism, both fusaric acid, a dopamine-β-hydroxylase inhibitor, and L-dopa decrease the increased serum TSH concentration. These findings suggest that norepinephrine may be stimulatory and dopamine inhibitory to TSH secretion in man, as in the rat. (For a review of regulation of TSH secretion, see Scanlon et al., 1978.)

Antithyroid Agents

A wide variety of chemical agents have the ability to inhibit one or more reactions required in the synthesis of thyroid hormones. When the effect of such agents is sufficient to reduce the secretion of thyroid hormones to subnormal levels, secretion of TSH is increased, and goiter ensues. Hence such agents are commonly termed goitrogens. In clinical practice, goitrogenic agents are encountered as drugs used in the treatment of hyperthyroidism, as pharmacologic agents used for other purposes but which happen to have antithyroid properties, and as goitrogens occurring naturally in foodstuffs. The present section will provide a classification of several varieties of antithyroid agents and their mode of action. Since the use of antithyroid drugs in the treatment of hyperthyroidism is discussed in a later section, special attention will be given here to those agents that are not used in the control of hyperthyroidism but may nonetheless be encountered clinically.

From the standpoint of the aspects of iodine metabolism which they inhibit, classic antithyroid agents can be grouped into two classes: agents that inhibit thyroid iodide transport and those that inhibit the complex of reactions involved in organic-binding and coupling processes. Without clear exception, inhibitors of iodide transport belong to the class of monovalent anions; of these, thiocyanate and perchlorate have been used clinically. Other anions that inhibit thyroid iodide transport have been discussed in the section on hormone biosynthesis. Because of their toxicity, neither thiocyanate nor perchlorate is any longer widely used in the treatment of hyperthyroidism, although they are usually effective agents in this respect. Inhibitors of iodide transport decrease hormone synthesis by limiting T:P concentration ratios for iodide, thereby reducing the intrathyroid iodide concentration. This is effective when the plasma iodide concentration is normal or low; however, should the patient be exposed to excessive amounts of iodine, hormone overproduction will resume. Thus control may be unpredictable and, furthermore, these agents cannot be used with iodine in preparing patients for subtotal thyroidectomy.

The second class of antithyroid agents consists of compounds that inhibit the thyroid organic-binding and coupling reactions. Although a great many compounds exert this effect, with few exceptions they can be classified into three main groups, according to their basic chemical struc-

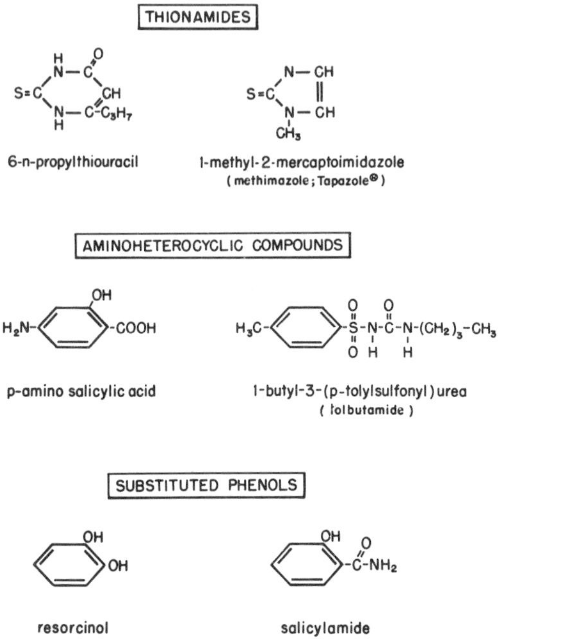

THIONAMIDES

6-n-propylthiouracil

1-methyl-2-mercaptoimidazole
(methimazole ; Tapazole®)

AMINOHETEROCYCLIC COMPOUNDS

p-amino salicylic acid

1-butyl-3-(p-tolylsulfonyl)urea
(tolbutamide)

SUBSTITUTED PHENOLS

resorcinol

salicylamide

Figure 4–13. Structural formulas of some representative antithyroid compounds.

ture: thionamides, aminoheterocyclic compounds, and substituted phenols (Fig. 4–13). In the case of the thionamides, it was initially thought that these agents exert their antithyroid action solely by inhibiting the initial oxidation and binding of iodide in the thyroid. Later it was learned that the inhibitory action of these agents is directed, in order of decreasing sensitivity, at the coupling of iodotyrosines, the iodination of MIT to form DIT, and lastly, the formation of MIT. Subsequent studies have shown a similar order of sensitivity in the action of all agents that ultimately (at their highest doses) inhibit organic binding per se.

As a class, the thionamide compounds, which include the classic antithyroid agents, are the most potent inhibitors of thyroid hormone formation known, and are characterized by the following substituent grouping

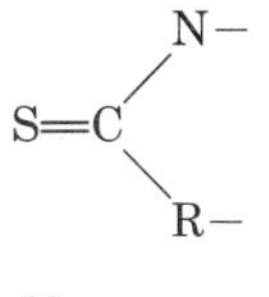

$$S=C \begin{array}{c} N- \\ \\ R- \end{array}$$

in which R may be a sulfur, oxygen, or nitrogen atom. In contrast to the action of agents that inhibit thyroid iodide transport, the action of the thionamides is not prevented by large doses of iodide, although it is decreased somewhat.

The aminoheterocyclic compounds are in general far less potent than the thionamides and are not used in the treatment of hyperthyroidism. Their effects on the thyroid are sometimes manifest, however, during their use in the treatment of other disease. Para-aminosalicylic acid, formerly used as an antituberculosis agent, is goitrogenic in rats, lowers RAIU in man, and occasionally produces goiter with or without hypothyroidism. The hypoglycemic sulfonylureas, tolbutamide and especially carbutamide, decrease RAIU in man, although they are not sufficiently potent to be goitrogenic in man. The goitrogenic effect of para-aminosalicylic acid and the sulfonylureas, like that of the thionamides, is slightly decreased by large amounts of iodine. An additional group of agents in this class is the sulfonamides. Although they have not been shown to be

goitrogenic in man, interest in them arises from the fact that their goitrogenic potency is usually increased by supplemental iodide. This and other evidence indicates that the mechanism of action of the sulfonamides differs from that of the thionamides and of other aminoheterocyclic compounds.

Another major category of antithyroid agents that inhibit organic binding is that of the substituted phenols. Agents of interest in this group include resorcinol, a cutaneous antiseptic that has produced goitrous hypothyroidism in man. Closely related to resorcinol are the congeners of salicylic acid. The latter is devoid of antithyroid action, although it does inhibit the binding of T_4 by TBPA. Several derivatives of salicylic acid, particularly those with an additional hydroxyl substitution, have moderate antithyroid potency and are also able to inhibit T_4 binding by TBPA. Agents of this class, such as salicylamide, are used clinically because of their antirheumatic, antipyretic, and especially their analgesic effects. Whether they exert a significant antithyroid action in ordinary clinical use is uncertain.

A number of other agents of diverse chemical nature also have antithyroid activity. Phenylbutazone decreases the thyroid uptake of I* and has been reported to produce goitrous hypothyroidism in man. Strangely, the latter effect is said to be transient. Large doses of iodides can, in some patients, act as a goitrogen. (See Braverman, 1978.) Iodopyrine, an antiasthmatic preparation containing iodine and antipyrine (phenazone), has been reported to produce goiter in about 30% of patients. This high incidence of goiter is due to a synergistic action of iodide upon the antithyroid effect of antipyrine, which is itself a goitrogen.

Lithium salts are potential goitrogens frequently encountered in clinical practice. Goiter, with or without hypothyroidism, is sometimes encountered in patients being treated with lithium, usually for bipolar manic-depressive psychosis. Like iodide, lithium inhibits thyroid hormone release, and, in high concentrations, can inhibit organic-binding reactions. At least acutely, iodide and lithium act synergistically in the latter respect. The mechanism underlying the several effects of lithium is uncertain. Also uncertain is what differentiates those patients who develop goiter during lithium therapy from those who do not. Underlying autoimmune thyroiditis may be at least one factor (Transbol et al., 1978).

Antithyroid agents also occur naturally in foods. These are widely distributed in the family Cruciferae or Brassicaceae, particularly in the genus Brassica. Included are cabbages, turnips, kale, kohlrabi, rutabaga, mustard, and a number of plants not eaten by humans but which serve as animal fooder. It is likely that some thiocyanate is present in such plants (particularly cabbage), especially in the leaves. In addition to some thiocyanate, the seeds, roots, and perhaps leaves also contain another variety of potential goitrogens or "progoitrins" in the form of various thioglycosides. The progoitrins are themselves not goitrogenic but become so when acted upon either by a heat-labile thioglycosidase, myrosinase, also present in the plant, or by the glycosidases liberated by intestinal bacteria. In the case of turnips, the active goitrogen has been shown to be L-5-vinyl-2-thiooxazolidone. Actively goitrogenic isothiocyanates have been isolated from other plants of the same family. Cassava meal, a dietary staple in many regions of the world, releases cyanide, which undergoes detoxification to thiocyanate. There is clear evidence that ingestion of cassava is a major factor in accentuating goiter formation in areas of endemic iodine deficiency. Except for thiocyanate, dietary goitrogens influence thyroid iodine metabolism in the same manner as do the thionamides, which they resemble chemically. The role of dietary goitrogens in the induction of disease in humans is uncertain; their effect may depend upon the concomitant iodine intake. Although humans rarely if ever eat goitrogenic foods in quantities sufficient to lead to goiter, the possibility of endemia due to transmission of sufficient quantities of the goitrogen in milk has been raised. An important contribution is the clear demonstration that water-borne, sulfur-containing goitrogens of mineral origin contribute to the development of endemic goiter in certain areas of the world. (See Ermans, 1980, and Gaitan, 1974, for discussions of the role of dietary and water-borne goitrogens in the genesis of endemic goiter.)

Sex and Sex Hormones

A relationship between the thyroid and the gonads is suggested by the far more frequent occurrence of thyroid disorders in women than in men and by the common appearance of goiter during puberty, pregnancy, and the menopause. This apparent relationship has engendered many studies to assess the effect of sex and of the administration of sex hormones on thyroid function.

In man, the administration of small doses of estrogens leads to an acute decrease in the serum TSH concentration, from which an escape occurs by the second or third day of continued administration. This effect of estrogens, which resembles that induced by glucocorticoids, appears to be exerted through an inhibition of endogenous TRH release. Testosterone and progesterone in essentially physiologic doses do not appear to influence TSH secretion.

The administration of estrogens or androgens has no consistent effect on the RAIU but causes alterations in the binding of thyroid hormones in plasma. Estrogens increase the concentration of TBG and elevate the serum T_4 and T_3 concentrations, whereas androgens induce converse effects, although they increase the concentration of TBPA. The kinetic consequences of these alterations in hormone transport have been discussed in an earlier section.

Thyroid function and the peripheral metabolism of the thyroid hormones appear to be essentially independent of the sex of the individual. There is no appreciable variation in RAIU during different phases of the menstrual cycle. The normal ranges for the serum T_4 and T_3 concentrations are the same in nonpregnant women and men. A clear difference between men and women exists, however, in the response of the serum TSH concentration to the administration of TRH. Responses are greater in women than in men, especially when comparisons are made in individuals over the age of 40. Estrogens appear to enhance the response to TRH, probably by increasing the number of TRH receptors in the thyrotroph, since responses tend to be increased in women receiving contraceptive steroids, and are greatest in normal women during the preovulatory phase of the menstrual cycle (See review by Scanlon et al., 1978). The basal metabolic rate (BMR) tends to be somewhat higher in men than in women, probably because of the relatively greater muscle mass in men.

Pregnancy and the Newborn State

Pregnancy affects virtually all aspects of thyroid hormone economy. The thyroid gland is enlarged, and a bruit, reflecting the increased blood flow, may be present. The RAIU and thyroid iodide clearance rate are increased. These alterations are largely due to the iodine deficiency state that occurs during pregnancy as a result of an increase in renal iodide clearance. The RAIU and the thyroid and renal iodide clearance rates return to nonpregnant levels within 6 weeks after delivery.

The serum T_4 concentration increases during the first month of pregnancy to values between 7 and 12 $\mu g/100$ ml and remains at this level until after delivery. The serum T_3 concentration also increases during pregnancy but to a lesser extent than does the serum T_4, with the result that the $T_4:T_3$ ratio in serum is greater than that in the nonpregnant state. The increase in serum T_4 and T_3 concentrations is due mainly to the increased concentration of TBG in plasma, resulting in all likelihood from the increased secretion of estrogens. The proportion of free T_4, whether assessed directly or indirectly by an uptake test *in vitro*, is decreased. Early in pregnancy, the free T_4 concentration is slightly increased. Subsequently, both the free T_4 concentration and free T_4 index are normal (see Yamamoto et al., 1979). The proportion of free T_3 is decreased, and the concentration of free T_3 is within, but often at the lower end of, the normal range. As a result of the decrease in the proportion of free T_4, the volume of distribution and fractional rate of turnover of T_4 are decreased, but the total daily disposal of hormone remains essentially unchanged. The serum T_4 and T_3 concentrations, as well as the concentration of TBG, return to nonpregnant levels within 6 weeks after delivery.

The serum TSH concentration is modestly decreased during the first trimester at a time when the concentration of human chorionic gonadotropin (hCG) is at its highest (see Yamamoto et al., 1979). This has been interpreted to suggest that hCG may play a role in supporting thyroid function in early pregnancy, but this is uncertain, since there is currently no consensus whether hCG is a stimulator of the human thyroid (Amir et al., 1980). Recent data indicate that a causative role cannot be ascribed to the so-called human chorionic thyrotropin (hCT) since its existence has been called into question. During the second and third trimesters, the serum TSH concentration is not appreciably different from that in the nonpregnant state, but the TSH response to TRH is accentuated relative to the nonpregnant state, very likely as a result of the hyperestrinemia that is present.

The basal metabolic rate (BMR) increases during the second trimester, and values of $+20$–30% are common at term. The increase in BMR is due to the increase in the total mass of body tissue.

In normal pregnancy at term, the concentration of T_4 in cord serum is only slightly less than that in serum, but because of a smaller increase in TBG relative to normal serum, the free T_4 concentration exceeds that in maternal serum. In addition, owing to the general inactivity of the fetal enzyme for converting T_4 to T_3, concentrations of total and free T_3 are far lower than those in maternal serum. Since it seems likely that any thyroid hormone that traverses the placenta would do so in the unbound or free form, these concentration differentials bespeak a very limited transplacental passage of T_4 and T_3 in either direction. As part of the low activity of iodothyronine 5'-monodeiodinase that characterizes fetal life, the concentration of rT_3 in cord serum at birth is far higher than that in maternal serum or that of normal adults. The concentration of TSH in cord serum also exceeds that in maternal serum (see Fisher, 1974).

After delivery, the serum TSH concentration in the neonate increases rapidly to a peak at 30 minutes of extrauterine life, returning to its initial value within 48 hours. This neotatal surge of TSH is believed to be due in part to the cooling that follows emergence into the extrauterine environment. Serum T_4 and T_3 concentrations increase rapidly during the first few hours after delivery and are in the distinctly hyperthyroid range by 24 hours of life. The increase in serum T_4 concentration can be accounted for by the surge in TSH secretion. While the TSH surge doubtless contributes to the increase in serum T_3 concentration, enhancement of the extrathyroid conversion of T_4 to T_3 is the major factor responsible. Recent work suggests that glucocorticoids may play a role in stimulating the conversion of T_4 to T_3 during the perinatal period. In contrast to T_4 and T_3, the elevated serum rT_3 concentration displays little change during the first 24 hours of postnatal life, but declines to normal values by the fifth postnatal day. By the tenth day or so, the serum T_4 and T_3 concentrations are lower, but still exceed normal adult values. (See Osathanondh et al., 1978, for references.)

The changes in thyroid function that accompany normal pregnancy are exaggerated in molar pregnancy. The serum T_4 and T_3 concentrations are usually distinctly increased, often very markedly so. The increase in serum TBG concentration in molar pregnancy is less than that in normal pregnancy, with the result that free T_4 and free T_3 concentrations in serum are usually elevated. When this is the case, responses to TRH are subnormal, indicating the presence of thyroid hormone excess. Nonetheless, though some patients with molar pregnancy are clinically thyrotoxic, most are not. The reason for this discordance is unclear (Nagataki et al., 1977). Thyroid hyperfunction in molar pregnancy clearly results from the elaboration by the abnormal trophoblast of an abnormal thyroid stimulator termed molar thyrotropin that is probably not hCG (Amir et al., 1980). Comparable abnormalities occur, though less frequently, in patients with choriocarcinoma or malignant trophoblastic tumor of the testis (see review by Hershman, 1978).

Age

The increased values for the serum T_4 concentration in the neonate (see preceding section) gradually decline, reaching the normal adult range toward the end of the first year. Values for the serum T_3 concentration remain higher through early adolescence than they are later in life.

Normative studies of the effects of aging on various aspects and laboratory indices of thyroid function are difficult to perform and the results difficult to evaluate, owing mainly to the difficulty in obtaining an elderly population free of significant disease and of medications that may influence the function being studied. This very likely accounts for the many significant inconsistencies in the data available in this field. Certain broad trends of change with age in several aspects of thyroid hormone economy can be discerned, nonetheless. From childhood through senescence, the serum T_4 concentration remains unchanged or decreases only slightly, while most, but not all, studies reveal a distinct decline in serum T_3 from middle age through senescence. When apparent, the decrease in serum T_3 is probably the result of decreased peripheral conversion of T_4 to T_3, but this may reflect the presence of mild illness, not an effect of aging itself. Free T_4 concentrations in the aged are somewhat low, on the average, and free T_3 concentrations at the lower end of the normal range for younger individuals (Hermann et al., 1974). The RAIU, thyroid clearance rate, and turnover rate decrease slightly with age, resulting in part from the decrease in the total daily disposal of T_4 that occurs with age and in part from an age-dependent decrease in renal iodide clearance. From infancy through senescence,

both the total daily disposal of T_4 and the BMR decrease progressively with age, probably reflecting alterations in the cellular metabolism of thyroid hormones. In some studies, mean serum TSH concentrations increase slightly during senescence (Sawin et al., 1979). In men, but apparently not in women, the peak increment in the response of the serum TSH concentration to TRH declines progressively with advancing age. The prevalence of circulating antithyroid antibodies increases with age. (For a comprehensive review of the effects of aging on thyroid hormone economy, see Ingbar, 1978b.)

Glucocorticoids

Both ACTH, through its action on the adrenal cortex, and glucocorticoids influence thyroid function. Early work demonstrated that pharmacologic doses of these agents decrease the thyroid RAIU, clearance rate, and turnover rate in man. In addition, it was demonstrated that these alterations could be reversed by the administration of exogenous TSH, suggesting that these agents suppress pituitary TSH secretion. This was confirmed by later studies in which it was shown that the administration of pharmacologic doses of glucocorticoid reduces serum TSH concentrations in both normal and hypothyroid patients. When glucocorticoids are withdrawn, the serum TSH concentration rebounds to values in excess of pretreatment values. With continued administration of glucocorticoids, there occurs an escape from the suppression of serum TSH concentration in some but not all patients. More recent studies have extended these findings by demonstrating that pharmacologic doses of glucocorticoid decrease the rate of TSH secretion in both normal and hypothyroid patients and depress the response of TSH, but not of prolactin, to exogenous TRH. In addition, it has been shown that reduction of serum cortisol concentration by metyrapone is accompanied by an increase in serum TSH concentration, indicating a suppressive influence of physiologic concentrations of glucocorticoid on TSH secretion (Re et al., 1976). The decrease in thyroid secretary rate resulting from the suppression of pituitary TSH secretion is in all likelihood responsible for the slight decrease in serum T_4 concentration that glucocorticoids induce in normal subjects, since no change in serum T_4 concentration is seen in hypothyroid patients maintained on a constant daily dose of exogenous hormone. On the other hand, pharmacologic doses of glucocorticoid induce a prompt and significant decline in serum T_4 concentration in hyperthyroid patients; the mechanism underlying this effect has not been ascertained, however (Williams et al., 1975).

Significant decreases in serum T_3 concentration are induced by pharmacologic doses of glucocorticoid in both normal and hyperthyroid patients. This phenomenon also occurs in hypothyroid patients maintained on replacement doses of exogenous T_4. This latter finding, as well as the fact that the decrease in serum T_3 concentration is accompanied by an increase in serum rT_3 concentration, provides compelling evidence that glucocorticoids inhibit monodeiodination of the outer ring of T_4 (and probably rT_3) in extrathyroid tissues. This is the converse of what is seen during the perinatal period, when glucocorticoids appear to result in an enhancement of the extrathyroid conversion of T_4 to T_3 (Osathanondh et al., 1978).

Pharmacologic doses of glucocorticoids decrease the concentration in serum of TBG and increase that of TBPA but do not affect the proportion or absolute concentration of free T_4. Consistent with the latter finding is the observation that glucocorticoids do not induce significant alterations in the metabolic disappearance of T_4. However, they do retard the distributive disappearance of T_4, probably by decreasing the hepatic binding of hormone.

Environmental Temperature

Exposure of human subjects to cold for several days results in an increase in serum T_4 concentration which is evident by 24 hours and which reaches a maximum by 3 days. The RAIU and clearance rate also increase. These alterations may represent a compensatory response to a depletion of the peripheral hormone pool, resulting from an increased rate of T_4 metabolism by the peripheral tissues. By contrast, short-term exposure to cold is not accompanied by an increased serum TSH concentration in adult subjects. In the newborn, on the other hand, brief cooling provokes an increase in serum TSH concentration, suggesting that the hypothalamus is initially responsive to the cold stimulus but becomes refractory with age.

Small seasonal variations in serum T_4 and T_3 concentrations have been noted in normal subjects. The values for both hormones appear to vary inversely with environmental temperature and are lowest in the summer (Smals et al., 1977).

Nutritional Influences

Alterations in nutritional state, whether short-term or chronic, and whether the result of underfeeding, overfeeding, or merely a change in substrate mix, affect various aspects of thyroid hormone economy, especially peripheral hormone metabolism. When euthyroid lean or obese subjects are starved, serum total and free T_3 concentrations decline abruptly, often into the clearly hypothyroid range. By contrast, the serum total T_4 concentration remains essentially unchanged, though the free T_4 concentration may increase slightly, owing to a modest decrease in the intensity of iodothyronine binding. Kinetic studies have demonstrated quite clearly that the decrease in serum T_3 concentration reflects a decrease in its peripheral generation from T_4, rather than a change in its metabolic clearance rate (Vagenakis et al., 1977). As serum T_3 concentrations decline, concentrations of rT_3 increase reciprocally, usually to values about twice normal. This is not the result of a major increase in the production of rT_3, but rather a decrease in its clearance rate. These changes have been ascribed to a selective inhibition of the outer-ring monodeiodination of both T_4 and rT_3, leading to decreased generation of T_3 from T_4 and increased accumulation of rT_3. (See Figure 4–4.) Similar changes have been observed *in vitro* in the liver of the starved rat. (For reviews of this topic see Ingbar and Braverman, 1975; Schimmel and Utiger, 1977; Cavalieri and Rapoport, 1978; Burman, 1978.)

Evidently, these aspects of peripheral iodothyronine metabolism are exquisitely sensitive to changes in the carbohydrate content of the diet. The abnormal T_3 and rT_3 concentrations in serum are quickly restored to normal, not only by refeeding with a balanced diet, but also by administration of small quantities (800 kcal) of pure carbohydrate. Similar quantities of protein have no effect on serum T_3 concentration, but may lower serum rT_3, and calories given as fat are ineffective. Other evidence of these relationships is that patients receiving hypocaloric diets composed principally of carbohydrate display little or no change in serum T_3 and rT_3 concentrations.

Despite the decrease in free T_3 concentration that occurs during starvation, the basal serum TSH concentration is unchanged, and the response to TRH is also unaffected, or even slightly depressed. Several factors could explain this apparent discordance. The pituitary may be responding to the normal or slightly increased concentration of free T_4; starvation may somehow alter the set-point of the feedback mechanism; or it may enhance the sensitivity of the feedback mechanism to T_3. Finally, the most intriguing possibility, supported by studies in the rat, is that feedback regulation of TSH secretion is largely conditioned by intrapituitary generation of T_3 from T_4, and that this continues unchanged during starvation.

Although measurements of the serum TSH concentration provide no evidence that the peripheral tissues of the starved subject experience a lack of thyroid hormone, other evidence suggests that they do. Basal oxygen consumption and heart rate decline, negativity of the nitrogen balance ultimately decreases, and peripheral steroid metabolism shifts toward the pattern seen in hypothyroidism. These changes are at least partly reversed by administration of exogenous T_3 while fasting continues. It is intriguing to speculate that the decrease in T_3-neogenesis that occurs during fasting is a beneficial, energy- and nitrogen-sparing adaptation, and that the mechanism that permits TSH secretion to remain normal, despite the decrease in serum T_3 concentration, allows this adaptation to persist. The recently observed decrease in the concentration of T_3 receptors in the liver of the fasted rat may also contribute to this adaptation (Schussler and Orlando, 1978).

Chronic malnutrition, as in protein-calorie malnutrition, and undernutrition, as in anorexia nervosa, are also associated with a decreased serum T_3 concentration. Serum T_4 concentrations tend to be slightly decreased, but serum TSH concentrations and their response to exogenous TRH are generally normal.

Overfeeding, particularly with carbohydrate, increases the T_3 production rate, increases serum T_3 concentration, lowers the serum rT_3 concentration, and induces an increase in basal thermogenesis (Danforth et al., 1979), an apparent converse of the adaptation to starvation.

Nonthyroid Illness

A diversity of abnormalities in thyroid hormone economy, some of them profound, can occur in patients with nonthyroid illness. Certain of these are common to any type of illness or other physiologic insult; others depend on the specific organ system involved. Most remarkable and consistent are abnormalities in the transport and peripheral metabolism of the thyroid hormones, and, as a consequence, in their total and free concentrations in the blood. Although the physiologic significance of these changes is as yet uncertain, they clearly have major implications for the diagnosis of thyroid disease in patients with moderate or severe intercurrent illness.

Three general patterns of change in peripheral thyroid hormone concentration and metabolism occur in euthyroid patients with nonthyroid illness. Common to all three is a decrease in serum T_3 concentration, sometimes to extremely low levels and usually accompanied by an increase in serum concentration of rT_3. These changes are similar to those that occur during starvation and, like them, have been ascribed to a coordinate reduction in the 5'-monodeiodination of T_4 and rT_3, so that both the formation of T_3 and the degradation of rT_3 are slowed. At least in patients with cirrhosis and chronic renal disease, kinetic studies have shown this to be the case. Despite a reduction in the intensity of iodothyronine binding, the free T_3 concentration is also subnormal, owing to the marked reduction in total T_3 concentration. Patients with these findings are commonly said to have the "low T_3 syndrome" or "sick euthyroid syndrome."

Changes of this type in serum T_3 and rT_3 concentrations evidently can be elicited by any physiologic stress of sufficient intensity, since they have been reported in so many otherwise differing states. Among acute illnesses included are febrile illnesses of all types, acute myocardial infarction, acute respiratory failure, uncontrolled diabetes and diabetic ketoacidosis, surgery, and even the administration of anesthesia alone. The same changes occur in chronic illness of moderate or severe degree, and, in both acute and chronic illness, the more severe the illness the lower the serum T_3 concentration. (See review by Cavalieri and Rapoport, 1977.)

Since the decrease in serum T_3 concentration and increase in serum rT_3 are common to all three categories of sick euthyroid syndrome, differentiation among them is based upon values of the serum total T_4 concentration. Most often, this is not appreciably changed. Binding of T_4 is decreased in intensity, but the factors responsible for this change are uncertain. The concentration of TBPA is almost always decreased, but the extent to which this contributes to the decrease in hormone binding is uncertain. Some reduction in the serum total concentration is seen, sometimes to levels that are almost unmeasurable. It occurs in extremely ill patients and mainly is seen, therefore, in a hospital setting. The extent of lowering in the serum total T_4 concentration correlates with the severity of illness and indeed, with the subsequent mortality. Serum T_3 concentrations are usually very low, and rT_3 concentrations are increased, though not usually to the extent seen in patients in whom serum T_4 concentrations are normal. Abnormalities in the binding of T_4 are similar to those that occur in other patients who are ill, but are generally more marked. Characteristically, the fraction of free T_4 is greatly increased. Together with the subnormal total T_4 concentration, this leads to values of the free T_4 concentration that are occasionally slightly low, are usually normal, but may occasionally be increased. Because values of the *in vitro* T_3 uptake tests are only slightly increased, free T_4 indices, calculated in the conventional manner, are usually subnormal. It is not clear whether the pronounced reduction in serum T_4 concentration seen in this category of patients reflects a greatly enhanced metabolic clearance rate of T_4, a decrease in T_4 production and secretion, or perhaps a combination of the two. (See Chopra et al., 1979.)

The third category of patients is less well defined, less well studied, and apparently less frequent. It comprises intrinsically euthyroid patients with systemic illness in whom serum T_3 concentrations are subnormal and serum T_4 concentrations increased during their illness, but return to normal thereafter. The few data available indicate that the free T_4 index is elevated and the free T_3 index, calculated as the product of the serum total T_3 concentration and *in vitro* T_3 uptake value, is slightly subnormal or at the lower end of the normal range. Owing to the elevation in serum T_4 concentration, these patients may be difficult to differentiate from those with "T_4-toxicosis," i.e., patients with hyperthyroidism in whom serum T_3 concentration is reduced into the normal range by the inhibition of T_3-neogenesis produced by intercurrent illness. (See Burrows et al., 1975.)

As in patients undergoing starvation, those with the sick euthyroid syndrome display normal or only slightly increased values of the serum TSH concentration. Responses to exogenous TRH are certainly not increased and, in the most severely ill patients, may be subnormal, particularly when considered in relation to prevailing serum T_3 and free T_3 concentrations. Virtually nothing is known of the periph-

eral metabolic state of the patient with the sick euthyroid syndrome or whether the changes in thyroid hormone metabolism are beneficial, detrimental, or neither.

Other aspects of thyroid hormone economy may also be affected in patients with severe nonthyroid illness. In patients with cirrhosis, the RAIU is often increased, reflecting the iodine-deficient state that may result from a salt-restricted or inadequate diet. Conversely, in patients with chronic renal failure, the reduction in renal iodide clearance may lead to an increase in plasma iodide which would result, in turn, in a retardation of the RAIU. In addition, there appears to be a greatly increased prevalence of goiter in patients with chronic renal failure; the pathogenesis of this abnormality has not been ascertained, however (Lim et al., 1977).

As mentioned earlier, a decreased concentration of TBG in plasma is often found in patients with severe chronic illness, particularly those with nephrosis and alcoholic cirrhosis. By contrast, an increased concentration of TBG in plasma, with a resulting increase in serum T_4 concentration, is often seen in patients with acute hepatitis or those with chronic active hepatitis or biliary cirrhosis. In the latter two diseases, free T_4 concentrations in serum may be subnormal, suggesting that the patients may be mildly hypothyroid, possibly owing to associated chronic thyroiditis. (See Schussler et al., 1978.)

LABORATORY TESTS OF THYROID HORMONE ECONOMY

In considering the patient with known or suspected thyroid disease, the physician should seek to arrive at two types of diagnosis, an etiologic or anatomic diagnosis and a functional diagnosis. The one encompasses an appreciation of the underlying cause or nature of the disorder, as well as the associated pathologic change in the gland. The other encompasses a decision whether the physiologic and metabolic state of the patient is being conditioned by an excess, normal, or insufficient supply of thyroid hormone. In many instances, obviously, the one diagnosis facilitates or influences the other. For example, a patient with a single nonfunctioning nodule in an otherwise normal gland is likely to be euthyroid, while a patient with a nodule that feels similar but who has clinical and laboratory evidence of thyroid hormone excess is likely to have a benign autonomous adenoma. On the other hand, many ambiguities are possible. An anatomic diagnosis of chronic thyroiditis is consistent with a metabolic state of hypothyroidism, euthyroidism, or thyrotoxicosis, either in different patients or in the same patient at different times. Conversely, clinical and laboratory evidence of thyrotoxicosis may follow from any of a great many causes. Consequently, a complete diagnosis in patients with thyroid disease, which is requisite for proper therapy, recognizes and exploits the interplay between the patient's history, symptoms, and signs; the findings on palpation or biopsy of the thyroid gland; and the results of laboratory tests.

In the ensuing section, the laboratory tests employed as aids in the diagnosis of thyroid disease will be discussed in substantial detail. The reasons for this emphasis are many. For one, the fact that so many tests are available is in itself a source of confusion (see classification of tests in Table 4–3). More important, however, is the fact that procedures of increasing specificity and sensitivity have made possible diagnosis of thyroid dysfunction in patients in whom clinical findings are marginal or are obscured by coincidental nonthyroid disorders. Further, even when the clinical picture seems clear and the diagnosis straightforward, the

Table 4–3.   COMMONLY EMPLOYED LABORATORY
TESTS OF THYROID HORMONE ECONOMY

1. *Direct Tests of Thyroid Function*
     Thyroid radioiodine uptake (RAIU)
2. *Tests Related to the Concentration and Binding of Thyroid Hormones in the Blood*
     Measurements of Hormone Concentration
         Serum total T_4
         Serum total T_3
         Serum free T_4
     Measurements of Hormone Binding
         Percent of free T_4 (%FT_4)
         Resin T_3 uptake *in vitro* (RT_3U)
         Thyroxine-binding globulin (TBG)
3. *Tests That Assess the Metabolic Impact of the Thyroid Hormones*
     Basal metabolic rate (BMR)
     Serum cholesterol concentration
     Specific serum enzyme concentration
     Systolic time intervals
4. *Tests That Assess the Mechanisms for Regulating Thyroid Function*
     Serum TSH concentration
     TRH-stimulation test
     Thyroid suppression test
5. *Miscellaneous Tests*
     TSH-stimulation test
     Antithyroid antibodies
     Serum thyroglobulin concentration
     Immunoglobulins of Graves' disease
     External scintiscanning
     Ultrasonography
     Thyroid biopsy

physician often seeks both the reassurance of confirmatory laboratory findings and the advantage of obtaining pretreatment baseline values. Finally, the very profusion of testing procedures indicates that each procedure has inherent limitations. Thus none is uniformly reliable in all disorders of thyroid function, and virtually all are subject to alteration by endogenous or exogenous factors that complicate their interpretation. Such factors may cause the several indices to diverge from their expected values in a confusing or conflicting way. Nevertheless, through an appreciation of the specific physiologic datum which each test provides and the factors that may influence the results obtained, it is usually possible, through careful selection and interpretation, to achieve at least a reasonably thorough understanding of the physiopathologic aberration present in specific diseases states or individual patients. It is to emphasize this dependence of clinical interpretation on physiologic understanding that laboratory procedures are not discussed immediately after the description of the disease states but rather here, immediately after reviewing the physiology and biochemistry of the thyroid and its hormones.

Laboratory procedures can be divided into four major categories: (1) direct tests of thyroid function that provide quantitative or qualitative information or both about hormone synthesis and secretion; (2) tests related to the concentration and binding of the thyroid hormones and other iodinated materials in the blood; (3) tests that assess the impact of the thyroid hormones upon the tissues (metabolic indices); and (4) tests that assess the mechanisms for regulating thyroid function. There are in addition a variety of miscellaneous tests that do not fit into the other categories.

Direct Tests of Thyroid Function

Although many tests exist from which the state of thyroid function can be inferred, it is only by means of *in vivo* procedures that employ a radioactive isotope of iodine as a tag for the body's stable form of iodine, ^{127}I, that the function of the thyroid gland can be directly measured. Among the many tests of this general type that have been devised, the most common by far is the measurement of the fractional uptake by the thyroid of a tracer (chemically inconsequential) dose of radioiodine, the thyroid radioactive iodine uptake or RAIU. In the past, the RAIU was frequently employed as a major aid in the diagnosis of hyperthyroidism or hypothyroidism, but in the last decade or so, several factors have combined to make this less and less the case. The first is the improvement in indirect methods for assessing thyroid status, either through specific measurement of the thyroid hormones in blood or through assessment of the state of mechanisms for regulating thyroid function. The second is the progressive decline in normal values for thyroid radioiodine uptake consequent to the widespread moderate increase in daily dietary iodine intake. The latter has greatly reduced the usefulness of measurements of thyroid radioiodine uptake in the diagnosis of hypothyroid states.

Nonetheless, measurements of thyroid radioiodine accumulation are of critical import in a number of circumstances. Indeed, there is a resurgence of interest in RAIU, owing to its unique value in the diagnosis of the several thyrotoxic states in which the RAIU is characteristically low, rather than elevated, as it is in classic hyperthyroidism. The former include the syndrome of chronic thyroiditis with transient hyperthyroidism; subacute thyroiditis; iodine-induced hyperthyroidism; thyrotoxicosis factitia; and thyrotoxicosis due to hyperfunction of ectopic thyroid tissue. The RAIU also retains its use in the thyroid suppression test, in the occasional assessment of the thyroid's response to exogenous TSH, and in the diagnosis or exploration of defects in the intrathyroid metabolism of iodine.

At present, two radioactive isotopes of iodine, ^{131}I and ^{123}I, are most commonly employed in a clinical setting. ^{125}I is extensively used as a tracer for *in vitro* procedures, such as radioimmunoassays, because of its long half-life (60 days) and the consequent long shelf-life of reagents labeled with it. ^{131}I (half-life 8.1 days) and ^{123}I (half-life 0.55 day) are both emitters of gamma radiation, which permits their external detection and quantitation at sites of accumulation, such as the thyroid. Physiologically they are indistinguishable, not only from one another, but also from the naturally occurring stable isotope of iodine, ^{127}I, which permits their use as valid tracers. Although ^{131}I has been the radioisotope predominantly used for decades, the shorter half-life of ^{123}I makes it preferable, since the radiation delivered to the thyroid per microcurie of administered ^{123}I is only about one one-hundredth of that delivered by ^{131}I. Logistical problems related to its short half-life and high relative cost have limited its use to date, but ^{123}I is increasingly employed, nonetheless.

Measurements of Thyroid Iodine Accumulation

Physiologic Basis.   When tracer quantities of inorganic radioiodine are administered either orally or intravenously, the isotope quickly becomes uniformly mixed with the endogenous stable iodide within the ECF. Immediately upon its entrance into the ECF, I* begins to be removed by its two major sites of clearance, the thyroid and the kidneys. As this process continues, the plasma concentration of I* declines exponentially. Normally, very low values are reached by 24 hours, and inorganic I* is virtually undetectable in the plasma by 72 hours after its administration. Since the quantity of I* that enters the thyroid (or urine) during any time period is proportional to the concentration of I* in the plasma, the thyroid content of I* increases rapidly during the early hours, then at a decreasing rate until a virtual plateau is reached. The proportion of administered I* ultimately accumulated by the thyroid is a function of the relative rates of clearance of iodide by the thyroid and kidneys. The relation is simply expressed as follows:

$$\text{RAIU at plateau (\%)} = \frac{C_T}{C_T + C_K} \times 100$$

where C_T represents the thyroid iodide clearance rate and C_K the renal iodide clearance rate. Since the normal thyroid iodide clearance rate is approximately 0.4 liter/hr and the renal iodide clearance rate 2.0 liters/hr, the ultimate uptake of I* normally approximates 17% of the administered dose (range, approximately 5–30%).

The plateau value of the percentage thyroid uptake of I* indicates the statistical likelihood that any molecule of iodide leaving the ECF will be accumulated by the thyroid and hence indicates the percentage of all the iodide removed from the ECF during any time period that is taken up by the thyroid. Measurements of the percentage RAIU are generally made at 24 hours not only as a matter of convenience but also because the value at 24 hours is usually near its plateau except in unusual circumstances noted below.

Usually, measurements of the RAIU are taken to indicate the rate of thyroid hormone synthesis and, by inference, the ongoing rate at which thyroid hormones are being released into the blood. In most instances, this is justified. However, interpretation of the RAIU in this manner is based on several assumptions which are not always valid. These are: (1) that the flux of iodide into and out of the ECF is occurring at a normal rate, i.e., that the concentration of iodide in the ECF is within the normal range; (2) that significant quantities of I* have not already been organified and secreted from the gland by the time the RAIU is being measured; (3) that the iodine being accumulated is being utilized in a normal manner for the synthesis of hormone; and (4) that it is not merely being utilized to replenish depleted thyroid hormone stores. Circumstances in which these assumptions are not valid and the means by which they can be tested will be discussed later.

RAIU. This is the most commonly used isotopic procedure for the assessment of thyroid function per se. The 24-hour interval is generally selected not only because of its convenience to the patient but also because the value is then at or near its plateau except in severe abnormal states. Except in the latter circumstances, when measurements are best made at a far different time interval, it is not necessary that the uptake be determined at precisely 24 hours. Little difference will be noted if the uptake is measured any time during the day following the day on which the isotope was administered.

The dose of I* is usually given orally. There is no requirement that the patient be fasting before receiving the isotope or that special dietary precautions be observed thereafter. No restrictions on the activity of the patient need be imposed, and no adverse reactions occur. At the designated time interval, the thyroid content of I* is determined with a suitable detector, and this is compared with the I* content of the administered dose (counting standard), positioned so as to simulate the geometric relationship of the patient's thyroid to the detector.

Because of the varying sensitivity of different counting devices to scattered or secondary radiation, variations in the geometry of the counting apparatus, and variations in

Table 4–4. FACTORS THAT INFLUENCE THE 24-HOUR THYROID I* UPTAKE

1. *Factors that Increase Uptake*
   Reflecting increased hormone synthesis
     Hyperthyroidism
     Response to glandular hormone depletion
       Recovery from thyroid suppression
       Recovery from subacute thyroiditis
       Antithyroid agents
     Excessive hormone losses
       Nephrosis
       Chronic diarrheal states
       Soybean ingestion
   Not reflecting increased hormone synthesis
     Iodine deficiency
       Dietary supply
       Excessive loss (dehalogenase defect, pregnancy)
     Hormone biosynthetic defects

2. *Factors that Decrease Uptake*
   Reflecting decreased hormone synthesis
     Primary hypofunction
       Thyroprivic hypothyroidism
       Antithyroid agents
       Some hormone biosynthetic defects
       Hashimoto's disease
       Subacute thyroiditis
     Secondary hypofunction
       Trophoprivic hypothyroidism
       Exogenous thyroid hormones
   Not reflecting decreased hormone synthesis
     Increased availability of iodine
       Dietary or pharmacologic supply
       Cardiac or renal insufficiency
     Increased hormone release
       Very severe hyperthyroidism (rare)

iodine intake, the range of normal values for the uptake at any time interval varies among laboratories and should be determined individually. In general, the range of normal values is approximately 5–30%. Higher values indicate thyroid hyperfunction; this usually but not always reflects hormone overproduction and a thyrotoxic state. Unfortunately, as with most other procedures, clinically difficult cases with mild hyperthyroidism often display values at or just above the upper limit of the normal range. (See Table 4–4 for a classification of factors that affect the RAIU.)

Sometimes under certain conditions it is best to measure the uptake before 24 hours after administration of the isotope. In states of severe thyroid hyperfunction, the uptake may be exceedingly rapid, plateau values being reached within a few hours or less. Thereafter, release of accumulated I*, either as true hormone in severe hyperthyroidism or as some hormonally inactive product, may be so rapid that the value for the uptake at 24 hours is well below its maximum and occasionally within the normal range. In hyperthyroidism this is rare, and the clinical manifestations in such cases are so clear as to make the diagnosis obvious. Nevertheless, some laboratories choose to measure the uptake at an earlier time when hyperthyroidism is suspected.

Thyroid Iodide Clearance Rate. Measurements of the thyroid iodide clearance rate are the most direct means of assessing the efficiency of the thyroid in extracting iodide from its perfusate. As with measurements of a renal clearance rate, the thyroid iodide clearance rate can be calculated as the quotient of the rate of entry of I* into the gland during any period of time and the plasma I* concentration during that period. Because the I* should be given intravenously, and because conjoint measurements of I* in thyroid and plasma are required, measurements of clearance rates are seldom made in a clinical setting, but remain valuable investigative tools.

Urinary Excretion of Radioiodine. Since the thyroid and kidneys together account for the removal of almost all iodide lost from ECF, the maximal urinary excretion of I* and maximal thyroid accumulation of I* should together approach 100% of the administered dose. In the past, accordingly, measurements of urinary I* excretion were employed as a means of estimating the RAIU. Currently, this is no longer done, but measurements of urinary I* excretion are occasionally of value nonetheless, principally when values of the RAIU are unexpectedly low. A clearly subnormal value for the sum of thyroid and urinary I*, assuming that the urine collection is complete, points strongly toward accumulation of I* in some ectopic focus or foci outside the thyroid area. These should be sought by external scintiscans performed with labeled pertechnetate or larger doses of radioiodine.

Absolute Iodine Uptake. As already mentioned, isotopic measurements of thyroid iodine accumulation provide information only about rates of movement (e.g., clearance rates) or proportionate distribution (e.g., percentage uptake) of iodine. Although isotopic procedures are widely used alone because of their relative simplicity, the information that both the clinician and the physiologist truly desire, i.e., the absolute rate of iodine accumulation, requires conjoint measurement of radioactive and stable iodine. Such measurements are not generally employed clinically but have nevertheless provided important information of both a clinical and physiologic nature. Furthermore, the principles upon which measurements of absolute iodine uptake are based are diagnostically applicable in the difficult clinical case.

All methods for measuring the absolute rate of thyroid iodine uptake or AIU are based on the inability of organs that metabolize iodine to distinguish between radioiodine and ^{127}I. The simplest method for measuring AIU is to administer I* and then, over any time period, to measure the thyroid uptake of I* and the urinary excretion of both I* and ^{127}I. AIU is then readily calculated from the following proportion:

$$\frac{\text{Thyroid } ^{127}I \text{ uptake (AIU)}}{\text{Thyroid I* uptake}} = \frac{\text{Urinary } ^{127}I \text{ content}}{\text{Urinary I* content}}$$

In a clinical setting, measurements of the AIU have value in determining whether or not discordances between the apparent clinical state and the value of the RAIU are due to abnormalities in iodine intake. For example, a hyperthyroid patient ingesting a few milligrams of iodine daily may have a normal RAIU, but measured values of the AIU will be elevated.

States Associated with an Increased RAIU

Although an increased RAIU may reflect the overproduction and ultimate release of excessive quantities of thyroid hormone, it is important to recognize that many other factors will produce a similar abnormality. An increase will occur whenever the thyroid iodide clearance rate is increased relative to that of the kidney. Such may reflect not hyperthyroidism but, for example, a compensatory response to factors tending to produce hypothyroidism. The following are the more important clinical states associated with an increased RAIU.

Hyperthyroidism. Except in the case of T_3 toxicosis (see below), hyperthyroidism is almost invariably associated with an increased RAIU, unless body iodide stores are in-

creased. Such increases in uptake are evident at all times of measurement except in patients with severe thyrotoxicosis, in whom release of hormone is so rapid that the thyroid content of I* has declined to the normal range by the time the measurement is made; this is rare and is usually associated with flagrant thyrotoxicosis. Unfortunately, in cases that are clinically marginal, values of the RAIU are often within or just above the upper limit of the normal range, as would be expected.

Aberrations in Hormone Synthesis. RAIU is increased in the absence of hyperthyroidism in a number of disorders in which accumulated iodine is inefficiently or ineffectively used to synthesize and secrete active hormone. Here, the impairment in iodine use leads to enhanced sensitivity to TSH, hypersecretion of TSH, or both; this in turn produces both goiter and stimulation of all steps in hormone synthesis capable of response. As a result, synthesis of normal quantities of hormone may resume; the patient will be metabolically normal but goitrous. Alternatively, secretion of hormone may remain inadequate, and the patient will display goitrous hypothyroidism. This sequence occurs as a consequence of defects in the organic-binding or coupling mechanisms or in the structure of the thyroglobulin molecule. It is also a consequence of disorders in which hormonally inactive products are released from the gland in the form of iodotyrosines (dehalogenase defect) or iodoproteins, including thyroglobulin. The magnitude of the increase in uptake and the time at which the plateau is achieved vary with the nature and severity of the disorder. (See Stanbury, 1978, for references and illustrated functional patterns.) Differentiation of the foregoing states from hyperthyroidism is generally not difficult since, in the former, clinical evidence of hyperthyroidism will be lacking and indeed hypothyroidism may be present. Furthermore, other indices of thyroid hormone production and thyroregulatory control will be concordant with the clinical state.

Iodine Deficiency. Increases in RAIU occur in response to acute or chronic iodine deficiency. Such can be demonstrated by measurement of urinary iodine excretion, values lower than 100 μg/day indicating a deficiency state. Chronic iodine deficiency is most often the result of an inadequate content of iodine in the food and water on which the patients subsist (endemic iodine deficiency). In regions of the world where iodine intake is sufficient, as in the United States, deficiency of iodine may also result from other than environmental factors. Patients with cardiac, renal, or hepatic disease may develop iodine deficiency if given diets severely restricted in salt, especially if diuretic agents are administered. Iodine deficiency not uncommonly occurs in patients with thyrotoxicosis treated with antithyroid drugs; this may forestall recurrence of thyrotoxicity when treatment is withdrawn (Harden et al., 1966). Thyroid hyperfunction in the normal pregnant woman is probably the result of increased renal iodide clearance. Iodine deficiency evidently plays a role in the goitrous hypothyroidism associated with deficiency of thyroid and peripheral iodotyrosine dehalogenase, in which large quantities of iodine are lost in the urine as iodotyrosines.

In severe iodine deficiency, in addition to the quantitative adjustments in thyroid avidity for iodide which the increased RAIU reflects, a qualitative adaptation occurs in which T_3 is preferentially synthesized and secreted. As a result, the ratio of T_3 to T_4 in the plasma is increased. This mechanism has important adaptive value, since for each atom of iodine secreted the caloric impact is approximately four times as great when the iodine is affixed to T_3 as when it is part of T_4.

Response to Thyroid Hormone Depletion. Withdrawal of factors that lead to thyroid hormone depletion is associated with a rebound increase in thyroid hormone synthesis without an associated increase in hormone release. If hormone depletion has been produced by factors that lead to decreased hormone supply to the tissues, such as antithyroid drugs, the rebound response may reflect in part enhanced TSH stimulation and in part an autoregulatory response to depletion of thyroid hormone stores. In other instances, only the latter mechanism appears responsible. Rebound increases in RAIU are seen after withdrawal of antithyroid therapy, after subsidence of transient or subacute thyroiditis, and after prolonged suppression of thyroid function by exogenous hormone. A striking increase in uptake is evident in patients with iodide-induced myxedema following cessation of iodide administration. The duration of the rebound is variable and probably depends on the time required to replenish thyroid hormone stores. Generally its duration is no longer than several weeks, but after withdrawal of prolonged thyroid suppression, an abnormally high uptake may persist for many weeks. Differentiation from thyrotoxicosis is evident from the history and from differences in the values of other conventional indices of thyroid function.

Excessive Hormone Losses.   Instances in which excessive losses of thyroid hormone occur may be associated with a compensatory increase in hormone synthesis that is, in turn, evident in an increased RAIU. The outstanding example of this sequence occurs in nephrosis, in which excessive losses of hormone in the urine in association with urinary loss of binding protein take place. In addition, diminished binding of T_4 in the plasma in nephrosis may lead to excessive loss of hormone via the feces. A similar sequence may occur when losses of hormone via the GI tract are abnormal, such as in chronic diarrheal states or during ingestion of soybean, which binds hormone in the gut.

States Associated with a Decreased RAIU

As indicated earlier, in the United States, the RAIU has largely lost its value in the diagnosis of the most common varieties of hypothyroidism, those that result from insufficient functioning thyroid tissue (thyroprivic hypothyroidism) or from inadequate stimulation of the thyroid (trophoprivic hypothyroidism). This is owing to a general increase in iodine intake that has made values of the RAIU in these disorders indistinguishable from those at the lower end of the normal range. In disorders characterized by aberrations in hormone synthesis, which are generally accompanied by goiter and sometimes by hypothyroidism, values of the RAIU are normal or increased.

Ironically, therefore, the major indication for measuring the RAIU is to establish not the diagnosis of hypothyroidism, but rather the diagnosis of those causes of thyrotoxicosis that are associated with decreased values of the RAIU. As discussed in detail subsequently, these are disorders in which the source of the excess thyroid hormone either is outside the thyroid gland or is a leakage of hormone from a gland that is not actively synthesizing hormone. In addition, the RAIU is subnormal in true hyperthyroidism associated with or actually caused by excessive iodine intake (Jod-Basedow phenomenon). The value of measurements of urinary stable iodine excretion in differentiating excess of iodine from other causes of subnormal RAIU cannot be overemphasized.

Hypothyroidism.   The technical problem involved in utilizing the RAIU as an aid to the diagnosis of hypothyroidism needs no further discussion. A special variety of thyroid failure is that which occurs when destruction of thyroid tissue by chronic inflammation or ablative treatment (surgery or ^{131}I) is incomplete. In this syndrome, often interchangeably termed "decreased thyroid reserve" or "subclinical hypothyroidism," mild symptoms of hypothyroidism may or may not be present. Values of the RAIU are often normal, but fail to increase after administration of exogenous TSH. The main diagnostic features of this syndrome are, however, evidence of predisposing causes and the presence of mild or moderate elevations of serum TSH concentration.

Exogenous Thyroid Hormone: Thyrotoxicosis Factitia.   Except in those disorders in which homeostatic control is disrupted or overridden (e.g., Graves' disease or autonomously functioning thyroid nodules), administration of exogenous thyroid hormone will suppress the TSH secretory mechanism and reduce the RAIU, usually to values below 5%. Suppression of uptake can be effected by adequate quantities of any thyroactive material and, depending on the dose administered, a normal or hypermetabolic state will be present. Suppression of the RAIU by physiologic quantities of hormone is, of course, the basis for the normal response in the thyroid suppression test, discussed later in this section. In the same way, lowering of the RAIU is often used as an index of the adequacy of suppressive therapy in nontoxic goiter, while, in this disease, failure of the RAIU to suppress nearly completely when adequate doses of exogenous hormone are administered signals the presence of foci whose function does not depend on TSH stimulation.

Low values of the RAIU in a patient who is clinically thyrotoxic may indicate the presence of thyrotoxicosis factitia, the syndrome produced by the ingestion, often surreptitious, of excess quantities of thyroid hormone. In the absence of preexisting goiter, an impalpable thyroid is often another clue. If the offending agent is levothyroxine (T_4) or thyroid extract, values for both the total and free T_4 and T_3 concentrations in serum will be increased. On the other hand, if liothyronine (T_3) is the hormone being consumed in excess, then the serum total and free T_4 concentrations will be decreased and the serum T_3 concentration increased. The response to exogenous TRH will be abolished in either instance.

Disorders of Hormone Storage.   Values of the RAIU are usually very low in two disorders of the thyroid, the early phase of subacute thyroiditis and the syndrome of chronic thyroiditis with transient hyperthyroidism. Here, inflammatory disease leads to follicular disruption, loss of the normal storage function of the gland, and leakage of hormone into the blood. In the early stage of the former disease, leakage of hormone accompanied by hormonally inactive iodoproteins is usually sufficient to suppress TSH secretion and decrease the RAIU greatly, and is often sufficient to produce thyrotoxicosis. Damage to the follicular epithelium also plays a role in some cases, since the RAIU may not respond well to exogenous TSH. In the latter syndrome, thyrotoxicosis is present, by definition, and TSH secretion is suppressed. In both disorders, the thyrotoxic phase is transient and should not be treated by the measures employed in patients who are hyperthyroid, in whom ongoing overproduction of hormone is present. Transient hypothyroidism often occurs late in both diseases, presumably when stores of preformed hormone are depleted; the RAIU may return to normal or increased values at that time. Histologic and clinical features of these diseases are discussed more fully in the later section on diseases associated with thyrotoxicosis.

Exposure to Excessive Iodine.   Exposure to excessive iodine and expansion of body iodide stores is probably the most common cause for a subnormal RAIU. Such decreases are "spurious" in the clinical sense, since they do not indicate decreased absolute iodine uptake and decreased hormone production. They are not spurious in the physiologic sense, however, since they reflect a desirable homeostatic response to overavailability of the iodide substrate.

The decreased fractional uptake of iodide resides in an autoregulatory inhibition of the iodide transport mechanism as a result of the increase in the glandular stores of organic iodine. In addition, when plasma iodide concentrations are sufficiently high, dilution of the administered isotope by stable iodide would lead to a decreased percentage accumulation of the isotope. As indicated in an earlier section, the compensatory response to excessive iodine stores is not perfect, and total iodine accumulation during continued overabundance of iodide will exceed normal values. Nevertheless, the excess iodine is not incorporated into active hormone but is organified and then lost from the gland largely as iodide itself.

A decreased RAIU can be produced by the introduction of excessive quantities of iodine into the body in any form — inorganic, organic, or elemental. Special offenders in this regard are organic iodinated dyes used as x-ray contrast media. The duration of suppression of the uptake varies from individual to individual and with the compound administered, depending on its rapidity of excretion or deiodination. In general, dyes used for pyelography are cleared relatively rapidly, while those used in cholecystography persist longer and may influence the uptake for several months. Inorganic iodide may be ingested directly, usually as an expectorant, and following a single large dose, a decreased uptake may persist for several days. Following chronic ingestion of iodide, depression of the uptake may persist for many weeks. It should be noted in this regard that Lugol's solution or saturated solution of potassium iodine (SSKI) in the dosage usually given will deliver up to about 500 mg of iodine daily. In addition to iodide per se and iodinated dyes, excessive quantities of iodine may be encountered in a variety of other forms, including vitamins and mineral preparations, vaginal or rectal suppositories, and iodinated antiseptics. Some preparations of barium sulfate used in x-ray diagnosis may contain substantial quantities of iodine. Very large quantities of iodine are ingested in the form of kelp by dietary faddists. Inhibition of uptake resulting from excess stable iodine is of shorter duration in hyperthyroid than in normal individuals.

The measurement of urinary iodine excretion is an invaluable means of establishing or excluding the existence of excessive body iodide stores. Such measurements should always be made when a low value of the RAIU is otherwise unexplained. Values in excess of several milligrams daily are sufficient in themselves to account for the low RAIU, while values less than 1000 μg daily, when the RAIU is low, strongly suggest the presence of one of the other disorders discussed in this section.

Measurements of Thyroid Radioiodine Turnover

Physiologic Basis. Following accumulation and organification of radioiodine, release from the thyroid of labeled products occurs. In a general way, the fractional rate of release or turnover of thyroid iodine can be inferred either from direct observation of the rate of radioiodine disappearance from the gland or from the rate of appearance of radioiodinated products in the blood. There are, however, several problems involved in drawing conclusions about the absolute rate of release of thyroid hormone from observations of the types just described. First, any inference concerning the quantity of hormone released requires knowledge of the iodine content of the pool or pools whose turnover is being measured; this is rarely available. Furthermore, the earlier, tacitly accepted concept that the entire thyroid behaves as a homogeneous entity is no longer tenable. Both anatomic and functional heterogeneity exists in the thyroid. Hence the iodine released is likely drawn from at least several pools of varying iodine content and turnover rate. Finally, other products (including iodide, iodotyrosines, and thyroglobulin or other iodoproteins) may be released. Their release would, of course, be reflected in the loss of ^{131}I from the gland or the appearance of radioiodinated materials in the blood.

Thyroid Release of ^{131}I. In this technique, a moderately large dose of ^{131}I (50 μCi or more) is administered and allowed to accumulate in the thyroid. Serial epithyroid counts will then reveal the rate of release of accumulated ^{131}I. This isotope, rather than ^{123}I, is used because its relatively long half-life permits prolonged observation. In order that the curve describing release of the initially accumulated ^{131}I not be obscured by reaccumulation of ^{131}I already secreted by the gland, completely blocking doses of an antithyroid agent are generally administered. When this is done, the curve of epithyroid counts closely conforms to a single exponential function of time, indicating the release of a constant fraction of thyroid ^{131}I unit time. When corrected for physical decay of the isotope, such observations indicate a rate of turnover of accumulated ^{131}I in normal humans of about 1% daily. The rate of glandular ^{131}I turnover is accelerated, often greatly so, in states associated with thyroid hyperfunction. In view of the considerable period of time and multiple observations required by this technique, it is rarely used for clinical diagnosis, particularly since indirect methods involving measurement of hormonal radioiodine in blood are available. The technique has, however, been very effectively employed in physiologic studies. TSH can be shown to enhance acutely, and iodide to retard acutely, the rate of iodine release (see Fig. 4–12).

Tests Related to the Concentration and Binding of Thyroid Hormones in Blood

Measurements of the concentration of thyroid hormones in serum, together with tests that assess the extent of their association with thyroid hormone–binding proteins, are the most commonly employed laboratory aids for differentiating among the hypothyroid, euthyroid, and thyrotoxic states. Several factors have combined to make such measurements almost always the first laboratory tests to which the physician turns in evaluating a patient's thyroid status. Among them are the declining utility of the RAIU in the diagnosis of thyroid hypofunction and the fact that tests performed on the patient's blood are by far the most convenient. Most important of all, however, is that such tests, when combined with a suggestive clinical picture, are sufficient to establish an accurate functional diagnosis in well over 90% of cases. Because of their general use and clinical importance, their physiologic interest, and the large number of factors that influence their interpretation, these tests will be discussed in considerable detail.

General Considerations

Sensitive and specific radioimmunoassays are widely available for measuring the serum concentrations of those thyroid hormones that are of major clinical importance, T_4, T_3, and in some instances rT_3. Moreover, the manner in which the concentration of these hormones is influenced by changes in the thyroid hormone–binding proteins, especially TBG, is generally well understood. This has been considered in detail in earlier sections, which the reader is advised to review. (See sections on Hormone Transport and Alterations in the Transport, Turnover, and Metabolism of the Thyroid Hormones.) What emerges from these considerations is that the metabolic state of the patient, over a wide range of clinical states, correlates much more closely with the free hormone concentration in serum than with the total hormone concentration. Hence, it is strongly recommended that the physician take account of this fact, at least in the initial evaluation of the patient, by obtaining some datum which provides evidence of the free hormone concentration. This can be a measurement of the free hormone concentration itself, an estimate thereof as in a free hormone index, or perhaps a measurement of the concentration of the major binding protein, TBG. As the ensuing section reveals, a profusion of tests exist by which any or all of these can be assessed. Thus, the physician has in hand both the knowledge and the tools that are needed for using measurements of the thyroid hormones in blood as an efficient and effective means for diagnosing thyroid dysfunction.

Nonetheless, some problems persist. First, the degree of abnormality in the tests employed is generally well correlated with the severity of the functional disturbance. Consequently, in patients with mild hypothyroidism or mild thyrotoxicosis, concentrations of the thyroid hormones in the serum, both total and free, may not be clearly different from normal values, and other types of diagnostic tests will be required. Further, many factors other than the supply or production of T_4 and T_3 and the concentration of TBG in plasma can influence the concentration of the two hormones, either singly or together. Acute and chronic illness, starvation, and a variety of drugs decrease serum T_3 concentration, but leave the serum T_4 unchanged or slightly increased. Some patients with a newly described disorder inherit an abnormal protein that binds T_4 but not T_3. They remain euthyroid, despite an elevated serum T_4 concentration, but unlike patients with an increased TBG, display no increase in serum T_3. Finally, some patients develop circulating antibodies against T_4 or T_3. These endogenous antibodies interfere with radioimmunoassays for their specific antigens, causing spurious values that are either much too high or much too low, depending on the details of the method employed.

In the section that follows, the thyroid and nonthyroid disorders that alter serum T_4 and T_3 concentrations, either together or separately, will be defined and discussed. Because of the diverse combinations of change that can be seen, and the many factors that produce them, no classification that is both comprehensive and completely consistent can be devised. Therefore, to assist the reader in locating a topic of interest, Table 4–6 contains an outline of the topics discussed and the major heading under which they will each be found.

Table 4–5. FACTORS THAT IMPAIR PERIPHERAL CONVERSION OF T_4 TO T_3

1. *Physiologic*
   Fetal and early neonatal life
   Old age?
2. *Pathologic*
   Fasting, malnutrition
   Systemic illness
   Trauma, postoperative state
3. *Pharmacologic*
   Drugs (propylthiouracil, dexamethasone, propranolol, aminodarone)
   Radiographic contrast agents

Measurements of Hormone Concentrations

For the thyroid hormones that are of principal clinical interest, T_4, T_3, and rT_3, total concentrations in the blood are almost always measured in whole serum by sensitive and specific radioimmunoassays, but enzyme-linked immunoassays, which are subject to automation, are receiving increasing attention. The quantities of serum required are small (10–100 μl). Commercial kits have greatly extended the availability and convenience of the assays. The tests are rapid; results are usually available within hours after the sample reaches the laboratory, and certainly the same day. Apart from the usual errors to which any measurement procedure or radioimmunoassay is susceptible, errors peculiar to tests for the thyroid hormones result from competition for the labeled antigen between the specific antibody and other binding proteins. This can occur if binding of the hormone-antigen to plasma proteins is not adequately inhibited by the agents used for this purpose, or if the patient's serum contains an endogenous antibody to the hormone that is being measured.

Serum T_4 Concentration. Measurement of the serum T_4 concentration, preferably with some means of evaluating the state of thyroid hormone binding, is the test the physician usually employs first as an aid in the diagnosis of hypothyroidism or thyrotoxicosis. The normal range in healthy, euthyroid adults lies between approximately 4 and 11 $\mu g/dl$, but small variations in the normal range among different laboratories and different methods should be taken into account. Serum T_4 concentrations at birth are higher than values in the normal adult, owing to the higher concentration of TBG in neonatal plasma; free T_4 concentrations are about the same as in normal adults. Values rise abruptly within a few hours after birth, peak at about 24 hours, and then gradually decline, but, until the age of about 5 years, remain somewhat higher than those present later in life. They then remain unchanged through the remainder of life, though small decreases have been observed by some in seemingly normal individuals undergoing senescence.

Serum T_3 Concentration. Measurements of the serum T_3 concentration are especially valuable in diagnosing hyperthyroidism and in following the course of therapy of this disorder. They are also useful adjuncts to clinical observation in avoiding overtreatment in patients with hypothyroidism being given synthetic T_4 (levothyroxine). In this respect, they may be more valuable than measurements of the serum T_4 concentration are; values of the latter are frequently elevated in patients receiving levothyroxine, even though they do not appear to be thyrotoxic.

Normal values of the serum T_3 concentration, like those of the serum T_4, vary among different laboratories and test procedures, but generally range between approximately 80 and 180 ng/dl. Serum T_3 concentrations normally display very marked age-related changes. At birth, concentrations are well below those found in normal adults. Within a few hours, however, the serum T_3 concentration rises abruptly, peaking at about 24 hours at values well into the thyrotoxic range for adults. Values gradually decline during the next few weeks, but are somewhat higher (by about 25%) than those in normal adults through early adolescence (see Westgren et al., 1976, and Fig. 4–14). An as yet unresolved question is whether serum T_3 concentrations decrease in the normal, euthyroid elderly, since data to the point are contradictory. Some reports describe a progressive decline with age throughout life, but others do not. Several suggest a decrease in serum T_3 concentration from the approximate age of 65 years onward, but some do not. The problem is complicated by the ability of even moderate nonthyroid

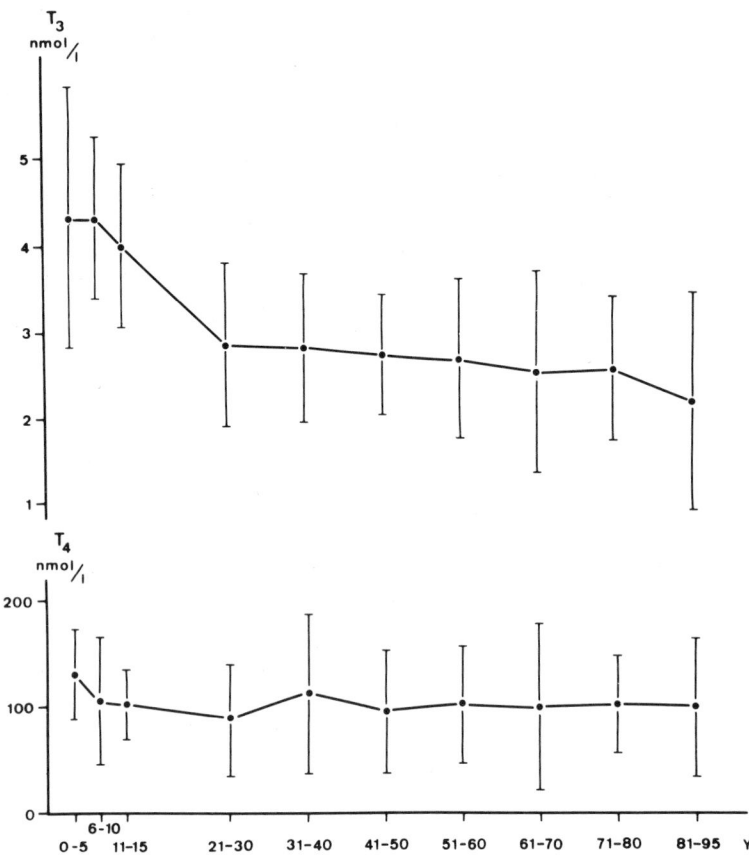

Figure 4–14. Changes with age in the serum concentrations of T_3 and T_4. (From Westgren, U., et al.: Blood levels of 3,5,3′-triiodothyronine and thyroxine: differences between children, adults, and elderly subjects. *Acta Med. Scand. 200*:493, 1976.)

illness to decrease the peripheral conversion of T_4 to T_3 and to lower the serum T_3 concentration. Thus, it is possible that the infirmities of old age, rather than old age itself, produce those age-related decreases in serum T_3 concentration that have been observed. Indeed, most of the studies of serum T_3 concentration in aging were carried out before the effects of illness and nutritional state on this function were recognized.

This problem is not one of mere idle interest, since it bears heavily on the question of the levels of the serum T_3 concentration that are diagnostic of thyrotoxicosis in elderly patients. While it may be true that serum T_3 concentrations do not decrease in the elderly if the subjects are meticulously selected, the authors' experience is that serum T_3 concentrations in randomly selected elderly individuals who are not especially ill are, nonetheless, often at the lower end of the normal range for younger adults. Consequently, values at the upper end of the usual normal range in patients in the seventh and especially the eight and ninth decades of life should be considered suggestive of thyrotoxicosis.

Serum rT_3 Concentration. Measurements of the serum rT_3 concentration are not yet widely available, though it is likely that increasingly they will become so owing to their value in selected clinical circumstances. The rT_3 in serum is present almost entirely as a result of its generation from T_3 in the peripheral tissues. Consequently, the quantity of T_4 available is an important determinant of the serum rT_3 concentration, so that it rises in thyrotoxicosis and declines in hypothyroidism. A second determinant of serum rT_3 concentration is, however, the rate of its metabolism, which proceeds mainly by 5′-monodeiodination to yield 3,3′-T_2. As a result, serum rT_3 concentrations are almost always elevated in euthyroid individuals subjected to those factors that inhibit the conversion of T_4 to T_3, a process that also involves 5′-monodeiodination (see Fig. 4–4 and Table 4—5). Therefore, increases in the serum rT_3 concentration may be helpful in differentiating the patient with the sick euthyroid syndrome (see earlier) whose serum T_4 and T_3 concentrations are low from the patient who is truly hypothyroid. In a patient with intercurrent illness whose serum T_4 concentration is elevated and serum T_3 concentration is normal or low, a greatly increased serum rT_3 concentration suggests that the patient is truly hyperthyroid and has T_4-toxicosis, rather than the transient hyperthyroxinemia sometimes associated with illness (Birkhauser et al., 1977).

Values for the concentration of rT_3 in serum are very low, owing to the rapid metabolic clearance of rT_3. Values differ greatly among different laboratories for reasons that are not understood, but normal means aggregate at about 20 ng/dl in some laboratories and about 40 ng/dl in others; this must be considered in interpreting any measurement. Serum rT_3 concentrations are greatly elevated at birth, but decline to stable values by about the fifth day of life. Values in the elderly tend to increase somewhat, possibly in accord with a concomitant decrease in serum T_3, but uncertainties regarding the frequency and cause of any such increase are entirely analogous to those already described in relation to the serum T_3 concentration.

Serum PBI. Although the mainstay of thyroid diagnosis for many years, measurements of PBI are now infrequently performed. The serum PBI measures iodine in T_4, the exceedingly small quantity of iodine in other iodothyronines, a great variety of iodinated materials of exogenous origin that are bound to protein, and a class of compounds, usually of endogenous origin, termed iodoproteins, in which iodine is covalently bound within the peptide sequence of the protein molecule. Hence, when exogenous contaminants are absent, the difference between the PBI and the T_4-iodine is an index of the iodine contained in iodoproteins. Such iodoproteins are commonly found in the sera of patients with Hashimoto's disease and subacute thyroiditis and may also be present in the sera of patients with nontoxic goiter and thyroid neoplasms. Here, measurement of the PBI–T_4-iodine difference may be of diagnostic value. Thus the PBI is no longer used as a measure of hormonal iodine but rather as a measure of nonhormonal iodine in the blood.

Measurements of Hormone Binding

As indicated earlier, the importance of tests that reflect hormone binding in serum stems from the fact that they afford the most convenient means of determining whether a change in the total concentration of hormone is due to a change in its binding or a change in its production rate. In the same sense, but put somewhat differently, they provide either direct or inferential evidence of whether an abnormality in the total concentration of a hormone in serum reflects a change in free hormone concentration. They assume critical importance, therefore, in differentiating hyperthyroidism and hypothyroidism from the euthyroid state.

Proportion and Concentration of Free T_4 and T_3. The absolute concentrations of free T_4 (FT_4) and free T_3 (FT_3) in serum are exceedingly low, and consequently have not been susceptible to direct measurement. As a result, such measurements have been performed by the difficult and cumbersome *dialysis* or *ultracentrifugation techniques*, particularly the former. Serum is enriched with a tracer concentration of the labeled hormone of interest. This quickly distributes itself between the free and bound forms to match the distribution of the endogenous hormone. The fraction of hormone that dialyzes or ultrafilters through a semipermeable membrane, which passes the free hormone but not the bound, is then measured. The absolute concentration of free hormone can then be a calculated simply as the product of the total hormone concentration and the fraction that is unbound or free.

Since methods of analysis differ in detail, normal values for the proportion of free T_4 have been variable, but generally range between 0.02 and 0.04% of the total. Because of the lesser affinity of T_3 for TBG, the proportion of free T_3 is normally about 10 times that of T_4, i.e., 0.30% of the total. Normal values for FT_4 approximate 2 ng/dl and for FT_3 about 0.4 ng/dl.

By means of very high-affinity antibodies, which are not generally available, it has become possible to measure chemical concentrations of FT_4 and FT_3 by *direct radioimmunoassay of dialysates*. Apart from the fact that they obviate the need to use radioisotopes, these methods appear to have no persuasive advantage over conventional dialysis techniques, since a cumbersome dialysis procedure is still required.

Considerable attention has been drawn recently to *commercially developed radioimmunoassay methods* for measuring FT_4 which are intended to supplant the far more cumbersome and time-consuming dialysis method. Although they do not truly measure the FT_4 directly, they yield values very similar to those found by dialysis in hypothyroidism and hyperthyroidism, as well as in patients with nonthyroid illness (Bayer and McDougall, 1980). Should they prove to have the same degree of reliability in all other states of interest, they will be extremely useful.

In Vitro Uptake Tests. Since direct measurements of the proportion of free T_4 and T_3 by dialysis are time-consuming and cumbersome, a variety of simpler methods have been devised. In common with measurements of the proportion of free T_4 and T_3, these provide evidence of the overall intensity of hormone binding in serum. They serve as an index, therefore, of the proportion of free T_4 and T_3. Such tests are performed by enriching the patient's serum with a tracer quantity of radioiodine-labeled hormone and incubating the serum with an insoluble particulate material that is capable of binding the hormone and competing with the binding proteins in the serum phase. After a standard interval, the proportion of labeled hormone bound by the particulate phase is determined. This varies inversely with the concentration and binding affinity of unoccupied binding sites on the individual binding proteins, principally TBG. Labeled T_3 is usually used in preference to labeled T_4 because of its less intense binding; this yields a higher uptake onto the particulate material, thereby reducing counting error. Variations in the techniques used stem principally from differences in the particulate material used. Most commonly an ion-exchange resin is employed, either in granular form or impregnated on a sponge, but coated charcoal and Sephadex are also used. The normal values must be determined for each laboratory in which the test is performed.

The product of the *in vitro* uptake value and the serum total T_4 concentration provides a so-called "free T_4 index" or FT_4I which is analogous to and varies with the FT_4 (Fig. 4–15). Such calculations can be performed regardless of

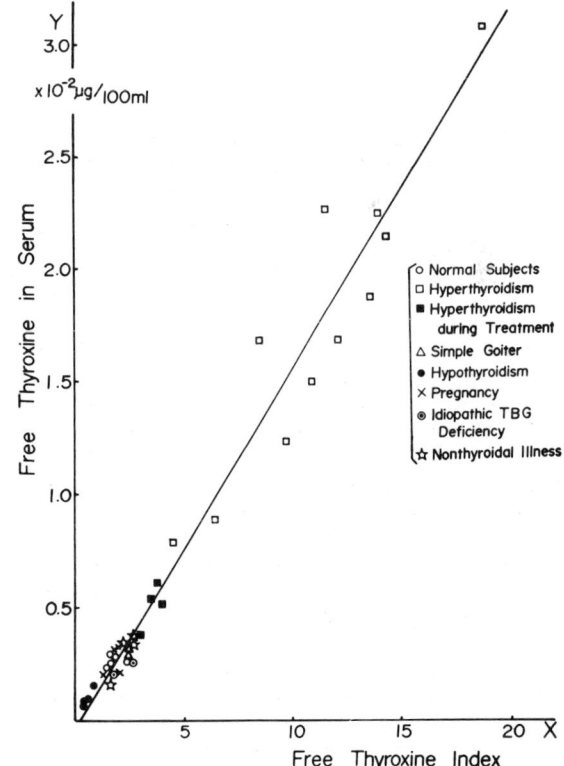

Figure 4–15. In the study from which this figure was derived, serum T_4 concentration was estimated from measurements of the PBI. The correlation between free T_4 concentration measured by dialysis and the free T_4 index is clearly demonstrated. Linearity of the relationship was achieved by calculating the free T_4 index as follows: PBI × RT_3U/1–0.6 RT_3U. Note that values for both functions in circumstances in which TBG is altered are in the normal range. (From Hamada, S., Nakagawa, T., et al.: Re-evaluation of thyroxine binding and free thyroxine in human serum by paper electrophoresis and equilibrium dialysis, and a new free thyroxine index. *J. Clin. Endocr.* 31:166, 1970.)

whether T_3 or T_4 was used as the labeled hormone, but normal values for the indices obtained with labeled T_3 will be much higher than those obtained with T_4.

Although values for the FT_4I vary from normal in the same direction as the FT_4 does, the correlation between the two when individual sera are studied is not linear. Divergence from linearity is especially evident when the FT_4 is low or particularly high. There has emerged, however, an appreciation that this is owing to the fact that the uptake value used in calculating the FT_4I has been traditionally calculated as the quotient of the quantity of labeled T_3 taken up by the resin and the total quantity added to the tube (free/total). This method is theoretically unsound. When, instead, the uptake value is calculated as the quotient of the labeled T_3 taken up by the resin and that which remains bound to the serum proteins (free/bound), the relation between calculated values of the FT_4I and the FT_4 becomes fully linear (Felicetta et al., 1977; Schussler et al., 1978).

In some laboratories, values of the *in vitro* uptake test are "normalized" by expressing them as a fraction of the uptake value in a standard normal serum. The "normalized FT_4I" calculated from the normalized uptake value has a numerical normal range similar to that of the serum total T_4 concentration, but, like any other value of the FT_4I, has no true dimensions or units. Kits have been developed which measure directly a value of the FT_4I that is internally "corrected" for variations in the concentration of TBG. Although such kits appear to yield satisfactory results, it is not recommended that one measure the FT_4I to the exclusion of the total T_4 concentration.

As with measurements of the free T_3 concentration, measurements of a free T_3 index have not been widely employed, though occasionally they may be useful, as in differentiating between T_4-toxicosis, in which they are likely to be elevated, and the transient elevation of serum T_4 seen in some euthyroid patients who are ill, in which they are normal or low (Gavin et al., 1979). Generally, the conjoint measurements of either the total and free T_4 or the total T_4 and an *in vitro* uptake test permit one to judge whether the concentration of TBG is abnormal, and this is taken into consideration in interpreting the serum concentration of T_3.

Concentrations of the T_4-Binding Proteins. An alternate approach to assessing the state of thyroid hormone binding in serum is to measure the activity or concentration of the T_4-binding proteins. With the aid of labeled T_4 and of filter paper electrophoresis to separate the individual binding proteins from one another, saturation analysis can be employed to determine the T_4-binding capacities of TBG and TBPA. These correlate closely with the actual concentration of the two proteins. In normal serum, the T_4-binding capacity of TBG averages approximately 20 μg T_4/dl; that of TBPA is much more influenced by the analytic technique, and varies between approximately 150 and 300 μg T_4/dl.

Electrophoretic analysis of T_4-binding capacities has become mainly a research tool, since an important role for binding of T_4 by TBPA has not been demonstrable, at least in the static sense, and since satisfactory radioimmunoassays for TBG have been developed. Normal concentrations of TBG measured by radioimmunoassay vary somewhat with the antibody and standard employed, are in the range of about 1.0–1.5 mg/dl, and tend to be slightly higher in women than men. The disorders associated with abnormalities in the concentration of TBG are shown in Table 4–2. Measurement of the serum TBG concentration can be employed in diagnosing hypothyroidism or thyrotoxicosis in one of two ways. First, calculation of a T_4/TBG or a T_3/TBG ratio yields values that correlate well with the FT_4I or FT_3I, and may be superior to it in differentiating euthyroid from abnormal functional states. (See Attwood, 1979.) In states such as pregnancy,

in which the increase in TBG is proportionately greater than the increase in total serum T_4 concentration, T_4/TBG ratios tend to be low, but this may be a reflection of a modest lowering of the free T_4 concentration in the pregnant state. Second, on the assumption that TBG is by far the major determinant of the overall intensity of T_4 binding, a calculated value of the FT_4 can be derived from the concentrations of TBG and total T_4 and the association constant for the interaction between the two. In most instances, values calculated in this manner correlate very well with FT_4 values directly determined. (See Glinoer et al., 1979.)

It does not appear that any of the foregoing methods for assessing the state of thyroid hormone binding in serum, or for measuring or estimating the FT_4, is clearly and consistently superior to the others. Consequently, in the authors' view, the choice among them should be made on the basis of precision, convenience, cost, and prevailing practice. It should be noted, however, that there are specific instances in which certain of the procedures are not reliable. Thus, in patients with severe nonthyroid illness, the FT_4I may seriously underestimate the true FT_4 concentration. Measurement of the T_4/TBG ratio would be misleadingly high in patients with the transient hyperthyroxinemia associated with illness or in those with familial isolated hyperthyroxinemia. The ratio would be misleadingly low as an indicator of FT_4 in patients with the sick euthyroid syndrome in whom serum T_4 concentrations are depressed proportionately more than the serum TBG concentration is. (See descriptions of these disorders in the discussion that follows.)

States Associated with Abnormal Hormone Concentrations in Blood

As indicated earlier, the concentrations of T_4 and T_3 in blood are the resultant of two factors, their individual rates of production or supply, which are usually a reflection of the level of thyroid function, and their rates of removal from the circulation, which are largely conditioned by their binding to plasma proteins. So many factors play upon the supply and disposal of T_4 and T_3, either singly or together, that a classification of disorders associated with abnormalities in serum T_4 or T_3 concentration that is both comprehensive and entirely consistent defies construction. In the last edition of this

Table 4–6. COMMON CAUSES OF CONCORDANT AND DIVERGENT ABNORMALITIES IN SERUM T_4 AND T_3 CONCENTRATIONS IN UNTREATED PATIENTS

1. *T_4 Increased, T_3 Increased*
   All varieties of thyrotoxicosis (see Table 4–7)
   Increased TBG (see Table 4–2)
2. *T_4 Increased, T_3 Normal or Low*
   T_4-toxicosis (thyrotoxicosis with decreased T_4 to T_3 conversion; see Table 4–5)
   Euthyroid elderly sick patient (?)
   Familial isolated hyperthyroxinemia
   Increased TBPA
   Radiographic contrast media
   Amiodarone
3. *T_4 Normal, T_3 Increased*
   T_3-toxicosis
   Thyrotoxicosis factitia (liothyronine)
   Iodine deficiency
4. *T_4 Normal, T_3 Decreased*
   Most causes of T_4 to T_3 conversion (see Table 4–5)
5. *T_4 Decreased, T_3 Normal*
   Mild or moderate thyroid failure
   Iodine deficiency
   Phenytoin
6. *T_4 Decreased, T_3 Decreased*
   Severe hypothyroidism
   Severe systemic illness (euthyroid patient)
   Decreased TBG

volume, an effort was made to classify disorders in relation to whether they produced concordant or discordant changes in the serum total T_4 and T_3 concentrations. In the present edition, this mode of classification is retained in Table 4–6. The table makes evident, however, the great heterogeneity of the disorders within each major category. Consequently, the following discussion of disorders that alter serum T_4 and T_3 concentrations is primarily organized according to the type of disorder, rather than the nature of the change in hormone concentrations. Consideration of the table and the text will provide, therefore, a vertical and horizontal view of the topic.

Disorders Associated with Thyrotoxicosis

Thyrotoxicosis is the syndrome that reflects the response of the peripheral tissues to an excess of thyroid hormone. The disorders that lead to thyrotoxicosis can be divided into two categories: those that are associated with true hyperthyroidism, i.e., ongoing overproduction of hormone by the thyroid gland, and those that are not. In the latter category, the excess hormone is either extrathyroid in origin or leaks from an inflamed, hypofunctioning thyroid gland. Classification of the causes of thyrotoxicosis into these two categories is useful, since their modes of treatment are very different.

Increased Serum T_4 and T_3. An increase in both the serum T_4 and T_3 concentrations is the usual pattern of change seen in patients with hyperthyroidism, regardless of whether this is caused by Graves' disease, toxic multinodular goiter, toxic adenoma, or those unusual varieties of thyroid hyperfunction caused by ectopic or inappropriate thyroid stimulators (molar pregnancy, choriocarcinoma in uterus or testis, hypothalamic-pituitary dysfunction, or pituitary tumor leading to hypersecretion of TSH). Serum T_4 concentrations range from values that are only slightly elevated, usually in patients with mild disease, to values in excess of 20 μg/dl in the most severe cases. Concentrations of T_3 are almost invariably increased, sometimes to levels that are many times the mean normal value. Usually, the increase in T_3 concentration is proportionately greater than the increase in serum T_4, so that the T_3/T_4 ratio in serum is almost always elevated. This stems from the fact that in hyperthyroidism the serum T_3 reflects not only peripheral generation from T_4 but also hypersecretion from the thyroid gland of a product with a high T_3/T_4 ratio.

Increased values for both the serum T_4 and T_3 concentrations are usually seen in those thyrotoxic states that are not associated with true hyperthyroidism: thyrotoxicosis factitia due to ingestion of large quantities of levothyroxine or thyroid extract; overproduction of hormone by ectopic thyroid tissue; and leakage of hormone from the gland in the early phase of subacute thyroiditis or in the syndrome of chronic thyroiditis with transient thyrotoxicosis. T_3/T_4 concentration ratios in serum are usually not as high as those seen in true hyperthyroidism. In the nonhyperthyroid varieties of thyrotoxicosis there is no abnormal thyroid stimulator, no excess of TSH, and no focus of autonomous function within the gland. Consequently, suppression of TSH secretion by the excess of hormone in the blood is reflected in subnormal values of the RAIU. Thyrotoxicosis in the presence of a decreased RAIU should also suggest the presence of iodine-induced hyperthyroidism (Jod-Basedow). This can be confirmed or excluded by measurement of the urinary iodine excretion.

In all of the foregoing disorders, owing to the increase in serum T_4 concentration, and frequently to a modest decrease in the concentration of TBG, the concentration of unoccupied binding sites on TBG is reduced, and the proportions of free

T_4 and free T_3, as well as their *in vitro* uptake values, are increased. Hence, values of the FT_4 and FT_3, as well as their corresponding indices, are increased even more markedly.

T_3-Toxicosis. Thyrotoxicosis associated with an increased serum T_3 concentration but a normal or occasionally low serum T_4 concentration is the entity termed T_3-toxicosis. It can occur in the course of any disorder that causes hyperthyroidism. Except for *thyrotoxicosis factitia* due to ingestion of liothyronine (T_3), it is very unlikely to occur in those thyrotoxic disorders that are not associated with true hyperthyroidism. The exact prevalence of T_3-toxicosis among patients initially diagnosed as being thyrotoxic is uncertain, but may be as high as 10%, or even higher in areas of iodine deficiency.

T_3-toxicosis almost certainly reflects a grossly predominant hypersecretion of T_3 by the thyroid, rather than an increase in the peripheral conversion of T_4 to T_3. Some patients with T_3-toxicosis, if left untreated, will develop the usual variety of hyperthyroidism in which the serum T_4 and T_3 concentrations are both increased. Similarly, in patients with Graves' disease who have been in remission following prior therapy, an increase in the serum T_3 concentration may herald recurrence of a thyrotoxic state.

Because of the higher affinity of TBG for T_4 than for T_3, the proportion of free T_4 is mainly determined by the interaction of TBG with T_4, rather than T_3. As a consequence, values for the proportion of free T_4 and *in vitro* uptake values are generally normal in patients with T_3-toxicosis, as are values for the FT_4 and FT_4I. Values for the FT_3 would, of course, be increased.

T_4-Toxicosis. Thyrotoxicosis in association with an elevated serum T_4 concentration and a normal or slightly decreased serum T_3 is the entity termed T_4-toxicosis. It is seen in patients with intercurrent illness, often the elderly, and often in patients who have recently been exposed to large quantities of iodine, as in x-ray contrast studies. (See Birkhauser et al., 1977.) The pathogenesis of T_4-toxicosis is not entirely clear, but the relatively low serum T_3 concentration may result from loss of that component contributed by peripheral conversion of T_4 to T_3, owing to inhibition of this process by intercurrent illness or, where applicable, by an iodinated contrast dye. Excess of iodine may also cause the thyroid secretory product to have a lowered T_3/T_4 ratio.

In patients with severe illness, the intensity of thyroid hormone binding in serum is often decreased. This results from a modest decrease in the concentration of TBG and perhaps from the appearance of an inhibitor of hormone binding. As a result of these factors, as well as the increase in serum T_4 concentration, the proportion of free T_4 in serum and values of *in vitro* uptake tests are increased; consequently, values of the FT_4 and FT_4I are distinctly elevated. The lesser intensity of thyroid hormone binding leads to values of the FT_3 that are increased, despite normal or somewhat low values of the total T_3 concentration. This may help to differentiate T_4-toxicosis from the isolated hyperthyroxinemia occasionally seen in association with illness in patients who are intrinsically euthyroid. Differentiation of the two is also abetted by elevation of the RAIU, marked elevation of the serum rT_3 concentration, and an absent response of the serum TSH to TRH administration, all of which suggest T_4-toxicosis.

Disorders Associated with Increased Hormone Binding

The foregoing section has discussed those disorders in which serum T_4 or T_3 concentration, or both, are increased as a result of an increase in hormone supply. Increased hormone binding is the other major cause of increases in the serum thyroid hormone concentrations. In the great majority of instances, this is due to an increase in the concentration of TBG. Much less commonly, other binding proteins are at fault.

Increased Serum T_4 and T_3: Increased TBG. Except in the rare syndrome of peripheral resistance to the action of thyroid hormones, concurrent elevations of the total T_4 and T_3 concentrations in serum, in the absence of thyrotoxicosis, are invariably due to an increase in serum TBG concentration. This occurs in a variety of clinical states (see Table 4–2), and in these situations, a number of secondary consequences occur (see Fig. 4–6). Most important clinically are secondary increases in the serum T_4 and T_3 concentrations, coupled both with decreases in the percentage of free T_4 and percentage of free T_3 and with lowered values of *in vitro* uptake tests. The extent of increase in the serum T_4 and T_3 concentrations varies with the increase in TBG, but typically, as in pregnancy, in which the concentration of TBG is approximately doubled, values of the serum T_4 concentration range between 7 or 8 and about 14 μg/dl. The FT_4 and FT_4I remain normal. The increase in serum T_3 concentration generally undergoes a smaller proportionate rise, with the result that values for the FT_3, though within the normal range, aggregate toward its lower end. Kinetically, decreases in the MCR of T_4 and T_3 are counterbalanced by the increase in serum concentrations, so that calculated production rates for the two hormones are normal and the patients remain euthyroid.

The most common causes of an increase in the concentration of TBG in plasma are those associated with hyperestrinemia, notably pregnancy and the taking of contraceptive steroid preparations. Increased TBG is also seen in women taking larger doses of natural or synthetic estrogens for the treatment of menopausal symptoms, and has been observed in some patients using topical estrogens and in some with estrogen-producing tumors. Estrogens increase the concentration of TBG in plasma by increasing the rate of synthesis of the protein.

The increase in TBG that occurs during normal pregnancy is detectable at about the third week after impregnation, is clearly evident several weeks thereafter, and persists throughout the remainder of gestation. Levels of TBG begin to decline immediately post partum and return to normal 4 to 6 weeks later. A similar time course of change follows administration and withdrawal of exogenous estrogens. As a result of abnormalities in the conceptus, likely accompanied by a subnormal secretion of estrogens, the increase of TBG in gravid patients who undergo spontaneous abortion by the tenth or twelfth week of pregnancy is absent or subnormal.

An increase in TBG is found in some patients with acute intermittent porphyria, especially women. The cause of this finding is unknown. Several diseases of the liver are associated with an increased concentration of TBG in the plasma. Among them are acute hepatitis, chronic active hepatitis, and biliary cirrhosis. In the latter two disorders, values of the FT_4 and FT_4I may be subnormal, indicating some degree of associated thyroid failure, possibly on an autoimmune basis (Schussler et al., 1978). Chronic abusers of heroin and methadone also display an increase in TBG, probably on the basis of associated liver disease.

Rarely, increased TBG is the result of a familial disorder that, with rare exception, is transmitted as an X chromosome–linked trait. This abnormality can be discovered during neonatal screening programs or in the screening of families of propositi known to have an elevated TBG. More commonly, it is recognized following the chance finding of an elevated serum T_4 concentration, with the consequence that some patients have been treated mistakenly for hyperthyroidism. The familial variety is not associated with hyperestrinism, and unlike the increase in TBG induced by estrogen, it is not accompanied by an increase in the serum concentration of other estrogen-sensitive transport proteins, such as ceruloplasmin and corticosteroid-binding globulin. The presence of a familial elevation in TBG does not exclude the possibility of associated thyroid disease. Indeed, true hyperthyroidism may be more common in patients with this disorder, and instances of associated hypothyroidism and of familial goiter have been reported.

Familial Isolated Hyperthyroxinema. Attention has been drawn recently to a new and extremely interesting syndrome, in which the patients display an increase, sometimes very marked, in the serum T_4 concentration without an accompanying increase in the serum T_3. (See Hennemann et al., 1979.) This disorder is apparently caused by the presence in plasma of an abnormal protein that migrates in the region of albumin during standard electrophoresis and that binds T_4 but not T_3. The other laboratory abnormalities associated with the disorder follow from this. With respect to T_4, they resemble in part those that accompany an increase in TBG, though concentrations of TBG are normal. The percentage of free T_4, directly determined, and the FT_4 are normal. However, because the abnormal binding protein does not bind T_3 appreciably, values of the *in vitro* uptake tests that use T_3 as the labeled hormone are normal. Hence, when calculated from such tests and the serum total T_4 concentration, values of the FT_4I are elevated, mistakenly suggesting thyrotoxicosis. In keeping with the normal values of FT_4 and the normal concentration and binding of T_3, the patients are not thyrotoxic and the response to TRH is normal. The mode of inheritance of this genetic disorder is uncertain, but it affects both males and females and may be transmitted as an autosomal dominant. Its prevalence is also uncertain, but in the short time since attention has been drawn to it, more than 10 families with the disorder have come to the authors' attention.

Hyperthyroxinemia with Increased TBPA. A single case, but one of exceptional interest, has recently been reported (Jacobsson et al., 1979). The patient, whose primary disease was a metastatic glucagon-secreting carcinoma of the pancreatic islet cells, had a serum T_4 concentration approximately twice normal, but a normal free T_4 concentration. This was associated with a three- to four-fold elevation of the serum concentration of TBPA. As would be expected from the negligible binding of T_3 by TBPA, the serum T_3 concentration was normal. TBPA was demonstrated in both tumor cells and in α-cells of normal human pancreatic islets by immunofluorescent techniques. This raises the likelihood that synthesis within the tumor was the cause of the high serum TBPA concentration seen in this patient. It further suggests that TBPA is normally either synthesized in or accumulated by the α-cells of the pancreas.

Disorders Associated with Hypothyroidism

The term hypothyroidism denotes the syndrome that follows upon an inadequate supply of active thyroid hormone to the peripheral tissues. Classically, the term implies failure of adequate production of hormone within the thyroid gland. However, in euthyroid individuals the most active thyroid hormone, T_3, is mainly generated in the peripheral tissues, and this process is inhibited in many abnormal situations generically designated as the "low T_3 syndrome." Thus, it is possible that in circumstances such as these the supply of active thyroid hormone to the tissues is inadequate and thyroid hormone–dependent functions are decreased, despite the absence of disease within the hypothalamic-pituitary-thyroid axis. Although many causes of the "low T_3 syndrome" are known, it is at present uncertain whether, and to what extent, they are associated with metabolic abnormalities due directly to thyroid hormone deficiency. For this reason, disorders associated with the low T_3 syndrome are not discussed here as a variety of hypothyroidism, but rather are considered in the section on States Associated with Altered T_3 Neogenesis (p. 158).

It should also be recognized that the manifestations of thyroid hormone lack are conditioned by both its severity and duration. Functional changes antecede structural changes, such as the classic integumentary changes seen in patients with myxedema, which are very slow to appear. In the discussion of hypothyroid states that follows, several of the disorders considered are associated with thyroid hypofunction that is mild or of short duration, or both. In these conditions, evidence of hypothyroidism is largely biochemical, rather than clinical.

Decreased Serum T_4 and T_3. In the absence of deficiency of TBG, subnormal concentrations of T_4 and T_3 in serum denote the presence of thyroid hypofunction. Severe thyroid failure is characteristically associated with decreases in both serum T_4 and T_3 concentrations, but in less severe hypothyroidism, the reduction in serum T_3 concentration is less dramatic than that in serum T_4. This results from the fact that the thyroid that has not totally failed and that is being stimulated by high concentrations of TSH very efficiently secretes a product with a high T_3/T_4 ratio. Thus, in mild or moderate hypothyroidism, low levels of the serum T_4 may be accompanied by an increased serum TSH concentration and by concentrations of T_3 that are near normal, normal, or even elevated. (See discussion of T_3-Euthyroidism that follows.)

When the serum T_4 concentration is low as a result of thyroid failure, the proportion of free T_4 and free T_3, as well as *in vitro* uptake tests, would be expected to be subnormal. Although this is often the case, a surprisingly high proportion of hypothyroid patients display values for the proportion of free T_4 and *in vitro* uptake tests that are within the normal range. The reason for this diagnostic overlap is uncertain, especially since the concentration of TBG is often slightly increased in hypothyroid patients. Even here, however, values for the FT_4 and FT_4I are subnormal because of the decrease in the serum total T_4 concentration.

Decreased serum T_4 and T_3 concentrations occur during the late phase of subacute thyroiditis and in some patients with chronic thyroiditis, especially post partum. In both disorders, decreased secretion of T_4 and T_3 is presumed to result from depletion of glandular hormone owing to earlier leakage of preformed hormone stores. This is consonant with the fact that the hypothyroid phase is often anteceded by a transient thyrotoxic phase in subacute thyroiditis, and probably in chronic thyroiditis as well.

Following the withdrawal of suppressive thyroid hormone therapy in euthyroid patients, serum thyroid hormone concentrations decline to subnormal levels, where they may remain for several weeks before returning to normal. During this period, basal serum TSH concentrations nonetheless remain low, and responses to exogenous TRH are absent or diminished. This clearly indicates that suppression of TSH secretion can be followed by a period of decreased TSH reserve and secondary hypothyroidism (see Vagenakis et al., 1975). The duration of this period varies with the length and completeness of previous suppression, and seems shorter when caused by T_3 than by T_4. Not suprisingly, a similar period of decrease, both in serum thyroid hormone concentrations and in responsiveness to TRH, sometimes of several months' duration, also follows relief of hyperthyroidism or treatment of autonomously functioning thyroid nodules. This transient phenomenon may account for some cases of hypothyroidism that appear soon after ablative therapy for hyperthyroidism. When doubt exists whether postablative hypothyroidism is likely to be transient or permanent, the physician can either withhold treatment and observe the patient or, preferably, treat the patient with liothyronine for some months and then withdraw the treatment and observe whether thyroid function recovers. Liothyronine is preferred in such cases, since, as already noted, the period of decreased TSH reserve following withdrawal of treatment is shorter with liothyronine than with preparations that contain T_4.

T_3-Euthyroidism. As indicated earlier, the thyroid gland that is hyperstimulated, whether by the normal stimulator of Graves' disease leading to hyperthyroidism, or by TSH in an effort to compensate for failing thyroid function, secretes a product with a high T_3/T_4 ratio. Consequent to this there are some patients with partial thyroid failure in whom serum T_4 concentrations are low, but serum T_3 concentrations are normal or even slightly increased. Most often this occurs in patients with Hashimoto's disease or patients whose hyperthyroidism has been treated surgically or with ^{131}I. They usually appear euthyroid from the clinical standpoint, and may be properly included among patients designated as having "subclinical hypothyroidism." Presumably, their normal or near-normal metabolic state is maintained by the normal quantity of T_3 in the circulation. Nonetheless, serum TSH concentrations in such patients display a better inverse correlation with the serum T_4 concentration than with the serum T_3. This gives credence to the view that the intrapituitary conversion of T_4 to T_3 plays a dominant role in the regulation of TSH secretion.

A special example of T_3-euthyroidism is that seen in patients with severe iodine deficiency. The relative or absolute hypersecretion of T_3 that this reflects constitutes an efficient mechanism for the defense of their metabolic status, since the calorigenic yield of an iodine atom secreted in T_3 is approximately four times that of an iodine atom secreted in T_4.

Disorders Associated with Decreased Hormone Binding

In view of the predominant role of TBG in the extracellular binding of both T_4 and T_3, it is not surprising that significant decreases in the concentrations of TBPA and albumin do not materially influence the concentrations of the hormones with which they can associate. Decreases in the rate of synthesis and plasma concentration of TBPA that accompany acute and chronic illness apparently are not responsible for occasional lowering of serum T_4 concentration seen in these circumstances. Further, although a decrease in serum T_4 concentration may occur in association with severe hypoalbuminemia, this probably reflects associated loss of TBG, as in nephrosis, or other effects of illness (see later). In two patients with hereditary analbuminemia studied by the authors, serum T_4 concentrations were not decreased. Hence, decreases in serum T_4 and T_3 concentrations that result from a decrease in their protein binding are seen in two varieties of disorder: conditions associated with a decrease in the concentration of TBG, and moderate or severe systemic illness. The latter category, in which an inhibitor of hormone binding may appear in the plasma, is discussed later. (See section of States Associated with Altered T_3-Neogenesis.)

Decreased Serum T_4 and T_3: Decreased TBG. The consequences of a decrease in the concentration of TBG are the direct antithesis of those associated with increased TBG (see Fig. 4–6 and Table 4–2). Patients are metabolically normal, although the serum T_4 and T_3 concentrations are in the hypothyroid range. In the majority of reported cases, thyroid function is normal. The proportions of free T_4 and T_3 are increased, as are values for *in vitro* uptake tests. The free T_4 and free T_3 concentrations are normal. With respect to the kinetics of hormone metabolism, the fractional rate of T_4 turnover and the T_4 clearance rate are increased, but daily T_4 disposal is normal. Similar kinetic changes occur in the case of T_3.

Pharmacologic doses of testosterone and several of its derivatives with predominant androgenic or anabolic activity decrease TBG greatly, usually to values one-half or one-third of normal. Values of the serum T_4 concentration decrease *pari passu,* but rarely decline into the frankly hypothyroid range. It is of interest that these agents also increase the binding capacity of TBPA. This may account for the failure of the serum T_4 concentration to decrease more markedly, since TBPA has been shown to increase the amount of its T_4 binding when TBG is decreased.

Very high doses of ACTH or glucocorticoids decrease TBG and increase TBPA. Values of the serum T_4 concentration often decline but do not reflect sustained thyroid hypofunction. Similar changes in TBG, TBPA, and serum T_4 concentration are seen in some patients with Cushing's syndrome.

Decreases in TBG are seen in some patients with active acromegaly. As in the case of glucocorticoid excess, the mechanism of this change is unknown. Urinary loss of TBG (and TBPA) occurs in nephrotic states; here, the decrease in serum hormone concentrations may also reflect some direct loss of hormone into the urine. Losses of TBG may also occur in patients with protein-losing enteropathy. Patients with hepatic cirrhosis may have a low concentration of TBG in their serum, and some decrease in serum TBG concentration is frequently seen in patients with other acute or chronic systemic illness, as is discussed later.

Occasionally, a decreased concentration of TBG in serum occurs as an X chromosome–linked heritable trait. In accord with the Lyon hypothesis, the extent of abnormality is more severe in males than in females. Findings in the blood with respect to the thyroid hormones are similar to those in other states associated with a decrease in TBG concentration, and patients are usually discovered by the demonstration of an anomalously low serum T_4 concentration. Data from neonatal screening programs indicate that inherited abnormalities in TBG occur in one of about every 2000 people, deficiency of TBG being much more common than excess. (See Fisher et al.,1976.)

States Associated with Altered T_3-Neogenesis

In patients with a normal thyroid gland, the majority of the T_3, and nearly all the rT_3, found in the plasma arises in the peripheral tissues through the monodeiodination of T_4, rather than from direct thyroid secretion. Consequently, unless the metabolic clearance rate of T_3 is concomitantly altered (which is not usually the case), any major change in the 5'-monodeiodination of T_4 (T_3-neogenesis) will produce a corresponding change in the serum T_3 concentration. In addition, though little is known of the factors that influence the 5-monodeiodination of T_4 to yield rT_3, it is clear that the enzyme that mediates the major pathway for the degradation of rT_3 is a 5'-monodeiodinase that is either the same as that which mediates T_3-neogenesis or is subject to very

similar regulatory control. Hence, factors that change the production rate of T_3 usually change the degradation rate of rT_3 in the same direction. As a result, in abnormal states, serum T_3 and rT_3 concentrations usually undergo reciprocal alterations. The following discussion describes the various conditions that are associated with changes in the absolute rate of T_3-neogenesis. (See Table 4–5). The great majority are associated with decreased formation of T_3 and a decreased serum T_3 concentration. The effect of these disorders on the serum T_4 concentration is variable, however. In some the serum T_4 is unchanged, in others it decreases, and in still others it is increased. (See further discussion of this topic under Alterations in the Transport, Turnover, and Metabolism of the Thyroid Hormones.)

Systemic Illness. From the standpoint of clinical diagnosis, the most important category of disorders that inhibit T_3-neogenesis is that which can be described broadly as systemic illness. Virtually any acute or chronic illness of sufficient severity, as well as accidental or surgical trauma, is likely to produce this effect, lowering the serum T_3 and increasing the serum rT_3 concentration. These physiologic insults are often associated with a modest decrease in the plasma concentration of TBG, and perhaps with the appearance in plasma of an inhibitor of hormone binding, so that the overall intensity of hormone binding, especially that of T_4, decreases. This is evident in an increase in the proportions of the serum T_4 and T_3 that are unbound or free. Despite this, free T_3 concentrations are depressed because of the severe reduction in serum total T_3 concentrations.

The level of the serum T_4 concentration allows patients with systemic illness to be classified into three different, though perhaps somewhat arbitrary, categories. In the less severely ill, the serum T_4 concentration is within normal limits, but the free T_4 concentration is increased. The laboratory findings in this group of patients are not likely to be confused with those of hypothyroidism or thyrotoxicosis. The second group of patients comprises those who are most severely ill, many of whom do not recover. Here, the serum T_4 concentration is decreased, sometimes to very low levels. In general, the lower the serum T_4 and T_3 concentrations, the less likely it is that the patient will recover. Because of the decrease in hormone binding, values of the serum free T_4 concentration approach or equal those in the normal range, or may even be increased. A most important point is that values for *in vitro* uptake tests that employ labeled T_3 as a tracer, when calculated in the traditional manner, do not increase as much proportionately as the directly determined percentage of free T_4 does. Therefore, the free T_4 index is spuriously low; this, together with low values of the serum T_4 and T_3 concentrations, suggests the presence of hypothyroidism. The serum TSH concentration is not elevated, however, and the response to exogenous TRH is normal or depressed. Further evidence against primary hypothyroidism is provided by the normality of the free T_4 concentration and the elevation of the serum rT_3 concentration. (See Chopra et al., 1979.)

In some patients with intercurrent illness, especially the elderly, the serum T_4 concentration is increased. The pathophysiology underlying this change is quite unclear, but the findings in this syndrome of isolated hyperthyroxinemia associated with illness may lead one to think that the patient has T_4-toxicosis. A diagnosis of T_4-toxicosis is favored, however, by higher values of the serum rT_3 concentration and elevated, rather than subnormal, values of the free T_3 concentration. An elevation of the RAIU will also indicate that the patient has T_4-toxicosis, but the RAIU will be subnormal if the hyperthyroidism is iodine-induced. Demonstration of a substantially increased urinary iodine excretion (> 1–2 mg daily) will suggest that the latter is the case. A subnormal, and particularly flat, response to exogenous TRH should indicate that the patient has T_4-toxicosis, but the differentiation may be less than completely clear, since the response to TRH declines in the elderly, especially in men.

Almost nothing is known of the true metabolic state of patients with systemic illness with respect to those aspects of metabolism that are thyroid hormone–responsive. Among other reasons, the inadequacy of metabolic indices that are currently available (see later) makes it unclear whether the lowered serum T_3 and free T_3 concentrations lead to peripheral thyroid hormone insufficiency. Moreover, it is uncertain whether particular tissues of the ill patient, such as the pituitary, continue to meet their own needs by generating T_3 from T_4 locally. (See earlier section on Pathways of Hormone Metabolism.) As a consequence, we remain quite ignorant of whether the alterations in thyroid hormone economy that accompany systemic illness are a beneficial or an adverse response and, if the latter, whether the apparent decrease in the availability of T_3 should be corrected with replacement therapy.

Drug-Induced Alterations. A number of pharmacologic agents in common use are capable of inhibiting T_3-neogenesis and decreasing, thereby, the serum T_3 concentration. These include propylthiouracil, but apparently not methimazole; propranolol; high doses of adrenal glucocorticoids; the antiarrhythmic agent amiodarone; and several iodinated dyes used as x-ray contrast media. The reductions in serum T_3 concentration produced by these agents are prompt and sustained, and are accompanied by increases in the serum rT_3 concentration. In most cases, serum T_4 and TSH concentrations remain essentially unchanged, but they may increase, along with the response to TRH, after the administration of amiodarone and contrast media. (See Suzuki et al., 1979.) The reason for these differing responses to the several agents that block overall T_3-neogenesis is unclear, but it may be that amiodarone and contrast dyes, unlike the other agents, block conversion of T_4 to T_3 within the pituitary. Both this and the lessened delivery of T_3 to the pituitary would result in an activation of TSH secretion. It is also possible that these agents inhibit the overall turnover of T_4 sufficiently to increase its concentration in the plasma significantly, despite a normal rate of T_4 production. Kinetic studies would enable an evaluation of the latter mechanism, but data to this point are lacking.

Phenytoin (diphenylhydantoin, DPH) is a drug with complex effects on multiple endocrine and metabolic systems, including the metabolism of thyroid hormones. Therapeutic doses of DPH lower the serum T_4 concentration, sometimes into the hypothyroid range. Although high concentrations are capable of inhibiting the binding of T_4 and T_3 by TBG, this effect probably cannot explain the lowering of the serum T_4, since free T_4 concentrations are also depressed. Rather, an effect of DPH on the activity of intracellular enzymes for T_4 degradation and disposal appears to be responsible. There is substantial disagreement as to the effect of DPH on the serum T_3 concentration. The majority of data indicate, however, that the serum total and free T_3 concentrations, as well as the serum TSH, are essentially unchanged, despite the reduction in serum T_4. This may reflect an action of DPH to enhance the conversion of T_4 to T_3, possibly within the liver. Serum rT_3 concentrations are decreased in proportion to the lowering of serum T_4. Either maintenance of the normal total and free T_3 concentrations or a direct effect of DPH on the pituitary may explain the normality of the serum TSH despite reduced concentrations of total and free T_4. (For references, see Rootwelt et al., 1978, and Cavalieri et al., 1979.)

From the few data available, it appears that therapeutic doses of phenobarbital, another agent that alters thyroid hormone binding in the plasma and also affects hepatic metabolism of the thyroid hormones in rats, has no clear effect on serum concentrations of total and free T_4 and T_3 (Rootwelt et al., 1978).

Nutritional Factors. Both acute and chronic alterations in nutritional state greatly influence the pathways of peripheral iodothyronine metabolism and, with them, the concentrations of the major initial metabolites of T_4, namely T_3 and rT_3. (See more extensive discussion in earlier section on Factors that Influence Thyroid Hormone Economy: Nutritional Influences.) Both complete fasting and reduced carbohydrate intake, sustained over days to weeks, are associated with decreased serum T_3 and increased serum rT_3 concentrations, owing beyond doubt to an overall inhibition of the $5'$-monodeiodination of T_4 and rT_3, respectively. Chronic malnutrition, as in anorexia nervosa or protein-calorie malnutrition, produces similar effects. Concentrations of T_4 in the serum are normal or slightly decreased, but because of a mild decrease in the intensity of hormone binding, values of the free T_4 concentrations are normal or increased. Serum TSH concentrations and responses to TRH are generally normal. Converse effects are produced by overfeeding.

Miscellaneous Disorders

Endogenous Antibodies Against T_4 and T_3. Antibodies directed against T_4, T_3, or both have been detected in a small percentage of patients with various thyroid diseases, most commonly patients with chronic thyroiditis, primary hypothyroidism, and diffuse toxic goiter. Endogenous antibodies of this type have also been detected in patients with nodular goiter, and in rare cases seem to have been associated with previous treatment with thyroid extract. Patients with non-Hodgkin's lymphoma of the thyroid constitute another group in which antihormone antibodies have been seen with inordinate frequency. This may reflect an association of this disease with chronic thyroiditis. Anti-T_4 and anti-T_3 antibodies are most commonly seen and are present in highest titers in sera that contain antibodies against thyroglobulin. Thyroglobulin may indeed have been the initiating antigen in most instances, since immunization with thyroglobulin can elicit antihormone antibodies, but this would not explain why such antibodies are not present in the blood normally, though low concentrations of thyroglobulin are. (See Ikekubo et al., 1978.)

Antibodies against T_4 and T_3 probably act to sequester the hormones within the intravascular space, acting in this regard like TBG. Hence, it is unlikely that they continue to impose demands upon the thyroid once a steady state with respect to the particular hormone that they bind has been reached. When present, however, they do assume major clinical importance by introducing artifacts into the measurement of the serum T_4 or T_3 concentration by RIA. Depending on specific details of the method employed, values can appear to be increased into the thyrotoxic range or lowered to subnormal or undetectable levels. How this takes place can be understood by considering the effect of an endogenous anti-T_3 antibody on the RIA for T_3. Its primary effect would be to bind a portion of the labeled T_3 added to the test serum as a tracer ligand. As a consequence, less of the tracer T_3 would be available to bind to the exogenous antibody and less would remain in the free form. Hence, in assays based on measurements of the proportion of tracer ligand bound to the exogenous antibody, as in solid-phase or double-antibody techniques, counts associated with the exogenous antibody would be spuriously low and measured concentrations of T_3 spuriously high. Contrariwise, in assays in which the free labeled ligand is measured, as in molecular-exclusion techniques that use coated charcoal or Sephadex, the fewer counts in the free fraction give the mistaken impression that the concentration of endogenous T_3 is low. Similar effects would occur, of course, in measurements of the serum T_4 concentration in sera that contain endogenous antibody against T_4.

Since endogenous antibodies against T_4 and T_3 appear to occur almost entirely in patients with underlying thyroid disease, the distortions of serum T_4 and T_3 concentrations they may produce are likely to be ascribed to the disease itself. Their presence should be suspected, however, when values of the serum T_4 or T_3 are grossly discordant with the patient's clinical state. Inordinately low values for an *in vitro* uptake test should also arouse suspicion, since they reflect the ability of the endogenous antibody to withhold its labeled antigen from the absorbing particle. Proof that such antibodies are present can be obtained by any protein-separative technique that permits one to demonstrate binding of added tracer antigen by the patient's immunoglobulins.

Resistance to Thyroid Hormones. A small number of patients have been reported whose peripheral tissues appear to be at least partially resistant to the actions of thyroid hormone. Principal evidence that this is the case is that serum total and free T_4 and T_3 concentrations are elevated, though clinical features of thyrotoxicosis are lacking, and that both basal serum TSH concentrations and the response to TRH are normal or increased. Clinical features in patients within this general category have varied widely. Some have been goitrous, others not. None has presented the clinical full-blown picture of hypothyroidism associated with thyroid failure, and some appear entirely euthyroid. Others, however, have displayed selected features of thyroid hormone lack, such as statural retardation, stippled epiphyses, delayed bone maturation, and deaf-mutism. Some degree of resistance to thyroid hormones at the pituitary level is evident in the combination of laboratory findings already described, but the ease of suppression of TSH secretion by exogenous hormone has varied. Theoretically, the syndrome may relate to that in which excessive secretion of TSH leads to frank hyperthyroidism, but, if so, the latter would appear to reflect resistance to thyroid hormone action at the level of the pituitary only. (For references on this topic, see Tamagna et al., 1979.)

Tests That Assess the Metabolic Impact of the Thyroid Hormones

Abnormalities in the supply of hormone to the peripheral tissues are associated with alterations in a vast number of metabolic processes. Among the many physiologic and biochemical changes that follow, some are susceptible, with greater or lesser ease, to measurement in a clinical setting. They provide, therefore, at least theoretically, a means of determining whether the supply of hormone to the tissues falls short of or exceeds their normal requirements. Tests of this type, often designated "metabolic indices," were for many years the only laboratory tests available for use in the diagnosis of thyroid disease, and they alone among test procedures remain the sole means of evaluating the metabolic impact of thyroid hormones within the peripheral tissues. Nevertheless, they have virtually no place in the current diagnostic armamentarium, having been supplanted by tests of generally greater sensitivity, specificity, and diagnostic accuracy. However, some metabolic indices are of historic interest, others are of current value in special circumstances, mainly for physiological exploration, and others are important to be aware of because they can be confused with metabolic changes that occur in other diseases. For these reasons, certain metabolic indices will be discussed here, though only briefly.

The negative view of metabolic indices reflects the reality of those indices that are currently known, not the substantial extent to which there remains an important role for test procedures that are clinically practical and that specifically and sensitively reflect the metabolic impact of thyroid hormone within the tissues. There are several reasons why such a need exists. First, mild degrees of hormone excess or insufficiency are difficult to detect clinically and are usually unaccompanied by clear-cut changes in the total and free T_4 and T_3 concentrations in the serum. Since the normal ranges for these concentrations are quite broad, values within the normal range may represent a significant abnormality for the individual patient. Further, a great many conditions are associated with divergent changes in serum T_4 and T_3 concentrations, and, in the light of current knowledge, reliable inferences cannot be drawn from them concerning the supply of active hormone to the tissues. Examples are those disorders in which the serum T_3 concentration is low and the serum T_4 normal, as in the sick euthyroid syndrome, or those in which the serum T_4 concentration is low and the serum T_3 normal, as in some patients with a failing thyroid gland. In addition, recognition of the role of T_3-neogenesis from T_4 within the pituitary as an important determinant of TSH secretion makes apparent the possibility that in some circumstances, as in starvation or the sick euthyroid syndrome, the serum TSH concentration may not accurately reflect an insufficiency of thyroid hormone in the other peripheral tissues. Finally, as judged from some patients with autonomous thyroid nodules or Graves' disease who appear euthyroid in all respects, feedback inhibition of the TSH-secretory mechanism is so finely poised that a flat response to exogenous TRH need not reflect a significant degree of thyroid hormone excess. Admittedly, the latter patients may indeed be experiencing a mild degree of thyroid hormone excess, but that is precisely the point, that by current techniques there is no way to make certain that this is the case.

In these and other circumstances, availability of a thyroid hormone–specific metabolic index would contribute immensely to clinical diagnosis and physiological understanding. It may be unrealistic to hope, however, that such an index can be discovered. Few metabolic processes are under the control of a single hormone or are unaffected by changes in regional blood flow or influences from the nervous system. Moreover, even if an entirely specific and clinically measureable response to thyroid hormone were found, it likely would (and should) reflect the severity of thyroid hormone excess or insufficiency and might, therefore, have limited value in the diagnosis of mild thyrotoxicosis and hypothyroidism.

Basal Metabolic Rate (BMR)

The classic metabolic action of the thyroid hormones is their calorigenic effect, increasing energy expenditure and heat production; this is manifest in the weight loss, increased caloric requirement, and heat intolerance of the thyrotoxic patient. The classic test that reflects this effect is the measurement of the basal metabolic rate or BMR. Since it is impractical to measure heat production directly, except in rare research facilities, the test actually measures oxygen consumption under specified basal conditions of fasting, rest, and tranquil surroundings. Under these conditions, the assumption is justified that the energy equivalent of 1 liter of oxygen (at standard temperature and pressure) is equivalent to 4.83 kCal, corresponding to a respiratory quotient of 0.82.

Under basal conditions, approximately 25% of oxygen consumption represents energy expenditure in visceral organs, including liver, kidney, and heart; 10% in brain; 10% in respiratory activity; and the remainder in skeletal musculature. Since energy expenditure is related to functioning tissue mass, the measured oxygen consumption is related to some index thereof, most often body surface area. Calculated in this way, basal oxygen consumption is higher in males than in females and it declines rapidly from infancy to the third decade and more slowly thereafter. Values in the patient, after normalization for surface area, are consequently calculated as a percentage of established normal means for sex and age. When calculated in this manner, normal values range between −15 and +5%. In severely hypothyroid patients, values may be as low as −40%. In thyrotoxic patients even greater deviations in excess of the norm can be seen. Abnormal, usually elevated, values are produced by a variety of technical factors and by a number of systemic disorders, notably febrile illnesses, pheochromocytoma, myeloproliferative disorders, anxiety, and disorders associated with involuntary muscular activity. (For an excellent discussion of the principles that underlie measurements of the BMR and the factors other than thyroid dysfunction that influence them, see Becker, 1978.)

Achilles Reflex Time

The duration of the deep tendon reflexes is prolonged in hypothyroidism and shortened in thyrotoxicosis. These differences are due not to differences in the neural component of the arc, but to differences in the speed of both muscular contraction and relaxation, particularly the latter. In about 90% of patients with hypothyroidism, this delay is readily visible. Several types of complex apparatus were developed, therefore, by means of which the duration of one or another component of the Achilles tendon reflex could be measured. Although they enjoyed a vogue for some time, they are not now used as primary diagnostic tools, even in hypothyroidism, because of extensive overlap of the values for defined intervals with those found in normal individuals. Adding to the problem is the delay in reflex relaxation that occurs in a variety of nonthyroid disorders, including diabetes mellitus, pernicious anemia, anorexia nervosa, edematous states, and peripheral vascular disease, and, most important, in hypothermia of any cause. Several drugs, including morphine, propranolol, quinidine, and procainamide, also prolong the relaxation time (for discussion and references, see Waal-Manning, 1969).

Delay in the relaxation of the deep tendon reflexes is a valuable clinical sign in hypothyroidism, but there appears to be little merit in attempts to quantify the measurement.

Enzymes in Blood and Other Metabolites

The concentrations in serum of several enzymes that apparently originate in skeletal muscle are usually elevated in hypothyroidism. The enzymes principally affected are the MM-variant of CPK, and less often LDH and SGOT. (See Jenkins, 1978, for references.) Concentrations of these enzymes may be slightly depressed in patients with thyro-

toxicosis. Such alterations are of negligible value in the diagnosis of thyroid dysfunction, but are important to recognize so that they are not confused with those due to other disease. Activities of a variety of erythrocyte enzymes are altered in the presence of thyroid dysfunction, but these changes are also not of primary diagnostic value (see Funakoshi and Deutsch, 1971, and Butenandt, 1972).

The serum cholesterol concentration is frequently elevated in patients with hypothyroidism and tends to be lowered in patients with thyrotoxicosis. Although once used as a major aid in the diagnosis of hypothyroidism, the breadth of the normal range and the many factors that influence the serum cholesterol concentration make it of no current value as a primary diagnostic measure, although it may have some value in following the response to therapy.

Although basal plasma cyclic AMP concentrations are not consistently affected by thyroid status, the increase in concentration that follows the administration of glucagon is greater than normal in patients with thyrotoxicosis and subnormal in those with hypothyroidism (Elkeles et al., 1972). Studies of urinary cyclic AMP excretion, either measured alone or in relation to creatinine excretion, have yielded variable results, but the increase in cyclic AMP excretion following administration of epinephrine appears to be greater than normal in patients with thyrotoxicosis. (For references, see Tucci and Kopp, 1976). The urinary pigment/creatinine ratio bears a linear relationship to basal metabolic rate and is increased in hypermetabolic states, including thyrotoxicosis, and decreased in hypothyroidism (see Franklin et al., 1971).

Noninvasive techniques for estimating the extent of thyroid hormone effect on myocardial contractility have been devised. The interval between the initiation of the QRS complex and the arrival of the pulse wave at the brachial artery at diastolic pressure (QKd), which is normally in the range of 200 msec, is shortened in thyrotoxicosis and lengthened in hypothyroidism, and the degree of abnormality appears to correlate well with the extent of thyroid dysfunction. However, values of the interval are decreased in high-output states, in conditions associated with increased adrenergic tone, and, owing to arterial inelasticity, in old age. Prolongation of the interval occurs in aortic stenosis, during β-adrenergic blockade, and in the presence of ventricular conduction defects. If extrathyroid factors such as these can be excluded, the QKd interval may be a reasonable means of evaluating the impact of thyroid hormone on a particularly critical organ, the heart. (See Young et al., 1976.) A related index of myocardial contractility, the preejection period (PEP), is shortened in patients with thyrotoxicosis, owing mainly to a decrease in the period of isovolumetric systole; lengthening of the PEP may occur in hypothyroidism. As with QKd, extrathyroid factors play upon this measurement, since the PEP is shortened in patients with aortic stenosis or insufficiency or by the administration of epinephrine (Parisi et al., 1974).

Tests That Assess the Mechanisms for Regulating Thyroid Function

Tests that provide information concerning the state of thyroregulatory control, i.e., whether the TSH-secretory mechanism is functioning normally, is activated, or is inhibited, have assumed a critical role in the diagnosis of thyrotoxicosis and hypothyroidism. The reason for this can be readily understood from a consideration of the role of thyroregulatory mechanisms in the causation of or response to thyroid hormone excess or insufficiency. Thyrotoxicosis, the clinical state that results from sustained thyroid hormone excess, can arise from a multiplicity of causes. In very rare cases, thyroid hyperfunction follows hypersecretion of TSH, owing either to the presence of a TSH-secreting pituitary tumor or to the fact that the feedback mechanism for control of TSH secretion is insensitive to thyroid hormones. Much more commonly, thyroid hormone excess results from one of the following: an abnormal thyroid stimulator whose secretion is not homeostatically regulated, as in patients with Graves' disease or trophoblastic tumor; one or more foci of autonomous hyperfunction within the thyroid gland; or entry into the blood of excess hormone owing to leakage from an inflamed gland, synthesis by autonomous ectopic thyroid tissue, or ingestion of exogenous hormone. In all of these latter varieties of thyrotoxicosis, the TSH-secretory mechanism is shut down, a response that is entirely appropriate to the prevailing excess of thyroid hormone. The relationships that pertain in hypothyroid states are analogous, though converse, to those in thyrotoxicosis. In trophoprivic hypothyroidism, primary disease in the hypothalamus or pituitary leads to insufficient production of biologically active TSH, with consequent thyroid atrophy and hypofunction. Much more commonly, insufficient hormone production arises at the level of the thyroid itself (thyroprivic hypothyroidism), reflecting destruction of thyroid tissue, iodine deficiency, abnormalities in the pathways of hormone synthesis and storage, or the action of exogenous goitrogenic agents. Here, the TSH-secretory mechanism is activated, a response that is again appropriate to the prevailing deficiency of thyroid hormone.

These considerations lead to a rule to which there are as yet no known exceptions, that all varieties of thyrotoxicosis or hypothyroidism are associated with changes in thyroregulatory function that represent either the primary cause of or an appropriate response to thyroid hormone excess or insufficiency. These changes in thyroregulatory function can invariably be demonstrated if appropriately sought, and consequently the tests by which they are demonstrated have great diagnostic value. These are measurements of basal serum TSH concentration, assessment of the TSH-secretory response to exogenous TRH, and the thyroid suppression test.

Serum TSH Concentration

Measurements of the serum TSH concentration are extremely valuable in the diagnosis and management of hypothyroidism and, when used as an index of response to exogenous TRH, in the diagnosis of thyrotoxicosis or the differentiation between hypothyroidism of thyroid origin and that due to disease in the pituitary or hypothalamus. (For reviews with extensive references, see Lamberg and Gordin, 1978, and Scanlon et al., 1978.) As with all radioimmunoassays, normal values obtained in different laboratories and with different reagents vary somewhat. With the materials currently available, the upper limit of the normal range is most commonly about 8 μU/ml, based on the Mill-Hill Human TSH Research Standard A, while the lower limit of the normal range cannot be defined, since it extends below the limit of the sensitivity of the assays, which is commonly about 1.0 μU/ml. In assays such as this, approximately 10% of normal individuals will have values that are unmeasurably low and that cannot be distinguished, therefore, from values that are pathologically decreased.

Continuous efforts to increase the sensitivity of the TSH assay have achieved some success. In assays of increasing sensitivity, the upper limit of the normal range also declines. A recently described assay, not yet widely applied, is

capable of measuring serum TSH concentrations as low as 0.33 μU/ml. With this assay, values in normal subjects ranged between 0.5 and 4.5 μU/ml, and could be clearly distinguished from the unmeasurable values found in the serum of patients with thyrotoxicosis (Wehmann et al., 1979). Detailed studies have revealed the existence of a circadian variation in TSH secretion that yields peak serum TSH concentrations just antecedent to sleep. This is superimposed on irregular, episodic peaks in serum TSH secretion which suggest that the hormone is secreted in a pulsatile manner. None of these variations carry the serum TSH concentration out of the normal range, however. (For a more extensive discussion of the physiology of TSH secretion in normal individuals, see the earlier section on Factors that Influence Thyroid Hormone Economy: Thyrotropin.)

The serum TSH concentration is invariably increased in patients with hypothyroidism of primary thyroid origin, the extent of increase correlating closely with the severity of the disease. (See Fig. 4–16.) Hence, values may range from those that are minimally elevated in very mild hypothyroidism to those that are in excess of 1000 μU/ml in patients with severe disease. In some patients with Hashimoto's disease and some who have been treated for hyperthyroidism with radioiodine or surgery i.e., patients with limited functioning thyroid mass, values for the serum TSH concentration are increased although the patients appear clinically euthyroid and serum T_4 and T_3 concentrations are within the normal range. Such findings are indicative of early thyroid failure associated with a compensatory increase in TSH secretion. Evidently, such compensation is complete, for when such patients develop frank hypothyroidism with the passage of time, as some but not all do, the serum TSH concentration increases further. A substantial problem arises in interpreting small increases in serum TSH concentration among the elderly. A recent study has revealed clear, though mild, elevations of the serum TSH concentration in approximately 7% of individuals older

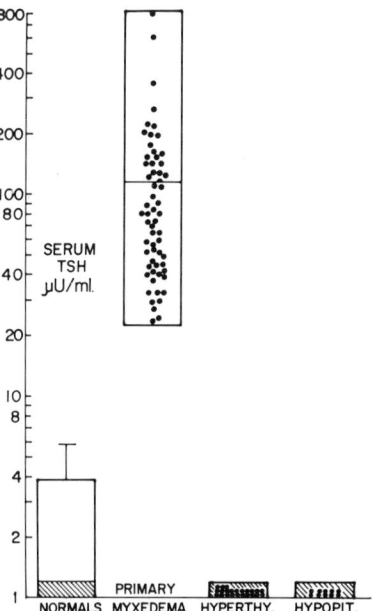

Figure 4–16. Serum TSH concentrations in various circumstances. Cross-hatched areas indicate values not distinguishable from zero. In primary hypothyroidism of mild degree, less marked elevations of serum TSH concentrations are observed. (From Hershman, J. M., and Pittman, J. A.: Utility of the radioimmunoassay of serum thyrotrophin in man. *Ann. Intern. Med.* 74:481, 1971.)

than 60 years of age. The finding was about two times more common in women than in men, and in about half of the group, serum T_4 concentrations and free T_4 indices were subnormal. These individuals appear to have some degree of thyroid failure. More problematic is the presence of slightly elevated values in a larger proportion of elderly patients (14.4%) in whom serum T_4 and T_3 concentrations were normal (Sawin et al., 1979). It is unclear whether this bespeaks a very mild degree of thyroid insufficiency, relative unresponsiveness of the thyroid to TSH, or the secretion with increasing age of an abnormal form of TSH, as some preliminary data suggest. Evidently, serum TSH concentrations are not infrequently increased in patients with primary adrenal insufficiency and decline following initiation of steroid replacement therapy (Topliss et al., 1980).

The association of a normal or undetectable serum TSH concentration with clear-cut hypothyroidism is indicative of trophoprivic hypothyroidism, but within this category, functional differentiation between the pituitary and hypothalamic varieties requires testing of the TSH response to TRH. It is important to recognize, however, that in as many as one-fourth of cases of hypothyroidism with proven disease in the pituitary or hypothalamus, serum immunoreactive TSH concentrations may be slightly elevated and the response of the serum TSH to TRH increased. Studies with an extremely sensitive cytochemical assay for TSH leave little doubt that this discrepancy stems from the secretion of an immunoreactive variant of TSH with reduced biologic activity. (See Faglia et al., 1979, for documentation and references.)

Except in the extremely rare cases of hyperthyroidism due to hypersecretion of TSH, the TSH-secretory mechanism is suppressed and serum TSH concentrations are subnormal in all patients with thyrotoxicosis, regardless of its cause. With the TSH assays currently available, values of the serm TSH concentrations are indeterminate, however, and documentation of the inhibition of TSH secretion requires either testing with TRH or performance of a thyroid suppression test. Among patients with TSH-induced hyperthyroidism, those with primary tumors have disproportionate increases in the concentration of α, but not β, subunits in the serum relative to the concentration of TSH, and fail to increase either serum TSH or subunit concentration after receiving TRH. In those lacking a pituitary tumor, the concentration of subunits relative to that of TSH is not high, and both TSH and subunit concentrations increase after administration of TRH. (See Kourides et al., 1977b.)

Although enhanced secretion of TSH is commonly implicated in its pathogenesis, simple or nontoxic goiter is not usually associated with an increased serum TSH concentration. However, when the pathogenetic factors that lead to simple goiter are sufficiently severe to produce hypothyroidism (goitrous hypothyroidism), then increased serum TSH concentrations emerge. In endemic goiter associated with severe iodine deficiency, serum TSH concentrations are often high and may be in part responsible for the hypersecretion of T_3 that occurs in these circumstances. In areas of less severe iodine deficiency, endemic goiter is associated with normal serum TSH concentrations, much as it is in sporadic nontoxic goiter discussed above. In the human neonate, the serum TSH concentration increases greatly during the first few hours following parturition, returning to normal values during the first day post partum. This response is thought to be due to the entry of the neonate into the relatively cool extrauterine environment. Cold exposure in the adult, however, has no apparent effect.

Except when massive doses of hormone are administered

acutely, treatment of patients with hypothyroidism progressively lowers the elevated serum TSH concentration, but normal levels are not attained for several weeks. Early in the course of replacement therapy, a paradoxical and unexplained increase in basal serum TSH concentration and, more often, in the peak response to TRH may occur (see Ridgeway et al., 1979). After withdrawal of replacement liothyronine in patients with hypothyroidism, a progressive increase in serum TSH concentration begins within a few days. By contrast, when patients have been treated for long periods with levothyroxine, return of the serum TSH concentration to elevated values may require a few weeks, even though the serum T_4 and T_3 concentrations have fallen to subnormal values in the interim.

TRH Stimulation Test

By providing a standard supraphysiologic challenge to the TSH-secretory mechanism within the thyrotroph, exogenous TRH makes it possible to determine, in appropriate cases, the intrinsic TSH-secretory reserve and, in others, the extent to which the mechanism is inhibited by thyroid hormones or other factors. Over a broad range, the extent of increase in serum TSH concentration induced by TRH is closely correlated with the basal serum TSH concentration. Hence, in most circumstances, exogenous TRH acts as an amplifier to exaggerate any abnormality in the rate of TSH secretion and hence in the plasma TSH concentration. In view of the insensitivity of current TSH immunoassays, stimulation with exogenous TRH is necessary to demonstrate the inhibition of TSH secretion that exists in patients with thyrotoxicosis, and it provides an extremely valuable diagnostic tool in this disorder when other tests are marginal.

TRH is effective in activating TSH secretion whether given orally, intramuscularly, or intravenously; however, the intravenous route is by far the most commonly used. A dose of 400 μg, which produces a maximal response, is administered as a single bolus. (See Fig. 4–17.) In normal individuals, the serum TSH concentration rises rapidly, reaches a peak in 20 to 30 minutes, and then declines more slowly, returning to basal values in 2 or 3 hours. In clinical practice, specimens for TSH analysis need be drawn only just before and 30 minutes after TRH administration. Unfortunately, the normal increment in serum TSH concentration varies broadly among different subjects and in the

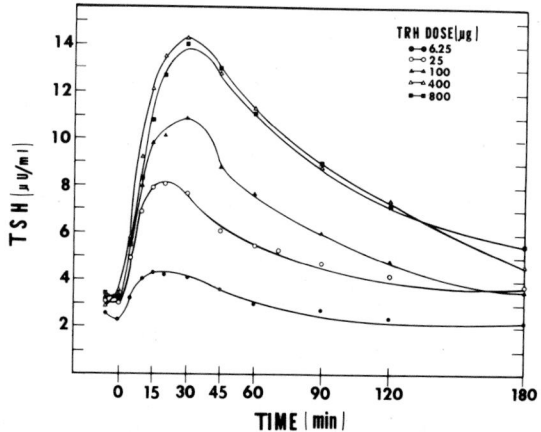

Figure 4–17. Response of serum TSH concentration to intravenous TRH in the dosage shown in normal subjects. (From Snyder, P. J., and Utiger, R. D.: Response to thyrotropin releasing hormone (TRH) in normal man. *J. Clin. Endocr.* 34:380, 1972.)

same subject from time to time. In general, normal increments range between 5 and 30 μU/ml, and average about 15 μU/ml. Responses in premenopausal women are slightly greater during the preovulatory phase of the menstrual cycle and are, in general, slightly greater than in men. These differences are not clinically significant, except in elderly men, in whom responsiveness to TRH declines. The poise of the negative feedback inhibition of TSH secretion and of TRH-responsiveness is extremely fine, so that very small doses of exogenous hormone, insufficient to increase the serum T_4 and T_3 concentrations appreciably, and certainly insufficient to bring them above the normal range, promptly and markedly decrease the response to TRH. Conversely, very small decreases in serum T_4 and T_3 concentration, such as those produced by large doses of iodides, are associated with increased basal serum TSH concentrations and an increased response to TRH. Indeed, in the clinical sense, the feedback mechanism may be too finely poised, since the response characteristic of thyrotoxicosis may be seen in patients with autonomously functioning nodules or in patients receiving replacement or suppressive doses of thyroid hormone, despite the fact that they are clinically euthyroid by all other criteria. This may account for the lack of response to TRH seen in some patients with euthyroid Graves' disease and ophthalmopathy, some patients who are apparently euthyroid after treatment of hyperthyroidism, and some apparently euthyroid relatives of patients with Graves' disease.

As would be expected, in hypothyroidism of primary thyroid origin, the response to TRH is accentuated; peak increments in serum TSH concentration are increased, often greatly so. An appreciably increased serum TSH concentration in a setting of proven or suspected hypothyroidism makes a TRH test unnecessary. Only when both the clinical picture and basal serum TSH concentration are marginal is a TRH test likely to be helpful. Among patients with subclinical hypothyroidism, which usually results from Hashimoto's thyroiditis or surgical or radioiodine treatment of hyperthyroidism, serum T_4 and T_3 concentrations are normal, but serum TSH concentrations are increased. The magnitude of this increase and of the response to TRH apparently are reliable predictors of the likelihood that frank hypothyroidism will supervene.

When hypothyroidism is present without an increase in basal serum TSH concentration, a diagnosis of suprathyroid (trophoprivic) hypothyroidism is indicated. The TRH test should then serve to distinguish between hypothyroidism of pituitary and of hypothalamic origin, and often it does. Classically, the patient whose disease arises in the pituitary displays a subnormal or absent response to TRH, while the patient with hypothalamic hypothyroidism displays a normal, but retarded, response, so that peak concentrations of serum TSH are not achieved until about 60 minutes after TRH administration. Quite frequently, however, a pattern contrary to that expected is seen, possibly because a lesion in the one site interferes anatomically or physiologically with the other. Some hypothyroid patients with disease in the hypothalamic-pituitary area have serum TSH concentrations, as measured by radioimmunoassay, that are slightly elevated and display an exaggerated response to TRH. This apparent paradox evidently results from the secretion of a TSH that has a low ratio of biologic activity to immunoreactivity (see Faglia et al., 1979). In patients with the rare syndrome of isolated TSH deficiency, TRH fails to elicit an increase in the serum TSH concentration, but the increase in serum prolactin concentration induced by TRH is normal.

By far the most frequent and most important use of the TRH test is its application to the diagnosis of thyrotoxicosis when the clinical findings are suggestive and the serum total and free T_4 and T_3 concentrations are equivocal. The TRH test has largely replaced the thyroid suppression test within this setting. Owing to the extreme sensitivity of the TSH-secretory mechanism to feedback inhibition, a normal response clearly excludes the possibility that the patient has thyrotoxicosis. A subnormal or flat response may be strongly suggestive or even conclusive if the clinical picture is strongly suggestive. However, subnormal or flat responses to TRH in association with a seeming euthyroid state are observed in most patients with hyperfunctioning thyroid adenomas; about 50% of patients with the ophthalmopathy of Graves' disease; many patients with treated hyperthyroidism in Graves' disease and some of their relatives; about 20% of patients with multinodular goiter; and many patients receiving replacement or suppressive therapy with exogenous thyroid hormone. Hence, a subnormal response to TRH is not pathognomonic of clinically significant thyrotoxicosis. Admittedly, patients of the types described above may be experiencing a slight excess of thyroid hormone, insufficient to produce clinical manifestations or to bring the serum T_4 and T_3 concentrations out of normal range. Hence, in patients with suspected thyrotoxicosis, judgment must always be the ultimate determinant of whether treatment should be instituted.

Apart from their use in the diagnosis of thyrotoxicosis, TRH tests may be valuable in establishing that Graves' disease is the cause of ophthalmopathy in a euthyroid patient. In this use, as opposed to its use in the diagnosis of thyrotoxicosis, an abnormal response provides strong evidence that the ophthalmopathy is related to Graves' disease, rather than an intracranial or intraorbital lesion. A negative test, in contrast, does not exclude the possibility that Graves' disease is the cause of ophthalmopathy. In patients with treated hyperthyroidism, persistence of an abnormal response to TRH is said to increase the likelihood of later recurrence. However, caution should be exercised in interpreting the results of TRH tests soon after restoration of a euthyroid state, since the TSH-secretory mechanism that has been suppressed for long periods of time by either replacement doses of exogenous hormone or excess quantities of endogenous hormone may be hyporesponsive to TRH for a few weeks or a few months, respectively.

Thyroid Suppression Test

When normal individuals are given thyroid hormone in quantities adequate to meet peripheral requirements, suppression of endogenous thyroid function occurs. Such suppression, which is the result of decreased secretion of TSH, is associated with both a decrease in the rate of hormone secretion and a decrease in the RAIU. This principle forms the basis for the thyroid suppression test, which has been of exceptional value in diagnosing suspected thyrotoxicosis and in establishing the presence of Graves' disease.

Implicit in the presence of hyperthyroidism is that normal thyroregulatory control has been overridden by some factor that permits the thyroid to hyperfunction in the absence of TSH stimulation. Without such disruption, overproduction of hormone could not persist. Since excessive quantities of endogenous hormone fail to suppress thyroid function, it would follow that exogenous hormone would be similarly ineffective. This line of reasoning has been so universally accepted and so uniformly borne out by clinical experience that virtually all agree that a normal suppressive response eliminates the possibility that the patient has active hyperthyroidism. The thyroid suppression test is therefore of special value in patients with marginal clinical findings and laboratory tests suggestive of mild hyperthyroidism. A normal suppressive response excludes the diagnosis of hyperthyroidism, and, as will be seen, an abnormal response is consistent with, but not pathognomonic of, hyperthyroidism.

An abnormal suppression test is found in hyperthyroidism, regardless of the underlying cause. Thus, it occurs in patients with the diffuse toxic goiter of Graves' disease, toxic adenoma, or toxic multinodular goiter. In none of these disorders is thyroid function TSH-dependent, and consequently exogenous hormone does not decrease thyroid function. Thus it is to be emphasized that an abnormal suppression test in the presence of hyperthyroidism does not dictate that the patient necessarily has Graves' disease. Other features, such as a diffusely active goiter or coexistent ophthalmopathy or both, would be necessary to make this diagnosis.

Although an abnormal suppression test in the presence of hyperthyroidism is not pathognomonic of Graves' disease, an abnormal suppression test in the absence of hyperthyroidism is almost always indicative of Graves' disease. It has been noted that abnormal suppression tests in Graves' disease may persist for varying periods, occasionally for many years, after thyrotoxicosis has been relieved either spontaneously or as a result of treatment (Fig. 4–18). Furthermore, abnormal suppression tests occur in about one-half of patients with active ophthalmopathy of Graves' disease, even when thyroid function is normal. Demonstration of an abnormal suppressive response in such patients greatly weighs in favor of the ophthalmopathy being due to Graves' disease, rather than to an intracranial or intraorbital lesion. The fact that an abnormal thyroid suppression test may occur in Graves' disease in the absence of frank hyperthyroidism indicates that this abnormal response is a reflection of a more basic pathogenetic element in this disorder.

The technique of carrying out the suppression test varies somewhat among different laboratories. Sodium T_3 (liothyronine) is universally used as the suppressive agent, and the lowering of the thyroid radioiodine uptake is most commonly employed as an index of suppression. The recommended dosage of liothyronine varies between 75 and 100

μg daily and the duration of administration between 8 days and 2 weeks. The authors prefer the larger dose of liothyronine in view of evidence suggesting that 75 μg daily may not constitute a full physiologic replacement dose. Others have suggested that suppressibility may be tested by the administration of a single 3-mg dose of L-thyroxine, thereby forestalling a spurious nonsuppression owing to failure of the patient to take the hormone. Side effects of this large acute dose do not seem to be a problem. (See Wenzel and Meinhold, 1974).

It is generally considered that a reduction of the RAIU to less than half of its initial value constitutes a normal response. Why the uptake should not be more completely suppressed is uncertain. Since the suppressive response to liothyronine is associated with a decrease in the secretion of T_4, a reduction in the serum T_4 concentration can also be used as an index of suppression. One disadvantage of the thyroid compression test is that when thyroid function is not suppressible, the hormone that continues to be secreted will add to that being administered so that adverse effects may result. Since the test is usually required in patients with mild hyperthyroidism, or some who are entirely euthyroid, this usually poses no significant risk. In the elderly, or in those with cardiac disease, who are likely to be especially susceptible to thyroid hormone excess, the suppression test should not be used, and the TRH test used instead.

It is commonly stated that an abnormal thyroid suppression test and an absent TSH-secretory response to exogenous TRH have the same significance, and that the two tests are interchangeable. In some sense this is true, and usually the results of the tests are entirely in accord with one another. There are, however, subtle differences between them in their physiologic bases. Complete or nearly complete suppression of thyroid function by exogenous thyroid hormone indicates that thyroid function is being sustained as a result of TSH stimulation. Conversely, failure of suppression, with very rare exception, indicates that thyroid function is independent of TSH stimulation, being truly autonomous or sustained by an abnormal stimulator. The suppression test does not, therefore, indicate how much thyroid hormone is available, merely whether or not thyroid function is being sustained by TSH. The response to TRH, on the other hand, is thought to indicate whether the level of available hormone is in excess of physiologic requirements, as judged from whether or not the TSH-secretory mechanism is shut down. Obviously, when thyroid function is controlled by TSH, and hormone production is normal, both tests will yield normal results. Conversely, when there is hyperthyroidism due to either thyroid autonomy or an abnormal thyroid stimulator, both tests will be abnormal. However, in certain circumstances results of the two tests will diverge. In the patient with Graves' disease who has been treated with ^{131}I or surgery, the abnormal stimulator may persist as the main source of thyroid stimulation. If, however, loss of thyroid tissue were sufficient and hormone production normal or somewhat decreased, the TSH-secretory mechanism would be at least normally active. Here, the suppression test would be abnormal and the response to TRH normal or increased. Instances of this type of discrepancy are not at all uncommon and are easily understood. Less common and less easily understood, but well documented, are instances in which the TRH test reveals a lack of response, indicating that an excess of hormone has suppressed the secretion of TSH, while the suppressive response to exogenous thyroid hormone is entirely normal, indicating that TSH is supporting thyroid function. This apparent paradox is unexplained, but

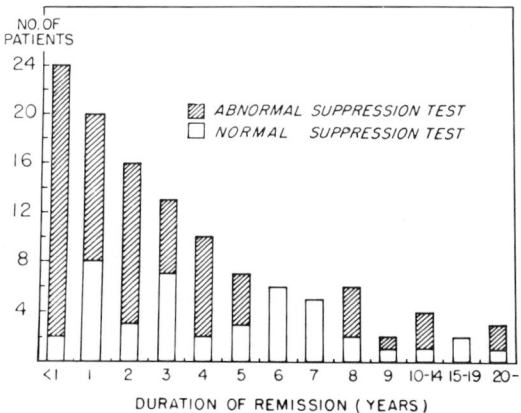

Figure 4–18. Persistence of abnormal T_3 suppression test following relief of thyrotoxicosis in patients with Graves' disease. Patients in this series had relief of thyrotoxicosis following surgical, radioiodine, or antithyroid therapy, or following spontaneous remission. Note the prolonged persistence of an abnormal suppression test in some patients despite maintenance of a normal metabolic state. (Figure constructed from data presented by Werner, S. C.: *J. Clin. Invest. 35*:57, 1956.)

suggests that our understanding of the true physiologic meaning of these responses is flawed. (See Smeulers et al., 1977; Tamai et al., 1978 and 1980a.)

Miscellaneous Tests

TSH Stimulation Test

The TSH stimulation test formerly played a prominent role in the diagnosis of several varieties of thyroid hypofunction. Currently, however, it need be applied in only a few selected conditions. The test depends on the fact that normal or potentially normal thyroid tissue can respond to an increase in TSH stimulation by increasing its rate of iodine accumulation and hormone release. On the other hand, a thyroid that is failing or has failed because of intrinsic diseases should already be maximally stimulated by endogenous TSH, provided that the TSH-secretory mechanism is intact. Thus the TSH test was formerly used mainly to differentiate between thyroprivic and trophoprivic hypothyroidism, and to demonstrate the presence of so-called decreased thyroid reserve. This term is used to denote the condition in which the maximal functional capacity of a failing thyroid gland has been evoked by an increased secretion of TSH, sufficient to yield a normal or near-normal rate of hormone secretion. These uses of the TSH stimulation test have been almost entirely supplanted, however, by the use of measurements of basal serum TSH concentration and the response to TRH.

The TSH stimulation test retains its utility in three major circumstances. The test can be used to determine whether the potential for thyroid function exists in a patient taking full replacement doses of thyroid hormone. Here, it may serve to establish or exclude a diagnosis of thyroprivic hypothyroidism without the need to withdraw hormone therapy. Stimulation by exogenous TSH can also be employed to determine whether areas of the thyroid that are not functioning, as indicated by scanning techniques, are capable of function. Scintiscans obtained after TSH administration can be employed to determine whether absence of I* accumulation in one lobe of the thyroid is due to hemiagenesis, or to demonstrate, prior to therapy, whether the extranodular thyroid tissue of a patient with a hyperfunctioning thyroid adenoma will be able to resume function after ablation of the nodule.

Several variants of the TSH stimulation test have been used. For the indications just noted, maximal stimulation seems desirable, since a single injection of TSH may not always activate thyroid tissue that has been dormant for a long period. After control studies have been carried out, 5 or 10 U of bovine TSH is administered once daily for 3 days. Approximately 24 hours after the last dose, the RAIU measurement is repeated if a quantitative evaluation of response is desired, the scintiscan is repeated if the functional capability of inactive areas is being evaluated, or a combination of the two procedures is carried out. Measurements of the serum T_4 and T_3 concentrations are not especially helpful when the TSH stimulation test is performed for these current indications.

Significant untoward reactions to TSH are quite uncommon. Virtually all patients experience some discomfort at the site of injection. Less common reactions include nausea and vomiting, pain and tenderness in the region of the thyroid or salivary glands, fever, urticaria, symptoms of thyrotoxicosis, dysrhythmias, and angina. In rare instances, anaphylactoid reactions have led to death. For this reason, the authors routinely perform intracutaneous tests for sensitivity to the bovine protein before the full intramuscular doses are administered. (For discussions of the responses and reactions to exogenous TSH, see Taunton et al., 1965, and Uller et al., 1973.)

Assessment of Organic Binding of Iodide

In normally functioning or generally hyperfunctioning thyroids, oxidation of iodide and organic binding are sufficiently rapid that relatively little free iodide is present in the thyroid at any time. Consequently, little loss of iodide from the normal thyroid can be demonstrated following the administration of agents, such as perchlorate, that inhibit iodide transport and thereby discharge accumulated iodide. When organic binding is incomplete, however, substantial accumulation of iodide occurs, and significant discharge follows inhibition of iodide transport. Two tests of the integrity of the organic-binding mechanism have been devised, the standard perchlorate discharge test and the iodide-perchlorate discharge test. In the former, a dose of radioiodine is allowed to accumulate in the thyroid, and after measurement of the thyroid I* content, a blocking dose of perchlorate is administered. A significant decrease in epithyroid radioactivity within 1 hour constitutes a positive response and indicates a defect in organic binding when the plasma stable iodide, and hence the intrathyroid iodide, concentration is normal or near-normal. The iodide-perchlorate discharge test affords a more severe challenge to the organic-binding mechanism, since an acute load of stable iodine is administered with the radioiodine. As a result, the concentration of intrathyroid iodide is greatly increased, and even a mild impairment of organic binding will leave a significant portion of thyroid radioiodine unbound and susceptible to discharge. Hence, subtle defects can be demonstrated by means of this test. However, the interpretation of the iodide-perchlorate discharge test is more complex than is that of the standard test. When entirely normal individuals are given sufficient quantities of stable iodide, an acute inhibition of organic binding (acute Wolff-Chaikoff effect) ensues, and a variable proportion of thyroid iodide becomes dischargeable. Although the dose of stable iodide used in the iodide-perchlorate discharge test is less than that required to induce an inhibition of organic binding in the normal gland, it may be sufficient to do so in the stimulated gland in which iodide transport activity is increased. This probably explains the positive tests that are seen in some patients with hyperthyroidism and in some normal individuals who have been given TSH. (For details of the testing procedures and further discussion of findings, see Suzuki and Mashimo, 1972.)

A positive response to the standard test is seen in patients with a genetically determined defect in organic binding, in some patients with Hashimoto's disease, and in patients with diffuse toxic goiter shortly after treatment with radioiodine. A positive response to the iodide-perchlorate discharge test is seen more commonly or more strikingly in all of the foregoing disorders, as well as in some patients with untreated hyperthyroidism and those previously treated surgically or with radioiodine or antithyroid drugs. A positive response to the iodide-perchlorate discharge test is thought to be a forerunner of thyroid failure and a likely indication that the patient will be prone to development of hypothyroidism if iodides are given chronically (Braverman et al., 1971).

Tssts for Antithyroid Antibodies

As is discussed more extensively later (see section on Graves' Disease), Graves' disease, Hashimoto's disease, and primary thyroprivic hypothyroidism compose the triad of interrelated autoimmune thyroid disorders. Among the several lines of evidence that support the role of autoimmunity in their pathogenesis is the frequency with which antibodies against one or another thyroid antigen can be demonstrated in the blood of patients with these diseases. Four types of antithyroid antibody have been demonstrated.

1. An antithyroglobulin antibody that is detectable by the agar gel diffusion precipitin technique, by the tanned red cell agglutination technique, by the fluorescent antibody technique using fixed sections of thyroid tissue, or by radioimmunoassay.

2. An antibody directed against a component of thyroid microsomes that is demonstrable by complement fixation, by the fluorescent antibody technique using unfixed tissue, by radioimmunoassay, and by tanned red cell agglutination. This antibody is probably the same as that which produces a cytotoxic effect in thyroid cells in tissue culture.

3. An antibody directed against a colloid antigen distinct from thyroglobulin, demonstrable by the fluorescent antibody technique using fixed tissue.

4. An antibody that reacts with a nuclear component of thyroid cells, detectable by the fluorescent antibody technique using unfixed sections of thyroid tissue.

These autoantibodies are immunoglobulins, and, except for the antinuclear antibody, are organ-specific. Only the antithyroglobulin and antimicrosomal antibodies have been used as diagnostic tools to any extent, owing to the fact that the tests for their detection in serum are more readily available.

Although radioimmunoassay techniques are the most sensitive tests for antithyroid antibodies available, both antithyroglobulin and antimicrosomal antibodies are most often measured by determining the highest dilution of the test serum capable of agglutinating sheep red cells that have been treated with tannic acid and coated with the appropriate antigen. The tests are simple and quite specific, and commercial kits by means of which they can be performed ave available. Of the two tests, that for the antimicrosomal antibody is the more useful, since it is more frequently positive and usually in higher titer. This is particularly the case in patients less than 20 years of age. Among young patients, positive tests for antithyroglobulin antibody are present in only about 50% of patients with other evidence of Hashimoto's thyroiditis, and titers are usually low, but the antimicrosomal antibody test is usually positive. Among adult patients with Hashimoto's disease, antimicrosomal antibodies are found in nearly all and antithyroglobulin antibodies in about 85%. (See Fig. 4–19.) Among patients with Graves' disease, the corresponding values are about 80% and 30%, respectively. A somewhat lower frequency of antithyroid antibodies is found in patients with primary hypothyroidism.

Sera of approximately 10% of seemingly normal individuals contain antimicrosomal or antithyroglobulin antibodies, or both, usually in low titer. The frequency increases with age, particularly in women. Antibody titers correlate with the presence of foci of lymphocytic infiltration within the thyroid, and positive tests within a normal population probably reflect the presence of some chronic thyroiditis. The frequency of antithyroid antibodies in the sera of patients with diseases other than Hashimoto's disease, Graves' disease, or primary myxedema is apparently no greater than that in an unselected population of patients who have no overt thyroid disease.

Tests for antithyroid antibodies have diagnostic value in several clinical situations. High titers are indicative of chronic thyroiditis, in a generic sense; with the appropriate clinical picture, they confirm the diagnosis of Hashimoto's disease. Antibodies in moderate titer appear transiently in patients with subacute thyroiditis, and may be present in patients with the syndrome of chronic thyroiditis associated with transient thyrotoxicosis (also referred to as hyperthyroiditis or painless thyroiditis). Demonstration of antithyroid antibodies may help to distinguish these disorders, in their thyrotoxic phase, from other disorders associated with a decreased RAIU, notably thyrotoxicosis factitia. Demonstrable antibodies also suggest that hypothyroidism is thyroid, rather than suprathyroid, in origin, and that ophthal-

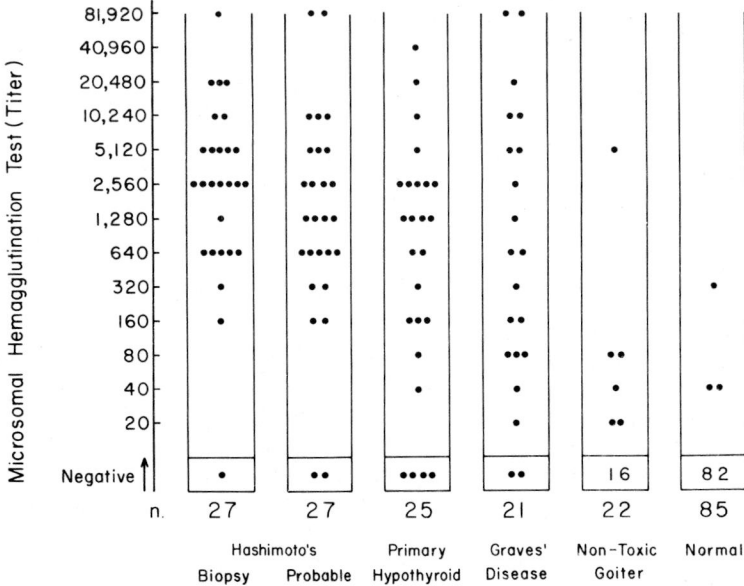

Figure 4–19. Titers of anti-microsomal antibodies in normal subjects and patients with various thyroid diseases. (From Abreau et al.: *Ann. Clin. Lab. Sci.* 7:73, 1977.)

mopathy in the absence of hyperthyroidism is related to Graves' disease, rather than an intraorbital or intracranial lesion.

Titers of antimicrosomal and antithyroglobulin antibodies in the serum of women with Hashimoto's disease or Graves' disease decrease progressively during pregnancy, and increase transiently thereafter, reaching their peak at 3 to 4 months post partum. This may explain the appearance of transient thyrotoxicosis or hypothyroidism in patients with chronic thyroiditis during the first several months after delivery. (For references to this topic and other aspects of antithyroid antibodies, see Amino et al., 1976 and 1978; Inada et al., 1979; and Abreau et al., 1977.)

Thyroglobulin

Contrary to long-standing belief, which held that thyroglobulin is normally a "sequestered antigen," sensitive radioimmunoassays have revealed that this protein is present in the sera of virtually all normal individuals. Concentrations are exceedingly low, ranging up to only 20 or 25 ng/ml; mean normal values vary with the particular assay used, but are on the order of 10 ng/ml. Concentrations tend to be somewhat higher in women than in men and are clearly, but moderately (several-fold), elevated in pregnant women and in the newborn. Distinctly elevated values are present mainly in three types of thyroid disorder: those associated with goiter and thyroid hyperfunction; those associated with inflammatory or physical injury to the thyroid; and differentiated thyroid tumors. Values are elevated in both endemic and sporadic nontoxic goiter and the degree of elevation varies in general with the thyroid size. Elevated values are also present in the serum of patients with hyperthyroidism. In Graves' disease, values tend to be lower when the disease is in remission, but not with sufficient frequency to afford a reliable prognostic index. Administration of exogenous TSH as well as the surge of TSH secretion that follows administration of TRH is followed by transient increases in the serum thyroglobulin concentrations. Transient elevations of the serum thyroglobulin concentration also occur in patients with subacute thyroiditis and as a result of trauma to the gland during thyroid surgery. Even low concentrations of antithyroglobulin antibodies interfere with measurements of the serum thyroglobulin concentration, as they are commonly carried out. Consequently, there are few data concerning the concentration of free thyroglobulin, if any does exist, in the serum of patients with Hashimoto's disease.

The major clinical value of measurements of the serum thyroglobulin concentration is in the management, but not the diagnosis, of differentiated thyroid carcinoma. Serum thyroglobulin concentrations are increased in patients with both benign and differentiated malignant tumors of the thyroid *in situ,* and do not serve to distinguish between the two. Following removal of the tumors, values decline into the normal range and remain normal if metastatic disease is not present. Those patients who either retain or develop demonstrable metastasis after treatment are found, however, to have either persistent or recurrent elevations of the serum thyroglobulin concentration. Such measurements are therefore a valuable adjunct to management, and may provide information of a type that cannot be obtained by other measures, including radioiodine scanning. (For references to measurement of serum thyroglobulin in diverse thyroid diseases, see review by Schneider and Ikekubo, 1979.)

Tests for Immunoglobulins Related to Graves' Disease

As discussed in the later section concerning the pathogenesis of Graves' disease, there is a general consensus that thyroid hyperfunction in this disorder results from the action on the gland of abnormal immunoglobulins that bind to the thyroid plasma membrane, activate adenylate cyclase therein, and induce thyroid growth, increased vascularity, and an increased rate of hormone production and secretion. Since the responsible immunoglobulins cannot at present be differentiated from others by chemical or immunologic means, demonstration of their presence is based upon tests of their bioactivity.

Three types of tests are most likely to be available. The first, a test for the long-acting thyroid stimulator (LATS), assesses the ability of IgG in the patient's serum to stimulate the release of radioiodine from the thyroid gland of the mouse whose thyroid has been prelabeled with radioiodine and then suppressed by administration of exogenous thyroid hormone. Assays for LATS are positive in only about half of patients with diffuse toxic goiter, a frequency of positive responses that is lower than that obtained with the other tests. The second category of test assesses the ability of IgG to inhibit the binding of ^{125}I-labeled TSH to its receptors in human thyroid membrane preparations (TSH-displacing antibody, TDA; TSH-binding inhibitory immunoglobulin, TBII). The frequency of positive responses in patients with active disease is on the order of 60 to 80%. The third type of test assesses the ability of IgG to stimulate adenylate cyclase or increase the concentration of cyclic AMP in human thyroid slices or membrane preparations (thyroid-stimulatory immunoglobulin, TSI). Tests of this type are positive in approximately 80% of patients with active Graves' disease, but, in some series, positive responses are obtained with IgG from the serum of patients with Hashimoto's disease.

None of these tests is available on a routine basis, but there are special circumstances in which efforts should be made to have them carried out in a specialized laboratory. Demonstration of the presence of Graves' disease–related IgG may be of great diagnostic value in the euthyroid patient with ophthalmopathy, especially when it is unilateral, and particularly when the thyroid suppression test has proved to be normal. High titers of bioactivity in the IgG of the pregnant woman with Graves' disease indicate the likelihood that neonatal thyrotoxicosis will be present in her offspring. The application of such tests that has the greatest potential importance, however, stems from recent observations, the preponderance of which suggest that the presence of these activities correlates well with the prognosis of patients with diffuse toxic goiter who have been given a course of treatment with antithyroid agents. (See reviews by Zakarija et al., 1980, and Kidd et al., 1980.)

External Scintiscanning

Localization of functioning or nonfunctioning thyroid tissue in the area of the thyroid gland or elsewhere is sometimes of great value in the diagnosis or management of the patient with thyroid disease, and is made possible by techniques of external scintiscanning. (For a comprehensive and well-illustrated consideration of thyroid imaging, see Johnson, 1978.) The general principle that underlies these techniques is that, with appropriate apparatus, isotopically labeled materials that are differentially accumulated by thyroid tissue can be detected and quantified *in situ* and the data transformed into a topologically accurate visual display. Two types of apparatus are available. The first, a rectilinear scanner, comprises a mechanical device that moves a highly collimated (focused) scintillation detector back and forth across the area of study in a series of parallel tracks moving progressively downward from above. A printing device that moves in concert with the detector is activated to record a mark whenever a predetermined number of counts have been received. In this way, a visual representation of the localization of radioactivity in the area being scanned is obtained, areas of greatest radioactivity corresponding to areas of greater density in the scan. Modifications of the foregoing apparatus make it possible to print a mark whose color varies with the counting rate, producing the so-called "color scan." Still other modifications make use of a light source that moves synchronously with the detector and whose intensity is proportional to the counting rate. The light exposes a sheet of x-ray film, and the degree of darkening of the final image corresponds roughly to the counting rate at the appropriate site in the thyroid ("photo scan"). The second type of apparatus is a stationary scintillation camera equipped with a pin-hole collimator that views the entire field of interest and translates the counting rates from specific areas of the field into photographic images or images on a fluorescent screen that can be viewed directly or photographed. Electronic and recording instruments permit the quantification of radioactivity in specific areas or the subtraction of extrathyroid radioactivity. Further, the information obtained can be recorded on tape for later study.

Several types of radioisotopes are employed in thyroid imaging. ^{99m}Tc-pertechnetate is a monovalent anion that, like iodide, is actively concentrated by the thyroid gland, but, unlike iodide, undergoes negligible organic binding. Thus, it is free to diffuse out of the thyroid as its concentration in the plasma declines. The short physical half-life of ^{99m}Tc (6 hours), together with its transient stay within the thyroid, makes the radiation delivered to the thyroid by a standard dose very low. Consequently very large doses (>1 mCi) can be administered, permitting high counting rates and often an adequate image of the thyroid when the fractional uptake is too low to permit scintiscanning with radioiodine. Pertechnetate is usually given as a single intravenous bolus, and imaging performed 4 to 6 hours later. With the scintillation camera, imaging can be begun almost immediately after administration of the tracer and serial images obtained thereafter. This makes possible studies of the dynamics of thyroid blood flow and isotope accumulation.

Three radioactive isotopes of iodine have been or are used in thyroid imaging, ^{131}I, ^{125}I, and ^{123}I. ^{131}I was the isotope most commonly used in the past, and it retains utility, particularly when functioning metastases of thyroid carcinoma are being sought. The physical half-life of ^{125}I (60 days) is much longer than that of ^{131}I (8 days), but its lower radiation energy results in a radiation dose to the thyroid per unit of radioactivity administered that is only about two-thirds that delivered by ^{131}I. The third radioactive isotope of iodine, ^{123}I, is in many respects ideal. Its short half-life and the absence of beta radiation result in a radiation dose to the thyroid that is about 1% that delivered by a comparable dose of ^{131}I. All three isotopes of iodine provide satisfactory images of the thyroid in its normal location.

Imaging of thyroid tissue is performed for a variety of indications. The technique can be used to provide some, though not accurate, evidence of overall thyroid size. Its most important use is to define areas of increased or decreased function ("hot" or "cold" areas, respectively) relative to function of the remainder of the gland, provided that these are 1 cm or more in diameter (Fig. 4–20). Small cold nodules may be obscured by overlying functioning tissue, but superior discrimination can be achieved if the gland is scanned in the lateral or oblique, in addition to the anterior-posterior, projection. Although the majority of nonfunctioning nodules do not prove to be malignant, lack of function increases the likelihood of malignancy, particularly if only one nodule is present. Conversely, functioning nodules, particularly if they are either more active than surrounding tissue or the sole functioning tissue ("hot nodule"), are quite unlikely to be malignant. Occasionally, irregularities in thyroid images occur in the absence of palpatory abnormalities. Irregularity of the image of the lateral margin of the thyroid lobe is particularly suspicious of tumor, but it is very important that images be interpreted judiciously, lest unnecessary surgery be performed.

Scintiscans obtained after administration of exogenous TSH may be useful in demonstrating conclusively the presence of hemiagenesis of the thyroid and in documenting the intrinsic functional capability of suppressed thyroid nodules. Conversely, scans performed after a period of exogenous thyroid hormone administration ("suppression scans") can reveal areas of autonomous function that may not have been detectable in baseline studies. Scintiscanning can also be used to demonstrate that substernal or intrathoracic masses represent thyroid tissue, and they are useful in detecting ectopic thyroid tissue in the tongue or ovary. A major clinical application is in the detection of functioning metastases of thyroid carcinoma (see later section on this topic).

Choice of the scanning agent for these various indications depends upon many factors. Pertechnetate is readily available in isotope laboratories, and since imaging is performed soon after administration of the scanning agent, the entire procedure requires only a single visit of the patient to the laboratory. Another major advantage is the very low radiation dose delivered to the thyroid. On the other hand, pertechnetate provides information only about the iodide-transport function of thyroid tissue, and not about organic binding or retention. Some tumors of the thyroid appear, therefore, to be functioning when examined with pertechnetate, but not with radioiodine. Because only the iodide-transport function is examined, the stay of pertechnetate within the thyroid is quite brief; imaging is done early, so that radiation from intravascular sources or from salivary tissue may obscure or confuse the findings. For the same reason, pertechnetate is an inappropriate agent for scans of substernal or intrathoracic goiter.

All three isotopes of iodine provide satisfactory thyroid scans, but many feel that superior scans are obtained with ^{123}I. The short half-life, which limits the radiation dose delivered to the thyroid, precludes its use in the search for functioning thyroid metastases. In the case of ^{125}I, its low-energy emissions preclude scanning from deep sources, such as substernal goiter or distant metastases, so that either ^{123}I or ^{131}I should be used in the former and ^{131}I in the latter.

Fluorescent Scans

An ingenious technique, but one that requires expensive instrumentation, is that of fluorescent scanning, which provides information concerning the content of stable iodine within the gland and its topologic distribution. In this technique, discrete zones of the thyroid are subjected to gamma radiation from a source of radioactive americium (^{241}Am). Upon encountering ^{127}I, this induces the emission of a fluorescent x-ray, which is appreciated by a suitable detector.

Thus, in contrast to gamma scintillation imaging, which localizes and quantifies ongoing accumulation of iodine, the fluorescent scan localizes and quantifies iodine stored within the gland. The technique has interesting research applications, but its clinical utility is limited. Nonfunctioning nodules generally have a low iodine content and are, therefore, "cold" on fluorescent scan. The technique may provide useful information in conditions in which isotopic scanning is either unsuccessful or contraindicated, as in iodine overload or during pregnancy. (See Hoffer et al., 1972, for a further discussion of this technique.)

Ultrasonography

Within recent years the technique of ultrasonography has been applied successfully to the thyroid gland for the purpose of revealing several aspects of its pathologic anatomy. (See

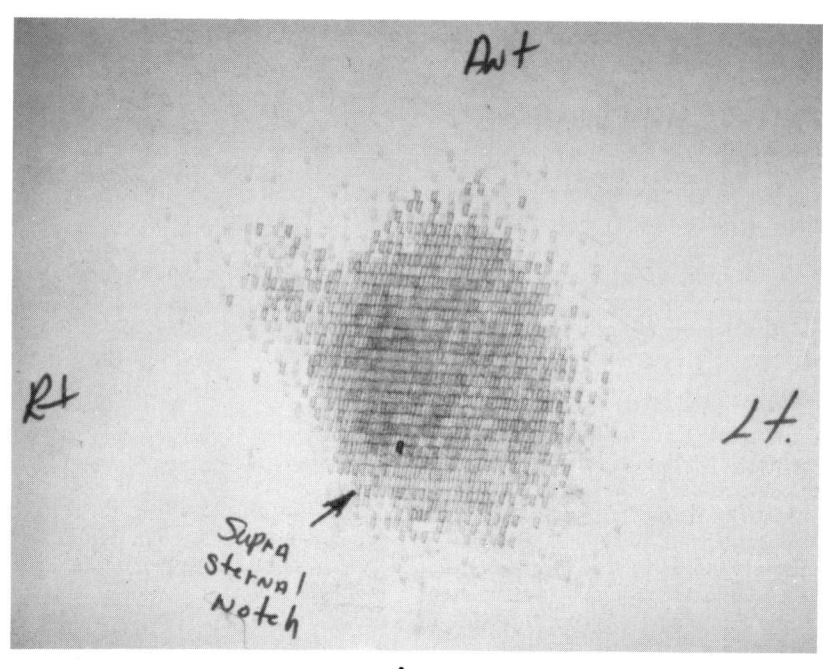

A

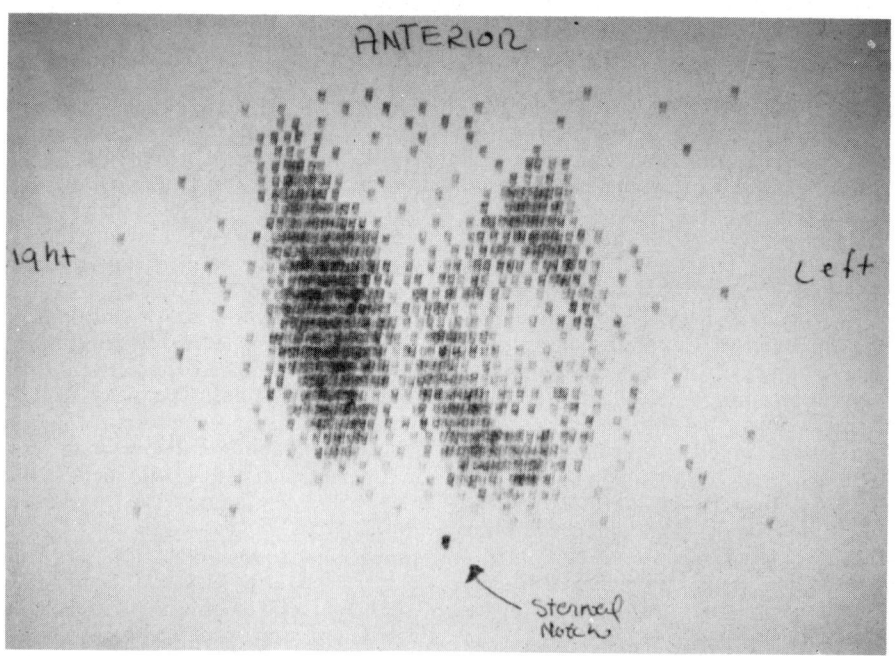

B

Figure 4–20. Scans of hyperfunctioning and nonfunctioning thyroid nodules. *A,* Scan of hyperfunctioning follicular adenoma arising at the junction of the isthmus and left lateral lobe. Function of the extranodular tissue is almost completely suppressed. *B,* Scan of nonfunctioning thyroid nodule in the corpus of the lateral left lobe. At operation, the lesion was a papillary carcinoma.

review by Rosen et al., 1979.) In ultrasonography, highly focused sound waves of extremely high frequency (greater than 1 million cycles per second) produced by a piezoelectric transducer are directed internally perpendicular to the skin surface. Echoes generated at interphases of differing acoustic impedance return to the apparatus and are detected and processed for visual display. A-mode scans are single-point recordings displayed in a linear format, in which echoes appear as spikes. The height of the spikes varies with the intensity of the echo, and the distance between them accurately indicates the distance between echoic interphases. In B-mode scans, the transducer is moved linearly across the neck in the horizontal plane and the data are processed to yield a transverse sonic laminogram. In gray-scale scans, the data are displayed in shades of gray across the spectrum from black to white in proportion to the intensity of the echoes generated. At the frequencies employed, ultrasonograms produce no tissue damage; they can be used, therefore, repeatedly and with impunity in children and pregnant women.

The normal thyroid produces a pattern of sparse, fine echoes in the paratracheal region. Ultrasonograms are capable of revealing diffuse or localized enlargements of the gland and provide an objective means of assessing changes in their size, as in the response to suppressive therapy. The greater value of ultrasonography is, however, in the differentiation of cystic from solid lesions of the gland. Purely cystic lesions are entirely sonolucent, creating echoes only at their anterior and posterior walls. Solid lesions, in contrast, create multiple echoes, owing to their multiple sonically active interphases, and they are often surrounded by a sonolucent halo. Mixed solid and cystic lesions are often encountered, and indeed many lesions that are predominantly solid are found to have small cystic areas, representing zones of focal degeneration. The demonstration that a nodule is purely cystic reduces, but does not eliminate, the likelihood that the lesion is malignant in nature. Mixed lesions have the same significance as solid lesions, but benign and malignant lesions cannot be differentiated from one another by ultrasonography alone. The manner in which ultrasonograms are integrated into the clinical approach to the management of the nodular thyroid gland is discussed in the appropriate subsequent section.

Thyroid Biopsy

Biopsy of the thyroid, particularly closed percutaneous needle biopsy, is a method increasingly employed to obtain an anatomic diagnosis in certain types of thyroid disease. Although biopsy can be applied to the diagnosis of a variety of thyroid disorders, such as subacute thyroiditis in atypical cases, Hashimoto's disease, or multinodular goiter, the major rationale for thyroid biopsy is to differentiate between benign and malignant thyroid nodules. Initially, open biopsy, a surgical procedure performed under general or local anesthesia, was the sole type of biopsy performed. In diseases involving the thyroid diffusely, a specimen was taken for histologic examination, but nodular lesions were usually removed *in toto*; hence, the procedure was often therapeutic, as well as diagnostic.

Subsequently, closed percutaneous biopsies intended to obtain a core of tissue for histologic diagnosis were introduced. In these office procedures, following local anesthesia, a large Vim-Silverman or Tru-cut needle (about 15-gauge) is introduced through a small nick in the skin, and one or more specimens for histologic examination are ob-

tained. In experienced hands, cutting needle biopsies are quite free of complications and a diagnostic accuracy of about 90% is obtained. (See Wang et al., 1976). In less experienced hands, however, such complications as hemorrhage, tracheal puncture, laryngoparalysis, and transient injury to the recurrent laryngeal nerve are less infrequent and specimens are more often insufficient for histologic diagnosis.

The major reasons for the growth of interest in and use of thyroid biopsy are a lessening fear of disseminating malignancy and the introduction of the fine-needle aspiration biopsy coupled with cytologic examination. (For a comprehensive review, beautifully illustrated, see Hamburger et al., 1979.) In this technique, which is simple and quite safe, the patient is placed in a supine position with the neck extended; local anesthesia is rarely required. The nodule is then penetrated with a fine (22- to 27-gauge) needle attached to a 20-ml syringe with a nozzle tip, and vigorous suction is applied manually. The contents of the needle are spread on a glass slide, dried or fixed, and stained.

Both large- and fine-needle biopsies have limitations. In both techniques, only a limited amount of tissue is obtained, and that may not be representative of the entire lesion. Neither technique is reliable in the diagnosis of differentiated follicular carcinoma, in which evidence of capsular or blood vessel invasion is required for diagnosis, and neither can reliably distinguish between Hashimoto's disease and lymphoma of the thyroid. In the case of fine-needle biopsy, the strongest caveat, however, is that slides be read not merely by an experienced cytologist, but by one who has specifically trained by comparing slides prepared from aspiration biopsies, obtained either preoperatively or at surgery, with those obtained following surgical excision of the lesion. When this is done, false-positive and false-negative readings are obtained in about 15% of cases.

Thyroid biopsy of any type should not be performed as an isolated diagnostic procedure, but rather should be integrated into a systematic approach to the management of the thyroid nodule that includes, in addition, careful clinical examination, scintiscanning, and ultrasonography. (See later section for the authors' recommendations in this regard.)

EFFECTS OF THYROID HORMONES ON METABOLIC PROCESSES

The thyroid hormones play upon a great multiplicity of metabolic processes, influencing the concentration and activity of numerous enzymes; the metabolism of substrates, vitamins, and minerals; the secretion and degradation rates of virtually all other hormones; and the response of their target tissues to them. As a consequence, it can truly be said that no tissue or organ system escapes the adverse effects of thyroid hormone excess or insufficiency.

In the sections that follow this one, the many physiologic and biochemical derangements that are expressed clinically in patients with hyperthyroidism or hypothyroidism will be discussed, together with the specific disease states that produce them. This section will first consider briefly the major metabolic effects of the thyroid hormones. For more detailed considerations of the truly voluminous literature bearing upon this topic, the reader is referred to several extensive reviews (Greenberg et al., 1974; Hoch, 1974; Bray and Jacobs, 1974; Freedberg and Hamolsky, 1974). The later portions of this section will summarize the main theories concerning the cellular and molecular basis of thyroid hormone action.

Effects on Calorigenesis

One classic action of the thyroid hormones is their stimulatory effect on calorigenesis. This is reflected in increased oxygen consumption in the whole animal or in isolated tissues *in vitro*. This response occurs after a latent period of several hours or days and is evident in most tissues, the spleen, brain, and testis being notable exceptions. T_3 causes a more prompt but somewhat shorter-lived effect than does T_4. The lag preceding these calorigenic responses has led to the suggestion that metabolic transformation of the thyroid hormones necessarily precedes induction of metabolic action. Other responses *in vivo*, however, such as increased heart rate, decreased cardiac glycogen content, and increased sensitivity to the lipolytic effect of epinephrine, precede any increase in oxygen consumption. Furthermore, several actions of the thyroid hormones *in vitro* that seem to bear a relationship to effects *in vivo* are demonstrable following a negligible lag.

The precise mechanism of the calorigenic effect of the thyroid hormones remains uncertain. As discussed subsequently, direct effects of the hormone on mitochondrial metabolism have been and remain a topic of interest. Major attention currently focuses, however, on the possibility that thyroid hormone–induced thermogenesis represents the energy expenditure of increased transport of sodium and potassium across the cell membrane by the enzyme Na^+-K^+-ATPase. As much as half of the increased energy expenditure involved in the transition from the hypothyroid to the euthyroid state, and approximately 80% of that involved in the transition from the euthyroid to the hyperthyroid state, has been ascribed to this mechanism. Enhanced enzyme activity in response to thyroid hormones has been detected in liver slices and liver cell monolayers, small intestine, kidney, muscle, and heart, and is evidently due to an increase in the number of enzyme units secondary to a stimulation of synthesis. Despite its attractiveness, this proposed mechanism is not universally accepted. Many studies have been performed with doses of thyroid hormone vastly in excess of physiologic requirement; other studies have failed to demonstrate any change in enzyme activity, even with very large doses of hormone; and still others indicate that the energy cost of sodium transport is less than that previously estimated, and is insufficient to account for the increased thermogenesis that thyroid hormones induce. Hence, the role of Na^+-K^+-ATPase in the calorigenic action of thyroid hormones remains an open question. (For further discussion and references, see Smith and Edelman, 1979; Biron et al., 1979; and Tobin et al., 1979.)

Effects on Protein Metabolism

The pronounced effects that the thyroid hormones exert on protein metabolism may be fundamental to many of the metabolic actions of the hormones. Stimulation of protein synthesis by thyroid hormones may be partly responsible for a portion of their calorigenic effect, while enhanced synthesis of specific enzymes may result in other metabolic sequelae. For example, thyroid hormones enhance the synthesis of lysozymal enzymes in muscle and are necessary for the catabolic response to a variety of stimuli in this tissue.

The effect of thyroid hormones on protein metabolism depends upon the metabolic state of the recipient organism and the size of the administered dose. In thyroidectomized rats, moderate doses of T_4 increase protein synthesis and decrease nitrogen excretion. Larger doses inhibit protein synthesis and increase the concentration of free amino acids in plasma, liver, and muscle. A similar biphasic response of protein synthesis has been noted in rabbit bone marrow slices incubated in varying concentrations of T_4 *in vitro*. In rats, optimal doses of thyroid hormone are necessary for the elicitation of the full growth response to growth hormone (GH); the nature of the interaction of these hormones is uncertain.

Variations in overall growth rate are probably the most general reflection of the effects of thyroid hormones on protein synthesis, and here too the effects are biphasic. In immature animals and young patients, growth is retarded by hypothyroidism, is restored by replacement doses, and is inhibited by excessive doses of hormone. In the thyrotoxic state, nitrogen excretion is increased, but it is not clear whether the catabolic response to thyroid hormones is an obligatory effect or is due to negative caloric balance. In adult patients with hypothyroidism, studies with ^{15}N-glycine indicate a decreased rate of protein synthesis, and observations with I*-labeled serum albumin indicate that the synthesis and degradation of this protein are retarded. These functions in the hypothyroid patient are restored to normal by replacement doses of thyroid hormone.

Effects on Carbohydrate Metabolism

Thyroid hormones affect virtually all aspects of carbohydrate metabolism. Many of their influences are dependent upon or modified by other hormones, in particular the catecholamines and insulin. Thyroid hormones appear to regulate the magnitude of the glycogenolytic and hyperglycemic actions of epinephrine, possibly by enhancing responsiveness of the adenylate cyclase–cyclic AMP system, and to potentiate the effects of insulin on glycogen synthesis and glucose utilization. Some of the effects of thyroid hormones depend upon the dose, and as a result, biphasic actions have been observed. For example, in rats, small doses of T_4 increase glycogen synthesis in the presence of insulin, whereas large doses increase hepatic glycogenolysis, causing glycogen depletion. This biphasic action of T_4 modifies the subsequent glycogenolytic response to epinephrine, small doses of T_4 enhancing and large doses depressing the response. Large doses of T_4 enhance gluconeogenesis by increasing the availability of precursors, such as lactate and glycerol. Thyroid hormones enhance the rate of intestinal absorption of glucose and galactose. They also increase the rate of uptake of glucose by adipose tissue and muscle and potentiate the effect of insulin in this respect. Insulin degradation appears to be increased by thyroid hormones, and this may account for the diminished sensitivity to exogenous insulin that is sometimes seen in thyrotoxicosis. The converse occurs in hypothyroidism.

Effects on Lipid Metabolism

Thyroid hormones appear to stimulate virtually all aspects of lipid metabolism, including synthesis, mobilization, and degradation. In general, degradation is affected more than synthesis, the net effect in states of hormone excess being a decrease in the stores of most lipids and usually their concentrations in plasma. This is true for triglycerides, phospholipids, and cholesterol. Converse changes are seen in states of thyroid hormone deficiency.

Most closely related to the changes in energy metabolism that accompany states of thyroid hormone excess or deficiency are changes in the metabolism of fatty acids at their sites of storage and degradation. Thyroid hormones increase lipolysis in adipose tissue both by a direct effect through the adenylate cyclase–cyclic AMP system and by sensitizing the tissue to other lipolytic agents, such as catecholamines, GH, glucocorticoids, and glucagon. In the case of glucagon, an increase in receptor number induced by thyroid hormone may be the responsible mechanism. Oxidation of FFA is also increased, and this enhancement may account for some of the calorigenic action of thyroid hormones.

Hepatic synthesis of triglycerides is increased, probably as a result of the increased availability of FFA and glycerol mobilized from adipose tissue. Concomitantly, removal of triglycerides from plasma is accelerated, possibly because of an increase in lipoprotein lipase.

A classic effect of thyroid hormones is to lower the concentration of cholesterol in plasma. This is probably the result of a variety of actions. Synthesis of cholesterol is enhanced at the stage of conversion of β-hydroxy-β-methylglutaryl-coenzyme A to mevalonate, probably by increasing the activity of the enzyme concerned. Thyroid hormone action on the elimination of cholesterol is effected by an increase in both the fecal excretion of cholesterol and its conversion to bile acids. A further effect of the thyroid hormones is to enhance the turnover of low density lipoprotein (LDL) to which are bound cholesterol and phospholipids. These effects may result from an action reflected by the ability of T_3 to stimulate the synthesis of LDL receptors and LDL degradation in fibroblasts *in vitro* (Chait et al., 1979).

Effects on Vitamin Metabolism

Because of their stimulatory effect on metabolic processes, thyroid hormones increase the demand for coenzymes and the vitamins from which they are derived. In hyperthyroidism, the requirements for water-soluble vitamins, such as thiamine, riboflavin, vitamin B_{12}, and vitamin C, are increased, and their tissue concentrations are reduced. The conversion of some water-soluble vitamins to the coenzyme form may be impaired in hyperthyroidism, possibly as a result of defective energy transfers. For example, phosphorylation of pyridoxine to pyridoxal-5-phosphate (codecarboxylase) and synthesis of pyridine nucleotides (NAD and NADP) from nicotinamide appear to be defective in tissues of hyperthyroid animals. On the other hand, the synthesis of some coenzymes from vitamin requires thyroid hormones. For example, the synthesis of flavin mononucleotide and flavin adenine dinucleotide from riboflavin requires the stimulatory effect of thyroid hormones on the enzyme flavokinase.

The metabolism of fat-soluble vitamins is also influenced by thyroid hormones. They are required for the synthesis of vitamin A from carotene and for the conversion of vitamin A to retinene, the pigment required for dark adaptation. In hypothyroidism, the serum carotene concentration is increased and may give the skin a yellow tint, and clinical manifestations of vitamin A deficiency may occur. In hyperthyroidism, the requirement for vitamin A is increased and the tissue concentration is reduced. Vitamins D and E appear to be deficient in hyperthyroid animals.

Interactions with the Sympathetic Nervous System

The similarities between many of the manifestations of thyrotoxicosis and those of sympathetic nervous system activation have long been recognized and long studied. Nonetheless, understanding of the nature and biochemical basis of the interaction between the thyroid hormones and the sympathetic nervous system is still incomplete. As judged from the plasma concentrations of epinephrine and norepi-

nephrine, as well as their urinary excretion and that of their metabolites, it is clear that the activity of the sympathetic nervous system is not increased in patients or animals with thyrotoxicosis. Another possibility is that thyroid hormones exert effects separate from, but similar and additive to, those of the catecholamines. This is true in the rat thymocyte, for example, in which epinephrine and T_3 *in vitro* independently and also additively increase cyclic AMP concentration. Similarly, in rat heart homogenate, thyroid hormones increase cyclic AMP concentration, and this effect is not blocked by adrenergic antagonists. This type of interaction would best explain why many of the sympathomimetic manifestations of thyrotoxicosis are only partly relieved by anti-adrenergic agents.

The most widely studied possibility is that thyroid hormones enhance tissue sensitivity to catecholamines. Whether this is the case is uncertain, and may depend upon the tissue in question. Although thyroid hormones clearly increase cardiac contractility, it is not yet certain that dose-response relationships for the stimulation of myocardial cyclic AMP concentration and contractility by catecholamines are altered. On the other hand, the evidence is entirely consistent that thyroid hormones increase the lipolytic response of adipose tissue to epinephrine and the response of hepatic glycogenolysis to epinephrine and glucagon.

The effects of thyroid hormones on plasma membrane receptors for catecholamines is a topic undergoing active exploration. In rat heart, chronic administration of thyroid hormones increases the number, but not the affinity, of β-adrenergic receptors. Another possibility, not yet fully explored, is that thyroid hormones alter the plasma membrane so that α-adrenergic receptors take on the properties of β-adrenergic receptors. Still another possibility is that thyroid hormones do not affect the number or affinity of catecholamine receptors, but increase the extent to which binding of agonist to the individual receptor is coupled to adenylate cyclase stimulation. This seems clearly to be the case in adipose tissue, but may be operative in other tissues as well, since the exaggerated increase in plasma cyclic AMP concentration that follows administration of epinephrine to thyrotoxic patients is also seen following administration of either glucagon or parathyroid hormone. (For reviews and references in this complex but important area, see Levey, 1976, and Landsberg, 1977.)

THEORIES CONCERNING THE MECHANISM OF ACTION OF THYROID HORMONES

There is an appealing parsimony in the concept that the manifold physiologic and biochemical effects of the thyroid hormones reflect a single action, or perhaps a few basic actions, at the cellular or molecular level. That this may be the case is suggested by the very diversity of hormonal effects, since it is very unlikely that a distinct mechanism is responsible for each. More likely, many of the effects observed are merely secondary consequences of one or more fundamental actions. Furthermore, most actions of the thyroid hormones are demonstrable only after a considerable latent period, suggesting that they are anteceded by some more proximal event. It is not surprising, therefore, that current research has been directed at uncovering what is often referred to as "*the* mechanism of action" of the thyroid hormones. Patterns of investigation have conformed to concepts standard to modern cell biology and applicable to studies of the mechanisms of action of other hormones. These involve a search for specific cellular receptors for hormone, for the signal(s) generated by binding of the hormone to its receptor, and for the manner in which generation of the signal results in the highly diverse, yet highly specific, manifestations of hormone action. Currently, varying amounts of evidence, summarized briefly in the ensuing discussion, support the existence of primary and independent actions of the thyroid hormones at several sites, including the nucleus, the mitochondrion, and the plasma membrane (see Fig. 4–20). For comprehensive discussions of this topic, amply referenced, the reader is referred to several reviews (DeGroot, 1979; Oppenheimer, 1979; Sterling, 1979; Segal and Ingbar, 1980).

The demonstration that thyroid hormones produce a relative prompt increase in RNA synthesis provided the first biochemical evidence of an action of thyroid hormones at a nuclear level. Major impetus to work in this area was provided, however, by the later demonstration of saturable, high-affinity binding sites for T_3 in the nuclei of rat pituitary gland. Subsequently, similar receptors have been identified in rat liver, brain, heart, kidney, and lymphocytes; in GH_1 cells, a rat pituitary cell line; and in human liver, kidney, and lymphocytes. The receptors in these various tissues resemble each other substantially in being acidic (nonhistone) chromatin proteins whose molecular weight is about 50,000 and whose affinity for T_3 is in the order of about 2–5×10^{11} M^{-1}, approximately ten times that for T_4. Unlike the binding of steroid hormones to nuclear receptors, that of T_2 and other thyroid hormones does not require initial binding of the hormone to a cytosolic receptor, with subsequent translocation of the complex to the nucleus. Instead, thyroid hormones appear to bind directly to nuclear chromatin, cytosolic binding proteins limiting, rather than facilitating, their entry.

A variety of nuclear events follow relatively shortly after administration of thyroid hormones. Among them are increases in the activity of RNA polymerases I and II, an increase in nuclear globulins and nonhistone proteins, and a change in the properties of the former. Nuclear phosphokinase activity is increased, and with it phosphorylation of nuclear proteins. Most important, however, are observations indicating that T_3 enhances the concentration of the specific mRNA for growth hormone, an effect seen in GH_1 cells, and for α-2μ globulin, an effect seen in rat liver, since synthesis of the corresponding protein is known to be increased by thyroid hormones.

The latter findings provide perhaps the strongest evidence that a primary action of thyroid hormones is exerted at the nuclear level to alter gene transcription. Additional evidence in favor of this view are instances in which nuclear occupancy by T_3 is correlated with metabolic response. There is, in general, a good concordance between the biologic potency of various thyroid hormone analogues and their binding to nuclear receptors, and some tissues that fail to respond to thyroid hormones with an increase in oxygen consumption display a relatively low concentration of nuclear receptors for T_3.

On the other hand, there are becoming known an increasing number of instances in which receptor number and thyroid hormone–related metabolic responses are dissociated, among them responses in neonatal rat brain and in rat liver following partial hepatectomy, glucagon administration, and starvation. Such discrepancies require the postulation of seemingly independent effects of thyroid hormones on post-transcriptional events. Further, discrepancies between the affinity of hormone analogues, such as triac and D-T_4, which bind strongly to the nuclear receptor, and their biologic potency, which is relatively low, have been ascribed to their rapid *in vivo* turnover, which limits their nuclear occupancy. It seems likely, however, that *in vivo* turnover rates also differ widely among those hormone analogues whose binding and biologic potency, relative to T_3, are in close accord. In addition, it is clear that nuclear receptors for T_3 are present in rat brain, including neonatal brain, though they are fewer in number than in most other tissues. This lesser number of receptors has been correlated with the failure of brain to increase its oxygen consumption in response to thyroid hormone, yet a biologic response to thyroid hormones is evident in the thyroid hormone–dependent maturation of brain that takes place while oxygen consumption is unresponsive. That being the case, the argument that failure of thyroid hormones to increase the oxygen consumption of testis and spleen is due to their lack of nuclear receptors should be challenged by a search for other biologic actions of the thyroid hormone in these tissues. All in all, it seems certain that the nuclear binding of T_3 is an initiating event for some aspects of thyroid hormone action, but how that action is brought about, what determines the specificity of hormone responses, and what other steps in the regulation of protein synthesis are also affected remain to be clarified.

In view of the fact that increased oxygen consumption is one of the cardinal effects of the thyroid hormones, great attention has been directed toward the effects of thyroid hormones on mitochondria, since they are the locus of terminal oxidation of metabolites and transfer of electrons to oxygen along the respiratory chain. It is here, too, that oxidations are most efficiently linked or coupled to the generation of the high-energy phosphate bonds of ATP, a form that can be utilized for the performance of physical or chemical work. An additional relevant feature of mitochondrial respiration is that the rate of generation of high-energy phosphate in some way regulates inversely the rate of substrate oxidation and oxygen utilization. Normally, the rate of oxidation is highly dependent upon the availability of ADP or other phosphate receptors. When this is the case, respiration is said to be "tightly controlled."

It is clear that uncoupling of oxidative phosphorylation is not the mechanism by which thyroid hormones increase oxygen consumption, as originally thought. However, a variety of other mitochondrial effects of the thyroid hormones have been observed. *In vivo*, T_4 induces an increase in the number and size of mitochondria and in the number of mitochondrial cristae. It induces swelling of mitochondria *in vitro* with loss of mitochondrial constituents, an effect seen in T_4-responsive tissues but not in tissues whose oxygen consumption fails to increase in response to T_4, such as brain, testis, and spleen. In hypothyroid animals, T_4 promptly stimulates mitochondrial respiration in the absence of added ADP (state 4 respiration) (Hoch, 1967), and later it stimulates ADP-dependent respiration (state 3) as well. Some evidence suggests that the stimulation of state 4 respiration may reflect the action of a specific mitochondrial protein whose synthesis is induced by thyroid hormones. T_4 and T_3, both *in vitro* and *in vivo*, promptly stimulate mitochondrial protein synthesis, and both, after several days, increase the carrier-mediated uptake of ADP by rat liver mitochondria, an effect thought to mediate enhanced ATP generation. It is not known whether or how the foregoing effects are interrelated, but their net result would presumably be an enhanced rate of oxygen consumption, an increased number of respiratory units, and an increased availability of high-energy phosphate (energy charge) within the cell.

The likelihood that the mitochondrion is a primary site of thyroid hormone action has been increased by the detection of high-affinity (10^{11} M^{-1}), limited-capacity binding of T_3 to specific mitochondrial components. The putative receptor is a lipoprotein derived from the inner mitochondrial membrane, the site of oxidative phosphorylations, and the intensity of its interaction with thyroid hormone analogues accords well with their biologic potency. Attention is further directed at the inner mitochondrial membrane by recent demonstrations that thyroid hormones alter its content of specific lipids and proteins. If recent claims that T_3 in low concentrations promptly and directly increases the oxygen consumption and ATP formation by mitochondria *in vitro* are substantiated, this will support strongly the likelihood that the mitochondrion, like the nucleus, is a primary site of thyroid hormone action.

Data are also accumulating which provide strong support for the postulate that thyroid hormones exert a primary effect at the level of the cell membrane. High-affinity, limited-capacity binding sites for T_3 have been found in highly purified plasma membrane fractions derived from rat liver and rat thymocytes. Thyroid hormones enhance the accumulation of exogenous free amino acids by rat muscle and brain *in vivo,* and increase amino acid accumulation *in vivo* in chick embryo cartilage and rat thymocytes. Inward transport of the sugar analogue 2-deoxyglucose (2-DG) is enhanced by T_3 *in vitro* in cultured myocardial cells of the chick embryo and in freshly isolated rat thymocytes. The latter response is the one best characterized in this area of study. The effect of T_3 on 2-DG accumulation by the thymocyte is very prompt in onset; is calcium-dependent; like all the aforementioned effects, does not require new protein synthesis; and in media supplemented with insulin and epinephrine is elicited by physiologic concentrations of T_3. The effect is apparently mediated by a T_3-induced increase in cellular cyclic AMP concentration, since T_3 increases cellular cyclic AMP within a few minutes, well before its effect on 2-DG uptake; since the effect of T_3 is mimicked by the addition of dibutyrylcyclic AMP; and since manipulations which block the cyclic AMP response to T_3, such as omission of calcium from the incubation medium or the addition of alprenolol, also block the effect of T_3 on 2-DG uptake. T_3 and epinephrine act synergistically in respect to cyclic AMP concentration and 2-DG uptake, furthering the likelihood that T_3 is producing its effects at the level of the plasma membrane.

On the basis of the foregoing evidence, the authors are persuaded that the thyroid hormones have primary actions at multiple sites within the cell, rather than a single site. Within this framework, one can visualize a coordinated metabolic response, in which action at the plasma membrane enhances substrate availability, action at the mitochondrion provides requisite metabolic energy, and action at the transcriptional and post-transcriptional level directs the synthesis of specific structural and functional components of the cell.

AN APPROACH TO THE CLINICAL DIAGNOSIS OF THYROID DISEASE

Diseases of the thyroid gland almost always manifest themselves through symptoms resulting from excessive or insufficient production of thyroid hormone, through local symptoms in the neck, principally goiter (but occasionally pain or compression of adjacent structures), or, in the case of Graves' disease, through exophthalmos. Although the physician's attention is directed initially at the major clinical evidence, he seeks ultimately to establish both a functional and an anatomic diagnosis; i.e., he seeks to define the patient's metabolic state and to ascertain the nature of the underlying disorder. These two aspects of the complete diagnosis are not arrived at independently, because the functional state will delimit the possible specific diagnoses and vice versa.

A functional diagnosis of thyroid disease is based upon a carefully taken history, a thorough search for the physical signs of hypothyroidism or thyrotoxicosis, and an intelligent appraisal of the results of laboratory tests. Characteristic alterations in these aspects will be found in the discussions of the various disease states. Although conditioned by the functional diagnosis, the anatomic diagnosis will depend largely upon the examination of the thyroid gland itself (Fig. 4–21).

Local examination of the neck is best accomplished with the patient seated in a good light with the neck moderately extended. The patient should be provided with a glass of water to facilitate swallowing. The physician should first inspect the neck from the front and sides. The presence of old surgical scars, distended veins, and redness or fixation of the overlying skin should be noted. If a mass is present, attention should be directed to its location and to whether or not it moves on swallowing. Movement on swallowing is a characteristic feature of the thyroid gland and is due to the fact that the gland is ensheathed by the pretracheal fascia; this feature distinguishes a goiter from most other masses arising in the neck. However, if a goiter is so large that it occupies all the available space in the neck, or if the thyroid gland is the seat of an invasive carcinoma or Riedel's thyroiditis that has led to fixation to adjacent structures, movement on swallowing may be lost. The physician should also inspect the dorsum of the tongue, which is the origin of the thyroglossal duct and occasionally the seat of a goiter (lingual goiter).

Palpation of the neck is best accomplished by standing behind the seated patient and palpating with the fingertips of both hands. The position of the cricoid cartilage is first determined; this is an important landmark, since the superior border of the isthmus lies just below it. The isthmus is a band of tissue crossing the front of the trachea and joining the two lateral lobes on either side of the trachea. The examiner then attempts to outline the thyroid gland and to determine the limits of the lower borders of the lateral lobes, while the patient swallows sips of water at appropriate intervals. A normal thyroid gland can usually be felt on palpation. The examiner should note the shape of the gland, its size in relation to normal, and its consistency. The normal gland feels rubbery. A literal rule of thumb is that the normal thyroid lobe has approximately the same size in frontal projection as the terminal phalanx of the thumb does. Whereas the diffuse colloid goiter and the hyperplastic gland of Graves' disease tend to be softer than normal, the gland of Hashimoto's disease tends to be firmer than normal, and the gland that is the seat of carcinoma or Riedel's thyroiditis may be "stony" hard. Irregularities of the surface, variations in consistency, and tender areas should be noted. If nodules are palpated, their shape, size, position, and consistency in relation to the surrounding tissue should be determined. A search should be made for the pyramidal lobe; this is a band of tissue extending upward from the isthmus to the right or left of the midline. The pyramidal lobe may be mistaken for the pretracheal or "delphian" lymph node that sometimes accompanies thyroid carcinoma or thyroiditis. Another midline mass that may lead to confusion is a thyroglossal cyst, but since this often remains attached to the base of the tongue by the obliterated thyroglossal duct, it moves upward when the tongue is protruded. During palpation a vascular thrill may be felt and, in the absence of cardiac disease, is very suggestive of hyperthyroidism. Finally, palpation should always include examination of the regional lymph nodes.

Auscultation of the neck should be performed since it gives some indication of the vascularity of the gland. A systolic or continuous bruit is commonly heard over a hyperplastic

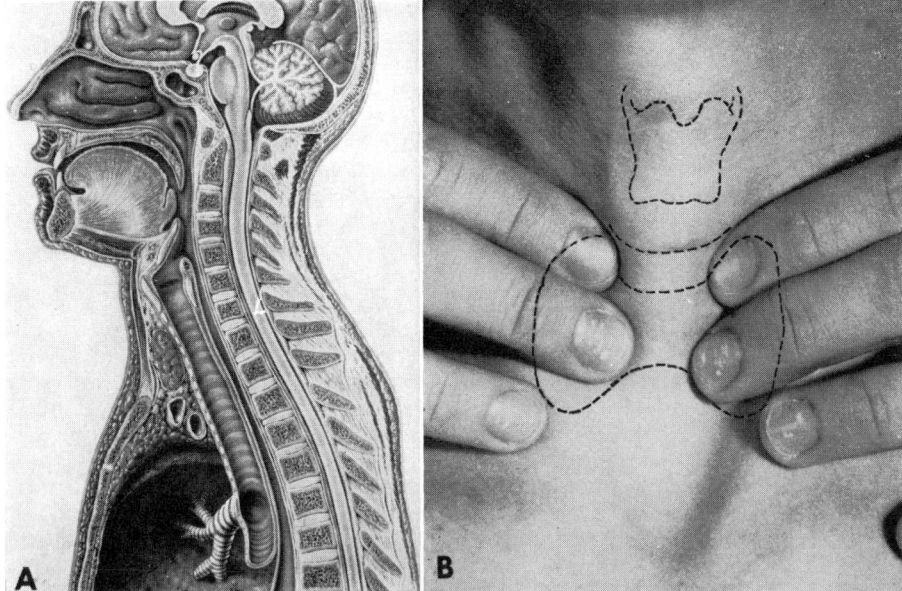

Figure 4–21. *A,* This sagittal section demonstrates the relations of the isthmus of the normal thyroid gland. The superior border is inferior to the cricoid cartilage. The inferior thyroid border is essentially at the level of the superior surface of the manubrium. The inferior portions of the lateral lobes (not shown) extend more inferiorly than the isthmus. (Reproduced by permission of Merck & Co., Inc.).

B, The cricoid cartilage is regarded as a very important landmark. Especially when the thyroid gland is suspected as being essentially normal or subnormal in size the cricoid should be located. This is easily accomplished. The index fingers are then inserted so that their superior portion rests against the inferior portion of the cricoid, while the inferior portion of these fingers is over the superior portion of the thyroid. The second and third fingers are rotated over other portions of the gland, evaluating its size, contour, consistency, possible adherence to surrounding structures, and other features. Since there is marked variation among different subjects in the length and thickness of the neck and in the length of the trachea superior to the level of the manubrium, there is variation in the relative position of the thyroid. In some cases, essentially all of the thyroid rests posterior to the sternum. In most instances, however, by having the patient extend his neck maximally (short of markedly tightening the neck muscles) and by having him swallow repeatedly, it is possible to palpate most or all of the gland. One point deserving emphasis is the fact that in spite of marked variations in neck-chest relations, thyroid tissue, when present, is found within 1 cm. of the cricoid. By concentrating the palpation meticulously in the area where the thyroid is normally found, with very rare exceptions it is possible to outline small as well as enlarged glands.

gland. However, care should be taken to distinguish a thyroid bruit from a murmur transmitted from the base of the heart or from a venous hum that can be obliterated by compression of the external jugular vein or by turning the head.

Two useful clinical maneuvers that are often neglected are transillumination and the arm-raising test. Transillumination is readily performed with a penlight and serves to distinguish between cystic and solid masses in the thyroid. Since the normal tissues of the neck transilluminate to some extent, the transillumination in the lesion should be compared with that in an indifferent area. The arm-raising test is useful in the patient in whom a retrosternal goiter is suspected. The basis for this maneuver is that if the size of the thoracic inlet is already reduced by a retrosternal goiter, raising both arms until they touch the sides of the head will further narrow the thoracic inlet and cause congestion of the face and respiratory distress (Pemberton's sign).

In addition to examination of the thyroid gland and regional lymph nodes, evidence of compression or displacement of adjacent structures should also be sought. Hoarseness may indicate compression of the recurrent laryngeal nerve, usually by a malignant thyroid neoplasm, and this should be confirmed by laryngoscopy. Displacement of the trachea may be evident, and inspiratory stridor may indicate compression of the trachea. Radiologic examination is a useful adjunct, since it may reveal retrosternal extension of a goiter, displacement or narrowing of the trachea, and, during a barium swallow, displacement of the esophagus.

Calcification in the thyroid gland may also be seen and, by its nature, aid in distinguishing between benign and malignant lesions.

THYROTOXICOSIS

The term thyrotoxicosis refers to the biochemical and physiologic complex that results when the tissues are pre-

Table 4–7. VARIETIES OF THYROTOXICOSIS

Disorder
1. Associated with Sustained Hormone Overproduction (Hyperthyroidism)*
   Increased TSH secretion (rare)
   Graves' disease
   Trophoblastic tumor
   Toxic multinodular goiter
   Toxic adenoma
   Iodine-induced (Jodbasedow)
2. Not associated with Hyperthyroidism†
   Thyrotoxicosis factitia
   Subacute thyroiditis
   Chronic thyroiditis with transient thyrotoxicosis ("painless thyroiditis," "hyperthyroiditis")
   Ectopic thyroid tissue (struma ovarii, functioning metastatic thyroid cancer)

*Except for iodine-induced hyperthyroidism, associated with increased values of the RAIU
†Associated with decreased values of the RAIU

sented with excessive quantities of the thyroid hormones. The authors prefer the general term thyrotoxicosis rather than hyperthyroidism to describe this syndrome, since it need not originate in the thyroid gland. The term hyperthyroidism is best reserved for those disorders in which thyrotoxicosis results from overproduction of hormone by the thyroid itself, Graves' disease being the most interesting and important among them. The various causes of thyrotoxicosis are listed in Table 4–7 and are discussed individually in the material that follows. The nature of the manifestations of thyrotoxicosis depends upon the severity of the syndrome, the age of the patient, and the presence or absence of disease in other organ systems. Additional clinical features are conditioned by the specific disorder producing the thyrotoxicosis.

Peripheral Manifestations of Thyrotoxicosis

Skin and Appendages

Thyrotoxicosis leads to a variety of changes in the skin and its appendages. Most characteristic is the warm moist feel of the skin that results from cutaneous vasodilation and excessive sweating as part of the hyperdynamic circulatory state. The hands are usually warm and moist, but the texture of the skin in this area is often altered by occupational or environmental factors; hence, texture is best assessed on the inner aspect of the arm or thigh or over the thorax. Classically, the elbows are smooth and pink. The complexion is rosy and the patient blushes readily. Palmar erythema, indistinguishable from "liver palms," is common, and there may be some telangiectasia. Increased diffuse pigmentation is found occasionally and may resemble that found in Addison's disease, but the authors have not noted buccal pigmentation in uncomplicated thyrotoxicosis. Patchy vitiligo may also occur. Increased pigmentation may result from hypersecretion of ACTH secondary to accelerated metabolism of cortisol.

The hair is fine and friable and does not retain a wave; some may fall out. The nails are often soft and friable. A characteristic finding is Plummer's nails, a term applied to separation of the distal margin of the nail from the nail bed with irregular recession of the junction (onycholysis). Dirt often accumulates under the nail. Usually these changes are best seen in the fourth finger and are frequently accompanied by a thin shiny appearance of the skin surrounding the nail.

Eyes

Retraction of the upper eyelid, evident as the presence of a rim of sclera between the lid and the limbus, is a very frequent manifestation of all forms of thyrotoxicosis, irrespective of the underlying cause. It is responsible for the bright-eyed "stare" of the patient with thyrotoxicosis. Accompanying lid retraction are the phenomena of lid lag, in which the upper lid lags behind the globe when the patient is asked to gaze slowly downward, and globe lag, in which the globe lags behind the upper lid when the patient gazes slowly upward. The movements of the lids are jerky and spasmodic, and a fine tremor of the lightly closed lids can often be observed. These ocular manifestations appear to be the result of increased adrenergic activity. It is important to differentiate these ocular manifestations, which occur in all forms of thyrotoxicosis, from those of infiltrative ophthalmopathy, which are characteristic of Graves' disease.

Cardiovascular System

Alterations in cardiovascular function are among the most prominent manifestations of thyrotoxicosis. Increased circulatory demands result from both the hypermetabolism and the need to dissipate the excess heat produced. At rest, peripheral vascular resistance is decreased, and cardiac output is increased as a result of an increase in both stroke volume and heart rate. Thyroid hormones in excess have a direct cardiostimulatory action, possibly mediated by alterations in the state of contractile proteins or in the function of sarcoplasmic reticulum. In addition, increased adrenergic activity also appears to be involved in the maintenance of the hyperdynamic circulatory state, since some amelioration of the hemodynamic manifestations accompanies treatment with adrenergic antagonists. This phenomenon may be related to the ability of thyroid hormones to increase the number of β-adrenergic receptor sites in tissues.

Clinically, tachycardia is almost always present, even at rest. Tachycardia during sleep (pulse rate greater than 90 beats/min) serves to distinguish tachycardia of thyrotoxic origin from that of psychogenic origin. The pulse pressure is widened as a result of both an increase in systolic and a decrease in diastolic pressure. The increased force of cardiac contraction is often felt by the patient as palpitation and is evident on inspection or palpation of the precordium. Owing to the diffuse and forceful nature of the apex beat, the heart often seems enlarged, but x-ray study generally does not confirm this impression. Heart sounds are loud and ringing, and a systolic or even a late diastolic or presystolic murmur may be present at the apex. A scratchy systolic sound along the left sternal border, resembling a pericardial friction rub, may also be heard. These physical signs abate when a normal metabolic state is restored.

Cardiac arrhythmias are common with thyrotoxicosis and are almost invariably supraventricular. Approximately 10% of patients with thyrotoxicosis manifest atrial fibrillation and a similar percentage of patients with otherwise unexplained atrial fibrillation prove to be thyrotoxic. Paroxysmal supraventricular tachycardia may be manifested or may be suggested by the history. Systolic time intervals are altered in thyrotoxicosis; the preejection period is distinctly shortened and the ratio of preejection period to left ventricular ejection time decreased.

The adequacy of the circulation is a question of great importance in the patient with thyrotoxicosis. The arteriovenous oxygen difference is generally normal, but the significance of this is obscured since, for purposes of heat loss, a considerable proportion of the cardiac output may be directed to the skin, in which relatively little oxygen consumption occurs. Although the cardiovascular cost of a standard work load or metabolic challenge is increased, this is adequately met if the patient is not or has not previously been in heart failure. Thus, in most patients without underlying heart disease, cardiac competence is maintained. Mild edema not uncommonly occurs in the absence of heart failure. Nevertheless, thyrotoxicosis may indeed lead to congestive heart failure, but even so, the circulation time may remain shortened. Heart failure usually occurs in patients with preexisting heart disease, but the presence of heart disease often cannot be determined until after thyrotoxicosis is relieved. There is little doubt that pure thyrocardiac disease does occur, but only uncommonly, and usually in association with atrial fibrillation. Since the latter decreases the efficiency of the cardiac response to any increased circulatory demand, it may play a prominent role in bringing about cardiac failure. Attempts to convert atrial fibrillation to sinus rhythm are usually of no avail while thyrotoxicosis is present. Regardless of the type of rhythm the response to digitalis is decreased, possibly because of accelerated metabolism of the drug, and large quantities may be required to produce a clinical effect. Resistance to digitalis, as well as failure of cardiac decompression to respond to a usually adequate regimen, should suggest the possibility of thyrotoxicosis.

The frequency of coronary artery disease in patients with thyrotoxicosis is uncertain. Frank myocardial infarction is uncommon; however, when angina pectoris is present, it is aggravated by thyrotoxicosis and relieved by treatment.

Respiratory System

Dyspnea is a common symptom of thyrotoxicosis and need not be due to heart failure. Studies of pulmonary function have revealed several factors that may contribute to this symptom. Vital capacity is commonly reduced; this appears to result mainly from weakness of the respiratory muscles, but decreased pulmonary compliance may also play a role. During exercise, ventilation is increased out of proportion to the increase in oxygen uptake; diffusing capacity of the lung is normal, however. The alterations in pulmonary function return to normal when a normal metabolic state is restored.

Alimentary System

Increase in appetite, both at mealtimes and between meals, is a common symptom of thyrotoxicosis, but the mechanism whereby this occurs is unknown. Except in unusual cases, increased intake of food is inadequate to meet the increased caloric requirements, and weight is lost at a variable rate. In the occasional, usually younger, patient with mild disease, weight gain may occur instead. Anorexia, rather than hyperphagia, sometimes accompanies severe forms of thyrotoxicosis. It also occurs in about one-third of elderly thyrotoxic patients and contributes to the picture of "masked" thyrotoxicosis.

The commonest symptoms referable to the alimentary tract are those related to bowel function. Frank diarrhea is rare; more often, stools are merely less well formed and the frequency of bowel movements is increased. In the authors' experience, patients may display intolerance to milk products while thyrotoxic. When constipation has anteceded the development of thyrotoxicosis, bowel function may return to normal. Anorexia, nausea, and vomiting are uncommon, but when they occur, it is usually in patients with severe disease. These symptoms, as well as abdominal pain, may be forerunners of thyroid storm. Gastric emptying and intestinal motility are increased in thyrotoxicosis and appear to be responsible for the slight malabsorption of fat. The mechanism underlying the gastrointestinal hypermotility has not been elucidated, but the hypermotility disappears when a normal metabolic state is restored. Gluten enteropathy and Graves' disease may coexist more frequently than can be accounted for by chance. A high proportion of patients display gastric achlorhydria. In the majority, acid secretion returns after relief of the thyrotoxicosis, but in some it does not. Circulating autoantibodies against gastric parietal cells are found in approximately one-third of patients with Graves' disease, and approximately 3% have been reported to have frank pernicious anemia. It is commonly thought that intestinal absorption is accelerated in thyrotoxicosis, but evidence for this is sparse. It is commonly stated that the oral glucose tolerance curve displays a high early peak in patients with thyrotoxicosis, but, in fact, the glycemic peak is frequently delayed.

Hepatic dysfunction occurs in thyrotoxicosis, particularly when the disease is severe; hypoproteinemia and increases in serum transaminase and alkaline phosphatase may occur. In milder cases, no dysfunction may be evident. In the most severe cases, hepatomegaly and jaundice may be found. Gynecomastia is present in about 5% of men with thyrotoxicosis. In thyrotoxicosis, splanchnic oxygen consumption is increased, while blood flow is essentially unchanged. As a result, the arteriovenous oxygen difference across the splanchnic bed is increased; hence, hypoxia may contribute to hepatic dysfunction. Hypoxia, together with the state of relative caloric deprivation, may partly account for the depletion of hepatic glycogen which is evident both in the response to glycogenolytic agents and on direct analysis. In the absence of severe thyrotoxicosis or congestive heart failure, the liver may appear normal on light microscopic examination. In severe cases, however, centrilobular fatty infiltration may occur, together with patchy portal fibrosis, lymphocytic infiltration, and proliferation of bile ducts. Ultramicroscopic examination of the liver reveals enlarged mitochondria and hypertrophic smooth endoplasmic reticulum. Graves' disease and chronic active hepatitis occur together more often than can be explained by chance.

Nervous System

Alterations in the function of the nervous system are an almost invariable accompaniment of thyrotoxicosis and are most commonly manifested by nervousness, emotional lability, and hyperkinesia. The nervousness of the thyrotoxic patient is not that of the patient who is chronically anxious but rather is characterized by restlessness, shortness of attention span, and a need to be moving around and doing, despite a feeling of fatigue. Unlike the patient with neurocirculatory asthenia, the thyrotoxic patient wishes to be active but is hampered by fatigability; he is tired from the neck down, rather than from the top of the head down. Fatigue may be a manifestation of muscle weakness and the insomnia of which patients with thyrotoxicosis commonly complain. In some patients, asthenia and fatigue are so severe the overall activity is decreased.

Emotional lability is also a prominent symptom. Patients lose their tempers easily and have episodes of crying without apparent reason. Crying may be evoked by merely questioning the patient about this symptom. In rare cases, severe psychic disturbance may occur; manic-depressive, schizoid, or paranoid reactions may emerge during thyrotoxicosis. These sometimes fail to regress when a normal metabolic state is restored.

The hyperkinesia of the thyrotoxic patient is characteristic to those who are familiar with the disease. During the interview, the patient cannot sit still; he drums on the table, taps his foot, or shifts positions frequently. Movements are quick, jerky, exaggerated and often purposeless. In children, in whom such manifestations tend to be more severe, Sydenham's chorea may be suggested. Examination also reveals a fine, rhythmic tremor of the hands, tongue, or lightly closed eyelids. With the aid of a magnifying glass, a tremor of the eyeballs may be seen. The tremor of thyrotoxicosis may sometimes mimic that of parkinsonism, while preexisting parkinsonian tremor is accentuated during thyrotoxicosis. In patients with convulsive disorders, the frequency of seizures is increased. The electroencephalogram reveals an increase in fast-wave activity, and in experimental animals, the convulsive threshold is decreased.

The physiologic basis of the findings referable to the nervous system is not well understood. In part, they may reflect increased adrenergic activity since some improvement occurs during treatment with adrenergic antagonists. Although the cerebral blood flow of thyrotoxic patients is increased, arteriovenous oxygen difference is diminished, and oxygen extraction is unchanged. This correlates well with the apparent inability of thyroid hormones to increase the oxygen consumption of brain tissue in animals. Nevertheless, failure of oxygen consumption to increase does not exclude the likelihood that other alterations in cerebral metabolism are induced by thyroid hormone.

Muscle

Weakness and fatigability are frequent complaints of the patient with thyrotoxicosis. In most instances, these are not accompanied by any objective evidence of local disease of muscle save for the generalized wasting that is associated with loss of weight. Often the weakness is most prominent in the proximal muscles of the limbs, with the result that the patient experiences difficulty in climbing stairs or in maintaining the leg in an extended position. The latter maneuver can be employed to assess the degree of muscle weakness. In occasional cases, involvement of muscles is associated with wasting that again tends to be proximal and is out of proportion to the overall loss of weight (thyrotoxic myopathy). Here, in the extreme form, the patient may be unable to rise from a sitting or lying position and may be virtually unable to walk. This disorder may resemble progressive muscular atrophy or polymyositis, but fasciculation is absent and, on biopsy, little if any inflammatory change is evident. Instead, atrophy of muscle and infiltration by fat cells and lymphocytes are present. Electron microscopy reveals abnormal mitochondria and focal dilations of the transverse tubular system. Electromyograms reveal a decreased duration of mean action potentials and an increased percentage of polyphasic potentials. The biochemical basis of the muscular weakness is uncertain but may be related to the impaired ability of thyrotoxic muscle to phosphorylate creatine. Creatinuria is present and creatine tolerance is diminished.

Myopathy affects men with thyrotoxicosis more commonly than women and may overshadow the other manifestations of the syndrome. In the most severe forms, the myopathy may involve the more distal muscles of the extremities, as well as muscles of the trunk and face. Although involvement of ocular muscles is unusual, the disorder may mimic myasthenia gravis. Graves' disease and myasthenia do occur together with inordinate frequency. In uncomplicated thyrotoxic myopathy, some improvement of muscular strength may follow administration of edrophonium, but, unlike that in myasthenia, the response is incomplete. Muscular strength returns to normal when a normal metabolic state has been restored, but muscle mass takes longer to recover.

Graves' disease occurs in about 3–5% of patients with myasthenia gravis, and about 1% of patients with Graves' disease develop myasthenia gravis. These associations are of interest in view of the frequent association of thymic enlargement with Graves' disease. Further, antibodies against specific receptors, i.e., the thyrotropin receptor and the acetylcholine receptor, appear to be important in the pathogenesis of the two diseases. Unlike thyrotoxic myopathy, the association of myasthenia gravis with Graves' disease has a distinct female sex preponderance similar to that of uncomplicated Graves' disease. The effect of both thyrotoxicosis and its alleviation on the course of myasthenia gravis is variable, but in the majority of instances, myasthenia is accentuated during the thyrotoxic state and improves when a normal metabolic state is restored.

Periodic paralysis of the hypokalemic type may occur together with thyrotoxicosis, and its severity is greatly accentuated by the latter disorder. The coincidence of the two disorders is particularly common in Japanese and Chinese patients, in whom the incidence of periodic paralysis has been reported to be as high as 13% in men and 0.4% in women with thyrotoxicosis. (See Engel, 1972, for a review of the musculoskeletal manifestations.)

Skeletal System: Calcium and Phosphorus Metabolism

Thyrotoxicosis is generally associated with increased excretion of calcium and phosphorus in urine and stool. Excessive loss of mineral is sometimes associated with radiologically demonstrable demineralization of bone and occasionally with pathologic fractures, especially in elderly women. In such instances, the histologic appearance of bone is variable, suggesting osteitis fibrosa, osteomalacia, or osteoporosis. Osteoporosis has been traditionally ascribed to loss of protein matrix, but severely negative calcium balance has been found in some patients who are in virtual nitrogen equilibrium, making this explanation unlikely. Urinary excretion of hydroxyproline is invariably increased in thyrotoxicosis, indicating increased turnover of collagen. Kinetic studies indicate an increase in the exchangeable calcium pool and acceleration of both bone resorption and accretion, the former especially so.

Hypercalcemia occurs in a significant proportion of patients with thyrotoxicosis. Total serum calcium concentration is reportedly increased in as many as 27% of patients and ionized serum calcium in 47% (Burman et al., 1976). The serum alkaline phosphatase concentration is also frequently increased. These findings are reminiscent of those of primary hyperparathyroidism, but the concentration of immunoreactive parathyroid hormone in serum is decreased in the vast majority of thyrotoxic patients with hypercalcemia. True primary hyperparathyroidism and thyrotoxicosis may sometimes coexist. In the occasional patient, hypercalcemia may be sufficient to induce anorexia, nausea, vomiting, polyuria, or even impairment of renal function. The alterations in calcium metabolism in thyrotoxicosis may be due to a direct effect of thyroid hormones in stimulating bone resorption, and are reversed when a eumetabolic state is restored.

The impact of thyroid hormone excess on vitamin D metabolism is still uncertain. Plasma 25-OH vitamin D concentrations are decreased in thyrotoxic patients, and this alteration could contribute to the decreased intestinal absorption of calcium and osteomalacia noted in some patients (Velentzas et al., 1977).

The average height is above normal in thyrotoxic children. Maturation of bone may be stimulated so that bone age is advanced, but usually this is not of marked degree.

Renal Function: Water and Electrolyte Metabolism

In the absence of associated hypercalcemia or diabetes mellitus, thyrotoxicosis produces no symptoms referable to the urinary tract save for mild polyuria. Nevertheless, rates of renal blood flow and glomerular filtration as well as tubular reabsorptive and secretory maxima are increased. Total body water and exchangeable potassium are decreased, possibly because of a decrease in lean body mass, but exchangeable sodium tends to be increased. Serum Na^+, K^+, and chloride concentrations are normal, however. In thyrotoxicosis, exchangeable magnesium is normal, but serum Mg^{2+} concentration is often decreased and urinary Mg^{2+} excretion increased.

Hematopoietic System

In most patients with thyrotoxicosis, the red cells are normal as judged by the usual indices, but red cell mass is increased. The increase in erythropoiesis appears to be due both to the direct effect of thyroid hormones on erythroid marrow mediated by a β_2-adrenergic receptor and to increased production of erythropoietin (Popovic et al., 1977). A parallel increase in plasma volume also occurs, with the result that the hematocrit remains normal in thyrotoxic patients. In thyrotoxicosis, oxygen release from hemoglobin is increased. This has been ascribed to the increased content of 2,3-diphosphoglyceric acid in the red cell in this disorder, since 2,3-diphosphoglyceric acid enhances the dissociation of oxygen from hemoglobin by virtue of its ability to bind to hemoglobin and stabilize its reduced form. Thyroid hormones increase the content of 2,3-diphosphoglyceric acid in normal red cells *in vitro*, perhaps by stimulating directly diphosphoglycerate mutase activity (Snyder and Reddy, 1970). Other red cell abnormalities in thyrotoxicosis include a reduced content of zinc and carbonic anhydrase I, and an increased content of Na^+, probably because activity of Na^+, K^+ ATPase is impaired.

Approximately 3% of patients with Graves' disease have pernicious anemia, and a further 3% are reported to have intrinsic factor autoantibodies with normal absorption of vitamin B_{12}. Circulating autoantibodies against gastric parietal cells have been reported to occur in about one-third of patients with Graves' disease. In thyrotoxicosis, requirements for vitamin B_{12} and folic acid appear to be increased. Rarely, thyrotoxicosis is associated with a mild, hypochromic anemia that is characterized by adequate stores of iron in the marrow and a response to large doses of pyridoxine.

In patients with thyrotoxicosis, the total white cell count is often low because of a decrease in neutrophils. The absolute lymphocyte count is normal or increased, leading to a relative lymphocytosis. Monocytes may also be increased, as may the absolute eosinophil count. Splenic enlargement occurs in about 10% of patients, and thymic and lymph node enlargement is said to be common. It is not known whether these abnormalities are a reflection of the autoimmune aspects of Graves' disease, but this is unlikely, since comparable alterations do not occur in Hashimoto's disease. Alternatively, these alterations may result from a direct effect of thyroid hormone on lymphoid tissue.

Blood platelets and the intrinsic clotting mechanism are normal. However, the concentration of factor VIII is often increased, and this returns to normal when the thyrotoxicosis is treated. The increase in factor VIII may reflect increased adrenergic activity, since infusion of epinephrine into normal subjects produces a similar effect.

Pituitary and Adrenocortical Function

In some respects, the thyrotoxic state imposes a challenge on pituitary and particularly adrenocortical function. In thyrotoxicosis, the metabolic transformations leading to the inactivation of cortisol are accelerated. These include reduction of the A ring, which is rapidly followed by conjugation, and oxidation of the 11-hydroxy group to a keto group as a result of an increase in 11β-hydroxysteroid dehydrogenase activity; the 11-keto compounds are less active than their 11-hydroxy precursors. As a result of these changes the disposal of cortisol is accelerated, but its rate of secretion is also increased so that plasma cortisol concentration remains normal. The concentration of corticosteroid-binding globulin in plasma is normal. The urinary excretion of 17-hydroxycorticosteroids (17-OHCS) is normal or slightly increased, whereas the urinary excretion of 17-ketosteroids (17-KS) may be moderately reduced.

The foregoing alterations require that some degree of adrenocortical hyperfunction be sustained in thyrotoxic patients but proof of increased secretion of ACTH is lacking. Pituitary-adrenal function is adequate for basal demands, as indicated by normal plasma cortisol concentrations, and the response to an acute challenge, such as is imposed by insulin-induced hypoglycemia, is generally adequate.

The rate of turnover of aldosterone is increased, but its plasma concentration is normal. Plasma renin activity is increased, and sensitivity to angiotensin II is reduced. (See Gordon and Southren, 1977, for a review of steroid metabolism in thyrotoxicosis.)

The response of plasma growth hormone (GH) concentration to insulin-induced hypoglycemia is subnormal in patients with thyrotoxicosis, particularly those with severe disease. This observation need not indicate deficient GH production but rather may reflect depletion of pituitary stores from prolonged caloric inadequacy or accelerated removal of GH from plasma. Suppression of plasma GH concentration by induced hyperglycemia has been reported to be incomplete in thyrotoxicosis; this may also reflect prolonged caloric deprivation.

Reproductive Function

Thyrotoxicosis beginning in early life may be associated with delayed sexual maturation, although general physical development is normal and skeletal growth is often accelerated. Thyrotoxicosis occurring after puberty also influences reproductive function, especially in women. An increase in libido sometimes occurs in both sexes, and in women menstrual function is usually disturbed. The intermenstrual interval may be either prolonged or shortened, while menstrual flow at first is diminished and ultimately ceases altogether. Fertility may be reduced, and if conception takes place, abortion may result.

In some patients, cycles are predominantly anovulatory, but in most ovulation occurs, as indicated by a secretory endometrium. In the former, a subnormal mid-cycle surge of luteinizing hormone (LH) may be responsible, but the cause of the menstrual abnormalities in the latter group is unclear. In premenopausal women with thyrotoxicosis, basal plasma concentrations of LH and TSH are reportedly normal and display normal responsiveness to gonadotropin-releasing hormone (GnRH) (Distiller et al., 1975).

In thyrotoxicosis, there occur both quantitative and qualitative alterations in the metabolism of gonadal steroids that may be of fundamental importance. With respect to the quantitative alterations, thyrotoxicosis, whether spontaneous or induced by T_3, is accompanied by a great increase in the concentration of testosterone-estradiol–binding globulin in plasma. As a result, the plasma concentrations of testosterone, dihydrotestosterone, and estradiol are increased, but their unbound fractions are decreased. The increased binding in plasma is responsible for the decreased metabolic clearance rate of testosterone and dihydrotestosterone. In the case of estradiol, however, the metabolic clearance rate is normal, suggesting that tissue metabolism of the hormone is increased. Converison rates of androstenedione to testosterone and to estrone and estradiol, and of testosterone to dihydrotestosterone, are increased. The increased rate of conversion of androgens to estrogens has been invoked as a mechanism for the gynecomastia that occurs in some thyrotoxic men.

With respect to the qualitative alterations, thyrotoxicosis favors metabolism of estradiol and estrone via 2-oxygenation over that via 16 α-hydroxylation, with the result that formation of 2-hydroxyestrone and its derivative, 2-methoxyestrone, is increased, while formation of estriol is decreased. In the case of androgens, thyrotoxicosis favors metabolism of testosterone to androsterone over that to etiocholanolone. These alterations occur in both spontaneous thyrotoxicosis and that induced by T_3, whereas the converse alterations occur in hypothyroidism. The physiologic significance of these alterations is uncertain, but it is of interest that androsterone has a hypocholesterolemic action, suggesting that some metabolic effects of the thyroid hormones may be mediated by alterations in the metabolism of other hormones. (For references, see Gordon and Southren, 1977.)

Catecholamines and Serotonin

An important association between the adrenergic nervous system and the thyroid hormones is evident in the thyrotoxic state. Many of the effects induced by excessive quantities of the thyroid hormones are reminiscent of those induced by epinephrine, including tachycardia, increased cardiac output, and enhanced glycogenolysis, lipolysis, and calorigenesis. Moreover, some of the clinical manifestations of thyrotoxicosis, among them eyelid retraction, tremor, excessive sweating, and tachycardia, are at least partly alleviated by adrenergic antagonists that either deplete tissue stores or block the action of catecholamines. These observations have been interpreted as indicating that a state of increased adrenergic activity exists in the thyrotoxic organism. This interpretation is supported by the observation that the plasma cAMP response to epinephrine and glucagon and the urinary cAMP response to parathyroid hormone are exaggerated in thyrotoxic patients (Guttler et al., 1977).

The mechanism ultimately responsible for the increased adrenergic activity is uncertain. The secretion rates of both epinephrine and norepinephrine, as well as their plasma concentrations, are normal in thyrotoxicosis (Coulombe et al., 1976 and 1977). Recent work suggests that the thyroid hormones increase the number of β-adrenergic receptor sites in the tissues and may in this manner enhance adrenergic responsiveness. (See reviews of this entire topic by Landsberg, 1976, and Levey, 1976.)

Some of the manifestations of thyrotoxicosis, such as flushing, sweating, tachycardia, and gastrointestinal hypermotility, are reminiscent of those of the carcinoid syndrome. However, plasma serotonin concentration, urinary 5-hydroxyindoleacetic acid excretion, and platelet monoamine oxidase activity have been reported to be normal in thyrotoxic patients.

Energy Metabolism: Protein, Carbohydrate, and Lipid Metabolism

The intrinsic effects of the thyroid hormones on intermediary metabolism are discussed in an earlier section. This section will deal largely with the manner in which these effects are clinically evident in the patient with thyrotoxicosis.

The stimulation of energy metabolism and heat production is reflected in the increased BMR, increased appetite, and heat intolerance and in the slightly elevated basal body temperature of the patient with thyrotoxicosis. Despite the increased food intake, however, a state of chronic caloric and nutritional inadequacy almost always ensues.

Both the synthesis and degradation of protein are increased, the latter to a relatively greater extent than the former, with the result that there is net degradation of tissue protein. This is evident in the negative nitrogen balance, loss of weight, muscle wasting and weakness, and mild hypoalbuminemia.

The oral glucose tolerance curve is often abnormal in patients with thyrotoxicosis and varies from one in which the peak glycemia is increased and somewhat delayed to one that is frankly diabetic in form. Plasma insulin concentrations, however, are increased, suggesting the existence of insulin antagonism. The pathogenesis of these alterations remains to be defined. Preexisting diabetes mellitus is aggravated by thyrotoxicosis, perhaps as a result of increased degradation of insulin.

Both the synthesis and degradation of triglycerides and of cholesterol are increased in thyrotoxicosis, but the net effect is principally one of lipid degradation. This is reflected in an increase in plasma free fatty acids (FFA) and glycerol and a decrease in serum cholesterol; serum triglycerides, however, may be variable but are usually slightly decreased. Post-heparin lipolytic activity has been reported as being both decreased and increased. The mobilization of FFA in response to fasting, catecholamines, and GH is accentuated, and the oxidation of FFA is enhanced. These alterations, which appear to be due to activation of adenylate cyclase, result in a tendency to ketosis and to fatty infiltration of the liver, depending upon the degree of caloric inadequacy. (See Nikkilä and Kekki, 1972, for a review of lipid metabolism in thyrotoxicosis.)

Composite Clinical Picture and Laboratory Tests in Thyrotoxic States

The immediately foregoing section described the effects of an excess of thyroid hormones on the major organ systems. While these effects are in general common to thyrotoxic states regardless of their underlying etiology, their frequency and intensity as well as the other findings with which they are associated are greatly influenced by the nature of the disorder underlying the thyrotoxicosis. To a large extent, the same may be said of the results of the laboratory tests. Consequently, it is propitious to consider the clinical picture, characteristic laboratory findings, and differential diagnosis of thyrotoxic states as they relate to each of the specific etiologies. This approach is undertaken not merely as a matter of literary convenience but to emphasize the differences among the various forms of thyrotoxicosis that have an important bearing upon the clinical course, diagnosis, and treatment.

Graves' Disease

The disease known as Graves' disease in the English-speaking world and as Basedow's disease on the continent of Europe has been known for over a hundred years, but in areas of iodine abundance it has remained the most enigmatic, and, from the clinical standpoint, the most important of all thyroid diseases.

Graves' disease is a multisystem disease characterized by diffuse goiter, thyrotoxicosis, infiltrative ophthalmopathy, and occasionally infiltrative dermopathy. In the individual patient, the thyroid disease and the infiltrative phenomena may occur singly or together, and run courses that are largely independent of one another. At least the thyroid component is closely related to that of two other thyroid diseases with strong autoimmune components, primary thyroid atrophy and especially Hashimoto's disease. Together, they form a triad of autoimmune thyroid disorders that relate to one another in certain aspects of their pathogenesis and clinical course. In Graves' disease, hyperthyroidism occurs in the presence of some degree of chronic thyroiditis and may ultimately be replaced by thyroid hypofunction. Conversely, hyperthyroidism may supervene in patients with preexisting Hashimoto's disease, and rarely can arise in a patient with preexisting primary myxedema. (For excellent reviews of autoimmunity and the pathogenesis of Graves' disease, see Doniach and Marshall, 1977; McKenzie and Zakarija, 1977 and 1978; Kidd et al., 1980.)

Evidence for the existence of humoral autoimmunity, i.e., for the presence of thyroid-sensitive B lymphocytes, in the three diseases of the triad is the regular occurrence in the serum of antibodies against thyroid microsomes and often against thyroglobulin, though titers tend to be highest in Hashimoto's disease and lowest in primary thyroid atrophy at the time it is diagnosed. All share evidence of cell-mediated immunity against thyroid antigen, evidence of sensitized T lymphocytes, as judged from a variety of criteria, including the ability of the lymphocytes to elaborate migration-inhibiting factor (MIF) when exposed to thyroid antigens. All three are characterized by lymphocytic infiltration of the thyroid gland or remnant thyroid bed, and they share, in patients or their relatives, the frequent clinical or serologic evidence of other disorders of presumed autoimmune origin, such as pernicious anemia, myasthenia gravis, idiopathic adrenal atrophy, and rheumatoid arthritis.

More nearly specific to Graves' disease are circulating immunoglobulins that appear to be antibodies to components of the thyroid cell membrane, that are capable of somehow inhibiting the binding of TSH to its specific receptor site in the cell membrane, and that are able to activate adenylate cyclase therein. But even these factors are sometimes found in the serum of patients who, by conventional criteria, appear to have Hashimoto's disease. These factors are discussed more fully later in this section.

Prevalence

The exact prevalence of Graves' disease is uncertain, but it has been estimated to occur in 0.4% of the population of the United States. It is the commonest cause of spontaneous hyperthyroidism in the patient under 40 years of age and, except perhaps in the elderly, it is several times more common than primary thyroprivic hypothyroidism, approaching Hashimoto's disease in frequency. Indeed, it has been estimated that the overall prevalence of autoimmune thyroid disease, comprising Graves' disease, Hashimoto's thyroiditis, and primary hypothyroidism, approaches that of diabetes mellitus.

Pathogenesis

There is almost universal, if somewhat tentative, agreement that the thyroid abnormalities characteristic of Graves' disease result from the action on the gland of immunoglobulins of the IgG class that may be antibodies against components or regions of the thyroid plasma membrane, possibly regions that include the specific receptor for TSH itself. These immunoglobulins are thought to bind to their complementary antigenic regions on the plasma membrane. As a consequence, they somehow activate adenylate cyclase within the membrane, thereby initiating a chain of reactions that leads to thyroid growth, increased vascularity, and hypersecretion of hormone.

A diversity of procedures has been developed to demonstrate the presence of these Graves' disease–related IgG in the blood. At present, it is not possible to detect them by chemical or immunochemical means; all assay procedures are, therefore, of a biologic nature, and detect an activity, not necessarily a specific compound or class of specific compounds. The terminology used in describing these assays has been extremely confusing, owing, in some cases, to the application of misnomers or to the application of different names to the same activity. For many years, the classic procedure for testing serum for Graves'-related IgG was to administer IgG to a mouse whose thyroid had been prelabeled with I*, and to seek evidence of a subsequent increase in thyroid hormone secretion in an increase in blood radioiodine concentration. Unlike the stimulation produced by TSH, which peaks at about 2 hours, that of Graves' IgG peaks at a much later time, around 16 hours. The IgG responsible for this activity were consequently designated long-acting thyroid stimulators or LATS (see Fig. 4–22). It is now recognized that LATS, which is demonstrable in the serum of about 50% of patients with active Graves' disease, is an IgG that happens to have the ability to stimulate the mouse thyroid gland (hence the suggestion that it be renamed the "mouse thyroid stimulator," MTS), but may not be able to stimulate the human thyroid. More recent attention has focused on Graves'-related IgG that interact in some way with human thyroid tissue. One such procedure stems from the observation that when IgG preparations containing LATS are incubated with a human thyroid particulate fraction (this would contain plasma membranes), LATS activity can be reversibly absorbed from IgG. Sera of a large percentage (approximately 90%) of patients with active Graves' disease, though they contain IgG that lacks LATS activity, are capable of preventing the absorption of LATS by the particulate fraction. The IgG responsible for this activity have been designated LATS-protector or LATS-p. Though sensitive, this assay is difficult and cumbersome, and has not been undertaken in many laboratories. IgG from the sera of many patients with Graves' disease are capable of stimulating colloid droplet formation when incubated with slices of human thyroid gland. The active factor(s) in this assay has been given the generic name "human thyroid stimulator" (HTS), but this assay is also technically difficult and has not been broadly used.

The two types of assay most recently developed are now the most widely employed. In the first, radioreceptor techniques are employed to demonstrate that IgG are capable of inhibiting the binding of ^{125}I-labeled bovine TSH to specific binding sites in human thyroid membranes. This is thought to result from competitive binding of IgG at or near the TSH receptor so as to preclude the receptor's binding of TSH. That this is the mechanism is uncertain, however, since it is possible that the responsible factor(s) acts elsewhere on the membrane, but, in so doing, induces a conformational change in the TSH receptor that prevents the binding of TSH. Although some have referred to the IgG which possess this activity as thyroid-stimulating immunoglobulins (TSI), the term is inappropriate, since the test does not evaluate the ability of the IgG to induce a functional stimulation. Alternate, and preferable, names include "TSH-displacing antibody" (TDA) and "TSH-binding inhibitory immuno-

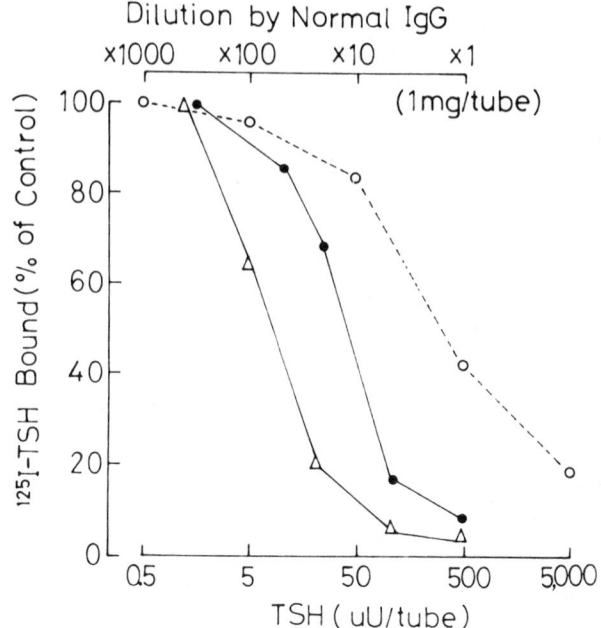

Figure 4–22. Inhibition of the binding of ¹²⁵I-TSH to receptors in human thyroid membranes by increasing concentrations of bovine TSH (o---o) and by increasing concentrations of IgG containing TSH binding inhibitory immunoglobulin (TBII) activity (●—● and △—△). (From Endo, K., et al.: *J. Clin. Endocrinol.* 46:734, 1978.)

cellular damage (cytotoxicity) that causes thyroid function in all of the three diseases to fail with variable degrees of rapidity. Others are capable of eliciting functional stimulation, and these would be most closely related to the clinical entity of diffuse toxic goiter. Even within the latter group, there is, however, substantial heterogeneity, so that some are capable of stimulating the thyroid of other species; some in some way interfere with binding of TSH to its receptor in the plasma membrane; some are agonists of the adenylate cyclase system; and some are antagonists to the agonistic action of other stimulators.

Cell-mediated immunity has also been invoked as a possible pathogenetic factor in the hyperthyroidism of Graves' disease. This would require that sensitized T lymphocytes infiltrate the thyroid and elaborate stimulatory lymphokines, but convincing evidence that this occurs is lacking. On the other hand, cooperativity between cell-mediated and humoral autoimmunity is suggested by the observation that the mitogen phytohemagglutinin stimulates the lymphocytes from patients with Graves' disease to elaborate thyroid-stimulating IgG.

The final link in the pathogenetic chain of the triad of autoimmune thyroid diseases is that which would explain why these autoimmune responses arise and, more impor-

globulin" (TBII). TBII activity is present in IgG derived from the serum of about 60% of patients with active Graves' disease (see Fig. 4–22).

In the remaining assay, IgG are tested for their ability to stimulate adenylate cyclase activity in human thyroid slices or particulate preparations. Active IgG have been designated human thyroid adenylate cyclase stimulators (HTACS) or, more simply, thyroid-stimulating immunoglobulins (TSI). TSI activity has been found in the IgG of approximately 80% of patients with active Graves' disease (see Fig. 4–23).

A distressing finding with respect to these tests is that the TBII activity and TSI activity in IgG from patients with Graves' disease do not correlate well with one another. Some sera potent in TBII activity display no TSI activity, and apparently the reverse is also the case. On the other hand, several recent studies have demonstrated a good correlation of one or another of these factors, usually TBII, with nonsuppressibility of thyroid function, with the degree of thyroid hyperfunction, and with relapse following withdrawal of antithyroid drug therapy (Clague et al., 1976; Davies et al., 1977; Endo et al., 1978; and O'Donnell et al., 1978). On the other hand, TBII are also detectable in approximately one-half of patients with euthyroid Graves' ophthalmopathy and occasionally in patients with Hashimoto's thyroiditis and in euthyroid relatives with Graves' disease. The absence of hyperthyroidism in these circumstances has been attributed either to limitation of thyroid responsiveness to stimulation or to dissociation between thyroid-stimulating and TSH-displacing activities. Indeed, a TSH-displacing IgG that inhibited TSH action has recently been described in a patient with Hashimoto's thyroiditis (Endo et al., 1978).

It seems increasingly clear that the thyroid-related IgG in autoimmune thyroid disease are a heterogeneous group of antibodies directed at varying sites within the thyroid cell membrane. Certain of them may be responsible for

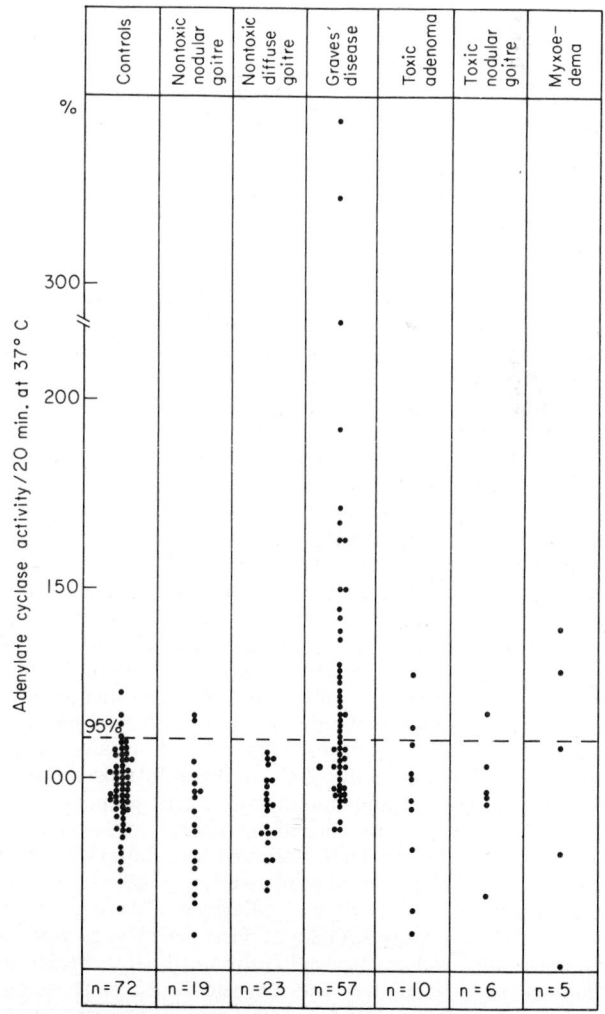

Figure 4–23. Stimulation of adenylate cyclase activity in human thyroid membranes by preparations of IgG from the serum of normal controls and patients with various thyroid diseases. (From Bech, K., and Nistrup Madsen, S. N.: Thyroid adenylate cyclase stimulating immunoglobulins in thyroid diseases. *Clin. Endocrinol.* 11:47, 1979.)

tant, persist. Evidence has emerged of cell-mediated as well as humoral thyroid autoimmunity during the course of subacute thyroiditis, but this abates when the disease becomes inactive. In chronic autoimmune thyroid disease, there is evidently a sustained, genetically determined disorder of immune surveillance which permits the persistence of clones of thyroid-sensitized immunocytes. The recent demonstration of deficient suppressor T cell activity in the lymphocytes of patients with Graves' disease or Hashimoto's disease supports this view.

The pathogenesis of the ophthalmopathy of Graves' disease is even more enigmatic. One hypothesis holds that an abnormal IgG acting in concert with an exophthalmos-producing factor composed in part of the β subunit of TSH induces mucopolysaccharide synthesis and edema formation in retro-orbital tissues (Kohn and Winand, 1975). Such a mechanism is difficult to reconcile, however, with the absence of measurable quantities of β subunit by radioimmunoassay of the sera of patients with ophthalmopathy. An intriguing alternative hypothesis has been proposed by Kriss and his associates, who have demonstrated the presence of thyroglobulin or a derivative thereof in extraocular muscle and have invoked lymphatic transport from the thyroid as its source (Mullin et al., 1977). They postulate that thyroglobulin in a retro-orbital location evokes an immune response, involving either immune-complex formation or infiltration of thyroglobulin-sensitized T cells, with exophthalmos as the end-result. The putative mechanism is in the early phase of its exploration, and conclusions concerning the pathogenesis of the ophthalmopathy of Graves' disease must be delayed. There has been no evident progress toward elucidation of the pathogenesis of the dermopathy of Graves' disease.

Constitutional Factors

Whatever its basic etiology, both the emergence of clinically evident Graves' disease and its subsequent course are modified by such factors as heredity, sex, and perhaps emotions. The role of heredity is manifest in several ways. Population studies reveal an increased frequency of haplotypes HLA-B8 in Caucasian, HLA-BW46 in Chinese, and HLA-BW35 in Japanese patients with Graves' disease. The tendency of Graves' disease to occur in several members of the same family and sometimes in several generations is well recognized. Several extensive studies have given statistical support to this concept (Martin and Fisher, 1945). In addition, a higher concordance rate of Graves' disease has been noted in monozygotic than in dizygotic twins. The foregoing statistics were based upon the appearance of overt thyroid disease in relatives. Studies conducted many years ago in the authors' clinic revealed a high incidence of abnormalities in iodine metabolism in euthyroid relatives, some of whom were goitrous. Thyroid ^{131}I uptakes were increased in approximately 20% of the relatives studied, especially in sisters and daughters of the propositi. An increase in the fractional rate of peripheral turnover of T_4 was noted, similar to that observed in clinically overt Graves' disease. More recent studies have revealed that IgG in the serum of some euthyroid relatives of patients with Graves' disease display LATS-p or TBII activity, as well as antimicrosomal and antithyroglobulin antibodies. Function studies reveal nonsuppressible thyroid function in some, hyporesponsiveness to TRH in some and hyperresponsiveness in others, and occasional elevations of serum T_3 concentration (Tamai et al., 1978).

The hereditary factor in Graves' disease also appears to involve autoimmune aspects. This is suggested by the increased incidence in patients with Graves' disease or in members of their families of other autoimmune disorders or manifestations, such as Hashimoto's disease or pernicious anemia, and of autoantibodies against thyroid tissue components, gastric parietal cells, and intrinsic factor.

A strong relationship also exists between sex and both the frequency and the clinical manifestations of Graves' disease. Overall, the disorder is many times more common in women than in men (approximately 7:1). Furthermore, it tends to become manifest during such times as puberty, pregnancy, and the menopause. Although men are less often affected, in them the disease tends to occur at a later age, to be more severe, and relatively more often to be accompanied by significant ophthalmopathy. It is not known whether the influence of sex in Graves' is a direct result of genetic determinants or of physiologic factors related to reproductive function. The female sex preponderance is consonant with the autoimmune aspects, since most disorders considered to be of an autoimmune nature occur most commonly in women. The foregoing evidence for the operation of autoimmune and genetic factors has led to a concept that Graves' disease is the result of a genetically determined defect of immunologic surveillance. This unifying concept, which implicates an immunologic defect as the inherited factor, ignores the absence of evidence of immunologic disorder in nontoxic goiter and thyroid carcinoma. Yet a marked preponderance of females is seen in both the latter disorders, and a familial relationship exists between nontoxic goiter and Graves' disease (see review by Skillern, 1972).

From the earliest descriptions of Graves' disease, the possible role of emotional factors in its emergence has been suggested. Those who see the disease frequently are repeatedly impressed by instances in which Graves' disease becomes evident either after a severe emotional stress, such as the actual or threatened separation from an individual upon whom the patient is emotionally dependent, or after an acute fright, such as an automobile accident. It has also been suggested that patients with Graves' disease may be drawn from a population with a characteristic pattern of personality, but some data do not support this hypothesis. The difficulties of conducting controlled studies in this field are obvious, but such are what is needed if conclusions concerning the role of emotional factors in the pathogenesis of overt Graves' disease are to be drawn. Beyond this, there would be required an elucidation of the physiopathologic mechanism whereby evocative emotional factors express their effect.

Natural History and Course

The course of the thyrotoxic component of untreated Graves' disease is variable and often erratic. In some patients the thyrotoxic component is persistent, though it may vary in severity; in others it may be cyclic, exhibiting exacerbations of varying frequency, intensity, and duration. This cyclic feature has an important bearing on the treatment of the disorder and must also be encompassed by any comprehensive theory of its pathogenesis. With the passage of time, which may be only a few months, but more often requires years, the thyrotoxic component tends to "burn itself out." In a recent study, approximately one-third of patients treated at least 20 years earlier with antithyroid agents were found to be hypothyroid (Wood et al., 1979).

Although the ophthalmopathy of Graves' disease often commences together with the thyrotoxic component, this association is frequently lacking. Thus thyrotoxic patients may be initially free of ophthalmopathy but may develop this manifestation months or years later or not at all. Conversely, the disease may begin with ophthalmopathy and only later, if at all, be associated with thyrotoxicosis. In this group of patients with "euthyroid Graves' diseaase," a small proportion show no evidence of thyroid abnormality, as judged from tests for LATS-p, thyroid suppressibility, or response to exogenous TRH. Others variously display thyroid nonsuppressibility and subnormal or elevated responses to exogenous TRH. Some become hypothyroid within a few years of initial observation and some hyperthyroid, while still others remain euthyroid, but alter their responses to exogenous T_3 or TRH. Many have evidence of chronic thyroiditis. (See Solomon et al., 1977, and Tamai et al., 1980a.) The important element that emerges is that most patients with euthyroid Graves' disease display some abnormality of thyroregulatory control, evidence of thyroid autoimmunity, or both. These considerations are important in establishing a positive diagnosis of thyroid-related eye disease. Of further clinical importance is recognition of the fact that the functional status of the thyroid in these patients is unstable.

Histopathology

A convenient designation for the thyroid gland of Graves' disease during the period of active thyrotoxicosis is the term *diffuse toxic goiter*, which denotes that the gland is both enlarged and uniformly affected. Diffuse toxic goiters vary in consistency from softer than normal to firm and rubbery. The outer surface is usually smooth but may be somewhat lobular; rarely, if ever, is it grossly nodular in the early stages of the disease prior to treatment. The cut surface is red and glistening. Microscopically, the follicles are small, are lined by hyperplastic columnar epithelium, and contain scant colloid that displays much marginal scalloping and vacuolization (Fig. 4–24). The nuclei are vesicular, are basally situated, and exhibit mitoses. Papillary projections of the hyperplastic epithelium into the lumina of the follicles are common. Vascularity is increased, and there is an infiltration to a varying degree of lymphocytes and plasma cells. These collect in aggregates forming lymphoid follicles. When the patient is treated with iodine, the thyroid undergoes a process termed *involution*, in which the hyperplasia and increased vascularity abate, the papillary projections recede, and the follicles enlarge and become filled with colloid. An extensive treatise on the fine structure of the thyroid in Graves' disease has been published (Heimann, 1966). No characteristic alterations have been described in the pituitary in Graves' disease.

In patients with *infiltrative ophthalmopathy*, the volume of the orbital contents is increased, owing to an increase in the retrobulbar connective tissue as well as to an increase in the mass of the extraocular muscles. Some of the increase

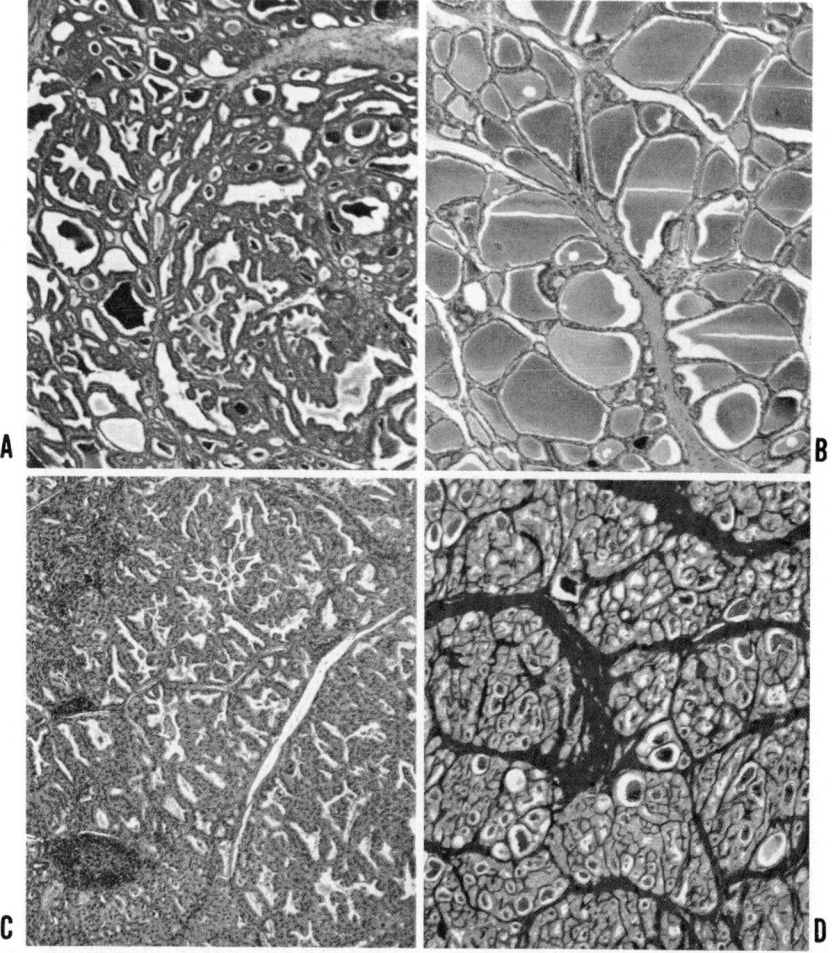

Figure 4–24. Sections of thyroid gland of four patients with Graves' disease. *A,* Untreated. *B,* After therapy with potassium iodide for 3 weeks. *C,* After treatment with thiouracil for 5 weeks. *D,* Three months after last of three treatments with radioiodine. Note the marked hypertrophy and hyperplasia of the acinar cells and scant amount of colloid in sections *A, C,* and *D.* A lymph follicle is present in *C.* Note the broad bands of scar tissue in *D.* Section *B* is almost normal in appearance. Each patient, except the first one, was euthyroid at the time of thyroidectomy.

in connective tissue is due to edema resulting from the increased content in the ground substance of hyaluronic acid, which is hydrophilic. The extraocular muscles are swollen, and the fibers display loss of striation, fragmentation, and lymphocytic infiltration. The lacrimal glands may also be involved. Ultimately, fibrosis of the tissues occurs.

In infiltrative dermopathy, the content of hyaluronic acid in the dermis is increased with resulting edema; the collagen fibers are separated and fragmented, and there is lymphocytic infiltration.

Pathophysiology

All aspects of thyroid hormone economy are abnormal in patients with diffuse toxic goiter. Thus, there occur disruptions of normal regulatory control of thyroid function; alterations in thyroid function itself; changes in the concentration, binding, and metabolism of thyroid hormones peripherally; and manifestations of thyroid hormone excess in the peripheral tissues. Abnormalities in all these aspects also occur in other disorders associated with thyrotoxicosis, but may differ in kind or amount.

An abnormality or override of normal regulatory control is inherent in the existence of any variety of thyrotoxicosis. In Graves' disease, as discussed in the section on Pathogenesis, normal regulatory mechanisms are overridden by the action of an abnormal stimulatory immunoglobulin. The resulting hyperfunction of the thyroid leads to an entirely appropriate suppression of the secretion of TSH that is reflected in the lack of response to TRH and the presence of an abnormal thyroid suppression test. Abnormal suppression and TRH tests can also be present in patients with euthyroid Graves' disease, relatives of patients with Graves' disease, or patients with diffuse toxic goiter in remission, indicating that an overriding of normal regulatory control is not necessarily associated with clinical thyrotoxicosis. Evidence of the intrinsic normality of regulatory control in almost all disorders associated with thyrotoxicosis is the reemergence of TSH secretion, or hypersecretion when appropriate, when thyrotoxicosis is relieved.

With respect to thyroid function, the disturbance is one that ultimately leads to hypersecretion of the thyroid hormones. Thyroid avidity for iodine is increased, so that thyroid iodide clearance rate is increased from its normal range of approximately 6–7 ml/min to values that vary with the severity of the disorder but that may approach 2 liters/min in the most severe cases. As a result, both RAIU and absolute uptake of iodine are enhanced. The great increase in iodide clearance rate must reflect enhanced thyroid blood flow, even if extraction of iodine is assumed to be complete. Hypervascularity of the thyroid in turn may be due to humoral or neurogenic mechanisms but is almost certainly due at least in part to the increased rate of energy metabolism in the gland itself. The enhanced thyroid iodide clearance rate is usually the result of an increase in both the overall glandular mass and its unit functional activity. Iodide transport and probably organic binding are accelerated. The increase in iodide transport is responsible at least in part for the enhanced susceptibility of the thyroid gland of Graves' disease to the inhibitory effects of iodide on organic-binding reactions; this is evident in a positive iodide-perchlorate discharge test (Suzuki and Mashimo, 1972). As judged from the normal ratio of iodotyrosines to iodothyronines, the rate of the coupling reaction must also be increased. The molar ratio of T_3 to T_4 in thyroglobulin is much higher than normal in Graves' disease. This disproportionate increase in T_3 production cannot be ascribed to intrathyroid iodine deficiency since the iodine content of thyroglobulin, as well as the number of T_4 residues per molecule, has been shown to be normal. It may reflect chronic hyperstimulation of the thyroid (Izumi and Larsen, 1977). The rate of turnover and release of the glandular iodine pool is increased, often greatly so. The major product of glandular secretion is T_4, but the ratio of T_3 to T_4 in the thyroid secretion is increased several-fold, reflecting disproportionate overproduction of T_3. In some instances, T_3 appears to be the major secretory product, with the result that the serum T_3 concentration alone is increased, the serum T_4 concentration being normal (T_3-toxicosis). Direct secretion of rT_3 may also occur, augmenting the increase in serum rT_3 concentration that reflects enhanced peripheral generation from T_4.

Thyroid hormone-protein interactions in the plasma are disturbed, the proportion of total T_4 and T_3 in the free or unbound state being increased. This change results from a decrease in the concentration of TBG, as well as from the increase in the concentrations of the two hormones. The fractional rates of turnover of T_4 and T_3 are increased, often greatly so, and this, together with the increased amounts of hormone in the peripheral pool, leads to an increase in total daily disposal of T_4 and T_3. In the most severe cases, values for this function may increase from the normal of approximately 80 μg of T_4 and 30 μg of T_3 daily to values in excess of 500 μg for both hormones. The total daily disposal of T_3 is disproportionately increased relative to that of T_4, indicating that the production rate of T_3 is disproportionately increased. Whether this results solely from a preferential increase in thyroid secretion of T_3 or whether there is in addition a disproportionate increase in the peripheral conversion of T_4 to T_3 is uncertain. In any event, since the metabolic potency of T_3 is about three times greater than that of T_4, T_3 is responsible for the bulk of thyroid hormone action in thyrotoxicosis. As judged from studies with the labeled hormones, the proportionate disposal of T_4 and T_3 by deiodination relative to fecal excretion is not altered.

The foregoing abnormalities in the kinetics of hormone turnover in the patient with active thyrotoxicosis irrespective of its underlying cause are probably the result of several factors, including both the disturbance in hormone binding and the hypermetabolism. In addition, in Graves' disease, several lines of evidence suggest that an intrinsic abnormality in the peripheral metabolism of T_4 exists. For example, an acceleration of the fractional rate of turnover of T_4 has been found in some patients long after the thyrotoxicosis had been relieved and also has been noted in some euthyroid relatives of patients with Graves' disease. Recently persistent acceleration of the fractional rate of turnover of T_3 has also been shown to be present in patients with Graves' disease after a normal metabolic state had been restored with treatment. The relationship of this abnormality to the other physiopathologic alterations in Graves' disease is unclear.

The many-fold physiological and biochemical abnormalities in peripheral tissues and their clinical manifestations have been discussed earlier. Particularly noteworthy among them, however, are those that reflect a hyperadrenergic state, since these can be ameliorated acutely by administration of the appropriate adrenergic blocking agents.

Clinical Picture

Graves' disease is most commonly manifest in patients in the third and fourth decades of life. The disease is rare before the age of 10 years, and although unusual, it is being diagnosed with increasing frequency in the elderly. Like other diseases of the thyroid, it displays a striking female sex preponderance of approximately 7:1. The whole syndrome comprises diffuse goiter, thyrotoxicosis, infiltrative ophthalmopathy, and occasionally infiltrative dermopathy. Since the infiltrative ophthalmopathy and dermopathy may occur independently of the former two manifestations, they will be discussed separately.

Diffuse Toxic Goiter. (Since hyperthyroidism occurs in diseases other than Graves' disease, and since Graves' disease may be present in the absence of thyrotoxicosis, the term diffuse toxic goiter is a convenient nosological entity in that it connotes the presence of thyrotoxicosis resulting specifically from Graves' disease.) Actual thyroid enlargement is its commonest manifestation, by definition, but is absent in a small percentage of cases. Most commonly, the symptoms of diffuse toxic goiter begin gradually, the patient noting nervousness, irritability, palpitation, fatigue, heat intolerance, weight loss, or change in menstrual pattern. Any one of these symptoms may predominate (Table 4–8). Enlargement of the thyroid may be noted as a fullness in the neck or rarely may produce obstructive symptoms. In about one-third of the cases, ocular manifestations begin coincidentally with the onset of thyrotoxicosis. Some of these are manifestations of thyrotoxicosis itself, whereas others are due to the ophthalmopathy and will be discussed later. Symptoms may remain mild or may progress to a florid state characterized by aggravation of the foregoing complaints together with weakness, insomnia, voracious appetite, and excessive sweating.

Several features of the foregoing symptoms merit further consideration. Nervousness, which is probably the most common symptom, may manifest itself in various ways, notably as a feeling of apprehension and inability to concentrate. Emotional lability and irritability may lead to difficulty in interpersonal relationships and to inappropriate spells of crying or euphoria. Fatigability frustrates the desire of the patient to be continuously active. Weakness is noted particularly on climbing stairs, and this activity, as well as others, is prone to produce breathlessness. Heat intolerance, associated with increased sweating, is also a prominent symptom and may be a cause of familial discord. The patient prefers a cooler environment than do others around him and may lower the thermostat, open the windows, sleep with fewer blankets, or kick off the covers while asleep. The patient usually prefers winter to summer and often finds hot weather intolerable. The change in menstrual pattern usually takes the form of oligomenorrhea

with a variable intermenstrual period, occasionally progressing to amenorrhea. Frank diarrhea is uncommon, but increase in the frequency of bowel movements and softening of the stools is often noted. Palpitation may be continuous or episodic, suggesting paroxysmal dysrhythmia. Although weight loss despite increase in appetite is common, the occasional patient notes a gain in weight, while in more severe cases the appetite may be decreased. Women may complain of excessive fineness of the hair and of its inability to hold a wave. The skin may become more pigmented. The ocular manifestations of thyrotoxicosis per se are due to spasm and retraction of the eyelids and are noted as a bright-eyed, staring appearance.

Although this symptom complex may develop over a period of months or even years before the patient is first seen, the disease is sometimes fulminant in its emergence, the florid clinical picture developing within a few weeks or less. In such patients, emotional stress may be a forerunner. In some patients with preexisting heart disease, mild or moderate thyrotoxicosis may precipitate heart failure, which then overshadows the manifestations of thyrotoxicosis. In others, severe weakness and wasting of muscles may dominate the clinical picture. The last two forms are often designated "masked" hyperthyroidism. This term is often taken to indicate that the characteristic clinical manifestations of thyrotoxicosis are lacking, but this is usually not the case, as a careful history and examination will disclose.

The characteristic physical signs in the patient with diffuse toxic goiter are manifold. Apart from the goiter and exophthalmos, which in themselves may suffice to establish a clinical diagnosis, other aspects of the patient's appearance and behavior may be virtually pathognomonic of thyrotoxicosis. The patient usually displays an exaggerated alertness, fidgets, responds quickly to questions or commands, is bright-eyed, may appear flushed, and often looks younger than would be expected from the chronological age.

The thyroid is enlarged in most patients but not invariably, since thyrotoxicosis in Graves' disease may occur in association with a gland of normal size in approximately 3% of patients, especially those who are elderly, in whom goiter may be absent in as many as 20%. The thyroid gland is most commonly two to three times normal size, but it may be massively enlarged (Fig. 4–25). Its consistency varies from one that is somewhat softer than normal to one that is firm

Table 4–8.   INCIDENCE OF SYMPTOMS AND SIGNS OBSERVED IN 247 PATIENTS WITH THYROTOXICOSIS

Symptom	Per Cent	Symptom	Per Cent
Nervousness	99	Increased appetite	65
Increased sweating	91	Eye complaints	54
Hypersensitivity to heat	89	Swelling of legs	35
Palpitation	89	Hyperdefecation (without diarrhea)	33
Fatigue	88	Diarrhea	23
Weight loss	85	Anorexia	9
Tachycardia	82	Constipation	4
Dyspnea	75	Weight gain	2
Weakness	70		

Sign	Per Cent	Sign	Per Cent
Tachycardia*	100	Eye signs	71
Goiter†	100	Atrial fibrillation	10
Skin changes	97	Splenomegaly	10
Tremor	97	Gynecomastia	10
Bruit over thyroid	77	Liver palms	8

*In other studies thyrotoxic patients with normal pulse rate have been observed.
†The data shown in this table are taken from Williams, R. H.: *J. Clin. Endocr.* 6:1, 1946. In the experience of the present authors, enlargement of the thyroid is lacking in approximately 3% of patients with thyrotoxicosis.

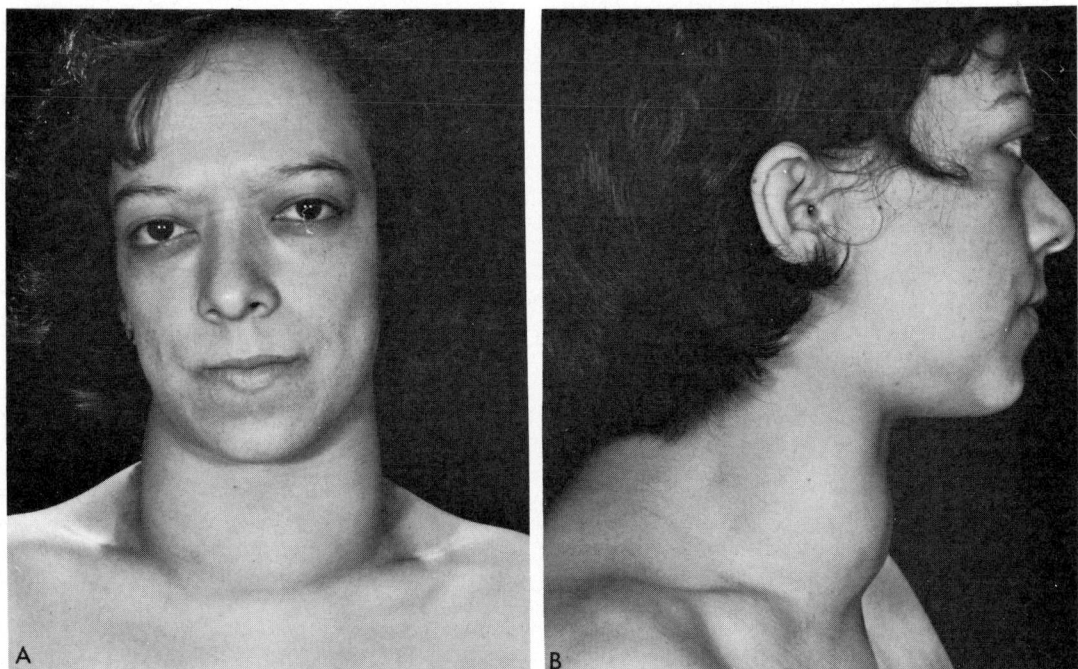

Figure 4–25. Massive thyroid enlargement due to diffuse toxic goiter. Note the sulcus between the thyroid and the lateral aspect of the neck in *B*, as well as the dilated veins overlying the thyroid gland. The patient was severely thyrotoxic and maintained a PBI of 40 μg/100 ml while receiving 1200 mg of propylthiouracil daily. The only ocular abnormality was slight widening of the right palpebral fissure, without true exophthalmos.

and rubbery. The enlargement is usually symmetrical, but sometimes the right lateral lobe is larger than the left. The surface of the gland is usually smooth but may feel lobular. Especially in more severe cases, a thrill may be felt, usually over the upper poles, and a bruit may be audible. This is usually continuous but may sometimes be heard only in systole and is most readily detected at the upper or lower poles. It should not be confused with a venous hum or murmur arising from the base of the heart. A thrill or bruit is highly suggestive but not pathognomonic of hyperthyroidism.

Spasm and retraction of the eyelids lead to widening of the palpebral fissure, with the result that sclera is exposed above the superior margin of the limbus. The retraction may be asymmetrical. When the patient looks downward, the upper lid lags behind the globe, exposing more of the sclera, and when he gazes upward the globe often lags behind the lid (lid lag and globe lag). The movements of the lids are jerky and spasmodic, and a tremor of the lightly closed lids can often be elicited.

The remaining peripheral manifestations of thyrotoxicosis were discussed in detail according to the individual organ systems in a previous section. Among these are the warm, smooth, moist texture of the skin, Plummer's nails, physical signs of a hyperdynamic circulation, tremor of the hands and tongue, muscular wasting, and hyperreflexia.

In general, men tend to develop the disease at a somewhat older age than women, and although the degree of thyroid hyperfunction is often more severe in men, the severity of the symptoms is often less. Men also seem especially prone to develop myopathy as well as the more severe forms of ophthalmopathy. In older patients the circulatory manifestations may predominate, while the nervous manifestations, which are especially prominent in children and young adults, are lacking. Ophthalmopathy is less common in the elderly patient, who is also more prone to display muscular weakness, prostration, and anorexia (apathetic hyperthyroidism).

Infiltrative Ophthalmopathy and Dermopathy. Ophthalmic changes are a major manifestation of Graves' disease. As has been suggested, it is important to differentiate between the ocular changes that result from thyrotoxicosis per se and those that not only are more proximately related to the disease process but also may pose serious problems in treatment and prognosis. It is the latter form which has been designated *infiltrative ophthalmopathy*. The thyrotoxic ocular manifestations have already been described. If present alone these usually abate when the thyrotoxicosis is relieved. Infiltrative ophthalmopathy on the other hand follows a course that is not uncommonly independent of the thyrotoxic aspect and is to a large extent uninfluenced by

its treatment (Fig. 4–26). Infiltrative ophthalmopathy is clinically evident in about 50% of patients. However, B-mode ultrasonographic examination of the orbits reveals changes, such as swelling of extraocular muscles and increased retro-orbital fat, in virtually all patients with Graves' disease, including those in whom the clinical changes are minimal or absent (Forrester et al., 1977). Occasionally, infiltrative ophthalmopathy occurs in the absence of diffuse toxic goiter, an entity that is termed euthyroid ophthalmic Graves' disease.

The symptoms associated with infiltrative ophthalmopathy are diverse and may appear in varying combinations. Early symptoms often include a sense of irritation in the eyes, resembling that caused by a foreign body, and excessive tearing that is often made worse by exposure to cold air or wind, especially if exophthalmos is present. Injection of the conjunctivae may be noted. Exophthalmos, which is frequently slightly asymmetrical but sometimes greatly so, may also be noted and may be accompanied by a feeling of pressure behind the globes. When exophthalmos is pronounced, the patient may be forced to sleep with his eyes partly open. Exophthalmos may be masked by periorbital edema, which is a common accompaniment and source of complaint. Patients frequently report that their vision is blurred and that their eyes tire easily. Double vision may be noted either in combination with the foregoing symptoms or alone. In severe cases, visual acuity may be decreased or lost, or the patient may display symptoms resulting from corneal ulceration or infection.

The ocular findings are quite variable (Fig. 4–27). Exophthalmos is probably the most common manifestation. This is usually bilateral but often is slightly asymmetrical. True unilateral exophthalmos is rare and usually occurs in the absence of thyrotoxicosis; most often the other eye is eventually affected. Exophthalmos is very frequently accompanied by periorbital edema which tends to obscure its degree. For this reason and because of their importance in following the course of the disease, objective measurements of the degree of exophthalmos must be made. These can be accomplished with the aid of either the Hertel or the Luedde exophthalmometer. These instruments conveniently and accurately permit measurement of the distance between the lateral angle of the bony orbit and an imaginary perpendicular tangent to the most anterior part of the cornea. Generally this distance does not exceed 16 mm, but 20 mm is considered the upper limit of normal. In severe exophthalmos, readings may be as high as 30 mm. A rough estimation of the degree of exophthalmos may be obtained by standing behind the seated patient and looking downward from above to ascertain the extent to which the eyes protrude beyond the plane of the forehead.

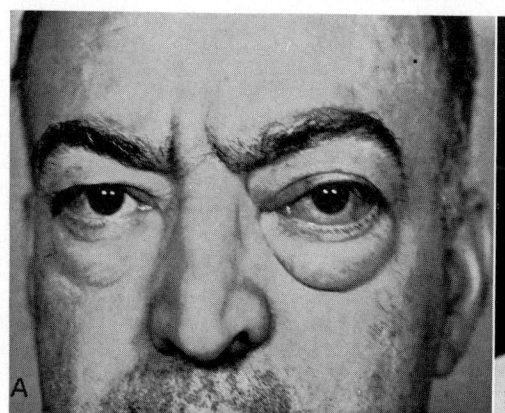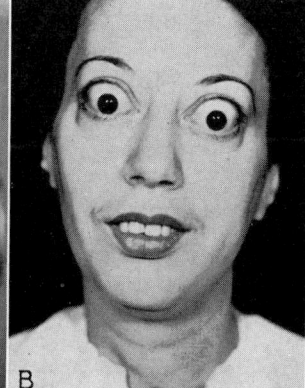

Figure 4–26. Patient *A* was euthyroid and had marked orbital swelling, exophthalmos, conjunctival injection, and chemosis. The proptosis, limitation of extraocular movements, edema, and other manifestations of infiltrative ophthalmopathy are much more marked in *A* than in *B*, who had mild hyperthyroidism, with slight diffuse enlargement of the thyroid, marked widening of the palpebral fissures, with marked stare and proptosis.

In addition to being edematous, the lids are often reddened, and enlarged lacrimal glands may cause a bulging of their surface. The extent to which the upper and lower lids can be completely apposed should be determined, since failure of apposition will promote drying and ulceration of the cornea. Injection of the bulbar conjunctiva is commonly seen and in more severe cases is accompanied by edema or frank chemosis, in which the edematous conjunctiva is seen to bulge from under the lids and around the corneal limbus.

Weakness of the extraocular muscles is an important finding that is most commonly evident in an inability to achieve or maintain convergence. Limitation of upward gaze and especially of superolateral gaze may be present.

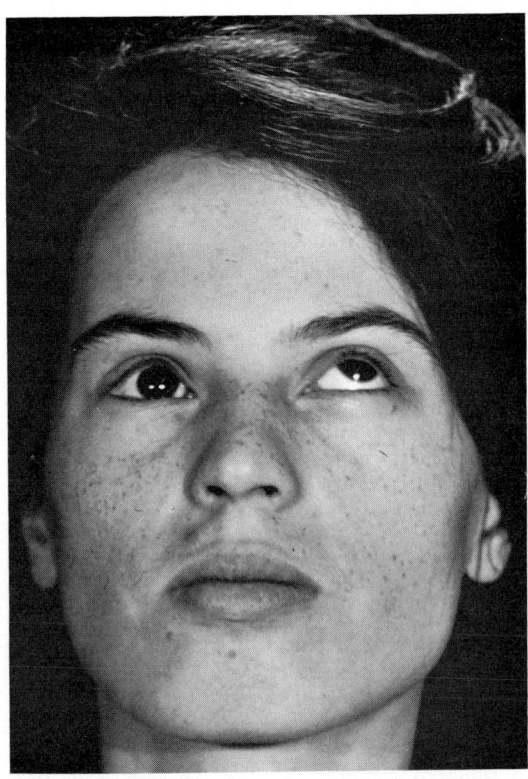

Figure 4–28. Ophthalmoplegia due to Graves' disease. The patient was severely hyperthyroid. Other than slight conjunctival injection, the only ocular abnormality was paralysis of upward gaze on the right.

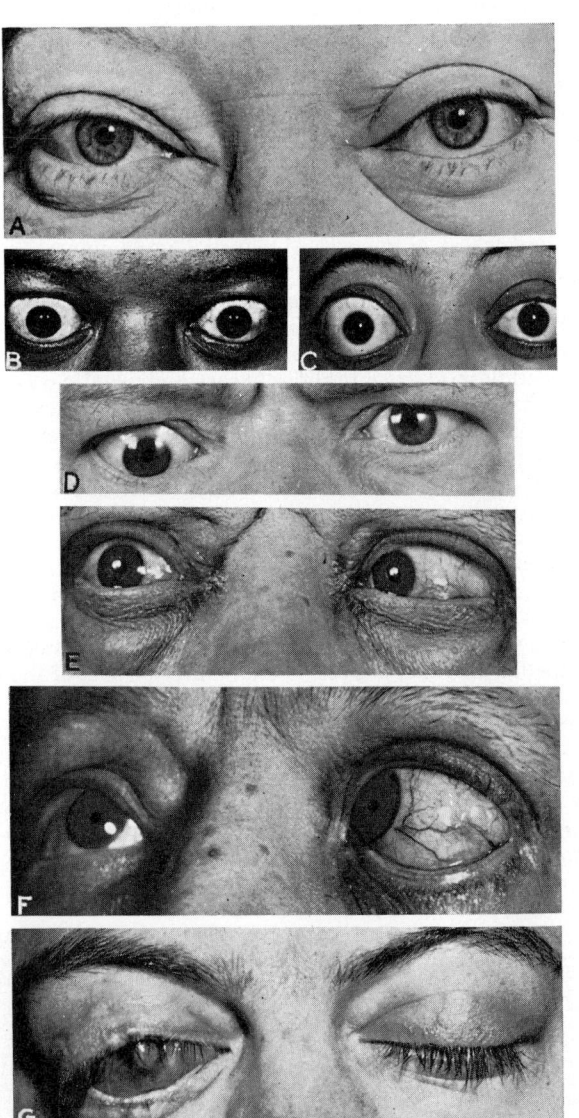

Figure 4–27. Infiltrative ophthalmopathy. *A,* Palpebral edema. This patient's eyeballs protruded anteriorly 1 cm. more than normal, but there is no "pop-eye" appearance, owing to edema of the surrounding structures. *B,* Marked widening of palpebral fissures; slight palpebral swelling. *C,* Unequal degrees of ophthalmopathy. *D,* Unilateral lid retraction. *E,* Palpebral swelling, due presumably to fat pads and edema; paralysis of right external rectus muscle. *F,* Marked conjunctival injection and chemosis, together with ophthalmoplegia. *G,* Failure to close lids on right due to marked exophthalmos, corneal scarring, and panophthalmitis; eye had to be enucleated.

Occasionally there is complete paralysis of upward gaze; in such cases, a characteristic position of the head is assumed in which the neck is extended to make possible a field of vision above the horizontal. Rarely is downward or inward gaze severely affected. Ophthalmoplegic manifestations usually occur in association with other signs of infiltrative ophthalmopathy but may occur alone. In some cases, only a single muscle is affected (Fig. 4–28).

Some indication of the severity of the infiltrative process in the orbit is provided by an assessment of intraorbital tension. Although an instrument for this purpose has been devised (orbitonometer), clinical assessment will usually suffice. This can be accomplished by having the patient close the eyes lightly and by determining the ease with which the globe can be displaced posteriorly by pressure from the thumb.

The manifestations of the most extreme form of ophthalmopathy or its complications are often catastrophic. These include subluxation of the globe and ulceration or infection of the cornea secondary to incomplete apposition of the lids. This may lead to panophthalmitis and destruction of one or both eyes. Ophthalmoscopic examination may reveal venous congestion and papilledema; these findings may be accompanied by visual field defects.

A classification of the eye changes of Graves' disease has been developed by a committee of the American Thyroid Association and has been in use for several years. As shown in Table 4–9, the first letters of each category constitute the mnemonic NO SPECS. NO connotes the absent or mild degree of involvement, whereas SPECS connotes the more serious degrees of involvement.

An uncommon manifestation of Graves' disease is *infiltrative dermopathy.* It occurs in about 5-10% of cases and is almost always accompanied by infiltrative ophthalmop-

Table 4–9. AMERICAN THYROID ASSOCIATION ABRIDGED CLASSIFICATION OF EYE CHANGES OF GRAVES' DISEASE

Class	Definition
0	No physical signs or symptoms
1	Only signs, no symptoms (signs limited to upper lid retraction, stare, lid lag, and proptosis to 22 mm)
2	Soft-tissue involvement (symptoms and signs)
3	Proptosis > 22 mm
4	Extraocular muscle involvement
5	Corneal involvement
6	Sight loss (optic nerve involvement)

athy, usually of severe degree. This lesion appears as a violaceous induration of the skin over the pretibial area (pretibial myxedema) and over the dorsa of the feet usually in the form of individual plaques but occasionally becoming confluent. Rarely it is seen on the face or dorsa of the hands. Clubbing of the digits and osteoarthropathy are occasionally associated manifestations (thyroid acropachy).

Laboratory Tests

In the classic case of moderate or severe diffuse toxic goiter, results of laboratory tests are clearly abnormal and are consonant with the pathophysiology of this disorder. The increase in thyroid iodide clearance rate is reflected in the increased RAIU, and hypersecretion of hormone leads to an increase in the concentrations in serum of T_4 and T_3, but the latter is disproportionately increased relative to the former. Occasionally, this discrepancy is exaggerated, the serum T_4 concentration being normal and the serum T_3 concentration alone being elevated (T_3-toxicosis); in this circumstance, the RAIU may also be within the normal range. In conjunction with the increased concentrations of T_4 and T_3 in the blood, a decrease of TBG produces an increase in both the proportions and absolute concentrations of free T_4 and T_3 and abnormally high values for the *in vitro* uptake test and free T_4 and T_3 indices. Metabolic indices, such as the BMR and serum cholesterol concentration, reflect the action of excessive amounts of thyroid hormone on the peripheral tissues.

An extensive discussion of the physiologic basis of these tests and the manner in which they are affected by factors other than thyroid disease has been presented in an earlier section. Nevertheless it is important to consider some practical aspects of the use of these tests in the diagnosis of diffuse toxic goiter. It is neither desirable nor usually feasible that all the major laboratory tests be used to assist in the diagnosis. Measurement of the serum T_4 concentration alone will probably establish or exclude the diagnosis in the great majority of cases. In order to exclude the possibility that the increase in serum T_4 concentration is the result of an increase in hormone binding in the blood, concomitant measurement either of the free T_4 concentration or free T_4 index should be made. If the latter functions are increased, a diagnosis of thyrotoxicosis is virtually assured. In the unusual instance in which values for the serum total or free T_4 concentrations are not increased, measurement of serum T_3 concentration should be performed.

Measurement of the serum T_3 concentration, together with some indicator of hormone binding, will establish or exclude the diagnosis of hyperthyroidism in an even greater proportion of patients than will values of the serum T_4 and free T_4 concentrations, and might, therefore, be regarded as the best initial approach. However, it is noteworthy that there are two thyrotoxic states in which the combination of an increased serum T_4 concentration and a normal serum T_3 concentration (T_4-toxicosis) may occasionally be encountered. The one circumstance is the association of thyrotoxicosis with severe intercurrent illness that impairs peripheral conversion of T_4 to T_3, and the other is the entity of iodine-induced thyrotoxicosis (Jod-Basedow phenomenon).

The diagnostic accuracy of the RAIU in hyperthyroidism may approach that of the serum T_4 concentration alone, but does not approach that of the free T_4 concentration or index or that of the serum T_3 concentration. Nevertheless, measurement of the RAIU is the most useful test for excluding thyrotoxicosis that is not due to active overproduction of hormone by the thyroid. Very low values of the RAIU in association with thyrotoxicosis signal the presence of thyrotoxicosis factitia, ectopic thyroid tissue, subacute thyroiditis, or the syndrome of chronic thyroiditis with transient thyrotoxicosis ("hyperthyroiditis"). A low value may also alert one to unsuspected iodine-induced hyperthyroidism, in which, of course, production of hormone by the thyroid gland is indeed increased.

It is in the borderline case of thyrotoxicosis that the laboratory tests are most greatly needed. In this circumstance, unfortunately, the values are likely to be only slightly abnormal, if at all. It is here that the tests of thyroregulatory mechanisms, the thyroid suppression test and the TRH stimulation test, have their greatest utility. Although an abnormal thyroid suppression test is not pathognomonic of thyrotoxicosis if the patient is known to have Graves' disease, a normal suppression test would clearly exclude thyrotoxicosis. On the other hand, a blunted or absent response to TRH would strongly suggest thyrotoxicosis. Because of its ease of performance and greater safety, particularly in the elderly patient or the patient with coexisting cardiac disease, the TRH stimulation test has largely superseded the thyroid suppression test.

The presence of IgG with TSI or TBII activity in the serum strongly suggests that the patient has Graves' disease, but does not always correlate with the presence of thyrotoxicosis. Measurement of these factors has its greatest utility in the pregnant patient and in the patient completing a course of antithyroid drug therapy. In the former, the presence of TSH or TBII predicts the likely occurrence of neonatal thyrotoxicosis in the offspring, while in the latter, absence of these factors augurs well for a long-term remission following withdrawal of therapy.

Differential Diagnosis

The patient who displays all the major manifestations of Graves' disease, namely thyrotoxicosis, goiter, and infiltrative ophthalmopathy, does not pose a diagnostic problem. In some patients, however, one of the major manifestations either dominates the clinical picture or is present alone, and the disorder may mimic some disease other than Graves' disease. Since the major manifestations are so different, the conditions from which they require differentiation will be considered separately.

A variety of disorders have features that resemble those of thyrotoxicosis in a general way. The most frequent disorder that simulates thyrotoxicosis is *neurasthenia*. As in Graves' disease, the commonest cause of thyrotoxicosis, the patient with neurasthenia is usually a young woman who complains of fatigue, palpitation, nervous irritability, and insomnia. Fatigue is pronounced and differs from that in thyrotoxicosis in that it is not accompanied by a desire to be active. The patient is both listless and fatigued and often feels tired on awakening. In the patient with neurasthenia, tachycardia is common during examination, but, in contrast to what is found in thyrotoxicosis, the sleeping pulse rate is normal. The palms are characteristically cool and clammy, rather than warm and moist. Hyperreflexia is present in both disorders. In neurasthenia, goiter is absent and laboratory indices of thyroid function are normal. *Chronic obstructive pulmonary disease* may require differentiation from thyrotoxicosis. Here, retention of carbon dioxide may lead to a warm flushed skin, tremulousness, and a bounding pulse. Mild exophthalmos may also be present. Very often these patients receive iodides as an expectorant, and this not only invalidates the RAIU but also may lead to goiter (iodide goiter). The BMR is increased by respiratory insufficiency. Nevertheless, the serum T_4 concentration will accurately reflect the metabolic state of the patient.

Pheochromocytoma may closely resemble thyrotoxicosis in that adrenergic overactivity and hypermetabolism are common to both. Similarities include nervous irritability, eyelid retraction, tremulousness, excessive sweating, and tachycardia. Like the patient with thyrotoxicosis, the patient with pheochromocytoma may have weight loss despite a good appetite, and hyperglycemia with glucosuria. However, in the patient with pheochromocytoma, diastolic hypertension is present, and urinary excretion of vanillylmandelic acid is increased, features that are lacking in thyrotoxicosis. In the patient with pheochromocytoma, goiter is absent, and, with very rare exceptions, the laboratory indices of thyroid function are normal.

In *diabetes mellitus*, weight loss despite a good appetite, polyuria, muscle wasting, and occasionally diarrhea may suggest thyrotoxicosis. Moreover, the incidence of goiter in patients with diabetes mellitus is higher than in the general population. However, other features of thyrotoxicosis are usually lacking, and laboratory indices of thyroid function are normal.

Myeloproliferative disorders are accompanied by hypermetabolism, which may be manifested by increased sweating and weight loss and by tachycardia, especially if anemia is present. This disorder, therefore, may bear a superficial resemblance to thyrotoxicosis, but goiter is absent and laboratory indices of thyroid function are normal.

Cirrhosis of the liver may require differentiation from thyrotoxicosis, since patients with cirrhosis often display weight loss, excessive sweating, a bounding pulse, and occasionally mild exophthalmos. Furthermore, the RAIU may be increased in cirrhosis as a result of iodine deficiency secondary to an inadequate diet. However, the serum T_4 concentration is normal, the serum T_3 concentration is often low, and goiter is generally absent. The RAIU returns to normal when a nutritious diet is given.

One disorder that simulates thyrotoxicosis clinically is unlikely to be encountered because of its rarity, but is nevertheless of great theoretical interest. A single case has been reported of a woman who displayed severe hypermetabolism (in the range of +200%), weight loss despite good appetite, profuse sweating, and progressive asthenia associated with myopathy. These symptoms had been present since childhood. Goiter was absent, and the RAIU was normal. The disorder was ascribed to structural abnormalities in the mitochondria leading to loosening of respiratory control (Luft et al., 1962).

Thyrotoxic myopathy may require differentiation from progressive muscular atrophy or polymyositis. In *progressive muscular atrophy*, fasciculation is present and the deep tendon jerks are diminished or absent. *Polymyositis* may resemble thyrotoxic myopathy, but muscle biopsy discloses inflammatory and degenerative changes. In both progressive muscular atrophy and polymyositis, other features of thyrotoxicosis are lacking and laboratory indices of thyroid function are normal.

The diffuse goiter of Graves' disease will rarely be confused with that of other thyroid diseases if thyrotoxicosis is present. Possible exceptions include the unusual case of Hashimoto's disease in which there is concurrent hyperthyroidism, the early stage of subacute thyroiditis, and the syndrome of painless thyroiditis. In subacute thyroiditis, asymmetry of the gland, tenderness, and systemic evidence of inflammation assist in the diagnosis. The subnormal RAIU aids in distinguishing this disease, as well as painless thyroiditis, from Graves' disease. When Graves' disease is in a latent or inactive phase and thyrotoxicosis is absent, the diffuse goiter usually persists and may require exclusion of Hashimoto's thyroiditis or simple nontoxic goiter as possible diagnoses. The goiter of Hashimoto's disease tends to be somewhat lobulated and firmer than that of Graves' disease. Antithyroid antibodies are more commonly found in the serum in Hashimoto's disease, and the titers are generally much higher. In the absence of thyrotoxicosis, the diffuse goiter of Graves' disease cannot be distinguished on clinical grounds from the diffuse stage of nontoxic goiter. An abnormal suppression test or the presence of TSI or TBII will indicate underlying Graves' disease, but their absence does not exclude Graves' disease.

The ophthalmopathy of Graves' disease, if bilateral and associated with thyrotoxicosis past or present, does not require differentiation from exophthalmos of other origin. However, unilateral exophthalmos, even when associated with thyrotoxicosis, should alert the physician to the possibility of a local cause. When exophthalmos occurs in the patient who has not been thyrotoxic, other diseases that may produce either unilateral or bilateral exophthalmos must be actively excluded. These include orbital neoplasms, caroticocavernous fistulae, cavernous sinus thrombosis, infiltrative disorders affecting the orbit, and pseudotumor cerebri. Mild bilateral exophthalmos, generally without infiltrative signs, is occasionally present on a familial basis and also sometimes occurs in patients with Cushing's syndrome, cirrhosis, uremia, chronic obstructive pulmonary disease, and superior vena caval syndrome. Ophthalmoplegia as the sole manifestation of the ophthalmopathy of Graves' disease requires exclusion of diabetes mellitus and other disorders affecting the brain stem and its connections. The demonstration of swelling of the extraocular muscles by orbital ultrasonography would strongly suggest that the ophthalmopathy is a manifestation of Graves' disease, as would the detection of TSI or TBII in serum or the demonstration of an abnormal TRH or thyroid suppression test.

Treatment of Thyrotoxicosis

Although considerable progress has been made in recent years toward an understanding of the pathogenesis of Graves' disease, this progress has not yet led to the development of therapeutic measures aimed at the basic pathogenetic factors in the disease. In a very real sense, existing therapies for both the thyrotoxic and the ophthalmopathic manifestations are merely palliative in that they may relieve but do not cure the disease. The lack of general agreement as to which of the several therapies is the best reflects the fact that, although they all may be satisfactory, none is ideal. Since the therapeutic problems posed by the thyrotoxicosis and the ophthalmopathy differ so widely and since they run independent courses, their treatment will be discussed separately.

As indicated earlier, the thyrotoxicosis of Graves' disease is due to an abnormal rate of hormone synthesis and release. All major forms of treatment exert their effects by imposing restraints on the rate of hormone secretion. This is accomplished either by means of chemical agents that inhibit one or more stages in hormone synthesis or release or by so reducing the quantity of thyroid tissue that overproduction of hormone is no longer possible.

Antithyroid Agents. The first stage in hormone biosynthesis that is susceptible to chemotherapeutic inhibition is the iodide transport mechanism. Both thiocyanate and perchlorate, agents that inhibit thyroid iodide transport, have been employed successfully. However, theoretical and practical disadvantages attend their use. The ameliorative effect of these agents in thyrotoxicosis depends upon their ability to decrease the net flux of iodide into the thyroid, thereby limiting the quantity of substrate available for subsequent steps in hormone biosynthesis. Such treatment, however, leaves the patient at the mercy of his iodine intake, since if plasma inorganic iodide concentration is increased, sufficient iodide can enter the thyroid by simple diffusion to permit reestablishment of an excessive rate of hormone formation. Furthermore, this consideration makes it impossible to use iodine together with these agents in the preparation of the patient for subtotal thyroidectomy. Serious adverse reactions, such as irreversible aplastic anemia, have led to abandonment of their use.

The major agents employed in the chemotherapy of thyrotoxicosis are drugs of the thionamide class having the chemical structure shown in Figure 4–13. The agents most commonly employed are propylthiouracil and methimazole (Tapazole) and the related drug, carbimazole (Neo-Mercazole). The mode of action of these agents on hormone biosynthesis is complex. Although initially considered to exert their antithyroid action solely by inhibiting the oxidation and organic binding of thyroid iodide, they are now known to inhibit the coupling of iodotyrosines primarily and the formation of DIT and MIT secondarily. Thus they are capable of producing an inhibition of hormone synthesis of far greater degree than the inhibition of total iodine accumulation. This fact is of importance in interpreting values for the RAIU during treatment with these drugs, since values may remain elevated despite the fact that the patient has been restored to a normal metabolic state. In addition to inhibiting hormone synthesis, propylthiouracil, but not methimazole, impairs the conversion of T_4 to T_3 in the peripheral tissues. Because of this additional action, propylthiouracil is generally used in preference to methimazole when rapid alleviation of severe thyrotoxicosis is sought.

Data concerning the distribution and metabolism of these agents are somewhat limited. The half-life in plasma of methimazole is about 6 hours, whereas that of PTU is about 1½ hours. However, the plasma concentration of drug may have little bearing on the duration of antithyroid action. Both drugs are accumulated by the thyroid, and a single 30-mg dose of methimazole may exert an antithyroid effect for longer than 24 hours. This provides a rational basis for the single daily dose regimen of methimazole in the patient with mild or moderate thyrotoxicosis.

An aspect of great importance in relation to the use of these drugs is that they cross the placenta, are excreted in breast milk, and are capable, therefore, of inhibiting thyroid function in the fetus and neonate. Recent work suggests that methimazole crosses the placenta more readily than propylthiouracil does (Marchant et al., 1977).

The initial dose of propylthiouracil most commonly employed by the authors is 100–200 mg given orally at intervals of 8 hours. Although this dosage is effective in most patients, in some no therapeutic response is seen. It is unlikely, however, that a true state of complete resistance to these agents ever occurs, although in some patients remarkably large doses of up to 1200 mg daily may be required. This relative lack of effect usually occurs in patients with severe thyroid hyperfunction and large thyroid glands, possibly because of a more rapid degradation of the drug either within the gland or extrathyroidally. When large doses are required, it is often advantageous to increase the frequency of administration to intervals of 4 hours instead of or in addition to the size. The response to effective antithyroid therapy invariably occurs only after a latent period. This follows from the fact that these agents inhibit the synthesis but not the release of hormone, and hence a reduction in the supply of hormone to the tissues must await depletion of glandular hormone stores. Although propylthiouracil differs from methimazole in additionally inhibiting the peripheral generation of T_3 from T_4, there appears to be little difference in the duration of the latent period when either of these agents is employed alone in the usual dosage.

Several factors influence the duration of the latent period. Among these are the quantity of hormone initially present in the thyroid, its inherent rate of release, and the degree of blockade of new hormone synthesis that is achieved. In the thyroid rich in iodine, such as occurs when the patient has received medications containing iodine, the clinical response to antithyroid agents may be delayed for long periods, even months. As would be expected, the latent period is shortened by the administration of large doses (more than 600 mg daily of propylthiouracil), and such should be used when a more rapid therapeutic response is required. Generally some improvement will occur within the first 2 weeks; the patient may note a decrease in nervousness and palpitations, an increase in strength, and a gain in weight during this period. Usually, a normal metabolic state can be restored within about 6 weeks. At this time, the dosage can often be reduced by approximately one-third and a normal metabolic state thereafter maintained.

During treatment, the size of the thyroid decreases in about one-third to one-half of the patients. In others it may remain unchanged, while in the remainder it enlarges. The latter change signals either an intensification of the disease process, which often requires that the dosage of drug be increased, or the production of hypothyroidism due to excessive dosage, which will be discussed shortly. Obviously, it is important to differentiate between these extremes. Clinical criteria should be the main guidelines by which the adequacy of treatment is judged, but confirmation may be sought in the serum T_4 and T_3 concentrations. Mild thyrotoxicosis may persist despite a serum T_4 concentration in the normal range, since the peripheral turnover of T_4 may remain accelerated for some time, and since the serum T_3 concentration may still be increased. The latter phenomenon may also account for the maintenance of a normal metabolic state in the face of a subnormal serum T_4 concentration. The response to TRH may remain subnormal, sometimes for months. Elevation of the RAIU may also persist despite adequate treatment, illustrating the primary action of the antithyroid agent on the later steps in hormone biosynthesis.

The antithyroid agents have the potential of inducing hypothyroidism if given in excessive quantities over prolonged periods. When this occurs, the patient often complains of excessive gain in weight, sluggishness, and fatigue. Signs of mild hypothyroidism may be present, especially a delay in the relaxation phase of the deep tendon jerks. Important signs of incipient hypothyroidism are enlargement of the thyroid gland and the appearance or accentuation of a bruit. These results from hypersecretion of TSH, together with hypothyroidism, can be reversed either by reducing the dosage of the antithyroid drug or by administering supplemental thyroid hormone. To forestall this development, which may have some adverse effects on preexisting ophthalmopathy, some physicians employ supplemental thyroid hormone routinely. Although the authors do not regularly prescribe this regimen, they see no contraindication to its use.

A central question in the long-term use of antithyroid drugs is the period over which treatment should be continued. No arbitrary answer can be given, but the problem is best understood in the light of the pathophysiology of the disorder. In the authors' opinion, there is no reason to believe that antithyroid therapy alters the course of the underlying disease process. If this is true, then persistence of remission following withdrawal of treatment will occur only if the disorder through its natural evolution has entered a latent or inactive phase, and this latter transition is more likely to occur the longer the course of treatment. This reasoning is the basis for the traditional practice of continuing antithyroid treatment for 12 months or longer. A recent study has suggested that the frequency of remission is as good when the antithyroid agent is withdrawn on attainment of a eumetabolic state as when the agent is continued for 12 months or longer (Greer et al., 1977). A later study indicates quite strongly, however, that this is not the case (Tamai et al., 1980b). Certain features may serve to indicate the likelihood of long-term remission following withdrawal of therapy (Table 4–10). The presence initially of T_3-toxicosis or of a small thyroid (less than 50 g) augurs well for a long-term remission. In addition, a decrease in the size of the thyroid and return of substantial suppressibility of thyroid function during treatment are favorable indicators, but, though reliable in a statistical sense, they are not reliable in the individual patient. Several recent studies strongly suggest that disappearance of circulating TSI or TBII during treatment of Graves' disease also portends a long-term remission following withdrawal of antithyroid (Davies et al., 1977; O'Donnell et al., 1978).

In the authors' clinic, treatment is continued for about 12 months and then withdrawn gradually. This permits an immediate exacerbation to be detected while some antithyroid effect is still maintained. Of the patients who relapse, about three-quarters will do so in the first 3 months following withdrawal of therapy and the bulk of the remainder during the subsequent 6 months. Elevation of the serum T_3 concentration, despite maintenance of a normal serum T_4, not infrequently signals exacerbation of the disease.

There is considerable uncertainty as to the frequency with which long-term remission occurs following withdrawal of antithyroid therapy. Until 10 years ago, there was nearly universal agreement that about one-half of patients with either diffuse or multinodular toxic goiter would experience a long-term remission. Several recent analyses have indicated a declining overall remission rate with time over the past 30 years, however (Wartofsky, 1973; Lumholz et al., 1977; Greer et al., 1977). This phenomenon does not appear to be due to the recent general increase in dietary iodine intake, as had been suggested, since it has also been observed to occur in a geographic region where iodine intake has remained constant and relatively low for the past 30 years. The foregoing has led to some disenchantment with antithyroid agents as the therapy of choice for thyrotoxicosis in Graves' disease. Nevertheless, it is the experience of the authors, as well as

Table 4–10. FACTORS FAVORING LONG-TERM REMISSION FOLLOWING ANTITHYROID THERAPY OF DIFFUSE TOXIC GOITER

T_3-toxicosis
Small goiter
Decrease in goiter size during therapy
Normal thyroid function test
Normal TRH-stimulation test
Negative tests for immunoglobulins of Graves' disease

others, that about one-third of patients will experience a lasting remission. Thus, a significant place for antithyroid agents as sole therapy in the treatment of thyrotoxicosis continues to exist.

Methimazole (Tapazole) is the alternative antithyroid agent most commonly used in the United States. Its potency is generally considered to be about 10 times that of propylthiouracil, and hence the doses given are one-tenth those described earlier. It is the authors' impression, however, that this ratio underestimates the potency of methimazole. Except for the dosage, the use of methimazole is similar in all respects to that of propylthiouracil. In many patients, methimazole can be administered as a single daily dose with good effect. This regimen will frequently enhance patient compliance when the latter has been a problem. Carbimazole is used more often than methimazole in Europe, and reportedly is less toxic, but differences between the two are difficult to understand, since carbimazole is very quickly converted to methimazole *in vivo*.

Adverse reactions occur in a small percentage of patients taking antithyroid drugs of the thionamide class (Table 4–11). The most significant of these is agranulocytosis, which occurs in a fraction of 1% of the patients. Agranulocytosis, like the other adverse reactions, generally occurs within the first few weeks or months of treatment. It is accompanied by fever and sore throat, and hence, when therapy is begun, the patient should be instructed to discontinue the drug and notify the physician immediately should these symptoms develop. This precaution is more important than the frequent measurement of leukocyte counts, since agranulocytosis may develop within a day or two. Should agranulocytosis occur, the drug should be discontinued immediately and the patient should be isolated and given glucocorticoids and antibiotics. Almost invariably recovery will occur. Lymphocytes of patients who have developed agranulocytosis while taking propylthiouracil undergo blast transformation when exposed *in vitro*, not only to propylthiouracil but also to methimazole. Consequently, such patients should never be given a thionamide drug again.

Granulocytopenia may also occur during antithyroid therapy and is sometimes a forerunner of agranulocytosis. On the other hand, mild granulocytopenia may be merely a manifestation of thyrotoxicosis. For this reason, granulocytopenia detected during the first few weeks of therapy may present the physician with a difficult decision — whether or not treatment should be continued. In this circumstance, serial measurements of the leukocyte count should be made,

Table 4–11. PER CENT INCIDENCE OF TOXIC REACTIONS

	All Reactions	Agranulocytosis
Methimazole	7.1	0.1
Carbimazole	1.9	0.8
Propylthiouracil	3.3	0.4
Methylthiouracil	13.8	0.5

and if these display a downward trend, the antithyroid drug should be discontinued. Usually, however, serial measurements will reveal a return of the white cell count to normal, and treatment need not be interrupted. Skin rash, which may take many forms, is the most common type of reaction, and in the authors' experience occurs more frequently with methimazole than with propylthiouracil. Some patients may display sun sensitization when taking propylthiouracil.

In addition to these reactions, others may occur, but fortunately even less frequently. These include arthralgia, myalgia, neuritis, hepatitis with evidence of cholestasis, thrombocytopenia, loss of or abnormal pigmentation of the hair, loss of taste sensation, enlargement of lymph nodes or salivary glands, edema, a lupus-like syndrome, and toxic psychoses. The nature of the pathologic disturbances underlying these reactions is not known, although some may disappear despite continuance of treatment. Nonetheless, it is the authors' view that appearance of any of these manifestations is an indication for abandonment of antithyroid therapy and recourse to surgery or [131]I.

Iodine. Iodine, which until 1943 was the major chemotherapeutic agent for thyrotoxicosis, is now rarely used as sole therapy. The mechanism of action of iodine in relieving thyrotoxicosis differs greatly from that of the thionamides. Although quantities of iodine in excess of several milligrams are capable of inducing an acute inhibition of organic binding (acute Wolff-Chaikoff effect), this is a transient phenomenon which, in all likelihood, does not contribute to the therapeutic action of iodine. Rather, the major action of iodine is to inhibit hormone release, as several lines of evidence indicate.

First, administration of iodine is associated with an increase in glandular organic iodine stores. Second, the beneficial effect of iodine is evident much more quickly than is the effect of even large doses of agents that inhibit hormone synthesis. Finally, in patients with diffuse toxic goiter, kinetic analysis demonstrates that iodine acutely retards the rate of secretion of T_4; this effect is rapidly lost when iodine is withdrawn. These features of its action provide both the disadvantages and advantages of iodine therapy. The enrichment of glandular organic iodine stores that occurs when this agent is given alone may greatly retard the clinical response to subsequently administered thionamide therapy, and furthermore, the decrease in RAIU that iodine produces will prevent the use of radioiodine as treatment for a period of weeks or more. In addition, if iodine is withdrawn, resumption of a rapid rate of release from an enriched glandular hormone pool may produce a severe exacerbation of thyrotoxicosis. Still another reason for not using iodine alone is that in some patients the therapeutic response is either incomplete or lacking and that, even if initially effective, iodine may lose its effect with time. (This phenomenon, which has been termed "iodine escape," should not be confused with the escape from the acute Wolff-Chaikoff effect; see section on Thyroid Autoregulation.) On the other hand, the rapid slowing of hormone release that iodine induces makes it a more effective agent than the thionamide drugs when rapid relief of thyrotoxicosis is mandatory. Therefore, aside from its use in the preparation of the patient for subtotal thyroidectomy, iodine is mainly useful for patients with actual or impending thyrotoxic crisis, severe thyrocardiac disease, or acute surgical emergencies — all conditions in which thyrotoxicosis is life-threatening.

If iodine is to be used in these circumstances, it is highly desirable that it be administered with large doses of a thionamide, as the severity of the thyrotoxicosis would itself indicate. The dose of iodine as iodide required for control of thyrotoxicosis is not entirely certain but has been estimated

to be approximately 6 mg daily, a quantity far less than that usually given. Six milligrams of iodide would be contained in approximately one-eighth of a drop of saturated solution of potassium iodide (SSKI) or eight-tenths of a drop of Lugol's solution; many physicians, however, prescribe 5–10 drops of one of these agents three times daily. Although it is advisable to administer amounts larger than the suggested minimal effective dose, the huge quantities of iodine commonly administered are distinctly disadvantageous in that they are more likely to produce adverse reactions, including iodide myxedema. The authors recommend the use of two drops of SSKI three times daily. In patients who are so ill that medications cannot be taken by mouth, antithyroid agents can be triturated and administered by stomach tube; iodine can be given by the same route. When use of a stomach tube is contraindicated, thionamide drugs cannot be administered, since preparations for parenteral use are not available. Here, the disadvantages attendant upon the administration of iodine may be accepted if the clinical situation is sufficiently serious, and a preparation of sodium iodide is available for intravenous use. Adverse reactions to iodine are unusual and, although varied, are generally not serious. These include skin rash, which may be acneiform, drug fever, sialadenitis, conjunctivitis and rhinitis, vasculitis, and a leukemoid eosinophilic granulocytosis. Sialadenitis may respond to reduction of the dosage; in the case of the other reactions, iodine should be withdrawn. As will be discussed later, iodine appears to be particularly effective when given after the administration of a therapeutic dose of [131]I. This combination may be very useful when rapid alleviation of thyrotoxicosis is required.

Like iodine, lithium carbonate also inhibits thyroid hormone secretion, but experience with this agent is limited. Unlike iodine, it has the advantage that it does not interfere with the accumulation of a subsequently administered dose of radioiodine.

Dexamethasone. This drug has become an important therapeutic adjunct when rapid alleviation of thyrotoxicosis is desired. Dexamethasone administered in a dosage of 2 mg every 6 hours inhibits both the glandular secretion of hormone and the peripheral conversion of T_4 to T_3 (Williams et al., 1975). With respect to the latter action, the inhibitory effect of dexamethasone is additive to that of propylthiouracil, suggesting different mechanisms of action. The concurrent administration of propylthiouracil, SSKI, and dexamethasone to the patient with severe thyrotoxicosis will effect a rapid reduction in serum T_3 concentration, often to

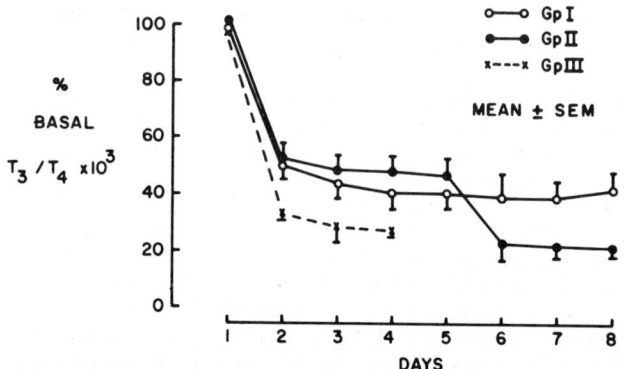

Figure 4–29. Combined drug therapy of hyperthyroidism: effects on the serum T_3/T_4 ratio. Group I treated with PTU and SSKI; Group II, with PTU and SSKI, followed by dexamethasone on day 5; and Group III, with PTU, SSKI, and dexamethasone from day 1. (From Croxson, M. S., et al.: Combination drug therapy for treatment of hyperthyroid Graves' disease. *J. Clin. Endocrinol. Metab. 45*:623, 1977. © 1977 The Endocrine Society.)

within the normal range in 24 to 48 hours (Croxson et al., 1977). (See Fig. 4–29.)

Adrenergic Antagonists. Agents that either deplete tissues of their catecholamine content (reserpine or guanethidine) or block the response to catecholamines at the receptor site (propranolol) are capable of antagonizing to a variable extent some of the manifestations of thyrotoxicosis. Hence they are useful adjuncts in the management of patients with this disorder. Tremulousness, palpitation, excessive sweating, eyelid retraction, and heart rate decrease. When administered in sufficient dosage, these agents have effects that are rapidly manifest and appear to be mediated largely through the adrenergic nervous system, although propranolol may impair to some extent the conversion of T_4 to T_3.

Adrenergic antagonists have their greatest use in patients with severe thyrotoxicosis, such as those with impending or actual thyrotoxic crisis (see section on Special Aspects of Thyrotoxicosis). They are also of value, however, in patients with less severe disease in whom tremor, tachycardia, palpitation, or nervousness is particularly troublesome. Adrenergic antagonists have also been used in patients with thyrocardiac disease in whom tachycardia of either sinus or ectopic origin is contributing to cardiac insufficiency. These agents should be used with caution, however, since by depressing myocardial contractility they may aggravate cardiac insufficiency. Moreover, since thyroid hormone also has a direct effect on the myocardium independent of the adrenergic nervous system, the authors prefer to use iodine in conjunction with propylthiouracil and dexamethasone for rapid control of thyrotoxicosis in the patient with severe thyrocardiac disease. Adrenergic antagonists should be considered as adjunctive rather than primary tools in the treatment of thyrotoxicosis. They are most frequently useful in the interval during which the response to thionamide or radioiodine therapy is being awaited.

Of the agents available, propranolol is the one of choice, as it is relatively free of adverse effects. It can be given either orally in a dose of 40–80 mg every 6 or 8 hours or, if indicated, intravenously in a dose of 2 mg with electrocardiographic monitoring. Propranolol is contraindicated in patients with asthma or chronic obstructive pulmonary disease since it aggravates bronchospasm. Because of its myocardial depressant action, it is also contraindicated in patients with heart block and in patients with congestive failure, unless severe tachycardia is a contributory factor. Finally, prolonged administration of propranolol is contraindicated in the pregnant patient in view of the reported association of its administration with a variety of abnormalities in the newborn, such as small size, low Apgar scores, and postnatal bradycardia and hypoglycemia (Gladstone et al., 1975; Tunstall, 1969).

Surgery. As mentioned earlier, there is no reason to believe that antithyroid therapy with a thionamide drug has any direct effect on the thyroid that persists after the treatment is discontinued. By contrast, the other major types of therapy, i.e., surgery and radioiodine, exert their effects through the permanent removal or destruction of thyroid tissue, rendering the gland incapable of producing excessive quantities of hormone. This effect is likely to be long-lasting, and hence these forms of ablative therapy are referred to as "definitive treatment." Thus, as regards their duration of effect, antithyroid therapy and ablative therapy are diametrically different, and their opposite properties may be considered advantageous or disadvantageous, depending upon one's point of view.

The impermanence of antithyroid therapy leads to a relatively frequent recurrence of thyrotoxicosis, while with abla-

Table 4–12. RANGE OF RESULTS OF SURGERY FOR HYPERTHYROIDISM, AS REPORTED FROM EIGHT CLINICS

	Per Cent
Mortality	0.0– 3.1
Recurrent hyperthyroidism	0.6–17.9
Vocal cord paralysis	0.0– 4.4
Permanent hypoparathyroidism	0.0– 3.6
Permanent hypothyroidism	4.0–29.7

From Hershman, J. M.: The treatment of hyperthyroidism. *Ann. Intern. Med. 64*:1306, 1966.

tive therapy recurrence is uncommon. On the other hand, antithyroid therapy never produces permanent hypothyroidism, while with ablative therapy the frequency of permanent hypothyroidism may be distressingly or unacceptably high. The effectiveness of surgery in relieving hyperthyroidism is unquestioned. In most series, the frequency of recurrent hyperthyroidism following subtotal thyroidectomy in adults is less than 10%. On the other hand, the combined prevalence of postoperative hypothyroidism and other surgical complications is relatively high, rendering surgery less than ideal as a form of treatment.

Table 4–12 is taken from a report in which the results of surgery for hyperthyroidism in eight series are summarized (Hershman, 1966). The major postoperative complication is permanent hypothyroidism, which in the series cited ranged between 4% and approximately 30%. It is worthy of note that the highest frequency of permanent postoperative hypothyroidism was reported from those clinics in which internists did the follow-ups on the patients. In a more recent study conducted by internists, a mean frequency of 28% was found in patients followed for 1–16 years, and the frequency in patients followed for 10 years was 43% (Nofal et al., 1966).

Although it has been assumed that hypothyroidism will usually develop within 1 year after operation if it is to occur at all, recently reported series indicate a progressive increase in the cumulative incidence with time similar to that produced by radioiodine but of lesser magnitude. It may be presumed that the overall frequency of some impairment of thyroid function is even higher than that of frank hypothyroidism since subtotal thyroidectomy is one important cause of decreased thyroid reserve. The increasing frequency of hypothyroidism with time may result from progressive restriction of blood supply or from autoimmune destruction of the thyroid remnant. If, as recently revealed, eventual thyroid failure is a frequent consequence of the Graves' disease process itself, the large increase in cumulative frequency of hypothyroidism with time that follows both surgery and radioiodine therapy is both expected and unavoidable. Treatment that destroys thyroid tissue would obviously accelerate the emergence of hypothyroidism resulting from the disease process itself.

It is generally agreed that an inverse relationship obtains between the frequency of recurrence and that of hypothyroidism, and that the relative frequency of the two partly depends upon the quantity of thyroid tissue left in place. What is more remarkable than the fact that some patients develop a recurrence and others hypothyroidism is that among patients whose thyroid glands vary greatly in size and degree of hyperfunction, and who are operated upon by surgeons whose techniques must vary to a considerable extent a normal metabolic state is restored, at least for long periods, in most patients. It has been held that this favorable outcome of surgery may result because the amount of tissue remaining after operation is alone insufficient to sustain a normal metabolic state and hence becomes stimulated by the necessary quantity of endogenous TSH. In this way, the patient's homeostatic mechanism provides the adjustment in thyroid function that the surgeon, quite naturally, could not. This hypothesis is supported by the return of TSH to the sera of patients restored to a normal metabolic state by surgery.

Bleeding into the operative site is the most serious postoperative complication, since it can rapidly produce death by asphyxia. This complication requires immediate evacuation of the hematoma and ligation of the bleeding vessel. Damage to the recurrent laryngeal nerve is one of the major complications of thyroid surgery and, if unilateral, it results in dysphonia that usually improves in a few weeks but which may leave the patient slightly hoarse. If damage is bilateral, obstruction of the airway will usually occur within a few hours, producing severe stridor; tracheostomy is then required, and at this time the nature of the damage to the nerves should be sought.

Hypoparathyroidism is another major complication; it may be either transient or permanent. Transient hypoparathyroidism results from two factors: inadvertent removal of some parathyroids and impairment of blood supply to those that remain. Depending upon the severity of these insults, symptoms and signs of hypocalcemia will appear, usually within 1–7 days after operation. The earliest indication of hypoparathyroidism may be anxiety and mental depression, followed by paresthesia and evidence of heightened neuromuscular excitability, such as Chvostek's and Trousseau's signs and carpopedal spasm. The serum calcium is subnormal and the inorganic phosphate increased, and the urine Sulkowitch test is negative. When hypoparathyroidism is first evident, if severe it should be treated with intravenous calcium gluconate or calcium chloride. Milder cases can be treated with oral calcium chloride in a dose of 1 g three times daily. Initially it is impossible to ascertain whether the hypoparathyroidism will be permanent or whether it will regress within a few weeks, as usually occurs.

Recently it has been suggested that the hypocalcemia that occurs in the thyrotoxic patient in the immediate postoperative period is not due to transient hypoparathyroidism, since it occurs more frequently here than after surgery for other thyroid disorders. Rather it has been ascribed to retention of calcium by bone in the thyrotoxic patient, but what initiates this phenomenon has not been determined (Michie et al., 1971). The frequency of permanent hypoparathyroidism varies in a general way with the proportion of the thyroid removed and hence with the frequency of postoperative hypothyroidism. The frequency of mild hypoparathyroidism (or diminished parathyroid reserve) detectable years after operation is probably greater than is generally supposed, and it may be as high as 24%. The treatment of permanent hypoparathyroidism is discussed in Chapter 19.

It is clear that the hazards of subtotal thyroidectomy are inversely related to the experience and skill of the surgical team. Consequently, as surgery is less frequently performed, the hazards attendant upon it increase. For these reasons, it is impossible to generalize about the frequency of complications, and statistics drawn from the former era in which surgery was commonly applied are probably no longer applicable. In the author's view, unless circumstances are otherwise compelling, thyroidectomy should not be performed by surgeons who carry out this operative procedure only occasionally.

Preoperative use of the antithyroid agents has greatly decreased the morbidity and mortality of surgery for diffuse toxic goiter. This results from the ability of these drugs to deplete glandular hormone stores and secondarily to restore the patient to an entirely normal metabolic state before operation. On the other hand, these agents do not have the favorable influence on the hyperplasia and hypervascularity of the gland that is exerted by iodine. Iodine induces a process termed involution that is characterized by a decrease in height of the follicular cells, enlargement of follicles with retention of colloid, and last, but most important, reduction of hypervascularity. Hence, the aim of preoperative management is to restore a normal metabolic state with antithyroid agents and then to bring about involution of the gland with iodine. Achievement of these objectives makes the patient a better operative and postoperative risk in all respects. In the authors' clinic, patients who are to undergo subtotal thyroidectomy are first given antithyroid therapy in the manner described earlier. Often, relatively large doses are given, either to hasten the clinical response or because the patients for whom surgery is recommended are frequently those with severe disease or very large goiters. After a normal metabolic state has been restored, SSKI is given as two drops three times daily for a further 7–10 days. During this period, a preexisting bruit or thrill may decrease in intensity or disappear entirely; the gland usually becomes firmer and may appear to have enlarged.

Within this general approach, there are several specific guidelines that should be followed. First, no definite date for surgery should be set until the patient has been restored to a normal metabolic state. Much too often, the operation is planned well in advance, and the patient is given a standardized regimen that is largely independent of his clinical progress. Second, therapy with iodine should not be started until metabolic control has been produced by the antithyroid drug; iodine should not be relied upon to complete an as yet incomplete response to antithyroid therapy. This is true because if the antithyroid drug is not entirely effective the additional iodine will enrich glandular hormone stores. Finally, for closely related reasons, antithyroid agents should not be withdrawn when therapy with iodine is begun.

Propranolol is a useful adjunct in controlling some symptoms (see earlier) while the patient is being prepared for surgery. It has also been advocated that it be used alone in the preoperative preparation of the patient in whom surgery is to be undertaken (Toft et al., 1978a). While this mode of therapy is reportedly safe and effective, the authors believe that restoration of the patient to a eumetabolic state, as outlined above, is desirable before the patient is subjected to the stress of general anesthesia and surgery.

Radioiodine. Radioiodine is a simple and economical means of treating thyrotoxicosis. It produces the ablative effects of surgery without the immediate operative and postoperative complications of the latter. The principal disadvantage attendant on the use of radioiodine is the high frequency of late hypothyroidism. Previously, there was concern that this form of therapy might also produce thyroid carcinoma, leukemia, or transmissible genetic damage. However, during the 30 years or so that radioiodine has been in use, no increased prevalence of thyroid carcinoma in patients so treated has been noted (Dobyns et al., 1974). Indeed, the prevalence may be lower than that in the general population, presumably because the radiation dose usually delivered to the thyroid interferes with cell replication. This phenomenon is to be contrasted with the increased prevalence of thyroid carcinoma in patients treated with much lower doses of radiation in childhood or adolescence. The prevalence of leukemia has also been shown to be no greater in patients treated with radioiodine (Saenger et al., 1968). Finally, the frequency of genetic damage in the offspring of patients treated earlier with radioiodine does not appear to be increased. Indeed, in this latter regard, it is worth noting that the conventional dose of radioiodine employed in the treatment of thyrotoxicosis delivers to the gonads a radiation dose approximately equivalent to that delivered by a barium enema examination or intravenous urogram. In view of the lack of evidence to date for significant carcinogenic, leukemogenic, or teratogenic effects of radioiodine in doses generally employed for treating hyperthyroidism, the age limit for the use of radioiodine has been lowered progressively from the initial limit of 40 years of age so that in some clinics it is employed regularly in children and adolescents. Nevertheless, the authors prefer to restrict this form of therapy to patients more than 30 years of age in view of the feeling that the duration of experience with respect to its radiation potential is still insufficient. Moreover, it is obvious that the greater the patient's life expectancy after radioiodine therapy, the greater the likelihood that hypothyroidism will develop.

During the early years of radioiodine therapy, attempts were made to standardize the radiation delivered to the thyroid gland by varying the dose of radioiodine according to the size of the gland, the uptake of ^{131}I, and its subsequent rate of release. It has become apparent, however, that such calculations do not provide uniform results, probably owing largely to variations in individual sensitivity. Hence most clinics have settled upon an arbitrary dose of approximately 140–160 μCi/g of estimated glandular weight.

Until the early 1960's most reports indicated that the frequency of postradioiodine hypothyroidism following doses of this magnitude was approximately 7–12%, most of this occurring during the first year or two after treatment. Although an occasional patient developed hypothyroidism later, this was considered an uncommon occurrence. In 1961, however, there appeared the first of several reports that by now have completely altered this view. Not only is the incidence of hypothyroidism higher during the first year or two after treatment than originally thought, but it continues to increase at a rate of approximately 3%/yr thereafter. Thus the incidence of postradioiodine hypothyroidism at 5 years is approximately 30% and at 10 years approximately 40%, although values as high as 70% have been reported (Dunn and Chapman, 1964; Nofal et al., 1966) (Fig. 4–30).

There is little doubt that the early beneficial effect of radioiodine and the early induction of hypothyroidism both depend upon radiation-induced destruction of thyroid parenchyma. Within the first few weeks after treatment, there occur epithelial swelling and necrosis, disruption of follicular architecture, edema, and infiltration with leukocytes (radiation thyroiditis). Resolution of the acute inflammation is followed by fibrosis, vascular narrowing, and lymphocytic infiltration. These structural changes account for the early response to radioiodine, be it favorable or excessive. In themselves, however, they do not appear sufficient to account for the increasing incidence of hypothyroidism with time, and more subtle factors appear to be operative. In some studies, the likelihood of hypothyroidism is increased by the presence of high titers of antithyroid antibodies at the time of treatment or by increasing age of the patient. The two predisposing factors may be related to one another.

A subtle functional abnormality is the defective organic binding of thyroid iodide that follows apparently successful therapy; this is evident in the frequently abnormal iodide-perchlorate discharge test and the enhanced susceptibility to iodide-induced hypothyroidism. This phenomenon may be but one of several abnormalities that eventually produce thyroid failure. Among these may be damage to the nucleus of the follicular cell, leading to failure of normal replication, progressive autoimmune destruction, or progressive restriction of blood supply. Such factors would summate with factors related to the disease process itself which lead to eventual thyroid failure.

In view of the foregoing, it is unlikely that the early ablative effects can be obtained free of subsequent late effects. If this is true, then doses of radioiodine sufficient to exert an early therapeutic action would inevitably be associated with a high frequency of delayed hypothyroidism.

This statement summarizes the therapeutic dilemma with respect to radioiodine therapy. From various clinics, several approaches to this dilemma have emerged. Some authorities continue to administer the conventional dose because of its relatively rapid and high effectiveness and because hypothyroidism, when it eventually occurs, is readily treated. A disadvantage of such an approach is that the onset and progression of hypothyroidism may be very insidious, that careful and prolonged follow-up of patients may not be possible, and that the patient may not associate symptoms arising as a complication of therapy long removed with that therapy. A rebuttal in favor of using this approach would be that the dangers of persistent or recurrent thyrotoxicosis in the patient lacking follow-up exceed those of hypothyroidism, especially if the patient is elderly.

A second approach seeks to forestall the eventual development of clinical hypothyroidism through the routine administration of replacement doses of thyroid hormone following radioiodine therapy. If this approach is to be used, it should be done only after a eumetabolic state has been achieved. It can be argued, however, that in anticipation of employing replacement therapy the physician may administer inordinately large doses of radioiodine hoping to obtain sure control of the thyrotoxicosis. Moreover, patients frequently tire of taking medication and discontinue it, despite urging to the contrary. The consequence of these factors would be a high frequency of hypothyroidism.

Other approaches have been undertaken in an attempt to minimize the frequency of hypothyroidism. One such approach involved the use of ^{125}I, rather than ^{131}I, on the basis that the lower energy and shorter path length of the β emission might permit irradiation of the apical portion of the thyroid cell with resulting impairment of hormone biosynthesis, while sparing the more distantly situated nucleus and its replicative machinery. However, long-term follow-up of a large series of patients treated with ^{125}I has revealed a frequency of hypothyroidism that is similar to that following

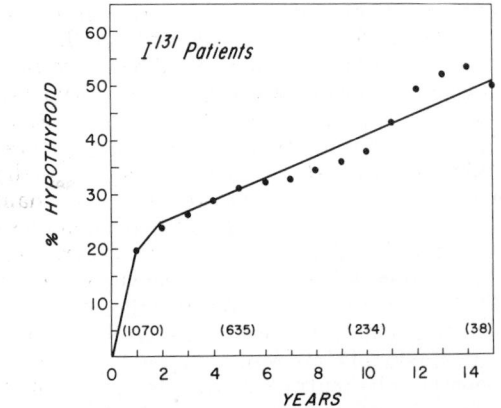

Figure 4–30. Incidence of postradioiodine hypothyroidism in relation to the duration of follow-up. Total number of patients followed for each of the indicated time periods is shown in parentheses. (From Dunn, J. T., and Chapman, E. M.: Rising incidence of hypothyroidism after radioactive-iodine therapy in thyrotoxicosis. *New Eng. J. Med.* 271:1037, 1964.)

[131]I (McDougall and Greig, 1976). Consequently, ^{125}I offers no advantages over [131]I.

A final approach employs smaller than usual doses of radioiodine. The rationale of such an approach is that the small dose may be sufficient to prevent both the high incidence of delayed hypothyroidism, which constitutes the chief disadvantage of conventional doses, and the late recurrence of thyrotoxicosis, which constitutes the chief disadvantage of antithyroid drug therapy. Although it is recognized that such small doses are likely insufficient to control thyrotoxicosis acutely, such control can be achieved by the administration of antithyroid drugs or stable iodine after radioiodine has been given (Smith and Wilson, 1967; Hagen et al., 1967).

The efficacy of this approach is not yet certain. Retrospective analysis indicates that the frequency of hypothyroidism varies directly with the magnitude of the dose used (Hershman, 1966). Moreover, in a controlled prospective study, the effects of a single conventional dose of approximately 140 μCi/g of estimated glandular weight were compared with the effects of half the dose (Smith and Wilson, 1967). Although the therapeutic effect of radioiodine appeared more slowly in the patients receiving the half-dose and a greater proportion required antithyroid drug therapy until this became apparent, the frequency of remission after 2 years was essentially the same as that in the patients receiving the conventional dose, and recurrence of thyrotoxicosis was no more common. Of great importance was the finding that with the full-dose group, the incidence of hypothyroidism was 8% at 1 year and 29% at 5 years, whereas in the half-dose group, the corresponding values were 4% and 7%. These results are in general agreement with those of another study (Hagen et al., 1967). However, recent data suggest that, although the use of low doses of ^{131}I reduces the incidence of hypothyroidism during the first few years, thereafter the cumulative frequency with time is similar to that observed with conventional doses (Malone and Cullen, 1976). It is apparent, therefore, that further observations of this type are required. The authors' viewpoints with regard to these approaches are discussed in the section concerning choice of therapy.

Several additional hazards may attend the use of radioiodine, particularly large doses. The parathyroids are exposed to radiation in patients treated with radioiodine, but the appearance of clinically overt hypoparathyroidism is rare. However, there is evidence to suggest that parathyroid reserve is diminished in some patients. The effect of radioiodine on other tissues that concentrate iodide, such as the salivary and gastric glands, has received little attention. Another potential hazard of radioiodine therapy, namely radiation thyroiditis, may influence the therapeutic regimen. This complication may lead to an exacerbation of thyrotoxicosis about 10–14 days after the radioiodine is administered. Serious consequences occasionally have resulted in patients with severe thyrotoxicosis or thyrocardiac disease; these include precipitation of thyrotoxic crisis and aggravation of cardiac insufficiency. In cases of this type, therefore, it is advisable to administer antithyroid drugs for several weeks before radioiodine is given in order to deplete glandular hormone stores. This prevents an outpouring of hormone should severe radiation thyroiditis occur. The antithyroid agent is withdrawn 2–3 days before administration of the radioiodine and, if the clinical condition warrants, it can be given again several days later.

Since ^{131}I administered to women during the first and second trimesters of pregnancy is likely to lead to irreversible hypothyroidism in the fetus, a pregnancy test should be carried out in all women of child-bearing age before they are given ^{131}I therapy.

General Measures. Several general measures often contribute substantially to the well-being of the thyrotoxic patient. Removal of the patient from what may be a troubled domestic or occupational environment to the restful atmosphere of a hospital may in itself be accompanied by a moderate decrease in thyrotoxic manifestations. In addition, a dietary regimen rich in protein, calories, and vitamins serves to repair the general and specific nutritional deficiencies that thyrotoxic patients frequently develop. Psychotherapy has been recommended, but whether its contribution to the patient's well-being is greater than it would be in other diseases is uncertain.

Choice of Therapy. The choice of therapy for thyrotoxicosis is often difficult in actuality, but it becomes even more difficult when considered in a hypothetical setting, since a variety of factors other than those immediately related to the disease itself interplay with the disease to modify the therapeutic decision. Among these are emotional attitudes, economic considerations, and factors within the family and home. Their impact will be discussed as they become pertinent to each of the therapeutic possibilities.

The authors' choice of therapy in diffuse toxic goiter is one which accommodates factors related to the natural history of the disease, the advantages and disadvantages of the several therapeutic modalities discussed above, and the factors pertinent to the population group in which the patient falls. It had been thought that the operative and immediate postoperative risks of surgery, as well as the discomfort and expense that surgery entails, were justified by the frequency with which a long-lasting remission of thyrotoxicosis could be achieved without a high frequency of hypothyroidism. However, the observation that the cumulative frequency of hypothyroidism increases to substantial values with time has modified this view. Admittedly it is likely that the incidence of postoperative hypothyroidism could be reduced if less thyroid tissue were removed at operation, but all available data suggest that the incidence of postoperative recurrence would increase as a result to an extent that is currently unpredictable. Hence the authors recommend surgery only in patients for whom shortcomings of other modes of therapy have special importance. As will be seen, this conclusion still leaves to surgery a significant role in the treatment of diffuse toxic goiter.

In the authors' opinion, therefore, radioiodine and antithyroid therapy become the mainstays of treatment, and the major choice rests between these two. The data currently available do not suggest that radioiodine carries an appreciable risk of thyroid carcinoma or leukemia. Furthermore, in patients who either by choice or by age will no longer become parents, the possibility of transmissible genetic damage induced by radioiodine does not exist. Consequently, the only tangible disadvantage to radioiodine therapy in such patients is the possibility that hypothyroidism will develop. Because of their relatively limited life expectancy and because of their susceptibility to serious complications of thyrotoxicosis, e.g., thyrocardiac disease, patients over 50 years of age should be given full or conventional doses of radioiodine. Supplemental thyroid hormone therapy is not routinely given for the reasons described earlier. Patients between 30 and 50 years of age are usually given the small-dose radioiodine regimen with supplemental antithyroid drug or iodine. Alternatively a conventional course of thionamide therapy alone may be used, especially if the disease is mild and the thyroid is small.

Considerations peculiar to the treatment of thyrotoxicosis in children and adolescents are discussed in a later section dealing with special aspects of thyrotoxicosis. Hence the remainder of this section will be confined to the choice of therapy in young adults. Although the genetic and carcinogenic risks of radioiodine do not appear significant, it should be remembered that it took approximately 20 years to recognize that radioiodine frequently produces hypothyroidism within 5-10 years after its administration. By analogy, it may require 40 years to detect more subtle complications that occur 20 years after treatment. These considerations impel the authors toward a general choice of antithyroid drug therapy in the younger age group.

This overall recommendation is modified by several factors, however. Many patients urgently wish to be freed of the manifestations of their disease as quickly as possible. Here surgery is advised if the patient persists in this desire after the relative risks of surgery have been explained. Surgery is also recommended in the young adult who, because of lack of compliance or other personal factors, is unwilling or unable to take medication or to be examined regularly. Such patients should be hospitalized until surgery has been performed, since they may avoid treatment altogether if left to their own devices. Surgery is also the treatment of choice for the young adult who has reacted adversely to both propylthiouracil and methimazole. Subtotal thyroidectomy is usually performed in young adults with severe disease or very large goiters (often accompanied by loud bruits), since in the experience of the authors and others these patients are less likely to experience a prolonged remission following withdrawal of antithyroid therapy. Surgery is also strongly considered for thyrotoxicosis that recurs after a single course of antithyroid therapy, and in this age group it will be recommended if two or more recurrences have taken place. The foregoing indications for surgical therapy in young adults are overruled, however, if a previous subtotal thyroidectomy has been performed, since the frequency of complications following secondary thyroid surgery is greatly increased. Finally, in the occasional young adult, it becomes necessary to remove a diffuse toxic goiter because of obstructive symptoms or cosmetic disfigurement.

These recommendations represent the general guidelines that the authors employ in selecting the mode of therapy in patients with diffuse toxic goiter. In view of the several approaches to treatment available, each with its advantages and disadvantages, it is incumbent upon the physician to explain these factors to the patient thoroughly, to indicate his or her own preference and the reasons for it, and to allow the final choice to rest with the patient.

Treatment of Infiltrative Ophthalmopathy and Infiltrative Dermopathy

Infiltrative ophthalmopathy varies in severity from a mild form, which is common, to a severe form that may threaten the vision and even the life of the patient. Fortunately the latter form is rare, since it presents difficult problems in the selection among and timing of many suggested modes of treatment. The variety of treatments that have been proposed and the continuing, often heated, discussion of their relative efficacy bespeak the general inadequacy of all, the most effective being merely palliative. The natural course of the disorder, which is highly variable and characterized by unaccountable exacerbations and remissions, makes conclusions about the efficacy of most treatments difficult or even dubious. This is all the more the case since the number of patients afflicted with the severe form is relatively small and since the severity of this form makes controlled studies difficult to perform. A further source of confusion is the variable terminology for describing the manifestations of ophthalmopathy and the lack of rigid criteria for defining

their severity. General use of the American Thyroid Association classification that defines these variables is therefore strongly recommended (see Table 4–9).

The first question that arises is the effect that various forms of treatment for thyrotoxicosis may have on the course of the ophthalmopathy. Although opinions vary widely, it does not appear that subtotal thyroidectomy, radioiodine therapy, or antithyroid therapy in themselves significantly influence the course of the ophthalmopathy except as they may lead to the development of hypothyroidism. Almost all would agree that hypothyroidism has an adverse effect upon the disorder and should be avoided. When hypothyroidism occurs it should be treated fully, but there is no evidence that exogenous thyroid hormone in the absence of hypothyroidism favorably influences the ophthalmopathy. Similarly, no evidence exists for a favorable action of iodine, once widely used. Indeed, in patients with Graves' disease, especially those treated with radioiodine, this agent may actually induce a hypothyroid state (iodide myxedema).

The measures used in treatment can be divided into those that are largely symptomatic (useful mainly in the mild form) and those that attempt to arrest or reverse the progression of the disorder, either by an attack on its presumed pathogenesis or by mechanical means. In milder forms of the disorder, little treatment is required. The patient who experiences photophobia and sensitivity to wind or cold air is benefited by wearing dark glasses, which also afford protection from foreign bodies. Elevation of the head of the bed at night and instillation of lubricants, such as 1% methylcellulose, may benefit the patient whose lids do not appose completely during sleep. Mild or moderate infiltrative changes may also be benefited by restriction of salt intake and administration of diuretics. Since the ophthalmic manifestations tend to be self-limited and the progression to a more severe form uncommon, such measures usually suffice to tide the patient over until the disorder regresses spontaneously.

The appearance of increasing proptosis, with increasing inability to appose the lids, or of such severe infiltrative manifestations as chemosis, indicates progression of the disorder and warrants the use of more vigorous therapeutic measures. In this stage of the disorder, when the condition is serious but not desperate, several methods of treatment have been proposed. It is in relation to the efficacy of these that the greatest doubt exists. Changes of this type, even when severe, may respond favorably and rapidly to the administration of prednisone in massive doses (120–140 mg daily). If improvement occurs, the daily dose is decreased to the lowest level at which improvement is maintained. The latter is still likely to be large, but it is hoped that a halt to the progression or actual regression of the disease will occur before untoward effects make withdrawal of the drug necessary. In an attempt to circumvent the inevitable side effects of large doses of glucocorticoids given systemically, periodic injection of depot preparations of glucocorticoids given subconjunctivally or into the retro-orbital space have been advocated. Such treatment may have a dramatic effect on irritative symptoms as well as on diplopia, but its efficacy varies, and mild systemic effects of the glucocorticoids are sometimes seen. Moreover, this treatment entails the risk of puncture of the globe or a retro-orbital hematoma.

As an alternative to glucocorticoid therapy, external radiation to the orbits or to the pituitary has been employed. The value of such treatment is not definitely established, since reported results have been variable. More recently, highly collimated supervoltage radiation of the retro-orbital space has been applied, with seemingly rapid and beneficial effects upon infiltrative and inflammatory manifestations (Donaldson et al., 1973). Relatively few patients have been treated, however, and this mode of therapy requires further evaluation.

On the basis of available evidence, there appears to be no merit to the suggestion that infiltrative ophthalmopathy is benefited or its progression retarded by total ablation of the thyroid, whether performed surgically or by radioiodine or by a combination of the two.

In view of the foregoing considerations, the authors recommend a trial of oral glucocorticoid therapy for patients with severe or progressive ophthalmopathy. If effective doses cannot be tolerated, a course of external radiation may be attempted. Local measures should be employed, along with these major forms of treatment. Ulceration and infection of the cornea should be treated with antibiotics, lubricants, and protective shields. An attempt to appose the lids by means of sutures (tarsorrhaphy) is often ineffective, as the sutures may tear out and result in scarring.

If glucocorticoid therapy and external radiation fail to halt progression of the disease, and if loss of vision is threatened either by ulceration or infection of the cornea or by changes in the retina or optic nerve, orbital decompression is performed. Classically this has involved removal of either the lateral wall or the roof of the orbit. More recently, good results have been reported with the transantral approach, in which the lateral wall of the ethmoid sinus and the roof of the maxillary sinus are removed (Ogura et al., 1971).

The management of the patient with severe ophthalmopathy should never be undertaken by the internist or endocrinologist or by the ophthalmologist acting alone. Close and coordinated observation with respect to the effects of medical therapy and the progress of the disease is necessary to determine whether and when the surgical approach to treatment, which almost invariably halts the progress of the disease and preserves vision if performed in time, should be employed.

Treatment of infiltrative dermopathy is seldom necessary. However, if this manifestation is severe, a topical glucocorticoid preparation along with an occlusive dressing will produce regression of the lesion.

Toxic Multinodular Goiter

Toxic multinodular goiter is a disorder in which hyperthyroidism arises in a multinodular goiter, usually of long standing. It is uncertain whether it represents one disease or whether it is the clinical expression of one of several pathogenetic factors. The authors feel it important to avoid the term "toxic nodular goiter," since this term encompasses both toxic multinodular goiter, as here described, and toxic adenoma of the thyroid gland, which will be discussed in a succeeding section.

Pathogenesis and Histopathology

The pathogenesis of toxic multinodular goiter cannot be considered apart from the clinical history of patients with this disorder or from the patterns of thyroid function with which it is associated. Here a nontoxic multinodular goiter, usually of long standing, invariably antedates development of hyperthyroidism. It is presumed that the pathogenesis and histopathology of the preexisting nontoxic goiter are those described in the later section dealing with this disorder. Recent work has shown that in general patients with nontoxic multinodular goiter have lower plasma TSH concentrations than patients with diffuse nontoxic goiter or

patients without goiter do (Toft et al., 1976a). Moreover, as many as one-quarter of patients with multinodular goiter whose serum T_4 and T_3 concentrations are within the normal range display a subnormal or absent TSH response to TRH (Gemsenjager et al., 1976; Dige-Petersen and Hummer, 1977). These observations suggest that functional autonomy develops in the evolution of multinodular goiter. Finally, in both endemic and sporadic nontoxic multinodular goiter, administration of iodine may lead to the development of thyrotoxicosis (Jod-Basedow phenomenon), implying that the potential for hyperfunction exists in areas of functional autonomy. What causes the preexisting nontoxic goiter to lose its normal homeostatic regulation, thereby making possible the development of hyperthyroidism, is unknown. The patterns of function displayed by toxic multinodular goiters, however, suggest that either of two mechanisms is responsible. In radioautographs and in scintiscans, two basic patterns are discernible. The first is a diffuse but somewhat uneven localization of radioisotope that is not appreciably altered by the administration of either TSH or exogenous thyroid hormone. Histopathologic examination reveals multiple aggregates of small follicles with hyperplastic epithelium, interspersed with variably sized nodules composed of large follicles that appear inactive and accumulate little radioiodine. The latter may represent the nodular areas of the preexisting nontoxic goiter. The functional characteristics suggest that, in this type of toxic multinodular goiter, all areas capable of functioning are functioning, and none is dependent upon TSH. Whether this autonomous function originates in the thyroid gland itself or is due to an external stimulator is not known. Studies in a small number of patients with toxic multinodular goiter have failed to demonstrate the presence in plasma of TBII (O'Donnell et al., 1978; Strakosch et al., 1978).

What appears to be the second type of toxic multinodular goiter is also distinguished by its functional pattern. Here radioiodine becomes localized in one or more discrete nodules, while iodine accumulation in the remainder of the gland is suppressed. No further suppression is produced by exogenous thyroid hormone, but TSH stimulates accumulation of iodine in the areas previously inactive. Histopathologically, the functioning areas resemble adenomas in being reasonably well demarcated from surrounding tissue. They generally consist of large follicles, sometimes with hyperplastic epithelium, but the correlation of architecture with functional state is not good. The remaining tissue appears inactive, and zones of degeneration are present in both functioning and nonfunctioning areas. These findings suggest that areas that are functioning can do so without TSH and may therefore be termed areas of "adenomatous hyperfunction." The remaining areas, in contrast, retain their dependency upon TSH, their function being suppressed as a consequence of hyperfunction in the autonomous zones. It is most unlikely that function in this type of gland is sustained by an external stimulator of normal or abnormal origin. Hence, from the pathophysiologic standpoint, this disorder resembles most closely the normal thyroid that harbors a solitary hyperfunctioning adenoma. Whether the hyperfunctioning areas represent true adenomas in a biologic sense is unknown.

Pathophysiology

Little careful work has been done to correlate other aspects of the pathophysiology of toxic multinodular goiter with the patterns of function that have been described. The major finding of certainty is the disruption of homeostatic regulation, regardless of its origin, that is evident in the failure of thyroid function to be suppressed by exogenous thyroid hormone. Several lines of evidence indicate that the extent of overproduction of thyroid hormone in toxic multinodular goiter is usually mild relative to that which occurs in classic Graves' disease. First, the clinical manifestations of thyrotoxicosis are rarely flagrant. Second, the serum T_4 and T_3 concentrations are often only marginally increased. Finally, the RAIU is not greatly increased and may even be within the normal range. The relative mildness of the hyperthyroidism is not inconsistent with either of its presumed pathogenetic origins. The effectiveness of any stimulus to hyperfunction may well be blunted in a thyroid that is the seat of a preexisting nontoxic goiter, since the latter disorder results from some inherent impairment in the efficiency of the gland with respect to hormone synthesis; this explanation is of course speculative.

Clinical Picture

Toxic multinodular goiter is a common complication of its nontoxic precursor, but its precise incidence in the latter disorder is unknown. It usually occurs after the age of 50 in patients who have had multinodular goiter for many years. Like its forerunner, it is many times more common in women than in men. Toxic multinodular goiter is almost never accompanied by infiltrative ophthalmopathy, but when it is, it doubtless represents the emergence of frank Graves' disease.

The clinical manifestations of thyrotoxicosis in toxic multinodular goiter tend to differ in predominance from those in the diffuse toxic goiter of Graves' disease. Cardiovascular manifestations tend to predominate, possibly because of the age of the patient. These may include atrial fibrillation or tachycardia, with or without heart failure. Frequently, a decreased response to digitalis first alerts the physician to the presence of thyrotoxicosis. Weakness and wasting of muscles are common. The nervous manifestations are less prominent than in the younger patient with thyrotoxicosis, but emotional lability may be pronounced. Because of the physical characteristics of the thyroid gland as well as its not infrequent retrosternal extension, obstructive symptoms are more common than in diffuse toxic goiter. On palpation, the characteristics of the goiter are the same as those of the more common nontoxic multinodular goiter discussed later. In as many as 20% of elderly patients with thyrotoxicosis, the thyroid gland is firm and irregular, but not palpably enlarged.

Laboratory Tests and Differential Diagnosis

The main clinical problem is to determine whether the patient with a multinodular goiter is thyrotoxic. Laboratory tests may or may not be of assistance in this regard. The RAIU may be of little value unless distinctly elevated, because thyrotoxicosis may exist in association with values that are normal or only slightly increased. Difficulty also arises from the fact that slight increases in the RAIU are seen in some patients with nontoxic multinodular goiter. Similar difficulties arise in connection with the serum T_4 concentration; often thyrotoxicosis is present in association with values that are only slightly increased or at the upper limit of normal. A value for the serum T_3 concentration that is at the upper limit of the usual normal range is highly suggestive of hyperthyroidism in the elderly, however, since the serum T_3 concentration usually decreases with advanc-

ing age. The thyroid suppression test may be of value, but should not be performed in the elderly patient or the patient with overt heart disease. It is in these situations that the TRH stimulation test has its greatest usefulness. A subnormal or absent response does not necessarily indicate the presence of hyperthyroidism, but suggests that production of thyroid hormone is at least equal to physiologic requirements, and that a trial of antithyroid therapy would be justified.

Treatment

Radioiodine appears to be the treatment of choice for the majority of patients with toxic multinodular goiter, despite the fact that there is considerable disagreement among the various clinics concerning the magnitude and number of doses required to achieve a therapeutic response. In general, the experience along the eastern seaboard of the United States indicates that the responsiveness to radioiodine of toxic multinodular goiter differs little from that of diffuse toxic goiter. On the other hand, in areas where goiter tends to be endemic, such as the Great Lakes area of the United States, toxic multinodular goiter is said to be very resistant to radioiodine. Although no correlative studies necessary to support this hypothesis have been reported, it might be suggested that the type that readily responds to radioiodine is that which resembles diffuse toxic goiter in displaying a relatively diffuse accumulation of iodine. The more resistant variety, on the other hand, may be that associated with adenomatous hyperfunction, in which focal accumulation of radioiodine occurs; here, tissue previously suppressed may regain function and ultimately achieve autonomy after the hyperactive tissue has been destroyed.

Because of the age of the patient and variations in sensitivity to radioiodine, the small-dose regimen that has been recommended by some clinics for the treatment of diffuse toxic goiter is not recommended for the treatment of toxic multinodular goiter. Instead, conventional doses should be administered. In any event, these are likely to be larger than those used in diffuse toxic goiter, because the percentage uptake of ^{131}I tends to be lower and the size of the gland greater. Many patients with this disorder have underlying heart disease. Therefore, it is recommended that the administration of radioiodine be preceded by a course of antithyroid therapy until a eumetabolic state is achieved. Medication is then discontinued for 3–5 days before radioiodine is administered. Several days thereafter, the antithyroid drug is reinstituted so that control of thyrotoxicosis is maintained until radioiodine exerts its effect. After 6–8 weeks, the antithyroid drug is gradually withdrawn, and if thyrotoxicosis recurs, a second course of therapy should be given. Surgical therapy is recommended after adequate preoperative preparation in patients in whom obstructive manifestations are present or in whom it is feared that such manifestations may result from the temporary enlargement of the thyroid that radioiodine sometimes produces.

Toxic Adenoma

A third and far less common form of hyperthyroidism is that sometimes produced by one or more autonomous adenomas of the thyroid gland. As herein employed, the term refers to adenomas present in a thyroid that is otherwise intrinsically normal, differentiating this lesion from areas of adenomatous hyperfunction within a toxic multinodular goiter. The disorder is usually caused by a single adenoma that is palpable as a solitary nodule and hence is sometimes referred to as "hyperfunctioning solitary nodule" or "toxic nodule." Occasionally, two or three adenomas of similar character are present.

Pathogenesis, Histopathology, and Pathophysiology

Toxic adenomas are true follicular adenomas of the thyroid gland (for histopathologic characteristics see section dealing with thyroid neoplasms); hence, their basic pathogenesis is unknown.

By definition, the adenoma is capable of functioning without stimulation by TSH, and assays reveal no abnormal thyroid stimulators in the blood (Strakosch et al., 1978). The natural course of the lesion is one of slow, progressive growth and increasing function evolving over many years. At first, it may be present as a small nodule or may be impalpable, but in either case, it may be detectable in the scintiscan as a localized area of increased radioiodine accumulation. Upon the administration of exogenous thyroid hormone the function of the remainder of the gland is suppressed, but function in the adenoma persists. Later, with further growth, a progressively increasing share of glandular function is assumed by the adenoma, with the result that the remaining tissue is increasingly suppressed. Ultimately, atrophy and complete suppression of the remainder of the gland occur, and the scintiscan reveals function only in the adenoma ("hot" nodule) (see Fig. 4–20). Although it is likely that continued growth of the adenoma is associated with secretion of excessive quantities of hormone, some time may pass before overt thyrotoxicosis is manifest. The extranodular tissue generally retains its capacity to function if TSH is provided, either by exogenous administration or as a result of ablation of the nodule. Some adenomas of this type secrete T_3 predominantly, and some, in addition to the normal thyroid hormones, secrete an iodinated protein that is measurable as protein-bound iodine (PBI), leading to a disproportionate elevation of the latter relative to T_4-iodine. Adenomas of this type not infrequently undergo infarction, changing from hyperfunctioning to hypofunctioning nodules; associated thyrotoxicosis may be relieved.

Clinical Picture

Toxic adenoma occurs in a younger age group than does toxic multinodular goiter, often being seen in patients in their thirties or forties. Frequently, a history of a long-standing, slowly growing lump in the neck is obtained. Rarely does the lesion develop sufficient function to produce thyrotoxicosis until it has achieved a diameter of 2.5–3 cm. Not infrequently, the lesion may undergo central necrosis and hemorrhage; as a result, the thyrotoxicosis may be relieved, the remainder of the thyroid may resume its function, and the adenoma may appear on the scintiscan as a cold area, suggesting a thyroid carcinoma. Calcification in the area of hemorrhage may take place and be evident on x-ray examination.

The peripheral manifestations of toxic adenoma are generally milder than those of diffuse toxic goiter and are notable for the absence of infiltrative ophthalmopathy and myopathy; cardiovascular manifestations, however, may be prominent. On examination, the nodule is usually felt as a smooth, well-defined, round or ovoid mass that is firm and moves freely on swallowing. Often, the remainder of the gland is not palpable. A bruit is never present.

Laboratory Tests

The results of laboratory tests depend upon the stage of the disorder. At first, laboratory indices are normal, except that the RAIU cannot be completely suppressed with exogenous thyroid hormone; the function that remains during suppression is localized in the adenoma, as shown by the scintiscan (Fig. 4–20). Later, suppressibility is lost as function is confined to the adenoma, but clear evidence of hyperfunction is lacking. At this stage, an increase in the RAIU may be found, but the serum T_4 and T_3 concentrations, as well as metabolic indices, will usually be normal. At this point, in view of the suppression of extranodular function, an absent response to TRH administration would be expected. When thyrotoxicosis supervenes, the RAIU is more greatly increased, the serum T_4 and T_3 concentrations are increased, and the metabolic indices are consistent with thyrotoxicosis. The degree of thyroid hyperfunction may not be accurately reflected by measurement of the RAIU. Measurement of the uptake at an earlier period, e.g., at 4 hours, frequently reveals a relatively greater increase in the uptake at this time. Occasionally, values for serum T_4 concentration are normal, and the serum T_3 concentration alone is increased (T_3-toxicosis). In this event, the RAIU may be normal. Relative to its overall rate of occurrence, toxic adenoma is the most frequent cause of T_3-toxicosis.

Treatment

The hyperfunctioning adenoma that has suppressed the remainder of the thyroid gland should be treated with ablative therapy, regardless of whether or not the patient is overtly thyrotoxic, since the likelihood of eventual thyrotoxicosis is high. Although the lesion may seem especially amenable to treatment with radioiodine because of the highly localized accumulation of iodine, the authors prefer excision of the adenoma unless surgery is contraindicated. Radioiodine frequently fails to eliminate the nodule entirely, whereas surgery in essence cures the disease. Furthermore, rare cases of hyperfunctioning thyroid carcinomas have been reported (Sung and Cavalieri, 1973). Before surgery, exogenous TSH should be administered in order that the scintiscan may verify the functional capability of the extranodular tissue; almost invariably, potential function is present. The rare instance in which the extranodular tissue is unresponsive to TSH may be analogous to the unresponsiveness sometimes found in long-standing hypopituitarism. In patients with this finding, replacement therapy with thyroid hormone will probably be required postoperatively, but in the great majority of patients, normal function will be reestablished in the residual tissue after the adenoma has been removed.

The thyroid that is the seat of a toxic adenoma is not diffusely hypervascular, and hence preoperative preparation with iodine is not required, but in the patient with overt thyrotoxicosis, restoration to a normal metabolic state with an antithyroid drug before surgery is desirable.

Hyperthyroidism in Trophoblastic Disease

Thyroid hyperfunction often accompanies hydatidiform mole, choriocarcinoma, or metastatic embryonal carcinoma of the testis. Such neoplasms, particularly hydatidiform mole, elaborate a thyroid stimulator that is distinct from pituitary TSH and that appears not to be hCG itself (Amir et al., 1980). Although some patients present with clinically overt thyrotoxicosis, in the majority clinical manifestations are not prominent and goiter is usually absent, despite frequent laboratory evidence of a severe hyperthyroid state (Miyai et al., 1976; Nagataki et al., 1977). The findings include an increased RAIU, increased serum total and free T_4 and T_3 concentrations, and abolition of the TSH response to TRH. The reason for this discordance between the clinical and laboratory indices is not known, but may be the relatively short duration of the thyroid hormone excess.

The possibility of a molar pregnancy should always be considered in a young woman with thyrotoxicosis, since the appropriate therapy would be evacuation of the uterus.

Hypersecretion of TSH

Rarely, hyperthyroidism results from hypersecretion of TSH. In most of the reported cases, a pituitary adenoma has been demonstrated and, in some, shown to be the probable source of TSH. Four additional patients have been reported in whom thyrotoxicosis with increased serum TSH concentration was not accompanied by evidence of a pituitary adenoma. In three of the patients, the serum TSH concentration responded in a qualitatively normal fashion to TRH and to exogenous thyroid hormone, but in the fourth no significant responses could be elicited. It was suggested that in the former instances the hypersecretion of TSH was the result of a higher than normal setting of the threshold for feedback control and that, in the latter instance, excessive TRH secretion was responsible. (See Tolis et al., 1978, for a review of TSH-secreting pituitary adenoma, and Novogroder et al., 1977, for a discussion of nonadenomatous hypersecretion of TSH.)

Iodine-Induced Hyperthyroidism

It has long been known that the administration of supplemental iodine to subjects with endemic iodine-deficiency goiter can result in overproduction of thyroid hormone. Although precise data are not available, experience in many areas of the world indicates that this response, termed iodine-induced hyperthyroidism or Jod-Basedow, occurs in only a small fraction of individuals at risk. The most recent and best studied experience with Jod-Basedow of this type emanates from Tasmania, where a pronounced, but temporary, increase in patients reporting for treatment of thyrotoxicosis followed shortly after the addition of small quantities of iodine to bread as a means of correcting iodine deficiency. Studies among the group thus affected revealed two major patterns of underlying thyroid disorder. In the first, especially common in older individuals, nodular goiter with areas of autonomous function were present and abnormal thyroid stimulators akin to those found in Graves' disease were not detectable in the blood. The second pattern typically occurred in younger individuals with diffuse goiter, and here thyroid-stimulating immunoglobulins were often present in the blood. These findings would indicate, as would be expected, that Jod-Basedow would occur only in those thyroid glands in which function was significantly independent of TSH stimulation. The occurrence of Jod-Basedow should not be construed as a reason for failing to treat endemic iodine deficiency. Apart from the many other benefits which accrue from the treatment and prophylaxis, it is certain that, over the long run, the frequency of spontaneous hyperthyroidism associated with the development of autonomous nodules is diminished.

Iodine-induced hyperthyroidism is an important disorder in areas of the world in which dietary iodine intake is quite sufficient. (For a review of iodine-induced hyperthyroidism, see Braverman, 1978.) In regions in which iodine intake is marginal but overt iodine deficiency is absent, moderate increments in iodine intake may induce hyperthyroidism in patients with autonomous thyroid nodules, and large pharmacologic doses of iodine, such as are employed in the treatment of pulmonary disease, can do so in geographic areas in which the iodine intake is more than adequate. Consequently, the physician must be alert to the possibility of inducing hyperthyroidism when large quantities of iodine are administered to patients with nodular goiter in the form of expectorants, x-ray contrast media, medications containing iodine, or in any other form. Since nodular goiter is generally a disease of the older population, induction of the Jod-Basedow phenomenon may have serious consequences, particularly since enrichment of the thyroid with iodine forestalls administration of ^{131}I and delays the response to antithyroid agents.

Jod-Basedow should be suspected in any patient with nodular goiter in whom hyperthyroidism has developed after known or suspected exposure to large quantities of iodine. In such patients, the serum T_3 concentration is sometimes normal, although the total and free T_4 concentrations are increased. Confirmation that the patient has been exposed to large quantities of iodine can be obtained by demonstrating that the RAIU is low and the urinary iodine excretion greatly increased (more than several milligrams per day).

Although physiological reasoning would dictate that the Jod-Basedow phenomenon could occur only when the thyroid is free of normal regulatory control, a number of patients with iodine-induced hyperthyroidism have been reported in whom thyroid function was normal, and normally suppressible, after iodine was withdrawn and a euthyroid state restored.

Thyrotoxicosis Without Hyperthyroidism

Several disorders are associated with thyrotoxicosis, i.e., with the manifestations of an excess of thyroid hormone at the level of the peripheral tissues, but without hyperthyroidism, i.e., ongoing overproduction of thyroid hormone. These disorders fall into two general categories: those in which the excess of hormone originates outside of the thyroid gland, as in thyrotoxicosis factitia and in ectopic hyperfunctioning thyroid tissue; and those in which inflammatory disease of the thyroid leads to loss of storage function and leakage of hormone into the blood, as in subacute thyroiditis and painless or silent thyroiditis. These disorders are recognized in part by the presence of low values of the RAIU, owing to suppression of TSH secretion, inflammatory injury to the gland, or a combination of the two.

Recognition of these forms of thyrotoxicosis is extremely important, since their treatment differs almost entirely from the treatment of those kinds of thyrotoxicosis associated with true thyroid hyperfunction.

Thyrotoxicosis Factitia

This term designates thyrotoxicosis that arises from the ingestion, usually chronic, of excessive quantities of thyroid hormone rather than from overactivity of the thyroid gland and is therefore an example of thyrotoxicosis without hyperthyroidism. The disorder usually occurs in women, often those with a background of underlying psychiatric disease, and especially in paramedical personnel who have access to thyroid hormone or in patients for whom thyroid hormone medication has been prescribed in the past. Generally, the patient is aware that she is taking thyroid hormone but may adamantly deny this to be the case. In other instances, large doses of thyroid hormone or other thyroactive material, such as iodocasein, may be given to the patient without her knowing their nature, usually as part of a regimen for weight reduction.

Symptoms are those typical of thyrotoxicosis and may be severe. In the absence of preexisting disease of the thyroid, diagnosis is made from the combination of typical thyrotoxic manifestations, together with thyroid atrophy and hypofunction. Infiltrative ophthalmopathy never occurs, but lid lag, stare, and other "thyrotoxic" eye signs may be present. Hypofunction of the thyroid gland is evidenced by subnormal values for the RAIU which can be increased by the administration of TSH. Values for the serum T_4 concentration are increased unless the patient is taking T_3, in which case they will be subnormal. Serum T_3 concentrations are increased in either case. Low, rather than elevated, values of the serum thyroglobulin concentration suggest that thyrotoxicosis results from exogenous hormone, rather than thyroid hyperfunction.

This disorder may be confused with other varieties of thyrotoxicosis associated with a subnormal RAIU and absence of goiter. These include the syndrome of chronic thyroiditis with transient thyrotoxicosis (also termed painless thyroiditis or "hyperthyroiditis") in which goiter may be lacking; ectopic thyroid tissue; and hyperfunctioning metastatic follicular carcinoma. Strong evidence for the two latter disorders can be obtained by the demonstration of low values for the sum of thyroid and urinary ^{131}I after a tracer dose and by localization of the ectopic focus or foci by external scintiscanning. Differentiation from painless thyroiditis may be very difficult. The presence of circulating antithyroid antibodies would point to painless chronic thyroiditis, while a nodular thyroid and a grossly elevated erythrocyte sedimentation rate would suggest the painless variant of subacute thyroiditis.

Treatment consists of withdrawing the offending medication. Psychotherapy may be desirable in certain instances.

Ectopic Thyroid Tissue

Thyroid tissue is not infrequently present in teratomas, especially in the ovary (struma ovarii), and such foci may produce thyrotoxicosis. Rarely, hyperfunctioning metastases of follicular carcinoma can produce thyrotoxicosis. The distinguishing features of such lesions are discussed in the section dealing with thyrotoxicosis factitia.

Silent or Painless Thyroiditis ("Hyperthyroiditis")

In a later section it is noted that thyrotoxicosis is associated with the early phase of subacute or giant-cell thyroiditis, in both its common painful and its far less common painless variants. Recently, attention has been drawn to the association of thyrotoxicosis associated with a painlesss form of thyroiditis in which biopsy of the thyroid reveals the histopathologic changes of lymphocytic thyroiditis rather than those of subacute thyroiditis (Gorman et al., 1978). This syndrome has variously been alluded to as silent or painless thyroiditis with thyrotoxicosis or as "hyperthyroiditis." This terminology is unfortunate, since it does not clearly distinguish the syndrome from the painless variant of subacute thyroiditis. A better name for the syndrome might be chronic thyroiditis with transient thyrotoxicosis.

As in subacute thyroiditis, the thyrotoxicosis in this syndrome is due to release of preformed hormone consequent to the disruption of follicular architecture and resolves spontaneously within 1 to 4 months. The thyroid gland may or may not be enlarged and is not tender to palpation. Laboratory indices include a very low value for RAIU and increased values for the serum T_4 and T_3 concentrations. Low titers of antithyroid antibodies may be present in the plasma, and these may persist after the thyrotoxicosis has resolved. The erythrocyte sedimentation rate is normal or only slightly increased, unlike the distinctly increased values that are commonly seen in subacute thyroiditis. Transition to a euthyroid state may involve passage through a phase of transient hypothyroidism, but permanent hypothyroidism is an uncommon sequel, at least for the period of time over which the natural history of this disorder has been observed.

Painless thyroiditis is not a rare disorder; in a recent series it accounted for 15% of the newly diagnosed cases of thyrotoxicosis in 1 year (Dorfman et al., 1977). Consequently, it is important to consider this disorder in any patient with thyrotoxicosis since antithyroid drug therapy and thyroid ablation by surgery or radioiodine are contraindicated. Rather, symptoms are ameliorated through the use of propranolol until the thyrotoxicosis regresses. Measurement of the RAIU will afford the necessary distinction, as will the subsequent course of the disease. Occasionally, thyrotoxic Graves' disease associated with a greatly expanded stable iodide pool or iodine-induced thyrotoxicosis may mimic painless thyroiditis from the laboratory standpoint, but urinary stable iodine excretion will be increased. Finally, when painless thyroiditis is not accompanied by goiter, thyrotoxicosis factitia must be considered.

Special Aspects of Thyrotoxicosis

T_3-Toxicosis

Concurrent measurements of T_4 and T_3 production rates have revealed a disproportionate increase in T_3 production in the majority of patients with spontaneous hyperthyroidism. Whether this phenomenon results solely from the preferential increase in the thyroid secretion of T_3 or whether there is in addition a disproportionate increase in the peripheral conversion of T_4 to T_3 is uncertain. In the extreme case, the production rate of T_3 alone is increased; the thyrotoxic state resulting therefrom has been designated T_3-toxicosis. In some patients, T_3-toxicosis may be the forerunner of the usual form of thyrotoxicosis in which both T_3 and T_4 production are increased, whereas in other patients it may persist as such. T_3-toxicosis may occur in association with Graves' disease, toxic multinodular goiter, or toxic adenoma. Its true prevalence is not known. In the authors' experience, it tends to be more common in the elderly population; consequently, in this age group especially, reliance should not be placed solely on the serum T_4 concentration to exclude the presence of thyrotoxicosis.

The diagnosis of T_3-toxicosis should be suspected in a patient with clinical manifestations of thyrotoxicosis in whom the serum T_4 concentration and free T_4 concentration or index are normal or decreased while the serum T_3 concentration and free T_3 index are increased. The frequently palpable goiter and normal or increased RAIU will exclude the presence of thyrotoxicosis factitia induced by ingestion of T_3. Preliminary experience suggests that patients with T_3-

toxicosis are more likely to enjoy a long-term remission following withdrawal of antithyroid drug therapy than patients with the usual form of thyrotoxicosis, in which production of both T_4 and T_3 is increased.

T_4-Toxicosis

Very recently, attention has been drawn to the entity termed T_4-toxicosis, i.e., thyrotoxicosis with an increased serum T_4 concentration and free T_4 concentration or index, but with a normal or decreased serum T_3 concentration. This phenomenon has been reported to occur in two circumstances. The one circumstance is that of iodine-induced thyrotoxicosis (Jod-Basedow phenomenon), discussed earlier. Here, as many as one-third of the patients will display a normal serum T_3 concentration and the remainder will display proportionate elevations of the serum T_3 and T_4 concentrations (Sobrinho et al., 1977). The presumption is that the availability to autonomous foci of abundant quantities of iodide will lead to increased production of both T_4 and T_3, but in the proportions in which they are normally synthesized. The second circumstance in which T_4-toxicosis may be seen is that of thyrotoxicosis accompanied by severe intercurrent illness. Here, that component of the serum T_3 usually contributed by peripheral T_3-neogenesis is decreased or lacking so that serum T_3 concentration, now sustained mainly or entirely by direct thyroid secretion, is normal or low, though the serum T_4 concentration is high. Concomitantly, serum rT_3 concentration is increased, often very markedly, owing to inhibition of its 5'-monodeiodination. With recovery from the intercurrent illness, serum rT_3 concentration declines and serum T_3 concentration increases into the thyrotoxic range (Engler et al., 1978). T_4-toxicosis of this type is to be differentiated from the elevation of serum T_4 concentration, with a low serum T_3 concentration, that occasionally occurs in the course of intercurrent illness in patients who are intrinsically euthyroid. Elevated values of the RAIU or diminished responsiveness to TRH may serve to distinguish those patients who are intrinsically hyperthyroid from those who are not.

Thyrotoxicosis in Childhood and Adolescence

Thyrotoxicosis in childhood and adolescence is almost always the result of Graves' disease. Although thyrotoxicosis in this age group makes up only a small proportion of all cases, it is worthy of special consideration because treatment is less satisfactory than it is in adults. Hence there is more uncertainty and greater disagreement concerning its optimal management. (For an excellent discussion of neonatal and childhood thyrotoxicosis, see Hayles, 1972.) Several factors weigh against the use of radioiodine in children. First, the enhanced carcinogenic potential of radiation in the thyroid gland of the infant or child seems clearly established by the very high correlation between childhood thyroid carcinoma and a history of x-ray therapy to the neck or chest in childhood (Favus et al., 1976). Second, among all patients with thyrotoxicosis, fear of transmissible genetic damage is most cogent among those treated in childhood or adolescence, although recent data suggest that this may not be significant (Safa et al., 1975). Finally, the authors consider postradioiodine hypothyroidism to be a particularly undesirable complication in children, since inadequate or interrupted therapy can have profound effects on growth and development and on scholastic performance. For these reasons, it is felt that radioiodine should not be used in the treatment of childhood thyrotoxicosis.

The choice between surgical and antithyroid therapy is a difficult one. The data indicate a lower frequency of long-term remission following antithyroid therapy than is the case in adults, although some believe that thyrotoxicosis often undergoes remission after adolescence. On the other hand, most surgical series reveal a relatively high frequency of postoperative hypothyroidism, which is no more desirable after surgery than after radioiodine administration. Recurrences are also more frequent, presumably as a result of attempts to avoid hypothyroidism. Furthermore, the occasional operative death seems more tragic in a child than in an adult, and such complications as hypoparathyroidism and recurrent laryngeal nerve damage need to be borne over a longer life span. On the basis of these considerations, the authors favor the use of antithyroid therapy and recommend a course of 1–2 years' duration. Supplemental thyroid hormone therapy is desirable, since it forestalls the possibility of therapeutic hypothyroidism and has no adverse side effects. In contrast to the recommendation in young adults, a second course of antithyroid therapy is regularly employed if recrudescence or relapse occurs after the first course. If sustained remission does not follow a second course of therapy and, particularly, if the patient has passed through adolescence during this period, surgery may be considered.

Thyrotoxicosis in Pregnancy

Thyrotoxicosis occurring during pregnancy is almost always due to Graves' disease. Difficulty in conception and fetal wastage are increased in women with thyrotoxicosis. Nevertheless, an occasional patient will become pregnant despite antecedent untreated hyperthyroidism. More commonly, a woman being treated for thyrotoxicosis will become pregnant, or hyperthyroidism will appear after pregnancy is under way. Whatever the sequence, the concurrence of thyrotoxicosis and pregnancy presents features of special concern from both the diagnostic and therapeutic standpoints.

Pregnancy and hyperthyroidism have many features in common. Both are accompanied by thyroid enlargement, manifestations of a hyperdynamic circulation, and hypermetabolism. Amenorrhea may occur in thyrotoxicosis not associated with pregnancy. In the two conditions, the serum T_4 and T_3 concentrations are increased, as is the RAIU, though radioiodine is not wittingly administered to pregnant women. Laboratory tests useful in this differentiation are measurements of the proportion of free T_4 in serum or in vitro uptake tests. These reflect the increased hormone binding in plasma in pregnancy and the decreased binding in thyrotoxicosis. A positive pregnancy test will complete the diagnostic differentiation. A more difficult diagnostic problem is whether or not a pregnant woman is mildly thyrotoxic. Increases in serum T_4 concentration above 12 μg/100 ml and failure of in vitro uptake tests to display their usual subnormal values, resulting in calculated values for the free T_4 index that are above the normal range are in accord with a diagnosis of thyrotoxicosis. In the borderline case, the TRH test will be helpful, since only slight increases in the quantity of hormone available to the tissues result in a decreased or absent response to TRH.

An even greater problem is posed by the management of thyrotoxicosis during pregnancy. Surgery during the last trimester and probably during the first trimester as well appears to be contraindicated because of the likelihood of inducing premature labor. Although surgery may be successful during the middle trimester, it is best to avoid any major surgical procedure during pregnancy if possible. Since antithyroid drug treatment poses no greater risk to the mother or fetus than does surgery, and possibly poses less risk, medical therapy is the method of choice. Furthermore, pregnancy appears to have an attenuating influence on the thyrotoxic state, possibly owing to a decrease in the concentration of thyroid-stimulating immunoglobulins, since titers of associated antithyroid antibodies decline (Amino et al., 1978). Consequently, the dosage of antithyroid drug required to control the disease is generally less than that required in the nonpregnant patient.

Certain aspects of placental permeability should be borne in mind in using antithyroid drugs to treat hyperthyroidism in the pregnant woman. First, propylthiouracil and methimazole readily cross the placenta, are concentrated in the fetal thyroid, and, if present in sufficient quantity, can produce goitrous hypothyroidism in the fetus. Second, there is strong evidence that little if any thyroid hormone passes from the circulation of the mother to that of the fetus. Consequently, thyroid hormone supplements given to the mother will not appreciably influence the thyroid hormone status of the fetus so as to prevent fetal goiter. For these reasons, the flux of antithyroid agent to the fetus should be limited by giving to the mother the smallest dosage of antithyroid agent that maintains the state consistent with normal pregnancy. The clinical manifestations of the mild hypermetabolism and the increased circulatory burden of normal pregnancy should not be construed as indicating inadequate treatment. The serum T_4 concentration should be maintained between 9 and 13 μg/dl and the free T_4 concentration or index in the upper normal range. As indicated earlier, this can generally be accomplished with a dosage of drug that is less than that required in the nonpregnant state. In any event, the daily maintenance dose should not exceed 200 mg in the case of propylthiouracil and 20 mg in the case of methimazole. In view of the evidence that methimazole crosses the placenta more readily than propylthiouracil, the latter is probably the agent of choice. Available data would suggest that children exposed to propylthiouracil *in utero*, under these guidelines for maternal therapy, do not differ appreciably from their nonexposed sibs with respect to intellectual development. However, if the daily maintenance dose of propylthiouracil required to control thyrotoxicosis exceeds 300 mg, the authors would recommend surgery in the middle trimester.

Iodine should not be used as adjunctive or sole therapy for any length of time in the pregnant woman. Iodine readily crosses the placenta and is capable of inducing in the fetus a very large goiter that may cause obstruction and even death. Propranolol is also contraindicated during pregnancy because of its association with intrauterine growth retardation and neonatal depression. (For a review of thyrotoxicosis in pregnancy, see Burrow, 1978.)

Mothers receiving antithyroid drugs post partum should not breast-feed their infants, since these drugs are excreted in the milk in quantities sufficient to produce goitrous hypothyroidism in the newborn.

Assays for TSI or TBII in the serum of pregnant women with known Graves' disease are of value, since neonatal thyrotoxicosis is prone to occur in the newborn when titers in the mother are high (see McKenzie and Zakarija, 1978).

Thyrotoxic Crisis

Thyrotoxic crisis or storm is an extreme accentuation of thyrotoxicosis. It is an uncommon but exceedingly serious complication, usually occurring in association with Graves' disease but sometimes with toxic multinodular goiter. Before the availability of adequate means for achieving full preoperative control, crisis frequently followed subtotal thyroidectomy ("surgical crisis"); currently "medical crisis" is the more common. Thyrotoxic crisis is almost always of abrupt onset and occurs in patients of any age and either sex in whom preexisting thyrotoxicosis has been treated either incompletely or not at all. Crisis is almost always evoked by a precipitating factor, such as infection, trauma, or surgical emergencies or operations. Less common precipitating factors include radiation thyroiditis, diabetic ketoacidosis, toxemia of pregnancy, and parturition. The mechanism whereby such factors lead to an accentuation of thyrotoxicosis has not been ascertained. The increases in serum T_3 concentration in crisis are not appreciably greater than those seen in uncomplicated thyrotoxicosis. The clinical picture is dominated by manifestations of severe hypermetabolism. Fever is almost invariably present and may be extreme; profuse sweating occurs. Marked tachycardia of sinus or ectopic origin may be accompanied by pulmonary edema or congestive heart failure. Early, tremulousness and restlessness are invariably present; delirium or frank psychosis occasionally occurs. Nausea, vomiting, and abdominal pain are common early manifestations. As the disorder progresses, apathy, stupor, and coma may supervene, and the blood pressure, which is initially well maintained, may fall to hypotensive levels. If the condition goes unrecognized, it is invariably fatal. This clinical picture in a patient either with a history of preexisting thyrotoxicosis or with goiter or exophthalmos or both is sufficient to establish the diagnosis, and treatment, which is urgently required, should not await laboratory confirmation.

There are no foolproof criteria by which severe thyrotoxicosis complicated by some other serious disease can be distinguished from thyrotoxic crisis induced by that disease. In any event, the differentiation between these alternatives is of no great significance, since treatment of the two is the same. Treatment of thyrotoxic crisis aims to correct both the severe thyrotoxicosis and the precipitating illness and to provide general supportive therapy. The therapy of crisis per se consists of efforts to inhibit both hormone synthesis and release and to antagonize the adrenergically mediated aspects of peripheral thyroid hormone action. Large doses of an antithyroid agent (200 mg of propylthiouracil every 4 hours) are given by mouth or stomach tube. Propylthiouracil is used in preference to methimazole since it possesses the additional action of inhibiting the peripheral generation of T_3 from T_4. The immediate administration of propylthiouracil serves to initiate therapy for the post-crisis period and to prevent enrichment of glandular hormone stores by the iodine, whose administration is of more immediate importance. The latter agent, administered either as SSKI (five drops every 6 hours) or as sodium iodide intravenously, is intended to retard acutely the release of hormone from the thyroid. Large doses of dexamethasone (2 mg orally every 6 hours) are also administered, since, in addition to providing glucocorticoid support, dexamethasone inhibits both the release of hormone from the thyroid and the peripheral generation of T_3 from T_4, synergizing with iodide and propylthiouracil, respectively, in regard to these actions. Indeed, the combined use of propylthiouracil, iodide, and dexamethasone will restore the serum T_3 concentration to within the normal range in 24 to 48 hours (Croxson et al., 1977). In the absence of significant cardiac insufficiency, propranolol, 40 to 80 mg orally every 6 hours, should be administered to antagonize the adrenergic component. If the patient cannot take medication by mouth, 2 mg of propranolol may be given intravenously, with electrocardiographic monitoring. Supportive measures that may be of great importance include the correction of the inevitable dehydration and possible hyponatremia. Glucose should be administered together with large amounts of vitamins of the B complex. A vigorous attack on the hyperpyrexia should be made. In milder cases, aspirin may suffice, but more often wet packs, fans, or ice packs may be required. If heart failure or pulmonary congestion is present, digitalis and diuretics are indicated.

Regimens similar to the foregoing have reduced the mortality rate in this disorder to approximately 20%, a figure that is still disturbingly high. When treatment is successful, improvement is usually manifest within 1–2 days, and recovery occurs within a week. At this time, iodide and dexamethasone are gradually withdrawn and plans for long-term management made.

THYROID HORMONE DEFICIENCY

A large number of structural or functional abnormalities may lead to deficient production of thyroid hormones. The clinical state resulting therefrom is termed hypothyroidism. A convenient classification of the causes of hypothyroidism is presented in Table 4–13. This classification divides the causes of hypothyroidism into three principal categories: (1) hypothyroidism resulting from loss or atrophy of thyroid tissue (thyroprivic hypothyroidism); (2) hypothyroidism due to insufficient stimulation of an intrinsically normal gland as a result of hypothalamic or pituitary disease (trophoprivic hypothyroidism); and (3) hypothyroidism associated with compensatory goitrogenesis as a result of defective hormone biosynthesis (goitrous hypothyroidism). Of the three categories, thyroprivic and goitrous hypothyroidism together account for approximately 95% of cases, only 5% or less being trophoprivic in origin.

A major advance in thyroidology, and a major contribution to health care, is the demonstration during very extensive neonatal screening programs in many areas of the world that hypothyroidism is present in one of every 4000–5000 newborns. Though screening programs are moderately costly (approximately $4000 per patient with hypothyroidism), the benefit/cost ratio of early diagnosis and treatment, in terms of costs of later institutional care saved and prevention of suffering, is enormous. (See Dussault et al., 1978, for a discussion of this important topic.) Population studies also indicate that unrecognized hypothyroidism may be present in a fairly large percentage of the elderly (Sawin et al., 1979). Thus, hypothyroidism may be much more common than has been thought. Some consideration should be given to the institution of screening programs for hypothyroidism in the elderly.

Peripheral Manifestations of Thyroid Hormone Deficiency

The clinical state of hypothyroidism is manifest in all organ systems. These manifestations are to a large extent independent of the underlying disorder in the thyroid gland, but are more closely related to the degree of hormone deficiency.

Skin and Appendages

In the dermis as well as in other tissues an accumulation of hyaluronic acid alters the composition of the ground substance. This material binds water, producing the mucinous edema that is responsible for the thickened features and puffy appearance of the patient with full-blown hypothyroidism and gives this severe degree of hypothyroidism its classic designation, *myxedema*. The myxedema is characteristically

Table 4–13. CLASSIFICATION OF THE CAUSES OF HYPOTHYROIDISM

1. *Thyroprivic*
   Postablative hypothyroidism
   Primary idiopathic hypothyroidism
   Sporadic athyreotic cretinism (thyroid aplasia or dysplasia)
2. *Trophoprivic*
   Sheehan's syndrome
   Infiltrative disorders of pituitary or hypothalamus
3. *Goitrous*
   Hashimoto's thyroiditis
   Endemic iodine deficiency
   Antithyroid agents (para-aminosalicylic acid, phenylbutazone, resorcinol, lithium; cruciferous plants; cassava)
   Iodide goiter and hypothyroidism
   Heritable defects in hormone biosynthesis and action
   Peripheral resistance to thyroid hormone (may be nongoitrous)

boggy and nonpitting and is most apparent around the eyes, on the dorsa of the hands and feet, and in the supraclavicular fossae. It causes enlargement of the tongue and thickening of the pharyngeal and laryngeal mucous membranes. A histologically similar type of deposit may occur in patients with Graves' disease usually over the pretibial area (infiltrative dermopathy or pretibial myxedema). In addition to having a puffy appearance, the skin in hypothyroidism is pale and cool as a result of cutaneous vasoconstriction. Anemia commonly accompanies hypothyroidism and contributes to the pallor; not uncommonly, hypercarotenemia gives the skin a yellow tint. The secretions of the sweat glands and sebaceous glands are reduced, leading to dryness and coarseness of the skin which, in extreme cases, may resemble that seen in ichthyosis.

Because of the skin's slow rate of growth, wounds of the skin tend to heal slowly. A bruising tendency is common in hypothyroidism and results from an increase in capillary fragility.

Characteristic changes are also seen in the skin appendages in hypothyroidism. Head and body hair is dry and brittle, lacks luster, and tends to fall out. Loss of hair from the temporal aspects of the eyebrows is a common feature. Growth of hair is greatly retarded so that haircuts and shaves are required less often. The nails are brittle and grow abnormally slowly.

In pituitary hypothyroidism, the changes in the skin and its appendages are less striking than in thyroprivic hypothyroidism. Although the skin is pale and cool, it tends to be thinner and finely wrinkled, and myxedematous infiltration of the tissues is less prominent than in thyroprivic hypothyroidism. Depigmentation of areas that are normally pigmented, such as the areolae, frequently occurs in pituitary but not thyroprivic hypothyroidism.

Histopathologic examination of the skin in hypothyroidism reveals hyperkeratosis with plugging of hair follicles and sweat glands. The dermis is edematous, and the connective tissue fibers are separated by an increase in the normal amount of metachromatically staining, PAS-positive mucinous material. This mucinous material consists of protein complexed with two mucopolysaccharides, hyaluronic acid and chondroitin sulfate B, especially the former. It is mobilized early during treatment with thyroid hormone, leading to an increase in the urinary excretion of nitrogen and hexosamines.

Cardiovascular System

In hypothyroidism, the cardiac output at rest is decreased because of a reduction in both stroke volume and heart rate,

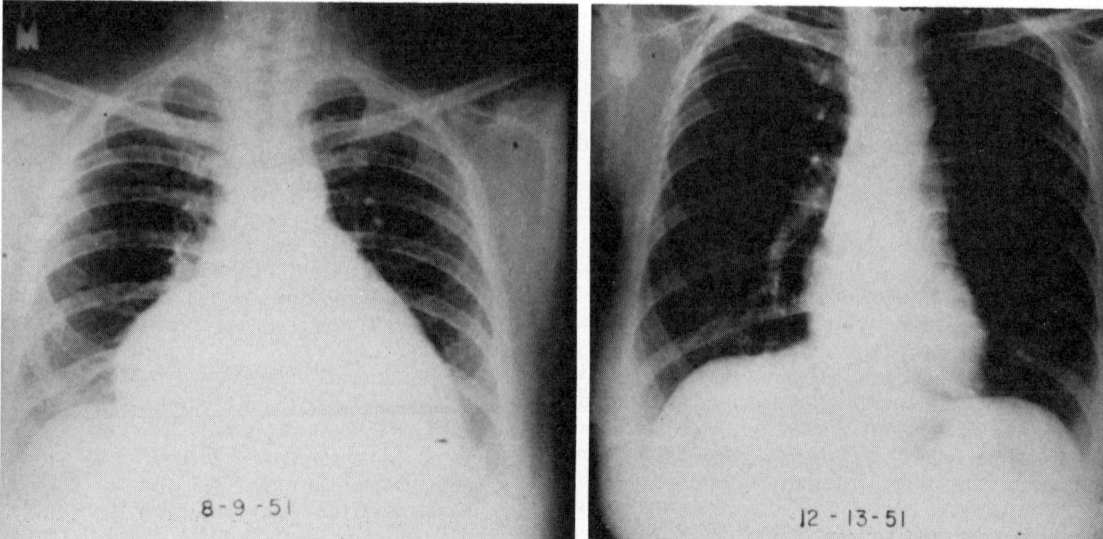

Figure 4–31. Chest roentgenograms in a patient with myxedema heart disease. The patient had signs of severe congestive heart failure and was treated with thyroid hormone alone. Within 4 months, the heart had returned to normal size and there was no evidence of underlying heart disease.

reflecting the loss of the inotropic and chronotropic effects of thyroid hormones. Peripheral vascular resistance at rest is increased, and blood volume is reduced. These hemodynamic alterations result in a narrowing of pulse pressure, a prolongation of circulation time, and a decrease in blood flow to the tissues. The decrease in cutaneous circulation is responsible for the coolness and pallor of the skin and the sensitivity to cold. In most tissues, the decrease in blood flow is proportional to the decrease in oxygen consumption, so that the mixed arteriovenous oxygen difference remains essentially normal. Despite the hemodynamic alterations at rest, which resemble those of congestive heart failure, cardiac output increases normally and peripheral vascular resistance decreases normally in response to exercise.

In thyroprivic hypothyroidism, the heart is enlarged (Fig. 4–31) and the heart sounds are diminished in intensity. These findings appear to be due largely to effusion into the pericardial sac of fluid rich in protein and mucopolysaccharides, but dilation of a "flabby" myocardium may also be a factor. Although pericardial effusion is common, it is very rarely of a degree sufficient to cause tamponade. In pituitary hypothyroidism, the heart is frequently small.

Angina pectoris is uncommon in hypothyroidism. Rarely is typical angina present in the hypothyroid state, and occasionally it disappears when the eumetabolic state is restored. More commonly, angina either appears or is worsened during treatment of the hypothyroid state with thyroid hormone. There has been much discussion as to whether the hypercholesterolemia that accompanies primary hypothyroidism accelerates the development of coronary atherosclerosis. Necropsy data suggest that the hypercholesterolemia of hypothyroidism predisposes to coronary atherosclerosis only in the presence of hypertension; in normotensive hypothyroid patients, the degree of coronary atherosclerosis appears to be no greater than that in age- and sex-matched normotensive control subjects (Steinberg, 1968).

Electrocardiographic (ECG) changes are common and include sinus bradycardia, prolongation of the PR interval, low amplitude of the P wave and QRS complex, alterations of the ST segment, and flattened or inverted T waves. Pericardial effusion is probably responsible in part for the ECG changes. Systolic time intervals are altered in hypothyroidism; the preejection period is distinctly prolonged and the ratio of preejection period to left ventricular ejection time increased.

The concentrations in serum of such enzymes as creatine phosphokinase, glutamic oxalacetic transaminase, and lactic dehydrogenase may be increased in hypothyroidism. Furthermore, the isoenzyme patterns sometimes suggest that the source of the increased creatine phosphokinase and lactic dehydrogenase is cardiac muscle.

In hypothyroidism, the large heart, together with the hemodynamic and ECG alterations and the serum enzyme changes, has been termed *myxedema heart*. There has been considerable discussion as to whether myxedema heart ever is the sole cause of heart failure. If it is, this must be quite rare, since in hypothyroidism the usual hemodynamic response to exercise differs from that observed in heart failure. Furthermore, the response of pulse pressure to the acute reduction in filling pressure induced by the Valsalva maneuver differs in the two situations. In the patient with hypothyroidism, as in the normal, the Valsalva maneuver leads to a decrease in pulse pressure, whereas in the patient with heart failure, the pulse pressure does not decrease, but displays a so-called "square-wave" response. In the absence of coexisting organic heart disease, treatment with thyroid hormone corrects the hemodynamic, ECG, and serum enzyme alterations of myxedema heart and restores heart size to normal (Fig. 4–31).

On pathologic examination, the pericardial sac contains an increased amount of fluid that is rich in protein and mucopolysaccharides. The heart is dilated and the myocardium is pale and flabby. Coronary atherosclerosis is commonly present. Histopathologic examination of the myocardium reveals interstitial edema and swelling of the muscle fibers with less of striations.

Respiratory System

Pleural effusions are common in hypothyroidism. Usually, these are evident only on radiologic examination but rarely may be of a degree sufficient to cause dyspnea. Lung volumes are usually normal in hypothyroidism, but maximal breathing capacity and diffusing capacity are reduced.

In severe hypothyroidism, myxedematous involvement of respiratory muscles as well as depression of the hypoxic ventilatory drive may lead to alveolar hypoventilation and carbon dioxide retention, which in turn may contribute to the development of myxedema coma. (See Zwillich et al., 1975, for a discussion of ventilatory control in hypothyroidism.)

Alimentary System

Although most patients show a modest gain in weight, the appetite is characteristically reduced. Contrary to popular conception, gross obesity is never a feature of hypothyroidism per se. Such weight gain as occurs is due largely to retention of fluid by the hydrophilic mucopolysaccharide deposits in the tissues. Peristaltic activity is decreased and, together with the decreased food intake, is responsible for the frequent complaint of constipation. The latter may be extreme, leading to fecal impaction. Gaseous distention of the abdomen may occur (myxedema ileus) and, if accompanied by colicky pain and vomiting, may mimic mechanical ileus. Clinically discernible ascites in the absence of other cause is unusual in hypothyroidism, but it may occur, usually in association with pleural and pericardial effusions. Like effusions into the other serous cavities, the ascitic fluid is rich in protein and mucopolysaccharides.

Achlorhydria after maximal histamine stimulation reportedly occurs in about one-half of patients with primary hypothyroidism. Even in the absence of overt anemia, many of these patients absorb vitamin B_{12} poorly and have low concentrations of vitamin B_{12} in serum. The impaired absorption of vitamin B_{12} is corrected by ingesting intrinsic factor. Circulating antibodies against gastric parietal cells have been found in about one-third of patients with primary hypothyroidism and probably reflect the presence of an atrophic gastric mucosa (Ardeman et al., 1966). Overt pernicious anemia is reported in about 12% of patients with primary hypothyroidism. The coexistence of pernicious anemia as well as other presumed autoimmune diseases with primary hypothyroidism supports the view that autoimmunity plays a primary role in the pathogenesis of primary hypothyroidism.

The effects of hypothyroidism on intestinal absorption are complex. Although the rates of absorption of many substances are decreased, the total amount that is eventually absorbed may be normal or even increased, because the decreased motility of the bowel may allow more time for absorption to occur. Overt malabsorption occasionally occurs.

Liver function tests are normal in hypothyroidism. Cholecystography often reveals a distended gallbladder that contracts sluggishly, but whether these changes predispose to the development of gallstones is unknown. Radiologic examination of the abdomen may reveal a greatly distended colon (myxedema megacolon).

Histopathologic examination frequently reveals atrophy of the gastric and intestinal mucosa and myxedematous infiltration of the bowel wall. The colon may be greatly distended. The volume of fluid in the peritoneal cavity is usually increased. The liver and pancreas are normal.

Nervous System

Thyroid hormone is essential for the development of the central nervous system (CNS). Deficiency of thyroid hormone beginning in fetal life or at birth results in retention of the infantile characteristics of the brain, hypoplasia of cortical neurons with poor development of cellular processes, retarded myelination, and reduced vascularity. (See review by Rossman, 1976.) If the deficiency is not corrected in early postnatal life, irreversible damage results. Deficiency of thyroid hormone beginning in adult life causes manifestations of lesser severity that usually respond adequately to treatment with thyroid hormone. The cerebral circulation shares in the hemodynamic alterations of hypothyroidism in that cerebral blood flow is reduced. Cerebral oxygen consumption, however, may be normal; this is in accord with the observation that the oxygen consumption in vitro of isolated brain tissue, unlike that of most other tissues, is not stimulated by administration of thyroid hormones. Consequently, the decrease in cerebral blood flow may lead to cerebral hypoxia.

One of the characteristic features of hypothyroidism is a general slowing of all intellectual functions, including speech. There is loss of initiative. Slow-wittedness and memory defects are common. Lethargy and somnolence are prominent. Dementia may occur and in the elderly patient may be mistaken for senile dementia. Psychiatric reactions are not uncommon and are usually of the paranoid or depressive type, but agitated states have also been described (myxedema madness). Headache occurs quite frequently. Cerebral hypoxia resulting from the circulatory alterations may predispose to confusional attacks and syncope. Syncope may be prolonged, leading to stupor or coma. Other factors predisposing to coma in hypothyroidism include exposure to severe cold, infection, trauma, hypoventilation with carbon dioxide retention, and depressant drugs. Epileptic fits have been reported and are especially liable to occur in myxedema coma (Jellinek, 1962). Night blindness is common and due to deficient synthesis of retinene, the pigment required for dark adaptation. Hearing loss of the perceptive type is frequently present. Perceptive deafness may also occur in association with a defect in the organic binding of thyroidal iodide (Pendred's syndrome) or with endemic cretinism, but in these instances, it is not due to hypothyroidism per se. Thick slurred speech and hoarseness are common and are due to myxedematous infiltration of the tongue and larynx, respectively. All movements are slow and clumsy, and pronounced ataxia of cerebellar type may occur. Numbness and tingling of the extremities are frequent complaints; in the fingers, these symptoms are often due to compression by mucinous deposits in and around the median nerve in the carpal tunnel (carpal tunnel syndrome). The tendon jerks are slow, especially during the relaxation phase, producing the characteristic "hung-up reflexes"; this phenomenon appears to result from a decrease in the rate of muscle contraction and relaxation, rather than from a delay in nerve conduction. The presence of extensor plantar responses or diminished vibration sense should alert the physician to the possibility of coexisting pernicious anemia with combined system disease.

Electroencephalographic changes are common and include a slow α-wave activity and general loss of amplitude. The concentration of protein in spinal fluid is often increased, but the pressure is normal.

On histopathologic examination, the nervous system is edematous, with mucinous deposits in and around nerve fibers. There may be foci of degeneration and an increase in glial tissue. The cerebral vessels commonly show atherosclerosis. (See review by Sanders, 1962, for an extensive discussion of the neurologic manifestations of myxedema.)

Muscle

Stiffness and aching of muscles are common complaints of the hypothyroid patient. Slowness of muscle contraction and relaxation is characteristic and is responsible for the slowness of movement and the delayed tendon jerks. These changes are aggravated by cold. Muscle strength is usually normal. Muscle mass may be slightly increased, and the muscles tend to be firmer than normal. Rarely, a great increase in muscle mass accompanied by slowness of muscular activity may be the predominant manifestation of hypothyroidism (the Kocher-Debre-Semelaigne or Hoffman syndrome).

Urinary excretion of creatine is reduced and creatine tolerance is increased, but these changes are generally not of a magnitude sufficient to afford a clear separation from normal values. The concentrations in serum of some enzymes of muscular origin, such as creatine phosphokinase and glutamic oxalacetic transaminase, are increased.

On histopathologic examination, the muscles appear pale and swollen. The muscle fibers may show swelling, loss of normal striations, and separation by mucinous deposits, but often no definite abnormalities are present.

Skeletal System: Calcium and Phosphorus Metabolism

Thyroid hormone is essential for the normal growth and maturation of the skeleton. The effect on growth appears to be due to a stimulation of protein synthesis as well as to a potentiation of both the secretion and action of GH. Before puberty, thyroid hormone is the major prerequisite for normal maturation of bone. Deficiency of thyroid hormone beginning in early life leads to both a delay in the development of and an abnormal, stippled appearance of the epiphysial centers of ossification (epiphysial dysgenesis). Linear growth is severely impaired, leading to dwarfism in which the limbs are disproportionately short in relation to the trunk. Bone age is always retarded in relation to chronological age.

Data concerning the effects of hypothyroidism on calcium and phosphorus metabolism in man are scanty. In general, urinary excretion of calcium is decreased, whereas fecal excretion of calcium and urinary and fecal excretion of phosphorus are variable. Calcium balance is also variable, and the changes reported are slight. The exchangeable pool of calcium and its rate of turnover are consistently reduced. These changes reflect decreases in the rates of bone formation and resorption. Aching and stiffness of the joints are not uncommon complaints, and joint effusions are occasionally seen.

Concentrations of calcium and phosphorus in serum are usually normal, but alkaline phosphatase is characteristically low in infantile and juvenile hypothyroidism. Bone density may be increased on radiologic examination. The radiologic appearances of the skeletal abnormalities of cretinism and juvenile hypothyroidism are discussed in the section dealing with these disorders.

Renal Function: Water and Electrolyte Metabolism

As part of the hemodynamic alterations that accompany hypothyroidism, renal blood flow and GFR are decreased, and tubular reabsorptive and secretory maxima are reduced. Blood urea nitrogen and serum creatinine, however, are normal. Urine flow is reduced, and the excretion of a water load may be delayed, resulting in a reversal of the normal diurnal pattern of urine excretion. The delay in water excretion appears to be due to decreased volume delivery to the distal diluting segment of the nephron as a result of the diminished renal perfusion as well as to disordered regulation of arginine vasopressin secretion (Skowsky and Kikuchi, 1978). It is reversed by treatment with thyroid hormone. The ability to concentrate urine may be slightly impaired. Proteinuria of mild degree may occur.

The impaired renal excretion of water along with retention of water by the hydrophilic deposits in the tissues results in an increase in total body water, even though plasma volume is reduced. This increase accounts for the hyponatremia that is commonly noted, since exchangeable Na^+ is increased in hypothyroidism. Exchangeable K^+ is usually normal in relation to lean body mass. The serum Mg^{++} concentration may be increased, but exchangeable Mg^{++} and urinary Mg^{++} excretion are decreased.

Hematopoietic System

In hypothyroidism, several hematologic abnormalities may occur. In response to the diminished oxygen requirements and decreased production of erythropoietin, the red cell mass is decreased; this is evident in the mild normocytic, normochromic anemia that often occurs. Less commonly, the anemia is macrocytic, and usually, though not invariably, this results from deficiency of vitamin B_{12}. Reference has already been made to the high incidence of pernicious anemia (and of achlorhydria and vitamin B_{12} deficiency without overt anemia) in patients with primary hypothyroidism (see Alimentary System). The defective absorption of vitamin B_{12} in primary hypothyroidism cannot be ascribed to lack of thyroid hormone per se, since it is not found to the same extent in the hypothyroid state that follows radioiodine treatment of thyrotoxicosis and is not corrected by treatment with thyroid hormone. In fact, defective absorption of vitamin B_{12} may develop or progress during treatment of hypothyroidism. Since this abnormality appears to be corrected by intrinsic factor, the macrocytic anemia that is sometimes seen in patients with primary hypothyroidism is more likely to be the result of deficiency of vitamin B_{12} than of thyroid hormone per se (Tudhope and Wilson, 1962). Nevertheless, thyroid hormone may be required for an optimal hematologic response to vitamin B_{12}. Folate deficiency resulting from malabsorption or dietary inadequacy may also be responsible for a macrocytic anemia. Both the frequent menorrhagia and the defective absorption of iron resulting from achlorhydria may lead to a microcytic, hypochromic anemia.

The total and differential white cell count is usually normal, and platelets are adequate in hypothyroidism though platelet adhesiveness is frequently depressed. An aspirate of bone marrow often has a gelatinous consistency, and the bone marrow may be hypocellular. If pernicious anemia or significant folate deficiency is present, the characteristic changes in the peripheral blood and bone marrow will be found. The intrinsic clotting mechanism may be defective because of decreased concentrations in plasma of factors VIII and IX, and this, together with an increase in capillary fragility and the decrease in platelet adhesiveness, may account for the bleeding tendency that sometimes occurs.

Pituitary and Adrenocortical Function

In long-standing hypothyroidism of thyroid origin, the pituitary gland is frequently enlarged and this can be detected radiologically in an increase in the volume of the pituitary fossa (Yamada et al., 1976). Rarely, such hypertrophy and hyperplasia of the thyrotrophs may be of such a degree that the function of other pituitary cells is compromised, resulting in pituitary insufficiency. Many patients with hypothyroidism display an increase in serum prolactin concentration which correlates with the increase in serum TSH concentration, and some patients display galactorrhea (Onishi et al, 1977). Treatment with thyroid hormone results in a decline in serum prolactin, as well as TSH concentration, and in disappearance of galactorrhea, if present. The mechanism underlying the hyperprolactinemia in hypothyroidism is uncertain, but it may be an enhanced sensitivity of the lactotrophs to TRH. In thyroprivic hypothyroidism, the responsiveness of growth hormone to provocative stimuli, such as insulin-induced hypoglycemia, is usually subnormal.

In hypothyroidism, the rate of turnover of cortisol is decreased. This alteration is due to a decrease in the rate of oxidation of cortisol to its inactive 11-keto metabolites as a result of a decrease in 11-β-hydroxysteroid dehydrogenase activity. As a result of the decreased rate of turnover of cortisol, the 24-hour urinary excretion of 17-OHCS and 17-KS is decreased, but the plasma cortisol concentration is usually normal. The responses of the urinary 17-OHCS to exogenous ACTH and metyrapone are usually normal in thyroprivic hypothyroidism, but occasionally sluggish responses are observed. The response of plasma cortisol to insulin-induced hypoglycemia may be impaired in some patients with thyroprivic hypothyroidism. In severe, long-standing, thyroprivic hypothyroidism, secondary depression of pituitary and adrenal function may occur, and adrenal insufficiency may be precipitated by stress or by rapid replacement therapy with thyroid hormone.

The rate of turnover of aldosterone is decreased, but the plasma concentration is normal. Plasma renin activity is decreased and sensitivity to angiotensin II is increased.

On histopathologic examination, the pituitary in thyroprivic hypothyroidism shows an increase in the number of actively secreting thyrotrophs. The adrenals are usually normal but occasionally show cortical atrophy. (See Gordon and Southren, 1977, for a review of steroid metabolism in hypothyroidism.)

Reproductive Function

In both sexes, thyroid hormone influences sexual development and reproductive function. Thyroprivic hypothyroidism from infancy, if untreated, leads to sexual immaturity, while hypothyroidism beginning before puberty causes a delay in the onset of puberty followed by anovulatory cycles. Thyroprivic hypothyroidism has been reported in association with precocious sexual development and galactorrhea.

In adult women, hypothyroidism is commonly associated with diminished libido and failure of ovulation. Secretion of progesterone fails and endometrial proliferation persists, resulting in excessive and irregular menstrual bleeding. These changes may be due to deficient secretion of luteinizing hormone (LH) (Distiller et al., 1975). In severe, long-standing, thyroprivic hypothyroidism, secondary depression of pituitary function may occur, leading to ovarian atrophy and amenorrhea. Fertility is reduced in hypothyroidism, but if conception does take place, abortion often results. In men, hypothyroidism may be accompanied by diminished libido, impotence, and oligospermia.

Values for urinary or plasma gonadotropins are usually in the normal range in thyroprivic hypothyroidism. In postmenopausal women with this disorder, these values are usually somewhat lower than in euthyroid women of the same age, but they are nevertheless distinctly increased.

This provides a valuable means of differentiating thyroprivic from pituitary hypothyroidism.

The metabolism of both androgens and estrogens is altered in hypothyroidism. Secretion of androgens is decreased, and the metabolic transformation of testosterone is shifted toward etiocholanolone rather than androsterone. In man, androsterone decreases serum cholesterol, but whether deficiency of androsterone in hypothyroidism is at all responsible for the increase in serum cholesterol remains to be determined. With respect to estradiol and estrone, hypothyroidism favors metabolism of these steroids via 16α-hydroxylation over that via 2-oxygenation, with the result that formation of estriol is increased at the expense of 2-hydroxyestrone and its derivative, 2-methoxyestrone. The binding activity of testosterone-estradiol binding globulin in plasma is decreased, with the result that the plasma concentrations of both testosterone and estradiol are decreased, but their unbound fractions are increased. The alterations in steroid metabolism disappear when the euthyroid state is restored. (See Gordon and Southren, 1977.)

Histopathologic examination of the ovaries and testes may reveal degenerative changes, especially if hypothyroidism began before puberty. In long-standing postpubertal hypothyroidism the ovaries may be atrophied.

Catecholamines and Serotonin

The plasma cAMP response to epinephrine is depressed in hypothyroid patients, lending support to the view that a state of decreased adrenergic activity accompanies thyroid hormone deficiency. In addition, the responses of cAMP to glucagon and parathyroid hormone are depressed, suggesting a general modulating influence of thyroid hormones on cAMP-mediated effects (Guttler et al., 1977). The mechanism underlying the decreased adrenergic responsiveness in hypothyroidism is uncertain. The secretion rate and plasma concentration of epinephrine are normal, but the corresponding functions in the case of norepinephrine are distinctly increased (Coulombe et al., 1976 and 1977). A possible mechanism is provided, however, by recent studies which suggest that thyroid hormones increase the number of β-adrenergic receptor sites. Plasma serotonin concentration, urinary 5-hydroxyindoleacetic acid excretion, and platelet monoamine oxidase activity are reportedly normal in hypothyroid patients.

Energy Metabolism: Protein, Carbohydrate, and Lipid Metabolism

The intrinsic effects of thyroid hormone on intermediary metabolism are discussed under Effects of Thyroid Hormones on Metabolic Processes. This section will deal with the manner in which these effects are clinically evident in the patient with hypothyroidism.

The decrease in energy metabolism and heat production of the hypothyroid patient is reflected in the low BMR, decreased appetite, cold intolerance, and slightly low basal body temperature.

In hypothyroidism, both the synthesis and degradation of protein are decreased, the latter especially so, with the result that nitrogen balance is usually slightly positive. The decrease in protein synthesis is reflected in retardation of both skeletal and soft tissue growth. In addition, thyroid hormone deficiency is accompanied by both a decrease in the secretion and a lessened effectiveness of GH.

Permeability of capillaries to protein is increased, ac-

Table 4–14. SYMPTOMATOLOGY OF MYXEDEMA
(77 Cases: 64 Women, 13 Men)

Symptom	Per Cent of Cases	Symptom	Per Cent of Cases
Weakness	99	Constipation	61
Dry skin	97	Gain in weight	59
Coarse skin	97	Loss of hair	57
Lethargy	91	Pallor of lips	57
Slow speech	91	Dyspnea	55
Edema of eyelids	90	Peripheral edema	55
Sensation of cold	89	Hoarseness or aphonia	52
Decreased sweating	89	Anorexia	45
Cold skin	83	Nervousness	35
Thick tongue	82	Menorrhagia	32
Edema of face	79	Palpitation	31
Coarseness of hair	76	Deafness	30
Pallor of skin	67	Precordial pain	25
Memory impairment	66		

After Means.

counting for the high concentration of protein in effusions into serous cavities and perhaps in spinal fluid. In addition, the total exchangeable albumin pool is increased, as a result of the relatively greater decrease in albumin degradation than in albumin synthesis. A greater than normal proportion and quantity of exchangeable albumin is localized in the extravascular space. The total concentration of serum proteins may be increased.

The oral glucose tolerance curve is characteristically flat and the insulin response delayed. These alterations may be due to a decreased rate of absorption of glucose from the gut. The disappearance from plasma of an intravenous load of glucose is delayed, reflecting the slow rate of uptake of glucose by the tissues. Degradation of insulin is slower than normal, with the result that there may be an increased sensitivity to exogenous insulin. This, as well as the decrease in appetite, presumably accounts for the diminished insulin requirement that occurs when hypothyroidism supervenes in a patient with preexisting diabetes mellitus.

Both the synthesis and degradation of lipid are depressed, the latter especially so, with the result that the net effect is one of lipid accumulation. The decrease in lipid degradation may reflect a decrease in post-heparin lipolytic activity, as well as a decreased delivery of lipid to degradative sites. Although an increase in serum cholesterol is the most commonly recognized abnormality of lipid metabolism in thyroprivic (but not pituitary) hypothyroidism, serum phospholipid phosphorus and serum triglycerides are also increased, and the concentration in serum of low-density lipoproteins

(LDL) is increased. Plasma FFA are decreased and the mobilization of FFA in response to fasting, catecholamines, and GH is impaired. (See Nikkilä and Kekki, 1972, for a review of lipid metabolism.)

Composite Clinical Picture of Hypothyroidism

Adult Hypothyroidism

The onset of hypothyroidism is usually so insidious that the classic clinical manifestations may take months or years to appear and frequently go unnoticed by persons well acquainted with the patient. The gradual development of the hypothyroid state is due to a slow progression both of thyroid hypofunction and of the clinical manifestations after thyroid failure is complete. This course is in contrast to the more rapid development of the hypothyroid state that occurs either when replacement therapy is discontinued in a patient with treated thyroprivic hypothyroidism or when the thyroid gland of a normal subject is surgically removed. In these circumstances, the BMR decreases to about −20%, and symptoms of mild hypothyroidism appear within 3 weeks. After 6 weeks, the BMR has decreased to −30%, and manifestations of frank hypothyroidism are present; by 3 months, full-blown myxedema is usually evident.

The early symptoms of hypothyroidism are variable and nonspecific (Table 4–14). Tiredness and lethargy are very common and lead to difficulty in performing a full day's

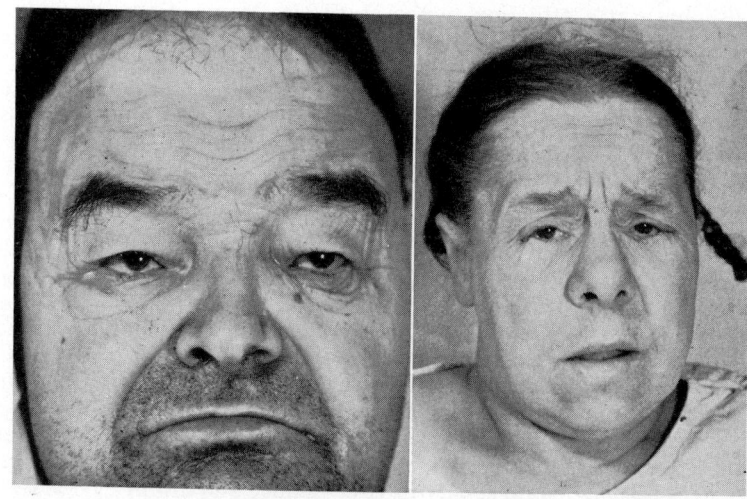

Figure 4–32. Typical facial appearance of myxedematous patients.

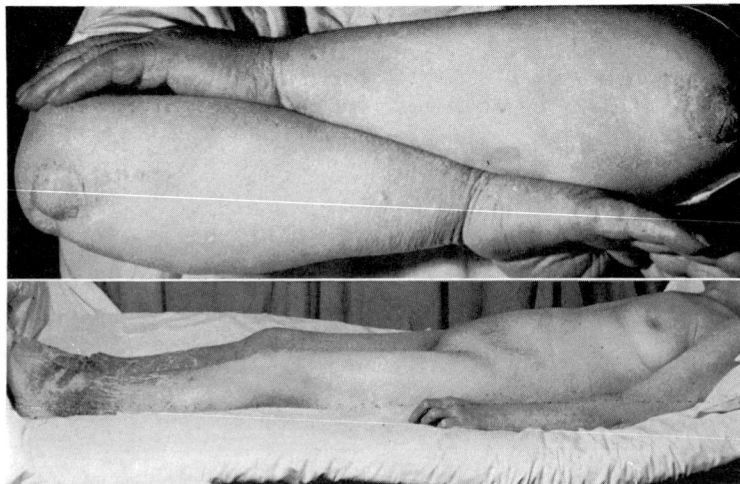

Figure 4–33. Dry, scaly skin with marked hyperkeratosis over the elbows and legs.

work. Constipation may either develop or, if already present, become worse. Sensitivity to cold may be an early manifestation; its presence is often suggested by the use of more blankets on the bed or a preference for warm weather. Women may complain of menstrual disturbance, especially menorrhagia, or difficulty in conceiving because of anovulatory cycles. Loss of libido occasionally occurs in both men and women. At this stage of the disease, the BMR is moderately decreased. With progression of the disease, the BMR falls to its minimal value, usually between −35 and −45%, but the clinical picture continues to evolve slowly. Drowsiness and slowing of intellectual and motor activity appear. The patient becomes apathetic and listless and loses interest in his work and environment. Women frequently complain of hair loss, brittle nails, and dry skin. Despite a reduction in appetite, modest weight gain often occurs. The voice becomes husky, which may be attributed to laryngitis. Periorbital puffiness may be noticed by the patient or his family (Fig. 4–32). Mucus collects in the eyes, and the lids are often stuck together when the patient awakens in the morning. Stiffness and aching of muscles are sometimes prominent symptoms and may be attributed to "rheumatism." Numbness and tingling of the fingers may occur. Progressive deafness may lead the patient to seek medical advice. Eventually, the picture of full-blown myxedema results, with thickened features, enlarged tongue, hoarseness, nonpitting edema, and extreme mental and physical lethargy. Mild hypothermia may call the physician's attention to the diagnosis. Many of the structural and functional manifestations presented in the preceding section become evident, but occasionally those arising in a particular organ predominate. The patient, if untreated, may remain in this state for many years, finally passing into a state of myxedema coma or succumbing to an intercurrent infection or a vascular occlusion.

Infantile Hypothyroidism and Cretinism

Hypothyroidism is seldom apparent at birth. The age at which symptoms of hypothyroidism appear will depend upon the degree of impairment of thyroid function in the infant. Severe hypothyroidism beginning in infancy is termed cretinism. As the age of onset increases, the clinical picture of cretinism merges imperceptibly with that of juvenile hypothyroidism. Retardation of mental development and growth is the hallmark of cretinism. Since these changes become manifest only in later infancy and are by

then largely irreversible, early recognition of the hypothyroid state is crucial and can be achieved by routinely measuring serum T_4 or TSH concentrations in the neonate. During the first few months of life, symptoms suggestive of hypothyroidism include feeding problems, failure to thrive, constipation, a hoarse cry, and somnolence. In succeeding months, especially in severe cases, protuberance of the abdomen, dry skin, poor growth of hair and nails, and delayed eruption of the deciduous teeth become evident. Retardation of mental and physical development is manifested by delay in reaching the normal milestones of development, such as holding up the head, sitting, walking, and talking.

Linear growth is severely impaired, resulting in dwarfism, with the limbs disproportionately short in relation to the trunk. Closure of the fontanelles is delayed, leading to a head that is large in relation to the body. The naso-orbital configuration of the infant is retained. Maldevelopment of the femoral epiphyses results in a waddling gait. The teeth are malformed and readily become carious. The appearance of the fully developed cretin is characteristic, with broad flat nose, widely set eyes, periorbital puffiness, large protruding tongue, sparse hair, rough skin, short neck, and protuberant abdomen with an umbilical hernia. Mental deficiency is always present and is usually severe.

Radiologic examination of the skeleton is diagnostic of cretinism. The skull shows a poorly developed base, delayed closure of the fontanelles, widely set orbits, and a short flat nasal bone. The pituitary fossa may be enlarged. Shedding of deciduous teeth and eruption of permanent teeth are delayed. A radiologic feature that is virtually pathognomonic of hypothyroidism in infancy and childhood is epiphysial dysgenesis. This abnormality may affect any center of endochondral ossification, depending on the age of onset of the hypothyroid state, but is usually best seen in larger centers, such as the femoral and humeral heads and the navicular bone of the foot. The center of ossification appears late, with the result that bone age is retarded in relation to chronological age. When the center eventually appears, instead of a single center, multiple small centers are scattered through a misshapen epiphysis. These small centers of ossification eventually coalesce, forming a single center that has an irregular outline and a stippled appearance ("stippled epiphysis"). Epiphysial dysgenesis is evident only in centers that would normally undergo ossification at a time after the onset of the hypothyroidism. After a normal metabolic state has been restored by treatment, development of

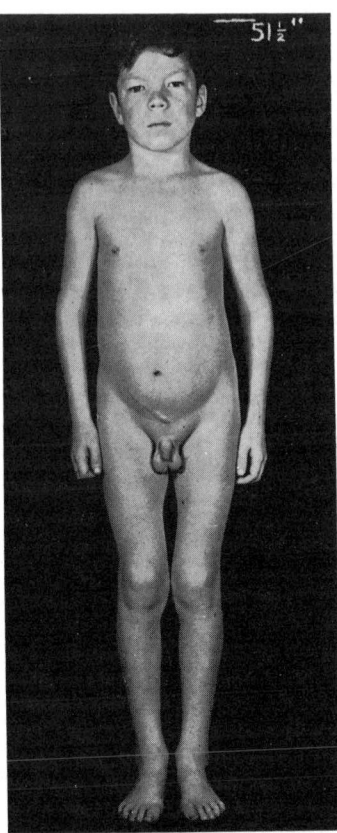

Figure 4–34. Juvenile hypothyroidism in a boy, aged 17. Dwarfism and delayed sexual development are apparent. Trunk is longer than legs. Appearance is youthful.

the centers destined to ossify at a later age proceeds normally.

Hypothyroidism beginning in childhood is termed juvenile hypothyroidism. The clinical manifestations of this state are intermediate between those of infantile and adult hypothyroidism, in that the developmental retardation is not as severe as that of cretinism and the manifestations of full-blown adult myxedema are rarely seen. Growth and sexual development are predominantly affected. Linear growth is severely retarded, resulting in dwarfism in which the limbs are disproportionately short in relation to the trunk. The rate of linear growth is characteristically less than that of weight gain. Maturation of the facial bones is impaired, so that the naso-orbital configuration of the infant or young child is retained. Eruption of permanent teeth is delayed. Sexual maturation is retarded, and the onset of puberty is delayed. The result is a child who appears much younger than his chronological age (Fig. 4–34). Rarely, precocious puberty and galactorrhea occur. Intellectual performance is distinctly poor, but the severe mental deficiency that characterizes cretinism is not found. The clinical manifestations of adult hypothyroidism are present to a varying, but usually milder, degree. On radiologic examination, epiphysial dysgenesis may be present, and epiphysial union is always delayed, resulting in a bone age that is retarded in relation to chronological age.

Laboratory Tests

A decrease in the secretion of the thyroid hormones is common to all varieties of hypothyroidism, irrespective of underlying etiology. The decrease in feedback inhibition of TSH secretion results in an increase in basal serum TSH concentration and increased serum TSH response to exogenous TRH if the hypothalamus and pituitary are intact. This the earliest laboratory abnormality in patients with intrinsic disease of the thyroid. With the passage of time, the serum T_4 and T_3 concentrations progressively approach subnormal values, the former more rapidly than the latter. This is owing to preferential synthesis and secretion of T_3 by residual functioning thyroid tissue under the influence of greatly increased plasma TSH concentrations. Accordingly, the serum T_3 concentration may be within the normal range at a time when the serum T_4 concentration is distinctly depressed. On the other hand, serum T_3 concentration is frequently decreased in euthyroid patients with severe systemic illness, and it normally declines with advancing age so that in the elderly it may be subnormal by usual standards. For these reasons, the serum T_3 concentration is less specific than the serum T_4 concentration in the diagnosis of hypothyroidism.

The decrease in circulating hormone concentrations, as well as a slight increase in the concentration of TBG, results in low values for *in vitro* uptake tests or the proportions of free T_4 and T_3. Calculated values for the free T_4 and T_3 indices are low, reflecting the decreased free hormone concentration.

The BMR is decreased in all varieties of hypothyroidism. The serum cholesterol concentration is increased to values usually in excess of 300 mg/100 ml, but in pituitary hypothyroidism the values may be normal or even low. In cretinism, hypercholesterolemia may not appear until late infancy; as a result, a normal value for serum cholesterol during the first several months of life does not exclude the diagnosis. Other manifestations of the hypothyroid state include both increased serum concentrations of such enzymes as creatine phosphokinase, SGOT, and LDH. In infantile and juvenile hypothyroidism, the serum alkaline phosphatase concentration does not display the usual increase seen during the period of active growth.

Tests that employ radioiodine and assess the function of the thyroid gland per se display a variable pattern, depending upon the underlying thyroid disorder. When the amount of thyroid tissue is reduced (thyroprivic hypothyroidism), the RAIU is subnormal. However, the diagnostic value of this finding is minimized by the recent decline in the range of normal values that has resulted from the increase in dietary iodine intake. On the other hand, in disorders in which hypothyroidism results primarily from biochemical rather than anatomic failure and in which compensatory goitrogenesis usually occurs, the RAIU may be normal or increased. Specific functional patterns are discussed later in relation to the several causes of hypothyroidism.

The differentiation of hypothyroidism due to intrinsic thyroid failure (thyroprivic and goitrous hypothyroidism) from that due to diminished TSH secretion as a result of hypothalamic or pituitary disease (trophoprivic hypothyroidism) is important, since failure to recognize the latter may have serious consequences for the patient when thyroid replacement is instituted. The serum TSH concentration is the most discriminating test since it is invariably increased in intrinsic thyroid failure, irrespective of underlying etiology, and is decreased in trophoprivic hypothyroidism. When basal serum TSH concentrations are not definitive, the response to exogenous TRH, which is usually subnormal in pituitary hypothyroidism and is normal rather than increased in hypothalamic hypothyroidism, may be of help.

In summary, laboratory confirmation of hypothyroidism

is best achieved through measurement of serum T_4 concentration in conjunction with an *in vitro* uptake test so that a free T_4 index can be derived. Alternatively, the free T_4 concentration can be measured directly. The additional measurement of serum TSH concentration will indicate whether the hypothyroidism is due to intrinsic disease of the thyroid or whether it is secondary to hypothalamic or pituitary disease.

Differential Diagnosis

The clinical picture of fully developed myxedema is usually characteristic enough to leave the diagnosis in little doubt. In its milder forms, hypothyroidism may require differentiation from several other states in which the appearance of the patient may be similar. The fact that these disorders, like hypothyroidism, tend to occur in elderly patients is partly responsible for any diagnostic uncertainty. In some elderly patients, slowing of mental and physical activity, dry skin, and loss of hair, especially from the lateral third of the eyebrows, may mimic similar findings in hypothyroidisim. Furthermore, elderly patients often become hypothermic on exposure to cold. In elderly patients, the results of the conventional laboratory tests, such as the RAIU and serum T_4 concentration, are not significantly different from those in younger individuals, but the overall turnover of thyroid hormone is substantially slowed. The serum T_3 concentration may be moderately depressed, reflecting reduced peripheral conversion of T_4 to T_3. The clinical features just described may reflect, therefore, a diminished flux of hormone to the tissues. In patients with chronic renal insufficiency, anorexia, torpor, periorbital puffiness, sallow complexion, and anemia may suggest hypothyroidism. However, retinopathy, azotemia, an abnormal urinalysis, and hypertension provide a clear differentiation between the two diseases. The differentiation of nephrotic states from hypothyroidism is more difficult. Here, waxy pallor, edema, hypercholesterolemia, and hypometabolism may suggest hypothyroidism. In addition, a decrease in serum T_4 concentration may occur if there is significant loss of TBG in the urine, but the free T_4 index will be normal or increased. The serum T_3 concentration is frequently decreased, suggesting impaired T_3-neogenesis from T_4, but the serum TSH concentration is not increased. In pernicious anemia, psychiatric abnormalities, a lemon-yellow tint of the skin, and numbness and tingling of the extremities may mimic similar findings in hypothyroidism. On the other hand, histamine-fast achlorhydria and mild macrocytosis in hypothyroidism may suggest pernicious anemia. Although there is a clinical and immunologic overlap between primary hypothyroidism and pernicious anemia, this association is not invariable, and when pernicious anemia occurs alone, it is not accompanied by specific clinical stigmata and laboratory evidence of thyroid hypofunction.

The presence of hypothyroidism is often suspected in patients who are severely ill, especially if they are elderly. In the ill patient, the serum T_3 concentration is almost invariably decreased, owing to decreased peripheral generation of T_3 from T_4. This should pose no problem, since measurements of the serum T_3 concentration should not be employed in the diagnosis of hypothyroidism. In the more severely ill patients, however, the serum T_4 concentration is also decreased, often markedly so. This is apparently due to a decrease in thyroid hormone binding and resulting rapid clearance of T_4 from the blood. *In vitro* T_3 uptake tests may be slightly increased, but values for the free T_4 index are usually subnormal. Nonetheless, perhaps because the binding of T_4 is more severely affected than that of T_3 is, values of the free T_4 concentration, directly determined, are normal or elevated. This, together with the absence of elevation of the serum TSH concentration, serves to differentiate the severely ill but intrinsically euthyroid patient from the patient with thyroprivic hypothyroidism.

Mongolism (Down's syndrome) resembles cretinism in that it is accompanied by retardation of mental development and shortness of stature. The differentiation of these two diseases is not difficult and can usually be made on clinical grounds alone. The infant with mongolism is more active, lacks the dry skin of the cretin, and displays specific stigmata, such as obliquely set eyes, epicanthal folds, white flecks in the iris (Brushfield's spots), inward-curving fifth fingers, and abnormal palmar and plantar creases. In addition, analysis of the chromosomes usually reveals either trisomy-21 or 15/21 translocation. Epiphysial dysgenesis and laboratory evidence of thyroidal hypofunction are lacking in mongolism. Dwarfism resulting from cretinism or juvenile hypothyroidism differs from dwarfism of other causes, such as hypopituitarism, rickets, and achondroplasia, in that it is accompanied by mental retardation and other manifestations of hypothyroidism, retarded bone age, and epiphysial dysgenesis. Replacement therapy with thyroid hormone restores growth in hypothyroid dwarfism but is ineffective in dwarfism due to other causes. The dysgenesis of the femoral epiphysis seen in hypothyroidism resembles that of Legg-Perthes' disease, but evidence of thyroid hypofunction is lacking in the latter disorder.

Thyroprivic Hypothyroidism

This section will deal with a variety of disorders characterized by loss or atrophy of thyroid tissue that results in decreased production of thyroid hormone despite presumably maximal stimulation of the thyroid remnant by TSH. The disorders that fall into this category include primary thyroid atrophy, the hypothyroid state that follows therapeutic ablation of the thyroid gland by surgery or radioiodine (postablative hypothyroidism), and sporadic athyreotic cretinism.

Primary Hypothyroidism

Although primary hypothyroidism may be an uncommon disorder, it is, after postablative hypothyroidism, the next most common cause of thyroid failure in the adult patient. It is several times more common in women than in men and occurs most often between the ages of 40 and 60. The cause is unknown. The presence of circulating thyroid autoantibodies in up to 80% of the patients as well as the clinical and immunologic overlap with presumed autoimmune diseases suggests, however, that it represents the end-stage of an autoimmune thyroiditis in which goiter either was absent or had gone unnoticed. Primary hypothyroidism may occur as part of an autoimmune syndrome of polyglandular failure in association with one or more of the following: idiopathic adrenal atrophy, idiopathic hypoparathyroidism, idiopathic hypogonadism, juvenile-onset-type diabetes mellitus, and pernicious anemia. In Caucasians, haplotype HLA-B8 is present with inordinate frequency in patients with this syndrome. Primary thyroid failure also occurs with inordinate frequency in patients with Hodgkin's disease who have been treated with mantle irradiation.

On histopathologic examination, the small thyroid remnant consists largely of fibrous tissue, with an occasional thyroid follicle and focus of lymphocytic infiltration.

The clinical manifestations and composite clinical picture of frank hypothyroidism have been discussed in an earlier section. In patients with this disorder, in contrast to the normal, the thyroid is usually impalpable, but occasionally a fibrous band may be felt in the region of the isthmus. Typical laboratory indices discussed earlier include a low serum T_4 concentration and a high serum TSH concentration that is hyperresponsive to TRH administration. Values for the *in vitro* uptake test and the proportion of free T_4 are often subnormal but may be in the normal range. Thyroid autoantibodies are detectable in the serum in up to 80% of the patients but may be absent in long-standing disease. The serum cholesterol concentration is usually increased.

In addition to spontaneous hypothyroidism, both surgical and radioiodine therapy (see below) may lead to a functional state of "decreased thyroid reserve" or "subclinical hypothyroidism," which represents a phase in the evolution of frank thyroid failure. During this phase, the patient is clinically eumetabolic with an increased serum TSH concentration, normal serum T_3 concentration, and normal or moderately decreased serum T_4 concentration.

Postablative Hypothyroidism

Postablative hypothyroidism is the commonest cause of thyroid failure in the adult. One type is that which follows total or subtotal thyroidectomy. Although functioning remnants may be present, as indicated by foci of radioiodine accumulation, hypothyroidism invariably develops after total thyroidectomy. This procedure, which is associated with a high frequency of recurrent laryngeal nerve palsy and postoperative hypoparathyroidism, is often performed in patients with thyroid carcinoma.

By far the most common type of postoperative hypothyroidism is that which follows subtotal resection of the diffuse goiter in Graves' disease. Its frequency is determined by the amount of tissue removed and varies inversely with the incidence of recurrent hyperthyroidism. In addition, autoimmune destruction of the thyroid remnant may sometimes be a factor, since a correlation has been shown to exist between the presence of circulating thyroid autoantibodies in thyrotoxicosis and the development of hypothyroidism after surgery (Green and Wilson, 1964). Hypothyroidism often becomes manifest during the first year after surgery, but, as in the case of postradioiodine hypothyroidism, there also occurs a progressively rising incidence with time. A survey of the surgical literature indicates a modal incidence of about 10%. However, since most patients who develop hypothyroidism seek medical rather than surgical advice, these figures may be an underestimation. In reports from clinics in which internists do the follow-up studies, the frequency may approach 30% or more (Hershman, 1966; Nofal et al., 1966). In some patients, mild hypothyroidism appears during the early postoperative period and then goes into remission. In adults, therefore, it may be justified to withhold replacement therapy for 1 or 2 months, provided that close observation is maintained. In children, treatment should be instituted whenever hypothyroidism supervenes.

Hypothyroidism following destruction of thyroid tissue with radioiodine is distressingly common and is the only verified disadvantage of this form of treatment for hyperthyroidism. Its frequency is determined in large part by the dose of radiation delivered to the thyroid, but it is also influenced by variations in individual susceptibility that are conditioned by other factors, including autoimmune phenomena (Green and Wilson, 1964). The incidence of postradioiodine hypothyroidism increases progressively with time. The data currently available indicate an incidence at 10 years of approximately 40%, although values as high as 70% have been reported. (See Dunn and Chapman, 1964, and Nofal et al., 1966, for data and references. See also the section on Graves' Disease.)

Sporadic Cretinism

Developmental defects of the thyroid are responsible for the remarkable frequency of hypothyroidism in the newborn, clearly shown to occur in one in every 4000–5000 births. These defects may take the form of complete absence of thyroid tissue or failure of the thyroid gland to descend properly during embryologic development. Thyroid tissue may then be found anywhere along its route of descent from the foramen cecum at the junction of the anterior two-thirds and posterior third of the tongue (lingual thyroid) to the normal site or below. Absence of thyroid tissue or its ectopic location, if present, can be ascertained by scintiscanning after administration of ^{99m}Tc pertechnetate. In a small percentage of patients, neonatal hypothyroidism results from biosynthetic defects in the thyroid or from pituitary or hypothalamic failure.

Even frank hypothyroidism is difficult to detect by clinical examination at birth or shortly thereafter. Suggestive signs are a high birth weight owing to postmaturity, enlargement of the posterior fontanelle, delay in the passage of meconium, persistence of neonatal jaundice, and hypothermia. When several of these signs are present, the diagnosis of hypothyroidism should be sought promptly in measurements of the serum T_4 and TSH concentrations.

Failure to institute therapy in patients with neonatal hypothyroidism will result in the patient's developing the full-blown picture of cretinism described earlier in this section. If treatment is initiated later than the first several weeks of life, the somatic manifestations of cretinism may be forestalled, but psychomotor development will be permanently impaired. This consideration highlights the urgency of routine screening of newborns for hypothyroidism, which can successfully be accomplished by routine measurements of serum T_4, TSH, or both, either in cord blood or in blood spots dried in filter paper, as in routine screening for phenylketonuria. In some cases, neonatal hypothyroidism is transient, and permanent hormone replacement therapy is not required. Rather than temporize, however, it is far better to initiate treatment early, during the critical period of central nervous system development, and to withdraw treatment some months later to see if continued therapy is needed (see Dussault et al., 1978, for a discussion of this important topic).

Trophoprivic Hypothyroidism

A thorough discussion of the evolution and clinical picture of pituitary insufficiency is presented in Chapter 3. This section will deal mainly with the features that may serve to differentiate hypothyroidism of primary thyroid origin from that arising from disease in higher centers. When the intrinsically normal thyroid gland is deprived of TSH stimulation as a result of hypothalamic or pituitary disease, partial atrophy of the thyroid and decreased production of thyroid hormones occur. In most cases, the hyposecretion of TSH is accompanied by decreased secretion of other pituitary hormones, with the result that evidence of gonadal and adrenocortical insufficiency is also present. Instances in which hyposecretion of TSH is the sole demonstrable abnormality (unitropic deficiency) are quite rare. Hypothyroidism resulting from pituitary insufficiency varies widely in severity, from instances in which it is mild and overshadowed by features of gonadal and adrenocortical failure to instances in which the features of the hypothyroid state are the predominant manifestations.

The differentiation of pituitary from thyroprivic hypothyroidism is important because, in the former, treatment with thyroid hormone alone fails to correct the associated endocrine abnormalities and, indeed, by precipitating acute adrenocortical insufficiency, may be dangerous. Three major aspects serve to differentiate pituitary from thyroprivic hypothyroidism: (1) features arising from the cause of the pituitary insufficiency itself; (2) differences in the clinical manifestations; and (3) differences in the laboratory indices.

In most cases, pituitary hypothyroidism results either from postpartal pituitary necrosis (Sheehan's syndrome) or from tumors of the pituitary or adjacent structures. The tumors most commonly responsible are chromophobe adenomas of the pituitary or craniopharyngiomas (suprasellar cysts). Postpartal pituitary necrosis is strongly suggested by a history of bleeding or shock after delivery necessitating blood transfusion, followed by deficient lactation, persistent amenorrhea, and loss of libido and of pubic and axillary hair. Symptoms of hypothyroidism may appear rapidly, in contrast to their usual slow evolution in thyroprivic hypothyroidism. Although these are the usual manifestations of Sheehan's syndrome, many years may elapse before symptoms of pituitary insufficiency appear. The presence of a tumor in the region of the pituitary is suggested by headache, especially if retro-orbital in location, by visual field defects, and by enlargement of the pituitary fossa. Intracranial pressure may be increased, and diverse neurologic manifestations may occur if the tumor extends widely beyond the pituitary fossa. Radiologic examination of the skull usually reveals enlargement of the pituitary fossa and erosion of the clinoid processes. Rarely, hyperplasia and hypertrophy of the thyrotropes as a result of long-standing thyroprivic disease may lead to radiologically demonstrable enlargement of the pituitary fossa. A craniopharyngioma is strongly suggested by suprasellar calcification. Cerebral angiograms may aid in the demonstration of a tumor or of an aneurysm of the internal carotid artery, which in rare instances may cause pituitary insufficiency.

The clinical manifestations of pituitary hypothyroidism tend to differ in certain respects from those of thyroprivic hypothyroidism. Although the skin is pale and cool, it tends to be thinner and finely wrinkled, and myxedematous infiltration of the tissues is less prominent than in thyroprivic hypothyroidism. Depigmentation of areas that are normally pigmented, such as the areolae, frequently occurs. The texture of the hair is finer than that in thyroprivic hypothyroidism. Enlargement of the tongue, which is a striking feature of thyroprivic hypothyroidism, is less prominent in pituitary hypothyroidism. Other differentiating features of pituitary insufficiency may result from inadequate secretion of other pituitary hormones, notably gonadotropins and corticotropin. In women of premenopausal age, amenorrhea rather than menorrhagia occurs, and the breasts are atrophic. As regards manifestations of adrenocortical hypofunction, some similarities may exist. Loss of axillary and pubic hair is common in women with either disease. In pituitary hypothyroidism, however, the heart is usually small, and the blood pressure is low. Furthermore, manifestations of hypoglycemia are not uncommon in pituitary hypothyroidism but are rare in thyroprivic hypothyroidism.

Very often, when the foregoing features are inconclusive, differentiation of pituitary from thyroprivic hypothyroidism will depend upon the results of laboratory tests. Indices of thyroid function tend to differ in the extent to which they are abnormal. In pituitary insufficiency, the serum T_4 concentration is usually not as low as in thyroprivic hypothyroidism, values at or near the lower limit of the normal range commonly being found. The same is true of the RAIU, but for reasons discussed earlier the test has little diagnostic value except as part of the TSH-stimulation test. The serum cholesterol concentration, which is usually increased in thyroprivic hypothyroidism, is low in pituitary hypothyroidism.

Measurement of serum TSH concentration by radioimmunoassay provides the most direct means of differentiating between pituitary and thyroprivic hypothyroidism. In pituitary hypothyroidism, serum TSH is usually undetectable and almost always within the normal range, whereas in thyroprivic hypothyroidism, the serum TSH concentration is invariably increased, often greatly so (Fig. 4–16). Measurements of the response of the serum TSH concentration to exogenous TRH are rarely required to make the diagnosis of thyroprivic hypothyroidism, but may provide useful information in patients with pituitary or hypothalamic disease. Subnormal responses would be expected in the former and normal, though perhaps delayed, responses in the latter. Not infrequently, however, the pattern is not that expected, probably because the disorder is not confirmed to one locus or another. Sometimes, in patients with pituitary or hypothalamic disease, basal serum TSH concentrations are increased and responses to TRH are augmented. These unexpected findings have been ascribed to secretion of a form of TSH that is immunoreactive but has little or not bioactivity. (See Faglia et al., 1979.)

Measurement of the urinary excretion or plasma concentration of gonadotropins can provide a means of differentiating pituitary from thyroprivic hypothyroidism. In postmenopausal women with thyroprivic hypothyroidism, the values may be somewhat lower than those found normally at the same age, but they remain, nevertheless, distinctly elevated. In women of premenopausal age, the values are less discriminatory, since they are normally much lower. In pituitary hypothyroidism, gonadotropins are usually absent from the plasma or urine.

Tests of the pituitary-adrenal axis are generally less useful. Although values for the basal 24-hour urinary excretion of 17-OHCS and 17-KS are characteristically reduced in hypopituitarism, subnormal values are also usually encountered in thyroprivic hypothroidism. The latter results, at least in large part, from decreased metabolic disposal of cortisol, with the result that the plasma cortisol concentration is usually normal despite a decreased rate of cortisol secretion. In pituitary hypothyroidism, the plasma cortisol concentration is usually low. Further evidence may be obtained by assessing the response of the urinary 17-OHCS to metyrapone. In thyroprivic hypothyroidism, the response is usually normal, the maximal increase in 17-OHCS occurring on the day after the administration of metyrapone. In some cases of thyroprivic hypothyroidism, however, the response is either subnormal or delayed, the maximal increase in 17-OHCS occurring 2 or 3 days after the administration of metyrapone. By contrast, in pituitary hypothyroidism, the response to metyrapone is usually subnormal, reflecting the diminished reserve of corticotropin. (See Bigas et al., 1978, for a careful study of pituitary function in hypothyroidism.)

In pituitary insufficiency, the increases in plasma GH and cortisol concentrations that normally occur in response to insulin-induced hypoglycemia either are blunted or fail to occur. Subnormal responses are also usually seen in thyroprivic hypothyroidism, and hence this test does not provide a useful means of differentiating between these two varieties of hypothyroidism.

Goitrous Hypothyroidism

This section will deal with a variety of disorders characterized by a relatively or absolutely impaired ability to synthesize thyroid hormone, either because of some extrinsic factor or because of an intrinsic, usually heritable, defect in hormone biosynthesis. Inadequate synthesis of hormone leads to hypersecretion of TSH, which in turn produces both goiter and stimulation of all steps in hormone biosynthesis capable of response. This compensatory response may be inadequate, and goiter with hypothyroidism or cretinism results. In many instances, however, the compensatory response overcomes the impairment in hormone biosynthesis, and the patient is eumetabolic but goitrous. The latter condition, termed simple or nontoxic goiter, will be discussed in a later section. Although Hashimoto's disease is the commonest cause of goitrous hypothyroidism in areas of iodine sufficiency, it is discussed in the section dealing with thyroiditis.

Endemic Goiter

The term endemic goiter denotes any goiter occurring in a region where goiter is prevalent. Classically, endemic goiter occurs in areas of environmental iodine deficiency and has been ascribed to this pathogenic factor; however, as will be indicated, other factors may also be operative. This disease is one of vast public health significance, since it has been estimated to afflict more than 200 million people throughout the world. Except perhaps in North America, it is prevalent on all continents, is most prevalent in mountainous areas, such as the Alps, Himalayas, and Andes, but may also occur in nonmountainous regions. In the United States, goiter was formerly common in the region around the Great Lakes, but here as in other areas of endemic disease, its incidence has been greatly reduced by the use of iodized salt. The belief that iodine deficiency plays a major role in the genesis of endemic goiter is supported by an inverse correlation between the iodine content of soil and water and the incidence of goiter, the kinetics of iodine metabolism in patients with this disorder, and a decrease in indicence with iodine prophylaxis. On the other hand, both the isolated geographic locale and the cultural patterns of some populations in areas of severe endemic incidence favor inbreeding, with the result that genetically determined abnormalities in hormonal biosynthesis may also play a role. The frequent occurrence of deaf-mutism, mental retardation, and motor defects in the populations of such areas also support this view. Furthermore, severe iodine deficiency and its associated abnormalities in the kinetics of iodine metabolism may occur in the absence of goiter. Endemic goiter may display a spotty incidence, even within an area of known iodine deficiency; the role of dietary minerals or naturally occurring goitrogens and of pollution of water supplies has been ques-

tioned in instances of this type. Indeed, in the Cauca valley of Columbia, water-borne goitrogens have been implicated. Increasing evidence indicates that in many areas of endemic iodine deficiency, consumption of cassava meal, which gives rise to thiocyanate, aggravates the iodine-deficient state by inhibiting thyroid iodide transport (Ermans et al., 1980).

A variety of abnormalities in iodine metabolism occur in patients with endemic goiter. The majority are consistent with the expected effects of iodine deficiency. Others, such as those indicating the existence of heterogeneous pools of thyroidal iodine and the secretion of butanol-insoluble iodinated products, are probably mere exaggerations of processes occurring in the normal gland but made more prominent by prolonged hyperfunction. To date, no abnormality clearly due to a primary defect in iodine metabolism has been described in endemic goiter. Thyroid iodide clearance rates and RAIU are increased inversely with the decrease in urinary stable iodine excretion. The absolute iodine uptake is normal or low. The thyroid hyperfunction can be suppressed by exogenous hormone, indicating that it represents a homeostatic compensatory response. In areas of only moderate iodine deficiency, the serum T_4 concentration is usually in the lower range of normal; in areas of severe endemia, however, the values may be distinctly decreased. Nevertheless, most patients in these areas do not appear to be clinically hypothyroid, a discrepancy that is due to an increase in the synthesis of the calorigenically more efficient hormone, T_3, at the expense of T_4 (Goslings et al., 1977).

The severity of goiter is not uniform among all inhabitants of an area of endemic incidence. As a group, goitrous inhabitants display lower serum T_4 concentrations and higher serum TSH concentrations than do nongoitrous inhabitants, indicating a less efficient adaptation to the iodine deficiency, but what underlies this difference in adaptive response is unclear. (For a discussion of the functional abnormalities in endemic goiter and references to earlier work, see Goslings et al., 1977.)

The gross and histopathologic appearance of endemic goiter depends upon the duration of the goiter and the severity of the pathogenetic insult. In the initial stages, the stimulus of iodine deficiency leads to hypertrophy and hyperplasia of the epithelial cells lining the follicles. The cells increase in height and number and may protrude into the follicular lumen, forming papillary projections. The amount of colloid in the follicles decreases. The hyperplasia is accompanied by an increase in vascularity. This is the diffuse hyperplastic goiter that is usually seen in children in endemic areas. If the iodine intake is increased, the hypertrophy and hyperplasia of the epithelial cells disappear, and colloid reaccumulates in the follicles. This process of involution leads to a return of the gland to normal size if the hyperplasia is of relatively short duration but probably results in a diffuse colloid goiter if the hyperplastic phase has been present for years. In long-standing goiter, repeated cycles of hyperplasia and involution eventually lead to the formation of nodules of involuted tissue surrounded by more hyperplastic tissue, and a multinodular goiter results. Localized hyperplasia with the formation of encapsulated adenomas (adenomatous hyperplasia) is a less common cause of nodularity in endemic goiter; it may be difficult to distinguish this lesion from true neoplasia. Nodules often undergo hemorrhagic or cystic degeneration and may become calcified or ossified.

The incidence and severity of endemic goiter, as well as the metabolic state of the goitrous patient, depend mainly on the degree of iodine deficiency. In the absence of hypothyroidism, the effects of the goiter are mainly disfiguring. When the goiter has become nodular, however, hemorrhage into a nodule may cause acute pain and swelling, mimicking subacute thryoiditis or neoplasia. Occasionally, a goiter may cause symptoms by compressing adjacent structures, such as the trachea, esophagus, and recurrent laryngeal nerves.

The development of hyperthyroidism is unusual in patients with endemic goiter. This is in contrast to the tendency of multinodular goiter in nonendemic regions to produce hyperthyroidism in later life. It seems likely that iodine deficiency protects some patients with endemic goiter from developing hyperthyroidism. The incidence of thyrotoxicosis in an endemic goiter region has been reported to increase following the introduction of measures to increase iodine intake (Connolly et al., 1970). The induction of iodine of hyperthyroidism in a patient with endemic goiter is known as the Jod-Basedow phenomenon. The incidence of thyroid carcinoma in endemic goiter is probably not increased; the suggestion that it may be increased seems largely due to the difficulty in distinguishing adenomatous hyperplasia from true neoplasia.

The incidence of endemic goiter has been greatly reduced in many areas by the introduction of iodized salt. In the United States, table salt is enriched with KI to a concentration of 0.01%, which, if the intake of salt is normal, would provide an iodine intake of approximately 500 μg daily, which is considered to represent the desired amount in an adult. In areas where the salt is crude and moist, iodine added as potassium iodide may be lost by sublimation; in this instance, potassium iodate is preferable since it is more stable. In primitive communities, an annual injection of iodized oil is an effective means of administering iodine.

The administration of iodine has little if any effect on a colloid or multinodular goiter, but it will cause the early hyperplastic goiter to regress. Similarly, thyroid hormone usually has no effect on goiters of long standing or on established mental or skeletal changes, but it should be given in full replacement doses if there is evidence of hypothyroidism; this is of paramount importance in pregnant women. Surgical treatment is indicated if the adjacent structures are compressed or if the goiter is either very large or enlarging rapidly.

Endemic Cretinism

Endemic cretinism is a specific developmental disorder that occurs in regions of severe endemic goiter. Both parents of an endemic cretin are usually goitrous. In addition to, or instead of, the classic features of hypothyroid cretinism described earlier, endemic cretins often display deaf-mutism, spasticity, and motor dysfunction. Thus, one can distinguish three types of cretins: hypothyroid cretins, neurologic cretins, and those with combined features of the two. The pathogenesis of neurologic cretinism is obscure, but may represent severe thyroid hormone deficiency during a critical phase of central nervous system development, with remission later.

Some cretins are goitrous, but often the thyroid is atrophic. This has been ascribed either to exhaustion atrophy, resulting from continuous overstimulation, or to a requirement for iodine of normal thyroid growth. Neither explanation seems wholly satisfactory, however.

Although the role of iodine deficiency, per se, in the pathogenesis of endemic cretinism has been questioned, there can be no question that iodine deficiency is somehow implicated, since cretinism appears to have been eradicated where maternal iodine supplementation has been undertaken. Of even greater import are recent observations indicating that some degree of psychomotor retardation is common in noncretinous children born in areas of severe iodine deficiency, and that this can be eliminated or alleviated by maternal iodine supplementation (Thilly et al., 1980).

Goiter Due to Antithyroid Agents

The ingestion of compounds with antithyroid potency is an occasional cause of goiter with or without hypothyroidism. Apart from the agents commonly used in the treatment of thyrotoxicosis, antithyroid agents may be encountered either as drugs used in the treatment of disorders unrelated to the thyroid gland or as agents occurring naturally in foodstuffs.

Of the drugs with potential goitrogenic action currently in use, lithium is the most important. Goiter with or without hypothyroidism is sometimes encountered in patients who are receiving lithium as treatment for a psychiatric disorder. Lithium, like iodide, decreases thyroid hormone synthesis. Surprisingly, lithium-induced hypothyroidism appears to be largely confined to women, particularly those over the age of 40 years, in whom as many as one-third will be hypothyroid. Many such women display evidence of thyroid autoimmunity, suggesting that coexisting autoimmune thyroid disease is a predisposing factor (Lindstedt et al., 1977; Transbol et al., 1978).

Other drugs that have occasionally been reported to produce goitrous hypothyroidism include para-aminosalicylic acid, phenylbutazone, and topically applied resorcinol. Like the commonly used antithyroid agents, these drugs exert their effect by interfering with both the organic binding of iodine and the later steps in hormone biosynthesis. Antithyroid agents readily cross the placenta and are excreted in breast milk. Consequently, administration of an antithyroid agent to a pregnant or lactating woman for the treatment of thyrotoxicosis may lead to goitrous hypothyroidism in the infant. The goiter and hypothyroidism in the infant are usually self-limited, disappearing soon after birth or after the child is weaned. Occasionally, however, a large neonatal goiter may cause respiratory distress and death from asphyxia.

Antithyroid agents, whose chemical nature has been discussed in an earlier section, occur naturally in certain plants, particularly those of the family Cruciferae. Some of these are eaten by man; among them rutabaga and white turnip appear to be richest in goitrogen. It is uncertain, however, whether goitrogenic quantities of such foods are ever directly ingested. Rather, such foods may accentuate the effects of dietary iodine deficiency, as is almost certainly the case with cassava meal.

Although soybean is not an antithyroid agent, soybean products in feeding formulas formerly led to goiter in children by enhancing fecal loss of hormone which, together with the low iodine content of soybean products, produced a state of iodine deficiency (Pinchera et al., 1965). Feeding formulas containing soybean products are now enriched with iodine.

Both the goiter and the hypothyroidism usually subside after the antithyroid agent is withdrawn, but if continued administration of pharmacologic goitrogens is required, replacement therapy with thyroid hormone will cause the disorder to regress.

Iodide Goiter and Hypothyroidism

Goiter and hypothyroidism, either alone or in combination, are sometimes induced by the chronic administration of large doses of iodine in either organic or inorganic form. This is seen most commonly in patients with chronic respiratory disease, since these patients are often given potassium iodide as an expectorant. Iodide goiter develops in only a small proportion of patients given iodine. By contrast, it has been reported that the incidence of goiter may be as high as 30% in asthmatic patients given iodopyrine, a compound of iodine and phenazone. This inordinately high incidence is due to a synergistic action of iodine upon the antithyroid effect of phenazone, which is itself a goitrogen. The development of iodide goiter has also been reported to follow the single administration of radiographic contrast media from which iodide is released slowly over a long period. Iodide goiter without hypothyroidism occurs endemically in Hokkaido, where seaweed is consumed in large quantity.

From the majority of reported cases, and from the fact that only a small percentage of patients who receive iodides chronically develop iodide goiter, it is clear that the disorder develops on a background of underlying thyroid dysfunction. Several categories of particularly susceptible patients have been identified, including those with Hashimoto's disease; those with Graves' disease, especially after treatment with radioiodine; and those with cystic fibrosis. Among these groups, many but not all patients display a positive iodide-perchlorate discharge test, indicating a defect in the thyroid organic-binding mechanism. However, intrinsic thyroid disease need not be present, since an inordinate propensity to develop iodide goiter and hypothyroidism has been demonstrated in patients who have undergone hemithyroidectomy for a solitary thyroid nodule and in whom the remaining lobe was histologically normal. In these patients, as in those with Hashimoto's disease or Graves' disease studied prospectively, patients with the highest basal serum TSH concentrations, even within the normal range, were those who developed iodide goiter.

Of particular importance is the fact that goiter and often hypothyroidism commonly occur in newborn infants of women given iodine during pregnancy, and death from neonatal asphyxia has been reported (Fig. 4–35). In such cases, the mother is usually free of goiter. Owing to the effects on the fetus, pregnant women should not be given large doses of iodine. It is not known whether iodide goiter in the newborn results from an inherent hypersensitivity of the fetal thyroid or from the fact that the placenta appears to concentrate iodide severalfold.

As was discussed in the section dealing with factors that influence thyroid hormone economy, large doses of iodine induce an acute inhibition of organic binding that in the normal individual abates, despite continued iodine administration (acute Wolff-Chaikoff effect and escape). Iodide goiter appears to result from a more pronounced inhibition of organic binding and a failure of escape to occur. As a consequence of decreased hormone synthesis, iodide transport is enhanced. Since inhibtion of organic binding is a function of the intrathyroidal concentration of iodide, a vicious circle, ultimately augmented by an increase in serum TSH concentration, is set in motion.

The disorder usually appears as a goiter with or without hypothyroidism; rarely, iodine may produce hypothyroidism unaccompanied by goiter. The disorder usually develops slowly. The thyroid is firm and diffusely enlarged, often greatly so. Histopathologic examination reveals hyperplasia that is often intense.

The laboratory indices in patients with iodide goiter are superficially confusing but in fact are entirely consistent with the physiopathology of this disorder. While iodine is being administered, the RAIU within the first few hours after radioiodine administration is often high, reflecting

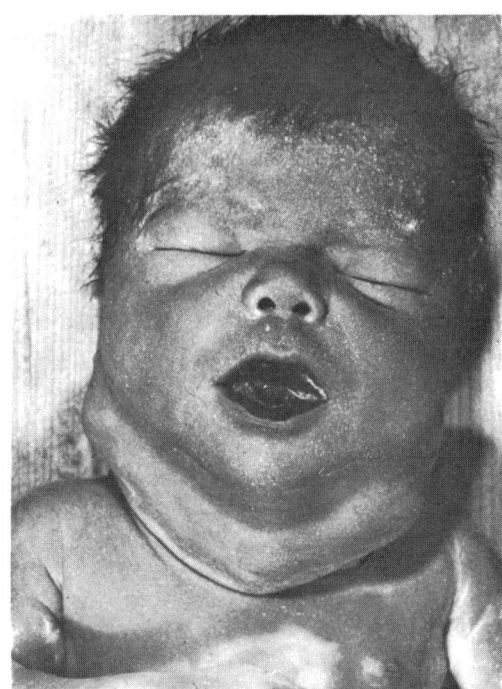

Figure 4–35. Large goiter in newborn which caused death by asphyxiation. The mother had received an iodine-containing medication for asthma during pregnancy. (From Galina, M. P., Avnet, N. L., et al.: Iodides during pregnancy. An apparent cause of neonatal death. *New Eng. J. Med.* 267:1124, 1962.)

both the large size of the thyroid and the hyperactive iodide transport mechanism. Since organic binding is inhibited, however, inorganic radioiodine is not retained and the thyroid uptake at 24 hours is subnormal. The serum TSH concentration is increased, while the serum T_4 concentration is normal or subnormal, in accord with the metabolic state of the patient. The 24-hour urinary iodine excretion and the serum inorganic iodide concentration are greatly increased.

The disorder regresses after iodine is withdrawn. Thyroid hormone may be given in addition to hasten regression. (For a more extensive discussion of iodide goiter and iodide myxedema, see Braverman, 1978.)

Defects in Hormone Biosynthesis

Genetically determined defects in hormone biosynthesis are rare but fascinating causes of goitrous hypothyroidism. Since an extensive review of this topic is available, these defects will be considered only briefly here (Stanbury, 1978). Several members of a family are usually affected. In most instances, the defect appears to be transmitted as an autosomal recessive characteristic. Individuals who display goitrous hypothyroidism are presumably homozygous for the abnormal gene, whereas euthyroid relatives with slightly enlarged thyroids are presumably heterozygous. In the latter, appropriate functional testing may disclose a milder abnormality of the same biosynthetic step that is grossly defective in the homozygous individual. In contrast to nontoxic goiter, which is many times more common in females than in males, these defects as a group affect females only slightly more commonly than males.

It is important to realize that although goiter may be present at birth, it more commonly does not appear until several years later. Therefore, the absence of goiter in a child with functioning thyroid tissue does not necessarily exclude the presence of hypothyroidism. Initially, the goiter is diffusely hyperplastic, often intensely so, suggesting papillary carcinoma; eventually, it becomes nodular. In general, the more severe the biosynthetic defect, the earlier the goiter appears, the larger it is likely to be, and the greater is the likelihood of the early emergence of manifestations of hypothyroidism. In severe cases, cretinism commonly results (sporadic goitrous cretinism).

Five specific defects in the pathways of hormone synthesis have been identified. (See Stanbury, 1978.)

Iodide Transport Defect. This defect, which is exceptionally rare, is characterized by nonfunction of the iodide transport mechanism which is specifically reflected in a very low RAIU. Impaired iodide transport is also demonstrable in other tissues, such as salivary gland and gastric mucosa, that share a similar embryologic origin with the thyroid and normally also transport iodide actively. The administration of iodine, by raising the plasma concentration of inorganic iodide, will increase the intrathyroidal concentration of iodide sufficiently to permit the production of normal quantities of hormone and will thereby cause regression of both goiter and hypothyroidism.

Organic-Binding Defect. This defect is characterized by a relative or absolute inability of the thyroid to carry out organic iodinations. The resulting goiter and enhancement of iodide transport lead to a rapid thyroid accumulation of I*, but this can be discharged almost completely by perchlorate. A milder form of this defect also occurs; when associated with nerve deafness, it is known as Pendred's syndrome. The deafness, which may either be present at birth or develop during early childhood, is not due to hypothyroidism per se, since most patients with this syndrome, though goitrous, are euthyroid.

Iodotyrosine Coupling Defect. In this defect, there appears to be an inability to couple iodotyrosines to form iodothyronines. The rate of thyroid accumulation of I* is very rapid, approaching 100% of the administered dose within the first 2 hours. Kinetic analysis reveals a very rapid turnover and recycling of thyroid iodine. Analysis of thyroid tissue in this disorder reveals little or no T_4 and T_3, most of the organic iodine being in the form of MIT and DIT. Of the several defects in hormone biosynthesis, this is the least well characterized, and indeed, some question has been raised whether the postulated abnormality truly exists.

Iodotyrosine Dehalogenase Defect. The pathogenesis of goiter and hypothyroidism in this defect is more complex than that in the other defects described. The major abnormality is an impairment of both intrathyroidal and peripheral deiodination of iodotyrosines, presumably because the enzyme is absent in these tissues. As a consequence of both intense thyroid stimulation and lack of intrathyroidal recycling of iodide derived from dehalogenation, I* is rapidly accumulated by the thyroid gland and rapidly released; labeled MIT and DIT are found in the blood and, together with their deaminated derivatives, in the urine. Hypothyroidism is presumed to result from an intense stimulation of the thyroid release mechanism, leading to the release of large quantities of MIT and DIT, together with iodine deficiency secondary to the loss of these iodotyrosines in the urine. The goiter and hypothyroidism are relieved by the administration of large doses of iodine. The most specific test for the presence of this defect is the appearance in the urine of a large proportion of unchanged MIT or DIT after their systemic administration. A milder defect of similar type is seen in some patients with nontoxic goiter and even in nongoitrous relatives of patients with the severe defect.

Abnormal Secretion of Iodoproteins. Release of abnormal iodinated proteins or polypeptides occurs in a variety of thyroid diseases, including Hashimoto's disease, benign adenomas, diffuse toxic goiter, thyroid carcinoma, and endemic goiter. In addition, release of similar compounds appears to be the sole or major physiopathologic abnormality leading to goiter with or without hypothyroidism. Goiter presumably develops because these calorigenically inactive compounds make up a major proportion of the products of hormone biosynthesis. They are collectively measured as protein-bound iodine (PBI), but not as T_4, thereby resulting in an abnormally large difference between the value for the PBI and the calculated value of the T_4-iodine; this discrepancy is the laboratory hallmark of the disorder. Reflecting the diversion of iodine into hormonally inactive iodoproteins, the RAIU is increased. Recent evidence suggests that a small quantity of similar iodoproteins is present in the serum of normal individuals. Hence the abnormality in the goitrous group appears to be quantitative rather than qualitative. In their physical properties, these compounds usually resemble serum albumin, but an iodoprotein resembling prealbumin has been described in some cases. A more extensive discussion of the nature of these iodoproteins and their relation to intrathyroidal proteins other than thyroglobulin appears in the section dealing with thyroid iodoproteins. Formation and release of these compounds are under the control of TSH, since exogenous TSH increases and exogenous thyroid hormone decreases their concentration in serum. The severity of the defect ranges from that sufficient to cause frank cretinism to that only sufficient to cause nontoxic goiter in the adult. At least in some instances the disorder is familial, but the frequency with which this is the case has not been established.

Hormone Resistance Syndromes. In addition to the foregoing biosynthetic defects, congenital hypothyroidism has been reported to result from an apparent inability of the thyroid to respond to TSH (Stanbury, 1978). Further, a rare entity of apparent resistance of the peripheral tissues to the action of thyroid hormones has been described in three members of a sibship resulting from consanguineous union (Refetoff et al., 1972). The syndrome included deaf-mutism, skeletal anomalies, goiter, and a euthyroid clinical state. The serum total and free T_4 and T_3 concentrations were increased in the presence of a detectable serum TSH concentration. Administration of large quantities of exogenous T_4 or T_3 resulted in only incomplete suppression of thyroid function, suggesting that the thyrotropes also shared in the resistance to the action of thyroid hormones. A deficiency of nuclear receptors for thyroid hormones is the probable explanation for the tissue resistance seen in these patients. The euthyroid clinical state at the time of testing reflects the adequacy of the compensatory increases in serum thyroid hormone concentrations. (For additional discussion of syndromes associated with thyroid hormone resistance, see earlier section on States Associated with Abnormal Hormone Concentrations in Blood: Miscellaneous Disorders.)

Treatment of Hypothyroidism

Treatment in the Adult

Hypothyroidism in the adult is generally one of the most gratifying diseases to treat because of the ease and completeness with which it responds to the administration of thyroid hormone. Treatment is carried out with one of two general types of preparations, either synthetic hormone or thyroprotein derived from animal thyroid glands. In the former category, sodium L-thyroxine (levothyroxine), sodium L-triiodothyronine (liothyronine), or a combination of the two (liotrix) has been employed. In the second category, thyroid extract, USP, is most commonly used. This preparation is a powder derived from dried, defatted thyroid glands that needs to be standardized only with respect to its organic iodine content (0.2%). A preparation of purified porcine thyroglobulin is also available, and its biologic activity is standardized according to its ability to inhibit propylthiouracil-induced goiter in the rat. The British Pharmacopoeia prescribes that thyroid extract be standardized according to "thyroxine" iodine content, i.e., the content of iodinated materials precipitated from a hydrolysate of the extract at pH 3.5. Some studies indicate that preparations of natural origin may vary considerably in regard to the proportion of total organic iodine present as T_4 and T_3, as well as the ratio between these hormones themselves. Consequently, variations in biologic potency may occur.

Over the years, there has been a distinct trend away from the use of the natural preparations and toward the newer synthetic preparations, in view of their uniform potency and, as a result, their more predictable effects. More recently acquired information has had a major impact upon the choice among synthetic agents. It was formerly believed that therapy with levothyroxine required the administration of doses sufficient to yield serum T_4 concentrations above the normal range, since the metabolic contribution normally provided by T_3 was felt to be lacking. This was considered a disadvantage of levothyroxine therapy in that the metabolic state of the patient and the serum T_4 concentration were thought to be partly dissociated. Indeed, liotrix was formulated with the intention of circumventing this difficulty. The recent demonstration that most of the T_3 in serum is derived from the metabolism of T_4 and, as a corollary, that serum T_3 concentrations are nearly normal in patients receiving replacement doses of T_4 has to a large extent eliminated the rationale for the use of liotrix, and has provided a rationale for the use of smaller maintenance doses of levothyroxine than formerly was the case. Disposal rates for T_4 and T_3 are considerably greater than normal when patients are given the maintenance dose of levothyroxine formerly prescribed, i.e., 300 μg daily (Braverman et al., 1973). Moreover, it has recently been shown that the oral dose of levothyroxine that abolishes the TSH response to exogenous TRH ranges from approximately 150 to 200 μg daily for most adult patients. Such a dose will result in undetectable values for serum TSH concentrations in samples obtained frequently during a 24-hour period (Hoffman et al., 1977).

Several positive advantages attend the use of levothyroxine. First, in contrast to the patient treated with liothyronine, the patient treated with levothyroxine develops a substantial peripheral pool of T_4 that turns over more slowly than does T_3 and that, therefore, provides a buffer against lapses in the ingestion of medication. Second, this pool of T_4 acts as a continuous source, thereby maintaining a constant serum T_3 concentration. This is in contrast to the recurrent peaks in serum T_3 concentration that attend the administration of thyroid extract, liotrix, or liothyronine (Surks et al., 1972). Such peaks make assessment of the proper dosage through measurement of hormone concentration extremely difficult and, moreover, may have adverse effects, especially in the older patient or in the patient with cardiac disease. This consideration accords with the experience of Smith et al. (1970), who noted a higher incidence of adverse effects with a combined T_4-T_3 preparation. In view of the foregoing, the authors believe that levothyroxine is the agent of choice in the maintenance therapy of hypothyroidism. For those who, despite the foregoing, wish to use a preparation other than levothyroxine, the approximate therapeutic equivalence of these agents when administered orally should be noted: levothyroxine, 100 μg; liothyronine, 25 μg; liotrix, 1 unit; and thyroid extract, 1 grain.

When first diagnosed, hypothyroidism is usually of long standing and seldom requires prompt reversal. Consequently, although a few authorities may disagree, the consensus is that the restoration of a normal metabolic state should be undertaken gradually. The untreated patient with hypothyroidism is inordinately sensitive to small doses of thyroid hormone. The initial daily dose, therefore, should not exceed 50 μg of levothyroxine, and often it is judicious to use even less. Caution is of paramount importance in the hypothyroid patient with heart disease and in the patient with severe long-standing hypothyroidism, because overenthusiastic treatment may precipitate heart failure or myocardial infarction in the former, or may provoke relative adrenocortical insufficiency in the latter. In these instances, an initial daily dose of 12.5 or 25 μg of levothyroxine is recommended. Thereafter, the daily dose is increased by increments of 25 or 50 μg at 2- to 3-week intervals until a normal metabolic state is attained. The final maintenance dose required is in the range of 2.2 to 2.5 μg/kg body weight, or about 150 μg daily.

The interval between the initiation of treatment and the appearance of the first evidences of improvement depends upon the size of the dose given. An early clinical evidence of response is the occurrence of diuresis, and this is accompanied by loss of weight and some regression of puffiness. Even earlier, the serum Na^+ increases if hyponatremia was present initially. Thereafter, pulse rate and pulse pressure increase; appetite improves, and constipation may disappear. Psychomotor activity increases, and the delay in the deep tendon jerks disappears. Hoarseness abates slowly, and the changes in the skin and hair generally require several months to disappear.

It is not always easy to define the optimal maintenance dose of thyroid hormone for the individual patient. The clinical state of the patient is generally the best means of determining when a satisfactory dose has been achieved. Nevertheless, even when the patient appears metabolically normal, a small increase in the dose may produce still further improvement without producing thyrotoxicosis. There is a tendency among physicians to rely too heavily upon the serum T_4 concentration as an indicator of the adequacy of treatment. This is true for several reasons. First, the normal range of the serum T_4 concentration is quite wide, and in the individual patient encompasses rather wide variations in the metabolic state. Second, in the case of levothyroxine, there are pronounced discrepancies in the literature concerning the level of serum T_4 concentration that is maintained by the smaller doses (150–200 μg) currently employed. All earlier studies at this dosage level indicated that serum T_4 concentrations were rarely above normal. (See Hoffman et al., 1977, for references.) However, recent studies in the author's laboratory, in which three separate assays were employed, have revealed wide variations in the serum T_4 concentration, values above the normal range being found in more than half of patients receiving levothyroxine at this dose level (Ingbar, J.C., in press). In the latter patients, the serum T_3 concentration appeared to correlate better with the metabolic state than the serum T4 concentration did, and indeed may be a better means of confirming adequacy of treatment.

A recent study has suggested that systolic time intervals obtained noninvasively by simultaneous recording of the ECG, phonocardiogram, and carotid pulse tracing may be very helpful in defining the optimal maintenance dose in the individual patient (Crowley et al., 1977). In the hypothyroid state, the preejection period (PEP) is prolonged, and the ratio of PEP to left ventricular ejection time (PEP/LVET) is increased. With progressive increments in dosage, PEP progressively shortens and the PEP/LVET decreases. Normal ranges for these indices have been established, and transition from the normal to hypermetabolic state is attended by further changes. Thus, systolic time intervals can serve as a means for objective monitoring of the metabolic response to replacement therapy. This aspect of management is of particular importance in the elderly patient with cardiac disease, in whom even slight excess of hormone must be avoided.

Several other interesting features attend the treatment of hypothyroidism. In contrast to what might be expected, there is no evidence that the requisite maintenance dose of thyroid hormone undergoes seasonal variation. In addition, patients with hypothyroidism display a great propensity to discontinue their medication when they are feeling better or when their supply of hormone is exhausted; this occurs even when the patient has been informed that treatment is required indefinitely. In this way, a single patient with myxedema may serve to familiarize successive groups of medical students with the features of this disease. A final feature of great interest is the fact that, in the usual patient with myxedema, manifestations of thyrotoxicosis are readily induced by doses of thyroid hormone only slightly in excess of those that provide optimal maintenance. This is in contrast to the relatively large doses of hormone that are required to induce thyrotoxicosis in the usual normal individual. The factors underlying this difference are unknown.

Restoration of a normal metabolic state, although the specific objective in treating hypothyroidism, is sometimes accompanied by adverse effects. These include production or aggravation of angina pectoris, heart failure, or, rarely, severe psychiatric disturbance. In such instances, the more general objective of therapy enunciated by Means should be sought, i.e., the maximal metabolic restoration consistent with the well-being of the patient.

Besides myxedema coma, which is discussed later, there are a few instances in which it seems mandatory to alleviate hypothyroidism rapidly. Inordinate sensitivity to CNS depressants and lack of sensitivity to pressor amines make the patient with hypothyroidism a very poor operative risk. In addition, such patients withstand acute infections poorly and may descend rapidly into myxedema coma as a result. Consequently, in these circumstances, rapid repletion of the peripheral hormone pool is necessary. This can be accomplished by a single intravenous dose of 500 μg of levothyroxine in the average adult. Alternatively, by virtue of its rapid onset of action, liothyronine can be used if the patient is able to take medication by mouth, as an intravenous preparation is not available. This is administered orally in a dose of 25 μg every 6 hours. With both regimens, the initial effect is achieved within several hours. Oral therapy with levothyroxine is instituted as soon as possible, as outlined earlier. Because of the possibility that acute increases in metabolic rate will overtax existing pituitary-adrenocortical reserve, supplemental glucocorticoid should be administered. Finally, in view of the tendency of hypothyroid patients to retain water, vigorous hydration with hypotonic or isotonic fluids should be avoided.

When hypothyroidism results from the administration of iodine or drugs with antithyroid activity, withdrawal of the offending agent will usually suffice to relieve both the hypothyroidism and the accompanying goiter.

Treatment in the Infant and Child

In the cretin, the critical factor determining eventual intellectual attainment is the age at which adequate treatment with thyroid hormone was begun. In general, if severe hypothyroidism did not begin *in utero,* the chances of normal intellectual development are good if vigorous treatment is begun before the age of 4 months. By contrast, normal physical development may occur even when treatment is begun later in infancy with doses of thyroid hormone that are inadequate for normal intellectual development. Thus, in assessing the response to treatment in infancy, it is essential that attention be paid to the ages at which the various milestones of development are attained. Because of its uniform potency, levothyroxine is the thyroid hormone preparation of choice. On a unit weight basis, infants and children require larger doses than do adults. Kinetically, this is reflected in a more rapid fractional rate of turnover of T_4. Treatment is begun with a daily dose of 25 μg of levothyroxine, and this is increased by increments of 25 μg at 1-week intervals, so that the infant will be receiving a daily dose of 100 μg after 3–4 weeks. Thereafter, the daily dose of levothyroxine is increased slowly so as to maintain the serum T_4 concentration between 9 and 12 μg/100 ml.; however, if the clinical response is unsatisfactory, even larger doses are administered. In the infant, intellectual development is the crucial guide to the adequacy of the treatment; it is better to give too much than too little hormone. In the older child, the rate of skeletal growth and maturation and the time of dental eruption and sexual maturation are important guidelines in treatment. Two recent studies have evaluated the dose of levothyroxine that will normalize serum TSH concentration and maintain normal growth rates in hypothyroid children ranging in age from 1 year to the mid-teens (Abassi and Aldige, 1977; Rezvani and DiGeorge, 1977). The dosages obtained in the two studies were very similar, averaging 3.5 μg/kg body weight daily in the one study and 3.8 μg daily in the other.

Special Aspects of Hypothyroidism

Mild Hypothyroidism, Metabolic Insufficiency, and Decreased Thyroid Reserve

The problem of mild hypothyroidism is one that has long vexed both the physician and the clinical physiologist. Until recently, it was uncertain that such a clinical state did in fact occur; this is now accepted. It is highly probable that the greatest proportion of thyroid hormone therapy administered in the United States is used in treating what is thought to be a mild rather than severe thyroid insufficiency. As will become evident, it is the authors' view that, in most instances, the disorders being treated are not truly thyroidal in origin or at least have not been conclusively shown to be so. From the evolution of hypothyroidism in patients with Hashimoto's disease or progressive thyroprivic hypothyroidism, the clinical picture resulting from clearly demonstrable but incomplete thyroid hormone deficiency can be derived. Symptoms include mild lassitude, fatigue, slight anemia, constipation, apathy, slight cold intolerance, menstrual irregularities, inability to conceive, dry skin, some loss of hair, and slight to moderate weight gain. These symptoms, however, are not pathognomonic of hypothyroidism since they also occur either singly or in varying combinations in other disorders of organic or psychogenic origin.

Many patients with such complaints have been treated with thyroid hormones. Frequently, adequate laboratory documentation of thyroid hormone deficiency is lacking, or at most, a moderately low BMR is demonstrable. The response to thyroid hormone therapy is sometimes gratifying, at least initially, but often symptomatic improvement disappears after a time, unless the dose is increased. In this way, the total dosage progressively increases until the amounts given exceed those required for complete hormone replacement in frank myxedema. Eventually, even such large doses may fail to alleviate the symptoms. This alone suggests that the symptoms do not arise from deficiency of thyroid hormone. Some patients report that omission of a single dose of thyroid hormone results in a rapid emergence (often within hours) of the previous symptoms and that these are equally rapidly relieved by a single dose. These responses are inconsistent with the time of onset and duration of action of thyroid hormones.

Despite the foregoing, it is clear that true mild hypothyroidism resulting from partial failure of T_4 secretion does exist. In such instances, a variety of adaptations occur. The first is an increase in serum TSH concentration, which stimulates the flagging thyroid and may permit maintenance of a serum T_4 concentration within the normal range. Some slight increase in T_3 secretion may also occur, so that the T_3/T_4 concentration ratio in serum is slightly increased. This combination of findings, whose hallmark is a slightly or moderately elevated serum TSH concentration, has been termed "subclinical hypothyroidism." It is seen most commonly in patients with Hashimoto's disease and those who have been treated for diffuse toxic goiter with ^{131}I or surgery; the remaining patients are presumed to be in an early stage of primary thyroprivic hypothyroidism. There has been much discussion, but no resolution. of the question whether or not patients with these findings are somewhat hypothyroid and whether or not they require replacement therapy. One view suggests that the patients are indeed hypothyroid since, if serum hormone concentrations were really normal, the serum TSH concentration would not remain increased. The other view suggests that the patients are fully compensated and metabolically normal, but only because the thyroid is being stimulated to an abnormal extent. The point is moot, since almost always the patient's true normal serum T_4 and T_3 concentrations are not known, and since objective means of evaluating the inadequacy or sufficiency of thyroid hormone supplies are not available. Although patients with subclinical hypothyroidism do not necessarily progress rapidly to frank hypothyroidism, it is the authors' bias to treat them with replacement doses of thyroid hormone, since the elevated TSH provides clear evidence that the thyroid is failing.

In some patients with more severe thyroid failure, enhanced TSH secretion may not be capable of restoring a normal rate of T_4 secretion, but does greatly enhance the secretion of T_3. Here, the serum T_4 concentration is depressed, the serum T_3 concentration normal or nearly so, and the apparent metabolic state of the patient normal. Despite the latter, the authors believe that these patients should receive treatment, for the reasons just discussed.

Not infrequently, the physician is confronted with a patient in whom the diagnosis of hypothyroidism, often mild, has already been made, and the patient has been given replacement therapy. In this circumstance, it is impossible to determine from the clinical or laboratory findings whether thyroid hormone replacement is truly required, since a normal thyroid would have been suppressed. Often, a strong indication that the patient is not truly hypothyroid can be obtained from the nature of his initial complaints or from peculiarities in the response to treatment, as already described. The best means of assessing whether replacement therapy is required is to withdraw thyroid hormone and determine serum T_4 and TSH concentrations approximately 6 weeks later. This latter period is based on two recent studies of the pattern of recovery following withdrawal of prolonged replacement therapy in patients with an intrinsically normal hypothalamic-pituitary-thyroid complex (Vagenakis et al., 1975; Krugman et al., 1975). During the first week or two following withdrawal, TSH is undetectable in serum and is unresponsive to TRH, despite a decline of serum T_4 and T_3 concentrations to subnormal values. Over the ensuing 2–3 weeks, serum TSH becomes detectable, responsiveness to TRH returns, and serum T_4 and T_3 concentrations return progressively to normal. This pattern of recovery suggests that prolonged replacement therapy results in depletion of pituitary TSH which is reversible when therapy is withdrawn.

Myxedema Coma

Myxedema coma is the ultimate stage of severe longstanding hypothyroidism in which mental obtundation and physiologic retardation are profound. This state, which invariably affects the elderly patient, occurs most commonly during the winter months and is associated with a very high mortality rate. It is usually, but not always, accompanied by a subnormal temperature, values as low as 23.3° C having been recorded. Since the ordinary clinical thermometer is graduated only to 32.4 or 34.5° C, and since a nurse may fail to shake down the mercury below 37° C the true depth of the hypothermia may not be appreciated. The external manifestations of severe myxedema, as well as bradycardia and severe hypotension, are invariably present. The characteristic delay in the deep tendon jerks may be lacking since the patient is often areflexic. Epileptic fits may accompany the comatose state (Jellinek, 1962).

Although the pathogenesis of myxedema coma is not known, several factors predispose to its development. Prominent among these are exposure to cold, infection, trauma, and CNS depressants. Alveolar hypoventilation, leading to carbon dioxide retention and narcosis, and dilutional hyponatremia resembling that seen during in appropriate secretion of antidiuretic hormone are common accompaniments of myxedema coma and may contribute importantly to the clinical state.

From the foregoing, it appears that the diagnosis of myxedema coma should be obvious. Nevertheless, this is not the case. Elderly patients may resemble patients with myxedema, and after a brainstem infarction, they may be both comatose and hypothermic. In addition, hypothermia of any cause, most commonly exposure of the elderly to cold, may induce physiologic alterations suggestive of myxedema, including a delay in the relaxation of the deep tendon reflexes. The importance of this difficulty in diagnosing myxedema coma is that a delay in therapy greatly worsens the prognosis. Consequently the diagnosis should be made on clinical grounds and therapy initiated without awaiting the results of confirmatory tests, such as the serum T_4 concentration.

The treatment of myxedema coma consists of the administration of thyroid hormone and of attempts to correct the associated physiologic disturbances. Because of the exceedingly sluggish circulation and severe hypometabolism, absorption of therapeutic agents from the gut or from subcutaneous or intramuscular sites is unpredictable; hence, all medications should be administered intravenously if possible. Thyroid hormone is best given as a single intravenous dose of 500 μg of levothyroxine. This serves to rapidly replete the peripheral hormone pool and is often followed by some improvement within several hours. Hydrocortisone (100 mg daily) should also be administered because of the likelihood of associated adrenocortical insufficiency, especially as the metabolic rate increases. Intravenous fluids should be administered cautiously because of the danger of water intoxication. Hypertonic saline and glucose may be required to alleviate severe dilutional hyponatremia and the occasional hypoglycemia. A critical element in therapy is support of respiratory function by means of assisted ventilation and controlled oxygen administration. External warming should be avoided since it may lead to vascular collapse, but further heat loss should be prevented. An increase in temperature is seen within 24 hours in response to levothyroxine. General measures applicable to the comatose patient, such as frequent turning, prevention of aspiration, and attention to fecal impaction and urinary retention, should be undertaken. Finally, the physician should be alert to the presence of coexisting disease, such as infection and cardiac or cerebrovascular disease. Ideally, the management of the patient with myxedema coma should be undertaken in an intensive care unit. As soon as the patient is able to take medication by mouth, treatment with oral levothyroxine should be instituted.

Although myxedema coma has carried a uniformly poor prognosis, survivals have been achieved with the therapeutic regimen outlined above. (See Royce, 1971, for an excellent review of myxedema coma.)

SIMPLE OR NONTOXIC GOITER: DIFFUSE AND MULTINODULAR

Simple or nontoxic goiter may be defined as any thyroid enlargement that is not associated with thyrotoxicosis or hypothyroidism and does not result from an inflammatory or neoplastic process. The term is usually restricted to that form which occurs sporadically, i.e, in nonendemic regions.

Pathogenesis and Pathophysiology

It is generally agreed that nontoxic goiter represents a compensatory response to any of a variety of factors that impair the efficiency of the thyroid in manufacturing adequate quantities of hormone. It had been thought that when such factors are operative, hypersecretion of TSH results, leading to a stimulation of thyroid growth and an increase in the activity of processes concerned with hormone biosynthesis that are capable of response. As a consequence of the resulting increases in thyroid mass and unit functional activity, a normal rate of hormone secretion is restored, and the patient is eumetabolic but goitrous. Thus, this disorder differs only in degree from goitrous hypothyroidism and can be presumed to result from the same specific etiologic factors. These have been discussed in the previous section.

This concept of the pathogenesis of nontoxic goiter is not supported, however, by several studies which have demonstrated that the serum TSH concentration is not increased in the majority of patients with nontoxic goiter (see Dige-Petersen and Hummer, 1977). Nonetheless, some participatory role of TSH in the maintenance of goiter is indicated by the regression of goiter that sometimes follows the administration of suppressive doses of thyroid hormone. Several

possible mechanisms may serve to accommodate these seemingly divergent findings. Of these, the one having the greatest experimental support derives from the observation that in hypophysectomized rats the response of thyroid weight to standard doses of TSH is augmented by prior thyroid iodine depletion (Bray, 1968). Hence, any factor that impairs normal iodine usage may lead to gradual development of goiter in response to normal concentrations of TSH. A second possibility is that the increase in serum TSH concentration is small and therefore not readily detected by the RIA methods that are generally available. A third possibility is that the nocturnal surge of TSH secretion is greater in patients with nontoxic goiter than in normal subjects and that this serves to maintain goiter, but data concerning this point are lacking. Finally, it may be that the primary goitrogenic stimulus is no longer present at the time of study, and that the residual normal TSH concentration is responsible for the maintenance of, but not the initiation, of the goiter.

Owing to the fact that the functional disturbance is milder than in goitrous hypothyroidism, the role of some contributory factors is more clearly evident. Prominent among these is the striking female sex preponderance (7–9:1). By contrast, as might be expected, the role of heredity is less readily apparent, although it is evident in some families and in large statistical studies. Owing to its more subtle nature, the functional defect is more difficult to define, and vigorous efforts directed at its elucidation are not justified. Although mild degrees of iodine deficiency can be readily detected, this is rarely a cause of sporadic nontoxic goiter in most areas of the world. In some areas of the world, dietary goitrogens have been implicated; in the remainder, the precise etiology is obscure but presumably resides in biosynthetic defects within the thyroid. Recent work has demonstrated that the majority of patients with sporadic nontoxic goiter have increased thyroglobulin concentrations and T_3:T_4 concentration ratios in serum (Pezzino et al., 1978). These abnormalities do not correlate with goiter size, serum TSH concentration, or urinary iodine excretion, and probably reflect defective iodination of thyroglobulin.

Nontoxic goiter seems to occur more commonly during adolescence or pregnancy. The pathogenetic relationship of these events to the development of goiter is unknown. In some patients, the goiter that appears at these times later regresses; in others, the goiter persists. Patients often have the impression that their thyroid enlarges during times of emotional stress or during the menses, but this is not well documented. During prolonged follow-up by the authors of a group of patients with nontoxic adolescent goiter, diffuse toxic goiter has supervened with an inordinately high frequency, in some cases even when suppressive doses of thyroid hormone were being administered. This suggests that some varieties of nontoxic diffuse goiter may be precursors of Graves' disease.

The evolution of the late multinodular form of nontoxic goiter from its earlier diffuse stage is similar to that described for endemic goiter. Once multinodular goiter has developed, patients often display evidence of thyroid functional autonomy, such as subnormal or absent TSH responsiveness to TRH (Dige-Petersen and Hummer, 1977). In such patients, thyrotoxicosis may develop spontaneously (toxic multinodular goiter) or may be induced by exposure to large quantities of iodine (Jod-Basedow phenomenon). In view of the latter, patients with nontoxic multinodular goiter should not be given medications that contain iodine and should be carefully observed after radiologic procedures that involve administration of iodinated contrast media.

Histopathology

The histopathologic evolution of nontoxic goiter from its initial diffuse form to its late multinodular stage is similar to that described for endemic goiter in the preceding section (Fig. 4–36).

Clinical Picture

The clinical features of nontoxic goiter are those that result from thyroid enlargement. Most commonly, the effect either is merely disfiguring or is felt as a tightening of garments worn about the neck. With larger goiters displacement or compression of the esophagus or trachea may occur, leading to dysphagia, a choking sensation, and inspiratory stridor. Narrowing of the thoracic inlet may compromise the venous return from the head, neck, and upper limbs sufficiently to produce venous engorgement. This obstruction is accentuated when the patient's arms are raised (Pemberton's sign); dizziness and even syncope may result. Compression of the recurrent laryngeal nerve leading to hoarseness suggests carcinoma rather than nontoxic goiter. Hemorrhage into a nodule or cyst produces acute, painful enlargement locally and, if crucially situated, can enhance or induce obstructive symptoms.

Laboratory Tests

In patients with nontoxic goiter, serum T_4 and T_3 concentrations are within the normal range, but the $T_3{:}T_4$ ratio is often increased, perhaps reflecting defective iodination of thyroglobulin. Serum thyroglobulin concentrations are increased in the majority of patients (Pezzino et al., 1978). The RAIU is usually normal, but in some patients may be increased, owing to either mild iodine deficiency or a biosynthetic defect. In patients with long-standing multinodular goiter, functional autonomy may develop and this would be reflected in diminished or absent responsiveness of the serum TSH concentration to TRH.

Differential Diagnosis

The differential diagnosis of nontoxic goiter can be considered from both functional and anatomic aspects. As indicated earlier, the same factors that lead to goitrous hypothyroidism can, if less severe, cause nontoxic goiter; consequently some patients with nontoxic goiter prove to be slightly hypothyroid. On the other hand, when multinodularity has developed, foci of autonomous function may appear. Consequently, in multinodular goiter, the spectrum of function can range from clinical euthyroidism with intact regulatory control, through clinical euthyroidism with some degree of functional autonomy, to frank thyrotoxicosis (toxic multinodular goiter).

From the anatomic standpoint, the diffuse stage of nontoxic goiter resembles most closely the thyroid of either Graves' disease or Hashimoto's disease. If the Graves' disease is not in an actively thyrotoxic phase and if the ocular manifestations are lacking, there is no way to differentiate the two disorders, save for demonstrating the presence of Graves'-specific IgG in the serum. Diffuse nontoxic goiter is sometimes difficult to differentiate from Hashimoto's disease. Functional patterns in the two may be quite similar. The thyroid of Hashimoto's disease is usually more firm, and its margins and surface are more irregular, but this is not invariably the case. Demonstration of high titers of antithyroid antibodies would indicate, however, the presence of Hashimoto's disease.

In its multinodular stage, nontoxic goiter may suggest the presence of thyroid carcinoma. The approach to differentiating between the two is discussed in the section dealing with thyroid neoplasms.

Treatment

Treatment of nontoxic goiter is directed at removing the stimulus to thyroid hyperplasia. This can be accomplished either by alleviating an external restraint to hormone formation or by supplying sufficient quantities of exogenous hormone to inhibit secretion of TSH, thereby putting the thyroid at rest. In the occasional instance, withdrawal of a pharmacologic goitrogen will suffice. Since iodine deficiency is not a common causative factor, at least in the United States, administration of iodine is generally ineffective, and its use is to be deplored in view of its demonstrated ability to induce thyrotoxicosis. As the etiology of the goiter is usually obscure, suppressive therapy with thyroid hormone is the treatment of choice, since its action is independent of the origin of the goiter. Successful therapy requires that doses of hormone sufficient to produce a maximal state of thyroid inactivity be given.

In the early stage of nontoxic goiter, before nodule formation has taken place, the requisite dose of thyroid hormone is easy to determine, and the response to treatment is generally good. Most patients with diffuse goiter are relatively young, so that adverse effects of suppressive therapy are unlikely to occur. Here, treatment can be initiated with 100 μg of levothyroxine daily, and the dosage increased by 50 μg daily at 2- or 3-week intervals to a maximum of 150 μg

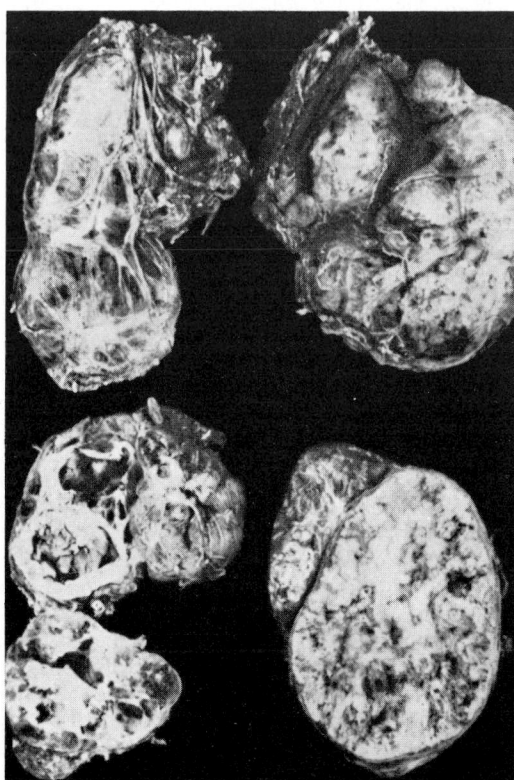

Figure 4–36. Outer and cut surface of a nontoxic nodular goiter observed by patient for 15 years. Note variations in size and structure of the nodules; there are thick areas of fibrous tissue, flecks of calcium, scattered areas of thyroid tissue, cysts, and small hemorrhages.

or 200 μg daily. Completeness of thyroid suppression can be verified by measurement of the RAIU, which should have decreased to a value of less than 5%. If complete thyroid suppression has not been obtained, it is often useful to perform a thyroid scintiscan, which may then reveal an impalpable focus of autonomous function.

The problem is somewhat more complicated in the patient with nodular nontoxic goiter, who tends, therefore, to be older and more susceptible to adverse effects of thyroid hormone excess. As an initial approach to the problem, all patients with nodular nontoxic goiter should undergo a thyroid scintiscan prior to treatment. This may reveal major or minor areas of disproportionately intense isotope accumulation, which often prove to be functionally autonomous. In most cases, the thyroid contains areas of TSH-supported, and hence suppressible, function intermixed with areas of functional autonomy. Unless the latter are strongly dominant, it is unlikely that suppressive doses of exogenous hormone will induce thyrotoxicosis, and treatment can be cautiously instituted. Two or three weeks after a maximal dose of 150 μg of levothyroxine has been achieved, the RAIU is measured again and, if suppression is complete, treatment continued. If complete suppression is not obtained, the scintiscan is repeated. Such "suppressions scans" will often reveal well-defined areas of autonomous function, cleared of the background previously created by areas of suppressible function. Evaluation of the clinical state at this time will permit a decision whether suppressive therapy should be continued. Whether or not it is, patients with major autonomous foci should be carefully observed for emergence of thyrotoxicosis, and exposure to large quantities of iodine avoided lest Jod-Basedow be induced.

In elderly patients with multinodular goiter or those with cardiovascular disease, particularly if the original scintiscan suggests predominance of autonomous foci, it may be hazardous to administer suppressive doses of thyroid hormone. In such cases, definitive evidence of either predominant functional autonomy or normal regulatory control should be sought by means of a TRH stimulation test. Lack of response to TRH will indicate that functional autonomy is complete or nearly so and that suppressive therapy should be avoided. To the contrary, ablation with ^{131}I should be considered as a means of eradicating autonomous foci and forestalling the likelihood of future thyrotoxicosis. In those patients, in contrast, in whom the TRH test indicates normal regulatory control, benefit may be obtained from suppressive therapy. Here, the initial dose of levothyroxine should not exceed 50 μg daily and increments should be undertaken gradually, partial rather than complete suppression of TSH secretion being the end-point. This can be ascertained by assuring that some TSH responsiveness to TRH is retained, and that generally requires that the dose of levothyroxine not exceed 150 μg daily.

Considerable variation is present in the reported results of suppressive therapy. In some clinics very favorable results are obtained, complete regression having been reported in 33% of diffuse and 24% of multinodular nontoxic goiters. Partial regression was noted in 34% of diffuse and over 50% of multinodular goiters (Astwood et al., 1960). Unfortunately, the experience of the present authors and others has not been as favorable. The diffuse form generally responds well, particularly when cases with Hashimoto's disease are excluded. In the multinodular stage, there is most commonly some decrease in overall thyroid size and occasionally in the size of individual nodules. Generally, however, regression of thyroid enlargement leaves most nodules unchanged or more prominent than they were before. Hence in the authors' view, the rationale for thyroid therapy in multinodular nontoxic goiter is to prevent further extension rather than to cause reversion of the pathologic process. By decreasing vascularity, suppressive therapy may also reduce the risk of hemorrhage. Furthermore, when symptoms of pressure are present, even a small decrease in thyroid size may afford relief. It is not known whether suppressive therapy forestalls the subsequent development of hyperfunction leading to thyrotoxicity in the multinodular nontoxic gland.

It is impossible to predict whether, as is sometimes the case, regression of goiter will persist if suppression is withdrawn; few if any data concerning this point are available. If, however, recurrence takes place, suppressive therapy should be reinstituted and continued indefinitely.

Surgery of simple nontoxic goiter is physiologically unsound, since it further restricts the ability of the thyroid to meet hormone requirements. Nevertheless, surgery may become necessary because of persistence of obstructive symptoms despite a trial of exogenous thyroid hormone. As discussed in the section dealing with thyroid neoplasms, surgery is sometimes indicated because a carcinoma is thought to be present in a multinodular goiter. It should never be performed for prophylaxis of carcinoma, however. In view of the physiopathology, surgery should always be followed by full replacement therapy with thyroid hormone in order to inhibit regrowth of the goiter.

THYROID NEOPLASMS

The subject of thyroid neoplasms is one that has received attention far beyond its importance as a cause of morbidity in the general population. As of the early 1970s, the incidence of thyroid cancer was estimated to be about 36 new cases per million population per year and the death rate only 9 per million per year. There are, however, several reasons why the diagnosis and management have been a focus for much concern. To begin with, thyroid cancer usually presents as an asymptomatic thyroid nodule in a euthyroid patient, and nontoxic nodular goiter is an extremely common disorder among the adult population of the United States, especially women. Estimates place its prevalence, as judged from clinical examination, at about 4%. (See Vander et al., 1968.) This, too, would pose no problem were it not for the fact that nodularity of the thyroid is an extremely nonspecific manifestation of a variety of thyroid diseases with widely differing implications for the patient's ultimate well-being. Further, in the absence of a histologic specimen, there is no means of differentiating benign from malignant nodules, and, until recently, that is, until the widespread acceptance of needle biopsy, this usually required the open surgery of excisional biopsy. Nonetheless, clinical criteria for the suspicion of malignancy have been sufficiently good, and selection of patients for surgery sufficiently reliable (Shimaoka et al., 1962), that surgical series have been biased to reveal a frequency of thyroid cancer in patients operated on that is higher than that present in the entire population of patients with nodular thyroids. Finally, the frequency of thyroid cancer has increased, probably by about 50% in 25 years, doubtless owing in large measure to the emergence of thyroid cancer after a long latent period and resulting from prior x-irradiation of the head and neck areas for a variety of reasons (see later).

The proper diagnosis and management of thyroid cancer, once diagnosed, has also been a controversial subject (and remains so to this time) because of wide variations in the biologic behavior of the tumors, some being extremely non-aggressive; because excisional biopsy, though required for diagnosis, was inherently a therapeutic measure; and because there was not available a sufficiently large series of patients with various thyroid tumors treated in differing ways to permit an analysis of the optimal mode of therapy for each. Thus, the vast literature that accumulated on this subject reflected not an abundant knowledge, but a considerable ignorance in this area. Fortunately, many of the problems cited above are undergoing resolution, so that the topic is less vexing than it formerly was. The authors' approach to the diagnosis and management of the nodular thyroid gland will be presented later in this section. First, it is necessary to consider the characteristics of that variety of thyroid nodule of greatest concern, the thyroid neoplasm.

Benign Neoplasms

Benign neoplasms of the thyroid gland are termed adenomas. The problem of their intrinsic causation and the biologic properties that cause their behavior to differ from that of normal tissue, on the one hand, or that of malignant neoplasms, on the other, are unknown but represent basic questions in oncology. Nevertheless, adenomas have the properties of being well encapsulated, of not invading adjacent tissues or metastasizing to noncontiguous areas, of displaying few mitoses, and, in the case of endocrine adenomas, of being at least relatively free of the usualy homeostatic restraints on growth and function. The most clear-cut lesions of the thyroid that display these properties are those that arise in glands that are otherwise entirely normal. Much of the confusion concerning thyroid nodules arises from the fact that lesions that are anatomically similar or identical (differing architecturally from surrounding tissue and separated therefrom by fibrous tissue) are found in the late stage of nontoxic multinodular goiter. Because of this similarity, they are often termed adenomas, and the disorder itself is termed *adenomatous goiter*. In most instances, it is not known whether these are true adenomas in the basic biologic sense and whether they arise *de novo* or as a consequence of the hyperplastic stimulus that is thought to underlie the pathogenesis of nontoxic goiter. Lacking such basic biologic criteria, the authors feel that the term adenoma, be it in a normal or an otherwise diseased gland, should be applied to lesions that display the anatomical properties just described, together with evidence of some degree of autonomy of growth and function. A further source of confusion, on the other hand, is the fact that, in the case of thyroid neoplasms, the architecture of benign and malignant lesions may be so similar that even careful histopathologic examination fails to reveal local evidence of malignancy, although the tumor displays evidence of malignancy by its clinical course. Finally, as is the case with neoplasms in other organs, it is uncertain whether benign neoplasms of the thyroid gland ever undergo malignant transformation.

The clearly defined benign neoplasms of the thyroid can be classified according to their histopathologic characteristics.

Histopathology (Fig. 4–37)

Embryonal Adenoma. Here, the histopathologic appearance resembles that of the embryonic thyroid prior to the development of follicles in that the cells are closely packed, forming a cordlike or trabecular pattern. For this reason, the lesion is sometimes termed a *trabecular adenoma*.

Fetal Adenoma. This lesion is characterized by an architecture that resembles the fetal thyroid in its stage of early follicle formation. The cells are arranged in a tubular pattern, but colloid is scant or absent.

Microfollicular Adenoma. This lesion is composed of small, closely packed follicles lined by a cuboidal epithelium and containing little colloid.

Macrofollicular Adenoma. Here well-formed follicles are present. These are usually large, well filled with colloid, and lined by a flat epithelium. Small follicles and areas of epithelial hyperplasia are often present. Another term applied to this lesion is *colloid adenoma*.

Papillary Cystadenoma. This lesion, although classified as an adenoma, is typically unencapsulated, merges into the adjacent tissue, and often cannot be distinguished on histopathologic grounds from low-grade papillary carcinoma. It is composed of columnar epithelium that is thrown into folds, forming papillary projections with connective tissue stalks and cystlike cavities. Follicular elements may be present to a varying degree.

Hürthle Cell Adenoma. This rare lesion is composed of large, pale, acidophilic cells that are usually arranged in a trabecular pattern.

The foregoing classification suggests that adenomas are uniform in structure, but in fact their architecture is often variegated; macrofollicular, microfollicular, and fetal elements are often found in the same lesion. In addition, multiple adenomas of differing histopathologic types are not infrequently present in the same gland, often in opposite lobes.

Clinical Picture and Laboratory Tests

The chief importance of thyroid adenomas lies in the need to differentiate them from carcinoma and in their ability in some instances to produce sufficient hormone to suppress the remaining thyroid tissue and induce a thyrotoxic state. The former problem is discussed later in this section in that part dealing with the management of the nodular thyroid gland, and the latter problem has been presented in the earlier section dealing with disorders that lead to thyrotoxicosis. However, some other features of thyroid adenomas merit consideration. The majority are predominantly follicular in type and are able to accumulate and retain radioactive iodine, a feature that aids in distinguishing them from most carcinomas. Functioning adenomas may retain their ability to respond to TSH but, as indicated earlier, are not dependent upon TSH for maintenance of their function. Such lesions tend to secrete abnormal iodoproteins that increase the serum PBI, causing the difference between the PBI and T_4-iodine concentration to widen. They are also prone to secrete T_3 in abnormally high proportion to T_4 and may be the source of T_3-toxicosis.

In general, adenomas grow slowly and produce no symptoms. When less than 1 cm in diameter, they are generally not palpable, but as they become larger they are likely to be noted as a lump in the neck. Not infrequently, however, they are the site of local hemorrhage that leads to acute painful enlargement, mimicking subacute thyroiditis. Resolution of the hemorrhage is often followed by loss of function and by development of either a cyst or a nodule of very

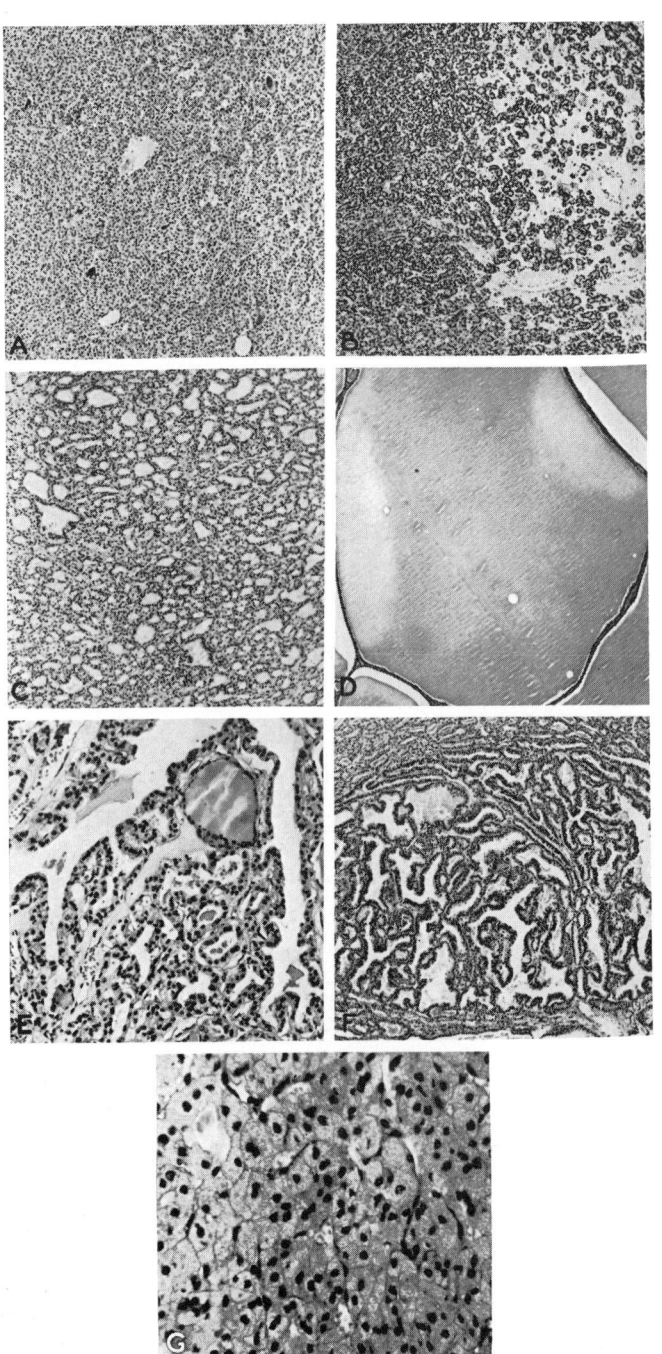

Figure 4–37. Thyroid adenomas. *A*, Embryonal (×80). *B*, Fetal (×80). *C*, Microfollicular (×80). *D*, Macrofollicular (×60). *E* and *F*, Papillary cystadenomas (×40). *G*, Hürthle cell (×450).

firm consistency that may be mistaken for carcinoma. Together with thyroid cysts, degenerated adenomas comprise the majority of nonfunctioning nodules of the thyroid.

Malignant Neoplasms

Virtually all malignant neoplasms of the thyroid are epithelial in origin and hence are carcinomas. Of these, two general types occur, those arising from follicular epithelium and, less often, those arising from parafollicular (C-cell) elements. Rarely, the thyroid is the seat of a metastatic deposit or of a fibrosarcoma or lymphosarcoma, both of which are highly malignant. Metastases of extrathyroid

cancers to the thyroid are probably more common than is usually appreciated and occasionally present a problem in diagnosis (Pillay et al., 1977).

Carcinoma of Follicular Epithelium: Histopathology and Clinical Features

A variety of classifications have been proposed, but the one most commonly used is that of Woolner and associates (1961). This classification demarcates three categories of carcinoma of follicular origin: papillary, follicular, and anaplastic (Fig. 4–38). A fourth category, that of medullary carcinoma with amyloid stroma, is discussed separately

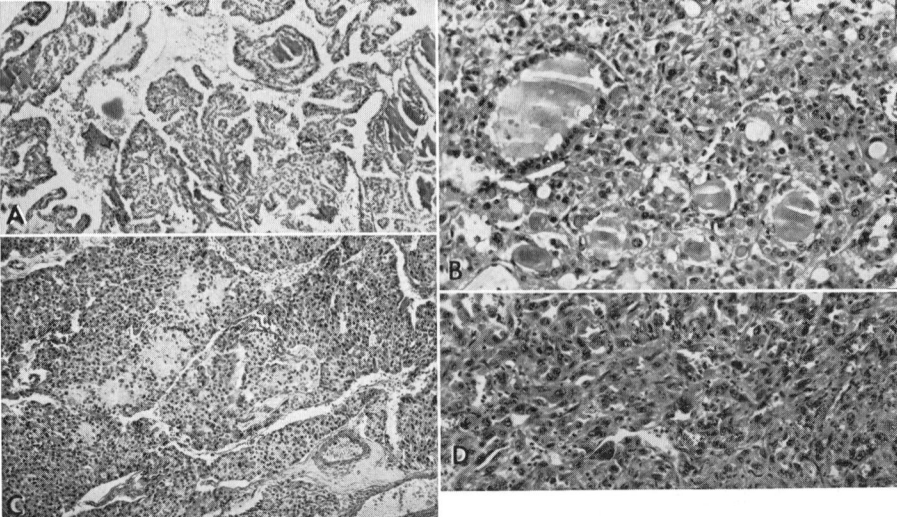

Figure 4–38. Thyroid carcinomas. *A,* Papillary carcinoma. *B,* Follicular carcinoma. *C,* Medullary carcinoma with amyloid stroma. (From Hazard, J. B., Hawk, W. A., et al.: Medullary (solid) carcinoma of the thyroid; a clinicopathologic entity. *J. Clin. Endocr.* 19:152, 1959.) *D,* Anaplastic carcinoma.

because of its parafollicular origin and distinctive manifestations.

Papillary Carcinoma. In most series, thyroid carcinoma that is either purely or predominantly papillary in structure is by far the most common, accounting for about one-half of all thyroid carcinomas. Papillary carcinoma may occur at any age, but it is seen more frequently in children and young adults than are the other types of thyroid malignancy; almost one-half of the cases occur before the age of 40 (Fig. 4–39). Women are affected two to three times more commonly than men. Young patients with this disease

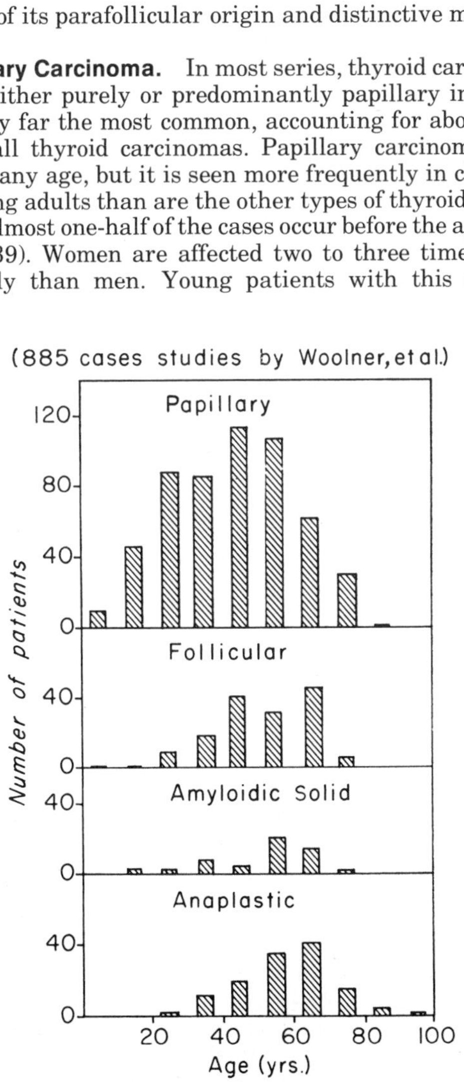

Figure 4–39. Age incidence of thyroid carcinoma of various types. (Taken from the data of Woolner, L. B., Beahrs, O. H., et al.: Classification and prognosis of thyroid carcinoma. A study of 885 cases observed in a thirty-year period. *Amer. J. Surg. 102*:354, 1961.)

sometimes give a history of having received x-ray therapy during childhood for cervical lymphadenitis or thymic enlargement, suggesting that radiation in the vicinity of the thyroid gland may play a pathogenetic role. In general, papillary carcinoma is the most slow-growing of all thyroid carcinomas, often remaining localized to the thyroid gland for many years. It tends to spread via the intraglandular lymphatics from its primary site to other parts of the thyroid and to the pericapsular and regional lymph nodes, where it may remain localized for years. Sometimes, the metastases in the cervical lymph nodes so overshadow the primary lesion that their true nature is overlooked. In the past, such lesions were thought to arise from the fourth pharyngeal pouch; these were called "lateral aberrant thyroids." Hematogenous spread to distant sites such as lung is uncommon. The growth of papillary carcinoma is thought by some to depend partly upon TSH stimulation; this view stems from the observation that the administration of suppressive doses of TH (thyroid hormone) sometimes leads to regression of metastases from a primary lesion that was predominantly papillary in type. It should be noted, however, that most papillary carcinomas contain follicular elements, and the metastases may be composed predominantly of the latter. Papillary carcinoma has a tendency to become more malignant with advancing age; indeed, it has been suggested that the highly malignant anaplastic carcinomas do not arise *de novo* but develop from preexisting low-grade papillary or follicular carcinomas (Russell et al., 1963). The age of the patient appears to be more important than any other factor in determining the prognosis in papillary carcinoma (McKenzie, 1971), and rarely does it cause death in young adults. Although the extra mortality owing to this tumor has been estimated at only 10 or 20% over several decades (Woolner et al., 1961), more recent estimates of survival rates in the general population suggest a greater lethality of this tumor (Beierwaltes, 1978).

Grossly, the carcinoma varies greatly in size and is usually unencapsulated. On histopathologic examination, it is composed of columnar epithelium that is thrown into folds, forming papillary projections with connective tissue stalks. There is frequently a mixed papillary and follicular pattern, the former predominating. Occasionally, there are foci of large cells with well-defined nuclei and pale, acidophilic cytoplasm (Hürthle cells). Concentrically layered deposits of calcium (psammoma bodies) are commonly found. There may be gross or microscopic foci of carcinoma in other parts of the gland, resulting from spread via the intraglandular lymphatics.

Clinically, papillary carcinoma usually appears either as an asymptomatic nodule in an otherwise normal thyroid or as an enlargement of the regional lymph nodes, sometimes without a palpable thyroid nodule. Invasion of adjacent structures and distant metastases are late manifestations.

Since papillary carcinoma accumulates iodine less efficiently than does the surrounding normal thyroid tissue, it will appear as a "cold" area in the thyroid scintiscan, provided that it is large enough to allow resolution by the scanner and is not surrounded by a large amount of functioning tissue (see Fig. 4–20). Radiologic examination of the neck may disclose concentrically layered calcium in the psammoma bodies.

Follicular Carcinoma.   In most series, thyroid carcinoma that is either purely or predominantly follicular in structure comprises about one-quarter of all thyroid carcinomas. It occurs in an older age group than papillary carcinoma, the majority of cases occurring after the age of 40 (Fig. 4–39). Women are affected two to three times more commonly than men. As in papillary carcinoma, there may be a history of radiotherapy to the neck area during infancy or childhood. Its degree of malignancy varies but generally exceeds that of papillary carcinoma. Follicular carcinoma seldom spreads to the regional lymph nodes, but invasion of blood vessels with hematogenous spread to distant sites, particularly bone, lung, and liver, often occurs relatively early. As is the case in primary papillary carcinoma, the metastases sometimes regress under the influence of suppressive doses of thyroid hormone. Follicular carcinoma occasionally becomes more malignant with advancing age.

Grossly, follicular carcinoma varies in size and is typically encapsulated. The histopathologic appearance of the lesion varies from area to area. In some areas, it resembles normal thyroid tissue except that the follicles are smaller and contain subnormal amounts of colloid, while in other areas it is composed of solid sheets of cells. The cells exhibit mitoses to a varying degree. There may be foci of Hürthle cells; rarely, these are the predominant type of cell. In many follicular carcinomas, papillary elements are present to a varying degree. Invasion of blood vessels and adjacent thyroid parenchyma is often observed. The degree of invasiveness, which is greatest in the older age group of patients (McKenzie, 1971), largely determines the prognosis in follicular carcinoma. In minimally invasive lesions, a 10-year survival rate of 86% has been reported, whereas the comparable figure for the more invasive variety is only 44% (Woolner et al., 1961). The metastases may display either a follicular or a mixed follicular and papillary pattern. In some cases, the histologic appearance of a metastatic lesion so closely resembles that of normal thyroid tissue that the term benign metastasizing struma was formerly applied to this lesion.

The clinical features of follicular carcinoma differ in several respects from those of the usual case of papillary carcinoma. In some patients, a goiter has been present for many years. The carcinoma usually consists of a single nodule or mass that is stony hard in consistency; sometimes it involves one whole lobe. Pain and invasion of adjacent structures are late manifestations. The regional lymph nodes are seldom enlarged. Occasionally, either a pathologic fracture due to a metastatic deposit in bone or a pulmonary metastatic nodule is the major manifestation.

Follicular carcinoma differs from the other types of thyroid malignancy in that it may accumulate iodine almost as efficiently as does the surrounding normal tissue. The metastatic deposits also may accumulate iodine if they are composed predominantly of follicular elements. Rarely, function in the metastases may be sufficient to produce thyrotoxicosis, including T_3-toxicosis (Sung and Cavalieri, 1973).

Anaplastic Carcinoma.   Anaplastic carcinoma comprises about 10% of all thyroid carcinomas. It usually occurs after the age of 50 and is slightly more common in women. It is a highly malignant lesion, rapidly invading adjacent structures and metastasizing extensively throughout the body.

Grossly, anaplastic carcinoma is unencapsulated and extends widely, distorting the shape of the thyroid. Its consistency varies, being stony hard in some areas and soft or friable in others. Evidence of invasion of adjacent structures, such as skin, muscle, nerve, blood vessels, larynx, and esophagus, is common. On histopathologic examination, the lesion is composed of atypical cells that exhibit numerous mitoses and form a variety of patterns. Spindle-shaped cells and multinucleate giant cells are usually the predominant types of cell. In some cases, small cells predominate; as a result, there may be difficulty in distinguishing the lesion from lymphosarcoma. Rarely, the lesion is composed of clear cells, resembling hypernephroma, or large epithelial cells (epidermoid carcinoma). Areas of necrosis and polymorphonuclear infiltration are frequently present. Sometimes elements of papillary or follicular carcinoma can be detected, suggesting that they may be the precursors of anaplastic carcinoma (Russell et al., 1963).

The usual clinical complaint is of a rapid, often painful enlargement of a mass that has been present in the thyroid gland for many years. The mass rapidly invades adjacent structures, causing hoarseness, inspiratory stridor, and difficulty in swallowing. On examination, the skin overlying the mass is often warm and discolored. The mass is large and tender and is often fixed to adjacent structures, with the result that it moves poorly on swallowing. It is stony hard in consistency, but some areas may be soft or fluctuant. The regional lymph nodes are enlarged, and there may be evidence of distant metastases. The patient usually succumbs within several months after the diagnosis has been made. In general, anaplastic carcinomas do not accumulate iodine. Rarely, extensive replacement of the thyroid parenchyma may produce hypothyroidism.

Carcinoma of Parafollicular Origin (Medullary Carcinoma)

This is the most distinctive type of thyroid carcinoma, although it comprises only about 5–10% of the cases. It usually occurs after the age of 50 and is slightly more common in women. It is more malignant than follicular carcinoma. Medullary carcinoma readily invades the intraglandular lymphatics, spreading to other parts of the gland and to the pericapsular and regional lymph nodes. In this respect it resembles papillary carcinoma, but unlike the latter it also spreads via the bloodstream to distant sites, particularly lung, bone, and liver.

Grossly, medullary carcinoma of the thyroid (MCT) is firm and usually unencapsulated. On histopathologic examination, it is composed of cells that vary widely in morphologic features and arrangement. Round, polyhedral, and spindle-shaped cells form a variety of patterns, but formation of papillary folds or follicles is not seen. The cells may appear undifferentiated and exhibit mitoses, but, unlike the findings in anaplastic carcinoma, necrosis and polymorphonuclear infiltration are absent. There is an abundant hyaline connective tissue stroma that gives the staining reactions for amyloid; apart from plasmacytoma, this feature is unique to solid thyroid carcinoma. Gross or microscopic foci of carcinoma are often evident in other parts of the gland. Invasion of blood vessels may be seen. The histopathologic appearance of the metastases closely resembles that of the primary lesion.

Clinically, MCT first appears either as a hard nodule or mass in the thyroid gland or as an enlargement of the regional lymph nodes. Occasionally, a metastatic lesion in a distant site is found first. Lesions are sometimes bilateral, and are usually localized to the upper two-thirds of the gland. Though some medullary carcinomas present as cold nodules, often, surprisingly, this is not the case.

MCT is an extremely interesting disease for several reasons. It arises from the parafollicular cells of the thyroid, rather than the follicular epithelium; it secretes a characteristic hormone, calcitonin (CT); it is frequently associated with one or more para-endocrine manifestations; it is often familial; and it provides an early biochemical signal, in hypersecretion of CT, that permits its early detection, treatment, and cure. (For reviews and references, see Landsberg, 1966, and Stepanas et al., 1979.)

This tumor of the thyroid occurs in both sporadic and familial forms, the latter comprising about 20% of the total. Of the two forms, the familial variety usually appears at a younger age, is more often bilateral, is less likely to have associated cervical metastases when diagnosed, and has a better survivorship. Most important, the familial variety is anteceded by a premalignant hyperplasia of the C-cells that is curable by total thyroidectomy. Survival in both the sporadic and familial forms is mainly determined by the presence or absence of metastases and the age of the patient at the time of diagnosis, older patients generally doing much less well. Overall, long-term survival is moderate, estimated at about two-thirds at 10 years.

A variety of symptoms, other than those due to mass lesions, are present in patients with MCT. The carcinoid syndrome and Cushing's syndrome may occur, owing to secretion of serotonin and ACTH, respectively. Prostaglandins, kinins, and vasoactive intestinal peptide may also be secreted and are variously responsible for the attacks of watery diarrhea that about one-third of patients experience. In patients with the familial variety, there is often clinical or laboratory evidence of hyperparathyroidism and pheochromocytoma (Sippel's syndrome; multiple endocrine adenomatosis, Type II). Hyperparathyroidism is most commonly due to parathyroid hyperplasia, rather than adenoma, with or without characteristic symptoms of hypercalcemia or those of nephrolithiasis or nephrocalcinosis. Pheochromocytomas are often bilateral, and are prone to secrete epinephrine, so that urinary total catecholamine and VMA excretion are normal. Specific measurements of urinary epinephrine excretion will often reveal some elevation, however. An apparent variant of the MEA II syndrome is one in which MCT, pheochromocytoma, and possibly parathyroid hyperplasia are associated with ganglioneuromas, mucosal neuromas ("bumpy lip" syndrome), a marfanoid habitus, and typical facies (MEA III).

In patients with the sporadic form of MCT, differentiation from other types of thyroid nodule on clinical grounds alone may be difficult. In patients with a family history of thyroid cancer, hypertension, and either hyperparathyroidism or nephrolithiasis, the MEA II syndrome should be suspected. In both, measurements of basal plasma calcitonin concentrations should be made, these being elevated in about one-third to two-thirds of patients with MCT. Infusions of pentagastrin or calcium elicit secretion of calcitonin, and the response is exaggerated in patients with MCT or the antecedent C-cell hyperplasia. Patients with MCT are usually normocalcemic; but those suspected of having the MEA II syndrome should be evaluated for hyperparathyroidism and for pheochromocytoma as well.

When the diagnosis of MCT has been made from calcitonin measurements, needle biopsy, or at surgery, total thyroidectomy with removal of regional nodes should be carried out. In patients with MEA II, pheochromocytomas should be treated first, and in patients in whom a diagnosis of MEA II has been made from the family history and who have been shown to have a pheochromocytoma or hyperparathyroidism, thyroidectomy should be performed, even in the absence of clinical abnormalities in the gland. Periodic measurements of basal plasma calcitonin concentration and the response to provocative stimuli should be carried out periodically to provide evidence of metastases, which function characteristically.

Members of the family of patients with MEA II, including small children, should be screened regularly, probably once yearly, for the emergence of one or more manifestations of the syndrome. Studies should include measurements of basal and stimulated calcitonin concentrations and tests for pheochromocytoma and hyperparathyroidism. Emergence of either of the latter two diagnoses, abnormalities in calcitonin concentration, or even rising concentrations of calcitonin alone are indications for prompt and total thyroidectomy.

Diagnosis and Management of the Nodular Thyroid Gland

In the last edition of this volume, the statement was made that benign and malignant thyroid nodules could not be differentiated from one another with absolute certainty on clinical grounds alone, and that cytopathologic examination was required for this purpose. This remains the case. It was also noted, however, that a reasonably accurate clinical judgment could be made as to whether a given nodule was probably benign or malignant, so that the likelihood of either leaving a carcinoma in place or performing an excisional biopsy of a benign nodule was reduced (Shimaoka et al., 1962). Obviously, this too remains the case (Miller et al., 1979). Nonetheless, the approach to the diagnosis and management of the nodular thyroid gland has been substantially modified in recent years, and the accuracy of diagnosis increased, by the application of two techniques, ultrasonography of the thyroid and cutting needle or aspiration biopsy. (See earlier section on Laboratory Tests of Thyroid Hormone Economy: Miscellaneous Tests.) This section will describe the clinical and laboratory criteria that can assist the physician in arriving at the first critical decision in the management of the patient with a nodular thyroid gland, whether or not the patient is to be operated upon. As is evident from the very extensive literature on this topic, not all authorities agree on the importance to be attached to certain findings or on the question of how often various diagnostic procedures should be applied. (For a very well referenced review of this and other aspects of thyroid cancer, see Van Herle and Uller, 1977; see also *World Jour-*

nal of Surgery Vol. 5, (1), January, 1981.) The authors' general approach to the management of patients with thyroid nodules will follow a discussion of the several sources of information that can be brought to bear upon the problem.

There is general agreement concerning the importance of several historical and physical findings. Especially important is a history of x-irradiation to the head or chest during infancy or childhood, since most would concur that prior irradiation of the thyroid increases the frequency of nodular disease and increases the proportion of nodules that are malignant. A history of thyroid carcinoma among other members of the patient's family suggests that a nodule is a medullary carcinoma, though rare instances of familial papillary carcinoma have been reported. The age of the patient is also an important consideration. In papillary carcinoma, by far the most common malignancy of the thyroid, almost half the cases are discovered in persons under the age of 40, yet most nonmalignant nodules in the thyroid occur in those beyond the age of 40. Hence, the younger the patient, the greater the likelihood that a nodular thyroid harbors a malignancy. Further to the point is the sex of the patient. The overall incidence of nodular goiter is greater in women than in men, but the sex ratio in carcinoma is lower. Hence, the ratio of malignant to benign nodules is much higher in men than in women.

The major consideration on physical examination is whether careful palpation reveals a single nodule in an otherwise normal gland, or whether the thyroid is generally enlarged and contains multiple nodules. The former is much more likely to be a neoplasm, either benign or malignant, and the latter a nontoxic multinodular goiter of the type discussed in an earlier section. This is true despite the facts, first, that a considerable proportion of thyroids that appear to contain a single nodule on external palpation prove to be multinodular at surgery, and, second, that thyroid carcinoma is not infrequently found at more than one site within the gland, owing to intraglandular lymphatic spread (Russell et al., 1963). Malignant nodules are most often, but not invariably, very firm or stony hard. Failure of a cervical mass to move with swallowing indicates that it lies outside the fascial plane occupied by the thyroid or is fixed to surrounding tissues. Such fixation, as well as vocal-cord paralysis, is highly suggestive of carcinoma. Extension of disease to cervical lymph nodes is especially likely to occur early in the course of papillary carcinoma in young patients. Nonetheless, this, as well as cord paralysis and fixation, is a late manifestation from the diagnostic standpoint, and the physician's decision should not await its appearance.

Standard laboratory tests, such as measurements of the RAIU or serum T_4 and T_3 concentrations, are rarely of help, as normal thyroid function is usually maintained in patients with thyroid carcinoma. Occasionally, a diffusely infiltrating carcinoma, most often one that is anaplastic in nature, will replace sufficient thyroid parenchyma to produce hypothyroidism. Apart from calcitonin, which serves as an indicator of medullary carcinoma, a search for tumor markers is unrewarding. A small proportion of patients with cancers of the thyroid have elevations of the plasma CEA concentration (Economidou et al., 1977). Though very helpful as a means of following patients known to have differentiated carcinoma of the thyroid, measurements of serum thyroglobulin are not useful for diagnosis, since elevations are seen in a variety of other thyroid disorders. (See the earlier section that described miscellaneous laboratory tests.)

Soft tissue films of the neck are sometimes helpful in patients with thyroid nodules that are suspect. Approximately half of all papillary carcinomas contain psammoma bodies, which may be demonstrable as cloudlike aggregations of finely stippled density (see Johannessen and Sobrinho-Simões, 1980). Calcifications in benign lesions usually follow hemorrhage, and are seen as more dense, chunky opacities, often surrounded by a ringlike shell of calcification.

For decades, the thyroid scintiscan has been a mainstay in evaluating the patient with a nodular thyroid gland for the question of malignancy. This follows from the fact that most malignant thyroid tumors, when discovered *in situ*, do not have the capacity to accumulate and organify significant quantities of radioiodine. Their appearance on scintiscan, therefore, is that of a nonfunctioning or "cold" nodule. The converse, i.e., that most cold nodules are thyroid carcinomas, is not the case, however. Although the reported frequency of cancer in cold nodules varies widely, a reasonable estimate is about 20%. The majority prove to be nonfunctioning, degenerated benign adenomas, cysts, or hypofunctioning colloid nodules in multinodular goiter. Nonetheless, when associated with any of the indications of malignancy described earlier, the finding of a cold nodule, particularly a solitary cold nodule, has been a strong impetus toward excision of the lesion.

The limitations that the size and location of a cold nodule impose on its detection by scintiscan have been discussed, and should be borne in mind. Also to be recognized is the fact that some thyroid carcinomas retain the capacity to transport iodide, but not to organify it. Such lesions will appear to be functioning or hyperfunctioning when examined with pertechnetate, but will appear cold when the radionuclide employed is an isotope of iodine (Turner and Spencer, 1976).

The principal value of ultrasonography is the differentiation among solid, cystic, and mixed cystic and solid nodules of the thyroid gland. (See review by Rosen, et al., 1979.) Solid and mixed lesions can be either benign or malignant but are, therefore, more likely to be benign, because only about 20% of nonfunctioning nodules are malignant. Small cysts, those less than 3 to 4 cm in diameter, are very rarely a result of carcinoma, but lesions of larger size are suspect. Cystic lesions of the thyroid should be aspirated and the fluid obtained examined. Clear, straw-colored fluid generally indicates a benign lesion, while fluid that contains fresh or old blood raises suspicion of malignancy. In any event, cytologic examination of the cyst contents should always be obtained, since malignant cells will occasionally be detected. Benign cysts will often remain collapsed when emptied of their fluid; in such cases, the problem is essentially terminated. When cysts rapidly or repeatedly reaccumulate fluid, they should be excised and subjected to careful pathologic examination.

Many physicians, when confronted with a solid single or dominant nodule in the thyroid gland, even one that is nonfunctioning, will choose to observe the response of the nodule to suppressive therapy. The rationale for this approach is that benign nodules, being TSH-dependent, are likely to decrease in size when secretion of TSH is suppressed, while malignant nodules, being less frequently or less obviously TSH-dependent, are unlikely to be suppressed during treatment. It is reasoned, moreover, that owing to the usual indolent nature of thyroid carcinoma, nothing is lost by a several-month trial of suppressive therapy, even if it proves to be unsuccessful. There is little to contradict this rationale or to contraindicate a 3- to 6-

month trial of full replacement doses of exogenous hormone. On the other hand, our own and others' experience has done little to encourage this approach, since only an occasional nodule has decreased significantly in size and only a very rare nodule has disappeared entirely (Miller et al., 1979). Moreover, findings on palpation may be misleading. Some nodules may become less prominent as the surrounding tissue undergoes atrophy, while others become more prominent for the same reason, like a sandbar rising from the sea at low tide. However, ultrasonography, a reproducible, noninvasive technique that produces no known tissue damage, can be employed to measure changes in the size of nodules that occur either spontaneously or as a result of suppressive therapy.

In an increasing number of clinics, in recent years, biopsy of the thyroid, particularly fine-needle biopsy, has become the final step in a diagnostic algorithm that determines whether the patient is to undergo thyroid surgery. Earlier fears that thyroid biopsy might lead to dissemination of a cancer appear to have been unfounded. Although a successful cutting needle biopsy provides a core of tissue that facilitates histologic diagnosis, complications of the procedure, such as tracheal puncture, hemorrhage, or transient injury to the recurrent laryngeal nerve, are possible, especially when the physician is lacking experience in the technique. For this reason, the major thrust has been toward the performance of fine-needle aspiration. This technique requires little experience for its performance; it is an office procedure that requires no cutaneous anesthesia and is apparently lacking in significant complications. The principal caveat is that the readings be performed by a cytopathologist especially interested and experienced in the interpretation of the resulting specimens. (See earlier section discussing miscellaneous tests.) A second concern, common to all biopsy procedures, is that a representative specimen be obtained. Failure to do so is a cause of false-negative biopsies, but such can be minimized by taking several samples from the same nodule. A further shortcoming of the aspiration biopsy is that readings are frequently indeterminate in well differentiated follicular tumors, in which the differentiation between benign and malignant lesions rests on the demonstration of capsular or vascular invasion. Clearly, this cannot be assessed in aspiration biopsies, and often not in cutting needle biopsies, either. Among the many reports that address the accuracy of fine-needle aspiration, results vary, but on the whole a 5 to 10% frequency of false-positives and false-negatives is indicated. False-negative readings are apparently more common than false-positives. The major impact of fine-needle aspiration, as documented in studies in which clinical impression, results of aspiration biopsy, and excisional biopsy have been compared, would appear to have been to decrease markedly the percentage of patients undergoing surgery for benign lesions and to increase the yield of carcinomas in operative specimens (Gershengorn et al., 1977; Miller et al., 1979). In addition, a clearly negative biopsy may facilitate a decision not to operate on a patient with a clinically suspect lesion in whom, as in the elderly, a surgical procedure is relatively contraindicated. Conversely, a positive biopsy may provide the impetus to operation when the patient or the physician is reluctant to have one performed. (For additional references on this subject, see Hamburger et al., 1979; Walfish et al., 1977; Lowhagen et al., 1981.)

One may well ask why, if thyroid biopsy is ultimately to be performed, additional or antecedent procedures, such as the scintiscan or ultrasonography should be carried out. There is merit to this question, but both of the latter procedures have independent value. With respect to the scintiscan, it may reveal a hyperfunctioning or "hot" nodule, in which instance it is extremely unlikely that the nodule is malignant, and further procedures directed toward the diagnosis of malignancy become unnecessary. In addition, the scan may reveal the typical patchy appearance of multinodular goiter, demonstrating hyperfunctioning or hypofunctioning areas not detectable by palpation, thereby decreasing the likelihood that the palpable nodule is carcinoma. In the latter case, the initial scan also provides a valuable baseline with which a "suppression" scan can be compared and areas of functional autonomy delineated. (See earlier section on Multinodular Goiter.) Like the scintiscan, the ultrasonogram also has potential independent value. When a cyst is known to be present, a larger needle can be used for evacuation of the cyst, making the procedure easier to complete. Further, knowing that a cystic lesion is present, the physician is likely to continue to probe the lesion until cyst fluid is found if none is initially obtained. In difficult cases, this can be facilitated by performing the aspiration with ultrasonic guidance.

On the basis of the foregoing considerations the authors have developed a general approach to the management of nodular thyroid disease. In the last analysis, in the great majority of patients, all paths ultimately lead either to long-term suppressive therapy without operation or to operation, usually followed by long-term suppressive therapy. As will be seen, there are few, if any, hard and fast values that determine which path the patient will be led to. Rather, the decision depends upon a series of factors, including the wishes of the informed patient, that are weighed in a balance that changes as new information is obtained.

In the patient with a clearly multinodular goiter, a scintiscan is uniformly indicated. If this reveals no major nonfunctioning focus; if none of the nodules is strongly dominant and none displays clinical features suggesting malignancy, such as recent growth; if there is no history of radiation to the head, neck, or chest; and if the patient is over 40 years of age, long-term suppressive therapy will be recommended. (See earlier section on Multinodular Goiter.) If one or more nodules then continue to grow, or if other signs suggesting carcinoma appear, further diagnostic measures will be undertaken.

All patients with seemingly solitary nodules are studied by scintiscan. If the nodule proves to be hyperfunctioning, the likelihood of malignancy is very greatly decreased. If the nodule comprises the sole functioning thyroid tissue, the remaining tissue being suppressed, the patient is carefully studied for the presence of thyrotoxicosis; if none is present, the patient is followed for its possible emergence. If a nodule appears hot but the remaining tissue retains some function, thyrotoxicosis is almost surely not present. In such instances, a short course of suppressive therapy followed by a suppression scan is carried out to prove that the nodule has functional autonomy.

If a single nodule proves to be hypofunctioning, institution of prolonged suppressive therapy without further diagnostic study is contraindicated, in our view. If the patient is young, and a male, and especially if worrisome clinical signs are present, surgery may be directly recommended. More often, however, an ultrasonogram will be obtained first to exclude the presence of a purely cystic lesion. In older patients with a solitary cold nodule, especially women, an ultrasonogram is obtained. Cystic lesions are dealt with as already discussed, and solid or mixed lesions are subjected to aspiration biopsy. Patients in whom biopsy indicates malignancy obviously proceed to surgery, as do patients in whom the specimen obtained is highly cellular or displays cellular atypia. Patients in whom biopsy results do not suggest malignancy are begun on long-term suppressive therapy. Growth of the lesion despite such treatment is an indication for either a repeat biopsy or surgical excision.

Surgery should be recommended, in our view, in essentially all patients with a clear history of x-irradiation to the head, neck, or chest during childhood and who present with nodular disease of the thyroid gland.

Occasional, usually older, patients with malignancy of or in the thyroid present with features suggesting subacute thyroiditis, including pain, elevation of the erythrocyte sedimentation rate, and decrease in the RAIU. Failure of symptoms to regress during treatment with salicylates or glucocorticoids provides a clue to the presence of "malignant pseudothyroiditis," as this syndrome has been termed. (See Rosen et al., 1978.) This suspicion should be confirmed by thyroid biopsy.

Treatment of Thyroid Carcinoma

Virtually no aspect of the treatment of differentiated thyroid carcinoma has been entirely free from controversy and uncertainty, even (or especially) among those most frequently concerned with the management of patients with this disease. Though few would disagree that proven carcinomas should be excised, substantial difference of opinion exists concerning the optimal surgical procedure to be employed under differing circumstances. Whether, when, and how radioiodine therapy should be undertaken, as well as its ultimate effectiveness, has also been a clouded issue. Similarly, the efficacy of suppressive thyroid therapy in the general population of patients with this disease has been uncertain, though its use involves no known risk to the patient. Many factors have contributed to this uncertainty. Among them are the relative infrequency of clinically significant disease and the frequency of clinically inapparent occult foci of tumor discovered incidentally or at autopsy; the variable and usually prolonged natural course of the disease following diagnosis; the influence of constitutional factors, such as age, on the behavior of histologically similar tumors; the fact that, until recently, definitive diagnosis has required surgical removal of the tumor, itself an effective therapeutic measure; and the potential morbidity associated with several modes of treatment. These problems and the uncertainties that they engender are fully documented in the literature. (For discussions and references, see Van Herle and Uller, 1977, and Mazzaferri et al., 1977. Multi-authored discussions of diverse aspects of problems related to the diagnosis and treatment of thyroid cancer are available in *Radiation-Associated Thyroid Carcinoma*, De-Groot, L.J. (ed.), New York, Grune and Stratton, 1976, and in *World Journal of Surgery*, Vol. 5 (1) January 1981.)

Because of the foregoing uncertainties and the differing needs of individual patients, treatment of thyroid carcinoma cannot always accord with a rigid algorithm. Nevertheless, the following general guidelines are those that the authors generally follow in patients with known or suspected papillary carcinoma. Surgery is the initial major therapeutic measure. Patients scheduled for surgery are often given suppressive thyroid therapy for several weeks preoperatively, the hope being to reduce the growth and aggressiveness of any tumor that may be disseminated during surgery. Vascularity of the thyroid is thereby reduced and some degree of atrophy of normal thyroid tissue may facilitate the identification of other abnormal foci within the gland at the time of operation. Surgery is performed under general anesthesia through a wide incision, and the suspected lesion is removed with a wide margin of surrounding tissue. Unless a clear diagnosis of carcinoma has been made preoperatively, as by thyroid biopsy, the suspected lesion is removed *in toto* with a wide range of surrounding tissue and is subjected to frozen section. In patients in whom carcinoma is present, the authors recommend a "near-total" thyroidectomy, i.e., removal of the affected lobe, isthmus, and contralateral lobe, with careful identification of the recurrent laryngeal nerves and with sufficient tissue left in association with the posterior capsule so that the parathyroid glands are spared. There is some disagreement whether as extensive a procedure as this should be performed in cases in which there is no evidence of intrathyroid multicentricity and no metastases to extrathyroid foci. In such cases, some would perform a lobectomy on the affected side, an isthmectomy, and perhaps a partial removal of the contralateral lobe, since the frequency of major surgical complications, particularly hypoparathyroidism, is unquestionably lower following the less extensive procedure. The rationale for the more extensive procedure is the frequency of multiple foci within the gland and data that demonstrate that both the frequency of recurrent disease and subsequent mortality rate are distinctly lower after total than after subtotal thyroidectomy. (See Mazzaferri et al., 1977.) Rarely is it the case that all thyroid tissue can be removed, judging from subsequent scintiscans, but the less tissue remaining, the more readily is complete ablation by radioiodine achieved, and this facilitates subsequent radioiodine treatment of metastatic disease. Data indicating that occult papillary thyroid carcinomas, usually defined as clinically inapparent tumors less than 1.5 cm in diameter, do not reduce subsequent life expectancy are often cited as favoring a lesser surgical procedure, but this is not really relevant to a discussion of the management of clinically apparent thyroid cancer. Moreover, more recently analyzed demographic data indicate that reduction in life expectancy does occur in occult thyroid carcinoma, though to a lesser extent than with larger or more aggressive tumors (Beierwaltes, 1976). In the last analysis, choice of the surgical procedure to be performed in patients with a clinically solitary papillary carcinoma, lacking metastases, should be most strongly conditioned by the skill of the surgeon performing the operation. It is highly desirable that, whenever possible, surgery for thyroid carcinoma be performed by one who is highly experienced and continually active in this field.

In patients in whom there is evidence of either multicentricity or metastatic spread, usually to the cervical lymph nodes, there is quite general agreement that near-total thyroidectomy should be performed. The same is true if there is evidence of local invasion, in which case as complete removal as possible is attempted.

In patients with unifocal disease seemingly confined to the thyroid, as judged from exploration of the regional nodes, prophylactic neck dissection is not recommended. In patients with metastatic disease, a modified neck dissection is performed. Radical, disfiguring neck dissections are not

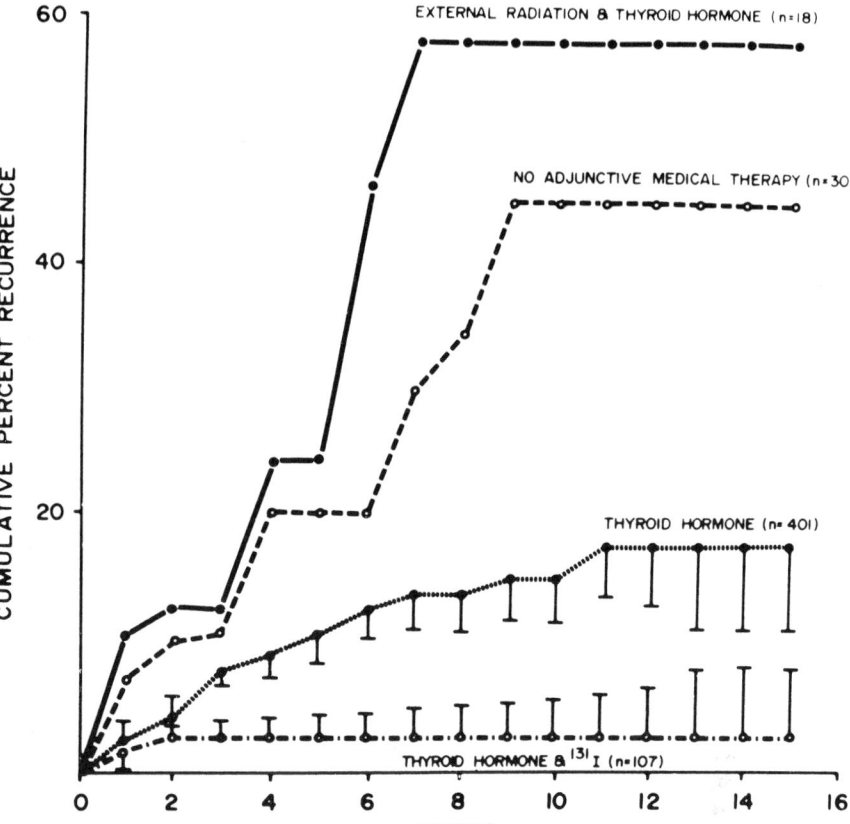

Figure 4–40. The influence of mode of therapy on the rate of postoperative recurrence in patients with papillary carcinoma of the thyroid. (From Mazzaferri, E. L., et al.: Papillary thyroid carcinoma: the impact of therapy in 576 patients. *Medicine 56*:171, 1977.)

indicated, particularly since the evidence indicates that the extent and nature of node dissection does not significantly influence either recurrence or survival.

Postoperative management of the patient is based upon several physiologic principles and upon evidence of the efficacy of the therapeutic measures that they dictate. Among the principles that apply is that accumulation of sufficient radioiodine within the tumor may eradicate the disease locally; that the efficiency of tumors with respect to radioiodine accumulation is less than that of normal thyroid tissue, but that it can be increased by high levels of circulating TSH; and that tumors may be TSH-reponsive with respect to growth and aggressiveness, as well as to iodine accumulation. The general regimen that grows out of these considerations is one in which: (1) total thyroidectomy is performed, both to remove competing thyroid tissue and to afford a basis for periodic elevations of endogenous TSH during which radioiodine therapy may be possible; and (2) effective suppression of TSH secretion is maintained at all other times. This combined approach has clearly been shown to reduce the frequency of recurrence of papillary carcinoma to a marked extent (see Figure 4–40 and Mazzaferri et al., 1977). A favorable effect of programs of radioiodine therapy is also described in other reports (Varma et al., 1970; Leeper, 1973; Beierwaltes, 1978). This can be achieved with only an occasional long-term adverse effect, principally development of leukemia.

The manner in which the foregoing principles are put into effect varies among different clinics. The authors' usual approach to postoperative management includes continuation of suppressive thyroid therapy, usually for 6 weeks after the operation. Once again, the intent is to

suppress any malignant cells distributed in the operative field or elsewhere during surgery. Preoperative, immediate postoperative, and long-term suppressive therapy is administered in the form of levothyroxine. Since the average optimal maintenance dose in patients with hypothyroidism is approximately 1 μg per pound body weight per day, we administer a dose approximately 50% greater, so as to assure a maximal suppressive effect. Approximately 3 weeks after operation, in preparation for radioiodine administration, liothyronine in a dose of 75–100 μg daily is substituted for levothyroxine during the next 3 weeks. The shorter duration of action of T_3 than of T_4, and possibly the intermittency of the T_3 effect, permits a more rapid resurgence of TSH secretion when T_3 therapy is withdrawn. We monitor serum TSH concentrations and prefer to allow serum TSH concentrations to reach approximately 50 μU/ml before radioiodine is administered. This usually requires 2 or 3 weeks. At that time, a large tracer dose of ^{131}I (1 μCi) is administered, and accumulation by residual tissue in the thyroid bed and in metastases is sought by external scanning at 24 and 72 hours. If evidence of residual thyroid tissue in the cervical bed is seen, as is usually the case at this point, but if no metastases are found, a thyroid-ablating dose of 50 mCi of ^{131}I is administered. If functioning metastases are seen, the dose is increased to 100 mCI. Suppressive therapy with levothyroxine is resumed 24 hours later.

Following this first course of ^{131}I administration, the patient is seen at 2- to 3-month intervals, and careful examination is made to ascertain whether local recurrence or regional node involvement has become manifest. If one or the other has, it is probably best treated surgically. If no evidence of recurrence develops, suppressive therapy is continued until the time for the next study with ^{131}I is due. These studies are carried out at 1-year intervals for several years if the preceding scan has not revealed metastases, and at 6 months if it has. In the light of convincing data concerning their value, measurements of the serum thyroglobulin concentration should be made at regular intervals, at the time of each examination, as this will provide evidence of incomplete ablation or recurrence of tumor. (See earlier section on miscellaneous laboratory tests.) It seems clear that elevations of serum thyroglobulin concentration can occur when radioiodine-accumulating metastases are not demonstrable (Pacini et al., 1980).

A similar regimen is employed in the management of follicular carcinoma of the thyroid. In this type of tumor, there is more general agreement that an extensive initial thyroidectomy should be performed. Metastases of follicular carcinoma are more likely than those of papillary carcinoma to accumulate radioiodine. Functioning metastases may respond very well to ^{131}I therapy; this is especially true of soft tissue lesions, less so in the case of those in bone.

Treatment of the several varieties of anaplastic carcinoma of the thyroid is extremely discouraging, since most patients with this disease will have died, usually by suffocation or by erosion of large vessels in the neck, within 6 months of diagnosis. Surgery is intended to remove as much tumor mass as possible and relieve existing obstruction, if possible. Anaplastic tumors cannot be treated with radioiodine, either. Bleomycin or adriamycin may delay death, and may be useful in the treatment of the late stage of differentiated thyroid cancers, as well. (See Van Herle and Uller, 1977, for references.)

Difficult as it may be, especially in the case of the small-cell variant, it is important that anaplastic tumors of the thyroid be differentiated from lymphoma involving the thyroid, as the latter may respond very well to therapy. (For a review of lymphoproliferative disorders of the thyroid, see Compagno and Oertel, 1980.)

THYROIDITIS

Hashimoto's Disease (Lymphocytic Thyroiditis, Struma Lymphomatosa)

The original description of this chronic disorder of the thyroid with its distinctive histologic appearance was given by Hashimoto in 1912. Until the demonstration of circulating antithyroid antibodies, Hashimoto's disease could be diagnosed with certainty only by biopsy of the thyroid. The demonstration of high titers of circulating antibodies in most patients with Hashimoto's disease, as well as evidence of cell-mediated immunity to thyroid antigens, has led to the use of the term *autoimmune thyroiditis* to describe this disorder.

Although its true prevalence is uncertain, Hashimoto's disease is very common and may be increasing in frequency. It affects women many times more often than men and occurs most commonly between the ages of 30 and 50, although no age is exempt. It is the most common cause of goitrous hypothyroidism in areas of iodine sufficiency. There is often a family history of Hashimoto's disease, goiter, hypothyroidism, or Graves' disease, and even in relatives without overt thyroid disease, circulating antithyroid antibodies may be detected. Other diseases with autoimmune components, such as pernicious anemia, idio-pathic adrenal atrophy, rheumatoid arthritis, chronic active hepatitis, and Sjögren's syndrome, appear to occur in patients with Hashimoto's disease and in their relatives more often than can be accounted for by chance. An association between Hashimoto's disease and angioimmunoblastic lymphadenopathy has also been noted.

Pathogenesis

The presence of lymphocytic infiltration of the thyroid, of circulating antithyroid antibodies, and of a clinical or immunologic overlap with other diseases in which autoimmune components are prominent provide compelling evidence that immunologic factors are involved in the pathogenesis of Hashimoto's disease. Indeed, it is generally agreed that Hashimoto's disease is one of the triad of autoimmune thyroid disorders that also includes Graves' disease and primary thyroid atrophy. What is unclear, however, is the manner in which immunologic factors bring about thyroid damage. A humorally mediated autoimmune mechanism has been suggested by the observation that antimicrosomal antibodies are cytotoxic to thyroid tissue *in vitro*. On the other hand, the extensive lymphocytic infiltration of the thyroid as well as the observation that lymphocytes from some patients with Hashimoto's disease elaborate migration inhibition factor when exposed to thyroid tissue *in vitro* has led to the suggestion that cell-mediated autoimmune mechanism is pathogenetically involved. A third mechanism for which there is some experimental support accommodates both of the foregoing by invoking lymphocyte-mediated cytotoxicity that is targeted and initiated by the antithyroid antibodies.

There is early, but increasing, evidence that these manifestations of autoimmunity in Hashimoto's disease, as in other autoimmune thyroid disorders, reflect a defect in immune surveillance, specifically a genetically determined deficiency of suppressor cells, that allows persistence of a forbidden clone of immunocytes directed against thyroid antigens. (For further discussion of the pathogenesis of autoimmune thyroid disorders, and especially of the relationship of Graves' disease to Hashimoto's disease, see the secton on the pathogenesis of the former disorder.)

Constitutional Factors

Reference has already been made to the female sex preponderance and to the familial predisposition to thyroid disease in Hashimoto's disease. Recent work has shown a significant association between Hashimoto's disease and the human leukocyte antigen HLA-DRW3 (Moens and Farid, 1978). The prevalence of this antigen is also significantly increased in patients with Graves' disease. These observations provide a genetic basis for the association between Hashimoto's disease and Graves' disease and for the familial predisposition to autoimmune thyroid disease. Hashimoto's disease occurs with unexpected frequency in patients with Down's syndrome and probably in those with Turner's syndrome, as well.

Histopathology

The glandular tissue is pale and firm. The histopathologic changes vary in type and extent but in general consist of a combination of diffuse lymphocytic infiltration, obliteration of thyroid follicles, and fibrosis (Fig. 4–41). In most cases, there is destruction of epithelial cells and degeneration and fragmentation of the follicular basement membrane. The remaining epithelial cells may be larger and show oxyphilic changes in the cytoplasm; these so-called Askanazy cells are virtually pathognomonic of this disease. In some cases epithelial hyperplasia may be a prominent feature. Colloid is sparse. The interstitial tissue is infiltrated with lymphocytes which may form typical lymphoid follicles with germinal centers. Plasma cells may be prominent. Fibrosis is generally present, especially in the older lesions, but not to the extent seen in Riedel's thyroiditis. Histologically, two variants can often be distinguished. The more common oxyphilic variant displays more oxyphilic change, less fibrosis, and more prominent infiltration with lymphocytes forming germinal centers. The fibrous variant is infiltrated mainly with plasma cells and displays more fibrosis. Important clinical differences between the two are described later.

Lymphocytic infiltration of a focal or diffuse nature may be found in the thyroid gland of Graves' disease, in thyroid neoplasms, and in simple or nontoxic goiter. In the past, a diagnosis of coexisting Hashimoto's disease was not made unless Askanazy cells or lymphoid follicles were present. Since the lymphocytic infiltration in these other diseases has been shown usually to be associated with circulating antithyroid antibodies, the pathogenetic mechanisms leading to lymphocytic infiltration in all these disorders may be similar. In the case of Graves' disease, lymphocytic infiltration and associated antibodies may favor the development of hypothyroidism after partial thyroidectomy or radioiodine therapy.

Pathophysiology

A variety of abnormalities in hormone biosynthesis may be seen in patients with Hashimoto's disease. These include a defect in organic binding of thyroid iodide, as evidenced by a positive perchlorate discharge test, and an accelerated turnover of a depleted organic iodine pool. In addition, abnormal release of iodoproteins occurs; in their physical properties, these may resemble either thyroglobulin or the albumin-like iodoprotein found in the sera of patients with other thyroid disorders. The foregoing abnormalities in hormone biosynthesis may occur in clinically normal individuals who either are relatives of patients with Hashimoto's disease or have circulating antithyroid antibodies.

Because of the faulty synthesis of hormone, hypersecretion of TSH results, producing functional evidence of thyroid hyperactivity without thyrotoxicosis. Maximal stimulation by endogenous TSH may take place, with the result that no further stimulation is brought about by exogenous TSH (decreased thyroid reserve).

A high proportion of patients with Hashimoto's disease develop iodide myxedema when iodide is taken chronically. Results of the iodide-perchlorate discharge test in such patients are abnormal, indicating an underlying defect in the organic-binding mechanism in the presence of an iodide load (Braverman et al., 1971).

Clinical Picture

Goiter is the outstanding clinical feature of Hashimoto's disease. It usually appears gradually and is often found during examination for some other complaint. In occasional instances, however, the thyroid enlarges rapidly, and when accompanied by pain and tenderness, the disorder may mimic de Quervain's or subacute thyroiditis. A moderate proportion of patients, especially those with the fibrous variant, are hypothyroid when first seen. The goiter is generally moderate in size and firm in consistency and moves freely when the patient swallows. Its surface is either smooth or scalloped, but well defined nodules are unusual. Both lobes are enlarged, but one is often larger than the other. Enlargement of the pyramidal lobe is common. Compression of adjacent structures, such as trachea, esophagus, and recurrent laryngeal nerves, occurs rarely. Enlargement of regional lymph nodes may be present but is unusual.

Although primary (thyroprivic) hypothyroidism is thought to be the end result of autoimmune destruction of the thyroid, the clinical entity of Hashimoto's disease has not been observed to progress to classic thyroprivic hypothyroidism in the individual patient. Indeed, the histopathologic picture tends to remain rather static, except for some increase in fibrous tissue. Clinically, the goiter tends either to remain unchanged or to enlarge gradually over many years if left untreated. The clinical features of hypothyroidism commonly develop over several years in those patients who are euthyroid when first seen. Although earlier studies had suggested that there is an increased prevalence of thyroid carcinoma in the thyroid of Hashimoto's disease, more recent observations do not support this association (Crile, 1978).

Patients with proven Hashimoto's disease may, in midcourse, develop typical manifestations of Graves' disease, including hyperthyroidism with evidence of ongoing thyroid hyperfunction. Other patients with chronic thyroiditis develop transitory thyrotoxicosis (painless thyroiditis with throtoxicosis; see section on Thyrotoxicosis). Here, evidence of ongoing thyroid hyperfunction is lacking, since the thyroid RAIU is depressed. A phase of transient hypothyroidism beginning several weeks post partum in women with chronic thyroiditis has been recognized increasingly. Often, there is a history suggesting mild thyrotoxicosis some time earlier (Amino et al., 1976). How the latter two syndromes are related, if they are, is unclear.

Hashimoto's disease may coexist with pernicious anemia, and even in the absence of overt anemia, circulating autoantibodies against gastric parietal cells may be found. Other diseases presumed to have an autoimmune basis, such as idiopathic adrenal atrophy, Sjögren's syndrome, rheumatoid arthritis, chronic active hepatitis, and systemic lupus erythematosus, appear to occur in patients with Hashimoto's disease or in their relatives more often than can be accounted for by chance.

Laboratory Tests

The results of the common tests of thyroid function are variable, depending on the stage of the disease. At first, the tests indicate the presence of thyroid hyperfunction, but without overproduction of active hormone. At this time, the serum TSH concentration and RAIU are often increased, but the serum T_4 and T_3 concentrations are normal. The serum protein-bound iodine (PBI) concentration may be slightly increased, however, reflecting the abnormal secretion of iodoproteins. At this stage, the patient is eumetabolic, indicating that the glandular response to TSH is adequate to compensate for the abnormalities in hormone biosynthesis. With the passage of time, the ability of the thyroid to respond to TSH diminishes, and the RAIU and

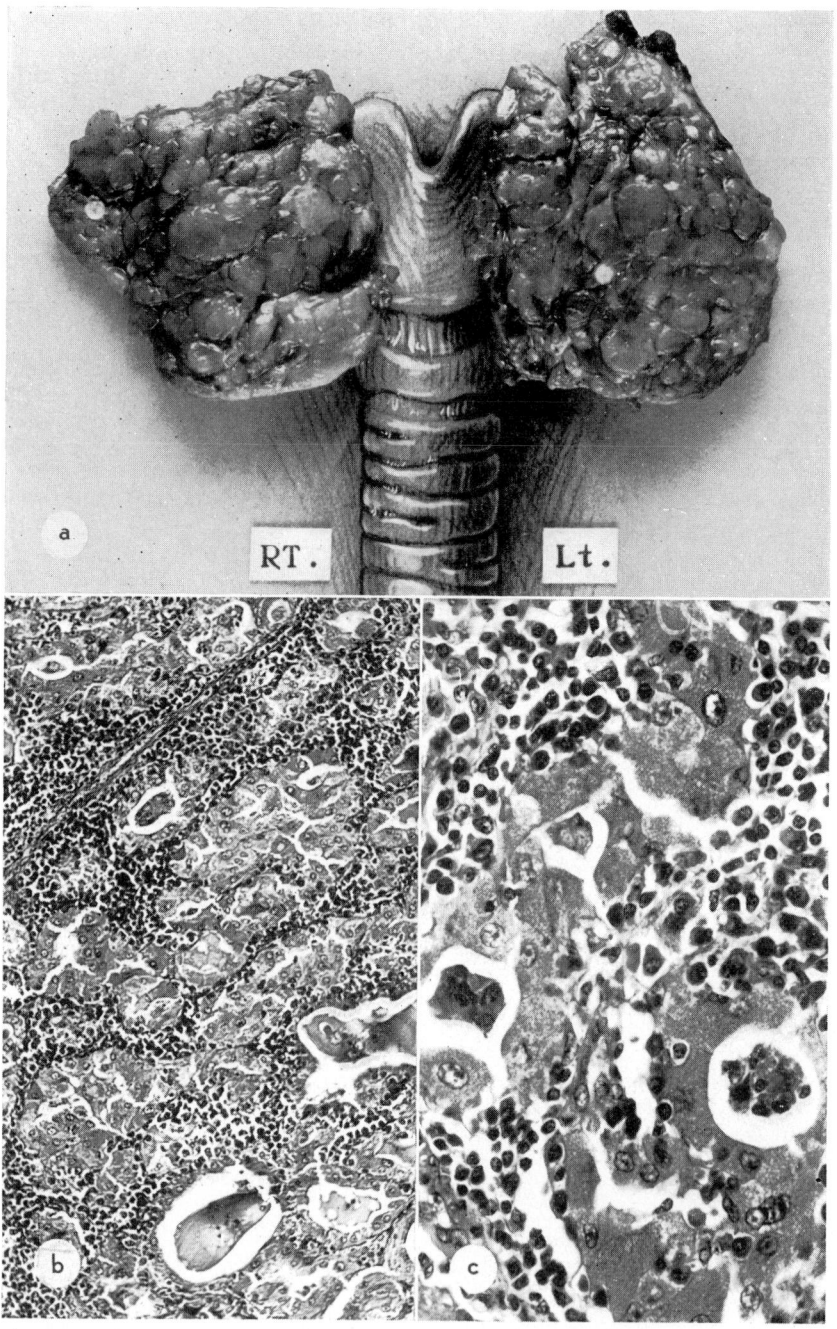

Figure 4–41.   Hashimoto's disease. *A,* Note exaggeration of normal lobular pattern. *B,* Interfollicular infiltration by lymphocytes and plasma cells. *C,* Granular, oxyphilic changes in the cytoplasm of the follicular epithelium (Askanazy cells). (From Woolner, L. B., McConahey, W. M., and Beahrs, O. H.: Struma lymphomatosa (Hashimoto's thyroiditis) and related thyroidal disorders. *J. Clin. Endocr. 19:*53, 1959.)

serum T_4 concentration progressively approach subnormal values. The serum T_3 concentration, however, may be slightly increased, reflecting in all likelihood maximal stimulation of the failing thyroid by the increased serum TSH concentration. The foregoing sequence in the evolution of complete thyroid failure reflects the development of what has been termed "diminished thyroid reserve" or "subclinical hypothyroidism." Ultimately, the serum T_3 concentration also declines to subnormal values, and the clinical state of the patient will be that of frank hypothyroidism.

The diagnosis of Hashimoto's disease is confirmed by the finding of antithyroid antibodies, usually of high titer, in the serum. Newly developed tanned red cell hemagglutination tests for antithyroglobulin and antimicrosomal antibodies have markedly enhanced our ability to detect these antibodies. Although circulating antibody titers tend to be higher in patients with the fibrous variant than in those with the oxyphilic type, almost all patients will display elevated titers of one or another, or both. In young patients, however, the presence of low antibody titers does not exclude the diagnosis.

Since the diagnosis of Hashimoto's disease in most patients can readily be confirmed by tests for antithyroid antibodies, needle biopsy is no longer an important adjunct in diagnosis. When a neoplastic lesion is suspected, fine-needle aspiration biopsy or open biopsy under general anesthesia can be undertaken.

Differential Diagnosis

The differentiation of Hashimoto's disease from other uncomplicated disorders of the thyroid has been greatly facilitated by the demonstration that high titers of antithyroid antibodies occur commonly in Hashimoto's disease but less frequently in other thyroid disorders. The frequent coexistence of hypothyroidism with Hashimoto's disease also serves to distinguish this disease from others, such as nontoxic goiter and thyroid neoplasm, from which it must be differentiated. Differentiation of Hashimoto's disease from diffuse nontoxic goiter is often difficult on clinical grounds, although the goiter in the latter disorder tends to be softer than that of Hashimoto's disease. In adolescent patients, the differentiation from a diffuse nontoxic goiter is even more difficult because in this age group Hashimoto's disease may not be accompanied by the high titers of antithyroid antibodies found in adult patients. Biopsy of the thyroid gland will then be necessary to establish the diagnosis. The presence of well defined nodules will generally serve to distinguish nontoxic multinodular goiter from Hashimoto's disease.

The differentiation between Hashimoto's disease and thyroid carcinoma can often be made on clinical grounds alone. A goiter that is the seat of a thyroid carcinoma is usually nodular and firm or hard and may become fixed to adjacent structures. Compression of the recurrent laryngeal nerve with consequent hoarseness is virtually pathognomonic of thyroid carcinoma. A history of a recent enlargement of the goiter is more frequent in thyroid carcinoma than in Hashimoto's disease. Enlargement of regional lymph nodes is common in thyroid carcinoma but unusual in Hashimoto's disease. Finally, in the case of thyroid carcinoma, external scintiscanning of the thyroid may reveal areas of nonfunction, whereas in Hashimoto's disease activity is usually present throughout the gland.

Treatment

In many patients, no treatment is required because the goiter is small and the disease asymptomatic. In other patients, treatment with thyroid hormone is directed at alleviating goiter or hypothyroidism or both. Treatment is indicated in patients in whom the goiter is pressing on adjacent structures or is unsightly. This is most likely to be effective in the patient with goiter of recent onset. In long-standing goiter, treatment with thyroid hormone is often ineffective, possibly because the gland is more fibrotic. Glucocorticoids cause regression of the goiter and decrease antibody titers, but in view of both their untoward side effects and the fact that the activity of the disease returns after treatment is withdrawn, these agents are not recommended in the management of the usual case. Full replacement doses of thyroid hormone should be given when frank hypothyroidism supervenes or when subclinical hypothyroidism has been demonstrated. Although surgery is a popular form of treatment in some centers, the authors feel that it is justified only if pressure symptoms or unsightly enlargement persists after a trial of suppressive therapy. Administration of hormone should be continued after surgery, because hypothyroidism inevitably results.

Subacute Thyroiditis

Subacute thyroiditis has been termed granulomatous, giant-cell, or de Quervain's thyroiditis. Considerable evidence suggests that it is caused by a viral infection of the thyroid gland. It often follows an upper respiratory illness, and a tendency to a seasonal and geographic aggregation of cases has been noted. The mumps virus has been implicated in some cases, there is some evidence suggesting that Coxsackie, influenza, and ECHO viruses and adenoviruses may also be etiologic agents, and viral isolation has been claimed in some cases (for references, see Stancek et al., 1975). Although evidence of thyroid autoimmunity is often present during the active phase of the disease (see Wall et al., 1976), this is usually transitory, except perhaps in the rare patient in whom the disease progresses to hypothyroidism.

This disease is uncommon, but it is likely that mild cases are mistakenly diagnosed as pharyngitis. Women are far more frequently affected than men, and the maximal incidence is in the fourth and fifth decades.

Histopathology (Fig. 4–42)

The histopathologic changes are distinctive and quite different from those seen in Hashimoto's disease. The lesions are patchy in distribution and characteristically vary in their stage of development from area to area. In affected areas, follicles are infiltrated with cells predominantly of the mononuclear type. These infiltrated follicles show disruption of epithelium, partial or complete loss of colloid, and fragmentation and duplication of the basement membrane. To this extent, the histopathologic appearance may resemble that seen in Hashimoto's disease. A more characteristic feature of the disease is seen in the well-developed follicular lesions and consists of a central core of colloid surrounded by the multinucleate giant cells, from which stems the designation "giant-cell" thyroiditis. Colloid may be found in the interstitium or within the giant cells (colloi-

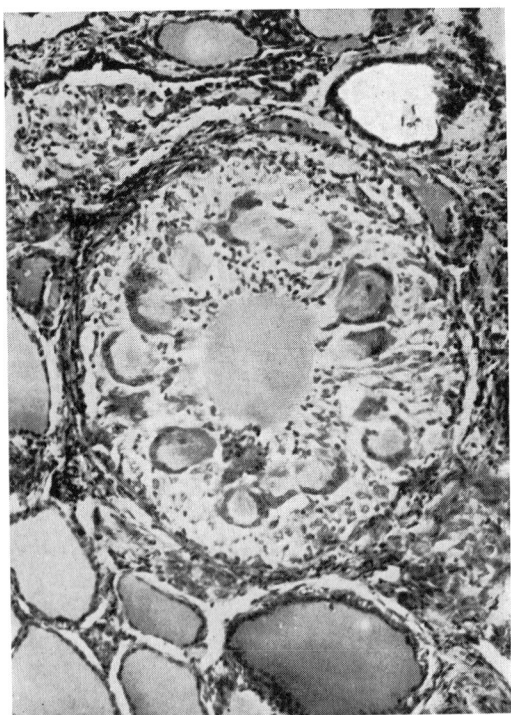

Figure 4–42. Subacute thyroiditis. Intrafollicular giant-cells surrounding a central core of colloid. (From Meachim, G., and Young, M. H.: De Quervain's subacute granulomatous thyroiditis: histological identification and incidence. *J. Clin. Path. 16*:189, 1963.)

dophagy). The follicullar changes progress to form granulomas. Interfollicular fibrosis and an interstitial inflammatory reaction are present to varying degrees. When the disease has subsided, an essentially normal histologic appearance is restored.

Pathophysiology

Destruction of follicular epithelium and loss of follicular integrity are the primary events in the pathophysiology of subacute thyroiditis. Preformed hormone is released, along with abnormal iodinated materials, often in quantities sufficient to elevate the serum T_4 and T_3 concentrations, produce clinical thyrotoxicosis, and suppress TSH secretion. As a result of the latter, thyroid function is decreased, the RAIU declines to low levels, and new hormone synthesis is interrupted. Destruction of the follicular epithelium contributes to the lowering of the RAIU and disruption of hormone synthesis, since TSH may fail to increase the RAIU appreciably. Later in the disease, when stores of preformed hormone are depleted, serum T_4 and T_3 concentrations decline, sometimes into the hypothyroid range, the serum TSH concentration rising, often to elevated values. As the disease becomes inactive, RAIU increases, and it may be greater than normal for a time, as glandular hormone stores are depleted. Ultimately, as hormone secretion resumes, serum T_4 and T_3 rise, and serum TSH declines, to normal values.

Clinical Picture

The characteristic feature of this disease is the gradual or sudden appearance of pain in the region of the thyroid

gland accompanied in severe cases by fever. The pain, which is aggravated by turning the head or swallowing, characteristically radiates to the ear, the jaw, or the occiput and may mimic disorders arising in these areas. Absence of pain does not exclude the diagnosis, since biopsy-proven painless subacute thyroiditis has been reported (Papapetrou and Jackson, 1975). Hoarseness and dysphagia may be present. Patients frequently complain of palpitation, nervousness, and particularly lassitude; lassitude is often extreme and unexpectedly great, considering the local nature of the disease. Although severe cases may appear with acute manifestations, in milder cases, which are often wrongly diagnosed, symptoms may have been present for months. On palpation, at least a part of the thyroid is slightly to moderately enlarged, firm, often nodular, and usually exquisitely tender, one lobe being generally more severely affected than the other. The overlying skin may be warm and red. Occasionally, the locus of maximal involvement migrates over the course of a few weeks to other parts of the gland. The disease usually subsides within a few months, leaving no residual deficiency of thyroid function. In rare cases, the disease may smolder with repeated exacerbations over many months, with hypothyroidism as the end result.

Laboratory Tests

The laboratory findings in patients with subacute thyroiditis vary substantially with the phase of the disease. During the active phase, the erythrocyte sedimentation rate is increased, often to a remarkable extent. Indeed, a diagnosis of active subacute thyroiditis is hardly tenable when the sedimentation rate is normal. The leukocyte count is normal or, at most, moderately increased.

Subacute thyroiditis is one of several causes of "low-uptake thyrotoxicosis," the others being so-called silent thyroiditis (see earlier), thyrotoxicosis factitia, and iodine-induced hyperthyroidism. For reasons described earlier, the RAIU is subnormal, despite the presence of normal, or often elevated, values of the serum T_4 and T_3 concentrations. If tested, the response to TRH will be subnormal during this phase. Subnormal values of the RAIU are found, even when only one portion of the gland seems involved clinically. Occasionally, especially in milder cases, some uptake of radioiodine may persist in unaffected portions of the gland, as revealed by scintiscan, but this is unusual, and a diagnosis of active subacute thyroiditis should be viewed with suspicion if the RAIU is normal.

In the hypothyroid phase of the disease, serum T_4 and T_3 concentrations are low and the serum TSH concentration appropriately elevated. With recovery, the RAIU returns to normal or high values, and normal values for the serum T_4 and T_3 concentrations are restored.

Differential Diagnosis

Subacute thyroiditis must be differentiated mainly from acute hemorrhagic degeneration in a preexisting thyroid nodule, from Hashimoto's disease of acute onset, and from acute pyogenic thyroiditis. Differentiation from hemorrhage into a nodule will present no difficulty when this occurs in a multinodular goiter, because other nontender nodules will be felt. Decision is more difficult when there is hemorrhage into a solitary nodule. In both varieties of hemorrhage, however, function in the remainder of the gland persists, and marked elevation of the sedimentation rate is rarely present. Hashimoto's disease of acute onset may be accompanied by pain and tenderness in the thyroid gland, but the gland is usually diffusely affected. Painless thyroiditis with thyrotoxicosis and a decreased RAIU, but with a histologic picture of chronic thyroiditis and no giant cells, often termed "hyperthyroiditis," may be difficult to distinguish from painless subacute thyroiditis. Lack of elevation of the erythrocyte sedimentation rate and high titers of antithyroid antibodies strongly suggest the former. Acute pyogenic thyroiditis is distinguished by the presence of a septic focus elsewhere, by a greater inflammatory reaction in the tissues adjacent to the thyroid, and by much greater leukocytic and febrile responses. In the authors' experience, a normal RAIU is preserved in acute pyogenic thyroiditis. Rarely, extensively infiltrating cancer of the thyroid can present with a clinical and laboratory picture almost indistinguishable from that of subacute thyroiditis (Rosen et al., 1978).

Treatment

Many forms of treatment have been recommended for subacute thyroiditis, including thionamide drugs, TSH, and suppressive doses of thyroid hormone. The evidence that these agents influence the course of the disease is unconvincing. In mild cases, aspirin is generally adequate to control the symptoms. In more severe cases, glucocorticoids (e.g., prednisone up to 40 mg daily) rapidly alleviate the clinical manifestations but do not influence the underlying disease process. Hence the symptoms may be exacerbated if treatment is withdrawn too early, but they will again respond if treatment is reinstituted. It has been suggested that a relapse can be avoided if glucocorticoid therapy is continued at a dose that maintains the patient in an asymptomatic state until the RAIU has returned to normal (Vagenakis et al., 1970). The application to the thyroid area of small doses of x-ray often produces clinical improvement and was formerly a popular mode of therapy.

Riedel's Thyroiditis

Riedel's thyroiditis is very rare and is observed chiefly in middle-aged women. The etiology is unknown. In the past, Riedel's thyroiditis was considered to be an advanced state of Hashimoto's disease, but it is now generally considered to be a separate disease entity. It is characterized by extensive fibrosis of the thyroid gland and adjacent structures and may be associated with fibrosis elsewhere, especially in the retroperitoneal area.

Symptoms develop insidiously and are related chiefly to compression of adjacent structures, in particular the trachea, esophagus, and recurrent laryngeal nerves. Constitutional symptoms of inflammation are uncommon. The thyroid gland is moderately enlarged and stony hard. The enlargement is usually asymmetrical. The stony hard consistency of the gland and the invasion of adjacent structures suggest carcinoma, but there is no enlargement of regional lymph nodes. The temperature, pulse, and leukocyte count are normal. Hypothyroidism occurs occasionally.

The RAIU may be normal or low. Some patients have circulating antithyroid antibodies, but much less frequently and in lower titer than is usually seen in Hashimoto's disease.

Treatment with thyroid hormone relieves the hypothy-

roidism but has no effect on the goiter. If pressure symptoms are prominent, partial thyroidectomy is indicated.

Miscellaneous Types of Thyroiditis

Acute pyogenic thyroiditis is a rare disorder that is due to an infection of the thyroid by pyogenic organisms, usually as a result of dissemination from a septic focus elsewhere. It is characterized by severe pain and tenderness in the region of the thyroid, with dysphagia, fever, and malaise. There are signs of acute inflammation in the gland and usually in the surrounding tissues. Needle biopsy of the thyroid should be performed so that the infecting organism can be identified and treatment with the appropriate antibody instituted. Surgical drainage is indicated only when fluctuation is present.

Rarely, the thyroid gland is the seat of tuberculosis or coccidioidal infection disseminated from some other focus.

REFERENCES

Abassi, V., and Adigi, C.: Evaluation of sodium L-thyroxine (T_4) requirement in replacement therapy of hypothyroidism. *J. Pediatr.* 90:298, 1977.

Abreu, C. M., Vagenakis, A. G., et al.: Clinical evaluation of a hemagglutination method for microsomal and thyroglobulin antibodies in autoimmune thyroid disease. *Ann. Clin. Lab. Sci.* 7:73, 1977.

Amino, N., Hagen, S. R., et al.: Measurement of circulating thyroid antibodies by the tanned red cell hemagglutination technique: Its usefulness in the diagnosis of autoimmune thyroid disease. *Clin. Endocrinol.* 5:115, 1976.

Amino, N., Kuro, R., et al.: Changes of serum anti-thyroid antibodies during and after pregnancy in autoimmune thyroid diseases. *Clin. Exp. Immunol.* 31:30, 1978.

Amino, N., Miyai, K., et al.: Transient hypothyroidism after delivery in autoimmune thyroiditis. *J. Clin. Endocrinol. Metab.* 42:296, 1976.

Amir, S. M., Sullivan, R. C., et al.: *In vitro* responses to crude and purified hCG in human thyroid membranes. *J. Clin. Endocrinol. Metab.* 51:51, 1980.

Attwood, E. C.: The T_3/TBG ratio and the biochemical investigation of thyrotoxicosis. *Clin. Biochem.* 12:88, 1979.

Bastomsky, C. H.: Thyroid iodide transport. In *Handbook of Physiology*, Section 7: *Endocrinology*. Vol. III, *Thyroid*. Greer, M. A., and Solomon, D. H. (eds.), Baltimore, Williams & Wilkins, 1974.

Bayer, M. F., and McDougall, I. R.: Radioimmunoassay of free thyroxine in serum: comparison with chemical findings and results of conventional thyroid-function tests. *Clin. Chem.* 26:1186, 1980.

Becker, D. V.: Tests of peripheral thyroid hormone action: metabolic indices. In *The Thyroid*. Werner, S. C., and Ingbar, S. H. (eds.), Hagerstown, Harper and Row, 1978.

Beierwaltes, W. H.: The natural history of thyroid cancer. In *Radiation-Associated Thyroid Carcinoma*. DeGroot, L. J. (ed.), New York, Grune and Stratton, 1976.

Beierwaltes, W. H.: The treatment of thyroid carcinoma with radioactive iodine. *Semin. Nucl. Med.* 8:79, 1978.

Bigos, S. T., Ridgway, E. C., et al.: Spectrum of pituitary alterations with mild and severe thyroid impairment. *J. Clin. Endocrinol. Metab.* 46:317, 1978.

Birkhauser, M., Burer, T., et al.: Diagnosis of hyperthyroidism when serum-thyroxine alone is raised. *Lancet* 2:53, 1977.

Biron, R., Burger, A., et al.: Thyroid hormones and the energetics of active sodium-potassium transport in mammalian skeletal muscles. *J. Physiol.* 297:47, 1979.

Borges, M., Labourene, J., et al.: Hepatic iodothyronine metabolism in the chick embryo. *Endocrinology* 107:1751, 1980.

Boyd, J. D.: Development of the human thyroid gland. In *The Thyroid Gland*. Pitt-Rivers, R., and Trotter, W. R. (eds.), Washington, Butterworths, 1964.

Braverman, L. E., Normal and abnormal responses to iodine: disorders of iodine excess. In *The Thyroid*. Werner, S. C., and Ingbar, S. H. (eds.), Hagerstown, Harper and Row, 1978.

Braverman, L. E., Ingbar, S. H., et al.: Conversion of thyroxine (T_4) to triiodothyronine (T_3) in athyreotic human subjects. *J. Clin. Invest.* 49:855, 1970.

Braverman, L. E., Vagenakis, A. G., et al.: Studies on the pathogenesis of iodide myxedema. *Trans. Assoc. Am. Physicians.* 84:130, 1971.

Braverman, L. E., Vagenakis, A. G., et al.: Effects of replacement doses of sodium L-thyroxine on the peripheral metabolism of thyroxine and triiodothyronine in man. *J. Clin. Invest.* 52:1010, 1973.

Bray, G. A., and Jacobs, H. S.: Thyroid activity and other endocrine glands. In *Handbook of Physiology,* Section 7: *Endocrinology.* Vol. III, *Thyroid.* Greer, M. A., and Solomon, D. H. (eds.), Baltimore, Williams & Wilkins, 1974.

Burman, K. D.: Recent developments in thyroid hormone metabolism: interpretation and significance of measurements of reverse T_3, $3,3'-T_2$, and thyroglobulin. *Metabolism* 27:615, 1978.

Burman, K. D., Monchik, J. M., et al.: Ionized and total serum calcium and parathyroid hormone in hyperthyroidism. *Ann. Intern. Med.* 84:668, 1976.

Burrow, G. N.: Hyperthyroidism during pregnancy. *New Engl. J. Med.* 298:150, 1978.

Burrows, A. W., Shakespear, R. A., et al.: Thyroid hormones in the elderly sick: "T_4 euthyroidism." *Br. Med. J.* 4:437, 1975.

Butenandt, O.: Erythrocytic enzyme activities in hypothyroid children. *Acta Haematol.* 47:335, 1972.

Cavalieri, R. R., Gavin, L. A., et al.: Serum thyroxine, free T_4, triiodothyronine, and reverse T_3 in diphenylhydantoin-treated patients. *Metabolism* 28:1161, 1979.

Cavalieri, R. R., and Rapoport, B.: Impaired peripheral conversion of thyroxine to triiodothyronine. *Ann. Rev. Med.* 28:57, 1977.

Chait, A., Bierman, E. L., et al.: Regulatory role of triiodothyronine in the degradation of low density lipoprotein by cultured human fibroblasts. *J. Clin. Endocrinol. Metab.* 48:887, 1979.

Chopra, I. J., Fisher, D. A., et al.: Thyroxine and triiodothyronine in the human thyroid. *J. Clin. Endocrinol. Metab.* 36:311, 1973.

Chopra, I. J., Solomon, D. H., et al.: Misleadingly low free thyroxine index and usefulness of reverse triiodothyronine measurement in nonthyroidal illnesses. *Ann. Intern. Med.* 90:905, 1979.

Clague, R., Mukhtar, E. D., et al.: Thyroid-stimulating immunoglobulins and the control of thyroid function. *J. Clin. Endocrinol. Metab.* 43:550, 1976.

Compagno, J., and Oertel, J. E.: Malignant lymphoma and other lymphoproliferative disorders of the thyroid gland. *Am. J. Clin. Path.* 74:1, 1980.

Connolly, R. J., Vidor, G. I., et al.: Increase in thyrotoxicosis in endemic goiter area after iodination of bread. *Lancet* 1:500, 1970.

Coulombe, P., Dussault, J. H., et al.: Catecholamine metabolism in thyroid diseases. I. Epinephrine secretion rate in hyperthyroidism and hypothyroidism. *J. Clin. Endocrinol. Metab.* 42:125, 1976.

Coulombe, P., Dussault, J. H., et al.: Catecholamine metabolism in thyroid disease. II. Norepinephrine secretion rate in hyperthyroidism and hypothyroidism. *J. Clin. Endocrinol.* 44:1185, 1977.

Crile, G., Jr.: Struma lymphomatosa and carcinoma of the thyroid. *Surg. Gynecol. Obstet.* 147:350, 1978.

Crowley, W. F., Jr., Ridgway, E. C., et al.: Noninvasive evaluation of cardiac function in hypothyroidism. *New Engl. J. Med.* 296:1, 1977.

Croxson, M. S., Hall, T. D., et al.: Combination drug therapy for treatment of hyperthyroid Graves' disease. *J. Clin. Endocrinol.* 45:623, 1977.

Dalovisio, J. R., Blonde, L., et al.: Subacute thyroiditis with increased serum alkaline phosphatase. *Ann. Intern. Med.* 88:505, 1978.

Danforth, E., Jr., Horton, E. S., et al.: Dietary-induced alterations in thyroid hormone metabolism during overnutrition. *J. Clin. Invest.* 64:1336, 1979.

Davies, T. F., Yeo, P. P. B., et al.: Value of thyroid-stimulating antibody in predicting short-term thyrotoxic relapse in Graves' disease. *Lancet* 1:1181, 1977.

DeGroot, L. J.: Mechanism of action of thyroid hormone. In *Free Thyroid Hormones.* Ekins, R., Faglia, G., Pennisi, F., and Pinchera, A. (eds.), Amsterdam, Excerpta Medica, 1979.

Dige-Petersen, H., and Hummer, L.: Serum thyrotropin concentrations under basal conditions and after stimulation with thyrotropin-releasing hormone in idiopathic non-toxic goiter. *J. Clin. Endocrinol. Metab.* 44:1115, 1977.

Distiller, L. A., Sagel, J., et al.: Assessment of pituitary gonadotropin reserve using luteinizing hormone-releasing hormone (LRH) in states of altered thyroid function. *J. Clin. Endocrinol.* 40:512, 1975.

Dobyns, B. M., Sheline, G. E., et al.: Malignant and benign neoplasms of the thyroid in patients treated for hyperthyroidism. A report of the cooperative thyrotoxicosis follow-up study. *J. Clin. Endocrinol. Metab.* 38:976, 1974.

Donaldson, S. S., Bagshaw, M. S., et al.: Supervoltage orbital radiotherapy for Graves' ophthalmopathy. *J. Clin. Endocrinol. Metab.* 37:276, 1973.

Doniach, D., and Marshall, N. J.: Autoantibodies to the thyrotropin (TSH) receptors on thyroid epithelium and other tissues. In *Autoimmunity.* Talal, N. (ed.), New York, Academic Press, 1977.

Dorfman, S. G., Cooperman, M. T., et al.: Painless thyroiditis and transient hyperthyroidism without goiter. *Ann. Intern. Med.* 86:24, 1977.

Dunn, J. T., and Chapman, E. M.: Rising incidence of hypothyroidism after radioactive-iodine therapy in thyrotoxicosis. *New Engl. J. Med.* 271:1037, 1964.

Dussault, J. H., Morissette, J., et al.: Modification of a screening program for neonatal hypothyroidism. *J. Pediatr.* 92:274, 1978.

Eckel, J., Rao, G. S., et al.: Uptake of L-triiodothyronine by isolated liver cells. *Biochem. J.* 182:473, 1979.

Economidou, J., Karacoulis, P., et al.: Carcinoembryonic antigen in thyroid disease. *J. Clin. Pathol.* 30:878, 1977.

Eleles, R. S., Lazarus, J. H., et al.: Plasma adenosine $3':5'$-cyclic monophosphate response to glucagon in thyroid disease. *Clin. Sci. Mol. Med.* 48:27, 1975.

Emerson, C. H., Dyson, W. L., et al.: Serum thyrotropin and thyroxine concentrations in patients receiving lithium carbonate. *J. Clin. Endocrinol. Metab.* 36:338, 1973.

Endo, K., Kasagi, K., et al.: Detection and properties of TSH-binding inhibitor immunoglobulins in patients with Graves' disease and Hashimoto's thyroiditis. *J. Clin. Endocrinol. Metab.* 46:734, 1978.

Engel, A. G.: Neuromuscular manifestations of Graves' disease. *Mayo Clinic Proc.* 47:919, 1972.

Engler, D., Donaldson, E. B., et al.: Hyperthyroidism with triiodothyronine excess: an effect of severe nonthyroidal illness. *J. Clin. Endocrinol. Metab.* 46:77, 1978.

Ermans, A. M., Mbulamoko, N. M., et al.: *Role of Cassava in the etiology of endemic goiter.* Ottawa, International Research Development Center, 1980.

Faglia, G., Bitensky, L., et al.: Thyrotropin secretion in patients with central hypothyroidism. Evidence for reduced biological activity of immunoreactive thyrotropin. *J. Clin. Endocrinol. Metab.* 48:989, 1979.

Favus, M. J., Schneider, A. B., et al.: Thyroid cancer occurring as a late consequence of head-and-neck irradiation. *New Engl. J. Med.* 294:1019, 1976.

Fawcett, D. W., Long, J. A., et al.: The ultrastructure of endocrine glands. *Recent Prog. Horm. Res.* 25:315, 1969.

Felicitta, J. V., Green, W. L., et al.: Thyroid function in patients with chronic renal disease treated by hemodialysis: with comments on the "free thyroxine index." *Metabolism* 28:756, 1979.

Field, J. B.: Pituitary thyrotropin: mechanism of action. In *The Thyroid.* Werner, S. C., and Ingbar, S. H. (eds.), Hagerstown, Harper and Row, 1978.

Fisher, D. A.: Thyroid function in the fetus. In *Handbook of Physiology,* Section 7: *Endocrinology.* Vol. III, *Thyroid.* Greer, M. A., and Solomon, D. H. (eds.), Baltimore, Williams & Wilkins, 1974.

Fisher, D. A., Burrow, G. N., et al.: Recommendations for screening programs for congenital hypothyroidism. *J. Pediatr.* 89:692, 1976.

Fisher, D. A., and Dussault, J. H.: Thyroid function in the fetus. In *Perinatal Thyroid Physiology and Disease.* Fisher, D. A., and Burrow, G. N. (eds.), New York, Raven Press, 1975.

Florsheim, W. H.: Control of thyrotropin secretion. In *Handbook of Physiology,* Section 7: *Endocrinology.* Vol. IV, *The Pituitary Gland and its Neuroendocrine Control.* Knobil, E., and Sawyer, W. H. (eds.), Baltimore, Williams & Wilkins, 1974.

Forrester, J. V., Sutherland, G. R., et al.: Dysthyroid ophthalmopathy: orbital evaluation with beta-scan ultrasonography. *J. Clin. Endocrinol.* 45:221, 1977.

Franklin, C. A. B., Galton, V. A., et al.: Urinary pigment/creatinine ratio in normal and molar pregnancy. *Obstet. Gynecol.* 37:761, 1971.

Freedberg, A. S., and Hamolsky, M. W.: Effects of thyroid hormones on certain nonendocrine organ systems. In *Handbook of Physiology,* Section 7: *Endocrinology.* Vol. III, *Thyroid.* Greer, M. A., and Solomon, D. H. (eds.), Baltimore, Williams & Wilkins, 1974.

Funakoshi, S., and Deutsch, H. F.: Human carbonic anhydrases. V. Levels in erythrocytes in various states. *J. Lab. Clin. Med.* 77:39, 1971.

Gaitan, E., Meyer, J. D., et al.: Environmental goitrogens in Colombia. In *Endemic Goiter and Cretinism: Continuing Threats to World Health.* Dunn, J. T., and Medeiros-Neto, G. A. (eds.), Washington, Pan American Health Organization, 1974.

Gavin, L. A., Hammond, M. E., et al.: $3,3'$-Diiodothyronine production, a major pathway of peripheral iodothyronine metabolism in man. *J. Clin. Invest.* 61:1276, 1978.

Gavin, L. A., Rosenthal, M., et al.: The diagnostic dilemma of isolated hyperthyroxinemia in acute illness. *JAMA* 242:251, 1979.

Gemsenjager, E., Staub, J., et al.: Preclinical hyperthyroidism in multinodular goiter. *J. Clin. Endocrinol. Metab.* 43:810, 1976.

Gershengorn, M. D., McClung, M. R., et al.: Fine-needle aspiration cytology in the preoperative diagnosis of thyroid nodules. *Ann. Intern. Med.* 87:265, 1977.

Gladstone, R., Hordf, A., et al.: Propranolol administration during pregnancy: effects on the fetus. *J. Pediatr.* 86:962, 1975.

Glinoer, D., Delange, F., et al.: Relationship between direct measurement of free T_4 and free T_4 index calculated from TBG. In *Free Thyroid Hormones.* Ekins, R., Faglia, G., Pennisi, G., and Pinchera, A. (eds.), Amsterdam, Excerpta Medica, 1979.

Gorbman, A.: Comparative anatomy and physiology. In *The Thyroid.* Werner, S. C., and Ingbar, S. H. (eds.), Hagerstown, Harper and Row, 1978.

Gordon, G. G., and Southren, A. L.: Thyroid-hormone effects on steroid-hormone metabolism. *Bull. N.Y. Acad. Med.* 53:241, 1977.

Gorman, C. A., Duick, D. S., et al.: Transient hyperthyroidism in patients with lymphocytic thyroiditis. *Mayo Clinic Proc.* 53:359, 1978.

Goslings, B. M., Djokomoeljanto, R,. et al.: Hypothyroidism in an area of endemic goiter and cretinism in Central Java, Indonesia. *J. Clin. Endocrinol. Metab.* 44:481, 1977.

Green, M., and Wilson, G. M.: Thyrotoxicosis treated by surgery or iodine-131. With special reference to development of hypothyroidism. *Brit. Med. J.* 1:1005, 1964.

Green, W. L.: Effects of 3-nitro-L-tyrosine on thyroid function in the rat: an experimental model for the dehalogenase defect. *J. Clin. Invest.* 50:2474, 1971.

Green, W. L.: Mechanisms of action of antithyroid compounds. In *The Thyroid.* Werner, S. C., and Ingbar, S. H. (eds.), Hagerstown, Harper and Row, 1978.

Greenberg, A. H., Najjar, S., et al.: Effects of thyroid hormone on growth, differentiation, and development. In *Handbook of Physiology,* Section 7: *Endocrinology.* Vol. III, *Thyroid.* Greer, M. A., and Solomon, D. H. (eds.), Baltimore, Williams & Wilkins, 1974.

Greer, M. A., and Haibach, H.: Thyroid secretion. In *Handbook of Physiology,* Section 7: *Endocrinology.* Vol. III, *Thyroid.* Greer, M. A., and Solomon, D. H. (eds.), Baltimore, Williams & Wilkins, 1974.

Greer, M. S., Kammer, H., et al.: Short-term antithyroid drug therapy for the thyrotoxicosis of Graves' disease. *New Engl. J. Med.* 297:173, 1977.

Guttler, R. B., Croxson, M. S. et al.: Effects of thyroid hormone on plasma adenosine 3',5'-monophosphate production in man. *Metabolism* 26:1155, 1977.

Hagen, G. A., Ouellette, R. P., et al.: Comparison of high and low dosage levels of I^{131} in the treatment of thyrotoxicosis. *New Engl. J. Med.* 277:559, 1967.

Hamada, S., and Nishimoto, M.: Inhibitory effect of certain drugs on thyroid hormone binding by human liver cytosol. *Acta Endocrinol.* 92:277, 1979.

Hamburger, J. I., Miller, J. M., et al.: *Clinical-Pathological Evaluation of Thyroid Nodules. Handbook and Atlas,* 1979 (limited edition, private publication).

Harden, R. M., Alexander, W. D., et al.: Quantitative studies of iodine metabolism after long-term treatment of thyrotoxicosis with antithyroid drugs. *J. Clin. Endocrinol. Metab.* 26:397, 1966.

Hayes, A. B.: Problem of childhood Graves' disease. *Mayo Clinic Proc.* 47:850, 1972.

Henneman, G., Docter, R., et al.: Raised total thyroxine and free thyroxine index but normal free thyroxine. A serum abnormality due to inherited increased affinity of iodothyronines for serum binding protein. *Lancet* 1:639, 1979.

Herrmann, J., Rusche, H. J., et al.: Free triiodothyronine (T$_3$) and thyroxine (T$_4$) serum levels in old age. *Horm. Metab. Res.* 6:239, 1973.

Hershman, J. M.: The treatment of hyperthyroidism. *Ann. Intern. Med.* 64:1306, 1966.

Hershman, J. M.: Hyperthyroidism caused by placental or pituitary thyrotropins. In *The Thyroid.* Werner, S. C., and Ingbar, S. H. (eds.), Hagerstown, Harper and Row, 1978.

Hoch, F. L.: Metabolic effects of thyroid hormones. In *Handbook of Physiology,* Section 7: *Endocrinology.* Vol. III, *Thyroid.* Greer, M. A., and Solomon, D. H. (eds.), Baltimore, Williams & Wilkins, 1974.

Hoffer, P. B., Gottschalk, A., et al.: Thyroid scanning technics: The old and the new. *Ann. Probl. Radiol.* 2:1, 1972.

Hoffman, D. P., Surks, M. I., et al.: Response to thyrotropin releasing hormone: an objective criterion for the adequacy of thyrotropin suppression therapy. *J. Clin. Endocrinol.* 44:892, 1977.

Ikekubo, K., Konishi, J., et al.: Anti-thyroxine and anti-triiodothyronine antibodies in three cases of Hashimoto's thyroiditis. *Acta Endocrinol.* 89:537, 1978.

Inada, M., Nishikawa, M., et al.: Post-partum transient thyrotoxicosis: report of two cases. *Endocrinol. Jpn.* 26:611, 1979.

Ingbar, S. H.: Effects of iodine: autoregulation of the thyroid. In *The Thyroid.* Werner, S. C., and Ingbar, S. H. (eds.), Hagerstown, Harper and Row, 1978a.

Ingbar, S. H.: The influence of aging on human thyroid hormone economy. In *Geriatric Endocrinology.* Greenblatt, R. (ed.), New York, Raven Press, 1978b.

Ingbar, S. H., and Borges, M.: Peripheral metabolism of the thyroid hormones. In: *Free Thyroid Hormones.* Ekins, R., Faglia, G., Pennisi, F., and Pinchera, A. (eds.), Amsterdam, Excerpta Medica, 1979.

Ingbar, S. H., and Braverman, L. E.: Active form of the thyroid hormone. *Ann. Rev. Med.* 26:443, 1975.

Izumi, M., and Larsen, P. R.: Triiodothyronine, thyroxine, and iodine in purified thyroglobulin from patients with Graves' disease. *J. Clin. Invest.* 59:1105, 1977.

Jacobsson, B., Pettersson, T., et al.: Prealbumin in the islets of Langerhans. *IRCS Med. Sci.* 7:590, 1979.

Jellinek, E. H.: Fits, faints, coma, and dementia in myxoedema. *Lancet* 2:1010, 1962.

Jenkins, D. J.: An investigation into creatine kinase and other plasma enzymes in thyroid disorders. *Clin. Chim. Acta* 85:197, 1978.

Johannessen, J. V., and Sobrinho-Simões, M.: The origin and significance of thyroid psammoma bodies. *Lab. Invest.* 43:287, 1980.

Johnson, P. M.: Radioisotopes and direct tests of thyroid function: thyroid and whole-body scanning. In *The Thyroid.* Warner, S. C., and Ingbar, S. H. (eds.), Hagerstown, Harper and Row, 1978.

Khandekar, J. D., and Scanlon, E. F.: Letter to the editor. *New Engl. J. Med.* 302:1149, 1980.

Kidd, A., Okita, N., et al.: Immunologic aspects of Graves' and Hashimoto's diseases. *Metabolism* 29:80, 1980.

Kohn, L. D., and Winand, R. J.: Exophthalmogenic activity of the beta subunit of thyrotropin. *Endocrinology* 96:1592, 1975.

Kourides, I. A., Re, R. N., et al.: Clearance and secretion rates of subunits of human thyrotropin. *J. Clin. Invest.* 59:508, 1977a.

Kourides, I. A., Ridgway, E. C., et al.: Thyrotropin-induced hyperthyroidism: use of alpha and beta subunits to identify patients with pituitary tumors. *J. Clin. Endocrinol. Metab.* 45:534, 1977b.

Krenning, E. P., Docter, R., et al.: The essential role of albumin in the active transport of thyroid hormones into primary cultured rat hepatocytes. *FEBS Lett.* 107:227, 1979.

Krugman, L. G., Hershman, J. M., et al.: Patterns of recovery of the hypothalamic-pituitary-thyroid axis in patients taken off chronic thyroid therapy. *J. Clin. Endocrinol. Metab.* 41:70, 1975.

Lamberg, B.-A., and Gordin, A.: Abnormalities of thyrotropin secretion and clinical implications of the thyrotropin releasing stimulation test. *Ann. Clin. Res.* 10:171, 1978.

Landsberg, L.: Catecholamines and the sympathoadrenal system. In *The Year in Endocrinology.* Ingbar, S. H. (ed.), New York, Plenum, 1976.

Landsberg, L.: Catecholamines and hyperthyroidism. *Clin. Endocrinol. Metab.* 3:697, 1977.

Larsen, P. R., and Silva, J. E.: Sources of pituitary nuclear T$_3$. In *Free Thyroid Hormones.* Ekins, R., Faglia, G., Pennisi, F., and Pinchera, A. (eds.), Amsterdam, Excerpta Medica, 1979.

Leeper, R. D.: The effect of ^{131}I therapy on survival of patients with metastatic papillary or follicular thyroid carcinoma. *J. Clin. Endocrinol. Metab.* 36:1193, 1973.

Levey, G. S.: The adrenergic nervous system in hyperthyroidism: therapeutic role of beta adrenergic blocking drugs. *Pharmacol. Ther.* 1:431, 1976.

Lim, V. S., Fang, V. S., et al.: Thyroid dysfunction in chronic renal failure. *J. Clin. Invest.* 60:522, 1977.

Lindstedt, G., Nilsson, L. A., et al.: On the prevalence, diagnosis and management of lithium-induced hypothyroidism in psychiatric patients. *Brit. J. Psychiatry* 130:452, 1977.

Lowhagen, T., Willems, J. S., et al.: Aspiration biopsy cytology in diagnosis of thyroid cancer. *World J. Surg.* 5:61, 1981.

Luft, R., Ikkos, D., et al.: A case of severe hypermetabolism of nonthyroid origin with a defect in the maintenance of mitochondrial control: a correlated clinical, biochemical, and morphological study. *J. Clin. Invest.* 41:1776, 1962.

Lumholtz, T. B., Loldrup-Paulsen, D., et al.: Outcome of long-term antithyroid treatment of Graves' disease in relation to iodine intake. *Acta Endocrinol.* 84:538, 1977.

Malone, J. F., and Cullen, M. J.: Hypothyroidism after ^{125}I therapy. *Ann. Intern. Med.* 86:823, 1977.

Marchant, B., Lees, J. F. H., et al.: Antithyroid drugs. *Pharmacol. Ther.* 3:305, 1978.

Maxon, H. R., Saenger, E. L., et al.: Clinically important radiation-associated thyroid disease. *JAMA* 244:1802, 1980.

Mazzaferri, E. L., Young, R. L., et al.: Papillary thyroid carcinoma: the impact of therapy in 576 patients. *Medicine* 56:171, 1977.

McDougall, I. R., and Greig, W. R.: ^{125}I therapy in Graves' disease. Long-term results in 355 patients. *Ann. Inter. Med.* 85:720, 1976.

McKenzie, A. D.: The natural history of thyroid cancer. *Arch. Surg.* 102:274, 1971.

McKenzie, J. M., and Zakarija, M.: LATS in Graves' disease. *Rec. Progr. Hormone Res.* 33:29, 1977.

McKenzie, J. M., and Zakarija, M.: Pathogenesis of neonatal Graves' disease. *J. Endocrinol. Invest.* 2:183, 1978.

Melander, A., Westgren, U., et al.: Influence of the sympathetic nervous system on the secretion and metabolism of thyroid hormone. *Endocrinology* 101:1228, 1977.

Michie, W., Stowers, J. M., et al.: Mechanism of hypocalcemia after thyroidectomy for thyrotoxicosis. *Lancet* 1:508, 1971.

Miller, J. M., Hamburger, J. I., et al.: Diagnosis of thyroid nodules. Use of fine-needle aspiration and needle biopsy. *JAMA* 241:481, 1979.

Miyai, K., Tanizawa, O., et al.: Pituitary-thyroid function in trophoblastic disease. *J. Clin. Endocrinol. Metab.* 42:254, 1976.

Moens, H., and Farid, N. R.: Hashimoto's thyroiditis is associated with HLA-DRW3. *New Engl. J. Med.* 299:133, 1978.

Mullin, B. R., Levinson, R. E., et al.: Delayed hypersensitivity in Graves' disease and exophthalmos. Identification of thyroglobulin in normal human orbital muscle. *Endocrinology* 100:351, 1977.

Nagataki, S.: Effect of excess quantities of iodide. In *Handbook of Physiology,* Section 7: *Endocrinology.* Vol. III, *Thyroid.* Greer, M. A., and Solomon, D. H. (eds.), Baltimore & Wilkins, 1974.

Nagataki, S., Mizuno, M., et al.: Thyroid function in molar pregnancy. *J. Clin. Endocrinol. Metab.* 44:254, 1977.

Nicoloff, J. T.: Thyroid hormone transport and metabolism: pathophysiologic implications. In *The Thyroid*. Werner, S. C., and Ingbar, S. H. (eds.), Hagerstown, Harper and Row, 1978.

Nikkila, E. A., and Kekki, M.: Plasma triglyceride metabolism in thyroid disease. *J. Clin. Invest.* 51:2103, 1972.

Nofal, M. M., and Beierwaltes, W. H.: Treatment of hyperthyroidism with sodium iodide I¹³¹ *JAMA* 197:605, 1966.

Novogroder, M., Utiger, R., et al.: Juvenile hyperthyroidism with elevated thyrotropin (TSH) and normal 24 hour FSH, LH, GH, and protein secretory patterns. *J. Clin. Endocrinol. Metab.* 45:1053, 1977.

O'Donnell, J., Trokoudes, K., et al.: Thyrotropin displacement activity of serum immunoglobulins from patients with Graves' disease. *J. Clin. Endocrinol. Metab.* 46:770, 1978.

Ogura, J., Wessler, S., et al.: Surgical approach to the ophthalmopathy of Graves' disease. *JAMA* 216:1627, 1971.

Onishi, T., Miyai, K., et al.: Primary hypothyroidism and galactorrhea. *Am. J. Med.* 63:373, 1977.

Oppenheimer, J. H.: Thyroid hormone action at the cellular level. *Science* 203:971, 1979.

Osathanondh, R., Chopra, I. J., et al.: Effects of dexamethasone on fetal and maternal thyroxine, triiodothyronine, reverse triiodothyronine and thyrotropin levels. *J. Clin. Endocrinol. Metab.* 47:1236, 1978.

Otten, J., Jonckheer, M., et al.: Thyroid albumin. II. *In vitro* synthesis of a thyroid albumin by normal human thyroid tissue. *J. Clin. Endocrinol. Metab.* 32:18, 1971.

Pacini, F., Pinchera, A., et al.: Serum thyroglobulin concentrations and ¹³¹I whole body scans in the diagnosis of metastases from differentiated thyroid carcinoma (after thyroidectomy). *Clin. Endocrinol.* 13:107, 1980.

Palmer, J. A., Mustard, R. A., et al.: Irradiation as an etiologic factor in tumours of the thyroid, parathyroid, and salivary glands. *Can. J. Surg.* 23:39, 1980.

Papapetrou, P. D., and Jackson, I. M. D.: Thyrotoxicosis due to "silent" thyroiditis. *Lancet* 1:361, 1975.

Parisi, A. F., and Hamilton, B. P.: The short cardiac pre-ejection period. An index to thyrotoxicosis. *Circulation* 49:900, 1974.

Parker, D. C., Pekary, A. E., et al.: Effect of normal and reversed sleep-wake cycles upon nyctohemeral rhythmicity of plasma thyrotropin: Evidence suggestive of an inhibitory influence in sleep. *J. Clin. Endocrinol. Metab.* 43:318, 1976.

Pezzino, V., Vigneri, R., et al.: Increased serum thyroglobulin levels in patients with nontoxic goiter. *J. Clin. Endocrinol. Metab.* 46:653, 1978.

Pierce, J. G.: Pituitary thyrotropin: chemistry. In *The Thyroid*. Werner, S. C., and Ingbar, S. H. (eds.), Hagerstown, Harper and Row, 1978.

Pillay, S. P., Angorn, I. B., et al.: Tumour metastasis to the thyroid gland. *S. Afr. Med. J.* 51:509, 1977.

Popovic, W. J., Brown, J. E., et al.: The influence of thyroid hormones on *in vitro* erythropoiesis. *J. Clin. Invest.* 60:907, 1977.

Re, R. N., Kourides, I. A., et al.: The effect of glucocorticoid administration on human pituitary secretion of thyrotropin and prolactin. *J. Clin. Endocrinol. Metab.* 43:338, 1976.

Refetoff, S., DeGroot, L. J., et al.: Studies of a sibship with apparent resistance to the intracellular action of thyroid hormone. *Metabolism* 21:723, 1972.

Reichlin, S.: Neuroendocrine control. In *The Thyroid*. Werner, S. C., and Ingbar, S. H. (eds.), Hagerstown, Harper and Row, 1978.

Rezvani, I., and DiGeorge, A. M.: Reassessment of the daily dose of oral thyroxine for replacement therapy in hypothyroid children. *J. Pediatr.* 90:291, 1977.

Ridgway, E. C., Kourides, I. A., et al.: Augmentation of pituitary thyrotropin response to thyrotropin releasing hormone during subphysiological triiodothyronine therapy in hypothyroidism. *Clin. Endocrinol.* 10:343, 1979.

Rootwelt, K., Ganes, T., et al.: Effect of carbamazepine, phenytoin and phenobarbitone on serum levels of thyroid hormones and thyrotropin in humans. *Scand. J. Lab. Invest.* 38:731, 1978.

Rosen, I. B., Strawbridge, H. G., et al.: Malignant pseudothyroiditis: a new clinical entity. *Am. J. Surg.* 136:445, 1978.

Rosen, I. B., Walfish, P. G., et al.: The ultrasound of thyroid masses. *Surg. Clin. North Am.* 59:19, 1979.

Rosman, N. P.: Neurological and muscular aspects of thyroid dysfunction in childhood. Pediatr. Clin. North Am. 23:575, 1976.

Roudebush, C. P., Asteris, G. I., et al.: Natural history of radiation-associated thyroid cancer. *Arch. Intern. Med.* 138:1631, 1978.

Royce, P. C.: Severely impaired consciousness in myxedema — a review. *Am. J. Med. Sci.* 261:46, 1971.

Russell, W. O., Ibanez, M. L., et al.: Thyroid carcinoma. Classification, intraglandular dissemination, and clinicopathological study based on whole organ sections of 80 glands. *Cancer* 16:1425, 1963.

Saenger, E. L., Thomas, G. E., et al.: Incidence of leukemia following treatment of hyperthyroidism. *JAMA* 205:855, 1968.

Safa, A. M., Schumacher, O. P., et al.: Long-term follow-up results in children and adolescents treated with radioactive iodine (¹³¹I) for hyperthyroidism. *New Engl. J. Med.* 292:167, 1975.

Sanders, V.: Neurologic manifestations of myxedema. *New Engl. J. Med.* 266:547 and 599, 1962.

Sawin, C. T., Chopra, D., et al.: The aging thyroid. Increased prevalence of elevated serum thyrotropin levels in the elderly. *JAMA* 242:247, 1979.

Scanlon, M. F., Smith, B. R., et al.: Thyroid-stimulating hormone: neuroregulation and clinical applications. *Clin. Sci. Mol. Med.* 55:1 and 129, 1978.

Schimmel, M., and Utiger, R. D.: Thyroidal and peripheral production of thyroid hormones. *Ann. Intern. Med.* 87:760, 1977.

Schneider, A. B., Favus, M. J., et al.: Letter to the editor. *New Engl. J. Med.* 302:1148, 1980.

Schneider, A. B., and Ikekubo, K.: Measurement of thyroglobulin in the circulation: clinical and technical considerations. *Ann. Clin. Lab. Sci.* 9:230, 1979.

Schussler, G. C., and Orlando, J.: Fasting decreases triiodothyronine receptor capacity. *Science* 199:686, 1978.

Schussler, G., Schaffner, F., et al.: Increased serum thyroid hormone binding and decreased free hormone in chronic active liver disease. *New Engl. J. Med.* 299:510, 1978.

Segal, J., and Ingbar, S. H.: Plasma membrane-mediated effects of thyroid hormones. In *Endocrinology 1980*. Cumming, I. A., Funder, J. W., Mendelsohn, F. A. O. (eds.), Canberra, Australian Academy of Sciences, 1980.

Shimaoka, K., Badillo, J., et al.: Clinical differentiation between thyroid cancer and benign goiter. *JAMA* 181:179, 1962.

Skillern, P. G.: Genetics of Graves' disease. *Mayo Clin. Proc.* 47:848, 1972.

Skowsky, W. R., and Kikuchi, T. A.: The role of vasopressin in the impaired water excretion of myxedema. *Am. J. Med.* 64:613, 1978.

Smals, A. G. H., Ross, H. A., et al.: Seasonal variation in serum T₃ and T₄ levels in man. *J. Clin. Endocrinol. Metab.* 44:998, 1977.

Smeulers, J., Docter, R., et al.: Response to thyrotropin-releasing hormone and triiodothyronine suppressibility in euthyroid multinodular goitre. *Clin. Endocrinol.* 7:389, 1977.

Smith, R. N., Taylor, S. A., et al.: Controlled clinical trial of combined triiodothyronine and thyroxine in the treatment of hypothyroidism. *Brit. Med. J.* 4:145, 1970.

Smith, R. N., and Wilson, G. M.: Clinical trial of different doses of I¹³¹ in treatment of thyrotoxicosis. *Brit. Med. J.* 1:129, 1967.

Smith, T. J., and Edelman, I. S.: The role of sodium transport in thyroid thermogenesis. *Fed. Proc.* 38:2150, 1979.

Snyder, L. M., and Reddy, W. J.: Mechanism of action of thyroid hormones on erythrocyte 2,3-diphosphoglyceric acid synthesis. *J. Clin. Invest.* 49:1993, 1970.

Sobrinho, L. G., Limbert, E. S., et al.: Thyroxine toxicosis in patients with iodine induced thyrotoxicosis. *J. Clin. Endocrinol. Metab.* 45:25, 1977.

Solomon, D. H., Chopra, I. J., et al.: Identification of subgroups of euthyroid Graves' ophthalmopathy. *New Engl. J. Med.* 296:181, 1977.

Stanbury, J. B.: Familial goiter. In *The Metabolic Basis of Inherited Disease*; 4th ed. Stanbury, J. B., Wyngaarden, J. B., Fredrickson, D. S. (eds.), New York, McGraw-Hill, 1978, p. 206.

Stancek, D., Stancekova-Gressnerova, M., et al.: Isolation and serological and epidemiological data on the viruses covered from patients with subacute thyroiditis de Quervain. *Med. Microbiol. Immunol.* 161:133, 1975.

Steinberg, A. D.: Myxedema and coronary artery disease — a comparative autopsy study. *Ann. Intern. Med.* 68:338, 1968.

Stepanas, A. V., Samaan, N. A., et al.: Medullary thyroid carcinoma. *Cancer* 43:825, 1979.

Sterling, K.: Thyroid hormone action at the cell level. *New Engl. J. Med.* 300:117 and 173, 1979.

Strakosch, C. R., Joyner, D., et al.: Thyroid stimulating antibodies in patients with autoimmune disorders. *J. Clin. Endocrinol. Metab.* 47:361, 1978.

Sung, L. C., and Cavalieri, R. R.: T₃ thyrotoxicosis due to metastatic thyroid carcinoma. *J. Clin. Endocrinol. Metab.* 36:215, 1973.

Surks, M. I., Schadlow, A. R., et al.: A new radioimmunoassay for plasma L-triiodothyronine: Measurements in thyroid disease and in patients maintained on hormonal replacement. *J. Clin. Invest.* 51:3104, 1972.

Suzuki, H., Kadena, N., et al.: Effect of three-day oral cholecystography on serum iodothyronines and TSH concentration: Comparison of the effects among some cholecystographic agents and the effect of ipanoic acid on the pituitary-thyroid axis. *Acta Endocrinol.* 92:477, 1979.

Suzuki, H., and Mashimo, K.: Significance of the iodide-perchlorate discharge test in patients with ¹³¹I-treated and untreated hyperthyroidism. *J. Clin. Endocrinol. Metab.* 34:332, 1972.

Tamagna, E. I., Carlson, H. E., et al.: Pituitary and peripheral resistance to thyroid hormone. *Clin. Endocrinol.* 10:431, 1979.

Tamai, H., Nakagawa, T., et al.: Changes in thyroid functions in patients with euthyroid Graves' disease. *J. Clin. Endocrinol. Metab.* 50:108, 1980.

Tamai, H., Suematsu, H., et al.: Responses to TRH and T_3 suppression tests in euthyroid subjects with a family history of Graves' disease. *J. Clin. Endocrinol. Metab.* 47:475, 1978.

Tata, J. R.: Growth and developmental action of thyroid hormones at the cellular level. In *Handbook of Physiology*, Section 7: *Endocrinology*. Vol. III, *Thyroid*. Greer, M. A., and Solomon, D. H. (eds.), Baltimore, Williams & Wilkins, 1974.

Taunton, O. D., McDaniel, H. G., et al.: Standardization of TSH testing. *J. Clin. Endocrinol. Metab.* 25:266, 1965.

Taurog, A.: Biosynthesis of iodoamino acids. In *Handbook of Physiology*, Section 7: *Endocrinology*. Vol. III, *Thyroid*. Greer, M. A., and Solomon, D. H. (eds.), Baltimore, Williams & Wilkins, 1974.

Thilly, C., Lagasse, R., et al.: Impaired fetal and postnatal development and high perinatal death rate in a severe iodine deficient area. Program of the VIII International Thyroid Conference, Sydney, February 3–8, 1980, p. 2.

Tobin, R., Berdanier, C. D., et al.: Effects of thyroxine treatment on the hepatic membrane ATPase activity in rats. *J. Environ. Pathol. Toxicol.* 2:1235, 1979.

Toft, A. D., Irvine, W. J., et al.: A comparison of plasma TSH levels in patients with diffuse and nodular non-toxic goiter. *J. Clin. Endocrinol. Metab.* 42:973, 1976a.

Toft, A. D., Irvine, W. J., et al.: Propranolol in the treatment of thyrotoxicosis by subtotal thyroidectomy. *J. Clin. Endocrinol. Metab.* 43:1323, 1976b.

Tolis, G., Bird, C., et al.: Pituitary hyperthyroidism. *Am. J. Med.* 64:177, 1978.

Topliss, D. J., White, E. L., et al.: Significance of thyrotropin excess in untreated primary adrenal insufficiency. *J. Clin. Endocrinol. Metab.* 50:52, 1980.

Transbol, I., Christiansen, C., et al.: Endocrine effects of lithium. 1. Hypothyroidism, its prevalence in long-term treated patients. *Acta Endocrinol.* 87:759, 1978.

Tucci, J. R., and Kopp, L.: Urinary cyclic nucleotide levels in patients with hyper- and hypothyroidism. *J. Clin. Endocrinol. Metab.* 43:1323, 1976.

Tunstall, M. E.: The effect of propranolol on the onset of breathing at birth. *Brit. J. Anaesth.* 41:792, 1969.

Turner, J. W., and Spencer, J. P.: Thyroid carcinoma presenting as a pertechnetate "hot" nodule, but without ^{131}I uptake: case report. *J. Nucl. Med.* 17:22, 1976.

Uchimura, H., Amir, S. M., et al.: Failure of organic iodine enrichment to influence the binding of bovine thyrotropin to rat thyroid tissue. *Endocrinology* 104:1207, 1979.

Ui, N.: Synthesis and chemistry of iodoproteins. In *Handbook of Physiology*, Section 7: *Endocrinology*. Vol. III, *Thyroid*. Greer, M. A., and Solomon, D. H. (eds.), Baltimore, Williams & Wilkins, 1974.

Uller, R. P., Van Herle, A. J., et al.: Comparison of alterations in circulating thyroglobulin, triiodothyronine and thyroxine in response to exogenous (bovine) and endogenous (human) thyrotropin. *J. Clin. Endocrinol. Metab.* 37:741, 1973.

Vagenakis, A. G., Braverman, L. E., et al.: Recovery of pituitary thyrotropic function after withdrawal of prolonged thyroid-suppression therapy. *New Engl. J. Med.* 293:681, 1975.

Vagenakis, A. G., Downs, P., et al.: Control of thyroid hormone secretion in normal subjects receiving iodides. *J. Clin. Invest.* 52:528, 1973.

Vander, J. B., Gaston, E. A., et al.: The significance of non-toxic thyroid nodules. Final report of a 15-year study of the incidence of thyroid malignancy. *Ann. Intern. Med.* 69:537, 1968.

Van Herle, A. J., and Uller, R. P.: Thyroid cancer classification, clinical features, diagnosis, and therapy. *Pharmacol. Ther.* 2:215, 1977.

Varma, V. M., Beierwaltes, W. H., et al.: Treatment of thyroid cancer. Death rates after surgery and after surgery followed by sodium iodide [131]I. *JAMA* 36:1143, 1970.

Velentzas, C., Oreopoulos, D. G., et al.: Vitamin-D levels in thyrotoxicosis. *Lancet* 1:370, 1977.

Visser, T. J.: A tentative review of recent *in vitro* observations of the enzymatic deiodination of iodothyronines and its possible physiological implications. *Mol. Cell. Endocrinol.* 10:241, 1978.

Waal-Manning, H. J.: Effect of propranolol on the duration of the Achilles tendon reflex. *Clin. Pharmacol. Ther.* 10:199, 1969.

Wall, J. R., Fang, S. L., et al.: Lymphocytic transformation in response to human thyroid extract in patients with subacute thyroiditis. *J. Clin. Endocrinol. Metab.* 43:587, 1976.

Walfish, P. G., Hazani, E., et al.: Combined ultrasound and needle aspiration cytology in the assessment and management of hypofunctioning thyroid nodule. *Ann. Intern. Med.* 87:270, 1977.

Wang, C., Vickery, A. L., Jr., et al.: Needle biopsy of the thyroid. *Surg. Gynecol. Obstet.* 143:365, 1976.

Wartofsky, L.: Low remission after therapy for Graves' disease: possible relation of dietary iodine with antithyroid therapy results. *JAMA* 226:1083, 1973.

Wehmann, R. E., Rubenstein, H. A., et al.: A sensitive, convenient radioimmunoassay procedure which demonstrates that serum hTSH is suppressed below the normal range in thyrotoxic patients. *Endocr. Res. Commun.* 6:249, 1979.

Wenzel, K. W., and Meinhold, H.: Evidence of lower toxicity during thyroxine suppression after a single 3-mg L-thyroxine dose: comparison to the classical L-triiodothyronine test for thyroid suppressibility. *J. Clin. Endocrinol. Metab.* 38:902, 1974.

Westgren, U., Burger, A., et al.: Blood levels of 3,5,3'-triiodothyronine and thyroxine: differences between children, adults, and elderly subjects. *Acta Med. Scand.* 200:493, 1976.

Williams, D. E., Chopra, I. J., et al.: Acute effects of corticosteroids on thyroid activity in Graves' disease. *J. Clin. Endocrinol. Metab.* 41:354, 1975.

Witt, T. R., Meng, R. L., et al.: The approach to the irradiated thyroid. *Surg. Clin. North Am.* 59:45, 1979.

Woeber, K. A., and Ingbar, S. H.: The interactions of the thyroid hormones with binding proteins. In *Handbook of Physiology*, Section 7: *Endocrinology*. Vol. III, *Thyroid*. Greer, M. A., and Solomon, D. H. (eds.), Baltimore, Williams & Wilkins, 1974.

Wood, L. C., and Ingbar, S. H.: Hypothyroidism as a late sequela in patients with Graves' disease treated with antithyroid agents. *J. Clin. Invest.* 64:1429, 1979.

Woolner, L. B., Beahrs, O. H., et al.: Classification and prognosis of thyroid carcinoma. A study of 885 cases observed in a thirty-year period. *Am. J. Surg.* 102:354, 1961.

Yamada, T., Tsukui, T., et al.: Volume of sella turcica in normal subjects and in patients with primary hypothyroidism and hyperthyroidism. *J. Clin. Endocrinol. Metab.* 42:817, 1976.

Yamamoto, T., Amino, N., et al.: Longitudinal study of serum thyroid hormones, chorionic gonadotropin and thyrotrophin during and after normal pregnancy. *Clin. Endocrinol.* 10:459, 1979.

Young, R. T., Van Herle, A. J., et al.: Improved diagnosis and management of hyper- and hypothyroidism by timing the arterial sounds. *J. Clin. Endocrinol. Metab.* 42:330, 1976.

Zakarija, M., McKenzie, J. M., et al.: Clinical significance of assay of thyroid-stimulating antibody in Graves' disease. *Ann. Intern. Med.* 93:28, 1980.

Zwillich, C. W., Pierson, D. J., et al.: Ventilatory control in myxedema and hypothyroidism. *New Engl. J. Med.* 292:662, 1975

CHAPTER 5

The Adrenals

By Grant W. Liddle

THE NORMAL ADRENAL CORTEX

Embryology

During the 4th to 6th weeks of fetal life, cells from the coelomic mesoderm of the posterior abdominal wall near the mesonephros form a cluster between the root of the mesentery and the genital ridge to establish the fetal adrenal cortex. Some 5 weeks later, small basophilic cells appear around the fetal cortex; these are the forerunners of the permanent adrenal cortex.

During the 7th week of embryonic development, the fetal adrenal cortex is invaded by cells migrating from the neural crest; these "sympathogonia" are forerunners of the adrenal medulla. They undergo further differentiation to form either ganglion cells or chromaffin cells; the latter secrete catecholamines.

The adrenal glands are relatively large structures during fetal life and undergo rapid involution during the first few months of extrauterine life.[1] Much of the bulk of the fetal adrenal cortex is attributable to an inner zone of large acidophilic cells arranged in anastomosing cords, separated by large, thin-walled sinusoidal capillaries. The fetal cortex is ACTH-dependent and is relatively small in the absence of a functioning pituitary.

Anatomy

The adrenal glands are paired, convoluted, somewhat pyramidal structures that, as their name implies, are situated atop the kidneys. The outer portion, or cortex (approximately 80 per cent by weight in the normal adult), is firm and golden yellow; the inner portion, or medulla, is soft and reddish brown in color. Normally, each gland weighs about 5 g; they are smaller in conditions associated with a deficiency of ACTH and may become as much as four times larger in response to a chronic excess of ACTH.

The adrenals are supplied by numerous small arteries arising from the phrenic arteries, the aorta, and the renal arteries and occasionally by branches from the ovarian, spermatic, or intercostal arteries as well. These vessels penetrate the gland along connective tissue trabeculae and break up into a network of sinusoidal capillaries that extend radially into large venous lacunae in the medulla. Venules collect into a large central vein that runs as an axis through the gland and empties on the left into the renal vein and on the right into the inferior vena cava. Anatomic variations are relatively common.

Histologically, the human adrenal has three zones; an outer *zona glomerulosa*, a middle *zona fasciculata*, and an inner *zona reticularis*, so named because of the arrangement of the cells in each zone (Fig. 5–1). The narrow subcapsular zona glomerulosa consists of relatively small, compact cells grouped in ill-defined clusters. Electron microscopy reveals elongated mitochondria with transverse shelflike infoldings of the inner mitochondrial membrane ("cristae"). The wider zona fasciculata consists of larger lipid-laden cells radially arranged in parallel cords. Here the mitochondria are more nearly spheric, and the cristae appear as short tubular invaginations of the inner membrane. The zona reticularis consists of anastomosing networks of cells that resemble those of the zona fasciculata except for the fact that they contain less lipid. Here the mitochondria are elongated and contain a mixture of tubular and flattened cristae. Differences in mitochondrial morphology are thought to be of aid in determining the origins of cells in adrenal neoplasms.

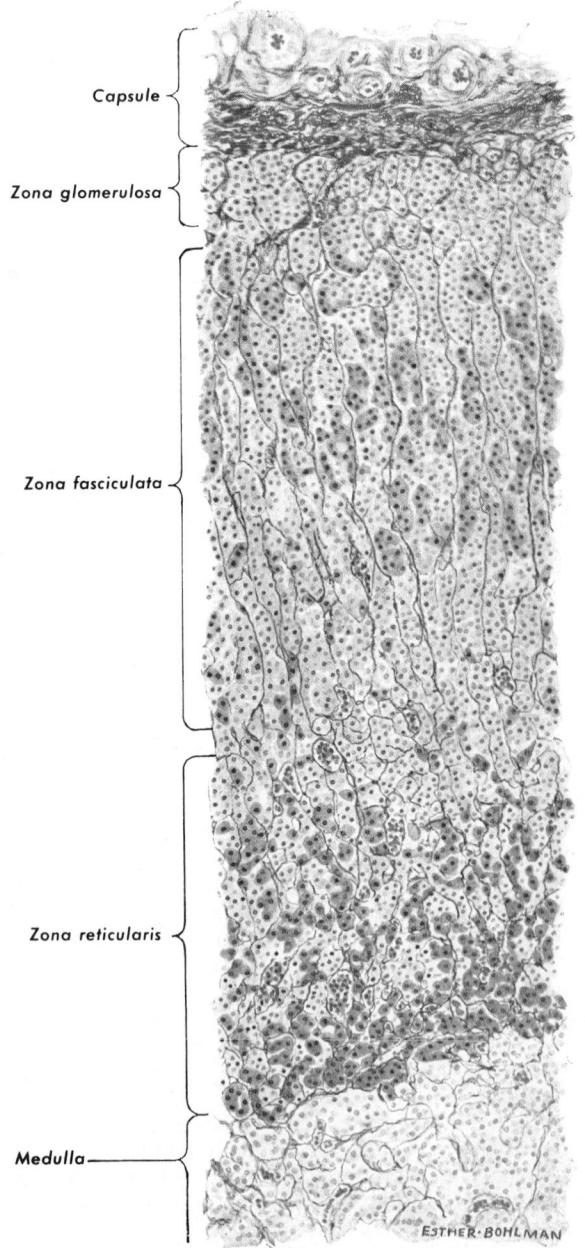

Capsule

Zona glomerulosa

Zona fasciculata

Zona reticularis

Medulla

ESTHER·BOHLMAN

Figure 5–1. Adrenal histology shown in cross section. Mallory-azan stain. (Modified from Maximow and Bloom.)

Biochemical Basis of Steroidogenesis

The adrenal cortex is able both to synthesize cholesterol and to take it up from the circulation. The cholesterol thus accumulated is then available for conversion into steroid hormones. The total process entails dozens of enzymatically governed chemical transformations. There is much that remains unknown about the natural processes of steroidogenesis because they are functions of subcellular organization, which is all too readily disrupted by experimental manipulation.

In certain cells, and presumably in the adrenal cortex, cholesterol is synthesized from acetate through a long series of reactions involving acetyl coenzyme A, mevalonic acid, squalene, lanosterol, zymosterol, and desmosterol as some of the intermediates. Whether cholesterol synthesis by the adrenal is as important quantitatively as cholesterol uptake from plasma has never been established with certainty, but both processes are known to occur, and under special circumstances it has been possible to demonstrate that the accumulation of cholesterol by the adrenal is stimulated by ACTH.[2] It has been demonstrated that cholesterol-rich lipoproteins in plasma become attached to specific receptors on the plasma membranes of adrenal cells. They then enter the cells through a process of endocytosis that is accelerated by ACTH. Within the cells much of the cholesterol is esterified with fatty acids and stored until utilized in steroidogenesis. As an early step in steroidogenesis, the droplets of cholesterol esters make contact with mitochondria and are hydrolyzed to free cholesterol. These processes, too, are stimulated by ACTH.

Normally, the rate-limiting step in biosynthesis of steroids is the conversion of cholesterol to pregnenolone.* Under all circumstances, an abundance of cholesterol is found in the adrenal cortex, most of it within cytoplasmic lipid droplets. Unless the adrenal cell is stimulated by one or another extra-adrenal regulator, there is little utilization of the available cholesterol, and the formation of adrenal cortical steroids is minimal. In the presence of an adrenal stimulator, however, cholesterol is utilized to form 20α-hydroxycholesterol, which is then converted to $20\alpha,22$-dihydroxycholesterol, which then undergoes scission between carbon atoms 20 and 22 to yield *pregnenolone* and isocaproic aldehyde. The best-known pathway of steroid biosynthesis involves the conversion of cholesterol to pregnenolone, which is readily transformed by a series of stable enzymes into the major biologically active corticosteroids.[3] The major steps involved in the derivation of these hormonal steroids are depicted in Fig. 5–2. In a side reaction, some cholesterol is converted to 17α-hydroxycholesterol, then to $17\alpha,20$-dihydroxycholesterol, then to 17α-hydroxypregnenolone, a possible precursor of the abundant but weak adrenal androgen, *dehydroepiandrosterone* (DHEA), as well as of the important glucocorticoid, *cortisol*.

The conversion of pregnenolone to cortisol by the zona fasciculata first entails the dehydrogenation of the 3β-hydroxyl group of pregnenolone to form pregn-5-ene-3,20-dione. This then undergoes isomerization, with a shift of the double bond from the 5–6 position to the 4–5 position, forming *progesterone*. Two closely related enzymes are necessary for the conversion of pregnenolone to progesterone. The first is 3β-hydroxysteroid dehydrogenase, which oxidizes the 3β-ol to a 3-oxo group. The second is a Δ^5-3-oxosteroid isomerase, which catalyzes the migration of the double bond from the 5–6 to the 4–5 position. Progesterone is converted to

*For the sake of convenience, commonly used trivial names are employed in this chapter. Their equivalents in standard chemical nomenclature are listed in Table 5–1.

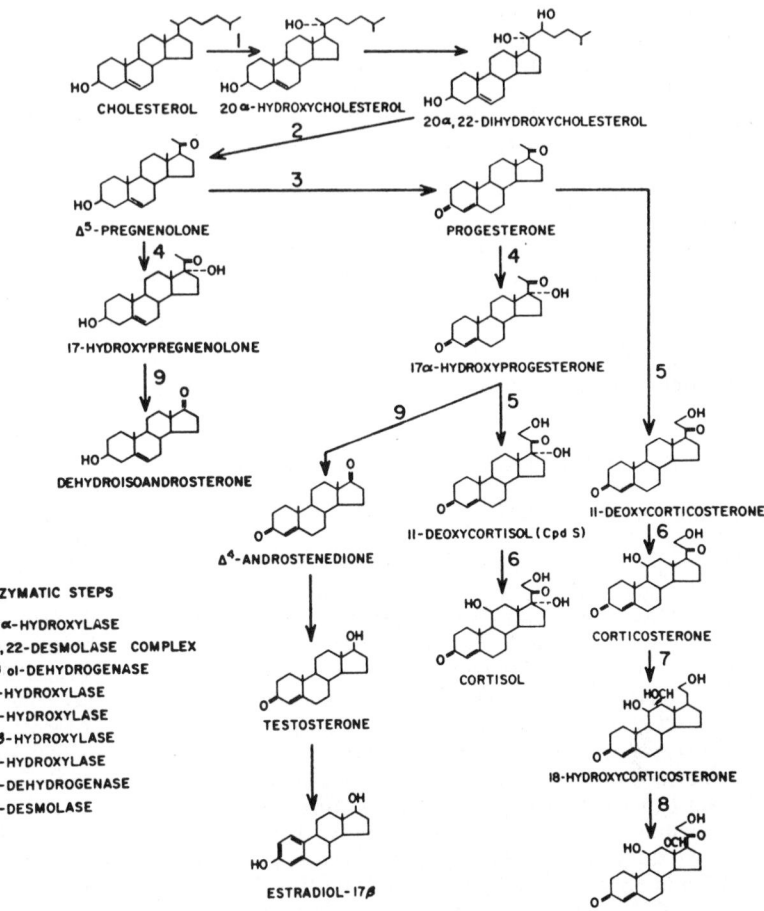

ENZYMATIC STEPS

1. 20 α-HYDROXYLASE
2. 20,22-DESMOLASE COMPLEX
3. 3β ol-DEHYDROGENASE
4. 17-HYDROXYLASE
5. 21-HYDROXYLASE
6. 11β-HYDROXYLASE
7. 18-HYDROXYLASE
8. 18-DEHYDROGENASE
9. 17-DESMOLASE

Figure 5–2. Major biosynthetic pathways for adrenal steroids. (From Temple, T. E., and Liddle, G. W.: Inhibitors of adrenal steroid biosynthesis. *Ann. Rev. Pharmacol. 10*:199, 1970.)

17α-hydroxyprogesterone by the action of a 17α-hydroxylase system. The 17α-hydroxyprogesterone is converted to a 17α,21-dihydroxyprogesterone (11-deoxycortisol or "substance S" of Reichstein) by the 21-hydroxylase system. Finally substance S is converted to cortisol (compound F) by the action of 11β-hydroxylase.

The zona fasciculata also forms a small amount of corti-

costerone as a by-product of cortisol synthesis. The pathway is identical except that progesterone escapes 17α-hydroxylation and proceeds directly to the 21-hydroxylase reaction and finally undergoes 11β-hydroxylation. It thus differs from cortisol only in that it lacks a 17α-hydroxyl group, but this structural difference accounts for a very great difference in the biologic potency of the two hormones.

The conversion of pregnenolone to aldosterone by the zona glomerulosa entails a series of enzymatically regulated steps similar to those involved in corticol synthesis but with three crucial differences. The zona glomerulosa lacks 17α-hydroxylase and therefore lacks the capacity to form 17α-hydroxyprogesterone; it is for this reason alone that the zona glomerulosa cannot synthesize cortisol. Instead it forms corticosterone, and some of this steroid is acted on by 18-hydroxylase to form 18-hydroxycorticosterone, and then by 18-hydroxysteroid dehydrogenase to form aldosterone. 18-hydroxysteroid dehydrogenase is found only in the zona gomerulosa, and this is the reason that only the zona glomerulosa has the capacity to synthesize aldosterone.

Although among the products of the human adrenal cortex only cortisol and aldosterone appear to be essential for good health, the adrenal also produces a number of by-products, including androgens and estrogens. Quantitatively, the most important of these is DHEA, which is derived from 17α-hydroxypregnenolone by the action of 17-desmolase, an enzyme that cleaves two adjacent hydroxylated carbon atoms, in this case [17]C and [20]C. Much of the DHEA formed by the adrenal is secreted without further modification, but a very small amount is converted to the classic androgens, androst-4-ene,3,17-dione and testosterone. Any of these can undergo 11β-hydroxylation, and

Table 5–1. TRIVIAL NAMES OF ADRENAL HORMONES AND RELATED SUBSTANCES

Cyclic AMP (cAMP): Adenosine-3′,5′-monophosphate
ACTH: Adenocorticotropic hormone, corticotropin
MSH: Melanocyte-stimulating hormone, melanotropin
CRF: Corticotropin-releasing factor
Aldosterone: 11β,21-Dihydroxy-3,20-dioxopregn-4-en-18-al
Androsterone: 3α-Hydroxy-5α-androstan-17-one
Cortisol: Hydrocortisone; 11β, 17α,21-Trihydroxypregn-4-ene-3,20-dione
Cortisone: 17α-21-Dihydroxy-4-pregn-ene-3,11,20-trione
Corticosterone: 11β,21-Dihydroxypregn-4-ene-3,20-dione
Cortol: α-Cortol; 5β-Pregnane-3α11β,17α,20α,21-pentol
Cortolone: 3α,17α,20α,21-Tetrahydroxypregnan-11-one
DHEA: Dehydroepiandrosterone, DHIA, dehydroisoandrosterone; 3β-Hydroxyandrost-5-en-17-one
DOC: Deoxycorticosterone, 11-deoxycorticosterone; 21-Hydroxypregn-4-ene-3,20-dione
Etiocholanolone: 3α-Hydroxy-5β-androstan-17-one
17-Hydroxypregnenolone: Pregn-5-ene-3β, 17α-diol, 20-one
17 α-Hydroxyprogesterone: 17α-Hydroxypregn-4-ene-3,20-dione
Pregnanetriol: Pregnane-3α,17α,20-triol
Pregnenolone: 3β-Hydroxypregn-5-en-20-one
Substance S: 11-Deoxycortisol, pregn-4-ene-17α,21-diol-3,20-dione
Tetrahydroaldosterone: Pregnane-3α,11β,21-triol-20-one-18-al
THE: Tetrahydrocortisone; 3α,17α,21-Trihydroxy-5β,pregnane-11,20-dione
THF: Tetrahydrocortisol; Pregnane-3α,11β,17α,21-tetrol-20-one
THS: Tetrahydro S; Pregnane-3α,17α,21-triol-20-one

any can appear as a sulfate esterified at the 3-position. Although the human adrenal can synthesize minute amounts of estrogen, the structural identity has been difficult to establish. There is evidence that adrenal "estrogens" are usually derived from adrenal androgens through extra-adrenal metabolism by tissues that possess enzymes necessary for aromatization of ring A.

Under normal circumstances, the enzymatic transformation of pregnenolone to cortisol, corticosterone, aldosterone, and DHEA occurs so rapidly that only these products accumulate in quantities sufficient to result in physiologically important secretion. As we shall see later, impairment of any of these enzymatic transformations can result in accumulation and secretion of biosynthetic intermediates in quantities sufficient to be of pathophysiologic importance.

Regulators of Adrenal Cortical Function

Adrenocorticotropic Hormone (ACTH)

The major regulator of adrenocortical growth and secretory activity is the anterior pituitary hormone, ACTH. This is one of many hormones now known to act through the mediation of cAMP. ACTH attaches to receptors on the surface of the adrenal cortical cell and activates the enzyme, adenylate cyclase, which converts adenosine triphosphate (ATP) to adenosine $3',5'$-monophosphate (cAMP). This interesting compound serves as a cofactor in activating key enzymes of the adrenal cortex, called protein kinases. The most thoroughly studied protein kinases are composed of two subunits that are metabolically inactive when combined with each other. One subunit serves as a receptor for cAMP and the other is potentially catalytic. The attachment of cAMP to the receptor results in dissociation of the receptor subunit from the catalytic subunit, which then acts to catalyze the transfer of phosphate groups from ATP to certain proteins. (By definition, "protein kinase" is an enzyme that catalyzes the transfer of phosphate radicals from ATP to a protein). When phosphorylated, these proteins take on biologic activities that would otherwise be inapparent. Presumably, these phosphorylated proteins, directly or indirectly, stimulate the rate-limiting step in steroidogenesis and, in addition, induce adrenocortical growth.

Although receiving little attention in most accounts of adrenal physiology, ACTH also enhances the activities of enzyme systems responsible for the postpregnenolone steps in steroid biosynthesis.

ACTH has also been demonstrated to have a number of effects on extra-adrenal tissues (Table 5–2), but their physiologic importance may be questioned inasmuch as they require high concentrations of ACTH. These extra-adrenal actions have also been shown to be mediated by cAMP.

Structure-Function Relationships of ACTH and Its Analogues

Peptide chemists of the past three decades have defined the structure of ACTH and have provided numerous modifications of the natural hormone that have been utilized in studies of structure-function relationships.[4,5] Several mammalian species have been found to produce corticotropic hormones that are single-chain polypeptides containing 39 amino acids (Fig. 5–3).

In all species that have been studied, the N-terminal 24 amino acids are the same, but minor species differences occur in amino acid composition in the 25–39 portion of the molecule.

The biologically active "core" of ACTH is its N-terminal 26 amino acids; this fragment of the hormone is almost equal to the complete molecule in biologic potency. In other words, as one shortens the 39-amino acid ACTH molecule by removing amino acids from the C-terminus, little or no change in potency occurs with removal of the C-terminal 13 amino acids. Thereafter, biologic potency is progressively reduced, so that the N-terminal 17-amino acid sequence has only about 5 per cent of that in the intact molecule. Removal of the 17th amino acid results in a 50-fold loss of potency. Further shortening of the sequence results in further loss of adrenal-stimulating activity. The shortest fragment that has been found to have adrenocorticotropic activity is the N-terminal 10-amino acid sequence, which has only about 0.002% of the biologic potency of the whole ACTH molecule.[5]

Comparatively minor modifications of the N-terminal portion of the ACTH molecule may severely reduce biologic potency. Oxidation of the N-terminal serine to a glyoxylyl residue virtually destroys the adrenal-stimulating activity of ACTH, but substitution of a glycyl residue for the N-terminal serine has little or no effect on biologic potency. From such observations, it has been inferred that an intact α-NH_2 group, though not necessarily a serine group, is requisite for biologic ACTH activity. Certain structural features of the ACTH molecule that were once thought to be essential for biologic activity are now known not to be absolutely essential. For example, the methionine residue in the fourth position from the N-terminus was formerly considered to be essential for full biologic activity, since its conversion to a sulfoxide by treatment with hydrogen peroxide was accompanied by loss of adrenal-stimulating activity. It is now known, however, that, in synthetic preparations of ACTH, an isoleucine can be substituted for the methionine without loss of biologic potency.

Several synthetic analogues of ACTH have had C-terminal amide groups rather than terminal carboxyl structures. In general, the amidated peptides have shown greater potency than their carboxylated congeners.

The fate of ACTH has been studied both in humans and in rats. Even though the adrenal cortex has high-affinity receptors for ACTH, only a very small proportion of the circulating hormone actually becomes attached to this target organ because the adrenal circulation represents such a small proportion of the total body circulation and because ACTH has a circulating half-time of only a few minutes. Even while it is circulating, ACTH is rapidly converted to a biologically inactive form that, nevertheless, retains for a time its reactivity with certain ACTH antibodies and retains approximately the same size as the active ACTH molecule. With the passage of several more minutes, however, even this inactivated ACTH is removed from the circulation by a number of organs (notably the liver and the kidneys) and is degraded into its constituent amino acids.[6]

Table 5–2. SOME EFFECTS OF ACTH

Adrenal

1. Maintenance of gland size
2. Depletion of ascorbic acid
3. Activation of adenylate cyclase
4. Accumulation of cholesterol
5. Conversion of cholesterol to pregnenolone
6. Maintenance of enzymes active in converting pregnenolone to hormonal steroids.

Extra-adrenal

1. Melanocyte stimulation
2. Activation of tissue lipase

α-MSH
Acetyl-Ser.Tyr.Ser.Met.Glu.His.Phe.Arg.Trp.Gly.Lys.Pro.Val-NH₂
        1   2   3   4   5   6   7   8   9   10   11   12   13

β-MSH
Ala.Glu.Lys.Lys.Asp.Glu.Gly.Pro.Tyr.Arg.Met.Glu.His.Phe.Arg.Trp.Gly.Ser.Pro.Pro.Lys.Asp
 1   2   3   4   5   6   7   8   9   10   11   12   13   14   15   16   17   18   19   20   21   22

ACTH
Ser.Tyr.Ser.Met.Glu.His.Phe.Arg.Trp.Gly.Lys.Pro.Val.Gly.Lys.Lys.Arg.Arg.
 1   2   3   4   5   6   7   8   9   10   11   12   13   14   15   16   17   18   Pro 19
                                                                                          Val 20
                                                                                          Lys 21

Phe.Glu.Leu.Pro.Phe.Ala.Glu.Ala.Ser.Glu.Asp.Glu.Ala.Gly.Asn.Pro.Tyr.Val
 39   38   37   36   35   34   33   32   31   30   29   28   27   26   25   24   23   22

Figure 5–3. Amino acid sequences of human adreno-corticotropic and melanocyte stimulating hormones.

The biosynthesis of ACTH by the pituitary is now thought to occur in a stepwise fashion. Initially, under the control of a particular species of messenger RNA, a large prohormone is synthesized that comprises a hydrophobic N-terminal segment, a middle segment that includes the 39-amino acid sequence known as ACTH, and a C-terminal segment consisting of the 91-amino acid sequence known as "β-lipotropin." β-lipotropin contains the sequences of β-MSH (a potent melanocyte-stimulating factor) and β-endorphin (a potent opiate). Subsequent to the synthesis of this large polypeptide and prior to its actual secretion into the circulation, the ACTH portion of the molecule is split off, presumably by the action of endopeptidases (though such endopeptidases have not been specifically identified). This postulated sequence of events provides an explanation for the observations that ACTH and "MSH" are always produced as "companion hormones," as are ACTH and endorphin; it also offers an explanation for the fact that these companion hormones are produced in approximately stoichiometric quantities.

Dynamics of Adrenal Response to ACTH

In animals, the adrenal response to ACTH can be evaluated in terms of (1) an increase in cyclic AMP content, which occurs almost instantly and reaches a maximum within 3 min; (2) an increase in steroid secretion, which appears within about 3 min after a "pulse" of ACTH, peaks at about 10 min, and wanes over a period of 10 min, or more, depending upon the dose of ACTH; (3) a decrease in adrenal ascorbic acid content, which is most marked 1 or 2 hours after the injection; or (4) an increase in adrenal size, which is apparent over a period of 1 day or more. In humans, the only practical way to appraise the adrenal response to ACTH is to measure steroids, particularly plasma cortisol or the urinary metabolites of cortisol, the so-called 17-hydroxycorticosteroids. Although other indices of the secretory response to ACTH have been employed in the past, they are little used at the present time.

If a subject with normal adrenals receives, on separate occasions, several intravenous infusions of ACTH, both the total magnitude and the duration of the adrenal secretory responses are directly proportional to the dose of ACTH. The family of curves describing this relationship are represented in Fig. 5–4.

A finite quantity of ACTH stimulates more cortisol secretion if it is administered slowly than if administered quickly. This is one of the main reasons underlying the development of depot preparations of ACTH for intramuscular injection. This relationship is represented in Fig. 5–5, showing that 32 U of ACTH infused intravenously over a 3-hour

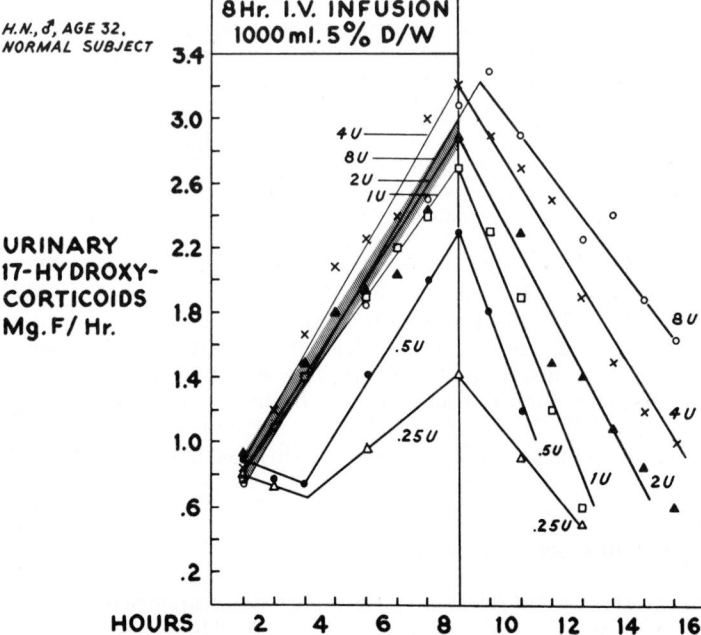

Figure 5–4. Hourly steroidogenic response to various doses of α-corticotropin (hog), administered by an 8-hour intravenous infusion. (From DiRaimondo, V. C., et al.: Improved steroidogenic assay of ACTH in man. *Metabolism* 4:110, 1955.)

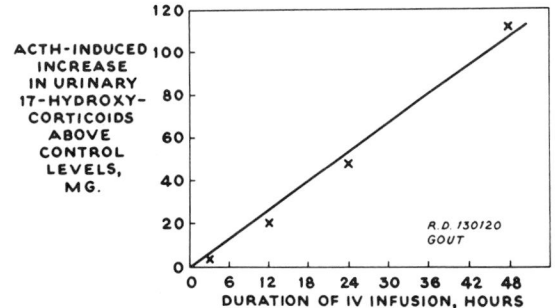

Figure 5–5. Steroidogenic effectiveness of ACTH as a function of duration of infusion (each infusion 32 USP units, x-5229).

period stimulates only a small increase in 17-hydroxy-corticosteroids on the day of injection. The same dose infused over a 12-, 24-, or 48-hour period stimulates proportionately larger increases in urinary 17-hydroxycorticosteroids.

Repetitive treatment with ACTH enhances the responsiveness of the adrenal to standard ACTH stimulation. For example, if one administers 50 U of ACTH as an 8-hour intravenous infusion on 5 successive days, urinary 17-hydroxycorticosteroids are likely to be about twice as high on the 5th day as on the 1st. The increase in responsiveness is retained only for a short time. It can still be demonstrated if one gives another infusion after a lapse of 1 or 2 days but will have disappeared if one waits more than 1 week before giving the next infusion of ACTH. Conversely, if one suppresses endogenous ACTH for a time by administering dexamethasone, there is a decrease in adrenal responsiveness. If one measures 17-hydroxycorticosteroids in response to a standard 8-hour infusion of ACTH on day 1, then gives dexamethasone on days 2 and 3, and tests the 17-hydroxycorticosteroid response to ACTH on day 4, the response will be only half as great as on day 1.

For practical considerations, there is a threshold dose of ACTH below which the adrenal response is almost imperceptible, and there is a larger dose that induces a "maximal" adrenal secretory response. This simply refers to the fact that, beyond a certain point in the dose-response curve, further increments in ACTH dosage do not induce further increments in cortisol secretion. Between these limits there is a rectilinear relationship between the log-dose of ACTH and the magnitude of the steroid secretory response. Perceptible stimulation of steroidogenesis occurs with plasma ACTH concentrations in the neighborhood of 0.1 mU/dl (10 pg/ml). Such concentrations can be achieved by the infusion (or secretion) of a mere 0.5 mU/min or 0.2 U over an 8-hour period. Almost maximal adrenal stimulation occurs with about 30 times this amount of ACTH, a plasma concentration of about 3 mU/dl resulting from an infusion of about 6 U/8-hour period. These facts have had many practical implications for our understanding of pituitary-adrenal relationships in many clinical disorders. A preliminary view of the plasma ACTH concentrations encountered under various normal and abnormal clinical conditions is presented in Fig. 5–6.

Regulation of ACTH Secretion

Since the normal adrenal secretes significant quantities of cortisol only in response to ACTH, it is possible to trans-

form the question, "What regulates cortisol," into the question, "What regulates ACTH secretion?" If one interrupts the portal vessels that pass from the hypothalamus to the anterior pituitary, pituitary-adrenal function usually diminishes to minimal levels. This plus the fact that hypothalamic extracts contain a "corticotropin releasing factor," or "CRF" has led to the concept that the secretion of ACTH is governed largely by the hypothalamus.[7] CRF is thought to act by stimulating cAMP formation within ACTH-secreting cells. This is not the whole story, however, for there is experimental and clinical evidence that corticosteroids act, at least in part, at the level of the anterior pituitary to suppress ACTH secretion. Recent experiments have suggested that the hypothalamic secretion of CRF is stimulated by cholinergic neurons and inhibited by adrenergic neurons.

For practical purposes, the secretion of ACTH by the normal pituitary may be considered to be governed by three factors: cortisol-like steroids, a "biologic clock," and stress. Each factor will be described separately, and some observations regarding their interaction will be summarized.

Negative Feedback Action of Corticosteroids. If other things are equal, the higher the level of cortisol-like steroids, the less ACTH is secreted. Of the products of the human adrenal cortex, only cortisol itself has much ACTH-suppressing activity. There are, however, a multitude of synthetic corticosteroids that share this along with the other biologic properties of cortisol. If cortisol levels are supraphysiologic, ACTH secretion is suppressed and the adrenal ceases its secretory activity until cortisol levels return to normal. Conversely, if cortisol levels are subnormal, the anterior pituitary is released from this suppressive influence, ACTH levels rise, and the adrenal secretes cortisol until normal blood levels are restored. This is a classic example of a negative feedback or "servomechanism," which is important in maintaining homeostasis.

Pituitary-Adrenal Rhythms. The normal individual has higher blood ACTH levels in the morning than in the evening. This accounts for the well-known diurnal rhythms in cortisol secretion, plasma cortisol concentration, and 17-hydroxycorticosteroid excretion. The regularity of this rhythm is a function of one's sleep-wake habits. Normal subjects who sleep regularly at the same hours each day develop ACTH-cortisol secretory patterns characterized by a sharp increase during the 3rd–5th hours of sleep, reaching a maximum shortly after the hour of awakening and falling

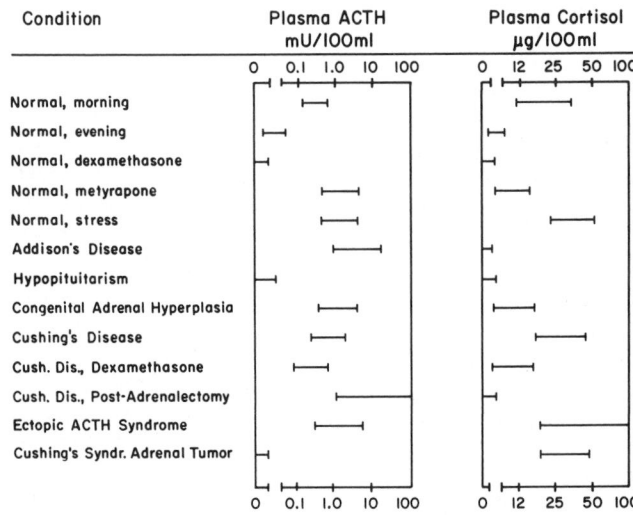

Figure 5–6. Typical values for plasma ACTH in various clinical states.

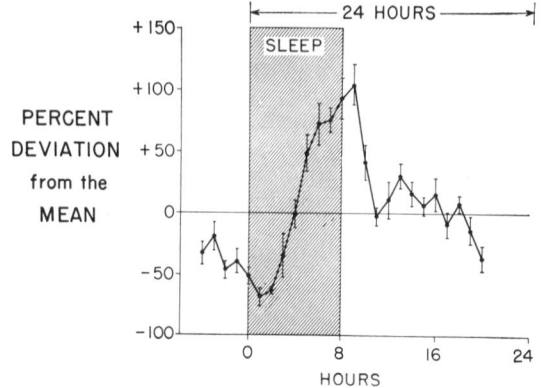

Figure 5–7. Temporal pattern of plasma cortisol concentrations in normal subjects who sleep at regular hours. (From Orth, D. N., Island, D. P., et al.: Experimental alteration of the circadian rhythm in plasma cortisol (17-OHCS) concentration in man. *J. Clin. Endocrinol. 27*:549, 1967.)

irregularly throughout the waking day to reach minimal values during the few hours before and after resumption of sleep (Fig. 5–7). The timing and duration of the pituitary-adrenal secretory cycle can be altered by consistent revision of the timing and duration of the sleep-wake schedule.[8] The presence of a rhythm in ACTH secretion has been demonstrated not only in subjects with normal adrenal function but also in patients with primary adrenal insufficiency.[9] Thus patients with Addison's disease who teleologically "need" more cortisol at all hours of the day, as evidenced by their round-the-clock elevations of ACTH, nevertheless have distinctly higher plasma ACTH levels in the morning than in the evening.

Pituitary-Adrenal Responses to Stress. Superimposed upon all other regulators of ACTH secretion is the stimulatory influence of *stress*. Regardless of the time of day and regardless of the level of plasma cortisol, the normal individual responds to a major stress (such as a laparotomy) with a brisk increase in ACTH secretion and a consequent increase in cortisol secretion. Among the stresses that have been shown to induce increased pituitary-adrenal activity are severe trauma, pyrogens, acute hypoglycemia, injections of histamine, electroconvulsive treatments, and acute anxiety. It has been observed that plasma cortisol concentrations are generally elevated in dying patients.

It appears that the "biologic clock" and "stress" work through the central nervous system to stimulate ACTH secretion and that cortisol works at the level of the pituitary (and possibly at CNS levels as well) to suppress ACTH secretion. Although much remains to be learned about the precise mechanisms through which each factor regulates ACTH secretion, it can be said that the three act as physiologic vectors. Other things being equal, the lower the plasma cortisol, the greater will be the secretion of ACTH. Other things being equal, the greater the stress, the greater will be the secretion of ACTH. And other things being equal, ACTH is secreted most abundantly during the late hours of sleep and the early hours of the waking day.

Secretion of ACTH by Neoplasms. As will be discussed in detail under the heading "Cushing's Syndrome," ACTH is sometimes secreted in unregulated fashion by tumors arising in various extrapituitary sites. These tumors appear to be unresponsive to stress. They fail to conform to the influence of biologic clocks. With very rare exceptions they appear to be uninfluenced by circulating corticosteroid levels.

Pituitary tumors often secrete ACTH in semiautonomous fashion. Their responses to stress are ambiguous: They seem to secrete ACTH in response to severe surgical stress but not in response to hypoglycemia or pyrogens. They do not conform to the influence of the normal biologic clock. They are somewhat suppressible, but not to a normal degree, by elevated concentrations of corticosteroids.

Measurement of ACTH

Extracts of pituitary tissue have long been assayable for their content of ACTH by a variety of methods that, though reliable and specific, lack the sensitivity needed to detect ACTH in plasma. Most of these methods have depended directly on an adrenal response to ACTH. In order to be certain that the assay animal was responding to the ACTH in the test material and not to endogenous ACTH secreted in response to stress, most assay methods employed hypophysectomized animals incapable of secreting endogenous ACTH. The adrenal responses that have provided quantitative indices of the amount of ACTH in the test dose have included the following:

1. *Adrenal weight.* ACTH prevents the loss of adrenal weight that would otherwise occur in the hypophysectomized animal.

2. *Adrenal ascorbic acid depletion.* ACTH stimulates the discharge of ascorbic acid from the adrenal gland of the hypophysectomized rat.

3. *Corticosteroid secretion.* ACTH stimulates increases in plasma cortisol, plasma corticosterone, urinary 17-hydroxycorticosteroids, and urinary 17-ketosteroids in various species.

4. *Thymic weight, liver glycogen, circulating eosinophils.* The corticosterone that is secreted in response to ACTH causes involution of the thymus gland, deposition of glycogen in the liver, and decreases in circulating eosinophils of the hypophysectomized rat.

In order to assay the ACTH content of plasma, it has generally been necessary to concentrate the hormone by some extraction procedure prior to assay.[10] This has been achieved by the use of agents such as oxycellulose, the cation exchange resin Amberlite IRC-50, or Quso. The ACTH content of 5–50 ml of plasma can then be assayed in one of the following systems:

1. Measurement of the acute increase in plasma corticosterone of the hypophysectomized rat.

2. Measurement of corticosterone production by freshly prepared suspensions of adrenal cells.

3. Radioimmunoassay: measurement of the degree of displacement of radioactive ACTH from specific ACTH antibodies by the nonradioactive ACTH in the test material.[11]

Recent improvements in the last two methods have made it possible to assay ACTH in unextracted plasma, but the procedures are not easy and, reliably performed, are of extremely limited availability.

The Renin-Angiotensin System

A major regulator of aldosterone production by the zona glomerulosa is the renin-angiotensin system.[12] Renin is an enzyme that is released into the circulation by the juxtaglomerular apparatus of the nephron. The action of renin is to cleave a plasma globulin, "renin substrate," to release the decapeptide, *angiotensin I*. This substance is further hydrolyzed to an octapeptide, "*angiotensin II*," by a "converting enzyme" that is found in abundance in the lung. Angiotensin II has been known for many years to be an extremely potent vasoconstrictor; in recent years it has been found to stimulate the formation of aldosterone.

Mode of Action and Temporal Aspects

The precise mechanism through which angiotensin stimulates aldosterone biosynthesis has not been elucidated. Whatever the mechanism of its action, angiotensin appears to stimulate the conversion of cholesterol to pregnenolone, which then serves as a precursor of the progesterone → desoxycorticosterone → corticosterone → 18-hydroxycorticosterone → aldosterone pathway.[13] The onset of action is rapid and is demonstrable within minutes of the time the adrenal is exposed to angiotensin; it ceases within minutes after angiotensin has been removed. If other factors are held constant, the aldosterone secretory response of the adrenal is proportional to the dose of angiotensin. In addition to its major action in stimulating the conversion of cholesterol to pregnenolone, angiotensin also has a minor stimulatory effect on later steps in the aldosterone biosynthetic pathway.

Angiotensin itself is a very labile peptide that, in plasma and tissues, is quickly destroyed by angiotensinases. The circulating half-time of angiotensin is only on the order of 1 min, in contrast to that of renin, which has a circulating half-time in humans of more than 10 min. Renin substrate appears to be abundantly available under all circumstances *in vivo*; plasma concentrations are particularly high during pregnancy and during treatment with supraphysiologic doses of estrogen (e.g., oral contraceptives) and glucocorticoids. Plasma renin activity (PRA) as it is ordinarily measured in clinical laboratories is elevated under these circumstances, as is the aldosterone secretion rate.[14]

Regulation of Renin Secretion

A whole host of circumstances leads to increased renin secretion, but many of them can be viewed as working through a smaller number of final common pathways.

Renal cell suspensions have been shown to increase their production of renin in the presence of cAMP, epinephrine, or norepinephrine.[15] It has been speculated that this effect of the catecholamines in renin-producing cells (like those in other tissues) might be mediated by cAMP. *In vivo,* exogenous epinephrine and norepinephrine stimulate renin release, and there is indirect evidence that endogenous catecholamines and the sympathetic nervous system may mediate the stimulation of renin secretion by painful stimuli, upright posture, and hypovolemia.[16]

One of the earliest facts established concerning the regulation of renin was that it is increased by compromising the blood flow to the kidney. This obviously occurs when a renal artery is constricted or becomes stenotic as a consequence of some disease, such as atherosclerosis or fibromuscular dysplasia. It occurs in a more subtle way whenever intravascular volume is reduced by exsanguination, dehydration, sodium depletion, or hypoalbuminemia. It can also occur when blood is sequestered on the venous side of the circulation by processes such as constriction of the vena cava, hepatic cirrhosis, or congestive heart failure. It has been shown experimentally that it is the decrease in perfusion pressure of the kidney rather than the decrease in the volume of blood flow that serves as the stimulus to renin release,[17] and it is considered likely that baroreceptors associated with the juxtaglomerular apparatus mediate this response.

The regulation of renin secretion is more intricate than this, however, for it has also been shown that the magnitude of sodium flux in the region of the macula densa of the ascending limb of Henle's loop is also a determinant of renin secretion. In many circumstances, a change in perfusion and a change in macula densa sodium flux work together to

regulate renin secretion, and it has been necessary to devise experiments of great elegance to demonstrate that the two mechanisms can operate independently of each other.[18]

A diurnal rhythm has been demonstrated in plasma renin activity. If other factors such as diet and posture are held constant, plasma renin activity is lower in the afternoon than in the forenoon in normal subjects who habitually sleep at night and are awake during the day. It seems probable that this rhythm is controlled by the nervous system, that it is related to a similar rhythm in renal function (glomerular filtration and solute excretion tend to be greater during the afternoon than during the forenoon), and that it in turn leads to a diurnal rhythm in aldosterone secretion, which is generally greater in the forenoon than in the afternoon.

A variety of other agents have also been shown to influence renin secretion. Angiotensin II itself has a direct inhibitory effect on renin secretion, thus completing the circuit in a "short loop" negative feedback system. Adrenergic blocking agents tend to decrease renin secretion. Agents that induce acute vasodilation, such as nitroprusside, increase renin secretion. Diazoxide, an arteriolar relaxant, increases renin secretion not only when administered systemically but also when injected directly into one renal artery. Potent diuretics such as furosemide induce acute increases in renin secretion. In general, if one wishes to appraise a patient's renin production in a meaningful way, it is best for him to receive no medications or to have the medications administered according to a well-standardized protocol.

From the standpoint of practical adrenal physiology, the most interesting determinant of renin secretion is aldosterone, which acts indirectly to suppress renin secretion and thus acts even more indirectly to suppress the further secretion of aldosterone, thus completing the circuit in a "long loop" negative feedback system. The relationships between renin and aldosterone are illustrated in Fig. 5–8. The administration of aldosterone or the autonomous secretion of aldosterone by an adrenal adenoma results in sodium retention that, in the presence of a normal osmoregulatory mechanism, necessarily results in water retention. The resultant expansion of the extracellular fluid compartment is associated with some expansion in blood volume, which is communicated to the arterial side of the circulation as an increase in "effective" blood volume. This brings about an increase in perfusion pressure of the kidney, resulting in suppression of renin secretion. Thus in "primary aldosteronism," one finds a combination of high aldosterone secretion rate and low plasma renin activity.[19] In contrast, there are several physiologic disorders in which there are decreases in effective blood volume. These are associated with increased secretion of renin and increased generation of angiotensin, which stimulates increased secretion of aldosterone. Again, the aldosterone promotes retention of sodium and water and

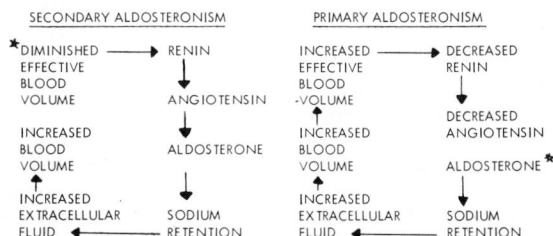

Figure 5–8. Typical relationships between renin and aldosterone secretion in secondary aldosteronism as contrasted with primary aldosteronism. In each part of the diagram, the asterisk represents the primary physiologic abnormality: diminished effective blood volume in secondary aldosteronism, and autonomous secretion of aldosterone in primary aldosteronism.

expansion of the extracellular fluid compartment, culminating in a compensatory increase in blood volume and effective blood volume. This sequence is commonly referred to as "secondary aldosteronism." These relationships between renin and aldosterone can be generalized. An increase in renin-angiotensin activity, regardless of the cause, tends to increase aldosterone secretion, and a primary excess of any mineralocorticoid tends to suppress renin production. (See also Ch. 22.)

Recently available pharmacologic antagonists of angiotensin II and pharmacologic inhibitors of the enzymatic conversion of angiotensin I to angiotensin II have made it possible to demonstrate the dependency of blood pressure and aldosterone secretion upon the presence of angiotensin II. The administration of such agents brings about a fall in blood pressure, a fall in aldosterone secretion, and a "compensatory" increase in renin secretion. In individuals in whom angiotensin is of little importance (such as those with primary aldosteronism or other low-renin states) these agents have relatively little effect on blood pressure, aldosterone, or renin.

Measurement of Renin and Angiotensin

Angiotensin can be assayed in terms of its pressor activity in anesthetized, nephrectomized, pentolinium-blocked rats.[20] Properly performed, this is a very sensitive and reliable assay method. It does not distinguish between angiotensin I and angiotensin II, since the former is quickly converted to the latter by a "converting enzyme" that is found in the lungs in very significant quantities. For most practical purposes, this distinction is unimportant.

The development of specific antibodies to angiotensin I and angiotensin II has made it possible to measure these peptides by radioimmunoassay.[21] Because the angiotensins are so labile in plasma and because they are generated in untreated plasma, great care must be taken in collection and storage of specimens for angiotensin assay, including special attention to the inactivation of renin and the inactivation of angiotensinases.

Renin can be assayed by incubating the specimen under standard conditions in the presence of the plasma α_2-globulin, "renin substrate," and then measuring the amount of angiotensin I that is generated. The angiotensin may be measured either by bioassay or radioimmunoassay. There is generally enough renin substrate in normal plasma so that renin can be assayed by incubating plasma without the special addition of substrate. When the assay is performed in this way, one ordinarily refers to the result as "plasma renin activity" (PRA). More specific assays of renin require kinetic analysis of the rate of generation of angiotensin I from precisely controlled quantities of renin substrate under standard conditions. Following the same principles, renin substrate can also be assayed by quantifying the rate of generation of angiotensin I that is catalyzed by a known quantity of renin.

Other Regulators of Adrenal Function

Electrolytes are of some practical importance in regulating the secretion of aldosterone, over and above their effects on extracellular fluid volume and renin production. Increases in potassium concentration stimulate and hypokalemia tends to minimize aldosterone biosynthesis.[22] Sodium concentration has also been shown to modify aldosterone secretion, at least in experimental situations; hyponatremia stimulates aldosterone secretion. One mechanism through which sodium and potassium influence aldosterone secretion may be modification of the number and the affinity of adrenal receptors for angiotensin II. Douglas, Catt, and their coworkers have reported that adrenal receptors for angiotensin are increased in rats treated with high-potassium or low-sodium diets and that the opposite occurs in response to potassium depletion and sodium loading. These ions tend to function as negative feedback regulators of aldosterone secretion, since potassium excretion is promoted by aldosterone and aldosterone secretion is in turn suppressed by potassium depletion, and sodium excretion is decreased by aldosterone and aldosterone secretion is in turn stimulated by hyponatremia. (It should be noted, however, that hyponatremia is often a consequence of persistent antidiuretic hormone action and is accompanied by bodily fluid expansion that tends to suppress rather than to stimulate aldosterone secretion. Thus the relationships just noted have often had to be demonstrated by carefully designed experiments in which one factor was held constant while the other was varied.)

Melanocyte-stimulating hormone (MSH) and its structural analogues have slight corticosterone-stimulating activity in the rat, and Rudman has even shown that, in the rabbit, β MSH has the same order of adrenal stimulating potency as ACTH.[23] It remains to be shown that MSH has significant adrenal-stimulating activity in human physiology. Certain prostaglandins have been shown by Kaplan's group to have steroidogenic activity in vitro.[24] Whether they have importance in normal physiology or in pathologic situations remains uncertain. In extremely large doses, vasopressin has direct adrenal-stimulating activity; it also stimulates the release of ACTH. Calcium ions are necessary for the steroidogenic action of ACTH, but as yet no clinical perturbation of calcium metabolism has been shown to be extreme enough to affect the rate of steroidogenesis.

Although it has no obvious effect on steroidogenesis, growth hormone (GH) has been demonstrated to promote an increase in adrenal size and, perhaps related to this, to stimulate ornithine decarboxylase activity in the adrenal. In both of these actions, GH acts synergistically with ACTH.

Other factors have been shown to modify adrenal function under experimental conditions, but their possible physiologic significance remains to be established.

Metabolic Fates of Adrenal Steroids

Transcortin: Steroid-Binding Globulin[25]

Once secreted, cortisol becomes associated with "transcortin," a plasma glycoprotein with high affinity for cortisol, progesterone, deoxycorticosterone, corticosterone, and some but not all synthetic corticosteroid analogues. Under most physiologic circumstances, about 75% of the plasma cortisol is tightly but reversibly bound to transcortin, one molecule of cortisol to one molecule of transcortin. About 15% of the plasma cortisol is loosely bound to albumin; about 10% of the plasma cortisol is unbound. It is this unbound fraction that is free to move into cells either to exert metabolic effects or to be transformed into an inactive metabolite. The reversibility of the binding of cortisol to transcortin is such that the transcortin-bound fraction and total plasma cortisol can fall from high normal values (e.g., 25 μg/dl) to low values (e.g., 5 μg/dl) within a period of less than 3 hours as the unbound fraction is cleared by the liver, provided there is no newly secreted cortisol to add to the pool size.

In normal pregnancy, and during treatment with supraphysiologic doses of estrogen, although cortisol secretion rates are not increased, plasma cortisol concentrations are increased two- to threefold, owing to increased plasma concentrations of transcortin.

Diseases characterized by hypoalbuminemia (e.g., the nephrotic syndrome) are usually characterized by subnormal plasma transcortin levels and correspondingly low plasma cortisol concentrations. Certain families have a genetically determined absence of transcortin and extremely low levels of plasma cortisol. These deviations from normal do not appear to have any serious consequences with regard to the efficacy of cortisol, the adrenal production of cortisol, or the ultimate metabolism of cortisol. The teleologic importance of transcortin is, therefore, open to doubt; nevertheless, its presence makes life easier for the adrenal physiologist, since it results in the development of higher (and therefore more readily measurable) plasma concentrations of cortisol than would occur otherwise.

In Cushing's syndrome (clinical hypercortisolism), the hypersecretion of cortisol tends to overload the binding capacity of transcortin, so that an abnormally high proportion of the plasma cortisol is unbound. Unbound cortisol is more readily excreted in the urine than is protein-bound cortisol; therefore, patients with Cushing's syndrome often have distinctly supernormal levels of urinary cortisol, a fact that has been turned to diagnostic use by some.

Transcortin concentrations, unlike cortisol concentrations, are quite constant throughout the day and from day to day. They are not affected by hyper- or hypocortisolism. When subjects are treated with estrogen, transcortin concentrations rise to a plateau within 3–5 days. After estrogen is withdrawn, transcortin decreases with a half-time of 4–5 days, and levels are normal within 2 weeks.

Although certain other steroids do have affinity for transcortin, they are ordinarily secreted in such small quantities that they do not seriously compete with cortisol for binding sites on the protein molecule. Aldosterone, for example, has some affinity for transcortin but less than that of cortisol; moreover, in comparison with cortisol, plasma concentrations are extremely low. DHEA, androstenedione, and the various steroid conjugates have little affinity for transcortin. Testosterone and estradiol have little affinity for transcortin but happen to have high affinity for yet another plasma protein (Chs. 6 and 7).

Extra-Adrenal Metabolism of Corticosteroids

The metabolic inactivation of hormonal steroids is, in the main, unrelated to the mechanism through which steroids exert their physiologic effects. The latter subject will be considered later. There is no evidence that the human body can destroy the basic steroid nucleus. Furthermore, intact, biologically active corticosteroids are excreted in various bodily fluids only in trace quantities. The general fate of corticosteroids is to undergo inactivation by enzymes that introduce oxygen or hydrogen atoms at one or more positions. They are then conjugated to form water-soluble derivatives that are excreted in the urine.

The major organ for inactivating steroids is the liver, and the major process through which corticosteroids are inactivated involves the enzymatic reduction of the 4–5 double bond in "ring A" to form the dihydrosteroid derivative, which is generally devoid of biologic activity. The dihydro derivative is quickly converted to a tetrahydro derivative by the enzymatic reduction of the 3-oxo group to a 3-hydroxyl group. This derivative is then readily conjugated with glucuronic acid, forming a water-soluble product that is rapidly excreted by the kidneys.

Thus a major derivative of cortisol is tetrahydrocortisol glucuronide (Fig. 5–9). A major derivative of aldosterone is tetrahydroaldosterone glucuronide. A major derivative of corticosterone is tetrahydrocorticosterone glucuronide. DOC is excreted as tetrahydro-DOC glucuronide, and 11-deoxycortisol (substance S) is excreted as tetrahydro-S glucuronide.

Cortisol can be converted to cortisone by the action of 11β-hydroxysteroid dehydrogenase, and cortisone is then metabolized and excreted as tetrahydrocortisone glucuronide. In similar fashion, corticosterone can be converted to its 11-oxo analogue, "compound A," which is then metabolized and excreted as tetrahydro-A glucuronide.

Cortisol and other steroids with 20-oxo groups can be acted on by enzymes that convert the 20-oxo to 20-hydroxyl groups. These steroids, too, are subject to ring A reduction, conjugation, and excretion as glucuronides. Thus cortisol can be converted to cortol glucuronide, progesterone to pregnanediol glucuronide, and 17-hydroxy-progesterone to pregnanetriol glucuronide.

A number of other pathways of metabolic inactivation are known. One involves a desmolase reaction that cleaves the 17–20 carbon linkage, yielding 17-ketosteroids (17-KS). This reaction is limited to steroids that have 17α-hydroxyl groups and 20-oxo groups. Cortisol is one such steroid, and approximately 5% of cortisol appears in the urine as a 17-KS.

A small proportion of cortisol is metabolized by hydroxylation at 6α-position. This pathway is greatly enhanced by drugs that induce hepatic 6α-hydroxylase, such as phenobarbital and o,p'-DDD (3,3 bis [p-aminophenyl] butanone-2). This pathway is also increased during pregnancy.

Aldosterone, in addition to being susceptible to ring A reduction, which results in the formation of tetrahydroaldosterone, is also susceptible to conjugation with glucuronic acid at the 18-oxo position. This is formed both in the liver and in the kidney. It is very water-soluble and is

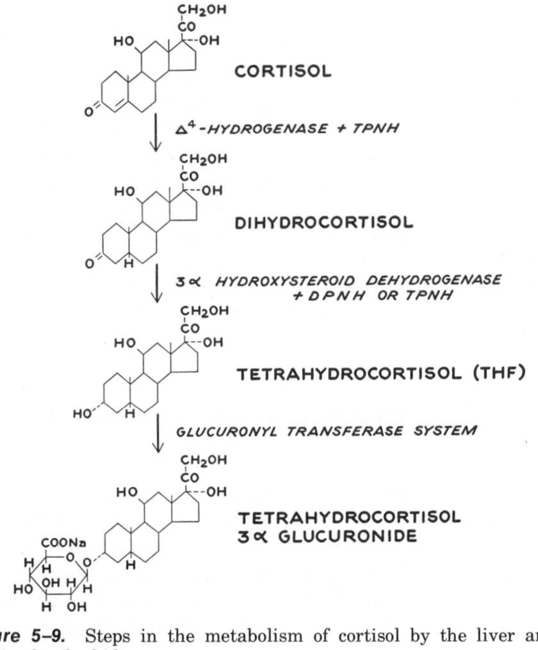

Figure 5–9. Steps in the metabolism of cortisol by the liver and its excretion by the kidney.

readily excreted into the urine. It can be cleaved by acid, yielding free aldosterone, and this fact is often used to advantage in the clinical measurement of urinary aldosterone.

DHEA, the major C-19 product of the human adrenal is, in the main, conjugated with sulfuric acid. DHEA sulfate is bound to plasma protein, and in this form it is not readily excreted but circulates in higher concentrations than any other steroid. DHEA is the principal precursor of the urinary 17-KS. Its metabolism is complex, but a major portion of the DHEA is oxidized at the 3-position to form androst-5-ene-3,17-dione. This is then acted on by an isomerase to form androst-4-ene-3,17-dione, which then undergoes the now familiar reduction of ring A to the tetrahydro derivatives, androsterone, and etiocholanolone. A portion of these metabolites are conjugated with glucuronic acid but a larger portion with sulfate. The urinary sulfates can be hydrolyzed enzymatically or with acid in order to liberate the water-insoluble steroids preparatory to their measurement as 17-KS. It will be noted that DHEA is metabolized to the same excretory end-products as testosterone. DHEA itself has little if any androgenic activity, but a small proportion of it is metabolized to testosterone and thus assumes biologic importance as an androgen. It has become traditional to minimize the value of urinary 17-KS as an index of androgen production; indeed, testosterone is such a potent androgen that it can induce full virilization without giving rise to enough urinary 17-KS to be clearly detectable. Nevertheless, when clear-cut virilization is due to an excess of *adrenal* steroids, DHEA is usually produced in sufficient quantities to elevate the urinary 17-KS. The measurement of urinary 17-KS, therefore, is of practical clinical value in evaluating patients with virilizing disorders.

Although the liver is the major extra-adrenal site of corticosteroid metabolism, it is not the only one. Other tissues, including muscle, skin, fibroblasts, intestine, and lymphocytes, can carry on oxidation-reduction reactions at the 3-, 11-, 17-, and 20-positions of the corticosteroid molecule, all positions where oxygen functions can exist as either oxo or hydroxyl groups.

The numerous minor pathways of corticosteroid metabolism lie beyond the scope of the present chapter. The interested reader will find a wealth of information on the entire subject of extra-adrenal metabolism of corticosteroids in an article by Peterson.[26]

Functions of Adrenal Steroids

Molecular Biology of Steroid Action

It is currently thought that steroids of all groups exert their biologic effects in the following way.[27] Steroid hormones experience little difficulty in traversing cell membranes and reaching the cytoplasm. A target tissue of a particular steroid has cytoplasmic receptor proteins that exhibit high affinity for the steroid in question. The steroid-receptor complex migrates into the nucleus, where it becomes attached to specific areas of the chromatin and serves to de-repress or activate certain genes, allowing their expression in the formation of new RNA. The new RNA controls the formation of new proteins, some of which are important in cell structure and some in cell replication. Some are enzymes regulating metabolic functions of the cells, and some are transported out of the target cells as secretory products. Certain steroids compete with others in their affinity for the cytoplasmic receptors

and, in doing so, act as biologic antagonists. In many instances, steroids that have similar biologic effects probably share the same receptor proteins and work through the same intracellular mechanisms. The mechanism just outlined requires a finite period of time to operate; therefore, there is a measurable latent period before the metabolic effects of a steroid can be observed, usually of hours duration.

It is known that some target tissues can metabolize tropic steroids, rendering them either more active or less active biologically. It has been suggested that testosterone is activated through its conversion to dihydrotestosterone by androgen-sensitive cells.[28] It is also probable that some steroid transformation products are devoid of biologic activity. This would represent one possible mechanism of limiting or terminating the effect of a steroid hormone within the target tissue. In any event, the duration of the stimulating effect of a steroid hormone is limited to a finite period of several hours (or perhaps a very few days in some cases). Unless there is a continuing supply of the steroid hormone, the formation of new RNA ceases, followed by disappearance of the associated proteins and cessation of the characteristic metabolic response of the target tissue.

The fact that certain tissues are "targets" for steroid hormone action and others are not apparently depends upon the fact that target tissues have cytoplasmic receptors for the particular steroid and others do not. The *type* of metabolic response is determined by the part of the genome that is functionally modified by the steroid-receptor complex and the type of RNA that is transcribed as a consequence.

Biologic Effects of Glucocorticoids[29]

The term "glucocorticoid" has been applied to steroids that have distinct effects on carbohydrate metabolism, including promotion of gluconeogenesis, promotion of liver glycogen deposition, and elevation of blood glucose concentrations. Of the naturally occurring steroids, only cortisol, cortisone, corticosterone, and 11-dehydrocorticosterone (compound A) have appreciable glucocorticoid activity. Of these, cortisol is the most potent. In certain species, such as the rat, that lack the capacity to synthesize cortisol, however, corticosterone is the most important glucocorticoid. Cortisone and compound A lack inherent glucocorticoid activity but are potentially active because they are convertible in the body to cortisol and corticosterone, respectively.

A large number of synthetic analogues of cortisol have been shown to have glucocorticoid activity; several are more potent than cortisol itself. Their relative potencies are listed in Table 5–3, and the structural features that

Table 5–3. RELATIVE POTENCIES OF STEROIDS

	Glucocorticoid Activity	Mineralocorticoid Activity
Cortisol	1	1
Cortisone	0.7	0.7
Corticosterone	0.2	2
11-Deoxycorticosterone	nil	20
Aldosterone	0.1	400
Fludrocortisone	10	400
Prednisone	4	0.7
Prednisolone	4	0.7
Dexamethasone	30	2
Triamcinolone	3	nil
6α-Methylprednisolone	5	0.5

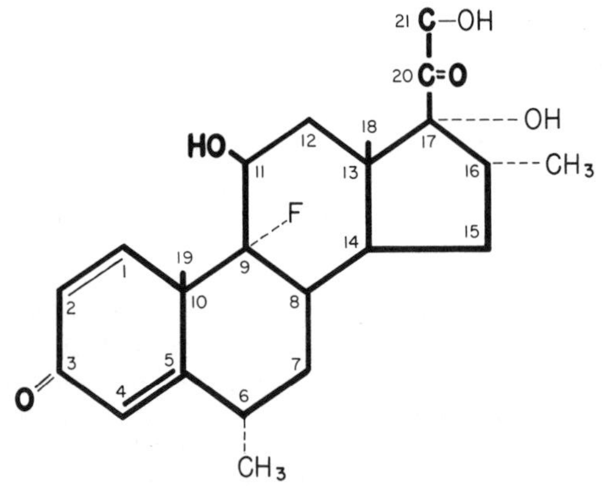

Figure 5–10. Structure-function relationships of corticosteroids. The bold lines and letters indicate the structure of pregn-4-ene, 11β-ol-3,20-dione, which is common to all steroids that have been shown to have glucocorticoid activity in humans. Substituents that individually are nonessential but that, if present, enhance glucocorticoid activity are represented by light lines and letters.

determine glucocorticoid potency are reviewed in Fig. 5–10.

More or less in proportion to their potency in affecting carbohydrate metabolism, all of the glucocorticoids also possess the following biologic properties, some of which are of considerable clinical importance:

1. *Protein-wasting activity.* Glucocorticoids accelerate the breakdown of proteins such as albumin. They inhibit amino acid uptake and protein synthesis by many extrahepatic tissues. Glucocorticoids accelerate the uptake of amino acids by the liver, which utilizes some of them to synthesize albumin. But the liver also deaminates amino acids to form urea and substrates for energy metabolism, and this process is accelerated by glucocorticoids (gluconeogenesis). If present chronically in supraphysiologic quantities, glucocorticoids suppress GH secretion and inhibit somatic growth; the latter effect cannot be completely overcome by the administration of GH.

2. *ACTH-suppressing activity.* All glucocorticoids suppress the synthesis and secretion of ACTH. There is experimental evidence indicating that this action of the steroids is exerted, at least partially, at the level of the pituitary itself, but it is possible that glucocorticoids also act to suppress CRF.

3. *Anti-inflammatory activity.* When present in supraphysiologic amounts, glucocorticoids inhibit inflammatory and allergic reactions. There are, of course, many components to the inflammatory response to tissue injury, and glucocorticoids act to suppress the response at multiple points. Glucocorticoids have been shown to stabilize lysosomes; these are intracellular packages of proteolytic enzymes that, when released as a consequence of cellular injury, cause damage to neighboring cells. Glucocorticoids inhibit the diapedesis of leukocytes across capillary walls and their migration through tissues. They inhibit granuloma formation. As a consequence of these actions, glucocorticoids may interfere with host responses to bacterial infection and suppress delayed sensitivity reactions.

Closely related to their anti-inflammatory actions are the immunosuppressive actions of the glucocorticoids. These steroids are lympholytic. They cause decreases in circulating lymphocytes and diminish the size of lymph nodes, thymus, and spleen. Antibody production is decreased.

4. *Miscellaneous activities.* Glucocorticoids also have a multitude of other activities, including the induction of several enzymes, stimulation of hematopoiesis, promotion of fat deposition in faciocervicotruncal areas, promotion of uric acid excretion, facilitation of free-water excretion, promotion of appetite, reduction of circulating eosinophils, and maintenance of muscular work capacity.

Biologic Effects of Mineralocorticoids

The term "mineralocorticoid" has been applied to steroids that have distinct effects on ion transport by epithelial cells, resulting in sodium conservation and loss of potassium. Many naturally occurring steroids have this property, but the most potent and, teleologically, the most useful is aldosterone. The second most potent is 11-deoxycorticosterone (DOC), followed in order of potency by 18-hydroxy-DOC, corticosterone, and cortisol.

A large number of synthetic corticosteroid analogues have been shown to have mineralocorticoid activity; some are even more potent than aldosterone. Their relative potencies are listed in Table 5–3. In addition, estrogens and androgens may promote sodium retention under certain circumstances, but the mechanism may be different from that of the mineralocorticoids.

Epithelial cells of the renal tubules, sweat glands, and glands of the alimentary system have enzymatically controlled mechanisms for transporting electrolytes across cell membranes. The electrolyte "pumps" respond to mineralocorticoids by conserving sodium and chloride and by wasting bodily potassium. A good example of such a system is found in the distal tubule of the mammalian nephron. Here, even in the absence of a mineralocorticoid, ion transport mechanisms bring about reabsorption of sodium ions from fluid in the lumen of the tubule and secretion of potassium and hydrogen ions into the lumen. These processes are accelerated by mineralocorticoids. Absence of mineralocorticoid activity may result in lethal wastage of sodium and retention of potassium. Sufficient mineralocorticoid helps the body to achieve electrolyte homeostasis, but an overabundance of mineralocorticoid can cause potassium depletion and excessive sodium retention, leading to edema, hypertension, and suppression of renal production of renin.

Biology of Adrenal Androgens and Estrogens

Under normal circumstances, adrenocortical production of androgen and estrogen is trivial in comparison with the production of these hormones by the gonads. A pathologic excess of adrenal androgen, however, can induce virilization (the development of masculine secondary sex characteristics). In the adult male, the effects of adrenal androgen escape notice since he is already fully virilized, but in the female or immature male they can be very conspicuous. Adrenal virilism in the female fetus can induce the formation of a urogenital sinus (rather than separate external orifices of the urinary and genital systems), labial fusion, and clitoral hypertrophy. Such ambiguity of the external genitalia is referred to as "pseudohermaphroditism." In children of either sex, an excess of adrenal androgen can cause phallic hypertrophy, increased muscularity, rapid somatic growth, and precocious development of pubic, axillary, and facial hair. In addition, the affected individual can develop acne, coarsening of the voice, and recession of scalp hair. The various manifestations of childhood virilism appear chronologically in the order listed previously. Women with adrenal virilism may experience clitoral hypertrophy, hirsutism, balding, coarsening of the voice, and suppression of estrogen effects, resulting in amenorrhea, infertility, and breast atrophy.

Feminization due to adrenal estrogen is extremely rare. It might be unnoticed in mature women, but in men and children it would lead to enlargement of the breasts and (in young girls) maturation of the uterus and vagina.

Although normal amounts of adrenal androgen and estrogen have trivial effects with respect to the development of secondary sex characteristics, they may have some importance in supporting the growth of certain tumors, specifically mammary and prostatic carcinomas. Some such tumors regress initially following gonadectomy and then again following adrenalectomy. Mammary tumors that respond to adrenalectomy can be identified in advance by demonstrating the presence of cytoplasmic estrogen-receptor proteins in biopsy specimens.[30] Synthetic steroids that compete at some point in the mechanism of action of estrogens or androgens are showing increasing promise as therapeutic agents in mammary and prostatic carcinomas.

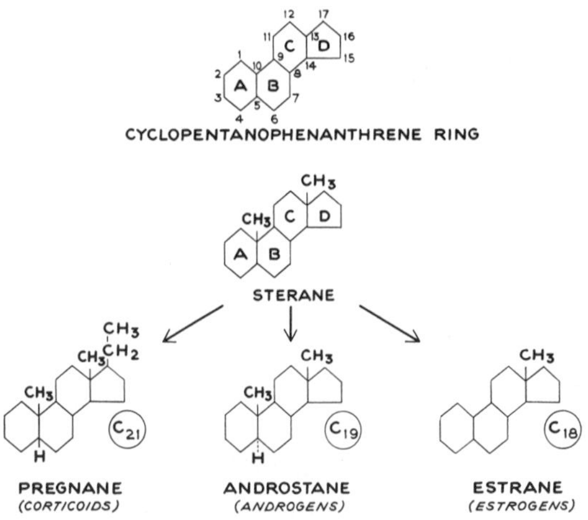

SUBSTITUENT	PREFIX	SUFFIX
NONE	NONE	-ANE
-OH	HYDROXY	-OL
=O	KETO	-ONE
UNSATURATION	DELTA n	-ENE

Figure 5–11. Basic concepts in steroid biochemistry and nomenclature.

Measurement of Adrenal Steroids

Steroids can be extracted from plasma, urine, or adrenal tissue with an organic solvent such as dichloromethane and then quantified by any of several procedures. Most of the quantification procedures are not entirely specific for one steroid; therefore, partial purification using differential solvent extraction or chromatography might be a necessary preliminary to quantification.

Cortisol

Cortisol, as well as certain related steroids, can be measured colorimetrically because its dihydroxy-acetone side chain reacts with phenylhydrazine in sulfuric acid to give a yellow color, the intensity of which is proportional to the amount of cortisol in the specimen. This method was developed by Porter and Silber[31]; therefore, the steroids measured by this procedure are often referred to as "Porter-Silber chromogens." These steroids are also referred to as "17,21-dihydroxy-20-ketosteroids," "17-hydroxycorticosteroids," or "17-OHCS." Since cortisol, cortisone, 11-deoxycortisol ("substance S"), and their tetrahydro derivatives all have 17,21-dihydroxy-20-keto side chains, they are all measurable as Porter-Silber chromogens (Figs. 5–11, 5–12, and 5–13). Of all these steroids, however, the only one that occurs in normal human plasma to any significant degree is cortisol. Cortisone will not be encountered unless it is administered as such. 11-deoxycortisol is normally barely detectable, but it is abundantly secreted in some cases of adrenal carcinoma, in subjects treated with an 11β-hydroxylase inhibitor (metyrapone), and in patients with congenital adrenal hyperplasia due to 11β-hydroxylase deficiency. The tetrahydro derivatives of cortisol, cortisone, and 11-deoxycortisol are so quickly converted to water-soluble glucuronides that they do not interfere with the measurement of cortisol. Therefore, for most practical purposes, measurements of plasma Porter-Silber chromogens are equivalent to measurements of plasma cortisol.

A rapid, relatively specific method for measuring cortisol is the fluorometric method of Mattingly,[32] based on the fact that cortisol fluoresces when incubated in ethanolic sulfuric acid. This property is shared by corticosterone, but the latter is present in human plasma in only about one tenth the concentration of cortisol. For most practical purposes, therefore, measuring fluorogenic steroids in human plasma is equivalent to measuring plasma cortisol.

A technically difficult but very sensitive method for measuring cortisol is the double isotope derivative method originally devised by Peterson. Recently, several groups have developed radioimmunoassays for cortisol that, although technically exacting, are so sensitive that they permit the measurement of cortisol in smaller specimens than possible heretofore.

As stated previously, unaltered cortisol appears in the urine in only very limited quantities. Even so, this has been turned to diagnostic use since there is a proportionately great increase in urinary cortisol in clinical hypercortisolism, when the amount of free plasma cortisol (as opposed to protein-bound cortisol) is excessive. Under these circumstances, urinary cortisol increases from its usual value of less than 150 μg/day to several hundred or even several thousand μg/day. After suitable extraction and purification, urinary cortisol can be measured by any of the procedures just described.

CH_2OH C=O C--OH	CH_2OH HCOH C--OH	CH_3 C=O C--OH	CH_3 HCOH C--OH
DIHYDROXYKETONE	GLYCEROL	17:20 KETOL	17:20 GLYCOL
CORTISONE CORTISOL	CORTOLONE CORTOL	17 α-HYDROXY-PROGESTERONE	PREGNANETRIOL
+	−	−	−
PORTER - SILBER REACTION (17-OHC)			
+	+	−	+
META-DINITROBENZENE REACTION AFTER $NaBiO_3$ OXIDATION (17-KGS)			

Figure 5–12. Characteristic side-chain groups and the practical tests specific for them. Note that only the steroids in the column on the left are 17-OHCS, whereas those in columns 1, 2, and 4 are 17-KGS.

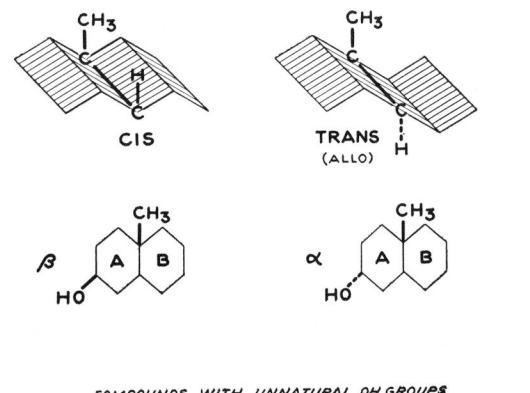

COMPOUNDS WITH UNNATURAL OH GROUPS
"EPI" OR "ISO"

Figure 5–13. Diagrammatic representation of stereoisomerism of the steroid molecule.

Urinary 17-Hydroxycorticosteroids (17-OHCS)

Although cortisol appears in the urine in only very limited quantities, its major metabolites, tetrahydrocortisol glucuronide and tetrahydrocortisone glucuronide, appear in quantities equivalent to about 30% of the cortisol secretory rate. These glucuronides are so water-soluble that they escape extraction with the organic solvents. Hydrolytic cleavage of the glucuronides with glucuronidase releases the free steroids, which can then be extracted with organic solvents and quantified as 17-OHCS by the Porter-Silber method. Urinary 17-OHCS determined in this way provide an extremely useful index of cortisol secretion. The method is not entirely specific for cortisol metabolites, however, since the tetrahydro derivative of 11-deoxycortisol, "tetrahydro S," is also excreted in the urine as a glucuronide, is liberated by glucuronidase, is extracted with organic solvents, and is measurable as a Porter-Silber chromogen. It is simple to distinguish "tetrahydro S" from cortisol metabolites, however, because the tetrahydro S is so nonpolar that it is extractable from urine with carbon tetrachloride; cortisol metabolites are not. By extracting the urinary glucuronidase-hydrolysate first with carbon tetrachloride and then with dichloromethane, one can readily fractionate the "total 17-OHCS" into 11-deoxycortisol metabolites and cortisol metabolites. In practice, there are occasions when it is important to know how much of the total 17-OHCS are derivatives of these two hormonal steroids, but there are other occasions (e.g., during metyrapone tests) when it is sufficient to know the total.

Aldosterone and Its Derivatives

Compared with cortisol, the measurement of aldosterone presents a technical challenge because of its much lower concentration in biologic fluids. Normal plasma concentrations are of the order of 10 ng/dl (compared with cortisol, which is normally present in concentrations of about 10 μg/dl). Urinary free aldosterone values are generally less than 1 μg/day. Aldosterone is unique in that a considerable portion (approximately 10%) of the hormonal steroid is excreted as a water-soluble 18-oxo-conjugate glucuronide).[33] When hydrolyzed by incubation with acid, aldosterone is released and can be extracted and measured by a variety of methods. The advantage of working with this metabolite rather than free aldosterone is that it appears in the urine in quantities of the order of 10 μg/day.

The double isotope derivative method[34] for measuring aldosterone involves the following steps. First, to the "unknown" specimen is added a trace amount of ^{3}H-labeled aldosterone to permit monitoring of recoveries at the conclusion of extensive purification. Second, the aldosterone-containing extract is subjected to various chromatographic procedures known to separate this from other steroids. Third, the "aldosterone fraction" is allowed to react with ^{14}C-labeled acetic anhydride under conditions that convert aldosterone (both ^{3}H-labeled aldosterone and that of biologic origin) to aldosterone-^{14}C-acetate. Fourth, the products of acetylation are then subjected to further chromatography, employing systems known to separate aldosterone acetates from other steroid acetates. Fifth, when repeated chromatography in various systems reveals that the ratio of ^{14}C to ^{3}H is constant, the purification is considered to be complete, and the quantity of aldosterone in the original specimen is computed from the amount of ^{3}H-labeled aldosterone added as tracer, the degree of "dilution" of ^{3}H-aldosterone-^{14}C-acetate with aldosterone-^{14}C-acetate, and the various dilutions and aliquots that were employed.

Recently, radioimmunoassays for aldosterone[35] have been developed with sensitivity comparable to that of the double isotope derivative method. Since antisera are rarely specific for any particular steroid, cross reactions with other structurally related steroids are common, and care must be taken to separate aldosterone from other potentially interfering steroids before quantification by radioimmunassay is attempted. The principles and techniques of radioimmunoassay have been described in detail elsewhere.

Another aldosterone metabolite, tetrahydro-aldosterone glucuronide, can also be measured following cleavage of the steroid from glucuronic acid using glucuronidase, extraction with dichloromethane, extensive purification, and measurement of "blue tetrazolium-reducing" activity.

17-Ketosteroids (17-KS)

The oldest practical chemical method for measuring adrenal steroids was that devised by Callow in 1940, employing the Zimmermann reaction for 17-KS. The most abundant urinary 17-KS are androsterone and etiocholanolone, which appear in the urine principally as water-soluble conjugates (largely sulfates). The main precursor of the urinary 17-KS is DHEA, but testosterone, androstenedione, and cortisol are included among a large number of minor precursors of this group of hormone metabolites. The steroid sulfates are hydrolyzed by exposure to acid. The steroids are then extracted with an organic solvent such as ether and estimated colorimetrically by the metadinitrobenzene ("Zimmermann") reaction. Although androsterone and etiocholanolone are derivatives of hormones originating in either adrenal or gonadal tissue, their 11-oxygenated analogues are derived exclusively from adrenal steroids. This distinction, if desired, can be made by chromatographic separation of the various 17-KS.

17-Ketogenic Steroids (17-KGS)

Not to be confused with 17-KS are the 17-*ketogenic* steroids — those that can be converted into 17-KS by treatment with the oxidizing reagent, sodium bismuthate.[36] These steroids include those with dihydroxyacetone side chains, glycerol side chains, or 17:20 glycol side chains attached to [17]C. The first group includes cortisol, cortisone, 11-deoxycortisol and their respective tetrahydro derivatives. The second group includes derivatives of these steroids that have undergone reduction of the 20-keto group (e.g., cortol and cortolone). The third group includes pregnanetriol. Interestingly, the precursor of pregnanetriol, 17α-hydroxyprogesterone, is *not* a 17-KGS. Due to its obvious lack of specificity, the 17-KGS method is not to be recommended when other methods are available.

Steroid Secretory Rates

An important new dimension in steroid methodology was developed during the late 1950's and early 1960's in the laboratories of Peterson, Lieberman, Tait, and Cope with the demonstration that production rates of many steroids can be measured if one has an isotopically labeled form of the steroid and if one can isolate and quantify some unique metabolite of the steroid in question. A known amount of the labeled steroid is administered. Urine is then collected over a sufficient period to allow the labeled steroid to mix with the body pool of secreted steroid and to be metabolized and excreted. The unique urinary metabolite is then quantified and its specific activity then provides a measure of the amount of steroid secreted during the period of the study, utilizing the principle that the secreted steroid, being unlabeled, would dilute the labeled steroid, thus decreasing its specific activity. The general formula is as follows:

$$\text{Secretory rate (mg)} = \frac{\text{Total counts of tracer injected (cpm)}}{\text{Specific activity of metabolite (cpm/mg)}}$$

This method must observe several rigorous conditions to give valid data, but it has proved extremely useful in providing information concerning production rates of cortisol, aldosterone, corticosterone, DOC, 11-deoxycortisol, and 18-hydroxycorticosterone.

It is also possible to measure the secretion rate of a steroid by the straightforward method of administering a tracer dose of the steroid and then determining the rate at which the labeled steroid is diluted with unlabeled steroid within the circulation. If one assumes that the metabolic clearance rate is the same for labeled and unlabeled steroid alike, then the decrease in specific activity of the steroid is a function of secretion of new, unlabeled steroid into the miscible pool.[37]

After a labeled steroid has been distributed throughout the miscible pool, it is characteristically cleared from the plasma at a relatively constant rate. This is referred to as the "metabolic clearance rate," and for most corticosteroids, it is normally of the order of 1000 l/day. The ratio of the secretion rate for a given steroid (μg/day) divided by the metabolic clearance rate (l/day) equals the mean plasma concentrations of the steroid throughout the day (μ/gl).[38]

Measurement of Other Steroids

Not only the steroids just listed but also several others have been measured by a variety of techniques. Thus DOC, 11-deoxycortisol, and progesterone in plasma have been measured by methods in which the steroids are first extracted from plasma, partially purified, and measured by a "competitive binding method" in which the endogenous steroid displaces labeled steroid from (or competes with it for) binding sites on transcortin. The principle is similar to that underlying radioimmunoassay except that a natural "binding protein" rather than an antibody is employed. Similar assays have been employed for certain estrogens and androgens using testosterone-binding globulin rather than transcortin. In addition, trace quantities of several steroids have been quantified by gas-liquid chromatography. Recently, radioimmunoassays have been developed for pregnenolone, 17-hydroxypregnenolone, and an increasing number of other steroids. The adaptability of these various methods for the measurement of various steroids seems to be unlimited.

Normal Values in Adults

Normal values for excretion rates of various steroids are listed in Table 5–4. It should be remembered that the actual values are functions of the physiologic state of the subject, the test conditions, the adequacy of collection and preservation of the specimens, and the care with which the laboratory procedure is performed. It is known that disparities between plasma and urinary steroid levels are common in pregnancy, estrogen therapy, hypothyroidism, hyperthyroidism, and hepatic insufficiency (Fig. 5–14). It

Table 5–4. SECRETION AND EXCRETION RATES OF CERTAIN STEROIDS BY NORMAL NONPREGNANT ADULTS

Steroid	Secretion Rate mg/day
Cortisol	12–30
Corticosterone	1–4
Aldosterone	0.05–0.15
DOC	0.05–0.2
DHEA	15–50

	Excretion Rate mg/day
17-OHCS	4–12
17-KS	7–20
Pregnanetriol	0.5–2.5

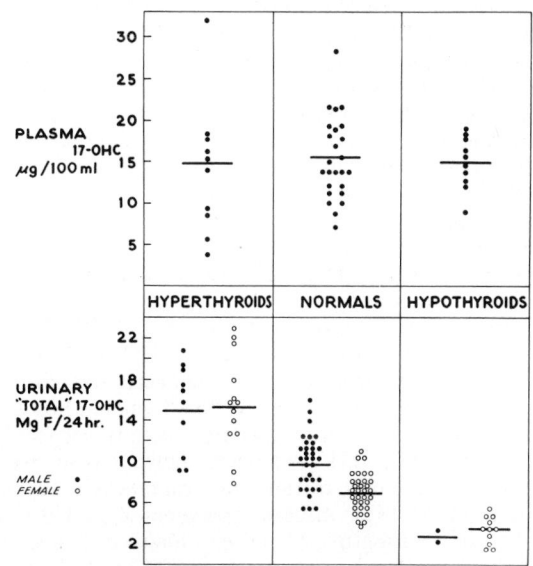

Figure 5–14. The effect of different thyroid states on adrenocortical function. Although plasma cortisol levels are essentially identical in all states, the urinary excretion is in the range of Cushing's syndrome in the group with hyperthyroidism and low in hypothyroidism. (After DiRaimondo and Sagan.)

is strongly recommended that the physician have full knowledge of the physiologic condition of the subejct and that he have a close working relationship with the laboratory so as to minimize the likelihood of misleading results.

Tests of Adrenal Reserve, Pituitary (ACTH) Reserve, and Pituitary-Adrenal Suppressibility

The normal pituitary-adrenal system has reserve capacity to secrete its hormones with more than ordinary intensity if properly stimulated. On the other hand, under appropriate conditions, it can be suppressed to such a degree that it virtually ceases to function. There are a number of clinical situations in which it is useful to know whether an individual has normal adrenal reserve, normal ACTH-secreting reserve, or normal pituitary-adrenal suppressibility. Therefore, standard tests of each of these functions have been developed.

Adrenal Reserve

The responsiveness of the adrenal to ACTH can be assessed by measuring plasma or urinary steroids before and again during the administration of ACTH. The most secure method of testing adrenal reserve is to infuse ACTH (corticotropin) intravenously at the rate of about 5 U/hour for 8 hours.[39] Plasma should be collected prior to the beginning of the infusion and again after at least 1 hour of the infusion but before the termination of the infusion. Urine should be collected for 24 hours prior to the ACTH infusion and again for 24 hours commencing with the start of the infusion. The time of day is not of critical importance in standardizing this test; however, the interpretation of control values should take into consideration the fact that plasma cortisol concentrations are normally in the range of 10–25 μg/dl in the morning and less than 10 μg/dl late in the evening. Regardless of the control values, however, the individual with normal adrenal reserve exhibits an increase of 10–25 μg/dl during the 1st hour and 15–40 μg/dl by the 8th hour of an ACTH infusion. Urinary 17-OHCS values are normally proportional to body size, and it is useful to relate them to urinary creatinine for individuals of all ages and sizes. Under control conditions, normal individuals should excrete 3–7 mg of 17-OHCS/g of creatinine. In response to a standard 8-hour infusion of ACTH, urinary 17-OHCS should increase to 12–25 mg/g of creatinine. In response to ACTH infusion, urinary 17-KS should increase by a factor of 1.5–2.5 relative to control values, which are normally 4–10 mg/g of creatinine under control conditions.

There are a number of modifications of the test for adrenal reserve, including the use of intramuscular injections rather than intravenous infusions of ACTH. One method is to inject 25 μg of synthetic $^{1\text{-}24}$ACTH (Cortrosyn) intramuscularly and to measure plasma cortisol before and 60 min following the injection; a normal response has a rise of 10–20 mg/dl. Yet another alternative is to inject 100 U of ACTH gel or zinc-ACTH suspension; normal responses to these depot-ACTH preparations are comparable to those observed when ACTH is infused intravenously, 5 U/hr for 8 hours. The critical feature of the test, however it might be performed, is that a substantial increase in adrenal steroids must occur in response to ACTH if one is to prove the existence of adrenal reserve. There have been cases in which adrenal insufficiency was mistakenly diagnosed when the

real difficulty was that the ACTH was of poor quality and was ineffective when administered intramuscularly.

Pituitary (ACTH) Reserve

If a particular individual's adrenals are responsive to exogenous ACTH (as described previously), then it is possible to utilize his adrenals to appraise changes in endogenous ACTH. In other words, by applying a stimulus to ACTH secretion and measuring changes in adrenal steroids, one can evaluate the integrity of the subject's ACTH secretory mechanism. If the individual responds normally to such a stimulus, it may be assumed that he possesses both pituitary reserve and adrenal reserve. If he responds normally to exogenous ACTH but not to the stimulus to ACTH secretion, it may be assumed that he lacks normal pituitary reserve. In the absence of intact adrenals, however, it is impossible to evaluate pituitary reserve using this group of tests.

Metyrapone is widely used in testing pituitary-adrenal reserve.[40] This drug inhibits 11β-hydroxylase, the enzyme that catalyzes the final step in cortisol biosynthesis. A metyrapone-induced decrease in cortisol secretion results in a compensatory increase in ACTH secretion that stimulates further steroid biogenesis. Since inhibition of 11β-hydroxylation is usually incomplete, the increased formation of cortisol precursors eventuates in partial restoration of cortisol secretion to normal, but this is accomplished only at the cost of increased pituitary secretion of ACTH and increased adrenal secretion of 11-deoxycortisol. An increase in 11-deoxycortisol alone does not mean that there has been an increase in pituitary-adrenal activity in response to metyrapone; it only means that cortisol secretion has been inhibited and that the cortisol precursor rather than cortisol itself is being released by the adrenal. An increase in total 17-OHCS, comprising cortisol, 11-deoxycortisol, and their respective metabolites, however, indicates that there has been an increase in ACTH secretion and a consequent increase in adrenal secretory activity (Fig. 5–15).

A standard test of pituitary-adrenal reserve is performed by administering metyrapone in oral doses of 10 mg/kg of ideal body weight every 4 hours for 6 doses. The normal response consists of a twofold (or greater) increase in total urinary 17-OHCS on either the day of treatment or on the subsequent day.

Various modifications of this test have been developed. In some, the metyrapone is given intravenously. In some, the test period is shortened. In some, the response is assessed in terms of increases in plasma ACTH, urinary 17-KGS, urinary 17-KS, plasma 11-deoxycortisol ("S"), or urinary "tetrahydro S." When critically performed, they all give essentially the same information. The most common mistakes have arisen from shortening the test so much that a full response is not elicited or from measuring "S" or its metabolites alone without taking into consideration the total adrenal output of 17-OHCS (see previous discussion).

Certain precautions should be taken in performing a metyrapone test. First, the patient should not simultaneously receive drugs that suppress ACTH secretion (exogenous glucocorticoids) or drugs that accelerate the metabolism of metyrapone (e.g., diphenylhydantoin).[41] Patients with manifestations of adrenal insufficiency should be observed closely during performance of a metyrapone test so that supportive treatment may be provided if the patient develops hypotension or vomiting. If absorbed too rapidly,

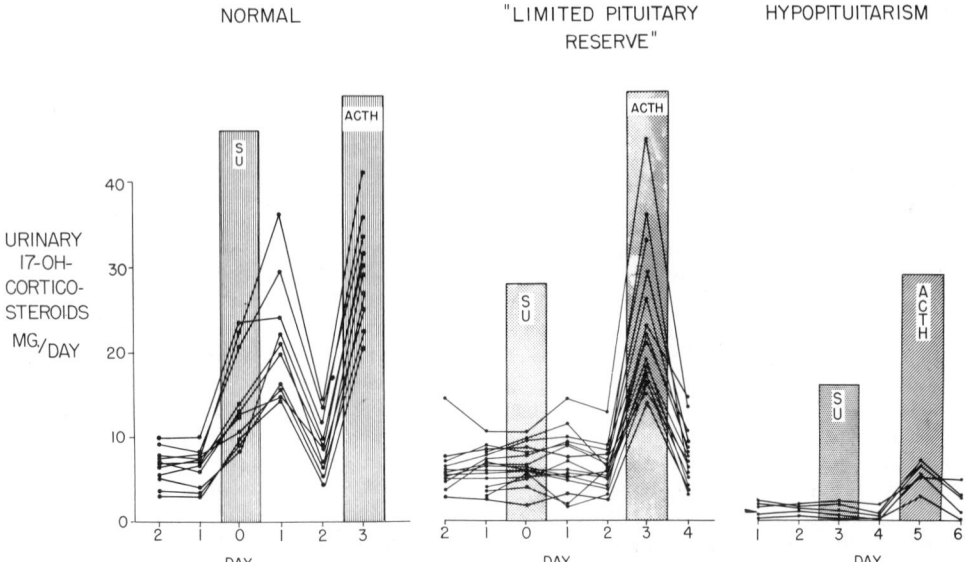

Figure 5–15. Typical responses of urinary 17-OHCS during treatment with standard doses of SU (metyrapone) or ACTH in normal subjects, in patients with limited pituitary reserve, and in patients with frank hypopituitarism. (From Liddle, G. W., Island, D., et al.: *Recent Progr. Hormone Res. 18:*125, 1962.)

metyrapone causes transient vertigo. This can be prevented by administering the tablets with a meal or 200 ml of milk.

A variety of mildly stressful stimuli have also been utilized in testing pituitary-adrenal reserve. These have included insulin-induced hypoglycemia, intravenous injection of pyrogens, and intravenous injection of vasopressin. The first causes sweating, tremulousness, and mental confusion. The second causes chills and fever. The third causes abdominal cramping. All of them cause increases in ACTH secretion, with consequent increases in plasma cortisol concentrations within approximately 1 hour. The ACTH simulation is so transient that urinary steroids are not appreciably affected. Despite the discomfort they cause, these stimuli have practical utility in that they permit relatively quick testing of pituitary-adrenal reserve.

Dexamethasone Suppression Tests

Glucocorticoids suppress the secretion of ACTH and thereby curtail the secretion of cortisol and its by-products. Thus, under normal circumstances, cortisol is self-regulating. In Cushing's syndrome, however, the pituitary-adrenal system loses its normal sensitivity to the suppressive action of glucocorticoids and, as a result, cortisol is excessively secreted. Standard pituitary-adrenal suppression tests have been developed to aid in the elucidation of this condition.[42] Dexamethasone is used as the suppressive agent because it is so potent biologically that only very small amounts of it are required to suppress ACTH. Such small amounts of the exogenous steroid do not interfere with the chemical measurement of endogenous steroids.

Normal nonstressed subjects respond to dexamethasone in doses of 0.5 mg every 6 hours with virtually complete cessation of ACTH and cortisol secretion (Fig. 5–16). Urinary 17-OHCS fall to less than 2.5 mg/day by the 2nd day of treatment, and plasma cortisol falls to less than 5 μg/dl. If in response to these small doses of dexametha-

sone, 16-OHCS are not profoundly suppressed, one must suspect the presence of Cushing's syndrome. The cause of the Cushing's syndrome can often be determined by the use of a "high-dose" suppression test in which dexamethasone is given in doses of 2.0 mg every 6 hours for 8 doses (see later). A screening test for Cushing's syndrome, employing a single 1-mg dose of dexamethasone, is described under the heading "Hypercortisolism."

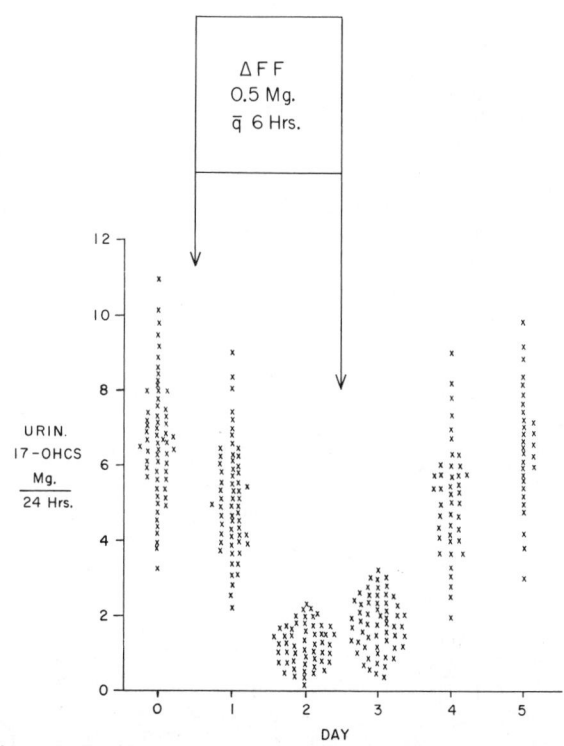

Figure 5–16. Normal responses of urinary 17-OHCS during treatment with standard doses of ΔFF (dexamethasone). (From Liddle, G. W., Island, D., et al.: *Recent Progr. Hormone Res. 18:*125, 1962.)

Pharmacologic Inhibition of Adrenal Steroid Biosynthesis

Several drugs have been shown to inhibit one or another of the enzymatically controlled steps through which cholesterol is converted to hormonal steroids.[43] Fig. 5–17 depicts structural formulas of the most important of these agents; some have yet to be assigned official pharmaceutical names. Enzyme inhibition results in decreased formation of steroids appearing in the pathway beyond the inhibited step and increased secretion of steroids occurring just prior to the inhibited step. If cortisol biosynthesis is inhibited, there ensues a compensatory increase in ACTH secretion, which results in accelerated formation of all steroids formed by the zona fasciculata. With increased formation of precursors, cortisol secretion may return toward normal, but this is achieved only at the cost of increased secretion of ACTH and increased biosynthesis of steroid precursors. Similarly, if mineralocorticoid secretion is impaired by an adrenal inhibitor, there will be a compensatory increase in renin-angiotensin production and increased formation of steroids appearing in the aldosterone biosynthetic pathway prior to the inhibited step. Thus pharmacologic inhibition of an adrenal enzyme may result in a distorted pattern of steroid secretion, and the biologic consequences of adrenal inhibition can be understood in terms of the biologic activities of steroids that are deficiently secreted and the biologic activities of steroids that are excessively secreted.

Amino-glutethimide has been shown to inhibit the conversion of cholesterol to pregnenolone, presumably by inhibiting the enzyme 20α-hydroxylase. It thus curtails the biosynthesis of all hormonal steroids and leads to accumulation of cholesterol within the adrenal cortex. Clinically, it has found limited use as an inhibitor of mineralocorticoid secretion in patients with steroid hypertension, as an inhibitor of cortisol secretion in patients with Cushing's syndrome, and as an inhibitor of estrogen precursors in patients with metastatic mammary carcinoma.

Cyanoketone and trilostane have been shown to inhibit the conversion of Δ^5-3β-ol steroids to Δ^4-3-oxo steroids, presumably by inhibitng the enzyme 3β-hydroxysteroid dehydrogenase. Consequently, pregnenolone cannot be converted efficiently to progesterone or its potent corticosteroid derivatives, all of which have Δ^4-3-oxo configurations.

SU-9055 and SU-8000 (Fig. 5–17) have been shown to inhibit 17α-hydroxylase and, thereby, to curtail the production of cortisol. They also inhibit aldosterone production by interfering with oxidation at carbon-18. As a consequence of the latter action, they induce sodium excretion in patients with primary or secondary aldosteronism.

Metyrapone and SKF-12185 (Fig. 5–17) have been shown to inhibit 11β-hydroxylase and thus to curtail the conversion of 11-deoxycortisol to cortisol and DOC to corticosterone. The former property has been exploited in establishing metyrapone as an agent for testing pituitary-adrenal reserve (see previously). These agents have also seen limited use in the treatment of hypercortisolism.

Heparin and heparinoids have been shown to alter the histochemical appearance of the zona glomerulosa and to inhibit aldosterone secretion. The precise mechanism is unknown. These agents have seen limited use in the treatment of primary and secondary aldosteronism.

The cells of the zona fasciculata and zona reticularis of dogs and humans are selectively destroyed by o,p'-DDD (also known as mitotane [Lysodren]), thus compromising the capacity of the adrenal to secrete cortisol. Although certain enzyme systems (e.g., 11β-hydroxylase) precede others in their loss of efficiency, it has not been shown that o,p'-DDD is a selective inhibitor of any particular enzyme in the same sense that metyrapone and cyanoketone

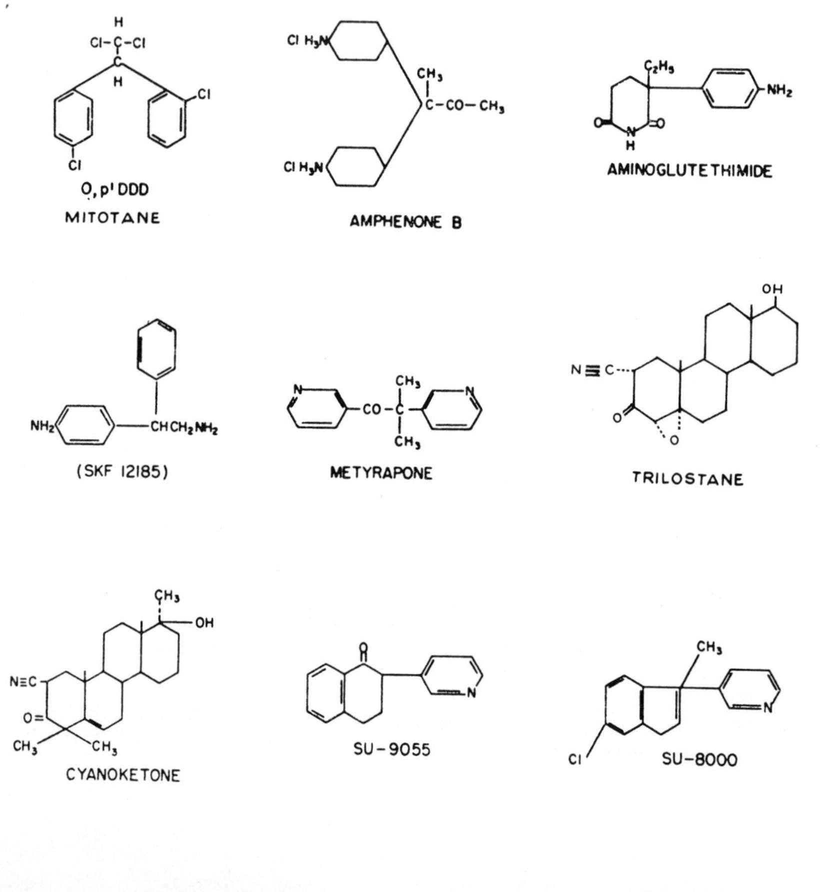

Figure 5–17. Structures of some adrenal inhibitors.

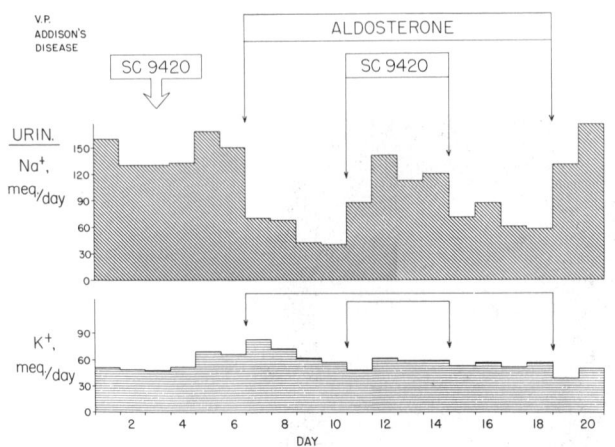

Figure 5–18. SC-9420 (spironolactone) is without discernible natriuretic effect in the absence of mineralocorticoids, as, for example, when it is administered to an addisonian patient who is maintained solely on a liberal sodium intake and a glucocorticoid. When the same patient is maintained on aldosterone, however, treatment with spironolactone exerts an obvious natriuretic effect.

are. This drug is of established value in the treatment of adrenocortical carcinoma and of Cushing's syndrome.

Amphenone B, one of the earliest known adrenal inhibitors, interferes with a number of steps in the steroid biosynthetic scheme. It has been used clinically to reduce aldosterone, cortisol, and adrenal estrogen production, but its clinical use has been abandoned because of its numerous side effects.

Aldosterone Antagonism

Certain steroids, even though lacking intrinsic corticosteroid activity, have the capacity of blocking the actions of corticosteroids. The best-known example of such a phenomenon is the action of spironolactone as an aldosterone antagonist. This is merely a particular instance of a more general phenomenon of mineralocorticoid antagonism by progesterone and a group of synthetic steroidal lactones.[44] These agents have little or no effect of their own on electrolyte excretion but, when administered in the presence of mineralocorticoids, they antagonize the sodium-retaining, potassium-losing actions of these steroids (Fig. 5–18). The steroidal lactones have been shown to promote sodium excretion and diminish potassium excretion in both primary and secondary aldosteronism and to correct edema, hypertension, and hypokalemia when these abnormalities are dependent upon mineralocorticoids. It has been suggested that the steroidal lactones compete with mineralocorticoids for attachment to their receptor proteins in target tissues and induce allosteric changes in the receptors that render them nonfunctional.

ADRENAL CORTICAL DISEASES

In the main, adrenal cortical diseases assume importance only when they lead to increased or decreased production of steroid hormones. Accordingly, this section will be organized in such a way as to give emphasis to the fact that the major endocrinopathies represent either overproduction or underproduction of particular hormones. By far the most important hormones of the human adrenal cortex are cortisol and aldosterone, and these hormones will

be given most attention, whereas others will be considered as by-products that only occasionally assume importance in clinical medicine.

Adrenal Cortical Hyperfunction

The hyperfunctioning adrenal cortex can produce syndromes of hypercortisolism, mineralocorticoid excess, virilism, or feminization. Mixed syndromes may occur.

Hypercortisolism (Cushing's Syndrome)

Although the medical literature had previously been sprinkled with reports of similar cases, it was not until Cushing's report[45] of cases of "pituitary basophilism" in 1932 that this clinical entity attracted major attention. In Cushing's view, the syndrome of central obesity, cutaneous striae, osteoporosis, weakness, hypertension, diabetes, plethora, and hirsutism was of pituitary origin, but others emphasized the role of the adrenal cortex in the pathogenesis of the syndrome. In 1942, Fuller Albright[46] pointed out that the distinctive features of Cushing's syndrome could best be attributed to the "sugar hormone" of the adrenal cortex, the hormone that favored gluconeogenesis, protein wasting, and diabetes; he contrasted this syndrome of glucocorticoid excess with that of adrenal androgen excess, in which there are conspicuous signs of protein anabolism. With Daughaday's development of a method for measuring formaldehydogenic steroids, it became possible to demonstrate that carbon–21 oxygenated steroids were elevated in the urine of patients with Cushing's syndrome. Subsequent evolution of more specific methods for measuring corticosteroids finally made it possible to demonstrate that the chemical common denominator of all cases of spontaneous Cushing's syndrome was an excess of cortisol. Cortisone and other synthetic glucocorticoids have given rise to iatrogenic Cushing's syndrome, but the only glucocorticoid produced in significant quantities by the human adrenal cortex is cortisol itself. Brief elevations of cortisol do not cause clinically recognizable Cushing's syndrome; rather, Cushing's syndrome is a result of a chronic excess of this steroid.

General Features of Hypercortisolism

Cushing's syndrome occurs sporadically in all races, all ages, and both sexes, but it has been reported with greatest frequency in women between the ages of 20 and 60. Typically it is characterized by weight gain, and, in contrast to certain other endocrinopathies such as acromegaly and virilism, the gain in weight is due principally to accumulation of adipose tissue, particularly in the facial, nuchal, truncal, and girdle areas. This is sometimes referred to as centripetal or "buffalo" obesity (Fig. 5–19).

Equally characteristic of hypercortisolism is evidence of protein wasting. In mild cases or those of only a few months' duration, this may amount to nothing more than a tendency to bruise easily. In more severe, chronic cases, the skin may be so thin and fragile that it is denuded by removal of a strip of adhesive tape or some other trivial injury. Insignificant trauma may result in formation of purpura, especially common on the dorsal aspects of the hands or forearms. Where the weakened integument is stretched by underlying accumulation of adipose tissue, it may become so thin that streaks of capillaries become visible — the pink or purple striae of classic Cushing's syndrome.

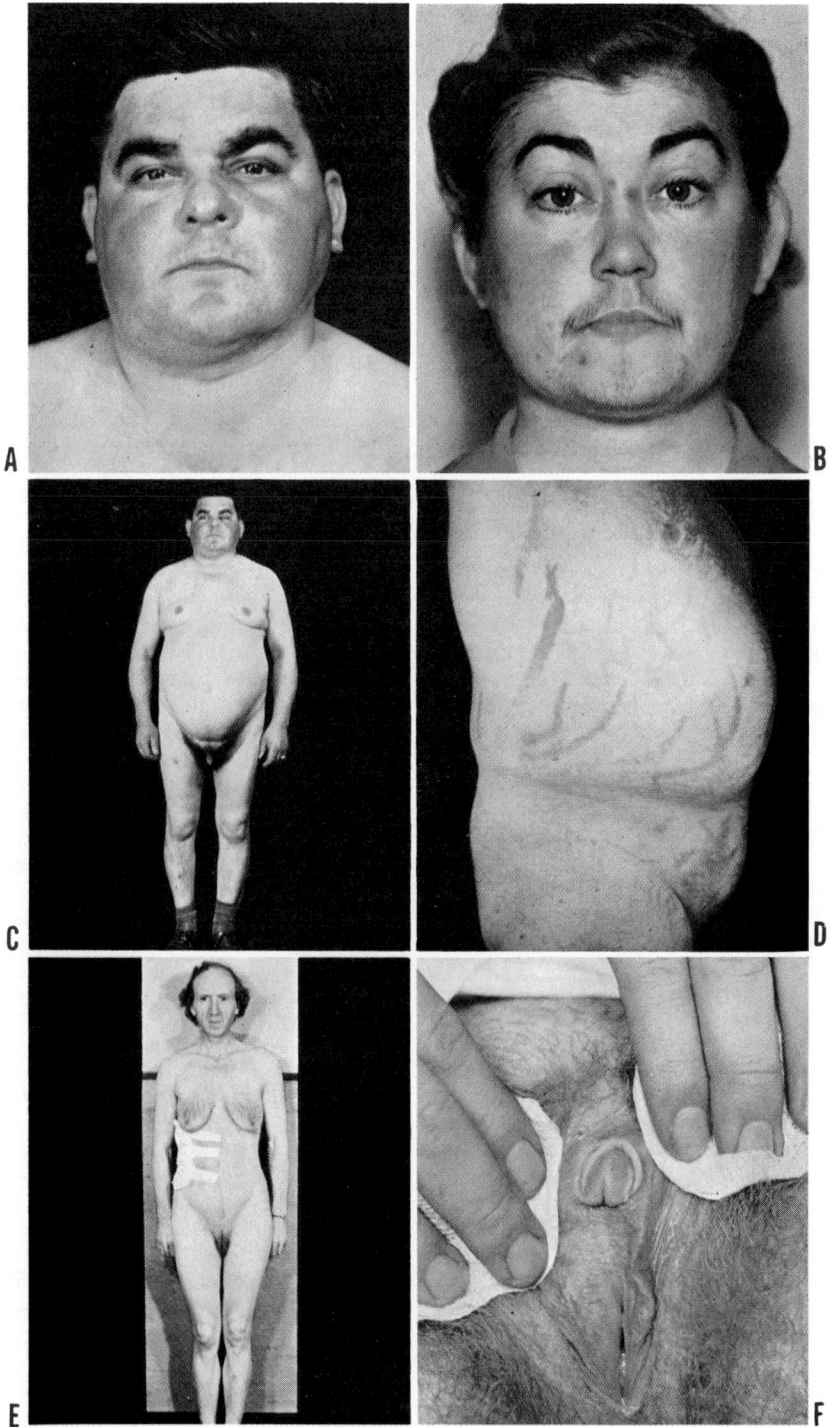

Figure 5–19.   *A* to *D*, Cushing's syndrome. *A*, Round, fiery-red face; short, thick neck. Typical moon face. *B*, Red moon face with hirsutism. *C*, Truncal obesity with prominent abdomen and relatively thin extremities. *D*, Purplish-red striae and protuberant abdomen. *E* and *F*, Adrenogenital syndrome. *E*, Masculine figure with prominent muscles, partial baldness, and excessive hair on the breasts. *F*, Enlarged clitoris in the same case.

Occasionally, muscle wasting progresses to the point at which it is objectively apparent; frequently it results in such severe weakness that the patient cannot rise from a deep-knee bend without assistance.

Attrition of bone matrix results in generalized osteoporosis. A particularly vulnerable part of the skeleton is the vertebral column, where weakening of the vertebral bodies may permit bulging of the intervertebral discs, giving a "codfish vertebrae" appearance in lateral radiographic views. Compression fractures may occur with anterior wedging of the vertebral bodies, resulting in kyphosis, loss of height, and backache. The osteoporotic process is generalized, and radiographic evidence of it is frequently encountered in the skull and extremities; pathologic fractures of the ribs and extremities have occurred in several cases.

Perhaps as a consequence of osteoporosis, modest hypercalciuria is common, with urinary calcium values of 150–300 mg/day. Renal stones occur in approximately 20% of long-standing cases of Cushing's syndrome.

Surgeons frequently find the tissues of patients with chronic or severe Cushing's syndrome to have poor tensile strength, so that they tear easily, retain sutures poorly, and heal slowly. Superficial wounds may also heal slowly and become sites of indolent infection and ulceration; this is especially common in pretibial areas.

Growth is arrested, and this is an important aspect of Cushing's syndrome in children and adolescents, for if the epiphyses of the long bones close before the Cushing's syndrome is corrected, short stature will be inevitable. As a rule, one can be fairly confident that an obese child who is growing rapidly does not have Cushing's syndrome, but the syndrome must be suspected in obese children who grow slowly.

In addition to centripetal obesity and protein wasting, the patient with Cushing's syndrome usually has impaired glucose tolerance. The usual pattern is not that of frank diabetes mellitus with glycosuria and elevated fasting blood glucose (these occur in about 20%) but rather a failure of the blood glucose to return to fasting levels during the 2nd and 3rd hours of a standard glucose tolerance test. Approximately 90% of patients with Cushing's syndrome will have at least mild impairment of glucose tolerance.

Whether it is owing entirely to hypercortisolism or partly to excessive secretion of associated steroids, the majority of patients with Cushing's syndrome have high blood pressure. In association with this, they may have left ventricular hypertrophy and increased susceptibility to occlusion of major arteries. Edema and hypokalemia (unprovoked by diuretics) occur in only a minority of patients with Cushing's syndrome, but these abnormalities are common in those patients whose steroid levels are especially high. A growing body of evidence indicates that one mechanism through which cortisol elevates the blood pressure is by increasing the level of circulating angiotensinogen.

Other common manifestations of hypercortisolism include heightened color of face and neck, downy hirsutism, oligomenorrhea, mild erythrocytosis, lymphopenia, and eosinopenia. About 30% of patients have superficial fungal infections such as tinea versicolor. Serum gamma globulin concentrations and serum protein-bound iodine concentrations are often slightly subnormal. Many patients with Cushing's syndrome are emotionally labile and easily irritated. A few are psychotic, and the psychotic patterns have most frequently resembled schizophrenia, hypomania, or depression. Patients with Cushing's syndrome often have difficulty in limiting the spread of infections.

In the past, death commonly resulted among patients with Cushing's syndrome from infections with pyogenic organisms, hypertensive-arteriosclerotic cardiovascular disease, and suicide.

Many patients with hypercortisolism have some associated excess of adrenal androgen. Unless the androgen excess is extreme, the clinical manifestations amount to nothing more than some hirsutism in androgen-sensitive areas, acne, and oligomenorrhea. Extreme excesses of adrenal androgen might result in temporal hair recession, coarsening of the voice, and clitoral hypertrophy.

Although a minority of patients with Cushing's syndrome present most of the clinical features just described, many of them present a less complete clinical picture. Rather than persisting in uncertainty and rather than devoting an inordinate amount of effort to nonspecific tests, it is often wise to proceed directly to the most efficient methods available for proving or disproving the diagnosis of hypercortisolism. For this purpose it is desirable to measure the cortisol in specimens of plasma obtained late in the evening and to measure 17-OHCS in 24-hour collections of urine. If the bedtime plasma cortisol concentration is greater than 7 μg/dl and if the urinary 17-OHCS are greater than 7 mg/g of creatinine, one should proceed with a "small-dose" dexamethasone suppression test (see before). If in response to dexamethasone, 0.5 mg every 6 hours for 2 days, plasma cortisol does not fall to less than 5 μg/dl and urinary 17-OHCS to less than 2 mg/g of creatinine, one is entitled to diagnose hypercortisolism.

An erroneous diagnosis of "non-Cushing's syndrome" might be made through laboratory errors or if the patient were almost normally sensitive to dexamethasone (perhaps 2% of cases). An erroneous diagnosis of Cushing's syndrome might be made (1) through laboratory error, (2) if the patient were severely stressed, (3) if the dexamethasone were not administered, or (4) if the patient were inadvertently given exogenous cortisol, ACTH, cortisone, or spironolactone (which interferes with chromogenic and fluorogenic measurements of cortisol).

Patients with Cushing's syndrome lack the normal diurnal rhythm in cortisol secretion. In contrast to normal individuals who have relatively high plasma cortisol values early in their waking day and low values as the hour of sleep approaches, patients with Cushing's syndrome have relatively high values at all hours.[47] It is decidedly unusual for patients with Cushing's syndrome to have any plasma cortisol values below 7 μg/dl. Plasma cortisol concentrations in Cushing's syndrome usually range from about 15–35 μg/dl regardless of the time of day. Obviously, this permits considerable overlap with normal morning values, which usually range from about 12–25 μg/dl. In contrast, there is usually clear separation of Cushing's syndrome values from the normal range of 1–8 μg/dl late in the evening. Therefore, in screening for Cushing's syndrome, there is little value in measuring plasma cortisol in the morning but great value in measuring it late in the evening.

Because certain factors modify the binding of plasma cortisol or alter the extra-adrenal metabolism of cortisol, it is advisable to employ more than one chemical dimension in establishing a diagnosis of Cushing's syndrome. One should demonstrate that plasma cortisol is relatively high and that it remains so late in the day, but one should also employ some index of cortisol production rate (such as urinary 17-OHCS excretion), and one should confirm the basic fact that there is abnormal resistance to suppression by performing a "small-dose" dexamethasone test (see before).

The following modification of the "small-dose" dexamethasone test deserves special mention because of its simplicity and economy in ruling out Cushing's syndrome when this diagnosis is considered improbable from the outset. By giving 1 mg of dexamethasone at midnight and sampling blood for cortisol measurement 8 hours later, one can, in about 90% of non-Cushing's syndrome patients, exclude the diagnosis of hypercortisolism by demonstrating a plasma cortisol value of less than 5 µg/dl. Patients whose plasma cortisol values are not so suppressible may then be tested further with the more discriminating 2-day test using dexamethasone, 0.5 mg every 6 hours for 8 doses.

Differential Diagnosis of Cushing's Syndrome

There are three major varieties of Cushing's syndrome. They are all characterized by the clinical features described in the preceding section as well as by increased production of cortisol, hypercortisolemia with loss of the normal diurnal rhythm, increased renal excretion of free cortisol, increased renal excretion of 17-OHCS, and abnormal resistance to the suppressive influence of small doses of dexamethasone. These features are present regardless of whether the primary cause of the hypercortisolism is autonomous function by an adrenal neoplasm, excessive stimulation of the adrenals by pituitary ACTH, or excessive stimulation of the adrenals by ectopic ACTH. The optimal treatment of each of these disorders is different; therefore, specific diagnosis is important. The differential diagnosis rests on the steroid secretory response to a "large-dose" dexamethasone test, the measurement of plasma ACTH, and a clinical appraisal for evidence of a neoplasm.

Adrenal Neoplasms That Secrete Cortisol Autonomously. Occasionally, clones of adrenal cortical cells lose their dependence upon ACTH and acquire the capacity to grow and secrete cortisol autonomously. Morphologically, these cells may behave like carcinomas that grow exuberantly, invade, and metastasize, or they may behave like benign adenomas. They are usually unilateral but rarely bilateral, or they may have the appearance of microadenomas in both adrenal glands. When the secretion of cortisol by such clones of cells exceeds that of normal adrenal glands, clinical and chemical hypercortisolism occurs, secretion of ACTH by the otherwise normal pituitary gland ceases, and the ACTH-dependent portions of the adrenals become atrophic.

In this disorder, the administration of large doses of dexamethasone is without effect on plasma cortisol or urinary 17-OHCS or 17-KS (Fig. 5–20). The explanation is simple: The only way in which dexamethasone has been shown to modify steroid secretion is by suppressing ACTH secretion. In patients with Cushing's syndrome due to autonomous cortisol secretion, ACTH is already suppressed, and dexamethasone has no way of affecting adrenocortical activity. Occasionally, one encounters an adrenal tumor that exhibits spontaneous day-to-day fluctuations in cortisol secretion, and inadequate study might lead one to the erroneous conclusion that dexamethasone had caused a fall in the steroid output by the tumor. There has never been a case of Cushing's syndrome due to an adrenal neoplasm in which steroid production has been shown to be reproducibly suppressed on repeated testing with dexamethasone.

Although valid measurements of plasma ACTH are not generally available, when these determinations have been performed, they have revealed that patients with Cushing's syndrome due to adrenal tumors have subnormal values. Indeed, any other finding would require special explanation.

A corollary to the rule that these patients have suppression of their ACTH secretory mechanisms is the extensively verified fact that they fail to respond to standard metyrapone tests of pituitary reserve. Unlike normal individuals, they do not exhibit increases in their *total* urinary 17-OHCS when given metyrapone to block the final step in cortisol biosynthesis.[40] The importance of focusing attention on changes in *total* 17-OHCS rather than "tetrahydro S" alone in interpreting the metyrapone test becomes obvious here. An adrenal tumor that autonomously secretes cortisol will, under the inhibitory influence of metyrapone, autonomously secrete 11-deoxycortisol ("S") in its stead. An increase in urinary "tetrahydro S," therefore, does not necessarily indicate an increase in pituitary-adrenal activity. In any event, a *failure* to respond to metyrapone with an increase in total 17-OHCS is a reliable diagnostic feature of Cushing's syndrome due to adrenal (tumor) autonomy.

To say that a group of adrenal cells can function autonomously in the absence of ACTH is not equivalent to saying that these cells would be unresponsive to ACTH if ACTH were present. About 50% of patients with Cushing's syndrome due to benign adrenal neoplasms show vigorous responses to standard ACTH tests. Proof that these responses come from the tumors themselves, rather than from the nontumorous portions of the adrenal, is based on the observation that surgical removal of the tumors results in adrenal insufficiency with subnormal responsiveness to ACTH. The remaining 50% of benign adrenal tumors and more than 90% of adrenal carcinomas are unresponsive to standard infusions of ACTH.[48]

Patients with hypercortisolism secondary to excess ACTH usually have elevated urinary 17-KS more or less in proportion to the elevation of their 17-OHCS. Patients with Cushing's syndrome due to autonomous adrenal tumors may have subnormal, normal, or supernormal 17-KS. A grossly disproportionate increase in "S" production or a grossly disproportionate degree of virilism relative to the severity of the hypercortisolism should make one alert to the probability of an adrenal carcinoma.

Until proved otherwise, a patient with elevated, arrhythmic plasma cortisol, elevated urinary 17-OHCS, absolute resistance to the suppressive influence of dexamethasone, unresponsiveness to metyrapone, and subnormal plasma ACTH must be considered to have an adrenal tumor. Usually, cortisol-secreting adrenal tumors can be located preoperatively by physical examination or radiographic studies. Most adrenal carcinomas are so inefficient in synthesizing cortisol that, by the time they have attracted medical attention through causing Cushing's syndrome, they are more than 6 cm in diameter. Some are massive enough to be palpable through the abdominal wall. Many are large enough to cause displacement of the kidney, as seen by intravenous urography. Most can be made visible by careful

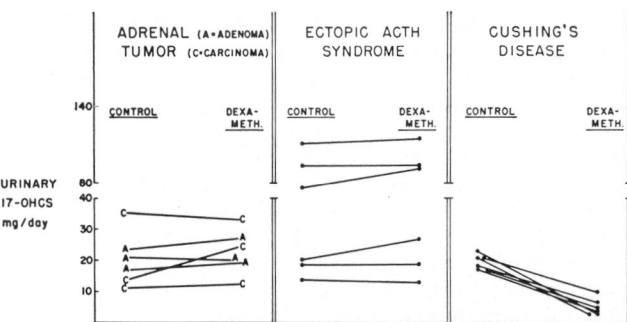

Figure 5–20. Results of dexamethasone suppression test, using 2 mg of dexamethasone every 6 hours for 2 days, in patients with hypercortisolism due to adrenal tumor, secretion of ectopic ACTH, or inappropriate secretion of pituitary ACTH. (From Liddle, G. W.: Cushing's syndrome, In *The Adrenal Cortex.* Eisenstein, A. B. (ed.), Boston, Little, Brown and Co., 1967.)

adrenal arteriography. Most benign adenomas that cause Cushing's syndrome are 2–6 cm in diameter and can usually be seen during adrenal arteriography or by computerized tomography. Other methods of revealing the tumors have also been used but are probably less reliable. Microadenomas less than 1 cm in diameter cannot be discerned with reliability by any available methods.

Unless the tumor is obviously nonresectable or the patient's general condition is too precarious to permit a major operation, every patient with a diagnosis of an adrenal tumor should be offered an adrenal exploration. A useful method is to have two surgeons operate simultaneously through bilateral flank incisions so that both adrenals can be examined before a decision is made regarding definitive therapy. If a tumor is found on only one side, as will be the case more than 90% of the time, that adrenal should be removed and the contralateral adrenal left intact. If bilateral adenomas are found, both adrenals should be removed. If no discrete adenomas are found, both adrenals should be removed in the expectation that they will show microadenomatosis. At this point it is obvious why the preoperative diagnosis of adrenal autonomy must be as firm as possible, since treatments other than adrenalectomy are usually preferable for the other varieties of Cushing's syndrome.[49]

It is imperative that a patient undergoing resection of adrenal tumors receive cortisol substitution therapy during and after the operation, until his remaining atrophic adrenal tissue has been demonstrated to be functioning adequately. Water-soluble esters of glucocorticoids should be given intravenously or intramuscularly until the patient can dependably take medications by mouth. If dexamethasone is used (in order to permit early evaluation of the completeness of removal of autonomous adrenal tissue), the dose should be 1/25 that suggested for hydrocortisone. On the day of the operation, the dose of steroid should be equivalent to 400 mg of hydrocortisone (100 mg every 6 hours, beginning with the operation). On each succeeding day, the dose may be decreased by a twofold factor until the total daily dose is 50 mg. This dose might well be given for 2 weeks, in two or three divided doses. Then one might give 30 mg daily for 2 months, 20 mg in the morning and 10 mg late in the day. Thereafter, one might give 20 mg once each morning for 6 months, by the end of which time pituitary-adrenal recovery should be demonstrable both clinically and chemically. To prove the latter, endogenous plasma cortisol concentrations should be at least 12 μg/dl 24 hours after the last morning dose of exogenous hydrocortisone. By giving the exogenous hydrocortisone in the amount of 20 mg/day, one can prevent symptoms of adrenal insufficiency; by giving it as a single dose only once each morning, one can avoid perpetuating the suppression of pituitary-adrenal function.

In the event that total adrenalectomy is necessary, lifelong treatment with glucocorticoids, sodium chloride, and usually mineralocorticoids must be employed, as outlined in the section on the treatment of primary adrenal insufficiency (Addison's disease).

Patients with adrenal carcinomas should be observed periodically for evidence of recurrence of the tumor. Recurrence after 12 years of clinical and chemical "cure" has been reported. A patient with definite evidence of a nonresectable adrenal carcinoma may be treated with the adrenocorticolytic drug, o,p'-DDD (mitotane [Lysodren]).[50] To date, this drug has never cured an adrenal carcinoma; nevertheless, it is the only agent that has been shown to have a selective effect in destroying adrenal tissue. In doses of 6–10 g/day, o,p'-DDD has been shown to induce objective regression of tumor size in about one third of patients with an adrenal carcinoma and to curtail steroid production not only in these but also in an additional one third. Objective remissions are usually of 3 months' to 3 years' duration. The side effects — anorexia, nausea, vomiting, diarrhea, lethargy, and ataxia — are often troublesome and may require reduction of dosage or even total withdrawal of the drug. If one has the good fortune of inducing a remission, it is possible that, with prolonged therapy, the zona fasciculata of the nontumorous adrenal may also be destroyed. Therefore, it is wise to add to the regimen a daily dose of dexamethasone, 0.5 mg in order to forestall possible adrenal insufficiency. Symptoms of the latter might be difficult to evaluate in patients receiving a drug that causes anorexia and nausea.

When the major symptoms of nonresectable adrenal carcinomas are due to the excessive production of corticosteroids, treatment with metyrapone can be employed to curtail the production of 11 β-hydroxysteroids such as cortisol. In doses of 1–3 g/day, metyrapone will usually bring plasma cortisol into an acceptable range of 10–20 μg/dl. In countries where it is marketed, aminoglutethimide can be employed to curtail the production of steroids of all classes. The usual dose of aminoglutethimide is 0.75–1.0 g/day; larger doses often cause ataxia.

Unless resected, an adrenal carcinoma sooner or later progresses relentlessly, invading the neighboring abdominal organs; occluding the inferior vena cava; metastasizing to the liver, where it may cause massive hepatomegaly; and metastasizing to the lungs, where it leads to progressive respiratory embarrassment. One rarely sees major involvement of bones, skin, brain, or other organs. The downhill course of the patient with an adrenal carcinoma is characterized by abdominal distention, ascites, edema of the lower extremities, anorexia, nausea, vomiting, dyspnea, wasting, weakness, and progressive debility. Occasionally, early or late, the patient's course may be punctuated by spontaneous rupture of the tumor, abdominal pain, and hemorrhagic shock.

In contrast to the salubrious prognosis of the patient with a benign adrenal tumor, in whom surgical care of the tumor and gradual recovery of normal pituitary-adrenal function is the rule, the prognosis of the patient with an adrenal carcinoma must remain guarded. Approximately one half of these tumors are incompletely resectable by the time the diagnosis is made. Another one fourth appear to be resectable initially but subsequently prove otherwise. The remaining one fourth can be cured by surgical removal of the primary adrenal tumor.

"Cushing's Disease": Hypercortisolism Secondary to Inappropriate Secretion of ACTH by the Pituitary. From a basic physiologic point of view, "Cushing's disease" stands in sharp contrast to hypercortisolism due to adrenal autonomy, although the clinical features of hypercortisolism are much the same in either disorder. "Cushing's syndrome" is the generic term applied to the constellation of clinical and chemical abnormalities resulting from a chronic excess of glucocorticoids. The more specific term, "Cushing's disease," is applied to those cases of Cushing's syndrome in which hypercortisolism is secondary to inappropriate secretion of ACTH by the pituitary. Patients with this disorder have *relatively* high plasma ACTH concentrations. Their adrenal secretory activity is at least partially suppressible with large doses of dexamethasone, and they have vigorous pituitary-adrenal responses to metyrapone. Furthermore, normalization of their plasma cortisol concentrations (by adrenalectomy followed by chronic cortisol substitution therapy) is followed by supernormal elevations of plasma ACTH. In all these respects,[51] patients with Cushing's disease differ from those with truly *primary* adrenal hyperfunction, i.e., those with adrenal neoplasms that autonomously secrete cortisol.

A diagnosis of Cushing's disease can be made with a high

degree of confidence if all the following criteria are satisfied: (1) there are definite clinical features of hypercortisolism, (2) plasma cortisol fails to fall to less than 8μg/dl late in the day, (3) urinary 17-OHCS are elevated under basal conditions and fail to fall to less than 2 mg/g of creatinine on the 2nd day of treatment with dexamethasone, 0.5 mg every 6 hours, (4) urinary 17-OHCS fall reproducibly in response to large doses of dexamethasone (2 mg every 6 hours for 2 days).

The dexamethasone suppression test can be of extremely great value[42] when used under controlled conditions and in combination with a specific method for measuring urinary 17-OHCS. In checking the validity of the methods one can, from time to time, carry out dexamethasone suppression tests in nonstressed subjects who do not have Cushing's syndrome. On either the small or the large dose of dexamethasone, urinary 17-OHCS should invariably fall to less than 2 mg/g of creatinine on the 2nd day of treatment. Failure to do so should alert one to the fact that a methodological problem exists; the possibilities include failure of the subject to take the dexamethasone, lack of specificity of the laboratory method for measuring 17-OHCS, or presence of interfering medications. In the last category one might include ACTH, cortisone, hydrocortisone, spironolactone, a variety of psychoactive drugs, and a few fungicides. Obviously, such sources of error should be scrupulously avoided in testing a patient suspected of having Cushing's syndrome.

The principal use of the "small-dose" dexamethasone test is to separate patients with true hypercortisolism from those without. Any nonstressed individual who does not show profound suppression of 17-OHCS in response to small doses of dexamethasone should be suspected of having Cushing's syndrome. It has sometimes been said that a "normal" response is a 50% (or greater) decrease below control 17-OHCS, but this is erroneous, for patients with Cushing's disease not infrequently qualify as "normal" under the "50% rule." For example, a decrease in urinary 17-OHCS from control values of 14 mg/g of creatinine down to 7 mg/g of creatinine during treatment with small doses of dexamethasone would be fairly typical of Cushing's disease.

The only purpose of the "large-dose" dexamethasone test is to separate patients with Cushing's disease from those with other varieties of Cushing's syndrome. Reproducible reduction of urinary 17-OHCS, on repeated testing with large doses of dexamethasone, should be interpreted to mean that adrenal function is pituitary-dependent. The degree of suppression is not crucial, as long as it is beyond the day-to-day

fluctuations observed during control periods. In response to large doses of dexamethasone, some patients with Cushing's disease exhibit decreases in urinary 17-OHCS to less than 2 mg/g of creatinine, and most exhibit decreases to less than 50% of their control values. A few, however, have been known merely to exhibit decreases to 70–80% of their control values.

If in response to *small* doses of dexamethasone, one observes *distinct* but incomplete suppression of 17-OHCS, it is not necessary to employ large doses. That is to say, in many patients with Cushing's disease one can demonstrate an abnormal degree of resistance to suppression yet the obvious presence of suppressibility with small doses of dexamethasone alone.

The following ancillary tests may be performed in characterizing the pituitary-adrenal function of the patient with Cushing's disease (Fig. 5–21): (1) *metyrapone test:* patients with Cushing's disease exhibit increases in *total* 17-OHCS, in contrast to patients with Cushing's syndrome due to adrenal neoplasms; (2) *ACTH infusion test:* patients with Cushing's disease exhibit distinct increases in 17-OHCS, in contrast to some patients with adrenal neoplasms; (3) *plasma ACTH assay:* patients with Cushing's disease have concentrations within the normal range or higher, in contrast to patients with adrenal neoplasms. These ancillary tests do not provide definitive information for separating patients with Cushing's disease from those with the ectopic ACTH syndrome (see later). This distinction must be based on the results of the dexamethasone test and morphologic evidence of a tumor.

Once a diagnosis of Cushing's disease has been established, it may be worthwhile to obtain radiographic views of the sella turcica in search of a pituitary tumor. At least 10% of patients with Cushing's disease have pituitary adenomas (usually chromophobic) that are large enough to cause sellar erosion.

Recent technical improvements in pituitary surgery, particularly the use of instruments that permit exploration of the gland with magnifying lenses via a transsphenoidal approach, have permitted several neurosurgeons to confirm Cushing's original belief that most patients with this disease have pituitary microadenomas.

Treatment of Cushing's Disease. The realization that Cushing's disease is usually caused by a pituitary microadenoma has led to the inference that the ideal method of treating this disease might be a selective removal of the microadenoma, leaving remaining pituitary structures un-

	NORMAL	ADRENAL TUMOR	"CUSHING'S DISEASE"	ECTOPIC ACTH SYNDROME
PLASMA CORTISOL	10-25 μg% RHYTHMIC	HIGH NO RHYTHM	HIGH, NO RHYTHM	HIGH, NO RHYTHM
PLASMA ACTH	0.1 - 0.4 mU%	LOW	HIGH	HIGH
17-OHCS RESPONSE TO ACTH	3-5 FOLD RISE	+,0	+	+,0
RESPONSE TO METYRAPONE	2-4 FOLD RISE	0	+	+,0
RESPONSE TO DEXAMETHASONE	0-3 mg/d	NO FALL	PARTIAL FALL	NO FALL
PLASMA ACTH AFTER ADRENALECTOMY, ON NORMAL CORTISOL	NORMAL	LOW	HIGH	HIGH

Figure 5–21. Typical ACTH, cortisol, and urinary 17-OHCS values in normal subjects and in subjects with various types of Cushing's syndrome under basal conditions and in response to various treatments. (From Liddle, G. W.: Pathogenesis of glucocorticoid disorders. *Am. J. Med. 53*:638, 1972.)

disturbed. In recent years a number of medical centers have reported success in this endeavor in 70–80% of their patients, using instruments that magnify the area being explored and approaching the pituitary gland via the transsphenoidal route. Removal of the microadenoma generally cures the Cushing's disease without inducing deficiencies of other pituitary hormones. An interesting observation that has been made repeatedly is that transient ACTH-cortisol deficiency may follow removal of the microadenoma, followed by gradual recovery of normal ACTH-cortisol relationships. This observation may be construed to mean that the primary cause of the patient's Cushing's disease was intrinsic to the ACTH-secreting microadenoma. For, if the primary cause had been hypersecretion of "hypothalamic corticotropin-releasing factor," the disease should have persisted or recurred as a consequence of hyperstimulation of ACTH-secreting cells that had escaped resection.

Twenty to 30% of the attempts to cure Cushing's disease by microadenomectomy are unsuccessful, either because an anatomic anomaly bars the neurosurgeon's access to the adenohypophysis or because a discrete, resectable adenoma cannot be found. In the latter circumstance, the neurosurgeon has the option of removing the entire adenohypophysis with the expectation of curing the Cushing's disease but at the price of producing hypopituitarism and, with it, lifelong dependence upon replacement therapy with cortisol, thyroxine (T_4), and sex hormones. This option, although acceptable in many cases, should not be exercised on patients who desire to have their own children.

An alternative to pituitary microadenomectomy is pituitary irradiation. The outcome of such therapy is in part a function of the age of the patient and in part a function of the dose of irradiation. For reasons that are unclear, irradiation of the pituitary with 4000–5000 rads has been found to cure 80% of juveniles (ages 7–16 years) with Cushing's disease but only about 20% of adults. In neither group is treatment with this dose associated with serious untoward effects; in particular, they do not develop deficiencies of any pituitary hormones.

Use of a proton beam permits the radiotherapist to deliver therapy to a more precisely circumscribed area and, therefore, to deliver higher doses of irradiation to the pituitary without incurring greater risks to neighboring structures. Proton beam therapy in doses of 8000–10,000 rads has been successful in curing approximately 70% of adults suffering from Cushing's disease. A sizeable minority of patients cured in this way develop hypopituitarism and require substitution therapy with cortisol, T_4, and sex hormones, however. Irradiation of this intensity is not, therefore, recommended for patients who desire to retain reproductive function.

Other methods that have been used with some success include cryohypophysectomy and implantation of radioactive gold or yttrium seeds via a transsphenoidal approach. Such procedures involve some risk of cerebrospinal fluid rhinorrhea and meningitis as well as some uncertainty as to the success of curing hypercortisolism without causing hypopituitarism. Hypophysectomy via craniotomy has had only limited use in the treatment of Cushing's disease. Although this method may cure the Cushing's disease, it does so at the price of causing hypopituitarism. In one reported case[52] of Cushing's disease, pituitary *stalk section* failed to correct the abnormalities of pituitary-adrenal function, even though it did induce hypopituitarism with respect to TSH and gonadotropin production. In general, procedures that carry a high risk of producing hypopituitarism are not ideal for growing children or for adults who wish to preserve reproductive potential.

Bilateral adrenalectomy has been employed as treatment for Cushing's disease ever since synthetic cortisone became generally available in 1950. It has the advantage of speed and certainty; the source of endogenous cortisol can be removed with only a very slight chance of late recurrence due to growth of accessory adrenal tissue. The main disadvantages are that (1) the operation itself is a major procedure, and this is of particular concern if the patient's condition is already precarious; (2) the patient is left dependent on steroid substitution therapy for the remainder of his life; and (3) there is risk of subsequent growth of a pituitary adenoma.

Unilateral adrenalectomy as the sole procedure is not adequate therapy for Cushing's disease; the pituitary merely secretes additional ACTH, and the remaining adrenal secretes approximately as much cortisol as the two adrenals had secreted prior to the operation. Subtotal adrenal resection, leaving a remnant of one adrenal, has occasionally been successful, but it is not recommended since the outcome is unpredictable. Some patients develop adrenal insufficiency, and others sooner or later experience recurrence of Cushing's syndrome. Re-exploration in an attempt to remove all adrenal tissue is then technically difficult and usually unsuccessful.

"Medical adrenalectomy" has been performed in selected cases of Cushing's disease by administering the adrenocorticolytic agent o,p′-DDD in doses of 2–5 g/day for several months.[53] In these doses, the side effects are usually tolerable. Plasma cortisol can be brought to within the desired range of 5–10 μg/dl without concomitant aldosterone deficiency. The degree of response is not totally predictable, and when plasma cortisol reaches normal, it is advisable to discontinue administration of o,p′-DDD and institute supportive treatment with dexamethasone 0.5 mg daily. The administration of o,p′-DDD alters the extra-adrenal metabolism of cortisol, and, for several weeks following a course of o,p′-DDD administration, urinary 17-OHCS are deceptively low.[54] Plasma cortisol levels must be followed as the index of adrenal function.

During and following any attempt at hypophysectomy or adrenalectomy, the patient should receive glucocorticoid substitution therapy until it has been established that his postoperative endogenous cortisol production is adequate.

Although mild cases of Cushing's disease do not require urgent treatment, severe cases should be treated without undue delay. While bringing the hypercortisolism under control, it is often desirable to minimize protein wasting by providing a high protein intake (at least 100 g/day). The desirability of a high-potassium, high-calcium, low-sodium intake should be considered. If frank diabetes exists, it should be brought under control with diet and insulin. Infections should be treated, when possible, with specific antibiotics. Hypomania may be treated with reserpine, 1 mg/day orally for up to a week. More serious psychiatric disturbances should receive the attention of a psychiatric consultant.

The Ectopic ACTH Syndrome. The third major variety of spontaneous hypercortisolism stems from the production of ACTH by a nonpituitary neoplasm and is usually referred to as "the ectopic ACTH syndrome."[55] In some cases, the clinical manifestations of this variety of hypercortisolism are indistinguishable from those of an adrenal neoplasm and Cushing's disease. Occasionally, the typical clinical features of Cushing's syndrome are remarkably severe in patients with the ectopic ACTH syndrome. In the majority of cases, however, the "typical" features of obesity, striae, plethora, osteoporosis, and renal stones are absent, and the clinical picture is dominated by wasting, weakness, and other manifestations of rapidly advancing malignancy. Often the condition is initially suspected on the basis of persistent hypokalemia in a patient with a tumor, and the suspicion is

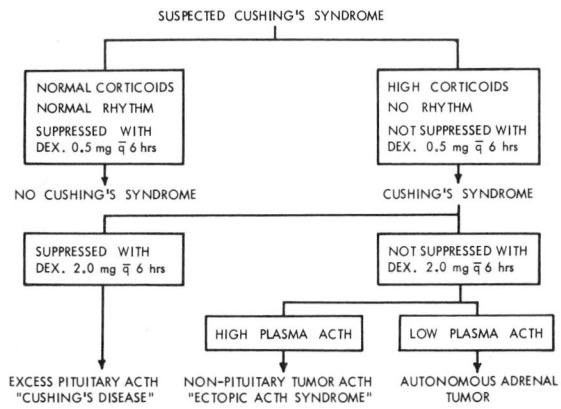

Figure 5–22. Diagnostic flow sheet employed in the diagnosis of Cushing's syndrome.

confirmed by finding extremely high plasma cortisol and urinary 17-OHCS. The clinical spectrum of the ectopic ACTH syndrome is extremely broad.

Final proof that a patient has the ectopic ACTH syndrome depends upon the demonstration that he has excessive cortisol production and that he has a nonpituitary tumor that contains a higher concentration of ACTH than is found in the plasma. A presumptive diagnosis of the ectopic ACTH syndrome may be based on the following findings: (1) high plasma cortisol and urinary 17-OHCS, (2) failure of dexamethasone in large doses to suppress the output of 17-OHCS reproducibly, and (3) "normal" or elevated plasma ACTH concentrations (Fig. 5–22).

If the patient appears to have the ectopic ACTH syndrome, a search for a tumor should be conducted. The majority of tumors will be found in the thorax, with "oat cell" (small-cell) carcinoma of the lung being the single most common variety. The search should not end there, however, for tumors arising in a wide variety of locations have been found to produce ectopic ACTH (Table 5–5). Even the adrenal should not be overlooked, for several ACTH-secreting tumors of the adrenal have been reported, including pheochromocytomas, one paraganglioma, and adrenocortical carcinoma. Approximately 10% of the reported cases of the ectopic ACTH syndrome have been cured by surgical removal of the tumor. In the others, the tumors proved to be incompletely resectable. This bleak statistic is weighted heavily by the fact that oat cell carcinoma of the lung, which is almost never curable, accounts for such a high percentage of the total number of cases. If surgical cure cannot be

effected, palliative treatment with adrenal inhibitors may be used to curtail the excessive secretion of cortisol and improve the metabolic status of the patient. If the course of the neoplastic disease is favorable enough to permit one to prognosticate survival for 1 year or more, bilateral adrenalectomy or its "medical equivalent" with o,p'-DDD might be considered as a method for controlling the hypercortisolism.

Virilism and Mineralocorticoid Excess Associated with Cushing's Syndrome. Even though the patient's clinical picture may be dominated by signs of virilism or by signs of mineralocorticoid excess rather than by typical features of Cushing's syndrome, it is important that every patient with such disorders be evaluated for possible hypercortisolism, for the choice of therapy will be critically affected by this information. When androgens or mineralocorticoids are produced in association with excess cortisol, the patient should be considered to have some variety of Cushing's syndrome and be managed according to the principles outlined previously. If there is excessive production of androgens or mineralocorticoids (particularly DOC) without hypercortisolism, however, the patient may have congenital adrenal hyperplasia, a condition that is best treated by administering cortisol; or he may have a neoplasm that can be treated by unilateral adrenalectomy or gonadectomy without danger of postoperative adrenal insufficiency. It is important to remember that all three varieties of Cushing's syndrome are often associated with some evidence of androgen or mineralocorticoid excess, and occasionally these features dominate the clinical picture in each variety of hypercortisolism.

Special Problems Related to Cushing's Syndrome

The Structure of Ectopic ACTH. Ever since the discovery that certain nonpituitary tumors synthesize "ectopic ACTH," attempts have been made to determine whether or not the tumor product has the same structure as pituitary ACTH. Through the use of ACTH antibodies and methods for separating polypeptides of different sizes, it has been demonstrated that tumors that make ectopic ACTH also make substances that share the immunoreactive properties of ACTH but differ from ACTH in molecular size and lack the biologic potency of ACTH. Orth has shown that the production of ectopic ACTH is accompanied by the production of smaller polypeptides that may be the C-terminal and N-terminal fragments of ACTH.[56] Berson and Yalow were the first to demonstrate the presence of "big" immunoreactive ACTH in association with the ectopic ACTH syndrome. Island, Orth, and Nicholson have shown that *biologically potent* tumor ACTH shares with pituitary ACTH all of the properties listed in Table 5–6. One way of reconciling all these observations is to postulate that certain nonpituitary neoplasms share with the pituitary corticotrope the capacity to synthesize the large glycoprotein precursor of ACTH and that various neoplasms have varying capacities to convert "pro-ACTH" to conventional ACTH.[57] Thus, the production of ectopic ACTH is accompanied by a variety of immunologically detectable ACTH analogues. The biologically active material that leads to the clinical "ectopic ACTH syndrome," however, is probably very similar in its chemical identity to conventional pituitary ACTH.[58]

Recovery from Pituitary-Adrenal Suppression. It has long been known that exogenous corticosteroids induce adrenal atrophy and that cortisol secreted by an adrenal tumor induces atrophy of the nontumorous portions of the adrenal cortex. The adrenal atrophy has been attributed to suppression of ACTH. It has been observed repeatedly that recovery from severe prolonged pituitary-adrenal suppression does not occur readily; in fact, it may be many months before the patient who has been cured of an adrenal adenoma recovers normal pituitary-adrenal function. The question of whether

Table 5–5. SOURCES OF ECTOPIC ACTH IN 100 CASES

Tumor	Number
Carcinoma of lung	52
Carcinoma of pancreas (including carcinoid)	11
Thymoma	11
Benign bronchial adenoma (including carcinoid)	5
Pheochromocytoma	3
Carcinoma of thyroid	2
Carcinoma of liver	2
Carcinoma of prostate	2
Carcinoma of ovary	2
Undifferentiated carcinoma of mediastinum	2
Carcinoma of breast	1
Carcinoma of parotid gland	1
Carcinoma of esophagus	1
Paraganglioma	1
Ganglioma	1
Primary site uncertain	3

Table 5-6. PROPERTIES COMMON TO PITUITARY
ACTH AND TUMOR ACTH

1. Stimulation of adrenocortical enlargement
2. Stimulation of corticosterone secretion in hypophysectomized rat
3. Stimulation of adrenal ascorbic acid depletion in hypophysectomized rat
4. Stimulation of cortisol, corticosterone, and 17-KS production in man
5. Melanocyte-stimulating activity *in vitro* in frog skin preparation and in hypophysectomized frog
6. Release of free fatty acids in adipose tissue incubates
7. Extractable from tissue with glacial acetic acid
8. Precipitable from acetic acid with acetone-plus-ether
9. Adsorbable onto IRC-50 from dilute acetic acid
10. Can be eluted from IRC-50 with 50% acetic acid
11. Adsorbable onto oxycellulose from dilute acetic acid
12. Can be eluted from oxycellulose with 0.1 N HCl
13. Behavior during counter-current distribution
14. Separable from MSH by chromatography on SE-Sephadex
15. Dialyzable only in acid medium
16. Inactivation by trypsin and chymotrypsin
17. Lability in unheated human plasma
18. Relative stability in acid and lability in alkali
19. Inactivated by hydrogen peroxide; reactivated by cysteine
20. Irreversibly inactivated by periodate
21. Neutralization by ACTH antisera
22. Stimulation of adrenal cAMP
23. Affinity for N-terminal ACTH antibody
24. Affinity for C-terminal ACTH antibody
25. Affinity for central ACTH antibody
26. Behavior on Sephadex G-50 Fine

the limiting factor in recovery is at the level of the pituitary or the adrenal was investigated by Graber,[59] who made serial measurements of plasma cortisol and ACTH in several patients before and after removal of adrenal tumors (Fig. 5–23). Prior to removal of the adrenal tumor, cortisol levels were supernormal and ACTH levels were suppressed. During the 1st month after removal of the tumor, cortisol levels were subnormal; despite this fact, ACTH levels also remained subnormal, indicating that the chronically suppressed pituitary did not readily return to normal after correction of hypercortisolism. During the ensuing 4 months, ACTH levels rose to normal and then to supernormal values, but cortisol values remained subnormal, indicating that adrenal responsiveness lags behind pituitary recovery. Finally, cortisol levels rose to normal and then ACTH levels fell back to normal. At this point, normal responses to metyrapone and ACTH were demonstrable. The entire recovery process required at least 9 months in patients who had suffered profound pituitary-adrenal suppression for periods in excess of

PATIENTS RECOVERING FROM
PROLONGED PITUITARY-ADRENAL SUPPRESSION

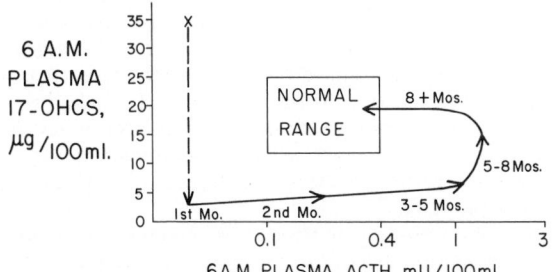

Figure 5–23. Relationship between plasma ACTH and plasma 17-OHCS (cortisol) concentrations during recovery from severe, prolonged pituitary-adrenal suppression with exogenous corticosteroids or autonomously secreted cortisol.

1 year. During this recovery period, patients may safely be supported by treatment with hydrocortisone, 5–20 mg each morning, until such time that their endogenous morning plasma cortisol concentrations are in the normal range.

Pituitary Tumors Following Bilateral Adrenalectomy. Prior to adrenalectomy, plasma ACTH levels are only modestly elevated in patients with Cushing's disease.[10] Apparently, pituitary production of ACTH is partially restrained, even in these patients, by the supraphysiologic levels of cortisol, for normalization of plasma cortisol (by bilateral adrenalectomy and subsequent administration of physiologic doses of cortisol) results in distinct elevation of ACTH levels to about 2–20 times the normal range.[60] In time, a minority of these patients will go on to develop astronomic elevations of plasma ACTH (100–1000 times normal). Such patients become deeply pigmented, and many of them can be demonstrated to have chromophobe adenomas that erode the sella turcica and occasionally impinge on the optic chiasm, expand into the third ventricle, or invade the cavernous or sphenoid sinus, sometimes causing death by occluding vessels of the circle of Willis. This complication of Cushing's disease has rarely been seen in patients who have received pituitary irradiation as their primary mode of therapy. Early transsphenoidal microadenomectomy as treatment for Cushing's disease should reduce the need for bilateral adrenalectomy and, beyond that, should reduce the occurrence of postadrenalectomy macroadenomas to a minimum. In view of the invasive tendencies of macroadenomas, it is probably wise to treat them aggressively by proton beam irradiation or surgical excision whenever they become evident, without waiting for them to invade adjacent structures. In summary, any patient with Cushing's disease who, following bilateral adrenalectomy, develops intense hyperpigmentation should have plasma ACTH assayed. If these values are astronomic despite adequate cortisol substitution therapy, the patient should have radiographic studies for a possible chromophobe adenoma. If an adenoma is found, it should be removed, if feasible.

Hormonal Basis of Hyperpigmentation in Cushing's Disease, the Ectopic ACTH Syndrome, and Addison's Disease. As long as the adrenal glands are intact, ACTH does not rise to extremely high levels; it could not do so without causing fulminant hyperadrenocorticism. Modest elevations in ACTH and associated melanocyte-stimulating substances usually cause little or no hyperpigmentation. Once the adrenal glands have been largely or totally resected or destroyed, however, ACTH and other melanocyte-stimulating compounds may rise to very high levels, leading to melanin deposition and striking hyperpigmentation. The hormonal basis of such hyperpigmentation was originally thought to be largely due to the action of β-MSH. There is now doubt that the highly potent substance "β-MSH" circulates as such, although it makes up part of the amino acid sequences of larger molecules that are measurable by immunoassay as "immunoreactive β-MSH." The biologic potencies of these larger moieties of "MSH" remain in doubt, however, and the precise hormonal basis of "addisonian pigmentation" remains confused, even though empirically the pigmentation is associated with chronic elevations of ACTH and its secretory by-products.

Paradoxical Responses to Dexamethasone. A few cases have been described in which patients with Cushing's syndrome have been observed to show paradoxical *increases* in adrenal function during treatment with dexamethasone. Since there is no known mechanism through which dexamethasone could directly stimulate steroid biosynthesis, these "paradoxical" increases have, until recently, remained unexplained. In a study of a patient with hypercortisolism and a "paradoxical response" to dexamethasone, Brown[61] discovered that the patient had enigmatic increases in adrenal function not only when treated with dexamethasone but also when observed during extended control periods. Detailed study revealed that this patient had striking periodic increases in cortisol secretion, with plasma and urinary steroids rising to extremely high peaks, then returning to modestly elevated levels, in cycles lasting about 11 days. ACTH concentrations were elevated. The patient proved to have a chromophobe adenoma that had extended into the third ventricle; removal of the adenoma and the pituitary cured the hypercorticism. Although there is no available explanation for the periodicity of pituitary-adrenal function, the very fact that such a phenomenon can occur might lead one to question whether apparently paradoxical responses to dexamethasone are really *responses* or merely *coincidences*. Perhaps the best way to solve this problem is to carry out protracted studies of patients with apparently paradoxical responses to dexamethasone in order to determine whether they might have spontaneous increases in adrenal function, even when they are not receiving dexamethasone, and to determine whether dexamethasone when given at irregular intervals invariably brings about increased adrenocortical function. Intermittent (if not periodic) hormonogenesis has been observed rarely in patients with hypercortisolism due to an adrenal neoplasm, to pituitary neoplasm, and to the ectopic ACTH syndrome. Such irregularities only serve to emphasize the fact that one must insist on reproducibility of a suppression or stimulation test before reaching a firm conclusion about the suppressibility or responsiveness of the pituitary-adrenal system in any particular case.

Hyperaldosteronism

Although aldosterone is physiologically useful in maintaining fluid and electrolyte homeostasis,[62] an excess can lead to potassium depletion and undesirable expansion of the extracellular fluid compartment; the latter may result in edema or hypertension. When hypersecretion of aldosterone occurs as a consequence of the adrenal-stimulating action of angiotensin, it is referred to as "secondary aldosteronism." When it occurs as a consequence of a primary adrenal abnormality (best illustrated by the autonomous function of an adrenal adenoma), it is referred to as "primary aldosteronism."

Atypical forms of hyperaldosteronism that do not fit neatly into either of these categories have been described. Laidlaw and coworkers[63] have described a familial disorder in which hypersecretion of aldosterone appeared to be ACTH-dependent. This is rare, however, and ordinarily ACTH has only a minor effect on aldosterone secretion, not one leading to clinical disease. It is also known that some patients with all the clinical and chemical features of primary aldosteronism have nonadenomatous adrenal glands, and this has raised the question of whether some factor other than angiotensin, ACTH, or potassium might be stimulating their aldosterone-secreting cells. At the moment, this entity remains idiopathic.[64]

Secondary Aldosteronism

As listed in Table 5–7, there are numerous clinical and experimental situations in which increased activity of the renin-angiotensin system results in secondary increases in aldosterone secretion. Anything that compromises the blood supply to the kidney is likely to bring about an increase in renin secretion. This is readily perceived as the mechanism through which experimental or pathologic constriction of the renal artery results in hyper-reninism. It may also be the

Table 5–7. STIMULI TO RENIN SECRETION

1. Dehydration
2. Sodium depletion
3. Serum albumin depletion
4. Exsanguination
5. Upright posture
6. Renal artery stenosis
7. Cardiac failure
8. Constriction of inferior vena cava
9. Hepatic cirrhosis
10. Surgical operations
11. Catecholamines
12. Renal nerve stimulation
13. Potassium depletion
14. Diazoxide and other direct vasodilators

mechanism through which a reduction in "effective" blood volume results in increased renin secretion. In general, those conditions that are associated with (1) depletion of extracellular fluid volume (severe water deprivation or sodium depletion), (2) reduction of plasma volume (hypoalbuminemia), or (3) sequestration of blood on the venous side of the circulation (caval constriction or hepatic cirrhosis) all result in increased renin and aldosterone production. Even the assumption of upright posture after a period of recumbency results in pooling of blood in the dependent portions of the body, decreased cardiac output, decreased renal blood flow, increased renin production, and increased secretion of aldosterone. In all the conditions just listed, the sympathetic nervous system may be an important mediator of the renin response to effective hypovolemia, and the renin-dependent increase in aldosterone secretion may be viewed, teleologically, as a compensatory mechanism designed to maintain effective blood flow to various organs, including the kidney. An increase in aldosterone promotes sodium retention, which is accompanied by water retention and expansion of the extracellular fluid compartment. The intravascular compartment participates in this volume expansion, and there is some increase in arterial pressure and blood flow to various organs. There may be so much expansion of extracellular volume that edema becomes apparent. The distribution of the edema will be determined by the nature of the primary circulatory disorder.

A special case of secondary aldosteronism is that of Bartter's syndrome, characterized by renal juxtaglomerular cell hyperplasia, hyper-reninemia, hyperaldosteronism, hypokalemia, and failure to thrive.[65] Blood pressure tends to be low and relatively unresponsive to exogenous angiotensin. There is uncertainty as to whether the primary abnormality is a sodium-wasting nephropathy or a refractoriness of blood vessels to the pressor action of angiotensin.

Another rare cause of secondary aldosteronism is that occurring in association with a renin-secreting tumor of the kidney.[66]

Increases in plasma renin activity and aldosterone secretion occur normally in pregnancy and during treatment with supraphysiologic doses of estrogen (e.g., with oral contraceptives). The increase in plasma renin activity is thought to be related to estrogen-induced increases in the hepatic production of renin substrate.[14] It has not been established that the hyper-reninism or hyperaldosteronism of pregnancy are deleterious. In fact, patients with pre-eclampsia tend to have lower plasma renin activity than do women with uncomplicated pregnancies.[67]

From the foregoing, it should be obvious that secondary aldosteronism is extremely common, occurring as it does in normal pregnancy, in healthy individuals in response to sodium loss, and in a wide variety of diseases. It should also be obvious that the diagnostic value of an aldosterone measurement is nil unless one knows a great deal about the physiologic status of the patient at the time the crucial specimen is collected.

Secondary aldosteronism is not a specific entity but rather a component of the pathophysiology of a multitude of clinical disorders. An appreciation of the role of aldosterone in various states is fundamental to a clear understanding of disturbed physiology, but secondary aldosteronism does not itself call for specific diagnosis and treatment. Although aldosterone plays a role in the pathogenesis of edema-forming disorders, it should be remembered that these are primarily circulatory disorders, that the hypersecretion of aldosterone is simply a response to the circulatory disorder, and that the distribution of edema fluid will be determined by the nature of the circulatory disorder. Therapeutic attention should generally be focused on the circulatory abnormality. Restriction of sodium intake and treatment with diuretics, although relieving certain congestive symptoms, may further compromise effective blood volume, calling forth even greater secretion of renin and aldosterone. Secondary aldosteronism rarely leads to potassium depletion unless the patient is treated with diuretics. With continued diuretic treatment of the edematous patient, increases in endogenous aldosterone may reduce the natriuretic effectiveness of diuretic agents while accentuating their effectiveness as kaliuretic agents. The mineralocorticoid antagonist, spironolactone, can be used to potentiate the natriuretic action of other diuretics while diminishing their kaliuretic effects.[68]

Although it is not necessary to prove that a patient has secondary aldosteronism in order to manage him properly, it has been of great academic interest to investigate aldosterone production and metabolism in various disorders. Normal well-hydrated adults secrete from 40–200 μg of aldosterone/day in response to plasma renin activity ranging from 100–800 ng/dl of plasma (the amount of angiotensin I generated during a 3-hour incubation). Higher aldosterone secretion rates may be said to represent hyperaldosteronism, and, if they are accompanied by higher levels of plasma renin activity, it may be assumed that they represent secondary aldosteronism. The combination of supernormal renin and subnormal aldosterone is seen in primary adrenal insufficiency. Conversely, an elevation of aldosterone accompanied by subnormal plasma renin activity is seen in primary aldosteronism. It is, therefore, the *combination* of high plasma renin activity and high aldosterone secretion rate that enables one to diagnose secondary aldosteronism with confidence. Plasma concentrations of aldosterone are ordinarily in excess of 20 ng/dl, and urinary excretion of the acid-hydrolyzable conjugate of aldosterone is ordinarily in excess of 20 μg/day in secondary aldosteronism. The quantitative relationships between secretion rates, plasma concentrations, and excretion rates are altered in certain diseases. Luetscher[69] has shown that patients with impaired hepatic blood flow or impaired hepatic function have diminished metabolic clearance rates of aldosterone; therefore, plasma concentrations of aldosterone in such patients can be high relative to the aldosterone secretion rate. Bledsoe[70] has shown that the liver and kidney compete with each other as sites for metabolism of aldosterone. The liver forms both tetrahydroaldosterone and the acid-labile conjugate of aldosterone, but the kidney forms only the latter. Hepatic insufficiency gives an advantage to the kidney, and for this reason patients with hepatic insufficiency excrete an abnormally high proportion of aldosterone as the acid-hydrolyzable conjugate. Therefore, urinary "aldosterone," as it is usually measured, is excessively high relative to aldosterone secretion rates or plasma aldosterone concentrations in patients with liver disease (Fig. 5–24).

METABOLISM OF ALDOSTERONE

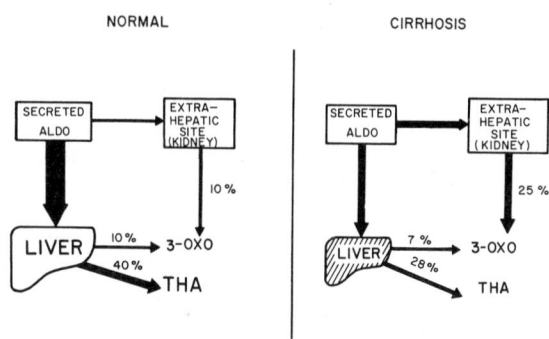

Figure 5–24. A diagrammatic representation of the concept that aldosterone is metabolized by the liver to two products, tetrahydroaldosterone (THA) and aldosterone-18-glucuronide (3-oxo); in addition, a small proportion of circulating aldosterone is converted by the kidney to 3-oxo. Cirrhosis decreases the capacity of the liver to metabolize aldosterone; therefore, more 3-oxo is formed by the kidney. The percentages should not be interpreted literally.

Primary Aldosteronism

Autonomous secretion of aldosterone gives rise to the clinical syndrome of primary aldosteronism. The term "primary" implies that the fundamental physiologic disorder is within the adrenal cortex itself, in contradistinction to "secondary" aldosteronism, in which the basically normal adrenal cortex secretes a superabundance of aldosterone in response to a stimulus originating outside of the adrenal. Usually the source of aldosterone is a solitary adrenal adenoma. Occasionally, there are multiple adenomas or the adrenal cortex appears hyperplastic or normal. In extremely rare instances, the source of aldosterone is an adrenocortical carcinoma.

The pathophysiology of primary aldosteronism[71] can be understood in terms of the known effects of this hormone on electrolyte metabolism. Aldosterone acts on epithelial cells of the nephron, sweat glands, salivary glands, and the gastrointestinal tract to promote the conservation of sodium chloride and the excretion of potassium. As a consequence of sodium retention, there is a modest expansion of extracellular fluid volume. Arterial blood pressure increases and may in time result in all the familiar features of hypertensive cardiovascular disease. Renin production is characteristically suppressed. As a consequence of potassium wastage, there may be hypokalemic alkalosis, alterations in myocardial electrophysiology, skeletal muscular weakness, and kaliopenic nephropathy. The hypokalemic alkalosis may give rise to tetany with muscle cramps and paresthesias. Cardiac abnormalities include depression of S-T segments and T waves and the appearance of U waves in the electrocardiogram. Premature ventricular contractions are frequently noted. The author has seen several patients who experienced near-fatal runs of ventricular fibrillation with repeated episodes of syncope before they were recognized as having the hypokalemia of primary aldosteronism. Skeletal muscular weakness may be so severe that the patient experiences episodic paralysis of the extremities associated with hyporeflexia. Kaliopenic nephropathy is characterized by loss of renal concentrating capacity; even after the injection of vasopressin, urine specific gravity might not exceed 1.020. Subjectively, the patient may note nocturia. It should be remembered that a majority of patients with primary aldosteronism do not have clear-cut *symptoms* of potassium depletion. The symptoms just listed are rare unless the hypokalemia is relatively severe (less than 3.0 mEq/1).

For practical purposes, the diagnosis of primary aldosteronism begins with the recognition that a patient has high blood pressure. Any hypertensive patient who has unprovoked hypokalemia should be evaluated carefully for primary aldosteronism. The diagnosis is established by demonstrating that, under standard conditions, aldosterone secretion (or excretion) is elevated and plasma renin activity is subnormal. Each of these points requires some elaboration.

Hypokalemia as a diagnostic criterion for primary aldosteronism is a convenience rather than a necessity. Primary aldosteronism can cause hypertension, can be diagnosed by measuring aldosterone and plasma renin activity, and can be cured by removing an adrenal adenoma in patients who have never been known to be hypokalemic.[72] Several studies have shown, however, that so-called "normokalemic" primary aldosteronism is a rare occurrence, whereas essential hypertension (from which it must be distinguished) is extremely common. It is generally not practical to carry out standard aldosterone studies in normokalemic hypertensives in search of the rare individual with normokalemic primary aldosteronism. It has been stated that only about 1% of patients with normokalemic hypertension have primary aldosteronism. In contrast, among the relatively small subset of patients with unprovoked hypokalemia and hypertension, one may expect that approximately 50% will prove to have primary aldosteronism.

Only "unprovoked" hypokalemia is of value in diagnosing primary aldosteronism. When a patient has lost potassium through vomiting, diarrhea, or the use of diuretics, potassium repletion should be accomplished and the patient observed further for the possible development of unprovoked hypokalemia.

Plasma renin activity (PRA) is characteristically subnormal in patients with primary aldosteronism. In order for it to be of diagnostic value, it is essential that the specimen be obtained under carefully controlled conditions. In anyone, sodium loading and recumbency will decrease renin production, and sodium depletion and upright posture will elevate renin production. In order to bring out the differences between patients with primary aldosteronism and those without it, it is best to stimulate renin production in a standard fashion. One method is to restrict sodium intake to 10 mEq/day kor 3 days and on the 3rd day have the patient upright (standing, sitting, or walking) for 3 hours prior to drawing blood for assay. Another method is to administer 40 mg of furosemide (a potent diuretic) at 6 AM and have the patient upright from 8 to 11 AM, at which time blood is drawn for assay. In either case, patients with primary aldosteronism still have low plasma renin activity levels after such maneuvers, whereas the majority of patients with other varieties of hypertensive disease will have clearly higher values. Each laboratory must standardize its own method and determine empirically what represents "normal" and what represents "suppressed' plasma renin activity. Under the conditions just described, the author's laboratory has found PRA values of less than 1 ng/ml (ng of generated angiotensin/hour incubation) in most patients with primary aldosteronism. Normal subjects and most hypertensive subjects studied under the same conditions have PRA values greater than 3. The finding of suppressed PRA has come to be a *sine qua non* in the diagnosis of primary aldosteronism.[73]

It has been proposed that measurement of PRA under standard conditions might be a useful screening procedure in searching for patients with primary aldosteronism. This proposal is not without merit, but it has been found that at least 20% of patients with essential hypertension have PRA levels comparable to those of patients with primary aldosteronism. Since this group of patients makes up 20% of the hypertensive population and primary aldosteronism only 1%, it is apparent that the PRA assay by itself is not a very efficient way of separating patients with primary aldosteronism from those without. It should be mentioned that PRA is suppressed not only in primary aldosteronism but also in other clinical disorders characterized by hypertension and potassium depletion, including pseudoaldosteronism,[74] licorice intoxication, and disorders characterized by DOC hypersecretion. In summary, although suppressed PRA is a *sine qua non* in the diagnosis of primary aldosteronism, the vast majority of patients with suppressed PRA do not have primary aldosteronism.

Aldosterone secretion rates, excretion rates, or *plasma concentrations* must be elevated under standard test conditions if one is to satisfy contemporary criteria for diagnosing primary aldosteronism. The standard test conditions for diagnosing primary aldosteronism include the administration of a diet containing at least 100 mEq of sodium/day for several days while withholding diuretics or other medications that might elevate aldosterone production. If, under these conditions, the aldosterone secretion rate exceeds 200 μg/day, aldosterone excretion exceeds 20 μg/day, or plasma aldosterone exceeds 20 ng/dl, primary aldosteronism must be seriously suspected. Although elevated aldosterone must be considered a *sine qua non* in diagnosing primary aldosteronism, it is not by itself sufficient, because, as stressed in foregoing paragraphs, secondary aldosteronism is far more common than primary aldosteronism. The combination of elevated aldosterone and low PRA is pathognomonic of primary aldosteronism. Ordinarily, the steps in diagnosis are the observation of hypertension, then hypokalemia, then suppressed PRA, then elevated aldosterone.

The standard treatment for primary aldosteronism is surgical removal of the adenoma (Fig. 5–25) or adenomas, if present, and removal of 1½ adrenal glands (in search of small adenomas) if none can be seen or palpated. If hyperaldosteronism persists following this operation or if the patient is not a satisfactory surgical candidate, the disorder can be controlled by chronic treatment with spironolactone, combined if necessary with other sodium-depleting, potassium-sparing measures. Such combinations minimize the side effects of spironolactone that may occur when this drug is employed alone in doses in excess of 100 mg/day for prolonged periods.

Role of the Adrenal Cortex in Essential Hypertension

"Essential hypertension" is, by definition, idiopathic. Yet there is increasing evidence that it is not a single disorder but rather a manifestation of a number of different disorders. Some patients with essential hypertension behave in many ways as though they have an excess of some mineralocorticoid. First, they have low PRA. Second, Woods and coworkers[75] demonstrated that these patients, but not those with hypertension and normal renin, experience amelioration of their hypertension when treated with aminoglutethimide, an inhibitor of steroid biosynthesis. Third, it has been shown by several groups that these patients experience amelioration of their hypertension when treated with spironolactone, an antagonist of mineralocorticoid actions (Fig. 5–26). Fourth, it has been shown by Gunnells and coworkers[76] that these patients experience amelioration of

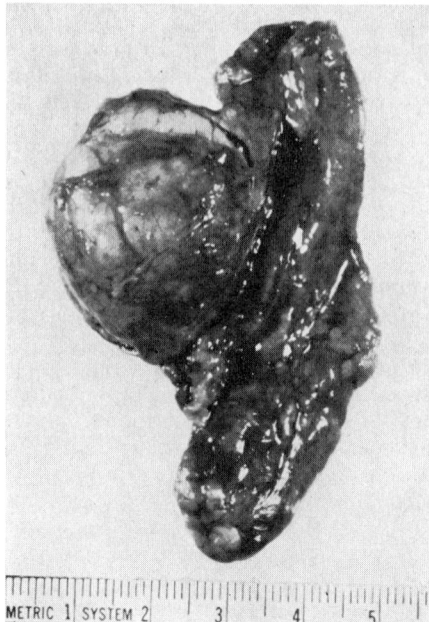
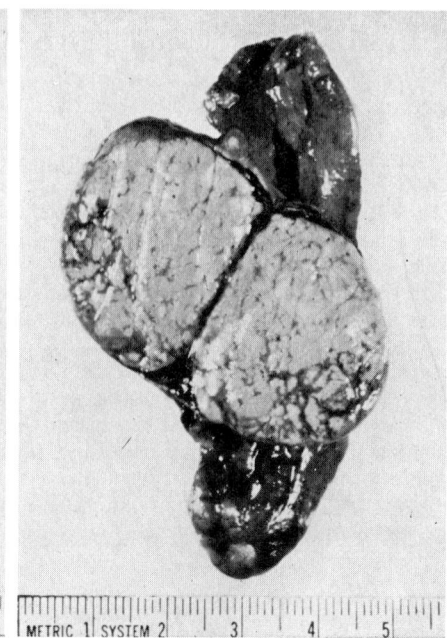

Figure 5–25. Typical aldosteronoma, canary yellow, weighing 5 g and measuring approximately 2 cm in diameter. Removal from patient led to regression of all the symptomatology within 4 weeks.

their hypertension following bilateral adrenalectomy. Finally, it has been shown by Adlin and coworkers[77] that these patients have lower salivary sodium/potassium ratios than do patients with essential hypertension and normal renin. It remains to be shown what mineralocorticoid (if any) is responsible for the syndrome of essential hypertension with suppressed renin. Nevertheless, patients who have been properly categorized in this way have approximately a 90% chance of responding to diuretics with significant reduction of their blood pressures.[78]

There is another disorder that has all the clinical hallmarks of primary mineralocorticoid excess, with hypertension, urinary wastage of potassium, and suppression of plasma renin activity, but that is clearly not due to an excess of mineralocorticoids. This is a familial disorder in which the renal tubules reabsorb sodium and excrete potassium excessively. The tendency to retain sodium results in hypertension, suppression of renin production, and suppression of aldosterone secretion to negligible values. The tendency to excrete potassium results in hypokalemic alkalosis. Because mineralocorticoid production is negligible, neither adrenal inhibitors nor mineralocorticoid antagonists are useful in favorably altering electrolyte excretion. Triamterene, a pteridine derivative that is not a mineralocorticoid antagonist but that does block sodium-potassium transport by the distal tubule, is used in the treatment of this disorder, which has been referred to as "pseudoaldosteronism."[74]

Virilizing Tumors, Feminizing Tumors, and "Nonfunctioning" Tumors of the Adrenal Cortex

Normal virilization and feminization are attributable to gonadal function, but when these phenomena occur inappropriately (virilization in women or children or feminization in men or children), they might alert the physician to the possibility of an adrenal neoplasm. As emphasized in foregoing paragraphs, any patient with signs of androgen excess should be studied for possible hypercortisolism, since proper understanding of the mechanisms involved and proper treatment will follow the lines outlined in Cushing's syndrome if hypercortisolism does in fact exist, regardless of the severity of the accompanying androgen excess. If cortisol levels are normal but urinary 17-KS are distinctly elevated and not suppressible to less than 5 mg daily after several successive days of treatment with dexamethasone, 0.5 mg every 6 hours, the probability of an adrenal or gonadal tumor is high enough to justify anatomic studies, such as culdoscopy in search of an ovarian tumor or adrenal arteriography in search of an adrenal tumor.

Feminizing adrenal tumors are extremely rare. Depending on the age and sex of the patient, they might enter into the differential diagnosis of Klinefelter's syndrome, precocious puberty, or ectopic gonadotropin production (see Chs. 6 and 7). Establishment of the diagnosis might be accomplished in the following steps: observation of abnormal feminization, then the demonstration of subnormal gonadotropin levels and supranormal estrogen levels, and, finally, radiographic demonstration of an adrenal mass.

Adrenal cortical tumors that are "nonfunctioning" in the

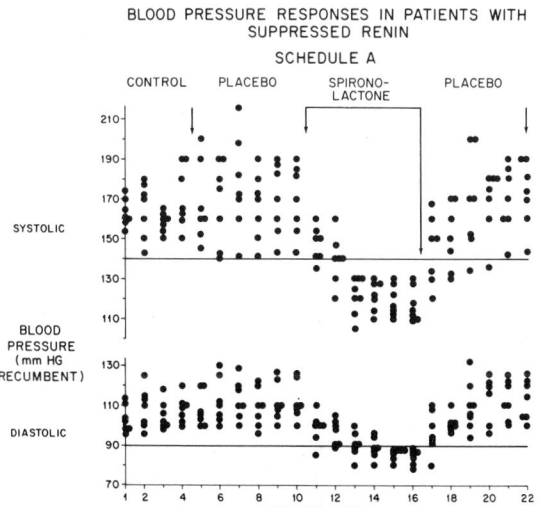

Figure 5–26. Effects of spironolactone, 400 mg/day, on the systolic and diastolic blood pressures of seven patients with the syndrome of essential hypertension and suppressed PRA.

sense that they produce no biologically active or chemically identifiable steroids are very rare. Most so-called nonfunctioning adrenal tumors that have been mentioned in the literature have not actually been carefully studied prior to their removal or the death of the patient. Some androgen-secreting adrenal tumors have been mistakenly considered to be nonfunctioning because they caused no symptoms; however, since the patients were already fully virilized men, there was no way in which an excess of adrenal androgen could express itself in terms of symptoms. The fact that the tumors were not truly nonfunctioning became clear when chemical measurements of steroids (e.g., urinary 17-KS) were performed. The more thoroughly one surveys patients with adrenal tumors, the more likely it is that the tumors will be found to secrete steroids, even though the steroids might cause no symptoms. It is conceivable that some adrenal tumors are truly "nonfunctioning" with respect to steroid secretion; a tumor that lacked the enzymatic machinery for converting cholesterol to pregnenolone might, for example, be considered to be truly nonfunctioning.

Hirsutism

The pattern of hair growth that distinguishes adults of either sex from children is attributable to the action of androgens. The relative sensitivity of various regions of the body to the hair-stimulating action of androgen can be brought to mind by referring to the course of new hair growth beginning at the time of puberty. Hair follicles in the pubic area are most sensitive to the action of androgens. Next in order of sensitivity are the hair follicles of the axillae, then the chin and upper lip, the cheeks and anterior neck, the sternal region and the linea alba, the forearms and legs, the thighs, the remainder of the anterior chest and abdomen, and, finally, the back and upper arms. Normal women secrete enough androgen to bring about development of pubic and axillary hair and trivial growth of hair in less sensitive regions. Normal men secrete enough androgen to bring about growth of hair on the face, neck, forearms, legs, thighs, anterior chest, and abdomen. With this much androgen there is some decrease in scalp hair, progressing from recession of temporal hairline to baldness of the crown and then the frontal areas. Only a few people develop remarkable quantities of hair on the back and upper arms.

The importance of recognizing this order of responsiveness to androgen is that one can assert with conviction that excessive hair growth is or is not androgen-dependent if it follows a particular sequence. For example, growth of hair on the back, shoulders, or face that is not preceded by development of pubic hair must be attributed to something other than androgens.

Hirsutism may only be a cosmetic problem, or it may be a clue to a disease that could have other pathophysiologic ramifications. One cannot be certain without the information derived from an accurate medical history, physical examination, and laboratory measurements of various steroids.

In the course of such an evaluation, one of the following diagnoses might be established:

1. Cushing's syndrome, with adrenal androgen overproduction occurring in association with hypersecretion of cortisol due to adrenal autonomy, ectopic ACTH, or an excess of pituitary ACTH.

2. Androgen-secreting neoplasm (benign or malignant) of adrenal cortex or gonad.

3. Virilizing congenital adrenal hyperplasia due to a deficiency of 21-hydroxylase or 11-hydroxylase.

4. Male pseudohermaphroditism, a condition in which an individual with an XY karyotype has intra-abdominal gonads that secrete too little androgen to induce fully masculine differentiation of the external genitalia but enough to induce some phallic hypertrophy, hirsutism, and coarsening of the voice.

5. Factitious hirsutism due to medicinal or surreptitious use of synthetic androgens.

All of the conditions just mentioned are described in detail elsewhere in this volume. After they have been ruled out by a careful history, physical examination, and precise laboratory studies, one will be left with a majority of hirsute patients still undiagnosed. In the past these patients have been said to have "idiopathic hirsutism" or "constitutional hirsutism." A large proportion have evidence of subtle abnormalities of ovarian function, with slightly excessive production of testosterone or androstenedione or both by their ovaries. Many of these women give histories of onset of mild hirsutism soon after the menarche, with very slow progression over the ensuing years. Oligomenorrhea and decreased fertility are common complaints. In some, the condition is familial. Various histologic abnormalities of the ovaries have been noted, including polycystic changes and hyperthecosis. In most cases it may be assumed that the steroidogenic enzymes of the ovaries are organized in such a way that, in the process of secreting normal quantities of estrogen, they secrete slightly excessive quantities of estrogen precursors, namely testosterone and Δ^4-androstenedione.

The great majority of patients with "idiopathic hirsutism" have well-developed breasts, indicating that they have had adequate estrogen activity at least for a considerable number of years.

It seems probable that what has been referred to as "idiopathic hirsutism" represents more than one pathophysiologic entity. As mentioned before, ovarian histology varies from normal, to hyperthecosis, to polycystic changes. Perhaps a majority, but not all, have modest elevations of androgen production, reflected in elevated blood levels of testosterone or Δ^4-androstenedione or both. It has been postulated that in at least some patients the skin has abnormal capacity for converting testosterone and androstenedione to dihydrotestosterone and that this results in a sort of cutaneous virilization without virilization of other organs (Meikle et al.). Without much in the way of supporting evidence, it has also been suggested that in some patients that problem resides in abnormal sensitivity of hair follicles to normal quantities of androgen, perhaps related to increased numbers of androgen receptors in the follicular cells.

It is important, of course, to keep "idiopathic hirsutism," with its subtle abnormalities of androgen metabolism, separate from the more flagrant varieties of virilism listed at the beginning of this section, in all of which there should be no difficulty in demonstrating distinct elevations of 17-KS (largely metabolites of dehydroepiandrosterone), testosterone, Δ^4-androstenedione, or a synthetic androgen. The role of the adrenal cortex is obvious in Cushing's syndrome, congenital adrenal hyperplasia, and virilizing tumors of that gland, but in addition, it has been suggested that the adrenal plays a supporting role even when there is an excess of ovarian androgen. According to this concept, the ovary that has enzymes that are relatively inefficient in converting androgens to estrogens will utilize precursor steroids coming from the adrenal via the general circulation and convert them to androgens more readily than to estrogens, in the same manner as when the precursor steroids are formed within the ovary itself.

Since the ovary is a major source of androgen in most cases of "idiopathic hirsutism," it is rational, and usually gratifying, to treat the condition with cyclic estrogens in order to suppress ovarian steroidogenesis to a major degree. The rate of new hair growth is usually greatly reduced by this treatment, and local measures, such as electrolysis are then increasingly satisfactory in eradicating hair that is already established. Chronic therapy is usually necessary in order to obtain ideal results. An alternative to ovarian suppressive therapy is the use of an estrogen antagonist such as cyproterone, which competitively inhibits the action of androgens at the level of the target cells, the hair follicles. Either ovarian suppression or androgen antagonism should be useful in curtailing hair growth whenever the latter is dependent upon ovarian androgens, regardless of the precise ovarian histology, regardless of whether the ovaries make use of precursor steroids of adrenal origin, and regardless of a cutaneous abnormality in which the hair follicle is excessively responsive to androgens or abnormally effective in converting testosterone to dihydrotestosterone.

It should be recalled that therapeutic suppression of ovarian androgen production is likely to be accompanied by suppression of ovulation. Therefore, women who desire to become pregnant must be advised to discontinue their ovarian suppressants until pregnancy has been established and carried to successful termination. During this interval one should not be surprised to witness a recrudescence of hirsutism. (For further discussion of Hirsutism, see Ch. 7.)

Adrenal Cortical Hypofunction

Adrenal insufficiency can occur as a result of a primary adrenal abnormality that impairs the capacity of this gland to secrete cortisol or aldosterone or both in response to adrenal stimulators, or it can occur as a result of the lack of adrenal stimulators. In certain disorders there are deficiencies of both cortisol and aldosterone; in other disorders production of only one hormone is impaired. A primary deficiency of cortisol results in a compensatory increase in ACTH production. In analogous fashion, a primary deficiency of aldosterone usually results in a compensatory increase in renin production.

Primary Adrenal Insufficiency (Addison's Disease)

Clinical and Chemical Features of Primary Adrenal Insufficiency

Destruction of the adrenal cortex, regardless of the nature of the underlying process, leads to Addison's disease. The major clinical manifestations are attributable to deficiencies of aldosterone (Table 5–8) and cortisol (Table 5–9). In addition, loss of adrenal androgen in women with Addison's disease may result in diminished growth of axillary hair.

Lack of aldosterone results in impaired ability to conserve sodium and excrete potassium. As long as the patient has a very high sodium intake (an occasional patient actually experiences salt craving), his lack of aldosterone may be of little consequence; however, on a moderate or restricted sodium intake, he soon becomes seriously depleted of sodium. This predicament can be quickly worsened if the patient experiences anorexia, vomiting, diarrhea, or excessive sweating. Without aldosterone substitution therapy, it is virtually impossible for the addisonian patient to diminish his urinary sodium to less than 50 mEq/day. Excretion of sodium in excess of intake results in decrease in extracellular fluid, weight loss, decrease in plasma volume, decrease in blood pressure, decrease in cardiac output, decrease in heart size, increase in renin production, decrease

Table 5–8. MANIFESTATIONS OF ALDOSTERONE DEFICIENCY

A. Inability to conserve sodium
  Decreased extracellular fluid volume
  Weight loss
  Hypovolemia
  Hypotension
  Decreased cardiac size
  Decreased cardiac output
  Decreased renal blood flow
  Prerenal azotemia
  Increased renin production
  Decreased pressor response to catecholamines
  Weakness
  Postural syncope
  Shock
B. Impaired renal secretion of potassium and hydrogen ions
  Hyperkalemia
    Cardiac asystole
  Mild acidosis

in renal blood flow, azotemia, generalized weakness, and postural syncope. Lack of aldosterone also favors the development of hyperkalemia and mild acidosis, in part due to diminished glomerular filtration rate and in part due to diminished ion transport by the distal convoluted tubule.

Lack of cortisol results in anorexia, abdominal pain, wasting of fat depots, apathy, weakness, fasting hypoglycemia, diminished ability to excrete free water, hyponatremia, increased production of ACTH and other melanocyte-stimulating hormones, hyperpigmentation (Fig. 5–27), and diminished ability to withstand a variety of physiologic stresses.

A combined deficiency of aldosterone and cortisol, therefore, culminates in the clinical picture so graphically described by Addison:[79]

The patient, in most of the cases I have seen, has been observed gradually to fall off in general health; he becomes languid and weak, indisposed to either bodily or mental exertion; the appetite is impaired or entirely lost; . . . the pulse small and feeble . . . excessively soft and compressible; the body wastes . . . slight pain or uneasiness is from time to time referred to the region of the stomach, and there is occasionally actual vomiting . . . it is by no means uncommon for the patient to manifest indications of disturbed cerebral circulation. . . . We discover a most remarkable, and, so far as I know, characteristic discoloration taking place in the skin — sufficiently marked indeed as generally to have attracted the attention of the patient himself, or of the patient's friends. . . . It may be said to present a dingy or smoky appearance, or various tints or shades of deep amber or chestnut brown. . . . The body wastes . . . the pulse becomes smaller and weaker, and . . . the patient at length gradually sinks and expires.

Formerly, the principal cause of Addison's disease was tuberculous destruction of the adrenal glands. In parts of the world where the incidence of tuberculosis has diminished in recent decades, idiopathic atrophy of the adrenals has become the most common cause of Addison's disease.

Table 5–9. MANIFESTATIONS OF CORTISOL DEFICIENCY

1. *Gastrointestinal:* anorexia, nausea, vomiting, hypochlorhydria, abdominal pain, weight loss
2. *Mental:* diminished vigor, lethargy, apathy, confusion, psychosis
3. *Energy metabolism:* impaired gluconeogenesis, impaired fat mobilization and utilization, liver glycogen depletion, fasting hypoglycemia
4. *Cardiovascular-renal:* impaired ability to excrete "free water," impaired pressor responses to catecholamines, hypotension
5. *Pituitary:* unrestrained secretion of ACTH and "MSH," resulting in mucocutaneous hyperpigmentation
6. *Impaired tolerance to stress:* any of the above manifestations might become more pronounced during trauma, infection, or fasting

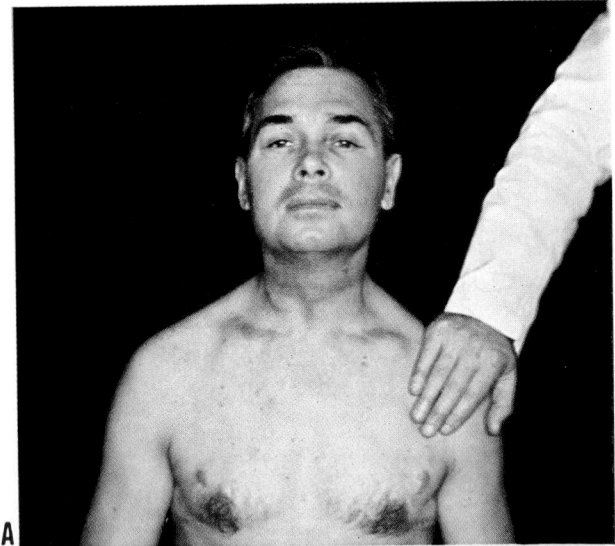

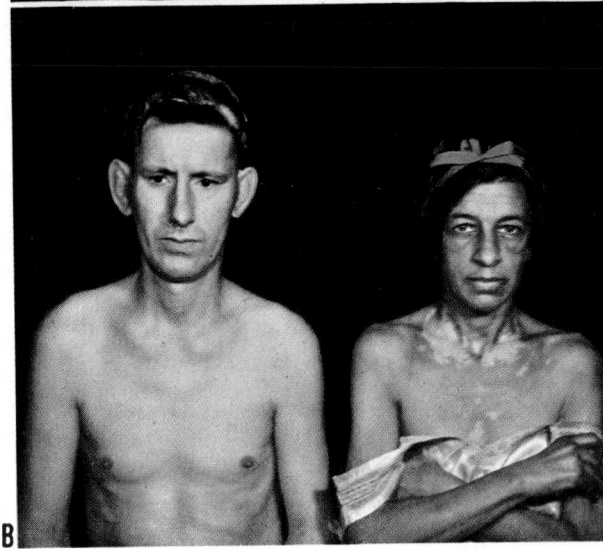

Figure 5–27. *A,* Addison's disease secondary to tuberculosis of the adrenals. Note diffuse brown pigmentation of variable intensity. The scars above and lateral to each breast are pigmented. *B,* Contrasting skin changes in two patients with adrenocortical insufficiency of differing etiology. Note the absence of pigmentation in the male suffering from a chromophobe adenoma of the pituitary contrasted with the presence of hyperpigmentation and vitiligo in the female with adrenocortical atrophy of unknown cause.

There is evidence suggesting that "idiopathic atrophy" might represent autoimmune destruction of the adrenal cortex.[80]

Patients with idiopathic adrenal atrophy are at increased risk with respect to "autoimmune" destruction of other tissues as well, and the physician should be alert to the possibility that they might in time develop hypothyroidism, diabetes mellitus, hypoparathyroidism, primary ovarian failure, or pernicious anemia. Conversely, patients with these disorders are at increased risk with respect to the development of Addison's disease.

In some regions where systemic fungal infections (such as histoplasmosis) are common, these may be as important as tuberculosis or autoimmune disease in the etiology of Addison's disease. Rare causes of Addison's disease include amyloidosis, adrenal apoplexy (Waterhouse-Friderichsen syndrome, Fig. 5–28), and metastatic carcinoma involving the adrenals. Nowadays, of course, bilateral adrenalectomy is performed in the treatment of several diseases, and this must be reckoned as a relatively common cause of the addisonian state. For the sake of completeness, one might mention that prolonged treatment with o,p'-DDD can result in adrenal atrophy and cortisol deficiency[81] and that treatment with heparinoids can result in structural changes in the zona glomerulosa and reversible aldosterone deficiency.[82] There is a familial disorder characterized by the combined abnormalities of diffuse demyelinization of the central nervous system (leukodystrophy) and Addison's disease, a disorder that appears to be limited to boys and young men. There have also been reports of children with congenital aplasia of the zona fasciculata and zona reticularis. Their miniature adrenal cortices are composed of zona glomerulosa cells that secrete aldosterone but not cortisol.

In most cases Addison's disease is insidious in its evolution, adrenal destruction is a gradual process, and compensatory increases in ACTH and renin enable the adrenal for a time to secrete enough cortisol and aldosterone to satisfy physiologic requirements in the absence of some intercurrent stress, such as vomiting, infection, trauma, or a surgical operation. When more than 90% of the adrenal cortex has been destroyed, however, homeostatic compensation can no longer be achieved, and the patient develops the clinical disease as it was seen by Addison. "Addisonian crisis" is the term applied to the patient whose hypotension progresses to shock and, if untreated, to death. Addisonian crisis is characterized by anorexia, vomiting, abdominal pain, apathy, confusion, and extreme weakness.

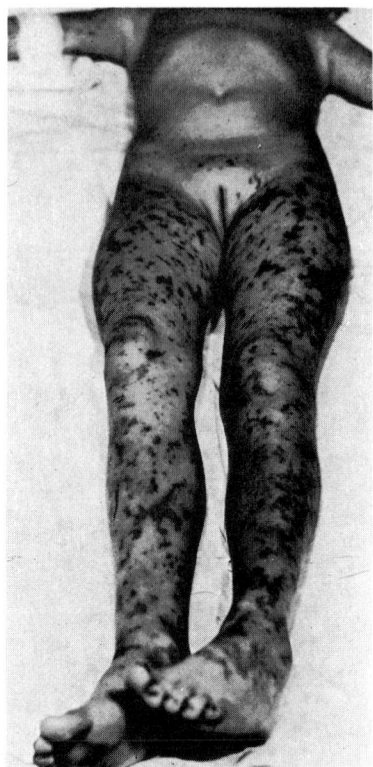

Figure 5–28. Waterhouse-Friderichsen syndrome of 2 days' duration. Note hemorrhagic lesions in the skin.

Diagnosis

The diagnosis of Addison's disease should be considered whenever one sees a patient with any of the features mentioned in the foregoing paragraphs. It should be strongly considered whenever one sees a patient with the tetralogy of hypotension, weight loss, anorexia, and weakness. Each of these manifestations is so characteristic of untreated Addison's disease that one can be fairly secure that a patient is not (at that moment) suffering from this disorder if one can be certain that the patient is hypertensive, that he is gaining weight, that he has a hearty appetite, or that he has normal vigor. Hyperpigmentation is not emphasized as much by contemporary endocrinologists as it was in Addison's original descriptions of this disease; its presence may be a useful clue, but its absence does not exclude the diagnosis of Addison's disease.

Modern methods make it possible to prove or disprove the diagnosis of Addison's disease without employing a large number of laboratory tests. It is only necessary to measure "adrenal reserve" by the technique outlined on p. 264. If the clinical suspicion of Addison's disease is correct, it may be highly desirable to institute treatment without delay. Fortunately, if one employs the following protocol it is possible to diagnose and treat Addison's disease simultaneously.

1. Draw 10 ml of blood for plasma cortisol assay.

2. Start a rapid intravenous infusion of physiologic saline; add (as soon as available) dexamethasone phosphate, 4 mg (1 ml of the pharmaceutical solution), and 25 IU corticotropin. This 1st liter of saline with dexamethasone and corticotropin should be infused within the 1st hour.

3. At the end of the infusion, draw a second 10-ml specimen of blood for plasma cortisol assay.

4. Administer additional 5% dextrose in saline as rapidly and as long as indicated for treatment of dehydration and shock.

5. Start a 24-hour urine collection for 17-OHCS assay.

6. Inject intramuscularly 80 IU of corticotropin (suspended in gelatin or complexed with zinc). As an alternative, one might add corticotropin to each liter of intravenous saline so that at least 3 IU are infused every hour for at least 8 hours.

7. Obtain a third blood specimen for plasma cortisol assay between the 6th and 8th hours of treatment with corticotropin.

If the patient does have Addison's disease, one should see distinct clinical improvement in response to treatment with saline and dexamethasone. In addition, all plasma cortisol values should be less than 15 μg/dl, including those obtained after the administration of corticotropin. Furthermore, the urinary 17-OHCS value should be less than 10 mg/24 hours, despite the administration of corticotropin. Steroid responses indicative of intact adrenocortical reserve exclude the diagnosis of Addison's disease. If one is to follow the combined diagnostic-therapeutic protocol outlined here, it is imperative that no hydrocortisone or cortisone be administered. These steroids will be detected in the assays for plasma cortisol and urinary 17-OHCS; dexamethasone will not. If dexamethasone is not available, the clinician must make a decision as to whether it is more important at the moment to follow the diagnostic protocol alone (giving ACTH with saline and measuring the steroid response) or to follow a modified therapeutic protocol by giving saline and hydrocortisone (or cortisone) and deferring the crucial diagnostic maneuvers until a later day.

In patients whose symptoms are so mild and stable that they do not seem to require urgent therapy, the diagnosis of Addison's disease can be established or excluded merely by testing adrenocortical reserve as outlined above.

Treatment of Primary Adrenal Insufficiency

Management of Addisonian Crisis.   Typical addisonian crisis is the outcome of combined cortisol deficiency, aldosterone deficiency, extracellular volume depletion, and (often) some precipitating stress. This is a life-threatening medical emergency that calls for rapid intravenous infusion of physiologic saline, parenteral administration of glucocorticoids, and specific treatment for any recognizable precipitating stress. It can usually be assumed that the patient in addisonian crisis is depleted of 20% of this extracellular fluid volume. Unless there is some obvious contraindication, this deficit should be corrected as rapidly as possible by intravenously infusing physiologic saline. An adult might require as much as 3 l of saline over a period of a few hours; a child might require proportionately less in terms of volume, but vigorous therapy is just as urgent as in the adult. One obviously cannot repair a sodium deficit without giving enough sodium. One does not depend upon sodium-*retaining* steroids to replenish sodium stores once they have become depleted. As long as one gives enough saline in treating addisonian crisis, it is relatively unimportant whether one establishes mineralocortoid substitution therapy immediately or waits until the patient's condition has stabilized. Such flexibility is not justified with respect to glucocorticoid replacement therapy. There is little to fear from giving intravenously a single 100-mg dose of hydrocortisone phosphate or a single 4-mg dose of dexamethasone phosphate, and such treatment immediately provides circulating glucocorticoid concentrations comparable to those of severely stressed patients with intact adrenal function. Such injections, therefore, are recommended routinely as part of the treatment for addisonian crisis. Once the addisonian patient has received enough saline to replenish his extracellular volume and enough glucocorticoid to mimic the normal adrenal response to severe stress, he should be considered for the moment to be "endocrinologically normal," and the remainder of his medical problems should be managed as they would be in patients without Addison's disease.

Management of Addisonian Patients During Surgical or Other Stresses. Patients undergoing adrenalectomy or addisonian patients who are subjected to surgical operations or other major stresses should be treated with adequate doses of cortisol; by "adequate" is meant at least as much as an endocrinologically normal individual would secrete in response to similar stresses. In response to major stresses, people with intact adrenals might secrete more than 100 mg/day but probably never more than 300 mg/day. Therefore, it is often recommended that severely stressed addisonian patients be given hydrocortisone phosphate in divided doses totaling not less than 300 mg on the day of stress. Since most surgical stresses are of brief duration, it is advisable to decrease the dose of hydrocortisone by 50% each day until the maintenance level has been reached (about 30 mg daily). Minor stresses or those of short duration might well be managed by administering a single 100-mg dose of hydrocortisone or an equivalent amount of some other glucocorticoid (Table 5–3).

In treating acute stresses it is permissible to err on the side of overtreatment, inasmuch as brief excesses of glucocorticoids are relatively innocuous and provide much security against any possibility of adrenal insufficiency. If stresses are protracted, however, one must consider the dangers of overtreatment as well as those of undertreatment. In treating the chronically stressed addisonian patient, one might give between 20 and 100 mg of hydrocortisone daily, depending upon the severity of the stress. If the stress is an infection, one might assume that glucocorticoid therapy is adequate if the temperature is less than 38° C but inadequate if it exceeds 39° C. In this situation, one would not wish to give too much glucocorticoid for fear of interfering with host defense mechanisms and of creating a false sense of security by masking signs of infection. On the other hand, one would not wish to give too little steroid and leave the patient vulnerable to the stress imposed by the infection.

Stressed patients usually cannot be relied upon to take full diets; therefore, in the absence of normal adrenal function, they may quickly become dangerously depleted of sodium. This can be avoided by giving any addisonian patient at least 1 l of physiologic saline intravenously every day until he is taking a full diet. Here it is wise to err on the side of oversolicitude, since ill patients may not consume full diets even though these are prescribed. Until the patient has fully demonstrated that he is eating heartily, he should continue to receive his daily liter of saline.

Management of Intercritical Addison's Disease. It is essential that the addisonian patient be thoroughly indoctrinated in how to care for himself during intervals between crises. With minor modifications, he should take cortisol (or its glucocorticoid equivalent) in doses of 20 mg each morning and 10 mg each evening, and fludrocortisone (Florinef) in doses of 0.1 mg/day. He should carry a sterile syringe containing 4 mg of dexamethasone phosphate (in 1 ml of water) for emergency injection. He should have an identification card giving his name, physician's name, and the following statement: "I have Addison's disease. In an emergency involving loss of consciousness, injury, or vomiting, I should immediately be given an intramuscular injection of dexamethasone phosphate (with my personal belongings).

Call a physician without delay." His diet should include a liberal amount of sodium (at least 150 mEq/day); moreover, in the event of diarrhea or profuse sweating, he should take supplemental sodium chloride. The dose of fludrocortisone should be cautiously decreased if the patient exhibits edema, hypertension, or hypokalemia and increased if he exhibits hypotension or hyperkalemia. Some patients who have had hypertension prior to the development of Addison's disease require no mineralocorticoid substitution therapy and may respond to ordinary doses of fludrocortisone by becoming hypertensive. Although some addisonian patients may not require mineralocorticoid therapy, they all require liberal intakes of sodium chloride.

It should be remembered that Addison's disease is often a complication of some other disease. If appropriate investigations reveal evidence of tuberculosis or disseminated histoplasmosis, these infections should be specifically treated. If the Addison's disease is thought to be due to autoimmune atrophy of the adrenals, the patient should be observed from time to time for evidence of hypothyroidism, hypoparathyroidism, or diabetes mellitus so that these conditions might be treated before they become incapacitating or life-threatening.

In growing children, it is of utmost importance that the dose of steroid employed in glucocorticoid substitution therapy be carefully regulated so as to avoid adrenal insufficiency on the one hand and retardation of linear growth on the other. Growth retardation is a very sensitive index of glucocorticoid excess and can occur in the virtual absence of obesity, impairment of glucose tolerance, ecchymoses, or other common signs of Cushing's syndrome. An initial maintenance dose of hydrocortisone might be 20 mg/m² of body surface /day (in two or three doses given principally in the morning), but one must be prepared to adjust the dosage from time to time according to the empirical requirements of the individual patient.

Secondary Adrenal Insufficiency

Cortisol deficiency can occur as a consequence of ACTH deficiency. The clinical manifestations of ACTH deficiency are listed in Table 5–9, with the exception that cutaneous hyperpigmentation is not present, since in this variety of adrenal insufficiency the pigmentary hormones ACTH and "MSH" are low rather than high.

Plasma cortisol concentrations and urinary 17-OHCS and 17-KS are characteristically subnormal and rise only sluggishly in response to standard test doses of ACTH. The fact that they rise at all, however, sets this condition apart from primary adrenal insufficiency, in which adrenocortical reserve is negligible. With prolonged treatment with ACTH, patients with secondary adrenal insufficiency can generate normal or supernormal adrenal steroid levels, but these cannot be maintained after exogenous ACTH has been withdrawn (Fig. 5–29).

The distinction between primary and secondary adrenal insufficiency is important for two practical reasons. First, in primary adrenal insufficiency, cortisol deficiency is usually accompanied by aldosterone deficiency; but in secondary adrenal insufficiency, the aldosterone-secretory mechanism is usually intact, and mineralocorticoid substitution therapy is not required. Second, although primary adrenal insufficiency should alert the physician to the possible coexistence of tuberculosis, histoplasmosis, amyloidosis, or autoimmune disorders, secondary adrenal insufficiency should alert the physician to the possibility that the patient might have deficiencies of multiple pituitary hormones as well as to the possibility that the disease leading to pituitary destruction

RESPONSE TO ACTH IN HYPOPITUITARISM

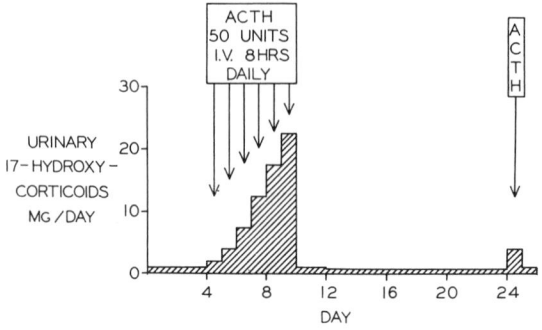

Figure 5–29. In patients with hypopituitarism, the adrenal steroidogenic response to a standard test dose of ACTH is subnormal. Repetitive treatment with ACTH enhances adrenal responsiveness, but if exogenous ACTH is withdrawn, adrenal reserve becomes subnormal again.

Table 5–10. RESULTS OF PITUITARY-ADRENAL EVALUATION IN 266 PATIENTS WITH VARIOUS ENDOCRINE-METABOLIC DISORDERS

| | Pituitary-Adrenal Status | | |
	Normal	Limited Pituitary Reserve	Frank Insufficiency
Pituitary dwarfism	0	2	5
Sheehan's syndrome	0	2	7
Craniopharyngioma	1	0	6
Chromophobe adenoma	12	26	6
Acromegaly	14	5	0
After pituitary irradiation	33	23	0
Low-FSH eunuchoidism	5	2	0
Metastases to pituitary	0	1	1
Cachexia	6	6	0
Post-traumatic diabetes insipidus	3	2	0
Cushing's syndrome, adrenal tumor	0	11	0
Cushing's syndrome, pituitary	29	1	0
Congenital adrenal hyperplasia (non–salt losers)	7	0	0
Primary aldosteronism	5	0	0
Primary hypothyroidism	34	2	0
Graves' disease	8	1	0

might endanger neighboring neural structures. The recognition of a pituitary tumor or cyst might lead to early treatment (either surgical or radiologic) in time to prevent encroachment on such structures as the optic chiasm or the circle of Willis. A detailed discussion of hypopituitarism is found in Chapter 2. In treating secondary adrenal insufficiency, one aims to provide exogenous glucocorticoids in quantities similar to those secreted by patients with intact adrenal function; the doses and indications are the same as those outlined for the treatment of primary adrenal insufficiency. As in the case of primary adrenal insufficiency, it is essential that the patient be well-educated as to his need for glucocorticoid therapy; he should carry an identification card and an emergency supply of injectable dexamethasone phosphate or hydrocortisone phosphate.

A special case of secondary hypocortisolism is that resulting from chronic suppression of ACTH by cortisol from an adrenal neoplasm or by exogenous glucocorticoids. There should be no difficulty in making this diagnosis since there will be a history of Cushing's syndrome following steroid withdrawal. Basal levels of plasma cortisol and urinary 17-OHCS are subnormal, and the adrenal cortical responses to standard test doses of ACTH are subnormal. In time, complete recovery of pituitary-adrenal function can be anticipated, but this may require as long as a year. During this period, the patient should receive protective doses of glucocorticoids during major stresses. Even in the absence of severe stress, some patients require daily steroid therapy in order to avoid symptoms of weakness, myalgia, anorexia, and despondency. Such steroid therapy should be given as single morning doses of hydrocortisone in order to minimize the possibility of continued suppression of ACTH secretion. As time passes, the daily dose of hydrocortisone can be diminished gradually and finally withdrawn altogether.

Limited ACTH Reserve

Any disease that can cause frank hypopituitarism can also cause a milder degree of pituitary dysfunction, a condition referred to as "limited pituitary reserve." Such patients secrete enough ACTH to maintain adrenal responsiveness to standard test doses of ACTH, but they are incapable of increasing their ACTH secretion normally in response to stress or in response to some stimulus designed to test ACTH reserve. In the latter category are insulin, pyrogens, and metyrapone (Fig. 5–15). Based on the results of standard metyrapone tests, patients with a variety of endocrin-

ologic disorders have been found to have limited pituitary reserve (Table 5–10).

Routine treatment of "limited pituitary reserve" is not necessary, but the physician should be prepared to administer glucocorticoids if the patient with "limited pituitary reserve" is subjected to a major stress.

Mixed Hypoadrenocorticism and Hyperadrenocorticism: Congenital Adrenal Hyperplasia

The secretion of the important adrenocortical hormones, cortisol and aldosterone, requires the integrity of biosynthetic pathways involving a long series of enzymatically regulated steps. If, through a genetic error, any one of these enzymes is defective, the corresponding biosynthetic step will be impeded, derivatives of that step will be diminished, and precursors immediately preceding the impeded step will accumulate in increased quantities. If the cortisol pathway is impeded, there will be a compensatory increase in ACTH secretion.[83] If mineralocorticoid production is impeded, there will be a compensatory increase in renin-angiotensin production. Increased stimulation of the adrenal by its tropic hormones results in increased formation of steroid precursors up to the impeded step. If the impediment is incomplete, then the increase in precursors may lead to normal or nearly normal production of cortisol or aldosterone, but this compensation will be accomplished at the price of a continuing increase in the production of tropic hormones and a continuing excess of preimpediment precursors and by-products. Some of these precursors and by-products have biologic activities that assume clinical importance when they are secreted in excessive amounts even through they are of little or no clinical importance when secreted in normal quantities. The clinical manifestations of a genetic error in adrenal metabolism depend upon the severity of the cortisol or aldosterone deficiency, on the one hand, and, on the other hand, upon the properties of the steroid precursors and by-products that are excessively secreted.

Because the inefficient adrenal glands are chronically stimulated by relatively high concentrations of adrenotropic hormones, they become hyperplastic. For this reason, these disorders have come to be grouped under the heading "congenital adrenal hyperplasia." The disorders appear to be inherited through autosomal recessive genes. In any one family, the affected siblings have similar adrenal steroid patterns and similar degrees of severity of the disorder.

There are now six known varieties of congenital adrenal hyperplasia, each attributable to inefficiency of a specific enzymatically regulated step in cortisol or aldosterone biosynthesis. Certain enzymes are unique to the cortisol pathway, others are unique to the aldosterone pathway, and still others are found in both. Therefore, in various types of congenital adrenal hyperplasia, one can find deficiencies of either cortisol or aldosterone or both, depending upon the specific biosynthetic error. Certain enzymes of the adrenal cortex are also found in the gonads. Inborn errors affecting these enzymes result not only in derangements of adrenal function but also of gonadal function.

Treatment of congenital adrenal hyperplasia is directed toward supplying physiologic quantities of the deficient steroids. Such treatment should restrain the overproduction of tropic hormones, thus correcting the adrenal hyperplasia and, to a large extent, correcting the hypersecretion of steroid precursors and by-product.[83] In patients with severe deficiences of cortisol and aldosterone, treatment with glucocorticoids, mineralocorticoids, and sodium chloride should be similar to that employed in Addison's disease, including special supplements during major stresses.

Deficiency of 20-Hydroxylase (Cholesterol Desmolase)

The earliest step in the conversion of cholesterol to hormonal steroids is hydroxylation at carbon-20, with subsequent cleavage of the 20–22 side chain (a desmolase reaction) to form pregnenolone. This process is thought to be essential for the formation of all adrenal and gonadal steroids. An inborn error in the enzyme system governing this reaction is thought to be the cause of a rare form of congenital adrenal hyperplasia, first described by Prader,[84] in which the adrenal glands are massively enlarged and laden with cholesterol. Infants with this disorder have female external genitalia even though they may have XY genotypes, and this has been taken as evidence that their gonads were incapable of synthesizing normal quantities of androgen. The poor survival of these infants has permitted little accumulation of biochemic data, but one would expect all steroids in blood and urine to be subnormal (Fig. 5–30)

and ACTH secretion to be abnormally high. Appropriate treatment should be directed at correcting the deficiencies of cortisol and aldosterone and should include, at the appropriate age, the use of estrogens and progestins.

Deficiency of 3β-Hydroxysteroid Dehydrogenase

An important step in the formation of all potent adrenal and gonadal steroids is dehydrogenation of the 3β-hydroxyl group of the Δ⁵ steroids. This facilitates the isomerase reaction through which the Δ⁵ double bond is shifted to the Δ⁴ position. Bongiovanni[85] was the first to describe a form of congenital adrenal hyperplasia caused by a defect in this process. Affected patients produce little in the way of Δ⁴ steroids, such as cortisol, but increased quantities of Δ⁵ steroids, such as DHEA (Fig. 5–31).

Clinically, patients with this disorder manifest cortisol and aldosterone deficiency; in addition, however, neonates of either sex have ambiguous external genitalia. Failure of the genetic males to develop normal external genitalia has been attributed to inability of their gonads to produce fetal androgen (presumably a Δ⁴ steroid, probably testosterone). Partial masculinization of the external genitalia of the genetic females has been attributed to their hypersecretion of weak adrenal androgens, possibly DHEA.

Treatment of this disorder is directed toward physiologic replacement of the deficient glucocorticoids and mineralocorticoids. Initially, glucocorticoid therapy might consist of cortisone acetate, 25 mg intramuscularly every 48 hours, and deoxycorticosterone pivalate, 25 mg intramuscularly once a month. Sodium chloride may be added to the formula or withheld, depending upon the state of hydration, blood pressure, and serum electrolyte concentrations.

The developmental aspects of sexual ambiguity, the differential diagnosis, and the therapeutic management are discussed in Chapter 9.

Deficiency of 17α-Hydroxylase

An essential step in the formation of cortisol, estrogens, androgens, and 17-KS precursors is 17α-hydroxylation of either progesterone or pregnenolone. This step is not involved in the biosynthesis of important mineralocorticoids. Because patients with genetic deficiencies of 17-

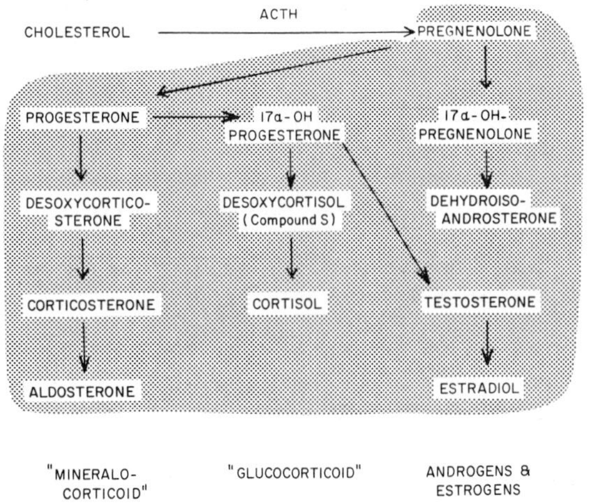

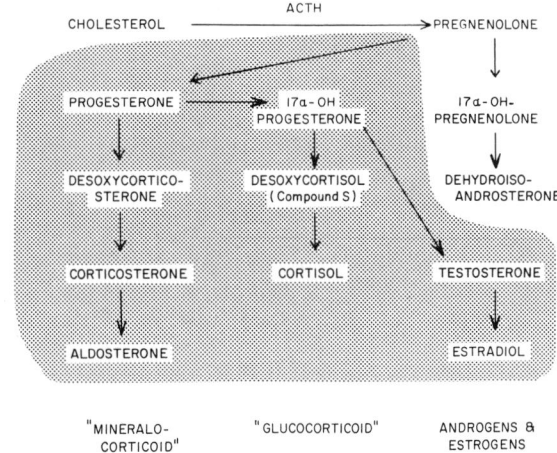

Figure 5–30. Consequences of impaired conversion of cholesterol to pregnenolone: a deficiency of all steroids within the shaded area.

Figure 5–31. Consequences of 3β-hydroxysteroid dehydrogenase deficiency: impaired formation of all steroids within the shaded area.

hydroxylase are incapable of secreting cortisol with normal efficiency, they have compensatory increases in ACTH secretion. Under the influence of high levels of ACTH, their adrenals synthesize large quantities of the 17-deoxycorticosteroids, DOC, and corticosterone.[86] In affected males, failure of the fetal testes to secrete androgen results in failure to develop masculine external genitalia. In females, failure of the ovary to secrete estrogen results in failure to develop secondary sex characteristics at the normal age of puberty.

Chemically (Fig. 5–32), this disorder is characterized by (1) subnormal levels of plasma cortisol, urinary 17-OHCS, and 17-KS; (2) supernormal levels of plasma ACTH, DOC, and corticosterone; (3) subnormal levels of plasma renin activity and aldosterone; (4) subnormal levels of estrogen and testosterone; and (5) supernormal levels of pituitary gonadotropins (after the normal age of puberty).

Clinically, this disorder is characterized by hypertension and sexual infantilism in phenotypic females.

Therapy is directed toward adequate replacement of glucocorticoids and estrogens. With adequate treatment, hypersecretion of DOC is suppressed and hypertension is corrected.

Deficiency of 21-Hydroxylase *(Fig. 5–33)*

This is the most common variety of congenital adrenal hyperplasia. An essential step in the biosynthesis of all glucocorticoids and mineralocorticoids is enzymatic hydroxylation at carbon-21. Because patients with 21-hydroxylase deficiency are incapable of synthesizing cortisol with normal efficiency, there is a compensatory increase in ACTH, leading to adrenal hyperplasia and excessive secretion of 17α-hydroxyprogesterone, the precursor of urinary pregnanetriol. The adrenal androgen, DHEA, is excessively secreted, leading to virilization and increased excretion of 17-KS. If the enzymatic defect is severe enough, it results in a frank deficiency of aldosterone, which in turn leads to hyperkalemia and to sodium depletion, dehydration, hypotension, and compensatory hyper-reninemia.

This disorder occurs in mild form in certain families and with life-threatening severity in others. The severe form is characterized by early virilization, leading, in female fetuses, to marked masculinization of the external genitalia with formation of a urogenital sinus, partial fusion of labioscrotal folds, and marked clitoral hypertrophy. The

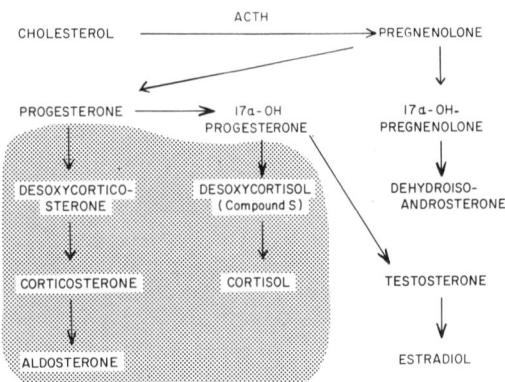

Figure 5–33. Consequences of 21-hydroxylase deficiency: impaired formation of all steroids within the shaded area.

condition is aptly described as "female pseudohermaphroditism," and the affected female infant may be mistaken for a male with bilateral cryptorchidism and hypospadias. The correct diagnosis can be made quickly by noting that an older sibling had virilizing congenital adrenal hyperplasia, that the karyotype is that of a normal female, that urinary pregnanetriol and 17-KS levels are elevated, and that, unless treated with sodium and mineralocorticoids, the child readily displays salt wasting and peripheral vascular collapse. In males, the diagnosis is not so obvious since the external genitalia are normal; unless there is a family history of the disorder, the diagnosis is often not suspected until the tendency toward salt-wasting becomes clinically evident. Salt-wasting congenital adrenal hyperplasia is often fatal unless diagnosed promptly and treated adequately with glucocorticoids, mineralocorticoids, and sodium chloride in much the same way as for Addison's disease.

Milder forms of virilizing congenital adrenal hyperplasia may be unnoticed (except, in some cases, for clitoral hypertrophy) until some time between the ages of 2 and 10 years when affected males or females attract attention because of rapid somatic growth, muscularity, early appearance of pubic and axillary hair, acne, coarsening of the voice, and cessation of linear growth due to closure of epiphyses of the long bones. Affected females do not develop normal secondary sex characteristics; they fail to menstruate, their breasts remain hypoplastic, and they develop facial hirsutism and temporal balding. Once glucocorticoid substitution therapy is instituted, the processes of virilization are arrested and normal feminization proceeds. If the female child has matured under the influence of adrenal androgen to such a degree that her bone age exceeds 13 years by the time glucocorticoid therapy is instituted, she is likely then to develop feminine secondary sex characteristics even though her chronologic age may be only 8 or 9 years. It thus appears that sex hormones exert a "positive feedback" effect on maturation of the gonadotropin-regulating mechanism. Infertility was the rule in congenital adrenal hyperplasia until glucocorticoid therapy was instituted to suppress excessive adrenal androgen production. With glucocorticoid therapy, patients with this disorder are now often able to have children.

Deficiency of 11β-Hydroxylase

The final step in the biosynthesis of cortisol and corticosterone is the introduction of a hydroxyl function in 11β-

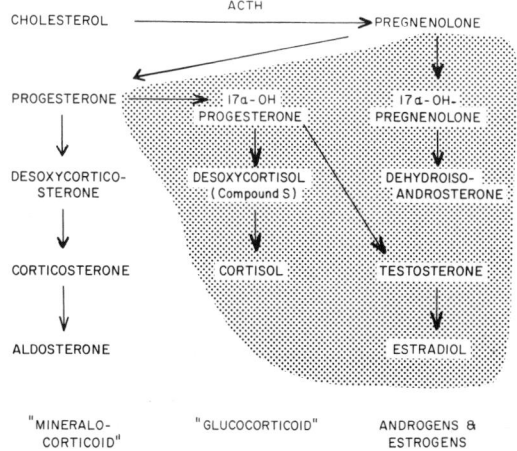

Figure 5–32. Consequences of 17α-hydroxylase deficiency: impaired formation of all steroids within the shaded area.

position. 11β-Hydroxylase is found only in the adrenal cortex. A deficiency of 11β-hydroxylase activity results in diminished secretion of cortisol, a compensatory increase in ACTH secretion, and a consequent increase in biosynthesis and secretion of 11-deoxysteroids.[88]

The chemical hallmarks (Fig. 5–34) of 11β-hydroxylase deficiency, then, are as follows:

1. *Subnormal plasma cortisol, urinary tetrahydrocortisol, and urinary tetrahydrocortisone.* Depending upon the severity of the enzymic defect, these steroids may be negligible, subnormal, or normal in quantity (the last situation representing a mild defect and fully effective homeostatic compensation).

2. *Supernormal plasma 11-deoxycortisol and DOC and supernormal urinary excretion of the tetrahydro derivatives of these steroids.*

3. *Supernormal excretion of 11-deoxy-17-KS.* These are derived largely from DHEA and appear in the urine as androsterone and etiocholanolone. Total urinary 17-KS are increased even though 11-oxygenated 17-KS are diminished.

4. *Supernormal plasma ACTH and "MSH."*

5. *Subnormal plasma renin activity and aldosterone secretion rates.*

The clinical manifestations of 11β-hydroxylase deficiency are as follows:

1. *Virilization.* This results from overproduction of adrenal androgen and may take the form of pseudohermaphroditism (in females), rapid somatic growth but early closure of epiphyses, phallic hypertrophy, early appearance of pubic and axillary hair, and (in females) mammary hypoplasia and amenorrhea.

2. *Hypertension.* This results from overproduction of DOC and can lead to the usual complications of hypertensive cardiovascular disease.

It is possible to mistake this disorder (with its virilism, hypertension, and elevated 17-OHCS) for Cushing's syndrome, but the latter is characterized by glucose intolerance, central obesity, and protein-wasting, none of which is characteristic of 11β-hydroxylase deficiency. In 11β-hydroxylase deficiency, 17-OHCS and 17-KS are profoundly suppressible with small doses of dexamethasone, in contrast to the resistance to suppression seen in patients with Cushing's syndrome or those with virilizing adrenal or ovarian tumors.

Treatment of 11β-hydroxylase deficiency consists of the administration of glucocorticoids in doses sufficient to suppress ACTH and thus suppress the secretion of DOC and adrenal androgens. Successful treatment leads, within several days, to correction of the hypertension and arrest of the virilization. As in other varieties of congenital adrenal hyperplasia, overtreatment with glucocorticoids might lead to inhibition of linear growth. Even though aldosterone production is subnormal, it is more than compensated for by DOC production, and mineralocorticoid substitution therapy is not a consideration in this variety of congenital adrenal hyperplasia.

Deficiency of 18-Hydroxysteroid Dehydrogenase

The final step in aldosterone biosynthesis is the removal of two hydrogen atoms from 18-hydroxycorticosterone, converting it to 18-aldo-corticosterone (aldosterone). The enzyme system that performs this function, 18-hydroxysteroid dehydrogenase, is limited to the zona glomerulosa and has no known function apart from the biosynthesis of aldosterone.

Deficiency of 18-hydroxysteroid dehydrogenase would be expected to result in aldosterone deficiency, sodium depletion, potassium retention, dehydration, hypotension, and increased plasma renin activity. As a consequence of the sodium depletion, hyperkalemia, and hyper-reninemia, one would expect accelerated biosynthesis of aldosterone precursors, culminating in supernormal secretion of 18-hydroxycorticosterone. Precisely this chemical-clinical syndrome has been described by Ulick[89] and has been attributed to 18-hydroxysteroid dehydrogenase deficiency (Fig. 5–35). Appropriate therapy consists of supplemental sodium chloride and mineralocorticoid substitution therapy, following the same principles advocated in the treatment of Addison's disease. Glucocorticoid substitution therapy is unnecessary.

PHARMACOLOGIC USE OF ACTH AND STEROIDS AS ANTI-INFLAMMATORY AND IMMUNOSUPPRESSIVE AGENTS

Although glucocorticoids are essential for survival and must be administered in the treatment of adrenal insufficiency, this represents only a very small portion of the total usage of such agents in contemporary medical practice. In

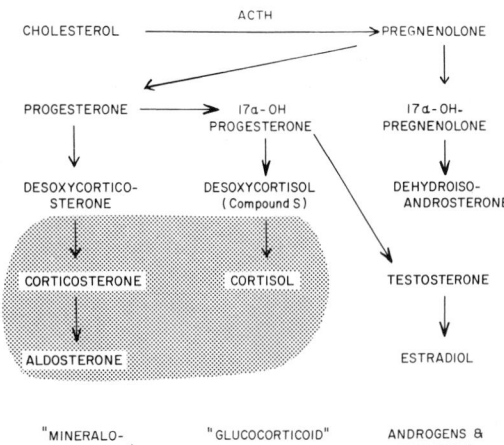

Figure 5–34. Consequences of 11β-hydroxylase deficiency: impaired formation of all steroids within the shaded area and increased formation of those not shaded.

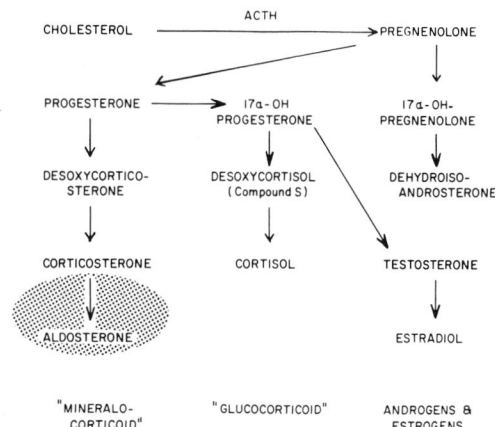

Figure 5–35. Consequences of 18-hydroxysteroid dehydrogenase deficiency: impaired formation of 18-hydroxycorticosterone with resultant impairment of aldosterone synthesis.

"supraphysiologic" doses, glucocorticoids have anti-inflammatory and immunosuppressive actions that have made them useful as therapeutic agents in a wide variety of diseases (Table 5–11). In addition to their uses as anti-inflammatory and immunosuppressive agents, glucocorticoids are efficacious in elevating the blood glucose in patients with hypoglycemia. Regardless of the therapeutic indication for which glucocorticoids are used, whenever they are given in supraphysiologic doses for prolonged periods of time they suppress inflammation and ACTH secretion; promote protein wasting; tend to antagonize the action of insulin; stimulate the deposition of fat in facial, cervical, and truncal depots; cause involution of lymphoid tissues; and inhibit antibody production. All available glucocorticoids share all these properties and differ from each other only with respect to potency (Table 5–3).

When injected into extravascular sites, various esters of the glucocorticoids have different rates of absorption and, therefore, different durations of action (Table 5–12). Those that are slowly absorbed are ideal when one desires a sustained effect but a low blood concentration. Those that are most rapidly absorbed can be used as alternatives to orally or intravenously administered steroids, providing peak blood concentrations quickly, followed by rapid dissipation of the steroids and their effects.

The untoward metabolic effects of corticosteroids are those of prolonged usage. There is no contraindication to a single dose of corticosteroid. In general, the briefer the course of corticosteroid therapy, the less likely one is to encounter any undesirable effects. In deciding whether or not to employ anti-inflammatory steroids for more than a few days, the physician must consider whether the disease he is attempt-

Table 5–11. NONENDOCRINE DISORDERS IN WHICH GLUCOCORTICOIDS ARE THERAPEUTICALLY EFFECTIVE

1. Rheumatoid arthritis
2. Psoriatic arthritis
3. Gouty arthritis
4. Bursitis and tenosynovitis
5. Systemic lupus erythematosus
6. Acute rheumatic carditis
7. Pemphigus
8. Erythema multiforme
9. Exfoliative dermatitis
10. Mycosis fungoides
11. Allergic rhinitis
12. Bronchial asthma
13. Atopic dermatitis
14. Serum sickness
15. Allergic conjunctivitis
16. Uveitis
17. Retrobulbar neuritis
18. Sarcoidosis
19. Löffler's syndrome
20. Berylliosis
21. Idiopathic thrombocytopenic purpura
22. Autoimmune hemolytic anemia
23. Lymphomas
24. Immune nephritis
25. Tuberculous meningitis
26. Urticaria
27. Chronic active hepatitis
28. Ulcerative colitis
29. Regional enteritis
30. Nontropical sprue
31. Dental postoperative inflammation
32. Cerebral edema
33. Subacute nonsuppurative thyroiditis
34. Malignant exophthalmos
35. Hypercalcemia
36. Trichinosis
37. Myasthenia gravis
38. Organ transplantation
39. Alopecia areata

Table 5–12. STEROID ESTERS FOR EXTRAVASCULAR INJECTION

Acid Group	Period of Absorption
Succinate	Minutes–hours
Phosphate	Minutes–hours
Acetate	Days–weeks
Diacetate	Days–weeks
Hexacetonide	Weeks
Pivalate	Weeks

ing to suppress is more dangerous than the Cushing's syndrome that he might induce. Corticosteroid therapy should supplement rather than supplant other standard therapeutic measures. When needed to save a life or prevent serious incapacitation, corticosteroids should be used without hesitation in whatever dosage is necessary.

Illnesses that are of short duration, such as urticaria, serum sickness, trichinosis, or other relatively acute allergic reactions will often respond dramatically to large doses of corticosteroids; moreover, if the illnesses are self-limited, treatment can be limited to a period of hours or days.

Certain other disorders can be controlled satisfactorily by giving corticosteroids intermittently, for example, a single large dose on alternate days or moderate doses for 3 consecutive days, followed by 4 days without steroids. In general, intermittent therapy is less likely than is continuous therapy to cause pituitary-adrenal suppression or the severe protein wasting of Cushing's syndrome. Intermittent therapy is not always effective in controlling inflammatory or immunologic disorders, however, and in each case it must be ascertained empirically whether the therapeutic objectives can be attained by using such a treatment schedule.

Whenever a disease process can be treated adequately by local administration of corticosteroids, this is ordinarily preferable to systemic treatment. Even if the administered steroid is ultimately totally absorbed into the systemic circulation, it will, nevertheless, be present in maximal concentrations at the point of application, thereby conferring a maximum of local benefit without necessarily producing commensurate systemic side effects. This principle has been used with some success in the treatment of certain ophthalmologic disorders, allergic dermatoses, allergic rhinitis, bronchial asthma, and arthritis.

Triamcinolone acetonide and fluorometholone are said to exhibit much higher ratios of potency (relative to hydrocortisone) when administered percutaneously than when administered systemically.

Certain groups of patients are especially vulnerable to the unwanted side effects of corticosteroids. Patients who are elderly, debilitated, or poorly nourished are especially vulnerable to the protein-wasting effects of corticosteroids. Supraphysiologic doses of corticosteroids cause growth retardation in children, a problem that has no counterpart in adults. Gonadectomized or postmenopausal women are especially likely to develop osteoporosis during treatment with glucocorticoids. Latent diabetes can be converted into frank diabetes by glucocorticoid therapy. Peptic ulcers may perforate or hemorrhage during treatment with glucocorticoids. Because of the special hazards accompanying corticosteroid therapy in these groups of patients, it is imperative that the therapeutic indications be clear cut and that the steroid dosage be kept as low as is consistent with achieving one's therapeutic objectives if one is to use steroids at all.

Because anti-inflammatory agents draw no distinction between the "useful" inflammation that walls off infection and "useless" inflammation, one should be reluctant to initiate steroid therapy for more than emergency purposes in patients who have infections for which specific antibiotics are not available. Even when specific antibiotic therapy is available, one should not use glucocorticoids in the presence of infection unless the therapeutic indications are compelling. A special dilemma arises whenever a patient who is already on steroid therapy acquires an infection. Here it is usually wise to continue steroids lest the stress of infection be poorly tolerated. Nevertheless, the dose of glucocorticoid should be held to the minimum that will forestall adrenal insufficiency and general clinical deterioration, and specific antibiotics should be employed without delay.

Although one can often safely treat diseases of brief duration with corticosteroids, there is a risk of incurring a long-term commitment when one treats a chronic disease such as rheumatoid arthritis or intractable bronchial asthma. What started as "short-term" therapy has often led to long-term therapy in such patients. When patients learn that steroids confer dramatic relief of their symptoms, they may be strongly tempted to abandon nonsteroidal therapeutic measures. If steroids must be used they should, if possible, be employed topically, briefly, intermittently, and in the lowest dosage consistent with achieving the desired objectives of preventing incapacitation due to inflammatory or immunologic disease.

Particularly after prolonged usage, abrupt withdrawal of corticosteroids may result in manifestations of adrenal insufficiency and exacerbation of inflammatory processes. Gradual withdrawal of steroids is, therefore, often advisable. Each week the daily dose may be decreased by an amount of steroid equivalent to 5 mg of hydrocortisone. Once physiologic levels are reached, the patient may be given a single daily dose of hydrocortisone, 20 mg each morning, for several months. This will not perpetuate the manifestations of Cushing's syndrome but will prevent adrenal insufficiency while permitting gradual recovery of normal pituitary-adrenal reserve.

Corticotropin (ACTH) may be used as an alternative to exogenous glucocorticoids in most of the conditions under consideration. Its anti-inflammatory, immunosuppressive action is mediated by the cortisol that is secreted in response to ACTH. The cortisol secretory response to ACTH is a function of the type of ACTH preparation, the route of administration, and the duration of treatment. ACTH can be absorbed after intranasal application, but the conventional routes of administration are intravenous or intramuscular. A pulse of ACTH given intravenously results in a brief increase in plasma cortisol lasting approximately 1 hour (more or less, depending upon the dose). A sustained intravenous infusion of ACTH results in a sustained cortisol secretory response lasting for the duration of the ACTH infusion plus 1 or two hours. The most convenient method of administering ACTH is by intramuscular injection. In this method, depot preparations of ACTH are most commonly employed. These are either gelatin suspensions or zinc hydroxide precipitates of ACTH. Depending upon the dose, they are absorbed from an intramuscular injection site over a period of about 8–16 hours.

In previously untreated patients with normal adrenals, 100 U of depot ACTH will result in the secretion of approximately 100 mg of cortisol during the ensuing 16 hours. Patients with adrenal atrophy secondary to prolonged steroid therapy will have much smaller responses, perhaps only 30 mg of cortisol during the ensuing 16 hours. Patients with adrenal hyperplasia secondary to prolonged ACTH therapy will have much larger responses, perhaps as much as 300 mg of cortisol during the ensuing 16 hours. One of the disadvantages of ACTH therapy compared with exogenous steroid therapy is the unpredictability of the cortisol secretory response. It should be apparent that there might be as

much as a 10-fold range of cortisol secretory responses to the same dose of ACTH depending upon the responsiveness of the adrenals. Another disadvantage of ACTH as compared with exogenous steroids is the fact that ACTH must be given parenterally, whereas steroids may conveniently be administered orally. An advantage of ACTH is that it maintains adrenal responsiveness rather than inducing adrenal atrophy, so that prolonged substitution therapy is not necessary after one elects to withdraw supraphysiologic doses of the hormone. As with cortisol itself, one often encounters an undesirable degree of sodium retention and potassium depletion when ACTH is used in high doses over prolonged periods. If there is a clinical indication for extremely large doses of glucocorticoids, such as in the treatment of the crises of disseminated lupus erythematosus, one should employ corticosteroids rather than ACTH since the adrenal glands are capable of secreting only 10–20 mg of cortisol/hour even with continuous maximum ACTH stimulation, and this may not be sufficient to control the inflammatory, immunologic disorder.

Although all available glucocorticoids are similar in suppressing inflammation, suppressing ACTH secretion, promoting protein wasting, elevating blood glucose, and promoting obesity, they differ significantly in their electrolyte-regulating properties. Cortisone and hydrocortisone ordinarily cause significant sodium retention and potassium depletion when administered in excess of 75 mg daily. Equivalent glucocorticoid doses of prednisone, prednisolone, and dexamethasone have only about 20% as much electrolyte-regulating activity as hydrocortisone, and triamcinolone has virtually no sodium-retaining activity.

REFERENCES

1. Villee, D. B.: The development of steroidogenesis. *Am. J. Med.* 53:533, 1972.
2. Gwynne, J., Mahaffe, D., et al.: Adrenal cholesterol uptake from plasma lipoproteins: Regulation by corticotropin. *Proc. Natl. Acad. Sci. U.S.A.* 73:4329, 1976.
3. Samuels, L. T., and Uchikawa, T.: Biosynthesis of adrenal steroids, In *The Adrenal Cortex*. Eisenstein, A. B. (ed.), Boston, Little, Brown, and Co., 1967, p. 61.
4. Hoffman, K.: Relations between chemical structure and function of adrenocorticotropin and melanocyte-stimulating hormones. In *Handbook of Physiology*, Section 7: Endocrinology. Vol. IV. American Physiological Society, Baltimore, Williams and Wilkins, 1974, pp. 29–58.
5. Ney, R. L., Ogata, E., et al.: Structure-function relationships of ACTH and MSH analogues, In *Endocrinology: Proceedings*. Second International Congress of Endocrinology. Part II. New York, American Elsevier Publishing Co., Inc., 1964, p. 1184.
6. Nicholson, W. E., Liddle, R. A., et al.: Adrenocorticotropic hormone biotransformation, clearance, and catabolism. *Endocrinology* 103:1344, 1978.
7. Krieger, D. T., and Ganong, W. F. (eds.): ACTH and related peptides. *Ann. N.Y. Acad. Sci. 297* , 1977.
8. Orth, D. N., Island, D. P., et al.: Experimental alteration of the circadian rhythm in plasma cortisol (17-OHCS) concentration in man. *J. Clin. Endocrinol.* 27:549, 1967.
9. Graber, A. L., Givens, J. R., et al.: Persistence of diurnal rhythmicity in plasma ACTH concentrations in cortisol-deficient patients. *J. Clin. Endocrinol.* 25:804, 1965.
10. Ney, R. L., Shimizu, N., et al.: Correlation of plasma ACTH concentration with adrenocortical response in normal human subjects, surgical patients, and patients with Cushing's disease. *J. Clin. Invest.* 42:1669, 1963.
11. Berson, S. A., and Yalow, R. S. (eds.): *Peptide Hormones.* Vol. 2: *Methods in Investigative and Diagnostic Endocrinology.* New York, American Elsevier Publishing Co., Inc., 1973.
12. Davis, J. O., Higgins, J. T., et al.: Relation of renin and angiotensin II to aldosterone secretion and sodium excretion. In *Aldosterone.* Baulieu, E. E., and Robel, P. (eds.), Oxford, Blackwell Scientific Publications, 1964, p. 175.
13. Kaplan, N. M., and Bartter, F. C.: The effect of ACTH, renin, angiotensin II and various precursors on biosynthesis of aldosterone by adrenal slices. *J. Clin. Invest.* 41:715, 1962.

14. Skinner, S. L.: Improved assay methods for renin "concentration" and "activity" in human plasma. *Circ. Res. 20*:391, 1967.

15. Michelakis, A. M., Caudle, J., et al.: *In vitro* stimulation of renin production by epinephrine, norepinephrine and cyclic AMP. *Proc. Soc. Exp. Biol. Med. 130*:748, 1969.

16. Gordon, R. D., Kuchel, O., et al.: Role of the sympathetic nervous system in regulating renin and aldosterone production in man. *J. Clin. Invest. 46*:599, 1967.

17. Vander, A. J.: Effect of catecholamines and the renal nerves on renin secretion in anesthetized dogs. *Am. J. Physiol. 209*:689, 1965.

18. Davis, J. O.: Mechanisms of renin release, In *Endocrinology: Proceedings.* Fourth International Congress of Endocrinology, Washington, D.C., June 18–24, 1972. Scow, R. (ed.), New York, American Elsevier Publishing Co., Inc., 1973.

19. Lever, A.: Discussion, In *Aldosterone.* Baulieu, E. E., and Robel, P. (eds.), Oxford, Blackwell Scientific Publications, 1964, p. 455.

20. Boucher, R., et al.: New procedures for measurement of human plasma angiotensin and renin activity levels. *Can. Med. Assoc. J. 90*:194, 1964.

21. Haber, E., et al.: Application of a radioimmunoassay for angiotensin I to the physiologic measurements of plasma renin activity in normal human subjects. *J. Clin. Endocrinol. 29*:1349, 1969.

22. Laragh, J. H., and Stoerk, H. C.: A study of the mechanism of secretion of the sodium-retaining hormone (aldosterone). *J. Clin. Invest. 36*:383, 1957.

23. Rudman, D., Del Rio, A. E., et al.: Effect of porcine beta melanocyte-stimulating hormone on blood lymphocyte count and serum corticosterone concentration of the rabbit. *Endocrinology 86*:1410, 1970.

24. Saruta, T., and Kaplan, N. M.: Adrenocortical steroidogenesis: the effects of prostaglandins. *J. Clin. Invest. 51*:2246, 1972.

25. Sandberg, A. A., and Slaunwhite, W. R., Jr.: Physical state of adrenal cortical hormones in plasma, In *The Human Adrenal Cortex.* Christy, N. P. (ed.), New York, Harper and Row, 1971, p. 69.

26. Peterson, R. E.: Metabolism of adrenal cortical steroids, In *The Human Adrenal Cortex.* Christy, N. P. (ed.), New York, Harper and Row, 1971, p. 87.

27. Feldman, D., Funder, J. W., et al.: Subcellular mechanisms in the action of adrenal steroids. *Am. J. Med. 53*:545, 1972.

28. Bruchovsky, N., and Wilson, J. D.: The conversion of testosterone to 5-alpha-androstan-17-beta-ol-3-one by rat prostate in vivo and in vitro. *J. Biol. Chem. 243*:2012, 1968.

29. Baxter, J. D., and Forsham, P. H.: Tissue effects of glucocorticoids. *Am. J. Med. 53*:573, 1972.

30. Jensen, E. V., and DeSombre, E. R.: Estrogen receptors in breast cancer. In *Endocrinology: Proceedings.* Fourth International Congress of Endocrinology, Washington, D.C., June 18–24, 1972. Scow, R. (ed.), New York, American Elsevier Publishing Co., Inc., 1973.

31. Porter, C. C., and Silber, R. H.: A quantitative color reaction for cortisone and related 17,21-dihydroxy-20-ketosteroids. *J. Biol. Chem. 185*:201, 1950.

32. Mattingly, D.: A simple fluorimetric method for the estimation of free 11-hydroxycorticoids in human plasma. *J. Clin. Pathol. 15*:374, 1962.

33. Underwood, R. H., and Tait, J. F.: Purification, partial characterization and metabolism of an acid-labile conjugate of aldosterone. *J. Clin. Endocrinol. 24*:1110, 1964.

34. Kliman, B., and Peterson, R. E.: Double isotope derivative assay of aldosterone in biological extracts. *J. Biol. Chem. 235*:1639, 1960.

35. Ito, T., et al.: A radioimmunoassay for aldosterone in human peripheral plasma including a comparison of alternate techniques. *J. Clin. Endocrinol. 34*:106, 1972.

36. Norymberski, J. K.: Determination of urinary corticosteroids. *Nature* (London) *170*:1074, 1952.

37. Peterson, R. E.: The miscible pool and turnover rate of adrenocortical steroids in man. *Recent Progr. Horm. Res. 15*:231, 1959.

38. Tait, J. F.: Review. The use of isotopic steroids for the measurement of production rates in vivo. *J. Clin. Endocrinol. 23*:1285, 1963.

39. Renold, A. E., Jenkins, D., et al.: The use of intravenous ACTH: a study in quantitative adrenocortical stimulation. *J. Clin. Endocrinol. 12*:763, 1952.

40. Liddle, G. W., Estep, H. L., et al.: Clinical application of a new test of pituitary reserve. *J. Clin. Endocrinol. 19*:875, 1959.

41. Jubiz, W., Levinson, R. A., et al.: Absorption and conjugation of metyrapone during diphenylhydantoin therapy. Mechanism of the abnormal response to oral metyrapone. *Endocrinology 86*:328, 1970.

42. Liddle, G. W.: Test of pituitary-adrenal suppressibility in the diagnosis of Cushing's syndrome. *J. Clin. Endocrinol. 20*:1539, 1960.

43. Temple, T. E., and Liddle, G. W.: Inhibitors of adrenal steroid biosynthesis. *Ann. Rev. Pharmacol. 10*:199, 1970.

44. Liddle, G. W.: Specific and non-specific inhibition of mineralocorticoid activity. *Metabolism 10*:1021, 1961.

45. Cushing, H.: The basophil adenomas of the pituitary body and their clinical manifestations (pituitary basophilism). *Bull. Johns Hopkins Hosp. 50*:137, 1932.

46. Albright, F.: Cushing syndrome. *Harvey Lect. 38*:123, 1942–1943.

47. Lindsay, A. E., et al.: The diagnostic value of plasma and urinary 17-hydroxycorticosteroid determinations in Cushing's syndrome. *Am. J. Med. 20*:15, 1956.

48. Scott, H. W., Jr., Foster, J. H., et al.: Cushing's syndrome due to adrenocortical tumor. *Ann. Surg. 162*:505, 1965.

49. Orth, D. N., and Liddle, G. W.: Results of treatment in 108 patients with Cushing's syndrome. *N. Engl. J. Med. 285*:243, 1971.

50. Hutter, A. M., Jr., and Kayhoe, D. E.: Adrenal cortical carcinoma. *Am. J. Med. 41*:581, 1966.

51. Liddle, G. W., Island, D., et al.: Normal and abnormal regulation of corticotropin secretion in man. *Recent Progr. Horm. Res. 18*:125, 1962.

52. Liddle, G. W.: Pathogenesis of glucocorticoid disorders. *Am. J. Med. 53*:638, 1972.

53. Temple, T. E., Jones, D. J., et al.: Use of o,p′DDD to correct hypercortisolism without inducing aldosterone deficiency in the treatment of Cushing's disease. *N. Engl. J. Med. 281*:801, 1969.

54. Bledsoe, T., Island, D. P., et al.: An effect of o,p-′DDD on the extra-adrenal metabolism of cortisol in man. *J. Clin. Endocrinol. 24*:1303, 1964.

55. Liddle, G. W., Nicholson, W. E., et al.: Clinical and laboratory studies of ectopic humoral syndromes. *Recent Progr. Horm. Res. 25*:238, 1969.

56. Orth, D. N., Nicholson, W. E., et al.: Biologic and immunologic characterization and physical separation of ACTH and ACTH fragments in the ectopic ACTH syndrome. *J. Clin. Invest. 52*:1756, 1973.

57. Bertagna, X. Y., Nicholson, W. E., et al.: Corticotropin, lipotropin, and β-endorphin production by a human nonpituitary tumor in culture: Evidence for a common precursor. *Proc. Natl. Acad. Sci. USA 75*:5160, 1978.

58. Lowry, P. J., Rees, L. H., et al: Chemical characterization of ectopic ACTH purified from a malignant thymic carcinoid tumor. *J. Clin. Endocrinol. Metab. 43*:831, 1976.

59. Graber, A. L., Ney, R. L., et al.: Natural history of pituitary-adrenal recovery following long-term suppression with corticosteroids. *J. Clin. Endocrinol. 25*:11, 1965.

60. Williams, W. C., Jr., Island, D., et al.: Blood corticotropin (ACTH) levels in Cushing's disease. *J. Clin. Endocrinol. 21*:426, 1961.

61. Brown, R. D., Van Loon, G. R., et al.: Cushing's syndrome with periodic hormonogenesis: one explanation for paradoxical response to dexamethasone. *J. Clin. Endocrinol. 36*:445, 1973.

62. Luetscher, J. A.: Studies of aldosterone in relation to water and electrolyte balance in man. *Recent Progr. Horm. Res. 12*:175, 1956.

63. Sutherland, D. J. A., et al.: Hypertension, increased aldosterone secretion and low plasma renin activity relieved by dexamethasone. *Can. Med. Assoc. J. 95*:1109, 1966.

64. Laragh, J. H., Ledingham, J. G. G., et al.: Secondary aldosteronism and reduced plasma renin in hypertensive disease. *Trans. Assoc. Am. Physicians 80*:168, 1967.

65. Bartter, F. C., et al.: Hyperplasia of the juxtaglomerular complex with hyperaldosteronism and hypokalemic alkalosis. Angiotensin II. *Am. J. Med. 33*:811, 1962.

66. Schambelan, M., and Biglieri, E. G.: Renin secreting tumor as a cause of hypertension, In *Endocrinology: Proceedings.* Fourth International Congress of Endocrinology, Washington, D.C., June 18–24, 1972. Scow, R. (ed.), New York, American Elsevier Publishing Co., Inc., 1973.

67. Brown, J. J., et al.: Plasma renin concentration in hypertensive disease of pregnancy. *Lancet 2*:1219, 1965.

68. Liddle, G. W.: Aldosterone antagonists. *Arch. Intern. Med. 102*:998, 1958.

69. Luetscher, J. A., Dowdy, A. J., et al.: Studies of secretion and metabolism of aldosterone and cortisol. *Trans. Assoc. Am. Physicians 75*:293, 1962.

70. Bledsoe, T., Liddle, G. W., et al.: Comparative fates of intravenously and orally administered aldosterone: evidence for extrahepatic formation of acid-labile conjugate in man. *J. Clin. Invest 45*:264, 1966.

71. Conn, J. W.: Primary aldosteronism, a new clinical syndrome. *J. Lab. Clin. Med. 45*:3, 1955.

72. Conn, J. W., Rovner, D. R., et al.: Normokalemic primary aldosteronism. *J.A.M.A. 195*:21, 1966.

73. Conn, J. W.: Plasma renin activity in primary aldosteronism. Importance in differential diagnosis and in research of essential hypertension. *J.A.M.A. 190*:222, 1964.

74. Liddle, G. W., Bledsoe, T., et al.: A familial renal disorder simulating primary aldosteronism but with negligible aldosterone secretion. *Trans. Assoc. Am. Physicians 76*:199, 1963.

75. Woods, J. W., Liddle, G. W., et al.: Effect of an adrenal inhibitor in hypertensive patients with suppressed renin. *Arch. Intern. Med. 123*:366, 1969.

76. Gunnells, C. J., et al.: Hypertension, adrenal abnormalities and alterations in plasma renin activity. *Ann. Intern. Med. 73*:901, 1970.

77. Adlin, E. V., Channick, B. J., et al.: Salivary sodium-potassium ratio and plasma renin activity in hypertension. *Circulation 39*:685, 1969.

78. Carey, R. M., Douglas, J. G., et al.: The syndrome of essential hypertension and suppressed plasma renin activity. *Arch. Intern. Med. 130*:849, 1972.

79. Addison, T.: On the Constitutional and Local Effects of Disease of the Suprarenal Capsules. London, Highley, 1855.

80. Blizzard, R. M., and Kyle, M.: Studies of the adrenal antigens and antibodies in Addison's disease. *J. Clin. Invest. 42*:1653, 1963.

81. Southren, A. L., Tochimoto, S., et al.: Remission in Cushing's syndrome with o,p-'DDD. *J. Clin. Endocrinol. 26*:268, 1966.

82. Laidlaw, J. C., Abbott, E. C., et al.: The influence of a heparin-like compound on hypertension, electrolytes and aldosterone in man. *Trans. Am. Clin. Climatol. Assoc. 77*:111, 1965.

83. Bartter, F. C., and Albright, F.: The effects of adrenocorticotropic hormone and cortisone in adrenogenital syndrome associated with congenital adrenal hyperplasia: An attempt to explain and correct its disordered hormonal pattern. *J. Clin. Invest. 30*:237, 1951.

84. Prader, V. A., and Gurtner, H. P.: Das syndrom des Pseudohermaphroditismus masculinus bei kongenitaler Nebennierenrinden-Hyperplasie ohne Androgenuberproduktion (adrenaler Pseudohermaphroditismus masculinus). *Helv. Paediatr. Acta 10*:397, 1955.

85. Bongiovanni, A. M., Eberlein, W. R., et al.: Disorders of adrenal steroid biogenesis. *Recent Prog. Horm. Res. 23*:375, 1967.

86. Biglieri, E. G., Herron, M. A., et al.: 17-Hydroxylation deficiency in man. *J. Clin. Invest. 45*:1946, 1966.

87. Bongiovanni, A. M., Eberlein, W. R., et al.: Disorders of adrenal steroid biogenesis. *Recent Progr. Horm. Res. 23*:375, 1967.

88. Eberlein, W. R., and Bongiovanni, A. M.: Plasma and urinary corticosteroids in the hypertensive form of congenital adrenal hyperplasia. *J. Biol. Chem. 223*:85, 1956.

89. Ulick, S., Gautier, E., et al.: An aldosterone biosynthetic defect in a salt-losing disorder. *J. Clin. Endocrinol. 24*:669, 1964.

Hirsutism

90. Givens, J. R.: Hirsutism and hyperandrogenism. *Adv. Intern. Med. 21*:221, 1976.

91. Kirschner, M. A., Zucker, I. R., and Jespersen, D.: Idiopathic hirsutism — an ovarian abnormality. *N. Engl. J. Med. 294*:637, 1976.

92 Meikle, A. W., Stringham, J. D., et al.: Plasma 5 alpha androstanediol: an androgen marker of hirsutism in women. *Trans. Assoc. Am. Physicians 89*:133, 1976.

CHAPTER 6

The Testes

By C. Wayne Bardin
and C. Alvin Paulsen

The two major functions of the testis, steroid hormone secretion and gametogenesis, are segregated anatomically, with androgen biosynthesis occurring in Leydig cells and spermatogenesis in the seminiferous tubules. The anterior pituitary participates in the control of both of these functions through its secretion of the gonadotropins, luteinizing hormone (LH) and follicle-stimulating hormone (FSH). The anterior pituitary is, in turn, regulated by multiple parts of the central nervous system which are coordinated via the hypothalamic secretion of gonadotropin-releasing hormone (GnRH). The interrelationship of the brain, the pituitary, and the testis is summarized in Figure 6–1. Although testosterone biosynthesis and spermatogenesis are intimately related, for convenience they will be discussed independently as the hypothalamo–pituitary–Leydig cell axis and the hypothalamo–pituitary–seminiferous tubular axis.

THE PHYSIOLOGY OF THE HYPOTHALAMO–PITUITARY–LEYDIG CELL AXIS

The Components of the Axis

The essential features of the hypothalamo–pituitary–Leydig cell axis are schematically shown in the left half of Figure 6–1. The components of this axis are described first, followed by a discussion of its integrated control.

The Hypothalamus and Gonadotropin-Releasing Hormone. Recent studies have emphasized the complexity of the microvasculature between the hypothalamus and the pituitary. The intimate association of the pituitary gland with the central nervous system offered by these blood vessels provides a pathway for releasing hormones from the brain to control anterior pituitary function. Although many parts of the brain may influence reproductive function, the hypothalamus may be viewed as the final common pathway through which the control of gonadotropin secretion and behavior are mediated. In addition, studies of several species have suggested that this vasculature is arranged in such a manner that pituitary secretions may be directed preferentially to the brain where they may modulate the regulatory functions of the central nervous system.

Testosterone and other sex steroids regulate gonadotropin secretion and reproductive behavior by their action on the brain. A series of studies on male animals using testosterone implants into the brain,[2] electrical stimulation,[3] and immunohistochemistry[3, 4] suggest that the medial basal hypothalamus is important for control of tonic gonadotropic secretion. Destruction of the arcuate nucleus in this area of the brain leads to decreased LH and testosterone secretion as well as to testicular atrophy.[2, 4] This portion of the hypothalamus contains a series of peptidergic neurons capable of secreting the hypothalamic hormone GnRH. Neurons arising from many parts of the central nervous system impinge upon this peptidergic system; the most important of these, which may control GnRH secretion directly or indirectly, are the catecholamine,[5, 6] endorphin-containing,[7] and dopa[8] fibers.

GnRH, like other hypothalamic peptides, is widely distributed in the central nervous system.[3, 4] The role of GnRH-containing neurons in portions of the brain other than the basal portion of the hypothalamus is not known. It is possible that they participate in the control of sexual behavior, as suggested by observations following systemic or intraventricular injections of exogenous GnRH in rats.[9, 10] Experiments with testosterone implanted into the brain indicate that male sexual behavior appears to be regulated by several portions of the hypothalamus, with the anterior hypothalamus apparently most important.[2]

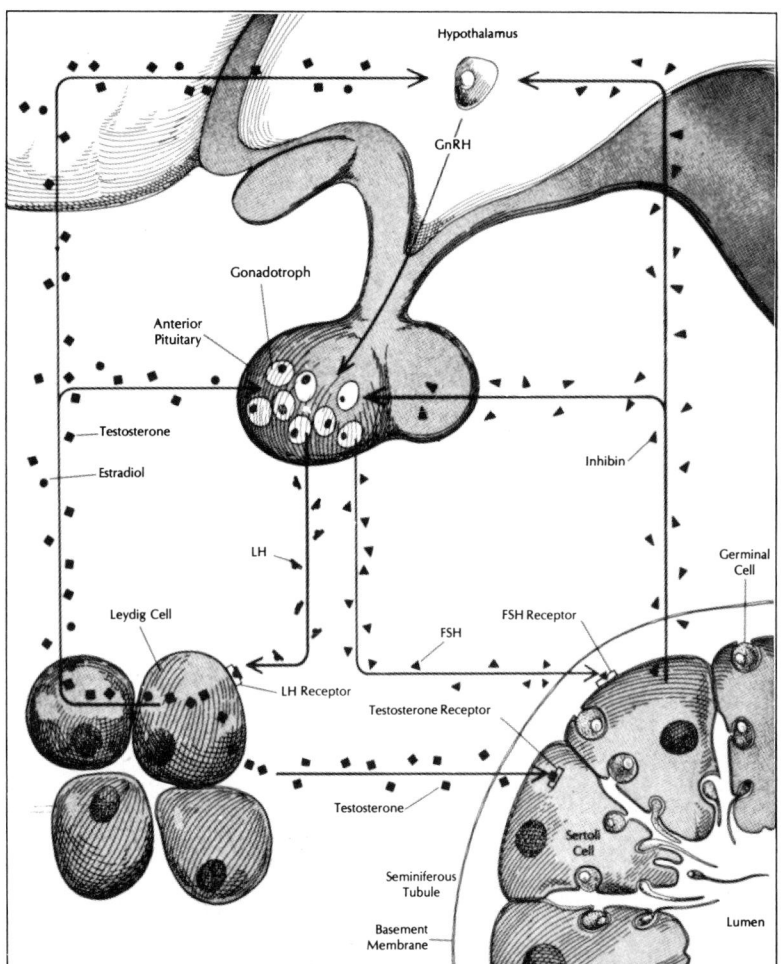

Figure 6–1. The hypothalamo-pituitary-testicular axis is composed of the hypothalamus and its neural connections with the rest of the brain, the gonadotropin-producing cells of the anterior pituitary, and the testis. The testis is functionally divided into interstitial tissue, which contains Leydig cells, and seminiferous tubules, which are, in turn, made up of Sertoli cells and their accompanying germinal cells. For the purpose of discussion, the hypothalamo–pituitary–Leydig cell axis, shown on the left, comprises the brain, pituitary, and the Leydig cells, along with their respective hormones, GnRH, LH, and testosterone and estradiol. The hypothalamo–pituitary–seminiferous tubular axis is shown on the right and is composed of the brain, pituitary, and Sertoli cells, along with their respective hormones, GnRH, FSH, and inhibin. Hypothalamic GnRH mediates pituitary release of LH and FSH. When LH binds to specific membrane receptors on testicular Leydig cells, a series of reactions is entrained, eventuating in secretion of testosterone and estradiol. As noted in the text and in Figure 6–8, most of the estrogen in men is produced at extraglandular sites from androgens. The sex steroids, in turn, act on brain and anterior pituitary, where they exert control of gonadotropin release via negative feedback mechanisms. Testosterone secreted by the Leydig cells binds to cytoplasmic receptors in the Sertoli cells of the seminiferous tubule, a critical event in spermatogenic differentiation. Binding of FSH to its membrane receptors on the Sertoli cells also is important for induction of spermatogenesis. Inhibin, released from Sertoli cells, reduces FSH secretion. (By Donner, C., from Bardin, C. W.: The neuroendocrinology of male reproduction. *Hospital Practice,* Vol. 14, No. 12, and from *Neuroendocrinology.* Krieger, D. K., and Hughes, J. C. (eds.), Sunderland, MA, Sinauer Associates, Inc., 1980, pp. 239–247. Reproduced with permission.)

Thus, testosterone and GnRH are only two of many possible hormones and neurotransmitters that appear to influence potency in man.

A better understanding of the neural control of gonadotropin secretion in man was facilitated by the isolation and structural elucidation of GnRH.[11, 12] The administration of this decapeptide, Pyro-Glu$_1$-His$_2$-Trp$_3$-Ser$_4$-Tyr$_5$-Gly$_6$-Leu$_7$-Arg$_8$-Pro$_9$-Gly$_{10}$-NH$_2$, stimulates the release of both LH and FSH from gonadotrophs by a Ca^{++}-dependent mechanism that is independent of cAMP or cGMP accumulation.[13, 14] The amount of each hormone released depends upon the age and hormonal milieu of the individual. After birth, the pituitary of infant primates reaches peak LH responsiveness to GnRH at 1–3 months of age. Thereafter sensitivity of the pituitary to this decapeptide declines, becoming relatively unresponsive to even repeated doses until the onset of puberty. The secretion of FSH (relative to LH) following GnRH administration is greater prior to puberty.[15] These age-related differences in sensitivity to GnRH in normal men and boys are important to understand for proper interpretation of provocative tests of the hypothalamo–pituitary–Leydig cell axis in hypogonadal patients.[16]

The metabolic clearance rate (MCR) of GnRH is 802 ± 74 (liters plasma/day/m^2) estimated during an infusion of 2.5 μg/m. The MCR of this peptide decreases progressively with increased dosage in a linear dose-dependent manner.[17] Immunoreactive metabolites of this peptide are excreted into the urine of subjects of all ages. Mean concentrations of urinary GnRH metabolites are lowest in infants and rise gradually in prepubertal boys, reaching a peak after 11 years. The amount of immunoreactive GnRH in the urine of men is highly correlated with LH and FSH secretion.[18] While these observations support the contention that GnRH is required for gonadotropin secretion, it is unlikely that measurements of immunoreactive releasing hormones will be widely used in clinical practice in the near future.

In addition to the native hormone, many potent agonists of GnRH have been synthesized. Among the many GnRH derivatives that have been prepared, those with substitution of D-amino acids at position 6 and replacement of the terminal glycine with ethylamide are noteworthy because of their enhanced potency.[19, 20] The increased biologic activities of the GnRH "superagonists" are related to their increased affinity for GnRH receptors and to their relative resistance to degradation. In addition to their actions on the pituitary, GnRH and its agonists have direct effects on the testis[21] and male reproductive tract.[22] In addition, antagonists of GnRH have been prepared by deletion of histidine from the 2 position and by substitution of D-amino acids in positions 2 and 3. These synthetic agonists and antagonists of GnRH not only are useful for study of the physiology of the pituitary gonadal axis, but also are potential agents for infertility and fertility control.[12]

The Pituitary and Luteinizing Hormone. This pituitary hormone derives its name from its action in the female where it facilitates ovulation and converts the ovulated follicle into a functioning corpus luteum. When the hormone was first discovered in the male it was called interstitial cell–stimulating hormone (ICSH) because of its effect on testicular Leydig cells. It is now recognized that LH and ICSH are identical, and the term "LH" is used in both sexes. Immunohistochemical studies indicate that LH and FSH are both secreted by the same PAS-positive basophilic cell in the pituitary.

LH, like several other glycoprotein hormones including FSH, thyroid-stimulating hormone (TSH), and human chorionic gonadotropin (hCG), contains two peptide chains designated α and β. The α-subunit of all these hormones from a given species appears to be identical. As a consequence, the β-subunit determines both the structural and the biologic differences between each of these proteins.[23] The evidence for these assertions is derived, in part, from studies in which hybrid proteins formed from a combination of the α-chain of TSH and the β-chain of LH possess the activity of LH. Similarly, combinations of α-LH and β-TSH result in a molecule that stimulates the thyroid.[24]

The structure of LH is virtually identical to that of hCG, except for an additional 30 amino acids on the carboxyl terminal end of the β-chain of hCG.[25] The gene for hCG-β appears to be a duplicated hLH-β gene with a mutation at its stop sequence. Thus hCG-β is larger because it must be read by RNA polymerase II to a new termination signal. The similarity in structure of LH and hCG undoubtedly accounts for the fact that they both stimulate testosterone synthesis and secretion by Leydig cells. It was once supposed that the major functional difference between these hormones was their sites of synthesis in the pituitary and placenta. Recent studies, however, have demonstrated that small amounts of immunoreactive material similar to hCG may be made in the testis, pituitary, and other normal tissues.[26-28] This suggests that the hCG gene may open in organs other than placenta. Once hCG-like activity was demonstrated in normal extraplacental tissues, several investigators identified this glycoprotein in tissues of many species, using both immunologic and radioreceptor assays. Subsequent studies have demonstrated that there are several possible explanations for the hCG-like material in normal tissues. In some instances, spurious hCG-like activity could be attributed to tissue proteases which degrade the radioactive tracers used in the immunological and receptor assays.[29] Another reason for apparent immunoreactive hCG is that there is a common amino acid sequence present in glycoprotein hormones and tissue proteases.[30] As a consequence, apparent hCG activity in normal tissue can also be related to cross-reactivity of hCG and LH antibodies, with all proteins bearing this common sequence. Furthermore, the identification of hCG bioactivity in unfractionated tissue extracts is not sufficient evidence for hCG identification since some enzymes can mimic hCG and LH by stimulating adenylate cyclase in vitro.[31] Taken together these observations indicate that radioimmunoassays, radioreceptor assays, and bioassays are not sufficient proof of the identity of a tissue hormone, particularly when it is present in very low concentrations. The ultimate identification must rest upon isolation of the active molecule, as was recently done for the hCG activity in bacteria.[32] At present, insufficient data are available to determine with certainty how much of the hCG-like activity of normal tissues is due to a gonadotropin and how much to enzymes.

The secretion of GnRH into the hypophyseal portal system is episodic rather than constant. Although the amount of this peptide has not been measured directly in

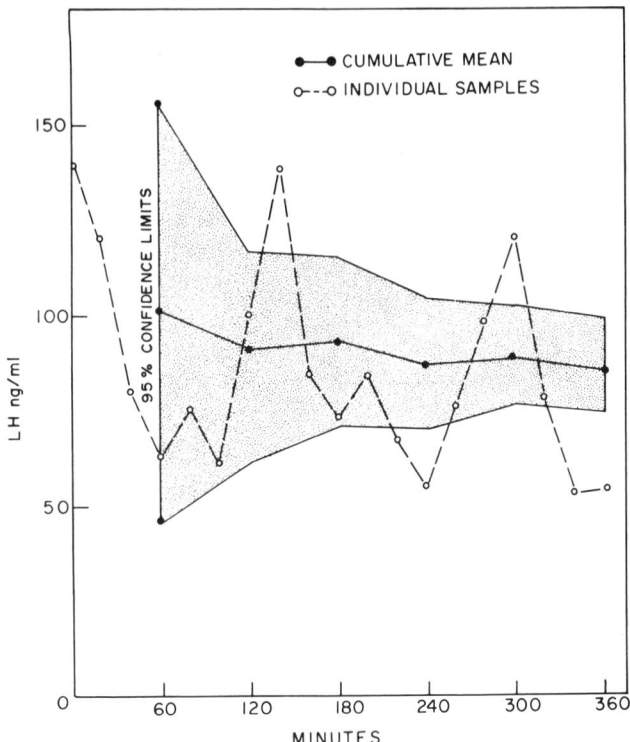

Figure 6–2. The secretory pattern of LH in a normal man. The cumulative mean LH level and its 95% confidence limits at hourly intervals for 6 hours are shown by the solid line in the shaded area. For comparison, the dashed line with open circles represents the actual estimates of serum LH in samples obtained at 20-minute intervals. (From Santen, R., and Bardin, C. W.: Episodic luteinizing hormone secretion in man. Pulse analysis, clinical interpretation, physiologic mechanisms. *J. Clin. Invest. 52*:2617, 1973. Reproduced by permission of the American Society for Clinical Investigation.)

the hypophyseal portal system of man, the estimates of < 30-300 pg/ml by Huseman and Kelch[17] are in accord with those observed in monkeys.[33, 34] The intermittent secretion of GnRH, in turn, results in the episodic release of LH into the blood.[35, 36] The pattern of LH secretion in normal men is illustrated in Figure 6–2. This glycoprotein is secreted in a series of secretory pulses which have amplitudes ranging from 35 to 270% of baseline. These pulses occur with a frequency of two to four per 6 hours.[37] A variety of studies have indicated that both the frequency and the amplitude of the LH secretory pulses can be attenuated by sex steroids and disease states.[38, 39] In addition, an infusion of low doses (2.5 μg/hr) of GnRH reduces the frequency and amplitude of the secretory pulses, whereas large amounts of this peptide appear to enhance the episodic fluctuations.[16, 17] Whether these latter observations can be explained as an intrinsic property of the pituitary gland *per se* remains to be established. A major problem posed by the variable secretion of LH is that a single serum sample cannot be used to evaluate gonadotropin physiology or to diagnose and manage endocrine disorders in patients. Proper assessment of LH secretion can be derived from hormone measurements in multiple serum samples or in timed urine specimens. Both these approaches provide a precise estimate of "mean" or "integrated" LH secretion.[40]

Part of the biologic responses of LH and hCG is related to their prolonged retention in the circulation compared to peptides like ACTH. Following administration of exogenous LH, disappearance from blood is described by two linear exponentials with a mean initial-phase half-time of 40 minutes and a second-phase half-time of 120 minutes.[37]

The hCG half-life is longer.[41] Prolonged retention of LH in the bloodstream relates in part to its sialic acid content. Several studies have demonstrated that asialoglycoproteins (including hCG) are rapidly cleared by the liver. As a consequence, asialo LH (hCG) has very little biologic activity when examined in *in vivo* bioassay systems in which prolonged action of the hormone is required for the response. By contrast, asialo hCG has a potency similar to that of the intact molecule when examined by immunoassay, radioreceptor assay, and *in vitro* bioassays in which short-term effects can be measured.[41] These and other studies suggest that heterogeneity of gonadotropins in plasma and urine is related to variation of carbohydrate and sialic acid on individual molecules. This, in turn, may account for variable estimates of potency depending upon the assay used.[42] Detailed studies of LH metabolism indicate that this hormone has a metabolic clearance rate of 25 ml/minute, which is unrelated to gonadal function.[43] Most of the LH secreted into the blood is degraded, since only a small fraction of its daily production rate appears in the urine.[44] The major action of LH is to stimulate testosterone biosynthesis and secretion by testicular Leydig cells.

Leydig Cells and Testosterone. The major site of testosterone synthesis in man is the Leydig cells (Fig. 6-3). These are polygonal cells (15-20 μ) in the interstitial areas which make up about 5% of total testicular volume.[45] These cells are characterized morphologically by typical plasma membranes which are frequently thrown into folds or microvilli. Their most prominent cytoplasmic organelle is the smooth endoplasmic reticulum (SER) consisting of interconnecting membrane tubules. These tubules are isolated from one another when viewed by electron micrography (Fig. 6-4). However, in three dimension within the living cell, the tubules apparently interconnect to form a continuous network throughout the cytoplasm. Scattered between the SER are patches of rough endoplasmic reticulum and mitochondria. The cytoplasm also contains lipid droplets, Reinke crystals, and lysosomes. Secondary lysosomes may contain lipofuscin pigment. The ultrastructure of the human Leydig cell has been extensively reviewed by Christensen.[46]

Leydig cells differentiate and secrete androgens during the seventh week of fetal life in the human.[47] The activation of Leydig cells correlates with the onset of androgen-dependent differentiation in the male fetus. Although the fetal pituitary secretes LH and FSH, if a gonadotropin is required for this initial differentiation, then it is probably hCG since functional Leydig cells develop in anencephalic infants born without pituitary glands. After birth, Leydig cells continue to secrete androgens for several months[48] and then revert to a relatively undifferentiated state until they are activated again at the time of puberty coincident with the increase in plasma and urinary GnRH and gonadotropins. Prior to puberty, Leydig cells are very responsive to hCG, and the magnitude of the testosterone response does not depend upon age. Concomitant with the onset of puberty there is an increased sensitivity of Leydig cells to hCG stimulation even before basal serum testosterone levels increase.[49] During fetal differentiation, in the pubertal boy, and following exogenous LH or hCG stimulation, androgen secretion correlates with the development of Leydig cell SER, which contains the majority of the enzymes necessary for steroid synthesis.[50]

LH stimulation of testosterone synthesis and secretion is initiated by LH binding to hormone-specific receptors on the Leydig cell membranes[51, 52] (Fig. 6-5). Leydig cells also have membrane receptors for prolactin, and this hormone potentiates the effects of LH.[53, 54] LH interaction with its receptor stimulates the membrane-bound adenylyl cyclase which catalyzes the synthesis of cAMP. In addition to LH, fluoride ion, cholera toxin, and guanyl nucleotides (GTP and its analogues) stimulate cAMP formation. Studies of these stimulators have led to the conclusion that the adenylyl cyclase system is composed of three distinct membrane-bound units (Fig. 6-5). These include the hormone receptor, which contains the specific site for recognition of LH; the catalytic unit of adenylyl cyclase, which converts ATP to cAMP and PP; and the guanyl nucleotide regulatory subunit, which binds GTP and couples the hormone receptor to adenylyl cyclase.[55] Once cAMP is released into the cytoplasm of the Leydig cell, it binds to the regulatory subunit of protein kinase which then dissociates from and, in turn, activates the catalytic subunit of this enzyme.[56] The catalytic subunit of Leydig cell protein kinase is believed to activate a product which, in turn, facilitates conversion of cholesterol to pregnenolone and subsequent androgen synthesis (Fig. 6-5). Following LH stimulation, there is a marked rise in total intracellular cAMP, with maximal testosterone production occurring after less than a 10% increase in nucleotide. The total amount of cAMP in Leydig cells, therefore, does not correlate with testosterone secretion. Recent experiments have indicated that steroid synthesis can be directly correlated with the occupancy of the regulatory subunit sites by cAMP.[57] Although the immediate effects of LH on steroid synthesis are mediated by the cAMP–protein kinase system, it remains to be established whether the growth-promoting and the differentiating effects of LH also are operative via this mechanism.

The ability of the polypeptide hormones to regulate the concentration of their specific sites on target cells has been demonstrated in numerous tissues after the observation that insulin and growth hormone receptor concentrations are inversely related to the prevailing amount of the homologous hormone.[58, 59] In the testis, receptors for LH decrease following administration of this exogenous gonadotropin. These receptor-depleted cells are desensitized in that they have a decreased responsiveness to LH in accordance with the severity of the receptor loss.[60, 61] Under normal conditions, only a small fraction of LH receptors need be occupied in order to evoke maximal testosterone synthesis. This indicates that Leydig cells can contain considerable excess of reserve or spare receptors which have full biologic potential for adenylyl cyclase activation.[62]

The presence of excess receptors above the number required to mediate acute and maximal steroid response to LH has several implications. One is that full LH responsiveness of the adenylyl cyclase system could recover more rapidly than testicular receptors after LH-induced loss. Even after the ability of Leydig cells to respond to LH with a rise of cAMP has recovered, testosterone synthesis is still depressed, indicating that large doses of LH down-regulate Leydig cell activity beyond the generation of this cyclic nucleotide.[51, 52] All of these effects may account for the lower than expected testosterone secretion in patients with markedly elevated levels of hCG.[63] In addition, large doses of GnRH and its analogues reduce the number of LH receptors.[64-66] The releasing hormone decreases FSH and prolactin receptors as well.[67] That many of these effects are also seen in hypophysectomized an-

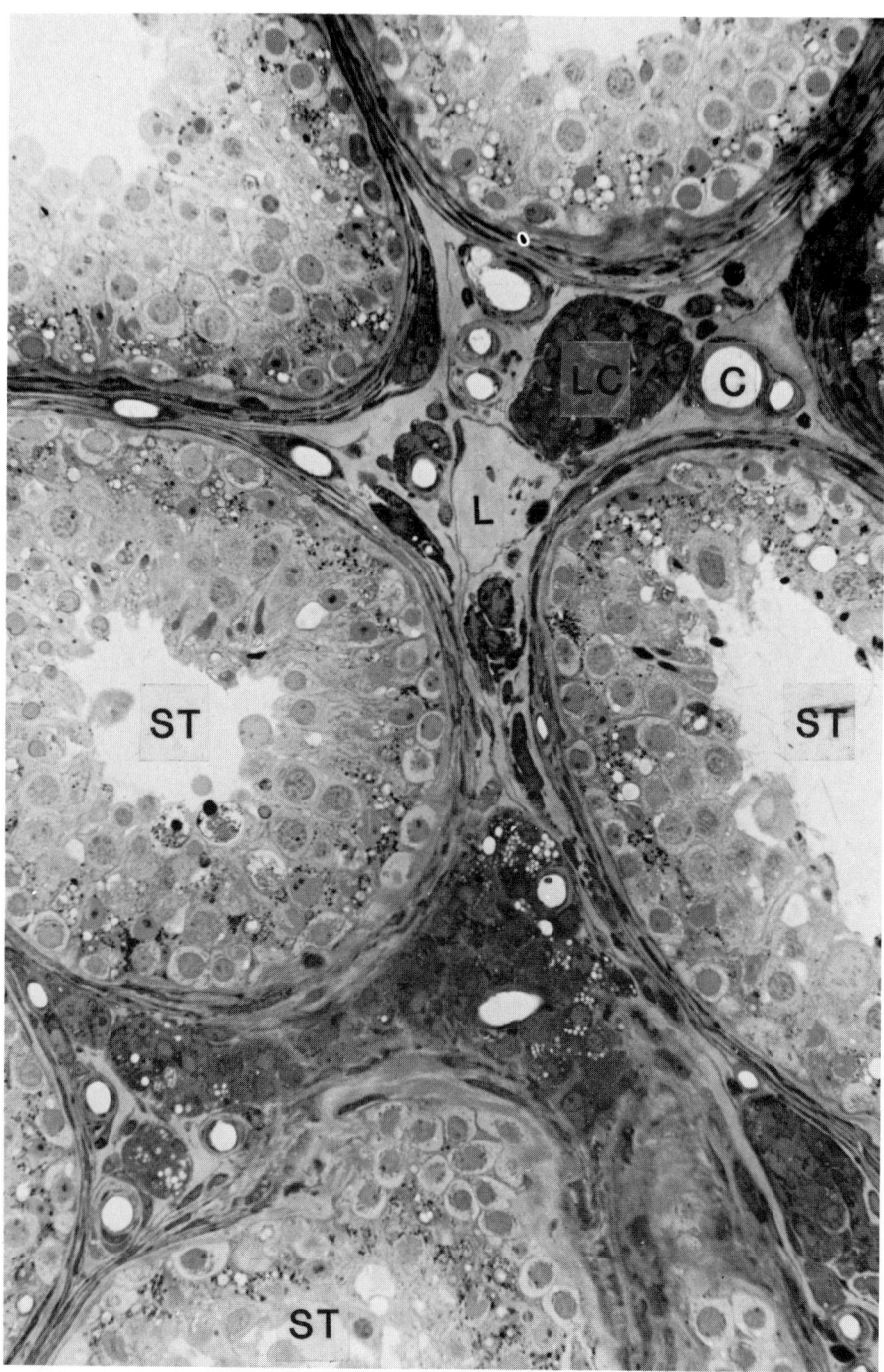

Figure 6–3. Light micrograph of human testis. Newly synthesized testosterone diffuses out of Leydig cell *(LC)* clusters to enter capillaries *(C)* and lymphatics *(L)*. This steroid also penetrates the seminiferous tubule *(ST)* to foster spermatogenesis. Leydig cells vary in the number of lipid droplets they contain. The droplets appear white in this micrograph since the lipid has been extracted during preparation for microscopy. A semi-thin Epon section fixed by perfusion with glutaraldehyde. The testis was removed from a 64-year-old man with prostate cancer. × 240. (From Christensen, A. K.: Leydig cells. In *Handbook of Physiology*, Section 7: Endocrinology. Vol. V: Male Reproductive System, Hamilton, D. W., and Greep, R. O. (eds.), Baltimore, Williams & Wilkins, 1975, pp. 57–94.)

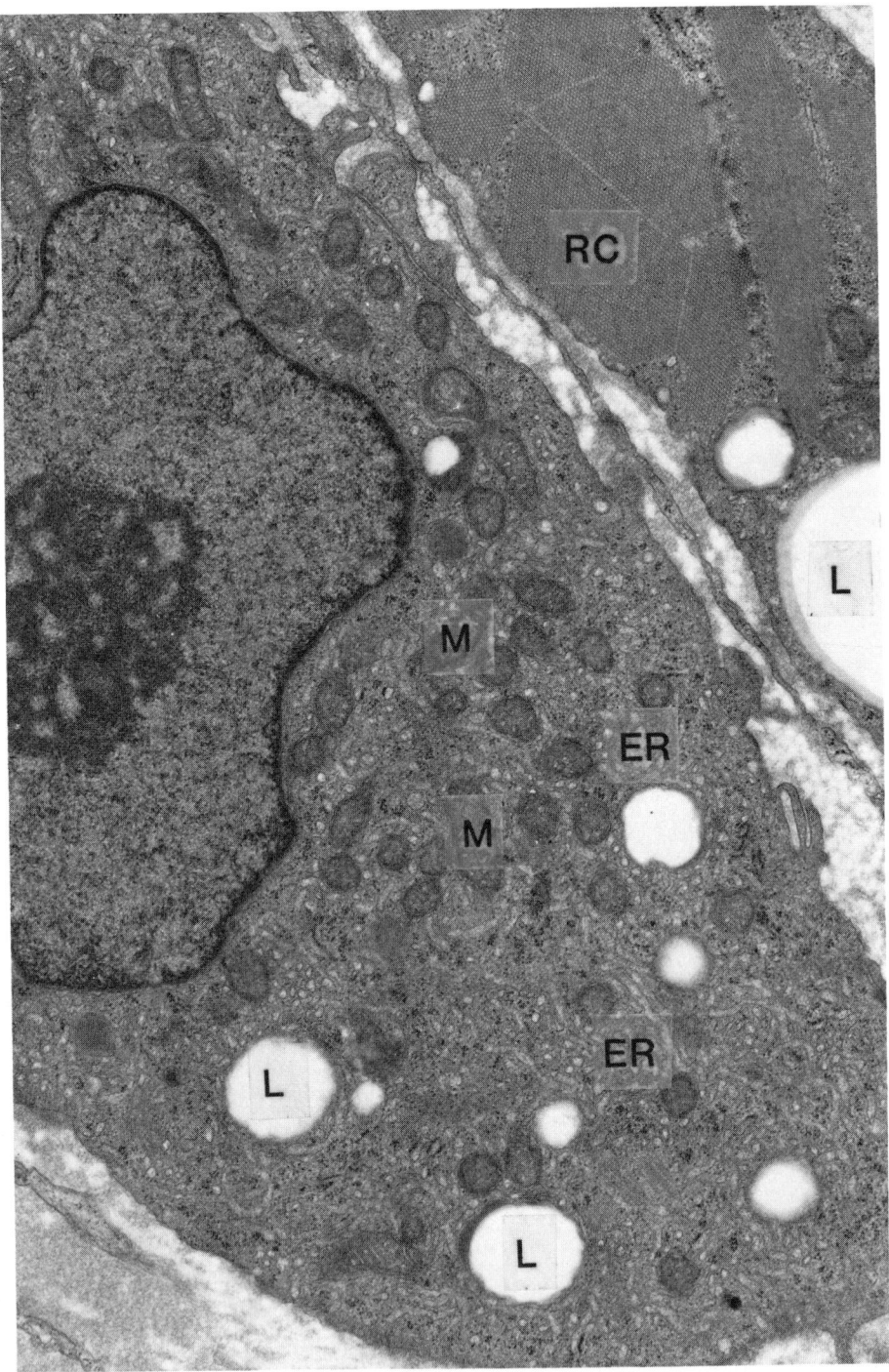

Figure 6–4. Cytoplasm of a human Leydig cell showing smooth endoplasmic reticulum *(ER)*, mitochondria *(M)*, and extracted lipid droplets *(L)*. The cell at the upper right includes an unusually large lipid droplet and several Reinke crystals *(RC)*. From a 22-year-old man with an ectopic testis. × 21000. (From Christensen, A. K.: Leydig cells. In *Handbook of Physiology*, Section 7: Endocrinology. Vol. V: Male Reproductive System, Hamilton, D. W., and Greep, R. O. (eds.) Baltimore, Williams & Wilkins, 1975, pp. 57–94.)

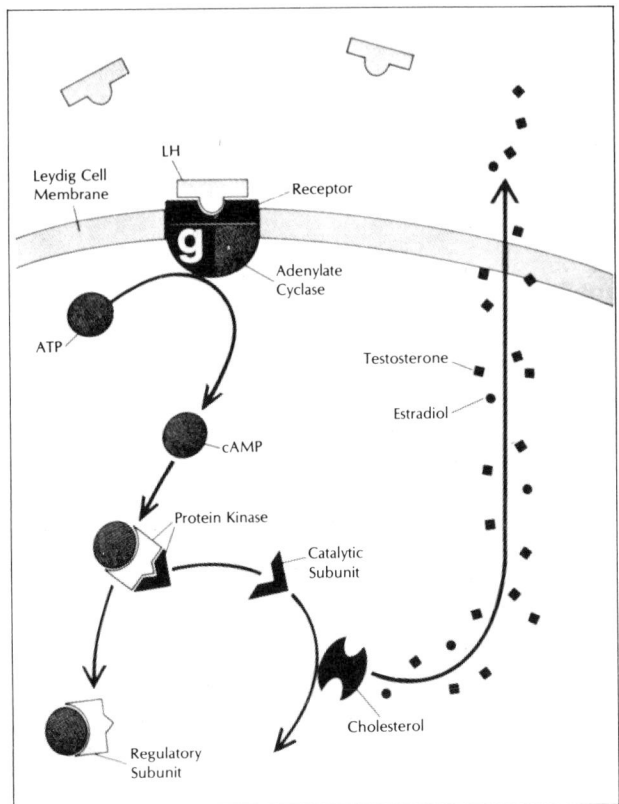

Figure 6–5. The action of LH on the Leydig cell. At the Leydig cell surface, LH interacts with a specific membrane receptor which is coupled to adenylyl cyclase by the guanyl nucleotide regulatory subunit (G). Adenylyl cyclase catalyzes the conversion of ATP to cAMP, which serves to activate a cytoplasmic protein kinase that is responsible for the conversion of cholesterol to sex steroids, primarily testosterone. A small amount of estradiol is also secreted by the Leydig cells, but in males most of the estrogen found in blood is made from testosterone in extragonadal tissue. (By Donner, C., from Bardin, C. W.: The neuroendocrinology of male reproduction. *Hospital Practice*, Vol. 14, No. 12, and from *Neuroendocrinology*. Krieger, D. K., and Hughes, J. C. (eds.), Sunderland, MA, Sinauer Associates, Inc., 1980, pp. 239–247. Reproduced with permission.)

imals has been taken as evidence that GnRH and its analogues have a direct effect on the testis in addition to their role on LH-mediated effects.[21]

In summary, the sensitivity of Leydig cells to LH can be regulated by prolactin, LH, and GnRH. Furthermore, *in vitro* studies indicate that vitamins and growth factors influence Leydig cell function.[68, 69] The fact that so many agents affect normal Leydig activity provides insight into how the activity of these cells can be altered in patients with a variety of systemic diseases.

Testicular Androgen Biosynthesis. Testosterone is the major androgen produced in the testis, and its primary site of synthesis is Leydig cells.[50] In these cells, cholesterol is synthesized from glucose and fatty acids. In addition, cholesterol can be accumulated from the blood. In the adrenal this pool of cholesterol is derived from low density lipoprotein and is a precursor of corticoids.[70] Recent studies indicate that the low density lipoprotein cholesterol may also be used in the testis. Leydig cell mitochondria, like those in the ovary and adrenal cortex, have the unique ability to cleave the cholesterol side chain to produce pregnenolone. This latter C-21 steroid is the precursor for steroid synthesis in all these organs. In the testis, pregnenolone is converted to testosterone by several microsomal enzymes, as shown in Figure 6–5. Although testosterone is the major secretory product of the testis, other intermediates are also produced, but they contribute very little to the overall androgen content in the blood of men.[50] This is in marked contrast to women, in whom dihydrotestosterone and androstenedione form a significant fraction of the total circulating androgens.[71, 72] Androstenedione (Fig. 6–6) is also secreted by the testis. This steroid is important as a precursor for blood estrogens in nonendocrine tissues. As noted below, androgens are the major origin of estrogens in men. Other testosterone precursors such as 17-hydroxyprogesterone and progesterone are also secreted by the testis, but their biologic function, if any, is not known. Mean blood levels of testosterone

Figure 6–6. Androgen biosynthesis in Leydig cells and estrogen production in nonglandular tissues. Cholesterol is synthesized in Leydig cells from acetate and is derived from low density lipoprotein (LDL) following its uptake by specific LDL receptors. In man the major pathway of biosynthesis is via the delta-5 pathway, including pregnenolone, 17-hydroxypregnenolone, and androstenediol. In other species, testosterone biosynthesis proceeds via the delta-4 pathway, including progesterone, 17-hydroxyprogesterone, and androstenedione. Testosterone and androstenedione are secreted into the blood and are converted to estrone and estradiol, respectively, at extraglandular sites in multiple tissues. The direct secretion of estradiol by the testis counts for only a small portion of this estrogen which enters the blood. In certain pathological conditions, such as Klinefelter's syndrome, the testicular secretion of estrogen is much more important. The concentrations of testosterone precursors secreted into the blood are shown in Table 6–1, and testosterone metabolism to products other than estrogens in peripheral tissue is shown in Figure 6–7. (From Bardin, C. W.: Pituitary-testicular axis. In *Reproductive Endocrinology*. Yen, S., and Jaffe, R. (eds.), Philadelphia, W. B. Saunders Co., 1978, pp. 110–125.)

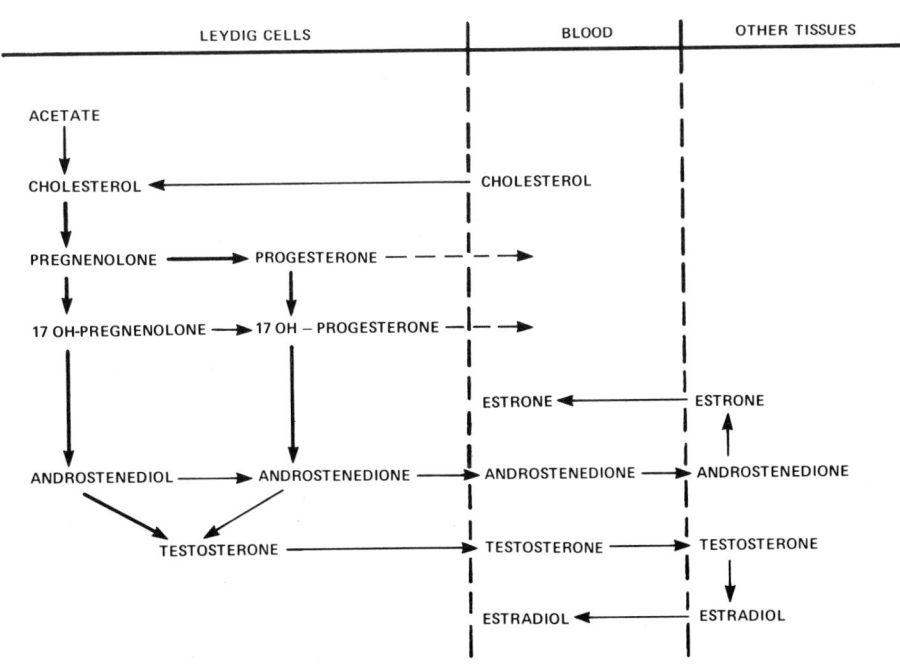

Table 6–1. THE PLASMA CONCENTRATION OF SPERMATIC AND PERIPHERAL VENOUS STEROIDS

Steroid	Spermatic Vein (ng/dl)	Peripheral Vein (ng/dl)
Testosterone	10,000–60,000	250–1,000
Dihydrotestosterone	60– 800	10– 45
Androsterone	40– 1,100	15– 40
Androstenedione	110– 1,200	40– 110
17α-Hydroxyprogesterone	110–10,000	40– 110
Progesterone	110– 1,100	10– 60
Pregnenolone	110– 1,200	30– 100

Blood samples from the spermatic vein were collected from patients with carcinoma of the prostate, hernia, varicocele, and hydrocele under local anesthesia. (From Hammond, G. L., et al.: The simultaneous radioimmuno-assay of seven steroids in human spermatic and peripheral venous blood. *J. Clin. Endocrinol. Metab.* 45:16–24, 1977.)

and its steroid precursors in spermatic and peripheral venous blood are summarized in Table 6–1. The daily production rates of the major sex steroids in man are summarized in Table 6–2.

Transport of steroids from the site of production through pericellular membrane structures to spermatic venous blood is not completely understood. Although testosterone can bind to albumin and steroid-binding globulins, it is not known whether these or other proteins from Leydig cells participate in androgen transport from the interstitial portion of the testis into blood. Since the flow of testicular lymph is only 0.01% that of blood flow and concentrations of testosterone in these fluids are similar, the major route for steroid exit from the testis into the general circulation is via the spermatic venous blood.[50]

In contrast to LH, the minute-to-minute oscillation of testosterone secretion is relatively small. It is difficult to define a "testosterone pulse" in man which corresponds to those of LH (see Fig. 6–2). There is evidence, however, for a circadian rhythm of testosterone secretion in young men. The acrophase of the rhythm is about the time of awakening and the nadir is in the evening; the amplitude is small (10–25%). It is established that there is a sleep-related rise in LH and testosterone levels during puberty in boys.[73] The circadian rhythm of testosterone may be a persistence of a sleep-related rise in this steroid in young adults[74] which ultimately disappears with advancing age.[39] In addition to the daily variations, 8- to 30-day cycles of testosterone levels have been described in 60% of men which range from 9 to 28% of the mean values.[75]

Testosterone Transport in Plasma. Once testosterone is secreted into the spermatic venous blood, it is eventual-

Table 6–2. ANDROGEN PLASMA LEVELS AND PRODUCTION RATES IN NORMAL MEN AND WOMEN

	Plasma Concentration (ng/dl)	Production Rate (μg/day)
Testosterone		
Men	700	7000
Women	40	300
Androstenedione		
Men	100	2500
Women	170	3500
Dihydrotestosterone		
Men	30	300
Women	20	60

ly bound to plasma proteins. One of the proteins that binds testosterone with high affinity is testosterone-estradiol–binding globulin (TeBG). This is a beta-globulin that is distinct from cortisol-binding globulin, the major transport protein for cortisol, corticosterone, and progesterone.[76]

The physical properties of TeBG have now been elucidated following its isolation in fully active form from plasma.[77, 78] TeBG is an 80,000–94,000 molecular weight protein that has 30–34% carbohydrate and one binding site per mole. Under denaturing conditions, TeBG separates into two subunits[79] with considerable microheterogeneity. This, in turn, is due to its variable sialic acid content.[80] As with other glycoproteins, removal of sialic acid leads to an increased rate of removal from blood.[81]

The concentration of TeBG in plasma is increased five to ten fold by estrogen and is decreased twofold in women by testosterone. In men, TeBG is higher than normal in hypogonadal patients, and the values decline following testosterone replacement. In addition, excess thyroid hormone increases TeBG, and decreased levels of this protein are found in hypothyroid individuals. Finally, TeBG is also elevated in the plasma of patients with cirrhosis and other metabolic disorders.[82] The clinical conditions associated with changes in TeBG concentration are summarized in Table 6–3.

In the blood of men, only 2% of testosterone is free; 30% is bound to TeBG, and 68% to albumin and other plasma proteins.[83] It was once assumed that free testosterone was the biologically important fraction of blood androgens. This postulate was supported by the observation that clinical androgenicity correlates with free testosterone in blood.[84, 85] However, studies by Vermeulen et al.[86] first suggested that in humans the rate of testosterone metabolism correlates directly with the quantity of free plus albumin-bound testosterone and inversely with the TeBG concentration in plasma. These observations show that TeBG-bound androgens are not readily available for *in vivo* metabolism. The fact that testosterone metabolism is required for expression of biologic activity in reproductive tissues and skin argues that both free and albumin-bound testosterone enter tissues where they are available for full biologic activity. These considerations question the current wisdom about the usefulness of free testosterone measurement to assess clinical androgenicity. In addition, recent *in vitro* studies on human prostate slices indicate that TeBG determines the metabolic rate of testosterone independent of its effect on plasma binding.[87] This may relate to the fact that TeBG may enter androgen-responsive cells.[88] Regardless of these considerations, the fact that TeBG is not present in the plasma of all species suggests that this binding protein does not play an essential role in the mechanism of action of androgens.[89] In species that synthesize this protein, including man, it is presumed that TeBG is made in the liver. The interesting relationship between TeBG and androgen-binding protein (ABP), a secretory protein of Sertoli cells, is discussed later.

The Metabolism of Testosterone and Other Androgens. The *in vivo* metabolism of testosterone or any other androgen may be defined as irreversible removal from the circulation as a result of enzymatic modification of steroid structure. It was once supposed that steroid metabolism served only as a method for hormone inactivation prior to excretion. Recent studies have indicated, however, that in some tissues testosterone metabolism is required as an essential step in the expression of its biologic activity. In view of this, it is not surprising to find that testosterone metabolism is altered in a variety of

Table 6–3. DIFFERENT WAYS OF ASSESSING TESTOSTERONE METABOLISM IN MEN AND WOMEN AND IN PATIENTS WITH VARIOUS DISEASES

Patients	MCR^T	TeBG	Skin 5α-Reductase Activity In Vitro		In Vivo	Androsterone: Etiocholanolone Ratio in Urine
			Pubic Skin	Genital Skin		
Normal men	+++	+	+++	++++	2.7	normal
Estrogen-treated men	+	+++	+	----	—	—
Hypogonadal boys	+	++	+	++++	1.0	normal
Androgen-treated boys	+++	+	+++	++++		
Normal women	+	++	++	++++	1.9	normal
Prepubertal girls	+			++++		normal
Hirsute women	+++	+	+++			
Complete Tfm	++	++	+++		1.0	
Partial Tfm	---		++			
5α-reductase deficiency			±	±	1.0	low
Acute intermittent porphyria	---	---	--	---	2.0	low
Barbiturate treatment	slight decrease	no change	--	---	—	low
Anorexia nervosa	---	---	--	---	—	low
Hypothyroid men and women	increase	+	--	---	—	low
Hyperthyroid men and women	decrease	+++	--	---	—	high
17-Alkylated androgen–treated women	+++	+	--	---	—	high
Flutamide-treated men	---	+	--	---	—	high
Cirrhosis	decrease	++	--	---	—	high
References	91, 92, 114, 115	92, 107, 109	100, 106, 108, 118	100, 106	99, 103, 107	102, 103, 109–112, 116

Abbreviations: MCR^T = metabolic clearance rate of testosterone; TeBG = testosterone-estradiol–binding globulin; Tfm = testicular feminization.

metabolic disorders and in clinical conditions involving masculinization. Although there are many enzymes that can modify testosterone, fluctuations of 5α-reductase and aromatase activities are the most relevant to the clinician. As a consequence, the discussion in this and the next section will emphasize the reactions catalyzed by these enzymes.

The metabolic clearance rate of testosterone (MCR^T) is one measure of irreversible removal or metabolism of this steroid.[90] The MCR^T is determined by measuring the rate of disappearance of radioactive testosterone from the blood. The MCR^T is greater in men than in women and prepubertal boys. Some of the clinical conditions associated with changes in MCR^T are summarized in Table 6–3. In women, androgen treatment and excess testosterone production secondary to adrenal or gonadal disease are associated with an increase in MRC^T. In view of this increased rate of metabolism, the plasma testosterone remains in the normal range in mildly virilized individuals (women with hirsutism) with only a one to two fold increase in testosterone production.[91] From studies involving hepatic vein catheterization it is possible to ascertain that almost all of the testosterone in women is cleared by the liver. In hirsute women and men, 30-50% of testosterone degradation occurs in extrahepatic sites,[92, 93] where its virilizing effects are manifest.

As already noted, MCR^T is in part determined by the binding of this steroid to plasma proteins. In effect, steroid-protein interactions will influence the rate at which testosterone leaves the extracellular compartment. As a general rule, when the concentration of TeBG is high, MCR^T is low, and vice versa (Table 6–3). Once in the cell, testosterone can reenter the extracellular space unchanged or it can be metabolized. Whether metabolism occurs depends upon the activities of enzymes that either oxidize or reduce steroids. Depending on the cell, testosterone may be metabolized (1) to a more active androgen that exerts its action on that cell or in some other tissue;

(2) to a less active or an inactive metabolite that is conjugated and excreted into the urine; or (3) to a steroid, such as estradiol, that has a different biologic activity than its precursor (estrogen formation from androgen is discussed in the next section). These examples of testosterone metabolism are summarized in Figures 6–6 and 6–7.

In one of the important pathways of androgen metabolism the biopotency of testosterone is amplified by 5α-reductase. In extrahepatic tissues such as the skin this enzyme reduces testosterone to dihydrotestosterone (5α-DHT). In addition, it participates in the conversion of androstenedione and dehydroepiandrosterone to 5α-DHT. This latter hormone is 2.5 times more potent than testosterone in several bioassay systems.[92] Dihydrotestosterone may be metabolized to the 5α-androstenediols (Fig. 6–7). Although these are also potent androgens, their biologic activities when administered systemically depend upon their conversion to 5α-DHT in the cell.[94] In the adult male, the production of the 5α-reduced androgens from testosterone occurs most notably in the male reproductive tract and skin where these steroids stimulate cell division. Since skin is one of the most accessible organs, much of our knowledge about the significance of 5α-reductase in humans has been derived from in vitro studies of testosterone metabolism in slices, homogenates, hair follicles, or fibroblast cultures prepared from this organ.[95-98] The metabolism of testosterone by skin has also been studied in vivo by an ingenious method devised by Mauvais-Jarvis and his colleagues[99] using the simultaneous percutaneous and intravenous administration of [^{3}H]-testosterone and [^{14}C]-testosterone, respectively. Using both in vitro and in vivo approaches, it has been possible to demonstrate that the activity of 5α-reductase varies with age, hormonal status, and anatomic location (Table 6–3). In the fetus, significant 5α-reductase activity is present in skin from the genital tubercle (phallus and scrotum) before the onset of testicular testosterone secretion. By contrast, this enzyme activity is low in the skin

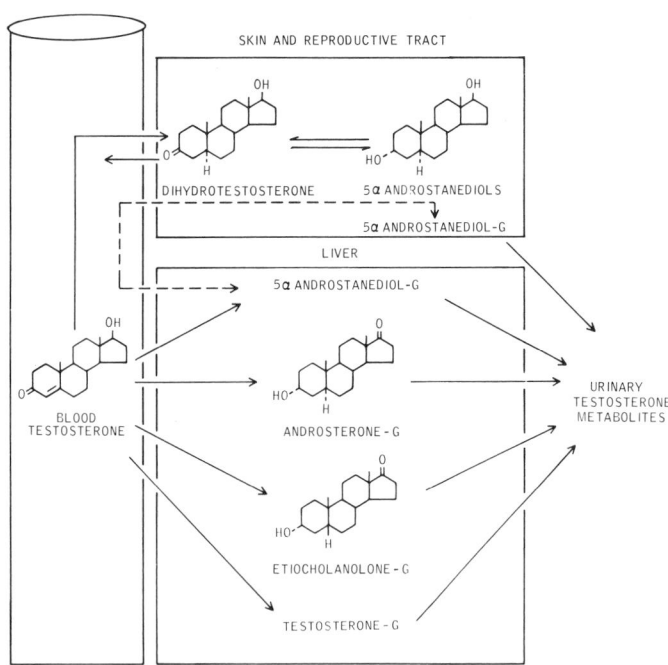

Figure 6–7. Testosterone and its important C-19 metabolites. In skin and reproductive tract, testosterone is metabolized by 5α-reductase to dihydrotestosterone which is, in turn, converted to 5α-androstanediol. The "diols" may be "back-converted" to dihydrotestosterone or may reenter the blood for subsequent hepatic metabolism. In the liver, testosterone is primarily converted to androsterone and etiocholanolone, which, along with other androgen metabolites, are conjugated to form glucuronides (G) or sulfates. These conjugates then reenter the blood and are excreted in the urine. Recent evidence indicates that a large fraction of the 5α-androstanediol formed in extrahepatic tissues is converted to the glucuronide at the site of synthesis rather than the liver (R. Horton, personal communication). This latter observation in part explains why urinary 5α-androstanediol-G is a good measure of extrahepatic androgen metabolism. Since 5α-reductase is androgen-dependent, urinary 5α-androstanediol-G is an index of virilization (see Table 6–6).

of other androgen-responsive sites prior to puberty, and it increases only after androgen exposure.[100, 101] As a consequence, total 5α-reductase activity in these tissues is lower in women, prepubertal children, and patients with testicular feminization than in men, androgen-treated hypogonadal boys, and hirsute women (Table 6–3). It is of interest that the increased enzyme activity in these latter groups correlates with the high extrahepatic clearance of testosterone.[92, 93]

Approximately 50% of the testosterone that enters this splanchnic circulation is metabolized in a single passage.[93] The major products of testosterone metabolism (60-70%) in the liver are androsterone and etiocholanolone, which are reduced in the 5α- and 5β-positions, respectively (Fig. 6–7). Both of these metabolites are excreted in the urine as glucuronides and sulfates. The ratio of androsterone to etiocholanolone in urine has been used as an index of hepatic 5α-reductase activity. Interestingly, patients with acute intermittent porphyria have a marked deficiency of hepatic but not cutaneous 5α-reductase activity.[102, 103] In this disorder the 5α-metabolites of testosterone and other steroids accumulate and are believed to make these individuals more susceptible to recurrent attacks. The relative activity of 5α-reductase in liver is also decreased in hypothyroidism, anorexia nervosa, and phenobarbital treatment (Table 6–3) and with advancing age, particularly in women.[104] An increase in the relative activity of hepatic 5α-reductase, as is suggested by an increase in urinary androsterone-etiocholanolone ratio, occurs in cirrhosis and following treatment with 17-alkylated androgens, flutamide, and thyroid hormones (Table 6–3).

Testosterone and 5α-androstanediol glucuronides are among the other androgen metabolites that are measured in urine (Fig. 6–7). Testosterone glucuronide originates predominantly in the liver from plasma testosterone, androstenedione, and dehydroepiandrosterone.[105] By contrast, 5α-androstanediol glucuronides arise as a consequence of testosterone metabolism in both the skin and liver. Since an increased 5α-reductase in skin and other extrahepatic tissues is produced by increased androgen secretion, the measurement of 5α-androstanediol glucuronides has been recommended as an index of clinical androgenicity.[100]

In summary, androgen metabolism in man has been examined with a variety of techniques including (1) estimation of the MCR^T, which is a measure of the rate of total body metabolism; (2) quantification of the rate of testosterone conversion to 5α-steroids by skin, which is an estimate of 5α-reductase activity; and (3) measurement of urinary testosterone metabolites, which are a reflection of hepatic metabolism with or without an extrahepatic component. It is significant that each of these approaches measures, to some extent, a different set of parameters of androgen metabolism, which are, in turn, modified by disease in different ways (Table 6–3). In general, a high MCR^T correlates with a low TeBG concentration and an increased 5α-reductase activity in extrahepatic tissues. Each of these, in turn, relates to increased androgen production. Finally, hepatic testosterone metabolism rarely correlates with that in other tissues except in the genetically determined 5α-reductase deficiency syndrome (Table 6–3).

Blood Androgens as the Origin of Blood Estrogens in Men. Estrone and estradiol are the important blood estrogens in men (see Fig. 6–6). Following orchiectomy, the levels of both of these steroid hormones decrease.[105] Furthermore, administration of hCG increases estrogen levels.[119, 120] These observations suggest that the testes secrete estrogens, and subsequent studies have indicated that both Leydig and Sertoli cells can synthesize these hormones.[121, 122] However, attempts to identify estrone and estradiol in spermatic venous blood indicated that only 10-20% of these steroids could be accounted for by gonadal secretion.[123, 124] Similarly, measurement of estrogens in adrenal venous blood suggested that this endocrine gland could account for only a small fraction of the total estrogens in the blood. The origin of the major portion of blood estrogens in men was first suggested by the observation that patients treated with large doses of testosterone for hypogonadism developed gynecomastia.[123] It was subsequently demonstrated that intravenously administered testosterone is converted to estradiol, which reenters the blood.[105] Many nonendocrine tissues, including brain,

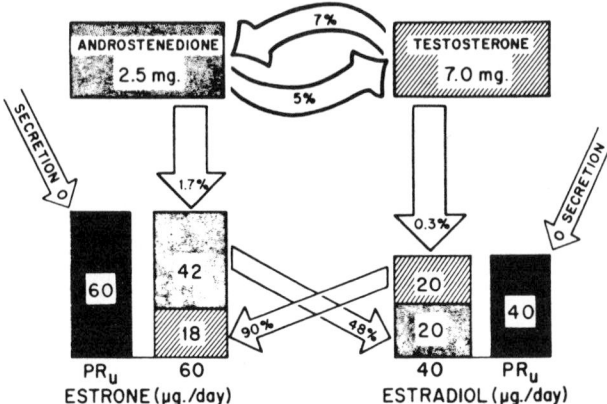

Figure 6–8. Analysis of androgen and estrogen production in normal men. The production rates of androstenedione (2.5 mg/day) and testosterone (7 mg/day) were determined from the product of the metabolic clearance rates times the plasma concentrations of each steroid. The production rates (PR$_u$) of estrone (60 μg/day) and estradiol (40 μg/day) were measured from the specific activity of a urinary metabolite following the administration of each of the [³H]-estrogens. The fraction of androstenedione (1.7%) and testosterone (0.3%) converted to each of the estrogens was also determined from the specific activity of a urinary metabolite. By using this technique the entire production of estrone and estradiol could be explained by synthesis in extraglandular tissue from androgens. This kinetic method is not sensitive enough to detect the small amount of each estrogen that is secreted. (From MacDonald, P. C., et al.: In *Gonadal Steroid Secretion.* Beard, D. T., and Strong, J. A. (eds.), Edinburgh, Edinburgh University Press, 1971, pp. 158–174.)

skin, fat, and liver, are known to have the cytochrome P-450–dependent aromatase required for conversion of androgens to estrogens, and whole-body kinetic experiments demonstrated conclusively that the major portions of blood estradiol and estrone in normal men are derived from blood testosterone and androstenedione, respectively.[124] The quantitative aspects of this extraglandular estrogen production from androgens are summarized in Figure 6–8.

The origin and mechanism of action of estrogen are even more complex in men with endocrinopathies that suggest estrogen dominance. First, it is worthy of note that normal men do not become feminized even though the production rates of estrogens are similar to those of women during the early follicular phase of the menstrual cycle. In some men, total estrogen production from all sources is normal and the only demonstrable abnormality is decreased testosterone secretion. In these individuals, feminization (as manifested by gynecomastia) relates to an increase in estrogen relative to androgen rather than to the absolute levels of these hormones.[126] These observations suggest that one of the actions of testosterone on tissues such as the breast is to diminish the action of estrogen. As a consequence, in these patients feminization occurs for lack of an effective masculinizing hormone at the end organ. Feminization also occurs in a number of clinical disorders in which there are blocked or abnormal androgen receptors. Testicular feminization is a notable example of the latter condition.[125, 127] In these individuals, marked breast development occurs as a result of unopposed estrogen action in a patient with end-organ insensitivity to androgens. As a consequence, patients with testicular feminization may be 10 times more sensitive to estrogens than normal individuals.[99] Commonly used drugs such as cimetidine, spironolactone, and digitalis reduce the effective androgen by competitively binding to androgen receptor.[128-131] This results in modest gyneco-

mastia in some men which is thought by some to represent mild feminization.

Other groups of patients become feminized because of increased amounts of estradiol and estrone in the blood. There are several reasons for increased production of these steroids, including: (1) increased glandular secretion of estrone or estradiol, as occurs from the testes in Klinefelter's syndrome;[132] (2) increased secretion of an estrogen precursor such as androstenedione from a feminizing adrenal tumor;[133] and (3) increased aromatase activity (with normal plasma precursor levels), as occurs prior to puberty and spontaneously in some apparently normal individuals.[134] Finally, obese men have increased estrogen production but do not become feminized, suggesting that they have an estrogen receptor defect.[135] The clinical conditions associated with abnormal estrogen production and action are summarized in Table 6–10 later in this chapter.

Androgen Action

Physiology of Androgens. The biologic actions of testosterone and its metabolites have been classified according to their sites of action. All effects that relate to growth of the male reproductive tract or to development of secondary sexual characteristics have been termed the "androgenic" action of this class of steroid, while the effects on somatic tissues, such as the liver, kidney, bone, and muscle, have been termed "anabolic." Earlier studies suggested that these might be two independent biologic actions of the same class of steroids.[136] Subsequent experiments, however, have suggested that these are organ-specific responses and that the molecular mechanisms that initiate androgen action are the same as or similar to those that stimulate anabolic responses. At present, it is therefore customary to classify the action of steroids according to their molecular mechanisms of action.[137] The importance of this approach may be illustrated by the fact that testosterone, progesterone, estradiol, cortisol, growth hormone, prolactin, insulin, and thyroxine have anabolic effects on several tissues, but each via a separate hormone receptor.

Testosterone and other androgens have some biologic activity on almost every organ in the body. These widespread effects as seen at puberty in boys are summarized in Table 6–4. All of the actions listed are considered phys-

Table 6–4. PUBERTAL CHANGES DUE TO TESTOSTERONE SECRETION

External genitalia
  The penis and scrotum increase in size and become pigmented. Rugal folds appear in the scrotal skin.

Hair growth
  Mustache and beard develop and scalp line undergoes recession. Pubic hair grows upward into the typical diamond-shape pattern of the male escutcheon. Axillary, body, extremity, and perianal hair appears.

Linear growth
  Until puberty, linear growth is fairly stable at about 2 inches per year. At puberty, there is a growth spurt which increases the rate to about 3 inches per year.

Accessory sex organs
  The prostate becomes palpable and the other organs, such as the seminal vesicles, enlarge over the next 4 to 5 years. Secretory activity develops.

Voice
  The voice pitch is lowered because of enlargement of the larynx and thickening of the vocal cords.

Psyche
  More aggressive attitudes are manifest; libido and sexual potentia develop.

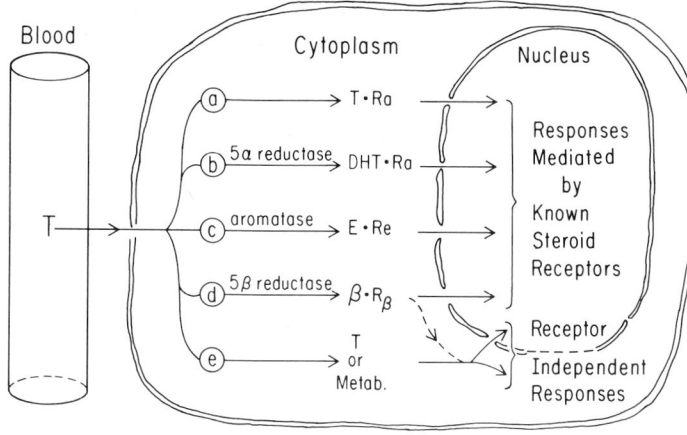

Figure 6-9. The mechanisms of action of testosterone (T). In the blood, T is transported by TeBG, albumin, and other proteins. Free and albumin-bound T are believed to enter the tissue by passive diffusion. The known pathways of T metabolism that lead to biologic activity in various tissues are summarized as though they occurred in a single cell. T leaves the blood and enters the cell by diffusion. In the cytoplasm, T can react in the following ways: (a) without being metabolized, T binds directly to the androgen receptor (Ra), and the steroid-receptor complex (T·Ra) is then transferred to nuclear acceptor sites in chromatin for initiation of the steroid-specific responses; (b) T is metabolized by 5α-reductase to 5α-dihydrotestosterone (DHT) which then binds to Ra, and the steroid-receptor complex (DHT-Ra) is bound in the nucleus where it initiates responses; (c) T is aromatized to estradiol (E) which binds to estrogen receptor (Re), and the E-Re complex is transferred and bound in nuclei as for (a) and (b); (d) T is metabolized to 5β-metabolites (β) which bind to the β-steroid receptor (Rβ), and the steroid-receptor complex (β-Rβ) presumably acts in the nucleus; (e) T or one of its metabolites (metab.) acts in the nucleus or cytoplasm by mechanisms which are independent of known receptors ("receptor-independent responses"). (From Bardin, C. W., and Catterall, J. F.: Testosterone: A major determinant of extragenital sexual dimorphism. *Science* 211:1285, 1981, Copyright 1981 by the American Association for the Advancement of Science.)

iologic responses of this group of steroids with the possible exception of the effect on behavior, which is considered to be a pharmacologic, or even a toxic, effect by some observers. The early steps in the testosterone activation of most tissues are summarized in Figure 6-9. In most tissues these actions are mediated by way of the androgen receptor with either testosterone or 5α-DHT as ligand. In addition, some of the effects of testosterone are also mediated by the estrogen receptor either before[138] or after aromatization. In tissue such as bone marrow the effects of testosterone are mediated by 5β-steroid receptor. Finally, intracellular effectors such as cAMP may also facilitate selected androgen responses in some tissues.[139]

The Importance of 5α-Reductase. As already noted, testosterone is metabolized by 5α-reductase to 5α-DHT. In adults, the activity of this enzyme is high in skin, prostate, seminal vesicle, and epididymis, so that 5α-DHT is the dominant intracellular androgen in these tissues (Fig. 6-9). The distribution of 5α-reductase activity in the adult is strikingly different from that in the fetus. In the developing embryo, there is very little 5α-reductase in wolffian ducts until after androgen-dependent differentiation of the primordial epididymis, seminal vesicle, and vas deferens. As a consequence, 5α-DHT cannot be important for differentiation of the wolffian ducts. By contrast, this latter steroid is essential for development of the prostate and the derivatives of the genital tubercle that have 5α-reductase activity well before the onset of androgen biosynthesis in the fetus.[125]

The importance of dihydrotestosterone as a differentiating androgen in the fetus was established following the description of men with inherited deficiency of 5α-reductase.[116, 118] This disorder has been particularly well studied in numerous related families living in an isolated community in the Dominican Republic. Males with this disorder are born with ambiguous genitalia; they have testes, epididymides, vasa deferentia, and seminal vesicles but lack well developed prostates, phalluses, and scrota. These individuals have normal testosterone levels, but cannot form 5α-reduced steroid metabolites. As a consequence, no tissue, including the male reproductive tract, is ever exposed to high levels of dihydrotestosterone. These observations are consistent with the hypothesis that in the male fetus 5α-DHT is required for differentiation of some tissues while testosterone will suffice for others. Since androgens do not have known functions in the differentiation of the female fetus, women with 5α-reductase deficiency are apparently normal.

The Importance of the Androgen Receptor. One of the first steps of androgen action is the binding of testosterone or dihydrotestosterone to an intracellular protein that is termed the androgen receptor (Fig. 6-9). The presence of this protein in a tissue is a major determinant of whether it will respond to androgens. Following the interaction with testosterone or dihydrotestosterone the steroid-receptor complex binds to specific sites on chromatin called the nuclear acceptor. Interaction of the steroid-receptor complex with its acceptor results in a striking increase in nuclear metabolism. This includes an increase in chromatin template activity, an increase in the activities of RNA polymerases, increases in the number of initiation sites on chromatin, and an increase in the synthesis of all classes of RNA. These events lead to transfer of messenger RNA to cytoplasm, which results in protein synthesis. This process (along with DNA synthesis in some tissues) results in growth and development of differentiated function.[139]

The necessity of the androgen receptor for the growth and differentiation is illustrated in animals and humans with the sex-linked recessive defect testicular feminization (Tfm/Y). Individuals with this disorder lack androgen-dependent development of wolffian duct derivatives and the external genitalia. As a consequence, genetic males with a complete form of this disorder appear as phenotypic females with abdominal testes. These male pseudohermaphrodites cannot be masculinized by large doses of either testosterone or dihydrotestosterone.[94]

Early studies demonstrated that rats and mice with Tfm/y could not transfer androgen bound to receptor to the nuclei of responsive tissues (Fig. 6-10). These observations suggested that there was an abnormality of the androgen receptor,[140, 141] and this was later shown to be the case (Fig. 6-10) not only in rodents but also in men. Some animals and humans with this disorder have a small amount of "residual receptor" with a variable ability to bind androgens;[142, 143] some individuals have a reduced amount of normal receptor; some, a receptor with a reduced binding affinity; and others, a receptor that will bind androgens normally but will not activate nuclear RNA metabolism.[144] At present none of these receptor defects have been uniquely associated with any of the clinical syndromes believed to arise because of androgen insensitivity, including complete and partial testicular feminization, Reifenstein's syndrome,[145] gynecomastia,[146] and oligospermia.[147] A more extensive discussion of androgen-dependent differentiation in male pseudoher-

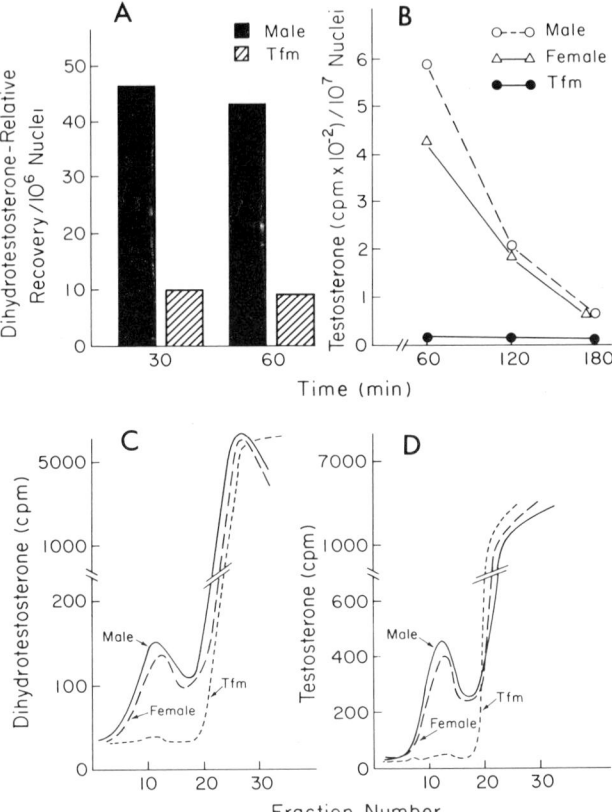

Figure 6-10. Androgen receptor deficiency in animals with testicular feminization (Tfm). *a*, The uptake of 5α-dihydrotestosterone in preputial gland nuclei of normal male and Tfm rats injected intravenously with [³H]-testosterone. The preputial gland is a skin derivative with 5α-reductase which is equally active in normal males and animals with Tfm. The reduced uptake of dihydrotestosterone in the nuclei of Tfm rats is due to reduced amounts of androgen receptor. *b*, Similarly, the uptake of [³H]-testosterone in kidney nuclei of Tfm mice is dramatically reduced below that of normal males and females. The mouse kidney has very little 5α-reductase activity so no dihydrotestosterone is detected. *c*, Binding of [³H]-dihydrotestosterone by preputial gland cytosols from male, female, and Tfm rats. *d*, Binding of [³H]-testosterone by kidney cytosols from male, female, and Tfm mice. Cytosols were incubated with [³H]-labeled steroids and analyzed on sucrose gradients. The androgen receptors in normal animals sedimented at 7S and 8S in fractions 10 to 14. Very little androgen receptor was detected in Tfm animals. (*a* from Bullock, L. P., and Bardin, C. W.: Decreased dihydrotestosterone retention by preputial gland nuclei from the androgen insensitive pseudohermaphrodite rat. *J. Clin. Endocrinol. Metab.* 31:113, 1970. *b* from Bullock, L. P., et al.: The androgen insensitive mouse: absence of intranuclear androgen retention in the kidney. *Biochem. Biophys. Res. Commun.* 44:1537, 1971. *c* and *d* From Bullock, L. P., and Bardin, C. W.: Androgen receptors in testicular feminization. *J. Clin. Endocrinol. Metab.* 35:935, 1972.)

maphrodites with 5α-reductase and androgen receptor deficiencies is presented in Chapter 9.

Hormonal Control of the Hypothalamo–Pituitary–Leydig Cell Axis

Negative and Positive Feedback of Luteinizing Hormone. The rate of testosterone synthesis and secretion by Leydig cells is primarily dependent upon the LH secreted into the blood. The secretion of this gonadotropin is reciprocally controlled by the action of sex steroids on the hypothalamus and pituitary. When either androgen or estrogen concentrations in the blood increase, LH levels decline, and this response is termed the "suppressive phase of negative feedback." When gonadal steroid levels decline, LH levels in-

crease. This has been termed the "recovery phase of negative feedback." The alternate suppression and recovery phases of the negative feedback control of LH secretion are regulated through the interaction of the hypothalamus, pituitary, and Leydig cells so that blood testosterone levels remain relatively constant from hour to hour. By contrast, "positive feedback" is a transient increase in LH occurring in response to prolonged exposure to estrogens. When this occurs LH secretion first decreases owing to elevated estrogen levels (negative feedback), and if the hormonal stimulus is maintained, then a large burst of LH secretion results as a positive response to estrogen. Positive feedback is readily observed in women as the stimulus for the midcycle LH surge, and in men it is most easily demonstrated in hypergonadotropic states. The features of negative and positive feedback control of LH are described in the following paragraphs.

Both testosterone and estradiol can inhibit LH secretion. It was, therefore, possible that the androgen effects on gonadotropin release were induced by estrogenic metabolites. This hypothesis was substantiated by the observations that brain tissue contains high concentrations of aromatase[148] and by the fact that estrogen receptors are partially filled in castrated animals following treatment with testosterone.[149] In spite of these considerations, a number of lines of evidence suggest that estradiol and testosterone exert independent negative feedback effects on LH secretion. First, acute infusions of estradiol (6–96 hours) reduced the amplitude and increased the frequency of the spontaneous LH discharges, whereas acute infusions of testosterone (6–96 hours) reduced the frequency of each LH discharge and increased its amplitude.[38, 150] These divergent effects of acute testosterone and estradiol administration on the pattern of LH secretion, along with the observation that the nonaromatizable androgens, dihydrotestosterone and fluoxymestrone,[38, 151, 152] can also suppress LH, indicate that androgen conversion to estrogen is not a prerequisite for its action on the hypothalamus and pituitary. This conclusion is supported by studies in patients with complete and partial androgen resistance (Tfm/Y). These individuals have significantly elevated plasma LH levels which are not suppressible by endogenous testosterone or administration of large amounts of dehydrotestosterone.[146] Interestingly, these patients have an increase in the number of LH secretory episodes (per 24 hours) suggestive of increased estrogen action. Even though estradiol production in these patients is moderately elevated, this is not sufficient to maintain LH levels in the normal range. Nonetheless, administration of additional exogenous estrogen will suppress this gonadotropin in Tfm/y rats and patients. These observations are consistent with the hypothesis that basal LH secretion is modulated independently by androgens and estrogens.[125, 153] Finally, it should be pointed out that the androgen resistance observed in Tfm/y is different from that of castrate males. In these latter individuals the negative feedback control of LH secretion is difficult to demonstrate with replacement doses of androgens. A similar resistance of the hypothalamo–pituitary–Leydig cell axis to androgen treatment has been observed in patients with hypergonadotropic hypogonadism such as Klinefelter's syndrome.[154, 155]

As noted earlier, the estrogen-induced positive feedback control of LH secretion is not as readily observed in men as it is in women. Prior to and during puberty in boys estradiol treatment produces negative but no positive feedback effect (Fig. 6–11). In men estrogen produces an initial suppression of LH which is followed by positive feedback in 50–60% of the individuals tested; in addition, the peak response does not exceed that of the initial pretreatment control levels of this

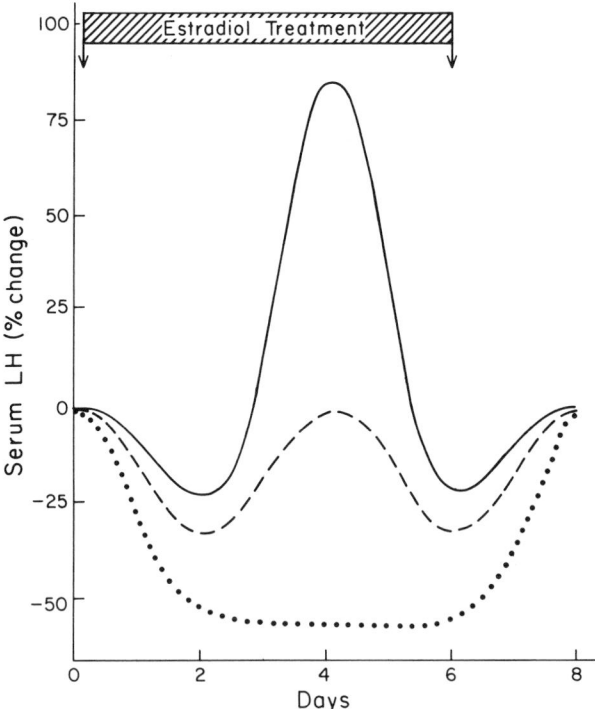

Figure 6–11. The effect of estradiol treatment on the plasma LH levels in normal prepubertal boys (lower dotted line), normal men (middle dashed line), and patients with primary testicular failure such as Klinefelter's and Sertoli-cell-only syndromes (upper solid line). During the first 3 days of estrogen treatment, negative feedback is observed in all three groups of individuals, with serum LH levels declining 25 to 50% below the untreated control values (baseline). In the normal boys, the serum LH levels remain suppressed throughout the estrogen treatment. In normal men, a rise of LH levels is noted (positive feedback) during continuous E_2 treatment, but the levels do not rise above the baseline. In men with primary testicular failure, a more exaggerated positive feedback is noted, with an increase of LH levels 100% above baseline.

gonadotropin.[156] By contrast, in patients with elevated gonadotropin associated with Klinefelter's and Sertoli-cell-only syndromes, a large positive feedback is observed in the presence of normal testosterone levels (Fig. 6–11). Finally, following orchiectomy and estrogen treatment, the positive effect of estradiol can be easily demonstrated in male monkeys.[157] In these latter studies the difference in the positive feedback noted in castrate male and female animals was normalized by long-term treatment of the males with a low dose of estrogen.

Action of Sex Steroids on the Hypothalamus and Pituitary. In the course of producing their feedback effects, testosterone and estradiol could regulate LH secretion either by influencing the amount of GnRH secreted by the hypothalamus or by modulating the sensitivity of pituitary cells to this peptide. The following observations suggest that both of these mechanisms may be determinants of gonadotropin secretion in normal and pathologic states. Following castration, hypothalamic GnRH content rapidly declines commensurate with the increased secretory rate of this hormone. Treatment with testosterone, dihydrotestosterone, or estradiol prevents the castration-induced depletion of GnRH by facilitating storage of this peptide.[158] These observations are consistent with a direct action of sex steroids on the central nervous system. In this regard, receptors for androgens and estrogens have been identified in various portions of the brain.

Direct action of androgens and estrogens on the pituitary has been studied by administering GnRH before and during treatment with these steroids. In normal men, the LH responsiveness of pituitary to GnRH progressively decreases during estrogen treatment.[38, 159, 160] In normal women, pituitary sensitivity to GnRH is initially reduced during the first 2–3 days of estrogen administration, but thereafter it is enhanced with continued treatment.[161-165] This latter increase in sensitivity is one of the important components of positive feedback. Acute testosterone administration does not alter the pituitary responsiveness to GnRH. However, prolonged treatment for 2–4 weeks does result in a striking decrease in the GnRH response similar to that observed with estradiol.[132, 166]

Since the suppressive effect of testosterone on GnRH responsiveness is observed only after weeks of treatment, it has not been studied extensively in patients. However, abnormalities of estrogen effects on the pituitary have been noted in a variety of conditions. Of particular interest is a study by Seyler et al.[167] demonstrating that female transsexuals seeking surgical conversion to the male phenotype exhibited a mean GnRH response following estrogen treatment which was intermediate between that of normal males and that of normal females. Early *in utero* androgen exposure was suggested as a possible mechanism for this interesting response in female transsexuals.

In summary, LH secretion is regulated by complex interaction of sex steroids and the neurons that secrete GnRH. As noted, these neurons may also be regulated by several other neurotransmitters such as DOPA, β-endorphin, and catecholamines. In the normal man, negative feedback is responsible for the day-to-day regulation of gonadotropins. In a variety of clinical disorders enhanced positive feedback and functional resistance to sex steroid may be observed.

THE PHYSIOLOGY OF THE HYPOTHALAMO–PITUITARY–SEMINIFEROUS TUBULAR AXIS

Components of the Axis

The essential features of the hypothalamo–pituitary–seminiferous tubular axis are schematically shown in Figure 6–1. A description of the components of this axis are presented, followed by a discussion of its integrated control.

The Hypothalamus and Pituitary. FSH is secreted from the same basophilic cells in the anterior pituitary that are believed to secrete LH. In prepubertal boys, there is a marked FSH response to GnRH which progressively declines during puberty so that in men the potency of this hypothalamic peptide for FSH release is only one-fifth that of its LH-releasing activity.[16] These observations alone are sufficient to indicate that the mechanism by which GnRH controls the minute-to-minute secretion of FSH is different from that for LH. Some studies suggest that there may be a separate FSH-releasing hormone; however, the existence of such a principle must await its isolation in pure form.[168]

As noted earlier, FSH, like the other glycoprotein hormones in man, is composed of two subunits. The species-specific α-subunit of FSH is virtually the same as the α-subunit of the other glycoprotein hormones, whereas the β-subunit is unique and determines the organ specificity of the intact hormone. The metabolic clearance rate of FSH in normal women (14 ml/minute) is similar to that of postmenopausal women.[169, 170] The clearance rates of this glycoprotein in men have not been determined. From estimates of production rate and the renal clearance, it is evident that only 3–5% of FSH appears in the urine each day in a biologically active form. Unlike LH, plasma levels of FSH do not fluctuate widely throughout the day. As a consequence, estimates of FSH in single plasma samples provide a reliable estimate of integrated FSH secretion.[37]

Germ Cells. The major mass of the testis is composed of tightly coiled seminiferous tubules which may reach 70 cm in length in man. Both ends of the tubules empty into the rete testis which discharges its contents into the caput epididymis via the efferent ductules. Large diploid spermatogonia are found against the basement membrane of the tubules. These cells undergo a series of mitotic divisions and finally differentiate into primary spermatocytes. During this stage DNA synthesis occurs, forming a tetraploid germ cell. The chromosomes thicken, pair off, and subsequently show a longitudinal split, except at the level of the centromere. It is at this stage that crossing over between paired chromosomes occurs, an event of enormous clinical and genetic import. In addition, this cell is extremely sensitive to toxic agents.[171] Thereafter, meiotic division occurs with members of the paired homologous chromosomes separating into two secondary spermatocytes, each containing 23 chromosomes. Since each of the chromosomes had doubled its DNA content, each of these cells still contains a diploid amount of DNA. They must, therefore, undergo a second "meiotic division" to produce haploid spermatids. These cells mature without further division into spermatozoa, which are released into the lumen of the seminiferous tubule.[171, 172]

From the foregoing discussion it is clear that the maintenance and growth of germ cells is a complex process. Studies of humans and animals having abnormal karyotypes with supernumerary sex chromosomes suggest that germ cells with an extra X chromosome cannot survive in the testis. For example, at birth both human and murine XXY males (Klinefelter's syndrome) have a normal number of primordial germ cells. However, their testes soon become devoid of spermatogonia so that Sertoli cells become the sole occupants of the seminiferous tubules. This is also the case of the sex-reversed (normal male with an XX karyotype) male that is heterozygous for an autosomal dominant gene, Sxr. Additional experiments establishing the importance of proper chromosomal make-up of germ cells were those by Cattanach et al.,[174] who observed that the testes of young adult XX male (Sxr/+), as well as XXY male, mice are totally devoid of germ cells. However, at about 300 days of age scattered regions in the seminiferous tubules of both groups of mice contain clones of male germ cells which complete spermatogenesis. Cytologic examination of these cells indicates that the first meiotic metaphase figures from these regions have XO sex chromosomes in the case of XX males and XY in the case of XXY males. A study of tetraparental XX/XY mosaic male mice further emphasizes the deleterious effect of an extra X chromosome on germ cell development. One would expect that these animals should have both XX and XY germ cell lines similar to those of the somatic cells. However, the XX germ cells are eliminated from the testis during the neonatal period, so that these animals transmit only the XY cell line to their progeny.[173] From these observations it was concluded that sterility in individuals with an extra X chromosome cannot be blamed on poor environment furnished by the somatic elements of the testes. It is, therefore, the presence of more than one X chromosome rather than the absence of the Y that is incompatible with further differentiation of testicular primordial germ cells to definitive spermatogonia.[175]

An understanding of the organization of germ cells within the seminiferous tubule of the human testis was provided by the studies of Clermont.[176] This investigator demonstrated

that the germinal epithelium is organized into six stages (Fig. 6–12). Each stage is composed of a specific cellular constellation representing a particular degree of maturation. The six stages are found in each functional unit of spermatogenesis. In humans, these functional units are arranged in interlocking groups or clones up and down the seminiferous tubule. Thus, the human germinal epithelium in individual seminiferous tubules lacks a uniform wave of spermatogenesis. As a consequence, when a single tubule is examined on cross section, two or more stages of spermatogenesis from two or more clones may be present side by side in a pie-shaped fashion. This is in striking contrast to the rodent testis, where a cross section contains only a single stage of spermatogenesis.

The duration of human spermatogenesis was determined by use of ^{3}H-thymidine.[177, 178] Each cycle lasts about 16 days and the individual stages occupy different periods in any given cycle. It appears that the beginning of spermatogenesis is at a midway point through stage 5 (Fig. 6–13). The end of spermatogenesis is some four cycles later, midway through stage 2. The interval is 74 ± 4.5 days. During this time the progeny of the relatively undifferentiated spermatogonia are converted into the highly specialized cell that has discarded half its chromosomes and acquired the machinery for motility and ovum penetration. Fully developed spermatozoa are released into the lumen of the seminiferous tubule, which is functionally the first portion of the male reproductive tract. The sperm cells are washed out of the tubules into rete testis and epididymis by a fluid drive provided by Sertoli cells. When spermatozoa enter the caput epididymidis they are nonmotile. Motility is acquired during their passage through the epididymis.[179] Although the exact role played by epididymal cells in this androgen-dependent maturational process is not understood[180] recent morphologic studies on nonmotile spermatozoa provided some insight into some of the structural components of sperm that are essential for motility. The major driving force for the sperm is provided by the axoneme of the axial filament complex, which consists of two central microtubules surrounded by a row of nine evenly spaced doublet microtubules (Fig. 6–13A). The occurrence of this nine plus two pattern in both flagella and cilia is remarkably constant throughout phylogeny.[181-183] The reasons for this phylogenetic stability undoubtedly relate to the fact that many of the essential structures of the axoneme are important for motility. This postulate is supported by the observation that axonemes with absent outer arms (Fig. 6–13B) or radial spokes and deranged or missing central fibers are not capable of motility.[184, 185]

The energy for motility is provided by an ATPase located in the dynein arms (Fig. 6–13A) on each doublet microtubule. The arms on one pair of tubules "walk along" the adjacent doublet in response to binding and hydrolysis of ATP.[186-189] This has been termed the sliding microtubule hypothesis of flagellar and ciliary motion. A variety of factors have been identified as possible physiologic regulators of sperm motility, including Ca^{++},[190-193] cAMP,[194-197] catecholamines,[198, 199] a protein motility factor,[200] and protein carboxyl-methylase.[201] How these factors regulate the force-generating ATPase is yet to be established.

Spermatozoa present in fresh ejaculate are not capable of fertilization despite their rapid motility. A further change occurs in the female reproductive tract, where the ability to fertilize is acquired through a process called capacitation.[202]

Sertoli Cells. The backbone of the seminiferous tubule is formed by the Sertoli cells which, along with spermatogonia, are the only cells that rest on the basal lamina (Fig. 6–14). All other germinal cells lie between Sertoli cells, surrounded

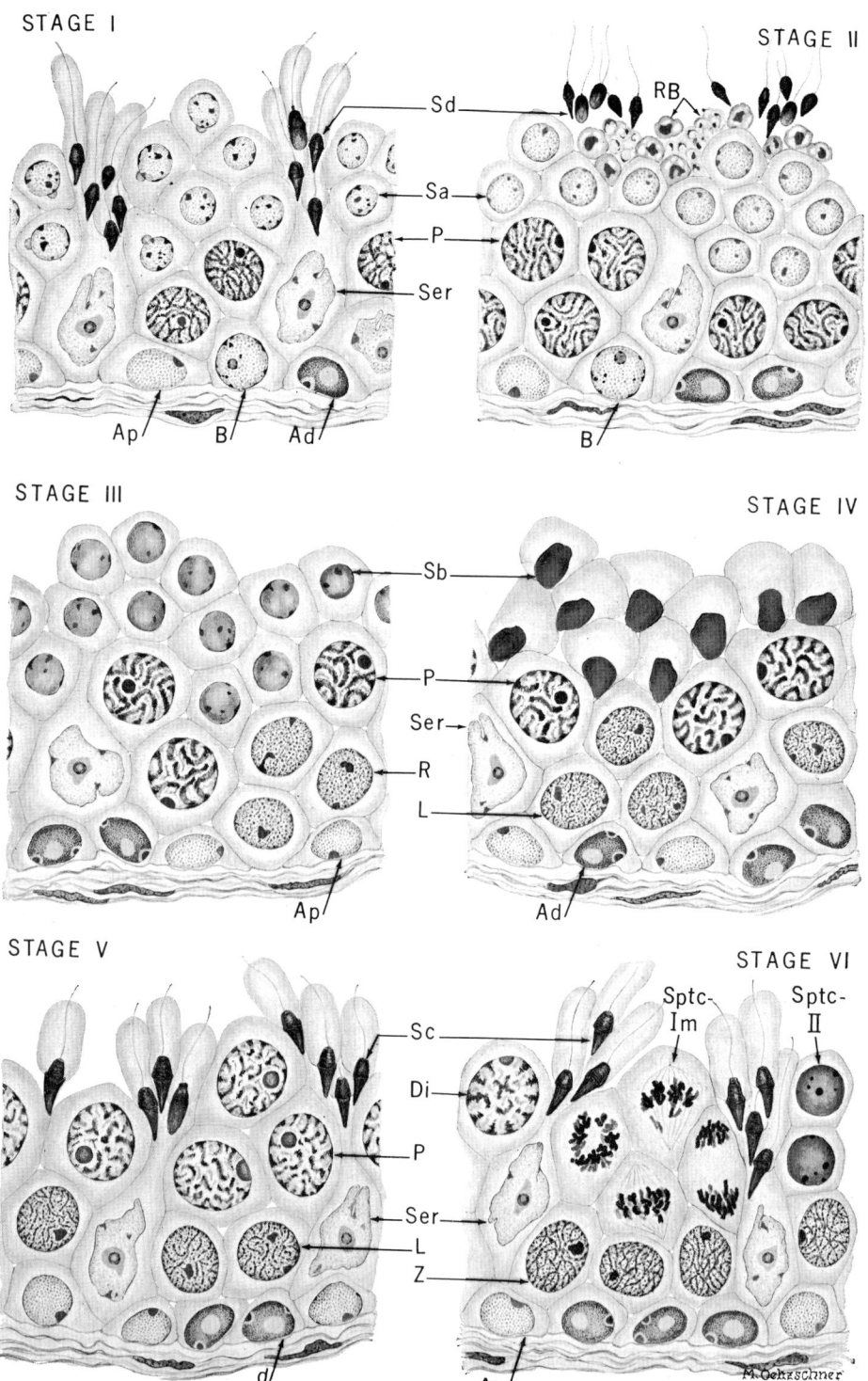

Figure 6–12. The six stages of spermatogenesis. Together these stages represent one cycle of the germinal epithelium. *Ser*, Sertoli cell; *Ad* and *Ap*, dark and pale type A spermatogonia; *B*, type B spermatogonia; *R*, resting or preleptotene spermatocytes; *L*, leptotene spermatocytes; *Z*, zygotene spermatocytes; *P*, pachytene spermatocytes; *Im*, primary spermatocytes in division; *II*, secondary spermatocytes; *Sa, Sb, Sc, Sd*, spermatids in various steps of spermiogenesis; and *RB*, residual bodies. Unlike the case in other mammals, the stages of spermatogenesis in the human are intermixed within the same tubule. (From Clermont, Y.: The cycle of the seminiferous epithelium in man. *Amer. J. Anat. 112*:35, 1963.)

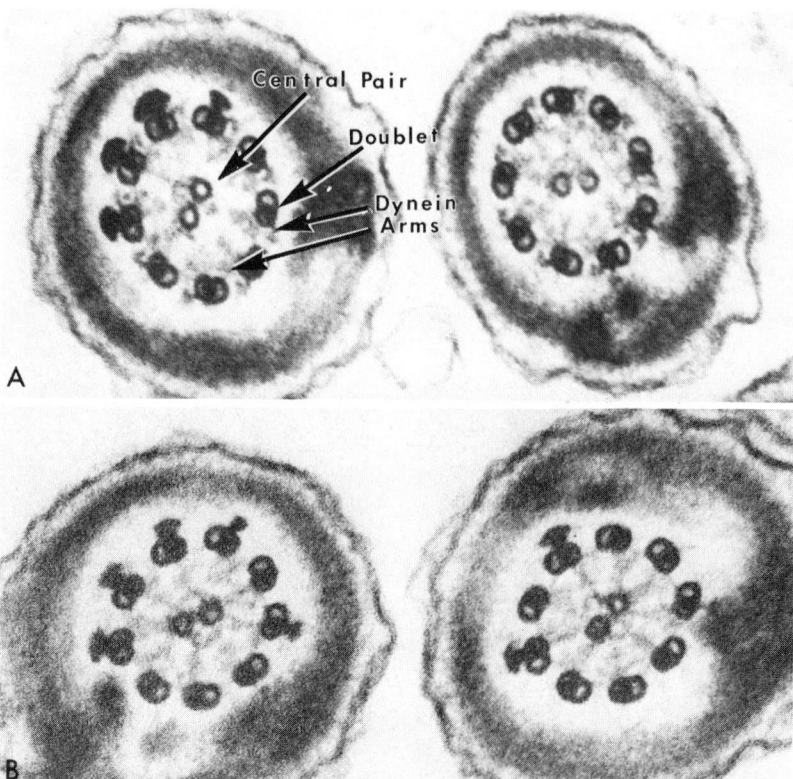

Figure 6–13. Electron micrographs of spermatozoa tails in cross section. *A,* The axoneme of the axial filament complex, consisting of the two central microtubules surrounded by a row of nine evenly spaced doublet microtubules, is shown. The dynein arms of the outer microtubules in normal spermatozoa are indicated by arrows. *B,* The axial filaments of nonmotile spermatozoa from a patient with Kartagener's syndrome. The outer dynein arms are missing. (Micrographs prepared by David M. Phillips.)

by their plasma membranes.[203] These latter cells are joined to one another above or on the luminal side of spermatogonia but below spermatocytes by specialized junctional complexes. These junctional complexes divide the seminiferous tubule into luminal and adluminal compartments. The arrangement of these cells is diagrammed in Figure 6–15. These Sertoli cell junctional complexes limit the transport of a variety of molecules from the interstitial space into the seminiferous tubular lumen. The functional significance of the anatomic arrangement of these cells was first suggested by studies in which a number of injected dyes could not be detected in the seminiferous tubules in histologic sections.[204] Subsequent studies have demonstrated that a variety of ions, proteins, hormones, and drugs have limited access into the seminiferous tubular lumen. These findings coupled with electron microscopic observations indicate that there is a blood-testis barrier functionally similar to that which exists between the vascular space and the brain.

The blood-testis barrier develops at the time of puberty and just prior to the beginning of spermatogenesis. One possible function of the barrier is to provide a unique environment in which sperm maturation and development can occur. It is perhaps significant that germ cells that remain outside the blood-testis barrier continue to divide by mitosis while those inside the barrier undergo meiosis. In addition, the blood-testis barrier serves to maintain germ cells in an immunologically privileged location since mature spermatozoa are very immunogenic if they are introduced into the systemic circulation.

In addition to maintaining the blood-testis barrier, Sertoli cells have a number of other important functions including: (1) phagocytosis of damaged germ cells; (2) nourishment of developing germ cells; (3) production of unique proteins that are secreted in the seminiferous tubular lumen; (4) maintenance of a potassium- and bicarbonate-rich tubular fluid that provides the major drive for flushing sperm from the testis into the epididymis; (5) acting as the site for hormone action on the testis; and (6) synthesis of estradiol from androgen precursors[205] (Fig. 6–15).

Increased understanding of the hormonal control of Sertoli cells is derived from studies of androgen-binding protein (ABP). This macromolecule is synthesized by Sertoli cells, is secreted primarily into the seminiferous tubular fluid, and is transported to the proximal portion of the caput epididymidis where it is absorbed and degraded.[205] Studies from several laboratories suggest that ABP and TeBG in rabbit and human are structurally and immunologically similar.[206, 207] Even though rabbit TeBG and ABP have been isolated in pure form, further structural studies are required to determine the distinctive features of these proteins.[208] The recent isolation of ABP in rat, a species without TeBG,[209] provided reagents for a sensitive radioimmunoassay which was used by Gunsalus et al.[210] to demonstrate that ABP is released into the blood. This was an unexpected observation; it was assumed that all Sertoli cell proteins are secreted into the seminiferous tubular lumen behind the blood-testis barrier. Even though the function of ABP in testicular physiology is not completely understood at present, this protein nonetheless serves as a marker for Sertoli cell function. Testosterone and FSH both stimulate ABP synthesis but by different mechanisms. FSH is also required for ABP secretion into the seminiferous tubular lumen.[205] ABP synthesis is affected by primary testicular disorders such as cryptorchidism and hereditary seminiferous tubular failure.[210, 211] Therefore, this and other specific Sertoli cell proteins could be an important tool for understanding the pathophysiology of the testis. The recent studies indicating that ABP is secreted into the blood establishes an important principle that testicular proteins can be measured in this compartment. The application of this principle to the human awaits the isolation of a unique testicular protein that can be measured in serum.[212]

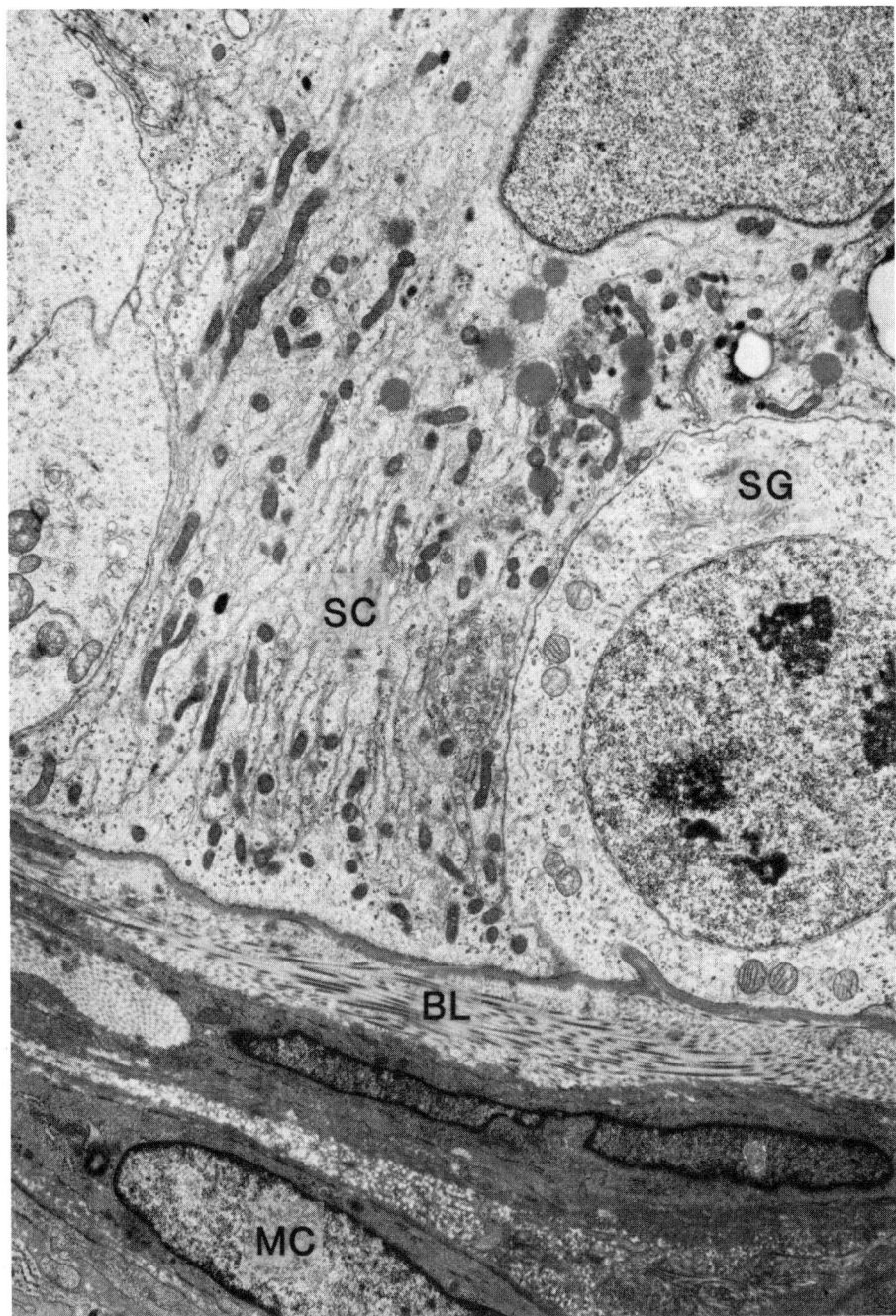

Figure 6–14. Electron micrograph of a human Sertoli cell *(SC)*. The Sertoli cell and the spermatogonia *(SG)* are the only cells of the seminiferous tubular epithelium that rest on the basal lamina *(BL)*. Two-thirds to three-fourths of the surface of the spermatogonia are in contact with the plasma membrane of Sertoli cells. The remainder of germ cells are surrounded by Sertoli cells on all sides (not shown). *MC* = myoid cells. (With permission of A.K. Christensen.)

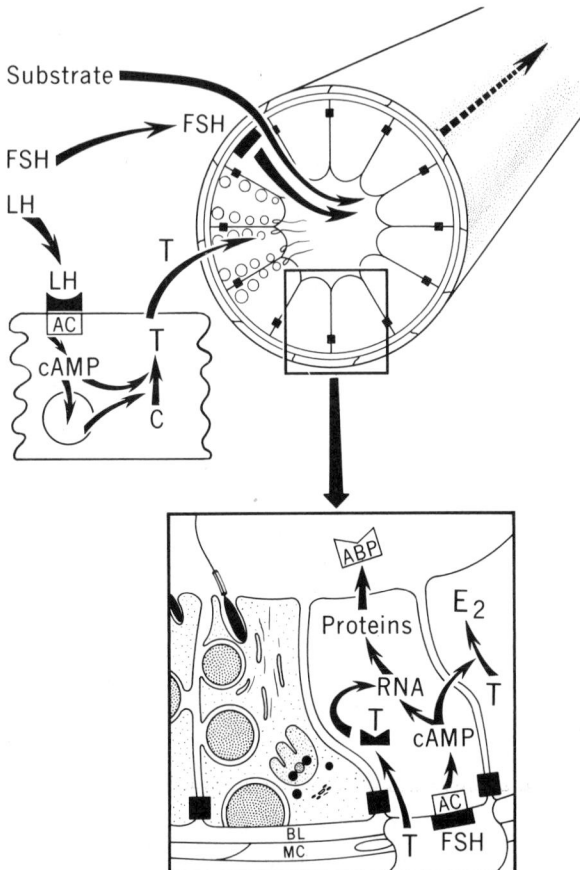

Figure 6–15. The mechanism of action of pituitary hormones and testosterone on the seminiferous tubule. In the upper panel, LH acts by way of its Leydig cell membrane receptors to stimulate cAMP formation, which facilitates the conversion of cholesterol to testosterone (for details, see Fig. 6–5). Both testosterone and FSH act directly on Sertoli cells to stimulate the transport of various substances (substrates) into the seminiferous tubular lumen. In the bottom panel two Sertoli cells are shown. On the left, germ cells (stippled circles) develop surrounded by Sertoli cell plasma membranes (compare with Fig. 6–14). On the right, testosterone and FSH stimulate Sertoli cell protein synthesis and secretion. One of these Sertoli cell products is androgen-binding protein (ABP). In addition, FSH stimulates the conversion of testosterone to estradiol (E_2). Black squares designate the junctional complexes; *AC,* adenylate cyclase; *BL,* basal lamina; *MC,* myoid cells. (From Bardin, C. W.: Pituitary-testicular axis. In *Reproductive Endocrinology.* Yen, S., and Jaffe, R. (eds.), Philadelphia, W. B. Saunders Co., 1978, pp. 110–125.)

Hormonal Control of Spermatogenesis

Studies from a number of laboratories indicate that both LH and FSH are required for spermatogenesis.[213] It is currently held that all of the effects of LH are mediated by way of testosterone from Leydig cells. As a consequence, testosterone and FSH are the hormones that act directly on the seminiferous tubular epithelium (see Figs. 6–1 and 6–15). An understanding of the hormonal requirements for sperm development is complicated by the fact that the initiation and maintenance of this process appear to be under independent control. At the time of puberty, initiation of spermatogenesis requires both testosterone and FSH. Once the normal germinal epithelium is established in the rat, testosterone alone can maintain sperm production in hypophysectomized animals provided treatment is begun immediately after removal of the pituitary. There are conflicting reports as to whether testosterone can maintain the seminiferous tubule in the primate. If, however, the seminiferous tubular epithelium is allowed to regress, then both testosterone and

FSH are again required to reinstitute sperm production.[214]

FSH action on the seminiferous tubules is initiated by binding to specific receptors on the plasma membranes of Sertoli cells.[215, 216] This interaction results in the stimulation of adenylate cyclase activity, which increases cAMP in the cell. In the Sertoli cell, as in other cells in which hormone stimulates cAMP, the adenylyl cyclase is probably coupled to the FSH receptor by a guanyl nucleotide regulatory subunit,[55] as is the case for LH (see Fig. 6–5). In the immature animal, cAMP appears to activate the cytoplasmic cAMP-dependent protein kinase. Following binding of cAMP to the regulatory subunit, the catalytic subunit is released so that it can phosphorylate a variety of proteins. The mechanism by which protein kinase regulates Sertoli cell function is still unresolved. An ultimate understanding of the FSH reaction will explain the mechanism by which this glycoprotein stimulates a variety of metabolic events in these cells, including RNA synthesis, DNA synthesis, protein secretion, cell movement, and testosterone conversion to estradiol.[217, 218]

The observations that 5α-reductase activity is low in adult testes and normal sperm development occurs in men with 5α-reductase deficiency indicate that dihydrotestosterone is not required for spermatogenesis.[116, 117] Androgen action on the seminiferous tubule is, therefore, believed to be mediated by testosterone, which is the major intranuclear androgen in this organ. Androgen receptors are present in testis that are similar to those in somatic tissues.[214] The action of androgen by way of its receptor is believed necessary for the formation of spermatogonia and for the second meiotic divisions that produce spermatids.[213, 214] An argument against this being an event mediated entirely by androgen receptor is the observation that the undescended testis of Tfm/y rats contains differentiating spermatogonia, as well as a large number of first-meiotic-prophase and some first-meiotic-metaphase figures.[94]

Hormonal Control of the Pituitary—Seminiferous Tubular Axis–The Negative Feedback of FSH

The fact that FSH secretion from the pituitary rises following orchiectomy indicates that a factor from the testis controls the secretion of this gonadotropin in much the same way that androgens and estrogens exert a negative feedback regulation of LH secretion. However, the facts that testosterone administration has little effect on FSH secretion in castrates and that very large doses of estrogen are required to suppress FSH suggest that another testicular secretory product is responsible for the control of FSH. McCullagh[220] first suggested the name "inhibin" for a water-soluble testicular product that could prevent the appearance of castration cells in the pituitary gland of gonadectomized animals. This name has subsequently been used for any nonsteroidal testicular factor that exerts a negative feedback effect on FSH secretion.[221] A variety of studies indicate that inhibin is a protein that may exist in multiple forms. The effect of inhibin is usually felt to be specific for inhibition of FSH release (see Fig. 6–1). Since no highly purified inhibin preparations are available at this writing, it is difficult to exclude an effect of inhibin on LH secretion.

Although initial observations suggested that inhibin was produced by germ cells, a variety of subsequent *in vivo* and *in vitro* studies indicate that the Sertoli cells are the most likely site of origin. The selective rise of FSH in individuals with damaged seminiferous tubules is presumably due to defective inhibin secretion from damaged Sertoli cells (Fig. 6–16). The fact that inhibin can be assayed on isolated

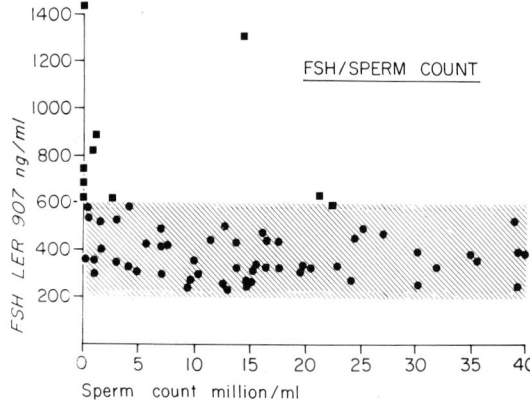

Figure 6–16. Mean sperm counts of patients with oligospermia or azoospermia compared with their serum FSH concentrations. (FSH levels are expressed with reference to standards of the National Pituitary Agency, LER 907.) Cross-hatched area indicates the normal range for serum FSH concentration in adult males. Note that the second highest FSH titer was present in a male with 15 million/ml mean sperm density. (From Leonard, J. M., et al.: Plasma and urinary follicle-stimulating hormone levels in oligospermia. *J. Clin. Endocrinol. Metab. 34*:209, 1972.)

pituitary cells indicates that it can inhibit FSH secretion directly. It is also possible that this hormone inhibits GnRH release. The status of inhibin isolation and assay has recently been reviewed by de Jong.[222]

THE ROLE OF PROLACTIN IN MALE REPRODUCTION

Prolactin Secretion

Although the existence of prolactin in rodents and sheep was recognized for many years, this protein was difficult to demonstrate in primates because its concentration in normal pituitaries is low and because human growth hormone is lactogenic.[223] Prolactin is associated with the female because it is lactogenic and required for establishing functional corpus luteum in some species. Specific radioimmunoassays demonstrated that this hormone circulates in the plasma of males as well as females. The prolactin concentration in neonatal boys is very high but declines and approaches the adult basal value by the sixth week of age; from this time until puberty there is no significant difference in the concentration of prolactin at various ages in either males or females.[224] Administration of estrogens, however, produces a rise in plasma prolactin. It is probably the secretion of this sex steroid at puberty that leads to the progressive increase in secretion in girls and ultimately accounts for the 50% higher levels in women.[224] There is a sleep-induced rise of prolactin that is not dependent upon puberty for its ontogeny.[225] Some other factors that control prolactin secretion are shown in Figure 6–17.

In contrast to LH and FSH, the hypothalamic control of prolactin is mediated by prolactin-inhibiting factor (PIF), which exerts a suppressive effect on secretion. Part of the evidence for this assertion is from the hyperprolactinemia that occurs following interruption of the hypophyseal portal system by pituitary stalk section.[226] The exact nature of PIF has not been identified, but it may be dopamine. In keeping with this, a variety of psychiatric and antihypertensive drugs that either block or deplete catecholamine stores markedly elevate prolactin secretion.[227] By contrast, dopaminergic agonists suppress prolactin secretion.[8]

There is an interesting relationship between prolactin and LH secretion. Clinical disorders and drugs that elevate prolactin secretion tend to lower plasma LH levels and vice

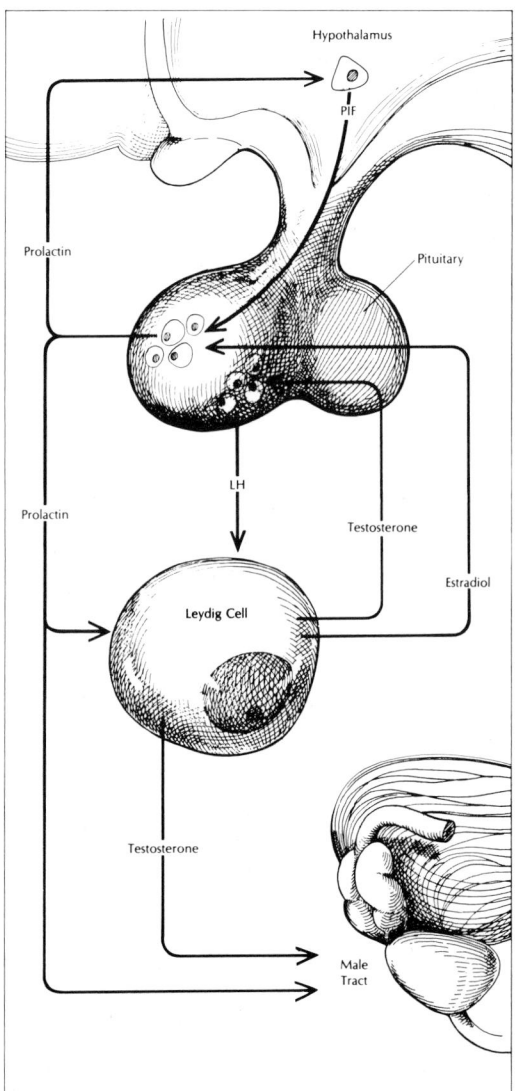

Figure 6–17. The mechanism of action and control of prolactin secretion. Prolactin-inhibiting factor (PIF) is secreted by the hypothalamus and partially inhibits prolactin release from the pituitary. Prolactin binds to specific receptors on Leydig cell membranes and facilitates secretion of testosterone by LH. Prolactin also synergizes with testosterone on the male reproductive tract. Testosterone and estradiol inhibit LH secretion, and estradiol facilitates prolactin secretion. There is some evidence to suggest that prolactin may also act directly on the brain to reduce pituitary secretion and to influence sex drive. (By Donner, C., from Bardin, C. W.: The neuroendocrinology of male reproduction. *Hospital Practice*, Vol. 14, No. 12, and from *Neuroendocrinology*. Krieger, D. K., and Hughes, J. C. (eds.). Sunderland, MA, Sinauer Associates, Inc., 1980, pp. 239–247. Reproduced with permission.)

versa. This relationship is seen with an α-adrenergic antagonist such as chlorpromazine, which suppresses the pulsatile secretion of LH in ovariectomized monkeys[228] and elevates prolactin secretion.[227] A similar reciprocal effect on LH and prolactin secretion was recently observed with naturally occurring and synthetic opiates and their antagonists. Opiates produce a rise in prolactin secretion,[229] and an opiate antagonist such as naloxone suppresses the basal secretion of this pituitary hormone.[230] The opposite effects on LH secretion are seen in men.[231]

Actions of Prolactin

One of the most convincing demonstrations that prolactin stimulates the male reproductive system is derived from experiments on hereditary dwarf mice by Bartke.[232] Two recessive mutations in the mouse, df and dw, result in the absence of the acidophil cells in the pituitary. As a result, animals homozygous (df/df; dw/dw) for either of these genes produce little or no prolactin and reproduce poorly. Treatment of male dwarf mice with purified prolactin increases sperm production and markedly improves fertility. One 17-year-old boy with short stature, delayed puberty, and isolated prolactin deficiency has been reported, but no treatment with prolactin was attempted.[233] Studies in hypophysectomized animals indicate that prolactin alone exerts very little effect on the male reproductive tract but significantly potentiates the effect of LH on Leydig cells (Fig. 6–17). Prolactin receptors have been identified not only on Leydig but also on adrenal and ovarian steroidogenic cells.[234, 235] It has been suggested that prolactin may control lipoprotein transport in these cells, thus assuring a constant supply of cholesterol for steroidogenesis.[232]

In addition to its action on the testis, prolactin works as an anabolic hormone in concert with testosterone on the male reproductive tract and other androgen-responsive tissues (Fig. 6–17). When prolactin is administered to castrate hypophysectomized animals it is essentially inactive. However, when given with testosterone there is a significant increase in the stimulatory effects on several organs.[236] The action of prolactin on androgen-responsive tissues is believed mediated through specific membrane receptors that act by a mechanism other than the cAMP-protein kinase system.[234] One of the ways that prolactin is able to facilitate androgen action is by increasing the amount of androgen-receptor complex that is transferred to the nuclei of responsive cells.[237]

Hyperprolactinemia and Impotence

As already noted, prolactin synergizes with LH and testosterone to increase reproductive function in the male. It was therefore of interest to find that a transplantable prolactin-producing pituitary tumor produces testicular involution and decreased testosterone levels in male rats. In these studies decreased reproductive function is associated with a prolactin-induced lowering of testosterone. Although the exact mechanism for this effect is not completely understood, it is possible that this has a direct effect on the Leydig cells, resulting in downregulation of gonadotropin receptors as described earlier for LH.[234]

Several series of men with hyperprolactinemia secondary to pituitary tumors have been reported recently.[238, 239] A striking finding in all these reports is the high incidence of impotence occurring in hyperprolactinemic individuals with both normal and low testosterone levels. Sexual function is restored by lowering prolactin levels with the dopa agonist bromergocryptine or by surgical removal of the pituitary tumor. Testosterone treatment is not usually effective in these individuals unless prolactin levels are lowered simultaneously.[239] Bromergocryptine treatment of impotent patients without hyperprolactinemia was not much more effective than placebo.[240] These latter observations suggest that prolactin can produce impotence independent of its action on testosterone secretion. Although the mechanism by which prolactin influences sexual drive is not known, it is intriguing to speculate that this pituitary hormone can act directly on the brain to influence behavior (Fig. 6–17).

METHODS FOR THE DIAGNOSIS OF HYPOGONADISM

Clinical Examination

If Leydig cell failure occurs before puberty, testosterone production will be low, the pubertal changes enumerated in Table 6–4 will not occur, and the patient will develop obvious features of eunuchoidism (Table 6–5). In addition to sexual infantilism, the delay in epiphysial closure allows continued long-bone growth, which results in the typical eunuchoidal habitus. These features are usually easy to recognize. However, the detection of Leydig cell failure occurring after puberty may be more difficult unless the testicular damage is severe, or unless sufficient time has elapsed to allow regression of the male secondary sex characteristics. After complete Leydig cell failure, the frequency of shaving will decrease gradually over many months, and it may take up to 10 years for the beard to completely disappear. If the beard and body hair are lost more rapidly (6–12 months), cortisol deficiency should be suspected. The symptoms of impotence and decreased libido that develop after Leydig cell failure in the adult are also encountered frequently in emotional disorders. This tends to limit their value as diagnostic points.

When damage to the seminiferous tubules occurs postpubertally, the testes become smaller and softer than normal, and infertility is usually the chief complaint. It should be emphasized that since the testes are elliptical in configuration, considerable damage has to occur before the external measurements are significantly reduced. Normally the testis measures 4.6 cm in length (mean value; range 3.6–5.5 cm) and 2.6 cm in width (range 2.1–3.2 cm). Age per se does not influence testicular size; therefore, the clinical significance of small testes in men over 50 years is the same as in younger adults.[1]

Examination of the Seminal Fluid

Functional evaluation of the seminiferous tubules is made by seminal fluid analysis. This examination has certain limitations which should be kept in mind. First, there is no direct method that has been fully validated which measures the fertilizing capacity of human sperm. Several investigators have reported their results with respect to using the zona-free hamster ova incubated with human sperm.[243-247] This in vitro test shows considerable promise but is not ready for routine use by the clinician. Next, the variability in sperm counts needs to be emphasized (Fig. 6–18). This variation does not follow a normal distribution, but efforts to establish the mathematical model for human sperm production are being actively studied.

Germ cell morphology appears to be a more constant area of measurement. Similarly, the seminal fluid volume remains fairly uniform for the same individual provided a set period of abstinence (2 or 3 days) is observed before each

---

Table 6–5. CLINICAL FEATURES OF EUNUCHOIDISM

Eunuchoidal skeleton
  Span more than 2 inches greater than height. Soles to symphysis more than 2 inches greater than symphysis to head. Delay in closure of epiphyses.

Lack of adult male hair distribution
  Sparse or absent facial and body hair. Scant pubic and axillary hair. Failure of scalp hair to recede.

High-pitched voice

Infantile genitalia
  Small penis, testes, and scrotum.

Poor muscular development
  Decreased muscle mass. Diminished endurance and strength.

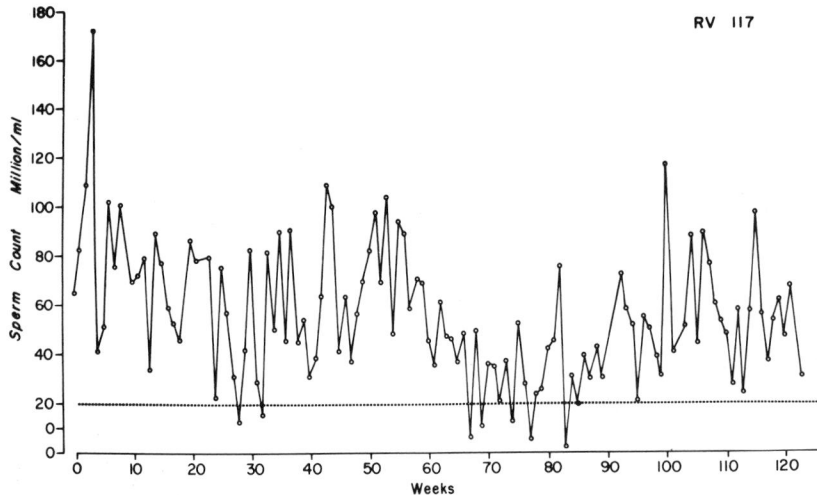

RV 117

Figure 6–18. Weekly seminal fluid sperm concentrations from one normal man over a period of 120 weeks. During this period the individual received no medication and reported no periods of febrile illness. Dotted line indicates 20 million/ml, which is generally considered to be the lower limit of normal range. (Paulsen, C. A.: Unpublished data.)

specimen is collected. The World Health Organization has recently prepared a laboratory manual in an effort to promote standardization of techniques,[248] a problem that has been addressed by many authors.[249-252] For practical purposes, the following criteria may be used as rough estimates of abnormality: (1) sperm counts persistently less than 20 million/ml in three separate specimens collected over a 2-month period; (2) less than 60% normal oval forms derived from properly stained seminal fluid smears; and (3) sperm motility less than 60% (wet drop examination).

Briefly, the procedure may be performed in the following manner: The only satisfactory way to obtain seminal fluid is to have the patient masturbate into a clean glass or suitable "snap-top" plastic container. The fresh specimen should be submitted for examination within an hour. Condom sheaths should not be used, since sperm motility decreases markedly upon contact with the sheath. Even the plastic sheaths are impractical since they irritate the female partner. In addition, immature germ cells and white cells tend to be removed from the seminal plasma since they adhere to the sheath. Interrupted coitus as a means of collecting seminal fluid is also unsatisfactory since the initial portion of the ejaculate, which contains the highest density of sperm, may be lost.

Immediately after ejaculation, coagulation of the seminal fluid occurs, followed in 15–30 minutes by liquefaction. In some specimens, liquefaction is incomplete or fails to occur. To these specimens several drops of Locke's solution with 5% α-amylase solution may be added to break up the coagulum.[253] This does not alter motility.

Estimation of motility is made by examining a drop of undiluted seminal fluid, using the 40× objective and recording the percentage of motile forms. Phase microscopy is preferred, but ordinary light microscopy may be used. The quality of motility can be graded 1 to 3. Spermatozoa with grade 3 motility tend to move rapidly across the field; grade 2 spermatozoa move aimlessly across the field, whereas spermatozoa with grade 1 motility remain in one spot exhibiting only tail motion. For research purposes, more elaborate techniques have been devised for evaluating motility.[254] Seminal fluid volume may be determined by use of a suitable graduated cylinder. The normal volume of the ejaculate ranges from 2.5 to slightly over 6.0 ml.

Sperm counts may be estimated by drawing thoroughly mixed seminal fluid up to the 0.5 mark of a standardized white cell pipet, and diluting to the 1.1 mark with a saline solution made as follows: 75 ml glacial acetic acid; 0.3 gm saponin dissolved in 2 ml saline then centrifuged for 20 minutes at 2000 rpm; 1500 ml saline; 165 ml 5% gentian violet. (Other solutions used are composed of $NaHCO_3$, formalin, and 1% methylene blue.[248]) Shake for 2 minutes, spread the diluted specimen over a 0.1-mm-deep Neubauer counting chamber, and estimate the number of spermatozoa per milliliter. For greater accuracy and efficiency, an electronic particle counter may be used to determine sperm concentration.[255-256] Although the apparatus is relatively expensive, many clinical laboratories use this method for counting blood cells. In order to process seminal fluid, a 50-μ-aperture tube is used instead of the 100-μ tube. The normal range for sperm counts is usually considered to be from 20 million to over 100 million/ml.

The importance of assessing germ cell morphology and the white blood cells in the seminal fluid should not be overlooked; for example, a relationship between an increase in tapered forms and a variocele exists in some infertile men. In short, the seminal fluid smear is prepared similar to the way a blood smear is made, but with special stains.[248] Data from the analysis of 602 ejaculates from 73 normal adult men showed the mean distribution of germ cell forms to be: normal oval form, 80.5%; large oval head, 0.3%; small oval head, 1.4%; tapering head, 0.4%; pyriform, 2.0%; duplicate head, 1.5%; amorphous head, 6.5%; tail defect, 5.2%; and cytoplasmic droplet, 2.2%.

With respect to the number of leukocytes in the ejaculate, 26% showed none and 54% showed 1×10^5 to 6×10^6 leukocytes per milliliter of seminal fluid. There are no complete data on the concentration of immature germ cells in the ejaculate but preliminary analyses from our laboratory show that normal male seminal fluid may contain as many as 4.6 $\times 10^6$ immature germ cells per milliliter. Clearly, more studies need to be carried out as to the importance of these various cell types in seminal fluid.

Testicular Biopsy

When oligospermia or azoospermia is present, a testicular biopsy specimen may be obtained and examined to allow full appreciation of the nature and extent of the defect. For example, when azoospermia is due to ductal obstruction, the biopsy specimen is normal. The appearance of the biopsy specimen also permits the physician to determine whether therapeutic measures are worthwhile in male infertility. Finally, it may be necessary to obtain testicular material for sex chromosomal analysis (see Klinefelter's syndrome). The aim is to establish the histologic basis of hypogonadism with precision and to define the effects of contraceptive, therapeutic, and other agents on testicular function. Quantification of the germinal epithelium is an important feature of the

biopsy examination. Techniques for this have been discussed by several authors.[257-260] The stages of the seminiferous epithelium in man are shown in Figure 6–12.

Testicular biopsy is not without some hazard. Studies in

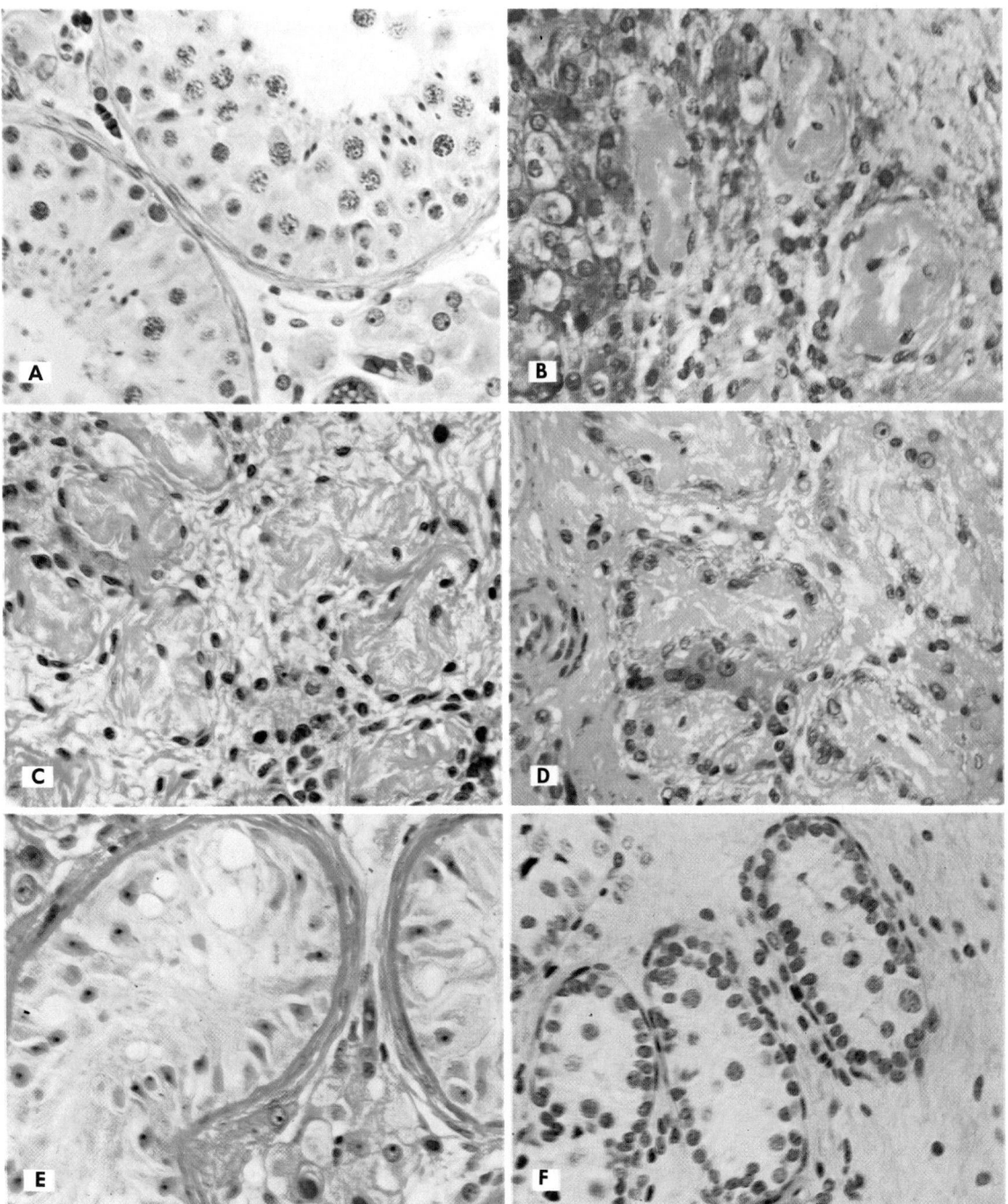

Figure 6–19. *A*, Normal testis: Germinal cells of the seminiferous tubules are undergoing active spermatogenesis. Sertoli cells; type A, B spermatogonia; zygotene, pachytene primary spermatocytes, and various types of spermatids can be readily identified. (Refer to Fig. 6–12 for characteristics of each cell type.) The basement membrane and tunica propria surround the tubules. Groups of Leydig cells may be seen in the interstitial spaces and are characterized by a prominent nucleolus and abundant cytoplasm (× 200).

B, Klinefelter testis: In this example, the tubules (blue) are devoid of germinal or Sertoli cells. The tubular membranes have undergone complete hyalinization. Leydig cells are in adenomatous "clumps." A portion of one such aggregate may be seen in the left-hand portion of the photomicrograph (× 200).

C, Klinefelter testis: In this case, the tubules are characteristically hyalinized but the Leydig cells are diffusely spread throughout the biopsy specimen (× 200).

D, Postmumps orchitis testis: Complete hyalinization of the seminiferous tubules has occurred. Although not shown, Leydig cells are grouped in adenomatous "clumps" similar to those observed in the usual case of Klinefelter's syndrome. However, in contrast to the picture noted in Klinefelter's syndrome (*B* and *C*), elastic and reticular fibers are present around the thickened tunica propria (× 200).

E, Sertoli-cell-only testis: The seminiferous tubules are somewhat reduced in size but the tubular membranes are not sclerosed. Sertoli cells, with their characteristic nucleoli and brush borders, are the only cells within the tubules. The Leydig cells appear normal (× 200).

F, Hypogonadotropic eunuchoid testis: Typical immature seminiferous tubules containing undifferentiated germinal epithelium can be seen. Mesenchymal precursors of Leydig cells are interspersed between the tubules (× 200).

normal volunteers demonstrate that sperm counts decrease in about 45% of men following testicular biopsy. This complication is usually temporary and the alteration in sperm production relatively minor. In our experience, patients and normal volunteers in research protocols have not been permanently harmed by a biopsy unless the epididymis was inadvertently entered. Therefore, careful attention to procedural details and proper selection of patients are important. Examples of biopsies from patients with various testicular disorders are shown in Figure 6–19.

A testicular biopsy can be readily performed under local anesthesia on an outpatient basis.[261, 262] The skin and subcutaneous tissue are infiltrated with a 2% procaine solution after premedication with meperidine (Demerol), atropine, and secobarbital. With one assistant holding the testis in proper orientation so as to avoid the epididymis, the operator makes a small incision in the scrotum. Next, the subcutaneous tissue and tunica vaginalis are incised and spread for exposure. With the sharp point of a scalpel blade, a 5-mm incision is made in the tunica albuginea. A small amount of seminiferous tubular tissue extrudes through the incision. This tissue is then excised with a razor blade. The razor blade is used to avoid crushing of the tubules. The specimen is immediately placed into freshly prepared Cleland's or Bouin's solution for fixation. Unless bleeding persists from the small vessels lying along the undersurface of the tunica albuginea, closure of this layer is not required. The tunica vaginalis and scrotum are closed and a Lister-type scrotal suspensory is used to support the testis and hold the dressing. The patient must be advised to avoid strenuous activities for the next week in order to prevent hematoma formation.

Buccal Smear and Karyotype

Examination of epithelial cells obtained by buccal smear is a practical screening method that provides evidence for the number of X chromosomes. In general, there is one chromatin or Barr body for every X chromosome in excess of one. When Barr bodies are present, the individual is said to be "chromatin-positive." If special stains and the fluorescent microscope are used, detection of the Y chromosome is possible. For difficult diagnostic problems or when chromosomal mosaicism is suspected, peripheral blood, fibroblasts, or gonadal tissue is submitted to short-term tissue culture for karyotype. This technique provides the physician an analysis of autosomal and sex chromosomal configuration. All of these procedures are discussed in detail in Chapters 9 and 27.

Hormone Assays

GnRH. As noted in a previous section of this chapter, immunoassays are available for GnRH. Most of the them are not capable of detecting the very small amounts of this peptide in peripheral blood, however. Procedures are available for detecting GnRH metabolites in urine.[18] The excretion of these peptides parallels that of the gonadotropins. Therefore, at present, their measurement offers no advantage to the clinician over that of LH and FSH.

Gonadotropins. The availability of sensitive radioimmunoassays makes the measurement of circulating levels of prolactin, LH, and FSH available to all clinicians. As noted earlier, LH is secreted in a pulsatile fashion, and this limits the value of a single determination in blood (see Fig. 6–2). Consequently, multiple blood samples are needed to determine the actual level of this hormone. LH is most accurately

assessed by measuring blood samples obtained at 20-minute intervals over a 3- or 6-hour period (see Fig. 6–2). In actual practice, however, a reasonable estimate of serum LH can be obtained by pooling four samples obtained at intervals of 20 minutes or greater. In this way only one pooled sample of serum is submitted for the estimation of LH.

Immunoassays are now used to measure LH and FSH in urine. With this procedure, the specimens are concentrated prior to assay and, as a result, they are useful for gonadotropin measurement in hypogonadal individuals and children.[263] Irrespective of the biologic specimen chosen for measurement (blood or urine), repeated basal hormone measurements performed over several months may be the most reassuring evidence of the actual status of the patient under consideration.

Prior to the advent of radioimmunoassay the only estimates of gonadotropins available were from bioassays of urinary extracts. The first widely used assay measured total gonadotropins in urine from changes in ovarian weight of the immature female rat or uterine weight of the immature female mouse. Unfortunately, the mouse uterine weight method was initially described as an "FSH assay." Thus, in the early literature, FSH levels were recorded which were, in fact, semiquantitative estimates of "total gonadotropins." Subsequently a number of investigators used specific bioassays for measuring urinary extracts. Biologically active FSH levels are measured using the Steelman-Pohley[264] method after kaolin-acetone precipitation.[265] When titers are expressed as IU/24 hr (Second International Reference Preparation, Second IRP), a typical normal adult male range is from 4 to 25 IU/24 hr. LH titers may be estimated in urine extracts by using immature hypophysectomized male rats as the assay model.[266] Increments in the prostate weight serve as the end point. The assay is extremely expensive and relatively insensitive to changes in LH titers. More recently bioassays have been developed that can detect LH in serum using testosterone production by isolated Leydig cells.

Sex Steroids. Radioimmunoassays for testosterone, estradiol, and estrone are now widely available from many commercial laboratories. A variety of clinical findings may be extremely useful when used in concert with these laboratory measurements. For example, an increase in sebum production is one of the earliest indications of androgen production in the child. Nitrogen retention, when the test is performed under careful balance conditions, provides a measure of endogenous effects of testosterone. Although these tests are not in routine clinical use, they may be extremely useful in detecting complete or partial end-organ unresponsiveness to androgens. In addition, urinary cytology can be used as an index of estrogen production in a hypogonadal male with gynecomastia.[263]

17-Ketosteroids. Prior to the advent of testosterone assays, urinary 17-ketosteroid assays were widely used by clinicians. Since more than 70% of 17-ketosteroids originate in the adrenal, they do not provide an index of gonadal status. Measurements of these steroids may be extremely useful, however, in the diagnosis of steroid-producing tumors and congenital adrenal hyperplasia. For this purpose, the measurements of serum androstenedione and DHA-sulfate have largely replaced ketosteroid measurements in urine.

Urinary Androstanediol (5α-androstane-3α,17β-diol) and Testosterone. Once assays for urinary testosterone glucuronide became available, it was not surprising to learn that they could be used to distinguish men from women. However, it was disappointing to note that urinary testosterone levels were often normal in mildly virilized women and pubertal boys who had clinical evidence of elevated testosterone production. The reason for this is that testos-

Table 6–6. URINARY EXCRETION OF ANDROSTANEDIOL AND TESTOSTERONE GLUCURONIDES

Subjects	Urinary* 5α-Androstanediol (μg/24 hr)	Urinary* Testosterone (μg/24 hr)
Normal men	133 ± 25	59 ± 16
Normal women	17 ± 6	6 ± 2
Testicular feminization	81	77
Women with hirsutism	88 ± 30	9 ± 4
Women with acne vulgaris	43 ± 14	6 ± 2

*Urinary steroids given in this table were measured by gas liquid chromatography by Mauvais-Jarvis et al.[267] Slightly lower values were reported by Doberne and New[268] using a radioligand method.

terone glucuronide is synthesized in the liver, not only from testosterone but also from a variety of other steroids such as androstenedione. Thus, the testosterone glucuronide in urine does not correlate with the testosterone production rate in women and children. As a consequence, an increase in testosterone production is not reflected by significant increase in testosterone glucuronide excreted into the urine. This has been discussed earlier in this chapter (see Fig. 6–7). An early effect of increased testosterone production in women or pubertal children is an increase of extrahepatic 5α-reductase (see Table 6–3). An increase in the urinary androstanediol out of proportion to urinary testosterone is believed to reflect this virilization.[267, 268] The excretion rates of androstanediol and testosterone glucuronides in men and women are summarized in Table 6–6.

Dynamic Tests of the Hypothalamo-Pituitary-Gonadal Axis

hCG Test. Human chorionic gonadotropin (4000 IU) administered to normal men or boys for 4 days produces at least a doubling in serum testosterone levels in 3 to 4 days. It should be noted that in prepubertal children this will not raise the testosterone into the range for normal men.[269] With the onset of puberty, however, the testes become particularly sensitive to hCG, and levels achieved in these boys equal or exceed those of men.[49] When hCG is administered to prepubertal or hypogonadal boys for 2 weeks or more (1500 IU/day), normal male testosterone levels are achieved. This latter approach is not useful as a routine test, however, since it takes multiple injections over a prolonged period.[270] Recently a number of investigators have recommended the use of a single-dose hCG test.[271, 272] In normal men testosterone levels peak at 2 to 4 hours, decline, and then rise again between 70 and 100 hours. While the simplicity of the procedure is attractive, wider experience must be gained in hypogonadal individuals before its utility can be assessed. The use of the hCG test is illustrated in Figure 6–32.

GnRH Test. As pointed out in a previous portion of this chapter, the pituitary gland changes its responsiveness to GnRH throughout puberty. This change is primarily in LH secretion since the quantitative response to FSH is relatively similar in children and adults. The amount of LH released after acute administration of GnRH probably reflects the amount of stored hormone in the pituitary, which, in turn, is related to the endogenous production of GnRH. A normal response to GnRH may provide reassuring information about pituitary function; it should be noted, however, that many hypogonadal individuals with pituitary tumors have normal responses to this releasing hormone. A negative or borderline response may be equally difficult to interpret since hypogonadotropic individuals may have blunted or absent responses until they have been treated with GnRH

for several days.[273] one type of GnRH test is illustrated in Figure 6–24.

Clomiphene Test. This procedure was first proposed prior to the development of the GnRH test. In the initial studies, 100 or 200 mg daily of clomiphene citrate increased plasma LH beginning on the second day. With the large dose, all normal individuals had a doubling of plasma LH levels by 6 days.[274] When normal men were treated for 51 days, increases of 200 to 700% in LH and of 70 to 360% in FSH were observed.[275] The slow increase in LH with clomiphene therapy had approximately the same time course as the increase in LH following gonadectomy.[276] After extended experience with this test, we recommend 50 mg twice a day for 10 days. Plasma LH and FSH are measured in four control samples (20 minutes apart) and in four similar samples after 10 days of treatment. The basis for this suggestion is shown in Figure 6–29.

Clomiphene citrate is a weak estrogen that has antiestrogenic activity on several end organs. It is therefore of interest to understand how this agent influences the pulsatile secretion of LH. In a recent study, Santen and Ruby[277] suggested that the antiestrogenic effect was mediated in the central nervous system; at this site clomiphene presumably blocks the action of estradiol, removing negative feedback, and allows GnRH secretion to increase. In the same experiment, it was demonstrated that clomiphene exerted an estrogenic effect on the anterior pituitary, as evidenced by blunting of the LH-releasing activity of exogenous GnRH.

The primary use of clomiphene is in patients who may have mild hypogonadism but whose plasma testosterone and gonadotropin levels are close to normal. The test may, therefore, be used in lieu of multiple sampling to detect mild abnormalities of the pituitary-gonadal axis. It is significant that this agent will produce very little change in gonadotropin levels in boys when their testosterone levels are below 100 ng/dl.[263] Therefore, clomiphene cannot be used to distinguish boys with delayed puberty from those with organic hypogonadotropism. As a consequence it is most useful in individuals in whom hypogonadotropism has developed after puberty.

MALE HYPOGONADISM

Male hypogonadism may be classified according to hormone concentrations, a known or suspected etiology, or anatomic site of the observed pathology. Thus, Klinefelter's syndrome could be classified as a hypergonadotropic, genetic, or primary testicular disorder. In practice, the clinician must adopt an approach to the patient which takes into account all methods of classification. In this presentation we will classify patients according to hypergonadotropic, hypogonadotropic, and eugonadotropic syndromes (Table 6–7). In considering patients in each of these categories, it is also useful to determine whether the testosterone concentrations are high, low, or normal. The hypergonadotropic syndromes usually refer to patients with severe primary testicular damage when observed after puberty. Sometimes selective elevations of either FSH or LH levels will be seen. In the hypogonadotropic syndromes, there are abnormalities of hypothalamo-pituitary function, with LH and FSH secretion that is inappropriately low. Occasionally there is selective involvement of LH and rarely of FSH. Moreover, the pituitary failure may be monotropic in nature (limited to gonadotropins) or may be more complicated, involving any combination of other tropic hormones. Finally, the term "eugonadotropic hypogonadism" has been added to the classification to focus attention on the fact that the majority of infertile men with oligospermia or, rarely, azoospermia

Table 6–7.   MALE HYPOGONADISM

Hypergonadotropic Syndromes
  Klinefelter's syndrome
    Classic form
    Variant forms
  XYY
  Myotonia dystrophica
  Noonan's syndrome
  Sertoli-cell-only syndrome
  Reifenstein's syndrome (androgen insensitivity)
  Functional prepuberal castrate (anorchia)
  Seminiferous tubular failure due to infection and toxic agents
    Parotitis
    Gonorrhea
    Leprosy
    Irradiation
  Gonadotropin-producing pituitary tumors
  Adult Leydig cell failure

Hypogonadotropic Syndromes
  Hypogonadotropic eunuchoidism
  Isolated LH deficiency
  Isolated FSH deficiency
  Panhypopituitarism
  Delayed puberty

Eugonadotropic syndromes
  Adult seminiferous tubular failure

demonstrate normal serum FSH, LH, and testosterone levels (see Fig. 6–16). Furthermore, these patients are characteristically free of endocrinopathy. This patient group represents a mild form of seminiferous tubule failure in which the normal interaction between central FSH secretory mechanisms and Sertoli cells is retained. It is likely that the condition of many of these patients will deteriorate with time, and eventually their FSH levels will rise. No data exist to confirm this contention. Several studies of infertile males indicate that FSH levels are not directly related to sperm counts; however, normal FSH levels are associated with lesser degrees of oligospermia.[278, 279] The exception to this is "obstructive" azoospermia. Normal FSH levels have also been observed in patients with minimal tubular membrane hyalinization and fibrosis with some evidence of active spermatogenesis, particularly in the early phases (i.e., spermatogonial cells are not grossly depleted in numbers). Finally, it should be noted that all three main categories of hypogonadism contain examples of acquired and hereditary disorders.

Hypergonadotropic Syndromes

Klinefelter's Syndrome

Definition and Incidence.   Various designations have been suggested for this disorder, including seminiferous tubule dysgenesis, pubertal seminiferous tubule failure, sclerosing tubular degeneration, and primary microorchidism. The authors prefer the term Klinefelter's syndrome for historical reasons since the other terms could apply equally well to other forms of primary testicular disease. For example, seminiferous tubule dysgenesis could refer to Klinefelter's syndrome or Sertoli-cell-only syndrome.

Klinefelter's syndrome represents one of the most common examples of male hypogonadism.[280, 281] It is characterized by varying degrees of seminiferous tubule failure and decreased Leydig cell function. In 1942, Klinefelter, Reifenstein, and Albright described a constellation of characteristics exhibited by a group of hypogonadal males.[282] As the pathogenesis has become better understood, the original description has been expanded to include additional fea-

tures.[283, 284] The presence of supernumerary X chromosomes is considered to be the fundamental underlying etiologic factor. Patients with Klinefelter's syndrome may be divided into two major categories, which include the classic and variant forms (Table 6–8). In the classic form, the salient features include small, firm testes, varying degrees of eunuchoidism (see Table 6–5), azoospermia, gynecomastia, mental abnormalities, elevated serum FSH and LH concentrations, chromatin-positive buccal smear, and an XXY sex chromosomal complement.

Males considered to have a variant form of Klinefelter's syndrome usually manifest different clinical features from those with the classic form. These differences include both number and severity of abnormal findings. The pathologic features are influenced by the presence of sex chromosomal patterns other than "pure" XXY and the specific tissue or tissues that contain the abnormal stem cell line(s). For example, in patients with sex chromosomal mosaicism (in which there is more than one stem cell line) gonadal function may be virtually normal if one of the cell lines is normal (XY).[281, 285] On the other hand, if more than one X chromosome and the Y chromosome are present in all the stem cell lines, the pathologic changes are more severe and widespread.[286]

As noted earlier, available data suggest that the presence of extra X chromosomes in testicular tissue is the focal point for the seminiferous tubular changes observed in Klinefelter's syndrome. Chromosomal analysis of skin or peripheral blood from some patients may reveal a normal chromosomal pattern, but if the testes contain a supernumerary X chromosomal complement, testicular dysgenesis typical of Klinefelter's syndrome develops. In this regard it is of note that some investigators have also classified patients with Klinefelter's syndrome as chromatin-positive or chromatin-negative (based on their buccal smear chromatin pattern).[287, 288] The presence or absence of sex chromatin (Barr body) in this instance indicates the number of X chromosomes in the buccal mucosa only and not in other tissues of the body such as the testes. Therefore, such a classification lacks precision.

Information about the incidence of Klinefelter's syndrome in the general population has been gathered primarily in surveys in which a chromatin-positive buccal smear was used to identify patients. In newborn infants, the incidence of chromatin-positive buccal smear patterns is 0.21%.[280] A similar incidence has been found in the adult male population (0.15–0.24%).[281, 289] That the frequency in the adult population is not decreased confirms that there is no lethal effect of this chromosomal abnormality. The incidence of Klinefelter's syndrome is significantly higher in mentally retarded individuals.[290, 291] The frequency varies from 0.45 to 2.38% in this segment of the population. One can appreciate from the foregoing figures that Klinefelter's syndrome represents a relatively common disorder. Furthermore, if one considers the variant forms that exhibit a chromatin-negative buccal smear and sex chromosomal mosaicism, the actual incidence of this syndrome is even higher.

Clinical Manifestations, Classic Form.   The finding of small, firm testes, gynecomastia, and decreased androgenicity suggests the presence of Klinefelter's syndrome (Figs. 6–20 and 6–21). Although the disorder is congenital, most of these relatively specific features are not evident prior to puberty. It has been suggested that the prepubertal Klinefelter testis contains fewer cellular elements in the undifferentiated germinal epithelium. Thus, these patients may have small testes by age 3. Since testicular size increases from age 6 until after puberty, the difference in the testes

Table 6–8. KLINEFELTER'S SYNDROME

Karotype and Clinical Features of Classic and Variant Forms

	Classic Form	XX Group	YY Group	Mosaicism	Poly X + Y Chromosome Group	
					Mosaicism	Poly X + Y Disorder
	XXY	XX	XXYY	XXY/XX	XXXY/XY	XXXY
				XXY/XY	XXXY/XXY	XXXYY
				XXY/XYY	XXXY/XXY/XY	XXXXY
				XXY/XXYY	XXXXY/XXXY	XXXxY
				XxY/XY/Yx	XXXXY/XXXXY/XXY	
Clinical and Laboratory Findings	1. Prepuberal: No definite decrease in germinal cells. Hyalinization or fibrosis of tubular membranes not present. 2. Cryptorchidism: Incidence not increased. 3. Subnormal intelligence (varying degrees — usually mild). 4. Bone abnormalities. Not consistent. 5. Buccal smear: One sex chromatin body.	This type is very uncommon. Patients possess the same features of the syndrome, except they may be somewhat shorter in height. The key laboratory findings to explain the male phenotype and testes is a positive H-Y antigen test.	Not common. Clinical and laboratory features similar to those seen in classic form except for the following: 1. More severe degree of mental retardation. 2. Tendency to be tall, e.g., over 6 ft. 3. Increased incidence of (a) "antisocial" behavior and (b) varicose veins.	Clinical and pathologic features vary. In patients with sex chromosomal mosaicism, spermatogenesis may be active and sperm present in the ejaculate. Thus the testes may be virtually normal in size. This is particularly true when the normal stem cell line (XY) is present in the testis. Patients with other forms of mosaicism usually demonstrate testicular damage that extends to that observed in the classic form.		1. Prepuberal: Definite decrease in immature germinal cells, with hypoplastic tubules and increased connective tissue stroma. 2. Cryptorchidism: Increased incidence. 3. Subnormal intelligence (severe). 4. Bone abnormalities: Radioulnar synostosis and other abnormalities of the elbow. 5. Buccal smear: 2 sex chromatin bodies in XXXY and XXXYY; 3 sex chromatin bodies in XXXXY.

Similar Postpuberal Features

1. Eunuchoidism (varying degrees).
2. Gynecomastia.
3. Azoospermia (oligospermia in XY mosaicism).
4. Elevated serum gonadotropins.
5. Small, firm testes (variable size in mosaicism).
   a. Hyalinization and fibrosis of seminiferous tubules (almost all tubules severely involved).
   b. Leydig cell hyperplasia and decreased function.
   c. Absence of elastic fibers around tunica propria of hyalinized tubules.

between patients with Klinefelter's syndrome and normal boys increases with age.[263] Certain signs, such as subnormal intelligence or a tendency toward eunuchoidal skeletal proportions, may be present before puberty, but these are not specific enough to aid in the diagnosis.

At puberty, when pituitary gonadotropin secretion increases, the testis undergoes typical pathologic changes. It fails to increase in size and becomes firmer in consistency. This is due to progressive fibrosis and hyalinization of the seminiferous tubules which ordinarily make up 85% of the volume of the normal testis (see Fig. 6–19B and C). The final testicular size in these patients rarely exceeds 2.0 × 1.5 × 1.5 cm. In contrast, the longest dimension of the normal adult testis is at least 3.5 cm.[242, 292] Leydig cell function is also impaired to varying degrees in these patients. Some patients have little androgen production, resulting in incomplete development of secondary sex characteristics. In others, the androgen deficiency is so subtle that superficial evaluation may result in the erroneous conclusion that testosterone production is normal. Indeed, a dichotomy between total serum testosterone levels and secondary sex characteristics exists in many patients. The reason for this may be related to observations that TeBG levels may be elevated in these patients, probably as a result of increased estrogen or decreased androgen secretion;[293] this results in a low "apparent free testosterone concentration" (AFTC) in men with Klinefelter's syndrome.[294] Wang et al.[295] found decreased testosterone metabolic clearance and secretion rates. These findings are all in keeping with the concept that metabolically active testosterone levels are low in these patients and that the "total" serum testosterone levels may be misleading.

Whereas androgen deficiency is the usual finding, the development of eunuchoidal skeletal measurements in Klinefelter's syndrome appears to be related to other factors. Usually, skeletal changes of this type are considered to arise from a delay in long-bone epiphysial closure secondary to testosterone deficiency. Normal thyroid, adrenocortical, and growth hormone production is also required. However, in most patients with Klinefelter's syndrome, the excessive long-bone growth is initiated prior to puberty,[269, 297] and the bone age is usually appropriate for the patient's chronologic age. Furthermore, linear growth of the long bones in the lower extremities is greater than it is in the upper extremities. This results in a span-height ratio of 1 or less. In patients whose eunuchoidal skeletal measurements are exclusively secondary to androgen deficiency, the situation is different. The long bones of the upper and lower extremities grow in a comparable fashion. This results in a span at least 2 inches greater than the height, and the ratio therefore is greater than 1. The basis for the skeletal changes in patients with Klinefelter's syndrome may be related to an abnormal sex chromosome constitution in the osseous tissue.

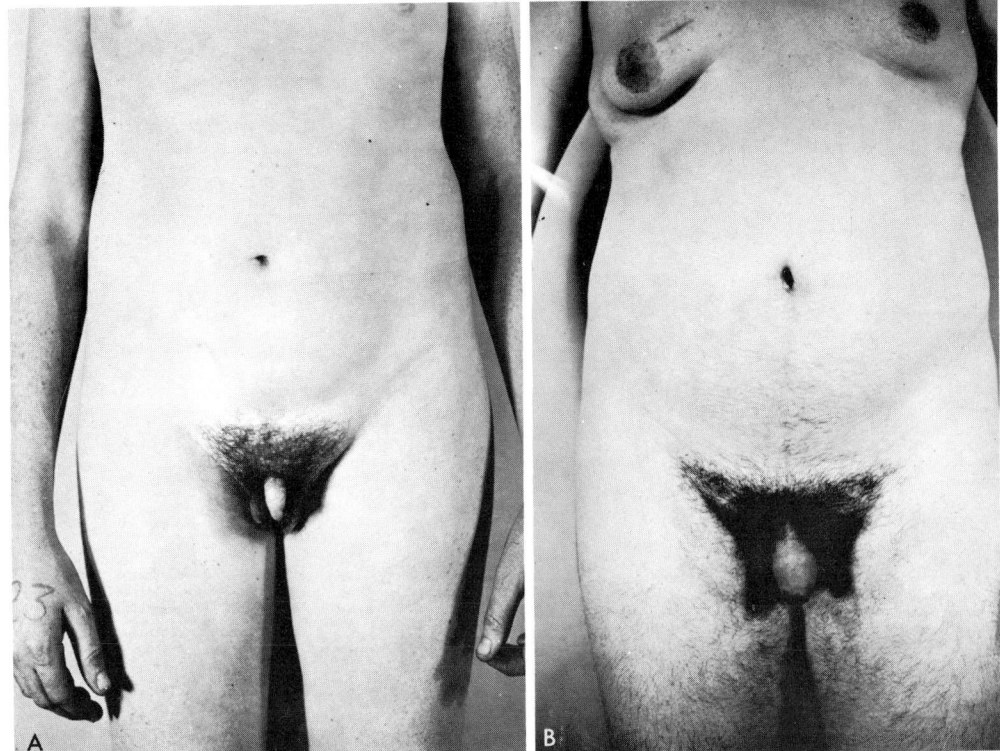

Figure 6–20.   Two untreated patients with Klinefelter's syndrome, who demonstrate the variations in Leydig cell function observed in this entity. *A*, The small penis accompanied by sparse pubic and body hair indicates minimal androgen secretion. *B*, Normal penile development and adequate pubic and body hair indicate normal androgen production by the testis. Gynecomastia is also present.

Bilateral gynecomastia is present in most patients with Klinefelter's syndrome. Usually this is evident either by inspection or by palpation. Microscopic examination of breast biopsy specimens sometimes is required for detection. When the gynecomastia is minimal, it may be overlooked by improper palpation. The cause of the gynecomastia remains obscure. It is known that patients with Klinefelter's syndrome secrete increased amounts of estrogens; however, the breast tissue is characterized microscopically by hyperplasia of the interductal tissue. In contrast, gynecomastia associated with systemic estrogen administration or increased endogenous estrogen production exhibits ductal hyperplasia. (See the discussion of gynecomastia later in this chapter for further details.)

Subnormal intelligence, defined as an IQ of less than 80, is evident in many patients with Klinefelter's syndrome.[298] When patients in the general population are considered, rather than those residing in mental institutions, the precise incidence is not known since detailed intelligence tests are not usually carried out. In some series of patients with Klinefelter's the incidence approaches 15–25%. Even though the remaining patients may demonstrate normal intelligence, many of them exhibit character or personality disorders. Whether this is genetic or acquired as a consequence of hypogonadism is difficult to decide. For example, when the affected boy reaches the age of puberty, he realizes he is different from his contemporaries. Physical exposure in communal locker rooms makes him vulnerable to ridicule because of his enlarged breasts or abnormal sexual development. The continued lack of androgens with consequent poor muscular development limits his physical capabilities. This tends to confirm in his mind that he is an inadequate individual. If his parents fail to understand the problem and do not seek proper medical advice, further difficulties in interpersonal relationships arise. Thus, it is not surprising that many of these patients have behavioral disorders, neuroses, or frank psychoses.

Witkin and colleagues[299] concluded that the increased criminality reported for patients with Klinefelter's syndrome and men with an XYY sex chromosomal pattern may be related to their low intelligence rather than to aggression *per se*. They studied all men over 184 cm in height who were born in Copenhagen between 1944 and 1947. They found a penal code violation in 9.3, 41.7, and 18.8% of normal (XY), XYY, and XXY men studied, respectively. Thus, it may be that these men have more difficulty in coping with society because of their mental dullness.

Occasionally a patient with a classic form of the syndrome may progress through puberty in reasonably normal fashion only to develop the typical pathologic changes in his testes at a later time. Such an individual may have complete maturation of his secondary sexual characteristics and may relate that his testes became smaller for no apparent reason or that the reduced testicular size resulted from trauma. This type of history naturally is misleading to the examiner unless further studies, such as buccal smear or a testicular biopsy, are performed. This type of patient may produce progeny prior to development of his testicular damage. Therefore, the history of having had children should not dissuade the physician from considering the possibility of Klinefelter's syndrome.

A greater incidence of other systemic disorders in patients with Klinefelter's syndrome has been suggested.[284, 300-302] These include diabetes mellitus, emphysema, chronic bronchitis, neoplasia, and various autoimmune or allergic disorders. Whether or not Klinefelter's syndrome is associated with a predisposition to these diseases awaits extensive epidemiologic study.

Variant Forms of Klinefelter's Syndrome — Poly X + Y.   The majority of male patients with more than two X

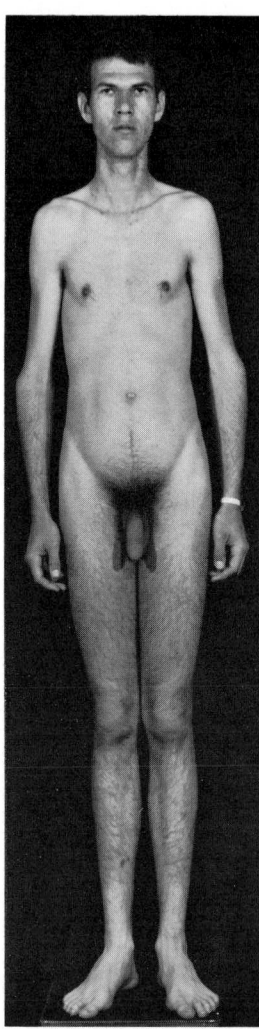

Figure 6–21.   Example of a variant of Klinefelter's syndrome; this 21-year-old patient demonstrates XXY/XY mosaicism in all tissue examined. Note the eunuchoidal skeletal features, particularly with regard to the lower extremities. Plasma testosterone levels were 420 ng/dl, which accounts for the virilization. The testes were somewhat larger than those encountered in patients with the classic form of the syndrome. Seminal fluid examination revealed a sperm count of 300,000/ml.

chromosomes have been discovered prepubertally by buccal smear surveys done in mental institutions; therefore, the overwhelming preponderance of mental retardation in these subjects may simply be a reflection of the method used for detection (see Table 6–8).

XXXXY Disorder.   The more constant features consist of severe mental retardation (highest IQ, 53), prepubertal testicular damage, scrotal hypoplasia, cryptorchidism, and various osseous abnormalities such as proximal radioulnar synostosis and overgrowth of the radial or ulnar heads or both. Somewhat more variable features include retarded linear growth, bone age, motor development, and coordination. These patients tend to be thin and may have epicanthal folds, hypertelorism, cubitus valgus, and incurving of the fifth digit.[286]

XXXY Disorder.   Patients afflicted with this chromosomal pattern present a clinical picture somewhere between that of the classic form of Klinefelter's syndrome and that of the XXXXY disorder.[303] The incidence and degree of mental retardation resemble those encountered in patients with the XXXXY disorder. Similarly, radioulnar synostosis and cryptorchidism are frequently present in these patients.

However, the prepubertal and postpubertal testes resemble those encountered in patients with the classic form of Klinefelter's syndrome (XXY).

Mosaicism.   The clinical picture is quite variable in patients with more than one stem cell line. In some, the damage is severe and resembles that seen in the classic form of the syndrome. However, the majority of patients with mosaicism exhibit less severe changes (Fig. 6–21), particularly if a normal stem cell line (XY) is present. Indeed, normal gonadal function during young adult life with successful fertility has been documented in this type of patient. Sometimes mental retardation may be the only clinical feature.

Clearly, then, the patient with the Klinefelter's variant that is associated with sex chromosomal mosaicism presents a great challenge insofar as detection and proper diagnosis are concerned. It is important to recall that all the tissues available for study (i.e., skin, blood, and testes) need not demonstrate the multiple stem cell pattern or even an abnormal stem cell line. For a more extensive discussion, the reader is referred to several review articles.[304-307]

YY Disorder.   Although this is not a common variant of the syndrome, patients in this category may have some characteristic clinical features.[308, 309] For example, they tend to be tall (over 6 feet) and have saphenous vein varicosities more frequently than expected. With respect to the increased height, Philip and coworkers found an increased number of sex chromosomal abnormalities in tall men when compared to newborn populations, and individuals with an XYY pattern outnumbered the individuals with an XXY pattern.[310] Whether this relationship holds true for the patients with an XXYY pattern requires verification by careful epidemiologic studies in different ethnic populations. Testicular damage and unstable behavior are similar to those observed in the classic form of XXY.

XX Disorder ("Sex Reversal").   Patients with a male phenotype and an XX karyotype have been termed sex-reversed males. Clinically they resemble patients with an XXY/XY mosaic pattern except they tend to be shorter.[311] There has been considerable speculation as to how phenotypic males can develop even imperfect testes without a Y chromosome. Serologic identification of the H-Y antigen in four such men suggests that a very small portion of the Y chromosome has been translocated to either an X chromosome or an autosome.[312] Alternatively, the Y chromosome could be intact in a mosaic stem cell line that does not grow well *in vitro.*[313] Actually, both explanations can apply. Approximately one in 9000 phenotypic males exhibits this abnormality.

Laboratory Findings.   Testicular biopsy specimens reveal two main features: hyalinization of the seminiferous tubular membranes and "adenomatous clumping" of the Leydig cells. In the usual case, virtually all the tubules are severely hyalinized and acellular (see Fig. 6–19B and C). Occasionally certain areas of the testes have tubules with spermatozoa. This finding is more common when sex chromosomal mosaicism of the XXY/XY variety is present. In all such cases it is probable that spermatozoa develop in a portion of the seminiferous tubule where the normal (XY) stem cell has survived and, as a result, the testicular damage associated with the extra X chromosome does not occur.[306] There are not sufficient data to conclude that the same condition holds true for Leydig cell function.[305, 306] In all forms of the syndrome, a disturbance in androgen biosynthesis is reflected by the adenomatous clumping of Leydig cells, which tend to be less granular than normal and to contain less lipid. Fibroblastic and intermediate forms of these cells are also increased. Before this syndrome was well recognized, these adenomatous clumps were sometimes mistaken for interstitial cell tumors. Rarely, the interstitial cells may be sparse and difficult to identify.[311, 312] Here, the transition to the fibroblastic forms may have been more rapid and complete.[313, 314] Special stains demonstrate the absence of elastic fibers in and around the thickened tunica propria. This finding supports the congenital nature of this entity, as elastic fibers normally appear during pubertal maturation.[315] Furthermore, it aids in differentiating Klinefelter's syndrome from mumps orchitis, myotonia dystrophica, and other disorders that may present a similar histologic pattern (see Fig. 6–19D).

Azoospermia is the characteristic finding in the classic form of Klinefelter's syndrome. Occasionally, as mentioned previously, spermatogenesis will be less damaged. This results in the finding of viable sperm in the ejaculate. Sperm counts in patients with XXY/XY mosaicism may be normal at some point, since fertility has been documented.[316, 317] However, in our experience, severe oligospermia is invariably present at the time of physician contact. The reason for this is obvious; examination of gonadal function is usually deferred until there are complaints referable to reproductive function. There are no unique diagnostic changes in the various constituents of the seminal plasma. In general, when androgen deficiency is severe, the volume of the ejaculate is small and the fructose and phosphatase content decreased.

In 1950, Plunkett and Barr[318] demonstrated a positive chromatin pattern in patients having this syndrome. Using a buccal smear to detect the condensed X chromosome is an invaluable aid to diagnostic screening for this syndrome. As mentioned previously, this laboratory test has limitations when sex chromosomal mosaicism is present.

Chromosome analysis by means of short-term tissue culture is the most accurate way of documenting the extra X chromosome(s) of Klinefelter's syndrome. However, this procedure is laborious and costly and should be reserved for the difficult diagnostic problems.

Patients with Klinefelter's syndrome have elevated serum gonadotropin levels. FSH is invariably elevated; on rare occasions, serum LH levels may fall within the normal adult male range.[319] We would expect that those patients whose pathologic features are delayed until later in life would probably pass through a phase when their levels of both gonadotropins are normal but this remains to be demonstrated.

Serum testosterone concentrations in patients with Klinefelter's syndrome range from low to low normal.[305] In our latest studies of 48 patients with either the classic or a variant form of the syndrome, serum testosterone levels varied from 50 to 860 ng/dl as compared to 300 to 1200 ng/dl in normal men. Seventeen of the 40 men with the classic form exhibited values below our mean value (670 ng/dl) for normal men, but were within the normal range.[319] Serum testosterone concentrations in the so-called chromatin-positive and chromatin-negative patients were not different. "Free" testosterone determinations by ammonium sulfate precipitation were found to be lower than normal in eleven patients with this syndrome.[295]

Administration of human chorionic gonadotropin (hCG) to stimulate Leydig cell function appears to have limited usefulness for diagnosing Klinefelter's syndrome. The original studies demonstrated that men with this disorder had decreased Leydig cell reserve.[320] When patients receive four daily injections of hCG there is some response on the first day but a limited increase on subsequent days.[305] It should be noted that many of the patients who have been tested have elevated gonadotropin levels. The possibility that high LH concentrations contribute to the "insensitivity" of the Leydig cells by downregulation of LH receptors has not been excluded.

Treatment of patients with Klinefelter's syndrome is directed toward correcting the androgen deficiency that is usually present. In this regard, androgen replacement therapy produces adequate sexual maturation. (See Androgen Replacement Therapy, later in this chapter.) The infertility is irreversible, and the gynecomastia is not amenable to medical therapy. When the latter is sufficient to cause social embarrassment, plastic surgery should be performed.

Early detection is an important goal in this syndrome. This may avoid many of the problems of social adjustment that otherwise develop for these patients. Furthermore, if the mental behavior is too disorganized, psychiatric care should be made available as early as possible. If early detection is to be achieved, Klinefelter's syndrome should be suspected in boys with one or more of the following: (1) scholastic problems; (2) inadequate and somewhat delayed sexual maturation; (3) long-leggedness; (4) behavioral problems at home or school or both; (5) genitalia smaller than normal for the individual's age.[321]

XYY Syndrome

The occurrence of XYY in the general population is estimated to be between 0.1 and 0.2%.[310, 322-326] Testicular function in terms of spermatogenesis may be normal, minimally impaired, or severely damaged.[327, 328] Retention of normal spermatogenesis in certain patients with an XYY pattern is considered to be related to the observation that the extra Y chromosome is usually deleted during spermatogonial mitosis.[329, 330] Thus, the genetic material within the germ cells regains "balance."

Histologically, there is no distinct pattern seen in the testicular biopsy specimen.[329] Some patients show spermatogenic arrest at the primary spermatocyte level. Others have more severe damage, with marked depletion of germ cells even to the point where tubules contain only Sertoli cells.[327, 329]

The serum testosterone levels are usually in the normal range.[329, 331] However, 10 men identified in a Danish study had higher testosterone levels than their age-matched controls (XY). Serum FSH and LH were also found to be elevated, but no seminal fluid studies were carried out.[332] Another study noted elevated FSH and LH titers in only one of seven men, and the testes were severely damaged in that patient. The reason for the modest elevation in testosterone in these patients is not known, but some investigators postulated that it is directly related to the YY karyotype. Clearly, this important point needs further study.

Additional features that are considered to be part of this syndrome include pustular acne;[333] increased height, which is apparently independent of the gonadal status;[310] and mental retardation and behavioral disorders, which have been mentioned previously. It is possible that the increased testosterone production provides the drive for the antisocial behavior in these patients.

No known treatment is available to improve fertility in those patients with impaired spermatogenesis.

Myotonia Dystrophica

This is a hereditary disorder characterized by myotonia (delayed relaxation after initial contraction). The major clinical features in addition to myotonia include lenticular opacities, frontal baldness, and testicular atrophy.[334, 335] Hypogonadism is present in approximately 80% of these patients. Clinically the testes are small and softer than normal. Pubertal development is usually normal, and the testicular damage occurs at varying times during adult life. Leydig cell function usually remains normal, and gynecomastia is not a characteristic finding.

The testicular biopsies from these patients reveal damage ranging from complete hyalinization and fibrosis of the seminiferous tubules to only moderate derangement of the seminiferous epithelium. Drucker et al.[334] concluded from their study that the hyalinized tubular membranes in these patients underwent more infolding than in Klinefelter's syndrome. This was believed to represent damage to previously normal seminiferous tubules. Leydig cells may tend to be clumped, but this is not a characteristic finding.

Although the testicular changes resemble those encountered in Klinefelter's syndrome, X chromosomal abnormalities are not an integral factor in the pathogenesis of this disorder. In 18 cases studied by Drucker et al.,[334] only one patient manifested a positive chromatin pattern. In some patients with myotonia, chromosomal gonadal dysgenesis may coexist.[336]

Despite the primary nature of the gonadal disorder, early studies suggested that urinary gonadotropin titers were not uniformly elevated.[334-336] This finding was due to the fact that total gonadotropin rather than specific FSH assays were employed. Subsequent studies have indicated that FSH concentrations in blood are uniformly increased. For example, Harper et al.[337] found serum FSH levels elevated (18.3–92.5 mIU/ml; their normal male range was 5.2–14.5 mIU/ml) in all 33 afflicted males studied, aged 15–44 years.

There is no known treatment for the infertility. Testosterone administration is not indicated since androgen production is usually normal.

Noonan's Syndrome (Male Turner's Syndrome)

This genetic disorder affects both males and females to almost an equal extent.[338] The abnormal features observed in these patients are similar to those seen in phenotypic females with "streak" ovaries and an XO sex chromosomal pattern (i.e., gonadal dysgenesis). These features include short stature, webbed neck, low-set ears, shieldlike chest, cubitus valgus, ocular abnormalities such as ptosis, and cardiovascular anomalies.[338-340] Pulmonary artery stenosis is very common. Many males with this disorder exhibit cryptorchidism, diminished spermatogenesis, and decreased Leydig cell function, but in others testicular function may be normal. Mental retardation of varying degrees is common.

In the limited number of patients studied, the testicular biopsy specimen has not shown a unique pattern. Some seminiferous tubules contain only Sertoli cells, whereas others have decreased numbers of germinal cells in various stages of maturation. Leydig cells may appear to be increased in number but do not show the characteristic adenomatous clumping seen in Klinefelter's syndrome.

Serum FSH and LH levels may be elevated in those patients who demonstrate diminished testicular function. Serum testosterone concentrations may be normal or decreased.

Originally, there was some question whether or not this disorder was associated with partial or complete deletion of an X chromosome in mosaic chromosomal pattern,[341] but the familial pattern of inheritance and the demonstration of male-to-male transmission clearly point to autosomal dominant inheritance with variable penetrance. Since this is not an abnormality of the X chromosome, the term Noonan's syndrome is preferred.

Treatment is directed toward correcting the androgen deficiency. Orchiopexy will not rectify any inherent spermatogenic abnormality. It is uncertain whether these patients carry the same risk for testicular carcinoma as a male with simple cryptorchidism or a greater risk.

Sertoli-Cell-Only Syndrome (Germinal Cell Aplasia)

This is an uncommon syndrome which may prove to have multiple etiologies. In its classic form the major features are testes of normal consistency but slightly smaller than normal, azoospermia, and elevated FSH titers. Androgen production usually remains intact. If so, LH concentrations are normal and the only presenting complaint is infertility. In certain patients with this disorder, serum testosterone levels are lower than normal and the serum LH levels are elevated along with the FSH titers.[342] Moreover, these patients may respond to hCG stimulation by showing a sluggish rise in serum testosterone concentration reminiscent of the diminished Leydig cell reserve in patients with Klinefelter's syndrome.[343] Gynecomastia is not a part of the clinical picture, but may occur with the same frequency and in the same magnitude as observed in normal males (see later). Abnormalities in sex chromosome configuration are uncommon.

The testicular biopsy specimen shows the seminiferous tubules to be moderately reduced in size and devoid of germ cells (see Fig. 6–19E). There may be some thickening of the tunica propria, but significant peritubular sclerosis and hyalinization are not present. Ultrastructural studies may show hypertrophy of the extracellular fibrillar network within the interstitial spaces.[344] In one instance interstitial fibrosis was detected by light microscopy. Leydig cells are morphologically normal, but may appear to be increased in number because of the decreased size of the seminiferous tubules. Adenomatous clumping does not occur.

Some workers have postulated that congenital absence of germ cells is the basis for this syndrome, but no direct evidence for this exists. Even though the biopsy specimen may uniformly demonstrate the absence of the germinal epithelium, an occasional patient will have a few sperm in his ejaculate.[314, 345] In other patients, an isolated tubule may be found containing some germinal elements. These variant features are usually observed in the younger individuals with this syndrome. Thus, the germinal epithelium may be essentially normal until puberty, when spermatogenesis is initiated. Then, the germinal cells, including spermatogonia, slough into the lumen so that finally the tubules are populated only by Sertoli cells. At this time electron microscopic examination shows evidence of damage of these cells.[346, 347] The disappearance of the germinal cells in some men may be secondary to some inherited defect in the Sertoli cells; studies of genetically determined infertility in animals support this concept.[348] In other patients, the disorder is associated with an XYY karyotype. This was detected in one of 10 patients in one report.[342] Extensive chromosomal studies have not been conducted in most clinics, but XYY as a causal factor is probably not common. Other chromosomal aberrations have been detected in a few men with Sertoli-cell-only syndrome.[349]

Serum gonadotropin assays and buccal smear examinations, including the use of fluorescent stains, are diagnostic aids in evaluating the patient with almost-normal-sized testes and azoospermia. The information obtained should enable the clinician to discriminate between patients with Sertoli-cell-only syndrome and those with a variant of Klinefelter's syndrome. It may be necessary to obtain a testicular biopsy to exclude the patient with ductal obstruction, especially when serum gonadotropins are in the high-normal range.

It should be emphasized that patients with other gonadal disorders may also have seminiferous tubules that contain only Sertoli cells.[350] However, in these individuals, in contrast to those with the Sertoli-cell-only syndrome, the testes are usually smaller, the microscopic pattern is not as uniform, and severe sclerosis and hyalinization are predominant features. For example, in Klinefelter's syndrome 90% of the tubules may be completely hyalinized and acellular, whereas 10% may be small and sclerotic and contain only Sertoli cells. Other conditions in which this variable pattern can be observed include mumps and gonococcal orchitis, cryptorchidism, adult seminiferous tubule failure, and damage due to irradiation or toxic agents.

Treatment cannot correct the infertility, which is permanent, and hormone replacement therapy is not needed.

Reifenstein's Syndrome (Partial Androgen Insensitivity)

Until recently it was not known why genetic males who have the capacity to synthesize testosterone fail to become masculinized. Increased knowledge of steroid hormone action indicated that an inherited defect of androgen receptors results in end-organ insensitivity to testosterone which, in turn, leads to feminization of individuals with an XY karyotype. Patients with receptor abnormalities may have a spectrum of phenotypes ranging from complete testicular feminization on one extreme to oligospermic masculinized males on the other. Patients with Reifenstein's syndrome represent an intermediate form of androgen insensitivity. See the discussion of androgen receptors earlier in this chapter (page 304).

Patients with Reifenstein's syndrome have hypospadias, gynecomastia, and varying degrees of diminished virilization.[145, 351, 352] Commonly, cryptorchidism is present and may be associated with a bifid scrotum. The prostate gland is usually smaller than normal and, in some patients, undetectable by palpation.

The hormonal findings are somewhat variable. For example, serum LH levels are elevated, but serum FSH levels may be within normal limits in some patients. The androgen levels (serum testosterone, dihydrotestosterone, and Δ-4 androstenedione) may be normal or elevated.[145, 146, 353-355] Serum estradiol levels are usually normal, but production rates of estradiol and estrone are elevated.[353] In contrast to patients with Klinefelter's syndrome, which this entity resembles, patients with Reifenstein's syndrome possess a normal XY sex chromosomal configuration in all tissues. Therefore, the buccal smear pattern is chromatin-negative.

The testicular histology in these patients reveals variable damage. Most of the seminiferous tubules are severely fibrosed or hyalinized, while others contain a reduced number of germ cells of all types. Elastic fibers are usually present in and around the hyalinized seminiferous tubules, which supports the contention that the testicular damage occurs postpubertally. Hyperplastic Leydig cells are observed in the interstitium. This finding corresponds to the presence of normal or elevated serum androgen levels in these patients.

Studies of androgen uptake by fibroblasts from patients with Reifenstein's syndrome indicate that the concentration of androgen receptor per cell is reduced. No qualitative abnormality has been demonstrated in the residual receptors in these patients. This is in contrast to subjects with testicular feminization with partial receptor deficiency; these latter patients have thermolabile receptors.[144] It should be emphasized that 5α-reductase activity is normal in patients with Reifenstein's syndrome.[353]

Genetic studies in three families suggest that this disorder is inherited as an X-linked recessive trait.[145, 351, 352] Analyses of the data indicate that there is not a close linkage with Xg^a but there might be such a linkage with the X locus for color blindness.[352] As noted earlier, these observations and similar studies in rats and mice suggest that a gene on the X chromosome regulates the synthesis or controls the activity of the androgen receptor.[194]

Treatment in patients with Reifenstein's syndrome is directed primarily toward surgical correction of the hypospadias and gynecomastia. Exogenous testosterone administration can overcome the partial androgen deficiency exhibited by these patients. Increased facial and body hair, as well as normal libido and sexual potentia, can be achieved. There is no known treatment for the abnormal spermatogenesis and infertility.

Functional Prepubertal Castrate Syndrome (Testicular Agenesis, Anorchia, "Vanishing" Testis Syndrome)

In these patients there is generally no recognizable testicular tissue.[356] Isolated reports have identified ectopic Leydig cells along the spermatic cord[357] or have measured significant testosterone levels within the spermatic vein despite the absence of testicular tissue.[358] Since these patients are phenotypic males without a uterus or uterine remnants, we presume that functioning testes are present until sometime around the fourteenth week of fetal life.[359-361] (See Chapter 9 for further details.)

Although the etiology of this condition remains unclear, genetic or chromosomal abnormalities do not appear to be involved. For example, this disorder has been documented in monozygotic twins of whom one of the brothers was affected and the other was normal.[362] In most instances testicular damage occurs in fetal life. Most investigators consider that severe bilateral testicular torsion is a likely cause. This is because incomplete testicular damage associated with torsion is frequently observed. Other disturbances must occur in fetal development to account for the finding of wolffian duct derivatives within the scrotum of certain patients. Finally, in a few patients fetal development was apparently normal and the damage occurred in early prepubertal life, resulting in complete atrophy. Surgical manipulations such as bilateral herniorrhaphy or orchiopexy, trauma, and infections have been suggested as causes of this disorder. In most instances, however, the etiology is obscure.

Somatic and visceral anomalies are not part of this syndrome; thus, these patients may readily be distinguished on clinical grounds from those who have Noonan's syndrome. Since there is no gonadal tissue to respond to endogenous or exogenous gonadotropins, puberty fails to occur. Therefore, these patients are characterized by sexual infantilism and appear to have an "empty" scrotum (Fig. 6–22). This latter feature frequently leads to the mistaken diagnosis of bilateral cryptorchidism with abdominal testes. On careful palpation, however, small, ill defined scrotal "masses" are usually encountered. Biopsy of these scrotal contents reveals remnants of wolffian duct derivatives or hyalinized prepubertal testes. These patients may be of short stature, or they may be typically eunuchoidal.

Serum testosterone levels are lower than normal for the patient's age. The serum LH and FSH concentrations are elevated even prior to puberty. At this time urinary LH and FSH measurements indicate that secretion is increased even before this is detectable by plasma assays.[263] After the age of puberty, serum LH and FSH concentrations rise into the true castrate range.

In men with anorchia no increase in testosterone occurs during hCG treatment. This is in contrast to the 3 to 12.5 fold increase in serum testosterone levels found in boys with bilateral cryptorchidism within 4 days following the administration of 2000 IU of hCG per day.[363] It is of note,

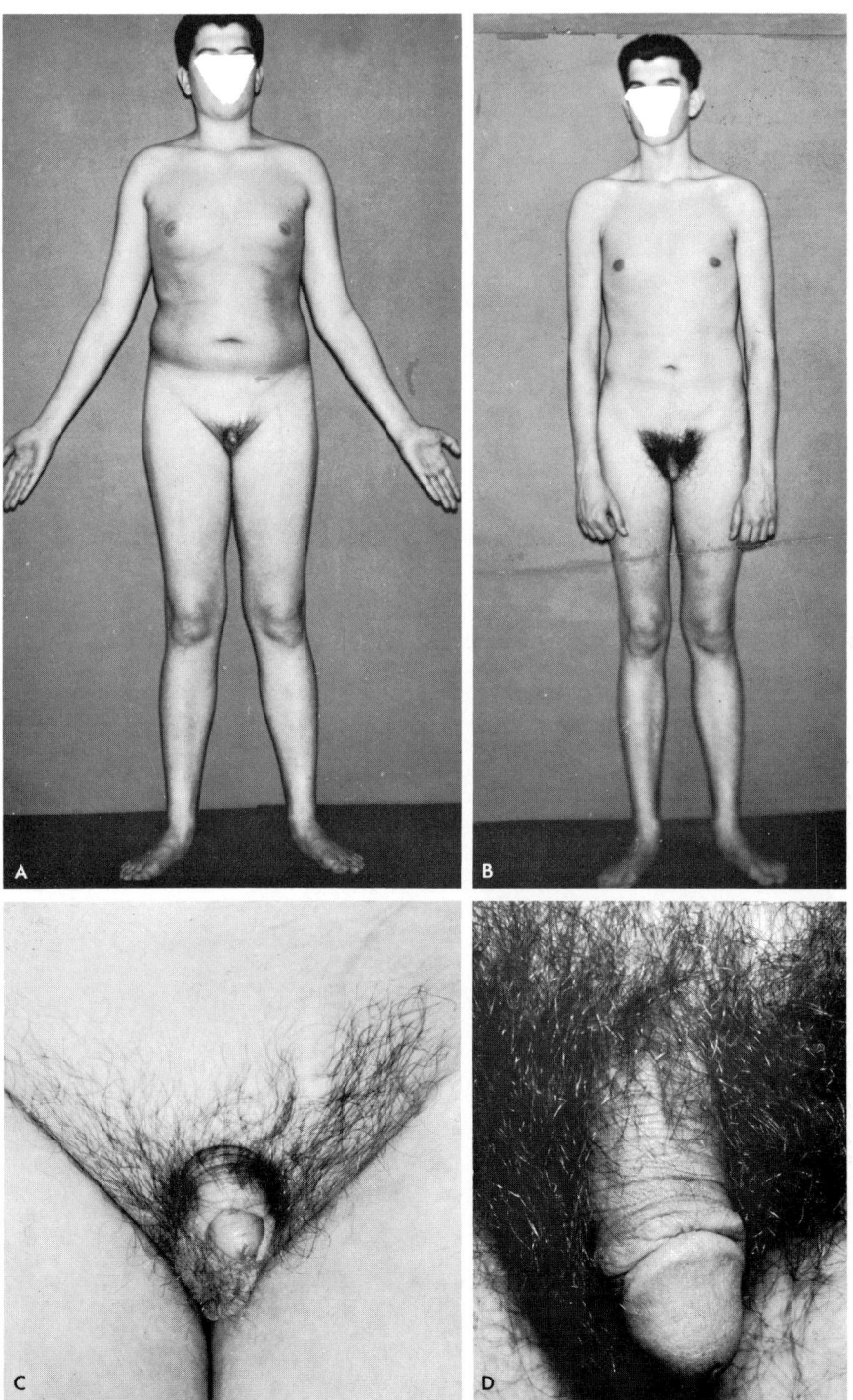

Figure 6–22. Functional prepubertal castrate. *A* and *C*, Before treatment. Note the "empty" scrotum, eunuchoidal features, and absence of somatic anomalies. No testicular tissue was found at the time of surgical exploration. *B* and *D*, After 15 years of testosterone therapy, scalp hair recession, penile development, and hair growth have occurred. The body habitus has attained masculine proportions, and muscle development is now that of a normal adult male.

however, that there is little or no increase in testosterone in patients in whom bilateral cryptorchidism is associated with hypogonadotropic eunuchoidism.[364] Thus caution should be exercised in concluding that testes are absent if there is no rise in testosterone levels during hCG administration unless one is confident of the pattern of gonadotropin secretion.

Androgen replacement therapy (page 335) should be instituted to produce full sexual maturation. Normal linear growth can be achieved provided treatment is initiated early.[360]

Seminiferous Tubular Failure Due to Infections and Toxic Agents

Orchitis with Epidemic Parotitis. About 15–25% of males with epidemic parotitis develop acute orchitis. Of those who have orchitis before puberty, most will recover completely, but when the pubertal or adult testes are involved, permanent damage to the seminiferous tubules usually results.[365] Even when only one testis is involved clinically, degenerative changes have been observed in the other.

During the acute phase, the pathologic findings vary from interstitial edema and cytoplasmic swelling of the germinal cells to complete sloughing of the germinal epithelium.[366] Chronic changes involve progressive tubular sclerosis and hyalinization. Sometimes the histologic picture resembles that seen in Klinefelter's syndrome, including the Leydig cell "clumping" (see Fig. 6–19B, C, and D). The full extent of the damage may not be evident until 10–20 years after the acute infection.

Leydig cell function usually remains intact, but in severe cases serum testosterone concentrations are low. Serum FSH titers may be normal or elevated. Semen analysis shows oligospermia or azoospermia. The testes are small and soft, and if androgen secretion is impaired, climacteric symptoms develop along with very slow regression of secondary sex characteristics.

Administration of estrogens during the acute phase has been advocated as a means of preventing permanent damage,[367] but long-term studies to establish the effectiveness of this treatment are lacking. Supposedly, estrogen therapy would be beneficial by suppressing spermatogenesis, thus making the germinal cells less vulnerable. But since it takes several weeks to significantly depress spermatogenesis and since the orchitis usually runs its course in 6–8 days, estrogen therapy does not appear logical. Prednisone treatment has not been uniformly effective during the acute phase, but observations on the chronic course are not available.[368] Probably the best treatment is still the supportive measures of bed rest and scrotal support.

Acute orchitis similar to that seen in parotitis is associated with gonorrheal infections. The sequelae are essentially the same. Progressive sclerosis of the tubular membranes resembling that of the Klinefelter testis also occurs in patients with chronic orchitis secondary to leprosy.

Irradiation. Exposure to x-rays, neutrons, and radioactive materials can cause germinal cell destruction.[369-371] After acute exposure, spermatogenesis may eventually recover, provided that the dose is not excessive. The maximal dose that permits full recovery is not known with certainty, but probably lies between 400 and 600 r[371] for a radiation source consisting of 250-kv x-ray energy.

Spermatogonia are quite sensitive to irradiation. Indeed, using 20 r gamma irradiation, Oakberg found significant cell destruction in the mouse.[372] Recent studies emphasize that the human testis is also quite sensitive to x-ray exposure. With 250-kv x-rays, spermatogenesis is temporarily damaged by dose levels as low as 15 r.[371, 373] These studies demonstrate that both "cell-kill" and "mitosis-halting" mechanisms occur after radiation exposure; the ED_{50} estimates for "cell kill" and "mitosis halting" are 75 and 27 r, respectively.[374] Histologic changes occur rapidly following exposure to radiation. As early as 27 days after 100-r x-ray, the reduction of all cell types except mature spermatids is striking (Fig. 6–23A and B).

In contrast, Leydig cell function is quite resistant to irradiation. The highest tolerated dose is not established, but it probably exceeds 800-r x-rays. Since Leydig cell function remains intact, testosterone levels as well as urinary LH excretion are normal.[373] FSH levels increase as a reflection of the impaired spermatogenesis. These levels return to normal when the germinal epithelium is replenished.

Although the importance of protecting gonadal function from accidental radiation exposure is self-evident, no pre-

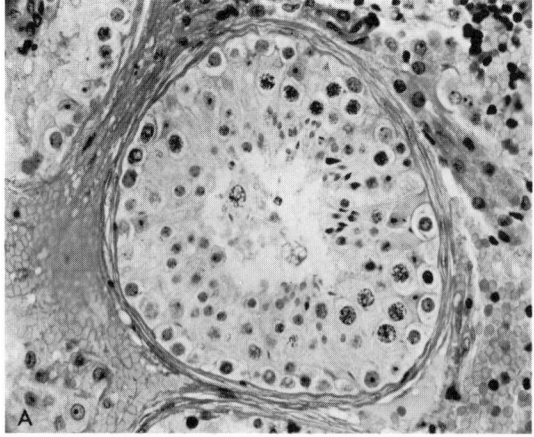
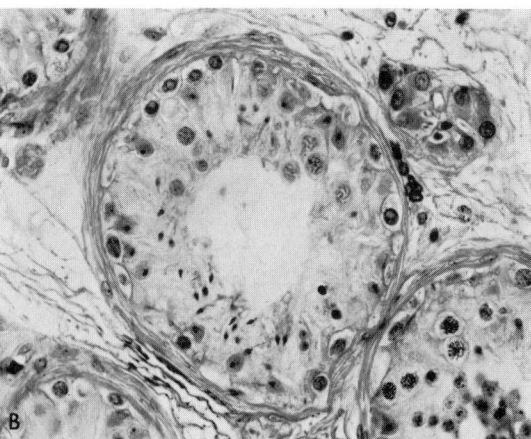

Figure 6–23. Effects of x-ray on the testis. A, Testicular biopsy specimen (× 64) from normal adult. Spermatogenesis is active and all germ cell types are present in normal numbers. B, Biopsy specimen (× 64) from same patient 27 days following exposure to 100 r x-ray. Only the mature spermatids are present in normal numbers. The progressive depletion of the germinal epithelium is due to lack of immature cell types undergoing maturation. The majority of spermatogonia were killed at the time of exposure. Note the absence of significant tubular membrane fibrosis. Leydig cells are normal.

ventive means are presently available except appropriate external shielding.

Gonadotropin-Producing Pituitary Tumors

In a recently reported series of pituitary adenomas, 12 of 50 patients had elevated serum concentrations of gonadotropins.[375] This suggested that gonadotropin-producing pituitary tumors may be more common than once suspected. Of the 21 known patients with this condition,[376] all had supernormal concentrations of serum FSH. Only one had a supernormal serum concentration of LH and testosterone and one other had a supernormal concentration of LH but not of testosterone. The other 19 patients had selective hypersecretion of FSH. Snyder and colleagues[376, 377] have investigated ways of distinguishing FSH-secreting pituitary adenomas from the hypersecretion of FSH associated with primary testicular disease. These investigators measured serum concentrations of FSH-α and FSH-β after GnRH administration. Both subunits increased after GnRH; however, only the rise in serum FSH-β could be used to distinguish patients with pituitary adenomas from primary testicular disease. Following GnRH, FSH-β rose 100% in patients with gonadotropin-producing adenomas and did not change in primary hypogonadism.[376] Better discrimination of these conditions was obtained following administration of TRH: after administration of this tripeptide, serum LH rose in 10 of 10 patients with FSH-secreting pituitary adenomas but not in patients with primary hypogonadism. TRH increased FSH secretion in only half of the tumor patients, however.[377]

At present there are no known patients with hypersecretion of FSH or LH from extrapituitary tumors. LH-secreting pituitary tumors must always be differentiated from neoplasms that produce hCG since this latter glycoprotein hormone is detected by all immunoassays and bioassays for LH.

Adult Leydig Cell Failure ("Male Climacteric")

In contrast to ovarian function, spermatogenesis and testosterone production do not suddenly decline at a certain point in the life of the male unless a pathologic process intervenes. Spermatogenesis is more vulnerable to metabolic and systemic disorders, but age per se does not appear to alter this process. This is supported in part by the presence of normal-sized testes in older men who have not sustained major disease.[242] Furthermore, fertility is not uncommon in the eighth and ninth decades, although extensive seminal fluid studies in this age group are lacking.

Testosterone production rates and metabolic clearance rates decline with increased age, but serum testosterone levels usually remain within the normal adult male range. An increase in serum TeBG concentrations may be responsible for normal serum testosterone levels even with the low production rate. The apparent free testosterone concentration is decreased. The physiologic significance of these findings requires further clarification, since routine androgen therapy in older men is not accompanied by convincing results.

When disease impairs Leydig cell function, and total serum testosterone levels decline, symptoms similar to those occurring in postmenopausal women appear; these are related to androgen withdrawal.[378] In addition to having hot flashes and decreased libido and sexual potentia, approximately half of these patients experience increased irri-

tability, inability to concentrate, and episodes of depression. This entity has been designated the "male climacteric."[379-381] This condition is associated with Klinefelter's syndrome, pituitary ablation (surgery or x-ray), idiopathic Leydig cell failure, and testicular atrophy (secondary to mumps orchitis or disruption of testicular blood supply during procedures such as bilateral herniorrhaphy). In our experience, the most common etiologic factor is Klinefelter's syndrome.

The age of onset is variable and depends on the pathogenesis. In those patients with Klinefelter's syndrome who have reasonably good Leydig cell function earlier in life, androgen production may decline sometime after age 40. The same sequence is observed in men who have severe mumps orchitis during early adult life. Although testicular blood supply can be interrupted at any age following surgery in that region, older men appear to be more vulnerable to this complication.

Establishing the correct diagnosis is less a problem when the aforementioned pathologic processes are responsible, since the clinician is alerted to the possibility of androgen failure by the presence of small, atrophic testes. Even testes that are smaller than normal should alert the clinician since testicular size does not diminish as a function of age. If Leydig cell failure is longstanding, the secondary sex characteristics may have regressed. Ideally, the diagnosis can be confirmed by determining plasma testosterone concentrations. The presence of a value less than 150 ng/dl is significant. In these patients, serum LH (and usually FSH) concentrations are markedly elevated (often into the range of the castrate). However, the use of isolated LH assays is not helpful since the concentrations of this hormone increase in many men after age 45 despite normal testosterone levels. This probably reflects decreased steroidogenic efficiency.

Difficulty usually arises in attempting to differentiate idiopathic Leydig cell failure from psychogenic impotence, which is seen much more frequently. Each can present the same clinical picture of vasomotor symptoms, fatigue, and decreased libido and sexual potentia. In both, sperm counts (if seminal fluid examination is possible) along with physical findings may be entirely normal. The serum testosterone concentrations are below the normal range (300–1200 ng/dl) but not down to castrate levels (40–70 ng/dl). For this situation, the "testosterone therapeutic test" may be helpful. Testosterone enanthate or cypionate is administered weekly for 4 weeks, in a dose of 200 mg/week. This is followed by four weekly injections of placebo (sesame oil). One to two weeks after the cessation of the last injection, the patient is interviewed. The test is considered positive for Leydig cell failure if amelioration of the "climacteric" symptoms occurred slowly, i.e., during the second week,[242] and relapse occurred gradually during the period of placebo injections.[378] The test is negative if no benefit results from the administered androgen or if the symptoms rapidly ameliorate and promptly return, coincident with the initiation and cessation of the androgen and the placebo injections. Further objectivity can be achieved by performing this test in a double-blind fashion. The nurse decides whether the androgen injections precede or follow the 4-week course of placebo injections. After the patient has been interviewed, the physician is informed of the schedule.

Once the diagnosis is established, maintenance androgen replacement therapy is given (page 335). In a few older patients, improvement of sexual function may not be important, but treatment should still be instituted to correct the negative nitrogen balance that exists. This will improve muscle strength and stamina, as well as the osteoporosis that is usually present. In psychogenic impotence, emotional problems are usually involved, and the patient should have a psychiatric evaluation.

Other factors responsible for decreased sexual potentia should not be neglected. These include vascular and neurogenic disorders. Since the ability to have an erection depends on an adequate blood supply to the penis, arteriosclerotic changes such as are observed in Leriche's syndrome may result in decreased sexual potentia. The finding of diminished femoral arterial pulsations or a history of gluteal claudication suggests the diagnosis. Patients with diabetes mellitus frequently complain of diminished sexual ability. In addition to the vascular changes seen in these cases, sympathetic neuropathies may occur. Since the integrity of the sympathetic fibers is necessary for sexual responses, such neurologic involvement may be responsible for the impotence seen in diabetes.

Androgen therapy does not improve the symptoms in the vascular or neurogenic disorders.

Hypogonadotropic Syndromes

Hypogonadotropic Eunuchoidism (Kallmann's Syndrome, Isolated Gonadotropin Deficiency)

Hypogonadotropic eunuchoidism (HE) represents a congenital, often familial, defect in gonadotropin secretion, involving both sexes.[382-386] Presumably, the reduction in gonadotropin release from the pituitary is secondary to hypothalamic dysfunction manifested by decreased or absent GnRH secretion. Direct evidence to verify this supposition is lacking since present radioimmunoassay methods are not sufficiently sensitive to measure GnRH levels in the peripheral circulation of normal individuals. Indirect evidence is supplied by the finding that GnRH stimulates LH and FSH secretion in these patients[387-390] (Fig. 6–24). Postmortem studies have shown hypothalamic lesions but normal pituitaries.[391, 392] There is no evidence of hypothalamic or pituitary dysfunction apart from the presumed GnRH deficiency.[269, 393] The original postulate that growth hormone deficiency could accompany the gonadotropin deficiency in some patients with this syndrome does not appear to be correct. When attention is given to the permissive role of estrogen and androgens, these patients display normal growth hormone secretion during arginine infusion or insulin administration.[269, 388]

Clinically, this syndrome presents as delayed puberty. Testosterone secretion is deficient and sexual maturation is absent. Since puberty in some normal boys may not begin until age 18 or 19,[394] the initial diagnosis of HE may be difficult unless the patient exhibits one of the congenital anomalies associated with this disorder, such as anosmia or hyposmia (Fig. 6–27).

The incidence of HE is not known with certainty, but it is one of the more common forms of hypogonadism aside from Klinefelter's syndrome and adult seminiferous tubular failure. Usually the disorder affects only a single member of a given family, but multiple individuals may be affected.

Data based on testing for the presence of anosmia, hyposmia, or normal sense of smell (Fig. 6–25), along with father-to-son transmission,[395] suggest that HE is inherited as an autosomal dominant disorder (Fig. 6–26). Examination of six kindreds suggests that there is either incomplete expression or genetic heterogeneity.[386] Some of the congenital abnormalities detected in these patients and the frequency of each are depicted in Figure 6–27. Skeletal abnormalities such as short fourth metacarpals have also been observed.[269, 396]

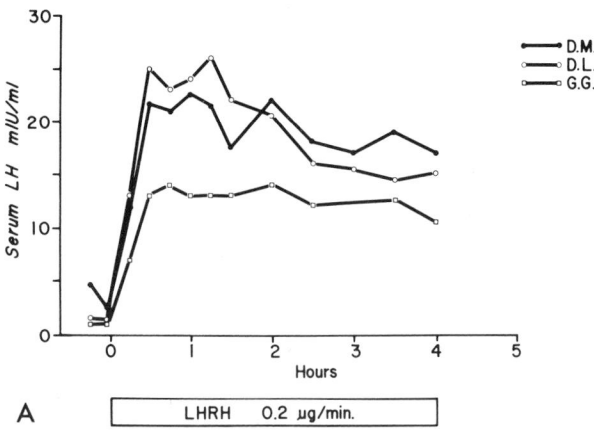

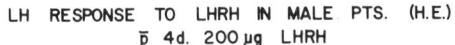

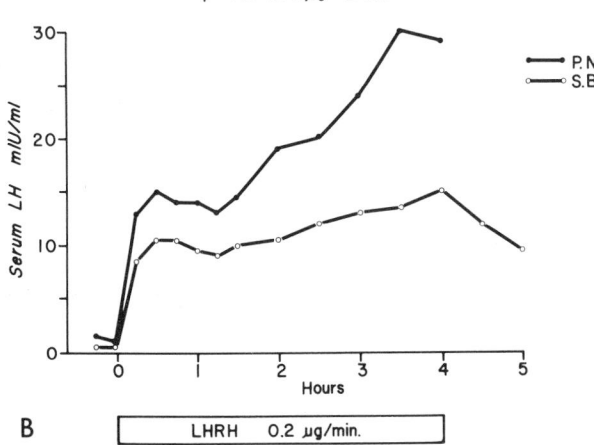

Figure 6–24.   Serum LH response to GnRH (LHRH) infusion in patients with hypogonadotropic eunuchoidism (HE) before *(A)* and after 4 days of subcutaneous LHRH administration *(B)*. In three patients with HE *(A)*, note the prompt increase of LH followed by a plateau pattern. After treatment with LHRH for 4 days *(B)*, the LH response during LHRH infusion in patient P.N. is biphasic, which is the pattern in normal adult males (not shown). Patient S. B. retains the monophasic immature pattern. (Adapted from data from Bremner, W. J., et al.: The effect of luteinizing hormone–releasing hormone in hypogonadotrophic eunuchoidism. *Acta Endocrinol.* 8:1, 1977.)

This syndrome is divided into two major categories on the basis of clinical and laboratory findings — the classic and the variant forms. Patients with the classic form present with evidence of decreased secretion of both LH and FSH, while patients with the variant forms are apparently deficient in either LH or FSH. Some investigators have recommended the assignment of additional subcategories based on the presence or absence of anosmia or hyposmia[397] or the patient's response to exogenous gonadotropin therapy.[398] In our experience the therapeutic response is not influenced by these factors[399] except when cryptorchidism coexists.[364]

Classic Form.   Clinically, these patients are usually tall or of normal stature and exhibit eunuchoidal features (Fig. 6–28). The testes are prepubertal in size and consistency. Gynecomastia occurs uncommonly in untreated patients.

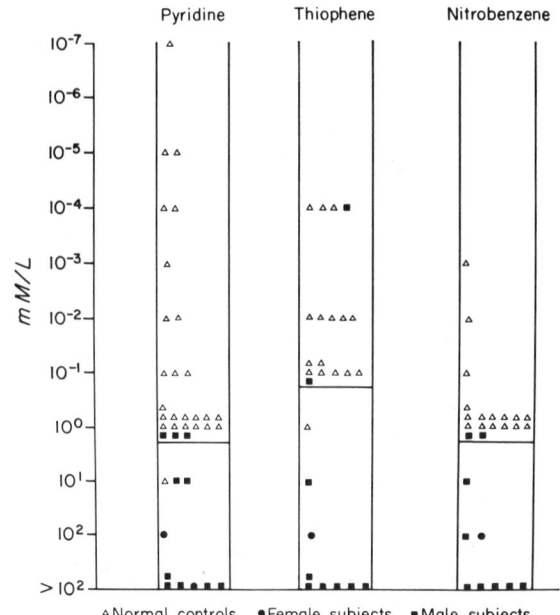

Figure 6–25. Olfactory threshold for normal adults and patients with hypogonadotropic eunuchoidism. Testing performed according to procedures outlined by Henkin (Henkin, R. I., and Bartter, F. C.: Studies on olfactory thresholds in normal man and in patients with adrenocortical insufficiency. *J. Clin. Invest.* 45:1631, 1966). Ordinate indicates molar concentrations of reagents used for testing. (From Santen, R. J., and Paulsen, C. A.: Hypogonadotropic eunuchoidism. I. Clinical study of the mode of inheritance. *J. Clin. Endocrinol. Metab. 36*:47, 1973.)

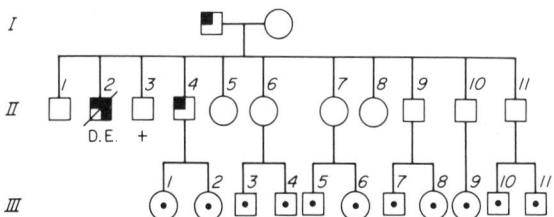

Figure 6–26. Kindred 1 studied for mechanism of genetic transmission of hypogonadotropic eunuchoidism. Opaque area in upper left-hand corner depicts anosmia. Note male-to-male transmission. Opaque area on entire right side depicts hypogonadism. Diagonal line indicates cryptorchidism. Central dot indicates prepubertal age. (From Santen, R. J., and Paulsen, C. A.: Hypogonadotropic eunuchoidism. I. Clinical study of the mode of inheritance. *J. Clin. Endocrinol. Metab. 36*:47, 1973.)

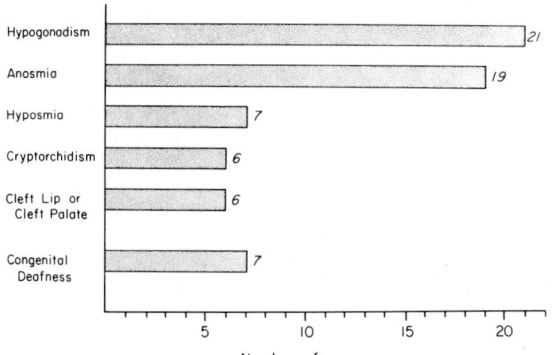

Figure 6–27. Incidence of abnormalities in 97 adult family members from six kindred studied, who either had hypogonadotropic eunuchoidism or were at risk because they were born to an affected or carrier parent. (From Santen, R. J., and Paulsen, C. A.: Hypogonadotropic eunuchoidism. I. Clinical study of the mode of inheritance. *J. Clin. Endocrinol. Metab. 36*:47, 1973.)

Since other facets of pituitary function are intact, secondary hypothyroidism and adrenal insufficiency do not occur. The congenital anomalies most commonly associated with HE are anosmia or hyposmia. The following are also associated with this disorder to a variable extent: congenital deafness, harelip, cleft palate, cryptorchidism, and skeletal defects including craniofacial asymmetry. Indeed, the correlation between anosmia and eunuchoidism is such that when the two defects are present together the diagnosis of hypogonadotropism is virtually assured. The presence of anosmia is not always appreciated by the physician. The reason for this is that the patient with an inadequate sense of smell may not volunteer this information. When asked, however, the patient and his family are aware that his olfactory capacity is reduced or absent. Hyposmia requires quantitative testing to be identified (see Fig. 6–25).

Microscopic examination of the testicular biopsy specimen reveals immature seminiferous tubules lined by Sertoli cells, spermatogonia, and occasional primary spermatocytes. There are no well defined Leydig cells; the interstitial spaces contain mesenchymal precursors of what will develop into Leydig cells (see Fig. 6–19*F*) when gonadotropins are administered. The histologic pattern is therefore that of the immature testis.

Serum and urinary FSH and LH concentrations are usually below the normal male range in patients with the classic form of this syndrome.[269, 364, 400] When serum gonadotropin levels overlap with normal values and some pubertal changes have occurred, so that the diagnosis is uncertain, clomiphene citrate may be administered as a test of pituitary-hypothalamic responsiveness[269, 401] (Figs. 6–29 and 6–30). Despite occasional reports to the contrary, patients with well documented hypogonadotropic eunuchoidism do not respond to clomiphene, even when it is administered on a long-term basis.[402, 403] Plasma testosterone levels are low.

If untreated, these patients will remain in their prepubertal state indefinitely. Testicular biopsy specimens from patients with hypogonadotropic eunuchoidism in their sixth decade demonstrate the same histologic findings as are encountered in younger patients (Fig. 6–31).

Since the absence of GnRH synthesis appears to be the basic defect, the most logical form of therapy would be the administration of this peptide. Mancini et al.[404] reported the use of this treatment in one patient. Full spermatogenesis and early sexual development were achieved. Mortimer et al.[405] induced spermatogenesis in two patients with GnRH treatment for 26–50 weeks. Even though chronic studies with GnRH are limited, small doses given every few hours to stimulate intermittent secretion of LH (see Fig. 6–2) are more likely to produce the best results; constant infusion of this peptide will down-regulate or desensitize the primate pituitary.[406] GnRH is not yet available commercially but should be in the near future.

Although expensive, treatment with human gonadotropins is the next logical choice if fertility is to be attained.[364, 384, 407-422] Two commercial preparations are available. hCG, which is purified from the urine of pregnant women, behaves like LH in the male by stimulating Leydig cell androgen secretion. Human menopausal gonadotropin (hMG) is purified from the urine of postmenopausal women. One marketed product contains 75 IU of FSH and 75 IU of LH per ampule. For optimal results, the following regimen is suggested. hCG should be started initially, since hMG alone does not stimulate the immature testis, at least with reasonable dose schedules. Also, because of its cost, hMG therapy is deferred until needed. The dosage of hCG is 2000–4000 IU three times a week. Clinical evidence of sexual maturation or serial serum testosterone determinations

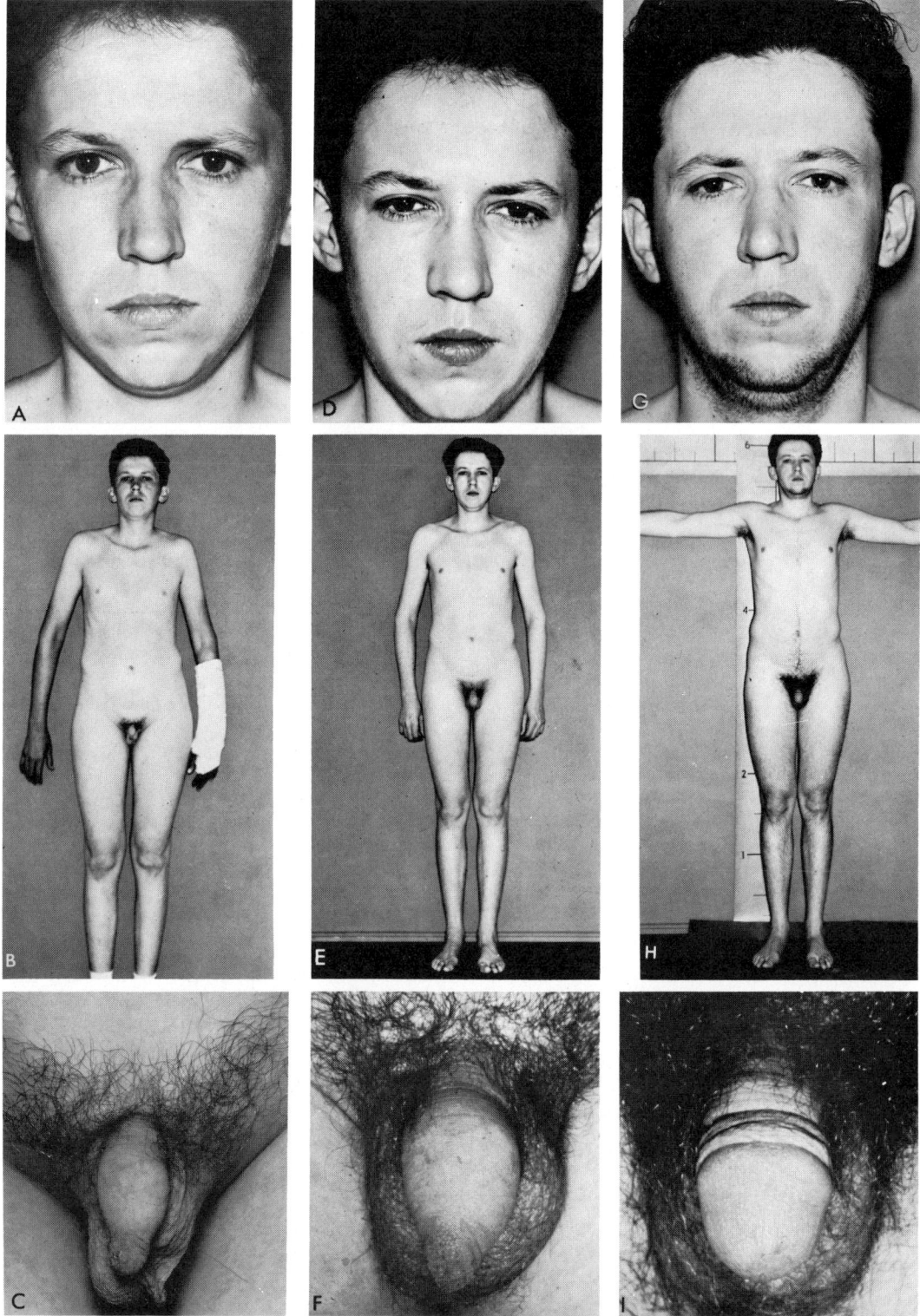

Figure 6–28. Example of a patient with hypogonadotropic eunuchoidism. *A*, *B*, and *C*, Pubertal development had not progressed past minimal pubic hair growth by age 22. *D*, *E*, and *F*, After 6 months of chorionic gonadotropin therapy, facial hair growth is evident on the upper lip and penile growth has occurred. Note the appearance of scrotal rugae. *G*, *H*, and *I*, After 5 years of intermittent chorionic gonadotropin therapy, full sexual maturation has been achieved. Note the increase in testicular size to near-normal dimensions.

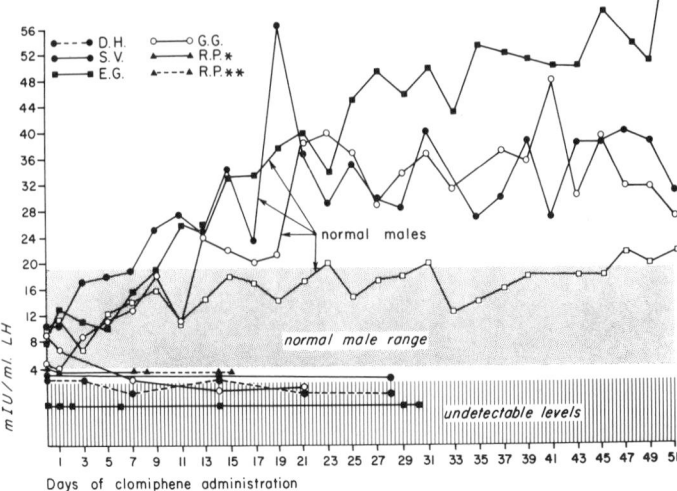

Figure 6-29. Serum LH concentrations during clomiphene citrate administration (50 mg bid × 51 days) to four normal adult men, four patients (D.H., S.V., E.G., and G.G.) with hypogonadotropic eunuchoidism, and one patient (R.P) with pituitary adenoma. The patient group received clomiphene 50 mg bid for 14 to 31 days, and R.P. was tested before* and after** pituitary irradiation. Stippled area depicts normal adult male range in basal state. These and similar observations indicate that a good test of pituitary function can be achieved with clomiphene citrate 50 mg bid for 10 days (see text). (From Santen, R. J., et al.: Short- and long-term effects of clomiphene citrate on the pituitary-testicular axis. *J. Clin. Endocrinol. Metab. 33*:970, 1971.)

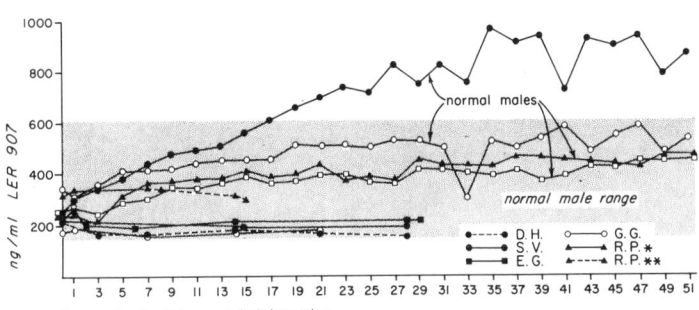

Figure 6-30. Serum FSH titers during clomiphene citrate administration to normal adult males and to patients with pituitary disease. Protocol and patients identical to those stated in legend for Figure 6-29. (From Santen, R. J., et al.: Short- and long-term effects of clomiphene citrate on the pituitary-testicular axis. *J. Clin. Endocrinol. Metab. 33*:970, 1971.)

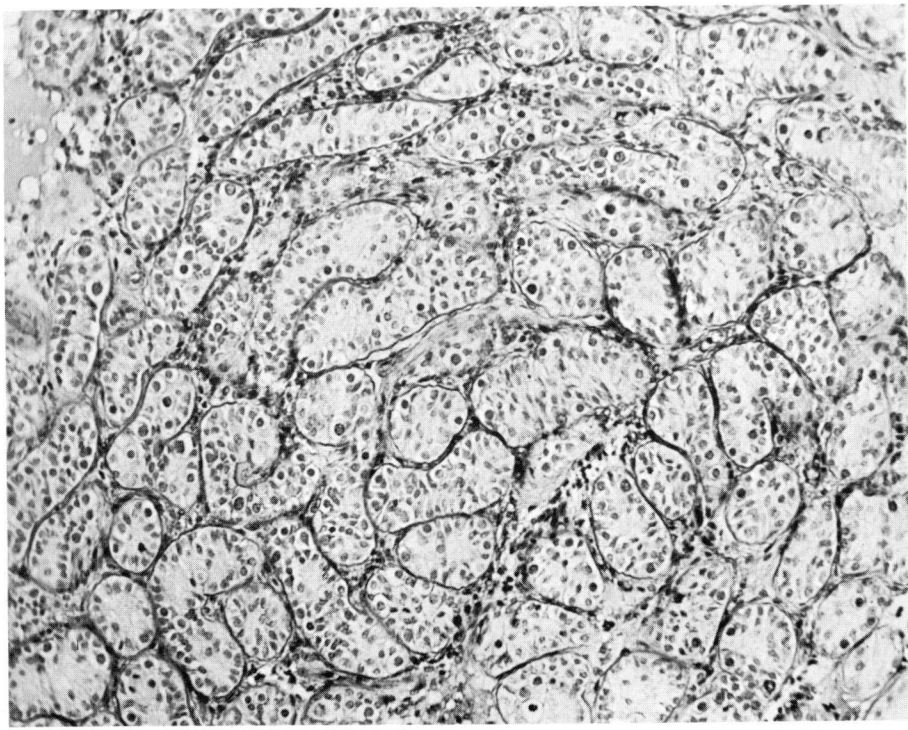

Figure 6-31. Testis from patient with hypogonadotropic eunuchoidism. This man was 52 years of age when studied. Note that the testicular histology of the biopsy specimen from this patient is similar to that of the prepubertal boy and that of the hypogonadotropic eunuchoid of an earlier age (compare with Fig. 6-19*F*) (× 64).

dictate the dose level required. During hCG therapy, Leydig cells mature, seminiferous tubules enlarge, Sertoli cells differentiate, and spermatogenesis begins and proceeds to varying degrees of "completeness." These seminiferous tubule changes are considered to be primarily due to the direct action of endogenous androgens. With prolonged treatment, sexual maturation can be achieved (see Fig. 6–28), and plasma testosterone rises to normal male levels in most patients. Some observations have suggested that the testes of some patients may not respond adequately to exogenous gonadotropin.[269, 272] In one long-term study the only patients who did not respond were those with bilateral cryptorchidism (Fig. 6–32).

Occasionally, hCG treatment by itself stimulates spermatogenesis sufficiently for sperm to appear in the ejaculate. However, most patients with the classic form of the syndrome require exogenous FSH to achieve more predictable and more complete testicular maturation. Therefore, when necessary, hMG, 150 IU three times a week, is given. hCG is still required since hMG by itself does not contain sufficient LH to maintain satisfactory Leydig cell function. The testicular development in a patient with sequential hCG and hCG plus hMG therapy is illustrated in Figure 6–33. After fertility is achieved with this general therapeutic plan, it is necessary to switch eventually to replacement testosterone therapy because of the expense of continuous gonadotropin administration. Although there are two case reports[423, 424] that indicate that testosterone alone induced normal spermatogenesis, our overall experience suggests that this does not occur in most patients.

Even though testosterone treatment will not stimulate spermatogenesis, many physicians use this steroid to induce sexual maturation in patients with HE. hCG could be used but the cost and inconvenience of this type of treatment tend to be prohibitive. When patients desire fertility, treatment is switched to exogenous gonadotropins. Earlier observations suggested that such a program might jeopardize the ability of the gonadotropins to stimulate the testosterone-exposed testis. Systematic studies have shown that this concern is not well founded. Indeed, both Leydig cell and germinal cell response is unimpaired in patients with HE and in patients with postpubertal pituitary failure.[425, 426]

Variant Forms of Hypogonadotropism

Isolated LH Deficiency ("Fertile" Eunuch). This interesting group of patients is characterized by eunuchoidism and effective endogenous FSH secretion.[364, 386, 427-429] The biologic evidence of FSH secretion ranges from well advanced spermatogenesis in the testicular biopsy (Fig. 6–34) to finding viable sperm in the ejaculate. Gynecomastia is likely to be present in the fertile eunuch, in contrast to patients with the classic form of the syndrome. The reason for this is not known. Serum LH and testosterone concentrations are low, while serum FSH levels are normal.[364, 430] Of interest is the observation that despite these normal FSH titers, clomiphene administration does not elicit any rise.

The approach to treatment is similar to that in patients with the classic form. Treatment with hCG is first employed, and this is more apt to induce full testicular maturation in these patients than in those with the classic form of the disorder. This is undoubtedly due to the presence of endogenous FSH. The lesion is permanent so that either hCG or androgen replacement therapy is required on a permanent basis.

Isolated FSH Deficiency. There are three reports of patients with isolated FSH deficiency, one in a female[431] and the others in males.[432, 433] In the latter patients, seminal fluid sperm concentration varied from azoospermia to normal. The patient with normal sperm concentration showed decreased sperm motility and an increase in immature forms. Histologic examination showed a variable pattern, i.e., germinal aplasia, hypospermatogenesis, and spermatogenic arrest. Leydig cells appeared uniformly normal and testosterone production was normal. The woman with FSH deficiency was successfully treated and became pregnant. There is, however, no experience with FSH treatment in men with this condition. It will be important to demonstrate a response to FSH as proof of deficiency, especially in patients with mature spermatozoa in their seminal fluid. This is of interest since many investigators feel that FSH is essential for the initiation of spermatogenesis, and studies in infrahuman primates indicate that spermatogenesis is suppressed by passive or active immunization against FSH.[434]

Pituitary Failure

Prepubertal Pituitary Failure (Pituitary Dwarfism). Lesions involving anterior pituitary or hypothalamus early in childhood result in a clinical syndrome in which short stature is associated with lack of growth hormone as well as decreased thyroid and adrenal function. In addition, puberty fails to occur owing to inability of the pituitary to increase LH and FSH secretion at the appropriate time. When this occurs, the testicular morphology resembles that of a normal prepubertal boy. Even though epiphysial closure is delayed, the skeletal measurements are not of eunuchoidal proportions. This is most likely due to the presence of growth hormone elaboration.

Since pituitary function is irreversibly damaged, chorionic gonadotropin stimulatory therapy is not practical for long-term treatment. Therefore, androgen replacement therapy is indicated in addition to thyroid, corticosteroids, and if possible, growth hormone.

Postpubertal Pituitary Failure. When pituitary function completely declines after sexual maturation, the testes are

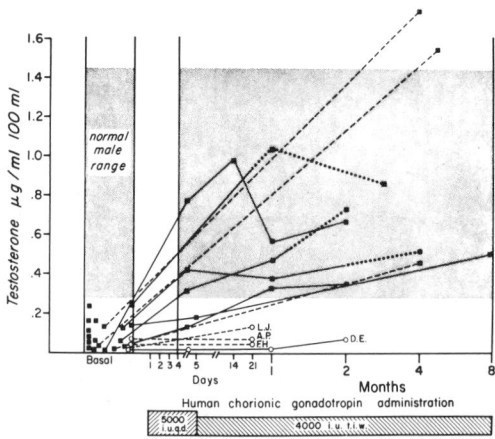

Figure 6–32. Plasma testosterone levels during acute and chronic hCG administration in 13 patients with hypogonadotropic eunuchoidism. Open circles denote four patients with bilateral cryptorchidism. Dashed lines refer to patients not tested acutely (e.g., 4 to 5 days). Dotted lines indicate nonconsecutive plasma sampling. Stippled area indicates normal basal levels for adult males. Note that all patients tested achieved normal testosterone levels within 1 month except those with bilateral cryptorchidism. Of five patients tested acutely, three achieved normal male levels. (From Santen, R. J., and Paulsen, C. A.: Hypogonadotropic eunuchoidism. II. Gonadal responsiveness to exogenous gonadotropins. *J. Clin. Endocrinol. Metab.* 36:55, 1973.)

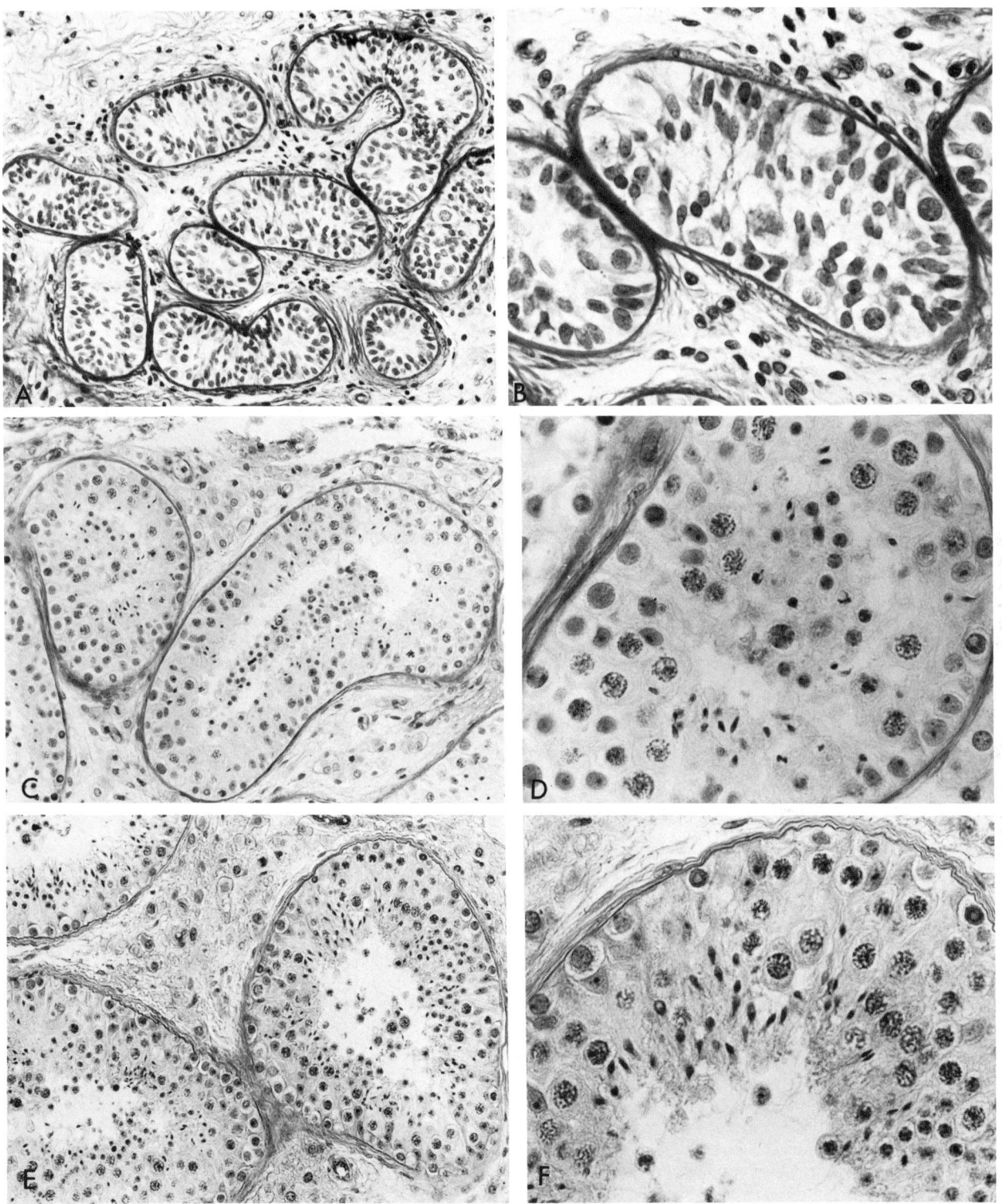

Figure 6-33. The effect of hCG followed by hCG plus hMG on the testes of a patient with hypogonadotropic eunuchoidism. Photomicrograph of testicular biopsy specimen at two magnifications *A* (× 64) and *B* (× 160). The specimen was obtained from patient J.P. before treatment. Note the immature germinal epithelium and mesenchymal cells within the interstitium. These mesenchymal cells are precursors to Leydig cells. *C* (× 64) and *D* (× 160), Specimen from patient J.P. 59 weeks after hCG therapy. Spermatogenesis is in progress and all germ cell types can be detected, up to and including Scd spermatids. *E* (× 64) and *F* (× 160), 31 weeks after combined hCG-hMG therapy. Note the increased numbers of all germ cells. Sperm counts at this time ranged from 10 to 13.6 million/ml.

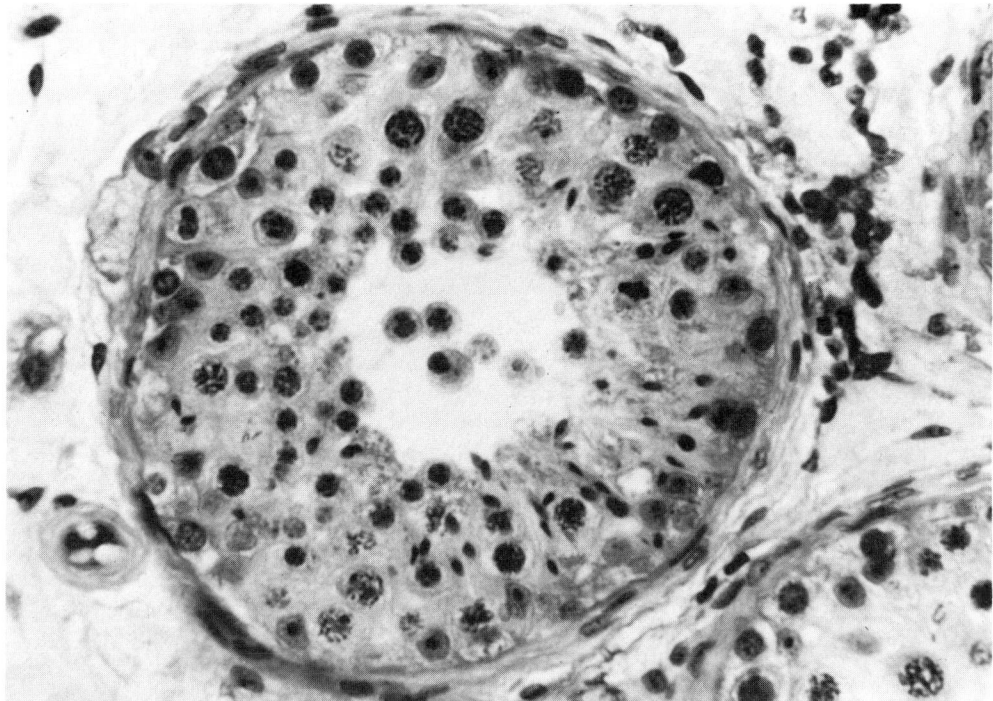

Figure 6–34. Testicular biopsy specimen (× 160) from patient D.H., aged 28 years, who is an example of the form of hypogonadotropism that has been termed "fertile eunuch." He had no previous treatment. His serum LH was low and FSH was normal; testosterone was low (100 ng/dl). Note that germ cells of each maturation phase are present, including Sc and Sd spermatids (see Fig. 6–12). Leydig cells could not be identified.

unable to maintain the germinal epithelium and testosterone secretion. This results in decreased libido, impotence, and a gradual regression of the secondary sex characteristics. The testes become small and soft, and varying degrees of damage are noted histologically. After normal puberty has been attained, the seminiferous tubules do not revert to a prepubertal state when pituitary failure occurs. Instead, disorganization and sloughing or total absence of the germinal epithelium may be seen. The tunica propria thickens, and peritubular proliferation develops. In some instances the testes may become hyalinized (Fig. 6–35). Leydig cells progressively decrease in numbers and show degenerative changes. One tends to find the most severe testicular damage in those patients with the longest history of hypopituitarism.

A variable amount of gonadotropin secretion is probably maintained in almost all patients. Serum FSH and LH levels may be low or in the low-normal male range. Although many may respond to GnRH, very few will respond to clomiphene.[269]

Adult patients who have acquired defects of gonadotropin secretion may be divided into two major groups, those with selective pituitary failure and those with panhypopituitarism.[435-439] Selective gonadotropin failure in a man who has undergone normal puberty is relatively uncommon. In our experience, hemochromatosis is frequently responsible. The diagnosis is made by finding abnormal liver function with serum ferritin levels in excess of 2000 ng/ml. Basal FSH and LH levels (but not other pituitary hormones) are low and usually do not rise following GnRH administration.[440] These patients almost always respond to exogenous gonadotropin administration, and resumption of normal fertility is possible.

In other patients, the cause of postpubertal selective gonadotropin failure is unknown. It should be emphasized,

however, that certain pituitary tumors may present as selective loss of LH and FSH. In these men, tumor expansion may cease before other tropic hormones are involved, or panhypopituitarism may gradually develop.

When the pituitary deficiency involves all the tropic hormones, the testes do not uniformly respond to exogenous

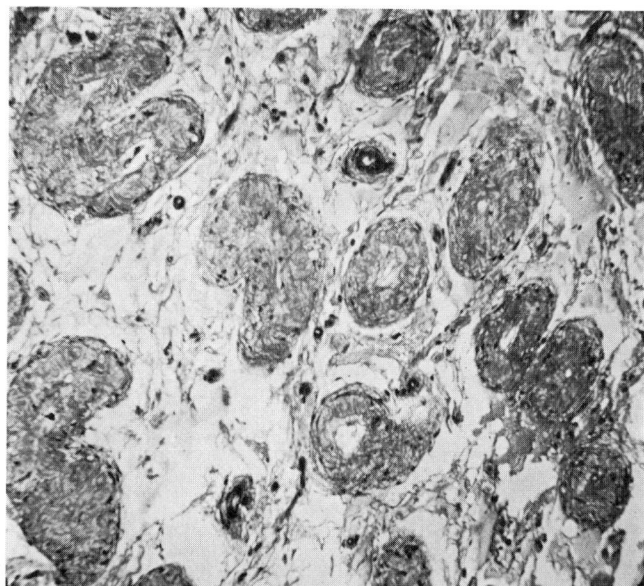

Figure 6–35. Testis from a patient with postpubertal pituitary failure. In this patient gonadotropin and ACTH secretion was not detected. Complete hyalinization of the seminiferous tubules is evident. Leydig cells are absent and only a few fibroblasts can be seen in the interstitium (× 160).

gonadotropin therapy. Presumably this failure to respond is due to complete testicular hyalinization (Fig. 6–35), and the interstitial fibroblastic elements are incapable of stimulation. How long after the onset of pituitary failure the testis remains potentially responsive is not known with certainty. MacLeod et al.,[441] Gemzell and Kjessler,[442] Mancini et al.,[443] and other workers[444] have demonstrated that hMG-hCG or hPG therapy may be effective in restoring spermatogenesis and Leydig cell function if treatment is instituted shortly after pituitary function is lost. We encountered an unresponsive testis 5 years after development of panhypopituitarism. In this instance, a basal skull fracture pinpointed the onset of the lesion. For practical purposes androgen replacement therapy is indicated unless fertility is an issue. This should be instituted as outlined later in this chapter and maintained for life.

Delayed Puberty

Puberty normally begins before age 15 years. When it is delayed beyond that time, the boy is classified as a "late bloomer." The reason for the phenomenon is not clear, but a familial pattern sometimes exists. If delayed puberty is the correct diagnosis, the boy will eventually achieve sexual maturity, usually by age 20–22 years. The main problem posed by boys with delayed puberty is our inability to distinguish them from patients with hypogonadotropic eunuchoidism who do not have anosmia, hyposmia, or a clear-cut genetic history. There was hope that the clomiphene test might be useful for this purpose, but prepubertal patients do not respond to this agent regardless of whether they will eventually undergo normal sexual maturation. In these patients clomiphene administration decreases gonadotropin concentrations.

Treatment for delayed puberty is reserved for those boys who experience social and psychologic problems related to their sexual underdevelopment. Therapy consists of a 12-week course of hCG (1500–4000 IU) intramuscularly three times a week. Therapy is then discontinued for 12 weeks. During this "waiting" period, maturation may progress, it may remain stationary, or it may regress. The status can usually be determined by interviews; occasionally serial serum testosterone determinations are required. If maturation does not progress, an additional course of hCG is given, followed by another "waiting" period. In our experience, patients with delayed puberty do not require more than three or four such courses of hCG treatment. Patients whose maturation regresses after multiple courses of hCG are likely to have hypogonadotropic eunuchoidism.

ANDROGEN REPLACEMENT THERAPY

When the testes are damaged to the extent that testosterone production is reduced, androgen replacement therapy with one of several preparations is indicated (Table 6–9). As mentioned in the section on hypogonadotropic eunuchoidism, gonadotropin therapy may prove impractical, so that the physician must rely on androgen treatment except when normal spermatogenesis is desired. For the same reason, androgen therapy is employed in managing patients with postpubertal pituitary failure.

Patients whose testicular disease has interfered with normal pubertal development need somewhat higher doses of testosterone to obtain full sexual maturation than the doses required for maintenance. The long-acting enanthate and cyclopentylpropionate esters of testosterone are preferred because of their potency and the steady response obtained. These preparations behave the same in terms of their pharmacokinetics.[445] The recommended dosage schedule is 200 mg intramuscularly every 1–2 weeks for a period of 2–3 years, at which time full development is usually attained. Then 100–200 mg is administered every 2–3 weeks for maintenance.

Intramuscular administration of an aqueous suspension of testosterone is ineffective or somewhat erratic. Testosterone propionate, a short-acting compound, is effective but not practical for long-term therapy. Oral medication in the form of methyltestosterone or fluoxymesterone elicits an androgenic response, but it does not approach the potency of testosterone enanthate or unconjugated testosterone pellets. One reason for this is the short half-life of methyltestosterone, which has been estimated to be about 2.7 hours.[446]

Androgen treatment is usually without complications, but several points should be kept in mind. Since testosterone may stimulate an existing prostatic carcinoma, the presence of this condition is a contraindication to therapy. Benign prostatic hyperplasia is not usually affected adversely.[447] However, in some patients over age 50 with longstanding androgen deficiency, the prostate gland may appear to be very sensitive to testosterone in that rapid enlargement and bladder neck obstruction occur. In this instance the apparent increased sensitivity is probably related to preexisting prostatic hyperplasia that regressed because of the androgen deficiency. In these men it is prudent to start with short-acting preparations, such as testosterone propionate, so that if obstruction does occur therapy can be rapidly withdrawn. If obstruction occurs, the physician must weigh the benefits of hormonal therapy against the problems of possible prostatic surgery.

Alterations in liver function may develop with methyltestosterone administration and, to a much lesser extent, with

Table 6–9. ANDROGEN PREPARATIONS

Medication	Dose (mg)	Route	Administration Schedule
Testosterone enanthate	200	IM	Every 1–2 weeks to complete puberty,
Testosterone cyclopentylpropionate	200	IM	then every 2–3 weeks for maintenance
Testosterone propionate	50	IM	Three times a week
Testosterone pellets* (unconjugated)	450	Subcutaneous	Every 4–6 months
Methyltestosterone† (linguets)	25–50	Buccal	Daily for maintenance
Fluoxymesterone†	5–10	Oral	Daily for maintenance

*Each pellet contains 75 mg unconjugated testosterone.

†At these doses, which have been recommended by other authors, the clinical response is less than that obtained with the long-acting esters.

fluoxymesterone therapy. The characteristic histologic abnormality is biliary capillary stasis with little, if any, parenchymal damage. Clinically, the findings are those of obstructive jaundice, and recovery is rapid and uneventful after steroid withdrawal.[448, 449] The reader is referred to suggested guidelines for monitoring certain patients who are receiving synthetic androgen treatment for potential hepatotoxic effects.[450] Finally, it should be emphasized that steroids with a 17α-alkyl group are primarily suspect for these adverse reactions, while the long-acting esters do not damage the liver.

An elevated hematocrit value due to stimulation of erythropoiesis is sometimes encountered in eunuchoidal males receiving testosterone. When this occurs the dose should be reduced. Elevated blood pressure, presumably secondary to salt retention, may also develop and dictate a reduction in dosage. For some individuals who seem unusually sensitive to testosterone, one may have to be satisfied with less than full replacement therapy.

Testosterone treatment may be associated with acne similar to that which occurs in normal puberty. In fact, the incidence of acne may be somewhat higher than in normal pubertal boys because testosterone blood levels are higher than normal for several days just after injection. Treatment of this complication is handled in the usual fashion with sun, soap, and antibiotics if necessary.

Although priapism has been stated to interfere with treatment in some hypogonadal males, strictly speaking this is not the case. Frequent erections to the point of disturbance do occur, but this problem can be overcome by adjusting the level of medication and conferring with the patient. It must be remembered that a eunuchoidal patient over 30 years of age may find even two erections per day troublesome. Thus, the physician has to provide guidance to individuals who undergo an "induced" puberty at a relatively late age. As in normal puberty, the patient learns to control his libido and sexual potentia, and the number of erections and incidence of masturbation decrease with time. It should also be emphasized that some males with severe androgen deficiency may be quite ambivalent toward treatment. In these patients a successful result can be achieved only by insisting on a definite therapeutic regimen.

CRYPTORCHIDISM

At birth, the incidence of undescended testes in all males is about 10%. During the first year testes descend in all but 1.7–3.0%,[451, 452] and before puberty the testes move into the scrotum in many of these. Patients with cryptorchidism can usually be distinguished from boys with so-called retractile testes (pseudocryptorchidism) by careful physical examination. At puberty the testes of boys with the latter disorder usually remain in the scrotum and thus present no problem in medical management. Postpubertally, about 0.3–0.4% of males have either unilateral or bilateral undescended testes. Failure of one testis to descend occurs four to five times as frequently as bilateral maldescent. The reader is referred to the works of Charny[451] and Jones and Scott[453] for detailed discussions of the mechanism involved in testicular descent.

It is important to remember that bilateral cryptorchidism may be the initial complaint of patients with a variety of types of hypogonadism such as the functional prepubertal castrate syndrome, Noonan's syndrome, and Reifenstein's syndrome. Other examples of hypogonadism, such as Klinefelter's syndrome, Sertoli-cell-only syndrome, and hypogonadotropic eunuchoidism, are associated with cryptorchidism to a variable extent and, therefore, should be kept in

mind when the patient with undescended testes is being evaluated. The following discussion of ectopic testes and "true" cryptorchidism assumes that these conditions have been excluded.

Ectopic testes apparently develop normally and begin their descent through the inguinal canal only to be diverted from their pathway before entering the scrotum. The reason for their abnormal location is poorly understood. Ectopic testes are located and classified as follows: perineal, femoral (crural), and superficial inguinal.[451, 453] Surgery is indicated when the diagnosis is established, since orchiopexy performed prior to puberty usually results in a normally functioning testis. This is probably due to the fact that ectopic testes contain inherently normal germinal epithelium and that the spermatic cords are of adequate length, which diminishes the likelihood of impaired testicular blood supply after orchiopexy.

In "true" cryptorchidism, the testes are situated intraabdominally or in the inguinal canal. A short spermatic artery is commonly encountered in these patients. This is believed to be a manifestation of poor testicular development (dysgenesis). Others have suggested that most retained testes are essentially normal until puberty, when exposure to internal body temperatures damages the germinal epithelium.[454, 455] However, the observations of Nelson[456] and Sohval[457] support the concept that testicular dysgenesis plays an important role in maldescent and also suggest that even if embryogenesis has been normal further testicular development may be retarded during the prepubertal years by virtue of the nonscrotal position. Mancini et al.,[458] in a detailed extension of their earlier work,[459] noted fewer immature spermatogonia in the cryptorchid testis prior to age 4 years. They compared the cytologic features of the cryptorchid testes with those of the contralateral scrotal testes and finally with those of the testes of a control population of similar age that did not exhibit cryptorchidism. Before sexual maturation, the changes were slight, but as the pubertal process progressed, the discrepancy in germinal cell maturation between the cryptorchid and scrotal testes increased markedly. Nelson's studies indicate that age 6–7 years may be the critical time for surgical intervention, whereas Mancini's study suggests that orchiopexy might be considered even earlier. It remains to be established whether early treatment will improve the "salvage" rate, however. In Charny's series of 61 patients with unilateral cryptorchidism subjected to orchiopexy at varying ages (either before or after puberty had started), not a single patient was observed to exhibit normal spermatogenesis in follow-up examination of testicular biopsy specimens.[460] Others report greater success, but as a general rule critical histologic evaluation has not been extensive.[461] The situation with respect to bilateral cryptorchidism appears to be different. For example, Gross and Jewett report "acceptable" fertility in 79% of their 38 cases.[462]

Whenever possible, unnecessary surgery on the migratory or pseudocryptorchid testes should be avoided. Therefore, until it is demonstrated that early treatment is clearly beneficial, surgical therapy should be delayed until the first signs of puberty. Sometimes an associated inguinal hernia will require correction prior to puberty. In this instance, orchiopexy can best be performed at the same time. The incidence of inguinal hernia in cases of cryptorchidism has been reported to range from 57 to 93%, but usually such hernias are of anatomic rather than clinical importance.

It may be desirable to determine in the prepubertal patient whether orchiopexy will be required at the time of sexual maturation. This can be accomplished by administering chorionic gonadotropin in a dose of 4000 IU three times a week for 3 weeks. Testicular descent will occur in the majority of patients during this test period. In some, the descent will be permanent, but in most the testis or testes will return to a nonscrotal position once treatment is discontinued. However, in these cases it can be predicted that at puberty permanent descent should occur and surgery will not be necessary. In patients who fail to respond, surgery will be indicated at the onset of puberty if spermatogenesis is to be preserved (provided that the potential is there). The dosage schedule as recommended here will not damage the testes, nor will undesirable androgenic effects occur.

When orchiopexy is performed, bilateral testicular biopsy specimens should be obtained even if there is only unilateral involvement. Then 18 months to 2 years later, repeat biopsy specimens should be obtained for study. If the once-cryptorchid testis shows abnormal spermatogenesis at this time, it is unlikely that active spermatogenesis will ever develop. Leydig cell function is usually normal, provided the blood supply to the testis is adequate.

The potential risk of development of testicular carcinoma in the cryptorchid testis has been shown to be as high as 8% in some populations.[463] The testicular malignancies occurred in the men examined despite the fact that orchiopexy had been performed 6 to 14 years previously. These observations substantiate the earlier concept that the "now-scrotal, once-cryptorchid" testis retains the increased chance of becoming malignant.[464-466] The clinician should, therefore, inform the patient and his parents of the need for long-term follow-up. If the repositioned testis does not demonstrate normal spermatogenesis within a reasonable period of time, unilateral orchidectomy should be considered. Apparently, the condition of bilateral cryptorchidism does not carry the same risk as unilateral cryptorchidism, but our information in that regard is fragmentary.

EFFECTS OF SPINAL CORD DAMAGE

More than 50% of males with paraplegia sustained by trauma exhibit decreased testicular function of varying degrees.[467-473] The commonest defect encountered is spermatogenic arrest associated with generalized hypoplasia of the germinal epithelium. Leydig cells usually appear normal, but nodular hyperplasia has been reported;[469, 470] serum FSH, LH, and testosterone levels have been found to be normal in one study, however.[472] Attempts have been made to correlate the level of the cord lesion with the incidence and extent of testicular damage. Although these studies have not indicated a precise relationship, observations to date suggest that when the lesion occurs in the lower cord segments less damage to the germinal epithelium is observed.

An increase in gonadal temperature is a possible factor in causing abnormal spermatogenesis in these patients. Studies in animals and humans have amply demonstrated the susceptibility of the germinal cells to increased temperature from 33° to 37° C. Scrotal skin temperatures increase when the lumbar sympathetics are interrupted. Furthermore, when the cremasteric reflex is absent, temperature regulation is hampered. The importance of the heat factor is emphasized by the observations of Bors and his associates,[473] who noted a relationship between segmented levels of sweat impairment and the severity of seminiferous tubule damage. Moreover, they observed an improvement in the sperm counts of one patient after daily application of ice bags to his scrotum for a period of 3 months.

Even if spermatogenesis remains normal, paraplegic men may be infertile because of retrograde ejaculation. In 84 patients studied by Munro and coworkers,[471] only 7% were able to produce a semen sample. They concluded that the ability to ejaculate effectively is most likely lost if the cord lesion is extensive and between T6 and L3. Some investigators have tried irrigating the bladder with sodium bicarbonate following orgasm to obtain viable sperm for insemination, but no systematic studies of this procedure have been carried out.

Paraplegia does not preclude normal fertility. However, in patients with impaired spermatogenesis and in those who have lost sexual potentia, the outlook for correction is poor. Endocrine therapy is directed toward correcting the negative nitrogen balance when present.

CLINICAL AND HORMONAL ASPECTS OF TESTICULAR NEOPLASMS

In general, testicular malignancies are an uncommon problem; the incidence in the total male population is only 0.002%. However, in males aged 20–35 years, tumors of the testis constitute one of the most common forms of malignancy. Moreover, since they usually metastasize early, prompt recognition and treatment are important in obtaining optimal results.

Morphologically, testicular neoplasms are divided into two major categories: germinal and nongerminal. The germinal tumors, which account for approximately 96% of the cases in most series, have been further classified by Mostofi and Price[474] as follows: (I) seminoma, (II) embryonal carcinoma, (III) embryonal carcinoma with teratoma, (IV) teratoma, (V) choriocarcinoma, and (VI) embryonal carcinoma, infantile. Several of these major categories are further subclassified; the reader is referred to reviews that discuss these in detail.[474-477]

With respect to early recognition, Skakkebaek has called attention to the entity of germinal cell carcinoma *in situ*. Originally this early form of carcinoma was recognized during a systematic survey of testicular biopsy specimens from a nonselected population of 555 infertile men.[478, 479] Six oligospermic men (incidence of 1.1%) demonstrated carcinoma *in situ*, and four of these men developed invasive carcinoma within 1.3 to 4.5 years of the initial testicular biopsy. Later, this entity was found in other groups of men[463, 480-482] who were known to be at greater risk for germinal cell carcinoma than age-matched controls by virtue of unilateral cryptorchidism, testicular feminization, or previous history of testicular carcinoma. Thereafter, carcinoma *in situ* was reported in patients[483-485] who were not at risk because of cryptorchidism or a previous testicular neoplasm. An example of such a patient from our own (CAP) infertility clinic is shown in Figures 6–36 and 6–37. Infertile men, therefore, present a worrisome clinical problem;[486] that is, there may be no evidence to alert the physician to carcinoma *in situ*. Tests must be developed that will assist in identifying these patients, but until this occurs it might be prudent to perform testicular biopsies more routinely in oligospermic men, particularly those patients who complain of spontaneous testicular pain.

Invasive germinal cell carcinoma usually presents with some enlargement or hardness of the involved testis. Pain may be an associated finding at this time. Careful palpation of the scrotal contents with proper identification of the intrascrotal parts is very important in the diagnosis, since in one large series the correct diagnosis was suspected in only 28% of the cases after the initial examination. Epididymitis was the most common incorrect diagnosis. Gynecomastia develops in approximately 30% of the patients and is usually, but not invariably, associated with choriocarcinomas or Leydig cell tumors.

Assays for hCG should be performed in patients with testicular tumors. Although hCG is invariably secreted by testicular choriocarcinomas, germinal cell malignancies of other cell types may also secrete this hormone. When assays are positive for hCG (radioimmunoassay utilizing β-subunit antisera), the patient should be considered at "high risk," and intensive chemotherapy should be started.

Radioimmunoassay of tumor markers such as α-fetoprotein has improved management of nonseminomatous germinal cell tumors. α-Fetoprotein is a normal α globulin that usually disappears from the circulation about the time of birth. It may be found not only in patients with testicular carcinoma but also in those with gastric, pancreatic, colonic, and bronchogenic carcinomas. Elevated β-hCG levels are also not specific for testicular tumors. Nonetheless, in some

series one or both of these tumor markers are elevated in germinal cell carcinomas. When present, they may be used to follow the course of therapy.

Treatment has improved during the last decade, in particular for patients with elements of choriocarcinoma. Some investigators[476] report 3-year survival rates of about 80%. The reader is referred to reviews[487-489] for details of radiation and chemotherapy.

Leydig cell tumors are the most important of the nongerminal testicular neoplasms. Functionally, these may be either virilizing[487] or feminizing.[490] When the androgen-producing type of tumor occurs in a prepubertal boy, precocious development of the penis, beard, and muscles occurs along with accelerated linear growth. When it occurs in an adult male, little change is noted since excess androgen in

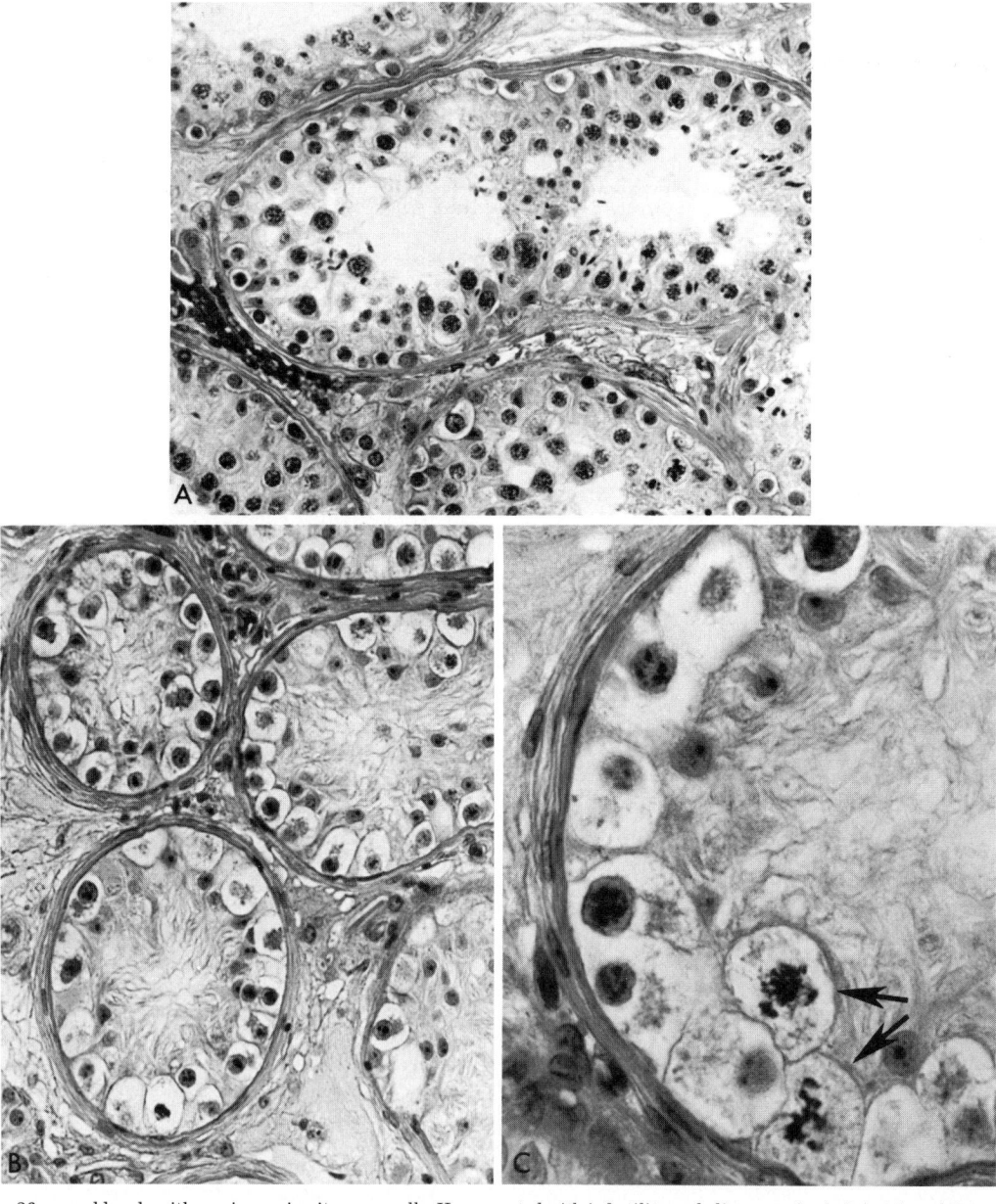

Figure 6–36. 26-year-old male with carcinoma-in-situ germ cells. He presented with infertility and oligospermia. *A, B* (×64), and *C* (×160). Photomicrographs of first testicular biopsy specimen. *A,* Left side. There is a decrease in germ cell type numbers, particularly the spermatids. *B* and *C,* Right side. Note the absence of active spermatogenesis. The abnormal "gonocytes" exclusively line the seminiferous tubules. They are characterized in general by presence of "swollen" cytoplasm, dark-staining nucleoli, and active mitosis.

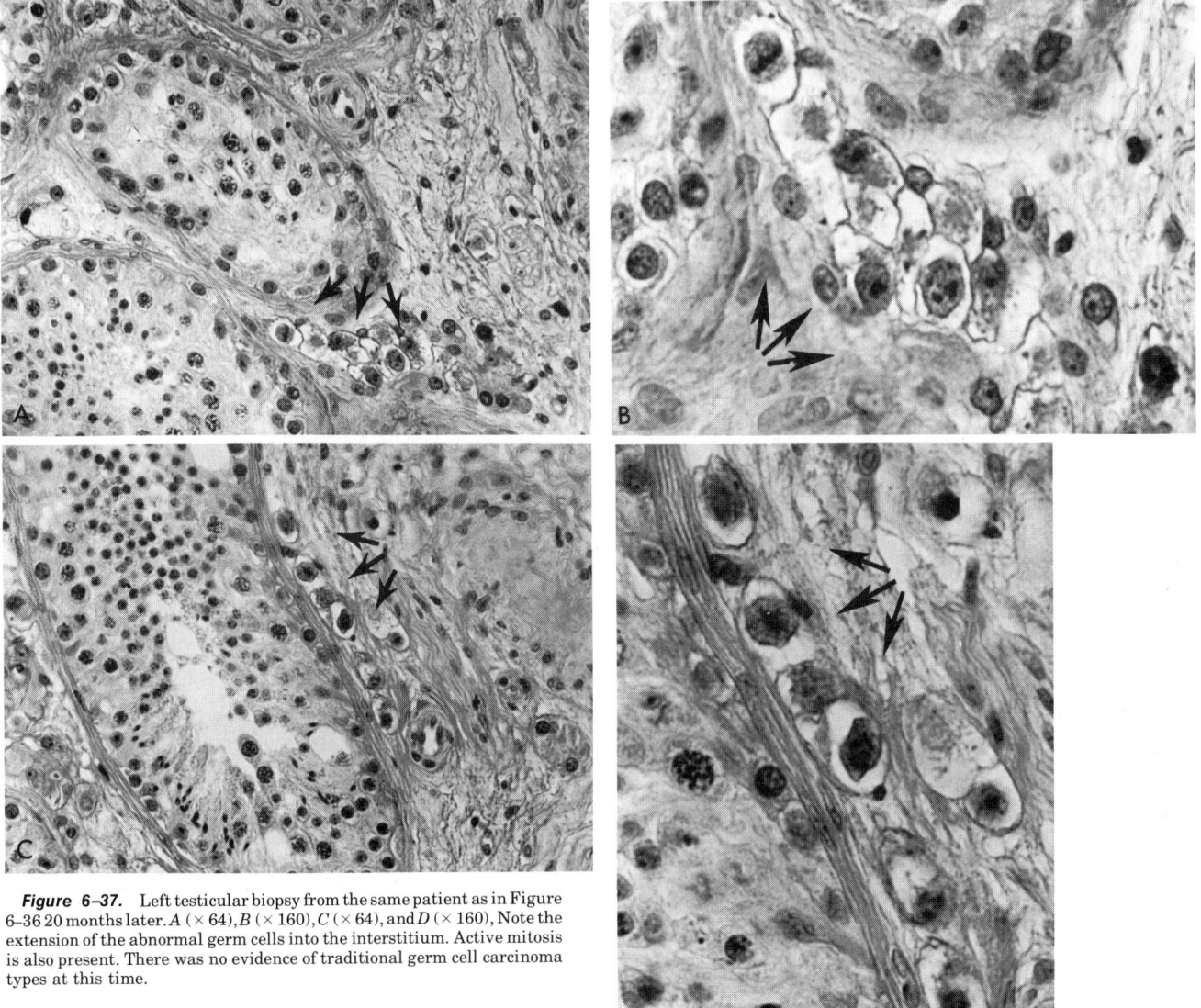

Figure 6–37. Left testicular biopsy from the same patient as in Figure 6–36 20 months later. *A* (×64), *B* (×160), *C* (×64), and *D* (×160), Note the extension of the abnormal germ cells into the interstitium. Active mitosis is also present. There was no evidence of traditional germ cell carcinoma types at this time.

the normal adult does not alter the secondary sex characteristics or increase libido and sexual potentia. Gynecomastia may develop, however.

Serum androgen levels, as well as urinary and plasma 17-ketosteroid levels, may be increased. These values drop to normal after surgery if metastases are not present. Occasionally in prepubertal boys the pattern of hormone production by Leydig cell tumors may be confused with that of congenital adrenal hyperplasia. In the latter condition, corticosteroid administration will suppress the excess androgen and 17-ketosteroid secretion. It is also important to distinguish testicular neoplasms from the adrenal tumors that develop adjacent to the testes in patients with excess ACTH secretion. Removal of the tumors, but not the testes, is recommended.

Leydig cell tumors that produce feminization are found only in adult males. Here, gynecomastia, impotence, and decreased hair growth result, and urinary estrogen excretion is high. These tumors must be distinguished from adrenal tumors which secrete similar steroids. Surgery is indicated for both types of Leydig cell tumors and, in contrast to the germinal cell neoplasms, they generally follow a more benign course.

GYNECOMASTIA

Gynecomastia, or "benign glandular" enlargement of the breast, occurs in the majority of males at some time during their life span. It is usually grossly evident but can be limited to microscopic changes. Clinically, it should be differentiated from other causes of breast enlargement including lipoma, carcinoma, neurofibromatosis, and obesity. Gynecomastia represents a concentric increase in glandular and stromal tissue. When the enlargement is grossly evident, it varies from a small "button" of subareolar tissue to full development indistinguishable from that of the adult female breast (Fig. 6–38). Bilateral gynecomastia is more common than unilateral involvement.

Microscopically, the normal male breast consists of a few scattered ducts containing low cuboidal epithelium. Strands of moderately dense collagenous tissue in the interlobular spaces support the ductal elements, and the periductal area is composed of scanty amounts of fiber-poor connective tissue. When gynecomastia is present, the histologic picture falls into either of two general patterns. In one, the major changes occur in the parenchymal elements so that ductal hyperplasia and lobular formation are the main features. In the other pattern, alterations in interlobular and periductal tissue predominate, with increases in dense collagenous fibers and adipose tissue, although ductal proliferation is also seen.[491, 492] The studies of Nicolis et al.[493] and Bannayan and Hajdu[494] suggest that the duration of the gynecomastia rather than etiologic factors dictates the histologic appear-

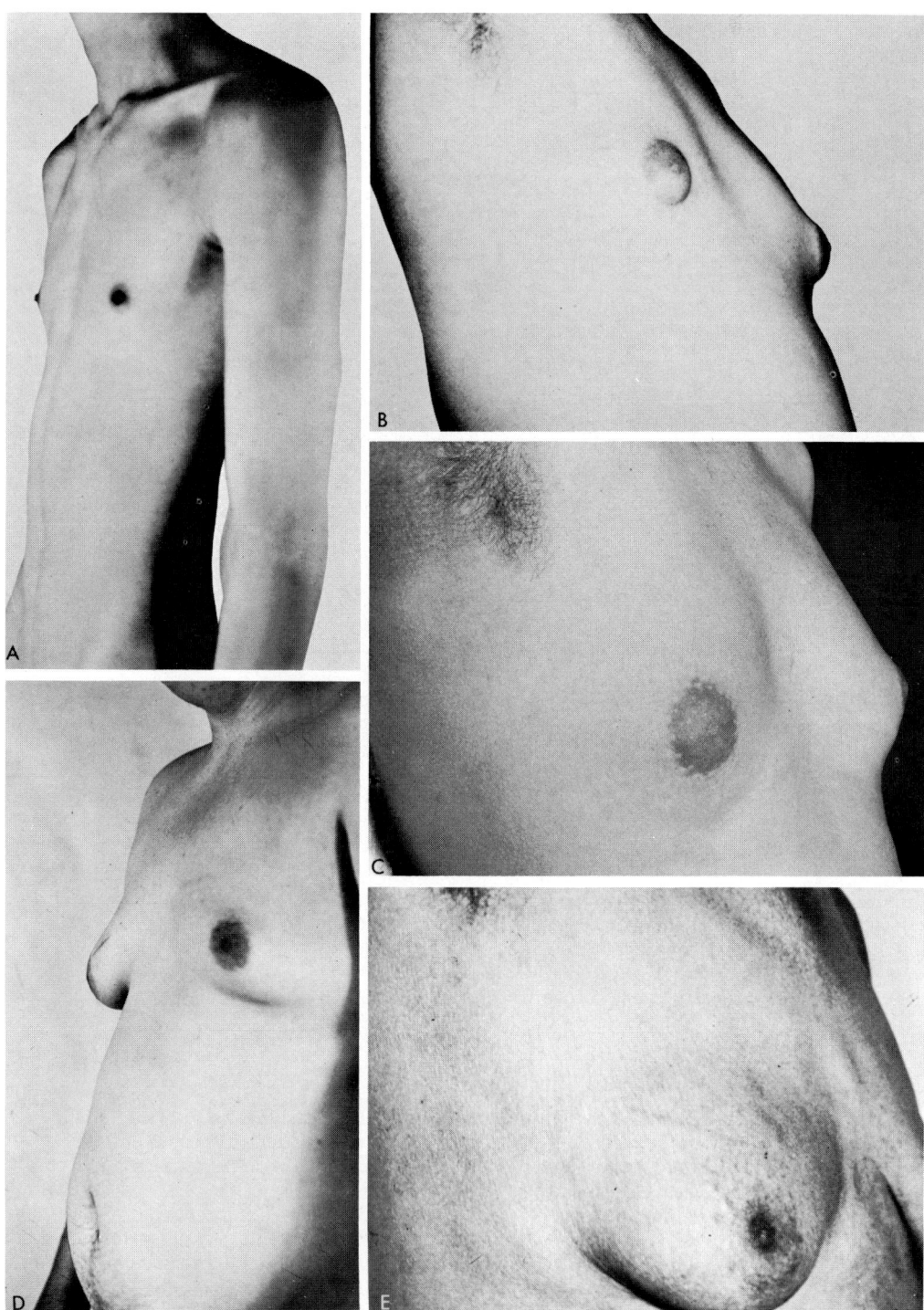

Figure 6–38. Examples of gynecomastia. *A*, Pubertal type. Note the plaquelike enlargement best seen in the lateral view of the right breast. *B, C, D,* and *E,* Gynecomastia of increasing severity in males with either Klinefelter's syndrome or the functional prepubertal castrate syndrome.

ance. The exception to this thesis may be the development of acini associated with estrogen ingestion or elevated endogenous estrogens.

Another interpretation is that the two basic microscopic patterns could imply different causal factors. The autopsy studies of Schwartz and Wilens support this contention.[492] These investigators detected acinar or lobular development only in those patients with gynecomastia who had received estrogen therapy for palliation of prostatic carcinoma. In the remaining cases, an increase in periductal connective tissue was the major feature and this was associated with either cirrhosis of the liver or a systemic disorder such as rheumatoid arthritis (with corticosteroid therapy), diabetes mellitus, chronic glomerulonephritis, or bronchogenic carcinoma. These observations agree with those of Morrione.[495] Thus, when parenchymal changes predominate, testosterone or estrogen alone or in combination may be primarily responsible, with prolactin playing a permissive role. When stromal changes predominate, unknown factors may be primarily responsible. It is possible that an increase in aromatase activity in breast tissue or an increased sensitivity to hormones may predispose certain patients to the development of gynecomastia despite a normal hormonal environment. These latter factors may be involved in some otherwise healthy patients who have gynecomastia in the absence of gonadal disease.[496]

One of the major problems confronting the clinician is that male breast enlargement is encountered commonly in apparently normal adult men. If the threshold for judging that the breast is enlarged is set at $\geq$ 2.0 cm in diameter, the incidence is 32–36% in normal men aged 17–58 years.[497-499] In these surveys most men were unaware that they had gynecomastia since symptoms such as tenderness were not present.

The other major problem is that gynecomastia is found in many patients with a variety of clinical conditions that seemingly have no common ground[500-505] (Table 6–10). Since estrogens stimulate breast development it is reasonable to assume that absolute or relative increases in effective concentration of these hormones result in gynecomastia. The theoretical basis of this concept is discussed in another portion of this chapter. Many clinical studies support this concept that estrogens play an important role in gynecomastia,[506-512] even though serum levels may not be increased in all patients.[513]

Androgens may also stimulate the male breast, but they differ from estrogens in their effect. For example, gynecomastia commonly develops during the initial phase of testosterone therapy for hypogonadism, but instead of increasing with continued steroid administration, it usually recedes gradually. Although testosterone is aromatized *in vivo* to estrogens, fluoxymesterone, which is not converted, may rarely produce gynecomastia. At puberty, steroids of testicular origin are responsible for the development of gynecomastia. This occurs transiently in approximately 70% of pubertal males and usually requires no treatment. Histologically, parenchymal stimulation is the major feature. A major cause of pubertal gynecomastia is believed to be the persistence of the high aromatase of childhood which results in high estrogen production.[132]

A peculiar type of gynecomastia has been documented[514-516] in men after release from prisoner-of-war camps. Painful breast enlargement occurred while they were recovering from malnutrition and not during the period of inanition, when there might have been derangement in liver function; hence the designation "refeeding" gynecomastia.[517] Since pituitary gonadotropin secretion is quite sensitive to protein deprivation, testicular function in these men during their period of severe weight loss was undoubtedly quiescent because of pituitary shutdown. When their diet improved and their metabolic processes returned to normal, pituitary gonadotropin secretion resumed, producing a "second puberty." This type of gynecomastia is probably more common than is appreciated and may explain the mechanism by which breast enlargement occurs in some patients who are recovering from a prolonged illness. The gynecomastia that develops during chronic hemodialysis for renal failure may be another example of this type.[518, 519] Hormonal studies have failed to find consistently elevated prolactin or estradiol levels. The same mechanism may also apply to the patient with liver disease, since the gynecomastia is commonly observed only after recovery from several episodes of decompensated liver function (Table 6–10).

In hypogonadism, gynecomastia is not common when gonadotropin secretion is below normal, as in the classic form, hypogonadotropic eunuchoidism. As stated previously, gynecomastia is seen frequently in the variant form "fertile eunuchoidism." Furthermore, it is seen quite regularly in hypergonadotropic syndromes such as Klinefelter's syndrome in which testosterone secretion is low and estrogen

---

Table 6–10. THE CLINICAL CONDITIONS AND SYNDROMES ASSOCIATED WITH GYNECOMASTIA

Increased estrogen secretion
1. Hypergonadotropism (Klinefelter's and Reifenstein's syndromes)
2. Leydig cell adenoma or carcinoma
3. Adrenocortical adenoma or carcinoma

Increased estrogen production in peripheral tissues
1. Normal puberty
2. Obesity
3. Increased secretions of an estrogen precursor such as androstenedione from testis or adrenal
4. Increased aromatase activity

Decrease in androgen secretion with normal or increased estrogen production
1. Klinefelter's syndrome
2. Testicular damage, i.e., mumps orchitis

End-Organ insensitivity to testosterone
1. Testicular feminization
2. Reifenstein's syndrome
3. Gynecomastia with normal external genitalia

Increased prolactin secretion
1. Pituitary tumors
2. Drugs (see below)

Increased gonadotropin secretion
1. Pituitary tumors (LH)
2. Choriocarcinoma (hCG)
3. Bronchogenic and other carcinoma (hCG)

Thyroid disease
1. Hyperthyroidism
2. Hypothyroidism

Drugs
1. Hormones — estrogens, androgens, hCG
2. Antiandrogens — cimetidine, spironolactone, marihuana, progestogens, flutamide, digitalis
3. Stimulators of prolactin — reserpine, hydroxyzine, phenothiazines

Chronic disease (sometimes the gynecomastia appears during recovery, but many factors may be involved)
1. Refeeding gynecomastia
2. Pulmonary tuberculosis
3. Diabetes mellitus
4. Cirrhosis
5. Congestive heart failure (digitalis)
6. Renal failure (hemodialysis)
7. Hodgkin's disease and other neoplasms

Breast tumors

The etiology of gynecomastia is complex and, as yet, not completely understood. In many patients there may be more than one cause. For example, patients with Reifenstein's syndrome are insensitive to testosterone and may also have increased estrogen production.

production is normal or slightly elevated. The histologic picture in these patients is characterized by stromal rather than parenchymal hyperplasia.

Drugs that affect the hypothalamus and other parts of the central nervous system have been associated with gynecomastia or galactorrhea or both. Some of these agents act by increasing prolactin secretion while others have a variety of effects on androgen action.[514-518] For example, spironolactone administration interferes with androgen synthesis[519] and, along with cimetidine and digitalis, has antiandrogenic properties.[129, 520] Since testosterone and estradiol have opposing actions on the breast, these antiandrogens increase the observed effects of estrogen on this tissue (Table 6–10).

From the above considerations, it is quite apparent that the precise etiology of gynecomastia is not known in many cases. Nonetheless, the clinician needs to evaluate each patient carefully so that the detection of serious diseases will not be overlooked. For example, gynecomastia may be the presenting complaint in patients with testicular germinal cell carcinoma or bronchogenic carcinoma. Indicators of recent breast enlargement are induration, pain, and tenderness.

There are a variety of diagnostic studies that may be useful. Hormone assays will be important in the following conditions: (1) serum hCG or β-hCG may be elevated in germinal cell, bronchogenic, hepatic, gastrointestinal, and mesothelial carcinomas; (2) serum estradiol and estrone may be increased in patients with feminizing adrenocortical carcinoma, interstitial cell tumor, and increased aromatase activity; and (3) serum prolactin may be modestly elevated with drugs; if the serum value is twice the upper limit of normal, a pituitary tumor should be considered. In addition to hormone measurement the following radiographic studies should be considered: (1) evaluation of the sella by polytomography or CAT scan, particularly with marked elevations of serum prolactin with or without galactorrhea; and (2) a general chest and organ survey if carcinoma is suspected. Finally, special studies will be required for diagnosis in certain patients, such as buccal smear and chromosomal studies (Klinefelter's syndrome), androgen receptors (Reifenstein's syndrome), and mammography or excision biopsy (breast carcinoma).

When breast enlargement is sufficient to disturb the patient, surgical removal is the only means of treatment. In particular, the clinician should understand the emotional impact of gynecomastia in the pubertal boy.

DISORDERS OF SEXUAL BEHAVIOR

Homosexuality, transvestism, and transsexualism are complex psychiatric disorders that are not known to be related to disturbances in sex hormone production. Although there have been suggestions that increased estrogen secretion or an altered androgen-estrogen ratio is responsible for these aberrations in phenotypic, genetic males, this has not been borne out by available data.[521-523]

It should be emphasized that estrogen administered to normal adult males results in impotence and decreased potentia, but the sexual preference remains unaltered. On the other hand, it could be argued that alterations in hormonal environment prior to puberty (i.e., any time from intrauterine life throughout prepubertal development) could affect sexual behavior. Patients with an XY karyotype and complete androgen insensitivity (testicular feminization) support such a contention except that they are completely feminized from birth and think of themselves as female. Patients with alterations in sex hormone production, such as genetic females with congenital adrenal hyperplasia, fail to support such an argument. Although these patients tend to be "tomboys," they follow their genetic and phenotypic lives with normal heterosexual behavior following appropriate suppression with corticoid suppressive treatment (see Chapter 9).

Kolodny et al.[524] point out that serum testosterone levels in a group of 30 homosexuals were significantly lower than those in 50 heterosexual males. A later publication revealed elevated serum LH titers.[525] Furthermore, many homosexual men studied demonstrated decreased sperm counts. Although these data are of interest, they could be secondary to the stress and emotional conflicts which these men are known to have. From a simplistic viewpoint, if testosterone levels are causally related to this problem, patients who occupy the "female" role should demonstrate lower testosterone levels than those patients who retain the "male" role.

Furthermore, if low androgen production were associated with homosexuality, then patients with hypogonadism associated with alterations in development of the external genitalia or gynecomastia should be susceptible. In fact, it is uncommon for these individuals to become overtly homosexual. We have found that most homosexuals have normal testicular function and sexual maturation. Careful psychiatric testing has demonstrated that many patients with Klinefelter's syndrome have subtle homosexual tendencies. Since it is beyond the scope of this discussion to deal with these findings, the reader is referred to the psychiatric literature for more details.

MALE CONTRACEPTION

During the past several years there has been renewed interest in developing new methods for male contraception. Reasons for this interest include: (1) sincere concern with possible adverse reactions associated with the use of the "pill" by women; (2) the definite social trend toward a sharing of responsibility for family planning between partners; and (3) the desire of many men to assume control over their own fertility. The methods currently available to men are interrupted coitus, condoms, and vasectomy. New surgical approaches have been tried to improve existing procedures. In order to expand the number of techniques, three medical approaches have been used to disrupt the male reproductive system: one used steroid or polypeptide hormones to inhibit the hypothalamic-pituitary-testicular axis; the second used drugs that act to inhibit spermatogenesis directly; and the third used agents that disrupt epididymal function.

Surgical Approaches to Contraception

Surgical studies have been designed to improve the procedures for interrupting the vas deferens, either by vasectomy or by introducing a "block" in the vas deferens. The aim has been to improve the potential for reversibility.[526-528] The pursuit of this goal has called attention to important gaps in our knowledge about the physiology and pathophysiology of the epididymis and vas deferens. For example, the entire issue of the immunologic consequences of vasectomy requires clarification. One concern is that sperm antibodies produced post vasectomy may interfere with spermatogenesis or post-testicular sperm maturation. If true, this could explain the reduced fertility rate following a technically successful reanastomosis of the vas deferens. Another point centers on the possibility that the immunologic response to vasectomy may accelerate the process of atherosclerosis.[529-531] There are several publications to which the reader may refer for greater detail concerning surgical approaches to male contraception.[526-528, 531]

Drugs that Inhibit the Hypothalamic-Pituitary-Testicular Axis

Observations made over the past 40 years have shown that the administration of either testosterone or synthetic progestins can inhibit pituitary gonadotropin secretion and lead to varying degrees of oligospermia or actual azoospermia.[532] This inhibitory effect on spermatogenesis has been considered to be completely reversible. The following single steroids and steroid combinations have been used in small-scale clinical trials: an androgen by itself; an androgen together with an impaired androgen, danazol; an antiandrogen; and several androgen-progestagen combinations.

Androgens. Several groups recently reexamined the role of testosterone administration on testicular function in normal men.[533-536] Data from one study showed that when tesosterone enanthate was given intramuscularly in doses of 200 mg/week, 50% of the men became azoospermic. An additional 39% of men became severely oligospermic. Treatment for 7 to 20 weeks was required to achieve azoospermia. Serum LH and FSH levels were usually depressed to undetectable levels. Increased levels of serum testosterone were found within 1 to 2 days following testosterone administration and gradually returned to basal levels after 7 days. The maximal elevation ranged from 1.5 to 3 times basal levels. In a second group of men, testosterone was administered in doses of 200 mg every 2 weeks. Forty-five per cent of these men achieved azoospermia within 7 to 27 weeks and an additional 23% became oligospermic within 4 to 31 weeks. Maintenance therapy was instituted in those men who had achieved azoospermia or oligospermia with weekly injections. Doses of 200 or 400 mg of testosterone enanthate given once a month failed to maintain suppression of spermatogenesis, and sperm production gradually increased to over 20 million/ml in 50% of the men.[537]

When testosterone administration was stopped, full recovery of sperm production occurred in every volunteer. Drug-related adverse reactions, which were minor in degree, included acne, weight gain, transient breast tenderness, and gynecomastia. Results of other clinical trials were similar in terms of inhibiting spermatogenesis and in the general lack of adverse reactions. Nevertheless, there are many potentially toxic effects of androgens, including effects on thrombosis and platelet aggregation.[538]

We conclude from these trials that it would be necessary to administer testosterone enanthate at intervals of every 7 to 10 days to achieve optimal suppression of spermatogenesis. This is clearly impractical and highlights the need to develop esters of testosterone with a longer duration of biologic action if this approach to male contraception is to be successful. Oral androgens, including methyltestosterone and testosterone undecanoate, have not proved to be effective contraceptives.[539, 540]

Androgen Plus an Impeded Androgen. Danazol exerts two effects on the male reproductive system. It has a direct effect on the testes to reduce testosterone secretion, and it also inhibits LH secretion.[541, 542] When relatively small amounts of testosterone are combined with danazol, sperm counts decrease sharply.[543] When testosterone enanthate, 200 mg/month, was administered with 400, 600, or 800 mg of danazol daily, azoospermia was achieved in 29, 33, and 43% of the men, respectively. The time required for maximal suppression of spermatogenesis varied between 4 and 48 weeks. Additional men in each group became severely oligospermic. Serum samples obtained just prior to the testosterone injections revealed decreases in LH and FSH levels.[534, 544] There were no changes in libido or sexual potency and no drug-related adverse reactions.

We conclude from these trials that for such a combination to be effective and economically practical more potent analogues of danazol would have to be synthesized.

Androgen-Progestagen Combinations. Synthetic progestational steroids when administered to men depress pituitary function and spermatogenesis.[545] However, testosterone levels are markedly depressed, so that typical androgen withdrawal symptoms of decreased libido and sexual potency occur. Moreover, some of these compounds are estrogenic and thus produce gynecomastia. Of the many progestin-androgen combinations that were tried, medroxyprogesterone acetate plus a testosterone ester was studied most extensively.[546-551] When 200 mg depo-medroxyprogesterone acetate plus 250 mg testosterone cypionate was given once monthly in one study, azoospermia was induced in 56% of men within 6 to 15 weeks. Most of the remaining men were oligospermic. The time required for recovery varied between 14 and 60 weeks. No significant adverse reactions apart from weight gain and minimal degrees of transient gynecomastia were noted. When the androgen and progestogen were administered orally, satisfactory suppression of spermatogenesis did not occur.[552]

Antiandrogens. Spermatozoa are known to mature within the epididymis, which is crucially dependent on androgens for normal function. Prasad et al.[553] treated rats with Silastic capsules containing cyproterone acetate and noted nonmotile sperm within 4 months, associated with sterile matings. No evidence of systemic androgen deprivation was observed. On the basis of these findings four clinical trials were conducted in which cyproterone acetate in daily doses of 5, 10, or 20 mg produced a reduction in serum gonadotropin testosterone levels and varying degrees of oligospermia.[554-558] The suppression of anterior pituitary function was undoubtedly related to the fact that cyproterone acetate possesses progestational as well as antiandrogenic properties.

We conclude from all the clinical trials in which steroids were used for sperm suppression, that they were able to induce azoospermia or oligospermia in most normal adult men. This can be accomplished without producing important adverse reactions. With present approaches, however, it does not appear that it will be possible to induce azoospermia in more than 70% of men. As a consequence, about 30% of such treated men may not be protected. Indeed, Barfield et al.[559] have documented fertility in subjects treated with testosterone and progestins with low sperm counts. These latter men may, therefore, be analogous to hypogonadotropic patients treated with hCG and hMG who become fertile with sperm counts of 5 million or less.

Analogues of Gonadotropin-Releasing Hormone. Animal studies have shown that several potent GnRH agonists produce changes in the GnRH and LH receptor sites of the pituitary and testis, respectively. This results in the phenomenon of "downregulation." That is, with chronic administration of the GnRH agonist, testicular stimulation changes to testicular suppression. Serum testosterone levels fall dramatically and spermatogenesis is disrupted. Pelletier has cautioned that testicular recovery, at least in rats, may not be complete.[560] Clearly, more animal studies will be required before extensive clinical trials can be performed.

Several antagonist analogues of GnRH have been synthesized and tested in experimental animals.[545, 561] Recently, a very potent antagonist has been reported to lead to a severe suppression of spermatogenesis in male rats.[561] Both the agonist and antagonist analogues of GnRH are known to inhibit testosterone production, so androgen replacement will be necessary if these analogues are used in clinical trials. Also, a delay of at least 1 to 2 months can be expected in suppression of spermatogenesis and in recovery after cessation of therapy.

Drugs that Act Directly on the Testis

Gossypol. Scientists in the People's Republic of China have conducted clinical trials in approximately 8800 men with gossypol,[562, 563] a substance extracted from cottonseed. Spermatogenesis in these men decreased markedly within 4 months, but testosterone levels remained unchanged. Animal studies have shown that early during drug exposure epididymal sperm are also affected and the mitochondria of spermatids become vacuolated and cystic.[564, 565] Side effects include hypokalemic paralysis in as many as 4.7% of men.[563] Studies *in vitro* suggest that the sodium-potassium ATPase system is inhibited and might be the cause of the hypokalemia.[566] Recovery of testicular function in men who have participated in these clinical trials has not yet been detailed. Further studies are required to determine whether gossypol will be useful as a male contraceptive agent.

Drugs that Alter Epididymal Function

Agents that alter the metabolism of the epididymis are attractive as contraceptives from at least two points of view. First, the latent period for such an antiepididymal agent to become effective would be relatively short, about 7 to 14 days. Furthermore, the potential for adverse genetic effects should be minimal since germ cells do not divide in this organ. Several compounds that alter epididymal function were identified. α-Chlorohydrin was first, and then aminochlorohydrin, and lastly a class of preparations designated as chlorinated sugars were examined. The mechanism by which these compounds produce their effect has not been clearly defined, but they probably interfere with the normal glucose metabolism within the epididymis. Aminochlorohydrin and one of the chlorinated sugars, 6-deoxy-6-chloro-D-glucose, were found to be effective in infrahuman primates.[567] Unfortunately, each of these compounds produced serious systemic toxic effects, and at this time no one has produced suitable nontoxic analogues.

REFERENCES

1. Bergland, R., and Page, R.: Can the pituitary secrete directly to the brain? *Endocrinology 102*:1325–1338, 1978.
2. Davidson, J. M., and Bloch, G. J.: Neuroendocrine aspects of male reproduction. *Biol. Repro. Supplement 1*:67–92, 1969.
3. Elde, R., and Hokfelt, T.: Distribution of hypothalamic hormones and other peptides in the brain. In *Frontiers in Neuroendocrinology*. Vol. 15. Ganong, W. F., and Martini, L. (eds.), New York, Raven Press, 1978, pp. 1–33.
4. Silverman, A. J., Krey, L. C., and Zimmerman, E. A.: A comparative study of the luteinizing hormone releasing hormone (LHRH) neuronal networks in mammals. *Biol. Reprod. 20*:98–110, 1979.
5. Negro-Vilar, A., Ojeda, S. R., and McCann, S. M.: Catecholaminergic modulation of luteinizing hormone-releasing hormone release by median eminence terminals *in vitro*. *Endocrinology 104*:1749–1757, 1979.
6. McCann, S. M.: Regulation of secretion of follicle-stimulating hormone and luteinizing hormone. In *Handbook of Physiology*, Section 7: Endocrinology. Greep, R. O., and Astwood, E. B. (eds.), Baltimore, Williams & Wilkins, 1975, p. 489.
7. Parvizi, N., and Ellendorff, F.: β-Endorphin alters luteinizing hormone secretion via the amygdala but not the hypothalamus. *Nature 286*:812–813, 1980.
8. Evans, W. S., Rogol, A. D., MacLeod, R. M., and Thorner, M. O.: Dopaminergic mechanisms and luteinizing hormone secretion. I. Acute administration of the dopamine agonist bromocriptine does not inhibit luteinizing hormone release in hyperprolactinemic women. *J. Clin. Endocrinol. Metab. 50*:103–107, 1980.
9. Pfaff, D. W.: Luteinizing hormone-releasing factor (LRF) potentiates lordosis behavior in hypophysectomized, ovariectomized female rats. *Science 182*:1148–1149, 1973.
10. Moss, R. L., and Foreman, M. M.: Potentiation of lordosis behavior by intrahypothalamic infusion of synthetic luteinizing hormone–releasing hormone. *Neuroendocrinology 20*:176–181, 1976.
11. Schally, A. V., Kastin, A. J., and Arimura, A.: The hypothalamus and reproduction. *Amer. J. Obstet. Gynecol. 114*:423–442, 1972.
12. Schally, A. V.: Aspects of hypothalamic regulation of the pituitary gland. *Science 202*:18–28, 1978.
13. Naor, Z., and Catt, K. J.: Independent actions of gonadotropin releasing hormone upon cyclic GMP production and luteinizing hormone release. *J. Biol. Chem. 255*:342–344, 1980.
14. Conn, P. M., Morrell, D. V., Dufau, M. L., and Catt, K. J.: Gonadotropin-releasing hormone action in cultured pituicytes: Independence of luteinizing hormone release and adenosine 3'5'-monophosphate production. *Endocrinology 104*:448–453, 1979.
15. Huhtaniemi, I. T., Koritnik, D. R., Korenbrot, C. C., Mennin, S., Foster, D. B., and Jaffe, R. B.: Stimulation of pituitary-testicular function with gonadotropin-releasing hormone in fetal and infant monkeys. *Endocrinology 105*:109–114, 1979.
16. Mortimer, C. H.: Gonadotropin-releasing hormone. In *Clinical Neuroendocrinology*. Martini, L., and Besser, G. M. (eds.), New York, Academic Press, 1977, pp. 213–236.
17. Huseman, C. A., and Kelch, R. P.: Gonadotropin responses and metabolism of synthetic gonadotropin-releasing hormone (GnRH) during constant infusion of GnRH in men and boys with delayed adolescence. *J. Clin. Endocrinol. Metab. 47*:1325–1331, 1978.
18. Bourguignon, J-P., Hoyoux, C., Reuter, A., and Franchimont, P.: Urinary excretion of immunoreactive luteinizing hormone-releasing hormone-like material and gonadotropins at different stages of life. *J. Clin. Endicrinol. Metab. 48*:78–84, 1979.
19. Vale, W., Rivier, C., and Brown, M.: Regulatory peptides of the hypothalamus. *Ann. Rev. Physiol. 39*:473–527, 1977.
20. Rivier, J. E., and Vale, W. W.: [D-pGlu¹,D-Phe²,D-Trp³·⁶]-LRF. A potent luteinizing hormone releasing factor antagonist *in vitro* and inhibitor of ovulation in the rat. *Life Sci. 23*:869–876, 1978.
21. Hsueh, A. J. W., and Erickson, G. F.: Extra-pituitary inhibition of testicular function by luteinizing hormone releasing hormone. *Nature 281*:66–67, 1979.
22. Wright, W., Chan, K., Sundaram, K., and Bardin, C. W.: New observations on androgen action: Androgen receptor stabilization and antisteroid effects on LHRH agonists. In *Hormones and Cancer*. Leavitt, W. W. (ed.), New York, Plenum Press, 1980 (in press).
23. Vaitukaitis, J. L., Ross, G. D., Braunstein, G. D., and Rayford, P. L.: Gonadotropins and their subunits: Basic and clinical studies. *Recent Prog. Horm. Res. 32*:289–331, 1976.
24. Pierce, J. G., Liao, T. H., Howard, S. M., Shome, B., and Cornell, J. S.: Studies on the structure of thyrotropin: Its relationship to luteinizing hormone. *Recent Prog. Horm. Res. 27*:165–212, 1971.
25. Bishop, W. H., Nureddin, A., and Ryan, R. J.: Pituitary luteinizing and follicle-stimulating hormones. In *Peptide Hormones*. Parsons, J. A. (ed.), Baltimore, University Park Press, 1976, pp. 273–298.
26. Braunstein, G. D., Rasor, J., and Wade, M. E.: Presence in normal human testes of a chorionic-gonadotropin-like substance distinct from human luteinizing hormone. *N. Engl. J. Med. 293*:1339–1343, 1975.
27. Chan, H.-C., Hodgen, G. D., Matsuura, S., Lin, L. J., Gross, E., Reichert, L. E., Jr., Birken, S., Canfield, R. E., and Ross, G. T.: Evidence for a gonadotropin from nonpregnant subjects that has physical, immunological and biological similarities to human chorionic gonadotropin. *Proc. Natl. Acad. Sci. USA 73*:2885–2889, 1976.
28. Borkowski, A., and Muquardt, C.: Human chorionic gonadotropin in the plasma of normal, nonpregnant subjects. *N. Engl. J. Med. 301*:298–302, 1979.
29. Maruo, T., Segal, S. J., and Koide, S. S.: Studies on the apparent human chorionic gonadotropin-like factor in the crab *Ovalipes ocellatus*. *Endocrinology 104*:932–939, 1979.
30. Kurosky, A., Markel, D. W., Peterson, J. W., and Fitch, W. M.: Primary structure of cholera toxin β-chain: A glycoprotein hormone analog? *Science 195*:299–301, 1977.
31. Richert, N. D., and Ryan, R. J.: Proteolytic enzyme activation of rat ovarian adenylate cyclase. *Proc. Natl. Acad. Sci. USA 74*:4857–4861, 1977.
32. Maruo, T., Cohen, H., Segal, S. J., and Koide, S. S.: Production of choriogonadotropin-like factors by a microorganism. *Proc. Natl. Acad. Sci. USA 76*:6622–6626, 1979.

33. Carmel, P. W., Araki, S., and Ferin, M.: Pituitary stalk portal blood collection in rhesus monkeys: Evidence for pulsatile release of gonadotropin-releasing hormone (GnRH). *Endocrinology* 99:243–248, 1976.

34. Neill, J. D., Patton, J. M., Dailey, R. A., Tsou, R. C., and Tindall, G. T.: Luteinizing hormone releasing hormone (LHRH) in pituitary stalk blood of rhesus monkeys: Relationship to level of LH release. *Endocrinology* 101:430–434, 1977.

35. Nankin, H. R., and Troen, P.: Repetitive luteinizing hormone elevations in serum of normal men. *J. Clin. Endocrinol. Metab.* 33:558–560, 1971.

36. Franchimont, P., and Roulier, R.: Gonadotropin secretion in male subjects. In *Clinical Neuroendocrinology.* Martini, L., and Besser, G. M. (eds.), New York, Academic Press, 1977, pp. 197–212.

37. Santen, R. J., and Bardin, C. W.: Episodic luteinizing hormone secretion in man: Pulse analysis, clinical interpretation, physiologic mechanisms. *J. Clin. Invest.* 52:2617–2628, 1973.

38. Santen, R. J.: Is aromatization of testosterone to estradiol required for inhibition of luteinizing hormone secretion in men? *J. Clin. Invest.* 56:1555–1563, 1975.

39. Baker, H. W. G., Santen, R. J., Burger, H. G., DeKretser, D. M., Hudson, B., Pepperell, R. J., and Bardin, C. W.: Rhythms in the secretion of gonadotropins and gonadal steroids. *J. Steroid Biochem.* 6:793–801, 1975.

40. Santen, R. J., and Kulin, H. E.: The male reproductive system. In *Practice of Pediatrics.* Vol. 1. Kelly, V. C. (ed.), Hagerstown, MD, Harper & Row, 1976, pp. 1–44.

41. VanHall, E. V., Vaitukaitis, J. L., Ross, G. T., Hickman, J. W., and Ashwell, G.: Effects of progressive desialylation on the rate of disappearance of immunoreactive hCG from plasma in rats. *Endocrinology* 89:11–15, 1971.

42. Solano, A. R., Dufau, M. L., and Catt, K. J.: Bioassay and radioimmunoassay of serum luteinizing hormone in the male rat. *Endocrinology* 105:372–381, 1979.

43. Kohler, P. O., Ross, G. T., and Odell, W. D.: Metabolic clearance and production rates of human luteinizing hormone in pre- and post-menopausal women. *J. Clin. Invest.* 47:38–47, 1968.

44. Keller, P. J.: The renal clearance of follicle-stimulating and luteinizing hormone in postmenopausal women. *Acta Endocrinol.* 53:225–233, 1966.

45. Ahmad, K. N., Lennox, B., and Mack, W. S.: Estimation of the volume of Leydig cells in man. *Lancet* 2:461–464, 1969.

46. Christensen, A. K.: Leydig cells. In *Handbook of Physiology,* Section 7: Endocrinology. Vol. V: Male Reproductive System. Hamilton, D. W., and Greep, R. O. (eds.), Baltimore, Williams & Wilkins, 1975, pp. 57–94.

47. Siiteri, P. K., and Wilson, J. D.: Testosterone formation and metabolism during male sexual differentiation in the human embryo. *J. Clin. Endocrinol. Metab.* 38:113–125, 1974.

48. Faiman, C., and Winter, J. S. D.: Gonadotropins and sex hormone patterns in puberty: Clinical data. In *Control of the Onset of Puberty.* Grumbach, M. M., Grave, G. D., and Mayer, F. E. (eds.), New York, John Wiley & Sons, 1974, pp. 32–61.

49. Forest, M. G.: Pattern of the response of testosterone and its precursors to human chorionic gonadotropin stimulation in relation to age in infants and children. *J. Clin. Endocrinol. Metab.* 49:132–137, 1979.

50. Eik-Nes, K. B.: Biosynthesis and secretion of testicular steroids. In *Handbook of Physiology,* Section 7: Endocrinology. Vol. V: Male Reproductive System. Hamilton, D. W., and Greep, R. O. (eds.), Baltimore, Williams & Wilkins, 1975, pp. 95–116.

51. Davies, T. F., Dufau, M. L., and Catt, K. J.: Gonadotrophin receptors: Characteristics and clinical applications. *Clin. Obstet. Gynecol.* 5:329–362, 1978.

52. Dufau, M. L., and Catt, K. J.: Gonadotropin receptors and regulation of steroidogenesis in the testis and ovary. *Vitam. Horm.* 36:461–592, 1978.

53. Aragona, C., and Friesen, H. G.: Specific prolactin binding sites in the prostate and testis of rats. *Endocrinology* 97:677–684, 1975.

54. Hafiez, A. A., Bartke, A., and Lloyd, C. W.: The role of prolactin in the regulation of testis function: Synergistic effects of prolactin and LH on the incorporation of [1-^{14}] acetate into testosterone and cholesterol by testes from hypophysectomized rats *in vitro. J. Endocrinol.* 53:223–230, 1972.

55. Abramowitz, J., Iyengar, R., and Birnbaumer, L.: Guanyl nucleotide regulation of hormonally-responsive adenylyl cyclases. *Mol. Cell. Endocrinol.* 16:129–146, 1979.

56. Podesta, E. J., Dufau, M. L., Solano, A. R., and Catt, K. J.: Hormonal activation of protein kinase in isolated Leydig cells: Electrophoretic analysis of cyclic AMP receptors. *J. Biol. Chem.* 253:8994–9001, 1978.

57. Catt, K. J., and Dufau, M. L.: Gonadotropin receptors and regulation of interstitial cell function in the testis. *Receptors Horm. Action* 3:291–339, 1978.

58. Kahn, C. R., Neville, D. M., and Roth, J.: Insulin-receptor interaction in the obese-hyperglycemic mouse: A model of insulin resistance. *J. Biol. Chem.* 248:244–250, 1973.

59. Lesniak, M. A., and Roth, J.: Regulation of receptor concentration by homologous hormone: Effect of human growth hormone on its receptor in IM-9 lymphocytes. *J. Biol. Chem.* 251:3720–3792, 1976.

60. Saez, J. M., Haour, F., and Cathiard, A. M.: Early hCG-induced desensitization in Leydig cells. *Biochem. Biophys. Res. Commun.* 81:552–558, 1978.

61. Haour, F., Sanchez, P., Cathiard, A. M., and Saez, J. M.: Gonadotropin receptor regulation in hypophysectomized rat Leydig cells. *Biochem. Biophys. Res. Commun.* 81:547–551, 1978.

62. Catt, K. J., and Dufau, M. L.: Spare gonadotrophin receptors in rat testis. *Nature [New Biol.]* 244:219–221, 1973.

63. Kirschner, M. A., Widner, J. A., and Ross, G. T.: Leydig cell function in men with gonadotropin-producing testicular tumors. *J. Clin. Endocrinol. Metab.* 30:504–511, 1970.

64. Auclair, C., Kelly, P. A., Coy, D. H., Schally, A. V., and Labrie, F.: Potent inhibitory activity of [D-Leu⁶,Des-Gly-NH₂¹⁰] LHRH ethylamide on LH/hCG and PRL testicular receptor level in the rat. *Endocrinology* 101:1890–1893, 1977.

65. Labrie, F., Auclair, C., Cusan, L., Kelly, P. A., Pelletier, G., and Ferland, L.: Inhibitory effect of LHRH and its agonists on testicular gonadotropin receptors and spermatogenesis in the rat. *Int. J. Androl.* (Suppl.) 2:303–318, 1978.

66. Vale, W., Rivier, C., Brown, M., and Rivier, J.: Pharmacology of thyrotropin releasing factor (TRF), luteinizing hormone releasing factor (LRF), and somatostatin. In *Hypothalamic Peptide Hormones and Pituitary Regulation.* Porter, J. C. (ed.), New York, Plenum Press, 1977, pp. 123–156.

67. Catt, K. J., Baukal, A. J., Davies, T. F., and Dufau, M. L.: Luteinizing hormone-releasing hormone-induced regulation of gonadotropin and prolactin receptors in the rat testis. *Endocrinology* 104:17–25, 1979.

68. Mather, J. P., and Sato, G. H.: The use of hormone-supplemented serum-free media in primary cultures. *Exp. Cell Res.* 124:215–221, 1979.

69. Mather, J. P.: Establishment and characterization of two distinct mouse testicular epithelial cell lines. *Biol. Reprod.* 23:243–252, 1980.

70. Kovanen, P. T., Schneider, W. J., Hillman, G. M., Goldstein, J. L., and Brown, M. S.: Separate mechanisms for the uptake of high and low density lipoproteins by mouse adrenal gland *in vivo. J. Biol. Chem.* 254:5498–5505, 1979.

71. Mahoudeau, J. A., Bardin, C. W., and Lipsett, M. B.: The metabolic clearance rate and origin of plasma dihydrotestosterone in man and its conversion to the 5α-androstanediols. *J. Clin. Invest.* 50:1338–1344, 1971.

72. Ito, T., and Horton, R.: The source of plasma dihydrotestosterone in man. *J. Clin. Invest.* 50:1621–1627, 1971.

73. Boyar, R. M., Rosenfeld, R. S., Kapen, S., Finkelstein, J. W., Roffwarg, H. P., Weitzman, E. D., and Hellman, L.: Human puberty: Simultaneous augmented secretion of luteinizing hormone and testosterone during sleep. *J. Clin. Invest.* 54:609–618, 1974.

74. Schiavi, R. C., Davis, D. M., White, D., Edwards, A., Igel, G., and Fisher, C.: Plasma testosterone during nocturnal sleep in normal men. *Steroids* 24:191–202, 1974.

75. Doering, C. H., Kraemer, H. C., Brodie, H. K. H., and Hamburg, D. A.: A cycle of plasma testosterone in the human male. *J. Clin. Endocrinol. Metab.* 40:492–500, 1975.

76. Corvol, P. L., Chramback, A., Rodbard, D., and Bardin, C. W.: Physical properties and binding capacity of testosterone-estradiol-binding globulin in human plasma, determined by polyacrylamide gel electrophoresis. *J. Biol. Chem.* 246:3435–3443, 1971.

77. Rosner, W., and Smith, R. N.: Isolation and characterization of the testosterone-estradiol-binding globulin from human plasma: Use of a novel affinity column. *Biochemistry* 14:4813–4820, 1975.

78. Iqbal, M. J., and Johnson, M. W.: Purification and characterization of human sex hormone binding globulin. *J. Steroid Biochem.* 10:535–540, 1979.

79. Mickelson, K. E., Teller, D. C., and Petra, P. H.: Characterization of the sex steroid binding protein of human pregnancy serum. Improvements in the purification procedure. *Biochemistry.* 17:1409–1415, 1978.

80. Mischke, W., Weise, H. C., Graesslin, D., Rusch, R., and Tamm, J.: Isolation of highly purified sex hormone binding globulin (SHBG): Evidence for microheterogeneity. *Acta Endocrinol.* 90:737–742, 1979.

81. Suzuki, Y., and Sinohara, H.: Hepatic uptake of desialylated testosterone-oestradiol-binding globulin in the rat. *Acta Endocrinol.* 90:669–679, 1979.

82. Rosner, W.: The binding of steroid hormones in human serum. In *Trace Components of Plasma, Isolation and Clinical Significance.* Vol. V. Jamieson, G. A., Greenwalt, T. J., and Liss, A. R. (eds.), New York, Alan R. Liss, Inc., 1976, pp. 337–395.

83. Nisula, B. C., and Dunn, J. F.: Measurement of the testosterone binding parameters for both testosterone-estradiol binding globulin and albumin in individual serum samples. *Steroids* 34:771–791, 1979.

84. Vermeulen, A., Stoica, T., and Verdonck, L.: The apparent free testosterone concentration, an index of androgenicity. *J. Clin. Endocrinol. Metab.* 33:759–767, 1971.

85. Rosenfield, R.: Plasma testosterone-binding globulin and indexes of the concentration of unbound plasma androgens in normal and hirsute subjects. *J. Clin. Endocrinol. Metab.* 32:717–728, 1971.

86. Vermeulen, A., Verdonck, L., Van der Straeten, M., and Orie, N.: Capacity of the testosterone-binding globulin in human plasma and influence of specific binding of testosterone on its metabolic clearance rate. *J. Clin. Endocrinol. Metab.* 29:1470–1480, 1969.

87. Mercier-Bodard, C., Marchuit, M., Perrot, M., Picard, M. T., Baulieu, E.-E., and Robel, P.: Influence of purified plasma proteins on testosterone uptake and metabolism by normal and hyperplastic human prostate in constant-flow organ culture. *J. Clin. Endocrinol. Metab.* 43:374–386, 1976.

88. Bordin, S., and Petra, P. H.: Immunocytochemical localization of the sex steroid-binding protein (SBP) of plasma in tissues of the adult monkey, *Macaca nemestrina. Proc. Natl. Acad. Sci. USA* 77:5678–5682, 1980.

89. Corvol, P., and Bardin, C. W.: Species distribution of testosterone binding globulin. *Biol. Reprod.* 8:277–282, 1973.

90. Tait, J. F.: Review: The use of isotopic steroids for the measurement of production rates *in vivo. J. Clin. Endocrinol. Metab.* 23:1285–1297, 1963.

91. Bardin, C. W., and Lipsett, M. B.: Testosterone and androstenedione blood production rates in normal women and women with idiopathic hirsutism or polycystic ovaries. *J. Clin. Invest.* 46:891–902, 1967.

92. Bardin, C. W., and Mahoudeau, J. A.: Dynamics of androgen metabolism in women with hirsutism. *Ann. Clin. Res.* 2:251–262, 1970.

93. Kirschner, M. A., and Bardin, C. W.: Androgen production and metabolism in normal and virilized women. *Metabolism* 21:667–668, 1972.

94. Bardin, C. W., Bullock, L. P., Sherins, R. J., Mowszowicz, I., and Blackburn, W. R.: Part II. Androgen metabolism and mechanism of action in male pseudohermaphroditism: A study of testicular feminization. *Recent Prog. Horm. Res.* 29:65–109, 1973.

95. Wilson, J. D., and Gloyna, R. E.: The intranuclear metabolism of testosterone in the accessory organs of reproduction. *Recent Prog. Horm. Res.* 26:309–336, 1970.

96. Takayasu, S., and Adachi, K.: The conversion of testosterone to 17β-hydroxy-5α-androstan-3-one (dihydrotestosterone) by human hair follicles. *J. Clin. Endocrinol. Metab.* 34:1098–1101, 1972.

97. Schweikert, H. U., and Wilson, J. D.: Regulation of human hair growth by steroid hormones. I. Testosterone metabolism in isolated hairs. *J. Clin. Endocrinol. Metab.* 38:811–819, 1974.

98. Mulay, S., Finkelberg, R., Pinsky, L., and Solomon, S.: Metabolism of 4-¹⁴C-testosterone by serially subcultured human skin fibroblasts. *J. Clin. Endocrinol. Metab.* 34:133–143, 1972.

99. Mauvais-Jarvis, P., Bercovici, J. P., Crepy, O., and Gauthier, F.: Studies on testosterone metabolism in subjects with testicular feminization syndrome. *J. Clin. Invest.* 49:31–40, 1970.

100. Mauvais-Jarvis, P.: Androgen metabolism in human skin: Mechanisms of control. In *Androgens and Antiandrogens.* Martini, L., and Motta, M. (eds.), New York, Raven Press, 1977, pp. 229–245.

101. Wilson, J. D., and Walker, J. D.: The conversion of testosterone to 5α-androstan-17β-ol-3-one (dihydrotestosterone) by skin slices of man. *J. Clin. Invest.* 48:371–379, 1969.

102. Bradlow, H. L., Gillette, P. N., Gallagher, T. F., and Kappas, A.: Studies in porphyria. II. Evidence for a deficiency of steroid Δ⁴-5α-reductase activity in acute intermittent porphyria. *J. Exp. Med.* 138:754–763, 1973.

103. Bradlow, H. L., Anderson, K., and Kappas, A.: Differences between cutaneous and hepatic steroid Δ⁴-5α-reductase in patients with acute intermittent porphyria. In *Porphyrins in Human Diseases.* Doss, M., and Lahn, M. (eds.), Basel, S. Karger, 1976, pp. 173–178.

104. Zumoff, B., Bradlow, H. L., Finkelstein, J., Boyar, R. M., and Hellman, L.: The influence of age and sex on the metabolism of testosterone. *J. Clin. Endocrinol. Metab.* 42:703–706, 1976.

105. Lipsett, M. B., Wilson, H., Kirschner, M. A., Korenman, S. G., Fishman, L. M., Sarfaty, G. A., and Bardin, C. W.: Studies on Leydig cell physiology and pathology: Secretion and metabolism of testosterone. *Recent Prog. Horm. Res.* 22:245–281, 1966.

106. Kuttenn, F., Mowszowicz, I., Wright, F., Baudot, N., Jaffiol, C., Robin, M., and Mauvais-Jarvis, P.: Male pseudohermaphroditism: A comparative study of one patient with 5α-reductase deficiency and three patients with the complete form of testicular feminization. *J. Clin. Endocrinol. Metab.* 49:861–865, 1979.

107. Mauvais-Jarvis, P., Crepy, O., and Bercovici, J. P.: Further studies on the pathophysiology of testicular feminization syndrome. *J. Clin. Endocrinol. Metab.* 32:568–571, 1971.

108. Kuttenn, F., Mowszowicz, I., Schaison, G., and Mauvais-Jarvis, P.: Androgen production and skin metabolism in hirsutism. *J. Endocrinol.* 75:83–91, 1977.

109. Hellman, L, Bradlow, H. L., Freed, S., Levin, J., Rosenfeld, R. S., Whitmore, W. F., and Zumoff, B.: The effect of flutamide on testosterone metabolism and the plasma levels of androgens and gonadotropins. *J. Clin. Endocrinol. Metab.* 45:1224–1229, 1977.

110. Kappas, A., Bradlow, H. L., Bickers, D. R., and Alvares, A. P.: Induction of a deficiency of steroid Δ⁴-5α-reductase activity in liver by a porphyrinogenic drug. *J. Clin. Invest.* 59:159–164, 1977.

111. Fishman, J., and Bradlow, H. L.: Effect of malnutrition on the metabolism of sex hormones in man. *Clin. Pharmacol. Ther.* 22:721–728, 1977.

112. Bradlow, H. L., Hellman, L., Zumoff, B., and Gallagher, T. F.: Interaction of hormonal effects: Influence of triiodothyronine on androgen metabolism. *Science* 124:1206–1207, 1956.

113. Zumoff, B., Levin, J., Bradlow, H. L., and Hellman, L.: The effect of 7β,17α-dimethyltestosterone (calusterone) on testosterone metabolism in women with advanced breast cancer. *J. Clin. Endocrinol. Metab.* 44:1203–1205, 1977.

114. Southren, A. L., Gordon, G. G., Olivo, J., Rafii, F., and Rosenthal, W. S.: Androgen metabolism in cirrhosis of the liver. *Metabolism* 22:695–702, 1973.

115. Gordon, G. G., Southren, A. L., Tochimoto, S., Rand, J. J., and Olivo, J.: Effect of hyperthyroidism and hypothyroidism on the metabolism of testosterone and androstenedione in man. *J. Clin. Endocrinol. Metab.* 29:164–170, 1969.

116. Imperato-McGinley, J., Guerrero, L., Gautier, T., and Peterson, R. E.: Steroid 5α-reductase deficiency in man: An inherited form of male pseudohermaphroditism. *Science* 186:1213–1215, 1974.

117. Peterson, R. E., Imperato-McGinley, J., Gautier, T., and Sturla, E.: Male pseudohermaphroditism due to steroid 5α-reductase deficiency. *Amer. J. Med.* 62:170–191, 1977.

118. Fisher, L. K., Kogut, M. D., Moore, R. J., Goebelsmann, U., Weitzman, J. J., Isaacs, H., Jr., Griffin, J. E., and Wilson, J. D.: Clinical, endocrinological, and enzymatic characterization of two patients with 5α-reductase deficiency: Evidence that a single enzyme is responsible for the 5α-reduction of cortisol and testosterone. *J. Clin. Endocrinol. Metab.* 47:653–664, 1978.

119. Maddock, W. O., and Nelson, W. O.: The effects of chorionic gonadotropin in adult men: Increased estrogen and 17-ketosteroid excretion, gynecomastia, Leydig cell stimulation and seminiferous tubule damage. *J. Clin. Endocrinol. Metab.* 12:985–1014, 1952.

120. Morse, W. I., Clark, A. F., MacLeod, S. C., Ernst, W. A., and Gosse, C. L.: Urine estrogen responses to human chorionic gonadotropin in young, old and hypogonadal men. *J. Clin. Endocrinol. Metab.* 22:678–682, 1962.

121. Valladares, L. E., and Payne, A. H.: Induction of testicular aromatization by luteinizing hormone in mature rats. *Endocrinology* 105:431–436, 1979.

122. Dorrington, J. H., and Armstrong, D. T.: Follicle-stimulating hormone stimulates estradiol-17β synthesis in cultured Sertoli cells. *Proc. Nat. Acad. Sci. USA* 72:2677–2681, 1975.

123. Kelch, R. P., Jenner, M. R., Weinstein, R., Kaplan, S. L., and Grumbach, M. M.: Estradiol and testosterone secretion by human, simian and canine testes in males with hypogonadism and in male pseudohermaphrodites with the feminizing testes syndrome. *J. Clin. Invest.* 51:824–830, 1972.

124. Weinstein, R. L., Kelch, R. P., Jenner, M. R., Kaplan, S. L., and Grumbach, M. M.: Secretion of unconjugated androgens and estrogens by the normal and abnormal human testis before and after human chorionic gonadotropin. *J. Clin. Invest.* 53:1–6, 1974.

125. Wilson, J. D., and MacDonald, P. C.: Male pseudohermaphroditism due to androgen resistance: Testicular feminization and related syndromes. In *The Metabolic Basis of Inherited Disease.* Stanbury, J. B., Wyngaarden, J. B., and Fredrickson, D. S. (eds.), New York, McGraw-Hill, 1978, pp. 894–913.

126. Aiman, J., Brenner, P. F., and MacDonald, P. C.: Androgen and estrogen production in elderly men with gynecomastia and testicular atrophy following mumps orchitis. *J. Clin. Endocrinol. Metab.* 50:380–386, 1980.

127. MacDonald, P. C., Madden, J. D., Brenner, P. F., Wilson, J. D., and Siiteri, P. K.: Origin of estrogen in normal men and in women with testicular feminization. *J. Clin. Endocrinol. Metab.* 49:905–916, 1979.

128. Corvol, P., Michaud, A., Menard, J., Freifeld, M., and Mahoudeau, J.: Antiandrogenic effect of spirolactones: Mechanism of action. *Endocrinology* 97:52–58, 1975.

129. Pita, J. C., Jr., Lippman, M. E., Thompson, E. B., and Loriaux, D. L.: Interaction of spironolactone and digitalis with the 5α-dihydrotestosterone (DHT) receptor of rat ventral prostate. *Endocrinology* 97:1521–1527, 1975.

130. Rifka, S. M., Pita, J. C., Jr., and Loriaux, D. L.: Mechanism of interaction of digitalis with estradiol binding sites in rat uteri. *Endocrinology* 99:1091–1096, 1976.

131. Funder, J. W., and Mercer, J. E.: Cimetidine, a histamine H₂ receptor

antagonist, occupies androgen receptors. *J. Clin. Endocrinol. Metab.* 48:189–191, 1979.

132. Siiteri, P. K., and MacDonald, P. C.: Role of extraglandular estrogen in human endocrinology. In *Handbook of Physiology,* Section 7: Endocrinology. Vol. II, Reproductive System — Female. Greep, R. O., and Astwood, E. B. (eds.), Baltimore, Williams & Wilkins, 1973, pp. 615–629.

133. Bardin, C. W., Lipsett, M. B., and French, A.: Testosterone and androstenedione production rates in patients with metastatic adrenal cortical carcinoma. *J. Clin. Endocrinol. Metab.* 28:215–220, 1968.

134. Hemsell, D. L., Edman, C. D., Marks, J. F., Siiteri, P. K., and MacDonald, P. C.: Massive extraglandular aromatization of plasma androstenedione resulting in feminization of a prepubertal boy. *J. Clin. Invest.* 60:455–464, 1977.

135. Schneider, G., Kirschner, M. A., Berkowitz, R., and Ertel, N. H.: Increased estrogen production in obese men. *J. Clin. Endocrinol. Metab.* 48:633–638, 1979.

136. Kochakian, C. D.: Definition of androgens and protein anabolic steroids. *Pharmacol. Ther.* 1:149–177, 1975.

137. Bardin, C. W., Bullock, L. P., Mills, N. C., Lin, Y.-C., and Jacob, S. T.: The role of receptors in the anabolic action of androgens. *Receptors Horm. Action* 2:83–103, 1978.

138. Rochefort, H., and Garcia, M.: Androgen on the estrogen receptor. I. Binding and *in vivo* nuclear translocation. *Steroids* 28:549–560, 1976.

139. Mainwaring, W. I. P., and Mann, T.: *The Mechanism of Action of Androgens.* New York, Springer-Verlag, 1976.

140. Bullock, L., and Bardin, C. W.: Decreased dihydrotestosterone retention by preputial gland nuclei from the androgen insensitive pseudohermaphrodite rat. *J. Clin. Endocrinol. Metab.* 31:113–115, 1970.

141. Bullock, L. P., and Bardin, C. W.: Androgen receptors in testicular feminization. *J. Clin. Endocrinol. Metab.* 35:935–937, 1972.

142. Attardi, B., and Ohno, S.: Cytosol androgen receptor from kidney of normal and testicular feminized (Tfm) mice. *Cell* 2:205–212, 1974.

143. Gehring, U., and Tomkins, G. M.: Characterization of a hormone receptor defect in the androgen insensitivity mutant. *Cell* 3:59–64, 1974.

144. Griffin, J. E.: Testicular feminization associated with a thermolabile androgen receptor in cultured human fibroblasts. *J. Clin. Invest.* 64:1624–1631, 1979.

145. Wilson, J. D., Harrod, M. J., Goldstein, J. L., Hemsell, D. L., and MacDonald, P. C.: Familial incomplete male pseudohermaphroditism, type 1: Evidence for androgen resistance and variable clinical manifestations in a family with the Reifenstein syndrome. *N. Engl. J. Med.* 290:1097–1103, 1974.

146. Boyar, R. M., Moore, R. J., Rosner, W., Aiman, J., Chipman, J., Madden, J. D., Marks, J. F., and Griffin, J. E.: Studies of gonadotropin-gonadal dynamics in patients with androgen insensitivity. *J. Clin. Endocrinol. Metab.* 47:1116–1122, 1978.

147. Aiman, J., Griffin, J. E., Gazak, J. M., Wilson, J. D., and MacDonald, P. C.: Androgen insensitivity as a cause of infertility in otherwise normal men. *N. Engl. J. Med.* 300:223–227, 1979.

148. Ryan, K. J., Naftolin, F., Reddy, V., Flores, F., and Petro, Z.: Estrogen formation in the brain. *Amer. J. Obstet. Gynecol.* 114:454–460, 1972.

149. McEwen, B. S.: Binding and metabolism of sex steroids by the hypothalamic-pituitary unit: Physiological implications. *Ann. Rev. Physiol.* 42:97–110, 1980.

150. Winters, S. J., Janick, J. J., Loriaux, D. L., and Sherins, R. J.: Studies on the role of sex steroids in the feedback control of gonadotropin concentrations in men. II. Use of the estrogen antagonist, clomiphene citrate. *J. Clin. Endocrinol. Metab.* 48:222–227, 1979.

151. Faiman, C., and Winter, J. S. D.: The control of gonadotropin secretion in complete testicular feminization. *J. Clin. Endocrinol. Metab.* 39:631–638, 1974.

152. Vigersky, R. A., Easley, R. B., and Loriaux, D. L.: Effect of fluoxymesterone on the pituitary-gonadal axis: The role of testosterone-estradiol-binding globulin. *J. Clin. Endocrinol. Metab.* 43:1–9, 1976.

153. Lacroix, A., McKenna, T. J., and Rabinowitz, D.: Sex steroid modulation of gonadotropins in normal men and in androgen insensitivity syndrome. *J. Clin. Endocrinol. Metab.* 48:235–240, 1979.

154. Capell, P. T., Paulsen, C. A., Derleth, D., Skoglund, R., and Plymate, S.: The effect of short-term testosterone administration on serum FSH, LH and testosterone levels: Evidence for selective abnormality in LH control in patients with Klinefelter's syndrome. *J. Clin. Endocrinol. Metab.* 37:752–759, 1973.

155. Winters, S. J., Sherins, R. J., and Loriaux, D. L.: Studies on the role of sex steroids in the feedback control of gonadotropin concentrations in men. III. Androgen resistance in primary gonadal failure. *J. Clin. Endocrinol. Metab.* 48:553–558, 1979.

156. Kulin, H. E., and Reiter, E. O.: Gonadotropin and testosterone measurements after estrogen administration to adult men, prepubertal and pubertal boys, and men with hypogonadotropism: Evidence for maturation of positive feedback in the male. *Pediatr. Res.* 10:46–51, 1976.

157. Karsch, F. J., Dierschike, D. J., and Knobil, E.: Sexual differentiation of pituitary function: Apparent difference between primates and rodent. *Science* 179:484–486, 1973.

158. Rudenstein, R. S., Bigdell, H., MacDonald, M. H., and Snyder, P. J.: Administration of gonadal steroids to the castrated male rat prevents a decrease in the release of gonadotropin-releasing hormone from the incubated hypothalamus. *J. Clin. Invest.* 63:262–267, 1979.

159. Gual, G., Scaglia, H. E., Midgley, R. A., Alcocer, J., Echeverria-Rivas, Y., and Lichtenberg, R.: Regulatory effects of steroids on the pituitary response to LH-RH. *J. Steroid Biochem.* 6:1067–1074, 1975.

160. D'Agata, R. S., Gulizia, S., Andó, S., Vitale, G., and Polosa, P.: Effect of oestradiol on gonadotrophin release induced by LHRH in men. *Clin. Endocrinol.* 5:393–397, 1976.

161. Yen, S. S. C., Vandenberg, G., and Siler, T. M.: Modulation of pituitary responsiveness to LRF by estrogen. *J. Clin. Endocrinol. Metab.* 39:170–177, 1974.

162. Jaffe, R. B., and Keye, W. R.: Estradiol augmentation of pituitary responsiveness to gonadotropin-releasing hormone in women. *J. Clin. Endocrinol. Metab.* 39:850–855, 1974.

163. Keye, W. R., Jr., and Jaffe, R. B.: Modulation of pituitary gonadotropin response to gonadotropin-releasing hormone by estradiol. *J. Clin. Endocrinol. Metab.* 38:805–810, 1974.

164. Keye, W. R., Jr., and Jaffe, R. B.: Strength-duration characteristics of estrogen effects on gonadotropin response to gonadotropin-releasing hormone in women. I. Effects of varying duration of estradiol administration. *J. Clin. Endocrinol. Metab.* 41:1003–1008, 1975.

165. Young, J. R., and Jaffe, R. B.: Strength-duration characteristics of estrogen effects on gonadotropin response to gonadotropin-releasing hormone in women. II. Effects of varying concentrations of estradiol. *J. Clin. Endocrinol. Metab.* 42:432–442, 1976.

166. Caminos-Torres, R., Ma, R. L., and Snyder, P. J.: Testosterone induced inhibition of the LH and FSH responses to gonadotropin-releasing hormone occurs slowly. *J. Clin. Endocrinol. Metab.* 44:1142–1153, 1977.

167. Seyler, L. E., Canalis, E., Spare, S., and Reichlin, S.: Abnormal gonadotropin secretory responses to LRH in transsexual women after diethylstilbestrol priming. *J. Clin. Endocrinol. Metab.* 47:176–183, 1978.

168. Igarashi, M., Nallar, R., and McCann, S. M.: Further studies on the follicle-stimulating hormone-releasing action of hypothalamic extracts. *Endocrinology* 75:901–907, 1964.

169. Coble, Y. D., Jr., Kohler, P. O., Cargille, C. M., and Ross, G. T.: Production rates and metabolic clearance rates of human follicle-stimulating hormone in premenopausal and postmenopausal women. *J. Clin. Invest.* 48:359–363, 1969.

170. Amin, H. K., and Hunter, W. M.: Human pituitary follicle-stimulating hormone: Distribution, plasma clearance and urinary excretion as determined by radioimmunoassay. *J. Endocrinol.* 48:307–317, 1970.

171. Setchell, B. P.: Spermatogenesis. In *The Mammalian Testis.* Setchell, B. P. (ed.), Ithaca, NY, Cornell University Press, 1978, pp. 181–185.

172. Steinberger, E., and Steinberger, A.: Spermatogenic function of the testis. In *Handbook of Physiology,* Section 7: Endocrinology. Vol. V.: Male Reproductive System. Hamilton, D. W., and Greep, R. O. (eds.), Baltimore, Williams & Wilkins, 1975, pp. 1–20.

173. Steinberger, E.: Hormonal control of mammalian spermatogenesis. *Physiol. Rev.* 51:1–22, 1971.

174. Cattanach, B. M., Pollard, C. E., and Hawkes, S. G.: Sex-reversed mice: XX and XO males. *Cytogenetics* 10:318–337, 1971.

175. Ohno, S.: Control of meiotic processes. In *The Testis in Normal and Infertile Men.* Troen, P., and Nankin, H. R. (eds.), New York, Raven Press, 1977, pp. 1–8.

176. Clermont, Y.: The cycle of the seminiferous epithelium in man. *Amer. J. Anat.* 112:35–51, 1963.

177. Heller, C. G., and Clermont, Y.: Kinetics of the germinal epithelium in man. *Recent Prog. Horm. Res.* 20:545–575, 1964.

178. Chowdhury, A. K., and Steinberger, E.: *In vitro* ³H-thymidine labeling pattern and topographic distribution of spermatogonia in human seminiferous tubules. In *The Testis in Normal and Infertile Men.* Troen, P., and Nankin, H. R. (eds.), New York, Raven Press, 1977, pp. 69–83.

179. Bedford, J. M.: Maturation, transport, and fate of spermatozoa in the epididymis. In *Handbook of Physiology,* Section 7: Endocrinology. Vol. V.: Male Reproductive System. Hamilton, D. W., and Greep, R. O. (eds.), Baltimore, Williams & Wilkins, 1975, pp. 303–318.

180. Orgebin-Crist, M. C., Danzo, B. J., and Davies, J.: Endocrine control of the development and maintenance of sperm fertilizing ability in the epididymis. In *Handbook of Physiology,* Section 7: Endocrin-

ology. Vol. V: Male Reproductive System. Hamilton, D. W., and Greep, R. O. (eds.), Baltimore, Williams & Wilkins, 1975, pp. 319–338.

181. Fawcett, D. W.: The mammalian spermatozoon. *Dev. Biol.* 44:394–436, 1975.

182. Phillips, D. M.: Mammalian sperm structure. In: *Handbook of Physiology*, Section 7: Endocrinology. Vol. V: Male Reproductive System. Hamilton, D. W. and Greep, R. O. (eds.), Baltimore, Williams & Wilkins, 1975, pp. 405–419.

183. Phillips, D. M.: Spermiogenesis. In *Ultrastructure of Cells and Organisms*. Lock, M. (ed.), New York, Academic Press, 1974, pp. 1–68.

184. Eliasson, R., Mossberg, B., Camner, P., and Afzelius, B. A.: The immotile-cilia syndrome: A congenital ciliary abnormality as an etiologic factor in chronic airway infections and male sterility. *N. Engl. J. Med.* 297:1–6, 1977.

185. Sturgess, J. M., Chao, J., Wong, J., Aspin, N., and Turner, J. A. P.: Cilia with defective radial spokes: A cause of human respiratory disease. *N. Engl. J. Med.* 300:53–56, 1979.

186. Afzelius, B. A.: Electron microscopy of the sperm tail. *J. Biophys. Biochem. Cytol.* 5:269–278, 1959.

187. Satir, P.: Studies on cilia. III. Further studies on the cilium tip and a sliding filament model of ciliary motility. *J. Cell Biol.* 39:77–94, 1968.

188. Summers, K. E., and Gibbons, I. R.: Effects of trypsin digestion on flagellar structures and their relationship to motility. *J. Cell Biol.* 58:618–629, 1973.

189. Satir, P.: Introductory remarks: Cilia, eukaryotic flagella and an introduction to microtubules. In *Cell Motility*. Vol. C. Goldman, R., Pollard, T., and Rosenbaum, J. (eds.), Cold Spring Harbor, NY, Cold Spring Harbor Laboratory, 1976, pp. 841–846.

190. Schmidt, J. A., and Eckert, R.: Calcium couples flagellar reversal to photostimulation in Chlamydomonas reinhardtii. *Nature* 262:713–715, 1976.

191. Brokaw, C. J.: Calcium induced asymmetrical beating of triton-demembranated sea urchin sperm flagella. *J. Cell Biol.* 82:401–411, 1979.

192. Gibbons, B. H., and Gibbons, I. R.: Calcium induced quiescence in reactivated sea urchin sperm. *J. Cell Biol.* 84:13–27, 1980.

193. Nelson, L., Young, M. J., and Gardner, M. E.: Sperm motility and calcium transport: A neurochemically controlled process. *Life Sci.* 26:1739–1749, 1980.

194. Garbers, D. L., Lust, W. D., First, N. L., and Lardy, H. A.: Effects of phosphodiesterase inhibitors and cyclic nucleotides on sperm respiration and motility. *Biochemistry* 10:1825–1831, 1971.

195. Hoskins, D. D., and Casillas, E. R.: Function of cyclic nucleotides in mammalian spermatozoa. In *Handbook of Physiology*, Section 7: Endocrinology. Vol. V: Male Reproductive System. Hamilton, D. W., and Greep, R. O. (eds.), Baltimore, Williams & Wilkins, 1975, pp. 453–460.

196. Lindemann, C. B.: A cAMP induced increase in the motility of demembranated bull sperm models. *Cell* 13:9–18, 1978.

197. Mohri, H., and Yanagimashi, R.: Characteristics of motor apparatus in testicular epididymal and ejaculated spermatozoa. *Exp. Cell Res.* 127:191–196, 1980.

198. Bavister, B. D., Chen, A. F., and Fu, P. C.: Catecholamine requirement for hamster sperm motility *in vitro. J. Reprod. Fertil.* 56:507–513, 1979.

199. Cornett, L. E., and Meizel, S.: Stimulation of *in vitro* activation and the acrosome reaction of hamster spermatozoa by catecholamines. *Proc. Natl. Acad. Sci. USA* 75:4954–4958, 1978.

200. Acott, T. S., and Hoskins, D. D.: Bovine sperm forward motility protein. *J. Biol. Chem.* 253:6744–6750, 1978.

201. Bouchard, P., Gagnon, C., Phillips, D. M., and Bardin, C. W.: The localization of protein carboxyl-methylase in sperm tails. *J. Cell Biol.* 86:417–423, 1980.

202. Austin, C. R.: Fertilization. Englewood Cliffs, NJ, Prentice-Hall, 1965, pp. 1–133.

203. Fawcett, D. W.: Ultrastructure and function of the Sertoli cell. In *Handbook of Physiology*, Section 7: Endocrinology. Vol. V: Male Reproductive System. Hamilton, D. W., and Greep, R. O. (eds.), Baltimore, Williams & Wilkins, 1975, pp. 21–56.

204. Setchell, B. P.: *The Mammalian Testis.* Ithaca, NY, Cornell University Press, 1978, pp. 223–284.

205. Hansson, V., Ritzen, E. M., French, F. S., and Nayfeh, S. N.: Androgen transport and receptor mechanisms in testis and epididymis. In *Handbook of Physiology*, Section 7: Endocrinology. Vol. V: Male Reproductive System. Hamilton, D. W., and Greep, R. O. (eds.), Baltimore, Williams & Wilkins, 1975, pp. 173–202.

206. Weddington, S. C., Bradtzaeg, P., Hansson, V., French, F. S., Petrusz, P., Nayfeh, S. N., and Ritzen, E. M.: Immunological cross reactivity between testicular androgen-binding protein and serum testosterone-binding globulin. *Nature* 258:257–259, 1975.

207. Vigersky, R. A., Loriaux, D. L., Howards, S. S., Hodgen, G. B., Lipsett, M. B., and Chrambach, A.: Androgen binding proteins of testis, epididymis, and plasma in man and monkey. *J. Clin. Invest.* 58:1061–1068, 1976.

208. Musto, N. A., Larrea, F., Cheng, S. L., Kotite, N., Gunsalus, G., and Bardin, C. W.: Extracellular androgen binding proteins: Species comparison and structure-function relationships. *Proc. NY Acad. Sci.* 1981 (in press).

209. Musto, N. A., Gunsalus, G. L., and Bardin, C. W.: Purification and characterization of androgen binding protein from the rat epididymis. *Biochemistry* 19:2853–2860, 1980.

210. Gunsalus, G. L., Musto, N. A., and Bardin, C. W.: Immunoassay of androgen binding protein in blood: A new approach for study of the seminiferous tubule. *Science* 200:65–66, 1978.

211. Gunsalus, G. L., Musto, N. A., and Bardin, C. W.: Bi-directional release of a Sertoli cell product, androgen binding protein, into the blood and seminiferous tubule. In *Testicular Development, Structure, and Function*. Steinberger, E., and Steinberger, A. (eds.), New York, Raven Press, 1980, pp. 291–297.

212. Koskimies, A. I., Kormano, M., and Alfthan, O.: Proteins of the seminiferous tubule fluid in man: Evidence for a blood-testis barrier. *J. Reprod. Fertil.* 32:79–86, 1973.

213. Steinberger, E.: Hormonal control of mammalian spermatogenesis. *Physiol. Rev.* 51:1–22, 1971.

214. Setchell, B. P., Endocrinology of the testis. In *The Mammalian Testis.* Setchell, B. P. (ed.), Ithaca, NY, Cornell University Press, 1978, pp. 109–180.

215. Castro, A. E., Alonso, A., and Mancini, R. E.: Localization of follicle-stimulating and luteinizing hormones in the rat testis using immunohistological tests. *J. Endocrinol.* 52:129–136, 1972.

216. Orth, J., and Christensen, A. K.: Localization of ^{125}I-labeled FSH in the testes of hypophysectomized rats by autoradiography at the light and electron microscope levels. *Endocrinology* 101:262–278, 1977.

217. Means, A. R.: Mechanisms of action of follicle-stimulating hormone (FSH). In *The Testis.* Johnson, A. D., and Gomes, W. R. (eds.), New York, Academic Press, 1977, pp. 163–184.

218. Means, A. R., Dedman, J. R., Tash, J. S., Tindall, D. J., van Sickle, M., and Welsh, M. J.: Regulation of the testis Sertoli cell by follicle stimulating hormone. *Ann. Rev. Physiol.* 42:59–70, 1980.

219. Baker, H. W. G., Bailey, D. J., Feil, P. D., Jefferson, L. S., Santen, R. J., and Bardin, C. W.: Nuclear accumulation of androgens in perfused rat accessory sex organs and testes. *Endocrinology* 100:709–721, 1977.

220. McCullagh, D. R.: Dual endocrine activity of the testes. *Science* 76:19–20, 1932.

221. Baker, H. W. G., Bremner, W. J., Burger, H. G., deKretser, D. M., Dulmanis, A., Eddie, L. W., Hudson, B., Keogh, E. J., Lee, V. W. K., and Rennie, G. C.: Testicular control of follicle-stimulating hormone secretion. *Recent Prog. Horm. Res.* 32:429–469, 1976.

222. de Jong, F. H.: Inhibin — fact or artifact. *Mol. Cell. Endocrinol.* 13:1–10, 1979.

223. Frantz, A. G., and Kleinberg, D. L.: Prolactin: Evidence that it is separate from growth hormone in human blood. *Science* 170:745–747, 1970.

224. Guyda, H. J., and Friesen, H. G.: Serum prolactin levels in humans from birth to adult life. *Pediatr. Res.* 7:534–540, 1973.

225. Finkelstein, J. W., Kapen, S., Weitzman, E. D., Hellman, L., and Boyar, R. M.: Twenty-four-hour plasma prolactin patterns in prepubertal and adolescent boys. *J. Clin. Endocrinol. Metab.* 47:1123–1128, 1978.

226. Nicoll, C. S., and Meites, J.: Estrogen stimulation of prolactin production by rat adenohypophysis *in vitro. Endocrinology* 70:272–277, 1962.

227. Turkington, R. W.: Prolactin secretion in patients treated with various drugs: phenothiazines, tricyclic antidepressants, reserpine, and methyldopa. *Arch. Intern Med.* 130:349–354, 1972.

228. Bhattacharya, A. N., Dierschke, D. J., Yamaji, T., and Knobial, E.: The pharmacologic blockade of the circhoral mode of LH secretion in the ovariectomized rhesus monkey. *Endocrinology* 90:778–786, 1972.

229. Tolis, G., Bent, R., and Guyda, H. J.: Opiates, prolactin and the dopamine receptor. *J. Clin. Endocrinol. Metab.* 47:200–203, 1979.

230. Gold, M. S., Redmond, D. E., and Donabedian, R. K.: The effects of opiate agonist and antagonist on serum prolactin in primates: Possible role for endorphins in prolactin regulation. *Endocrinology* 105:284–289, 1979.

231. Cicero, T. J., Meyer, E. R., and Bell, G. A.: Effects of morphine and methadone on serum testosterone and luteinizing hormone levels and on the secondary sex organs of the male rat. *Endocrinology* 98:367–372, 1976.

232. Bartke, A.: Pituitary-testis relationship: Role of prolactin in the regulation of testicular function. In *Progress in Reproductive Biology.* Vol. 1. Hubinont, P. O. (ed.), Basel, S. Karger, 1976, pp. 136–152.

233. Spitz, I. M., Landau, H., Almaliach, U., Rosen, E., Brautbar, N., and

Russell, A.: Diminished prolactin reserve: A case report. *J. Clin. Endocrinol. Metab.* 45:412–418, 1977.

234. Barkey, R. J., Shani, J., and Barzilai, D.: Regulation of prolactin binding sites in the seminal vesicle, prostate gland, testis and liver of intact and castrated adult rats: Effect of administration of testosterone, 2-bromo-α-ergocryptine and fluphenazine. *J. Endocrinol.* 81:11–18, 1979.

235. Davies, T. F., Katikineni, M., Chan, V., Harwood, J. P., Dufau, M. L., and Catt, K. J.: Lactogenic receptor regulation in hormone-stimulated steroidogenic cells. *Nature* 283:863–865, 1980.

236. Antliff, H. R., Prasad, M. R. N., and Meyer, R. K.: Action of prolactin on seminal vesicle of guinea pig. *Proc. Soc. Exp. Biol. Med.* 103:77–80, 1960.

237. Baker, H. W. G., Worgul, T. J., Santen, R. J., Jefferson, L. S., and Bardin, C. W.: Effect of prolactin on nuclear androgens in perfused male accessory sex organs. In *The Testis in Normal and Infertile Men.* Troen, P., and Nankin, H. R. (eds.), New York, Raven Press, 1977, pp. 379–385.

238. Thorner, M. O., Edwards, C. R. W., Hanker, J. P., Abraham, G., and Besser, G. M.: Prolactin and gonadotropin interaction in the male. In *The Testis in Normal and Infertile Men.* Troen, P., and Nankin, H. R. (eds.), New York, Raven Press, 1977, pp. 351–366.

239. Carter, J. N., Tyson, J. E., Tolis, G., Van Vliet, S., Faiman, C., and Friesen, H. G.: Prolactin-secreting tumors and hypogonadism in 22 men. *N. Engl. J. Med.* 299:847–852, 1978.

240. Ambrosi, B., Rossella, B., Travaglini, P., Weber, G., Peccoz, P. B., Rondena, M., Elli, R., and Faglia, G.: Study of the effects of bromocriptine on sexual impotence. *Clin. Endocrinol.* 7:417–421, 1977.

241. Hammond, G. L., Ruokonen, A., Kontturi, M., Koshela, E., and Vihko, R.: The simultaneous radioimmunoassay of seven steroids in human spermatic and peripheral venous blood. *J. Clin. Endocrinol. Metab.* 45:16–24, 1977.

242. Lubs, H. A., Jr.: Testicular size in Klinefelter's syndrome in men over 50: report of a case with XXY/XY mosaicism. *N. Engl. J. Med.* 267:326, 1962.

243. Yanagimachi, R., Yanagimachi, H., and Rogers, B. J.: The use of zona-free animal ova as a test-system for the assessment of the fertilizing capacity of human spermatozoa. *Biol. Reprod.* 15:471, 1976.

244. Rogers, B. J., Van Campen, H., Ueno, M., Lambert, H., Bronson, R., and Hale, R.: Analysis of human spermatozoal fertilizing ability using zona-free ova. *Fertil. Steril.* 32:6, 1979.

245. Barros, C., Gonzales, J., Herrera, E., and Bustos-Obregon, E.: Fertilizing capacity of human spermatozoa evaluated by actual penetration of foreign eggs. *Contraception* 17:87, 1978.

246. Barros, C., Gonzales, J., Herrera, E., and Bustos-Obregon, E.: Human sperm penetration into zona-free hamster oocytes as a test to evaluate the sperm fertilizing ability. *Andrologia* 11:197, 1979.

247. Rudak, E., Jacobs, P. A., and Yanagimachi, R.: Direct analysis of the chromosome constitution of human spermatozoa. *Nature* 274:913, 1978.

248. Belsey, M. A., Eliasson, R., Callegos, A. H., Moghissi, K. S., Paulsen, C. A., and Prasad, M. R. N. (eds.): *Laboratory Manual for the Examination of Human Semen and Semen-Cervical Mucus Interaction.* Singapore, Press Concern, 1980.

249. MacLeod, J., and Gold, R. Z.: The male factor in fertility and infertility. VI. Semen quality and certain other factors in relation to ease of conception. *Fertil. Steril.* 4:10, 1953.

250. Eliasson, R.: Standards for investigation of human semen. *Andrologia* 3:49, 1971.

251. Couture, M., Ulstein, M., Leonard, J. M., and Paulsen, C. A.: Improved staining method for differentiating immature germ cells from white blood cells in human seminal fluid. *Andrologia* 8:61, 1976.

252. Amelar, R. D., and Dubin, L.: Semen analysis. In *Male Infertility.* Amelar, R. D., Dubin, L., and Walsh, P. C. (eds.), Philadelphia, W. B. Saunders Co., 1977.

253. Bunge, R. G., and Sherman, J. K.: Liquefaction of human semen by alpha-amylase. *Fertil. Steril.* 5:353, 1954.

254. Jouannet, P., Volochine, B., DeGuent, P., Serres, C., and David, G.: Light scattering determination of various characteristic parameters of spermatozoa motility in a series of human sperm. *Andrologia* 9:36, 1977.

255. Gordon, D. L., Moore, D. J., Thorslund, T., and Paulsen, C. A.: The determination of size and concentration of human sperm with an electronic particle counter. *J. Lab. Clin. Med.* 65:506, 1965.

256. Gordon, D. L., Herrigel, J. E., Moore, D. J., and Paulsen, C. A.: Efficacy of Coulter counter in determining low sperm concentrations. *Amer. J. Clin. Path.* 47:226, 1967.

257. Tjioe, D. Y., Steinberger, E., and Paulsen, C. A.: A simple method for quantitative analysis of seminiferous epithelium in human testicular biopsies. *J. Albert Einstein Med. Ctr.* 15:56, 1967.

258. Steinberger, E., and Tjioe, D. Y.: A method for quantitative analysis of human seminiferous epithelium. *Fertil. Steril.* 19:960–970, 1968.

259. Rowley, M. J., and Heller, C. G.: Quantitation of the cells of the seminiferous epithelium of the human testis employing the Sertoli cell as a constant. *Z. Zellforsch.* 115:461–472, 1971.

260. Barr, A. B., Moore, D. J., and Paulsen, C. A.: Germinal cell loss during human spermatogenesis. *J. Reprod. Fertil.* 25:75–80, 1971.

261. Gordon, D. L., Barr, A. B., Herrigel, J. E., and Paulsen, C. A.: Testicular biopsy in man. I. Effect upon sperm concentration. *Fertil. Steril.* 16:522, 1965.

262. Hotchkiss, R. S.: Male factor in fertile and barren marriage. *NY State J. Med.* 41:564, 1941.

263. Santen, R. J., and Kulin, R. E.: The male reproductive system. In *Practice of Pediatrics.* Vol. 1. Hagerstown, MD, Harper and Row, 1976, pp. 1–43.

264. Steelman, S. L., and Pohley, F. M.: Assay of the follicle stimulating hormone based on the augmentation with human chorionic gonadotropin. *Endocrinology* 53:604, 1953.

265. Albert, A., Derner, I., Leiferman, J., Stellmacher, V., and Barnum, J.: Studies on the biologic characterization of human gonadotropins. VII. Urinary gonadotropins of men, postmenopausal women and eunuchs. *J. Clin. Endocrinol. Metab.* 21:839–848, 1961.

266. Greep, R. O., Van Dyne, H. B., and Chow, B. F.: Use of anterior lobe of prostate gland in the assay of metakentrin. *Proc. Soc. Exp. Biol. Med.* 46:644–649, 1941.

267. Mauvais-Jarvis, P., Charransol, G., and Bobas-Masson, F.: Simultaneous determination of urinary androstanediol and testosterone as an evaluation of human androgenicity. *J. Clin. Endocrinol. Metab.* 36:452–459, 1973.

268. Doberne, Y., and New, M. I.: Urinary androstanediol and testosterone in adults. *J. Clin. Endocrinol. Metab.* 42:152–154, 1976.

269. Bardin, C. W., Ross, G. T., Rifkind, A. B., Cargille, C. M., and Lipsett, M. B.: Studies of the pituitary-Leydig cell axis in young men with hypogonadotropic hypogonadism and hyposmia: Comparison with normal men, prepubertal boys, and hypopituitary patients. *J. Clin. Invest.* 48:2046–2056, 1969.

270. Saez, J. M., and Betrand, J.: Studies on testicular function in children: Plasma concentrations of testosterone, dehydroepiandrosterone and its sulfate before and after stimulation with human chorionic gonadotropins. *Steroids* 12:749, 1968.

271. Saez, J. M., and Forest, M. G.: Kinetics of human chorionic gonadotropin-induced steroidogenic response of human testis. I. Plasma testosterone: Implications for human chorionic gonadotropin test. *J. Clin. Endocrinol. Metab.* 49:278–283, 1979.

272. Okuyama, A., Namiki, M., Koide, M., Itatani, H., Mizutani, S., Sonoda, T., Aono, T., and Matsumoto, K.: A simple hCG stimulation test for normal and hypogonadal males. In *Archives of Andrology.* Vol. 6. New York, Elsevier/North Holland, 1981, pp. 75–81.

273. Tomita, M.: Consecutive administration of synthetic LRH in the evaluation of gonadotrophin reserve in children. *Acta Endocrinol.* 94:289–296, 1980.

274. Bardin, C. W., Ross, G. T., and Lipsett, M. B.: Site of action of clomiphene citrate in men: A study of the pituitary-Leydig cell axis. *J. Clin. Endocrinol. Metab.* 27:1558–1564, 1967.

275. Santen, R. J., Leonard, J. M., Sherins, R. J., Gandy, H. M., and Paulsen, C. A.: Short- and long-term effects of clomiphene citrate on the pituitary-testicular axis. *J. Clin. Endocrinol. Metab.* 33:970, 1971.

276. Walsh, P. C., Swerdloff, R. S., and Odell, W. D.: Feedback regulation of gonadotropin secretion in men. *J. Urol.* 110:84, 1973.

277. Santen, R. J., and Ruby, E. B.: Enhanced frequency and magnitude of episodic luteinizing hormone-releasing hormone discharge as a hypothalamic mechanism for increased luteinizing hormone secretion. *J. Clin. Endocrinol. Metab.* 28:315, 1979.

278. Leonard, J. M., Bremner, W. J., Capell, P. T., and Paulsen, C. A.: Male hypogonadism: Klinefelter's and Reifenstein's syndromes. Presented at the 1974 Birth Defects Conference, Newport Beach, Calif. In *Genetics of Hypogonadism.* Bergsma, D. (ed.), New York, National Foundation, March of Dimes, 1975, pp. 17–22.

279. de Kretser, D. M., Burger, H. G., Fortune, D., Hudson, B., Long, A. R., Paulsen, C. A., and Taft, H. P.: Hormonal, histological and genetic studies in male infertility. *J. Clin. Endocrinol. Metab.* 35:392, 1972.

280. Maclean, N., Harnden, D. G., et al.: Sex chromosome abnormalities in newborn babies. *Lancet* 1:286, 1964.

281. Paulsen, C. A., de Souza, A., Yoshizumi, T., and Lewis, B. M.: Results of a buccal smear survey in noninstitutionalized adult males. *J. Clin. Endocrinol.* 24:1182, 1964.

282. Klinefelter, H. G., Jr., Reifenstein, E. C., Jr., and Albright, F.: Syndrome characterized by gynecomastia, aspermatogenesis without a-Leydigism and increased excretion of follicle-stimulating hormone. *J. Clin. Endocrinol. Metab.* 2:615, 1942.

283. Heller, C. G., and Nelson, W. O.: Hyalinization of the seminiferous tubules associated with normal or failing Leydig-cell function. Discussion of relationship to eunuchoidism, gynecomastia, elevated gonadotrophins, depressed 17-ketosteroids and estrogens. *J. Clin. Endocrinol. Metab.* 5:1, 1945.

284. Becker, K. L., Hoffman, D. L., et al.: Klinefelter's syndrome. Clinical and laboratory findings in 50 patients. *Arch. Intern. Med. 118*:314, 1966.

285. Barr, M. L., Carr, D. H., et al.: An XY/XXXY sex chromosome mosaicism in a mentally deficient male patient. *J. Ment. Defic. Res. 6*:65, 1962.

286. Day, R. W., Levinson, J., et al.: An XXXXY male; case report and review. *J. Pediatr. 63*:589, 1963.

287. Stewart, J. S. S., Mack, W. S., et al.: Klinefelter's syndrome. Clinical and hormonal aspects. *Quart. J. Med. 28*:561, 1959.

288. Nowakowski, H., and Lenz, W.: Genetic aspects in male hypogonadism. *Recent Progr. Horm. Res. 17*:53, 1961.

289. Kaplan, N. M., and Norfleet, R. G.: Hypogonadism in young men (with emphasis on Klinefelter's syndrome). *Ann. Intern. Med. 54*:461, 1961.

290. Ferguson-Smith, M. A.: The prepubertal testicular lesion in chromatin-positive Klinefelter's syndrome (primary micro-orchidism) as seen in mentally handicapped children. *Lancet 1*:219, 1959.

291. de la Chapelle, A.: Sex chromosome abnormalities among the mentally defective in Finland. *J. Ment. Defic. Res. 7*:129, 1963.

292. Raboch, J.: Thirty-one men with female sex chromatin. *J. Clin. Endocrinol. Metab. 17*:1429, 1957.

293. Wieland, R. G., Zorn, E. M., et al.: *J. Clin. Endocrinol. Metab. 51*:1199, 1980.

294. Vermeulen, A., Stoica, T., and Verdonck, L.: The apparent free testosterone concentration, an index of androgenicity. *J. Clin. Endocrinol. Metab. 33*:759, 1971.

295. Wang, C., Baker, H. W., et al.: Hormonal studies in Klinefelter's syndrome. *Clin. Endocrinol. 4*:399, 1975.

296. Stewart, J. S. S.: Medullary gonadal dysgenesis (chromatin-positive Klinefelter's syndrome): a genetically determined condition with eunuchoid measurements but early epiphyseal closure. *Lancet 1*:1176, 1959.

297. Tanner, J. M., Prader, A., et al.: Genes on the Y chromosome influencing rate of maturation in man; skeletal age studies in children with Klinefelter's (XXY) and Turner's (XO) syndromes. *Lancet 2*:141, 1959.

298. Raboch, J., and Sipova, I.: The mental level in 47 cases of true Klinefelter's syndrome. *Acta Endocrinol. 36*:404, 1961.

299. Witkin, H. A., Mednick, S. A., Schulsinger, F., Bakkeström, E., Christiansen, K. O., Goodenough, D. R., Hirschhorn, K., Lundsteen, C., Owen, D. R., Philip, J., Rubin, D. B., and Stocking, M.: Criminality in XYY and XXY men. *Science 193*:547, 1976.

300. Rohde, R. A.: Klinefelter's syndrome with pulmonary disease and other disorders. *Lancet 2*:149, 1964.

301. Bomers-Marres, A. J. M. L.: Klinefelter's syndrome with asthma. *Lancet 2*:364, 1964.

302. Nielsen, J.: Diabetes mellitus in parents of patients with Klinefelter's syndrome. *Lancet 1*:1376, 1966.

303. Carr, D. H., Barr, M. L., et al.: An XXXY sex chromosome complex in Klinefelter subjects with duplicated sex chromatin. *J. Clin. Endocrinol. Metab. 21*:491, 1961.

304. Ford, C. E.: Mosaics and chimeras. *Brit. Med. Bull. 25*:104, 1969.

305. Paulsen, C. A., Gordon, D. L., Carpenter, R. W., Gandy, H. M., and Drucker, W. D.: Klinefelter's syndrome and its variants: A hormonal and chromosomal study. *Recent Progr. Horm. Res. 24*:321, 1968.

306. Gordon, D. L., Krmpotic, E., Thomas, W., Gandy, H. M., and Paulsen, C. A.: Pathologic testicular findings in Klinefelter's syndrome 47,XXY vs 46,XY/47,XXY. *Arch. Intern. Med. 130*:726, 1972.

307. Frøland, A.: Klinefelter's syndrome. Clinical, endocrinological and cytogenetical studies. *Dan. Med. Bull. 16*(Suppl. 6): 1, 1969.

308. Muldal, S., and Ockey, C. H.: The "double male": A new chromosome constitution in Klinefelter's syndrome. *Lancet 2*:492, 1960.

309. Court Brown, W. M., Harnden, D. G., et al.: Abnormalities of the sex chromosome complement in man. M. R. C. Special Report Series No. 305, London, Her Majesty's Stationery Office, 1964.

310. Philip, J., Lundsteen, C., and Owen, D.: The frequency of chromosome aberrations in tall men with special reference to 47,XYY and 47,XXY. *Amer. J. Hum. Genet. 28*:404, 1976.

310a. de la Chapelle, A.: Analytic review: Nature and origin of males with XX sex chromosomes. *Amer. J. Hum. Genet. 24*:71, 1972.

310b. Wachtel, S. S., Koo, G. C., Breg, W. R., Thaler, H. T., Dillard, G. M., Rosenthal, I. M., Dosik, H., Gerald, P. S., Saenger, P., New, M., Lieber, E., and Miller, O. J.: Serologic detection of a Y-linked gene in XX males and XX true hermaphrodites. *New Engl. J. Med. 295*:750, 1976.

310c. Harvey, D., Wachtel, S. S., et al.: *JAMA 236*:2505, 1976.

311. Augustine, J. R., and Jaworski, Z. F.: Unusual testicular histology in "true" Klinefelter's syndrome. *Arch. Pathol. 66*:159, 1958.

312. Ford, C. E., Jones, K. W., et al.: The chromosomes in a patient showing both mongolism and the Klinefelter's syndrome. *Lancet 1*:709, 1959.

313. Nelson, W. O., and Heller, C. G.: Hyalinization of the seminiferous tubules associated with normal or failing Leydig cell function; microscopic picture in the testis and associated changes in the breast. *J. Clin. Endocrinol. Metab. 5*:13, 1945.

314. Sniffen, R. C., Howard, R. P., et al.: The testis. III. Absence of germ cells, sclerosing tubular degeneration, "male climacteric." *Arch. Pathol. 51*:293, 1951.

315. de la Balze, A., Bur, G. E., et al.: Elastic fibers in the tunica propria of normal and pathologic human testes. *J. Clin. Endocrinol. Metab. 14*:626, 1954.

316. Warburg, E.: A fertile patient with Klinefelter's syndrome. *Acta Endocrinol. 43*:12, 1963.

317. Court Brown, W. M., Mantle, D. J., et al.: Fertility in an XY/XXY male married to a translocation heterozygote. *J. Med. Genet. 1*:35, 1964.

318. Plunkett, E. R., and Barr, M. L.: Cytologic tests of sex in congenital testicular hypoplasia. *J. Clin. Endocrinol. Metab. 16*:829, 1956.

319. Leonard, J. M., Paulsen, C. A., Ospina, L. F., and Burgess, E. C.: The classification of Klinefelter's syndrome. Presented at the 1976 Birth Defects Conference, Albany, NY. In *Genetic Mechanisms of Sexual Development.* New York, Academic Press, 1979, pp. 407–423.

320. Lipsett, M. B., David, T. E., et al.: Testosterone production in chromatin-positive Klinefelter's syndrome. *J. Clin. Endocrinol. Metab. 25*:1027, 1965.

321. Caldwell, P. D., and Smith, D. W.: The XXY (Klinefelter's) syndrome in childhood: Detection and treatment. *J. Pediatr. 80*:250, 1972.

322. Sergovich, F., Valentine, G. H., et al.: Chromosome aberrations in 2159 consecutive newborn babies. *N. Engl. J. Med. 280*:171, 1969.

323. Ratcliffe, S. G., Stewart, A. L., et al.: Chromosome studies on 3500 newborn male infants. *Lancet 1*:121, 1970.

324. Lubs, H. A., and Ruddle, F. H.: Chromosomal abnormalities in the human population: estimation of rates based on New Haven newborn study. *Science 169*:495, 1970.

325. Hamerton, J. L., Ray, M., et al.: Chromosome studies in a neonatal population. *Can. Med. Assoc. J. 106*:776, 1972.

326. Friedrich, V., and Nielson, J.: Chromosome studies in 5,049 consecutive newborn children. *Clin. Genet. 4*:333, 1973.

327. Santen, R. J., de Kretser, D. M., et al.: Gonadotrophins and testosterone in the XYY syndrome. *Lancet 2*:371, 1970.

328. de la Chapelle, A.: Sex chromosome abnormalities among the mentally defective in Finland. *J. Ment. Defic. Res. 7*:129, 1963.

329. Skakkebaek, N. E., Hultén, M., et al.: Quantification of human seminiferous epithelium. II. Histological studies in eight 47,XYY men. *J. Reprod. Fertil. 32*:391, 1973.

330. Melnyk, J., Thompson, H., et al.: Failure of transmission of the extra chromosome in subjects with 47,XYY karyotype. *Lancet 2*:797, 1969.

331. Hudson, B., Burger, H., et al.: Plasma testosterone and luteinising hormone in XYY men. *Lancet 2*:699, 1969.

332. Schiavi, R. C., Owen, D., et al.: Pituitary-gonadal function in XYY and XXY men identified in a population survey. *Clin. Endocrinol. 9*:233, 1978.

333. Vorhees, J. J., Hayes, E., et al.: XYY chromosomal complement and nodulocystic acne. *Ann. Intern. Med. 73*:271, 1970.

334. Drucker, W. D., Blanc, W. A., et al.: The testis in myotonic muscular dystrophy: a clinical and pathologic study with a comparison with the Klinefelter syndrome. *J. Clin. Endocrinol. Metab. 23*:59, 1963.

335. Clarke, G. B., Shapiro, S., et al.: Myotonia atrophica with testicular atrophy: urinary excretion of interstitial-cell-stimulating (luteinizing) hormone, androgens, and 17-ketosteroids. *J. Clin. Endocrinol. Metab. 16*:1235, 1956.

336. Bassöe, H. H.: Familial congenital muscular dystrophy with gonadal dysgenesis. *J. Clin. Endocrinol. Metab. 16*:1614, 1956.

337. Harper, P., Penny, R., et al.: Gonadal function in males with myotonic dystrophy. *J. Clin. Endocrinol. Metab. 35*:852, 1972.

338. Collins, E., and Turner, G.: The Noonan syndrome — a review of the clinical and genetic features of 27 cases. *J. Pediatr. 83*:941–950, 1973.

339. Baird, P. A., and DeJong, B. P.: Noonan's syndrome (XX and XY Turner phenotype) in three generations of a family. *J. Pediatr. 80*: 110–114, 1972.

340. Noonan, J. A.: Hypertelorism with Turner phenotype. *Amer. J. Dis. Child. 116*:373–380, 1968.

341. Chaves-Carballo, E., and Hayles, A. B.: Ullrich-Turner syndrome in the male: review of the literature and report of a case with lymphocytic (Hashimoto's) thyroiditis. *Proc. Staff Meet. Mayo Clin. 41*:843, 1966.

342. de Kretser, D. M., Burger, H. G., et al.: Hormonal, histological and chromosomal studies in adult males with testicular disorders. *J. Clin. Endocrinol. Metab. 35*:392, 1972.

343. de Kretser, D. M., Burger, H. G., Hudson, B., and Keogh, E. J.: The HCG stimulation test in men with testicular disorders. *Clin. Endocrinol. 4*:591, 1975.

344. de Kretser, D. M., Kerr, J. B., and Paulsen, C. A.: The peritubular tissue in the normal and pathological human testis: An ultrastructural study. *Biol. Reprod. 12*:317, 1975.

345. Howard, R. P., Sniffen, R. C., et al.: Testicular deficiency: clinical and pathologic study. *J. Clin. Endocrinol. Metab. 10*:121, 1950.

346. Chemes, H. E., Dym, D. W., Fawcett, D. W., Jayadpour, N., and Sherins, R. J.: Patho-physiological observations of Sertoli cells in patients with germinal aplasia or severe germ cell depletion. Ultrastructural findings and hormone levels. *Biol. Reprod. 17*:108, 1977.

347. de Kretser, D. M., Kerr, J. B., et al.: Evaluation of the ultrastructural changes in the human Sertoli cell in testicular disorders and the relationship of the changes to the levels of serum FSH. *Int. J. Androl.* 1981 (in press).

348. Musto, N. A., Santen, R. J., Huckins, C., and Bardin, C. W.: Abnormalities of the pituitary-gonadal axis of H^re rats: A study of animals with an inherited disorder of seminiferous tubular and Leydig cell function. *Biol. Reprod. 19*:797–806, 1978.

349. Kjessler, B.: *Karyotype, Meiosis and Spermatogenesis in a Sample of Men Attending an Infertility Clinic.* Basel, S. Karger, 1966, p. 56.

350. Heller, C. G., Paulsen, C. A., Mortimore, G. E., Jungck, E. C., and Nelson, W. O.: Urinary gonadotrophins, spermatogenic activity and classification of testicular morphology — their bearing on the utilization hypothesis. *Ann. NY Acad. Sci. 55*:685, 1952.

351. Bowen, P., Lee, C. S. N., et al.: Hereditary male pseudohermaphroditism with hypogonadism, hypospadias, and gynecomastia (Reifenstein's syndrome). *Ann. Intern. Med. 61*:252, 1965.

352. Bremner, W. J., Ott, J., Moore, D. J., and Paulsen, C. A.: Reifenstein's syndrome: Investigation of linkage to X-chromosomal loci. *Clin. Genet. 6*:216, 1974.

353. Amrhein, J. A., Klingensmith, G. J., Walsh, P. C., McKusick, V. A., and Migeon, C. J.: Partial androgen insensitivity: Reifenstein syndrome revisited. *N. Engl. J. Med. 297*:350, 1977.

354. Walsh, P. C., Madden, J. D., et al.: Familial incomplete male pseudohermaphroditism, type 2. Decreased dihydrotestosterone formation in pseudovaginal perineoscrotal hypospadias. *N. Engl. J. Med. 291*:944, 1974.

355. Lacroix, A., McKenna, T. J., et al.: Sex steroid modulation of gonadotropins in normal men and in androgen insensitivity syndrome. *J. Clin. Endocrinol. Metab. 48*:235, 1979.

356. Heller, C. G., Nelson, W. O., et al.: Functional prepuberal castration in males. *J. Clin. Endocrinol. Metab. 3*:573, 1943.

357. Amelar, R. D.: Anorchism without eunuchoidism. *J. Urol. 76*:174, 1956.

358. Kirschner, M. A., Jacobs, J. B., and Fraley, E. E.: Bilateral anorchia with persistent testosterone production. *N. Engl. J. Med. 282*:240, 1970.

359. Jost, A.: Sur le rôle des gonades foetales dans la différentiation sexuelle somatique de l'embryon de lapin. *C. R. Assoc. Anat. 34*:255, 1947.

360. Jost, A.: Recherches sur la différentiation sexuelle de l'embryon de lapin. III. Role des gonades foetales dans la différentiation sexuelle somatique. *Arch. Anat. Microsc. Morphol. Exp. 36*:271, 1947.

361. Raynaud, A., and Frilley, M.: Destruction des glandes génitales de l'embryo de souris par une irradiation au moyen des rayons X, à l'age de 13 jours. *Ann. Endocrinol. 8*:400, 1947.

362. Aynsley-Green, A., Zachmann, M., Illig, R., Rampini, S., and Prader, A.: Congenital bilateral anorchia in childhood: A clinical, endocrine and therapeutic evaluation of twenty-one cases. *Clin. Endocrinol. 5*:381, 1976.

363. Winter, J. S. D., Taraska, S., et al.: The hormonal response to HCG stimulation in male children and adolescents. *J. Clin. Endocrinol. Metab. 34*:348, 1972.

364. Santen, R. J., and Paulsen, C. A.: Hypogonadotrophic eunuchoidism. II. Gonadal responsiveness to exogenous gonadotropins. *J. Clin. Endocrinol. Metab. 36*:55, 1973.

365. Ballew, J. W., and Masters, W. H.: Mumps, a cause of infertility. I. Present consideration. *Fertil. Steril. 5*:536, 1954.

366. Gall, E. A.: The histopathology of acute mumps orchitis. *Amer. J. Path. 23*:637, 1947.

367. Savran, J.: Diethylstilbestrol in prevention of orchitis following mumps. *Rhode Island Med. J. 29*:662, 1946.

368. Mongon, E. S.: The treatment of mumps orchitis with prednisone. *Amer. J. Med. Sci. 237*:749, 1959.

369. Oakberg, E. F., and Clark, E.: Species comparison of radiation response of the gonads. In *Proceedings of the International Symposium on Effects of Ionizing Radiation in the Reproductive System.* Oxford, Pergamon Press, 1963, pp. 11–24.

370. Paulsen, C. A.: In Panel Discussion, Effects of ionizing radiation on reproduction in the male. In *Effects of Ionizing Radiation on the Reproductive System.* Carlson, W. D., and Gassner, F. X. (eds.), New York, Macmillan, 1964, pp. 305–307.

371. Heller, C. G., Wootton, P., et al.: Action of radiation upon human spermatogenesis. In *Proceedings of the 6th Pan-American Congress*

of Endocrinology, International Congress Series 112. Amsterdam, Excerpta Medica Foundation, 1966.

372. Oakberg, E. F.: Initial depletion and subsequent recovery of spermatogonia of the mouse after 20 r of gamma-rays and 100, 300 and 600 r of x-rays. *Radiat. Res. 11*:700, 1959.

373. Paulsen, C. A.: The study of irradiation effects on the human testis: including histologic, chromosomal and hormonal aspects. Final progress report of AEC contract AT(45–1)-2225, Task Agreement 6. RLO-2225–2, 1973.

374. Thorslund, T. W., and Paulsen, C. A.: Effects of x-ray irradiation on human spermatogenesis. In *Proceedings of the National Symposium on Natural and Manmade Radiation in Space.* Warman, E. A. (ed.), NASA Document TM X-2440, 1972, pp. 229–232.

375. Snyder, P. J., Bigdell, H., Gardner, D. F., Mihailovic, V., Rudenstein, R. S., Sterling, F. H., and Utiger, R. D.: Gonadal function in fifty men with untreated pituitary adenomas. *J. Clin. Endocrinol. Metab. 48*:309–314, 1979.

376. Snyder, P. J., Johnson, J., and Muzyka, R.: Abnormal secretion of glycoprotein alpha-subunit and follicle-stimulating hormone (FSH) beta-subunit in men with pituitary adenomas and FSH hypersecretion. *J. Clin. Endocrinol. Metab. 51*:579–748, 1980.

377. Snyder, P. J., Muzyka, R., Johnson, J., and Utiger, R. D.: Thyrotropin-releasing hormone provokes abnormal follicle-stimulating hormone (FSH) and luteinizing hormone responses in men who have pituitary adenomas and FSH hypersecretion. *J. Clin. Endocrinol. Metab. 51*:744–748, 1980.

378. Heller, C. G., and Myers, G. B.: The male climacteric, its symptomatology, diagnosis and treatment. *JAMA 126*:472, 1944.

379. Werner, A. A.: The male climacteric. *JAMA 112*: 1441, 1939.

380. McCullagh, E. P.: Climacteric — male and female. *Cleveland Clin. Quart. 13*:166, 1946.

381. Werner, S. C.: Clinical syndrome associated with gonadal failure in men. *Amer. J. Med. 3*:52, 1947.

382. Kallmann, F., Schonfeld, W. A., et al.: The genetic aspects of primary eunuchoidism. *Amer. J. Ment. Defic. 48*:203, 1944.

383. de Morsier, G.: Etudes sur les dysraphies crânioencéphaliques; agénésie des lobes olfactifs (télencéphaloschizis latéral) et des commissures calleuse et antérieure (télencéphaloschizis médian); la dysplasie olfacto-génitale. *Neurochirurgie Psychiatr. 74*:309, 1954.

384. Heller, C. G., and Nelson, W. O.: Classification of male hypogonadism and a discussion of the pathologic physiology, diagnosis and treatment. *J. Clin. Endocrinol. Metab. 8*:345, 1948.

385. Bartter, F. C., Sniffen, R. C., et al.: Effects of chorionic gonadotropin (APL) in male "eunuchoidism with low follicle-stimulating hormone": aqueous solution versus oil and beeswax suspension. *J. Clin. Endocrinol. Metab. 12*:1532, 1952.

386. Santen, R. J., and Paulsen, C. A.: Hypogonadotropic eunuchoidism. I. Clinical study of the mode of inheritance. *J. Clin. Endocrinol. Metab. 36*:47, 1973.

387. Naftolin, F., and Harris, G. W.: Effect of purified luteinizing hormone releasing factor on normal and hypogonadotrophic anosmic men. *Nature 232*:296, 1971.

388. Hashimoto, T., Miyai, K., Izumi, K., and Kumahara, Y.: Isolated gonadotropin deficiency with response to luteinizing-hormone-releasing hormone. *N. Engl. J. Med. 287*:1059, 1972.

389. Yoshimoto, Y., Moridera, K., and Imura, H.: Restoration of normal pituitary gonadotropin reserve by administration of luteinizing-hormone-releasing hormone in patients with hypogonadotropic hypogonadism. *N. Engl. J. Med. 292*:242, 1975.

390. Bremner, W. J., Fernando, N. N., and Paulsen, C. A.: The effect of luteinizing hormone-releasing hormone in hypogonadotrophic eunuchoidism. *Acta Endocrinol. 86*:1–14, 1977.

391. Gauthier, G.: Olfacto-genital dysplasia (agenesis of the olfactory lobes) with absence of gonadal development at puberty. *Acta Neuroveg. 21*:345, 1960.

392. de Morsier, G., and Gauthier, G: La dysplasie olfacto-génitale. *Pathol. Biol. 11*:1267, 1963.

393. Winters, S. J., Mecklenburg, R. S., et al.: Hypothalamic function in men with hypogonadotropic hypogonadism. *Clin. Endocrinol. 8*:417, 1978.

394. Greulich, W. W., Dorfman, R. I., et al.: Somatic and endocrine studies of puberal and adolescent boys. Washington, D.C., Society for Research in Child Development, National Research Council, 1942, Vol. 7, p. 85.

395. Merriam, G. R., Beitins, I. Z., and Bode, H. H.: Father-to-son transmission of hypogonadism with anosmia: Kallmann's syndrome. *Amer. J. Dis. Child. 131*:1216, 1977.

396. Bardin, C. W.: Hypogonadotropin hypogonadism in patients with multiple congenital defects. *Birth Defects: Original Article Series 7*:175–178, 1971.

397. Hamilton, C. R., Henkin, R. I., Weir, G., and Kliman, B.: Olfactory status and response to clomiphene in male gonadotrophin deficiency. *Ann. Intern. Med. 78*:47, 1973.

398. Check, J. H., Caro, J. F., et al.: Leydig cell responsiveness with germinal cell resistance to gonadotropin therapy in Kallmann's syndrome. *Amer. J. Med.* 67:495, 1979.

399. Paulsen, C. A., Espeland, D. H., and Michals, E. L.: Effects of HCG, HMG, HLH and HGH administration on testicular function. In *The Human Testis.* Rosemberg, E., and Paulsen, C. A. (eds.), New York, Plenum Press, 1970, p. 547.

400. Boyar, R. M., Finkelstein, J. W., et al.: Studies of endocrine function in isolated gonadotropin deficiency. *J. Clin. Endocrinol. Metab.* 36:64, 1973.

401. Santen, R. J., Leonard, J. M., Sherins, R. J., Gandy, H. M., and Paulsen, C. A.: Short- and long-term effects of clomiphene citrate on the male pituitary-testicular axis. *J. Clin. Endocrinol. Metab.* 33:970, 1971.

402. Schroffner, W. G., and Furth, E. D.: Hypogonadotropic hypogonadism with anosmia (Kallmann's syndrome) unresponsive to clomiphene citrate. *J. Clin. Endocrinol. Metab.* 31:267, 1970.

403. Hashimoto, T., Miyai, K., Onishi, T., Matsumoto, K., and Kumahara, Y.: Comparison of short- and long-term treatment with synthetic LH-releasing hormone and clomiphene citrate in male hypothalamic hypogonadism. *J. Clin. Endocrinol. Metab.* 41:905, 1975.

404. Mancini, R. E.: In *Hypothalamic Hypophysiotropic Hormones, Physiological and Clinical Studies.* Proceedings of the Serono Research Foundation Conference, Acapulco, Mexico, 1972. Amsterdam, Excerpta Medica Foundation, 1973.

405. Mortimer, C. H., McNeilly, A. S., Fisher, R. A., Murray, M. A. F., and Besser, G. M.: Gonadotrophin-releasing hormone therapy in hypogonadal males with hypothalamic or pituitary dysfunction. *Brit. Med. J.* 4:617, 1974.

406. Belchetz, P. E., Plant, T. M., Yakai, Y., Keogh, E. J., and Knobil, E.: Hypophysial responses to continuous and intermittent delivery of hypothalamic gonadotropin-releasing hormone. *Science* 202:631, 1978.

407. Paulsen, C. A.: The effect of human menopausal gonadotrophin on spermatogenesis in hypogonadotrophic hypogonadism. In *Proceedings of the Sixth Pan American Congress of Endocrinology, Mexico City, 1965.* Amsterdam, Excerpta Medica Foundation, 1966, pp. 398–402.

408. Paulsen, C. A.: Effect of human chorionic gonadotrophin and human menopausal gonadotrophin therapy on testicular function. In *Gonadotropins 1968.* Rosemberg, E. (ed.), Palo Alto, Geron-X, Inc., 1968, p. 491.

409. Mancini, R. E.: Immunological aspects of male infertility. In *The Human Testis.* Rosemberg, E., and Paulsen, C. A. (eds.), New York, Plenum Press, 1970, p. 529.

420. Paulsen, C. A., et al.: In *The Human Testis.* Rosemberg, E., and Paulsen, C. A. (eds.), New York, Plenum Press, 1970.

421. Joel, C. A.: Treatment of azoospermia by human gonadotropins. *Harefuah* 71:281, 1966.

422. Lunenfeld, B., Mor, A., and Mani, M.: Treatment of male infertility. I. Human gonadotropins. *Fertil. Steril.* 18:581, 1967.

423. Hurxthal, L. M., Bruns, H. J., et al.: Development of spermatogenesis in hypogonadism. *J. Clin. Endocrinol. Metab.* 9:1245, 1949.

424. Werner, S. C.: Spermatogenesis and apparent fertility in eunuchoid male in eleventh year of androgen therapy. *J. Clin. Endocrinol. Metab.* 11:612, 1951.

425. Berger, H. G., de Kretser, D. M., Hudson, B., and Wilson, J. D.: Effects of preceding androgen therapy on testicular response to human pituitary gonadotropin in hypogonadotropic hypogonadism: A study of three patients. *Fertil. Steril.* 35:64, 1981.

426. Ley, S. B., Leonard, J. M., Paulsen, C. A., and Leach, R. B.: Exogenous gonadotropins following prolonged androgen therapy: Testicular response in hypogonadotropic eunuchoidism. Abstract from 1981 Endocrine Society Meeting.

427. Pasqualini, R. Q., and Bur, G. E.: Sindrome hipoandrogenico con gametogenesis conservada. *Rev. Asoc. Med. Argent.* 64:6, 1950.

428. McCullagh, E. P., Beck, J. C., et al.: A syndrome of eunuchoidism with spermatogenesis, normal urinary FSH and low or normal ICSH (fertile "eunuchs"). *J. Clin. Endocrinol. Metab.* 13:489, 1953.

429. Pasqualini, R. W., and Bur, G. E.: Hypoandrogenic syndrome with spermatogenesis. *Fertil. Steril.* 6:144, 1955.

430. Faiman, C., Hoffman, R. J., et al.: The "fertile eunuch" syndrome: demonstration of isolated luteinizing hormone deficiency by radioimmunoassay technique. *Mayo Clin. Proc.* 43:661, 1968.

431. Robin, D., Spitz, I., et al.: Isolated deficiency of follicle-stimulating hormone. *N. Engl. J. Med.* 287:1314, 1972.

432. Stewart-Bentley, M., and Wallack, M.: Isolated FSH deficiency in a male. *Clin. Res.* 24:96A, 1975.

433. Maroulis, G., Parlow, A. F., et al.: Isolated follicle-stimulating hormone deficiency in man. *Fertil. Steril.* 28:818, 1977.

434. Wicklings, E. J., and Nieschlag, E.: Suppression of spermatogenesis over two years in Rhesus monkeys actively immunized with follicle-stimulating hormone. *Fertil. Steril.* 34:269, 1980.

435. Paschkis, K. E., and Cantarow, A.: Hypopituitarism: studies in pituitary tumors and Simmonds' disease. *Ann. Intern. Med.* 34:669, 1951.

436. Maddock, W. O., Leach, R. B., et al.: Selective pituitary failure: an example characterized by deficient ACTH and gonadotrophin secretion with intact thyrotrophin secretion. *Amer. J. Med. Sci.* 226:509, 1953.

437. McCullagh, E. P., Gold, A., et al.: Alterations in testicular structure and function in organic disease of the pituitary. *J. Clin. Endocrinol. Metab.* 10:871, 1950.

438. Albert, A., Underdahl, L. O., et al.: Male hypogonadism. V. The testis in adult patients with multiple defects in pituitary functions. *Proc. Staff Meet. Mayo Clin.* 29:317, 1954.

439. Albert, A., Underdahl, L. O., et al.: Male hypogonadism. VI. The testis in gonadotropic failure in adults. *Proc. Staff Meet. Mayo Clin.* 29:368, 1954.

440. Leonard, J. M., and Milder, M. S.: Pituitary origin of hypogonadism in idiopathic hemochromatosis (I. H.). *Clin. Res.* 26:106A, 1978.

441. MacLeod, J., Pazianos, A., et al.: Restoration of human spermatogenesis by menopausal gonadotrophins. *Lancet* 1:1196, 1964.

442. Gemzell, C., and Kjessler, G.: Treatment of infertility after partial hypophysectomy with human pituitary gonadotrophins. *Lancet* 1:644, 1964.

443. Mancini, R. E., Vilar, O., et al.: Effect of human urinary FSH and LH on the recovery of spermatogenesis in hypophysectomized patients. *J. Clin. Endocrinol. Metab.* 33:888, 1971.

444. World Health Organization Technical Report Series No. 514: Agents Stimulating Gonadal Function in the Human. Geneva, World Health Organization, 1973.

445. Schulte-Beerbühl, M., and Nieschlag, E.: Comparison of testosterone, dihydrotestosterone, luteinizing hormone and follicle-stimulating hormone in serum after injection of testosterone enanthate or testosterone cypionate. *Fertil. Steril.* 33:201, 1980.

446. Alkalay, D., Khemani, L., et al.: Sublingual and oral administration of methyltestosterone. A comparison of drug bioavailability. *J. Clin. Pharmacol.* 13:142, 1973.

447. Lesser, M. A., Vore, S. N., et al.: Effect of testosterone propionate on the prostate gland of patients over 45. *J. Clin. Endocrinol. Metab.* 15:297, 1955.

448. Werner, S. C., Hanger, F. M., et al.: Jaundice during methyltestosterone therapy. *Am. J. Med.* 8:325, 1950.

449. Wood, J. C.: Jaundice due to methyltestosterone therapy. JAMA 150:1484, 1952.

450. Boyer, J. L., Preisig, R., Zbinden, G., de Kretser, D. M., Wang, C., and Paulsen, C. A.: Guidelines for assessment of potential hepatotoxic effects of synthetic androgens, anabolic agents and progestagens in their use in males as antifertility agents. *Contraception* 13:461, 1976.

451. Charny, C. W., and Wolgen, W.: *Cryptorchidism.* New York, Paul B. Hoeber, 1957.

452. Bishop, P. M. F.: Studies in clinical endocrinology. V. The management of the undescended testicle. *Guy's Hosp. Rep.* 94:12, 1945.

453. Jones, H. W., Jr., and Scott, W. W.: *Hermaphroditism, Genital Anomalies and Related Endocrine Disorders.* Baltimore, Williams & Wilkins, 1958.

454. Anderson, H., Andreassen, M., et al.: Testicular biopsies in cryptorchidism. *Acta Endocrinol.* 18:567, 1955.

455. Hand, J. R.: Undescended testes: report of 153 cases with evaluation of clinical findings, treatment, and results on followup up to thirty-three years. *Trans. Am. Assoc. Genitourin. Surg.* 47:9, 1955.

456. Nelson, W. O.: Mammalian spermatogenesis: effect of experimental cryptorchidism in the rat and non-descent of the testis in man. *Recent Progr. Horm. Res.* 6:29, 1951.

457. Sohval, A. R.: Histopathology of cryptorchidism: study based upon comparative histology of retained and scrotal testes from birth to maturity. *Amer. J. Med.* 16:347, 1954.

458. Mancini, R. E., Rosemberg, E., et al.: Cryptorchid and scrotal human testes. I. Cytological, cytochemical and quantitative studies. *J. Clin. Endocrinol. Metab.* 25:927, 1965.

459. de la Balze, F. A., Mancini, R. A., et al.: Histological study of the undescended human testis during puberty. *J. Clin. Endocrinol. Metab.* 20:286, 1960.

460. Charny, C. W.: Spermatogenic potential of undescended testis before and after therapy. *J. Urol.* 83:697, 1960.

461. Hortling, H., de la Chapelle, et al.: An endocrinologic follow-up study of operated cases of cryptorchism. *J. Clin. Endocrinol. Metab.* 27:120, 1967.

462. Gross, R. E., and Jewett, T. C.: Surgical experience from 1222 operations for undescended testes. *JAMA* 160:634, 1956.

463. Krabbe, S., Berthelsen, J. G., et al.: High incidence of undetected neoplasia in maldescended testes. *Lancet* 1:999, 1979.

464. Sumner, W. A.: Malignant tumor of testis occurring 29 years after orchiopexy. *J. Urol.* 81:150, 1959.

465. Patton, J. F., and Mallis, N.: Tumors of the testis. *J. Urol.* 81:457, 1959.

466. Linke, C. A., and Kiefer, J. H.: Occurrence of testis tumor in undescended testes. *J. Urol.* 82:347, 1959.

467. Cooper, I. S., Rynearson, E. H., et al.: Metabolic consequences of spinal cord injury. *J. Clin. Endocrinol. Metab.* 10:858, 1950.

468. Cooper, I. S., and Hoen, T. I.: Gynecomastia in paraplegic males: report of seven cases. *J. Clin. Endocrinol. Metab. 9:*457, 1949.
469. Horne, H. W., Paull, D. P., et al.: Fertility studies in the human male with traumatic injuries of the spinal cord and cauda equina. *N. Engl. J. Med. 239:*959, 1958.
470. Stemmerman, G. H., Weiss, L., et al.: A study of the germinal epithelium in male paraplegics. *Amer. J. Clin. Path. 20:*24, 1950.
471. Monro, D., Horne, H. W., Jr., et al.: The effect of injury to the spinal cord and cauda equina on the sexual potency of men. *N. Engl. J. Med. 239:*903, 1958.
472. Kikuchi, T. A., Skowsky, W. R., El-Toraei, I., and Swerdloff, R.: The pituitary-gonadal axis in spinal cord injury. *Fertil. Steril. 27:*1142, 1976.
473. Bors, E., Engle, E. T., et al.: Fertility in paraplegic males. *J. Clin. Endocrinol. Metab. 9:*457, 1949.
474. Mostofi, F. K., and Price, E. B., Jr.: In *Atlas of Tumor Pathology*, Second Series, Fascicle 8. Washington DC, Armed Forces Institute of Pathology, 1973, p. 1.
475. Bar, W., and Hedinger, C.: Comparison of histopathologic types of primary testicular germ cell tumors with their metastases: consequences for the WHO and British Nomenclatures? *Virchows Arch. [Pathol. Anat.] 370:*41, 1976.
476. Nochomovitz, L. E., De La Torre, R. F. E., et al.: Pathology of germ cell tumors of the testis. *Urol Clin. North Am. 4:*359, 1979.
477. Nochomovitz, L. E., and Rosai, J.: Current concepts on the histogenesis, pathology, and immunochemistry of germ cell tumors of the testis. *Pathol. Annu. 13:*327, 1978.
478. Skakkebaek, N. E.: Possible carcinoma-in-situ of the testis. *Lancet 2:*516, 1972.
479. Skakkebaek, N. E.: Carcinoma-in-situ of the testis: frequency and relationship to invasive germ cell tumours in infertile men. *Histopathology 2:*157, 1978.
480. Berthelsen, J. G., Skakkebaek, N. E., Mogensen, P., and Sørensen, B. L.: Incidence of carcinoma-in-situ of germ cells in contralateral testis of men with testicular tumours. *Brit. Med. J. 2:*363, 1979.
481. Skakkebaek, N. E.: Carcinoma-in-situ of testis in testicular feminization syndrome. *Acta Pathol. Microbiol. Scand.* Sect. A 87:87, 1979.
482. Skakkebaek, N. E.: Atypical germ cells in the adjacent "normal" tissue of testicular tumours. *Acta Pathol. Microbiol. Scand.* Sec. A 83:127, 1975.
483. Waxman, M.: Malignant germ cell tumor in situ in a cryptorchid testis. *Cancer 38:*1452, 1976.
484. Williams, T. R., and Brendler, H.: Carcinoma in situ of the ectopic testis. *J. Urol. 117:*610, 1977.
485. Nuesch-Bachmann, I. H., and Hedinger, C.: Atypische Spermatogonien als Präkanzerose. *Schweiz. Med. Wochenschr. 107:*795, 1977.
486. Skakkebaek, N. E., and Berthelsen, J. G.: Carcinoma-in-situ of testis and orchiectomy. *Lancet 2:*204, 1978.
487. Rubin, P.: Cancer of the urogenital tract: testicular tumors. *JAMA 213:*89, 1970.
488. Anderson, T., Waldmann, T. A., Javadpour, N., and Glatstein, E.: Testicular germ-cell neoplasms: Recent advances in diagnosis and therapy. *Ann. Intern. Med. 90:*373, 1979.
489. Fraley, E. E., Lange, P. H., and Kennedy, B. J.: Germ cell testicular cancer in adults. *N. Engl. J. Med. 301:*1370, 1420, 1979.
490. Savard, K., Dorfman, R. I., et al.: Clinical morphological and biochemical studies of a virilizing tumor in the testis. *J. Clin. Invest. 39:*534, 1960.
491. Nelson, W. O., and Heller, C. C.: Hyalinization of the seminiferous tubules associated with normal or failing Leydig cell function; microscopic picture in the testis and associated changes in the breast. *J. Clin. Endocrinol. Metab. 5:*13, 1945.
492. Schwartz, I. S., and Wilens, D. L.: The formation of acinar tissue in gynecomastia. *Amer. J. Pathol. 43:*797, 1963.
493. Nicholis, G. L., Modlinger, R. S., et al.: A study of the histopathology of human gynecomastia. *Gynecomastia 32:*173, 1971.
494. Bannayan, G. A., and Hajdu, S. I.: Gynecomastia: clinicopathologic study of 351 cases. *Amer. J. Clin. Pathol. 57:*431, 1972.
495. Morrione, T. G.: Effect of estrogens in testis in hepatic insufficiency. *Arch. Pathol. 37:*39, 1944.
496. Wallach, E. E., and Garcia, C. R.: Familial gynecomastia without hypogonadism: a report of three cases in one family. *J. Clin. Endocrinol. Metab. 22:*1201, 1962.
497. Nuttall, F. Q.: Gynecomastia as a physical finding in normal men. *J. Clin. Endocrinol. Metab. 48:*338, 1979.
498. Ley, S. B., Mozaffarian, G. A., Leonard, J. M., Higley, M., and Paulsen, C. A.: Palpable breast tissue versus gynecomastia as a normal physical finding. *Clin. Res. 28:*24A, 1980.
499. Carlson. H. E.: Gynecomastia. *N. Engl. J. Med. 303:*795, 1980.
500. Treves, N.: Gynecomastia. *Cancer 11:*1083, 1958.
501. Rosewater, S., Weinup, G., et al.: Familial gynecomastia. *Ann. Intern. Med. 63:*377, 1965.
502. Krant, M. J.: Estrogen hyperexcretion in a patient with nonendocrine cancer. *Arch. Intern. Med. 115:*464, 1965.

503. Jull, J. W., and Dossett, J. A.: Hormone excretion studies of gynaecomastia of puberty. *Brit. Med. J. 2:*795, 1964.
504. Jull, J. W., Bonser, G. J., et al.: Hormone excretion studies of males with gynaecomastia. *Brit. Med. J. 2:*797, 1964.
505. Fusco, F. D., and Rosen, S. W.: Gonadotropin-producing anaplastic large cell carcinomas of the lung. *N. Engl. J. Med. 275:*507, 1966.
506. MacDonald, P. C., Madden, J. D., Brenner, P. F., Wilson, J. D., and Siiteri, P. K.: Origin of estrogen in normal men and in women with testicular feminization. *J. Clin Endocrinol. Metab. 49:*905, 1979.
507. Vigersky, R. A., Kono, S., Sauer, M., Lipsett, M. B., and Loriaux, D. L.: Relative binding of testosterone and estradiol to testosterone-estradiol-binding globulin. *J. Clin. Endocrinol. Metab. 49:*899, 1979.
508. Kirschner, M. A., Cohen, F. B., and Jesperson, D. C.: Estrogen production and its origin in men with gonadotropin-producing neoplasms. *J. Clin. Endocrinol. Metab. 39:*112, 1974.
509. Hemsell, D. L., Edman, C. D., Markes, J. F.: Massive extranglandular aromatization of plasma and androstenedione resulting in feminization of a prepubertal boy. *J. Clin. Invest. 60:*455, 1977.
510. Gordon, G. C., Altman, K., Southren, A. L., Rubin, E., and Lieber, C. S.: Effect of alcohol (ethanol) administration on sex-hormone metabolism in normal men. *N. Engl. J. Med. 295:*793, 1976.
511. Aiman, J., Brenner, P. F., and MacDonald, P. C.: Androgen and estrogen production in elderly men with gynecomastia and testicular atrophy after mumps orchitis. *J. Clin. Endocrinol. Metab. 50:*380, 1980.
512. Baker, H. W. G., Burger, H. G., de Kretser, D. M., Dulmanis, A., Hudson, B., O'Connor, S., Paulsen, C. A., Purcell, N., Rennie, G. C., Seah, C. S., Taft, H. P., and Wang, C.: A study of the endocrine manifestations of hepatic cirrhosis. *Quart. J. Med. 177:*145, 1976.
513. Marynick, S. P., Nisula, B. C., Pita, J. C., Jr., and Loriaux, D. L.: Persistent pubertal macromastia. *J. Clin. Endocrinol. Metab. 50:*128, 1980.
514. Canfield, C. J., and Bates, R. W.: Nonpuerperal galactorrhea. *N. Engl. J. Med. 273:*897, 1965.
515. Ayd, F. J., Jr.: Thorazine and serpasil treatment on private neuropsychiatric patients. *Amer. J. Psychiat. 113:*16, 1956.
516. Sulman, P. G., and Wennik, H. Z.: Hormonal effect of chlorpromazine. *Lancet 1:*161, 1950.
517. Pettinger, W. A., Horwitz, D., et al.: Lactation due to methyldopa. *Brit. Med. J. 1:*1460, 1963.
518. Robinson, B. A.: Breast changes in the male and female: lactation with chlorpromazine. *Med. J. Aust. 2:*239, 1957.
519. Rose, L. I., Underwood, R. H., Newmark, S. R., Kisch, E. S., and Williams, G. H.: Pathophysiology of spironolactone-induced gynecomastia. *Ann. Intern. Med. 87:*398, 1977.
520. Winters, S. J., Banks, J. L., and Loriaux, D. L.: Cimetidine is an antiandrogen in the rat. *Gastroenterology 76:*504, 1978.
521. Friedman, R. C., Wollesen, F., et al.: Psychological development and blood levels of sex steroids in male identical twins of divergent sexual orientation. *J. Nerv. Ment. Dis. 163:*282, 1976.
522. Friedman, R. C., Dryenfurth, I., Linke, D., Tendler, R., and Fleiss, J. L.: Hormones and sexual orientation in men. *Amer. J. Psychiat. 134:*571, 1977.
523. James, S., Carter, R. A., and Orwin, A.: Significance of androgen levels in the aetiology and treatment of homosexuality. *Psychol. Med. 7:*429, 1977.
524. Kolodny, R. C., Masters, W. H., Hendryx, J., and Toro, G.: Plasma testosterone and semen analysis in male homosexuals. *N. Engl. J. Med. 285:*1170, 1971.
525. Kolodny, R. C., Jacobs, L. S., Masters, W. H., Toro, G., and Daughaday, W. H.: Plasma gonadotrophins and prolactin in male homosexuals. *Lancet 2:*18, 1972.
526. Johnson, D. S.: Reversible male sterilization: current status and future directions. *Contraception 5:*327–338, 1972.
527. Lee, H. Y.: Observations of the results of 300 vasovasostomies. *J. Androl. 1:*11–15, 1980.
528. Silber, S. J.: Vasectomy and vasectomy reversal. *Fertil. Steril. 29:*125–140, 1978.
529. Alexander, N. J., and Clarkson, T. B.: Vasectomy increases the severity of diet-induced atherosclerosis in Macaca fascicularis. *Science 201:*538–541, 1978.
530. Clarkson, T. B., and Alexander, N. J.: Long-term vasectomy: effects on the occurrence and extent of atherosclerosis in rhesus monkeys. *J. Clin. Invest. 65:*15–25, 1980.
531. Lepow, I. H., and Crozier, R. (eds.): *Vasectomy: Immunologic and Pathophysiologic Effects in Animals and Man.* New York, Academic Press, 1979.
532. Frick, J., Bartsch, F., and Weiske, W. H.: The effect of monthly depot medroxyprogesterone acetate and testosterone on human spermatogenesis. I. Uniform dosage level. *Contraception 15:*649–668, 1977.
533. Cunningham, G. R., Silverman, V. E., and Kohler, P. O.: Clinical evaluation of testosterone enanthate for induction and mainte-

nance of reversible azoospermia in man. In *Hormonal Control of Male Fertility*. Patanelli, D. J. (ed.). DHEW Publication No. (NIH) 78–1097, 1978, pp. 71–87.

534. Patanelli, D. J. (ed.): *Hormonal Control of Male Fertility*. DHEW Publication No. (NIH) 78–1097, 1978.

535. Steinberger, E., and Smith, K. D.: Testosterone enanthate, a possible reversible male contraceptive. *Contraception* 16:261–268, 1977.

536. Swerdloff, R. S., Palacios, A., McClure, R. D., Campfield, L. S., and Brosman, S. A.: Clinical evaluation of testosterone enanthate in the reversible suppression of spermatogenesis in the human male: efficacy, mechanism of action and adverse effects. In *Hormonal Control of Male Fertility*. Patanelli, D. J. (ed.). DHEW Publication No. (NIH) 78–1097, 1978, pp. 41–63.

537. Paulsen, C. A., Leonard, J. M., Burgess, E. C., and Ospina. L. F.: Male contraceptive development: re-examination of testosterone enanthate as an effective single entity agent. In *Hormonal Control of Male Fertility*. Patanelli, D. J. (ed.). DHEW Publication No. (NIH) 78–1097, 1978, pp. 17–36.

538. Ramwell, P.: Discussion: endocrine approach to contraception. *Int. J. Androl*. Suppl. 2, part 2:729–739, 1978.

539. Paulsen, C. A., and Leonard, J. M.: Clinical trials in reversible male contraception. In *Regulatory Mechanisms of Male Reproductive Physiology*. Spilman, C. H., Lobl, T. J., and Kirton, K. T. (eds.), Amsterdam, Elsevier Excerpta Medica, 1976, pp. 197–208.

540. Nieschlag, E., Hoogen, H., Bulk, M., Schuster, H., and Wickings, E. J.: Clinical trial with testosterone undecanoate for male fertility control. *Contraception* 18:607–614, 1978.

541. Sherins, R. J., Gandy, H. M., Thorslund, T. W., and Paulsen, C. A.: Pituitary and testicular function studies. I. Experience with a new gonadal inhibitor, 17 alpha-pregn-4-en-20-yno (2,3-d) isoxazol-17-ol (danazol). *J. Clin. Endocrinol. Metab*. 32:522–532, 1971.

542. Barbieri, R. L., Tanick, J. A., and Ryan, K. J.: Danazol inhibits steroidogenesis in the rat testis *in vitro*. *Endocrinology* 101:1676–1682, 1977.

543. Skoglund, R. D., and Paulsen, C. A.: Danazol-testosterone combination: a potentially effective means for reversible male contraception: a preliminary report. *Contraception* 7:357–365, 1973.

544. Leonard, J. M., and Paulsen, C. A.: Contraceptive development studies for males: oral and parenteral steroid hormone administration. In *Hormonal Control of Male Fertility*. Patanelli, D. J. (ed.). DHEW Publication No. (NIH) 78–1097, 1978, pp. 223–238.

545. Bremner, W. J., and de Kretser, D. M.: The prospects for new, reversible male contraceptives. *N. Engl. J. Med*. 295:111–117, 1976.

546. Brenner, P. F., Mishell, D. R., Jr., Bernstein, G. S., and Ortiz, A.: Study of medroxyprogesterone acetate and testosterone enanthate as a male contraceptive. *Contraception* 15:679–691, 1977.

547. Føgh, M., Damgaard-Pedersen, F., Gormsen, J., Knudsen, J. B., and Schou, G.: Oral levo-norgestrel-testosterone effects on spermatogenesis hormone levels, coagulation factors and lipoproteins in normal men. *Contraception* 21:381–393, 1980.

548. Føgh, M., Nichol, K., Petersen, I. B., and Schou, G.: Clinical evaluation of long-term treatment with levo-norgestrel and testosterone enanthate in normal men. *Contraception* 21:631–640, 1980.

549. Frick, J., Bartsch, G., and Weiske, W. H.: The effect of monthly depot medroxyprogesterone acetate and testosterone on human spermatogenesis. II. High initial dose. *Contraception* 15:669–677, 1977.

550. Lee, H. Y., Kim, S. I., and Kwon, E. H.: Clinical trial on reversible male contraceptive with long-acting sex hormones. *Seoul J. Med*. 20:1–18, 1979.

551. Schearer, S. B., Alvarez-Sanchez, F., Anselmo, J., Brenner, P., Coutinho, E., Latham-Faundes, A., Frick, J., Heinild, B., and Johanson, E. D. B.: Hormonal contraception for men. *Int. J. Androl*. Suppl. 2:680–712, 1978.

552. Bain, J., Rochlis, V., Robert, E., and Khait, Z.: The combined use of oral medroxyprogesterone acetate and methyltestosterone in a male contraceptive trial programme. *Contraception* 21:365–380, 1980.

553. Prasad, M. R. N., Singh, S. P., and Rajalakshmi, M.: Fertility control in male rats by continuous release of microquantities of cyproterone acetate from subcutaneous silastic capsules. *Contraception* 2:165–178, 1970.

554. Koch, U. J., Lorenz, F., Danehl, K., Ericsson, R., Hasan, S. H., Keyserlingk, D. V., Lubke, K., Mehring, M., Rommler, A., Schwartz, U., and Hammerstein, J.: Continuous oral low-dosage cyproterone acetate for fertility regulation in the male? — a trend analysis in 15 volunteers. *Contraception* 14:117–135, 1976.

555. Roy, S., Chatterjee, S., Prasad, M. R. N., Poddar, A. K., and Pandey, D. C.: Effects of cyproterone acetate on reproductive functions in normal human males. *Contraception* 14:403–420, 1976.

556. Moltz, K., Rommler, A., Post, K., Schwartz, V., and Hammerstein, J.: Medium dose cyproterone acetate (CPA): Effects on hormone secretion and on spermatogenesis in men. *Contraception* 21:393–414, 1980.

557. Føgh, M., Corker, C. S., Hunter, W. M., McLean, H., Philip, J., Schou, G., and Skakkebaek, N. E.: The effects of low doses of cyproterone acetate on some functions of the reproductive system in normal men. *Acta Endocrinol*. 91:545–552, 1979.

558. Wang, C., and Yeung, K. K.: Use of low-dosage oral cyproterone acetates as a male contraceptive. *Contraception* 21:245–272, 1980.

559. Barfield, A., Melo, J., Coutinho, E., Alvarez-Sanchez, F., Faundes, A., Brache, V., Leon, P., Frick, J., Bartsch, G., Weiske, W. H., Brenner, P., Mishell, D., Jr., Bernstein, G., and Ortiz, A.: Pregnancies associated with sperm concentrations below 10 million/ml in clinical studies of a potential male contraceptive method, monthly depot medroxyprogesterone acetate and testosterone esters. *Contraception* 20:121–172, 1979.

560. Pelletier, G., Cusan, G. L., Belanger, A., Seguin, C., Kelly, P. A., and Labrie, F.: Further studies on the inhibitory effect of (D-Ala⁶ des-gly-NH₂¹⁰) LHRH ethylamide on spermatogenesis and steroidogenesis in the rat: reversibility and effect of androgen administration. *J. Androl*. 1:171–181, 1980.

561. Rivier, C., Rivier, J., and Vale, W.: Antireproductive effects of a potent gonadotropin-releasing hormone antagonist in the male rat. *Science* 210:93–95, 1980.

562. National Coordinating Group on Male Antifertility Agents: Gossypol — A new antifertility agent for males. *Chinese Med*. 4:417-428, 1978.

563. Qian Shaozhen, Xu Ye, and Jing Guang-Wei: The potassium-depleting effect of gossypol on isolated rabbit heart and its possible mechanisms. *Acta Pharmacol. Sinica* 14:216, 1979.

564. Dai Rong-xi and Gong Rong-Hua: Studies on antifertility effect of gossypol. I. An experimental analysis by epididymal ligature. *Acta Biol. Exp. Sinica* 11:15–22, 1978.

565. Dai Rong-xi, Pang Shih-Nee, and Liu Zhen-Lian: Studies on the antifertility effect of gossypol. II. A morphological analysis of the antifertility effect of gossypol. *Acta Biol. Exp. Sinica* 11:27–30, 1978.

566. Qian Shaozhen, Jing Guang-Wei, Wu Xianoyun, Xu Ye, Li Yaoqing, and Zhou Zhibong: Clinico-pharmacological studies on gossypol-related hypokalemia. *Acta Pharmacol. Sinica* 14:1–11, 1979.

567. Ford, W. C. L., and Waites, G. M. H.: Chlorinated sugars: a biochemical approach to the control of male fertility. *Int. J. Androl*. Suppl. 2, part 1:541–564. 1978.

CHAPTER 7

The Ovaries and the Breasts*

By Griff T. Ross,

Raymond L. Vande Wiele,

and Andrew G. Frantz

Part I: The Ovaries

By Griff T. Ross

and Raymond L. Vande Wiele

THE NORMAL OVARY

Morphology

Grossly the human ovary is a reniform structure attached to the posterior surface of the broad ligament by a peritoneal fold called the mesovarium. Nerves, blood vessels, and lymphatics traverse the mesovarium and penetrate the ovary at its hilum. In normal women, the combined weight of the ovaries during the reproductive years is 10–20 g, averaging 14 g.

Microscopic Anatomy

Microscopically the ovary consists of three distinct regions: an outer cortex, a central medulla, and an inner hilum around the point of attachment of the ovary to its mesentery. None of these areas are structurally homogeneous, and microscopic appearance varies with age, principally in terms of relative amounts of cellular constituents. The principal components consist of a covering by coelomic epithelium, follicles in varying stages of either maturation or degeneration, supportive tissues collectively referred to as stroma, and blood vessels and lymphatics. To appreciate changes occurring during fetal or postnatal development of the ovary, more detailed

*The authors are grateful to Mesdames A. Ross, O. Monger, and E. Donohue for skillful assistance in the preparation of the manuscript.

consideration must be given to cellular composition of follicles and stroma.

The Follicle

Maturation. Morphologically, the follicle changes as it matures. The most immature stage is referred to as a *primordial follicle* (Fig. 7–1A). The primordial follicle, separated from surrounding stroma by an inconspicuous but definite basal lamina (basement membrane), contains a primary oocyte in attenuated prophase of the first meiotic division. The oocyte is surrounded by a single layer of spindle-shaped cells and protoplasmic processes that form a desmosomal union with the plasma membrane of the oocyte, providng a route for transfer of nutrients to the oocyte.

When the flat, spindle-shaped cells inside the basal lamina of a primordial follicle become cuboidal (Fig. 7–1 A and B), the term *primary follicle* is applied. Successive mitotic divisions of the cuboidal cells give rise to a multilayered stratum granulosum or zona granulosa, and a band of mucoid substance, secreted by the granulosa cells and called the zona pellucida, separates the cuboidal granulosa cells from the oocyte (Fig. 7–1B and C). Protoplasmic processes from adjacent granulosa cells traverse the zona pellucida to establish contact with the plasma membrane of the oocyte. The contents of the follicle

within the basal lamina remain avascular until after ovulation, and transfer of nutrients must occur by diffusion.

Coincident with proliferation of granulosa cells bounded by the basal lamina, adjacent stromal cells outside the basal lamina become arranged in concentric perifollicular layers, in which density of nuclei is less than that of stroma further removed from the follicle. This layer of differentiated and uniquely oriented cells constitutes the *theca* (Fig. 7–1B and C). That portion of the theca adjacent to the basal lamina is called *theca interna*; that portion merging with surrounding stroma is called *theca externa*. As numbers of granulosa cells continue to increase, some of the spindle-shaped cells in the theca interna acquire increased amounts of cytoplasm and appear rounded or epithelioid (Fig. 7–1C). Capillaries and lymphatic spaces, which terminate at the basal lamina, appear among these cells.

Hypertrophy and epithelioid transformation of the theca interna are followed by the appearance of cleftlike fluid-filled spaces among the granulosa cells. These spaces become confluent to give rise to a fluid-filled *antrum*, a distinctive feature of *graafian follicles* (Fig. 7–1D). The fluid consists of a plasma transudate containing secretory products of granulosa cells, including sex steroid hormones in concentrations that are orders of magnitude greater than those in peripheral blood. As the antral follicle enlarges, the quantity of fluid progressively increases, and the oocyte, surrounded by a hillock of granulosa cells called the

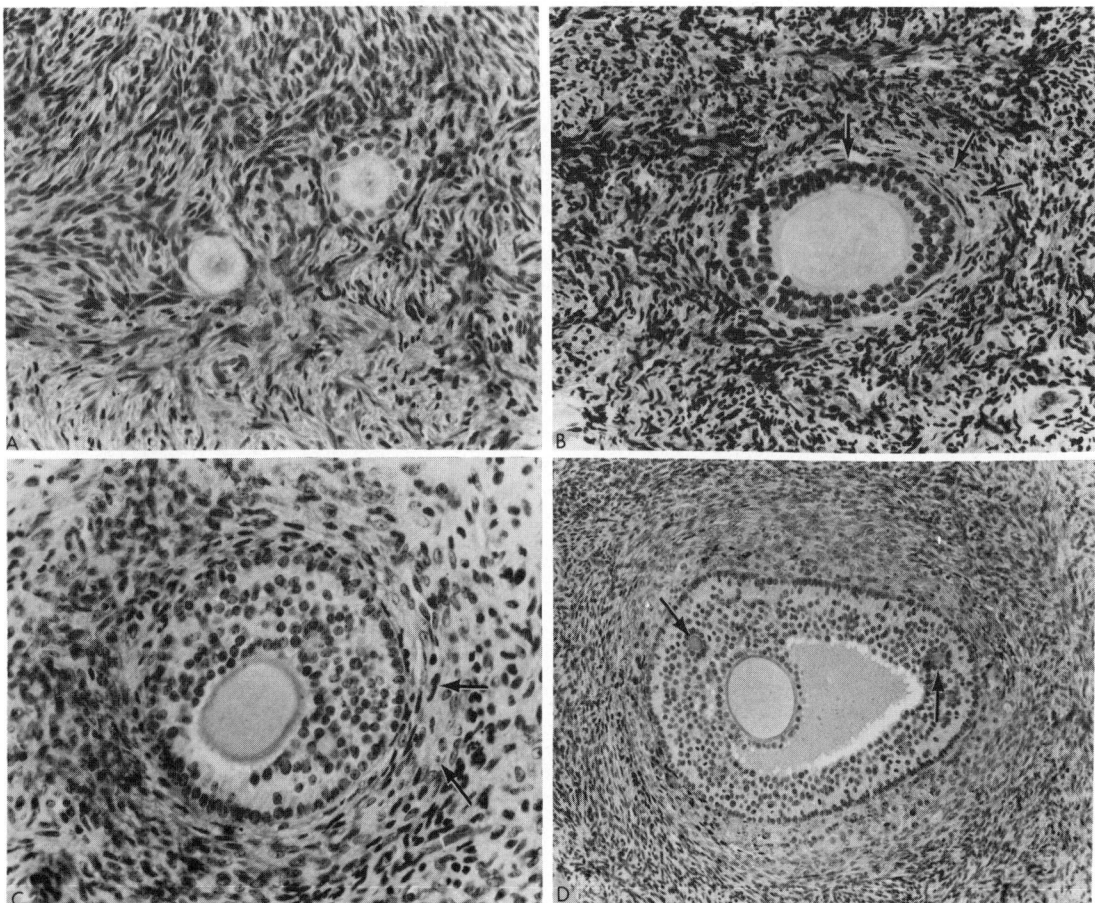

Figure 7–1. *A*, Primordial follicle (lower left) and primary follicle (upper right) in human ovary. *B*, Primary follicle with 3 layers of granulosa cells and incipient differentiation of theca (arrows) from surrounding stroma. *C*, Primary follicle with multiple layers of granulosa cells and beginning epithelioid transformation of the theca (arrows). *D*, Graafian follicle. Note the epithelioid character of theca cells and Call-Exner bodies (arrows) among granulosa cells.

cumulus oophorous, comes to occupy a polar eccentric position within the follicle.

Although the follicle continues to enlarge until just prior to ovulation, the oocyte ceases to enlarge around the time of antrum formation. Thus, despite the fact that follicle diameters increase 200- to 400-fold (from 50μ to $10,000-20,000\mu$), the oocyte diameters increase only 6- to 10-fold (from $15-20\mu$ to 150μ) as maturation progresses from the primordial to the preovulatory follicle.

Atresia.   Prior to the menarche, all maturing follicles undergo a degenerative process called atresia that may occur at any stage of follicular development. As a result of atresia, the oocyte and all other cells within the lamina basalis die and are replaced by fibrous tissue, producing a structure referred to as a corpus candicans. In contrast to cells within the lamina basalis, thecal cells outside the lamina basalis do not die but "dedifferentiate" and return to the stromal pool of interstitial cells. (See later.)

After the menarche, atresia persists but one follicle ovulates per cycle. Since not all follicles mature to the same extent before undergoing atresia and only one ovulates per cycle, it seems likely that local factors must participate in determining the fate of individual follicles. Recent observations suggest that regulation of both peptide and steroid hormone concentrations in the environment of individual follicles may be involved.

Ovulation.   Beginning with the menarche and continuing until the menopause, one (or rarely more than one) of the maturing follicles enlarges rapidly during the second half of the follicular phase of the cycle. Following the preovulatory LH surge, this follicle ruptures, extruding an oocyte surrounded by its cumulus oophorous.

About the time of rupture, the first meiotic division is resumed and completed with extrusion of the first polar body, leaving a secondary oocyte surrounded by granulosa cells of the cumulus oophorous. After the follicle has ruptured, vessels from the theca interna penetrate the basal lamina and form a corpus luteum (see later), which incorporates the granulosa cells remaining inside the collapsed postovulatory follicle and surrounding thecal cells. A new corpus luteum is formed in each menstrual cycle, and in subsequent cycles the epithelial cells of the older corpora lutea degenerate and are ultimately replaced by acellular, avascular connective tissue. The residual structure is called a corpus albicans; these structures accumulate in the medullary portion of the ovary.

The Stroma

Generically two types of cells compose the ovarian stroma. The first consists of connective tissue cells similar to those serving supportive functions in other tissues. In the ovary, as elsewhere, these cells are distinguishable histologically with special connective tissue stains. The second generic type, called interstitial cells, consists of eight or more morphologically distinctive types of cells that secrete sex steroid hormones and undergo morphologic changes in response to the interstitial cell–stimulating hormones, hCG and LH. Hormonally stimulated morphologic changes in interstitial cells are particularly noteworthy in the ovaries of pregnant women in whom high levels of hCG in the blood continuously perfuse the ovaries.

The Hilar Cells

The hilus of the ovary is the portal of entry and exit of blood and lymphatic vessels and of nerves. These structures and the supportive connective tissue are the most impressive components of the hilar region. Careful examination of serial sections of the hilus of ovaries from sexually mature and postmenopausal women, however, reveals the presence of another variety of cells, morphologically indistinguishable from Leydig cells, including crystalloids of Reinke, but referred to as hilar cells. These cells are scattered around and sometimes among the fibers of nonmyelinated nerves that traverse the hilus of the ovary. Hilar cells are less conspicuous and more difficult to identify in ovaries examined from the first year of life until puberty. Occasionally, hyperplastic or neoplastic changes in these cells result in virilizing syndromes associated with production of excessive amounts of testosterone. Otherwise, the origin and function of these cells remain obscure.

Morphologic Changes During Growth and Development and with Aging

The Fetal Ovary

Details of gonadal differentiation are discussed in Ch. 8. Briefly, bipotential gonadal anlagen, which may give rise to either ovaries or testes, can be identified in human embryos around the 30th postovulatory day. Histologically, these consist of layers of coelomic epithelial cells overlying primitive mesenchymal cells, blastemic cells of the mesonephros, and primordial germ cells. Although coelomic epithelial, mesenchymal, and blastemic cells arise in situ, the primordial germ cells arise in the yolk sac in the region of the hindgut and migrate into the genital ridge. There, successive mitotic divisions of these primordial germ cells give rise to oogonia that continue to proliferate. Baker (1963) has estimated that the 600,000 oogonia present by the 8th week give rise to 6 to 7 million oogonia by the 20th week of gestation. Although it is clear that oogonia give rise to oocytes (see later) and coelomic epithelial cells give rise to the germinal epithelium in the definitive ovary, the fetal progenitors of other cells composing follicle complexes in the mature ovary remain to be defined with certainty.

Between the 8th and 13th week meiosis is initiated in some oogonia, converting these to primary oocytes. In turn, these primary oocytes become surrounded by precursors of granulosa cells, giving rise to primordial follicles, the morphologic markers of fetal ovarian differentiation. Experimental evidence suggests that diffusible substances, produced by the fetal rete ovarii, are required for initiating meiosis and for subsequent follicle formation (Byskov, 1975).

The nucleus of the oocyte in the primordial follicle remains in the diplotene stage of prophase of the first meiotic division until that division is resumed and completed by extrusion of the first polar body around the time of ovulation. (See before.)

Conversion of oogonia to oocytes and incorporation of the latter into primordial follicles are not completed until the 6th month post partum. Oocytes failing to be incorporated into primordial follicles degenerate. Thus, of the estimated 6 million oogonia present in the fetal ovaries at 20 weeks, only an estimated 2 million have been incorporated into follicles that persist at birth. Furthermore, there is no convincing evidence that additional oocytes arise from germinal epithelium of the human ovary postnatally.

The temporal sequence of morphologic changes in the human fetal ovaries, described by Van Wagenen and Simpson (1965), is summarized in Fig. 7–2. Although not

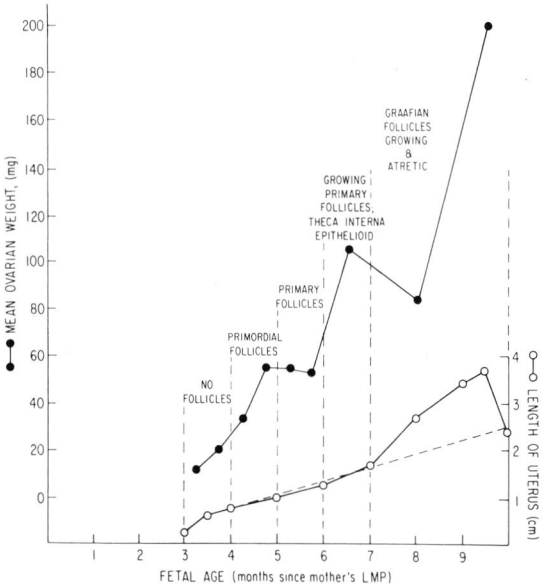

Figure 7–2. Changes in human fetal ovarian weight and morphology (adapted from data of Van Wagenen, G., and Simpson, M. E.: *Embryology of the Ovary and Testis–Homo Sapiens and Macaca Mulatta.* New Haven, Yale University Press, 1965) and human fetal uterine length (adapted from data of Scammon, R. E.: *Proc. Soc. Exp. Biol. Med.* 23:687, 1926) during gestation.

observed in their material until the 5th month of gestation, primordial follicles appear earlier. Initially, these are found deep in the cortex, adjacent to the medulla, while oogonial divisions continue to occur in the outer cortex. These primordial follicles progressively increase in number, and between the 5th and 6th months of gestation, some of them become transformed into primary follicles containing growing oocytes. Between the 6th and 7th months, the growing oocyte in some primary follicles comes to be surrounded by several layers of cuboidal granulosa cells, and epithelioid theca interna cells are first observed at this time. Concomitantly, atretic changes are noted in some primary follicles in the region of the corticomedullary junction.

After the 7th month of gestation, many developing primary follicles with hypertrophied epithelioid theca interna, a few graafian follicles, and follicles of both types undergoing atresia have been found regularly when serial sections of fetal ovaries have been examined. Maturation does not progress to the graafian follicle stage in the absence of gonadotropic stimulation postnatally.

Recently, indirect evidence has been adduced that is consistent with similar requirements for follicle growth in fetal ovaries. Thus, hypoplasia of the gonads and failure of normal progression of follicle maturation have been described in studies on ovaries from anencephalic fetuses surviving until term. All these fetuses have hypoplastic anterior pituitary glands that contain less gonadotropin than pituitaries of normal fetuses of equivalent gestational age, suggesting that the hypoplastic ovaries result from gonadotropin deficiency. Furthermore, FSH and LH/hCG have been measured in specimens of normal human fetal blood recovered as early as the 5th month of gestation.

Recent studies of fetal rhesus monkeys have provided more direct evidence for a role of the fetal pituitary in supporting follicle growth in fetal ovaries. Gulyas and colleagues (1977) examined ovaries from rhesus monkeys born at term following total surgical hypophysectomy around the 100th day of gestation (roughly equivalent to the 7th month of human gestation). They found hypoplas-

tic ovaries in which orderly progression of follicle growth and oogenesis had been disrupted. Moreover, not only was the total number of follicles reduced but also more of the extant follicles were undergoing atresia. Although the nature of the pituitary hormones required remains to be determined, it is clear that the fetal hypophysis is essential for maintenance of normal follicle growth in fetal ovaries.

George and Wilson (1978) have shown that the capacity to produce estrogens by aromatizing androgens appears in human fetal ovaries during the 8th–10th week of gestation. In addition, histochemical evidence for 3β hydroxysteroid dehydrogenase activity in granulosa cells indicates that human fetal ovaries have some other enzymes required for steroid hormone synthesis. There is no convincing evidence that fetal ovaries secrete steroid hormones, however.

The Premenarcheal Ovary

From birth to menarche, mean ovarian weight increases progressively with age (Fig. 7–3). Histologic studies of ovaries recovered at postmortem examination following sudden death of infants and children from accidents or acute illnesses reveal that active follicle growth and atresia occur throughout infancy and childhood. Moreover, these histologic studies reveal that three processes, all related to follicle growth and atresia, contribute to the age-related increase in ovarian weight. The first process is a progressive increase in the quantity

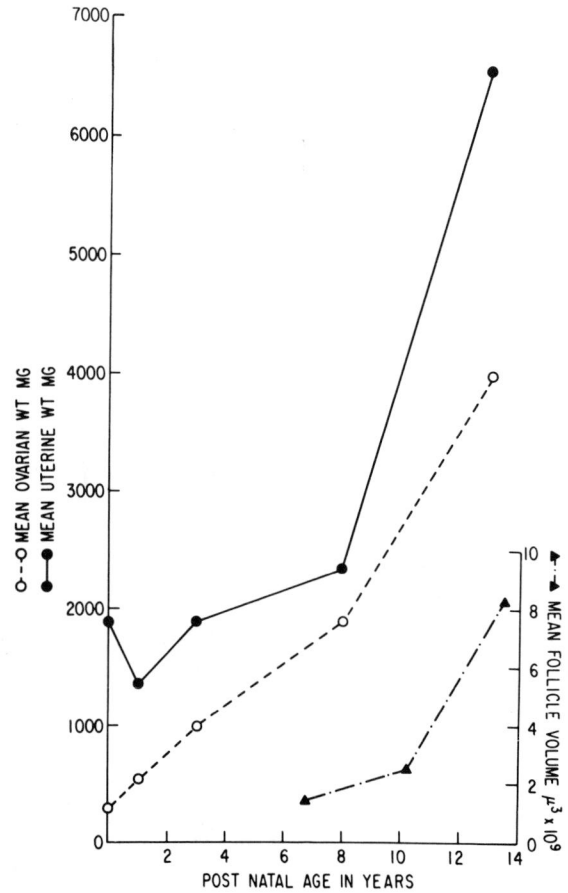

Figure 7–3. Increments in ovarian and uterine weights (adapted from data of Wehefritz, E.: *Z. Ges. Anat.* 9:161, 1923) and volumes of largest atretic follicle (adapted from data of Parini, F., and Molla, W.: *Ann. Obstet. Gynec.* 62:1629, 1940) in human ovaries from birth to 14 years.

of medullary stroma, representing the residue accumulating after maturation and atresia of successive groups of follicles. The second is an age-related increase in diameter (and thus in volume) achieved by maturing follicles prior to atresia (Fig. 7–3). The third is an age-related increase in numbers of follicles attaining this larger size prior to atresia. These last two processes are illustrated dramatically in Fig. 7–4A, B, C.

Age-related changes in blood gonadotropin and estrogen concentrations, occurring concomitantly with changes in ovarian weight and morphology, are shown in Fig. 7–5. Since mean serum gonadotropin levels rise after 6–8 years, there is a concomitant increase in the maximum size attained and in the number of follicles reaching that size prior to atresia and an increase in mean serum estradiol levels. This association suggests that gonadotropins stimulate follicle growth and estrogen synthesis in premenarcheal ovaries.

Additional evidence consistent with the interdependence of gonadotropins, follicle growth, and estrogen production in premenarcheal ovaries is adduced from studies of blood hormone concentrations and ovarian morphology in girls with olfactogenital dysplasia and gonadotropin deficiencies. Small ovaries, retarded follicle growth, and low serum estradiol levels are characteristically seen in girls with this syndrome. Moreover, ovarian follicle growth and estrogen production are stimulated following treatment of these girls with gonadotropins. In summary then, studies of hormonal, morphologic, and functional correlates in premenarcheal girls provide evidence that gonadotropins stimulate follicle maturation and sex steroid hormone secretion by premenarcheal ovaries.

The Postmenarcheal Ovary

Around the time of the menarche, unknown factors result in the initiation of cyclic ovulation while atresia

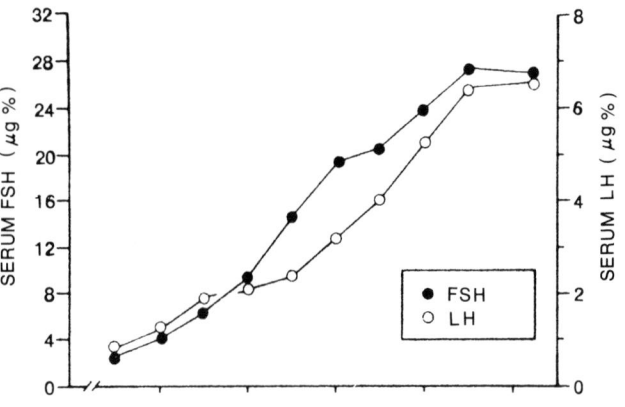

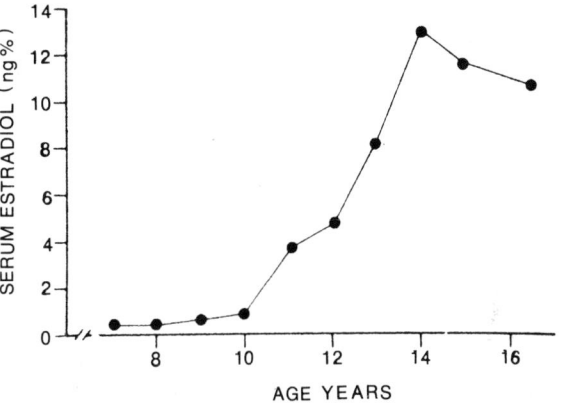

Figure 7–5. Age-related trends in blood FSH, LH, and estradiol prior to and during pubescence. (Reproduced with permission of the authors and publishers of *Clin. Endocrinol. Metab.* 7:513, 1978.)

continues. Although follicle growth and maturation beyond the primary stage appear to be dependent upon gonadotropic stimulation, the period of time required for a primordial follicle to reach maturity once growth is initiated is not known for the human. Women whose ovaries contain follicles not advanced beyond the primary stage, however, can be made to ovulate with exogenous gonadotropins administered over a period not exceeding the follicular phase of the spontaneous ovulatory cycle. On the basis of such observations, it is reasonable to suppose that complete follicular maturation, beginning with a primary follicle, can be completed in 10–12 days. Details of morphologic changes will be presented in connection with the discussion of hormonal control of follicle growth.

After ovulation, one of the more dramatic ovarian morphologic changes occurring during the cycle relates to the formation of a corpus luteum. This structure arises by transformation of granulosa cells remaining behind after extrusion of the ovum and involves profound morphologic changes in cellular appearance as well as in the cytoplasmic organelles. The mitochondria, the endoplasmic reticulum, and the Golgi apparatus all acquire the properties of cells secreting steroid hormones. These intracellular changes are accompanied by vascularization of the corpus luteum with capillaries from the theca interna that penetrate the basal lamina. Cells, called K cells, morphologically distinct from the majority of granulosa cells, are thought by some to originate in the theca interna (White et al., 1951) and appear to be incorporated into the corpus luteum. In the formation of a corpus luteum, the succession of morphologic changes and the time required for completion of these is sufficiently characteristic that an

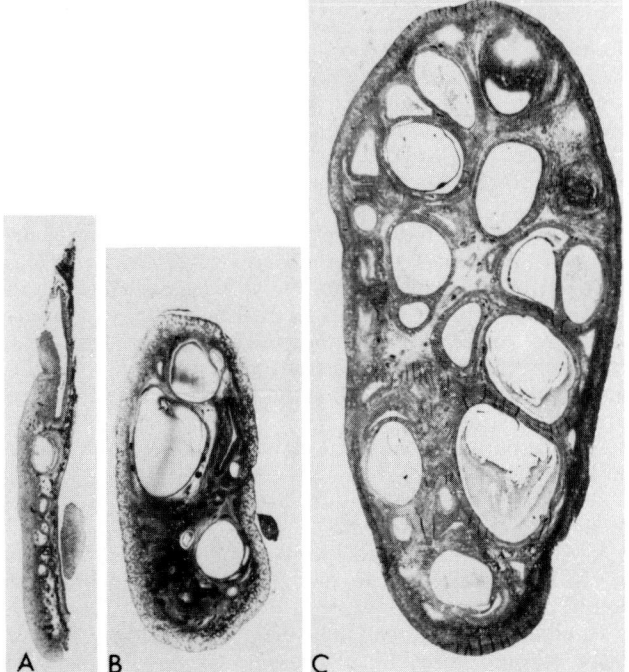

Figure 7–4. Ovaries of (*A*) newborn and (*B*) 10 month infant; (*C*) ovary of a 9 year old girl. All × 6.5. (Reproduced with permission of the authors and publishers of *Clin. Endocrinol. Metab.* 7:469, 1978.)

experienced pathologist is able, by histologic criteria, to assign an age (in days of an idealized 28-day cycle) to the corpus luteum.

The Postmenopausal Ovary

Successive cycles of ovulation and atresia deplete what Hertig (1944) has called the "ovarian capital" of oocytes. One of the associated changes is a progressive decline in ovarian weight from an average of about 14 g in the 4th decade to about 5 g in the 5th, 6th, and 7th decades.

Grossly, the postmenopausal ovary is a yellowish, lusterless structure with a wrinkled surface. Microscopically, the wrinkled appearance is seen to be associated with undulating gyrus-like formations in the cortex. The germinal epithelium persists and follows the undulations, during some of which connection of the epithelium with the surface is lost. This phenomenon, coupled with epithelial metaplasia, gives rise to either inclusion cysts, lined with epithelium, or islands of metaplastic epithelium.

Primordial follicles have largely disappeared from the cortex of the postmenopausal ovary. Rarely, a few immature follicles undergoing maturation and atresia may be seen at the corticomedullary junction for up to 5 years after the last menses. Occasional, small follicular cysts not containing oocytes are also found.

Striking changes occur in the cortical stroma, which becomes hyperplastic in ovaries of women after the age of 40. The extent of the process may vary from multinodular proliferations in the periphery of the ovary, in its milder form, to an enlarged ovary consisting almost entirely of hyperplastic nodules, in its most florid form.

Stromal hyperplasia and two other histologic lesions with which it is associated are of interest because of an increased frequency of these changes said to occur in ovaries from women with carcinomas of the endometrium or of the breast. The first of these other lesions consists of foci of cells containing lipid, referred to as "lutein cells," interspersed with areas of stromal hyperplasia. The second have been called cortical granulomas by Woll et al. (1948) and contain lipoids, lymphocytes, other mononuclear cells, and multinucleate giant cells arranged as in inflammatory tubercles. Whether cortical stromal hyperplasia can be equated with hormone synthesis by the postmenopausal ovary remains problematic, since estrone, the principal estrogen produced after the menopause, has been shown to be derived from extraovarian, extraadrenal aromatization of androstenedione. (See later.) Indeed, blood production rate of estrone remains unchanged after oophorectomy of some postmenopausal women, suggesting an adrenal origin of the precursor androgen.

Relative to the cortex, the medullary portion of the ovary, the repository of corpora albicantia and corpora candicantia, is proportionally larger in the postmenopausal ovary. As in the cortex, the stromal elements of the medulla become fibrotic, and blood vessels traversing this region become sclerotic and their lumens reduced.

Finally, hilar cells seem to be more readily apparent in ovaries from postmenopausal women. Indeed, virilizing syndromes secondary to hilar cell hyperplasia and neoplasia are more commonly seen in postmenopausal women. (See later.)

Function

Introduction

Normal ovarian function results in two major classes of products: sex steroid hormones and ova. Both are products of the follicular apparatus interacting with surrounding stromal elements under the stimulus of hormones secreted by the pituitary, which is controlled in turn by hypophysiotropic hormones. Developmentally, the hormones, especially the estrogens, are produced long before ovulation occurs for the first time, and these substances play an important role in stimulating both somatic and genital growth prior to the menarche. During the reproductive epoch, as we shall see, the estrogens act locally to mediate some of the effects of gonadotropins in stimulating follicular maturation and peripherally via the hypothalamus to modulate anterior pituitary gonadotropin secretion. In addition to their role in modulating gonadotropin secretion, the sex steroid hormones play a fundamental role in gamete transport and thus in fertilization as well as in conditioning the uterus for implantation of the zygote.

Biochemical, Physiologic, and Clinical Manifestations of Normal Ovarian Function

Before the Menarche

Indirect evidence suggests that gonadal-hypothalamic-pituitary interactions, mediated in part by sex steroid hormones, occur prior to puberty. Mean serum and urinary gonadotropin concentrations are higher after puberty than before, and it is generally agreed that these reflect changes in the degree to which a given quantity of exogenous or endogenous estrogen inhibits or stimulates pituitary gonadotropin secretion.

Recently, it has been found that the patterns differ when gonadotropin concentrations in blood collected from prepubertal, peripubertal, and postpubertal girls during sleep are compared. Perhaps this nocturnal variability will be shown to be an important factor in inducing pubertal changes.

Premenarchal ovarian function is manifest in accelerated linear growth (the pubertal growth "spurt") and by the appearance of the secondary sexual characteristics, including development of breasts, maturation of the genitalia, and appearance of pubic and axillary hair. When the ovary is absent or functions inadequately, puberty either fails to occur or progresses very slowly. Pubertal changes in these girls can be effectively reproduced by giving continuous estrogen alone, initially, followed by cyclic estrogen and progestogen treatment, indicating that sex steroid hormones mediate the role of the ovary (Ch. 9).

Age at onset of pubertal changes and their rates of progression are subject to a number of variables, so that no universally applicable normative values exist. Ideally, the data should be derived from longitudinal studies of representative subjects in the population under evaluation. When such information is available, according to Marshall and Tanner (1969), it is helpful in answering three clinical questions.

1. Is a patient's pubertal development within normal limits for her age?

2. Once puberty has begun, are breasts and pubic hair developing at a normal rate?

3. Are breasts and pubic hair developing in unison and in the proper relation to the growth spurt and to menarche?

Marshall and Tanner (1969) have described the ages at onset of, and rates of progression of, development for breasts and pubic hair, the ages of achievement of maximal velocity in linear growth, and the ages at menarche

Table 7-1. CORRELATIONS OF DEVELOPMENT OF BREASTS AND PUBIC HAIR WITH EACH OTHER AND WITH MAXIMAL LINEAR GROWTH AND MENARCHE

Tanner Stage	% in Stage at Time of Maximal Linear Growth		% in Stage at Time of Menarche		Stage of Pubic Hair	% in Stage for Breasts			
	For Breasts	For Pubic Hair	For Breasts	For Pubic Hair		2	3	4	5
1	0	23 (23)*	0	1	1	61	22	4	0
2	26 (26)	28 (51)	1 (1)	4 (5)	2	29	28	10	2
3	51 (77)	36 (87)	26 (27)	19 (24)	3	8	33	24	7
4	23 (100)	13 (100)	62 (89)	63 (86)	4	2	16	51	36
5	0 (100)	0 (100)	11 (100)	14 (100)	5	0	1	11	56

*Cumulative percentage.
Adapted from Marshall, W. A., and Tanner, J. M.: Variations in pattern of pubertal changes in girls. *Arch. Dis. Child. 44*:291, 1969.

observed in longitudinal studies at 3-month intervals of 192 British girls living in family groups in a children's home. Although Marshall and Tanner have not regarded these as universally applicable, we have found ourselves returning to this paper again and again in relation to specific constellations seen in the clinic. We have found the relationships among different events and the probabilities of concomitance described to be helpful in deciding whether to temporize or to undertake a complicated and expensive series of studies. For this reason, in Tables 7–1 and 7–2 we have reorganized the data from Marshall and Tanner in the fashion in which they have been useful to us.

To use the tabulated information effectively, the clinician must be familiar with the stages 1–5 for development of breasts and pubic hair shown in Figs. 7–6 and 7–7. Although these were evaluated from photographs in the study of Marshall and Tanner (1969), they are easily applicable to the clinical examination. The criteria that we have found useful for breasts are modified from those described by Marshall and Tanner as follows:

Stage 1: No palpable glandular tissue; areola not pigmented. Except for nipple, breast does not project from anterior chest wall.

Stage 2: Glandular tissue is palpable at least coextensively with the diameter of the areola; nipple and breast project as a single mound from the anterior chest wall.

Stage 3: Increased glandular tissue to palpation; breasts enlarged; areola increasing in diameter and becoming more darkly pigmented, but contours of breast and areola remain in a single plane.

Stage 4: Further enlargement; increased areola pigmentation; areola and nipple form a secondary mound above level of the breast.

Stage 5: Areola and nipple no longer project but have receded to make a smooth contour in profile view.

The stages for pubic hair related to change in quality, quantity, and distribution as follows:

Stage 1: None.

Stage 2: Occasional wispy strands, usually along the labia.

Stage 3: More, darker, coarser hair extending superiorly over the pubis.

Stage 4: Dark, coarse, curly hair, covering the mons pubis in the adult pattern, but not extending to medial aspects of thighs.

Stage 5: Mature; extends to thighs but otherwise remains in female pattern.

In Tables 7–1 and 7–2, the significance of ages has been minimized, in view of the variability from population to population. Mean ages at achievement of Tanner stages 1–5 for development of breasts and pubic hair are included to indicate the following:

1. Breast changes usually constitute the first signs of puberty, becoming apparent earlier on the average than the appearance of pubic hair. Once initiated, however, maturation of pubic hair progresses more rapidly.

2. The time required for completion of maturation averages approximately 4 years for breasts and approximately 3 years for pubic hair.

Rates of progression from one stage to another are very similar for breasts and pubic hair, averaging from 0.5 to 0.9 year from beginning through stage 4, but rate of advancement from stage 4 to 5 is more variable. In Table 7–1 it can be seen that appearance of breast changes heralds the onset of the pubertal growth spurt (maximal rate of linear growth). By the time breast development had reached stage 3, maximal rate of linear growth had been achieved by about 75% of the girls.

Finally, in Table 7–2 it can be seen that completion of maturation of the breasts before the appearance of pubic hair is an uncommon event. Similarly, completion of the

Table 7-2. MEAN AGE ± STANDARD DEVIATIONS AT ACHIEVEMENT OF STAGE AND MEAN TIME ± STANDARD DEVIATIONS FOR COMPLETION OF INDICATED STAGES OF DEVELOPMENT OF BREASTS AND PUBIC HAIR

Tanner Stage	Mean Age ± S.D. in Years at Achievement of Stage		Mean Time (95th–5th Percentile) in Years for Completion of Stage	
	For Breasts	For Pubic Hair	For Breasts	For Pubic Hair
1	Prepubertal	Prepubertal	Prepubertal	Prepubertal
2	11.15 ± 1.10	11.69 ± 1.21	0.86 (1.03–0.21)	0.63 (1.27–0.16)
3	12.15 ± 1.09	12.36 ± 1.10	0.89 (2.19–0.13)	0.51 (0.93–0.18)
4	13.11 ± 1.15	12.95 ± 1.01	1.96 (6.82–0.12)	1.30 (2.37–0.57)
5	15.33 ± 1.74	14.41 ± 1.12	Mature	Mature

Adapted from Marshall, W. A., and Tanner, J. M.: Variations in pattern of pubertal changes in girls. *Arch. Dis. Child. 44*:291, 1969.

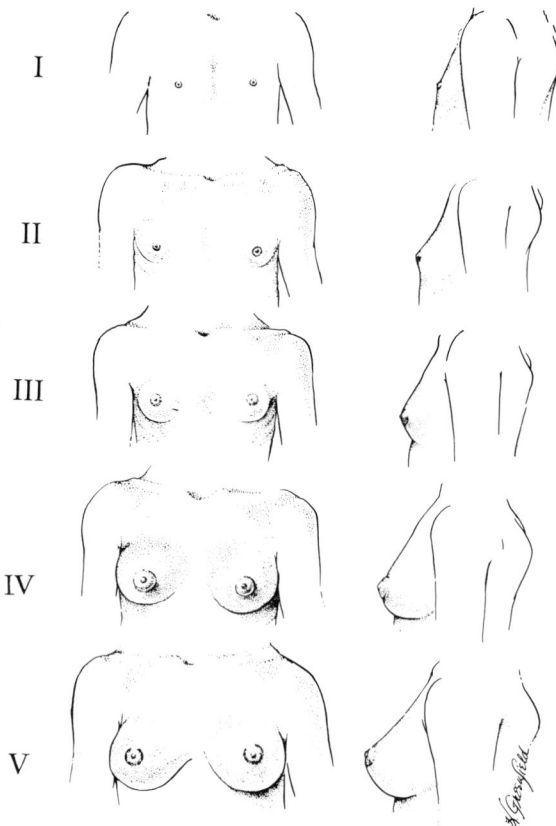

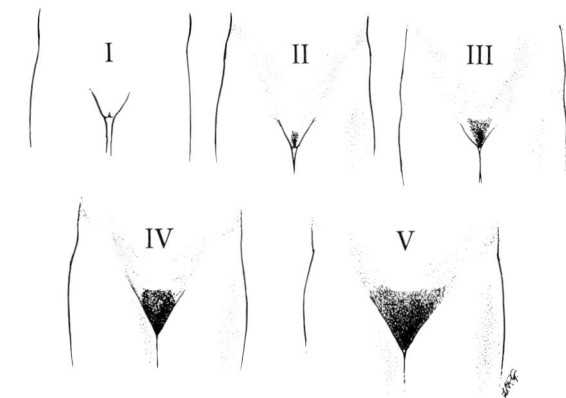

Figure 7–7. Diagrammatic representation of Tanner stages I to V for development of human pubic hair (adapted from Marshall, W. A., and Tanner, J. M.: *Arch. Dis. Child. 44*:291, 1969).

Figure 7–6. Diagrammatic representation of Tanner stages I to V of human breast maturation (adapted from Marshall, W. A., and Tanner, J. M.: *Arch. Dis. Child. 44*:291, 1969).

maturation of pubic hair before initiation of breast development is unusual. The former suggests a syndrome such as testicular feminization (Ch. 9), and the latter some virilizing syndrome.

It should be emphasized that wide individual differences are included within the spectrum of "normal" pubertal development. Further, evaluation of a number of indices has been shown to provide the most accurate measure of the progress of an individual in relation to others with respect to the chronology of maturation.

The Menarche

Data on ages at menarche and other pubertal milestones among North American girls were reported by Zacharias and coworkers (1970). The data were obtained from responses to questionnaires completed by 6217 students enrolled in 65 nursing schools in 35 states in the United States. Average ages at appearance of some secondary sexual characteristics, including menses, calculated for 4844 persons whose health records were judged to be normal are summarized in Table 7–3. The mean age at menarche for the entire group was 152 months (12.65 years) with a standard deviation of 14.1 months (1.17 years). Adding or subtracting three standard deviations of the mean age at menarche results in a range of from 9.14 to 16.16 years for individuals. After the menarche, occurrence of "regular" and "painful" menses, presumptive indicators of ovulatory cycles, was delayed by an average of 14 and 24 months respectively.

During pubescence, appearance of pubic hair either preceded or coincided with breast budding in girls from all

geographic regions. When ages for appearance of these two milestones are known for an individual, the nomogram in Fig. 7–8 may be used to predict an approximate age for onset of menses.

When the data from women with abnormal health records were stratified on the basis of the medical reasons for their exclusion from the normal group, obesity was found to be the only factor significantly affecting age at menarche. Menarche occurred earlier among girls whose body weight exceeded normal by up to 30%, consistent with the long-held impression that menarcheal girls tend to be heavier (and taller) than premenarcheal girls of the same age.

Additional evidence that body weight is related to age at menarche was adduced by Frisch and her colleagues, who analyzed data on growth and development collected in three separate studies involving a total of 169 girls. They observed that mean body weight (circa 48 kg) did not change

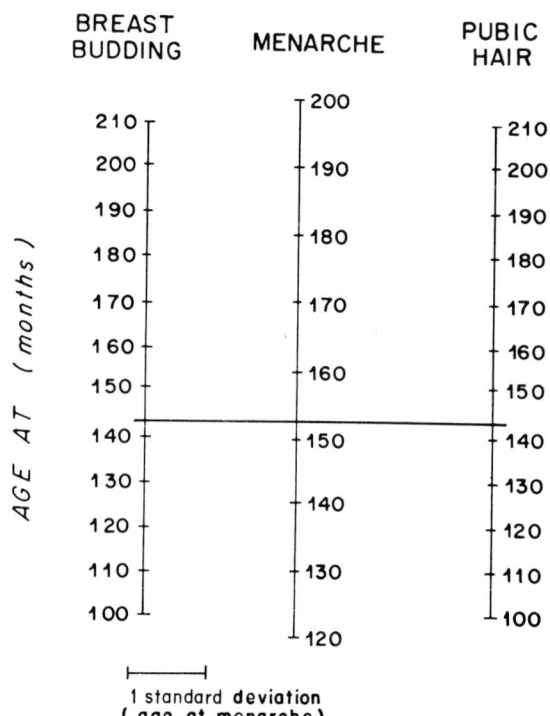

Figure 7–8. Nomogram for estimating age at menarche when age at appearance of breast budding and pubic hair is known. (From Zacharias, L., et al.: *Am. J. Obstet. Gynecol. 108*:833, 1970.)

Table 7-3. AVERAGE AGES (MONTHS) FOR APPEARANCE OF SEVERAL SECONDARY SEXUAL CHARACTERISTICS AMONG PUBESCENT GIRLS FROM REGIONS INDICATED

Geographical Regions*	No.†	Pubic Hair	Breast Budding	Axillary Hair	Menarche	Regular Menses	Painful Menses
East Central	239	141.0	141.7	143.5	149.1	161.1	170.7
Middle Atlantic	1,265	141.4	142.2	144.1	151.0	164.7	173.1
New England	644	142.1	143.1	145.6	151.5	164.2	175.6
North Central	438	142.4	143.6	145.2	152.1	165.3	176.0
Southeast	579	143.4	143.4	144.7	152.3	166.3	176.3
Southwest	449	142.3	143.1	145.6	152.5	165.5	180.0
Midcentral	672	143.7	143.4	145.5	152.9	166.5	175.7
Northwest	558	143.9	143.7	145.4	153.0	165.6	177.5
Total Normal		142.5	143.0	144.9	151.8	165.2	175.4
Standard Deviation		13.9	14.5	15.1	14.1	24.2	29.8
Standard Error		0.21	0.21	0.23	0.20	0.39	0.65
Sample Size	4,844	4,390	4,683	4,395	4,844	3,830	2,072

* Geographical regions: East Central–Illinois, Kentucky, Ohio, West Virginia; Middle Atlantic–District of Columbia, Maryland, New Jersey, New York, Pennsylvania; New England–Connecticut, Massachusetts, New Hampshire, Rhode Island, Vermont; North Central–Michigan, Minnesota, Wisconsin; Southeast–Alabama, Florida, Louisiana, Mississippi, Tennessee, Virginia; Southwest–Arizona, Southern California, Oklahoma, Texas, Utah; Midcentral–Iowa, Kansas, Missouri, North Dakota; Northwest–Northern California, Montana, Oregon, Washington.

†No.–number of subjects.

From Zacharias, L. et al.: Sexual maturation in contemporary American girls. *Amer. J. Obstet. Gynecol.* 108:833, 1970.

significantly as menarcheal age increased and interpreted this "unvarying mean weight at menarche" to be consistent with "a direct relation between body weight and menarche." Subsequently, Frisch and coworkers have proposed that a critical body weight (about 48 kg) corresponding to a critical metabolic rate that is related in turn to a critical proportion of body fat acts as a "trigger" for the menarche.

A mean body weight of 47.2 kg at menarche, similar to the "critical weight" proposed by Frisch and associates, was noted by Zacharias and coworkers (1976) in a prospective longitudinal study of physical growth and maturation among 633 girls in Newton, Massachusetts. This mean represented a wide range of body weights, however, and comparisons of correlation coefficients showed menarcheal age to be more closely related to height than to weight. Among girls of the same height at menarche, younger ones tended to be heavier or stouter and older ones tended to be lighter or thinner, suggesting that age at menarche might correlate better with "shape" than with height or weight. Indeed, a highly significant correlation coefficient was found for age at menarche with a measure of shape called a ponderal index, obtained by dividing height by the cube root of weight.

In summary, although the question of whether a cause and effect relationship exists between body weight and age at menarche remains debatable, existence of a correlation between the two seems to be established. Moreover, the "trigger" for pubescence and the menarche remains obscure.

After the Menarche: The Normal Menstrual Cycle

Events in the normal menstrual cycle result from interactions among the hypothalamus, pituitary, ovaries, and genital tract. Understanding how the ovaries coordinate these interactions is essential for diagnosis and rational therapy of disordered ovarian function in sexually mature women. Accordingly, the relation of normal ovarian function to events occurring at each of these loci will be considered in detail in the following sections.

Length. Folklore associates the length of the menstrual cycle with the duration of a lunar cycle, but there is no evidence to support this association, and in fact the woman with a 28-day cycle is the exception rather than the rule. There are numerous studies of the temporal aspects of the "normal" menstrual cycle: The most recent and most comprehensive one is that of Vollman. The large majority of the cycles fall between 25 and 30 days in length, but the distribution within this range is skewed toward cycles with 30 days. The greatest variability is found in the years following menarche and the years immediately preceding the menopause, during which the cycle length is greatly increased mainly because of the frequency of anovulation and of prolonged proliferative phases. The smallest variability is found between the ages of 20 and 30, but, interestingly enough, in all studies in which this factor was evaluated, there was a clear-cut decrease in the length of the cycle with increasing age. There have been several studies of the relative length of the proliferative and secretory phases, all of them indicating that the secretory phase is remarkably constant in duration and lasts approximately 13 days, while the length of the preovulatory phase is much more variable. In one study, 79.6% of the cycles had a preovulatory phase lasting 10–16 days, whereas 95% of the luteal phases fell within this range. There was a poor correlation between the length of two consecutive cycles, but when the length of six preceding cycles is known, the length of subsequent cycles can be accurately predicted. Hormonal determinants of the length of the menstrual cycle will be described in connection with corpus luteum function.

Blood Hormone Levels During the Normal Menstrual Cycle

Ovarian Steroid Hormones. Most of the earlier information about the secretion of the ovarian hormones was derived from studies of the excretion of their urinary metabolites. There are major limitations to this approach, however, since urinary metabolites represent only a small and variable fraction of their secreted precursors. More importantly, most of these metabolites are derived from multiple precursors, thereby making deductions about levels and secretory processes hazardous, if not impossible. The advent of the radioimmunoassays made it possible to measure blood steroids, and these methods have rapidly supplanted the urinary methods. The situation, however, remains complicated by the fact that most of the ovarian steroids are also secreted by the adrenal, or derived from adrenal secretory products. In many clinical situations, then, it is difficult if not impossible to determine what comes from the adrenal and what from the ovary. Much has been learned in this respect from patient studies in which the contribution by either the ovary or the adrenal can be ignored (i.e., following ovariectomy or adrenalectomy), but this does not solve the problem in the individual patient. Clinically, the question of the relative contributions of the adrenal and the ovary is most frequently of importance in the patient with evidence of hypersecretion of androgens when the answer to this question is critical for therapy. In such clinical situations, suppression of ovarian or adrenal function by the administration by gonadal or adrenal steroids has often been used to resolve the question of the origin of the increased androgens. This approach, however, must be used with caution since often it will lead to confusing and misleading results. Theoretically, the preferred approach to the solution of this problem is direct catheterization of the ovarian or adrenal vein. Unfortunately, this approach remains technically difficult to carry out and is not without danger.

The Concept of the Prohormone in Gonadal Physiology and Pathology. The application of isotopic dilution methods to the estimation of the secretion rates of the ovarian hormones, besides offering quantitatively more reliable solutions, has brought forward new insights into the complexity of the processes involved in the secretion and the metabolism of these hormones. It also has led to the formulation of novel concepts, such as production rates (PR) distinct from secretory rates (SR) and metabolic clearance rates (MCR). More importantly, these studies have led us to a clearer realization of the importance of the prohormone concept in gonadal physiology and pathology. Since familiarity with these concepts is of importance to the serious student of ovarian function, a short consideration of them is useful.

The secretory rate of hormone $A(SR_A)$ is the amount of A released by the endocrine gland into the circulation per unit of time. Hormone A may, however, also be derived from the peripheral conversion of a second hormone, B, secreted either by the same or by another endocrine gland. (Refer to Fig. 7–9, in which the example of peripheral conversion of Δ_4-androstenedione [hormone B] to estrone [hormone A] has been depicted.) Hormone B, in this instance, is said to be a prohormone of A, and this pathway of formation of A will be referred to as the prohormone pathway.

The production rate in the blood of $A(PR_A)$ is the total rate at which A enters *de novo* into the circulation; conversely, in a steady state, it can also be defined as the rate by which the hormone is irreversibly removed from the circulation. When a hormone derives exclusively from glandular secretion, the SR and the PR are obviously the same, but when the hormone originates from peripheral metabolism as well as from secretion, the PR will be higher than the SR.

The MCR is a concept related to that of the blood PR; it equals the volume of blood that, per unit of time, is irreversibly cleared of the hormone. It follows from this definition that the blood PR will equal the MCR multiplied by the concentration (c) of the hormone in the blood (PR = MCR × c). For different hormones, the MCR may be very different, but it is relatively constant for individuals within a specific clinical group. Consequently, within such a group PR's of a hormone may be assumed to vary as their concentrations. SR's and PR's of steroid hormones can be measured by several experimental approaches. The most frequently used approach involves the intravenous infusion of a radioactive hormone until equilibrium of radioactivity in the blood has been obtained. At this time the total entry of the hormone into the circulation can be calculated (its PR) from the experimental data. In cases in which a plasma steroid is derived from more than one precursor, infusions of each of the precursors make it possible to calculate the relative contribution of each of these to the blood PR of the hormone.

The concept of the prohormone and the prohormone pathways is perhaps of more importance for the study of the ovarian hormones than for any other endocrine function. It is of special importance for the origin of the estrogens in the circulation. In women with normal ovarian function most of the estradiol in the circulation derives from the direct secretion of estradiol by the growing follicle or the corpus luteum. Little, if any, estradiol originates via the prohormone pathway (from the conversion of testosterone to estradiol). Estrone, on the other hand, is secreted only to a minor extent, and most of the estrone in the circulation originates from prohormones: estradiol (to a minor extent) and androstenedione.

In normal men and women, approximately 1% of the secreted androstenedione is converted to estrone. The site of this conversion of androgens to estrogens is not completely known, but it is important to emphasize that it is independent of the presence of ovaries, testes, or adrenal or pituitary glands. A major site of the conversion of androstenedione to estrone is in the fat, and in a significant number of obese women, the conversion of androstenedione to estrone is significantly greater. Other factors that influence the

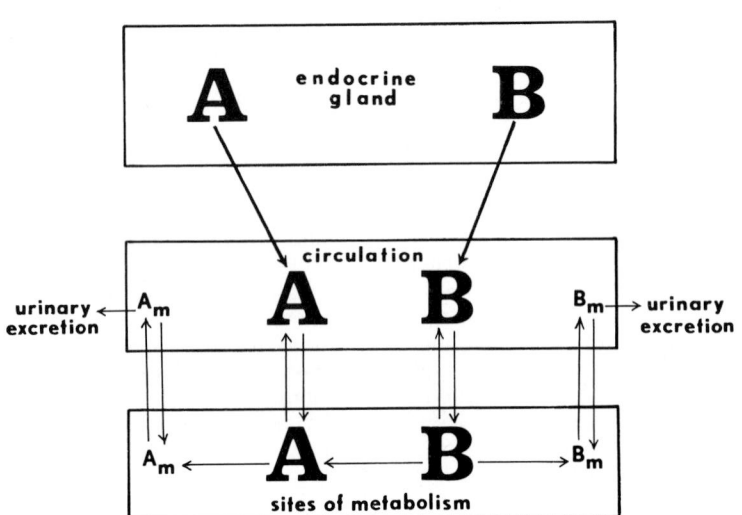

Figure 7–9. A or B may be secreted by the ovaries or adrenal. A_m and B_m represent inactive metabolites of A and B, respectively.

conversion of androstenedione to estrone are age, liver function, heart failure, and thyroid dysfunction.

Two examples will suffice to illustrate the importance of the prohormone pathway in ovarian physiopathology.

1. Ovaries of menopausal women do not secrete estrogens, yet menopausal women have significant levels of estrone in their circulation. Most, if not all, of the estrone originates via the prohormone pathway, specifically from the peripheral conversion of androstenedione secreted by the adrenals. Estrone has low biologic activity and the amounts of estrone circulating in normal menopausal women are insufficient to prevent the appearance of hot flashes and other symptoms of estrogen deprivation resulting from the cessation of ovarian function. In certain circumstances, such as in obese women for instance, the fraction of androstenedione converting to estrone increases, yielding enough of the estrogen to produce endometrial proliferation and bleeding.

2. In normal women, the sequence of events during the menstrual cycle is dependent upon the continuous interplay between stimulation of the ovaries by the gonadotropins and feedback of the estrogens to the hypothalamus and the pituitary. Under normal circumstances the amount of estrone generated by the prohormone pathway is small and does not play a significant role in the feedback, but under abnormal conditions (e.g., obesity) the amount may become sufficient to interfere with normal feedback mechanisms and produce disturbances of the ovarian cycle.

Table 7–4 summarizes the concentrations, the MCR's, the PR's, and the ovarian SR's of steroids in normal women.

Changes in the Ovarian Steroids During the Normal Menstrual Cycle

Estrogens. Fig. 7–10 illustrates the changes in the plasma estradiol during the normal menstrual cycle. In the early period of follicular development (during menses), the levels of estradiol remain low. Approximately 1 week before the LH peak there is an initial slow and then a more rapid rise of estradiol, reaching a peak the day before the LH peak or, less frequently, coinciding with it. There is a sudden drop in the estrogen concentrations concomitant with the ovulatory rise in LH. Since rupture of the follicle occurs approximately 24–36 hours after the LH peak, the estrogen drop actually precedes ovulation. During the luteal phase, estradiol (E_2) rises again, reaching a maximum approximately 5–8 days after the rupture of the follicle.

The changes in estrone (E_1) are similar but E_2/E_1 ratios change appreciably during the menstrual cycle due to the fact that most of the estrone in the circulation is derived from prohormones other than estradiol (Fig. 7–11). A small fraction of the estrone level in the plasma is derived from the metabolism of secreted estradiol, but the majority of estrone in circulation is derived from the conversion to estrone of androstenedione (of adrenal or ovarian origin). Consequently, the ratio of estradiol to estrone will fluctuate depending on the relative contribution of each of these pathways. As an example, at the time of menstruation when the secretion of estradiol by the follicles is minimal, most of the estrone is derived from adrenal precursors producing low E_2/E_1 ratios.

Recent studies of estradiol and estrone concentrations in the venous effluent from the two ovaries have shown that the rise of estradiol reflects almost completely the secretion of estrogen by the dominant follicle. Similarly, the rising levels of estrogen during the luteal phase reflect secretory activity of the ovary containing the corpus luteum (Fig. 7–12).

Progesterone and Related Substances. The changes in progesterone during the normal menstrual cycle are illus-

Table 7–4. CONCENTRATION, METABOLIC CLEARANCE RATES, PRODUCTION RATES, AND OVARIAN SECRETION RATES OF STEROIDS IN BLOOD

Compound	"MCR"* of Compound in Peripheral Plasma, liters/day	Phase of Menstrual Cycle	Concentration in Plasma, μg/100 ml	PR** of Circulating Compound, mg/day	SR† by Both Ovaries, mg/day
Estradiol	1,350	Early follicular	0.006	0.081	0.07
		Late follicular	0.033–0.070	0.445–0.945	0.4–0.8
		Midluteal	0.020	0.270	0.25
Estrone	2,210	Early follicular	0.005	0.110	0.08
		Late follicular	0.015–0.030	0.331–0.662	0.25–0.50
		Midluteal	0.011	0.243	0.16
Progesterone	2,200	Follicular	0.095	2.1	1.5
		Luteal	1.13	25.0	24.0
20α-hydroxyprogesterone	2,300	Follicular	0.05	1.1	0.8
		Luteal	0.25	5.8	3.3
17-hydroxyprogesterone		Early follicular	0.03	0.6	0–0.3
	2,000	Late follicular	0.20	4.0	3–4
		Midluteal	0.20	4.0	3–4
Androstenedione	2,010		0.159	3.2	0.8–1.6
Testosterone	690		0.038	0.26	
Dehydroisoandrosterone	1,640		0.490	8.0	0.3–3

*Metabolic clearance rate.
**Production rate.
†Secretion rate.

From Tagatz, G. E., and Gurpide, E.: Hormone secretion by the normal human ovary, In *Handbook of Physiology*, Sect. 7: Endocrinology. Vol. II, Pt. 1. American Physiological Society, Greep, R. O., and Astwood, E. B. (eds.), Baltimore, Williams & Wilkins, 1973, pp. 603–613.

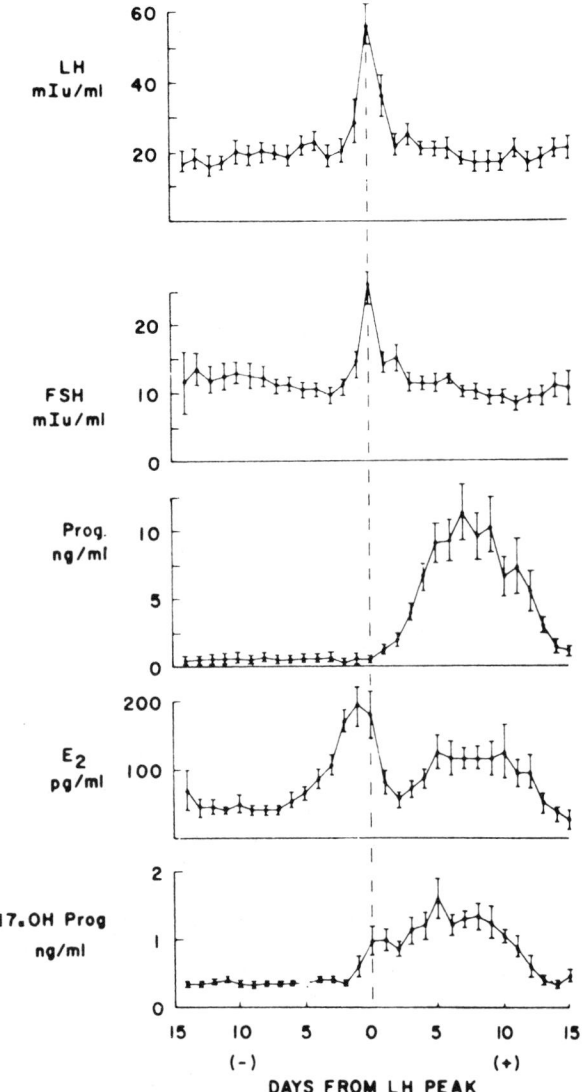

Figure 7–10. Mean LH, FSH, progesterone, estradiol, and 17-OH progesterone levels in blood specimens collected daily throughout presumptively ovulatory menstrual cycles from normal women. Cycle days were synchronized around the day of the LH peak = day 0. (Reproduced with permission of the authors and publishers of *Am. J. Obstet. Gynecol.* 111:947, 1971.)

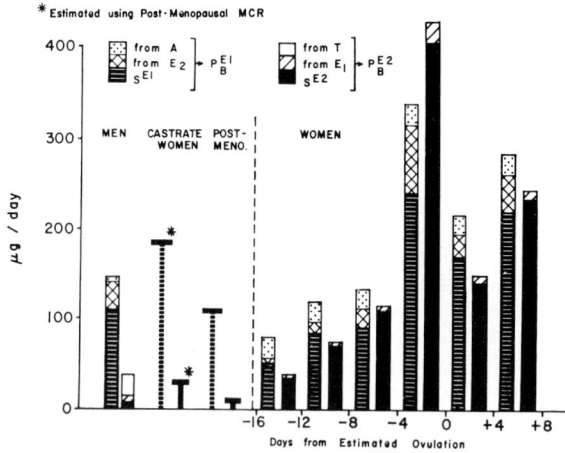

Figure 7–11. Metabolic clearance rates and blood production rates of estrone and estradiol, indicating relative amounts derived from ovarian secretion and from peripheral conversion of precursors. (From Baird, D. T., et al.: *Recent Progr. Hormone Res.* 25:611, 1969.)

trated in Fig. 7–10. Small amounts of progesterone are present in the circulation prior to the LH surge, and some of these may be of ovarian origin since large amounts of progesterone are found in the follicular fluid of the preovulatory follicle. (See later.) The bulk of progesterone in the circulation during the proliferative phase, however, appears to be derived from extraglandular conversion of adrenal pregnenolone and pregnenolone sulfate to progesterone and also from the secretion of small amounts of progesterone by the adrenals. At the beginning of the LH surge, there is a small initial increase in the concentration of progesterone, followed by a second major increase that parallels the increase in estrogens during the luteal phase. The timing of the early rise in progesterone makes it likely that this rise is the result of a direct effect of the high levels of LH upon granulosa cells of the yet unruptured but luteinizing ovarian follicle; the mechanism by which the progesterone secreted is turned on and the estrogen secretion is turned off remains unknown.

Comparisons of steroid hormone levels in specimens of ovarian and peripheral venous blood collected simultaneously have shown that throughout the cycle progesterone is secreted in small amounts by both ovaries. From the middle to late follicular phase, however, concentrations are higher in venous blood from the ovary containing the dominant follicle, and throughout the luteal phase, levels are higher in venous blood from the ovary containing the corpus luteum.

Although peripheral blood levels remain relatively constant, antral fluid progesterone levels rise as preovulatory follicle growth progresses during the last half of the follicular phase. Results of *in vitro* studies are consistent with the concept that granulosa cells in preovulatory follicles, responding to LH, secrete progesterone into antral fluid during preovulatory follicle growth. The amount produced is insufficient to alter peripheral blood levels significantly until after ovulation, however.

Rising peripheral blood levels of 17α-hydroxyprogesterone during the late follicular phase also reflect the secretory activity of the ovary containing the dominant follicle. Blood levels of 17α-hydroxyprogesterone throughout the luteal phase reflect the secretory activity of the ovary containing the corpus luteum. Although 20α-dihydroxyprogesterone is secreted by the ovary, the contribution of secreted hormone to blood levels is not known. There is no evidence that 20β-dihydroprogesterone is secreted by the ovary, although significant amounts of this compound circulate during the luteal phase; it is assumed that 20β-dihydroprogesterone is derived from secreted progesterone.

Changes in serum concentrations of Δ-5-pregnenolone and of 17α-OH-Δ-5-pregnenolone throughout the normal menstrual cycle have been reported. Both compounds were found to be lower in the follicular phase than in the luteal phase.

Androgens

Androstenedione. Androstenedione is secreted both by the ovary and by the adrenal, and the relative contribution of these two sources to plasma androstenedione changes with the time of the day and the phase of the ovarian cycle. Adrenal androstenedione exhibits a *diurnal* rhythm paralleling that of cortisone, but there seems to be no variation of the adrenal secretion of androstenedione during the menstrual cycle. The growing graafian follicle secretes androstenedione, which is reflected by an elevation of plasma androstenedione (and a twofold increase in its production) near the midcycle (Fig. 7–13). During the luteal phase there

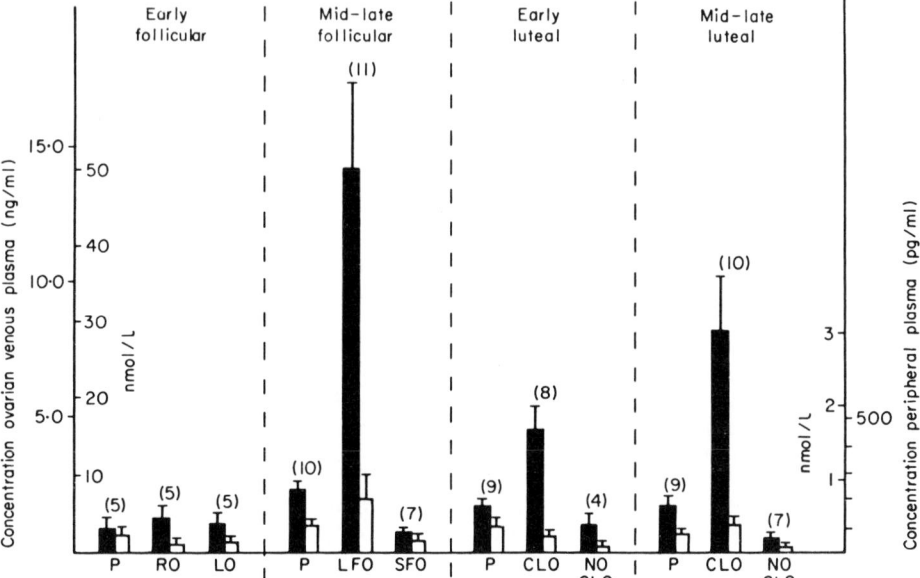

Figure 7–12. Concentrations of estradiol (solid bars) and estrone (open bars) in peripheral (P) and ovarian (O) venous plasma from ovary containing dominant follicle (LFO), the contralateral ovary (SFO), the ovary containing corpus luteum (CLO) or no corpus luteum (No CLO) sampled during follicular or luteal phases. (Reproduced with permission of the author and publishers of *Clin. Endocrinol.* 4:259, 1975.)

is a second peak in this secretion of androstenedione reflecting the secretion of androstenedione by the corpus luteum.

Testosterone. Studies of the ovarian venous and adrenal venous effluent have demonstrated that both the ovary and the adrenal secrete small amounts of testosterone. The majority of the testosterone in the circulation derives from the metabolism of androstenedione, however, and fluctuations during the menstrual cycle are minimal.

Dihydrotestosterone. Dihydrotestosterone is secreted by the ovary in small amounts, but the majority of dihydrotestosterone in the circulation derives from the conversion of

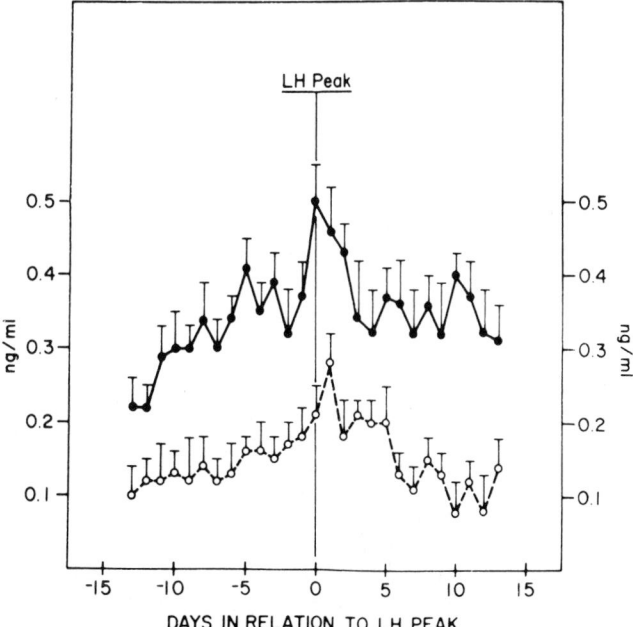

Figure 7–13. Mean daily levels of serum androstenedione during consecutive cycles in six premenopausal women. In one cycle (open circles) 0.5 mg dexamethasone was given four times daily to suppress adrenal steroid hormone secretion; in the other (closed circles) no treatment was given. Values have been synchronized around day 0, the day of the preovulatory LH surge. Bars represent one standard error of the mean. (Reproduced with permission of the author and publishers of *J. Clin. Endocrinol. Metab.* 39:340, 1974.)

androstenedione and testosterone to dihydrotestosterone. In the male, testosterone conversion accounts for approximately 70% of plasma dihydrotestosterone, but in the female the major prohormone for plasma dihydrotestosterone appears to be androstenedione.

Δ-5-androstenediol is an intermediate in the conversion of dehydroisoandrosterone (dehydroepiandrosterone) to testosterone. Small amounts of Δ-5-androstenediol are secreted by the ovary and the adrenal, but the vast majority is derived from secreted dehydroepiandrosterone (DHEA).

DHEA and DHEA Sulfate. There are only minor fluctuations in blood DHEA and DHEA sulfate levels during the menstrual cycle. This is not unexpected since small amounts of DHEA and DHEA sulfate are secreted by the ovary, and the bulk comes from the adrenal. The biologic role of DHEA in women appears uncertain. It serves as a prohormone for the production of Δ-5-androstenediol and, to a minor extent, for the production of androstenedione.

It is of interest to note that in women receiving glucocorticoid replacement therapy following adrenalectomy or for Addison's disease, the cycle proceeds normally and that the adrenal androgens are therefore not necessary for normal reproductive function.

Estrogens and androgens in the circulation are bound to a specific steroid hormone–binding globulin (SHBG), and it is assumed that the protein-bound hormone is inactive. SHBG is assumed to be synthesized in the liver, and its synthesis is increased by estrogen and thyroid hormone but decreased by testosterone and thyroid hormone deficiency. Dihydrotestosterone has the highest binding affinity for SHBG; estradiol and testosterone have approximately one third of the affinity of dihydrotestosterone, Δ-5-androstenedione binds also but less tightly to SHBG; androstenedione and DHEA are not bound. Progesterone is not bound to SHBG.

There are other hormonal changes during the normal menstrual cycle that are secondary to the effects of ovarian steroids on other endocrine glands. During the luteal phase, there is an increase in aldosterone that probably is a compensatory mechanism to overcome the inhibitory effect of progesterone upon the sodium-retaining activity of aldosterone. Renin, on the other hand, has a midcycle maximum, and available evidence indicates that this is secondary to estrogen changes.

Peptide Hormones

Gonadotropins and Prolactin. Daily patterns of FSH and LH have been determined in large groups of normal women. Although individual characteristics disappear in averaging the values for a group of women, characteristic patterns, as shown in Figs. 7–10 and 7–14, are obtained when the daily values are synchronized around the day of the midcycle preovulatory peak of LH and the means of these are calculated. LH levels rise slightly through the follicular phase, increase dramatically during the midcycle surge, and decline during the luteal phase. FSH levels begin to rise progressively during the late luteal phase of the preceding cycle, reach maximum levels in the first half of the proliferative phase, and decline during the preovulatory period. At midcycle, there is a modest surge of FSH, usually coinciding with the LH surge, temporarily interrupting the decline in FSH, which then resumes and reaches a low point during the luteal phase to rise again prior to menses.

No characteristic changes have been reported to occur in the blood levels of prolactin (PRL) during spontaneous ovulatory cycles. Recently, some of the earlier controversies have been resolved, and it appears that PRL levels are consistently higher during the luteal phase than during the follicular phase.

Other Pituitary Hormones. There have been several studies of growth hormone (GH) in the course of the menstrual cycle, but definitive conclusions are difficult to make. There seems to be a peak at midcycle, but other changes are seen inconsistently. In one study ACTH levels were found to be declining during the follicular phase to a nadir 2 days prior to the midcycle LH surge period following a significant peak coinciding with the LH surge. In the same study, no significant changes in TSH were observed. Recent studies indicate that in monkeys as well as humans, neurophysin levels exhibit a maximum at midcycle, either coinciding

with or following the midcycle LH peak. This finding is of interest since estrogen neurophysin is a hypothalamic secretory product and therefore may reflect hypothalamic activity.

Miscellaneous Hormones

Melatonin. Recent studies of melatonin during normal cycles in women have shown a biphasic pattern with high levels at the onset of the cycle and low levels extending from a few days before to a few days after the LH rise.

Relaxin. More than 50 years ago, relaxin was first isolated from sow corpora lutea and later from corpora lutea of other species. The hormone has been purified to near homogeneity; it is a polypeptide with a molecular weight of approximately 6000 and is capable of eliciting a specific immune response. During gestation, relaxin increases in the tissues and blood of several animals, including humans. It was not detected in plasma of nonpregnant women even during the late luteal phase, however. Although recent studies suggest that human relaxin inhibits myometrial contractions, its role in human physiology remains in doubt.

Hormonal Control of the Normal Menstrual Cycle

Hormonal Control of Gonadotropin Secretion. Based on the frequency of their fluctuations in the blood, three types of gonadotropin secretions may be distinguished:

1. The low-frequency changes during the normal menstrual cycle have already been discussed in detail. Because they recur approximately every 30 days, these have been called "trigintan" or "circatrigintan."

2. The gonadotropins also exhibit high-frequency changes superimposed on these low-frequency changes, with pulses repeating themselves approximately every 70–100 min. These have been called "circhoral" changes by Knobil since they repeat themselves approximately every hour.

3. In addition to the "trigintan" and "circhoral" changes in the gonadotropins, there are changes of intermediate frequency, called "diurnal" because they recur every 24 hours in a fashion similar to the diurnal changes in the adrenal steroid levels. In normal women, the magnitude of these changes is small, but in young women going through puberty, the diurnal changes are very marked and characterized by important peaks in LH and FSH during sleep. Little is known about the factors controlling the diurnal changes, and they will not be discussed further.

The "trigintan" and "circhoral" changes in the gonadotropin secretion are the result of a dynamic interplay between the central nervous system, which puts out a pulsatile signal, and the ovarian steroids, which modify this signal. These changes will be discussed in detail.

Central Nervous System Control. Knobil, Ferin, and others have shown that the area in the central nervous system of the rhesus monkey (and presumably of humans) that is responsible for the control of gonadotropin secretion resides in a small circumscribed part of the hypothalamus, the medial basal hypothalamus. When this area is isolated from the rest of the central nervous system by creating a hypothalamic-pituitary island the cycle continues and negative and positive feedback operate normally. Similarly, the "circhoral" pulses continue unchanged, suggesting that all elements necessary for normal ovarian function are contained within this island. These studies do not exclude the possibility that input from other parts of the brain modifies gonadotropin secretion, however. In fact, both experimental work in animals and clinical data suggest that other parts of the central nervous system have both positive and negative effects upon gonadotropin secretion.

Although evidence for other hormones remains controversial, a single hormone, the gonadotropin-releasing hor-

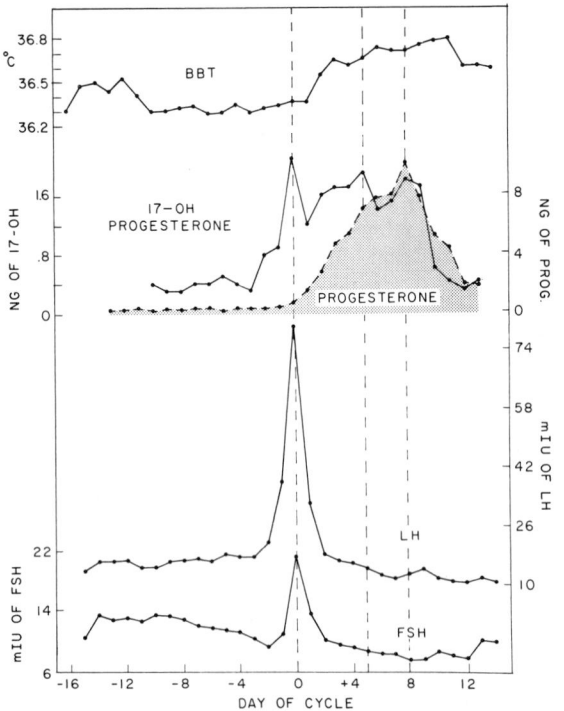

Figure 7–14. Mean daily plasma FSH, LH, progesterone, and 17α-OH progesterone concentrations and basal body temperatures during 16 presumptively ovulatory cycles from 15 young women. (Adapted from Ross, G. T., et al.: *Recent Progr. Hormone Res.* 26:1, 1970.)

mone (GnRH) secreted by the medial basal hypothalamus and reaching the pituitary via the hypothalamic-pituitary portal system, controls pituitary synthesis and release of both FSH and LH. GnRH is synthesized within neurons in the medial basal hypothalamus and is secreted into the capillaries of the hypothalamic portal system. GnRH has been localized in other parts of the brain, and it is assumed that in these parts GnRH may function as a neurotransmitter. Recent studies involving the collection of hypothalamic-pituitary portal venous blood have shown that GnRH is secreted in a pulsatile fashion, though the exact frequency of these pulses remains to be determined.

Recent work from the laboratories of Knobil and Ferin has demonstrated that the pulsatile pattern of secretion of GnRH is fundamental for the control of gonadotropin secretion. This concept arises from attempts to reactivate gonadotropin secretion following either destruction of the arcuate nucleus or complete stalk section. Knobil and associates have shown that pituitary secretion of FSH and LH could not be reactivated by the administration of GnRH unless the hormone was administered in a pulsatile fashion (6 min on and 54 min off). A continuous infusion of GnRH or pulses of a frequency much less than the ideal frequency failed to stimulate the gonadotropes to secrete FSH and LH (Fig. 7–15). Similarly, the positive and negative feedback effects of the estrogens could be restored only following reactivation of gonadotropin secretion by pulsatile administration of GnRH. In fact, normal cycles could be produced without changing the amplitude or frequency of the pulses in such animals.

Ovarian Sex Steroid Control. The circhoral pulses of GnRH and of FSH and LH are inherent to the operation of an endogenous clock mechanism within the medial basal hypothalamus. The magnitude and the frequency of the pulses, however, are modulated by feedback from the ovarian hormones.

Negative Feedback. It has been known for a long time that ovarian steroids, principally estrogens, modulate the secretion of gonadotropins. This is evident from the well-known increase in FSH and LH as estrogens decline after castration or during the menopause, and the decrease in FSH and LH following the administration of estrogens to castrate or postmenopausal women. Although progesterone and androgens in large amounts will produce a negative feedback upon gonadotropin secretion, it is likely that the estrogens are the most important component in the negative feedback effect of the ovarian steroids.

Positive Feedback. In addition to a negative feedback effect upon FSH and LH secretion, gonadal hormones also exert a positive effect on gonadotropin secretion. This positive effect is a cardinal factor in the regulation of the menstrual cycle, since the LH surge preceding ovulation is triggered by the rising level of estrogen in the late proliferative phase. The observation made by Hohlweg in 1934 that estrogen injections induce ovulation in immature rats may be regarded as the first evidence for a positive feedback of estrogens on LH secretion. Recent work has conclusively established the effect of estrogen on LH secretion and has added much qualitative and quantitative information about the nature of this relationship. The positive feedback effect of estrogen upon gonadotropin secretion is more marked for LH than for FSH, and in a number of experimental conditions, the effect of estrogens upon the gonadotropins is limited to LH. Progesterone, on the other hand, appears equally effective in its positive feedback effect upon FSH and LH. It is likely that the small rise in progesterone at the time of ovulation enhances and prolongs the feedback of estrogens upon FSH and LH, but at other times estrogen appears to be the critical determinant in the feedback process. In contrast to the negative feedback of estrogens, which operates within minutes, the positive feedback of estrogens upon FSH and LH requires sustained estrogen stimulation, and a significant rise in the LH is not seen before 24 hours.

The exact locus of the feedback effect of the ovarian steroids remains in doubt. Results of earlier work involving the direct instillation of estrogen into the hypothalamus favored a hypothalamic site. More recent work from the laboratories of Knobil and Ferin suggests, however, that the primary locus of estrogen action is the pituitary rather than the hypothalamus. Although at this time it is difficult to reconcile all experimental results, it is likely that estrogens exert their feedback effect by a dual mechanism, by modulating the frequency and magnitude of the GnRH pulses, and by regulating pituitary sensitivity to GnRH stimulation.

In addition to sex steroid hormones, there is evidence that classic neurotransmitters may modulate gonadotropin secretion. Thus, experiments in rodents have clearly indicated a role for catecholamines, norepinephrine, and dopamine in the control of gonadotropin secretion. Although it is likely that catecholamines play the same role in the monkey and in the human, the nature of this control and its pathways remain obscure.

The recent discovery of the endorphins suggests the possi-

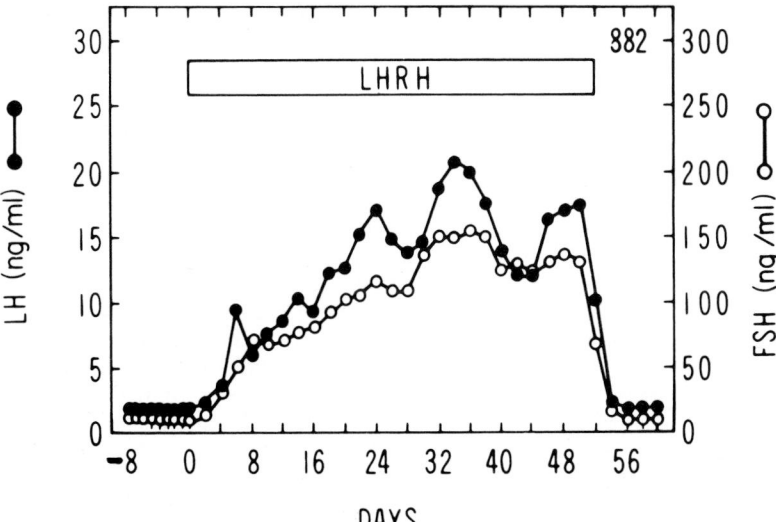

Figure 7–15. Blood LH (closed circles) and FSH (open circles) prior to, during, and following intermittent intravenous infusion of 1 μg of GnRH for 6 minutes of every hour in an ovariectomized rhesus monkey in which gonadotropin secretion had been abolished with a hypothalamic lesion. (Reproduced with permission of the authors and publishers of *Endocrinology 102:*1008, 1978.)

bility of an additional control for the gonadotropins. Since endorphins appear to play an important role in the secretion of PRL, they may exert an effect on gonadotropin by modulating PRL secretion.

Hormonal Control of Preovulatory Follicle Growth and Atresia. How are the cyclic changes in blood steroid hormone levels related to follicle growth and atresia in normal women? Hormonal requirements for preovulatory follicle growth and atresia have been studied extensively in hypophysectomized female rats, and circumstantial evidence has been adduced that these are relevant to requirements for similar functions in human ovaries. In hypophysectomized immature female rats (HIFR), the gonadotropins, both FSH and LH, were required for preovulatory growth to proceed normally. The effects of the gonadotropins were mediated, however, by estrogens that stimulated granulosa cell proliferation and inhibited atresia and by androgens that inhibited granulosa cell proliferation and stimulated atresia. The role of progestogens has not been determined.

Both FSH and LH were required for estrogen synthesis, and quantities of the steroid produced were dependent upon relative proportions once minimal effective doses of gonadotropins had been achieved. FSH-induced aromatase activity and LH stimulated the synthesis of androgens that served as substrate for estrogen synthesis.

In addition to its roles in stimulating preantral follicle growth and estrogen synthesis, FSH was required for antrum formation and preovulatory follicle growth. *Pari passu*, estradiol and FSH induced membrane receptors for LH in granulosa cells of preovulatory antral follicles. In summary then, gonadotropins stimulated synthesis of estrogens, androgens, and progestogens within the ovary. In turn, these steroid hormones acted to mediate the stimulatory effects of gonadotropins on atresia, preovulatory follicle growth, and induction of receptors required for subsequent actions of gonadotropins and steroids during ovulation and oogenesis.

How do hormones act in regulating follicle growth and atresia? According to current theories on the mechanism of hormone action, membrane and cytosolic receptors are required for direct effects of sex steroid hormones and gonadotropins on their respective target cells. Granulosa cells from preantral follicles in immature rat ovaries have cytosolic receptors for estrogens and androgens and progestogens. Furthermore, nuclear translocation of androgens and estrogens has been shown to occur in these cells *in vivo* and *in vitro*. These observations are consistent with a receptor-mediated role of estrogens in stimulating and of androgens in inhibiting granulosa cell proliferation during gonadotropin stimulation of preantral follicle growth in rodent ovaries. Again, the role of progestogens remains to be elucidated.

The numbers and distribution of membrane receptors for peptide hormones change during preovulatory follicle growth in rodent ovaries. Prior to antrum formation, membrane receptors for LH/hCG are confined to thecal and other types of interstitial cells outside the lamina basalis of the follicle complex. In contrast, FSH receptors are confined to granulosa cells inside the lamina basalis of preantral follicles. After antrum formation, LH/hCG receptors appear in granulosa cells within the lamina basalis. Furthermore, both antrum formation and LH/hCG receptor induction require exposure to FSH in the presence of estrogens, and effects of both hormones are mediated via the appropriate receptors.

What is the evidence that these observations are relevant to follicle growth in human ovaries? Although both ethical and practical constraints limit studies of the relationships

of hormones to preovulatory follicle growth and atresia in normal women, two lines of evidence are available. The first is purely circumstantial and is based upon an examination of cyclic changes in follicle morphology during the normal menstrual cycle. In Fig. 7–16, the changes in follicular properties during the menstrual cycle from the studies of Block (1951) have been replotted to coincide temporally with changes in pituitary gonadotropic hormone concentrations occurring during presumptive ovulatory cycles in normal young women and synchronized around day 0, the day of the LH surge at midcycle.

There are two "peaks" in numbers of graafian follicles greater than 1 mm in diameter, one occurring around the time of ovulation and the other in midluteal phase. Each of these "peaks" in numbers of normal follicles is associated with a reciprocal "trough" in numbers of follicles undergoing atresia expressed as the percentage of the volume of the ovary occupied by atretic follicles (Fig. 7–16). The peak in numbers of normal follicles seen during the luteal phase occurs coincident with declining concentrations of gonadotropins but high concentrations of estrogens (Fig. 7–10), suggesting that in human ovaries, as in ovaries of some other mammals, estrogens may act locally to enhance follicular responsiveness to gonadotropins. (See later.)

Recently, McNatty (1978) has shown that the mean diameter of the largest antral follicles found early in the preovulatory phase of the cycle is smaller than that of follicles seen during the luteal phase (Fig. 7–17). In the light of this observation, it seems likely that the large antral follicles

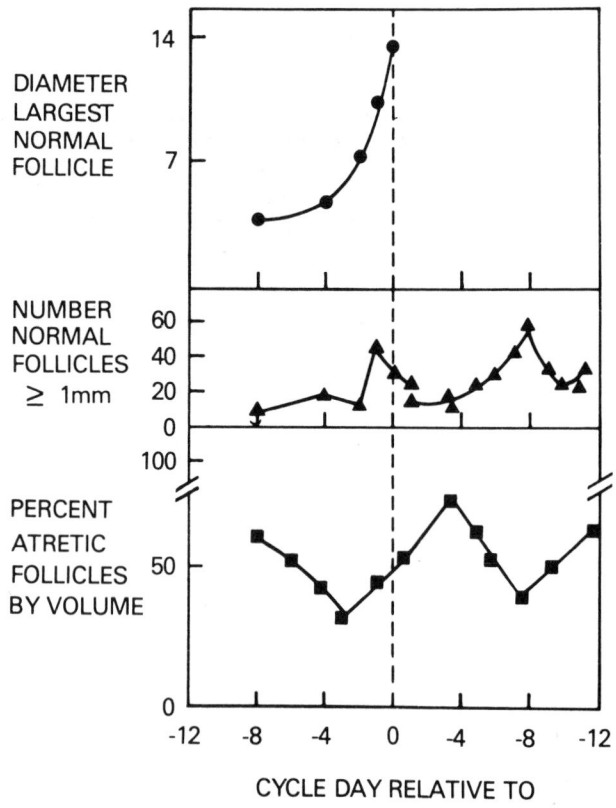

Figure 7–16. Changes in diameter of the largest normal follicle, numbers of normal follicles equal to or greater than 1 mm in diameter, and % of atretic follicles (by volume) as a function of time in the menstrual cycle synchronized around the day of the LH peak (day 0). (Modified from the data of Block, 1951).

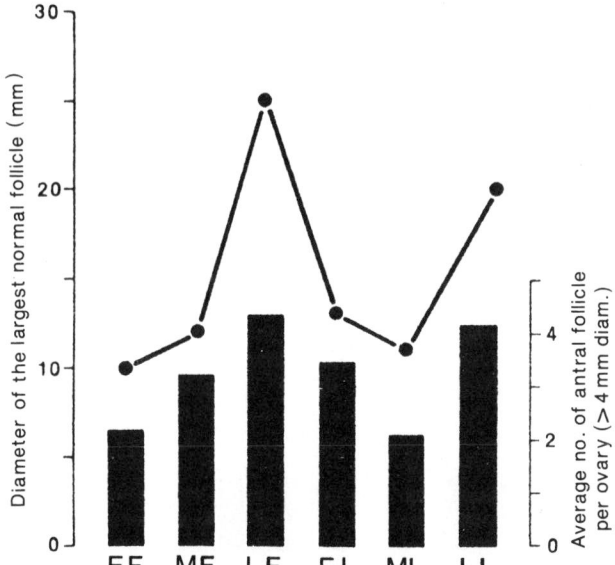

Figure 7–17. Changes in the diameter of the largest normal follicle and average numbers of follicles greater than 4 mm in diameter per ovary in specimens recovered surgically from normal women during early (EF), middle (MF), and late (LF) follicular phase and early (EL), middle (ML), and late (LL) luteal phase of the menstrual cycle. (Reproduced with permission of the author and publishers of *Clin. Endocrinol. Metab.* 7:577, 1978.)

seen in ovaries during the middle to late luteal phase undergo atresia, perhaps as a result of declining levels of gonadotropins. It follows then that the follicle destined to ovulate in the next cycle must be drawn from a "pool" of smaller follicles present during the luteal phase. Numbers of preantral follicles equal to or greater than 100μ in diameter were greatest in ovaries recovered during the midluteal phase of the cycle in Block's specimens. Hormonally dependent maturation of these preantral follicles might be initiated by estrogens and then stimulated further by rising levels first of FSH and then of LH, beginning late in the luteal phase and continuing into the follicular phase of the succeeding cycle.

During the last half of the follicular phase, the diameter of the follicle destined to ovulate increases rapidly to values around 20 mm (Fig. 7–16). Coincident with this period of rapid growth, reflecting proliferation of granulosa cells and accumulation of antral fluid, blood estradiol concentrations rise rapidly (Fig. 7–10), and recent studies of steroid hormone concentrations in ovarian venous effluent have shown that most of the estradiol comes from the ovary containing the dominant follicle. Thus, in human ovaries, estrogens are not only required for preovulatory follicle growth, as in rodent ovaries, but are also markers of the adequacy of that growth.

The second line of evidence for similarities in hormonal requirements for preovulatory follicle growth in rats and in humans is more direct. Follicle maturation has been shown not to progress normally either when gonadotropins are deficient or when gonadotropic stimulation fails to elicit estrogen synthesis in women with disorders of ovarian function. Moreover, hormonal changes similar to those occurring during normal menstrual cycles have been reproduced during induced ovulatory cycles. These observations are consistent with the concept that roles of gonadotropins and sex steroid hormones in stimulating preovulatory follicle maturation are similar in rats and humans.

What about receptors and their cellular distribution in human ovaries? Although receptors have not been demon-

strated in every case, progesterone secretion by granulosa cells removed from large preovulatory follicles of monkey and human ovaries has been shown to be stimulated by adding FSH and LH to the incubation medium *in vitro*. Moreover, these steroidogenic effects are accompanied by increased cyclic AMP (cAMP) production and constitute *prima-facie* evidence for the presence of membrane receptors for FSH and hCG in these cells from human and monkey ovaries, as in cells from rodent ovaries.

Although hormone concentrations are identical in blood perfusing the two human ovaries, ovulation occurs in only one of them during each menstrual cycle. Moreover, among follicles maturing in that ovary during that cycle, only one ovulates, while the remaining ones of that vintage in both ovaries undergo atresia. To account satisfactorily for the discrepant behavior between ovaries and among follicles, one must suppose that some process is acting at the level of individual follicles and individual cellular components of the follicular complex to determine the fate of individual maturing follicles. Evidence that such controls exist in human ovaries has been adduced from measurements of sex steroid hormones, FSH, LH, and PRL concentrations in antral fluid from follicles of varying sizes recovered from normal ovaries at different times during the menstrual cycle. Some typical results, stratified on the basis of time in the cycle and follicle size, are shown in Fig. 7–18A, B.

On the basis of antral fluid steroid levels, two populations were identified (Fig. 7–18A). In the one, estrogen and progestogens predominated, and in the other, androgens predominated. Estrogen predominance was found commonly among follicles greater than 8 mm in diameter but uncommonly among smaller follicles in which androgen predominance was characteristic. In general, FSH was detected in antral fluid from follicles in which estrogens and progestogens were predominant (larger follicles) but not in follicles in which androgens predominated (smaller follicles). In larger follicles containing predominantly estrogens and progestogens, antral fluid FSH levels were rising while blood FSH levels were declining. In contrast, in follicles in which androgens predominated, changes in antral fluid FSH levels tended to decline as blood levels declined in middle to late follicular phase (Figs. 7–10 and 7–18B).

LH concentrations were usually below the limit of detection except for the periovulatory period (Fig. 7–18B). If the role of LH in modulating follicular growth during the remainder of the cycle depends upon its antral fluid levels, the quantities required would seem to be very small.

In addition to those of LH and FSH, PRL concentrations in antral fluid also vary with respect to the size of the follicle, time in the cycle, and steroid hormone profiles. Very high levels in early follicular phase decline in late follicular phase, more impressively in larger (estrogen-progestogen–predominant) than in smaller (androgen-predominant) follicles. These observations indicate that FSH, LH, and PRL do not diffuse freely into antral fluid of every follicle but that the process is regulated.

What were the functional correlates of differences in intrafollicular hormone levels among follicles? *In vivo* granulosa cells were more numerous in estrogen-progestogen–predominant follicles, and *in vitro* these cells synthesized estradiol *de novum* and secreted more progesterone than did cells from androgen-predominant follicles. Furthermore, after incubation for 48 hours *in vitro* oocytes from estrogen-dominant follicles resumed meiosis and completed the first meiotic division; this did not occur in oocytes from androgen-dominant follicles. Collectively, the data suggested that androgen dominance was associated with atresia and was consistent with a role for antral fluid sex steroid hormone levels in determining whether a maturing follicle

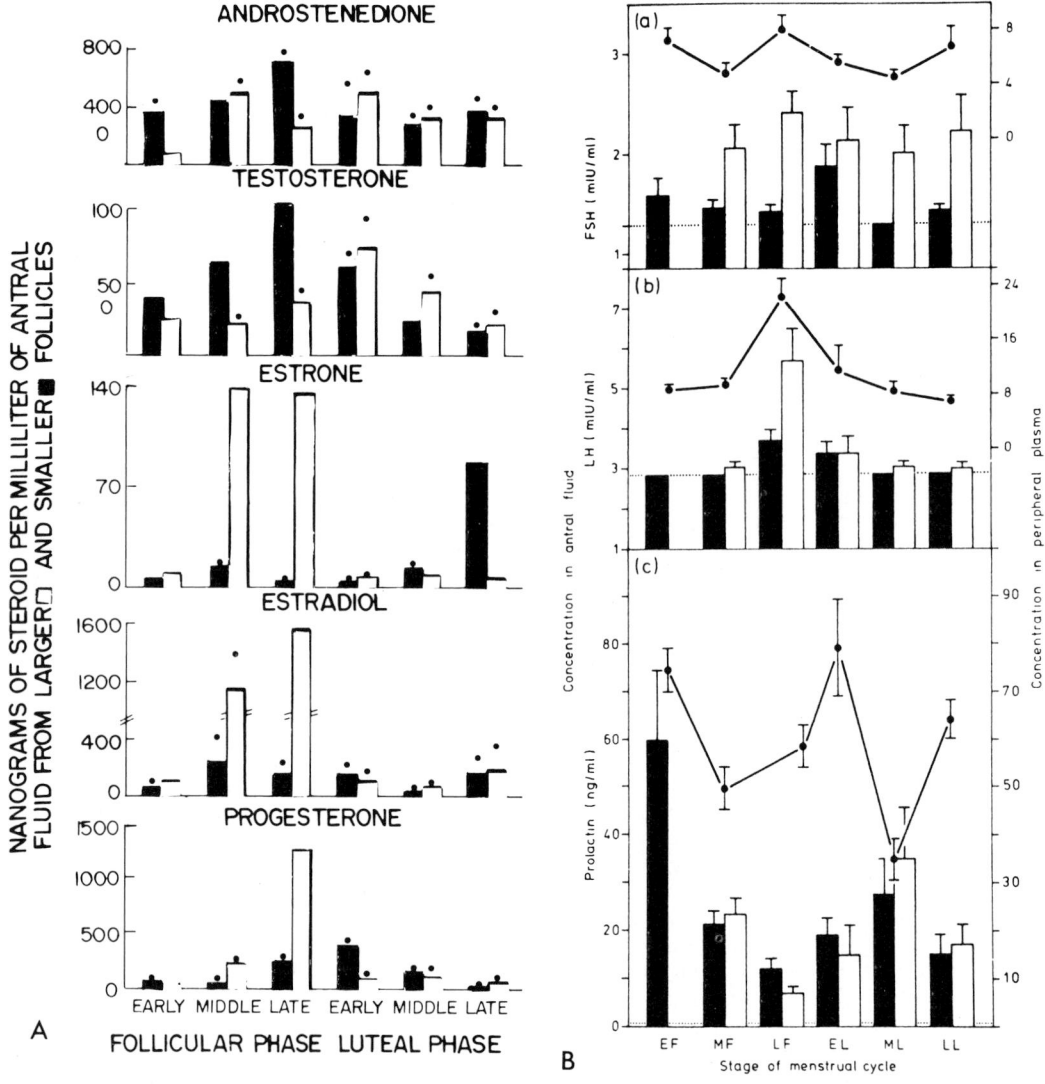

Figure 7–18. *A*, Concentrations of steroid hormones in antral fluid from follicles greater than 8 mm in diameter (open bars) and less than 8 mm in diameter (closed bars) sampled, at times indicated, during follicular and luteal phases of normal menstrual cycles. (Adapted from McNatty et al., 1975, 1976.) *B*, Concentrations of FSH, LH, and prolactin in antral fluid from follicles greater than 8 mm in diameter (open bars) and less than 8 mm in diameter (closed bars) sampled, at times indicated, during follicular and luteal phases of normal menstrual cycles. (Reproduced with permission of the author and publishers of *Clin. Endocrinol. Metab.* 7:577, 1978.)

ovulates or becomes atretic in human ovaries, as in rodent ovaries.

In summary then, irrespective of how differences in hormone profiles among follicles are achieved, the evidence seems convincing that the intraovarian hormonal milieu in human ovaries is regulated follicle by follicle. Moreover, the evidence is consistent with a role for these differences in determining whether follicle maturation, stimulated by gonadotropins, terminates in ovulation or atresia.

Hormonal Control of Ovulation and Oogenesis. In mammalian ovaries, once follicles reached maturity, LH stimulated ovulation and formation of a corpus luteum. When LH was given concomitantly with indomethacin, an inhibitor of prostaglandin synthetase, both ovulation and cortical migration of mature follicles were inhibited in rat ovaries. In some follicles, failure to migrate to a cortical position was associated with extrusion of the oocyte into the surrounding interstitial spaces, and in others, the oocyte was "trapped." Both FSH and LH stimulated prostaglandin synthesis by granulosa cells. Furthermore, both gonadotropins and prostaglandins stimulated granulosa cells to secrete an activator that converts plasminogen derived from plasma into plasmin, a protease that may be important in the dissolution of the lamina basalis during ovulation.

The mechanisms involved in hormonal stimulation of ovulation remain obscure. Increased intrafollicular pressure, ovarian contractions and enzymic dissolution of the follicle wall have all been postulated to be precipitating events in hormonally stimulated follicle rupture at ovulation.

The role of increased follicular pressure in precipitating follicle rupture at ovulation has been discredited recently. First, direct measurements have shown that basal levels of intrafollicular pressure, in the range of 10–15 mm Hg, remain stable throughout the latter half of the follicular phase and do not rise prior to rupture. Furthermore, follicular rupture, observed endoscopically in women and other primates, is not explosive, as would be expected if increased intrafollicular pressure were responsible for rupture.

The phenomenon of ovarian contractility and its relationship to ovulation have been the subject of a recent critical review (Espey, 1978). Although there is convincing evidence that ovarian contractions occur, their functional significance is controversial. Moreover, it is not clear that these are required for ovulation.

The concept that enzymic digestion is involved in ovulatory rupture of the follicle wall remains attractive. Morphologic changes in the ovulatory follicle provide indirect evidence consistent with this concept. These changes include dissociation of the granulosa cell layer, degenerative changes in the overlying germinal epithelium, loosening of the tunica albuginea and theca, and ultrastructural changes in the connective tissue matrix of the follicle wall.

Recently, more direct evidence has been adduced for a role of enzymic digestion in ovulation. Thus, follicular rupture, similar to ovulation, has been noted following microinjection of proteases into antral fluid. Moreover, the tensile strength of strips of follicle wall has been shown to be reduced following incubation in solutions containing proteases. Until recently, no protease with the required properties had been identified in ovarian tissue. Considerable circumstantial evidence has accumulated to suggest that the protease, plasmin, might have the required properties. First, antral fluid has been shown to contain plasminogen, presumably derived from serum. Second, granulosa cells from antral follicles secrete a plasminogen activator, antral fluid concentrations of which increase as ovulation approaches. Third, FSH, cAMP, and prostaglandins of the E series stimulate granulosa cell secretion of the activator. Finally, exposure to plasmin reduces the tensile strength of follicle wall strips. Thus, if protease digestion is required for ovulation, the enzyme plasmin may be a suitable candidate for this role.

Recently, the spontaneous resumption of meiosis in cumulus-free rat or pig oocytes *in vitro* was shown to be inhibited by peptides extracted from antral fluid of porcine and human follicles. Moreover, similar inhibition was observed when granulosa cells were cocultured with cumulus-free oocytes, suggesting that substances produced by granulosa cells participate in regulating oocyte maturation.

Hormonal Control of the Corpus Luteum Function. Luteinization and rupture of the follicles are induced by LH (or hCG, which can be used as its surrogate in cases when ovulation is induced), but recent studies have emphasized the role of follicle rupture and expulsion of the ovum and follicular fluid on the process of luteinization. There is evidence to suggest that the follicular fluid may contain a substance or substances that inhibit luteinization prior to the rupture of the follicle. Attempts to isolate and characterize these substances have not been successful, however, and the status of luteinization-inhibitory substances remains uncertain at this time. Luteinization is accompanied by a rapid drop of estradiol and of 17α-hydroxyprogesterone, whereas progesterone slowly rises. As the corpus luteum becomes functional, progesterone rises further, and in the human there is a parallel rise of the estrogens and 17α-hydroxyprogesterone. Although studies of ovarian venous blood clearly indicate that in women the estrogens secreted during the luteal phase are secreted by the corpus luteum, in many other species the corpus luteum does not secrete estrogens. The question of whether or not the corpus luteum secretes estrogens appears to correlate with the presence of luteinized thecal cells as part of the functioning corpus luteum.

The mechanisms that control the secretion of steroids by the corpus luteum and determine its remarkably constant lifespan of 14 days (outside of pregnancy) are not completely understood. The role of LH as a luteotropic agent is well established by studies showing that when ovulation is induced in hypophysectomized women, the life span of the corpus luteum is abbreviated unless repeated injections of LH are administered. Similarly, in women and in rhesus monkeys, progesterone secretion by the corpus luteum can be stimulated and prolonged by the administration of hCG. Finally, the presence of specific LH/hCG receptors in membrane preparations of human corpus luteum cells and the demonstration that LH stimulates cAMP production and

progesterone secretion by the human corpus luteum cells, are consistent with the luteotropic role of LH. On the other hand, the role, if any, of FSH in the luteal phase is unknown.

It is increasingly evident that adequate follicle maturation in the preovulatory phase is an important determinant of the function of the corpus luteum. Women with abnormal corpus luteum function have low levels of estradiol and of 17α-hydroxyprogesterone during the preovulatory phase. Since the levels of these steroids are considered to be markers of follicle maturation, these changes have been interpreted as indicating incomplete follicle maturation. Concomitant with the low levels of steroids, the serum levels of FSH are reduced while the LH levels are normal. Taken together, these observations indicate that inadequate preovulatory FSH stimulation and its consequence, insufficient follicle maturation, result in inadequate corpus luteum function.

In rodents, PRL is a potent luteotropic factor, but in women, its role in the regulation of corpus luteum function remains controversial. As noted earlier, in the normal menstrual cycle, PRL levels in the peripheral blood undergo only trivial changes, and these are most likely the result of fluctuation in estrogens. On the other hand, as mentioned previously, there are dramatic changes in the content of antral fluid, with high levels of PRL in immature follicles and very low levels of PRL in the immediately preovulatory follicle when progesterone is also high. Further evidence for a role of PRL in controlling progesterone secretion is derived from the studies of McNatty, who showed that in tissue culture the addition of PRL to granulosa cells significantly inhibited progesterone secretion. This inhibition of progesterone secretion by PRL was not overcome by the addition of LH or FSH. The fact that treatment with FSH or LH induced normal follicle growth, ovulation, and corpus luteum function in hypophysectomized women who had unmeasurable levels of PRL, however, militates against a significant role of PRL in the menstrual cycle. On the other hand, abnormal corpus luteum function is frequently observed in women with abnormally high levels of PRL. Whether the effects of the hyperprolactinemia on corpus luteum function result from alteration in follicular growth during the proliferative phase rather than from a direct effect upon the corpus luteum is uncertain, but the former appears to be more likely.

Much less is known about the mechanisms that limit the life span of the corpus luteum to 14 days unless pregnancy intervenes. Although a potent luteotropic agent in the earlier part of the postovulatory phase, LH progressively loses this capacity in later stages of the luteal phase, so that increasingly larger doses of LH must be administered to maintain progesterone secretion and prevent the involution of the corpus luteum. This has led to the concept that the life span of the corpus luteum is dependent upon a balance between luteotropic and luteolytic processes. Such a situation prevails in many domestic animals, in which prostaglandin $F_2\alpha(PGF_2\alpha)$, synthesized and released by the uterus, is responsible for the regression of the corpus luteum. This mechanism appears not to be operative in the human since, in contrast to the situation in domestic animals, hysterectomy does not prolong the survival of the corpus luteum. There are several lines of evidence implicating estrogens as a luteolytic agent in humans. Estradiol, implanted into the ovary containing the corpus luteum in women undergoing a laparotomy during the early secretory stages of the menstrual cycle, significantly shortened the length of the luteal phase. On the other hand, estradiol implanted in the contralateral ovary did not modify the cycles, suggesting that the effect of estradiol was a local intraovarian one. In women and other primates, systemic administration of estrogens has a luteolytic effect, and in monkeys it was shown that the luteolytic effect persisted in the absence of changes in the serum levels, further suggesting a local rather than a systemic effect. It is likely that luteolytic effects of estrogens are mediated by the action of prostaglandins since, in women, the venous effluent from the corpus luteum–bearing ovary contains significantly higher levels of $PGF_2\alpha$.

It is also likely that the estrogen secreted by the corpus luteum plays a significant role in determining the length of the subsequent preovulatory phase and, therefore, the timing of the next ovulation. In animals whose corpora lutea do not secrete estrogen, the proliferative phase is significantly shorter than it is in humans and other primates. Studies involving luteectomy in primates indicate that removal of the corpus luteum, and therefore of the progesterone and estrogens, advances the timing of the next ovulation by approximately the numbers of days by which the postovulatory phase was shortened. In humans and other primates, it must be assumed that the estrogens secreted during the postovulatory phase inhibit LH and FSH secretions to levels inadequate to sustain growth in extant antral follicles (which then undergo atresia) or to initiate growth of new preantral follicles. Consequently, a new set of follicles will only start growing when, at the very end of the luteal phase, the inhibitory effects of estrogen disappear, and the next ovulation will not occur until 14 days later, the time required for maturation of the ovulatory follicles.

Hormonal Control of Changes in Genital Tract Epithelium During the Normal Cycle. The cyclic changes in ovarian morphology and in gonadotropic and sex steroid hormone secretion having been described, consideration will now be given to the cyclic changes in the epithelia of the genital tract. These have been systematically studied and elegantly documented by Papanicolaou and his associates (1948). A schematic representation of their observations, coupled with measurements of pituitary and sex steroid hormones, is shown in Fig. 7–19, which depicts the changes described in the following sections.

The Endometrium. The uterine mucosa consists of a surface layer of columnar epithelial cells and an underlying stroma composed of spindle-shaped cells permeated by blood vessels. The continuity of the surface layer is interrupted by crypts called "glands" lined by similar epithelial cells in a tubular arrangement that dip into the stromal layer. Some of the columnar epithelial cells are ciliated; others are nonciliated and appear to be secretory cells. Normal cyclic changes affecting the morphology of epithelium, stroma, and blood vessels are sufficiently stereotyped to make microscopic evaluation of these valuable in diagnosing disorders of ovarian function. (See later.)

During the preovulatory phase of the cycle and under the influence of the estrogens, dominant changes are due to mitotic proliferation of the epithelium and the stroma. As a consequence, the mucosa thickens, and the tubular glands lengthen but remain straight. Nuclei of individual epithelial cells tend to be in a position midway between the basal and the luminal borders of the cell. Under the influence of progesterone produced by the corpus luteum, marked coiling of the glands, "loosening" (suggestive of edema), and increased vascularity of the stroma are characteristic changes. These gross changes are accompanied by reduction in mitotic activity, vacuolization of the cytoplasm, and increase in glycogen content of the epithelial cells, the nuclei of which take up a more basal position. The most superficial stromal cells now come to resemble decidual cells characteristic of early pregnancy; intermediate and deeper layers show no such changes. Coincident with declining function of the corpus luteum reflected in decreasing plasma concentration of estrogens and progestogens, necrotic changes occur in the mucosa, resulting in multifocal and progressive exfoliation

of all save the cells lining the depths of the tubular glands. Necrosis of blood vessels opens vascular channels with resultant menstrual bleeding.

The mechanisms resulting in the necrosis of the blood vessels remain obscure, but necrosis is preceded by intense vasospasm that is thought to be a prostaglandin effect. Prostaglandins are present in large amounts in secretory endometrium and in menstrual blood. Also, infusions of $PGF_2\alpha$ produce endometrial necrosis and bleeding. The hypothesis has been proposed that the release of prostaglandins is the result of a decrease in the stability of the lysosomal membranes in the endometrial cell due to the decrease in estrogen and progesterone. This lysosomal reaction results in the liberation of phospholipids with subsequent synthesis of $PGF_2\alpha$. After menstruation, the surface epithelium of the uterine mucosa is reconstituted by the proliferation of epithelial cells in the depths of the glandular crypts and the cycle is repeated.

Estrogen and progesterone effects upon the endometrial cells are mediated via cytosol receptors, and recent studies, in animals as well as in humans, have shown that estrogens themselves are the stimulus to the synthesis of the estrogen receptors. Progesterone receptor synthesis is also induced by estrogens, but interestingly enough, it appears that the turnover of the progesterone receptors is accelerated by progesterone.

The Endocervical Glands. The epithelium of the endocervical glands undergoes cyclic changes more closely correlated with changes in the vaginal epithelium than with changes in the endometrium. Of greater interest and more easily evaluated, however, are the cyclic changes in both quantity of and physical characteristics of the mucus secreted by these glands. During the first week after onset of the menses, small amounts of viscous mucus are produced. Coincident with rapid follicular growth and increasing plasma estrogen concentration in the second half of the follicular phase of the cycle, the quantity of mucus produced increases by up to 30-fold. Qualitatively, this mucus is more watery, more viscous, and more elastic. With increasing estrogen, the elasticity, usually referred to as "spinnbarkeit," of endocervical mucus increases, so that a long, fine thread is generated by stretching a small drop of secretion. Stretching is maximal just before ovulation when estrogen production is maximal. In addition, a characteristic ferning or palm leaf arborization is observed on microscopic examination when endocervical secretions aspirated with a clean pipette are spread as a thin film onto a clean glass slide and permitted to dry. This pattern is the result of crystallization of sodium chloride from dilute solutions containing proteins and polypeptides. As progesterone secretion rises after ovulation, the quantity, the viscosity, and the elasticity of the cervical mucus decline. In castrate women, injections of estrogen reproduce the changes in cervical mucus seen in the second half of the follicular phase of a spontaneous menstrual cycle. Concomitant injections of progesterone reverse the estrogenic effects on cervical mucus. These changes in water content, viscosity, and elasticity secondary to changes in steroid hormone secretion provide the basis for simple, effective indirect tests of ovarian function. (See later.)

The Vaginal Epithelium. The human vagina is lined by stratified squamous epithelium that consists of superficial, intermediate, inner, parabasal, and basal layers. The morphologic properties of cells from each of these layers as seen in films of vaginal secretions stained with polychrome stains and in biopsies of vaginal mucosa were described by Papanicolaou and coworkers. More recently, uniform morphologic and tinctorial criteria for identification of cells from each of the five layers have been agreed upon by cytologists.

Proliferation and maturation of vaginal epithelium is

influenced by estrogens and progestogens. When ovarian estrogen secretion is low, prepubertally and postmenopausally, vaginal epithelium is thin and susceptible to infection that may be accompanied by vaginal bleeding. Following either local application or systemic administration of estrogen, epithelial proliferation is stimulated and the tinctorial and morphologic properties of the exfoliated cells change. Early in the follicular phase of the cycle, basophilic cells with vesicular nuclei predominate, but increasing ovarian estrogen secretion stimulates both proliferation and keratinization, and acidophilic cells with pyknotic nuclei come to predominate.

During the postovulatory phase of the cycle, regressive changes appear in both acidophilic and basophilic cells; the percentage of acidophilic cells decreases, and increasing numbers of polymorphonuclear leukocytes appear.

The Urethral Epithelium. The character of cells exfoliated from the urethra changes with alterations in the sex steroid hormonal milieu. Properly prepared stained smears of epithelial cells in fresh urinary sediment reflect cyclic alterations in estrogen and progesterone levels in sexually mature women. These cells are more accessible than vaginal epithelial cells of infants and children and have been studied for diagnostic screening when excessive estrogen production is suspected.

After the Menopause

The basic ovarian event in the menopause is the cessation of cyclic ovarian function. Although a few follicles, usually quiescent, have been shown to persist for as long as 5 years after the last menses (see previously), functional changes can be attributed to depletion of follicles. Initially this is marked clinically by decreasing frequency of ovulation, sometimes associated with irregular menses or variable periods of amenorrhea, and later by decreasing estrogen secretion. Thus ovulation and menses, last to appear at menarche, cease first, and estrogen production, first to appear at menarche, is last to decline at menopause.

Some years before the final cessation of menstruation, there is a decrease in the responsiveness of the ovary to gonadotropins. Recent studies indicate that in women who are in the perimenopausal age group but who still have ovulatory periods, mean concentrations of FSH and LH are increased over levels seen in younger women while the levels of estrogens and progesterone throughout the cycle are decreased. The results were variable, however, and in the earlier part of the perimenopausal period, the characteristic change was an increase in FSH without a concomitant increase in LH.

After the menopause, concentrations of estrogens in both ovarian venous blood and in peripheral blood decline to very low levels, and removal of the ovaries frequently fails to alter the quantities of estrogens excreted in the urine of postmenopausal women. It is assumed that after the menopause most of the estrogens are derived from peripheral conversion of androgenic precursors secreted principally by the adrenals (see previously). Concentrations of testosterone and of androstenedione in ovarian venous blood from ovaries of postmenopausal women are higher than are concentrations in samples of peripheral blood collected simultaneously. These observations allow for the possibility that the postmenopausal ovary may secrete small amounts of androgens that are aromatized and converted to estrogens peripherally.

The declining estrogen secretion is accompanied by signs and symptoms of hormone deficits in the estrogen-dependent target organs, including the pituitary, uterus, cervix, vagina, and breasts. Pituitary gonadotropin secretion rises and is reflected by increased quantities of gonadotropin in blood and urine; the endometrium becomes atrophic, myometrial mass decreases, and the vaginal epithelium becomes thin and deficient in glycogen and fails to become keratinized.

Metabolic Effects of Sex Steroid Hormones. The use of estrogens and progestogens as contraceptive steroids has made us increasingly aware of the widespread effects of the gonadal hormones upon many metabolic processes. Much confusion remains, however, and most of what we know relates to the synthetic rather than to the natural steroids. Since there are quantitative and qualitative differences between the physiologic effects of these two classes, evidence from studies in which synthetic steroids were used, often in unphysiologic doses, must be interpreted with caution. Even so, a number of facts appear to be well established. Estrogens enhance the insulin response to carbohydrate loads and decrease the sensitivity to insulin. Because of a concomitant increase in GH and cortisol, the net effect may be a decrease in carbohydrate tolerance. This effect will obviously be more pronounced in women whose pancreata have a limited capacity to secrete insulin. Progesterone, at least in physiologic doses, appears to have little influence upon carbohydrate metabolism.

Estrogens augment plasma triglycerides mainly via an increase in the triglyceride-rich pre-β-lipoproteins (βLPH). Lipoprotein lipase, as measured by postheparin lipolytic activity, is decreased. Progesterone has little effect, but some synthetic progestogens, such as norethindrone acetate, a progestogen with inherent androgenic activity, will decrease triglyceride levels in patients with hyperlipidemia.

Estrogens increase plasma proteins that bind steroids such as cortisol, progesterone, and thyroxine (T_4) as well as plasma steroids that bind serum iron and copper. Recently, it has been established that in addition to an increase in bound cortisol, estrogens also produce a moderate increase in unbound, and therefore physiologically active, cortisol. Estrogens reduce the secretory capacity of the liver for certain organic anions, such as bromsulfophthalein. Increases in liver enzymes and hyperbilirubinemia can occur, as well as idiosyncratic biliary secretory failure. If a disorder of biliary excretion is present, estrogens will aggravate the problem. Mention has already been made of the effect of estrogens upon plasma renin, angiotensin, and aldosterone and of the resulting changes in these substances during the normal menstrual cycle. The role of estrogens in electrolyte regulation is complex, with an initial natriuresis followed by a period of sodium retention. Progesterone may also cause natriuresis, but its effects are transient.

Tests of Ovarian Function

Indirect — Evaluation of Target Organ Responses. The vaginal epithelium, the mucous secretions of the endocervical glands, the epithelium of the urethra, and the endometrium, are easily accessible target organs of the estrogens and progesterone. In our experience, the evaluation of these target organ responses is a much better guideline for the evaluation of the patient with abnormal ovarian function than are the biochemical assays for the plasma levels of estrogens or progesterone. At the same time, it is important to realize the limitations of the "bioassay" approach. As in all bioassays, the change in the genital epithelium resulting from stimulation with estrogens or progesterone can only be used as a quantitative index of the hormonal titer within a rather narrow range. As an example, the disappearance of basal cells in the vaginal mucosa or the appearance of cervical mucus in patients treated with gonadotropin is a most convenient index of the initial response of the ovary. In later stages of the treatment, however, when estrogens rise

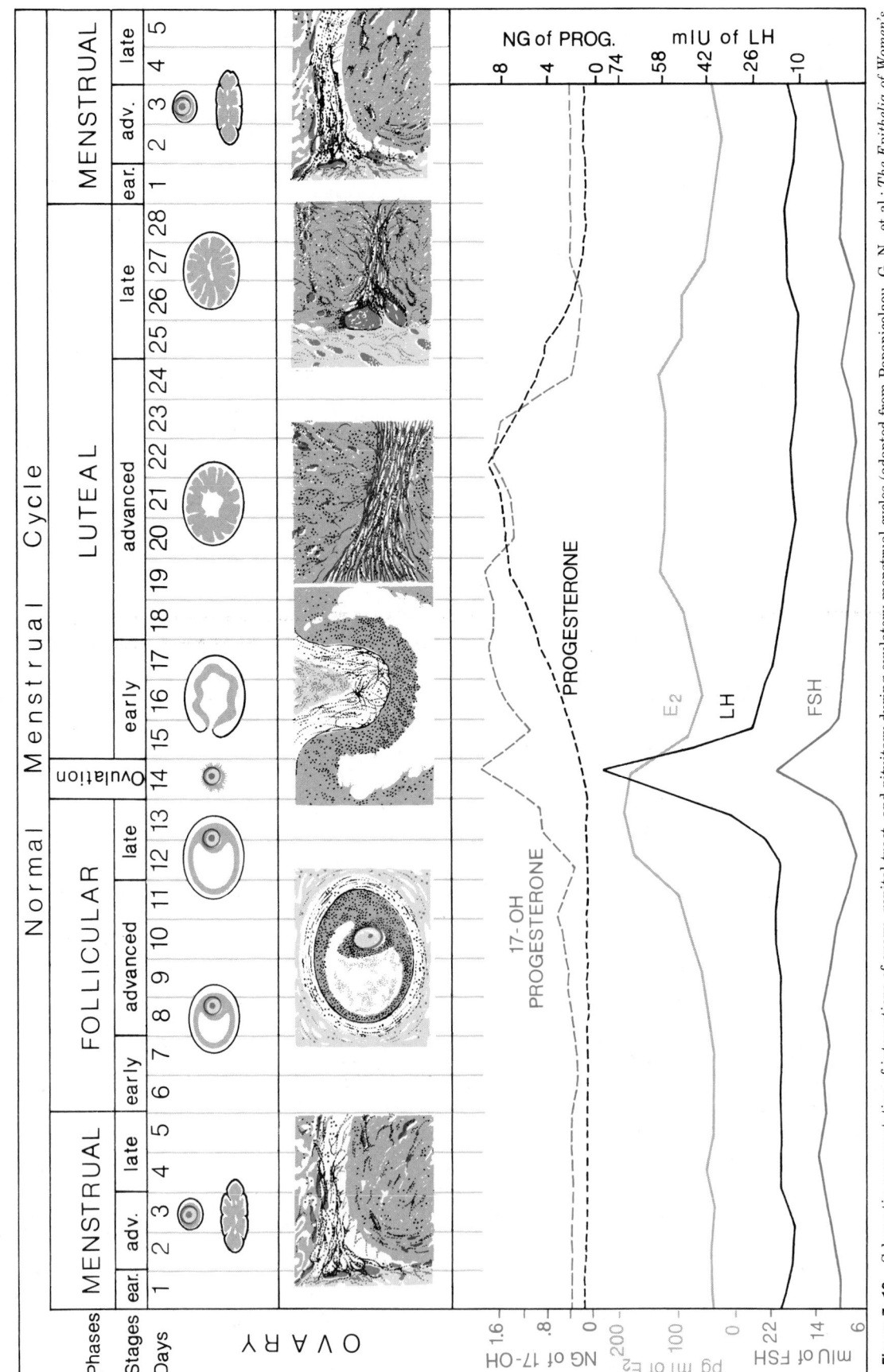

Figure 7–19. Schematic representation of interactions of ovary, genital tract, and pituitary during ovulatory menstrual cycles (adapted from Papanicolaou, G. N., et al.: *The Epithelia of Women's Reproductive Organs.* New York, Commonwealth, 1948, and Ross, G. T.: *Recent Progr. Hormone Res.* 26:1, 1970.)

Illustration continued on opposite page.

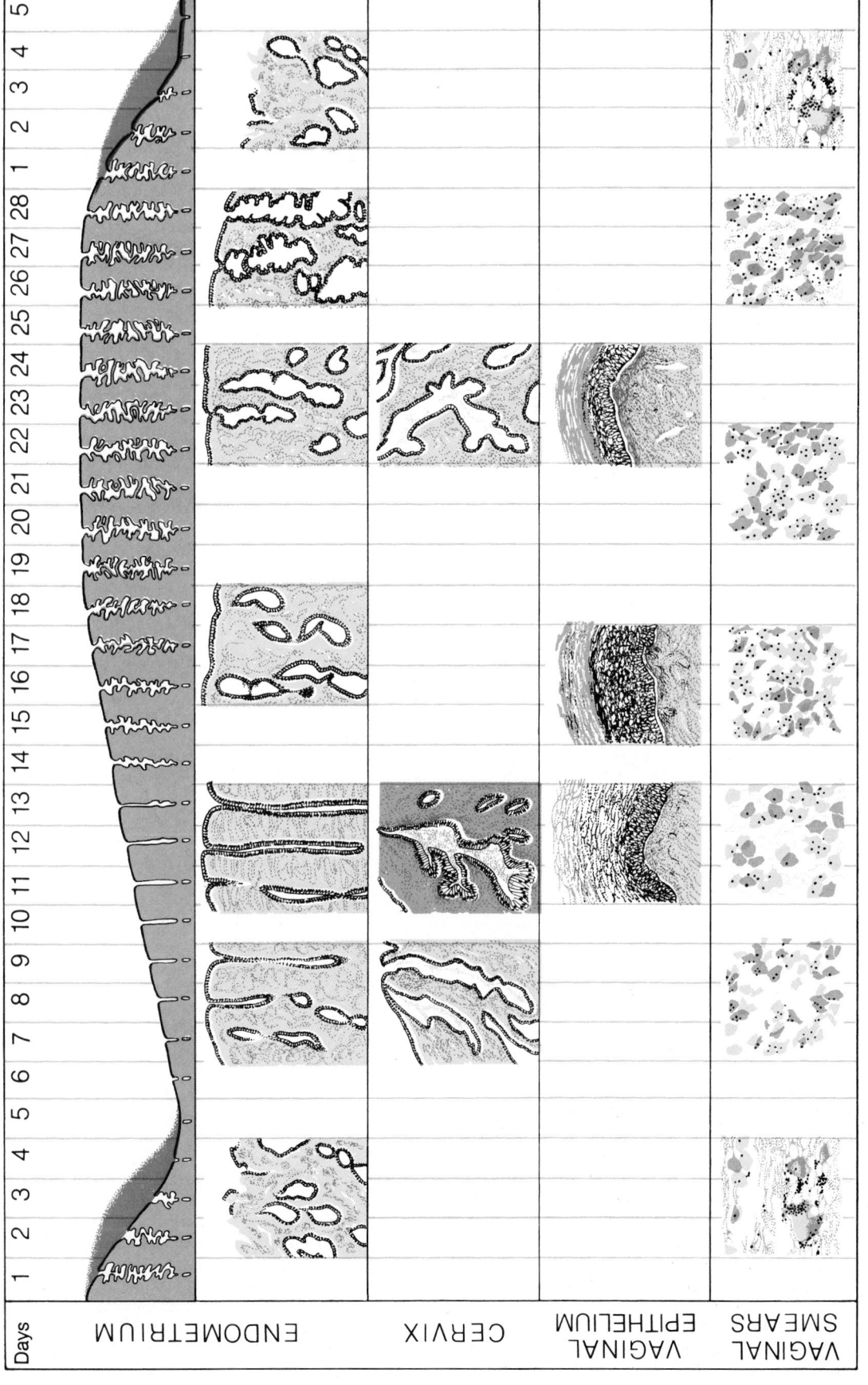

Figure 7–19. *Continued.*

to preovulatory levels neither of these endpoints can be used as the quantitative index of estrogen levels.

Vaginal Epithelium. Steroid hormone–dependent cyclic changes in the morphology of the vaginal epithelium described earlier provide the basis for a reasonably accurate and rapid screening assessment of ovarian steroid hormone production. The major usefulness of the vaginal smear for evaluation of ovarian function is when estrogens are low and routine assays are not sufficiently sensitive. Often, too much reliance is given to the quantitative aspects of the changes in the vaginal smears, such as in determining a "maturation index." Conclusions derived from such an index are often misleading, since many factors other than the estrogen level will determine the ratio of basal, intermediate, and precornified cells.

Endocervical Mucus. The presence of cervical mucus is a most convenient index for the presence of estrogens and the absence of progesterone. The presence of cervical mucus rules out pregnancy, since the presence of cervical mucus requires a ratio of estrogens to progesterone that is incompatible with normal pregnancy. On the other hand, when mucus is absent, distinction must be made between two possibilities: either estrogens are absent or estrogens and progesterone are present. The first possibility can be ruled in or ruled out by doing a vaginal smear.

The Endometrium. As noted earlier, the morphologic changes in the endometrium throughout the menstrual cycle are sufficiently stereotyped to make microscopic examination of endometrial biopsies useful in studies of ovarian function. Criteria have been established for "dating" secretory endometrium, assuming that ovulation occurs on day 14 of a 28-day cycle. In our experience, endometrial biopsies are a much better index of the adequacy of the postovulatory phase than the determination of progesterone, even at multiple intervals.

Indeed, changes in the endometrial histology depend not only on progesterone but also on the integrated effect of estrogens, progesterone, and androgens, not only at the time of the biopsy but also during the days preceding it.

A practical test of ovarian function based upon endometrial reactions is the progesterone withdrawal test, consisting of the intramuscular injection of 50–100 mg of progesterone. Vaginal bleeding within a week following the injections implies that (1) the endometrium is responsive to both estrogens and progesterone, (2) the ovary is responsive to FSH and LH stimulation and secretes sufficient amounts of estrogen to produce endometrial proliferation, (3) the pituitary secretes FSH and LH. A positive response therefore indicates at least partial integrity of hypothalamic-pituitary-ovarian-uterine function. Mishell and colleagues have recently shown that patients responding to progesterone have a mean level of estradiol of 60 pg/ml, whereas patients who do not respond have a mean level of 15 pg/ml. The negative response therefore indicates a more profound disturbance of the hypothalamic-pituitary-ovarian axis and suggests a more aggressive diagnostic approach.

The Basal Body Temperature. Perhaps the most widely used presumptive indicator of ovarian progesterone production is the so-called thermogenic shift detected by daily measurements of basal body temperatures. Thermometers especially designed for the purpose are used to measure either oral or rectal temperatures daily before arising. Ovarian production of progesterone, presumably reflecting function of the corpus luteum, results in a "shift" of the basal body temperatures upward around the time of ovulation (Fig. 7–14). This thermogenic response results from a direct effect of progesterone upon the thermoregulatory center in the hypothalamus and can be shown in postmenopausal or castrate women and in men.

The thermogenic shift merely reflects progesterone secretion and therefore is only a presumptive test of ovulation. Indeed luteinization of the follicle and progesterone secretion may occur in the absence of rupture of the follicle and expulsion of the ovum. Another limitation of the use of the temperature chart lies in the fact that the amounts of progesterone that are adequate to produce a maximal increase in the basal body temperature chart are less than the amounts necessary to induce a transformation of the endometrium sufficient to allow implantation. Biphasic temperature charts therefore, although good indexes of the presence of ovulation, do not prove that the postovulatory phase was normal. Finally, there have been several recent reports indicating that a small number of patients who ovulate do not have a biphasic temperature chart, and this limitation of the use of the thermogenic shift for the diagnosis of ovulation must be kept in mind.

Mention must be made of a number of other tests that in our experience, although occasionally interesting, are only of limited value in the diagnosis and classification of patients with ovarian dysfunction. One was devised to test the integrity of the positive feedback mechanisms. Estradiol benzoate is administered, and blood is taken on 3 subsequent days to determine whether administered estrogen will induce an LH surge. One other method developed to test the feedback mechanisms is to administer clomiphene. Although of some interest in the investigation of the controlling mechanisms of the ovarian cycle, we have found these tests to be of very limited use in the clinical world.

Direct—Measurements of Gonadotropins and Steroid Hormones in Blood and Urine. With rare exceptions, radioligand binding assays for peptide and steroid hormones in blood have replaced the more cumbersome assays of 24-hour urine specimens. Moreover, *in vitro* biologic assays for LH/hCG, equivalent in sensitivity to radioligand binding assays, have made it possible to compare potencies obtained by immunoassay of aliquots from the same specimens of blood. The significant variations in amplitude and frequency of pulses of peptide hormone secretion minimize the diagnostic value of a single determination by any of these methods. Hence, to obtain an accurate estimate of blood levels requires either repetitive blood samples or alternatively timed urine collections that minimize effects of pulsatile secretion and reflect an "average" level during the sampling period.

THE ABNORMAL OVARY

Introduction

There is no completely satisfactory system for the etiologic classification of ovarian diseases. None of them, including the one we shall propose, can encompass all the nuances that may be associated with the protean manifestations of ovarian dysfunction. In the preceding discussion of normal ovarian function, however, we emphasized the central role of sex steroid hormones in mediating ovarian function during growth, development, and aging. Moreover, if we have accomplished our goals, it should be clear to the reader that the clinical evidence of normal ovarian function varies with the menarcheal status of the person being examined. Thus, premenarcheally, appearance and progression of secondary sexual characteristics and somatic growth and development are regulated in part by ovarian sex steroid hormones. Postmenarcheally, sex steroid hormones coordinate interaction of ovaries, hypothalamus, pituitary, and genital tract during the ovulatory menstrual cycle. Finally, factors regulating extraovarian conversion of adrenal precursors to sex steroid hormones are the major determinants of target tissue responses in postmenopausal women. In this context, then, events resulting from sex steroid hormone actions on target tissues, consistent with those for physiologically normal peers, constitute *prima-facie* evidence of normal ovarian function at any time in life. Conversely, peripheral effects of sex steroid hormones, inappropriate for the peer group, constitute *prima-facie* evidence of abnormal ovarian function at any time in life. To assist the physician in using these concepts for diagnosing and treating disorders of ovarian function we will outline methods useful in determining whether target responses to ovarian sex steroid hormones are appropriate for the menarcheal status of the patient under consideration.

Syndromes of Ovarian Dysfunction

In Infancy and Childhood

As noted earlier, ovarian sex steroid hormones participate in development of secondary sexual characteristics during childhood.

Two extremes of pubescence — precocious initiation and delayed achievement — provide the framework for discussion of syndromes of pathophysiologic ovarian function in infancy and childhood. It should be noted that these syndromes are encountered rarely outside of referral centers specializing in diagnosis and treatment of endocrine disorders in children. Nonetheless, when such problems arise, some understanding of their implications provides a basis for rational management by the physician who first sees the patient.

Precocious Puberty and Pseudopuberty

Introduction. Puberty is defined as the state of physical development when sexual reproduction first becomes possible, and in primate females, this is marked by the menarche. Normally, the acquisition of reproductive capability occurs *pari passu*, with development of estrogen-dependent secondary sexual characteristics, including maturation of the breasts, development of pubic and axillary hair, and accelerated linear skeletal growth. Pathophysiologically, however, development of secondary sexual characteristics may occur without concomitant maturation of the gametogenic function of the ovaries.

In either case, development of estrogen-dependent secondary sexual characteristics in girls under 9 years implies an aberration in ovarian function. If the abnormality results from premature activation of cyclic hypothalamic-pituitary function, sex steroid hormone secretion is accompanied by follicular maturation and ovulation, and these processes appear to be regulated in a manner identical to that occur-

ring in women during their reproductive years. Indeed, among such children ovulation with or without pregnancy has been demonstrated repeatedly, so that the syndromes are described appropriately as *precocious puberty*, or sometimes as *true precocious puberty*. In contrast, when the aberration consists of secretion of sex steroid hormones in the absence of pituitary gonadotropic stimulation and without ovulation, the syndrome should be referred to as *precocious pseudopuberty*, sometimes called *pseudoprecocious puberty*, since reproductive capability has not been attained. Though both are rare, precocious puberty is seen 5–6 times more frequently than precocious pseudopuberty.

Making the distinction between precocious puberty and precocious pseudopuberty is important clinically for two reasons, both of which relate to treatment. Firstly, although the cause of precocious puberty remains unknown in most instances, it is not regarded as primarily ovarian in origin, whereas primary ovarian abnormality is the basis for disease in most children with precocious pseudopuberty, with adrenal disease accounting for the remainder. Thus, making the distinction helps to establish the locus of disease. Secondly, the clinical course and consequences of the two processes differ. The clinical course is benign in most children with precocious puberty, but in about 10% of them, premature activation of cyclic hypothalamic-pituitary function can be shown to be associated with potentially life-threatening intracerebral diseases, including neoplasms. In contrast to the usually benign course of precocious puberty, precocious pseudopuberty is more frequently symptomatic of potentially life-threatening diseases, which may be curable if recognized early and treated appropriately. Failure to make the distinction between puberty and pseudopuberty may, then, result in delay of treatment, with important implications for survival of patients with pseudopuberty.

Making the distinction between puberty and pseudopuberty is complicated by the fact that the clinical signs of the two entities are similar in the absence of ovulation, which may not occur until late in the course of precocious puberty. Not uncommonly, screening diagnostic procedures fail to provide a definitive basis for making this distinction, so that the physician must decide whether to temporize or to pursue more complex diagnostic procedures; with either course, intrinsic morbidity and cost are significant. When the probability of a life-threatening disorder can be minimized simply, expectant waiting is justified and unlikely to increase morbidity significantly or to affect prognosis adversely.

Syndromes of Precocious Puberty. Syndromes of precocious puberty, both idiopathic and secondary to disease of the CNS, are discussed in Chapter 11. Pseudopubertal variants, premature thelarche, and premature adrenarche are discussed in Ch. 26. Some salient features, useful in differential diagnosis, are summarized in Table 7–5.

Table 7–5. PHYSICAL FINDINGS AMONG PATIENTS WITH VARIOUS SYNDROMES OF PRECOCIOUS PUBERTY AND PSEUDOPUBERTY

Findings	Premature Thelarche	Premature Adrenarche	Precocious Puberty				Precocious Pseudopuberty					
							Isosexual			Heterosexual		
			Idiopathic	Central Nervous System Tumor	McCune-Albright Syndrome	Hypothyroid	Ovarian Tumors	Adrenal Tumors	Factitious	Ovarian Tumors	Adrenal Tumors	Adrenal Hyperplasia
Breast enlargement	Yes	No	Yes	Yes	Yes	Yes	Yes	Yes	Yes	Yes	Yes	Yes
Pubic hair	No	Yes	Yes	Yes	Yes	Unusual	Yes	Yes	Yes	Yes	Yes	Yes
Vaginal bleeding	No	No	Yes	Yes	Yes	Yes	Yes	Yes	Yes	Yes	Yes	Yes
Virilizing signs	No	No	No	No	No	No	No	Yes	No	Yes	Yes	Yes
Bone age	Normal	Normal to Minimally Advanced	Advanced	Advanced	Advanced	Normal or Retarded	Advanced	Advanced	Advanced	Advanced	Advanced	Advanced
Neurologic deficit	No	No	No	Yes	Yes	No	No	No	No	No	No	No
Abdomino-pelvic mass	No	No	Occ'l	No	No	Occ'l	Usually	No	No	Occ'l	No	No

Syndromes of Precocious Pseudopuberty. When secondary sexual characteristics develop prematurely in the absence of maturation of the gametogenic function of the ovary, the syndrome is called *precocious pseudopuberty*. If secondary sexual changes seen in precocious pseudopuberty are consistent with those expected on the basis of the genetic sex of the child, the syndrome is referred to as *isosexual precocious pseudopuberty*. On the other hand, when virilizing signs characteristic of pubescent genetic males occur in girls, the syndrome is called *heterosexual precocious pseudopuberty*. Accelerated linear growth, breast development, appearance of pubic and axillary hair, genital maturation, and periodic vaginal bleeding, appearing in the same sequence as in normal puberty, have been observed in girls with isosexual precocious pseudopuberty. These changes may also occur in girls with heterosexual precocious pseudopuberty, but in addition, virilizing signs, such as acne, hirsutism, and clitorimegaly, may occur in children whose diseases result from ovarian or adrenal neoplasms producing a combination of androgens and estrogens.

Precocious Pseudopuberty Due to Adrenal and Ovarian Diseases. Adrenal tumors producing estrogens and androgens in children before the age of expected puberty are rare. Diagnostic procedures are discussed in detail in Ch. 5.

Primary ovarian lesions, including neoplasms and non-neoplastic cysts, though rare, are more commonly encountered than are adrenal neoplasms among children with isosexual and heterosexual precocious pseudopuberty. Granulosa cell tumors producing signs and symptoms of isosexual pseudopuberty account for about 60% of cases. The remainder are distributed approximately equally among arrhenoblastomas, lipoid cell tumors, chorioepitheliomas, and benign ovarian cysts.

In a comprehensive review of precocious pseudopuberty of ovarian origin, Serment and coworkers (1970) summarized findings in 234 cases of precocious pseudopuberty occurring in girls under 9 years of age. Among 148 patients with isosexual pseudopuberty secondary to granulosa cell tumors of the ovary for whom satisfactory data were available, enlargement of the breasts occurred in 138, pubic hair appeared in 131, and genital bleeding was noted in 120.

In 18 instances of arrhenoblastomas, Sertoli cell tumors, and lipoid cell tumors occurring in girls under 9 years of age, breast enlargement was observed in 10, eight of whom also had vaginal bleeding. Hirsutism and clitorimegaly were observed in about half of these girls.

For reasons that are not apparent, ectopic section of hCG by hepatoblastomas, which results in pseudopuberty in boys, has never been recognized in girls. In girls, then, pseudopuberty secondary to tumors producing hCG is limited to primary ovarian choriocarcinomas, which, though rare, usually occur in children and young adolescents. These tumors progress rapidly to a fatal issue, usually less than 1 year after onset of symptoms that lead to diagnosis. It is not surprising, therefore, that signs and symptoms of pseudopuberty frequently do not progress beyond minimal breast enlargement or the appearance of small amounts of pubic hair. Although spotty bleeding has been observed, copious vaginal bleeding is unusual.

Benign ovarian cysts occur commonly in the ovaries of prepubertal and peripubertal girls. When these are of sufficient size to enlarge the ovary of a child with signs of precocious puberty, surgical exploration is required to distinguish a benign cyst from a malignant ovarian tumor. In a limited number of patients in whom a non-neoplastic cyst has been encountered at laparotomy, excision of the cyst has resulted in regression of secondary sexual characteristics until pubescence occurred at a normal age. More commonly, excision of these cysts has failed to alter the course of pubertal change among girls with idiopathic precocious puberty. The virtue of the exploration, then, derives from eliminating the possibility that a resectable ovarian neoplasm underlies the precocious pseudopuberty rather than from the likelihood of altering the clinical course of pubertal changes.

There is a paucity of information about preoperative laboratory studies in children with precocious pseudopuberty due to ovarian tumors. Consequently, the usefulness of such studies in differentiating pseudopuberty from puberty remains to be established.

Urinary estrogen has been measured in 23 children with precocious pseudopuberty secondary to granulosa cell tumors. In 15 instances, values were equal to or less than those seen in sexually mature women during their reproductive years; in 8, levels were markedly elevated to 60–720 $\mu g/24$ hr. In 22 of 24 patients studied, vaginal smears showed evidence of estrogenic effects. In all instances, urinary estrogen excretion ultimately declined after ablation of the tumor.

Urinary 17-ketosteroid (17-KS) excretion is not invariably elevated in girls with precocious pseudopuberty secondary to arrhenoblastomas and lipoid cell tumors of the ovary. In contrast, when heterosexual precocious pseudopuberty results from adrenal tumor or from congenital adrenal hyperplasia, urinary 17-KS excretion has been found to be elevated in virtually 100% of cases. Thus, normal 17-KS excretion suggests an ovarian tumor, but elevated values do not differentiate between ovarian and adrenal tumors in a child with heterosexual pseudopuberty. Although determinations of plasma and urinary testosterone have been reported only rarely in children with such tumors, it is reasonable to suppose that values will be found to be elevated, as they are in sexually mature women with similar tumors.

In view of the well-established negative feedback of estrogens on pituitary gonadotropin excretion in sexually mature women, it might be supposed that measurements of gonadotropins in urine or blood would be useful in distinguishing precocious pseudopuberty from precocious puberty in children. Urinary gonadotropin excretion, usually the result of a single determination by bioassay, has been reported for very few children with granulosa cell tumors producing estrogen, however. In 13 of 14 patients in one series, values were 3–10 mouse uterine units/24 hr whereas a value of 40 mouse uterine units was reported for a single patient, so that these determinations did not distinguish children with precocious pseudopuberty from those with precocious puberty. Urinary gonadotropin excretion in children with virilizing ovarian tumors has been studied too rarely to merit discussion. Urinary gonadotropins have been invariably markedly elevated in only one syndrome of precocious pseudopuberty — the syndrome secondary to ovarian tumors secreting chorionic gonadotropin.

Measurements of immunoreactive gonadotropins in a limited number of serum and urine specimens from girls with precocious pseudopuberty have not provided information useful in distinguishing these children from children with precocious puberty or from normal children.

Factitious Precocious Pseudopuberty. Very rarely, inadvertent ingestion of or topical application of estrogens has been reported to induce breast enlargement, appearance of pubic hair, and onset of vaginal bleeding in girls less than 8 years old. Sources of exogenous estrogens include foods, drugs, and cosmetics. Examples include ingestion of the hormone by a child playing with a jar of cleansing cream containing estrogen, topical application of creams marketed for control of "diaper rash," and use of vitamin preparations and a variety of other drugs contaminated with estrogen during manufacture. Identification of these sources of estrogens depends upon a carefully taken history, followed by either chemical or biologic detection of hormone in the suspected source. Laboratory studies reported have been too limited to be meaningful.

Clinical Evaluation of the Patient with Signs of Precocious Puberty and Pseudopuberty. Some of the diagnostic features of the syndromes of precocious puberty and pseudopuberty that can be determined by history and physical examination are summarized in Table 7–5. A scheme for further evaluation based upon findings at genital examination is shown in Fig. 7–20. The objective of the scheme is to distinguish between pseudopuberty and puberty, and this distinction is based primarily on the presence or absence of virilizing signs and the presence or absence of an adnexal mass.

The History. A carefully taken history may provide diagnostically useful information. First, one should inquire about possible inadvertent ingestion or topical application of estrogens. Mothers should be questioned carefully about medications taken and cosmetics, creams, and powders used for the child or by women with whom the child has repeated and frequent contact, including older siblings, maids, aunts, and grandmothers. It may be helpful to have the mother produce cosmetic containers, since laws in most countries require labeling of preparations containing hormones.

Second, mothers should be questioned carefully about behavioral changes or psychomotor equivalents of seizures. Evidence obtained in this way has led in our experience to

identification of an intracerebral neoplasm underlying true precocious puberty.

Third, when medical advice is sought late in the course of precocious puberty, careful dating of events may be helpful. Some authorities express the opinion that progression of changes from earliest evidence of breast maturation to onset of vaginal bleeding is more rapid when a tumor, secreting steroid hormones, is the basis of the process, but no firm data have been published to support this impression. If breast enlargement or appearance of pubic hair is to be followed by menarche, the rate of progression is similar to that seen in physiologic pubescence. (See Tables 7–1 and 7–2.) On the other hand, if the process represents premature thelarche or premature adrenarche, advancement will be delayed and menarche will occur at the expected age.

When vaginal bleeding occurs, a history of cyclicity suggests that the process may be under hypothalamic-pituitary control, leading to a diagnosis of precocious puberty. This is not definitive, however, since periodic genital bleeding has been observed in patients with pseudopuberty secondary to ovarian and adrenal neoplasms secreting sex steroid hormones.

The Extragenital Physical Examination. The skin should be carefully inspected for café-au-lait spots. These lesions have been seen in instances of precocious puberty associated with phakomatosis and with the McCune-Albright syndrome. Cutaneous manifestations of hypothyroidism are suggestive of the syndrome of precocious puberty secondary to hypothyroidism. Excessive facial hirsutism and facial acne are suggestive of heterosexual precocious pseudopuberty. Facial asymmetry or skeletal deformity are pathog-

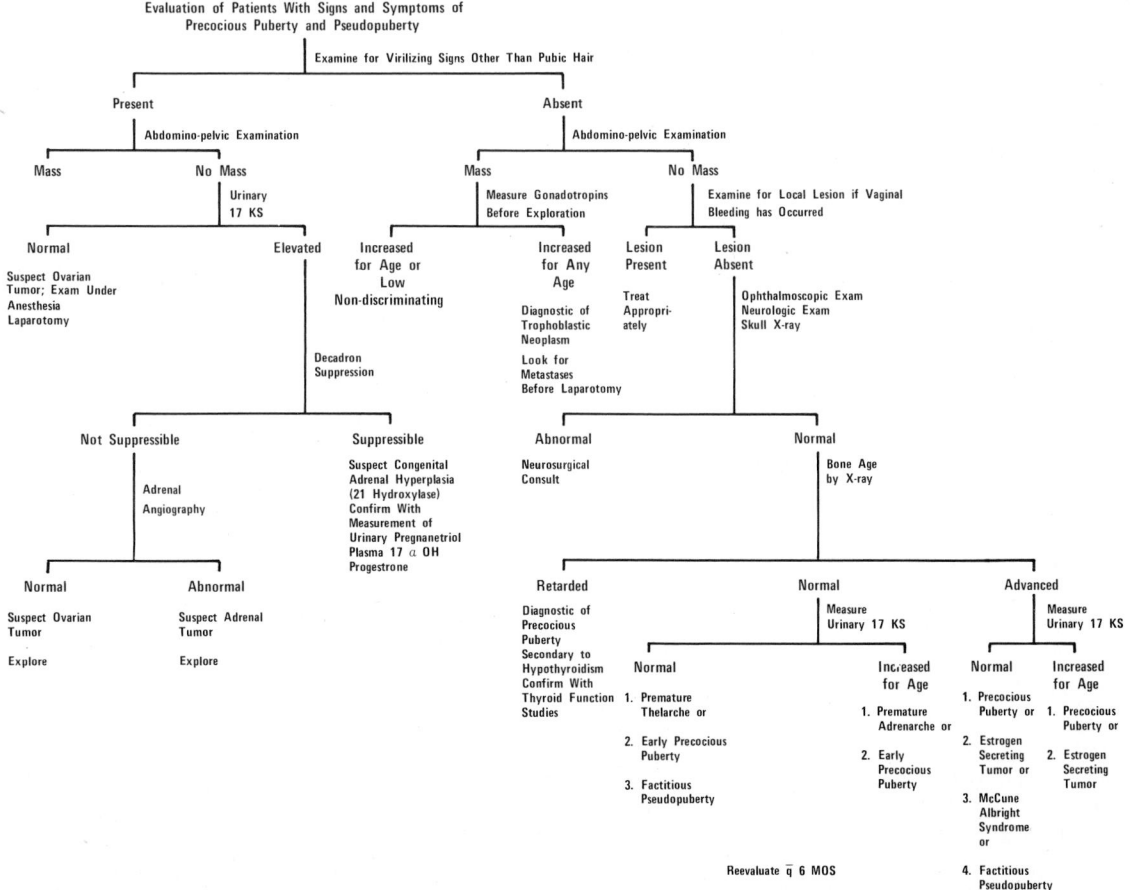

Figure 7–20. Outline for diagnostic evaluation of patients with signs and symptoms of precocious puberty and pseudopuberty.

nomonic of the McCune-Albright syndrome. Neurologic deficits are seen in precocious puberty due to disease of the CNS and may be seen in the McCune-Albright syndrome as well. In the latter, these are more commonly cranial nerve deficits, thought to be secondary to sclerotic changes in the base of the skull.

The Genital Examination and Further Studies.   Attention is directed to Fig. 7–20. A careful search for evidence of virilization is an important part of the physical examination of children in whom appearance of pubic hair is the first sign of precocious puberty or pseudopuberty. One should look for acne, extragenital hirsutism, and clitoromegaly in these instances.

When virilizing signs are present, failure to palpate a pelvic or an abdominal mass after a satisfactory abdominorectal examination, under sedation or anesthesia if necessary, makes an ovarian source of the virilization an unlikely possibility, although rarely such tumors do not become palpable until late in the course of the disease. When no mass is palpated, urinary 17-KS excretion should be measured. If quantities are found to be normal in a 24-hour urine collection, an ovarian source of androgen is probable, even in the absence of a palpable mass, and abdominal exploration should be undertaken. In contrast, if urinary 17-KS excretion is elevated, a dexamethasone suppression test (Ch. 5) should be performed. If urinary 17-KS excretion is not suppressible, adrenal angiography, accompanied by measurement of DHEA in adrenal venous effluent, may lead to a preoperative diagnosis of a unilateral adrenal neoplasm and obviate the need to explore both adrenals. If neither angiography nor adrenal venous hormonal concentration is abnormal, an ovarian tumor too small to be palpated should be suspected and sought at laparotomy. When elevated urinary 17-KS excretion is suppressible with dexamethasone, a diagnosis of congenital adrenal hyperplasia due to a 21-hydroxylase deficiency should be suspected. The finding of increases in either plasma 17-hydroxyprogesterone or its urinary metabolite, pregnanetriol, provides confirmatory evidence for the diagnosis.

When virilizing signs are absent in a girl under study for signs and symptoms of precocious puberty and pseudopuberty, an ovarian cause for the disease is rendered improbable but not excluded by failure to palpate an adnexal mass. On the other hand, palpating an adnexal mass does not establish an ovarian etiology of the disorder. When a mass is palpated, abdominal exploration is indicated, but results of measurements of gonadotropins in serum or urine should be obtained preoperatively. When gonadotropins are in excess of those attributable to pituitary secretion, a trophoblastic neoplasm should be suspected and appropriate studies for metastatic spread initiated before laparotomy. Gonadotropin levels that are minimally elevated, normal, or low for age provide no other discriminating diagnostic information, so that a functioning ovarian neoplasm should be suspected and the nature of the mass determined by laparotomy.

When vaginal bleeding has been observed in the absence of an ovarian or adrenal mass and in the absence of other signs and symptoms of precocious puberty or pseudopuberty, local lesions resulting in vaginal bleeding should be sought. Causes of these include vaginal infections, foreign bodies, and tumors. When no local lesion is found, ophthalmoscopic examination and neurologic and x-ray examinations of the skull should be performed. When these are abnormal, further evaluation should be made under the supervision and direction of a neurosurgeon.

When no abnormalities are found by either skull x-ray or funduscopic or neurologic examination, x-ray determination of bone age will provide a useful basis for proceeding with further studies. If bone age is retarded, precocious puberty

secondary to hypothyroidism should be suspected and confirmed by appropriate studies of thyroid function (Ch. 4).

When bone age is found to be normal or advanced for chronologic age, urinary 17-KS excretion should be measured. Among girls with *normal bone age and normal urinary 17-KS excretion,* diagnosis of premature thelarche, early precocious puberty, and factitious pseudopuberty should be considered if breast enlargement is the only sign of precocious maturation of secondary sexual characteristics. The diagnosis of premature thelarche can be eliminated if breast enlargement is accompanied by appearance of pubic hair or vaginal bleeding.

When *bone age is normal but urinary 17-KS excretion is increased for chronologic age,* findings are consistent with premature adrenarche if pubic hair is the sole evidence of precocious puberty. A diagnosis of early precocious puberty should be considered if breast enlargement accompanies the appearance of pubic hair.

When *bone age is advanced but urinary 17-KS excretion is normal or advanced for age,* precocious puberty is the most probable diagnosis. Rarely, factitious pseudopuberty or an ovarian tumor secreting estrogen, but not palpable, could be present. Re-examination at intervals of 3–6 months should make the distinction possible.

Delayed Menarche and Primary Amenorrhea

Introduction.   Delayed initiation and progression of puberty, including delayed menarche, constitute a second group of syndromes of abnormal ovarian function in childhood. As noted earlier, the range of ages at menarche extends from 9 to 16 years, normally. When menarche has not occurred by age 16, delayed menarche is an appropriate diagnosis. Since changes in vaginal smears, growth of breasts, and appearance of pubic hair usually precede first menses, the absence of these early signs of puberty at age 16 should suggest a tentative diagnosis of primary amenorrhea, as opposed to delayed menarche. Since primary amenorrhea is an objective manifestation of a pathophysiologic state, the underlying disorder must be identified.

Etiology.   Primary amenorrhea is an uncommon disorder that results from fetal errors in gonadal, gonaductal, and genital development in about 60% of cases. Of these, one half are due to the syndromes of gonadal dysgenesis, one third are due to mullerian dysgenesis, and one sixth are due to errors in genital development. The remaining 40% of women have primary amenorrhea due to hypogonadotropic states, other endocrinopathies, sclerocystic ovaries, follicles insensitive to gonadotropins, idiopathic delayed puberty, and endometrial synechiae. Thus, it is apparent that primary ovarian disease accounts for the disorder in about half the patients with primary amenorrhea.

Clinical Evaluation of the Patient with Primary Amenorrhea.   Prior to approaching the patient with primary amenorrhea, the physician should review the sequences and velocities of pubertal changes described earlier in this chapter. These changes become indirect tests of ovarian sex steroid hormone secretion and thus, tests of prepubertal and pubertal ovarian function. Although recall is not always reliable, careful questioning about these features, including age at onset, progression, and synchrony of pubescent events frequently provides the physician with a presumptive diagnosis and thereby with definite indications for critical diagnostic tests. For example, the constellation of normal age at onset, normal progression, and completely normal maturation of all secondary sexual characteristics except menses indicates that ovarian function is normal and suggests that mullerian dysgenesis is the basis for the amenorrhea. Similarly, maturation of breasts without maturation of axillary and pubic hair suggests that testicular feminization is the cause of the amenorrhea. Conversely, maturation of axillary and pubic hair in a male pattern associated with failure of breasts to develop is suggestive of the syndrome of male pseudohermaphroditism due to 5α reductase deficiency.

When the history of progression of pubertal changes is not helpful, features of value in discriminating among the various etiologic bases of primary amenorrhea should be sought during the physical examination. In addition to appraising the indirect indicators of ovarian function, special attention should be paid to extragenital features such as inguinal hernias or masses, stature, habitus, musculoskeletal anomalies, and cutaneous lesions. For example, since inguinal hernias are uncommon in women, inguinal hernias with or without inguinal masses in an amenorrheic woman with female external genitalia suggest a diagnosis of male pseudohermaphroditism. Musculoskeletal anomalies, cutaneous lesions, and short stature are commonly observed among patients with gonadal dysgenesis.

Tables 7–6 A and B and 7–7 A and B contain the diagnostically useful information that should be obtained from the history and physical examination for suspecting, and the anticipated results of tests essential for confirming, the diagnosis of syndromes associated with primary amenorrhea. The tables reveal nothing distinctive about delayed menarche. How is the syndrome diagnosed then?

A diagnosis of delayed menarche is a diagnosis made first by excluding other pathophysiologic bases for failure of menses to appear and second by the subsequent spontaneous occurrence of the menarche. Progression of pubertal changes over time is consistent with the diagnosis, and the observation of such changes may encourage the physician, the parents, and the patient to persist in expectant waiting as opposed to premature therapy.

Although constraints imposed by the format make it impractical to include all exceptions that may be encountered, it is thought that effects of these on diagnostic accuracy will be minimal. For additional information the reader should turn to the appropriate chapters in this or other texts in which the syndromes are described in greater detail.

Treatment of Primary Amenorrhea. Since primary amenorrhea is a sign of an underlying disorder of the hypothalamic-hypophyseal-gonadal-genital axis, rational therapy depends upon correct diagnosis of the pathophysiologic basis for the disorder. For those in whom the ovarian-genital portion of the axis is intact but the disorder is in the hypothalamic and pituitary units, replacement therapy for maturation of secondary sexual characteristics consists in the use of sex steroid hormones as described in Chapter 9. When pregnancy is desired, ovulation induction with exogenous gonadotropins can be attempted. (See later.)

When the basis for the disorder is primarily gonadal or genital in origin, surgical correction should be undertaken when feasible, primarily to provide socially acceptable, functional genitals. Optimally, as noted earlier and discussed in Chapter 9, need for these procedures will have been recognized perinatally and their timing planned to conform with development of the peer group in the case of persons born with ambiguous genitalia. For the most part, fertility is an unrealistic goal for the majority of these patients, and the patient should be informed of this deficit as gently as possible.

After the Menarche: Secondary Amenorrhea

Secondary amenorrhea is defined as the absence of menses in patients who have menstruated before, whereas patients with primary amenorrhea have never menstruated. To a large extent this distinction is artificial, since many conditions usually associated with primary amenorrhea will occasionally produce secondary amenorrhea. Even in congenital disorders, such as gonadal dysgenesis, the patient may have periods, and in some cases even ovulate and conceive, only to develop amenorrhea after months of cyclic menstrual function. Conversely, a condition such as the polycystic ovary syndrome may develop early enough during puberty to block ovarian function before the first menstrual bleeding. In fact, the difference between primary and secondary amenorrhea is often only a quantitative matter, the former occurring when estrogen levels remain below, the latter when estrogen levels exceed at any one time the threshold level for endometrial proliferation and subsequent necrosis. Even so, the distinction remains useful since most congenital conditions will fall in the category of primary amenorrhea. Until more is known about the mechanisms controlling normal ovarian function, it is impossible to present a completely consistent etiologic classification of secondary amenorrhea. The classification illustrated in Table 7–8 goes a long way toward this goal and has the advantage of offering a practical approach and requiring a minimum of laboratory tests.

Not included in Table 7–8 are the physiologic causes of secondary amenorrhea. It is important to stress that in patients with secondary amenorrhea the first diagnosis to be considered is pregnancy, and this must be weighed until it can be ruled out. Too often in doing this, one relies upon pregnancy tests or one of the classic signs of early pregnancy, such as uterine enlargement, bluish discoloration of the cervix, or softening of the isthmic part of the uterus — tests that all too often fail to yield a clear-cut answer. In most instances, an unequivocal answer can be obtained without delay by a simple examination of the cervix for mucus. If mucus is present the patient is not pregnant, since this indicates a ratio of estrogen to progesterone that is incompatible with normal pregnancy. The two other major physiologic causes of secondary amenorrhea, puerperal amenorrhea and normal menopause, can be easily ruled out by history.

In discussing the various types of secondary amenorrhea and their causes, it is important to stress that amenorrhea is only the end in a continuum of conditions that range from apparent normal function to total absence of ovarian function. In its milder form or in an early stage, the ovarian abnormality that will produce amenorrhea later on may manifest itself only by the presence of infertility while, at least by the usual criteria, the cycle is completely normal. In a more advanced form, the cycle remains ovulatory, but the luteal phase is more or less abnormal. Abnormal luteal function need not produce gross abnormalities in the menstrual cycle. The basal body temperature chart may be normal, and only careful study of the endometrium and of the hormones secreted by the corpus luteum will bring the abnormality to light. As the condition progresses the patient becomes anovulatory, but the ovary continues to secrete estrogens, occasionally cyclically, and the individual may still have fairly normal cycles. More often, however, there is oligomenorrhea, and in this stage of ovarian dysfunction, excessive bleeding may alternate with episodes of amenorrhea. As the ovarian disturbance becomes more and more severe, the ovary secretes less and less estrogen until finally estrogen secretion ceases. The patient complains of amenorrhea and progressive symptoms of estrogenic deficiency with full atrophy of the vaginal mucosa in extreme cases. The differential diagnosis shown in Table 7–8 applies to mild as well as to severe forms.

A schematic outline for clinical evaluation of patients

Table 7-6, A CLINICAL CORRELATES

PATHOPHYSIOLOGIC BASIS	SYNDROME(S)	History			Physical Examination		
		Pubertal Changes		Other	Secondary Sexual Characteristics	Genitalia	Miscellaneous
		Onset	Progression				
	1. Male pseudohermaphroditism due to deficient testosterone synthesis						
	(A) 20, 22-desmolase	Unknown	Unknown	Neonatal adrenal cortical insufficiency	Immature female	Female or anomalous	Inguinal mass(es); inguinal hernia(s)
	(B) 3β-hydroxy-steroid dehydrogenase	Normal or minimally delayed	Minimal with virilization	Neonatal adrenal cortical insufficiency	Variably virilized with gynecomastia	Female or anomalous	Nothing distinctive
	(C) 17 α-hydroxylase	Delayed	Minimal	Nothing diagnostic	Gynecomastia only; no axillary or pubic hair	Female or anomalous	Hypertensive
	(D) 17, 20-desmolase	Delayed	Minimal	Nothing diagnostic	Immature female	Anomalous	Inguinal masses
	(E) 17-ketosteroid reductase	Normal	Minimal with virilization	Nothing diagnostic	Variably virilized with gynecomastia	Female or anomalous	Inguinal masses
Fetal errors in genital differentiation	2. Male pseudohermaphroditism due to 5α reductase deficiency	Normal or minimally delayed	Virilization of genitalia; no gynecomastia	Family history of sexual immaturity, infertility	Male breasts; axillary and pubic hair normal	Anomalous	Habitus female
	3. Male pseudohermaphroditism due to androgen resistance						
	(A) Complete testicular feminization	Normal or minimally delayed	Maturation of breasts advanced relative to axillary and pubic hair	Family history of sexual immaturity, infertility	Female breasts with immature nipples and hypopigmented areolae; scant to absent axillary and pubic hair	Immature female external genitalia; patent vagina with no cervix	Inguinal mass(es); inguinal hernia(s)
	(B) Incomplete testicular feminization	Normal or minimally delayed	Maturation of axillary and pubic hair advanced relative to breasts	Family history may not be helpful	Female breasts; axillary and pubic hair normal	Partial labioscrotal fusion; clitorimegaly; patent vagina with no cervix or urogenital sinus	Inguinal mass(es); inguinal hernia(s)
	(C) Familial incomplete male pseudohermaphroditism (type 1)	Normal or minimally delayed	Maturation of axillary and pubic hair advanced relative to breasts	Family history of sexual immaturity, infertility	Male breasts with gynecomastia; axillary and pubic hair normal	Variable: from female with clitorimegaly to anomalous male	Inguinal mass(es); hernia(s); signs of virilism
	4. Female pseudohermaphroditism with fetal and postnatal androgen excess	May be precocious	Maturation of axillary and pubic hair advanced relative to breasts	Family history of neonatal adrenal cortical insufficiency	Axillary and pubic hair advanced relative to breasts	External genitalia female with clitorimegaly	Short stature

Table 7-6, B

RESULTS OF DIAGNOSTIC STUDIES

SYNDROME(S)	Cytogenetic — Nuclear Sex† Barr Bodies	"F" Bodies	Karyotype	Pituitary Function — Basal Gonadotropin Secretion Relative to Peers	Other Hormones	Gonadal Visualization And Biopsy	Miscellaneous Diagnostic Studies	TREATMENT
1. Male pseudohermaphroditism due to deficient testosterone synthesis								
(A) 20, 22-desmolase	− A	+ A	XY A	Not described B	Normal C	Testes A	Low serum and urinary hydroxycorticoids A	Remove testes; glucocorticoid replacement; sex steroid hormone replacement
(B) 3-hydroxy-steroid dehydrogenase	− A	+ A	XY A	Normal (?) B	Normal C	Testes A	Low serum and urinary hydroxycorticoids; plasma testosterone low normal A	Glucocorticoid replacement
(C) 17 α-hydroxylase	− A	+ A	XY A	Elevated B	Normal C	Testes A	High serum progesterone, desoxycorticosterone**; hypokalemia A	Glucocorticoid replacement; sex steroid hormone replacement
(D) 17, 20-desmolase	− A	+ A	XY A	Elevated B	Normal C	Testes A	Low serum or urinary DHEA A	Remove testes; sex steroid hormone replacement
(E) 17-ketosteroid reductase	− A	+ A	XY A	Elevated B	Normal C	Testes A	High serum androstenedione, estrone; low testosterone A	Removes testes; sex steroid hormone replacement
2. Male pseudohermaphroditism due to 5 α reductase deficiency	− A	+ A	XY A	Normal or elevated B	Normal C	Testes A	Low urinary androsterone	Remove testes; clitoridectomy; sex steroid hormone replacement
3. Male pseudohermaphroditism due to androgen resistance								
(A) Complete testicular feminization	− A	+ A	XY A	Normal or elevated B	Normal C	Testes A	Abdominal plain film; serum testosterone in normal male range	Remove testes; postoperative sex steroid hormone replacement
(B) Incomplete testicular feminization	− A	+ A	XY A	Elevated B	Normal C	Testes A	Abdominal plain film; serum testosterone in normal male range or elevated	Remove testes; postoperative sex steroid hormone replacement
(C) Familial incomplete male pseudohermaphroditism (type 1)	− A	+ A	XY A	Elevated A	Normal C	Testes A	Serum testosterone may be normal or high; vaginoscopy; urethroscopy; cystoscopy if required A	Remove testes; postoperative sex steroid hormone replacement
4. Female pseudohermaphroditism with fetal and postnatal androgen excess*	+ A	− C	XX C	Normal or elevated B	ACTH** secretion increased A	Ovaries	Bone age advanced; steroid hormone levels consistent with etiology** A	Glucocorticoid replacement therapy as indicated

A — Results essential for diagnosis and treatment
B — Of interest, but not essential
C — Not indicated
** — Associated with congenital adrenal hyperplasia
∴ — Results of glucocorticoid suppression tests are diagnostic
† — When nuclear sex is consonant with genital sex, further cytogenetic study is optional; when nuclear sex is not consonant with genital sex, further study is mandatory

Table 7-7, A CLINICAL CORRELATES

PATHOPHYSIOLOGIC BASIS	SYNDROME(S)	History — Pubertal Changes — Onset	History — Pubertal Changes — Progression	History — Other	Physical Examination — Secondary Sexual Characteristics	Physical Examination — Genitalia	Physical Examination — Miscellaneous
Fetal errors in gonadal development	1. True hermaphroditism	Normal or delayed	Virilization	Nothing diagnostic	Variably virilized	Usually anomalous	Nothing diagnostic
	2. Gonadal dysgenesis with stigmata of Turner's syndrome	Delayed	None to minimal	Edema of extremities in neonatal period	Immature female	Immature female	Short stature; musculoskeletal, cutaneous, osseous anomalies
	3. Mixed gonadal dysgenesis	Normal	Minimal with virilization	Nothing diagnostic	Variably virilized	Usually anomalous	Nothing diagnostic; normal stature
	4. Pure gonadal dysgenesis	Delayed	None to minimal	Family history of sexual immaturity, infertility	Immature female	Immature female; may have clitorimegaly	Habitus may be eunuchoidal; stature normal
Fetal errors in gonaductal development	Mullerian dysgenesis	Normal	Normal	Cyclic abdominal pain	Maturing or mature female	Vagina absent or not patent	Congenital musculoskeletal malformations; abdominal masses; endometriomas
Ovarian follicles insensitive to gonadotrophins	17 α-hydroxylase deficiency	Delayed	Minimal	Family history of sexual immaturity	Immature female	Immature female	Hypertensive
	"Resistant Ovaries"	Delayed	Minimal	Nothing diagnostic	Immature female	Immature female	Normotensive
Hypothalamic-pituitary diseases	Familial hypogonadotropic hypogonadism	Delayed	Minimal	Family history of anosmia, mid-line defects and hypogonadism in boys and girls	Immature female	Immature female	Anosmia, mid-line defects
	Pituitary and parapituitary tumors; idiopathic panhypopituitarism	Normal or delayed	None, minimal, or interrupted	Failure to grow; other signs and symptoms of anterior pituitary failure, diabetes insipidus	Immature female	Immature female	Short stature; other signs of hypopituitarism
Unknown	Polycystic ovaries (chronic anovulation)	Normal	Variable virilization	Nothing diagnostic	Variably virilized	Female; may have clitorimegaly	Hirsutism; diabetes; acanthrosis nigricans
	Delayed menarche	Delayed	Minimal	Nothing diagnostic	Immature female	Immature female	May have short stature
	Systemic diseases	Delayed	Minimal	Signs and symptoms of systemic disease	Immature female	Immature female	Appropriate to systemic disease

Table 7-7, B

RESULTS OF DIAGNOSTIC STUDIES

SYNDROME(S)	Cytogenetic			Pituitary Function		Gonadal Visualization And Biopsy	Miscellaneous Diagnostic Studies	TREATMENT
	Nuclear Sex[†]		Karyotype	Basal Gonadotropin Secretion Relative to Peers	Other Hormones			
	Barr Bodies	"F" Bodies						
1. True hermaphroditism	+ or − / A	+ or − / A	XX, XY or mosaics / A	Normal or elevated / B	Normal / C	Testis, ovary and ovotestis in varying combinations / A	Vaginoscopy, urethroscopy, cystoscopy, if required / A	Preservation of gonadal tissue consistent with sex of rearing
2. Gonadal dysgenesis with stigmata of Turner's syndrome	+ or − / A	+ or − / A	45, X or mosaics; all varieties of breakage, with or without reunion / A	Elevated / A	Normal / C	Bilateral streaks devoid of germ cells / A or B ††	X-rays for skeletal malformations; urinary tract anomalies / A	Sex steroid hormone replacement
3. Mixed gonadal dysgenesis	− / A	+ or − * / A	X/XY / A	Normal or elevated / B	Normal / C	Unilateral streak, contralateral testis or tumor / A	Vaginoscopy, urethroscopy / C	Remove tumors; timing of gonadectomy controversial
4. Pure gonadal dysgenesis	+ or − / A	+ or − / A	XX,XY / A	Elevated / A	Normal / C	Bilateral streaks devoid of germ cells / A or B	Nothing of diagnostic or therapeutic value / C	Sex steroid hormone replacement
Mullerian dysgenesis	+ / C	− / C	XX / C	Normal / C	Normal / C	Normal ovaries / C	Examination under anesthesia, if necessary / A	Surgery appropriate to lesion: hymenotomy, vaginoplasty or opening cervical canal to vagina
17 α-hydroxylase deficiency	+ / C	− / C	XX / C	Elevated / A	ACTH** secretion increased; but suppressible / A	Small ovaries containing unstimulated follicles / B	Elevated serum** progesterone, desoxycorticosterone; hypokalemia / A	Sex steroid hormone replacement; glucocorticoid replacement
"Resistant Ovaries"	+ / B	B or C	XX / C	Elevated / A	Normal / C	Small ovaries containing unstimulated follicles / A	Nothing diagnostic	Sex steroid hormone replacement if indicated
Familial hypogonadotropic hypogonadism	+ / A	− / C	XX / C	Low / A	Normal / C	Small ovaries containing unstimulated follicles / B	Tests of smell / A	Sex steroid hormone replacement or ovulation induction if pregnancy is desired
Pituitary and parapituitary tumors; idiopathic panhypopituitarism	+ / A	− / C	XX / C	Normal or low / A	Abnormal / A	Small ovaries containing growing follicles / C	X-rays of sella, other neuroradiologic studies as indicated / A	Sex steroid hormone replacement or ovulation induction if pregnancy is desired
Polycystic ovaries	+ / C	− / C	XX / C	LH/FSH ratio may be elevated / B	Normal / C	Sclerocystic ovaries / A	Blood testosterone may be elevated / A	Cyclic progesterone; ovulation induction if pregnancy is desired
Delayed menarche	+ / A	− / C	XX / A	Normal or low / A	Normal / C	Small ovaries containing growing follicles / C	Progesterone withdrawal; clomiphene test	Expectant waiting
Systemic diseases	+ / A	− / C	XX / C	Normal or low / B	May be normal / B	Small ovaries containing growing follicles / C	Tests appropriate to systemic disease suspected	Appropriate therapy for primary disease; replacement therapy if indicated

A — Results essential for diagnosis and treatment
B — Of interest, but not essential
C — Not indicated
* — Failure to demonstrate "F" bodies is not conclusive evidence for absence of a Y chromosome
** — Results of glucocorticoid suppression tests are diagnostic
† — When nuclear sex is consonant with genital sex, further cytogenetic study is optional; when nuclear sex is not consonant with genital sex, further study is mandatory
†† — Essential if X/XY mosaicism is found on cytogenetic study

Tables 7-6, A, B and 7-7, A, B. Adapted from data of Ross, G. T., In DeGroot, L. J., et al. (eds.): *Endocrinology.* New York, Grune & Stratton, 1979, pp. 1419–1433.

with secondary amenorrhea is depicted in Fig. 7–21. Coupled with Tables 7–8 and 7–9, this scheme will facilitate diagnosing the pathophysiologic and etiologic basis of most cases of ovarian dysfunction.

The first step in the diagnosis of secondary amenorrhea lies in a precise characterization of ovarian steroid production. The questions to ask and to answer are as follows: (1) Do the ovaries make progesterone; i.e., is the patient ovulatory? (2) Do the ovaries secrete normal amounts of estrogens? (3) Do they secrete normal amounts of androgens? Approaches to these questions have been outlined in earlier sections of this chapter, and it must be stressed that in almost all cases the answer can be obtained easily by a simple evaluation of a few hormonal target organs with the vaginal smear, cervical mucus, endometrial biopsy, the basal body temperature and by carrying out a progesterone withdrawal test. In interpreting these tests, it is essential to keep in mind the limitations of their interpretations that have been discussed previously.

As an example, the sensitivity to estrogens of the vaginal mucosa, cervical mucus, and endometrium is remarkably different, the vaginal mucosa being the most sensitive to estrogens, the cervical mucus intermediate, and the endometrium the least sensitive. Similarly, the significance of the progesterone withdrawal test must be well understood. Progesterone withdrawal implies a level of estrogens sufficient to produce proliferation of the endometrium and therefore a relatively high level of estrogens. Since the test is an all or none test, two patients having the same condition but with slightly different levels of estrogens and, therefore, different degrees of endometrial proliferation may respond in opposite ways to progesterone. Similarly, a patient may respond to a first progesterone injection with a

positive response and fail to respond to a second injection a few weeks later. By relying too much on the progesterone withdrawal test as the only discriminant, there is the danger of separating into different categories patients that are qualitatively identical and only quantitatively different. Following a careful assessment of their ovarian steroid production, patients with secondary amenorrhea can be put in one of the three major categories (Fig. 7–21 and Table 7–8):

1. Patients with normal ovarian steroid production
2. Patients with decreased ovarian steroid production
3. Patients with increased ovarian steroid production

With Normal Ovarian Steroid Production

In a few women with secondary amenorrhea, ovarian function is normal; although menses have been absent for a prolonged period, the presence of a biphasic temperature chart or of cyclic fluctuations in the secretion of ovarian hormone indicates that the ovaries are functioning normally. Since normal ovarian steroid production requires normal function of the hypothalamus, pituitary, and ovaries, the cause of the amenorrhea is to be found in the lower genital tract, mainly in the uterus, and additional diagnostic tests will address themselves to this area when ovarian steroid production is normal. In most of these patients, the amenorrhea is due to the presence of intrauterine synechiae or adhesions, resulting in a more or less complete obliteration of the endometrial cavity. The diagnosis is easily made by establishing normal ovarian function in a patient with amenorrhea and is confirmed by hysterosalpingography or hysteroscopy. In most instances, uterine synechiae result from a postabortal or postpartum

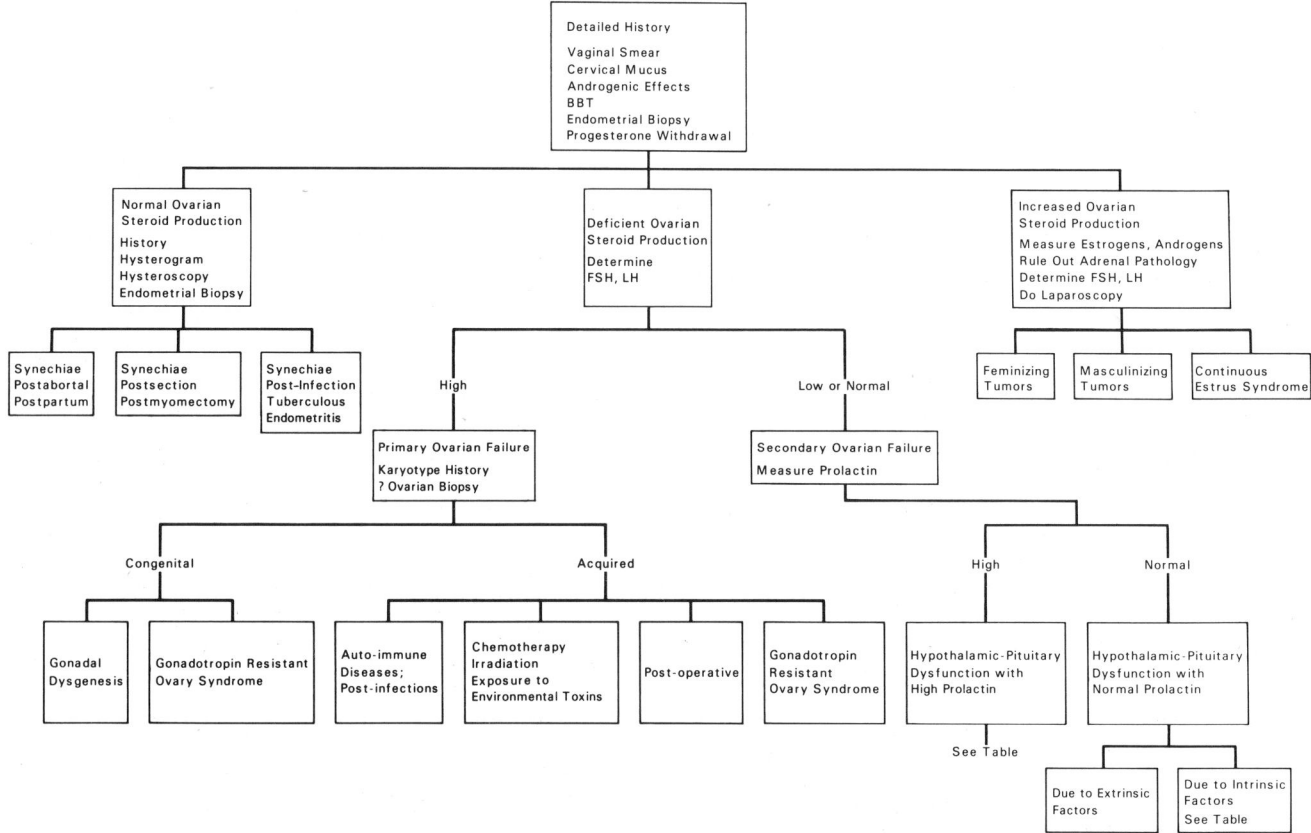

Figure 7–21. A schema for the clinical evaluation of patients with secondary amenorrhea.

Table 7–8. CLASSIFICATION OF CAUSES OF
SECONDARY AMENORRHEA

I. With Normal Ovarian Steroid Production
  A. Intrauterine synechiae (Asherman's syndrome)
    1. Following postabortal or postpartum infection and trauma
    2. Following myomectomy or cesarian section
    3. Tuberculous endometritis
  B. Hysterectomy

II. With Decreased Ovarian Steroid Production
  A. With high gonadotropins (primary ovarian failure)
    1. Congenital
      a. Gonadal dysgenesis
      b. Gonadotropin-resistant ovary syndrome
    2. Acquired: premature primary ovarian failure
      a. Autoimmune diseases
      b. After chemotherapy (cytoxan, etc.)
      c. After irradiation
      d. Postinfection (mumps)
      e. Environmental toxins (smoking)
      f. Gonadotropin-resistant ovary syndrome
      g. Postoperative
  B. With low or normal gonadotropins (secondary ovarian failure)
    1. Hypothalamic-pituitary dysfunction with high PRL, with or without galactorrhea (See Table 7–9)
    2. Hypothalamic-pituitary dysfunction with normal PRL, with or without galactorrhea
      a. Hypothalamic-pituitary dysfunction due to intrinsic factors
        (1) Hypothalamus
          (a) tumors
          (b) head trauma
          (c) following CNS surgery
          (d) following irradiation
        (2) Pituitary
          (a) intrinsic pituitary disease
          (b) chromophobic tumors
          (c) other pituitary tumors
          (d) surgery
          (e) x-ray
          (f) Sheehan's syndrome
          (g) empty sella syndrome
      b. Hypothalamic-pituitary dysfunction due to extrinsic factors
        (1) Psychogenic amenorrhea
        (2) Starvation amenorrhea, anorexia nervosa
        (3) Post-pill amenorrhea without galactorrhea
        (4) Excessive extraovarian production of estrogen
          (a) obesity
          (b) age
          (c) other factors leading to increased conversion of androgens to estrogen (thyroid dysfunction)
        (5) Extraovarian endocrine disease
          (a) thyroid
          (b) adrenal
          (c) pancreas
        (6) Intercurrent disease
          (a) acute
          (b) chronic
        (7) Unknown

III. With Increased Ovarian Steroid Production
  A. Feminizing ovarian tumors
  B. Masculinizing ovarian tumors
  C. Continuous estrus syndrome (polycystic ovary syndrome)

Table 7–9. DIFFERENTIAL DIAGNOSIS OF
GALACTORRHEA-AMENORRHEA SYNDROMES

I. Inhibition of Dopamine Activity
  A. Drug-induced
    a. dopamine receptor blockade
      1. phenothiazines
        chlorpromazine
        butaperazine maleate
        trifluoperazine hydrochloride
        perphenazine
        prochlorperazine
        thiethylperazine
        thioridazine
      2. thioxanthines
        thiothixene
      3. butyrophenones
        haloperidol
      4. diphenylbutylpiperidines
        pimozide
      5. dibenoxazapines
        loxapine succinate
      6. dihydroindolones
        molindone hydrochloride
      7. procainamide derivatives
        metoclopramide
        sulpiride
    b. catecholamine-depleting agents
      reserpine
      α-methyldopa
  B. Central Nervous System Disease
    a. encephalitis, postencephalitis
    b. craniopharyngioma
    c. tumors of the pineal gland
    d. aneurysms
    e. hypothalamic tumors, primary, metastatic
    f. pseudotumor cerebri

II. Inhibition of Dopamine Transport
  A. Pituitary stalk resection

III. Tumors that Secrete PRL
  A. Pituitary tumors
    a. chromophobe adenoma
    b. eosinophilic adenoma
    c. basophilic adenoma
  B. Tumors other than of pituitary (very rare, see V., A., f)

IV. Hyperplasia of the Lactotrophs
  A. Thyroid abnormalities
    a. hypothyroidism
  B. Gonadal abnormalities
    a. during treatment with estrogen/progestin combinations
    b. following withdrawal of estrogen/progestin combinations

V. Neural Stimulation
  A. Disorders of the chest wall and of thorax
    a. thoracotomy
    b. mastectomy
    c. thoracoplasty
    d. burns of chest wall
    e. herpes zoster
    f. bronchogenic tumors
    g. bronchiectasis and chronic bronchitis
  B. Nipple stimulation
    a. chronic inflammatory disease
    b. stimulation of the nipples
  C. Laparotomy
  D. Spinal cord
    a. tabes dorsalis
    b. syringomyelia
  E. Psychogenic
    a. pseudocyesis
    b. ? stress

endometritis. It has been thought by some that too vigorous curettage, with removal of most of the endometrium, causes amenorrhea, but the fact that lysis of the adhesions restores normal menstrual function demonstrates that this is not true. Tuberculous endometritis is another cause for the development of uterine synechiae, but this form of tuberculosis is infrequently seen in the United States.

Treatment of uterine synechiae consists of lysis of the adhesions, preferably under direct vision during hysteroscopy or in advanced cases following hysterotomy. The prognosis in terms of restoration of menstrual function is excellent but less favorable in terms of fertility, since following conception a significant number of patients will have early or late abortions or even an intrauterine fetal demise.

With Decreased Ovarian Steroid Production

In patients with decreased ovarian steroid production, the next important step lies in the determination of the level of gonadotropins. If the gonadotropins are in the menopausal range, one is dealing with primary ovarian failure;

when they are low or in the normal preovulatory or post-ovulatory range, the patient has secondary ovarian failure. In some instances, a single determination of plasma gonadotropins will allow a distinction between these two categories. In many cases, because of the episodic nature of gonadotropin secretion, multiple determinations are necessary to provide definitive information. The distinction between primary and secondary ovarian failure is critical, both in terms of etiology and in terms of prognosis and therapy. In primary ovarian failure in which the etiology lies in the ovary, the condition is almost always irreversible, and there is little hope of successful therapy. On the other hand, in secondary ovarian failure, in which the immediate cause is to be found in the hypothalamic-pituitary axis, spontaneous reversal is frequent and therapy is successful in most cases.

With High Gonadotropins (Primary Ovarian Failure). Gonadal dysgenesis, commonly associated with primary amenorrhea, is included in this differential diagnosis, since occasionally this syndrome produces secondary amenorrhea. Gonadal dysgenesis is discussed in detail in Chapter 9.

Cessation of ovarian function due to exhaustion of the supply of oocytes normally occurs between ages 48 and 52 but can occur at an earlier age and has been reported in teenaged girls. Some authors apply to this condition the term of premature menopause, but this terminology is unfortunate because of its implications of aging. Also, it implies that the etiology of the condition is the same as in the natural menopause, an assumption that is not always warranted. For this reason the term premature primary ovarian failure, although somewhat awkward, is preferred. The diagnosis is based on finding elevated gonadotropins and atrophy of the target organs of the estrogens. Since little is known about the factors controlling the rate of follicular atresia, the etiology of premature ovarian failure remains unknown, but recently a number of causes for this condition have been identified.

In some cases, immunologic mechanisms have been implicated, and in some of these women antibodies that react with cells from corpora lutea and theca interna of mature graafian follicles have been found. Interestingly enough, in some of these women antibodies were also found that reacted with steroid hormone-producing cells in all three layers of human adrenal cortices, and in others, with interstitial cells in human testes and with human trophoblastic epithelium.

Chemotherapy of leukemia and lymphomas has been associated with amenorrhea due to premature depletion of oocytes in some young women. Moreover, the extent of depletion depends upon doses received and duration of treatment. Similarly, inclusion of ovaries in fields exposed to irradiation in x-ray therapy for abdominal neoplasms has resulted in oocyte depletion and amenorrhea. Recently, smoking has been implicated in the etiology of oocyte depletion and early menopause. Furthermore, regional increments in the incidence of amenorrhea following exposure to noxious chemicals such as insecticides suggest that oocytes in human ovaries may be susceptible to deleterious effects of these substances. Excessive resection of ovarian tissue in therapy of sclerocystic ovaries or in excision of ovarian cysts or of benign neoplasms has been implicated in premature menopause.

Recently, several cases of premature ovarian failure have been reported in which ovarian biopsies revealed the presence of morphologically normal, although immature, follicles. The high gonadotropin in the presence of diminished or absent ovarian follicle response has been thought to suggest an insensitivity of the ovarian follicle, hence the name of the syndrome, gonadotropin-resistant ovaries. In some cases, treatment with high doses of gonadotropins overcame the relative insensitivity of the follicles and in fact induced ovulation. The etiology of the condition that in some patients may produce primary and in others secondary amenorrhea remains uncertain, but the suggestion has been made that the insensitivity of the follicle to gonadotropin secretion may be due to a deficient gonadotropin-receptor mechanism.

With Low or Normal Gonadotropins. A low or normal level of gonadotropins in the face of deficient ovarian hormone production implies hypothalamic-pituitary unit dysfunction or failure. In some cases, the secondary amenorrhea can be attributed to a specific lesion within the hypothalamic-pituitary unit. In the vast majority of cases, however, this cannot be done and the amenorrhea must be considered either to be owing to a hypothalamic-pituitary dysfunction, nature unknown, or to be induced by factors extrinsic to the hypothalamic-pituitary unit. When gonadotropin releasing hormone (GnRH) became available, it was thought that this would lead to methods allowing differentiation between pituitary and hypothalamic amenorrheas. The assumption was that patients having normal LH release following administration of GnRH could be assumed to have hypothalamic amenorrhea, and vice versa. Unfortunately, this hope was not borne out. For instance, in patients with pituitary tumors, the response to GnRH may be perfectly normal or even exaggerated. In general terms, it is becoming increasingly evident that the dose of GnRH is not the only, or even the most important, factor determining the rate of release of LH, but that other variables, such as earlier stimulation with GnRH, estrogens, and so on, are more important modulators of the stimulatory effect of GnRH upon LH release. Hopes were also raised that radioimmunoassays for GnRH would be developed that would be sensitive enough to detect GnRH in the peripheral circulation. Again, this hope has not been borne out. Even if such methods were available, it is unlikely there would be a correlation between the levels of GnRH in the peripheral circulation and its concentration in the hypothalamic-pituitary portal system.

If gonadotropins are normal or low and ovarian steroid production is deficient, the clinician arrives at a third important diagnostic branching point, dividing the patients into two categories depending on the presence or absence of an elevated PRL level or of galactorrhea. Approximately 20% of patients with secondary amenorrhea have elevated levels of PRL. Due to the episodic nature of PRL secretion, a single determination of PRL may not always be an adequate discriminant. It must be noted that a significant number of patients with high PRL do not have galactorrhea, and vice versa.

Some pathophysiologic and etiologic bases of high PRL and secondary amenorrhea are listed in Table 7–9. These conditions are considered in more detail in the section on the breasts and will not be considered further. Some of the syndromes in the high PRL or galactorrhea, or both, group appear again in the next category (with normal PRL). Why the same condition will be associated with galactorrhea in some women and not in others is not known.

In patients with normal PRL, intrinsic hypothalamic or pituitary conditions such as tumors, granulomata, and so on, should be considered but only very rarely will this be found and, if so, the neurologic symptoms in most instances will predominate and the secondary amenorrhea will be incidental.

In a significant number of patients, although the immediate cause of the amenorrhea is hypothalamic-pituitary dysfunction, the dysfunction is secondary to factors extrinsic to the hypothalamic-pituitary-ovarian axis. Psychologic reasons for amenorrhea are known to be quite frequent, but in most cases a diagnosis can only be made by exclusion since there is no characteristic pattern for this type of amenorrhea. The earlier assertion that low levels of LH in the presence of normal levels of FSH are diagnostic for psychogenic amenorrheas is no longer tenable since this pattern is found in most cases of advanced secondary ovarian failure.

In a diet-conscious society, weight loss is becoming a frequent cause of amenorrhea. One interesting form is the amenorrhea seen in anorexia nervosa, a condition characterized by weight loss and amenorrhea most frequently occurring in pubertal girls. In addition to emaciation and amenorrhea, hallmarks of this diagnosis include severe constipation, bradycardia, and hypothermia. The endocrine picture is most characteristic: low serum T_4 and normal T_3 levels, low to absent levels of LH in the presence of normal levels of FSH, and elevated plasma corticoids. Although plasma corticoids are elevated, their secretion rate is actually decreased. This discrepancy between secretion rates and plasma levels is due to a markedly increased half-life of plasma cortisol. The characteristic combination of low gonadotropins and elevated blood corticoids makes it easy to differentiate anorexia nervosa from other types of secondary amenorrhea. A similar and probably identical symptom complex, however, is observed in all patients who are losing weight, whether it be for psychologic, cosmetic, or other reasons, and therefore it is preferable to combine all these conditions under one name, that of starvation-amenorrhea.

An interesting cause of secondary amenorrhea is that due to excessive extraovarian production of estrogens. In some patients with obesity, for example, as a result of the increased fat cell mass, there is an increased conversion of androstenedione to estrone. The increased levels of estrogen by their inappropriate feedback produce an imbalance in the hypothalamic-pituitary-ovarian relationships.

Acute and chronic disease will often produce menstrual disturbances by central mechanisms and interference with the hypothalamic-pituitary axis. Acute infections (including infections of the reproductive tract, such as pelvic inflammatory disease) will rarely produce amenorrhea but in most cases merely postpone ovulation or cause irregular bleeding due to the occurrence of one or more anovulatory cycles. In contrast, chronic diseases such as tuberculosis or cancer will occasionally produce amenorrhea.

Diseases of the other endocrine glands, such as the thyroid, adrenal, and pancreas, are frequently the cause of secondary amenorrhea. Usually the symptoms of the primary disease will rapidly lead to the correct diagnosis, and effective treatment will result in return of normal ovarian function.

In a majority of cases of secondary amenorrhea with low or normal gonadotropins, no organic disease can be found. To a small extent this may be due to the fact that pituitary tumors are too small to be detected by classic means, but it is unlikely that this can account for a significant fraction of the secondary amenorrheas without known etiology. It is more likely that in most patients the cause of amenorrhea lies in a functional disarrangement of the control mechanisms that govern the relationship between the hypothalamic-pituitary axis and the ovary.

With Increased Ovarian Steroid Production

Very rarely, secondary amenorrhea may result from ovarian tumors. Ovarian dysfunction has been associated with primary tumors arising in the ovary, with tumors metastasizing to the ovary from a primary site in another organ, and with tumors ectopically secreting gonadotropins. Both primary and secondary tumors, intrinsically, without endocrine function, may alter ovarian function by mechanisms that remain to be elucidated. In addition to gonadotropins, some ovarian tumors secrete other substances, such as serotonin and T_4, which are not usually regarded as secretory products of normal ovarian tissue, so that such tumors may be included among those associated with so-called "ectopic hormone production." Primary ovarian tumors that produce hormones and their important clinical features are listed in Table 7–10.

Tumors Producing Estrogens

Granulosa-Theca Cell Tumors.   These are the most common functioning ovarian neoplasms and are referred to as "granulosa-theca cell tumors" or alternatively, as "feminizing mesenchymomas." Collectively, these tumors account for 15–20% of all solid ovarian neoplasms. Careful microscopic examination of multiple sections reveals that granulosa-theca cell tumors are rarely composed exclusively of either granulosa cells or theca cells, so that attempts to classify them separately have not seemed useful. Although these tumors are commonly thought of as producing estrogen excess, signs of virilism are frequent. This is not unexpected in view of the fact that in addition to small amounts of estrogens, they mainly secrete androstenedione, while the bulk of the circulating estrogens derive from the peripheral conversion of androstenedione to estrone. It should be noted that 80% or more of feminizing tumors are palpable on pelvic examination.

Tumors Producing Androgens.
These tumors include arrhenoblastomas, dysgerminomas, gonadoblastomas, lipoid cell tumors, and adrenal-like and hilar cell tumors.

Despite the fact that arrhenoblastomas are the most common among the ovarian tumors secreting androgens, they occur rarely, accounting for less than 1% of the solid ovarian tumors. Although arrhenoblastomas have been found in all age groups, about 70% occurred in women less than 40 years of age. The majority of arrhenoblastomas are large enough to be palpated, but many are much smaller and may even escape detection at the time of laparoscopy. Rapid and profound virilization and significant elevations of testosterone in the face of normal or slightly elevated 17-KS are diagnostic of arrhenoblastomas.

Gonadoblastomas are observed in genetic males with female external genitalia.

The term lipoid cell tumor has been used by Morris and Scully to describe rare virilizing ovarian tumors of two kinds. The most commonly applied synonyms for the first of the two kinds are adrenal rest tumors or adrenal-like tumors, but the terms masculinovoblastoma, luteoma, hypernephroma, and androblastoma diffusum have also been used. Tumors of the second kind have been called hilar cell tumors and Leydig cell tumors. The variety of names is explained in part by the fact that tumors of the first group consist of cells reminiscent of adrenal cortical cells, luteinized ovarian stromal cells, or clear cells in hypernephroma, whereas those of the second group resemble hilar or Leydig cells. The cells giving rise to these tumors have not been conclusively identified, and the question remains whether they are really different. Hilar cell tumors are more common in older women.

Adrenal-like tumors tend to be more malignant, have more frequently significantly elevated 17-KS, and more often than not are palpable. Although some women with adrenal-like tumors may have symptoms reminiscent of Cushing's syndrome, neither elevated plasma cortisol nor increased urinary free cortisol excretion have ever been

Table 7-10. CLINICAL FEATURES OF HORMONE-PRODUCING OVARIAN TUMORS

| Tumor | Hormones Produced* | Incidence | | Malig-nancy | Bilater-ality | Size Range in cm (% Palpable) | Miscellaneous |
		Peak	Range				
Arrhenoblastoma	Androgens, Estrogens	20–40	4–69	20%	rare	<5->25 (85)	Most common virilizing ovarian neoplasm
Dysgerminoma	Androgens, Chorionic gonadotropin	10–30	6–76	100%	15%	3–50 (60)	
Gonadoblastoma	Androgens, Estrogens	10–30	6–38	50%	40%	<1->30 (?)	Usually occur in genetic males with female external genitalia
Granulosa-Theca cell	Estrogens, Androgens, Progestogens	30–70	<1–92	5–20%	10–15%	<1->30 (80–90)	Most common functioning ovarian neoplasm
Lipoid cell (Hilar cell type)	Androgens, Estrogens	45–75	4–86	rare	rare	1–9 (50)	Hypertension in 50% Diabetes in 50%
Lipoid cell (adrenal-like)	Androgens, Estrogens	20–50	6–78	20%	rare	0.5–30	Diabetes associated with lesion in 50%
Teratomas, benign cystic	Serotonin, Thyroxine	10–40	<1–78	rare	10%	2–45 (90)	
Teratomas, malignant	Chorionic gonadotropin	6–15	6–42	100%	rare	>5 (100)	

*When more than one hormone is secreted, the major one is underlined.

reported in patients with lipoid cell tumors. One possible exception was a girl of age 8 who suffered from congenital adrenal hyperplasia and whose ovary on laparotomy was found to contain a tumor resembling an adrenocortical adenoma, which was shown by biochemic, morphologic, and histochemical investigation to be of true adrenocortical origin.

Miscellaneous Tumors Associated with Virilization and Feminization. Signs and symptoms of virilization and feminization have been found to be associated with many nonfunctioning ovarian tumors such as dysgerminomas, Brenner tumors, and simple cystadenomas and cystadenocarcinomas. They have also been found with some tumors metastatic to the ovary from primary sites in breast, stomach, and colon. When any of these tumors are associated with virilizing syndromes, foci of luteinized cells, variable in extent, are observed in the stroma of the ovary bearing the tumor. Examination of the tumor venous effluent demonstrates that these tumors secrete mainly androstenedione and that the occasional association of virilism and estrogen excess is owing to the conversion of androstenedione to estrone.

Tumors Producing Nonsteroidal Hormones

Tumors Producing Chorionic Gonadotropin. Occasionally, a dysgerminoma and, more rarely, a malignant ovarian teratoma secretes a gonadotropin immunologically and biologically similar to hCG, produced by normal trophoblastic tissue. More recently, the observation has been made that a number of other tumors secrete small amounts of hCG that can only be detected by sensitive and specific radioimmunoassay. Most recently, evidence has been published indicating that small amounts of hCG occur in the serum and urine of normal women who are not pregnant.

Tumors Producing Serotonin and Thyroxine. Benign cystic teratomas or dermoids have occasionally contained foci of chromaffin tissue producing serotonin; others consisted almost exclusively of thyroid tissue (struma ovarii) sufficiently differentiated to produce thyroxine.

Polycystic Ovary Syndrome. Although pathophysiologically of great interest, ovarian tumors are numerically unimportant causes of secondary amenorrhea. The most frequent cause of secondary amenorrhea associated with increased estrogen production is the polycystic ovary syndrome.

The polycystic ovary syndrome probably comprises a number of different syndromes. The symptom complex as reported in the literature is indeed too variable to assume that there is only one nosologic entity. Certain cases, however, have sufficient biochemic and pathologic features in common to constitute a specific clinical syndrome, and we should limit the diagnosis of polycystic ovary syndrome to these. The term polycystic ovaries is misleading, since the ovaries are studded with atretic follicles, not with cysts. A more appropriate name for the symptom complex would be the continuous estrus syndrome, since the hallmark of the condition is anovulation and unopposed estrogen stimulation. The following features appear characteristic. In most instances, the menstrual disturbance dates back to puberty. The menstrual picture is variable, ranging from long-term amenorrhea to oligomenorrhea with episodes of menometrorrhagia, but the common denominator is anovulation, which is a *sine qua non* of the diagnosis. Essential also for the diagnosis is the uninterrupted production of estrogens as evidenced by the continuous formation of copious amounts of cervical mucus and the persistence of a well-developed proliferative endometrium. In a few cases, adenomatous hyperplasia of the endometrium has been reported, and in some of these the lesion had advanced to the point at which the diagnosis of adenocarcinoma *in situ* was warranted. The second cardinal symptom of the syndrome is the evidence of androgen overproduction. Virilization is not often seen, but hirsutism is frequent and appears to be more frequent with increased duration of the disease. In adequately studied cases, there is always biochemic evidence of androgen overproduction, even when clinical hirsutism is not present. 17-KS are in the normal range (but most of the time high normal range), and when a group of patients with the syndrome is compared to a group of properly matched controls, the mean levels of 17-KS in the continuous estrus group are higher than those in the controls. Dexamethasone suppression will decrease the 17-KS, but the residual level remains clearly above the level seen in the control patients, indicating the ovarian source of the excessive 17-KS. Plasma levels of androstenedione and, to a lesser extent, of testosterone are increased, as are production rates of these steroids. In the ovarian veins, androstenedione levels are found to be greatly elevated but estrogen levels are strikingly low. Most of the estrogens in the peripheral circulation then are derived from the peripheral conversion of androgens to estrogens. Although the rate of conversion is normal in these patients, estrogen production is high because of the high production rate of androstenedione.

In many but not all cases, the ovaries are enlarged to several times normal size. In typical cases, the ovary is globular, with a thickened, glistening capsule, often with characteristic telangiectasia (Fig. 7–22). Beneath the capsule there are many small follicular cysts in various stages of atresia, often with hyperplastic and luteinized thecal cells.

The cause of the continuous estrus syndrome remains unknown. Polycystic ovaries have been reported in association with Cushing's syndrome, congenital adrenal hyperplasia, and central nervous system pathology, but these associations are exceptions and in virtually all cases there is no overt pathology outside the ovary. Minimal increases in adrenal androgens have been reported in some patients with the continuous estrus syndrome, but it is not clear whether these changes are primary or secondary. Available evidence is compatible with the hypothesis that the pathogenesis of the continuous estrus syndrome is to be found in a derangement of the relationship between the ovarian and hypothalamic-pituitary signal.

Reference has been made in an earlier part of this chapter to the role of the intraovarian microenvironments in the control of the follicle growth. Excessive formation of ovarian androgens, or excessive concentrations of androgens in the ovary due to adrenal hypersecretion of androgens, will increase follicular atresia that, because of the resulting increase in the thecal cell mass, will increase androstenedione production. Increased production of androstenedione will result in increased formation of estrone via the prohormonal pathway that, in turn, will stimulate the hypothalamic-pituitary axis to secrete more LH, resulting in further hyperplasia and hypersecretion of the thecal cells. After some time, therefore, the syndrome continues autonomously, even when the abnormal external stimulus disappears. There is also the possibility that initially the ovary is normal but the response of the hypothalamic-pituitary axis to the ovarian signal is abnormal. Evidence for this possibility derives from an animal model that has many features in common with the human continuous estrus syndrome. In rats (in which the hypothalamic-pituitary axis does not mature until several days after birth), the administration of testosterone to newborn female rats permanently modifies the feedback relationship between the hypothalamic-pituitary axis and the ovary. At puberty, an animal so treated will not display cyclic ovarian function but instead will enter into a state of continuous estrus: The ovaries contain many cystic follicles, and there is biologic evidence that production of androgens and estrogens is increased. Although the analogy between the experimental model and the polycystic ovary syndrome is striking, caution must be exercised in translating data from studies with rodents to women.

Hirsutism of Ovarian Origin. As noted, excessive androgen secretion may be associated with hirsutism, acne, clitoral hypertrophy, temporal hair recession, and deepening of the voice. The vast majority of women with androgen excess have only hirsutism and acne, whereas clitoral hypertrophy and other signs of virilization are seen only in a few cases, mostly women with tumors. Many women, with hirsutism as the only sign of excessive androgen secretion, do not fit in any of the previous categories and have been diagnosed as having idiopathic hirsutism.

Hair growth in the androgen-sensitive areas of the face, breast, and pubic, sacral, and perineal areas depends to a

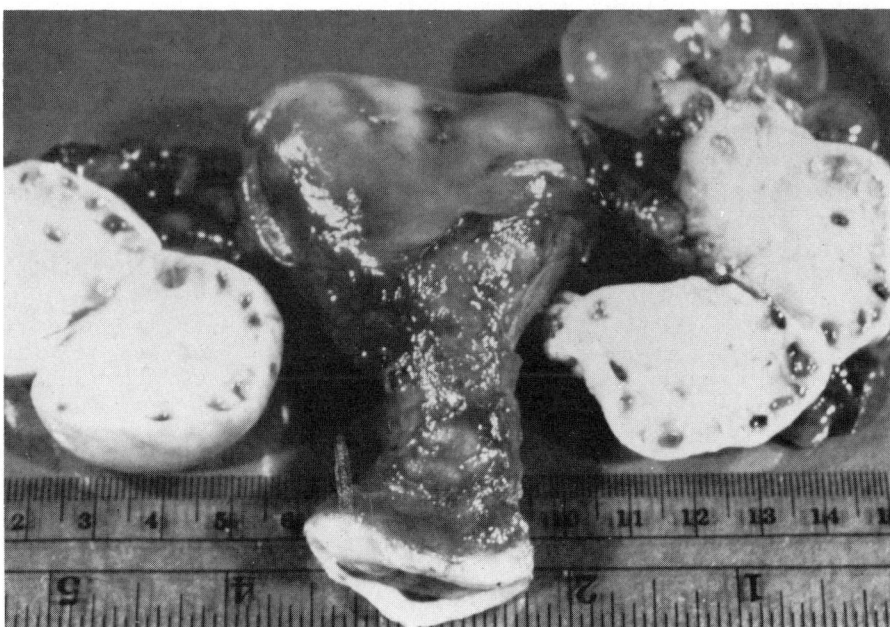

Figure 7–22. Uterus and ovaries removed from patient with polycystic ovaries. Note the glistening white color, the thickened capsule, and the multiple cortical cysts in the bivalved ovaries.

significant degree on racial factors, and because of important variations among normal populations, borderline cases of excessive hair growth are often difficult to classify as normal or abnormal. Whether hirsutism (other than that due to racial factors) exists in the absence of hypersecretion of androgens remains uncertain, but the possibility must be considered that in women with normal androgen secretion, hirsutism may be due to excessive conversion of testosterone to dihydrotestosterone at the target organ level. Whatever the case may be, as more and more precise and specific methods have become available to measure androgens, increased androgen secretion has been documented in women with hirsutism, and the diagnosis of idiopathic hirsutism has been made less frequently. Clinical signs of androgen excess correlate best with the levels of free testosterone. Increased testosterone may be due to increased ovarian or adrenal secretion of testosterone, but more frequently abnormal testosterone levels result from the peripheral conversion of androgen prohormones, such as androstenedione to testosterone.

Making the distinction between adrenal and ovarian sources of excess androgen is not always easy and in some ovarian cases, there is evidence of excess androgen secretion by the adrenal as well. In these cases, whether the adrenal abnormality is primary rather than secondary is not known. Significant elevations of DHEA sulfate and consequently of its metabolites, the urinary 17-KS, indicate adrenal pathology, and often other symptoms and signs of adrenal hyperactivity, such as increased cortisol levels, are found. On the other hand, low levels of 17-KS or their precursors strongly suggest ovarian pathology. In doubtful cases, as noted earlier, suppression of ACTH with a glucocorticoid may be attempted but the results are not always reliable, since administration of glucocorticoids may inhibit ovarian steroidogenesis as well. Suppression of gonadotropins with estrogens and progestins while adrenal suppression is maintained may yield additional useful information. This approach is not entirely reliable since the changes to be expected following gonadotropin inhibition are small, however. Also, it is important to recall that estrogens, by stimulating steroid hormone binding globulin (SHBG) production, will alter the ratio of free to total testosterone; consequently, during estrogen suppression tests, total testosterone may remain unchanged or even increase while free testosterone levels decrease. Direct catheterization of the ovarian or adrenal veins is a useful technique to pinpoint the origin of the abnormal androgen secretion but is not without significant side effects. In addition to hormone manipulations, imaging by ultrasonography, isotopic screening, and computerized axial tomography or direct visualization by endoscopy may be required to exclude the diagnosis of an ovarian or adrenal tumor.

Hirsutism of ovarian origin appears to be much more frequent than adrenal hirsutism. The vast majority of women with ovarian hirsutism have chronic anovulation and signs and symptoms of the continuous estrus syndrome; ovarian tumors as a cause of hirsutism are extremely infrequent. (See previously.) A few cases have been published in which there was increased testosterone secretion while the remaining ovarian function was normal.

A few women with hirsutism will be found to have congenital adrenal hyperplasia, and the diagnosis in these patients is easy to make because of the increased levels of 17α-hydroxyprogesterone. Most women with adrenal hirsutism have adrenal hyperplasia with increased secretion of DHEA. In a few women, adrenal catheterization demonstrated increased levels of testosterone without any other abnormalities of adrenal function. Adrenal tumors associated with virilization are infrequent and easy to diagnose because of the massive increases in 17-KS or their precursors.

Most recently, increased secretion of DHEA by the adrenal has been reported in women with elevated PRL levels. In some of these, there was clinical virilization, and the increased levels of DHEA could be suppressed by the administration of ergocryptin.

Hirsutism as a complication of drug therapy is infrequent. Testosterone is rarely used in women and testosterone derivatives, such as in contraceptive mixtures, are used in doses insufficient to produce significant symptoms. Diphenylhydantoin (Dilantin) is often associated with increased hair growth, but the distribution is more generalized than that seen with androgens.

Therapy for hirsutism is discussed in the section dealing with inhibition of androgen secretion.

Treatment of Ovarian Dysfunction

Introduction

In the vast majority of patients with secondary amenorrhea, the defective link can be identified to be the hypothalamic-pituitary unit, but most of the time the ultimate cause of the disturbance will remain unknown. Treatment in most patients, therefore, is symptomatic rather than causal, but even so, as far as the patient is concerned, it is very successful. Whether the patient complains of absence of sexual development, hot flashes, vaginal atrophy, acne, and hirsutism or of anovulation and sterility, there is hardly a symptom of ovarian dysfunction that cannot be corrected by appropriate therapy. The only real exception is the anovulation and infertility of the patient with primary ovarian failure.

In a few cases, therapy can attack the cause of the reproductive dysfunction and restore cyclic ovarian function. This is mainly the case in patients in whom the ovarian abnormality is secondary to a disturbance outside the reproductive axis, such as thyroid disease, adrenal disease, psychologic stress, or intercurrent nonendocrine disease. An exception applies to patients with polycystic ovarian disease, in whom wedge resection may restore cyclic function, occasionally for the rest of the patient's reproductive life, but the mechanism by which this occurs is unknown.

In considering therapy, it is essential to treat symptoms rather than signs. For example, mere absence of menses is not necessarily a sufficient indication for treatment, and withdrawal bleeding need not be induced unless the amenorrhea is of concern to the patient because of fear of pregnancy or identification of menses as a sign of good health and femininity. Similarly, there is no reason to induce ovulation in an anovulatory patient unless she wants to conceive. After finishing the workup of a patient with ovarian dysfunction, it is our custom to have a final conference with the patient (and mother or husband, as appropriate) to discuss in some detail ovarian physiology and the degree to which her own ovarian function differs from the normal. The problem of therapy can be approached in a logical fashion by asking the patient what symptoms she wishes to have corrected and by treating only these symptoms. Such an approach very often will result in a final decision that no therapy is necessary and in all cases will assure that therapy will be adjusted to the real needs of the patient. In using this approach, it is essential that symptoms about which the patient may not be presently complaining, but which may develop in subsequent years, be fully discussed. As an example, in women whose ovaries are not secreting any estrogens, the problem of chronic calcium loss and the possibility of late development of osteoporosis as well as other metabolic consequences of estrogen deficiency must be discussed.

Varieties of Therapy

Therapy of sex steroid hormone deficiency or excess can be divided into two main categories:

1. Substitution therapy: In this type of therapy, hormones are administered to substitute for the failure of secretion of the gonadal hormones.

2. Inhibition therapy: In this category, therapy aims at the inhibition of unwanted ovarian secretion.

Therapy of Sex Steroid Hormone Deficiency or Excess

Substitution Therapy

Estrogens. Although there is a large choice of estrogen preparations, we limit ourselves almost completely to the use of two: ethinyl estradiol (or its methyl ether) and conjugated estrogens (e.g., Premarin). We do not use injectable and long-acting estrogens unless there is a contraindication for the use of oral preparations. Topical applications of estrogens are used by some in cases such as atrophic vaginitis with the hope of limiting the effect of estrogens on the vagina and avoiding the systemic effects of the estrogens. Estrogens, however, are rapidly absorbed through the vaginal mucosa, and equally good results with less side effects may be obtained with smaller doses of estrogen administered orally.

In estimating the dose to be administered, it is useful to keep as a yardstick the rule that in an average patient 50–100 μg of ethinyl estradiol or 2–4 mg of Premarin administered daily for 1–2 weeks produce well-developed proliferative endometrium and consequently produce withdrawal bleeding, even in the completely estrogen-deficient patient. In many instances (e.g., in castrate and menopausal patients), the dose can and should be maintained below the level that produces withdrawal bleeding. Hot flashes, for instance, can easily be controlled by the administration of 0.3 mg of conjugated estrogens, a dose below the threshold for withdrawal bleeding unless progestins are added for the last 5 days of treatment. Similarly, recent evidence indicates that increased calcium loss observed in postmenopausal women can be prevented by the administration of 0.3 mg of conjugated estrogens. It must be noted that even such small doses may produce systemic effects. As an example, 0.3 mg of conjugated estrogens will produce an increase in CBG and 0.6 mg of estrogens will result in significant changes in lipids. On the other hand, when estrogens are given for their hemostatic effects (e.g., in dysfunctional bleeding), it may be necessary to give much higher doses, and it is generally advantageous to combine them with progestogens. When given for extended periods, they should always be administered in cyclic fashion. It is doubtful whether there is an advantage to administering progestogen together with estrogen as long-term therapy — for example, to produce sexual development in women with primary amenorrhea — although there is some evidence that progestogen may counteract some of the undesirable metabolic side effects of estrogen (e.g., alteration in carbohydrate and lipid metabolism).

Often the gynecologic endocrinologist will be consulted by women concerned about the small size of their breasts.

Indications and contraindications for giving estrogens are discussed in the section on the breasts.

The long-term administration of estrogen to postmenopausal women remains controversial. There is a clear-cut indication for such therapy when hot flashes are a problem, when vaginal atrophy interferes with marital function, or in women with a tendency for osteoporosis. Other indications are much more controversial, and whenever estrogens are administered, the benefits must be weighed against possible risks, mainly that of endometrial cancer. We feel that if estrogens are administered to menopausal women, endometrial biopsies must be taken at regular intervals, and provided such precaution is taken, a patient can be reassured about this danger of chronic administration of estrogens. At this time, it is uncertain whether a concomitant administration of progestogens can offset the increase of endometrial cancer seen in patients taking estrogens.

The use of estrogen to arrest growth in young girls in an effort to prevent excessive height remains controversial. The data in the literature are difficult to evaluate. The extent of inhibition achieved has to be judged on the basis of projected growth, estimated from standard tables of chronologic and bone ages, or even less securely from the height of the mother and other siblings. A number of authors doubt that significant inhibition can be achieved. There is agreement that if treatment is to be successful, estrogen must be started soon after the earliest signs of puberty, and that high doses (e.g., 10 mg ± of conjugated estrogens) are necessary. Some authors object to this treatment, because they fear that the high doses during this phase of development of the child may have long-term effects on subsequent menstrual function.

Progestogens. Some of the advantages of using progestogens have been mentioned in discussing indications for estrogen therapy. Progesterone or some other progestogen is mainly used to produce regular withdrawal bleeding in women with chronic anovulation. In these women, one frequently sees episodes of amenorrhea alternating with episodes of profuse or prolonged bleeding. Such forms of dysfunctional bleeding can easily be prevented by the administration of a progestogen every 4–6 weeks. The induction of withdrawal bleeding with progestogens has often been referred to as "medical curettage." The conditions necessary for progesterone withdrawal bleeding have been discussed previously. To produce withdrawal bleeding, we administer 100 mg of progesterone in oil, but one of the oral progestational agents (e.g., aceto-medroxy-progesterone, 10 mg/day for 3 or 5 days) may be used and is preferable in chronic conditions.

Recently, topical progesterone (either in an alcoholic solution or in a cream) has been suggested for the treatment of acne. The rationale for this treatment is that progesterone acts as a competitive inhibitor for the conversion in the skin of testosterone to dihydrotestosterone, thereby preventing the biologic effect of testosterone. Few controlled studies of this therapy have been carried out, but in our experience this treatment appears to be useful in minor forms of acne.

Androgens. There are few indications for the use of androgen in women with ovarian dysfunction. Occasionally, in women with primary amenorrhea, androgen can be administered to induce pubic and axillary hair growth. In our opinion, androgens have no place in the treatment of dysfunctional bleeding or dysmenorrhea.

Earlier evidence derived from studies in which androgen was given to women with breast cancer clearly shows that large doses of androgen increase libido. It was not clear in these studies whether the effect was owing to direct action upon the central nervous system or to congestion of the external genitalia (more specifically of the clitoris), however. We are unaware of any "controlled" study in which the effect upon libido of nonvirilizing doses of androgen have been tested in normal women, and this indication for androgen remains controversial.

Inhibition Therapy

Contraception. By far the most frequent indication for the inhibition of ovarian function is contraception. In 1974, when the popularity of this method of contraception was at its peak, 17.1% of all women in the United States used steroid contraception. In 1977, 12.2% of all women were still using steroid contraception. Table 7–11 lists the composition of the oral contraceptives currently used in the United States. The doses of estrogens and progesterone now employed are much lower than those used when steroid contraception first became popular. The main pressure to reduce the dose of oral contraceptives was generated by a legitimate concern about the serious side effects described in a very small fraction of women taking oral contraceptives. This concern was and is legitimate, but the present disenchantment of a significant fraction of the medical profession with steroid contraception appears to be an overreaction, often based upon incomplete knowledge of the physiology and pathology of the contraceptive steroids and not

infrequently upon medicolegal considerations. Qualitatively, the metabolic effects of the synthetic contraceptive steroids are the same as those of the ovarian hormones. These were briefly discussed earlier in this chapter. In 1979, sufficient information accumulated to allow an assessment of the safety of the contraceptive steroids. Table 7–12 illustrates the frequency of the most important side effects of the contraceptive steroids and compares them with the incidence of these symptoms in patients using other methods of contraception. This table also contrasts them with the frequency of some of the beneficial effects of steroid contraception.

The most important area of concern lies in that of cardiovascular diseases. It appears well established that oral contraceptive users die of vascular disease at a higher rate than nonusers. Whereas the initial concern dealt mainly with thrombosis and embolism, recent information has broadened the range of the diseases involved. Frank hypertension is infrequently seen in patients on contraceptive steroids, but in most women on contraceptive steroids there is an admittedly very small but still significant increase in blood pressure. Most people who develop a significant increase in blood pressure will develop it in the 1st month of therapy and experience has shown that after stopping therapy blood pressure reverts back to normal, and in some

Table 7–11. ORAL CONTRACEPTIVES (U.S. 1973)*

| Agent | Composition | | Manufacturer | Type |
	Estrogen	Progestogen		
Oracon	Ethinyl estradiol 0.100 mg.	Dimethisterone 25 mg.	Mead-Johnson	Sequential
Ortho-Novum 10	Mestranol 0.060 mg.	Norethindrone 10 mg.	Ortho	Combination
Ortho-Novum 2	Mestranol 0.100 mg.	Norethindrone 2 mg.	Ortho	Combination
Ortho-Novum 1/50	Mestranol 0.050 mg.	Norethindrone 1 mg.	Ortho	Combination
Ortho-Novum 1/80	Mestranol 0.080 mg.	Norethindrone 1 mg.	Ortho	Combination
Ortho-Novum SQ	Mestranol 0.080 mg.	Norethindrone 2 mg.	Ortho	Sequential
Micronor		Norethindrone 0.35 mg.	Ortho	Progestogen only
Norlestrin 2.5	Ethinyl estradiol 0.050 mg.	Norethindrone acetate 2.5 mg.	Parke-Davis	Combination
Norlestrin 1	Ethinyl estradiol 0.050 mg.	Norethindrone acetate 1 mg.	Parke-Davis	Combination
Demulen	Ethinyl estradiol 0.050 mg.	Ethynodiol diacetate 1 mg.	Searle	Combination
Enovid 5	Mestranol 0.075 mg.	Norethynodrel 5 mg.	Searle	Combination
Enovid-E	Mestranol 0.100 mg.	Norethynodrel 2.5 mg.	Searle	Combination
Ovulen	Mestranol 0.100 mg.	Ethynodiol diacetate 1 mg.	Searle	Combination
Norinyl 2	Mestranol 0.100 mg.	Norethindrone 2 mg.	Syntex	Combination
Norinyl 1/50	Mestranol 0.050 mg.	Norethindrone 1 mg.	Syntex	Combination
Norinyl 1/80	Mestranol 0.080 mg.	Norethindrone 1 mg.	Syntex	Combination
Norquen	Mestranol 0.080 mg.	Norethindrone 2 mg.	Syntex	Sequential
NOR-Q.D.		Norethindrone 0.35 mg.	Syntex	Progestogen only
Ovral	Ethinyl estradiol 0.050 mg.	Norgestrel 0.5 mg.	Wyeth	Combination

*Most contraceptive products now on the market belong to the combination type. In this type, estrogens and progestogens are combined and taken for a specified number of days of the cycle (20 or 21 days). In the sequential type of steroid contraception, an estrogen is taken during the first 14 or 16 days of the cycle, while for the subsequent 5 or 6 days, a combination of estrogen and progestogen is taken. In the progestogen-only type of contraceptive regimens, small amounts of a progestogen are taken continuously. The incidence of breakthrough bleeding in the latter type of contraception is much higher than in the combined or sequential types. The pregnancy rate is also much higher and presently is reported as 3 in 100 woman years. Recently, most contraceptive packages contain, in addition to the hormone-containing tablets, seven inert tablets. In this fashion, it is easier for the patient to keep track of her schedule, since she takes one tablet a day without interruption.

Table 7–12. ANNUAL NUMBER OF BIRTH-RELATED, METHOD-RELATED, AND TOTAL DEATHS, BY METHOD OF FERTILITY CONTROL, IN A HYPOTHETICAL COHORT OF 100,000 U.S. WOMEN

	Age in Years					
Regimen	15–19	20–24	25–29	30–34	35–39	40–44
No control						
Birth-related	5.3	5.8	7.2	12.7	20.8	21.6
Abortion only						
Method-related	1.0	1.9	2.4	2.3	2.9	1.7
OCs only/nonsmokers						
Birth-related	0.1	0.2	0.2	0.4	0.6	0.4
Method-related	0.6	1.1	1.6	3.0	9.1	17.7
Total deaths	0.7	1.3	1.8	3.4	9.7	18.1
OCs only/smokers						
Birth-related	0.1	0.2	0.2	0.4	0.6	0.4
Method-related	2.1	4.2	6.1	11.8	31.3	60.9
Total deaths	2.2	4.4	6.3	12.2	31.9	61.3
IUD's only						
Birth-related	0.1	0.2	0.2	0.4	0.6	0.4
Method-related	0.8	0.8	1.0	1.0	1.4	1.4
Total deaths	0.9	1.0	1.2	1.4	2.0	1.8
Barrier methods only						
Birth-related	1.1	1.5	1.9	3.3	5.0	4.0
Barrier methods, plus abortion						
Method-related	0.1	0.3	0.4	0.4	0.4	0.2

Modified from Tietze and Lewit.

women, even to less than the earlier value. Of concern also is the fact that according to some studies the risk not only increases with length of use but also persists even years after the steroids have been abandoned. The absolute risk in young women (below 35) remains very small if not insignificant, but with increasing age the risk is a significant one. Most important is the finding that smoking acts synergistically to increase the risk, and at the present time, there is almost uniform agreement that women over 40 who smoke should not take oral contraceptives. The initial impression that the risk for vascular disease increased with the amount of estrogen in the contraceptive mixture has not been borne out, and it appears that the progesterone content plays an equally significant role.

The initial fear that extensive use of contraceptive steroids might lead to a significant increase in the rate of reproductive cancers has not been borne out. Recent studies do not indicate any increase in the incidence of malignant breast disease and show a very significant decrease in the incidence of benign breast disease. Earlier hopes that, by decreasing the amount of steroid administered, it would be possible to reach a level at which the metabolic effect would become negligible while preserving an acceptably low pregnancy rate have not been borne out. At the levels at which the metabolic effect of the steroids disappear, pregnancy rates increase and breakthrough bleeding becomes annoyingly frequent. Even so, it is imperative in choosing a contraceptive agent to choose the agent with the lowest level of estrogen compatible with the patient's symptoms.

Efforts have also been made to optimize the ratio of side effects to contraception by changing the route of administration. It was thought that this might be possible by the delivery of the contraceptive mixture by a subcutaneously implanted Silastic capsule, through which small amounts of hormone would be released at a constant rate. Most recently, plastic devices containing progestogens have been implanted into the cervix or into the uterus in order to deliver the hormone directly to one of its target sites. None of these methods, however, have fulfilled the initial expectations.

Inhibition of Ovulation for Dysmenorrhea. The old dictum "nulla dysmenorrhea sine ovulation" is still valid, and when dysmenorrhea becomes incapacitating, blocking of ovulation with estrogens or a combination of estrogens and progestogens is almost always successful. In patients with premenstrual tension, however, results are disappointing most of the time.

Inhibition of Androgen Secretion. Rational therapy begins with identifying the source of excess androgen correctly. In women with hirsutism, we decry the empiric "trial of therapy" approach to treatment since objective regression of excess hair occurs slowly even with rational therapy. As a result, patients frequently become discouraged and prematurely abandon treatment that would have been effective if pursued longer.

At the outset of treatment, the patient should be informed that 6–12 months will be required for maximal benefits to become apparent. Moreover, the patient should be instructed in the appropriate use of such supplementary cosmetic regimens as bleaching, regular shaving, mechanical depilation, and electrolysis for symptomatic treatment. Some patients are encouraged by following changes in hair growth by shaving and weighing the hair removed from a unit area of skin at regular intervals. Once the suppressible ovarian source of excess androgen has been identified, we have found combinations of estrogens and progestins to be effective suppressants. For this purpose, we have given a combination of mestranol (0.1 mg) and norethynodrel (2.5 mg) twice daily for the first 3–4 months and once daily for the remaining period of up to 12 months. Any excessive hair failing to regress after 12 months of treatment should be destroyed by electrolysis.

When acne is a major symptom of ovarian androgen excess, improvement to the point of cure often follows effective suppressive therapy.

Regimens for suppressing adrenal cortical production of androgenic precursors have been described in the chapter on steroids.

Therapy of Anovulation

Women who are anovulatory often revert spontaneously to ovulatory cycles, and the first evidence that they have returned to normal ovarian function may well be pregnancy. For a condition that has about a 20% tendency to resolve spontaneously, any treatment will have a significant chance of success, which may explain the transient popularity of such treatments as thyroid hormone, cyclic therapy with estrogen with or without progestogen, and many others. At the present time, there are four main ways to induce ovulation: ovarian wedge resection, clomiphene, gonadotropins, and the ergolins. The efficacy of these modes of therapy is very high, and it may be said that, excluding patients with primary ovarian failure, ovulation can be induced in virtually all patients with anovulation. Obviously, when anovulation is secondary to a disturbance with a known etiology (i.e., intercurrent disease), therapy must, if possible, be directed to the cause of the disturbance rather than to the symptoms.

Thyroid Hormones. Many women are still being treated with thyroid hormone merely because they are anovulatory. Although tests of thyroid function are normal, it is assumed that certain patients have a mild form of hypothyroidism manifesting itself only by the presence of anovulation. This is not a reasonable treatment and should not be based only on anovulation.

Glucocorticoids. In patients with biochemically proven forms of adrenal hyperplasia, anovulation is the rule, and treatment should obviously be directed to suppression of adrenal hyperactivity. Glucocorticoids have also been administered to women with anovulation in whom the adrenal origin of the abnormality could not be unequivocally established. In our hands, this treatment has met with very little success, and we believe that adrenal suppression with glucocorticoids should be limited to patients in whom there is a biochemic reason to suspect adrenal hyperplasia. One situation in which glucocorticoids may be used to induce ovulation is in patients in whom the anovulation or amenorrhea is owing to inappropriate feedback of estrogens derived from the peripheral conversion of androstenedione to estrone. (See Table 7–8.) In such cases (as in obese women), the administration of glucocorticoids by decreasing the level of the adrenal prohormone will decrease circulating estrone levels and restore normal feedback relationships resulting in ovulation.

Clomiphene. Clomiphene, a nonsteroidal compound with weak estrogenic activity, is one of the most effective agents for inducing ovulation. Clomiphene has antiestrogenic activity and probably acts by competing with circulating estrogen for estrogen receptor sites in the hypothalamus and the pituitary. In the presence of clomiphene, the negative feedback effect of the estrogens is blocked, and consequently the pituitary begins to secrete increased amounts of FSH and LH, thus initiating follicular maturation (Fig. 7–23). The resulting rise in circulating estrogen triggers an LH surge that induces ovulation. If this concept of the action of clomiphene is correct, it should be expected that clomiphene will be most effective in anovulatory women whose ovaries are still secreting estrogens and whose pituitary remains sensitive to the positive feedback effect of the estrogens. Extensive clinical experience has shown this to be true, and in only very exceptional cases will clomiphene treatment be successful in women with signs of estrogenic insufficiency. For these reasons, withdrawal bleeding that follows progesterone therapy is an excellent indication that the patient is likely to respond to clomiphene.

Before starting treatment, it is important to ascertain that the ovaries are not enlarged and that the patient is not pregnant. Initially, treatment consists of one 50-mg clomiphene tablet daily for 5 days. If no response occurs after two 5-day courses of clomiphene, the dose is doubled (100 mg daily for 5 days). In grossly obese women, it may be worthwhile to use a higher dose, but if an average patient does not ovulate after two or three courses at the 100 mg level, it is unlikely that she will respond to a higher dose, and the risk of complications increases at higher dose levels. In a few patients, the administration of hCG at the time of the expected endogenous LH surge will induce ovulation and assure a normal luteal phase in patients who otherwise would not have ovulated or would have had a short luteal phase. The major complication of both clomiphene and gonadotropin treatment is ovarian hyperstimulation. This complication is discussed later.

No serious toxic reactions have followed clomiphene therapy. A few patients have experienced blurring of vision, but this is reversible, and there are no reports of lens changes such as occurred with triparanol, a parent compound of clomiphene. Nevertheless, visual symptoms prompt immediate discontinuance of treatment. Abnormal sulfobromophthalein retention has also been observed in a few patients, and therefore liver damage is a contraindication to the use of clomiphene. The antiestrogenic effect of the drug probably accounts for the fairly common occurrence of hot flashes.

It is possible to induce ovulation in more than 70% of patients with anovulation despite their capacity to secrete estrogen. In our experience, 20–30% have become pregnant as a result of clomiphene therapy. About 10% of these pregnancies have resulted in multiple births, usually twins, in contrast to a general incidence of about 1%. Clomiphene has also been used in ovulatory patients who were having difficulties in conceiving. Rather than enhance fertility, clomiphene given to ovulatory women will often induce abnormal luteal phases, and its use is therefore contraindicated. There have been claims that there is an increase in fetal malformations in patients who conceive following clomiphene. Careful analysis of the published data does not bear out these claims.

Gonadotropins. Gonadotropins are effective in inducing ovulation in most patients in whom clomiphene has failed. Since clomiphene acts via its antiestrogenic activity, it is ineffective in patients with low estrogen levels, and it will obviously not work in patients whose pituitary has lost its secretory capacity. The only patient who obviously cannot be expected to respond to gonadotropins is the patient with primary ovarian failure: Levels of gonadotropins in the menopausal range are therefore a contraindication to gonadotropin therapy.

Treatment with gonadotropin is a two-step treatment; in the first phase, follicular maturation is induced with a preparation having a high FSH to LH ratio. When sufficient follicular maturation is obtained, ovulation is induced with a luteinizing agent. For this purpose, hCG has been the agent of choice in most cases, but purified human LH of pituitary origin has also been used. FSH-LH is given intramuscularly, 75–150 IU/day for 10–15 days. The patient must be examined frequently to determine the ovarian response.

This response is evaluated by observing changes in cervical mucus, vaginal cytologic changes, the size of the ovaries, and most importantly, the level of plasma or urinary estrogens. When no response is obtained within 4–6 days, higher doses may be injected, but in these cases extreme caution should be exercised to avoid hyperstimulation. Human CG is withheld until there is evidence of complete follicular maturation and until adequacy of insemination is demonstrated by the postcoital test. Ovulation can be expected in almost 100% of patients treated in this manner, and

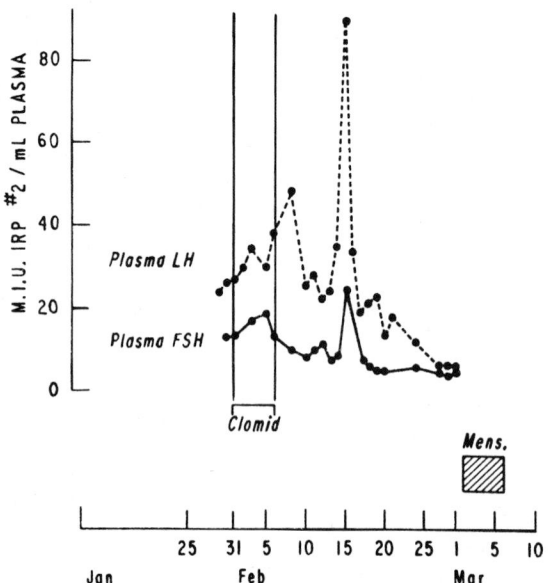

Figure 7–23. Plasma FSH and LH levels in a patient who ovulated in response to a 5-day course of clomiphene. (Adapted from Lipsett, M. B., et. al.: *Ann. Intern. Med.* 72:933, 1970.)

pregnancy in about 60%, provided that there are no other causes of infertility.

Although extremely effective in inducing ovulation, treatment with gonadotropins has a number of drawbacks. As with clomiphene, the risk of hyperstimulation is always present. In its mild form, hyperstimulation mainly produces abdominal pain and distention, nausea, and malaise. The full-blown syndrome, however, is manifested by massive enlargement of the ovaries, ascites, hydrothorax, and occasionally an ileus-like syndrome. Hyperstimulation is a complication of the second stage of treatment with gonadotropins and will never occur until ovulation. Most cases of hyperstimulation can be avoided by judicious selection of patients and careful adjustment of the dose to the response. Estrogens should be monitored throughout the last days of the FSH-LH treatment, and ovulation should not be induced in women whose estrogens are excessive. In these cases, hCG is not administered, and after withdrawal bleeding, treatment is started at a lower level.

If severe hyperstimulation develops, treatment is conservative and consists of bed rest and careful maintenance of the electrolyte balance. A laparotomy is not indicated unless there is evidence of intra-abdominal bleeding or of ovarian necrosis, which may be the result of twisting of the ovarian pedicle. Intra-abdominal bleeding appears to have been almost always a consequence of pelvic examination, which should be done with the utmost caution in patients with massively enlarged ovaries.

A second drawback in gonadotropin therapy lies in the frequency of multiple pregnancies, which is even higher than that seen in patients treated with clomiphene. Multiple pregnancies result in a higher abortion rate and even more seriously, in a catastrophic fetal mortality due to prematurity in cases in which there are more than two fetuses. Although severe hyperstimulation can be avoided by careful monitoring of the treatment, multiple pregnancies cannot be completely avoided. Because timing is a critical factor in gonadotropin therapy, and treatment is expensive and time-consuming, it should not be undertaken unless laboratory facilities are available for determinations of estrogen levels and of the other parameters indicative of ovulation.

Ergolins. In the amenorrhea-galactorrhea syndrome, the preferred therapy is the administration of bromoergocriptine, a derivative of ergotrate. Bromoergocriptine, a dopamine agonist, inhibits the secretion of PRL by a direct effect upon the pituitary. Whether restoration of gonadotropic function is secondary to the lowering of the PRL levels or results from a direct effect of bromoergocriptine upon GnRH secretion, remains unknown. Side effects at the therapeutic dose levels are minimal, mainly constipation, and since bromoergocriptine induces ovulation by restoration of normal gonadotropic function, the danger of hyperstimulation and multiple pregnancies, the major drawbacks of clomiphene citrate (Clomid) and gonadotropin, are absent. Bromoergocriptine is also an effective treatment for the few patients having a short luteal phase and high PRL. Bromoergocriptine has also been used in patients with anovulation or amenorrhea and normal levels of PRL. In some of these, ovulation was induced, but sufficient experience is not available to determine whether this was coincidence or cause and effect.

Bromoergocriptine should not be administered without a careful endocrine workup of the patient, including an x-ray polytomography of the sella turcica. Most investigators feel that pregnancy is contraindicated in women with an enlarged sella turcica because of the danger of further enlargement during pregnancy. There is evidence that treatment with bromoergocriptine will decrease the size of pituitary adenomata, but at the time this chapter was written, insuf-ficient evidence was available to decide whether bromoergocriptine can be given to patients who wish to conceive and have an enlarged sella turcica. Although there is evidence from animal studies suggesting that bromoergocriptine may have a teratogenic effect, extensive experience in humans has not borne out this fear.

Vitamin B_6 in very large amounts (75 mg or more/day) has been reported to induce ovulation in a few patients with amenorrhea-galactorrhea syndromes. Within our experience, this treatment has been disappointing.

Gonadotropin Releasing Hormone (GnRH). The availability of GnRH has raised the hope of a more direct approach to inducing ovulation in patients whose anovulation was due to hypothalamic disturbance. Unfortunately at this time this hope has not been borne out.

Reference has been made before that in physiologic conditions GnRH is secreted in a pulsatile fashion and that the magnitude and the frequency of these pulses are critical for the response of the pituitary to GnRH. It is possible that by mimicking the physiologic situation, GnRH treatment can be made more effective.

Estrogens. In the normal menstrual cycle, estrogens serve as a trigger for the preovulatory LH surge, and it should therefore be possible to induce ovulation by the administration of estrogens. In anovulatory patients, estrogens will often induce a significant LH surge, but ovulation is only infrequently seen because the necessary sequence in follicular maturation → secretion of estrogens → LH surge has not been followed, and an immature follicle will not respond to LH.

Ovarian Wedge Resection. Before clomiphene and gonadotropins were available, ovarian wedge resection was one of the few successful ways to induce ovulation in anovulatory women. This is still an acceptable form of therapy and, in our view, continues to be indicated occasionally. The major drawback of ovarian wedge resection is that it involves major surgery, but it has the significant advantage that, if successful, it will restore ovulation for years, if not for the rest of the patient's reproductive life. In contrast, treatment with clomiphene or with gonadotropins, even following a successful pregnancy, will rarely be followed by a resumption of spontaneous cycles.

X-Ray Irradiation. This treatment was used until some time ago and was often considered as an alternative to wedge resection. With the availability of other methods to induce ovulation, it is no longer an acceptable treatment for infertility in view of the obvious genetic hazards.

Therapy of the Short Luteal Phase. The therapy of the short luteal phase remains controversial and in general terms unsatisfactory. To a significant extent the discrepancy between the claims of various authors reflects differences in their criteria of diagnosis. Temperature charts cannot be relied upon for diagnosis nor can an isolated low value of progesterone. The diagnosis is to be based on well-timed endometrial biopsies that, in at least two consecutive cycles, must be out of phase with the stage of the cycle.

In a few women with short luteal phases, high levels of PRL have been reported and in these, as expected, treatment with bromoergocriptine is often successful. In patients with normal PRL, treatment is often disappointing. Since (see previously) most women with short luteal phases have low preovulatory FSH values, a rational therapy would be to administer FSH in the preovulatory phase. Results of such treatments, however, have not been encouraging. For a number of years attempts have been made to correct short luteal phases by administration, during postovulatory phase, of either hCG or progesterone, but few well-controlled studies are available and in our hands, the treatment has been disappointing.

Part II: The Breasts

By Andrew G. Frantz

NORMAL DEVELOPMENT

Fetal Life Through Adolescence

Early in fetal life, epithelial cells, derived from the epidermis in the area that will later become the areola, proliferate into the underlying mesenchyme. In the human, 20 or so short cords are formed that later develop lumina to become ducts that are connected to the nipple and open to the surface. Surrounding the ducts is a network of myoepithelial cells, destined ultimately to serve in the expulsion of milk. In the later stages of gestation, the blind ends of the ducts undergo some budding to form alveolar structures, and a small amount of secretory activity, resulting in the formation of so called "witch's milk," may be present in the human fetus at term. After parturition, with the decline in circulating fetal PRL and estrogen and progesterone of placental origin, there is a cessation of secretory activity and regression of the breast to a resting stage composed essentially of a small number of scattered ducts. Shortly before menarche, with increased secretion of ovarian estrogen, lengthening and branching of the ducts begin, accompanied by budding of the terminal ends and also by increased formation of underlying fat and connective tissue. With the onset of menses, further growth takes place in the cyclic fashion, some regression occurring at the end of each cycle.

Pregnancy

During pregnancy, the maternal breast is exposed to high levels of circulating estrogen and progesterone, as well as to a concentration of PRL from the maternal pituitary that increases steadily throughout gestation, presumably as a consequence of estrogenic stimulation. There are also increasing quantities of human placental lactogen. Under these stimuli a dramatic augmentation of breast growth

takes place, characterized by increasing branching of ducts and differentiation of their end buds to form alveoli; these group in clusters known as lobules. Toward the end of pregnancy, secretory vacuoles are seen within the epithelial cells, and some secretory material may be present in the ducts, though actual lactation does not occur until after parturition. The secretory material has many components, including fat, protein (casein, lactalbumin, lactoglobulin), and lactose.

HORMONAL REGULATION OF BREAST DEVELOPMENT

Optimum development of the breast requires the coordinated action of many hormones: PRL, estrogen, progesterone, adrenal steroids, insulin, GH, and thyroid hormone. A broadly simplified summary view has been to consider that estrogen promotes primarily duct growth, whereas PRL and progesterone are necessary for lobuloalveolar development, and PRL alone governs lactation. In spite of enormous work, however, the precise roles of each hormone have been difficult to delineate because one hormone, besides having actions of its own, may also regulate both the secretion and the activity of other hormones. *In vitro* findings have not always paralleled those *in vivo,* and species differences make uncertain the application of some observations to the human, which has been studied relatively less than other species.

Prolactin

Of all hormones, PRL appears to be the dominant one governing the breast. Its importance in all phases of breast development was clearly shown in the careful studies of Lyons, Li, and Johnson. Using hypophysectomized, adrenalectomized, gonadectomized rats, these workers found that estrogen alone is completely ineffective in inducing any degree of ductal or other mammary growth. If administered together with PRL and GH, however, or if administered to animals with intact pituitaries, estrogen was an effective promoter of ductal growth. Some degree of ductal and lobuloalveolar growth with high doses of PRL alone in the triply operated rat has been reported by Talwalker and Meites, though it would seem that ordinarily PRL requires estrogen to function as a stimulator of epithelial cell proliferation. With the addition of progesterone, PRL particularly fosters lobuloalveolar development. Its growth-promoting properties in various animal preparations have been substantiated by DNA measurement in addition to microscopic observation. PRL is also the controlling hormone regulating many steps of the secretory process, including the formation of the milk proteins, casein and α-lactalbumin. Their measurement, along with that of other secretory products, has been used as a specific and quantitative index of PRL activity both *in vitro* and *in vivo*. PRL *receptors* have been demonstrated in mammary tissue of several species, including the human, and appear to increase in number during gestation. Their hormonal regulation has been less well studied in the breast than in certain other tissues, e.g., rat liver, in which it has been shown that estrogen treatment augments the number of PRL receptors and that PRL itself may do the same. Whether these hormones have a similar action on PRL receptors in the breast is uncertain. A *decrease* in PRL receptors after estrogen treatment has been reported in rat mammary tumors.

The chorionic hormone *placental lactogen* (hPL) also circulates in large amounts in maternal blood during human pregnancy. It appears to have essentially the same action as PRL. Although of slightly lesser potency than PRL on a weight basis, it is present in considerably greater quantities and therefore must be regarded along with PRL as being a major contributor to breast growth during gestation.

Estrogen

The role of estrogen is complex. Although a highly potent mammogen, it is ineffective by itself in the absence of anterior pituitary hormones. Administration of estrogen to intact animals promotes the formation of lactotroph cells in the pituitary and increases the secretion of PRL. In humans it also increases GH secretion. In the presence of these two hormones estrogen acts on breast tissue to promote primarily ductal development.

Although helping to prepare the breast for eventual milk formation, estrogen inhibits actual lactation, and in this respect appears to act as an antagonist to PRL. It is largely because of the high levels of circulating estrogen (and progesterone) that women do not lactate during pregnancy, and it is the abrupt withdrawal of these two hormones following the expulsion of the placenta that triggers the onset of lactation. As just noted, estrogen may act to regulate the number of PRL receptors in breast tissue, though this action requires further definition. As with actions of estrogen on other tissues, dose considerations are probably important, and differential actions of estrogen, depending on blood or tissue levels, may well exist. Of interest is the finding that the fat cells of breast tissue, like fat cells elsewhere, have power to form estrogens by aromatization of circulating androgens, e.g., androstenedione and testosterone. The relative importance of this local source of estrogen production in breast tissue is unknown.

Estrogen receptors, both cytoplasmic and nuclear, have been demonstrated in normal as well as in tumorous breast tissue. Concentrations of cytoplasmic receptors rise during later pregnancy and the first part of lactation. The signifi-

cance of this rise and the factors that regulate estrogen receptor synthesis are still largely unknown.

Progesterone

Like estrogens, progesterone has no effect on the breast in the absence of anterior pituitary hormones. Even in the presence of PRL, progesterone has little or no effect unless there is concomitant or preceding estrogen stimulation. Under these conditions progesterone acts principally to synergize with PRL in promoting lobuloalveolar development. Like estrogen, progesterone inhibits actual lactation, which begins after the decline of progesterone that follows parturition. Exogenously administered progesterone is considerably less effective than is estrogen in stopping lactation once the process has become established. Progesterone *receptors* exist in breast tissue but little is known about their regulation.

Growth Hormone

GH appears to synergize with PRL, and may be able to substitute for it in promoting certain phases of breast growth, such as ductal development. Different animal GH's possess different degrees of PRL-like activity in homologous and heterologous species. Although GH seems to improve the degree of breast growth obtainable with combinations of other hormones in hypophysectomized animals, its essentiality for breast growth is questionable, at least in humans. Despite the fact that human and primate GH's have strong intrinsic PRL-like activity, the fact that ateliotic dwarfs — who are essentially completely lacking in GH — develop breasts and lactate normally post partum, suggests that GH is not important for lactation in the human.

Insulin

Insulin is necessary for PRL and other hormones to exert their effects on breast tissue *in vitro*, and insulin or serum factors resembling it are probably necessary *in vivo* as well. The importance of insulin as a mitogenic agent has been emphasized by the studies of Topper. Insulin *receptors* have been demonstrated in breast tissues. Although necessary for breast growth and lactation, insulin probably does not play a regulatory role in any of these processes by virtue of changes in its concentration.

Adrenal Steroids

Like insulin, corticosteroids appear to be necessary for most phases of breast growth and secretion, both *in vitro* and *in vivo*. The requirement is probably for a glucocorticoid (hydrocortisone) or steroid having glucocorticoid activity (e.g., aldosterone), rather than for a mineralocorticoid. Cytoplasmic glucocorticoid *receptors* have been demonstrated in lactating mammary tissue. As with insulin, corticosteroids probably exert a permissive rather than a regulatory role.

Thyroid Hormone

Thyroid hormone does not appear to be essential for either breast development or lactation, although both processes may be adversely affected in states of thyroid hormone deficiency or excess.

HORMONAL CONTROL OF LACTATION

Lactation begins when the maternal breast, primed by long exposure to high levels of PRL, estrogen and progesterone, experiences the sudden withdrawal of the latter two placental hormones. Thereafter, lactation proceeds in an environment of relatively high (though declining) PRL and low estrogen and progesterone. Suckling provides an essential stimulus for the release of both oxytocin (OT) and PRL.

Oxytocin

A necessary component of effective lactation is expulsion of the milk from the alveoli and ducts. This is caused by contraction of the myoepithelial cells, which surround these structures, under the influence of OT. OT secretion can be caused by purely psychic factors, such as anticipation of nursing or by sensory stimuli arising from the nipple during the act of nursing. It is experienced by the mother as a sensation of milk "let-down," and by appearance of milk sometimes rather forcibly ejected at the nipple. Uterine cramps are also occasionally experienced during nursing. OT secretion can be inhibited (with marked impairment of milk yield) by stress and by psychic factors, e.g., fright, that appear to involve activation of the sympathetic nervous system and release of norepinephrine and epinephrine.

Prolactin: Effect of Suckling

Suckling in postpartum women is a powerful stimulus for the release of PRL. Unlike OT, which is also released by nipple stimuli transmitted via dorsal nerve roots to the hypothalamus, PRL does not respond to anticipatory psychic stimuli. Release of the two hormones is quite independent, and one may be liberated without the other (Fig. 7–24). In the first few weeks postpartum, maternal serum PRL levels are continuously high and undergo marked further evaluation (5- to 10-fold) with each nursing episode. Later on, somewhere between the 3rd and 7th week after parturition, internursing concentrations of PRL fall to the point where they are within the normal range (less than 25 ng/ml) most of the time. Some degree of PRL rise during each suckling

episode persists in most women, however, even many months post partum (Fig. 7–25), and this nursing-induced rise is probably important in maintaining the breast in an actively lactating state. Thus, for the initiation of lactation, high levels of PRL appear to be necessary, but once breast enzyme systems have become adapted to secrete milk, lactation can go on with mean PRL concentrations that are slightly, if at all, elevated. Even at these levels, however, PRL remains essential for maintenance of lactation. If its concentrations are further lowered by ergot drugs, or by hypophysectomy in animals, lactation stops abruptly.

Of interest is the fact that human GH is low throughout the lactation and does not rise with nursing (Fig. 7–25), further indicating its lack of participation in this process. TSH is also unaffected by nursing, a strong indication that the PRL rise of nursing is not mediated by TRH.

Breast Stimulation in Normal Subjects

In normally menstruating, nonpostpartum women, manual stimulation of the breast and nipple causes a PRL rise of twofold or greater in about one third of subjects (Noel et al., 1974). The factors that differentiate women who respond from those who do not are unclear. Men uniformly show no PRL response to breast stimulation. It appears that the reflex for this type of response is present at least in latent form in all women and is somehow turned on or enhanced by the hormonal events of pregnancy and parturition.

CLINICAL CONSIDERATIONS IN POSTPARTUM LACTATION

Suppression of Lactation

If a woman does not nurse or empty her breasts postpartum, lactation usually stops spontaneously in a week or two, accompanied by rapid involution of much of the recently differentiated lobuloalveolar structure of the breast. Stasis of milk in the ducts and alveoli and a rise in intramammary pressure leading to some degree of alveolar rupture and cell necrosis are major factors in causing cessation of lactation, but the detailed mechanisms are not altogether clear. PRL levels revert quickly to normal, and menses usually resume in 4–12 weeks (occasionally not until 6 months), the mean

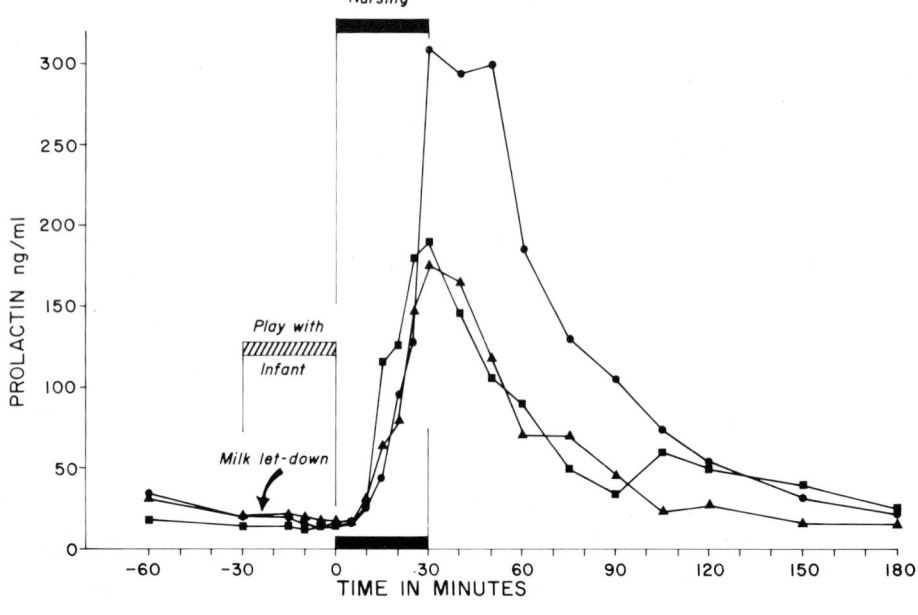

Figure 7–24. Plasma prolactin concentrations during anticipation of nursing and course of nursing in three women who were between 22 and 26 days post partum. The women played with their infants for 30 minutes before suckling began. Milk letdown, an oxytocin-mediated phenomenon, occurred in each case approximately 25 minutes before suckling. Prolactin levels did not rise until there was contact with the breast itself. (Reprinted with permission of the authors and publishers of *J. Clin. Endocrinol. Metab.* 38:413, 1974.)

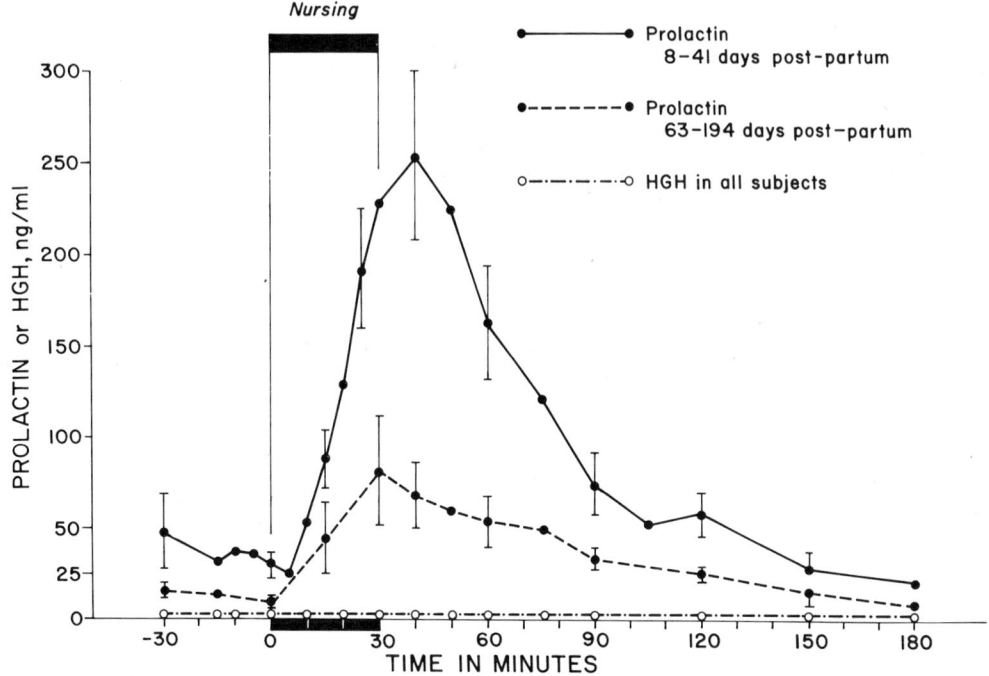

PROLACTIN AND GROWTH HORMONE DURING NURSING
Effect of Time Post-Partum

Figure 7–25. Plasma prolactin and growth hormone concentrations during nursing in postpartum women. Eight women were studied 8–41 days post partum and six women were studied 63–194 days post partum. Prenursing prolactin levels in the latter group are within the normal range. Plasma growth hormone showed no change in any of the subjects during nursing. (Reprinted with permission of the authors and publishers of *J. Clin. Endocrinol. Metab.* *38*:413, 1974.)

being 8 weeks. During the first week or two post partum, there is a variable amount of discomfort caused by engorgement of the breast, which can usually be treated satisfactorily by simple measures such as ice packs, tight binder, and analgesics. In women who do not wish to nurse their babies, lactation can be effectively suppressed in most patients and discomfort avoided by a single intramuscular injection of a long-acting estrogen-androgen combination (e.g., 2 or 3 ml of Deladumone containing 4 mg estradiol valerate and 90 mg testosterone enanthate/ml) given during labor. The drug is less effective if administered after lactation has begun. The androgen synergizes with the estrogen in inhibiting breast secretion and helps minimize later recurrence of lactation. Despite the wide use of this and similar preparations for many years, growing awareness of the potential toxicity of estrogen preparations has led to a decline in their use, and for most patients they are best avoided. Bromocriptine nesylate (Parlodel), 2.5 mg bid, has been effective in preliminary studies in stopping postpartum lactation through its PRL lowering effects, and ergot derivatives seem likely to become the agents of choice for pharmacologic suppression of lactation.

Failure of Lactation

The only common or generally recognized endocrine disorder associated with failure of lactation is Sheehan's syndrome. This disorder, caused by vascular injury to the pituitary at the time of delivery, frequently first manifests itself by lack of postpartum milk production, presumably due to low circulating PRL. Other signs of pituitary hormone deficiency, e.g., failure of menses to resume, hypothyroidism, and sparse regrowth of shaved pubic hair, may later become apparent. The pattern of individual hormone deficiencies in Sheehan's syndrome may be spotty, and spontaneous amelioration may later occur. Otherwise deficiency of PRL, whether congenital or acquired, appears to be a rare condition. The possibility of using PRL-stimulating drugs, e.g., sulpiride, to augment milk yields (Aono et al., 1979) in nursing mothers requires further investigation. Most cases of insufficient lactation have been generally considered to be due to emotional factors. These could conceivably operate via noradrenergic pathways to inhibit OT secretion, but adequate endocrine studies to support this or other etiologies in such patients are still lacking.

Lactation-Associated Infertility

If postpartum nursing is prolonged, amenorrhea will usually continue for at least 4–6 months and frequently much longer, but return of menses has been reported in two thirds of women by 9 months post partum, despite continued lactation. The mechanisms of lactation-associated amenorrhea clearly relate in part to the antigonadotropin effects of hyperprolactinemia, but other factors, particularly in the later postpartum period, may also be operative. For practical purposes it must be emphasized that amenorrhea does not guarantee infertility, many instances being known of conception occurring post partum without an intervening menstrual period. Therefore, conception, if desired, should begin soon after delivery, at least before the 5th week post partum, whether the mother nurses her child or not. If oral contraceptives are used in a nursing mother, a low-dose estrogen preparation should be chosen to minimize inhibitory effects on milk yield. It is of interest that in many species other than primates prolonged lactation is no barrier to rapid resumption of ovulatory cycles. Insemination of domestic cows is frequently undertaken 3 months or less post partum, despite copious lactation that proceeds, if milking continues, throughout ensuing gestation.

GALACTORRHEA

Galactorrhea may be defined as a persistent discharge from the breast that looks like milk and that either does not occur in relation to parturition or else persists post partum for several months (e.g., more than 6) in the absence of nursing. Formerly regarded as rare, it has been recently recognized as fairly common, particularly if one accepts minimal degrees of secretion that may be evident only when specifically looked for by squeezing the breast. Doubt as to whether the secretion represents milk may be resolved by doing fat stains or, for greater specificity, tests for specific milk products such as α-lactalbumin, casein, or lactose; clinically, such tests are rarely necessary. Nonmilky types of nipple discharge (e.g., serous, purulent, and sanguineous) also occur, but these are rarely if ever reflective of an endocrine disturbance. In the past, such discharges, particularly colored ones, were thought to be suggestive of cancer, but recent studies suggest that most are not associated with malignancy, though fibrocystic disease may be present. A careful search for breast nodules should nevertheless be made in patients with such discharges. True galactorrhea is not associated with an increased incidence of cancer.

Galactorrhea occurs in a wide variety of endocrine and nonendocrine disorders. (See Table 7–9.) The largest series (235 patients) reported to date is that of Kleinberg, Noel and Frantz (1977); the discussion that follows is based on this series, the findings of which are in general agreement with those of other observers.

Galactorrhea with Pituitary Tumors

Clinically, the most important diagnostic consideration in galactorrhea is pituitary tumor. Twenty per cent of all our patients with galactorrhea and 34% of women with associated amenorrhea had pituitary tumors. The true prevalence of tumors may be even higher because of failure to detect some small microadenomas radiologically. The histology is almost always that of a chromophobe adenoma, with increased lactotrophs visible by special stains. A small minority of patients will have associated acromegaly; these have all had evident clinical stigmata of acromegaly as well as elevated serum GH.

As a group, patients with tumors have the highest serum PRL values (Fig. 7–26), and the likelihood of finding a tumor is directly proportional to the level of the PRL. All patients with values of over 300 ng/ml, in our experience, have had tumors, and any value of more than 75–100 ng/ml should be regarded with great suspicion. Of the few patients with tumors who had normal serum PRL's, all but two either had acromegaly or had had prior treatment. Amenorrhea is very common (greater than 80%) in patients with galactorrhea and tumors and was primary in 10% of our patients. Menses, if present, are apt to be irregular; only 3 of 48 patients with tumors in our series had regular menses.

Idiopathic Galactorrhea with Menses

Although most women with galactorrhea were formerly thought to have associated amenorrhea, the largest single category of galactorrhea patients, in our experience, comprises those with regular menses and no associated endocrine disease. Galactorrhea is often overlooked because these patients do not think it worth reporting. In over half of such women galactorrhea represents a residue of postpartum lactation that never altogether disappeared despite resumption of menses. The great majority of these patients have PRL levels that are within the normal range (Fig. 7–26), and their fertility is usually normal. In this group of women the abnormality is probably not primarily a hormonal one but rather an excessive sensitivity of the breast tissue itself — perhaps due to increased PRL receptors — to normal levels of circulating PRL. From a clinical standpoint, the combination of regular menses and a normal serum PRL is strong evidence against the presence of pituitary tumor, though skull x-rays should be obtained in such patients.

Idiopathic Galactorrhea with Amenorrhea: The Role of Hyperprolactinemia

An appreciable minority of women with galactorrhea have associated amenorrhea, no history of drug ingestion, and normal skull x-rays. Most such women have hyperprolactinemia (Fig. 7–26). It seems likely that most of these women have occult pituitary tumors, the likelihood rising with the level of the serum PRL. It is also probable that the hyperprolactinemia, in these as in other patients with galactorrhea and amenorrhea, is causing the amenorrhea since any treatment that lowers PRL close to or into the normal range is likely to restore menses. Possible mechanisms include an interference by PRL at the hypothalamic level with the tonic or cyclic release of LRH, a partial desensitization of the pituitary of the action of LRH, and an interference with the steroidogenic action of gonadotropins at the ovarian level. Evidence for all three mechanisms exists, but currently a hypothalamic or pituitary site of interference appears most probable.

Chiari-Frommel Syndrome

The so-called Chiari-Frommel syndrome, defined as galactorrhea and amenorrhea persisting more than 6 months post partum in the absence of nursing without evident pituitary tumor, is still not a well-understood phenomenon. Some of these patients probably harbor occult microadenomas, stimulated by the hormones of pregnancy, that may later become radiologically evident. In about half of such patients, however, menses eventually return in a matter of months to 2 or 3 years. Serum PRL is elevated in some but not all patients (Fig. 7–26).

Post–Oral Contraceptive Galactorrhea

Post-pill galactorrhea is somewhat less common than post-pill amenorrhea, with which it is usually associated. Both are uncommon in relation to the large number of women who have used oral contraceptives. As with Chiari-Frommel syndrome, some of these patients may eventually develop radiologically evident tumors, though most in our experience do not. In this syndrome, as in the postpartum woman, milk production is triggered by estrogen and progesterone withdrawal after a period of stimulation by these hormones (and also by some estrogen-enhanced PRL secretion). Despite the much lower hormone levels and shorter duration of stimulation involved in the post-pill galactorrhea syndrome than in postpartum lactation, the fundamental mechanisms of the two conditions may be similar.

Hypothyroidism

Galactorrhea is a rare accompaniment of primary hypothyroidism in children — in whom it may be associated with precocious puberty (Van Wyk and Grumbach) — and in

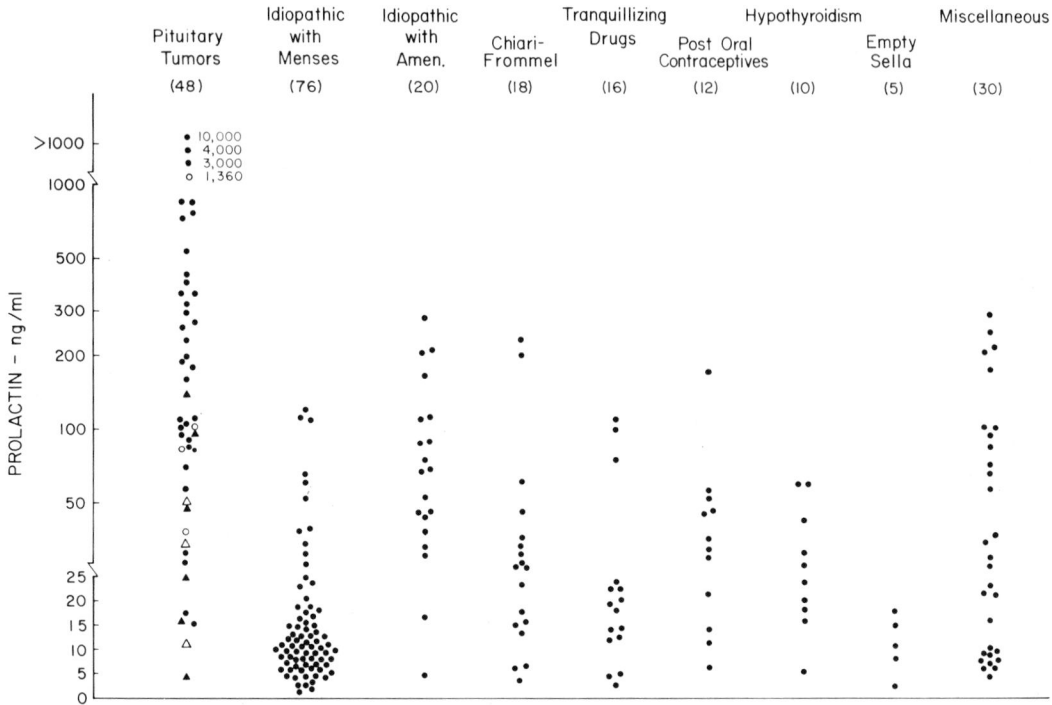

Figure 7–26. Plasma prolactin in 235 patients with galactorrhea of varying causes. Among the patients with tumor, triangles denote patients with acromegaly. Open circles or triangles denote patients studied only after radiotherapy or surgical resection. Normal female levels of prolactin are considered to be less than 25 ng/ml. (Reproduced with permission of the authors and publishers of *New Engl. J. Med. 296*:589, 1977.)

adults. In the latter group PRL levels may be slightly more than a given patient's normal mean but are often within the normal female range or only slightly elevated (Fig. 7–26). Administration of thyroid hormone to restore euthyroidism stops the galactorrhea and lowers the PRL somewhat; in children it may also cause precocious menses if present to stop until the normal time of menarche. The precise underlying mechanisms in these cases are not clear and may involve complex alterations of PRL and gonadotropin production and degradation rates, as well as changes in breast tissue sensitivity. Administration of thyroid hormone to patients with other forms of galactorrhea who are euthyroid has no effect on the galactorrhea.

Drug Administration

Galactorrhea has been associated with a wide variety of drugs that raise serum PRL levels, including phenothiazines, butyrophenones, reserpine, α-methyldopa, tricyclic antidepressants, estrogens, and various narcotics (Table 7–9). Many of these agents appear to act as antidopaminergic agents, decreasing dopamine-mediated inhibition of PRL secretion at the level of the pituitary or hypothalamus or both.

Chest Wall Disease: Breast Stimulation

Galactorrhea has occasionally been reported in diseases affecting the chest wall, e.g., herpes zoster, or after thoracotomy, presumably secondary to stimulation of PRL secretion by sensory impulses from nerves leading from the breast and areola. Although stimulation of a woman's breasts by herself or by her husband is a theoretical predisposing cause of galactorrhea, we have not personally encountered this phenomenon in any of our patients. Efforts to induce a PRL rise by breast stimulation were unsuccessful in 8 of 9 women

with established galactorrhea, and in the 9th patient only a modest rise was obtained. We were also unsuccessful in inducing either galactorrhea or any breast engorgement in two normal young women who underwent self-stimulation of the breast four times a day for half an hour for a period of 2 weeks (Noel et al., 1974). Anecdotal accounts exist of nonlactating, sometimes postmenopausal, women, usually in primitive tribes, who are able to initiate lactation when placed in contact with an infant to be nursed. These should be viewed with skepticism, despite a total of 13 such cases since the year 1900 cited in a report by Richardson (1970).

Miscellaneous

Conditions occasionally associated with galactorrhea include various hypothalamic and pituitary diseases (sarcoidosis, Schuller-Christian disease, craniopharyngioma, Cushing's disease); head trauma; major surgery, including cholecystectomy and oophorectomy; isoniazid administration; and refeeding after starvation (Kleinberg, Noel, and Frantz, 1977).

Males

Galactorrhea is far less common in men than in women (13 of our 235 patients were men), presumably because the breast has received less estrogenic priming. PRL-secreting pituitary tumors are the most common cause, followed by drug ingestion of various kinds.

Role of Prolactin in Galactorrhea

Though serum PRL concentrations are often elevated in galactorrhea, sometimes extremely so, they were within the normal range in 46% of our patients. Thus galactorrhea can be present without hyperprolactinemia, as well as hyperprolactinemia without galactorrhea. In the latter case the absence of galactorrhea may be due to inadequacy of estrogenic and progestational priming (as in most males) or lack of a suitable triggering event involving estrogen withdrawal (oophorectomy, abortion, cessation of estrogen or oral contraceptive medication). In many cases of galactorrhea, however, no triggering event is evident from the history. In patients with galactorrhea and normal serum PRL, it is conceivable that an earlier transient period of hyperprolactinemia may have existed at the time of onset of the galactorrhea. As with nursing mothers many months postpartum, milk secretion once established can continue with what appear to be normal PRL levels. In these patients galactorrhea remains PRL-dependent, however; lowering of their normal serum PRL concentrations with ergot drugs stops the galactorrhea. In summary, it may be said that though PRL is essential for milk production, the serum levels of the hormone show very little correlation with the copiousness of milk flow among galactorrhea patients as a group.

CLINICAL CONSIDERATIONS IN GALACTORRHEA

Diagnosis

A careful history is essential with attention to menses, drug ingestion, and symptoms suggestive of pituitary or hypothalamic disease (headaches, visual disturbances, abnormalities of temperature, thirst, or appetite regulation), as well as thyroid or adrenal dysfunction. On physical examination the physician should check visual fields by confrontation, eye movements, skin texture, pigmentation, degree of hirsutism, and possible stigmata of acromegaly, hypothyroidism, Cushing's syndrome, and hyperthyroidism. The breast should be examined for nodules and gently but firmly compressed by the physician or patient to assess the degree of galactorrhea. A serum PRL and polytomograms of the sella turcica should be ordered on all patients, and serum gonadotropins on those with amenorrhea. Serum T_4 is also worth measuring on all patients but other hormonal measurements, e.g., GH and adrenal steroids, are not necessary in the absence of clinical indications. At one time it seemed possible that PRL stimulation and suppression tests, with such agents as TRH, L-dopa, phenothiazines, and metoclopramide, might prove valuable in distinguishing pituitary tumors from other causes of galactorrhea or hyperprolactinemia, but extensive experience in our own and other institutions has indicated that such tests are too variable in their results to be worth the time and expense necessary. The diagnosis of pituitary tumor rests essentially on the height of the serum PRL and on the skull x-rays. Future experience may indicate that the newer high resolution computerized tomographic (CT) scans may offer a satisfactory substitute for polytomograms, but this has not been our experience with CT scans to date.

Treatment

In most cases the galactorrhea is not so copious or troublesome as to require treatment for its own sake. If fertility is not desired, and if there is no evidence of pituitary tumor, treatment for elevated PRL (if present) is not necessary, since there is no evidence that prolonged hyperprolactinemia by itself is deleterious. If there are minimal indications of a microadenoma, such as slight sellar asymmetry on polytomography, but fertility is not

desired, it is currently questionable whether surgery should be advised. Although transsphenoidal hypophysectomy for minimal tumors by experienced neurosurgeons is associated with a mortality or serious morbidity that is probably less than 1%, the natural history of these tumors is still not well known. A majority may well show little or no progression for many years, and a good case can be made for watchful waiting with serum PRL determinations at 6-month to yearly intervals and polytomograms less frequently, e.g., at 2- to 5-year intervals, depending on duration of disease and absence of change in symptoms or serum PRL levels. For large or obviously growing tumors, pituitary surgery with or without radiotherapy is currently the most popular treatment. Radiotherapy alone, however, has been effective in many cases in the past in arresting tumor growth and in gradually lowering PRL levels over a period of months to years. With either surgery or radiotherapy, restoration of menses and complete cessation of galactorrhea depend largely on whether serum PRL is lowered to within or close to the normal range. Size of tumor is also a factor. With large tumors, or with serum PRL values of over 200 ng/ml, restoration of menses will probably occur after either treatment in only 50% or less of patients.

The *ergot derivatives*, especially bromoergocriptine, have been more effective than any other form of treatment in lowering serum PRL, stopping galactorrhea, and restoring ovulatory menses in patients with hyperprolactinemia, whether due to tumor or other cause. The usual dose is 2.5 mg/day for 1 week, increased to 2.5 twice or three times a day thereafter. Initial nausea is experienced by many patients but usually wears off. Postural hypotension and nasal stuffiness may also occur but rarely require discontinuation of the drug. In the great majority of cases the drug is effective only for the duration of its administration; hyperprolactinemia and the other associated abnormalities tend to recur as soon as it is withdrawn. If ergot drugs are used to restore fertility in a patient with a clearly enlarged sella turcica, it currently seems advisable to perform preliminary surgery, or possibly radiotherapy, to minimize the risk of rapid tumor growth during pregnancy. In cases in which only mild sellar asymmetry, without enlargement, is present, it is doubtful whether preliminary surgery should be advised before the use of ergot drugs to induce fertility (Gemzell and Wang, 1979). In most reported cases to date, surgery has not been done and complications during pregnancy have been few. There is also evidence that bromoergocriptine itself will shrink some tumors (George et al., 1979). The extent of this phenomenon will require further exploration.

OTHER BREAST DISORDERS

Hypoplasia

Hypoplasia or aplasia of the breasts due to delayed or absent sexual maturation, as in Turner's syndrome, will usually respond satisfactorily to cyclic estrogen-progesterone therapy. The same is also true of the breast atrophy that follows premature menopause. Occasionally one sees partial or total failure of breast development, sometimes only one-sided, in a woman who is having regular menses and appears to be endocrinologically normal. The problem in such cases seems to be a relative insensitivity of breast tissue itself to normal hormonal stimulation. Estrogen or other hormone therapy should not be used to augment breast size in these patients. Estrogens are unlikely to have any significant effect in doses close to the physiologic range, and the pharmacologic doses that might conceivably produce slight improvement carry unacceptable risks of thrombo-embolism and other toxicity.

Macromastia

Progressive enlargement of the female breasts to tremendous size, often accompanied by pain and sometimes ulceration of the stretched overlying skin, is a rare and still poorly understood disorder. Sometimes the enlargement is rapidly progressive over a period of weeks or months; such cases are most commonly encountered either in adolescence or during the course of pregnancy, but can occur at other times. Galactorrhea is usually not present and hormone levels, including PRL, are probably most often within the normal range, though no large or well-studied series of such patients has been reported. That excess PRL secretion by itself is not responsible is indicated by the fact that severe hyperprolactinemia, such as occurs with some pituitary tumors, is not characteristically associated with any increase in breast size. It seems reasonable to assume that excessive sensitivity of the breast itself to normal levels of circulating hormones, or to the combined hormone elevation seen in pregnancy, is the major factor in most cases. Those cases that occur during pregnancy may regress after parturition or abortion but may recur during a later pregnancy. Though there are few indications as yet that such treatment is likely to be successful, a therapeutic trial of bromoergocriptine may be warranted — especially in cases of recent onset — before considering the more drastic alternative of reduction mammoplasty.

Mastalgia

Many women complain at times of pain in the breasts. In the large series studied by Preece (1976) the pain was most commonly diffuse and subject to cyclic premenstrual induction or exacerbation. A smaller group had well-localized pain ascribed to ductal ectasia and periductal mastitis. Tietze's syndrome, trauma, and cancer were diagnoses in smaller numbers of cases. Preliminary reports, requiring confirmation, have suggested that bromoergocriptine may give relief to some patients with diffuse pain, but whether this drug is more effective than a placebo requires further investigation.

REFERENCES

Morphology

Baker, T. G.: A quantitative and cytological study of germ cells in human ovaries. *Proc. Roy. Soc.* (B) *158*:417, 1963.

Beers, W. H., et al.: Ovarian plasminogen activator: relationship to ovulation and hormonal regulation. *Cell 6*:387, 1975.

Blandau, R. L.: Follicular growth, ovulation, and egg transport, In *The Ovary.* Mack, H. C. (ed.), Springfield, Charles C Thomas, 1968.

Block, E.: Quantitative morphological investigations of follicular system in women: variations in different phases of sexual cycle. *Acta Endocrinol. 8*:33, 1951.

Byskov, A. G.: The role of the rete ovarii in meiosis and follicle formation in different mammalian species. *J. Reprod. Fertil. 45*:201, 1975.

Corner, G. W., Jr.: Histological dating of human corpus luteum of menstruation. *Am. J. Anat. 98*:377, 1956.

Edwards, R. G.: Follicular fluid. *J. Reprod. Fertil. 37*:189, 1974.

Espey, L. L.: Ovarian proteolytic enzymes and ovulation. *Biol. Reprod. 10*:216, 1974.

Espey, L. L.: Ovarian contractility and its relationship to ovulation: a review. *Biol. Reprod. 19*:540, 1978.

George, F. W., and Wilson, J. D.: Conversion of androgen to estrogen by the human fetal ovary. *J. Clin. Endocrinol. Metab. 47*:550, 1978.

Gulyas, B. J., Hodgen, G. D., et al.: Effects of fetal or maternal hypophysectomy on endocrine organs and body weight in infant rhesus monkeys (*Macaca mulatta*) with particular reference to oogenesis. *Biol. Reprod. 16*:216, 1977.

Hertig, A. T.: The aging ovary — a preliminary note. *J. Clin. Endocrinol. 4*:581, 1944.

Kaplan, S. L., and Grumbach, M. M.: Pituitary and placental gonadotrophins and sex steroids in the human and sub-human primate fetus. *Clin. Endocrinol. Metab. 7*:487, 1978.

Merrill, J. A.: Ovarian hilus cells. *Am. J. Obstet. Gynecol. 78*:1258, 1959.

Morris, J. M., and Scully, R. E.: *Endocrine Pathology of the Ovary.* St. Louis, C. V. Mosby, 1958.

Mossman, H. W., and Duke, K. L.: *Comparative Morphology of the Human Ovary.* Madison, University of Wisconsin Press, 1973.

Ohno, S., Klinger, H., et al.: Human oogenesis. *Cytogenetics 1*:42, 1962.

Parini, F., and Molla, W.: Contributo anatomo-istologico al significato biologico dell'atresia folliculare. *Ann. Obstet. Gynecol. 62*:1629, 1940.

Peters, H., Byskov, A. G., et al.: Follicular growth in fetal and prepubertal ovaries of humans and other primates. *Clin. Endocrinol. Metabol. 7*:469, 1978.

Polhemus, D. W.: Ovarian maturation and cyst formation in children. *Pediatrics 11*:588, 1953.

Ross, G. T., and Lipsett, M. B.: Hormonal correlates of normal and abnormal follicle growth after puberty in humans and other primates. *Clin. Endocrinol. Metab. 7*:561, 1978.

Sauramo, H.: Histology, histopathology and function of the senile ovary. *Ann. Chir. Gynaecol. Fenn. 41* (Suppl. 1):1, 1952.

Scammon, R. E.: The prenatal growth and natal involution of the human uterus. *Proc. Soc. Exp. Biol. Med. 23*:687, 1926.

Sternberg, W. H.: Morphology, androgenic function, hyperplasia and tumors of the human ovarian hilus cells. *Am. J. Pathol. 25*:493, 1949.

Strickland, S., and Beers, W. H.: Studies on the role of plasminogen activator in ovulation. *J. Biol. Chem. 251*:5694, 1976.

Tsafriri, A., Lindner, H. R., et al.: Physiological role of prostaglandins in the induction of ovulation. *Prostaglandins 2*:1, 1972.

Van Wagenen, G., and Simpson, M. E.: *Embryology of the Ovary and Testis: Homo Sapiens and Macaca mulatta.* New Haven, Yale University Press, 1965.

Wehefritz, E.: Systematische Geiwichtsuntersuchungen am Ovarien mit Beruecksichtigung anderer Druesen mit inner Sekretion. *Z. Ges. Anat. 9*:161, 1923.

Winter, J. S. D., Faiman, C., et al.: Sex steroid production by the human fetus: its role in morphogenesis and control by gonadotropins. *Birth Defects 12*:41, 1977.

Witschi, E.: Embryology of the ovary, In *The Ovary.* Grady, H. G., and Smith, D. E. (eds.), Baltimore, Williams & Wilkins, 1963, p. 1.

Woll, E., Hertig, A. M., et al.: Ovary in endometrial carcinoma, with notes on morphological history of aging ovary. *Am. J. Obstet. Gynecol. 56*:617, 1948.

Puberty

Boyar, R., Finkelstein, J., et al.: Synchronization of augmented LH secretion with sleep during puberty. *N. Engl. J. Med. 287*:582, 1972.

Frisch, R. E., and McArthur, J. W.: Menstrual cycles: Fatness as a determinant of minimum weight for height necessary for their maintenance at onset. *Science 185*:949, 1974.

Hansen, J. W., Hoffman, P., et al.: Monthly gonadotropin cycles in premenarcheal girls. *Science 190*:161, 1975.

Kulin, H. E., Moore, R. G., et al.: Circadian rhythms in gonadotropin secretion in prepubertal and pubertal children. *J. Clin. Endocrinol. Metab. 42*:770, 1976.

Marshall, W. A., and Tanner, J. M.: Variations in pattern of pubertal changes in girls. *Arch. Dis. Child. 44*:291, 1969.

Penny, R., Ocambiwannu, N. O., et al.: Episodic fluctuation of serum gonadotropins in pre- and post-pubertal boys and girls. *J. Clin. Endocrinol. Metab. 45*:307, 1977.

Styne, D. M., and Grumbach, M. M.: Puberty in the male and female: its physiology and disorders, In *Reproductive Endocrinology.* Yen, S. S. C., and Jaffe, R. B. (eds.), Philadelphia, W. B. Saunders, 1978, p. 189.

Winter, J. S. D., Faiman, C., et al.: Gonadotropins and steroid hormones in the blood and urine of prepubertal girls and other primates. *Clin. Endocrinol. Metab. 7*:513, 1978.

Zacharias, L., Wurtman, R. J., et al.: Sexual maturation in contemporary American girls. *Am. J. Obstet. Gynecol. 108*:833, 1970.

Zacharias, L., Rand, W. H., et al.: A prospective study of sexual development and growth in American girls: the statistics of the menarche. *Obstet. Gynecol. Surv. 31*:325, 1976.

Cyclic Changes in Genital Tract Epithelium and Tests of Ovarian Function

Castellanos, H., and Sturgis, S. H.: Urinary cytology in the endocrine evaluation of the normal female. *Progr. Gynecol. 4*:98, 1963.

Collett-Solberg, P. R., and Grumbach, M. M.: A simplified procedure for evaluating estrogenic effects and the sex chromatin pattern in exfoliated cells in urine: Studies in premature thelarche and gynecomastia of adolescence. *J. Pediatr. 66*:883, 1965.

Davis, M. E., and Fugo, N. W.: Cause of physiologic basal temperature changes in women. *J. Clin. Endocrinol. 8*:550, 1948.

Gaudefroy, M.: Cytologic criteria of estrogen effect. *Acta Cytol. 2*:347, 1958.

Goldenberg, R. L., Grodin, J. M., et al.: Withdrawal bleeding and luteinizing hormone secretion following progesterone in women with amenorrhea. *Am. J. Obstet. Gynecol.* 115:193, 1973.

Israel, S. L.: *Menstrual Disorders and Sterility.* 5th ed. New York, Hoeber Medical Division, Harper and Row, 1967.

Israel, S. L., and Schneller, O.: Thermogenic property of progesterone. *Fertil. Steril.* 1:53, 1950.

Noyes, R. W., Hertig, A. T., et al.: Dating endometrial biopsy. *Fertil. Steril.* 1:3, 1950.

Papanicolaou, G. N.: Sexual cycle in human female as revealed by vaginal smears. *Am. J. Anat.* 52:519, 1933.

Papanicolaou, G. N., Traut, H. F., et al.: *The Epithelia of Women's Reproductive Organs.* New York, Commonwealth, 1948.

Preeyasombat, C., and Kenny, F. M.: Urocytograms in normal children and various abnormal conditions. *Pediatrics* 38:436, 1966.

Rebar, R. W.: Practical evaluation of hormonal status, In *Reproductive Endocrinology.* Yen, S. S. C. and Jaffe, R. B. (eds.), Philadelphia, W. B. Saunders, 1978, p. 469.

Rock, J.: Medical progress: physiology of human conception. *N. Engl. J. Med.* 240:804, 1949.

Weid, G. L., and Keebler, C. M.: Vaginal cytology of female children. *Ann. N.Y. Acad. Sci.* 142:646, 1967.

Menopause

Jaffe, R. B.: The menopause and perimenopausal period, In *Reproductive Endocrinology.* Yen, S. S. C. and Jaffe, R. B. (eds.), Philadelphia, W. B. Saunders, 1978, p. 261.

Korenman, S. G., Sherman, B. M., et al.: Reproductive hormone function: the perimenopausal period and beyond. *Clin. Endocrinol. Metab.* 7:265, 1978.

Gonadotropin and Steroid Measurements

Abraham, G. E.: Radioimmunoassay of steroids in biological materials. *Clin. Biochem.* 7(3):193, 1974.

Berson, S. A., and Yalow, R. S. (eds.): *Peptide Hormones.* New York, American Elsevier, 1973.

Cameron, E. H. D., Hillier, S. G., et al. (eds.): *Steroid Immunoassay.* (Proceedings of the 5th Tenovus Workshop, 1974, Cardiff, Wales), Cardiff, Alpha Omega, 1975, p. 334.

Jaffe, B. M., and Behrman, H. (eds.): *Methods of Hormone Radioimmunoassay.* 2nd ed. New York, Academic Press, 1979.

Gupta, D. (ed.): *Radioimmunoassay of Steroid Hormones.* Weinheim, Verlag Chemie, 1975, p. 224.

Wide, L., Nillius, S. J., et al.: Radioimmunosorbent assay of follicle-stimulating hormone and luteinizing hormone serum and urine from men and women. *Acta Endocrinol.* [Suppl.] (Kbh) 174:3, 1973.

Menstrual Cycle

Abraham, G. E., and Chakmakjian, Z. H.: Serum steroid levels during the menstrual cycle in a bilaterally adrenalectomized woman. *J. Clin. Endocrinol. Metab.* 37:581, 1973.

Baird, D. T., and Guevara, A.: Concentration of unconjugated estrone and estradiol in peripheral plasma in nonpregnant women throughout the menstrual cycle, castrate and postmenopausal women and in men. *J. Clin. Endocrinol.* 29:149, 1949.

Baird, D. T., Horton, R., et al.: Steroid prehormones. *Perspect. Biol. Med.* 3:384, 1968.

Baird, D. T., Horton, R., et al.: Steroid dynamics under steady state conditions. *Recent Progr. Hormone Res.* 25:611, 1969.

Carmel, P. D., Araki, S., et al.: Prolonged stalk portal blood collection in rhesus monkeys. Pulsatile release of gonadotropin-releasing hormone (GnRH). *Endocrinology* 99:243, 1976.

Dyrenfurth, I., Jewelewicz, R., et al.: Temporal relationships of hormonal variables in the menstrual cycle, In *Biorhythms and Human Reproduction.* Ferin, M., Halberg, F., et al. (eds.), New York, John Wiley & Sons, 1973.

Fishman, J.: The cathechol estrogens. *Neuroendocrinology* 4:363, 1976.

Goodman, A. L., Nixon, W. E., et al.: Regulation of folliculogenesis in cycling rhesus monkey: Selection of dominant follicle. *Endocrinology* 100:155, 1977.

Grodin, J. M., Siiteri, P. K., et al.: Source of estrogen production in menopausal women. *J. Clin. Endocrinol.* 36:207, 1973.

Gurpide, E., and Gandy, H.: Dynamics of hormone production, In *Endocrinology of Pregnancy.* Fuchs, F., and Klopper, A. (eds.), New York, Harper and Row, 1971, p. 1.

Henzl, M. R., Smith, R. E., et al.: Lysosomal concept of menstrual bleeding in humans. *J. Clin. Endocrinol. Metab.* 34:860, 1972.

Johansson, E. D., Wide, L., et al.: Luteinizing hormone (LH) and progesterone in plasma and LH and oestrogens in urine during 42 normal menstrual cycles. *Acta Endocrinol.* 68:502, 1971.

Judd, H. L., and Yen, S. S. C.: Serum and androstenedione and testosterone levels during menstrual cycle. *J. Clin. Endocrinol. Metab.* 36:475, 1973.

Knobil, E.: On the control of gonadotropin secretion in the rhesus monkey. *Recent Prog. Hormone Res.* 30:1, 1974.

Leyendecker, G., Wildt, L., et al.: Experimental studies on the positive feedback effect of progesterone, 17-hydroxyprogesterone and 20-dihydroprogesterone on the pituitary release of LH and FSH in the human female. *Arch. Gynaekol.* 221:29, 1976.

Louvet, J.-P., Harman, S. M., et al.: Evidence for a role of androgen in follicular maturation. *Endocrinology* 97:366, 1975.

MacDonald, P. C., Grodin, J. M., et al.: The utilization of plasma androstenedione for estrone production in women, in *Progress in Endocrinology.* Gual, C. (ed.), Amsterdam, Excerpta Medica Foundation, 1969.

McNatty, K. P., Hunter, W. M., et al.: Changes in the concentration of pituitary and steroid hormones in the follicular fluid of human graafian follicles throughout the menstrual cycle. *J. Endocrinol.* 64:555, 1975.

McNatty, K. P., Baird, D. T., et al.: Concentrations of oestrogens and androgens in human ovarian venous plasma and follicular fluid through the menstrual cycle. *J. Endocrinol.* 71:77, 1976.

McNatty, K. P.: Cyclic changes in antral fluid hormone concentrations in humans. *Clin. Endocrinol. Metab.* 7:577, 1978.

Mikhail, G.: Hormone secretion by the human ovaries. *Gynecol. Invest.* 1:5, 1970.

Presser, H. B.: Temporal data relating to the human menstrual cycle, In *Biorhythms and Human Reproduction.* Ferin, M., Halberg, F., et al. (eds.), New York, John Wiley & Sons, 1974, p. 145.

Ross, G. T., Cargille, C. M., et al.: Pituitary and gonadal hormones in women during spontaneous and induced ovulatory cycles. *Recent Progr. Hormone Res.* 26:1, 1970.

Salhanick, H. A., Vande Wiele, R. L., et al. (eds.): Metabolic effects of contraceptive steroids. *Proceedings of Conference on Metabolic Effects of Gonadal Hormones and Contraceptive Steroids,* Boston, 1968. New York, Plenum Press, 1969.

Schally, A. V., Arimura, A., et al.: Isolation and properties of the FSH and LH-releasing hormone. *Biochem. Biophys. Res. Commun.* 43:393, 1971.

Speroff, L., and Vande Wiele, R. L.: Regulation of the human menstrual cycle. *Am. J. Obstet. Gynecol.* 109:234, 1971.

Tagatz, G. E., and Gurpide, E.: Hormone secretion by the normal human ovary, In *Handbook of Physiology* Section 7: *Endocrinology.* American Physiological Society. Greep, R. O., and Astwood, E. B. (eds.). Baltimore, Williams & Wilkins, 1973.

Tait, J.: Review of the use of isotopic steroids for the measurement of production rates *in vivo, J. Clin. Endocrinol.* 23:1285, 1963.

Thorneycroft, I. H., Sribyatta, B., et al.: Measurement of serum LH, FSH, progesterone, 17-hydroxyprogesterone, and estradiol levels at 4-hour intervals during the periovulatory phase of the menstrual cycle. *J. Clin. Endocrinol. Metab.* 39:754, 1974.

Treloar, A. E., Boynton, R. E., et al.: Variation of the human menstrual cycle through reproductive life. *Intern. J. Fertil.* 12:77, 1967.

Vande Wiele, R. L., Bogumil, J., et al.: Mechanisms regulating the menstrual cycle in women. *Recent Progr. Hormone Res.* 26:63, 1970.

Vande Wiele, R. L., and Dyrenfurth, I.: Gonadotropin-steroid interrelationships. *Pharmacol. Rev.* 25:2, 1973.

Vekemans, M., Delvoye, P., et al.: Serum prolactin levels during the menstrual cycle. *J. Clin. Endocrinol. Metab.* 44:989, 1977.

Vollman, R. F.: *The Menstrual Cycle.* Philadelphia, W. B. Saunders, 1977.

Yen, S. S. C.: The human menstrual cycle (integrative functions of the hypothalamic-pituitary-ovarian-endometrial axis), In *Reproductive Endocrinology.* Yen, S. S. C., and Jaffe, R. B. (eds.), Philadelphia, W. B. Saunders, 1978.

Yen, S. S. C., Lasley, B. L., et al.: The operating characteristics of the hypothalamic-pituitary system during the menstrual cycle and observations of biological action of somatostatin. *Recent Prog. Hormone Res.* 31:321, 1975.

Yen, S. S. C., VandenBerg, G., et al.: Causal relationship between the hormonal variables in the menstrual cycle. In *Biorhythms and Reproduction.* Ferin, M., Halberg, F., et al. (eds.), New York, John Wiley and Sons, 1974, p. 219.

Steroid Hormones

Brown, J. B., and Matthew, J. D.: The application of urinary estrogen measurements to problems in gynecology. *Recent Progr. Hormone Res.* 18:337, 1962.

Korenman, S. G., Perrin, L. E., et al.: A radio-ligand binding assay system for estradiol measurement in human plasma. *J. Clin. Endocrinol.* 29:879, 1969.

Loraine, J. A., and Bell, E. T.: Hormone excretion during the normal menstrual cycle. *Lancet* 1:1340, 1963.

Strott, C. A., and Lipsett, M. B.: Measurement of 17-hydroxyprogesterone in human plasma. *J. Clin. Endocrinol.* 28:1426, 1968.

Yoshimi, T., and Lipsett, M. B.: The measurement of plasma progesterone. *Steroids* 11:527, 1968.

Neoplastic Diseases

Allander, E., and Wagenmark, J.: Leydig cell tumors of the ovary. *Acta Obstet. Gynecol. Scand.* 48:433, 1969.

Asadourian, L. A., and Taylor, H. B.: Dysgerminoma. An analysis of 105 cases. *Obstet. Gynecol.* 33:370, 1969.

Audet-Lapointe, P, and Vauclair, R.: Les tumeurs de la granulosa. Revue de la littérature et présentation de 7 cas. *Bull. Cancer* 55:457, 1968.

Berge, T., and Borglin, N. E.: Brenner tumors. Histogenetic and clinical studies. *Cancer 20*:308, 1970.

Blanc, B.: Les gonadoblastomes. Revue Generale. *Rev. Franc. Endocr. Clin. 11*:529, 1970.

Boivin, Y., and Richart, R. M.: Hilus cell tumors of the ovary. A review with a report of 3 new cases. *Cancer 18*:231, 1965.

Breen, J. L., and Neubecker, R. D.: Ovarian malignancy in children with special reference to the germ-cell tumors. *Ann. N. Y. Acad. Sci. 142*:658, 1967.

Brown, P. A., and Richart, R. M.: Functioning ovarian carcinoid tumors. Case report and review of the literature. *Obstet. Gynecol. 34*:390, 1969.

Burger, J. P., Schlaeder, G., et al.: Le chorioépithelioma primitif de l'ovarie. *Rev. Franc. Gynecol. 64*:351, 1969.

Chen, H-C, Hodgen, G. D., et al.: Evidence for a gonadotropin from nonpregnant subjects that has physical, immunological, and biological similarities to human chorionic gonadotropin. *Proc. Natl. Acad. Sci. USA 73*:2885, 1976.

Costin, M. E., Jr., and Kennedy, R. L. J.: Ovarian tumors in infants and in children. *Am. J. Dis. Child. 76*:127, 1948.

Diddle, A. W.: Granulosa and theca cell ovarian tumors: Prognosis. *Cancer 5*:215, 1952.

Dockerty, M. B., and MacCarty, W. C.: Granulosa cell tumors, with report of 34 pound specimen and a review. *Am. J. Obstet. Gynecol. 27*:425, 1939.

Dunihoo, D. R., Grieme, D. L., et al.: Hilar cell tumors of the ovary. Report of 2 new cases and a review of the world literature. *Obstet. Gynecol. 27*:703, 1966.

Eberlein, W. R., Bongiovanni, A. M., et al.: Ovarian tumors and cysts associated with sexual precocity. *J. Pediatr. 57*:484, 1960.

Ein, S. H., Darte, J. M., et al.: Cystic and solid ovarian tumors in children: A 44-year review. *J. Pediatr. Surg. 5*:148, 1970.

Fox, L. P., and Stamm, W. J.: Krukenberg tumor complicating pregnancy; report of a case with androgenic activity. *Am. J. Obstet. Gynecol. 92*:702, 1965.

Gross, R. E.: Neoplasms producing endocrine disturbances in childhood. *Am. J. Dis. Child. 59*:579, 1940.

Hodgson, J. E., Dockerty, M. B., et al.: Granulosa cell tumor of ovary; a clinical and pathological review of 62 cases. *Surg. Gynecol. Obstet. 81*:631, 1945.

Hughesdon, P. E.: Ovarian lipoid and theca cell tumors; their origins and interrelations. *Obstet. Gynecol. Surv. 21*:245, 1966.

Lipsett, M. B., Kirschner, M. A., et al.: Malignant lipid cell tumor of the ovary: clinical, biochemical and etiologic considerations. *J. Clin. Endocrinol. 30*:336, 1970.

Malkasian, G. D., Jr., Dockerty, M. B., et al.: Functioning tumors of the ovary in women under 40. *Obstet. Gynecol. 26*:669, 1965.

Marcus, C. C., and Marcus, S. L.: Struma ovarii. A report of 7 cases and a review of the subject. *Am. J. Obstet. Gynecol. 81*:752, 1961.

Mannubini, G.: Primary chorionepithelioma of the ovary. *Acta Obstet. Gynecol. Scand. 28*:251, 1949.

Moore, J. G., Schifrin, B. S., et al.: Ovarian tumors in infancy, childhood, and adolescence. *Am. J. Obstet. Gynecol. 99*:913, 1967.

Norris, H. J., and Taylor, H. B.: Prognosis of granulosa-theca tumors of ovary. *Cancer 21*:255, 1968.

Norris, H. J., and Taylor, H. B.: Virilization associated with cystic granulosa tumors. *Obstet. Gynecol. 34*:629, 1969.

Novak, E. R., Facog, J. K., et al.: Feminizing gonadal stromal tumors. *Obstet. Gynecol. 38*:701, 1971.

Pedowitz, P., and Pomerance, W.: Adrenal-like tumors of the ovary. Review of the literature and report of two new cases. *Obstet. Gynecol. 19*:183, 1962.

Peterson, W. F., Prevost, E. C., et al.: Benign cystic teratomas of ovary; clinico-statistical study of 1007 cases with a review of the literature. *Am. J. Obstet. Gynecol. 70*:368, 1955.

Taylor, H. B., and Norris, H. J.: Lipid cell tumors of the ovary. *Cancer 20*:1953, 1967.

Thompson, J. P., Dockerty, M. B., et al.: Ovarian and paraovarian tumors in infants and children. *Am. J. Obstet. Gynecol. 97*:1059, 1967.

Scully, R. E.: Gonadoblastoma. A review of 74 cases. *Cancer 25*:1340, 1970.

Shuster, M., Mendoza-Divino, E., et al.: Carcinoid tumor metastasizing to the ovaries. *Obstet. Gynecol. 36*:515, 1970.

Smith, F. G.: Pathology and physiology of struma ovarii. *Arch. Surg. 53*:603, 1946.

Spadoni, L. R., Lindberg, M. C., et al.: Virilization coexisting with Krukenberg tumor during pregnancy. *Am. J. Obstet. Gynecol. 92*:981, 1965.

Vaitukaitis, J. L., Ross, G. T., et al.: Gonadotropins and their subunits: basic and clinical studies. *Recent Prog. Hormone Res. 32*:289, 1976.

Zangeneh, F., and Kelly, V. C.: Granulosa-theca-cell tumor of the ovary in children. *Am. J. Dis. Child. 115*:494, 1968.

Autoimmune Diseases

Irvine, W. J., Moira, M. W., et al.: The further characterization of autoantibodies reactive with extra-adrenal steroid-producing cells in patients with adrenal disorders. *Clin. Exp. Immunol. 4*:489, 1969.

Ruehsen, M., Blizzard, R. M., et al.: Autoimmunity and ovarian failure. *Am. J. Obstet. Gynecol. 112*:693, 1972.

Precocious Puberty and Pseudopuberty

Albright, F., Butler, A. M., et al.: Syndrome characterized by osteitis fibrosa disseminata, areas of pigmentation and endocrine dysfunction, with precocious puberty in females; report of 5 cases. *N. Engl. J. Med. 216*:727, 1937.

Beas, F., Vargas, L., et al.: Pseudoprecocious puberty in infants caused by a dermal ointment containing estrogens. *J. Pediatr. 75*:127, 1969.

Capraro, V. J., Bayonet-Rivera, N. P., et al.: Premature thelarche (review). *Obstet. Gynecol. Surv. 26*:2, 1971.

Cloutier, M. D., and Hayles, A. B.: Precocious puberty. *Advances Pediatr. 17*:125, 1970.

Dresch, C., Arnal, M., et al.: Étude de 22 cas de développement prémature isolé des seins ou "premature thelarche." *Helv. Paediat. Acta 15*:585, 1960.

Ferrier, P., Shephard, T. H., et al.: Growth disturbances and values for hormone excretion in various forms of precocious sexual development. *Pediatrics 28*:258, 1961.

Hall, R., and Warrick, C.: Hypersecretion of hypothalamic releasing hormones: a possible explanation of the endocrine manifestations of polyostotic fibrous dysplasia (Albright's syndrome). *Lancet 1*:1313, 1972.

Hertz, R.: Ingestion of estrogens by children. *Pediatrics 21*:203, 1958.

Jenner, M. R., Kelch, R. P., et al.: Hormonal changes in puberty. IV. Plasma estradiol, LH, and FSH in prepubertal children, pubertal females and in precocious puberty, premature thelarche, hypogonadism, and in a child with a feminizing ovarian tumor. *J. Clin. Endocrinol. 34*:521, 1972.

Kenney, F. M., Midgley, A. R., Jr., et al.: Radioimmunoassayable serum LH and FSH in girls with sexual precocity, premature thelarche and adrenarche. *J. Clin. Endocrinol. 29*:1272, 1969.

McCune, D. J.: Ostetitis fibrosa cystica: The case of a nine year old girl who also exhibits precocious puberty. *Am. J. Dis. Child. 52*:743, 1936.

Ramos, A. S., and Bower, B. F.: Pseudoisosexual precocity due to cosmetic ingestion. *J.A.M.A. 207*:368, 1969.

Rosenfeld, R. L.: Plasma 17-ketosteroids and 17-beta hydroxysteroids in girls with premature development of sexual hair. *J. Pediatr. 79*:260, 1971.

Royer, P.: La précocité-isoséxuelle. *Rev. Franc. Endocr. Clin. 8*:217, 1967.

Serment, H., Piana, L., et al.: Puberté précoce d'origine ovarienne. *Rev. Franc. Endocr. Clin. 11*:489, 1970.

Sigurjonsdottir, T. J., and Hayles, A. B.: Precocious puberty. A report of 96 cases. *Am. J. Dis. Child. 115*:309, 1968.

Sigurjonsdottir, T. J., and Hayles, A. B.: Premature pubarche. *Clin. Pediatr. 7*:29, 1968.

Silverman, S. H., Migeon, C., et al.: Precocious growth of sexual hair without other secondary sexual development; "premature pubarche," constitutional variation of adolescence. *Pediatrics 10*:426, 1952.

Steiner, M. M.: Enlargement of breasts during childhood. *Pediatr. Clin. North Am. 2*:575, 1955.

Talbot, N. B., Sobel, E. H., et al.: *Functional Endocrinology from Birth through Adolescence.* Cambridge, Harvard University Press, 1952.

Thamdrup, E.: Precocious sexual development. A clinical study of 100 children. *Danish Med. Bull. 8*:140, 1961.

Van Wyk, J. J., and Grumbach, M. M.: Syndrome of precocious menstruation and galactorrhea in juvenile hypothyroidism: an example of hormonal overlap in pituitary feedback. *J. Pediatr. 57*:416, 1960.

Wilkins, L.: *The Diagnosis and Treatment of Endocrine Disorders in Childhood and Adolescence.* 3rd ed. Baltimore, Williams & Wilkins, 1965.

Wood, L. C., Olichney, M., et al.: Syndrome of juvenile hypothyroidism associated with advanced sexual development: Report of two new cases and comment on the management of an associated ovarian mass. *J. Clin. Endocrinol. 25*:1289, 1965.

Zurbruegg, R. P., and Gardner, L. I.: Urinary C_{19} steroids in two girls with precocious sexual hair. *J. Clin. Endocrinol. 23*:704, 1963.

Delayed Menarche and Primary Amenorrhea

Bjoro, K.: Primary amenorrhea. A study with special reference to the morphology of the genital organs. *Acta Obstet. Gynecol. Scand. 44* (Suppl.):1, 1965.

Bjoro, K.: Amenorrhea. A study with particular attention to the problems of ovarian failure. *Acta Obstet. Gynecol. Scand. 45* (Suppl. 1):69, 1966.

Black, W. P., and Govan, A. D. T.: Laparoscopy and gonadal biopsy for assessment of gonadal function in primary amenorrhea. *Br. Med. J. 1*:672, 1972.

Canales, E. S., and Zarate, A.: Primary amenorrhea associated with polycystic ovaries. Endocrine, cytogenetic and therapeutic considerations. *Obstet. Gynecol. 37*:205, 1971.

Caspersson, T., Zech, L., et al.: Analysis of human metaphase chromosome set by aid of DNA-binding fluorescent agents. *Exp. Cell Res. 62*:490, 1970.

Counseller, V. S.: Congenital absence of vagina. *J.A.M.A. 136*:861, 1948.

Grover, S., Solanki, B. R., et al.: A clinicopathologic study of Müllerian duct aplasia with special reference to cytogenetic studies. *Am. J. Obstet. Gynecol. 107*:133, 1970.

Hauser, G. A., and Kumschick, F.: Die primare Amenorrheae. *Gebürtshilfe Frauenheilkd.* 26:645, 1966.

Henzl, M., Presl, J., et al.: Practical possibilities for classification of primary amenorrhea with special reference to the use of pneumopelvigraphy. *Am. J. Obstet. Gynecol.* 93:79, 1965.

Hertz, R., Odell, W. D., et al.: Diagnostic implications of primary amenorrhea. *Ann. Intern. Med.* 65:800, 1966.

Jacobs, P. A., Harnden, D. G., et al.: Cytogenetic studies in primary amenorrhea. *Lancet* 1:1183, 1961.

Jagiello, G. M., Kaminetsky, H. A., et al.: Primary amenorrhea. A cytogenetic and endocrinologic study of 18 cases. *J.A.M.A.* 198:30, 1966.

Jones, G. S., and de Moraes-Ruehsen, M.: A new syndrome of amenorrhea in association with hypergonadotropism and apparently normal ovarian follicular apparatus. *Am. J. Obstet. Gynecol.* 104:597, 1969.

Kadotani, T., Ohama, K., et al.: A preliminary cytogenetic survey in primary amenorrhea. *Jap. J. Hum. Genet.* 13:278, 1969.

Kinch, R. A. H., Plunkett, E. R., et al.: Primary ovarian failure; a clinicopathological and cytogenetic study. *Am. J. Obstet. Gynecol.* 91:630, 1965.

Lewis, A. C. W.: Chromosomal aspects of primary amenorrhea. *Proc. R. Soc. Med.* 63:297, 1970.

Morin, J. P., Sudan, J. P., et al.: Amenorrhees primaires par synechies uterines d'origine tuberculeuse. *Rev. Franc. Gynec. Obstet.* 64:539, 1969.

Pearson, P. L., Bobrow, M., et al.: Technique for identifying Y chromosomes in human interphase nuclei. *Nature* (London) 226:78, 1970.

Philip, J., Sele, V., et al.: Primary amenorrhea. A study of 101 cases. *Fertil. Steril.* 16:795, 1965.

Polishuk, W. Z., Sharf, M., et al.: Primary amenorrhea due to intrauterine adhesions. *Gynaecologia* (Basel) 154:181, 1962.

Reschini, E., Giestina, G., et al.: Radioimmunoassayable plasma luteinizing hormone in primary amenorrhea. *Am. J. Obstet. Gynecol.* 111:173, 1971.

Ross, G. T.: Diagnosis and treatment of primary amenorrhea, secondary amenorrhea, and dysfunctional uterine bleeding, In *Endocrinology*. DeGroot,. L. J., et al. (eds.), New York, Grune & Stratton, 1979, p. 1419.

Ross, G. T., and Tjio, J. H.: Cytogenetics in clinical endocrinology. *J.A.M.A.* 192:977, 1965.

Shearman, R. P.: A physiological approach to the differential diagnosis and treatment of primary amenorrhea. *J. Obstet. Gynaec. Brit. Emp.* 75:1101, 1968.

Starup, J., Sele, V., et al.: Amenorrhea associated with increased production of gonadotropins and a morphologically normal ovarian follicular apparatus. *Acta Endocrinol.* 66:248, 1971.

Steele, S. J., Beilby, J., et al.: Visualization and biopsy of the ovary in the investigation of amenorrhea. *Obstet. Gynecol.* 36:899, 1970.

Turunen, A.: Ueber kongenitales Fehler der Scheide. *Ann. Chir. Gynaecol. Fenn.* 46:125, 1957.

Weiser, P.: Beobachtungen bei atresei von Uterus und Vagina. *Gebürtshilfe Frauenheilkd.* 26:1388, 1966.

Zourlas, P. A., and Comninos, A. C.: Primary amenorrhea with normally developed secondary sex characteristics. *Obstet. Gynecol.* 38:298, 1971.

Secondary Amenorrhea

Bardin, C. W., and Lipsett, M. B.: Testosterone and androstenedione blood production rates in normal women and women with idiopathic hirsutism or polycystic ovaries. *J. Clin. Invest.* 46:891, 1967.

Bassi, F., Fiusti, G., et al.: Plasma androgens in women with hyperprolactinemic amenorrhea. *Clin. Endocrinol.* 6:5, 1977.

Bergh, T., Nillius, S. J., et al.: Bromocriptin treatment of 42 hyperprolactinemic women with secondary amenorrhea. *Acta Endocrinol.* 88:435, 1978.

Bergh, T., Nillius, S. J., et al.: Bromocriptin treatment of seven women with primary amenorrhea and prolactin-secreting pituitary tumors. *Clin. Endocrinol.* 10:145, 1979.

Besser, G. M., Thorner, M. O., et al.: Therapeutic use of bromocriptin and growth hormone release inhibiting hormone. *Progr. Reprod. Biol.* 2:261, 1977.

Blizzard, R. M., Chee, D., et al.: The incidence of adrenal and other antibodies in the sera of patients with idiopathic adrenal insufficiency (Addison's disease). *Clin. Exp. Immunol.* 1:119, 1966.

Change, R. J., Keye, W. R., et al.: Detection, evaluation, and treatment of pituitary microadenomas in patients with galactorrhea and amenorrhea. *Am. J. Obstet. Gynecol.* 128:356, 1977.

DeVane, G. W., Czekala, N. M., et al.: Circulating gonadotropins, estrogens and androgens in polycystic ovarian disease. *Am. J. Obstet. Gynecol.* 121:496, 1975.

Garcia, J., Jones, G. S., et al.: The use of clomiphene citrate. *Fertil. Steril.* 28:707, 1977.

Goldzieher, J. W.: Polycystic ovarian disease, In *Progress in Infertility*. Behrman, S. J., and Kistner, R. W. (eds.), Boston, Little, Brown and Co., 1968, p. 351.

Gruen, P. H., Sachar, E. J., et al.: Prolactin responses to neuroleptics in normal and schizophrenic subjects. *Arch. Gen. Psychiatry* 35:108, 1978.

Hardy, J.: Transsphenoidal surgery of hypersecreting pituitary tumors, diagnosis and treatment of pituitary tumors, In *International Congress Series No. 303*, Kohler, P. W., and Ross, G. T. (eds.). Amsterdam, Excerpta Medica. 1973, p. 179.

Irvine, W. J., Chan, M. M. W., et al.: Immunological aspects of premature ovarian failure associated with idiopathic Addison's disease. *Lancet* 2:883, 1968.

Jewelewicz, R.: Management of infertility resulting from anovulation. *Am. J. Obstet. Gynecol.* 122:909, 1975.

Jewelewicz, R., Khalaf, S., et al.: Obstetric complications after treatment of intrauterine synechiae (Asherman's syndrome). *Obstet. Gynecol.* 47:701, 1976.

Kirschner, M. A., and Jacobs, J. B.: Combined ovarian and adrenal vein catheterization to determine the site(s) of androgen overproduction in hirsute women. *J. Clin. Endocrinol.* 33:199, 1971.

Kirschner, M. A., Zucker, I. R., et al.: Idiopathic hirsutism — an ovarian abnormality. *N. Engl. J. Med.* 294:637, 1976.

Lachelin, G. C. L., Abu-Fadil, S., et al.: Functional delineation of hyperprolactinemic amenorrhea. *J. Clin. Endocrinol. Metab.* 44:1163, 1977.

Lachelin, G. C. L., and Yen, S. S. C.: Hypothalamic chronic anovulation. *Am. J. Obstet. Gynecol.* 130:825, 1978.

Lloyd, C. W., Lobotsky, J., et al.: Plasma testosterone and urinary 17-ketosteroids in women with hirsutism and polycystic ovaries. *J. Clin. Endocrinol.* 26:314, 1966.

Mecklenburg, R. S., Loriaux, D. L. et al.: Hypothalamic dysfunction in patients with anorexia nervosa. *Medicine* 53:147, 1974.

Mishell, D. R., Jr., Kletzky, O. A., et al.: The effect of contraceptive steroids on hypothalamic-pituitary function. *Med. J. Obstet. Gynecol.* 128:60, 1977.

Oelsner, G., Serr, D. M., et al.: The study of induction of ovulation with menotropins: analysis of results of 1897 treatment cycles. *Fertil. Steril.* 30:538, 1978.

Shearman, R. P., and Cox, R. I.: The enigmatic polycystic ovary. *Obstet. Gynecol. Surv.* 21:1, 1966.

Slade, P. D., and Russell, G. F. M.: Awareness of body dimensions in anorexia nervosa: Cross-sectional and longitudinal studies. *Psychol. Med.* 3:188, 1973.

Thorner, M. O., Besser, G. M.: Bromocriptin treatment of hyperprolactinemic hypogonadism. *Acta Endocrinol.* [Suppl.] (Kbh) 216:131, 1978.

Tolis, G., Somma, M., et al.: Prolactin secretion in sixty-five patients with galactorrhea. *Am. J. Obstet. Gynecol.* 118:91, 1974.

Warren, M. P., and Vande Wiele, R. L.: Clinical and metabolic features of anorexia nervosa. *Am. J. Obstet. Gynecol.* 117:435, 1973.

Whitelaw, M. J., Nolan, V. F., et al.: Irregular menses, amenorrhea, and infertility following synthetic progestational agents. *J.A.M.A.* 195:780, 1966.

Yen, S. S. C.: Chronic anovulation, In *Reproductive Endocrinology*, Yen, S. S. C., and Jaffe, R. B. (eds.): Philadelphia, W. B. Saunders, 1978.

Yen, S. S. C., Vela, P., et al.: Inappropriate secretion of follicle-stimulating hormone and luteinizing hormone in polycystic ovarian disease. *J. Clin. Endocrinol.* 30:435, 1970.

Treatment of Ovarian Dysfunction

Cullberg, J.: Mood changes and menstrual symptoms with different gestagen/estrogen combinations. A double blind comparison with a placebo. *Acta Psychiatr. Scand.* 236 (Suppl.):1, 1972.

Engel, T., Jewelewicz, R., et al.: Ovarian hyperstimulation syndrome. Report of a case with notes on pathogenesis and treatment. *Am. J. Obstet. Gynecol.* 112:1052, 1972.

Gemzell, C. A.: Induction of ovulation with human gonadotropins. *Recent Prog. Hormone Res.* 21:179, 1965.

Judd, H. L., Rigg, L. A., et al.: The effects of ovarian wedge resection on circulating gonadotropin and ovarian steroid levels in patients with polycystic ovary syndrome. *J. Clin. Endocrinol. Metab.* 43:347, 1976.

Kistner, R. W.: Induction of ovulation with clomiphene citrate. In *Progress in Infertility*. Behrman, S. J., and Kistner, R. W. (eds.), Boston, Little, Brown and Co., 1968.

Salhanick, H. A., Vande Wiele, R. L., et al. (eds.): *Metabolic Effects of Contraceptive Steroids*. New York, Plenum Press, 1968.

Vande Wiele, R. L., and Turksoy, R. N.: Treatment of amenorrhea and of anovulation with human menopausal and chorionic gonadotropins. *J. Clin. Endocrinol. Metab.* 25:369, 1965.

Vande Wiele, R. L.: Treatment of infertility due to ovulatory failure. *Hosp. Pract.* 7:119, 1973.

Breast Development—Morphology and Hormonal Influences

Anderson, R. R.: Endocrinological control, In *Lactation. A Comprehensive Treatise.* Larson, B. L., and Smith, V. R. (eds.), New York, Academic Press, 1974, p. 97.

Ceriani, R. L.: Hormones and other factors controlling growth in the mammary gland: A review. *J. Invest. Dermatol.* 63:93, 1974.

Cowie, A. T., Tindal, J. S., et al.: The induction of mammary growth in the hypophysectomized goat. *J. Endocrinol.* 34:185, 1966.

Djiane, J., Durand, P., et al.: Evolution of prolactin receptors in rabbit mammary gland during pregnancy and lactation. *Endocrinology* 100:1348, 1977.

Freeman, C. S., and Topper, Y. J.: Progesterone is not essential to the differentiative potential of mammary epithelium in the male mouse. *Endocrinology* 103:186, 1978.

Holdaway, I. M., and Friesen, H. G.: Hormone binding by human mammary carcinoma. *Cancer Res.* 37:1946, 1977.

Hsueh, A. J., Peck, Jr., E. J., et al.: Oestrogen receptors in the mammary gland of the lactating rat. *J. Endocrinol.* 58:503, 1973.

Hunt, M. E., and Muldoon, T. G.: Factors controlling estrogen receptor levels in normal mouse mammary tissue. *J. Steroid Biochem.* 8:181, 1977.

Kledzik, G. S., Bradley, C. J., et al.: Effects of high doses of estrogen on prolactin-binding activity and growth of carcinogen-induced mammary cancers in rats. *Cancer Res.* 36:3265, 1976.

Kleinberg, D. L., Todd, J., et al.: Prolactin stimulation of α-lactalbumin in normal primate mammary gland. *J. Clin. Endocrinol. Metab.* 47:435, 1978.

Lyons, W. R., Li, C. H., et al.: The hormonal control of mammary growth and lactation. *Recent Prog. Hormone Res.* 14:219, 1958.

Nimrod, A., and Ryan, K. J.: Aromatization of androgens by human abdominal and breast fat tissue. *J. Clin. Endocrinol. Metab.* 40:367, 1975.

Posner, B. I., Kelly, P. A., et al.: Prolactin receptors in rat liver: possible induction by prolactin. *Science* 188:57, 1975.

Salazar, H., Tobon, H., et al.: Developmental, gestational and postgestational modifications of the human breast. *Clin. Obstet. Gynecol.* 18:113, 1975.

Shyamala, G.: Specific cytoplasmic glucocorticoid hormone receptors in lactating mammary glands. *Biochemistry* 12:3085, 1973.

Talwalker, P., and Meites, J.: Mammary lobulo-alveolar growth induced by anterior pituitary hormones in adreno-ovariectomized and adreno-ovariectomized-hypophysectomized rats. *Proc. Soc. Exp. Biol. Med.* 107:880, 1961.

Topper, Y. J., and Oka, T.: Some aspects of mammary gland development in the mature mouse, In *Lactation. A Comprehensive Treatise.* Larson, B. L., and Smith, V. R. (eds.), New York, Academic Press, 1974, p. 327.

Wagner, R. K., and Jungblut, P. W.: Oestradiol- and dihydrotestosterone receptors in normal and neoplastic human mammary tissue. *Acta Endocrinol.* 82:105, 1976.

Lactation and Suckling

Aono, T., Shioji, T., et al.: Augmentation of puerperal lactation by oral administration of sulpiride. *J. Clin. Endocrinol. Metab.* 48:478, 1979.

Cooke, I., Foley, M., et al.: The treatment of puerperal lactation with bromocriptine. *Postgrad. Med. J.* 52(Suppl.):75, 1976.

Kolodney, R. C., Jacobs, L. S., et al.: Mammary stimulation causes prolactin secretion in non-lactating women. *Nature* 238:284, 1972.

Noel, G. L., Suh, H. K., et al.: Prolactin release during nursing and breast stimulation in postpartum and nonpostpartum subjects. *J. Clin. Endocrinol. Metab.* 38:413, 1974.

Vorherr, H.: Suppression of lactation, In *The Breast: Morphology, Physiology, and Lactation.* Vorherr, H. (ed.), New York, Academic Press, 1974, p. 198.

Galactorrhea

Boyd III, A. E., and Reichlin, S., et al.: Galactorrhea-amenorrhea syndrome: diagnosis and therapy. *Ann. Intern. Med.* 87:165, 1977.

Friesen, H. G., and Tolis, G.: The use of bromocriptine in the galactorrhea-amenorrhea syndromes: the Canadian cooperative study. *Clin. Endocrinol.* (Oxf.) 6 (Suppl.):91s, 1977.

Kleinberg, D. L., Noel, G., et al.: Galactorrhea: A study of 235 cases, including 48 with pituitary tumor. *N. Engl. J. Med.* 296:589, 1977.

Richardson, G. S.: Reflex lactation (thoracotomy) and reflex ovulation (intercostal block): case report, review of the literature, and discussion of mechanisms. *Obstet. Gynecol. Surv.* 25:1021, 1970.

Rimsten, A., Skoog, B., et al.: On the significance of nipple discharge in the diagnosis of breast disease. *Acta Chir. Scand.* 142:513, 1976.

Tolis, G., Somma, M., et al.: Prolactin secretion in sixty-five patients with galactorrhea. *Am. J. Obstet. Gynecol.* 118:91, 1974.

Prolactin and Hyperprolactinemia

Antunes, J. L., Housepian, E. M., et al.: Prolactin-secreting pituitary tumors. *Ann. Neurol.* 2:148, 1977.

Balagura, S., Frantz, A. G., et al: The specificity of serum prolactin as a diagnostic indicator of pituitary adenoma. *J. Neurosurg.* 51:42, 1979.

Besser, G. M., and Thorner, M. O.: Bromocriptine in the treatment of the hyperprolactinaemia-hypogonadism syndromes. *Postgrad. Med. J.* 52 (Suppl. 1):64, 1976.

Bohnet, H. G., Dahlen, H. G., et al.: Hyperprolactinemic anovulatory syndrome. *J. Clin. Endocrinol. Metab.* 42:132, 1976.

Franks, S., Murray, M. A. F., et al.: Incidence and significance of hyperprolactinaemia in women with amenorrhea. *Clin. Endocrinol.* (Oxf.) 4:597, 1975.

Frantz, A. G.: The assay and regulation of prolactin in humans. *Adv. Exp. Med. Biol.* 80:95, 1977.

Frantz, A. G.: Prolactin. *N. Engl. J. Med.* 298:201, 1978.

Gemzell, C., and Wang, C. F.: Outcome of pregnancy in women with pituitary adenoma. *Fertil. Steril.* 31:363, 1979.

George, S. R., Burrow, G. N., et al.: Regression of pituitary tumors, a possible effect of bromergocryptine. *Am. J. Med.* 66:697, 1979.

Hwang, P., Guyda, H., et al.: A radioimmunoassay for human prolactin. *Proc. Nat. Acad. Sci.* (USA) 68:1902, 1971.

McNatty, K. P., Sawers, R., et al.: A possible role for prolactin in control of steroid secretion by the human Graafian follicle. *Nature* 250:635, 1974.

Nicoll, C. S.: Physiological actions of prolactin, In *Handbook of Physiology.* Greep, R. O. (ed.), Baltimore, Williams & Wilkins, 1974, Vol. IV, Part 2, p. 253.

Pepperell, R. J., Evans, J. H., et al.: A study of the effects of bromocriptine on serum prolactin, follicle stimulating hormone and luteinizing hormone and ovarian responsiveness to exogenous gonadotrophins in anovulatory women. *Br. J. Obstet. Gynecol.* 84:465, 1977.

Zimmerman, E. A., Defendini, R., et al.: Prolactin and growth hormones in patients with pituitary adenomas: A correlative study of hormone in tumor and plasma by immunoperosidase technique and radioimmunoassay. *J. Clin. Endocrinol. Metab.* 38:577, 1974.

Mastalgia

Mansel, R. E., Preece, P. E., et al.: Bromocriptine for severe mastalgia. *Br. Med. J.* 1:1356, 1977.

Palmer, B. V., and Monteiro, J. C. M.: Bromocriptine for severe mastalgia. *Br. Med. J.* 1:1083, 1977.

Preece, P. E., Mansel, R. E., et al.: Clinical syndromes of mastalgia. *Lancet* 2:670, 1976.

Macromastia

Hollingsworth, D. R., and Archer, R.: Massive virginal breast hypertrophy at puberty. *Am. J. Dis. Child.* 125:293, 1973.

Kullander, S.: Effect of 2 Br-alpha-ergocryptin (CB 154) on serum prolactin and the clinical picture in a case of progressive gigantomastia in pregnancy. *Ann. Chir. Gynaecol.* 65:227, 1976.

Van der Meulen, A. J.: An unusual case of massive hypertrophy of the breast. *S. Afr. Med. J.* 48:1465, 1974.

CHAPTER 8

Endocrinology of Pregnancy

By Evan R. Simpson, Ph.D.
and Paul C. MacDonald, M.D.

The endocrine alterations that accompany human pregnancy are among the most remarkable recorded in human physiology or pathophysiology. Consider the following. In the pregnant woman at or near term there is a daily production of 15–20 mg of estradiol 17β, 50–100 mg of estriol, 250–300 mg of progesterone, 1–2 mg of aldosterone, and 3–8 mg of deoxycorticosterone (DOC). Furthermore there are strikingly increased levels of plasma renin, angiotensinogen, and angiotensin II, together with the daily production of 1 g of human placental lactogen (hPL); massive quantities of human chorionic gonadotropin (hCG); and likely human chorionic thyrotropin (hCT), chorionic ACTH, and possibly chorionic TRH, LHRH, and somatostatin. Thus the most remarkable physiologic event of pregnancy may be the establishment of mechanisms by which the gravid woman and her fetus adapt to this unusual endocrine milieu.

ESTROGEN FORMATION DURING HUMAN PREGNANCY

During the course of normal human pregnancy, very large quantities of estrogens are produced (Fig. 8–1). It is now established that after the first 3–4 weeks of human pregnancy nearly all the estrogens produced are synthesized in the trophoblasts of the placenta. The mechanism by which estrogen is produced in the placenta is unique, however. The placenta appears to lack steroid 17α-hydroxylase activity, and consequently is incapable of converting C$_{21}$-steroids to C$_{19}$-steroids. Thus, progesterone is not metabolized further within the placenta except to 5α-dihydroprogesterone (in limited amounts) and to 20α-dihydroprogesterone (little of which is secreted by the placenta). More than 20 years ago, however, Ryan[1] demonstrated that placental tissue pos-

sessed a remarkable capacity for the aromatization of C$_{19}$-steroids. He found that androstenedione, testosterone, and dehydroepiandrosterone (DHEA) were efficiently converted to estrone and estradiol 17β by placental tissue minces, placental microsomes, or both. At that time, however, another enigma existed, since it was also known that there was a disproportionate amount of estriol in the urine of pregnant women. Whereas in nonpregnant women the ratio of urinary estriol to estrone plus estradiol 17β is approximately 1, in pregnant women this ratio reaches 10 or more. It was known that this disproportionate excretion of estriol could not be due to an alteration in the metabolism of estrone or estradiol 17β in the maternal compartment or to the formation of estriol from estrone or estradiol 17β in the placenta. This obtained since it was shown that the fractional conversion of intravenously administered estrone and estradiol 17β to estriol was the same in pregnant and nonpregnant persons, and the placenta has little or no 16α-hydroxylase enzyme activity. Thus two questions were posed. First, what is the source of the C$_{19}$-steroids utilized by the placenta for estrogen biosynthesis; and second, what is the mechanism by which the disproportionate amount of estriol arises in pregnant women? It seemed likely that the fetus was involved in placental estrogen biosynthesis, since Frandsen and Stakeman[2] found that urinary estrogen levels were very low in women pregnant with an anencephalic fetus.

Placental Aromatization of Circulating C$_{19}$-Steroids

In 1963, several groups of investigators demonstrated that the placenta depends upon circulating C$_{19}$-steroid precursors for estrogen biosynthesis. From the results of a number of

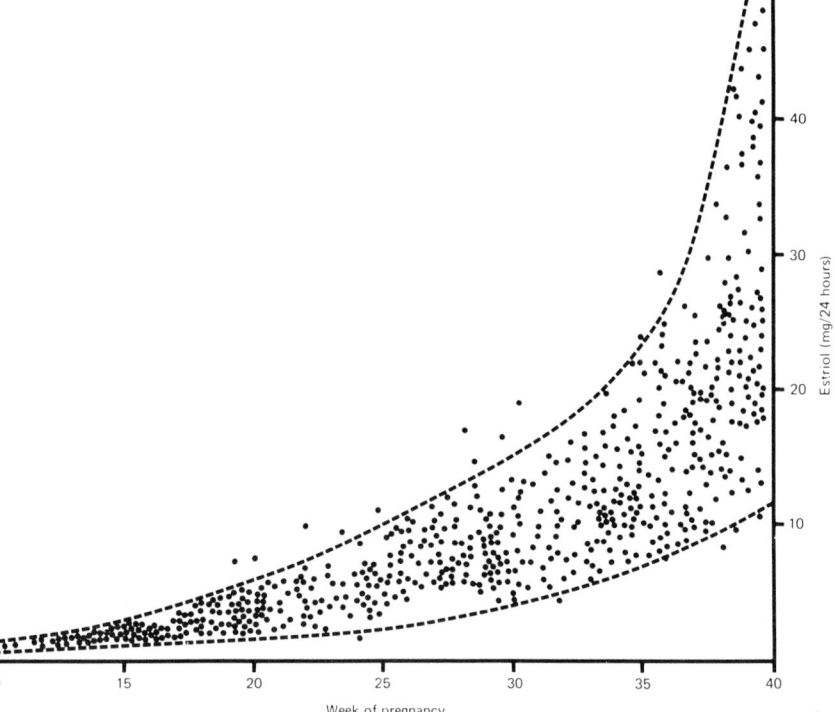

Figure 8-1. Urinary excretion of estriol-16-glucuronide in 31 healthy pregnant women followed throughout pregnancy. The upper and lower dashed lines are the 95% confidence limits. (Reprinted from Beling, C.: Estrogens. *Endocrinology of Pregnancy;* 2nd ed. Fuchs, F., and Klopper, A. (eds.), New York, Harper and Row, 1977, p. 88.

studies conducted by these investigators, it was shown that the principal precursor of placental estradiol 17β is circulating DHEA sulfate[3-5] (Fig. 8-2). Moreover, it was demonstrated that the reason for the disproportionate amount of estriol in maternal plasma and urine was the secretion of estriol by the placenta. Estriol is formed in the placenta by the aromatization of circulating 16α-hydroxydehydroepiandrosterone (16α-hydroxy DHEA) sulfate.[6, 7]

DHEA sulfate circulating in both fetal and maternal plasma is utilized by the placenta in the formation of estradiol 17β and estrone. The product of the aromatization of DHEA sulfate that enters the maternal compartment is principally estradiol 17β. It is not yet clear whether the principal product entering the fetal circulation is estrone or estradiol 17β. However, it appears that both estradiol 17β and estrone are secreted into the fetal compartment or else estradiol 17β is converted to estrone by fetal erythrocytes. Near term, approximately one half of the estradiol 17β synthesized in the placenta is derived from the utilization of precursors in the fetal circulation and one half is derived from the utilization of precursors in the maternal circulation.[7] On the other hand, estriol is derived principally from the utilization of 16α-hydroxyDHEA sulfate in the fetal plasma. DHEA sulfate, secreted by the fetal adrenal cortex, is converted extensively to 16α-hydroxyDHEA sulfate, principally in the fetal liver. It is likely that some 16α-hydroxyDHEA sulfate is also secreted by the fetal adrenal glands. In any event, it has been computed that approximately 90% of the estriol that is excreted into maternal urine is derived from the placental aromatization of fetal plasma 16α-hydroxyDHEA sulfate.[7] Importantly, the steroid sulfatase activity in the placenta is great.[8, 9] Thus the entry of DHEA into the trophoblast as the sulfoconjugate presents no obstacle to the utilization of this precursor in estrogen biosynthesis.

Placental Sulfatase Deficiency

A number of cases of placental sulfatase deficiency have been reported.[10] In this disorder there is a failure to hydrolyze DHEA sulfate or 16α-hydroxyDHEA sulfate and thus there is a deficiency in estrogen formation by the placenta. In such instances the levels of estriol in maternal plasma and urine are quite low. Indeed the levels of estriol are so low that one might expect such levels to be associated with death of the fetus. On the contrary, however, the infants born of such pregnancies usually are normal. Interestingly, all such infants have been male. It is also considered important that in many pregnancies associated with placental sulfatase deficiency, there is a delay in the onset of parturition and a refractoriness to the induction of labor by the intravenous administration of oxytocin (OT). Many women with pregnancies involving placental sulfatase deficiency have been hypertensive. Presently, however, there is no reason to believe that the placental sulfatase deficiency *per se* is associated with a predisposition for the development of pregnancy-associated hypertension. Rather, it is more likely that estriol levels were being monitored in such women because they were hypertensive.

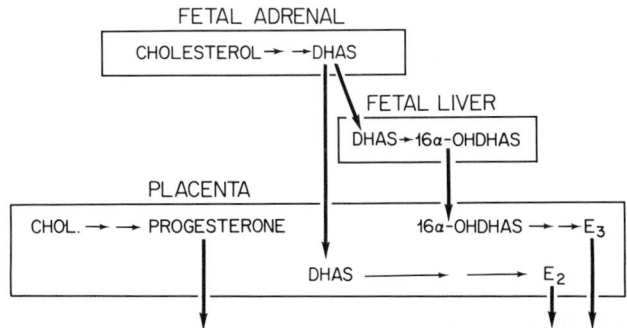

Figure 8-2. Schematic representation of steroid hormone biosynthesis in the fetal-placental unit. DHAS, dehydroisoandrosterone sulfate; E_2, estradiol; E_3, estriol.

Role of the Fetal Adrenal in Placental Estrogen Biosynthesis

The human is one of few mammals in whom estrogens are produced in large quantities during pregnancy, and the fetal adrenal of the human appears to be unique among mammals. The human fetal adrenals at term are as large as those of adults, weighing 10 g or more[11] (Fig. 8–3). Morphologically, however, the fetal adrenal differs strikingly from that of the adult. The human fetal adrenal is comprised principally of an inner fetal zone that constitutes 85% of the gland. The outer neocortex, i.e., the structure that will develop into the adult adrenal cortex, occupies 15% or less of the total volume of the organ. In addition to its relatively enormous size, the human fetal adrenal possesses a remarkable capacity for steroidogenesis. It can be computed that in some fetuses near term, the adrenals secrete 100–200 mg of steroids per day. The principal secretory product of the human fetal adrenal is DHEA sulfate. Indeed many, if not most, of the steroids secreted by the fetal adrenal are secreted as sulfoconjugates.

In addition to its role in providing the precursors for placental estrogen formation, many believe that the fetal adrenal cortex serves a central role in effecting the biochemic events that lead to the initiation of parturition and to fetal lung maturation.[12, 13] Therefore the control of the rate of steroidogenesis by the human fetal adrenal has become an important consideration for those who study the endocrinology of human pregnancy. Many investigators have reasoned that the fetal adrenal is subject to more than one trophic stimulus. This proposition is based upon several observations. ACTH levels in human fetal blood decline as gestation advances.[14] Paradoxically, the rate of growth of the fetal adrenal increases strikingly at a time when ACTH levels are falling. Moreover, the pattern of steroid secretion by the fetal adrenal is considerably different from that of the adult. For these reasons and more, a role for various peptides such as growth hormone (GH), chorionic gonadotropin (CG), prolactin (PRL), placental lactogen (PL), and α-MSH as trophic agents for the fetal adrenal has been proposed. Although each of these compounds has been found by some to stimulate steroid production by fetal adrenal tissue, there is little convincing evidence to date that any of these protein hormones serve a crucial role in directly stimulating growth or steroidogenesis in the fetal adrenal cortex.

Recently, another approach to this problem was taken.

The question was asked, what is the precursor of the steroid hormones synthesized by the fetal adrenal? Some investigators have suggested that circulating progesterone and pregnenolone of placental origin serve as precursors for fetal adrenal steroidogenesis. Based upon the level of pregnenolone in umbilical venous blood, however, it can be computed that this source of steroid precursor could account for no more than 1% of the DHEA sulfate secreted by the fetal adrenal. Possibly a portion of fetal adrenal cortisol is formed through the utilization of progesterone produced within the placenta. This important question is presently unresolved. In any event, it has been shown that the fetal adrenal possesses the capacity for *de novo* synthesis of cortisol and thus it is unlikely that under normal circumstances placental steroids are important, quantitatively, in fetal adrenal steroidogenesis. Rather, it is more likely that the principal precursor utilized for fetal adrenal steroid biosynthesis is cholesterol. If this were true, then the question arises as to the source of cholesterol utilized in fetal adrenal steroidogenesis. There are two possible sources of cholesterol. First, cholesterol could be formed by *de novo* synthesis from 2-carbon precursors in the fetal adrenal. Second, cholesterol could be assimilated by the fetal adrenal cells from plasma lipoproteins. It has been demonstrated that many tissues take up cholesterol from circulating lipoproteins. For example, human fibroblasts in culture derive most of their cholesterol from low-density lipoprotein (LDL).[15] This is also known to be the case in mouse adrenal tumor cells in culture.[16] In addition, it has been shown that the adult rat adrenal assimilates cholesterol from high-density lipoprotein (HDL).[17] Importantly, LDL-cholesterol in cord blood of newborn infants is extremely low[18]; the level of cholesterol in LDL is approximately 30 mg/dl, a value one-fourth to one-fifth that found in the plasma of normal adults.

An important question was asked. Is the level of circulating LDL in the fetal plasma low because of its rapid utilization by the fetal adrenal for steroidogenesis? It can be computed that the LDL-cholesterol present in the entire plasma volume of the fetus near term is only 30 mg of cholesterol. Thus if LDL were the principal source of cholesterol precursor for fetal adrenal steroidogenesis, the turnover of LDL in fetal plasma would be very rapid compared with that of the adult. In studies conducted by Simpson and colleagues,[19] it was demonstrated that fetal adrenal tissue fragments maintained in organ culture preferentially utilized lipoprotein-cholesterol for steroidogenesis. By 6 days in culture, fetal

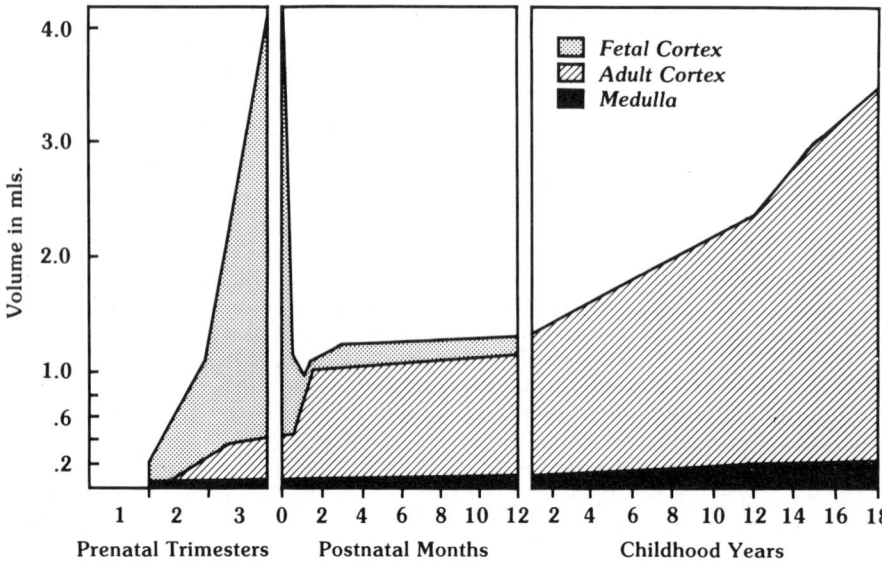

Figure 8–3. Size of the adrenal gland and its component parts *in utero*, during infancy, and during childhood. (Adapted from Bethune, J.E. (ed.): *The Adrenal Cortex, A Scope Monograph.* Kalamazoo, Michigan, Upjohn Co., 1974, p. 11.)

adrenal fragments maintained in the presence of ACTH preferentially used lipoprotein-cholesterol for the biosynthesis of pregnenolone sulfate, DHEA sulfate and cortisol. In these studies it was computed that at a minimum 50–80% of the steroids secreted were derived from lipoprotein-cholesterol compared to cholesterol produced *de novo*.[19]

Carr and coworkers[20] also found that the preferred lipoprotein utilized by the fetal adrenal is LDL. HDL was much less effective in maintaining steroidogenesis in fetal adrenal tissue fragments maintained in the presence of ACTH, and very low–density lipoprotein (VLDL) was relatively ineffective. The regulation of cholesterol metabolism by the human fetal adrenal is presented in Fig. 8–4. Based on these observations, it appears possible that the rate of fetal adrenal steroidogenesis may be determined, in part, by the concentrations of LDL in the fetal plasma, and hence by the rate of synthesis of plasma lipoproteins in the fetus.

Another major question arises. What is the source of lipoproteins in the fetus? It appears that no more than 20% of fetal cholesterol is derived from the maternal circulation.[21] Recalling that LDL is derived from VLDL through the action of lipoprotein lipase to hydrolyse the triglyceride portion of VLDL, one can envision that the fetal lung may be important in LDL formation. This obtains since there is little adipose tissue in the human fetus prior to the 36th week of gestation. Lipoprotein lipase activity is known to be present in fetal rat lung tissue and PRL is known to stimulate lipoprotein lipase in other tissues.[22] Thus, it is possible that PRL acts to facilitate adrenal steroidogenesis through stimulation of the conversion of VLDL to LDL in fetal tissues. Importantly, fetal plasma PRL levels increase in a fashion parallel to the rate of increase of the size of the fetal adrenal cortex. Thus PRL may yet be found to serve as a second trophic agent for the fetal adrenal, even though PRL does not seem to stimulate fetal adrenal steroidogenesis directly.

Secretion of Placental Estrogen into the Maternal and Fetal Compartments

The estrogens synthesized in the trophoblast preferentially enter the maternal circulation. In fact, Gurpide and coworkers[23] have shown that more than 90% of the estradiol 17β and estriol formed in the trophoblast is secreted into the maternal compartment. The same is true of progesterone formed in the trophoblast. Specifically, Gurpide and coworkers[24] found that 85% or more of trophoblastically formed progesterone enters the maternal compartment and that little of the progesterone in the maternal circulation enters the fetus.

PROGESTERONE FORMATION

During the latter few weeks of pregnancy, the placenta secretes 250 mg or more of progesterone per day (Fig. 8–5). Indeed, it can be computed that in some pregnancies involving multiple fetuses, up to 600 mg of progesterone are formed per day. Hellig and associates[25] and Bloch[26] demonstrated that progesterone formed by the human placenta was derived from the utilization of circulating maternal cholesterol. The fetus does not contribute to progesterone formation by the placenta. This was demonstrated by showing that following ligation of the umbilical cord there was no immediate reduction in plasma progesterone or in the levels of pregnanediol in maternal urine.[27] Hellig and coworkers,[25] in a study of women pregnant with an anencephalic fetus, demonstrated that after the administration of radiolabeled cholesterol for sufficient time to achieve steady state conditions, the specific activity of plasma progesterone and that of pregnanediol in maternal urine were similar to that of circulating cholesterol. Thus a major question arose. What is the form of circulating cholesterol utilized by the placenta for progesterone formation?

Mechanism of Placental Progesterone Formation

In near-term pregnant women, the amount of progesterone formed per day is equivalent to one fourth to one third of the daily cholesterol turnover rate in nonpregnant adults. In spite of this, the rate of incorporation of [14C]acetate into cholesterol by trophoblastic tissue is low, and the activity of

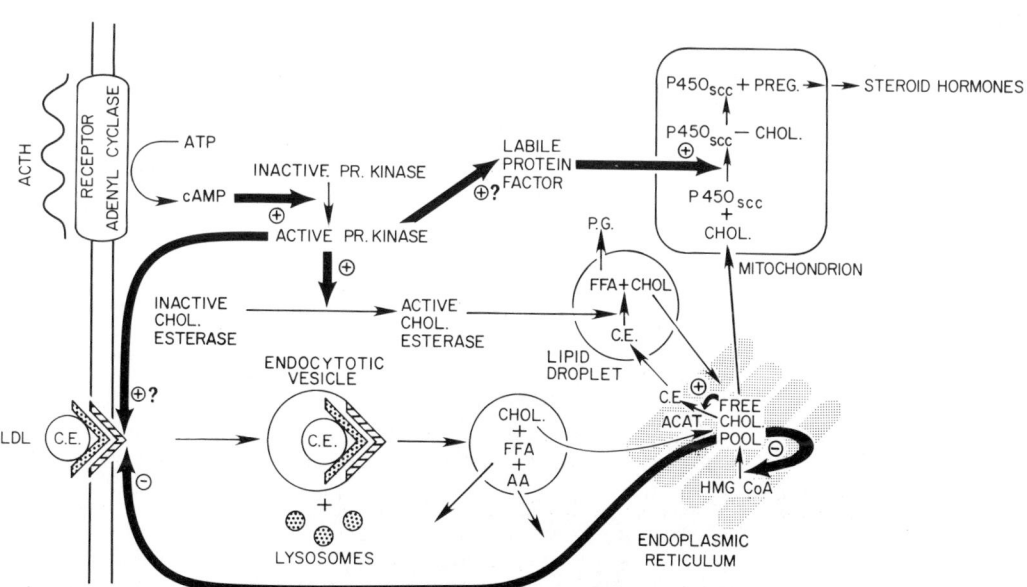

Figure 8–4. Pathways of cholesterol metabolism and its regulation in the human fetal adrenal. C.E., cholesteryl esters; Chol., cholesterol; FFA, free fatty acids; AA, amino acids; HMG CoA, 3-hydroxy-3-methylglutaryl coenzyme A; ACAT, acyl coenzyme A:cholesterol acyltransferase; P.G., prostaglandins; P450scc, cholesterol side chain cleavage cytochrome P450. (Reprinted from Simpson, E.R.: Cholesterol side-chain cleavage, cytochrome P450, and the control of steroidogenesis. Elsevier-North Holland Scientific Publications, Inc., *Mol. Cell Endocrinol. 13:*213, 1979).

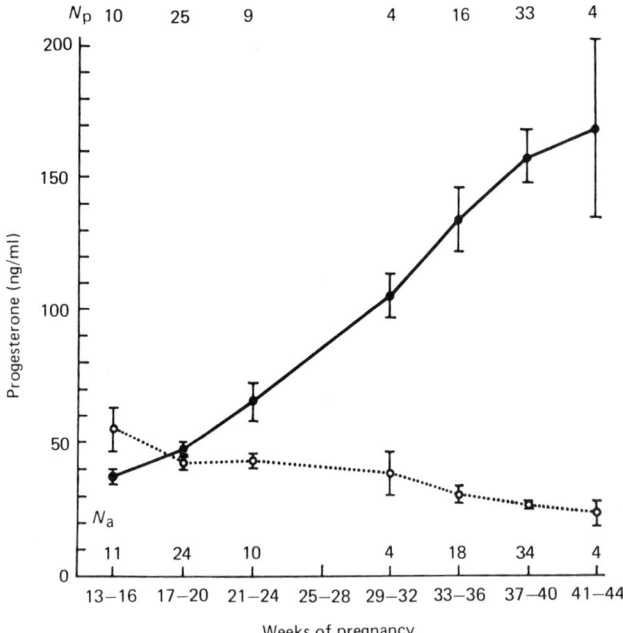

Figure 8–5. Progesterone levels in maternal plasma (—) and amniotic fluid (......) from the same subjects. The values were grouped in 4-week periods. N_p indicates the number of plasma samples and N_a the number of amniotic fluid samples in each period. (Reprinted from Johansson, E.D., and Johansson, L.E.: Progesterone levels in amniotic fluid and plasma from women. I. Levels during normal pregnancy. *Acta Obstet. Gynecol. Scand.* 50:339, 1971.)

3-hydroxy-3-methyl glutaryl coenzyme A (HMG CoA) reductase in human placental microsomes is also low. Therefore it must be concluded that ordinarily the rate of *de novo* synthesis of cholesterol in the human placenta is also low. Employing choriocarcinoma cells in monolayer culture as a model for the study of trophoblastic tissue cholesterol metabolism and steroid biosynthesis[28] and employing dispersed trophoblasts obtained by trypsin treatment of normal human term placental tissue, Simpson and colleagues have shown that lipoproteins are the principal source of cholesterol utilized by trophoblastic cells in culture. The lipoprotein preferred as a source of circulating cholesterol by human trophoblasts is LDL. These investigators demonstrated that LDL became bound to a saturable population of trophoblastic cell plasma membrane receptors possessing high affinity for LDL. Following binding of LDL to the trophoblastic cell surface receptor, the lipoprotein was internalized through a process of adsorptive endocytosis. The endocytotic vesicles appeared to fuse with lysosomes, and the lysosomal enzymes effected hydrolysis of the lipoprotein. Hydrolysis of the protein moiety of LDL gave rise to amino acids while the hydrolysis of the cholesteryl esters gave rise to fatty acids and cholesterol. The liberated cholesterol was then available to serve as a precursor for pregnenolone formation in mitochondria and thence the pregnenolone was converted to progesterone in the endoplasmic reticulum. The mechanism of progesterone biosynthesis from circulating LDL is illustrated diagrammatically in Fig. 8–6.

Ordinarily, the uptake of LDL by a tissue is associated with an increase in cholesteryl ester synthesis through stimulation of acylCoA:cholesterol acyl transferase (ACAT) activity.[29] Paradoxically, however, trophoblastic tissue contains little or no cholesteryl esters. The explanation for this apparent paradox came from the findings of a study of the effect of progesterone on ACAT activity[30, 31] in which it was demonstrated that progesterone inhibits ACAT activity. Indeed, employing concentrations of progesterone similar to those one can compute to be present in trophoblastic cells, ACAT activity is inhibited almost completely. Such inhibition might be useful physiologically to ensure a continuing supply of cholesterol for utilization in progesterone biosynthesis by preventing the sequestration of cholesterol into an inappropriate storage form, namely cholesteryl esters. It will be interesting to follow future developments in this field. It is possible that amino acids derived from the hydrolysis of the protein component of LDL constitute a source of essential amino acids for the fetus, and the fatty acids derived from hydrolysis of the cholesteryl esters of LDL, principally linoleic acid, may represent an important source of essential fatty acid for the fetus.

Presently there is no evidence that any class of steroid other than estrogens and progesterone is formed or secreted by the placenta. Specifically, there is no evidence for glucocorticosteroid or mineralocorticosteroid production by the trophoblasts of the human placenta.

TRANSFER OF STEROID HORMONES FROM THE MATERNAL TO THE FETAL COMPARTMENT

Generally speaking, little of the steroids circulating in the maternal compartment reach the fetal compartment. This obtains for several reasons. The much greater size of the maternal compartment together with the rapid clearance of steroids from maternal plasma precludes the likelihood of

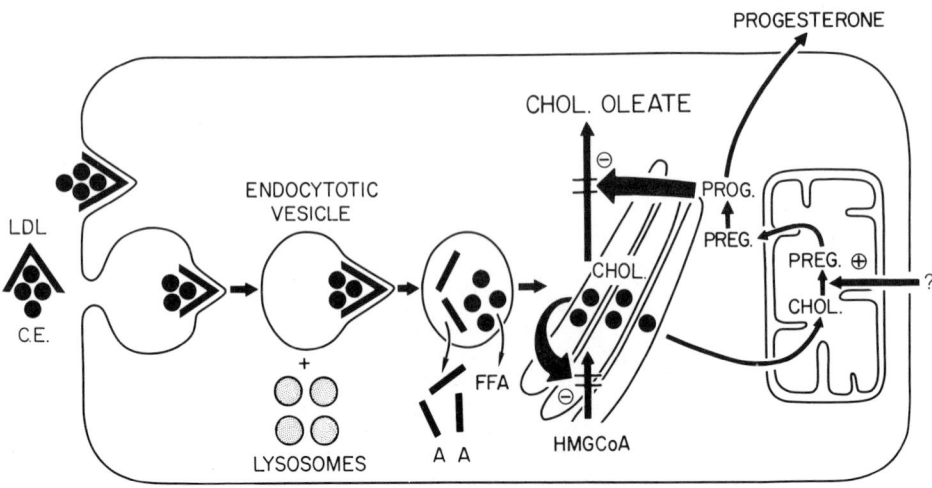

Figure 8–6. Pathways of cholesterol metabolism and its regulation in the human placenta. Preg., pregnenolone; prog., progesterone.

accessibility of large quantities of circulating maternal steroids to the trophoblastic cells. In addition, once in the trophoblast the steroids are more likely to re-enter the maternal compartment than to enter the fetal compartment. Let us consider several examples. Little maternal circulating cortisol enters the trophoblast. Even less cortisol in the trophoblast is available to the fetus both because steroids in trophoblastic cells are preferentially secreted into the maternal compartment and because cortisol within the trophoblast is converted largely to cortisone.[32] Thus most of the cortisol in the maternal compartment that enters the fetal compartment would do so in the form of cortisone. Fortunately, circulating C_{19}-steroids in the maternal compartment, *viz.*, DHEA sulfate, DHEA, androstenedione, and testosterone, usually do not escape into the fetal compartment in significant quantities because of the very large capacity of the aromatase enzyme system of the trophoblast for the conversion of C_{19}-steroids to estrogens. Indeed it has been shown that in most circumstances the aromatase system of the human trophoblast is not a rate-limiting step in the rate of formation of estrogen from circulating maternal C_{19}-steroids. This obtains since it has been shown that the fractional conversion of circulating C_{19}-steroids to estradiol 17β is not altered by wide fluctuations in the levels of C_{19}-steroids in the maternal circulation.[33] This likely constitutes a protective mechanism that prevents virilization of the female fetus of women who have or who develop androgen-secreting tumors of the ovary during pregnancy. In many women with strikingly increased rates of production of testosterone, virilization of the female fetus does not occur. It is likely that fetuses who are virilized because of excessive androgen formation in the maternal compartment are virilized by the action of C_{19}-steroids that are not estrogen prehormones, for example, dihydrotestosterone or 5α-androstanedione, or else such fetuses become virilized during early pregnancy before the placenta can efficiently clear testosterone by aromatization.

PROTEIN HORMONES OF THE PLACENTA

Very early in human pregnancy, perhaps from the day of nidation, several protein hormones are produced by the human trophoblast. Among these are hCG, hPL, hCT,[34] and possibly chorionic ACTH.[35-37] In addition, it appears that there may be a hierarchy of control of protein hormone secretion by the placenta, inasmuch as it has been shown that the trophoblast produces LHRH[38] and TRH.[39]

Human Chorionic Gonadotropin

It is believed that hCG is secreted by the syncytiotrophoblast. At least most evidence points to the syncytiotrophoblast as the cell of origin of hCG. Employing immunofluorescent techniques, it has been found that hCG is concentrated in syncytiotrophoblasts. Interestingly, however, the maximum rate of secretion of hCG coincides with the time that cytotrophoblasts are present in the placenta in greatest abundance (Fig. 8–7). Since it is believed that the cytotrophoblast is the progenitor of the syncytiotrophoblast, it may be that the rate of formation and secretion of CG is related more to the age of the syncytiotrophoblast than to a possible origin for hCG in the cytotrophoblast. The rate of secretion of hCG increases rapidly in the first few weeks of pregnancy, and the maximum levels in maternal blood and urine are attained at approximately 10 weeks' gestation. Thereafter, the levels of hCG in both maternal serum and maternal urine decline slowly, reaching a nadir at approximately 120 days of gestation. After this time hCG levels in maternal plasma persist at a level of approximately 20 IU/ml.

Increased levels of hCG are found in women with multiple fetuses and in women with hydatidiform mole and choriocarcinoma. Late in pregnancy, rising levels of CG also may be observed in women whose pregnancies are complicated by Rh isoimmunization with an affected fetus and in some women whose pregnancies are complicated by diabetes mellitus. Importantly, in these last two circumstances, a reappearance of cytotrophoblasts is found in the placenta late in gestation. At approximately 10 weeks of gestation, when the maximum levels of hCG are attained, the mean level in the plasma of most pregnant women is 100 IU/ml. In plasma of women with hydatidiform mole, enormous levels of CG may be observed. In fact, if the levels of hCG rise about 500 IU/ml of plasma, the diagnosis of hydatidiform mole is virtually assured. Unfortunately the reverse is not the case. Namely, levels below 500 IU/ml of serum do not exclude the possibility of neoplastic trophoblastic disease. Interestingly, increased levels of hPL do not exist in subjects with neoplastic

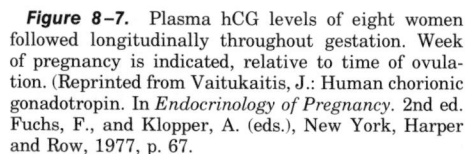

Figure 8–7. Plasma hCG levels of eight women followed longitudinally throughout gestation. Week of pregnancy is indicated, relative to time of ovulation. (Reprinted from Vaitukaitis, J.: Human chorionic gonadotropin. In *Endocrinology of Pregnancy*. 2nd ed. Fuchs, F., and Klopper, A. (eds.), New York, Harper and Row, 1977, p. 67.)

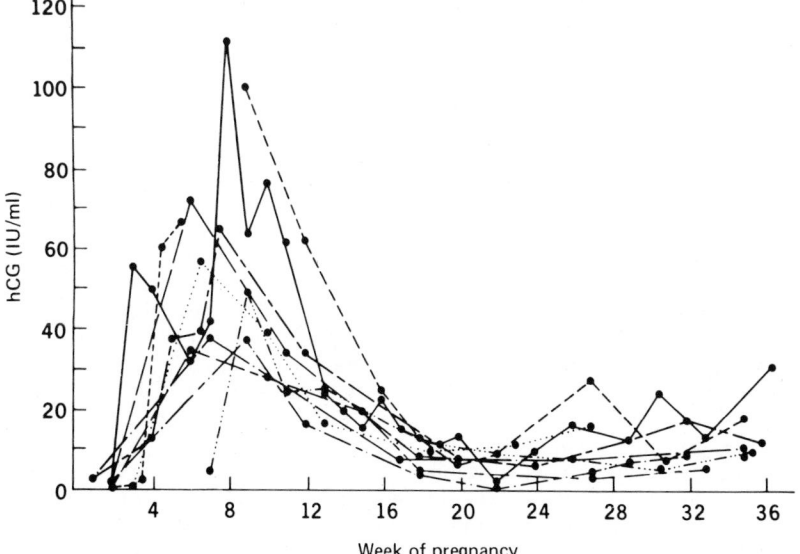

trophoblastic disease. In fact it has been suggested that the finding of high levels of hCG together with low levels of hPL is indicative of neoplastic trophoblastic disease. The finding of theca-lutein cysts of the ovary during pregnancy is indicative, generally, of high levels of hCG, and these lesions are found most often in women with hydatidiform mole and less often in women whose pregnancies are complicated by multiple fetuses, diabetes, or Rh isoimmunization.

The role of hCG in human pregnancy is not fully defined. It is likely, as pointed out in Chapter 7, that hCG is a luteotropin in the human; i.e., hCG maintains the corpus luteum, and hCG action is responsible for the conversion of the corpus luteum of menstruation to the corpus luteum of pregnancy through an extension of its life span and through stimulation of progesterone secretion by this organ. It also seems reasonable, as pointed out in Chapter 9, that hCG stimulates the fetal testes to secrete testosterone at a time prior to the secretion of LH by the fetal pituitary. Some investigators have also envisioned a role for hCG in the provision of immunologic protection to the trophoblast.[40] Others have questioned whether hCG serves this role or whether it is subserved by a contaminant in hCG preparations.[41]

It is possible that the hyperstimulation of the maternal thyroid that occurs in some women with molar pregnancy comes about through the action of hCG.[42] It has also been suggested that excessive secretion of hCT by neoplastic trophoblasts is responsible for the strikingly increased serum levels of thyroxine (T_4) found in some women with hydatidiform mole. The role of placental hormones on the function of the maternal thyroid is considered in detail in Chapter 4.

Because of the biologic and immunologic similarity between hCG and LH, it was difficult previously to distinguish between these two gonadotropins. With the recognition that each is composed of an α and β subunit and that the β subunits of the two compounds differ, however, it was possible to develop antibodies specifically against the β subunit of hCG; consequently, it is now possible to distinguish between pituitary LH and hCG. The measurement of hCG employing antibodies developed against the β subunit has facilitated the monitoring of subjects with hydatidiform mole and choriocarcinoma and the monitoring of the efficacy of treatment of such persons through the sequential measurement of the level of hCG in blood or urine.[43]

Human Placental Lactogen

Human placental lactogen (hPL) is also secreted by the syncytiotrophoblast, and the secretion of hPL also may commence on the day of nidation. The pattern of secretion of hPL, however, is strikingly different from that of hCG (Fig. 8–8). The rate of secretion of hPL increases slowly and the levels in maternal blood appear to parallel placental mass. Maximum levels of hPL in maternal blood are attained sometime after the 32nd week of gestation and remain relatively constant after that time. The rate of secretion of hPL in pregnant women is the greatest of any protein hormone known in man. Rates of secretion of hPL of 1 g or more occur late in normal pregnancy. It has both lactogenic and somatotrophic properties. However, hPL possesses only approximately 1/100th of the potency in promoting growth as does pituitary GH. Nonetheless, because of the remarkable amount of hPL produced during human pregnancy, it is believed that this hormone exerts significant physiologic effects in the pregnant woman. Little hPL enters the fetal circulation. The principal role of hPL in human pregnancy is believed to be mediated by its action as an insulin antagonist, and it is

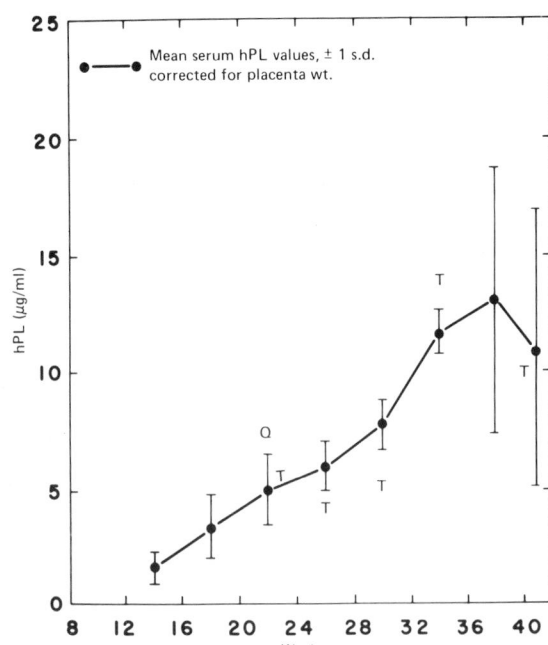

Figure 8–8. Change in mean serum hPL concentration during 4-week periods during pregnancy. T, values from twin pregnancies; Q, values from a quintuplet gestation. (Reprinted from Javert, C.T. (ed.): *Spontaneous and Habitual Abortion.* New York, McGraw-Hill, 1957.)

believed that the action of hPL may be responsible for the development of diabetic ketoacidosis in pregnant women who were not known to have diabetes before they became pregnant and who did not require insulin after the pregnancy was terminated.

Human Chorionic Thyrotropin

Several molecular species of hCT have been isolated from extracts of placental and hydatidiform mole tissue.[34] None of these species appear to be identical to that of TSH produced by the anterior pituitary. The principal component of hCT is more similar to bovine TSH. The role of hCT is unclear. It is not known what the circulating levels of hCT are in either the fetal or the maternal compartment. Excessive amounts of hCT are found in neoplastic trophoblastic tissue. The impact of pregnancy on maternal thyroid function is discussed in Chapter 4.

Chorionic ACTH

Several groups of investigators have isolated an ACTH-like compound from extracts of placental tissue.[35-37] Such ACTH appears to be biologically active and immunoreactive with antibodies prepared against human pituitary ACTH. At this time, it is not established absolutely that the placenta produces chorionic ACTH and if it does so what is the pattern of production during the course of human pregnancy, however.

Luteinizing Hormone and Thyrotropin Hormone Releasing Hormones

It has been demonstrated that extracts of placental tissues contain LHRH-like[38] and TRH-like[39] substances. Moreover, it has been found that placental tissue maintained in culture secretes LHRH.[39] These findings are suggestive of a hierarchy of control for the elaboration of hCG and hCT by tropho-blastic tissue. At this time, however, this proposition is highly speculative and the role of releasing factors produced by the human placenta awaits the results of further investigation.

THE MEASUREMENT OF PLACENTAL HORMONES AS AN INDEX OF FETAL WELL-BEING

For decades physicians have sought to evaluate the well-being of the fetus by monitoring the levels of various hormones that arise in the placenta or fetal placental unit. It was reasoned that alterations in placental function could be assessed by the measurement of such hormones and that alterations in the levels would reflect changes in the well-being of the fetus. With such knowledge, it was hoped that information could be gained that would allow intervention in high-risk pregnancies in order to effect premature delivery when the intrauterine environment was deteriorating.

Estriol

Determination of the levels of estriol in maternal plasma or urine is one of the most popular indices utilized for monitoring fetal well-being for the following reasons: (1) Estriol is formed in the placenta, and (2) estriol is formed principally by utilization of fetal adrenal C_{19}-steroids; therefore, a decrease in estriol in the maternal plasma or urine would be reflective of a decline in fetal well-being. Moreover, it has been well documented that following fetal death there is a striking reduction in the levels of estriol in maternal plasma and urine. Indeed, the diagnosis of fetal death can be established with some degree of reliability by the measurement of estriol levels in the maternal compartment. Moreover it has been shown that in many high-risk pregnancies, i.e., pregnancies in which the fetus is primarily at risk, marked reductions in estriol levels, or persistently low levels of estriol, are predictive of impending fetal demise. With such a background of information it would seem, superficially, that the measurement of estriol in the maternal compartment would constitute a reliable index of fetal well-being. Unfortunately, this is not universally true. For example, in some pregnancies in which the fetus is undoubtedly at risk, there may be no reduction in estriol values. Examples of such high-risk pregnancies include those complicated by Rh isoimmunization with an affected fetus and those complicated by maternal diabetes mellitus, type A, B, or C. In such pregnancies the level of estriol in the maternal compartment may be even greater than normal.

There are several enigmas concerning the utility of estriol measurements in the selection of an optimal management plan for the pregnancy unit in which the fetus is believed to be at risk. First, it is not clear how the fetus responds to "stress." In most cases, fetal "stress" or fetal hypoxia is the result of decreased uteroplacental blood flow, e.g., in women whose pregnancies are complicated by chronic hypertension, pregnancy-induced hypertension (preeclampsia–eclampsia), placental insufficiency (due to unknown causes), fetal growth retardation (for unknown reasons) and diabetes mellitus types D and R. Unfortunately fetal "stress" has been equated with stress in the adult that involves the "flight or fight" phenomenon associated with increased ACTH secretion. If pituitary ACTH secretion were increased in the "stressed" fetus, one would anticipate that estriol in the maternal compartment would rise, not fall. This obtains since the principal precursor of placental estriol is circulat-ing fetal 16α-hydroxyDHEA sulfate that arises from DHEA sulfate secreted by the fetal adrenal. Thus if fetal pituitary secretion of ACTH were to increase, the secretion of fetal adrenal DHEA sulfate should increase, giving rise ultimately to increased 16α-hydroxyDHEA sulfate and thence to increased levels of estriol. Such is not the case. Rather it seems more reasonable to assume that during times of fetal hypoxia there is a decrease in the secretion of fetal pituitary ACTH, a decrease in the rate of secretion of fetal adrenal DHEA sulfate and thence a decrease in the rate of estriol secretion. For these reasons it is not tenable to equate "stress" of the fetus with the "flight or fight" type of response to stress that is observed in the adult. In fact, during times of fetal hypoxia, one observes decreased fetal body[44] and tho-racic movements,[45] findings that suggest that during times of hypoxia there are longer sleep periods for the fetus. In support of this view we have found recently that the cord blood levels of plasma LDL of newborns of mothers with chronic and pregnancy-induced hypertension were significantly higher than those of newborns of normotensive mothers. This finding, together with the finding that the fetal adrenal preferentially utilizes LDL-cholesterol for steroidogenesis *in vitro*, is supportive of the view that during fetal hypoxia there is decreased fetal adrenal utilization of circulating LDL for steroidogenesis.

Let us return to the principal question, i.e., does the measurement of estriol in maternal plasma or urine constitute an index of fetal well-being that will provide insight to the physician who must choose the ideal timing of delivery of a fetus whose intrauterine environment is compromised? The physician may be required to choose between prematurity on the one hand and a deteriorating intrauterine environment for the fetus on the other. It is our view that the results of measurements of estriol levels in maternal blood or urine do not provide new and meaningful information over and above that available from clinical assessment of the pregnancy unit.[46] Clinical assessment is accomplished by determination of the rate of fetal growth by clinical and sonographic criteria, by systematic evaluation of maternal blood pressure, and by the evaluation of the mother's renal function or the status of carbohydrate metabolism in pregnant women with diabetes mellitus. It is not difficult to conclude that the fetus is at risk when maternal hypertension is worsening. It is not difficult to conclude that the fetus is at risk in the diabetic whose carbohydrate metabolism is not controlled. It is easy to recognize that the fetus is at risk when the biparietal diameter of the fetal head fails to grow at a proper rate. These considerations, together with the fact that estriol levels fluctuate widely in the same pregnant subject and from subject to subject, have led us to the view that more harm than good can come from the timing of delivery on the basis of the level of estriol in the maternal compartment. Many other investigators do not share this view. They argue that the measurement of estriol levels can be of value if these are assessed in the context of the total information available in any given pregnancy in which the fetus is at risk. To date there has been only one controlled, prospective study of the utility of estriol measurements, and in this investigation it was found that estriol values did not provide new and meaningful information.[46]

Estetrol

Estetrol, 15α-hydroxyestriol, is formed uniquely in the fetal compartment by 15α hydroxylation of estriol or following 16α hydroxylation of 15α-hydroxylated estrogens.[47] The finding that 15α-hydroxylation occurred uniquely in the fetal compartment prompted several groups of investigators to evaluate estetrol levels in the maternal plasma or urine as an index of fetal well-being. Since the placental estrogen precursors arise in the fetal adrenal cortex and since 15α-hydroxylation is unique to the fetus, it seemed reasonable to presume that estetrol levels may be a better index of fetal well-being than are estriol levels. Unfortunately this has not proved to be the case. All of the reservations concerning the utility of estriol measurements in the management of complicated obstetric problems are applicable to the measurement of estetrol as well. Moreover, there are other factors involved in the biosynthesis of estetrol and its entry into the maternal compartment that mitigate its value in the evaluation of fetal well-being.

Human Placental Lactogen Measurements as an Index of Fetal Well-Being

Since hPL is secreted by the trophoblast and since the rate of its secretion is generally proportional to placental mass, many investigators have measured hPL in maternal plasma in attempts to evaluate placental function and, indirectly, fetal well-being. Again, the objective of such measurements was to gain insight into the well-being of fetuses of complicated pregnancies in order to best determine pregnancy management, i.e., to choose the ideal time for delivery of the adversely affected fetus. In some high-risk pregnancies, especially those complicated by chronic or pregnancy-induced hypertension, there is a reasonable correlation between levels of hPL and newborn outcome.[48] Unfortunately, however, this correlation is no better than, and likely not as good as, that between the level of estriol and fetal well-being and fetal outcome. As in the case of estriol measurements, the measurement of hPL in maternal plasma does not provide information over and above that available from clinical evaluation alone to assist in a better timing of the delivery of the fetus at risk.

Placental Clearance of Maternal Plasma Dehydroepiandrosterone Sulfate Through Estradiol 17β Formation and Dehydroepiandrosterone Loading Test

Taking advantage of the fact that the placenta does not possess the capacity for *de novo* synthesis of estrogen but depends rather upon circulating C_{19}-steroids for estradiol 17β formation, a technique was developed for evaluating placental clearance by measuring the placental clearance (PC) of maternal plasma DHEA sulfate (DS) through placental estradiol 17β (E_2) formation (PC-DSE$_2$).[49] In order to do so, the metabolic clearance rate of maternal plasma was measured as well as the fractional conversion of maternal plasma DS E_2. The product of these two values is the volume of maternal plasma cleared of DS by the placenta through the formation of E_2 per unit time. It is believed that such measurements are reflective of uteroplacental blood flow. Employing this technique it has been demonstrated that the placental clearance of DS is reduced strikingly in primagravid women with pregnancy-induced hypertension and in ambulatory women with chronic hypertension[50] (Fig. 8–9). Moreover, the PC-DSE$_2$ is reduced during sodium deprivation in normal pregnant women and in women with pregnancy-induced and chronic hypertension and is reduced even further during diuretic administration to normal pregnant women and those with hypertension.[51] For these reasons and others, most investigators suggest that salt deprivation and diuretic administration should not be employed in most pregnant women. Certainly, salt depriva-

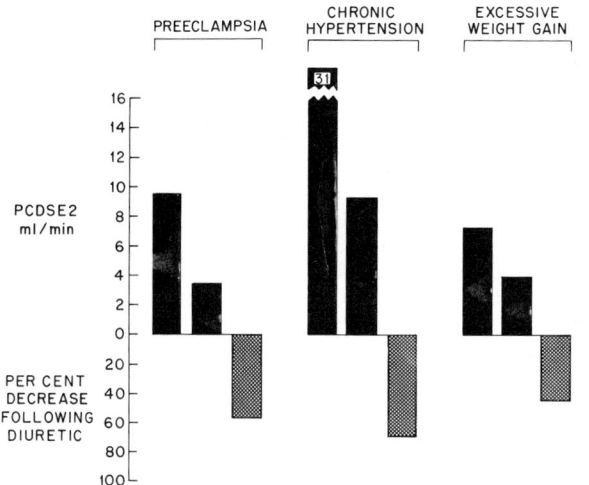

Figure 8–9. Placental clearance of dehydroepiandrosterone sulfate through estradiol formation and the effect of diuretic therapy.

tion and diuretic administration should not be employed in women who have simple edema of pregnancy and pregnancy-induced hypertension (preeclampsia) and in the majority of pregnant women with chronic hypertension. Generally speaking, salt deprivation and diuretic administration should be utilized only in pregnant subjects with pulmonary edema and congestive heart failure. In unusual instances of chronic hypertension in which the woman is being treated with diuretics before she conceives, it may be reasonable to continue diuretic therapy if the hypertension does not abate, as it commonly does, during the second trimester of pregnancy.

The measurement of the placental clearance of DS through E_2 formation, however, is cumbersome and expensive and requires several weeks of laboratory testing. For these reasons, and perhaps others, this measurement has no apparent utility in the clinical management of high-risk pregnancies. Other investigators have sought to measure the increase in E_2 following the administration of a loading dose of DS.[52] Employing such tests it was reasoned that an indirect assessment of placental clearance of maternal DS through either E_2 or estriol formation could be obtained by measuring the change in the levels of the estrogens in the maternal compartment following the administration of the loading dose of the placental estrogen precursor. The results of such studies have been similar to those employing the placental clearance of DS through E_2 formation. To date there are no prospective studies on the utility of such measurements in determining optimum management of the high-risk pregnancy, however.

MATERNAL ADAPTATIONS TO PREGNANCY

As stated at the outset of this chapter, one of the most remarkable features of human pregnancy is the successful physiologic adaptation of a woman to the enormous endocrine changes effected by the steroid and protein hormones produced by the placenta. The woman is one of few mammals that experience considerable blood loss at delivery. On the average, blood loss with vaginal delivery is 500 ml; with cesarean section, 1000 ml; and with cesarean section-hysterectomy, 1500 ml.[53] On the average, however, the pregnant woman increases her blood volume from nonpregnant values of 3500 ml to 5000 ml by the latter part of pregnancy. In spite of this striking increase in blood volume, high levels of plasma renin activity, increased angiotensin II, and aldosterone secretory rates that are 10–40 times those of nonpregnant women, the systolic and diastolic blood pressures ordinarily are lower during pregnancy than before or after. This remarkable process of adaptation is not understood fully, but many of the individual components of the mechanism appear to have been clarified. Estrogen stimulates the hepatic synthesis of angiotensinogen, the precursor of angiotensin I that is converted to angiotensin II. Estrogen or progesterone or a combination of the two stimulates the secretion of renin, the enzyme that catalyzes the conversion of angiotensin substrate to angiotensin I. Thus the hormones of the placenta stimulate the synthesis of angiotensin II, and pregnancy also produces a dichotomy in tissue responsiveness to angiotensin II. On the one hand, the zona glomerulosa of the maternal adrenal remains responsive to tropic action of angiotensin II — aldosterone secretion increases strikingly during human pregnancy — but on the other hand the maternal vasculature becomes refractory to the pressor effects of angiotensin II. These two events, acting in concert, likely are responsible for the expansion of blood volume that accompanies normal pregnancy. Refractoriness to the pressor effect of angiotensin II develops early in pregnancy and persists throughout gestation in gravidas who do not develop pregnancy-induced hypertension (preeclampsia–eclampsia). In normal men and nonpregnant women, the intravenous infusion of angiotensin II at a rate of 7 ng/kg body weight/min will cause a 20 mm Hg rise in diastolic pressure. On average, more than 16 ng/kg body weight/min is required to effect a similar pressor response in pregnant women, and in some gravidas there is little response to 40 ng angiotensin II. The alterations in the vasculature that lead to pressor refractoriness are not fully understood, but the *in situ* formation of prostaglandin or a prostaglandin-like substance is believed to mediate the process, since prostaglandin synthetase inhibitors, e.g., indomethacin and aspirin, abolish the refractoriness of pregnant women to the pressor effect of angiotensin II.[54] Although the physiologic adaptation to pregnancy is remarkable, the failure of such adaptation may be catastrophic. In a prospective study of young primigravid women considered to be at risk of developing pregnancy-induced hypertension, Gant and colleagues[55] found that the women who ultimately developed preeclampsia did become refractory to the pressor effects of angiotensin II early in pregnancy. These women began to lose refractoriness to angiotensin II — in some as early as 22 weeks of gestation — long before hypertension developed, however. This failure in the adaptive process of pregnancy is believed to be important in the pathophysiology of pregnancy-induced hypertension. With the development of hypertension, the levels of renin, angiotensin II, and aldosterone in the plasma of pregnant women fall, sometimes to values only slightly greater than those found in nonpregnant women. The rate of production of deoxycorticosterone (DOC) does not behave in a similar manner, however. The levels of DOC in plasma increase strikingly in women during pregnancy,[56, 57] the increase occurring principally during the last trimester. The production of DOC in pregnant women is not controlled by the same mechanisms that modulate the secretion of aldosterone or cortisol. Indeed, the administration of ACTH or dexamethasone to near-term pregnant women does not bring about a change in the levels of DOC in the plasma of pregnant women.[57] These findings led to the belief that the increased levels of DOC in the maternal compartment arose by transfer of DOC from the fetus to the mother. The levels of DOC in umbilical cord plasma are higher than those in the maternal plasma. Based on the umbilical artery–venous difference in concentration of DOC,[56] however, this source of DOC cannot account for the levels of DOC found in maternal plasma. The levels of DOC sulfate in the fetal circulation are even greater than those of DOC. The contribution of circulating DOC sulfate in the fetus to DOC in the maternal compartment is unknown, however. Recently we found that circulating progesterone is converted to DOC in nonadrenal tissue.[58] Moreover, the fractional conversion of plasma progesterone to DOC was similar in men and in nonpregnant and pregnant women. Thus the rate of extra-adrenal DOC formation is proportional to the plasma concentration of progesterone. Based on these observations, extra-adrenal 21 hydroxylation of progesterone to form DOC must be added to a growing list of reactions leading to hormone formation from circulating precursors in extra-glandular tissues. Interestingly, the fractional conversion of circulating progesterone to DOC, unlike the fractional conversion of other steroid hormones to metabolites, varies widely among persons (0.002–0.03). It may be that with high progesterone secretion (e.g., midluteal phase of the ovarian cycle [30 mg/24 h] or during pregnancy [250 mg/24 h]) the impact of DOC formation from plasma progesterone could vary widely depending on the fractional conversion of plasma progesterone to DOC in a given person. In some pregnant women, 7.5 mg or more of DOC could be produced each day from circulating progesterone.

The levels of cortisol in plasma are strikingly increased in pregnant women, presumably because of the threefold to fourfold increase in the levels of transcortin.[59] The rate of secretion of cortisol by the maternal adrenal is not increased in pregnant women. Rather, the rate of clearance is decreased; i.e., the $t_{1/2}$ is prolonged, and this accounts for the increase in plasma concentration of cortisol. ACTH levels are suppressed during pregnancy,[60] presumably owing to the action of estrogen and progesterone[61]; however, the lowest levels are found early in pregnancy and the highest levels are found in women between 26 weeks and term.[60]

The rate of secretion of DHEA sulfate by the maternal adrenal has not been studied systematically in pregnant women. The concentration of DHEA sulfate in plasma declines appreciably[62] during pregnancy, but this is believed to be due to the striking increase in the metabolic clearance rate of this compound through (a) utilization by the placenta for estradiol 17β formation and (b) extensive 16α-hydroxylation in the maternal liver. PRL secretion increases steadily during pregnancy, levels in plasma of 150–250 ng/ml being observed in near-term pregnant women. The role of PRL in adrenal function, if any, is not defined, however.

The physiologic adaptation of the mother during pregnancy seems to be designed in such a manner that the fetus is assured of the placental transfer of nutrients required for growth and development and the mother is protected from the trauma of delivery by a mechanism that provides for considerable expansion of her blood volume, ordinarily without a concomitant increase in arterial pressure.

REFERENCES

1. Ryan, K. J.: Aromatization of steroids. *J. Biol. Chem.* 234:268, 1959.
2. Frandsen, V. A., and Stakeman, G.: The site of production of oestrogenic hormones in human pregnancy. Hormone excretion in pregnancy with anencephalic fetus. *Acta Endocrinol.* 38:383, 1961.
3. Siiteri, P. K., and MacDonald, P. C.: The utilization of circulating dehydroisoandrosterone sulfate for estrogen synthesis during human pregnancy. *Steroids* 2:713, 1963.

4. Baulieu, E. E., and Dray, F.: Conversion of ³H-dehydroisoandrosterone (3β-hydroxy-Δ⁵-androsten-17-one) sulfate to ³H-estrogens in normal pregnant women. *J. Clin. Endocrinol. Metab.* 23:1298, 1963.

5. Bolté, E., et al.: Studies on the aromatization of neutral steroids in pregnant women: I. Aromatization of C-19 steroids by placentas perfused in situ. *Acta Endocrinol.* 45:535, 1964.

6. Magendantz, H. G., and Ryan, K. J.: Isolation of an estriol precursor, 16α-hydroxydehydroepiandrosterone, from human umbilical sera. *J. Clin. Endocrinol. Metab.* 24:1155, 1964.

7. Siiteri, P. K., and MacDonald, P. C.: Placental estrogen biosynthesis during human pregnancy. *J. Clin. Endocrinol.* 26:751, 1966.

8. Pulkkinen, M. O.: Arylsulphatase and the hydrolysis of some steroid sulphates in developing organism and placenta. *Acta Physiol. Scand.* 52 (Suppl. 180)1, 1961.

9. Warren, J. C., and Timberlake, C. E.: Steroid sulfatase in the human placenta. *J. Clin. Endocrinol.* 22:1148, 1962.

10. Tabei, T., and Heinrichs, W. L.: Diagnosis of placental sulfatase deficiency. *Am. J. Obstet. Gynecol.* 124:409, 1976.

11. Spector, W. S. (ed.): Handbook of Biological Data. Philadelphia, W. B. Saunders, 1956, p. 353.

12. Liggins, G. C.: Premature delivery of foetal lambs infused with glucocorticoids. *J. Endocrinol.* 45:515, 1969.

13. MacDonald, P. C., et al.: Initiation of parturition in the human female. *Semin. Perinatol.* 2:273, 1978.

14. Winters, A. J., et al.: Plasma ACTH levels in the human fetus and neonate as related to age and parturition. *J. Clin. Endocrinol. Metab.* 39:269, 1974.

15. Goldstein, J. L., and Brown, M. S.: Binding and degradation of low density lipoproteins by cultured human fibroblasts. *J. Biol. Chem.* 249:5153, 1974.

16. Faust, J. R., et al.: Receptor-mediated uptake of low-density lipoprotein and utilization of its cholesterol for steroid synthesis in cultured mouse adrenal cells. *J. Biol. Chem.* 252:4861, 1977.

17. Anderson, J. M., and Dietschy, J. M.: Regulation of sterol synthesis in 15 tissues of rat. II. Role of rat and human high and low density plasma lipoproteins and of rat chylomicron remnants. *J. Biol. Chem.* 252:3652, 1977.

18. Gleuck, C. J., et al.: Low and high density lipoprotein cholesterol interrelationships in neonates with low density lipoprotein cholesterol above the 10th percentile and in neonates with high density lipoprotein cholesterol below the 90th percentile. *Pediatr. Res.* 11:957, 1977.

19. Simpson, E. R., et al.: The role of serum lipoproteins in steroidogenesis by the human fetal adrenal cortex. *J. Clin. Endocrinol. Metab.* 49:146, 1979.

20. Carr, B. R., et al.: The role of low density, high density, and very low density lipoprotein in steroidogenesis by the human fetal adrenal gland. *Endocrinology* (submitted).

21. Lin, D. S., et al.: Placental transfer of cholesterol into the human fetus. *Am. J. Obstet. Gynecol.* 128:735, 1977.

22. Zinder, O., et al.: Effect of prolactin on lipoprotein lipase in mammary gland and adipose tissue of rats. *Am. J. Physiol.* 226:744, 1974.

23. Gurpide, E., et al.: Fetal and maternal metabolism of estradiol during pregnancy. *J. Clin. Endocrinol. Metab.* 26:1355, 1966.

24. Gurpide, E., et al.: Fetomaternal production and transfer of progesterone and uridine in sheep. *Am. J. Obstet. Gynecol.* 113:21, 1972.

25. Hellig, H., et al.: Steroid metabolism from plasma cholesterol. I. Conversion of plasma cholesterol to placental progesterone in humans. *J. Clin. Endocrinol. Metab.* 30:624, 1970.

26. Bloch, K.: Biological conversion of cholesterol to pregnanediol. *J. Biol. Chem.* 157:661, 1945.

27. Cassmer, O.: Hormone production of the isolated human placenta. Studies on the role of the foetus in the endocrine functions of the placenta. *Acta Endocrinol.* (Kbh) 32 (Suppl.)45:1, 1959.

28. Simpson, E. R., et al.: Uptake and degradation of plasma lipoproteins by human choriocarcinoma cells in culture. *Endocrinology* 104:8, 1979.

29. Brown, M. S., et al.: Cholesterol ester formation in cultured human fibroblasts. *J. Biol. Chem.* 250:4025, 1975.

30. Simpson, E. R., and Burkhart, M. F.: AcylCoA:cholesterol acyltransferase activity in human placental microsomes: Inhibition by progesterone. *Arch. Biochem. Biophys.* (in press).

31. Simpson, E. R., and Burkhart, M. F.: Regulation of cholesterol metabolism by human choriocarcinoma cells in culture: Effect of lipoproteins and progesterone on cholesteryl ester synthesis. *Arch. Biochem. Biophys.* (in press).

32. Murphy, B. E. P., et al.: Conversion of maternal cortisol to cortisone during placental transfer to the human fetus. *Am. J. Obstet. Gynecol.* 118:538, 1974.

33. MacDonald, P. C., and Siiteri, P. K.: Origin of estrogen in women pregnant with an anencephalic fetus. *J. Clin. Invest.* 44:465, 1965.

34. Hennen, G. P.: Detection and study of a human chorionic thyroid stimulating factor. *Arch. Int. Physiol. Biochim.* 73:689, 1965.

35. Rees, L. H., et al.: Possible placental origin of ACTH in normal human pregnancy. *Nature* 254:620, 1975.

36. Liotta, A., et al.: Presence of corticotropin in human placenta: Demonstration of in vitro synthesis. *Endocrinology* 101:1552, 1977.

37. Odagiri, E., et al.: Human placental immunoreactive corticotropin lipotropin and β-endorphin. Evidence for a common precursor. *Proc. Natl. Acad. Sci. USA* 76:2027, 1979.

38. Siler-Khodr, T. M., and Khodr, G. S.: Luteinizing hormone releasing factor content of the human placenta. *Am. J. Obstet. Gynecol.* 130:216, 1978.

39. Gibbons, J. M., et al.: In vitro biosynthesis of TSH- and LH-releasing factors by human placenta. *Am. J. Obstet. Gynecol.* 121:127, 1975.

40. Adcock III, E. W., et al.: Human chorionic gonadotropin: Its possible role in maternal lymphocyte suppression. *Science* 181:845, 1973.

41. Golbus, M. S., and Siiteri, P. K.: Effects of human chorionic gonadotropin preparations on amino acid uptake and incorporation into protein in vitro. *Endocrine Res. Commun.* 3:273, 1976.

42. Kenimer, J. G., et al.: The thyrotropin in hydatidiform moles in human chorionic gonadotropin. *J. Clin. Endocrinol. Metab.* 40:482, 1975.

43. Herz, R.: Choriocarcinoma and Related Gestational Tumors in Women. New York, Raven Press, 1978.

44. Boddy, K., and Mantell, C. D.: Observations of fetal breathing movements transmitted through maternal abdominal wall. *Lancet* 2:1219, 1972.

45. Pearson, J. F., and Weaver, J. B.: Fetal activity and fetal well-being: An evaluation. *Br. Med. J.,* 1:1305, 1976.

46. Duenhoelter, J. H., et al.: An analysis of the utility of plasma immunoreactive estrogen measurements in determining delivery time of gravidas with a fetus considered at high risk. *Am. J. Obstet. Gynecol.* 125:889, 1976.

47. Gurpide, E., et al.: Fetal and maternal metabolism of estradiol during pregnancy. *J. Clin. Endocrinol. Metab.* 26:1355, 1966.

48. Spellacy, W. N., et al.: Distribution of human placental lactogen in the last half of normal and complicated pregnancies. *Am. J. Obstet. Gynecol.* 120:214, 1974.

49. Madden, J. D., et al.: The pattern and rates of metabolism of maternal plasma dehydroisoandrosterone sulfate in human pregnancy. *Am. J. Obstet. Gynecol.* 125:915, 1976.

50. Worley, R. J., et al.: Placental clearance of dehydroisoandrosterone sulfate and pregnancy outcome in three categories of hospitalized patients with pregnancy-induced hypertension. *Gynecol. Invest.* 6:28, 1975.

51. Worley, R. J., et al.: Fetal considerations: Metabolic clearance rate of maternal plasma dehydroisoandrosterone sulfate. *Semin. Perinatol.* 2:15, 1978.

52. Pupkin, M. J., et al.: The dehydroisoandrosterone loading test. III. A possible placental function test. *Am. J. Obstet. Gynecol.* 134:281, 1979.

53. Pritchard, J. A. (ed.): In *Williams Obstetrics,* 15th Ed., New York, Appleton-Century-Crofts, 1976, p. 183–186.

54. Everett, R. B., Worley, R. J., et al.: Effect of prostaglandin synthetase inhibitors on pressor response to angiotensin II in human pregnancy. *J. Clin. Endocrinol. Metab.* 46:1007, 1978.

55. Gant, N. F., Daley, G. L., et al.: A study of angiotensin II pressor response throughout primagravid pregnancy. *J. Clin. Invest.* 52:2682, 1973.

56. Brown, R. D., Strott, C. A., et al.: Plasma deoxycorticosterone in normal and abnormal human pregnancy. *J. Clin. Endocrinol. Metab.* 35:736, 1972.

57. Nolten, W. E., Linheimer, M. D., et al.: Deoxycorticosterone in pregnancy: Sequential studies of the secretory patterns of deoxycorticosterone, aldosterone and cortisol. *Am. J. Obstet. Gynecol.* 132:414, 1978.

58. Winkel, C. A., et al.: Conversion of plasma progesterone to deoxycorticosterone in men, nonpregnant and pregnant women, and adrenalectomized subjects: Evidence for steroid 21-hydroxylase activity in non-adrenal tissues. *J. Clin. Invest.* (submitted).

59. Doe, R. P., et al.: Measurement of corticosteroid-binding globulin in man. *J. Clin. Endocrinol. Metab.* 24:1029, 1964.

60. Carr, B. R., et al.: Maternal plasma adrenocorticotropin (ACTH) and cortisol relationships throughout human pregnancy. *Am. J. Obstet. Gynecol.* (Submitted).

61. Vale, W., et al.: Effects of purified hypothalamic corticotropin-releasing factor and other substances on the secretion of adrenocorticotropin and β-endorphin-like immunoreactivities in vitro. *Endocrinology* 103:1910, 1978.

62. Milewich, L., et al.: Dehydroisoandrosterone sulphate in peripheral blood of premenopausal, pregnant and postmenopausal women and men. *J. Steroid Biochem.* 9:1159, 1978.

CHAPTER 9

Disorders of Sex Differentiation

By Melvin M. Grumbach
and Felix A. Conte

In our culture, the distinction between male and female is expected to be absolute, and these terms are often used to epitomize opposites. Usually the components of an individual's sexual makeup are indeed dominantly of one gender and conform to the chromosomal pattern established in the zygote at the time of fertilization. Most sexual characteristics, however, emerge from identical bipotential precursors in the embryo, and a spectrum of differentiation is possible at each level of sexual organization.

The remarkable accumulation of knowledge over the past two decades and new insights in the field of sex determination and sex differentiation represent major landmarks in biomedical science. No aspect of prenatal development is better understood. Advances in experimental embryology, steroid and molecular biochemistry, cytogenetics and genetics, endocrinology, immunology and transplantation biology, cell biology, and the behavorial sciences all have contributed richly to the present state of our knowledge of anomalies of sex in man and to the clinical management of these disorders. Of note are the major contributions that have stemmed from studies in patients with abnormalities of sex differentiation; in many instances, animal counterparts for these human disorders have been identified or experimentally induced. It is clear that failure at any of the sequential stages of sex development, whether the cause is genetic or environmental, can have a profound effect on the phenotype and lead to complete sex reversal, various degrees of ambisexual development, or less overt abnormalities in sexual function that first become apparent after sexual maturity.

NORMAL SEX DETERMINATION AND SEX DIFFERENTIATION

Sex determination and differentiation is a sequential process that involves successively the establishment of chromosomal (and genetic) sex in the zygote at the moment of conception, the determination of gonadal (primary) sex by the genetic sex, and the regulation by gonadal sex of the differentiation of the genital apparatus and, hence, the phenotypic sex. At puberty the development of sex specific secondary sex characteristics reinforces and provides more visible phenotypic manifestations of this sexual dimorphism. Sex determination is concerned with the control of the primary or gonadal sex, and sex differentiation with all of the events that entrain subsequent to gonadal organogenesis. These processes are regulated by at least 30 specific genes located on sex chromosomes or autosomes that act through a variety of mechanisms, including organizing factors, sex steroid and peptide secretions, and specific tissue receptors. Both male and female embryos possess indifferent, common primordia that have an inherent tendency to feminize unless there is active interference by masculinizing factors: an ovary differentiates unless the indifferent embryonic gonad is diverted by a testis-organizing factor (H-Y antigen) regulated by the Y chromosome; female differentiation of the somatic sex structures (the internal and external genital tract) occurs independent of gonadal hormones and will emerge in the absence of fetal testes whether ovaries are present or not. Thus, the sexual dimorphism in phenotype that results from sex differentiation in placental mammals is mediated by the fetal testis and its secretions, and not by the ovary (Table 9–1). Further, male differentiation takes place despite an environment in which the concentration of circulating estrogens and progestins is high.

Before discussing the genetic control of sex determination and gonadogenesis, we shall consider some aspects of cytogenetics of importance to our understanding of abnormalities of sex differentiation.

Chromosomal Sex and X- and Y-Chromatin

A systematized array of metaphase chromosomes from a single cell is known as a karyotype (14). The meaning of this term is usually extended to imply that the chromosomal pattern in that cell typifies all of the diploid cells of that individual or even of that species, although, as will be seen, this is by no means always true. When the 22 autosomes and two sex chromosomes (two X chromosomes or an X and a Y) are arrayed and serially numbered according to size, the X chromosome(s) are identified by their resemblance to the larger autosomes in the medium-sized group with submedian centromeres (group 6–12). The Y chromosome resembles the very short acrocentric autosomes in group 21–22 (14) (Fig. 9–1).

Positive identification of all the pairs of chromosomes can be made by the use of chromosome staining techniques (14). The pattern of DNA replication in human chromosomes is disclosed by pulse labeling cell cultures with tritiated thymidine and preparing autoradiographs of the chromosomal spreads (15, 16), or by the more recent and less laborious BrdU (bromodeoxyuridine) dye technique (17). It was shown that one of two X chromosomes in the human female replicates late (15, 16), and that this characteristic is responsible for the distinctive X chromatin body seen in female somatic cells (vide infra).

Major advances in cytogenetics have come from the discovery of chromosome staining techniques which differentially stain segments along the length of the chromosome. Caspersson and his associates (18, 19) introduced fluorescence staining with substances such as quinacrine mustard or quinacrine hydrochloride (Atabrine). Now referred to as the Q-staining method, this staining procedure gives a distinctive fluorescent banding pattern (Q bands) for each chromosome (Fig. 9–2) and for many of the arms of individual chromosomes. The distal portion of the Y chromosome is intensely fluorescent. Shortly thereafter, Pardue and Gall reported a Giemsa staining technique which preferentially stained only the centromeric regions of the chromosome (20). These areas of constitutive (centromeric) heterochromatin are known as C bands (14). Stimulated by this finding, various workers modified the Giemsa staining technique (21), using a multitude of pretreatment procedures on fixed metaphase chromosomes (e.g., hypertonic saline, NaOH, variation of pH temperature, cation concentration, and proteolytic enzymes), which produced Giemsa-stained bands in human chromosomes identical (with minor exceptions) to the Q bands described by Caspersson (18); this method gives permanent preparations for conventional light microscopy (Fig. 9–2). The resulting bands are designated G bands (14). More recently, R-banding has been described (14), which is a Giemsa staining method that produces a reverse pattern of chromosome banding to either the Q or G bands. The structural components of the chromosome that give rise to the banding patterns are uncertain but the differential distribution of base composition and the state of condensation of the chromatin appear to be involved. There is evidence that the Q bands result from binding of quinacrine stains to adenine- and thymine (A-T)–rich regions of

Table 9–1. ONTOGENY OF SEXUAL CHARACTERISTICS

Characteristic	How Identified	Origin	Factors Determining Differentiation

Chromosomal sex	Karyotype analysis	Sex chromosomes of parental germ cell	Normal: chromosomal composition of sperm
			Abnormal:
			    Nondisjunction during meiotic divisions of parental germ cells
			    Nondisjunction or anaphase lag in early mitotic divisions of the zygote
			    Structural errors due to chromosome breakage

X-chromatin	Buccal smear; neutrophil spreads; smears or sections of other peripheral tissues	Late replicating (hetero-chromatized) X chromosome	Partial inactivation and heterochromatization of all X chromosomes in excess of one
Y-body	Same as for X-chromatin; also seen in sperm	Y chromosome	Distal segment of the long arm of the Y
Gonadal sex	Histologic appearance	Testis	Testis: H-Y antigen; synthesis and secretion regulated by genes on the Y and X chromosome. Specific receptors for H-Y antigen on gonadal cells
		Ovary	Ovary: Sex determining genes on two X chromosomes, ? H-O antigen
Genital ducts	Pelvic examination; pelvic exploration	Müllerian and wolffian ducts	Intrinsic tendency to feminize; müllerian involution requires peptide duct inhibitory factor from fetal Sertoli cells; testosterone stimulates male duct development

External genitalia	Inspection; investigation of urogenital sinus by urethroscopy and/or x-ray contrast study	Genital tubercle, urethral folds, labio-scrotal folds, and urogenital sinus	Intrinsic tendency to feminize; masculinization requires androgenic stimulation before twelfth fetal week
			    Normal male: testosterone from fetal testes converted to dihydro-testosterone at the end organ
			    Virilized female: adrenal hyperplasia (21- and 11-hydroxylase deficiency); maternal androgen
			    Incompletely differentiated male: insufficient testosterone secretion by fetal testes; 5α-reductase insufficiency; end organ insensitivity

Hormonal sex	*Secondary sex characteristics*
	    Male: sexual hair pattern; voice; muscularity; phallic size
	    Female: breast development; rounding of the contours; growth of reproductive tract; menstruation; ovulation
	Hormonal patterns
	    Male: testosterone secretion from testes; tonic gonadotropin release
	    Female: cyclic secretion of gonadotropins, estrogen and progesterone
		Hypothalamus and other neural centers; luteinizing hormone releasing factor
		Pituitary gonadotropin
		Secretory cells of testes, ovaries and adrenals
			Hypothalamus and neural centers: gonadotropin releasing factor
			Pituitary: gonadotropin release governed by pulsatile secretion of hypothalamic releasing factor and circulating levels of sex steroids
			Gonads: differentiation of secretory cells and biosynthetic enzymes; stimulation N by pituitary gonadotropins
			Hormonal expression may be modified by end organ sensitivity

Gender role	Social comportment; mannerism and dress; direction of sex drive	Neuter at birth	Psychological environment during early years of paramount importance in establishing gender identity:
			    Attitudes of parents
			    Interactions of both sexes
			    Conformity of genitalia and secondary sex characteristics at puberty to assigned sex
			Hormonal factors: adult sexual postures in lower species conditioned by hormonal factors in perinatal period

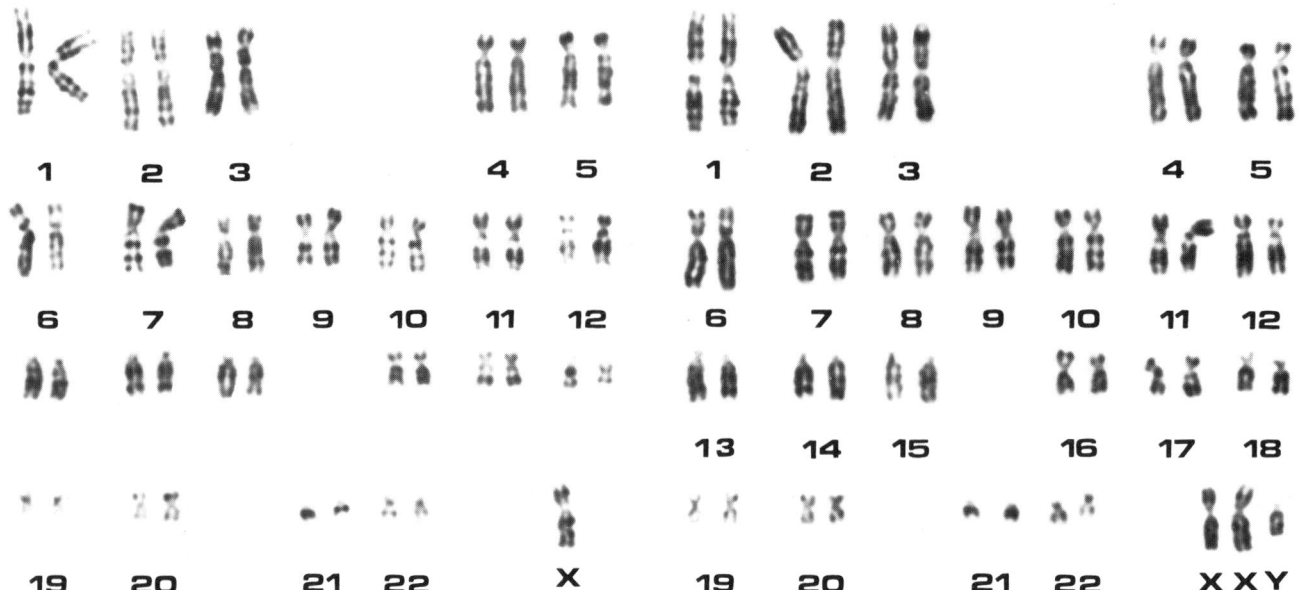

Figure 9–1. Typical "G" banded karyotype from patients with abnormal gonadal differentiation. The XO karyotype on the left is from a patient with streak gonads, short stature, and the physical stigmata of Turner syndrome. The XXY karyotype on the right is from a phenotypic male with seminiferous tubule dysgenesis (Chromatin positive Klinefelter syndrome).

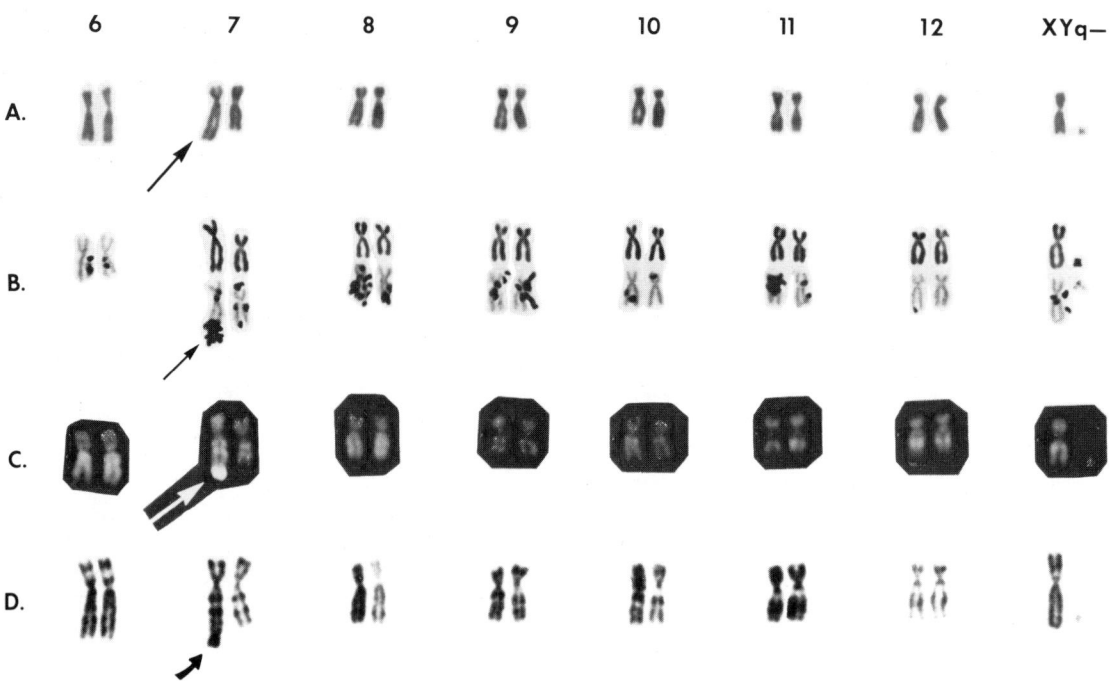

Figure 9–2. *Upper,* Partial karyotype of the C group (chromosome number 6–12) and the X and Y in a patient with a 46,t (Yq — ,7q+) karyotype. Standard Giemsa staining, autoradiography, and fluorescent (Q) and Giemsa (G) banding techniques were used to identify the chromosome anomaly. *A,* The standard staining technique for karyotype analysis revealed an enlarged C-group chromosome and a deleted G-group chromosome. *B,* Autoradiography after incubation of the lymphocyte culture with tritiated thymidine showed a late-labeling segment on the distal arms of the C chromosome and the absence of a late-labeling segment on the deleted long arm of the presumptive Y. *C,* Quinacrine hydrochloride staining and fluorescent microscopy demonstrated translocation of the brightly fluorescent segment of the long arm of the Y chromosome to the long arm of chromosome No. 7. *D,* Giemsa banding confirmed that the C-group chromosome involved in the translocation was chromosome No. 7.

Table 9–2. NOMENCLATURE FOR DESCRIBING THE HUMAN KARYOTYPE PERTINENT TO DESIGNATING SEX CHROMOSOME ABNORMALITIES

Paris Conference	Description	Former Nomenclature
46,XX	Normal female karyotype	XX
46,XY	Normal male karyotype	XY
47,XXY	Karyotype with 47 chromosomes including an extra X chromosome	XXY
45,X	Monosomy X	XO
45,X/46,XY	Mosaic karyotype composed of 45,X and 46,XY cell lines	XO/XY
p	Short arm	p
q	Long arm	q
46,X, del (X) (:p21 qter)	Deletion of the short arm of the X-distal to band Xp21	Xp–
46,X, del (X) (pter q21:)	Deletion of the long arm of the X-distal to band Xq21	Xq–
46,X,i(Xq)	Isochromosome of the long arm of X	Xqi
46,X,i(Xp)	Isochromosome of the short arm of X	Xpi
46,X,r(X)	Ring X chromosome	Xr
46,X,del(Y) (pter→q11:), t(7;Y) (7pter 7q36::Yq11→ Yqter)	Translocation of the distal fluorescent portion of the Y chromosome to the long arm of chromosome 7	46,XYt(Yq–,7q+)

DNA; guanine- and cytosine (G-C)–rich regions of the chromosome quench the fluorescence. The G bands appear to be a consequence of differential dye binding by nonhistone protein overlying the A-T–rich regions.

In any event, the chromosome banding procedures have provided precise methods for the identification of each chromosome and for the accurate analysis of chromosome abnormalities, including complex chromosome rearrangements (Fig. 9–2). Recommendations for a standard nomenclature for the identification and designation of individual chromosomes, chromosome regions and bands, and structurally altered chromosomes are embodied in the report of the 1971 Paris Conference on Standardization in Human Cytogenetics (14). Table 9–2 summarizes the nomenclature applied to sex chromosome anomalies.

Within a short span of years, a vast literature has emerged, attempting to correlate sex chromosome abnormalities with both sexual and somatic abnormalities. It is clear that anomalies in number and structure of sex chromosomes occur with far greater frequency than was pre-viously suspected and that these anomalies are of such variety that they cannot be attributed to any single mechanism or stage of cellular replication. Although many confusing and contradictory findings have been reported, cytogenetic studies have shed considerable light on the biologic roles of the X and Y chromosomes.

Mechanisms of Chromosomal Anomalies

Chromosomal errors can arise from faulty replication of the germ cells during spermatogenesis or oögenesis, or they can arise from faulty mitotic division of cells in the zygote after fertilization. Aneuploid cells are those which contain a different number of chromosomes from that characteristic of the species.

Aneuploidy. One mechanism of producing aneuploidy is nondisjunction, a process which may occur during either mitotic or meiotic division. Nondisjunction is charac-

ORIGIN OF CHROMOSOMAL ERRORS IN ZYGOTE
MITOTIC NONDISJUNCTION

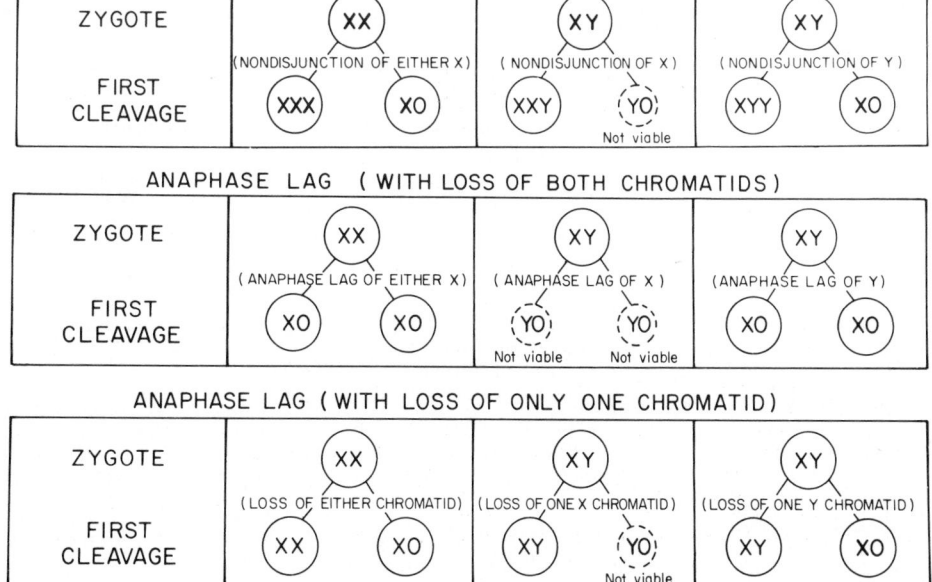

Figure 9–3. Daughter cell lines that can arise from mitotic nondisjunction or anaphase lag during the first mitotic division in the zygote. More complex mosaicism can result if the zygote is aneuploid or if replication errors arise beyond the one-cell stage. In females, nondisjunction or anaphase lag may involve either the maternal or paternal X chromosome. Deductions regarding the origin of X chromosomes in aneuploid patients can sometimes be made by correlating sex-linked traits with those in the parents.

terized by failure of either a pair of sister chromatids or members of a pair of homologous chromosomes to separate during anaphase. Thus, one daughter cell receives an extra chromosome while the other remains one short (Fig. 9–3). Aneuploidy may also be caused by anaphase lag, in which there is a simple loss of a chromosome from one or both of the two daughter cells. Presumably this is caused by failure of one chromosome to become properly oriented at the equatorial plate during metaphase. If both chromatids are extruded, both daughter cell lines will be lacking in this chromosome. If, however, only one member of the chromatid pair is subsequently lost, the descendants from one daughter cell will be normal, while the other will be one short (Fig. 9–3).

Mosaicism. Mosaicism is the term applied to individuals with two or more cell lines, differing in chromosomal constitutions but originating from a single zygote. Although this condition can arise only from errors in mitosis after fertilization has occurred, embryos derived from gametes of abnormal chromosomal makeup are prone to further errors of replication. Mosaicism has been found to be much more common than was first supposed from early karyotypic analysis, and many of the seeming paradoxes between genotype and phenotype are attributable to studies that have lacked sufficient data to exclude this explanation. The difficulties of detecting or, especially, excluding sex chromosome mosaicism are often formidable. When mosaicism is present, the sex chromosome constitution may vary in different tissues and even in different areas of the same tissue (22). For this reason, it may be necessary to examine cell lines from a variety of tissues. The following additional factors must be considered when attempting to establish the presence of sex chromosome mosaicism:

1. even in normal individuals, a small percentage of metaphase cells gain or lose chromosomes (usually the latter) for purely technical reasons.

2. a gradual and slight increase in the proportion of aneuploid cells with age, especially in females, has been observed by Jacobs et al. (23). In males, the aneuploidy is mainly due to the loss of the Y chromosome and in females to the loss of an X chromosome. By the age of 75 years this selective loss of a sex chromosome may involve as many as 5% of the metaphase figures in lymphocytes cultured from peripheral blood. This age-related aneuploidy is not a significant factor in assessing sex mosaicism before late adult life.

Chimerism. Chimerism is the term applied to individuals with more than one cell line, each of which has a different genetic origin. In the classic case of the freemartin, a common form of hermaphrodism in cattle, chimerism is derived by admixture of hemopoietic and primordial germ cells between biovular twins of opposite sex through anastomotic placental channels. Although it may be difficult to recognize the presence of chimerism if the separate cell lines have the same karyotype, the presence of cell lines of different sex will be marked by an XX/XY karyotype. Ford has discussed mechanisms by which XX/XY chimerism could also result from (a) double fertilization (dispermy) of a binucleate ovum, (b) fusion of two complete zygotes or morulae before implantation, or (c) fertilization by separate sperms of an ovum and its polar body (24). It should be emphasized that the difference between mosaicism and chimerism depends solely on whether the different cell lines are of the same or different genetic origin.

Structural Errors. With the increased facility to identify the morphologic characteristics of human chromo-

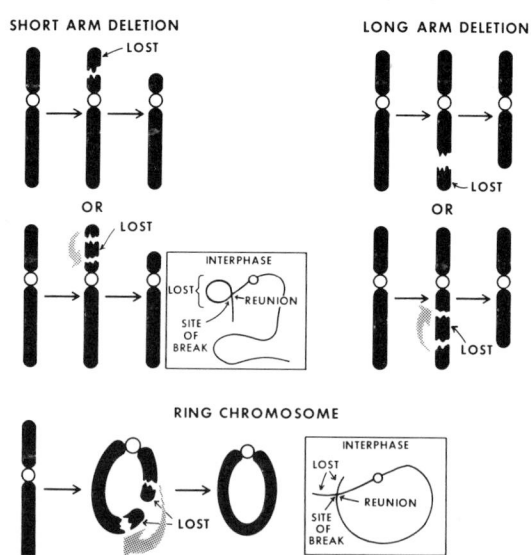

PRODUCTION OF SOME STRUCTURAL ABNORMALITIES OF A CHROMOSOME

SHORT ARM DELETION

LONG ARM DELETION

LOST

LOST

OR

OR

LOST

LOST

INTERPHASE

LOST — REUNION

SITE OF BREAK

RING CHROMOSOME

LOST

INTERPHASE

LOST — REUNION

SITE OF BREAK

Figure 9–4. Diagram of chromosome breakage and recombination to form long- and short-arm deletions and ring chromosomes. The deleted segments also may be transposed to the terminal portions of other chromosomes as additions, or there may be reciprocal translocations of deleted segments with those from another chromosome.

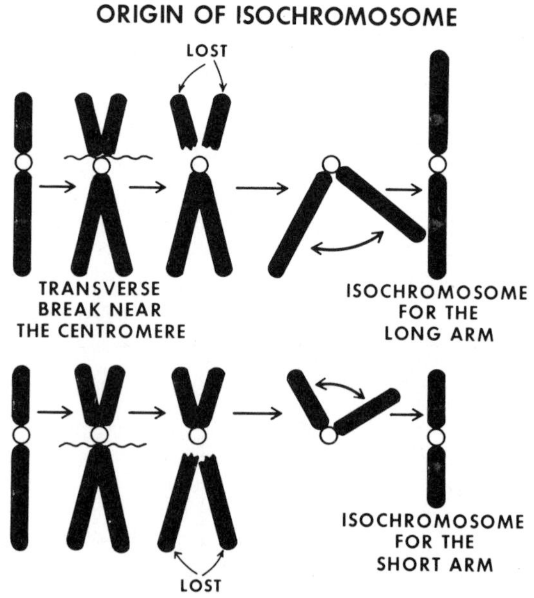

somes provided by banding techniques, subtle as well as more obvious abnormalities of structure have been described. Structural errors are due to breakage or partial deletion, often followed by improper reunion of the fragments (Fig. 9–4). Most of the structural abnormalities

ORIGIN OF ISOCHROMOSOME

LOST

TRANSVERSE BREAK NEAR THE CENTROMERE

ISOCHROMOSOME FOR THE LONG ARM

ISOCHROMOSOME FOR THE SHORT ARM

LOST

Figure 9–5. X isochromosomes are thought to arise from transverse rather than longitudinal division of the centromere during the second meiotic division of germ cells in either parent or during mitosis in the zygote. Although two daughter cell lines might be expected, one with isochromosomes for the long arm and another for the short arm, this form of mosaicism has not been recognized. It is probable, however, that the break rarely occurs through the centromere, and the chromosomal segment which lacks a centromere is lost.

that are sufficiently distinctive to be made visible by the light microscope are characterized by an abnormally long or short chromosome. Chromosomal fragments lacking a centromere or acquiring an additional centromere are usually eliminated from the cell. The nomenclature recommended by the Chicago and Paris Conferences for designating the human karyotype with reference to sex chromosome abnormalities is shown in Table 9–2 (14, 25). The following are the more common structural abnormalities:

Isochromosomes are chromosomes with identical arms. They have been thought to arise by horizontal rather than longitudinal division of the chromosome (Fig. 9–5). The isochromosome may consist of either two long arms (e.g., Xqi) or two short arms (Xpi). Recent data indicate that isochromosomes may have either one or two centromeric bands, and some isochromosomes may exhibit subtle differences in the banding pattern and size of the two arms. Thus, the origin of this chromosome may not be as simple as previously proposed. *Deletion* is characterized by detachment and loss of a portion of a chromosome. The superscript q− refers to deletion of a portion of the long arm and p− to deletion of a portion of the short arm. *Duplication* occurs when a deleted segment is incorporated into another chromosome, usually the other member of a homologous pair. *Translocations* are characterized by exchanges of chromosomal segments between two chromosomes. *Ring chromosomes* (Xr) arise by deletions from the ends of a chromosome with reunion of the new distal portions to form a ring.

The larger the involved segment in structural errors, the more likely are polygenic abnormalities and resultant sterility. However, many visible chromosomal anomalies are compatible with fertility and are transmitted in a manner simulating mendelian laws of inheritance. Indeed, the distinction between congenital anomalies due to mutant genes and those due to chromosomal errors is based primarily on whether the disordered chromosomal structure is of sufficient size to be identified with current procedures for karyotype analysis.

Mutant genes or structural abnormalities of sex chromosomes, similar to those just described but involving chromosomal segments that are too short to be seen with the light microscope, may account for certain discrepancies between the sex chromosomes and the gonadal morphology.

Biologic Functions of the Y Chromosome

Until the advent of human chromosome analysis, it was believed by many that the Y chromosome was inert and that male determiners were carried on the autosomes. The finding of an XXY pattern in some patients with Klinefelter syndrome has provided convincing demonstration that the Y chromosome carries powerful male-determining genes which can induce testicular development in the presence of two or more X chromosomes. Subsequent work has amply confirmed this conclusion, especially the recent discovery of H-Y antigen, the putative testis morphogenetic factor, and the role of a Y-

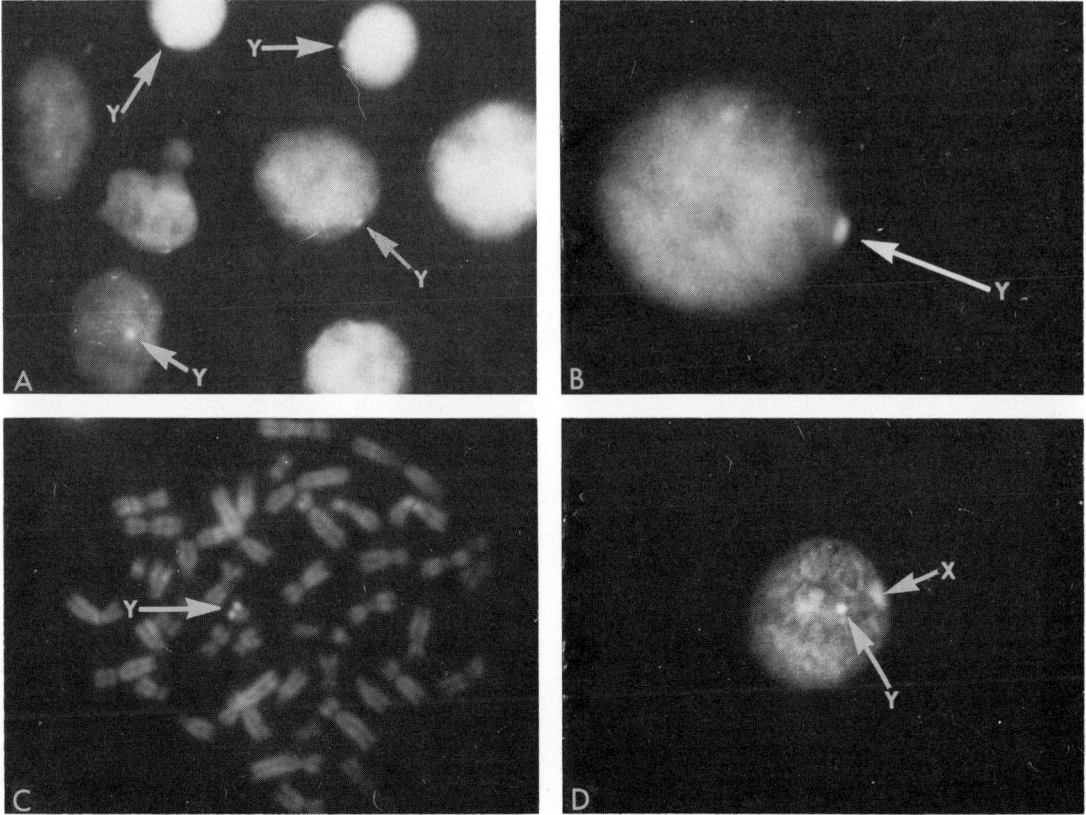

Figure 9–6. *A,* Quinacrine hydrochloride staining and fluorescent microscopy of interphase cells from a normal male, illustrating typical Y bodies. *B,* Enlarged photograph of one cell, showing the fluorescent Y body at the periphery of the nucleus. *C,* Metaphase chromosomes from a normal male, illustrating the brightly fluorescent distal segment of the long arm of the Y chromosome. *D,* An interphase nucleus in the buccal smear of a patient with a 47,XXY karyotype. A brightly fluorescent Y body, as well as an X chromatin body (which exhibits much weaker fluorescence) were identified by quinacrine staining and fluorescent microscopy.

linked gene in its expression (reviewed in 8, 26). The presence of a Y chromosome leads to testicular differentiation even in individuals with an XXXXY sex chromosome constitution, whereas no testicular differentiation occurs in XO individuals. In addition to its role in gonadal differentiation, the Y is essential to spermatogenesis in man.

The size of the human Y chromosome varies considerably—as much as threefold in length in normal men. The length and morphology of the Y is heritable, relatively constant in male relatives, and exhibits racial variation. Most of this variation is limited to the length of the long arm and its distal brilliantly fluorescent segment in quinacrine(Q)-stained preparations (Fig. 9–6). As this polymorphism in the size of the fluorescent portion as well as loss of part of the distal nonfluorescent portion of the long arm is consistent with normal male sex differentiation and not associated with any specific phenotypic effects, it is quite likely that a large segment of the long arm of the Y is not engaged in gene transcription (27). The long arm of the Y contains highly repetitious Y-chromosome specific and non-Y specific sequences of DNA; these repetitious sequences are distributed throughout its length and are not confined to the distal fluorescent segment.

The major function of the Y chromosome is to direct the bipotential embryonic gonad to differentiate as a testis; otherwise, few gene loci have been assigned to the Y (27). Either a regulatory or a structural gene locus for H-Y antigen (the testis-organizing factor), possibly in multiple or repetitious copies of the gene locus, is situated on the short arm of the Y close to the centromere and possibly the pericentromeric region of the long arm (28).

It has also been adduced that the Y contains loci homologous to those on the short arm of the X, since the presence of a Y chromosome with a normal X prevents the short stature and the somatic abnormalities found in Turner syndrome (22, 29). Karyotype-phenotype correlations for the Y chromosome have been especially difficult and are tentative at best. The presence of tall stature in XYY individuals suggests that this trait is transmitted through loci on the Y, and evidence from deletion mapping of the Y supports the localization of genes that influence stature, tooth size and spermatogenesis to the proximal portion of the long arm (27).

Y Chromatin (Y Body). The fluorescent end of the Y chromosome in human male metaphases, stained with the fluorochrome quinacrine hydrochloride or its mustard derivative, is represented as a small, brightly fluorescent body (Y body) in a high proportion of diploid interphase nuclei of the male, frequently located close to the nuclear membrane. The technique of fluorescence has been used to detect the Y body in interphase nuclei in a variety of tissue preparations, including buccal mucosal smears, lymphocytes and polymorphonuclear leukocytes in peripheral blood smears, hair root sheath cells, and cells grown in culture (21). In XY males, a single body, sometimes bipartite in structure, is present in interphase nuclei (Fig. 9–6), whereas two Y bodies are detectable in over 15% of nuclei in XYY and XXYY males (Table 9–3). Of interest are the reports of Pearson et al. (30) and others of the occurrence of a Y body in slightly less than 50% of mature sperm. In a small percentage of normal males (<0.05%) with a small Y chromosome that lacks all or most of the distal fluorescent segment, a Y body is absent in somatic nuclei. Fluorescence of quinacrine-stained X-chromatin bodies has been observed in cultured fibroblasts and certain other tissues from females, but the intensity of the fluorescent X body is less and the size 3–5 times larger than the Y body (Fig. 9–9).

Biologic Functions of the X Chromosome

The biologic functions of the large paired X chromosomes are more complex. Genes on the X have a critical influence on sex determination in both the female and male and on the differentiation of the somatic sex structures in the male. In addition, over 150 gene loci unrelated to sex development are known to be X-linked (4).

The X chromosome contains a locus on the short arm for either a regulatory or a structural gene for H-Y antigen (8). Two X chromosomes are required in the human being for normal ovarian differentiation; XO individuals have bilateral streak gonads. Studies of patients with various types of deletions of one of the two X chromosomes suggest that loci on both the long and short arms are involved in ovarian differentiation (31, 32, 33). Further, the gene that codes for the cytosol androgen receptor and thus is a major regulator of male differentiation of the genital tract and of male secondary sex characteristics is located on the X (34).

The X chromosome also harbors genes active on both X's that prevent short stature and many of the somatic abnormalities found in the syndrome of gonadal dysgenesis. They appear to be located mainly on the short arm of the X. Similar genetic loci are situated on the short arm of the Y chromosome. Further, on the X chromosome, there are a large number of unpaired genes, missing on the Y, that are responsible for a wide variety of X-linked traits. Using the techniques of somatic cell hybridization, pedigree analysis, and cytogenetic banding methods for chromosome identification, recent studies have assigned the loci for hypoxanthine guanine phosphoribosyl transferase and glucose-6-phosphate dehydrogenase to the terminal segment of the long arm; phosphoglycerate kinase, α-galactosidase, color blindness, and hemophilia A to the long arm (35); and steroid sulfatase and the XG blood group gene, both of which escape inactivation, to the short arm (36).

Whereas the Y chromosome is one of the smallest of human chromosomes and is mainly concerned with testis organogenesis, the X chromosome is the eighth longest and contains about 5% of the total DNA content of a haploid set (X + 22 autosomes). Furthermore, the X chromosome contains genetic coding for functions involving every system in the body. Since females have twice the amount of this genetic material in their cells as do males, the biologic differences between the sexes should be far greater than is indeed the case. Theories that have been proposed to explain this paradox are an outgrowth of the pioneer observations of Barr of the X chromatin body in somatic cells of females.

X Chromatin (X or Barr Body) (6). In 1949, Barr and Bertram described the presence of a stainable chromatin mass at the periphery of the nucleus in resting ganglion cells of female cats but not of male cats (37). This distinguishing characteristic of the female sex was subsequently found to be present in the peripheral cells of most mammalian species. Since 1953, this nuclear difference has been used as a cytologic means of assessing the number of X chromosomes in humans with various errors of sex differentiation (Fig. 9–7).

The X chromatin body is usually planoconvex, with its flattened side in apposition to the inner surface of the nuclear membrane; in some nuclei, it has a bipartite struc-

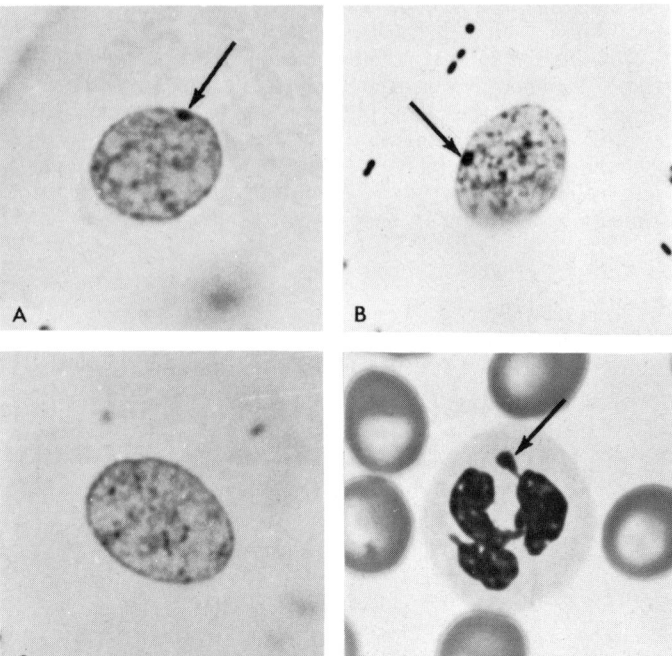

Figure 9–7. *A* and *B*, X chromatin body (Barr body) in nucleus of buccal mucosal cells obtained from normal female (thionine stain, × 2000). Such cells are found in about 25% of well-preserved nuclei. *C*, Buccal mucosal cell from normal male, illustrating absence of this body. *D*, A typical "drumstick" nuclear appendage found in a variable proportion of leukocytes of female subjects.

ture. It measures about 1 μ in diameter and stains positively for DNA. In certain tissues, e.g., amniotic membrane, almost every interphase nucleus is chromatin-positive. In buccal mucosal smears, the most commonly used preparation for determining the X chromatin pattern, the proportion of X chromatin-positive nuclei in females may be lower than in other somatic tissues, but in most laboratories they are present in no less than 20% of well-preserved nuclei.

This sexual dimorphism in polymorphonuclear leukocytes takes a different form; in females, 1–15% of neutrophils (mean 2.5%) have a drumstick-shaped, dense chromatin accessory nuclear appendage that is not found in normal males (Fig. 9–7, *D*). These appendages have the same significance as X chromatin in other somatic tissues.

In patients with more than two X chromosomes, the

maximum number of X chromatin bodies in any diploid nucleus is one less than the total number of X chromosomes. In XXX females or XXXY males, for example, a maximum of two Barr bodies are present in diploid nuclei, whereas XY and XO individuals are X chromatin–negative (Table 9–3). Abnormalities in shape and size of the X chromatin body can often be correlated with structural abnormalities of the X chromosome. An abnormally small X chromatin body has been found in females with one normal X and one deleted X (XXp–) or with one ring X chromosome (XXr). A large X body is associated with a large X isochromosome (Xqi). When a structurally abnormal X is present, it is the aberrant X chromosome that replicates late and gives rise to the X chromatin (except in the rare unbalanced X autosome translocations or when the sex chromosome complement consists of two structurally abnormal X chromosomes).

X Chromatin and Gene Expression. In 1959, Ohno reported the first evidence that X chromatin arises from only one of the two X chromosomes in the interphase nuclei of female somatic cells (38). The staining characteristics of such nuclei arise from the fact that a portion of one X chromosome is highly condensed (heteropycnotic); the other X does not contribute to the heterochromatic material since, like the autosomes, it is extended and filamentous (39). This difference in staining quality also betokens a striking difference in the functional roles of the two X chromosomes. By studying the sequence of incorporation of ^{3}H thymidine into replicating chromosomes, Morishima, Grumbach, and Taylor showed that the X that gives rise to X chromatin completes its DNA synthesis later than does any other chromosome in the cell and that the maximum number of X chromatin bodies in a single diploid nucleus is equal to the number of late-replicating X chromosomes (Fig. 9–8) (15, 16). These observations and the incisive genetic studies of Mary Lyon, Beutler, and other workers have led to the concept (Lyon hypothesis) that only one X chromosome per cell is genetically active during interphase; the other, which retains its heterochromatic properties, is genetically inactive for many of

Table 9–3. SEX CHROMOSOME COMPLEMENT CORRELATED WITH X CHROMATIN AND Y BODIES IN SOMATIC INTERPHASE NUCLEI*

	Maximum Number in Diploid Somatic Nuclei	
Sex Chromosomes	X Bodies	Y Bodies
45,XO	0	0
46,XX	1	0
46,XY	0	1
47,XXX	2	0
47,XXY	1	1
47,XYY	0	2
48,XXXX	3	0
48,XXXY	2	1
48,XXYY	1	2
49,XXXXX	4	0
49,XXXXY	3	1
49,XXXYY	2	2

*The maximum number of X chromatin bodies in diploid somatic nuclei is one less than the number of X's, whereas the maximum number of Y fluorescent bodies is equivalent to the number of Y's in the chromosome constitution.

its functions (40, 41). Lyon has critically and comprehensively reviewed X chromosome inactivation (42).

The change in state (heterochromatinization) of one of the X chromosomes in each female cell appears to be induced during the late blastocyst stage, between the twelfth and the eighteenth day in the human embryo (6). The female germ cells beyond the stage of oögonia are the only cell lines known to be exempted from heterochromatinization, a finding in keeping with the requirement for a second X chromosome for normal ovarian differentiation to take place. Epstein has provided evidence that both X chromosomes in mouse oöcytes are active and code for the X-linked genes, glucose-6-phosphate dehydrogenase and hypoxanthine-guanine phosphoribosyl transferase (43). This observation has been confirmed in human fetal and postnatal oöcytes (44). In each of the other cells, it is by random chance whether the maternally or the paternally derived X chromosome becomes the inactive one. Once

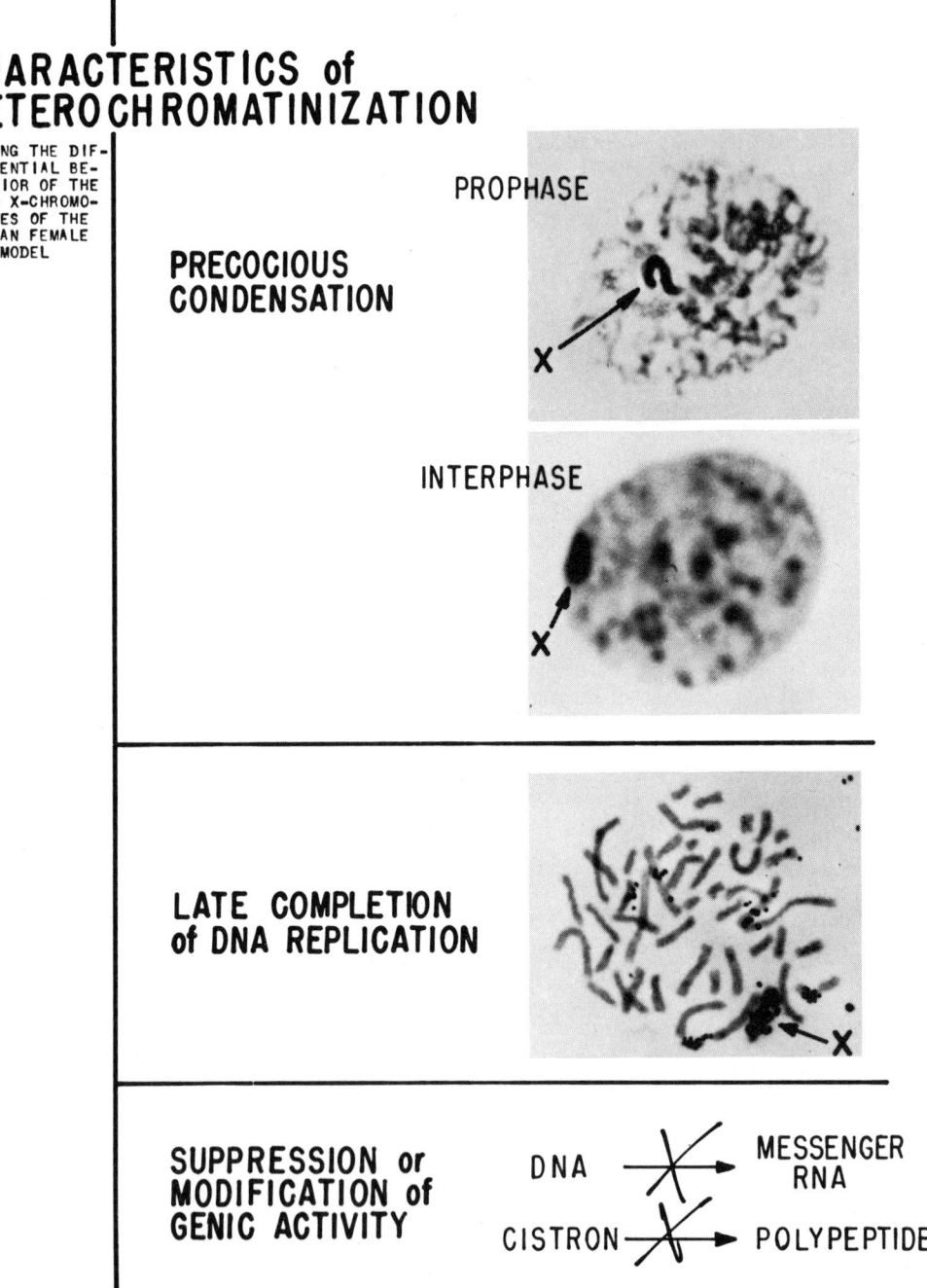

Figure 9–8. Characteristics of heterochromatinization as exemplified by the differential behavior of the two X chromosomes of the female in somatic cells. *1*, Precocious condensation of a large part of one of the two X chromosomes in prophase and the formation of the X chromatin body in interphase nuclei; *2*, delayed replication of DNA in one of the X chromosomes (the arrow indicates silver grains overlying one X chromosome in the autoradiogram of metaphase chromosomes from a normal female exposed to tritiated thymidine late in the synthetic period); *3*, suppression or modification of genic activity in the heterochromatinized portions of one X chromosome. (From Grumbach, M. M.: *Second International Conference on Congenital Malformations.* New York, International Congress, Ltd., 1963, p. 63.)

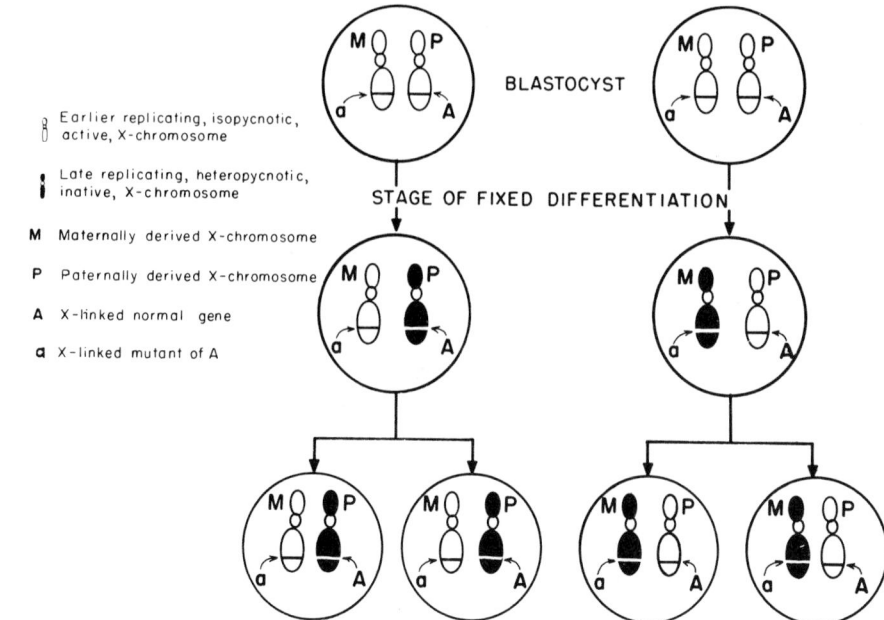

Figure 9–9. Diagrammatic representation of the fixed differentiation or Lyon hypothesis of X chromosome behavior in somatic cells of the human female. At the late blastocyst stage (the time when X chromatin can first be identified), one of the two X chromosomes becomes heterochromatinized in each cell and gives rise to an X chromatin body; it is by random chance in each cell whether this differentiation involves the maternally derived X (X^M) or the paternally derived X (X^P). Once the differentiation has occurred, this characteristic is fixed in succeeding generations of somatic cells. The genes on the heterochromatinized portion of an X chromosome are suppressed or inactivated, thus serving as a means of "dosage compensation" for the increased number of X-linked genes in the female relative to the male. This mechanism has an important bearing on the expressivity and penetrance of an X-linked mutant gene in a heterozygous female. In the diagram, the maternally derived X carries a mutant gene (a) which is only expressed in cells in which this X is the isopycnotic, euchromatic active X (white X^M). Although the heterochromatinized X (black X) in this diagram is represented as being wholly inactive, it should be emphasized that some loci on the heterochromatinized X do remain active and exert genetic effects. It should also be noted that the female germ-cell line beyond the oögonia stage is exempted from heterochromatinization. (From Grumbach, M. M., In *Biologic Basis of Pediatric Practice.* Cooke, R. E. (ed.), New York, McGraw-Hill, 1967.)

this transformation is established, however, the inactive state of that particular X chromosome is transmitted to all descendants of that cell. This control system appears to function as a mechanism of dosage compensation by which each female somatic cell functions as if it had virtually only one genetically active X chromosome (42). The female, therefore, in effect, has no more active genetic material than does the male. This hypothesis is variously referred to as the "inactive X theory," the "Lyon hypothesis," or the "fixed differentiation hypothesis of X chromosome behavior."

The implication that normal females function as genetic mosaics insofar as X-linked traits are concerned has found its strongest support in studies of the mouse (45) and in studies of X-linked traits in man (41). Davidson, Nitowsky, and Childs demonstrated two populations of cells in females who were heterozygous for a mutant form of the X-linked gene, glucose-6-phosphate dehydrogenase, which has an electrophoretic mobility different from the normal form (46) (Fig. 9–9). Heterochromatinization of all

X chromosomes in excess of one also provides an explanation for the relatively minor phenotypic changes seen in women with more than two X chromosomes, since the supernumerary X chromosomes are also heterochromatinized and therefore relatively inactive (Fig. 9–10). By way of contrast, strikingly severe changes are usually associated with trisomy for an autosome as small as chromosome No. 21, as in the case of Down syndrome. Little is known about the molecular basis of X-chromosome inactivation (15, 41); changes in the structure of DNA or of DNA-protein interactions that alter chromatin conformation may be involved. Modification of DNA by methylation is a possible mechanism of segmental inactivation of the second X chromosome (45). New knowledge of the structure and molecular chemistry of chromosomes and the development of methods to isolate single X chromosomes and to analyze gene sequences by recombinant DNA techniques may clarify fundamental aspects of the X-inactivation process.

It should be emphasized that in man, in contrast to the

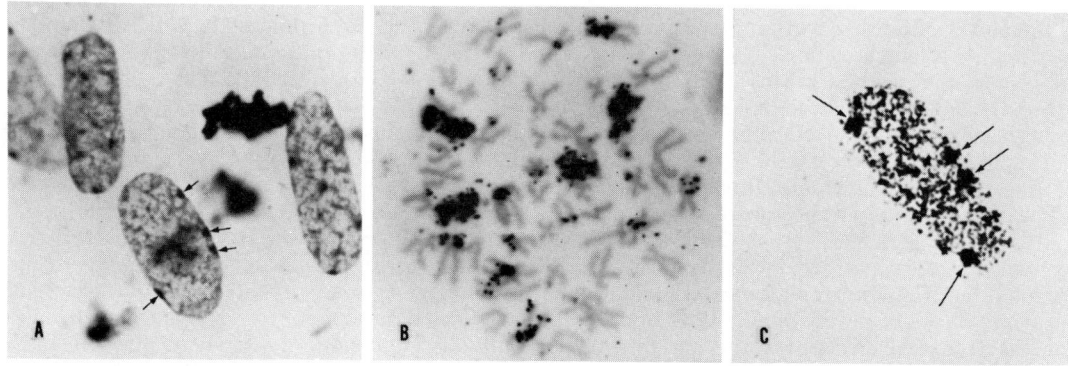

Figure 9–10. Diploid somatic cells from a girl with a 49,XXXXX karyotype. *A* Four X chromatin bodies in an interphase nucleus from a culture of skin fibroblasts. *B*, Autoradiogram of metaphase chromosomes, illustrating four areas of high grain density overlying four of the five X chromosomes. *C*, Autoradiogram of an interphase nucleus in a culture of skin fibroblasts; the four peripheral "hot" areas (indicated by arrows) of high grain density overlie four X chromatin bodies and provide direct evidence that each X chromatin body is derived from one late-labeling X chromosome. (From Grumbach, M. M., Morishima, A., et al.: *Proc. Nat. Acad. Sci. USA* 49:581, 1963, and Grumbach, M. M.: *Second International Conference on Congenital Malformations.* New York, International Congress, Ltd., 1963, p. 63.)

mouse, the inactivation of an X chromosome does not involve the entire chromosome. The heteropycnotic X in the human female is not completely, only segmentally, inactive genetically. Individuals with XO or XXY constitutions, for example, have abnormalities both in their sexual development and in somatic features unrelated to sex. Further, the red cell antigen Xg and the steroid sulfatase loci escape inactivation and are active on both X chromosomes in the female; both of these genes have been mapped to the distal part of the short arm of the X (47). This suggests that in normal individuals there are loci on both the heteropycnotic X and on the Y chromosome which are paired with a locus on the active X and which express a dosage effect.

While the female germ cell requires two active X chromosomes to give rise to normal oocytes (in contrast to the inactivation of one X chromosome in the somatic tissues), the X chromosome must be inactivated prior to meiosis in male germ cells for normal spermatogenesis to occur.

Genes and Testicular Organogenesis

H-Y Antigen and Testis-Determining Genes

The genetic sex of the zygote is established by the fertilization of a normal ovum by an X- or Y-bearing sperm. However, the mechanisms involved in the translation of genetic sex into a testis or an ovary are still poorly understood. The Y chromosome contains testis-determining gene(s) in its pericentromeric region which act in a dominent fashion and lead to differentiation of the bipotential gonad as a testis. Until recently little was known about how the Y chromosome regulated testicular morphogenesis.

Lately, a discovery with profound implications for sex determination emerged from the field of transplantation biology and the study of histocompatibility antigens in the mouse. In 1955, Eichwald and Silmser discovered the H-Y (histocompatibility Y) antigen, a male-specific cell membrane component in males of a highly inbred strain of mice that caused the uniform rejection by female mice of skin grafts from male donors of the same strain; grafts exchanged between other sex combinations were accepted (48). Antibodies to H-Y antigen were identified serologically in male-grafted female mice by Goldberg et al. in 1971 (49), and applied by a combined absorption and sperm cytotoxicity test to the semi-quantitation of H-Y antigen. In the cytotoxicity test, anti H-Y sera generated in the mouse or rat are absorbed with the target cells (e.g., peripheral lymphocytes or cultured fibroblasts from a male or a female). Unabsorbed anti H-Y serum and antiserum, absorbed with female cells, killed male sperm in the cytotoxicity test; the residual killing potency after absorption with male cells was reduced or lost as a result of removal by absorption of H-Y antibodies. In addition to mouse sperm, epidermal cells from the rat tail, and one human cell line, Raji human male Burkitt lymphoma cells, among others, are used as the source of cells in the cytotoxicity test. Other serologic assays for H-Y antigen are based on the direct or indirect detection of anti H-Y bound to target cells. The determination of H-Y antigen is still in an early phase of development. It is important to emphasize the technical difficulties and the questions concerning the specificity and reproducibility of the various serologic tests for H-Y antigen in man. There are uncertainties about the role of the major histocompatibility antigens in the serologic reaction (8, 50), and the relation of the immunoreactive and bioactive sites on H-Y antigen

to the serologic potency and specificity of a given mouse or rat antiserum to H-Y. One must not be unmindful of these caveats in the critical evaluation of the provocative and rapidly expanding literature on H-Y antigen, especially the clinical applications of the qualitative serologic tests for H-Y.

Following the development of the sperm cytotoxicity assay, Wachtel, Koo, and Boyse (51) discovered the invariant association of H-Y antigen with the heterogametic sex in a wide range of vertebrates, including mammals, birds, amphibians, and bony fish. In mammals, H-Y antigen is expressed in the heterogametic XY male but not the homogametic XX female; in birds the female is the heterogametic sex (ZW), and H-Y (or HW) antigen appears to act as an ovary organizer (26). The striking conservation throughout evolution of this ubiquitous cross-reacting minor plasma membrane histocompatibility antigen, its appearance early in embryonic development (in the mouse, pre-implantation male embryos at the 8-cell stage are H-Y antigen positive [52]), and its association with the heterogametic sex led Wachtel and Ohno and their associates to suggest that the phylogenetically conserved H-Y antigen is the factor responsible for inducing testicular organogenesis and that it is a product of the testis-organizing gene.

Support for this hypothesis was quickly obtained. XYY and XXYY men express increased amounts of H-Y antigen (26). XX sex-reversed sterile males in man, mouse, goat, and dog are H-Y antigen positive, as are XX true hermaphrodites and chromosomal males with testicular feminization (26, 53). In addition, the gonad of the bovine freemartin (the intersex XX twin of a male fetus) is positive for H-Y antigen (8). Further, these studies indicated that even in the absence of a discrete Y chromosome or karyotypic evidence of a Y to X chromosome or Y to autosome translocation or insertion, the presence of testicular tissue was invariably associated with a positive test for H-Y antigen (54). Evidence was adduced for the existence in multiple copies of either a structural or regulatory gene for the expression of H-Y antigen on the pericentromeric region of the Y-chromosome (26).

There is evidence in the Scandinavian wood lemming, that the expression of H-Y antigen is under the control of an X-linked gene; in the absence of serologically reactive H-Y antigen, XY animals develop as fertile females. This species shows a striking departure from the usual 1:1 male to female sex ratio. Fertile females can be XX or XY; the XY females produce only female offspring. Fredga et al. have shown that an X-linked gene in the fertile XY female wood lemming suppresses the expression of the testis-determining action of the Y chromosome, which previously had been functional in the male parent (55, 56). Later, Wachtel reported that these fertile XY females were H-Y antigen-negative (57). Two explanations have been considered: 1) a mutation of a regulatory gene on the X-chromosome restrains or suppresses the expression of the H-Y gene by the Y (or possibly an autosome); or 2) the structural gene is on the X-chromosome and a mutation at this locus prevents the expression of H-Y antigen despite the presence of the Y chromosome and its regulatory locus or loci for H-Y antigen. In any event, an X-linked gene seems essential for the production of H-Y antigen. In one form of familial XY gonadal dysgenesis, affected individuals are H-Y antigen negative (53, 58); as in the wood lemming, apparently an X-linked mutant gene in man prevented or suppressed H-Y antigen expression and, thus, testicular organogenesis (29).

Hence, the critical factor in testis organogenesis is not

the presence or absence of a detectable Y-chromosome *but the expression of H-Y antigen.*

Properties of H-Y Antigen and Its Receptors

According to Ohno, biologically active H-Y antigen is a protein composed of hydrophobic peptide subunits, each with a molecular weight of 16,500 to 18,000, which are linked by intersubunit disulfide bonds (54). The only gonadol cell known to disseminate antigen is the primitive Sertoli cell (8). H-Y antigen has been detected in all cell membranes from normal XY males except immature germ cells (8). There are apparently two receptors for H-Y antigen. Ohno (8, 26, 54) has proposed that one receptor is non-specific and ubiquitous and represents the stable cell membrane anchorage sites for H-Y antigen in all male cells; the anchorage site is conceived as an association of major histocompatibility complex cell surface antigens (HLA) with β_2-microglobulin. The second receptor is found only on gonadal cells, both male and female, and binds H-Y antigen with higher affinity than the non-specific anchorage site. The nature of the gonad-specific receptors that react with H-Y antigen to induce testis differentiation of the indifferent gonad is not known, but it is not dependent upon β_2-microglobulin. In addition to the H-Y negative form of familial XY gonadal dysgenesis, an H-Y positive form has been described (53). In these latter patients there is presumptive evidence of failure of the specific gonadal receptor to bind H-Y antigen as a result of defective or absent gonad-specific H-Y receptors; alternatively, the H-Y antigen in these patients may be immunoreactive but biologically inactive as a testis organizer.

Regulation of H-Y Antigen

A major uncertainty in the H-Y antigen story is the location of the H-Y structural gene, the gene that codes for H-Y antigen. Initially, the evidence tended to favor Y-linkage, possibly in multiple copies of the gene (8). As more knowledge was gained, alternative explanations have been advanced. The XY fertile female wood lemming (56, 57) provided strong support for an X-linked gene, either structural or regulatory, that is essential for the production of H-Y antigen. Studies of H-Y antigen positive familial forms of XX males in several species raised the possible role of an autosomal gene in the regulation of H-Y antigen (26, 53). A testis-determinant in XX males acts as an autosomal recessive gene in some human kinships (59) and in the goat (60), and as an autosomal dominant in other affected human families and in the dog (61) and the sex-reversed mouse (62). Excluding the forms of human XX males that may be due, for example, to hidden mosaicism for a Y-bearing cell line or a non-detectable translocation of the Y, the XX male has been interpreted by some as evidence for the presence of an H-Y regulatory gene locus or possibly a structural locus on an autosome. Alternative interpretations are at least equally plausible, namely the postulate of Ohno and Wachtel of translocation or insertion of some of the putative multiple copies of the testis-determining gene on the Y-chromosome, in some pedigrees to an autosome and in other kindreds to an X-chromosome (8, 26).

The present evidence tends to favor the Y- or X-linkage of the H-Y structural gene, in which case the opposite sex chromosome would contain the locus for an activator of the H-Y gene; in addition, the possible presence of a repressor of the H-Y structural gene on an autosome has not been excluded. Further, the alternative of multiple structural genes coding for H-Y on more than one chromosome remains a possibility. These issues will remain unresolved and speculative until the structural gene locus, or loci, for H-Y is established.

Exceptional or Anomalous Expression of "H-Y Antigen" in Man

Recently, several groups of workers have reported the detection of H-Y antigen in unexpected circumstances. H-Y antigen positive serologic tests were described in some patients with XO gonadal dysgenesis, and in association with an autosome translocation in a phenotypic female with primary hypogonadism as well as with other structural abnormalities of the X chromosome (usually a long arm isochromosome of the X) in phenotypic females with the syndrome of gonadal dysgenesis (50). None of these individuals had testicular tissue or a detectable Y chromosome. Two groups have reported the presence of H-Y antigen in some female-to-male transsexual patients and the lack of H-Y antigen in some male-to-female transsexuals, none of whom had inappropriate gonads for their chromosomal sex (63, 64). These observations, if confirmed, would be of interest, but the specificity and reliability of current serologic tests for H-Y antigen have been seriously challenged; thus far, the possibility that at least some of the findings are the result of false positive or negative serologic tests for H-Y antigen is highly likely. It must be emphasized that only a limited number of normal males and females have been tested for H-Y antigen, especially by the qualitative serologic tests used in these reports. Rat anti H-Y sera and the Raji lymphoma cell was the serologic test system in most of these studies. Questions of the specificity, reproducibility, and quantification of these technically difficult serologic tests for H-Y antigen must be addressed before one can interpret these discrepancies between a putative immunoreactive H-Y antigen and the gonadal and chromosomal sex. Ohno and Stapleton (65) suggest that some H-Y antisera may cross-react, even after extensive absorption, with major histocompatibility complex (MHC) antigens; further, H-Y antibodies usually recognize H-Y antigen associated with altered MHC antigen complexes and not H-Y antigen alone. Conversely, H-Y antigen "not in strong association" with MHC antigens of certain haplotypes may not be recognized by H-Y antibodies. The development of potent, highly specific H-Y monoclonal antibody and improved and reliable quantitative serologic tests would permit wider clinical application of assays for H-Y antigen and resolve many of the discrepancies, uncertainties, and controversies in the field.

Effect of H-Y Antigen on Gonadogenesis

A hypothesis for the organogenesis of the indifferent embryonic gonad as testis based on the observations of Wachtel and Ohno can be summarized as follows: The pericentromeric region of the Y-chromosome contains a locus (or loci) which either codes for the plasma membrane H-Y antigen or regulates its expression. The H-Y antigen is disseminated by cells in the gonadal blastema (possibly Sertoli cell precursors [66]), binds to gonad-specific H-Y receptors, and induces differentiation of the primitive

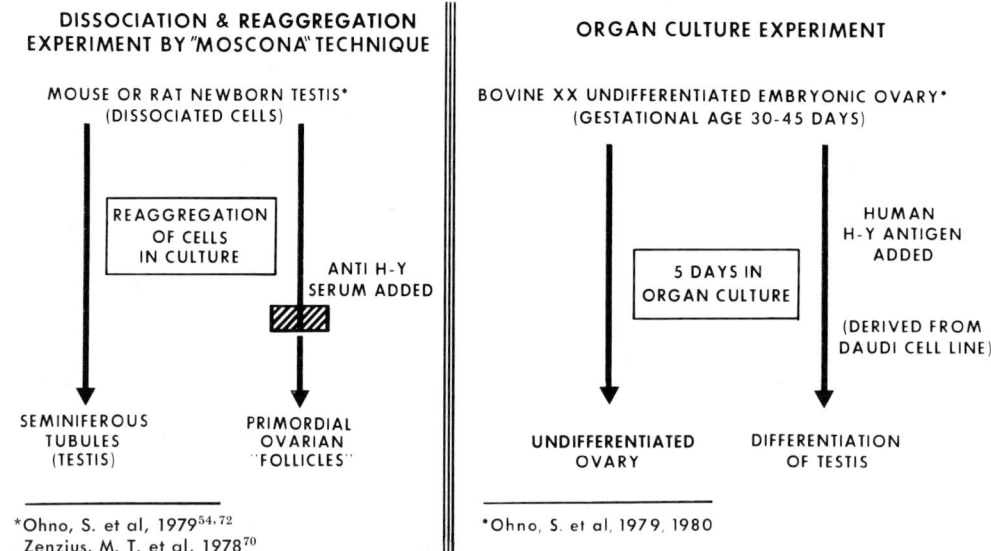

Figure 9–11. Diagrammatic scheme summarizing experimental evidence that supports H-Y antigen as the inducer of the testis in gonadal organogenesis. *Left panel*: In 1978 Ohno et al.[67] and Zenzes et al.[68] reported that a free suspension of newborn mouse or rat testicular cells when incubated in Moscona-type rotary cultures reaggregated to form seminiferous tubule-like structures. However, when the dissociated testicular cells were exposed to an excess of H-Y *antibody* (which leads to formation of a cap of specific cell surface antigen-antibody complexes over a pole of the cell and the subsequent autophagocytosis of the complexes by lysosomes — a process known as lysostripping), the cells formed ovarian primordial follicle-like aggregates but not seminiferous tubules. *Right panel*: In a series of converse experiments by Ohno et al.[54, 72] and Zenzes[70] et al., dispersed newborn rat ovarian cells and bovine fetal ovarian cells incubated in a medium containing H-Y *antigen* reassociated to form seminiferous tubule-like structures. In a critical experiment demonstrating the testis-organizing property of H-Y antigen, Ohno et al. showed that the indifferent gonads of chromosomally verified XX bovine embryos (25–30 mm in crown-rump length, about 40–45 days gestational age) maintained for 5 days in organ culture and incubated in a culture medium which contained concentrated human H-Y antigen "underwent complete and very precocious testicular differentiation" beginning with the formation of seminiferous tubules and by day 5, a tunica albuginea. XX indifferent gonads cultured in a control medium remained in the indifferent state. The H-Y antigen was purified from the media of a Daudi human male Burkitt lymphoma cell line that was β_2 microglobulin and HLA negative, and thus lacked the putative plasma membrane anchorage sites for H-Y antigen.

gonad as a testis. The embryonic gonad has an inherent tendency to form an ovary in the absence of H-Y antigen or its specific gonad receptor.

All of the evidence discussed previously in support of the testis-organizing function of H-Y antigen is indirect and circumstantial. However, recent experimental data provide more direct support for this hypothesis. In a series of experiments, Ohno and his associates (67) and Zenzes et al. (68) have reported cell dissociation and reaggregation experiments on newborn rat and mouse gonads (Fig. 9–11). Using the Moscona technique (69), a suspension of single cells from newborn mouse and rat testes was obtained. The free cell suspension was exposed to excess anti-HY serum and incubated in rotation culture. The H-Y antibody treated dissociated testicular cells reaggregated to form ovarian "primordia-like follicles," whereas untreated testicular cells reorganized as seminiferous tubules. In a converse group of experiments, free cell suspensions of rat newborn (70) or bovine fetal ovarian cells (54, 71, 72) exposed to H-Y antigen reorganized to form "seminiferous tubule-like" structures. Ohno et al. (54, 72) purified H-Y antigen from the culture media of a Daudi human male Burkitt lymphoma cell line which lack the putative H-Y anchorage site (β_2-microglobulin-MHC antigen dimers). Bovine fetal indifferent gonads (30-45 days of gestation) or known chromosomal sex were incubated for 5 days in media that contained purified H-Y antigen. The XX indifferent gonad exhibited testicular differentiation by the fourth day (54). These two types of experiments — 1) transformation of dissociated XY newborn rodent testes cells into ovarian follicle-like structures by treatment with H-Y antibody and 2) the induction of testicular differentiation in XX indifferent gonads by exposure to human or rat HY antigen — provide the most direct evidence in mammals for the testis-organizing function of H-Y antigen. It would appear that the capacity of H-Y antigen to induce the indifferent embryonic XX or

XY gonad primordium to differentiate as a testis is a consequence of the presence of gonad-specific H-Y *receptors* in both sexes.

Genes and Ovarian Organogenesis

As early as 1957 (73) it was suggested that two X chromosomes are required for differentiation of the indifferent gonad as a normal ovary, in contrast to the mouse and certain lower mammals in which an XO sex chromosome constitution does not prevent the development of a fertile ovary (42) (although it leads to accelerated atresia of ovarian follicles). Over the years there has been continued support for this postulate in man. Genes for normal ovarian differentiation are located on both the long and short arms of the human X chromosome, proximal to the telomeric portion of each arm. In XO individuals, oöcytes usually do not survive meiosis and folliculogenesis fails to occur or is defective; this leads to loss of germ cells and development of the gonads as streaks. In addition to genes on the X chromosome, the occurrence of familial XX gonadal dysgenesis, which is transmitted as an autosomal recessive trait, suggests that an autosomal gene, possibly expressed through its direct or indirect action on the germ cell, is essential for ovarian organogenesis. Among the latter possibilities, a mutant autosomal gene that leads to a defect in development of the "rete ovarii" or the synthesis or action of its meiosis-stimulating factor described by Byskov (74, 75) could result in familial XX gonadal dysgenesis.

Whether a counterpart to the H-Y antigen exists in the female and is involved in ovarian differentiation is uncertain. Preliminary studies by Wachtel and Hall (76) and Zenzes et al. (77) provide some support for this notion. A supernatant of the fetal rat or dog ovary, but not of adult ovarian cells, may contain a factor(s) which inhibits testicular organogenesis. More studies are needed before one can assess the significance of this potential ovarian-organizing factor.

Gametogenesis

Origin of Primordial Germ Cells. Primordial germ cells have been identified in the human in the 24-day embryo, at which time they are located in the dorsal endoderm of the yolk sac close to the allantoic evagination. From this site, the germ cells, increasing in number by mitosis, migrate during the fourth and fifth weeks to the hindgut wall and then through the dorsal mesentery to the primordial gonad in the urogenital ridge (78). In the complete absence of gonocytes, sterile gonadal ridges develop (31).

Spermatogenesis. During early testicular differentiation, the primordial germ cells become distributed throughout the primitive seminiferous tubules as progenitors of spermatogonia. During childhood the primordial germ cells remain quiescent and do not differentiate further until late in the prepubescent period. With the onset of adolescence, the basement membrane becomes lined by proliferating spermatogonia which have arisen by the mitotic division of primitive germ cells (79). The spermatogonia in turn give rise by mitotic division to primary spermatocytes. In striking contrast to the oöcyte, male germ cells do not enter meiosis until puberty.

The formation of haploid secondary spermatocytes from the euploid primary spermatocytes is accomplished by a special form of cell division known as meiosis. Whereas in mitotic division both daughter cells receive duplicates of each of the 46 parental chromosomes, in the first meiotic division each daughter cell receives only 23 chromosomes, one from each of the homologous pairs (Fig. 9–12). Thus half of the secondary spermatocytes contain 22 autosomes and an X chromosome, and the other half 22 autosomes and a Y chromosome. Each haploid daughter cell receives by random chance either the maternally or paternally derived chromosomes of each homologous pair, but not both. This process ensures great diversity in the genetic composition of the gametes, since by independent assortment and recombination of the paternal and maternal chromosomes constituting the 23 pairs it is possible to obtain 2^{23} different kinds of gametes. This was not the only mechanism for ensuring genetic variation, however, since the special nature of the prophase during this reduction division facilitates exchanges of DNA (crossing over) between homologous chro-

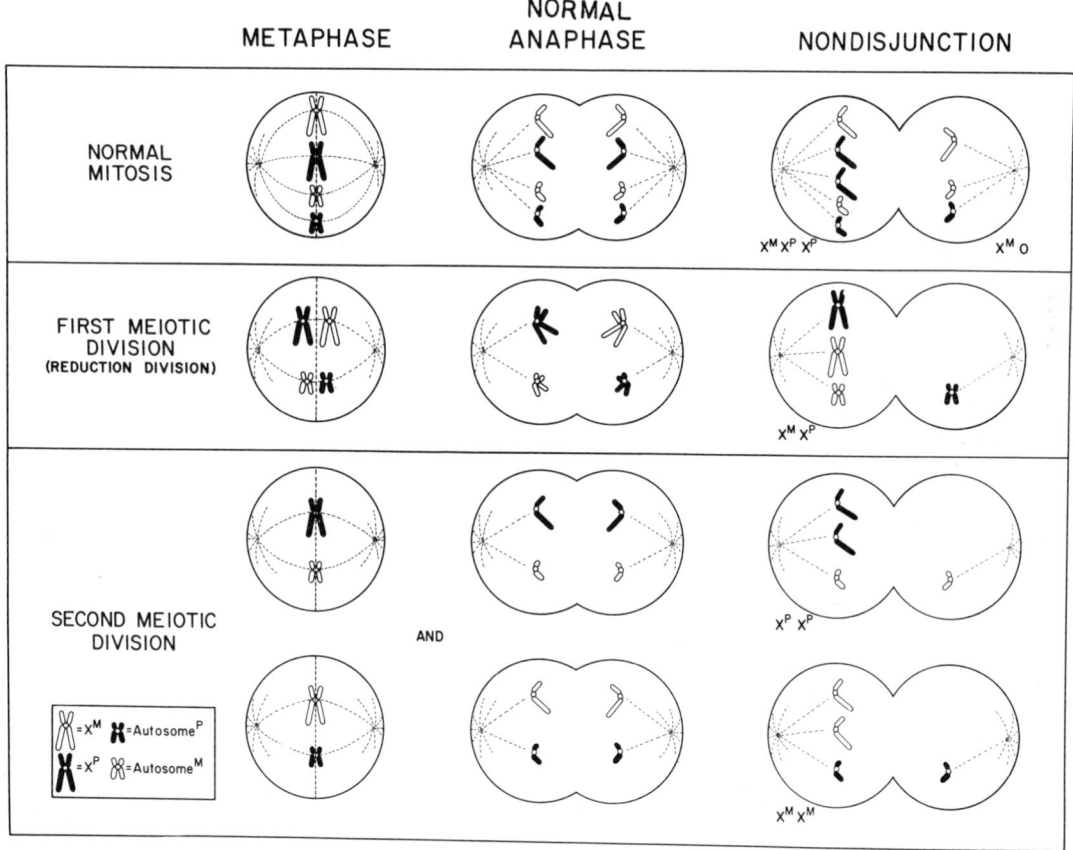

Figure 9–12. *Mitosis*, Diagram of female somatic cell undergoing mitosis. Represented at the metaphase plate are the two homologous C chromosomes and two homologous autosomes of the group 21–22. Division occurs through the centromere, giving two daughter cells of identical chromosomal composition. Replication of each arm into two chromatids takes place while the chromosomes are extended and prior to the next metaphase. *First Meiotic Division*, The first meiotic division involves pairing of homologous chromosomes. The centromere does not divide in this cell division. It is by random chance whether the maternal or the paternal member of each pair goes to the respective daughter cells. During the complex prophase of the first meiotic division (not shown), multiple chiasmata are formed between the chromosomes of each pair, thus facilitating exchanges of chromosomal segments (crossing over) between them. These peculiarities of the first meiotic division result in gametes with an almost infinite number of combinations of maternal and paternal genes. *Second Meiotic Division*, During the second meiotic division, the centromere again divides, giving daughter cells identical with the parent cell. This division more nearly resembles mitosis than the first meiotic division. *Nondisjunction*, Nondisjunction can take place either in mitosis or in the first or second meiotic division. Representative examples are illustrated.

mosomes. The details of this complex process are recounted in standard genetics texts.

Secondary spermatocytes give rise to spermatids by a second meiotic division, but this division is more analogous to mitosis than to the first meiotic division, since daughter cells are again produced by a longitudinal split of the two chromatid filaments comprising each of the unpaired chromosomes (Fig. 9–12). Thus the haploid number is not altered.

Spermatids do not undergo further division but rather develop into spermatozoa by a complex process of metamorphosis. Germ cells in the adult male are continually being renewed and undergoing maturation. Heller and Clermont have shown by labeling studies with tritiated thymidine that in adult males the complete cycle from spermatogonium to mature sperm requires about 74 ± 5 days (80).

Oögenesis.   Female germ cells pursue a considerably different course from that of the male. During ovarian differentiation, the primary germ cells undergo vigorous replication and successive differentiation into oögonia and primary oöcytes. The period of oögonial proliferation results in a peak population of about 6–7 million germ cells in the two ovaries at 5 months, including oögonia, oöcytes in various stages of prophase, and degenerating germ cells (81). Formation of oögonia from primary germ cells has ceased by the seventh month of gestation and is never again resumed. Some of the oöcytes remain in undifferentiated nests, whereas others form primordial follicles (78). The number of primordial follicles in the ovary is greatest at the time of birth, and from then on the number rapidly diminishes. In the germ cells that survive, the oöcyte is arrested at late prophase of its first meiotic division (diplotene state) and remains in this state from before birth until ovulation occurs many years later. The long life span of female germ cells, as contrasted with those of the male, may have an important bearing on the increased prevalence of certain chromosomal anomalies with advanced maternal age.

Just before ovulation, the first polar body is extruded, thus completing the first meiotic division. The haploid secondary oöcyte immediately begins its second meiotic division but remains in metaphase and does not extrude the second polar body until the ovum is penetrated by a sperm cell. The frequent finding of triploidy in spontaneously aborted fetuses can be explained either by failure of the second polar body to be extruded (polygyny) or by double fertilization (polyspermy).

Differentiation of the Testis and Ovary (3, 10, 82–86)

The gonads of both sexes develop from anlagen located on the medioventral border of the urogenital ridge, adjacent to the kidney and primitive adrenal (Fig. 9–13). Until the 12-mm. stage (approximately 42 days of gestation), the gonads of the male and female are indistinguishable on morphologic grounds and, indeed, could potentially differentiate either as a testis or as an ovary. The close ontogenic relationship between gonadal and adrenal cells at this early stage is noteworthy since, as differentiation proceeds, nests of adrenal cells frequently separate off with the gonad and are found as adrenal rests in the hilum of the mature ovary or testis. Such rests may become a problem in patients with long-standing untreated adrenal hyperplasia. Testicular rests, in particular, may later enlarge under persistent ACTH stimulation and be mistaken for tumors or true testicular enlargement.

The primitive undifferentiated gonad is derived from pro-

liferation of the mesodermal coelomic epithelium, the mesenchymal cell mass on the urogenital ridge, and from mesonephric elements (3, 82, 86, 87). Also in the primitive gonad are found the large alkaline phosphatase-containing primordial germ cells which have migrated from the posterior endoderm of the yolk sac through the mesenchyme of the mesentery to the gonad (86). By about 42 days, 300-1300 primordial germ cells have seeded the undifferentiated gonad. These large cells will later become either oögonia or spermatogonia. Lack of these germ cells is incompatible with ovarian differentiation but apparently does not prevent testicular morphogenesis. The role of the primordial germ cells in testis differentiation is still unsettled. The origin of the Sertoli cell of the testis and its counterpart in the ovary, the granulosa cell, is not established in the human being. The gonadal mesenchyme, coelomic epithelium, and mesonephric tubules all have been suggested and none can be excluded. In the mouse the rete ovarii, a derivative of the mesonephric tubules, seems to give rise to the first granulosa cells (10, 75).

There is a striking sex difference in the timing of gonadal differentiation. Under the influence of H-Y antigen, testis organization begins at about 45 days' gestation (6 to 7 weeks). On the other hand the ovary does not emerge from the indifferent stage until 3 months, when the earliest sign appears — the beginning of meiosis as marked by the maturation of oögonia to oöcytes (3, 10, 84).

Testis.   Until recently, some embryologists believed that the testis is derived primarily from the medullary portion of the primitive gonad, whereas the ovary is derived primarily from the cortical portion. According to this concept, the testis and ovary are not strictly homologous, since they differentiate from different primordial structures. Witschi (88) suggested that in genetic males the medullary portion secretes an inductor substance that stimulates development of seminiferous tubules and inhibits cortical development; conversely, the cortex of genetic females was thought to secrete an inductor substance that inhibited testicular development and resulted in ovarian dominance.

Jost (85), Jirásek (3), and van Wagenen and Simpson (86), among others, have recently called into question the older histologic descriptions of gonadal differentiation that served as the basis for these theories. After carefully examining numerous early embryos, Jost (85) and Jirásek (3) concluded that it was impossible to identify primary sex cords as such prior to the 15-mm stage (about 45 days), when epithelial cords derived from the coelomic epithelium, the gonadal blastema, and the germ cells, antecedents of the seminiferous tubules, are already apparent in the male. With the onset of testicular differentiation induced by H-Y antigen (p. 435) and the incorporation of the germ cells into the primitive seminiferous cords, proliferation of the germ cells is suppressed, and differentiation beyond the primitive spermatogonial stage is arrested. This may be mediated by a Sertoli cell meiosis-inhibiting factor or by the isolation of the primordial germ cell from the meiosis-stimulating factor secreted by the rete testis (74). After testicular differentiation (43-50 days gestational age) occurs (3), the male could also be recognized by beginning atrophy of the primitive müllerian ducts (30-mm stage, about 60 days) and the differentiation of male external genitalia (40-mm stage, 65-77 days).

An early endocrine function of the fetal testis is the secretion by the Sertoli cells of the müllerian duct inhibitory factor, a glycoprotein, which functions as a paracrine secretion and by diffusion passes to the paired müllerian ducts and induces their dissolution (89). The versatile Sertoli cell also secretes H-Y antigen and inhibitor, nurtures the germ cells, synthesizes an androgen-binding protein, and, as noted, prevents meiosis.

Leydig cells are first found in 32- to 35-mm fetuses (about 60 days) and rapidly proliferate during the third month, after differentiation of the primitive testicular cords, and during the first half of the fourth month (3, 86); during this period the interstitial spaces between the seminiferous tubules are conspicuously crowded with Leydig cells. By the onset of testosterone biosynthesis at about 9 weeks, the Leydig cell has acquired hCG-LH cell membrane receptors, which are apparently induced by H-Y antigen (90). The Leydig cells, which have an active 3β-hydroxysteroid dehydrogenase, secrete testosterone, the regulator of male dif-

ferentiation of the wolffian ducts, urogenital sinus, and external genitalia. The plasma concentration of testosterone in the male fetus correlates with the biosynthetic activity of the fetal testes (91). Peak concentrations in the fetal circulation (200–600 ng/dl) are reached by about 16 weeks of gestation, comparable to values in the adult male (92, 93). Between 16 and 20 weeks the testosterone level falls to about 100 ng/dl; after 24 weeks the concentration of testosterone is low (in the early pubertal range). Testosterone in amniotic fluid shows a similar pattern (94). hCG secreted by the syncytiotrophoblast stimulates testosterone secretion during the critical period of male sex differentiation (93, 95). Whether hCG is required to initiate testosterone secretion in man is not known, and this aspect is com-

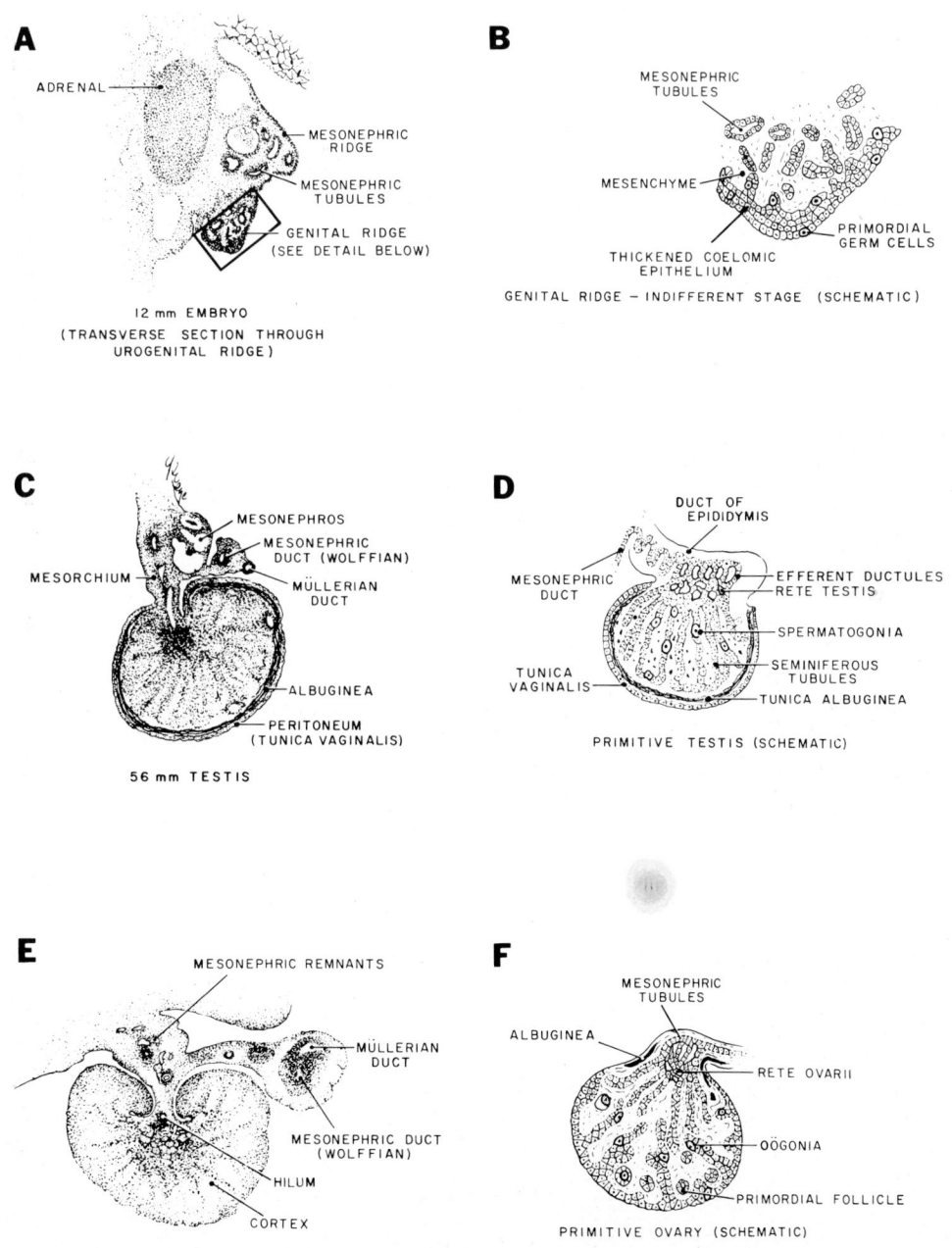

Figure 9–13.   Anatomic and schematic representations of gonadal differentiation. *A* and *B*, Transverse section through urogenital ridge at stage of indifferent gonad. Note proximity of large fetal adrenal to hilar portion of gonad. *C* and *D*, Transverse section through fetal testis at 56-mm. stage. *E* and *F*, Transverse section through fetal ovary at 60-mm. stage. In ovarian development, the coelomic epithelium continues to proliferate for a much longer period. (Redrawn from Arey[494] and Witschi.[495])

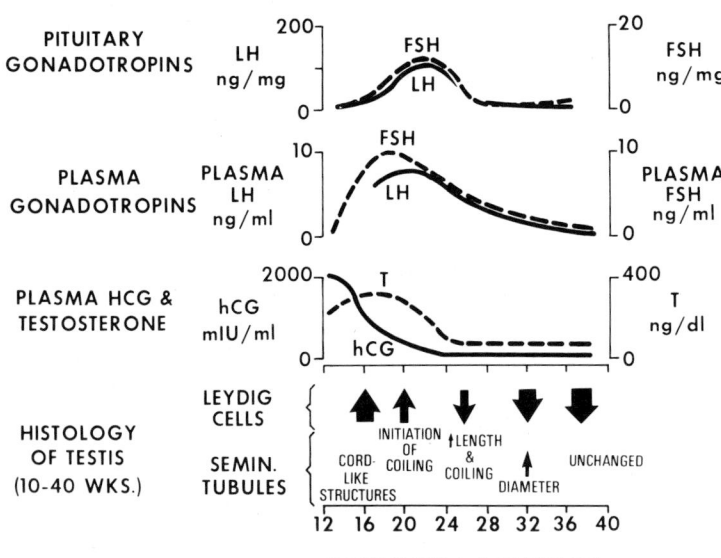

Figure 9–14. A comparison of the pattern of change of serum testosterone, chorionic gonadotropin (hCG), and serum and pituitary LH (LER 960) and FSH (LER 869) in the human male fetus during gestation in relation to the morphologic changes in the fetal testis. (From Kaplan and Grumbach.[93])

plicated by the discovery of hGH-like material in the fetal testis (96). The pattern of testosterone secretion early in gestation follows that of hCG (92, 93). The number of Leydig cells declines after 18 weeks and few cells show Leydig cell characteristics in the interstitium of the testis at birth. However, a low level of testosterone secretion is maintained after 15 weeks' gestation by both fetal pituitary LH and hCG (93, 97). Fetal pituitary gonadotropins are essential for the continued growth and function of the fetal testis after the critical period of sex differentiation. Fetal pituitary LH seems necessary in concert with hCG for the normal growth of the differentiated penis and scrotum and for the descent of the testes (97). The male fetus with anencephaly or congenital hypopituitarism often has hypoplastic male external genitalia and undescended testes; the testes have a decreased number of Leydig cells (93, 97).

Figure 9–14 correlates the pattern of testosterone, hCG, and fetal pituitary FSH and LH during gestation with the histologic changes in the fetal testis.

In sum, organogenesis of the testis involves successively the differentiation of the seminiferous cords with primitive Sertoli cells enveloping the extragonadal-derived germ cells, and the development of the tunica albuginea; the subsequent appearance of Leydig cells; and finally, differentiation of the mesonephric tubules into the ductuli efferentes which connect the seminiferous tubules and rete network with the epididymis to provide the pathway for sperm into the excurrent duct system.

Ovary. In the absence of H-Y antigen, the gonadal primordium has an inherent tendency to develop as an ovary, provided that germ cells are present and survive. The indifferent stage persists in the female fetus weeks after testis organogenesis begins. There is, however, continued proliferation of the coelomic epithelium and primordial germ cells, which gradually enlarge and become oögonia. Despite the discordance in the histologic appearance of the primordial testis and ovary, George and Wilson (98) have noted the simultaneous development at 8 weeks of gestation of the capacity of the fetal testis to synthesize testosterone and of the exclusive synthesis of estradiol by the fetal "ovary." Although the gonads of both male and female fetus have 3β-hydroxysteroid dehydrogenase activity at this stage, the activity of this enzyme is more than 50-fold greater in the fetal testis (98). While testosterone is synthesized by the fetal Leydig cell, the site of synthesis of estradiol in the primordial ovary is not known. However, Gondos has identified,

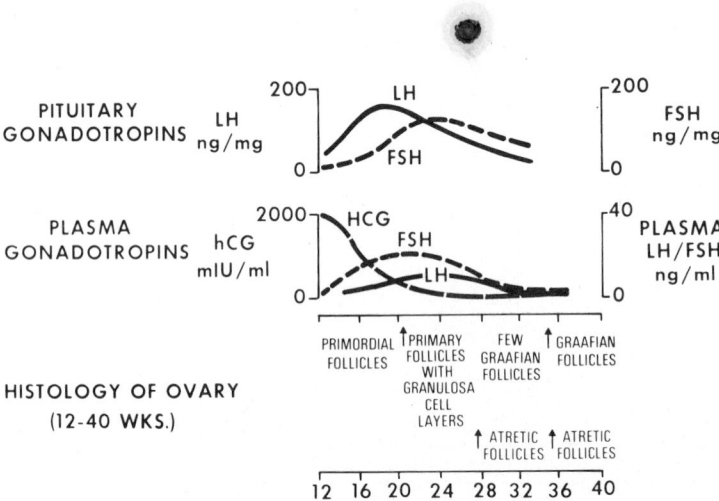

Figure 9–15. A comparison of the pattern of serum FHS, LH, hCG and pituitary FSH and LH in the human female fetus during gestation with the developmental histology of the fetal ovary. (From Kaplan and Grumbach.[93])

HUMAN SEX DIFFERENTIATION

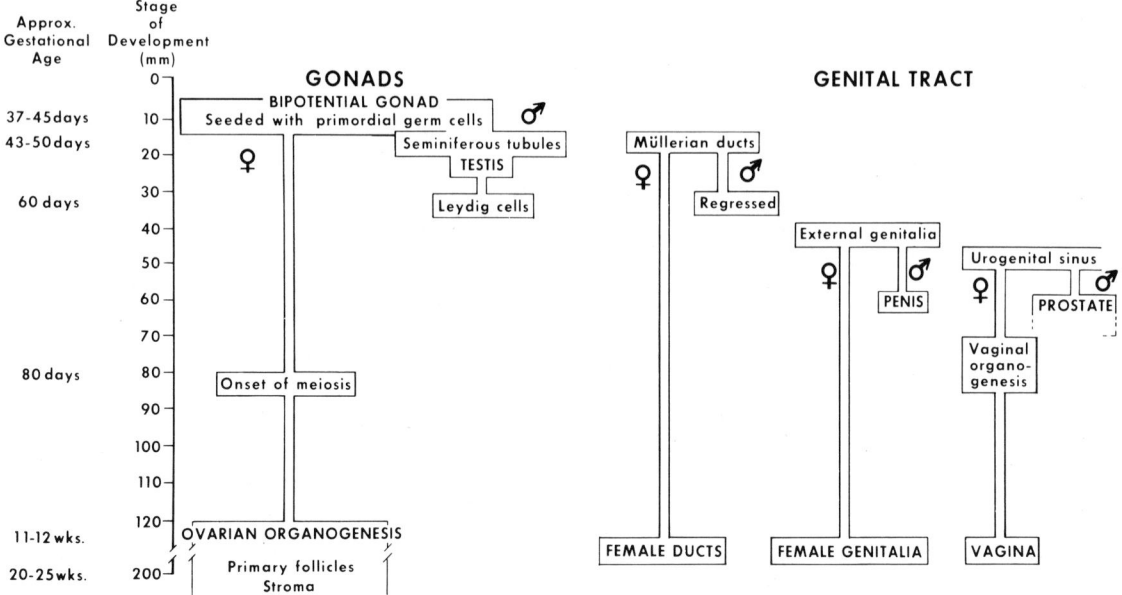

Figure 9–16. The sequence of sexual differentiation in the human fetus, as schematically depicted here, emphasizes that testicular development in the male fetus precedes all other forms of sexual dimorphism. There is an inherent propensity of the gonads, genital ducts, and external genitalia to feminize, whereas masculinization requires Y chromosome-mediated differentiation of the fetal testes. (Modified from Jost.[87])

at about 12 weeks of gestation, interstitial cells in the ovarian primordium that have the ultra-structural characteristics of steroidogenic cells (99). The fetus is bathed in estrogens of placental origin, and it is unlikely that the fetal ovary contributes significantly to circulating estrogens in the fetus. The ovary has no role in sex differentiation of the female genital tract.

During the ninth week the rete ovarii arises from the hilar mesonephric tubules and infiltrates the gonad as a syncytium of tubules and cords (10). About the eleventh to twelfth week (80 mm stage), long after differentiation of the testis in the male fetus, a significant number of germ cells begin to enter meiotic prophase, which characterizes the transition of oögonia into oöcytes; this event marks the onset of ovarian differentiation from the indifferent stage. The oögonia in the most central part of the ovary are the first to come in contact with the rete ovarii and the first to enter meiosis. According to Byskov (74, 75) the rete secretes a meiosis-inducing factor. The formation of primordial follicles (in which the oöcyte is enveloped by a single layer of flat granulosa cells) reaches a maximum during the twentieth to the twenty-fifth week of gestation; it is during this period that the plasma concentration of fetal pituitary FSH attains its peak (93, 97) and the first primary follicles are formed (Fig. 9–15). Hence, by the twentieth to the twenty-fifth week, the gonad has the morphologic characteristics of a definitive ovary. As discussed on p. 438, the maximum number of germ cells declines from between 6 and 7 million to 2 million at term. The last oögonia enter meiosis at 7 months of gestation. In the anencephalic female fetus, the ovaries are small and exhibit a decreased number and hypoplasia of primary follicles (93, 97). While the meiosis-inducing factor of the rete may be essential for meiosis and the formation of primordial follicles, the growth, development and maintenance of folliculogenesis are influenced by fetal pituitary gonadotropins, mainly FSH (93, 97).

The sequence and time of events in gonadal organogenesis and the relationship to the differentiation of certain male and female somatic sex characteristics are shown in Figure 9–16.

Differentiation of the Genital Ducts

At the seventh week of intrauterine life, the fetus is equipped with primordia of both male and female genital ducts derived from the mesonephros. The müllerian ducts serve as the anlagen of the uterus and fallopian tubes, whereas the mesonephric or wolffian ducts have the potentiality of differentiating further into the epididymis, vas deferens, seminal vesicles, and the ejaculatory duct of the male. During the third fetal month either the müllerian or wolffian ducts complete their development while involution occurs simultaneously in the opposite structures (Fig. 9–17).

It has been clearly demonstrated by Alfred Jost in classic experiments that secretions from the fetal testis play a decisive role in determining the direction of genital duct development (100, 101). In the presence of functional testes, the müllerian structures involute while the wolffian ducts complete their development, whereas in the absence of testes the wolffian ducts are resorbed and the müllerian structures mature (Fig. 9–18). These two events, the retrogression of the müllerian ducts and the stabilization and differentiation of the wolffian ducts, are mediated by two different fetal testicular secretions: (1) a glycoprotein müllerian duct inhibitory factor secreted by the Sertoli cells (89); and (2) the steroid testosterone synthesized by the Leydig cells.

Female development is not contingent on the presence of an ovary, since equally good development of the uterus and tubes will take place if no gonad is present. However, the müllerian duct fails to differentiate in the absence of the mesonephric ducts; commonly, renal aplasia and absent uterus is associated with a hypoplastic fallopian tube and uterus and vaginal agenesis (see p. 500).

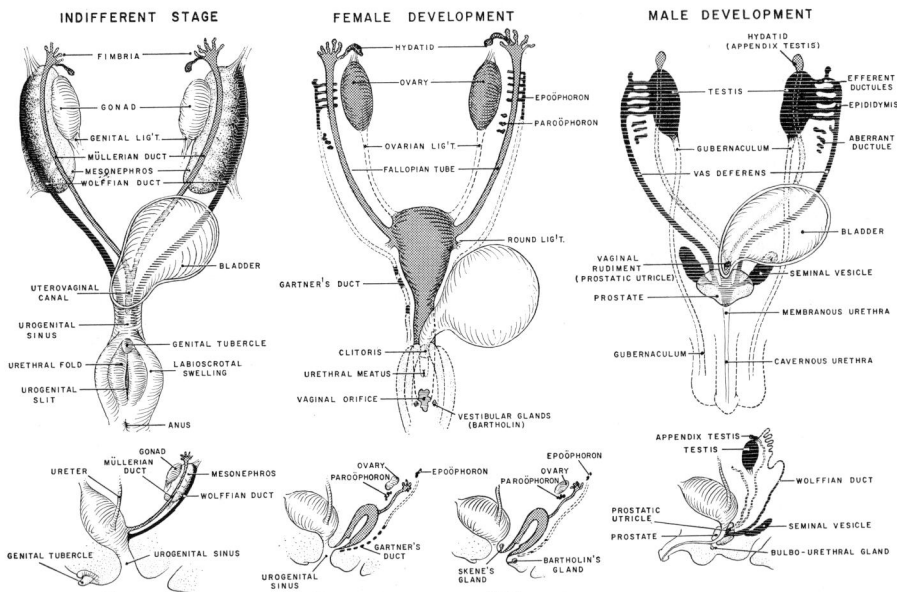

Figure 9–17. Embryonic differentiation of male and female genital ducts from wolffian and müllerian primordia. *A*, Indifferent stage showing large mesonephric body. *B*, Female ducts. Remnants of the mesonephros and wolffian ducts are now termed the epoöphoron, paraoöphoron, and Gärtner's duct. *C*, Male ducts before descent into scrotum. The only müllerian remnant is the testicular appendix. The prostatic utricle (vagina masculinus) is derived from the urogenital sinus. (Redrawn from Corning[492] and Wilkins.[493])

The influence of a fetal testis on duct development is exerted locally and unilaterally since, if one testis is removed at an early stage of development, the oviduct will develop normally on that side, whereas müllerian regression will occur on the side with the intact testis (101).

The systemic administration of androgen to an early embryo has under no conditions been observed to cause regression of müllerian structures. Even when high doses of androgen have been implanted locally in the gonadal region of female fetuses, the müllerian ducts have undergone no atrophy, although the wolffian ducts showed signs of stimulation (100, 101). On the other hand, if a testis is grafted onto an ovary, müllerian regression occurs on that side (Fig. 9–18). For these reasons, Jost proposed that the fetal testis secretes a müllerian duct-inhibiting substance that is distinct from ordinary androgens.

Nathalie Josso has studied the influence of the fetal testis on müllerian duct inhibition in organ culture (89, 102).

Direct contact between the testis and the müllerian anlage was not necessary to bring about this inhibition. By separating the testis from the müllerian ducts by dialysis membranes, she concluded that the material secreted from the testis was macromolecular and not a steroid. She also demonstrated that the human fetal testis, irrespective of its age, inhibits the müllerian ducts of 14.5-day-old fetal rats in similar organ culture studies, whereas the human postnatal testis has no müllerian duct-inhibiting activity. Using bovine fetal testes in which the tubules and interstitial tissue were isolated and assayed separately, she showed that müllerian duct-inhibiting activity was largely derived from the fetal seminiferous tubules rather than from the Leydig cells. Josso subsequently reported that the fetal Sertoli cell synthesizes and secretes the müllerian duct inhibitory factor (anti-müllerian hormone), a glycoprotein with an estimated molecular weight of about 125,000 (89, 103). The mechanism of action of this factor is not known

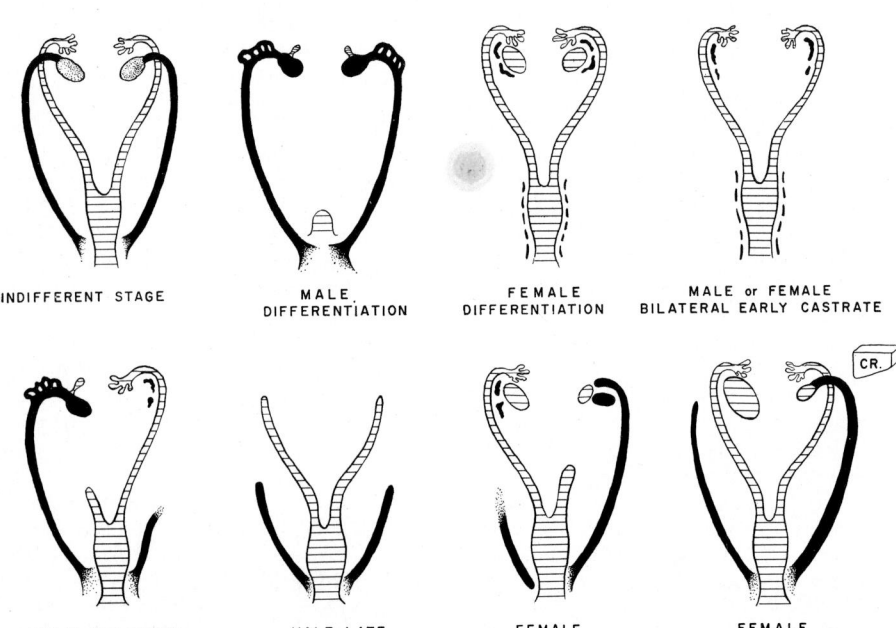

Figure 9–18. Schematic summary of Jost's experiments with rabbit embryos.[82] The fetal testis plays a decisive role in determining the differentiation of genital ducts. Testosterone stimulates wolffian development but fails to effect involution of müllerian structures.

but it appears to act through its effect on the underlying mesenchyme rather than the epithelium (104).

Studies of humans with various forms of hermaphrodism have abundantly confirmed that a nonsteroidal substance secreted locally by the fetal testis is the decisive factor in causing regression of the müllerian ducts. In patients with rudimentary gonads, the uterus and fallopian tubes develop normally regardless of the chromosomal sex. In true hermaphrodites who have a testis on one side and an ovary on the other, regression of the müllerian ducts is most marked on the side of the testis. Similarly, müllerian derivatives are notably absent in males with the syndrome of testicular feminization, a condition characterized by unresponsiveness of peripheral tissues to the action of androgenic hormones. Conversely, early intrauterine exposure of human female fetuses to high levels of androgenic hormones (as in the adrenogenital syndrome) fails to hinder normal development of the uterus and fallopian tubes.

Although müllerian involution is not an androgen-dependent process, the stimulation of primitive wolffian ducts to differentiate into epididymis, vas deferens, and seminal vesicles requires testosterone and the cytosol androgen receptor . Androgen-insensitive XY human beings, mice, and rats treated with cyproterone acetate (an agent which blocks androgen action) show the expected regression of the müllerian ducts, but structures derived from wolffian ducts remain vestigial (105). Jost showed that the implantation of a crystal of testosterone adjacent to the fetal rabbit ovary stimulated the differentiation of male ducts on that side, but to a much lesser extent on the contralateral side; similar results were observed by grafting a fetal testis adjacent to the ovary (101) (Fig. 9–18).

The lateralization of these effects suggests that higher local concentrations of androgen are required for male duct stimulation than are required for masculinization of the external genitalia and derivatives of the urogenital sinus. Unlike the masculinization of the urogenital sinus and external genitalia, in which testosterone reaches these target tissues systemically via the circulation (a classic endocrine effect), the local diffusion of testosterone from the testis induces stabilization and differentiation of wolffian duct derivatives. This effect of an inducing-factor from one cell source on neighboring cells by local dissemination is referred to as a paracrine action.

A further feature of male duct differentiation is that during organogenesis these tissues lack the 5α-reductase which converts testosterone to dihydrotestosterone. Thus testosterone (not dihydrotestosterone) binds to the cytosol androgen receptor in the wolffian duct cells during the critical period of sex differentiation and induces the development of male duct derivatives. This is in striking contrast to the urogenital sinus and genital tubercle, which acquire this enzyme even before the testis has developed the capacity to synthesize testosterone (106). Dihydrotestosterone mediates the masculinization of the urogenital sinus and external genitalia.

In human patients with ambiguous genitalia, well-differentiated male genital ducts are seen only in those patients who have testes. Female patients with congenital adrenal hyperplasia do not display this development, even though their external genitalia may be highly virilized *in utero*. Patients with asymmetric gonadal differentiation likewise have asymmetric male duct development which correlates very well with the degree of testicular differentiation on that side.

If the critical role of the testis in male duct development is to provide a high local concentration of testosterone, it would be anticipated that male duct development would be deficient, even though testes are present, in patients with absolute defects in steroid biosynthesis (type VI congenital adrenal hyperplasia, p. 487) or in XY patients whose tissues are highly unresponsive to testosterone (complete syndrome of testicular feminization (p. 491). The epididymides and vasa deferentia of these patients are indeed hypoplastic or rudimentary. During sex differentiation testosterone and the müllerian duct inhibitory factor may mediate their morphogenetic action on the underlying mesenchymal cells rather than by a direct effect on the epithelial cells (107). The action of the hormone-stimulated mesenchyme on the epithelial cells appears to be a major factor in the morphogenesis of the male ducts and the retrogression of the müllerian ducts (103, 107).

Differentiation of External Genitalia and Urogenital Sinus

Origin of the External Genitalia

At the eighth fetal week the external genitalia of both sexes are identical and have the capacity to differentiate in either direction. They consist of a urogenital slit that is bounded by paired urethral folds, and, more laterally, by labioscrotal swellings. The urogenital slit is surmounted by a genital tubercle consisting of corpora cavernosa and glans (Fig. 9–19). The mucosa-lined urethral folds may remain separate, in which case they are called labia minora, or they may fuse to form a corpus spongiosum enclosing a phallic urethra. The fleshy labioscrotal swellings may remain separate to form labia majora, or they may fuse in the midline to form a scrotum and the ventral epidermal covering of the penis. The distinction between a clitoris and penis is based primarily on size and whether or not the labia minora have fused to form a corpus spongiosum.

By the 50 mm crown-rump stage, male and female fetuses can be distinguished by inspection of the external genitalia; in the male, the urethral folds have fused completely in midline to form the cavernous urethra and corpus spongiosum by 12 to 14 weeks of gestation. Penile length seems to increase linearly, at about 0.7 mm per week, from 10 weeks to normal term; a 12-fold increase occurs from 0.3 cm at 10 weeks to 3.5 cm at term, a rate of growth about 3.5 times that of the clitoris (108).

Origin of the Vagina

The urogenital sinus separates from a common cloaca in very early fetal life. There is disagreement about the relative contribution of the müllerian duct and the urogenital sinus to the vagina. However, the contact and interaction of the fused müllerian ducts with the urogenital sinus is essential for normal development of the vagina (109, 110). In normal female development, proliferation of the vesico-vaginal septum pushes the vaginal orifice posteriorly so that it acquires a separate external opening; thus no urogenital sinus as such is preserved. In male development the vaginal pouch is usually obliterated when the müllerian ducts are resorbed, although by appropriate techniques a vestigial blind vaginal pouch known as the prostatic utricle can sometimes be demonstrated.

The prostate gland and bulbourethral glands of Cowper in the male are outgrowths of the urogenital sinus; their differentiation is mediated by dihydrotestosterone and requires the presence of cytosol androgen receptors. In the female, the paraurethral glands of Skene and the vestibular glands of Bartholin have homologous origins (Table 9–4).

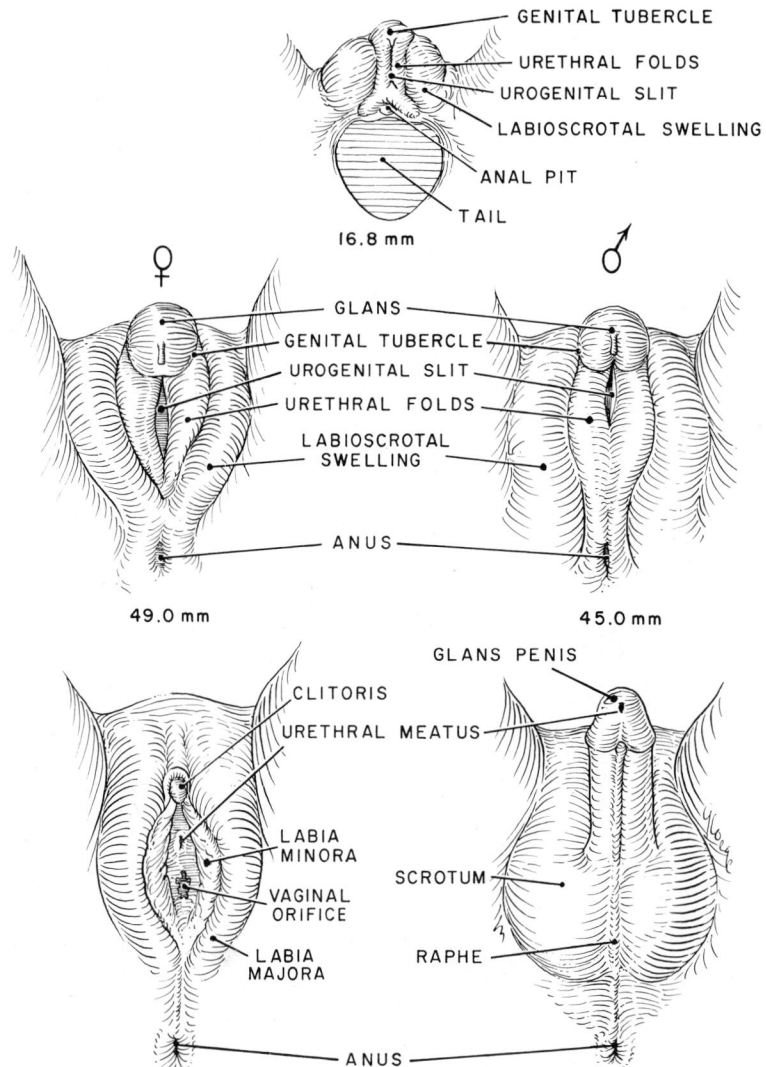

Figure 9–19. Differentiation of male and female external genitalia from indifferent primordia. Male development will occur only in the presence of androgenic stimulation during the first 12 fetal weeks. (Redrawn after Spaulding.[496])

Table 9–4. HOMOLOGIES BETWEEN MALE AND FEMALE SEXUAL STRUCTURES

Male Derivative	Primordial Structure	Female Derivative
	Gonad	
	Indifferent Gonad derived from	
Seminiferous Tubules	Coelomic Epithelium	Graafian Follicles
Sertoli cells	Mesenchymal Cell Mass	Granulosa Cells
Leydig Cells	Mesonephric Elements	Theca Cells
		Interstitial Cells
Rete Testes		Rete Ovarii
Septa and Tunica Albuginea		
Tunica Vaginalis		
Spermatogonia→Sperm	Primordial Germ Cells	Oögonia→Ova
	Genital Ducts	
Ductuli Efferentes	Mesonephric Tubules	Epoöphoron
Aberrant Ductules		Paraoöphoron
Epididymis	Mesonephric (Wolffian) Ducts	Gartner's Ducts
Vas Deferens		
Seminal Vesicles		
Ejaculatory ducts		
Appendix Testis (hydatid)	Müllerian Ducts	Fallopian Tubes
		Uterus
		Upper Vagina
	External Genitalia	
Penis	Genital Tubercle	Clitoris
Corpora Cavernosa		Corpora Cavernosa
Glans Penis		Glans Clitoris
Corpus Spongiosum (enclosing penile urethra)	Urethral Folds	Labia Minora
Scrotum & Ventral Epidermis of Penis	Labio-scrotal Swellings	Labia Majora
Prostate	Urogenital Sinus	Para-Urethral Glands (of Skene)
Bulbo-Urethral Glands (of Cowper)		Bartholin's Glands
Prostatic Utricle (vagina masculinus)		Vagina (lower)

Mechanism of Androgen Action (111, 112)

Our understanding of the action of steroid hormones has increased enormously over the past two decades. The target cells for a steroid hormone contain specialized protein molecules known as receptors that bind the hormone and mediate its effects on the cell. The central dogma of the mechanism of action of sex steroid hormones dictates the entry of testosterone into the cell by diffusion; conversion of testosterone to dihydrotestosterone in the cytoplasm by the enzyme 5α-reductase; the binding of dihydrotestosterone to a specific high affinity cytosol protein receptor; a conformation change in the hormone-receptor complex; the translocation of the activated complex to the nucleus where it binds to chromatin acceptor sites composed of DNA and non-histone chromosomal proteins in the target genome (Fig. 9–20). The interaction of the hormone-receptor complex with the chromatin of the cell nucleus activates gene transcription. After transcription and processing of the messenger RNA the specific RNA moves to the cytoplasm and is translated on cytoplasmic ribosomes; translation results in the synthesis of new androgen-induced proteins. The androgen receptor is regulated by a gene on the X chromosome (35), and this receptor, which has a high binding affinity for testosterone as well as dihydrotestosterone, is present in androgen-sensitive target tissues (and other somatic tissues, e.g., fibroblasts) of both males and females. Thus both sexes have the cellular apparatus for androgen action; the limiting factor is the plasma concentration of testosterone. A defect at any of the sequential steps in the action of androgen in a male fetus could result in impaired masculinization of the internal and external genitalis (Fig. 9–21).

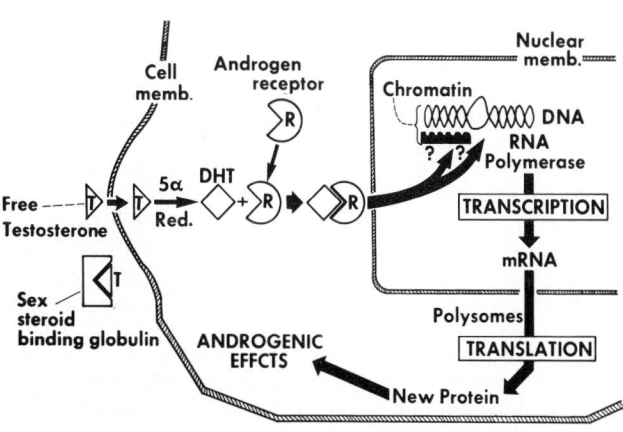

Figure 9–20. Diagrammatic representation of the mechanism of action of testosterone at the target organ. 5-α-Red = 5-α-reductase. DHT = dihydrotestosterone.

Role of Androgens in the Differentiation of External Genitalia and Urogenital Sinus

In contrast to the wolffian ducts, the induction of male differentiation of the external genitalia and urogenital sinus is effected by dihydrotestosterone, the 5α-reduced product of testosterone. Testosterone is the pro-hormone

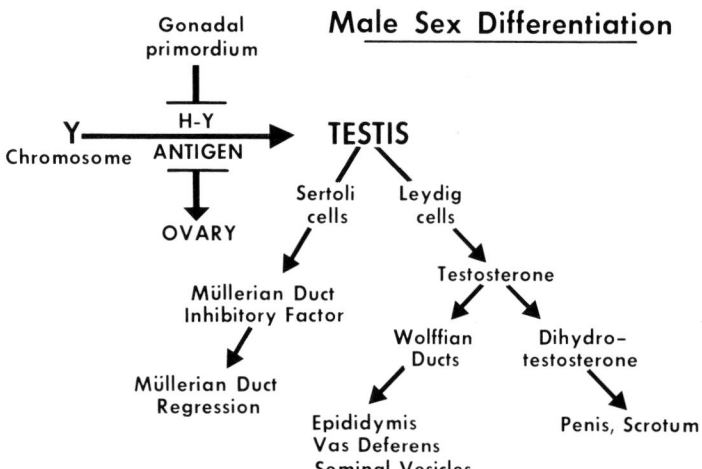

Figure 9–21. Scheme of male sex differentiation. (From Grumbach, M. M. In *Genetic Mechanisms of Sexual Development,* Vallet, H. L., and Porter, I. H. (eds.) New York, Academic Press, 1979.)

and is delivered to these target tissues by the blood stream. The cytosol of their anlagen is rich in the enzyme 5α-reductase and can convert testosterone to dihydrotestosterone, even before the fetal testis secretes testosterone (106). Dihydrotestosterone binds to the cytosol androgen receptor which is coded by an X-linked structural gene, and, after translocation to the nucleus, initiates the events that lead to androgen action. As in the case of the genital ducts, there is an inherent tendency for the external genitalia and urogenital sinus to feminize, without the intervention of fetal gonadal secretions. Male differentiation of the external genitalia and urogenital sinus occurs only if the androgenic stimulus is received during the critical period of sex differentiation early in fetal life. Dihydrotestosterone stimulates growth of the genital tubercle and induces fusion of the urethral folds and labioscrotal swellings. It also induces differentiation of the prostate and inhibits growth of the vesicovaginal septum, thereby preventing the development of the vaginal derivative of the urogenital sinus. These morphogenetic effects of androgen seem to be mediated by the specific mesenchyme of these tissues and not the overlying epithelium (107). After about the twelfth week, when the vagina has already separated from the urogenital sinus, fusion of the labioscrotal folds and urethral groove will not occur, even under an intense androgenic stimulus (113). Androgenic stimulation will cause clitoral hypertrophy, however, at any time during fetal life as well as after birth. The male fetus with 5α-reductase deficiency and thus impaired conversion of testosterone to 5α-dihydrotestosterone has defective masculinization of the external genitalia and urogenital sinus including absence or hypoplasia of the prostate. However, at puberty, virilization of the external genitalia takes place under the influence of testosterone. Although this failure of testosterone to masculinize the fetal external genitalia has been ascribed to the inability of the target tissues to form dihydrotestosterone which binds to the cytosol androgen receptors, other explanations are possible. The androgen receptor has a high affinity for testosterone itself; as the fetal environment is rich in estrogen and progestins, the effect of 5α-reductase deficiency on the binding of testosterone to the androgen receptor and its action in the male fetus and at puberty may be different.

Whereas in lower species fetal pituitary gonadotropins are required to sustain the secretion of testosterone by the fetal testes, in the human, placenta chorionic gonadotropin also stimulates Leydig cell development. This probably explains why the external genitalia of male babies with anencephaly or hypopituitarism and pituitary gonadotropin deficiency usually differentiate normally in contrast to those of lower mammals hypophysectomized *in utero*. Incomplete fusion of the labial folds and retention of the vaginal pouch in male infants may therefore be attributed to a primary testicular defect leading to deficient androgen secretion or to failure of the target tissues to respond to androgenic stimulation. Conversely, if female infants are subjected *in utero* to androgenic stimulation from some extragonadal source, their external genitalia can exhibit any degree of masculinization, ranging from simple clitoral hypertrophy to the formation of a normal-appearing penis. Thus identical external abnormalities can be produced in the male by androgen deficiency (or failure of the target tissues to respond) or in the female by exposure to androgen from some pathologic source in the fetus or mother.

Endocrine and Paracrine Control Mechanisms in Sex Differentiation

The regulation of sex differentiation by chemical messengers involves two types of control mechanisms. One is the classic endocrine mechanism: a cell, usually in a discrete endocrine gland, secretes a peptide, steroid, or other molecule into the bloodstream where it is transported to a distant target tissue to regulate or induce differentiation. In this context, a striking example of an endocrine secretion is testosterone: testosterone secreted by the fetal Leydig cell is delivered via the circulation to the anlagen of the external genitalia and urogenital sinus. Another is chorionic gonadotropin (hCG), which is synthesized by the syncytiotrophoblast and acts on the Leydig cell to stimulate testosterone secretion.

The second type of control mechanism in sex differentiation is mediated by paracrine secretion. This local and more primitive regulatory mechanism involves the dissemination of a peptide or steroid from its site of synthesis to its target cell or tissues by local diffusion through the extracellular space. Examples of this delivery system for chemical messengers are the action of müllerian duct inhibitory factor on the müllerian duct, the action of testosterone on the wolffian duct (in this instance testosterone is a paracrine secretion), and the dissemination of H-Y antigen within the gonadal blastema. Table 9–5 lists some of the chemical messengers involved in sex differentiation and classifies their effect as mediated by an endocrine or paracrine control mechanism.

Table 9–5. PARACRINE AND ENDOCRINE MECHANISMS IN SEX DIFFERENTIATION

| | Paracrine Mechanisms | | | Endocrine Mechanisms | |
Agent	Source	Target	Agent	Source	Target
			Testes		
H-Y antigen	Sertoli cell	Gonadal blastema (specific H-Y cell membrane receptors)	Chorionic gonadotropin	Synctio-trophoblast	Leydig cell (cell membrane receptor)
Meiosis-inhibiting factor	Sertoli cell	Spermatogonia	Testosterone (dihydro-testosterone)	Leydig cell	Urogenital sinus and external genitalia (cytosol androgen receptors)
Müllerian duct inhibitory factor	Sertoli cell	Müllerian ducts			
Testosterone	Leydig cell	Wolffian ducts (cytosol androgen receptors)			
			Ovaries		
? Ovary-inducing factor	?	Gonadal blastema (cell membrane receptors)			
Meiosis-inducing factor	Rete ovarii	Initiation of meiosis in oögonia	Fetal FSH	Fetal pituitary gonadotrope	Primordial follicle Folliculogenesis and maintenance of primary oöcyte
? Meiosis-inhibiting factor	Granulosa cell	Primary oöcyte			

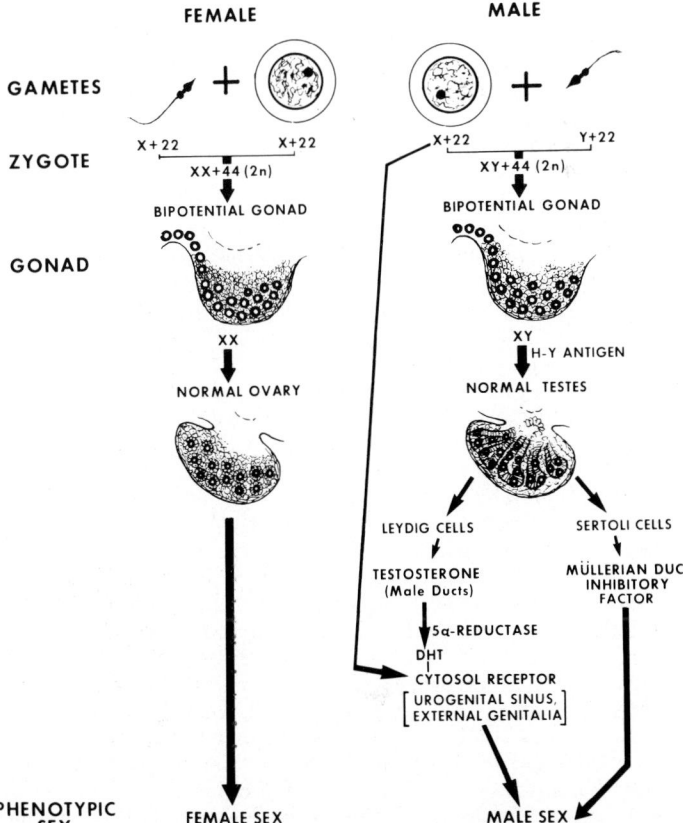

Figure 9–22. A diagrammatic representation of human sex determination and differentiation. Intrinsic or extrinsic factors adversely affecting any stage of these processes can lead to anomalies of sex.

Hormonal Sex Differentiation

Sex differentiation is not completed until the secondary sex characteristics have developed, fertility is attained, and the ultimate goal, procreation, becomes possible (Fig. 9–22). These developments occur during puberty. In the past we regarded puberty as a *de novo* event because of the dramatic changes brought about by the maturation of the gonads and the increased secretion of sex steroids. However, the development of gonadal function can now be viewed as a continuum extending from sex differentiation of the gonad and the ontogeny of the hypothalamic-pituitary-gonadal system in the fetus, through puberty, to the attainment of full sexual maturation and fertility. Puberty is not an isolated event but rather a critical stage in a sequence of complex maturational changes. The hypothalamic-pituitary gonadotropin unit (including the pulsatile secretion of the hypothalamic gonadotropin-releasing factor and of FSH and LH) matures in the fetus, is suppressed to a low level of activity during childhood for about a decade, and is reactivated at the onset of puberty. The hormonal changes and the neuroendocrinology of puberty, including adrenarche and gonadarche, are reviewed elsewhere (114, 115).

Sexual Differentiation in the Hypothalamus

Although in both sexes the control of gonadal function is mediated by both FSH and LH, the secretory patterns of the gonadotropins are very different in males and females. In man and many other species, the male pituitary gland characteristically secretes both FSH and LH in a pulsatile but relatively constant and sustained manner — so-called tonic release, whereas in the adult female, secretion of FSH and LH is cyclic and is characterized by a preovulatory surge which leads to ovulation.

In 1936, Pfeiffer reported studies in the rat suggesting that during the early postnatal period the pituitary becomes differentiated according to the nature of the gonads present in the individual (116). Subsequently it was shown, however, that the cyclic secretory pattern characteristic of the female pituitary is not an innate property of the pituitary itself. The pituitary of a male animal, when grafted under the hypothalamus of an adult female, is fully able to sustain the rhythm of repeated estrus cycles. When the male pituitary is grafted elsewhere in the recipient, ovulation fails to occur. Observations such as these suggest that the hypothalamus or higher neural centers function differently in the two sexes (117, 118, 119). It is now clear from the contributions of many workers that in the rat, mouse, hamster, guinea pig, and sheep there is an apparently inherent tendency toward the development of a female neurohypophysial pattern of gonadotropin release and that this pattern is converted to a male pattern if the newborn animal is exposed to androgens or estrogens during the neonatal period (117, 118, 119); in the guinea pig and sheep the androgen must be administered prenatally. Once the male pattern has been imprinted on sex centers in the hypothalamus (usually by testicular androgens), the potential for cyclic activity on the part of the hypophysis is irrevocably lost. In the rat, the critical period is the first 10 days of life. Female rats given as little as 1 μg. of testoterone during this period exhibit structural changes in certain regions of the hypothalamus (120, 121) and develop permanent sterility, since gonadotropin secretion at maturity is sustained rather than cyclic, and ovulation does not occur. The ovaries of these rats develop multiple follicular cysts and no corpora lutea. Similarly, if male rats are castrated during the first few days of life, later ovarian implants form corpora lutea in a normal female manner.

In contrast, in man and subhuman primates, sex differentiation of the CNS mechanism mediating gonadotropin secretion does not occur even though testosterone has been administered to pregnant monkeys beginning early in gestation. Further evidence in support of species differences is the observation that most females with congenital virilizing adrenal hyperplasia, or females who have been exposed to androgens *in utero*, later develop a female-type FSH response to the administration of gonadotropin-releasing factor (122) and normal ovulatory cycles, although cystic ovaries have been reported in rare patients (123). Moreover, in both castrate men and male monkeys (124, 125), the acute rise in concentration of serum estradiol following estrogen administration has elicited a surge in LH secretion; this suggests that in primates the potential for cyclic gonadotropin secretion is intact and that androgen-induced differentiation of the gonadotropin regulatory mechanism comparable to that described in rodents and sheep is not applicable to man.

Psychosexual Differentiation (Gender Role) (126)

By gender role is implied not only a person's legal and social designation of sex but also his psychosexual identification of himself in relation to other members of his own and the opposite sex. Outward manifestations of gender role are the dress, mannerisms, social comportment, and orientation of sexual impulses.

In lower species, the sexual role adopted at maturity is determined by the hormonal environment in early life (5, 127). As is the case with other forms of sex differentiation, there appears to be an innate tendency toward the development of female sexual postures. Eventual development of male patterns of sexual behavior, on the other hand, is influenced to a large extent by whether there has been exposure to androgen in the prenatal period. This organizing capacity of certain androgens administered at a "critical stage" of development has been localized to specific areas in the brain. Once this has occurred, later castration of the male or exposure of the female to androgens may modify the intensity of the sexual drive but may not alter its pattern.

In contrast, the role of prenatal exposure to sex hormones on adult human sexual behavior is uncertain, and the evidence that exists is indirect. The behavioral changes attributed to prenatal exposure to androgens and progestins in females and to estrogens in males are subtle, do not appear to affect gender identity, and are within the broad range of normal although they may modify the cultural stereotype for sex behavior of normal males and females (126). On the other hand, testosterone has a potent influence on sexual behavior and drive at the time of puberty. Imperato-McGinley and Peterson et al. reported an effect of testosterone on gender identity and a reversal of gender role at puberty in a small group of pseudohermaphrodites with 5α-reductase deficiency reared in isolated villages in the Dominican Republic (128).

Studies of humans who have been reared in a sex opposite to their own chromosomal or gonadal sex provide strong evidence that the gender role is not itself coded on the sex chromosomes, nor need it necessarily be concordant with the gonadal or hormonal sex (5, 129, 130). Social and environmental influences during the early years of life exert such a strong impact on subsequent gender identity that some authors have discounted the importance of organic or hormonal influences. According to this concept, a newborn infant is neuter at birth, and the gender role is learned through early childhood experiences. A child is continually reminded of his sexual identification by the words and attitudes of those around him, by the clothes he wears, and by comparison of his own genitalia with those of others. In the absence of ambiguous attitudes on the part of the parents, sexual identity is well established by 18–30 months of age, even though there may exist some external genital discrepancy. Even the subsequent development of paradoxical secondary sexual characteristics and hormonal patterns characteristic of the opposite sex *may* not shake this conviction of sexual identity if it has been fixed with sufficient strength early in life. However, this does not preclude an important influence of sex hormones at puberty on human sexual behavior. The study of Imperato-McGinley et al. (128) is a serious challenge to the hypothesis of Money that gender identity is usually irreversibly fixed by environmental factors alone by two years of age. The apparent plasticity of gender identity in the cultural isolate that she studied has important implications for our understanding of the effects of sex hormones on psychosocial differentiation. It must not be applied, however, to the assignment of sex in patients with abnormalities of sex differentiation, since in our cultural setting the weight of evidence strongly supports environmental factors as the principal determinant of gender identity (126). These considerations have an important bearing on the management of children born with ambiguous sexual characteristics.

In recent years, there has been a tendency to give stronger credence to the role of early hormonal influences on the patterning of adult sexual behavior in the human (126). Diamond (127) has reexamined the "neutrality at birth" hypothesis and presented arguments that humans, like other species, are already at birth, or very soon thereafter, predisposed to a male or female gender orientation, depending on whether or not an androgenic imprint has been left on the critical neural centers. Most observers have failed to detect any evidence of hypogonadism or diminished virility in the majority of male homosexuals (5). This conclusion has recently been challenged by several studies which suggest that a substantial number of male homosexuals have abnormally low plasma testosterone levels. In 1971, Kolodny et al. (131) reported that, among a population of normal and homosexual college men, approximately 25% of the latter group had plasma testosterone levels below the lowest recorded values in a normal control group. Similarly, the group with the lowest testosterone levels ranked among the most extreme on Kinsey's 6-point rating scale for homosexuality. Many of these men had low sperm counts as well. These findings might possibly be attributable to some poorly classified form of congenital hypogonadism resulting in incomplete masculinization of the neural centers controlling sexual behavior. Other explanations, however, are equally plausible. Psychologic factors exercise an important influence on both sperm counts and testosterone levels. Both fall markedly during depressive episodes, and conceivably homosexuality per se or some consequence of homosexuality could be responsible for the diminished gonadal function observed in these patients, rather than the reverse.

If prenatal exposure to androgen predisposes to a male gender role in humans, it might be expected that female infants who were virilized *in utero* might display male sexual attitudes and postures in later life. Ehrhardt et al. (132) have found that prenatal virilization due to adrenal hyperplasia or maternal ingestion of progestogens does indeed influence the subsequent development of behavior, although to a limited extent. Such girls display tomboy behavior and greater interest in competitive sports than is usually expected of girls. They are often more interested in careers than romance and lack a strong interest in maternal doll play. However, the well managed patients have not displayed loss of feminine gender identity, and most of them eventually achieve a satisfactory female sexual role in marriage (reviewed in 126).

The eventual outcome of this "nature" versus "nurture" controversy is of practical importance, since it might possibly alter the attitude of society towards transvestism and homosexuality. The evidence obtained in both hypogonadal males, the syndrome of feminizing testes, and prenatally virilized girls supports the thesis that exposure to androgens before birth does play a role in programming a male gender role in later life. In both groups, however, there is abundant evidence that these hormonal factors are rarely decisive and that the most important element in the development of gender role is the assigned sex of rearing and the reinforcement that this receives during the period of infancy and early childhood and by hormone replacement therapy with the sex steroid appropriate to the sex of rearing at the normal age of puberty. If this reinforcement is weak because of ambiguous attitudes in the parents, the outlook for attaining a normal gender identity in adult life is greatly diminished. These interpretations are strongly supported by the empirical evidence obtained from the use of a pragmatic approach to the assignment of sex in patients with ambiguous genitalia. This approach, as outlined on page 501, has proven to be eminently successful and should not be lightly discarded.

CLASSIFICATION OF ERRORS IN SEX DIFFERENTIATION (Table 9–6)

In the past, individuals with hermaphrodism have been classified according to their gonadal morphology. In the terminology of Klebs, a true hermaphrodite is a person who possesses both ovarian and testicular tissue. A male pseudohermaphrodite is one whose gonads are exclusively testes but whose genital ducts or external genitalia, or both, exhibit the phenotypic characteristics of a female or incompletely differentiated male. A female pseudohermaphrodite is a person with exclusively ovarian gonadal structures whose external genitalia exhibit some masculine characteristics. Utilizing the rapidly advancing knowledge of chromosome and biochemical defects, we have classified errors in sex differentiation by a modification and expansion of this broad framework. We have attempted to blend etiologic mechanisms and clinical entities into a simplified rational classification. The striking clinical and etiologic heterogeneity of syndromes presenting with similar anatomic findings merits emphasis.

DISORDERS OF GONADAL DIFFERENTIATION AND SEX CHROMOSOME ANOMALIES

Not all patients with anomalies of their sex chromosomes have abnormal gonads and, conversely, congenital defects in gonadal differentiation cannot always be ascribed to chromosomal errors. The association is so frequent, however, that these topics are inseparable. Exceptions to this association are of special importance in defining the genetic and chromosomal determinants of gonadogenesis.

Table 9–6. CLASSIFICATION OF ANOMALOUS SEXUAL DEVELOPMENT

I. Disorders of gonadal differentiation
   A. Seminiferous tubular dysgenesis (Klinefelter syndrome)
   B. Syndrome of gonadal dysgenesis and its variants (Turner syndrome)
   C. Complete and incomplete forms of XX and XY gonadal dysgenesis
   D. True hermaphrodism

II. Female pseudohermaphrodism
   A. Congenital virilizing adrenal hyperplasia
   B. Androgens and synthetic progestins transferred from maternal circulation
   C. Associated with malformations of intestine and urinary tract (non-androgen-induced female pseudohermaphrodism)
   D. Other teratologic factors

III. Male pseudohermaphrodism
   A. Testicular unresponsiveness to hCG and LH
   B. Inborn errors of testosterone biosynthesis
      1. Enzyme defects affecting synthesis of both corticosteroids and testosterone (variants of congenital adrenal hyperplasia)
         a. Cholesterol desmolase complex deficiency (congenital lipoid adrenal hyperplasia)
         b. 3β-hydroxysteroid dehydrogenase deficiency
         c. 17α-hydroxylase deficiency
      2. Enzyme defects primarily affecting testosterone biosynthesis by the testes
         a. 17,20-desmolase (lyase) deficiency
         b. 17β-hydroxysteroid oxidoreductase deficiency
   C. Defects in androgen-dependent target tissues
      1. End organ insensitivity to androgenic hormones (androgen receptor and post receptor defects)
         a. Complete syndrome of androgen insensitivity and its variants (testicular feminization and its variant forms)
         b. Incomplete syndrome of androgen insensitivity and its variants (Reifenstein syndrome)
         c. Androgen insensitivity in infertile men
      2. Defects in testosterone metabolism by peripheral tissues
         a. 5α-reductase deficiency—male pseudohermaphrodism with normal virilization at puberty (familial perineal hypospadias with ambiguous development of urogenital sinus and male puberty; pseudovaginal perineoscrotal hypospadias)
   D. Dysgenetic male pseudohermaphrodism
      1. X chromatin-negative variants of the syndrome of gonadal dysgenesis (e.g., XO/XY,XYp—)
      2. Incomplete forms of XY gonadal dysgenesis
      3. Associated with degenerative renal disease
      4. "Vanishing testes" (embryonic testicular regression syndrome; XY agonadism; XY gonadal agenesis; rudimentary testes; anorchia)
   E. Defects in synthesis, secretion, or response to müllerian duct inhibitory factor
      1. Female genital ducts in otherwise normal men—"uteri herniae inguinale;" persistent müllerian duct syndrome
   F. Maternal ingestion of estrogens and progestins

IV. Unclassified forms of abnormal sexual development
   A. In males
      1. Hypospadias
      2. Ambiguous external genitalia in XY males with multiple congenital anomalies
   B. In females
      1. Absence or anomalous development of the vagina, uterus, and fallopian tubes (Rokitansky-Küstner syndrome)

Seminiferous Tubule Dysgenesis: Klinefelter Syndrome and Its Variants

XXY Seminiferous Tubule Dysgenesis (Typical Klinefelter Syndrome)

Seminiferous tubule dysgenesis is one of the most common forms of primary hypogonadism and infertility in the male, with an increased prevalence in mentally retarded males. Concepts of this syndrome have been modified considerably since 1942, when it was first defined as a clinical entity by Klinefelter, Reifenstein, and Albright. As originally described, the characteristic features, which first become manifest during adolescence, were gynecomastia, a variable degree of eunuchoidism, small atrophic testes with hyalinization of the seminiferous tubules, aggregation of Leydig cells, aspermatogenesis, and increased urinary excretion of gonadotropin. In 1956, several groups found that a high proportion of patients with this syndrome were X-chromatin-positive in contrast to their phenotypic male appearance. Soon thereafter, the syndrome was separated into a chromatin-positive form and a less common chromatin-negative form. Although the clinical features of the two groups were similar, subtle differences were found in the histologic structure of the testes in the two forms. Mental retardation is associated primarily with the chromatin-positive group (X chromatin-negative patients usually have a normal XY karyotype; the present discussion is concerned primarily with the X chromatin-positive group).

In 1959, Jacobs and Strong (133) and Ford et al. (134) first reported an XXY sex chromosome constitution in patients with this disorder, thus explaining the positive chromatin pattern. More recently, a variety of other sex chromosome complexes, including mosaicism, have been described. Virtually all these variants have in common the presence of at least two X chromosomes and a Y chromosome, except for the rare group which has only an XX sex chromosome complement by karyotype analysis of multiple tissues.

Table 9–7.   SALIENT FEATURES OF KLINEFELTER SYNDROME

Karyotype: 47,XXY

Inheritance: Sporadic; associated with advanced maternal age; non-disjunction during first or second meiotic division in either parent (67% maternal, 33% paternal); mitotic non-disjunction.

Genitalia: Male

Wolffian duct derivatives: Normal

Müllerian duct derivatives: Absent

Gonads: Small, firm testes; seminiferous tubule dysgenesis; azoospermia; Leydig cell hyperplasia

Habitus: Poor to normal virilization at puberty; gynecomastia; disproportionately long legs.

Hormone profile: Testosterone levels variable but usually ↓; ↑ levels of plasma LH and FSH postpubertally.

The differentiation of testes and lack of ovarian differentiation in patients with XXY, and more strikingly, an XXXXY complement, indicates that a single Y chromosome and the expression of H-Y antigen are sufficient to bring about testicular oranogenesis and male sex differentiation in the presence of as many as four X chromosomes (8).

Clinical Features (135, 136, 137). The only constant clinical features of chromatin positive seminiferous tubule dysgenesis are small, firm testes that measure less than 3 cm in length (and often less than 1.5 cm), azoöspermia, and a male phenotype (Fig. 9–23). The clinical profile of 63 patients with an XXY karyotype ascertained by chromosome analysis of newborn infants indicates that children with this karyotype as a group have lower birth weights than controls; an increased incidence of major and minor congenital anomalies, especially clinodactyly; height percentiles that increase with age; a lower verbal I.Q. than

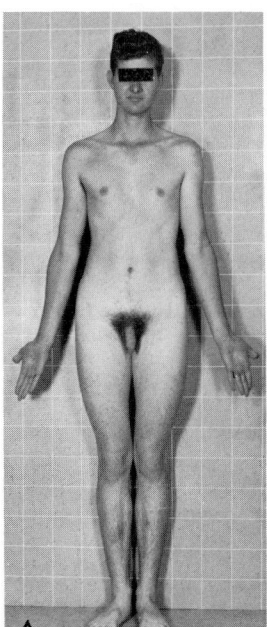
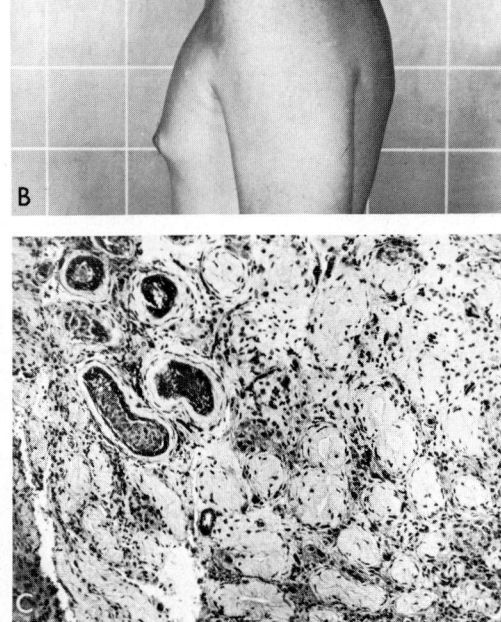
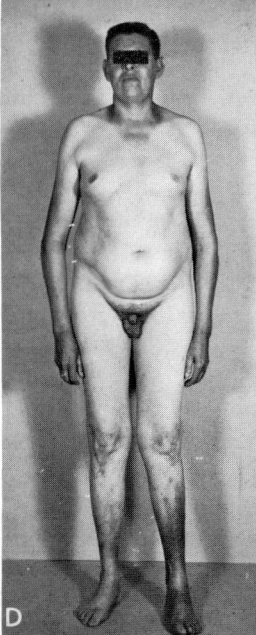

Figure 9–23. *A*, 19 year old phenotypic male with chromatin positive seminiferous tubule dysgenesis (Klinefelter syndrome). His karyotype was XXY, gonadotropins were elevated and testosterone levels were low normal. Note normal virilization with long legs and (*B*) gynecomastia. The testes were small and firm and measured 1.8 × 0.9 cm. Testicular biopsy (*C*) revealed a severe degree of hyalinization of his seminiferous tubules and Leydig cell "hyperplasia." *D*, 48 year old male with chromatin-positive Klinefelter syndrome who came to medical attention because of severe leg varicosities.

normal boys; and, more frequently than in a control population, delayed emotional development and poor gross motor control (138). The disorder should be suspected in prepubertal males with abnormally small testes and in boys who have personality and behavioral disorders with or without intellectual subnormality (139). Gynecomastia, as well as signs of androgen deficiency such as diminished facial and body hair, a female escutcheon, a small phallus, poor muscular development, and a enuchoidal body habitus occur postpubertally with increased frequency in affected patients (135, 136, 137).

Patients with an XXY karyotype tend to be taller than average, mainly because of the disproportionate length of their legs (140, 141). This finding is often present before clinical signs of puberty are evident and may not be accompanied by a proportional increase in span. The prepubertal onset of enuchoidal proportions suggests that it is not solely related to androgen deficiency and delayed epiphyseal closure. Androgen deficiency after the age of puberty augments the prepubertal deviation in skeletal porportions (141).

Prepubertally, the plasma concentration of FSH and LH and the response to luteinizing hormone releasing factor are within the normal range (142). With the onset of puberty, progressive histologic changes and a decreased capacity of the Leydig cells to synthesize testosterone become apparent. Thus, in postpubertal patients the concentration of testosterone (137) tends to be low, while the levels of urinary and plasma gonadotropins are elevated. Diminished potency is common in the adult patient and Leydig cell reserve is impaired, which is reflected in a subnormal increase in the concentration of serum testosterone following the administration of hCG (137, 143). The testosterone production rate, the total and free levels of testosterone, and the metabolic clearance rates of testosterone and estradiol tend to be low, while plasma estradiol levels are normal or elevated (144). The testicular failure in Klinefelter syndrome progresses with age. The gynecomastia which occurs in about 90% of patients is quite likely secondary to an increased ratio of serum estradiol to testosterone.

An increased frequency of mental retardation and psychopathology, including antisocial behavior and delinquency, is found in patients affected with this problem although the exact risk is uncertain.

Associated Abnormalities. Abnormalities in thyroid function have been reported, including a diminished thyroid response to TSH, decreased uptake of radioactive iodine and a subnormal increase in serum TSH following the administration of thyrotropin-releasing factor (145). Clinically significant thyroid disease is uncommon. An increased incidence of thyroid antibodies is not found in this disorder, in contrast to patients with the syndrome of gonadal dysgenesis.

The frequency of mild diabetes mellitus is increased. Nielsen et al. reported that in a group of 157 patients, 19% had impaired glucose tolerance and 8% had frank diabetes (146). The prevalence of diabetes mellitus was increased in their parents. The patients with diabetes mellitus were usually under 50 years of age and their diabetes was generally mild.

XXY patients with gynecomastia have an increased predisposition to cancer of the breast. In a survey of 187 males with breast cancer, eight patients with chromatin-positive seminiferous tubule dysgenesis were detected, about 18 times the expected prevalence (147). There is some evidence to suggest that chronic pulmonary disease and varicose veins may also be more prevalent in adults with Klinefelter syndrome. Although statistical studies are lacking, it is the impression of some observers that these patients are uncommonly prone to a variety of somatic ailments. Recently, sexual precocity due to an hCG-secreting intrathoracic polyembryoma was reported in six XXY boys (148). The diagnosis was suggested by the association of small testes with sexual precocity in the absence of a virilizing adrenal disorder.

Frequency. Surveys of the prevalence of XXY fetuses by karyotype analysis of unselected newborn infants indicate an incidence of about one per 1000 males (149). No racial or geographic predilection has been observed (150). Whereas 10% of clinically recognizable spontaneous abortions have an XO constitution, only 0.1% have a 47,XXY karyotype (149).

Testicular Lesion. The changes in the histologic structure of the testis which occur with age in XXY individuals are noteworthy (151, 152). Blanc and Grumbach studied the testes of a chromatin-positive premature male infant, weighing 1700 g and found that the histology was normal, including the complement of germ cells and the appearance of the seminiferous tubules and Leydig cells. Subtle changes were detected in the testes of other XXY patients in later infancy and childhood, the main feature at this stage of development being a diminished number of spermatogonia (153). In considering the pathogenesis of the testicular lesion in XXY seminiferous tubule dysgenesis, it seems that a normal or near-normal complement of spermatogonia is present until late in fetal life. During the late prenatal period and early infancy, a drastic loss of germ cells apparently ensues. This reduction in the germ cell complement in XXY individuals may represent an exaggeration of the normal degeneration of spermatogonia that occurs in the perinatal period. Excessive germ cell loss could occur either because of defective maturation or from failure of the germ cells to migrate to the periphery of the tubule and to align themselves in apposition to the basement membrane.

With the approach of adolescence, and even before pubertal signs are well advanced, the action of pituitary gonadotropins on the intrinsically defective testis induces progressive hyalinization of the seminiferous tubules and pseudoadenomatous clumping of Leydig cells. Despite this clumping, however, the mean volume of Leydig cells is usually normal (154). After pubescence, the testes are characterized by small dysgenetic tubules which have undergone arrested development and often early fibrosis and hyalinization. Peritubular elastic tissue is usually absent in the small dysgenetic tubules or diminished (151). That gonadotropin secretion plays a direct or indirect role in bringing about this change was illustrated in a 7-year-old XXXY male with precocious puberty and elevated urinary gonadotropins. Unlike the relatively normal architecture that is found in most boys of this age with Klinefelter syndrome, the testes of this boy exhibited extensive hyalinization and fibrosis of the tubules and clumping of Leydig cells (Fig. 9–24). Conversely, XXY patients who have gonadotropin deficiency do not exhibit these changes in testicular histology.

Hyalinization of the tubules is usually extensive but varies considerably in degree from patient to patient and even between the testes of the same patient. The fibrosis tends to progress with age, and in some older patients few tubules can be identified. Conversely, in an occasional patient, the tubules are lined by Sertoli cells, tubular fibrosis is relatively slight, and the histologic appearance closely resembles that of germinal cell aplasia. Rarely, spermatogenesis is found in isolated tubules, and there have been sporadic reports of alleged paternity; most of these cases have

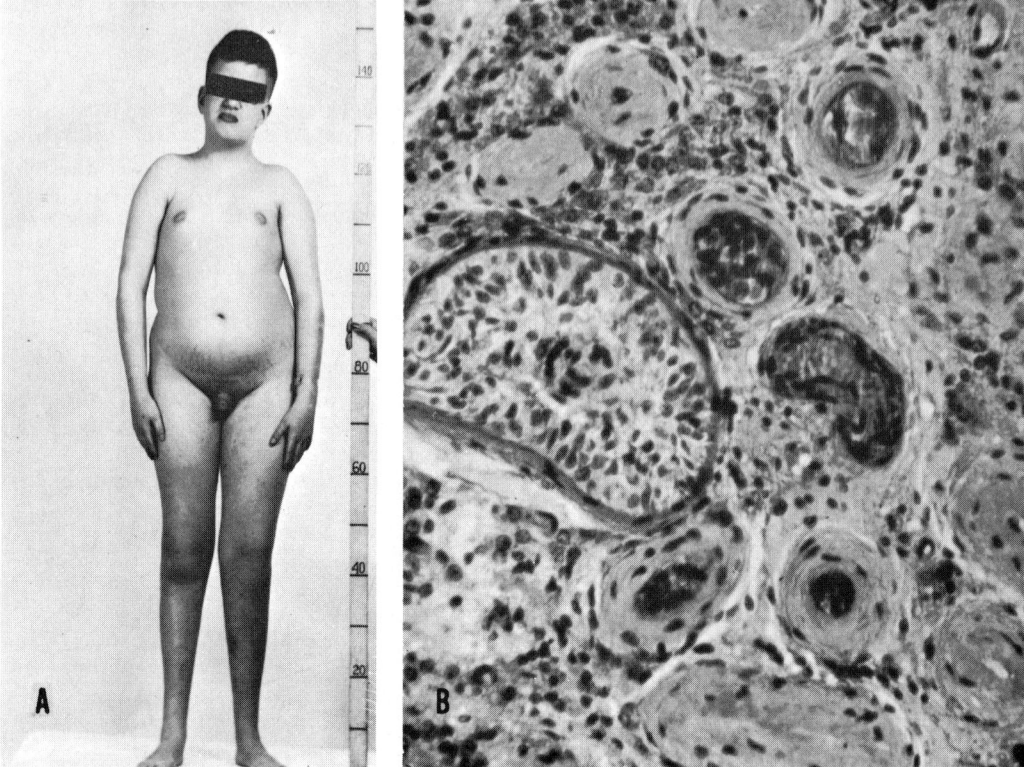

Figure 9–24. *A,* An 8 8/12-year-old boy with an XXXY sex chromosome constitution, mental retardation, precocious sexual development, and accelerated growth. Appearance of pubic hair noted at age 6. By 8 years acne, a deep voice, tall stature, and axillary hair were present. Height 148 cm. (+2.9 SD); weight 47.7 kg (+3.9 SD); span 140 cm.; upper segment/lower segment =0.87. Testes measured 2.1 × 1.3 cm. Note long legs, prognathism, small hands and feet, and the gynecomastia and secondary sexual characteristics. IQ 62. Urinary 17-KS 3.2 mg./day; urinary gonadotropins > 10 m.u., < 50 m.u./day. Bone age 13½ years. Buccal smear contained diploid nuclei with a maximum of two X chromatin bodies. Karyotype of cells derived from skin and blood was 48, XXXY. *B,* Testicular biopsy showed hyalinized tubules and clumping of Leydig cells; germ cells were absent. The findings suggest that the precocious puberty, with stimulation of the juvenile testes by pituitary gonadotropin, led to the premature appearance of the typical histologic changes of seminiferous tubule dysgenesis. (From Grumbach, M. M., Morishima, A., et al.: Unpublished data.)

proven to have had sex chromosome mosaicism; in others, acceptable documentation of paternity has not been provided. Those fertile patients who were proven to have XY/XXY mosaicism often lacked features that otherwise distinguished them from typical Klinefelter syndrome. The XY/XXXY patient of Barr et al. who was detected in a survey of mentally retarded males had normal-sized testes with active spermatogenesis (155). Cultures of the peripheral blood lymphocytes grew out only an XY cell line, but cultures of the skin and testes revealed the mosaicism.

Origin of XXY Constitution. XXY males may develop from nondisjunction of the sex chromosomes during either the first or second meiotic division in either parent or, less commonly, from mitotic nondisjunction in the zygote at the time of or following fertilization (Figs. 9–3 and 9–12). Fertilization of either an XX ovum by a Y-bearing sperm or of an X ovum by an XY-bearing sperm would yield an XXY zygote. Mitotic nondisjunction of the sex chromosomes in an XY zygote could yield an XXY and a YO daughter cell (Fig. 9–25). Since the YO cell line is nonviable, only the XXY cell line would survive.

The abnormalities of meiosis just discussed almost always occur in a parent with a normal sex chromosome constitution. However, Rosenkranz has described two XXY patients, one of whose mother was XXX and the other's an XX/XXX mosaic (156). Whether an XXY karyotype is derived more frequently from a polysomic X constitution in the mother than previously suspected remains to be determined.

Pedigree studies using X-linked markers, such as color

vision, Xg blood group, serum Xm group, and glucose-6-phosphate dehydrogenase have disclosed that, in informative pedigrees, both X's are of maternal origin (X^MX^MY) in 67% of cases and one X is paternal (X^MX^PY) in 33% (33, 157, 158). Similar observations have been made in mice (158a).

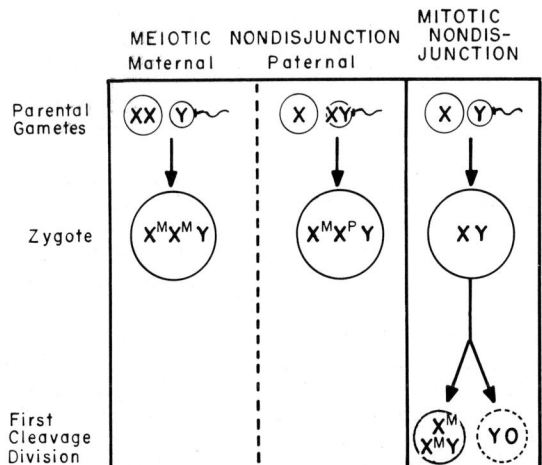

Figure 9–25. The origin of an XXY sex chromosome constitution. The superscripts M and P designate respective matriclinous and patriclinous X chromosome. The interrupted circle indicates a nonviable cell line. (From Grumbach, M. M., In *Cecil-Loeb Textbook of Medicine,* 13th ed. Beeson, P. B., and McDermott, W. (eds.), Philadelphia, W. B. Saunders Company, 1971, p. 1811.)

Ferguson-Smith et al. (159) and others (135) have reported a positive association with advanced maternal age in XXY patients, although this association is less marked than in trisomy 21. These data suggest that a high proportion of X^MX^MY cases may result from nondisjunction during oögenesis rather than from mitotic nondisjunction in the first cell division of an XY zygote. Data in the X^MX^PY group support the view that paternal nondisjunction is not dependent on age (159), a finding also reminiscent of autosomal trisomies.

Rarely, Klinefelter syndrome has been associated with a supernumerary X chromosome that is structurally abnormal, e.g., an X-autosome translocation or an isochromosome for the long arm of the X.

Etiologic Factors. The most important factor so far imputed in the etiology of an XXY sex chromosome constitution is advanced maternal age (135, 159). As discussed previously, the maternal age effect in chromosome abnormalities may be a consequence of the long diplotene stage of human ova. Ova remain suspended in prophase of the first meiotic division from birth to ovulation, which may not occur for 40 years or longer. The defective segregation of the two X chromosomes could be caused, at least in part, by reduction of the length of the chiasma between certain chromosomes as the length of the diplotene stage increases. As in gonadal dysgenesis, there is suggestive evidence that the prevalence of twinning in sibships of XXY individuals is increased.

Genetic factors that predispose to nondisjunction may also be important and have been demonstrated in lower species. While chromosome abnormalities are usually sporadic, a number of pedigrees have been reported in which leukemia and various chromosome abnormalities have occurred in siblings and relatives. In addition, patients with two coexisting forms of trisomy seem to be found more frequently than expected by chance alone. The role of radiation and viruses as predisposing factors is not known.

Diagnosis and Treatment. The diagnosis of Klinefelter syndrome is suggested by the typical phenotype and hormonal changes. It is confirmed by the finding of a positive buccal sex chromatin pattern and subsequently a XXY karyotype or a variant sex chromosome complement in blood, skin, or gonads. Treatment of Klinefelter syndrome is directed toward androgen replacement therapy when there is evidence of androgen deficiency. In general, parenteral preparations are more effective in virilizing the patient and are safer. Hepatic tumors and abnormalities in liver function studies have been associated with chronic administration of oral androgen analogues that have substitutions at the 17α position (e.g., a methyl group). This has not been a problem with testosterone ester preparations such as propionate or enanthate. Testosterone enanthate in oil, 200 mg IM every 2 weeks, is recommended for full replacement therapy. It is wise to begin therapy at a lower dose to avoid rapid virilization and bone maturation especially in adolescent males. A possible side effect of androgen therapy is salt and water retention with resultant edema. In general, gynecomastia, if present, does not diminish significantly as a result of androgen replacement. Severe or psychologically disturbing gynecomastia can be corrected by reduction mammoplasty.

Variant Forms of Klinefelter Syndrome: XY/XXY Mosaicism

Second only to the XXY constitution, XY/XXY mosaicism is the most frequent karyotype encountered in phenotypic males with X chromatin-positive patterns. The presence of a normal XY cell line in these patients can modify the clinical expression of the XXY cell line. Thus, in general, these patients manifest a lesser degree of gynecomastia, androgen deficiency, and testicular pathology. As a group they are older (mean age 45 years) at the time of diagnosis than patients with XXY Klinefelter syndrome. Symptoms of decreased libido and potency may not appear until the fourth or fifth decades. At the time of diagnosis, serum FSH levels are elevated while serum testosterone concentrations are often in the normal range. Secondary sex characteristics are less affected than in patients with XXY karyotypes. Seminiferous tubules exhibiting spermatogenesis are much more common than in XXY patients (137). At least four patients with XY/XXY mosaicism have been fertile (137).

The diagnosis of XY/XXY mosaicism can be established by the finding of at least 5% XY cells in blood, skin, or gonads in which the second cell line is XXY. XY/XXY mosaicism may result from nondisjunction or anaphase lag in an XXY zygote.

XXYY. Over 60 patients with a 48,XXYY karyotype have been described (12). Affected individuals not only have the typical features of Klinefelter syndrome but often exhibit several additional characteristics. They comprise about 3% of chromatin-positive males, and most of the reported patients have been mentally retarded. The XXYY karyotype is usually associated with tall stature (the mean height of 26 patients was 181 cm compared with 172 cm for XXY males), disproportionately long lower extremities, gynecomastia, often delinquent behavior, and unusual dermatoglyphic patterns. Peripheral vascular disease, especially varicose veins and stasis dermatitis, are prevalent in this group. Secondary sexual characteristics are poorly developed, and testicular histology is similar to that in XXY patients. The sex chromatin pattern is indistinguishable from that of the XXY groups; however, two fluorescent Y bodies are present in a high proportion of somatic nuclei.

In order to have two Y chromosomes, nondisjunction must occur in paternal meiosis. In two informative matings the Xg blood groups indicated that the father contributed an X as well as two Y's, which suggests that fertilization of an X ovum by an XYY sperm (arising from successive nondisjunction in the first and second meiotic divisions) is the usual origin of XXYY individuals. The XXYY karyotype in a patient whose mother was XXX (160) could have arisen by the fertilization of an XX ovum by a YY sperm.

XXXY and XXXYY. All of the reported patients with an XXXY karyotype have been mentally retarded, usually to a more severe degree than in XXY patients (12). In addition, they have had small testes and signs of androgen deficiency. With an increase in the number of X chromosomes, an increase in severity and frequency of somatic anomalies is noted, such as short neck, epicanthal folds, radioulnar synostosis, and clinodactyly.

Mental retardation, somatic anomalies, and small testes were features of XXXYY patients (161).

XXXXY. This karyotype has been reported in over 70 patients since the first report of Fraccaro et al. in 1960 (162, 163). The diagnosis may be suspected from the clinical picture. In addition to mental deficiency, often of a severe degree, these patients tend to exhibit certain phenotypic similarities including a) a variety of skeletal abnormalities, especially radioulnar synostosis, and b) hypoplastic external genitalia with a small penis, underdeveloped scrotum, and very small and frequently undescended testes; the appearance of the external genitalia may be ambiguous, owing to hypospadias, bifid scrotum, hypoplastic phallus, and cryptorchidism. In adult patients, gynecomastia is absent and androgen deficiency is severe. Before puberty, the testes often contain hypoplastic seminiferous tubules. Other described anomalies include congenital heart disease, cleft palate, strabismus, and microcephaly. The facies not infrequently has a characteristic appearance: mandibular prognathism, hypertelorism, strabismus, and myopia. These patients have three chromatin bodies in a proportion of their diploid nuclei.

XX Males. Over 100 cases of phenotypic males with a 46,XX karyotype have been described since 1964; this disorder occurs in about 1 per 32,000 males. de la Chapelle analyzed 45 cases and found that their clinical features and hormonal values were similar to those of X-chromatin-positive Klinefelter syndrome (157). However, XX males are shorter (mean height 168 cm) than those with an XXY karyotype or normal males, but taller than normal females. In addition, unlike males with Klinefelter syndrome, their skeletal proportions are usually normal. Intellectual subnormality, behavior disorders, and mental illness seemed to occur less frequently than with XXY seminiferous tubule dysgenesis. Mean maternal age was not advanced. The histology of the testes is usually similar to that of XXY males; seminiferous tubules are decreased in size and number, germinal cells are usually absent, and peritubular and interstitial fibrosis occurs. Leydig cells appear hyperplastic. In some patients the morphology was that of germinal cell aplasia or intermediate between it and semiferous tubule dysgenesis. At least 10% of XX males have been reported to have hypospadias which can be attributed to fetal Leydig cell deficiency. Approximately one-third have clinically apparent gynecomastia postpubertally. There is no significant association of somatic anomalies. Extensive investigation of multiple tissues has not usually resulted in the finding of a Y-bearing cell line. However, all XX males have been H-Y antigen positive (8, 164).

Three theories have been advanced to explain this rare example of sex reversal and the presence of H-Y antigen: 1) cryptic sex chromosome mosaicism in an XX male with an undetected cell line containing a Y chromosome; 2) interchange or translocation between a Y and an X chromosome or autosome which results in the location of masculinizing genes on an X chromosome or on an autosome; and 3) a mutant autosomal gene that leads to the differentiation of testes in an XX embryo as in the "Saanen" goat and the sex reversed mouse (SxrXX). There is evidence that each of these abnormalities may be involved.

The distribution of blood group Xg^a positive and negative individuals in 33 cases suggested that in some instances the two X chromosomes were maternal in origin, consistent with an XXY cell line which was undetected (157). Recently, 17% of a group of XX males were reported to have a small proportion of XXY cells in cultured skin, blood, or testis (165). However, it may be questioned whether a small proportion of XXY or XY cells in "hidden" mosaicism can induce bilateral testicular differentiation.

In support of the second possibility, a translocation of a minute segment of the Y to an X or an autosome, is the detection of H-Y antigen in a human XX male who had a discrepancy in the size of the short arms of his two X chromosomes (164) and the results of studies of G- and R-banded chromosome preparations from XX males in which no evidence of sex chromosome mosaicism or of a discrete Y chromosome was found. In 8 of 12 XX males, Evans et al. (166) found a heteromorphism in the banding profile and length of the short arm of one X chromosome. A Y-specific DNA fragment in DNA digests was detected in one of three XX males, suggesting a translocation involving the short arms of the X and Y chromosome (166). The evidence suggests that some XX males may occur as a consequence of the

inheritance of a paternal Y to X interchange product which contains the testis-determining genes. Moreover, Y to X and Y to autosome interchange has been documented karyotypically in humans (167, 168) in whom the highly fluorescent portion of the Y chromosome has been translocated to an X or an autosome. The small size and non-specific banding of the pericentromeric region of the Y chromosome (putative site of a gene(s) locus for expression of H-Y antigen) makes the cytologic confirmation of a translocation involving this region difficult to verify.

The third possibility, that of a mutant gene which leads to the expression of H-Y antigen, is supported by familial cases of XX males. de la Chapelle et al. reported three XX males in a single pedigree (59). All three XX males were H-Y antigen positive and their mothers expressed a reduced and variable amount of H-Y antigen. This observation is consistent with an autosomal recessive mode of sex determination in the kinship (59, 60). Ohno has suggested that the regulatory gene for H-Y antigen is on the Y chromosome and has undergone gene duplication and therefore exists in multiple copies; if this is so, then there is the possibility that translocation of subthreshold or subcritical portions of the gene copies for testis determination on the Y to an autosome a) could lead to autosomal recessive transmission in some pedigrees or b) could behave as an autosomal dominant in other pedigrees if sufficient copies of the gene were transmitted to an autosome or X chromosome (60). With present techniques, there are major limitations to quantifying the amount of H-Y antigen. Further, the chromosomal site (X, Y or possibly an autosome) of the structural gene for H-Y antigen is uncertain (see p. 435). Thus, it is necessary to reserve judgment on whether some XX men arise as a consequence of a submicroscopic Y to autosome or Y to X chromosome transfer or insertion, or as a result of an autosomal mutant gene that leads to expression of H-Y antigen. Our present knowledge of the regulation of H-Y antigen does not permit this distinction, and either or both of the alternatives are possible. Familial evidence of XX males, all of whom expressed H-Y antigen, have been described in a number of species including the sex reversed mouse (Sxr) (62), where it behaves as an autosomal dominant, and in the XX Saanen goat homozygous for the autosomal dominant gene for hornlessness (polled) (60), and the XX male cocker spaniel, in which the gene for testis differentiation was transmitted as an autosomal recessive trait (61). In the human being, goat and dog, XX males and XX true hermaphrodites can occur in the same pedigree, which suggests a link between these two disorders. Both are disorders of gonadogenesis in an XX gonad in which differentiation of testicular tissue occurs in H-Y antigen positive individuals in the absence of a discrete Y chromosome.

In sum, it is likely that the pathogenesis of this syndrome is heterogenous. Evans et al. estimated that 70% of cases are attributable to X-Y interchange, 20% to hidden mosaicism, and the remaining 10% to a single mutant gene (166).

The Syndrome of Gonadal Dysgenesis: Turner Syndrome and Its Variants (12, 22, 31, 32, 169, 170, 171, 172)

In 1938, Turner described seven phenotypic females who exhibited dwarfism, sexual infantilism, webbing of the neck, and cubitus valgus. Subsequent studies of this intriguing syndrome and its variants have contributed more to the evolution of our current concepts of sex differentiation than have studies in any other group of patients.

In the early 1940's Albright et al. and associates found that the excretion of urinary gonadotropin was increased in affected adolescents and adults. Wilkins and Fleischmann soon thereafter described the gonads as bilateral, pale "streaks" of connective tissue situated in the mesosalpinges and devoid of any germ cells. In 1950, Wilkins proposed, in the light of Jost's fetal castration experiments in the rabbit, that some of these functionally agonadal patients might be genetic males, since fetal castration of either sex invariably leads to a female phenotype. The discovery in 1954 that many of these patients, contrary to their phenotype, were X chromatin-negative seemed initially to confirm the hypothesis that some of these patients were indeed genetic males. However, in 1959, soon after techniques became available to determine the actual chromosome constitution, Ford et al. reported that the sex chromosome constitution in a 14-year-old phenotypic female with this syndrome was XO rather than XY (173). Work in many laboratories has now defined more precisely the chromosomal basis of this and related disorders (32, 170, 22).

The absence of a second sex chromosome (X chromosome monosomy) is associated with four cardinal features: 1) female phenotype; 2) short stature; 3) sexual infantilism owing to rudimentary gonads; and 4) a variety of associated somatic abnormalities. Any or all of these features may be modified by the presence of lesser degrees of sex chromosome deficiency. It is therefore useful to consider the syndrome of gonadal dysgenesis and its variants as a continuum of clinical features ranging from those of the typical XO phenotype to a normal female or male. The functional importance of chromosomal additions to the basic XO pattern can be deduced from the extent to which they modify toward normal, in at least some cases, the dwarfism, sexual infantilism, and somatic anomalies that typify the patient with complete sex chromosome monosomy.

Partial sex chromosome monosomy may be attributed to a structurally abnormal second sex chromosome (X or Y), sex chromosome mosaicism involving an XO cell line, or both a structural abnormality and mosaicism. It is important to emphasize, however, that even though the modified clinical forms are almost invariably associated with partial sex chromosome monosomy, the contrary is not necessarily true; apparently identical partial sex chromosome monosomies may be associated with the typical clinical picture found in XO patients. For this reason, classifications of these variants based solely on their sex chromosome constitution tend to be confusing. Subdivision of these variants according to their X chromatin pattern, however, is helpful, since this test is readily available and immediately discloses the presence or absence of X chromosome additions to the monosomic X. X chromatin-positive patients tend to fall within the clinical spectrum ranging from sexually infantile females to normal females, whereas X chromatin-negative patients usually range between sexually infantile females and hypogonadal males. There are numerous exceptions to these generalizations, however, most of which may be explained by sex chromosome mosaicism.

Typical Turner Syndrome (XO Gonadal Dysgenesis) (2, 12, 22, 171, 172)

Of those cases displaying all the cardinal features that typify sex chromosome monosomy, the X chromatin pattern is negative in about 80%; most of these have an XO sex chromosome constitution.

Associated Somatic Stigmata. The typical patient (Fig. 9–26) is often recognizable by her distinctive facies in which micrognathia, epicanthal folds, prominent, low-set or deformed ears or both, a fishlike mouth, and ptosis are

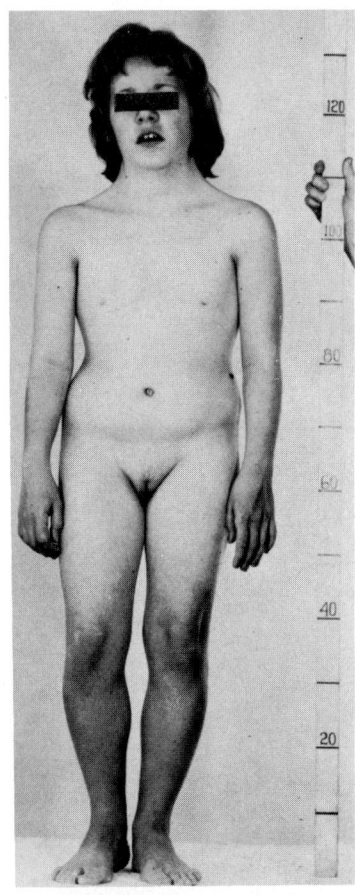

Figure 9–26. A 14 10/12-year-old patient with the typical form of the syndrome of gonadal dysgenesis (Turner syndrome). The X chromatin pattern is negative and the karyotype is 45, XO. She is short (height 134.5 cm; height age 9 5/12 years), sexually infantile except for the appearance of sparse pubic hair, and exhibits characteristic stigmata of the syndrome. There is the short webbed neck, shield-like chest with widely separated nipples, bilateral short 4th metacarpals, puffiness over the dorsum of the fingers, cubitus valgus, and increased number of pigmented nevi. The facies is characteristic and the ears are low set. The bone age is 13 6/12 years; urinary 17-KS 5.1 mg/day; plasma and urinary gonadotropins were elevated. Vaginal smears and the urocytogram showed an immature pattern in which cornified squamous cells were absent. With estrogen therapy, female secondary sex characteristics were induced; the cyclic administration resulted in periodic estrogen-withdrawal bleeding.

Table 9–8. SALIENT FEATURES OF XO GONADAL DYSGENESIS: TURNER SYNDROME

Karyotype: 45,XO

Inheritance: Sporadic; meiotic or mitotic non-disjunction

Genitalia: Female

Wolffian duct derivatives: Absent

Müllerian duct derivatives: Normal female

Gonads: Streak

Habitus: Short stature; sexual infantilism at puberty, somatic stigmata

Hormone profile: ↑ plasma LH and FSH concentrations; ↓ plasma estradiol levels

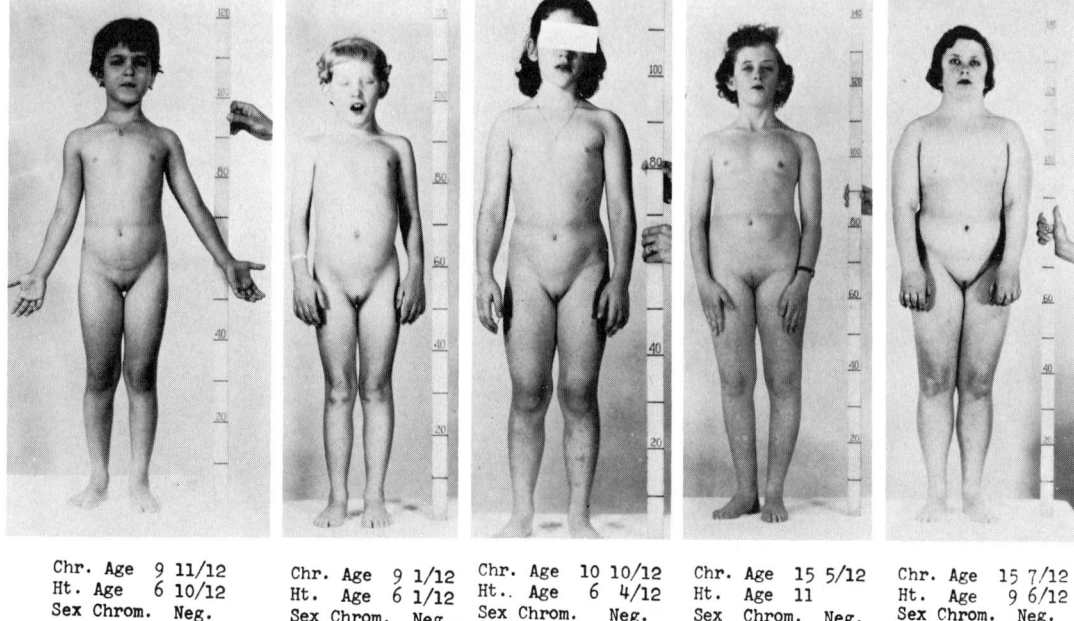

Chr. Age	9 11/12	Chr. Age	9 1/12	Chr. Age	10 10/12	Chr. Age	15 5/12	Chr. Age	15 7/12
Ht. Age	6 10/12	Ht. Age	6 1/12	Ht. Age	6 4/12	Ht. Age	11	Ht. Age	9 6/12
Sex Chrom.	Neg.	Sex Chrom.	Neg.	Sex Chrom.	Neg.	Sex Chrom.	Neg.	Sex Chrom.	Neg.

Figure 9-27. Variation in physical appearance in five patients with typical form of the syndrome of gonadal dysgenesis (Turner syndrome). All these patients had an XO karyotype, and all had differences between their height age and chronological age of 3 years or more. (From Grumbach, M. M., In *Clinical Endocrinology, I.* Astwood, E. B. (ed.), New York, Grune & Stratton, 1960, p. 407.)

present with varying degrees of frequency. The chest is usually square and shieldlike with microthelia. The neck is short and often broad with a low hairline in back. Webbing of the neck is present in about 40% of the patients and coarctation of the aorta in 10–20%. Those with coarctation almost universally also have webbing of the neck. Additional anomalies include cubitus valgus, congenital lymphedema of the feet and hands (30%) (Fig. 9–27) or, more frequently, puffiness of the dorsum of the fingers, short fourth metacarpal (50%), renal abnormalities (60%), high-arched palate, a variety of skeletal anomalies, an excessive number of pigmented nevi, tendency to keloid formation, hypoplastic nails, recurrent otitis media which may result in conductive hearing loss, unexplained hypertension, and rarely, gastrointestinal bleeding secondary to intestinal telangiectasia. The incidence of mental retardation is not increased significantly. Money (129) has reported that impairment of directional sense and space-form recognition is a common occurrence; this perceptual disability results in a lower mean performance IQ than is found in the general population, whereas verbal ability is not affected. Severe psychopathic manifestations are uncommon, in contrast to the XXY individuals who also exhibit an increased frequency of mental retardation.

The eponym "Bonnevie-Ullrich syndrome" has been applied to phenotypic female infants who have lymphedema of the distal extremities and loose folds of skin over the back of the neck in addition to the other classic features of gonadal dysgenesis (Fig. 9–28). In the neonate, pleural effusions and ascites that clear spontaneously are not uncommon (174) and, rarely, pericardial effusion has been reported. The serous effusions, as well as the lymphedema, are attributable to hypoplasia and other defects of the lymphatic system. XO abortuses commonly exhibit generalized edema and a large hygroma of the neck (175). The latter abnormality results in webbing of the neck postnatally.

In addition to coarctation of the aorta, the commonest cardiovascular abnormalities, aortic stenosis and bicuspid aortic valve, may occur as conjoint or separate defects.

Coarctation and cystic medial necrosis of the aorta may lead to dissecting aneurysm. Other cardiovascular anomalies are uncommon, in contrast to the situation in pseudo-Turner's syndrome (p. 000).

The most common renal abnormalities are rotation of the kidney, horseshoe kidney, duplication of the renal pelvis and ureter, and hydronephrosis secondary to ureteropelvic obstruction. Abnormal differentiation of the kidneys and

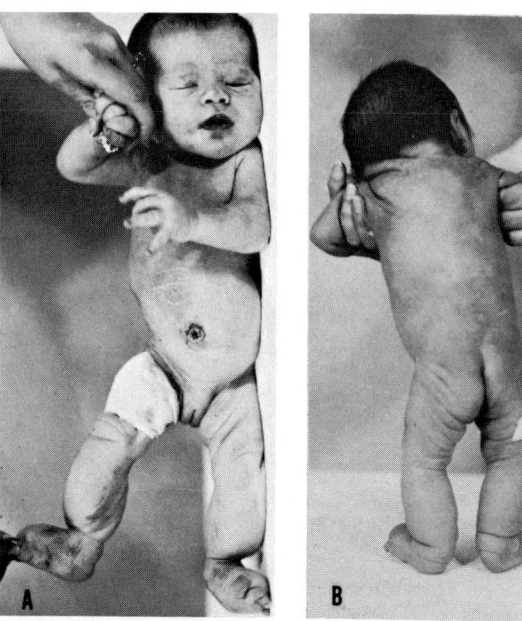

Figure 9-28. Infant with the syndrome of gonadal dysgenesis (karyotype XO) and associated lymphedema of the extremities. The term Bonnevie-Ullrich's syndrome is applied when this characteristic swelling of the feet or hands, or both as associated with other features of Turner's syndrome. (From Grumbach, M. M., and Barr, M. L.: *Recent Progr. Hormone Res. 14:*335, 1958.)

upper collecting system is found so commonly in this syndrome that routine intravenous urography is warranted.

Skeletal maturation is normal or only slightly delayed in childhood but lags in adolescence. In most cases, the skeleton exhibits localized areas of rarefaction, especially of the hands and feet, elbow, and upper femur (176). Adults who are not treated with estrogen often develop a severe form of the postmenopausal type of osteoporosis and may suffer from collapse of vertebrae. Osteochondrosis-like changes in the spine are commonly seen (176). In addition to the metacarpal sign (shortening of the fourth metacarpal), Kosowicz described a "carpal sign" characterized by a more acute angular configuration of the proximal row of carpal bones (177). The knee may show deformities of the medial tibial epicondyles, with obliquely tipped tibial epiphyses and medial projections of the tibial metaphyses. The pelvis tends to have a male-type inlet. An "empty sella" was noted on C-T scan in two of our patients.

Short Stature. Short stature is an invariant feature in XO individuals. The mean final height of patients is 142 cm, with a range from 133 to 153 cm (178); the ratio of sitting height to height is frequently increased by late childhood and reflects the greater retardation in growth of the legs. Intrauterine growth retardation is not uncommon in XO infants, and their average birth weight (2.81 kg) and length (47.6 cm) are significantly below the mean for normal infants of a comparable gestational age (179).

Postnatally, the growth pattern is variable. In general, they grow at a slow velocity (10th to 25th percentile) (179) when compared to normal peers, and by 5 years of age they are invariably 2.5 SD below the mean height for age (22). The mean height at 11 years of age is 124 cm and no pubertal growth spurt ensues (179) (Fig. 9–29 A, B). The bone age is retarded after 11 years of age.

Current data suggest that the short stature in patients with the syndrome of gonadal dysgenesis is not attributable to a deficiency of growth hormone (180), somatomedin (181), or adrenal and gonadal sex steroids (182). A positive correlation has been documented between final height in this syndrome and mean parental height (178). As yet, the etiology of the progressive growth failure in the syndrome has not been defined. We postulate that the abnormality resides in the cellular response to somatomedin.

Sexual Infantilism. The genital ducts and external genitalia in this syndrome are entirely female in character but immature. Located in the mesosalpinges parallel to the fallopian tubes are long, attenuated, pale, fibrous streaks of connective tissue. Typically, these streak-like or spindle-shaped structures consist of fibrous stroma arranged in whorls similar to those found in ovarian stroma, but they lack primordial follicles or seminiferous tubules. Vestigial medullary elements and rudimentary mesonephric tubules like those found deep in the primitive genital ridge are common at the hilus. After puberty, aggregates of epithelioid cells resembling Leydig or hilus cells are found in variable quantity.

Singh and Carr studied the gonadal ridge of eight spontaneously aborted embryos and fetuses ranging in the gestational age from 5 weeks to 4 months (175). Primordial germ cells were observed in all eight specimens. Until the third month of gestation, no appreciable differences were noted between these gonads and those from XX fetuses; after that, an increase in connective tissue stroma and impaired formation of follicles were found. These observations suggest that primordial germ cells seed the primitive gonad in XO individuals, but many degenerate during oöcyte formation and folliculogenesis, and the surviving oöcytes undergo accelerated atresia (183). Jirásek has re-

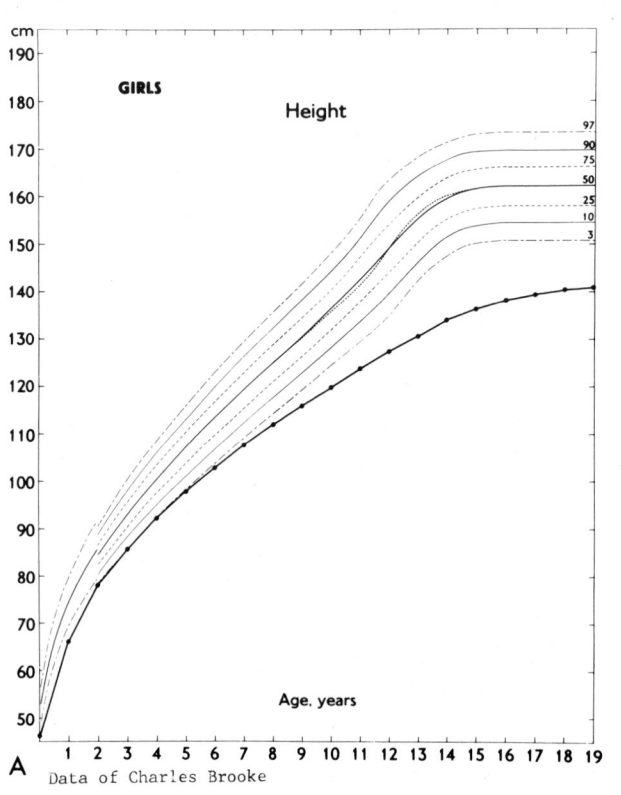

A
Data of Charles Brooke

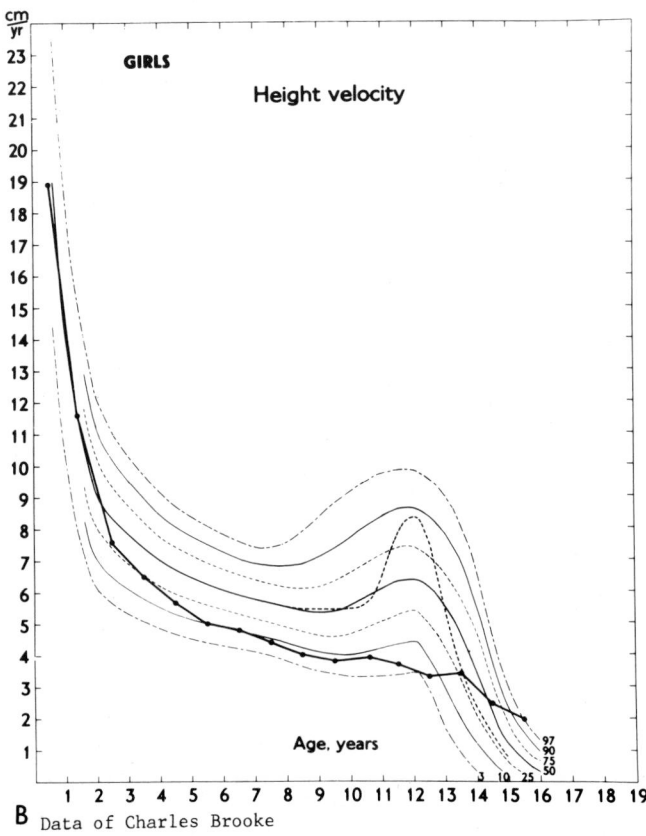

B
Data of Charles Brooke

Figure 9–29. A, Mean height in 38 untreated patients with 45,XO karyotypes. B, Mean yearly height velocities from data on 36 untreated patients with 45,XO karyotypes. Note the absence of a pubertal growth spurt. (A and B from Brook, C. G. D., et al.[179])

ported that in patients with an XO karyotype, oöcytes degenerate shortly after formation of the primary follicle (184). Apparently, two active X chromosomes are required in the human for the normal development of oögonia and oöcytes. The presence of a few follicles in the gonadal streaks in XO infants is probably not unusual at birth, although it is an uncommon finding by late childhood and adolescence.

Longitudinal studies of both basal and LRF evoked gonadotropin secretion in patients with gonadal dysgenesis demonstrate a lack of feedback inhibition of the hypothalamic-pituitary axis by the dysgenetic gonad in affected infants and young children (185, 186). Basal levels of LH and FSH were studied in 58 patients ages 2 days to 20 years. An elevation in the concentration of plasma FSH was noted as early as 5 days after birth. Plasma FSH levels between 2 days and 4 years of age were strikingly elevated and fell to normal to high normal values at 5 to 10 years of age (Fig. 9–30). After 10 years of age, plasma FSH rose again into the castrate range. Thus, the pattern of plasma FSH followed a diphasic curve qualitatively similar to, but quantitatively higher than, that in normal infants and children. The pattern of change in LH levels was similar but the concentrations were one-third to one-tenth that of FSH. LRF-induced LH and FSH responses exhibited a diphasic pattern with age, similar to that for basal levels. In patients under 5 years of age both the mean basal and the rise in gonadotropins induced by the administration of LRF were significantly increased over normal values for age. Between 5 and 10 years of age, mean basal concentration of FSH and LH as well as LRF evoked responses were significantly less than values for patients with gonadal dysgenesis under 5 years of age. In some patients between 6 and 10 years of age, both FSH and LH concentrations and the LRF induced gonadotropin responses were comparable to values in normal children. After 11 years of age a striking rise in basal and readily releasable LH and FSH was observed. Thus, between 5 and 10 years of age, basal as well as LRF elicited gonadotropin responses may not reflect the functional status of the gonads in all patients with gonadal dysgenesis.

Although streak gonads are the rule in XO gonadal dysgenesis, exceptions have been well documented. Primary follicles have been described in the ridges of some XO individuals in adolescence, and this correlates with the rare occurrence of menarche and a variable but attenuated period of regular menses (187). In 11 women, conceptions have been documented despite extensive karyotypic studies revealing only an XO cell line in multiple tissues (187, 188). One possible explanation for the presence of oögonia in XO individuals is that a certain number of XO germ cells may undergo mitotic non-disjunction with the formation of XX oögonia. This process normally occurs in the female creeping vole and serves as a sex-determining mechanism in this species. Alternatively, some fertile XO patients may be unrecognized sex chromosome mosaics. In women harboring an XO cell line there is increased fetal wastage and an increased number of chromosomally abnormal live-born infants (188, 189).

Clitoral enlargement is another rare finding in patients with an XO karyotype. Enlargement of the clitoris may be present at birth or first become manifest at puberty. Secretion of androgens by "Leydig cells" in the gonadal streak is a possible cause, as is the presence of an undetected Y cell line.

Incidence in Abortuses, Newborns and Twins. The incidence of XO newborns is about one per 10,000 females (149). There is, however, a considerable loss of XO embryos and fetuses. About 10% of all clinically recognizable sponta-

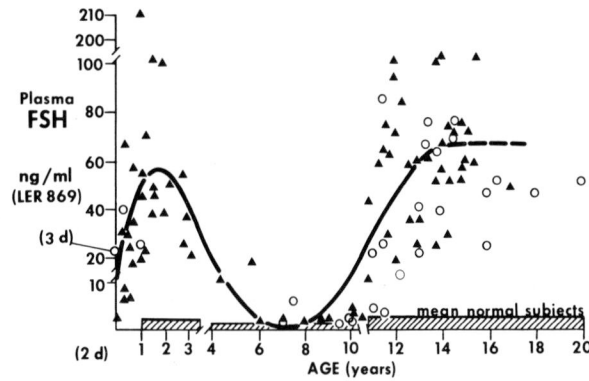

Figure 9–30. Pattern of plasma FSH (concentration) in relation to age in 58 patients with the syndrome of gonadal dysgenesis ▲ = XO karyotype; ○ = patients with structural abnormalities of the X chromosome and mosaics. The hatched area indicates the mean range for FSH values in normal females. (From Conte, F. A., Kaplan, S. L., and Grumbach, M. M.[185])

neous abortuses have an XO constitution (149). It is estimated that the frequency of XO zygotes is 0.8%, probably the commonest chromosome anomaly in man, but less than 3% of XO conceptuses survive to term (190). An increased incidence of XO conceptuses has been reported in teenage pregnancies (191).

There is some evidence to suggest that the prevalence of twinning is increased in XO individuals and their siblings. The occurrence of both monozygotic twinning and aneuploidy suggests that a single postfertilization event was responsible for both (190).

Associated Disorders. Engel and Forbes studied the association between gonadal dysgenesis and other selected metabolic and endocrine disorders in 48 adult patients (mean age 42 years) (169). Positive associations were found with obesity, hypertension due to causes other than coarctation of the aorta, diabetes mellitus, Hashimoto's thyroiditis, precocious aging, achlorhydria, cataracts, and corneal opacity or scarring. There is an increased incidence of thyroid antibodies and clinically manifested hypothyroidism even during childhood and adolescence (192, 193). Early diagnosis of Hashimoto's thyroiditis may be facilitated by following thyroid antibody levels and TRH induced TSH responses in these patients. Rheumatoid arthritis as well as inflammatory bowel disease is increased in patients with an XO karyotype (194). Decreased glucose tolerance is common in patients over 16 years of age (169). In a survey of 289 patients with Turner stigmata, Wertelecki found eight patients with nongonadal tumors, suggesting a possible increased risk of malignancy (195).

Origin of XO Constitution. An XO chromosome constitution may arise by a variety of chromosome errors (Figs. 9–3, 9–12). It may be a consequence of nondisjunction or chromosome loss during gametogenesis in either parent, resulting in a sperm or ovum lacking any sex chromosome. Although errors of mitosis in a normal zygote often lead to mosaicism, a purely XO constitution may arise at the first cleavage division from anaphase lag with loss of a sex chromosome or, less likely, mitotic nondisjunction with failure of the complementary XXX or XYY cell line to survive (Fig. 9–3). There is indirect evidence to suggest that loss of one X or a Y chromosome between fertilization and the first cleavage division may be a frequent but not the only cause of the XO embryo (22).

Several lines of evidence support a mitotic error in this syndrome: 1) the lack of association with advanced maternal age, in contrast to chromatin-positive Klinefelter syndrome

(170); 2) the prevalence of sex chromosome mosaicism; 3) the increased frequency of twinning in sibships with an XO individual; and 4) the occurrence of an XY monozygotic co-twin of an XO individual.

Family studies of such X-linked traits as color blindness and the Xg blood group indicate that loss of the paternally derived sex chromosome is more common than would be expected if either the maternally or paternally derived sex chromosome were lost randomly (158); recent estimates indicate that in informative pedigrees 77% of XO individuals have loss of the paternal sex chromosome (X^PO), and 23% loss of the maternal X chromosome (X^MO). An excess of X^MO over X^PO in mice has been found by Russell and Chu, who considered sex chromosome loss as the most likely mechanism (158a).

The underlying cause of this sex chromosome abnormality is not known. An increased incidence of XO mice was noted by Russell, following irradiation of the mother soon after mating (158a). An increased frequency of thyroid autoimmunity in patients with the syndrome of gonadal dysgenesis and also in their parents has been observed. This suggests that the genetic predisposition to develop autoantibodies in one or both parents is associated with an increased prevalence of an XO constitution and certain other chromosomal abnormalities in their offspring. Of note is the report of three patients with gonadal dysgenesis born following artificial insemination (196). The familial occurrence of XO gonadal dysgenesis is exceedingly rare.

Diagnosis and Treatment.   Phenotypic females with the following features should have a buccal smear for sex chromatin: 1) short stature (greater than 2.5 S.D. below the mean value for age); 2) somatic stigmata associated with the syndrome of gonadal dysgenesis; and 3) delayed adolescence and increased plasma or urinary gonadotropins. Normal females have between 20 to 30% sex chromatin positive cells at all ages, including the neonatal period. XO patients lack an X-chromatin body in interphase nuclei, while XO/XX mosaics usually have between 3 and 19% chromatin-positive cells. While determination of the X-chromatin pattern is a rapid method of screening, karyotype analysis is the definitive procedure. Plasma gonadotropins, especially FSH levels, are useful in assessing the functional status of the gonads. It is important in patients with Turner syndrome to perform an intravenous pyelogram to exclude a renal anomaly; to assess cardiovascular function; to evaluate thyroid function regularly; and to determine glucose tolerance after adolescence.

Therapy of patients with the syndrome of gonadal dysgenesis has been directed toward attempts to augment stature, to correct somatic anomalies, and to induce secondary sexual characteristics and menses. As noted, the short stature in Turner syndrome is not related to a deficiency of growth hormone, thyroid hormone, or adrenal and gonadal sex steroids. Although the administration of exogenous human growth hormone produces nitrogen retention in these patients, the increase in linear growth has been modest. Acromegaly has been described by Willemse in a woman with typical Turner syndrome; her growth increased from 139 cm to 154 cm between ages 18 and 28 (197). Some studies have reported a growth spurt and an augmentation in height in a small number of patients who were treated with the "anabolic" steroid oxandrolone (198). However, in a well controlled study, treatment with the "anabolic" steroids nandrolone phenproprionate and methandrostenolone did not increase final height above that achieved with estrogen therapy or in untreated patients (199). At present there appears to be no effective therapy for *significantly* augmenting final height in patients with gonadal dysgenesis. In addition, androgens and anabolic steroids may produce the undesirable effect of virilization.

Estrogen therapy has commonly been deferred until after 15 years of age or later on the assumption that treatment at an earlier age leads to rapid skeletal maturation and a diminished height. This premise has been based largely on the fact that pharmacologic doses of estrogens can accelerate bone age and lead to premature epiphyseal fusion without a proportionate increase in height. We examined the effect of low dose, early conjugated estrogen therapy on linear growth, bone age and the development of secondary sex characteristics in a group of patients with gonadal dysgenesis (178). Twelve patients were started on therapy with 0.3 mg of conjugated estrogens at a mean age of 13.6 years. The administration of 0.3 mg of conjugated estrogens was associated with an increase in mean growth rate from 2.2 cm/year to 6.2 cm/year (p < .001). However, the acceleration was not sustained and a return to pretherapy growth velocity was observed in less than 18 months. The final height in these patients was 142 ± 5.8 cm, which is not significantly different from that in untreated and androgen-treated patients. The patients developed breasts within 3 months and usually experienced withdrawal bleeding within 8 months of the start of estrogen therapy.

Serious psychological effects are frequently associated with a prolonged delay in the treatment of the sexual infantilism in patients with the syndrome of gonadal dysgenesis (200, 201). The institution of low dose, conjugated estrogen or synthetic estrogen therapy within the normal age range of puberty (about 12 to 13 years) elicits a growth spurt without inordinate advancement of skeletal maturation or reduction in final height, and induces the development of secondary sex characteristics at an age more comparable to normal peers, thereby obviating the undesirable psychological consequences of a prolonged delay in sexual maturation.

Thirteen instances of endometrial carcinoma have been reported in patients with the syndrome of gonadal dysgenesis (202). The evidence suggests that estrogens, especially when unopposed by progesterone, can produce a progression of histologic changes from endometrial hyperplasia to invasive carcinoma. In an attempt to clarify the relationship between estrogen therapy and endometrial pathology in gonadal dysgenesis, Rosenwaks et al. studied 41 patients on estrogen replacement therapy (203). The increased risk of an abnormal endometrial history correlated with 1) a lifetime dosage of conjugated estrogens of greater than 2500 mg; 2) greater than 7 years of estrogen therapy; and 3) a daily dose of conjugated estrogens greater than 1.25 mg. Progestins can modify the effect of estrogens on endometrial histology. It is therefore prudent to treat patients with gonadal dysgenesis with low dose estrogen replacement therapy administered in a cyclical fashion, with progestin administered at the end of each cycle.

Replacement Therapy.   We routinely initiate therapy at 12 to 13 years of age with 0.3 mg (or less) of conjugated estrogen, or ethinyl estradiol, 5 μg by mouth, for the first 21 days of the calendar month. Thereafter the dose of estrogen is gradually increased over the next 2-3 years to 0.6 to 1.25 mg conjugated estrogens or 10 to 20 μg of ethinyl estradiol daily for the first 21 days of the month. The patient is maintained on the minimum dose of estrogen needed to maintain secondary sex characteristics and withdrawal bleeding. Medroxyprogesterone acetate, 5 mg daily, is given on the twelfth through the twenty-first day of the month to ensure more physiologic menses and possibly to reduce the risk of endometrial carcinoma.

Partial Sex Chromosome Monosomy and Clinical Variants of the Syndrome of Gonadal Dysgenesis

Sex chromosome abnormalities that can be regarded as examples of partial sex chromosome monosomy may or may not modify the expression of the classic XO phenotype (22, 32). Approximately 20% of patients with the typical syndrome of gonadal dysgenesis are X chromatin-positive. This group usually has a structurally abnormal X chromosome and, more commonly, sex chromosome mosaicism involving an XO cell line. Chromatin-positive and chromatin-negative clinical variants of the syndrome of gonadal dysgenesis will be discussed in relation to the more usual types of sex chromosome aberrations with which they may be associated. A diagrammatic scheme interrelating the variable effect of partial sex chromosome monosomy on the cardinal clinical features of the syndrome is shown in Figure 9–31.

In patients with sex chromosome mosaicism, the ratio in each gonad of XO primordial germ cells and blastemal components to those with a normal XX or XY constitution is probably the major determinant of whether the ultimate gonadal structure will be a streak, a dysgenetic or hypoplastic ovary or testis, or a relatively normal gonad (22, 32). The weight of evidence supports the notion that, after migration into the primitive gonad, primordial germ cells that bear an XO constitution degenerate more rapidly than do XX cells, resulting in a streak, hypoplastic, or normal ovary. Similarly, if the gonadal blastemal components do not contain an appropriate number of XY cells and H-Y antigen, testicular development will not take place (Fig. 9–32).

The quantitative relation in peripheral tissues between XO cells and those with an XX or XY pattern may also be responsible for the variable effect of mosaicism on stature and associated somatic stigmata (22).

In patients with single cell lines of structurally abnormal sex chromosomes, the somatic and gonadal consequences appear to be related to the nature and degree of the short- or long-arm deficiency of the second X or the Y chromosome. Table 9–9 summarizes the correlation between structural abnormalities of the X and Y chromosomes and the clinical manifestations. The use of deletion mapping of the human sex chromosomes to clarify the relation of phenotype to karyotype has limitations. Structural abnormalities are often associated with mosaicism, owing to loss of the structurally abnormal sex chromosome from the stem-cell line. Further, structural rearrangements of chromosomes are more complex than previously thought and may not represent simple terminal deletions of the long and short arms of the X chromosome. However, the advent of chromosome banding techniques has greatly facilitated the analysis of structurally abnormal sex chromosomes. At present, the data suggest that 1) gonadal determiners are located on both the long and short arm of the X chromosome; patients with short arm deletions proximal to band Xp21 or long arm deletions proximal to band Xq27 usually have streak gonads and sexual infantilism (204, 205); and, 2) the short arm of the X chromosome contains loci which if deleted result in short stature and the somatic stigmata of the syndrome of gonadal dysgenesis. Therman et al. (206) have provided a provocative analysis of the pathogenesis of somatic stigmata in X chromosome aberrations.

X Chromatin-Positive Variants of Gonadal Dysgenesis (22, 32, 171, 172)

XO/XX; XO/XXX; and XO/XX/XXX Mosaicism. XO/XX mosaicism is the most common finding in patients with chromatin-positive gonadal dysgenesis and is second in frequency only to XO. Patients with these forms of mosaicism usually exhibit fewer of the associated somatic anomalies, are not invariably short, and may menstruate and even be fertile. One gonad may be of the streak type and the contralateral gonad either a hypoplastic or normal ovary, or both ovaries may be either normal or hypoplastic. During a fami-

Figure 9–31. Range of phenotypic and gonadal expression, which occurs in the variants of the syndrome of gonadal dysgenesis, and its relationship to the sex chromosome constitution. The typical phenotypic and gonadal findings in monosomic XO gonadal dysgenesis may be modified by the presence of a mosaic chromosomal constitution or by the presence of a structurally abnormal second sex chromosome. For example, XO/XX, XO/XXX mosaicism may be associated on the one hand with normal stature, minimal somatic features of Turner syndrome, and some degree of ovarian differentiation, or on the other hand with a clinical picture indistinguishable from classic XO gonadal dysgenesis. The phenotype and gonadal differentiation apparently depend upon the proportion of XO to XX or XXX cell lines in the somatic and germ cells during differererentiation. Similarly, the presence of a structurally abnormal X chromosome frequently alleviates some features of the classic syndrome. When XO/XY mosaicism or a structurally abnormal Y chromosome is present, varying degrees of testicular differentiation may be found. The spectrum of clinical findings may thus extend from that of a phenotypic male through pseudohermaphrodism to a phenotypic female, depending upon the degree of fetal testicular insufficiency. In addition, the beneficial effects of the normal XY cell line or the presence of some part of a Y chromosome may lead to normal stature and a modification of somatic defects associated with XO monosomy. (From Grumbach, M. M., In *Biologic Basis of Pediatric Practice.* Cooke, R. E. (ed.), New York, McGraw-Hill, 1967.)

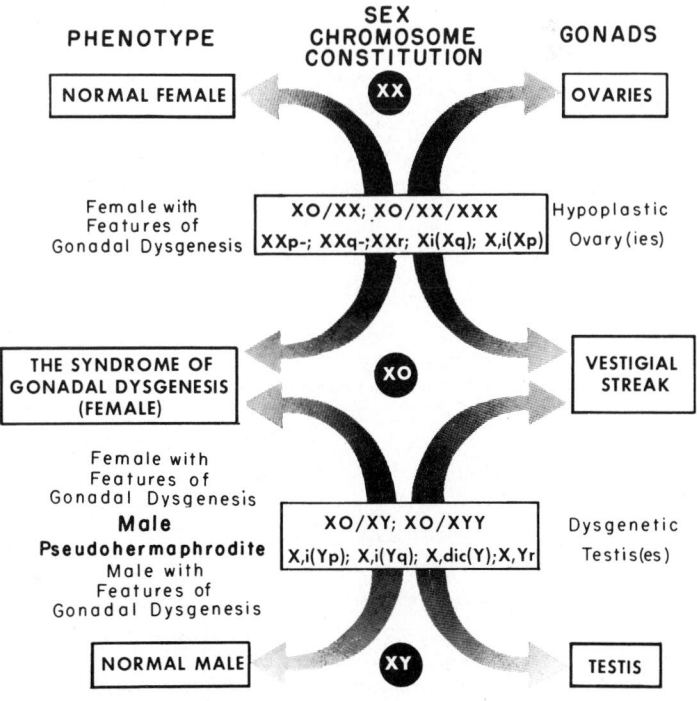

PHENOTYPE — SEX CHROMOSOME CONSTITUTION — GONADS

NORMAL FEMALE — XX — OVARIES

Female with Features of Gonadal Dysgenesis — XO/XX; XO/XX/XXX / XXp-; XXq-;XXr; Xi(Xq); X,i(Xp) — Hypoplastic Ovary(ies)

THE SYNDROME OF GONADAL DYSGENESIS (FEMALE) — XO — VESTIGIAL STREAK

Female with Features of Gonadal Dysgenesis / **Male Pseudohermaphrodite** / Male with Features of Gonadal Dysgenesis — XO/XY; XO/XYY / X,i(Yp); X,i(Yq); X,dic(Y);X,Yr — Dysgenetic Testis(es)

NORMAL MALE — XY — TESTIS

- =deletion, i=isochromosome, r=ring q=long arm, p=short arm, dic=dicentric

THE PRIMORDIAL GERM CELLS, THE SEX CHROMOSOMES AND GONADOGENESIS

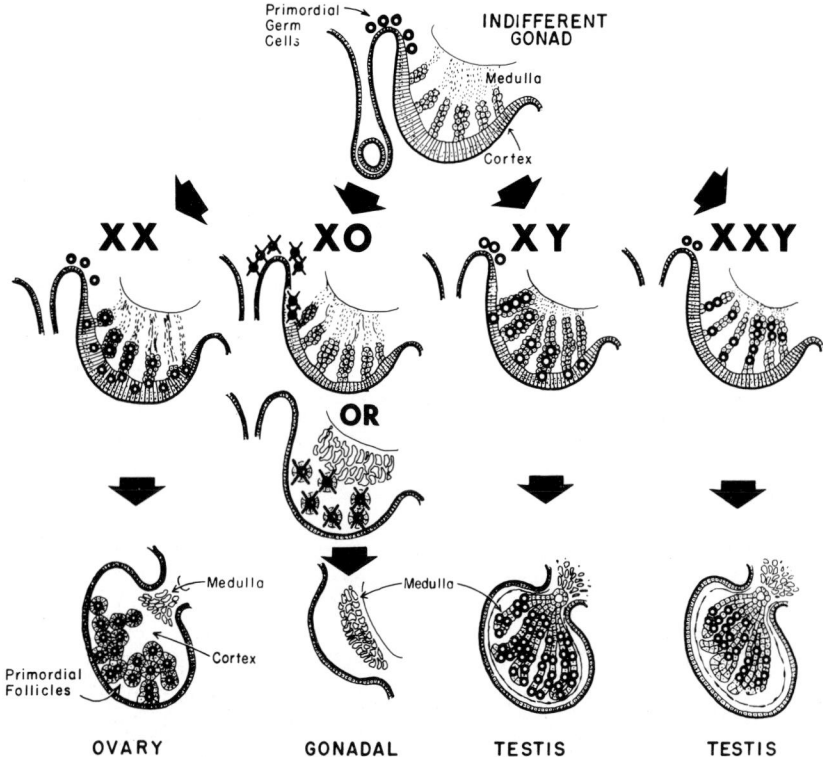

Figure 9–32. The primordial germ cells, the sex chromosomes, and gonadogenesis. Loss of germ cells during migration to or after seeding of the indifferent gonad in an XO individual would give rise to a gonadal streak, as germ cells are necessary for ovarian development of the indifferent gonad; recent evidence suggests that the loss occurs after the germ cells implant. In the presence of XO/XX mosaicism, gonadal differentiation may vary from that of an ovary to that of a gonadal streak. Similarly in XO/XY mosaics, depending on the sex chromosome constitution of the germ cells and of the gonadal blastema, gonadal differentiation may vary from that of a testis to that of a gonadal streak. In XXY individuals, germ cells become implanted in the primitive testis, but a marked loss of spermatogonia seems to occur in the perinatal period. (From Grumbach, M. M., In *Biologic Basis of Pediatric Practice.* Cooke, R. E. (ed.), New York, McGraw-Hill, 1967.)

ly survey for a leukocyte anomaly, Briggs et al. fortuitously discovered a normal grandmother with XO/XX/XXX mosaicism. Some appreciation of the variable clinical features may be gleaned from nine patients with these forms of mosaicism studied by Morishima and Grumbach (22). All had female external genitalia. Of seven who attained pubertal age, four showed some development of female secondary sex characteristics, and two menstruated regularly. One of these two has had three pregnancies. In some, no important somatic abnormalities were detected, and two were of normal stature. One of the XO/XX patients had a webbed neck, coarctation of the aorta, and a variety of other stigmata but was of normal stature and has menstruated regularly since

puberty. A 12-year-old XO/XX/XXX patient had primary hypothyroidism and Hashimoto's thyroiditis.

The X-chromatin pattern may provide clues to the presence of mosaicism. The proportion of X chromatin-positive cells often is less than in normal females, although this is not a consistent finding. The buccal smear, as well as smears from other tissues, may vary from chromatin-negative to a normal proportion of X chromatin-positive nuclei. If the patient harbors an XXX cell line, nuclei with duplicate X chromatin bodies may be found.

XXqi and XO/XXqi. Patients with the Xqi structural abnormality (presumptive isochromosome for the long arm of the X) have been thought to have an X chromosome that

Table 9–9. RELATIONSHIP OF STRUCTURAL ABNORMALITIES OF THE X AND Y TO CLINICAL MANIFESTATIONS OF THE SYNDROME OF GONADAL DYSGENESIS

Type of Sex Chromosome Abnormality	Karyotypes	Phenotype	Sexual Infantilism	Shortness of Stature	Somatic Anomalies of Turner's Syndrome
Loss of an X or Y	XO	Female	+	+	+
*Deletion of short arm of an X	XXqi	Female	+ (occ.±)	+	+
	XXp–	Female	+, ±, or –	+ (–)	+ (–)
*Deletion of long arm of an X	XXpi	Female	+	–	– or (±)
	XXq–	Female	+	– (+)	– or (±)
Deletion of both arms of an X (ring X)	XXr	Female	– or +	+	+ or (±)
Loss of short arm of Y	XYp–	Ambiguous	+	+	+

*In Xp – and Xq –, the extent and site of the deleted segment are variable.

Xqi = isochromosome for long arm of an X; Xp–= deletion of short arm of an X; Xpi = isochromosome for short arm of an X; Xq–= deletion of long arm of an X; Xr = ring chromosome derived from an X; Yp–= deletion of the short arm of the Y chromosome.

consists of two long arms (Xq) but lacks a short arm (Xp) (Fig. 9–33), as the result of division of the centromere in a transverse rather than longitudinal plane. Recent studies utilizing C and G banding techniques have demonstrated X isochromosomes that are both monocentric and dicentric (207). In one series 26 of 43 patients with an XXqi had an XO cell line and in most of the mosaics the long arm isochromosome was dicentric (i.e., it had two "C" bands). It has been suggested that dicentric X isochromosomes are more unstable than the monocentric form, and usually result in sex chromosome mosaicism through loss of the heteromorphic X chromosome. Isochromosome for the long arm of the X is the most common form of structural rearrangement of the X chromosome.

Patients with a long arm X isochromosome are invariably short, and have stigmata of the syndrome of gonadal dysgenesis and streak gonads (22, 32, 170) although some individuals have been reported to have menstruated spontaneously (208). Coarctation of the aorta and severe lymphedema of the hands and feet are conspicuously absent in XXqi patients. Webbing of the neck, if present, is usually only slight. The findings in these patients suggest that absence of the short arm on the second X, even in the presence of an X chromosome composed of two long arms, leads to shortness of stature, failure of ovarian development, and some somatic stigmata of Turner syndrome. The prevalence of Hashimoto's thyroiditis, decreased glucose tolerance, and inflammatory bowel disease may be higher in patients with structural abnormalities of the X chromosome, especially XXqi, than XO individuals.

Structurally abnormal X chromosomes are usually late replicating (except in balanced X-autosome translocations) and they give rise to the X chromatin body. Thus, X chromatin bodies are larger than normal in patients with an XXqi constitution, but their increased size may be less evident in buccal smears than in other tissues. Chromosome analysis reveals a metacentric X chromosome with two arms of equal length whose banding pattern is similar to the long arm of the normal X chromosome.

XXpi. Isochromosome for the short arm of the X chromosome is a rare anomaly of the X chromosome which has been infrequently reported (209, 210, 211). Two putative cases have been re-evaluated and found to represent long arm deletions (212, 213). All cases have had primary amenorrhea, sexual infantilism, normal stature, and few stigmata of the syndrome of gonadal dysgenesis. These patients are of special interest because they support the hypothesis that genes located on both the long and short arms of the X chromosome affect gonadogenesis, while loci that influence stature and prevent the expression of the major somatic abnormalities appear to be situated mainly on the short arm of the X.

XXr or XO/XXr. A ring X chromosome (Xr) usually occurs as part of XO/XXr mosaicism or a more complex karyotype (Fig. 9–32) (170, 214). Short stature is present in the majority of patients, and most have minor stigmata of Turner syndrome; none had either a webbed neck or coarctation of the aorta. Approximately one-third of the reported cases had spontaneous menstruation and developed secondary sexual characteristics.

The proportion of X chromatin-positive cells is decreased in patients with a ring X chromosome, and the X chromatin bodies are small. The ring X chromosome with rare exception exhibits late DNA replication (22).

The ring X chromosome arises by loss of both ends of a chromosome with union of the proximal breaks; as a consequence, a variable amount of chromatin material is lost from each arm (Fig. 9–4). Ring chromosomes are especially unstable and there is commonly a considerable variability in the size of the ring chromosome in different cells. In relation to the syndrome of gonadal dysgenesis, patients with a ring X chromosome provide evidence that loss of both terminal ends (telomere) of an X chromosome need not lead to the development of streak gonads.

XXp- and XO/XXp-. Deletions of the short arm of the X chromosome (Xp-) are rare and are frequently associated with XO mosaicism. Phenotypic-karyotypic correlations suggest that *terminal* deletions of the X chromosome (distal to band p21) can result in females who have normal ovarian function and no stigmata of the syndrome of gonadal dysgenesis, except possibly for short stature (204, 215, 216a). Usually, patients with deletions of the short arm of the X chromosome proximal to band 21, with and without XO cell lines, have clinical findings comparable to those observed in the XO karyotype. They are short and exhibit variable stigmata of the syndrome of gonadal dysgenesis (Fig. 9–34).

The abnormal X chromosome in these patients is usually

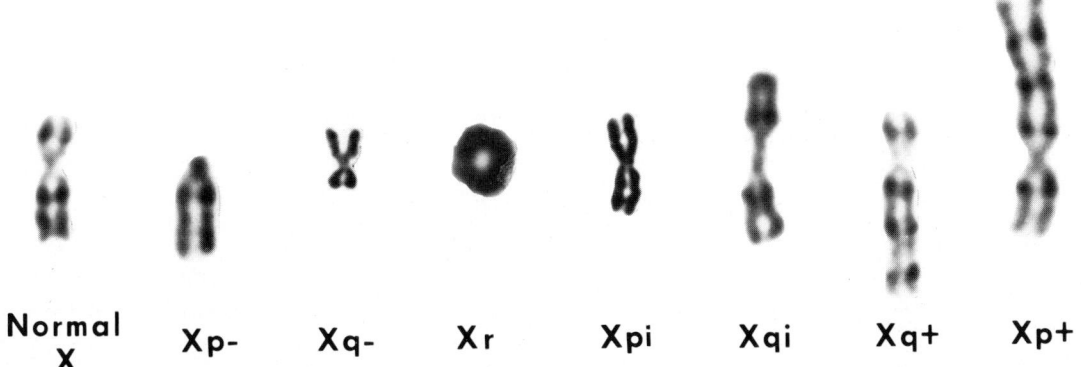

Normal X   Xp-   Xq-   Xr   Xpi   Xqi   Xq+   Xp+

Figure 9–33. Structural anomalies of the X chromosome. The normal X is on the left and is "G" banded; there is a dark band on the short arm and there are two major dark bands on the long arm. The Xq-, Xr, and Xpi are not banded. These structurally abnormal X chromosomes were ascertained by their late replicating patterns with tritiated thymidine. The Xqi is "G" banded. Note the apparent presence of two centromeres and the identical "G" banding patterns of both arms of the long arm isochromosome. The Xq+ is "G" banded and has an extra band on the long arm of the X chromosome. The extra chromosomal material appears to be a "suppressed" centromere, and the short arms of an X chromosome. The Xp+ chromosome has 6 major "G" bands (the normal 3 plus 3 more on the p arm of the X). This entire chromosome replicates late, it forms equal size bipartite X chromatin bodies, and by "C" banding exhibits two centromeric bands — one near the centromere and the other on the p+ arm. This chromosome is presumably an X-X translocation with telomeric fusion of two X chromosomes, short arm to short arm; despite the extra "C" band (centromeric chromatin), the second centromere is suppressed ("isodicentric").

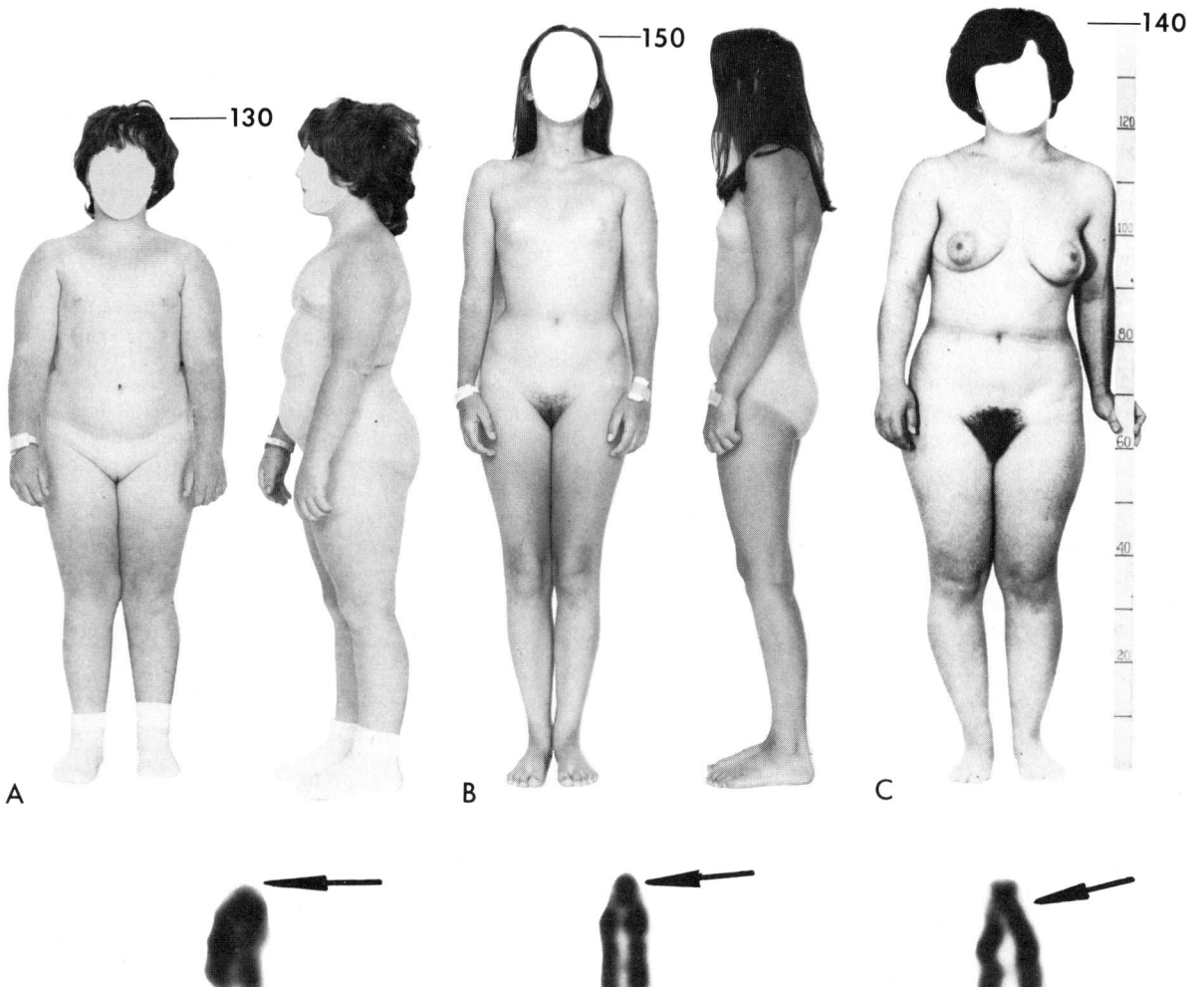

Figure 9–34. The variable gonadal function and phenotypic stigmata in three patients with a deletion of the short arm of the X chromosome (XXp −) of differing degree. *A*, A 13-year-old phenotypic female of short stature (− 3.5 SD), with low-set ears, a high-arched palate, a low hair line, a broad chest with wide-spaced areolae, cubitus valgus, puffy hands and feet, and short 4th metacarpals. There was no evidence of secondary sexual characteristics at 13 years of age. Plasma gonadotropins were elevated; LH 1.6 ng./ml. (LER-960), and FSH 26 ng./ml. (LER-869). Plasma estradiol was less than 6 pg./ml. The buccal smear contained a normal proportion of X chromatin bodies in the interphase nuclei which were conspicuously small. Karyotype analysis and autoradiography revealed a 46,XXp — karyotype. The abnormal X chromosome appeared to lack the entire short arm. *B* A 17 4/12-year-old phenotypic female with stigmata of the syndrome of gonadal dysgenesis. Her height was 151 cm. (− 3 S), and she had multiple nevi, cubitus valgus, and a short 4th metacarpal on the right hand. At age 13, the patient noted the spontaneous onset of breast development which did not progress. Plasma gonadotropins were elevated; LH 7.3 mg./ml. (LER-960), and FSH 53 ng./ml. (LER-869). The concentration of plasma estradiol was 19 pg./ml. On buccal smear the cells had a normal proportion of X chromatin bodies which appeared small. Karyotype analysis and autoradiography indicated a 46,XXp — chromosome had been deleted close to the centromere, but a small segment of the short arm is visible distal to the centromere. *C*, A 20-year-old phenotypic female with a chief complaint of dysfunctional uterine bleeding. She had short stature, slight puffiness of her hands and feet, and short 4th metacarpals. Female secondary sexual characteristics appeared at 11 years of age, and menarche at 13 years was followed by regular menses which later became irregular. The buccal smear exhibited nuclei with a normal proportion of small sex chromatin bodies. Bilateral ovaries were identified grossly and histologically during an appendectomy. The karyotype was 46,XXp —. The extent of deletion of the short arm of the abnormal X chromosome in this patient is less than that seen in patients A and B. A segment of the short arm is readily discernible above the centromere.

It appears that, in these three patients with XXp- karyotypes, the somatic and gonadal manifestations of the "syndrome of gonadal dysgenesis" correlated with the magnitude of the deletion of the short arm of the X chromosome.

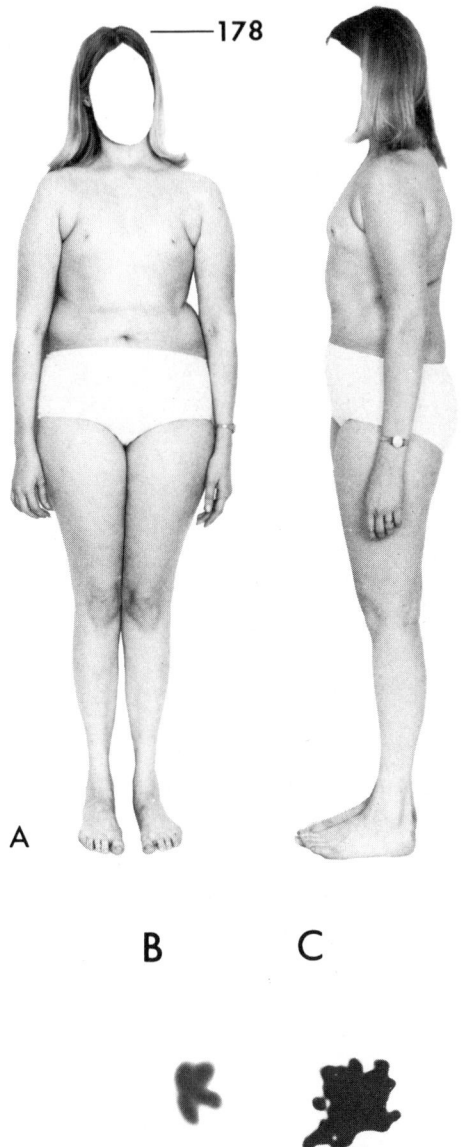

—178

A

B   C

Figure 9–35. *A*, A 22 year old, tall female with a chief complaint of primary amenorrhea who has a deletion of the long arms of one X chromosome Xq-. At 12 years of age she developed sparse pubic hair. Breast development did not occur and she remained sexually infantile. Height 178 cm (+2.6 SD); weight 70 Kg (+1.2 SD). No somatic stigmata of the syndrome of gonadal dysgenesis were noted. Plasma gonadotropins were elevated: LH 5.6 ng/ml (LER960), and FSH 36.5 ng/ml (LER869). The buccal smear showed a normal proportion of X chromatin bodies that were slightly small. Karyotype analysis: 46,XXq-. A Giemsa stained Xq- (*B*) is shown which exhibited the late labeling pattern characteristic of an X chromosome (*C*).

the late DNA replicating X chromosome and is the origin of the small X chromatin body found in interphase nuclei in these patients. Of interest is the report of a familial group of 7 patients with the syndrome of gonadal dysgenesis secondary to a deletion of the short arm of an X chromosome in which the disorder was transmitted by carriers of a balanced translocation between the X and chromosome number 1 (217).

XXq- and XO/XXq-. A small number of patients have been reported with this X-chromosome anomaly (Xq- designates a deletion of the long arm of the X chromosome). In general these patients are normal in stature and exhibit few if any stigmata of Turner syndrome, but have primary amenorrhea, sexual infantilism, and streak gonads. We

have studied two patients with 46,XXq-karyotypes and the findings in one patient are summarized in Figure 9–35. Exceptions to the rule that XXq- patients lack stigmata of Turner syndrome and are of normal height were reported before chromosome banding techniques became available. Such cases may represent either hidden mosaicism or complex structural rearrangements of the X chromosome, including inversions and interstitial rather than terminal deletions.

X-X Translocation and X-Autosome Translocations (205). Summitt has reviewed the reports of X-autosome translocations (205). The pattern of X inactivation observed in these karyotypes usually preserves a single active X in the genome of the cell. Dysgenetic gonads were present in patients with breaks in the X chromosome located between bands Xq13 and Xq27. This suggests that this region of the long arm of the X chromosome contains loci that affect gonadal differentiation. Cases of putative unbalanced X-autosome translocations associated with Turner syndrome are probably X-X translocations or duplications and not X-autosome translocations (205).

Recently, Mirzayants et al. reviewed the reported cases with X-X translocations (218). These are large, late-replicating X chromosomes which are joined by either their long or short arms (Fig. 9–32, Xp+). This karyotype is frequently associated with an XO cell line. These large X chromosomes have two C bands but only one functional centromere (isodicentric) and tend to form large bipartite sex chromatin bodies. Patients with long arm to long arm translocations usually lack stigmata of Turner syndrome but have primary gonadal failure, whereas short arm to short arm X-chromosome translocations have short stature, somatic stigmata, and streak gonads.

X Chromatin-Negative Variants of the Syndrome of Gonadal Dysgenesis

The pattern of sex chromosome mosaicism and structural abnormalities of the Y chromosome is similar to that described for the X chromosome, although the chromatin-negative variants are less common. Usually as a consequence of its effect on gonadal differentiation, a Y-bearing cell line modifies the classic female phenotype of the syndrome by leading to a variable degree of masculine differentiation of the genital tract.

XO/XY; XO/XYY; XO/XY/XYY, and Related Abnormalities (Table 9–10). A highly diverse phenotype is encountered in

Table 9–10. SALIENT FEATURES OF XO/XY MOSAICISM

Karyotype: 45,XO/46,XY

Genitalia: Female→ambiguous→male

Wolffian duct derivatives:	Duct differentiation, contingent upon functional integrity of homolateral fetal gonad, i.e. streak →uterus, fallopian tubes; dysgenetic testis→variable structures; testis→wolffian duct derivatives
Müllerian duct derivatives:	

Gonad: Streak gonads→dysgenetic testes→normal testes; ↑risk gonadal neoplasm (gonadoblastoma)

Habitus: Variable; streak gonads→sexual infantilism; testes (dysgenetic) →virilization; if gonadoblastoma present, may → gynecomastia 2° to estradiol secretion

Hormone profile: ↑ plasma FSH, LH and ↓ testosterone concentrations

H-Y antigen positive (may be decreased from that in XY males)

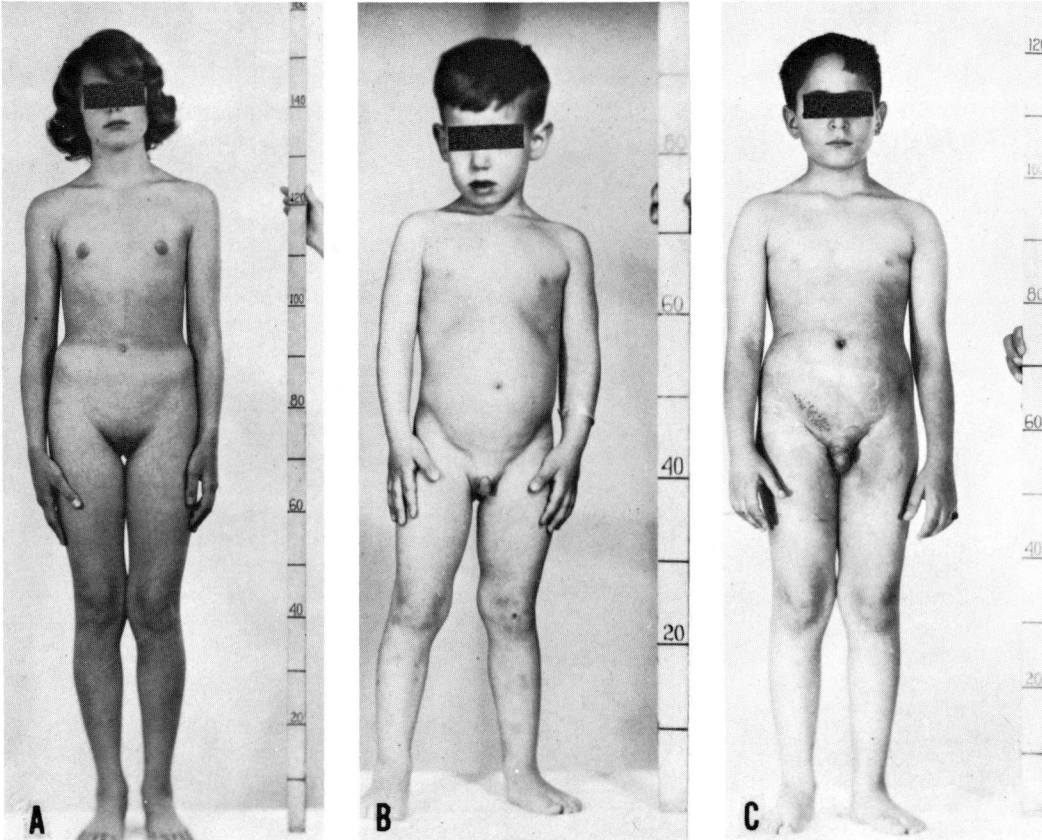

Figure 9–36. Three patients with XO/XY sex chromosome mosaicism who illustrate the highly varied phenotype in this variant of the syndrome of gonadal dysgenesis. (Patient numbers refer to designation in Table 9–11.) *A*, Patient 1, a phenotypic female, was 15 4/12 years of age. She had shortness of stature (— 3.1 SD), increased number of pigmented nevi, puffiness over the dorsum of the fingers, and broad and short hands, and was sexually infantile (the breast development seen in the photograph followed estrogen therapy), except for sparse pubic and axillary hair. The titer of urinary gonadotropin was > 80 m.u./day. *B*, Patient 3, a 3 1/12-year-old child, has ambiguous external genitalia, perineal hypospadias, and undescended gonads. He was of average height and had a broad chest and a duplication of the left kidney. *C*, Patient 9, an 8 1/12-year-old phenotypic male with a penile urethra and unilateral undescended gonad, was of average height and had cubitus valgus, short fourth metacarpals, and puffiness of the dorsum of the fingers. By 15 years of age, male secondary sexual characteristics were well advanced, and the scrotal testis, which was normal in histologic appearance, measured 4.0 × 2.4 cm.

these forms of mosaicism (22, 219). Such individuals may appear as phenotypic females, as individuals with ambiguous external genitalia, or as phenotypic males (Fig. 9–36). As in XO/XX mosaicism, short stature and the associated somatic abnormalities, while frequently present, are inconsistent features and may vary independently of each other and of gonadal differentiation. Zäh et al. reviewed 111 patients with XO/XY mosaicism (219). Two-thirds had been reared as females.

Of nine patients with XO/XY or XO/XY/XYY mosaicism studied by Morishima and Grumbach (22), one was a phenotypic female, one was a phenotypic male, and seven had ambiguous external genitalia (Table 9–11). The differentiation of the gonads varied from presumed bilateral streaks in the phenotypic female to bilateral dysgenetic testes. In others the development was asymmetric: one patient had a streak in one mesosalpinx and a rudimentary testis on the contralateral side (so called mixed gonadal dysgenesis); another patient had a normal testis in the scrotum and a herniated streak, fallopian tube, and a vestigial uterus (hernia uteri inguinale) in the contralateral inguinal region. In at least one reported case in infancy, the streak gonad contained a few primordial follicles. The development of the genital ducts, urogenital sinus, and external

genitalia usually correlates well with the extent of testicular differentiation and, consequently, fetal testosterone production.

The restricted local or paracrine action of the testes on the differentiation of genital ducts is well demonstrated in patients with asymmetric gonadal development. In such patients, the development of male ducts and involution of the müllerian structures are also asymmetric and parallel the degree of testicular development on each side. As discussed on page 443, local action of the testis on müllerian regression is mediated through a müllerian duct-inhibiting protein, whereas unilateral stimulation of male ducts is through mechanisms which serve to concentrate high local levels of testosterone in the wolffian ducts and their derivatives. The presence of Sertoli cells in the ipsilateral gonad correlates with the absence of müllerian structures on the same side in patients with XO/XY mosaicism (220). This observation is consistent with the secretion of müllerian duct inhibitory factor by embryonic and fetal Sertoli cells. Male differentiation of the external genitalia, however, would be brought about by testicular tissue in either fetal gonad, as masculinization of these structures is responsive to systemic androgens, and these may be secreted by either testis. The phenotype may range from simulant female with only slight

Table 9–11.   GENITAL STRUCTURES IN NINE PATIENTS WITH XO/XY SEX CHROMOSOME MOSAICISM*

Case	External Genitalia	Uro-genital Sinus	Phallic En-large-ment	Gonads	Genital Ducts Female		Genital Ducts Male	
1	Female	−	−	Rt. streak?	Rt. fallopian tube?		Rt.	−
				Lt. streak?	Lt. fallopian tube?	uterus	Lt.	−
2	Ambiguous	+	+	Rt. testis	Rt. fallopian tube		Rt. vas deferens	
				Lt. streak	Lt. fallopian tube	uterus	Lt.	−
3	Ambiguous	+	+	Rt. not found	Rt. fallopian tube		Rt.	−
				Lt. streak	Lt. fallopian tube	uterus	Lt.	−
4	Ambiguous	+	+	Rt. dysgenetic testis	Rt. fallopian tube		Rt. vas deferens	
				Lt. dysgenetic testis	Lt. fallopian tube	vestigial uterus	Lt.	−
5	Ambiguous	+	+	Rt. dysgenetic testis	Rt. fallopian tube		Rt. vas deferens	
				Lt. dysgenetic testis	Lt. fallopian tube	uterus	Lt. vas deferens	
6	Ambiguous	+	+	Rt. dysgenetic testis	Rt. fallopian tube		Rt.	−
				Lt. dysgenetic testis	Lt. fallopian tube	uterus	Lt.	−
7	Ambiguous	+	+	Rt. dysgenetic testis	Rt.	−	Rt. vas deferens	
				Lt. dysgenetic testis	Lt.	−	Lt. vas deferens	
8	Ambiguous	+	+	Rt. dysgenetic testis	Rt. fallopian tube		Rt. vas deferens	
				Lt. streak	Lt. fallopian tube	uterus	Lt.	−
9	Male	−	Normal penis	Rt. streak	Rt. fallopian tube		Rt.	−
				Lt. testis	Lt.	−	vestigial uterus Lt. vas deferens	

*From Morishima, A., and Grumbach, M. M.: *Ann. N.Y. Acad. Sci. 155*:695, 1968.

clitoral hypertrophy to a completely male configuration. XO/XY mosaicism has been reported in a few patients with the phenotype of the "male Turner syndrome." Although in most patients the secretion of androgenic hormones at adolescence is predictable from the degree of masculinization of the external genitalia *in utero,* virilization has occurred at puberty in some patients with a predominantly female phenotype. Breast development at or after the age of puberty occurs in about one-fourth of cases, and is usually associated with a gonadal neoplasm. We studied two adolescent XO/XY patients who exhibited breast development and had pubertal levels of plasma estradiol; at laparotomy a gonadoblastoma was found that secreted estradiol (Fig. 9–37).

The propensity of patients with XO/XY mosaicism to develop gonadal tumors is much increased, and prophylactic removal of the streak gonads or dysgenetic undescended testes is indicated. Gonadoblastoma, a complex tumor composed of large germ cells, Sertoli cells, and stromal derivatives, is the neoplasm most often found; it can give rise to the malignant germinoma. Thus, after the removal of the gonds, serial sections should be examined for evidence of a tumor. The risk of a gonadal tumor is about 20% overall (221) and is age-related. Sonography of the pelvis is a useful procedure for screening for gonadal neoplasms. Computerized tomography can demonstrate calcification in gonadoblastomas not visible on routine X-ray films of the pelvis.

A useful clue to the presence of functional testicular elements before puberty is the detection of a rise in the concentration of serum testosterone above prepubertal values following a course of human chorionic gonadotropin (1000–2000 units intramuscularly, every 3 days for 3 doses).

Patients have been reported with XO/XY or XO/XXY mosaicism in whom the brightly fluorescent portion of the Y chromosome was absent. Caspersson et al. (222) noted the absence of bright fluorescence of the Y chromosome in 4 of 7 patients he studied. In one of his patients, a putative Y to chromosome 2 translocation during gametogenesis was suspected. In other patients (223, 224), no evidence of translocation or deletion of the Y was present. Fluorescence as well as C banding and replication of the Y chromosome was altered when compared to normal. Analysis of these cases suggests the possibility that the primary lesions in these patients is a molecular alteration in the Y-specific DNA sequences of an XY zygote, resulting in mitotic loss of the Y and the production of an XO cell line and mosaicism. Our limited experience with patients who have had a nonfluorescent Y chromosome is that they may have a reduced overall risk of gonadal malignancy below that for the general group.

Mixed, asymmetric, or *atypical gonadal dysgenesis* is a term that has sometimes been used to describe patients with a streak gonad on one side and a testis on the other. It is important to emphasize that, while this association is common in XO/XY mosaicism, these gonadal findings are not specific for XO/XY mosaicism, and occur with an XY karyotype (e.g., in familial XY gonadal dysgenesis).

XO/XY mosaicism probably arises through anaphase lag. However, XO/XY mosaicism is frequently associated with structurally abnormal Y chromosomes. Thus, interchromosome rearrangements with loss of the structurally abnormal

Y may be a common mechanism for the production of XO/XY mosaicism with structurally abnormal Y chromosomes (223, 224).

Rarely, patients who have male or ambiguously male genitalia have been reported to have only an XO karyotype in the tissues studied (225, 226). H-Y antigen was found to be positive in two cases in which it was examined (225, 226). Cryptic mosaicism or a translocation of Y- material appears to be the most likely etiology of this condition (225).

Treatment. The diagnosis of XO/XY mosaicism is established by the demonstration of XO/XY mosaicism in blood, skin, or gonadal tissue. A Y chromosome lacking the distal fluorescent portion of its long arm can be recognized as a Y by its size, morphologic appearance (parallel long arms and short, fuzzy short arms), and lack of a C band. The decision as to the sex of rearing should be based on the potential for normal function of the external genitalia. In patients assigned a female gender role, the gonads should be removed, and the external genitalia repaired by clitoral recession, vaginoplasty, and labioscrotal reduction. Estrogen therapy, initiated at the age of normal puberty, is necessary to induce female secondary sex characteristics (see p. 460). In affected infants in whom a male gender assignment is selected, all gonadal tissue except that which appears histologically normal and is in the scrotum should be removed and prosthetic testes placed in the reconstructed scrotal sac. In these patients, removal of the müllerian duct remnants is indicated, as is repair of the hypospadias. Androgen replacement therapy is usually necessary at adolescence depending on the functional capacity of the testis to secrete testosterone. Because of the increased risk of neoplasm in dysgenetic testes, especially in adults, patients raised as males in whom a testis is retained must be examined regularly (227).

Structural Abnormalities of the Y Chromosome (27, 228). Structural abnormalities of the Y chromosome, which are of clinical significance in regard to sex differentiation and the syndrome of gonadal dysgenesis, are much rarer than those involving the X chromosome. This may be because the deleted Y chromosome, being much smaller than most structural abnormalities of the X chromosome, is more readily lost from the cell during mitosis. Some XO individuals may therefore arise as a consequence of a structural abnormality of the Y that is lost at an early cleavage division.

The small size of the Y chromosome and the inability to

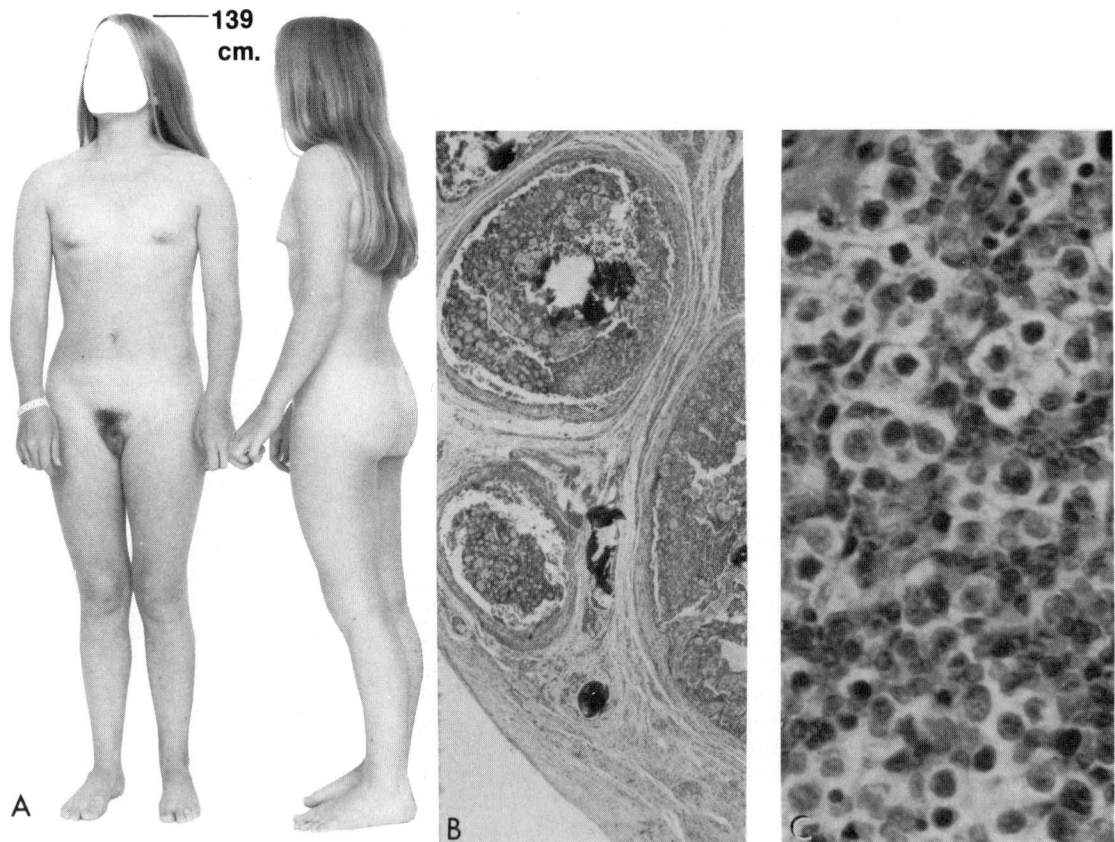

Figure 9–37. XO/XY mosaicism with a feminizing gonadoblastoma. *A*, A 20-year-old female with many of the stigmata of the syndrome of gonadal dysgenesis, including short stature, multiple nevi, cubitus valgus, and hyperconvex, small nails. The buccal smear was X chromatin-negative; on fluorescent microscopy, 30% of the interphase nuclei had a single Y body. The karyotype was XO/XY. The patient had spontaneous development of pubic and axillary hair at 12 years of age. At 18 years of age, breast development was noted. Her height was 139 cm. (− 5.1 SD) and weight 39 kg. (− 2.5 DS). The bone age was 17 years; an intravenous pyelogram was normal. The concentration of plasma gonadotropins at 20 years of age was elevated; plasma LH 8 ng./ml. (LER-960), and FSH 50 ng./ml. (LER-869). A urocytogram showed a "moderate" estrogen effect. The concentration of plasma estradiol was 26 pg./ml. and of estrone 32 pg./ml.; plasma testosterone was less than 20 ng./100 ml. On exploratory laparotomy, normal-appearing fallopian tubes and uterus were found. The right gonad was a typical "streak," with whorls of fibrous connective tissue. *B*, The left gonad was replaced by a 1.3 × 1 × 1-cm. tumor mass which, on histologic section, revealed well-defined nests and islands of Sertoli-Leydig-like cells and germ cells, as well as calcification consistent with the diagnosis of "gonadoblastoma." *C*, Higher magnification illustrates the aggregates of germ cells and smaller epithelial cells resembling immature Sertoli cells, as well as cells indistinguishable from Leydig cells.

completely characterize the short arm of the Y (Yp) and the proximal portions of the long arm (Yq) by banding techniques complicate the localization of the testis-determining gene(s) on the Y chromosome. Koo et al. recently examined 17 patients with structurally abnormal Y chromosomes varying in composition from long arm deletions to ring and minute Y chromosomes (28) and concluded that the testis-determining loci are located in the pericentromeric region of the Y chromosome, most likely on neighboring segments of both the long and short arms of the Y chromosomes. The highly fluorescent heterochromatic distal portion of the Y chromosome contains little or no genetically active material since its absence has been reported in normal males. Patients with minute Y chromosomes or small rings invariably have testicular tissues supporting the pericentromeric location of the testicular determining genes (229, 230).

Of interest is a patient recently reported to have a short arm deletion of the Y chromosome (XYp-) without an XO cell line who had ambiguous genitalia, stigmata of Turner syndrome, and intermediate levels of H-Y antigen (231). The findings in this patient support earlier evidence that patients with extensive deletions of the short arms of X and Y chromosomes have the stigmata of Turner syndrome, while long arm deletions of the X and Y chromosomes do not result in these somatic anomalies. Most patients with an isochromosome, ring, or dicentric Y chromosome are sex chromosome mosaics and have an associated XO cell line. Their phenotype is highly variable and extends from that of a normal adult male through individuals with ambiguous genitalia and male pseudohermaphrodism to patients with infantile female external genitalia and bilateral streak gonads. The variation in phenotype is best explained by the effect of the XO cell line and the magnitude of the loss of active segments of the Y chromosome. Several instances of Y-autosome translocations are known (168, 232); usually there is translocation of the distal heterochromatic region of the long arm of the Y chromosome to an autosome, and male sex differentiation is normal (Fig. 9–2). Buhler has reviewed recent information regarding the Y chromosome and has attempted to assign different functions and genes to different regions of the Y chromosome (27).

Pure Gonadal Dysgenesis

This term has been applied to phenotypic females with a 46,XX or 46,XY karyotype who have rudimentary streak gonads and remain sexually infantile, but who are of normal or tall stature and lack the somatic stigmata of Turner syndrome. At puberty, they exhibit the usual effects of prepubertal castration, and their plasma and urinary gonadotropin values are increased. The X chromatin pattern may be either positive or negative. The X chromatin-negative patients occasionally have clitoral enlargement, which may be present at birth or first becomes manifest at puberty; clitoral enlargement is rarely present in X chromatin-positive patients.

The designation "pure gonadal dysgenesis" was introduced by Harden and Stewart in 1959 in their report of a 19-year-old phenotypic female with the described phenotype and an XY karyotype (233). This represented an elaboration of the concept of gonadal dysgenesis in normal appearing females which had been proposed earlier by Hoffenberg et al. It is now known that a variety of etiologic factors may lead to the development of this clinical picture. We have chosen to restrict the term "pure gonadal dysgenesis" to those patients with XX and XY gonadal dysgenesis (see below).

Familial XX Gonadal Dysgenesis and Its Incomplete Forms (Table 9–12). XX gonadal dysgenesis is characterized by normal stature, sexual infantilism, bilateral streak gonads (similar in structure to those of XO gonadal dysgenesis), normal female internal and external genitalia, primary amenorrhea, elevated gonadotropins, absence of the somatic stigmata of the syndrome of gonadal dysgenesis, and a 46,XX karyotype (12).

The habitus is often eunuchoid. Rare cases have had a few somatic abnormalities including cubitus valgus, but not the classic phenotypic manifestations of Turner syndrome. McDonough et al. reviewed the phenotypic and cytogenetic findings in 82 phenotypic female patients with primary gonadal failure. Sex chromosome anomalies were found in association with ovarian failure in 52/82 patients, all of whom were less than 63 inches tall. Conversely, all patients with ovarian failure greater than 63 inches tall had either a 46,XX or 46,XY karyotype (234). Occasionally, patients with clitoral enlargement, hirsutism, and other signs of virilization are reported; the concentration of serum testosterone was increased above the range for normal women in such a patient reported by Judd et al. (235). The streak gonads in their patient secreted testosterone, presumably from the nests of hilus cells which were found on histologic examination. It is assumed that in this case, the high concentration of gonadotropins led to hilus cell hyperplasia and a modest increase in circulating androgens which, in the presence of meager estrogen production, had more potent biological action.

Families in which multiple siblings have been affected are not uncommon (12). Within families, the expression of the

Table 9–12.   XX GONADAL DYSGENESIS AND VARIANT FORM

	Complete	Incomplete
Karyotype:	46,XX	
Inheritance:	Autosomal recessive in familial cases (sensorineural deafness in about 10%)	
Genitalia:	Normal female	
Wolffian duct derivatives:	Absent	
Müllerian duct derivatives:	Normal female	
Gonads:	Bilateral streak gonads	Hypoplastic ovary and streak or bilateral hypoplastic ovaries
Habitus:	Normal stature, no somatic stigmata of Turner syndrome	
	Sexual infantilism	Incomplete puberty, premature ovarian failure
Hormone profile:	↑ plasma FSH and LH concentration	Plasma estradiol variable: decreased or normal

disease may vary in affected siblings. The gonads may range from bilateral streak gonads to hypoplastic ovaries with varying degrees of ovarian function. In the familial cases transmission is consistent with an autosomal recessive trait. Autosomal recessive XX gonadal dysgenesis provides evidence that a mutant gene on a pair of autosomes can lead to a profound disturbance of ovarian differentiation, and, alternatively, that an autosomal gene has an important role in the differentiation of normal ovaries. The abnormal gonadogenesis may be the consequence of the effect of a mutant gene on germ cell migration, the gonadal blastema, the rate of germ cell attrition, or a defect in the putative ovary-organizing factor or its receptor.

In five families 46,XX gonadal dysgenesis has been associated with sensorineural deafness (12). Genetic heterogeneity is suggested by concordance of the gonadal defect with deaf mutism in these families and by four other families in which short stature, XX gonadal dysgenesis, microcephaly, and arachnodactyly occurred in affected siblings (12). Hamet et al. reported three sisters with renal failure, adrenal hyperplasia, hypertension, sensorineural deafness, and primary hypogonadism (236). A kindred with cerebellar ataxia and hypergonadotropic hypogonadism as well as another with mental retardation, streak gonads, myopathy, and various neurological abnormalities have been described (237).

Sporadic cases of XX gonadal dysgenesis may represent a heterogenous group. For example, ovarian hypoplasia has been associated with trisomy 13 and trisomy 18. XX gonadal dysgenesis should be distinguished from ovarian failure as a consequence of infection, such as mumps in childhood, or autoimmune oöphoritis, and from patients with antibodies to gonadotropin receptors, a biologically inactive FSH, or gonadotropin insensitive ovaries, as well as from patients with biosynthetic errors that affect estrogen formation (e.g., 17α-hydroxypase deficiency).

In contrast to XY gonadal dysgenesis, gonadal neoplasms are rare in XX gonadal dysgenesis. The diagnosis of XX gonadal dysgenesis is based on finding a normal karyotype in a sexually infantile phenotypic female with hypergonadotropic hypogonadism. In sporadic cases, it is important to confirm the presence of streak or hypoplastic gonads by sonography or laparoscopy. Replacement therapy with estrogen is similar to that for patients with XO gonadal dysgenesis (p. 460).

Familial XY Gonadal Dysgenesis and Its Incomplete Forms. XY gonadal dysgenesis was first described by Swyer (238). This syndrome in its complete form is characterized by a female phenotype, normal to tall stature, bilateral dysgenetic gonads, sexual infantilism with primary amenorrhea, eunuchoid habitus, and a 46, XY karyotype. Somatic features of Turner syndrome are inconspicuous or absent. The internal structures are female with bilateral tubes, a uterus, and a vagina. Clitoral enlargement is not uncommon, and the frequency of gonadal neoplasms, especially gonadoblastoma and germinoma (seminoma, dysgerminoma) is high. Breast development after the normal age of puberty strongly suggests the presence of an estrogen-secreting gonadal tumor, especially a gonadoblastoma. Plasma gonadotropins and the excretion of urinary gonadotropins are increased. In some patients the level of serum testosterone is increased above prepubertal and normal female values, presumably because of the secretion of androgens from the hilus cells of the streak gonads. A male proportion of single fluorescent Y bodies is present in interphase nuclei. In an isolated case the Y chromosome was non-fluorescent (239). Excluded from this syndrome are patients with variants of the syndrome of gonadal dysgenesis, such as XO/XY mosaicism and structural abnormalities of the Y chromosome.

Familial aggregates as well as sporadic cases have been described (12, 240). Simpson reviewed 15 affected pedigrees and confirmed the general view that the disorder is transmitted as an X-linked or male limited autosomal dominant trait. Familial cases may vary in the appearance of the external genitalia and the development of secondary sex characteris-

Table 9-13. SALIENT FEATURES OF XY GONADAL DYSGENESIS AND VARIANT FORM

	Complete	Incomplete
Karyotype:	46,XY	
Inheritance:	Familial cases consistent with X-linked (or male inheritance limited autosomal dominant)	
Genitalia:	Female	Ambiguous
Wolffian duct derivatives:	Absent	Rudimentary → hypoplastic
Müllerian duct derivatives:	Normal	Variable, rudimentary → hypoplastic
Gonads:	Bilateral streak gonads	Bilateral dysgenetic testes or streak gonad + dysgenetic testes (mixed gonadal dysgenesis)
	↑ risk of gonadal tumor, gonadoblastoma, especially if H-Y antigen positive	
Habitus:	Sexual infantilism at puberty	Variable degree of virilization at puberty
	Breast development suggests presence of gonadal tumor	
	↑ plasma FSH and LH and ↓ testosterone concentrations	
Hormone profile:	70% H-Y antigen positive or intermediate: 30% H-Y antigen negative	H-Y antigen positive

tics. Usually the external and internal genital tract is completely female and the patient is sexually infantile (complete form); however, affected siblings may have ambiguous external genitalia and development of the genital ducts and urogenital sinus (incomplete or variant form). The spectrum of genital ambiguity suggests that the mutant gene(s) exhibits variable expressivity. In a family reported by Chemke et al., two siblings had XY gonadal dysgenesis with bilateral streak gonads and another had the incomplete form with genital ambiguity, bilateral dysgenetic testes, and müllerian derivatives (241). We studied the infant born to the "normal" 46,XX sister in the Chemke propositi. This 46,XY patient had ambiguous external genitalia, bilateral dysgenetic testes, and müllerian derivatives. Inheritance in this family is consistent with an X-linked or male-limited autosomal dominant trait. Other forms of inheritance of XY gonadal dysgenesis have been described. Of note is the association of XY gonadal dysgenesis with camptomelic dwarfism, an autosomal recessive form of lethal dwarfism (242). In XX females with this type of lethal dwarfism, the gonadal histology is normal. A new familial syndrome of XY gonadal dysgenesis with anomalies of ectodermal and mesomelic structures has been reported (243).

Both H-Y antigen positive and H-Y antigen negative forms (58, 244, 245) have been described and reflect the genetic heterogeneity of the syndrome. For example, a familial case of 46,XY gonadal dysgenesis has been described in which H-Y antigen studies were negative and a structural abnormality of the X chromosome was present (246). This case is similar to that described in the Scandinavian wood lemming, in that both a structurally abnormal X chromosome and the absence of H-Y antigen expression were found in 46,XY "females" (55, 57, 247). Evidence reviewed earlier in the Scandinavian wood lemming suggests that the expression of H-Y antigen is under control of a gene on the X chromosome as well as the Y (p. 434). Part of the normal mechanism of sex determination in this species includes not only fertile XX females and XY males but also fertile XY *females*; the latter produce only female offspring. Wachtel et al. showed that these fertile XY females are H-Y antigen negative (57). Thus, some forms of familial XY gonadal dysgenesis may be due to an X-linked mutant gene that suppresses H-Y antigen elaboration and dissemination (248, 249). The lack of H-Y antigen, despite the XY sex chromosome constitution, leads to failure of the bipotential gonad to develop as a testis. Unlike the XY female wood lemming, which has fertile ovaries, streak gonads are present in patients with XY gonadal dysgenesis. As discussed before, in man two X chromosomes are required for normal ovarian development; in the absence of a second X chromosome, despite the lack of H-Y antigen, functional ovaries would not be expected in the human.

H-Y antigen-positive patients have been reported in both familial and sporadic cases of XY gonadal dysgenesis (244, 248). Thus, the expression of serologically detectable H-Y antigen does not ensure differentiation of testes. It has been postulated that the H-Y antigen-positive patients with XY gonadal dysgenesis have either defective receptors for H-Y antigen on gonadal cells or are producing an abnormal H-Y antigen which has a low affinity for its gonadal receptor (249). Even in relation to the expression of H-Y antigen, XY gonadal dysgenesis is a heterogeneous disorder.

Three loci appear to be involved in H-Y antigen synthesis and expression: a locus on the short arm of the X chromosome; one or more loci in the pericentromeric region of the Y chromosome; and possibly a locus on an autosome. XY gonadal dysgenesis may result from a mutant gene that affects the expression of H-Y antigen (H-Y negative), a defect in the gonad specific H-Y antigen receptor (H-Y positive), and possibly the elaboration of a serologically reactive but abnormal H-Y antigen which lacks affinity for the H-Y antigen receptors on gonadal cells (H-Y positive) (249).

There is a high prevalence of gonadal tumors, especially gonadoblastoma and germinoma, in this syndrome. The tumors may be bilateral and can occur in more than one affected sibling. Hence, bilateral prophylactic gonadectomy is indicated and can be performed when the diagnosis is established. In the first affected member of a family, this is usually at the age of puberty in the complete form and in infancy in patients with ambiguous external genitalia (incomplete form).

Sex of rearing in patients with the incomplete form of XY gonadal dysgenesis is determined by the extent of genital ambiguity and the age at diagnosis. Patients raised as females should be placed on estrogen replacement therapy at 12–13 years of age and eventually be cycled monthly with both estrogen and progesterone (see p. 460). In patients raised as males, testosterone replacement therapy is begun at the age of puberty (see p. 454).

So-Called "Male Turner Syndrome"

Many phenotypic males have been reported with short stature, webbed neck, and other somatic abnormalities associated with the syndrome of gonadal dysgenesis in whom the testes were hypoplastic and frequently undescended. The resemblance of these males to phenotypic females with XO gonadal dysgenesis suggested a pathogenetic parallelism or Turner syndrome in the male and the female. However, with rare exceptions, this interrelationship is no longer tenable (31). A few patients with the phenotypic features of male Turner syndrome have had a sex chromosome abnormality, such as XO/XY mosaicism, and they represent a partial sex chromosome monosomy variant of Turner syndrome. In all the other karyotypic studies of these patients, the sex chromosome constitution was XY. The XY cases form a heterogeneous clinical group in which there may be multiple causes. Unless partial sex chromosome monosomy can be demonstrated, these patients ought not to be considered as the clinical parallel in the male of Turner syndrome in phenotypic females. Many of the cases previously categorized as "male Turner syndrome" are examples of the syndrome of webbed neck, ptosis, hypogonadism, and short stature usually associated with congenital heart disease and mental retardation (31, 250, 251, 252) discussed below.

Syndrome of Webbed Neck, Ptosis, Hypogonadism, Congenital Heart Disease, and Short Stature (XX and XY Turner Phenotype, Pseudo-Turner Syndrome, Noonan Syndrome, Ullrich Syndrome)

Among the group of phenotypic males previously classified as "male Turner syndrome," a distinctive clinical entity was identified which led to the identification of its counterpart in the female and its distinction from the syndrome of gonadal dysgenesis. A variety of eponyms has been applied to this syndrome, but we prefer to exclude Turner from the designation in order to avoid confusion with Turner syndrome, which is a consequence of partial or complete sex chromosome monosomy. It is of interest that in 1938, the year Henry Turner's paper appeared, Bizarro reported a phenotypic female with the features of this "pseudo-Turner" syndrome. Table 9–14 lists the clinical features in 2 phenotypic males and 12 phenotypic females with this entity studied by us. These patients have a characteristic facies

Table 9–14. SUMMARY OF CLINICAL FINDINGS IN 14 PATIENTS WITH THE SYNDROME OF
WEBBED NECK, PTOSIS, HYPOGONADISM, CONGENITAL HEART DISEASE, AND SHORT STATURE*

Clinical Characteristics	Males	Females	Clinical Characteristics	Males	Females
Short stature (> 2 SD below mean)	2/2	8/12	Both PS and ASD	2/2	3/10
			Patent ductus arteriosus (PDA)	0/2	2/10
			Undiagnosed heart disease	0/2	2/10
Typical facies	2/2	12/12	Incompletely evaluated	0/2	2/12
Triangular shape of face	2/2	7/12			
Prominent brow	2/2	12/12	Extremities		
Hypertelorism	2/2	12/12	Cubitus valgus	2/2	9/12
Epicanthus	2/2	9/12	Gracile fingers	1/2	8/12
Antimongoloid palpebral slant	2/2	10/12	Short stubby fingers	1/2	2/12
Ptosis	2/2	12/12	Lymphedema	0/2	3/12
Depressed nasal bridge	1/2	2/12	Dystrophic nails	2/2	2/12
Broad apex nasi	2/2	11/12	Shortened fourth metacarpal(s)	0/2	3/12
			Clinodactyly of fifth finger(s)	1/2	2/12
Low-set and/or malformed ears	2/2	8/12	Palmar simian crease	1/2	1/12
High-arched palate	2/2	8/12	Undescended testes	2/2	—
Neck					
Short	2/2	10/12	Delayed puberty	1/1	3/3
Webbing	2/2	10/12			
Low hairline	2/2	10/12	Skeletal retardation	2/2	8/10
Chest			Mental development		
Shieldlike	1/2	11/12	Retarded	2/2	4/12
Wide-spaced nipples	2/2	11/11	Borderline	0/2	5/12
Pectus excavatum	2/2	5/12	Normal	0/2	3/12
Cardiac abnormalities	2/2	11/12	Intrauterine growth retardation	1/2	4/12
Pulmonic stenosis (PS)	2/2	5/10			
PS and ventricular septal defect	0/2	1/10	Renal collecting system		
Atrial septal defect (ASD)	2/2	6/10	Normal	2/2	7/8
ASD with anomalous pulmonary			Abnormal	0/2	1/8
venous return	0/2	1/10			
Endocardial cushion defect (ECD)	0/2	2/10	Normal karyotype	2/2	12/12
ECD + patent ductus arteriosus					
and mitral insufficiency	0/2	1/10			

*After Grumbach, Morishima, and Liu (250).

and, frequently, a webbed neck and short stature (Fig. 9–38); in 12 of 14 cases, congenital heart disease was present. The most common cardiac malformations have been pulmonic stenosis (approximately 50%) and atrial septal defect, or both; ventricular septal defect, patent ductus arteriosus, and ventricular hypertrophy also have been found. Coarctation of the aorta and aortic stenosis, the most common cardiovascular anomalies in the syndrome of gonadal dysgenesis, have occurred but are infrequent findings. Pectus excavatum, cubitus valgus, and impaired mental development are often present. Lymphedema has been reported to occur in 15% of patients (253). The chromosome constitution is normal, and the direction of gonadal differentiation is appropriate for the phenotypic and chromosomal sex. In males, cryptorchidism is common, and the testes may be hypoplastic and exhibit germinal aplasia. Androgen deficiency is not uncommon at puberty. However, some affected males have normal testicular function, including fertility. At present, we prefer to limit this diagnosis to patients with four or more of the cardinal features of the syndrome and a normal chromosome constitution. The females have functioning ovaries, and although the onset of puberty may be delayed, female secondary sexual characteristics eventually emerge.

The incidence of this syndrome is approximately 1/8000 and 7 of 8 patients are thought to arise as a spontaneous mutation (253). Since the diagnosis of this syndrome is based upon a constellation of clinical findings, it is possible that sporadic cases are not all new mutations but appear so because of incomplete ascertainment due to the variable phenotype.

Familial clusters have been described consistent with autosomal dominant inheritance (253, 254, 255). The in-

creased abnormality of gonadal function in males with this syndrome as well as the higher incidence of congenital heart disease in males may play a part in the apparent higher maternal transmission of the mutant gene. However, we as well as others have studied familial cases transmitted through the male.

The diagnosis is based upon the constellation of stigmata, the most prominent of which are short stature, webbed neck, ptosis, and right-sided congenital heart disease in a patient with a normal sex chromosome constitution. At puberty affected males may require testosterone replacement therapy. We have not observed an increased prevalence of renal anomalies in affected patients.

True Hermaphrodism (9, 256–258)

Definition

The diagnosis of true hermaphrodism requires the presence of both ovarian and testicular tissue in either the same or opposite gonads. Failure to adhere to this definition has led to considerable confusion. Gonadal stroma arranged in whorls, similar to those found in the ovary but lacking oöcytes, should not be considered as sufficient evidence to regard the rudimentary gonad as an ovary. Similarly, when testicular tissue is present in the contralateral gonad, the presence of a few oöcytes in a streak gonad is not considered by the authors to be adequate evidence for the diagnosis of true hermaphrodism. Since rare female-type germ cells may be found in patients with XO gonadal dysgenesis, it seems of little value from the clinical, cytogenetic, embryologic, or

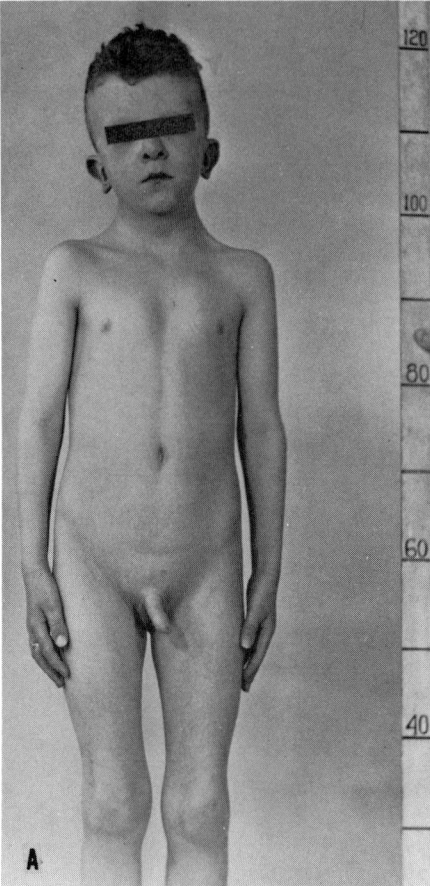
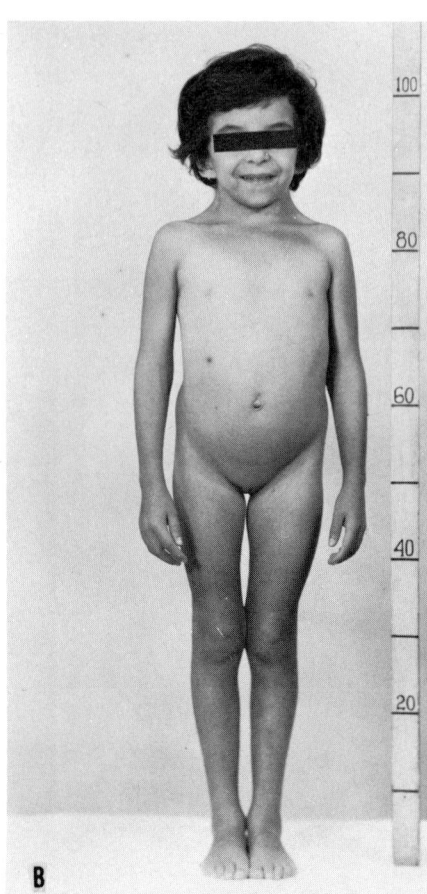

Figure 9–38. A phenotypic male and female with the syndrome of webbed neck, ptosis, congenital heart disease, short stature, and hypogonadism (Pseudo-Turner syndrome; Noonan syndrome). *A*, A 9 7/12-year-old boy who exhibited the characteristic abnormalities: triangular facies, prominent brow, hypertelorism, ptosis, antimongoloid slant of palpebral fissures, broad apex nasi, low set ears, webbed neck, pectus excavatum, pulmonic stenosis and atrial septal defect, short stature (— 3.5 SD), bilateral undescended testes, and high grade mental retardation. At 18 years of age, he was 154.0 cm. in height (height age: 12 5/12 years); the boy had Leydig cell hypofunction. Biopsy of the testes showed germinal aplasia. 46,XY chromosome constitution with a normal karyotype. (From Grumbach, M. M., and Barr, M. L.: *Recent Progr. Hormone Res. 14*:335, 1958.) *B*, An 8-year-old girl with similar features. Height 106.2 cm. (height age 4 4/12 years). Pulmonic stenosis was present. 46,XX karyotype.

nosologic standpoint to classify as true hermaphrodites those XO/XY mosaics in whom a dysgenetic testis is present with exceedingly rare oöcytes. Similarly, the status of the internal and external genitalia, while invariably exhibiting some degree of ambisexual development, should not be used as a criterion for the classification of an individual as a true hermaphrodite.

Classification

True hermaphrodism is an uncommon disorder, although it has been reported in over 350 patients (257). Patients with this syndrome may be subclassified clinically according to the type and location of the gonads.

Lateral. The arrangement of testis on one side and an ovary on the other occurs in about 30 per cent of patients. The ovary is found more frequently on the left side.

Bilateral. Testicular and ovarian tissue is found bilaterally, usually as ovotestes; this disposition occurs in about 20 per cent of patients.

Unilateral. Testicular and ovarian tissue on one side and a testis or ovary on the other; this occurs in slightly less than one-half of the cases. A testis or ovotestis may be situated along the normal pathway of descent of a testis, but an ovary lies almost invariably in its normal position.

Clinical Features (Table 9–15)

The differentiation of the genital tract and the development of secondary sexual characteristics are highly variable (Fig. 9–39). The external genitalia may simulate those of either a male or a female. Often they are ambiguous, and three-fourths of the patients have been reared as males because of the size of their phallus. Almost all the subjects have hypospadias, which varies in extent from perineal to penile, with incomplete fusion of the labioscrotal folds. In rare cases a penile urethra is present. Cryptorchidism is common, and an inguinal hernia, which may contain a gonad or uterus, is present in about one-half of the cases. In virtually all cases there is a uterus. The differentiation of the genital ducts usually follows that of the gonads. The ovotestes is the most common gonad found in true hermaphrodites, followed by the ovary and, least commonly, the testes.

Table 9–15. TRUE HERMAPHRODISM

Karyotype: 46,XX (most common), 46,XX/46,XY or 46,XY (rare)

Inheritance: Familial cases (autosomal recessive, autosomal dominant transmission) rare.

Genitalia: Ambiguous; cryptorchidism frequent; ovotestis may be located in labio-scrotal fold.

Wolffian ducts: Duct differentiation follows that of the
Müllerian ducts: homolateral gonad.

Gonad: Testis, ovary or ovotestes.

Habitus: Breast development and virilization common at puberty.

Hormone profile: Variable; H-Y antigen positive but serologic expression is usually reduced.

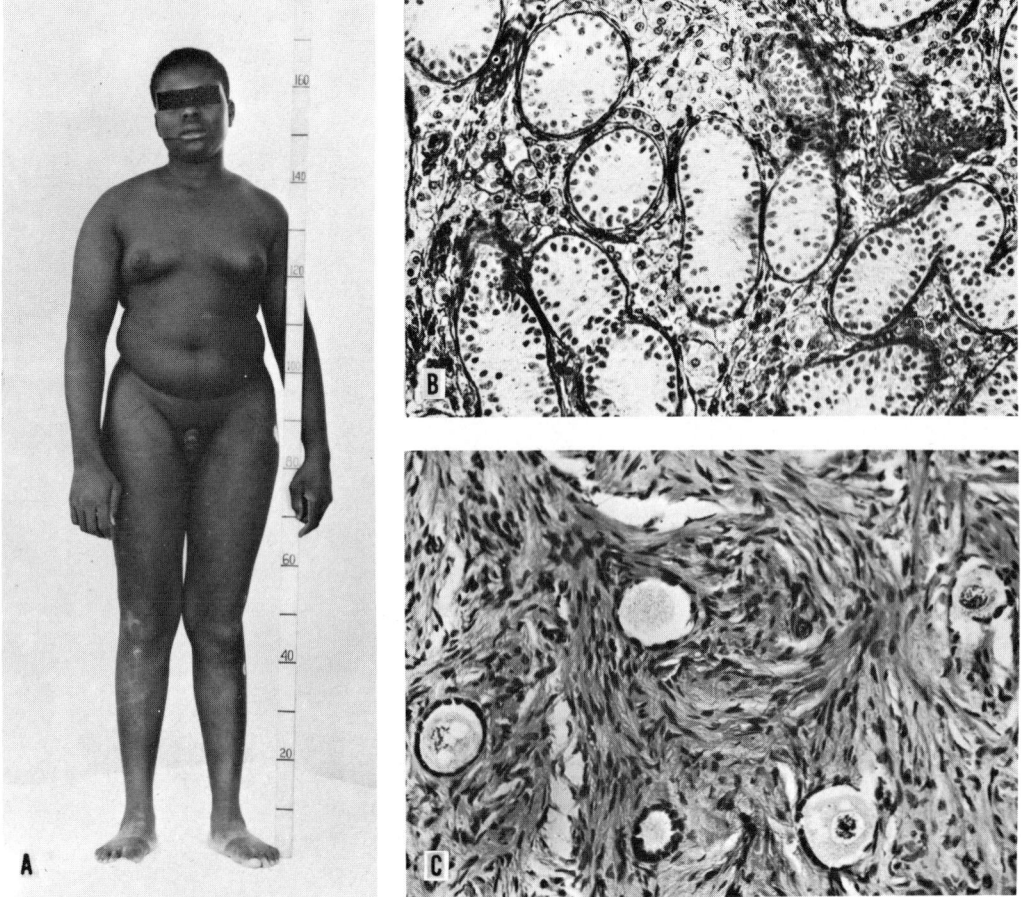

Figure 9–39. *A*, A 17-year-old true hermaphrodite with bilateral scrotal ovotestes and an XX sex chromosome constitution in cultures of the peripheral blood and skin, a perineal hypospadias (partially repaired in the photograph), moderate bilateral gynecomastia and pubic hair (recently shaved in the picture), sparse axillary hair, a high-pitched voice, and absent facial hair. Height 66 inches. Urinary 17-KS 1.3 mg./day; urinary gonadotropin > 10 m.u., < 80 m.u./day. At operation there was a male type of urethra, bilateral scrotal fallopian tubes and ovotestes, and a rudimentary bicornate uterus and vagina attached to the posterior urethra.

Photomicrograph showing histopathology of the demarcated ovarian and testicular portion of one ovotestis: *B*, immature seminiferous tubules lined with Sertoli cells and spermatogonia and Leydig cells; *C*, ova and follicles. (From Grumbach, M. M., and Barr, M. L.: *Recent Progr. Hormone Res. 14*:335, 1958.)

In the patients with a testis on one side and an ovary on the other, the development of the homolateral duct is usually consistent with that of the gonad, despite the varied appearance of the external genitalia. Most patients with an ovotestis have predominantly female development of the genital ducts. The relationship between gonadal structure and differentiation of the genital tract in true hermaphrodism provides added evidence for the essentially local effect of the müllerian duct inhibitory protein secreted by the Sertoli cells of the embryonic and fetal testes.

Breast development is common during puberty in true hermaphrodites, and menses occur in over half the patients. Periodic hematuria due to menstruation is a late clue to the diagnosis. While spermatogenesis is rare, ovulation is not uncommon, and pregnancy and childbirth have been reported in several patients with an XX karyotype (259).

Few studies of hypothalamic-pituitary-gonadal function have been carried out in true hermaphrodites. Whereas an ovary or ovarian portion of an ovotestis may function normally, with rare exceptions the testis or testicular portion of the ovotestis is dysgenetic (260). A cyclical pattern of FSH and LH secretion similar to that in normal women can

occur (261). As in males with gynecomastia, a low testosterone/estradiol ratio in plasma plays a role in the breast development that is seen frequently in post-pubertal true hermaphrodites (262).

Chromosomal Findings

About 70% of true hermaphrodites are X chromatin-positive. Van Niekerk analyzed the cytogenetic findings in 148 patients; 89 patients were 46,XX, 18 had a 46,XY karyotype, 21 were XX/XY chimeras, and the remainder were sex chromosome mosaics (257, 258).

Previously, the absence of a discrete Y chromosome in patients with testicular tissue seemed contrary to the prevailing concept of sex determination. However, the discovery of H-Y antigen and the observation that all true hermaphrodites are H-Y antigen positive, irrespective of their karyotype, have considerably clarified this apparent paradox. Undetected mosaicism with a Y-bearing cell line is undoubtedly present in some of the reported cases. In support of this contention are the various types of sex chromosome mosaicism with a Y-bearing cell line that have been described in true hermaphrodites (257, 258).

Origin of True Hermaphrodism

True hermaphrodism may result from a) sex chromosome mosaicism, b) chimerism, c) Y-autosome or Y-X chromosome translocation or interchange, or d) an autosomal mutant gene. There is evidence to support each of these possibilities in the pathogenesis of this clinically and anatomically heterogenous syndrome, and all would lead to the expression of H-Y antigen. XX/XXY mosaicism may arise by loss of a Y chromosome at an early cleavage division of an XXY zygote, whereas the XX/XXYY and XX/XXY/XXYYY patterns could be a consequence of mitotic nondisjunction in an XXY zygote. However, chimerism (24, 263) arising as a consequence of double fertilization or possible fusion of two normally fertilized ova is the more likely cause of XX/XY mosaicism, and this has been demonstrated by genetic studies in some cases. XX/XY chimeric individuals have two distinct populations of cells, each of which has a different genetic origin. The first case of XX/XY chimerism, a 2½-year-old true hermaphrodite with an ovary and ovotestis and iris heterochromia, was reported by Gartler et al. (264). The patient had two populations of red blood cells with multiple blood group antigenic differences. The father, who was heterozygous at two loci (MNSs and Rh), contributed both alleles to the patient, whereas inheritance of these loci from the mother was the same in each of the two red cell populations. These observations provided evidence for the fertilization of a binucleate ovum by two sperms, one bearing an X and the other a Y. The segregation of the haptoglobin phenotype in the XX/XY true hermaphrodite of Josso et al. leads to a similar interpretation (265). All patients with whole body chimerism do not have true hermaphrodism. The XX/XY patient described by Zuelzer et al. was a phenotypic male without evidence of true hermaphrodism; a likely mechanism for the chimerism (mosaicism) in this case, based on the blood group studies and other findings, is fusion of two zygotes or fertilization of an ovum and its polar body.

In addition to true hermaphrodism and the patient of Zuelzer who had a normal male phenotype, XX/XY chimerism has been associated with 1) a female phenotype with female secondary sexual characteristics but primary amenorrhea, female duct development, a dysgerminoma replacing the left gonad, and a streak gonad on the right side and 2) ambiguous external genitalia with a dysgenetic testis containing a gonadoblastoma.

The experiments of Tarkowski using XX and XY blastocytes demonstrate that random fusion of two blastocytes *seldom* produces XX/XY true hermaphrodism (266). Fused mouse blastocysts usually result in testicular organogenesis rather than ovarian development or both (ovotestes). Ohno has suggested that XY cells may have a selective advantage over XX gonadal cells when confronting one another because of 1) their ability to disseminate H-Y antigens, and 2) the ability of XX cells to bind free H-Y antigen (8). These factors may account for the increased frequency of testes found in XX/XY chimeric mice and humans. Indeed, then, if one accepts this scheme of gonadal organogenesis, it is easy to understand the formation of ovarian tissue in XX/XY chimeras as the result of paucity of XY cells (i.e., H-Y antigen disseminating cells) either in a gonad or a particular region of the gonad (ovotestis). Winter et al. have demonstrated just this phenomenon (267). Fibroblast cultures obtained from each pole of an ovotestis from an XX true hermaphrodite showed that the cells from the testicular portion were XY

and H-Y antigen positive, while those from the ovarian portion were XX and H-Y antigen negative (267). Thus, an ovotestis may result from failure of dissemination of H-Y antigen in the ovarian part of an ovotestis or possibly may be due to the direct or indirect effect of a postulated ovarian inhibitor of H-Y antigen to gonadal cells (268).

XX True Hermaphrodism. The problem of excluding mosaicism in karyotype studies is a formidable one, especially in true hermaphrodites in whom only X-bearing cell lines are detected. However, even though there may be good reason to suspect that some of the XX true hermaphrodites may harbor an XY or other Y-bearing cell line, especially in the testicular tissue, the detection of H-Y antigen positive patients has provided new explanations for the occurrence of the most commonly found form of true hermaphrodism.

So far, all XX true hermaphrodites studied have been H-Y antigen positive; however, in some patients the expression of H-Y antigen is less than in normal males (164, 269). Similar to the evidence for the heterogenous origin of XX males described on p. 455, in addition to hidden sex chromosome mosaicism for a Y-containing cell line, XX true hermaphrodism may result from transfer of testis-organizing gene(s) from the Y to either an X chromosome or an autosome, or from an autosomal recessive or dominant mutant gene. There is cytologic support for the translocation hypothesis. On the other hand, some familial forms of XX true hermaphrodism (261, 270, 271) are consistent with autosomal recessive inheritance; in the family described by Fraccaro et al. (269) autosomal dominant transmission was suggested. Ohno and Wachtel have proposed that the autosomal sex determining mechanism in these patients and in the XX intersex dog and hornless goat (polled) results from the transfer to an autosome of some of the multiple copies of the gene that regulates expression of H-Y antigen (26). Quantitative variations in the gene dosage effect on the synthesis of H-Y antigen then could lead to either a recessive or a dominant pattern of inheritance. Further, the degree of expression of H-Y antigen would determine whether partial or complete reversal of ovarian differentiation to a testis or ovotestis occurred. The reports of XX males and XX true hermaphrodites in the same kinship (272, 273) may be manifestation of the abnormal inheritance of H-Y antigen. Alternatively, Fraccaro et al. postulate that the structural gene for H-Y antigen is on an autosome and not the Y, and therefore an autosomal mutation affecting the structural gene for H-Y antigen results in the differentiation of a testis or ovotestis in an XX individual (269). We mentioned earlier that the locus of the structural gene for H-Y antigen is not known. Until this is ascertained and the sites of the putative regulatory genes that may affect the expression of H-Y are determined, one can only speculate about the pathogenesis of true hermaphrodism in relationship to H-Y antigen synthesis and action.

The pathogenesis of XY true hermaphrodism is not clear. One possibility is hidden mosaicism or chimerism for an XX cell line.

Diagnosis and Therapy

The diagnosis of true hermaphrodism should be considered in all patients with ambiguous genitalia. An XX/XY karyotype in a patient with ambiguous external genitalia strongly suggests the diagnosis of true hermaphrodism; a 46,XX or 46,XY karyotype does not exclude the diagnosis. The finding of a gonad in the labioscrotal fold (especially on the right side) with a lobulated bipolar consistency compatible with an ovotestis is suggestive. If all other forms of male and female pseudohermaphrodism have been appropriately rule out, the diagnosis of true hermaphrodism should be confirmed by the histologic demonstration of both ovarian and testicular tissues.

The management of true hermaphrodism is contingent on the age at diagnosis and a careful assessment of the functional capacity of the internal and external genitalia. In infants in whom gender identity has not already been established, either a male or female assignment of sex can be made. If a male gender role is assigned, all müllerian and ovarian structures should be removed. The testis or testicular component of an ovotestis is usually dysgenetic and the risk of malignant transformation is increased. Thus, in XX true hermaphrodites raised as males we recommend gonadectomy, the insertion of prosthetic testes, and hormone replacement at puberty. However, in XX/XY chimeras and XY true hermaphrodites, especially when a testis is present on one side and an ovary on the other and the size of the phallus is adequate, the possibility should be weighed of retaining a histologically normal-appearing testis in the scrotum and raising the patient as a male, even though the risk of malignancy may be increased. In true hermaphrodites reared as females, surgery and removal of all testicular tissue is indicated. Normal ovarian function and, in rare instances, pregnancy have been reported in true hermaphrodites, usually of the 46,XX variety; however, there may be an increased risk of neoplasm in the retained ovarian tissue or ovary in these patients (274). In older patients gender identity is the major consideration; usually it conforms to the sex of rearing. The discordant gonad and dysgenetic gonadal tissue should be removed and plastic repair of the external genitalia carried out. Appropriate sex hormone replacement therapy is recommended at the age of puberty.

Sex Chromosome Abnormalities Unassociated with Gonadal Defects

Four sex chromosome abnormalities that are not accompanied by a typical gonadal defect but in which mental retardation is frequent will be discussed.

XXX. This is a common sex chromosome abnormality; the frequency is about 1 per 1000 newborn female infants (149). The prevalence of XXX individuals in institutions for the mentally retarded is 4.3 per 1000 (275), suggesting an increased risk for this complication in polysomy X. While a few patients have had delayed menarche or premature ovarian failure, most XXX females have normal ovarian function. XXX females can give birth to XXY sons, but this is rare (156). Recently, the subtle clinical features in a group of young females ascertained by karyotype analysis in the neonatal period were described and included the following: a tendency to low birth weight; advanced mean parental age; an increased incidence of clinodactyly; normal postnatal growth patterns; an increased risk of speech and language problems; and a lower mean I.Q. than their siblings or a control group (138).

The diagnosis of XXX can be confirmed by the finding of two sex chromatin bodies in interphase cells and by the demonstration of a 47,XXX karyotype by the use of appropriate banding techniques. Because of the increased risk in the offspring of a sex chromosomal abnormality (XXY in males, and XXX in females), prenatal counseling and amniocentesis should be considered in XXX females who are pregnant.

XXXX. This is a rare sex chromosome anomaly. Over 30 patients with this karyotype have been reported (276, 277). Considerable phenotype heterogeneity exists among tetra-X individuals, making identification of such persons by clinical means difficult. The most constant feature of this condition is a variable degree of mental retardation affecting most prominently the speech (277). Ovarian function has been normal except in rare cases (277). The diagnosis can be suspected by finding three sex chromatin bodies in a proportion of somatic nuclei and confirmed by karyotype analysis.

XXXXX (12, 278). The penta-X syndrome occurs quite rarely. Since 1963, when it was first described, 14 other cases have been reported (279). Severe prenatal and postnatal growth delay and mental retardation are invariable findings. In addition, other somatic stigmata include hypertelorism, epicanthal folds, upslanted palpebral fissures, depressed nasal bridge, abnormal dentition, short neck, congenital heart disease, clinodactyly, and overlapping toes. The external genitalia are usually normal and gonadal function has been reported to be compromised (277). A proportion of interphase nuclei are found to contain four X-chromatin bodies.

XYY. The first patient reported by Sandberg et al. (280) was an essentially normal fertile male of average intelligence. He was detected only because he had a daughter with Down syndrome. Surveys in penal institutions have disclosed an increase in prevalence of this anomaly, especially in tall prisoners. The early reports gave rise to an underserved stereotype which has been greatly modified by later studies (281, 282). Among 43 XYY boys, 1 to 12 years of age, ascertained by routine karyotype analysis in the newborn period, no clear-cut XYY syndrome emerged in childhood (139). No major deviations were evident that could be attributed to an extra Y chromosome, with the possible exception of a skew to the left in I.Q. scores. Data indicate that XYY individuals have a 1% risk of exhibiting criminal behavior as opposed to a 0.1% risk in XY males (12). XYY is one of the more common sex chromosome abnormalities, occurring in 1 per 1000 male births. Among the features that have been associated with this karyotype are tall stature, antisocial behavior, nodulocystic acne, and skeletal anomalies, especially radioulnar synostosis. These individuals rarely show any abnormality in sexual development. A few reports have described hypospadias in XYY patients, but this may be coincidental. The diagnosis of XYY syndrome should be suspected in tall males with nodulocystic acne who exhibit antisocial behavior. It can be confirmed by demonstrating two fluorescent Y bodies in somatic interphase nuclei stained with quinacrine and by karyotype analysis.

XYYY. A rare karyotype, the reported cases have had multiple somatic abnormalities and mental retardation (283). The diagnosis is based on finding three fluorescent Y bodies in interphase nuclei and by karyotype analysis.

Gonadal Neoplasms in Dysgenetic Gonads (284–287)

The prevalence of gonadal neoplasms is greatly increased in patients with certain types of dysgenetic gonads, in particular all those with a Y bearing cell line (285–288). Germinoma (dysgerminoma, seminoma), teratoma, and gonadoblastoma have been found most frequently. Cryptorchid testes, even when not associated with intersexuality, have an increased risk of malignancy. The probability that cryptorchid testes will undergo malignant degeneration is difficult to assess but it is many times greater than for normally descended testes (289, 290). Eleven per cent of males with testicular neoplasms have been or are cryptorchid (289). In addition, 33% of cryptorchid-associated carcinoma of the testis occurred after orchiopexy, and in patients with unilateral cryptorchidism 25% of tumors were located in the contralateral descended testes (290). The management of cryptorchid testes (291, 292, 293) is discussed in Chapter 6.

Gonadal neoplasms are uncommon in patients with XYY seminiferous tubule dysgenesis; a small number of patients with gonadal or extra-gonadal germ cell tumors have been reported (148, 294). Similarly, gonadal tumors are rare in the streak gonads of XO patients and in XO mosaics with a structurally abnormal X chromosome in the second cell line. There is one report of an XO patient with a germinoma, but sex chromosome mosaicism was not excluded (295). Three XO/XX mosaics with gonadal tumors have been reported; one had a pseudomucinous cyst adenocarcinoma (296), another had bilateral gonadoblastoma (297), and a third had a hilus cell tumor with signs of virilization (298).

Gonadoblastomas are tumors usually composed of three elements — large germ cells, sex cord derivatives (Sertoligranulosa cells), and stromal elements (theca cells, Leydig cells). They may be microscopic or large masses, and often are calcified. A comprehensive review of gonadoblastoma has been published by Scully (288) (Fig. 9–36). In 27 of his 74 cases, a tumor was found in both gonads. Thirty patients were under 15 years of age when the tumor was first diagnosed, and 10 patients were less than 10 years old. A third of these tumors were detected incidentally on histologic examination of dysgenetic gonads removed for other indications. In patients in whom chromosomal studies had been carried out, the predominant karyotypes were XO/XY and XY. Although 80% of these patients had been reared as females, most of them displayed some degree of clitoromegaly or hirsutism; rarely, these tumors secrete enough estrogen to induce breast development (Fig. 9–36). Even though the gonadoblastoma itself is rarely if ever malignant, these tumors frequently contain germinomas (dysgerminoma or seminoma) or other malignant tumors that can metastasize and cause death. Teter and Boczkowski (299) have emphasized the increased risk of gonadal neoplasms in dysgenetic gonads and reviewed its familial occurrence in patients with XY gonadal dysgenesis. The strikingly disparate propensity for neoplastic transformation in the streak or dysgenetic gonads of patients with XY gonadal dysgenesis (20–30%) in contrast to XX gonadal dysgenesis must be emphasized.

In view of the now well-documented malignant potential of dysgenetic gonads, the question of prophylactic gonadectomy merits serious attention. The neoplasms are infrequently detected in childhood (300), but the risk rises appreciably in young adults. It is possible that high gonadotropin levels play a role in their growth, and that substitution therapy with sex steroids might afford some protection. A prudent course is to advise laparotomy and castration of all patients with XY gonadal dysgenesis (complete and incomplete forms), and all patients with the syndrome of gonadal dysgenesis who have a cell line with a normal or a structurally abnormal Y chromosome or who exhibit some degree of virilization regardless of the apparent karyotype. Rare exceptions to this rule may occur in patients who have been

Table 9–16. CLASSIFICATION OF FEMALE PSEUDOHERMAPHRODISM

A. Androgen-induced
  1. Fetal Source
    a. Congenital virilizing adrenal hyperplasia
      i. Virilism only, defective adrenal 21-hydroxylation
      ii. Virilism with salt-losing syndrome, defective adrenal 21-hydroxylation
      iii. Virilism with hypertension, defective adrenal 11β-hydroxylation
      iv. Virilism with adrenal insufficiency, deficient 3β-hydroxysteroid dehydrogenase
  2. Maternal Source
    a. Iatrogenic
      Testosterone and related steroids
      Certain synthetic oral progestins and rarely stilbestrol
    b. Virilizing ovarian or adrenal tumor
    c. Virilizing luteoma of pregnancy
    d. Congenital virilizing adrenal hyperplasia in the mother
  3. Undetermined source
    ?Virilizing luteoma of pregnancy
B. Nonandrogen-induced disturbances in the differentiation of urogenital structures

assigned a male gender role in whom a histologically normal gonad is found in the scrotum. The fact that a gonad is scrotally located and palpable does not guarantee against a disastrous result, since seminomas tend to metastasize at an early stage before a local mass is obvious. Patients with XO Turner syndrome who have no suggestion of clitoromegaly are not at risk. The risk of gonadal tumors in patients with only X chromosome abnormalities, such as XO/XX, XXr, and XXq-, is low; these patients, however, should be examined at regular intervals and followed by sonography of the pelvis for signs of gonadal neoplasm.

FEMALE PSEUDOHERMAPHRODISM
(Table 9–16)

Female pseudohermaphrodism is the easiest of the sexual anomalies to comprehend, as the ovaries and müllerian derivatives are normally developed and anatomical ambisexuality is limited to the external genitalia. Since, in the absence of testes, there is an inherent tendency for the external genitalia to feminize, a female fetus will be masculinized only if subjected to an environment of androgens from some extragonadal source. The degree of fetal masculinization is determined by the stage of differentiation at the time of exposure. Once the vagina has separated from the urogenital sinus (about the twelfth fetal week), androgens will cause only clitoral hypertrophy (Fig. 9–40). Even with severe masculinization of the external genitalia, the uterus and fallopian tubes remain normal, since the regression of the primordia for these structures, the müllerian duct, requires the secretion of the müllerian duct-inhibiting protein by fetal testes, and this action cannot be mimicked by androgenic steroids. Although the presence of virilized genitalia usually provides *prima facie* evidence of an androgenic

Figure 9–40. Female pseudohermaphrodism induced by prenatal exposure to androgens. Exposure after the twelfth fetal week leads only to clitoral hypertrophy (diagram on left). Exposure at progressively earlier stages of differentiation (depicted from left to right in drawings) leads to retention of the urogenital sinus and labioscrotal fusion. If exposure occurs sufficiently early, the labia will fuse to form a penile urethra. (From Grumbach, M. M., and Ducharme, J. R.: *Fertil. Steril.* 11:157, 1960.)

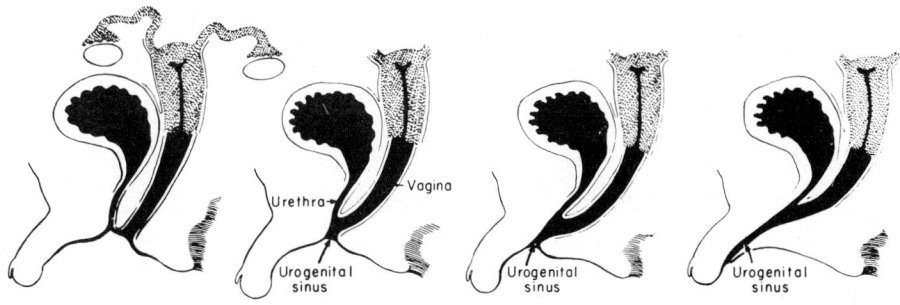

influence during early gestation, ambiguous genitalia, superficially resembling those produced by androgen, are an occasional feature of other, more generalized teratologic malformations.

Congenital Adrenal Hyperplasia (301, 302)

Congenital virilizing adrenal hyperplasia accounts for most of the cases of female pseudohermaphrodism and approximately half of all patients with ambiguous external genitalia.

Biochemical Variants of Congenital Adrenal Hyperplasia (Fig. 9–41)

Six major types of congenital adrenal hyperplasia (CAH) have been described, each with its distinctive clinical picture and specific biochemical lesion (301). All are transmitted as an autosomal recessive trait. The common denominator in all six biochemical types is impaired cortisol formation with consequent hyperplasia of the adrenal cortex due to hypersecretion of ACTH through the negative feedback mechanism. Only types I, II, and III, however, are predominantly virilizing disorders. In these types, the most striking abnormality of the sexual phenotypes is prenatal masculinization of the female fetus due to overproduction of adrenal androgens and androgen precursors. Affected males have no abnormalities of their genitalia at birth. Hence, these disorders will be discussed in this chapter as causes of female pseudohermaphrodism.

Biochemical types IV, V, and VI have in common defects in steroid hormone synthesis, which not only block cortisol synthesis but also impair the production of sex steroids by the gonads as well as by the adrenal glands. Hence, affected males exhibit varying degrees of male pseudohermaphrodism due to deficient androgen production by the fetal Leydig cells, whereas affected females may or may not exhibit virilization. If present, virilization in females is usually considerably less than in types I, II and III. These forms of congenital adrenal hyperplasia in the male will be discussed in a later section as causes of male pseudohermaphrodism. The administration to the pregnant rat of selective synthetic inhibitors of the enzymes involved in adrenal and testicular steroid biogenesis has produced abnormalities of sex differentiation in the offspring which are the counterparts of congenital adrenal hyperplasia in man and has served to clarify further the role of steroidogenic enzymes in the control of fetal sex differentiation (303).

Type I. C_{21} Hydroxylase Defect Affecting Hydroxylation in the Zona Fasciculata (Simple Virilization). This deficiency is the most common cause of ambiguous genitalia in infants as well as the most common form of adrenogenital syndrome. It is inherited (as are the other forms) as an autosomal recessive (304). Recent data indicate that the gene which codes for 21 hydroxylation is located on the short arm of chromosome number 6 in close proximity to the locus for the histocompatibility gene HLA-B (305) (Fig. 9–42). Levine et al. have used HLA typing to detect heterozygotes and cryptic homozygotes in families with affected individuals, and for the prenatal diagnosis of affected fetuses (305) when the HLA genotyping of amniotic cells indicates that the fetus has the same HLA genotype as a previously affected sib (Fig. 9–43).

In the United States and Europe the incidence of this disease in Caucasians is estimated to be between 1 in 4000 to 1 in 15,000 (306); the gene frequency appears to vary in different ethnic groups. For example, the prevalence of

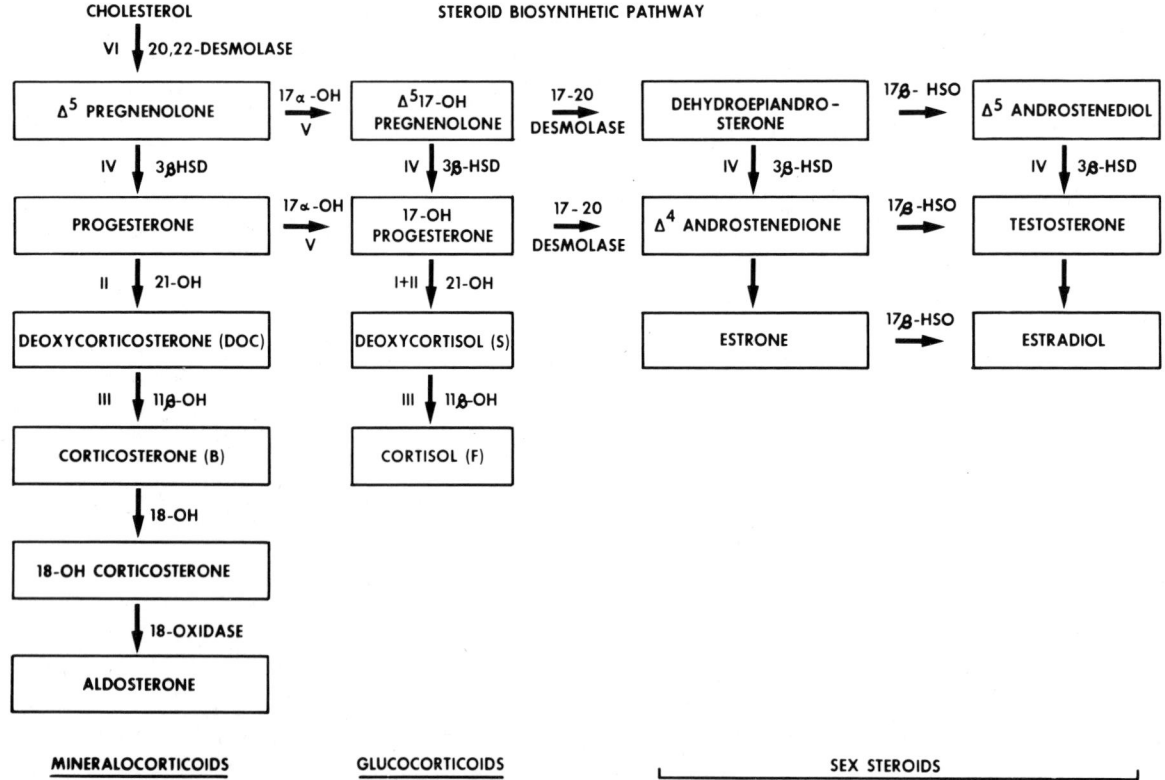

Figure 9–41. Diagrammatic representation of the steroid biosynthetic pathways. I to VI correspond to the numbers used for the specific biosynthetic defects that result in congenital adrenal hyperplasia. OH = hydroxylase, 3β-HSD = 3β-hydroxysteroid dehydrogenase Δ⁵ isomerase, and 17-β-HSO = 17-β-hydroxysteroid oxidoreductase.

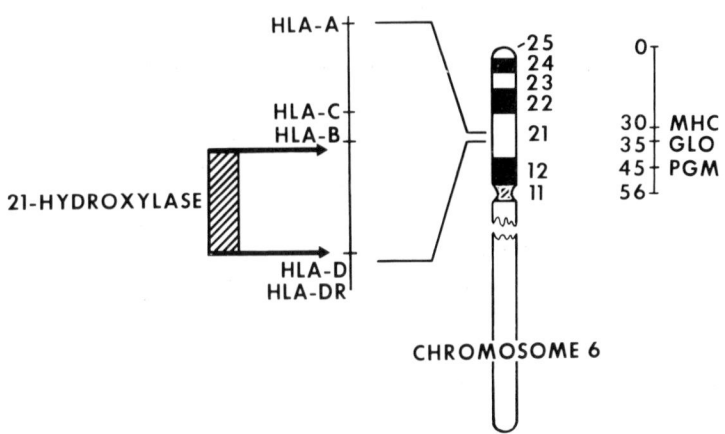

Figure 9–42. A diagrammatic representation of chromosome number 6. Only the banding pattern of the short arm is shown. The numbers 11 to 25 delineate the bands according to the Paris nomenclature. To the right of the chromosome, the sites of the genes for the major histocompatibility complex (MHC), glyoxalase I (GLO), and phosphoglucomutase (PGM) on a recombinant unit scale are indicated. To the left is a scheme of the genes in the major histocompatibility complex. By linkage analysis, the gene for 21 hydroxylation is closely linked to HLA-B and most likely resides between the HLA-B and HLA-D loci.

C_{21}-hydroxylase deficiency is 1 per 490 in the Yupik Eskimos of Alaska (307).

The abnormality in adrenal biosynthesis in patients with type I, C_{21}-hydroxylase deficiency is defective C_{21} hydroxylation of 17-hydroxyprogesterone, which results in increased production of 17-hydroxyprogesterone and decreased synthesis of cortisol. As a consequence of defective cortisol synthesis, there is hypersecretion of ACTH with resultant addisonian-like pigmentation, and the adrenal is stimulated to produce increased amounts of cortisol precursors, including androgens and androgen precursors, proximal to the block in the biosynthetic pathway. The concentration of plasma 17-hydroxyprogesterone is usually greatly increased and the plasma levels of androstenedione and testosterone are elevated in affected patients. Postnatally, metabolites of these steroids result in the increased excretion of urinary 17-ketosteroids and of pregnanetriol and 11-keto-pregnanetriol. Prenatally, excess adrenal androgen synthesis in the female fetus results in elevated circulating testosterone levels. Prior to the 12th week of gestation, high fetal androgen levels lead to a varying degree of labioscrotal fusion and clitoral enlargement in the female fetus; exposure to androgen after 12 weeks induces clitoromegaly alone. Postnatally, secretion of testosterone by the adrenal gland, as well as the conversion of androstenedione to testosterone in peripheral tissues, results in continued virilization of the untreated patient. In contrast to the salt-wasting form (type II) only the 21 hydroxylation of C_{21} 17-hydroxysteroids and

17-deoxysteroids by the fasciculata is impaired. Untreated patients with simple C_{21}-hydroxylase deficiency usually have normal aldosterone secretion rates (308). In untreated patients the increased androgen production leads to accelerated growth during childhood and to disproportionate acceleration of skeletal maturation, which results in premature closure of the epiphyses and short stature in adolescence and adulthood (309).

The genitalia of females with the virilizing forms of CAH (types I, II, III) may exhibit a spectrum of masculinization from simple enlargement of the clitoris to complete labioscrotal fusion with a penile urethra (Fig. 9–34). In most cases the urogenital sinus is preserved and serves as a common outlet for both the urethra and vagina. Presumably, the hypersecretion of androgens and androgen precursors begins before the twelfth week of gestation, especially in the patients who manifest more than simple clitoromegaly. The uterus, tubes, and ovaries, however, are normally formed, except in rare cases. The spectrum of virilization in females with adrenal hyperplasia varies with the nature and degree of the biochemical defect.

Type II: Complete C_{21} Hydroxylation Defect (Virilization with Salt Wasting. In type II patients with C_{21}-hydroxylase deficiency, both virilization and salt loss occur. This variant is thought to be due to a defect in 21 hydroxylation that involves both the zona fasciculata and glomerulosa and which leads to impaired cortisol (fasciculata) and aldosterone (glomerulosa) secretion. This results in aldosterone

Figure 9–43. The pedigrees of two families with children who are affected with 21-hydroxylase deficiency. The HLA haplotypes for HLA-A, HLA-B, and HLA-C are indicated for each individual. a, b (½ hatched symbol) indicates the paternal haplotypes and c, d (½ hatched symbol) the maternal haplotypes. The parents are heterozygotes for 21-hydroxylase deficiency. Haplotype a, c, (hatched symbol) indicates the patients with homozygous 21 hydroxylase deficiency. Haplotype b, d (unhatched symbol) indicates a child who has two normal genes for 21 hydroxylase activity. (Redrawn from Levine L., et al.[305])

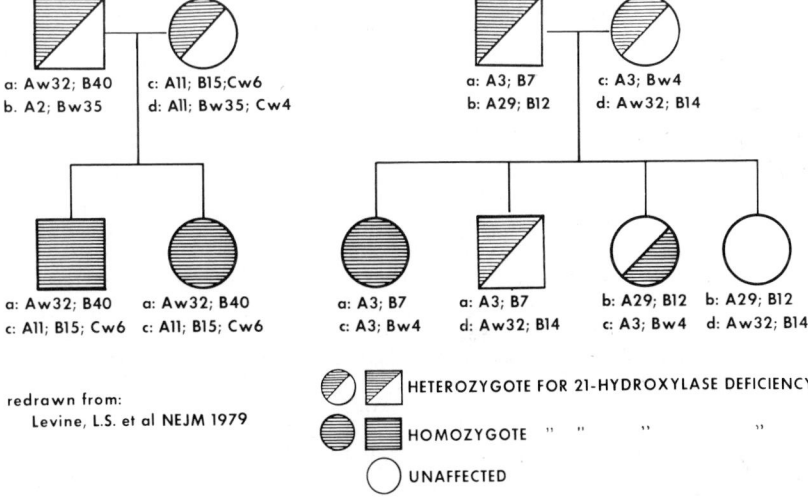

redrawn from:
Levine, L.S. et al NEJM 1979

deficiency and increased plasma renin activity. Electrolyte and fluid losses result in hyponatremia, hyperkalemia, acidosis, dehydration, and vascular collapse. About 50% of patients have their first salt-losing crisis between the 6th and 14th days of age; it is infrequent before age 6 days. Masculinization of the external genitalia and urogenital sinus in affected females tends to be more severe in type II C_{21}-hydroxylase deficiency than in simple C_{21}-hydroxylase or C_{11}-hydroxylase deficiency. Without specific therapy, death can ensue secondary to hyperkalemia, dehydration, and shock. In the affected male whose genitalia are normal, the differential diagnosis includes sepsis, pyloric stenosis, gastroenteritis, and congenital heart disease.

Recent data have demonstrated the heterogeneity of 21-hydroxylase deficiency. Siblings and parents of "affected patients" have been shown by HLA typing and steroid analysis to have asymptomatic 21-hydroxylase deficiency (310). These data suggest that classic adrenal hyperplasia, "acquired" adrenal hyperplasia, and "cryptic" adrenal hyperplasia are all forms of 21-hydroxylase deficiency with a wide range of clinical and biochemical abnormalities (310).

Diagnosis. The diagnosis of C_{21}-hydroxylase deficiency should always be considered in 1) patients with ambiguous genitalia and the features of female pseudohermaphrodism, 2) apparent cryptorchid males, 3) infants who present in shock or a severely dehydrated condition, and 4) males and females with signs of virilization prior to puberty. The family history may reveal a previously affected sibling, an unexpected death in infancy, or a male sibling with sexual precocity. The initial step in the evaluation of any infant with ambiguous genitalia is a buccal smear for sex chromatin analysis. A karyotype can be performed to confirm the sex chromatin analysis. The excretion of urinary 17-ketosteroids and pregnanetriol and the elevated concentration of 17-hydroxyprogesterone establish the diagnosis in affected infants and children. The most useful test is the determination of plasma 17-hydroxyprogesterone (17-OHP) (311). The concentration of 17-OHP is normally elevated in umbilical cord blood (mean 1640 ng/dl) but rapidly decreases to 100–200 ng/dl after 24 hours of age (Fig. 9–44). Recent data indicate that in affected infants the concentration of 17-OHP in cord blood, in contrast to samples at a few days of age, may not be diagnostic of 21-hydroxylase deficiency (94). After 24 hours of age both 17-OHP and Δ^4-androstenedione (A) levels usually distinguish infants with 21-hydroxylase deficiency from normal infants. However, "sick" unaffected infants may have elevated A and 17-OHP levels which can confound the diagnosis of 21-hydroxylase deficiency (312).

In affected patients 17-OHP values usually range from 3000–40,000 ng/dl depending upon age and severity of the defect in 21 hydroxylation. Patients with "mild" 21-hydroxylase deficiency and heterozygotes may have a borderline or non-diagnostic level of 17-OHP. In these instances, determining the effect of ACTH on the rise of 17-OHP and the 17-OHP/cortisol ratio often will identify affected infants (305). In a kinship with an affected infant, HLA genotyping can be used to distinguish between heterozygosity and a mild form of the disorder in a homozygous patient.

The striking elevation in the concentration of plasma 17-hydroxyprogesterone is such a distinctive marker of 21-hydroxylase deficiency that prenatal diagnosis has been attempted by determination of its concentration in amniotic fluid in pregnancies at risk (313, 94). We have studied the concentration of 17-hydroxyprogesterone in amniotic fluid between 14 and 20 weeks of gestation and in amniotic fluid from seven pregnancies at risk for 21 hydroxylase deficiency. In six of the latter, amniotic fluid 17-hydroxyprosterone

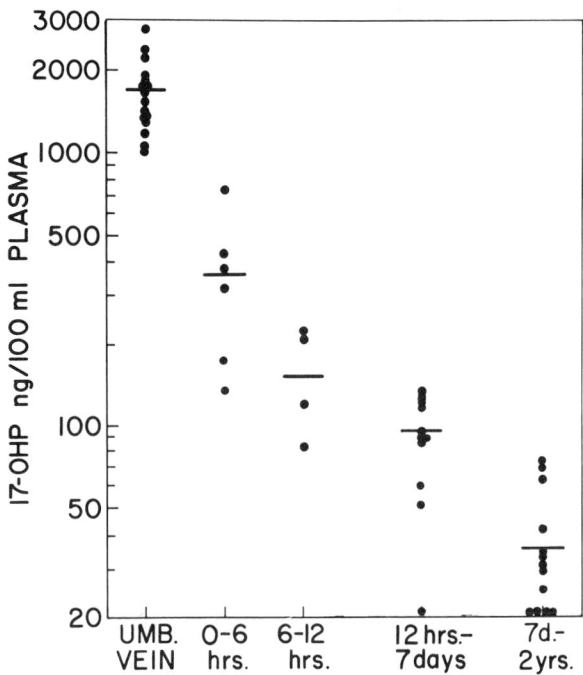

Figure 9–44. Normal plasma 17-hydroxyprogesterone values in nanograms per deciliter in non-stressed infants from birth to 2 years of age. (From Jenner, M. R., Grumbach, M. M., and Kaplan, S. L.[311])

levels were within the normal range and the infants were normal at birth. The seventh gestation, which had a five-fold increase in amniotic fluid 17-OHP, resulted in an infant with 21-hydroxylase deficiency confirmed at birth. Similar results have been obtained by others. Recently, Levine and co-workers have utilized HLA typing of cells obtained from amniotic fluid of mothers who had a previously affected offspring to identify fetuses who were homozygous or heterozygous for 21-hydroxylase deficiency (314).

In the past, the diagnosis of 21-hydroxylase deficiency has been based on the assessment of the excretion of urinary 17-ketosteroid and pregnanetriol. The excretion of 17-ketosteroids varies with age. In the first few days of life, the excretion of 17-ketosteroids in unaffected infants can be as high as 2–4 mg/24 hours. After one month of age, urinary 17-ketosteroids decrease to an upper limit of approximately 0.5 mg/year of age until the onset of adrenarche. Pregnanetriol, the urinary metabolite of 17-OHP, is a "hallmark" of 21-hydroxylase deficiency. However, in the neonatal period, the values of urinary pregnanetriol may be normal in affected infants. Thereafter, the levels rise and are useful diagnostically.

Infants with salt wasting usually have clinical evidence of frank or incipient adrenal insufficiency or crises after the sixth day of life and especially during the second week. The early diagnosis of the salt-losing form of congenital adrenal hyperplasia is usually based on the clinical signs of poor appetite, weight loss, and vomiting, and the finding of hyponatremia and hyperkalemia. Although the plasma concentration and the excretion of aldosterone are low while plasma renin activity is high, these tests are usually not useful in the prompt diagnosis of salt wasting. Mild salt losers may have normal electrolytes under basal conditions, but exhibit elevated plasma renin activity and hyponatremia, hyperkalemia, and inappropriate natriuresis with salt restriction.

Treatment. Therapy for patients with congenital adrenal hyperplasia can be divided into two phases: acute and chronic.

In acute adrenal crises in infants and children with the salt-losing form of 21-hydroxylase deficiency, both cortisol and aldosterone are deficient. This rapidly leads to dehydration, hypoglycemia, electrolyte imbalance, hypotension, and, consequently, vascular collapse and cardiac arrest. An intravenous infusion of 5% glucose in isotonic saline should be started immediately and fluids calculated upon estimates of deficiency and maintenance of both electrolytes and water. In the first hour, restoration of intravascular volume is imperative. If the patient is hypotensive, 20 ml/kg of 5% glucose in isotonic saline is administered by rapid infusion. 50 mg/m² of hydrocortisone sodium succinate should be given as a bolus intravenously and another 50–100 mg/m² added to the infusion fluid over the first 24 hours. When hyponatremia and hyperkalemia are present, deoxycorticosterone acetate (DOCA) is given (1–3 mg IM, depending on age) every 12–24 hours. The frequency and amount of DOCA, as well as the amount and sodium concentration of intravenous fluids, are adjusted in light of the serum electrolytes, state of hydration, body weight, and blood pressure. Excess DOCA and salt can result in hypertension, congestive heart failure, and hypertensive encephalopathy, while too little salt and DOCA will not correct the electrolyte imbalance. Severe hyperkalemia may result in life-threatening cardiac arrhythmias. Under these circumstances, intravenous sodium bicarbonate and calcium as well as rectal cation exchange resins are useful to reduce the serum potassium levels.

After diagnosis and stabilization, maintenance therapy is begun. During the first 2 years of life, we prefer to treat infants with intramuscular cortisone acetate. This avoids the problems of regurgitation and the variable absorption of oral medication. The initial suppressive dose in infants is 20 to 25 mg of cortisone acetate intramuscularly, daily for 5 days. Thereafter, cortisone acetate is injected every 3 days in a dose (15–20 mg), which approximates the daily requirement of 12 ±3 mg/m² per 24 hours. With stress, febrile episodes, acute gastrointestinal disorders, and surgery, the dose is tripled by giving the injection daily rather than every 3 days. This regimen of glucocorticoid replacement is usually continued until 18–24 months of age.

The dose of glucocorticoids (see Table 9–17) is empirical and must be adjusted for each patient by assessing bone age, linear growth, the 24 hour excretion of 17-ketosteroids, and clinical signs of glucocorticoid deficiency or excess. Plasma levels of testosterone, androstenedione, and 17-hydroxyprogesterone have not been found to be more useful than urinary 17-ketosteroids in assessing the adequacy of therapy in infants and children.

After 18 to 24 months of intramuscular therapy, we change to oral glucocorticoids. The oral dose of cortisone acetate is approximately 22 mg/m²/day (for hydrocortisone, 18 mg/m²/day), and is divided into three equal doses (309). These doses of cortisone acetate and hydrocortisone have been found to permit normal growth and development (309). Adjustment of the oral dose of the more potent and longer-acting glucocorticoids such as methylprednisolone and dexamethasone is more difficult in infants and children, and not infrequently their use has resulted in overtreatment manifested by growth suppression and "cushingoid features." Thus, we tend to avoid these potent glucocorticoid analogues in the treatment of infants and young children. On the other hand, glucocorticoid analogues are useful in post-pubertal females, since their long action leads to less fluctuation in adrenal suppression and often facilitates normal hypothalamic-pituitary-gonadal function and menses (315). Many affected women when treated appropriately have given birth to "normal" children. Polycystic ovaries and sterility have been reported in certain forms of adrenal hyperplasia, although the frequency of this finding is not known (123).

Patients with salt wasting require therapy with both mineralocorticoid and salt. After the infant has been diagnosed and stabilized, the DOCA (1 to 2 mg per day) and salt supplements (1 to 3 gm per day by mouth) are adjusted to maintain normal electrolytes, blood pressure and plasma renin activity. In the past, we have preferred to implant one or two 125 mg DOCA pellets — the number of pellets depends on the severity of salt loss, as judged by the daily DOCA and salt required to maintain the weight, electrolytes, and blood pressure within the normal range. These pellets are absorbed slowly and provide a constant level of mineralocorticoid activity. After DOCA pellet implantation, a few days of close observation are necessary to assess the need for added salt or excessive fluid retention. If the latter occurs, sodium chloride intake is restricted; overtreatment with mineralocorticoid rarely necessitates pellet removal. The pellets last 6–9 months and should be replaced before the onset of clinical mineralocorticoid deficiency. We routinely use DOCA pellets during the first 1–2 years of life. If DOCA pellets are not available, 9 α-fluorohydrocortisone tablets (0.05–0.15 mg/day) may be substituted.

Table 9–17. MEAN ESTIMATED OPTIMAL DOSE OF GLUCOCORTICOIDS FOR GROWTH IN PATIENTS WITH CONGENITAL ADRENAL HYPERPLASIA, COMPARED WITH ANTI-INFLAMMATORY POTENCIES*

	ACTUAL DOSE IN mg/m²/24hrs	EQUIVALENT DOSE	REPORTED POTENCY BASED ON ANTI-INFLAMMATORY EFFECT
Dexamethasone	0.23	1	1
Methylprednisolone	2.4	10	5
Prednisone	3.7	16	7
Hydrocortisone	18.4	80	27
Cortisone Acetate (I.M.)	13.9	60	17
Cortisone Acetate (P.O.)	22.0	96	33

*From Styne, D. D., Grumbach, M. M., et al. in *Congenital Adrenal Hyperplasia*, Lee, P. A., et al. (eds), Baltimore, University Park Press, 1977.

Plasma renin activity determinations are a useful index of the adequacy of mineralocorticoid replacement therapy. Recent data indicate that insufficient mineralocorticoid and salt therapy not only results in hypovolemia, hyperkalemia, and hyponatremia but also can lead to increased secretion of glucocorticoid precursors and adrenal androgens (316). For optimal therapy, and to ensure normal growth and development, we recommend that all salt losers be maintained on mineralocorticoid therapy; the dosage should be assessed periodically, and especially before an increase in the maintenance dose of glucocorticoid therapy is instituted. By 2–3 years of age, the patients with salt wasting can regulate their dietary salt intake.

Long term follow up data over the past 25 years are accumulating on the effects of glucocorticoid and mineralocorticoid replacement in patients with congenital adrenal hyperplasia (309, 317, 318, 319). The adult height of both males and females tends to be shorter than unaffected siblings. Although puberty and even fertility have been reported in untreated adult males with congenital adrenal hyperplasia, we recommend that all patients continue treatment with a glucocorticoid and, if indicated, a mineralocorticoid (Fig. 9–45).

Plastic repair of the external genitalia of female infants with ambiguous external genitalia should be initiated after the patient is stabilized and before 12 months of age. Clitoral recession or clitoroplasty rather than clitorectomy is preferred (320). It is of critical importance to reassure the parents that with appropriate treatment and compliance their child will grow and develop into a normal, functional adult. Fertility in males as well as feminization, menstruation, and fertility in females can be expected in the adequately treated patient. Psychologic guidance and support by the physician are an essential component of long-term management.

Type III: C₁₁ Hydroxylase Defect (Virilization with Hypertension) (321).

A defect in hydroxylation at C_{11} leads to hypersecretion of 11-deoxycorticosterone (DOC) and 11-deoxycortisol (compound S) in addition to adrenal androgens. Defective 11 β-hydroxylation in the glucocorticoid (fasciculata) pathways results in increased DOC secretion, which causes salt and water retention and consequent hypertension with low renin levels. Thus, such patients exhibit hypertension in addition to virilization. Of note, even though 11 β-hydroxylation (and 18-hydroxylation) is deficient in the zona fasciculata, the mineralocorticoid 11-β

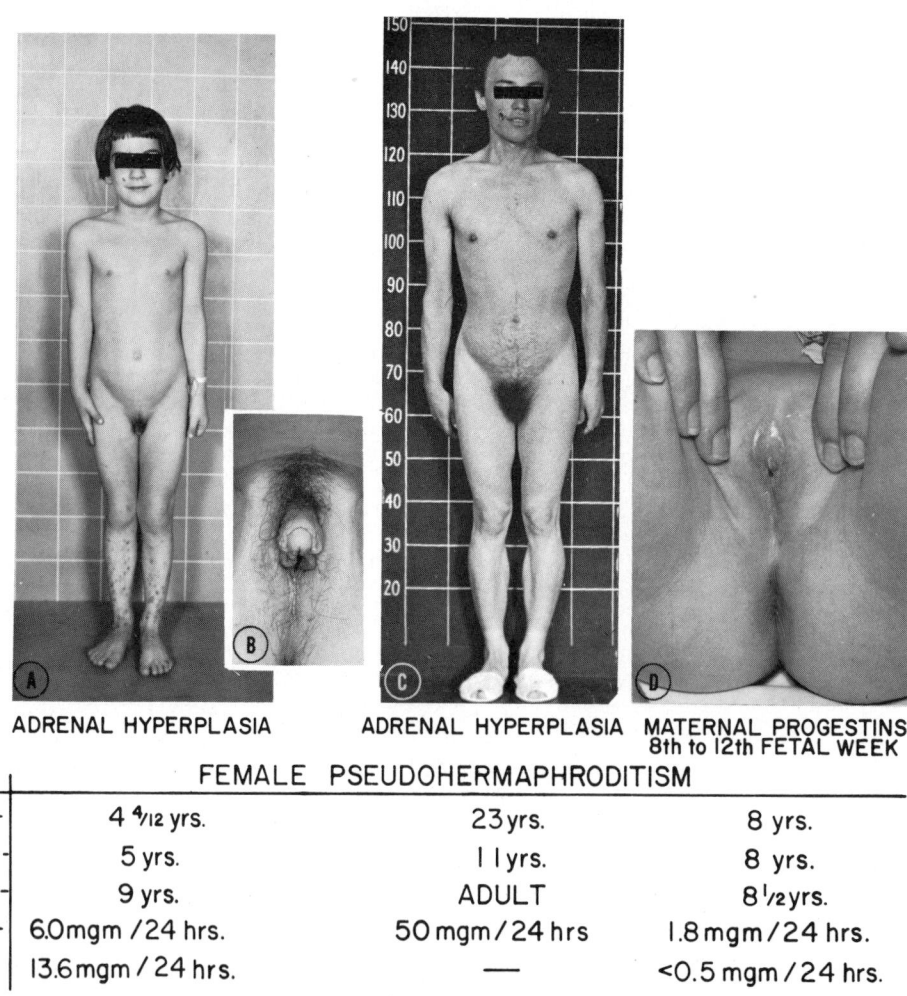

FEMALE PSEUDOHERMAPHRODITISM

	ADRENAL HYPERPLASIA	ADRENAL HYPERPLASIA	MATERNAL PROGESTINS 8th to 12th FETAL WEEK
AGE	4 4/12 yrs.	23 yrs.	8 yrs.
HT. AGE	5 yrs.	11 yrs.	8 yrs.
BONE AGE	9 yrs.	ADULT	8½ yrs.
17 K.S.	6.0 mgm / 24 hrs.	50 mgm / 24 hrs	1.8 mgm / 24 hrs.
Pregnanetriol	13.6 mgm / 24 hrs.	—	<0.5 mgm / 24 hrs.

Figure 9–45. *A* and *B*, Untreated girl with relatively mild form of congenital adrenal hyperplasia. Androgens caused disproportionate acceleration of bone maturation as compared with stature. *C*, Virilized adult female with adrenal hyperplasia. Patient had deep voice, shaved daily, and wore a toupee for baldness. After treatment with cortisone her 17-KS fell to normal levels, her breasts enlarged, she underwent a normal menarche, and hair regrew on her head. Note short stature and short extremities. (From Wilkins, L.: *The Diagnosis and Treatment of Endocrine Disorders in Childhood and Adolescence.* 3rd ed. Courtesy of Charles C Thomas, Publisher, 1965.⁴⁹³) *D*, Female pseudohermaphrodism due to maternal ingestion of oral progestational compound from eighth to twelfth week of pregnancy. Labioscrotal fusion is sufficient to obscure vaginal orifice and create urogenital sinus. The clitoris is enlarged. There is no progressive virilizing tendency, and adolescent normal female development and fertility can be expected.

and 18 hydroxylase pathway in the zona glomerulosa is functional and normal amounts of aldosterone can be secreted under the influence of the renin-angiotension system (306). The excessive secretion of DOC in the untreated patient suppresses the concentration of plasma renin and hence aldosterone secretion. The aldosterone pathway is activated following glucocorticoid treatment and the decrease in the ACTH-stimulated abnormal DOC secretion. As in other forms, the defect is sometimes partial and hypertension may either be absent or may not appear until late childhood or adulthood. The gene for 11 β-hydroxylase is not linked to the HLA loci. In most large series in the United States the disorder is about 1/5 to 1/10 as frequent as 21 hydroxylase deficiency; but in certain Middle Eastern populations (e.g., Moroccan Jews) defects in 11 and 21 hydroxylation are equally prevalent.

Female infants with this syndrome manifest ambiguity of the genitalia, while males have normal external genitalia at birth. Progressive virilization, increased growth, and skeletal maturation occur in the untreated patient. There are reports of 11 β-hydroxylase deficiency, which first manifests clinical signs in adolescence with hirsutism, menstrual disturbance, acne, deepening of the voice, and variable hypertension (322). Salt loss leading to hyponatremia and hyperkalemia can occur transiently, especially in infants, with 11 β-hydroxylase deficiency as a result of the suppression of DOC secretion by glucocorticoid therapy as a consequence of the suppression of ACTH stimulated DOC secretion soon after the initiation of glucocorticoid therapy, before the inhibited renin-angiotensin-aldosterone system has had time to recover (323).

The diagnosis of 11 β-hydroxylase deficiency can be confirmed by the finding of elevated plasma concentrations of 11-deoxycortisol (compound S) and DOC, and increased excretion of their metabolites in urine (mainly tetrahydro S) and their suppression by glucocorticoid therapy. When hypertensive, these patients characteristically have an increased deoxycorticosterone (DOC) plasma concentration and secretion rate, but low levels of plasma renin activity and aldosterone. The treatment of this form of CAH is similar to that of simple 21-hydroxylase deficiency. Cortisol therapy suppresses ACTH secretion and the increased secretion of adrenal androgens, their precursors and 11-deoxycosterone (DOC). This results in a decrease in hypertension, usually into the normal range, and the arrest of virilization. The disorder can be detected prenatally (see p. 505).

Type IV: 3β-Hydroxysteroid Dehydrogenase Defect (Male or Female Pseudohermaphrodism and Adrenal Insufficiency).

This disorder, first described by Bongiovanni, is due to a deficiency of the enzyme 3β-hydroxysteroid dehydrogenase (324). This enzyme acts at an early stage in steroid biosynthesis and is required by both the adrenals and gonads for the synthesis of their respective biologically active steroids. A deficiency of the enzyme results in an inability to convert 3β-hydroxy-Δ^5-steroids to 3-keto-Δ^4-steroids. The defect leads to defective synthesis of aldosterone, cortisol, and the potent androgens and estrogens. In addition to adrenal insufficiency, affected females exhibit slight to moderate clitoral enlargement, whereas affected males have varying degrees of male pseudohermaphrodism. The mild virilization observed in 46,XX females has been attributed to a modest increase in adrogen production in the fetus. Mild forms of 3β-hydroxysteroid dehyrogenase deficiency may not become clinically apparent until adolescence (325).

The concentration of plasma dehydroepiandrosterone and its sulfate and C$_{21}$ steroids with a 3β-hydroxy-Δ^5 configuration are greatly elevated, as well as urinary 17-ketosteroids, predominantly dehydroepiandrosterone sulfate and other C$_{19}$-Δ^5-β-hydroxysteroids. Suppression of the increased plasma and urinary 3β-hydroxysteroids by glucocorticoids distinguishes 3β-hydroxysteroid dehydrogenase deficiency from a virilizing adrenal tumor. Therapy is similar to that for patients with type II C$_{21}$-hydroxylase deficiency. The mortality in infancy has been high in patients with this disorder.

Type V: 17α-Hydroxylase Defect (Male Pseudohermaphrodism, Sexual Infantilism, Hypertension and Hypokalemic Alkalosis).

17α-hydroxylase deficiency was initially reported by Biglieri in 46,XX females with hypertension, hypokalemia, and sexual infantilism (326). Subsequently, this defect has been described in 46,XY infants, children, and adults with male pseudohermaphrodism (327–333).

The defect in 17 hydroxylation results in impaired synthesis of 17-hydroxyprogesterone, and 17-hydroxypregnenolone and, thus, of cortisol and sex steroids (e.g., testosterone and estradiol). The secretion of large amounts of corticosterone and 11-deoxycorticosterone (DOC) leads to hypertension, hypokalemia, and alkalosis and to suppression of the renin-angiotensin system and aldosterone secretion.

The clinical manifestations are a consequence of the defect in adrenal and gonadal steroid biosynthesis. XX females with this defect have normal female development, both internally and externally. However, their ovaries cannot secrete estrogens at puberty and thus, affected females exhibit sexual infantilism and hypogonadism with elevated FSH and LH levels. In males, impaired testosterone synthesis by the fetal testes results in male pseudohermaphrodism (333). The external genitalia may be that of a phenotypic female or exhibit an ambiguous appearance. In males, female duct derivatives are absent, since the secretion of müllerian duct inhibitory factor by the fetal Sertoli cells is not impaired.

Diagnosis. 17α-hydroxylase deficiency should be considered in patients with ambiguous external genitalia or phenotypic females with sexual infantilism who have hypertension associated with hypokalemic alkalosis. Elevated levels of progesterone, Δ^5-pregnenolone, deoxycorticosterone (DOC) and corticosterone (compound B) in plasma and increased excretion of their urinary metabolities establish the diagnosis.

Glucocorticoid therapy similar to that in C$_{21}$-hydroxylase deficiency results in suppression of DOC and corticosterone secretion (see p. 481). With correction of the excess circulating mineralocorticoids, the blood pressure and serum potassium return to normal. At puberty, both males and females require sex steroid replacement.

Type VI: Cholesterol Desmolase Complex Defect (Male Pseudohermaphrodism, Sexual Infantilism, and Adrenal Insufficiency).

The first step in synthesis of steroids in both the adrenal and gonads is the conversion of cholesterol to Δ^5-pregnenolone. 20,22 hydroxylation of cholesterol side chain cleavage and conversion to pregnenolone requires a complex mitochondrial mixed-function oxidase system including the enzyme cytochrome pigment 450 (P-450). Recently, a decrease in the adrenal mitochondrial content of cytochrome P-450 was shown in patients with this defect (334). These patients have congenital lipoid adrenal hyperplasia owing to a primitive biosynthetic defect in the conversion of cholesterol to any biologically active steroid.

Prader first described this form of adrenal hyperplasia associated with severe glucocorticoid and mineralocorticoid deficiency in which no C$_{21}$, C$_{19}$ or C$_{18}$ steroids are elaborated by the adrenal glands or gonads (335). As a consequence, affected males usually have female external genitalia with a

Table 9–18. CLINICAL MANIFESTATIONS OF VARIOUS TYPES OF CONGENITAL ADRENAL HYPERPLASIA

ENZYMATIC DEFECT	CHOLESTEROL DESMOLASE SYSTEM (CHOLESTEROL 20α-HYDROXYLASE)		3β-HYDROXYSTEROID DEHYDROGENASE		17α-HYDROXYLASE		11β-HYDROXYLASE		21α-HYDROXYLASE	
TYPE	VI		IV		V		III		II & I	
CHROMOSOMAL SEX	XX	XY	XX	XY	XX	XY	XX	XY	XX	XY
EXTERNAL GENITALIA	female	female	female (clitoromegaly)	ambiguous	female	female or ambiguous	ambiguous	male	ambiguous	male
POSTNATAL VIRILIZATION	(sexual infantilism at puberty)		±	mild to moderate	(sexual infantilism at puberty)		+		+	
ADDISONIAN CRISES	+		+		−		−		+ in 40% (type II)	
HYPERTENSION	−		−		+		+		−	

From Grumbach & van Wyk, Williams. Textbook of Endocrinology. ed. 5 (1974)

blind vaginal pouch but absent müllerian duct derivatives. Females with this disorder have a normal internal and external genital tract. At autopsy the adrenals are strikingly enlarged and lipid laden. At least 16 patients with this defect have been described (336–340). Most patients have died in infancy of adrenal insufficiency, although at least two have survived to adolescence with replacement therapy.

In patients with this defect, little or no C_{21} or C_{19} steroids are detectable in plasma or urine. In XX females, the differential diagnosis includes congenital adrenal hypoplasia. Radiographic demonstration of enlarged adrenals readily differentiates these two entities. Therapy is directed toward replacement with glucocorticoids and mineralocorticoids, with the addition of estrogen at puberty. Affected males are raised as females and require gonadectomy and estrogen replacement therapy at puberty. Few affected children have survived infancy owing to the severe cortisol and aldosterone deficiency.

The clinical manifestations of each of these forms of congenital adrenal hyperplasia are summarized in Table 9–18.

Maternal Androgens and Progestins

Masculinization of the external genitalia of female infants has been frequently observed following the maternal ingestion of testosterone or synthetic progestational agents during the first trimester of pregnancy (341–343) (Fig. 9–45D). If the exposure occurs after the 12th week of gestation, fusion of the labioscrotal folds does not occur, although there may be clitoral enlargement. Severe virilization may be caused by methyltestosterone in dosages as small as 3 mg daily, even though androgenic effects are not noticeable in the mother.

Since progesterone itself is only very slightly active when administered orally, various synthetic derivatives which may be taken by mouth have frequently been prescribed in the past for women with habitual or threatened abortion. Most of these compounds are intrinsically androgenic to some degree and regularly produce virilization of female fetuses in experimental animals. Before this potential complication was publicized, norethindrone (Norlutin) and various commercial forms of ethisterone (Pranone, Lutocylol, Progesterol) have been responsible for most cases, but female pseudohermaphrodism also has been induced by norethynodrel and medroxyprogesterone acetate (343). Ishi-

zuka found some degree of masculinization of the external genitalia in 2.75% of female infants whose mothers received progestins of various types during pregnancy (344).

Bongiovani, Di George, and Grumbach collected four similar cases of female pseudohermaphrodism in which the mother had received only stilbestrol in large dosages (345). The mechanism of virilization in these cases is obscure, but it may be related to inhibition of adrenal 3β-hydroxysteroid dehydrogenase by this compound. Recently, maternal ingestion of stilbestrol and other chemically related nonsteroidal synthetic estrogens during pregnancy has been associated with an increased prevalence of clear-cell adenocarcinoma of the vagina and cervix in adolescent and young adult females. Transplacental carcinogenesis by stilbestrol was implicated in at least 46 of 66 cases of this rare tumor by Herbst et al. (346); in light of these findings, stilbestrol and related analogues should not be given to pregnant women.

In rare instances, masculinization of the female fetus may occur if the mother is suffering from a virilizing ovarian (usually arrhenoblastoma or Krukenberg tumor) or adrenal tumor, a virilizing form of congenital adrenal hyperplasia, or if she develops virilism from some other cause during the course of her pregnancy (342, 347–349). Luteoma of pregnancy, an ovarian pseudotumor composed of hyperplastic luteinized thecal cells, which regress postpartum, has been associated with masculinization of the external genitalia of female infants (350). Ovarian lutein cysts in pregnancy *(hyperreactio luteinalis)*, which are considered by some as a ciated with masculinization of the external genitalia of female infants (350). Overian lutein cysts in pregnancy (hyperreactio luteinalis), which are considered by some as a cystic form of luteoma, are less frequently associated with maternal virilization and, rarely, with fetal masculinization (351). Placental aromatization of androgens may protect the mother and especially the fetus from virilization (351). Some of the rare cases of non-adrenal female pseudohermaphrodism of undetermined etiology may have been a consequence of a luteoma of pregnancy that regressed spontaneously after neoplasm, but the clinical features are compatible with ingestion of potentially androgenic steroids and the postpartum course of the mother is inconsistent with a virilizing neoplasm, but the clinical features are more compatible with fetal exposure to androgens. The absence of virilism in the mother does not exclude a maternal source of androgen in these children, however, since the quantities required to masculinize the external genitalia of an early female fetus may be less than those that cause overt manifestations in the mother (342).

Female pseudohermaphrodism arising from the transfer of androgenic steroids in the mother is the most easily treated of all types of ambisexual development. No hormonal therapy is necessary, postnatal virilism does not occur, and female secondary sexual characteristics can be expected to emerge at the usual age of adolescence. Surgical correction of the external genitalia restores feminine appearance and permits normal sexual function.

Malformations of the Intestine and Urinary Tract

Genital abnormalities are frequently associated with imperforate anus, renal agenesis, and other congenital malformations of the lower intestine and urinary tract (352). Carpentier and Potter reviewed the findings in such infants and suggested the term "nonspecific female pseudohermaphrodism" (353). Some, but not all of these anomalies are incompatible with life. Renal failure, often accompanied by pyelonephritis, is frequently present and may confuse the picture with that of salt-losing congenital adrenal hyperplasia. In contrast with other forms of female pseudohermaphrodism, the internal genital ducts may also be malformed. The findings in these patients may be quite bizarre, and persistence of a primitive cloaca is not infrequent. The pathogenesis of these anomalies is different from other types of ambisexual development and should be considered in the context of other forms of teratology. Familial occurrence of nonadrenal female pseudohermaphrodism with multiple anomalies has been reported (354).

MALE PSEUDOHERMAPHRODISM

Definition and Classification

Male pseudohermaphrodism is a heterogenous condition in which the gonads are exclusively testes but the genital ducts or external genitalia are incompletely masculinized and exhibit to a varying degree the phenotypic characteristics of a female. The clinical spectrum varies from individuals in whom the configuration of the external genitalia is female to mild forms as represented by hypospadias, cryptorchidism, and minimal ambiguity of the external genitalia.

With the elucidation of etiologic mechanisms, systems of nomenclature based on phenotype have become less important. There are at least six major etiologic categories of male psueodhermaphrodism with many subtypes, all of which are associated with incomplete masculinization of the fetal gential tract and/or incomplete regression of the müllerian ducts.

In this section, forms of "male pseudohermaphrodism" in XY individuals with relatively normal embryonic differentiation of their testes will be discussed. In such patients, defective male development must be ascribed to a more specific failure of the fetal testes to overcome the inherent tendency to feminize the somatic sex structures. This failure may stem either from a secretory failure of the testes themselves during the critical period of sex differentiation or from a failure of target tissues to respond normally to androgen stimulation. The classification of male pseudohermaphrodism outlined in Table 9–19 reflects an attempt to classify the many forms of male pseudohermaphrodism on the basis of etiology, insofar as that is known.

The ability of the testes to virilize the patient at adoles-

Table 9–19. MALE PSEUDOHERMAPHRODISM

A. Testicular unresponsiveness to hCG and LH
B. Inborn errors of testosterone biosynthesis
 1. Enzyme defects affecting synthesis of both corticosteroids and testosterone (variants of congenital adrenal hyperplasia)
  a. Cholesterol desmolase complex deficiency (congenital lipoid adrenal hyperplasia)
  b. 3β-hydroxysteroid dehydrogenase deficiency
  c. 17α-hydroxylase deficiency
 2. Enzyme defects primarily affecting testosterone biosynthesis by the testes
  a. 17,20-desmolase (lyase) deficiency
  b. 17β-hydroxysteroid oxidoreductase deficiency
C. Defects in androgen-dependent target tissues
 1. End-organ insensitivity to androgenic hormones (androgen receptor and post-receptor defects)
  a. Complete syndrome of androgen insensitivity and its variants (testicular feminization and its variant forms)
  b. Incomplete syndrome of androgen insensitivity and its variants (Reifenstein syndrome)
  c. Androgen insensitivity in infertile men
 2. Defects in testosterone metabolism by peripheral tissues
  a. 5α-reductase deficiency—male pseudohermaphrodism with normal virilization at puberty (familial perineal hypospadias with ambiguous development of urogenital sinus and male puberty; pseudovaginal perineoscrotal hypospadias)
D. Dysgenetic male pseudohermaphrodism
 1. X chromatin-negative variants of the syndrome of gonadal dysgenesis (e.g., XO/XY,XYp−)
 2. Incomplete form of XY gonadal dysgenesis
 3. Associated with degenerative renal disease
 4. "Vanishing testes" (embryonic testicular regression syndrome; XY agonadism; XY gonadal agenesis; rudimentary testes; anorchia)
E. Defects in synthesis, secretion, or response to müllerian duct inhibitory factor: Female genital ducts in otherwise normal men— "uteri hernia inguinale"; persistent müllerian duct syndrome.
F. Maternal ingestion of estrogen and progestins

cence is frequently a recapitulation of their capacity to masculinize the external genitalia *in utero.* The greater the development of the phallus, the greater likelihood that male secondary sex characteristics will emerge. Individuals with ambiguous genitalia may remain eunuchoid, exhibit mild virilism, or develop breast enlargement and other feminine secondary sex characteristics. Those with an external female phenotype will usually either feminize or remain sexually infantile. These are only approximate guides, however, and the paradoxical development of sexual characteristics at adolescence is encountered especially in incomplete androgen insensitivity and patients with 5α-reductase deficiency.

Male pseudohermaphrodism can result from deficient testosterone secretion by the male fetus as a consequence of a) testicular unresponsiveness to hCG and LH and Leydig cell hypoplasia; b) a specific and familial defect in testosterone biosynthesis; c) familial end-organ insensitivity to androgen owing to abnormalities in the cytosol receptor for testosterone and dihydrotestosterone and post-receptor defects; d) defects in the intracellular metabolism of testosterone; e) aberrations in testicular organogenesis (dysgenetic male pseudohermaphrodism); f) defective synthesis, secretion, or response to müllerian duct inhibitory factor; and g) maternal ingestion of progestins or estrogens. Except for dysgenetic male pseudohermaphrodism and the persistent müllerian duct syndrome, all other forms of male pseudohermaphrodism are characterized by the absence of müllerian duct derivatives. Except for some variants of dysgenetic male pseudohermaphrodism and the maternal ingestion of progestins and estrogens, all forms of male pseudohermaphrodism are familial and characterized by genetic heterogeneity. No doubt many subtypes will be defined and characterized in the future by refined biochemical techniques. Although we have previously discussed dysgenetic male pseudohermaphrodism — the group of disorders associated with defective organogenesis of the testes on p. 470 — it is convenient to include it under male pseudohermaphrodism, since it must be considered by the clinician in the differential diagnosis of male pseudohermaphrodism.

Testicular Unresponsiveness to hCG and LH (Leydig Cell Agenesis or Hypoplasia)

The production of testosterone by fetal Leydig cells is critical to male sexual differentiation of the wolffian ducts and the external genitalia. Leydig cell agenesis or hypoplasia, or a receptor abnormality resulting in Leydig cell unresponsiveness to hCG-LH, would result in male pseudohermaphrodism. Berthezene (355), Brown (356) and Perez-Palacios (357) and their associates have described a new form of male pseudohermaphroditism with Leydig cell hypoplasia. These 46,XY patients had a female phenotype, sexual infantilism, small inguinal or intra-abdominal testes composed of infantile seminiferous tubules lined by Sertoli cells, and rare spermatogenia. Leydig cells were absent despite elevated gonadotropin levels. The external genitalia were female except for slight posterior labial fusion, and clitoromegaly in the patient reported by Brown et al. (356). Separate vaginal and urethral openings were present, but no müllerian structures (uterus and fallopian tubes) were identified; male duct differentiation (epididymis and vas deferens) were present in two patients but

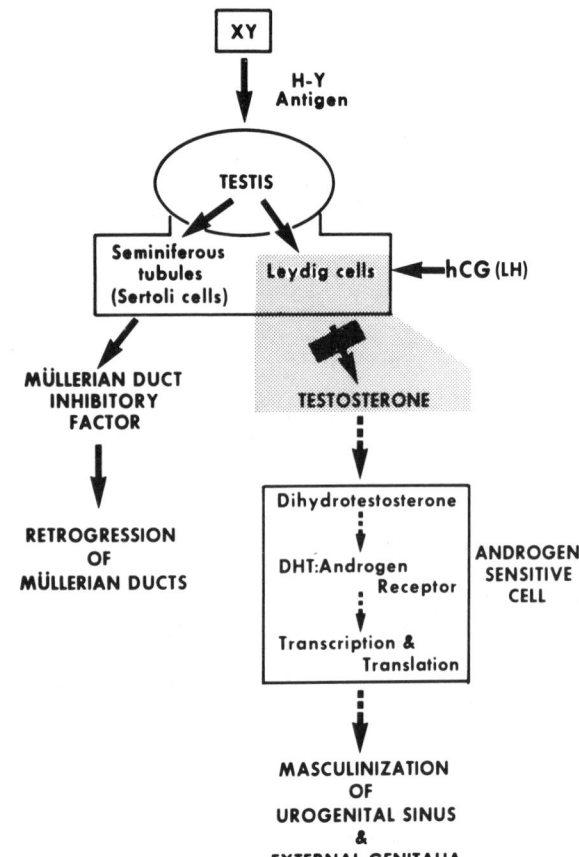

Figure 9–47. Diagrammatic scheme of male sex determination and differentiation showing the consequences of an enzymatic block in the biosynthesis of testosterone that results in male pseudohermaphrodism.

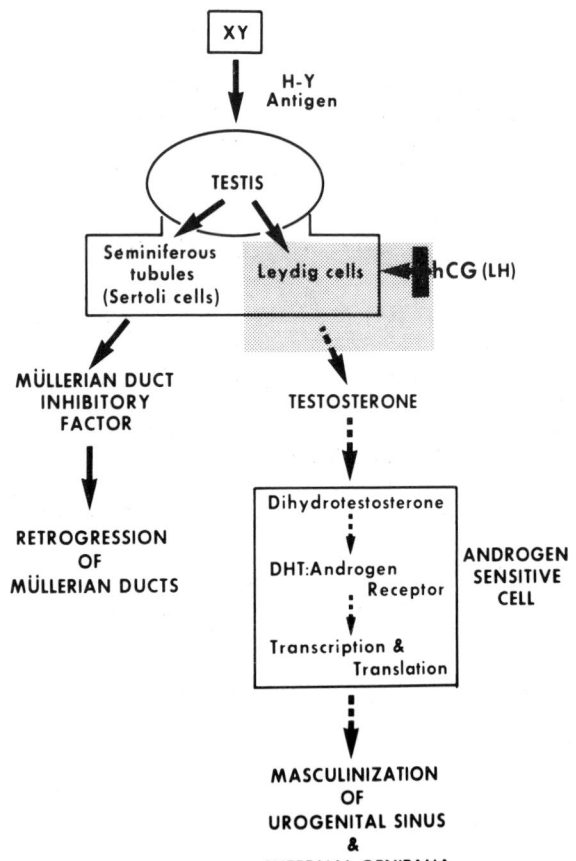

Figure 9–46. Diagrammatic scheme of male sex determination and differentiation showing a defect in Leydig cell responsiveness to hCG (LH) resulting in male pseudohermaphrodism. The solid bar (▮) delineates the defect, and the hatched area designates the general site of the defect. Interrupted lines indicate that the subsequent processes may be completely or partially affected.

absent in the three cases reported by Perez-Palacios. The concentration of plasma LH was elevated, and FSH levels were normal or increased. Plasma testosterone levels were low, and treatment with human chorionic gonadotropin did not elicit an increase in plasma testosterone, androstenedione, or dehydroepiandrosterone. While this disorder initially had been attributed to primary Leydig cell agenesis, we suggested that the findings in these patients could be explained by end-organ unresponsiveness to hCG and LH, most likely owing to a deficiency or abnormality of the hCG-LH receptor on the plasma membrane of the fetal and postnatal Leydig cell (Fig. 9–46) (29). In these patients, fetal testosterone deficiency results in poorly masculinized external genitalia, but müllerian duct regression is complete, since the secretion of müllerian duct inhibitory factor by the fetal Sertoli cells is intact. Of interest is the paradoxical finding of wolffian derivatives, which are testosterone-dependent in some patients despite little or no masculinization of the external genitalia (only posterior labial fusion). One possibility is that the initial differentiation and function of fetal Leydig cells may be autonomous of hCG (29, 98); however, this possibility would not explain the absent male duct differentiation in some affected individuals. A more likely explanation is that the defect in the hCG-LH receptor is of variable severity. During the ambiguous and early fetal period, sufficient testosterone may have been secreted locally to induce male duct development, but the concentration in the fetal circulation was too low to evoke male differentiation of the external genitalia and urogenital sinus. hCG stimulation is necessary for

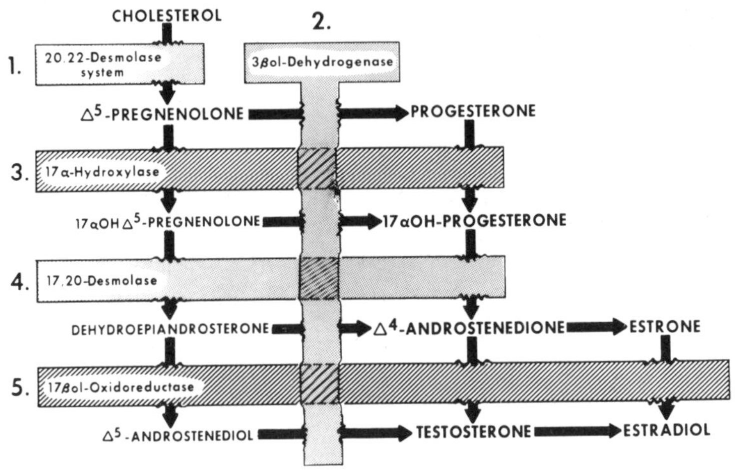

Figure 9–48. Enzymatic defects in the biosynthetic pathway for testosterone. All five of the enzymatic defects cause male pseudohermaphrodism in affected males. Even though all of the blocks affect both gonadal and adrenal cortical steroidogenesis, those at steps 1, 2, and 3 are associated with major abnormalities in the biosynthesis of glucocorticoids and mineralocorticoids.

sustained Leydig cell formation and growth. The resistance of the undifferentiated embryonic and fetal Leydig cells to hCG would result in fetal testosterone deficiency and thus, to female or predominantly female differentiation of the external genitalia (29). Alternatively, the elevated hCG concentration early in gestation may have been sufficient to overcome the end-organ resistance and to influence Leydig cell differentiation. Bardin has described a counterpart to this disorder in the rat, the vestigial testes syndrome, in which he obtained evidence of an LH receptor defect (358). More recently, similar evidence was obtained by *in vivo* and *in vitro* studies in three patients with this disorder, including lack of binding of ^{125}I labeled LH to Leydig cells (357).

In the human male fetus, the deficient fetal pituitary gonadotropin secretion associated with anencephaly, hypothalamic hypopituitarism, and isolated gonadotropin deficiency (Kallmann syndrome) is not associated with ambiguous genitalia, although undescended testes and a microphallus are commonly present (97). These clinical observations are consistent with the important role of hCG in testosterone secretion by the human fetal testis during the critical period of male sex differentiation; fetal pituitary FSH and LH are not required for differentiation of testes or male external genitalia but do play a role in their growth at a later stage.

Inborn Errors of Testosterone Biosynthesis

Enzyme Defects Affecting Both Corticosteroid and Testosterone Biosynthesis (Variants of Congenital Adrenal Hyperplasia) (Fig. 9–47)

Five familial enzymatic defects in testosterone biosynthesis have been described, one at each of the enzymatic steps required for the conversion of cholesterol to testosterone (Fig. 9–48). Three of the defects (cholesterol desmolase complex deficiency, 3β-hydroxysteroid dehydrogenase, and 17α-hydroxylase) involve enzymes affecting both glucocorticoid and sex steroid biosynthesis; these errors in steroid biosynthesis are discussed in part in the section on congenital adrenal hyperplasia (p. 483).

Cholesterol Desmolase Complex Deficiency (Lipoid Adrenal Hyperplasia (Table 9–20). Infants with this defect, first described by Prader, present with severe adrenal insufficiency and enormous accumulations of lipid in the cells of both the adrenal cortex and gonads. Affected males have female or ambiguous external genitalia with a blind vaginal pouch and hypoplastic male genital ducts but no uterus or fallopian tubes; the genitalia of affected females are normal. In males, the testes may be abdominal, inguinal, or in the labia. Glucocorticoid and mineralocorticoid insufficiency are usually severe and if untreated usually results in death. However, three male pseudohermaphrodites survived the perinatal period without therapy and presented at 6 weeks, 12 weeks, and 8½ months of age (339, 340, 359). The patient reported by Grumbach et al. in the previous edition is now 12 years old and entirely well on glucocorticoid and mineralocorticoid replacement therapy.

The diagnosis of cholesterol desmolase complex deficiency should be suspected in patients with male pseudohermaphrodism who manifest adrenal insufficiency. The diagnosis can be confirmed by low or absent mineralocorticoids, glucocorticoids, and sex steroids and their metabolites in plasma and urine. As with other forms of congenital adrenal hyperplasia, this enzymatic defect is inherited as an autosomal recessive trait. Therapy is directed toward glucocorticoid and mineralcocorticoid replacement. All affected XY males have been reared as females. Estrogen replacement therapy at puberty is indicated, as is prophylactic orchidectomy.

3β-Hydroxysteroid Dehydrogenase Deficiency (Table 9–21). Male pseudohermaphrodism associated with adrenal insufficiency is the usual finding in affected males with 3β-hydroxysteroid dehydrogenase Δ^5 isomerase deficiency. Since the block occurs at an early stage of steroid biosynthesis, both adrenal steroidogenesis and testosterone

Table 9–20. SALIENT FEATURES OF CHOLESTEROL DESMOLASE COMPLEX DEFICIENCY

Karyotype: 46,XY

Inheritance: Autosomal recessive

Genitalia: Female → (Ambiguous)

Wolffian duct derivatives: Absent → (Hypoplastic)

Müllerian duct derivatives: Absent

Gonads: Testes

Habitus: Severe adrenal insufficiency in infancy, little or no virilization at puberty

Hormone profile: ↓ or absent glucocorticoids, mineralocorticoids, and sex steroids in plasma and urine, ↑ plasma LH and FSH

Table 9–21. SALIENT FEATURES OF 3β-HYDROXYSTEROID DEHYDROGENASE DEFICIENCY

Karyotype: 46,XY

Inheritance: Autosomal recessive

Genitalia: Hypospadiac male

Wolffian duct derivatives: Normal

Müllerian duct derivatives: Absent

Gonads: Testes

Habitus: Severe adrenal insufficiency in infancy; poor virilization at puberty with gynecomastia

Hormone profile: $\uparrow$ concentrations of Δ^5C_{21} and C_{19} steroids (e.g., dehydroepiandrosterone and its sulfate) in urine and plasma

secretion by the fetal Leydig cells are impaired. Unlike affected males with the cholesterol desmolase complex defect, 3β-hydroxysteroid dehydrogenase/Δ^5 isomerase deficient males exhibit incomplete masculinization of the external genitalia. The external genitalia of the affected male usually exhibit a small phallic structure with second or third degree hypospadias, partial fusion of the labioscrotal folds, a urogenital sinus and a blind vaginal pouch (Fig. 9–49). Wolffian duct differentiation is normal. As with other enzymatic blocks in testosterone biosynthesis or defects in androgen-dependent target tissues, müllerian structures are absent. Although most of the cases reported originally died in infancy, an increasing number of male pseudo-hermaphrodites with 3β-hydroxysteroid dehydrogenase deficiency who survived infancy and entered puberty have been described; at least some of these patients have a partial deficiency of the enzyme. All had ambiguous external genitalia and developed gynecomastia at puberty (360–365). The gynecomastia and masculinization at puberty may be related to the increased testicular secretion of Δ^5-androstenediol. In the older XY patients, low normal concentrations of plasma testosterone increased estrogen levels, and the appearance of C_{21} steroids such as pregnenetriol in the urine has been attributed to the maturation of a

hepatic enzyme under different genetic control with the capacity to convert C_{21} and C_{19} 3β-hydroxysteroids to Δ^43-ketosteroids.

The diagnosis of 3β-hydroxysteroid dehydrogenase deficiency should be suspected in all XY males with ambiguous genitalia and adrenal insufficiency. The hormonal characteristics of this disorder are the increased concentrations of Δ^5C_{21} and C_{19} steroids (e.g., dehydroepiandrosterone and its sulfate) and their derivatives in plasma and urine. However, the diagnosis in early infancy can be confounded by the elevation of Δ^5-3β-hydroxy C_{21} and C_{19} steroids that is found in normal premature and full-term infants during the first few weeks of life. Thus, in early infancy it is essential to interpret the increased concentration of C_{21} and C_{19} 3β-hydroxysteroids in relation to normal values for age. Therapy involves replacement of glucocorticoids and mineralocorticoids as in salt-wasting patient with 21-hydroxylase deficiency.

The disorder is transmitted an an autosomal recessive trait. The clinical and biochemical variability in the expression of the enzyme defect suggests genetic heterogeneity.

17α-Hydroxylase Deficiency (Table 9–22). The phenotype of affected males with 17α-hydroxylase deficiency, a defect which involves both adrenal and gonadal steroidogenesis, has varied from that of a male pseudohermaphrodite with normal appearing female external genitalia and a blind vaginal pouch, to a hypospadic male with a small phallus. The magnitude of the impaired masculinization of the external genitalia in the male fetus correlates with the severity of block in 17α-hydroxylation and, hence, testosterone synthesis (332, 333, 366–371). The testes may be intra-abdominal, in the inguinal canal, or in the labioscrotal folds. Müllerian structures are absent and wolffian derivatives are usually hypoplastic. The excessive secretion of 11-deoxycorticosterone and corticosterone, the consequence of the failure to 17-hydroxylate C_{21} steroids, leads to hypertension and hypokalemia. As sex steroid secretion is low, the severely affected patients fail to develop secondary sex characteristics, including pubic and axillary hair at puberty, and plasma and urinary FSH and LH values are elevated. In the patient reported by New et al., a partial deficiency of 17-hydroxylase was present, and prominent gynecomastia and incomplete development of male secondary sex characteristics occurred at puberty (333).

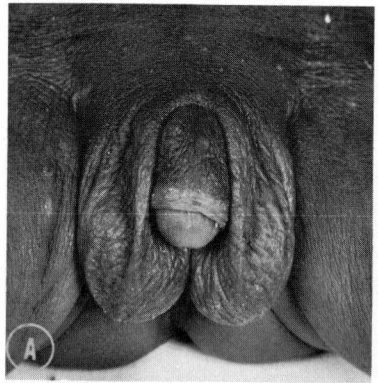
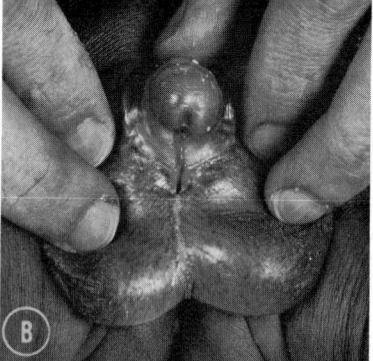

NCMH #11-74-13   3 MO. MALE   KARYOTYPE: XY

CONGENITAL ADRENAL HYPERPLASIA DUE TO
3-β HYDROXY-STEROID DEHYDROGENASE DEFICIENCY
17 KS : 3.2 mgm / 24 hrs
"pregnanetriol" : 1.4 mgm / 24 hrs.

Figure 9–49. Genitalia of male infant with congenital adrenal hyperplasia due to 3 β-hydroxysteroid dehydrogenase deficiency. This boy was admitted at 9 days of age in a salt-losing crisis and died at 3 months of unexplained muscular paralysis. Paresis, resembling that of the Werdnig-Hoffmann syndrome, became progressively more severe even though adrenal replacement therapy was adequate and blood electrolytes were normal. The biochemical findings revealed a severe block in the conversion of Δ-5,3 β-hydroxysteroids to Δ-4,3 ketones. The findings in this boy were reported by Bongiovanni (Case IV).[324]

Table 9–22. SALIENT FEATURES OF 17α-HYDROXYLASE DEFICIENCY

Karyotype: 46,XY

Inheritance: Autosomal recessive

Genitalia: Female → Ambiguous → Hypospadiac male. Blind vaginal pouch

Wolffian duct derivatives: Absent → Hypoplastic

Müllerian duct derivatives: Absent

Gonads: Testes

Habitus: Absent or poor virilization at puberty, gynecomastia
Hypertension with hypokalemic alkalosis

Hormone profile: ↓ plasma testosterone; ↑ plasma LH and FSH levels;
↑ plasma DOCA, corticosterone and progesterone concentrations; ↓ plasma renin level

The diagnosis of 17α-hydroxylase deficiency should be suspected in male pseudohermaphrodites, including XY phenotypic females, with hyporeninemic hypertension and hypokalemic alkalosis. Plasma concentrations of ACTH, 11-deoxycorticosterone, corticosterone, and progesterone are elevated whereas the levels of aldosterone, 17-hydroxyprogesterone, cortisol, and the sex steroids are low. Replacement therapy with physiologic doses of cortisol or its analogues results in suppression of 11-deoxycorticosterone and corticosterone secretion and the return of serum potassium and blood pressure to normal. At puberty, appropriate sex steroid replacement therapy is indicated, as is gonadectomy in the XY patients who have been assigned a female sex of rearing.

Enzyme Defects Primarily Affecting Testosterone Biosynthesis by the Testes (Table 9–23)

17,20-Desmolase (Lyase) Deficiency. Zachmann et al. (372) studied three patients — two first cousins and a maternal aunt — with a familial form of male pseudohermaphrodism which they ascribed to a partial defect in the conversion of the C_{21} steroids 17α-hydroxyprogesterone and 17α-hydroxypregnenolone to the C_{19} steroids testosterone, androstenedione, and dehydroepiandrosterone by the testes and adrenal glands. The patients had ambiguous external genitalia, inguinal or intraabdominal testes, and an XY sex chromosome constitution. Both first cousins had severe hypospadias but a male-type urethra and male duct development. The aunt, who was sexually infantile, had a laparotomy and bilateral orchidectomy previously and was reputed to have a vagina and some rudimentary müllerian derivatives in addition to a vas deferens and epididymis. The cousins, who were studied at 1.8 and 2.2 years of age, excreted appropriate amounts of 17-KS and 17-OHCS for their age. The excretion of urinary pregnanetriol was normal, but pregnenetriol and 11-ketopregnanetriol were increased, suggesting elevated plasma levels of 17α-hydroxyprogesterone and 17α-hydroxypregnenolone. Following the administration of hCG, urinary testosterone glucuronide was unchanged in contrast to that in age-matched normal males, but there was a striking increase in 11-ketopregnanetriol. After ACTH administration, the excretion of dehydroepiandrosterone remained undetectable, but urinary 11-ketopregnanetriol increased four-fold and 17 hydroxycorticoids rose normally. A sample of testicular tissue from one patient was studied in vitro with appropriate C_{21} steroid precursors, and a defect in the conversion of C_{21} steroids to testosterone (C_{19} steroids) was demonstrated. These results are consistent with a deficiency of adrenal and testicular 17,20-desmolase. In this family, the first described, the familial aggregation suggests male-limited autosomal dominant or X-linked recessive inheritance.

Goebelsmann et al. subsequently reported a sexually infantile 16-year-old phenotypic female with a 46,XY karyotype (373). This patient had normal prepubertal female external genitalia without clitoromegaly or labial fusion. A 7 cm vagina ended blindly and gonads were not palpable in the labia or inguinal canals. At laparotomy no müllerian structures were found, but atrophic wolffian derivatives and bilateral abdominal testes were present. No signs of sexual maturation were present. Plasma gonadotropins were elevated while plasma testosterone and estradiol values were low. Testosterone administration resulted in positive nitrogen balance and signs of virilization, excluding androgen insensitivity. Basal and ACTH induced rises in plasma steroids indicated normal secretion of glucocorticoids and mineralocorticoids. The low concentrations of dehydroepiandrosterone, its sulfate, and androstenedione, and their minimal response to ACTH in the light of the normal rise in serum C_{21} steroids strongly suggested a defect in 17,20-desmolase. Direct confirmation of this hypothesis was not possible as the testes had been removed previously.

The diagnosis of 17,20-desmolase deficiency should be considered in male pseudohermaphrodites with absent müllerian derivatives, and XX phenotypic females who do not have an abnormality in glucocorticoid or mineralocorticoid synthesis but at puberty fail to develop secondary characteristics, and have elevated FSH and LH values. In male pseudohermaphrodites before the age of puberty, 17,20-desmolase deficiency needs to be distinguished from the incomplete forms of androgen insensitivity, 5α-reductase deficiency, and 17-oxidoreductase deficiency.

The diagnosis can be established by demonstrating the inability of the adrenals and gonads to convert C_{21} to C_{19} steroids in vivo and in vitro, e.g., 17-hydroxyprogesterone to androstenedione and Δ^5 17-OH-pregnenolone to dehydroepiandrosterone. ACTH and hCG stimulation tests facilitate the diagnosis, especially in prepubertal patients, by bringing out more sharply the abnormal ratio of C_{21} to C_{19} steroids.

The age at diagnosis and the degree of masculinization of the external genitalia are important determinants of the

Table 9–23. SALIENT FEATURES OF 17-20-DESMOLASE DEFICIENCY

Karyotype: 46,XY

Inheritance: Familial; ? X-linked or autosomal recessive

Genitalia: Female → male with perineal hypospadias

Wolffian duct derivatives: rudimentary → normal

Müllerian duct derivatives: Absent

Gonads: Testes

Habitus: Normal stature; sexual infantilism

Hormone profile: ↓ plasma testosterone androstenedione, dehydroepiandrosterone, and estradiol concentrations; abnormal ↑ in plasma 17OH progesterone and 17OH pregnenolone and ↑ ratio of 17OH C_{21} deoxysteroids to C_{19} steroids (T,Δ^4A) after hCG stimulation test; plasma LH and FSH elevated

sex of rearing. Sex steroid therapy is necessary in both sexes at the age of puberty, while gonadectomy is recommended in 46,XY patients raised as females.

17β-Hydroxysteroid Oxidoreductase (17β-Hydroxysteroid Dehydrogenase) Defect (Table 9–24). A familial form of male pseudohermaphrodism caused by a partial block in the last step of androgen and estrogen biosynthesis by the testis, the reduction of androstenedione to testosterone and of estrone to estradiol (374–385), was first described by Saez et al. (374, 375). At birth these XY patients have female external genitalia or subtle ambiguity, testes (usually located in the inguinal canal), male genital duct derivatives only, and a blind vagina. Puberty is characterized by progressive clitoral enlargement and virilism, amenorrhea, and commonly gynecomastia. Whether breast development occurs is quite likely related to the severity of the enzymatic defect and the relative plasma concentrations of androgens and estrogens; the estrogens arise from direct secretion by the testes and the peripheral metabolism of C_{19} steroids from the adrenal and testes (mainly androstenedione) to estrone.

At puberty the concentration of testosterone is low for a male and does not rise above the levels found in early male puberty, but the plasma androstenedione and estrone are strikingly elevated and fall after gonadectomy or testicular suppression with synthetic androgens. There is impaired conversion of androstenedione to testosterone and of dehydroepiandrosterone to androstenediol by testicular tissue. Histologic examination of the testes after the age of puberty reveals Leydig cell hyperplasia. Absent or deficient germ cells in the seminiferous tubules are found on microscopic examination of the testes.

We studied four XY male pseudohermaphrodites with this defect (386). Plasma androstenedione and estrone values were strikingly elevated in the postpubertal patients; testosterone and estradiol levels were low but not absent. This resulted in a reversal of the usual testosterone/androstenedione and estradiol/estrone ratios. The reversal was especially striking in the testicular venous effluent. As low concentrations of testosterone and estradiol were measurable in the plasma, either the block in 17-oxidoreductase was incomplete in these patients or the enzymatic reduction of the 17-ketosteroids androstenedione and estrone to their 17-hydroxylated analogues, testosterone and estradiol, occurred in peripheral tissues, or both mechanisms were operative. Plasma dehydroepiandrosterone levels were not elevated, indicating that DHEA to androstenedione conversion was not impaired, and there was appropriate 3β-hydroxysteroid dehydrogenase activity in the gonads and adrenal. Basal FSH and LH values and LRF-induced LH and FSH responses were elevated. All four patients appeared to have greater impairment in the conversion of estrone to estradiol than of androstenedione to testosterone. All four patients exhibited virilization at puberty, and two of the four had gynecomastia.

17-α-hydroxysteroid oxidoreductase deficiency should be considered in 1) male pseudohermaphrodites with absent müllerian derivatives who have no abnormality in glucocorticoid or mineralocorticoid synthesis and 2) male pseudohermaphrodites who virilize at puberty, especially if gynecomastia is also present. Virilization at puberty in association with gynecomastia occurs in a variety of subtypes of male pseudohermaphrodism. The absence of müllerian structures distinguishes patients with defective testosterone biosynthesis or androgen insensitivity from those with dysgenetic male pseudohermaphrodism. In the prepubertal patient or young adolescent, plasma androstenedione and estrone levels may not be elevated. However, at any age the defect in testosterone biosynthesis can be demonstrated by an hCG stimulation test (1000 to 2000 units intramuscularly of 72 hours × 3). A disproportionate rise in plasma androstenedione and estrone in comparison to testosterone and estradiol occurs in affected patients. 17-oxidoreductase deficiency has been documented in a one-month-old XY infant with genital ambiguity in this manner (387). The disorder is transmitted as an autosomal recessive trait.

In patients with this disorder reared as females (the usual case), the appropriate treatment is castration followed by estrogen substitution at puberty. In the patient with ambiguous genitalia reared as a male, plastic repair of the external genitalia is required and replacement therapy with testosterone is necessary to achieve full masculinization at puberty. A plausible explanation for the absence of spermatogenesis in these patients, aside from cryptorchidism, is the low local concentration of testosterone in the testis.

Defects in Androgen-Dependent Target Tissues

Earlier (p. 445) we discussed the complex mechanism of action of androgens at the target tissue within the cell (111) (Fig. 9–20). A defect at any site from 5α-reduction of testosterone, receptor function, translocation of the steroid receptor complex, activation of nuclear binding sites, transcription, or translation could lead to impaired androgen action and result in male pseudohermaphrodism. Two major forms have been identified: end-organ insensitivity to androgenic hormones (the androgen receptor defects and receptor-positive forms) and errors in testosterone metabolism by peripheral tissues, as illustrated by 5α-reductase deficiency.

End Organs Insensitivity to Androgenic Hormones (Androgen Receptor and Post-Receptor Defects) (388, 389)

Several forms of androgen insensitivity have been identified. The spectrum of phenotypes in XY individuals with androgen insensitivity syndromes varies from individuals with normal female external genitalia through patients with genital ambiguity to those with a normal male phenotype and infertility. As yet, no invariable correlation between androgen receptor activity and phenotype has been

---

Table 9–24. SALIENT FEATURES OF 17β-HYDROXYSTEROID OXIDOREDUCTASE DEFICIENCY

Karyotype: 46,XY

Inheritance: Autosomal recessive

Genitalia: Female → ambiguous; blind vaginal pouch

Wolffian duct derivatives: Hypoplastic

Müllerian duct derivatives: Absent

Gonads: Testes

Habitus: Virilization at puberty (phallic enlargement, deepening of voice, and development of facial and body hair); gynecomastia variable

Hormone profile: ↑ plasma estrone and androstenedione; ↓ ratio of plasma testosterone/androstenedione and estradiol/estrone; after hCG stimulation test; ↑ plasma FSH and LH levels

established. Both qualitative and quantitative defects in the cytosol androgen receptor are known, as are receptor-positive forms.

Complete Syndrome of Androgen-Insensitivity and Its Variants (Testicular Feminization, Feminizing Testes) (Table 9–25)

The term "testicular feminization," coined by Morris, has been applied to a highly distinctive X-linked disorder in which affected males are phenotypic females and develop female secondary sex characteristics at puberty, but fail to menstruate (390). That they are indeed genetic males is attested to by their 46,XY karyotype and male level of H-Y antigen. Phenotypically, these patients present with entirely female external genitalia, a blind vaginal pouch with absent müllerian structures (uterus and tubes), testes located in the labial or inguinal region or intraabdominally, and absent or vestigial wolffian derivatives (Fig. 9–50). Histologically, the gonads are testes, and before puberty they are difficult to distinguish from normal prepubertal testes. Postpubertally, small seminiferous tubules with few spermatogonia and absent spermatogenesis are seen (391, 392). The Leydig cells are hyperplastic and tend to form adenomatous clumps. The testes are predisposed to malignant transformation (390). It is generally agreed that the risk of neoplasia is low prior to age 25 (287), after which age it increases significantly. However, the overall risk of malignancy in patients with testicular feminization may be only moderately greater than that for neoplastic transformation in otherwise normal men with cryptorchid testes (286).

At birth and in childhood the diagnosis should be suspected in phenotypic females with an inguinal hernia and a testes-like mass in the inguinal region, or in the labia. At adolescence, female secondary sexual characteristics develop including well developed breasts, and female body habitus, but no menses. Pubic and axillary hair is usu-

Table 9–25. SALIENT FEATURES OF COMPLETE ANDROGEN INSENSITIVITY

Karyotype: 46,XY

Inheritance: X-linked recessive

Genitalia: Female with blind vaginal pouch

Wolffian duct derivatives: Usually absent; less commonly, rudimentary or hypoplastic

Müllerian duct derivatives: Absent

Gonads: Testes

Habitus: Scanty or absent pubic and axillary hair; breast development and female habitus at puberty; primary amenorrhea ("hairless woman")

Hormone profile: ↑ plasma LH and testosterone concentration; ↑ estradiol (for men); FSH levels often low or normal.
Resistance to the androgenic and metabolic effects of testosterone.
Androgen receptor studies: Genetic heterogeneity:
  a) Low or undetectable amount of normal receptor (receptor negative)
  b) Unstable receptor (thermolabile, partial receptor deficiency)
  c) Receptor-positive form (? abnormal receptor or post-receptor defect)

ally sparse and is completely lacking in about one-third of patients. Slight vulval hair is usually present. The clitoris is normal or small, the vagina is shallow and ends in a blind pouch, and the labia minora tend to be underdeveloped. Approximately 10% of patients have exhibited slight ambiguity of the external genitalia at birth (partial fusion of the labioscrotal folds and modest clitoromegaly). Wolffian duct derivatives are absent, vestigial, or hypoplastic; no müllerian structures are found, presumably because of the secretion of müllerian duct inhibitory factor by the fetal Sertoli cells. In some patients in whom wolffian duct derivatives are hypoplastic, slight clitoromegaly and virilization occurs at puberty, as does the appearance of pubic and axillary hair and feminization (breast development and

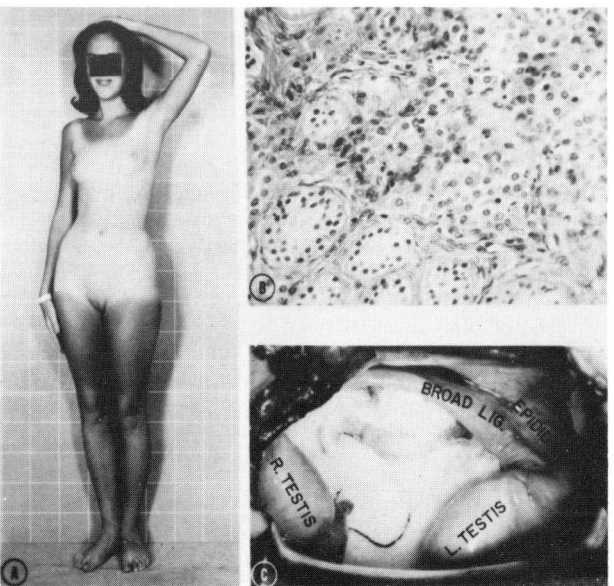

COMPLETE FORM OF SYNDROME

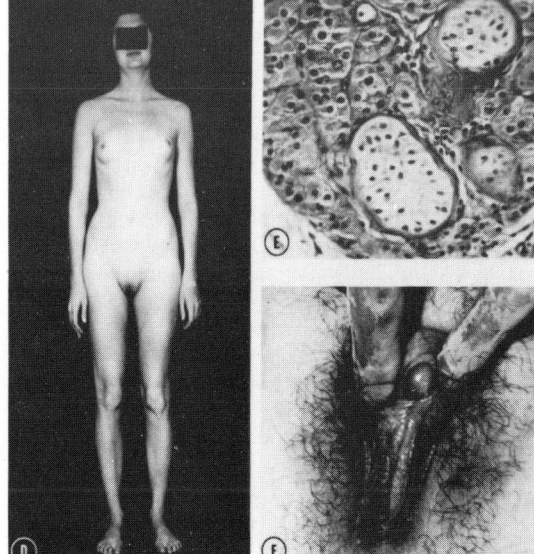

VARIANT FORM OF SYNDROME

Figure 9–50. The complete syndrome of androgen insensitivity and its variant form. *A*, Seventeen-year-old patient with the complete syndrome. The phenotypic female is chromatin negative, has a 46,XY karyotype, and has total absence of sexual hair with female secondary sexual characteristics. A small vagina ended blindly. *B*, The testes exhibited Leydig cell hyperplasia and the seminiferous tubules lacked germinal elements. *C*, At laparotomy abdominal testes, rudimentary wolffian structures and no müllerian structures were found. *D*, The variant form of the syndrome in a 25-year-old female. Sexual hair is present though sparse. *E*, The testes exhibit Leydig cell hyperplasia. *F*, The clitoris is hypertrophied but there is no labial fusion. A shallow vagina ended blindly. At laparotomy, hypoplastic wolffian structures and absent müllerian structures were found.

a female habitus) (393). We prefer to classify these patients as a variant form of complete testicular feminization. Intelligence is normal; there are no associated clinical anomalies. Gender identity is that of a normal female with strong maternal instincts. Estimates of prevalence vary from 1:20,000 to 1:64,000 male births.

Pathophysiology and Hormonal Profile (Fig. 9–51). *The Androgen Receptor.* Our understanding of the pathogenesis of this syndrome has advanced rapidly over the past few years. In 1950, Wilkins first suggested that failure of androgenization of the male fetus and the development of female rather than male secondary sex characteristics at puberty could be explained by end-organ unresponsiveness to androgen. Further studies by subsequent workers supported this contention by failing to demonstrate a clinical or metabolic response to testosterone administration in patients with the complete form of this syndrome (394). This X-linked disorder has been described in several mammalian species including the mouse, rat, bull, and chimpanzee (395).

Studies in two animal models, the tfm/y mouse and rat by Bardin et al. (395), Gehring, Tompkins and Ohno (396), and Goldstein (397) et al. first indicated that the primary defect was a deficient number of cytosol androgen receptors for dihydrotestosterone (DHT) and testosterone. Soon thereafter, Keenan and Migeon et al. reported an undetectable or low amount of cytosol androgen receptors by demonstrating absent or diminished high affinity DHT binding sites in cultured fibroblasts from the genital skin of patients with this disorder (398). They provided definitive evidence of its transmission as an X-linked recessive trait (35).

Subsequent studies from Migeon's laboratory and others indicated that genetic heterogeneity in the defect exists within the group of patients with complete androgen insensitivity (399, 400). Cytosol and nuclear binding of DHT was found to be entirely normal in a second group of patients with the phenotype of complete androgen insensitivity (399, 400). These receptor-positive patients presumably represent an as yet undefined post-receptor defect or a subtle qualitative abnormality in the androgen receptor itself (401). In receptor-positive patients with clinically complete androgen resistance syndrome who have been studied, the affinity of the receptor for androgen (402) and the capacity of the receptor complex to translocate from the cytoplasm to the nucleus appeared normal (403).

Griffin recently described a third mutant form characterized by a qualitatively abnormal androgen receptor in patients with complete androgen insensitivity (404). The clinical features in this group of patients were heterogenous in that they manifested the complete or the variant form of complete androgen insensitivity. The amount of androgen receptor was about half normal at 37°C and decreased further at 42°C. The thermolability indicated a structural abnormality that results in an unstable androgen receptor. Pinsky et al. have reported a similar receptor abnormality in two patients with complete androgen insensitivity (405).

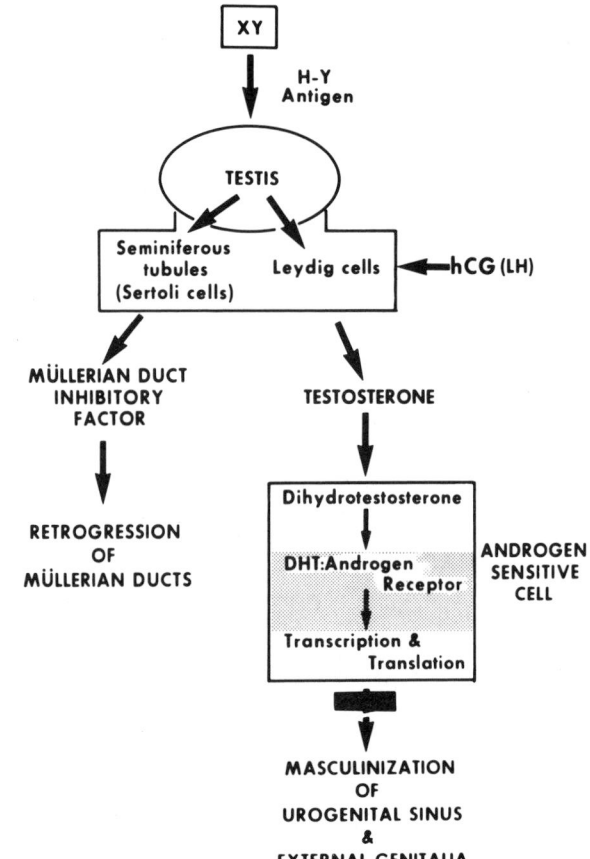

Figure 9–51. Diagrammatic scheme of male pseudohermaphrodism due to complete or incomplete androgen insensitivity.

Thus, in the complete form of androgen insensitivity, two definite abnormalities in the androgen receptor have been defined: 1) an undectable or low amount of androgen receptor and 2) an unstable androgen receptor. A third group of patients are receptor positive and may represent a post-receptor abnormality (Table 9–26).

In patients with the variant form of complete androgen insensitivity two types of molecular abnormalities have been defined: 1) an intermediate amount of androgen receptor and 2) an unstable androgen receptor.

The heterogeneity of molecular defects leading to complete androgen insensitivity is similar to the phenotypes described by Tompkins in dexamethasone-resistant clones of S-19 mouse lymphoma cells. He described various types of defects including: 1) a variant in which the receptor was absent or an abnormality in binding was present; 2) a nuclear transfer-deficiency type; and 3) a variant in which cytosol and nuclear binding were normal but no response to dexamethasone was elicited. Types 1 and 3 are similar to

Table 9–26. ANDROGEN RECEPTOR STUDIES IN ANDROGEN INSENSITIVITY SYNDROMES

Disorder	Level of Quality of Androgen Receptor
Complete androgen insensitivity and its variants	1) Receptor negative or low, or 2) Structurally abnormal receptor (thermolabile), or 3) Receptor positive
Incomplete androgen insensitivity and its variants	1) Partial deficiency of receptors, or 2) Receptor positive
Infertile men	1) Partial deficiency of receptor

the abnormalities in the androgen receptor in complete androgen insensitivity. One may anticipate the discovery of new defects in the mechanism of action of androgens in the testicular feminization syndrome, either at the level of the receptor, the level of activation, or a post-receptor defect in the "final response."

Hormone Profile. Hormonal studies in post-pubertal patients with complete androgen insensitivity indicate that plasma testosterone levels as well as testosterone production rates are higher than those of normal men (388, 406). This results from the increased concentration of plasma LH, apparently due to the lack of normal sensitivity of the hypothalamic-pituitary unit to feedback inhibition by testosterone. The concentrations of plasma estradiol and the estradiol production rates are higher than in normal men (407). The estradiol arises from peripheral conversion of testosterone and androstenedione and by direct secretion of estradiol by the testes (407, 408). The concentration of plasma FSH has been variable; it may be normal or slightly elevated (408–410). Thus, androgen insensitivity in the hypothalamic-pituitary apparatus leads to elevated LH levels, which in turn increase androgen and estrogen production. As long as the testes remain *in situ,* LH concentrations fail to reach the high levels found after castration, since the hypothalamic-pituitary unit is sensitive to estrogen.

Androgen insensitivity during embryogenesis blocks stabilization of the wolffian ducts and masculinization of the external genitalia. Secretion of müllerian duct inhibitory factor by the fetal Sertoli cells leads to involution of the müllerian ducts. At puberty, androgen insensitivity results in augmented LH secretion and elevated levels of testosterone and estradiol. Androgen insensitivity coupled with increased estradiol production induces the development of female secondary sex characteristics at the expected age of puberty.

Diagnosis. The diagnosis of complete androgen insensitivity (testicular feminization) can be established by clinical criteria alone in the post-pubertal patient and can be strongly suspected in the prepubertal individual. The patients may present with an inguinal hernia or labial mass, primary amenorrhea despite female secondary sex characteristics, and a history of an affected sister, aunt or cousin. A phenotypic female with primary amenorrhea, breast development, scant or absent pubic and axillary hair, a shallow vagina and absent cervix on gynecologic examination, and an X chromatin-negative chromatin pattern on buccal smear (or an XY karyotype) has the complete form of androgen-insensitivity. Similarly, the detection of an XY karyotype or X chromatin-negative pattern in a female infant or child with an inguinal or labial testes-like mass suggests the diagnosis. Absence of the uterus can be confirmed by sonography. Prepubertally, the differential diagnosis includes defects in testosterone biosynthesis and 5α-reductase deficiency. In the prepubertal patient, the family history, phenotype, endocrine evaluation including the androgen response to hCG and ACTH, the determination of androgen cytosol receptor activity, and, if necessary, the metabolic response to testosterone are used to establish the diagnosis.

XX females heterozygous for the androgen receptor-deficient form of complete androgen insensitivity are ascertainable by receptor analysis of fibroblast clones derived from genital skin (35). Theoretically, affected 46,XY fetuses could be detected by DHT receptor studies on cells from amniotic fluid.

Treatment. Therapy in patients with complete androgen insensitivity includes affirmation and reinforcement of their female phenotype and gender identity. Prepubertal

orchidectomy is indicated when the testes of patients with complete androgen insensitivity are located in the inguinal region or the labia majora and are associated with a hernia. Otherwise, we usually defer castration until late adolescence to allow the patient to undergo spontaneous feminization at puberty and follow the size of intra-abdominal testes by periodic sonograms of the pelvis. Patients with the variant form of complete androgen insensitivity (with clitoromegaly and/or posterior fusion) may exhibit mild virilization as well as feminization at puberty; in these patients, it is prudent to remove the testes prepubertally. If the testes are removed, estrogen substitution is necessary to promote secondary sex characteristics at the expected age of puberty (see p. 460). The vagina may be adequate in length for sexual intercourse, but in patients with a short vaginal pouch, manual dilatation with a prosthesis is effective in adolescence.

Incomplete Syndrome of Androgen Insensitivity and Its Variants (Reifenstein Syndrome)

A heterogenous group of incomplete or partially androgen-insensitive XY individuals has been described (388, 401, 411) (Table 9–27). The external genitalia are predominantly male or ambiguous. The pedigree analysis is consistent with an X-linked recessive trait. The patients described in the past by Lubs, Gilbert-Dreyfus, Reifenstein, Rosewater, Walker, and their associates quite likely represent variant forms of incomplete androgen insensitivity (388, 412). The variability in the degree of masculinization of affected males within and between kinships is well illustrated by the studies from Wilson's laboratory (413, 414). In a family studied by Wilson, 11 males were affected; two had a relatively mild defect in masculinization of the external genitalia (small penis and bifid scrotum), eight had perineal hypospadias, and one affected male had hypospadias, a urogenital sinus with a blind vaginal pouch, and absent vas deferens. All lacked müllerian structures. In contrast, in the complete form of testicular feminization within families there is little variability in the expression of the mutant gene. The most common presentation in infancy is an apparent male with a third-degree hypospadias (the urethral orifice is located at the base of the phallus), a small penis,

Table 9–27. SALIENT FEATURES OF INCOMPLETE ANDROGEN INSENSITIVITY

Karyotype: 46,XY

Inheritance: X-linked recessive

External genitalia: Ambiguous with blind vaginal pouch
→ hypoplastic male → normal male with infertility

Wolffian duct derivatives: Rudimentary → hypoplastic → normal

Müllerian duct derivatives: Absent

Gonads: Testes

Habitus: ↓ to normal axillary and pubic hair, beard growth and body hair; gynecomastia common at puberty

Hormone profile: ↑ plasma LH and testosterone concentrations; ↑ estradiol (for men); FSH levels may be normal
Partial resistance to the androgenic and metabolic effects of testosterone
Androgen receptor studies: Genetic heterogeneity:
  a) Partial deficiency of normal receptor
  b) Receptor-positive form (? abnormal receptor or post-receptor defect)

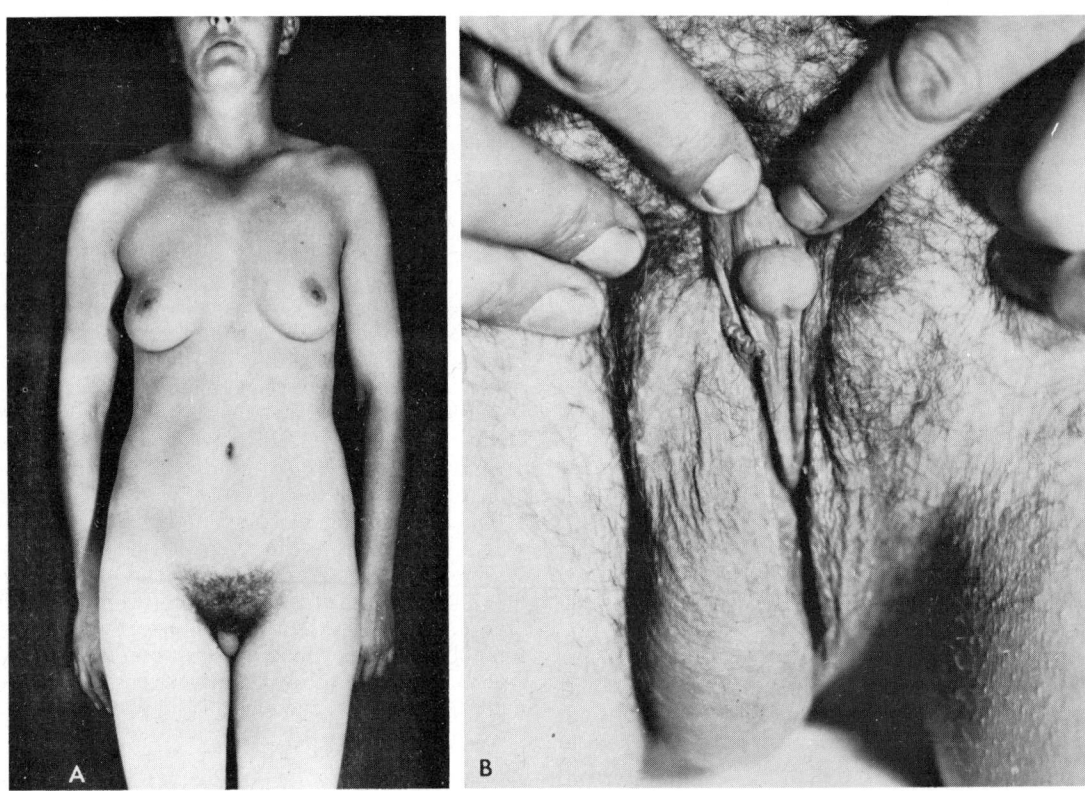

Figure 9–52.   Patient with incomplete androgen insensitivity (Reifenstein syndrome). Both the patient and his brother had hypospadias, poor masculinization and marked gynecomastia. Both he and his brother had a normal 46,XY karyotype, normal wolffian duct derivatives and no müllerian structures. (From
Bowen, P., et al.:[413] Courtesy of Dr. E. C. Reifenstein, Jr.)

and frequently cryptorchidism. Müllerian duct derivatives are absent; in some patients wolffian duct derivatives are present but usually hypoplastic. At puberty, pubic and axillary hair as well as gynecomastia usually appear, male secondary sex characteristics are poorly developed, the testes remain small and exhibit azoospermia due to germinal cell arrest beyond the primary stage. Similar to other patients with androgen insensitivity, the concentrations of plasma LH and testosterone are elevated, whereas in most cases the FSH level is normal; the high LH concentrations are resistant to suppression by exogenous testosterone. Estradiol and testosterone secretion rates are increased. However, the degree of feminization at puberty despite the elevated estradiol secretion is less than in the complete form of androgen insensitivity (Fig. 9–52).

Although a single biochemical defect has been suspected as an explanation for the clinical findings in these disorders, it was not until the reports from Wilson's and Migeon's laboratories that the pathogenesis was clarified (414–416). Studies of dihydrotestosterone binding by cultured fibroblasts from genital skin have shown two patterns: 1) Some patients have reduced high affinity binding of dihydrotestosterone to the cytosol androgen receptor, a quantitative or partial deficiency of the androgen receptor; 2) Other familial and sporadic cases had receptor positive androgen resistance; skin fibroblasts from these patients showed high affinity cytosol and nuclear binding of dihydrotestosterone (389, 416, 417). Only one of the two patterns occurred within an affected family. In neither of the two genetic variants was a qualitative defect in the receptor demonstrated. As in the androgen receptor-positive form of complete testicular feminization, the molecular defect in the receptor-positive patients with incomplete androgen insensitivity is uncertain. However, the receptor-positive cases may represent a subtle qualitative abnormality in the androgen receptor in which the activated steroid-receptor complexes bind to nuclear chromatin ("acceptor sites") but fail to elicit the events subsequent to nuclear binding that mediate the cellular response to androgen. Alternatively, the defect could be the result of a post-receptor abnormality such as in transcription of the DNA into RNA, in the levels of steroid regulated specific messenger RNA's, or in the processes of RNA translation. Future studies, no doubt, will bring to light new genetic defects in the action of androgen on target cells.

There are fundamental gaps in our knowledge of the mechanism of androgen action. As yet undefined cellular factors, apart from receptors, may influence the response of the target tissues to androgen. This is well illustrated by the wide variation in phenotype in patients with incomplete androgen insensitivity, by the lack of correlation of the severity of the defect in masculinization of the external genitalia, with the magnitude of the receptor abnormality *in vitro,* and by the variation in androgen insensitivity within different target tissues in the same patient (the hypothalamic-pituitary-gonadotropin complex versus the external genitalia).

Androgen Insensitivity in Infertile Men

Aiman et al. recently described a new and specific cause of infertility in three unrelated men with uninformative family histories as a consequence of a partial deficiency of the androgen receptor (389, 411). Two of the men had a normal adult male phenotype; one had slight gynecomastia, decreased body hair, and a modest reduction in testicular size. All were infertile and had severe oligospermia or azoospermia. The striking hormonal findings were elevated serum concentrations of testosterone in the presence of elevated to normal LH levels. Two of the three men had increased plasma production for testosterone, androstenedione, and estradiol. The decreased high-affinity cytosol binding capacity for dihydrotestosterone in genital skin fibroblasts was consistent with a partial deficiency of the androgen receptor. These observations strongly suggest that infertility in otherwise normal men may be the only clinical manifestation of incomplete androgen insensitivity and represents one end of the highly variable phenotypic expression of androgen insensitivity in patients with a comparable deficiency in androgen receptors by *in vitro* studies. High intratesticular concentrations of testosterone are required for normal spermatogenesis; thus, the infertility in these patients is quite likely a consequence of the androgen insensitivity, since testosterone levels were not decreased in these patients. Although the pattern of inheritance is uncertain, indirect evidence suggests that an X-linked recessive trait is the most likely mode. The prevalence of this new cause of male infertility is not known but screening infertile men for increased plasma concentrations of testosterone and LH or a high testosterone × LH product promises to shed light on this question.

Diagnosis. The diagnosis of incomplete or partial androgen insensitivity cannot be made from the phenotype alone. Errors in testosterone biosynthesis can result in an XY patient with a hypoplastic, hypospadiac phallus, incomplete fusion of the labioscrotal folds, a blind vaginal pouch, and gynecomastia at puberty. However, the pattern of inheritance and measurement of plasma LH, and of testosterone and its precursors before and after the administration of hCG, will serve to distinguish patients with androgen insensitivity. Studies of cytosol and nuclear binding of DHT in cultured fibroblasts from genital skin may show either a partial deficiency of androgen receptors or a normal number of androgen receptors. The demonstration of a poor or absent metabolic and clinical response to testosterone can serve as a useful adjuvant in the diagnosis of partial androgen resistance.

There is no specific therapy for partial androgen resistance. Sex of rearing is dependent on age at diagnosis and degree of genital ambiguity. In view of the limited response to testosterone in patients with this condition and the gynecomastia which is apparent at puberty, it may be prudent to raise all patients with this syndrome who have ambiguous genitalia as females. In patients assigned a female gender identity, plastic repair of the genitalia and gonadectomy are indicated before 6 months of age. Estrogen substitution therapy at puberty is required.

Defects in Testosterone Metabolism by Peripheral Tissues

5α-Reductase Deficiency; Male Pseudohermaphrodism with Normal Virilization at Puberty (Familial Perineal Hypospadias with Ambiguous Development of Urogenital Sinus and Male Puberty; Pseudovaginal Perineoscrotal Hypospadias)

Nowakowski and Lenz described in 1961 a familial type of male pseudohermaphrodism, which they termed "pseudovaginal perineoscrotal hypospadias" and which was transmitted as an autosomal recessive trait (418). These patients resemble those with other forms of male pseudohermaphrodism by having an XY karyotype, normally differentiated testes, male internal ducts, and ambiguous external genitalia. At puberty striking but selective signs of masculinization appear.

In 1974, Walsh et al. (419) and Imperato-McGinley and

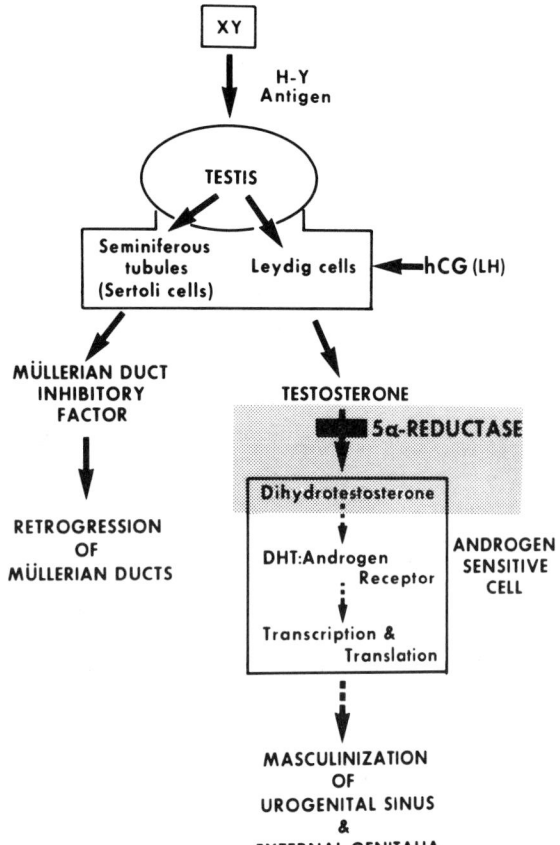

Figure 9-53. Diagrammatic scheme of male pseudohermaphrodism due to 5α reductase deficiency.

Table 9-28. SALIENT FEATURES OF 5α-REDUCTASE DEFICIENCY

Karyotype: 46,XY

Inheritance: Autosomal recessive

Genitalia: Usually ambiguous with small, hypospadiac phallus; blind vaginal pouch

Wolffian duct derivatives: Normal

Müllerian duct derivatives: Absent

Gonads: Normal testes

Habitus: Virilization at puberty without gynecomastia; ↓ facial and body hair, no temporal hair recession; prostate not palpable

Hormone profile: ↓ ratio of 5α/5βC$_{21}$ and C$_{19}$ steroids in urine; ↑ plasma T/DHT ratio before and after hCG stimulation; modest ↑ plasma LH ↓ conversion of T → DHT *in vivo*

Genetic heterogeneity of 5 α-reductase deficiency:
a) Severe 5α-reductase deficiency — defective binding of T
b) Unstable 5α-reductase — intermediate activity with decreased affinity of enzyme for cofactor NADPH
c) Unstable 5α-reductase with decreased affinity for substrate (T) and cofactor

Peterson et al. (420–422) reported a defect in the conversion of testosterone to its 5α-reduced metabolite dihydrotestosterone in patients with this syndrome (Fig. 9–53). Imperato-McGinley and Peterson described studies in a genetic isolate from villages in the southwestern part of the Dominican Republic. In 24 families, 33 male pseudohermaphrodites were identified, 24 of whom were postpubertal (422) (Table 9–28). The typical features of this form of male pseudohermaphrodism in infancy include a clitoris-like, hypospadiac phallus bound in chordee of variable degree, a bifid scrotum,

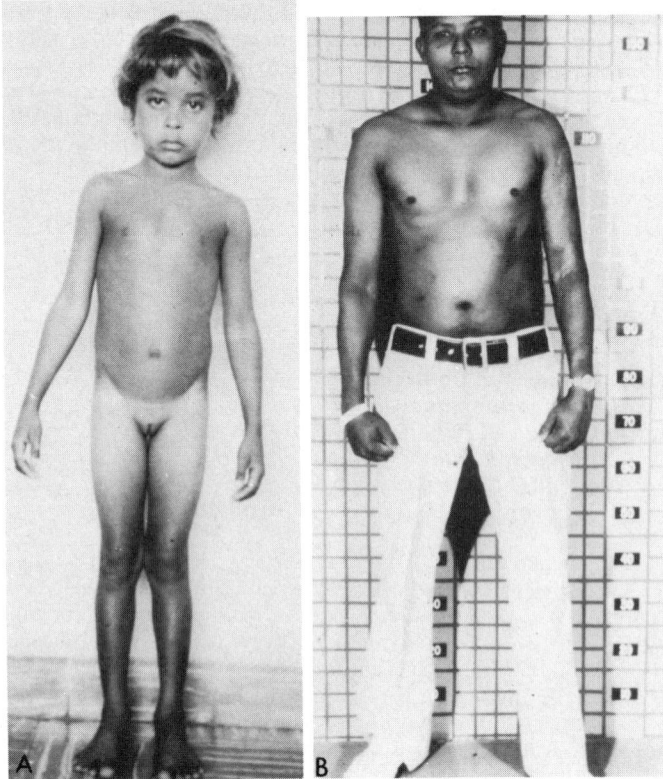

Figure 9-54. *A*, Prepubertal XY child with 5α reductase deficiency raised as a female. *B*, Post-pubertal male with 5α reductase deficiency who has virilized and changed gender identity. (From Peterson, R. E., et al.[422])

and a urogenital sinus which opens on the perineum. The blind vaginal pouch opens either into the urogenital sinus or into the urethra. The testes are well differentiated and are located either in the inguinal canal or the labioscrotal folds. No müllerian structures are present. The wolffian structures (epididymis, vas deferens, and seminal vesicle) are well differentiated; the ejaculatory ducts usually terminate in the blind vaginal pouch. At puberty, plasma testosterone increases into the adult male range while dihydrotestosterone levels remain quite low. Affected males virilize without gynecomastia: the voice deepens, muscle mass increases, and the phallus, although bound in chordee of variable severity, enlarges to 4–8 cm in length. The bifid scrotum becomes rugated and pigmented, and the testes enlarge and descend into the labioscrotal folds. However, none of the postpubertal affected males exhibited acne, more than sparse facial or body hair, temporal hair recession, or enlargment of the prostate. Semen analysis in one patient revealed 40 million sperm per ml, and testicular biopsy from another affected male exhibited complete spermatogenesis (422). One of the interesting aspects was the observation that although 18 of 38 affected male patients were raised "unambiguously" as females, 17 of these 18 changed to a male gender identity and 16 changed to a male gender role after the onset of puberty (128) (Fig. 9–54A, B).

The hormonal profile in these patients is consistent with defective 5α-reduction of testosterone to dihydrotestosterone in androgen target tissues (419). After the onset of puberty, the plasma testosterone levels are normal to elevated and the dihydrotestosterone levels significantly decreased in affected males (422, 423). The testosterone/dihydrotestosterone ratio in peripheral blood is increased to 35–84 in affected adult males in contrast to the normal male ratio of 8–16 (423). Prepubertally, because of the low levels of plasma androgens, the testosterone/dihydrotestosterone ratio may be normal in affected males under basal conditions (424); however, after hCG stimulation of testosterone secretion, an abnormal ratio can be readily demonstrated (424). Postpubertally, plasma LH concentrations are usually elevated and plasma FSH values tend to be higher than in age-matched controls (423). Thus, affected postpubertal males exhibit an important biochemical hallmark of peripheral androgen ineffectiveness — elevated plasma LH and testosterone values. Additional features of 5α-reductase deficiency are diminished ratios of urinary 5α-reduced to 5β-reduced C_{19} and C_{21} steroids and deficient or abnormal 5α-reductase activity in cultured fibroblasts from genital skin (the preferred source for in vitro studies) (423). The level of androgen receptor is normal. Adult females homozygous for the defect have no clinical manifestations (423). Heterozygotes for 5α-reductase deficiency have intermediate ratios of urinary 5α-reduced to 5β-reduced C_{19} steroids (e.g., androsterone/etiocholanolone) (423).

5α-reductase deficiency is inherited as an autosomal recessive trait and causes abnormal sex differentiation and other clinical manifestations only in males homozygous for the trait. The enzyme defect exhibits genetic heterogeneity. At present, three types of mutations that affect the 5α-reductase enzyme in this disorder have been described (389, 423, 425). In the first reports, including the families from the Dominican Republic, enzyme studies on genital biopsy specimens and fibroblast cultures derived from genital skin indicated a very low level of 5α-reductase activity due to an abnormality in the enzyme that affects its capacity to bind steroid substrate (e.g., testosterone) (423). More recently, a second type of defect, an alteration of the stability of the enzyme, has been described by Wilson and Griffin and by Imperato-McGinley and her associates in some affected families (389, 425, 426). In one kinship, 5α-reductase activity

was low in fresh biopsy specimens of genital skin but in the low normal range in cultured fibroblasts. The enzyme bound testosterone normally, but had a low affinity for the cofactor nicotinamide adenine dinucleotide phosphate (NADPH); as a consequence, the 5α-reductase was unstable and had a very rapid turnover. A variant 5α-reductase in another affected family had decreased affinity for both the substrate testosterone, and the cofactor NADPH; the activity and the stability of the enzyme were reduced in cultured fibroblasts.

The phenotype of patients with 5α-reductase deficiency supports the hypothesis that testosterone induces differentiation of the male ducts, while dihydrotestosterone causes male differentiation of the urogenital sinus, prostate, and external genitalia. Peterson has postulated that the increased muscle mass, deepening of the voice, spermatogenesis, and male sex drives seen at puberty in these patients are testosterone mediated, while acne, temporal hair recession, facial hair, and prostatic enlargement are dihydrotestosterone dependent (423). The growth of the phallus at puberty, despite the presence of severe 5α-reductase deficiency and incomplete masculinization of the external genitalia during fetal life, is not well explained. Since the dihydrotestosterone receptor also binds testosterone, but with a lower affinity, the sustained high levels of circulating testosterone attained at puberty may be a factor in the growth of the phallus. In addition, the enzyme defect is incomplete, and at puberty the plasma concentration of dihydrotestosterone, while low, is detectable; also, the hormonal environment is markedly different at puberty in that large quantities of competitive steroids, such as estrogen and progestins, are not present as they are in utero. These patients do not manifest gynecomastia at puberty; the production rate of estrogen is not increased.

Imperato-McGinley and Peterson et al. (128) have reported a provocative study of gender identity and gender identity transformation of the patients with 5α-reductase deficiency in the three rural villages in the southwestern part of the Dominican Republic. Among 38 affected individuals, 18 had been reared "unambiguously" as females. During or after puberty with the development of male secondary sex characteristics including phallic enlargement and increased muscle mass, 16 of 18 changed their assigned sex and sex of rearing from female to male, and 17 of 18 were assessed as having a male gender identity. Those who assumed a male gender role behaved as men. Despite the uniqueness of this genetic isolate and social setting, this study raises important questions about the relative influence and interaction of male sex hormones, sex of rearing, social conditions, and learning on psychosexual development. Although these observations are regarded by some as a serious challenge to the hypothesis of an early critical period of gender identity imprinting in infancy and early childhood, advanced by Money, Hampson, and Hampson (129), they are insufficient to warrant a revision of the recommendations for early sex assignment and the clinical management of infants and children with intersexuality.

Diagnosis. The diagnosis of 5α-reductase deficiency should be suspected in all prepubertal male pseudohermaphrodites with perineoscrotal hypospadias and a blind vaginal pouch, and male pseudohermaphrodites who virilize at puberty without evidence of gynecomastia. Virilization at puberty and the absence of gynecomastia in male pseudohermaphrodites is not unique to 5α-reductase deficiency. For example, 17-oxidoreductase deficiency and incomplete androgen insensitivity may present in this manner, but they can be distinguished biochemically from 5α-reductase deficiency. The diagnosis of 5α-reductase deficiency can be confirmed prepubertally as well as postpubertally by demonstrating an abnormally high testosterone/dihydrotestosterone ratio in peripheral blood before and following hCG administration (421, 426). The T/DT ratio under basal conditions in postpubertal affected males is 35 to 84, while the ratio in normal males is 8 to 16 (421). In infant males, when testosterone and dihydrotestosterone are detectable, the ratio of T/DHT ranges from 1.7 to 17 (mean 4.9 ± 2.85 SD) (424). In view of the low levels of testosterone and dihydrotestosterone in prepubertal males, the administration of hCG (1000–2000 units IM q 72 hours × 3) usually is necessary to demonstrate the defect. Affected patients with 5α-reductase deficiency have high T/DHT ratios after hCG. Following a course of hCG, the T/DHT ratio is 5.2 ± 1.5 SD in normal infant males (17 days–6 months) and 11 ± 4.4 SD in normal prepubertal males (6 months–14 years) (424). Similarly, the ratio of $5\alpha/5\beta$ metabolites of testosterone in urine is a marker both prepubertally and postpubertally of 5α-reductase deficiency (420, 421). An abnormal $5\alpha/5\beta$ C_{19} steroid ratio also occurs in hypothyroidism, Cushing syndrome, and acute intermittent porphyria (420, 421). Less available, but more direct studies which can be used to confirm the diagnosis include determination of the *in vitro* conversion of testosterone to dihydrotestosterone by genital skin fibroblasts (420, 421, 427) and of the blood production rate of dihydrotestosterone (428).

The early diagnosis of 5α-reductase deficiency is important because of its bearing on the assignment of sex in the affected infant. In view of the natural history of this syndrome, we recommend that these infants be reared as males and undergo appropriate plastic repair of their external genitalia. Testosterone or dihydrotestosterone therapy can be given to augment phallic size and to facilitate surgical repair. We believe that individuals who are diagnosed after infancy, in whom gender identity is unequivocally female, should have a prophylactic orchidectomy prior to puberty to prevent virilization, a clitoroplasty, and estrogen therapy at the age of puberty.

Dysgenetic Male Pseudohermaphrodism (Ambiguous Genitalia Due to Dysgenetic Gonads (429, 430)) (Fig. 9–55)

Ambiguous development of the genital ducts, urogenital sinus, and external genitalia as a consequence of defective testicular gonadogenesis occurs in patients with X chromatin-negative variants of the syndrome of gonadal dysgenesis, e.g., XO/XY mosaicism or certain structural abnormalities of the Y chromosome (see p. 465), and in patients with familial forms of XY gonadal dysgenesis (see p. 470). These disorders are classified as disorders of gonadal differentiation but are also included as a subgroup of male pseudohermaphrodism. Patients with faulty testicular differentiation are found with the clinical syndrome of male pseudohermaphrodism, and this must be considered in the differential diagnosis. We have used the designation "dysgenetic male pseudohermaphrodism," a term suggested by Federman, to describe this group of patients whose gonadal development is often asymmetric and on either side varies from a gonadal streak to a dysgenetic testis to a normal testis. The prevalence of malignant gonadal tumors in dysgenetic male pseudohermaphrodism is strikingly increased (p. 476).

Associated with Degenerative Renal Disease

Several cases are recorded of male pseudohermaphrodism associated with congenital or early onset renal disease

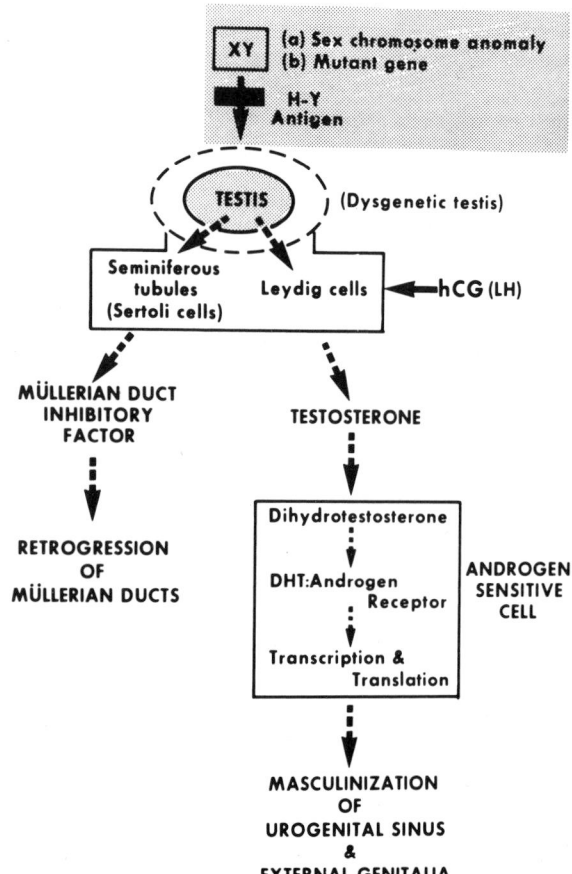

Figure 9–55. Diagrammatic representation of the pathogenesis of dysgenetic male pseudohermaphrodism. The scheme illustrates that this condition can result from a sex chromosome anomaly or from a mutant gene which affects the expression of H-Y antigen (H-Y negative) or the plasma membrane receptor for H-Y antigen (H-Y positive). The degree of masculinization is dependent upon the functional ability of the dysgenetic gonad to produce müllerian duct inhibitory factory and testosterone.

(chronic glomerulonephritis) and variably with a Wilms tumor (431–434). The association suggests a common developmental aberration during organogenesis of the testes and kidney of undetermined origin and multifactoral etiology.

The "Vanishing Testes Syndrome" (Embryonic Testicular Regression Syndrome; XY Agonadism; Rudimentary Testis Syndrome; Congenital Anorchia)

A variety of terms have been used to describe the spectrum of genital anomalies resulting from cessation of testicular function during the critical stages of male sexual differentiation, *i.e.*, 8–14 weeks' gestation. We first used the term "vanishing testes syndrome" to describe this heterogeneous group of male pseudohermaphrodites in 1957 because the genitalia in these cases suggested that the fetal testicular deficiency occurred and the testes "vanished" (for an obscure reason) before the completion of male sexual differentiation. These patients have an XY karyotype. Gonadal elements are absent and the differentiation of the genital ducts, urogenital sinus, and external genitalia is highly variable. At one end of the spectrum is the group of patients with female external and internal genitalia in whom the deficiency of embryonic testicular function presumably occurred before 8 weeks of gestation (435). Lack of function in fetal testes beginning between 8 and 10 weeks of gestation would lead to ambiguous genitalia and variable development of the genital ducts, from complete absence of both müllerian and wolffian ducts to partial development of either. This form of dysgenetic male pseudohermaphrodism has been referred to by some as the "XY gonadal agenesis syndrome" (436–438). Loss of testicular function occurring after the critical phase of male differentiation (14 weeks) results in "anorchia" — a syndrome characterized by the finding of normal male differentiation both internally and externally but no gonadal tissue. Unilateral and bilateral anorchia as well as familial cases, including monozygotic twins concordant and discordant for anorchia, have been described (439, 440, 441). Fetal testicular insufficiency and incomplete regression of the fetal testes between 11 and 14 weeks would be expected to produce a syndrome similar to that described by Bergada (442, 443), i.e., small rudimentary testes with microphallus and male ejaculatory ducts.

The nature of the underlying defect, which in some cases leads to absence or repression of genital ducts as well as testes, is not known. Several sibships with multiple affected individuals have been described. Josso et al. reported two siblings, one of whom was a normally differentiated male with a microphallus and anorchia (444). The other patient had an XY karyotype but was raised as a female. She had a clitoris which was not enlarged, fused labioscrotal folds, a single perineal opening that led into a urogenital sinus, and a vagina. At laparotomy, absent gonads with coexistent müllerian and wolffian structures were found. This patient's phenotype was compatible with a diagnosis of "XY gonadal agenesis." In spite of their "absent gonads," the patients had marked phenotypic differences in their internal and external genitalia. The coexistence of "XY gonadal agenesis" and "anorchia" in the same sibship suggests that both disorders are related and are due to embryonic testicular repression occurring at different stages of male development *in utero*; this also suggests the operation of a rare, single gene mutation in at least some cases of this syndrome.

The diagnosis of "anorchia" can be suspected in normally differentiated males with apparent cryptorchidism and elevated gonadotropins. This finding in conjunction with a failure of testosterone response to hCG (1000–2000 units I. M. q 72 hours × 3) assures the diagnosis and obviates the need for laparotomy.

Defects in Synthesis, Secretion, or Response to Müllerian Duct Inhibitory Factor

Persistent Müllerian Duct Syndrome (Female Ducts in Otherwise Normal Men — Uteri Herniae Inguinale)(Fig. 9–56)

More than 80 men and boys have been described with relatively well-developed testicular morphology and male external genitalia who possess well-developed müllerian structures in addition to their male ducts (445–447). The diagnosis is often unsuspected until the uterus and fallopian tubes prolapse through an inguinal hernia, or the problem is encountered in the course of abdominal surgery. The vasa deferentia are often attached to, or embedded in, the uterus; these structures, as well as the epididymis and the tunica albuginea of the testes, may exhibit developmental abnormalities. The retention of the müllerian structures can be attributed to the failure of the fetal Sertoli cells to synthesize and secrete müllerian duct inhibiting factor, a structurally abnormal inhibitory factor, or to a defect in the duct response to this factor. Unilateral or bilateral cryptorchidism is a common finding; in some patients the testes are hypo-

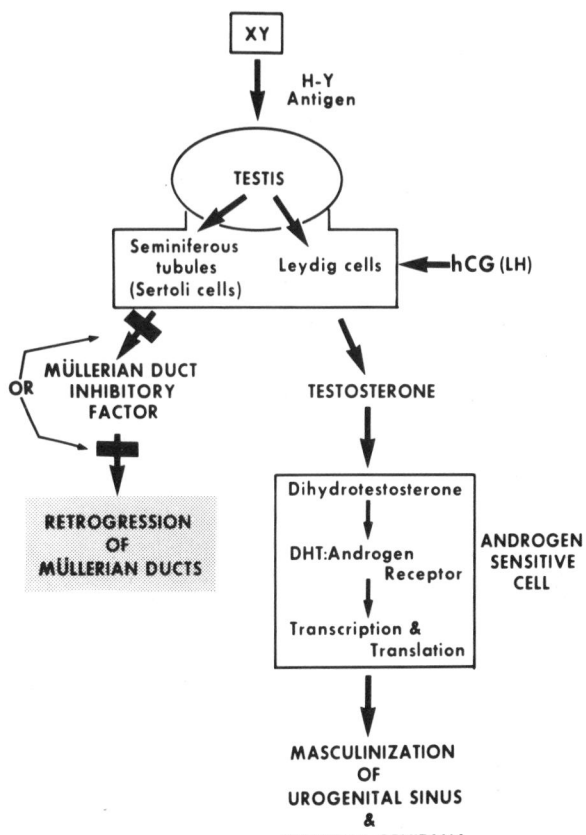

Figure 9–56. Diagrammatic representation of the pathogenesis of persistent müllerian duct syndrome.

plastic. These patients usually virilize well at adolescence, and fertile patients have been reported. The testes have a propensity to undergo malignant degeneration, and an increased prevalence of seminoma and other germ cell tumors has been reported (286). At least 10 sibships with affected brothers are known, including two studied by the authors. Pedigree analysis favors transmission as a sex-linked autosomal recessive trait; however, X-linked recessive inheritance and genetic heterogeneity have not been excluded (447).

Maternal Ingestion of Progestins and Estrogens

Progestins and synthetic estrogens alone and in combination have been implicated but not proven as a rare cause of male pseudohermaphrodism. Courrier and Jost in 1942 were the first to experimentally demonstrate an antiandrogen effect on the male fetus induced by a synthetic progestin, ethisterone (448). Newmann et al. observed that relatively high doses of progesterone or of synthetic progestins impaired urethral groove fusion in a low percentage of fetal male rats (105). Aarskog has reported 130 patients with hypospadias, studied retrospectively (449). A history of maternal ingestion of oral progestins in early pregnancy was obtained in 11 cases. In six cases the progestin was administered for threatened abortion and in five cases progestin in combination with estrogens was given as a pregnancy test

(449). Hypospadias occurred anywhere from the glans to the base of the penile shaft; the location correlated with the week in gestation that progestin therapy was initiated. Several other studies have suggested an association between progestins and hypospadias (450, 451).

Aarskog postulated that maternal progestins might inhibit testosterone synthesis by the fetal testes or the reduction of testosterone to dihydrotestosterone at the target tissue, and thus lead to failure of urethral groove fusion and hypospadias. Recent *in vitro* studies have shown that progestins can inhibit 5α-reductase activity (452). Inhibition of this enzymatic activity at an early fetal stage, through placental transfer of oral progestins given to the mother, for example, could result in impaired masculinization of the male external genitalia. Alternatively, progestins may bind to androgen receptors and block androgen expression.

Kaplan (453) has described male pseudohermaphrodism in a boy whose mother received large doses of diethylstilbestrol during early pregnancy.

Because of the report of Herbst (346) linking maternal diethylstilbestrol therapy during pregnancy with vaginal and cervical adenocarcinoma in daughters, abnormalities in the genital tract have been sought in sons (454, 455). An increased incidence of meatal stenosis, epididymal cysts, hypoplastic testes, and induration of the testicular capsule was observed in two studies, but hypospadias has not been reported. Thus the relationship between diethylstilbestrol administration during pregnancy and male pseudohermaphrodism is still to be confirmed.

Unclassified Forms of Abnormal Sexual Development

A significant advance in our understanding of male pseudohermaphrodism and its heterogeneity has occurred since the first edition of this book. The major subgroups are now defined, including recognition of enzyme defects in testosterone biosynthesis not associated with clinical abnormalities of adrenocortical functions. Nonetheless, there are forms of male pseudohermaphrodism that are not readily categorized and others in which the pathogenesis is obscure.

Sexual Abnormalities of Unknown Cause in Males

Hypospadias.   When hypospadias occurs as an isolated finding (about 1:700 newborn males), it is, by definition, a mild form of male pseudohermaphrodism; however, this is an impractical and unfortunate designation for those individuals who ultimately masculinize fully and achieve fertility. Although, on theoretical grounds, deficient virilization of the external genitalia implies subnormal Leydig cell function *in utero* or a mild degree of androgen insensitivity of the end organ, in most patients there are few grounds in adult life for suspecting either mechanism, and non-endocrine factors which affect differentiation of the primordia may be responsible for the anomaly. About 40 per cent of cases have associated anomalies of the urogenital tract; most of these are mild. Hypospadias as an isolated anomaly is occasionally observed in multiple members of families. Sörenson found familial occurrence in 38 per cent of cases and a concordance rate in twins of about 50 per cent (456). In addition, hypospadias is a feature of over 20 malformation syndromes (252, 447, 457).

Aarskog (458) has carried out a careful prospective study of 100 consecutive patients with hypospadias without other somatic anomalies, the majority of whom were referred from a plastic and reconstructive surgery clinic. No familial cases were encountered. One patient was a genetic female with congenital virilizing adrenal hyperplasia, five patients had sex chromosomal abnormalities (XO/XY or XX/XY), one had the incomplete form of XY gonadal dysgenesis, and nine were from pregnancies during which the mother had taken exogenous progestational compounds during the first trimester. Hence, in 15 per cent of these patients, a pathogenic mechanism was found or suspected.

Cryptorchidism.   Undescended testes, the commonest urogenital abnormality in malformation syndromes, is associated with over 40 such syndromes (457). Although normal testes may fail to descend into the scrotum because of coincidental anatomical abnormalities, in many instances cryptorchidism is due to a defective testis. Recent evidence indicates that fetal pituitary gonadotropin deficiency, either partial or complete, may play a role in cryptorchidism as well as microphallus (292, 459–461). Cryptorchidism and its management are considered in greater detail in Chapter 6.

Ambiguous Genitalia in XY Males with Multiple Anomalies.   Ambiguous genitalia are associated with several malformation syndromes including those associated with autosomal abnormalities (447, 457). In malformation syndromes such as the Aarskog and Opitz syndromes, the genital anomaly is of diagnostic significance (457).

Other reports of rare causes of male pseudohermaphrodism include that of a patient with a putative biologically inactive, but immunologically reactive LH (462). A group of familial cases in which a defect was postulated in fetal Leydig cell maturation with inadequate fetal testosterone production and impaired differentiation of germinal elements has also been reported (463). These patients had ambiguous genitalia at birth but normal virilization at puberty.

Sexual Abnormalities of Unknown Cause in Females

Absence of or Anomalous Development of the Vagina Associated with Variable Abnormalities of the Müllerian Structures.   Congenital absence of the vagina in association with abnormal or absent müllerian structures has been recognized as a syndrome for over 100 years (464–466) and is usually known as the Mayer-Rokitansky-Kustner-Hauser syndrome. Congenital absence of the vagina occurs in 1 in 5000 female births (464). It was the second most common cause of primary amenorrhea in a series of 538 patients reviewed by Ross and van de Wiele (467). The principal features of the syndrome are primary amenorrhea in XX females with well-developed female secondary sex characteristics, an absent or hypoplastic vagina, and müllerian derivatives that vary from a normal uterus to bicornuate cords to absence of the uterus. Ovarian function is usually normal and exhibits cyclic gonadotropin secretion with ovulation (468). The syndrome may be associated with renal, skeletal and other congenital anomalies (469). Clitoromegaly is not a feature of the Mayer-Rokitansky-Kustner-Hauser syndrome, which distinguishes it from the adrenal and non-adrenal forms of female pseudohermaphrodism; the positive X-chromatin pattern, XX karyotype, and plasma sex steroid values are some of the features that differentiate this disorder from testicular feminization.

Ultrasound scan and computerized tomography are useful for determining the presence of a uterus and its structure.

Hematocolpos is a preventable complication if surgical reconstruction is begun before puberty is advanced (470). Vaginal lubrication, orgasm, and marital relations have been reported to be satisfactory in adults who have had vaginal reconstruction (471).

MANAGEMENT OF PATIENTS EXHIBITING AMBISEXUAL DEVELOPMENT

Considerations Governing Choice of Sex for Rearing

With proper assignment of sex for rearing and appropriate subsequent management, individuals with ambiguities of their genitalia should be able to lead well-adjusted lives and ultimately attain the goal of a satisfactory sex life. To obtain this favorable result, it is incumbent upon the attending physician to make a correct diagnosis as early as possible and to reach a firm decision on the sex for rearing. We look upon the detection of genital ambiguity in a newborn infant as a neonatal, psychosocial emergency. Once the sex for rearing is assigned, the gender role is thereafter reinforced by the appropriate employment of whatever surgical, hormonal, and psychologic measures are indicated.

Deeply ingrained in our culture is the concept that some innate biologic difference between males and females is responsible for the behavioral differences between boys and girls as well as for the sexual orientation as adults. Studies of patients reared in a sex discordant with their chromosomal sex, gonadal sex, hormonal sex, and even external genital organs have clearly shown, however, that no one parameter can be used infallibly as a basis upon which to assign sex for rearing. This choice should therefore be governed principally by the possibilities that exist for achieving unambiguous and sexually useful genital structures.

The hormonal sex expected at maturity and the possibilities for fertility are of secondary importance except in cases of patients with female pseudohermaphrodism, in whom the abnormality is limited to a surgically correctable ambiguity of the external genitalia. Also, in affected males with 5α-reductase deficiency, the dramatic virilization which takes place at puberty and the reports of normal spermatogenesis support the assignment of a male sex of rearing as a rational and appropriate decision.

With the exception of female pseudohermaphrodites, males with 5α-reductase deficiency, and rare true hermaphrodites, ambiguities of the external genitalia are caused by lesions that invariably render the person sterile. Thus, the major consideration in these patients should be the possibility for achieving cosmetic and functionally normal external genitalia by surgical and endocrinological means. In considering a decision to recommend a male sex of rearing, it is our belief that greater emphasis should be directed to the size of the shaft and glans and to its potential for growth rather than to the degree of labioscrotal fusion. All phenotypic males with microphallus (penile length less than 2.5 cm at birth) should be given, after appropriate measures to exclude a sex anomaly, a trial of testosterone enanthate in oil, 25–50 mg IM monthly × 3 doses, to ascertain the potential of the phallus for further growth before a decision on sex of rearing is made (460). No significant increase in phallic length (mean response = 2.0 cm. ± 0.6 cm SD) suggests that the phallus lacks the capacity for growth in later childhood and at puberty, and raises for consideration a female sex assignment (472). Principles governing the differential diagnosis and the surgical, hormonal, and psychological management of patients with genital ambiguity are treated more extensively in the following sections.

Differential Diagnosis of Ambisexual Development in Infancy

Abnormalities of sex differentiation should be suspected not only in infants with grossly ambiguous genitalia but also in apparent females with inguinal masses, inguinal herniae, or slight clitoral enlargement. Apparent males with cryptorchidism, hypospadias, or unusually small genitalia or gonads likewise deserve close scrutiny. Sufficient investigation should be carried out in the newborn period to permit the assignment of sex with enough firmness to preclude future uncertainty. An accurate determination of the X chromatin pattern, or preferably karyotype analysis, is an imperative first step in all such newborns, since the presence of X chromatin bodies in the nuclei of oral mucosal cells or an XX karyotype should suggest the need for additional studies to determine whether or not female pseudohermaphrodism is present (Fig. 9–57).

Infants with X Chromatin-Positive Nuclear Pattern

All infants with sexual ambiguity and a positive X chromatin pattern should receive sufficient study in the neonatal period to differentiate the various forms of female pseudohermaphrodism from true hermaphrodism or variants of gonadal dysgenesis.

Congenital Adrenal Hyperplasia.   If female pseudohermaphrodism is secondary to congenital adrenal hyperplasia, the excretion of 17-KS should be elevated. During the first 4 weeks of life, the values of normal infants may be as high as 4 mg/24 hours. If the 17-KS values are equivocal, the finding of significant quantities of pregnanetriol (Ch. 00) may settle the diagnosis; however, the excretion of urinary pregnanetriol glucuronide usually is not increased during the first few weeks of life. Recently, a strikingly increased concentration of plasma 17-hydroxyprogesterone has been demonstrated in patients with defective 21 hydroxylation; values over 3000 ng/dl in an infant with ambiguous genitalia who is 24 hours of age or older are virtually diagnostic of the type I and II forms of congenital adrenal hyperplasia in infants who are not acutely ill from some other cause, such as sepsis. Any infant with ambiguous external genitalia who fails to thrive or who develops vomiting and dehydration during the first few weeks of life is highly suspect for the salt-losing type of adrenal hyperplasia. If such an infant is found to have hyperkalemia associated with acidosis and hyponatremia, the diagnosis is virtually assured, and vigorous therapy with glucocorticoids, salt, and mineralocorticoids should be instituted on an urgent basis to prevent collapse and sudden death. Once the diagnosis of adrenal hyperplasia is established, glucocorticoid therapy should be instituted and continued for life.

Other Forms of Female Pseudohermaphrodism.   X chromatin-positive infants may be presumed to have simple female pseudohermaphrodism if adrenal hyperplasia has been excluded and if there is a reliable history that the mother received androgens or progestational hormones during pregnancy, or if she developed some virilizing tendency. These children will require no further hormonal medication during childhood and will feminize normally at adolescence. The diagnosis of female pseudohermaphrodism can likewise be made with some confidence in X chromatin-positive infants if gross anomalies of the lower intestine or urinary tract are present. Such children should be studied for the presence of pyelonephritis and anomalies in other systems. Patients with female pseudohermaphrodism usually have a normal uterus and fallopian tubes with ovaries situated in the normal location. For this reason, the diagnosis should be

History: family history, pregnancy (hormones, virilization inspection)
Palpapation of inguinal region, labioscrotal folds & rectal examination
X chromatin pattern; karyotype analysis
Initial studies: Urinary 17-ketosteroids & pregnanetriol; plasma 17-hydroxyprogesterone
Serum electrolytes & urocytogram
Provisional Dx:

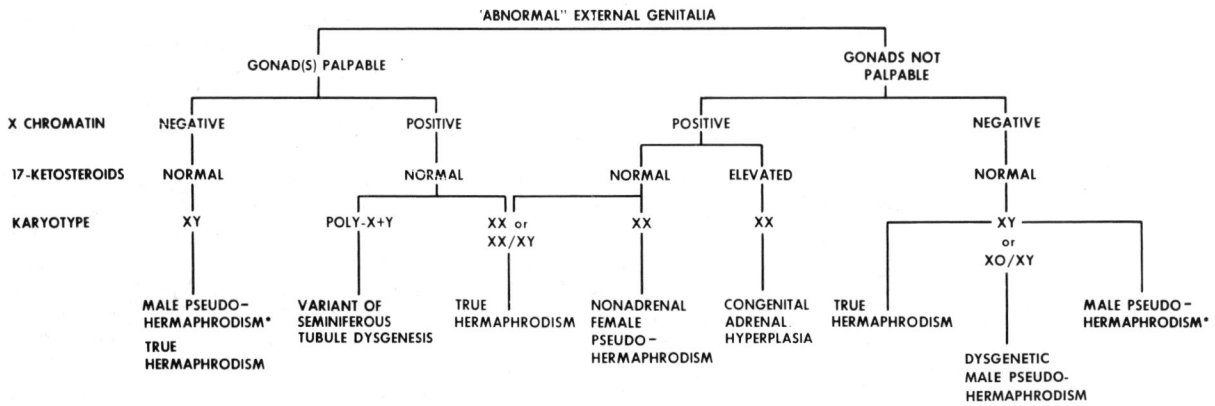

"Vaginogram" (urogenital sinogram): selected cases
    Endoscopy, laparotomy, gonadal biopsy: restricted to suspected male pseudohermaphrodites,
    true hermaphrodites, & selected instances of nonadrenal female pseudohermaphrodism

*17-ketosteroids are elevated in male pseudohermaphrodites with congenital
adrenal hyperplasia due to a defect in 3β-hydroxysteroid dehydrogenase

Figure 9–57.   Steps in the diagnosis of intersexuality in infancy and childhood. (Adapted from Grumbach, M. M., In *Pediatrics*. 13th ed. Holt, L. E., Jr., McIntosh, R., and Barnett, H. L. (eds.), New York, Appleton-Century-Crofts, 1962.)

viewed with suspicion if there is an inguinal hernia or if gonad-like masses are palpable in the groin. Such patients more frequently have testes. The presence of a uterus can often be detected in the newborn period by digital examination via the rectum. If there is uncertainty, an ultrasound scan of the pelvis is a useful procedure. It is often possible to confirm the presence of endometrial tissue by cytologic means after expressing mucoid secretions from a urogenital sinus by bimanual manipulation of the suspected uterus. Once the physiologic hyperplasia of the uterus, present at birth, has regressed, the interpretation of a rectal examination may be inconclusive.

True Hermaphrodism.   Seventy per cent of patients with true hermaphrodism are X chromatin positive, and it may be difficult to distinguish some of them from the rare idiopathic cases of female pseudohermaphrodism. True hermaphrodites, however, often have gonads located in their labia or inguinal canals; a bipartite gonad is highly suggestive of an ovotestes. In all of these cases, the assignment of sex should be deferred until the nature of the internal genital structures and gonads can be determined by sonography, urethroscopy, radiologic study with contrast media, and pelvic exploration, if necessary. Karyotype analysis is necessary for the detection of the patients with sex chromosome abnormalities. The assignment of sex to a true hermaphrodite should be based on the possibilities for surgical correction of the external genitalia. Not infrequently, the heterologous gonadal tissue can be removed. It is important to emphasize the risk of malignant degeneration of the dysgenetic testicular tissue that is retained. In general, assignment of a female sex and an attempt to preserve an ovary or ovarian tissue is the preferable approach.

X Chromatin-Positive Seminiferous Tubule Dysgenesis (Klinefelter's Syndrome).   A positive X chromatin pattern is found in approximately one of every 1000 newborn phenotypic males. Most of these infants will have an XXY karyotype and will not come to attention during infancy because their external genitalia exhibit normal male development and only rarely hypospadias.

Infants with X Chromatin-Negative Nuclear Pattern

A negative X chromatin pattern is found in all patients with male pseudohermaphrodism (by current definition), in approximately 80 per cent of those with the syndrome of gonadal dysgenesis, and in about 30 per cent of true hermaphrodites. In many of these patients, the phenotype will be so clearly male or female that the sex for rearing will not be in question. Nonetheless, efforts should be made, insofar as possible, to establish an etiologic diagnosis, since this may have an important bearing on subsequent management. A detailed family history with construction of a pedigree should not be neglected, since many sexual abnormalities are hereditary in nature, and this type of historical information is not readily volunteered. For example, a history of "aunts" who have never menstruated or of an inguinal hernia or labial mass in a phenotypic female may suggest the diagnosis of the androgen-insensitivity syndrome. The mother, likewise, should be queried about drugs or hormones that she may have received during the early part of pregnancy.

Studies during the newborn period should always include an examination of the karyotype. A sufficient number of metaphase plates should be examined to reduce the possibility of overlooking mosaicism. The morphology of the Y chromosome should be examined with the Giemsa and quinacrine-banding techniques.

An ultrasound scan, roentgenologic studies of the urogenital sinus following the injection of contrast media from a syringe with a blunt tip so placed in the single perineal orifice as to prevent leakage of dye, and fiberoptic endoscopic examination aid in this initial evaluation. Laparotomy is usually not necessary during the neonatal period since, in choosing the sex for rearing, primary emphasis should be placed on the external genitalia and the possibilities for ultimately obtaining adequate sexual function. However, before recommending a sex assignment, the anatomical findings need to be assessed in the light of karyotype studies, the pattern of plasma sex steroids before and following hCG stimulation, and other measures to identify a specific type of male pseudohermaphrodism.

Urinary steroids as well as plasma androgens before and after ACTH and hCG (1000–2000 units IM q 72 hours × 3) should be determined in patients with male pseudohermaphrodism in order to ascertain whether the patient has a block in testosterone metabolism or 5α-reductase deficiency. The testosterone response to hCG may result in significant phallic enlargement. Thus, in addition to providing objective information on the functional capacity of the Leydig cells to respond to this stimulus and secrete testosterone, it may provide evidence for the capacity of androgen-sensitive target tissues to respond to this stimulus. In the patient with male pseudohermaphrodism with no evidence of a testosterone biosynthetic error, 5α-reductase deficiency, or dysgenetic male pseudohermaphrodism, clinical or metabolic evidence of testosterone responsiveness should be demonstrated before a sex assignment is made.

The problem of sex assignment in the male infant with a micropenis is particularly vexing. Males with congenital hypopituitarism frequently have diminished genitalia and unilateral or bilateral cryptorchidism, and this diagnosis should be excluded by appropriate pituitary function studies before considering the possibility of sex reassignment. It is our view that all male infants with microphallus should be given a trial administration of adequate doses of testosterone, parenterally, before concluding that the phallus lacks the capacity for growth. The administration of a dose of 25–50 mg of testosterone enanthate intramuscularly once a month for 3 months should provide an adequate androgen stimulus to make this assessment (460). This treatment may cause a slight advancement of the skeletal age, but this consideration is trivial when weighed against the momentous question of deciding the child's future sex of rearing.

In most patients a precise etiologic diagnosis and sex assignment can be made on the basis of the criteria stated above. In the rare patient in whom no evidence of defective testosterone synthesis, end organ unresponsiveness to androgen, or testicular dysgenesis can be found, true hermaphrodism should be considered. In these patients laparotomy and the demonstration of both ovarian and testicular tissue will establish the diagnosis.

Once the decision is made to rear the infant as a boy or girl, there should be no further indecision in the minds of either the physician or parents. It is nevertheless required in most patients to carry out surgical exploration to determine the structure of the internal genital ducts and gonads. This pelvic exploration can be deferred until such time that plastic procedures on the external genitalia are undertaken.

Reassignment of Sex after the Newborn Period

Frequently children are assigned a totally inappropriate sex because of errors in diagnosis or because of ignorance of the principles that should properly govern this choice. In such cases, the knotty decision to change the sex of rearing or to leave matters undisturbed is largely dependent upon the age of the child and the degree to which the gender role has been established. Money et al. (472) have shown that a change in the sex for rearing is feasible until the age of 1½ years and is sometimes successful until 2½ years, but thereafter, in our culture, serious and sometimes calamitous psychiatric and social consequences may be encountered. Although these concepts are now being challenged, change of sex after 18 months should be undertaken only after a painstaking review of possible alternatives and only if provision has been made for close supervision and long-term counseling of the patient, parents, and siblings.

After adolescence, the patient himself may reach the decision that he or she has been reared in the wrong sex and may request assistance in changing his or her sex of assignment. If there is sufficient anatomical grounds for this belief, the request should be seriously considered and honored if possible. Such patients may have serious psychiatric disturbances, and both psychiatric and legal counsel should be sought.

Reconstructive Surgery

Since the presence of ambiguous external genitalia is likely to reinforce doubt regarding the sexual identity of the infant or child, it is desirable to initiate reconstructive surgery as early as is medically and surgically feasible. Money's group (472) has stressed the importance of both early genital operation and psychological support for the family in ensuring a successful outcome. Thus, it is highly desirable that surgery on the external genitalia be initiated prior to 12 months of age, if not sooner. Certainly, in patients with non-adrenal forms of female pseudohermaphrodism and male pseudohermaphrodites assigned a female sex, genital reconstruction should be undertaken as soon as possible in the neonatal period.

The management of clitoromegaly in female pseudohermaphrodites and male pseudohermaphrodites being raised as females has been a controversial issue. Three different operative approaches have been recommended: clitorectomy (473), clitoral recession (474), and clitoroplasty (475–477). Recent observations on the role of the clitoris as an erotic organ in females (478) have made it clear that clitorectomy should be avoided if at all possible. We have recommended the clitoral recession procedure as introduced by Lattimer (474). Follow-up data in a group of 12 patients with clitoral recession indicated that 11 of 12 patients had good to excellent cosmetic results (320). Five out of five patients who admitted sexual experience reported normal erectile clitoral function and erotic sensation associated with stimulation of the clitoris. One patient developed painful enlargement of the clitoris, necessitating excision. Although "recession" seems a reasonable approach, clitoromegaly with painful erection may occur, especially in patients with androgen excess (479). "Clitoroplasty," as recommended by Allen (475) and Shaw (476), requires excision of the shaft and corpora with retention of the glands. Long-term data will be necessary to evaluate the efficacy of this procedure with respect to appearance and sexual function.

The extent of the initial repair of the urogenital sinus and vagina depends in large part on the skill and experience of the surgeon. Even in the most experienced hands it is not uncommon for patients who have had vaginoplasties performed at 1½ years or earlier to require secondary operations because of stenosis (479). We feel that reconstruction of a vagina in male pseudohermaphrodites reared as females can be deferred until adolescence or until requested by the patient. A small vaginal pouch can often be enlarged by daily manipulations with a suitable mold (480). Even if the vagina remains too shallow for satisfactory sexual relations, manual dilatations make it easier to carry out subsequent surgical correction.

A male with hypospadias will usually require multiple operations to create a phallic urethra. This is a major surgical undertaking and should not be regarded lightly (481). Circumcision should be avoided to preserve as much tissue as possible. Pelvic exploration can be undertaken (if necessary) simultaneously with the initial operation to correct chordee. It is often desirable to insert prosthetic testes to give the scrotum dependency and to improve cosmetic appearance. These may be changed to adult size prostheses in adolescence.

Removal of the Gonads

A high incidence of gonadal tumors in patients with certain forms of gonadal dysgenesis and various other forms of hermaphrodism makes it mandatory that an evaluation of this risk be given priority over other considerations in deciding if and when the gonads should be removed. Currently available information on the incidence of tumors in the various forms of gonadal dysgenesis is reviewed on p. 000. Although the incidence of gonadoblastomas and germinomas (seminoma or dysgerminoma) increases near the normal time of adolescence, a significant number of these tumors have been discovered during the first decade. As temporizing serves no useful purpose and may expose the child to hormone secretions inappropriate to the chosen sex for rearing, it is advisable to proceed with gonadectomy concurrently with the initial repair of the external genitalia in patients who are at risk. At present, we are evaluating the use of ultrasonic scan of the pelvis every one to two years to screen for a gonadal neoplasm in children at risk. Similarly, gonadectomy and removal of the uterus should be carried out as early as possible in the rare cases of female pseudohermaphrodism who have been mistakenly reared as boys and in whom change of sex is inadvisable.

Although Morris reported a 9 per cent incidence of gonadal tumors in his 1953 review of 85 cases of testicular feminization, it is quite possible that some of these patients who developed tumors actually had atypical forms of gonadal dysgenesis. The incidence of gonadal malignancy prior to 25 years appears to be relatively low. Although gonadectomy should ultimately be carried out in these patients, it is often desirable to leave the gonads *in situ* until after puberty, in the hope that testicular estrogens will bring about the development of normal feminine sexual characteristics. This greatly reinforces the patient's concept of her sexual identity, and castration to prevent malignancy is then more easily explained and readily accepted.

There is a high risk of some degree of virilization at the time of puberty in patients with the incomplete form of androgen insensitivity and with other forms of male pseudohermaphrodism in which a female sex for rearing has been assigned; castration in childhood is desirable. In other forms of male pseudohermaphrodism in which a male sex for rearing has been selected, it can be anticipated that at least partial development of male secondary sex characteristics will occur with the onset of puberty. Provided that the testes are not dysgenetic and are sufficiently descended to permit palpation, it is reasonable to leave the testes *in situ*. Such patients should be carefully examined at regular intervals for the presence of a tumor.

Hormonal Substitution Therapy

Hormonal substitution therapy in hypogonadal patients should be prescribed in such a way that secondary sexual characteristics emerge appropriately in both timing and sequence. The goal of therapy should be to approximate normal adolescent development as closely as possible.

In females, hormonal substitution therapy (including patients with the syndrome of gonadal dysgenesis) is initiated with low doses of estrogen (0.3 mg conjugated estrogens or 5 μg ethinyl estradiol) daily by mouth, for the first 21 days of the month. This therapy is continued for a period of time. Breast enlargement and growth of the uterus frequently occur within 3 months. Usually, cyclic therapy with estrogen and an oral progestin is begun after about 6 months of continuous estrogen therapy or sooner, if breakthrough bleeding occurs (see p. 460 for more detailed discussion).

More adequate virilization is usually obtained by repository injections of testosterone than by oral preparations. Methyltestosterone has the added disadvantage of predisposing to biliary stasis and jaundice and hepatic tumors. However, sudden virilization is often inadvisable, and it is preferable to bring about adolescent changes gradually over a period of many months in a manner similar to that in normal boys. Due regard should be given to the fact that the effect of sex steroids on skeletal maturation is dosage-related, whereas the effect on linear growth is less so. Thus, at the inception of therapy, the relation between attained stature and skeletal maturation as well as the dosage of androgen prescribed will determine the ultimate effect of this therapy on the adult height. An initial dose of 50 mg of testosterone enanthate or other long-acting testosterone ester, intramuscularly, may be given monthly, beginning at 12 to 13 years of age. Thereafter the dose should be gradually increased over 3–4 years to the adult replacement dose of 200 mg every two weeks.

Psychological Management

Few people are sufficiently sophisticated to accept a sex for rearing discordant with their chromosomal or gonadal sex. For this reason, it is advisable to avoid such a disclosure at the beginning and to present the issues in more readily comprehended terms. There should never be any doubt in the mind of parent or patient that a child is being reared in his or her own "true sex," although it is best to admit uncertainty regarding the "true sex," and urge the parents not to assign a surname or send out birth announcements until sufficient studies have been completed. This approach is completely honest if the physician himself fully recognizes that sex is not a single biologic entity with one decisive parameter but rather the net expression of many morphologic characteristics and functional potentialities. Thus, in the strictest sense, an infant's "true sex" is in fact the one to which he or she is assigned after these many factors have been thoroughly evaluated. A simple embryologic explanation of the double set of sexual organs present in early life is useful, since it lays the groundwork for the concept that sex differentiation is often not completed *in utero*. An analogy to other congenital malformations such as cleft lip or congenital heart disease is accurate and easily understood. The parents should be reassured that their child does not have a "reversed sex" nor is he "half boy and half girl." It should be clearly stated that the anatomical abnormalities in sexual development do not predispose to homosexual drives.

Children reared in an atmosphere in which their sex for rearing is accepted with conviction need not have catastrophic psychological problems. With proper surgical reconstruction and hormonal substitution, when required, most individuals with ambisexual development should reach adulthood as well-virilized men or as feminine women capable of achieving satisfactory sexual relationships, although usually infertile.

PRENATAL DIAGNOSIS OF ABNORMALITIES OF SEXUAL DIFFERENTIATION (AND ADRENAL FUNCTION) (TABLE 9–29)

With the advent of amniocentesis, antenatal monitoring and diagnosis of genetic disorders is now an integral part of perinatology. Abnormalities involving sex chromosome number and structure are readily amenable to diagnosis by karyotype analysis of banded chromosomes from amniotic fluid cells obtained as early as 14 to 16 weeks of gestation (482). Sex chromosome abnormalities are usually sporadic, and the prenatal diagnosis of these abnormalities usually results from accidental ascertainment for indications such as advanced maternal age.

The measurement of steroid hormones in amniotic fluid provides information about fetal steroidogenesis in the fetal testis as well as the fetal adrenal cortex. The plasma concentration of testosterone is higher in the male fetus during the second trimester of pregnancy (483), owing to the secretion of testosterone by the fetal testes. This sex difference is reflected as well in amniotic fluid testosterone values between 14 and 20 weeks of gestation (483). Attempts have been made to use the concentration of testosterone in amniotic fluid to "sex" the fetus. Even though the values differ according to sex (males 0–370 pg/ml, females 0–130 pg/ml at 14–20 weeks' gestation) there is a significant overlap, and in a few normal male fetuses testosterone was not detected in amniotic fluid (94). Thus, a low amniotic fluid testosterone concentration is not diagnostic either of a female fetus or of an abnormality in fetal Leydig cell function. A sex difference in the concentration of amniotic fluid FSH also has been reported (484). In male fetuses the concentration of FSH is usually less than 1 mIU/ml from 8–20 weeks, while in the female fetuses the values have ranged from 1–10 mIU/ml (484).

Amniotic fluid steroid values have been used to ascertain prenatally the 21-hydroxylase deficient form of congenital virilizing adrenal hyperplasia (485, 486). Amniotic fluid 17-hydroxyprogesterone and androstenedione concentrations were elevated in affected male and female fetuses in studies carried out between 14 and 20 weeks of gestation (94, 485, 486). Recently the gene for 21-hydroxylase has been shown to be closely linked to the HLA locus on the short arm of chromosome number six. Homozygous (affected), heterozygous (carriers) and fetuses lacking the mutant gene can be identified by HLA typing of amniotic fluid cells in pregnancies known to be at risk because of the previous birth of an affected child (314). The combined use of HLA typing, 17-hydroxyprogesterone and androstenedione concentrations in amniotic fluid permits the definitive prenatal diagnosis of 21-hydroxylase deficiency. Similarly, a fetus affected with 11 β-hydroxylase deficiency can be detected by measurement of 11-deoxycortisol in amniotic fluid (487, 488) or by the determination of 11-deoxycortisol and its metabolites in maternal plasma and urine. Theoretically, other forms of congenital adrenal hyperplasia, such as a 20, 22 desmolase complex deficiency, could be detected prenatally by finding low estriol values in maternal plasma and urine.

It is possible that the androgen receptor deficient forms of androgen insensitivity could be ascertained by assay of cytosol androgen receptor activity in cultured amniotic fluid cells, but this remains to be established. As significant

Table 9–29. PRENATAL DIAGNOSIS OF ABNORMALITIES OF SEXUAL DIFFERENTIATION

	Determination	Comments
Determination of fetal sex:	Karyotype analysis on cells in amniotic fluid.	
	Amniotic fluid { Males: High T, low FSH / Females: Low T, high FSH	Overlap between male and female fetuses, as well as low T in some normal male fetuses; fetal sexing by sonography, 100% accurate after 28 weeks of gestation. Karyotype analysis is the most accurate method
Sex chromosome disorders: (e.g., XO; XXY; XO/XY)	Karyotype analysis of amniotic fluid cells	
Congenital adrenal hyperplasia: a) 21 hydroxylase deficiency	Amniotic fluid concentrations of 170HP and $\triangle^4$ androstenedione are elevated between 14 and 20 weeks of gestation. HLA typing of amniotic fluid cells in an informative family can identify affected, heterozygous and normal fetus.	
b) 11 β-hydroxylase	Elevated value of 11-deoxycortisol and its metabolites in amniotic fluid and maternal plasma and urine.	No HLA linkage
Male pseudohermaphrodism: a) Androgen insensitivity	Karyotype analysis of amniotic fluid cells will identify males at risk. ? Androgen cytosol receptor analysis of amniotic fluid cell cultures. Ultrasonography and/or fetoscopy to confirm genital ambiguity	Androgen-receptor analysis of amniotic fluid cell cultures have not yet been reported. Further, the receptor-positive form of androgen insensitivity is not distinguishable from normal by androgen receptor studies
b) 5α-Reductase deficiency	Karyotype analysis will identify males at risk. ? In vitro determination of T to DHT conversion by amniotic fluid cell cultures. Ultrasonography and/or fetoscopy to confirm genital ambiguity.	DHT to T conversion by normal amniotic fluid cells has not yet been established
c) Enzymatic defects in testosterone biosynthesis	Karyotype analysis to identify XY males at risk	Amniotic fluid testosterone concentration overlap between male and female fetuses, as well as low T in some normal male fetuses; fetal sexing by sonography, 100% accurate after 28 weeks
d) Familial XY gonadal dysgenesis	Testosterone concentrations in amniotic fluid.	Serological tests for H-Y antigen using amniotic fluid cells have not been reported

quantities of dihydrotestosterone are not present in amniotic fluid, the absence of this steroid cannot be used to prenatally diagnose 5α-reductase deficiency. However, the analysis of the in vitro conversion of testosterone to dihydrotestrone by amniotic fluid cells might be useful for this purpose.

Direct visualization of the fetal genitalia by non-invasive as well as invasive techniques can aid in the diagnosis of abnormalities of sexual differentiation. Fetal sexing by ultrasonography is now possible with 100 per cent accuracy after 28 weeks of gestation (489). Direct fetoscopy before 20 weeks has been used to exclude various developmental disorders characterized by morphological abnormalities and also to sample fetal blood and skin. However, at present, fetoscopy is limited by the state of the art. With advances in instrumentation, fetoscopy may become more useful for the identification of an abnormality in the development of the fetal genitalia before 20 weeks of gestation.

Estriol concentrations in maternal plasma and its secretion in urine reflect the functional integrity of the fetal adrenal and the placenta. Disorders of fetal hypothalamic-pituitary-adrenal function can lead to low maternal estriol values in the plasma and urine (490). These abnormalities include anencephaly, hypothalamic hypopituitarism, pituitary aplasia, some forms of congenital adrenal hyperplasia (e.g., 20, 22 desmolase complex deficiency), familial unre-

sponsiveness to ACTH, and congenital adrenal hypoplasia. Low estriol values in urine are also found prenatally in affected male fetuses with X-linked steroid sulfatase deficiency, an enzyme defect associated with ichthyosis (491).

REFERENCES

1. Hamerton, J. L.: *Human Cytogenetics, General Cytogenetics*, Vol. 1. New York, Academic Press, 1971.
2. Hamerton, J. L.: *Human Cytogenetics, Clinical Cytogenetics.* Vol. 2. New York, Academic Press, 1971.
3. Jirásek, J. E.: *Development of the Genital System and Male Pseudohermaphrodism.* Baltimore, Johns Hopkins Press, 1971.
4. McKusick, V. A.: *Mendelian Inheritance in Man.* 5th ed. Baltimore, Johns Hopkins Press, 1978.
5. Money, J., and Ehrhardt, A. A.: *Man and Woman, Boy and Girl: The Differentiation and Dimorphism of Gender Identity from Conception to Maturity.* Baltimore, Johns Hopkins Press, 1972.
6. Moore, K. L.: *The Sex Chromatin.* Philadelphia, W. B. Saunders Co., 1966.
7. Ohno, S.: *Sex Chromosomes and Sex-linked Genes.* Berlin, Springer-Verlag, 1967.
8. Ohno, S.: *Major Sex Determining Genes.* Berlin, Springer-Verlag, 1979.
9. Overzier, C. (ed.): *Intersexuality.* New York, Academic Press, 1963.
10. Peters, H., and McNatty, K. P.: *The Ovary.* Berkeley, University of California Press, 1980.
11. Rimoin, D. L., and Schimke, R. N.: *Genetic Disorders of the Endocrine Glands.* St. Louis, C. V. Mosby Co., 1971.

12. Simpson, J. L.: *Disorders of Sexual Differentiation:* Etiology and Clinical Delineation. New York, Academic Press, 1976.
13. Vallet, H. L., and Porter, I. H. (eds.): *Symposium on Genetic Mechanisms of Sexual Development.* New York, Academic Press, 1979.
14. Hamerton J. L., et al. (ed.), Paris Conference (1971): Standardization in human cytogenetics. *Birth Defects: Orig. Art. Ser., 8*(7), 1973.
15. Grumbach, M. M., et al.: Human sex chromosome abnormalities in relation to DNA replication and heterochromatinization. *Proc. Natl. Acad. Sci. 49*:581, 1963.
16. Morishima, A., et al.: Asynchronous duplication of human chromosomes and the origin of sex chromatin. *Proc. Natl. Acad. Sci. 48*:756, 1962.
17. Latt, S. A.: Patterns of late replication in human X chromosomes. *In Genetic Mechanisms of Sexual Development.* Vallet, H. L., and Porter, I. H. (eds.): New York, Academic Press, 1979.
18. Caspersson, T., et al.: Identification of human chromosomes by DNA-binding fluorescent agents. *Chromosoma 30*:215, 1970.
19. Caspersson, T., and Zech, L.: Chromosome identification by fluorescence. *Hosp. Practice 7*:51, 1972.
20. Pardue, M. L., and Gall, J. G.: Chromosomal localization of mouse satellite DNA. *Science 168*:1356, 1970.
21. Pearson, P.: The use of new staining techniques for human chromosome identification. *J. Med. Genet. 9*:264, 1972.
22. Morishima, A., and Grumbach, M. M.: The interrelationship of sex chromosome constitution and phenotype in the syndrome of gonadal dysgenesis and its variants. *Ann. N.Y. Acad. Sci. 155*:695, 1968.
23. Jacobs, P. A., et al.: Change of human chromosome count distributions with age: evidence for a sex difference. *Nature 197*:1080, 1963.
24. Ford, C. E.: Mosaics and chimeras. *Brit. Med. Bull. 25*:104, 1969.
25. Bergsma, D., Hamerton, J. L., and Klinger, H. P. (eds.), Chicago Conference: Standardization in Human Cytogenetics. *Birth Defects: Orig. Art. Ser. 2*(2), 1966.
26. Wachtel, S. S., and Ohno, S.: The immunogenetics of sexual development. *In Progress in Medical Genetics. Vol. III,* Steinberg, A. G. (ed.), New Series, 1979. Philadelphia, W. B. Saunders Co., 1979.
27. Bühler, E. M.: A synopsis of the human Y chromosome. *Hum. Genet. 55*:145, 1980.
28. Koo, G. C., et al.: Mapping the locus of the H-Y gene on the human Y chromosome. *Science 198*:940, 1977.
29. Grumbach, M. M., Genetic mechanisms of sex differentiation. *In Genetic Mechanisms of Sexual Development.* Vallet, H. L., and Porter, I. H. (eds.), New York, Academic Press, 1979.
30. Pearson, P. L., et al.: Technique for identifying Y chromosomes in human interphase nuclei. *Nature 226*:78, 1970.
31. Grumbach, M. M.: Male reproductive tract-development, anatomy, physiology and disorders. *In Biologic Basis of Pediatric Practice.* Cooke, R. E., (ed.), New York, McGraw-Hill, 1968.
32. Ferguson-Smith, M. A.: Karyotype-phenotype correlations in gonadal dysgenesis and their bearing on the pathogenesis of malformations. *J. Med. Genet. 2*:142, 1965.
33. Jacobs, P. A., and Ross, A.: Structural abnormalities of the Y chromosome in man. *Nature 210*:352, 1966.
34. Meyer, W. J. III, et al.: Locus on the X chromosome for dihydrotestosterone receptor and androgen insensitivity. *Proc. Natl. Acad. Sci. USA 72*:1469, 1975.
35. de la Chapelle, A., and Miller, O. J.: Report of the committee on the genetic constitution of chromosomes 10, 11, 12, X and Y. *Cytogenet. Cell Genet. 25*:47, 1979.
36. Mohandas, T., et al.: Regional assignment of the steroid sulfatase X-linked ichthyosis locus: Implications for a non-inactivated region on the short arm of the human X-chromosome. *Proc. Natl. Acad. Sci. USA 76*:5779, 1979.
37. Barr, M. L., and Bertram, E. G.: A morphological distinction between neurones of the male and female, and the behavior of the nucleolar satellite during acceleration of nucleoprotein synthesis. *Nature 163*:676, 1949.
38. Ohno, S., et al.: Formation of the sex chromatin by a single X-chromosome in liver cells of *Rattus norvegicus. Exper. Cell Res. 18*:415, 1959.
39. Grumbach, M. M., and Morishima, A.: Sex chromatin and the sex chromosomes: On the origin of sex chromatin from a single X chromosome. *Acta Cytol. 6*:46, 1962.
40. Beutler, E., et al.: The normal human female as a mosaic of X-chromosome activity: Studies using the gene for G-6-PD deficiency as a marker. *Proc. Natl. Acad. Sci. 48*:9, 1962.
41. Lyon, M. F.: X-chromosome inactivation and developmental patterns in mammals. *Biol. Rev. 47*:1, 1972.
42. Lyon, M. F.: Mechanism and evolutionary origins of variable X-chromosome activity in mammals. *Proc. Roy. Soc.* London (Biol) *B187*:243, 1974.
43. Epstein, C. J.: Expression of the mammalian X chromosome before and after fertilization. *Science 175*:1467, 1972.
44. Gartler, S. M., and Andrina, R. J.: Mammalian X-chromosome inactivation. In *Advances in Human Genetics.* Harris, H., and Hirschhorn, K. (eds.), New York, Plenum Press, 1976.
45. Riggs, A. D.: X inactivation, differentiation, and DNA methylation. *Cytogenet. Cell Genet. 14*:9, 1975.
46. Davidson, R. G., et al.: Demonstration of two populations of cells in the human female heterozygous for glucose-6-phosphate dehydrogenase variants. *Proc. Natl. Acad. Sci. 50*:481, 1963.
47. Shapiro, L. J., et al.: Non-inactivation of an X-chromosome locus in man. *Science 204*:1224, 1979.
48. Eichwald, E. J., and Silmser, C. R.: Communication. *Transpl. Bull. 2*:148, 1955.
49. Goldberg, E. H., et al.: Serological demonstration of H-Y (male) antigen on mouse sperm. *Nature 232*:478, 1971.
50. Haseltine, F. P., and Ohno, S.: Mechanisms of gonadal differentiation. *Science,* in press 1981.
51. Wachtel, S. S., et al.: Evolutionary conservation of H-Y ("male") antigen. *Nature 254*:270, 1975.
52. Krco, C. J., and Goldberg, E. H.: H-Y male antigen: detection on eight-cell mouse embryos. *Science 193*:1134, 1976.
53. Wachtel, S. S.: The genetics of intersexuality: Clinical and theoretic perspectives. *Obstet. Gynecol. 54*:671, 1979.
54. Ohno, S., et al.: Testis-organizing H-Y antigen and the primary sex-determining mechanism of mammals. *Rec. Prog. Horm. Res. 35*:449, 1979.
55. Fredga, K., et al.: Fertile XX- and XY- type females in the wood lemming (Myopus schisticolor). *Nature 261*:255, 1976.
56. Fredga, K., et al.: A hypothesis explaining the exceptional sex ratio in the wood lemming (Myopus schisticolor). *Hereditas 85*:101, 1977.
57. Wachtel, S. S., et al.: H-Y antigen and the origin of XY- female wood lemmings (Myopus schisticolor). *Nature 264*:638, 1976.
58. Ghosh, S. N., et al.: Absence of H-Y antigen in XY females with dysgenetic gonads. *Nature 276*:180, 1978.
59. de la Chapelle, A., et al.: Recessive sex-determining genes in XX male syndrome. *Cell 15*:837, 1978.
60. Wachtel, S. S., et al.: Recessive male-determining genes. *Cell 15*:279, 1978.
61. Selden, J. R., et al.: Genetic basis of XX male syndrome and XX true hermaphroditism: Evidence in the dog. *Science 201*:644, 1978.
62. Bennett, D., et al.: Serological evidence for H-Y antigen in Sxr,XX sex reversed phenotypic males. *Nature 265*:255, 1977.
63. Eicker, W., et al.: H-Y antigen in trans-sexuality. *Lancet 2*:1137, 1979.
64. Engel, W., et al.: H-Y antigen in transsexuality, and how to explain testis differentiation in H-Y antigen-negative males and ovary differentiation in H-Y antigen-positive females. *Hum. Genet. 55*:315, 1980.
65. Ohno, S., and Stapleton, D. W.: Associative recognition of testis organizing H-Y antigen and immunological confusion. In press, 1981.
66. Zenzes, M. T., et al.: Studies on H-Y antigen in different cell fractions of the testis during pubescence. Immature germ cells are H-Y antigen negative. *Hum. Genet. 45*:297, 1978.
67. Ohno, S., et al.: Testicular cells lysostripped of H-Y antigen organize ovarian follicle-like aggregates. *Cytogenet. Cell Genet. 20*:351, 1978.
68. Zenzes, M. T., et al.: Studies on the function of H-Y antigen: Dissociation and reorganization experiments of rat gonadal cells. *Cytogenet. Cell Genet. 20*:365, 1978.
69. Moscona, A. A., and Hausman, R. E.: Biological and biochemical studies on embryonic cell-cell recognition. *In Cell and Tissue Interactions.* Lash, J. W., and Burger, M. M. (eds.), New York, Raven Press, 1977.
70. Zenzes, M. T., et al.: Organization *in vitro* of ovarian cells into testicular structures. *Hum. Genet. 44*:333, 1978.
71. Ohno, S., et al.: Hormone-like role of H-Y antigen in bovine freemartin gonad. *Nature 261*:597, 1976.
72. Nagai, Y., et al.: The identification of human H-Y antigen and testicular transformation induced by its interaction with the receptor site of bovine fetal ovarian cells. *Differentiation 13*:155, 1979.
73. Grumbach, M. M., and Barr, M. L.: Cytologic tests of chromosomal sex in relation to sexual anomalies in man. *Rec. Prog. Horm. Res. 14*:255, 1958.
74. Byskov, A. G.: Regulation of initiation of meiosis in fetal gonads. *Int. J. Andrology (Suppl)2*:29, 1978.
75. Byskov, A. G.: The anatomy and ultrastructure of the rete system in the mouse ovary. *Biol. Reprod. 19*:720, 1978.
76. Wachtel, S. S., and Hall, J. L.: H-Y binding in the gonad: Inhibition by a supernatant of the fetal ovary. *Cell 17*:327, 1979.
77. Zenzes, M. T., et al.: Inhibition of testicular organization *in vitro* by newborn rat ovarian cell supernatants. *Differentiation 16*:193, 1980.
78. Witschi, E.: Embrology of the ovary. *In The Ovary.* Grady, H. G., and Smith, E. D. (eds.) Baltimore, Williams & Wilkins Co., 1963.
79. Mancini, R. E., et al.: Origin and development of the germinative epithelium and Sertoli cells in the human testis: Cytological, cytochemical and quantitative study. *Anat. Rec. 136*:477, 1960.
80. Heller, C. G., and Clermont, Y.: Kinetics of the germinal epithelium in man. *Rec. Prog. Horm. Res. 20*:545, 1964.

81. Baker, T. G.: A quantitative and cytological study of germ cells in human ovaries. *Proc. Roy. Soc. (B) 148*:417, 1963.

82. Jost, A., et al.: Studies on sex differentiation in mammals. *Rec. Prog. Horm. Res. 29*:1, 1973.

83. Gondos, B.: Testicular development. *In The Testis,* Vol. 4. San Francisco, Academic Press, 1977.

84. Gondos, B.: Oogonia and oocytes in mammals. *In The Vertebrate Ovary: Comparative Biology and Evolution.* Jones, R. E. (ed.), New York, Plenum Press, 1978.

85. Jost, A.: A new look at the mechanism controlling sex differentiation in mammals. *Johns Hopkins Med. J. 130*:38, 1972.

86. van Wagenen, G., and Simpson, M. E.: *Embryology of the Ovary and Testis, Homo Sapiens and Macaca Mulatta.* New Haven, Yale University Press, 1965.

87. Jost, A.: Hormonal factors in the sex differentiation of the mammalian fetus. *Trans. Roy. Soc. (B) 259*:119, 1970.

88. Witschi, E., et al.: Genetic, developmental and hormonal aspects of gonadal dysgenesis and sex inversion in man. *J. Clin. Endocrinol. Metab. 17*:737, 1957.

89. Josso, N., et al.: The antimüllerian hormone. *Rec. Prog. Horm. Res. 33*:117, 1977.

90. Müller, U., et al.: Appearance of hCG-receptor after conversion of newborn ovarian cells into testicular structures by H-Y antigen *in vitro. Hum. Genet. 45*:203, 1978.

91. Siiteri, P. K., and Wilson, J. D.: Testosterone formation and metabolism during male sexual differentiation in the human embryo. *J. Clin. Endocrinol. Metab. 38*:113, 1974.

92. Reyes, F. I., et al.: Studies in human sexual development II. Fetal and maternal serum gonadotropins and sex steroid concentration. *J. Clin. Endocrinol. Metab. 38*:612, 1974.

93. Kaplan, S. L., and Grumbach, M. M.: Pituitary and placental gonadotropins and sex steroids in the human and sub-human primate fetus. *Clin. Endocrinol. Metab. 7*:487, 1978.

94. Pang, S., et al.: Amniotic fluid concentrations of Δ^5 and Δ^4 steroids in fetuses with congenital adrenal hyperplasia due to 21 hydroxylase deficiency and in anencephalic fetuses. *J. Clin. Endocrinol. Metab. 51*:223, 1980.

95. Huhtaniemi, I. T., et al.: hCG binding and stimulation of testosterone biosynthesis in the human fetal testis. *J. Clin. Endocrinol. Metab. 44*:963, 1977.

96. Huhtaniemi, I. T., et al.: Content of chorionic gonadotropin in human fetal tissues. *J. Clin. Endocrinol. Metab. 46*:994, 1978.

97. Kaplan, S. L., et al.: The ontogenesis of pituitary hormones and hypothalamic factors in the human fetus: Maturation of central nervous system regulation of anterior pituitary function. *Rec. Prog. Horm. Res. 32*:161, 1976.

98. George, F. W., and Wilson, J. D.: The regulation of androgen and estrogen formation in fetal gonads. *Ann. Biol. Anim. Biochem. Biophys. 19(4B)*:1297, 1979.

99. Gondos, B., and Hobel, C. S.: Interstitial cells in the human fetal ovary. *Endocrinology 93*:736, 1973.

100. Jost, A.: Problems of fetal endocrinology: The gonadal and hypophyseal hormones. *Rec. Prog. Horm. Res. 8*:379, 1953.

101. Jost, A.: Embryonic sexual differentiation. (Morphology, physiology, abnormalities.) *In Hermaphroditism, Genital Anomalies and Related Endocrine Disorders.* Jones, H. W., and Scoot, W. W. (eds.), Baltimore, Williams & Wilkins Co., 1971.

102. Josso, N.: Interspecific character of the müllerian-inhibiting substance: Action of the human fetal testis, ovary and adrenal on the fetal rat müllerian duct in organ culture. *J. Clin. Endocrinol. Metab. 32*:404, 1971.

103. Picard, J. Y., et al.: Biosynthesis of labelled anti-müllerian hormone by fetal testes: Evidence for the glycoprotein nature of the hormone and for its disulfide-bonded structure. *Molec. Cell. Endocrinol. 12*:17, 1978.

104. Dyche, W. J.: A comparative study of the differentiation and involution of the müllerian duct and wolffian duct in the male and female fetal mouse. *J. Morphology 162*:175, 1979.

105. Neumann, F., et al.: Aspects of androgen-dependent events as studied by anti-androgens. *Rec. Prog. Horm. Res. 26*:337, 1970.

106. Wilson, J. D., and Siiteri, P. K.: Developmental pattern of testosterone synthesis in the fetal gonad of the rabbit. *Endocrinology 92*:1182, 1973.

107. Cunha, G. R., et al.: Stromal-epithelial interactions in sex differentiations. *Biol. Reprod. 22*:19, 1980.

108. Feldman, D. W., and Smith, D. W.: Fetal phallic growth and penile standards for newborn male infants. *J. Pediatr. 86*:395, 1975.

109. Forsberg, J.-G.: Origin of vaginal epithelium. *Obstet. Gynecol. 25*:787, 1965.

110. Cunha, G. R.: The dual origin of vaginal epithelium. *Amer. J. Anat. 143*:387, 1975.

111. Chan, L., and O'Malley, B. W.: Mechanism of action of the sex steroid hormones. (3 parts.) *N. Engl. J. Med. 294*:1322, 1372, 1430, 1976.

112. Liao, S.: Molecular actions of androgens. *In Biochemical Actions of Hormones.* Vol. 4. Litwack, G. (ed.), New York, Academic Press, 1978.

113. Grumbach, M. M., and Ducharme, J. R.: The effects of androgens on fetal sexual development. Androgen-induced female pseudohermaphrodism. *Fertil. Steril. 11*:157, 1960.

114. Grumbach, M. M.: The neuroendocrinology of puberty. *Hosp. Prac. 15*:51, 1980.

115. Styne, D., and Grumbach, M. M.: Puberty in the male and female: Its physiology and disorders. *In Reproductive Endocrinology.* Yen, S. S. C., and Jaffee, R. B. (eds.), Philadelphia, W. B. Saunders, Co., 1978.

116. Pfeiffer, C. A.: Sexual difference of the hypophyses and their determination by the gonads. *Amer. J. Anat. 58*:195, 1936.

117. Donovan, B. T., and Van Der Werff Ten Bosch, J. J.: *Physiology of Puberty.* London, E. Arnold, 1965.

118. Gorski, R. A.: Gonadal hormones and the perinatal development of neuro-endocrine function. *In Frontiers of Neuroendocrinology.* Martini, L., and Ganong, W. F. (eds.), London, Oxford Univ. Press, 1971.

119. Harris, G. W.: Sex hormones, brain development and brain function. *Endocrinology 75*:627, 1964.

120. Raisman, G., and Field, P.: Sexual dimorphism in the neuropil of the preoptic area of the rat and its dependence on neonatal androgen. *Brain Res. 54*:1, 1973.

121. Brawer, J. R.: Effects of a single injection of estradiol valerate on the hypothalamic arcuate nucleus and on reproductive function in the female rat. *Endocrinology 103*:501, 1978.

122. Reiter, E. O., et al.: The response of pituitary gonadotropins to synthetic LRF in children with glucocorticoid-treated congenital adrenal hyperplasia: Lack of effect of intrauterine and neonatal androgen excess. *J. Clin. Endocrinol. Metab. 40*:318, 1975.

123. Sizonenko, P. C., et al.: Gonadotrophins, testosterone and oestrogen levels in relation to ovarian morphology in 11β-hydroxylase deficiency. *Acta Endocrinol 71*:539, 1972.

124. Karsch, F. J., et al.: Sexual differentiation of pituitary function: Apparent difference between primates and rodents. *Science 179*:484, 1973.

125. Barbarino, A., et al.: Presence of positive feedback between oestrogen and LH in patients with Klinefelter's syndrome and Sertoli-cell-only syndrome. *Clin. Endocrinol. 10*:235, 1979.

126. Baker, W. S.: Psychosexual differentiation in the human. *Biol. Reprod. 22*:61, 1980.

127. Diamond, M.: A critical evaluation of the ontogeny of human sexual behavior. *Quart. Rev. Biol. 40*:147, 1965.

128. Imperato-McGinley, J. L., et al.: Androgens and the evolution of male-gender identity among male pseudohermaphrodites with 5α-reductase deficiency. *N. Engl. J. Med. 300*:1233, 1979.

129. Money, J., et al.: An examination of some basic sexual concepts: the evidence of human hermaphroditism. *Bull. Johns Hopkins Hosp. 97*:301, 1955.

130. Money, J., et al.: Visual constructional deficit in Turner's syndrome. *J. Pediatr. 69*:126, 1966.

131. Kolodny, R. C., et al.: Plasma testosterone and semen analysis in male homosexuals. *N. Engl. J. Med. 285*:1170, 1971.

132. Ehrhardt, A. A., et al.: Fetal androgens and female gender identity in the early-treated adrenogenital syndrome. *Johns Hopkins Med. J. 122*:160, 1968.

133. Jacobs, P. A., and Strong, J. A.: A case of human intersexuality having a possible XXY sex-determining mechanism. *Nature* (London)*183*:302, 1959.

134. Ford, C. E., et al.: The chromosomes in a patient showing both Mongolism and the Klinefelter syndrome. *Lancet 1*:709, 1959.

135. Frøland, A.: Klinefelter's syndrome. Clinical, endocrinological and cytogenetical studies. *Dan. Med. Bull. 16*(Suppl 6):1, 1969.

136. Hsueh, W. A., et al.: Endocrine features of Klinefelter's syndrome. *Medicine 57*:447, 1978.

137. Leonard, J. M., et al.: The classification of Klinefelter's syndrome. *In Symposium on Genetic Mechanisms of Sexual Development.* Vallet, H. L., and Porter, I. H. (eds.), New York, Academic Press, 1978.

138. Robinson, A., et al.: Summary of clinical findings: Profiles of children with 47,XXY, 47,XXX, and 47,XYY karyotypes. *Birth Defects: Orig. Art. Ser. 15*:1, 261, 1979.

139. Caldwell, P. D., and Smith, D. W.: The XXY Klinefelter syndrome in childhood: Detection and treatment. *J. Pediatr. 80*:250, 1972.

140. Schibler, D., et al.: Growth and body proportions in 54 boys and men with Klinefelter's syndrome. *Helv. Paediatr. Acta 29*:325, 1974.

141. Smals, A. H. G., et al.: Body proportions and androgenicity in relation to plasma testosterone levels in Klinefelter's syndrome. *Acta Endocrinol. 77*:387, 1974.

142. Illig, R., et al.: LH and FSH responses to synthetic LH-RH in children and adolescents with Turner's and Klinfelter's syndrome. *Helv. Paediatr. Acta 30*:221, 1975.

143. Smals, A. H. G., et al.: Effect of short and long term human chorionic

gonadotrophin (hCG) administration of plasma testosterone levels in Klinefelter's syndrome. *Acta Endocrinol.* 77:753, 1974.

144. Wang, C., et al.: Hormonal studies in Klinefelter syndrome. *Clin. Endocrinol.* 4:399, 1975.

145. Smals, A. H. G., et al.: The pituitary-thyroid axis in Klinefelter's syndrome. *Acta Endocrinol.* 84:72, 1977.

146. Nielsen, J.: Diabetes mellitus in patients with aneuploid chromosome aberrations and in their parents. *Humangenetik* 16:165, 1972.

147. Harnden, D. G., et al.: Carcinoma of the breast and Klinefelter's syndrome. *J. Med. Genet.* 8:460, 1971.

148. Chaussain, J. L., et al.: Klinefelter syndrome, tumor and sexual precocity. *J. Pediatr.* 97:607, 1980.

149. Jacobs, P. A.: The incidence and etiology of sex chromosome abnormalities in man. *Birth Defects: Orig. Artic. Ser.* 15(1):3, 1979.

150. Hook, E. B., and Hamerton, J. L.: The frequency of chromosome abnormalities detected in consecutive newborn studies — difference between studies — results by sex and severity of phenotypic involvement. In *Population Cytogenetics, Studies in Humans.* Hook, E. B., and Porter, I. H. (eds.), New York, Academic Press, 1977.

151. Ferguson-Smith, M. A.: The prepubertal testicular lesions in chromatin positive Klinefelter's syndrome (primarily micro-orchidism) as seen in mentally handicapped children. *Lancet* 1:219, 1959.

152. Grumbach, M. M., et al.: Sex chromatin pattern in seminiferous tubule dysgenesis and other testicular disorders: Relationships to true hermaphrodism and to Klinefelter's syndrome. *J. Clin. Endocrinol. Metab.* 17:703, 1957.

153. Teter, J., and Boczkowski, K.: Occurrence of tumors in dysgenetic gonads. *Cancer* 20:1301, 1967.

154. Ahmad, K. N., et al.: Leydig cell volume in chromatin positive Klinefelter's syndrome. *J. Clin. Endocrinol. Metab.* 33:517, 1971.

155. Barr, M. L., et al.: An XY/XXXY sex chromosome mosaic in a mentally defective male patient. *J. Ment. Defic. Res.* 6:65, 1965.

156. Rosenkranz, V.: Klinefelter Syndrome bei Kindern von Frauen mit Geschlechtschromosomen-Anomalien. *Helv. Paediat. Acta* 20:359, 1965.

157. de la Chapelle, A.: Nature and origin of males with XX sex chromosomes. *Amer. J. Hum. Genet.* 24:71, 1972.

158. Sanger, R., et al.: Xg groups and sex chromosome abnormalities in people of northern European ancestry: an addendum. *J. Med. Genet.* 14:210, 1977.

158a. Russell, L. B.: Chromosome aberrations in experimental mammals. In *Progress in Medical Genetics.* Vol. 2. Steinberg, A. B., and Bearn, A. G. (eds.), New York, Grune & Stratton, 1962.

159. Ferguson-Smith, M. A., et al.: Parental age and source of the X chromosomes in XXY Klinefelter's syndrome. *Lancet* 1:46, 1964.

160. Zizka, J., et al.: XXYY son of a triple X mother. *Humangenetik* 26:159, 1975.

161. Lecluse-Van Der Bilt, F. A., et al.: An infant with an XXXYY karyotype. *Clin. Genet.* 5:263, 1974.

162. Fraccaro, M., et al.: A child with 49 chromosomes. *Lancet* 2:899, 1960.

163. Terheggen, H. G., et al.: Das XXXXY Syndrom. Bericht uber 7 neue Fälle und Literaturübersicht. *Z. Kinderheilkd.* 115:209, 1973.

164. Wachtel, S. S., et al.: Serologic detection of a Y-linked gene in XX males and XX true hermaphrodites. *N. Engl. J. Med.* 295:705, 1976.

165. Miro, R., et al.: Mosaicism in XX males. *Hum. Genet.* 45:103, 1978.

166. Evans, H. J., et al.: Heteromorphic X chromosomes in 46,XX males: Evidence for the involvement of X-Y interchange. *Hum. Genet.* 49:11, 1979.

167. van den Berghe, H., et al.: Y to X translocation in man. *Hum. Genet.* 36:129, 1977.

168. Develing, A., et al.: A Y-autosome translocation 46,Xt(Yq−:7q+) associated with multiple congenital anomalies. *J. Pediatr.* 82:495, 1976.

169. Engel, E., and Forbes, A. P.: Cytogenetic and clinical findings in 48 patients with congenitally defective or absent ovaries. *Medicine* 44:135, 1965.

170. Linsten, J.: *The Nature and Origin of X Chromosome Aberrations in Turner Syndrome. A Cytogenetical and Clinical Study of 57 Patients.* Stockholm, Almqvist and Wiksell, 1963.

171. Mattevi, M. S., et al.: Cytogenetic, clinical and genealogical analysis in a series of gonadal dysgenesis patients and their families. *Humangenetik* 13:126, 1971.

172. Palmer, C. G., and Reichman, A.: Chromosomal and clinical findings in 110 females with Turner syndrome. *Hum. Genet.* 35:35, 1976.

173. Ford, C. E., et al.: A sex chromosome anomaly in a case of gonadal dysgenesis (Turner's syndrome). *Lancet* 2:711, 1959.

174. Gordon, R. R., and O'Neill, E. M.: Turner's infantile phenotype. *Brit. Med. J.* 1:483, 1969.

175. Singh, R. F., and Carr, D. H.: The anatomy and histology of XO human embryos and fetuses. *Anat. Rec.* 155:369, 1966.

176. Preger, L., et al.: Roentgenographic abnormalities in phenotypic females with gonadal dysgenesis. A comparison of chromatin positive patients and chromatin negative patients. *Amer. J. Roentgenol. Radium. Ther. Nucl. Med.* 104:899, 1968.

177. Kosowicz, J.: The roentgen appearance of the hand and wrist in gonadal dysgenesis. *Amer. J. Roentgenol. Radium. Ther. Nucl. Med.* 93:354, 1965.

178. Alexander, R. L., et al.: The effects of initiating estrogen treatment early in adolescence in the syndrome of gonadal dysgenesis. In press.

179. Brook, C. G. D., et al.: Growth in children with 45,XO Turner's syndrome. *Arch. Dis. Child.* 49:789, 1974.

180. Kaplan, S. L., et al.: Growth and growth hormone. I. Changes in serum level of growth hormone following hypoglycemia in 134 children with growth retardation. *Pediatr. Res.* 2:43, 1968.

181. Saenger, P., et al.: The interaction of growth hormone, sommatomedin, and oestrogen in patients with Turner's syndrome. *Acta Endocrinol.* 81:9, 1976.

182. Sklar, C., et al.: Lack of effect of estrogens on adrenal androgen secretion. *Clin. Endocrinol.* 14:311, 1981.

183. Weiss, L.: Additional evidence of gradual loss of germ cells in the pathogenesis of streak ovaries in Turner's syndrome. *J. Med. Genet.* 8:540, 1971.

184. Jirásek, J.: Principles of reproductive embryology. In *Disorders of Sexual Differentiation.* Simpson, J. L. (ed.), New York, Academic Press, 1976.

185. Conte, F. A., et al.: A diphasic pattern of gonadotropin secretion in patients with the syndrome of gonadal dysgenesis. *J. Clin. Endocrinol. Metab.* 40:670, 1975.

186. Conte, F. A., et al.: Correlation of luteinizing hormone-releasing factor induced luteinizing hormone and follicle-stimulating hormone release from infancy to 19 years with the changing pattern of gonadotropin secretion in agonadal patients: Relation to restraint of puberty. *J. Clin. Endocrinol. Metab.* 50:163, 1980.

187. Kohn, G., et al.: Two conceptions in a 45,X woman. *Amer. J. Med. Genet.* 5:339, 1980.

188. King, C. R., et al.: Pregnancy and the Turner syndrome. *Obstet. Gynecol.* 52:617, 1978.

189. Dewhurst, J.: Fertility in 47,XXX and 45,X patients. *J. Med. Genet.* 15:132, 1978.

189a. Reyes, F. I., et al.: Fertility in women with gonadal dysgenesis. *Am. J. Obstet. Gynecol.* 126:668, 1976.

190. Carr, D. H.: Chromosome and abortion. In *Advances in Human Genetics.* Harris, H., and Hirschhorn, K. (eds.), New York, Plenum Press, 1971, Vol. 2.

191. Warburton, D.: Monosomy X: A chromosomal anomaly associated with young maternal age. *Lancet* 1:167, 1980.

192. Fialkow, P. J., and Uchida, I. A.: Autoantibodies in Down's syndrome and gonadal dysgenesis. *Ann. N.Y. Acad. Sci.* 155:759, 1968.

193. Pai, G. S., et al.: Thyroid abnormalities in 20 children with Turner syndrome. *J. Pediatr.* 91:267, 1978.

194. Price, W. H.: A high incidence of chronic inflammatory bowel disease in patients with Turner's syndrome. *J. Med. Genet.* 16:263, 1979.

195. Wertelecki, W., et al.: Nongonadal neoplasia in Turner's syndrome. *Cancer* 26:485, 1970.

196. King, C. R., and Maginis, E.: Turner syndrome in the offspring of artificially inseminated pregnancies. *Fert. Steril.* 30:604, 1978.

197. Willemse, C. H.: A patient suffering from Turner's syndrome and acromegaly. *Acta Endocrinol.* 39:204, 1962.

198. Moore, D. C., et al.: Studies of anabolic steroids. VI. Effect of prolonged administration of oxandrolone on growth in children and adolescents with gonadal dysgenesis. *J. Pediatr.* 90:462, 1977.

199. Lev-Ran, A.: Androgens, estrogens and the ultimate height in XO gonadal dysgenesis. *Amer. J. Dis. Child.* 131:648, 1977.

200. Perheentupa, J., et al.: Hormonal treatment of Turner's syndrome. *Acta Pediatr. Scand. (Suppl)* 256:24, 1975.

201. Ehrhardt, A. A.: Behavioral effects of estrogens in the human female. *Pediatrics* 62:1166, 1978.

202. Levine, L. S.: Treatment of Turner's syndrome with estrogen. *Pediatrics* 62:1178, 1979.

203. Rosenwaks, Z., et al.: Endometrial pathology and its relation to estrogen therapy in patients with hypogonadism. *Pediatrics* 62:1184, 1979.

204. Fraccaro, M., et al.: Women heterozygous for deficiency of the (p21-pter) region of the X chromosome are fertile. *Hum. Genet.* 39:283, 1977.

205. Summitt, R. L., et al.: X-autosome translocation: A review. *Birth Defects* 14(6C):219, 1978.

206. Therman, E., et al.: X chromosome constitution and the human female phenotype. *Hum. Genet.* 54:133, 1980.

207. Fujita, H., et al.: Cytological findings of 10 cases of I(Xq) and one with dic (X). *Hum. Genet.* 39:147, 1977.

208. Stafford, T. M., et al.: Gonadal dysgenesis with isochromosome X and menstruation. *Amer. J. Obstet. Gynecol.* 116:886, 1973.

209. Caspersson, T. A., et al.: The nature of structural X chromosome aberrations in Turner's syndrome as revealed by quinacrine mustard fluorescent analysis. *Hereditas* 66:287, 1970.

210. Van den Berge, H., et al.: 46,XXip karyotype in a woman with normal stature and gonadal dysgenesis without other anomalies. *Humangenetik* 20:163, 1973.

211. Keogh, E. J., et al.: Isochromosome for the short arm of the X with primary amenorrhea and a pituitary tumor. *Aust. N.Z. J. Med.* 3:617, 1973.

212. Grumbach, M. M., and Van Wyk, J.: Disorders of sex differentiation. *In Textbook of Endocrinology.* Williams, R. H. (ed.), 5th ed., Philadelphia, W. B. Saunders Company, 1974.

213. de la Chapelle, A. L., et al.: Reappraisal of a 46,Xi(Xp) karyotype as 46,X,del(Xq). *Hereditas* 80:137, 1975.

214. Hagemeijer, A., et al.: Late replicating ring X-chromosome identified by R-banding after Brdu pulse. Three new examples of 45,XO/46,Xr(X). *Hum. Genet.* 34:45, 1976.

215. Hoo, J. J.: A note on Xp−. *Hum. Genet.* 50:339, 1979.

216. Herva, R., et al.: Inherited interstitial del(X)p with minimal consequences. *Amer. J. Med. Genet.* 3:43, 1979.

216a. Kalousek, D., et al.: Partial short arm deletions of the X chromosome and spontaneous pubertal development in girls with short stature. *J. of Pediatr.* 94:891, 1979.

217. Leichtman, D. A., et al.: Familial Turner syndrome. *Ann. Int. Med.* 89:473, 1978.

218. Mirzayants, G. G., and Baranovskaya, L. I.: X-X translocation in a patient with gonadal dysgenesis and the problem of phenotypic-karyotypic correlations. *Hum. Genet.* 40:249, 1978.

219. Zäh, W., et al.: Mixed gonadal dysgenesis. *Acta Endocrinol. (Suppl) (Kbh)* 79(197):1, 1975.

220. Bonaventura, L., et al.: The Sertoli cell in mixed gonadal dysgenesis. *Obst. Gynecol.* 53:324, 1979.

221. Simpson, J. L.: Male pseudohermaphroditism: Genetics and clinical delineation. *Hum. Genet.* 44:1, 1978.

222. Caspersson, T. A., et al.: Translocation causing non-fluorescent Y chromosomes in human XO/XY mosaicism. *Hereditas* 68:317, 1971.

223. Kluzewski, B., et al.: A theory explaining the abnormality in 45,X/46,XY mosaicism with non-fluorescent Y chromosome. Presentation of 3 cases. *Ann. Genet.* 21:5, 1978.

224. Madan, K., et al.: Three cases of sex chromosome mosaicism with a nonfluorescent Y. *Hum. Genet.* 46:295, 1979.

225. Koo, G. C., et al.: Mapping the locus of H-Y antigen. *Birth Defects* 12(7):175, 1976.

226. Forabasco, A., et al.: H-Y antigen in a male with a 45,X karyotype. *Lancet* 2:313, 1978.

227. Donahoe, P. K., et al.: Mixed gonadal dysgenesis, pathogenesis and management. *J. Pediatr. Surg.* 14:287, 1979.

228. Yanagisawa, S.: Structural abnormalities of the Y chromosome and abnormal external genitals. *Hum. Genet.* 53:183, 1980.

229. Tiepolo, L., and Zuffardi, O.: Localization of factors controlling spermatogenesis in the non-fluorescent portion of the human Y chromosome long arm. *Hum. Genet.* 34:119, 1976.

230. Yunis, E., et al.: Yq deletion, aspermia and short stature. *Hum. Genet.* 39:117, 1977.

231. Rosenfeld, R., et al.: Sexual and somatic determinants of the human Y chromosome: Studies in a 46,XYp− phenotypic female. *Amer. J. Hum. Genet.* 31:458, 1979.

232. Kohdr, G., et al.: Y-autosome translocation, gonadal dysgenesis, and gonadoblastoma. *Amer. J. Dis. Child.* 133:277, 1979.

233. Harden, D. G.: The chromosomes in a case of pure gonadal dysgenesis. *Brit. Med. J.* 2:1285, 1959.

234. McDonough, P. G., et al.: Phenotypic and cytogenetic findings in eighty-two patients with ovarian failure — changing trends. *Fertil. Steril.* 28:638, 1977.

235. Judd, H. L., et al.: Pure gonadal dysgenesis with progressive hirsutism; Demonstration of testosterone production by gonadal streaks. *N. Engl. J. Med.* 282:881, 1970.

236. Hamet, P., et al.: Hypertension with adrenal, genital and renal defects, and deafness. *Arch. Int. Med.* 131:563, 1973.

237. Skre, H., et al.: Cerebellar ataxia and hypergondotropic hypogonadism in two kindreds. Chance occurrence, pleiotropism, or linkage. *Clin. Genet.* 9:234, 1976.

238. Swyer, G. I. M.: Male pseudohermaphrodism: A hitherto undescribed form. *Brit. Med. J.* 2:709, 1955.

239. Gaal, M., et al.: 46,XY pure gonadal dysgenesis with non-fluorescent Y chromosome. *Clin. Genet.* 14:83, 1978.

240. German, J., et al.: Genetically determined sex reversal in 46,XY humans. *Science* 202:53, 1978.

241. Chemke, J., et al. Familial XY gonadal dysgenesis. *J. Med. Genet.* 7:105, 1970.

242. Hofnagel, D., et al.: Camptomelic dwarfism associated with XY- gonadal dysgenesis and chromosome anomalies. *Clin. Genet.* 13:489, 1978.

243. Brosman, P. G., et al.: A new familial syndrome of 46,XY gonadal dysgenesis with anomalies of ectodermal and mesodermal structures. *J. Pediatr.* 97:586, 1980.

244. Wolf, U.: XY gonadal dysgenesis and the H-Y antigen. *Hum. Genet.* 47:269, 1979.

245. Dorus, E., et al.: Clinical, pathologic and genetic findings in a case of 46, XY pure gonadal dysgenesis (Swyer's syndrome). II. Presence of H-Y antigen. *Amer. J. Obstet Gynecol.* 127:829, 1977.

246. Bernstein, R., et al.: Abnormality of the X chromosome in human 46,XY female siblings with dysgenetic ovaries. *Science* 207:768, 1980.

247. Herbst, E., et al.: Cytologic identification of two X chromosome types in the wood lemming (Myopus schisticolor). *Chromosoma* 69:185, 1978.

248. Wachtel, S. S.: H-Y antigen in 46,XY gonadal dysgenesis. *Hum. Genet.* 54:25, 1980.

249. Wachtel, S. S.: The dysgenetic gonad: Aberrant testicular differentiation. *Biol. Reprod.* 22:1, 1980.

250. Grumbach, M. M., et al.: A distinctive clinical entity simulating Turner's syndrome in boys and girls associated with congenital heart disease, appropriate gonadal differentiation and a normal sex chromosome constitution. *J. Pediatr.* 67:966, 1965 (abst.).

251. Noonan, J.: Hypertelorism with Turner phenotype. A new syndrome with associated congenital heart disease. *Amer. J. Dis. Child.* 116:373, 1968.

252. Smith, D. W.: *Recognizable Patterns of 160 Human Malformations: Genetic, Embryonic and Clinical Aspects.* 2nd ed., Philadelphia, W. B. Saunders, 1976.

253. Miller, M., et al.: Noonan syndrome in an adult family presenting with chronic lymphedema. *Amer. J. Med.* 65:379, 1978.

254. Char, F., et al.: The Noonan syndrome — a clinical study of 45 cases. In Proceedings of the Fourth Conference on the Clinical Delineation of Birth Defects. XV, The Cardiovascular System. *Birth Defects* 8:110, 1972.

255. Collins, E., et al.: The Noonan syndrome — a review of the clinical and genetic features of 27 cases. *J. Pediatr.* 83:941, 1973.

256. Jones, H. W., and Scott, W. W.: *Hermaphroditism, Genital Anomalies, and Related Endocrine Disorders.* 2nd ed. Baltimore, Williams & Wilkins Co., 1971.

257. van Niekerk, W. A.: True hermaphroditism. An analytic review with a report of 3 new cases. *Amer. J. Obstet. Gynecol.* 126:890, 1976.

258. van Niekerk, W. A.: *True Hermaphrodism.* Hagerstown, Harper and Row, 1974.

259. Kim, M. H., et al.: Pregnancy in a true hermaphrodite("es"). *Obstet. Gynecol.* 53(3 Suppl.):40S, 1979.

260. Shannon, R., and Nicolaides, N. J.: True hermaphrodism with oogenesis and spermatogenesis. *Aust. N. Z. J. Obstet Gynecol.* 13:184, 1973.

261. Armendares, S., et al: Familial true hermaphrodism in three siblings: Clinical, cytogenetic, histologic and hormonal studies. *Humangenetik* 29:99, 1975.

262. Aiman, J., et al.: Production and origin of estrogen in two true hermaphrodites. *Amer. J. Obstet. Gynecol.* 132:401, 1978.

263. Benirschke, K., et al.: True hermaphroditism and chimerism. *Amer. J. Obstet. Gynecol.* 113:449, 1972.

264. Gartler, S. M.: An XX/XY human hermaphrodite resulting from double fertilization. *Proc. Natl. Acad. Sci.* 48:332, 1962.

265. Josso, N.: True hermaphrodism with XX/XY mosaicism, probably due to double fertilization of the ovum. *J. Clin. Endocrinol. Metab.* 25:114, 1965.

266. Tarkowski, A. K.: Mouse chimera developed from fused eggs. *Nature (London)* 190:857, 1961.

267. Winters, S. J., et al.: H-Y antigen mosaicism in the gonad of a 46,XX true hermaphrodite. *N. Engl. J. Med.* 300:745, 1979.

268. Wachtel, S. S., and Hall, J. L.: H-Y binding in the gonad: Inhibition by a supernatant of the fetal ovary. *Cell* 17:327, 1979.

269. Fraccaro, M., et al.: Familial XX true hermaphrodism and the H-Y antigen. *Hum. Genet.* 48:45, 1979.

270. Clayton, G. W., et al.: Familial true hermaphrodism in pre- and post-pubertal genetic females. Hormonal and morphological studies. *J. Clin. Endocrinol. Metab.* 18:1349, 1958.

271. Mori, Y., and Mitzutami, S.: Familial true hermaphrodism in genetic females. *Jpn. J. Urol.* 59:857, 1968.

272. Berger, R., et al.: Hermaphrodisme vrai et <<Garcon XX>> dans une fratrie. *Rev. Eur. Etud. Clin. Biol.* 15:330, 1970.

273. Kasdan, R., et al.: Paternal transmission of maleness in XX human beings. *N. Engl. J. Med.* 288:539, 1973.

274. Schwartz, I. S.: Dysgerminoma of the ovary associated with true hermaphroditism. *Obst. Gynecol.* 56:102, 1980.

275. Barr, M. L., et al.: The triple-X female. An appraisal based on a study of 12 cases and a review of the literature. *Can. Med. Assoc. J.* 101:247, 1969.

276. Nielsen, J., et al.: Women with tetra-X (48,XXXX). *Hereditas* 85:151, 1977.

277. Collen, R. J., et al.: A 48,XXXX female with absent ovaries. *Amer. J. Med. Genet.* 6:275, 1980.

278. Cirillo-Silengo, M., et al.: The 49,XXXXX syndrome. Report of a case with 48,XXXX/49,XXXXX mosaicism. *Acta Paediatr. Scand.* 68:769, 1979.

279. Toussi, T., et al.: Renal hypodysplasia and unilateral ovarian agenesis in the penta-X syndrome. *Amer. J. Med. Genet.* 6:153, 1980.

280. Sandberg, A. A., et al.: An XYY human male. *Lancet, 2*:488, 1961.

281. Hook, E. B.: Extra sex chromosome and human behavior: The nature of the evidence regarding XYY, XXY, XXXY, and XXX genotypes. In *Genetic Mechanisms of Sexual Development.* Vallet, H. L., and Porter, I. (eds.), New York, Academic Press, 1979.

282. Owen, D. R.: Psychological studies in XYY men. In *Genetic Mechanisms of Sexual Development.* Vallet, H. L., and Porter, I. (eds.), New York, Academic Press, 1979.

283. Ridler, M. A. C., et al.: An adult male with XYYY sex chromosomes. *Clin. Genet.* 4:69, 1973.

284. Melicow, M. M., and Uson, A. C.: Dysgenetic gonadomas and other gonadal neoplasms in intersexes: Report of 5 cases and review of the literature. *Cancer 12*:522, 1959.

285. Schellhas, F.: Malignant potential of the dysgenetic gonad. *Obstet. Gynecol. 44*:298 (Part I) and 455 (Part II), 1974.

286. Simpson, J. L., and Photopulas, G.: The relationship of neoplasia to disorders of abnormal sexual differentiation. In *Cancer and Genetics, Birth Defects: Orig. Art. Ser. 12*(1):15, 1976.

287. Manuel, M., et al.: The age of occurrence of gonadal tumors in intersex patients with a Y chromosome. *Amer. J. Obstet. Gynecol. 124*:293, 1976.

288. Scully, R. E.: Gonadoblastoma. A review of 74 cases. *Cancer 25*:1340, 1970.

289. Mostafi, F. K., et al.: Testicular tumors: Epidemiologic, etiologic and pathologic features. *Cancer 32*:1186, 1973.

290. Gehring, G. G., et al.: Malignant degeneration of cryptorchid testes following orchiopexy. *J. Urol. 112*:354, 1974.

291. Hinman, F. Jr.: Unilateral abdominal cryptorchidism. *J. Urol. 122*:715, 1979.

292. Leavitt, S., et al.: The impalpable testis: A rational approach to management. *J. Urol. 120*:515, 1978.

293. Hinman, F. Jr.: Orchiopexy: Contraindications. *Amer. J. Surg. 138*:37, 1979.

294. Sogge, M. R., et al.: The malignant potential of the dysgenetic germ cell in Klinefelter's syndrome. *Amer. J. Med. 66*:515, 1979.

295. Greenblatt, R. B., et al.: The spectrum of gonadal dysgenesis: A clinical, cytogenetic and pathologic study. *Amer. J. Obstet. Gynecol. 98*:151, 1967.

296. Goldberg, M. B., et al.: Gonadal dysgenesis in phenotypic female subjects: A review of 87 cases, with cytogenetic studies in 53. *Amer. J. Med. 45*:529, 1968.

297. Patel, S. K., and Prentice, S. A.: Gonadoblastoma, distinctive ovarian tumor. *Arch. Pathol. 94*:165, 1972.

298. Warren, J. C., et al.: Hilus cell adenoma in a dysgenetic gonad with XX/XO mosaicism. *Lancet 1*:141, 1964.

299. Boczkowski, K., et al.: Sibship occurrence of XY gonadal dysgenesis with dysgerminoma. *Amer. J. Obstet. Gynecol. 113*:952, 1972.

300. Isurugi, K., et al.: Prepubertal XY gonadal dysgenesis. *Pediatrics 59*:569, 1977.

301. Bongiovanni, A. M.: Congenital adrenal hyperplasia and related conditions. In *Metabolic Basis of Inherited Disease.* 4th ed. Stanbury, J. B., and Wyngaarden, J. B., et al. (eds.), New York, McGraw-Hill, 1977.

302. Migeon, C. J.: Diagnosis and treatment of adrenogenital disorders. In *Endocrinology.* Vol. 2, De Groot, L. (ed.), New York, Grune & Stratton, 1979.

303. Goldman, A. S.: Animal models of inborn errors of steroidogenesis and steroid action. In *Colloq. Biol. Chem. Sect. 2. Reproduction.* Gibian, H., and Plotz, E. J. (eds), 1970.

304. Childs, B., et al.: Virilizing adrenal hyperplasia: A genetic and hormonal study. *J. Clin. Invest. 35*:213, 1956.

305. Levine, L. S., et al.: Genetic mapping of the 21-hydroxylase deficiency gene within the HLA linkage group. *N. Engl. J. Med. 299*:911, 1979.

306. New, M. I., et al.: An update of congenital adrenal hyperplasia. *Recent Prog. Hormone Res.* (in press).

307. Hirschfeld, A. J., and Fleshman, J. K.: An unusually high incidence of salt-losing congenital adrenal hyperplasia in the Alaskan Eskimo. *J. Pediatr. 75*:492, 1969.

308. Kowarski, A., et al.: Aldosterone secretion rate in congenital adrenal hyperplasia: A discussion of the theories on the pathogenesis of the salt-losing form of the syndrome. *J. Clin. Invest. 44*:1505, 1965.

309. Styne, D. M., et al.: Growth pattern in CAH: Correlation of glucocorticoid therapy with stature. In *Congenital Adrenal Hyperplasia.* Lee, P. A., Plotnick, L. P., and Kowarski, A. A. (eds), Baltimore, University Park Press, 1975.

310. Levine, L. S., et al.: Cryptic 21-hydroxylase deficiency in families of patients with classical adrenal hyperplasia. *J. Clin. Endocrinol. Metabl. 51*:1316, 1980.

311. Jenner, M. R., et al.: Plasma 17-OH progesterone in maternal and umbilical cord plasma in children and in congenital adrenal hyperplasia (CAH): Application to neonatal diagnosis of CAH. (Abst.) *Pediatr. Res. 4*:380, 1970.

312. Pang, S., et al.: Serum androgen concentrations in neonates and young infants with congenital adrenal hyperplasia due to 21 hydroxylase deficiency. *Clin. Endocrinol. 11*:575, 1979.

313. Frasier, S. D., et al.: Elevated amniotic fluid concentration of 17α-hydroxyprogesterone in congenital adrenal hyperplasia. (Letters to the editor.) *J. Pediatr. 86*:310, 1975.

314. Pollack, M., et al.: Prenatal diagnosis of CAH due to 21 hydroxylase deficiency by HLA typing of amniotic fluid cells. (Abst.) *Pediatr. Res. 13*:384, 1979.

315. Richards, G. E., et al.: Plasma sex steroids and gonadotropins in pubertal girls with CAH: Relation to menstrual disorders. In *Congenital Adrenal Hyperplasia.* Lee, P. A., Plotnick, L., and Kowarski, A. A. et al. (eds.), Baltimore, University Park Press, 1975.

316. Horner, J., and Hintz, R.: The role of renin and angiotensin in salt-losing, 21 hydroxylase deficient congenital adrenal hyperplasia. *J. Clin. Endocrinol. Metab. 48*:776, 1979.

317. Urban, M. D., et al.: Adult height and fertility in men with congenital virilizing adrenal hyperplasia. *N. Engl. J. Med. 299*:1392, 1978.

318. Brook, C. G. D., et al.: Experience with long-term therapy in congenital adrenal hyperplasia. *J. Pediatr. 85*:12, 1974.

319. Klingensmith, G. J., et al.: Glucocorticoid treatment of girls with congenital adrenal hyperplasia: Effects on height, sexual maturation and fertility. *J. Pediatr. 90*:996, 1977.

320. Sotiropoulos, A., et al.: Long term assessment of genital reconstruction in female pseudohermaphrodites. *J. Urol. 115*:599, 1976.

321. Eberlein, W. R., and Bongiovanni, A. M.: Congenital adrenal hyperplasia with hypertension: Unusual steroid pattern in blood and urine. *J. Clin. Endocrinol. Metab. 15*:1531, 1955.

322. Cathelineau, G., et al.: Adrenocortical 11-β-hydroxylation defect in adult women with post menarcheal onset of symptoms. *J. Clin. Endocrinol. Metab. 51*:287, 1980.

323. Holcombe, J. A., et al.: Neonatal salt loss in the hypertensive form of congenital adrenal hyperplasia. *Pediatrics 65*:777, 1980.

324. Bongiovanni, A. M.: The adrenogenital syndrome with deficiency of 3-β-hydroxysteroid dehydrogenase. *J. Clin. Invest. 41*:2086, 1964.

325. Rosenfield, R. L., et al.: Pubertal presentation of congenital Δ⁵-3β-hydroxysteroid dehydrogenase deficiency. *J. Clin. Endocrinol. Metab. 51*:345, 1980.

326. Biglieri, E. G., et al.: 17-hydroxylation deficiency in man. *J. Clin. Invest. 45*:1946, 1966.

327. Goldsmith, O., et al.: Hypogonadism and mineralocorticoid excess: The 17-hydroxylase syndrome. *N. Engl. J. Med. 277*:673, 1967.

328. Miura, K., et al.: A case of glucocorticoid-responsive hyperaldosteronism. *J. Clin. Endocrinol. Metab. 28*:1807, 1968.

329. Mallin, S. R., et al.: Congenital adrenal hyperplasia secondary to 17 hydroxylase deficiency: Two sisters with amenorrhea, hypokalemia, hypertension and cystic ovaries. *Ann. Int. Med. 70*:69, 1969.

330. Linquette, M., et al.: Déficit en 17-hydroxylase: A propose d'une observation. *Annales d'Endocrinol* (Paris) *32*:574, 1971.

331. Tronchette, F., et al.: Troubles surréno ovariens par déficit enzymatiques. *Actualities Endocrinologiques 13 eme Serie.* L'Expansion Editions (Paris), 1973, pp. 78–88.

332. Heremans, G. F. P., et al.; Female phenotype in a male child due to 17α-hydroxylase deficiency. *Arch. Dis. Child. 51*:721, 1976.

333. New, M. I.: Male pseudohermaphrodism due to 17α-hydroxylase deficiency. *J. Clin. Invest. 49*:1930, 1970.

334. Koizumi, S., et al.: Cholesterol side-chain cleavage enzyme activity and cytochrome P-450 content in adrenal mitochondria of a patient with congenital lipoid adrenal hyperplasia (Prader disease). *Clin. Chem. Acta 77*:301, 1977.

335. Prader, A., and Gurtner, H. P.: Das Syndrom des Pseudohermaphroditismus masculinus bei kongenitaler Nebennierenrinden-Hyperplasia ohne Androgenuberproduktion (adrenaler Pseudohermaphroditismus masculinus). *Helv. Paediatr. Acta 10*:397, 1955.

336. O'Doherty, N. J.: Lipoid adrenal hyperplasia. *Guy's Hospital Rep. 113*:368, 1963.

337. Moragas, A., and Ballaheja, A.: Congenital lipoid adrenal hyperplasia of the fetal adrenal gland. *Helv. Paediatr. Acta 24*:226, 1969.

338. Tsutsui, Y., et al.: An autopsy case of congenital lipoid hyperplasia of the adrenal cortex. *Acta Pathol. Jap. 20*:227, 1970.

339. Camacho, A. M.: Congenital adrenal hyperplasia due to a deficiency of one of the enzymes involved in biosynthesis of pregnenolone. *J. Clin. Endocrinol. Metab. 28*:153, 1968.

340. Kirkland, R. T., et al.: Congenital lipoid adrenal hyperplasia in an eight year old phenotypic female. *J. Clin. Endocrinol. Metab. 56*:488, 1973.

341. Grumbach, M. M., et al.: On the fetal masculinizing action of certain oral progestins. *J. Clin. Endocrinol. Metab. 19*:1369, 1959.

342. Grumbach, M. M., and Ducharme, J. R.: The effects of androgens on fetal sexual development: Androgen-induced female pseudohermaphrodism. *Fertil. Steril. 11*:157, 1960.

343. Wilkens, L.: Masculinization of the female fetus due to the use of orally given progestins. *J.A.M.A. 172*:1028, 1960.

344. Ishizuka, N., et al.: Statistical observations in genital anomalies of newborns following the administration of progestin to their mothers. *Obstet. Gynecol. Surv. 19*:496, 1964.

345. Bongiovanni, A. M., et al.: Masculinization of the female infant asso-

ciated with estrogen therapy alone during gestation. Four cases. *J. Clin. Endocrinol. Metab.* 19:1004, 1959.

346. Herbst, A. L., et al.: Clear cell adenocarcinoma of the genital tract in young females. *N. Engl. J. Med.* 287:1259, 1972.

347. Mürset, G., et al.: Male external genitalia of a girl caused by a virilizing adrenal tumor in the mother. *Acta Endocrinol.* 65:627, 1970.

348. Novak, D. J., et al.: Virilization during pregnancy. *Amer. J. Med.* 49:281, 1970.

349. Kai, H., et al.: Female pseudohermaphrodism caused by maternal congenital adrenal hyperplasia. *J. Pediatr.* 95:418, 1979.

350. Malinak, L. R., et al.: Bilateral multicentric ovarian luteomas of pregnancy associated with masculinization of a female infant. *Amer. J. Obstet. Gynecol.* 91:251, 1965.

351. Hensleigh, P. A., et al.: Fetal protection against masculinization with hyperreactio luteinalis and virilization. *J. Clin. Endocrinol. Metab.* 40:816, 1975.

352. Park, I. J., et al.: Special female hermaphroditism associated with multiple disorders. *Obstet. Gynecol.* 39:100, 1972.

353. Carpentier, P. J., et al.: Nuclear sex and genital malformations in 48 cases of renal agenesis, with especial reference to non-specific female pseudohermaphrodism. *Amer. J. Obstet. Gynecol.* 78:235, 1959.

354. Fraser, G. R.: Our genetical "load." A review of some aspects of genetic malformations. *Ann. Hum. Genet.* 25:387, 1962.

355. Berthezéne, F., et al.: Leydig cell agenesis: a cause of male pseudohermaphroditism. *N. Engl. J. Med.* 295:969, 1976.

356. Brown, D., et al.: Leydig cell hypoplasia: A cause of male pseudohermaphrodism. *J. Clin. Endocrinol. Metab.* 46:1, 1978.

357. Perez-Palacios, G., et al.: Inherited deficiency of gonadotropin receptors in Leydig cells: A new form of male pseudohermaphrodism. (Abst). *Amer. J. Hum. Genet.* 27:71a, 1975.

358. Bardin, C. W., et al.: Androgen metabolism and mechanism of action in male pseudohermaphrodism: A study of testicular feminization (Part II). *Rec. Prog. Horm. Res.* 29:65, 1973.

359. Grumbach, M. M., and Van Wyk, J.: Disorders of sex differentiation. In *Textbook of Endocrinology.* 5th Ed., Williams, R. H., (ed), Philadelphia, W. B. Saunders Co., 1974.

360. Jänne, O., et al.: Plasma and urinary steroids in an eight-year-old boy with 3β-hydroxysteroid dehydrogenease deficiency. *J. Clin. Endocrinol. Metab.* 31:162, 1970.

361. Zachmann, M., et al.: Unusual type of congenital adrenal hyperplasia probably due to deficiency of 3β-hydroxysteroid dehydrogenase. Case report of a surviving girl and steroid studies. *J. Clin. Endocrinol. Metab.* 30:719, 1970.

362. Parks, G. A., et al.: Pubertal boy with the 3β-hydroxysteroid dehydrogenase defect. *J. Clin. Endocrinol. Metab.* 33:269, 1971.

363. Kenny, F. M., et al.: Partial 3β-hydroxysteroid dehydrogenase (3β-HSD) deficiency in a family with congenital adrenal hyperplasia: Evidence for increasing 3β-HSD activity with age. *Pediatrics* 48:756, 1971.

364. Jänne, O., et al.: Testicular endocrine function in a pubertal boy with 3β-hydroxysteroid dehydrogenase deficiency. *J. Clin. Endocrinol. Metab.* 39:206, 1974.

365. Schneider, G., et al.: Persistent testicular Δ⁵-isomerase-3β-hydroxysteroid dehydrogenase (Δ⁵-3β-HSD deficiency in the Δ⁵-3β-HSD form of congenital adrenal hyperplasia. *J. Clin. Invest.* 55:681, 1975.

366. Mantero, F., et al.: Hypertension artérielle, alcalose hypokaliemique et pseudohermaphrodisme mâle par défit en 17α-hydroxylase. *Schweiz. Med. Wochenschr.* 101:38, 1971.

367. Bricaire, H., et al.: A new male pseudohermaphroditism associated with hypertension due to a block of 17α-hydroxylation. *J. Clin. Endocrinol. Metab.* 35:67, 1972.

368. Alvarez, M. N., et al.: Male pseudohermaphroditism due to 17α-hydroxylase deficiency in two siblings. *Pediatr. Res.* (Abstract) 7:325, 1973.

369. Kershnar, A. K., et al.: Studies in a phenotypic female with 17α hydroxylase deficiency. *J. Pediatr.* 89:395, 1976.

370. Tourniaire, J., et al.: Male pseudohermaphroditism with hypertension due to a 17α-hydroxylation deficiency. *Clin. Endocrinol.* 5:53, 1976.

371. Ito, S.: The 17α-hydroxylase deficiency found in genotypically female and male siblings both phenotypically female. *Jap. J. Hum. Genet.* 21:247, 1977.

372. Zachmann, M., et al.: Steroid 17,20-desmolase deficiency. A new cause of male pseudohermaphroditism. *Clin. Endocrinol.* 1:369, 1972.

373. Goebelsmann, U., et al.: Male pseudohermaphrodism consistent with 17,20-desmolase deficiency. *Gynecol. Invest.* 7:138, 1976.

374. Saez, J. M., et al.: Familial male pseudohermaphroditism with gynecomastia due to a testicular 17-ketosteroid reductase defect. I. Studies *in vivo. J. Clin. Endocrinol. Metab.* 32:604, 1971.

375. Saez, J. M., et al.: Further *in vivo* studies in male pseudohermaphroditism with gynecomastia due to a testicular 17-ketosteroid reductase defect (compared to a case of testicular feminization). *J. Clin. Endocrinol. Metab.* 34:598, 1972.

376. Goebelsmann, U., et al.: Male pseudohermaphroditism due to testicular 17β-hydroxysteroid dehydrogenase deficiency. *J. Clin. Endocrinol. Metab.* 36:867, 1973.

377. Knorr, D., et al.; Reifenstein's syndrome, a 17β-hydroxysteroid oxydoreductase deficiency? *Acta Endocrinol.* (Kbh) (Suppl) 173:37, 1973.

378. Tourniaire, J., et al.: Pseudohermaphrodisme male familial par déficit testiculaire en 17-ceto-steroide-réductase. *Ann. Endocrinol.* 34:440, 1973.

379. Givens, J. R., et al.: Familial male pseudohermaphroditism without gynecomastia due to deficient testicular 17-ketosteroid reductase activity. *N. Engl. J. Med.* 291:938, 1974.

380. Zübrugg, R.: Inborn errors in testosterone biosynthesis with special reference to 17-oxosteroid reductase deficiency. *Helv. Paediatr. Acta* 29(Suppl 34:63), 1974.

381. Goebelsmann, U., et al.: *In vitro* steroid metabolic studies in testicular 17β-reduction deficiency. *J. Clin. Endocrinol. Metab.* 41:1136, 1975.

382. Harkness, R. A., et al.: 17β-hydroxysteroid oxydoreductase deficiency causing male pseudohermaphrodism in a child. *J. Endocrinol.* 67:16, 1975.

383. Schiason, G., and Sitruk, L. R.: Male pseudohermaphrodism due to a testicular 17-ketosteroid reductase deficiency. *Horm. Metabl. Res.* 8:307, 1976.

384. Pittaway, D. E., et al.: Deficient 17β-hydroxysteroid oxidoreductase activity in testes from a male pseudohermaphrodite. *J. Clin. Endocrinol. Metab.* 43:457, 1976.

385. Akesode, F. E., et al.: Male pseudohermaphrodism with gynecomastia due to testicular 17-ketosteroid reductase deficiency. *Clin. Endocrinol.* 7:443, 1977.

386. Reiter, E. O., et al.: Pubertal onset of gynecomastia and virilization in phenotypic females with male pseudohermaphroditism due to a deficiency of testicular 17β-hydroxysteroid oxidoreductase. (in press)

387. Levine, L. S., et al.: Male pseudohermaphroditism due to 17-ketosteroid reductase deficiency diagnosed in the newborn period. (Abstract) *Pediatr. Res.* 14(4) Part 2):480, 1980.

388. Wilson, J. D., and MacDonald, P. C.: Male pseudohermaphroditism due to androgen resistance: Testicular feminization and related syndromes. In *Metabolic Base of Inherited Disease.* Stanbury, J. B. (ed.), New York, McGraw-Hill, 1978.

389. Griffen, J. E., and Wilson, J. D.: The syndrome of androgen resistance. *N. Engl. J. Med.* 302:198, 1980.

390. Morris, J. M., and Mahesh, V. B.: Further observations on the syndrome, "testicular feminization." *Amer. J. Obstet. Gynecol.* 87:731, 1963.

391. O'Leary, J. A.: Comparative studies of the gonad in testicular feminization and cryptorchidism. *Fertil. Steril.* 16:813, 1965.

392. Ferenczy, A., and Richart, R. M.: The fine structures of the gonads in the complete form of testicular feminization syndrome. *Amer. J. Obstet. Gynecol.* 113:399, 1972.

393. Madden, J. D., et al.: Clinical and endocrinologic characterization of a patient with the syndrome of incomplete testicular feminization. *J. Clin. Endocrinol. Metab.* 41:751, 1973.

394. French, F. S., et al.: Further evidence of a target organ defect in the syndrome of testicular feminization. *J. Clin. Endocrinol. Metab.* 26:493, 1966.

395. Bardin, C. W., et al.: Androgen metabolism and mechanism of action in male pseudohermaphrodism: A study of testicular feminization. *Rec. Prog. Hormone Res.* 29:65, 1973.

396. Gehring, U., et al.: Effect of the androgen-insensitivity mutation on a cytoplasmic receptor for dihydrotestosterone. *Nature (New Biol.)* 232:106, 1971.

397. Goldstein, J. L., and Wilson, J D.: Studies on the pathogenesis of the pseudohermaphroditism in the mouse with testicular feminization. *J. Clin. Invest.* 51:1647, 1972.

398. Keenan, B. S., et al.: Syndrome of androgen insensitivity in man: Absence of 5α-dihydrotestosterone binding protein in skin fibroblasts. *J. Clin. Endocrinol. Metab.* 38:1143, 1974.

399. Amrhein, J. A., et al.: Androgen insensitivity in man: Evidence for genetic heterogeneity. *Proc. Natl. Acad. Sci. USA* 73:891, 1976.

400. Kaufman, M., et al.: Complete androgen insensitivity with a normal amount of 5α-dihydrotestosterone-binding activity in labium majus skin fibroblasts. *Amer. J. Med. Genet.* 4:401, 1979.

401. Migeon, C. J., et al.: The syndrome of androgen insensitivity in man: Its relation to our understanding of male sex differentiation. In *Genetic Mechanisms of Sexual Development.* Vallet, H. L., and Porter, I. (eds.), New York, Academic Press, 1979.

402. Griffen, J. E., and Wilson, J. D.: Studies on the pathogenesis of the incomplete forms of androgen resistance in man. *J. Clin. Endocrinol. Metab.* 45:1137, 1977.

403. Collier, M. E., et al.: Intranuclear binding of [³H] dihydrotestosterone by cultured human fibroblasts. *Endocrinology* 103:1499, 1978.

404. Griffen, J. E.: Testicular feminization associated with a thermolabile

androgen receptor in cultured fibroblasts. *J. Clin. Invest. 64*:1624, 1979.

405. Pinsky, L.: Androgen insensitivity (AI) due to a kinetically abnormal 5α-dihydrotestosterone receptor. (Abstract 344) *Pediatr. Res. 14*:483, 1980.

406. Tremblay, R. R., et al.: Plasma concentration of testosterone, dihydrotestosterone, testosterone-oestradiol binding globulin, and pituitary gonadrotropins in the syndrome of male pseudohermaphroditism with testicular feminization. *Acta Endocrinol. 70*:331, 1972.

407. MacDonald, P. C., et al.: Origin of estrogen in normal men and in women with testicular feminization. *J. Clin. Endocrinol. Metab. 49*:905, 1979.

408. Kelch, R. P., et al.: Estradiol and testosterone secretion by human, simian, and canine testes, in males with hypogonadism and in male pseudohermaphrodites with the feminizing testes syndrome. *J. Clin. Invest. 51*:824, 1972.

409. Faiman, C., and Winter, J. S. D.: The control of gonadotropin secretion in complete testicular feminization. *J. Clin. Endocrinol. Metab. 39*:631, 1974.

410. Boyar, R. M., et al.: Studies on gonadrotropin-gonadal dynamics in patients with androgen insensitivity. *J. Clin. Endocrinol. Metab. 47*:1116, 1978.

411. Aiman, J., et al.: Androgen insensitivity as a cause of infertility in otherwise normal men. *N. Engl. J. Med. 300*:223, 1979.

412. Reifenstein, E. C., Jr.: Hereditary familial hypogonadism. *Clin. Res. 3*:86, 1947.

413. Bowen, P., et al.: Hereditary male pseudohermaphroditism with hypogonadism, hypospadias, and gynecomastia (Reifenstein's syndrome). *Ann. Intern. Med. 62*:252, 1965.

414. Wilson, J. D., et al.: Familial incomplete male pseudohermaphrodism, type I. *N. Engl. J. Med. 290*:1097, 1974.

415. Griffin, J. E., et al.: Dihydrotestosterone binding by cultured human fibroblasts: Comparison of cells from control subjects and from patients with hereditary male pseudohermaphroditism due to androgen resistance. *J. Clin. Invest. 57*:1342, 1976.

416. Amrhein, J. A., et al.: Partial androgen insensitivity: The Reifenstein syndrome revisited. *N. Engl. J. Med. 297*:350, 1977.

417. Keenan, B. S., et al.:Male pseudohermaphroditism with partial androgen insensitivity. *Pediatrics 59*:224, 1977.

418. Nowakowski, H., and Lenz, W.: Genetic aspects in male hypogonadism. In *Recent Progress in Hormone Research*. Pincus, G. (ed.), *17*:53, 1961.

419. Walsh, P. C., et al.: Familial incomplete male pseudohermaphroditism, type II: Decreased dihydrotestosterone formation in pseudovaginal perineoscrotal hypospadias. *N. Engl. J. Med. 291*:944, 1974.

420. Imperato-McGinley, J. L., et al.: Steroid 5α-reductase deficiency in man: An inherited form of male pseudohermaphrodism. *Science 186*:1213, 1974.

421. Imperato-McGinley, J. L., and Peterson, R. E.: Male pseudohermaphroditism: The complexities of male phenotypic development. *Amer. J. Med. 61*:251, 1976.

422. Peterson, R. E., et al.: Male pseudohermaphroditism due to steroid 5α-reductase deficiency. *Amer. J. Med. 62*:170, 1977.

423. Peterson, R. E., et al.: Hereditary steroid 5α-reductase deficiency: A newly recognized cause of male pseudohermaphrodism. In *Genetic Mechanisms of Sexual Development*. Vallet, H. L., and Porter, I. H. (eds.), New York, Academic Press, 1979.

424. Pang, S., et al.: Dihydrotestosterone and its relationship to testosterone in infancy and childhood. *J. Clin. Endocrinol. Metab. 48*:821, 1979.

425. Fisher, L. K., et al.: Clinical, endocrinological, and enzymatic characterization of two patients with 5α-reductase deficiency: Evidence that a single enzyme is responsible for the 5α-reduction of cortisol and testosterone. *J. Clin. Endocrinol. Metab. 47*:653, 1978.

426. Saenger, P., et al.: Prepubertal diagnosis of steroid 5α-reductase deficiency. *J. Clin. Endocrinol. Metab. 46*:627, 1978.

427. Pinsky, L., et al.: 5α-reductase activity of genital and nongenital skin fibroblasts from patients with 5α-reductase deficiency, androgen insensitivity or unknown forms of male psueodhermaphrodism. *Amer. J. Med. Genet. 1*:407, 1978.

428. Griffen, J. E., and Wilson, J. D.: Hereditary male pseudohermaphroditism. *Clinics in Obstetrics and Gynecology 5*:457, 1978.

429. Simpson, J. L.: Male pseudohermaphrodism: Genetics and clinical delineation. *Hum. Genet. 44*:1, 1978.

430. Rajfer, J., et al.: Dysgenetic male psueodhermaphrodism. *J. Urol. 119*:525, 1978.

431. Bain, A. D., and Scott, J. S.: Renal agenesis and severe urinary tract dysplasia. A review of 50 cases, with particular reference to the associated anomalies. *Brit. Med. J. 1*:841, 1960.

432. Drash, A., et al.: A syndrome of psueodhermaphroditism, Wilm's tumor, hypertension and degenerative renal disease. *J. Pediatr. 76*:585, 1970.

433. Barakat, A. Y., et al.: Pseudohermaphroditism, nephron disorder, and Wilm's tumor: A unifying concept. *Pediatrics 54*:366, 1974.

434. Gotloib, L., et al.: Infantile nephrotic syndrome due to glomerulonephritis in a male pseudohermaphrodite. *Israel J. Med. Sci. 12*:52, 1976.

435. Cleary, R. E., et al.: Endocrine and metabolic studies in a patient with male pseudohermaphrodism and true agonadism. *Amer. J. Obstet. Gynecol. 128*:862, 1977.

436. Sarto, G. E., and Opitz, J. M.: The XY gonadal agenesis syndrome. *J. Med. Genet. 10*:288, 1973.

437. Edman, C. D., et al.: Embryonic testicular regression. A clinical spectrum of XY agonadal individuals. *Obstet. Gynecol. 49*:208, 1977.

438. Coulam, C. B.: Testicular regression syndrome. *Obstet. Gynecol. 53*:44, 1979.

439. Goldberg, L. M., et al.: Congential absence of the testes: Anorchism and monorchism. *J. Urol. 111*:840, 1974.

440. Hall, J. G., et al.: Familial congenital anorchia. In *Genetic Forms of Hypogonadism Birth Defects: Orig. Art. Ser. 11*(4):115, 1974.

441. Green, A. A., et al.: Congenital bilateral anorchia in childhood: A clinical, endocrine and therapeutic evaluation of 21 cases. *Clin. Endocrinol. 5*:381, 1976.

442. Bergada, C., et al.: Variants of embryonic testicular dysgenesis: Bilateral anorchia and the syndrome of rudimentary testes. *Acta Endocrinol.* (Copenhagen) *40*:521, 1962.

443. Najjar, S. S., et al.: The syndrome of rudimentary testes: Occurrence in five siblings. *Pediatrics 84*:119, 1974.

444. Josso, N., and Briad, M.: Embryonic testicular regression syndrome: Variable phenotypic expression in siblings. *J. Pediatr. 97*:200, 1980.

445. Brook, C. G. D., et al.: Familial occurrence of persistent müllerian structures in otherwise normal males. *Brit. Med. J. 1*:771, 1973.

446. Weiss, E. B., et al.: Persistent müllerian duct syndrome in male identical twins. *Pediatrics 61*:797, 1978.

447. Summitt, R. L.: Genetic forms of hypogonadism in the male. In *Progress in Medical Genetics*, New Series, Vol. III, 1979.

448. Courrier, R., et al.: Intersexualitié tóetale provoqué par la pregnéninolone au cours de la grossesse. *Soc. Biol.* (Paris) *136*:395, 1942.

449. Aarskog, D., : Maternal progestins as a possible cause of hypospadias. *N. Engl. J. Med. 300*:75, 1979.

450. Sweet, R. A., et al.: Study of the incidence of hypospadias in Rochester, Minnesota, 1940–1970, and a case control comparison of possible etiologic factors. *Mayo Clinic Proc. 49*:52, 1974.

451. Lorber, C. A., et al.: Is there an embryo-fetal exogenous sex steroid exposure syndrome (EFESSES)? *Fertil. Steril. 31*:21, 1979.

452. Voight, W., et al.: Further studies on testosterone 5α-reductase of human skin: Structural features of steroid inhibitors. *J. Biol. Chem. 248*:4280, 1973.

453. Kaplan, N. M.: Male pseudohermaphrodism: Report of a case, with observations on pathogenesis. *N. Engl. J. Med. 261*:641, 1959.

454. Gill, W. B., et al.: Structural and functional abnormalities in sex organs of male offspring of mothers treated with diethylstilbestrol. *J. Reprod. Med. 16*:147, 1976.

455. Henderson, B. E., et al.: Urogenital tract abnormalities in sons of women treated with diethylstilbesterol. *Pediatrics 58*:505, 1976.

456. Sörenson, H. R.: *Hypospadias with Special Reference to aetiology*. Copenhagen, Munksgaard, 1953.

457. Buyse, M., et al.: Syndromes associated with abnormal external genitalia. In *Genetic Mechanisms of Sexual Development*. Vallet, H. L., and Porter, I. H. (eds.), New York, Academic Press, 1979.

458. Aarskog, D.: Clinical and cytogenetic studies in hypospadias. *Acta Paediatr. Scand.* (Suppl) *203*:1, 1970.

459. Walsh, P. C., et al.: Clinical and endocrinological evaluation of patients with congenital microphallus. *J. Urol. 120*:90, 1978.

460. Burstein, S., et al.: Early determination of androgen-responsiveness is important to the management of microphallus. *Lancet 2*:983, 1979.

461. Lovinger, R. D., et al.: Congenital hypopituitarism associated with neonatal hypoglycemia and microphallus: Four cases secondary to hypothalamic hormone deficiency. *J. Pediatr. 87*:1171, 1975.

462. Park, I. J., et al.: A case of male pseudohermaphrodism associated with elevated LH, normal FSH and low testosterone possibly due to the secretion of an abnormal LH molecule. *Acta Endocrinol. 83*:173, 1976.

463. Meyer, W. J., et al.: Familial male pseudohermaphroditism with normal Leydig cell function at puberty. *J. Clin. Endocrinol. Metab. 46*:593, 1978.

464. Griffin, J. E., et al.: Congenital absence of the vagina. The Mayer-Robitansky-Huster-Hauser syndrome. *Ann. Intern. Med. 85*:224, 1976.

465. Pinsky, L.: A community of human malformation syndromes involving müllerian ducts, distal extremities, urinary tract and ears. *Teratology 9*:65, 1974.

466. Michels, V. V., and Caskey, C. T.: Müllerian aplasia with hypoplastic thumbs: Two case reports. *Int. J. Gynaecol. Obstet. 17*:6, 1979.

467. Ross, G. T., and van de Wiele, R. L.: The Ovaries. In *Textbook of Endocrinology*. 5th ed., Williams, R. A. (ed.). Philadelphia, W. B. Saunders, 1974.

468. Fraser, I. D., et al.: Cyclical ovarian function in women with congenital absence of the uterus and vagina. *J. Clin. Endocrinol. Metab. 36*:634, 1973.

469. Ducan, P. A., et al.: The MURSC association: Müllerian duct aplasia, renal aplasia and cervicothoracic somite dysplasia. *J. Pediatrics 95*:399, 1979.

470. Garcia, J., and Jones, H. W.: The split thickness graft technique for vaginal agenesis. *Obstet. Gynecol. 49*:328, 1977.

471. Hecker, B. R., and McGuire, L. S.: Psychosocial function in women treated for vaginal agenesis. *Amer. J. Obstet. Gynecol. 129*:453, 1977.

472. Money, J., et al.: Hermaphroditism: recommendations concerning assignment of sex, change of sex, and psychologic management. *Bull. Johns Hopkins Hosp. 97*:284, 1955.

473. Gross, R. E., et al.: Clitorectomy for sexual abnormalities: Indications and technqiues. *Surgery 59*:300, 1966.

474. Lattimer, J. K.: Relocation and recession of the enlarged clitoris with preservation of the glands: An alternative to amputation. *J. Urol. 86*:113, 1961.

475. Spense, H. M., and Allen, T. D.: Genital reconstruction in the female with adrenogenital syndrome. *Brit. J. Urol. 45*:126, 1973.

476. Shaw, A.: Subcutaneous reduction clitoroplasty. *J. Ped. Surg. 12*:331, 1977.

477. Rosenfield, R. L., et al.: The diagnosis and management of intersex. In *Current Problems in Pediatrics.* Vol. 10, #7, Gluck, L. (ed.), Year Book Medical Publishers, May 1980.

478. Masters, W. H., and Johnson, V. E.: *Human Sexual Response.* Boston, Little, Brown & Co., 1966.

479. Jones, H. W., et al.: Necessity for and the technique of secondary surgical treatment of masculinized external genitalia of patients with virilizing adrenal hyperplasia. In *Congenital Adrenal Hyperplasia.* Lee, P. A., et al. (eds.), Baltimore, University Park Press, 1977.

480. Wabrek, A. J., et al.: Creation of a neovagina by the Frank nonoperative method. *Obstet. Gynecol. 37*:408, 1971.

481. Kelalis, P. P., and King, L. R. (eds.): *Clinical Pediatric Urology.* Philadelphia, W. B. Saunders Company, 1976.

482. Milunsky, A.: *Genetic Disorders and the Fetus.* New York, Plenum Press, 1979.

483. Belisle, S., and Tulchinsky, D.: Amniotic fluid hormones. In *Maternal-Fetal Endocrinology.* Tulchinsky, D., and Ryan, K. (eds.). Philadelphia, W. B. Saunders Company, 1980.

484. Belisle, S., et al.: Amniotic fluid testosterone and follicle stimulating hormone in the determination of fetal sex. *Amer. J. Obstet. Gynecol. 128*:514, 1977.

485. Nagamani, M., et al.: Maternal and amniotic fluid 17α hydroxyprogesterone levels during pregnancy. Diagnosis of congenital adrenal hyperplasia *in utero. Amer. J. Obstet. Gynecol. 130*:791, 1978.

486. Milunsky, A., and Tulchinsky, D.: Prenatal diagnosis of congenital adrenal hyperplasia due to 21 hydroxylase deficiency. *Pediatrics 59*:768, 1977.

487. Schumert, Z., et al.: 11-deoxycortisol in amniotic fluid: Prenatal diagnosis of congenital adrenal hyperplasia due to $11\text{-}\beta$-hydroxylase deficiency. *Clin. Endocrinol. 12*:257, 1980.

488. Rösler, A., et al.: Prenatal diagnosis of $11\text{-}\beta$-hydroxylase deficiency congenital adrenal hyperplasia. *J. Clin. Endocrinol. Metab. 49*:546, 1979.

489. LeLann, D.: Diagnostic échographique antinátal du sexe masculin et feminin. *La Nouvelle Presse Medicale 8*:34, 2760, 1979.

490. Davies, J.: The fetal adrenal. In *Maternal-Fetal Endocrinology.* Tulchinsky, D., and Ryan, K. (eds.), Philadelphia, W. B. Saunders Company, 1980.

491. Ryan, K. J.: Placental synthesis of steroid hormones. In *Maternal-Fetal Endocrinology.* Tulchinsky, D., and Ryan, K. (eds.), Philadelphia, W. B. Saunders Company, 1980.

)2. Corning, H. K.: *Lehrbuch der Entwicklungsgeschichte des Menschen.* Munich, J. F. Bergmann, 1921.

493. Wilkins, L.: *The Diagnosis and Treatment of Endocrine Disorders in Childhood and Adolescence.* 3rd ed. Springfield, Ill., Charles C Thomas, 1965.

494. Arey, L. B.: *Developmental Anatomy.* 7th ed. Philadelphia, W. B. Saunders Company, 1965.

495. Witschi, E.: *Development of Vertebrates.* Philadelphia, W. B. Saunders Company, 1956.

496. Spaulding, M. H.: *Carnegie Inst. Contrib. Embryol. 13*(61):69, 1921.

CHAPTER 10

The Endocrinologic Function of Selected Autacoids: Catecholamines, Acetylcholine, Serotonin, and Histamine*

By Kenneth L. Melmon

*This work was supported in part by NIH training grant GM-07065

AUTACOIDS

In previous editions of this text, catecholamines and the adrenal medulla composed a section in one chapter, serotonin and carcinoid tumors were described in another, polypeptides were mentioned in both, and histamine was included to describe its contrasting effects to serotonin and polypeptides in patients with carcinoid tumors and in patients with mastocytosis. In this edition, these substances plus acetylcholine (ACh) will be grouped in one chapter. Their structures differ and their physiologic and pharmacologic activities are disparate, but they are grouped together here for several reasons: (1) they share common natural occurrences in the body, (2) they often have coordinated interactions that subserve physiologic and pathologic processes, (3) their direct effects often mimic or complement each other, and (4) drugs that affect the synthesis or function of one often affect the body's response to the others. This chapter thus contains a motley group of substances, all of which have endocrinologic and intense pharmacologic activity.

These different substances have been variously described as *local hormones, autopharmacologic agents,* and the like, but a generic term that is at once shorter, more accurate, and euphonious is *autacoid,* a word derived from the Greek *autos* ("self") and *akos* ("medicinal agent" or "remedy"). This term was devised by Sir Edward Schäfer in 1917,[476] later Sharpey-Schäfer, as a substitute for Starling's word *hormone,* which, being derived from the Greek *hormaein* (meaning "to stir up"), is a misnomer for the inhibitory substances that also came to be embraced by this designation. However, Starling's term *hormone,* albeit unsatisfactory from the etymologic standpoint, has won the day, and Schäfer's has passed into limbo. As Douglas has stated, such a good word deserves a better fate.[140a]

What is the significance of autacoids? What is their endocrinologic role in the body? What is their value as drugs? What is their place in therapeutics? Unfortunately, only rather imprecise answers can be given to these questions. The very fact that the substances have been classified under the noncommittal title of *autacoids* is, in a sense, a confession that current evidence does not permit a more precise and functional classification, such as, for example, hormone or neurohumor. This is not to say that such functions are foreign to the autacoids. On the contrary, as evidence concerning their possible roles in the body unfolds, it is apparent that both such functions may be displayed by the substances under consideration. But the core of the matter is that, although the autacoids possess an astonishingly wide range of physiologic and pharmacologic activities at vanishingly small concentrations (with the exception of catecholamines), there are comparatively few instances in which a physiologic role can be stated with assurance. Nevertheless, it is generally agreed that each of the autacoids to be discussed is important to the body's economy. All are agents that the body uses to execute various functions in health and disease: they clearly are part and parcel of the physiologic and pathologic phenomena that provide the rationale for drug therapy, and their existence provides numerous possibilities for therapeutic intervention by the use of drugs that mimic or antagonize their action or interfere in one way or another with their metabolism.[140a]

CATECHOLAMINES

Catecholamines are dihydroxylated phenolic amines. The most prominent members of this family are 3, 4-dihydroxyphenethylamine (dopamine), norepinephrine, and epinephrine (Fig. 10-1). Each of the three has different and characteristic physiologic functions, pharmacologic actions, sites of production, and pathways of metabolism. As a group they are synthesized in the brain, in sympathetic nerve ends, and in cells of neural crest origin throughout the body. This chapter will focus on the dynamics and effects of these autacoids in areas outside of the brain. In Ch. 11 their role in central nervous system (CNS) endocrinology will be discussed. When released from storage sites in nerve endings and in the adrenal medulla, they have profound effects on smooth muscle, adipose tissue, myocardium, liver, brain, formed elements of the blood, a number of hormone-producing organs, and myometrium. All effects are exaggerated when catecholamines are administered or released in unusually large quantities. During certain diseases small quantities may produce an exaggerated effect, as, for instance, in patients with sympathetic denervation of any cause, including neurogenic orthostatic hypotension,[333, 401, 404, 615] cardiomyopathies, or some dietary deficiency syndromes. Conversely, the effects of catecholamines are diminished in patients with endocrinopathies such as myxedema and Addison's disease. Alterations of responses in diseases such as asthma may be a reflection of an abnormal complement of receptors, caused by treating the patients with drugs,[193] or apparent abnormalities of tissue responsiveness to catecholamines.[244]

In the last 25 years scientists have elucidated the biochemical nature, the modes of synthesis and degradation, and the physiologic significance of catecholamines, as well as the pathologic changes they induce. All the enzymes involved in the synthesis of catecholamines have been isolated. Characterization of the enzymes has permitted identification of rate-limiting steps and observations on responses to drugs that interfere with catecholamine synthesis, breakdown, or peripheral effects. The information integrated from these sources has enabled us to distinguish between drugs that interfere with the catecholamine effects or synthesis and drugs that must be incorporated into the pathways of synthesis and transformed to false neurotransmitters before they can produce pharmacologic effects. We can now undertake a rational and methodical search for agents that can predictably alter catechol synthesis, release, or tissue response or that can produce effects that in part mimic the actions of catecholamines. In addition, we can begin to understand the symptoms, biochemical alterations, and complications produced by tumors that elaborate excessive amounts of catecholamines.

It is hard to think of any field in biology that has moved more rapidly or has been more applicable to

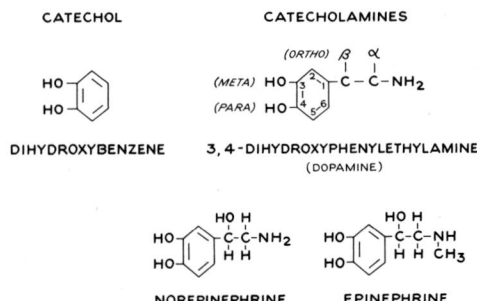

Figure 10-1. Biochemic structure of a catechol (left) and of the endogenous catecholamines (right). Carbon chain and phenolic ring positions are indicated on the dopamine structure.

humans. We now can define the molecular nature of catecholamine effects and practically can change at will the synthesis, storage, release, reuptake, metabolism, and elimination of the amines. We can even begin to change specific functions of specific amines in individual tissues.[375, 570] We also have become aware of many of the interrelationships of catecholamines with other endocrine systems, and we are attuned to the possibility of highly selective and therapeutically effective alteration of endocrine systems via perturbation of the catecholamine system. Now an endocrinologist must become familiar with all aspects of catecholamine physiology, chemistry, and pathology in order to understand the functions of many endocrine organs.

This section primarily summarizes the well-founded data on the synthesis, degradation, and pharmacologic and physiologic significance of catecholamine substances, the diseases characterized by extreme sensitivity or insensitivity to catecholamines, the unusual interrelationships between catecholamines and other biologically active substances, the diseases produced by tumors derived from cells of neural crest origin, and the rationale for the use or the avoidance of certain agents during the treatment of pheochromocytoma. In addition, the extraordinarily exciting (even if in some cases less firmly established) developments related to each of these areas are discussed. For instance, new discoveries suggest possibilities for understanding both the chemical basis and the implications of interrelationships of catecholamines with leukocytes. A feasible search for drugs that will alter autonomic nervous system function in given areas of specific organs can be initiated.

In other sections of this chapter, ACh, serotonin, and histamine are presented as mediators and modifiers of physiologic and pathologic endocrinology, and diseases characterized either by unusual production of the substances or by unusual responses to them are described.

Synthesis

Catecholamine synthesis occurs exclusively in the brain, sympathetic nerve endings, and chromaffin tissue, including the adrenal medulla, organ of Zuckerkandl, and ectopic rests of neural crest tissue. The main mammalian pathway starts with tyrosine, which usually is abundant in human tissue and is derived either from the diet (the probable main source) or via parahydroxylation of phenylalanine by phenylalanine hydroxylase, mainly in the liver (Fig. 10–2). The concentration of tyrosine in local tissue sites, particularly the brain, may modulate the production of catecholamines.[198] Only recently has the interplay between phenylalanine hydroxylase and norepinephrine been appreciated. As norepinephrine accumulates in tissues, it inhibits formation of tyrosine. The inhibition is competitive with respect to one cofactor (pteridine) and noncompetitive with respect to the substrate, phenylalanine. In diseases such as phenylketonuria, accumulation of phenylalanine may interfere with the action of tyrosine hydroxylase, the rate-limiting enzymatic step in the synthesis of catecholamines.

Subsequent steps in the mammalian synthesis of catecholamines include the meta-hydroxylation of tyrosine to 4, 5-dihydroxyphenylalanine (dopa) (by tyrosine hydroxylase), decarboxylation of dopa to dopamine (by L-amino acid decarboxylase), and β-hydroxylation of dopamine to norepinephrine (by dopamine β-oxidase). The latter step may also be rate-limiting in some circumstances but does not seem as critical as the conversion of tyrosine to dopa. Norepinephrine can be converted to epinephrine by the N-methylating enzyme, phenylethanolamine-N-methyl transferase, found only in the adrenal medulla or organ of Zuckerkandl (and in very small amounts in the brain). The regulation of each of these enzymes appears to be genetically controlled.[89] Some alternate pathways in the synthesis of catecholamines have been proposed and demonstrated in subprimates. Tyramine can be a direct precursor of catecholamines and has been found in sympathetic nerve endings[534] and in the blood of patients with cirrhosis.[168] Although many alternate pathways are postulated to exist in humans they have not been proved.

Figure 10–3 illustrates the distribution within the neuron of the enzymes for synthesis of catecholamines. Note that the rate-limiting enzyme (tyrosine hydroxylase) is located in the mitochondria within the cytoplasm and is separated from the end product of synthesis (norepinephrine) by the granules containing dopamine β-hydroxylase. The distribution of the enzymes implies that (1) sufficient quantities of tyrosine must be transported to the site of the tyrosine hydroxylase enzyme before dopa can be formed, (2) dopamine must be actively transported into the granule before norepinephrine can be synthesized, and (3) either norepinephrine must be released from the granule or extraneuronal norepinephrine must

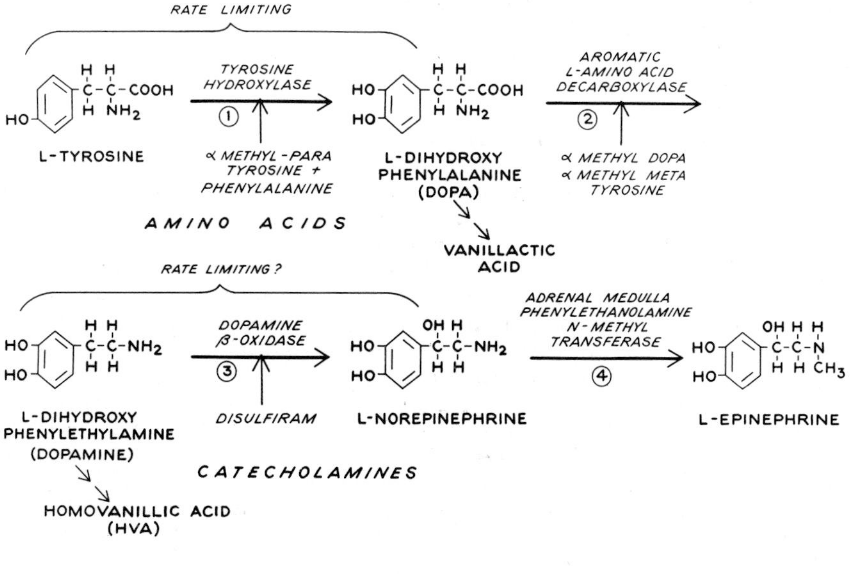

Figure 10–2. Biosynthesis of catecholamines in the brain, adrenal medulla, and sympathetic nerve endings. Rate-limiting steps are those in which only minimal inhibition of enzymes will result in significantly diminished synthesis (1 and ?3). Heavy horizontal arrows represent major steps documented in man. Vertical arrows represent inhibition of specific steps.

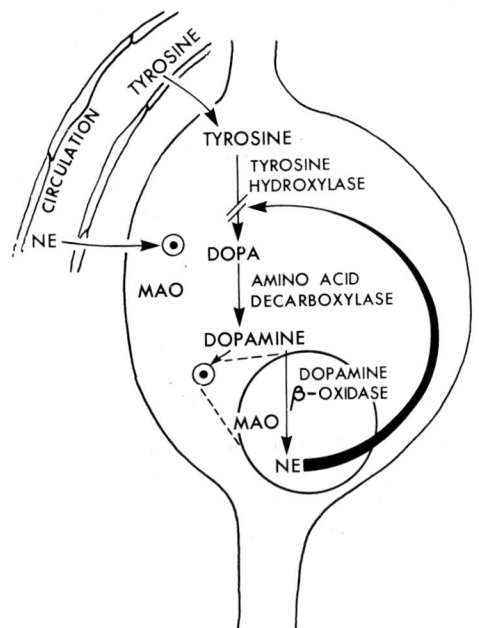

Figure 10–3. The biosynthesis of norepinephrine in the sympathetic nerve. Abbreviations: NE, norepinephrine; MAO, monoamine oxidase. (Reproduced from Axelrod, J., and Kopin, I. J. The uptake, storage, release, and metabolism of noradrenaline sympathetic nerves, In *Mechanisms of Synaptic Transmission, Progress in Brain Research*, Vol. 31. Akert, K., and Wasser, P. G. [eds.], Amsterdam, Elsevier, 1969, Fig. 2, p. 24.)

be taken up into the cytoplasm if there is to be either feedback inhibition of the rate-limiting step in synthesis or the production of epinephrine. The only important intraneuronal degradative enzyme for catecholamines is cytoplasmic monoamine oxidase (MAO).

The major pathway described previously normally occurs in all tissues that synthesize catecholamines. However, local conditions in each organ apparently regulate the rate of synthesis, release, uptake, and metabolism of the catecholamines. In most tissues, the control of synthesis depends on the rate of turnover (e.g., increased during sympathetic nerve stimulation) of catecholamines in that tissue. In brain and in the adrenal medulla, a number of physiologic factors in addition to nerve stimulation may profoundly influence rates of synthesis. For practical purposes, it is reasonable to think of the synthesis, release, effects, and metabolism of catecholamines in the CNS as being independent of their counterparts in the peripheral sympathetic nervous system. The system in the CNS is described in Ch. 11.

Tyrosine Hydroxylase

Tyrosine hydroxylase can be found in the adrenal medulla, brain, and sympathetically innervated tissues. The enzyme, purified from several tissues, including a pheochromocytoma,[420] and even crystallized from bacteria, has similar characteristics in various animal tissues. It requires oxygen to incorporate into tyrosine to form dopa, a reduced pteridine cofactor (oxygen also affects the affinity of pteridine for the enzyme), and perhaps iron (Fe^{++}). Experiments *in vitro* in which perfusions of guinea pig hearts were used demonstrated that the rates of tyrosine conversion to norepinephrine were dependent on the concentration of tyrosine and were maximal at substrate concentrations of $5 \times 10^{-4}M$ tyrosine. The apparent K_m for

the overall reaction (tyrosine → norepinephrine) was comparable to that observed for conversion of tyrosine to dopa by purified tyrosine hydroxylase.[338] When isolated guinea pig heart was perfused in turn with varying concentrations of radiolabeled tyrosine, dopa, and dopamine, the conversion to norepinephrine reached ordinary maximum rates only with the first of these substrates. Furthermore, in some studies, it was found that the actual and calculated degrees of tyrosine hydroxylase inhibition *in vivo* were almost identical, a circumstance that can only be explained if the enzyme is rate-limiting. The absence of appreciable amounts of dopa or dopamine in most sympathetically innervated tissues provides further evidence for the rate-limiting activities of tyrosine hydroxylase.

Synthesis may be slowed by manipulations other than limitation of substrate availability. The level of the pteridine cofactor may be critically controlled by shifting concentrations of dihydropteridine reductase; catecholamines at relatively low concentrations ($2 \times 10^{-5}M$) initially can markedly inhibit tyrosine hydroxylase. (The later effects actually increase the rate of formation of tyrosine hydroxylase.)[228] However, increased tissue concentrations of dihydropteridine reductase can overcome enzyme inhibition by catecholamines. Thus at least three endogenous factors seem to influence the usual rate of production of catecholamines: (1) tyrosine concentration in the intraneuronal site, which depends on an active transport system that may be altered by disease, unnatural extracellular accumulation of large quantities of alternate amino acids that may compete for the same transport system, or toxic levels of some drugs that interfere with transport; (2) concentration of the pteridine cofactor; and (3) concentration of norepinephrine in the milieu of the enzyme.

Physiologic and pharmacologic manipulations that release catecholamines from their storage sites may also influence the rate of synthesis.[593] Stimulation of the sympathetic nerves to a variety of organs releases catecholamines and may be associated with a considerable increase in synthesis of norepinephrine.[266, 505] Neither the actual depolarization of the nerve nor any blood-borne factor seems to trigger the acceleration of norepinephrine synthesis. The increased synthesis does not depend on tyrosine transport or effector organ activity. Rather, the synthesis rate appears to rise as the newly formed norepinephrine, composing the majority of readily released catecholamines, is released from the cells (Fig. 10–4).[195, 543] The increase in rate of synthesis is not necessarily accompanied by an overall depletion of intracellular norepinephrine or by an increase in the total amount of tyrosine hydroxylase in the stimulated nerve. The rapid synthesis is probably due to removal of the feedback inhibition of existing tyrosine hydroxylase as cytoplasmic (not total) concentrations of catecholamine fall. Recent information shows that cyclic 3′, 5′-adenosine monophosphate (cAMP) activation of protein kinase that phosphorylates, and thereby activates, tyrosine hydroxylase can increase production of catecholamines.[273, 442, 447, 580, 587, 594] Because there may be a panoply of receptors (including those for catecholamines) on appropriate nerve bodies that mediate production of cAMP, this mechanism is but one example of not only how the effects of one autacoid can add to the pharmacologic and physiologic effects of another autacoid but also how autacoids can modulate the rates of synthesis of each other.

When nerve stimulation is intense or protracted (hours), when nervous stimulation is provoked by drugs that block sympathetic action, or when partial chemical or surgical sympathectomy is performed, the increased

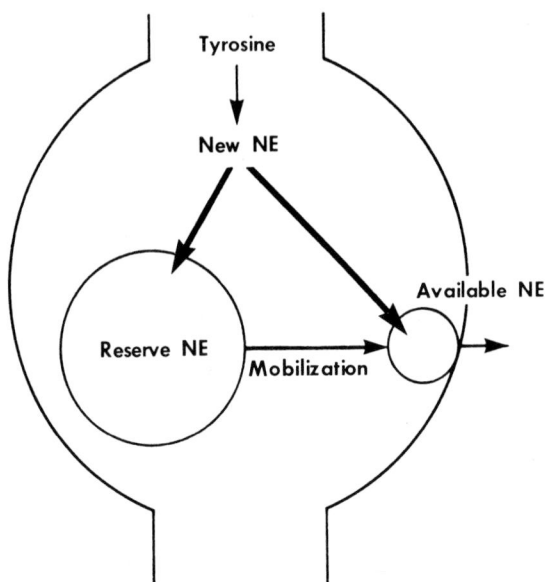

Figure 10–4. Selective release of newly synthesized norepinephrine (NE). NE, which is released by nerve stimulation, comes from a small, immediately "available" store. Both newly synthesized NE and NE mobilized from the reserve stores are used to replenish the NE in the available store. Although new NE can also enter the reserve store, it is a greater fraction of the smaller available store. (Reproduced from Axelrod, J., and Kopin, I. J. The uptake, storage, release, and metabolism of noradrenaline in sympathetic nerves, In *Mechanisms of Synaptic Transmission, Progress in Brain Research*. Vol. 31. Akert K., and Wasser, P. G. [eds.], Amsterdam, Elsevier, 1969, Fig. 4, p. 28.)

rate of catecholamine synthesis in the affected nerves or residual nervous system is accompanied by an increase in the activity of tyrosine hydroxylase.[388, 541, 616] This additional compensatory mechanism for catecholamine synthesis can be blocked by agents inhibiting protein synthesis and, therefore, presumably is due to an increase in the rate of synthesis of tyrosine hydroxylase.[391] In summary, a prime stimulatory factor in the synthesis of catecholamines probably is reduction of the concentration of cytoplasmic norepinephrine. A second factor involves increased synthesis of the rate-limiting enzyme. The molecular stimulus for increased enzyme synthesis is not known. However, several intriguing facts led Axelrod and his coworkers to suggest, and others to confirm, that in the adrenal medulla there may be a cholinergic receptor or an unidentified neurotransmitter that mediates the increase in tyrosine hydroxylase.[390, 413]

At one time it was thought that catecholamines were synthesized primarily in the nerve bodies of the sympathetic neuron and gradually migrated down the axon. Although this may be true, another explanation seems plausible. The induction of tyrosine hydroxylase by reserpine in various segments of sciatic nerves indicates a proximal to distal transport of the enzyme. The apparent rate of enzyme transport is not sufficient to account for the total increase in enzyme in the nerve terminals. Thus local synthesis *de novo* of both enzyme and catecholamines may account for the catecholamines in the nerve terminals.[542]

Once tyrosine hydroxylase was established as the rate-limiting factor in the physiologic pathway for catecholamine synthesis, progress was rapid: (1) specificity of the enzyme was found to be quite high, (2) derivatives of tyrosine were correctly predicted as inhibitors, and (3) α-methyltyrosine was discovered as a potent competitive inhibitor of catecholamine synthesis *in vitro* and *in vivo*

(Fig. 10–2).[509] In addition, halogenated derivatives of tyrosine, one a precursor of thyroid hormone (3-iodotyrosine), were found to inhibit tyrosine hydroxylase, a fact that potentially linked synthesis of thyroxine (T_4) with synthesis of catecholamines. Also, it was found that serotonergic neurons in the CNS could augment the activation of tyrosine hydroxylase,[442] while 5-halogenated tryptophan could inhibit tyrosine hydroxylase, thus linking the catecholamine pathway with serotonin. Finally, catechol derivatives themselves have significant inhibitory effects on tyrosine hydroxylase.

Aromatic L-Amino Acid Decarboxylase

Aromatic L-amino acid decarboxylase is found in large quantities in the cytoplasm of many tissues and has high affinity for a number of primary phenolic L-amino acids also found in tissues. The enzyme requires pyridoxal 5-phosphate as a cofactor. Unlike the production of dopa, which may be severely impaired by minor decreases in concentration of the substrate for tyrosine hydroxylase, decarboxylation of dopa proceeds at a high rate even when concentrations of dopa are low. Under ordinary circumstances, the rate of dopa formation by tyrosine hydroxylase cannot approach the capacity of the decarboxylase to rapidly convert the amino acid into the first catecholamine, dopamine. Because of the enzyme's high affinity for its substrate and a high V_{max} (maximum velocity), even very potent inhibitors do not decrease the rate of catecholamine synthesis *in vivo*. Therefore, the enzyme plays a negligible role in regulating the synthesis of norepinephrine.

As with inhibitors of tyrosine hydroxylase, among the earliest known decarboxylase inhibitors were derivatives of the substrate dopa (i.e., α-methyldopa and α-methyldopa hydrazine). Because the decarboxylase lacked the substrate specificity of tyrosine hydroxylase, other derivatives of native L-amino acids were tried. Thus, α-methylmetatyrosine, tryptophan derivatives, and a host of hydrazine compounds were found capable of decreasing decarboxylase activity *in vitro* and *in vivo*. Those that have proved most useful clinically are α-methyldopa and α-methyldopa hydrazine. Both drugs substantially inhibit decarboxylase activity *in vivo*, but neither used alone decreases catecholamine synthesis. An additional recent finding is that some decarboxylase inhibitors predominantly affect the enzyme in peripheral tissues but are insufficiently distributed to central nervous tissues to inhibit the enzyme there. When, for instance, α-methyldopa hydrazine is administered to humans, it blocks decarboxylase activity outside the brain. If the amino acid dopa is then administered, far more than the ordinary amount reaches the brain; less than normal amounts of dopamine and its metabolites are made in the periphery, but excessive dopa, dopamine, and metabolites accumulate in the brain.[213, 421, 508] Coadministering a peripheral inhibitor of decarboxylase with L-dopa has been therapeutic for some patients with parkinsonism; far lower doses of L-dopa are required than would be needed to manage the disease with the amino acid alone, thereby decreasing or eliminating some of the unwanted peripheral effects of L-dopa.

Dopamine β-Hydroxylase

Once dopamine has been formed, it is actively transported by an adenosine triphosphatase (ATP)–dependent mechanism into "cytoplasmic particles" present in sympathetic nerve endings and the adrenal medulla. The transport can be inhibited by norepinephrine itself.[523] The particles or granules harbor dopamine β-hydroxylase, a copper-containing mixed-function oxidase enzyme that requires ascorbic acid and oxygen to hydroxylate dopamine to norepinephrine. The enzyme has been purified, crystallized, and characterized, and antibodies to it have been produced.[146, 295, 613] The antibodies have been used to assay the enzyme and to detect genetic differences in the biosynthesis of the enzyme. The dopamine β-hydroxylase apparently is contained on the inner surface of the saclike granule or vesicle that, surrounded by a semipermeable membrane, behaves as an osmotic system. At least 40% of the enzyme is in association with the granule wall protein. This portion has much higher activity than does a water-insoluble portion that is not associated with the granule membrane but is within the granule. In the granule, the enzyme is associated with a macromolecule (MW 2.9×10^5) termed chromogranin A.[242, 243] This water-insoluble substance may be composed of subunits of dopamine β-hydroxylase, and when it comes in contact with ATP, the enzyme and chromogranin become solubilized, and the enzyme becomes activated. ATP also has a functional relationship to storage of catecholamines in the granules.

A number of assays for dopamine β-hydroxylase have been devised. The enzyme has been found in human and rat plasma; its concentration seems somewhat dependent on the integrity and activity of the sympathetic nervous system.[269] When the sympathetic nervous system is destroyed or its function is inhibited by preventing release of catecholamines from storage sites, the amount of circulating enzyme is low. Increased sympathetic nervous activity has the opposite effect. The characteristics of the circulating enzyme are similar to those of enzyme obtained from the adrenal medulla and sympathetic nerves. If evidence suggesting that catecholamines are released by a process of exocytosis involving extrusion of the whole vesicle including the membrane was true (see the following), then the assay of circulating dopamine β-hydroxylase might complement direct measurements of catecholamines in the blood. If exocytosis is operative both in the nerve endings and in the adrenal medulla, such measurements could reflect the functional state of the sympathetic nervous system in physiologic and disease states.[450] In many diseases in which abnormalities of the autonomic nervous system are suspected (idiopathic orthostatic hypotension, familial dysautonomia, hypertension, and infantile hypoglycemia), measurements of circulating catecholamines or their metabolites are not sufficiently accurate to indicate with certainty that a lesion exists. In addition, some diseases of the autonomic nervous system may indicate primary alterations of enzymatic contents of the storage vesicle that would not be reflected in routine measurements of the end products.

The control of synthesis of dopamine β-hydroxylase seems related to the same factors favoring synthesis of tyrosine hydroxylase. Modifiers of synaptic function appear to regulate the enzyme by affecting its rate of synthesis, while hypophyseal hormones (including adrenal corticotropic hormone [ACTH] appear to regulate its rate of degradation.[90] Unlike tyrosine hydroxylase, the dopamine-converting enzyme is lost from the neuron when catecholamines are released.[309, 397] It is not surprising, therefore, that factors that increase release of catecholamines from the neuron also stimulate the synthesis of dopamine β-hydroxylase.[91] As is the case with any of the enzymes in the synthetic or metabolic pathway for catecholamines, the actual chemical signal for initiating or stopping synthesis of dopamine β-hydroxylase is not known.

There is little substrate specificity of dopamine β-hydroxylase; it will hydroxylate many phenylethylamines including epinine, forming epinephrine and octopamine. Tyramine is probably a better substrate for the enzyme than dopamine is, and this amine has been identified and located in the sympathetic nerves as a naturally occurring substance. Substrate activity occurs only in the presence of an aromatic ring, with a side chain of two or three carbon atoms terminating with an amino group. Phenylalkylamines with two carbon side chains are better substrates than are those with three carbon atoms, and primary amines are better than secondary.

There is considerable pragmatic importance to the nonspecificity of many of the steps in the transport of substrates and the synthesis of intermediates of catecholamines. Amino acid transport into the neuron is active but nonspecific with regard to eventual substrates for L-amino acid decarboxylase; once in the cytoplasm, a number of amino acids will be decarboxylated to their corresponding amines. Many of these can be actively transported into the vesicle containing dopamine β-hydroxylase, where some will be converted into β-hydroxylated products; these intragranular amines may not be catecholamines (e.g., a natural noncatecholamine is tyramine) but many have pharmacologic properties. Some displace norepinephrine (the natural neurotransmitter) from storage sites. Others, if bound within the granule, may be released by nerve stimulation and produce their own characteristic effects. These latter unnatural substances have become classified as "false" neurotransmitters, but they have considerable pharmacologic importance themselves.

There are several natural endogenous inhibitors of dopamine β-hydroxylase. These are of low molecular weight (MW 750–1200) and contain carbohydrate, phosphate, and trace amounts of nitrogen. They have a distinctive ultraviolet spectrum and apparently work by chelation of enzyme-bound Cu^{++}. They are found in many tissues and probably in blood. We know little about the controls for their synthesis or their physiologic importance. It is likely that they have physiologic or pathologic importance, since, in many circumstances, dopamine β-hydroxylase appears to be rate-limiting in the synthesis of catecholamines.

The rate-limiting characteristics of dopamine β-hydroxylase have been revealed by use of competitive inhibitors (derivatives of phenylethylamines) that are themselves substrates for the enzyme. In certain experimental settings, these inhibitors result in decreased content of tissue (primarily brain) norepinephrine with a reciprocal but nonstoichiometric increase in dopamine. The incomplete replacement of norepinephrine by dopamine has been taken to indicate that binding of dopamine in the neuronal vesicle is not as avid as binding of norepinephrine. Another interpretation may be that other unidentified substances accumulate in the nerve ending as a result of inhibition of the enzyme. With stimulation of the affected neurons, release of dopamine and norepinephrine is in perfect proportion to their ratios in the involved neurons. This further indicates that release of amines is in quanta by extrusion of intact vesicles from the nerve.[540] The ability to selectively deplete norepinephrine from the CNS helped to elucidate its individual role in the CNS.

A caveat related to inhibitors of dopamine β-hydroxylase seems warranted. Disulfiram (Antabuse) is an inhibitor of dopamine β-hydroxylase.[209] *In vivo,* the drug is reduced to a chelating agent and has been reported to decrease norepinephrine levels in the heart and brain. One interpretation of these results would be that dopamine β-hydroxylase is a rate-limiting step. However, the chelating properties affect Fe^{++} and thereby also inhibit tyrosine hydroxylase, a known rate-limiting step. These results should serve as a reminder that many drugs have multiple actions that must be investigated. An additional example concerns another "dopamine β-hydroxylase inhibitor," 5-butylpicolinic acid (fusaric acid). When given to animals, it decreases their brain norepinephrine levels, increases serotonin (which should be unaffected by the inhibitor) by 25%, but does not change dopamine concentrations. The combination of decreased norepinephrine, normal dopamine, and raised serotonin cannot be fully explained on the basis of inhibition of dopamine β-hydroxylase. Further investigations may reveal additional useful actions of the inhibitor that are not obvious today.

Phenylethanolamine-N-Methyl Transferase

In selected tissues, synthesis of catecholamines can continue beyond norepinephrine to epinephrine. In humans, only the chromaffin cells nearest the adrenal cortex (and some in the brain) appear to have the cytoplasmic enzyme capable of N-methylating norepinephrine.[164, 433] This enzyme, because it has relatively nonspecific requirements for substrate, was named phenylethanolamine-N-methyl transferase (PNMT) by Axelrod,[23] who first characterized it. It predominantly methylates phenylethanolamines, which include endogenous β-hydroxycatecholamines (e.g., norepinephrine and octopamine), their methoxyamine metabolites (e.g., normetanephrine), drugs structurally related to phenylethanolamine (e.g., norephedrine and amphetamine), and even some secondary β-hydroxylated amines (e.g., epinephrine and neosynephrine). The substrate with the lowest K_m is norepinephrine, the apparently preferred substrate.

The sulfhydryl-containing enzyme has an absolute requirement for a methyl-group donor (S-adenosylmethionine), oxygen, and probably Mg^{++}. Norepinephrine and most of its substrates competitively inhibit the function of the enzyme but its product, epinephrine, is its most potent and noncompetitive inhibitor. Epinephrine also may inhibit synthesis of PNMT.[66] Ordinary concentrations of unbound epinephrine in the cell cytoplasm are probably sufficient to regulate the minute-to-minute function of the enzyme. The details of the affinity of PNMT for various substrates, of its chemical and physical properties, of its synthesis and action, and of its distribution in mammals still are under investigation.[92, 189, 207, 224, 433, 559]

False Neurotransmitters

General Concepts

We have begun to realize that norepinephrine and epinephrine are not the only physiologic transmitters released from sympathetic nerve endings during physiologic stimulation. Few doubt that the amines are transmitters released from nerves or that they can produce the majority of changes associated with activation of the sympathetic system.[148, 270]

However, the process of synthesis of catecholamines is nonspecific at a number of steps; unnatural amino acids[307] can be transported into the neuron, where they can be decarboxylated (Fig. 10–5) and the resulting amines often can serve as unnatural substrates for dopamine β-hydroxylase (Fig. 10–6). As will be discussed, the process of storage and release of the catecholamines also is nonspecific. Therefore, the unnatural amines conceivably can be used as substitute or false neurotransmitters.

The criteria for a false neurotransmitter have been reviewed frequently and are now adequately summarized in standard texts of pharmacology. Generally, although they are not normally present in the sympathetic neurons in significant quantity, they can be made to accumulate in the nerve endings at the same site as the natural transmitter. The accumulation may follow administration of the sub-

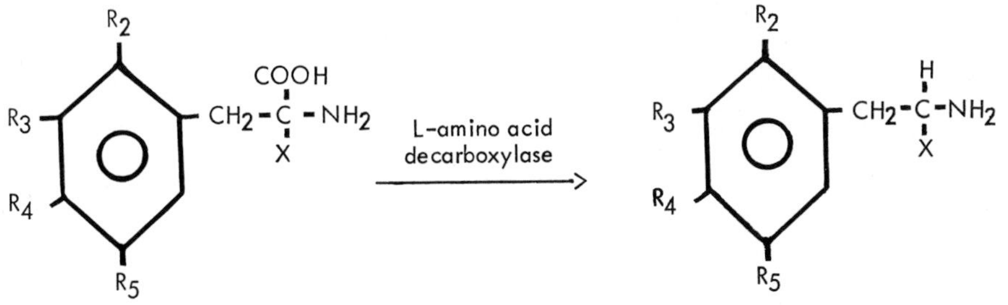

Figure 10–5. Substrates for aromatic L-amino acid decarboxylase and the product that would be produced in the cell. (Reproduced with modification from Kopin, I. J.: Unnatural amino acids as precursors of false transmitters. *Fed. Proc. 30*:904, 1971, with permission.)

Substitutes in Position					Product
R_2	R_3	R_4	R_5	X	
-	-	OH	-	-	Tyramine
-	OH	-	-	-	m-Tyramine
-	OH	OH	-	-	Dopamine
OH	-	OH	OH	-	6-Hydroxydopamine
-	OH	OH	OH	-	5-Hydroxydopamine
-	OH	OCH_3	OH	-	3,5-Dihydroxy-4-methoxyphenylethylamine
-	OH	-	-	CH_3	α-Methyl-m-Tyramine
-	OH	OH	-	CH_3	α-Methyl Dopamine
OH	-	-	-	-	0-Tyramine

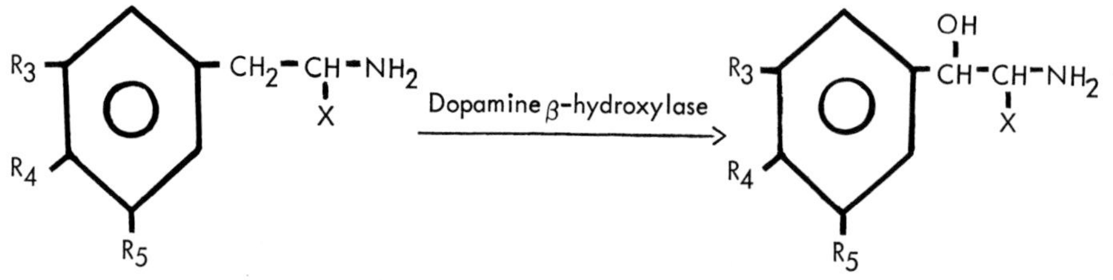

	Substitutes in Position			Product
R_3	R_4	R_5	X	
–	–	–	–	Phenylethanolamine
–	OH	–	–	Octopamine
OH	–	–	–	m-Octopamine
OH	OH	–	–	Norepinephrine
OH	OH	OH	–	5-Hydroxynorepinephrine
–	OH	–	CH_3	α-Methyloctopamine
OH	–	–	CH_3	Metaraminol
OH	OH	–	CH_3	α-Methylnorepinephrine
–	–	–	CH_3	Norephedrine
OH	OH	OCH_3	–	5-Methoxynorepinephrine
OH	OCH_3	OH	–	4-Methoxy-3,5-dihydroxyphenylethanolamine

Figure 10–6. Phenylethanolamine-type substrates that can gain access to the intraneuronal vesicle containing dopamine beta-hydroxylase. The products will only be found in the sympathetic nerve or adrenal chromaffin cell where the enzyme is exclusively harbored. Only the beta-hydroxylated amines are released as transmitters during nerve stimulation.[155] (Reproduced with modification from Kopin, I. J.: Unnatural amino acids as precursors of false transmitters. *Fed. Proc. 30*:904, 1971, with permission.)

stance itself, a precursor, or a drug that allows an endogenous compound to form the false neurotransmitter. The false neurotransmitter must be held in the same storage sites, released by the same nerve stimulation, and depleted by drugs that deplete the physiologic neurotransmitter norepinephrine. The released substance does not, however, have to have the same pharmacologic properties as the native transmitter. In addition, the pharmacologic effects of a false neurotransmitter may not be due to its activity as a stimulator of an effector cell but rather to its effect on synthesis, storage, or release of the native transmitter.[552] Only selected drugs and transmitters that have been found clinically useful will be discussed. As might be expected, they affect the cardiovascular system and clinically have so far been used in the management of hypertension. The heuristic qualities (both positive and negative) of the false neurotransmitter concept will be weighed in this section. Following the history of research into the actions of some antihypertensive drugs should lead the reader to understanding of the practical importance of the concept.

α-Methyldopa (Methyldopa) and α-Methylnorepinephrine

Methyldopa was first studied as an antihypertensive drug because it inhibited aromatic L-amino acid decarboxylase *in vitro*. The effects in animals were discouraging, but Oates and coworkers[335, 411] found that the L- or S-enantiomer inhibited decarboxylase, decreased tissue stores of norepinephrine, and lowered arterial pressure in patients with essential hypertension. The latter two actions were considered to be caused by diminished catecholamine synthesis at step 2 in Fig. 10–2 (the conversion of dopa to dopamine). Then it was discovered that (1) depletion of norepinephrine produced by methyldopa exceeds the duration of decarboxylase inhibition; (2) metabolism of catecholamines as reflected by vanillylmandelic acid (VMA) excretion in urine was not significantly changed after administration of methyldopa; and (3) agents producing more profound decarboxylase in-

hibition did not alter the rate of synthesis, size of stores, or turnover of catecholamines, nor did they affect arterial blood pressure. Because decarboxylation is not a rate-limiting step in the biosynthesis of catecholamines, its inhibition cannot be expected to affect the net synthesis of the end product.

After effective doses of methyldopa were administered to animals, α-methylnorepinephrine was found in brain tissue. α-Methyldopa presumably is taken into the sympathetic neurons where it undergoes decarboxylation and subsequent β-hydroxylation to α-methylnorepinephrine by the same enzymes that convert dopa to norepinephrine (Figs. 10–2 and 10–7).[500] The newly formed α-methylnorepinephrine then can displace norepinephrine and other normal mediators, can be stored in the storage granules, and can be released in place of norepinephrine by nerve stimulation.[75]

Although the false neurotransmitter concept is scientifically valuable and has practical implications, it has failed to explain satisfactorily the mechanism of action of methyldopa. α-Methylnorepinephrine is almost as potent a vasoconstrictor and cardioaccelerating agent as norepinephrine when tested in many animals, but in humans it may be somewhat less potent than norepinephrine. The peripheral sympathetic blockade produced by methyldopa may be related to inhibition of tyrosine hydroxylase in the nerve ending by α-methylnorepinephrine. As we have seen, inhibition of this rate-limiting step in the synthesis of catecholamines results in a decrease in the amount of transmitter available for release.[305] Another possibility is that α-methylnorepinephrine, although less available for release by nerve stimulation, is nevertheless capable of displacing the native neurotransmitters from binding sites within the cell. Recent studies of the effects of α-methyldopa at steady-state on the concentrations of brain amines show that the concentrations and turnover rates of α-methyldopamine, rather than α-methylnorephinephrine, correlate best with the decrease in blood pressure that is produced by the drug.[186] None of these observations proves the actual mechanisms of action. Indeed, it is likely that methyldopa has

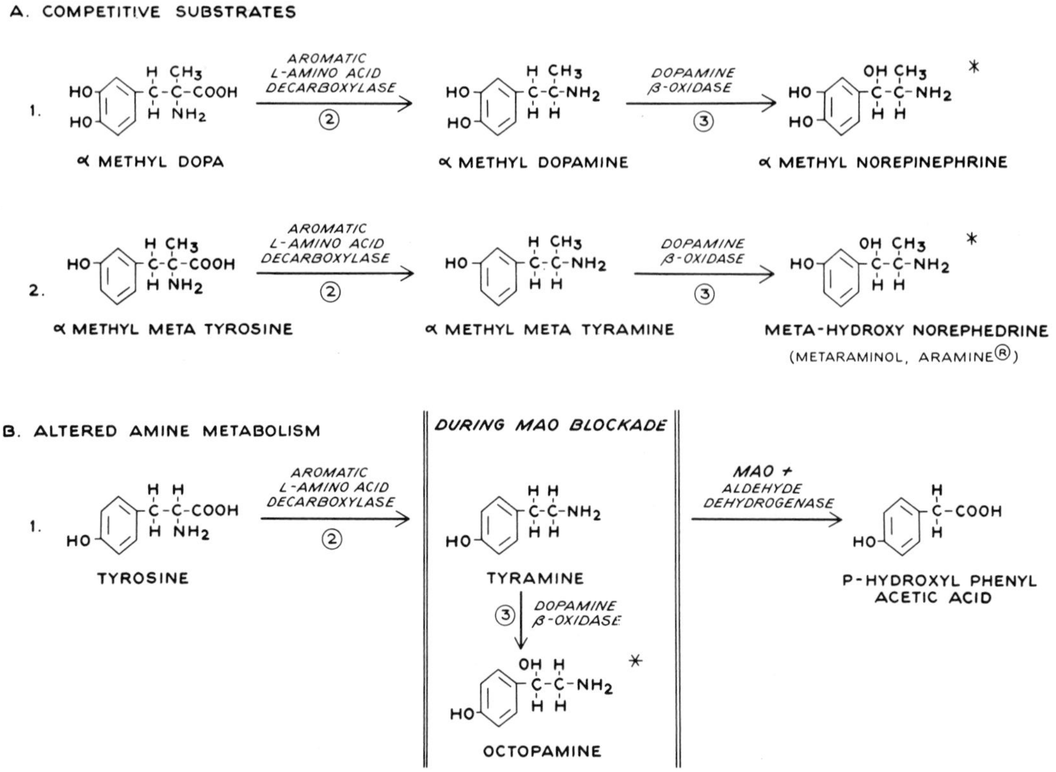

Figure 10-7. Formation of false neurotransmitters (indicated by asterisk). Some are formed by incorporation of a pharmacologic compound into the metabolic pathway for catecholamine synthesis (A.1 and A.2); others are formed independently of catecholamine production (B.1).

important additional effects on arterial blood pressure through direct dilation of peripheral vessels, through inhibiting the secretion of renin, and through its actions on the CNS.[593]

α-Methylmetatyrosine and Metaraminol

After the discovery that α-methylnorepinephrine qualified as a false neurotransmitter, the breadth of the concept was tested in a prospective manner. Additional analogs of tyrosine, dopa, dopamine, and norepinephrine were investigated. α-Methylmetatyrosine was found to be transported into the nerve endings and brain and transformed into meta-hydroxynorephedrine (metaraminol) by the same enzymes that form norepinephrine from tyrosine (Figs. 10–2 and 10–7). The endogenously formed metaraminol is a false neurotransmitter: it stoichiometrically displaces norepinephrine from the storage sites and is released by stimulation of nerves.[93] Such findings emphasize the assets of a hypothesis in helping to design studies on the mechanism of action of a drug.

Infused metaraminol is taken up by the adrenergic neuron and directly displaces norepinephrine from the granules. When clinically useful doses are rapidly infused, metaraminol is initially an effective pressor agent. However, tachyphylaxis (loss of responsiveness to a constant signal) to the pressor effects of metaraminol occurs later, an effect that can be explained by the false neurotransmitter hypothesis. Metaraminol has less than 5% of the potency of norepinephrine; when most of the norepinephrine in the nerve ending has been replaced, stimulation of the nerve results in minimal release of native transmitters, and a partial blockade of the sympathetic nervous system

is established. Further doses of metaraminol fail to release adequate amounts of norepinephrine, resulting not only in lack of pressor responses to metaraminol but also in the appearance of a new drug effect, hypotension. Patients treated with metaraminol have large concentrations of the drug in their sympathetic tissues.[107] An infusion of norepinephrine reestablishes the stores of norepinephrine and restores the hypertensive response to metaraminol.

Metaraminol given in repeated small doses does not produce hypertension because the quantity of catecholamines released after a single dose is small, but eventually the cumulative effects seriously deplete stores of catecholamines and reduce the blood pressure of patients with essential hypertension. Although use of metaraminol as an antihypertensive drug is not seriously suggested, knowledge of its mechanism of action can help explain an otherwise paradoxical response. Both metaraminol and α-methylmetatyrosine, therefore, can be antihypertensive agents in humans, depending on the details of administration. Again, a valid hypothesis not only may explain an observed effect but also may be used to predict future observations (regardless of how unexpected they may seem). If the hypothesis fails to predict a response, either the hypothesis or the observation is incorrect. Usually the hypothesis is more vulnerable.

Observing the effects of metaraminol allows us to define further the usefulness of the false neurotransmitter hypothesis:

1. Metaraminol does not cross the blood-brain barrier; therefore, attention can be focused entirely upon peripheral mechanisms of sympathetic blockade.

2. Metaraminol has only one hydroxyl group on the aromatic ring, proving that the catechol (dihydroxyphenyl) structure is not an absolute requirement for a false neuro-

transmitter. Indeed in recent years, many drugs that are noncatecholamines but that behave pharmacologically as adrenergic agents have been shown to be capable of acting as false neurotransmitters.

Monoamine Oxidase Inhibitors

Originally used as antidepressants, MAO inhibitors were found to produce postural hypotension that correlated with the degree of inhibition of MAO *in vivo*. Although MAO does not primarily inactivate circulating catecholamines, it does metabolize the amines accessible to it in the cytoplasm. Interest in MAO inhibitors as possible therapeutic agents has been rekindled by the discovery that there are isozymes of MAO, that these isozymes have different substrate specificities, and that they can be inhibited selectively.[474] Isozymes of MAO have been physically separated and evidence suggests that the active sites of the isozymes are identical to each other. The different properties of the enzymes appear to be related to the lipid environment in which the enzyme is situated.[257, 546] The two isozymes are termed MAO-A and MAO-B. In original descriptions of these isoenzymes it was postulated that MAO-A was localized in neuronal tissue and that MAO-B was localized elsewhere; this generalization has not held. Rat liver and brain contain approximately equal portions of the two isozymes. Rat superior cervical ganglion and spleen contain MAO-A almost entirely. Intestinal MAO is almost 70% of the A type, and human platelets and striatum contain MAO-B. MAO-A preferentially deaminates physiologic substrates such as serotonin, norepinephrine, epinephrine, metanephrine, and normetanephrine. It also deaminates other β-hydroxylated phenylethylamines such as octopamine. Preferential substrates for MAO-B include benzylamine, tryptamine, 5-0-methyltryptamine, and phenylethylamine. Tyramine, dopamine, and 3-0-methyltyramine are metabolized to similar degrees by both isozymes. Taking advantage of these relative differences in substrate specificity has led to the development of therapeutically useful agents that block only one type of MAO. When MAO is blocked, the amount of norepinephrine as well as other amines (e.g., octopamine) in the storage granules increases. When these amines enter the granule, they become potential false neurotransmitters that might either compete with norepinephrine for release or act in the nerve ending to disrupt normal catecholamine synthesis, storage, or release. Octopamine may be the key false neurotransmitter during MAO inhibition. It is formed by β-hydroxylation of tyramine, the product of decarboxylation of tyrosine, and is less than 1% as potent as norepinephrine (Fig. 10–7). Normally, tyramine and octopamine are rapidly destroyed by MAO, but, when protected from oxidation during MAO inhibition, both can accumulate. Thus after any standard nerve stimulation, a finite amount of transmitter leaves the nerve ending, but the amount of potent transmitter may be diluted by the impotent false neurotransmitter, octopamine. The resulting sympathetic blockade appears to account for the antihypertensive action of MAO inhibition.

Infused tyramine in normal persons releases norepinephrine from nerve endings and results in a brief rise of arterial pressure. Because tyramine is rapidly destroyed by MAO, its effects are transient. Furthermore, under ordinary circumstances ingested tyramine is oxidized by MAO as it crosses the intestinal mucosa. When catecholamine stores are increased, as in patients with pheochromocytomas, an infusion of tyramine produces a brief but exaggerated rise of arterial blood pressure. When catecholamine stores are increased and tyramine is protected from destruction by administration of nonspecific MAO inhibitors, relatively small amounts of infused or ingested tyramine can provoke severe prolonged hypertension. Hypertensive reactions have been reported in patients taking MAO inhibitors after they ingest tyramine-containing foods, including aged cheese, wine, beer, marmite, pickled herring, broad beans, or chicken liver. In addition to tyramine-containing foods, commonly used catecholamine-releasing drugs (amphetamine, ephedrine, phenylpropanolamine, mephentermine, metaraminol, methylphenidate, and phenmetrazine) can produce hypertensive reactions during MAO inhibition.

Clorgyline, which is closely related structurally to pargyline, is a selective inhibitor of MAO-A.[275] A chemically similar compound, deprenyl, is a selective inhibitor of MAO-B and can inhibit 90% of MAO-B activity in humans.[299, 611] Phenelzine and isocarboxazid may inhibit type B more than type A, but they generally are not selective inhibitors. In striking contrast to the known nonspecific MAO inhibitors (e.g., phenelzine and isocarboxazid), deprenyl does not result in profound and potentially lethal potentiation of the effects of catecholamines when the inhibitors are administered concurrently with a centrally effective amine. For example, a patient receiving deprenyl may eat cheese or take levodopa without danger.[298] However, administration of deprenyl inhibits the intracerebral metabolic degradation of dopamine. The resultant preservation of dopamine in the basal ganglia appears to maximize the therapeutic efficacy of levodopa.[457] Consequently, when deprenyl is added to the therapeutic regimen, the dose of levodopa may be reduced without loss of therapeutic benefit. Although preliminary clinical trials with this compound are encouraging, deprenyl is not yet generally available in the United States.

Guanethidine

Guanethidine has many properties common to the false neurotransmitters. Its closely related congeners that have combined a basic guanidine or amidine moiety (similar to that in guanethidine) with an aromatic ring constituent (similar to that in bretylium) include bethanidine and debrisoquin. The properties of guanethidine are generally shared by these other drugs. Each is actively transported into the nerve ending by the transport system for norepinephrine. Like norepinephrine, their uptake is blocked by cocaine, imipramine and its derivatives, and amphetamine. The drugs are bound to the norepinephrine storage sites; they release norepinephrine from the nerve ending, and because they do not inhibit MAO in the nerve, the net effect is depletion of catecholamines. Guanethidine-like drugs can be released by reserpine or by nerve stimulation and their effects are prevented or reversed by imipramine, cocaine, ephedrine, amphetamine, tyramine, or metaraminol, the same list of drugs that either release or block uptake of norepinephrine.

In spite of their similarity to classic false neurotransmitters, guanethidine-like drugs produce sympathetic inhibition prior to major decreases in catecholamine stores, and the sympathetic inhibition disappears before the amine content is noticeably repleted. They probably not only deplete but also interfere with release of norepinephrine during physiologic stimulation of the nerve. They may cause a persistent and direct depolarization of the sympathetic nerve ending, which in turn initially discharges catecholamines and results in adrenergic inhibition. This hypothesis is consistent with the observation that large parenteral doses of guanethidine and its congeners release enough norepinephrine to induce hypertension while simultaneously blocking the response to postganglionic nerve stimulation. Hypertensive response to agents that deplete adrenergic neuronal stores of norepinephrine should be expected, particularly in patients with expanded stores of catecholamines (e.g., caused by a pheochromocytoma, neuroblastoma, or MAO inhibitor), and should be treated when necessary with the most specific therapy: α-adrenergic blocking agents. Comprehensive reviews of antihypertensive agents and false neurotransmitters along with discussions of the possible role of the sympathetic nervous system in essential hypertension are included in the works cited in references 47, 408, and 593.

6-Hydroxydopamine

Drugs that affect the sympathetic nervous system as false neurotransmitters are useful not only to the clinician. Selective and specific methods of manipulating the autonomic nervous system yield specific lessons. For instance, surgical ablation of a spinal cord gives considerably less information about the specific function of the autonomic nervous system than does a surgical sympathectomy. On the other hand, information about the sympathetic nervous system was gained from the finding that antisera to a sympathetic nerve growth factor could ablate the entire sympathetic system in newborn animals.[268] Certain drugs (e.g., reserpine, methyldopa, α-methylmetatyrosine) can alter stores of catecholamines and give an idea of the function of sympathetic nerve endings;[182] a major advance was the realization that 6-hydroxydopamine was one of the unnatural substances that could be transported into the nerve ending and could interfere with uptake, synthesis, storage, and release of the native transmitter.

When the amine is given to animals, it specifically enters adrenergic neurons. When given intraperitoneally, it produces a selective peripheral sympathectomy, sparing the adrenal gland and the CNS. Within hours of administration, it begins to destroy the nerve ending in a characteristic fashion; a rapid depletion of endogenous norepinephrine is associated with a preferential release of microsomal contents of the neuron (containing the catecholamine storage vesicles) and loss of tyrosine hydroxylase. After the loss of the neurotransmitter, the actual nerve ending degenerates. This stage of diminished uptake of exogenous catecholamines correlates with hypersensitivity of the effector organs to the amine. The interesting mechanism of the supersensitivity to catecholamines has been studied by administering 6-hydroxydopamine while the noradrenergic nerve terminals are being destroyed; the density of β-adrenergic receptors on the effector sites is greatly increased.[513] The ontogeny of the postsynaptic β receptor does not seem to be dependent on the presence of presynaptic input; the absence of the presynaptic component does not lead to more β receptors in relation to adenylate cyclase, which apparently accounts for hypersensitivity to β-adrenergic agonists. The rate of synthesis of receptors appears normal, both in the presence and in the absence of the presynaptic terminals.[232]

The late effects of 6-hydroxydopamine are to allow some neurons to regenerate, and their ability to take up (and therefore biologically inactivate) catecholamines returns before synthesis of the catechols is reestablished at normal rates.

When given intracisternally, the drug is also taken up into specific sites in the brain but produces no peripheral effects. Although some doses exhaust both norepinephrine and dopamine, careful regulation depletes norepinephrine sites more than dopaminergic sites. Serotonergic sites are not affected. The study of behavioral changes correlated with isolated changes in norepinephrine or dopamine content of brain has helped to identify both the presence and the function of specific sets of adrenergic neurons. Although these findings may not directly interest the nonbiologic investigator, they suggest the best use, and therapeutic effects, of catecholamine precursors in patients with Parkinson's disease.

The mechanism of action of 6-hydroxydopamine has been partially elucidated. When given to animals, the precursor 6-hydroxydopa enters primarily the peripheral sympathetic nerves and must be decarboxylated to be effective. Although the amine enters the catecholamine storage vesicle, this is not essential for its action. Perhaps its biochemical effects are related to its ability to generate hydrogen peroxide.[239] The peroxide damages biogenic amine uptake systems in synaptosomes (pinched-off nerve endings), and both peroxide generation and effects of 6-hydroxydopamine are partially prevented by catalase. Of interest is the fact that vinblastine appears to have the same selective destructive effects on adrenergic nerves as does 6-hydroxydopamine.[229] The pharmacology of 6-hydroxydopamine has been reviewed by Thoenen and Tranzer[539] and Kostrzewa and Jacobowitz.[311]

Physiologic Factors That Affect Catecholamine Synthesis

As methods for studying the synthesis and disposition of catecholamines have developed, physiologic controls of synthesis have come to light. Nerve stimulation has been mentioned as a vital factor in catecholamine synthesis. Mild stimulation increases tyrosine hydroxylase activity by releasing the most recently synthesized pool of catecholamines, thus reducing feedback inhibition of the activity of the enzyme. Intense or protracted stimulation increases synthesis of both tyrosine hydroxylase and dopamine β-hydroxylase and is in part responsible for intensified production of catecholamines.[383] The counterpart of nerve stimulation to the peripheral adrenergic neurons is light stimulation, which affects the synthesis of serotonin and catecholamines in the pineal.[125]

The physiologic factors of moment-to-moment control of the synthesis in the brain seem more complex. There is a diurnal variation (control mechanism unknown) in concentration of catecholamines in the brain and perhaps in peripheral tissues. The pool of catecholamines in the brain is greatest at night, and the amines seem to have a function (not fully defined) in such cyclic processes as sleep, arousal, temperature regulation, and even eating and drinking.[324] There is some evidence that the functions of one subcategory of nerve ending (e.g., a serotonergic or dopaminergic ending) can control the functions of another subcategory (e.g., one containing norepinephrine).[431] What other factors enter into the control of brain amine synthesis and whether similar factors control synthesis in both the brain and the peripheral tissues remains to be seen.

The basal rate of synthesis of catecholamines seems to be variably affected by the function of "unassociated" endocrine systems. Normal maintenance of adrenal tyrosine hydroxylase requires ACTH;[389] follicle stimulating hormone (FSH) but not luteinizing hormone (LH) controls the turnover of norepinephrine in selected parts of the brain,[10] and dopamine and serotonergic nerves apparently regulate release of LH in rats.[480] Angiotensin may have a stimulative effect (perhaps by releasing some of the newly synthesized norepinephrine or by inhibiting its uptake into nerve endings)[51, 122, 419, 429] on norepinephrine production in the peripheral sympathetic nerves.

When humans[211, 617] or other animals are subjected to extraordinary stresses (e.g., childbirth, burns, cold, hypoxia, immobilization, isolation, or physical exercise), the rate of synthesis of catecholamines increases greatly. The increase is associated with an increase in production of synthesizing enzymes and sometimes may be limited by the availability of substrate for the enzymes.[531] The rate of synthesis is integrated with, but not entirely dependent upon, production of ACTH, corticosteroids, and perhaps other trophic hormones produced by the pituitary.[316, 428] At least two additional mechanisms may influence the overall synthesis and effect of the catecholamines: (1) as the stress continues, the sensitivity of effector organs to catecholamines may gradually increase, requiring less and less released catecholamine to elicit any given effect;[314] and (2) metabolic compensatory responses related to such factors as heat production may alter (increase or decrease) the need for release of catecholamines.[315, 317, 532] Any loss of the nerves from the sympathetic nervous system — by accident, surgery, chemical ablation, or perhaps some diseases affecting the integrity of the nerves — will increase production of the catecholamines in the remaining intact areas.[318, 388]

Many commonly used drugs, common diseases, or complex physiologic activities such as fighting alter the synthesis of catecholamines. However, their actions are often complex, affecting not only synthesis but also storage, release, metabolism, and excretion of the amines. They will therefore be discussed after an explanation of these other factors.

Storage and Release of Catecholamines

The presence of "cytoplasmic particles" in the adrenal medulla and sympathetic nerve endings was reported first by Blaschko and Welch in 1953[48] and confirmed shortly afterward by von Euler and Hillarp. In addition to their important role in the synthesis of catecholamines, these granules also play a major role in the storage and biologic inactivation of catecholamines. Storage of catecholamines is probably related to hydrogen bonding of the catecholamines to the phosphorus moiety of ATP and to a specific intragranular protein.[575] These granules then are a storehouse of potentially active catecholamines, which, if left free in the cytoplasm, would be metabolized by MAO.

The biochemical composition of the granules (their complement of amino acids, electron carriers, lipids, and electrolytes), as well as their morphologic characteristics and appearance on electron microscopy, is remarkably constant regardless of the organ or species of origin. Even neoplastic tissue (pheochromocytoma) has "normal" granules. The development of the granules in the early embryologic life of rats correlates with the ability to take up and then synthesize catecholamines.[101] The granules are almost certainly responsible for the major part (more than 80%) of binding of catecholamines in any tissue, although some tissues (e.g., skeletal muscle) may be able to bind the amines at extragranular sites. The granules are found only in chromaffin-derived cells and are physically distinct from the mitochrondria and lysosomes. Although the granules have similar physical properties, some evidence indicates that their function varies, depending on their location in specific organs.[35, 72] For example, granules obtained from different segments of the same blood vessel will have different amine content.

The granules are relatively nonspecific as to the amines they will transport and bind[538] (see "False Neurotransmitters"). The concentrating process in all granules studied is active and energy-consuming, shows preference for the L-isomers of the respective amines, is dependent on Na^+, ATP, and Mg^{++}, and is inhibited by ouabain (an inhibitor of the Na-K ATPase pump), K^+, and Ca^{++}. Despite the pump's ability to transport an amine against a concentration gradient, low levels of amine in a fluid perfusing a tissue will result in disproportionately low final concentrations in the granule. In a perfusate containing low concentrations, the transported amines are rapidly metabolized, and accumulation will be apparent only when large quantities are transported. The pump is stimulated by O-methylated metabolites of catecholamines, a fact that might encourage conservation of the amines after a sudden burst or sustained release.[267] As more is known about transport processes, it appears that specific drugs may be designed to selectively inhibit transport into either dopamine- or norepinephrine-containing neurons.[254] Finally, in some diseases such as pheochromocytoma the ratio of norepinephrine plus epinephrine to ATP is increased,[484, 524] which tends to promote a leak of catechols and a more rapid than normal turnover of formed catecholamines.[106]

Two pools of catecholamines have been postulated:[24] one that is kept from active metabolism by cytoplasmic enzymes and has a half-life approaching 24 hours, and a second smaller pool that is readily available for release from the nerve ending and has a half-life of only 2 hours. The second pool has been termed the "easily releasable" pool because it is readily diminished by physiologic stimulation and pharmacologic agents such as tyramine.[69] It is composed primarily of the most recently synthesized amines[37, 308] and is probably concentrated in peripheral portions of nerve endings; it equilibrates only slowly with the first or "tightly bound" pool. There is no convincing evidence that the two pools are anatomically separate.

Ordinarily nerve stimulation is necessary to release catecholamines from both functional storage sites into the plasma.[248] The actual chemical mediation of the release appears to be linked either to the presence of ACh or to the influx of calcium ions into the granule, or both.[67, 140, 291, 472] The process is energy-dependent, requiring glycolysis or oxidative metabolism.[471] Not all catecholamine release is via stimulation of sympathetic nerves; at least a small reserve can be released by stimulation of the vagus nerve.[569] In fact, recent data demonstrate that a major point for interaction of autacoids is at the site where the release of norepinephrine is regulated consequent to nerve stimulation. Whereas extracellular calcium is required for neurotransmitter release caused by stimulation of adrenergic and other neurons, a large number of substances modify the amount of norepinephrine released per nerve impulse.[325, 518, 600] Generally, cyclic nucleotides (see later), β-adrenergic agonists, cholinergic nicotine agonists, and angiotensin enhance release, whereas α-adrenergic agonists, cholinergic muscarinic agonists, prostaglandins of the E series, opiates, enkephalins, dopamine, and adenosine inhibit release. Table 10–1 summarizes known interactions. Whether all of these agents work by a final common mechanism, i.e., via modulation of the production or effects of cyclic nucleotides, is not known. A recent symposium covers this area.[517]

One mechanism of release from both sympathetic nerves and the adrenal medulla appears similar to the secretory process of a number of exocrine glands.[479] The hormone can be released in quanta along with the chemical constituents

Table 10–1. INTERACTIONS OF PHYSIOLOGIC REGULATORS OF RELEASE OF NOREPINEPHRINE*

Modulator	Receptor	Effect on Release	Effect on Tissue cAMP	Tissue cAMP
Norepinephrine	α_2	↓	↑ CNS†, ↓ other	↑ cerebellum
Norepinephrine or epinephrine	β	↑	↑ CNS; ↑ other	
Dopamine	?	↓	↑ CNS; SCG‡	no change SCG
Prostaglandin E series		↓	↑ CNS; ↑ other	
Acetylcholine	Muscarinic	↓	↓ neuroblastoma	↑ heart, smooth muscle
	Nicotinic	↑	↑ adrenal medulla	
Adenosine		↓	↑ CNS	
Morphine, enkephalin		↓	↓ neuroblastoma	↑ neuroblastoma

Adapted from Weiner, N.: *Fed. Proc.* 38:2193, 1979.

*Although many of the autacoids have not yet been tested for their effects on this system, they are known to modulate concentrations of cyclic nucleotides in tissues that are critical to this function.

†CNS = central nervous system

‡SCG = superior cervical ganglion

of the vesicle.[46] The migration of the vesicle to the cell surface, where it is extruded by exocytosis, seems dependent on contraction of the microfibrils of the cells;[437] the microfibrils may perform a similar function in the release of histamine from mast cells, insulin from the pancreas, and granules from leukocytes during phagocytosis. Release of catecholamines is inhibited by colchicine, vinblastine, and vincristine (all of which interfere with the microtubules) and is potentiated by deuterium oxide, which also potentiates histamine and insulin release. The release of catecholamines from the adrenal gland can be selective: in humans, release of epinephrine is not necessarily associated with concomitant release of norepinephrine. How the adrenal receives signals to call for release of one amine instead of the other is not known. The quantal release of catecholamines by a process of exocytosis and the presence of dopamine β-hydroxylase in the wall of the granules has led some to measure the concentration of the dopamine β-hydroxylase in plasma and to consider that measurement as indicative of the activity of the sympathetic nervous system. Although some correlation between the concentrations of catecholamines and the concentrations of enzyme in plasma can exist, several studies show that the release of the enzyme can be dissociated from the release of catecholamine. In addition, differences in the half-lives of the two substances in plasma make it difficult to interpret ratios of their concentrations.[263, 269, 463]

Apparently not all release involves exocytosis;[46, 478] not only is there a constant leak of catecholamines into the circulation, but some unusual chemicals such as acetaldehyde, which accumulates during metabolism of alcohol or in diabetics, can promote release of catecholamines without exocytosis.[478] These situations are not associated with protein release from the granules, though they appear to depend on the direct action of chemicals on the granules. Whether or not acidemia or hypoxemia provokes release of catecholamines entirely by reflex stimulation of nerves is unknown but is not likely.[400]

Sympathomimetic amines such as tyramine and amphetamine release bound norepinephrine from the storage vesicles, indirectly causing a rise in blood pressure.[68] Tyramine and reserpine both reduce catecholamine (or false neurotransmitter) content in tissues but by different mechanisms. The tyramine rapidly releases relatively large quantities of catecholamines that leave the nerve unmetabolized and produce a pressor effect. The tyramine is metabolized later.[306] On the other hand, reserpine both abolishes the ability of the nerve vesicle to bind norepinephrine[253] and releases catecholamines more slowly than tyramine. The released catecholamines are likely to be oxidized in the

nerve ending by intraneuronal MAO, and the metabolites that are physiologically inactive produce no pharmacologic effects when they are released from the axon.

Once the catecholamines are released, they act on effector sites[528, 529] and are then rapidly destroyed by plasma enzymes, rebound by granules, or excreted in the urine. As will be recounted below, feedback loops can exist only when released catecholamines stimulate a presynaptic receptor (either an α_2-adrenergic or dopaminergic receptor) and thereby decrease the amount of neurotransmitter released by subsequent physiologic or pharmacologic stimulation.[325, 394, 440, 545] In addition, other substances, such as amino acids, local hormones (such as thyroid and progesterone), the mediator itself (and in combination with adenosine and ATP that may be released with norepinephrine), other autacoids (e.g., serotonin), and drugs, can modulate the release of norepinephrine into the synapse area.[237, 260, 424, 492, 589] What is known of the physiochemical mechanism of action of catecholamines has been described in a comprehensive review.[31]

Inactivation of Catecholamines

Reuptake of Catecholamines

Four mechanisms biologically inactivate catecholamines. Probably the most important is the "reuptake" of the catecholamines by postganglionic neuron storage granules,[248] a fact supported by two observations: (1) agents (e.g., guanethidine, cocaine, imipramine) that block reuptake of catecholamines into sympathetic nerve endings potentiate the response of tissues to sympathetic nerve stimulation or catecholamine infusion (Fig. 10–8); and (2) when tissues have been deprived of sympathetic innervation and, therefore, of postganglionic neuron storage granules, the response of the effectors to administered catecholamines is enhanced.

The granules bind catecholamines without destroying the molecule, thus allowing later release of the same catecholamines. The process of uptake by transport across the neuronal membrane and into the nerve vesicle is distinct from the process of storage in the vesicle. Drugs that interfere with one may have little or no effect upon the other. Reserpine, which interferes with storage of norepinephrine, affects uptake minimally, and cocaine and tricyclic antidepressants (imipramine) that block uptake have no obvious effect on storage. A third separate process is synthesis. Drugs that influence synthesis need not also influence uptake or storage of catecholamines. Only inhibition of uptake

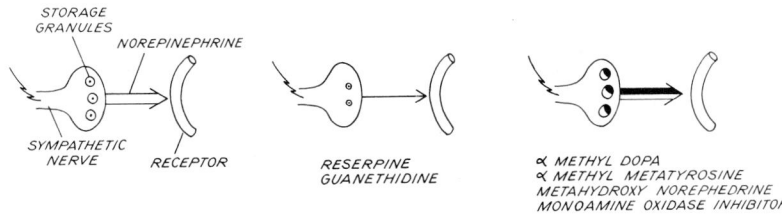

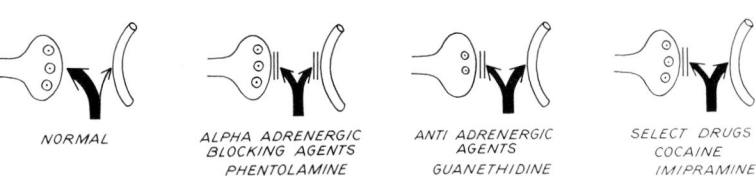

Figure 10–8. Schematic diagram of the mechanism by which pharmacologic agents alter the effect of endogenous or exogenous catecholamines. Some agents (*top*) act by diminishing the stores of catecholamines in nerve endings (guanethidine), by promoting formation of false neurotransmitters (methyldopa), or by being accumulated themselves as false neurotransmitters (metahydroxy norephedrine). Other agents (*bottom*) act by inhibiting uptake of catecholamines into storage sites or into both storage and effector sites (phentolamine, Dibenzyline). When uptake into storage sites is blocked (imipramine), uptake into effector sites is greatly increased.

is associated with striking supersensitivity to norepinephrine.

Metabolism of Norepinephrine and Epinephrine by Peripheral Tissues

Two of the mechanisms of inactivation are enzymatic. For some time, the physiologic importance of these two metabolic pathways has been controversial. Apparently, however, catechol-O-methyl transferase (COMT), which is found in plasma, liver, kidneys, red blood cells, the endothelium of blood vessels, and the cytoplasm of myocardial cells, is responsible for the initial enzymatic inactivation of physiologic amounts of circulating catecholamines[350] (Fig. 10–9). The content of enzyme in human red blood cells is determined as an autosomal recessive trait.[595] When COMT is inhibited by an agent such as pyrogallol, O-methylation of the catecholamines is blocked, and the effect of sympathetic nerve stimulation or of administered catecholamines is somewhat prolonged.

Such is not the case when MAO is inhibited. Blockage of MAO, although it alters the response to sympathetic stimulation, does not change the degree or duration of tissue reaction to administered catecholamines.[220] Despite its presence in plasma and the fact that it may be induced by the presence of substrate, apparently MAO plays a minor role in the metabolism of circulating catecholamines. MAO is thought to be responsible for the rapid inactivation of catechols in the cytoplasm of the nerve endings. Inhibition of MAO by pargyline or equivalent agents results in an increase in stored catecholamines and other biologically important amines (see discussion on false neurotransmitters).

Regardless of which of the two groups of enzymes, COMT or MAO, accounts for the initial inactivation of catecholamines, VMA is the end product. Conjugated forms of normetanephrine or metanephrine make up a relatively small portion of the metabolized catecholamines.

The fourth, and minor, mechanism for the biologic inactivation of physiologic amounts of catecholamines is their metabolism or their excretion, unaltered by the kidney.

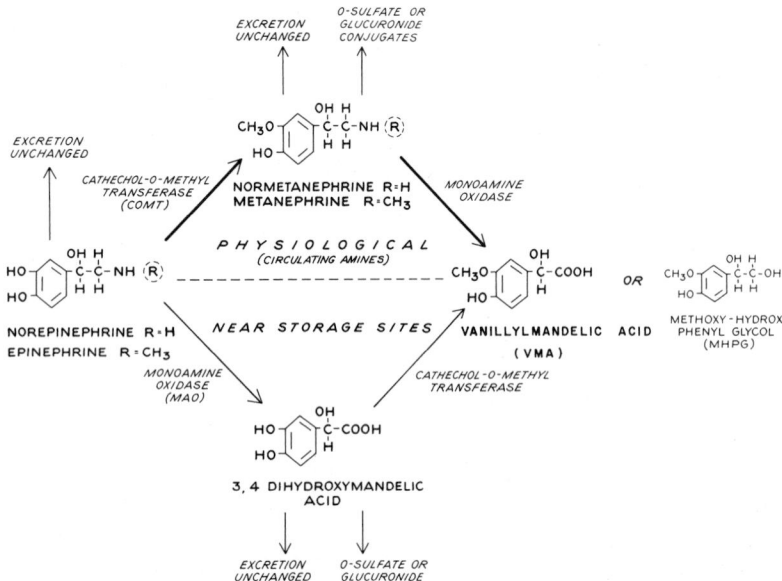

Figure 10–9. Biochemic pathways for the metabolism of catecholamines. Heavy diagonal arrows indicate the major sequence of metabolism of catecholamines released into the circulation. Light diagonal arrows indicate the sequence of metabolism of catecholamines released intracellularly. Vertical arrows indicate minor mechanism of excretion or metabolism of specific intermediary products.

The synthesis and metabolism of catecholamines in the CNS, their effects, and the drugs that can modulate them are described in Ch. 11. Only recently have we come to realize the importance of the role of catecholamines in the brain.

Pharmacologic and Physiologic Actions of Catecholamines

General Considerations

Norepinephrine and epinephrine circulate in quantities sufficient for biologic activity. Concentrations in arterial blood usually are less than those in venous blood.

The two major sources of circulating norepinephrine are the sympathetic nerve endings and, to a much lesser degree, the adrenal medulla.[54] The sympathetic nerve endings constantly "leak" norepinephrine into the venous blood, but the most profound increases in venous concentration occur during intense sympathetic nerve stimulation. Norepinephrine also is released from nerve endings and the adrenal medulla by endogenous hormones, such as bradykinin, histamine, and, in some settings, serotonin; many drugs, including tyramine; many clinically useful pressor agents, such as metaraminol (Aramine), mephentermine (Wyamine), and ephedrine; and some of the hypotensive agents, such as reserpine, α-methyldopa, and guanethidine.

Epinephrine is intermittently released almost exclusively by the adrenal medulla. The CNS, although it contains large amounts of catecholamines, neither contributes substantially to the circulating catecholamines nor receives them readily across the blood-brain barrier.

Once released into the circulation, catecholamines have a short half-life, rarely exceeding two or three circulation times.[25] In studies in humans, infused ^{3}H-norepinephrine has a half-life (in tissues) of about 8 hours, and its metabolite VMA a half-life of about 11–16 hours.[130] These studies provided reasonably valid assay systems for determining the kinetics of catecholamines in humans; they indicated that assays of total urinary norepinephrine plus normetanephrine excretion per day should be a reasonable measure of peripheral sympathetic nerve activity, perhaps more useful than measurements of dopamine β-hydroxylase in plasma.[352] The techniques are now being used to study possible alterations of uptake, binding, release, or metabolism in disease states such as hypertension and familial dysautonomia.[7, 59, 121, 200, 212, 223, 320, 395] There are at least two advantages to such an approach over the techniques of simply measuring concentrations of amine in blood or excretion of amine or metabolites in urine: (1) the studies of kinetics are more likely to be sensitive to small but physiologically important lesions; and (2) careful analysis of data might pinpoint the etiology of a lesion (i.e., uptake, binding, release, synthesis, metabolism, or excretion).

Catecholamines in circulation either bind to receptor sites in various organs, where they produce their physiologic effect, or are inactivated. Their fate depends on enzyme composition and innervation of the organ to which they are distributed, acid-base balance in the body, presence or absence of a disease capable of modifying their effect, and the pharmacologic state of the body at the time of their release. Although the duration and magnitude of effect vary with different doses, catecholamines elicit a predictable response. Pharmacologists have separated these responses into a spectrum of α and β receptor-mediated effects.

Receptors for Catecholamines

The idea that a released neurotransmitter resulted in a physiologic change, via its interaction with a specific portion of the effector cells, came from Cannon and Rosenbleuth.[73] They postulated that a single transmitter (or, in modern terms, first messenger) contacted effector cells and produced one of two substances, sympathin E if the response was "excitatory" or sympathin I if the response was "inhibitory." The concept of a single transmitter was questioned when two transmitters (epinephrine and norepinephrine) were found to be released from various sympathetic nerve tissues. The concept was abandoned when it was decided that the tissue membranes probably were the most important discriminatory factors in any given response.

Ahlquist noted that different tissues produced their characteristic responses when exposed to any of a number of sympathomimetic agents.[5] The responses were reproducible in any given tissue; the potency ranking of the agents was also reproducible. This led him to a tentative conclusion, that at least two types of receptors existed for catecholamines. He defined the α receptor as one that was found in a tissue that responded most to epinephrine or norepinephrine and least to equimolar doses of isoproterenol (epinephrine > norepinephrine >> isoproterenol) and the β receptor as one that was found in a tissue that responded most to isoproterenol and less to equimolar concentrations of epinephrine or norepinephrine, with phenylephrine being the least potent sympathomimetic amine in this series (isoproterenol >> epinephrine or norepinephrine > phenylephrine).

The theory gained additional attention from the fact that ergot and its derivatives specifically blocked the effects of the sympathomimetic drugs in tissues with α receptors but could not inhibit responses to the same drugs in tissues with β receptors. Such observations are remarkable in view of the very complex pharmacologic actions of ergots, which even today are being revealed.[332] Later it was discovered that derivatives of isoproterenol — first those whose phenyl hydroxyl groups were replaced by chloride (DCI) and then the derivatives, propranolol and pronethalol, which did not stimulate tissues themselves — could block β, but not α, receptor reactions to stimulation.[461]

Despite Ahlquist's warnings, many medical scientists concluded that the receptors were concrete identifiable structures (an assumption that appears to be coming true), that only α receptors were stimulated by norepinephrine or phenylephrine, and that only β receptors were stimulated by isoproterenol (assumptions that clearly are not true).

All drugs tested produced some effects on each tissue tested. That is, isoproterenol, norepinephrine, and epinephrine, if used in sufficient concentration, could stimulate both α and β receptors. Therefore, the response to a single agent (particularly *in vivo*) could not characterize the receptors that are stimulated to produce the effect. Also, although the classic α blockers (such as phentolamine, dihydroergotamine, and phenoxybenzamine) and β blockers (such as propranolol and pronethalol) specifically blocked their respective receptors, their actions *in vivo* or at high concentrations *in vitro* might be nonspecific and depend on some other pharmacologic property. Thus, although propranolol may have a salutary effect on some clinical condition (e.g., tachycardia), the response *per se* does not mean that the drug is working by its receptor-blocking qualities nor that the pathogenesis of the clinical condition lies in an abnormality of the sympathetic nervous system or the receptors.[55, 192]

Using two procedures, pharmacologists have begun to rigorously classify responses of various tissues. They first determine the concentration-response curves of a given effector system (cell, tissue, organ, or organ system) for a series of sympathomimetic drugs. Then they establish the quantitative capacity of a series of antagonists to reduce the sensitivity of the responding tissues to an agonist.[192, 385.] By the latter procedure, they establish a series of dissociation constants (K_B) for the receptor-antagonist complexes.[192] Major advantages have attended this careful approach.

The chemical characteristics of receptors began to be understood. The α receptors, previously thought to be strikingly similar regardless of the tissue or species of origin in which they were found, are now becoming known as a spectrum of receptors. Likewise, the β receptors seem to represent a broad spectrum of chemical or physical types; the potency orders of agonists and K_B vary in different tissues, or even in the same tissue, when different responses are studied. On this basis, and on the basis of the study of the distribution of specifically bound radiolabeled antagonists of α-adrenergic receptors (e.g., ^{3}H-dihydroergocryptine) or β-adrenergic receptors (e.g., ^{131}I-hydroxybenzylpindolol or ^{3}H-dihydroalprenolol), we have come to a new and medically useful classification of α- and β-adrenergic receptors.[8, 16, 17, 21, 137, 405, 430, 548, 556, 557, 563, 565, 605] In fact, we can attach fluorescent molecules to β-adrenergic antagonists to identify the receptors in intact tissues, and methods have been designed that measure receptors in whole (intact) and suspended cells.[16, 264, 368] Lands and coworkers[322, 323] categorized β receptors as either β_1 or β_2; β_1-adrenergic receptors are predominant in cardiac tissues, whereas β_2 receptors are predominant primarily in smooth muscle and glandular cells. However, different tissues may possess both β_1 and β_2 receptors in varying proportions.[380] A similar heterogeneity also applies to α receptors. Those designated α_1 are predominant at postsynaptic effector sites of smooth muscle and glandular cells; α_2 receptors, which are proposed to exist on nerve terminals, are believed to mediate the presynaptic feedback inhibition of neural release of norepinephrine and, perhaps, ACh. Activating such α_2 receptors on cholinergic nerve terminals may contribute to the inhibition of intestinal activity that is caused by α-adrenergic agonists by limiting release of norepinephrine from nerve endings in the gut. Many of the adrenergic receptors in the CNS, and those that mediate certain metabolic responses to catecholamines, have not yet been definitively classified.[115, 191, 518]

The relative sensitivities of these adrenergic receptors to the three major catecholamines (epinephrine, norepinephrine, and isoproterenol) are as follows: (1) at sites with α_1 receptors, epinephrine is equal to or more potent than norepinephrine, which in turn is much more potent than isoproterenol (see previously); (2) at sites with α_2 receptors, epinephrine is either more or less potent than norepinephrine, depending on the tissue, and isoproterenol is ineffective; (3) at sites with β_1 receptors, isoproterenol is more potent than epinephrine, which is equipotent with norepinephrine; and (4) at sites with β_2 receptors, isoproterenol is equal to or more potent than epinephrine, which is more potent than norepinephrine. A number of drugs selectively activate or block these receptors. Particularly notable has been the development of β_1- and β_2-adrenergic agonists and of β_1 antagonists.

Generally, the effect of activating α_1 receptors in smooth muscle is excitatory, whereas the effect of activating β_2 receptors at such sites is inhibitory, although this is not an absolute distinction. In other tissues, β-adrenergic receptors can mediate stimulatory effects. Thus, activation of β receptors results in stimulation of various secretions (such as that of insulin), and the stimulatory effects of catecholamines on the heart are mediated by β_1 receptors.

Catecholamines inhibit propulsive contraction, and they reduce the tone of most intestinal smooth muscle; these effects appear to be mediated by both α- and β-adrenergic receptors. Activating β receptors located on smooth muscle cells relaxes them. α Receptors appear to inhibit gastrointestinal motility by a presynaptic action. Thus, activation of α receptors on cholinergic nerve terminals within the intestinal wall is associated with inhibition of the release of ACh. This is consistent with the observation that an α and a β blocking agent are both required to prevent completely the inhibitory effect of epinephrine on the intestine.[4]

An important factor in the response of an organ to sympathomimetic amines is the proportion and density of α and β receptors in the tissue. Norepinephrine has little effect on bronchial air flow because the receptors in bronchial smooth muscle appear to be largely of the β_2 type. In contrast, isoproterenol and epinephrine are potent bronchodilators. Cutaneous blood vessels possess α receptors almost exclusively, so that norepinephrine and epinephrine cause marked constriction of such vessels, and isoproterenol has little effect. The smooth muscle of blood vessels supplying skeletal muscles has both β receptors, the activation of which by low concentrations of epinephrine causes vasodilatation, and α receptors, which allow epinephrine to constrict these vessels. In this tissue the threshold concentration of epinephrine for activation of β_2 receptors is lower, but when both types of receptors are activated the response to α receptors predominates.

The Role of Receptor Stimulation or Blockade in Release of Catecholamines

Many sympathomimetic drugs, such as *amphetamine* and *ephedrine*, exert a large fraction of their effects by releasing norepinephrine from storage sites in the sympathetic nerves to the effector organ. The responses they elicit are therefore similar to those of norepinephrine but are slower in onset and generally longer lasting than those of a single equipressor dose of norepinephrine. They also exhibit tachyphylaxis; that is, repeated injections or continuous infusions of these indirectly acting drugs become less effective as the norepinephrine in releasable stores is depleted. Many sympathomimetic drugs owe part of their effect to release of norepinephrine, and they also act directly on adrenergic receptors. These agents generally are called "mixed"-acting sympathomimetic amines.

α-Adrenergic *agonists* can profoundly inhibit the release of norepinephrine by postganglionic neurons.[114, 115, 153, 226, 521] Conversely, when the sympathetic nerve to a tissue is stimulated in the presence of an α-adrenergic *antagonist*, such as phentolamine, tolazoline, or prazosin, there is a marked increase in the amount of norepinephrine released per nerve impulse.[62, 128] The inhibitory effect of norepinephrine on its release from noradrenergic nerve terminals appears to be mediated by a presynaptic α receptor.[520] As mentioned previously, these presynaptic α receptors are pharmacologically distinct from those found at postsynaptic sites. Yohimbine has been reported to be a relatively selective inhibitor of α_2-adrenergic receptors. It enhances neural release of norepinephrine at concentrations less than those required to block postsynaptic α_1 receptors.[518] Certain drugs, such as α-methylnorepinephrine and clonidine, are more potent agonists at sites with α_2 receptors than at sites with α_1 receptors, and, at appropriate concentrations, they preferentially inhibit the release of norepinephrine. A component of the antihypertensive effect of these agents may rely on this action.[36, 519] Phenylephrine and methoxamine, in contrast, activate postsynaptic α_1 receptors at much lower concentrations than are required to inhibit the release of transmitter.[325, 518] Agonists that stimulate β-adrenergic receptors (e.g., isoproterenol) appear to enhance the release of norepinephrine from neurons, but the intensity of this effect *in vivo* is under debate.[2, 135, 169] Regardless of whether β-adrenergic effects on release of mediator occur *in vivo*, they are modest when compared with the powerful inhibitory actions of α agonists. The clinician can now use drugs that will selectively effect only certain functions of the effectors (Table 10–2).

By insolubilizing some drugs with a high affinity for receptors, we can isolate the chemical components of cells that make up the receptor.[174, 331] Furthermore, we have already begun to separate those cells with receptors to specific agonists from suspensions of cells with similar morphologic characteristics.[371, 374, 596] Thus the functions of those agonists in cells previously not known to respond to catecholamines are being more readily defined.

Finally, we are beginning to understand and apply data that define the molecular interactions of catecholamines with other hormones (e.g., corticosteroids), with drugs (e.g., tolbutamide),[165, 501] and with the components of the receptor-adenylate cyclase system,[39, 61, 230, 294, 330, 339, 483, 488] as well as to understand how these components contribute to the overall responsiveness to adrenergic agonists,[259, 288] and how we might reconstitute those components in a cell hybrid.[483, 485] The next interesting steps in our understanding of receptors and their membrane and intracellular machinery will be learning how to reconstitute all components in a cell-free system. Many groups are working with this goal in mind.

Table 10–2. α-ADRENERGIC AND β-ADRENERGIC BLOCKING DRUGS*

	Receptors Blocked	Type of Blockade
α-Adrenergic Blocking Agents		
Phenoxybenzamine	Relatively selective for α_1	Noncompetitive
Dibenamine	Relatively selective for α_1	Noncompetitive
Prazosin	Relatively selective for α_1	Competitive
Phentolamine	Nonselective	Competitive
Tolazoline	Nonselective	Competitive
Yohimbine	Selective for α_2	Competitive
β-Adrenergic Blocking Agents		
Propranolol	Nonselective	Competitive
Alprenolol	Nonselective	Competitive
Oxyprenolol	Nonselective	Competitive
Pindolol	Nonselective	Competitive
Penbutolol	Nonselective	Competitive
Timolol	Nonselective	Competitive
Metoprolol	Relatively selective for β_1	Competitive
Atinolol	Relatively selective for β_1	Competitive
Acebutolol	Relatively selective for β_1	Competitive
Tolamolol	Relatively selective for β_1	Competitive
Butoxamine	Relatively selective for β_1	Competitive

*For reviews of the pharmacology of these drugs see Nies, A.: In *Clinical Pharmacology: Basic Principles in Therapeutics.* Melmon, K. L., and Morrelli, H. F. (eds.), New York, Macmillan Publishing Company, 1978, p. 142, 155; Prichard, B. N. C.: *Br. J. Pharmacol.* 5:379, 1978; Weiner, N.: In *The Pharmacological Basis of Therapeutics.* Goodman, L. S., and Gilman, A. S. (eds.), New York, Macmillan Publishing Company, 1980, Chs. 7, 8, and 9.

Physiologic and Pathologic Factors that Modify Availability of Adrenergic Receptors

Many physiologic and pathologic states can contribute to the responsiveness to a sympathetic or sympathomimetic stimulus; one such determinant is age itself.[571] As we have already stressed, the mechanisms of altered *in vivo* responsiveness are protean. Recently, because of our ability to measure chemically the presence of a receptor without necessarily awaiting a biologic response, we have begun to realize that one mechanism of altered responsiveness to constant hormonal signals is the modification of the availability of receptors.

Hormonal determinants of the availability of receptors include the effects of estrogens on α receptors in the uterus. α-Adrenergic binding sites increase more *in uteri* from animals treated with estrogen alone, than when progesterone is given after treatment with estrogen.[458] The hormones do not alter the availability of β-adrenergic receptors. The myocardium of rats treated with thyroid hormone greatly increases its complement of β-adrenergic receptors while the number of available α-adrenergic receptors decreases.[88, 603] When propylthiouracil is given to the hyperthyroid animals, the number of β receptors declines, but the decrease in α receptors is greater than when thyroid hormone is given alone. Of the receptors that are left, the binding affinity for agonist increases. Some feel that these observations help to explain the changes in the ability of these animals to respond to catecholamines. Other steroids, namely cortisone, can decrease availability of β-adrenergic receptors and may account for some of the altered responses to catecholamines in patients being given steroids (e.g., during shock).[609]

Temperature changes can alter the affinity of a receptor for its agonist. Cooling of peripheral veins may increase the affinity of the α receptors of the vessel for catecholamines and thus increase their responsiveness to the adrenergic stimulus.[271] Some have observed that temperature changes actually may contribute to the interconversion of α- and β-adrenergic receptors.[286] Aging also appears to play a role in decreasing availability of β receptors in the rat's erythrocyte and even perhaps in humans.[40, 48, 70]

Studies in which radioactive specific ligand markers are used to determine the type and number of adrenergic receptors on tissues are just now enabling us to realize that some diseases, such as leukemia, may reduce β-adrenergic receptor availability of the affected cells,[493] whereas other disease states, such as adrenocortical tumors, may create receptors for, and responsiveness to, β-adrenergic agonists because the tumor cells develop receptors that were not apparent on their normal progenators.[604]

The effects of drugs on receptors will be discussed in the section on tachyphylaxis (see below).

A few representative responses produced by catecholamines are listed in Table 10–3. An exhaustive list of the pharmacologic actions of catecholamines and a classification of their α and β mediation is beyond the scope of this chapter but is well reviewed[593] and is the subject of a number of other chapters in this book.

Mechanisms of "Receptor Activation"

A number of different studies have shown that the response of a cell to catecholamines is determined by whether or not receptors to α- and β-adrenergic agonists are available.[503] Early studies described the dose-response relationship for an agonist and an effector cell, as well as the relationship of agonists to antagonists in terms of availabil-

Table 10-3. CLASSIFICATION OF MAJOR α-ADRENERGIC AND β-ADRENERGIC RESPONSES ELICITED BY CATECHOLAMINES

Effects	α	β
Vascular		
Constriction, veins and arteries	+	0
Dilatation, arteries	0	+
Cardiac		
Increase in heart rate	0	+
Increase in atrial contractility and		
conduction rate	0	+
Increase in conduction velocity of A-V node	0	+
Increase in ventricular contractility,		
automaticity, and conduction velocity	0	+
Pulmonary		
Dilatation of bronchial musculature	0	+
Liver		
Glycogenolysis, gluconeogenesis	0	+
Pancreas		
Acinic—decreased secretion	+	0
Islets—decreased secretion	+	0
increased secretion	0	+
Fat cells		
Lipolysis	0	+
Salivary glands		
Potassium and water secretion	+	0
Amylase secretion	0	+
Pineal gland		
Melatonin synthesis	0	+

ity of receptors. In these studies, many tissues appeared to contain receptors in excess of the number required for a full response to most agonists ("spare receptors"). A considerable proportion could be irreversibly inactivated before the tissue was rendered incapable of a maximal response. With increasing doses of the blocking agent, the dose-response curve for an agonist shifts progressively to the right while the number of available receptors is reduced. When the number of functional receptors is reduced to a degree that makes the original maximal response no longer attainable with a full agonist, the dose-response curve does not shift further to the right; further blockage of the receptor leads to a depression in the maximal response. The reduction in maximal response is then proportional to further irreversible blockage of the remaining receptors.

Changes in the availability of receptors to an agonist has helped us to explain one major mechanism of tachyphylaxis. Several mechanisms may be involved, but one is the apparent disappearance of receptors for catecholamines from the cell surface.[139, 185, 292, 302, 340, 345, 378, 392, 393] This process of desensitization to the pharmacologic effects of catecholamines may involve internalization of receptors or some type of ill-defined prolonged high affinity relationship of the receptor with the agonist. The process appears to depend to some extent on synthesis of proteins.[132] In leukocytes, the loss of receptors appears to be dependent on the presence, but not the activation, of adenylate cyclase.[491] Apparently, neither the direct effects of cAMP nor the indirect effects of activation of cAMP-dependent protein kinase are involved in the loss of availability of receptors for the agonist. Furthermore, only the agonist and *not* the antagonist produces the apparent loss of receptors.[231] The loss of receptors is specific for the agonist and does not reduce the effects of other agonists that require adenylate cyclase for their biologic effects. Antagonists actually appear to increase receptor availability.[202]

Other mechanisms contribute to tachyphylaxis.[84, 271] Among them is the mechanism by which the second messenger (see below) activates a protein kinase that is dependent upon its presence. The kinase in turn activates (presumably by phosphorylation) specific enzymes or substrates for enzymes that mediate a variety of biologic events stimulated by catecholamines. One such enzyme, phosphodiesterase, metabolizes intracellular cAMP and thereby limits any continued intracellular message provoked by the catecholamines.[369] To what precise extent each of the two described mechanisms accounts for all of the tachyphylaxis and whether other factors also contribute to tachyphylaxis in a single cell remains to be determined.

In tissues that are more complex than suspended cells, many additional factors can contribute to tachyphylaxis. They include, but are not limited to, the relative distribution of α versus β receptors on the tissue, the altered regional blood flow caused by a drug, the degree of oxygenation of tissues and the blood, the alterations in pH at the site of drug action, the metabolic viability of responding cells, and the state of responsiveness of the body or local nerves to homeostatic reflex drives.

A group of studies elegantly elucidates one likely molecular mechanism by which the β agonist allies the β receptor with adenylate cyclase and thus initiates the production of cAMP. Axelrod and his coworkers have used rat erythrocyte membranes that contain β receptors to demonstrate a two-step process of initiation of hormone-caused effects. They have shown that erythrocyte membranes synthesize phosphatidylcholine from phosphatidylethanolamine by two steps involving two separate enzymes. The first enzyme is localized on the cytoplasmic side of the membrane, and it methylates phosphatidylethanolamine to phosphatidyl-N-monomethyl-ethanolamine. It has a high affinity for the methyl donor (S-adenosyl-L-methionine) and requires magnesium. The second enzyme is localized on the cell surface near the receptor; it accepts the first product and transfers two additional methyl groups to it, thus converting it to phosphatidylcholine. The second enzyme has a low affinity for the methyl donor and does not require magnesium. The spatial segregation of the two enzymes facilitates the rapid transfer of phospholipids across the membrane as methylations occur (Fig. 10–10). This in turn presumably causes profound changes in membrane fluidity. The complex but well-defined process that might enhance membrane fluidity is stimulated by a β-agonist, such as isoproterenol, and is crucial to the coupling of the β-adrenergic receptor to adenylate cyclase.[22] How and whether the process also relates to the role of guanyl nucleotides in helping to link receptor to adenylate cyclase and to activate the latter remains for further study.[549-551, 564] It seems likely that these studies on the erythrocyte will translate to other cells. Whether the same process contributes to mobility of receptors produced by agonists is not known.

For general references and new information related to adrenergic receptors refer to the works cited in references 190, 278, 341, 456, 526, and 602.

Cyclic 3',5'-Adenosine Monophosphate and Catecholamines

Knowing what the catecholamines can do and that the various responses are mediated through α or β receptors does not mean that the actual mechanism of their effect is known. There are several determinants of the response of a cell: the catecholamine must be released and make its way to the cell; the cell must possess a proper receptor to accept the messenger; the initial response of the cell to the messenger appears to be dependent on some intracellular second messenger; and the ultimate response depends on the transfer of the second message to the cellular machinery that carries on the response.

In some cells, a response may go unnoticed because we do not know what to measure (e.g., the effects of catechola-

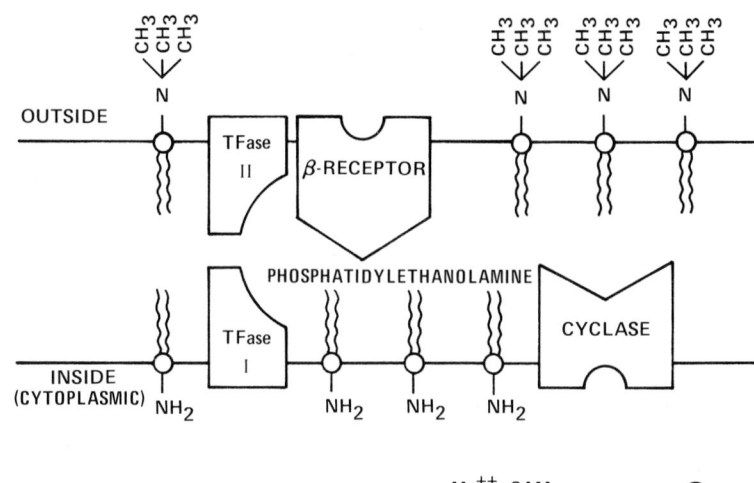

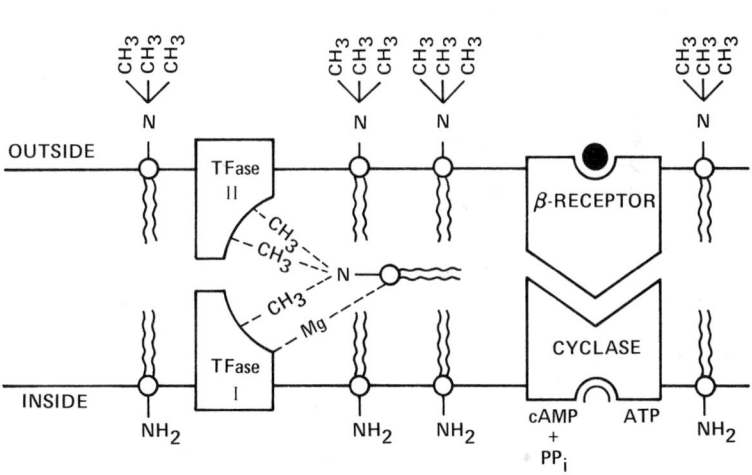

Figure 10–10. *A proposed mechanism of stimulation of phospholipid methylation by isoproterenol-facilitated coupling of the beta-adrenergic receptor and adenylate cyclase.* TFase I = phosphatidylethanolamine-N-methyltransferase; TFase II: Phosphatidylcholine forming enzyme; SAM = S-adenosyl-L-methionine; ● is L-isoproterenol. Note the transfer of the phosphatidylethanolamine from the cytoplasmic side of the membrane to the outer surface. Simultaneous with this is the likely alignment of the hormone-occupied receptor with adenylate cyclase. (Adapted from Hirata, F., Strittmatter, W. J., and Axelrod, J.: *Beta*-adrenergic receptor agonists increase phospholipid methylation, membrane fluidity and *beta*-adrenergic receptor-adenylate cyclase coupling. *Proc. Natl. Acad. Sci. USA 76:* 368-372, 1979.)

mines on avian or amphibian red blood cells); however, in most instances the *effect* is known, but the mechanism of its initiation is not. The second messenger for at least some responses to catecholamines is cAMP. As discussed in this and other chapters, cAMP appears to be a key second messenger for a variety of hormones, including the other autacoids that we are now considering.

cAMP was discovered during studies of the effects of epinephrine on hepatic glycogenolysis. cAMP is now established as a likely second messenger after receptor stimulation by catecholamines. Studies have convincingly linked the production of glucose by the liver with stimulation of the β receptor and accumulation of cAMP. The present minimal criteria for determining whether cAMP mediates the effect of any catecholamine include the following: the agonist drug or hormone must produce a specific effect, which is specifically blocked by an antagonist, and the stimulation should correlate with (1) a rise in intracellular cAMP; (2) a drop in cAMP when the response is blocked; (3) a mimicking of the effect of the agonist by cAMP or a derivative, dibutyryl cAMP, more capable of entering cells; and (4) the ability of drugs (e.g., xanthine derivatives such as theophylline) that prevent intracellular enzymatic breakdown of cAMP to potentiate the effects of the agonist at doses that only potentiate accumulation of intracellular cAMP. In recent years one more test has occasionally been added: nonspecific stimulants of adenylate cyclase that result in accumulation of intracellular cAMP (e.g., cholera toxin, which

stimulates adenylate cyclase in all tissues in which it has been tested) should produce the same cellular effect as the agonist. Of course, the ultimate aim of investigators is to isolate the cell machinery and to show that cAMP initiates the effect in a cell-free system. In the case of the hepatocyte, such has been done (see previous discussion).

The majority of the criteria just mentioned have been applied to a few select actions of catecholamines on β receptors, including (1) hepatic glycogenolysis, (2) lipolysis in the adipocyte, (3) the positive inotropic response in the heart, (4) relaxation of uterine muscle, (5) release of insulin from the pancreas, (6) inhibition of leukocytic release of histamine provoked by IgE, of cytolysis of mast cells by sensitized lymphocytes, and of antibody release from some lymphocytes, and (7) decreases in ornithine and S-adenosylmethionine decarboxylase activities.[618] The latter may indicate that we are beginning to understand some anti-inflammatory actions of catechol and indole amines.[12, 13, 215]

It is likely that more effects of catecholamines mediated by stimulation of β receptors will be linked to cAMP (e.g., calorigenic effects of catecholamines, vascular and bronchial dilation, lactic acid production by skeletal muscle, effects on some hormone-producing glands such as the pineal, and many of the actions of catecholamines on brain) (see Ch. 11). The nucleotide has a host of pharmacologic effects that, if listed, might supply an outline for a text of endocrinology.[233] Although there are several theoretic reasons why

Table 10–4. SOME CELLS AND TISSUES IN WHICH ADENYLATE CYCLASE IS STIMULATED BY CATECHOLAMINES

Liver	Adipose tissue
Spleen	Pancreatic islets
Cardiac muscle	Avian and amphibian but not
Skeletal muscle	human erythrocytes
Smooth muscle	Leukocytes
Brain	Parotid gland
Pineal	Lung

the receptor *per se* may not be adenylate cyclase alone, it already seems apparent that, at least in myocardial tissue, the β receptor is intimately and physically associated with some components of the cAMP-generating system.[331] Additional evidence clearly shows that the receptor and cyclase have different genetic determinants.[265] Table 10–4 lists some tissues in which adenylate cyclase is stimulated by catecholamines.

Sympathomimetic amines do not stimulate α receptors via a mediating step involving activation of cellular adenylate cyclase. In fact, the opposite perhaps occurs. Stimulation of α receptors in the pancreas limits insulin release, in the adipocyte inhibits lipolysis, in the dorsal frog skin antagonizes skin darkening effect, in the platelet inhibits platelet aggregation, and in toad bladder reduces permeability to water. In each preparation, stimulation and the effect are associated with reduction of cAMP concentrations. The mechanism of this reduction is not known. It was probably fortunate that responses to β stimulation were studied before those to α stimulation were studied. In a number of experimental settings in the study of the α receptor, pharmacologic manipulations first had to be performed to raise concentrations of cAMP. Only then could stimulation of the α receptor be correlated with noticeable decreases in cAMP. Such observations make it less easy to accept cAMP as the second messenger for α receptor stimulation than it is to accept it as the second messenger for β stimulation. Perhaps a decrease in the nucleotide concentration could be a signal for activity in the cells; perhaps another mediator is the true messenger. One candidate that has been considered for years but that has not yet been established is cyclic guanosine monophosphate (cGMP).

Finally, it is important to realize that the response of tissues to catecholamines can be modulated by other chemically unrelated hormones. For instance, estrogenic steroids and progesterones modify the response of the uterus to catecholamines during the normal menstrual cycle (described previously). Glucocorticoids modify the response of adipocytes and vascular tissue to catecholamines by entirely different mechanisms.[280, 482] The effects of some steroids on the oviduct and the prostate can be reversed by β blocking drugs at reasonable doses (>10^{-4} to 10^{-5}M.).[45] Serotonin and dopamine may modify the effects of sympathomimetic agents on insulin release.[445] Many of these interactions are discussed in other chapters but are mentioned here to draw attention once again to the complexity of interrelationships that must always be considered when interpreting the action of catecholamines *in vitro* and attempting to apply them *in vivo*.

Pharmacologic Effects of Dopamine and Dobutamine

No longer can dopamine be considered only as a chemical precursor of norepinephrine. It also appears to have specific physiologic roles in the CNS, the carotid body, and the kidney.[74, 597] The pharmacologic effects of the amine and its congeners have been studied, and they are distinct from those of norepinephrine and epinephrine. Receptors for dopamine are also distinguishable from those for α- and β-adrenergic agonists.[205] The differences between the pharmacologic properties of dopamine and those of the two endogenous catecholamines may have some clinical importance.

Peripheral Effects

Dopamine has positive inotropic effects on the myocardium and acts as an agonist at sites of β_1 receptors. It also has the capacity for releasing norepinephrine from nerve terminals, and thus contributes to β_2-like effects. Tachycardia is less likely to occur when relatively small amounts of dopamine are infused and more likely to occur when small amounts of isoproterenol are infused. Dopamine appears to increase both systolic and pulse pressures, and it either has no effect on or only slightly increases diastolic blood pressure. Total peripheral resistance usually is unchanged by low or intermediate therapeutic doses. This is probably because dopamine can reduce regional arterial resistance in the mesentery and the kidney, while mildly increasing it in other regional beds. The effects of dopamine on the renal vasculature and CNS appear to be mediated by specific pre- and postsynaptic dopaminergic receptors.[303, 399] When infused in relatively low doses, dopamine is associated with increased glomerular filtration rate, renal blood flow, and sodium excretion. On this basis, dopamine theoretically could be especially useful in managing cardiogenic, traumatic, or hypovolemic shock when major increases in the sympathetic activity may disproportionately compromise renal function. Because dopamine is a potent sympathomimetic agent, its use in life-threatening states of shock must be monitored as carefully as the use of other catecholamines. As the doses increase, the predominant α-adrenergic effects must be carefully monitored in order to avoid inordinately elevated blood pressure and also to avoid reducing renal function as a consequence of renal vasoconstriction. Many aspects of the pharmacology of dopamine have been reviewed by Goldberg and his coworkers.[204]

Although there are specific dopaminergic receptors in the CNS, parenterally administered dopamine probably does not affect the CNS because it does not easily or rapidly cross the blood-brain barrier (see below).

Although dopamine does not produce the majority of metabolic effects associated with its β-hydroxylated relatives, what metabolic effects it does have (e.g., on inhibition of insulin release) are mediated by its ability either to release catecholamines or to mimic the effects of norepinephrine. Its ability to inhibit insulin release is in turn blocked by α-adrenergic blocking drugs. When given intravenously (e.g., as in the treatment of shock in humans), dopamine may produce a transitory increase in blood pressure by the same mechanism by which it affects release of insulin. This arterial constriction can be prevented by giving the drug slowly, administering an α blocking agent, or, as has been noted, administering the drug as the amino acid, L-dopa.[178] A series of blockers that is able to interfere selectively with dopamine has been identified and is reviewed in standard texts of pharmacology.[332, 593]

L-Dopa generally produces the same cardiovascular and metabolic effects as dopamine. The amino acid is readily decarboxylated, particularly in non-CNS tissues. If decarboxylation is inhibited, the majority of the direct pharmacologic effects of L-dopa are also inhibited.[416] The drug, unlike dopamine, can enter the brain. There its amine (produced both by enzymatic and nonenzymatic decarboxylation) produces minor negative inotropic and chronotropic effects on the heart.[416] The effects of L-dopa on the function of certain areas of the brain are profound, however, and its proper use has resulted in one of the most exciting therapeutic stories, involving dopamine and Parkinson's syndrome (see below).

Dobutamine resembles dopamine chemically but possesses a bulky aromatic substituent on the amino group. Despite the absence of a β-OH group, dobutamine is a direct-acting agent with selectivity for β_1 receptors; its indirect actions are slight.[506]

Dobutamine appears to be relatively more effective in enhancing the contractile force of the heart than it is in increasing heart rate, and it does not produce peripheral vasodilatation.[560, 561] The drug therefore appears to be a relatively specific β_1 agonist when producing its inotropic effect. Although dobutamine does enhance the automaticity of the sinus node in humans, this action is not as prominent as that produced by isoproterenol. Dobutamine does not appear to affect atrial conduction velocity in humans, although it does augment conduction velocity through the atrioventricular node. It has little or no effect on ventricular impulse conduction. In contrast to dopamine, dobutamine does not have an effect on the dopaminergic receptors in the renal vasculature, and, therefore, does not produce renal vasodilatation.[204]

In animals, dobutamine, administered at a rate of 2.5–15 μg/kg/min, increases cardiac contractility and cardiac output. Total peripheral resistance is not notably affected. The heart rate increases only modestly when the rate of administration of dobutamine is maintained at less than 20 μg/kg/min. After β-blocking agents are administered, infusion of dobutamine fails to increase cardiac output but total peripheral resistance increases, which suggests that dobutamine does have modest direct effects on α receptors in the vasculature. Reflex tachycardia associated with isoproterenol-induced hypotension cannot explain the greater chronotropic effect of isoproterenol as compared with dobutamine because neither vagotomy nor agents that interfere with the function of sympathetic neurons eliminate the difference in the chronotropic effects of the two drugs.

Dopamine and the Central Nervous System

The diversified work leading to the present use of L-dopa in the treatment of Parkinson's disease is an instructive scenario for modern pharmacology and neuroendocrinology. The critical steps in that work follow.

Initially, study of the function of the basal ganglia was carried out by physiologists who were more or less limited to creating surgical lesions and studying the functional results. Few if any useful models of parkinsonism were developed. By chance, pharmacologists discovered that a number of drugs could create a condition similar to Parkinson's syndrome. These drugs (haloperidol, reserpine, and phenothiazines) were dissimilar in chemical structure but all had effects on the CNS that only recently have been mechanistically defined. Simultaneously, as investigations of these three drugs progressed, evidence began to indicate a role for ACh in the CNS.

Belladonna was given 75–100 years ago to some patients with Parkinson's disease and was sometimes beneficial. Neither the reason it worked in some but not others nor its mechanism of action was known. Investigation at first was limited to screening of drugs. A number of additional anticholinergic drugs were tried with variable but more or less useful results. Later, cholinomimetic drugs (e.g., trem-

orine) were injected into the CNS, where they reproduced a tremor similar to that in Parkinson's disease. Until 1967, no one was sure whether the beneficial effects of the antiparkinsonism drugs (anticholinergic drugs) were based on their effects on the CNS. Then it was clearly shown that physostigmine given centrally reproduced the syndrome, and only those anticholinergic drugs that were transported into the CNS (e.g., benztropine and scopolamine but not quarternary anticholinesterases) would ameliorate symptoms.

Working with these drugs, Duvoisin made a major breakthrough when he pinpointed the corpus striatum as the locale of their beneficial effects. Later, this area was found to contain the highest concentrations of choline acetylase, ACh, and acetylcholinesterase of any region in the brain. Duvoisin was among the first to conclude that cholinergic activity was important in ordinary function of the extrapyramidal areas and to suggest that the influence of the cholinergic system was probably balanced by another chemical in the brain — dopamine.

Investigation of the function of the adrenergic neurons in the CNS paralleled study of the function of ACh. Some expected that the functions of dopamine, which had been determined in the CNS, would be different from those of the other adrenergic neurotransmitter, norepinephrine. In the cardiovascular system, the effects of dopamine were different from those of norepinephrine and epinephrine, and in the brain dopamine composed about 50% of the total catecholamines. It did not seem logical that so much should be there simply as a substrate for catecholamine synthesis when the rate-limiting step in synthesis was tyrosine hydroxylase, not dopamine β-oxidase. The turnover of dopamine was faster in areas where it was concentrated than in areas where norepinephrine was predominant.[138] The opposite would have been expected if the dopamine were serving only as a precursor to norepinephrine. Then Carlsson's group and others found that most of the dopamine in the brain was concentrated in very few areas, primarily in the corpus striatum where the ratio of dopamine to norepinephrine was 100/1. In the caudate nucleus of some animal species, dopamine concentration was 10 μg/g, and norepinephrine was 0.1 μg/g. Conversely, in the hypothalamus of the same animals, the ratio was reversed, 1/10.

In studies in which fluorescent staining techniques were used, catecholamines (norepinephrine and dopamine) were found in the neuron bodies of the substantia nigra of nonprimates, but not in the corpus striatum. These same studies showed that lesions in the substantia nigra produced degeneration of nerves in that area, loss of dopamine from axons of the corpus striatum, and a tremor that resembled parkinsonism; analogous experiments in subhuman primates produced the same results. Furthermore, stimulation of the nerves of the substantia nigra resulted in release of dopamine from the area of the corpus striatum, while chlorpromazine could block uptake of dopamine in the receptor areas of the nerves. Pharmacologic inhibition (by haloperidol) of the effects of dopamine produced a tremor. Reserpine depleted dopamine and norepinephrine, and dopamine-like drugs (apomorphine) had beneficial effects in patients with Parkinson's syndrome.[100]

A hypothesis linking dopamine to the function of the extrapyramidal system was developing. In some experiments reserpine and other drugs selectively replenished dopamine in the brain of the mouse while also reawakening the animal and restoring normal extrapyramidal function.[103] It remained only to find that humans with parkinsonism had consistent lesions in the substantia nigra. The same area showed abnormally low concentrations of dopamine and its metabolite, homovanillic acid (HVA), without profound depletion of norepinephrine and serotonin. The pathogenesis seemed certain.

It was later found that the decarboxylase enzyme and amine-metabolizing enzymes remained in the area of the lesions and that administration of dopa (which crossed the blood-brain barrier) could reverse the central effects of reserpine and chlorpromazine (an adverse drug reaction had proved beneficial).[251] The way was paved for a proper therapeutic trial with dopa in humans.[370] When prolonged high doses of dopa were administered to patients with Parkinson's disease, most were noticeably improved and some "cured." They became indistinguishable from normal individuals until the drug was withdrawn, at which time the symptoms returned.[448]

The present hypothesis proposed that ACh and dopamine interact to control the function of the extrapyramidal system. The system can be rebalanced either by returning the malfunctioning component to normal (ideal) or by inhibiting the function of the normal component to bring it into harmony with the other (e.g., use of anticholinergic drugs in parkinsonism). Combinations of both approaches are rational and efficacious. It would be foolish to say that such advances could have been made or understood without knowing the details of catecholamine synthesis, storage, release, effect, and metabolism.

L-Dopa is well absorbed. It must be given in large doses to ensure that adequate amounts will penetrate the brain;[610] it must be spontaneously or enzymatically decarboxylated before it works, and its effects are consistent with its inhibitory function.[343, 344] The deficiency of tyrosine hydroxylase that produces the lesion in parkinsonism need not be inherited. Any abnormality that results in degenerative lesions of the adrenergic nerves will decrease the tissue content of tyrosine hydroxylase (see synthesis of catecholamines).[210, 359] In a great number of patients with Parkinson's disease or syndrome, L-dopa is effective; it even works in those patients with magnesium poisoning that results in physical and chemical lesions similar to those in parkinsonism.[98]

There are unwanted side effects from use of the drug, apparently including some peripheral effects of dopamine and its common and uncommon[547] metabolites. If the peripheral effects of dopamine were detrimental, decarboxylase inhibitors might be expected to preferentially inhibit metabolism of dopa in non-brain tissues. Such tests of decarboxylase inhibition will have to be carefully watched because there is evidence that some beneficial effects of dopa are mediated by the peripheral effects of some of its metabolites. In addition, it has been learned that diets of patients taking dopa should probably be controlled[591] and that MAO inhibitors can cause hypertension in these people.[262] When dopamine is formed rapidly, it accumulates and probably displaces norepinephrine from its storage sites in the same way as would tyramine (see section on false neurotransmitters).

Hypotension may also be a problem during chronic administration of the drug. The mechanism of action is not certain but could include arterial dilation of the renal vascular system, the naturetic effects of dopa, and its central negative inotropic and chronotropic actions. Also actions of unusual metabolites of the drug or amine may cause the hypotension. We are a long way from fully understanding all we need to know about the action of the drug. If the hypotension is related to the peripheral actions of dopamine or its metabolites, perhaps peripheral decarboxylase inhibitors will counter it. Otherwise, decreasing the dose of dopa and adding adjunctive drugs seems inevitable.[56] One adjunctive drug may be a dopamine derivative that crosses the blood-brain barrier and has no peripheral effects.[28, 434]

Others might be drugs like amantadine, which, though not a catecholamine, seems to enhance accumulation of dopamine in the brain.[578] Still others might be the anticholinergic drugs having a mechanism of action very different from that of dopa. Finally, combinations of drugs have been used that allow smaller doses of L-dopa and that minimize its decarboxylation outside of the brain and the deamination of dopamine inside the brain. The combination requires an inhibitor of L-amino acid decarboxylase that does enter the brain, plus an inhibitor of MAO-B (see above). These combinations have become clinically useful.

There are at least two additional clinical applications of our knowledge of the chemistry and pharmacology of dopa and dopamine.

1. The decreased renal arterial vascular resistance and lack of major peripheral vascular pressor effects from dopamine may explain the relative infrequency of hypertension in patients with neuroblastomas, tumors frequently associated with increased urinary excretion of dopamine and its metabolite, HVA.

2. In cases of suspected neural crest tumors, increased excretion of dopamine or HVA or both may herald the malignant spread of a pheochromocytoma or of tumors of more primitive types (discussed later).[99]

Alterations During Disease and Drug Therapy

In several pathologic states, the responses to endogenous or exogenous catecholamines may be altered (Table 10–5). For example, in patients with various types of cardiomegaly, the increased mass of myocardium may "dilute" nerve endings that are capable of biologically inactivating catecholamines, whereas effector sites remain stable.[179] This explanation, although plausible, is unproved and chemical

Table 10-5. SOME CONDITIONS CHARACTERIZED BY ALTERED SENSITIVITY TO CATECHOLAMINES

Conditions Associated with Increased Sensitivity
Cardiomegaly
  Congestive heart failure
  Hypertrophy—secondary to physical obstruction or increase in peripheral vascular resistance
  Myocardiopathy of various etiologies
Thyrotoxicosis (?)*
Sympathetic denervation
  Diabetes mellitus
  Surgical or anesthetic procedures
  Orthostatic hypotension
Nutritional abnormalities
  Scurvy
Unclassified diseases
  Hyperkinetic cardiovascular disorders
  Familial dysautonomia
Drugs
  Imipramine
  Some antiadrenergic drugs (e.g., guanethidine and reserpine)
Conditions Associated with Decreased Sensitivity
Acidosis—metabolic or respiratory
Myxedema
Adrenal insufficiency
Conditions Associated with Paradoxical Effects
Diseases
  Carcinoid syndrome
Drug administration
  Phenothiazines

---

*There is considerable debate about the sensitivity of patients with thyrotoxicosis to catecholamines. The rate of turnover and the binding properties by the neurons may be altered, and excessive adrenergic activity may result. However, recently acquired data makes it unlikely that there is true hypersensitivity in response to exogenous catecholamines.[334]

alterations in binding sites as well as defects in synthesis of catecholamines have been detected in some cardiac disease (e.g., congestive heart failure). The increased sensitivity to catecholamines after surgical sympathetic denervation or in disease states such as diabetes mellitus also may be related to a decrease in the uptake of catecholamines into storage sites.[246] The same phenomenon occurs in patients taking drugs that do block catecholamine uptake into storage sites but that do not affect receptor areas,[247, 515, 610] and this may be an operative factor in thyrotoxicosis or during administration of thyroid hormone.[334] Not all drugs that alter the effects of catecholamines are similar in chemical structure of catecholamines, nor are they all used for their effects on the sympathetic nervous system (Fig. 10–8).

Major alterations in the receptor tissue could cause increased or decreased responsiveness to catecholamines, as in such diseases as metabolic or respiratory acidosis, myxedema, and adrenocortical insufficiency. In rare clinical conditions and during administration of certain drugs, catecholamines may elicit a hypotensive rather than hypertensive response. The occurrence of such paradoxical effects is seen most strikingly in the carcinoid syndrome.

For many years, it has been suspected that some abnormality of the sympathetic nervous system or change in the sensitivity of effector organs for the actions of catecholamines might participate in the pathogenesis of essential hypertension in humans.[7, 104, 121, 123, 223, 376, 395] Although there is evidence that abnormal storage of catecholamines in the CNS of a strain of rats may result in familial hypertension, there is little if any evidence that such abnormalities are shared by hypertensive humans.[310] Catecholamines may influence the production of angiotensin[607] or other vasoactive peptides that may affect blood pressure.[358] However, though various abnormalities in storage, synthesis, or release of catecholamines have been described in experimental and human hypertension, neither these abnormalities nor consistent abnormalities of the sympathetic nervous system have been etiologically related to essential hypertension in humans.[249, 408, 586]

Evidence of Functional Interrelationships in the Physiologic and Pharmacologic Effects of Autacoids

In the 4th edition of this text, a section (albeit short) was devoted to the interrelated effects of histamine, catecholamines, serotonin, and vasoactive polypeptides. In the last edition, that section was dropped, mainly because the data linking the various autacoids in pharmacologic and physiologic events were not convincing. Now they are convincing, and they have been alluded to many times in the preceding section. In this chapter we have already described the multiple factors, including a spectrum of autacoids themselves, that impact on physiologic net storage of catecholamines in, and their release from, nerve endings. These interrelationships can be applied to other situations and now appear to have unequivocal pharmacologic and physiologic meaning; knowing about them should heuristically affect both the endocrinologist and the student.

Autacoids can interact simultaneously at multiple levels. That is, the mechanisms by which they interact can be direct, indirect, or some combination thereof. They may be additive or antagonistic: if additive the effects may serve either to augment or to inhibit a physiologic event; if antagonistic the effects may be to nullify opposing forces that therefore are never expressed biologically unless one force is withdrawn from the setting. Because so many drugs are available and so many diseases have been identified that selectively intensify or inhibit the release or effect of autacoids, one should be aware of the challenges to homeostasis, as well as to correct interpretation of the effects that the use of these agents, or the appearance of specific diseases, present. It was not our intention to recount all of the known interactions of the autacoids in this chapter. In fact, many of their crucial interactions take place in the CNS and are discussed in Ch. 11. Nevertheless, some are demonstrable in the periphery, and they illustrate the known interconnections that must be taken into account in therapy and diagnosis.

Interactions between catecholamines, ACh, histamine, and serotonin are all that we will consider, but many other substances entwine themselves into these relationships. The interactions can be a result of the *direct actions of the hormones*. For instance, ACh and histamine both can act, but through separate receptors, on bronchial smooth muscle to produce additive bronchoconstriction.[144] This interaction may exist in patients with asthma, thus resulting in recent reconsiderations of atropine as an adjunctive drug in the management of patients with asthma. The direct actions of ACh can summate with the effects of serotonin on the esophagus and relax its sphincters.[449] Similarly, ACh may intensify the effects of α-adrenergic stimulation on the parotid gland.[415] In addition, β-adrenergic stimulation may provoke production of serotonin.[63] Conversely, the additive effects of epinephrine, histamine, and prostaglandins of the E series may summate *to inhibit or to antagonize* IgE-mediated release of histamine from basophils or mast cells.[53] In catecholamines, α-mimetic effects counter β-mimetic effects in secretion of insulin and illustrate direct actions that inhibit each other, as do opposing effects of α-mimetic amines (constrictor effects) versus histamine (dilator effects) on vascular smooth muscle, the effects of epinephrine (dilator) versus histamine and ACh (constrictor) on bronchial musculature, or the effects of epinephrine (positive inotropic) versus ACh (negative inotropic) on the heart.[293] The inhibitory effects may not work through classic receptors. For instance, epinephrine may antagonize the effects of histamine on lymph flow, but the effects of the catecholamines are not inhibited by α-adrenergic blocking agents.[357] Many autacoids affect the amount of transmitter that is released after stimulation of the sympathetic nervous system. Norepinephrine, ACh, histamine, and serotonin will inhibit release of norepinephrine, whereas angiotensin II and some prostaglandins augment the release.[492]

The additive effects may be due to *indirect actions* of one or each autacoid. For example, serotonin and its precursor amino acid may facilitate the release of a number of neurotransmitters at the synapse and thus augment the effects of what ordinarily would be expected from nerve stimulation.[32, 406, 588] Similarly, the effects provoked when ACh releases multiple neurotransmitters from the same, or various, tissues as well as the ability of histamine both to be released by, and to release, catecholamines from their respective neuronal storage areas are well known.

The interrelationships of autacoids are not necessarily defined simply by the effects of what are considered selective antagonists. For instance, phentolamine and phenoxybenzamine can do more than simply antagonize α-adrenergic agents. In recent examples, phenoxybenzamine can antagonize the effects of opiates,[511] and phentolamine was shown to have anticholinergic actions that modulated histamine-mediated reflex vasodilation in a dog.[453] Finally, some endogenous substances can modify the effects of autacoids, e.g., endogenous opiates can block inhibition by dopamine of prolactin (PRL) secretion in *in vitro* models.[163]

Finally, the interrelated effects can express themselves

at multiple tiers of an event. For instance, epinephrine can directly modulate (by inhibiting) the release of parathyroid hormone (PTH). Because PTH regulates calcium and calcium in turn may modify the pharmacologic expression of the effects of catecholamines on the myocardium, we can see the difficulty in understanding such an overtly simple, but occult and truly complex, series of events in one biologic action.[50] The same challenges arise when one considers the effects of estrogen and progesterone on the effects of serotonin on central blood flow, or the effects of centrally mediated serotonin action on coronary artery control.[150, 504]

In summary, complex interactions between autacoids, between autacoids and more classic hormones, and between autacoids and reflex compensatory events clearly exist. They are important to physiologic, pathologic, and therapeutic endocrinology. Understanding that these interrelationships exist should awe and challenge us to unravel their complexities and should warn us that physiologic or pharmacologic manipulation of an obvious action may manipulate more than one system, and we should not assume that the observed effect of an endocrinologic disease or therapy is a direct effect until it is proved to be so. We should look for and accept the meaning and the cause of an unanticipated or unpredicted event when it occurs (particularly when treating an endocrinologic disorder) in order to discover biologically and medically important relationships that are not yet known.

ACETYLCHOLINE

Acetylcholine was first synthesized in 1867 by a German chemist named Adolf von Baeyer, who previously had discovered choline in the human brain. Von Baeyer was never able to realize the significance of his discovery primarily because, as a chemist, he represented a field that medical men of his time feared, and he was not versed in anatomy. For these reasons, he was refused a chair by the medical faculty and never pursued his research on the chemistry of the brain. Perhaps this incident in history protracted physiologic and pharmacologic studies of ACh. Perhaps not.[95] Forty years would pass before pharmacologic interest in ACh would be revived. But in the meantime, other substances were studied, including arecoline (derived from the seed of the *Areca catechu* — betel nut) and pilocarpine (obtained from the leaves of *Pilocarpus jaborandi*). Arecoline was found to produce weak nicotine-like effects, and, before the reappearance of ACh, it played an important role in eliciting parasympathomimetic muscarinic-like symptoms. Pilocarpine was the regularly available compound to mimic stimulation of the parasympathetic, also until the reappearance of ACh, some time after which its use was found in ophthalmology.[252]

Methods were sought to standardize pharmacologic products derived from plants, and ergot became the forerunner. Henry Wellcome decided to compete with Parke, Davis and Co., who had standardized products from ergot, and inadvertently prompted studies that would extend our knowledge of cholinergic mechanisms. In 1904, he employed Henry Dale in the Wellcome Physiological Research Laboratories, providing the catalyst for basic pharmacologic observations upon which this entire chapter is based. For an exciting account of some of the most masterful pharmacologic research, including the first identification of ACh in the brain, see W. S. Feldberg[172] and Henry H. Dale.[118]

Subsequent discovery of methods by which to measure ACh[272] and the discovery that ACh is a neurotransmitter have led to physiologically, pharmacologically, and medically important advances.

Neurohumoral transmission left the theoretic stage more than 50 years ago. One can no longer doubt that nerves transmit their impulses across most synapses and neuroeffector junctions by means of specific chemical agents such as the catecholamines (for most sympathomimetic events) and ACh (for ganglionic and parasympathomimetic events, both muscarinic and nicotinic). (See standard textbooks for the division of the autonomic nervous system.) The actions of most drugs that affect smooth muscle and glandular cells result from mimicking or modifying the synthesis, release, or actions of the neurotransmitters that are released by autonomic fibers.

The earliest concrete proposal of a neurohumoral mechanism was made shortly after the turn of the 20th century. Lewandowsky[342] and Langley[326] noted independently the similarity between the effects of injection of extracts of the adrenal gland and stimulation of sympathetic nerves. In 1905, T. R. Elliot,[151] while a student at Cambridge, England, extended these observations and postulated that sympathetic nerve impulses release minute amounts of an epinephrine-like substance in immediate contact with effector cells.[151] He considered this substance to be the chemical step in the process of transmission. He also noted that long after sympathetic nerves had degenerated, the effector organs still responded characteristically to the hormone of the adrenal medulla. In 1905, Langley suggested that effector cells have excitatory and inhibitory "receptive substances," and that the response to epinephrine depended on which type of substance was present. In 1907, Dixon was so impressed by the similarity between the effects of the alkaloid muscarine and the responses to vagal stimulation that he advanced the important idea that the vagus nerve liberated a muscarine-like substance that acted as a chemical transmitter of its impulses.[134] In 1914, Dale thoroughly reinvestigated the pharmacologic properties of ACh.[119] He was so intrigued with the remarkable fidelity with which this drug reproduced the responses to stimulation of parasympathetic nerves that he introduced the term *parasympathomimetic* to characterize its effects. Dale also noted the brief duration of the action of this chemical and proposed that an esterase in the tissues rapidly splits ACh to acetic acid and choline, the latter being a much less potent compound.

The brilliant research of Otto Loewi, begun in the winter of 1921, established the first real proof of the chemical mediation of nerve impulses by the peripheral release of specific chemical agents.[347] Loewi's studies deserve description because the technic used is basic to investigations in this field. He stimulated the vagus nerve of a perfused (donor) frog heart and allowed the perfusion fluid to come into contact with a second (recipient) frog heart that was being used as a test object. A substance liberated from the first organ slowed the rate of the second. Loewi referred to this chemical substance as *Vagusstoff* ("vagus-substance": parasympathin); subsequently, Loewi and Navratil[348] identified the substance as ACh. Loewi also discovered that an accelerator substance similar to epinephrine was liberated into the perfusion fluid in summer, when the action of the sympathetic fibers in the frog's vagus, a mixed nerve, predominated over that of the inhibitory fibers. Loewi's discoveries were eventually confirmed and are now universally accepted.

Evidence that the cardiac vagus-substance is also ACh in mammals was presented in 1933 by Feldberg and Krayer.[173] Many other investigations established quite conclusively that, in mammals, a chemical mediator, ACh, is instrumental in the transmission of parasympathetic impulses to other structures, including the iris, salivary glands, stomach, and small intestine.

In addition to its role as the neurohumoral transmitter of all postganglionic parasympathetic fibers and of a few postganglionic sympathetic fibers, such as those to the sweat glands and the sympathetic vasodilator fibers, ACh also functions as a transmitter in three other classes of nerves: (1) preganglionic fibers of both the sympathetic and the parasympathetic systems, (2) motor nerves to skeletal muscle; and (3) certain neurons within the CNS.

The role of catecholamines as neurotransmitters has already been discussed.

Test Criteria for the Role of Acetylcholine in Biologic Events

Although chemical tests for detecting ACh have improved, many pharmacologic tests are still used to determine the presence and action of ACh on organized tissues. In 1933, Chang and Gaddum described the minimum criteria for suspicion of ACh as a mediator of biologic events.[82] They include (1) inhibition of cholinesterase (ChE) in the test object, which usually increases the response obtained; (2) the presence of blood or tissue can decrease or destroy the activity of ACh, a destruction that is prevented by ChE inhibitors; (3) the ACh is quickly destroyed by hydrolysis in an alkaline medium; (4) boiling the ACh for several minutes in weakly acidic solution does not destroy the ACh; (5) atropine, curare, and nicotine individually block certain specific pharmacologic actions of the ACh, but they do not interfere significantly with its release at nerve terminals; and (6) the responses of various biologic indicators to ACh bear a definite quantitative relation to each other, and the chemical mediator being studied gives these same relative values. The cholinergic mediator at most sites fulfills all the requirements mentioned. Still other reasons for identifying it as ACh are that both are dialyzable, both are soluble in alcohol but not in ether, and both are restored to activity by acetylation after inactivation by ChE's.

Chang and Gaddum's pharmacologic tests for ACh have subsequently been considerably modified and expanded. Procedures have been developed for concentrating and purifying extracts so that the active substance can be applied to single neurons by microiontophoresis, in the case of ionized compounds such as ACh, or by electro-osmosis for nonionized compounds. Remarkable sensitivity has been achieved. By means of its iontophoretic application to the denervated motor end-plate of frog muscle, it is possible to detect as little as 5×10^{-15} mol of ACh.[402] The same level of sensitivity has been obtained by a much more simple procedure with a clam heart as the test object.[97]

Properties of choline acetyltransferase, the enzyme that catalyzes the acetylation of choline with acetylcoenzyme A in the production of ACh, have been well characterized,[469] as has acetylcholinesterase, the enzyme that inactivates ACh.[300]

Storage and Release of Acetylcholine

Fatt and Katz[170] recorded at the motor end-plate of skeletal muscle and observed the random occurrence of small (approximately 0.1–3.0 mv) spontaneous depolarizations at a frequency of approximately one per second. The magnitude of these miniature end-plate potentials (mepps) is considerably below the threshold required to fire a muscle action potential (AP): that they are due to the release of ACh is indicated by their enhancement by neostigmine and their blockage by d-tubocurarine. This was the first evidence that ACh is stored in and released from motor-nerve

endings in constant amounts or quanta. The morphologic counterpart of this phenomenon was discovered shortly thereafter in the form of synaptic vesicles noted in electron micrographs of nerve terminals by De Robertis and Bennett.[131] The storage and release of ACh was investigated most extensively at motor end-plates; nevertheless, most of the principles discovered at this locus probably apply to other sites of cholinergic transmission as well and, in many respects, to noncholinergic transmission.[312, 382]

The release of ACh by exocytosis through the prejunctional membrane is similar to the process of release of catecholamines. The release of ACh is inhibited by the toxin produced by *Clostridium botulinum*, one of the most potent toxins known. A small number of molecules of this toxin bind irreversibly to their sites of action, essentially irreversibly blocking all cholinergic junctions.[281] Death results from respiratory failure. Black widow spider toxin has a similar site of action as botulinum toxin but has an opposite effect. Clumping of vesicles at the prejunctional membrane is associated with the release of excessive amounts of ACh.[188, 443] When an AP arrives at the motor-nerve terminal, there is an explosive release of 100 or more quanta (or vesicles) of ACh, after a latent period of approximately 0.75 millisecond (msec).[289] The intermediate steps appear to be as follows: The depolarization of the terminal permits the influx of calcium ions, which hypothetically then bind to negative charges or other sites on the internal surface of the terminal axoplasmic membrane. This could facilitate fusion of axonal and vesicular membranes, resulting in the extrusion of the contents of the vesicles. The presence of calcium ion in the extracellular fluid is essential for the release of ACh elicited by the nerve impulse, and this effect is in turn antagonized by magnesium ions.[96, 382]

Although there is general agreement regarding certain steps involved in the storage and release of ACh, many of the details are still moot or unknown, as reference to the reviews listed previously will disclose. Estimates of the ACh content of the synaptic vesicles range from 1000 to more than 50,000 molecules per vesicle, and it has been calculated that a single motor-nerve terminal contains 300,000 or more vesicles. In addition, an uncertain but significant amount of ACh is present in the extravesicular cytoplasm. Applying mathematics to the data obtained from postsynaptic recording at the motor end-plate during the continuous application of ACh to resting muscle has permitted estimation of the potential change induced by a single molecule of ACh (3×10^{-7} v); from such calculations, it is evident that even the lower estimate of the ACh content per vesicle (1000 molecules) is sufficient to account for the magnitude of the mepps.[290]

In the superior cervical ganglion of the cat, approximately 85% of the total ACh is stored in a releasable "depot" form that, like catecholamines, is subdivided into more readily and less readily releasable reservoirs. The remaining 15% of the extractable ACh is in a "stationary" form and is perhaps located centrally to the axonal terminals. An additional "surplus" portion that may exceed the total depot of ACh accumulates in the presence of an anticholinesterase (anti-ChE) agent. The ganglion is able to support a remarkably high rate of ACh synthesis and release: When it is perfused with plasma and stimulated supramaximally at a frequency of 20 cycles per second, the amount of ACh released during 1 hour is approximately six times the original amount.[44]

The characteristics of cholinergic transmission at the neuromuscular end-plate, the cardiovascular conduction system, the autonomic ganglia, and the prejunctional and postjunctional sites appear to be the same. The functions of receptors for ACh in some sites, e.g., uninnervated vascular smooth muscle and leukocytes,[214] have not been biologically defined. Only the role of ACh in the ganglion will be discussed here, as a prototype of the effects of ACh elsewhere. The effects of ACh on the CNS are discussed in Ch. 11.

The Role of Acetylcholine at the Ganglion

Neurotransmission in the ganglia is based largely on the availability or action of the primary neurotransmitter, ACh. The passage of impulses in autonomic ganglia can be influenced by drugs that (1) interfere with the storage and synthesis of the transmitter (e.g., hemicholinium); (2) prevent the liberation of ACh from the preganglionic nerve endings (e.g., botulinum toxin, local anesthetics); (3) inactivate ganglionic ChE's (e.g., physostigmine); and (4) either mimic or prevent the interactions between ACh and its ganglionic (nicotinic) cholinergic receptor sites.

Neurotransmission in autonomic ganglia has long been recognized to be a far more complex process than the single neurotransmitter-receptor system, and intracellular recordings reveal at least four different changes in potential that can be elicited by stimulation of the preganglionic nerve.[147, 409, 589] The primary pathway involves the depolarization of postsynaptic sites by ACh. The receptors are classified as nicotinic, and the pathway is sensitive to classic nondepolarizing blocking agents, such as hexamethonium. Activation of this primary pathway gives rise to an initial excitatory postsynaptic potential (EPSP).

An AP is generated in the postganglionic neuron when the initial EPSP attains critical amplitude. In mammalian sympathetic ganglia *in vivo*, it may be necessary for multiple synapses to be activated before transmission is effective. The initial EPSP (and the initial depolarization that can be evoked experimentally by ionophoretic application of ACh to the postganglionic neuron) can be attributed to increases in the conductances of sodium and potassium. Because this event is rapid, it is necessary to envision a tightly coupled relationship between occupation of the receptor and activation of the channel that gives rise to the enhanced conductance. In this sense, the mechanism of generation of the initial EPSP parallels that seen at the neuromuscular junction.

Stimulation of preganglionic nerve fibers increases the content of cAMP and cGMP in sympathetic ganglia. These changes in the concentrations of cyclic nucleotides result from activation of postsynaptic muscarinic receptors.[363, 590] Catecholamines only increase the concentration of cAMP. However, other procedures that affect the generation or availability of cyclic nucleotides in ganglia do not cause the changes in permeability or potential that would be expected if the cyclic nucleotides served as obligatory mediators of the electrophysiologic responses.[194, 444, 589] Thus, the role of cyclic nucleotides in the regulation of the slow changes in potential remains to be established.

Other synaptic mediators appear to influence ganglionic transmission, but their precise sites of action remain to be ascertained. Furthermore, the relative importance of the secondary pathways, and even the nature of the modulating transmitters, appears to differ among individual ganglia and between parasympathetic and sympathetic ganglia. It should be emphasized that the secondary synaptic events serve to modulate the initial EPSP. Conventional ganglionic blocking agents can inhibit ganglionic transmission completely; the same cannot be said for muscarinic antagonists or α-adrenergic agonists.[573, 589]

Drugs that stimulate cholinergic receptor sites on autonomic ganglia can be grouped into two major categories. The first group consists of drugs with nicotinic specificity,

including *nicotine* itself. Their excitatory effects on ganglia are rapid in onset, are blocked by nondepolarizing ganglionic blocking agents, and mimic *the initial EPSP*. The second group is composed of drugs such as *muscarine* and *methacholine* and, in part, anti-ChE agents. Their excitatory effects on ganglia are delayed in onset, blocked by atropine-like drugs, and mimic *the late EPSP*.

Ganglionic blocking agents impair transmission by actions at the primary nicotinic receptor and also may be classified into two groups. The *first group* includes those drugs that initially stimulate the ganglia by an ACh-like action and then block because of a persistent depolarization (e.g., nicotine): Prolonged application of nicotine results in desensitization of the cholinergic receptor site and continued blockade. The blockade of autonomic ganglia produced by the *second group* of blocking drugs, of which hexamethonium can be regarded as a prototype, does not involve prior ganglionic stimulation or changes in the ganglionic potentials. Such agents impair transmissions by competing with ACh for ganglionic cholinergic receptor sites and, in a manner analogous to the blockade of transmission at the neuromuscular junction by curare, prevent the development of the postsynaptic depolarization (initial EPSP). Some evidence indicates that these drugs also may block the channel that is associated with the activated receptor. Compounds in this group do not affect nerve conduction or the release of transmitter substance from the nerve terminals. This class of conventional ganglionic blocking agent is used in therapy.

The Cholinergic Receptor Site

The concept of cholinergic nicotinic and muscarinic receptors is equivalent to that described for α- and β-adrenergic receptors. However, studies that clarified the chemical structure and molecular nature of the cholinergic receptor, with its similarities and differences as compared to the active sites of acetylcholinesterase, were the first to convince pharmacologists that tangible receptor systems existed for low molecular weight hormones.[6, 241, 297, 403, 496, 592] In many ways, pharmacologists and endocrinologists approach research on receptors with the same techniques used to define cholinergic receptors, and they have come to extrapolate what is known about the receptor for ACh and apply it to receptors for other neurotransmitters. Thus has the ACh receptor come to be known as the "prototype receptor."

By taking advantage of specialized evolutionary events related to cholinergic neurotransmission, it has been possible in recent years to isolate and characterize the cholinergic nicotinic receptor. The electric organs from the aquatic species of *Electrophorus* and, especially, *Torpedo* are rich sources of receptor. The electric organ is derived embryologically from myoid tissue, but in contrast to skeletal muscle, a significant fraction of the surface of the membrane is excitable and contains cholinergic receptors.[33] In vertebrate skeletal muscle, motor end-plates occupy 0.1% or less of the cell surface. The discovery of seemingly irreversible antagonism of neuromuscular transmission by an α-toxin from venoms of the krait, *Bungarus multicintis*, or varieties of the cobra, *Naja naja*,[81] offered a suitable marker for identification of the receptor. The α-toxins are peptides of around 8000 MW that can be isolated and labeled with radioisotopes. The interaction of α-toxins with the receptor was initially applied to an assay for identification of the isolated cholinergic receptor *in vitro* by Changeux and colleagues in 1970.[83] The α-toxins have extremely high affinities to, and slow rates of dissociation from, the receptor, yet the interaction is noncovalent. *In situ* and *in vitro* their behavior resembles that expected for a high affinity antagonist.

In parallel studies, a site-directed, irreversible sulfhydryl labeling reagent, *maleimidobenzyl trimethylammonium*, was used, and a 40,000 dalton peptide was identified in the preparations that contained receptors, the labeling of which is protected by an agonist.[284] This peptide also predominates in preparations that were subsequently purified by use of the α-toxin assay.[285] Thus, two separate approaches that rely on distinctly different aspects of receptor specificity identified the same protein (or peptide therefrom) as the cholinergic receptor. Further evidence that the isolated protein was the receptor came from immunologic studies,[426] after initial attempts at reconstitution of receptor function in isolated membranes met with only marginal success. More recently, several of the expected properties of receptor function have been reconstituted by adding soluble receptor to phospholipid vesicles. The immunologic approach has continued to yield critical information on the location and membrane disposition of the receptor. Furthermore, immunization of experimental animals with receptor results in an autoimmune response and a syndrome that in many ways resembles the human disease, *myasthenia gravis* (see below).

Because of their high affinity and selectivity for the receptor, the α-toxins were initially used to isolate a receptor. Their added value as markers for examination of the biosynthesis, location, and turnover of the receptor is also now clear.[166, 238, 427]

Despite its relative paucity in muscle, the nicotinic receptor has also been isolated from mammalian skeletal muscle; it has virtually the same biochemical properties as does the receptor found in the electric fish.[136, 187] Subcellular fractions that bind α-toxins have been extracted from brain[584] and a cultured pheochromocytoma.[425] In the latter cells, the ACh receptor that mediates changes in ion permeability is distinct from the α-neurotoxin binding entity. This is not unexpected, because the nicotine receptor of cells that originate from the neural crest (which gives rise to autonomic ganglia) has a different pharmacologic specificity than does the receptor of the neuromuscular junction. Thus, α-toxins may be specific markers only for nicotinic receptors, the embryonic origin of which is skeletal muscle.

The isolated receptor is an asymmetrical (14 nm × 8 nm) molecule of 250,000 daltons. It is composed of multiple subunits of 40,000–69,000 daltons with two α-toxin and one or two agonist-antagonist binding sites per receptor molecule.[238] The agonist-antagonist recognition site is on the 40,000 dalton peptide, and the functional role played by the other peptides remains unknown. Measurement of the number of receptors per unit area and the membrane conductance has demonstrated that roles of ion translocation are sufficiently rapid (5×10^7 ions/second) to require movement through an open channel, rather than rotation of the carrier of ions.[283] Moreover, agonist-mediated changes in ion permeability (inward movement of sodium and outward movement of potassium) apparently can occur through a single class of channels.[133] Thus, the agonist binding site appears to be intimately coupled with an ion channel; binding of agonist results in a rapid conformational change that opens the channel.

Many studies are under way to determine the points of similarity and variance of the muscarinic and nicotinic receptors. At present we know that there are many similarities between the receptors (e.g., antibodies against one cross-react with others) but that there must also be differences (the nicotinic receptor lacks requirements for stereospecificity while the muscarinic receptor is highly stereoselective).[240] Pharmacologic intervention to block muscarinic (e.g., with atropine) or nicotinic (e.g., with *d*-tubocurarine) receptors is possible, as well as the use of

ChE inhibitors to increase local concentrations of ACh, and therefore initially augment but later diminish ACh-like effects. The latter event is caused in part by the same type of desensitization that is caused by α- or β-adrenergic agonists on their respective adrenergic receptors (discussed previously). The diverse factors that contribute to regulation of the ACh receptors are described in the works cited in references 216, 364, 410, and 446.

Atropine and Related Drugs as Antagonists of Muscarinic Receptors

Much evidence supports the notion that atropine and related compounds compete with muscarinic agonists for identical binding sites on muscarinic receptors.[58, 261, 612] Based on an extensive study of the affinities of agonists and antagonists for muscarinic receptors in membranes prepared from rat cerebral cortex, Birdsall and coworkers have proposed that there are two major populations of binding sites with different affinities for agonists and a third minor population with an extremely high affinity for muscarinic agonists.[42] In contrast, only one type of binding site for muscarinic antagonists was demonstrated in these preparations.[261] The low affinity agonist binding site and the antagonist binding site closely resemble the muscarinic binding site that has been studied by ligand binding technics in peripheral smooth muscle (guinea pig ileum).[612] Birdsall and associates[43] proposed that there may be only a single muscarinic binding site in the cerebral cortex and that it is identical to that found in peripheral smooth muscle. This binding site is presumably coupled to effector systems that mediate the contractile response. A hypothetical consequence of the energy expended in this coupling reaction is that the affinity constant for ligand binding to the receptor is thought to be less for the coupled than for the uncoupled receptor. In contrast, affinity constants for antagonists are proposed to be the same for all populations of receptors because antagonists do not alter the effector system. According to this hypothesis, only a fraction of the receptors in the cerebral cortex are coupled to effector systems, which accounts for the heterogeneity of affinities for the binding of agonists.[41, 43]

Diseases Caused by Abnormalities of the Receptor for ACh

Just as the ACh receptor has come to be the prototype for predicting characteristics for other receptors, so has a disease of ACh receptors, myasthenia gravis, come to be the prototype for predicting the pathogenesis of diseases characterized by abnormal function of the sympathetic nervous system or abnormal effects of sympathomimetic agents. A description of myasthenia gravis follows.

Myasthenia Gravis

Myasthenia gravis is a neuromuscular disease that is characterized by weakness and marked fatigability of skeletal muscle;[141, 222] exacerbations and partial remissions occur frequently. Its clinical manifestations were described before the turn of the century.[71, 276] Jolly noted the similarity between the symptoms of myasthenia gravis and the symptoms of curare poisoning in animals and suggested that *physostigmine*, an agent then known to antagonize curare and now known to cause that action by inhibiting acetylcholinesterase, might be of therapeutic value. Forty years elapsed before his suggestion was given systematic trial.[581] Remen[451] and Walker[582] independently noted that *neostigmine* was useful in the management of patients with this disease, and although *pyridostigmine* is frequently used today, neostigmine remains the standard for comparison of new agents.

The defect in myasthenia gravis has been proved to be in synaptic transmission at the neuromuscular junction but not in the release of ACh. When a motor nerve of a normal subject is stimulated at 25 Hertz (Hz), electrical and mechanical responses are well-sustained. A suitable margin of safety exists for maintenance of neuromuscular transmission. Initial responses in the myasthenic patient may be normal, but they diminish rapidly, which explains the difficulty in maintaining voluntary muscle activity for more than brief periods. When the patient is given an appropriate dose of neostigmine, the response to tetanic stimulation is improved, along with symptomatic improvement in muscle strength. The same dose of neostigmine in control subjects leads to a *reduced* response to tetanic stimulation, accompanied by fasciculations, local weakness, and repetitive AP's in response to a single stimulus.[222] Elmqvist and his coworkers[152] observed that the amplitude of mepps was reduced in patients with myasthenia gravis and, because they were unable to demonstrate reduced receptor sensitivity, postulated that the change was due to a decrease in the number of ACh molecules per quantum of stimulation. The relative importance of prejunctional and postjunctional defects was a matter of considerable debate until Patrick and Lindstrom[426] found that rabbits immunized with the nicotinic receptor purified from electric eels slowly developed muscular weakness and respiratory difficulties that resembled the symptoms of myasthenia gravis. The rabbits also exhibited decremental responses after repetitive nerve stimulation, enhanced sensitivity to curare, and symptomatic and electrophysiologic improvement of neuromuscular transmission after administration of anti-ChE agents. Although this *experimental immune-based* myasthenia gravis differs somewhat from the naturally occurring disease, particularly in the marked acute phase in the experimental condition, this critical development of an animal model prompted speculation that the natural disease represented an autoimmune injury directed toward the ACh receptor. Antireceptor antibody was soon identified in patients with myasthenia gravis.[9] Receptor binding antibody has been detected in sera of 87% of patients with myasthenia gravis, although the clinical status of the patients does not correlate precisely with the antibody titer.[346] Nevertheless, plasmapheresis of very ill patients can substantially reverse the disease by lowering the titer of antibody to the receptor. Passive transfer of antibody, by the use of an immunoglobulin fraction prepared from myasthenic patients, produces the myasthenic syndrome in recipient animals.[553] By use of the snake α-neurotoxins that were also essential for the purification and characterization of the isolated nicotinic receptor from eel, Fambrough and associates[167] were able to detect a 70–90% reduction in the number of receptors per end-plate in myasthenic patients. This finding provided crucial support for the hypothesis that a decrease in receptors in the postsynaptic membrane accounts for the defects of the disease.

The picture that ultimately emerges is that myasthenia gravis is caused by an autoimmune response to the ACh receptor at the postjunctional end-plate. Antibodies, which are also present in plasma, reduce the number of receptors that can be detected either by toxin binding assays or by electrophysiologically measuring sensitivity to ACh.[141, 142]

In these patients, immune complexes have been detected in the postsynaptic membrane, along with marked ultrastructural abnormalities in the synaptic cleft.[155] The latter appear to be a consequence of the destructive autoimmune reaction.

Diagnosis. Although the diagnosis can usually be made from the patient's medical history and the signs and symptoms, its differentiation from certain neurasthenic, infectious, endocrine, neoplastic, and degenerative neuromuscular diseases may sometimes be difficult. However, myasthenia gravis is the only condition in which the aforementioned deficiencies can be improved dramatically by anti-ChE medication. The *edrophonium test* is performed by injecting intravenously 2 mg of edrophonium chloride, followed 45 seconds later by an additional 8 mg if the first dose has no effect; a positive response consists of a brief improvement in strength, unaccompanied by lingual fasciculation (which generally occurs in nonmyasthenic patients).

An excessive dose of an anti-ChE drug results in a *cholinergic crisis.* The condition is characterized by weakness resulting from excessive depolarization of the motor end-plate; other features result from overstimulation of muscarinic receptors. The weakness resulting from blockade caused by depolarization may closely resemble *myasthenic weakness,* which is due to insufficient anti-ChE medication. Making the distinction is clinically crucial because the former is treated by withholding and the latter by administering the anti-ChE agent. When the edrophonium test is performed cautiously, limiting the dose to 1 or 2 mg, and with facilities for respiratory resuscitation immediately available, a further decrease in strength indicates cholinergic crisis, while improvement signifies myasthenic weakness. *Atropine sulfate,* 0.6 mg or more intravenously, should be given immediately if a severe muscarinic reaction ensues (for complete details see works cited in references 417 and 418).

If the patient suspected of having myasthenia gravis exhibits minimal symptoms at the time of examination, a provocative test can be performed by injecting intravenously 0.1–0.5 mg of *d*-tubocurarine chloride. A positive response consists in the rapid precipitation of the characteristic weakness and associated symptoms: It should be reversed by the immediate intravenous injection of 2.0 mg of neostigmine methylsulfate. The *d*-tubocurarine test is a potentially hazardous procedure: It should be performed only with an anesthesiologist present and with facilities for respiratory and cardiovascular resuscitation immediately at hand. A regional curare test involving intra-arterial injection into one limb has been developed and involves less risk.[255]

Treatment. *Neostigmine, pyridostigmine,* and *ambenonium* are the standard anti-ChE drugs used in the symptomatic treatment of myasthenia gravis. All can increase the response of myasthenic muscle to repetitive nerve impulses, primarily by preserving endogenous ACh. Receptors over a greater cross-sectional area of the end-plate are then presumably exposed to concentrations of ACh that are sufficient for stimulation. In a normal end-plate, the density of receptors is sufficient so that recruiting additional receptors is unnecessary.

In cases in which administering anti-ChE agents at optimal doses is not sufficient to enable near-normal motor activity, other therapeutic measures must be considered. Controlled studies reveal that *corticosteroids* provide clinical improvement in a high percentage of patients.[154, 258, 356] When treatment with steroids is continued over a prolonged period, however, several undesirable side effects may result. The contraindications and side effects are typical of chronic steroid treatment. Gradual lowering of maintenance doses and alternate-day regimens are used to minimize side effects.[258, 489] In addition, initiation of steroid treatment augments muscle weakness, but as the patient improves with continued administration of steroids, doses of anti-ChE drugs can be reduced.[141] The immunosuppressive activity of corticosteroids is likely of primary importance because antireceptor activity is diminished in circulating lymphocytes after such treatment.[1]

Thymectomy should be considered when the myasthenia gravis is associated with a thymoma or when the disease is not adequately controlled by anti-ChE agents. An improved prognosis after thymectomy is likely and apparent remissions have been observed in some cases.[65] The relative risks and benefits of the surgical procedure versus anti-ChE and corticosteroid treatment require careful assessment in each case, however.[366] Because the thymus contains myoid cells, it has been suggested that the disease arises in this tissue;[141] however, the thymus is not required for perpetuation of the condition. Treatment with plasmapheresis of antibody is being tested with some encouraging signs of success.

Anticholinergic Intoxication by Anticholinergic Drugs

Many of the peripheral and central effects of poisoning by atropine and related antimuscarinic drugs can be reversed by intravenous injection of physostigmine. Many other drugs, such as the phenothiazines, antihistamines, tricyclic antidepressants, and benzoquinamide have central, as well as peripheral, anticholinergic activity, and *physostigmine salicylate* may be useful in reversing the central anticholinergic syndrome produced by overdosage or an unusual reaction to these drugs.[11, 473] An initial intravenous dose of 0.5–2 mg of physostigmine is indicated, with additional increments given as necessary.

Other etiologies (e.g., abnormal reactions to penicillamine) have now been associated with the development of antibodies to ACh receptors and with the clinical development of a myasthenic-like syndrome in humans.[362] For interesting and complete reviews on the actions of ACh see the works cited in references 353 and 585.

DISEASES ASSOCIATED WITH ABNORMALITIES OF THE ADRENAL MEDULLA

No known diseases are caused by adrenal medullary insufficiency. After bilateral adrenalectomy, urinary excretion of epinephrine falls rapidly, but excretion of norepinephrine and its metabolic products remains relatively unchanged. The physiologic function of the adrenal medulla is difficult to determine because it is a minor source of catecholamines. Tumors at that site often produce distinct and clinically important syndromes. The most prominent tumor, the pheochromocytoma, has served as a model for applying the previously discussed facts to life-threatening clinical disease.

Pheochromocytoma

Pheochromocytomas (or functioning paragangliomas),[337, 512] although found in less (perhaps much less) than 1% of the hypertensive population,[124, 245, 558] have several clinically important aspects:

1. Associated hypertension is usually curable.

2. The presence of these tumors may herald other occult, potentially fatal but curable diseases.

3. Their manifestations may suggest other diseases of altered metabolism such as diabetes mellitus, hypercalcemia, thyrotoxicosis, anxiety states, severe infection,[396] Cushing's syndrome, and the carcinoid syndrome.

4. A rational, specific approach to diagnosis and therapy is available.

5. Family studies disclose a high incidence of pheochromocytoma in kindreds, inheritance as an autosomal dominant trait, a very high prevalence of multiple endocrine neoplasia, and need for genetic counseling. Questions regarding gene expressivity and the etiology of certain types of neoplasia may be answered by further investigation of such families.

Pathogenesis of the Symptoms of Pheochromocytoma

The common manifestations of a pheochromocytoma (Table 10–6) may result directly from the physical presence of the tumor (e.g., syringomyelia associated with von Hippel-Lindau disease, or Brown-Séquard syndrome as the tumor invades the spinal cord).[381] More often, manifestations relate to increased production of catecholamines. The numerous reasons for increased production of catecholamines in tumor tissue have been studied. In some studies, abnormally rapid turnover rates, particularly in tumors in children and in small tumors in adults, were noted. The biochemical properties of the chromaffin cells and granules of the tumor are remarkably similar to those of the normal cell. The storage mechanisms as far as they have been studied are also normal. Therefore, the unusual production and secretion rates must be linked to lack of ordinary control mechanisms regulating synthesis or release of norepinephrine or its precursors. Sometimes drugs given for treatment of hypertension increase the synthesis and release of catecholamines. Both antihypertensive drugs, which release catecholamines from normal storage sites, and drugs

Table 10–6. COMMON MANIFESTATIONS OF PHEOCHROMOCYTOMAS AND UNUSUAL COMBINATIONS OF SYMPTOMS LEADING TO ERRONEOUS DIAGNOSIS*

Signs and Symptoms Attributable to Secretion of Catecholamines

Hypertension	
Sweating	
Paroxysmal attacks of blanching or flushing	
Palpitations, tachycardia and/or myocardiopathy	Commonly found in
Headache	pheochromocytomas
Anorexia, weight loss, psychic changes	
Evidence of hypermetabolism, increased fasting blood glucose level	
Decrease gastrointestinal motility	
Postural hypotension	
Increased blood pressure, palpitations, headache, sweating, evidence of hypermetabolism and psychic changes	Suggesting toxemia of pregnancy
Increased fasting blood glucose level and abnormal results in glucose tolerance tests	Suggesting diabetes mellitus
Psychosis, tremulousness, increased respiratory rate	Suggesting functional hyperventilation
Decreased gastrointestinal motility and resultant constipation to severe colitis and watery diarrhea	Suggesting Hirschsprung's disease
Increased basal metabolic rate, increased oxygen consumption, weight loss, psychosis, tremulousness, increased respiratory rate	Suggesting thyrotoxicosis

*Data obtained from review of 91 consecutive patients with pheochromocytomas seen at the University of California Medical Center and Stanford University School of Medicine.

such as phentolamine or clonidine, which block presynaptic α receptors (disallowing catecholamine-induced inhibition of release of catecholamines), can increase the amount of catecholamines released into the circulation.[18] A malignant tissue may be autonomous, but other phenomena may explain the excessive production of amines:

1. Ordinary concentrations of norepinephrine in the tumor cell do not seem to inhibit tyrosine hydroxylase.[398, 470] This could mean that the enzyme is unusual (has a different K_m for its substrate) or that once the amines are formed they are held in compartments that do not allow feedback inhibition of normal enzymes.[608] The relative contribution of each factor to the abnormalities of synthesis has not been determined.

2. The tumor metabolizes a substantial proportion of the amines it produces. These metabolites can prevent ordinary feedback inhibition of tyrosine hydroxylase by norepinephrine.[267]

Most symptoms can be readily explained on the basis of the pharmacologic effects of catecholamines. The metabolic effects of the catecholamines are well known and usually do not produce symptoms. Some direct effects of catecholamines on the parathyroid and other actions can produce hypercalcemia that may be the only presenting symptom in a patient with a pheochromocytoma.[127, 196, 423] Increased peripheral vascular resistance is a well-recognized aspect of the disease. The hypertension may be sustained or paroxysmal, probably depending on whether the secretion of catecholamines, particularly norepinephrine, from the tumor into the blood is sustained or comes in "spurts."[384] In some patients, high rates of excretion of catecholamines are not accompanied by hypertension or by symptoms that can be attributed to catecholamines;[536] their blood pressure may be intermittently abnormal, but the concentrations of catecholamines in blood and of metabolites in urine can be elevated consistently or only intermittently. One of the most common symptoms is sweating,[183, 441] which may be episodic and associated with profound flushing or blanching, or continuous and subtle, provoking a need for frequent showers and shampoos. Palpitations and tachycardia are also prominent symptoms. Weight loss, tremulousness, and other evidence of hypermetabolism may be the direct result of increased production of catecholamines. Headaches seem to be caused by sudden changes in the concentrations of catecholamines in the circulation rather than by steady elevations of blood pressure.[32] Less easy to explain, but an important symptom, is the existence of postural hypotension in the untreated hypertensive patient.[112] The most plausible explanation is a catecholamine-induced decrease in plasma and total blood volumes. Such reductions in plasma volume, however, are less frequent than the orthostatic hypotension.[499] In contrast, postural hypotension occurs frequently in aldosteronism, a disease characterized by increases in plasma volume.[38] Hyperaldosteronism may accompany pheochromocytoma.[572] The analogy with the aldosterone-producing tumor can be extended, since patients with such tumors also have impaired sympathetic reflexes as a result of decreased total body potassium.[38] Severe potassium deficiency, however, has been found infrequently in patients with a pheochromocytoma. Another mechanism that may contribute to the orthostatic hypotension is the ganglionic blocking activity of excessive amounts of catecholamines.

The basis for the CNS manifestations of a pheochromocytoma is not clear. Catecholamines can affect the CNS, producing changes in sleep patterns,[412] psychosis, tremulousness, and hyperventilation. Although little is known about the total concentration of catecholamines in the brains of patients with pheochromocytoma, an increase could be expected despite the fact that circulating catecholamines have difficulty passing the blood-brain barrier. Over long periods, the increased concentrations of catecholamines in blood could alter the usual equilibrium of catecholamines in the CNS.

Catecholamines produce myocarditis and myocardial necrosis in patients with pheochromocytomas; the mechanism is unknown. The lesion may be so severe that the presenting symptoms of the patient may not be hypertension but congestive heart failure. At least one effect of high catecholamine (isoproterenol) concentrations on the heart is to create a defective storage of endogenous amines.[387] In addition, high concentrations of free fatty acids caused by the metabolic activity of catecholamines may contribute to myocardial lesions.[250] Myocarditis, which may be manifested by arrhythmia or congestive failure and nonspecific electrocardiographic changes, may be a direct toxic effect of catecholamines or may be mediated by the increased work demanded of the myocardium.[86, 162, 296, 502, 533, 568] Arrhythmia may also be caused by the direct chronotropic effects of the catecholamines, by reflex baroreceptor-mediated bradycardia secondary to sudden increases in blood pressure,[126] or, rarely, by sudden decreases in blood pressure after spontaneous necrosis of the tumor.[181]

Whether catecholamines can have effects on the bowel analogous to those on the heart is unknown. However, severe enterocolitis with peritonitis has been reported in a child with pheochromocytoma. All gastrointestinal lesions disappeared after the tumor was removed.[171] Catecholamines ordinarily depress motility of the gastrointestinal tract, and a predominant gastrointestinal symptom of a patient with a pheochromocytoma can be severe constipation, or even the appearance of a Hirschsprung-like disease (described later). However, the tumor can produce vasoactive intestinal peptide (VIP), which may cause watery diarrhea.[555]

The cells of origin of pheochromocytomas and similar tumors have a pluripotential endocrine capacity similar to that of the cells composing the carcinoid tumor. In addition to VIP, pheochromocytomas can produce ACTH and calcitonin (or a calcitonin-like substance). They can either directly elaborate PTH or indirectly release it through a humoral substance that is made in the tumor.[34, 236, 279, 414, 507] Thus, symptoms of hypercalcemia, hypocalcemia, or Cushing's syndrome can be caused by the tumor, although not by catecholamines. Furthermore, excessive production of corticosteroids may induce adrenal phosphoethanolamine-N-methyltransferase or may add to salt and fluid retention, which can contribute to the effects of catecholamines.[117] Identifying and removing an underlying pheochromocytoma will reverse both the catecholamine- and noncatecholamine-induced signs and symptoms. If the unusual symptoms of a pheochromocytoma are not recognized and acted upon before the patient is subjected to potentially morbid procedures or undergoes surgery, the patient may suffer needlessly.[110]

Spontaneous or drug-induced adrenergic crisis can occur in patients with pheochromocytoma.[544] These crises resemble a thyroid storm. They apparently are caused by the release of catecholamines secondary to breakdown of the tumor or by the direct effects of some drugs used to treat pheochromocytoma, e.g., α-adrenergic antagonists.[18] By blocking presynaptic α receptors, the α-antagonists can incite increased release of catecholamines through nerve endings that are already engorged with releasable catecholamines. They also may have direct or reflex-derived abilities to release catecholamines from normal storage sites. Similarly, the use of antagonists of angiotensin II in patients with pheochromocytoma has led to adrenergic crisis. In one case, for example, saralasin (1-sar-8-ala-angiotensin II) rapidly antagonized the excessive effects of angiotensin in some patients and led to what probably was reflex hyper-release of catecholamines.[145, 567] Lower doses of the drug would not necessarily produce a crisis.[462] Other drugs that can directly release catecholamines from storage sites (e.g., metoclopramide) should not be given to patients with pheochromocytoma because they can produce the same type of crisis.[487] Occasionally, after a spontaneous crisis caused by hemorrhage into the tumor, the remaining tumor undergoes avascular necrosis and the patient can experience a spontaneous remission.[19]

Differential Diagnosis

A pheochromocytoma may be manifested by relatively few symptoms or by an unusual combination of symptoms, leading at times to an erroneous diagnosis (Table 10–6). For example, the occurrence of polyuria (on the basis of the ADH secreting activity of norepinephrine) or polydipsia (in association with an increase in the fasting blood glucose level) in a patient without hypertension or other symptoms characteristic of a pheochromocytoma may lead to a diagnosis of nonketotic diabetes mellitus. Similarly, a diagnosis of functional hyperventilation syndrome has been made in patients with a pheochromocytoma because their initial symptoms were psychosis, nervousness, or hyperventilation in the absence of sustained hypertension. Symptoms of hypermetabolism can be mistakenly interpreted to indicate hyperthyroidism, neurotic behavior, and even severe infection. Severe constipation resulting from the inhibitory effects of catecholamines on intestinal motility, although unusual, also may be a manifestation of a pheochromocytoma. This finding has been interpreted to indicate Hirschsprung's disease and has led to unnecessary and hazardous operative procedures. Conversely, watery diarrhea caused by catecholamine-induced enteritis or by excessive production of VIP may be the sole presenting symptom.

Some patients without pheochromocytoma can have symptoms that would seem to indicate a pheochromocytoma. Thus patients with diencephalic epilepsy may have episodes of hypertension, tachycardia, and flushing that are associated with wide swings in the concentration of catecholamines in plasma. These symptoms may be difficult to distinguish from symptoms of pheochromocytoma.[377]

When combinations of symptoms are incorrectly interpreted, diabetes mellitus, thyrotoxicosis, or even toxemia of pregnancy may be considered the most "obvious" diagnosis. Because their manifestations can be mimicked in part by the pharmacologic effect of catecholamines, such diseases must be considered in the differential diagnosis of a pheochromocytoma.

Associated Diseases

Certain diseases are frequently associated with a pheochromocytoma but may be occult at the time the tumor is detected. For example, the incidence of neuroectodermal syndromes is increased in this select hypertensive population. Neurofibromatosis, the most common of these conditions, and perhaps optic nerve gliomas,[180] are found in about 5% of patients with pheochromocytomas. Patients with Lindau's disease, which is characterized by retinal hemangioblastomas, cerebellar, medullary, and spinal cord hemangioblastomas, and cysts in the lung, liver, pancreas, kidneys, and epididymis, as well as by hypernephromas, also have a high incidence of pheochromocytomas.[256, 373]

Sturge-Weber disease, hereditary cerebellar ataxia with telangiectasia of the conjunctiva, and tuberous sclerosis are other neuroectodermal syndromes whose manifestations may coexist with those of neurofibromatosis and Lindau's disease. Most of these diseases are familial and are inherited in the same genetic pattern as pheochromocytomas (autosomal dominant trait), and at least one (ataxia telangiectasia) has an immunologic pathogenesis.[475] An increased incidence of pheochromocytomas might be expected in such patients. Therefore, when any one of these syndromes is diagnosed, the patient and his family should be carefully screened both for other manifestations of the primary disease and for a pheochromocytoma.

In 1961, Sipple noted a 14-fold increase in the frequency of pheochromocytoma in patients with medullary carcinoma of the thyroid. This tumor is derived from the parafollicular or C-cells of the thyroid, which are of neuroectodermal origin and synthesize and release calcitonin.[77, 149, 598] These patients also have an increased incidence of hyperparathyroidism, but it is still debated as to whether those with hyperplasia of the glands (as opposed to adenomas) have developed the lesion primarily or as a result of protracted secretion of calcitonin. The disease is familial and it is inherited as an autosomal dominant lesion. In fact, the intriguing data of Balin and his colleagues[29] indicate that some of these patients have multiple tumors of a single clonal cell origin. This would contrast with the multiclonal origin of most genetic tumors. Sipple's syndrome is one of the multiple endocrine neoplasia syndromes (MEN) and has been classified as multiple endocrine neoplasia (MEN) type IIa. (Type I, or Wermer's syndrome, involves tumors of the pituitary, pancreas, and parathyroid glands, and type IIb includes medullary carcinoma of the thyroid and pheochromocytomas that are associated with mucosal neuromas but rarely with parathyroid disorders.) Excellent pictures of the various lesions can be found in the monograph by Manger and Gifford.[355] Patients with Sipple's syndrome often have bilateral, multicentric, and malignant pheochromocytomas. They resemble patients with the carcinoid syndrome in that they can secrete ACTH and autacoids in addition to catecholamines. The autacoids secreted include histamine, prostaglandins, and serotonin. In fact, some of these patients, particularly those with type IIb, can present to a physician with diarrhea, difficulty with feeding, projectile vomiting, cramping abdominal pain, and loud borborygmi.[76, 78] Conversely, their presentation sometimes can be quite subtle, with hypertension as the only overt manifestation of the syndrome.[486]

Measurement of calcitonin can be a clinical marker for the presence of medullary carcinoma of the thyroid and MEN II. If basal concentrations in plasma are not high, a series of provocative tests is suggested. These tests vary from carefully executed 4-hour calcium infusion tests[422] to the use of pentagastrin or cholecystokinin[599] to the simple ingestion of whiskey.[537] Hypercalcitoninemia may strongly suggest the possibility of MEN II and pheochromocytoma, but it does not definitively establish the diagnosis. The thyroid disease may remain remarkably benign in some families but ravage others. The possibility of a pheochromocytoma should be considered in all members of a family with a proven MEN syndrome.

The pheochromocytoma may elaborate an erythrocyte-stimulating factor, causing an absolute increase in red blood cell mass.[467] In rare cases, pheochromocytoma is associated with an astrocytoma in the brain (which may account for headache in some patients) or with xanthine oxidase deficiency, as reported by Engelman and coworkers.[162] Unusual patterns of development of pheochromocytoma may appear in families. For instance, hydroureter and hydronephrosis have presaged pheochromocytoma in two generations of a family.[514] In similar cases, an aggressive search for an asymptomatic pheochromocytoma seems justified.

Physical Examination

The findings by physical examination are relatively non-specific. Pheochromocytomas may occur at any age, although the majority of patients are in the 4th to 6th decade. There is no sex predilection. Most patients seek medical advice because of symptoms associated with hypertension or other pharmacologic effects of catecholamines. In the 5% who also have neuroectodermal disorders, the most striking physical findings may be associated with these diseases. These findings include neurofibromas, café-au-lait spots, "port wine" nevi, telangiectasia over the conjunctiva, and CNS disturbances referable to the cerebellum, medulla, or spinal cord. The latter may include compression by the tumor or syringomyelia. The common physical findings directly attributable to the pheochromocytoma are sticky and moist hair, profuse sweating, retinal changes consistent with hypertension, nodules in the thyroid as part of the manifestations of MEN II, rapid heart rate with a left ventricular thrust, and enlargement of the heart if catechol myocardiopathy or congestive heart failure is present. Abdominal organs usually are not palpable unless coexistent Lindau's disease has produced significant cystic disease of the liver or pancreas.

The tumor is present in the abdominal cavity in 95% of affected patients but is palpable in only about 15%. In about 50%, however, pressure on the abdomen will produce a rise in blood pressure or an increase in sweating. If the primary tumor is in the neck, it usually can be palpated; if it is in the chest, it can be detected in most instances by roentgenography. If the primary tumor is in the bladder or pelvic region, it may be manifested by micturition syncope or paroxysms of hypertension associated with micturition. In some cases, palpation over the bladder may provoke these symptoms. When the tumor has metastasized into bone, it can often be palpated in the rib area, or pain may be evoked when pressure is applied over the affected skeletal parts.

Neurologic findings are relatively nonspecific and include psychotic manifestations of the disease, focal abnormalities due to metastatic or associated primary lesions in the brain, and metabolic encephalopathy associated with secondary hyperparathyroidism or hyperaldosteronism. Parkinson's disease is not seen with pheochromocytoma or neuroblastoma, however, and dopamine levels in various brain areas have not been measured.

In summary, the diagnosis of a pheochromocytoma is dependent on the physician's awareness of the subtleties of its manifestations. Thus any patient of any age should be suspected of having a pheochromocytoma if he has moderate to severe sustained or intermittent hypertension with or without excessive sweating, orthostatic hypotension, headache, hypermetabolism, weight loss, psychic changes, or an elevated fasting blood glucose level. A full spectrum of symptoms may not be apparent when the patient is first seen, and in many cases the initial diagnosis is essential hypertension, hyperthyroidism, diabetes mellitus, psychoneurosis, idiopathic orthostatic hypotension, or functional bowel problems. *Every patient with suspected essential hypertension should at some point in his or her care undergo simple, effective, and inexpensive screening for a pheochromocytoma.*[26] That more attention must be paid to "insignificant" symptoms is emphasized by the high mortality during operative procedures on patients with unsuspected pheochromocytoma.

Diagnostic Procedures

The diagnosis may be suspected on the basis of the history and initial physical findings but cannot be definitive until laboratory tests have been performed.

Routine Laboratory Tests. Routine laboratory data may heighten the physician's suspicion. The hematocrit may be increased because of (1) a decrease in plasma volume and relative increase in red cell mass due to the direct effects of catecholamines; or (2) the elaboration by the tumor of large amounts of erythrocyte-stimulating factor (ESF). The latter, although relatively infrequent, has been well demonstrated by Rosse and Waldmann.[467] The presence of a coexistent tumor may also result in an increase in red cell mass. For example, in a patient with a pheochromocytoma and Lindau's disease, excessive amounts of ESF may be produced by a cerebellar hemangioblastoma with associated cysts or by an associated hypernephroma, which is more common in patients with Lindau's disease than in the general population.[373] There are no consistent abnormalities in leukocyte or platelet counts, although leukocytosis is not rare and can be caused by catecholamines.[522] For unknown reasons, but probably because the hypertension is of short duration, chemical tests on blood do not usually reveal evidence of renal failure, although proteinuria is found in up to 65% of patients with persistent hypertension.[354] The urine may contain glucose if the blood glucose level is sufficiently increased.

Increased fasting blood glucose and free fatty acid levels[158] also help to increase the suspicion of the diagnosis. Serum concentrations of electrolytes and alkaline phosphatase may be altered if hyperparathyroidism is present. Decrease in serum potassium levels have been noted in some patients. In one of five patients studied, the serum potassium concentration was consistently below 3 mEq/liter. The mechanism of the decrease has been discussed above; it probably is related to aldosterone abnormalities.

Roentgenography. Roentgenographic studies help to locate the tumor and thus are of importance in preoperative evaluation.[99, 129, 454, 583] Routine x-ray films of the chest, together with oblique views, may reveal a paravertebral tumor mass. Scout films of the abdomen will locate the tumor in about 20% of patients. Intravenous pyelograms with or without tomography of the perirenal area will place the tumor in about 50% of cases. Retroperitoneal infusion of carbon dioxide is occasionally useful. Because it is laborious to perform and is associated with a low but definite incidence of complications (e.g., hypertensive crisis), gas insufflation should be reserved for selected patients whose tumors have escaped surgical detection or are by chemical tests judged to be small and cannot be detected by retrograde venography, arteriography, [131]I-19-iodocholesterol scintigraphy, or computerized axial tomography (CAT) scans. Selective arteriography and venography have been used to demonstrate primary and metastatic lesions but, like retroperitoneal gas studies, should be limited to difficult cases. These procedures may be successful because pheochromocytomas are often highly vascular and the tumor will appear as a "blush" in arteriograms and venograms. When a pheochromocytoma is suspected, clinicians understandably want to locate the tumor before surgery. The value of standard arteriography has been considerably enhanced by the addition of retrograde venography, selective arteriography, and "subtractive techniques" to the routine radiographic studies. Some series show that such radiographic techniques help to locate at least one tumor in about 75% of patients who eventually are found to have a pheochromocytoma.[562] In one series, 14 patients with 16 pheochromocytomas were studied over 7 years, and the tumor site was identified by roentgenography in 15 instances. However, enormous expertise is required, as 6 of the 15 tumors were quite subtle. Furthermore, the procedures can be dangerous in that one half of the studies provoked hypertension even though the patients were taking α-blocking drugs.[87]

In one patient who was studied recently by Dr. Lee Goldman and the author at the University of California Medical Center, an intravenous pyelogram (IVP) revealed a right kidney of 13.8 cm and a left kidney of 15.6 cm. A 3.5- × 3.0-cm soft tissue density was noted above the right kidney. No abnormalities were seen above the left kidney, and arteriograms confirmed both the mass on the right and the normality on the left. At surgery, an 87-gm mass measuring 10 × 6 × 3.5 cm was found in the left adrenal. A much smaller mass also was removed from the right adrenal. Because a tumor was not expected on the left side, surgeons favored a right flank incision. Had this been done, the patient almost surely would have been subjected to a second surgical procedure. Thus there can be perils in overreliance on preoperative radiologic procedures. A comparison of the relative values of the radiologic versus the chemical techniques that can be used to diagnose and locate a pheochromocytoma follows.

Computerized Axial Tomography.   The CT or CAT scan has been useful in locating retroperitoneal tumors. Most major medical centers have used the procedure to locate pheochromocytomas, but we do not yet know its relative value in the diagnostic work-up of these patients.

Radioisotopic Study of the Adrenal Glands.   Scintography of the adrenal gland with ^{131}I-19-iodocholesterol recently has been added to radiologic techniques in adrenal imaging and has been used successfully to demonstrate anatomical and functional disorders of the adrenals in a variety of clinical situations. Although the procedure is not designed primarily to locate adrenal medullary tumors, it has successfully located at least three pheochromocytomas in the adrenal gland.[554] The procedure would not be expected to be valuable if the tumor were in extra-adrenal sites.

There are studies that compare the relative value of ultrasound, scintography, and arteriography in locating adrenal lesions. Biochemically suspected adrenal lesions appear to be equally well studied by sonography and scintography. Arteriography usually is reserved for settings in which the diagnosis is inconclusive and extra-adrenal sites for a pheochromocytoma are suspected.[294]

Definitive Chemical Tests.   Although routine procedures are useful in locating a primary tumor or areas of metastases, they are not specific for pheochromocytomas. Certain chemical tests, however, provide unequivocal data for a definitive diagnosis of pheochromocytomas. Concentrations of catecholamines in blood can now be accurately ascertained, but with technical difficulty and at considerable expense.[11, 57] Similarly, some patients with pheochromocytoma have elevated concentrations of dopamine β-hydroxylase in their plasma, but the finding is not consistent enough to make this measurement clinically useful.[20, 525] All these tests can be modulated by drugs that have ACh- or caffeine-like effects.[217, 218, 459] The clinician usually can gain much information from standard quantitative measurements of the urinary excretion of catecholamines and their metabolites metanephrine, normetanephrine, and VMA. Experience at the University of California Medical Center has shown that the most reliable methods are those of Crout and Pisano and their collaborators.[105, 108, 435, 436] The normal range of catecholamine concentrations in urine, blood, and adrenal medulla and of urinary VMA and normetanephrine are listed in Table 10–7.

Table 10–7.   NORMAL RANGE OF CATECHOLAMINE AND METABOLITE CONCENTRATIONS*

Urine
Catecholamines††
 Norepinephrine: 10 to 70 μg. per 24 hr.
 Epinephrine: 0 to 20 μg. per 24 hr.
Normetanephrine and metanephrine:
 <1.3 mg. per 24 hr.
Vanillylmandelic acid: 1.8 to 9.0 mg. per 24 hr.
Dopamine: <200 μg. per 24 hr.
Blood (Plasma)
Catecholamines: <1 μg. per liter
Norepinephrine: 0.2 ± 0.08 μg. per liter plasma**
Epinephrine: 0.05 ± 0.03 μg. per liter plasma**
Dopamine beta-hydroxylase: 116 ± 1.8 N moles per ml. per 20 min.†
Adrenal Medulla
Norepinephrine: 0.04 to 0.16 mg. per g.
Epinephrine: 0.22 to 0.84 mg. per g.

---

*Since the values obtained in different laboratories vary considerably, only a general range can be given.
**Engelman, K., and Portnoy, B.: *Circ. Res.* 26:53, 1970.
†Weinshilboum, R., and Axelrod, J.: *Circ. Res.* 28:307, 1971.
††In most patients with pheochromocytomas, total catecholamine excretion is >300 μg per day.

For determinations on urine, 24-hour specimens are collected in 15 ml of 6 N hydrochloric acid. Because a variety of tests exist and because the methods used in different laboratories differ in specificity, certain drugs and foods should be withdrawn before urine specimens are collected. Administration of exogenous catecholamines such as vasopressors, even for nasal stuffiness, highly fluorescent compounds (e.g., tetracyclines), and certain antihypertensive drugs (such as α-methyldopa), which are catechols themselves or form catecholamines, may influence the results of determinations of catecholamines. Such drugs, however, have no appreciable effect on VMA and metanephrine determinations and, if clinically advisable, need not be withdrawn before such tests. Long-term administration of reserpine or guanethidine usually has no significant effect on the results of such assays. MAO inhibitors, however, may result in a misleading increase in urinary metanephrine and a decrease in VMA excretion. Because several of the screening tests for VMA also detect other phenolic acids, the patient should omit coffee, vanilla, certain vegetables and citrus fruits, and chocolates from the diet before his or her urine is tested for VMA. Other drugs used in the therapy of hypertension and its complications, including hydrochlorothiazide, hydralazine, and digitalis, do not affect the assay. α-Methyldopa in patients with no pheochromocytoma may lower VMA excretion. Phentolamine, phenoxybenzamine, and propranolol have not substantially interfered with the chemical tests and may be used during diagnostic procedures.

What are the most reliable chemical tests for the detection of a pheochromocytoma? Sjoerdsma and coworkers,[499] in evaluating the data on 24-hour urinary excretion of catecholamines and methoxylated metabolites in 62 patients with pheochromocytomas, found normal or near-normal values for VMA (in three cases), for metanephrine (in two cases), and for catecholamines (in two cases). In the three cases of normal VMA excretion, metanephrine and catecholamine levels were abnormally high. One of the two patients with normal catecholamine levels excreted abnormally high amounts of catecholamines for short periods after administration of histamine and after spontaneous attacks of hypertension; total 24-hour catecholamine levels for this patient, however, appeared normal, the normal or subnormal periods of excretion compensating for the periods of abnormally high "spurts." In another series of 91 patients with pheochromocytomas studied at the University of California Medical Center, the only six who excreted normal amounts of VMA showed increased urinary catecholamine excreted over 24 hours. If a 24-hour urine collection cannot be obtained, single voided urine metanephrine assays may be useful in screening for patients with pheochromocytomas because the rate of excretion appears to be constant and to be unaffected by diurnal variation.[282] Secretion of dopa in some patients with a pheochromocytoma also may be of diagnostic value, particularly if the patient appears to be normotensive most of the time.[349]

In some patients, it is preferable to collect timed samples during a period of hypertension and to express the excretion rates of the catecholamines and their metabolites in μg/hour. Normal rates (μg/hour) are as follows: total free catecholamines, 2.5 ± 0.8 with 22% being epinephrine; total free and conjugated metanephrines and normetanephrines, 16±5 with 35% being metanephrine; VMA 240±120 (means ± one standard deviation). Excretion of catecholamines in excess of 10 μg/hour, metanephrine in excess of 60 μg/hour, or VMA in excess of 500 μg/hour should be taken to indicate a pheochromocytoma until proved otherwise. In some patients under severe stress or with other diseases characterized by excessive sympathetic nervous system activity (e.g., congestive heart failure, acute myocardial infarction, or recent surgical procedures), the "normal" values will be exceeded.

Dividing the 24-hour urine collection into day and night samples may be useful in detecting pheochromocytomas, because normally the patient's upright position during the day is more likely to increase catecholamine excretion than is the supine position at night;[235] in patients with pheochromocytomas, there should be little difference between the two periods of collection.

In summary, the initial screening test for pheochromocytomas should estimate the 24-hour excretion of VMA or normetanephrine-metanephrine. In 80 or 90% of patients, either test will confirm the diagnosis of a pheochromocytoma. These tests are cheaper, more reliable, and technically less difficult than determinations of urinary catecholamines. Negative results in a suggestive clinical setting would justify repeating the tests, and, if necessary, determining urinary catecholamine excretion. If all three tests give negative results but the diagnosis is still suspect, urine collected over a 2- or 3-hour period after a spontaneous attack of hypertension or after administration of histamine with or without simultaneous use of an α-blocking agent should be assayed for catecholamine content. The use of prostaglandins instead of histamine might become preferable for the same purpose.[225] In such cases a control sample should be tested for comparison.

After a definitive diagnosis of pheochromocytoma has been made, the ratio of norepinephrine to epinephrine in the urine may aid in locating the tumor. The N-methylating enzyme for the conversion of norepinephrine to epinephrine is found predominantly in the adrenal medulla and the organ of Zuckerkandl.[23, 203] Therefore, when epinephrine constitutes more than 20% of the total catecholamines in the urine, the tumor is almost invariably located in one of these two sites.[351] When norepinephrine alone is increased, the tumor probably will be found in the adrenal gland, possibly in other intra-abdominal sites, and occasionally in extra-abdominal sites.

The pattern of excretion of catecholamines and metabolites in the urine varies considerably from patient to patient, although it depends in part on the size of the pheochromocytoma. Thus the ratio of urinary norepinephrine plus epinephrine to metabolites, particularly VMA,

may predict the size of the mass.[109] A low ratio of urinary VMA to norepinephrine plus epinephrine will indicate a tumor with a low content of norepinephrine and epinephrine (less than 100 mg), usually weighing less than 5 g. Such tumors rapidly synthesize catecholamines and, for some reason, readily release the amines as biologically active norepinephrine or other catecholamines into the circulation. Patients with such tumors will manifest symptoms before the mass becomes large. Tumors with a high content of catecholamines (100 mg to 10 g) bind amines well (probably by virtue of near-normal ATP concentrations), have a slow rate of catecholamine turnover, metabolize catecholamines within the tumor substance, and release metabolites as well as catecholamines into the circulation. Symptoms in such patients will not appear until sufficient amounts of active catecholamines have been released into the blood. By the time symptoms occur, the tumor is large (weighing 50 g or more) and the ratio of VMA to norepinephrine plus epinephrine in the urine usually is high.

Two additional substances are helpful for diagnosis in families with medullary carcinoma of the thyroid and bilateral pheochromocytomas. High concentration of calcitonin in plasma provides evidence of the medullary thyroid carcinoma;[535] increased concentrations of histaminase or diamine oxidase in plasma may indicate metastasis.[30]

Pharmacologic Testing. In recent years, pharmacologic tests have become safer but less necessary and less popular for screening purposes. If the patient is hypertensive, phentolamine (Regitine), an α-blocking agent, may be used in both a diagnostic and a therapeutic capacity to lower the blood pressure. If a pheochromocytoma is present, however, even small doses of phentolamine, 1 mg or less, may produce profound and prolonged hypotension (Fig. 10–11), creating a risk of cerebral or myocardial infarction. Therefore, instead of the recommended dose of 5 mg, the initial dose of phentolamine in patients with suspected pheochromocytomas should be less than 1 mg. A fall in blood pressure of 35/25 mm Hg, lasting at least 4 min but persisting up to 2 or 3 hours, suggests a pheochromocytoma. The test is only 75% accurate; false positive results are frequent, especially in patients with azotemia or in those under sedation or being treated for hypertension. Some of the false positive tests may be eliminated by also measuring changes in circulating insulin and blood glucose. When the phentolamine is given, patients with pheochromocytomas will show a rise in insulin and a fall in glucose that accompany the fall in blood pressure.[510]

In a normotensive patient, either of two pharmacologic agents may be used to provoke an attack of hypertension or, in the presence of α-adrenergic blockade, increase excretion of urinary catecholamines. Both histamine (by producing reflex sympathetic discharge) and tyramine (by direct action) release the catecholamine stores of normal sympathetic nerve endings. In a patient with a pheochromocytoma, these stores are increased because the nerve endings constantly are exposed to abnormally high concentrations of catecholamines in plasma. The uptake process expands their releasable store. Because pheochromocytoma tissue probably is not innervated, histamine would not be expected to affect the tumor itself. Although the effect of tyramine on tumor tissue has not been defined, its direct action on release of catecholamines from tissues would likely effect their release from the tumor.

The clinical usefulness of the histamine test currently is limited to patients with negative urinary catecholamine tests or those on whom other diagnostic tests could not be performed during spontaneous hypertension. Although histamine can be used to provoke an attack, the initial dose

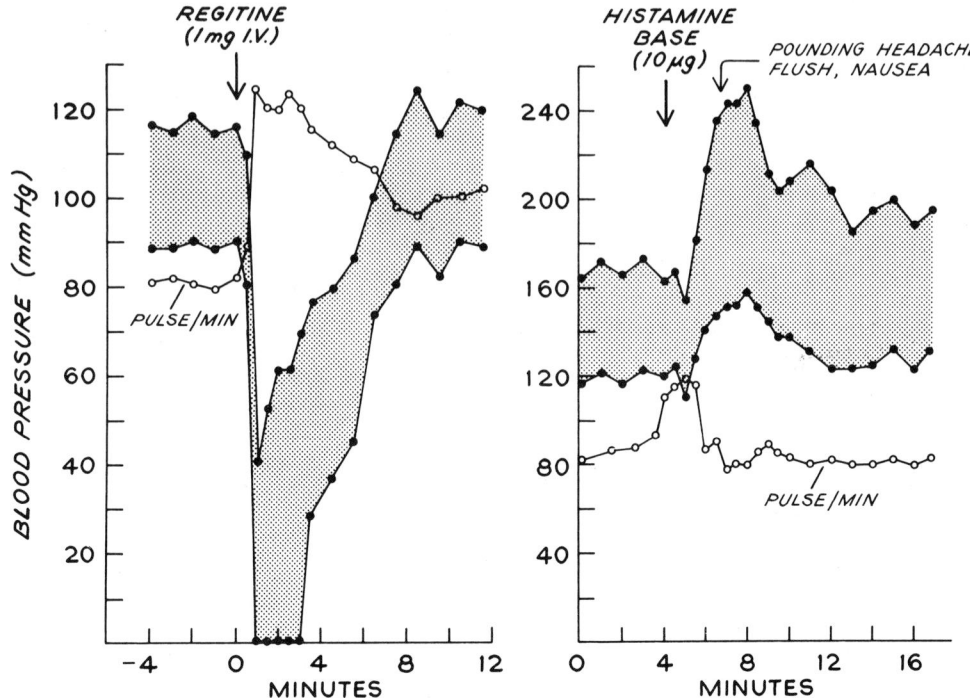

Figure 10-11. Responses to administration of phentolamine (Regitine) (1 mg) and histamine (10 μg) in patients with pheochromocytoma, showing that even small amounts of these agents (20 per cent of the doses usually recommended for pharmacologic testing) can cause profound changes in blood pressure.

should be smaller (less than 25 μg) than the usual amount recommended for pharmacologic testing. An α blocking agent should be used immediately for any large unexpected rise in blood pressure (Fig. 10–11). Urine collected for a 2-hour period before and after the histamine test should be assayed for catecholamines (but not for metabolites). The histamine test rarely gives false negative results.

The tyramine test depends on direct release of catecholamines from nerve endings.[156, 160, 499] Rapid intravenous administration of tyramine in graded doses of up to 2 mg will produce an increase in blood pressure within 45 to 60 sec, which reaches a peak at 1 to 1½ min. The response lasts less than 3 min. A rise of 20 to 80 mm Hg in systolic pressure and about 40 mm Hg in diastolic pressure is considered a positive response (Fig. 10–12). If the increase is prolonged or unusually or dangerously high, phentolamine will reverse it rapidly. False negative results are seen in about 25% of patients with pheochromocytomas, most frequently in those with the familial variety of the tumor associated with a medullary carcinoma of the thyroid, precisely the setting for which a simple screening test would be most desirable. False negative results are also possible in the patient taking hydrochlorothiazide or phenoxybenzamine. Nevertheless, the tyramine test may be preferable to the histamine test that often produces untoward effects.

A third test in the normotensive patient involves administering glucagon. The peptide is normally released from pancreatic islet cells during hypoglycemia. Its release or administration is associated with considerable increases in catecholamines in the peripheral and adrenal venous blood.[329] False positive results are not common; however, it has not been tried in enough patients with pheochromocytomas to determine either its value or the likelihood of false negative tests. If the effects of glucagon are limited to the adrenal, it would likely affect tumors only in that site and would not influence the same pools of catecholamines that are affected by histamine and tyramine. Further study will

determine where glucagon fits in the diagnostic armamentarium.

Pharmacologic tests are also important in excluding pheochromocytomas in patients with hypertension before they are treated with antiadrenergic drugs. As shown in Fig. 10–8, many agents frequently used in treating hyper-

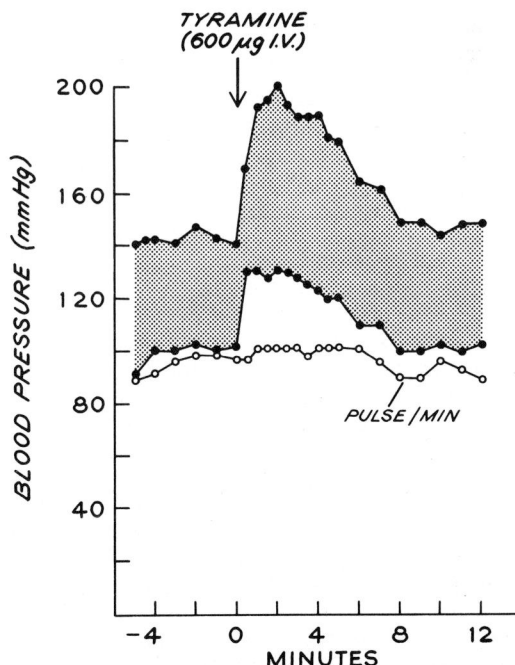

Figure 10-12. Results of a tyramine test in a patient with pheochromocytoma, showing a positive response (rise of about 80 mm Hg in systolic pressure and 40 mm Hg in diastolic pressure within 45–60 sec after intravenous administration of the drug).

tension, such as reserpine, α-methyldopa, guanethidine, and clonidine have in common the property of releasing stored catecholamines. In normotensive human subjects, administering guanethidine in large amounts has resulted in paradoxical hypertension instead of hypotension. Even less potent catecholamine releasers such as reserpine and α-methyldopa have produced pressor responses in normal individuals.[94, 336] Since abnormally large stores of catecholamines are characteristic in a patient with pheochromocytoma, affected patients can be expected to react adversely to these drugs. Therefore, when patients with moderate to severe hypertension are seen for the first time, they should be tested for a pheochromocytoma before treatment with these drugs is instituted. If a patient is hospitalized because of malignant acceleration of hypertension but has not been seen previously, he should be tested with phentolamine before other antihypertensive treatment is attempted. If the test is positive, phentolamine can be continued until further studies can be completed (see section on therapy). If the phentolamine test is equivocal, potent, rapid-acting ganglionic blocking agents (e.g., trimethaphan) should be administered rather than antiadrenergic agents that can release catecholamines. (The trimethaphan would not be expected to affect circulating catecholamines. However, it would be beneficial in a patient, even one with a pheochromocytoma, in whom the majority of catecholamines were released from normal nerve endings. If the majority of amines were coming from the adrenal tumor [a postganglionic structure] the ganglionic blocker would probably not be of help.) Some centrally active drugs (e.g., propranolol) and those that directly and indirectly reduce peripheral arterial resistance (e.g., nitroprusside, hydralazine, and prazosin) should all be useful in treating patients with pheochromocytoma.[113] When the phentolamine test is negative, antiadrenergic agents can be administered with relative safety.

To summarize, about 90% of pheochromocytomas can be diagnosed by a single test for urinary norepinephrine and epinephrine, normetanephrine plus metanephrine, or VMA levels. The size of the tumor can be estimated from the ratio of urinary VMA to norepinephrine plus epinephrine, and the location of the tumor can be predicted if large amounts of epinephrine are secreted. Pharmacologic tests and estimations of the concentrations of catecholamines in plasma are adjuvants to diagnosis for the other 10% of pheochromocytomas. Tyramine and histamine tests should be performed cautiously; ordinarily they are not used in patients with blood pressure above 170/100 mm Hg. Adrenergic blocking agents, which act by inhibiting the effects of circulating catechols at the receptor site, should be used only when the blood pressure is high.

Special Procedures. Blood volume determinations may indicate the need for fluid replacement before and during removal of the tumor. Previously, reduced blood and plasma volumes were assumed to be the major cause of the orthostatic or postoperative hypotension frequently seen in patients with pheochromocytomas. Sjoerdsma and coworkers[499] altered this assumption; only 4 of their 15 patients with pheochromocytomas showed a decrease in plasma volume greater than 2 standard deviations below the mean value in normal subjects. In addition, when ^{51}Chromium labeled red cells were used, only 3 of the 15 showed a reduction in total blood volume greater than 2 standard deviations below normal. Nevertheless, replacement or even overreplacement of blood deficits estimated by preoperative testing or lost at operation can be of major importance in preventing postoperative hypotension and surgical mortality.[64, 206] Biskin, Meyer, and Beadner[45] reported that profound hypotension develops in more than 50% of patients after resection of a pheochromocytoma and will be a frequent cause of death if pressor agents alone are used for its control.

Determining concentrations of catecholamines in the blood at different levels during catheterization of the inferior or superior vena cava is a useful procedure in the rare cases in which the tumor cannot be located by other means.[355, 412, 495] It is a difficult technical procedure, and the data must be interpreted skillfully. The findings may be misleading because of intermittent secretion of catecholamines by the tumor or falsely elevated or lowered catecholamine concentrations caused by laminar flow in different vessels. The test can falsely suggest only a single tumor if most of the increased concentration of catecholamines is localized in a narrow portion of the vessel, when actually the single vein is draining multiple tumors. Remember that 80% of all pheochromocytomas originate in the adrenal glands, and 95% are located in the abdominal or pelvic regions. Remember also that in 10% of adult patients, and a greater percentage of children, the tumors arise bilaterally or from multiple foci. These observations indicate that most if not all surgical procedures must be designed to explore the entire abdominal cavity. The catheterization procedure for determining concentrations of catecholamines in the blood should be restricted to those cases in which a tumor is not found by careful exploration of the abdomen or is suspected to be elsewhere than in the abdominal cavity.

The Relative Values of Chemical Versus Radiologic Procedures for Diagnosing Pheochromocytoma. The impressive value of chemical diagnostic tests has been defined above and supports the assumption that screening for excretion of catecholamines and their metabolites in urine is a highly selective and sensitive means for establishing the presence, or absence, of a pheochromocytoma at a very reasonable cost. Even the anatomical location and size of the tumor(s) have been predicted with reasonable accuracy by determining the dominant type of catecholamine excreted (norepinephrine or epinephrine) and the ratio of excretion of catecholamines to metabolites. No matter what the discriminative and localizing power of chemical tests, however, their use can never justify precluding a thorough exploration of the abdominal cavity at the time of surgery. Only after such exploration can we reasonably assess whether more than one tumor exists.

Despite the beliefs of Moorhead,[384] the pharmacologic provocation of the tumor by histamine, tyramine, or glucagon tests is diagnostically unreliable and can be hazardous. In the last decade at the Moffitt Hospital at the University of California, San Francisco, provocative tests have been used only 11 times in 9 patients, all of whom eventually proved to have pheochromocytomas. Ten of the 11 tests were considered to be positive, but all 9 patients also had diagnostic elevations of urinary catecholamines or their metabolites. One patient suffered an acute myocardial infarction during a hypotensive reaction to phentolamine. Sheps and his colleagues[494] noted that only 75% of their patients with documented pheochromocytomas had positive histamine tests and only 40% had positive phentolamine tests. At least two patients from the University of California have had positive phentolamine tests but have had no evidence of pheochromocytoma by chemical or diagnostic radiographic procedures. In the absence of pheochromocytoma, urinary VMA is rarely (virtually never) elevated in noncomatose patients who are on diets low in VMA and catecholamine content or who are taking no drugs that would interfere with the tests.[432, 494] Sheps and his colleagues[494] recorded only 2 of 148 occasions when estimations of VMA were falsely positive; neither of the patients with abnormal VMA had any other urinary abnormality.

False positive metanephrines were more common (11%), but the abnormal values were never greater than twice normal.

In the large Mayo Clinic series, preoperative diagnostic work-up often included an IVP and/or arteriography or venography. Nephrotomography localized up to 74% of suprarenal pheochromocytomas; the diagnostic accuracy was felt to be especially good if the tumors were larger than 2.5 cm.[452] Zelch and his coworkers,[614] however, were able to find only 12 of 37 (32%) pheochromocytomas by IVP and nephrotomography. At the University of California only 11 of the last 23 (48%) adrenal pheochromocytomas have been detected before surgery by such studies. Of our last four patients who had bilateral pheochromocytomas, in only one was the second tumor suspected before surgery, although all patients had IVPs. The second tumor in the other three was found during surgery. Early in our series, retroperitoneal air insufflation located only three of five adrenal pheochromocytomas. We no longer use this procedure for diagnosing pheochromocytomas because of the relatively high morbidity associated with its use and the lack of demonstrable benefits over other radiographic procedures. However, even though the morbidity of an IVP is not as great as that of a retroperitoneal gas insufflation, the discriminatory powers of the IVP are not impressive. It is useful when it reveals a lesion but it is probably overused. Any interpretation of the IVP should not preclude a thorough exploration at laparotomy.

The use of arteriography for diagnosing pheochromocytomas is controversial. Early reports of the danger of this procedure overemphasized the risk; all three reported deaths were associated with the translumbar approach and all occurred before 1960.[52] Since 1966, more than 60 reported cases of pheochromocytoma have been localized by arteriography. Agee and his coworkers[3] found 11 of 13 tumors by using aortography. A 12th patient had 2 negative arteriograms before a selective venous catecholamine blood sampling revealed the site at which excessive concentrations of catecholamines were produced. A final selective arteriogram, which was done in the anatomical vicinity of the elevated concentrations of catecholamines in the venous blood, located the tumor, but with considerable expense. Zelch and his colleagues,[614] using arteriography, correctly located tumors in 29 of 35 patients. An additional five pheochromocytomas were found by venography. Zelch and his coworkers also noted that 19 of their patients experienced hypertensive reactions during angiography. Meaney and Buonocore[367] suggested that angiography was a useful provocative study based on the fact that one of their patients who had a normal angiogram also experienced wide fluctuations in blood pressure during the test. Later, the pheochromocytoma was found, but only because a laparotomy was performed. At the University of California, arteriography has correctly localized six of nine pheochromocytomas. Selective catheterizations have accurately localized a tumor in three of four patients. In these patients, four of five tumors were accurately located. One patient experienced a hypertensive crisis during the procedure but no residual morbidity. Data from Rossi and his colleagues[468] also show that hypertensive reactions occur in less than half of the patients with pheochromocytoma who undergo angiography. Also, angiography should not be used as a provocative test because the blood pressure of patients who undergo the test is usually not monitored carefully; they are not easily given pharmacologic treatment to reverse an unexpected surge in blood pressure; and safer, less invasive diagnostic tests are available.

Although pheochromocytomas frequently are demonstrated by angiography, Zelch and his coworkers[614] report

that only about 70% of the tumors are vascular enough to show clearly on arteriograms. Less vascular pheochromocytomas would require venography (which is of unproven reliability) or selective sampling of venous blood for catecholamine analysis, which, when used by Agee and his colleagues,[3] gave three false positive localizations in seven attempts. Because chemical analyses are so reliable for making or excluding the diagnosis, it follows that angiograms are generally not needed for the diagnosis of pheochromocytomas. Over the last several years, three patients at the University of California who had normal concentrations of catecholamines and metabolites in their urine were subjected to angiography. All three patients had negative angiograms; none has subsequently been found to have a pheochromocytoma. On the other hand, if a patient persistently has abnormal urine chemistries and has not been comatose or ingested substances that could interfere with the chemical tests, he almost surely will have to undergo surgical exploration regardless of the angiographic findings.

A presumably important proposed use for angiography is to localize a tumor before surgery is performed. However, analysis of the three largest recent series,[3, 452, 614] as well as of our own 70 cases (a total of 256 patients with pheochromocytomas), indicates that at least 90% of pheochromocytomas are located in the adrenal glands and that another 8% are located in the renal hilus, the organ of Zuckerkandl, or the para-aortic sympathetic chain. Zelch and his coworkers[614] report one case in which the tumor was retrocaval. Three of the 138 pheochromocytomas in the Mayo Clinic series were in the subdiaphragmatic region.[452] All tumors from the combined three series were in the abdominal cavity. Thus, a negative adrenal arteriogram is as likely to give a false negative (about 10–15% in the recently reported larger series) as it is to indicate that a pheochromocytoma is truly extra-adrenal. Also, as shown in a case report,[80] angiography seems even more unlikely to visualize extra-adrenal pheochromocytomas. In addition, because of the high incidence of multiple tumors (about 10% in most large series) even a positive angiogram does not alter the need for thorough surgical exploration of the abdomen.

Among our 70 patients, the only "recurrent" pheochromocytomas occurred in patients who underwent unilateral flank surgical approaches in the late 1950's. Both patients underwent surgery in the mid 1960's to remove a pheochromocytoma on the other side. Four other patients who were thought, because of results from an IVP with tomography (three) or angiography (one), to have unilateral tumors were properly explored by an anterior abdominal approach and were found to have bilateral tumors. Thus, full exploration is mandatory even when clinical events, such as intraoperative blood pressure returning to normal after the initial tumor has been removed, suggest a single tumor.

In summary, because medical costs are escalating, all tests on patients must be necessary, not just interesting. The estimated cost of a search for secondary causes of hypertension is well above $2,000.[175, 365] With this in mind, the following diagnostic approach for patients suspected of having pheochromocytomas is suggested: (1) the diagnosis should hinge primarily on pathognomonic chemical assays of the urine; (2) the extremely rare extra-abdominal pheochromocytoma should be ruled out preoperatively to a comfortable pragmatic extent by historical features of the patient, the physical examination, and the film of the chest; and (3) if an IVP, arteriogram, or venogram is done, the results should never be used to preclude surgery or a careful examination of both adrenals, the adrenal hilar areas, the organ of Zuckerkandl, and the para-aortic sympathetic chain. Surgeons should use a midline abdominal approach after the patient's blood pressure has been preoperatively controlled with phenoxybenzamine or propranolol, or both, and after the blood volume is known to be normal (see below).

Angiography may occasionally be of use in the seriously ill patient. It could shorten the amount of time needed for the operation. However, multiple tumors may not be apparent on angiography. The surgeon may initially be assisted by a positive angiogram, but the fact remains that angiography produces false negative findings 10–15% of the time and that at least 98% of pheochromocytomas can be found by a surgical approach.

Therapy. *General.* Therapy for the patient with a pheochromocytoma has two distinctive phases: (1) the preparation of the patient for surgical removal of the tumor, and (2) the chronic management of the patient with a malignant pheochromocytoma or the patient unable to undergo a definitive surgical procedure. Effective control of blood pressure, blood volumes, and myocardial damage enables the patient to sustain the surgical and postsurgical course. Untreated patients frequently die from cardiovascular complications directly related to the pheochromocytoma.

Two major classes of drugs are used. The most widely used are the α-adrenergic blocking agents, which inhibit the effects of catecholamines but do not alter their synthesis or degradation. Both phentolamine, a short-acting agent, and phenoxybenzamine hydrochloride (Dibenzyline), a haloalkylamine that must be metabolized before it becomes an effective α blocker, are used. The choice of agents for presurgical therapy appears relatively unimportant. If the patient is generally well and requires only moderate control of blood pressure for a short time, phentolamine is the drug of choice. When given intravenously, phentolamine acts quickly and for short periods, allowing minute-to-minute control of the effects of catecholamines. When given orally, however, it has several disadvantages for prolonged use. It is well absorbed but may produce severe nausea or gastric irritation; it must be given every 4–6 hours, which requires waking the patient during the night; and its effect may be uneven, resulting in variations in blood pressure from normotensive to severely hypertensive. Therefore, in most medical centers, phenoxybenzamine is given instead in single oral doses (40–100 mg) every 12 hours. Despite initial fears, experience has indicated that this drug can be given until the time of operation without causing severe hypotension that might be unresponsive to adrenergic pressor agents after the tumor is removed and without totally inhibiting telling increases in blood pressure as the surgeon palpates the tumor mass.

With both drugs, therapy can be considered effective when blood pressure returns to normal, when hypertensive attacks cease, when sweating decreases, and, in many instances, when concentrations of fasting blood glucose and plasma free fatty acid return to normal.[566] Most patients should be treated for 10 days to 2 weeks before surgery, although patients with severe catecholamine-induced cardiomyopathy may require longer preoperative treatment. Two of the patients described by Engelman and Sjoerdsma[159, 162] required up to 6 months of presurgical treatment. The drugs may block some but not all of the effects of catecholamines. In several clinical cases, these agents have blocked the cardiovascular effects of catecholamines but not their gastrointestinal effects.[499] In other patients, concentrations of free fatty acid and fasting blood glucose and consumption of oxygen did not return to baseline, although palpitations disppeared and peripheral vascular resistance returned to normal.[566] Thus the disadvantage of α blocking agents lies in their apparent inability to reverse all the

β receptor–mediated effects of catecholamines. The potential value of drugs that affect the central sympathetics by diminishing the activities of the peripheral sympathetic nervous system (e.g., clonidine) or of drugs that affect presynaptic α-adrenergic receptors and alter small arterial vessel resistance (e.g., prazosin) has not been evaluated in patients with pheochromocytoma but probably will be.[47]

The β-adrenergic blocking agents may be very helpful in patients with cardiac arrhythmia who are not responsive to α-adrenergic blocking agents or efforts to reduce blood pressure. Neither our own clinical experience nor publications dealing with β-blocking drugs have convincingly documented a routine need for propranolol in the preoperative management of patients with pheochromocytoma.[606] Patients with pheochromocytomas can be extraordinarily sensitive to both α- and β-adrenergic blocking agents. A patient should be started on 20 mg of phenoxybenzamine daily and the dose increased by 10–20 mg/day until the cardiovascular manifestations are controlled. If arrhythmia persists after a maximally tolerable dosage schedule of the α blocking agent, propranolol in low doses of 10–40 mg may control the arrhythmia. Propranolol should not be used until an effective regimen of phenoxybenzamine has been established. If propranolol were used alone, severe hypertension could result because the α-mimetic activity of the circulating catecholamines would continue unopposed by the blocking agent and unbalanced by β receptor–mediated vasodilation.

A second major class of drugs, now available for the treatment of pheochromocytomas, acts at the rate-limiting step in the biosynthesis of catecholamines. The effect of these drugs is to decrease total catecholamine synthesis and, at least theoretically, prevent symptoms caused by excessive production of catechols. One such agent, α-methyltyrosine, inhibits tyrosine hydroxylase.[509] Engelman, Sjoersdma, and their collaborators used the drug on 19 patients with pheochromocytomas, including 4 with malignant pheochromocytomas.[161, 498] They found decreases in the synthesis of catecholamines by the tumor and reductions of up to 70–80% in urinary excretion of catecholamines and their metabolites. We obtained similar results with α-methyltyrosine in the treatment of three patients with malignant pheochromocytomas. The drug has been used successfully in one child whose symptoms of pheochromocytoma were not sufficiently ameliorated by α-adrenergic blocking agents.[460] The decreased excretion of catecholamines was accompanied by general improvement in the clinical status of the patient and decreases in blood pressure, pulse rate, sweating, and oxygen consumption. The drug has been further tested.[157, 201] The initial impressions of its effectiveness in patients with pheochromocytoma hold true. Some have used it to inhibit synthesis of catecholamines only when conventional adrenergic blocking agents were inadequate to control the effects of catecholamines. Not surprisingly, α-methyltyrosine has little effect on patients who have essential hypertension and in whom synthesis of catecholamines appears to be normal. As the drug inhibits synthesis of catecholamines, undesirable effects seem inevitable. Sedation is common and is followed by insomnia when the drug is withdrawn. Anxiety, diarrhea, and galactorrhea are common. Tremors similar to those seen in Parkinson's disease have been observed during chronic administration of the drug. For the present, conservative and sparing use of the drug appears warranted.

To repeat, β-blocking agents and inhibitors of the synthesis of catecholamines are useful for the short-term preoperative care of patients with pheochromocytomas, for patients with malignant lesions, and for those who cannot tolerate operative procedures. If metastasis has occurred, symptomatic treatment is the only alternative. No data have been reported that strongly support the use of antitumor agents in this disease. Because of the neural crest origin of the tumor cells, pheochromocytomas would be expected to be highly resistant to radiation and most antitumor drugs, and thus far they have proved so.[143, 227]

After the patient has been asymptomatic for 10 days to 2 weeks and ancillary diagnostic procedures have defined the presence, probable location, and biochemical characteristics of the tumor, surgical resection is the next step. Because patients with pheochromocytomas often have gallstones, gallbladder function should be evaluated before the operation. Simultaneous cholecystectomy and removal of a pheochromocytoma have been reported,[499] but it would seem prudent to perform the procedures separately. If a patient is pregnant at the time the pheochromocytoma is discovered, special considerations are necessary. Phentolamine and propranolol can be given to these patients indefinitely. Effective, surgically assisted delivery can be accomplished, but with relatively high morbidity and mortality of both patients.[328, 477]

Enemas should be avoided before removing an abdominal pheochromocytoma because they may induce a hypertensive crisis. However, because the colon must be manipulated during the abdominal exploratory procedure, it may be reasonable to have the patient take a clear fluid diet for 1–2 days before surgery. Antibiotics also have been used to prepare the bowel.

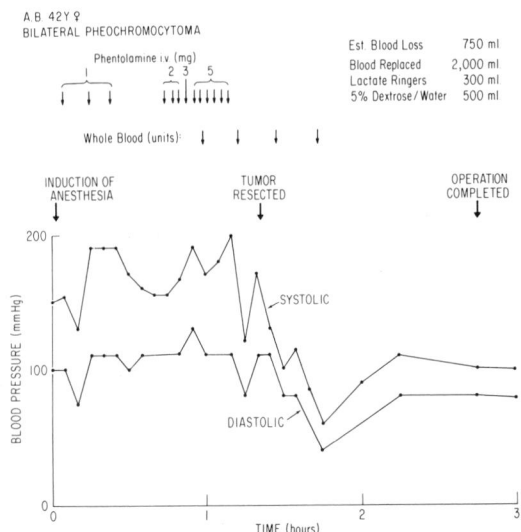

Figure 10–13. Effect of repeated doses of phentolamine on blood pressure levels of a patient with bilateral pheochromocytoma during surgical removal of the tumors. (Reproduced from Sjoerdsma, A., Engelman, K., et al.: *Ann. Intern. Med.* 65:1302, 1966, by permission of authors and publisher.)

Anesthetic Considerations

A narcotic analgesic used in conjunction with scopolamine has been used frequently for preanesthetic medication. Atropine is occasionally followed by tachycardia, which may be a direct effect of the drug on the heart.[465] Phenothiazines can produce shock,[60] and both drugs should therefore be avoided.

Before intubation or induction of anesthesia, an intra-arterial needle should be inserted into either the radial or brachial artery to allow constant monitoring of blood pressure. Electrocardiographic leads and a Swan-Ganz catheter for measuring cardiac output and determining total peripheral resistance should also be positioned for use. Careful monitoring of pressures is particularly important during early induction of anesthesia and tracheal intubation, when the blood pressure may rise. During periods of increased blood pressure, repeated doses of 1–5 mg of phentolamine should be given intravenously (Fig. 10–13). β-Blocking agents such as propranolol have been helpful in controlling arrhythmia.[606]

The type of anesthetic probably is inconsequential. Halothane has been used at the National Institutes of Health because it elicits little or no sympathoadrenal activity as measured by changes in plasma norepinephrine levels. It has the drawback, however, of being able to potentiate catecholamine-induced arrhythmia and probably should not be used unless an effective β-blocking agent is available. If such agents are not available, lidocaine may be given intravenously if ventricular arrhythmia occurs. Droperidol has some theoretical advantage over halothane in that it antagonizes the pressor effects and the arrhythmogenic effects of catecholamines.[516, 527] Anesthetics known to cause increased sympathetic activity and possible hypertension (e.g., ether and cyclopropane) probably should be avoided. In most hospitals, thiopental sodium and nitrous oxide are reasonable choices because neither is known to release catecholamines or to potentiate the arrhythmic effects of catecholamines. Curare can be used for muscle relaxation. Theoretical reasoning aside, the practical choice of anesthetics varies widely, and no particular agent is uniquely safe or hazardous. Paying attention to the fundamentals of oxygenation and proper

intravascular fluid volume leads to relatively favorable responses regardless of the anesthetic used. Replacement of blood should be started soon after anesthesia and surgical intervention and continued at a rate that will not dangerously increase pulmonary artery wedge pressures.

Surgical Considerations

Most surgeons choose an abdominal incision for a patient with a possible pheochromocytoma. When the pheochromocytoma is found in the adrenal, a "radical" adrenalectomy, with removal not only of the gland but also of adjacent areolar tissue (often the site of neural crest rests or other primary tumors), is the preferred procedure. Episodes of hypertension may occur during intubation, induction of anesthesia, peritoneal incision, manipulation and isolation of the tumor, and palpation of other organs that may contain tumor masses. Such episodes can be readily managed by repeated injection of phentolamine, as described previously, or constant infusions of phentolamine. The surgeon should palpate the gallbladder for the presence of stones or evidence of chronic cholecystitis. With the exception that pheochromocytomas in children often are bilateral and multiple, the principles of management are not different from those applied to the adult.[49, 197]

If blood volume has been adequately maintained and the patient well managed during surgery, there is little risk of postoperative hypotensive episodes that cannot be controlled by further replacement of blood or by the use of small amounts of pressor agents.[277] Of the 46 patients with pheochromocytomas operated on most recently at the University of California Medical Center and Stanford University School of Medicine, use of pressor agents has been required in very few. Corticosteroid replacement must be planned if a bilateral adrenalectomy is carried out.

The surgeon should be aware that whether or not the tumor is malignant it can seed in local tissue sites. Therefore, great care should be exercised to keep the tumor from touching normal tissue.[497]

Several days after the operation, 24-hour urinary excretion of catecholamines and metabolites should be measured to determine whether the surgical procedure has been successful. If concentrations of VMA are still abnormally high after the first postoperative week, further evaluation is indicated, and additional surgical procedures should be considered. Once the concentrations of urinary catecholamines and metabolites return to normal, the patient can be discharged. The patient should be reevaluated at regular intervals because additional primary pheochromocytomas may occur. This is particularly true in young patients, in families in which more than one member has had a pheochromocytoma, or in patients in whom multiple endocrine neoplasia has been found. For comprehensive reviews of pheochromocytoma see the works cited in references 234, 354, and 355.

Other Tumors Arising from Sympathetic and Adrenal Medullary Tissue

Because it is derived from neural crest tissue, the adrenal medulla occasionally is the site of tumors other than pheochromocytomas. Although found most commonly in the adrenal medulla, they may occur in other retroperitoneal and retropleural sites. Such tumors also occur in other sites of neural crest origin, such as the brain, sympathetic ganglia, and celiac plexus. The neoplasms are of two main types: neuroblastomas and ganglioneuromas (Fig. 10–14). The neuroblastomas are usually large. They occur in the neonate and child, and rarely in the adult. The young also are predisposed to the ganglioneuroma, but it occurs more frequently in the adult. There may be a familial predisposition to neuroblastomas.[85] The tumor cells of both neoplasms are small and round, have hyperchromatic nuclei, and are dispersed in rosettes among more highly differentiated cellular elements. They derive chiefly from sympathogonia and sympathoblasts. Because pheochromoblasts and sympathoblasts are difficult to differentiate, neuroblastomas may arise from both cell types. Such tumors metastasize early, either by direct spread into contiguous tissues or by embolization to lymph nodes, liver, other abdominal organs, and bone. The most common symptom of neuroblastomas (and occasionally ganglioneuromas) is diarrhea.[464] Hypertension, although it does occur, is infrequent. For the neuroblastoma, early radical surgical resection, radiation therapy, and administration of antitumor agents may result in a cure.[327, 530, 574] Treatment is most successful when metastasis is confined to the abdomen, but occasional instances of very widespread disease may have a favorable prognosis after vigorous therapy.[120]

The ganglioneuroma is derived from sympathetic ganglion cells and is composed of organized, mature cells. This tumor usually develops during youth but also occurs frequently in adulthood. If detected early enough, it can be treated successfully by surgical extirpation, but it may become anaplastic and degenerate into a malignant neuroblastoma. Pathologists have classified a tumor with cellular elements intermediate between those of neuroblastoma and ganglioneuroma as a ganglioneuroblastoma.[379] This differentiation is largely on a histologic basis. The ganglioneuroblastoma may behave either as a ganglioneuroma or as a neuroblastoma. There have been instances of actual maturation of a neuroblastoma to a ganglioneuroma.[14]

The pheochromocytoma, neuroblastoma, ganglioneuroblastoma, and ganglioneuroma have a common embryologic origin. Therefore, the finding by Mason and coworkers[360] of increased excretion of pressor amines in the urine of an infant with a neuroblastoma is not surprising. Later studies have shown that patients with neuroblastomas as well as neuroblastoma cells[208] frequently excrete a variety of chemical precursors of catecholamines and their metabolic products.[27, 199, 219, 319, 576, 577] In one reported series of 73 patients with neuroblastoma,[287] increased urinary excretion of VMA was found in 69 patients; excretion of dopamine was increased in 32 of 36 patients tested; and the oxidation product of dopamine, HVA, was increased in 24 of 36. Subsequent experience has confirmed the usefulness of measuring urinary catecholamines both to detect the tumor and to follow the effects of therapy in patients with neuroblastoma.[177, 386] The radiologic techniques used to discover pheochromocytomas are applicable to neuroblastomas and ganglioneuromas.

Experience with neural crest tumors other than pheochromocytomas has led to two important observations. First, it appears that the more primitive the tumor cell, the more likely it is that the tumor will elaborate the precursors of catecholamines and their metabolic products. Thus the neuroblastoma is associated almost invariably with a high urinary output of VMA and frequently with elaboration of dopamine and HVA.[287] In contrast, dopamine and HVA usually are not excreted by patients with pheochromocytomas unless the tumors have become malignant.[287, 577] Second, as the cell type approaches a more mature form of differentiation, the frequency with which biologically active substances are excreted diminishes. In the histologically primitive tumor, the tumor cells actually may be able to produce catecholamines, but the binding properties of the cells are impaired. A good rule of thumb is that increased excretion of dopa, dopamine, or HVA suggests the malignant rather than the benign form of the neural crest tumors; in the case of the neuroblastoma and the ganglioneuroma, the more primitive form is more likely to be associated with increased excretion of VMA. An exception to the rule is the finding that urinary excretion of dopa and its metabolites may be elevated in patients with melanomas.[579] When excretion of dopa is increased in a patient with any neural crest tumor, hypotensive or normotensive blood pressures are likely.

Another point of interest is that apparently little or no correlation exists between the clinical symptoms, such as chronic diarrhea, hypertension, or abnormalities in serum glucose levels,[490] and the excretion of known catecholamines or their metabolites in patients with either neuroblastomas or ganglioneuromas. One possible explanation for the lack of correlation may be the metabolism of most of the biologically active amines within the tumor cells. However, a more likely explanation is that we have not identified all the biologically active substances that the tumor cells can produce or the various autacoids and other substances to which the tumor can respond.[455] As we have discussed, some authorities believe that the pheochromocytoma may be an incomplete

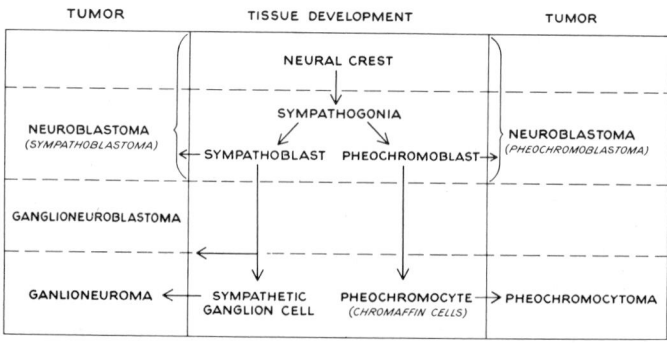

Figure 10–14. Embryologic derivation of endocrinologically functioning tumors of neural crest origin. The ganglioneuroblastoma is derived from cell types intermediate between those of the neuroblastoma and pheochromocytoma.

expression of pluriglandular adenomatosis because it is associated with other endocrinopathies. The pheochromocytoma is capable of producing more than one class of endocrine hormone. It seems equally possible that neuroblastomas and ganglioneuromas may produce their symptoms by elaborating a biologically active substance as yet unidentified. The tumors apparently are responsible for the symptoms, because removal of the primary or metastatic masses is followed by lessening of the diarrhea and hypertension, and often the patient becomes asymptomatic.[301, 304] Thus such tumors may be analogous to the carcinoid tumor, which can elaborate a spectrum of biologically active substances. The neural crest tumors may be able to produce hormones by some mechanism completely unrelated to their usual cell function. That such a phenomenon can occur is shown by the description of tumors that are histologically unrelated to the carcinoid tumor but that produce symptoms indistinguishable from those of the carcinoid syndrome. Whether the symptoms result from the release of endogenous vasoactive substances by the tumor or whether the tumor actually produces biologically active compounds remains to be determined.

SEROTONIN

Mammalian physiologists have known for about a century that a vasoconstrictor material appears in serum when blood is allowed to clot. This unidentified vasoconstrictor material, which went by a variety of names such as *vasotonin*, was a frequent nuisance in perfusion experiments in which defibrinated blood was used, although physiologists discovered empirically that it could be eliminated by passing the blood through the lungs, a phenomenon now understood to be due to uptake and enzymatic destruction. In the late 1940's, the substance appeared in another context during a search for humoral pressor agents such as angiotensin that might explain arterial hypertension. In this work the serum vasoconstrictor was a "pest," to be eliminated before the other inquiry could proceed. In 1948, investigators at the Cleveland Clinic isolated this vasoconstrictor substance as a crystalline complex and named it *serotonin*;[907] shortly thereafter Rapport[906] deduced that the active moiety of this complex (for which he retained the name *serotonin*) was 5-hydroxytryptamine (5-HT). This compound, when prepared synthetically by Hamlin and Fischer[785] and others, proved to have all the properties of natural serotonin.

Quite independently, studies had been proceeding in Italy that would soon reveal 5-HT as an autacoid whose occurrence and activities ranged far beyond the cardiovascular system. This work was begun in the 1930's by Erspamer and his colleagues, whose original purpose was to extract and characterize the substance that imparts peculiar histochemical properties to enterochromaffin cells of the gastrointestinal mucosa. Their experiments led them to discover, first in the mucosa and later in other tissues, a gut-stimulating factor of a basic nature, which they termed *enteramine*. By the late 1940's, Erspamer had accumulated a great deal of information on the pharmacologic activity of enteramine, had shown that it was present in many tissues of vertebrates and invertebrates, and had suggested that it was an indole alkylamine.[729] In 1952, Erspamer and Asero identified enteramine as 5-HT.[730]

Thus, by the time 5-HT had been recognized as such, there already existed a mass of evidence indicating that it was widely distributed in nature and that it possessed a variety of pharmacologic, and possibly physiologic, actions. It is therefore not surprising that the introduction of synthetic 5-HT in 1951 touched off an explosion of research. This was further fueled when 5-HT was discovered in the brain,[629, 977] when lysergic acid diethylamide (LSD) and other potent hallucinogens were recognized to be structurally similar to 5-HT and were found to block smooth muscle responses to 5-HT,[749, 993] and when the potent tranquilizing drug reserpine was observed to lower concentrations of 5-HT in the brain.[667] All this suggested that 5-HT serves as a neurotransmitter, a function now established, and attention was focused on a possible role for 5-HT in mental illnesses.[992]

Chemical Synthesis and Storage

Serotonin (chemical name: 3-[β-aminoethyl]-5-hydroxyindole) is widely distributed in the plant and animal kingdoms. Its production depends upon hydroxylation of the amino acid tryptophan to form 5-hydroxytryptophan (Fig. 10–15). Tryptophan hydroxylase has been isolated from tumors and normal animal tissues, including the brain stem, pineal gland, and liver of the rat, dog, cow, and mouse, and the mouse mast cell tumor. The enzyme was difficult to isolate as it was sometimes confused with phenylalanine hydroxylase, but it has been well characterized.[836] It appears to originate from either the cell cytoplasm or the mitochondria and has an absolute requirement for oxygen, a reduced pteridine, and ferrous iron. In most preparations, the K_m for the substrate is reasonably low (3×10^{-4} to 4×10^{-5}), but it has been characterized as responsible for the rate-limiting step in the synthesis of serotonin and melatonin. The enzymatic production of 5-hydroxytryptophan can be accelerated by increasing availability of substrate[740] and inhibited by either norepinephrine or phenylalanine[836] or by decreasing the availability of substrate.[921]

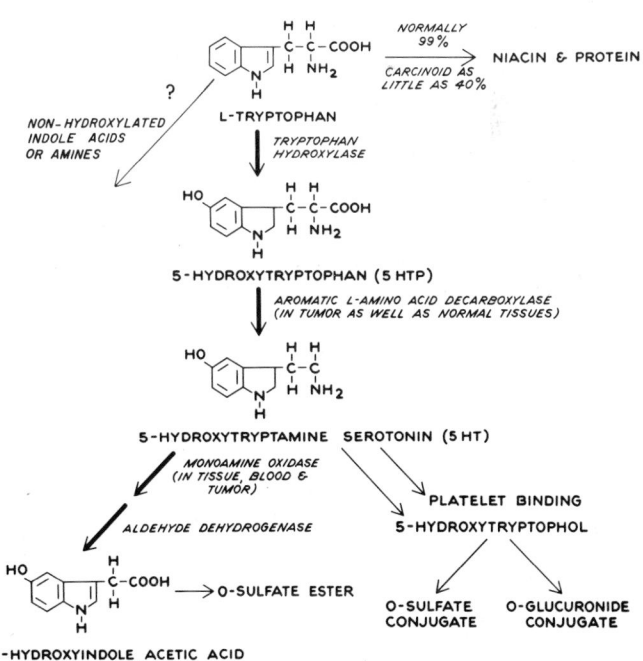

Figure 10–15. Metabolism of tryptophan in a patient with carcinoid syndrome. Heavy arrows indicate the shunting of tryptophan away from its usual metabolic pathway to form niacin and protein. Heavy arrows leading from serotonin show the major metabolites of serotonin excreted in the urine. Several gastric and some bronchial tumors lack aromatic L-amino acid decarboxylase and release large amounts of 5-hydroxytryptophan into the blood. Metabolites in the urine then include 5-hydroxytryptophan, 5-hydroxytryptamine, and less 5-hydroxyindole acetic acid than is expected.

There is no feedback inhibition of tryptophan hydroxylase by serotonin as there is of tyrosine hydroxylase by norepinephine,[833] and the enzyme is not sensitive to steroidal or thyroid hormones.[815] There is a complex relationship between the turnover rates of serotonin and norepinephrine, however.[633, 736, 933, 999] Generally speaking, it is inverse: When synthesis of catecholamines decreases or stores of catecholamines are depleted, the rate of synthesis of serotonin increases and the amine accumulates. When the catecholamines are stored in an area that contains serotonin-N-acetyltransferase (an enzyme that participates in producing melatonin from serotonin), stimulation of β-mimetic receptors contributes to increased activity of the enzyme and a subsequent decrease in the concentration of serotonin in the vicinity.[637, 669, 703, 704] The rate of synthesis of serotonin is dependent on the availability of tryptophan, thus diet and the state of liver function may substantially influence the synthesis of serotonin.[741, 921, 978] The unusual mental symptoms in some patients with carcinoid tumors may be explained by their diets or by the relative availability in the brain of substrate for tryptophan hydroxylase. Perhaps the functional states of the circulation or the liver can alter distribution of an amino acid to various parts of the CNS so as to alter significantly the synthesis of serotonin.

The fact that phenylalanine inhibits tryptophan hydroxylase in the majority of tissues in which the enzyme is found is clinically important.[836] In fact, the reason for the low rates of synthesis of 5-hydroxytryptophan in liver preparations apparently is that the liver enzyme is phenylalanine hydroxylase and not tryptophan hydroxylase. Derivatives of phenylalanine have been synthesized, and not surprisingly they inhibit tryptophan hydroxylase. The inhibition is noncompetitive and involves inactivation of the enzyme. It also is associated with decreased concentration of serotonin in brain and decreased rates of synthesis. One derivative, parachlorophenylalanine, has been used clinically to inhibit synthesis of serotonin.[698, 723, 923, 939] Although it decreases diarrhea in patients with the carcinoid syndrome, it also induces psychiatric effects, implying that serotonin deficiency in the brain may in part be responsible for some affective illnesses. As expected, the drug also inhibits phenylalanine hydroxylase *in vivo,* resulting in substantial rises in concentrations of serum phenylalanine.[969] Whether the phenylalanine itself contributes to any of the effects of parachlorophenylalanine is not known.

Besides diet, liver function, and general availability of tryptophan to the enzyme, other factors participate in regulating the synthesis of serotonin. Psychologic stress increases the rate of both synthesis and metabolism of serotonin in the brain;[988] the serotonin-associated physiologic events that accompany stress seem dependent on a small portion of the total pool, predominantly the portion most recently synthesized.[765, 768, 771] It is likely that stress or stimulation of the midbrain induces synthesis of tryptophan hydroxylase, accounting for the rapid rates of synthesis of serotonin.[719] Synthesis of serotonin in the pineal gland has a circadian rhythm that is dependent on the amount of light that the animal can visually appreciate.[634, 947] The serotonin thus synthesized has important relationships to a number of endocrine functions, including secretion of luteinizing hormone (LH)[998] and the circadian rhythm of 17-hydroxycorticoids.[821]

Effects of Drugs

A number of drugs also affect the synthesis, action, or metabolism of serotonin. Reserpine depletes serotonin from a variety of tissue stores in the same manner as it affects stores of norepinephrine and dopamine.[973] MAO inhibitors promote retention of amine and expansion of amine stores in a variety of tissues. Lithium can either increase or decrease the turnover rate of serotonin in various areas of the brain; it presumably does so by altering the storage of serotonin.[691, 796] Morphine also seems to affect synthesis and metabolism of serotonin. Tolerance to morphine may, in part, be related to its effects on synthesis of serotonin.[847, 935, 995] Chlorpromazine, which has a profound effect on transport and synthesis of catecholamines, appears to block the peripheral effects of serotonin (i.e., it may prevent serotonin action in the same way that adrenergic blocking agents inhibit the effects of catecholamines on effector organs).[766] Drugs that allow release or prevent reuptake of β-mimetic catecholamines can influence the rate of transformation of serotonin to melatonin.[799]

Origin, Uptake, and Storage

Although considerable 5-HT is present in the diet, much is metabolized as it crosses the intestinal wall, and most of the rest is destroyed by the liver and lungs.[757] The 5-HT found in enterochromaffin cells, neurons, and most other 5-HT-containing cells is synthesized *in situ* from tryptophan. Platelets, an important exception, acquire 5-HT from their environment. 5-HT, whether synthesized or acquired (as by platelets), is taken up into secretory granules (or vesicles) and stored therein as a nondiffusible complex with ATP and other substances to await the signal for secretion. The molecular events involved in pumping the amine into its granular storage sites and sequestering it there are presumably similar to those involved in the storage of the catecholamines. Drugs that disrupt the storage of catecholamines (such as reserpine) impair the storage of 5-HT similarly.[751] Platelets take up 5-HT during their passage through the intestinal blood vessels, where they encounter relatively high concentrations of 5-HT that result from its secretion by enterochromaffin cells and possibly other sources. A high-affinity uptake mechanism allows 5-HT to accumulate in spite of an enormous concentration gradient. This high-affinity uptake mechanism is also present in tryptominergic nerve endings, thereby permitting them to recapture released transmitter. These uptake mechanisms are also similar, but not identical, to those for reuptake of catecholamines by adrenergic and dopaminergic neurons;[887, 945] for example, both are influenced by the tricyclic antidepressant drugs. Because platelets are relatively easy to isolate and study, they are often used as models for the study of such processes.[946, 962] (For recent reviews on the metabolism of 5-HT and drugs affecting it, see the works cited in references 662 and 751.)

The turnover of serotonin is rapid: Approximately all body stores of the amine are replenished each day.

Mechanisms of Action

Receptors for serotonin, which are located on the cell surface, are less well characterized than are those for catecholamines and histamine, but they are distinctive and specific.[650, 686] They can be located and quantitated with the use of ^{3}H-spiroperidol,[697] and their dynamics are affected by serotonin or serotonergic neurons in ways analogous to the receptors for other autacoids.[878, 948]

As with other autacoids, transduction of receptor occupancy into a functional response seems often to involve changes in permeability of the membrane to inorganic ions (which thereby influence ion fluxes), membrane potential, excitability, and spiking activity or a change in the intracellular concentration of free calcium ions, which is critical to excitation-contraction coupling[985] and stimulus-secretion coupling.[714, 715] In neurons of mollusks, in which the most detailed studies of the effects of 5-HT on membrane properties have been performed, excitation results from two independent actions of 5-HT: The first increases conductance to Na^+, the second reduces conductance to K^+. Similarly, 5-HT–induced inhibition may arise from an increase in K^+ conductance or from an increase in Cl^- conductance.[695, 754] In vertebrates, events may be simpler, with excitation and inhibition perhaps involving only increased conductance to Na^+ and K^+, respectively. A depolarizing action leading to influx of Ca^{2+} seems to account for the stimulatory effect of 5-HT on chromaffin cells[718] and on certain cells in the adenohypophysis (pars intermedia), where 5-HT elicits action potentials.[716] Smooth muscle contraction elicited by 5-HT reduces the free intracellular concentration of Ca^{2+}.[966] In smooth muscle, evidence points to an association between elevated concentrations of cAMP and relaxation on the one hand and elevated concentrations of cGMP and contraction on the other. Nevertheless, there are many discrepancies that suggest that these nucleotides are not mandatory intermediates in such responses of smooth muscle.[709] The possible involvement of cyclic nucleotides in other 5-HT–sensitive systems has been reviewed.[651, 657, 814, 879] (For further discussion of cyclic nucleotides and of protein phosphorylation as they may relate to the action of 5-HT, see the works cited in references 693 and 774.)

Pharmacologic and Physiologic Effects

Serotonin (5-HT) stimulates or inhibits a variety of smooth muscles and nerves. These and other actions result in a wide spectrum of responses involving, in particular, the cardiovascular, respiratory, and gastrointestinal systems. Characteristically, responses to 5-HT are variable; they differ not only between species but also between animals of the same species and even in successive tests in the individual. This variability, which is responsible for many discrepant reports and much controversy, is attributable in large part to two factors: (1) many of the effects of 5-HT are reflexly mediated and hence subject to influences such as patterns of innervation, route and speed of injection, anesthetic state, and spontaneous tone; and (2) tachyphylaxis is common when tests are made at frequent intervals. Detailed accounts of the pharmacologic actions of serotonin can be found in the Handbook edited by Erspamer[727] and in the series of monographs edited by Essmann.[731-734]

Respiratory System

Intravenous injection of 5-HT in dogs and in humans commonly causes a short-lived increase in respiratory minute volume accompanied by variable changes in respiratory rate. With lower doses, the effect is due to stimulation of carotid and aortic chemoreceptors. With higher doses, other ill-defined effects contribute to the responses observed. Sometimes, particularly in cats and in humans, respiratory movements are inhibited through stimulation of vagal afferent fibers. In humans, brief periods of apnea can result from intravenous injection of the amine.

Bronchoconstriction

5-HT causes bronchoconstriction in many animals but rarely in humans, except in patients with asthma. The effect is partly reflex but is caused mainly by direct stimulation of bronchial smooth muscle.[919]

Cardiovascular System

The effects of 5-HT on this system are uniquely complex. By acting directly on vascular smooth muscle, the drug may evoke vasoconstriction or vasodilatation, depending on the vascular bed, its resting tone, and the dose given. By its actions on a variety of sensory nerve endings, it activates pressor and depressor reflexes; by direct and reflex mechanisms, it either stimulates or depresses cardiac output, and in high doses, it influences ganglionic transmission, adrenal medullary secretion, and the release of transmitters from nerve endings.

Blood Vessels

Direct vasoconstriction is a classic effect of 5-HT and is responsible for the synonyms *vasotonin* and *serotonin*. The effect of 5-HT in animals who have no reflex responses to its effects is to cause a prompt uncomplicated rise in blood pressure, which lasts several minutes. The splanchnic and renal beds are particularly affected, and in some laboratory animals necrosis of the renal cortex results. Placental, uterine, and umbilical vessels also constrict. Cerebral blood vessels are powerfully constricted in several species.[720] Pulmonary vasoconstriction is prominent in dogs and cats and less prominent in humans.

Vasodilatation occurs in skeletal muscle, especially with lower doses of 5-HT. The drug acts directly on the smooth muscle, but it can also reduce the release of norepinephrine from sympathetic nerve terminals. In the forearm, where muscle is preponderant, vasodilatation tends to increase blood flow. Superficial vessels of the human skin also dilate after intradermal or intra-arterial injection of 5-HT. The resulting flush, at first bright red, assumes a dusky hue, indicating stagnation, probably as a result of venoconstriction. The overall response to 5-HT given intra-arterially is a rise in cutaneous vascular resistance, however. In the hand, where skin is preponderant, this effect reduces blood flow.

Capillary permeability is not much affected by 5-HT, except in rats, in which it increases.

Heart

5-HT has positive inotropic and chronotropic effects of varying intensity. These are evident in isolated preparations and they reflect in part direct actions on cardiac tissue and indirect actions that are mediated by the release of norepinephrine from sympathetic nerve terminals. *In vivo*, such effects are commonly blunted or overshadowed by autonomic reflexes arising from changes in blood pressure or direct actions of 5-HT on baroreceptors, chemoreceptors, and vagal endings in the coronary bed. The latter action is particularly noteworthy. It initiates the coronary chemoreflex (Bezold-Jarisch reflex), characterized by inhibition of sympathetic outflow and increased activity of the cardiac (efferent) vagus, which leads to profound bradycardia and hypotension. Occasionally cardiovascular collapse and fainting occur from such causes when 5-HT is given to humans. No significant changes in the electric properties of the heart have been attributed to 5-HT.

Blood Pressure

In contrast to the pithed animal, intact animals respond to an intravenous injection of 5-HT with changes in blood pressure that are notoriously variable because they represent the outcome of several opposed and capricious influences, both direct and reflex. In most species, including humans, it is nevertheless possible to discern three successive phases: a brief depressor phase immediately after the injection; a succeeding pressor phase; and finally, within 1 or 2 min of the injection, a prolonged depressor phase. The early depressor phase results from the coronary chemoreflex; it is abolished by cutting the vagi (which contain both the afferent and the efferent limbs of the reflex) or by the administration of a combination of parasympathetic and sympathetic blocking agents. The pressor phase is due mainly to the direct effects of 5-HT increasing the total peripheral resistance and cardiac output. The late depressor phase is attributable mainly to the direct vasodilator effects of 5-HT, principally in skeletal muscle; it persists after block of sympathetic outflow.

Veins are strongly constricted by 5-HT, and intense venospasm commonly accompanies intravenous infusions. This action probably is responsible for the frequent inability to draw venous blood from patients with the carcinoid syndrome.

Kidney and Antidiuresis

In most species, including dogs and humans, effects of 5-HT on renal blood flow and formation of urine are minor and inconstant. Feeble antidiuretic responses accompanied by diminished glomerular filtration rate are most commonly observed. There is no evidence of increased secretion of antidiuretic hormone (ADH) or of aldosterone, although the secretion of aldosterone can increase in response to 5-HT in isolated adrenals.[623]

Platelets

5-HT promotes aggregation of platelets without inducing the "release action." The effect, which is small and reversible, seems to be due to activation of specific receptors on the platelet surface.[661]

Exocrine Glands

Intravenous infusion of 5-HT in the dog reduces the volume, acidity, and pepsin content of gastric juice secreted spontaneously or in response to vagal activation, cholinergic drugs, or histamine, but at the same time it increases the production of mucus. Somewhat similar effects have been described in humans and various other species and apparently involve reflex as well as direct actions.[972] Variable effects on salivary, pancreatic, and other exocrine secretions have been reported in mammals.

Nerve Endings

Stimulatory effects of 5-HT on various sensory nerve endings have been mentioned above in connection with respiratory and circulatory reflexes. These are but illustrations of a general property of 5-HT, shown also by its tendency, when administered intravenously, to produce pain at the site of injection, as well as to produce gasping, hyperventilation, substernal "pressure," coughing, and "tingling and prickling all over."[798] Stimulatory effects of 5-HT on autonomic efferent nerves, with release of norepinephrine or ACh, seem to participate in the responses of some tissues (e.g., the heart and gut),[619] although inhibition of the release of transmitters at nerve endings has also been noted.[852]

Autonomic Ganglia

In high doses, 5-HT fires ganglion cells; lower doses facilitate or inhibit ganglionic transmission, depending on experimental conditions.[924]

Adrenal Medulla and Other Endocrine Glands

High doses of 5-HT cause secretion of catecholamines from the adrenal gland by depolarizing chromaffin cells.[718] The drug has capricious stimulatory or inhibitory effects on many other endocrine systems, including the adrenal cortex, pancreatic β cells, and adenohypophyseal cells; in the latter the action may be to modulate action potentials.[716]

Serotonin may modulate ACTH (by increasing the amount released) and may alter glucose tolerance by additional mechanisms.[901] Release of insulin can be inhibited by serotonin, and competitive blockers of 5-HT can reverse this inhibition.[739] As a result, antiserotonin agents may reverse abnormal glucose tolerance in patients with the carcinoid syndrome.[738, 902] The same 5-HT stimulus that inhibits the release of insulin may also independently stimulate growth hormone (GH), and, indeed, hypoglycemia may be associated with increased release of 5-HT.[655] Finally, indoles may inhibit the breakdown of insulin in the liver by inhibiting the activity of the protease for insulin.[670]

Smooth Muscle (Alimentary Tract)

Intravenous injections of 5-HT augment the rate of progression of peristalsis and the intraluminal pressures of the intestine. Humans are particularly sensitive and often respond to doses insufficient to affect the cardiovascular or respiratory system: Typically, the response consists of an initial intense spasm followed first by heightened tone with rhythmic propulsive contractions and then by a period of inhibition of spontaneous activity. Motility of the stomach and large intestine may also be increased by 5-HT, but in most animals, and in humans, the usual response is inhibition. Isolated segments of gastrointestinal tract in vitro generally exhibit responses qualitatively similar to those obtained in vivo, namely, contraction, inhibition, or mixtures of these. The complexity of the pattern is in large measure due to the variety of elements, both neural and muscular, that respond to 5-HT. The direct action is blocked by 5-HT antagonists such as LSD, methysergide, and cyproheptadine (see below). The stimulation of neural transmission through ganglion cells is countered by tetrodotoxin or cocaine, both of which block the nerves; by atropine, which blocks the action of the ACh that the neurons liberate; and by morphine, which has the dual property of opposing the excitatory effect of 5-HT on the ganglion cells and of diminishing the output of ACh from their terminals. In addition, 5-HT can increase peristaltic activity by stimulating or sensitizing intramural nerve endings. There is growing evidence that tryptaminergic nerve fibers may be present in mammalian gut.[748, 755]

Central Nervous System and Serotonin

During studies in animals of the drugs that altered the production, stores, and metabolism of serotonin, many of the pharmacologic effects that are observed began to be linked to serotonin.[873] We now realize that perhaps the most important physiologic function of serotonin is to serve as a chemical transmitter in neurons within the brain (i.e., tryptaminergic or serotonergic neurons). In addition, 5-HT serves as a precursor of melatonin.

States of serotonin deprivation were induced in laboratory animals with parachlorophenylalanine; they were associated with affective disorders, retardation of passive-avoidance learning, suppression of rapid eye movements during sleep, and increases in sexual activity. In humans, serotonin is strongly indicated as an influence in the CNS on a variety of behavioral patterns including sleep, perception of pain, arousal, emotionality, and social behavior.[658, 673, 809, 834, 845, 851, 959]

Although serotonin does not cross the blood-brain barrier, factors in the periphery may influence the brain. If, for example, tryptophan is shunted from normal pathways in the periphery, less amino acid than usual will reach the brain; this may occur in patients with the carcinoid tumor. Because synthesis is dependent on availability of substrate, a relative depletion of serotonin in the brain may result. Treatment with parachlorophenylalanine could yield the same effect because parachlorophenylalanine reduces synthesis of serotonin in the brain and in the peripheral tissues. Chlorpromazine may block the central as well as the peripheral effects of serotonin. The central effects of serotonin are fully discussed in Ch. 10. They include modification of hypothalamic-anterior pituitary function, as has been alluded to above.[641, 820]

Metabolism

Serotonin is oxidatively deaminated by MAO and subsequently oxidized by aldehyde dehydrogenase to 5-hydroxyindoleacetic acid (5-HIAA). Its metabolism by patients with the carcinoid tumor is described under the heading "Carcinoid Syndrome and Mastocytosis." About 2–20 mg of 5-HIAA is excreted in the human urine each day, as are relatively small amounts of 5-hydroxytryptophol.[662] The pattern of metabolism of 5-HT is strikingly affected by ingestion of ethyl alcohol, which diverts 5-hydroxyindoleacetaldehyde from the normally predominant oxidative route to the reductive pathway because of the elevated concentration of reduced NADH. This greatly reduces excretion of 5-HIAA.[662, 961]

Drugs That Affect Serotonin

Drugs that alter the effects, synthesis, storage, or release of serotonin fall into seven categories: (1) a precursor of 5-HT, tryptophan, which can increase endogenous concentrations of the amine[994] and may be of value in phenylketonuria; (2) inhibitors of synthesis, which include p-chlorophenylalanine (PCPA), which block the rate-limiting enzyme tryptophan hydroxylase. PCPA is a valuable experimental tool but is too toxic for clinical use. Another inhibitor of this enzyme is p-chloroamphetamine (PCA): this agent is less specific and more complex in its actions. The amino acid analog 6-fluorotryptophan is a more specific tryptophan hydroxylase inhibitor; (3) inhibitors of membrane uptake, which include the tricyclic antidepressant drugs, which also inhibit catecholamine uptake. The tertiary amines chloroimipramine, imipramine, and amitriptyline preferentially block 5-HT uptake over narrow concentration ranges. All of these are more effective in blocking the uptake of 5-HT than are the secondary amines of this class, but, like the latter, they also inhibit the uptake of catecholamines. A more potent and selective inhibition of 5-HT uptake is obtained with fluoxetine;[825] (4) inhibitors of granule uptake and storage, which include reserpine, tetrabenazine, and other benzoquinolizines, all of which decrease storage of 5-HT. A long-lasting depletion of 5-HT can also be achieved

with fenfluramine: the mechanism of its action is uncertain;[968] (5) inhibitors of degradation, which include principally the MAO inhibitors; (6) neurotoxins that preferentially destroy 5-HT-containing neurons, which include 5, 6-dihydroxytryptamine (5,6-DHT) and 5,7-DHT. Their action is complex;[968] and (7) antagonists of 5-HT at the level of the receptor, which include ergot alkaloids, methysergide, and cyproheptadine.

HISTAMINE

Histamine, bradykinin, and prostaglandins are also elaborated by endocrine tumors. These autacoids, like catecholamines, ACh, and serotonin, are involved in diverse physiologic and pathologic processes. One or more participates in physiologic functions such as neurotransmission (histamine and bradykinin), inflammation and immunity (all three), and gastric secretion (at least histamine), and possibly all three affect the CNS. Understanding of their biology and chemistry has burgeoned as drugs that can modulate their synthesis, release, or effects have become available. So much has been written about them in conveniently available resource texts that only a sketch will be offered here in order to create a milieu for understanding their role in two endocrine diseases, the carcinoid tumor and mastocytosis. Reviews are cited for those interested in more detailed information.

Synthesis, Storage, and Release of Histamine

Histamine is widely but unevenly distributed throughout the tissues of humans. Every mammalian tissue that contains histamine is capable of synthesizing it from histidine by virtue of its content of a decarboxylase specific for the L-amino acid. In most tissues the chief storage site for histamine is the mast cell or, in the blood, the basophil. These cells synthesize histamine and store it in secretory granules. The mechanism of release of histamine from these granules is analogous to that of catecholamines from their storage granules. The turnover rate of histamine is slow, and, when tissues rich in mast cells are depleted of their stores of histamine, it may take weeks before concentrations of the autacoid return to normal. Sites of histamine formation or storage, other than the mast cell and basophil, include cells of the human epidermis, enterochromaffin-like cells in the rat gastric mucosa, cells within the CNS (probably neurons), and cells in regenerating or rapidly growing tissues. At these sites turnover is rapid, because the histamine is continuously released rather than stored. This contributes significantly to the daily excretion of histamine and its metabolites in the urine. Because the enzyme L-histidine decarboxylase is inducible by a number of physiologic stresses, histamine-forming capacity at such non–mast cell sites is subject to regulation by various physiologic and pathologic factors. Conjecture on the functions of non–mast cell histamine is abundant.

Of interest are the facts that histamine can augment the uptake of L-histidine into the cell via its actions on an H_1 receptor,[955] and can restrict its own release via an H_2 receptor.[663] Imidazoleacetic acid, produced by the action of histaminase on histamine, can inhibit the specific release of histaminase from human granulocytes (hence, modulation of enzyme release is via the activity of the enzyme itself).[791] These factors illustrate the complexity of the regulation of the synthesis, the release, and the intensity and duration of the effects of histamine by histamine itself.

Mechanism of Effect

Histamine exerts most if not all of its effects on cell receptors that apparently are located on the cell surface. The receptors appear to be dividable into two main classes: H_1 receptors that subserve such functions as histamine-induced bronchoconstriction and contraction of the gut; and H_2 receptors that mediate the changes in gastric acid secretion as well as various functions of immunocytes. For a complete review of histamine receptors see the works cited in references 644 and 996.

Recently, radiolabeled mepyramine (a classic H_1 receptor blocker) has been used to mark and quantitate H_1 receptors in the brain.[684, 975] Whether markers can be used to detect the receptors elsewhere, and whether we can develop labels for H_2 receptors, is not certain. Nonetheless, the pharmacodynamic effects of histamine on a variety of tissues make it likely that the behavior of histamine receptors will parallel that of catecholamines and ACh receptors.[803, 971]

The two classes of histamine receptors are also revealed by differential responses to various histamine-like agonists. Thus, 2-methylhistamine preferentially elicits responses mediated by H_1 receptors, whereas 4-methylhistamine has a correspondingly preferential effect mediated through H_2 receptors.[656] These compounds represent two newly recognized classes of histamine-like drugs, the H_1- and H_2-receptor agonists. The availability of these H_1 and H_2 agonists and of the corresponding antagonists has greatly enriched understanding of the pharmacology and physiology of histamine and has allowed new therapeutic approaches. This is reflected in a recent handbook edited by Rocha é Silva;[913] also see the works cited in references 644, 682, 795, 965, 967.

The molecular mechanisms by which histamine causes its effects are uncertain. Broadly speaking, two principal lines of evidence have a bearing on the problem of stimulus-response coupling for histamine, as well as for most other autacoids and many drugs. The first line concerns actions leading to altered permeability of the plasma membrane to common inorganic ions, particularly increased permeability to sodium and calcium, which allows them to enter the cell, usually along electrochemical gradients; these actions also tend to promote elevation of the concentration of free intracellular calcium. The intracellular concentration of free calcium ions is a critical factor in determining muscle tension[985] and secretion.[714, 715] Changes in permeability to ions in response to histamine are reflected in the smooth muscle depolarizing responses that accompany contraction, in the depolarization of chromaffin cells, in the generation of nerve impulses, and in an increased calcium component of the cardiac AP during the positive inotropic effect.

The second line of evidence concerning stimulus-response coupling relates to effects of extracellular regulators on adenylate cyclase and, perhaps, on guanylate cyclase. Several effects of histamine, including secretion of gastric acid, stimulation of cardiac contraction, and inhibition of secretion from basophils, have all been associated with elevated concentrations of cAMP.[663, 813, 891] These responses are mediated through H_2 receptors. It is also of interest that histamine stimulates the accumulation of cAMP in brain tissue by acting on H_2 receptors.[775] Whether smooth muscle relaxation, which again involves H_2 receptors, also involves a rise in the concentration of cAMP is uncertain. Although elevated concentrations of cGMP have been demonstrated in smooth muscle contracted through H_1 receptors, the physiologic actions of this nucleotide are unknown. Of course, the two lines of evidence may converge, because cAMP may modulate ionic permeability, and calcium may

regulate the activity of enzymes responsible for the synthesis and degradation of cyclic nucleotides.[644, 913] There are many uncertainties concerning the involvement of cAMP and cGMP in mediating various cellular responses to histamine and other autacoids.[675, 693, 708, 709, 804]

Selected Physiologic and Pharmacologic Effects of Histamine of Importance to the Endocrinologist

Cardiovascular System

In humans and in most other animals, histamine characteristically exerts a predominantly dilator effect on the vasculature that involves the finer blood vessels; this results in flushing, lowered total peripheral resistance, and a fall in systemic blood pressure. The vasodilation is mediated by both H_1 and H_2 receptors.[779] In addition, histamine tends to increase capillary permeability. Its effects on the heart are generally less important. For extensive reviews on the cardiovascular actions of histamine and the involvement of the different receptors see the works cited in references 889, 913, and 915.

"Capillary" dilatation is the most characteristic action of histamine on the vascular tree and one of the most important in humans. It results from a direct action of histamine on the blood vessels that is mediated by both H_1 and H_2 receptors, and thus is independent of innervation.

Increased "Capillary" Permeability

This is the second of the classic effects of histamine on the fine vessels and results in outward passage of plasma protein and fluid into the extracellular spaces, increased flow of lymph and its protein content, and formation of edema. H_1 receptors are clearly important for the response; participation of H_2 receptors is uncertain. This effect results from dilatation of small vessels, but the most crucial effect of the histamine is to actively contract and shrink the endothelial cells.[627, 840]

Heart

Histamine increases both the rate and the force of myocardial contraction, as well as cardiac output. It also tends to slow atrioventricular (A-V) conduction and, especially in high concentrations, may cause various arrhythmias. H_2 receptors seem to be largely responsible for positive chronotropic effects. They (along with H_1 receptors) participate in the positive inotropic effects, and they contribute importantly to the arrhythmias. Slowed A-V conduction mainly involves H_1 receptors. In addition to acting directly on cardiac tissue, histamine also appears to stimulate sympathetic nerve endings to release norepinephrine and thus elicit indirect effects.

When humans are given conventional doses of histamine, direct cardiac effects are not prominent and tend to be overshadowed by receptor reflexes elicited by the reduced blood pressure, which in turn stimulates heart rate and force by enhancing sympathetic outflow. Such effects, coupled with some constriction of the large veins and augmented venous return, may cause a prompt but transient rise in cardiac output; thereafter, cardiac output is generally little altered and may even fall when blood pools in the periphery.

Blood Pressure

Only small depressor responses to histamine are effectively inhibited by H_1 antagonists, which have only modest effects on responses to larger doses of the autacoid. The residual effects can be blocked by adding an H_2 blocker, however. Thus both H_1 and H_2 receptors are involved, and both must be used simultaneously in order to effect a blockade (e.g., to modify the vascular effects of sudden release of histamine in patients with systemic mastocytosis).[889]

Regional Vascular Responses

Responses to histamine vary in different vascular beds. For the most part, the differences are quantitative and reflect varying degrees of dilatation in the skeletal, mesenteric, coronary, cerebral, and renal beds. Within the pulmonary circulation, both constrictor and dilator effects (involving H_1 and H_2 receptors, respectively) have been demonstrated. Variable effects on pulmonary arterial pressure have also been noted; some of the variability (like the corresponding effects on pulmonary venous pressure) may reflect changes in venous return and cardiac output rather than local vascular actions. In humans, a fall in pulmonary arterial pressure has been demonstrated after subcutaneous injection of histamine.[889, 956]

Extravascular Smooth Muscle

Histamine stimulates or, more rarely, relaxes various smooth muscles. Contraction is due to activation of H_1 receptors, and relaxation for the most part is due to activation of H_2 receptors. Responses of different tissues, species, and even individuals vary widely.

Exocrine Glands *(Gastric Glands)*

Histamine is a powerful gastric secretagogue. It evokes a copious secretion of gastric juice of high acidity in doses below those that influence the blood pressure. In humans, the output of pepsin and intrinsic factor is increased along with that of acid. Although these actions are believed to be exerted directly on the gland cells (both parietal and chief), the presence of an intact vagus nerve permits a higher rate of secretion. After cholinergic blockade by atropine, the response to histamine is reduced. It appears that a "background" of cholinergic effects on the secretory cells enhances their responsiveness to histamine. A similar potentiating effect can be shown with gastrin. From all this it has been concluded that gastric secretagogues are mutually interdependent.[949] This interaction appears to be responsible for producing a flush in patients with gastric carcinoid tumors that produce histamine.

The effects of histamine on glands outside of the stomach are relatively unimportant; they include mild stimulatory actions on salivary, lacrimal, pancreatic, intestinal, and bronchial secretions. Histamine also stimulates secretion of bile.[808]

Nervous System

Histamine can trigger the release of norepinephrine from sympathetic nerve endings.[853] It can alter behavior and elevate blood pressure, heart rate, and secretion of ADH while lowering body temperature and causing arousal via its central H_1 and H_2 receptor effects.[773, 931]

White Blood Cells

In recent years, H_2 receptors for histamine have been found to be nonrandomly distributed on the leukocytes of mice, rats, and humans. In most instances, they modify the function of the leukocytes by inhibiting the secretion of substances that would ordinarily contribute to the immune or inflammatory related processes of the leukocyte. In neutrophils, histamine prevents the release of lysosomal enzymes during phagocytosis of zymogen granules or antigen-antibody complexes. In an analogous manner, histamine inhibits the release of antibody from B cells and the release of lymphokines from T cells; it prevents cytolysis of allogeneic target cells by T-effector cells; and it reverses the suppressor function of selected T-suppressor cells. The dominant net effect that histamine exerts on an *in vivo* immune response depends primarily on when it is introduced in relation to when the antigen is introduced and on whether the antigen provokes a cell-mediated or humorally mediated response. The amine can augment the humoral antibody response if it is introduced at the same time as the antigen, but it can also prevent the release of formed antibody from B cells if it is introduced late in the course of response to antigen. Conversely, the cell-mediated event is suppressed by histamine regardless of the time the amine is introduced in relation to antigen.

Of general interest has been the hypothesis that mediators of inflammation may, by virtue of inhibition of various biologic responses (e.g., IgE-induced release of histamine from basophils and mast cells), play an anti-inflammatory role (see below). In addition, it now appears likely that mediators of inflammation, plus β-mimetic catecholamines and selected prostaglandins, may modulate the immune process. The major clinical implication of these recent findings is that antihistaminics might augment inflammatory processes and modify immune processes in a manner previously considered unlikely. In fact, recent data seem to verify the ability of antihistaminics to augment, rather than ameliorate, delayed hypersensitivity in humans.[632]

Finally, it is now apparent that other mediators of inflammation can modify the availability of histamine at the site of active inflammation. For instance, the C3b fragment of complement will stimulate release of histaminase (one of two important histamine-catabolizing enzymes) from neutrophils. The complement fragment is produced during active inflammation.[792] For excellent articles on the role of histamine as a modifier of inflammation see the works cited in references 663, 843, 854, 855, 899, 900, 917, 918, 934, and 983.

Anaphylaxis and Allergy

Although histamine is not the only mediator of inflammation that is associated with anaphylaxis and allergy, its participation and mechanism of release in the anaphylactic response is important. The principal target cells of the hypersensitivity reactions of the immediate type are the mast cells and the basophils. Within the secretory granules of these cells, histamine is stored along with a heparin-protein complex to which it is loosely bound by ionic forces involving carboxyl groups. The secretion (or "release") of histamine from sensitized mast cells or basophils in response to specific antigen is believed to be initiated when the antigen combines with and bridges adjacent molecules of IgE that have become attached to the cell surface.[635, 802] The ensuing perturbation seemingly sets in motion a series of reactions that show a critical requirement for calcium and metabolic energy and terminate in the extrusion of the contents of secretory granules by the process of exocytosis.

With respect to several of these properties, secretion by mast cells and basophils is identical with that of exocrine and endocrine cells. The specific secretory response to antigen is an active process that must be distinguished from the passive process that involves loss of histamine and that may occur in response to cytolysis.

When studies on endocrine, exocrine, and other secretory cells led to the concept of stimulus-secretion coupling in which secretagogues of different sorts are thought to act by promoting an influx of calcium into their target cells and thereby inducing exocytosis, the suggestion was made that specific antigen acting on its sensitized target cells might release histamine in the same way.[715, 717] In this view, the agonist or secretagogue (in this case, specific antigen) combines with its receptors (here, membrane-bound IgE molecules) to promote an increase in membrane permeability and the influx of calcium ions. Considerable evidence now sustains this hypothesis: (1) the secretory response to antigen fails if extracellular calcium is absent; (2) calcium chelators arrest ongoing secretion if added during the response to antigen; (3) in the absence of calcium the interaction of antigen and cell-bound IgE still proceeds to the extent that calcium will elicit histamine secretion when subsequently introduced; (4) exposure to antigen causes increased uptake of calcium; and (5) various other procedures that promote calcium influx or otherwise raise intracellular concentrations of calcium (e.g., microinjection of calcium or exposure to calcium ionophores) are sufficient to initiate histamine secretion by exocytosis.[714, 745, 831, 872]

As in other secretory systems, further details on the cellular events involved in stimulus-secretion coupling and the critical function of calcium are obscure. There have been suggestions that changes in concentrations of cyclic nucleotides may participate, because reduced cAMP or increased cGMP both favor secretion, but this is controversial.[708] There are indications that crucial protein phosphorylation reactions are activated by calcium[937] and that arachidonic acid and its metabolites may be involved.[958] Despite these uncertainties, it is evident that considerable modulation of the secretion of histamine from mast cells and basophils can be achieved with drugs that regulate concentrations of cyclic nucleotides. Thus, some inhibition can be achieved with epinephrine (acting through β-adrenergic receptors) and with theophylline (acting through inhibition of phosphodiesterase), both of which have long been used in the therapy of allergic states such as asthma, although their main benefit probably reflects their dilator actions on smooth muscle. Moreover, as stated above, histamine itself also tends to restrict its own release, acting through H_2 receptors, thereby suggesting a negative feedback mechanism; the potentiating effects of H_2 blockers on the release of histamine are consistent with this observation. All these inhibitory responses may involve an elevation of the concentrations of cAMP.[663] In addition, disodium cromoglycate, by an ill-defined mechanism, clearly reduces allergic secretion of mast cells in the lungs. In contrast, cholinergic drugs, acting through muscarinic receptors, appear to potentiate allergic secretion, possibly by elevating concentrations of cGMP.

Limitations of the Histamine Hypothesis of Hypersensitivity Reactions

Involvement of Other Autacoids

It is now evident that the classic histamine hypothesis provides only a partial explanation for the effects that accompany hypersensitivity (antigen-antibody) reactions. During such reactions numerous other autacoids are liberated or produced. They include slow-reacting substance of anaphylaxis (SRS-A), prostaglandins and other products of arachidonic acid metabolism, kallikrein and kinins, eosinophilic leukocyte chemotactic factor, and (in some animals) 5-HT and dopamine. The nature and relative importance of these substances vary with species and with tissue, and this accounts largely for the widely variable efficacies of histamine antagonists in combating allergic responses.[631, 635]

The mechanisms by which drugs or destruction of tissues can trigger the release of histamine and the physiologic roles the amine may have in the growth of tissue are reviewed in standard texts.

Blockers of histaminic effects are divided into two categories and are illustrated in Fig. 10–16. Their pharmacology

REPRESENTATIVE H_1 & H_2 HISTAMINE RECEPTOR BLOCKERS

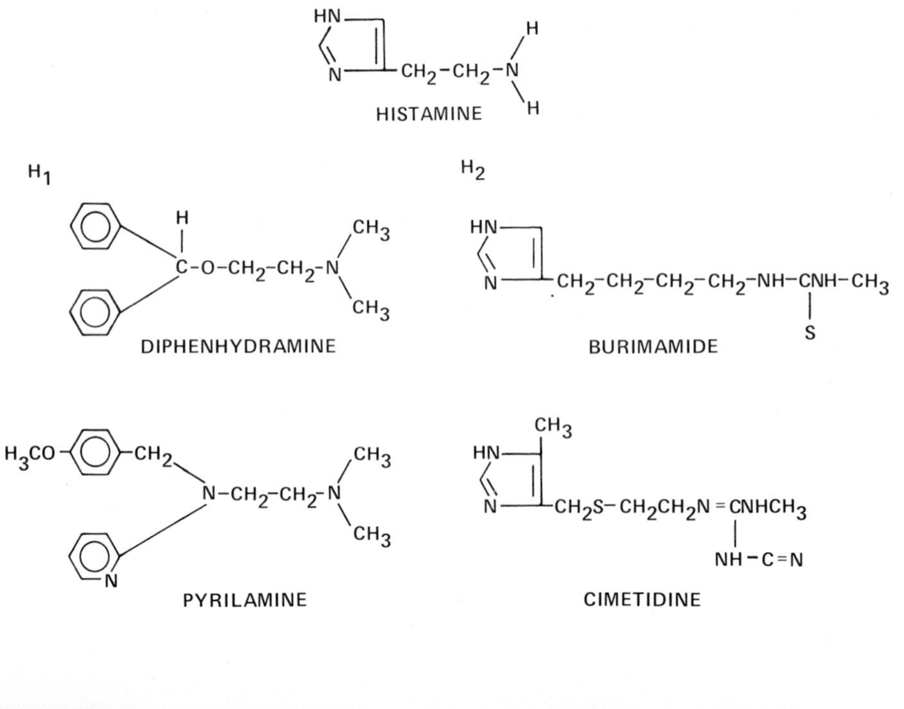

Figure 10–16.

will be discussed under "Mastocytosis." Their general pharmacology is discussed by Douglas.[713]

KININ PEPTIDES

Kinins (lysyl-bradykinin and bradykinin) are produced by the action of the enzyme kallikrein on an α_2-globulin substrate kininogen (Fig. 10–17). Kallikrein is normally found as an inactive enzyme in plasma and in many tissues, including the gut. The kallikrein in plasma is chemically distinct from kallikreins derived from other tissues. Plasma kallikrein, in a manner similar to trypsin and snake venoms, forms bradykinin from a kininogen of high ($\approx 100,000$) MW. Glandular and other tissue kallikreins form the decapeptide kallidin from a kininogen of lower ($\approx 50,000$) MW. Activation of plasma kallikrein usually depends on activation of either a component of the clotting system or critical components of complement or upon some unusual functions of the granulocyte. Plasma kallikrein probably has nothing to do with production of kinin in patients with the carcinoid syndrome.

In tissues such as the submaxillary gland, kallikrein appears to be stored in granules.[753] In the same granules, or at least in similar cells, renin-like activity also has been found. The activation of glandular kallikrein is not well understood. Because it exists in granules, it is likely that a secretory process is involved, but whether this depends on exocytosis is not known. The enzyme can be released by hormones such as catecholamines. It has been implicated in dissimilar dysfunctions such as hypertension,[841] the dumping syndrome,[744] reactions to antilymphocytic globulin,[665] and anaphylaxis,[880] and in mediating a number of abnormalities after gastric surgery.[700] It also is involved in physiologic neural transmission.[694]

The peptides produced by kallikrein are potent vasodilators: They may release catecholamines from nerve endings, and they have been implicated as mediators of various aspects of the inflammatory process. They normally are present in plasma in concentrations of less than 2.5 ng/ml and they have a half-life of less than 15 sec.[856] In a single passage through the pulmonary bed, some 60–90% of the peptides are degraded, and no less than five peptide bonds are broken. Other tissues, as well as plasma, also rapidly degrade kinins. There are two principal kininases: kininase I (carboxypeptidase-N or arginine carboxypeptidase), which removes the C-terminal arginine, and kininase II, which removes the C-terminal dipeptide Phe-Arg. Either cleavage yields virtually inactive peptides. Kininase II is the same enzyme as peptidyl dipeptidase (PDP), an enzyme that converts angiotensin I to angiotensin II. Kinins are the preferred substrate for this enzyme (Km 10^{-7} for bradykinin as opposed to 10^{-5} for angiotensin I). It follows that the substances sometimes referred to as converting enzyme inhibitors (e.g., teprotide and captopril) inhibit kininase II. Kininase I is not inhibited by inhibitors of PDP, but it is inhibited by some substituted succinic acid derivatives that inhibit pancreatic carboxypeptidase B. The synthesis and destruction of kinins has been extensively reviewed.[724-726, 897, 898, 925]

Normal blood contains all essential ingredients for the formation of massive amounts of pharmacologically active bradykinin. Usually very little bradykinin is formed, however, mainly because plasma kallikrein is present in its inactive form, prekallikrein. However, prekallikrein is readily converted to kallikrein (and bradykinin is subsequently formed) by various factors that disturb the equilibrium of plasma. These factors include substantial changes in pH or temperature and contact with negatively charged surfaces. Such surfaces occur on glass and kaolin *in vitro* and on biologic material such as the collagen of vascular and other basement membranes, which is readily exposed by damage to tissue *in vivo*. Many of the events that activate kallikrein involve coagulation and fibrinolysis that has been initiated by Hageman factor (HF). Thus, formation of bradykinin can involve a cascade of enzymatic reactions that has been triggered by activation of HF. The three systems not only share this factor but they also overlap and integrate. Two other essential components of the bradykinin-forming cascade, high molecular weight (HMW) kininogen and prekallikrein, are critical to HF-dependent coagulation and fibrinolysis.

Kallikrein is the principal activator of HF in the fluid phase of plasma, and it rapidly cleaves HF to fragments that are particularly potent activators of prekallikrein. Thus, a mechanism of positive feedback that stimulates production of kinin is defined. Additionally, HMW kininogen facilitates cleavage of HF by kallikrein, and it also increases the rate of activation of prekallikrein by HF fragments. Besides these excitatory factors, plasma also contains several proteins that tend to restrain the system by complexing with, and thus inactivating, kallikrein. These include the C_1-esterase inhibitor ($\overline{C1}$-INH) of the complement system and other plasma protease inhibitors, such as α_2 macroglobulin and α_1 antitrypsin. Moreover, some *negative* feedback when HF is activated is provided by products of HMW kininogen that have been cleaved by kallikrein.[786] Some of the interrelations between the formation of kinin and other functions involving HF and complement are detailed in reviews.[681, 689, 692, 712, 724]

Hundreds of congeners of the kinins have been synthesized, and a considerable amount of information comparing their activities and their structures has emerged. The minimal effective compound is the nonapeptide in which arginine is essential both at position 1 and at position 9. In contrast to comparable studies on angiotensin II, the work on congeners of kinins so far has not led to the discovery of one with kinin-blocking activity.[638, 898]

The pharmacologic properties of kinin that are most prominent in endocrinologic disease include their ability to increase permeability of capillaries, their ability to produce marked vasodilatation and flushing in humans, and their ability to evoke pain and to alter bronchial resistance.[682, 724-726, 925] Abnormal generation of kinin appears to occur during some forms of hypertension; during angioedema;[712] in the carcinoid syndrome (see "Carcinoid Syndrome and Mastocytosis"); in episodic flushing syndromes associated with hyperbradykininemia;[957] in septic and anaphylactic shock; in inflammatory disorders, including arthritis; and in some

Figure 10–17. Kinin production and destruction in the human. The pharmacologic actions listed have been produced by kinins in man and other species. The role of the kinins in the carcinoid syndrome is related to vasodilatation in some patients. Their role in other symptoms of the syndrome is pharmacologically possible but as yet is unproved.

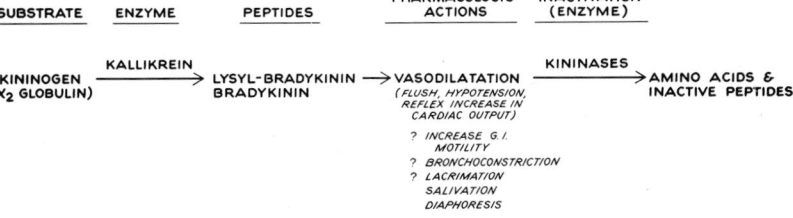

immune reactions. It may participate in some circulatory readjustments of the neonate, and in the mitogenesis that occurs when a wound is healing, and in granulomatous conditions. For reviews of data supporting the role of kinins in diverse physiologic and pathologic conditions see the works cited in references 692, 724–726, 780, 881, 898, 914, 925, 936.

Mechanism of Action

Peptide antagonists with a high affinity for the kinin receptor, which could be used as a receptor probe, have not been found. Neither have agonists been identified that could aid in the search for the kinin receptor. All that is known at present about the receptors is that they can be pharmacologically distinguished from receptors for other peptides.[638] Some responses to kinins appear to be mediated by the generation of prostaglandins, apparently after phospholipase A_2 has been stimulated. Such a relationship between two autacoids appears to be critical for the effects of oxygen on neonatal circulatory adaptation. The oxygen releases bradykinin, which in turn activates synthesis of prostaglandin in the newborn. The combined effects of these two autacoids appear to be vital for readjustment of the neonate's circulatory system to extrauterine life.[858] Release of prostaglandins in response to bradykinin was first demonstrated in guinea pig lung,[896] where the prostaglandins contribute to bronchoconstriction. A similar mechanism may underlie the later phases of vasodilatation, the slowly developing nocioceptive responses, and other effects of kinins, including the prominent renal dilator effects that are reduced by inhibitors of the synthesis of prostaglandins. Both cAMP and cGMP may mediate some kinin-induced responses.[724, 725, 881, 964]

Kinins and Clinical Medicine

Therapeutic interest in the kinins, as with most other autacoids, focuses mainly on modulation of their metabolism *in vivo*. Although no therapeutic use has been found for the kinins, slowing the destruction of bradykinin (therefore allowing kinins to accumulate) may prove to be a clinically useful effect of inhibitors of angiotensin converting enzyme (PDH inhibitors). Captopril, for example, blocks kininase II. Therefore, besides its effect on angiotensin formation, captopril will slow kinin destruction and tend to raise levels of kinin in tissues or in the circulation, contributing, *inter alia*, to the hypotensive action of the inhibitor. The full significance and usefulness of such actions have not yet been defined, but the recent development of effective inhibitors of kininase I makes this approach increasingly interesting.

The opposite approach, that of blocking the endogenous kinin system, has obvious clinical applications because of the excess kinins that are involved in various clinical settings. The lack of specific kinin-antagonists that would be comparable to the effective antagonists of angiotensin II is an obstacle to this approach. Nevertheless, in some settings in which kinins have been implicated, such as inflammatory states and the carcinoid syndrome, some of the beneficial effects of aspirin and other nonsteroidal anti-inflammatory agents may reflect the kinin-initiated suppression of the synthesis of prostaglandins, and, for this reason, these anti-inflammatory agents can be regarded as indirect kinin antagonists. The increasing evidence that several of the effects of kinins are mediated by prostaglandins, or aided by concurrent kinin-induced prostaglandin formation, indicates that such inhibitors of the synthesis of prostaglandins may have broader, albeit nonspecific, anti-kinin activity than has been suspected. Blockade of kinin formation by kallikrein inhibitors is another theoretical but clinically unproven approach. A kallikrein inhibitor, *aprotinin* (Trasylol, etc.), which seems identical to the polyvalent protease inhibitor of Kunitz, has been used with dubious success in acute pancreatitis,[976] carcinoid syndrome, and other conditions involving excess formation of kinins.[780]

Other Active Polypeptides

Erspamer and his colleagues documented the existence of many small polypeptides in a wide range of nonmammalian species. These polypeptides have remarkable pharmacologic activity. Some resemble the mammalian kinins already described. A second group, which contains polypeptides that also are active vasodilator and hypotensive agents, resembles substance P. A third group resembles mammalian gastrointestinal hormones such as CCK-PZ. A fourth group uniquely stimulates (by releasing) mammalian gastrointestinal hormones and has recently been found in the mammalian gastrointestinal tract.[652] A remarkable feature of these comparative studies is that they have not only revealed substances of pharmacologic activity and of interest in their own right, but they have also emphasized the common distribution of active peptides in the animal kingdom, have provided valuable clues to mammalian physiologists and endocrinologists, and have offered potentially valuable therapeutic agents. The importance of such discoveries is heightened by the concurrently developing awareness that many, and perhaps most, peptides that have been isolated from the gastrointestinal tract and associated there with endocrine function are also found in the brain (and vice versa) and (as mentioned above) are suspected of subserving neurotransmitter, as well as neuroendocrine, function. Some examples include CCK-PZ, somatostatin, enkephalin, and gastrin, as well as VIP and substance P; the latter two peptides are discussed in the works cited in references 879 and 892. All the pharmacologically active peptides in this general family are discussed in recent reviews.[652, 865, 898, 925]

CARCINOID SYNDROME AND MASTOCYTOSIS

Introduction

Carcinoid tumors are composed of enterochromaffin cells. These cells, which contain granules and often have an affinity for silver salts (argentaffin cells), are easily found throughout the gastrointestinal tract, bronchus, gallbladder, biliary tract, and ducts of the pancreas. They can also be found in the thymus, thyroid, ovary, uterus, and salivary glands, and carcinoid tumors may arise in any of these sites. The tumors are thought to derive from common neural cells called Kulchitsky's cells. Considering the pervasive nature of these cells, it is not surprising to find carcinoid tumors in the gut and in a number of endocrine organs, including the breast, testes, and uterus.[835, 905, 920, 960] Nor is it surprising to find carcinoid tumors with endocrine potential or in association with the MEN syndromes.[625, 648, 666, 687, 707, 781, 801, 816, 909, 987] Although the physiologic role of Kulchitsky's cells is poorly understood, it is known that they are innervated cells and that they contain several biologically active substances.[654] Wherever Kulchitsky's cells are found, a high concentration of 5-HT is often detected. The cells are identified in various tissues by a specific formaldehyde-induced fluorescence test,[894] and they appear to give rise to all carcinoid tumors in a variety of locations.[990] Because of the common origin of the Kulchitsky's cells, Williams and Sandler have classified carcinoid tumors on the basis of the original location of the cell of the primary tumor.[990] The ileal carcinoid tumor (the most common) derives from midgut cells and contains a high concentration of 5-HT. The tumor is associated with the classic carcinoid syndrome. On the other hand, carcinoid tumors arising from the hindgut, especially the rectum, have different staining characteristics than their midgut relatives, only very rarely contain serotonin, and have not been associated with a syndrome related to release of hormone. Carcinoid tumors derived from cells of the foregut (bronchial, pancreatic, duodenal, and gallbladder areas) are particularly interesting. Cells from this area contain only small amounts of serotonin; however, because there is often high excretion of 5-HIAA in the urine of patients with the tumor, a rapid release or intratumor oxidation of synthesized amine is indicated. Foregut-derived tumors are able to make a variety of hormones and are frequently associated with atypical carcinoid syndromes (Table 10–8).

The incidence of carcinoid tumors has been computed in closed populations that may or may not represent the general population. In a Swedish population that was studied over a 12-year period, the tumors were found in a little more than 1% of 16,294 patients at autopsy. Of these, the bronchial tumor accounted for 0.1% of the total. About 90% of all carcinoid tumors were found incidentally at autopsy. The prevalence of the tumor averaged 8.4 per 100,000 people.[649] Only one patient with the tumor exhibited the carcinoid syndrome. Thus, although this syndrome cannot be considered common, it has taught us many lessons in endocrinologic physiology and pathophysiology.

In the United States, the disease occurs most often in black males.[759] Survival seems to be determined by the location of the primary tumor: 99% of patients with appendiceal tumors survive for more than 5 years, but only 33% of patients with tumors in the sigmoid colon survive for the same period.[759] Carcinoid tumors are rarely familial except when associated with multiple endocrine neoplasia syndromes.[868]

The endocrine potential of carcinoid tumors was not recognized until 1953, when Lembeck discovered that they contained large amounts of 5-HT.[824] Almost simultaneously, three independent investigating teams defined a syndrome associated with the presence of malignant carcinoid tumors of the ileum. The most prominent features included flushes, bronchial constriction, lesions of the valves of the heart, and diarrhea, not all of which could be due to serotonin.[974] Although hypertension was initially considered to be common in patients with the carcinoid syndrome, it is now known that most patients are normotensive and in fact develop severe hypotension during flushes. These tumors can produce histamine, catecholamines, prostaglandins, vasoactive peptides, and more complex peptides similar, if not identical, to substance P, ACTH, melanocyte-stimulating hormone (MSH), parathyroid hormone, calcitonin, and insulin.[628, 646, 660, 702, 794, 838]

The spectrum of pharmacologically active substances produced by the tumor relates to the pathogenesis of different manifestations of the syndrome.[940] 5-HT is not the only agent that produces manifestations of the carcinoid syndrome. The syndrome in any patient at any given time is the sum of effects of the active substances being elaborated by the tumor. In addition, tumors that arise in primary sites other than the small intestine may produce characteristic syndromes that are distinct from the classic carcinoid syndrome.

Classic Carcinoid Syndrome

Morbid Anatomy

The primary tumor usually derives from the enterochromaffin cells of the midgut, and it is usually located in the terminal ileum (Fig. 10–18). The tumor can be as small as a few millimeters in diameter, and it rarely is large enough to produce symptoms of intestinal obstruction (Fig. 10–19).[787, 970] The tumor is usually yellow and firm and consists of regularly dispersed epithelial cells that have little evidence of mitosis and that are surrounded by well-defined fibrous borders (Fig. 10–20). The epithelial cells frequently contain intracellular granules that stain with silver salts. The average period of time before a primary tumor metastasizes is unknown, but it has been estimated that 38% of extra-appendiceal tumors, or approximately 1–6% of all carcinoid tumors, have metastasized at the time of discovery. Metastatic lesions first involve the mesenteric lymph nodes and then the liver (Fig. 10–21). The right lobe of the liver, which receives most of the venous drainage from the ileum, enlarges more frequently than does the left lobe. With only one possible exception,[764, 769] the carcinoid syndrome does not appear until after metastases have occurred in the liver and after biochemical substances produced by the tumor have bypassed the portal circulation. The metastatic lesions usually are confined to the abdominal cavity.

Cutaneous lesions associated with the carcinoid syndrome include *telangiectasia of the skin* over the cheeks and the bridge of the nose. Mast cells sometimes infiltrate the area of telangiectasia.[954] However, because human mast

Table 10–8. CHARACTERISTICS OF CARCINOID TUMORS DERIVED FROM DIFFERENT EMBRYONIC DIVISIONS OF THE GUT

	Foregut	Midgut	Hindgut
Histologic structure	Tendency to be trabecular; may differ widely from classic pattern	Characteristic	Tendency to be trabecular
Argentaffin and diazo reactions	Usually negative	Positive	Often negative
Association with the carcinoid syndrome	Frequent	Frequent	None
Tumor 5-HT content	Low	High	Not detected
Urinary 5-HIAA	High	High	Normal
5-HTP secretion	Frequent	Rare	Not detected
Metastases into bone (usually osteoblastic) and skin	Common	Unusual	Common
Association with other endocrine secretion	Frequent	Not described	Not described

5-HT, 5-hydroxytryptamine; 5-HIAA, 5-hydroxyindole acetic acid; 5-HTP, 5-hydroxytryptophan.

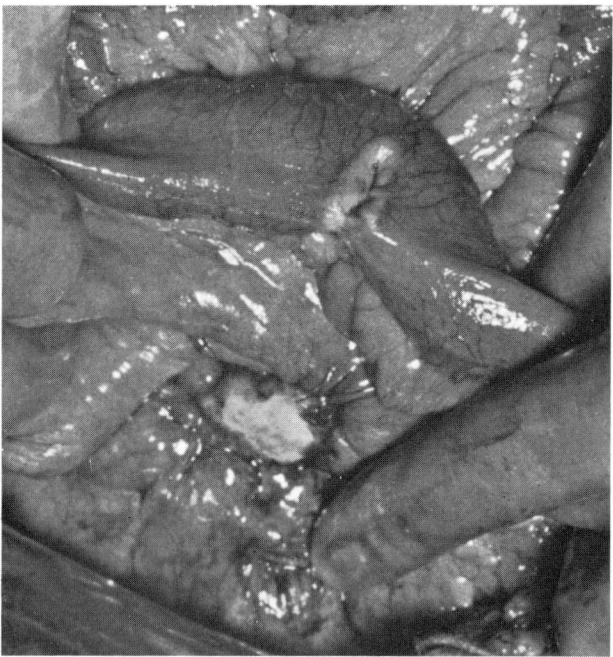

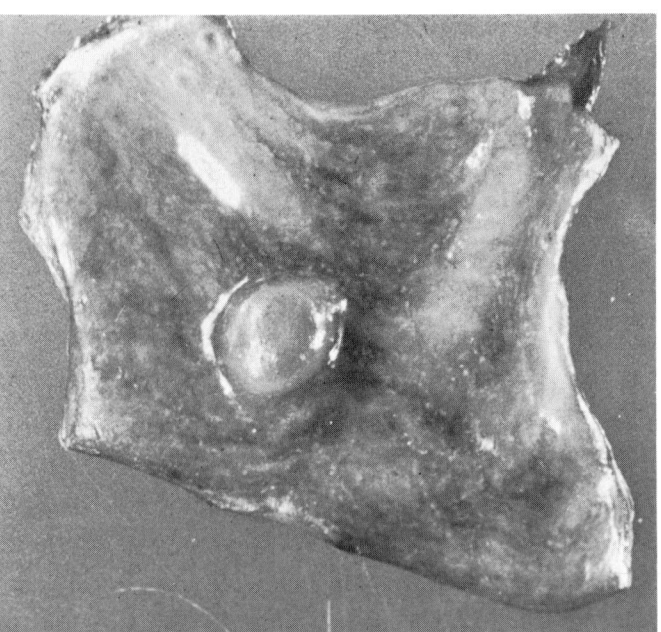

Figure 10–18. A primary ileal carcinoid tumor that has already metastasized to a regional mesenteric lymph node.

Figure 10–19. A typical primary ileal lesion that was only 3 mm in diameter and was not located until the bowel was examined carefully during autopsy. Although the tumor was quite small, it had metastasized extensively to the peritoneum and liver (Figs. 10–20 and 10–21).

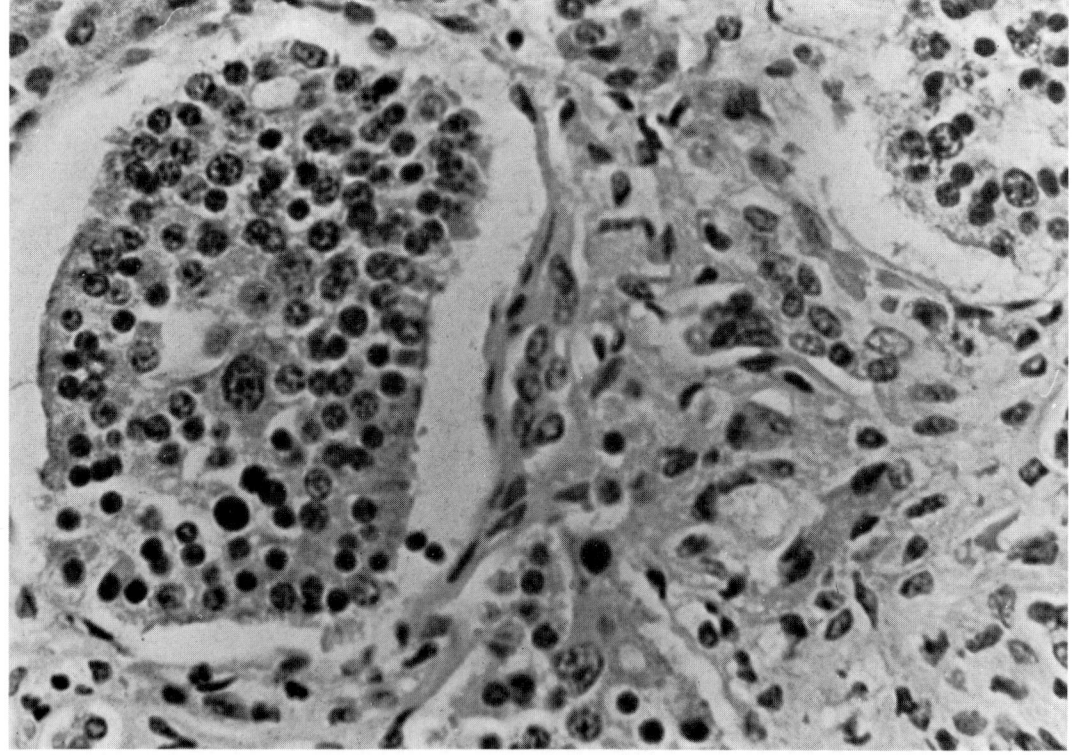

Figure 10–20. Carcinoid tumor illustrated in Fig. 10–19. Nests of evenly dispersed epithelial cells are surrounded by bands of fibrous tissue. This tumor was argentaffin-negative but produced and contained large amounts of serotonin. (Hematoxylin and eosin stain, original magnification × 340.)

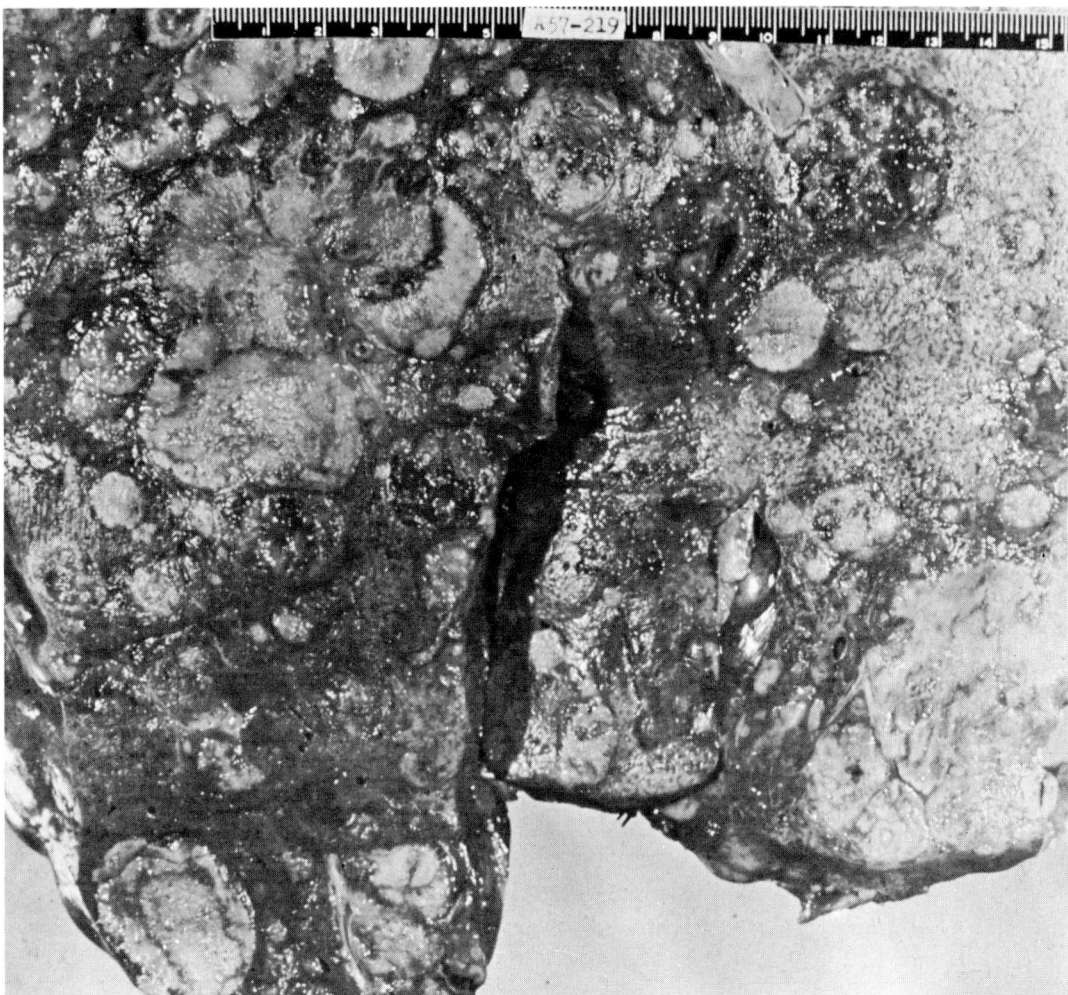

Figure 10–21. A carcinoid tumor which has metastasized from the ileal primary tumor (shown in Fig. 10–19) to the liver. Despite massive replacement of liver parenchyma, hepatic function was normal by usual parameters.

cells do not contain serotonin, the substance cannot be incriminated in the pathogenesis of the skin lesion.

The *lesions of the heart* are confined to the endocardial surface and are highly specific.[911] Deposits of collagen are most prominent in the chambers of the right side and often extend to the intima of the great veins and arteries. The deposits may involve the valve leaflets and chordae tendineae and may produce valvular stenosis or insufficiency. Although the tricuspid and pulmonic lesions are most prominent, the subendocardium of the chambers on the left side can be affected and may become clinically important when an atrial septal defect with right-to-left shunting is present.[783, 911] The myocardium is separated from the fibrotic process by the intact internal elastic membrane, a feature that makes the lesion quite specific (Fig. 10–22).[735] Severe fibrotic lesions in other areas of the body have been reported with the carcinoid tumor. Lesions involving the *peritoneum and mesentery of the small bowel,* which result in extensive matting and fibrous adhesions, may occur spontaneously[783] but usually occur after abdominal surgery. These adhesions may obstruct the intestine. Because they so characteristically occur after any abdominal incision, indications for laparotomy must be especially clear. Thirty-three of 49 small bowel obstructions in patients with carcinoid syndrome were caused by fibrosis around the bowel after a surgical procedure that usually did not involve the bowel itself.[869]

The location of the endocardial lesions suggests that a circulating humoral substance mediates the fibrosis. Administering indole precursors of serotonin or serotonin alone has not produced similar pathologic changes in rats. However, prolonged administration of serotonin to tryptophan-deficient guinea pigs whose livers were damaged by a hepatotoxin was associated with proliferative fibroplasia of the endocardium.[953] These conditions simulated the major biochemical abnormalities seen in patients with carcinoid tumors, in which excessive use of tryptophan for the production of serotonin occurs by metastatic hepatic lesions. Because bradykinin, histamine, and prostaglandins also can contribute to fibrosis in an inflammatory lesion and because they are produced by some of these tumors, they too could be in part responsible for the abnormalities found in the heart and blood vessels of patients with the carcinoid syndrome. Nevertheless, their pathogenetic role has not been evaluated.

Clinical Features

Most symptoms of the syndrome result from the pharmacologic or endocrinologic effects of the tumor, not from its size or its replacement of normal tissues. Although there is a distinct complex of symptoms that constitutes the complete syndrome, most patients have few or only one of these

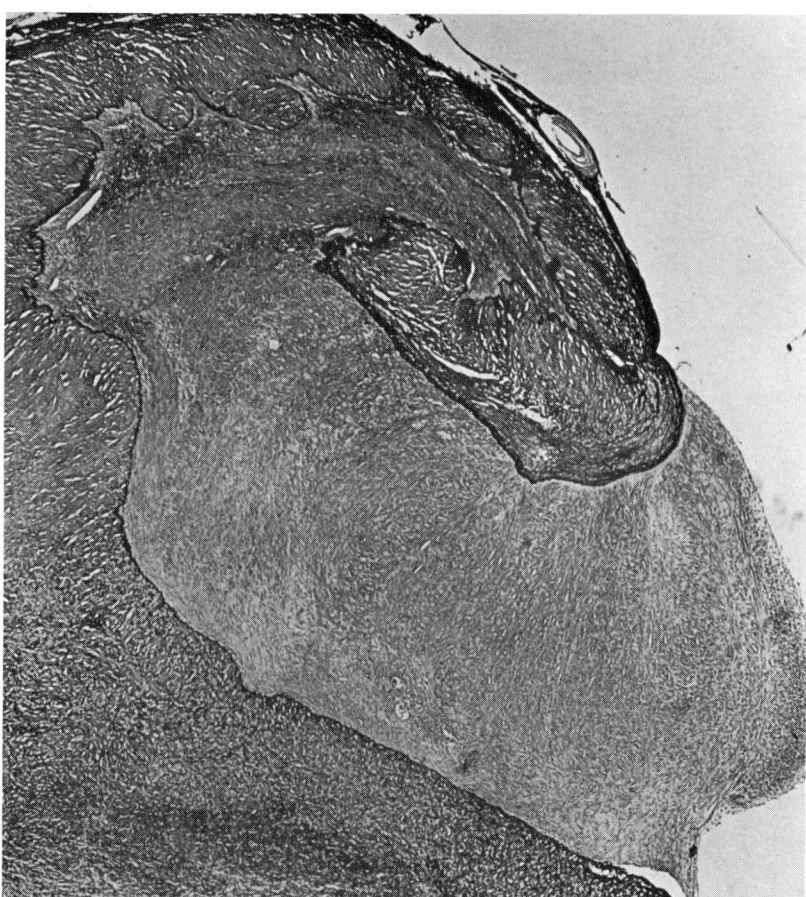

Figure 10–22. The collagenous deposit on the pulmonary valve of a patient with carcinoid syndrome is separated from the muscular tissue by the intact internal elastic membrane. (Hematoxylin and eosin stain, original magnification × 100.)

symptoms as an indication of the presence of tumor. Because the symptoms appear and disappear, and because the course of the disease is so long, the physician may care for a patient with "bizarre complaints" for several years before the correct diagnosis is made.

The unique *vasomotor phenomena* are the most dramatic features of the carcinoid syndrome. They may develop gradually, and the only hint of disease may be slow development (over a year or two) of telangiectasia associated with a chronic cyanotic hue over the blush area. Most patients, however, experience several cyanotic, tricolored, or bright red *flushes* over the face and upper chest. These may be caused by stimuli that activate the autonomic nervous system; i.e., anger, tension, severe exercise, sudden change in position, or the Valsalva maneuver may predictably provoke a flush. Administration of exogenous catecholamines (see "Diagnosis") also may provoke flushes in these patients, as will ingestion of food and alcohol. Catecholamines and alcohol provoke flushes by indirect effects. Their actions are delayed for several seconds or minutes after injection or ingestion, respectively. The flush-provoking activity of the drugs is inhibited by α-adrenergic blocking agents.[621, 622] Both catecholamines and alcohol work in part by the release from the tumor of kallikrein, which produces bradykinin from plasma substrates. The flushes may occur as infrequently as once a month or may occur 20–30 times a day. Flushes generally last for minutes and may be associated with a feeling of warmth, perspiration, and increased lacrimation and salivation. They also may be associated with remarkable hypotension, tachycardia, bronchial constriction, increased respiratory rate, increased gastrointestinal motility (borborygmus), and occasionally diarrhea. If

flushes are prolonged, periorbital and facial edema as well as oliguria may occur.

The *pulmonary manifestations* of the syndrome are less frequently observed than earlier work suggested.[769] Hyperventilation may occur during the flush. Evidence of asthma may be present between flushes and may exacerbate during them. Most frequently, however, patients do not have pulmonary symptoms, and evidence of bronchial constriction is found only during flushing attacks. It is not at all unusual to find patients with no signs or symptoms of pulmonary disease. If bronchoconstriction does become a threatening problem, therapeutic measures must be carefully considered. Intravenously administered catecholamines usually will exacerbate both the flush and the bronchoconstriction. Aerosol sprays of isoproterenol or other β-adrenergic mimetic drugs may be used sparingly to distribute the drug to the affected area in reasonable concentrations. By such a route, the amount reaching the peripheral circulation is minimized and usually insufficient to continue the old flush or to initiate a new one.

Cardiac manifestations of the syndrome may be of two varieties. The most prominent are associated with stenosis or insufficiency of the pulmonary or tricuspid valves. These lesions can lead to intractable right-sided congestive heart failure. The presence of deposits of collagen immediately beneath other areas of the endocardium usually is not apparent clinically. If there is evidence of mitral or aortic valve disease, the possibility of an atrial septal defect with right-to-left shunting of blood, a bronchial carcinoid with direct venous drainage to the left side of the heart, or acquired or congenital valvular defects unrelated to the carcinoid tumor should be considered.[911] In addition to the anatomical abnormalities of the heart, a high cardiac output at rest has been recorded in patients during their flushes. This functional abnormality does not seem to be related to an excess of serotonin but has been attributed to the release of a vasodilator substance by the tumor.[930]

The *gastrointestinal symptoms* may represent the most debilitating aspect of the carcinoid syndrome. Probably the most common initial complaint is abdominal discomfort and frequent diarrheal stools. There is considerable evidence that serotonin is the mediator of the diarrhea and intestinal hypermotility. Serotonin is found mainly in two areas of the body, the gastrointestinal tract and the brain. (It is also present in high concentration in the lungs and platelets.) In the gut and brain, the amine is synthesized and stored in nerve endings.[671, 980] When the preganglionic myenteric nerves are stimulated, serotonin is released as a neurotransmitter. The existence of specific serotonergic nerves in the brain has been established.[980] The nerves are not part of the adrenergic system, and they specifically take up and release serotonin. Any degenerative lesion of the nerves, either physical or chemical (e.g., by a drug, 6-hydroxytryptamine, which works by being specifically transported into serotonergic nerves and selectively destroying them),[640, 642] results in a major depletion of the stores of serotonin. In the gut, serotonin seems to have a role in peristalsis and perhaps absorption of fats.

Serotonin is released into the venous effluent of the normal intestine when the serosal surface is scratched, when ACh is administered intra-arterially, or when intraluminal pressure is increased.[674] Evidence that the amine reaches specific receptors in various tissues is abundant, but there are few data regarding its second messenger. In the gut, serotonin may reduce the threshold of excitation of mucosal sensory nerve endings, so that a lower than usual increase in intraluminal pressure will elicit a peristaltic reflex.[672, 793, 890] The amine also directly stimulates an increase in the tone and motility of the small intestine[788, 875] and inhibits the motility of the stomach and colon.[647, 742, 789] The pattern of diarrhea in patients with the carcinoid syndrome is quite consistent with the effects of serotonin.[864] It would be important to know whether the stores of serotonin in the specific serotonergic neurons of the gut are expanded in patients with the carcinoid syndrome. If they are, normal stimulation of the nerves would result in exaggerated release and effects of serotonin. Thus the amine could produce effects on the gut whether or not it was released from the tumor into blood. An analogy with the pheochromocytoma seems appropriate: The pheochromocytoma slowly releases catecholamines into the blood. The amines are taken up into usable stores of the adrenergic nerve endings as one process of biologic inactivation. The stores in the nerve thus are expanded, and more catecholamines can be released after normal or pharmacologic (e.g., tyramine) stimulation of the nerves. Stores of serotonin are expanded in platelets in patients with the carcinoid syndrome. It would be logical to assume that stores are also expanded in other sites[701] where active transport mechanisms for the indolamines are found.

Indirect pharmacologic data also implicate serotonin in the mediation of diarrhea and perhaps in the malabsorption found in a number of patients.[721, 818, 862, 876] Agents that retard inactivation of serotonin (e.g., MAO inhibitors) will increase diarrhea,[810] whereas drugs that are pharmacologic antagonists of serotonin (e.g., methysergide) usually ameliorate the abdominal cramps, diarrhea, or malabsorption.[862] In addition, parachlorophenylalanine, an effective inhibitor of the synthesis of serotonin, alleviates diarrhea in patients with the carcinoid syndrome.[723] In practice, however, these are not necessarily the most useful drugs for

modifying this symptom. The antagonists and inhibitors of the synthesis of serotonin do not decrease the other symptoms and signs of carcinoid syndrome — the flush, heart lesions, or asthma. Moreover, during an acute flushing episode accompanied by hyperperistalsis, serotonin is released infrequently into the blood.[912] Both bradykinin and prostaglandins are found in high concentration in the circulation during a flush.[922] Both have direct pharmacologic effects on the gut and could contribute to changes in intestinal motility during acute flushes. Their role in intestinal motility of these patients is not known.

There are two additional abdominal symptoms in patients with carcinoid syndrome:

1. The *acute abdominal "crisis"* (abdominal pain, fever, leukocytosis, and thrombocytosis) is usually associated with necrosis of metastatic lesions in the liver. Tumor necrosis is thought to occur when the tumor outgrows its blood supply. Indeed, the crisis can be precipitated by occlusion of the hepatic artery, which has occurred in some patients after perfusion of hepatic arteries with antitumor agents.[874] The symptoms may be due to the release of pharmacologically active substances by the metastasis and distention of the liver capsule by hemorrhage. The crisis may end with marked pulmonary complications (pleural effusions and pneumonia) secondary to immobilization and irritation of the diaphragm overlying the liver. These crises are often difficult to distinguish from true small bowel obstruction, which does not occur often unless there has been abdominal surgery and sufficient time for fibrous adhesions to develop. Spontaneous fibrosis also may produce small bowel obstruction, retroperitoneal fibrosis,[678, 782, 871] or, apparently, pericardial fibrosis. Peptic ulcer occurs with high incidence when the primary tumor is in the stomach.[885]

2. *Deficiency syndromes* may develop in patients with the carcinoid syndrome. Normally, hydroxylation of tryptophan accounts for about 1% of the dietary intake of the amino acid. If the tumors are sufficiently large, more than half the dietary tryptophan can be converted to serotonin, thereby diverting this amino acid from forming niacin and protein. Thus patients may have hypoalbuminemia and pellagra. Questions have been raised as to whether diversion of 50% of tryptophan into unusual pathways would be sufficient to cause pellagra[690, 857] and whether the only abnormality of metabolism of tryptophan was the increased synthesis of 5-hydroxytryptophan, serotonin, and their metabolites. Some 5,6-hydroxylated products of tryptophan and tryptamine have been found in normal animal tissues. They could conceivably produce biologic effects, but they have not been screened for in normal individuals or in patients with the carcinoid syndrome.[826] Williams and coworkers have demonstrated, in 3 of 11 patients with biopsy-proven carcinoid tumors and some symptoms of the syndrome, that non-hydroxylated products of tryptophan can be abnormally elevated and could participate both in the shunt of tryptophan away from protein synthesis and in its keinurenic pathway, and perhaps in the symptoms of the disease.[991] These studies indicate that when the three patients with unusual patterns of excretion of indole acid were given tryptophan loads, the biochemical abnormality became pronounced, and, during the loading, unusual psychologic features, such as anxiety, depression, amnesia, and, in one patient, visual hallucinations, occurred. These psychologic features were not seen in the other eight patients with classic increased 5-hydroxylated products but did mimic some of the spontaneous symptoms the three patients had previously described. A major function of this section is to present the multipotential qualities of the carcinoid tumor and the scientific and clinical drawbacks of concentrating on one obvious abnormality (e.g., excess production of sero-

tonin) and concluding that it alone is responsible for all symptoms.[767, 769, 770, 882] The data discussed above serve as an example of one of the many lessons in biochemistry, pharmacology, and endocrinology that the carcinoid tumor is likely to teach us.

Evidence of *hepatic insufficiency* is relatively rare in the carcinoid syndrome until extensive metastases have developed. Then hyperbilirubinemia, hypoprothrombinemia, hypoalbuminemia, and hepatic coma may occur. Hypoalbuminemia also may result from excessive loss of the protein from the gut. The mechanism may include the passive congestive effects of right-sided heart failure on the gut mucosa, and it may be dependent on the pharmacologic effects of the autacoids that are produced by the tumor.[842] Like others suffering from neoplastic disease, patients with carcinoid tumors may become cachectic before death.

Perhaps abnormalities in *glucose tolerance and metabolism* were to be expected in the presence of the carcinoid tumor. The metastatic tumor grows to massive sizes, and some tumors replace almost all of the liver. Some tumors of foregut origin (bronchial and pancreatic carcinoid tumors) produce ACTH, GH, and insulin.[620, 844] Even an ileal tumor can make and inappropriately release enough insulin to cause symptomatic hypoglycemia. Finally, abnormal concentrations of some amino acids such as tyrosine and tryptophan might alter the release or effects of insulin.[737] All the factors just mentioned could contribute to abnormal handling of glucose. Symptoms of hypoglycemia, unusual patterns of hunger and eating, or osmotic diuresis related to high concentrations of glucose in the blood should be sought and objectively documented in patients with the carcinoid syndrome. During medical evaluation in three patients (two with ileal carcinoids and one with bronchial carcinoid) with symptoms of hypoglycemia and a craving for foods with high sugar content, we were surprised to find normal glucose tolerance and rates of metabolism. Further evaluation did little more to define the pathogenesis of the symptoms other than to reveal that the three patients had normal to low basal circulating levels of immunoreactive insulin.[645] When challenged with orally or intravenously administered glucose, the K values of glucose disappearance were normal, *but* release of immunoreactive insulin was minimal or absent. Response of GH was appropriate. We can only begin to understand these phenomena with the information available. Serotonin may inhibit glucose-induced release of insulin[827] and perhaps contribute, in ill-defined ways, to maintenance of normal concentrations of glucose in plasma.[938] Whether these activities of serotonin operate in these patients is as yet unknown. Even more puzzling is the possibility that the tumor may be making an unidentified noninsulin substance capable of promoting transport of glucose into tissues.[844] Again, the carcinoid syndrome challenges us to understand fundamental facts related to endocrinology.

Abnormal Chemistry and Pathogenesis

Synthesis and Metabolism of Serotonin (Fig. 10–15)

The 5-hydroxytryptophan produced by tryptophan hydroxylase is stereospecific and has a high affinity (K_m 2×10^{-5}) for aromatic-L-amino acid decarboxylase.[772] This enzyme converts 5-hydroxytryptophan to 5-HT. Of the indoles produced by the carcinoid tumor, serotonin is one of the most pharmacologically active. It may be metabolized by MAO in the tumor (in which case it produces little pharmacologic effect) or in the blood after release from the tumor. Serotonin

is oxidized to 5-hydroxyindole acetaldehyde, which is converted to 5-HIAA by aldehyde dehydrogenase. Small amounts of circulating serotonin are inactivated by ATP-dependent binding to platelets or by conversion to the alcohol, 5-hydroxytryptophol, or its conjugates, 5-hydroxytryptophol-O-sulfate and 5-hydroxytryptophol-O-glucuronide. Most of the 5-HIAA is excreted in the urine as the free acid, although small amounts may be conjugated to the O-sulfate ester before excretion. Patients with the carcinoid syndrome usually have an expanded pool of serotonin,[941] a two- to tenfold increase in concentrations of serotonin in blood and platelets, and 5-HIAA in the urine.

It is important to note that some patients with the "carcinoid syndrome" do not have elevated concentrations of 5-HIAA in the urine.[828] In contrast, patients with carcinoid tumors but without the syndrome may have marked elevations of the acid in the urine.[984] The absence of symptoms during excessive excretion of 5-HIAA may indicate that the metabolism of serotonin is occurring within the tumor substance and that only biologically inactive metabolites are being released from the tumor. Conversely, it is possible that a tumor could rapidly produce and release critical amounts of amine only at the times symptoms are caused. If the tumor sporadically releases serotonin but does not metabolize or release oxidation products of serotonin, the total amount of 5-HIAA in the urine over a day could be minimally elevated or even normal. An analogous situation was discussed under the heading "Pheochromocytoma." Even very small pheochromocytomas may produce symptoms without elevating excretion of the metabolites of catecholamines in the urine. In such an instance, the turnover of catecholamines is rapid, little amine is bound or metabolized in the tumor, and sufficient amine is released from the tumor to create symptoms. The only abnormality associated with the symptoms is an elevated concentration of amines, but not their metabolites, either in blood or urine.

The concentration of serotonin in the urine is not routinely measured in patients with carcinoid syndrome. We do not know whether symptoms in patients with normal concentrations of 5-HIAA in the urine are associated with changes in the concentrations of serotonin in the urine or blood. When serotonin is released from the tumor into the blood, the severity of the gastrointestinal aspects of the syndrome frequently correlates with the quantity of the amine produced.

Other Amines and the Carcinoid Tumor

Other amines have been found in the urine of carcinoid patients. Excretion of histamine is frequently and consistently elevated in patients with gastric carcinoid tumors and inconsistently elevated in patients with ileal tumors. Studies on these patients indicate that the amine is not made in mast cells and is most often seen in tumors that lack aromatic-L-amino acid decarboxylase, i.e., gastric and bronchial carcinoids. Concentrations of catecholamines and their metabolites in the urine also have been elevated in some patients with the carcinoid syndrome.[981] This abnormality is unusual and has not been correlated with specific symptoms or tumor locations.

Mediators of the Flush and Bradykinin

Evidence indicates that serotonin is not the only biologically active substance that mediates the flush in the carcinoid syndrome: (1) intravenous injection of 5-HT does not reproduce the typical spontaneous attacks of flushing in carcinoid patients; (2) there is little correlation between concentrations of free 5-HT in the plasma and flushing episodes; (3) although infusion of epinephrine or norepinephrine provokes typical flushing attacks, it is not often accompanied by elevation of 5-HT in blood taken from either the hepatic vein or the brachial artery; (4) the carcinoid syndrome with flushing is not always accompanied by increased excretion of 5-HIAA; and (5) metastatic carcinoid tumors can be present without the syndrome, even though excretion of 5-HIAA is increased.[984]

A group of vasodilator peptides has been implicated among the mediators of the flush in some patients. Because kallikrein normally is present in gut tissue, which gives rise to the carcinoid tumor, and because it may be released by catecholamines, which also may provoke a flush, the role of kinins in the carcinoid flush was investigated. When synthetic bradykinin was rapidly infused into patients with the carcinoid syndrome, the resultant flush closely mimicked spontaneous flushes.[746, 883] Bradykinin was elevated in the hepatic venous blood of some patients during spontaneous and epinephrine-induced flushes.[884] Tumors have been extracted from patients with the carcinoid syndrome and prominent flushing, and most contained a type of tissue kallikrein.[860] These results have been broadly confirmed.[621, 752, 848, 944] In addition, kallikrein has been located in a carcinoid tumor by immunofluorescent techniques.[636] Finally, in several patients with carcinoid flush, the release of kallikrein has correlated with production of the flush, with an increase in the flow of blood in the forearm, and with a decrease in systemic arterial pressure (Fig. 10–23).[621, 848, 849, 944]

It is now believed that the flush in any given patient with the carcinoid syndrome can be caused by a variety of biologically active substances.[904] Those known to contribute to the flush include prostaglandins, histamine, lysyl bradykinin, and bradykinin. Others, although not yet identified, are substances that can be released by pentagastrin or gastrin.[747] From available data, it would appear that flush-provoking stimuli, such as epinephrine, sympathetic discharge, and ingestion of alcohol, liberate kallikrein from the tumor (Fig. 10–24). The mechanisms by which the kallikrein is released are not known. Once in the blood, kallikrein splits lysyl-bradykinin from kininogen. The lysyl-bradykinin is rapidly converted to bradykinin. Both lysyl-bradykinin and bradykinin are capable of producing profound vasodilation, systemic hypotension, edema, tachycardia, and increased salivation, lacrimation and cardiac output.

In addition, in some species the kinins are bronchial constrictors and, as mediators of inflammation, may participate in fibrosis. It is conceivable that they may be contributing to the asthma and increased fibrosis that occur in patients with the carcinoid syndrome.

Just as serotonin is not likely to be the only mediator of the flush, there is evidence that bradykinin is not either. The most convincing evidence is from three separate laboratories including our own: Abnormally high concentrations of bradykinin cannot be detected in the venous blood of every patient who has a carcinoid flush. In addition, substances such as histamine and prostaglandin can be released from some tumors and certainly are capable of influencing a carcinoid flush. In fact, recent data indicate that in some patients with gastric carcinoids, histamine may be the sole direct mediator of the flush. A combination of H_1 and H_2 receptor blockers was required to suppress the flush fully.[910] When H_1 blockers were used alone, only the frequency but not the duration of the flush was affected. The H_2 blocker by itself decreased the duration of the flushes without decreasing the rate of occurrence. In some patients, antihistaminics do not affect the flush in any way. In others, the only

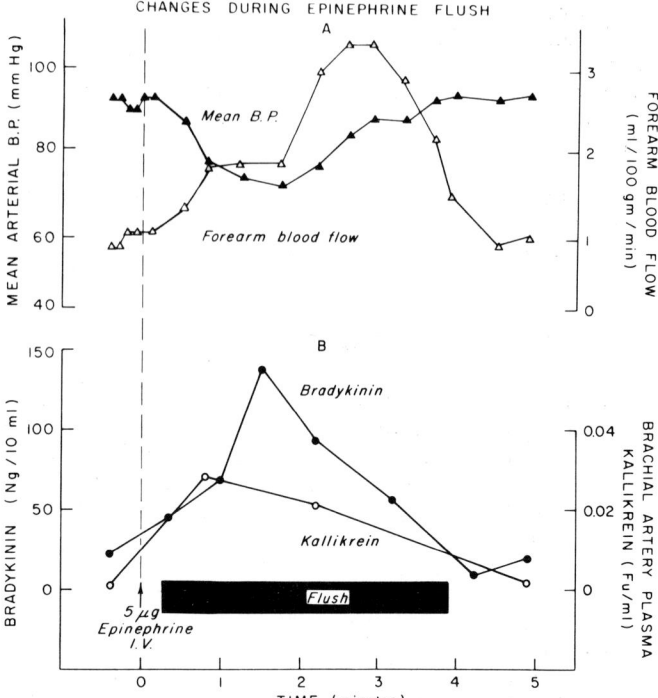

Figure 10–23. Serial determination of mean arterial pressure (B.P.) (solid triangles) and forearm blood flow (open triangles), top panel (*A*), and of bradykinin (closed circles) and kallikrein (open circles), bottom panel (*B*), before and after injection of epinephrine into a patient with carcinoid syndrome. The subnormal control values for forearm blood flow are compatible with the fact that the patient was in congestive heart failure. (From Mason, D. T., and Melmon, K. L.: Abnormal forearm vascular responses in the carcinoid syndrome: the role of kinins and kinin-generating system. *J. Clin. Invest.* 45:1691, 1966.)

efficacious drug for flushes and diarrhea may be aspirin at doses sufficient to inhibit the synthesis of prostaglandins.[705,747,910] Possibly not all the vasoactive agents that surface during a given flush come from the tumor; excesses of one substance may release other hormones from normal tissues (see above). Although a tumor may produce a

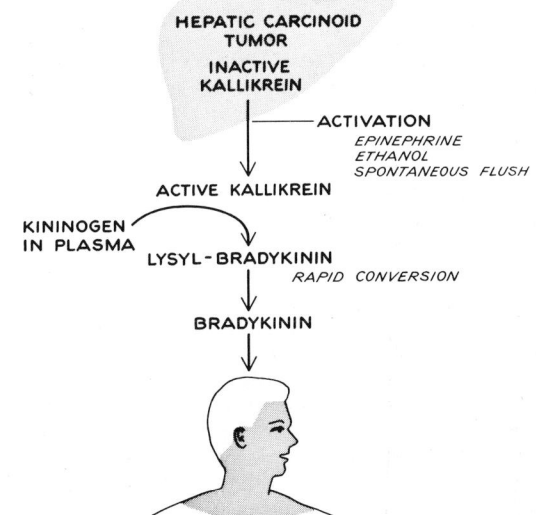

Figure 10–24. Summary of present concepts by which kallikrein and kinins may contribute to the carcinoid flush. The flush mechanism, however, is complex; in some patients, kinin levels are normal. (From Melmon, K. L.: Kinins in medicine—present and future. *Physiol. Pharmacol. Physicians,* *1*:6, 1966.)

substance at one time, it does not follow that the same carcinoid will continue to produce the same amount or the same quality of hormone indefinitely. The physician should constantly reassess the chemicals produced by each patient, particularly if a previously successful regimen fails. The inconstancy of the hormone markers in carcinoid tumors is characteristic of other tumors with endocrine potential.[643] Knowing the particular chemical abnormality responsible for a flush in any given patient may be critical for designing effective therapy.

Additional Biologically Active Compounds Produced by or Associated with the Tumor

There is strong evidence that carcinoid tumors may be ectopic sites for production of ACTH. These tumors produce a syndrome similar to Cushing's syndrome, and they usually occur in sites other than the ileum. The ACTH probably is secreted intermittently. At least one patient with Cushing's syndrome secreted excessive corticosteroids on a cyclical basis.[680] To date, the only tumors found to contain ACTH-like material (by bioassay[784] and immunofluorescence studies[807]) were carcinoids unassociated with the classic carcinoid syndrome. The carcinoid tumor can produce and release insulin, and the syndrome may appear concomitantly with tumors of the pancreas that release a substance with insulin-like activity.[711, 943] The carcinoid tumor may be associated with MEN or, alternatively, may simultaneously produce a variety of substances that ordinarily would remind the physician of MEN (see above). One tumor produced GH, another appeared to secrete a GH-releasing substance.[951] It seems reasonable to assume, by analogy with other polypeptide hormone–producing neoplasms, that substances such as ADH, erythrocyte-stimulating factor, or other vasodilatory peptides may also be produced by these tumors but have simply remained undetected to date. The precedent for the manufacture of some of these biologically active substances by other tumors, such as oat cell carcinomas, cerebellar hemangioblastomas, and pheochromocytomas, has already been established.[643, 664]

The hormones produced at various ectopic sites are similar if not identical to the natural hormones made by normal tissues.[664, 832] Production of hormone appears to be a highly organized and biochemically economical function of tumor tissue.

The differentiation of cells ultimately is an expression of their genetic instructional material.[777, 778] Any cells capable of differentiation may theoretically develop any form or function within the range and competence of their genetic information. The inappropriate biochemical behavior of carcinoid tumors suggests that a large amount of genetic knowledge is retained in neoplastic cells and is derepressed in the process of autonomous control of growth. Such reactivation of latent information is relatively common in a variety of malignant tissues.[989] The most direct evidence to support such an explanation comes from experiments in which nuclei from normal intestinal epithelial cells of an adult frog were transplanted into enucleated eggs of *Xenopus laevis*. Normal adult frogs resulted. In addition, nearly normal tail-bud tadpoles can be produced by transplanting nuclei from renal adenocarcinoma cells to enucleated eggs of *Rana esculenta*.[777, 778] Some argue that nuclei of differentiated somatic cells do not generally undergo restrictive changes that affect the genetic material itself.[777, 778]

A variety of tumors, including adenocarcinoma of the pancreas, nonbeta islet-cell carcinoma of the pancreas, small cell carcinoma of the lung, ovarian neoplasms, carcinoma of the gallbladder, and anaplastic carcinomas of unknown ori-

gin, may produce clinical syndromes resembling the carcinoid syndrome.[762, 866] Most of these tumors produce typical flushes, and many patients have experienced diarrhea and bronchial constriction. At least two oat cell carcinomas have been associated with the fibrous subendocardial lesions typical of carcinoid tumor.[639] Although these tumors frequently are associated with an increased production of 5-HIAA, few have demonstrated evidence of abnormal indole metabolism. Kallikrein activity has been found in at least one patient with oat cell carcinoma of the bronchus.[710] The discovery of additional biologically active substances that might be elaborated by these tumors is the object of current research. A number of the noncarcinoid, endocrine-active tumors have been examined by electron microscopy. Beusch and coworkers postulated the existence of Kulchitsky's cells in at least the bronchial tumors.[653] They concluded that, in the case of small cell carcinoma, some hormonal production could be under the control of "ectopically" placed Kulchitsky's cells and even went so far as to suggest that the bronchial carcinoid tumor is a more benign form of the small cell carcinoma. Others have compared the histology of the cells that compose the bronchial carcinoid tumors to Type I and II pneumocytes or to muscle cells.[659, 688]

There is no need to accept the pluripotential cell theory over the ectopic cell theory of unnatural production of hormones. A reasonable and rational compromise has been proposed by Weichert.[986] He suggests that the enterochromaffin cell system is derived from cells of the neuroectoderm, which probably migrate into the primitive alimentary tract during embryonic development. These neuroectodermal "stem" cells may migrate with endocrine glands developing from the embryonic foregut — the anterior pituitary, thyroid, parathyroid, and pancreatic islets. These cells may also form the chromaffin cell system of the adrenals and paraganglia, the autonomic ganglia, and the cells in the hypothalamus, which produce posterior pituitary hormones. Weichert suggests that ectopic hormone-producing tumors and tumors in the syndrome of MEN arise from cells with a common neuroectodermal embryonic precursor. Their capacity to synthesize a variety of peptide and amine hormones may be revealed as their genetic material is derepressed during neoplastic transformation. This theory (as described above in discussing the origin of the Kulchitsky's cells) seems quite plausible.

The precise role of each of the biologically active substances produced by the carcinoid tumor in each instance is not well defined, but certainly serotonin is not the exclusive mediator of the symptoms of the carcinoid syndrome.

Variants of the Classic Carcinoid Syndrome

Deviations from the classic syndrome include: (1) unusual syndromes associated with a carcinoid tumor in a location other than the small bowel (Table 10–9), and (2) syndromes resembling the classic carcinoid syndrome but caused by a heterogeneous group of neoplasms that have no histologic relation to carcinoid tumor (described above). Variant forms of the carcinoid syndrome may sometimes be managed with specific medical therapy.

The Gastric Carcinoid Tumor

The gastric carcinoid syndrome is distinguishable from the classic syndrome by the pattern of flushes. They are patchy and extend over the face and neck to the arms, trunk, and legs. The flush has a geographic distribution with sharply delineated serpentine borders (Fig. 10–25). The patches of

Table 10-9. COMPARATIVE FEATURES OF THE SYNDROME ASSOCIATED WITH PRIMARY CARCINOID TUMORS IN VARIOUS SITES

Features	Tumor Site		
	Ileal	*Gastric*	*Bronchial*
Flush	Brief, multiple, occurs over head and neck areas	Generalized, bright red, geographic distribution	Prolonged, severe, may include anxiety, tremulousness, periorbital and facial edema, lacrimation, salivation, diaphoresis, fever, and oliguria
Heart lesions	Right sided	May be rare	Frequently left-sided, with pulmonary edema during flushing
Metastases	Rarely beyond abdominal cavity	Rarely beyond abdominal cavity	Widespread metastases with osteoblastic bone lesions
Chemistry	Urinary 5-HIAA accounts for more than 90% indole products; elevation histamine inconstant	Tumor often lacks decarboxylase enzyme. Therefore, 5-HIAA may account for less than 90% of indoles and 5-HT and 5-HTP are frequently elevated. Urinary histamine is often continuously elevated	Often has large amounts of 5-HTP as well as 5-HIAA in urine
Association with other disorders	Rare	High frequency of peptic ulceration	High incidence of other endocrine disorders
Treatment	Determined by symptoms and specific chemical abnormalities	Aromatic-L-amino acid decarboxylase inhibitors may be helpful	Corticosteroids may have unique and dramatic effects on symptoms
Prognosis	Fair: 10–15 year survival not unusual	Fair	Very poor

5-HIAA, 5-hydroxyindole acetic acid; 5-HT, 5-hydroxytryptamine; 5-HTP, 5-hydroxytryptophan.

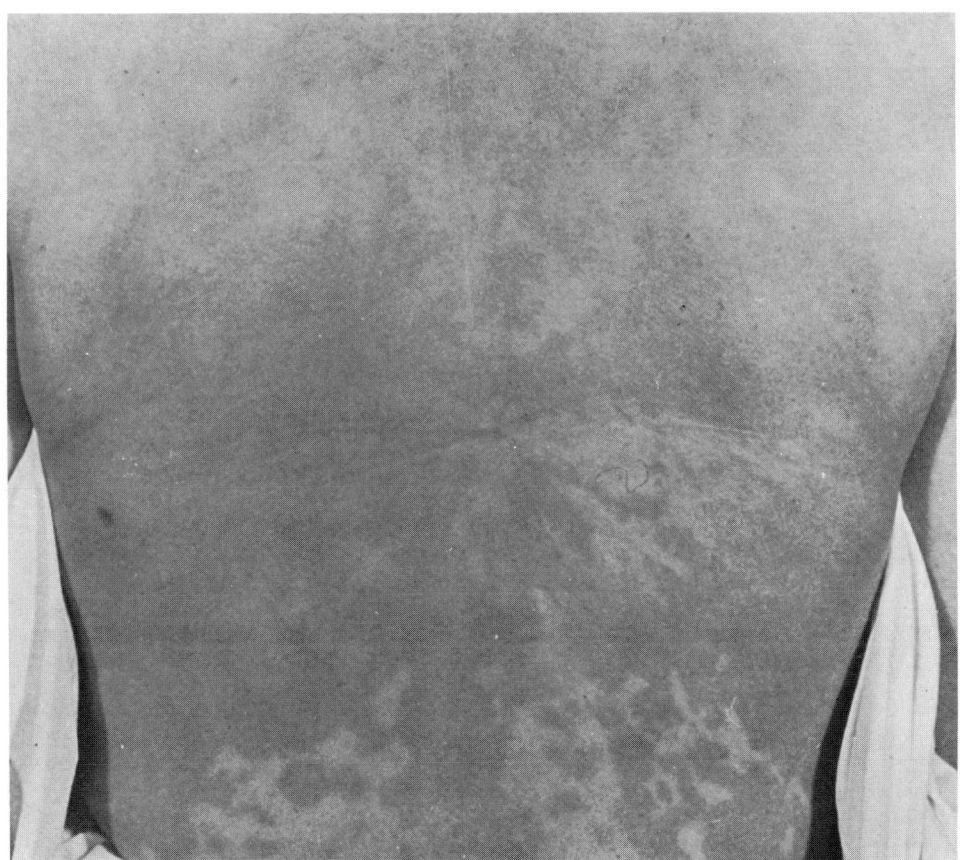

Figure 10-25. A generalized flush with geographic distribution and sharply delineated serpentine borders as seen in a patient with a gastric carcinoid tumor.

discoloration will become confluent if the attacks last long enough. Characteristic production of large amounts of histamine may contribute to the geographic pattern of the flushes. In these patients only, the combined use of H_1 and H_2 receptor blockers can totally ablate the flushes.[910] The excessive histamine may also be responsible for the increased production of gastric acid and hence peptic ulcers in these patients. Again, cimetidine (an H_2 antagonist) can be helpful. Other gastrointestinal symptoms are less common in these patients, whose primary tumor is in the stomach, than in patients with the classic lesion.

In addition to fairly consistent increases in the concentrations of histamine in the blood and in the urine, the pattern of excretion of indoles can be distinct for the patient with gastric carcinoid syndrome. The tumor usually lacks aromatic-L-amino acid decarboxylase and consequently releases unconverted 5-hydroxytryptophan rather than 5-HT into the blood. Thus platelet serotonin values are normal and the concentration of 5-hydroxytryptophan is elevated in the urine. A portion of the 5-hydroxytryptophan is decarboxylated in the kidney, resulting in elevated concentrations of serotonin in the urine. There is a concomitant decrease in the fraction of indoles (to less than 90% of the total amount of indoles in the urine) excreted as 5-HIAA because serotonin is not available for oxidation.

Oates and Sjoerdsma state that patients with gastric carcinoid are less likely to have cardiac lesions than are those with ileal tumors.[885] Perhaps the decreased production of serotonin is responsible for the absence of both prominent cardiac lesions and gastrointestinal symptoms. The decarboxylase inhibitor α-methyldopa can be therapeutically used to diminish substantially the production of 5-HT in other parts of the body, and its use is accompanied by less severe flushing episodes. This clinical response to α-methyldopa is unusual in patients with the classic carcinoid syndrome.

The Bronchial Carcinoid Tumor

The bronchial tumors produce the most striking clinical variants of the carcinoid spectrum and serve as the best example of the multiple endocrine functions of the carcinoid tumor.[861]

By far the most important clinical features that separate the bronchial syndrome from the ileal are the acute episodes of flushing. The flushes may be severe and prolonged, lasting as long as 3 or 4 days. They are often preceded by disorientation, anxiety, and tremulousness of the hands. They are associated with periorbital and facial edema and striking increases in lacrimation (Fig. 10–26 A and B), salivation, sweating, temperature, and heart rate. The nausea, vomiting, explosive diarrhea, dyspnea, and wheezing common to the flush period are usually totally absent between flushes. The flushes may be associated with profound hypotension, oliguria, and, if left-sided cardiac lesions are present, pulmonary edema. The attacks of pulmonary edema may be fatal. Other unusual and prominent features of the syndrome are the prevalence of mitral rather than pulmonic and tricuspid valve lesions, the appearance of hypoventilation of a single lobe due to physical obstruction of a bronchus by the tumor[790] or diffuse pulmonary infiltrates caused by the tumor,[942] and associated, seemingly unrelated, disorders. For example, the increased incidence of Cushing's syndrome,

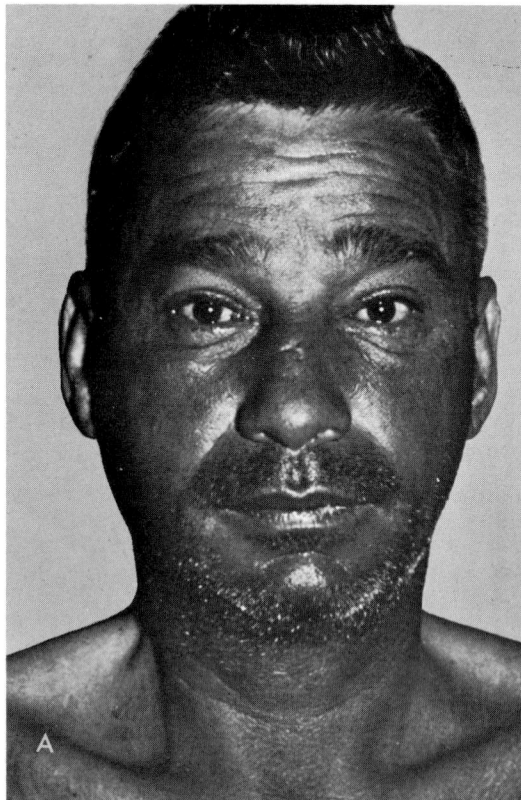
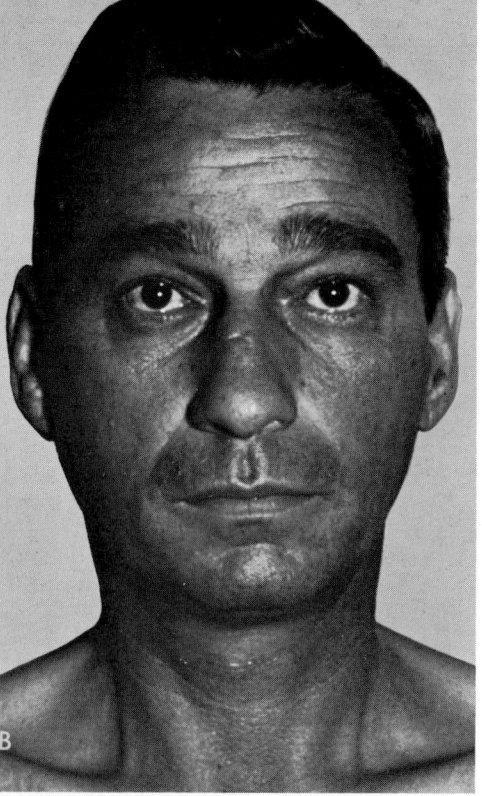

Figure 10–26. A, Appearance of patient during a severe and prolonged flush associated with a bronchial carcinoid tumor. Note the periorbital and facial edema, glistening of the eyes due to lacrimation, and parotid swelling. B, After recovery, patient appears normal and asymptomatic. (From Melmon, K. L., Sjoerdsma, A., et al.: Distinctive clinical and therapeutic aspects of the syndrome associated with bronchial carcinoid tumors. *Am. J. Med. 39:*568, 1965.)

pluriglandular adenomatosis, and acromegaly may be due to trophic proteins elaborated by the tumor itself or to the co-existence of other endocrine-producing tumors. The tumors may produce large amounts of 5-hydroxytryptophan as well as serotonin. The association of increased excretion of 5-HIAA with an *asymptomatic* pulmonary "coin" lesion, discovered during routine roentgenologic examinations, has encouraged Warner and coworkers to suggest the use of 5-HIAA as a screening test in these individuals.[984]

It is generally believed that patients with bronchial carcinoids seem to have a poorer prognosis than do those with the usual carcinoid tumor, although some recent data challenge this belief[886] and indicate that the prognosis for many patients with carcinoid tumors is poor. Widespread metastases are more common and include osteoblastic bone lesions and involvement of lymph nodes, heart, lungs, kidneys, gallbladder, pancreas, adrenal and thyroid glands, and even the optic nerve.[743] However, the symptoms of these patients may respond dramatically to treatment with corticosteroids. Such treatment has permitted patients with regular and life-threatening flushes to remain asymptomatic for as long as 2 years. One patient first examined because of increased salivation and lacrimation, and later for severe flushes, was given a therapeutic trial of 15 mg of prednisone a day. Because of her dramatic response to corticosteroids, the patient was suspected of having a bronchial carcinoid tumor, and a previously overlooked pulmonary density was then observed in chest roentgenograms. Several months later the patient died; an autopsy revealed the bronchial carcinoid tumor. The reason for the dramatic response of patients with bronchial carcinoids to steroid therapy is not understood.

Diagnosis

General

When a patient has a fully developed clinical syndrome, the diagnosis may be easy. However, a patient seldom has all the features of the carcinoid syndrome, and the disease should be suspected in patients with only a single feature of the syndrome, such as unexplained intermittent diarrhea, development of telangiectasia over the face, episodes of flushing, bronchial constriction, or psychosis appearing late in life. A physical examination may disclose little, not even isolated hepatomegaly or bronchoconstriction, as a clue to the underlying pathologic changes. If the primary tumor can be removed before metastases occur, the patient can be cured. Female patients with suggestive symptoms and signs should be accorded special attention because an ovarian carcinoid or teratoma may give rise to symptoms before it has metastasized.[797] Similarly, early discovery of a bronchial lesion may permit a complete cure.

Routine clinical laboratory tests are seldom helpful. However, thrombocytosis and leukocytosis during abdominal crisis may occur. Liver function tests may show elevated alkaline phosphatase without hyperbilirubinemia — signs consistent with neoplastic involvement of this organ. Hypoalbuminemia may occur in the later course of the disease. The ^{99}Tc sulfur colloid "liver scan" is helpful, but not completely reliable, for detecting early hepatic involvement. Liver biopsy can aid in the proper diagnosis in a patient with or without evidence of hepatomegaly or chemical evidence of abnormal liver function. In seven patients without other evidence of metastatic spread or chemical abnormalities that could be attributed to involvement of the liver by the tumor, the biopsy revealed positive involvement of the liver with typical carcinoid tumor.

Determination of concentrations of cholesterol, carotene, and vitamin A in plasma and the results of xylose tolerance tests as well as quantitation of stool fat while the patient is on controlled fat intake may expose occult malabsorption or steatorrhea, even in the absence of diarrhea.[862]

Roentgenographic studies may help detect a bronchial carcinoid tumor or metastases, peptic ulcer or primary gastric neoplasm. The barium upper gastrointestinal series with small bowel follow-through rarely reveals a primary ileal tumor but may show swollen mucosal folds, edema of the intestinal wall, and evidence of mesenteric retraction, presumably as a function of the effects of the autacoid on the intestines. An additional finding may be rapid transit of the barium meal through the small bowel.[800, 929] On rare occasions, angiography has revealed a carcinoid tumor, but this technique is not recommended.[839]

Sigmoidoscopy may detect a rectal carcinoid, but because these tumors so rarely produce a syndrome, they usually are discovered by serendipity.

Special Studies

Excessive excretion of 5-HIAA continues to be the most useful indicator of the carcinoid tumor. The qualitative test is rapidly obtainable and is positive if the excretion of 5-HIAA exceeds 25–30 mg/day. Because some carcinoid tumors will not produce enough serotonin to elevate 5-HIAA above 15 mg/day, it is worthwhile to perform a quantitative determination of this indole metabolite when the diagnosis is strongly suspected. Elevations in the range of 9–25 mg/day can be seen either with carcinoid syndrome or with nontropical sprue.[819] The acid may be deceptively low when the patient has a gastric carcinoid tumor. In such a patient, 5-HT and 5-hydroxytryptophan should be sought by paper chromatography of the urine. Low excretion of 5-HIAA can occur during either diet-induced or spontaneous pyridoxal phosphate deficiencies.[679, 750] Then the decarboxylation of tryptophan and other amino acids may be inhibited by lack of the essential cofactor. Some have advocated, but generally on relatively weak grounds, that diets that are deficient in vitamin B_6 and that contain inhibitors of pyridoxal phosphate might be therapeutic for patients with the carcinoid syndrome. Falsely negative results may occur in patients with carcinoid tumors that do not excrete excessive 5-HIAA. Patients with intestinal obstruction or small intestinal resection also may have unusually low excretions of 5-HIAA. Falsely negative results also may occur when patients are taking phenothiazine drugs. Eating bananas, walnuts, or other foods containing serotonin may elevate excretion of 5-HIAA in the absence of a tumor. Some proprietary cough medications containing glyceryl guaiacolates may produce falsely positive results. Therefore, urine specimens should be collected after the patient has stopped taking drugs for 3 or 4 days. Concentrations of histamine, of catecholamines, and of metabolites in the urine may be elevated, but this is not specifically related to carcinoid tumors.[846] Determination of the amount of 5-HT in whole blood, plasma, or platelets may help to confirm the diagnosis. Measurements of kinins, tumor-kallikrein, histamine, and prostaglandins, released into the peripheral circulation are feasible, but the methods are specialized and laborious.

Provocation of a flush by intravenously administering small doses of epinephrine, orally administering a few ounces of ethyl alcohol, or intravenously administering pentagastrin may help detect a carcinoid tumor in patients complaining of flushes.[829, 893] A flush similar in quality to those that the patient experiences spontaneously, as well as conjunctival suffusion and increased lacrimation and respiratory rate, may be seen 1–2 min after administering 1–5

μg of epinephrine. The epinephrine test also may be positive in patients who have not experienced or been aware of flushes in the past.[828] The incidence of falsely positive and falsely negative results has not been determined, but in general this test, when done in a carefully controlled manner, has been a useful adjunct to the chemical screening tests.

Treatment and Prognosis

Surgical removal of an isolated primary tumor is apparently the best treatment and may be curative. However, the diagnosis is seldom made before metastasis has occurred. After metastasis has occurred, surgical removal of the primary tumor is justified only if the tumor is large or is causing mechanical obstruction. In rare instances, resection of large, isolated, hepatic lesions has substantially but only temporarily eased the patient's symptoms. Such procedures are associated with considerable morbidity and mortality.[997] There are reports of symptomatic relief after the surgical ligation or the arteriographic embolization of branches of the hepatic artery supplying major metastatic deposits.[626, 874] If metastases are extensive, the treatment should be tailored to the patient's symptoms, the defined chemical abnormalities, and the location of the primary tumor. Even after metastasis of the tumor, supportive and symptomatic treatment is extremely important; some patients, particularly those with ileal carcinoid tumor, have lived as long as 23 years and others may live 10 or more years after the syndrome appears. Although the disease can be relatively unaggressive, the prognosis frequently is much poorer than past impressions have led us to believe. Nevertheless, the clinician should not necessarily be discouraged by excretion of large quantities of 5-HIAA in the urine. There is no correlation between the amount of indole acid excreted and the prognosis.

There are some reports that antitumor agents, e.g., 5-fluorouracil (5-FU), cyclophosphamide and adriamycin or either agent separately may be effective in decreasing tumor burden and in providing symptomatic relief in patients with metastatic disease.[769, 823, 863, 867, 874, 882, 908, 950] Recently, some have suggested that streptozotocin, particularly when combined with 5-FU, may have positive effects in patients with carcinoid tumors.[926-928] Treatment with these drugs must be studied further and probably should be used when other forms of medication have failed or when the major clinical problem results from a rapidly growing tumor. At present there is little evidence that these toxic agents significantly alter the long-term prognosis, nor has treatment with radiation been strikingly successful.[776]

When directed at specific chemical abnormalities, specific pharmacologic therapy may be very helpful, although only palliative. Thus, if excretion of 5-HIAA is elevated and gastrointestinal symptoms are the major complaint of the patient, antiserotonin agents (either competitive inhibitors, e.g., methysergide, or cyproheptadine, or inhibitors of synthesis of serotonin, e.g., parachlorophenylalanine) may diminish abdominal cramps and diarrhea and may even reverse steatorrhea.[862] The effect of antiserotonin agents on flushes is inconsistent. These drugs appear not to control the growth of the tumor, development of heart lesions, or bronchial manifestations of the syndrome. Agents such as methysergide and cyproheptadine will antagonize the peripheral effects of serotonin without altering its synthesis or metabolism. Because methysergide may produce retroperitoneal fibrosis and even pericardial fibrosis, prolonged use must be carefully supervised or avoided.[677, 763, 888] Decarboxylase inhibitors such as α-methyldopa may be helpful in ameliorating the symptoms of some patients with gastric carcin-

oid tumors but generally are not useful therapeutic agents. When the patient's prime symptoms are flushes, antiserotonin agents rarely help. Phenothiazine drugs, which are effective α-adrenergic blocking agents as well as antikinin agents, may control flushes.[916] Phenoxybenzamine, an α-adrenergic blocking drug, but not propranolol, a β-adrenergic blocking drug, appears to help control the flushes in some patients.[769] In the bronchial carcinoid patient, corticosteroids may be immensely helpful (see "The Bronchial Carcinoid Tumor") and in patients with gastric carcinoid tumors H_1 and H_2 blockers may play a very positive role. Aspirin or indomethacin might be useful in patients whose flushes do not respond to other measures and that, by a process of elimination, may be found to have been caused by excessive production of prostaglandin.

Hypotension may be difficult to manage during surgical procedures. In such a situation it is important to avoid pressor agents that are catecholamines (e.g., norepinephrine or epinephrine) or that primarily act by release of endogenous catecholamines (e.g., metaraminol). These agents quite likely will produce further hypotension by activating tumor-kallikrein or by releasing other as yet unidentified vasodilator substances. Methoxamine or angiotensin, whose major action is direct constriction of arterioles, will increase peripheral vascular resistance and effectively raise blood pressure in carcinoid patients without causing a flush. Dopamine and dobutamine have not been assessed in patients with carcinoid syndrome, but it would be difficult to imagine that their effects would vary noticeably from the β-mimetic catechols.

Supportive therapy must include good nutrition and vitamin supplements (particularly niacin when there is evidence of pellagra or when excretion of 5-HIAA exceeds 200–300 mg/day). Deodorized tincture of opium may be used alone or in conjunction with antiserotonin agents in the management of severe diarrhea. When therapy is administered rationally, it is often quite effective. In the last edition of this text, I stated my hope that, as we learned more about the endocrine potential of these tumors, therapy would become more specific and successful; it has, but much remains to be learned.

Mastocytosis

Comparisons with the Carcinoid Syndrome

Recurrent severe diarrhea, occasionally in association with intestinal malabsorption, flushing in association with tachycardia and hypotension, telangiectatic lesions of the skin, hepatomegaly, and bone lesions are common both to the carcinoid syndrome and to systemic mastocytosis. Waldenström was first to point out the analogy between the diseases.[815] This analogy has been supported by the finding of mast cell infiltration beneath the telangiectatic lesions of patients with carcinoid syndrome and the presence of large numbers of mast cells in some carcinoid tumors.[722] Despite the similar signs and symptoms, however, the two diseases are distinct entities, differing in etiology and pathogenesis[699, 1000] (Table 10–10).

Mastocytosis may occur during childhood as a benign, self-limited disease, or commonly in adulthood as a systemic disease (Table 10–11). Occasionally, solitary tumors in the lungs may resemble plasmacytomas.[685, 850] In the child, the most common clinical manifestation is an accumulation of mast cells in the skin, either in the form of a single fairly well circumscribed nodule, 2–3 cm in diameter, or as multiple smaller, diffuse infiltrates that blister and urticate after minor trauma. This form of proliferation of mast cells usually

Table 10-10. COMPARISON OF SYSTEMIC MASTOCYTOSIS AND CARCINOID TUMORS

	Mastocytosis	Carcinoid Tumor
Pathogenesis	Increased infiltration of "normal" mast cells; rarely malignant	Malignant enterochromaffin cell tumor
Symptoms		
Skin		
Pruritus	Prominent	
Cardiovascular		
Flush	Childhood	Any age
Tachycardia and hypotension	Common	Common
Gastrointestinal		
Diarrhea	Common	Common
Steatorrhea	Rare	Rare
Ulcers	Common	High incidence, especially with primary gastric tumors
Pulmonary		
Wheezing	Infrequent	Infrequent
Signs		
Skin		
Telangiectasia	Generalized	Localized
Dermatographism	Common	Rare
Pellagra		Rare
Lymph node enlargement	Common	
Cardiovascular		
Valvular lesions		Common
Abdominal		
Liver enlargement	Common (mast cell infiltration)	Common (metastasis)
Spleen enlargement	Common	
Skeletal		
Osteoblastic lesions	Diffuse osteosclerosis or isolated osteoblastic lesions	Common, especially with primary bronchial tumors
Other	Osteoporosis and isolated osteoclastic lesions	
Chemical Mediators		
Known		
Histamine	+	+
Serotonin	±	+
Kinins	?	+
Catecholamines	−	+
Heparin	+	−
Prostaglandins	?	+
Other, suspected	+	+

regresses spontaneously before or shortly after puberty. In systemic mastocytosis, the proliferating mast cells invade multiple organs of the reticuloendothelial system (skin, lymph nodes, liver, spleen, bone marrow), where they produce and release certain biologically active substances in sufficient quantity to cause dermatographism, pruritus, bronchial spasm, and peptic ulceration of the pylorus and stomach in addition to the symptoms already described. Recent attempts to correlate the signs and symptoms of systemic mastocytosis with the anatomy of the mast cell, its distribution, and its known biochemical contents have revealed that some symptoms and signs (e.g., development of osteoporosis and osteosclerosis or cognitive changes) cannot be explained by what is known about the pharmacologically active substances that can be made by the cell.[811] Despite the extensive infiltration of mast cells required to produce these abnormalities, prognosis usually is good, and the disease progresses to a malignant or "pseudoleukemic" phase in only a small number of patients. Because mast cells multiply and produce symptoms by release of their hormones, they, like enterochromaffin cells, have become the subject of intensive biochemical research.

Table 10-11. CLASSIFICATION OF MASTOCYTOSIS

Classification	Age at Time of Onset	Comment
Benign		
Solitary lesions (mastocytoma)	Birth or shortly after; rarely in adult	
Multiple lesions (urticaria pigmentosa)	Infancy or early childhood	
Multiple lesions	Late childhood, adolescence, or adulthood	Approximately 20% of cases progress to systemic mastocytosis
Malignant		
Systemic mastocytosis	Adulthood	May be associated with amyloidosis, Hodgkin's disease, or intestinal carcinoma

Biochemistry of the Mast Cell

Mast cells from different species have different biochemical capabilities.[932] The mast cells of all species are relatively large and contain cytoplasmic granules that stain metachromatically with thiazine dyes such as toluidine blue. Cells from several species synthesize heparin, 5-HT, histamine,[895] and kinins. They are able to take up and store dopamine and other catecholamines,[722] and they contain proteolytic enzymes, as well as tryptophan hydroxylase, phenylalanine hydroxylase, and carbonic anhydrase.[817, 822, 837] Human mast cells synthesize and store heparin and histamine and can manufacture kinins.[859] Recent data have revealed the elaborate biochemical potential of the mast cell for producing eosinophil chemotactic factor of anaphylaxis (ECF-A), ECF-oligopeptide, high MW neutrophilic chemotactic factors (NCF), chymase and macromolecular heparin. Each of these substances is released when noncytotoxic degranulation is initiated by immunologic mechanisms. In addition, when ECF-A and high MW NCF are released, three new substances are formed. They include SRS-A, a platelet activating factor (PAF) that can release serotonin from platelets, and a lipid chemotactic factor. Serotonin may be present in low concentrations in the mast cell, but it is not synthesized in the cell.[728] Despite the low concentration or complete absence of serotonin in the cells, trauma to the skin of patients with urticaria pigmentosa may result in increased excretion of 5-HIAA in the urine,[706] possibly caused indirectly by release of serotonin from platelets by PAF. Whether the human mast cell contains a kallikrein or releases kinin as a mediator of the flush and hypotension of systemic mastocytosis remains to be determined. Recent data, however, indicate that intravenous injection of epinephrine into patients with mastocytosis does not result in flushes.[979] Presumably, neither kallikrein nor bradykinin causes the spontaneous flushes. The physiologic and pathologic interrelationships between the biologically active contents of the mast cell have been reviewed.[830]

In patients with mastocytosis, the occurrence of urticaria, itching, diarrhea, nausea, vomiting, peptic ulceration of the pylorus and stomach, syncope, shock, and even malabsorption, correlates roughly with the release of histamine, and perhaps other mediators, that the mast cell contains.[676, 706] Heparin probably is released also,[676] judging from the prolonged clotting time of venous blood obtained directly from a lesion; apparently, however, it is not released in sufficient quantities to cause systemic blood-clotting abnormalities. When gross bleeding does occur in patients with mastocytosis, it can usually be attributed to thrombocytopenia associated with infiltration of the bone marrow by the cells.

No data indicate that the production and release of the mediators by the cell is abnormal. Normal mast cells depend on oxygen, glucose, compounds with disulfide linkage, magnesium, and a critical concentration of SH groups as requisites for release of histamine.[870, 895] Degranulation of normal cells can occur during antigen-antibody reactions (predominantly IgE-related), during anaphylaxis, and after exposure to certain pharmacologic agents. Perhaps analogous situations occur in patients with mastocytosis whose gastrointestinal symptoms resemble celiac disease but apparently depend on degranulation of the mast cells.[630] Whether any of these mechanisms are involved in the release of histamine in mastocytosis is not known. Perhaps once histamine is released, other vasoactive substances (e.g., serotonin, kinins) are liberated from normal tissues and contribute to the symptoms. As with the carcinoid syndrome, it cannot be assumed that all the biochemical mediators of the symptoms in mastocytosis have been identified.

Diagnosis and Treatment

The disease should be suspected in any patient with flushing, tachycardia, gastrointestinal complaints, and headaches. The demonstration of excessive amounts of histamine or its metabolite, 1,4-methylimidazole acetic acid, in the urine will help to confirm the diagnosis. A definitive diagnosis, however, must be based on histologic examination of a biopsy specimen of the red-brown macules or slightly raised papules. Repeated biopsies may be required to detect the characteristic extensive concentrations of mast cells in the upper corium. When the disease is widespread (systemic mastocytosis), the cells will be found in a variety of organs of the reticuloendothelial system. If bone is involved, either discrete isolated lytic or sclerotic lesions or generalized osteoporosis or osteosclerosis may be present. Such bone involvement is associated at times with bone pain, anemia secondary to hypoplasia of cellular elements, or bleeding secondary to thrombocytopenia.

Because the disease usually is self-limiting, symptomatic treatment is often sufficient. Since there is no evidence to indicate that the abnormality in patients with mastocytosis is anything more than an increase in the number of mast cells, most investigators have assumed that their functions can be controlled in a manner that would control normal cells. Thus, it seems prudent for patients to avoid sensitizing agents and for physicians to prevent unnecessary inflammatory lesions[758] or skin trauma.[760, 761] Drugs that can release histamine should be avoided (e.g., opium alkaloids, and perhaps corticosteroids[624]). Additional measures that might be tried in these patients include attempts to increase the cAMP content of their mast cells.[663, 812]

Use of β-adrenergic agonists such as isoproterenol might reduce bronchospasm and at the same time increase the cAMP content of the cells, thus reducing the release of a host of intracellular substances that might mediate some symptoms of the disease. The E series of the prostaglandins theoretically could have the same effects on the cells, but they have not been evaluated in patients with the disease. Induction of relative hypoxia, hypoglycemia, or hypomagnesemia might theoretically limit the release of the contents of the mast cells.[668] These measures are untested and unevaluated and carry potential risks to the patient, however. Continued hypomagnesemia also might prevent the reaccumulation of histamine in the mast cell.

A recent double-blind and controlled crossover study in which disodium chromoglycate was administered to several patients with systemic mastocytosis clearly demonstrated the efficacy of this drug.[952] The dominant positive effects were to ameliorate the gastrointestinal symptoms, presumably because the highest concentrations of the drug went to the gut. Although the drug is presumed to produce some effects by inhibiting the calcium-dependent coupled activation-secretion response of mast cells by blocking calcium channels, its efficacy in patients with mast cell disease is not associated with return to normal of the concentrations of histamine in blood or urine. Presumably, other undefined properties of the drug contribute positive effects. Drugs that control the exocytotic processes of the cell (e.g., colchicine) have not yet been evaluated in this disease. Neither have drugs that prevent formation of histamine (e.g., inhibitors of histidine decarboxylase) been found to be helpful in the management of patients with mastocytosis.

If it is eventually found that the release of mediators from mast cells cannot be prevented adequately, the physician must resort to adjunctive or exclusive treatment that indirectly or directly blocks the effects of circulating histamine. In the former category, isoproterenol or other bronchodilators may antagonize bronchospasm; norepinephrine, phenylephrine, or other vasoconstrictors may antagonize hypotension and shock; antacids can neutralize the effects of histamine-induced secretion of gastric acid; and antispasmotics could reverse some of the effects of hypermotility of the gut. Nevertheless, these drugs are not ideal as long-term therapeutic agents for patients with systemic mastocytosis, and a great deal of recent attention has been focused on the use of competitive antagonists of histamine for patients whose diseases are caused by excessive effects of histamine.

The general pharmacologic properties of histamine were described in a preceding section. In patients with systemic mastocytosis we would expect H_1 effects to mediate the symptoms and signs related to contraction of the stomach and ileum, to bronchoconstriction, to some aspects of vasodilation and increased vascular permeability, and to those actions that invoke the synthesis and subsequent effects of prostaglandins.[683, 803, 903] Thus, conventional antihistaminics that contain a substituted ethylamine moiety and tertiary amino groups linked to two aromatic substituents (e.g., mepyramine, diphenhydramine, and tripelennamine) would be expected to and do competitively block a substantial number of these effects.

However, the effects of histamine on the H_2 receptors can also be clinically important and can lead to expression of impressive and debilitating features of the disease.[656] These could include the effects of histamine on uterine contraction, chronotropic effects on the heart, provocation of ulcers by excessive secretion of gastric acid, vasodilation and increased vascular permeability in addition to the H_1 effects, and alteration of the immune and inflammatory effects of leukocytes. Cimetidine (an H_2 blocker) reverses these actions on the basis of competitive blockade. But the lesson we have learned in controlling the histamine-induced flush of patients with gastric carcinoid tumor probably should be applied to patients with systemic mastocytosis. Both H_1 and H_2 blockers are required to nullify the vascular effects of histamine. They probably should be given simultaneously if the vascular-related effects of histamine are causing severe symptoms in patients with mastocytosis.

Words of caution seem appropriate. Largely because mastocytosis is so rare, we do not know the efficacy of antihistaminics. Theoretically, they do have a role, but there are other facts that must be considered in this theory. Most patients with the disease have consistently elevated concentrations of histamine in their plasma, even when symptoms are not prominent. Perhaps tachyphylaxis, or the constant stimulation by the autacoid (analogous to the effects of isoproterenol on β-adrenergic receptors), could explain why symptoms do not directly correlate with absolute concentrations of histamine but may be more related to the flux in those concentrations. In addition, not all of the effects of histamine are detrimental. For example, histamine can inhibit its own release from mast cells.

Thus, when the physician chooses to use antihistaminics for patients with mastocytosis, he must be prepared to look for and to manage the possible negative consequences of withdrawal. The prolonged use of antihistaminics may have the same effect on histamine receptors as antagonists of β-adrenergic receptors (e.g., propranolol) appear to have on adrenergic receptors. Use of propranolol will encourage build-up of adrenergic receptors, which, once the blockers are discontinued, may lead to inordinate responses to relatively low concentrations of agonists. If the same appears to be true of the effects of antagonists of histamine on receptor build-up, then sudden withdrawal of H_1 and H_2 blockers could lead to inordinate histamine-related symptoms if the concentrations of histamine are high in the region of the receptors. Those concentrations would be expected to be higher after use of H_2 blockers than before their use because the histamine-induced feedback inhibition of release would be nullified by the H_2 blockers. Therefore the patient should be warned to keep a good supply of H_1 and H_2 blockers available and to discontinue their use only under the advice of the physician. If discontinuation is necessary, the drug should be withdrawn gradually and, again, only under the supervision of the physician. If the symptoms return as the drugs are tapered, the doses should be increased slightly but it would still be likely that over time they could be discontinued. Such discontinuation would be dependent upon re-equilibration of receptor number toward normal and re-establishment of limited release of histamine by virtue of its direct effects on the mast cell.

Protamine is of little value in therapy because the amount of heparin released is usually not sufficient to cause bleeding. Splenectomy is indicated if hypersplenism threatens life.

No known treatment has altered the prognosis of systemic mastocytosis. Although radiation therapy may ameliorate pain in sites of local bone or soft tissue involvement, neither radiation nor antitumor agents have produced objective long-term benefits; in addition, such measures may result in massive release of histamine and in death.

REFERENCES

1. Abramsky, O., Aharonov, A., et al.: *Arch. Neurol. 32*:684, 1975.
2. Adler-Grashinsky, E., and Langer, S. Z.: *Br. J. Pharmacol. 53*:43, 1975.
3. Agee, O. F., Kaude, J., et al.: *Acta Radiol. 14*:545, 1973.
4. Ahlquist, R. P., and Levy, B.: *J. Pharmacol. Exp. Ther. 127*:146, 1959.
5. Ahlquist, R. P.: *Am. J. Physiol. 153*:586, 1948.
6. Alberts, P., and Bartfai, T.: *J. Biol. Chem. 251*:1543, 1976.
7. Alexander, N., and Velasquez, M. T.: In *Proceedings of the Fourth International Catecholamine Symposium.* Vol. 1. Usdin, E., Kopin, I. J., et al. (eds.), New York, Pergamon Press, 1978, p. 903.
8. Alexander, R. W., Cooper, B., et al.: *J. Clin. Invest. 61*:1136, 1978.
9. Almon, R. R., Andrew, C. G., et al.: *Science 186*:55, 1974.
10. Anton-Tay, F., Pelham, R. W., et al.: *Endocrinology 84*:1489, 1969.
11. Aquilonius, S. M.: In *Cholinergic Mechanisms and Psychopharmacology.* Jenden, D. J. (ed.), New York, Plenum Press, 1977, p. 817.
12. Assem, E. S. K., Pickup, P. M., et al.: *Br. J. Pharmacol. 39*:212P, 1970.
13. Assem, E. S. K., and Schild, H. O.: *Br. J. Pharmacol. 42*:620, 1971.
14. Aterman, K., and Schueller, E. F.: *Am. J. Dis. Child. 120*:217, 1970.
15. Atlas, D., and Levitzki, A.: *Proc. Natl. Acad. Sci. USA 74*:5290, 1977.
16. Atlas, D., and Levitzki, A.: *Biochem. Biophys. Res. Commun. 69*:397, 1976.
17. Atlas, D., Steer, M. L., et al.: *Proc. Natl. Acad. Sci. USA 73*:1921, 1976.
18. Atuk, N. O., and Westfall, T. C.: *Lancet 1*:259, 1977.
19. Atuk, N. O., Kuldeep, T., et al.: *Arch. Intern. Med. 137*:1073, 1977.
20. Aunis, D., Miras-Portugal, M.-T., et al.: *Clin. Chim. Acta 70*:455, 1976.
21. Aurbach, G. D., Fedak, S. A., et al.: *Science 185*:1223, 1974.
22. Hirata, F., Strittmatter, W. J., et al.: In *Proceedings of the Fourth International Catecholamine Symposium.* Vol. 1. Usdin, E., Kopin, I. J., et al. (eds.), New York, Pergamon Press, 1978, p. 501.
23. Axelrod, J.: *J. Biol. Chem. 237*:1657, 1962.
24. Axelrod, J.: In *Clinical Chemistry of Monamines.* Varley, H., and Gowenlock, A. H. (eds.), New York, American Elsevier Publishing Company, 1963, p. 5.
25. Axelrod, J., Weil-Malherbe, H., et al.: *J. Pharmacol. Exp. Ther. 127*:251, 1959.
26. Baer, L.: *Bull. N. Y. Acad. Med. 52*:690, 1976.
27. Barontini de Gutiérrez Moyano, M., Bergadá, C., et al.: *J. Pediatr. 77*:239, 1970.
28. Bartholini, G., Kuruma, I., et al.: *Nature* (Lond.) *230*:533, 1971.
29. Baylin, S. B., Gann, D. S., et al.: *Science 193*:321, 1976.
30. Becker, J. M., Schneider, K. M., et al.: *Progr. Clin. Cancer 4*:382, 1970.
31. Belleau, B.: *Pharmacol. Rev. 18*:131, 1966.
32. Bennett, J. P., Jr., and Snyder, S. H.: *Fed. Proc. 37*:137, 1978.
33. Bennett, M. V. L.: *Annu. Rev. Physiol. 32*:471, 1970.
34. Berenyi, M. R., Singh, G., et al.: *Arch. Pathol. Lab. Med. 101*:32, 1977.
35. Berkowitz, B. A., Tarver, J. H., et al.: *J. Pharmacol. Exp. Ther. 177*:119, 1971.
36. Berthelsen, S., and Pettinger, W. A.: *Life. Sci. 21*:595, 1977.
37. Besson, M. J., Cheramy, A., et al.: *Proc. Natl. Acad. Sci. USA 62*:741, 1969.

38. Biglieri, E. G., and McIlroy, M. B.: *Circulation 33*:78, 1966.
39. Bilezikian, J. P., Spiegel, A. M., et al.: *Mol. Pharmacol. 13*:786, 1977a.
40. Bilezikian, J. P., Spiegel, A. M., et al.: *Mol. Pharmacol. 13*:775, 1977b.
41. Birdsall, N. J. M., Burgen, A. S. V., et al.: In *Receptors.* Jacob, J. (ed.), New York, Pergamon Press, 1979, p. 23.
42. Birdsall, N. J. M., Burgen, A. S. V., et al.: *Mol. Pharmacol 14*:723, 1978a.
43. Birdsall, N. J. M., Burgen, A. S. V., et al.: In *Cholinergic Mechanisms and Psychopharmacology.* Jenden, D. J. (ed.), New York, Plenum Press, 1978b. p. 25.
44. Birks, R. I., and MacIntosh, F. C.: *Can. J. Biochem. 39*:787, 1961.
45. Biskind, G. R., Meyer, M. A., et al.: *J. Clin. Endocrinol., 1*:113, 1941.
46. Bittner, G. D., and Kennedy, D.: *J. Cell Biol. 47*:585, 1970.
47. Blaschke, T. F., and Melmon, K. L.: In *The Pharmacological Basis of Therapeutics.* 6th ed. Goodman, L. S., Gilman, A., et al. (eds.), New York, Macmillan Company, 1980, Ch. 32, (in press).
48. Blaschko, H., and Welch, A. D.: *Arch. Exp. Pathol. Pharmakol. 219*:17, 1953.
49. Bloom, D. A., and Fonkalsrud, E. W.: *J. Pediatr. Surg. 9*:179, 1974.
50. Blum, J. W., Fischer, J. A., et al.: *J. Clin. Invest. 61*:1113, 1978.
51. Boadle, M. D., Hughes, J., et al.: *Nature 222*:987, 1969.
52. Boijsen, E., Williams, C. M., et al.: *Am. J. Roentgenol. Radium Ther. Nucl. Med. 98*:225, 1966.
53. Bourne, H. R., Lichtenstein, L. M., et al.: *Science 184*:19, 1974.
54. Bourne, H. R., and Melmon, K. L.: *Ration. Drug. Ther. 5*:#4, 1971.
55. Bourne, H. R., Thomson, P., et al.: *Arch. Intern. Med. 125*:1063, 1970.
56. Braham, J.: *Br. Med. J. 2*:540, 1970.
57. Bravo, E. L., Tarazi, R. C., et al.: *N. Engl. J. Med. 301*:682, 1979.
58. Brimblecombe, R. W.: *Drug Actions on Cholinergic Systems.* Baltimore, University Park Press, 1974.
59. Broberger, O., and Zetterstrom, R.: *J. Pediatr. 59*:215, 1961.
60. Brody, I. A.: *J.A.M.A. 169*:1749, 1959.
61. Brown, E. M., Fedak, S. A., et al.: *J. Biol. Chem. 251*:1239, 1976.
62. Brown, G. L., and Gillespie, J. S.: *J. Physiol. 138*:81, 1957.
63. Brownstein, M., Holz, R., et al.: *J. Pharmacol. Exp. Ther. 186*:109, 1973.
64. Brunjes, S., Johns, V. J., Jr., et al.: *N. Engl. J. Med. 262*:393, 1960.
65. Buckingham, J. M., Howard, F. M., et al.: *Ann. Surg. 184*:543, 1976.
66. Burke, W. J., Davis, J. W., et al.: In *Proceedings of the Fourth International Catecholamine Symposium.* Vol. 1. Usdin, E., Kopin, I. J., et al. (eds.), New York, Pergamon Press, 1978, p. 168.
67. Burn, J. H.: *Nature* (Lond.) *231*:237, 1971.
68. Burn, J. H., and Rand, M. J.: *Br. J. Pharmacol. 15*:56, 1960.
69. Burn, J. H., and Rand, M. J.: *J. Physiol.* (Lond.) *144*:314, 1958.
70. Bylund, D. B., Tellez-Inon, M. T., et al.: *Life Sci. 21*:403, 1977.
71. Campbell, H., and Bramwell, E.: *Brain 23*:277, 1900.
72. Campos, H. R., and Crout, J. R.: *Fed. Proc. 29*:545, 1970.
73. Cannon, W. B., and Rosenbleuth, A.: *Autonomic Neuroeffector Systems.* New York, Macmillan Publishing Company, 1948.
74. Carey, R. M., Thorner, M. O., et al.: *J. Clin. Invest. 63*:727, 1979.
75. Carlsson, A., Lundberg, P., et al.: *J. Pharmacol. Exp. Ther. 158*:175, 1967.
76. Carney, J. A., and Hayles, A. B.: *Mayo Clin. Proc. 52*:543, 1977.
77. Carney, J. A., Sizemore, G. W., et al.: *Am. J. Clin. Pathol. 66*:279, 1976a.
78. Carney, J. A., Go, V. L. W., et al.: *N. Engl. J. Med. 295*:1287, 1976b.
79. Cartaud, J., Benedetti, E. C., et al.: *J. Cell Sci. 29*:313, 1978.
80. Case Reports of the Massachusetts General Hospital. *N. Engl. J. Med. 293*:1085, 1975.
81. Chang, C. C., and Lee, C. Y.: *Arch. Int. Pharmacodyn. Ther. 144*:241, 1963.
82. Chang, H. C., and Gaddum, J. H.: *J. Physiol.* (Lond.) *79*:255, 1933.
83. Changeux, J.-P., Kasai, M., et al.: *Proc. Natl. Acad. Sci. USA 67*:1241, 1970.
84. Charness, M. E., Bylund, D. B., et al.: *Life Sci.* 1979 (in press).
85. Chatten, J., and Voorhess, M. L.: *N. Engl. J. Med. 277*:1230, 1967.
86. Cheng, T. O., and Bashour, T. T.: *Chest 70*:397, 1976.
87. Christenson, R., Smith, C. W., et al.: *Am. J. Roentgenol. Radium Ther. Nucl. Med. 126*:567, 1976.
88. Ciraldi, T., and Marinetti, G. V.: *Biochem. Biophys. Res. Commun. 74*:984, 1977.
89. Ciaranello, R. D., Hoffman, H. J., et al.: *J. Biol. Chem. 249*:4528, 1974.
90. Ciaranello, R. D., Wooten, C. F., et al.: *J. Biol. Chem. 250*:3204, 1975.
91. Ciaranello, R. D., Wooten, G. F., et al.: *Brain Res. 113*:349, 1976.
92. Ciaranello, R. D.: In *Proceedings of the Fourth International Catecholamine Symposium.* Vol. 1. Usdin, E., Kopin, I. J., et al. (eds.), New York, Pergamon Press, 1978, p. 162.
93. Cohen, D. H., and Ratner, M.: *Science 168*:854, 1970.
94. Cohn, J.: *N. Engl. J. Med. 275*:643, 1966.
95. Comroe, J. H., Jr.: *Retrospectroscope. Insights into Medical Discovery.* Menlo Park, CA, Von Gehr Press, 1977.
96. Cooke, J. D., Okamoto, K., et al.: *J. Physiol.* (Lond.) *228*:459, 1973. (See also immediately preceding papers by same group on pages 377, 407, and 435.)
97. Cottrell, G. A., Powell, B., et al.: *Br. J. Pharmacol. 40*:866, 1970.
98. Cotzias, G. C.: *Hosp. Pract.* 35, 1969.
99. Cotzias, G. C., and Papavasiliou, P. S.: *J.A.M.A. 207*:1353, 1969.
100. Cotzias, G. C., Papavasiliou, P. S., et al.: *N. Engl. J. Med. 282*:31, 1970.
101. Coyle, J. T., and Axelrod, J.: *J. Neurochem. 18*:2061, 1971.
102. Crandell, D. L., and Myers, R. T.: *J.A.M.A. 187*:12, 1964.
103. Creveling, C. R., Daly, J., et al.: *Biochem. Pharmacol. 17*:65, 1968.
104. Crout, J. R.: In *Hormones and Hypertension.* Manger, W. M. (ed.), Springfield, Ill., Charles C Thomas, 1966, p. 3.
105. Crout, J. R.: In *Standard Methods of the American Association of Clinical Chemists.* Vol. III. Seligson, D. (ed.), New York, Academic Press, Inc., 1960, p. 62.
106. Crout, J. R.: *Pharmacol. Rev. 18*:651, 1966.
107. Crout, J. R., and Brown, B. R., Jr.: *Anesthesiology 30*:29, 1969.
108. Crout, J. R., Pisano, J. J., et al.: *Am. Heart J. 61*:375, 1961.
109. Crout, J. R., and Sjoerdsma, A.: *J. Clin. Invest. 43*:94, 1964.
110. Crowe, J., Bottomly, K., et al.: *Endoscopy 9*:58, 1977.
111. Cryer, P. E.: *Diabetes 25*:1071, 1976.
112. Cryer, P. E.: *Arch. Intern. Med. 137*:783, 1977.
113. Csánky-Treels, J. C., Lawick, W. P., et al.: *Anaesthesia 31*:60, 1976.
114. Cubeddu, L. X., and Weiner, W.: *J. Pharmacol. Exp. Ther. 192*:1, 1975a.
115. Cubeddu, L. X., and Weiner, N.: *J. Pharmacol. Exp. Ther. 193*:105, 1975b.
116. Cubeddu, L. X., Langer, S. Z., et al.: *J. Pharmacol. Exp. Ther. 188*:368, 1974.
117. Daggett, P., and Franks, S.: *Br. Med. J. 1*:84, 1977.
118. Dale, H. H.: *Adventures in Physiology.* London, Wellcome Trust, 1965.
119. Dale, H. H.: *J. Pharmacol. Exp. Ther. 6*:147, 1914.
120. D'Angio, G. J., Evans, A. E., et al.: *Lancet 1*:1046, 1971.
121. Da Prada, M., Picotti, G. B., et al.: In *Proceedings of the Fourth International Catecholamine Symposium.* Vol. 1. Usdin, E., Kopin, I. J., et al. (eds.), New York, Pergamon Press, 1978, p. 915.
122. Davila, D., and Khairallah, Ph.A.: *Arch. Int. Pharmacodyn. Ther. 193*:307, 1971.
123. de Champlain, J., Cousineau, D., et al.: In *Proceedings of the Fourth International Catecholamine Symposium.* Vol. 1. Usdin, E., Kopin, I. J., et al. (eds.), New York, Pergamon Press, 1978, p. 909.
124. De Graeff, J., and Horak, B. J. V.: *Acta Med. Scand. 176*:583, 1964.
125. Deguichi, T., and Axelrod, J.: *Proc. Natl. Acad. Sci. USA 70*:2411, 1973.
126. Delaney, J. P., and Paritzky, A. Z.: *N. Engl. J. Med. 280*:1394, 1969.
127. De Plaen, J. F., Boemer, F., et al.: *Br. Med. J. 2*:734, 1976.
128. De Potter, W. P., Chubb, I. W., et al.: *Arch. Int. Pharmacodyn. Ther. 193*:191, 1971.
129. DeQuattro, V., Margolin, A. H., et al.: *J. Clin. Endocrinol. 30*:138, 1970.
130. DeQuattro, V., and Sjoerdsma, A.: *J. Clin. Invest. 47*:2359, 1968.
131. De Robertis, E., and Bennett, H. S.: *J. Biophys. Biochem. Cytol. 1*:47, 1955.
132. De Vellis, J., and Brooker, G.: *Science 186*:1221, 1974.
133. Dionne, V. E., Steinbach, J. H., et al.: *J. Physiol.* (Lond.) *281*:421, 1978.
134. Dixon, W. E.: *Med. Mag.* (Lond.) *16*:454, 1907.
135. Dixon, W. R., Mosimann, W. F., et al.: *J. Pharmacol. Exp. Ther. 209*:196, 1979.
136. Dolly, J. O., and Barnard, E. A.: *Biochemistry 16*:5053, 1977.
137. Dolphin, A., Adrien, J., et al.: *Mol. Pharmacol. 15*:1, 1979.
138. Dorris, R. L., and Shore, P. A.: *J. Pharmacol. Exp. Ther. 179*:15, 1971.
139. Douglas, J. S., Lewis, A. J., et al.: *Eur. J. Pharmacol. 42*:195, 1977.
140. Douglas, W. W., and Rubin, R. P.: *J. Physiol.* (Lond.) *159*:40, 1961.
140a. Douglas, W. W.: In *The Pharmacological Basis of Therapeutics.* 6th ed. Goodman, L. S., Gilman, A., et al. (eds.), New York, Macmillan Company, 1980, Chs. 26 and 27 (in press).
141. Drachman, D. B.: *N. Engl. J. Med. 298*:136, 186, 1978.
142. Drachman, D. B., Angus, C. W., et al.: *N. Engl. J. Med. 298*:1117, 1978.
143. Drasin, H.: *West. J. Med. 128*:106, 1978.
144. Drazen, J. M., and Schneider, M. W.: *J. Clin. Invest. 61*:1441, 1978.
145. Dunn, F. G., De Carvalho, J. G. R., et al.: *N. Engl. J. Med. 295*:605, 1976.
146. Dunnette, J., and Weinshilboum, R.: In *Proceedings of the Fourth International Catecholamine Symposium.* Vol. 1. Usdin, E., Kopin, I. J., et al. (eds.), New York, Pergamon Press, 1978, p. 147.
147. Eccles, R. M., and Libet, B.: *J. Physiol.* (Lond.) *157*:484, 1961.

148. Edis, A. J., and Shepherd, J. T.: *Arch. Intern. Med. 125*:716, 1970.
149. Editorial: *Lancet 1*:939, 1977.
150. Eidelman, B. H., Mendelow, A. D., et al.: *Am. J. Physiol. 234*:(3):H300, 1978.
151. Elliot, T. R.: *J. Physiol.* (Lond.) *32*:401, 1905.
152. Elmqvist, D., Hoffman, W. W., et al.: *J. Physiol.* (Lond.) *174*:417, 1964.
153. Enero, M. A., Langer, S. Z., et al.: *Br. J. Pharmacol. 44*:672, 1972.
154. Engle, W. K.: *Ann. N.Y. Acad. Sci. 274*:623, 1976.
155. Engle, A. G., Lambert, E. H., et al.: *Mayo Clin. Proc. 52*:267, 1977.
156. Engelman, K., Horwitz, D., et al.: *N. Engl. J. Med. 278*:705, 1968.
157. Engelman, K., Horwitz, D., et al.: *J. Clin. Invest. 47*:577, 1968.
158. Engelman, K., Mueller, P. S., et al.: *N. Engl. J. Med. 270*:865, 1964.
159. Engelman, K., and Sjoerdsma, A.: *Ann. Intern. Med. 61*:229, 1964.
160. Engelman, K., and Sjoerdsma, A.: *J.A.M.A. 189*:81, 1964.
161. Engelman, K., and Sjoerdsma, A.: *Circ. Res. 18* (Suppl. 1):104, 1966.
162. Engelman, K., Watts, R. W. E., et al.: *Am. J. Med. 37*:839, 1964.
163. Enjalbert, A., Ruberg, M., et al.: *Nature* (Lond.) *280*:595, 1979.
164. Erdelyi, E., Ciaranello, R. D., et al.: In *Proceedings of the Fourth International Catecholamine Symposium.* Vol. 1. Usdin, E., Kopin, I. J., et al. (eds.), New York, Pergamon Press, 1978, p. 174.
165. Fain, J. N.: *Fed. Proc. 29*:1402, 1970.
166. Fambrough, D.: *Physiol. Rev. 59*:165, 1979.
167. Fambrough, D. M., Drachman, D. B., et al.: *Science 182*:293, 1973.
168. Faraj, B. A., Fulenwider, J. T., et al.: *J. Clin. Invest. 64*:413, 1979.
169. Farnebo, L.-O., and Hamberger, B.: *J. Pharm. Pharmacol. 26*:644, 1974.
170. Fatt, P., and Katz, B.: *J. Physiol.* (Lond.) *117*:109, 1952.
171. Fee, H. J., Fonkalsrud, E. W., et al.: *Ann. Surg. 185*:448, 1977.
172. Feldberg, W. S.: *Biographical Memoirs of Fellows of the Royal Society, London 16*:77, 1970.
173. Feldberg, W., and Krayer, O.: *Naunyn Schmiedebergs Arch. Pharmakol. 172*:170, 1933.
174. Feldman, J. M., and Lebovitz, H. E.: *J. Pharmacol. Exp. Ther. 179*:56, 1971.
175. Ferguson, R.: *Ann. Intern. Med. 82*:761, 1975.
176. Fertuck, H. C., and Salpeter, M. M.: *J. Cell. Biol. 69*:144, 1976.
177. Finklestein, J. Z., and Gilchrist, G. S.: *Calif. Med. 116*:27, 1972.
178. Finlay, G. D., Whitsett, T. L., et al.: *N. Engl. J. Med. 284*:865, 1971.
179. Fischer, J. E., Horst, D. W., et al.: *Nature* (Lond.) *207*:951, 1965.
180. Fledelius, H., and Eldrup-Jørgensen, P: *Br. J. Ophthalmol. 61*:240, 1977.
181. Forde, T. P., Yormak, S. S., et al.: *Am. Heart J. 76*:388, 1968.
182. Forsyth, R. P.: *Fed. Proc. 31*:1240, 1972.
183. Foster, K. G., Ginsburg, J., et al.: *Clin. Sci. 39*:823, 1970.
184. Franco-Morselli, R., Baudouin-Legros, M.: In *Programs and Abstracts for Proceedings of the Fourth International Catecholamine Symposium.* Vol. 1. Usdin, E., Kopin, I. J., et al. (eds.), New York, Pergamon Press, 1978, p. 54.
185. Franklin, T. J., and Twose, P. A.: *FEBS Lett. 66*:225, 1976.
186. Freed, C. R., Quintero, E., et al.: *Life Sci. 23*:313, 1978.
187. Froehner, S. C., Reiness, C. G., et al.: *J. Biol. Chem. 252*:8589, 1977.
188. Frontali, N., Ceccarelli, B., et al.: *J. Cell Biol. 68*:462, 1976.
189. Fuller, R. W., Perry, K. W., et al.: In *Proceedings of the Fourth International Catecholamine Symposium.* Vol 1. Usdin, E., Kopin, I. J., et al. (eds.), New York, Pergamon Press, 1978, p. 186.
190. Furchgott, R. F.: *Fed. Proc. 113*:178, 1978.
191. Furchgott, R. F.: In *Catecholamines.* (Handbook of Experimental Pharmacology, Vol. 33.) Blaschko, H., and Muscholl, E. (eds.), New York, Springer-Verlag, 1972, p. 283.
192. Furchgott, R. F.: *Fed. Proc. 29*:1352, 1970.
193. Galant, S. P., Duriseti, L., et al.: *N. Engl. J. Med.,* 1979, (in press).
194. Gallagher, J. P., and Shinnick-Gallagher, P.: *Science 198*:851, 1977.
195. Gewirtz, G। P., and Kopin, I. J.: *J. Pharmacol. Exp. Ther. 175*:514, 1970.
196. Ghose, R. R., Winsey, H. S., et al.: *Postgrad. Med. J. 52*:593, 1976.
197. Gibbs, M. K., Carney, J. A., et al.: *Ann. Surg. 185*:273, 1977.
198. Gibson, C. J., and Wurtman, R. J.: *Biochem. Pharmacol. 26*:1137, 1977.
199. Gitlow, S. E., Bertani, L. M., et al.: *Cancer 25*:1377, 1970.
200. Gitlow, S. E., Bertani, L. M., et al.: *Pediatrics 46*:513, 1970.
201. Gitlow, S. E., Pertsmlidis, D., et al.: *Am. Heart J. 82*:557, 1971.
202. Glaubiger, G., and Lefkowitz, R. J.: *Biochem. Biophys. Res. Commun. 78*:720, 1977.
203. Glenn, F., and Gray, G. F.: *Ann. Surg. 183*:578, 1976.
204. Goldberg, L. I., Hsieh, Y.-Y., et al.: *Prog. Cardiovasc. Dis. 19*:327, 1977.
205. Goldberg, L. I.: *Biochem. Pharmacol. 24*:651, 1975.
206. Goldfien, A.: *Anesthesiology 24*:462, 1963.
207. Goldstein, M., Sauter, A.: In *Proceedings of the Fourth International Catecholamine Symposium.* Vol. 1. Usdin, E., Kopin, I. J., et al. (eds.), New York, Pergamon Press, 1978, p. 159.
208. Goldstein, M., Anagnoste, B., et al.: *Science 160*:767, 1968.
209. Goldstein, M., Anagnoste, B., et al.: *Life Sci. 3*:763, 1964.
210. Goodall, McC., and Alton, H.: *J. Clin. Invest. 48*:2300, 1969a.
211. Goodall, McC., and Alton, H.: *J. Clin. Invest. 48*:1761, 1969b.
212. Goodall, McC., Gitlow, S. E., et al.: *J. Clin. Invest. 50*:2734, 1971.
213. Goodwin, F. K., Brodie, H. K., et al.: *Lancet 2*:908, 1970.
214. Gordon, M. A., Cohen, J. J., et al.: *Proc. Natl. Acad. Sci. USA 75*:2902, 1978.
215. Gözsy, B., and Kátó, L.: *Int. Arch. Allerg. 30*:553, 1966.
216. Greene, L. A.: *Nature* (Lond.) *268*:501, 1977.
217. Greene, L. A., and Rein, G.: *Nature* (Lond.) *268*:349, 1977a.
218. Greene, L. A., and Rein, G.: *Brain Res. 129*:247, 1977b.
219. Greenberg, R. E., and Gardner, L. I.: *J. Clin. Invest. 39*:1729, 1960.
220. Griesemer, E. C., Barsky, J., et al.: *Proc. Soc. Exp. Biol. Med. 84*:699, 1953.
221. Grob, D.: In *Cholinesterases and Anticholinesterase Agents.* (Handbook of Experimental Pharmacology, Vol. 15.) Koelle, G. B. (ed.), New York, Springer-Verlag, 1963a, p. 989.
222. Ibid., 1963b, p. 1028.
223. Grobecker, H., Saavedra, J. M., et al.: In *Proceedings of the Fourth International Catecholamine Symposium.* Vol. 1. Usdin, E., Kopin, I. J., et al. (eds.), New York, Pergamon Press, 1978, p. 906.
224. Grunewald, G. L., Vincek, W. C., et al.: In *Proceedings of the Fourth International Catecholamine Symposium.* Vol. 1. Usdin, E., Kopin, I. J., et al. (eds.), New York, Pergamon Press, 1978, p. 189.
225. Gutman, Y., and Boonyaviroj, P.: *Prostaglandins 12*:487, 1976.
226. Haggendahl, J.: In *Bayer Symposium II. New Aspects of Storage and Release Mechanisms of Catecholamines.* Schumann, H. J., and Kroneberg, G. (eds.), New York, Springer-Verlag, 1970, p. 100.
227. Hamilton, B. P. M., Cheikh, I. E., et al.: *Arch. Intern. Med. 137*:762, 1977.
228. Hanbauer, I., Kopin, I. J., et al.: *J. Pharmacol. Exp. Ther. 193*:95, 1975.
229. Hanbauer, I., Jacobowitz, D. M., et al.: *Br. J. Pharmacol. 50*:219, 1974.
230. Hanski, E., Rimon, G., et al.: *Biochemistry 18*:846, 1979.
231. Hanski, E., and Levitzki, A.: *Life Sci. 22*:53, 1978.
232. Harden, T. K., Wolfe, B. B., et al.: *J. Pharmacol. Exp. Ther. 203*:132, 1977.
233. Hardman, J. G., Robison, G. A., et al.: *Ann. Rev. Physiol. 33*:311, 1971.
234. Harrison, T. S.: *Johns Hopkins Med. J. 139*:137, 1976.
235. Harrison, T. S., Bartlett, J. D., et al.: *N. Engl. J. Med. 277*:725, 1967.
236. Heath, H., III, and Edis, A. J.: *Ann. Intern. Med. 91*:208, 1979.
237. Hedqvist, P., and Fredholm, B. B.: In *Proceedings of the Fourth International Catecholamine Symposium.* Vol. 1. Usdin, E., Kopin, I. J., et al. (eds.), New York, Pergamon Press, 1978, p. 256.
238. Heidmann, T., and Changeux, J. P.: *Annu. Rev. Biochem. 47*:317, 1978.
239. Heikkila, R., and Cohen, G.: *Science 172*:1257, 1971.
240. Heilbronn, E.: In *Cholinergic Mechanisms.* Waser, P. G. (ed.), New York, Raven Press, 1975, p. 343.
241. Heinemann, S., Bevan, S., et al.: *Proc. Natl. Acad. Sci. USA 74*:3090, 1977.
242. Helle, K. B.: *Biochim. Biophys. Acta 245*:80, 1971.
243. Helle, K. B., and Brodtkorb, E.: *Biochim. Biophys. Acta 245*:94, 1971.
244. Henderson, W. R., Shelhamer, J. H., et al.: *N. Engl. J. Med. 300*:642, 1979.
245. Hermann, H., and Mornex, R.: *Human Tumours Secreting Catecholamines.* New York, Pergamon Press, 1964.
246. Hertting, G., Axelrod, J., et al.: *Nature* (Lond.) *189*:66, 1961.
247. Hertting, G., Axelrod, J., et al.: *J. Pharmacol. Exp. Ther. 134*:146, 1961.
248. Hertting, G., Potter, L. T., et al.: *J. Pharmacol. Exp. Ther. 136*:289, 1962.
249. Hickler, R. B., and Vandam, L. D.: *Anesthesiology 33*:214, 1970.
250. Hoak, J. C., Warner, E. D., et al.: *Arch. Pathol. 87*:332, 1969.
251. Hollister, L. E.,: In *Clinical Pharmacology. Basic Principles in Therapeutics.* Melmon, K. L., and Morrelli, H. F. (eds.), New York, Macmillan Publishing Company, 1972, pp. 842, 874.
252. Holmstedt, B.: In *Cholinergic Mechanisms.* Waser, P. G. (ed.), New York, Raven Press, 1975, p. 1.
253. Holzbauer, M., and Vogt, M.: *J. Neurochem. 1*:8, 1956.
254. Horn, A. S., Coyle, J. T., et al.: *Mol. Pharmacol. 7*:66, 1971.
255. Horowitz, S. H., Genkins, G., et al.: *Neurology* (Minneap.) *26*:410, 1976.
256. Horton, W. A., Wong, V., et al.: *Arch. Intern. Med. 136*:769, 1976.
257. Houslay, M. D., and Tipton, K. F.: *Life Sci 19*:467, 1976.
258. Howard, F. M., Jr., Duane, D. D., et al.: *Ann. N. Y. Acad. Sci. 274*:596, 1976.
259. Howlett, A. C., Van Arsdale, P. M., et al.: *Mol. Pharmacol. 14*:531, 1978.

260. Hsu, C.-Y., Brooker, G., et al.: *Science 187*:1086, 1975.
261. Hulme, E. C., Birdsall, N. J. M., et al.: *Mol. Pharmacol. 14*:737, 1978.
262. Hunter, K. R., Boakes, A. J., et al.: *Br. Med. J. 3*:388, 1970.
263. Huttunen, J. K., Pispa, J., et al.: *Hypertension 1*:47, 1979.
264. Insel, P. A., and Stoolman, L. M., *Mol. Pharmacol. 14*:549, 1978.
265. Insel, P. A., Maguire, M. E., et al.: *Mol. Pharmacol. 12*:1062, 1976.
266. Iuvone, P. M., Galli, C. L., et al.: *Mol. Pharmacol. 14*:1212, 1978.
267. Iversen, L. L.: *Eur. J. Pharmacol. 10*:408, 1970.
268. Iversen, L. L., Glowinski, J., et al.: *Nature* (Lond.) *206*:1222, 1965.
269. Jacobs, T. P., Henry, D. P., et al.: *Am. J. Physiol. 234*:E600, 1978.
270. James, T. N., Bear, E. S., et al.: *Arch. Intern. Med. 125*:512, 1970.
271. Janssens, W. J., and Vanhoutte, P. M.: *Am. J. Physiol. 234*(4):H330, 1978.
272. Jenden, D. J.: In *Cholinergic Mechanisms.* Waser, P. G. (ed.), New York, Raven Press, 1975, p. 87.
273. Joh, T. H., Park, D. H., et al.: In *Proceedings of the Fourth International Catecholamine Symposium.* Vol. 1. Usdin, E., Kopin, I. J., et al. (eds.), New York, Pergamon Press, 1978, p. 43.
274. Johnson, G. I., and Bourne, H. R.: *Biochem. Biophys. Res. Commun. 78*:792, 1977.
275. Johnston, J. P.: *Biochem. Pharmacol. 17*:1285, 1968.
276. Jolly, F.: *Neurol. Zbl. 14*:34, 1895.
277. Juno, P.: *Minn. Med. 60*:22, 1977.
278. Kahn, C. R.: *J. Cell Biol. 70*:261, 1976.
279. Kalager, T., Glück, E., et al.: *Br. Med. J. 2*:21, 1977.
280. Kalsner, S.: *Circ. Res. 24*:383, 1969.
281. Kao, I., Drachman, D. B., et al.: *Science 193*:1256, 1976.
282. Kaplan, N. M., Kramer, N. J., et al.: *Arch. Intern. Med. 137*:190, 1977.
283. Karlin, A.: *Fed. Proc. 32*:1847, 1973.
284. Karlin, A.: *J. Gen. Physiol. 54*:245S, 1969.
285. Karlin, A., and Cowburn, D. W.: *Proc. Natl. Acad. Sci. USA 70*:3636, 1973.
286. Karow, A. M., Jr.: *Fed. Proc. 36*:2569, 1977.
287. Kaser, H.: *Pharmacol. Rev. 18*:659, 1966.
288. Kaslow, H. R., Farfel, Z., et al.: *Mol. Pharmacol. 15*:472, 1979.
289. Katz, B., and Miledi, R.: *Proc. R. Soc. Biol.* (Lond.) *161*:483, 1965.
290. Katz, B., and Miledi, R.: *J. Physiol.* (Lond.) *224*:665, 1972.
291. Katz, R. I., and Kopin, I. J.: *J. Pharmacol. Exp. Ther. 169*:229, 1969.
292. Kebabian, J. W., Zatz, M., et al.: *Proc. Natl. Acad. Sci. USA 72*:3735, 1975.
293. Keely, S. L., Jr., Lincoln, T. M., et al.: *Am. J. Physiol. 234*(4):H432, 1978.
294. Kehlet, H., Blichert-Toft, M., et al.: *Br. Med. J. 2*:665, 1976.
295. Klein, R. L., Yang, W.-H., et al.: In *Proceedings of the Fourth International Catecholamine Symposium.* Vol. 1. Usdin, E., Kopin, I. J., et al. (eds.), New York, Pergamon Press, 1978, p. 141.
296. Kline, I. K.: *Am. J. Pathol. 38*:539, 1961.
297. Kloog, Y., Egozi, Y., et al.: *Mol. Pharmacol 15*:545, 1979.
298. Knoll, J.: *J. Neural Transm. 43*:177, 1978.
299. Knoll, J.: In *Monoamine Oxidase and Its Inhibition.* (CIBA Foundation Symposium 39). New York, Excerpta Medica Foundation, 1976, p. 135.
300. Koelle, G. B.: In *The Nervous System.* Tower, D. B. (ed.), New York, Raven Press, 1975, p. 363.
301. Kogut, M. D., and Kaplan, S. A.: *J. Pediatr. 60*:694, 1962.
302. Kolata, G. B.: *Science 196*:747, 1977.
303. Komiskey, H. L., Bossart, J. F., et al.: *Proc. Natl. Acad. Sci. USA 75*:2641, 1978.
304. Kontras, S. B.: *Cancer Chemother. Rep. 16*:443, 1962.
305. Kopin, I. J.: *Annu. Rev. Pharmacol. 8*:377, 1968.
306. Kopin, I. J.: *Proc. 3rd Intl. Pharmacol. Mtg. 10*:83, 1966.
307. Kopin, I. J.: *Fed. Proc. 30*:904, 1971.
308. Kopin, I. J., Breese, G. R., et al.: *J. Pharmacol. Exp. Ther. 161*:271, 1968.
309. Kopin, I. J.: *Ann. Intern. Med. 85*:211, 1976.
310. Kopin, I. J.: *Ann. Intern. Med. 88*:671, 1978.
311. Kostrzewa, R. M., and Jacobowitz, D. M.: *Pharmacol. Rev. 26*:199, 1974.
312. Krnjević, K.: *Physiol. Rev. 54*:418, 1975.
313. Krnjević, K., Morris, M. E.: *Can. J. Physiol. Pharmacol. 52*:736, 1974.
314. Kvetnansky, R., Gewirtz, G. P., et al.: *Am. J. Physiol. 220*:928, 1971.
315. Kvetnansky, R., Gewirtz, G. P., et al.: *Endocrinology 89*:50, 1971.
316. Kvetnansky, P., Gewirtz, G. P., et al.: *Endocrinology 87*:1323, 1970.
317. Kvetnansky, R., Silbergeld, S., et al.: *Psychopharmacologia 20*:22, 1971.
318. Kvetnansky, R., Weise, V. K., et al.: *Endocrinology 87*:744, 1970.
319. LaBrosse, E. H.: *J. Clin. Endocrinol. 30*:580, 1970.
320. Lagercrantz, H., Bistoletti, P., et al.: In *Proceedings of the Fourth International Catecholamine Symposium.* Vol. 1. Usdin, E., Kopin, I. J., et al. (eds.), New York, Pergamon Press, 1978, p. 912.
321. Lance, J. W., and Hinterberger, H.: *Arch. Neurol. 33*:281, 1976.
322. Lands, A. M., Arnold, A., et al.: *Nature* (Lond.) *214*:597, 1967a.
323. Lands, A. M., Luduena, F. P., et al.: *Life Sci. 6*:2241, 1967b.
324. Landsberg, L. L., and Young, J. B.: *N. Engl. J. Med. 298*:1295, 1978.
325. Langer, S. Z.: *Br. J. Pharmacol. 60*:481, 1977.
326. Langley, J. N.: *J. Physiol.* (Lond.) *27*:237, 1901.
327. Langman, M. J. S.: *Arch. Dis. Child. 45*:385, 1970.
328. Leak, D., Carroll, J. J., et al.: *Can. Med. Assoc. J. 116*:371, 1977.
329. Lefebvre, P. J., Cession-Fossion, A., et al.: *Lancet 2*:1366, 1966.
330. Lefkowitz, R. J.: *Ann. Intern. Med. 91*:450, 1979.
331. Lefkowitz, R. L., and Haber, E.: *Proc. Natl. Acad. Sci. USA 68*:1773, 1971.
332. Lemberger, L.: *Fed. Proc. 37*:2176, 1978.
333. Leveston, S. A., Shah, S. D., et al.: *J. Clin. Invest. 64*:374, 1979.
334. Levey, G. S.: *Am. J. Med. 50*:413, 1971.
335. Levine, R. J., and Sjoerdsma, A.: *J. Pharmacol. 146*:42, 1964.
336. Levine, R. J., and Strauch, B. S.: *N. Engl. J. Med. 275*:946, 1966.
337. Levit, S. A., Sheps, S. G., et al.: *N. Engl. J. Med. 281*:805, 1969.
338. Levitt, M., Spector, S., et al.: *J. Pharmacol. Exp. Ther. 148*:1, 1965.
339. Levitzki, A.: *Biochem. Biophys. Res. Commun. 74*:1154, 1977a.
340. Levitzki, A.: In *Receptors and Recognition.* (Series A, Vol. 3). Cuatrecasas, P., and Greaves, M. F. (eds.), New York, John Wiley and Sons (Halstead press), 1977b, p. 2.
341. Levitzki, A.: In *Receptors and Recognition.* (Series A, Vol. 2). Cuatrecasas, P., and Greaves, M. F. (eds.), New York, John Wiley and Sons (Halstead Press), 1976, p. 201.
342. Lewandowsky, M.: *Zentbl. Physiol. 12*:599, 1898.
343. Libet, B.: *Fed. Proc. 29*:1945, 1970.
344. Libet, B., and Tosaka, T.: *Proc. Natl. Acad. Sci. USA 67*:667, 1970.
345. Lin, C.-S., Hurwitz, L., et al.: *J. Pharmacol. Exp. Ther. 203*:12, 1977.
346. Lindstrom, J. M., Seybold, M. E., et al.: *Neurology* (Minneap.) *26*:1054, 1976.
347. Loewi, O.: *Pflügers Arch. Ges. Physiol. 189*:239, 1921.
348. Loewi, O., and Narratil, E.: *Pflügers Arch. Ges. Physiol. 214*:678, 1926.
349. Louis, W. J., Doyle, A. E., et al.: *Br. Med. J. 4*:325, 1972.
350. Lowe, M. C., and Creveling, C. R.: In *Proceedings of the Fourth International Catecholamine Symposium.* Vol. 1. Usdin, E., Kopin, I. J., et al. (eds.), New York, Pergamon Press, 1978, p. 219.
351. Lulu, D. J.: *Arch. Surg. 99*:641, 1969.
352. Maas, J. W., and Landis, D. H.: *J. Pharmacol. Exp. Ther. 177*:600, 1971.
353. MacIntosh, F. C.: In *Basic Neurochemistry.* 2nd ed. Siegal, G. J., et al. (eds.), Boston, Little, Brown and Co., 1976, p. 180.
354. Manger, W. M., and Gifford, R. W., Jr.: *Cardiovasc. Med. 289*, 1978.
355. Manger, W. M., and Gifford, R. W.: *Pheochromocytoma.* New York, Springer-Verlag, 1977.
356. Mann, J. D., Johns, T. R., et al.: *Ann. N. Y. Acad. Sci. 274*:608, 1976.
357. Marciniak, D. L., Dobbins, D. E., et al.: *Am. J. Physiol. 234*(2):H180, 1978.
358. Margolius, H. S., Geller, R., et al.: *Lancet 2*:1063, 1971.
359. Martin, W. E.: *Lancet 1*:1050, 1971.
360. Mason, G. A., Hart-Mercer, I., et al.: *Lancet 2*:322, 1957.
361. Masserano, J., and Weiner, N.: In *Proceedings of the Fourth International Catecholamine Symposium.* Vol. 1. Usdin, E., Kopin, I. J., et al. (eds.), New York, Pergamon Press, 1978, p. 100.
362. Masters, C. L., Dawkins, R. L., et al.: *Am. J. Med. 63*:689, 1977.
363. McAfee, D. A., Schunderet, M., et al.: *Science 171*:1156, 1971.
364. McConnell, M. G., and Simpson, L. L.: *J. Pharmacol. Exp. Ther. 198*:507, 1976.
365. McNeil, B. J., Varady, P. D., et al.: *N. Engl. J. Med. 293*:216, 1975.
366. McQuillen, M. P., and Leone, M. G.: *Neurology* (Minneap.) *27*:1103, 1977.
367. Meaney, T. F., and Buonocore, E.: *Radiology 87*:309, 1966.
368. Melamed, E., and Lahav, M.: *Nature* (Lond.) *261*:420, 1976.
369. Melmon, K. L., and Insel, P. A.: *Johns Hopkins Med. J. 141*:15, 1977.
370. Melmon, K. L.: *Calif. Med. 117*:77, 1972.
371. Melmon, K. L., Bourne, H. R., et al.: *Science 177*:707, 1972.
372. Melmon, K. L., Goldfien, A., et al.: Unpublished data.
373. Melmon, K. L., and Rosen, S. W.: *Am. J. Med. 36*:595, 1964.
374. Melmon, K. L., Weinstein, J., et al.: *J. Clin. Invest. 53*:22, 1974.
375. Melmon, K. L., Verlander, M. S., et al.: In *Proceedings of the Fourth International Catecholamine Symposium.* Vol. 1. Usdin, E., Kopin, I. J. (eds.), New York, Pergamon Press, 1978, p. 474.
376. Mendlowitz, M., Wolf, R. L., et al.: *Am. Heart J. 79*:401, 1970.
377. Metz, S. A., Halter, J. B., et al.: *Ann. Intern.Med. 88*:189, 1978.
378. Mickey, J., Tate, R., et al.: *J. Biol. Chem. 250*:5727, 1975.
379. Mindell, H. J., and Kupic, E. A.: *Am. J. Roentgenol. 106*:208, 1969.
380. Minneman, K. P., Hegstrand, L. R., et al.: *Mol. Pharmacol. 15*:286, 1979.
381. Miyamori, I., Yamamoto, I., et al.: *Cancer 40*:402, 1977.
382. Miyamoto, M. D.: *Pharmacol. Rev. 29*:226, 1978.
383. Molinoff, P. B., and Brimijoin, S., et al.: *Proc. Natl. Acad. Sci. USA 66*:453, 1970.
384. Moorhead, E. L., Caldwell, J. R., et al.: *J.A.M.A. 196*:1107, 1966.

385. Moran, N. C.: *Ann. N. Y. Acad. Sci. 139*:545, 1967.
386. Moyano, M. B., Bergada, C., et al.: *J. Pediatr. 77*:239, 1970.
387. Mueller, R. A., and Axelrod, J.: *Circ. Res. 23*:771, 1968.
388. Mueller, R. A., Thoenen, H., et al.: *Science 158*:468, 1969.
389. Mueller, R. A., Thoenen, H., et al.: *Endocrinology 86*:751, 1970.
390. Mueller, R. A., Thoenen, H., et al.: *Eur. J. Pharmacol. 10*:51, 1970.
391. Mueller, R. A., Thoenen, H., et al.: *Mol. Pharmacol. 5*:463, 1969.
392. Mukherjee, C., and Lefkowitz, R. J.: *Proc. Natl. Acad. Sci. USA 73*:1494, 1976.
393. Mukherjee, C., Caron, M. G., et al.: *Proc. Natl. Acad. Sci. USA 72*:1945, 1975.
394. Mulder, A. H., de Langen, C. D. J., et al.: In *Proceedings of the Fourth International Catecholamine Symposium.* Vol. 1. Usdin, E., Kopin, I. J., et al. (eds.), New York, Pergamon Press, 1978, p. 259.
395. Murphy, D. L., Lake, C. R., et al.: In *Proceedings of the Fourth International Catecholamine Symposium.* Vol. 1. Usdin, E., Kopin, I. J., et al. (eds.), New York, Pergamon Press, 1978, p. 918.
396. Myers, M. G., and Arshinoff, S. A.: *J.A.M.A. 237*:2095, 1977.
397. Naftchi, N. E., Wooten, G. F., et al.: *Circ. Res. 35*:850, 1974.
398. Nagatsu, T., Yamamoto, T., et al.: *Biochim. Biophys. Acta 198*:210, 1970.
399. Nagy, J. I., Lee, T., et al.: *Nature* (Lond.) *274*:278, 1978.
400. Nahas, G. G., Zagury, D., et al.: *Am. J. Physiol. 213*:1186, 1967.
401. Nanda, R. N., Johnson, R. H., et al.: *Lancet 2*:1164, 1976.
402. Nastuk, W. L., and Levine, L.: *Proc. Soc. Exp. Biol. Med. 106*:502, 1961.
403. Nelson, P. G.: *Fed. Proc. 37*:1999, 1978.
404. Neubauer, B., and Christensen, N. J.: *Diabetes 25*:6, 1976.
405. Newman, K. D., Williams, L. T., et al.: *J. Clin. Invest. 61*:395, 1978.
406. Ng, L. K. Y., Chase, T. N., et al.: *Brain Res. 45*:499, 1972.
407. Nies, A.: In *Clinical Pharmacology. Basic Principles in Therapeutics.* Melmon, K. L., and Morrelli, H. F. (eds.), New York, Macmillan Publishing Company, 1978, p. 155.
408. Nies, A. S.: In *Clinical Pharmacology. Basic Principles in Therapeutics.* Melmon, K. L., and Morrelli, H. F. (eds.), New York, Macmillan Publishing Company, 1972, p. 142.
409. Nishi, S., and Koketsu, K.: *J. Neurophysiol. 31*:109, 1968.
410. Noble, M. D., Brown, T. H., et al.: *Proc. Natl. Acad. Sci. USA 75*:3488, 1978.
411. Oates, J. A., Gillespie, L., et al.: *Science 131*:1890, 1960.
412. Odell, W. D.: *Calif. Med. 117*:32, 1972.
413. Oka, M., Isosaki, M., et al.: In *Proceedings of the Fourth International Catecholamine Symposium.* Vol. 1. Usdin, E., Kopin, I. J., et al. (eds.), New York, Pergamon Press, 1978, p. 70.
414. O'Neal, L. W., Kipnis, D. M., et al.: *Cancer 21*:1219, 1968.
415. Oron, Y., Kellogg, J., et al.: *Mol. Pharmacol. 14*:1018, 1978.
416. Osborne, M. W., Wenger, J. J., et al.: *J. Pharmacol. Exp. Ther. 178*:517, 1971.
417. Osserman, K. E., and Genkins, G.: *Ann. N. Y. Acad. Sci. 135*:312, 1966.
418. Osserman, K. E. Foldes, F. F., et al.: In *Neuromuscular Blocking and Stimulating Agents.* Vol. 2. (International Encyclopedia of Pharmacology and Therapeutics: Section 14). Cheymol. J. (ed.), New York, Pergamon Press, 1972, p. 561.
419. Palaic, D., and Khairallah, P. A.: *Biochem. Pharmacol. 16*:2291, 1967.
420. Park, D. H., and Goldstein, M.: *Life Sci. 18*:55, 1976.
421. Parks, L. C., Watanabe, A. M., et al.: *Lancet 2*:1014, 1970.
422. Parthemore, J. G., Bronzert, D., et al.: *J. Clin. Endocrinol. 39*:108, 1974.
423. Passwell, J., Biochis, H., et al.: *Am. J. Dis. Child. 131*:1011, 1977.
424. Paton, D. M.: In *Proceedings of the Fourth International Catecholamine Symposium.* Vol. 1. Usdin, E., Kopin, I. J., et al. (eds.), New York, Pergamon Press, 1978, p. 253.
425. Patrick, J., and Stallcup, B.: *J. Biol. Chem. 252*:8629, 1977.
426. Patrick, J., and Lindstrom, J.: *Science 180*:871, 1973.
427. Patrick, J., Heinneman, S., et al.: *Annu. Rev. Neurosci. 1*:417, 1978.
428. Paul, M. I., Kvetnansky, R., et al.: *Endocrinology 88*:338, 1971.
429. Peach, M. J., Bumpus, F. M., et al.: *J. Pharmacol. Exp. Ther. 167*:291, 1969.
430. Peroutka, S. J., Greenberg, D. A., et al.: *Mol. Pharmacol. 14*:403, 1978.
431. Persson, T., and Waldeck, B.: *Eur. J. Pharmacol. 11*:315, 1970.
432. Pertsemlidis, D., Gitlow, S. E., et al.: *Ann. Surg. 169*:376, 1969.
433. Phyall, W., and Lovenberg, W.: In *Proceedings of the Fourth International Catecholamine Symposium.* Vol. 1. Usdin, E., Kopin, I. J., et al. (eds.), New York, Pergamon Press, 1978, p. 180.
434. Pinder, R. M.: *Nature* (Lond.) *228*:358, 1970.
435. Pisano, J. J.: *Clin. Chim. Acta 5*:406, 1960.
436. Pisano, J. J., Crout, J. R., et al.: *Clin. Chim. Acta 7*:285, 1962.
437. Poisner, A. M., and Bernstein, J.: *J. Pharmacol. Exp. Ther. 177*:102, 1971.
438. Potter, L., and Smith, D. S.: *Tissue Cell 9*:585, 1977.
439. Prichard, B. N. C.: *Br. J. Clin. Pharmacol. 5*:379, 1978.
440. Printz, M. P., Wallis, C. J., et al.: In *Proceedings of the Fourth International Catecholamine Symposium.* Vol. 2. Usdin, E., Kopin, I. J., et al. (eds.), New York, Pergamon Press, 1978, p. 1419.
441. Prout, B. J., and Wardell, W. M.: *Clin. Sci. 36*:109, 1969.
442. Pujol, J. F., McRae-Degueurce, A., et al.: In *Proceedings of the Fourth International Catecholamine Symposium.* Vol. 1. Usdin, E., Kopin, I. J., et al. (eds.), New York, Pergamon Press, 1978, p. 52.
443. Pumplin, D. W., and Reese, T. S.: *J. Physiol.* (Lond.) *273*:444, 1977.
444. Quenzer, L., Yahn, D., et al.: *J. Pharmacol. Exp. Ther. 208*:31, 1979.
445. Quickel, K. E., Jr., Feldman, J. M., et al.: *Endocrinology 89*:1295, 1971.
446. Quinton, P. M.: *Nature* (Lond.) *279*:549, 1979.
447. Raese, J. D., Edelman, A. M., et al.: In *Proceedings of the Fourth International Catecholamine Symposium.* Vol. 1. Usdin, E., Kopin, I. J., et al. (eds.), New York, Pergamon Press, 1978, p. 46.
448. Rao, N. S.: *Lancet 2*:470, 1970.
449. Rattan, S., and Goyal, R. K.: *Am. J. Physiol. 234*(3):E273, 1978.
450. Redick, J. A., Thomas, J. A., et al.: *Neuropharmacology 13*:1005, 1974.
451. Remen, L.: *Dt. Z. Nerv Heilk, 128*:66, 1932.
452. Remine, W. H., Chang, G. C., et al.: *Ann. Surg. 179*:740, 1974.
453. Rengo, F., Trimarco, B., et al.: *Am. J. Physiol. 234*(3):H305, 1978.
454. Reuter, S. R.: *N. Engl. J. Med. 278*:1423, 1968.
455. Richelson, E.: *Science 201*:69, 1978.
456. Rickenberg, H. V.: *Biochemistry of Mode and Action of Hormones.* (International Review of Biochemistry: Vol. 20). Baltimore, University Park Press, 1978.
457. Riederer, P., Youdim, M. B. H., et al.: In *Advances in Biochemical Psychopharmacology.* Vol. 19. Roberts, P. J., Woodruff, G. N., et al. (eds.), New York, Raven Press, 1978, p. 377.
458. Roberts, J. M., Insel, P. A., et al.: *Nature* (Lond.) *270*:624, 1977.
459. Robertson, D., Frölich, J. C., et al.: *N. Engl. J. Med. 298*:181, 1978.
460. Robinson, R. G., DeQuattro, V., et al.: *J. Pediatr. 91*:143, 1977.
461. Robinson, G. A., and Sutherland, E. W.: *Circ. Res. 27* (Suppl. 1):147, 1970.
462. Röckel, A., Heidland, A., et al.: *N. Engl. J. Med. 296*:50, 1977.
463. Roizen, M. F., Thoa, N. B., et al.: *Anesthesiology 44*:54, 1976.
464. Rosenstein, B. J., and Engelman, K.: *J. Pediatr. 63*:217, 1963.
465. Ross, E. J., Prichard, B. N. C., et al.: *Br. Med. J. 1*:191, 1967.
466. Ross, M. J., Klymkowsky, M. W., et al.: *J. Mol. Biol. 116*:635, 1977.
467. Rosse, W. F., and Waldmann, T. A.: *Blood 24*:739, 1964.
468. Rossi, P., Young, I. S., et al.: *J.A.M.A., 205*:547, 1968.
469. Rossier, J.: *Int. Rev. Neurobiol. 20*:283, 1977.
470. Roth, R. H., Stjarne, L., et al.: *J. Lab. Clin. Med. 72*:397, 1968.
471. Rubin, R. P.: *J. Physiol.* (Lond.) *202*:197, 1969.
472. Rubin, R. P.: *Pharmacol. Rev. 22*:389, 1970.
473. Rumack, B. H.: *Pediatrics 52*:449, 1973.
474. Sandler, M., and Youdim, M. B. H.: *Pharmacol. Rev. 24*:331, 1972.
475. Saxon, A., Stevens, R. H., et al.: *N. Engl. J. Med. 300*:700, 1979.
476. Schäfer, E. A.: *Lancet 1*:80, 1917.
477. Schenker, J. G., and Chowers, I.: *Survey 26*:739, 1971.
478. Schneider, F. H.: *J. Pharmacol. Exp. Ther. 177*:109, 1971.
479. Schneider, F. H., Smith, A. D., et al.: *Br. J. Pharmacol. 31*:94, 1967.
480. Schneider, H. P. G., and McCann, S. M.: *Endocrinology 86*:1127, 1970.
481. Schocken, D. D., and Roth, G. S.: *Nature* (Lond.) *267*:856, 1977.
482. Schonhofer, P. S., Skidmore, I. F., et al.: *Naunyn Schmiedebergs Arch. Pharm. 273*:267, 1972.
483. Schramm, M., Orly, J., et al.: *Nature* (Lond.) *268*:310, 1977.
484. Schumann, H. J.: *Klin. Wochenschr. 38*:11, 1960.
485. Schwarzmeier, J. D., and Gilman, A. G.: *J. Cyclic Nucleotide Res. 3*:227, 1977.
486. Scully, R. E., Galdabini, J. J., et al.: *N. Engl. J. Med. 293*:1085, 1975.
487. Sever, P. S.: *Lancet 1*:703, 1977.
488. Sevilla, N., and Levitzki, A.: *FEBS Lett. 76*:129, 1977.
489. Seybold, M. E., and Drachman, D. B.: *N. Engl. J. Med. 290*:81, 1974.
490. Shapiro, R. G.: *Br. Med. J. 3*:403, 1970.
491. Shear, M., Insel, P. A., et al.: *J. Biol. Chem. 251*:7572, 1976.
492. Shepherd, J. T.: *Fed. Proc. 37*:179, 1978.
493. Sheppard, J. R., Gormus, R., et al.: *Nature* (Lond.) *269*:693, 1977.
494. Sheps, S. G., Tyce, G. M., et al.: *Circulation 34*:473, 1966.
495. Shoback, D. (ed.): *Johns Hopkins Med. J. 139*:131, 1976.
496. Shorr, R. G., Dolly, J. O., et al.: *Nature* (Lond.) *274*:283, 1978.
497. Sivula, A.: *Acta Chir. Scand. 140*:334, 1974.
498. Sjoersma, A., Engelman, K., et al.: *Lancet 2*:1092, 1965.
499. Sjoersma, A., Engelman, K., et al.: *Ann. Intern. Med. 65*:1302, 1966.
500. Sjoersma, A., Vendsalu, A., et al.: *Circulation 28*:492, 1963.
501. Skidmore, I. F., Schonhofer, P. S., et al.: *Pharamacology 6*:330, 1971.
502. Smith, H. J., Roche, A. H. G., et al.: *Am. Heart. J. 91*:792, 1976.
503. Snyder, S. H.: *N. Engl. J. Med. 300*:465, 1979.

504. Sole, M. J., Van Loon, G. R., et al.: *Science 201*:620, 1978.
505. Sole, M. J., Wurtman, R. J., et al.: *J. Mol. Cell. Cardiol. 9*:225, 1977.
506. Sonnenblick, E. H., Frishman, W. H., et al.: *N. Engl. J. Med. 300*:17, 1979.
507. Spark, R. F., Connolly, P. B., et al.: *N. Engl. J. Med. 301*:416, 1979.
508. Spector, S.: *Pharmacol. Rev. 18*:599, 1966.
509. Spector, S., Sjoerdsma, A., et al.: *J. Pharmacol. Exp. Ther. 147*:86, 1965.
510. Spergel, G., Levy, L. J., et al.: *J.A.M.A. 211*:266, 1970.
511. Spiehler, V., Fairhurst, A. S., et al.: *Mol. Pharmacol. 14*:587, 1978.
512. Spitzer, R., Borrison, R., et al.: *Radiology 98*:577, 1971.
513. Sporn, J. R., Harden, T. K., et al.: *Science 194*:624, 1976.
514. Spring, D. B., and Palubinskas, A. J.: *Br. J. Radiol. 50*:596, 1977.
515. Stafford, A.: *Br. J. Pharmacol. 21*:361, 1963.
516. Stamenković, L., and Spierdijk, J.: *Anesthesia 31*:941, 1976.
517. Standaert, F. G., et al.: *Fed. Proc. 38*:2182, 1979.
518. Starke, K.: *Rev. Physiol. Biochem. Pharmacol. 77*:1, 1977.
519. Starke, K., and Altmann, K. P.: *Neuropharmacology 12*:339, 1973.
520. Starke, K.: *Naunyn Schmiedebergs Arch. Pharmacol. 274*:18, 1972.
521. Starke, K.: *Naturwissenschaften 58*:420, 1971.
522. Steel, C. M., French, E. B., et al.: *Br. J. Haematol. 21*:413, 1971.
523. Stjarne, L.: *Acta Physiol. Scand. 67*:441, 1966.
524. Stjarne, L., Von Euler, U. S., et al.: *Biochem. Pharmacol. 13*:809, 1964.
525. Stone, R. A., Lilley, J. J., et al.: *Clin. Endocrinol.* (Oxf.) *5*:181, 1976.
526. Straub, R. W., and Bolis, L.: *Cell Membrane Receptors for Drugs and Hormones: A Multidisciplinary Approach.* New York, Raven Press, 1978.
527. Sumikawa, K., and Amakata, Y.: *Anesthesiology 46*:359, 1977.
528. Sutherland, E. W., and Rall, T. W.: *Pharmacol. Rev. 12*:265, 1960.
529. Sutherland, E. W., and Robison, G. A.: *Pharmacol. Rev. 18*:145, 1966.
530. Sutow, W. W., Gehan, E. A., et al.: *Pediatrics 45*:800, 1970.
531. Sved, A. F., Fernstrom, J. D., et al.: *Proc. Natl. Acad. Sci. USA 76*:3511, 1979.
532. Svensson, T. H.: *Naunyn Schmiedebergs Arch. Pharmacol. 271*:111, 1971.
533. Szakacs, J. E., and Cannon, A.: *Am. J. Clin. Pathol. 30*:424, 1958.
534. Tallman, J. F., Saavedra, J. M., et al.: *J. Pharmacol. Exp. Ther. 199*:216, 1976.
535. Tashjian, A., Howland, B., et al.: *N. Engl. J. Med. 283*:890, 1970.
536. Taubman, I., Pearson, O. H., et al.: *Am. J. Med. 57*:953, 1974.
537. Telenius-Berg, M.: *Acta Med. Scand. 597* (Suppl.):1, 1976.
538. Thoa, N. B., Johnson, D. G., et al.: *Eur. J. Pharmacol. 15*:29, 1971.
539. Thoenen, H., and Tranzer, J. P.: *Annu. Rev. Pharmacol. 13*:169, 1973.
540. Thoenen, H., Haefely, W., et al.: *J. Pharmacol. Exp. Ther. 156*:246, 1967.
541. Thoenen, H., Mueller, R. A., et al.: *Nature* (Lond.) *221*:1264, 1969.
542. Thoenen, H., Mueller, R. A., et al.: *Proc. Natl. Acad. Sci. USA 65*:58, 1970.
543. Thoenen, H., Mueller, R. A., et al.: *J. Pharmacol. Exp. Ther. 169*:249, 1969.
544. Thomas, D. J. B., MacDougall, C. N., et al.: *Br. Med. J. 1*:688, 1977.
545. Thureson-Klein, Å., Klein, R. L., et al.: In *Proceedings of the Fourth International Catecholamine Symposium.* Vol. 1. Usdin, E., Kopin, I. J., et al. (eds.), New York, Pergamon Press, 1978, p. 262.
546. Tipton, K. F.: In *Handbook of Physiology*, Section 7: Endocrinology. Vol. VI. Blaschko, H., Sayers, G., et al. (eds.), American Physiological Society, Baltimore, Williams and Wilkins, 1975, p. 677.
547. Tissot, S. E., Gregg, F. J., et al.: *J.A.M.A. 182*:152, 1962.
548. Titeler, M., and Seeman, P.: *Proc. Natl. Acad. Sci. USA 75*:2249, 1978.
549. Tolkovsky, A. M., and Levitzki, A.: *Hormones and Cell Regulation 2*:89, 1978a.
550. Tolkovsky, A. M., and Levitzki, A.: *Biochemistry 17*:3795, 1978b.
551. Tolkovsky, A. M., and Levitzki, A.: *Biochemistry 17*:3811, 1978c.
552. Torchiana, M. L., Porter, C. C., et al.: *Arch. Int. Pharmacodyn. Ther. 174*:118, 1968.
553. Toyka, K. V., Drachman, D. B., et al.: *Science 190*:397, 1975.
554. Troncone, L., Galli, G., et al.: *Br. J. Radiol. 50*:340, 1977.
555. Trump, D. L., Livingston, J. N., et al.: *Cancer 40*:1526, 1977.
556. Tsai, B. S., and Lefkowitz, R. J.: *J. Pharmacol. Exp. Ther. 204*:606, 1978a.
557. Tsai, B. S., and Lefkowitz, R. J.: *Mol. Pharmacol. 14*:540, 1978b.
558. Tucker, R. M., and Labarthe, D. R.: *Mayo Clin. Proc. 52*:549, 1977.
559. Turner, B. B., Katz, R. J., et al.: In *Proceedings of the Fourth International Catecholamine Symposium.* Vol. 1. Usdin, E., Kopin, I. J., et al. (eds.), New York, Pergamon Press, 1978, p. 183.
560. Tuttle, R. R., Hillman, C. C., et al.: *Cardiovasc. Res. 10*:452, 1976.
561. Tuttle, R. R., and Mills, J.: *Circ. Res. 36*:185, 1975.
562. Tuynman, F. H. B., and van Voorthuisen, A. E.: *Radiologia Clin. 45*:202, 1976.

563. U'Prichard, D. C., Snyder, S. H.: *Eur. J. Pharmacol. 51*:145, 1978a.
564. U'Prichard, D. C., and Snyder, S. H.: *J. Biol. Chem. 253*:3444, 1978b.
565. U'Prichard, D. C., Charness, M. E., et al.: *Eur. J. Pharmacol. 50*:87, 1978.
566. Vance, J. E., Buchanan, K. D., et al.: *J. Clin. Endocrinol. 29*:911, 1969.
567. van Hoogdalem, P., Donker, A. J. M., et al.: *Acta Med. Scand. 201*:395, 1977.
568. Van Vliet, P. D., Burchell, H. B., et al.: *N. Engl. J. Med. 274*:1102, 1966.
569. Vassalle, M., Mandel, W. J., et al.: *Am. J. Physiol. 218*:115, 1970.
570. Venter, J. C.: *Mol. Pharmacol. 14*:562, 1978.
571. Vestal, R. E., Alastair, J. J., et al.: *Clin. Pharmacol. Ther. 26*:181, 1979.
572. Vetter, H., Vetter, W., et al.: *Am. J. Med. 60*:866, 1976.
573. Volle, R. L.: *Annu. Rev. Pharmacol. 9*:135, 1969.
574. *Am. J. Dis. Child. 119*:308, 1970 (by an author group).
575. von Euler, U. S., Lishajko, F., et al.: *Acta Physiol. Scand. 59*:495, 1963.
576. Von Studnitz, W.: *Scand. J. Clin. Lab. Invest. 12* (Suppl. 48):58, 1960.
577. Von Studnitz, W.: *Klin. Wochenschr. 40*:163, 1962.
578. von Voigtlander, P. F., and Moore, K. E.: *Science 174*:408, 1971.
579. Voorhess, M. L.: *Cancer 26*:146, 1970.
580. Vulliet, P. R., Langan, T. A., et al.: In *Proceedings of the Fourth International Catecholamine Symposium.* Vol. 1. Usdin, E., Kopin, I. J., et al. (eds.), New York, Pergamon Press, 1978, p. 94.
581. Walker, M. B.: *Lancet 1*:1200, 1934.
582. Walker, M. B.: *Proc. R. Soc. Med.* (Lond.) *28*:759, 1935.
583. Wallace, J. H., Hill, C. S., et al.: *Radiol. Clin. North Am. 8*:463, 1970.
584. Wang, G., Molinaro, S., et al.: *J. Biol. Chem. 253*:8507, 1978.
585. Waser, P. G. (ed.): *Cholinergic Mechanisms.* New York, Raven Press, 1975.
586. Watson, R. D. S., Hamilton, C. A., et al.: *Hypertension 1*:341, 1979.
587. Waymire, J. C., Haycock, J. W., et al.: In *Proceedings of the Fourth International Catecholamine Symposium.* Vol. 1. Usdin, E., Kopin, I. J., et al. (eds.), New York, Pergamon Press, 1978, p. 40.
588. Weight, F. F.: *Fed. Proc. 38*:2078, 1979.
589. Weight, F. F., Schulman, J. A., et al.: *Fed. Proc. 38*:2078, 1979.
590. Weight, F. F., Petzold, G., et al.: *Science 186*:942, 1974.
591. Weil-Malherbe, H., and van Buren, J. M.: *J. Lab. Clin. Med. 74*:305, 1969.
592. Weiland, G., and Taylor, P.: *Mol. Pharmacol. 15*:197, 1979.
593. Weiner, N.: In *The Pharmacological Basis of Therapeutics.* 6th ed. Goodman, L. S., Gilman, A., et al. (eds.), New York, Macmillan Company, 1980, Chs. 7, 8, and 9 (in press).
594. Weiner, N., Posiviata, M., et al.: In *Proceedings of the Fourth International Catecholamine Symposium.* Vol. 1. Usdin, E., Kopin, I. J., et al. (eds.), New York, Pergamon Press, 1978, p. 49.
595. Weinshilboum, R.: In *Proceedings of the Fourth International Catecholamine Symposium.* Vol. 1. Usdin, E., Kopin, I. J., et al. (eds.), New York, Pergamon Press, 1978, p. 216.
596. Weinstein, Y., Melmon, K. L., et al.: *J. Clin. Invest. 52*:1349, 1973.
597. Welsh, M. J., Heistad, D. D., et al.: *J. Clin. Invest. 61*:708, 1978.
598. Wells, S. A., Jr., and Ontjes, D. A.: *Annu. Rev. Med. 27*:263, 1976.
599. Wells, S. A., Jr., Ontjes, D. A., et al.: *Ann. Surg. 182*:362, 1975.
600. Westfall, T. C.: *Physiol. Rev. 57*:659, 1977.
601. Whitby, L. G., Hertting, G., et al.: *Nature* (Lond.) *187*:604, 1960.
602. Williams, L. T., and Lefkowitz, R. J.: *Receptor Binding Studies in Adrenergic Pharmacology.* New York, Raven Press, 1978.
603. Williams, L. T., Lefkowitz, R. J., et al.: *J. Biol. Chem. 252*:2787, 1977a.
604. Williams, L. T., Gore, T. B., et al.: *J. Clin. Invest. 59*:319, 1977b.
605. Williams, L. T., Snyderman, R., et al.: *J. Clin. Invest. 57*:149, 1976.
606. Williams, R. L., and Melmon, K. L.: In *Beta-adrenergic Blockade, A New Era in Cardiovascular Medicine.* New York, American Elsevier, 1978, p. 89
607. Winer, N., Chokshi, D. S., et al.: *Circ. Res. 29*:239, 1971.
608. Winkler, H., and Smith, A. D.: *Lancet 1*:793, 1968.
609. Wolfe, B. B., Harden, T. K., et al.: *Proc. Natl. Acad. Sci. USA 73*:1343, 1976.
610. Wurtman, R. J., Chou, C., et al.: *J. Pharmacol. Exp. Ther. 174*:351, 1970.
611. Yahr, M. D.: *J. Neural. Trans. 43*:227, 1978.
612. Yamamura, H. I., and Snyder, S. H.: *Mol. Pharmacol. 10*:861, 1974.
613. Yang, W.-H., Gasparis, M. S., et al.: In *Proceedings of the Fourth International Catecholamine Symposium.* Vol. 1. Usdin, E., Kopin, I. J., et al. (eds.), New York, Pergamon Press, 1978, p. 135.
614. Zelch, J. V., Meaney, T. F., et al.: *Radiology 111*:279, 1974.
615. Ziegler, M. G., Lake, C. R., et al.: *N. Engl. J. Med. 296*:293, 1977.
616. Zigmond, R. E., Chalazonitis, A., et al.: In *Proceedings of the Fourth International Catecholamine Symposium.* Vol. 1. Usdin, E.,

Kopin, I. J., et al. (eds.), New York, Pergamon Press, 1978, p. 58.

617. Zuspan, F. P.: *J. Clin. Endocrinol. 30*:357, 1970.
618. Insel, P. A., and Fenno, J.: *Proc. Natl. Acad. Sci. USA 75*:862, 1978.
619. Adam-Vizi, V., and Vizi, E. S.: *J. Neural Transm. 42*:127, 1978.
620. Adamson, A. R., Grahame-Smith, D. G., et al.: *Br. Med. J. 3*:93, 1971.
621. Adamson, A. R., Grahame-Smith, D. G., et al.: *Am. Heart J. 81*:141, 1971.
622. Adamson, A. R., Grahame-Smith, D. G., et al.: *Lancet 2*:293, 1969.
623. Adler, S.: In *Serotonin in Health and Disease: Clinical Correlates*, Vol. 4. Essman, W. B. (ed.), New York, Spectrum Publications, 1976, p. 99.
624. Akcasu, A., and Unna, K. R.: *Eur. J. Pharmacol. 13*:103, 1970.
625. Albores-Saavedra, J., Larraza, O., et al.: *Cancer 38*:2328, 1976.
626. Allison, D. J., Modlin, I. M., et al.: *Lancet 2*:1323, 1977.
627. Altura, B. M., and Halevy, S.: In *Histamine 11 and Anti-Histaminics: Chemistry, Metabolism and Physiological and Pharmacological Actions.* (Handbook of Experimental Pharmacology, Vol. 18, Part 2.) Rocha é Silva, M. (ed.), New York, Springer-Verlag, 1978, p. 1.
628. Alumets, J., Håkanson, R., et al.: *Histochemistry 52*:217, 1977.
629. Amin, A. H., Crawford, T. B. B., et al.: *J. Physiol.* (Lond.) *126*:596, 1954.
630. Ammann, R. W., Vetter, D., et al.: *Gut 17*:107, 1976.
631. Assem, E. S. K.: *Med. Biol. 54*:369, 1976.
632. Avella, G., Binder, H. G., et al.: *Lancet 1*:624, 1978.
633. Axelrod, J.: In *Mechanisms of Release of Biogenic Amines.* von Euler, U.S. (ed.), New York, Pergamon Press, 1966, p. 189.
634. Axelrod, J., and Wurtman, R. J.: *Adv. Pharmacol. 6*:157, 1968.
635. Bach, M. K.: *Immediate Hypersensitivity. Modern Concepts and Developments.* New York, Marcel Dekker, 1978.
636. Bach, N.: In *Symposium on Hypotensive Peptides.* Erdos, E. G., Bach, N., et al. (eds.), Berlin, Springer-Verlag, 1966.
637. Bäckström, M., Olson, L., et al.: *Acta Physiol. Scand. 99*:9, 1977.
638. Barabé, J., Drovin, J.-N., et al.: *Can. J. Physiol. Pharmacol. 55*:2170, 1977.
639. Bates, H. R., Jr.: *Lancet 1*:1111, 1967.
640. Baumgarten, H. G., Bjoerklund, A., et al.: *Acta Physiol. Scand.* [Suppl.] *373*:1, 1971.
641. Baumgarten, H. G., Bjoerklund, A., et al.: *Neural Hormones and Reproduction:* Proceedings, 3rd International Symposium on Brain-Endocrine Interaction, Wurgberg, July, 1977. Scott, D. E., Kozlowski, G. P., et al. (eds.), Basel, S. Karger, 1978, p. 327.
642. Baumgarten, H. G., Evetts, K. D., et al.: *J. Neurochem. 19*:1587, 1972.
643. Baylin, S. B., Weisburger, W. R., et al.: *N. Engl. J. Med. 299*:105, 1978.
644. Beaven, M. A.: *Histamine: Its Role in Physiological and Pathological Processes.* Kallos, P. (ed.), Basel, S. Karger, 1978.
645. Becker, N., Burrill, K., et al.: *Clin. Res. 19*:186, 1971.
646. Bennett, A., Del Tacca, M., et al.: *Br. J. Cancer 35*:881, 1977.
647. Bennett, A., and Whitney, B.: *Gut 7*:307, 1966.
648. Bergdahl, L.: *Aust. N. Z. J. Surg. 46*:136, 1976.
649. Berge, T., and Linell, F.: *Acta Pathol. Microbiol. Scand. 84*:322, 1976.
650. Berridge, M. J.: *J. Exp. Biol. 56*:311, 1972.
651. Berridge, M. J.: *Adv. Cyclic Nucleotide Res. 6*:1, 1975.
652. Bertaccini, G.: *Pharmacol. Rev. 28*:127, 1976.
653. Beusch, K. G., Corrin, B., et al.: *Cancer 22*:1163, 1968.
654. Beusch, K. G., Gordon, G. B., et al.: *J. Ultrastruct. Res. 12*:668, 1965.
655. Bevins, C. H., Lebovitz, H. E., et al.: *N. Engl. J. Med. 289*:236, 1973.
656. Black, J. W., Duncan, A. M., et al.: *Nature* (Lond.) *235*:385, 1972.
657. Bloom, F. E.: *Rev. Physiol. Biochem. Pharmacol. 74*:1, 1975.
658. Boelkins, C.: Unpublished manuscript, Stanford University School of Medicine, Stanford, California, 1971.
659. Bonikos, D. S., Bensch, K. G., et al.: *Cancer 37*:1977, 1976.
660. Bonikos, D. S., and Bensch, K. G.: *Am. J. Med. 63*:765, 1977.
661. Born, G. V. R., and Michal, F.: In *Biochemistry and Pharmacology of Platelets.* (CIBA Foundation Symposium, Vol. 35). New York, Excerpta Medica Foundation, 1975, p. 287.
662. Bosin, T. R.: In *Serotonin in Health and Disease: Availability, Localization, and Deposition,* Vol. 1. Essman, W. B. (ed.), New York, Spectrum Publications, 1978, p. 181.
663. Bourne, H. R., Lichtenstein, L. M., et al.: *Science 184*:19, 1974.
664. Bower, B. F., and Gordon, G. S.: *Ann. Rev. Med. 16*:83, 1965.
665. Bradley, J., Mason, K., et al.: *Lancet 2*:578, 1971.
666. Briselli, M., Mark, G. J., et al.: *Cancer 42*:2870, 1978.
667. Brodie, B. B., and Shore, P. A.: *Ann. N. Y. Acad. Sci. 66*:631, 1957.
668. Broitman, S. A., McCray, R. S., et al.: *Am. J. Med. 48*:382, 1970.
669. Brownstein, M., Saavedra, J. M., et al.: *Mol. Pharmacol. 9*:605, 1973.
670. Brush, J. S.: *Biochem. Pharmacol. 26*:2349, 1977.

671. Bulbring, E., and Gershon, M. D.: *Adv. Pharmacol. 64*:323, 1968.
672. Bulbring, E., and Lin, R. C. Y.: *J. Physiol. 140*:381, 1958.
673. Bunney, W. E., Jr., Murphy, D. L., et al.: *Lancet 1*:1022, 1970.
674. Burks, T. F., and Long, J. P.: *Am. J. Physiol. 211*:619, 1966.
675. Busis, N. A., Weight, F. F., et al.: *Science 200*:1079, 1978.
676. Caplan, R. M.: *J.A.M.A. 194*:1077, 1965.
677. Carr, R. J., and Biswas, B. K.: *Br. Med. J. 2*:1116, 1966.
678. Cater, D. B., and Taylor, C. R.: *Br. J. Cancer 20*:517, 1966.
679. Chabner, B. A., DeVita, V. T., et al.: *N. Engl. J. Med. 282*:838, 1970.
680. Chajek, T., and Romanoff, H.: *Arch. Intern. Med. 136*:441, 1976.
681. Chan, J. X. C., Burrowes, C. E., et al.: *Agents Actions 8*:65, 1978.
682. Chand, N., and Eyre, P.: *J. Pharm. Pharmacol. 29*:387, 1977.
683. Chand, N., and Eyre, P.: *Agents Actions 5*:277, 1975.
684. Chang, R. S. L., Tran. V. T., et al.: *Eur. J. Pharmacol. 48*:463, 1978.
685. Charrette, E. E., Mariano, A. V., et al.: *Arch. Intern. Med. 118*:358, 1966.
686. Christian, S. T., and Smythies, J. R.: In *Serotonin in Health and Disease: Availability, Localization, and Disposition,* Vol. 1. Essman, W. B. (ed.), New York, Spectrum Publications, 1978, p. 363.
687. Churg, A., and Warnock, M.: *Cancer 37*:1469, 1976.
688. Churg, A.: *Arch. Pathol. Lab. Med. 101*:216, 1977.
689. Cochrane, C. G.: In *The Role of Immunological Factors in Infectious, Allergic, and Autoimmune Processes.* Beers, R. F., and Bassett, E. G. (eds.), New York, Raven Press, 1976, p. 237.
690. Cohen, R. M.: *Calif. Med. 114*:1, 1971.
691. Collard, K. J., and Roberts, M. H. T.: *Neuropharmacology 16*:671, 1977.
692. Colman, R. W., and Wong, P. Y.: *Thromb. Haemostas. 38*:751, 1977.
693. Conference (various authors): *Third International Conference on Cyclic Nucleotides.* Greengard, P., and Robison, G. A. (eds.), *Adv. Cyclic Nucleotide Res. 9*:1, 1978.
694. Corrêa, F. M. A., Innis, R. B., et al.: *Proc. Natl. Acad. Sci. USA 76*:1489, 1979.
695. Cottrell, G. A.: *Neuroscience 2*:1, 1977.
696. Cottrell, G. A.: *Nature* (Lond.) *225*:1060, 1970.
697. Creese, I., and Snyder, S. H.: *Eur. J. Pharmacol. 49*:201, 1978.
698. Cremata, V. Y., and Koe, B. K.: *Clin. Pharmacol. Ther. 7*:768, 1966.
699. Cryer, P. E., and Kissane, J. M. (eds.): *Am. J. Med. 61*:671, 1976.
700. Cuschieri, A., and Onabanjo, O. A.: *Br. Med. J. 3*:565, 1971.
701. DaPrada, M., and Pletscher, A.: *Life Sci. 8*:65, 1969.
702. Deftos, L. J., McMillan, P. J., et al.: *Metabolism 25*:543, 1976.
703. Deguchi, T.: *Science 203*:1245, 1979.
704. Deguchi, T., and Axelrod, J.: *Mol. Pharmacol. 9*:612, 1973.
705. Delmont, J., and Rampal, P.: *Br. Med. J. 4*:165, 1975.
706. Demis, D. J.: *Ann. Intern. Med. 59*:194, 1963.
707. Devitt, P. G.: *Br. Med. J. 2*:327, 1978.
708. Diamant, B., Kazimerczak, W., et al.: *Allergy 33*:50, 1978.
709. Diamond, J.: *Adv. Cyclic Nucleotide Res. 9*:327, 1978.
710. DiMattei, P.: *Biochem. Pharmacol. 16*:909, 1967.
711. Dollinger, M. R., Ratner, L. H.: et al.: *Arch. Intern. Med. 120*:575, 1967.
712. Donaldson, V. H., Rosen, F. S., et al.: *Trans. Assoc. Am. Physicians 90*:174, 1977.
713. Douglas, W.: In *The Pharmacological Basis of Therapeutics.* 6th ed. Goodman, L. S., Gilman, A., et al. (eds.), New York, Macmillan Company, 1980, Chs. 26 and 27.
714. Douglas, W. W.: In *Respiratory Tract Mucus.* CIBA Foundation Symposium *54*:61, 1974.
715. Douglas, W. W.: *Br. J. Pharmacol. 34*:451, 1968.
716. Douglas, W. W., and Taraskevich, P. S.: *J. Physiol.* (Lond.) *280*:13P, 1978.
717. Douglas, W. W., and Rubin, R. P.: *J. Physiol.* (Lond) *159*:24P, 1961.
718. Douglas, W. W., Kanno, T., et al.: *J. Physiol.* (Lond.) *188*:107, 1967.
719. Eccleston, D., Ritchie, I. M., et al.: *Nature* (Lond.) *226*:84, 1970.
720. Edvinsson, L., and Mackenzie, E. T.: *Pharmacol. Rev. 28*:275, 1977.
721. Egan, T. J.: *Israel J. Med. Sci. 3*:587, 1970.
722. Enerbäck, L.: *Acta Pathol. Microbiol. Scand. 64*:491, 1965.
723. Engelman, K., Lovenberg, W., et al.: *N. Engl. J. Med. 277*:1103, 1967.
724. Erdös, E. G. (ed.): *Bradykinin, Kallidin and Kallikrein.* (Handbook of Experimental Pharmacology, Vol. 25) New York, Springer-Verlag, 1979.
725. Erdös, E. G.: *Biochem. Pharmacol. 25*:1563, 1976.
726. Erdös, E. G.: *Bradykinin, Kallidin, and Kallikrein.* (Handbook of Experimental Pharmacology, Vol. 25), New York, Springer-Verlag, 1970.
727. Erspamer, V. (ed.): *Handbook of Experimental Pharmacology,* Vol. 19. New York, Springer-Verlag, 1966.
728. Erspamer, V.: *Progr. Drug Res. 3*:151, 1961.
729. Erspamer, V.: *Arch. Sci. Biol. 31*:86, 1946.
730. Erspamer, V., and Asero, B.: *Nature* (Lond.) *169*:800, 1952.
731. Essman, W. B.: In *Serotonin in Health and Disease.* Vol. 1. New York, Spectrum Publications, 1978.

732. Ibid., Vol. 2.
733. Ibid., Vol. 3.
734. Ibid., Vol. 4, 1977.
735. Farrans, V. J., and Roberts, W. C.: *Human Pathol.* 7:387, 1976.
736. Feer, H., and Wirz-Justice, A.: *Experientia* 27:885, 1971.
737. Feldman, J. M., and Plonk, J. W.: *Metabolism* 25:97, 1976.
738. Feldman, J. M., Plonk, J. W., et al.: *Diabetes* 24:664, 1975.
739. Feldman, J. M., and Lebovitz, H. E.: *Trans. Assoc. Am. Physicians* 85:279, 1972.
740. Fernstrom, J. D., and Wurtman, R. J.: *Science* 173:149, 1971.
741. Fernstrom, J. D., and Wurtman, R. J.: *Nature* [New Biol.] 234:62, 1971.
742. Fishlock, D. J., and Parks, A. G.: *Br. J. Pharmacol.* 28:164, 1966.
743. Fishman, M. L., and Rosenthal, S.: *Br. J. Ophthal.* 60:583, 1976.
744. *Can. Med. Assoc. J.* 96:1282, 1967.
745. Foreman, J. C., Garland, L. G., et al.: *Sym. Soc. Exp. Biol.* 30:193, 1976.
746. Fox, R. H., Goldsmith, R., et al.: *J. Physiol.* (Lond.) 157:589, 1961.
747. Frölich, J. C., Bloomgarden, Z. T., et al.: *N. Engl. J. Med.* 299:1055, 1978.
748. Furness, J. B., and Costa, M.: *Cell Tissue Res.* 188:527, 1978.
749. Gaddum, J. H.: *J. Physiol.* (Lond.) 121:15P, 1953.
750. Gailani, S., Roque, A. L., et al.: *Ann. Intern. Med.* 65:1044, 1966.
751. Garattini, S., and Samanin, R.: In *Serotonin in Health and Disease: Physiological Regulation and Pharmacological Action*, Vol. 2. Essman, W. B. (ed.), New York, Spectrum Publications, 1978, p. 247.
752. Gardner, B., Dollinger, M., et al.: *Surgery* 61:846, 1967.
753. Geipert, F., and Erdös, E. G.: *Experientia* 27:912, 1971.
754. Gerschenfeld, H. M., and Paupardin-Tritsch, D.: *J. Physiol.* (Lond.) 243:427, 1974.
755. Gershon, M. D., Dreyfus, C. F., et al.: *Proc. Natl. Acad. Sci. USA* 74:3086, 1977.
756. Gershon, M. D., and Altman, R. F.: *J. Pharmacol. Exp. Ther.* 179:29, 1971.
757. Gillis, C. N., and Roth, J. A.: *Biochem. Pharmacol.* 25:2547, 1976.
758. Glovsky, M. M., Hugli, T. E., et al.: *J. Clin. Invest.* 64:804, 1979.
759. Godwin, J. D., II: *Cancer* 36:560, 1975.
760. Gold, W. M.: *Am. Rev. Resp. Dis.* 115:127, 1977.
761. Gold, W. M., Meyers, G. L., et al.: *J. Appl. Physiol.* 43:271, 1977.
762. Gowenlock, A. H., Platt, D. S., et al.: *Lancet* 1:304, 1964.
763. Graham, J. R., Suby, H. I., et al.: *N. Engl. J. Med.* 274:359, 1966.
764. Grahame-Smith, D. G., and Ferriman, D. G.: *Proc. R. Soc. Med.* 68:701, 1965.
765. Grahame-Smith, D. G.: Unpublished report. St. Mary's Hospital Medical School, London, 1971.
766. Grahame-Smith, D. G.: *Br. J. Pharmacol.* 43:856, 1971.
767. Grahame-Smith, D. G.: *Gut* 11:189, 1970.
768. Grahame-Smith, D. G.: *J. Neurochem.* 18:1053, 1971.
769. Grahame-Smith, D. G.: *Hosp. Med.* 4:556, 1968.
770. Grahame-Smith, D. G.: *Am. J. Cardiol.* 21:376, 1968.
771. Grahame-Smith, D. G.: Unpublished report. St. Mary's Hospital Medical School, London, 1971.
772. Grahame-Smith, D. G.: *Biochim. Biophys. Acta* 86:175, 1964.
773. Green, J. P., Johnson, C. L., et al.: In *Psychopharmacology: A Generation of Progress.* Lipton, M. A., DiMaseio, A., et al. (eds.), New York, Raven Press, 1978, p. 319.
774. Greengard, P.: In *Distinguished Lecture Series of the Society of General Physiologists.* Vol. 1. New York, Raven Press, 1978.
775. Greengard, P.: *Nature* (Lond.) 260:101, 1976.
776. Gunderson, L. L.: *Clin. Gastroenterol.* 5:743, 1976.
777. Gurdon, J. B.: *Q. Rev. Biol.* 38:54, 1963.
778. Gurdon, J. B.: In *Advances in Morphogenesis.* Abercrombie, M., and Bracket, J. (eds.), New York, Academic Press, 1964, p.1.
779. Guth, P. H., and Smith, E.: *Am. J. Physiol.* 234:E370, 1978.
780. Haberland, G. L.: *Klin. Wochenschr.* 56:325, 1978.
781. Habib, A., Kaneko, M., et al.: *Cancer* 43:535, 1979.
782. Hale, J. F., and Lane-Mitchell, W.: *Cent. Afr. J. Med.* 10:162, 1964.
783. Hallen, A.: *Lancet* 1:746, 1964.
784. Hallwright, G. P., North, A. K., et al.: *J. Clin. Endocrinol.* 24:496, 1964.
785. Hamlin, K. E., and Fischer, F. E.: *J. Am. Chem. Soc.* 73:5007, 1951.
786. Han, Y. N., Kato, H., et al.: *J. Biochem.* 83:213, 1978.
787. Haqqani, M. T., and Williams, G.: *J. Clin. Pathol.* 30:473, 1977.
788. Haverback, B. J., and Davidson, J. D.: *Gastroenterology* 35:570, 1958.
789. Hendrix, T. R., Atkinson, M., et al.: *Am. J. Med.* 23:886, 1957.
790. Hepper, N. G., Payne, W. S., et al.: *Am. Rev. Res. Dis.* 115:351, 1977.
791. Herman, J. J., Brenner, J. K., et al.: *Science* 206:77, 1979a.
792. Herman, J. J., Rosner, I. K., et al.: *J. Clin. Invest.* 63:1195, 1979b.
793. Hiatt, R. B., Goodman, I., et al.: *Am. J. Surg.* 119:527, 1970.
794. Hirata, Y., Sakamoto, N., et al.: *Cancer* 37:377, 1976.
795. Hirschowitz, B. I.: *Annu. Rev. Pharmacol. Toxicol.* 19:203, 1979.
796. Ho, A. K. A., Loh, H. H., et al.: *Eur. J. Pharmacol.* 10:72, 1970.
797. Hoch, A., Lichtig, C., et al.: *Am. J. Obstet. Gynecol.* 110:1141, 1971.
798. Hollander, W., Michelson, A. L., et al. (eds.): *Circulation* 16:246, 1957.
799. Holz, R. W., Deguichi, T., et al.: *J. Neurochem.* 22:205, 1974.
800. Hudson, H. L., and Margulis, A. R.: *Am. J. Roentgenol.* 91:833, 1964.
801. Ishii, T., Iri, H., et al.: *Am. J. Gastroenterol.* 67:171, 1977.
802. Ishizaka, T., and Ishizaka, K.: *J. Immunol.* 120:800, 1978.
803. Jacobs, S., and Cuatrecasas, P.: *N. Engl. J. Med.* 297:1383, 1977.
804. Jacobson, E. D., and Thompson, W. J.: *Adv. Cyclic Nucleotide Res.* 7:199, 1976.
805. Janoff, A., Schaefer, S., et al.: *J. Exp. Med.* 122:841, 1965.
806. Jaques, L. B.: *Gen. Pharmacol.* 6:235, 1975.
807. Jarrett, L., Lacy, P. E., et al.: *J. Clin. Endocrinol.* 24:543, 1964.
808. Jones, R. S., and Meyers, W. C.: *Annu. Rev. Physiol.* 41:67, 1979.
809. Jouvet, M.: *Science* 163:32, 1969.
810. Kabakow, B., Weinstein, J. B., et al.: *Fed. Proc.* 17:382, 1958.
811. Kaliner, M. A.: *N. Engl. J. Med.* 301:498, 1979.
812. Kaliner, M. A.: *J. Clin. Invest.* 60:951, 1977.
813. Kanoff, P. D., and Greengard, P.: *Mol. Pharmacol.* 15:445, 1979.
814. Kebabian, J. W.: *Adv. Cyclic Nucleotide Res.* 8:421, 1977.
815. Kizer, J. S., Palkovits, M., et al.: *Endocrinology* 98:743, 1976.
816. Kojiro, M., Ohishi, H., et al.: *Cancer* 38:1636, 1976.
817. Korhonen, L. K., and Korhonen, E.: *Experientia* 21:628, 1965.
818. Kowlessar, O. D., Law, D. H., et al.: *Am. J. Med.* 27:673, 1959.
819. Kowlessar, O. D., Williams, R. C., et al.: *N. Engl. J. Med.* 259:340, 1958.
820. Krieger, D. T.: In *The Central Nervous System.* Vol. 3. Serotonin in Health and Disease. Essman, W. B. (ed.), New York, Spectrum Publications, 1978, p. 51.
821. Krieger, D. T., and Rizzo, F.: *Am. J. Physiol.* 217:1703, 1969.
822. Lagunoff, D., and Benditt, E. P.: *Ann. N. Y. Acad. Sci.* 103:185, 1963.
823. Legha, S. S., Valdivieso, M., et al.: *Cancer Treat. Rev.* 61:1699, 1977.
824. Lembeck, F.: *Nature* (Lond.) 712:910, 1953.
825. Lemberger, L., Rowe, H., et al.: *Clin. Pharmacol. Ther.* 23:421, 1978.
826. Lemberger, L., Axelrod, J., et al.: *J. Pharmacol. Exp. Ther.* 177:169, 1971.
827. Lernmark, A.: *Horm. Metab. Res.* 3:305, 1971.
828. Levine, R. J., Elsas, L. J., et al.: *J.A.M.A.* 186:905, 1963.
829. Levine, R. J., and Sjoerdsma, A.: *Ann. Intern. Med.* 58:818, 1963.
830. Lewis, R. R., and Austen, K. F.: *Fed. Proc.* 36:2676, 1977.
831. Lichtenstein, L. M., and Austen, K. F.: *Asthma, Physiology, Immunopharmacology and Treatment.* New York, Academic Press, 1978.
832. Liddle, G. W., Nicholson, W. E., et al.: *Recent Progr. Hormone Res.* 25:283, 1969.
833. Lin, R. C., Neff, N. H., et al.: *Life Sci.* 8:1077, 1969.
834. Lipton, M. A.: In *Neurobiological Aspects of Psychopathology.* New York, Grune & Stratton, 1969, p. 310.
835. Lokich, J. J., and Li, F.: *Ann. Intern. Med.* 89:364, 1978.
836. Lovenberg, W., Jequier, E., et al.: *Adv. Pharmacol.* 6:21, 1968.
837. Lovenberg, W., Levine, R. J., et al.: *Biochem. Pharmacol.* 14:887, 1965.
838. Lowry, P. J., Rees, L. H., et al.: *J. Clin. Endocrinol. Metabol.* 43:831, 1976.
839. MacIntosh, C. E., and Newman, J.: *J. R. Coll. Surg. Edinb.* 21:233, 1976.
840. Majno, G., Shea, S. M., et al.: *J. Cell Biol.* 42:647, 1969.
841. Margolius, H. S., Geller, R., et al.: *Lancet* 2:1063, 1971.
842. Mariani, G., Strober, W., et al.: *Cancer* 38:854, 1976.
843. Marks, R., and Greaves, M. W.: *Br. J. Clin. Pharmacol.* 4:367, 1977.
844. Marks, V.: *Clin. Endocrinol. Metabol.* 5:769, 1976.
845. Marsden, C. A., and Curzon, G.: *Neuropharmacology* 16:489, 1977.
846. Marshall, P. B.: *J. Pharm. Pharmacol.* 18:764, 1966.
847. Maruyama, Y., Hayashi, G., et al.: *J. Pharmacol. Exp. Ther.* 178:20, 1971.
848. Mashford, M. L., and Zacest, R.: *Aust. Ann. Med.* 16:326, 1967.
849. Mason, D. T., and Melmon, K. L.: *J. Clin. Invest.* 45:1685, 1966.
850. McBride, T. I., McDonald, G. A., et al.: *Postgrad. Med. J.* 43:176, 1967.
851. McGinty, D. J., Harper, R. M., et al.: In *Serotonin Behavior.* Barchas, J., and Usdin, E. (eds.), New York, Academic Press, 1973, p. 267.
852. McGrath, M. A.: *Circ. Res.* 41:428, 1977.
853. McGrath, M. A., and Shepherd, J. T.: *Fed. Proc.* 37:195, 1978.
854. Melmon, K. L., and Insel, P. A.: *Johns Hopkins Med. J.* 141:15, 1977.
855. Melmon, K. L., Weinstein, Y., et al.: In *Immunopharmacology.* Hadden, J. W., Spreafico, F., et al. (eds.), New York, Plenum Press, 1977, p. 331.
856. Melmon, K. L.: *Physiol. Pharmacol. Physicians* 1:1, 1966.
857. Melmon, K. L.: *Calif. Med.* 114:33, 1971.

858. Melmon, K. L., Cline, M. J., et al.: *J. Clin. Invest. 47*:1295, 1968.
859. Melmon, K. L., and Cline, M. J.: In *International Symposium on Vasoactive Peptides, Bradykinin and Related Kinins*. Rocha é Silva, M., and Rothschild, H. A. (eds.), Sao Paulo, Brazil, Livraria Editora Flamboyant Ltds., 1967, p. 223.
860. Melmon, K. L., Lovenberg, W., et al.: *Clin. Chim. Acta 12*:292, 1965.
861. Melmon, K. L., Sjoerdsma, A., et al.: *Am. J. Med. 39*:568, 1965.
862. Melmon, K. L., Sjoerdsma, A., et al.: *Gastroenterology 48*:18, 1965.
863. Mengel, C. E.: *Ann. Intern. Med. 62*:587, 1965.
864. Misiewicz, J. J., Waller, S. L., et al.: *Gut 7*:208, 1966.
865. Modlin, I. M., Bloom, S. R., et al.: *Adv. Exp. Med. Biol. 106*:195, 1978.
866. Moertel, C. G., Beahrs, O. H., et al.: *N. Engl. J. Med. 273*:244, 1965.
867. Moertel, C. G.: *Cancer 36*:675, 1975.
868. Moertel, C. G., and Dockerty, M. B.: *Ann. Intern. Med. 78*:389, 1973.
869. Moertel, C. G., Sauer, W. G., et al.: *Cancer 14*:901, 1961.
870. Mongar, J. L., and Perera, B. A. V.: *Immunology 8*:511, 1965.
871. Morin, L. J., and Zuerner, R. T.: *J.A.M.A. 216*:1647, 1971.
872. Morrison, D. C., and Henson, P. M.: In *Immediate Hypersensitivity: Modern Concepts and Developments*. Bach. M. K. (ed.), New York, Marcel Dekker, Inc., 1978, p. 431.
873. Mouret, J., Bobillier, P., et al.: *Eur. J. Pharmacol. 5*:17, 1968.
874. Murray-Lyon, I. M., Parsons, V. A., et al.: *Lancet 2*:172, 1970.
875. Murrell, T. G. C., Wangel, A. G., et al.: *Gastroenterology 51*:656, 1966.
876. Nash, D. T., and Borin, M.: *N. Y. J. Med. 64*:1128, 1964.
877. Nathanson, J. A.: *Physiol. Rev. 57*:157, 1977.
878. Nelson, D. L., Herbert, A., et al.: *Mol. Pharmacol. 14*:983, 1978.
879. *Neuropeptide Symposium. Approaches to the Cell Biology of Neurons.* Cowan, W. H., and Ferrendelli, J. A. (eds.), Bethesda, MD., Society Neurosciences, 1977, p. 241.
880. Newball, H. H., Berninger, R. W., et al.: *J. Clin. Invest. 64*:457, 1979.
881. Nustad, K., Ørstavik, T. B., et al.: *Gen. Pharmacol. 9*:1, 1978.
882. Oates, J. A.: *Adv. Pharmacol. 5*:109, 1967.
883. Oates, J. A., Melmon, K. L., et al.: *Lancet 1*:514, 1964.
884. Oates, J. A., Pettinger, W. A., et al.: *J. Clin. Invest. 45*:173, 1966.
885. Oates, J. A., and Sjoerdsma, A.: *Am. J. Med. 32*:333, 1962.
886. Okike, N., Bernatz, P. E., et al.: *Ann. Thorac. Surg. 22*:270, 1976.
887. Omenn, G. S., and Smith, L. T.: *J. Clin. Invest. 6262*:235, 1978.
888. Orlando, R. C., Moyer, P., et al.: *Ann. Intern. Med. 88*:213, 1978.
889. Owen, D. A. A.: *Gen. Pharmacol. 8*:141, 1977.
890. Page, I. H.: *Serotonin*. Chicago, Year Book Publishers, 1968.
891. Palacios, J. M., Garbarg, M., et al.: *Mol. Pharmacol. 14*:971, 1978.
892. Pearce, A. G. E.: *Med. Biol. 55*:115, 1977.
893. Peart, W. S., Robertson, J. I. S., et al.: *Lancet 2*:715, 1959.
894. Pentilla, A., and Lempinen, M.: *Gastroenterology 54*:375, 1968.
895. Perera, B. A. V., and Mongar, J. L.: *Immunology 8*:519, 1965.
896. Piper, P. J., and Vane, J. R.: *Nature* (Lond.) *223*:29, 1969.
897. Pisano, J. J.: In *Proteases and Biological Control*. Cold Spring Harbor Laboratory, 1975, p. 199.
898. Pisano, J. J., and Austen, K. F. (eds.): *Chemistry and Biology of the Kallikrein-Kinin System in Health and Disease*. Fogarty International Center Proceedings No. 27, DHEW Publ. No. (NIH) 76-791, 1977.
899. Plaut, M., and Lichenstein, L. M.: In *Histamine Receptors*. Yellin, T. D. (ed.), New York, SP Medical and Scientific Books, 1979a, p. 351.
900. Plaut, M., and Roszkowski, W.: In *Histamine Receptors*. Yellin, T. D. (ed.), New York, SP Medical and Scientific Books, 1979b, p. 361.
901. Plonk, J., and Feldman, J. M.: *J. Clin. Endocrinol. Metabol. 42*:291, 1976.
902. Plonk, J., and Feldman, J. M.: *Metabolism 24*:1035, 1975.
903. Powell, J. R., and Brody, M. J.: *J. Pharmacol. Exp. Ther. 196*:1, 1976.
904. *Lancet 1*:404, 1968.
905. Rao, U., and Takita, H.: *Thorax 32*:771, 1977.
906. Rapport, M. M.: *J. Biol. Chem. 180*:961, 1949.
907. Rapport, M. M., Green, A. A., et al.: *J. Biol. Chem. 176*:1243, 1948.
908. Reed, M. L., Kuipers, F. M., et al.: *N. Engl. J. Med. 269*:1005, 1963.
909. Robboy, S. J., Scully, R. E., et al.: *Obstet. Gynecol. 49*:203, 1977.
910. Roberts, L. J., II, Marney, S. R., et al.: *N. Engl. J. Med. 300*:236, 1979.
911. Roberts, W. C., and Sjoerdsma, A.: *Am. J. Med. 36*:5, 1964.
912. Robertson, J. I. S., Peart, W. S., et al.: *Q. J. Med. 31*:103, 1962.
913. Rocha é Silva, M.: In *Handbuch du Experimentellen Pharmakologie*. Vol. 18, Part 2, Berlin, Springer-Verlag, 1978, p. 295.
914. Rocha é Silva, M., and Garcia Leme, J.: *Chemical Mediators of the Acute Inflammatory Reaction*. New York, Pergamon Press, 1972.
915. Rocha é Silva, M. (ed.). In *Handbuch du Experimentellen Pharmakologie*. Vol. 18, Part 1, Berlin, Springer-Verlag, 1966.
916. Rocha é Silva, M., and Garcia Leme, J.: *Med. Exp. 8*:287, 1963.
917. Rocklin, R. E., Greineder, D., et al.: *Cell. Immunol. 37*:162, 1978.
918. Rocklin, R. E.: *J. Clin. Invest. 57*:1051, 1976.
919. Rodbard, S., and Kira, S.: *Angiology 23*:188, 1972.
920. Rosai, J., Levine, G., et al.: *Eng. Pathol. Ann. 11*:201, 1976.
921. Sahakian, B. J., Wurtman, R. J., et al.: *Nature* (Lond.) *279*:731, 1979.
922. Sandler, M., Karim, S. M. M., et al.: *Lancet 2*:1053, 1968.
923. Satterlee, W. G., Serpick, A., et al.: *Ann. Intern. Med. 72*:919, 1970.
924. Saum, W. R., and de Groat, W. C.: *J. Pharmacol. Exp. Ther. 185*:70, 1973.
925. Schachter, M., and Barton, S.: In *Endocrinology: Metabolic Basis of Clinical Practice*. Cahill, G., Jr., and de Groot, L. J. (eds.) New York, Grune & Stratton (in press).
926. Schein, P. S.: *Cancer 30*:1616, 1972.
927. Schein, P. S., O'Connell, M. J. O., et al.: *Cancer 34*:993, 1974.
928. Schein, P. S., Kahn, R., et al.: *Arch. Intern. Med. 132*:555, 1973.
929. Schlangan, J. T.: *Radiol. Clin.* (Basel) *45*:105, 1976.
930. Schwaber, J. R., and Lukas, D. S.: *Am. J. Med. 32*:846, 1962.
931. Schwartz, J.-C.: *Annu. Rev. Pharmacol. Toxicol. 17*:325, 1977.
932. Selye, H.: *The Mast Cells*. New York, Appleton-Century-Crofts, 1965, p. 320.
933. Shaskan, E. G., and Snyder, S. H.: *J. Pharmacol. Exp. Ther. 175*:404, 1970.
934. Shearer, G. M., Melmon, K. L., et al.: *J. Exp. Med. 136*:1302, 1972.
935. Shen, F.-H., Loh, H. H., et al.: *J. Pharmacol. Exp. Ther. 175*:427, 1970.
936. Sicuteri, F., Back, N., et al.: *Adv. Exp. Med. Biol. 70*:1, 1976.
937. Sieghart, W., Theoharides, T. C., et al.: *Nature* (Lond.) *275*:329, 1978.
938. Sirek, A., Geerling, E., et al.: *Am. J. Physiol. 211*:1018, 1966.
939. Sjoerdsma, A., Lovenberg, W., et al.: *Ann. Intern. Med. 73*:607, 1970.
940. Sjoerdsma, A., Lovenberg, W., et al.: *Ann. Intern. Med. 73*:607, 1970.
940. Sjoerdsma, A., and Melmon, K. L.: *Gastroenterology 47*:104, 1964.
941. Sjoerdsma, A., Weissback, H., et al.: *Am. J. Med. 23*:5, 1957.
942. Skinner, C., and Ewen, S. W. B.: *Thorax 31*:212, 1976.
943. Sluys, V. J., Chonfoer, J., et al.: *Lancet 1*:1416, 1964.
944. Smith, A. N., and Zeitlin, I. J.: *Br. J. Surg. 53*:867, 1966.
945. Smith, L. T., Hanson, D. R., et al.: *Brain Res. 146*:400, 1978.
946. Sneddon, J.: *Prog. Neurobiol. 1*:153, 1973.
947. Snyder, S. H., Axelrod, J., et al.: *J. Pharmacol. Exp. Ther. 158*:206, 1967.
948. Sole, M. J., Van Loon, G. R., et al.: *Science 201*:620, 1978.
949. Soll, A., and Walsh, J. H.: *Annu. Rev. Physiol. 41*:35, 1979.
950. Solomon, A., Sonoda, T., et al.: *Cancer Treat. Rev. 60*:273, 1976.
951. Sönksen, P. H., Ayres, A. B., et al.: *Clin. Endocrinol. 5*:503, 1976.
952. Soter, N. A., Austen, K. F., et al.: *N. Engl. J. Med. 301*:465, 1979.
953. Spatz, M.: *Lab. Invest. 13*:288, 1964.
954. Steiner, K.: *Arch. Derm. 84*:477, 1961.
955. Stewart, J., and Kay, A. B.: *Nature*, (Lond.) 1980 (in press).
956. Storstein, O., Calabresi, M., et al.: *Yale J. Biol. Med. 32*:197, 1959.
957. Streeten, D. H. P., Kerr, L. P., et al.: *Lancet 2*:1048, 1972.
958. Sullivan, T. J., and Parker, C. W.: *J. Immunol. 122*:431, 1978.
959. Sulser, F., Vetulani, J., et al.: *Biochem. Pharmacol. 27*:257, 1978.
960. Sundström, C., and Wilander, E.: *Acta Path. Microbiol. Scand. 84*:311, 1976.
961. Symposium (Various authors): *Adv. Pharmacol. 6A*:1, *6B*:1, 1968.
962. Symposium (Various authors): *Biochemistry and Pharmacology of Platelets*. (CIBA Foundation Symposium.) Vol. 35. New York, Excerpta Medica Foundation, 1975, p. 1.
963. Symposium (Various authors): Serotonin — New Vistas: Histochemistry and Pharmacology. Costa, E., Gessa, G. L., et al. (eds.), *Adv. Biochem. Psychopharmacol. 10*:1, 1974.
964. Symposium (Various authors): Kinins, Renal Function and Blood Pressure. McGiff, J. C. (Chairman), *Fed. Proc. 35*:172, 1976.
965. Symposium (Various authors): *Proceedings of the Second International Symposium on Histamine H₂-Receptor Antagonists. Cimetidine*. Burland, W. L., and Simkins, M. A. (eds.), New York, Excerpta Medica Foundation, 1977a, p. 1.
966. Symposium (Various authors): *Proceedings of the International Symposium on Excitation Contraction Coupling in Smooth Muscle and the Erwin-Riesch Symposium*. Casteels, R., Godfraind, T., et al. (eds.), New York, Elsevier/North Holland Biomedical Press, 1977b.
967. Symposium (Various authors): Third Symposium on Histamine H₂-receptor Antagonists: Clinical Results with Cimetidine. Fordtran, J. S., and Grossman, M. I. (eds.), *Gastroenterology 7*:1, 1978a.
968. Symposium (Various authors): Serotonin Neurotoxins. Jacoby, J. H., and Lytle, L. D. (eds.), *N. Y. Acad. Sci. 305*:1, 1978.
969. Szeinberg, A., Shani, M., et al.: *Israel J. Med. Sci. 6*:475, 1970.
970. Taub, S. J., Greenwald, R. A., et al.: *J.A.M.A. 239*:2686, 1978.
971. Taylor, J. E., and Richelson, E.: *Mol. Pharmacol. 15*:462, 1979.
972. Thompson, J. H.: *Res. Commun. Chem. Pathol. Pharmacol. 2*:687, 1971.
973. Thompson, J. H., and Campbell, L. B.: *Experientia 23*:826, 1967.
974. Thorson, A., Biork, G., et al.: *Am. Heart. J. 47*:795, 1954.

975. Tran, V. T., Chang, R. S. L., et al.: *Proc. Natl. Acad. Sci. USA* 75:6290, 1978.
976. Trapnell, J. E.: In *Chemistry and Biology of the Kallikrein-Kinin System in Health and Disease*. Pisano, J. J., and Austen, K. F. (eds.), DHEW Publ. No. (NIH) 76-791, 1977, p. 573.
977. Twarog, B. M., and Page, I. H.: *Am. J. Physiol.* 175:157, 1953.
978. Tyce, G. M., Flock, E. V., et al.: *Biochem. Pharmacol.* 16:979, 1967.
979. Vaidya, A. B., Wustrack, K. O., et al.: *Ann. Intern. Med.* 74:711, 1971.
980. van Praag, H. M.: *Psychiatr. Neurol. Neurochir.* (Amst.) 73:9, 1970.
981. von Studnitz, W.: *Scand. J. Clin. Lab. Invest.* 11:309, 1959.
982. Waldenström, J.: *Acta Endocrinol.* 17:432, 1954.
983. Wang, S. R., and Zweiman, B.: *Cell. Immunol.* 36:28, 1978.
984. Warner, R. R. P., Kirschner, P., et al.: *J.A.M.A.* 178:1175, 1961.
985. Weber, A. M., and Murray, J. M.: *Physiol. Rev.* 53:612, 1973.
986. Weichert, R. F.: *Am. J. Med.* 49:232, 1970.
987. Weitzner, S., and Robison, J. R.: *J. Urol.* 116:821, 1976.
988. Welch, A. S., and Welch, B. L.: *Biochem. Pharmacol.* 17:699, 1968.
989. Williams, E. D.: *Lancet* 2:1108, 1969.
990. Williams, E. D., and Sandler, M.: *Lancet* 1:238, 1963.
991. Williams, H. E., Wilson, K. M., et al.: *Clin. Res.* 18:541, 1970.
992. Woolley, D. W.: *The Biochemical Basis of Psychoses; or, The Serotonin Hypothesis About Mental Illness*. New York, John Wiley & Sons, 1962.
993. Wooley, D. W., and Shaw, E.: *Science* 119:587, 1954.
994. Wurtman, R. J., and Fernstrom, J. D.: *Biochem. Pharmacol.* 25:1691, 1976.
995. Yarbrough, C. G., Buxbaum, D. M., et al.: *Life Sci.* 10:977, 1971.
996. Yellin, T. O. (ed.): *Histamine Receptors*. New York, SP Medical & Science Books, 1979.
997. Zeegen, R., Rothwell-Jackson, R., et al.: *Gut* 10:617, 1969.
998. Zenker, N., Hanker, J. S., et al.: *Science* 159:1104, 1968.
999. Zweig, M., and Axelrod, J.: *J. Neurobiol.* 1:87, 1969.
1000. Demis, D. J. (ed.): *Clinical Perinatology*, Vol. 1. New York, Harper and Row, 1974, Units 4–11.

CHAPTER 11

Neuroendocrinology

By Seymour Reichlin

INTRODUCTION

Neural regulation of glandular secretion is exerted by two mechanisms: one secretomotor and the other neurosecretory (Fig. 11–1). Secretomotor control is mediated through nerve terminals ending directly on secretory cells. Neurosecretory control is mediated through secretory products released into the circulation from nerve terminals. Examples of secretomotor control are the regulation of the

flow of saliva, of tears, and of gastric acid by acetylcholine released from cholinergic nerves. Examples of neurosecretory control are the regulation of renal function by vasopressin (VP) secreted by axon terminals in the neurohypophysis and the regulation of anterior pituitary function by releasing factors secreted by neurons of the hypothalamus.

Anterior pituitary hormones in turn have myriad effects on bodily functions directly or by way of the adrenal cortex, thyroid gland, and gonads.

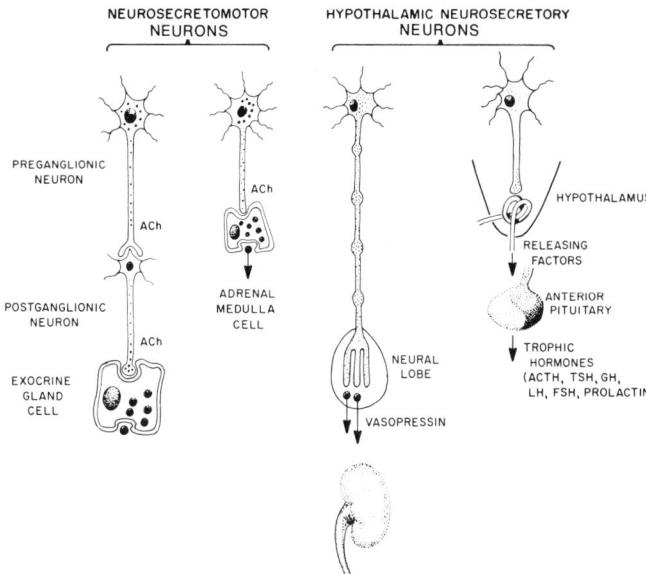

Figure 11–1. Types of neuroendocrine transducer systems. *Left,* Neurosecretomotor neurons. Postganglionic or preganglionic sympathetic fibers make direct synaptic contact with hormone-secreting cells. *Right,* Hypothalamic neurosecretory neurons. Neurosecretory neurons of the supraoptic system release ADH (vasopressin) into the systemic blood stream. Hypothalamic tuberoinfundibular neurons release hypophysiotrophic hormones (releasing factors) into the pituitary portal system to regulate secretion of hormones from the anterior pituitary. Abbreviations: ACh, acetylcholine; ACTH, adrenocorticotropin; TSH, thyroid-stimulating hormone (thyrotropin); GH, growth hormone (somatotropin); LH, luteinizing hormone; FSH, follicle-stimulating hormone. (From Martin, J. B., Reichlin, S., et al.: *Clinical Neuroendocrinology.* Philadelphia, F. A. Davis, 1977, p. 5, with permission.)

In turn, virtually all circulating hormones modify the function of the nervous system. In some instances, these effects are part of a feedback control loop, as for example regulation of antidiuretic hormone (ADH) secretion by plasma osmolality. In other instances, as for example with thyroid hormone, brain effects are incidental to other metabolic actions of the hormone. The study of the interaction between the central nervous and the endocrine systems is the subject of neuroendocrinology. Neuroendocrine interactions regulate most homeostatic activities and are essential for the control of reproductive function.

NEUROSECRETION

The idea that a neuron could possess secretory function was proposed by Ernst Scharrer in 1928 and was based on morphologic study of certain hypothalamic cells in fish. Later, he and his colleagues observed analogous structures in the mammalian hypothalamus, recognized that the appearance of certain groups of neurons was modified by changes in state of hydration, and showed that extracts of the hypothalamus contained bioassayable ADH. They proposed that the secretions of the neural lobe actually arose in the hypothalamus. At first, the concept of neurosecretion was highly controversial because it was based mainly on nonspecific histologic staining reactions, but later developments validated the concept. Most important were the discovery of the phenomenon of axoplasmic flow, which is the transport of constituents of cytoplasm and organelles from the body of the nerve cell to the axon terminal, and the demonstration that secretory products of the neurohypophysis accumulate proximal to section or ligation of the pituitary stalk.

Neurosecretion is now recognized to be but one example of the general property of all nerve cells to form bioactive products in the cell body and to release them from nerve endings (Fig. 11–2).

The ultimate route taken by the secretory product of an axon depends upon its special topographic relationships. Secretory products may be released in juxtaposition to a capillary plexus to be blood borne, and thence act as a hormone, or may be released in proximity to another neuron body or neuron process. Such contacts may take place at synaptic junctions or, more diffusely, may modify neuron function. Some neurosecretions may be looked upon as true neurotransmitters, others as "neuromodulators." See Bloom 1979 for discussion.

The discovery of the endogenous opiates (see later) and of the widespread distribution of extrahypothalamic peptidergic neuron systems has led to the recognition that many important brain functions are modulated by the secretions of specific neurons. Guillemin (1978b) has referred to this insight as "the new endocrinology of the neuron." In fact, there is growing use of the term "neurosecretion" to apply to all peptide and protein axonal secretions regardless of their site of release. Peptide secretions, the product of "peptidergic" neurons, are synthesized on endoplasmic reticulum, as is the case for more obviously glandular cells such as those of the parathyroid gland or pancreatic islet cells. Synthesis is directed by the genetic program of the cell; the secretory product is packaged into granules in the Golgi apparatus; the granules are transported by axoplasmic flow and are released from nerve endings by reverse pinocytosis in response to a propagated action potential (Figs. 11–3 and 11–4).

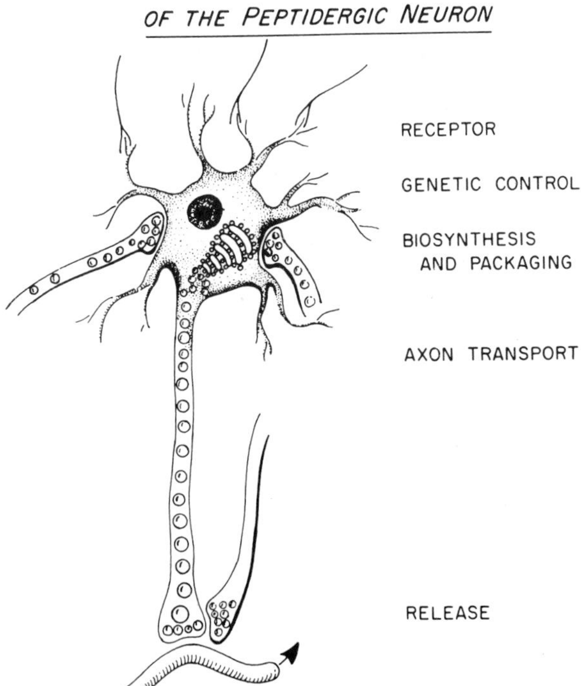

NEUROBIOLOGY OF THE PEPTIDERGIC NEURON

RECEPTOR

GENETIC CONTROL

BIOSYNTHESIS AND PACKAGING

AXON TRANSPORT

RELEASE

Figure 11–2. Neurobiology of the peptidergic neuron. Neurosecretory neurons can be looked upon as having secretory functions in many ways analogous to gland cells. A secretory product, formed on endoplasmic reticulum under the direction of mRNA, is packaged in granules and transported along the axon by axoplasmic flow to reach nerve terminals, where they are released. Virtually all neurons carry out similar functions: Some secrete neurotransmitters, such as acetylcholine or noradrenaline; others, such as motor nerves, secrete myotrophic factors. In all neurons there is a constant orthograde (forward) flow of cytoplasm and formed elements such as mitochondria. Retrograde flow also takes place to bring substances that enter nerve endings back to body of the cell. (From Reichlin, S.: In *Brain Peptides: A New Endocrinology.* Gotto, A. M., Jr., Peck, E. J., Jr., et al. [eds.]. New York, Elsevier-North Holland Biomedical Press, 1979, p. 397, with permission.)

Neurosecretory cells retain the functional and structural properties of neurons. They display electrophysiologic characteristics similar to other neurons, have neuron-type organelles and other cell constituents, are acted upon by other neurons through synapses and membranes, and react to neural transmitter substances such as acetylcholine. The specialized neural structures that possess endocrine function serve as the major links by which the brain regulates metabolic and reproductive activities. Wurtman and Axelrod applied the term "neuroendocrine transducer" to these nerve cells because they are capable of translating neural activity to a hormonal output. Neurons affecting glandular function are in turn governed by other neurons and by their metabolic and hormonal environments. Specialized neuronal receptors sensitive to changes in both the internal and the external environments can thus modulate endocrine function. These receptors also serve to generate adaptive and sexual behavior. At the highest level, the central nervous system integrates the varied neural and hormonal mechanisms to maintain the integrity of the individual organism and the perpetuation of the species.

This chapter deals with the endocrine function of the neurohypophysis and hypothalamus and the brain as a secretory organ. In addition, several other intracranial structures will be considered, including the pineal gland and the periventricular organs, all of which are derived embryologically from ependyma and possess secretory functions. The adrenal medulla, a secretory organ of neural crest origin, is dealt with in Chapter 10 and the role of the neurohypophysis in water balance in Chapter 20.

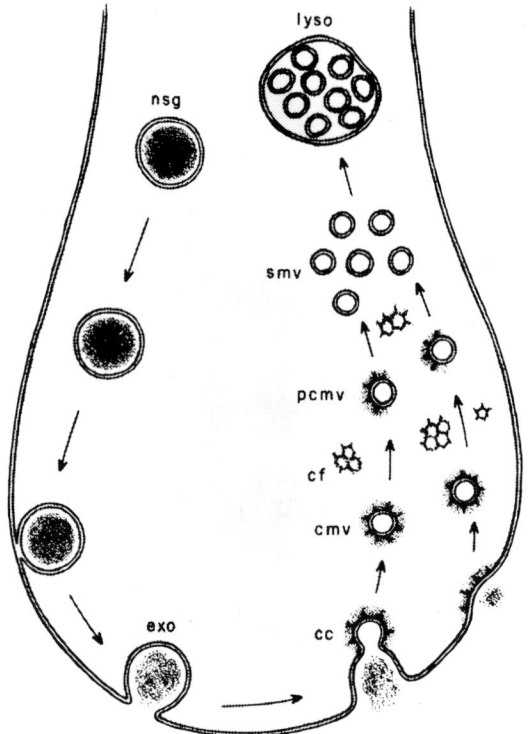

Figure 11–3. Release of stored neurosecretory granules from nerve terminals in the neural lobe. According to Douglas and collaborators, exocytosis takes place by fusion of the neurosecretory granule (nsg) membrane and the cell membrane, with extrusion of granule content into the extracellular space. Granule membrane is retrieved from the terminal's surface by micropinocytosis-like activity (vesiculation), producing coated caveolae (cc) that pinch off as coated microvesicles (pcmv) and, finally, smooth (synaptic) microvesicles (smv). These in turn are incorporated in lysosome bodies (lyso), presumably where they are degraded, and contents recycled. (From Douglas, W. S.: Mechanism of release of neurohypophysial hormones: stimulus-secretion coupling, In *Handbook of Physiology,* Section 7: *Endocrinology:* American Physiological Society. Greep, R. O., and Astwood, E. B. [eds.], Baltimore, Williams and Wilkins, 1974, p. 211, with permission.)

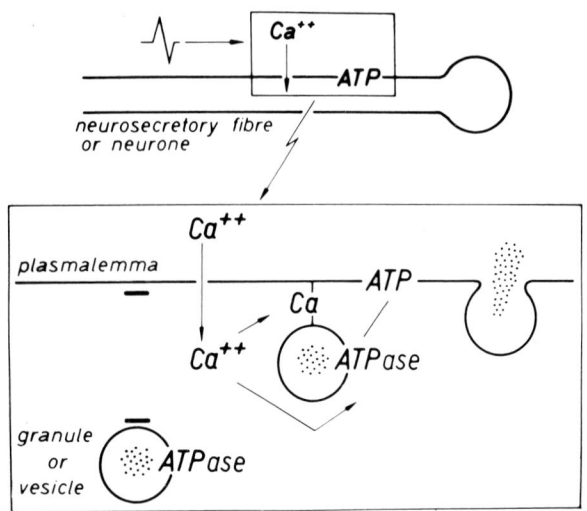

Figure 11–4. Proposed molecular basis of neurosecretion from neurohypophysis that may be applicable to other neurosecretory neurons, and other nerve endings. In response to a propagated action potential, membrane depolarization takes place, permitting entry of Ca^{++} into the nerve terminal. Within the cell, Ca^{++} is postulated by Douglas to have two effects. One effect is to neutralize the negative charge on the inner face of the plasma membrane (plasmalemma) and on the secretory granule membrane and form a cationic bridge, permitting the physical apposition of these two structures in anticipation of secretion (see also Fig. 11–3). Ca^{++} also activates granule ATPase with release of plasma membrane ATP, which in turn induces fusion of the two membranes, and extrusion of the secretory product. Contractile elements in the nerve terminal analogous to those of muscle actomyosin are activated by ATP in the presence of Ca^{++}. The most recent work suggests that Ca^{++} combines with a brain-specific calcium-binding protein (calmodulin) to form a complex that is itself an activating moiety. (From Douglass, W. W.: How do neurons secrete peptides? Exocytosis and its consequences, including synaptic vesicle formation, in the hypothalamoneurohypophyseal system. *Prog. Brain Res. 39:*21, 1973, with permission.)

HYPOTHALAMIC-PITUITARY UNIT

Anatomic Overview

The pituitary gland is divided into the adenohypophysis (anterior lobe, pars distalis, pars glandularis), the intermediate lobe (pars intermedia), and the neural lobe (posterior pituitary, infundibular process) (Figs. 11–5 and 11–6). The intermediate lobe is rudimentary in man, making up less than 0.8% of total gland weight. This figure underes-

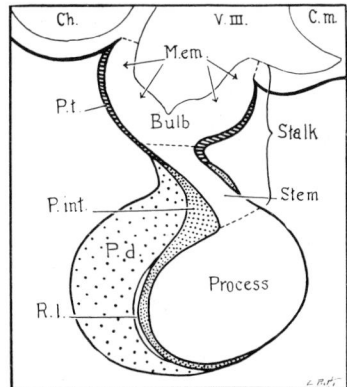

Figure 11–5. The structure and standard nomenclature of the hypothalamic-pituitary unit are outlined in this diagram of the hypophysis of a macaque monkey (*Macaca mulatta*). Bulb, infundibular "bulb" or "infundibulum"; Ch., optic chiasma; C.m., mammillary body; M.em., median eminence; P.d., pars distalis; P.t., pars tuberalis; P. int., pars intermedia; Process, infundibular process (neural lobe); R.l. residual lumen; Stem, infundibular stem; V.III., third ventricle. (Reproduced from Rioch, D. M., Wislocki, G. B., et al.: Précis of preoptic, hypothalamic and hypophyseal terminology with atlas. *Assoc. Res. Nerv. Ment. Dis. Proc.* [*1939*] 20:3, 1940, with permission.)

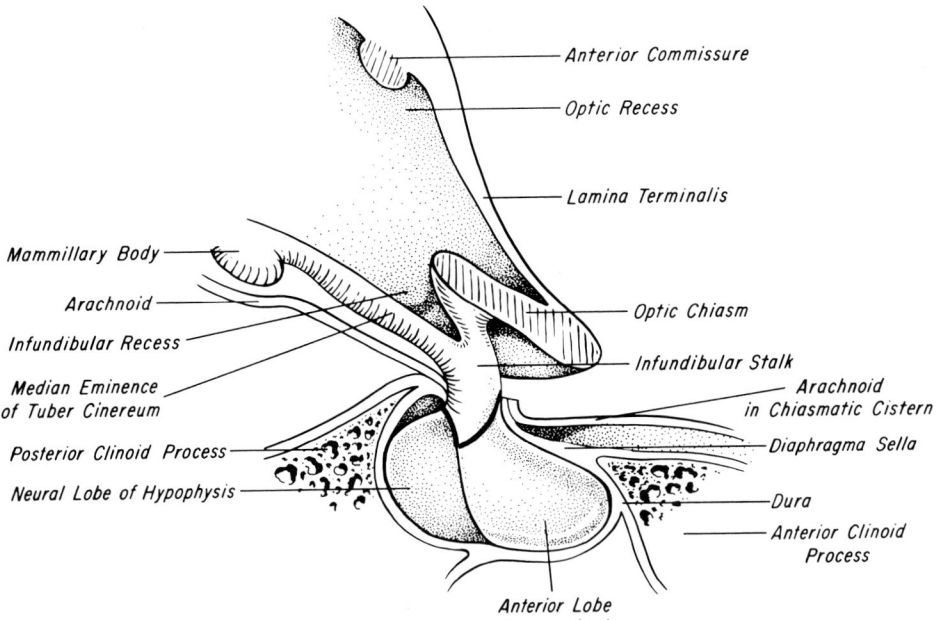

Figure 11–6. The human hypothalamic-pituitary unit to show relationship to sella turcica, brain membranes, and optic chiasm.

timates the mass of intermediate lobe cells, however, because a significant number of them are distributed diffusely in the adenohypophysis and neural lobe. The neurohypophysis consists of specialized tissue at the base of the hypothalamus, together with the neural stalk and the neural lobe. The neurohypophyseal portion of the hypothalamus (which forms the base of the third ventricle) is funnel-shaped, which gave rise to the term *infundibulum* and to

Vesalius' hypothesis that cerebrospinal fluid drained mucus ("pituita") from the brain into the nose via this structure. The central portion of the infundibulum is enveloped from below by the pars tuberalis portion of the anterior pituitary gland and is penetrated by numerous capillary loops of the primary portal plexus of the hypophyseal-portal circulation. This neurovascular complex forms a small but conspicuous structure at the base of the hypothalamus that is

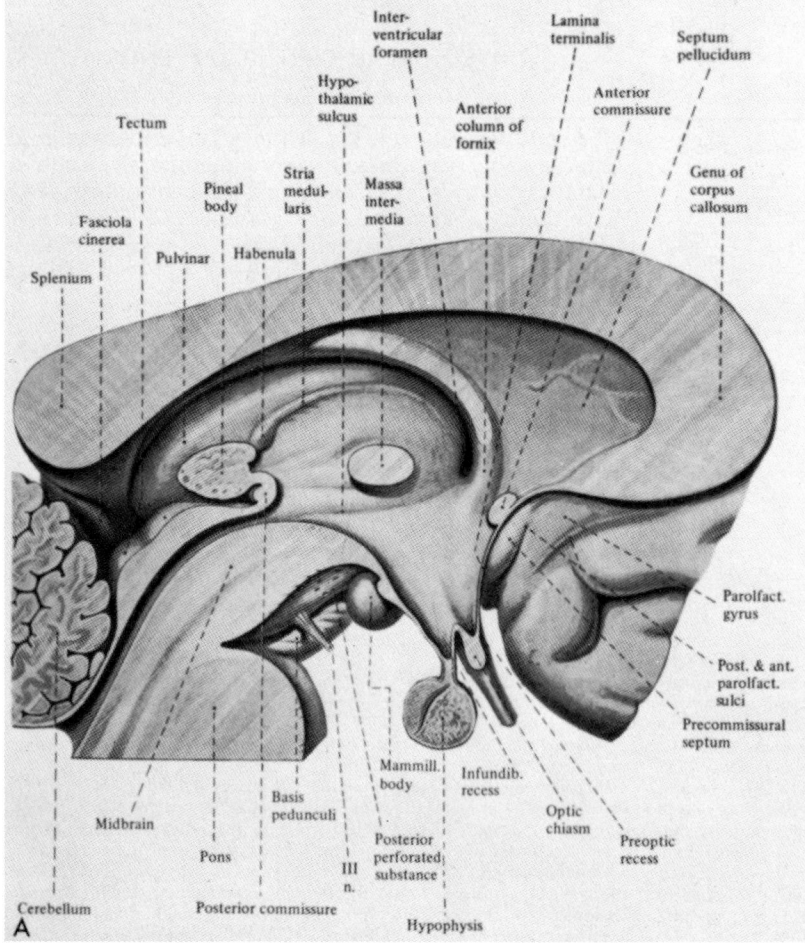

Figure 11–7. *A*, Midsagittal view of the human brain showing the hypothalamus and neighboring structures.

Illustration continued on opposite page

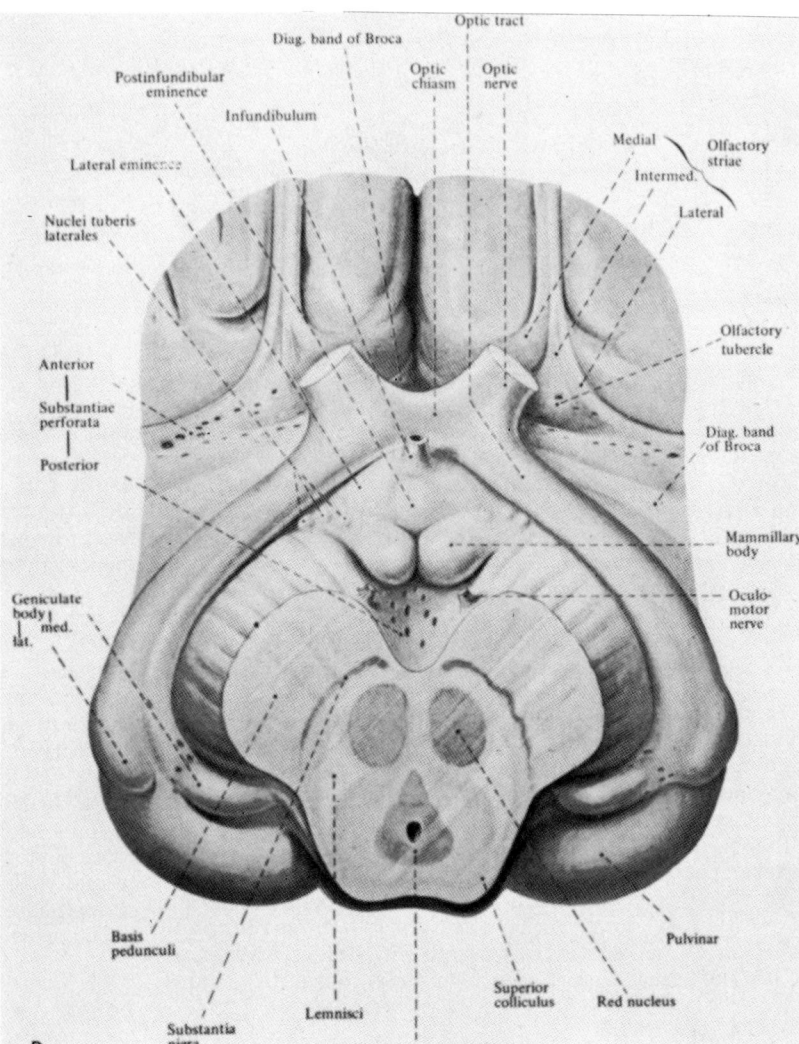

Optic tract

Diag. band of Broca

Optic chiasm · Optic nerve

Postinfundibular eminence

Infundibulum

Lateral eminence

Medial · Olfactory striae

Intermed.

Lateral

Nuclei tuberis laterales

Olfactory tubercle

Anterior
|
Substantiae perforata
|
Posterior

Diag. band of Broca

Mammillary body

Oculomotor nerve

Geniculate body med. lat.

Basis pedunculi

Pulvinar

Substantia nigra

Lemnisci

Superior colliculus

Red nucleus

Periaqueduct. gray matter

B

Figure 11–7 (continued). B, The base of the human brain, showing the hypothalamus and neighboring structures. (From Haymaker, W., Anderson, E., et al.: *The Hypothalamus,* Springfield, Ill., Charles C Thomas, 1969, p. 137, with permission.)

termed the *median eminence* of the *tuber cinereum* (see later).

The hypothalamus is readily outlined by several landmarks visible on gross inspection (Fig. 11–7) Anteriorly, it is bound by the optic chiasm, and laterally, by the sulci formed with the temporal lobes. The mamillary bodies are the posterior portion of the hypothalamus. The smooth, rounded base of the hypothalamus is termed the *tuber cinereum,* and its central region, from which descends the *pituitary stalk,* is termed the median eminence. In fresh specimens (with blood-filled vessels) or India ink–perfused specimens, the extent of the median eminence can be easily determined because it is coextensive with the distribution of the primary plexus of the hypophyseal-portal circulation. Dorsally, the hypothalamus is delineated from the thalamus by the hypothalamic sulcus.

The Neurohypophysis

Anatomy

The neural lobe develops embryologically as a downgrowth from the ventral diencephalon and retains its neural character in the adult life. The dominating features of the neurohypophysis are the supraopticohypophyseal and paraventriculohypophyseal nerve tracts (Fig. 11–8). These unmyelinated nerve tracts descend through the infundibulum and the neural stalk to terminate in dilated endings in

the neural lobe (Fig. 11–9). Capillaries supplying the neurohypophysis are fenestrated and thus resemble the structure of capillaries in other endocrine glands.

Cells of origin of these tracts are strikingly large (hence called magnocellular) and are consolidated into well-characterized groups situated in paired nuclei above the optic tract (supraoptic) and on each side of the ventricle (paraventricular) (Fig. 11–10). A few cells of this system are also distributed between the two nuclei. The other nerve cells of the hypothalamus are relatively small (parvicellular) and do not have any obvious distinguishing characteristics by conventional microscopy. Because they are conspicuous neurohypophyseal cell bodies, they have been the subject of study for many years and have been shown to be richly endowed by capillaries whose fenestrated endothelia are characteristic of endocrine glands generally. The principal projections of the two nuclei terminate in the neural lobe. Newer specific histochemical methods have shown an additional pathway of neurophysin (the neurohypophyseal hormone carrier protein) containing nerve endings located within the median eminence in relation to the primary plexus of the hypophyseal-portal circulation. It has been inferred therefore that neurohypophyseal neurons may have a role in anterior pituitary regulation, as well as in neural lobe secretion. Neurophysin-containing fibers have also been found to project from the hypothalamus to the brain stem and spinal cord, where they produce as yet unrecognized regulatory effects on neural function (Sofroniew and Weindl). Most of the cell bodies in

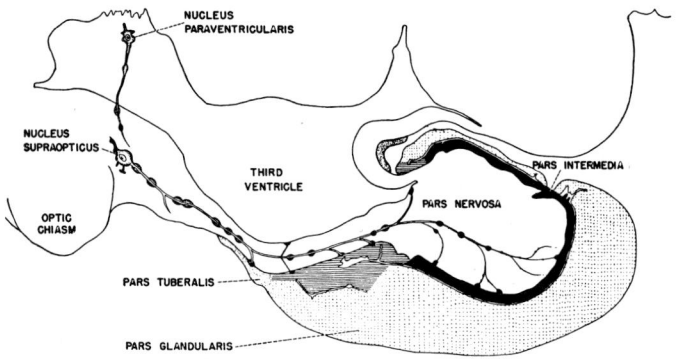

Figure 11–8. Course of the neurosecretory substance from hypothalamic cell body, along neural stalk to neurohypophysis. This diagram illustrates the concept of cell body formation of oxytocin-vasopressin and passage of the material down the stalk to a storage site in the neural lobe. The dilated areas on the axons have been thought in the past to represent extraneuronal accumulation of neurosecretory material (NSM). Electron microscopy now shows that all of the NSM is within the axon itself. (Reproduced from Bargmann, W., and Scharrer, E.: *Am. Sci. 39:*225, 1951, with permission.)

the supraoptic nucleus contain vasopressin (VP), but some contain oxytocin (OT). A somewhat smaller percentage (but still the majority of stainable cells) in the paraventricular nucleus also contain VP. Cells contain either one peptide or the other, but a few cells may contain both hormones (Defendini and Zimmerman, 1978).

Secretions of the Neurohypophysis

As late as 1889, the neural lobe of the pituitary was regarded as a "rudimentary organ without physiological function" (see H. Heller, for early history of neurohypophyseal research). The earliest physiologic studies of the neurohypophysis carried out in the last decade of the 19th century gave results that tended to confuse, rather than to illuminate, its function. Neural lobe extracts were found to exert a pressor effect and, paradoxically, to stimulate diuresis. The true significance of the neurohypophysis as an organ of water conservation first came to light as the result of clinical investigation of patients with diabetes insipidus (DI). The association of pathologic conditions of the neural stalk and pituitary with this syndrome prompted two physicians, Farini and Von den Velden, to postulate independently that DI was a deficiency disease. They reported in 1913 the therapeutic antidiuretic effect of neural lobe extracts in patients with DI. In 1924, Starling and Verney identified the locus of the effect of posterior pituitary extracts on water excretion by perfusing the isolated kidney. In the early 1930's, Verney demonstrated the physiologic effects of hyperosmolar stimuli on antidiuresis, and the neuroanatomic basis of neurohypophyseal secretion was established by Fisher and collaborators in 1935. Extensive efforts to identify the active principles of the neural lobe led, in 1950, to the elucidation of the structure of OT and, in 1954, VP. For this pioneering work in the history of peptides, du Vigneaud was awarded a Nobel Prize. Du Vigneaud's demonstration that it was possible to synthesize brain peptides was the inspiration for Guillemin and Schally and their collaborators to institute efforts to similarly characterize the hypophysiotropic peptides TRH and LRH.

The principal biologically active substances isolated from

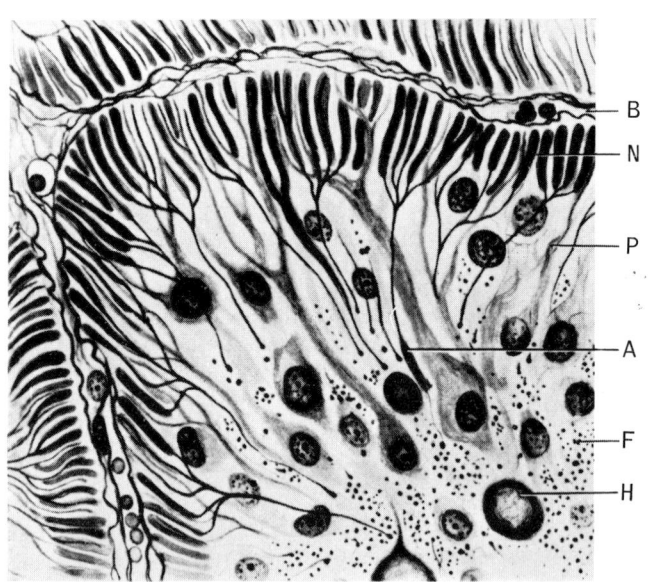

Figure 11–9. Pattern of nerve endings in the neurohypophysis of the opossum (*Didelphis virginiana*). Simple form of opossum neurohypophysis allows easy demonstration of enlarged, clublike dilations of supraopticohypophyseal nerve endings in relation to blood vessels of the neural lobe. B, blood vessel-collagenous septal layer; N, palisade zone, formed by nerve fiber terminals; P, pituicyte fibers; A, axons with neurosecretion; F, nerve fibers from the supraopticohypophyseal tract; H, Herring bodies. (Reproduced from Bodian, D.: Nerve endings, neurosecretory substance and lobular organization of neurohypophysis. *Bull. Johns Hopkins Hosp. 89:*354, 1951, with permission.)

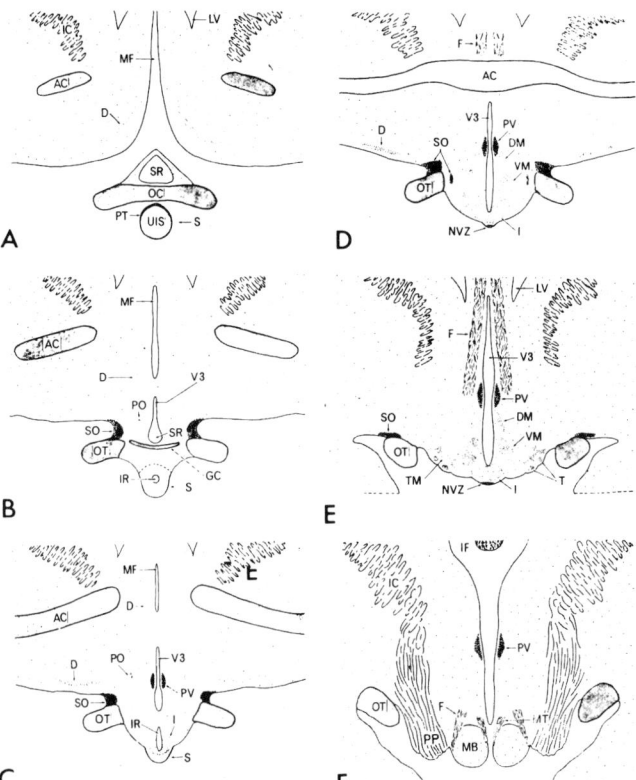

Figure 11–10. Frontal section through the hypothalamus of man to show the paraventricular nucleus, a triangle-shaped nucleus in the midline.

neural lobes are classified as having antidiuretic (water-conserving) activity and oxytocic (uterus-contracting) activity. Vasopressin (VP), so called because it was recognized at first by its ability to raise blood pressure through vasoconstruction when given in relatively large doses, is also referred to as ADH. Oxytocin (OT) is the principal oxytocic substance. Both VP and OT are nonapeptides containing 9 amino acids; both have a Cys-Cys bridge in the 1–6 position (Table 11–1). In most vertebrates more primitive than mammals, only one neurohypophyseal peptide, arginine vasotocin, is found. Sawyer has suggested that this compound is the phylogenetic precursor of both OT and VP. A single point mutation in vasotocin in position 8 (arginine to leucine) gives rise to OT. A single point mutation in position 3 (isoleucine to phenylalanine) gives rise to VP. Vasotocin is also found in mammals but, curiously, only in the pineal gland, not the neurohypophysis. VP's found in all mammals, with the exception of the pig, have identical amino acid sequences (arginine VP); in swine, arginine in position 9 is substituted by lysine. In keeping with a common phylogenetic origin of neurohypophyseal nonapeptides is the finding that there is some degree of cross-over of biologic activity, VP manifesting minimal oxytocic activity and OT minimal antidiuretic activity. Biologic activity depends upon the presence of a carboxy terminal amide group, as in the case for many peptide hormones. Three other biologically active peptides — somatostatin, thyrotropin releasing hormone (TRH) and substance P (see later) — are also found in the neurohypophysis. Their function at this site is unknown. In addition to the nonapeptides VP and OT, neural lobe extracts are also rich in proteins (neurophysins) with a minimum molecular weight of 10,000 that have the special property of binding both OT and VP by noncovalent bonds. The neurophysins are associated with OT and VP in secretory granules combined in a stoichiometric ratio and are released simultaneously with the nonapeptides. In virtually all species that have been studied, including the human, it has been possible to identify at least two major classes of neurophysins that differ somewhat in physicochemical properties and amino acid composition. Vasopressin and oxytocin are each associated with a distinct neurophysin now recognized to be part of common precursor hormones termed by Brownstein and his colleagues pro-pressophysin and pro-oxyphysin. Individual cells contain both the nonapeptide and the appropriate neurophysin. (Dierickx and Vandesande). In man, the two principal forms of neurophysin are immunologically distinct. As shown by Robinson (1975), different factors control their secretion. "Nicotine-stimulated neurophysin" is probably associated with vasopressin, while "estrogen-stimulated neurophysin" is probably associated with oxytocin.

Although evidence suggesting a common precursor for the neurophysin and the nonapeptides is strong, not all work supports this view; in one experiment, a vasopressin-producing oat cell carcinoma studied in tissue culture synthesized no neurophysin.

Hormone Synthesis, Transport, and Secretion

VP and OT are synthesized in the cell bodies of the supraoptic and paraventricular neurons as part of a prohormone. Like all neurosecretions, they are transported in membrane-bound vesicles through the axons to the neural lobe, where they are stored and later released (Figs. 11–3, 11–4, 11–9). Within the granule, they are bound to neurophysin. Some VP may also exist in a free, non-granule–bound form.

Nerve action potentials arising in the cell body are propagated along the axon and trigger hormone discharge (Fig. 11–4). The neurohypophyseal hormones leave the cell together with neurophysin in fixed ratio, thus accounting for the finding that plasma neurophysin levels rise under conditions of increased neurohypophyseal activity.

The function of neurohypophyseal neurons is in turn directly controlled by cholinergic and noradrenergic neurotransmitters and by several neuropeptides. Acetylcholine stimulation releases VP and OT, thus explaining the antidiuretic effects of tobacco smoking as a response to nicotinic acid receptor stimulation. Application of acetylcholine onto single supraoptic neurons markedly accelerates firing rate. Adrenergic influences, in contrast, are inhibitory to both hormone secretion and electric activity. Pharmacologic analysis has shown that the response is β-adrenergic. It is likely that the stress-induced inhibition of the "milk let-down" reflex (see later), well known from both animal husbandry and human nursing experience, is due to β-adrenergic inhibition of OT release. The same kind of reaction may be responsible for stress-induced diuresis.

Secretion of VP and electrophysiologic activation of supraoptic neurons are also stimulated by the administration of angiotensin II. This peptide is the mediator of an integrated homeostatic system for water conservation (see later). Neurohypophyseal neurons are also stimulated by endogenous opiates (endorphins). The well-known antidiuretic action of morphine is due to the release of VP, an effect that can be duplicated by the intracerebroventricular administration of β-endorphin. That the endorphins may be involved in VP secretion regulation is further supported by the observation that naloxone, an endorphin antagonist, reverses neurogenically inappropriate ADH secretion in some cases. Supraoptic nuclei contain many other active compounds: dopamine, serotonin, histamine, substance P, TRH, somatostatin, and α-MSH (Brownstein, 1978).

Table 11–1. PRINCIPAL PEPTIDES OF THE NEUROHYPOPHYSIS

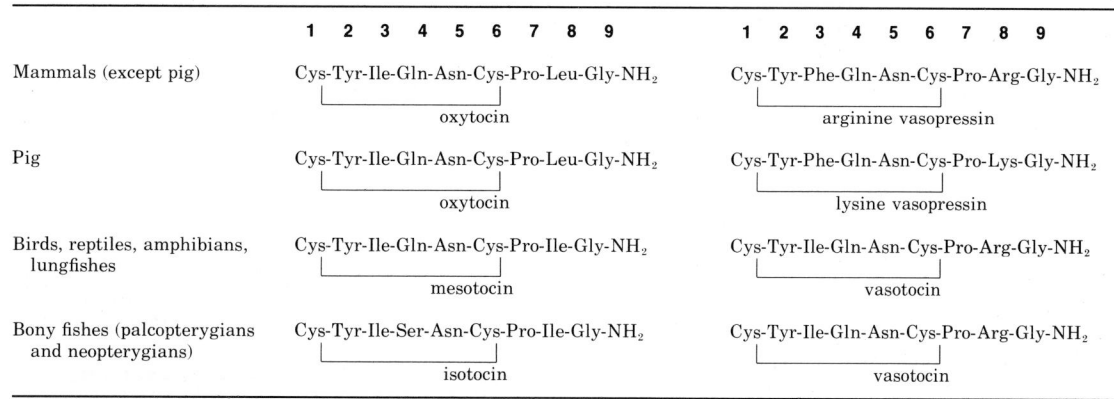

	1 2 3 4 5 6 7 8 9	1 2 3 4 5 6 7 8 9
Mammals (except pig)	Cys-Tyr-Ile-Gln-Asn-Cys-Pro-Leu-Gly-NH₂ oxytocin	Cys-Tyr-Phe-Gln-Asn-Cys-Pro-Arg-Gly-NH₂ arginine vasopressin
Pig	Cys-Tyr-Ile-Gln-Asn-Cys-Pro-Leu-Gly-NH₂ oxytocin	Cys-Tyr-Phe-Gln-Asn-Cys-Pro-Lys-Gly-NH₂ lysine vasopressin
Birds, reptiles, amphibians, lungfishes	Cys-Tyr-Ile-Gln-Asn-Cys-Pro-Ile-Gly-NH₂ mesotocin	Cys-Tyr-Ile-Gln-Asn-Cys-Pro-Arg-Gly-NH₂ vasotocin
Bony fishes (palcopterygians and neopterygians)	Cys-Tyr-Ile-Ser-Asn-Cys-Pro-Ile-Gly-NH₂ isotocin	Cys-Tyr-Ile-Gln-Asn-Cys-Pro-Arg-Gly-NH₂ vasotocin

Physiologic Regulation of Neurohypophyseal Hormone Release

Vasopressin Secretion

The most important factors regulating VP secretion are plasma osmolarity and "effective" circulating blood volume. Blood pressure, nausea, and emotional stress also influence VP release.

Osmolarity. Maintenance of normal blood water concentration is the major homeostatic function of the neurohypophysis. Blood osmolarity is jealously guarded over a relatively narrow range (±1.8%). Detailed studies of osmotic control of VP release by Miller and Moses (1977) and by Robertson (1977) have shown that the mean set point of plasma osmolality for normal individuals is 281.7 mOsm/kg and that VP release was initiated after infusion of hypertonic saline had led to an increase to 287.3 mOsm/kg, a value termed the osmotic threshold. Above this value, VP secretion increases rapidly and progressively with increasing plasma osmolarity (Fig. 11–11). Water loading inhibits VP release. This precise regulatory system operates through a hypothalamic osmoreceptor neuron system. As first shown by Verney, intracarotid perfusion with hypertonic saline led to antidiuresis, an effect blocked by lesions of the neurohypophysis. This finding is proof that some form of osmoreceptor exists within the perfusion area of the carotid. More specific localization was made by Andersson, who induced VP release by infusing minute amounts of hypertonic saline into the third ventricles of goats (Andersson et al., 1975). The precise mechanisms of osmoreceptor control have not been established with certainty. A number of neurons in both supraoptic and paraventricular nuclei, including some that project directly to the neural lobe (hence are hormone-secreting), show increased frequency of electric discharge immediately following intracarotid injections of hypertonic saline. This finding would suggest that supraopticohypophyseal and paraventriculohypophyseal neurons are intrinsically osmoreceptive. The possibility also exists, however, that another population closely related to osmoreceptor cells may activate the VP-secreting cells transsynaptically. Under some conditions, osmoreceptor control of VP secretion can be lost while other forms of control remain, a finding that reinforces the suggestion that there is a distinct population of osmoreceptor cells. The neuronal nature of the osmoreceptive process remains obscure. Any osmotically active particle that does not enter nerve cell bodies can stimulate VP release.

Volume Regulation. Hemorrhage or decreased blood volume due to any cause, if sufficient in degree, is followed by release of VP. As shown by Robertson (1977), only substantial hypovolemia is sufficient to stimulate VP secretion. For example, phlebotomy, which reduces blood volume by 6–9%, and assumption of the upright posture, which reduces central blood volume by 10–15%, had no effect on VP release. A change of between 10 and 25%, which can be produced by the combination of phlebotomy and assumption of the erect position, will bring about VP release. Under usual conditions, plasma osmolality is the prime determinant of VP secretion, but severe volume depletion can override the osmoreceptor control. With less severe degrees of volume change, osmotic control is precisely exerted, but there is a shift of "osmotic set point" so that a lower osmotic threshold is required to trigger VP secretion in the volume-depleted animal.

Receptors for volume control are located in the left atrium and in the baroreceptors of the carotid sinus and perhaps elsewhere. Modest degrees of volume depletion, insufficient to lower blood pressure, activate the atrial receptors, while depletion sufficient to cause hypotension mobilizes baroreceptor reflexes. Reflex VP release may have pressor homeostatic function in this setting. Hypertension inhibits VP release.

Neural reflexes involved in volume and pressure control reach the brain stem by way of cranial nerve afferents, ascend through multisynaptic pathways, and ultimately impinge upon the nuclei of the neurohypophyseal system. Presumably, the principal activating pathways are mediated by cholinergic neurotransmitters, but other pathways could be involved in view of the wealth of potential neurotransmitters in the supraoptic nucleus.

Stress and Nausea. The secretion of VP is affected by inputs from various parts of the "visceral brain" and the reticular activating system regions involved in the maintenance of consciousness and in emotional expression. Nausea is accompanied by intense VP release, presumably by reflex from the medullary vomiting center.

When Verney began his studies of water regulation in the dog, he was struck by the marked effect of emotional stress on antidiuretic activity. It has been generally believed that humans and rats also release VP in response to emotional stress, but Robertson (1977) has recently shown by using immunoassay methods that pain or other stresses incidental to physiologic experiments in man rarely influences plasma VP levels, nor does deliberately applied severe stress in rats. Nevertheless, the influence of "higher" neural centers on VP secretion can be demonstrated by the experimental induction of diuresis or antidiuresis by hypnotic suggestion in man or by psychologic conditioning of dogs.

Inappropriate Secretion of Antidiuretic Hormone. Excessive and inappropriate VP secretion not infrequently

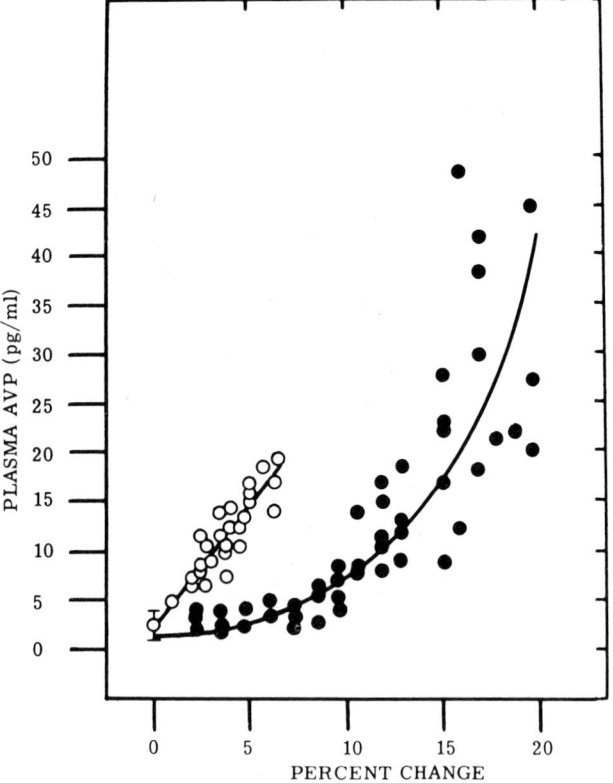

Figure 11–11. The relationship of plasma arginine vasopressin (AVP) to % *increase* in blood osmolality (○) or *decrease* in blood volume (●) in conscious rats. Plasma AVP is a linear function of percentage change in blood volume; virtually no change in AVP is detectable until there has been a 10–15% change in blood volume. (From Dunn, M. J., et al.: *J. Clin. Invest.* 52: 3212, 1973, with permission.)

arises in a variety of spontaneously occurring brain disorders in humans (see Chapter 20). It is likely that such cases are due to loss of normal tonic inhibitory influences on the neurohypophyseal neurons. Experimentally induced lesions involving the anterior margin of the supraoptic nucleus have been reported to cause increased neuronal activity in the supraopticohypophyseal pathway and to give rise to inappropriate VP release (Anderson et al., 1975).

Relation Between Vasopressin Secretion and Drinking Behavior. Drinking behavior, like VP secretion, is also regulated by plasma osmolarity and circulating blood volume, integrated by hypothalamic mechanisms, and designed to maintain the constancy of the internal milieu. The sensation of thirst (as contrasted with the sensation of dry mouth) results from an internally perceived signal arising from the hypothalamus. As with VP secretion, thirst can be generated by inducing local hyperosmolarity in the hypothalamus and by severe hemorrhage. The thirst mechanism is in some way integrated with the VP controlling mechanism. Both are activated by hypothalamic osmoreceptors that may or may not be the same. Drinking behavior and VP release can be activated neuropharmacologically by intrahypothalamic administration of acetylcholine analogues, thus suggesting that there may be a common neuromediator pathway for the two functions. There is less certainty about the role of the hypothalamic angiotensin II system in VP regulation, although it has been well established as an important regulatory factor in drinking behavior. All the biochemical ingredients and enzyme systems for the formation of angiotensin II occur *in situ* in the hypothalamus, and angiotensin II–containing neurons have been demonstrated in the region, as have angiotensin II binding sites. Local injection of angiotensin II gives a dose response–related stimulation of drinking behavior in the rat (Fig. 11–12), and drinking by dehydrated rats is blocked by local administration of saralasin, an angiotensin II receptor antagonist. Angiotensin II also stimulates VP release, both after local hypothalamic injection and upon addition to tissue cultures of neurohypophysis, but the precise dose response characteristics of this effect in relation to drinking dose response have not been adequately worked out so as to show how the two water-safeguarding

activities are integrated. Central angiotensin receptors are also responsive to angiotensin II synthesized outside the brain, thus accounting at least in part for the severe thirst sometimes seen in renovascular hypertension and in hypovolemic shock. (See also discussion of subfornical organ later on.)

Neural Control of Oxytocin Secretion

Milk Let-Down Reflex. When a hungry infant begins to nurse from its mother's breast, it does not obtain milk immediately. Rather, milk appears at the nipple after a delay of one half minute or so. This response is termed milk "let-down" and was first recognized in dairy animals. The stimulus of suckling initiates a neurogenic reflex transmitted from afferent nerve endings in the nipple that is conducted through the spinal cord, midbrain, and finally hypothalamus, where it triggers release of OT from the neurohypophysis. The released OT causes contraction of the myoepithelial cells that encircle mammary acini and thence expel the milk into the nipple. In the absence of this reflex contraction, milk cannot be obtained from even a full breast. Nursing rats, for example, cannot obtain milk from mothers previously subjected to removal of the neural lobe until injections of OT are given. The milk let-down reflex is accompanied by changes in hypothalamic neuronal function and can be blocked by specific neural lesions and also by certain types of neural stimuli. In cows, let-down can be abolished by a strange or threatening environment, and similar blockade has been noted in painfully stressed rabbits. Pain or fright inhibits milk let-down in the rabbit by adrenergic stimulation. In women, milk let-down occurs in response to suckling and in some women can be conditioned by the crying of a hungry baby. Milk let-down can be inhibited by emotional stress and triggered by sexual excitement and orgasm. OT has been administered therapeutically in some women with failure to show normal milk let-down.

Oxytocin Secreted in Relation to Labor. Although the uterus-contracting activity of OT was the first of its actions to be recognized and is a biologic activity that has been utilized to induce labor and manage obstetric hemorrhage, there is still considerable question about its importance in the initiation and maintenance of normal labor in the human.

Labor is said to be relatively normal in women with DI, even in those in whom OT deficiency can be demonstrated. Complicating the interpretation of this finding is the fact that the fetal neural lobe secretes OT and that fetal OT can gain access to the uterus. Once labor has been instituted in normal women, maternal OT secretion, which takes place in spurts, increases and reaches a maximum at the time of delivery (Chard, 1977). Reflexes arising from the contracting uterus trigger OT release, thus providing a powerful positive feedback control of the process of labor.

Secretion of VP and of OT are independent. For example, in lactating women, ADH secretion can be achieved by hypertonic saline infusion without producing let-down, and the suckling stimulus induces let-down without accompanying antidiuresis.

The Median Eminence and Tuberhypophyseal Neurons

Anatomy (Figs. 11–13 to 11–18)

The median eminence consists of a neural component (the infundibulum of the hypothalamus), a vascular component

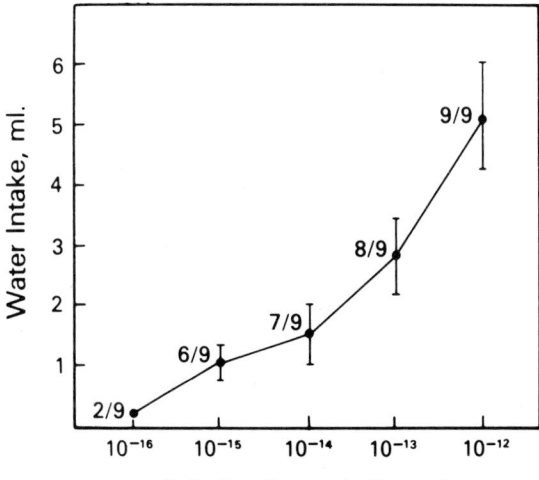

Figure 11–12. Dose-response curve of drinking produced by injection of angiotensin II directly into the subfornical organ, a structure located in the dorsal anterior wall of the third ventricle (see under "Periventricular Organs"). (From Simpson, J. B., Epstein, A. N., et al.: The localization of receptors for the dipsogenic action of angiotensin II in the suffornical organ of rat. *J. Comp. Physiol. Psychol. 92:*581, 1978, with permission.)

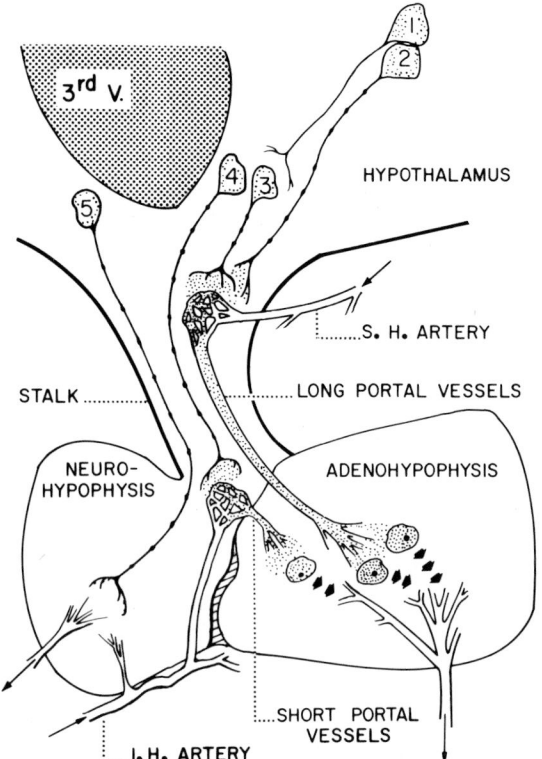

Figure 11–13. Neural control of pituitary gland. This figure summarizes the types of neural input into pituitary regulation. Neuron 5 represents the peptidergic neurons of the supraopticohypophyseal and paraventriculohypophyseal tracts, with hormone-producing cell bodies in the hypothalamus and nerve terminals in the neural lobe. Neurons 4 and 3 are the neurons of the tuberohypophyseal tract that secrete the hypophysiotropic hormones into the substance of the median eminence in anatomic relationship to the primary plexus. Neuron 1 represents a monoaminergic neuron ending in relation to the cell body of the peptidergic neuron. Neuron 2 represents a monoaminergic neuron ending on terminals of the peptidergic neuron to give axo-axonic transmission, as proposed by Schneider and McCann. Neurons 1 and 2 are the functional links between the remainder of the brain and the peptidergic neuron. (From Gay, V. L.: The hypothalamus: physiology and clinical use of releasing factors. *Fertil. Steril.* 23:50, 1972, with permission.)

unlike most of the brain is permeable to molecules such as thyroxine (T_4), trypan blue, and growth hormone (GH). Most workers believe that there are no morphologically demonstrable synapses or axons in the median eminence. As Joseph and Knigge (1978) point out:

The extracellular and perivascular space of the median eminence would appear to be a medium of remarkable composition. . . large pools of nerve terminals and nonneuronal elements are bathed in an interstitial fluid containing a multitude of hormones, and excitatory and inhibitory neurotransmitters.

Although most axons of the supraopticohypophyseal and paraventriculohypophyseal tracts pass through the median eminence on their way from cells of origin in the hypothalamus to termination in the neural lobe, a distinct population of paraventricular neurons project to the median eminence. In this location they may have an anterior pituitary regulatory role.

The form of the blood vessels in the primary plexus varies somewhat from species to species. In humans, capillaries form loops that are part of complex spiral structures termed *gomitoli*. These penetrate the infundibulum and stalk. Arterioles of the stalk and median eminence of humans have highly muscular walls, suggesting that hemodynamic changes in these vessels might affect pituitary function, but evidence to support this point of view is lacking. Reflex constriction of these vessels following postpartum hemorrhage has been suggested as a factor in the genesis of pituitary infarction.

Blood reaches the plexus of the median eminence and upper stalk by way of the superior hypophyseal artery, a branch of the internal carotid (see Ch. 3). This plexus is drained by the long portal veins that run along the stalk and finally reach the pituitary sinusoids. The capillary plexus in the lower portion of the stalk is supplied by the inferior hypophyseal artery and is drained by short portal veins that enter the pituitary almost directly. Although classic studies have demonstrated that the direction of blood flow in the long portal vessels is from the hypothalamus to the pituitary, more recent work indicates that flow of blood from pituitary to median eminence can also occur by way of the short portal vessels that drain both anterior and posterior pituitary. One consequence of this "circular" flow is that the hypothalamus is exposed to exceedingly high concentrations of the secretions of both anterior and posterior pituitary lobes (Fig. 11–14).

The third component of the median eminence, the pars tuberalis, is a thin glandular sheath around the infundibulum and pituitary stalk. In some animals, the epithelial component may make up as much as 10% of the total glandular tissue of the pituitary, and several pituitary tropic hormones have been extracted from this region. Moreover, nerve fibers can be traced to the pars tuberalis. These findings to the contrary, the bulk of studies indicate that the pars tuberalis does not have an important physiologic function but serves merely as the region through which arteries and veins of the hypophyseal-portal circulation are conducted.

(the hypophyseal-portal capillaries and veins), and an epithelial component (the pars tuberalis of the adenohypophysis). Electron microscopic studies show that the infundibulum is composed mainly of densely packed nerve endings; capillaries with conspicuous perivascular spaces; supporting cells; and ependymal cells, including one type, the tanycyte, that traverses the median eminence from the lumen of the third ventricle to the outer mantle plexus. The nerve endings are the terminals of the tuberohypophyseal neurons, which arise chiefly in the ventral hypothalamus; the capillaries form the primary plexus of the portal circulation.

Two classes of tuberhypophyseal neurons project to the median eminence. Some are peptidergic (for example, TRH, LRH and somatostatin) and others are bioaminergic, the most important being dopaminergic.

Relationships of nerve endings, basement membrane, interstitial space, and capillary wall are identical in plan to those in the neural lobe, and the release of neuropeptides can be stimulated by exposure to high K^+ concentration in the presence of Ca^{++}. Thus the process of secretion at median eminence terminals is analogous to the stimulus-secretion mechanism of the neurohypophysis. The large, perivascular space contact area and the peculiar vessels in this region, which have fenestrations typical of those seen in ordinary endocrine glands, account for the observation that the neurohypophysis, including the median eminence,

Portal Vessel–Chemotransmitter Control

The hypophyseal portal vessel–chemotransmitter hypothesis of pituitary control was introduced as an explanation of how the anterior pituitary gland, which is devoid of secretomotor nerve fibers, could be influenced by the nervous system.

Several workers, including Hinsey and Markee (1933) and Friedgood (1936), had postulated a neurohumoral con-

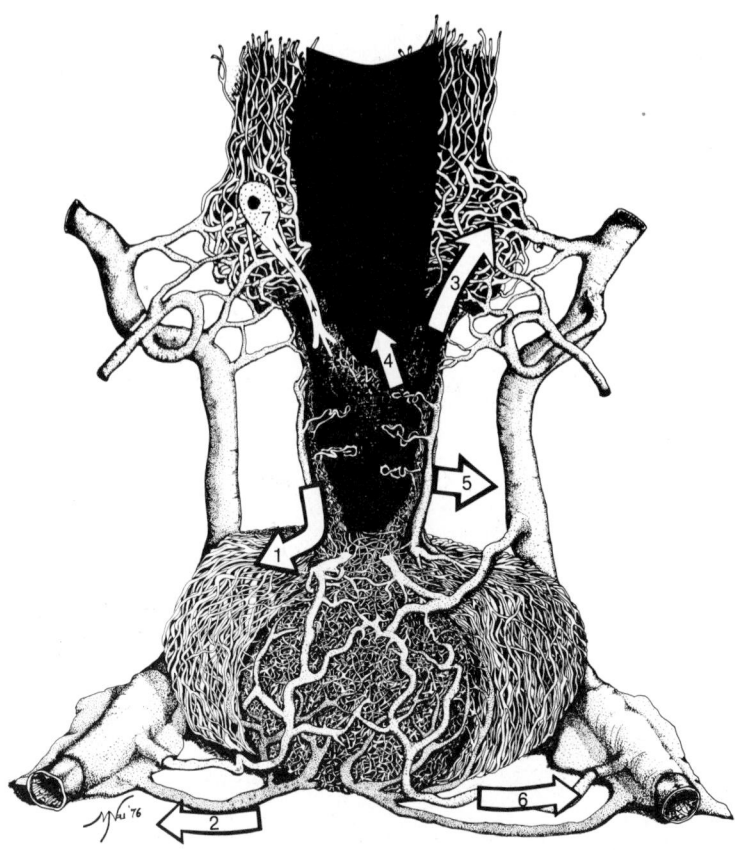

Figure 11–14. In this drawing of a pituitary vascular cast, the posterior portion of the infundibulum has been removed. The arrows demonstrate the potential efferent routes from the neurohypophysis: (1) Portal vessels may convey blood to the adenohypophysis; (2) confluent pituitary veins may carry blood to the cavernous sinus; (3) blood may flow from the infundibulum to the hypothalamus via connecting capillaries; (4) tanycytes may transport some substances into the ventricle; (5) substances may leak through the endothelial fenestrations of portal vessels into the subarachnoid space; (6) certain hypophyseal arteries may under certain conditions serve as efferent vascular channels; and (7) retrograde axonal flow may carry substances from the neurohypophysis to the hypothalamus. Five of these routes are directed toward the brain. (Reprinted by permission of the authors and publisher of Endocrinology, from Bergland, R. M., and Page, R. B. Can the Pituitary Secrete Directly to the Brain? (Affirmative Anatomical Evidence) *Endocrinology 102*:1326, 1978.)

trol system for the anterior pituitary by the mid-1940's, but it is Geoffry Harris and John Green who are generally given credit for the modern formulation of this theory (Green and Harris, 1947). The studies by Harris and his collaborators on the function of the vascular component of the pituitary stalk were crucial in popularizing the hypophyseal portal–chemotransmitter concept and stimulated a wealth of physiologic and anatomic experiments. Definitive

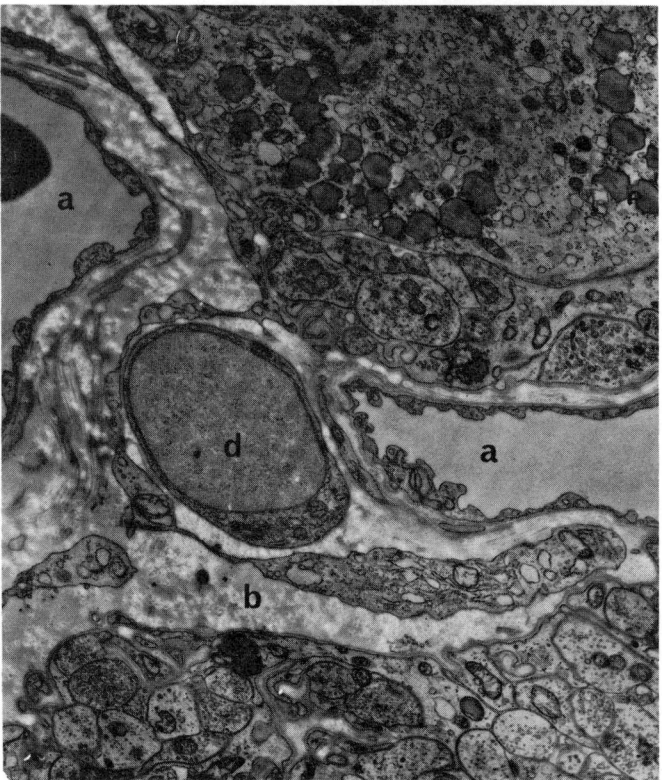

Figure 11–15. Electron micrograph of hamster median eminence. The median eminence is made up of densely packed nerve endings distributed in relation to the perivascular space of the primary portal capillaries in a schema resembling in principle the distribution of nerve endings in the neurohypophysis. The nerve endings shown here in cross-section profiles contain a variety of vesicles, both large and small, of differing electron density, some of which contain neurosecretions and others are thought to be recycled membrane vessels (see Fig. 11–13). Mitochondria are also found. Note that nerves end in close relation to a basement membrane. The path of secretion is from nerve endings, through axon basement membrane and finally endothelium. This is the characteristic arrangement of glandular cells throughout the endocrine system. Symbols: a, capillary lumen; b, perivascular space; c, nerve endings; d, nucleus of supporting (connective tissue) cell. (Courtesy of Karl M. Knigge, unpublished, 1966.)

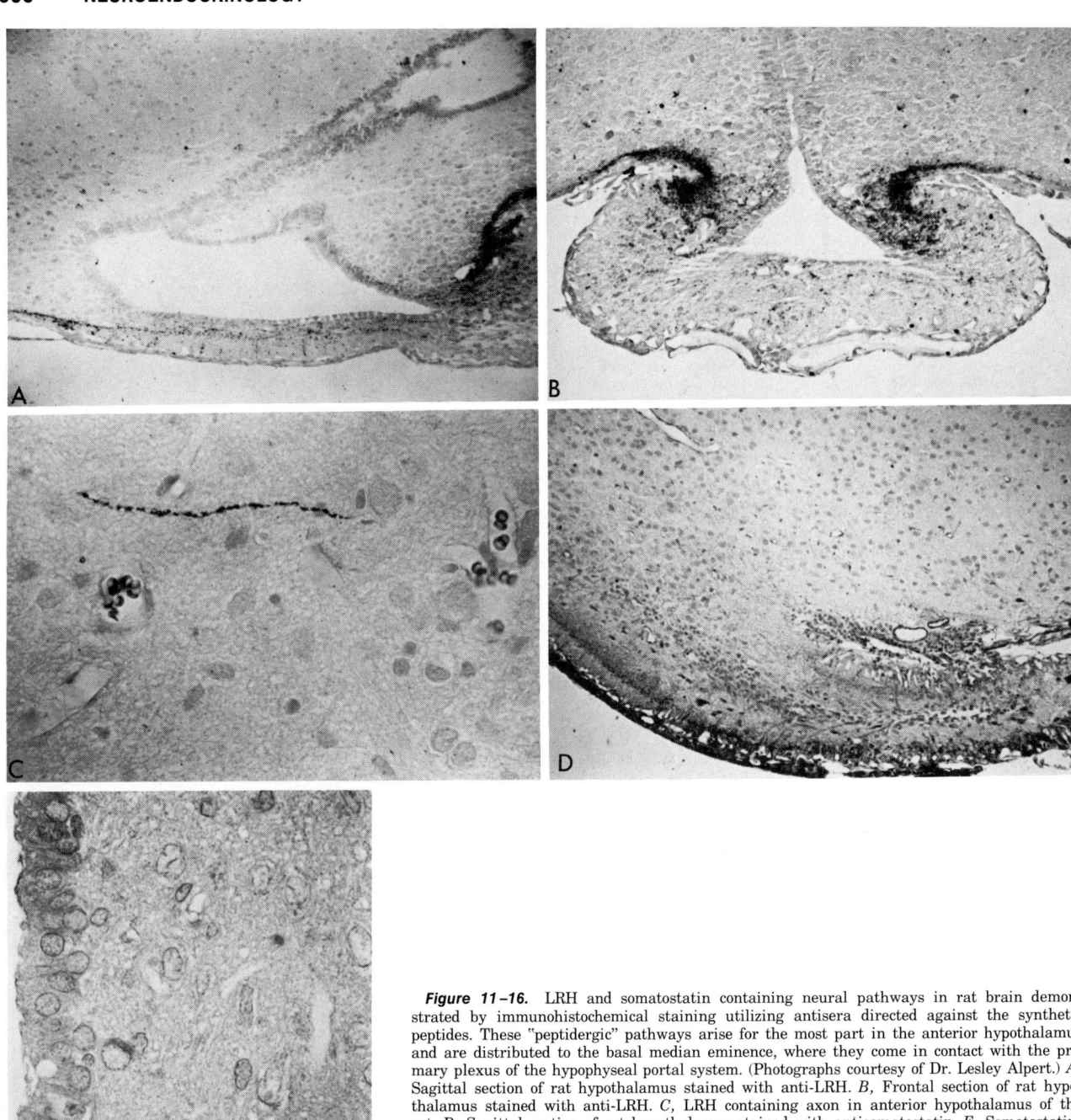

Figure 11–16. LRH and somatostatin containing neural pathways in rat brain demonstrated by immunohistochemical staining utilizing antisera directed against the synthetic peptides. These "peptidergic" pathways arise for the most part in the anterior hypothalamus and are distributed to the basal median eminence, where they come in contact with the primary plexus of the hypophyseal portal system. (Photographs courtesy of Dr. Lesley Alpert.) *A*, Sagittal section of rat hypothalamus stained with anti-LRH. *B*, Frontal section of rat hypothalamus stained with anti-LRH. *C*, LRH containing axon in anterior hypothalamus of the rat. *D*, Sagittal section of rat hypothalamus stained with antisomatostatin. *E*, Somatostatin-containing cells in rat anterior hypothalamus.

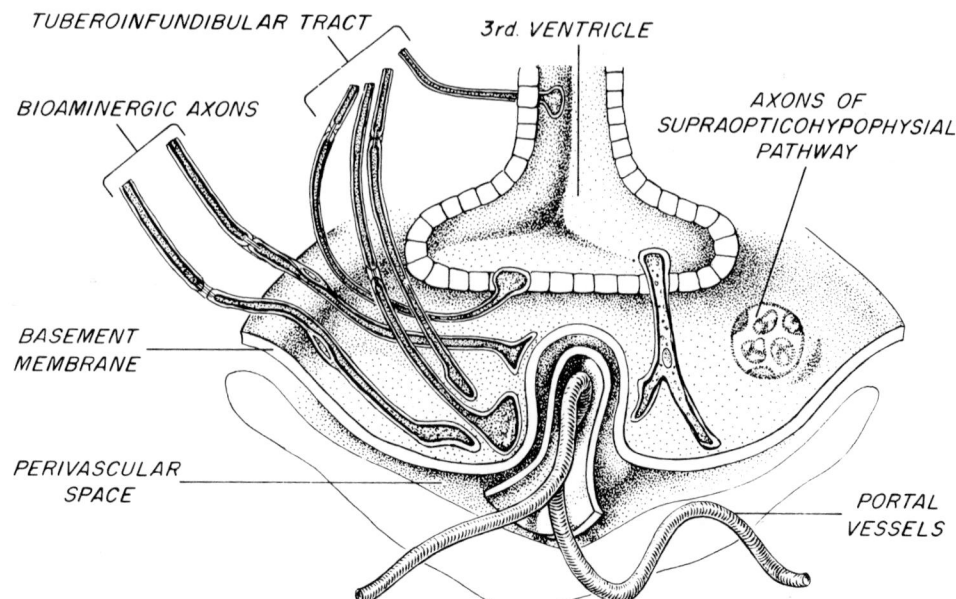

Figure 11–17. Diagram of anatomic relationships of important secretory structures in the median eminence, visualized as if one were looking rostrally at a cut section. The interstitial space in which all the nerve endings terminate is a free pool without a blood-brain barrier. It is separated from the lumen of the third ventricle by ependyma whose tight junctions prevent direct diffusion from medial eminence to third ventricle lumen. Tuberoinfundibular neurons, some peptidergic, some bioaminergic, end in the interstitial space; many, but not all, end directly on capillary loops. Few if any true axo-axonic synapses are found here. Stretching between lumen and outer third of median eminence are tanycytes, specialized cells that may have transport functions. The supraopticohypophyseal pathway is shown as a cut section of fibers in passage, but it should be recognized that some of the neurohypophyseal neurons end in the median eminence.

proof finally came when TRH and LRH were chemically identified and shown to be present in hypophyseal-portal blood. These findings, together with the demonstration of neurosecretory tuberohypophyseal neurons, allow us to conclude that the portal vessel–chemotransmitter hypothesis has been fully validated. For their work in the elucidation of the chemistry of the hypophysiotropic hormones, Roger Guillemin and Andrew Schally were awarded Nobel Prizes in 1977. (See Guillemin, 1978, Schally, 1977, Fink, 1976, and Flerk, 1980.)

Hypophysiotropic Hormones of the Hypothalamus

The search for hypothalamic neurohormones with anterior pituitary regulating properties focused upon extracts of stalk median eminence (SME) and hypothalamus. Such hypophysiotropic materials have been called releasing *factors* after the first description of corticotropin releasing factor (CRF). This term was introduced by Saffran and Schally (1955) to describe a substance extracted from hypothalamic tissues that stimulated the release of ACTH from pituitary fragments maintained in organ culture. At the present time, the term "releasing *factor*" is still applied to hypothalamic substances of unknown chemical nature, whereas substances with established chemical identity, such as TRH and LRH (thyrotropin releasing hormone and luteinizing releasing hormone), are referred to as releasing *hormones*. The chemical structures of the three peptide hypophysiotropic hormones thus far identified are shown in Fig. 11–19. Dopamine can also be included as a hypophysiotropic hormone because it is present in hypophyseal-portal vessel blood in concentration sufficient to duplicate all its known

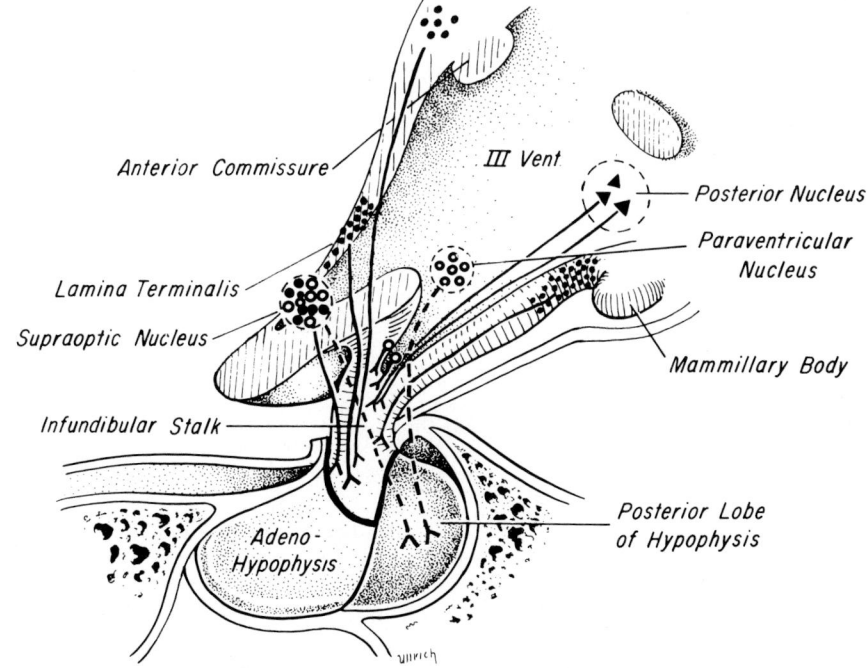

Figure 11–18. Hypophysiotropic peptide pathways in the human hypothalamus. This semi-schematic diagram is a composite drawing based on several reports in the literature that describe the localization of LRH, TRH and somatostatin in the human hypothalamus. (Sources: J. Barry, Characterization and topography of LH-RH neurons in the human brain, *Neuroscience Letters, 3*:287–291, 1976, J. Barry., Immunofluorescence study of LRF neurons in man, *Cell Tiss Res. 181*:1, 1977. C. Buganon, D. Fellman, B. Bloch. Immunocytochemical study of the ontogenesis of the hypothalamic somatostatin-containing neurons in the human fetus, *Cell Tiss Res 183*:319, 1977, E. Okon, Y. Koch, Localization of gonadotropin-releasing and tyrotropin-releasing hormones in human brain by radioimmunoassay, *Nature 263*:345, 1976. Diagram prepared through the courtesy of Dr. Mark Molitch.)

pyroGlu-His-Pro-NH$_2$

TRH, Thyrotropin-releasing hormone

pyroGlu-His-Trp-Ser-Tyr-Gly-Leu-Arg-Pro-Gly-NH$_2$

LHRH, Luteinizing hormone-releasing hormone, gonadotropin-releasing
hormone, GnRH

```
               ┌──────────── S–S ────────────┐
               │                             │
H-Ala-Gly-Cys-Lys-Asn-Phe-Phe-Trp-Lys-Thr-Phe-Thr-Ser-Cys-OH
```

Somatostatin, SRIF

Figure 11–19. Structural formulas of the established hypophysiotropic hormones.

effects on the pituitary gland. Structures of CRF, GH releasing factor (GHRF) are unknown. There are several candidates for prolactin (PRL) releasing factors (see later). The many other active peptides found in the hypothalamus are listed in Table 11–2. Releasing factors also have stimulatory effects on other pituitary functions, such as differentiation and hormone synthesis.

Certain hypothalamic factors exert significant inhibitory actions on anterior pituitary function. Inhibitory factors interact with the respective releasing factor to exert dual control of secretion of PRL, GH, TSH, and to a lesser extent, the gonadotropins. These are discussed later in relation to control of specific anterior pituitary secretions. Contrary to expectations, the action of each of the hypophysiotropic hormones is not limited strictly to a single pituitary hormone. For example, TRH is a potent releaser of PRL and, under some circumstances, releases ACTH and GH. LRH releases both LH and FSH. Somatostatin inhibits secretion of GH, TSH, and a wide variety of other nonpituitary hormones (see later). The principal inhibitor of PRL secretion is dopamine, but this potent bioamine acting directly on the pituitary also inhibits TSH and gonadotropin secretion and, under some circumstances, also inhibits GH secretion.

Thyrotropin Releasing Hormone

Chemistry and Effects on the Pituitary

The chemical structure of TRH was elucidated by investigators working in association with Roger Guillemin and Andrew Schally. Their work, which was the culmination of more than a decade of effort to identify the nature of the thyrotropin releasing activity of crude hypothalamic extracts, made neuroendocrinology credible to the general scientific and clinical community. It also made possible the introduction of TRH into clinical medicine, vastly widened the scope of understanding of TRH in other biologic systems, and gave a powerful incentive to efforts to identify other biologic activities in hypothalamic extract.

TRH is relatively simple substance, a tripeptide amide (pyro) glu-His-Pro-NH$_2$ (Fig. 11–19). Although some substituent forms are potent, an intact amide and the cyclized glutamic acid terminus are essential for activity. TRH is chemically stable but is rapidly degraded in plasma by enzymatic action. Following injection in humans or in rats, blood TSH levels rise rapidly and dramatically, a change being detected within 3 min; peak values are attained between 10 and 20 min. after injection in normal individuals (Fig. 11–20), somewhat later in patients with hypothyroidism. TRH is very potent, as little as 15 mcg giving detectable responses and maximal effects being achieved by a dose of 400 mcg. The standard clinical dose commonly administered as a bolus is 500 mcg. Transient mild nausea, sense of urinary urgency, and mild decreases or increases in blood pressure occur as side effects of injection in an appreciable number of patients, but no serious or life-threatening complications have been reported. The surge of TSH release induced by TRH injection leads to a readily detected rise in plasma triiodothyronine (T$_3$), and an increase in T$_4$ release that may not be large enough to produce significant increase in plasma levels of this hormone. The clinical applications of TRH testing are covered in detail in Ch. 4 (The Thyroid Gland), and its role in neuroendocrine regulation of TSH secretion is discussed in this chapter.

One of the most important aspects of TRH action on the pituitary is that its effects are blocked by prior treatment with thyroid hormone. In fact, it is the interaction of the negative feedback action of thyroid hormone on the pituitary with the stimulating effects of TRH that is the main basis of the integrated neuroendocrine control system of TSH secretion (see later).

In addition to bringing about TSH release, TRH is also a potent PRL releasing factor (Fig. 11–21). The time course of response of blood PRL levels to TRH, dose response characteristics, and suppressibility by thyroid hormone pretreat-

Table 11–2.   SEVERAL HYPOTHALAMIC PEPTIDES WHOSE STRUCTURES AND ACTIONS ARE KNOWN BUT WHOSE PHYSIOLOGIC FUNCTIONS ARE NOT FULLY UNDERSTOOD

Name	Structure
Substance P	Arg-Pro-Lys-Pro-Gln-Gln-Phe-Phe-Gly-Leu-Met-NH$_2$
Neurotensin	pGlu-Leu-Tyr-Glu-Asn-Lys-Pro-Arg-Arg-Pro-Tyr-Ile-Leu-OH
Angiotensin II	Asp-Arg-Val-Tyr-Ile-His-Pro-Phe
Leu-enkephalin	Tyr-Gly-Gly-Phe-Leu-OH
Met-enkephalin	Tyr-Gly-Gly-Phe-Met-OH
α endorphin	Tyr-Gly-Gly-Phe-Met-Thr-Ser-Glu-Lys-Ser-Gln-Thr-Pro-Leu-Val-Thr-OH
β endorphin	Tyr-Gly-Gly-Phe-Met-Thr-Ser-Glu-Lys-Ser-Gln-Thr-Pro-Leu-Val-Thr-Leu-Phe-Lys-Asn-Ala-Ile-Val-Lys-Asn-Ala-His-Lys-Lys-Gly-Gln-OH
γ endorphin	Tyr-Gly-Gly-Phe-Met-Thr-Ser-Glu-Lys-Ser-Gln-Thr-Pro-Leu-Val-Thr-Leu-OH
Vasoactive intestinal peptide	His-Ser-Asp-Ala-Val-Phe-Thr-Asp-Asn-Tyr-Thr-Arg-Leu-Arg-Lys-Gln-Met-Ala-Val-Lys-Lys-Tyr-Leu-Asn-Ser-Ile-Leu-Asn-NH$_2$
Gastrin (17-I)*	pGlu-Gly-Pro-Trp-Leu-Glu-Glu-Glu-Glu-Glu-Ala-Tyr-Gly-Trp-Met-Asp-Phe-NH$_2$

Cholecystokinin-pancreazymin	Lys-Ala-Pro-Ser-Gly-Arg-Val-Ser-Met-Ile-Lys-Asn-Leu-Gln-Ser-Leu-Asp-Pro-Ser-His-Arg-Ile-Ser-Asp-Arg-Asp-Tyr-Met-Gly-Trp-Met-Asp-Phe-NH$_2$
	                                  |
	                                 SO$_3$H

Bombesin	pGlu-Gln-Arg-Leu-Gly-Asn-Gln-Trp-Ala-Val-Gly-His-Leu-Met-NH$_2$

All peptides listed above have been reported to occur in hypothalamus and many other parts of the brain. Localization in perykarya, nerve ending, and tracts suggests a role in brain function. In addition, several polypeptides have been identified in brain, including ACTH and related peptides, insulin, GH, PRL, TSH, and neurotensin.

* There are three forms of gastrin in man. Shown here is Gastrin 17-I (mw 2096).

From Li, C. H., and Chung, D.: Primary structure of human β-lipoprotein. *Nature* 260:622, 1976.

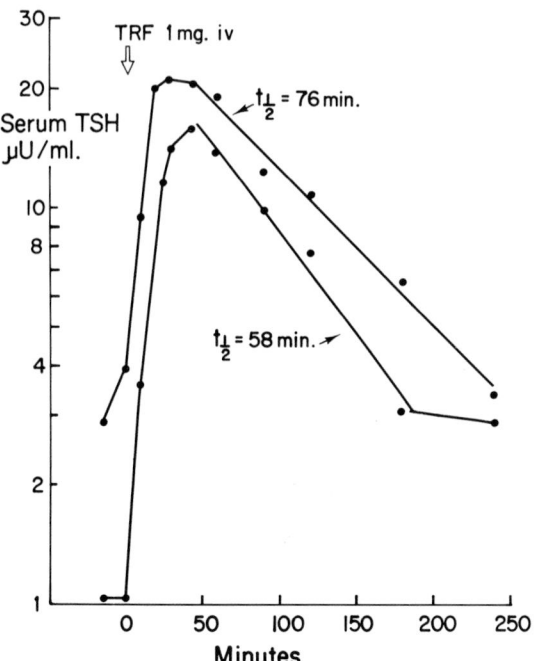

Figure 11-20. Effect of intravenous injection of TRF on plasma TSH in the human. (Reproduced from Hershman, J. M., and Pittman, J. A., Jr.: Control of thyrotropin secretion in man. *N. Engl. J. Med.* 285:997, 1971, with permission.)

ment (all of which parallel changes in TSH secretion) make it appear almost a certainty that TRH is involved in the regulation of PRL secretion. It has been stated facetiously that if PRL release bioassays had been used to isolate TRH, it would have been called PRF (PRL releasing factor).

Despite these striking overlapping effects it is unlikely that TRH plays more than a modulatory role in PRL regulation under normal circumstances. The PRL response to nursing in women and in experimental animals is unaccompanied by changes in plasma TSH, thus indicating that this neurogenic reflex does not involve TRH release. Most workers (but not all) have found that the administration of

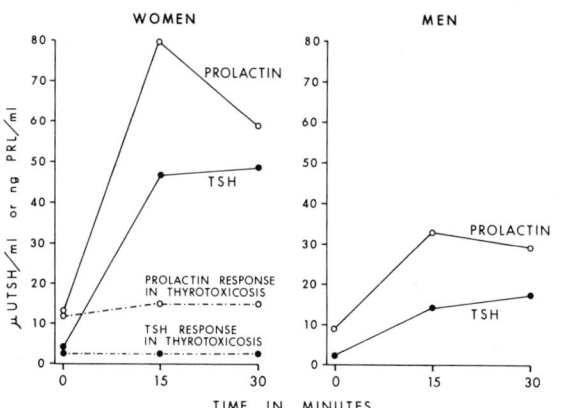

Figure 11-21. PRL and TSH secretory response to injection of TRH in humans. This figure shows that TRH induces discharge of both PRL and TSH, that the effect in females is greater than it is in males (presumably owing to estrogen sensitization of the pituitary), and that thyrotoxicosis inhibits the response of both PRL and TSH to TRH. The inhibitory effect on TRH response is noted at the upper limit of the normal range of thyroid hormone levels and is a very sensitive test of minor degrees of thyroid hormone excess. Although TRH is a potent PRF, there is evidence that there is another PRF material physiologically connected to PRL regulation. (Replotted from data of Bower, S., Friesen, H. G., et al.: *Biochem. Biophys. Res. Comm.* 45:1033, 1972.)

anti-TRH antibody to rats which neutralizes endogenous TRH, has no effect on plasma PRL levels. The PRL release–stimulating actions of TRH may be responsible for the occasional occurrence of hyperprolactinemia (with or without galactorrhea) in patients with hypothyroidism, however. This finding has been attributed to an increased sensitivity of PRL-secreting cells to TRH in the hypothyroid state, to an increase in TRH secretion, or to the hypothyroidism-induced inhibition of secretion of PRL inhibitory factors (see "Prolactin Regulatory Factors" later on).

In normal individuals, TRH has no influence on pituitary hormone secretions other than TSH and PRL. Under special circumstances, however, it exerts a number of other effects on pituitary secretion, including the release of ACTH in some patients who have Cushing's disease and the release of GH in some patients with acromegaly. These responses are thought to be due to the presence on pituitary cell membranes of TRH receptors ordinarily obscured by the normal regulatory processes of the pituitary or appearing as a consequence of "derepression" of the adenoma to a more primitive cell resembling an ancestral pituitary stem cell. TRH also releases GH in some patients with uremia, hepatic disease, and anorexia nervosa, in children with hypothyroidism, and in some patients with psychotic depression. TRH inhibits sleep-induced GH release through a central nervous system mechanism and has other central nervous system effects as well (see later).

Extrahypothalamic Distribution and Neuromodulator Function of Thyrotropin Releasing Hormone

One of the most surprising consequences of the development of specific methods for detection of TRH was its demonstration in brain tissue outside of the classic "thyrotropic area" of the hypothalamus. TRH has been found by immunoassay or immunohistochemistry in virtually all parts of the brain, including the cerebral cortex and spinal cord, in nerve endings abutting the ventral horn motor cells, in the circumventricular structures (see later), in the neurohypophysis, and in the pineal. (See Jackson, 1979 and Reichlin, 1979, for review.) TRH has also been found in pancreatic islet cells and in various parts of the gastrointestinal tract. Although present in low concentrations in these areas, the aggregate in extrahypothalamic tissues far exceeds the total amount in the hypothalamus. As the phylogenetic scale is descended, the concentration of TRH found in neural tissues outside the hypothalamus increases, so that in the frog, for example, the concentration in all the extrahypothalamic brain is fully half that in the hypothalamus. In some species of frogs, TRH is found in the skin in concentrations higher than those found in the hypothalamus, an association presumed to be related to the embryologic origin of skin cells in neuroectoderm. TRH has been detected in the most primitive vertebrate, the larval form of the lamprey; in the amphioxus, a provertebrate; and in snail nerve ganglia. Since the lamprey probably does not synthesize TSH and amphioxi and snails lack a pituitary gland, it seems that the TRH molecule appeared in evolutionary development as a primitive neurosecretion prior to the evolution of TSH and that the pituitary has "co-opted" TRH as its regulatory hormone. The same might be said for dopamine, which first appears in the nervous nets of the sponge, a primitive invertebrate.

The extensive extrahypothalamic distribution of TRH, its localization in nerve endings, and the presence of TRH receptors in brain tissue strongly suggest that TRH serves as a neurotransmitter or neuromodulator outside the hypothalamus. See Table 11–3 for a summary of the neural effects of TRH.

Neuropharmacologic tests in experimental animals (even those hypophysectomized) indicate that TRH has a general stimulant activity. TRH also induces hyperthermia upon central administration in the rat, suggesting a role in central thermoregulation. A number of authors have reported that TRH has a beneficial psychologic effect in some depressed patients, but others have failed to confirm these findings. Although a possible effect of TRH in depression is still controversial, virtually all experiments indicate that the pituitary TSH response to TRH is blunted significantly in many depressed patients. Several other effects of TRH on brain functions have now been described, but the physiologic role of TRH as a neuroregulator remains to be defined.

Gonadotropin Releasing Hormone
(GnRH, LRH)

Chemistry and Effects on Pituitary

It has been known for more than 20 years from the work of McCann and of Harris and their respective collaborators that extracts of hypothalamic tissue contained a biologically active substance(s) capable of stimulating the release of gonadotropic hormones from the pituitary. This material was isolated in almost pure form from the hypothalami of stockyard animals by Guillemin and by Schally and their collaborators, and the structure was finally elucidated by Schally's group in 1971. Only 200 nanomoles of material were available for structural studies that showed that the LRH in porcine hypothalami was a decapeptide (Fig. 11–19). Like TRH, the amino terminal is a pyroglutamic acid residue and the carboxy terminal is a substituted amide. A terminal amide group is also characteristic of a number of other small peptide hormones, including VP, OT, calcitonin, gastrin and glucagon, and is needed for full hormonal activity in all the hormones.

Following intravenous injection, the naturally occurring LRH, or its synthetic form, brings about a prompt dose-related release of LH, and follicle stimulating hormone (FSH) in humans and in all vertebrate species in which it has been tested (Fig. 11–22). The onset of effect on FSH release after a single bolus injection is somewhat delayed, as compared with effects on LH secretion, the values peaking at 10–30 min after injection. The response to LRH is

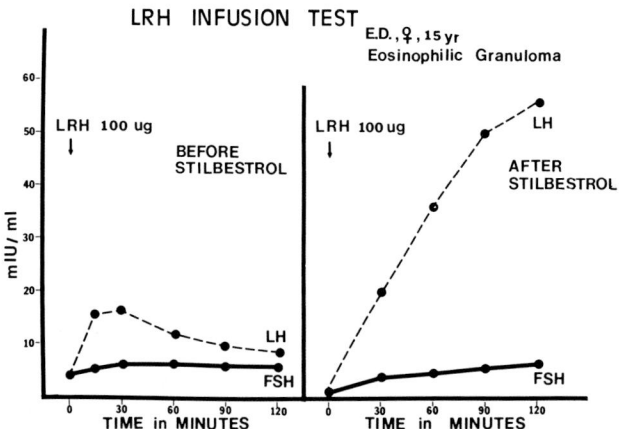

Figure 11–22. Gonadotropin secretory response to LRH "bolus" infusion (100 mcg) in patient with hypothalamic hypopituitarism. Note that LH response is greater than FSH response and that the peak response is somewhat delayed. After estrogen treatment, there was marked sensitization of response, characteristic of the "positive" feedback effect of estrogens on hypothalamic-pituitary gonadotropin secretion. (Reprinted by permission from Reichlin, S.: Regulation of the endocrine hypothalamus. *Med. Clin. North Am.* 62:235, 1978.)

markedly influenced by the prior LRH secretory state; by the steroid milieu of the patient; by gonadal function; by time course of LRH injection, i.e., single dose, multiple pulse, or constant infusion; and by the patient's genetic sex. Through secondary effects of pituitary activation and under appropriately defined conditions, LRH can induce spermatogenesis and testosterone production in men with hypothalamic hypogonadotropic hypogonadism and ovulation in women with hypothalamic amenorrhea. The role of LRH in gonadotropin regulation is discussed in the section "Reproduction," its use as a diagnostic agent is dealt with in Chs. 3 and 7, and its function as a neuromodulator is covered in the next section.

Until the LRH decapeptide had been isolated in pure form and synthesized, there had been some uncertainty as to whether FSH releasing factor (FRF) was distinct from LRH. Earlier workers had demonstrated that biologic activities of LRH could be partly separated from FRF in partially purified hypothalamic extracts and that LH and FSH secretion could be dissociated in a variety of conditions. Most, but not all, reproductive neuroendocrinologists believe that the LRH decapeptide is the only peptide gonadotropin regulator and that observed dissociations of secretion are due to the interacting effects of prior hormone status, steroid pretreatment, and history of exposure to LRH, however. One of the most convincing lines of evidence in support of this view is the demonstration that antisera prepared against the LRH decapeptide block ovulation in the female rat and lower blood levels of both LH and FSH in castrated animals. Although reports of a separate FRF still appear in the literature from time to time, the unitary hypothesis (initially advanced by White) is widely accepted, and there is a growing tendency to use the term gonadotropin releasing hormone (GnRH) instead of LRH. The most cautious view, however, is that there is an outside possibility that a distinct FRF exists.

Extrahypothalamic Distribution and Function of Gonadotropin Releasing Hormone

Unlike TRH and somatostatin, almost all of the GnRH in the brain is restricted to the hypothalamus and related neural structures. Small amounts are found in the circumventricular organs, including the pineal gland. Recently

Table 11–3. CENTRAL NERVOUS SYSTEM MEDIATED ACTIONS OF THYROTROPIN RELEASING FACTOR

Increases spontaneous motor activity
Alters sleep patterns
Produces anorexia
Inhibition of conditioned avoidance behavior
Head-to-tail rotation
Opposes actions of barbiturates on sleeping time, hypothermia, lethality
Opposes actions of ethanol, chloral hydrate, chlorpromazine, and diazepam on sleeping time and hypothermia
Enhances convulsion time and lethality of strychnine
Increases motor activity in morphine-treated animals
Potentiates DOPA-pargyline effects
Amelioration of human behavioral disorders?
Central inhibition of morphine-mediated secretion of growth hormone and prolactin
Alteration of brain cell membrane electrical activity
Increases norepinephrine turnover
Releases norepinephrine and dopamine from synaptosomal preparations
Enhances disappearance of norepinephrine from nerve terminals
Potentiates excitatory actions of acetylcholine on cerebral cortical neurons

From Vale, W., Rivier, C., and Brown, M.: Regulatory peptides of the hypothalamus. *Ann. Rev. Physiol.* 39:473–527, 1977.

LRH has been reported to have a neurotransmitter function in frog sympathetic ganglia. It has also been found in milk, suggesting that the breast, a dermal-derived structure, may have embryologic origins analogous to the primitive neuroectoderm, the source of neuroendocrine cells. Upon direct application to individual nerve cells, LRH can enhance or depress certain populations. Despite the fact that this peptide is found in a very restricted area, responding cells are localized in many other areas of the brain. The most important neural effects of LRH appear to be those involved in regulation of mating behavior. Direct injection of LRH into the hypothalamus has been reported to enhance female sexual responsivity, even in animals without a pituitary and hence incapable of responding with gonadotropin-ovarian activation. Clinical trials of LRH as a stimulator of sex drive have given conflicting results (Moss, 1979).

Growth Hormone Regulating Factors

Growth Hormone Releasing Factor* (Releasing Factor, SRF)

Injection of crude or partially fractionated extracts of hypothalamic tissue or the addition of such extracts to pituitary cells has been shown by many workers to stimulate the release of GH. Despite much effort, however, the chemical nature of GH releasing factor (GHRF) has not been elucidated. Many peptides found in the hypothalamus are capable of stimulating GH release when administered to whole rats either systemically or by direct injection into the third ventricle. These peptides include the endorphins, substance P, neurotensin, VP, glucagon, parathyroid hormone (PTH), and α MSH. None are effective when applied directly to the pituitary, however, and must therefore be acting through the GHRH mechanism. The principal biogenic amines of the hypothalamus, dopamine, serotonin, and norepinephrine, are also capable of releasing GH after intrahypothalamic injection, but they too are ineffective when applied locally to the pituitary.

Somatostatin†

Chemistry and Effects on Pituitary. During the course of efforts to isolate GHRF from hypothalamic extracts, Krulich and McCann discovered a fraction that inhibited GH release from pituitary incubates *in vitro* (Krulich et al., 1968). They named the factor growth hormone–release inhibiting factor and postulated that GH secretion was regulated by a dual control system, one stimulatory, the other inhibitory. Relatively little attention was paid to this bioactivity when first described because it was thought by most workers to be a relatively nonspecific effect. Several years later, however, Brazeau (1973) and a number of collaborators working in Guillemin's laboratory on the attempted isolation of GHRF again observed the inhibitory factor and, with the background in methodology gained from earlier studies of TRH and LRH, were able in a relatively short time to isolate and identify a potent peptide from hypothalamic extracts that inhibited GH release (Fig. 11–19). The material, to which the name somatostatin (SRIF) was applied, is a 14-amino acid peptide, lacking the amide and pyroglutamic acid termini characteristic of LRH and TRH but containing a S-S cyclic bridge similar to that of VP and OT. That SRIF is important as a physiologic regulator of

*Somatotropin release inhibiting factor (SRIF).
†Called also somatotropin releasing factor (SRF).

Table 11–4. BIOLOGIC ACTIONS OF SOMATOSTATIN OUTSIDE THE CENTRAL NERVOUS SYSTEM

Inhibits Hormone Secretion of:	Other Gastrointestinal Actions
Pituitary gland	*Inhibits:*
TSH, GH	Gastric acid secretion
Gastrointestinal Tract	Gastric secretion
Gastrin	Gastric emptying
Secretin	Pancreatic bicarbonate
Gastrointestinal polypeptide	Pancreatic enzyme secretion
Motilin	Intestinal absorption
Enteroglucagon	Gastrointestinal blood flow
Vasoactive intestinal peptide	Genitourinary tract inhibits renin
Pancreas	VP-stimulated water transport
Insulin	(to bladder)
Glucagon	

GH release is shown by studies in which the somatostatinergic pathways are damaged or endogenous SRIF neutralized by treatment with antisomatostatin antibody.

Shortly after chemically synthesized SRIF became available for study, it was found to inhibit the secretion of TSH, glucagon, and insulin. Subsequently, SRIF has been shown to inhibit the secretions of many other secretory structures in the body, including virtually all the glands of the gastrointestinal tract (Table 11–4). Studies of SRIF content of body tissues carried out by radioimmunoassay and immunohistochemistry show that almost every tissue that is acted upon by SRIF contains this peptide in specialized cells. Thus, SRIF, originally isolated from the hypothalamus, has been shown to be a widely distributed tissue component that in some settings acts as a paracrine secretion ("control of one cell by secretions of an adjacent tissue") and in others as a neuroendocrine secretion (as in the tuberohypophyseal neurons of the hypothalamus). Somatostatin is found in gastric juice and is effective when given by mouth. This kind of action has been termed "lumone," i.e., a chemical regulatory message delivered by way of the GI tract. Thyroid parafollicular cells contain both somatostatin and calcitonin. Since somatostatin inhibits calcitonin secretion, its action may be regarded as "autocrine."

The role of SRIF in pancreatic regulation is dealt with in Chapter 15 and in the gastrointestinal tract in Chapter 14.

Extrahypothalamic Distribution. Of the hypophysiotropic hormones thus far isolated, SRIF has the highest extrahypothalamic concentration, both in other parts of the central nervous system and in extraneural structures, especially the gastrointestinal tract (see Ch. 14). In general, the major direct effect of SRIF on nerve cells is to depress spontaneous activity. In some sites, SRIF seems to increase nerve activity, but this may be due to suppression of tonic inhibitory interneurons. Applied locally to the brain, SRIF has a sedative effect, as shown by extension of barbiturate sleeping time. It also has a hypothermic effect. In dorsal root ganglia it appears to modify centrally directed pain impulses by regulating substance P release in the dorsal root entry zone of the spinal cord. The physiologic role of SRIF in brain function remains to be elucidated.

Corticotropin Releasing Factor

Although corticotropin releasing factor (CRF) was the first of the releasing factors to be recognized and named (Saffran and Schally, 1955), its chemical nature is still unknown. A substance acting to release ACTH has been isolated from blood draining the primary portal plexus. Evidence has also been presented that CRF enters the general circulation and the cerebrospinal fluid. This material

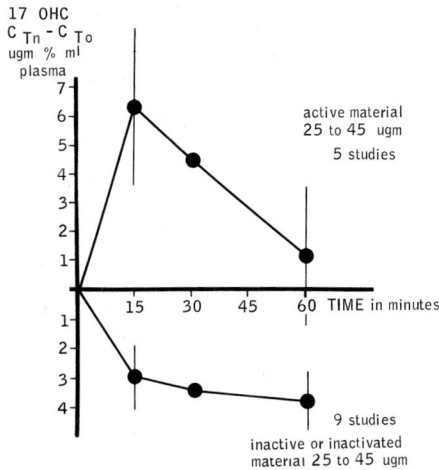

Figure 11–23. Variations of the plasma 17-OH corticoid concentration in normal individuals receiving a single intravenous injection of purified corticotropin releasing factor (electrophoretic fraction DΔ). Bottom of diagram, control studies. (Reproduced from Guillemin, R.: Hypothalamic control of the anterior hypophysis and its metabolic implications. *Diabetes* 8:352, 1959, with permission.)

disappears after destruction of the "adrenotropic" region of the hypothalamus. Stress also has been shown to deplete the median eminence of CRF activity, and a few patients treated with purified hypothalamic fractions have responded with a rise in plasma corticoid levels, an effect due to induced ACTH release (Fig. 11–23).

VP was initially thought by some to be CRF because it is secreted during stress and releases ACTH both *in vivo* and *in vitro* and because hypothalamic lesions that cause DI also block reflex ACTH discharge. More recent work has shown high concentrations of VP in portal vessel blood. Several lines of evidence indicate that although VP may under certain circumstances serve as *a* CRF, it is not *the* CRF. The secretion of ACTH and of VP, though usually occurring under similar circumstances, is independent under certain conditions such as hypoglycemic stress or intracarotid hypertonic saline injection. The most convincing evidence that VP is not essential for ACTH discharge comes from studies of rats with hereditary DI. Such animals are incapable of synthesizing VP yet have nearly normal adrenocortical responses to stress. Similar studies have been made in humans with idiopathic DI. Microinjections of VP in threshold amounts trigger ACTH release when introduced into the median eminence but not the anterior pituitary, providing further evidence that VP is *not* CRF. Under certain circumstances, VP sensitizes pituitary ACTH release in response to hypothalamic extract, thus suggesting that VP may have a permissive role in ACTH regulation.

Prolactin Regulatory Factors

Prolactin Inhibiting Factor

In keeping with the observation that the hypothalamus exerts an *inhibitory* effect on PRL secretion (see later) is the finding that crude hypothalamic extracts inhibit PRL release. This bioactivity was termed "PIF" by Meites (1966) and collaborators. PRL inhibiting factor (PIF) has been identified in portal vessel blood by Kamberi, Porter, and their collaborators (1971), again satisfying one of the critical requirements for proof of physiologic significance for a hypophysiotropic hormone.

Extensive efforts to determine the chemical structure of

PIF have been carried out in several laboratories. Dopamine is the most important PIF. This biogenic amine, the secretory product of the tuberohypophyseal dopaminergic pathways, is present in hypophyseal-portal vessel blood in sufficient concentration to inhibit PRL release. Gamma aminobutyric acid (GABA), a constituent of hypothalamic extracts, is also an active PIF, but its presence in portal vessel blood in appropriate concentrations has not as yet been established. Several groups have also claimed that there is at least one additional PIF activity, distinct from the two that have already been mentioned. The third "PIF" may be histidyl-proline diketopiperazine, a cyclic degradation product of TRH formed by incubation with hypothalamic tissue. There may be additional PIF's as well, but the relative importance of each remains for future elucidation. It must be emphasized that all of the known PRL inhibitory *functions* of the hypothalamus can be explained by dopamine only, though not all the PIF activity of hypothalamic extracts can be so explained.

Prolactin Releasing Factor

Although the stalk section and transplantation experiments indicate that the predominant effect of the hypothalamus on PRL secretion is inhibitory, the acute release of PRL seen after suckling and acute stress have raised the possibility that there may also be a PRL releasing factor(s) (PRF). Indeed, as noted previously, TRH is a potent PRF. Bioassay studies of hypothalamic fractions suggest that there may be other factors with PRF activity, but they have not been chemically characterized. Neuropharmacologic analysis (see later on) suggests that the PIF functions are generally under dopaminergic control, whereas PRF influences are mediated via serotonergic systems.

Melanocyte Stimulating Hormone Regulatory Factors

In considering mechanisms for regulation of melanocyte stimulating hormone (MSH) secretion, it is important to emphasize that the cells of the intermediate lobe (unlike the anterior lobe) receive direct bioaminergic secretomotor nerve supply from the hypothalamus and are not perfused directly by hypophyseal-portal vessel blood.

Several groups of workers have isolated hypothalamic factors that influence the secretion of MSH from the pituitary glands of experimental animals, including frogs and rats. The one that has received the most attention is a tripeptide, Pro-Leu-Gly-NH$_2$, which is formed by enzymic breakdown of OT and appears in some studies to inhibit MSH release from the rat pituitary *in vivo*. The physiologic role of this compound is still uncertain. In humans, and other species that do not have a distinct intermediate lobe, neither α nor β MSH are secreted as such into the peripheral blood, and the tripeptide (so-called MIF) would not be expected to have any effect on MSH secretion and has in fact been shown to have none. In lower forms, studies of whole animal responses as compared with *in vitro* pituitary incubation experiments have given conflicting results, and there is no general agreement as to their significance. MSH releasing factors have also been described to be active in the rat, but their chemical nature is also unclear. The neuroendocrine regulation of the intermediate lobe is discussed later. Although there is controversy as to the physiologic role of Pro-Leu-Gly-NH$_2$, numerous studies indicate that this substance has significant neurophysiologic and behavioral effects. (See Sandman et al., 1978, for review.)

REGULATION OF SECRETION OF THE TUBEROHYPOPHYSEAL NEURONS: NEUROPHARMACOLOGY OF HYPOTHALAMIC REGULATION

As outlined in previous sections, the tuberohypophyseal neurons are the "final common pathway" of neural control of the anterior pituitary. This group of neurons is acted upon by neurotransmitters; by the feedback effects of hormones secreted by target glands, such as the sex steroids, thyroid hormone, and cortisol; by pituitary peptide hormones (short-loop feedback control); and by neuropeptide modulators. This complex set of controls is integrated at the neuron level for the regulation of anterior pituitary secretion (Fig. 11–24).

Neurotransmitter Regulation of Hypophysiotropic Neurons

The function of central bioaminergic neurotransmitters is relevant to psychiatric disease, to behavior, and to affect as well as to pituitary regulation. Consequently they have been studied a great deal.

The structures of the important hypothalamic neuro-transmitters are illustrated in Fig. 11–25. Their mechanisms of synthesis are summarized in Table 11–5 and in Ch. 10, and their overall effects are summarized in Table 11–6.

Dopaminergic Pathways

An important group of bioaminergic neurons involved in anterior pituitary regulation arise mainly in the arcuate nucleus of the hypothalamus and are distributed to the median eminence (Fig. 11–26). This grouping, termed the dopaminergic tuberohypophyseal system, is mainly important for its function in direct control of anterior pituitary secretion.

Two other relatively independent dopaminergic systems have also been identified. The best known, and the earliest to be recognized by neurologists, is that involved in extra-pyramidal control, namely, the nigrostriatal pathways that arise in the substantia nigra in the hindbrain and are distributed to the caudate nucleus and other structures in the forebrain. Parkinson's disease is due to defects in this system. The third dopaminergic system arises in cells adjacent to the hypothalamus and projects to several hypothalamic regulatory areas. Dopaminergic neurotransmitters

A MEMBRANE RECEPTORS

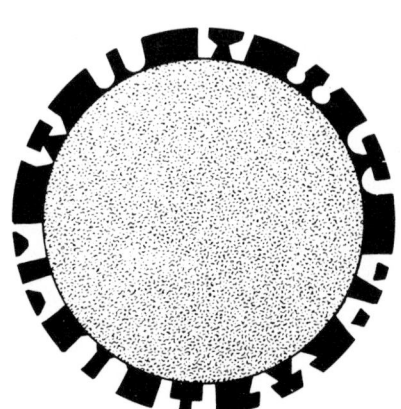

1. NEUROTRANSMITTERS

   DOPAMINE   SEROTONIN   NOREPINEPHRINE   ACETYLCHOLINE

   ? HISTAMINE   ? EPINEPHRINE   ? GABA

2. NEUROPEPTIDES

   LH RH (ULTRA-SHORT-LOOPFEEDBACK)   ENDORPHINS (GH, PRL)

   VASOPRESSIN (RECURRENT COLLATERAL INHIBITION)

   ANGIOTENSIN II (B VASOPRESSIN RELEASE, ? CRF RELEASE)

   ENDORPHINS (GH, PRL), SUBSTANCE P (GH, PRL),
        NEUROTENSIN (GH, PRL)

   ? BOMBESIN, VASOACTIVE INTESTINAL PEPTIDE (VIP), CCK

3. PEPTIDE HORMONES

   GH PRL ACTH LH FSH ? TSH

B CYTOPLASMIC-NUCLEAR RECEPTORS

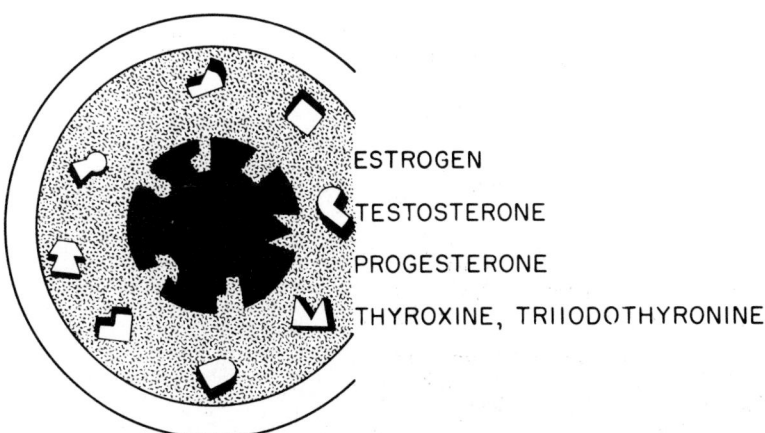

ESTROGEN

TESTOSTERONE

PROGESTERONE

THYROXINE, TRIIODOTHYRONINE

Figure 11–24. Schematic outline of the various known or suggested types of membrane (*A*) and nuclear (*B*) receptors that may regulate hypophysiotropic neuron function. (Reproduced by permission, from A. M., Jr., Peck, E. J., Jr., et al. [eds.]: *Brain Peptides: A New Endocrinology.* New York, Elsevier-North Holland Biomedical Press, 1979.)

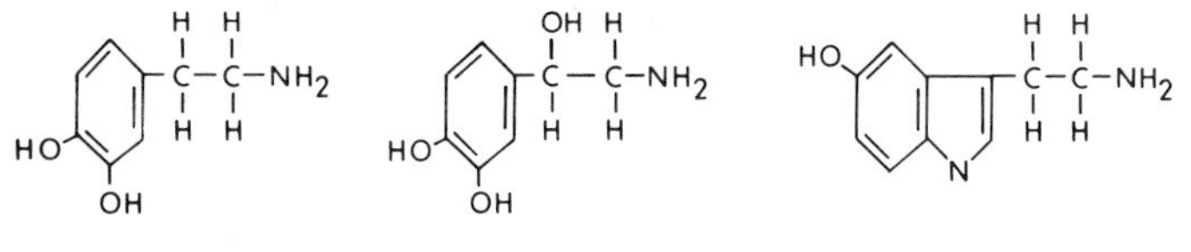

Figure 11–25. Structures of the three major monoaminergic neurotransmitters involved in regulation of the hypophysiotropic (peptidergic) neurons. For descriptions of pathways of synthesis and degradation of the catecholamines, dopamine and norepinephrine, and indoleamines, see Ch. 10 and Table 11–5.

DOPAMINE   NOREPINEPHRINE   SEROTONIN

may be of importance by producing either direct effects on the pituitary or indirect effects on other tuberoinfundibular neurons, or both. This complexity of input underlines the problem encountered when dopamine agonists and antagonists are used to analyze the neuropharmacologic coding of anterior pituitary regulation.

Noradrenergic Pathways

All the cell bodies of origin of the noradrenergic pathways arise outside of the hypothalamus in several nuclear groups in the hindbrain, the most conspicuous being the locus ceruleus in the floor of the fourth ventricle (Fig. 11–26). From the locus ceruleus, noradrenergic fibers ascend to the

Table 11–5. SUMMARY OF FUNCTION OF CENTRAL CATECHOLAMINERGIC NEURONS: SITES OF ACTION OF NEUROPHARMACOLOGIC AGENTS

Step 1: Uptake of amino acids into aminergic neurons: tyrosine, precursor of dopamine, norepinephrine, epinephrine
Drug: No drug known to interfere with tyrosine uptake
Step 2: Enzymic synthesis
   Tyrosine is hydroxylated by tyrosine hydroxylase to form L-dopa. L-Dopa is decarboxylated to form dopamine (DA), which in turn is hydroxylated to form norepinephrine. Norepinephrine is methylated to form epinephrine
Drug: α-Methyltyrosine blocks L-dopa synthesis. Disulfiram (Antabuse) blocks dopamine conversion to norepinephrine
Step 3: Storage phase
   Norepinephrine (NE), dopamine, and epinephrine (E) are stored in specific granules within nerve terminals
Drug: Reserpine blocks storage of NE, DA, and E.
Step 4: Release of preformed granules
   In response to neuronal depolarization, granules are extruded from the nerve ending
Drug: Amphetamines may act, at least in part, on release of NE
Step 5: Interaction of catecholamine with receptor located on postsynaptic neuron

   The extruded bioamine binds to specific receptors
Drug: Noradrenergic effects are duplicated by α receptor agonist clonidine, β receptor agonist isoproterenol; α receptors are blocked by phentolamine, β receptors by propranolol

   Dopamine effects are duplicated by agonists apomorphine, and bromocriptine and blocked by the antagonists phenothiazines, pimozide
Step 6: Re-uptake process
   Following release of preformed hormone, free neurotransmitter in the synaptic cleft that has not reacted with receptor is taken up into the presynaptic nerve ending
Drug: Cocaine, tricyclic antidepressants make NE more available by blocking re-uptake
Step 7: Degradation of neurotransmitter and dopamine
   Norepinephrine bound to postsynaptic membranes or free in the presynaptic nerve ending is destroyed by the enzyme monoamine oxidase

   The enzyme catechol-O-methyl transferase is also responsible for inactivating these amines
Drug: Monoamine oxidase inhibitors (pargyline, isocarboxizide, tranylcypromine) make more neurotransmitter available to the postsynaptic cell

Adapted from Cooper, J. R., Bloom, F. E., and Roth, R. H.: The Biochemical Basis of Neuropharmacology. 3rd Ed. New York, Oxford University Press, 1978; and Martin, J. B., Reichlin, S., and Brown, G. M.: Clinical Neuroendocrinology. Philadelphia, F. A. Davis Co., 1977.

hypothalamus and other midbrain and forebrain structures and descend into the spinal cord. The bulk of noradrenergic fibers involved in neuroendocrine control arise from areas adjacent to the locus ceruleus and from cells anatomically close to the nucleus of the vagus nerve. These ascend in defined anatomic pathways and terminate on cell bodies of tuberohypophyseal neurons and neurohypophyseal neurons and within the median eminence itself.

Serotonergic Pathways

Most of the serotonergic neurons project to the hypothalamus from cell bodies located in the brainstem (raphe nuclei) (Fig. 11–21). They are extensively distributed to hypothalamic neurons, and to a lesser extent to the median eminence and ependymal cells. Serotonin-containing nerves ramify over the ventricular surface of the brain. An intrinsic serotonin pathway within the hypothalamus analogous to the tuberohypophyseal dopamine pathway probably exists as well.

Dopamine, serotonin, and noradrenalin pathways are the principal biogenic amine control systems, but recent work has demonstrated the presence of adrenergic and histaminergic neural control systems as well. The cell bodies of origin of these pathways arise for the most part in hindbrain regions, but there are also smaller bioaminergic systems self-contained in the hypothalamus.

Cholinergic Control

Choline acetyltransferase, an enzyme marker of acetylcholine synthesis, is distributed in all defined nuclei in the hypothalamus, including the arcuate, and in the median eminence, two regions especially related to anterior pituitary control. Because only small changes have been noted

Table 11–6. NEUROTRANSMITTERS AND ANTERIOR PITUITARY SECRETION

	NE	DA	5-HT	ACH	H	GABA
ACTH	↓	↓	↑	↑	↑	↓
TSH	↑	↓	↓	→	↑	–
LH-FSH	↑	↑↓	↓	↑	↑	↑
GH	↑	↑	↑	→	→	↑
PRL	↑↓	↓	↑	↑↓	↑	↑↓

The effects of various neurotransmitters is inferred from neuropharmacologic studies using agonists, antagonists, and precursors. It must be *emphasized* that there are many inconsistencies and contradictions in the literature. These are due in part to species differences, prior functional status, lack of specificity of some drugs, and direct pituitary effects differing from hypothalamic effects.

Symbols: ↑ = increase; ↓ = decrease; → = no change; – = not known.

Adapted from Müller, E. E., Nistico, G., and Scapagnini, U. (eds.): Neurotransmitters and Anterior Pituitary Function. New York, Academic Press, 1977; and Weiner, R. I., and Ganong, W. F.: Role of brain monoamines and histamine in regulation of anterior pituitary secretion. *Physiol. Rev.* 58:905–976, 1978.

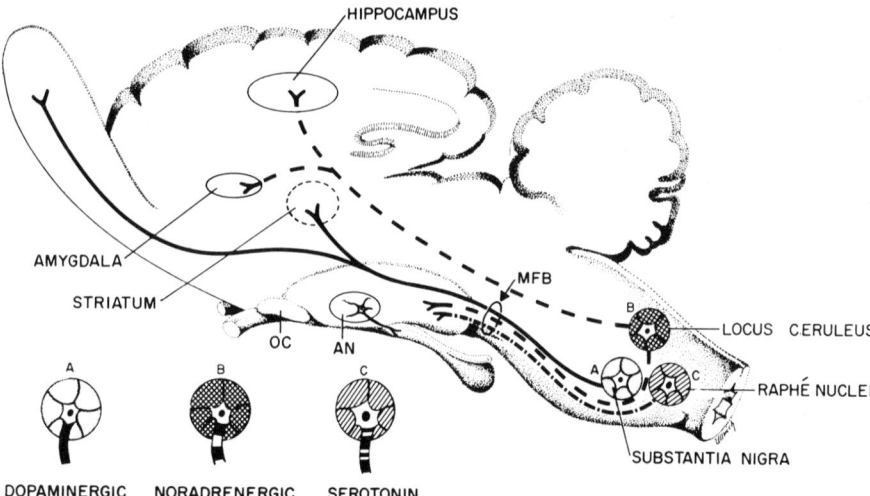

Figure 11–26. Simplified diagram to show the major distribution of the ascending mono-aminergic pathways in mammalian brain. Principal source of all three major biogenic amines in the brain are nuclei in the brain stem. Locus ceruleus, the source of most noradrenergic fibers; raphe nucleus, the source of most serotonin fibers; and substantia nigra, the source of most dopaminergic fibers. An important dopaminergic pathway arises in the arcuate nucleus of the hypothalamus and is the principal source of dopamine to the hypophyseal circulation. (Reprinted by permission, from Reichlin, S., Baldessarini, R., et al. [eds.]: *The Hypothalamus, Vol. 56,* New York, Raven Press, 1977.)

in medial basal hypothalamic concentration of choline acetyltransferase after surgical isolation of this region of the brain, it has been proposed that there is "a cholinergic tuberoinfundibular pathway similar to the dopaminergic one, which may be responsible for the neuroendocrine effects of cholinergic agents" (Müller et al., 1977). Anatomic analysis of the hypothalamus (and other parts of the brain) by the technique of microiontophoresis onto individual nerve cells by Bloom and his collaborators (Cooper et al., 1978) has revealed an extensive distribution of acetylcholine responsive neurons, some of which are excited and others inhibited by this neurotransmitter. Whether or not these are tuberoinfundibular is not known.

Gamma Aminobutyric Acid

Gamma aminobutyric acid (GABA) has also been demonstrated in fairly high concentration in the hypothalamus and median eminence, and the presence of GABA-sensitive neurons has been demonstrated by microiontophoresis in the hypothalamic ventromedial nucleus as well as at other sites in the "endocrine hypothalamus." Immunohistochemical methods utilizing antisera developed against glutamic acid decarboxylase (the GABA synthesizing enzyme) reveal dense networks of nerve endings in virtually all hypothalamic nuclei. GABA in the median eminence is not reduced by surgical isolation of the hypothalamus, thus providing evidence for an intrinsic GABA-secreting neuron system.

Endocrine Significance of Neuropeptides

In addition to the enkephalins and the hypophysiotropic peptides (see later), a number of other peptides have been demonstrated to occur in neurons distributed in the hypothalamus and other brain regions (Table 11–7). Almost all

are represented in characteristic glandular cells of the gastrointestinal tract, believed to arise in embryologic life from the primitive neuroectoderm (APUD system). (See Pearse, 1978, and Ch. 4.)

Substance P is present in high concentration in the hypothalamus as well as other brain areas. Little is present in the median eminence, suggesting that there is no direct tuberoinfundibular input, but the rich innervation of most hypothalamic nuclei suggests a regulatory role for this peptide nevertheless.

Other neuropeptides with hypothalamic distribution of nerve endings are meth-enkephalin (an endorphin), angiotensin II, neurotensin, gastrin, and cholecystokinin. The findings of meth-enkephalin–containing cell bodies in the hypothalamus and a median eminence distribution support the presence of an intrinsic hypothalamic control system for this peptide as well as a system with projections from other parts of the brain.

These neuropeptides have been found to exert changes in brain function, homeostasis, and some endocrine activities. Whether the central neuropeptides influence pituitary function by direct action on hypophysiotropic or intermediary neurons is not known.

When called upon to explain neural control of anterior pituitary secretion, the contemporary neuroendocrinologist suffers from an embarrassment of riches with regard to potential neurohumoral mediators. Summarized in Tables 11–6 and 11–7 are the overall effects of the various classes of neurotransmitters and other hypothalamic regulators on anterior pituitary regulation. It should be borne in mind that a given effect of an agonist or antagonist may be due to direct or indirect effects on other regulatory systems and that many of the findings are not uniform in all studies in all mammals and under all conditions.

ENDOGENOUS OPIATES*

Discovery of the endogenous opiates and recognition of their importance in brain function, homeostasis, and neuro-

Table 11–7.   ENDOCRINE EFFECTS OF CENTRAL ACTION OF NEUROPEPTIDES

ADH	Stimulates release of ACTH
TRH	Blocks GH release
LRH	May suppress LRH secretion
Somatostatin	Inhibits TRH release
Substance P	Increases PRL and GH release
Neurotensin	Increases PRL and GH release
Vasoactive intestinal peptide	Increases PRL and GH release
Angiotensin II	Releases ADH

* The rapid accumulation of knowledge in this area has been accompanied by terminological confusion. The term "endorphin," standing for endogenous morphine-like substance, was devised by Eric Simon as a general designation for all opiate-like compounds occurring naturally in the brain. Usage of this term is now restricted to the specific sequenced peptides α, β, and γ endorphin. The term enkephalin is restricted to the two pentapeptides, leu- and met-enkephalin. Any peptide with opioid activity of known or unknown sequence is referred to as an "opioid peptide" (see Uhl, Childers, Snyder, 1978).

endocrine regulation has been one of the most exciting episodes in modern biology. Search for these compounds was instituted in several laboratories when it had been established that morphine and its analogues bind to specific receptors in brain and in peripheral target tissues, such as the intestine and vas deferens. It was reasoned that the presence of morphine binding sites could not be a fortuitous occurrence and must be associated with the presence of an endogenous ligand to be bound by the receptor. As pointed out by Kosterlitz (1978), this idea was strongly supported by the observation that the antinociceptive (antipain) effects of electric stimulation of certain regions of the midbrain were reversed by administration of the morphine antagonist naloxone. ". . . this phenomenon was best explained by the assumption that the electrical stimulation released an endogenous substance with morphine-like actions, the effect of which was reversed by the antagonist naloxone."

The first endogenous opiates to be isolated from brain extracts were called enkephalins by their discoverers Hughes and Kosterlitz and collaborators in 1975 (see Kosterlitz, 1978 and Garfield, 1979 for historical reviews). The enkephalins (met-enkephalin, leu-enkephalin) are pentapeptides (Fig. 11–27). Morris, the protein chemist who established their structure, recognized that the amino acid sequence of met-enkephalin corresponded to an identical sequence in the pituitary hormone β lipotropin (LPH) that had been isolated previously by Li in 1964 but had no previously known physiologic function (Fig. 11–27).

The structure of the enkephalins was rapidly confirmed by Snyder and collaborators, who had developed morphine receptor assays for the brain. Study of endogenous opiates in pituitary extracts was initiated by Goldstein and by Guillemin within weeks of the report that the enkephalin sequence was part of a pituitary hormone. Research findings, which have come as a dizzying pace, reveal that the molecule β LPH is the prohormone of several endogenous opiates (Fig. 11–27), the most potent of which was named β endorphin, a polypeptide corresponding to the sequence 61–91 of the β LPH molecule that has 91 amino acid residues. Two other endorphins have been described: α endorphin (residues 61–76) and γ endorphin (61–77). β LPH also includes a sequence 41–58 corresponding to β MSH. The entire molecule is synthesized together with ACTH in a large prohormone that has been called 31K on the basis of its molecular weight. There is good evidence that β LPH and ACTH are formed in the same cell (whether in pituitary or

brain). In the anterior pituitary the secretion of both ACTH and β LPH is regulated similarly by the feedback action of glucocorticoids and discharged simultaneously by exposure to hypothalamic extracts rich in CRF. The virtually complete molecular structure of bovine ACTH-β LPH, "proopiocorticotropin," has been elucidated by Nakanishi and colleagues (1979) by genetic recombination methods. Although the sequence of leu-enkephalin is an intrinsic part of the β LPH molecule (leu-enkephalin corresponds to β LPH (61–65), there is good evidence to indicate that leu-enkephalin is not the product of β LPH breakdown but arises independently, presumably from another prohormone. A prohormone for met-enkephalin has not as yet been identified. Cells that synthesize β lipotropin-ACTH are distinct from those that synthesize the enkephalins.

Enkephalin-containing neurons, which account for the bulk of endorphins in the brain, are widely distributed in regions correspondingly rich in opiate receptors. In these locations, the peptides are in cell bodies and nerve endings. β endorphin makes up most of the remaining fraction of opiate activity, but recent reports suggest that there are other endorphins, including one that has the immunologic characteristics of morphine and one even more potent than β endorphin.

Regional concentrations of the endorphins correspond to regionally specialized functions (Fig. 11–28). In spinal cord, opiate receptors and enkephalins are in highest concentration in the dorsal gray matter, corresponding to the centrally directed nerve endings of primary sensory neurons. These are believed to modulate pain perception at the cord level by suppressing activity of substance P–containing nerve endings that also arise in sensory ganglia. Vagal nuclear localization corresponds to the emetic effects of morphine and its antitussive properties. Localization of enkephalins in the locus ceruleus (the principal site of origin of ascending noradrenergic fibers) may account for the euphoria-producing actions of morphine and, through projections to the hypothalamus, for the regulation of some pituitary functions. The amygdala is also considered a prime site for morphine-generated euphoria. Rich concentrations of enkephalin and opiate receptors in the hypothalamus and in the locus ceruleus may account for the effects of endorphins on the stimulation of the release of PRL and GH and the suppression of TSH and gonadotropin release.

In sharp contrast to the distribution of enkephalin, the principal localization of β endorphin is in the pituitary

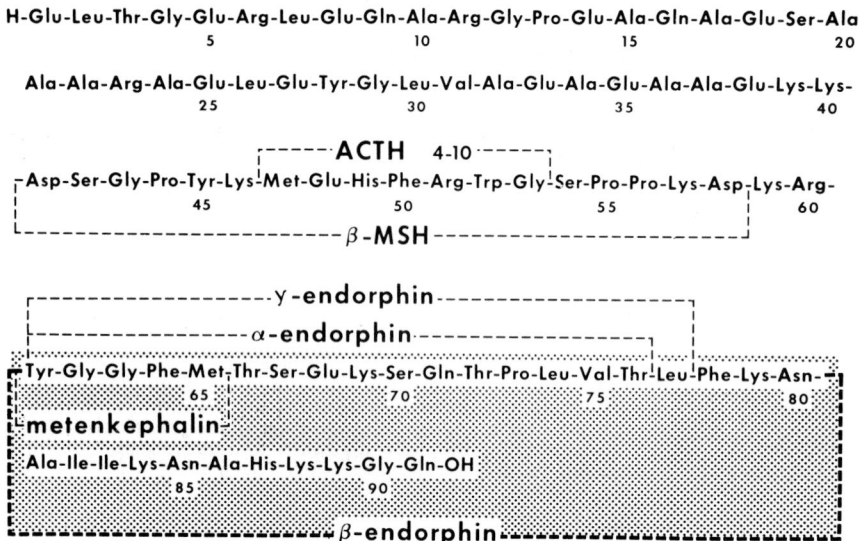

H-Glu-Leu-Thr-Gly-Glu-Arg-Leu-Glu-Gln-Ala-Arg-Gly-Pro-Glu-Ala-Gln-Ala-Glu-Ser-Ala-
         5   10   15   20

Ala-Ala-Arg-Ala-Glu-Leu-Glu-Tyr-Gly-Leu-Val-Ala-Glu-Ala-Glu-Ala-Ala-Glu-Lys-Lys-
    25   30   35   40

            ACTH 4-10
Asp-Ser-Gly-Pro-Tyr-Lys-Met-Glu-His-Phe-Arg-Trp-Gly-Ser-Pro-Pro-Lys-Asp-Lys-Arg-
         45   50   55   60
           β-MSH

          γ-endorphin
          α-endorphin
Tyr-Gly-Gly-Phe-Met-Thr-Ser-Glu-Lys-Ser-Gln-Thr-Pro-Leu-Val-Thr-Leu-Phe-Lys-Asn-
         65   70   75   80
metenkephalin
Ala-Ile-Ile-Lys-Asn-Ala-His-Lys-Lys-Gly-Gln-OH
         85   90
β-endorphin

Figure 11–27. Homologies in structures of sheep β-lipotropin with the ACTH fragment (4–10), β-MSH (41–58), methionine enkephalin (61–65), α endorphin (61–76), γ-endorphin (61–77) and β-endorphin (61–91). (Reprinted with permission, from Martin, J., Reichlin, S., et al.: *Clinical Neuroendocrinology* Philadelphia, F. A. Davis, 1977.)

SCHEMATIC DISTRIBUTION OF ENDORPHINS AND RELATED PEPTIDES IN RAT BRAIN

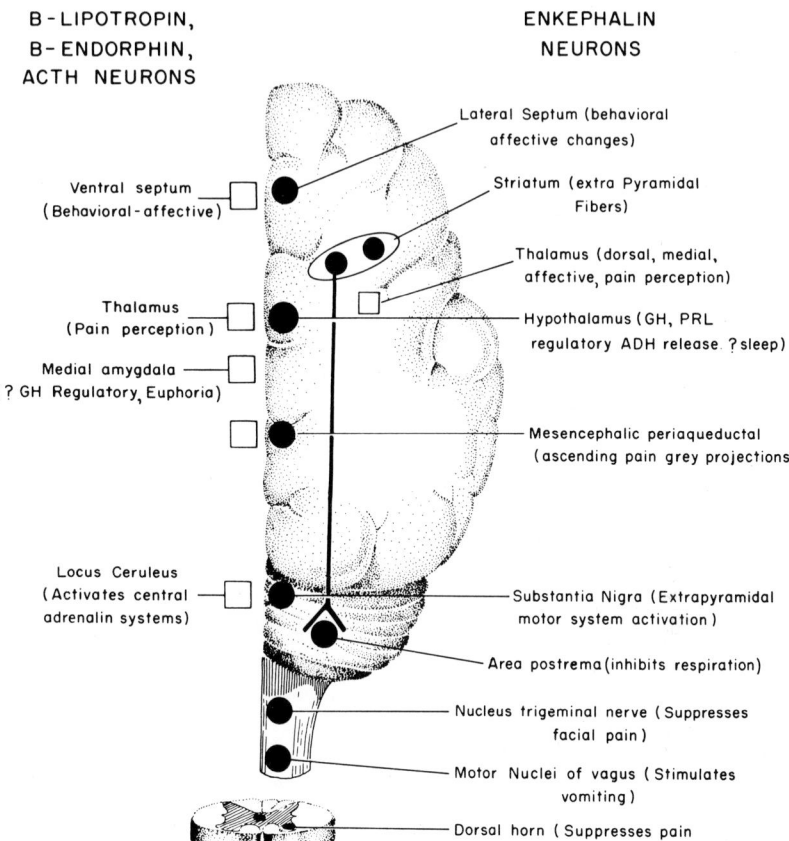

B-LIPOTROPIN,
B-ENDORPHIN,
ACTH NEURONS

ENKEPHALIN
NEURONS

Lateral Septum (behavioral affective changes)

Striatum (extra Pyramidal Fibers)

Ventral septum (Behavioral-affective)

Thalamus (dorsal, medial, affective, pain perception)

Thalamus (Pain perception)

Hypothalamus (GH, PRL regulatory ADH release ? sleep)

Medial amygdala (? GH Regulatory, Euphoria)

Mesencephalic periaqueductal (ascending pain grey projections)

Locus Ceruleus (Activates central adrenalin systems)

Substantia Nigra (Extrapyramidal motor system activation)

Area postrema (inhibits respiration)

Nucleus trigeminal nerve (Suppresses facial pain)

Motor Nuclei of vagus (Stimulates vomiting)

Dorsal horn (Suppresses pain perception)

Figure 11–28. Regional concentrations of endorphins in the central nervous system. (Diagram modified from Barchas, J. D.: *Science, 200*:964, 1978.)

gland, especially in the intermediate lobe. Less is found in the hypothalamus, and still smaller amounts elsewhere. Brain tissue homogenates can break down β LPH of pituitary origin to form β endorphin, but the content of β lipotropin in the brain is unaltered by hypophysectomy. Although there is a distinct set of intrinsic neurons in the hypothalamus that contain β endorphin (together with ACTH), there is no evidence that brain function is directly controlled by pituitary β LPH. Brain and pituitary endorphin systems probably are distinct, although the interactions of the two cannot be excluded.

Important physiologic actions of the endogenous opiates are to raise the threshold of pain, to produce sedation, and to influence extrapyramidal motor activity. Electric stimulation of the periaqueductal gray of the spinal cord in humans, which causes analgesia, is associated with an increase in the concentration of enkephalins in the cerebrospinal fluid. Contrariwise, it has been reported that pain-prone individuals have lower than normal concentrations of bioassayable opiates in their lumbar spinal fluid.

Opiate addiction and tolerance are other important consequences of endogenous opiate actions. It has been postulated that morphine causes euphoria by intense stimulation of opiate receptors in specific areas. Addiction has been postulated to be the result of suppression of secretion (or synthesis) of endogenous opiates from presynaptic nerve endings, possibly related to local feedback inhibition. Following discontinuation of morphine treatment, absolute or relative endogenous opiate deficiency may ensue, lasting until the induced deficiency state is restored to normal. Symptoms of morphine withdrawal, such as prostration, malaise, restlessness, anxiety, sweating, tachycardia, and abdominal distress, can be attributed to the loss of endogenous opiate effects on central vegetative functions together with an autonomic nervous system reaction to this loss.

The virtual absence of reaction to administration of morphine antagonists in normal individuals suggests that the endogenous opiate system may only become significant under conditions of activation, such as stress or pain.

It must be emphasized that there may be several classes of endorphin receptors (analogous to the γ and β noradrenergic and H-I and H-II histamine receptors) and that naloxone and other presently available blockers may not block all such receptors.

NEUROENDOCRINE ASPECTS OF CONTROL OF SPECIFIC PITUITARY TROPIC HORMONES

General Considerations: Servoengineering Concepts in Neuroendocrinology

For each of the pituitary control systems, one can identify hormonal feedback effects exerted on the pituitary or hypothalamus or both and interactions with relevant behavioral and homeostatic functions.

In the literature of neuroendocrinology, servoengineering concepts and formulations have been liberally applied to describe endocrine control systems. To clarify these terms, a brief account of feedback control is presented in this section together with a review of specific controls for hormonal systems described in following sections.

Most hormonal systems form part of a homeostatic feedback loop in which the controlled variable (generally the plasma hormone level or some function of it) determines the rate of secretion of the hormone. Most hormonal systems are, in fact, negative feedback control systems (see later), but examples of positive feedback control can be cited. All the negative and positive feedback systems in which the pituitary is involved have nervous system inputs that either alter the "set point" of the feedback control system or introduce an "open loop" element of control.

Some definitions used in feedback control models should be clarified; they are largely borrowed from servoengineering. The mathematic modeling of these systems provides an important tool for the analysis and investigation of endocrine function. The mathematic basis of feedback systems is useful, particularly for research; the concepts are relatively simple and can be grasped at an intuitive level.

A *system* is a set of components related in such a way as to act as a unit.

A *control system* is so arranged as to regulate itself or another system.

An *input* is the stimulus applied to a control system from a source outside of the system so as to produce a specified response from the control system.

An *output* is the actual response of a control system.

An *open loop* control system is one with the control action independent of output.

A *closed loop* control system is one in which the control action depends upon (is a function of) output.

A *negative feedback* system is one in which the control action is a function of output in such a way that the *output* inhibits the control action.

A *positive feedback* system is a closed loop control system in which the output *accelerates* the control action.

All negative feedback systems have a "controlled variable" that is the factor (in the case of homeostatic functions) the system is designed to maintain. For example, thyroid hormone levels are the controlled variable of the pituitary-thyroid axis, blood calcium is the controlled variable of the parathyroid-calcitonin-skeleton axis, blood glucose is the controlled variable in the pancreas-liver axis.

All feedback systems, negative or positive, have a "sensor element" capable of detecting the concentration of the controlled variable. Information gained by the sensor is used to determine the output of the controlling system. In *engineering* formulations of feedback, there are three elements of "executive" control of the controlled variable. There is a "sensing" element, which detects the concentration of the controlled variable; there is a "reference input," which may be defined as an absolute measure of what the controlled variable should be; and there is an "error signal," which is a function of the difference between what the sensor senses the controlled variable to be and what the reference input determines it *should* be. The magnitude of the error signal and the direction of its deviation (negative or positive) determine the output of the system. The reference input can be considered the "set point" of the system. An example of these terms can be found in the common household thermostat. The reference input is the preferred temperature to which the thermostat is set. The sensor is a thermometer that detects the actual room temperature. When the tem-

perature sensed by the detector is different from the reference input, the furnace is turned either off or on until the error signal is minimized. In common furnace applications, the error signal is either off or on, but in more complex systems it is apparent that the error signal might determine output in a more sophisticated way. For example, a large error signal might call for a large initial burst of heat, and a small error signal might call for a small burst of heat; the rate of heating may be programmed as a complex function.

Hormonal feedback control systems resemble their engineering analogues in that the concentration of the hormone in the blood (or some function of the hormone) regulates the output of the controlling gland. Hormonal feedback control systems differ from the engineering formulation system in that the sensor element and the reference input element are not readily distinguishable. Rather than having a reference input signal with which the controlled variable is compared, thus providing an error signal to determine gland output, the controlled variable has a more or less direct regulatory influence on the secretory process.

Thyrotropic Hormone Regulation

The secretion of TSH is regulated by two interacting elements: negative feedback by thyroid hormone and neural control by hypothalamic hypophysiotrophic factors (Fig. 11–29). TSH secretion is also modified by other hor-

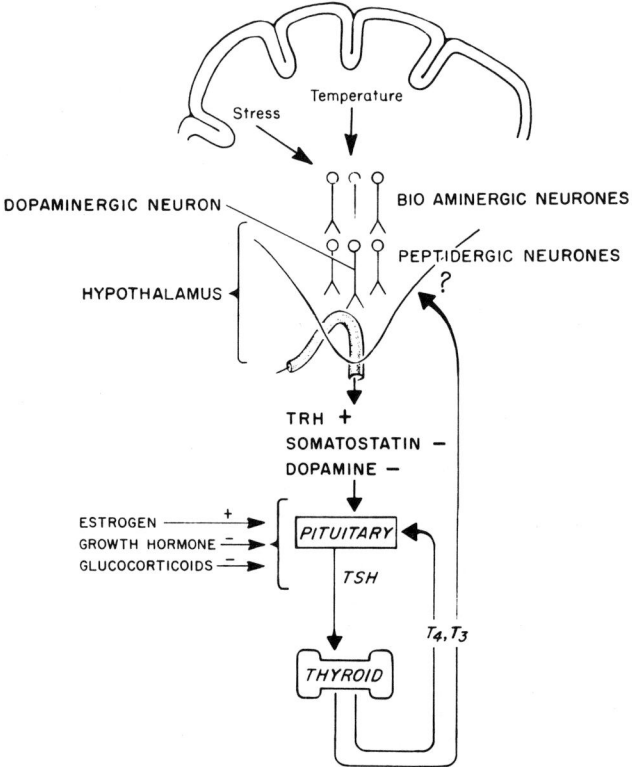

Figure 11–29. Schematic outline of the neural elements involved in regulation of TSH secretion as they interact with pituitary-thyroid feedback control. Three hypothalamic regulating factors, all secretory products of the tuberohypophyseal neuron system, are involved—one stimulatory, TRH, and two inhibitory, somatostatin and dopamine. In turn these tuberohypophyseal neurons are regulated by bioaminergic neurons. The endorphins are inhibitory to this system. Shown also is the negative feedback effect of thyroid hormone (T$_4$, T$_3$) on the pituitary and the inhibitory effect of GH and glucocorticoids. Inhibitory effects of GH may be exerted through stimulation of somatostatin rather than by direct action on the pituitary. Estrogenic hormones potentiate the releasing effects of TRH. The pituitary thyroid axis is a closed loop negative feedback system with open loop neural control transients, i.e., stress, cold.

mones, especially estrogens and glucocorticoids, and may also be influenced by GH. Aspects of the pituitary-thyroid axis are considered in Chs. 3 (The Adenohypophysis) and 4 (The Thyroid Gland). Neuroendocrine mechanisms will be reviewed in this chapter.

The Pituitary-Thyroid Axis

For more than a century it has been known that the function of the pituitary is linked in some manner to the function of the thyroid gland. As early as 1851, Nièpce had noted that the pituitaries of cretins observed at autopsy were grossly enlarged; the contemporary clinician can demonstrate enlargement of the sella turcica in the skull x-rays of cretins and of others with hypothyroidism of long standing.

Modern views of pituitary-thyroid control are the culmination of many experimental steps, including the demonstration that pituitary extracts stimulate the thyroid and that thyroid extract inhibits thyroid gland growth and function.

The "pituitary-thyroid axis," first christened by Salter, is an example *par excellence* of a classic negative feedback system. Hoskins described the system as follows in 1949:

When the titer of circulating thyroxine rises, the anterior pituitary is selectively inhibited and the discharge of thyrotropin is thereby decreased. Contrarywise, episodic or persistent thyroxine deficiency, if sufficient in degree, results in augmented thyrotropic production with resulting tendency for the production of more thyroid hormone. (Quoted in Reichlin, 1966.)

This statement, supplemented by more recent views about both neural control and the tissue-effective form of the circulating thyroid hormone, is now accepted as a virtually unchallengeable principle of endocrinology.

Thyroid hormone level in blood, or the concentration of its unbound fraction, can be looked upon as the controlled variable. The "set point" of pituitary-thyroid function is the normal resting level of plasma thyroid hormone. The main-

tenance of this level requires a specific level of TSH. Secretion of TSH is inversely regulated by the level of thyroid hormone, so that deviations from the set point of control lead to appropriate, graded changes in the rate of TSH secretion (Fig. 11–30). A number of additional factors determine the rate of TSH secretion required to maintain a given level of thyroid hormone. These include the rate of peripheral degradation of both TSH and thyroid hormone. Disappearance times for both are affected by changes in peripheral tissue metabolic activity.

Feedback control by thyroid hormone through effects at the pituitary level is remarkably precise. Small doses of T_3 and T_4, administered daily for 3–4 weeks to normal individuals in amounts insufficient to raise measured plasma thyroid hormone levels significantly, nevertheless inhibit TSH response to TRH. As a complementary finding, barely detectable decreases in plasma thyroid hormone levels produced by administration of iodide are sufficient to sensitize the pituitary to TRH. These results could mean that the fine adjustment of TSH secretion is mediated at the pituitary level by the feedback effect of the thyroid hormones (Vagenakis, 1979). Effects of TRH are almost immediate; increases in plasma TSH levels are detectable within a minute or two after intravenous administration of TRH in both rats and humans. On the other hand, inhibition of TSH secretion following T_4 and T_3 administration shows a distinct lag period of several hours. The mechanism underlying these responses is considered later under TRH action.

Both T_4 and T_3 inhibit pituitary TSH secretion. Labeled T_3 appears in the pituitary after the systemic injection of labeled T_4, a finding attributable to both an active pituitary monodeiodinating system and the presence of high-affinity binding sites for T_3 that act to concentrate this hormone from the blood and from the products of local conversion. Data obtained using rat pituitary tumor cell cultures of the GH-PRL–secreting type indicate that both T_4 and T_3 can bind to distinctly different classes of receptors on pituitary cells.

Studies in this tumor line have further shown that the stimulation of GH secretion and inhibition of PRL release

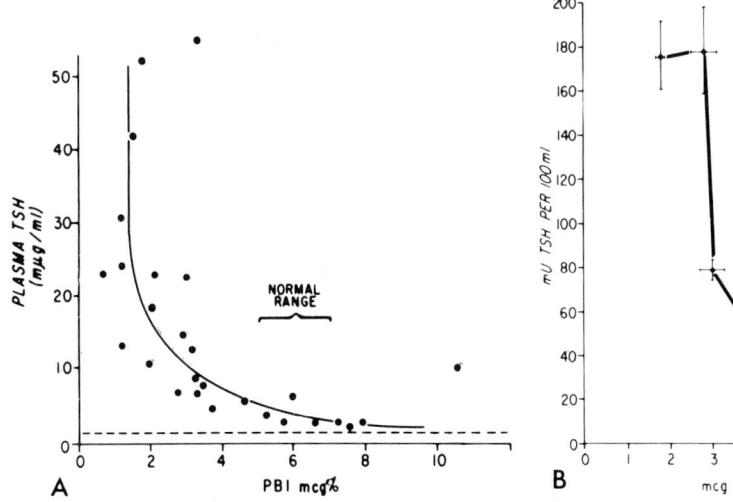
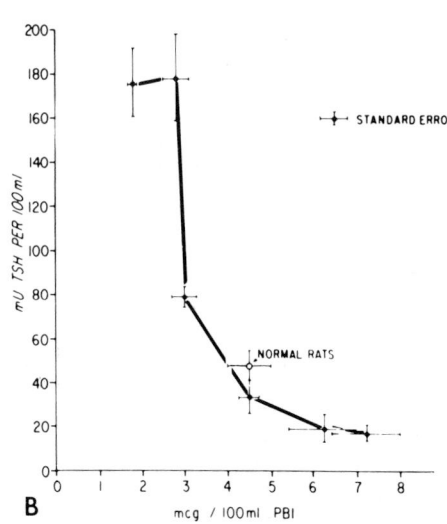

Figure 11–30. The relationship between plasma TSH and thyroid hormone (as determined by plasma PBI measurements in man and in the rat). These curves illustrate in the human (*A*) and the rat (*B*) that plasma TSH levels are a curvilinear function of plasma thyroid hormone level. Human studies were carried out by giving myxedematous patients successive increments of thyroxine at approximately 10-day intervals. Each point represents simultaneous measurements of plasma PBI and plasma TSH at various times in the six patients studied. The rat studies were done by treating thyroidectomized animals with various doses of thyroxine for two weeks prior to assay of plasma TSH and plasma PBI. These curves illustrate that the secretion of TSH is regulated over the entire range of thyroid hormone levels. At the normal set point for T_4, the small changes above and below the controlled level are followed by appropriate increases or decreases in plasma TSH. (*A*: From Reichlin, S., and Utiger, R. D.: Regulation of the pituitary thyroid axis in man: Relationship of TSH concentration to concentration of free and total thyroxine in plasma. *J. Clin. Endocrinol. Metab.* 27:251, 1967. *B*: From Reichlin, S., Martin, J. B., et al.: Measurement of TSH in plasma and pituitary of the rat by a radioimmunoassay utilizing bovine TSH: Effect of thyroidectomy or thyroxine administration on plasma TSH levels. *Endocrinology* 87:1022, 1970, with permission.)

can be induced by either T_3 or T_4 and that the relative potency of these thyroid hormones is paralleled by the relative binding of the two hormones to isolated cell nuclei.

Growth and differentiation of the pituitary may be influenced by the thyroid hormone at a critical stage of development. Administration of high doses of T_3 or T_4 to newborn rats (neonatal hyperthyroidism) leads to permanent disturbance in pituitary-thyroid function. These animals grow subnormally, and as adults have decreased plasma levels of T_4 and TSH. That the defect is in the pituitary is suggested by the finding that responses to exogenous TRH are subnormal. These observations have been interpreted to mean that the "set point" of pituitary-thyroid feedback control may be regulated by thyroid hormone concentration during a critical "imprinting" period.

Neural Control of Pituitary-Thyroid Function

A long period of speculation based on erroneously interpreted clinical observations preceded the emergence of current concepts of the role of the nervous system in the control of thyroid function. Thyrotoxicosis has classically been described as "frozen fright" and was classified as a neurotic disorder in the 19th century. Numerous clinical studies, including Parry's first report in 1825, noted that the disease or its relapses occurred in a setting of chronic or acute psychic trauma. This observation notwithstanding, Graves' disease is not caused by brain-induced TSH hypersecretion. With the exception of a few rare cases, plasma TSH levels are low or undetectable in Graves' disease. Normal pituitary secretion is usually suppressed in Graves' disease and is in fact an "innocent bystander" to the thyroid hypersecretion caused by an immunologic thyroid stimulator whose source is outside the pituitary.

Even though Graves' disease can no longer be looked upon as a model of stress-induced TSH hypersecretion, however, the nervous system plays a major role in the regulation of the pituitary-thyroid axis. In all situations in which the pituitary is deprived of input from the median eminence region of the hypothalamus, TSH secretion is reduced below normal. This occurs after section of the pituitary stalk, after transplantation of the pituitary to a remote site, after the production of lesions of the "thyrotropic area," and in pituitary cells in culture.

Although basal secretion of TSH is reduced when the pituitary is deprived of hypothalamic input, appropriate secretory responses are elicited by alterations in thyroid hormone concentration. For example, in response to thyroidectomy, animals with lesions of the thyrotropic area show increased TSH levels, but at a still-reduced level. Thyroid hormone administration is followed by inhibition of TSH secretion (Fig. 11–30).

These and numerous other observations have led to the postulation that the function of the hypothalamus in pituitary-thyroid interplay is to determine the "set point" of feedback control around which the usual feedback regulatory responses are elicited. Even massive lesions in the "thyrotropic area" do not destroy all TRH-secreting elements in the hypothalamus of the rat, however. Pituitary-thyroid regulation in animals with hypothalamic lesions is thus conditioned by some, albeit reduced, TRH influence. In humans, some patients with spontaneously occurring hypothalamic disease have TSH deficiency as severe as that seen after hypophysectomy.

Hypothalamic lesions were initially used to identify the region of the brain involved in pituitary regulation. Later, it became possible to map regions of the hypothalamus electrically excitable for TSH release. Both kinds of study have outlined areas of the hypothalamus capable of modifying TSH secretion. Most recently, bioassay and immunoassay methods have delineated regions of the hypothalamus rich in TRH.

The anatomic region involved in TSH regulation is largely confined to the medial basal hypothalamus ("hypophysiotropic area"), which shows a concentration gradient of TRH from dorsal hypothalamus to median eminence, reflecting the convergence of TRH-containing nerve fibers and storage granules toward the pituitary stalk region. In rats in which the medial basal hypothalamus is isolated from the rest of the brain by surgical means, there is reduction of TRH within the isolated region, suggesting that some neurons arise outside of the medial basal hypothalamus or that other kinds of neural inputs are involved in regulating TRH secretion in this region. Such animals show relatively normal basal TSH secretion but lose both normal circadian TSH secretory rhythms and cold-induced TSH responses. The location of TRH-containing structures has also been determined in the human brain (Fig. 11–18).

The most anteriorly situated TSH regulatory area in the rat is the preoptic region, functionally important because it is the site of temperature-sensitive neurons; activation by local cooling is capable of stimulating TSH release, neurogenic heat conservation responses, and increased eating.

It has been postulated that this region of the brain integrates all visceral homeostatic mechanisms maintaining body heat. Several extrahypothalamic regions, including the pineal gland, have also been implicated in TSH regulation. Some workers have suggested that the pineal exerts a predominately inhibitory influence on TSH release through melatonin secretion, but not all have confirmed these observations. It is of interest, but of uncertain significance in relation to pituitary-thyroid control, that the pineal glands of several species of animals, including the rat and the frog, contain TRH. In the frog, altered light and dark regimens are followed by altered TRH concentrations, the hypothalamic concentrations of TRH remaining constant.

Hypophysiotropic Factors in Thyrotropic Hormone Regulation (Fig. 11–29)

TRH is the major hypothalamic hormone stimulating TSH release, but other hypothalamic hormones also influence its secretion. The most important of these is SRIF, which is a potent inhibitor of TRH-induced TSH secretion. This conclusion is based on experiments in rats in which endogenous SRIF is inactivated by pretreatment with anti-SRIF antisera. Such animals show an increase in basal TSH levels, an enhanced TSH response to cold exposure, and an enhanced response to injections of TRH. The role of SRIF secretion in regulation of human TSH secretion is unknown, but it has been postulated that the inhibitory effect of GH on TSH secretion and the TSH secretory response to TRH may be due to increased SRIF secretion, the result of activation of "short loop" feedback control by GH.

Dopamine, the secretion of the dopaminergic tuberohypophyseal system, also appears to inhibit TSH secretion in humans through a direct action on the pituitary.

The relative importance of TRH, SRIF, and dopamine in determining the "set point" of the pituitary-thyroid axis has not been fully determined, but it is important to re-emphasize that, in the absence of all hypothalamic input, TSH secretion is markedly reduced. Still uncertain is the effect of thyroid status on the secretion of TRH, SRIF, and dopamine. The direct injection of thyroid hormones into the hypothalamus has recently been shown to inhibit TSH secretion in the monkey, but it has not been determined whether this is owing to inhibition of TRH secretion or to activation of secretion of SRIF or another inhibitory hypothalamic factor.

The effect of biogenic amines on TSH secretion (other than the direct dopaminergic inhibition of the pituitary) has received much study. The bulk of data now available suggests that release of TRH is inhibited by drugs that deplete central catecholamines and stimulated by norepinephrine, acting through central α receptors. Serotonin appears to inhibit TRH release. Contradictory findings have been reported by some workers, however, and histamine has been claimed to be a releaser of TRH secretion *in vitro*. Endorphinergic pathways also inhibit TRH release.

Although an extensive network of central pathways capable of modifying TRH secretion exists and much work indicates that thyroid function in most experimental animals is activated by cold exposure and inhibited (rarely activated) by stress, human pituitary-thyroid function shows only modest evidence of neuroendocrine control other than the regulation of basal TRH levels. The most important manifestations of neural control of TSH secretion in the human are cold-induced TSH release (seen only in the newborn) and the circadian rhythms of TSH release. The 24-hour plasma TSH profile as described by Patel and coworkers is characterized by a circadian periodicity with a maximum between 2115 and 0530 hours and a minimum between 1602 and 1848 hours. Superimposed on the circadian rhythm pattern are smaller TSH peaks occurring every 2–4 hours. These short-term oscillations typify an ultradian rhythm and have been attributed to episodic secretion of TRH, although periodic release of SRIF as the modulating influence cannot be excluded. Severe physical stress (usually accompanied by chronic illness and malnutrition) can lead to inhibition of TSH secretion presumably as a neurally mediated response, but this has not been established with absolute certainty. In rats, stress-induced TSH inhibition is due to somatostatin release.

Corticotropin Secretion

Any theory designed to explain how ACTH secretion is regulated must account for several important features of pituitary-adrenal function. These features include the occurrence of a circadian rhythm entrained to both sleep-wake and light-dark cycles, the occurrence of spontaneous bursts of release (ultradian rhythm), the inhibition by glucocorticoid administration, the enhanced secretion after adrenalectomy, and the release induced by stress (see Ch. 5). These varied kinds of secretory patterns are explained best by a dual control system involving the interaction of two mechanisms, one a closed loop negative feedback mediated by circulating glucocorticoids and the other an open loop control system involving the brain and mediated by the hypothalamic hormone CRF (Fig. 11–31).

Feedback effects of glucocorticoids are directed both at the pituitary adrenotrope cell and on the secretion of CRF. Evidence that the pituitary is a target for feedback effects comes from studies of isolated glands in culture; basal and CRF-stimulated ACTH secretion is inhibited by cortisol added to the media. Neural sites of feedback are demonstrated by the inhibitory responses that follow intracerebral implants of glucocorticoids and by release of CRF from incubated hypothalamic fragments. A further indication that both neural and pituitary sites are involved in feedback control is the finding of glucocorticoid receptors in both pituitary and brain. Two different classes of receptors mediate feedback control in both brain and pituitary; one responds promptly (within a few minutes) and is sensitive to

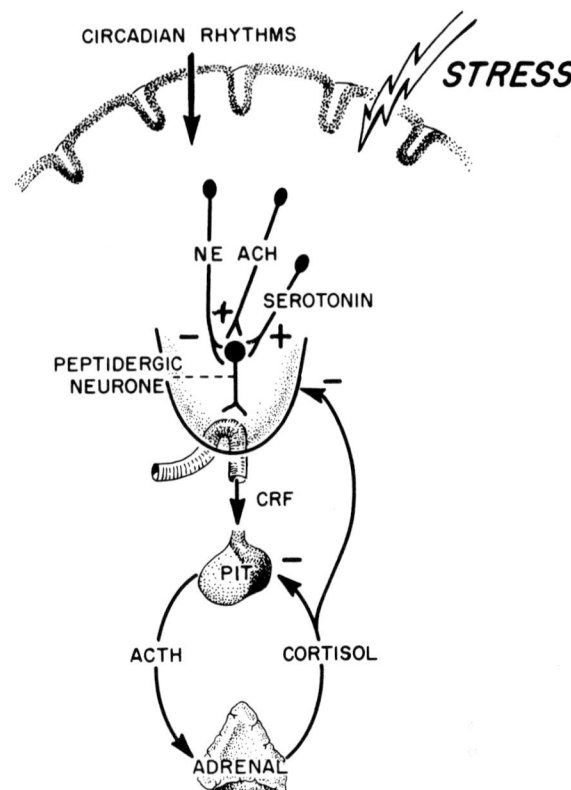

Figure 11–31. Regulatory elements of the hypothalamic-pituitary-adrenal cortical system for regulation of cortisol secretion, a closed loop negative feedback control system with open loop transients. Secretion of ACTH is stimulated by CRF (corticotropin releasing factor) and inhibited at the pituitary level by cortisol. Cortisol also acts on the hypothalamus or other parts of the brain to inhibit secretion of CRF. CRF secretion is regulated by neurotransmitter effects on the CRF neuron. Acetylcholine (ACH) is excitatory; norepinephrine is inhibitory, as is gamma aminobutyric acid (GABA), not shown. Serotonin is illustrated as an excitatory neurotransmitter, but Jones (1978) suggests that it acts by stimulating cholinergic activity. (Reprinted with modifications from Martin, J., Reichlin, S., et al.: *Clinical Neuroendocrinology.* Philadelphia, F. A. Davis, 1977.)

rapid increases in glucocorticoids; the other is subject to a several hour delay before inhibition of ACTH release is noted. Because the delayed effects are blocked by agents that interfere with RNA transcription or translation, glucocorticoids are believed to modulate the genome (as is the case for glucocorticoid effects in several parenchymal tissues) (Chs. 2 and 5). The short-term inhibitory effects very likely involve direct changes in membrane function of CRF-secreting neurons and pituitary adrenotrope cells. Early nongenomic effects of glucocorticoids on neural function have been demonstrated by electrophysiologic techniques. Most glucocorticoid receptor cells lie outside the hypothalamus in areas including the hippocampus, septum, and amygdala. These structures are part of the "visceral brain" that is involved in the manifestations of emotional state. It is likely therefore that the neural component of feedback is directed at the very regions involved in stress-induced ACTH release. Moreover, it is likely that the emotional disturbances that sometimes follow glucocorticoid administration may involve abnormal function of these regions (see Ch. 12).

Owing to the fact that the chemical identity of CRF is still unknown, pathways of the CRF-secreting neurons have not been elucidated with the same degree of immunohistochemical elegance as has been the case of SRIF and LRH. Nevertheless, it appears likely that CRF is secreted by tuberohypophyseal neurons located in the medial basal hypothalamus and that the releasing factor is transported to the median eminence, as is the case for the other hypothalamic hypophysiotropic hormones. The CRF neuron receives regulatory signals from many parts of the brain. Important excitatory inputs are from the suprachiasmatic nucleus (the regulator of circadian rhythms), from the amygdala, and from the raphe nuclei of the brainstem. Inhibitory inputs of CRF secretion arise in the hippocampus and in the locus ceruleus of the midbrain. These anatomic inputs are neurotransmitter coded; excitatory influences are both cholinergic and serotonergic. Inhibitory influences are noradrenergic (Fig. 11–31).

A plausible model of the way in which neural and feedback factors are integrated to influence ACTH secretion can be developed along lines analogous to the regulation of the pituitary-thyroid axis.

It is proposed that the set point of plasma cortisol feedback is determined by the central nervous system through modulation of the rate of CRF release. In the presence of high CRF levels, high concentrations of cortisol are required to inhibit ACTH release. Contrariwise, when CRF secretion is low (as in the late afternoon) or in individuals with hypothalamic lesions, the brain-pituitary controlling mechanism is highly susceptible to steroid suppression. The brain thus determines the set point of the "adrenostat," located both in pituitary and in part in brain. Unlike the secretion of TSH, which becomes completely unresponsive to the hypothalamic hormone TRH if thyroid hormone levels are sufficiently high, severe neurogenic stress can "break through" the feedback inhibition by glucocorticoids. In evaluation of ACTH secretion control in humans with hypothalamic-pituitary disorder (see Ch. 5), it is well to recognize that tests of secretory reserve do not of themselves distinguish between pituitary and hypothalamic sites of disease because normal ACTH secretion requires normal function of both brain and pituitary.

In addition to the feedback effects exerted by glucocorticoids on ACTH secretion, evidence has accumulated for the existence of a "short loop" feedback exerted on ACTH secretion by ACTH itself. Several workers have shown that the administration of ACTH to adrenalectomized animals maintained on a fixed dose of glucocorticoid suppresses ACTH secretion. This observation has been interpreted to mean that ACTH inhibits its own secretion. Until recently, there has been little insight as to possible mechanisms of the effect. The most important new observations that may aid in interpretation of this finding are the demonstration of high concentrations of ACTH in blood reaching the hypothalamus by "reflux" from the pituitary, the identification of a population of clearly defined ACTH-containing (and synthesizing) neurons in the medial basal hypothalamus and related areas, and the finding that a radiolabeled analogue of ACTH when injected into the pituitary can be recovered in the hypothalamus. Conditions exist therefore that allow high concentrations of ACTH to reach regions of the brain involved in ACTH regulation. The relative importance of this possible mode of regulation has not been elucidated.

ACTH-containing pathways may also be responsible for some of the effects on high brain function noted after injection of ACTH or its analogues (see Ch. 12).

Comment should also be made about the role of central endorphinergic pathways in ACTH regulation. It has been known for many years that acute administration of morphine stimulates the release of ACTH and that chronic administration blocks ACTH release induced by a wide variety of stresses. These observations have been interpreted to suggest that endorphinergic fibers are part of the "stress" pathway. Because opiate antagonists do not block stress-induced ACTH release, the endorphin system can be looked upon as being *one* of the inputs into ACTH regulation, rather than *the* essential mediator.

Prolactin Regulation

The secretion of PRL, like that of GH and ACTH, is responsive to a wide variety of external stimuli, including suckling and emotional and physical stresses, and to internal rhythms related to the sleep cycle (Table 11–8). In contrast to all of the other anterior pituitary secretions, the predominant effect of the hypothalamus on PRL secretion is that of tonic suppression. Secretion of PRL is also responsive to alterations in the hormonal milieu of the pituitary, especially to the stimulatory action of estrogenic hormones (Fig. 11–32).

Hypothalamic control of PRL secretion is mediated by two or more regulatory hormones synthesized by tuberohypophyseal neurons. The single most important regulatory hypophysiotropic hormone is dopamine, the neurohormonal product of one set of neurons of the arcuate nucleus that terminates in the median eminence. Secreted into the hypophyseal-portal blood, dopamine exerts a direct inhibitory control on pituitary lactotrope cells by way of cell membrane dopamine receptors. In addition to dopamine, there may be other PRL inhibiting factors (PIF's), including GABA and an as yet uncharacterized peptide(s). It is the loss of tonic hypothalamic control by these factors that leads to hypersecretion of PRL after connections between pituitary and median eminence have been interrupted. PRF's are also found in the hypothalamus, the best-characterized being TRH. This substance releases PRL from normal pituitaries and follows the same dose response pattern as for TSH release (Fig. 11–21). Yet TRH is probably not the only PRF. Hypothalamic extracts bring about PRL release even when the TRH content has been inactivated or separated chromatographically. PRL regulation is not altered by treatment with anti-TRH antibody in most (but not all) experiments, and suckling, which brings about a sharp rise in plasma PRL, is without effect on TSH secretion. The chemical nature of the authentic PRF has not been elucidated.

The hypothalamic PRL regulatory system is governed by two major bioaminergic control systems and by peptidergic inputs as well. Dopamine, acting in the hypothalamus, releases PIF(s) that suppress PRL secretion. Serotonin, acting centrally, stimulates PRL release. There is much evidence from the use of neurotransmitter agonists and antagonists to support the postulation that PRL stimulation is under serotonergic control and inhibition is under dopaminergic control. (See Table 11–6 for summary of pharmacologic effects of neurotransmitters on PRL regulation.) Lesions of the ascending serotonin pathways and of arcuate dopaminergic pathways give rise to changes in PRL secretion that confirm the studies using drugs. PRL regulation is also influenced by central neuropeptide pathways, including the endorphinergic system, which stimulates PRL release. (See Table 11–7 for summary of central peptidergic effects on PRL release.)

The most important of the influences on PRL regulation is exerted by PRL itself and constitutes a feedback element of short loop control. The best evidence that PRL exerts negative feedback effects on PRL secretion comes from studies in which PRL pellets were placed within the hypothalamus in experimental animals. PRL secretion inhibition by this procedure is evidenced by a lowering of plasma PRL levels and suppression of normal lactational response to suckling. Effects of PRL appear to be mediated by changes in the activity of the tuberohypophyseal dopamine neurons shown by measurements of dopamine turnover that are increased in PRL-treated rats and concentration in portal vessel blood. Short loop feedback of PRL and LRH secretion is also responsible for the gonadotropin inhibition that occurs in women who are nursing and in patients with PRL-secreting adenomas of the pituitary.

Table 11–8. FACTORS THAT INFLUENCE SERUM PROLACTIN LEVELS IN HUMANS

Physiologic	Pathologic	Pharmacologic
Increase in Serum Prolactin		
1. Pregnancy	1. Prolactin-secreting pituitary tumors	1. TRH
2. Postpartum	2. Hypothalamic-pituitary disorders:	2. Psychotropic drugs
a. Non-nursing mothers (days 1–7)	a. ("functional"?)	a. Phenothiazines
b. Nursing mothers after suckling	b. Tumors (craniopharyngioma) metastases	b. Reserpine
3. Nipple stimulation (males and females)	c. Histiocytosis X	3. Oral contraceptives
4. Coitus (some subjects)	d. Inflammation-sarcoidosis	4. Estrogen therapy
5. Stress	3. Pituitary stalk section	5. α-Methyl-dopa
6. Exercise	4. Hypothyroidism	
7. Neonatal period (2–3 months)	5. Renal failure	
8. Sleep	6. Ectopic production by malignant tumors	
Decrease in Serum Prolactin		
1. Water loading	1. Isolated pituitary prolactin deficiency	1. L-Dopa
		2. Apomorphine
		3. Bromocryptine

Adapted from Martin, J. B., Reichlin, S. et al. (eds.): *Clinical Neuroendocrinology.* Philadelphia, F. A. Davis Co., 1977.

All forms of external and internal stimuli that modify PRL release converge on the tuberohypophyseal neurons that secrete PIF(s) and PRF(s). Anatomic pathways involved in the suckling reflux have been well characterized in experimental animals and are presumed to be similar in humans. These arise in nerves innervating the nipple, enter the cord by way of spinal afferent neurons, ascend the spinal cord to the midbrain, and enter the hypothalamus by way of the medial forebrain bundle. For the greatest part of the pathway, nerves regulating the milk let-down response (see earlier discussion) accompany those involved in PRL regulation; at the level of the paraventricular nuclei, fibers

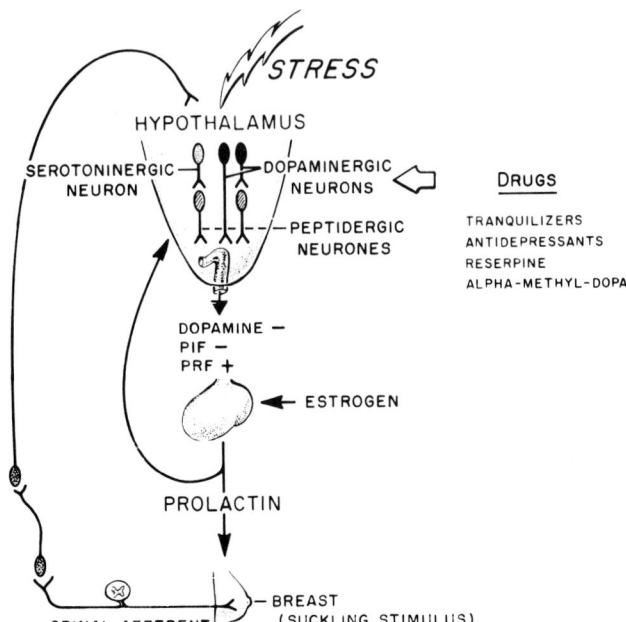

Figure 11–32. Hypothalamic regulation of PRL secretion. Many control elements are involved in PRL regulation. The predominant effect of the hypothalamus is inhibitory, an effect mediated by at least one PRL inhibitory factor (PIF), which is dopamine, secreted by the tuberohypophyseal dopaminergic system. There may be at least one additional PIF, under central dopaminergic control. PRL releasing factors (PRF) (one is TRH, and others may exist) can stimulate PRL release in response to stimuli (?) stress, (?) suckling. The PRF component appears to be under serotonergic control. Hypothalamic elements are modified by neuroleptic agents: dopamine agonists inhibit, serotonin agonists stimulate PRL secretion. Estrogen effects exerted on the pituitary sensitize it to PRF's. Neurologic stimuli from the periphery trigger suckling induced PRL release. PRL feeds back on the hypothalamus to regulate its own secretion and increases dopamine secretion.

influencing OT release spin off. There is reason to believe that the suckling reflex may bring about a release of PRF as well as the inhibition of PIF activity. The consequent increase in PRL, as noted before, has an inhibitory effect on PRL release and on gonadotropin secretion, thus explaining the anovulatory state observed in women who are nursing their babies.

The PRL release reflex has broad biologic implications. From an evolutionary point of view, the development of PRL release and of milk let-down reflex provides a mechanism by which the infant can regulate its mother's milk production and milk delivery to the nipple. The complementary suckling reflex of the infant, a response to tactile stimulation of the lips, presumably developed in a parallel fashion. These complex behavioral and neuroendocrine mechanisms involving mother and infant, evolved over untold generations, are requirements for the successful survival of the mammal.

The PRL secretory response to breast stimulation also has major implications for human ecology. In most societies, lactation-induced suppression of ovulation is the principal means by which pregnancies are spaced.

The PRL regulatory system and its bioaminergic control have received much attention in recent years because of the recognition of important syndromes of PRL hypersecretion and the difficulty of diagnosis of occult pituitary adenomas (see Ch. 3 and later in the chapter). In this context, it is important to emphasize that both pituitary and hypothalamus have PRL inhibitory dopamine receptors; response to dopamine receptor stimulation and blockade does not distinguish between central and peripheral actions of the drug. One means that has been used to differentiate among these sites of action is the use of drugs, such as carbidopa, that interfere with the conversion of L-dopa to dopa; some of these drugs appear to act only beyond the blood-brain barrier.

Another important recent impetus to study of PRL secretion in relation to biogenic amines has been the recognition of the effects of commonly used neuroleptic drugs on PRL secretion. Phenothiazines, including chlorpromazine, haloperidol, tricyclic antidepressants, and reserpine all bring about the release of PRL by interference with tonic dopamine receptor stimulation. In addition to the practical problem of lactation and amenorrhea, which may be induced in such patients, it has been recognized that the PRL response may be a good index of the antipsychotic properties of a given agent. Further, the idea has been expressed in recent neurologic and psychiatric experiments that PRL secretion, reflecting as it does central dopaminergic activity, may serve as a "window to the hypothalamus." It must be emphasized that PRL secretion reflects a balance between serotonin and dopamine activity and that there is no proof that the pathways involved in pituitary regulation are the same as those involved in affective state. Moreover, the role of central peptidergic pathways in PRL regulation has not been fully characterized.

Growth Hormone Regulation

Secretion of GH is modified by a wide variety of external stimuli and by endogenous neural rhythms (Tables 11–9 and 11–10). The more important naturally occurring events that trigger GH release are exercise, physical and emotional stresses, high protein intake, and carbohydrate-rich meals (during the descending limb of blood glucose levels). The most important endogenous modifications of GH release are the surges of secretion that occur within an hour or two of falling asleep and others that occur randomly through the day and night, apparently unrelated to any identifiable extrinsic or internal event. All of these changes are determined by the central nervous system acting through the hypothalamus. In addition to the crucially important neural control system, GH secretion is modified by the hormonal milieu of the pituitary; enhanced in the presence of estrogens, testosterone, and thyroid hormone; and suppressed by abnormally high levels of glucocorticoids (see Ch. 3).

Hypothalamic influences are mediated by two hypophysiotropic hormones: the one, GH releasing factor (GHRF), the chemical nature of which has still not been identified despite nearly two decades of effort in many laboratories, and the other, somatostatin (GH inhibiting factor — SRIF or GHIF) (Fig. 11–33). The predominant influence of the hypothalamus on GH release is stimulatory, as evidenced by the fact that damage to the hypothalamic pituitary connection, such as occurs with section of the pituitary stalk or lesions of the basal hypothalamus, is followed by profound inhibition of both basal and induced GH release. In situations in which the inhibitory somatostatinergic component is inactivated, basal GH levels are higher than normal, and responses to the usual provocative stimuli are more exuberant. It has been suggested that the paradoxical release of GH that

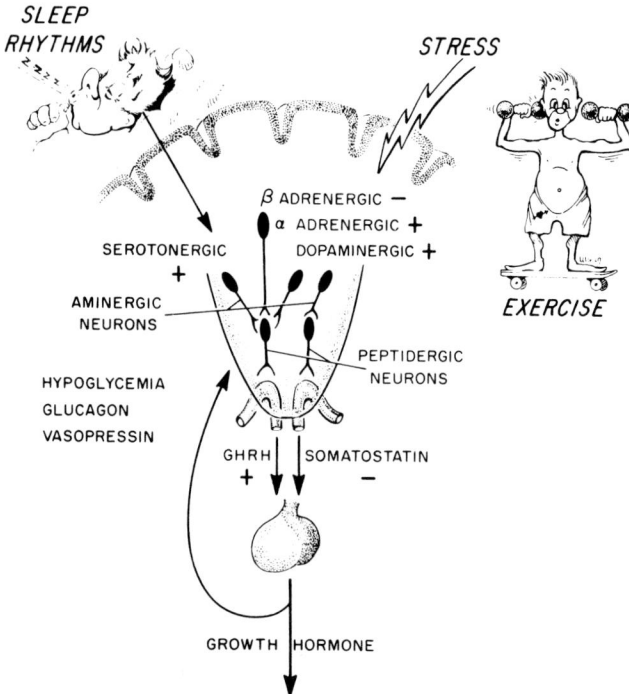

Figure 11–33. Neuroendocrine factors in GH regulation. GH secretion is completely dependent upon the hypothalamic secretion of GH releasing factor (GHRF, GHRH), but there is also an inhibitory input from somatostatinergic fibers. GHRF-secreting neurons are stimulated by three classes of biogenic aminergic neurons—serotonin, dopamine, and the α-adrenergic component of noradrenaline. β-adrenergic influences are inhibitory. Somatostatin is also controlled by biogenic aminergic neurons, but the pharmacologic coding is not worked out well. Sleep rhythms, exercise, stress, blood sugar levels, and vasopressin and glucagon effects are all mediated indirectly through the hypothalamus.

follows glucose injection in some patients with optic nerve glioma (a lesion compressing the anterior hypothalamus) and various forms of metabolic encephalopathy, including uremia and hepatic coma, is due to functional inactivation of the somatostatinergic inhibitory control system. Lacking

---

Table 11–9. FACTORS THAT STIMULATE GROWTH HORMONE SECRETION IN PRIMATES

Physiologic	Pharmacologic	Pathologic
1. Episodic, spontaneous	1. Insulin hypoglycemia	1. Acromegaly
2. Exercise	a. 2-Deoxyglucose	a. TRH
3. Stress	2. Amino acid infusions	b. LRH
a. Physical	a. Arginine	c. Glucose
b. Psychological	b. Leucine	d. Arginine
4. Sleep	c. Lysine, etc.	2. Pyrogens
5. Postprandial glucose decline	3. Small peptides	3. Protein depletion
	a. ADH	4. Fasting and starvation
	b. α MSH	5. Anorexia nervosa
	c. ACTH (1–24)	
	d. Glucagon	
	4. Monoaminergic stimuli	
	a. Epinephrine, α receptor stimulation	
	b. L-dopa	
	c. Apomorphine	
	d. 2-Bromocryptine	
	e. Clonidine	
	f. 5-hydroxytryptophan	
	g. Fusaric acid (dopa-β-hydroxylase inhibitor)	
	h. Propranolol	
	i. Melatonin	
	5. Nonpeptide hormones	
	a. Estrogens	
	b. Diethylstilbestrol	
	6. Potassium infusion	
	7. Dibutyryl-cAMP	

Table 11–10. FACTORS THAT INHIBIT GROWTH HORMONE SECRETION IN PRIMATES*

Physiologic	Pharmacologic	Pathologic
1. Postprandial hyperglycemia	1. Melatonin	1. Acromegaly
2. Elevated free fatty acids (?pharmacologic)	2. Serotonin antagonists	a. L-dopa
3. Elevated GH levels	a. Methysergide	b. Apomorphine
	b. Cyproheptadine	c. Phentolamine
	3. Phentolamine	d. 2-bromocriptine
	4. Chlorpromazine	2. Hyperthyroidism
	5. Morphine	3. Hypothyroidism
	6. Zn-tetracosactin	
	7. Progesterone	
	8. Theophylline	

*In many instances, the inhibition can only be demonstrated as a suppression of GH release induced by a pharmacologic stimulus.
Reprinted with modifications with permission from Martin, J. B., Brazeau, P., et al.: Neuroendocrine organization of growth hormone regulation, In *The Hypothalamus.* Reichlin, S., Baldessarini, R. J., et al. (eds.), New York, Raven Press, 1978, pp. 329–357.

specific immunohistochemic reagents to identify the pathways of the GHRF neuron, it has not been possible to delineate these pathways with precision, but they are probably located in the tuberohypophyseal neuron system and terminate (as do all the other tuberohypophyseal neurons) in the median eminence.

Corresponding to the complexity of stimuli to which it responds, the neuron system regulating GHRF and SRIF release receives a variety of neural inputs (Figs. 11–34 and 11–35). Impulses arising in the hippocampus (presumed to be linked to the sleep cycle) are excitatory, whereas those arising in the amygdaloid nuclei can be both excitatory (basolateral amygdala) and inhibitory (corticomedial amygdala). The amygdala is a part of the visceral brain involved in the generation of emotion and stress responses and is probably a component of the pathways responsible for stress-induced GH release. The inhibitory inputs are presumed to activate SRIF release via the anterior somatostatinergic pathway; the stimulatory pathway is by way of the ventromedial nucleus.

The association of the ventromedial (VM) nucleus with GH release is important for the regulation of carbohydrate metabolism. The VM nucleus contains glucoreceptors capable of influencing insulin secretion as well as GH release and, in addition, generates the drive for food consumption (see Ch. 18). This region has also been shown to contain insulinergic nerve pathways and insulin and SRIF receptors. Although the details have not been fully worked out, it appears likely that the hypothalamus, especially the VM nucleus, integrates the secretion of important glucoregulatory hormones with eating.

The GH regulatory neuron system also receives impulses from each of the three principal ascending monaminergic systems — dopaminergic, noradrenergic and serotonergic; the control attributed to hippocampus and amygdala may in fact be mediated at least in part by way of these aminergic

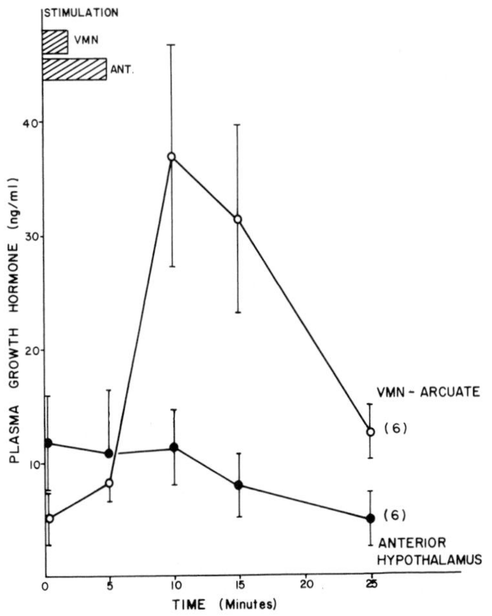

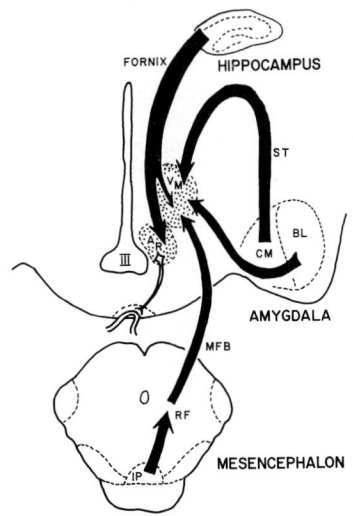

Figure 11–34. Effect on plasma GH of electrical stimulation of the ventromedial hypothalamic nucleus of the rat. This figure shows the marked increase in plasma GH levels that follows electrical stimulation of the ventromedial nucleus of the rat. The ventromedial nucleus and ventral-basal hypothalamus are the only regions of the hypothalamus that are capable of this response, although certain extrahypothalamic sites may also cause this change (see Fig. 11–35). Note the very short latent period of the response. The ventromedial nucleus is also important in that it has an effect on insulin secretion and satiety sensation and is the site of glucoreceptors. (Reproduced from Martin, J. B.: Plasma growth hormone (GH) response to hypothalamic or extrahypothalamic electric stimulation. *Endocrinology 91*:107, 1972, with permission.)

Figure 11–35. Neural pathways involved in GH regulation. This diagram illustrates the varied pathways by which impulses from the limbic system (visceral brain) ultimately impinge upon the ventromedial nucleus, which in turn is capable of stimulating GH release through the mediation of GHRF. Pharmacologic blocking studies show that the pathways between the extrahypothalamic regions and the ventromedial nucleus are catecholaminergic, whereas those between the ventromedial nucleus and the stalk-median eminence region are not catecholaminergic. (Reproduced from Martin, J. B.: Plasma growth hormone (GH) response to hypothalamic or extrahypothalamic electric stimulation. *Endocrinology 91*:107, 1972, with permission.)

systems. The first clue to a central dopaminergic control system was the observation that administration of L-dopa (converted to dopamine in the brain) led to a release of GH. Soon thereafter it was shown that hypoglycemia-induced GH release was blunted by α receptor blockers. Current views are that dopamine stimulates GHRF both by direct action on central dopamine receptors and by stimulation of α receptors after conversion to norepinephrine. Norepinephrine, acting centrally, is an extremely potent GH release stimulator, as is serotonin. It is important to emphasize that each class of neurotransmitter may be involved in a specific set of physiologic stimuli to GH secretion. For example, sleep-induced GH release is mainly mediated by serotonergic fibers, whereas hypoglycemia-induced GH release, as well as that due to exercise, VP and most stresses, is mediated by α-adrenergic (noradrenergic) pathways. The relative importance of the three aminergic control systems is different from species to species, as is the character of response to specific stimuli, such as hypoglycemia and stress. Studies based on rats and even monkeys cannot be extrapolated freely to humans.

In addition to the monaminergic control system, several central peptidergic neuron nets are involved in GH regulation. Endorphin receptor stimulation, either by morphine administration or by third ventricular injection of β endorphin, stimulates GH release. Since these agents have no effect on GH secretion from the pituitary when applied *in vitro,* the effect appears to be secondary to activation of the GHRF neuronal system. Other peptides recently shown to stimulate GH release are vasoinhibitory peptide (VIP) and neurotensin. Substance P inhibits GH release when injected into the third ventricle by inducing SRIF secretion. TRH has paradoxical inhibitory and excitatory effects on GH secretion. When introduced directly into the brain, it inhibits GH release and, by systemic injection in humans, inhibits the GH secretory surge that normally follows early sleep. These findings are interpreted to mean that central TRH pathways are inhibitory to the GH regulatory process. On the other hand, under several circumstances, such as malnutrition, and in acromegaly, TRH acts directly on the pituitary to stimulate GH secretion (see the discussion under "Thyrotropin Releasing Hormone").

Unlike the pituitary secretions that are influenced by feedback from peripheral target glands, GH secretion is regulated by GH itself or by a GH-dependent factor. The observations on which this concept is based are the prior treatment with GH either by systemic injections (humans and rhesus monkeys) or direct implantation into the hypothalamus (rats) inhibits the GH secretory response to various stimuli. Several elements of this control system have not been elucidated. It is not known whether the effect on the brain is mediated by GH or by a GH-dependent factor like somatomedin. One clue to suggest that somatomedin is the necessary intermediary is that in conditions in which plasma somatomedin concentration is low (Laron-type dwarf, anorexia nervosa, Kwashiorkor), plasma GH levels are generally elevated.

Reproduction: Neuroendocrine Aspects of the Regulation of Sexual Function (Figs. 11–36 and 11–37)

Every component of the patterned reproductive activity of the higher vertebrates depends upon a close interplay between neural and endocrine events. Perpetuation of the species obviously requires the accurate correlation of overt mating behavior with the internal events of gametogenesis in ovary and testis. This correlation of behavior and readi-

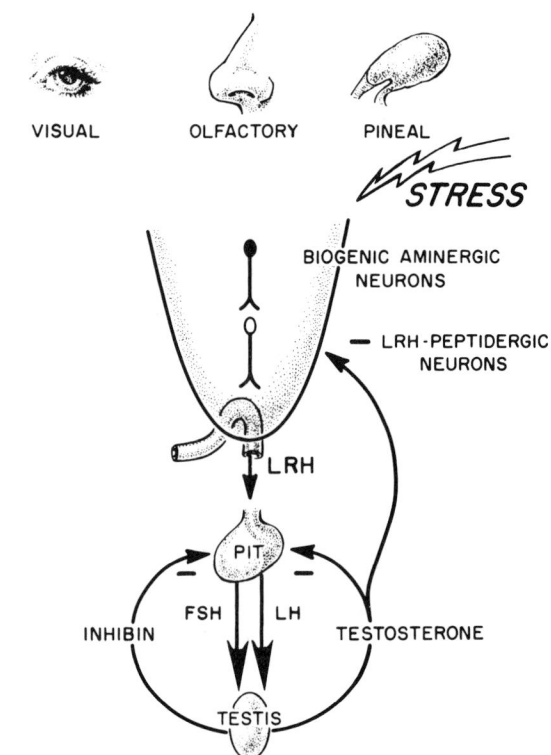

Figure 11–36. Regulation of gonadotropin secretion in the male. Schematic diagram of gonadotropin control system in the male, showing the interactions of neural and hormonal feedback controls. Pituitary and testis are connected by a negative feedback link. Secretion of testosterone by the testis is stimulated by LH, whereas maturation and growth of the tubule cells are stimulated by FSH. The secretion of testosterone in turn inhibits the secretion of LH. It is likely that the major target of negative feedback is the hypothalamus; testosterone administration in humans does not interfere with the effectiveness of LRH (pituitary sensitivity is relatively unaltered). A newly discovered peptide secretion of the testis, "inhibin," is believed to be secreted by tubular epithelium and to exert a direct inhibitory effect on FSH secretion. It is not known whether inhibin affects the hypothalamus directly. The LRH-peptidergic neurons are in turn regulated by a biogenic amine neural system that links gonadotropin regulation to the remainder of the brain. Through this system a wide variety of impulses can be exerted on reproductive function. Stimuli affecting male gonadotropic secretion have been well demonstrated in experimental animals, though they are not as worked out well in the human. Visual influences include light-induced changes in seasonal breeders such as domestic cattle, deer, and birds. Olfactory signals in male rats influence gonadal function. The pineal glands in many species of animals inhibit gonadotropin secretion by direct effects of pineal secretions on either the hypothalamus or the pituitary. The role of the pineal in human reproduction control has not been established. (From Martin, J., Reichlin, S., et al. in *Clinical Neuroendocrinology,* Philadelphia, F. A. Davis, 1977, with permission.)

ness for insemination is achieved by complex neuroendocrine mechanisms involving the brain, the pituitary, and the sex steroid hormones. The role of the nervous system in regulating pituitary-gonadal function extends beyond the integration of reproductive behavior and the production of reproductive cycles, however. Neuroendocrine influences also determine the timing of onset of puberty, are involved in initiating and maintaining lactation, and, in most vertebrates, determine parental behavior.

The influence of the brain on sexual function in the human has been recognized for many centuries. Pseudocyesis (false pregnancy) was known to the ancients, and menstrual abnormalities are common in psychologically disturbed women. Spontaneously occurring disease of the hypothalamus has long been known to be a cause of gonadal insufficiency, and neuroleptic agents interfere with ovulation. These occurrences are just a few of the kinds of observations that emphasize the role of neural factors in various aspects of reproductive regulation.

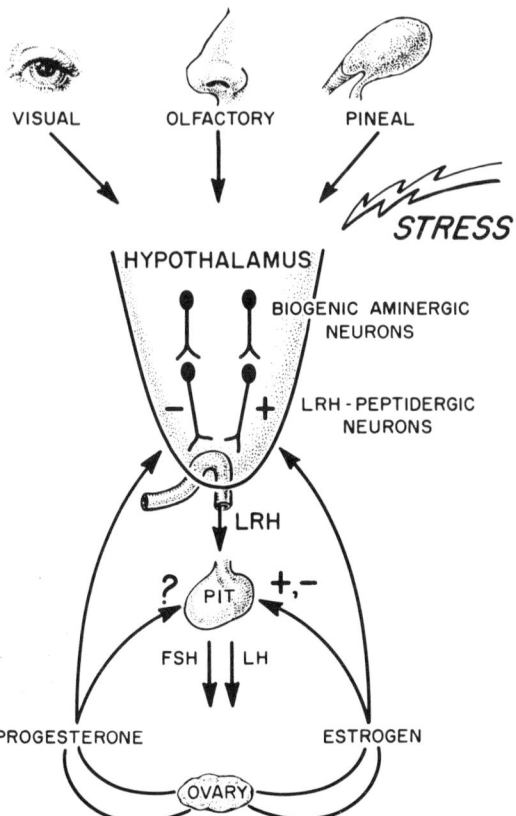

Figure 11–37. Regulation of gonadotropin secretion in the female. Schematic diagram of gonadotropin control systems in female showing the interactions of neural and hormonal feedback controls. The development of the ovarian follicle is largely under control of FSH. Ovulation is brought about by LH. Estrogenic hormones have complex effects on the feedback control mechanism of LH and FSH secretion. Depending upon dose, time course, and prior hormonal status, estrogens can either inhibit or stimulate the secretion of LH through effects at both hypothalamic and pituitary levels. Thus, there is evidence for both negative and positive feedback control. Progesterone also can either stimulate or inhibit LRH secretion, depending upon the setting in which it is given, but its effects at the pituitary level are relatively insignificant. Secretions of the LRH peptidergic neurons are in turn regulated by the biogenic-aminergic system, through which a variety of nonhormonal signals can influence reproductive function. Visual stimuli in many lower animals can influence onset of sexual function (as in seasonal breeders). Olfactory signals through "pheromones" influence estrus cycles in many rodents, and may do so in women. Pineal factors in lower animals delay onset of puberty. (From Martin, J., Reichlin, S., et al.: In *Clinical Neuroendocrinology.* Philadelphia, F. A. Davis, 1977, with permission.)

Pituitary gonad function is regulated by the feedback effects of gonadal hormones and by the hypothalamus. All three classes of steroid secretions of the gonad — estrogens, progestins and androgens — bind to specific receptors in the pituitary and influence gonadotropin secretion directly. Steroid receptors are also demonstrable in some brain cells, where they are involved in the regulation of sexual behavior and also in the regulation of secretion of the gonadotropin releasing hormone (LRH).

Hormones other than the gonadal steroids and the gonadotropins are also involved in regulation of reproductive function. These include inhibin, a newly recognized peptide of gonadal origin believed to exert selective inhibitory effects directly on pituitary FSH-secreting cells; PRL, which is inhibitory to the release of LRH; and dopamine, a hypothalamic neurosecretion that under some circumstances is directly inhibitory to LH secretion. Thyroid hormone also influences gonadotropin secretion. Imposed upon the steroid regulatory inputs from the gonad, the hypothalamic secretion of LRH is modulated by neural impulses from other parts of the brain.

In view of the large number of regulatory factors involved, it is not surprising that many find neuroendocrine control of gonadotropin secretion confusing. This system becomes more easy to understand if one considers control in three categories: (1) negative feedback, (2) positive feedback, and (3) neural open loop component.

Negative Feedback

In the presence of a normally functioning hypothalamus, the secretion of LH and FSH by both sexes is suppressed by the administration of constant doses of estrogens and androgens and is increased following castration (or administration of antiestrogen or antiandrogen drugs) (Fig. 11–38). Negative feedback effects involve both the pituitary and the hypothalamus. If the hypothalamic component of control is inactivated (for example, by destruction of the medial basal hypothalamus, by pituitary stalk section, or by transplantation of the pituitary away from the brain), basal gonadotropin secretion falls dramatically, and the pituitary hypersecretory response to castration is blunted markedly or completely. A functioning hypothalamus is required for the expression of normal response to gonadectomy, but it is not known with certainty whether there is an increase in LRH secretion or whether the effect is the response of the pituitary in the presence of some permissive level of LRH secretion (or some combination of these). Suppression of pituitary secretion by sex steroids also involves both neural and pituitary components, is somewhat different in men as compared with women, and is determined by both dosage and time-dependent variables. In women with normal cycles, the administration of "physiologic" doses of estrogenic hormone leads to suppression of basal levels of both LH and FSH. For the first 1–3 days after initiation of treatment, pituitary responsiveness to test doses of LRH is reduced, thus indicating that the suppressive effects of the estrogen have been exerted, at least in part, by direct inhibition of the pituitary. After approximately 3 days (and despite the fact that basal levels of LH and FSH remain depressed), the pituitary becomes more responsive than normal to test doses of LRH (see Ch. 7). Therefore, at this time, it must be assumed that estrogens have suppressed gonadotropin secretion by inhibition of LRH release. Estrogen-treated men also show a reduction in plasma LH and FSH and a persistent suppression of pituitary responsiveness to LRH. These findings indicate that an important component of negative feedback effects of estrogen in men is exerted at the level of the pituitary, although inhibitory effects on the hypothalamus cannot be excluded. Men treated with testosterone also show a fall in basal gonadotropin secretion unaccompanied, at least initially, by change in pituitary responsivity to LRH. These findings are interpreted to mean that negative feedback under these circumstances involves the hypothalamus. Long-term administration of either estrogens or testosterone in both sexes leads to suppression of pituitary responsiveness to LRH. It can be concluded that the overall effects of chronic exposure to sex steroids is to suppress gonadotropin secretion by inhibition of either the pituitary or the hypothalamus, and perhaps in some cases by both, but the hypothalamic and pituitary components do not always follow similar time course of response. Negative feedback effects of estrogens can be demonstrated in men and women with hypogonadism.

Negative feedback directed at the FSH-secreting cell is also exerted by inhibin, a peptide hormone derived from germinal cells of ovary and testis. In situations in which germinal activity is reduced (as in prepubertal girls and boys or after cyclophosphamide destruction of the germinal epi-

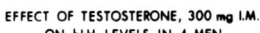

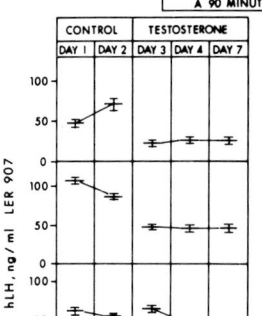

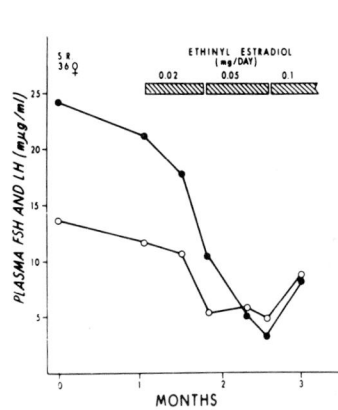

Figure 11–38. Inhibitory effects of sex steroids on LH secretion. The administration of estrogen to hypogonadal (menopausal) women (*left*) or of testosterone to men (*right*) results in a fall in plasma LH, demonstrating the negative feedback control. (Left figure from Schalch, D. S.: Gonadotropin secretion in the human, In *Neuroendocrinology of Human Reproduction.* Mack, H. C., and Sherman, A. E. (eds.), Springfield, Ill., Charles C Thomas, 1971, with permission.)

thelium of the testis and ovary), plasma FSH levels are disproportionately elevated as compared with LH levels, and the FSH secretory response to LRH is also exaggerated.

Positive Feedback

Under certain circumstances in sexually mature women, estrogenic hormones are capable of sensitizing the pituitary gonadotropin response to LRH and of stimulating the release of gonadotropic hormones. This effect requires an intact, normally functioning, postpubertal hypothalamus and a particular time sequence of delivery of estrogen that resembles, in general, the pattern of change in plasma estrogen normally occurring during the midcycle, preovulatory estradiol "surge" (Ch. 7). The crucial element in the pattern is the appearance in the blood of a pulse of high estrogen activity superimposed on a background of chronic lower dose estrogen exposure (Fig. 11–39). Pituitary sensitivity to test doses of LRH is markedly increased immediately following the estrogen pulse. Since enhanced pituitary sensitivity and enhanced secretion of LH and FSH can be induced in monkeys by estrogen administration under circumstances in which LRH is held constant (for example, by pituitary stalk section plus chronic infusion of LRH), the effect does not necessarily depend upon an increase in LRH secretion from the hypothalamus. Analogous results have been seen in a woman with hypogonadotropic hypogonadism due to hypothalamic disease. When such patients are treated with repeated injections of LRH over time, basal levels of LH and FSH rise gradually, an estrogen surge is induced, and this induces sufficient LH secretion to cause ovulation. These kinds of observations had led Knobil and his collaborators to suggest that the timing of ovulation in primates is due to an ovarian signal (Knobil and Plant, 1978). This makes good sense teleologically, because it provides the means by which the ripening ovary can signal the hypothalamic-pituitary axis that it is ready to be stimulated by an ovulatory surge of gonadotropic hormone.

In addition to the estrogen signal, there is evidence, albeit conflicting, that LRH secretion is stimulated by the preovulatory release of estrogens.

Neural Components of Control

The secretion of both LH and FSH is stimulated by LRH secreted by the LRH peptidergic neurons of the hypothalamus. If the medial basal hypothalamus (or pituitary stalk) is

destroyed, the "final common pathway" for LRH transfer to the pituitary circulation is lost, and complete gonadotropin deficiency with consequent gonadal inadequacy is produced. Electric stimulation of the hypothalamus causes an increase in LH and FSH secretion. These observations indicate that normal basal gonadotropin secretion depends upon the con-

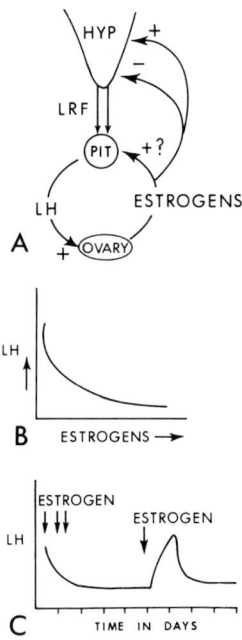

Figure 11–39. Pituitary-gonad axis: closed loop negative feedback system with positive feedback elements and open loop neural transients. The level of estrogen in plasma is observed in control LH secretion (*A*) negative feedback. When plasma estrogens are elevated, LH secretion is inhibited. When plasma estrogen levels are low, the secretion of LH is enhanced. Thus plasma LH can be shown to be a negative function of plasma estrogen concentration (*B*). The precise target for estrogen in bringing out this negative inhibition is still not firmly established, but most work indicates the effect is mediated at the hypothalamic level (there designated as a [−]), presumably through inhibition of the secretion of LRF. *B*, Positive feedback. Estrogen transients (such as occur after administration of estrogens in animals or humans and in the spontaneous phases of the estrus [cycle]) are capable of stimulating the release of LH (*C*). The site of action of the positive hormone transient has not been fully established. There is evidence that the positive feedback element may be exerted at the level of the pituitary (by sensitizing the LH-releasing mechanism to estrogens) or at the hypothalamic level. In addition, the secretion of LRF by the hypothalamus is subject to open loop neural transients, such as sexual stimulation, which in some species, including the human, can inhibit LH secretion.

tinued secretion of LRH and that increased LRH secretion can stimulate the pituitary to further hormone release. In primates, the principal site of the LRH neurons appears to be in the medial basal hypothalamus because both basal and estrogen-stimulated LH and FSH secretion are normal in rhesus monkeys in which the region is isolated from the rest of the brain. On the other hand, in the rat (the most widely used experimental animal for studies of reproduction), the capacity to develop a positive feedback response to estrogens depends upon a more extensive LRH pathway arising in the preoptic hypothalamus. The anterior LRH pathway is responsible for the light-dark entrained reproductive cycles characteristic of the rodent and for regulation of timing of puberty.

LRH pathways receives innervation from other neural sites capable of either stimulating or inhibiting LRH secretion. It is through these inputs that gonadal function responds to changes in light-dark cycle, emotional stress, and, in some species, to sexual stimuli. Various parts of the "visceral brain," including hippocampus and amygdala, project to the LRH pathways. The former region is inhibitory and the latter excitatory. In addition, LRH neurons receive an important pathway from the midbrain (locus ceruleus).

Several pharmacologic classes of neurotransmitters modify central control of gonadotropin secretion. Most important is the noradrenergic input (α-adrenergic). Injection of noradrenalin into the medial basal hypothalamus triggers LH release in the rat; α-adrenergic blockers prevent the usual ovulatory response of both rat and rabbit. Cholinergic impulses are also important for gonadotropin regulation. In fact, from a historical point of view, the demonstration by Sawyer and his colleagues that atropine in large doses blocked reflex ovulation in the rabbit was the first study to show the importance of neurotransmitters in anterior pituitary regulation.

The role of central catecholamines in gonadotropin regulation is important clinically because of the frequent occurrence of ovulatory disorder following the use of drugs that interfere with hypothalamic aminergic activity. Further, the finding that turnover of hypothalamic catecholamines is markedly altered by changes in gonadal steroids and gonadotropins suggests that one component of feedback control at the level of the hypothalamus is attributable to changes in secretion of catecholamine pathways.

Neuroendocrine Aspects of the Midcycle Ovulatory LH Surge: The Female Brain

Both a normally functioning hypothalamus and a normally developing ovary are required for the appearance of normal midcycle ovulatory surge of gonadotropins (see Ch. 7). The factors that bring this about include two, and possibly three, elements. The first (as noted previously) is that estrogens are capable of sensitizing the pituitary to the effects of LRH. The second is that LRH is capable of sensitizing the pituitary to subsequent exposure to LRH (self-priming action of LRH), a response that requires the presence of estrogens. Finally, there may be an increase in secretion of LRH at midcycle. As noted before, this effect is not essential for ovulation to occur in primates. The capacity to develop an increase in LH secretion at midcycle, or "positive feedback," is characteristic of female animals. Positive feedback is exerted at the level of both the pituitary and the hypothalamus. In the rodent, there is good evidence that the appearance of "positive feedback" depends upon the hormonal milieu at a critical stage of development. The normal development of the capacity to show positive feedback is lost in normal males, or in females treated with androgens

during the first 5 days of life (neonatal androgenization). Corresponding to the loss of positive feedback responsivity is a variety of sex-specific morphologic changes in the structure of the preoptic hypothalamus and in patterns of sexual behavior. The functional sex behavioral differences in gonadotropin regulation and their morphological concomitants have led to the designation of the "female" and the "male" brain (see Ch. 12). There is much uncertainty as to whether comparable male-female differences occur in primate brain. Under certain circumstances (estrogen priming of castrated male monkeys followed by a bolus of estrogen) positive feedback can be elicited, and several experiments in men have given somewhat analogous results (Karsch et al., 1973, Stearns et al., 1973). It may well be that the capacity for steroid-induced organization of brain cells mediating sexual reproduction is much less developed in the primate than in the rodent. This corresponds to the greater susceptibility of reproduction in the rodent to be influenced by lighting and olfactory cues.

Timing of Puberty

An additional level of neural control imposed on the secretions of the LRH pathway determines the time of onset of puberty. Long before puberty begins, the gonads and secondary sex accessories are capable of being stimulated by gonadal steroids, and the pituitary is capable of releasing gonadotropins when stimulated by LRH. In human females, the positive feedback response to estrogens develops at the time of puberty. Prior to that time, only negative feedback control can be demonstrated.

Clinical analysis of hypothalamic disease and destruction of various parts of the brain in experimental animals have shown that certain regions of the hypothalamus tonically inhibit gonadotropin secretion before puberty. Donovan and van der Werff ten Bosch (1965) have argued that since feedback control of gonadotropin secretion from estrogens appears to involve hypothalamic and not pituitary receptors, the fundamental change in the advance toward sexual maturity is a reduction in hypothalamic sensitivity to feedback effects of gonadal hormone. According to this interpretation, the infantile hypothalamus is more sensitive to estrogens and androgens and therefore maintains the low gonadotropin levels characteristic of the prepubertal state. As the brain matures, this sensitivity to the inhibitory actions of gonadal steroids decreases, allowing the secretion of gonadotropin to increase. Maturation toward decreasing sensitivity to hormone feedback is analogous to other maturational changes in the developing brain, which include changes in behavior, intelligence, and personality. McCann (1974) suggests that hypothalamic lesions, both clinical and experimental, bring on precocious puberty by reducing the size of the area from which pituitary-inhibiting stimuli arise. Such an interpretation agrees well with clinical data on destructive lesions of the hypothalamus (see later).

Pubertal development in the human female is accompanied by the capacity to respond to estrogen with increased LH secretion. The time of onset of pubertal brain function depends upon genetic and environmental factors. In humans, the secular trend for decreasing age of onset of puberty demonstrable by study of records over the past century and comparisons of different population groups indicates that the trigger for puberty is a critical factor related to body size. This probably explains why improved nutrition and freedom from disease have been followed by decreasing age of onset of menarche. Moderately obese girls have earlier puberties than do girls of normal weight, and individuals (or rats) with malnutrition fail to develop normal pituitary-ovarian function.

Effect of Sex Steroids on the Brain

Not only does feedback action of sex steroids on the central nervous system play an important role in regulating gonadotropin secretion, but also the direct effects of sex steroids on the brain markedly alter sexual behavior. (See Ch. 12 for discussion of sex steroids in human behavior.) After castration, female cats refuse to mate and the genital tract becomes atrophic, both responses resulting from estrogen lack and both readily reversed by systemic replacement treatment. Minute implants in certain hypothalamic regions restore normal sexual behavior with amounts of sex hormone that do not reverse atrophic genital changes. These observations indicate that the cat's brain is sensitive to estrogens and capable of inducing the full range of sexual behavior. Estrogen chemoreceptor function of the hypothalamus can also be demonstrated by radioautographic localization of labeled estrogenic hormones after systemic administration, estrogen concentrating in areas corresponding to those from which physiologic effects are obtained after local implantations. Specific cytoplasmic and nuclear estrogen-binding proteins analogous to those found in the uterus have been identified in this region. It is apparent that sex drive is generated by a neural signal from an estrogen receptor located within the hypothalamus. This generation of a basic drive is analogous to hunger drive in hypoglycemia, to thirst following hyperosmolarity, and to temperature-safeguarding behavior following central cooling or heating.

Progesterone blocks the ovulatory surge of LH release but, by itself, does not inhibit either FSH or the tonic component of LH secretion. The effect on ovulation is one basis for the use of the oral contraceptive progestational agents. Adding small, otherwise ineffective, amounts of estrogen to progesterone leads to complete inhibition of LH secretion. Neurophysiologic studies indicate that progesterone acts on certain hypothalamic neurons to decrease their rate of spontaneous firing and to elevate their threshold of excitability to reflex stimulation from the uterine cervix. In this regard, it should be recalled that progesterone in the human acts on the hypothalamus to raise body temperature. This mechanism is responsible for the postovulatory rise in basal body temperature commonly used as an index of ovulation. The hypothalamus is not the only structure in which excitability is decreased by progesterone. Spontaneous and electrically or pharmacologically stimulated contractions of the uterus are also inhibited by progesterone.

Although it has appeared reasonable to believe that the suppressive effects of progesterone are exerted on the hypothalamic component of control, a number of recent studies have indicated that progesterone and synthetic gestagens of the type used in a contraceptive (i.e., chlormadinone) block the effect of LRF at the pituitary level rather than in the hypothalamus. Progesterone action is thus analogous to thyroid hormone and cortisol feedback. Although progesterone has many inhibitory actions, under certain conditions it can also elicit gonadotropin stimulatory responses. For example, progesterone can hasten the onset of puberty and induce an ovulatory LH surge if given to an estrogen-primed woman. Factors determining the nature and direction of the gonadotropic response to progesterone and the site of its action in each of these activities remain to be clarified.

Pheromones

Every owner of a female dog in heat becomes unpleasantly aware of the fact that the dog emits a scent infinitely attractive to male dogs in the neighborhood. This phenomenon is an example of a response mediated by a pheromone, the term applied to chemical substances secreted by one animal that arouse either behavioral or hormonal changes in another individual or the same species. In nonvertebrate forms such as moths, pheromones are of great importance in regulating many aspects of activity and behavior. In sheep and goats, the onset of estrus behavior and ovulation is accelerated if males are placed with the flock. In the female mouse, gonadotropic function is very strikingly altered by the presence of a male. When female mice are housed in cages without males, their estrus cycles tend to be irregular and may be prolonged. In the presence of the male, sexual cycles become synchronized, and on the third night after contact with the male, estrus behavior and mating occur. This response, termed the "Whitten" effect, can be induced merely by exposing the females to the urine-contaminated bedding of the male. The "Bruce effect" refers to the phenomenon that female mice successfully mated with familiar males will fail to carry pregnancy to term if permitted to come in contact with the urine of a strange male or a male from a different strain of mice. Female rats deprived of their olfactory bulbs will not build nests for their young or retrieve them. In monkeys, fatty acids formed in the vagina at estrus, presumably as a consequence of hormonally altered bacterial flora, arouse grooming behavior in the male.

Little is known about the role of pheromones in human sexual activity. Perfumes have been used since antiquity for purposes of enhancing the sexual attractiveness of women. Interestingly, certain of the ingredients used in perfumes (musk and civet) are derived from the glands of animals who use these secretions as sexual attractants. The ability to detect certain kinds of smells is hormone-dependent in women and is heightened at midcycle. There is a statistically significant correlation between the timing of the menstrual cycle in women living together as roommates compared with that of those who are separated. The basis of this synchronization of cycles is unknown, but the role of pheromones in this response is strongly suggested. It should be emphasized that a pheromone may act without the individual being consciously aware of the stimulus. The role of pheromones in human function is largely unknown but may prove to be more important than is generally recognized.

THE PINEAL GLAND AND PERIVENTRICULAR ORGANS

Lining the ventricles of the brain and the central canal of the spinal cord are ependymal cells that in most places form cuboidal, usually ciliated epithelium. In several areas of the third ventricle, and the fourth ventricle, the simple single-layered lining has become modified into secretory structures that are of actual or presumptive neuroendocrine interest (Fig. 11–40). Most important of these is the pineal gland, derived embryologically from ependymal cells of the roof of the third ventricle. Others in the third ventricle are the subcommissural organ (SCO), the subfornical organ (SFO), the organum vasculosum of the lamina terminalis (OVLT), and the specialized ependyma of the median eminence. At the posterior margin of the lip of the roof of the fourth ventricle is found another periventricular organ, the area postrema (AP). All of the structures mentioned have well-developed interstitial tissue spaces into which relatively large molecules circulating in the blood can penetrate, thus indicating that in this region the usual "blood-brain" barrier does not exist. Further, nerve endings in these regions, with the associated blood vessels, form "neurohemal" organs. Despite close contiguity with the ventricles, the periventricular organs, with the exception of the SCO (see later),

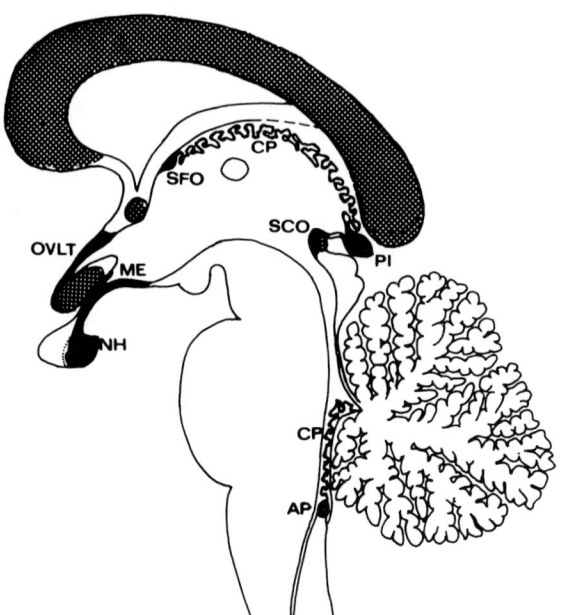

Figure 11–40. Median sagittal section through the human brain to show the circumventricular organs outlined in black: AP, area postrema; ME, median eminence; NH, neurohypophysis; OVLT, organum vasculosum of the lamina terminalis; PI, pineal body; SFO, subfornical organ; SCO, subcommissural organ; CP, choroid plexus. (From Weindl, A.: Neuroendocrine aspects of circumventricular organs, In *Frontiers in Neuroendocrinology.* Ganong, W. F., and Martini, L. (eds.), New York, Oxford University Press, 1973, with permission.)

probably do not secrete their products into the cerebrospinal fluid (CSF). This interference is based on the electron microscopic demonstration of "tight junctions" at the ventricular boundary. Rather, these structures permit brain secretions to enter peripheral blood and have been called, somewhat romantically, windows to the brain. The choroid plexus, also an ependymal derivative, forms melatonin, a characteristic secretion of the pineal gland.

The Pineal Gland

Structure

Few if any brain structures as small as the pineal gland (which in the human weighs only 0.1–0.18 gm) have been the subject of so much speculation, and for such a long time. First described nearly 2300 years ago by Herophilus, an Alexandrian anatomist, the pineal from the first has been associated with mental functions. Separated by the relatively thin tectal plate from the aqueduct of Sylvius, as it lies in the groove between the superior colliculi (Fig. 11–7), the pineal could obstruct the flow of CSF in the ventricular system if enlarged. Perhaps this is why it was regarded by early Green anatomists as the "valve that controlled the flow of memories, stored in the rear brain ventricle, forward to the consciousness-serving part of the brain" (Altschule, 1975). The emphasis given to the pineal in later times was the result of the teaching of the 17th century philosopher Descartes, whose contribution to science was the introduction of the idea of mechanism into physiologic thinking. According to Rolleston (1936), "Descartes regarded the human body as an earthly machine presided over by the 'rational soul' which occupied the pineal gland, 'the little gland in the middle of the substance of the brain.' The search for a physical embodiment of the soul was a preoccupation of philosophers at the time and "there was no particular reason for placing the soul in the pineal gland

except that it happened to be a single or unpaired organ" (Rolleston). Even today, the function of the pineal gland in humans is still the subject of speculation, but research has confirmed that it is indeed a true secretory structure, that it contains an extraordinary number of biologically active substances, and that it is the occasional site of significant human disease.

The pineal, so called because it resembles a pine cone, arises in embryologic development from the ependyma lining the roof of the third ventricle. In all vertebrate forms, the pineal gland contains biologically active materials and is made up of cells with anatomic features suggesting neurosecretory functions. In lower vertebrates, like fish and amphibia, pineal cells form a true eyelike, light-sensitive structure, but in higher vertebrates, including mammals, all vestiges of light receptor function have disappeared and the secretory activities emerge as the dominant feature. Early in phylogenetic development (when still a light-sensitive organ), the pineal is connected to the roof of the brain by sensory nerves, but in mammals all direct nerve connection to the brain is lost and is replaced by a new form of nervous innervation, a postganglionic sympathetic nerve supply from the superior sympathetic ganglia (Fig. 11–41). Detailed anatomy of this system has been studied chiefly in the rat. The preganglionic fibers in the superior sympathetic chain arise in turn in the lateral cell column of the spinal cord. These sympathetic nerve cells are regulated by supraspinal nerve impulses, some of which arise (either directly or via intermediate synapses) from a paired nucleus located in the hypothalamus just above the optic chiasm termed the suprachiasmatic nucleus. The suprachiasmatic nucleus receives a direct nerve input from the retina, the retinohypothalamic tract, that conveys information about light and dark independent of conscious perception. It is by way of this neural pathway that external light regulates pineal activity. In the absence of light input, pineal rhythms persist, but they are no longer entrained to the external light-dark cycle. The free-running rhythms are attributed to the intrinsic function of the suprachiasmatic nucleus believed to serve as an internal "clock" or biologic oscillator. Signals that cue the internal clock are called "zeitgeibers" (time givers); light-dark shifts are the most important for the pineal.

Crucial to the regulation of pineal function is its sympathetic nerve innervation consisting of noradrenergic fibers that end in the interstitial space of the gland or on the plasma membrane of pinealocytes. Pinealocytes are true secretory cells, organized into cords and resting on a basement membrane in relationship to an interstitial space.

Endothelium of the pineal gland is fenestrated, thus permitting the exit and entry of relatively large molecules from and to the interstitial space of the gland. In this regard, the pineal differs from the bulk of brain in not having a blood-brain barrier, but it resembles other periventricular glands, such as median eminence, SFO, and SCO (see previous discussion), all of which, like the pineal, are derived from ependyma.

All neuroendocrine functions of the pineal parenchymal cells are regulated by β-adrenergic receptors. Section of the sympathetic innervation or use of β-adrenergic antagonists inhibits pineal cell metabolic activity (see Fig. 11–3).

Physiologic Function of the Pineal Gland

Since the report by Huebner in 1898 of precocious puberty in a boy aged 4, the bulk of research on pineal function has dealt with its role in the regulation of sexual function, and most clinical reports have stressed its relationship to

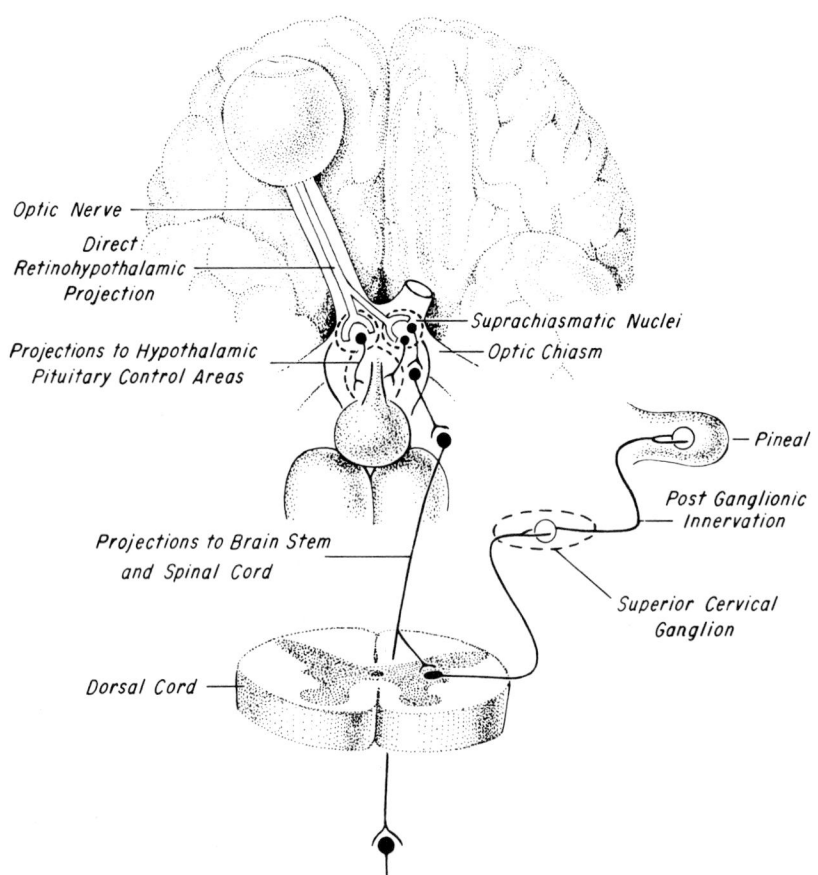

Optic Nerve

Direct
Retinohypothalamic
Projection

Projections to Hypothalamic
Pituitary Control Areas

Suprachiasmatic Nuclei

Optic Chiasm

Pineal

Post Ganglionic
Innervation

Projections to Brain Stem
and Spinal Cord

Superior Cervical
Ganglion

Dorsal Cord

Figure 11–41. Schematic diagram of neural structures regulating pineal function. The principal regulator of pineal functions is the light-dark cycle that innervates paired suprachiasmatic nuclei. These in turn project to the cervical cord to synapse in cell bodies of the sympathetic nervous system in the lateral column. Preganglionic fibers regulate postganglionic impulses that reach the pineal by way of sympathetic inflow accompanying blood vessels of the pineal. The suprachiasmatic nucleus has an intrinsic circadian oscillation that determines pineal and other circadian rhythms; the input from the retina serves to entrain the intrinsic rhythm to extensive rhythms. Light thus acts as a "zeitgeber" (time-giver). (Adapted from Moore, R. Y.: Central neural control of circadian rhythms, In *Frontiers of Neuroendocrinology*, Vol. 5. Ganong, W. F., and Martini, L. (eds.), New York, Raven Press, 1978, p. 195, with permission.)

sexual development. It is fair to say that all data relating the pineal to physiologic function in the human is still inferential. The most consistent effect observed in animal studies is that under certain well-defined circumstances, gonadotropin secretion is suppressed by the pineal gland. Extirpation of the pineal leads to precocious puberty in several species, but the effect is modest. Much more convincing than the fact that the pineal inhibits gonadotropin secretion is the effect of pinealectomy in reversing the gonadal involution that follows exposure to constant darkness or shortened photoperiods in both rats and hamsters. If blinded or exposed to constant darkness, male rats show a reduction in testis weight and delayed growth of accessory sex organs secondary to testosterone deficiency. Similarly, in female rats, gonadotropin secretion is inhibited and ovarian growth is impaired. These effects are completely reversed by pinealectomy, thus indicating that exposure to darkness has stimulated the secretion of some pineal factor. Section of neural pathways to the pineal produces the same effects as pinealectomy.

Other actions of the pineal (as inferred from removal) have been less clear cut. It has been claimed that the diurnal rhythm in PRL secretion is abolished by pinealectomy, but this finding has not been confirmed by all workers. Changes in GH, adrenal, and thyroid functions have also been observed, but reports from various laboratories have been inconsistent.

The Secretions of the Pineal

The pineal contains many biologically active substances. These include biogenic amines (norepinephrine, serotonin, histamine, melatonin and other related indoleamines, do-

pamine, and octopamine) and peptides (LRH, TRH, SRIF, and vasotocin, an analogue of OT). The pineal also contains the inhibitory neurotransmitter GABA, a protein that resembles neurophysin, and another protein that is different from neurophysin to which the term epiphysin has been given. In addition to these substances, there is evidence of other, as yet uncharacterized, factors, peptide in nature, that may mediate the gonadotropin inhibitory actions of the pineal. There is no shortage of candidate pineal hormones.

Of numerous biologically active materials present in the pineal gland, melatonin has been studied most intensively, although it is still far from certain that it is the only, or even the principal, gonadotropin-regulating hormone of the pineal. Melatonin was the first unique biologically active compound to be identified in the pineal. This discovery (1958) was the result of the effort by Lerner and his colleagues to isolate from mammalian pineals the factor that caused lightening of amphibian skin. Melatonin is synthesized from tryptophan within pineal parenchymal cells by three well-characterized enzymic steps (Fig. 11–42) that include the formation of the intermediates 5-hydroxytryptamine, serotonin, N-acetylserotonin, and finally melatonin. The enzyme mediating the formation of N-acetylserotonin from serotonin (serotonin-N-acetyltransferase) is thought to be the principal rate-limiting enzyme in formation of melatonin, but the final synthetic reaction involving O-methylation by hydroxyindole-O-methyl-transferase (HIOMT) to form melatonin may also be rate limiting. For a long time the pineal was thought to be unique in having HIOMT, but more recently this enzyme has been found in the retina, choroid plexus, and harderian glands (orbital structures of unknown function). The role of these other structures in melatonin secretion is unknown, but the presence of this enzyme outside the pineal may explain the fact that mela-

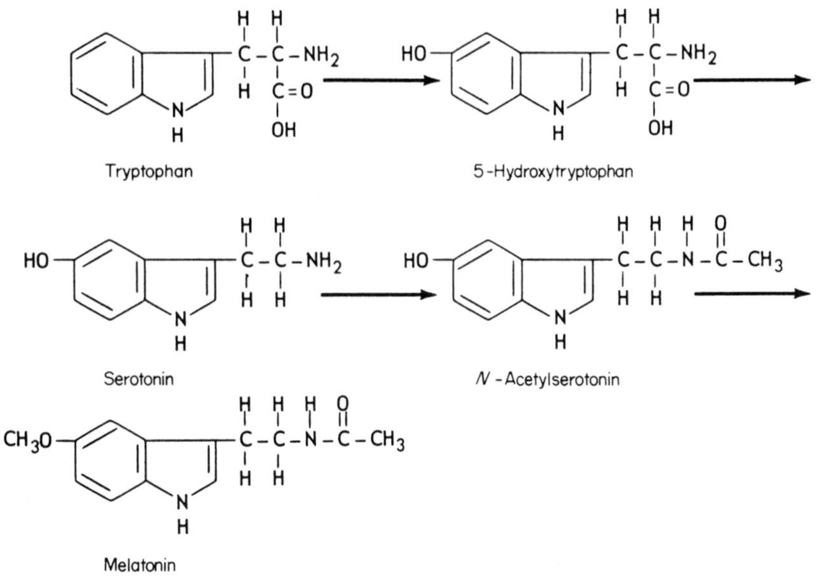

Figure 11–42. Biosynthesis of melatonin from tryptophan in the pineal gland. Step 1 is catalyzed by tryptophan hydroxylase; step 2 by L-aromatic amino acid decarboxylase; step 3 by N-acetylating enzyme; and step 4 by HIOMT. (From Wurtman, R. J., Axelrod, J., et al.: *The Pineal.* New York, Academic Press, 1968, p. 60, with permission.)

tonin excretion persists at about 25% of basal levels after pinealectomy.

One of the most important advances in pineal physiology came from the use of enzyme assay for determination of pineal regulation even before it was certain that the pineal had an external secretion. Rhythms in enzyme concentration are now known to reflect the rate of secretion of melatonin and are readily modified by manipulations of lighting, denervation, or neuropharmacologic agents that lead to altered noradrenergic input into the pinealocyte. During the night, when melatonin secretion is highest, the content of melatonin in the pineal gland is high and that of serotonin (its precursor) is low. When melatonin secretion is high, the concentration of N-acetyltransferase is high; the reverse is also true. Changes in N-acetyltransferase content are dramatic — marked increases of 25 to 100-fold are evident within a few minutes of the signal "lights off." Administration of a β-adrenergic blocking agent or exposure to light will cause a sharp decline in enzyme activity with a rapid fall (t ½ = 3½ min). Detailed analysis of this reaction, carried out by Klein and collaborators (1978) indicates that β-adrenergic activation is mediated by a classic cyclic AMP (cAMP) reaction and a cascade of both transcription and translation. The effects of enzyme activation are blocked by actinomycin D (a blocker of transcription) and by cycloheximide (a blocker of translation).

Factors that Influence Pineal Secretion

Any manipulation causing an activation of the sympathetic nervous system can increase the concentration of melatonin-synthesizing enzymes in the pineal, and therefore presumably the secretion of melatonin. These factors include immobilization or hypoglycemia stress. Administration of L-dopa, a precursor of L-dopamine, also increases melatonin synthesis in rats.

Use of newly developed bioassay and immunoassay methods has shown that light-altered changes in melatonin secretion are exactly the same as those that had been predicted from studies of changes in pineal enzyme activity.

Recent technical advances have made it possible to show that melatonin is in fact released into the general circulation (Fig. 11–43). In humans, and in domestic animals and rats, melatonin secretion is activated almost immediately after exposure to darkness and is turned off upon exposure to light. In humans, there are also occasional bursts of secretion unrelated to changes in lighting or apparent stress. As summarized by Wurtman and Moskowitz (1977), the rhythm in melatonin excretion in urine can be entrained by the light-dark cycle and by other factors, such as sleep, diet, posture, and activity. The characteristic melatonin rhythms are unaffected by sleep deprivation or sustained light exposure in untrained volunteers for a single night, but a group of women who had been trained to sleep at odd hours were capable of shifting melatonin secretory patterns.

A critical question with respect to pineal and melatonin secretions is the route by which the hormone reaches pituitary and hypothalamus, its putative targets. Detailed anatomic study of the mammalian pineal led Kappers, one of the leading workers in this field, to conclude that all secretions must leave the gland by way of the venous drainage into the peripheral circulation. He pointed out that there is no direct conduit from pineal to third ventricle and that the pineal, though in part located in the subarachnoid space, has a fairly thick capsule that would militate against direct subarachnoid release. On the other hand, anatomic differences among species do exist, and in primates the pineal forms part of the roof of the third ventricle. In calves and young children, the concentration of melatonin in spinal fluid is higher than that in blood, but in adult humans and monkeys, levels of CSF melatonin are lower than are levels in blood. These findings suggest that, in adult primates, melatonin enters CSF from blood. The relative concentrations are attributable to the concentration of melatonin-binding protein, which is higher in blood than in CSF. When injected into the hypothalamus, melatonin has been found to inhibit gonadotropin secretion, but a direct effect on the pituitary has also been shown. In concentrations equivalent to that found in the blood (10^{-8} M), melatonin almost completely inhibited pituitary LH response to LRH *in vitro,* an effect that was markedly dependent upon the age of rat from which the pituitary was obtained. It is thus possible that melatonin acts on both hypothalamus and pituitary to inhibit gonadotropin secretion. In addition to its effects at these sites, melatonin has been found to localize at receptors in the ovary, suggesting still another locus of action.

Efforts to show that melatonin administration reverses the effects of pinealectomy (and thereby complete the clas-

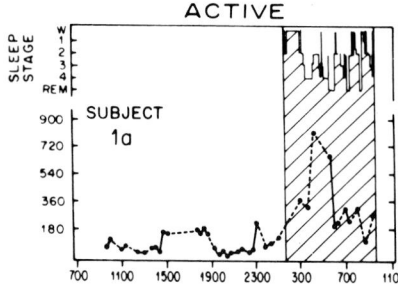

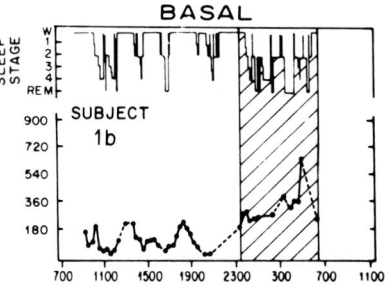

Figure 11–43. Pattern of melatonin secretion in a normal subject when active and at rest. Lights off shown in dashed area brought about a release of melatonin. Note also that spontaneous release of melatonin also takes place. (From Weinberg, U., Eletto, R. D., et al.: Circulating melatonin in man: episodic secretion throughout the light-dark cycle. *J. Clin. Endocrinol. Metab. 48:* 114, 1979.)

sic requirements for proof of the endocrine function of a gland) have not been uniformly successful. It may be that failure to show inhibition of gonadal function after melatonin (equivalent to that seen after blinding or dark exposure) is due to inadequate dosage, but this alone cannot be the reason because melatonin injection can bring about either inhibition or stimulation of gonadal secretion depending upon the timing of administration.

Failures to show that melatonin injection duplicates all effects of functional activation of the pineal have led to efforts to identify other gonad inhibitory substances. Pineal extracts free of melatonin have been shown to produce gonadal inhibition in a number of assay systems. Vasotocin, a constituent of mammalian pineals, is another candidate gonadotropin inhibitory hormone, but it has not been proved that the doses used are equivalent to the levels found under physiologic circumstances. Further, several workers have shown that pineal extracts from which both melatonin *and* vasotocin have been removed still retain potent gonadal inhibitory effects. Vasotocin is especially interesting because it is a normal constituent of the posterior lobe of birds but is found in mammals only in the pineal gland. Thus, the nature of the pineal gonadotropin inhibitory factors remain uncertain. Serotonin is also synthesized in pineal parenchymal cells and taken up by sympathetic nerve endings in the gland.

With the exception of dopamine and norepinephrine, which are also present in sympathetic nerve termini, the physiologic function of the other biologically active substances in the pineal are unknown. Whether the TRH, SRIF, and LRH present in the pineal of some species of animals are secreted into the peripheral blood is unknown, but it has been shown that SRIF is released by pineals in organ culture when subjected to depolarizing conditions, thus suggesting that it is regulated by biologically excitable cells. Since TRH and SRIF have effects on neural structures and on some glands, it is possible that they act in the pineal as local modulators of pineal hormone secretion.

Effects of Melatonin in Humans

Melatonin administered to normal volunteers causes a lowering of plasma LH levels; suppresses GH secretion; and induces sleepiness, changes in the electroencephalogram (EEG) (mainly an increase in alpha waves), increases in rapid eye movement (REM) sleep, and, in a few cases, "a sensation of well being and moderate elation" (Watson and Maden IV). Relatively large amounts may produce headaches and abdominal cramps (Lerner and Nordlund). Since melatonin is secreted in response to darkness, it is an attractive hypothesis (though unproved) that melatonin release contributes to drowsiness noted in students and others when the lights are turned down. When administered to depressed patients, melatonin was found to increase self-ratings of depression and, paradoxically, to increase the

degree of insomnia. Relevance of any of these findings to normal, or abnormal, brain function is still unknown. Melatonin has no beneficial effect on patients with depression, schizophrenia, parkinsonism or Huntington's chorea.

Calcification of the Pineal

The pineal is clinically significant as a marker of the midline (as a consequence of its calcification) and as a rare site of tumor formation (see later). Calcification begins early in childhood and becomes increasingly evident by x-ray beginning in the second decade of life. Its frequency is different in several racial groups. Calcification has no known effect on pineal function, as inferred from the fact that the concentrations of characteristic enzymes of the pineal (hydroxy-O-methyltransferase, monoamine oxidase, and histamine N-methyltransferase) are relatively constant throughout life. An apatite form of calcium phosphate crystals is laid down in a matrix of ground substance secreted by pinealocytes to form nodules termed acervuli. It has been proposed that calcium deposition is in some manner related to cell function because section of the nerves to the pineal of the hamster reduces the growth rate of acervuli.

Periventricular Organs

The Subcommissural Organ (Fig. 11–40)

The subcommissural organ (SCO) is a poorly understood structure that has persisted through evolutionary development from fish to human. The SCO is a collection of columnar cells lining the roof of the caudal end of the third ventricle, where it enters the aqueduct connecting the third and fourth ventricles. This region is beneath the habenular commissure and is adjacent to the pineal recess (to the apex of which is attached the pineal gland). Cells of the SCO differ from the usual ependymal cell in being much taller and in containing secretory granules that stain selectively with various histochemic reagents. An outstanding peculiarity of the SCO in animals studied so far (except for the human) is that the cells secrete into the lumen of the aqueduct a substance relatively insoluble in CSF. This secretion forms a cordlike structure (Reissner's fiber) that is extruded through the aqueduct and through the fourth ventricle and spinal cord lumen to terminate in the caudal spinal canal.

Reissner's fiber contains mucopolysaccharides and apparently breaks down at its termination in the sacral spinal cord, but in some species, such as the rat, the tip of the fiber forms a coil much as a rope would under similar mechanical circumstances. In humans, intracellular secretory granules are identifiable in the SCO but Reissner's fiber is absent. The SCO secretion in humans is therefore presumed to be relatively more soluble than in other animals and is absorbed directly from the CSF. In addition to drainage into the CSF, which is characteristic of ependyma in general, there may be drainage into regional capillaries. The SCO has no direct nerve supply, and its anatomic location adjacent to the pineal gland does not appear to be functionally significant.

The Subfornical Organ (Fig. 11–40)

The subfornical organ (SFO) is another "neurohemal" ependymal structure of suspected neuroendocrine function. It consists of both neurosecretory neurons and modified ependymal cells found at the junction between the lamina terminalis and the tela choroidea of the third ventricle. Its name is derived from its location under the fornices. The neurons of the SFO receive cholinergic innervation that has been traced to cells in the midbrain. Electron microscopic study of the SFO suggests a neurosecretory gland. The intensity of staining of the neurosecretory material is modified by anesthesia, stress, hyperosmotic challenge, alcohol injection, and estrogen administration. The histologic changes are of unknown significance and have been related by some workers to the control of salt and water balance by the central nervous system. A role for the SFO in salt and water regulation is supported by recent studies of the effects of injection of angiotensin II in the region of the SFO, although the localization of effect cannot be regarded as being entirely specific. Such injections lead to the release of VP and the stimulation of drinking behavior. The effects of angiotensin II injection are potentiated by hypertonic saline (see before). The endothelium of this region, as in other parts of the brain and peripheral endothelia, contains the converting enzyme that synthesizes angiotensin I to angiotensin II.

Organum Vasculosum of the Lamina Terminalis*

This structure lies in the midline of the lamina terminalis of the third ventricle between the anterior commissure and the optic chiasm. Its external surface is in contact with the CSF of the prechiasmatic cistern, and its internal surface is in contact with the CSF of the brain. Electron microscopic study and experiments utilizing horseradish peroxidase have shown that large molecules are prevented from entering the CSF by the presence of "tight junctions" between the ependymal cells, a finding analogous to that of the median eminence. The structure has its own arterial and venous circulation independent from that of other circumventricular organs. Large molecules readily penetrate the OVLT, indicating that the blood-brain barrier does not exist here. The OVLT is richly innervated by nerve endings containing LRH and SRIF and neurophysin. The function of these particular neuropeptides in this region is unknown. It is important to recognize that the region of the OVLT in the rat is the site of estrogen receptor neurons, and from this region direct estrogen application or electric stimulation is capable of stimulating ovulation. Moreover, injection of LRH in the same area is reported to increase sexual drive in rats, even in those that have been hypophysectomized and maintained on a constant replacement dose of steroid hormone. This region therefore appears to be an important sex-regulating area in the rat. Its function in primates is unknown.

---

*Organum vasculosum of the lamina terminalis (OVLT) (Supraoptic crest).

NEUROENDOCRINE DISEASE

General Considerations

Clinical manifestations of disordered hypothalamic control of anterior pituitary function resemble those due to intrinsic pituitary disease (see Ch. 3). Decreased secretion is the usual finding, but in some instances a hypothalamic deficit may appear as a hypersecretory state because there has been loss of a usual inhibitory control. Examples are hypersecretion of PRL following damage to the PIF control system and precocious puberty due to loss of normal restraint over gonadotropin maturation. Deficits in inhibitory control of the neurohypophysis at a supranuclear level can lead to the syndrome of inappropriate ADH secretion (SIADH) (see also Ch. 20). Other more subtle abnormalities in secretion may take place owing to selective impairment of the control system. For example, loss of normal circadian rhythm of ACTH secretion may occur before loss of pituitary-adrenal secretory reserve, and paradoxical responses to usual physiologic stimuli are sometimes observed. Because there is no direct way to measure hypophysiotropic hormone secretion and because most pituitary hormones are regulated by complex multilayered controls, the measurement of pituitary hormones in blood does not necessarily give a meaningful picture of what is really happening at the hypothalamic and higher levels. The etiology of hypothalamic disorder is summarized in Table 11–11, and a classification of hypothalamic-pituitary syndromes is given in Table 11–12.

Disorders of the hypothalamic-pituitary unit can be viewed as taking place at many levels of function. At the lowest level, defects can arise from destruction of the pituitary itself (as by tumor or infarct) or from a genetically determined deficiency of a particular pituitary cell, as occurs in rare cases of isolated FSH deficiency, or the selective loss of thyroid hormone feedback control for TSH. At a higher level, disorders may arise through disruption of the SME vascular contact zone, or the stalk itself, or of nerve termini of the tuberohypophyseal system. Such destruction of the "final common path" of anterior pituitary regulation occurs after surgical stalk section, in tumors of the stalk region, and in some inflammatory diseases. At the next higher level, that of input into the tuberohypophyseal system, one can see loss of tonic inhibitory and excitatory inputs, manifested for example by loss of circadian rhythms or by precocious puberty. At the highest level of control, that related to the effects of symbolic stress and emotional disorder, one may see activation of the stress response and suppression of normal gonadotropin secretion (psychogenic amenorrhea) and of GH secretion (maternal deprivation syndrome) (Ch. 12). Various levels of deficit will be considered in the following paragraphs. Intrinsic disease of the pituitary is extensively reviewed in Ch. 5.

Pituitary Stalk Interruption in Humans

Destructive lesions of the pituitary stalk, rupture as after head injury, surgical transection, or spontaneous disease (tumor, granuloma) produce a characteristic pattern of pituitary secretion. Diabetes insipidus (DI) is the most prominent abnormality. DI develops in approximately 80% of cases, the crucial factor in its occurrence being the level at which the stalk has been sectioned. If the stalk is cut close to the hypothalamus, DI is almost always produced, whereas if the section is low on the stalk, the incidence is less. The extent to which neurohypophyseal nerve terminals in the upper stalk are preserved determines the clinical

Table 11–11. ETIOLOGY OF HYPOTHALAMIC DISEASE
BY AGE

1. Premature infants and neonates:
   Intraventricular hemorrhage
   Meningitis: bacterial
   Tumors: glioma, hemangioma
   Trauma
   Hydrocephalus, kernicterus
2. 1 month–2 years:
   Tumors
     Glioma, especially optic glioma
     Histiocytosis X
     Hemangiomas
     Hydrocephalus, meningitis
     "Familial" disorders: Laurence-Moon-Biedl, Prader-Labhart-Willi
3. 2–10 years:
   Tumors
     Craniopharyngioma
     Glioma, dysgerminoma, hamartoma, histiocytosis X, leukemia
     Ganglioneuroma, ependymoma, medulloblastoma
   Meningitis
     Bacterial
     Tuberculous
   Encephalitis
     Viral and demyelinating
     Various viral encephalides and exanthematous demyelinating
       encephalitides
     Disseminated encephalomyelitis
     "Familial" disorders: diabetes insipidus, etc.
4. 10–25 years:
   Tumors
     Craniopharyngioma
     Glioma, hamartoma, dysgerminoma
     Histiocytosis X, leukemia
     Dermoid, lipoma, neuroblastoma
   Trauma
     Subarachnoid hemorrhage, vascular aneurysm, arteriovenous
       malformation
     Inflammatory diseases, meningitis, encephalitis, sarcoid, tuberculosis
     Associated with midline brain defects: agenesis of corpus callosum
     Chronic hydrocephalus or increased intracranial pressure
5. 25–50 years:
   Nutritional: Wernicke's disease
   Tumors
     Glioma, lymphoma, meningioma
     Craniopharyngioma, pituitary tumors
     Angioma, plasmacytoma, colloid cysts
     Ependymoma, sarcoma, histiocytosis X
   Inflammatory
     Sarcoid
     Tuberculosis, viral encephalitis
   Subarachnoid hemorrhage, vascular aneurysm, arteriovenous
     malformation
   Damage from pituitary radiation therapy
6. 50 years:
   Nutritional: Wernicke's disease
   Tumors
     Sarcoma, glioblastoma, lymphoma
     Meningioma, colloid cysts, ependymoma, pituitary tumors
   Vascular
     Infarct, subarachnoid hemorrhage
     Pituitary apoplexy
   Infections: encephalitis, sarcoid, meningitis

From Plum, F., and Van Uitert, R.: In Reichlin, S., Baldessarini, R. J.,
et al. (eds.): *The Hypothalamus.* New York, Raven Press, 1978, with
permission.

course. The classic triphasic syndrome of initial polyuria,
followed by normal water control and then by ADH deficiency, occurring over a period of approximately 1 week to
10 days, is observed in about half the patients. The sequence described is attributed to an initial loss of neurogenic control of the neural lobe followed by autolysis of the
neural lobe with release of active ADH into the circulation
and later by complete loss of ADH. In other cases, DI alone
may develop at some time after stalk injury without a
recognizable transitional phase. Injury to the neurohypophysis or stalk, as may occur during the course of surgical

exploration of the pituitary, can sometimes give rise to
transient *inappropriate* secretion of ADH. When DI occurs
after head injury or operative trauma, recovery can take
place even after many months or even a year.

Menses cease following both stalk section and hypophysectomy, but gonadotropic failure is less severe in the stalk-
sectioned patients. Unlike the situation after hypophysectomy, gonadotropins may still be detectable in urine. Urinary excretion of 17-hydroxysteroids and 17-ketosteroids
and plasma hydroxysteroid levels fall after both hypophysectomy and stalk section, but the change is slower after
stalk section and there may sometimes be a transient increase in adrenal cortical secretion, postulated to be due to
release of preformed stores of ACTH. ACTH response to
lowering of blood corticoid levels is markedly reduced by
stalk section, but the stress response may still be retained
in some patients. These changes have been attributed to the
release into the circulating blood of hypothalamic factors,
and possibly similar factors from other parts of the brain
and elsewhere. The most striking difference between patients with secretions of the pituitary stalk and those with
hypophysectomy relates to the secretion of GH and PRL.
Basal GH level is in the low normal range in stalk-
sectioned patients, but the response to hypoglycemic stimulation is impaired. In hypophysectomized individuals, basal
levels are depressed below normal and GH responses absent. Stalk-sectioned individuals develop hyperprolactin-

Table 11–12. ETIOLOGY OF ENDOCRINE SYNDROMES
OF HYPOTHALAMIC ORIGIN

Hypophysiotropic Hormone Deficiency:
Surgical pituitary stalk section
Basilar meningitis and granuloma, sarcoidosis, tuberculosis, sphenoid
  osteomyelitis, eosinophilic granuloma
Craniopharyngioma
Hypothalamic tumor
  Infundibuloma
  Teratoma (ectopic pinealoma)
  Neuroglial tumors, particularly astrocytoma
Maternal deprivation syndrome
Isolated GHRF deficiency
Hypothalamic hypothyroidism
Panhypophysiotropic failure
Disorders of Regulation of LRH:
Female
  Precocious puberty
  Delayed puberty
  Neurogenic amenorrhea
  Pseudocyesis
  Anorexia nervosa
  "Functional amenorrhea"
  "Functional oligomenorrhea"
  Drug-induced amenorrhea
Male
  Precocious puberty
  Fröhlich's syndrome
  Olfactory-genital dysplasia (Kallmann's syndrome)
**Disorders of Regulation of Prolactin-Inhibiting Hormone
(nonpuerperal galactorrhea):**
Tumor
Sarcoid
Drug-induced
Reflex
Herpes zoster of chest wall
Post-thoracotomy
Nipple manipulation
Spinal cord tumor
"Psychogenic"
Chiari-Frommel syndrome
Hypothyroidism
CO_2 narcosis
Disorders of Regulation of CRF:
Paroxysmal ACTH discharge (Wolff's syndrome)
Loss of circadian variation
Depression

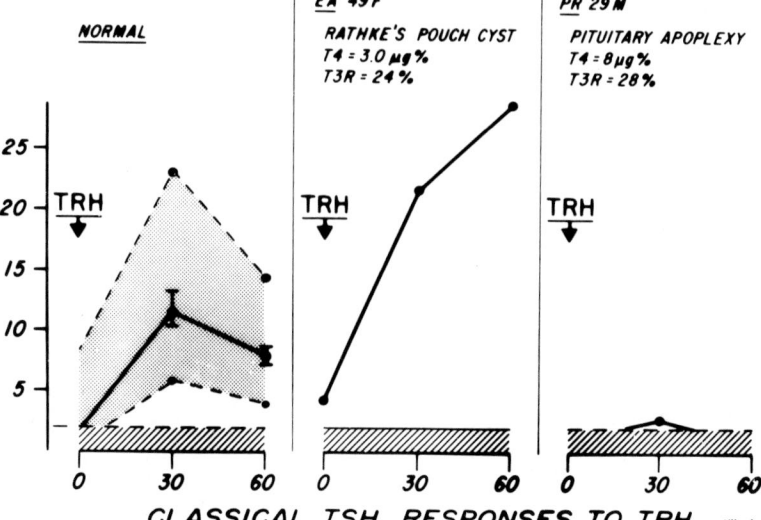

Figure 11–44. "Classic" pituitary responses to TRH administration in patients with hypothalamic-pituitary disease that has caused hypothyroidism. If due to intrinsic pituitary damage, response is abnormally low. If due to hypothalamic damage, response is normal or exaggerated. It must be emphasized that some patients with hypothalamic disease may not respond to TRH and that some patients with pituitary disease may respond to TRH.

emia and, in a few, galactorrhea. Of course this does not occur in hypophysectomized individuals. Spontaneously arising disease of the median eminence region also causes the stalk interruption syndrome.

Hypophysiotropic Hormone Deficiency

Deficiency of TRH secretion gives rise to the syndrome of "hypothalamic hypothyroidism," also called tertiary hypothyroidism. This condition may be seen in any form of hypothalamic disease and apparently rarely also as an isolated defect of hypothalamic function. From a clinical point of view, one can distinguish hypothalamic causes from pituitary causes of TSH deficiency by a consideration of the anatomic site of the responsible lesion, by the pattern of other pituitary deficits, and, to a certain extent, by the use of the TRH test (see later). The "classic" pituitary response to TRH administration in patients with TRH deficiency is an enhanced and somewhat delayed peak (Fig. 11–44), whereas the response to TRH in patients with intrinsic pituitary TSH failure is subnormal. In actual practice, there is a considerable overlap in responses, so that patterns in an individual case (and in the absence of other data) cannot alone be used to classify the type of TSH failure. It is generally true that persistent failure to demonstrate responses to TRH is good evidence for the presence of intrinsic pituitary disease, but a response does not mean that the pituitary itself is normal. The diagnosis of true hypothalamic hypothyroidism is difficult to establish with certainty, and some cases so called in the literature may be misclassified.

LRH deficiency accounts for the gonadotropin disturbances of "panhypophysiotropic failure" but can also be an isolated deficit. The best example is Kallman's syndrome (gonadotropin deficiency with associated hyposmia — see also Chs. 3 and 6). These patients have agenesis of the olfactory lobe on a heredofamilial basis and are believed to have abnormal development of the LRH neural pathways, although specific studies of the brains of such patients have not been carried out. Malformations of the midline structures, such as absent septum pellucidum, sometimes are associated with various defects in gonadotropin regulation, the most common of which is hypogonadotropic hypogonadism, but precocious puberty has also been observed in this syndrome. The LRH test often gives seemingly inappropriate results in patients with hypothalamic hypogonad-

ism. One would predict that such cases would show gonadotropin secretory responses resembling the normal, since the pituitary itself is preserved. Many such cases show little or no response to an initial test dose, however, and only after repeated injection does pituitary response return to normal (Fig. 11–45). This phenomenon is due to the fact that LRH sensitizes the pituitary to LRH; long-standing LRH deficiency is postulated to lead to a loss of pituitary LRH receptors. In the case of hypogonadotropic failure due to intrinsic pituitary disease, response to LRH may be absent or within the normal range. Because of these differences in response, a single injection of LRH does not constitute an adequate means for distinguishing between hypothalamic and pituitary disorders. Recent work using prolonged infusions, repeated injections, or sex steroid priming may lead to more precise diagnostic tools.

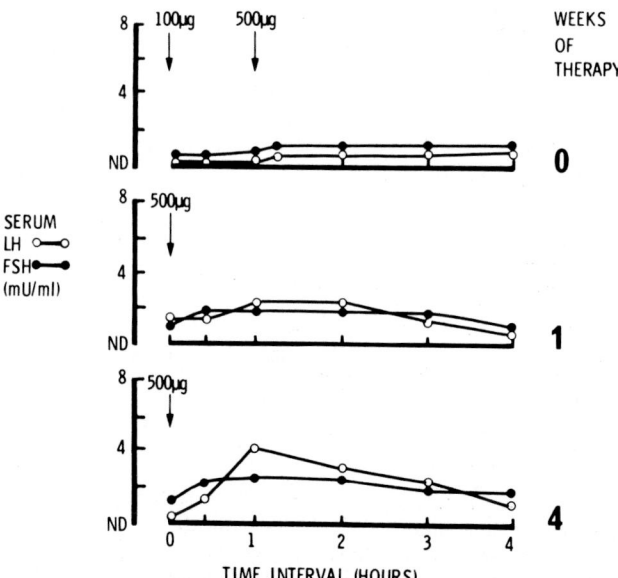

Figure 11–45. Demonstration of increasing responsivity of gonadotropin secretion to LRH after repeated administration of the hormone in a prepubertal boy with a craniopharyngioma. The hormone was administered s.c. in a dose of 500 μg twice daily for 4 weeks and was tested with intravenous doses. Note that there was little or no response initially, but after a period of treatment, responsivity gradually rose. (From Mortimer, C. H.: Gonadotropin-releasing hormone, In *Clinical Neuroendocrinology*, Martini, L., and Besser, G. M. (eds.), New York, Academic Press, 1977, p. 213, with permission.)

GHRF deficiency appears to underlie the GH deficit in the bulk of patients with idiopathic dwarfism (see also Ch. 3). The frequent association of hypophysiotropic deficiency with abnormal EEG's and a history of birth trauma in some cases suggests an analogy with other forms of birth injury. Deficiency of PIF secretion leads to hyperprolactinemia.

Nonendocrine Manifestations of Hypothalamic Disease

In considering the clinical presentation of patients with hypothalamic disease, it is well to keep in mind that the hypothalamus is also involved in the regulation of visceral functions and of behavior. These are listed in Tables 11–13 and 11–14. Psychic abnormalities are common in hypothalamic disease, including attacks of rage, laughing, and crying; disturbed sleep patterns; excessive sexuality; and antisocial behavior. Somnolence, or pathologic wakefulness, has been observed, as have bulemia and malignant anorexia. The abnormal eating patterns in humans are analogous to the syndromes of hyperphagia and loss of food drive produced in the rat by destruction of the ventromedial nucleus and lateral hypothalamus respectively. Patients with hypothalamic damage may show hyperthermia, hypothermia, and unexplained fluctuations in body temperature. Occasionally they may present as "fever of unknown origin." Pathologic disturbance of sweating, acrocyanosis, and loss of sphincter control can all occur. Diencephalic epilepsy is a rare manifestation. One of the most distressing aspects of hypothalamic damage is the loss of recent memory, believed to require intact mamillothalamic pathways. The profound impact of hypothalamic damage on higher brain functions is of great importance to endocrinologists who deal with pituitary problems, because severe memory loss, obesity, and personality changes (apathy, loss of ability to concentrate, aggressive antisocial behavior) may follow suprasellar extension of tumors, or damage incurred by surgical attempts to remove the tumor. This issue is especially important in the management of suprasellar tumors and should be weighed carefully with the neurosurgeon, the patient, and his or her family in planning the therapeutic approach. Hypothalamic lesions growing slowly may reach surprisingly large size without producing much disturbance of behavior or homeostasis, but surgical manipulation (of a much less extensive extent) can produce striking immedi-

Table 11–14. SYMPTOMS AND SIGNS OF HYPOTHALAMIC DISEASE*

Symptoms and Signs	Number of Cases
Sexual abnormalities (hypogonadism or precocious puberty)	43
Diabetes insipidus	21
Psychic disturbance	21
Obesity or hyperphagia	20
Somnolence	18
Emaciation, anorexia	15
Thermodysregulation	13
Sphincter disturbance	5

*From a review of 60 autopsy-proven cases.
Adapted from Bauer, H. G.: Endocrine and other clinical manifestations of hypothalamic disease: A survey of 60 cases with autopsies. *J. Clin. Endocrinol. Metab. 14*:13, 1954.

ate functional abnormalities. Presumably this is because the slowly developing lesions permit compensatory responses to take place.

Neuroendocrine Disease of Gonadotropin Regulation

True Precocious Puberty

The term "precocious puberty" is used when otherwise normal pituitary-gonad function appears at an abnormally early age. In boys this means the onset of androgen secretion and spermatogenesis before the age of 9 or 10 years, and in girls onset of estrogen secretion and cyclic ovarian activity before the age of 8 years. The general subject of precocious puberty and its diagnosis is dealt with in several other chapters in this volume (the Adrenals, Ch. 5; The Testes, Ch. 6; and The Ovaries and Breasts, Ch. 7). Considered here are neurogenic causes of precocious puberty. True precocious puberty always arises from disturbed neural function, which may or may not have an identifiable structural basis. Pseudoprecocious puberty, which refers to premature sexual development due to excessive secretion of androgens or estrogenic hormones by tumors (both gonadal and extragonadal), is considered elsewhere as primary endocrine gland disturbance.

Idiopathic Sexual Precocity

This is the largest category of true precocity. Familial occurrence is uncommon, but there is a hereditary form, largely confined to males. In the study of Liu and coworkers (1965), girls with true precocity were found to have a high incidence of abnormal EEG's and behavioral disturbance suggesting the presence of underlying or associated brain damage, but Beirich (1975) disputes this contention and claims that idiopathic precocious puberty is unaccompanied by even occult brain changes. The pathogenesis of this disorder therefore remains a matter of controversy, although it is still reasonable to postulate that the crucial factor responsible is related to hypothalamic development.

Neurogenic Precocious Puberty with Structural Disease

The site of hypothalamic lesions that influence the timing of puberty in the human is not as well established as it is in the rat. In the classic compilation of Weinberger and Grant, approximately two thirds of the cases in which anatomic

Table 11–13. NEUROLOGIC MANIFESTATIONS OF NONENDOCRINE HYPOTHALAMIC DISEASE

Disorders of Temperature Regulation
  Hyperthermia
  Hypothermia
  Poikilothermia
Disorders of Food Intake
  Hyperphagia (bulimia)
  Anorexia, aphagia
Disorders of Water Intake
  Compulsive water drinking
  Adipsia
  Essential hypernatremia
Disorders of Sleep and Consciousness
  Somnolence
  Sleep rhythm reversal
  Akinetic mutism
  Coma

Disorders of Psychic Function
  Rage behavior
  Hallucinations
Periodic Disease of Hypothalamic Origin
  Diencephalic epilepsy
  Kleine-Levin syndrome
  Periodic discharge syndrome of Wolff
Disorders of the Autonomic Nervous System
  Pulmonary edema
  Cardiac arrhythmias
  Sphincter disturbance
Hereditary Hypothalamic Disease
  Laurence-Moon-Biedl syndrome
Miscellaneous
  Prader-Willi syndrome
  Diencephalic syndrome infancy
  Cerebral gigantism

correlations could be made had destruction of the posterior hypothalamus, but it must be recognized that by the time most patients came to autopsy, damage had been extensive. In the rat, precocious puberty is regularly produced by localized lesions in the preoptic hypothalamus. Electric stimulation of the amygdala delays puberty, thus suggesting that, in the rodent at least, the timing of puberty is determined by a dual control system — hypothalamic and extrahypothalamic. Specific lesions that have been recognized to cause precocity include craniopharyngioma (although delayed puberty is more common), astrocytoma, pineal tumors (see later), encephalitis, miliary tuberculosis, tuberous sclerosis, Sturge-Weber syndrome, porencephaly, craniostenosis, microcephaly, hydrocephalus, and Tay-Sachs disease.

One category of neoplasm of the hypothalamus that produces precocious puberty by a unique mechanism is the hamartoma. This lesion is an exception to the generalization that tumors of the brain cause precocious puberty by destructive effects on regions that normally suppress gonadotropin secretion. A hamartoma can be defined neuropathologically as "a tumor-like collection of normal nerve tissue lodged in an abnormal location." One type of hypothalamic hamartoma consists of a sharply encapsulated nodule of nerve tissue attached to the posterior hypothalamus at a point between the anterior portion of the mamillary body and the posterior region of the tuber cinereum. These differ from locally invasive glial tumors that may occupy the same region.

The hypothalamic hamartoma grows into the cisternal space between the cerebral peduncles, adapting itself to the pyramidal shape of the cisterna, and it may produce precocious puberty before other neural effects occur. Tumors of this type are exceedingly rare, fewer than 50 having been reported up to 1972, but miniature "hamartomatous" nodular formations of the tuber cinereum have been seen not uncommonly in normal brains. Not all hypothalamic hamartomas cause precocious puberty. It has been proposed by Richter (1951) that precocious puberty occurs when the cells of the hamartoma make specific connections with the median eminence, and thus serve as an "accessory hypothalamus." That the tumor may secrete LRH was first proposed by Beirich (1975), who found LRH in the spinal fluid of three such patients. The hypothesis has been supported more firmly by the direct demonstration of LRH peptidergic pathways in an excised hamartoma by Judge and collaborators (1977), and a second case has been observed by Hochman and his collaborators (unpublished). We may postulate with some reason that LRH secretion by ectopically placed LRH peptidergic neurons is not subject to the normal restraining influences of the anterior hypothalamus and that early development is the consequence of this unrestrained LRH secretion.

The clinical presentation in patients with hamartomas is not different from other known cerebral causes of precocity. They occur in either sex, have been seen as early as 3 months of age, and usually are fatal before the age of 20, although one case surviving into the 7th decade has been reported. Early in the course of illness, precocity is the only sign; later, hypothalamic compression causes severe local disturbances.

Hypothyroidism

Hypothyroidism is listed here as a cause of neurogenic precocious puberty without proof that the disordered gonadotropin secretion is really due to hypothalamic disturb-

ance. This condition, sometimes associated with hyperprolactinemia and galactorrhea, is a "functional" disorder of gonadotropin regulation completely reversible by thyroid hormone replacement. One explanation, expressed by Van Wyck and Grumbach, is that there is cross specificity in negative feedback control of TSH, LH, and FSH, all glycoprotein hormones secreted by basophil cells. I hold an alternative theory that proposes that hypothyroidism causes hypothalamic hypothyroid encephalopathy with resultant deficits in the usual tonic-suppressing actions of the hypothalamus on gonadotropin release. The high PRL levels that sometimes accompany this disorder can also be looked upon as being due to a deficiency in PIF secretion. Alternative explanations, such as increased secretion of TRH and increased sensitivity of the pituitary to tonic TRH secretion, are also tenable on the basis of current knowledge.

Tumors of the Pineal Gland

Pathology. Pineal tumors are uncommon, composing 0.2–1% of brain neoplasms in Caucasians and 4% in Japanese. Though rare, they have attracted a great deal of interest because of a variety of lesions, complexity of classification, variability of growth pattern, problems in management, and possible relationship to endocrine disorder. The various types of lesions found in the pineal region (including the posterior third ventricle) are summarized in Table 11–15, taken from the work of DeGirolami (1977). The term pinealoma refers to a tumor of the pineal parenchymal cell and can be a pineoblastoma or pineocytoma, according to its degree of differentiation. In one series of pineal tumors, only 9 of 53 fitted this category, and there were 13 glial tumors, including astrocytomas and glioblas-

Table 11–15. CLASSIFICATION OF TUMORS OF THE PINEAL REGIONS

A. Germ Cell Tumors
  1. Germinoma
    a. Posterior third ventricle and pineal
    b. Anterior third ventricle, suprasellar or intrasellar
    c. Combined lesions in anterior and posterior third ventricle, apparently noncontiguous, with or without foci of cystic or solid teratoma
  2. Teratoma
    a. Evidencing growth along two or three germ lines in varying degrees of differentiation
    b. Dermoid and epidermoid cysts with or without solid foci of teratoma
    c. Histologically malignant forms with or without differentiated foci of benign, solid, or cystic teratoma—teratocarcinoma, chorioepithelioma, embryonal carcinoma (endodermal-sinus tumor or yolk-sac carcinoma), combinations of these with or without foci of germinoma, chemodectoma (Smith et al.).
B. Pineal Parenchymal Tumors
  1. Pineocytes
    a. Pineocytoma
    b. Pineoblastoma
    c. Ganglioglioma and chemodectoma
    d. Mixed forms exhibiting transitions between these
  2. Glia
    a. Astrocytoma
    b. Ependymoma
    c. Mixed forms and other less frequent gliomas (glioblastoma, oligodendroglioma, etc.)
C. Tumors of Supporting or Adjacent Structures
  1. Meningioma
  2. Hemangiopericytoma
D. Non-Neoplastic Conditions of Neurosurgical Importance
  1. "Degenerative" cysts of the pineal lined by fibrillary astrocytes
  2. Arachnoid cysts
  3. Cavernous hemangioma (Hubschmann)

From: DeGirolami, U.: In *Pineal Tumors*, Schmidek, H. H. (ed.), New York, Masson Pub. U.S.A., Inc., 1977.

tomas (DeGirolami and Schmidek, 1977). The commonest tumors of the pineal region are not pinealomas at all. Most are germinomas, so designated because of their presumed origin in germ cells. Some germinomas, histologically indistinguishable from those of the pineal region, may arise in the anterior hypothalamus or floor of the third ventricle. They have traditionally been classified as atypical teratomas (D. Russell, 1963) or as ectopic pinealomas (germinoma-like lesions arising outside of the pineal). They have also been called "seminomatous pinealomas" by pathologists because they resemble testicular tubules. Identical tumors can be found in the testis and anterior mediastinum. Intracranial germinomas have a tendency to spread locally, to infiltrate the hypothalamus, to metastasize to the spinal cord (or other brain regions), and to appear in CSF. Even extracranial metastases (to the skin or liver) have been observed rarely (Tompkins et al.). Teratomas containing structures derived from two or more germ cell layers also are found in the pineal region. Chorionic tissue in such teratomas may secrete human chorionic gonadotropin (hCG) in sufficient amounts to cause gonadal maturation (see later). A possible viral etiology for pinealoma was proposed by Kuramado and associates on the basis of their finding of virus-like particles in one case.

Relation to Precocious Puberty. The relationship of pineal tumors to precocious puberty has been much studied in an effort to determine whether the pineal is truly involved in the regulation of sexual function in humans. Contrary to generally held conceptions, precocious puberty is not a uniform, or even a common, finding in pineal disease. In 65 pineal tumors studied by Ringertz and colleagues (1954), not a single case of sexual precocity was noted; only 7 of these patients were younger than 11 years of age. Pineal disease is not common before puberty, and when present before puberty, advanced sexual maturation is not common. In a study of 177 patients by Bing and coworkers (1938), 56 were less than 15 years of age and of these only one third had sexual precocity. In their analysis, neuroanatomic evidence pointed to extensive damage beyond the pineal region in all cases of precocious puberty. They concluded that puberty was due to the effects of tumor on function of the adjacent hypothalamus and further emphasized that clinical overt evidence of hypothalamic involvement, such as DI, polyphagia, somnolence, obesity, or behavioral disturbance, was noted in 71% of cases. These workers suggest that pineal neoplasms caused precocious puberty by mechanisms similar to that caused by other brain lesions. With the rarest of exceptions, precocious puberty associated with pineal lesions is seen only in boys.

One of the most important compilations and analyses of the relationship of the pineal to abnormal puberty is that of Kitay (1954), who reviewed 46 published cases of precocious puberty associated with pineal tumor and formulated a humoral hypothesis. Ten were associated with "parenchymal" tumors; 36 were associated with "nonparenchymal" tumors despite the overall equal frequency of nonparenchymal and parenchymal tumors in their collected cases. Because nonparenchymal tumors were postulated to destroy pineal parenchyma, these workers reasoned that the tumors interfered with the normal pineal suppression of the appearance of puberty. Included in the list of tumors were teratomas, supporting tissue tumors, germinomas, and other less common neoplasms. Unfortunately, these cases were all studied before the introduction of modern assay methodology, and it is now recognized that some pineal germinomas and teratomas secrete hCG.

The few cases of pineal choriocarcinoma that have been studied with modern methods have shown high hCG and decreased or normal FSH blood levels. Human hCG alone can stimulate testosterone secretion from the testis but does not stimulate estrogen secretion from the ovary. It would be expected therefore, as emphasized by several authors, including Axelrod, that precocious puberty caused by pineal tumors would be more frequently seen in males than in females. This is in fact the case. Kubo and collaborators claim to have seen the first such case in a female, a 5-year-old child in whom specific immunoassays documented the presence of high plasma hCG, normal FSH levels in blood, and hCG in tumor extracts. The incidence of gonadotropin secretion in tumors of the pineal causing precocious puberty is unknown, but the occurrence of this group of cases seriously detracts from the argument that nonparenchymal tumors cause precocious puberty by damage to normally functioning pineal tissue. Furthermore, the recent demonstration that the pineal contains LRH suggests another potential (though not proven) mechanism by which a tumor could stimulate gonadotropin secretion.

Even less well understood are those rare pineal tumors that are associated with delayed puberty. As reviewed by Kitay and Altschule, parenchymal tumors were responsible for 20 of 30 cases of pineal tumor–related hypogonadism culled from the literature. It is in this group that the postulation of a gonadotropin inhibitory hormone of pineal origin is most reasonable. As yet, no studies of gonadotropin inhibitory factors or circulating melatonin in such cases have been reported, but in two cases (not necessarily associated with delayed puberty), assays of tumor tissue (in one case a third ventricular pinealoma and in another a cutaneous metastasis) have demonstrated characteristic melatonin-forming enzymes (Wurtman, 1966).

Because many other signs of pituitary insufficiency, including DI, are common in pineal tumors, it is likely that some significant proportion of such cases may have tumor-induced hypothalamic lesions rather than intrinsic pineal secretory disorder.

DI, visual impairment, and anterior pituitary insufficiency are the characteristic triad of finding in germinomas of the floor of the third ventricle. Were it not for the fact that tumors of identical morphologic structure may arise in the region of the pineal, and that tumors of the pineal can spread to the base of the brain, there would be no place for the discussion of this disorder in the chapter on the pineal.

Neurologic Manifestations of Pineal Tumors. The classic neurologic manifestation of tumors compressing the optic tectum in the region of the pineal gland is Parinaud's syndrome, which consists of paralysis of upward gaze, pupillary areflexia (to light), paralysis of convergence, and wide-based gait (Table 11–16). Wray has presented an analysis of the ocular finding in pinealomas (Table 11–17), and

Table 11–16. PINEALOMAS: FREQUENCY (%) OF PRESENTING SYMPTOMS AND SIGNS

1. Increased intracranial pressure	85
2. Spasticity	35
3. Ataxia	30
4. Parinaud's syndrome	25
5. Cerebellar type nystagmus	25
6. Syncope	20
7. Vertigo	20
8. Cranial nerve palsy (other than CN VI,VIII)	20
9. Intention tremor	15
10. Scotoma	10
11. Tinnitus	10
12. Other	10

From Brady, W. L.: In *Pineal Tumors*. Schmidek, H. H. (ed.), New York, Masson Pub. U.S.A., Inc., 1977.

Table 11–17. OCULAR SYMPTOMS AND SIGNS IN 22 CASES OF PINEALOMA

		No. Patients
Symptoms	Diplopia	7
	"Blurred vision"	4
	Reading difficulty	1
Signs	Upward gaze palsy	12
	Pupils: Areflexic to light, near response retained	13
	Accommodative control disorder	3
	Convergent-retraction nystagmus	10
	Convergence paretic	3
	Downward gaze palsy	0
	Collier's sign	0
	Skew deviation	5
	Third nerve palsy	0
	Fourth nerve palsy (bilateral)	1
	Sixth nerve palsy	3
	Fundi: Normal	8
	Papilledema	10
	Optic atrophy	4
	Vision: Reduced acuity	8
	Visual fields: Normal	15
	Constricted	3
	Bitemporal	4

Wray, S. H.: In *Pineal Tumors.* Schmidek, H. H. (ed.), New York, Masson Pub. U.S.A., Inc., 1977.

detailed ophthalmologic evaluation of such cases. Classic Parinaud's syndrome occurs in about half of the cases of pinealoma.

Treatment of Pineal Tumors. Management of tumors in the pineal region is somewhat controversial. The earlier literature emphasizes the great danger involved in biopsy and attempted removal, and operative mortality of 14–37% in different series having been reported (Schmidek). On the other hand, an aggressive approach to pineal region has been emphasized by Stein (1979). Citing his own experience with only one perioperative death in 22 consecutive cases operated on with a supracerebellar-infratentorial approach utilizing the operating microscope, Stein emphasizes the need for making a histologic diagnosis, the variety of pathologic disorders found in this region, the possibility of removal of an encapsulated lesion, and the possible use of cytotoxic chemotherapy for certain lesions such as germinoma and choriocarcinoma.

More than 70% of tumors in the posterior third ventricle are radiosensitive and, according to Brady, should respond to adequate courses of radiation therapy within 3–6 months after treatment. Radiotherapy is combined with shunting procedures when indicated by presence of hydrocephalus.

In contrast to the controversial question of surgical approach to the pineal tumor, ectopic pinealomas in the chiasmal region should in general be explored surgically, the tumor decompressed if possible, and biopsy diagnosis made. This recommendation is based on the relative safety of these procedures and the incidence of many other lesions that are not amenable to x-ray but are amenable to surgical removal. It is important to recognize that germinomas are exceedingly radiosensitive, in contrast to most other tumors in the region of the third ventricle. In the large series of 18 cases studied by Takeuchi and collaborators in Kyoto, 15 underwent irradiation; of these, one was surviving after 16 years, three were alive with a 10-year follow-up, and 8 others (with shorter follow-up periods) were still alive. Deaths occurred in three, one of unknown cause, one of hypothalamic necrosis following repeated courses of x-ray therapy, and one after metastases to the spinal cord. Thus, the designation of Rubin and Kramer that these lesions are potentially curable must be borne in mind. It is also important to point out that the diagnosis can sometimes be made by cytologic

study of the spinal fluid, by radioimmunoassay of spinal fluid for hCG, or by specific serum radioimmunoassays that will show high β-hCG levels. The use of prophylactic whole skull and spine x-ray must be considered in patients with either pineal or chiasmal germinomas because of the high incidence of neuroaxis seeding by tumors. Histologic study of CSF is indicated, and chemotherapeutic approaches are now being evaluated.

Neurologic Approach to the Patient with True Precocious Puberty

In the child with precocious development of secondary sex characteristics, the first requirement is to determine whether mature germ cells are being formed. Clues to normal testicular development in boys include enlargement to adult size, the appearance of sperm in overnight voided urine specimens and after seminal vesicle and prostate massages, and, if necessary, biopsy of the testicle. Excessive secretion of androgenic hormones by adrenal or other tumors usually leads to small, prepubertal-sized testes, but rarely, testicular enlargement can occur owing to adrenal rests, or even adrenal hypersecretion. Other reasons why testes may appear to be of adult size in pseudoprecocious puberty are because testosterone secretion by ectopic tumors may stimulate tubular growth and because of chorionic gonadotropic hormone secretion arising from a teratoma located elsewhere, such as the mediastinum or pineal region. The laboratory is helpful in distinguishing these forms of abnormality (see Ch. 6). Once the diagnosis of neurogenic precocity is made in the male, the high frequency with which intracranial disease is found requires that the patient undergo complete neurologic evaluation. Conventional roentgenogram study, polytomography, and CAT scans are indicated. Spinal fluid should be examined for hCG and for cells to identify the presence of germinoma. If no abnormalities are noted, continued regular follow-up is strongly indicated. Complete pituitary work-up is indicated as well.

In females, the appearance of regular menses is suggestive of normal pituitary-gonad axis (see Ch. 7). Neurologic evaluation should include skull films, CAT scans, and EEG's. If there are no abnormal neurologic findings and pituitary function is otherwise normal, including tests for DI and GH secretory reserve, it is likely that the patient has "idiopathic" sexual precocity and need not be kept under such close surveillance as the male.

Management of True Precocity

If a neurologic lesion is demonstrable, surgery should be carried out if possible to remove tumor or to establish the diagnosis by biopsy with the possible exception of pineal region tumors (see earlier). X-ray therapy obviously must be considered, since many lesions that are not resectable may be radiosensitive. Whether it is due to a resectable lesion or not, drug therapy may also be indicated to delay or reverse pubertal development. The standard approach used currently is to administer medroxyprogesterone acetate (MPGA). In girls this drug usually inhibits ovulation and causes a regression of breast hypertrophy and menses. In general, this therapy does not delay the early and premature closure of epiphyses with ultimate short stature, however. A potential new approach to the management of precocity is treatment with newly developed "super LRH agonists." These peptide analogues of LRH, some of which have been synthesized by Vale and colleagues, have the ability to suppress gonadotropin secretion when given continuously and in high doses. The mechanism underlying this response is thought to be a "down regulation" of pituitary LRH receptors. I am unaware of any clinical trials of the LRH analogues for this purpose, and such an approach would clearly have to be regarded as an experimental procedure at this time.

Psychologic management of the sexually precocious is of great importance. (See Ch. 12 and papers by Money and Hampson, 1955; Money and Alexander, 1969; and Ehrhardt and Meyer-Bahlburg for a discussion of this aspect.)

Psychogenic Amenorrhea

Cessation of normal menstrual cycles in young, nonpregnant women who have no demonstrable structural abnormalities of brain, pituitary, or ovary occurs in several clinical syndromes. These syndromes are pseudocyesis (false pregnancy), anorexia nervosa, a large group of poorly defined conditions loosely called "psychogenic" or "hypothalamic" amenorrhea, and hyperprolactinemia due to an occult adenoma (see Ch. 3) or to otherwise unexplained excessive PRL secretion. This entire group of disorders is often associated with gross psychopathology or with psychic stress and is usually temporary. Depending upon the degree and type of gonadotropin deficiency present, the ovarian abnormality in these cases ranges from failure of ovulation to severe degrees of estrogen loss. Abnormalities in the timing of ovulation represent the mildest form of this disorder. All of these disorders probably arise from functional abnormalities in the hypothalamic gonadotropin regulating areas. Certain tranquilizer drugs, such as reserpine and chlorpromazine, may block ovulation and delay menses. These disorders are considered in detail in Ch. 12.

Neurogenic Hypogonadism in the Male

Since gonadotropin secretion in the male as well as in the female is regulated by the hypothalamus, hypogonadotropic hypogonadism might be expected to arise sometimes from neurogenic causes. Indeed, organic disorders of the hypothalamus, such as tumor, encephalitis, microcephaly, Friedreich's ataxia, and demyelinating disorders, can cause gonadal failure, but the largest proportion of men with hypogonadotropic hypogonadism do not have *clinically* detectable structural disease of the pituitary gland and have otherwise normal pituitary function (see Ch. 12). Experimental work in animals fosters the speculation that such cases may be due not only to intrinsic defects in pituitary gonadotrope cells but also to failure of proper maturation of hypothalamic gonadotropin regulating areas.

This speculative view cannot be confirmed in most cases, but in one category of gonadotropin deficiency reasonable evidence exists for a primary neurogenic disorder. In this disease, called Kallmann's syndrome or "olfactory-genital dysplasia," hypogonadism is associated with anosmia or hyposmia and often with other neurologic defects, such as color blindness and nerve deafness. Dystrophic bone changes also occur. Pathologic examination of the brains of such individuals reveals that the olfactory defect is due, in some instances, to agenesis or maldevelopment of the olfactory lobes. In view of the close anatomic and physiologic connections between the rhinencephalon and sex-regulating areas of the hypothalamus (described earlier), failure to develop gonadotropic function is very probably due to maldevelopment of the hypothalamus. Kallmann's syndrome is a genetic disorder thought to be inherited as an X chromosome–dominant gene with incomplete penetrance. In such pedigrees, one may find males with hyposmia but with normal male sexual development and females with hyposmia who usually have normal gonadotropic function. In other more usual forms of pituitary hypogonadism, sensitivity of the sense of smell is enhanced. This clinical difference between gonadotropin failure due to pituitary disease and that associated with Kallmann's syndrome has been stated to be of value in differential diagnosis. Sporadic cases without family history also occur. An unexplained accompaniment of hypogonadotropism is the relative nonresponsiveness of the testes to exogenous gonadotropins (as compared with usual gonadotropin deficiency). Bardin and colleagues (1969) have noted that "both ends of the pituitary-gonad axis are abnormal." Pituitary responses to LRH injection may also be much below normal in some but not all cases.

Psychogenic impairment of testicular function has received little study.

A well-established neurogenic cause of hypogonadism is that observed following inflammatory or traumatic lesions of the spinal cord, occasionally in association with gynecomastia. Such cases are associated with loss of sensation in the genital area. Since LH secretion can be triggered in certain animals by stimulating the uterine cervix and since the secretion of PRL in the human can be induced by irritative lesions of the thoracic spinal nerves, maintenance of gonadotropic function may reasonably be expected to depend somewhat upon neural stimuli from the genital region. Convincing data in the human on this point have not been published.

In any discussion of hypogonadotropic hypogonadism, mention must be made of Fröhlich's syndrome (adiposogenital dystrophy). As first reported in 1901, the affected patient, a boy, had hypogonadism and obesity due to a pituitary tumor. A similar syndrome can readily be produced in experimental animals by damaging the median eminence and the ventromedial nuclei of the hypothalamus, clearly the result of disturbed FSH and LH release together with loss of sense of satiety. In humans, tumors and various inflammatory or degenerative lesions can produce the same disorder.

On the other hand, the overwhelming majority of obese children with delayed sexual development brought to endocrinologists do not have any structural damage to the hypothalamus. In some, the seeming failure of penile growth may be due merely to the presence of a large pubic fat pad. In most, the problem is constitutional delayed puberty in association with obesity of the usual type. Whether there is a functional disorder of the hypothalamus in these cases is not known. Many endocrinologists suspect that obesity in some way can delay onset of puberty. It is important to reassure the patient and his parents about the benign nature of this condition. The use of testosterone or CG injections is sometimes indicated for psychologic reasons, but the administration of these hormones without a strict weight reduction regimen does not ameliorate the obesity (see Ch. 6).

Neurogenic Disorders of Prolactin Regulation

One of the most significant developments in clinical endocrinology over the past decade has been the recognition of the frequency with which hyperprolactinemia occurs and the hitherto unsuspected incidence of PRL-secreting microadenomas (see Ch. 5). It should be borne in mind that neurologic disturbances may also underlie hypersecretory states (see Table 11–18). Important neurogenic causes in-

Table 11–18. DIFFERENTIAL DIAGNOSIS OF GALACTORRHEA AND/OR HYPERPROLACTINEMIA*

A. Structural Hypothalamic Lesions with Damage to Ventral Hypothalamus or Pituitary Stalk:

craniopharyngioma	metastatic or primary neoplasms
sarcoidosis	Rathke's pouch cyst
encephalitis	surgical stalk section
irradiation	ectopic pinealoma
head trauma	histiocytosis X
ectopic pinealoma	

B. Structural Pituitary Lesions

Prolactin-producing pituitary tumors	pituitary angiosarcoma
empty sella syndrome	acromegaly
combined prolactin-growth hormone producing pituitary tumors	
Cushing's disease	

C. Drug-Induced

Compazine**	Stelazine**	Prolixin	Amphetamines
Thorazine**	Mellaril**	Equanil	Elavil
Perlactin	Reserpine	Aldomet	Pimozide
Metochlopramide	Prostaglandins	Estrogens	Androgens
Miltown	Sulpiride		

D. Endocrine-Metabolic

Hypothyroidism (50% with myxedema have increased prolactin but only 5% have galactorrhea, usually with amenorrhea)

Addison's disease	Nelson's syndrome	Sheehan's syndrome
adrenal carcinoma	adrenal hyperplasia	diabetes
liver disease	chronic renal failure	

E. Irritative Lesions of the Chest Wall

herpes zoster	thoracotomy	thoracic burns
tight garments	mastectomy	cystic breast disease
chest trauma	atopic dermatitis	mammoplasty

F. Hypothalamic Biochemical Lesions with Presumed Decrease of Prolactin-Inhibitory Factor or Increase of Prolactin Releasing Factor†

G. Other Described Causes

pseudotumor cerebri	syringomyelia	pseudocyesis
tabes dorsalis	male hypogonadism	pneumonencephalo-
choreoepithelioma of testis	Stein-Leventhal	gram
hysterectomy	syndrome	IUD use
dilatation/curettage	ovarian resection	
	neck surgery	

H. Lesions of Upper Spinal Cord

extrinsic tumors	cervical ependymoma

I. Ectopic Prolactin Production

bronchogenic CA	hypernephroma

* Compiled by Dr. Bruce Biller .

**NB: 25% of psychiatric patients on phenothizine derivatives will have galactorrhea, but many will have normal PRL; amenorrhea may also occur and both may persist for several years after medication is stopped.

†NB: Diagnosis of exclusion — patients may still have a biochemical and radiologically undetectable prolactin-producing pituitary tumor that will only become apparent as time goes on.

clude irritative lesions of the chest wall (herpes zoster, post-thoracotomy) presumed to act by chronic stimulation of nipple afferent nerves; excessive tactile stimulation of the nipple, usually to relieve breast congestion or less commonly as a source of erotic pleasure; and lesions within the spinal cord such as ependymoma. Prolonged mechanical stimulation of the nipples by suckling or the use of a breast pump can initiate lactation in some women who are not pregnant and even in women who have never been pregnant. A foster mother may thus be enabled to suckle her adopted child. Any lesion that can interrupt the hypothalamic-pituitary connection can also cause hyperprolactinemia. The use of neuroleptic agents, especially the phenothiazines, tricyclic antidepressants, reserpine, and alpha methyldopa (Aldomet) must be excluded as a cause.

Still obscure is the role of psychogenic factors in the pathogenesis of hyperprolactinemia. Psychogenic galactorrhea had been a commonly applied diagnosis in the past, but it was often a diagnosis by exclusion. With the current recognition of the frequency of microadenomas, the very existence of hyperprolactinemia as a psychogenic disorder is now in question (see also Ch. 12).

Because the nervous system exerts profound effects on PRL secretion, it has been reasonable to postulate that patients with hyperprolactinemia (including those with adenomas) have a deficit of PIF or an excess of PRF activity. The most reasonable way to test this hypothesis is to carry out detailed studies of PRL secretory dynamics in patients apparently cured by removal of microadenomas. In one such series studying patients before and after adenomectomy by Goodman and collaborators, all patients achieving normal PRL levels had normal PRL secretory dynamics after surgery. Still unresolved is the cause of the persistent hyperprolactinemia and secretory disturbance in those cases unsuccessfully treated by surgery. Does this group include incomplete removal (as is likely in the larger tumors) or abnormal function in the remaining part of the gland? Many prolactinomas when studied by tissue culture methods show secretion of other hormones, including GH and ACTH. I believe it unlikely that disturbed PRF's could give rise to abnormalities of more than one cell type and for this reason think that prolactinomas are intrinsic diseases of the pituitary, although they may require the presence of hypothalamic function in the early stages of their development.

Neurogenic Disorders of Growth Hormone Secretion

Growth Hormone Insufficiency: Hypothalamic Disease

Loss of GH secretory responses to provocative stimuli and of the normal nocturnal increase in GH secretion occurs early in the course of hypothalamic disease of any etiology and is usually the most sensitive endocrine indicator of hypothalamic dysfunction. (See Table 11–20 for specific etiologies of hypothalamic disease.) Developmental abnormalities associated with anatomic malformations of midline cerebral structures have been documented in which GH secretion is abnormal, presumably owing to failure to develop normal GH regulatory structures. Some of the associated disorders include optic nerve dysplasia and midline prosencephalic malformations (absence of the septum pellucidum, abnormal third ventricle, and lamina terminalis). In one series of six patients, all had GH deficiency and four of the six had more than one pituitary disturbance, presumably due to deficiency of the appropriate hypothalamic hypophysiotropic hormone. Idiopathic hypopituitarism was considered earlier, under the heading "Hypophysiotropic Hormone Deficiency."

Maternal Deprivation Syndrome (Psychosocial Deprivation Syndrome)

Many reports have appeared documenting GH secretory impairment in children with growth failure occurring in a setting of severe emotional deprivation. Deficient GH release in response to stimuli such as insulin-induced hypoglycemia or arginine infusion and, in a smaller proportion, deficiency in the release of ACTH and gonadotropins are noted. This disorder is rapidly reversed by placing a child in a supportive hospital milieu; growth and neuroendocrine GH responses return rapidly. Excessive β-adrenergic inhibitory effects may be one of the causative factors in the syndrome. In one reported patient, normal GH secretion was restored immediately by treatment with propanolol, a β blocker.

Inhibition of GH release is the usual pattern of response to stress in the rat, and in this species, effects of stress are blocked by treatment with antisera to SRIF. It is believed, therefore, that in the rat stress brings about the release of SRIF. The extent to which increase in SRIF secretion and suppression of GHRF secretion are involved in the human response to deprivation is unknown.

Several more recent studies of the maternal deprivation syndrome have emphasized the importance of stress-induced malnutrition rather than psychologic factors causing growth failure; each case should be carefully evaluated from this point of view. Finally, it has been suggested that the growth retardation in a series of "deprived" children was a function of stress-induced sleep disturbance.

Hypersecretion of Growth Hormone due to Neurogenic Causes

The role of the hypothalamus in the pathogenesis of acromegaly and gigantism is still controversial, the main points at issue being the incidence of microadenomas in patients who have no other evidence of pituitary tumor and the role of the hypothalamus in bringing about pituitary dysfunction. This question has been reviewed in detail by Daughaddy et al., 1973 and Reichlin, 1980 and is considered in Ch. 5. In general, acromegalic patients lose normal circadian rhythms of GH secretion but may show intermittent surges of secretion, suggesting continued influences from the brain. Many patients show the normal suppressive effect on GH by glucose administration (but not to a normal degree), and some release GH after hypoglycemic stress, but these findings may mean only that an intrinsic pituitary disorder retains some physiologic control. Acromegalics show, in addition, a high frequency of paradoxical GH regulatory responses that do not occur in normal individuals. These include the release of GH after glucose administration, release of GH after TRH administration, and suppression of release by bromocriptine and other dopamine receptor stimulators. Only a few patients have been studied in detail before and after resection of a microadenoma; these have shown a restitution to completely normal physiologic GH secretory status. In such cases, an underlying hypothalamic defect could not have been present.

Further evidence against the hypothalamic hypothesis of acromegaly is the finding that four out of eight of the tumors studied by Zimmerman and collaborators (1974) had PRL-secreting cells as well as GH-secreting cells. It is unlikely that hypersecretion of a GHRF could cause PRL cell stimulation as well.

Several authors have reported findings of GHRF-like activity in the blood of patients with acromegaly. Although this finding could be taken as evidence for hypersecretion of hypothalamic factors, evidence specifically linking the abnormality to hypothalamic secretion has not been adduced. Mention should be made of the production of GHRF-active fractions by tumors of the APUD series, principally carcinoids. Several reports have appeared that document the remission of acromegaly after removal of the tumors. Some cases are due to overproduction of GH by the tumor, but others are due to the presence of a substance that releases GH from pituitaries. The relationship between GHRF of hypothalamic origin and that of tumor origin has not been characterized adequately as yet.

Cachexia and emaciation may be the presenting complaint in infants and children with tumors in and around the third ventricle. A striking feature in most reported cases of *diencephalic syndrome* is the alert appearance and seeming euphoria of the children despite their wasted state.

A variety of associated neurologic abnormalities have been identified in these children (Table 11–9), and the varied etiologies have been summarized by Burr and collaborators (1976) (Table 11–20). Somewhat less than one third of such patients have lesions in the region of the optic nerve. Many such cases have elevated GH levels, often with paradoxical responses to administration of glucose and with hypoglycemia. Deficits of pituitary-adrenal regulation are often observed.

Neurogenic Disorders of Adrenocorticotropin Regulation

Of all pituitary hypersecretory disorders, Cushing's disease comes closest to fitting the theoretic prediction of what a disease caused by primary excess of hypophysiotropic hormone secretion ought to be. "Set point" for plasma cortisol is elevated, as manifested by an excessively high threshold for feedback inhibition, and high plasma ACTH levels are elevated. Following adrenalectomy, the operation of the negative feedback control loop is manifested by excessive increase in ACTH secretion. Patients with Cushing's disease may show spontaneous fluctuations in the severity of their disease and lose normal sleep-related ACTH and GH secretory patterns. Moreover, as emphasized by Krieger, treatment with cyproheptidine, a serotonin receptor blocker, produces a clinical remission in some cases of Cushing's disease and has been reported to arrest Nelson's syndrome in at least one patient. Further, the paradoxical ACTH stimulatory response to TRH seen in Cushing's disease is reversed by cyproheptidine (Krieger et al., 1971). (See Chs. 3 and 5.) Despite this wealth of highly suggestive data, recently acquired evidence indicates that most patients with Cushing's disease have pituitary adenomas, and results of studies in detail show that ACTH regulatory function returns to normal after adenomectomy. If there is a form of Cushing's disease due to primary hypersecretion of CRF, it will prove to be relatively uncommon. Critical proof will require the measurement of CRF secretion by such patients.

Table 11–19. CLINICAL FEATURES OF DIENCEPHALIC SYNDROME (POOLED DATA OF 67 ANATOMICALLY DEFINED TUMORS)

Clinical Features	%
Emaciation	100
Alert appearance	87
Increased vigor and/or hyperkinesis	72
Vomiting	68
Euphoria	59
Pallor	55
Nystagmus	55
Irritability	32
Hydrocephalus*	33
Optic atrophy	24
Tremor	23
Sweating	15
Large hands/feet	5
Large genitals	5
Polyuria	5
Papilledema	5
Positive pneumoencephalogram	98
Endocrine anomalies**	90
CSF protein	64
CSF abnormal cells	23

*Hydrocephalus includes clinical plus pneumoencephalographic findings.
** Positive in 9 of 10 with adequately recorded investigation. (Occasionally patients had electrolyte and blood pressure anomalies and eosinophilia.)
From Burr, I. M., et al.: Diencephalic syndrome revisited. *J. Pediatr.* 88: 429, 1976.

Table 11–20. HISTOLOGY OF TUMORS PRODUCING
DIENCEPHALIC SYNDROME

Tumors	No. of Patients	
Gliomas	56	
Astrocytoma		37
Not subclassified		10
Spongioblastoma		5
Astroblastoma		1
Oligodendroglioma		1
Mixed astrocytoma/spongioblastoma		1
Mixed astrocytoma/oligodendroglioma		1
Ependymoma	2	
Ganglioglioma	1	
Dysgerminoma	1	
No histology	10	

From Burr, I. M., et al.: Diencephalic syndrome revisited. *J. Pediatr.*
*88:*429, 1976.

In contrast to the unsettled situation with Cushing's disease, there is at least one case of ACTH hypersecretion that is likely due to central nervous system causes. This syndrome, afflicting a single individual, was described by Wolff and collaborators (1964) under the title of periodic hypothalamic discharge. It is part of a recurring cyclic disorder characterized by high fever and paroxysm of glucocorticoid hypersecretion accompanied by paroxysmal EEG disturbance. When first seen at the age of 14, the patient, a male, had cushingoid features, and pneumoencephalogram showed some dilation of the left lateral ventricle and cortical atrophy. In an attempt to inhibit central neurotransmitters regulating CRF secretion, he was placed on chlorpromazine, with complete remission as a result. Since that time (follow-up period of 17 years), he has remained in remission as long as he continues to take chlorpromazine (personal communication, Sheldon Wolff) and has shown no evidence of progressive neurologic abnormality.

REFERENCES

Introduction

Bloom, F. E.: Contrasting principles of synaptic physiology: Peptidergic and non-peptidergic neurons. In *Central Regulation of the Endocrine System.* Fuxe, K., Hökfelt, T., and Luft, R. (eds.), New York Plenum Press, 1979, pp. 173–187.

Boyar, R. M.: Sleep-related endocrine rhythms, In *The Hypothalamus, Vol. 56,* Reichlin, S., Baldessarini, R. J., et al. (eds.), New York, Raven Press, 1978, pp. 373–386.

Collu, R., Barbeau, A., Ducharme, J., and Rochefort, J.-G. (eds.): *Central Nervous System Effects of Hypothalamic Hormones and Other Peptides.* New York, Raven Press, 1979.

Everett, J. W.: The mammalian hypothalamo-hypophysial system, In *The Endocrine Hypothalamus.* Jeffcoate, S. L., and Hutchinson, J. S. M. (eds.), New York, Academic Press, 1978, pp. 1–34.

Fuxe, K., Hökfelt, T., and Luft, R. (eds.): *Central Regulation of the Endocrine System.* New York, Plenum Press, 1979.

Gainer, H. (ed.): *Peptides in Neurobiology.* New York, Plenum Press, 1977.

Gotto, A. M., Jr., Peck, E. J., Jr., et al.: *Brain Peptides: A New Endocrinology.* New York, Elsevier-North Holland Publishing Co., 1979.

Green, J. D., and Harris, G. W.: Observation of hypophysioportal vessels of the living rat. *J. Physiol. 108:*359, 1949.

Guillemin, R.: The brain as an endocrine organ. *Neurosci. Res. Program Bull. 16*(Suppl.):1, 1978a.

Guillemin, R.: Biochemical and physiological correlates of hypothalamic peptides. The new endocrinology of the neuron. In *The Hypothalamus, Vol. 56.* Reichlin, S., Baldessarini, R. J., et al. (eds.), New York, Raven Press, 1978b, pp. 155–194.

Harris, G. W.: Neural control of the pituitary gland. *Physiol. Rev. 28:*139, 1948.

Hayward, J. N.: Functional and morphological aspects of hypothalamic neurons. *Physiol. Rev. 57:*574, 1977.

Iverson, L. L., Nicoll, R. A., et al.: Neurobiology of peptides. *Neurosci. Res. Program Bull. 16*(2):211, 1978.

Jeffcoate, S. L., and Hutchinson, J. S. M. (eds.): *The Endocrine Hypothalamus.* London, Academic Press, 1978.

Knigge, K. M., Scott, D. E., et al. (eds.): *Brain-Endocrine Interaction. Median Eminence: Structure and Function.* I (International Symposium on Brain-Endocrine Interaction, Munich, 1971.) White Plains, N. Y., A. J. Phiebig, B. Karger, Basel, 1972.

Knobil, E., and Sawyer, W. H. (eds.): The pituitary gland and its neuroendocrine control, In *Handbook of Physiology, Section 7: Endocrinology, Vol. IV, Pt. 1, 2.* American Physiological Society. Greep, R. O., and Astwood, E. B. (eds.), Baltimore, Williams & Wilkins, 1973.

Martin, J. B., Reichlin, S., et al.: *Clinical Neuroendocrinology.* Philadelphia, F. A. Davis Co., 1977.

Martini, L., and Ganong, W. F. (eds.): *Neuroendocrinology.* New York, Academic Press; Vol. 1, 1966, Vol. 2, 1967.

Martini, L., and Ganong, W. F. (eds.): *Frontiers in Neuroendocrinology.* New York, Oxford University Press; Vol. 1 (Ganong and Martini), 1969; Vol. 2 (Martini and Ganong), 1971; Vol. 3 (Martini and Ganong), 1973; Vol. 4 (Martini and Ganong), New York, Raven Press, 1976; Vol. 5 (Ganong and Martini), 1978.

Martini, L., and Besser, G. M.: *Clinical Neuroendocrinology.* New York, Academic Press, 1977.

Moore, R. Y.: Neuroendocrine regulation of reproduction, In *Reproductive Endocrinology: Physiology, Pathophysiology and Clinical Management.* Yen, S. S. C., and Jaffe, R. B. (eds.), Philadelphia, W. B. Saunders Co., 1978, pp. 3–33.

Naftolin, F., Ryan, K. J., et al. (eds.): Subcellular mechanisms in reproductive endocrinology. (Symposium on subcellular mechanisms in reproductive neuroendocrinology, Jamaica Plain, Mass., 1975.) New York, Elsevier-North Holland Pub. Co., 1976.

Pearse, A. G. E.: Diffuse neuroendocrine system: peptides common to brain and intestine and their relationship to the APUD concept, In *Centrally Acting Peptides.* Hughes, J. (ed.), Baltimore, Md., University Park Press, 1978, pp. 49.

Porter, J. C. (ed.): Hypothalamic peptide hormones and pituitary regulation. (Workshop on Peptide-Releasing Hormones, National Institutes of Health, 1976.) New York, Plenum Press, 1977.

Sawyer, C. H.: Neuroendocrine regulation: The peptidergic neuron, introduction and historical background, In *Central Regulation of the Endocrine System.* Fuxe, K., Hökfelt, T., et al. (eds.), New York, Plenum Press, 1978, pp. 3–8.

Stumpf, W. E., and Grant, L. D. (eds.): *Anatomical Neuroendocrinology:* Proceedings. (Conference on Neuroendocrinology, Chapel Hill, N. C.) White Plains, N. Y., A. J. Phiebig (Basel, S. Karger,) 1975.

Szentagothai, J., Flerko, B., et al.: *Hypothalamic Control of the Anterior Pituitary.* New York, Grune & Stratton, 1968.

Tolis, G., Labrie, F., Martin, J. B., and Naftolin, F. (eds.): *Clinical Neuroendocrinology.* New York, Raven Press, 1979.

Weitzman, M. (ed.): *Bibliographica Neuroendocrinologica.* New York, Albert Einstein School of Medicine, Department of Anatomy, published periodically.

Neurosecretion

Jeffrey, P. P. L., and Austin, L.: Axoplasmic transport, In *Progress in Neurobiology.* Kerkut, G. A., and Phillis, J. W., (eds.), Oxford, Pergamon Press, 1973.

Livett, B. G.: Axonal transport and neuronal dynamics: Contributions to the study of neuronal connectivity, In *Neurophysiology II,* Vol. 10. Porter R. (ed.), Baltimore, University Park Press, 1976, pp. 37–124.

Ochs, S., and Worth, R. M.: Axoplasmic transport in normal and pathological systems, In *Physiology and Pathology of Axons.* Waxman, S. G. (ed.), New York, Raven Press, pp. 251–264.

Pickering, B. T.: The neurosecretory neurone: A model system for the study of secretion, In *Essays in Biochemistry,* Vol. 14. 1978, pp. 45–81.

Sawyer, C. H.: Neuroendocrine regulation: The peptidergic neuron. Introduction and historical background. In *Central Regulation of the Endocrine System.* Fuxe, K., Hökfelt, I., and Luft, R. (eds.), New York, Plenum Press, 1978, pp. 3–8.

Scharrer, E., and Scharrer, B.: Secretory Cells within the hypothalamus, In *The Hypothalamus.* Association for Research on Nervous and Mental Disease. New York, Hafner Publishing Company, Inc., 1940, p. 170.

Wurtman, R. J., and Axelrod J.: The pineal gland. *Sci. Am. 213:*50–60, 1965.

Hypothalamic-Pituitary Unit

NEUROHYPOPHYSIS

Anatomy

Defendini, R., and Zimmerman, E. A.: The magnocellular neurosecretory system of the mammalian hypothalamus, In *The Hypothalamus, Vol. 56.* Reichlin, S., Baldessarini, R. J., et al. (eds.), New York, Raven Press, 1978, pp. 137–152.

Dierickx, K., and Vandesande, F.: Immunocytochemical demonstration of separate vasopressin-neurophysin and oxytocin-neurophysin neurons in the human hypothalamus. *Cell Tissue Res. 196:*203, 1979.

Sofroniew, M. V., and Weindl, A.: Extrahypothalamic neurophysin-containing perikarya, fiber pathways and fiber clusters in the rat brain. *Endocrinology 102:*334–337, 1978.

Secretions of the Neurohypophysis

Acher, R.: Chemistry of the neurohypophysial hormones: An example of molecular evolution, In *The Pituitary Gland and Its Neuroendocrine Control,* Part I, Washington, D.C., American Physiological Society, 1974, pp. 119–130.

Chard, T.: Oxytocin, In *Clinical Neuroendocrinology,* Martini, L., and Besser, G. M. (eds.), New York, Academic Press, 1977, pp. 569–583.

Edwards, C. R. W.: Vasopressin, In *Clinical Neuroendocrinology.* Martini, L., and Besser, G. M. (eds.), New York, Academic Press, 1977, pp. 527–567.

Heller, H.: History of neurohypophysial research. In *Handbook of Physiology, Endocrinology.* Vol. 4, Part I. Washington, D. C., American Physiological Society, 1974, 103–117.

Pickering, B. T.: Neurohypophysial Hormones—Comparative Aspects. 1978 In Jeffcoate, S. L., and Hutchinson, J. S. M. (eds.), *The Endocrine Hypothalamus.* London, Academic Press, pp. 213–227.

Robinson, A. G.: Isolation, assay and secretion of individual human neurophysins. *J. Clin. Invest. 55*:360, 1975.

Robinson, A. G.: Neurophysins, In *Clinical Neuroendocrinology.* Martini, L., and Besser, G. M. (eds.), New York, Academic Press, 1977, pp. 585–602.

Hormone Synthesis, Transport, and Secretion

Brownstein, M. J., Russell, J. T., and Gainer, H.: Synthesis, transport, and release of posterior pituitary hormones. *Science 207*:373–378, 1980.

Thorn, N. A., Russel, J. T., et al.: Activation of release and mechanism of release of neurohypophyseal hormones, In *Central Regulation of the Endocrine System.* Fuxe, K., Hökfelt, T., et al. (eds.), New York, Plenum Press, 1978, pp. 49–60.

Physiologic Regulation of Neurohypophyseal Hormone Release

Andersson, B., Leksell, L. G., et al.: Perturbations in fluid balance induced by medially placed forebrain lesions. *Brain Res. 99*:261, 1975.

Fitzsimmons, J. T.: Thirst. *Physiol. Rev. 52*(2):468, 1972.

Fitzsimmons, J. T., Epstein, A. N., et al.: The peptide specificity of receptors for angiotensin-induced thirst, In *Central Actions of Angiotensin and Related Hormones.* Buckley, J. P., and Ferrario, C. M. (eds.), New York, Plenum Press, 1977, pp. 405–415.

Miller, M., and Moses, A. M.: Clinical states due to alteration of ADH release and action, In *Neurohypophysis.* (International Conference, Key Biscayne, Florida, 1976) White Plains, N. Y., A. J. Phiebig (Basel, S. Karger), 1977.

Phillips, M. I., and Felix, D.: Specific angiotensin II receptive neurons in the cat subfornical organ. *Brain Res. 109*:531, 1976.

Robertson, G. L.: The regulation of vasopressin function in health and disease. *Recent Progr. Horm. Res. 33*:333, 1977.

MEDIAN EMINENCE AND TUBEROHYPOPHYSEAL NEURONS

Anatomy

Brownstein, M. J.: Distribution of LHRH and SRIF in the Central Nervous System, In *Central Nervous System Effects of Hypothalamic Hormones.* Collu, R., Barbeau, A., et al. (eds.), New York, Raven Press, 1978, pp. 325–330.

Hokfelt, T., Elde, R., et al.: Aminergic and peptidergic pathways in the nervous system with special reference to the hypothalamus, In *The Hypothalamus, Vol. 56.* Reichlin, S., Baldessarini, R. J., et al. (eds.), New York, Raven Press, 1978, pp. 69–135.

Jackson, I. M. D.: Extrahypothalamic and phylogenetic distribution of hypothalamic peptides, In *The Hypothalamus, Vol. 56.* Reichlin, S., Baldessarini, R. J., et al. (eds.), New York, Raven Press, 1978, pp. 217–231.

Joseph, S. A., and Knigge, K. N.: The endocrine hypothalamus: recent anatomical studies, In *The Hypothalamus, Vol. 56.* Reichlin, S., Baldessarini, R. J., et al. (eds.), New York, Raven Press, 1979, pp. 15–47.

Knigge, K. M., Joseph, S. A., et al.: Organization of LRF and SRIF neurons in the endocrine hypothalamus, In *The Hypothalamus, Vol. 56.* Reichlin, S., Baldessarini, R. J., et al. (eds.), New York, Raven Press, 1978, pp. 49–67.

Pelletier, G.: Immunohistochemical localization of hypothalamic hormones and other peptides in the central nervous system, In *The Central Nervous System Effects of Hypothalamic Hormones.* Collu R., Barbeau, A., et al. (eds.), New York, Raven Press, 1979, pp. 331–344.

Renaud, L. P.: Neurophysiological organization of the endocrine hypothalamus, In *The Hypothalamus, Vol. 56.* Reichlin, S., Baldessarini, R. J., et al. (eds.), New York, Raven Press, 1978, pp. 269–301.

Renaud, L. P., Blume, H. W., et al.: Neurophysiology and neuropharmacology of the hypothalamic tuberoinfundibular system, In *Frontiers in Neuroendocrinology,* Vol. 5. Ganong, W. F., and Martini, L. (eds.), New York, Raven Press, 1978, pp. 135–162.

Zimmerman, E. A., Hsu, K. C., et al.: Localization of gonadotropin-releasing hormone (GnRH) in the hypothalamus of the mouse by immunoperoxidase technique. *Endocrinology 95*:1, 1974.

Portal Vessel–Chemotransmitter Control

Adams, J. H., Daniel, P. M., et al.: Some effects of transection of the pituitary stalk. *Br. Med. J. 2*:1619, 1964.

Bennett, G. W., Edwardson, J. A., et al.: Release of somatostatin from rat brain synaptosomes. *J. Neurochem. 32*:1127, 1979.

Berelowitz, M., Hudson, A., et al.: Subcellular localization of growth hormone release inhibiting hormone in rat hypothalamus, cerebral cortex, striatum and thalamus. *J. Neurochem. 31*:751, 1978.

Bergland, R. M., and Page, R. B.: Pituitary-brain vascular relations: a new paradigm. *Science 204*:18, 1979.

Correa, F. M. A., Innis, R. B., et al.: Bradykinin-like immunoreactive neuronal systems localized histochemically in rat brain, *Proc. Natl. Acad. Sci. 76*:1489, 1979.

Epelbaum, J., Brazeau, P., et al.: Subcellular distribution of radioimmunoassayable somatostatin in rat brain. *Brain Res. 126*:309, 1977.

Fink, G.: The development of the releasing factor concept. *Clinical Endocrinology,* 1976, *5* (Suppl.): 245s–260s.

Friedgood, H. B.: Studies on the sympathetic nervous control of the anterior hypophysis with special reference to a neuro-humoral mechanism, Symposium on endocrine glands, Harvard Tercent. celebration, 1936, reprinted in *J. Reprod. Fertil. 10*(Suppl.):3.

Green, J. D., and Harris, G. W.: Neurovascular link between neurohypophysis and adenohypophysis. *J. Endocrinol. 5*:136, 1947.

Hinsey, J. C., and Markee, J. E.: Pregnancy following bilateral section of the cervical sympathetic trunks in the rabbit. *Proc. Soc. Exp. Biol. N.Y. 31*:270–271, 1933.

Hökfelt, T., Elde, R., et al.: Immunohistochemical evidence for the presence of somatostatin, a powerful inhibitory peptide in some primary sensory neurons. *Neurosci. Lett 1*:231, 1975.

Hökfelt, T., Elde, R. P., et al.: Immunohistochemical evidence for separate populations of somatostatin-containing and substance P-containing primary afferent neurons. *Neuroscience I*:131, 1976.

Hökfelt, T., Elfvin, L. G., et al.: Occurrence of somatostatin-like immunoreactivity in some peripheral sympathetic noradrenergic neurons, *Proc. Natl. Acad. Sci. 74*(8):3587, 1977.

Jan, Y. N., Jan, L. Y., et al.: A peptide as a possible transmitter in sympathetic ganglia of the frog. *Proc. Natl. Acad. Sci. 76*:1501, 1979.

Oliver, C., Mical, R. S., et al.: Hypothalamic-pituitary vasculature: evidence for retrograde blood flow in the pituitary stalk. *Endocrinology 101*(2):598, 1977.

Samson, W. K., Said, S. I., et al.: Radioimmunologic localization of vasoactive polypeptide (VIP) in hypothalamic and extrahypothalamic sites in the rat brain, *Neuroscience Letter 12*:265, 1979.

Wise, P. M., Rance, N., et al.: Further evidence that luteinizing hormone-releasing hormone also is follicle-stimulating hormone-releasing hormone. *Endocrinology 104*:940, 1979.

HYPOPHYSIOTROPIC HORMONES OF THE HYPOTHALAMUS

Burgus, R., Dunn, T. F., et al.: Structure moléculaire du facteur hypothalamique hypophyisiotrope TRF d'origine ovine; mise en évidence par spectrométrie de masse de la séquence PCA-His-Pro-NH$_2$ C. R., *Acad. Sci.* (Paris) *269*:1870, 1969.

Bowers, C. Y., Friesen, H. G., et al.: Prolactin and thyrotropin release in man by synthetic pyroglutamyl-histidyl-prolinamide. *Biochem. Biophys. Res. Commun. 45*(4):1033, 1971.

Bowers, C. Y., Schally, A. V., et al.: Porcine thyrotropin releasing hormone is (pyro)glu-his-pro (NH$_2$). *Endocrinology 86*:1143, 1970.

Brazeau, P., Vale, W., et al.: Hypothalamic polypeptide that inhibits the secretion of immunoreactive pituitary growth hormone. *Science 179*:77, 1973.

Brodish, A.: Extra-CNS corticotropin-releasing factor. *Ann. N.Y. Acad. Sci. 297*:420, 1977.

Brownstein, M.: Biologically active peptides in the mammalian central nervous system, In *Peptides in Neurobiology.* Gainer, H. (ed.), New York, Plenum Press, 1977, pp. 145–170.

Ehrensing, R. H., and Kastin, A. J.: TRH: clinical investigations for non-endocrine actions in man, In *Clinical Neuroendocrinology.* Martini, L., and Besser, G. M. (eds.), New York, Academic Press, 1978, pp. 133–142.

Frohman, L. A., Newer understanding of human hypothalamic-pituitary disease obtained through the use of synthetic hypothalamic hormones, In *The Hypothalamus, Vol. 56.* Reichlin, S., Baldessarini, R. J., et al. (eds.), New York, Raven Press, 1978, pp. 387–413.

Gay, V. L.: The hypothalamus: physiology and clinical use of releasing factors. *Fertil. Steril. 23*:50, 1972.

Guillemin, R.: Peptides in the brain: The new Endocrinology of the neuron. *Science 202*:390–402 (Nobel Prize Lecture 1977), 1978.

Guillemin, R., and Gerich, J.: Somatostatin: physiological and clinical significance. *Annu. Rev. Med. 27*:379, 1976.

Hershman, J. M.: Clinical application of thyrotropin-releasing hormone. *New Engl. J. Med. 290*(16):886, 1974.

Jackson, I. M. D.: The releasing factors of the hypothalamus. In Barrington, E. J. W. (ed.), *Hormones and Evolution,* Huntington, N. Y., Robert Krieger 1979, pp. 723–789.

Jackson, I. M. D., and Reichlin, S.: Distribution and biosynthesis of TRH in the nervous system, In *Central Nervous System Effects of Hypothalamic Hormones.* Collu R., Barbeau, A., et al. (eds.), New York, Raven Press, 1978, pp. 3–34.

Jones, M. T., and Hillhouse, E. W.: Neurotransmitter regulation of corticotropin-releasing factor in vitro. *Ann. N.Y. Acad. Sci. 297*:536, 1977.

Kamberi, I. A., Mical, R. S., et al.: Hypophyseal portal vessel infusion:in vivo demonstration of LRF, FRF, and PIF in pituitary stalk plasma. *Endocrinology 89*:1042, 1971.

Koch, Y., Goldhaber, G. G., et al.: Suppression of prolactin and thyrotropin secretion in the rat by antiserum to thyrotropin-releasing hormone. *Endocrinology 100*:1476, 1977.

Krieger, D. T., and Zimmerman, E. A.: The nature of CRF and its relationship to vasopressin, In *Clinical Neuroendocrinology*. Martini, L., and Besser, G. M.(eds.), New York, Academic Press, 1978, pp. 364–391.

Krulich, L., Dhariwal, A. P., et al.: Stimulatory and inhibitory effects of purified hypothalamic extracts on growth hormone release from rat pituitary in vitro. *Endocrinology 83*:783, 1968.

Marks, N.: Biotransformation and degradation of corticotropins, lipotropins and hypothalamic peptides, In *Frontiers in Neuroendocrinology*, Vol. 5. Ganong, W. F., and Martini, L. (eds.), New York, Raven Press, 1978, pp. 329–377.

Meites, J.: Control of mammary growth and lactation, In *Neuroendocrinology*. Vol. 1, Martini, L., and Ganong, W. F. (eds.), New York, Academic Press, 1966–1967, pp. 669–707.

Mortimer, C. H.: Growth hormone release-inhibiting hormone (GH-RIH, somatostatin), In *Clinical Neuroendocrinology*. Martini, L., and Besser, G. M. (eds.), New York, Academic Press, 1978, pp. 279–294.

Mortimer, C. H.: Gonadotropin-releasing hormone, In *Clinical Neuroendocrinology*. Martini, L., and Besser, G. M. (eds.), New York, Academic Press, 1978, pp. 213–236.

Mortimer, C. H., et al.: The luteinizing hormone and follicle stimulating hormone-releasing hormone test in patients with hypothalamic-pituitary-gonadal dysfunction. *Br. Med. J. 4*:73, 1974.

Moss, R. L.: Actions of hypothalamic-hypophysiotropic hormones on the brain. *Ann. Rev. Physiol.* 41:617–631, 1979.

Moss, R., Riskand, P., et al.: The effects of LHRH on sexual activities in animals and man, In *Central Nervous Systems Effects of Hypothalamic Hormones*. Collu, R., Barbeau, J., et al. (eds.), New York, Raven Press, 1978, pp. 345–367.

Prange, A., Jr., Nemeroff, C. B., et al.: Behavioral effects of thyrotropin-releasing hormone in animals and man: a review, In *Central Nervous System Effects of Hypothalamic Hormones*. Collu, R., Barbeau, A., et al. (eds.), New York, Raven Press, 1978, pp. 75–96.

Roth, J. C., Grumbach, M. M., et al.: Effect of synthetic luteinizing hormone-releasing factor on serum testosterone and gonadotropins in prepubertal, pubertal and adult males. *J. Clin. Endocrinol. Metab. 37*:680, 1973.

Saffran, M.: Chemistry of hypothalamic hypophysiotropic factors. In *Handbook of Physiology-Endocrinology*, Vol. 4, Pt. 2, Washington D.C., American Physiological Society, 1974, pp. 563–586.

Saffran, M., Schally, A. V., et al.: Stimulation of the release of corticotrophin from the adenohypophysis by neurohypophyseal factor. *Endocrinology 57*:439, 1955.

Sandow, J., and König, W.: Chemistry of the hypothalamic hormones, In *The Endocrine Hypothalamus*. Jeffcoate, S. L., and Hutchinson, J. S. M. (eds.), New York, Academic Press, 1978, pp. 150–212.

Schally, A. V.: Aspects of hypothalamic regulation of the pituitary gland. Its implications for the control of reproductive processes. *Science 202*: 18–28 (Nobel Prize Lecture 1977), 1978.

Schally, A. V., and Arimura, A.: Physiology and nature of hypothalamic regulatory hormones, In *Clinical Neuroendocrinology*. Martini, L., and Besser, G. M., (eds.), New York, Academic Press, 1978, pp. 2–42.

Schally, A. V., Arimura, A., et al.: Hypothalamic hormones regulating pituitary (and other) functions: their physiology and biochemistry as well as recent studies with their synthetic analogues, In *Central Regulation of the Endocrine System*. Fuxe, K., Hökfelt, T., et al. (eds.), New York, Plenum Press, 1979, pp. 9–30.

Schally, A. V., Kastin, A. J., et al.: Hypothalamic follicle-stimulating hormone (FSH) and luteinizing hormone (LH)-regulating hormone: structure, physiology and clinical studies, *Fertil. Steril. 22*:703, 1971.

Schally, A. V., Nair, R. M., et al.: Isolation of the luteinizing hormone and follicle-stimulating hormone-releasing hormone from porcine hypothalami. *J. Biol. Chem. 246*:7230, 1971.

Siler, T. M., Vanderberg, G., et al.: Inhibition of growth hormone release in humans by somatostatin. *J. Clin. Endocrinol. Metab. 37*:632, 1973.

Snyder, J. J., Jacobs, L. S., et al.: Diagnostic value of thyrotrophin-releasing hormone in pituitary and hypothalamic diseases: assessment of thyrotrophin and prolactin in 100 patients. *Ann. Intern. Med. 81*:751, 1974.

Vale, W., Brazeau, P., et al.: Somatostatin. *Recent Progr. Horm. Res. 31*:365, 1975.

Vale, W., Grant, G., et al.: Chemistry of the hypothalamic releasing factors: studies on structure-function relationships, In *Frontiers in Neuroendocrinology*. Ganong, W. F., and Martini, L. (eds.), New York, Oxford University Press, 1973, pp. 375–413.

Vale, W., Rivier, C., et al.: Regulatory peptides of the hypothalamus. *Annu. Rev. Med. 39*:473, 1977.

Vale, W., Rivier, C., et al.: Pharmacology of thyrotropin releasing factor

(LRF) and somatostatin, In *Hypothalamic Peptide Hormones and Pituitary Regulation*. Porter, J. C. (ed.), New York, Plenum Press, 1977, pp. 123–156.

Vale, W., Rivier, J., et al.: Effects of purified CRF and other substances on the secretion of ACTH and β endorphin like immunoactivity by cultured anterior or neurointermediate pituitary cells, In *Central Nervous System Effects of Hypothalamic Hormones*. Collu, R., Barbeau, A., et al. (eds.), New York, Raven Press, 1978, pp. 163–176.

Winokur, A., and Utiger, R. D.: Thyrotropin-releasing hormone in the central nervous system: distribution and degradation, In *Central Nervous System Effects of Hypothalamic Hormones*. Collu R., Barbeau, A., et al. (eds.), New York, Raven Press, 1978, pp. 35–64.

Melanocyte-Stimulating Hormone Regulatory Factors

Kastin, A. J., Viosca, S., et al.: Regulation of melanocyte-stimulating hormone release, In *Handbook of Physiology*, Section 7: *Endocrinology*. Vol. IV, Pt. 2. Greep, R. O., and Astwood, E. B. (eds.), American Physiological Society. Baltimore, Williams & Wilkins, 1974, pp. 551–562.

Sandman, C. A., Kastin, A. J., et al.: Central nervous system actions of MSH and related pituitary peptides, In *Clinical Neuroendocrinoloy*. Martini, L., and Besser, G. M., (eds.), New York, Academic Press, 1978, pp. 443–469.

Taleisnik, S.: Control of melanocyte-stimulating hormone (MSH) secretion, In *The Endocrine Hypothalamus*. Jeffcoate, S. L., and Hutchinson, J. S. M. (eds.), New York, Academic Press, 1978, pp. 421–438.

Regulation of Secretion of Tuberhypophyseal Neurons: Neuropharmacology of Hypothalamic Regulation

Hutchinson, J. S. M.: Control of the Endocrine hypothalamus, In *The Endocrine Hypothalamus*. Jeffcoate, S. L., and Hutchinson, J. S. M. (eds.), New York, Academic Press, 1978, pp. 75–106.

Livett, B. G.: Histochemical visualization of peripheral and central adrenergic neurons. *Br. Med. Bull.* 29:93, 1973.

NEUROTRANSMITTER REGULATION OF HYPOPHYSIOTROPIC NEURONS

Boyd, A. E., Lebovitz, H. E., et al.: Stimulation of human-growth-hormone secretion by L-dopa. *New Engl. J. Med. 283*:1425, 1970.

Brown, M., and Vale, W.: Central nervous system effects of hypothalamic peptides. *Endocrinology 96*(5):1333, 1975.

Carraway, R., and Leeman, S. E.: The isolation of a new hypotensive peptide, neurotensin, from bovine hypothalami. *J. Biol. Chem. 248*(19):6854, 1973.

Collu, R.: Role of central cholinergic and aminergic neurotransmitters in the control of anterior pituitary hormone secretion, In *Clinical Neuroendocrinology*. Martini, L., and Besser, G. M. (eds.), New York, Academic Press, 1978, pp. 44–65.

Cooper, J. R., Bloom, F. E., et al.: *The Biochemical Basis of Neuropharmacology*. 3rd ed. New York, Oxford University Press, 1978.

del Pozo, E., and Lancranjan, I.: Clinical use of drugs modifying the release of anterior pituitary hormones. *Frontiers in neuroendocrinology 5*: 209–247.

Dupont, A., Cusan, L., et al.: Evidence for a role of endorphins in the control of prolactin secretion, In *Central Nervous System Effects of Hypothalamic Hormones*. Collu. R., Barbeau, A., et al. (eds.), New York, Raven Press, 1978, pp. 283–300.

Fuxe, K., Andersson, K., et al.: Neurotransmitter mechanisms in the control of the secretion of hormones from the anterior pituitary, In *Central Regulation of the Endocrine System*. Fuxe, K., Hökfelt, T., et al. (eds.), New York, Plenum Press, 1979, pp. 349–380.

Ganong, W. F.: Neurotransmitters involved in ACTH secretion: catecholamines. *Ann. N.Y. Acad. Sci. 297*:509, 1977.

Kanazawa, I., Emson, P. C., et al.: Evidence for the existence of substance P-containing fibres in striato-nigral and pallido-nigral pathways in rat brain. *Brain Res. 119*:447, 1977.

Krieger, D. T.: Serotonin regulation of ACTH secretion. *Ann N.Y. Acad. Sci. 297*:527, 1977.

Labrie, F., Beaulieu, M., et al.: Control of prolactin secretion at the pituitary level: A model for postsynaptic dopaminergic systems, In *Central Nervous System Effects of Hypothalamic Hormones*. Collu, R., Barbeau, A., et al. (eds.), New York, Raven Press, 1978, pp. 207–236.

Leeman, S. E., and Mroz, E. A.: Substance P. *Life Sci.* 15:2033, 1974.

Martini, L., Celotti, F., et al.: Feedback effects on central mechanism controlling neuroendocrine functions, In *Central Regulation of the Endocrine System*. Fuxe, K., Hökfelt, T., et al. (eds.), New York, Plenum Press, 1979, pp. 273–296.

McCann, S. M., Kruølich, et al.: Neurotransmitters in the control of anterior pituitary function, In *Central Regulation of the Endocrine System*. Fuxe, K., Hökfelt, T., et al. (eds.), New York, Plenum Press, 1979, pp. 329–348.

McCann, S. M., and Moss, R. L.: Putative neurotransmitters involved in discharging gonadotropin-releasing neurohormones and the action of LH-releasing hormones on the CNS. *Life Sci.* 16:833, 1975.

Montoya, E., Wilber, J. F., et al.: Catecholaminergic control of thyrotropin secretion. *J. Lab. Clin. Med.* 93:887, 1979.

Müller, E. E., Nistico, G., et al. (eds.): *Neurotransmitters and Anterior Pituitary Function.* New York, Academic Press, 1977.

Pearse, A. G. E.: Diffuse neuroendocrine systems: Peptides common to brain and intestine and their relationship to the APUD concept. In *Centrally Acting Peptides.* Hughes, J. (ed.), University Park Press, Baltimore, 1978, 49–58.

Rivier, C., Vale, W., et al.: Stimulation in vivo of secretion of prolactin and growth hormone by β-endorphin. *Endocrinology* 100:238, 1977.

Snyder, S. H.: Peptide neurotransmitter candidates in the brain: focus on enkephalin, angiotensin II and neurotensin, In *The Hypothalamus, Vol. 56.* Reichlin, S., Baldessarini, R. J., et al. (eds.), New York, Raven Press, 1978, pp. 233–243.

Snyder, S. H., and Bennett, J. P.: Neurotransmitter receptors in the brain: biochemical indentification. *Annu. Rev. Physiol.* 38:153, 1976.

Vernikos-Danellis, J., Kellar, K. J., et al.: Serotonin involvement in pituitary-adrenal function. *Ann. N.Y. Acad. Sci.* 297:518, 1977.

Weiner, R. I., and Ganong, W. F.: Role of brain monoamines and histamine in regulation of anterior pituitary secretion. *Physiol. Rev.* 58:905–976, 1978.

The Endorphins

Barchas, J. D., Akil, H., Elliott, G. R., Holman, R. B., and Watson, S. J. Behavioural neurochemistry: Neuroregulators and behavioural states. *Science* 200:964–973, 1978.

Garfield, E.: Current comments. Controversies over opiate receptor research typify problems facing awards committees. *Current Contents* 20:5–18, May 14, 1979.

Goldstein, A.: Opioid peptides (endorphins) in pituitary and brain. *Science* 193:1081, 1976.

Hughes, J., Kosterlitz, H. W., et al.: Pharmacological and biochemical aspects of the enkephalins, In *Centrally Acting Peptides.* Hughes, J. (ed.), Baltimore, University Park Press, 1978, p. 179.

Hughes, J., Smith, T. W., et al.: Identification of two related pentapeptides from the brain with potent opiate agonist activity. *Nature* 258:577, 1975.

Kosterlitz, H. W.: Endogenous opioid peptides: historical aspects, In *Centrally Acting Peptides.* Hughes J. (ed.), Baltimore, University Park Press, 1978, p. 157.

Krieger, D. T., and Liotta, A. S.: Pituitary hormones in brain: Where, how, and why. *Science* 205:366, 1979.

Lazarus, L. H., Ling, N., et al.: Beta-lipotropin as a prohormone for morphinometic peptides, endorphins and enkephalins. *Proc. Natl. Acad. Sci.* 73:2156, 1976.

Li, C. H., Barnafi, L., et al.: Isolation and amino acid sequence of β-LPH from sheep pituitary glands. *Nature* 208:1093, 1975.

Liotta, A. S., Gildersleeve, D., et al.: Biosynthesis in vitro of immunoreactive 31,000-dalton corticotropin/β-endorphin-like material by bovine hypothalamus. *Proc. Natl. Acad. Sci.* 76(1):1448, 1979.

Lord, J. A. H., Waterfield, A. A., et al.: Endogenous opioid peptides: Multiple agonists and receptors. *Nature* 367:495, 1977.

Mains, R. E., Eipper, B. A., et al.: Common precursor to corticotropins and endorphins. *Proc. Natl. Acad. Sci.* 74:3014, 1977.

Meites, J., Bruni, J. F., et al.: Effects of endogenous opiate peptides on release of anterior pituitary hormones, In *Central Nervous System Effects of Hypothalamic Hormones.* Collu, R., Barbeau, A., et al. (eds.), New York, Raven Press, 1978, pp. 261–272.

Miller, R. J., Chang, K. J., Cuatrecasas, P.: Distribution and pharmacology of the enkephalins and related opiate peptides, In *Centrally Acting Peptides.* Hughes, J. (ed.), Baltimore, University Park Press, 1978, p. 195.

Nakanishi, S., Inoue, A., et al.: Nucleotide sequence of cloned cDNA for bovine corticotropin-β-lipotropin precursor. *Nature* 278:423, 1979.

Neill, J. D.: Prolactin: its secretion and control, In *Handbook of Physiology, Section 7: Endocrinology. Vol. IV, Pt. 2.* American Physiological Society, Greep, R. O., and Astwood, E. B. (eds.), Baltimore, Williams and Wilkins, 1974, pp. 469–488.

Rivier, C., Brown, M., et al.: Effect of neurotensin, substance P and morphine sulfate on the secretion of prolactin and growth hormone in rat. *Endocrinology* 100:751, 1977.

Rivier, C., Rivier, J., et al.: The effect of bombesin and related peptides on prolactin and growth hormone secretion in the rat. *Endocrinology* 102:519, 1978.

Rossier, J., Vargo, T., et al.: Regional dissociation of β-endorphin and enkephalin contents in rat brain and pituitary. *Proc. Natl. Acad. Sci.* 74:5162, 1977.

Simantov, R., Kuhar, M. J., et al.: Opioid peptide enkephalin: immunohistochemical mapping in rat central nervous system. *Proc. Natl. Acad. Sci.* 74:2167, 1977.

Simon, E. J.: Opiate receptor binding with H-Etorphine. Neurosci. *Neurosci. Res. Program Bull.* 13:43–50, 1975.

Snyder, S. H.: Opiate receptors and internal opiates. *Sci. Amer.* 236(3):44–56.

Tache, Y., Charpenet, G., et al.: Role of serotonergic pathways in hormonal changes induced by opioid peptides, In *Central Nervous System Effects of Hypothalamic Hormones.* Collu, R., Barbeau, A., et al. (eds.), New York, Raven Press, 1978, pp. 301–316.

Terenius, L.: The opioid receptors and their ligands, In *The Central Regulation of the Endocrine System.* Fuxe, E., and Hökfelt, T. (eds.), New York, Plenum Press, 1977, pp. 137–148.

Terenius, L., and Wahlstrom, A.: Physiological and clinical relevance of endorphins, In *Centrally Acting Peptides.* Hughes, J. (ed.), Baltimore, University Park Press, 1978, p. 161–178.

Uhl, G. R., Childers, S. R., and Snyder, S. H.: Opioid peptides and the opiate receptor. *Frontiers in Neuroendocrinology* 5:289–328, 1978.

Vijayan, E., and McCann, S. M.: In vivo and in vitro effects of substance P and neurotensin on gonadotropin and prolactin release. *Endocrinology* 105(1):64, 1979.

Vijayan, E., Samson, W. K., et al.: Vasoactive intestinal peptide (VIP): Evidence for a hypothalamic site of action to release growth hormone, luteinizing hormone and prolactin in conscious ovariectomized rats. *Endocrinology* 104:53, 1979.

Neuroendocrine Aspects of Control of Specific Pituitary Tropic Hormones

Aron, C.: Mechanisms of control of the reproduction function of olfactory stimuli in female mammals. *Physiol. Rev.* 59(2):229, 1979.

Bardin, C. W.: Pituitary-testicular axis, In *Reproductive Endocrinology: Physiology, Pathophysiology and Clinical Management.* Yen, S. S. C., and Jaffe, R. B. (eds.), Philadelphia, W. B. Saunders, 1978, pp. 110–125.

Burger, H. G., and Patel, Y. C.: TSH and TRH: their physiological regulation and the clinical applications of TRH, In *Clinical Neuroendocrinology.* Martini, L., and Besser, G. M. (eds.), New York, Academic Press, 1978, pp. 67–131.

Chan, V., Jones, A., et al.: The relationship between circadian variations in circulating thyrotropin, thyroid hormones and prolactin. *Clin. Endocrinol.* 9:337, 1978.

Cryer, P. E., and Daughaday, W. H.: Growth hormone, In *Clinical Neuroendocrinology.* Martini, L., and Besser, G. M., (eds.), New York, Academic Press, 1978, pp. 243–277.

Donovan, B. T., and van der Werff ten Bosch, J. J.: *Physiology of Puberty.* Baltimore, Williams and Wilkins, 1965.

Franchimont, P., and Roulier, R.: Gonadotropin secretion in male subjects, In *Clinical Neuroendocrinology.* Martini, L., and Besser, G. M. (eds.), New York, Academic Press, 1978, pp. 197–212.

Ganong, W. F., Alpert, L. C., et al.: ACTH and the regulation of adrenocortical secretion. *New Engl. J. Med.* 290(18):1006, 1974.

Gudelsky, G. A., and Porter, J. C.: Release of dopamine from Tuberoinfundibular neurons into pituitary stalk blood after prolactin or haloperidol administration. *Endocrinology* 106:526, 1980.

Hershman, J. M., and Pittman, J. A.: Control of thyrotropin secretion in man. *New Engl. J. Med.* 285(18):997, 1971.

Job, J. C.: The neuroendocrine system and puberty, In *Clinical Neuroendocrinology.* Martini, L., and Besser, G. M. (eds.), New York, Academic Press, 1978, pp. 488–501.

Jones, M. T.: Control of corticotrophin (ACTH) secretion. In *The Endocrine Hypothalamus.* Jeffcoate, S. L., and Hutchinson, J. S. M. (eds.), New York, Academic Press, 1978, pp. 386–420.

Karsch, F. J., Dierschke, D. J., and Knobil, E.: Sexual differentiation of pituitary function: Apparent difference between primates and rodents. *Science* 179:484–486, 1973.

Knobil, E., and Plant, T. M.: The hypothalamic regulation of LH and FSH secretion in the Rhesus monkey, In *The Hypothalamus, Vol. 56.* Reichlin, S., Baldessarini, R. J., et al. (eds.), New York, Raven Press, 1978, pp. 359–372.

Labrie, F., Drouin, J., et al.: Interactions between hypothalamic and peripheral hormones at the anterior pituitary level, In *Central Regulation of the Endocrine System.* Fuxe, K., Hökfelt, T., et al. (eds.), New York, Plenum Press, 1979, pp. 85–198.

Lembeck, F.: Substance P: a historical account, In *Centrally Acting Peptides.* Hughes, J. (ed.), Baltimore, University Park Press, 1978, p. 119.

Liddle, G. W., Island, D., et al.: Normal and abnormal regulation of corticotropin secretion in man. *Recent Progr. Horm. Res.* 18:125, 1962.

Martin, J. B.: Neural regulation of growth hormone secretion. *New Engl. J. Med.* 288(26):1384, 1973.

Martin, J. B., Brazeau, P., et al.: Neuroendocrine organization of growth hormone regulation, In *The Hypothalamus, Vol. 56.* Reichlin S., Baldessarini, R. J., et al. (eds.), New York, Raven Press, 1978, pp. 329–357.

McCann, S. M.: Regulation of secretion of follicle-stimulating hormone and luteinizing hormone, In *Handbook of Physiology, Section 7: Endocrinology. Vol. IV, Pt. 2.* Greep, R. O., and Astwood, E. B. (eds.), American Physiological Society. Baltimore, Williams and Wilkins, 1974, pp. 489–518.

McEwen, B. S., Davis, P. G., et al.: Steroid hormone receptors in brain and pituitary, In *Central Regulation of the Endocrine System.* Fuxe, K., Hökfelt, T., et al. (eds.), New York, Plenum Press, 1979, pp. 261–272.

McEwen, B. S., Krey, L. C., et al.: Steroid hormone action in the neuroendocrine system: When is the genome involved? In *The Hypothalamus, Vol. 56.* Reichlin S., Baldessarini, R. J., et al. eds.), New York, Raven Press, 1978, pp. 255–268.

Meites, J.: Control of mammary growth and lactation, In *Neuroendocrin-*

ology. Martini, L., and Ganong, W. F. (eds.), New York, Academic Press, 1966, pp. 669–707.

Molitch, M. E., Edmonds, M., et al.: Specificity of short-loop feedback of luteinizing hormone in the rabbit. *Neuroendocrinology* 29:49, 1979.

Nillius, S. J.: Normal gonadotropin secretion in females, In *Clinical Neuroendocrinology.* Martini, L., and Besser, G. M. (eds.), New York, Academic Press, 1978, pp. 144–174.

Palkovits, M.: Neural pathways involved in ACTH regulation, *Ann. N.Y. Acad. Sci., 297:*455, 1977.

Palkovits, M.: Neural pathways involved in ACTH regulation, In *ACTH and Regulated Peptides: Structure, Regulation and Action.* (Annals of the New York Academy of Sciences), N.Y. Acad. Sci., 1977.

Pecile, A., and Olgiati, V. R.: Control of growth hormone secretion, In *The Endocrine Hypothalamus.* Jeffcoate, S. L., and Hutchinson, J. S. M. (eds.), New York, Academic Press, 1978, pp. 362–385.

Pfaff, D. W.: Peptide and steroid hormones and the neural mechanisms for female reproductive behavior, In *The Hypothalamus, Vol. 56.* Reichlin, S., Baldessarini, R. J., et al. (eds.), New York, Raven Press, 1978, pp. 245–253.

Rees, L. H.: Human adrenocorticotropin and lipotropin (MSH) in health and disease, In *Clinical Neuroendocrinology.* Martini, L., and Besser, G. M. (eds.), New York, Academic Press, 1978, pp. 402–404.

Reichlin, S.: Control of thyrotropic hormone secretion. In *Neuroendocrinology.* Margini, L. and Ganong, W. F. (eds.), New York, Academic Press, pp. 445–536.

Reichlin, S.: Regulation of somatotropic hormone secretion, In *Handbook of Physiology. Section 7: Endocrinology, Vol. IV.* American Physiological Society, Greep, R. O., and Astwood, E. B. (eds.), Baltimore, Williams and Wilkins, 1974, pp. 405–447.

Reichlin, S., Martin, J. B., et al.: The hypothalamus in pituitary-thyroid regulation. *Recent Progr. Horm. Res.* 28:229, 1972.

Reichlin, S., Martin, J. B., et al.: Regulation of thyroid-stimulating hormone (TSH) secretion, In *The Endocrine Hypothalamus.* Jeffcoate, S. L., and Hutchinson, J. S. M. (eds.), New York, Academic Press, 1978, pp. 230–270.

Schwartz, N. B.: A model for the regulation of ovulation in the rat. *Recent Progr. Horm. Res.* 25:1, 1969.

Sharp, P. J., Fraser, H. M.: Control of reproduction, In *The Endocrine Hypothalamus.* Jeffcoate, S. L., and Hutchinson, J. S. M. (eds.), New York, Academic Press, 1978, pp. 271–332.

Smals, A. G. H., Kloppenborg, P. W. C., et al.: Modulation of the gonadotropin response to constant luteinizing hormone-releasing hormone infusion by acute and chronic testosterone administration in Klinefelters syndrome. *J. Clin. Endocrinol. Metab.* 48:148, 1979.

Stearns, E. L., Winter, J. S. D., and Faiman, C.: Positive feedback effect of progestin upon serum gonadotropins in estrogen-primed castrate men. *J. Clin. Endocrinol.* 37:635–638, 1973.

Styne, D. M., and Grumbach, M. M.: Puberty in the male and female: its physiology and disorders, In *Reproductive Endocrinology: Physiology, Pathophysiology and Clinical Management.* Yen, S. S. C., and Jaffe, R. B. (eds.), Philadelphia, W. B. Saunders, 1978, pp. 189–240.

Thorner, M. O.: Prolactin: clinical physiology and the significance and management of hyperprolactinemia, In *Clinical Neuroendocrinology.* Martini, L., and Besser, G. M. (eds.), New York, Acadmic Press, 1978, pp. 320–361.

Tindal, J. S.: Control of prolactin secretion, In *The Endocrine Hypothalamus.* Jeffcoate, S. L., and Hutchinson, J. S. M. (eds.), New York, Academic Press, 1978, pp. 333–361.

Vagenakis, A. G.: Regulation of TSH secretion. In *Clinical Neuroendocrinology: A Pathophysiological Approach.* Tolis, G. et al. (eds.), New York, Raven Press, 1979, pp. 329–343.

Vande Wiele, R. L., Bogumil, J., et al.: Mechanisms regulating the menstrual cycle in women. *Recent Prog. Horm. Res.* 26:63, 1970.

Yates, F. E., and Maran, J. W.: Stimulation and inhibition of adrenocorticotropin release, In *Handbook of Physiology, Section 7: Endocrinology. Vol. IV, Pt. 2.* American Physiological Society. Greep, R. O., and Astwood, E. B. (eds.), Baltimore, Williams and Wilkins, 1974, pp. 367–404.

Yen, S. S. C.: The human menstrual cycle (integrative function of the hypothalamic-pituitary-ovarian-endometrical axis), In *Reproductive Endocrinology: Physiology, Pathophysiology, and Clinical Management.* Yen, S. S. C., and Jaffe, R. B. (eds.), Philadelphia, W. B. Saunders, 1978, pp. 126–151.

Yen, S. S. C.: Physiology of human prolactin, In *Reproductive Endocrinology: Physiology, Pathophysiology and Clinical Management.* Yen S. S. C., and Jaffe, R.B (eds.), Philadelphia, W. B. Saunders, 1978, pp. 152–170.

Yen, S. S. C.: Neuroendocrine aspects of the regulation of cyclic gonadotropin release in women, In *Clinical Neuroendocrinology.* Martini, L., and Besser, G. M. (eds.), New York, Raven Press, 1978, pp. 175–196.

The Pineal Gland and Periventricular Organs

Akert, K.: The mammalian subfornical organ. *J. Neurovisc. Relat. 31*(Suppl 9):8, 1969.

Altschule, M. D. (ed.): *Frontiers of Pineal Physiology.* Cambridge, MIT Press, 1975, pp. 1–4.

Brownstein, M. J.: The pineal gland. *Life Sci. 16:*1363–374, 1975.

Daniel, P. M., and Treip, C. S.: The pathology of the hypothalamus. *Clin. Endocrinol. Metab.* 6(1):3, 1977.

Kappers, J. Ariens, Smith, A. R., and De Vries, R. A. C.: The mammalian pineal gland and its control of hypothalamic activity. In *Progress in Brain Research.* Swaab, D. F., and Schade, J. P. (eds.), Vol. 41, Elsevier Scientific Publishing Co., Amsterdam, 1974, pp. 149–174.

Kawakami, M., Kimura, F., et al.: Involvement of the circumventricular organ in the regulation of gonadotropin and prolactin, In *Biological Rhythms in Neuroendocrine Activity.* Kawakami, M. (ed.), Tokyo, Igaku-Shoin, Ltd., 1974, pp. 167–186.

Klein, D. C.: The pineal gland: a model of neuroendocrine regulation, In *The Hypothalamus, Vol. 56.* Reichlin, S., Baldessarini, R. J., et al. (eds.), New York, Raven Press, 1978, pp. 303–327.

Lerner, A. B., and Nordlund, J. H.: Melatonin: Clinical pharmacology. *J. Neural Transmission* 13(Suppl.):339–347, 1978.

Lerner, A. B., Case, J. D., Takahashi, Y., Lee, T. H., and Mori, W.: Isolation of melatonin, the pineal factor that lightens melanocytes. *J. Am. Chem. Soc.* 80:2587, 1958.

Moskowitz, M. A., and Wurtman, R. J.: Pathological states involving the pineal, In *Clinical Neuroendocrinology.* Martini, L., and Besser, G. M. (eds.), New York, Academic Press, 1977, pp. 503–526.

Reiter, R. J.: Pineal regulation of hypothalamicopituitary axis: Gonadotropins. In *Handbook of Physiology, Endocrinology, Vol. 4, Part 2.* Knobil, E. and Sawyer, W.H. (eds.), Washington, D. C., American Physiologica! Society, 1974.

Rolleston, Sir Humphrey Davy: *The Endocrine Organs in Health Disease with an Historical Review.* Oxford, University Press, 1936, p. 452.

Rudman, D., Del Rio, A. E., et al.: Comparison of lipolytic and melanotropic factors in bovine choroid plexus and in bovine pineal gland. *Endocrinology* 90:1139, 1972.

Seyler, L. E., Jr., Canalis, E., Spare, S., and Reichlin, S.: Abnormal gonadotropin secretory responses to LRH in transsexual women after diethylstilbestrol priming. *J. Clin. Endocrinol. Metab.* 47:176–183, 1978.

Watson, S. J., and Maden, J.: IV, Melatonin and other pineal substances: Psychiatric and neurological implications, In *Neuroregulators and Psychiatric Disorders.* Usdin, Earl, Hamburg, D. A., and Barchas, J. D. (eds.), New York, Oxford University Press, 1977, pp. 193–200.

Weinberg, U., Eletto, R. D., et al.: Circulating melatonin in man: Episodic secretion throughout the light-dark cycle. *Clin. Endocrinol. Metab.* 48: 114–118, 1979.

Weindl, A., and Joynt, R. J.: The median eminence as a circumventricular organ, In *Brain-Endocrine Interaction: I Median Eminence: Structure and Function: Proceedings. International Symposium on Brain-Endocrine Interactions, Munich, 1971.* Knigge, K., et al. (eds.), White Plains, N.Y., A. J. Phiebig (Basel, S. Karger), 1972, pp. 280–297.

Wetterberg, L.: Melatonin in humans: physiological and clinical studies. *J. Neurol. Trans.* 13(Suppl.):289, 1978.

Wurtman, R. J., and Moskowitz, M. A.: The pineal organ. *N. Engl. J. Med.* 296:1329, 1977.

Neuroendocrine Disease

Adams, J. H., Daniel, P. M., and Pritchard, M. D.: Transection of the pituitary stalk in man: Anatomical changes in the pituitary gland. *J. Neurol. Neurosurg. Psychiatry* 29:545–555, 1966.

Antaki, A., and Somma, M.: Hypothalamic pituitary function in the olfactogenital syndrome. *J. Clin. Endocrinol. Metab.* 38(6):1083, 1974.

Anthony, G. J., Van Wyk, J. J., et al.: Influence of pituitary stalk section on growth hormone, insulin and TSH secretion in women with metastatic breast cancer. *J. Clin. Endocrinol. Metab.* 29:1238, 1969.

Axelrod, L.: Endocrine dysfunction in patients with tumors of the pineal region. In *Pineal Tumors.* H. H. Schmidek (ed.), New York, Masson Publishers, 1977, pp. 61–77.

Bagshawe, K. D., and Harland, S.: Immunodiagnosis and monitoring of gonadotropin-producing metastases in the central nervous system. *Cancer* 38(7):112, 1976.

Bardin, C. W., Ross, G. T., et al.: Studies of the pituitary-Leydig cell axis in young men with hypogonadotropic hypogonadism and hyposmia: comparison with normal men, prepuberal boys, and hypopituitary patients. *J. Clin. Invest.* 48:2046, 1969.

Bauer, H. G.: Endocrine and other clinical manifestations of hypothalamic disease; a survey of 60 cases, with autopsies. *J. Clin. Endocrinol. Metab.* 14:13, 1954.

Berlinger, F. G., Ruder, H. J., et al.: Cushing's syndrome associated with galactorrhea, amenorrhea, and hypothyroidism, a primary hypothalamic disorder. *J. Clin. Endocrinol. Metab.* 45(6):1205, 1977.

Bierich, J. R.: Sexual precocity. *J. Clin. Endocrinol. Metabol.* 4:107, 1975.

Bing, J. F., Globus, J. H., et al.: Pubertas praecox: a survey of the reported cases and verified anatomical findings. *Mt. Sinai J. Med. N.Y.* 4:935, 1938.

Boyar, R. M.: The effect of clomiphene citrate in anosmic hypogonadotrophism. *Ann. Intern. Med.* 71:1127, 1969.

Brady, L. W.: The role of radiation therapy, In *Pineal Tumors.* H. H. Schmidek, (ed.), Masson Publ. U.S.A., Inc., New York, 1977, pp. 99–113.

Braunstein, G. D., and Kohler, P. O.: Pituitary function in Hand-Schüller-

Christian disease. Evidence for deficient growth hormone release in patients with short stature. *New Engl. J. Med.* 286:1225, 1972.

Castleman, B., and McNeely, B. U.: Case 25– 1971 (germinoma). Case records of the Massachusetts General Hospital. *New Engl. J. Med.* 284:1427, 1971.

Burr, I. M., et al.: Diencephalic syndrome revisited. *J. Pediatr.* 88:429, 1976.

Costom, B. H., Grumbach, M. M., et al.: Effects of thyrotropin-releasing factor on serum thyroid stimulating hormone: an approach to distinguishing hypothalamic from pituitary forms of idiopathic hypopituitary dwarfism. *J. Clin. Invest.* 50:2219, 1971.

Daughaday, W. H., Cryer, P. E., and Jacobs, L. S.: The role of the hypothalamus in the pathogenesis of pituitary tumors. In *Diagnosis and Treatment of Pituitary Tumors.* Kohler, P. O., and Ross, G. T. (eds.), Amsterdam and New York, Excerpta Medica, 1973, pp. 26– 34.

Daughaday, W. H.: Cushing's disease and basophilic microadenomas. *New Engl. J. Med.* 298(14):793, 1978.

DeGirolami, U., and Schmidek, H. H.: Clinicopathological study of 53 tumors of the pineal region. *J. Neurosurg.* 39:455, 1973.

DeGirolami, U.: Pathology of tumors of the pineal region. In *Pineal Tumors.* H. H. Schmidek, (ed.), New York, Masson Publishers, 1977, pp. 1– 19.

Dugger, G. S., Van Wyk, J. J., et al.: The effect of pituitary-stalk section on thyroid function and gonadotropic-hormone secretion in women with mammary carcinoma. *J. Neurosurg.* 19:589, 1962.

Ehni, G., and Eckles, N. E.: Interruption of the pituitary stalk in the patient with mammary cancer. *J. Neurosurg.* 16:628, 1959.

Ehrhardt, A. A., and Meyer-Bahlburg, H. F. L.: Psychologic correlates of abnormal pubertal development. In Disorders of Puberty, *Clinics in Endocrinology and Metabolism, No. 4.* Bierich, J. (ed.), Philadelphia, W. B. Saunders Co., 1975, pp. 207– 222.

Fehm, H. L., Voigt, K. H., et al.: Adrenal insufficiency secondary to hypothalamic corticotropin releasing factor (CRF) insufficiency with hyperpigmentation: a case report. *Horm. Metab. Res. 8*(6):470, 1976.

Feldman, J. M., Plonk, J. W., et al.: Inhibitory effect on serotonin antagonists on growth hormone release in acromegalic patients. *Clin. Endocrinol.* 5:71, 1976.

Fine, S. A., and Frohman, L. A.: Loss of central nervous system component of dopaminergic inhibition of prolactin secretion in patients with prolactin-secreting pituitary tumors. *J. Clin. Invest.* 61(4):973, 1978.

Futterweit, W., and Goodsell, C. H.: Galactorrhea in primary hypothyroidism: report of two cases and review of the literature. *Mt. Sinai J. Med. N.Y.* 37:584, 1970.

Gates, R. B., Friesen, H., et al.: Inappropriate lactation and amenorrhea: pathological and diagnostic considerations. *Acta Endocrinol.* 72:101, 1973.

Gomez-Pan A., Tunbridge, W. M. G., et al.: Hypothalamic hormone interaction in acromegaly. *Clin. Endocrinol.* 4:455, 1975.

Goodman, R., Biller, B., Moses, A. C., Molitch, M., Feldman, S., and Post, K.: Restoration of normal prolactin secretory dynamics after surgical cure of prolactinoma is evidence against underlying hypothalamic dysregulation. Proceedings of 61st Annual Meeting, Endocrine Society, Anaheim, California, June, 1979.

Green, J. R., Buchan, G. C., et al.: Hereditary and idiopathic types of diabetes insipidus. *Brain* 90:707, 1967.

Hampson, J. G., and Money, J.: Idiopathic sexual precocity in the female. Report of 3 cases. *Psychosom. Med.* 17:16, 1955.

Haynes, B. F., and Fauci, A. S.: Diabetes insipidus associated with Wegener's granulomatosis successfullly treated with cyclophosphamide. *New Engl. J. Med.* 299(14):764, 1978.

Herbai, G., and Werner, I.: Sheehan's syndrome of hypothalamic origin in a woman with juvenile diabetes mellitus. *Acta Med. Scand.* 199:539, 1976.

Hökfelt, B., and Luft, R.: The effect of suprasellar tumours on the regulation of adrenocortical function. *Acta Endocrinol.* 32:177, 1959.

Iba, K., Hamada, N., et al.: A female case of Kallmann's syndrome. *Endocrinol. Jpn.* 23:289, 1976.

Ihalainen, O.: Psychosomatic aspects of amenorrhoea. *Acta Psychiatr. Scand.* 262(Suppl.):1, 1975.

Jolly, H.: *Sexual Precocity.* Springfield, Illinois, Charles C Thomas, 1955.

Judge, D. M., Kulin, H. E., et al.: Hypothalamic hamartoma. A source of luteinizing-hormone-releasing factor in precocious puberty. *New Engl. J. Med.* 296:7, 1977.

Kahana, L., Kahana, S., et al.: Endocrine manifestation of intracranial extrasellar lesions, In *An Introduction to Clinical Neuroendocrinology.* Bajusz, E. (ed.), Baltimore, Williams and Wilkins, 1967, pp. 254– 272.

Katz, J. L., and Weiner, H.: A functional, anterior hypothalamic defect in primary anorexia nervosa? *Psychosom. Med.* 37(2):103, 1975.

Kawakami, M., Kimura, F., and Yanase, M.: Involvement of the circumventricular organ in the regulation of gonadotropin and prolactin. In *Biological Rhythms in Neuroendocrine Activity.* Kawakami, M. (ed.), Igaku Shoin Ltd., Tokyo, pp. 167– 186.

Killeffer, F. A., and Stern, W. E.: Chronic effects of hypothalamic injury. Report of a case of near total hypothalamic destruction resulting from removal of a craniopharyngioma. *Arch. Neurol.* 22:419, 1970.

Kitay, J. I.: Pineal lesions and precocious puberty: a review. *J. Clin. Endocrinol. Metab.* 14:622, 1954.

Kleinberg, K. L., Noel, G. L., et al.: Galactorrhea: a study of 235 cases, including 48 with pituitary tumors. *New Engl. J. Med.* 296(11):589, 1977.

Krieger, D. T., Glick, S., et al.: A comparative study of endocrine tests in hypothalamic disease. Circadian periodicity of plasma 11-OHCS and growth hormone response to insulin hypoglycemia and metyrapone responsiveness. *J. Clin. Endocrinol. Metab.* 28:1589, 1968.

Krieger, I., and Mellinger, R. C.: Pituitary function in the deprivation syndrome. *J. Pediatr.* 79:216, 1971.

Kubo, O., Yamasaki, N., Kamijo, Y., Amano, K., Kitamura, K., and Demura, R.: Human chorionic gonadotropin produced by ectopic pinealoma in a girl with precocious puberty. *J. Neurosurg.* 47:101– 105, 1977.

Kurmado, K., and Mori, W.: Virus-like particles in human pinealoma. *Acta Neuropathol.* (Ber) 37:273– 276, 1976.

Lerner, A. B., and Norlund, J. H.: Melatonin: clinical pharmacology. *J. Neural Trans. 13*(Suppl.):339, 1978.

Li, M. C., Rall, J. E., et al.: Thyroid function following hypophysectomy in man. *J. Clin. Endocrinol. Metab.* 15:1228, 1955.

Liddle, G. W.: Cushing's syndrome. *Ann. N.Y. Acad. Sci.* 297:594, 1977.

Lipsett, M. B., West, C. D., et al.: Adrenal function after hypophysectomy in man. *J. Clin. Endocrinol Metab.* 17:356, 1957.

Liu, N., Grumbach, M. M., et al.: Prevalence of electroencephalographic abnormalities in idiopathic precocious puberty and premature pubarche: bearing on pathogenesis and neuroendocrine regulation of puberty. *J. Clin. Endocrinol. Metab.* 25:1296, 1965.

Lovinger, R. D., Kaplan, S. L., et al.: Congenital hypopituitarism associated with neonatal hypoglycemia and microphallus: four cases secondary to hypothalamic hormone deficiencies. *J. Pediatr.* 87:1171, 1975.

Lowry, W. S.: Late effects of pituitary irradiation. *New Engl. J. Med.* 289:658, 1970.

Martin, L. G., Martul, P., et al.: Hypothalamic origin of idiopathic hypopituitarism. *Metabolism* 21(2):143, 1972.

Matuk, F., and Kalyanaraman, K.: Syndrome of inappropriate secretion of antidiuretic hormone in patients treated with psychotherapeutic drugs. *Arch. Neurol.* 34:374, 1977.

McClintock, M. K.: Menstrual synchrony and suppression. *Nature* 229:224, 1971.

McLanahan, C. S., and Tindall, G. T.: Amenorrhea, hyperprolactinemia and pituitary tumors. *New Engl. J. Med.* 294(16):904, 1976.

Merriam, G. R., Beitins, I. Z., et al.: Father-to-son transmission of hypogonadism with anosmia. Kallmann's syndrome. *Am. J. Dis. Child. 131*:1216, 1977.

Mitsuma, T., Shenkman, L., et al.: Hypothalmic hypothyroidism: diminished thyroidal response to thyrotropin-releasing hormone. *Am. J. Med. Sci.* 265(4):315, 1973.

Money, J., and Alexander, D.: Psychosexual development and absence of homosexuality in males with precocious puberty. *J. Nerv. Ment. Dis.* 148:111, 1969.

Money, J., and Hampson, J. G.: Idiopathic sexual precocity in the male: management: report of a case. *Psychosom. Med. 17*:1, 1955.

Mortimer, C. H., and McNeilly, A. S.: Gonadotrophin-releasing hormone therapy in hypogonadal males with hypothalamic or pituitary dysfunction. *Br. Med. J.* 4:617, 1974.

Naftolin, F., Harris, G. W., et al.: Effect of purified luteinizing hormone releasing factor on normal and hypgonadotropic anosmic men. *Nature* 232:496, 1971.

Obrador, S., Soto, M., et al.: Surgical management of tumours of the pineal region. *Acta Neurochir.* 34:159, 1976.

Oppenheimer, J. H.: Abnormalities of neuroendocrine functions in man, In *Neuroendocrinology, Vol. 2.* Martini, L., and Ganong W. F. (eds.), New York, Academic Press, 1967.

Peake, G. T., and Daughaday, W. H.: Disturbances of pituitary function in central nervous system disease. *Med. Clin. North Am.* 52:357, 1968.

Pittman, J. A., Jr., Haigler, E. D., et al.: Hypothalamic hypothyroidism. *New Engl. J. Med.* 285:844, 1971.

Plum, F., and Van Uitert, R.: Nonendocrine diseases and disorders of the hypothalamus, In *The Hypothalamus, Vol. 56.* Reichlin, S., Baldessarini, R. J., et al. (eds.), New York, Raven Press, 1978, pp. 415– 473.

Powell, G. F., Brasel, J. A., et al.: Emotional deprivation and growth retardation simulating idiopathic hypopituitarism. II. Endocrinologic evaluation of the syndrome. *New Engl. J. Med.* 276:1279, 1967.

Randall, R. V., Clark, E. C., et al.: Polyuria after operation for tumors in the region of the hypophysis and hypothalamus. *J. Clin. Endocrinol. Metab.* 20:1614, 1960.

Reichlin, S.: Etiology of pituitary adenomas. In *Pituitary Adenoma.* Post, K., Jackson, I. M. D., and Reichlin, S. (eds.), New York, Plenum Publishing Corp., 1980.

Reiter, R. J.: Pineal regulation of hypothalamicopituitary axis: gonadotropins, In *Handbook of Physiology, Section 7: Endocrinology. Vol. 4, Pt. 2.* American Physiological Society. Greep, R. O., and Astwood, E. B. (eds.), Baltimore, Williams and Wilkins, 1974.

Reeves, A. G., and Plum, F.: Hyperphagia, rage and dementia accompanying a ventromedial hypothalamic neoplasm. *Arch. Neurol.* 20:616, 1969.

Richter, R. B.: True hamartoma of the hypothalamus associated with pubertas praecox. *J. Neuropathol.* 10:368, 1951.

Ringertz, N., Nordestam, H., et al.: Tumors of the pineal region. *J. Neuropathol. 13*:540, 1954.

Roth, J. C., Grumbach, M. M., et al.: Effect of synthetic luteinizing hormone-releasing factor on serum testosterone and gonadotropins in prepubertal, pubertal and adult males. *J. Clin. Endocrinol. Metab. 37*:680, 1973.

Russell, D. S., Rubinstein, L. J., et al.: Pineal neoplasms, In *Pathology of Tumours of the Nervous System.* 2nd ed. Russell, D. S., and Rubinstein, L. J. (eds.), Baltimore, Williams and Wilkins, 1963, pp. 173–183.

Santen, R. J., and Paulsen, C. A.: Hypogonadotropic enuchoidism. I. Clinical study of the mode of inheritance. *J. Clin. Endocrinol. Metab. 36*(1):47, 1973.

Schally, A. V., and Coy, D. H.: Regulatory and inhibitory analogs of luteinizing hormone releasing hormone (LHRH). In *Hypothalamic Peptide Hormones and Pituitary Regulation.* Porter, J. C. (ed.), New York, Plenum Press, 1977.

Schmidek, H. H.: Surgical management of pineal region tumors. In *Pineal Tumors.* Schmidek, H. H. (ed.), New York, Masson Publishing, 1977, pp. 99–113.

Schneider, H. P. G., Bohnet, H. G., et al.: Hypothalamic amenorrhea: an approach to diagnosis and therapy with LH-releasing hormone, In *Basic Applications and Clinical Uses of Hypothalamic Hormones: Proceedings.* International Symposium on Basic Applications and Clinical Uses of Hypothalamic Hormones, 1st, Madrid, 5–7 May, 1975. Charro Salgado, A. L., et al. (eds.), New York, American Elsevier Publishing Co., Inc., 1976, pp. 261–269.

Sherman, B. M., Halmi, K. A., et al.: LH and FSH response to gonadotropin-releasing hormone in anorexia nervosa: effect of nutritional rehabilitation. *J. Clin. Endocrinol. Metab. 41*(1):135, 1975.

Spiegel, A. M., DiChiro, G., et al.: Diagnosis of radiosensitive hypothalamic tumors without craniotomy. Endocrine and neuroradiologic studies of intracranial atypical teratomas. *Ann. Intern. Med. 85*:290, 1976.

Stein, B. M., Supracerebellar-infratentorial approach to pineal tumors. *Surg. Neurol. 11*:331, 1979.

Tagataz, G., Fialkow, P. J., et al.: Hypogonadotropic hypogonadism associated with anosmia in the female. *New Engl. J. Med. 283*:1326, 1970.

Takeuchi, J., Handa, H., and Nagata, I.: Suprasellar germinoma. *J. Neurosurg. 49*:41–48, 1978.

Tompkins, V. N., Haymaker, W., and Campbell, E. H., Metastatic pineal tumors. *J. Neurosurg. 7*:159–169, 1950.

Turkington, R. W., Underwood, L. E., et al.: Elevated serum prolactin levels after pituitary stalk section in man. *New Engl. J. Med. 285*:707, 1971.

Vale, W., Rivier, C., Brown, M., and Rivier, J.: Pharmacology of thyrotropin releasing factor (TRF), luteinizing hormone releasing factor (LRF), and somatostatin, In *Hypothalamic Peptide Hormones and Pituitary Regulation.* Porter, J. C. (ed.), New York, Plenum Press, 1976, pp. 123–156.

Van Wyk, J. J., Dugger, G. S., et al.: The effect of pituitary stalk section on the adrenal function of women with cancer of the breast. *J. Clin. Endocrinol Metab. 20*:157, 1960.

Van Wyk, J. J., and Grumbach, M. M.: Syndrome of precocious menstruation and galactorrhea in juvenile hypothyroidism: An example of hormonal overlap in pituitary feedback. *J. Pediat. 57*:416, 1960.

Vigersky, R. A., Loriaux, D. L., et al.: Delayed pituitary hormone response to LRF and TRF in patients with anorexia nervosa and with secondary amenorrhea associated with simple weight loss. *J. Clin. Endocrinol Metab. 43*(4):893, 1976.

Weinberg, U., Eletto, R. D., et al.: Circulating melatonin in man: episodic secretion throughout the light-dark cycle. *J. Clin. Endocrinol. Metab. 48*:114, 1979.

Weinberger, L. M., and Grant, F. C.: Precocious puberty and tumors of the hypothalamus. *Arch. Int. Med. 67*:762–792, 1941.

Weinstein, R. L., and Reitz, R. E.: Pituitary-testicular responsiveness in male hypogonadotropic hypogonadism. *J. Clin. Invest. 53*:408, 1974.

Whitten, C. F., Pettit, M. G., et al.: Evidence that growth failure from maternal deprivation is secondary to undereating. *J.A.M.A. 209*:1675, 1969.

Wiele, R. L. V.: Anorexia nervosa and the hypothalamus. *Hosp. Prac. 12*:45, 1977.

Wilkins, L.: The diagnosis and treatment of endocrine disorders in childhood and adolescence. Springfield, Illinois, Charles C Thomas, 1965.

Wolff, S. M., Adler, R. C., et al.: A syndrome of periodic hypothalamic discharge. *Am. J. Med. 36*:956, 1964.

Wood, L. C., Olichney, M., et al.: Syndrome of juvenile hypothyroidism associated with advanced sexual development: report of two new cases and comment on the management of an associated ovarian mass. *J. Clin. Endocrinol. Metab. 25*:1289, 1965.

Wray, S. H.: The neuro-ophthalmic and neurologic manifestations of pinealomas. In *Pineal Tumors.* Schmidek, H. H. (ed.), New York, Masson Publishing, 1977, pp. 61–77.

Wurtman, R. J. and Kammer, H.: Melatonin synthesis by an ectopic pinealoma. *N. Engl. J. Med. 274*:1233, 1966.

Yoshimoto, Y., Moridera, K., et al.: Restoration of normal pituitary gonadotropin reserve by administration of luteinizing-hormone-releasing hormone in patients with hypogonadotropic hypogonadism. *New Engl. J. Med. 292*(5):242, 1975.

Zacharias, L., and Wurtman, R. J.: Age at menarche. Genetic and environmental influences. *New Engl. J. Med. 280*(16):868, 1969.

Zimmerman, E. A., Defendini, R., et al.: Prolactin and growth hormone in patients with pituitary adenomas: a correlative study of hormone in tumor and plasma by immunoperoxidase technique and radioimmunoassay. *J. Clin. Endocrinol. Metab. 38*:577, 1974.

CHAPTER 12

Psychoendocrinology

By Robert M. Rose
and Edward Sachar

The fact that this edition of the textbook has a specific chapter on psychoendocrinology reflects the growing appreciation of the interplay between higher central nervous sytem (CNS) function and endocrinology. Although a large body of data has been available on the CNS control of pituitary and other endocrine function — neuroendocrinology — it is only more recently that there has been widespread appreciation of the importance of psychological influences on endocrine secretion as well as how hormones influence behavior in man.

Although the scope of this chapter is large, it is far from complete. There is usually much better information available from animal research than that for humans, e.g, profound and long-lasting influences of prenatal hormones or the endocrine influences on behavioral changes during puberty. Much of our appreciation of the influence of endocrine dysfunction on behavior is based primarily on clinical observation or anecdote, with more rigorous assessment of these behavioral abnormalities or psychiatric disorders just beginning. The disorders of endocrine control and regulation associated with the major mental disorders has been under serious, systematic study for less than a decade. When we turn to the behavioral effects of the short peptides, such as endorphins or enkephalins, systematic research began only 2–3 years ago.

Despite such serious gaps in our knowledge, the large picture is clear. The brain does function as a master endocrine organ, controlling secretion downstream and integrating feedback information from most hormonal systems. Thus we must turn our attention to this fascinating interplay between psychological functioning and endocrine secretion.

BEHAVIORAL INFLUENCES OF PRENATAL HORMONES

Organizational and Activational Influences

Research in animals has conclusively demonstrated the crucial role of sex steroids on the developing nervous systems. These hormonal influences act during a specific period of brain development, prenatally in the guinea pig, monkey, and man and during the first 10 days after birth in the rat. These prenatal or neonatal *organizational* effects are to be differentiated from the effects of androgens, estrogens, and progestins observed later in life, during puberty or adulthood, that are referred to as *activational* influences. The activational effects of various sex steroids, such as inducing mounting in normal male rats, are significantly modified by the earlier organizational action of these same steroids. Thus, a male rat castrated neonatally fails to respond to the activational stimulation of testosterone given when adult, whereas a female rat given testosterone neonatally not only fails to secrete gonadotropin cyclically when adult, referred to as neonatal sterilization, but also responds to testosterone when given as adult with mounting behavior similar to that observed with normal males.

Nonsexual behavior in animals is also effected by the early organizational action of hormones. Goy and Resko (1972) observed that genetic female rhesus monkeys, androgenized *in utero* by administration of testosterone propionate to their mothers during pregnancy, are behaviorally quite different from controls. These females showed masculinized external genitalia but normal female internal reproductive structures. The females from treated mothers exhibited more malelike behavior in terms of increased frequency of threatening peers, greater initiation of rough and tumble play, as well as increased frequency of mounting behavior. The frequency of these behaviors seen in treated females was greater than that of female controls, but less than that observed in normal males. Unlike rats, female monkeys treated with androgens during the crucial period of brain development are not sterile and do develop normal menstrual cycles, although they may be delayed in onset.

The increased rough and tumble play observed in treated female monkeys is an example of a behavior pattern influenced by the organizational action and does not require additional activational influence later, i.e., administration of testosterone after birth. Similarly, the normal male dog's posture for urination may be influenced organizationally and does not require additional activation. There are gender differences in learning tasks and open field behavior observed in rats that do require the later activational action of hormones as well as being influenced neonatally.

It is reasonable to assume that sex steroids also have important organizational influences in man. Our current knowledge is still most fragmentary, however, and, as most experimental studies in this area would be unethical, knowledge derives primarily from congenital abnormalities such as congenital adrenal hyperplasia (CAH) or testicular feminization syndrome and the effects of steroids on the developing fetus administered during pregnancy to prevent spontaneous abortion, and so on.

Androgens

Fetal Androgenization

Girls who are exposed to an excess of adrenal androgens, secondary to CAH, show many similar characteristics with the female rhesus monkeys treated with high doses of testosterone *in utero*. They are born with masculinized external genitalia, usually surgically corrected in the first weeks of life. The administration of corticosteroids suppresses the excess androgens, and normal development will ensue.

Several studies of these girls are now available, including observations of some into their 20's. There is consensus that they have increased physical energy expenditure in sports, a preference for boys as playmates, and a low interest in doll care and baby care. There is also a higher frequency of tomboyism among these girls compared to various control groups. All studies report that these girls have normal female gender *identity*, however, even though there is considerable evidence of their gender *role* or sexually dimorphic behavior being somewhat closer to males.

There is not consensus about their sexual *orientation*, i.e., erotic attraction to one sex or another. Initially it was reported that there was no increased incidence of homosexuality or bisexuality of these women compared to various control groups. There is now some question that there may be an increased incidence of bisexuality as well as statistically less frequent marriage occurring among this group, however. These conclusions must be replicated by future studies.

There are no consistent behavioral differences observed in boys who were exposed to increased levels of adrenal androgens during fetal life. Boys with CAH did not show increased aggressiveness or other differences in play behavior compared with other males. The juvenile male with CAH may show signs of precocious puberty with an early growth start and start early sexual development, but most aspects of masculine behavior development in such children are not affected by hormone androgen excess.

Progestogen Administration

Certain synthetic C-19 progestins such as 17-αethinyltestosterone, or 17-αethinyl-19-nortestosterone, have been observed to induce genital masculinization in a minority of female newborns, even though infants from the majority of progestogen-treated pregnancies are born with normal genitalia. Several authors, however, have reported significant behavioral differences among treated females, in the same direction as observed in females with CAH. These girls are reported to have more masculine interests, more tomboyism, and less interest in doll play. More recently it has been noted that the progestin-treated group tended to marry earlier than the CAH exposed females, however. There were also fewer cases of bisexuality or homosexuality in the progestin group. The issue of alterations in sexual orientation, however, for either group is still unclear.

Testicular Feminization Syndrome (Androgen Insensitivity)

It is clear from animal studies that in the absence of the organizing influence of androgens, differentiation and development is female. The syndrome of androgen insensitivity or testicular feminization syndrome, provides confirmatory evidence for this conclusion in man.

These genetic males show typical female gender identity as well as showing female gender role behavior, and their sexual orientation is consistently heterosexual. Thus for these individuals sex of rearing parallels endocrine state.

In those cases with partial insensitivity, some masculinization occurs and sex of rearing may be of either gender. In most cases in which genetic sex (chromosomal) or endocrine influence is at variance with sex of rearing, however, sex of rearing tends to be the predominate influence on primary gender identification. For these individuals in whom endocrine stimulation is disparate from sex of rearing, however, hormonal factors may significantly influence sexual role behavior or sexual orientation.

Estrogens

Animal data regarding the organizational effects of estrogen are not as clear as those for the role of androgens. As noted, female rats appeared to mature normally in the absence of any estrogen. Aministration of large amounts of estrogen tends to masculinize female rats, whereas in males large doses interfere with normal masculinization. Whether these paradoxical effects are a result of the aromatization of testosterone to estrogen is not yet clear.

The behavioral effects of prenatal estrogen administration in man are not well understood, not only because of the relative paucity of data but also because of the fact that estrogens have been given in pregnancy in combination with progestational agents. There is some evidence of decreased athletic ability and assertiveness in two groups of 20 males, exposed *in utero* to administered estrogens and progestins, although appropriate controls were not studied.

Progesterone

The possible action of progesterone and C-19 analogs, used previously for the relief of pre-eclampsia, on the behavior of offspring has also been studied. In general, progesterone appears to have an antiandrogen effect. Girls exposed to progesterone showed less tomboyism and more traditional feminine behavior in childhood. Medroxyprogesterone acetate has also been observed to produce similar effects in girls who were exposed prenatally, but was without effect in boys. There are conflicting reports on the effects of prenatal progesterone or prenatal androgens on intelligence. Early studies show a positive effect of these steroids in IQ testing, but later reports with children compared to their own siblings failed to show such significantly increased IQ scores.

In summary, there is evidence that excess androgen can influence later behavioral propensities in females but not in males. There is less convincing evidence about the effects of excess prenatal estrogens or progestogens on gender role functioning or sexual orientation.

PUBERTY

The endocrinologic changes in puberty have been increasingly well described in the last 10–15 years with the advent of radioimmunoassay. It is not yet clear what constitutes the crucial initiating event leading to the onset of puberty that influences the rise of LRH, which in turn stimulates the early increase in gonadotropins seen first during sleep. However, psychosocial stimuli have been shown in animal studies to significantly advance or retard the onset of puberty.

In female rodents, stressful stimuli, acting via increased secretion of adrenal steroids, lead to earlier vaginal canalization. Opposite results have been obtained with male rhesus monkeys. Acute trauma, such as loss of an eye or a broken leg, has been observed to delay the pubertal increase in testosterone usually seen in the breeding of the 3rd–4th year. Similarly, the presence of large numbers of more dominant adolescent or adult males may delay the endocrine and behavioral change usually observed by age 3–4. Puberty can be advanced in both male and female rodents by exposure to urine containing pheromones from oppositely sexed animals.

Animal studies clearly show the importance of rising gonadal steroids in activating latent behavioral differences in males and females. Receptivity in female rats, characterized by the lordosis response and subsequent mounting by the male, is dependent on appropriate endocrine influences being present during puberty, as well as the presence or absence of testosterone during perinatal development. However, we have much less information about the precise role rising gonadal steroids play in humans in evolving the dramatic behavioral changes associated with adolescence.

The various behavioral changes in puberty, such as increased aggression, lability of mood, increased interest in and concern about sexual functioning, have been described in the clinical psychiatric and psychological literature. Unfortunately, despite the wealth of endocrine information available, there are no studies that correlate behavioral changes during puberty in either sex with the very rapidly and profoundly changing endocrine picture. Studies of the psychoendocrinology of puberty or normal adolescents are badly needed, and until work is undertaken to capture some of the rich strategies that are available to elucidate how endocrine factors may affect behavior we will remain unable to understand the interaction between social and endocrinologic events that shape the very prominent alterations seen in psychological functioning during pubertal development.

In any prospective psychoendocrine study of puberty, however, it must be kept foremost in mind that social influences are very important in determining the change in behavior that adolescents exhibit. For example, in a careful study conducted in West Germany it was found that in individuals born from 1936 to 1946, an average of only 7–8% of males had their first experience of intercourse by age 16, compared with 38% of males born in 1953 and 1954. Similar figures for females rise from 3% to 26%. In any evaluation of the sexual behavior of adolescents one must evaluate the social context in which the behavior occurs as well as the dramatic alterations in endocrine status.

Precocious Puberty

Many parents of boys and girls with precocious puberty are anxious about the possible impact of their child's premature physical development on their social and sexual behavior. Often parents are fearful of any early onset of heterosexual activity leading to promiscuity or pregnancy. It is now clear from several studies that such fears are not warranted and physicians caring for such children can reassure their parents that sexual activity generally does not parallel their early endocrine maturation period. Masturbation and sex play in childhood do not appear to be enhanced among these children. Because of their early growth spurt along with premature development of their sex characteristics, however, school acceleration is often helpful in reducing the discrepancy these children experience in comparison with their age mates. In general, counseling is most helpful to reassure the child that he or she is not grossly abnormal but just an early developer, along with sex education appropriate to the physical and not chronological age.

Delayed Puberty

Delayed puberty can lead to rather serious psychological problems, not only during the teen-age years but also over a long-term period. This is especially true for males, as delayed puberty in females, if not extremely delayed, seems to have less impact on self-esteem, peer acceptance, or performance. The late-developing male who is short, puny, less able to compete athletically, and teased by peers has a significant psychological handicap. Long-term follow-up into adulthood of late-developing males indicates they are significantly less represented in leadership positions, making lower salaries, and usually delay marriage. Workers in the field such as Ehrhardt and Meyer-Bahlburg (1975) strongly suggest that boys who are significantly delayed in the onset of puberty and with significant psychological symptoms, such as hypochondriacal complaints, withdrawal from peers and social contact, poor school performance, dropping out of sports, or school absenteeism, should receive combined psychological counseling and endocrine treatment to "mainstream" them back to maturational development consistent with their age.

MALE SEXUAL BEHAVIOR

Normal Males

Possibly one of the oldest areas of interest in endocrinology has been in the relationship between gonadal hor-

mones and changes in sexual activity in men, especially to explain and possibly correct the fall in libido often seen in later years. Consequently there have been several studies attempting to correlate sexual activity in normal men with plasma testosterone levels. Generally the studies have been negative, and there is no close relationship between plasma levels of testosterone and sexual activity or interest in individuals *whose testosterone is in the normal range.* This is true both for men in the earlier decades after puberty and for those who show mild to more moderate declines in both testosterone and sexual activity after age 50–60.

Studies in animals suggest that significantly less testosterone than that normally secreted in adult males is necessary to maintain adequate sexual function. In rats, testosterone levels between one-tenth and one-third the mean plasma levels of intact animals were sufficient to maintain normal sexual behavior and activity. No increase in sexual activity was found by giving larger amounts of testosterone to these animals. Similar results have been found when normal males with adequate testosterone levels are given large doses of testosterone; there is no significant increase in sexual activity or interest.

In addition, men who report more frequent intercourse, e.g., several times per week, do not have higher levels of plasma testosterone than those who report less frequent sexual activity. In summary, many studies have reported no relationship between varying levels of testosterone in eugonadal males and differences in the frequency of coitus or intensity of sexual interests, such as fantasies and daydreams.

There is some suggestion, however, that *anticipation* of sexual activity elicited either by viewing sexually explicit films or by anticipation of actual sexual relations may serve as a stimulus to increase testosterone levels in normal males. The effect of anticipation seems to be independent of the actual act of intercourse, which has not been found to lead consistently to an increased level of testosterone either during or after coitus. The anticipation of sexual activity, however, which may evoke sexual fantasies, may explain the observation that masturbation can lead to a slight increase in testosterone, along with the larger increases in adrenal androgens. Viewing of sexually explicit movies has also been shown to lead to increased testosterone secretion. It also has been reported that male monkeys and rats show an increase in sexual activity with parallel increases in testosterone when exposed to receptive females who are unfamiliar to these males.

Effects of Diminished Androgens

Castration

Several studies have reported on the effects of castration on patients and men institutionalized as sexual offenders. These reports indicate that, parallel with animal data, castrated individuals showed a decrease in sexual activity following castration regardless of the direction or orientation of sexual interest, i.e., heterosexuality, homosexuality, pedophilia. In addition, these men also reported a fall in sexual interest and sexual fantasy life parallel with diminished sexual activity.

Studies with cats and monkeys have shown that the rate of fall in sexual activity following castration is dependent upon the past history of the animal, with more experienced males showing a slower decline.

Antiandrogens

Cyproterone acetate, perhaps the most potent antiandrogen, has been used in Europe in the treatment of hypersexuality. Studies generally have reported a decline in libido and potency during the administration of this drug, but some patients were reported to have increased sexual activity following cessation of the drug.

Ethinyl estradiol and medroxyprogesterone have also been used to inhibit sexual behavior, the latter sometimes employed with individuals with a history of imprisonable sex offenses. There is not a close relationship reported between the fall in sexual activity and the individual's plasma levels of testosterone, however. Medroxyprogesterone markedly diminishes plasma testosterone, whereas estradiol leads to an increase in total plasma levels but a fall in free testosterone secondary to its stimulation of sex-steroid binding globulin.

Thus it can be concluded that lowering available testosterone by castration or antiandrogens does affect sexual behavior and sexual interest although there is not a close parallel between exact rate of change in testosterone and fall in sexual behavior.

Hypogonadism

In contrast to the lack of relationship of sexual libido and gonadotropin or testosterone levels in eugonadal males, men who have hypogonadism from a variety of causes do show a significant diminution of the sexual libido or potency or both. In individuals with tumors in the region of the sella turcica, a significant correlation has been demonstrated between levels of testosterone and libido, as shown in Fig. 12–1. Males with hyperprolactin-

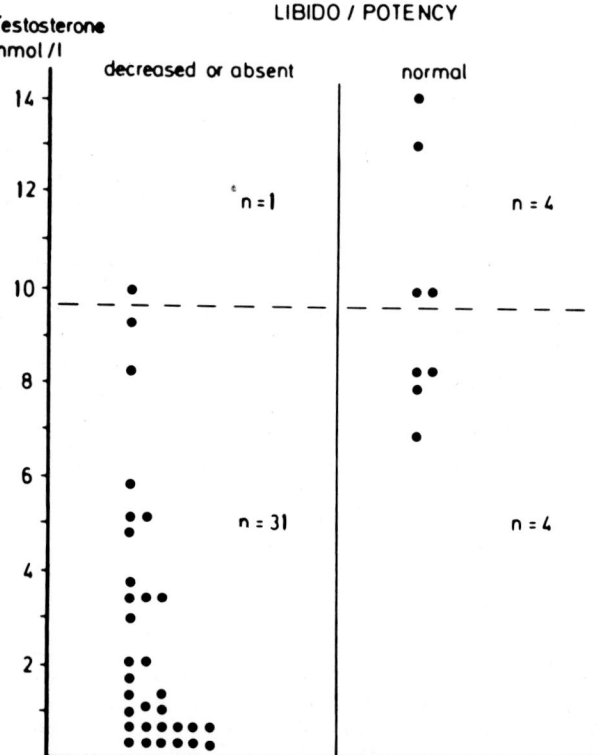

Figure 12–1. Serum testosterone concentrations in 40 men with tumors in the region of the sella turcica and with normal, decreased, or absent libido/potency. (From Lundberg, P. O., and Wide, L.: Sexual function in males with pituitary tumors. *Fertil. Steril.* 39:175, 1978. Reproduced with the permission of the authors and the publisher, the American Fertility Society, Birmingham, Alabama.)

emia are also likely to have sexual dysfunction with diminished sexual feelings as well as diminished ability to maintain erections. This may be due to prolactin (PRL) or melatonin blocking of gonadotropin-induced gonadal secretions or possibly to the high levels of PRL interfering with the conversion of testosterone into dihydrotestosterone.

Although hypogonadal males have been treated for years with depot testosterone, many workers have questioned the specific therapeutic efficacy of testosterone in increasing sexual libido or impotency. A recent double-blind, placebo study by Davidson and coworkers (1979) demonstrated a dose-response relationship between testosterone and the frequency of erections, as shown in Fig. 12–2, indicating a specific effect beyond placebo activity. These workers also raised questions about the adequacy of once monthly administration of testosterone in maintaining sexual behavior in hypogonadal men.

Impotence

Consistent with the lack of relationship between levels of testosterone and sexual behavior in eugonadal males, most studies indicate that the administration of exogenous testosterone to men with impotence, but with plasma testosterone values clearly in the normal range, yields conflicting and inconsistent results. An exception to this may be with individuals with varicoceles and symptoms of sexual inadequacy who show depressed testosterone levels. Following surgical repair of varicoceles, testosterone levels were found to rise, along with a return of sexual potency.

In recent years there have been a number of studies that have reported the effects of the administration of LRH on sexual potency in males. In individuals with evidence of hypothalamic-pituitary disease resulting in clinical hypogonadism, there is a significant sexual response to LRH, but at times even before there is a rise in testosterone. This observation suggests that the rapid return of potency in these hypogonadal patients may be due to direct action of LRH on the brain and is not mediated secondarily by the rise in testosterone. This observation is consistent with the numerous reports indicating direct CNS effects of the hypothalamic hypophysiotrophic hormones. These results are still preliminary and need to be repeated with more placebo controls before the use of LRH in hypogonadal patients is well established.

The use of LRH in impotent males in whom there is no clinical endocrine pathology is much less promising. In all studies that employed a double-blind cross-over design, there is a strong placebo effect that reflects the importance of psychological expectation on sexual performance. Nevertheless, some authors do report an improvement of sexual performance and interest with LRH, although not in double-blind studies, but delayed in onset until 2 or more months after treatment. Other studies have not confirmed the enhancement of sexual performance of libido above and beyond that obtained by the prominent placebo effect.

In summary, individuals who show significantly depressed testosterone levels for a variety of causes are more likely to show an increase in sexual libido and performance with the administration of either testosterone or LRH. The degree of depression of testosterone that must be present before a therapeutic response is obtained, however, has not yet been established, although one report suggests levels lower than 150 ng/dl (Davidson et al., 1979) respond to 400 mg of testosterone enanthate once

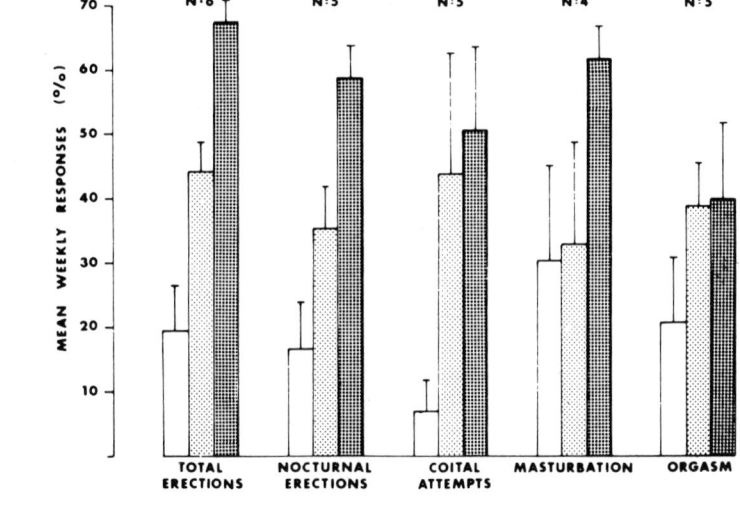

Figure 12-2. Effects of testosterone dose on mean (±SE) frequencies during the first treatment cycle of diurnal and nocturnal erections, coitus (including unsuccessful attempts), masturbation, and orgasms. All responses were normalized by expressing them as a percentage of the maximum weekly performance of that subject during the course of the cycle. Normalized data were averaged over the 4 weeks of each treatment period. Only subjects reporting a given response at least once during the study were included. Thus, for some responses n is <6. (From Davidson, J. M., Camargo, C. A., and Smith, E. R.: Effects of androgen on sexual behavior in hypogonadal men." *J. Clin. Endocrinol. Metab.* 48:957, 1979.)

every 3 or 4 weeks, depending on blood levels. Individuals whose testosterone levels are clearly in the normal range without evidence of hyperprolactinemia or other endocrine pathology are much less likely to respond to the administration of either testosterone or LRH, although there is insufficient data with the use of this peptide and longer-acting analogs may show greater clinical efficacy. Because of the strong placebo effect consistently reported, the reader must keep in mind the very important psychological component that functions in impotence, even in individuals with pituitary-gonadal pathology.

Homosexuality

The possibility of an endocrine abnormality in male homosexuality was suggested by the finding of an abnormal androsterone:etiocholanole ratio in homosexuals, followed the next year by a report of diminished testosterone levels in homosexuals. Earlier studies also found differences in FSH and LH levels in homosexuals. More than a dozen reports published in the last 8–9 years have failed to replicate these initial findings, however. In general, there is consensus that basal plasma testosterone levels in male homosexuals are not significantly different from those of men who report heterosexual preferences. Recently, several authors have reported lower levels of *unbound* testosterone or higher levels of estrogens in male homosexuals, however. These results are still unconfirmed, as is the finding that male homosexuals show a different response in plasma LH following suppressive doses of estrogens. The lack of consistent and significant differences in gonadal steroids or gonadotropin levels in male homosexuals raises a serious question about the endocrine basis of homosexuality. There may be a subgroup of individuals who do show abnormal endocrine levels or altered endocrine responsivity to tropic stimulation. This group is yet to be defined, however. No authors have been able to correlate specific psychologic or behavioral characteristics, i.e., degree of effeminate behavior, with testosterone levels or any differences in sexual preference among homosexuals with differences in testosterone or estrogen levels. The lack of significant endocrine differences is paralleled by the failure to find a significantly increased frequency of homosexuality in individuals with hypogonadism or who suffer from an androgen deficiency syndrome from a variety of causes.

These findings suggest that we must search elsewhere for a more comprehensive explanation of homosexuality than a strict endocrine basis. Nevertheless, the ability to study a representative sample of homosexuals in an unbiased and scientific manner will be facilitated by the general change in attitude about homosexuality. There is also a possibility, extrapolating from animal studies, that homosexuality may be secondary to inadequate androgenization *in utero*. There are no studies in man that report data relevant to this hypothesis.

FEMALE SEXUAL BEHAVIOR

Attractiveness, Proceptivity, Receptivity

Our understanding of female sexual behavior, including the importance of endocrine determinants of this behavior, has been seriously hampered until very recently. In most studies, female sexual behavior has been inferred from the performance of males, and it has been assumed that the height of female sexual receptivity coincides with periods of enhanced male libido. Recently, Beach (1975), in reviewing studies in rodents, nonhuman primates, and humans, has suggested that our understanding of female sexual behavior would be considerably facilitated by separating it into three component parts: *attractiveness* (the effectiveness of the female as a sexual stimulus), *proceptivity* (the extent to which the female seeks out the male and elicits sexual behavior), and *receptivity* (willingness to receive a male in copulation). Most observations or studies with humans have failed to differentiate between attractiveness, proceptivity, and receptivity. Consequently, we may have been drawing erroneous conclusions in this perspective of confusing female behavior with that of males.

Very few studies have reported concurrent endocrine findings with reported changes in sexual behavior or libido in women during the menstrual cycle, pregnancy, menopause, or puberty. In those studies in which sexuality has been reported, most often endocrine assays have not been made and levels of estrogens, progesterone, or androgens have only been inferred. Consequently there is relatively little data available to assess hormonal influences on female sexual behavior, especially in healthy women.

Menstrual Cycle

Although a great deal has been written about changes in sexuality during the menstrual cycle, most of these studies have been without concomitant measures of gonadal hormones, and hormonal levels have usually been inferred from cycle day. Survey studies based on reported sexual activity have yielded conflicting results. One report by Udry and Morris (1968) did find increased frequency of sexual intercourse during the midcycle, with a drop during the menstrual period, but a reanalysis of the data indicated that increased sexual behavior may also occur earlier in the follicular phase. Recently, a study by Adams and Gold (1978) appeared in which individuals were asked to indicate whether sexual activity was initiated by the female or by the male. These authors reported that both frequency of female-initiated heterosexual activities as well as autosexual activities increased around the estimated time of ovulation. Women who were taking a variety of oral contraceptives failed to show this increase of sexual activity in the periovulatory phase of the cycle. This suggests that the increase in female-initiated sexual behavior (proceptivity) may be related to the rise in estrogens seen about the time of ovulation or perhaps to the peak of testosterone also reported to increase in the periovulatory period. Other recent investigations of women followed longitudinally throughout the cycle, however, suggest that there is no relationship between the frequency of various female-initiated sexual behaviors, the frequency of sexual intercourse, or the level of sexual arousal and changes in plasma estradiol. In order to clarify the endocrine influences on female sexuality during other periods of life, such as during puberty or menopause, it would be important to identify which aspect of female sexual behavior is being investigated, as has been done most recently in studies of sexual behavior during the menstrual cycle.

Menopause

The endocrine changes associated with the menopause have generally been well described. There are differences whether menopause is associated with aging or secondary to surgical castration. Nevertheless, there is a rise in FSH and LH along with changes in the ultradian rhythm (frequencies of 60–90 min.) of gonadotropins following the fall in the ovarian secretion of estrogens. It is clear that estrogen production in postmenopausal women is in part accountable by extraglandular conversion of plasma δ_4 androstenedione.

Many of the symptoms that are often attributed to the menopause, however, are not clearly related to the fall in estrogen levels. The physical symptoms that are most related to hypoestrogenism are those described as hot flashes, although the frequency and duration of these vasomotor symptoms vary considerably from patient to patient. In addition, there are significant anatomic and physiologic changes related to the atrophy of the epithelium in the vulva and vagina. Vaginal lubrication decreases and the time interval required to produce significant vaginal secretions in response to sexual stimulation gradually increases. Perhaps the most controversy relates to the psychologic changes that are often attributed to the menopause *per se*. Most authors now agree that it is difficult to separate many of these psychological changes from that of aging, and that patient symptomatology must be evaluated in the context of the life events associated with changes in the 40's and 50's in most women.

There is no evidence to suggest that there is an increased risk for serious psychiatric illness in the *menopause,* although the frequency and severity of mood disorders, particularly depression, *increase with increasing age.* There is no evidence that women, including those with surgically induced menopause, are at a greater risk for depression or presenile brain syndromes because of involution of the female reproductive system.

There is general consistency in various studies reporting a decrease in libido occurring in menopausal women. Careful analysis of these data strongly suggests that the change in sexual interest may be related to changes in the individual's psychosocial environment, however, i.e., change in her husband's libido, rather than to specific effects of the fall in estrogen levels. Administration of conjugated estrogenic hormones (Premarin), especially when assessed in double-blind studies, failed to reverse any decrease in libido that women report in the menopause.

The treatment of the symptoms of anxiety and depression reported by women with associated menopausal vasomotor and genitourinary changes is more complicated. The wide use of minor tranquilizers, such as benzodiazepines, to treat anxiety and depression in this group may serve to mask more serious depressive symptoms that should be treated more appropriately with antidepressants. Administration of estrogens has not consistently been found to alleviate symptoms of depression and anxiety in these patients. In addition, there has been no correlation observed between presenting symptoms of loss of libido in menopausal patients and the plasma level of the androgens or estrogens in these patients. Many studies report a very large placebo effect, which points to the need for general support for the emotional problems reported by some women during this period.

Adrenalectomy, Hypophysectomy, and Oophorectomy

There has been general consensus that adrenal androgens or testosterone derived from ovarian sources are the more important endocrine influences on libido or sexual activity in females. More recent work, especially with monkeys, however, has raised some doubts about this conclusion. Nevertheless, studies of women following hypophysectomy or adrenalectomy have generally reported decreases in sexual function compared to an absence of such changes following a bilateral oophorectomy. Most of these older studies can be faulted because they included patients with serious medical problems and most did not include data from appropriate controls.

More recently, a number of women were studied by Johansson and associates (1975) 40 years after bilateral oophorectomy, and most reported no changes in their sexual behavior following removal of the ovaries. An additional finding was that those who had a good sexual adaptation before the operation also reported adequate sexual functioning following surgery.

Some insight might be achieved into the role of various hormones in initiating and maintaining female sexual behavior from studies carried out in rhesus monkeys. There is considerable evidence indicating that androgens from the adrenal or testosterone from exogenous sources or endogenously secreted significantly increase female monkey *proceptivity* (the extent to which the female seeks out the male and elicits sexual behavior). There is some evidence that female proceptivity may also be enhanced by estrogens, and this effect of estrogens to enhance female proceptivity may account for the observation noted earlier in the chapter by some workers of an increased frequency of human female-initiated sexual activity during the periovulatory state of their menstrual cycle.

Progesterone reduces the sexual *attractivity* of females to males, probably by antagonizing the action of estrogens in stimulating vaginal secretions, which appear to have a positive pherhormonal action. *Receptivity* of the female is enhanced by estrogen and also possibly by androgens, although receptivity of the female appears to be under less consistent and direct endocrine influence than can be demonstrated for proceptivity.

It should also be emphasized that a variety of other stimuli in addition to hormones modulate the sexual behavior of all primates, including nonhuman primates such as rhesus monkeys. Such factors as partner preference, social stimuli, and social history are very important determinants of sexual interest and behavior in monkeys as well as in man.

Homosexuality and Transsexualism

Most studies of endocrine levels of homosexual or transsexual females report no significant differences from controls (Meyer-Bahlburg, 1979). About one third of these studies, however, do report elevated androgens among some individuals, but often the higher average levels are due to a relatively few subjects. There are also preliminary reports of an altered response among transsexual females to LRH stimulation, but the numbers are small and require replication.

Larger numbers of both homosexual females and women seeking transsexual surgery must be gathered and more careful investigation of any differences in psychologic characteristics and orientation should be obtained along with attempts to investigate any differences in levels or secretion of androgens.

PREMENSTRUAL TENSION SYNDROME

Definition and Prevalence

There is a great deal of controversy about the nature and prevalence of premenstrual symptoms in women. Part of this is definitional in that there is no consistency among various investigators as to what symptoms are essential and required before the diagnosis can be made. In addition, there is further confusion as to how severe various symptoms must appear before individuals should be described as suffering from the premenstrual tension syndrome.

Many symptoms have been listed as composing the premenstrual tension syndrome. These include the presence of depression or anxiety, fatigue, irritability, swelling of legs and abdomen, tenderness of the breasts, significant weight gain, increased acneiform eruptions, as well as the degree to which symptoms interfere with school or work.

A review of information gathered by questionnaires and surveys on approximately 10,000 women over the last 15 years reveals that there is a preponderance of younger women in these studies and the format has been to ask the respondent whether she experiences any of a list of symptoms. The magnitude of distress or intensity of symptoms is rarely investigated. A significant percentage of women report some degree of depression or anxiety, fatigue, irritability, or swelling immediately prior to the onset of menses. Although there is considerable variability, a summary figure of approximately 25–30% of women

report one symptom. A smaller number report combinations of two or more. It is unlikely that the percentages reflect the real prevalence of the premenstrual tension syndrome, but rather the frequency of one mild or moderate symptom. A more accurate estimate of the prevalence of the syndrome is probably closer to 5% of the women surveyed, extrapolating from those who reported multiple and severe symptoms.

We know that many individuals over-report in responding to questions regarding the presence of premenstrual symptoms. This phenomenon has been described extensively in the psychologic literature on attribution theory. Careful studies in which individuals are followed prospectively, either daily or repeatedly throughout the menstrual cycle, fail to yield a high number of women being affected by premenstrual symptoms. In a classic study in 1937, McCance and coworkers reported on 167 women who filled out daily questionnaires during approximately six menstrual cycles. Only 3–6% of the 167 women studied over 1932 cycles showed an increase of depression before the onset of menses.

Individuals' propensities to exaggerate their symptoms during days they identify as premenstrual have been reported in numerous studies. When one group of women was led to believe they were premenstrual, they reported significantly more pain, symptoms of swelling, and change in eating habits compared with others who were told they were not premenstrual. Both groups were at the same stage of their cycles. It is clear that social influences, expectation, or belief systems may significantly alter reporting of symptoms ascribable to premenstrual distress.

Individuals may be defined as having the premenstrual tension syndrome by requiring that they have one or more psychologic symptoms of depression, anxiety, crying easily, or increased fatigability, as well as showing one or more of the following physical symptoms of swelling of the legs and abdomen, tenderness of the breasts, or significant weight gain, *and* these symptoms are of a moderate or severe nature. When utilizing these more stringent criteria, there is some evidence that some individuals with the premenstrual tension syndrome show an increased risk of having future psychiatric problems, especially with disturbances of affect, such as depression. It is clear, however, that many individual women who suffer significantly with severe and repetitive symptoms of a premenstrual tension syndrome are without other psychiatric diagnoses or disabilities.

Etiology

The most common hypothesis involves the relationship between changes in estrogen and progesterone during the premenstrual period. One theory suggests that diminished progesterone, either absolutely or in relation to estrogen levels, is responsible for premenstrual symptoms. The estrogen dominance theory, however, has not been supported by studies in which estrogen and progesterone were measured, comparing patients with and without premenstrual symptoms. Furthermore, there is no evidence to indicate that individuals with premenstrual syndrome experience a more rapid fall in the levels of either hormone before menses. Another hypothesis has suggested that there is increased activation of the renin-angiotensin-aldosterone enthusiasm; this has not been substantiated by carefully controlled metabolic studies of the relationship between psychologic symptoms and water and salt retention.

Other theories postulating premenstrual hypoglycemia, or a specific menstrual toxin, have not been supported. Recently, hyperprolactinemia has been suggested as a cause of premenstrual tension syndrome. Several studies have found that women with premenstrual distress have higher PRL during the late luteal phase compared with levels in the follicular phase and higher levels than those in women without the premenstrual syndrome. In addition, when treated with bromocriptine (an active dopamine agonist) individuals with premenstrual tension were found to have a significant improvement in breast symptoms, reduction in weight, and improvement in mood, compared with controls. A second double-blind clinical trial failed to replicate the efficacy of bromocriptine compared to placebo, however.

It also has been suggested that individuals who manifest the premenstrual syndrome are more neurotic or manifest more neurotic traits; however, this is not a consistent finding.

Treatment

Many treatments have been utilized for premenstrual distress, with diuretics being more common. Despite the fact that clinicians report success using diuretics, there are no controlled studies supporting this treatment. There is no consistent evidence suggesting that the disorder or mood, whether it be depression, anxiety, irritability, or fatigue, can be related to changes in weight during the menstrual cycle or to changes in renin-angiotensin-aldosterone secretion.

Another treatment has been the use of progesterone. One study of 320 women suggests that there is a small subgroup of women whose symptoms are hormone-dependent and exacerbated by estrogens and improved with progestational oral contraceptives. Contradictory data abounds, however, and it is by no means clear that placing patients on oral contraceptives will eliminate premenstrual tension in those patients so affected. Similarly, controlled studies do not support the use of synthetic progestogens. No consistent results have been obtained and double-blind cross-over studies are not available alternating progesterone with placebo in patients with premenstrual tension. Plasma progesterone levels following progesterone administration failed to show any relationship between levels of progesterone and therapeutic benefit. The use of bromocriptine for the treatment of premenstrual syndrome is only recently reported and studies are not consistent, as noted previously.

Summary

There still is a great deal of controversy regarding the nature and extent of premenstrual symptomatology. Survey data exaggerate the true prevalence of premenstrual symptomatology. Nevertheless, there are significant numbers of women, possibly as high as 5% of the general population, who show significant premenstrual symptomatology and suffer from a true premenstrual tension syndrome. The etiology of this condition is as yet unclear, as is the preferred treatment. Patients who come to the physician seeking relief of premenstrual symptoms might be treated with diuretics or minor tranquilizers, or even placed on oral contraceptives. All these treatments have advocates, although none have survived more vigorous double-blind control studies. Individuals with very severe symptoms might be placed on bromocriptine, although this is still in an experimental stage. It is clear that some women are severely affected premenstrually, whose symptoms remit dramatically upon the onset of menses and whose ability to function is compromised by the existence of the premenstrual tension syndrome. What is most confusing has been extrapolating from these patients to all women who menstruate and asserting that they are regularly and periodically incapacitated by virtue of having menstrual periods.

ENDOCRINE RESPONSES TO STRESS

As reviewed in the previous chapter on "Neuroendocrinology," our knowledge of the physiological substrate for CNS influence on endocrine secretion has expanded enormously over the last decade, or since previous editions of this textbook. All pituitary hormones are thus susceptible to regulation from the hypothalamus and hence other structures including, of course, input from the cerebral cortex. Careful delineation of the nature of psychological stimuli that have been observed to effect hormone secretion has proceeded more slowly than description of the relevant pathways in brain, including neurotransmitter regulation, the isolation and purification of hypothalamic hormones, and, more recently, the role of brain peptides. Nevertheless, a growing body of data exists describing changes in a number of endocrine systems, and, indeed, some scattered reports are now available about psychological influences or the effects of stressful stimuli on almost all endocrine products. A significant amount of data, however, is available for a limited number of hormones, and hence this review is restricted to those more widely studied systems. This restriction, however, is not to indicate that other hormones, such as insulin or thyroxine (T_4), are not susceptible to CNS or psychological input, but rather that significantly less data is available for these hormone products.

Cortisol

Over the past quarter century a very large literature has been published documenting the responsiveness of the adrenal cortex to a wide variety of stressful stimuli. The adrenal cortex, in human and nonhuman primates, responds with increased cortisol secretion (in rodents corticosterone rises), stimulated by the increased secretion of ACTH from the pituitary, which responds to increased ACTH releasing factor (CRF).

Early studies were limited to measuring changes in the weight of adrenals, or in humans, increased adrenal activity was inferred from the fall in blood eosinophils. Later studies measured the group of urinary metabolites of cortisol, referred to as 17-hydroxycorticosteroids (17-OHCS), metabolites with the dihydroxyacetone side chain at the 17 position (Porter-Silber chromagens). During the last 10 years, investigators have relied increasingly on the direct measurement of plasma cortisol. In general, the findings obtained by urinary measures have been replicated by plasma cortisol assays or by determining secretory rate via isotope dilution methods. In addition, when investigated, the rise in plasma cortisol has been found to be due to increases in secretion, and not due to a fall in metabolic clearance rate. In certain conditions, such as stress-induced gastrointestinal (GI) bleeding, the increase in cortisol secretion is intensified by a fall in transcortin levels, leading to even higher free cortisol levels.

Most early studies of the response of the adrenal to a variety of stressful stimuli focused on a *situational* definition of stress. There are numerous reports of the increase in cortisol during surgery. Other studies included responses to rowing, marathon running, or sudden exposure to heat or cold. The underlying assumption was that most subjects would experience these stimuli as arousing or stressful, similar to surgery. As we begin to investigate adrenal responses to the *anticipation* of surgery, exposure to novel environment such as admission to the hospital, examinations, provocative movies, or a variety of other stimuli, however, significant differences were observed between individuals. Some individuals showed very brisk increases in cortisol, whereas others showed little or no response.

One observation reported by many authors provided an important clue to understanding these individual differences in responses to presumably identical stimuli. If the individual was repeatedly exposed to the same stimulus, the adrenal soon showed no response. Thus the *novelty* of the stimulus for that individual was one important determinant of how provocative or stressful the stimulus was. The issue of how individuals *adapted* to stimuli was but one psychologic variable that could explain individual differences in response to *potentially* threatening or distressing stimuli.

Further work was done to clarify why certain individuals showed adrenal corticoid responses and others did not when exposed to a variety of stimuli, primarily psychological in nature. Observations of the emotional state of these individuals or their reports of how difficult or threatening they found the environment were useful in predicting adrenal responses.

Differences in levels of adrenal activity measured by 17-OHCS excretion could be predicted in parents of children dying of leukemia by estimates of how disturbed or how intensely these events impacted on each parent during this very upsetting or potentially stressful period in their lives. Similar estimates of psychological state, referred to as defensive reserve, of women awaiting breast biopsy after discovery of a lump, were predictive of the individual's cortisol secretory rate. In another study of young male recruits during the 1st month of basic training in the Army, significant differences in their excretion of 17-OHCS were found, as shown in Fig. 12–3. Psychological ratings of how negative or aversive each man found basic training were predict-

ive of adrenal activity. In another study significant differences were found among a group of soldiers anticipating an attack from the enemy in Vietnam. The captain and radio operator showed a significant increase during the period of anticipated attack, whereas the enlisted personnel showed a fall in excretion of 17-OHCS. The latter group expressed eager anticipation of the encounter; the captain was concerned about his team performance and was in constant contact with his commanding officer.

Reinvestigation of various physical stimuli has also emphasized the importance of differences in the individual's past experience or perception of the environment. Experienced athletes exercising moderately below 70% of maximum O_2 consumption failed to show adrenocortical activation compared with less experienced athletes. This raises the question of how stressful physical stimuli are in and of themselves. Many studies purporting to investigate the stressful nature of a variety of physical stimuli may have only been observing how exposure to a *novel* stimulus provokes adrenal secretion.

Until recently, the study of cortisol or other endocrine responses to stressful stimuli has yielded perplexing and inconsistent results. This has been due, in part, to the fact that individuals do not respond to the same stimulus as "stressful." When investigators have taken into consideration that individuals differ in how they interpret the amount of stress inherent in any given situation, prediction of cortisol responses can be made, and results are no longer confusing.

Endorphins

As noted in the chapter on neuroendocrinology, β-endorphin and ACTH appear to be synthesized in the same cells in the pituitary. It is now clear that a variety of stressful stimuli, studied mostly in the rat, provoke a parallel increase in β-endorphin and ACTH, as shown in Fig. 12–4. It also appears that the control of β-endorphin secretion from the pituitary closely parallels that for ACTH. Thus, both rise following adrenalectomy, and both are inhibited following administration of dexamethasone.

Increased tolerance to pain has also been observed following stress, and the question arises whether this tolerance is related directly to the increased β-endorphin secretion from the pituitary. Preliminary evidence does not indicate a parallel rise in *hypothalamic* β-endorphin during stress. It is possible, though as yet not demonstrated, that there may be a parallel rise in enkephalins in other sites in the brain that parallels the rise in pituitary β-endorphin during stress (Barchas et al., 1968). There also is preliminary evidence that the endorphin system may itself modulate the response of other endocrine systems to stressful stimuli. Naltrexone, which inhibits endorphin action, prevents the rise in PRL seen in foot shock in the rat but will not block the rise in PRL following administration of a dopamine antagonist (haloperidol), suggesting an interaction of endorphins and dopamine neurons.

It is clear that the endorphins are a major pepidergic influence in the brain and their participation in modification of endocrine responses to stress is just beginning to be appreciated.

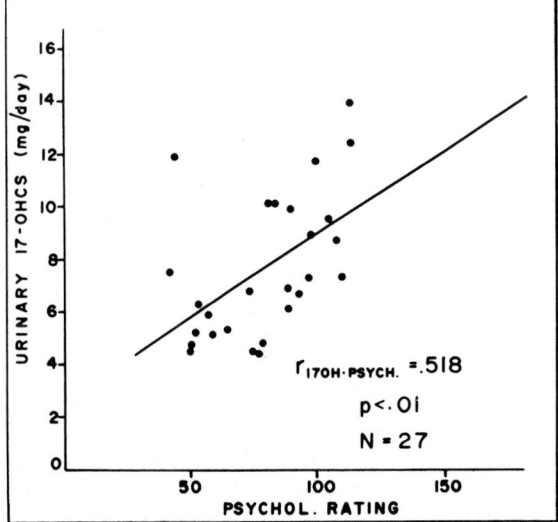

Figure 12–3. Individual mean urinary 17-OHCS and psychological rating. (From Rose, R. M., et al.: Psychological state and body size as determinants of 17-OHCS secretion. *Arch. Intern. Med. 121*:406, 1968.)

Growth Hormone

Although the literature is not as extensive as studies involving cortisol, it is now well established that growth hormone (GH) is also responsive to stressful stimuli. Eleva-

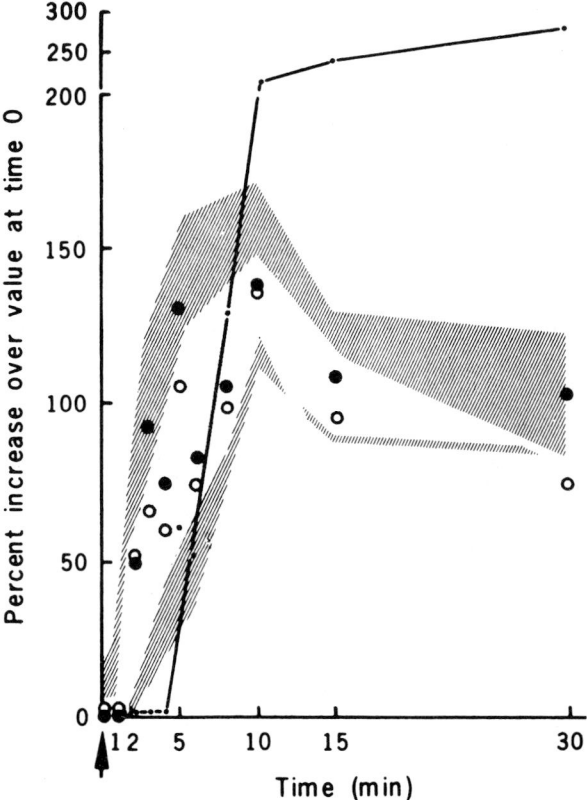

Figure 12–4. Plasma levels of ACTH (closed circles) and β-endorphin (open circles) measured by radioimmunoassays in trunk blood obtained from rats killed at times shown on the abscissa; acute stress occurred at time zero. Solid line shows plasma levels of adrenal corticosterone measured by fluorometry. Shaded areas show confidence limits of the measurements. The correlation coefficient—p—between the two populations of ACTH and β-endorphin concentrations is 0.9708 for values of means (df = 20) and 0.7785 for all individual values (df = 64). (From Guillemin, R., et al.: Beta-endorphin and adrenocorticotropin are secreted concomitantly by the pituitary gland. *Science* 197:1367, 1977.)

tions of GH occur during surgery, cardiac catheterization, electroshock therapy, gastroscopy, physical exercise, and other physical stimuli. Increased GH secretion is also associated with exposure to stimuli of a more psychological nature. Perhaps the earliest such report involved the elevation of GH in a medical student who was anticipating the hypoglycemic effect of an insulin tolerance test, and although he received only saline, he showed a brisk elevation in GH. Other psychological stimuli that can provoke GH secretion are examinations, viewing of violent or sexually arousing films, *anticipation* of exhausting exercise, and performance tests designed to evoke anxiety or distress.

Dissociations between cortisol and GH response to both physical and psychological stimuli are frequent, suggesting a separate mechanism controlling the secretion of these two stress labile hormones. In most situations, GH responses are usually not found unless there is a significant rise in cortisol secretion. Rises in cortisol occur often in the absence of GH. Thus fewer subjects in any given study show elevations of both GH and cortisol than cortisol alone, suggesting that a more intense response of the subject is required to provoke GH secretion.

Growth hormone is secreted episodically and the rate of change in blood levels is very rapid, with large changes occurring in 5–10 min. These large episodic bursts, however, are relatively infrequent during the day, but because of these abrupt elevations and falls, baseline levels are diffi-

cult to obtain and responses of individuals to a variety of stimuli are difficult to interpret. The episodic nature of GH secretion has complicated the interpretation of insulin tolerance tests, responses to arginine or lysine vasopressin (VP) or ingestion of protein, as well as GH responses to a variety of stressful stimuli.

GH responses to stressful stimuli are not mediated by changes in blood glucose. This is true whether the stimulus is surgery or exposure to examination. Similar to studies of cortisol responses, there are significant individual differences in GH response. As noted GH responses occur less frequently than cortisol responses, and most elevations in GH are found only in those individuals who show increased cortisol levels. Patients who were found to be anxious, but observed to be interacting with medical personnel during cardiac catheterization showed elevations in cortisol, while anxious patients who were withdrawn and not communicating with others showed elevations in both cortisol and GH.

Catecholamines

The importance of catecholamine response to arousing or stressful stimuli was established by Cannon's research and generalized into his "fight or flight" hypothesis. It has been well established that peripheral catecholamines increase rapidly when the organism is confronted by a variety of provocative stimuli, and there are many physiologic sequelae to the sudden rise of epinephrine and norepinephrine, including increased heart rate and cardiac output, shunting of blood away from the viscera to muscle and brain, increase in blood glucose, and so on, all of which subserve either fight or flight.

In many ways, stimuli that increase the secretion of cortisol also function to increase catecholamine secretion. Thus, stimuli that appear threatening, distressing, or novel increase both catecholamines as well as corticoids. There is some evidence to suggest that adaptation occurs more rapidly with cortisol, however, and this response dampens more rapidly than that for catecholamines. Therefore, it appears that when *vigilance* or *increased effort* are required, even though the stimulus has lost its novelty dimension, catecholamines remain elevated, even though cortisol fails to respond. There is also evidence that intense, pleasurable, or erotic stimuli associated with more positive effects, such as winning at games or viewing of sexually explicit films, lead to catecholamine secretion. Thus, the intensity of affect rather than its direction seems to be related to the magnitude of catecholamine excretion.

Most stimuli that are effective in raising catecholamine levels stimulate both epinephrine and norepinephrine. Large increases in epinephrine are associated with increases in *uncertainty* and *arousal* similar to those qualities of stimuli associated with increased cortisol secretion, however. Increases in norepinephrine have been reported to be related to more effort or vigilance.

Several years ago the ratio of epinephrine to norepinephrine was thought to be associated with the amount of aggression exhibited by differing animal species or by different individuals. This hypothesis has not been confirmed by subsequent studies, however. Part of this confusion may relate to the fact that although urinary epinephrine is clearly derived from the adrenal medulla, individuals differ in how much norepinephrine is derived from the medulla and how much from peripheral sympathetic ganglia.

Increased catecholamine secretion following myocardial infarction carries with it a greater risk for later complications. This appears to be related not to the severity of the infarction, but rather is a reflection of how disturbed or psychologically aroused the individual is during the period immediately following his infarction.

Prolactin

There are now numerous studies documenting the response of PRL to stressful stimuli. PRL clearly rises during surgery. It has also been reported to increase associated with other procedures, such as gastroscopy, proctoscopy, and pelvic examination. The fact that women may respond to gynecologic examination with an increase in PRL may lead to a misdiagnosis of hyperprolactinemia and to inappropriate treatment with bromocriptine.

There are relatively few studies of PRL response to psychologically disturbing stimuli. Although it has been reported to rise during parachute jumping or after induction of motion sickness, it has not been observed to increase following venipuncture. Similar to the observation that cortisol and GH responses may dissociate, PRL has been reported to show little change following exercise compared to a larger increase in GH. Although there is insufficient evidence at this time, it does appear as if PRL, similar to GH, requires a more intensely disturbing or provocative stimulus compared to that leading to an increase in cortisol or catecholamine levels.

PRL appears to be responsive to sexual stimuli, especially in women following stimulation of the nipple or areola. This is probably related to the stimulation of PRL observed during nursing, i.e., mechanical stimulation of the nipple by suckling.

Testosterone

Unlike cortisol, catecholamines, GH, or PRL, testosterone levels fall following exposure to stressful stimuli. Initially observed in the rat following ether anesthesia, the fall in testosterone has been reported in monkeys and man as a result of exposure to a variety of different stimuli. Surgery has been reported by several investigators to induce a fall in testosterone. The mechanism, however, remains unclear. LH or FSH levels have not been observed to parallel the fall in testosterone. As LH has been reported to fall following surgery in the rat, or to be suppressed by social subordination in the monkey, the absence of such a fall in LH in man is confusing. It has been suggested that

the drop in testosterone during surgery may be secondary to increased corticoids acting to suppress either LH release by the pituitary or LH action in stimulating steroidogenesis in the testis. With the latter mechanism there should be a rebound increase in LH, however, secondary to the diminished negative feedback of falling testosterone. As this has not been observed, the mechanism leading to suppression of testosterone remains unclear.

Psychological stimuli have also been reported to lead to a fall in testosterone. Individuals during the first several weeks of basic combat training in Officer Candidate School showed a significant drop in testosterone levels that returned to normal following completion of their course, as shown in Fig. 12–5. Individuals engaged in a rigorous 5-day combat training mission also experienced a significant fall in testosterone, associated with a rise in testosterone binding globulin, which would lead to an even greater fall in free testosterone levels. The fall in testosterone associated with defeat, observed in rhesus monkeys, may last for many weeks, if the animals are isolated following defeat and permitted no opportunity for social interaction. A large fall in testosterone associated with combat maneuvers or combat training may function adaptively in diminishing sexual libido, which would be considered inappropriate at such times.

In summary, early work in the field emphasized the ubiquity of endocrine responses to a wide variety of stressful stimuli, as if stress response represented one final common pathway. This conclusion fails to take into account the very large role that novelty played even when exposing individuals to presumably physical stimuli, such as heat or cold. Since different physical demands would require different metabolic responses for adaptation, it is unlikely that there is just one pattern of endocrine responses for all stressful stimuli. Rather, much of the early work can be characterized by observing the psychoendocrine response to novelty.

The other "lesson" learned from observing how individuals differ in response to the same stressful stimuli emphasizes the relevance of whether or not the individual perceives the event as potentially threatening or challenging. If this is not so he fails to become aroused and there is no endocrine response. The now well-established critical role of the brain in controlling endocrine secretion not only makes the interpretation of the importance of psychological events influencing endocrine activity feasible, but also establishes hormonal response as one of the three major effector systems of the CNS (motor, autonomic, endocrine).

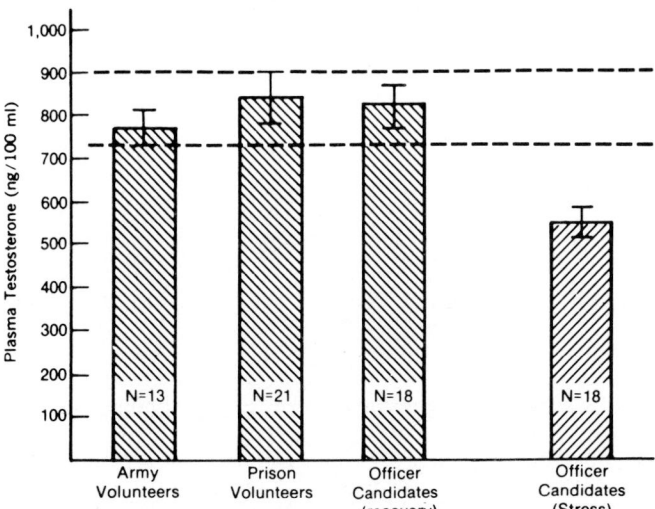

Figure 12–5. Mean plasma testosterone levels (with standard error of the mean) for officer candidates during the early, stressful period of training contrasted with levels for the same group later in training (recovery). Levels for two other nonstressed groups of men are also included. (From Kreuz, L. E., et al.: Suppression of plasma testosterone levels and psychological stress. *Arch. Gen. Psychol.* 26:480, 1972. Copyright 1972, American Medical Association.)

ENDOCRINE DISTURBANCES IN PSYCHIATRIC DISORDERS

Major Depressive Disorders

According to current diagnostic criteria, major depressive disorders are defined by: (1) a pervasive dysphoric (unpleasant) mood or loss of interests and pleasure, or both and (2) at least four of the following symptoms: anorexia, sleep disturbance, loss of energy, loss of libido, inappropriate guilt, psychomotor agitation or retardation (slowing), and suicidal ideas. Such patients often also manifest autonomic disturbances (dry mouth, constipation), and a diurnal variation in symptomatology (worse in the morning).

An overwhelming body of evidence points to a major biologic component to this form of depressive illness. This evidence includes the heritability of the disorder; rapid responsivity to antidepressant medication or electroconvulsive therapy, with lack of responsivity to conventional psychotherapy; an absence of significant psychosocial precipitants in at least two-thirds of the episodes; and the relapsing course of the disorder. The current view of the psychobiological disturbance is that it involves a deficit in brain noradrenergic or serotonergic (or both) activity. With many clinical signs implicating hypothalamic function (disturbances of mood, sleep, appetite, sexual drive, and autonomic activity), it is not surprising that neuroendocrine function is also affected. (It should be emphasized, however, that there are other depressive disorders that do not meet criteria for major depressions, and little is known yet about hormone function in these cases.)

Hypersecretion of Cortisol

During illness, approximately 50–60% of patients with major depressive disorder hypersecrete cortisol and ACTH, with reversion to normal after clinical recovery. There is no change in the biologic half-life of cortisol in these cases, and the excessive secretion of cortisol has been verified by isotopic dilution methods, indicating that the hypersecretion is probably secondary to increased hypothalamic CRF activity.

In the hypersecreting cases, both 24-hour cortisol production rate and mean 24-hour plasma cortisol concentration are elevated about 50% above normal. Analysis of the circadian pattern of plasma cortisol, determined every 20 min by blood sampling through an indwelling cannula, reveals a relative flattening of the diurnal curve: relative to the normal subjects, or to the same patients after clinical recovery, the depressive secrete more cortisol in the afternoon, evening, and early morning hours (Fig. 12–6).

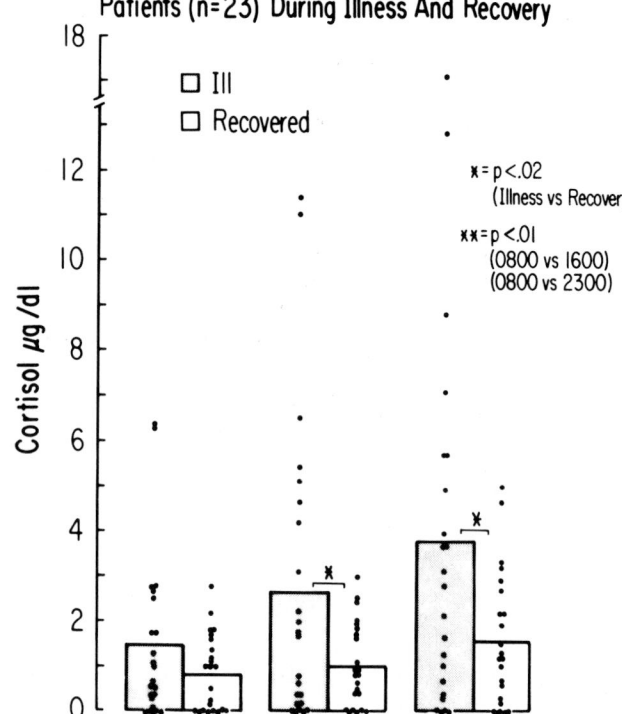

Figure 12–7. Plasma cortisol following dexamethasone (2 mg po administered previous day at 2300 hrs) in 23 endogenous depressed patients, during illness and after recovery. (From Sachar, E. J., Halbreich, M., et al.: Neurotransmitter regulation of cortisol secretion in depression. Studies of the response to dextroamphetamine, In *Neuroactive Drugs in Endocrinology: Physiologic, Diagnostic and Therapeutic Applications.* Muller, E. E., (ed.), New York, Elsevier-North Holland, in press.)

Depressed patients also manifest resistance to cortisol suppression by dexamethasone. After 2 mg of dexamethasone administered at 11 PM, nearly all depressed patients show cortisol suppression at 8 AM the next day, but 20–40% of patients manifest "escape" of plasma cortisol above 6 μg/dl at 4 PM or 11 PM (Fig. 12–7). The dexamethasone-resistant patients are those who hypersecrete cortisol, but only about half of hypersecreting patients are dexamethasone-resistant to this dose.

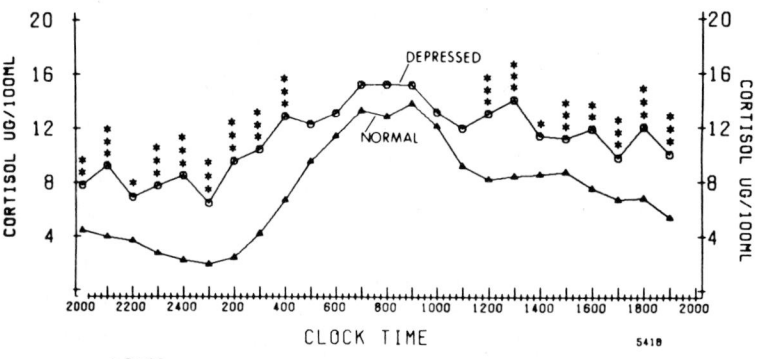

Figure 12–6. Mean hourly plasma cortisol levels in 7 unmedicated depressed patients and in 54 normal subjects. Differences between depressed patients and normals: x = p <.05; xx = p <.01; xxx = p <.001. (From Sachar, E. J., Halbreich, M., et al.: hemotransmitter regulation of cortisol secretion in depression. Studies of the response to dextroamphetamine, In *Neuroactive Drugs in Endocrinology: Physiologic, Diagnostic and Therapeutic Applications.* Muller, E. E. (ed.), New York, Elsevier-North Holland, in press.)

It is quite unlikely that cortisol hypersecretion in depressive illness reflects a stress response. The flattened circadian pattern is not reproduced in psychiatrically normal subjects experiencing severe emotional stress or prolonged sleep deprivation. The hypersecretion in depressed patients is not diminished by anxiolytic drugs such as diazepam, barbiturates, or chlorpromazine. The excessive secretion is not limited to waking periods but persists during EEG-verified sleep, and the hypersecreting pattern is also found in unanxious apathetic depressives. The resistance to cortisol suppression by dexamethasone is only rarely found in other acutely disturbed psychiatric cases. Indeed, it is possible that the dexamethasone suppression test, or measures of cortisol secretion, may eventually be useful as laboratory aids in the diagnosis of major depression.

Thus far, it has not been possible to identify clinical characteristics within the group of patients with major depressions that reliably predict those who are cortisol hypersecretors, although very recent evidence suggests that it occurs more frequently in older patients and those with "primary" depressions, i.e., "pure" depressions without a history of other psychiatric disorders.

Presumably, the hypersecretion reflects an underlying hypothalamic neurotransmitter abnormality. Since noradrenalin tonically inhibits (in animals) hypothalamic CRF secretion, it is possible that the hypothesized deficit in noradrenergic activity in major depression results in a disinhibition of CRF, ACTH, and cortisol secretion. Small intravenous doses of dextroamphetamine, which releases brain noradrenalin, have been shown to rapidly suppress cortisol levels in major depressives (Fig. 12–8).

Despite their increased production of cortisol, often for weeks or months, depressed patients never manifest physical signs of Cushing's syndrome. The reasons are unknown but may relate to the fact that the diurnal cortisol curve, although relatively flattened, is still partially preserved or to the fact that the extremely high cortisol secretion rates usually seen in Cushing's syndrome are rarely achieved in depressives. Free (unbound) cortisol levels may also be greater in Cushing's syndrome.

Deficient Human Growth Hormone Responses

About half of patients with major depressions have diminished human GH (HGH) responses to insulin-induced hypoglycemia, compared with control subjects matched for age, sex, and degree of hypoglycemia. In one study of nonobese, postmenopausal women with primary major depressions, half failed to achieve a 5 ng/ml rise in HGH after insulin tolerance tests (0.1 U/kg of regular insulin IV).

Insulin Resistance

About 30–50% of medically healthy, nonobese, depressed patients manifest a relative resistance to hypoglycemia during the standard insulin tolerance test (0.1 U/kg regular insulin IV), failing to have a 50% drop from baseline blood glucose levels or a nadir of less than 50 mg%. Depressed patients as a group have a significantly larger hypoglycemic response after clinical recovery than during illness (Fig. 12–9). The reason for this relative insulin resistance during depression is probably the increased afternoon and evening secretion of cortisol, since it occurs primarily in the cortisol-hypersecreting patients. A clinical corollary of this observation is that diabetic patients who suffer episodes of major depression may, while depressed, have an increased insulin requirement.

Thyrotropin Response to Thyrotropin-Releasing Hormone

Depressed patients as a group have a blunted thyrotropin (TSH) response to an infusion of a standard dose (500 μg) of thyrotropin-releasing hormone (TRH), compared with normal subjects matched for age and sex. About 50% of depressed patients fail to have an increase of 6 ng/ml after

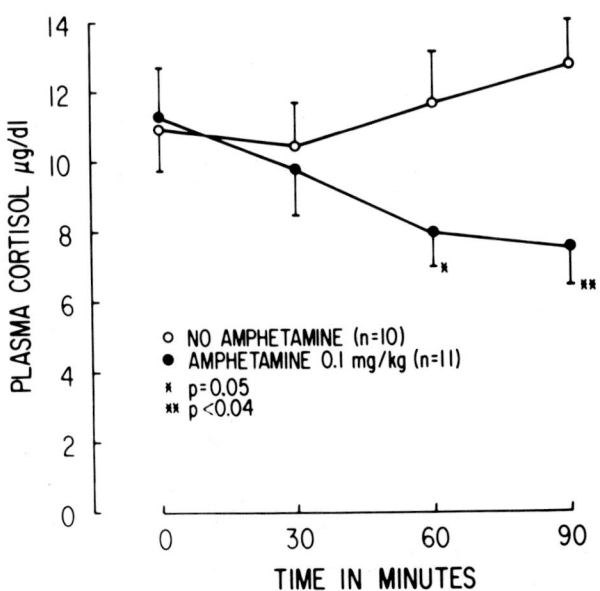

MORNING PLASMA CORTISOL IN 21 DEPRESSED PATIENTS WITH AND WITHOUT AMPHETAMINE

Figure 12–8. Plasma cortisol between 0930 and 1100 hours in 11 depressed patients receiving amphetamine (0.1 mg/kg IV) at 0 time and in 10 depressed patients receiving no amphetamine. (From Sachar, E. J., et al., *Arch. Gen. Psychiatry,* in press.)

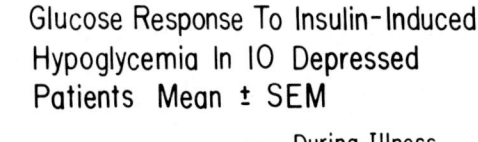
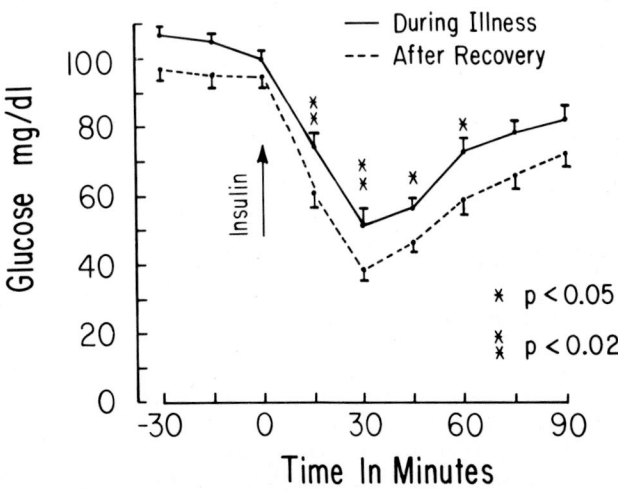

Figure 12–9. Mean hypoglycemic responses to insulin (0.1 U/kg IV) in depressed patients during illness and after recovery.

TRH infusion. Immediately after clinical recovery, the mean TSH response is significantly increased, compared with that achieved by the same subjects during illness, but some patients continue to show blunted responses. The cause of the blunted TSH response is unknown, since depressed patients show no other abnormality in thyroid function. It has been suggested that it may be secondary to the increased circulating levels of cortisol seen in many depressives, but one study found no such relation.

Summary

Although the elucidation of the causes of the various hormonal abnormalities in major depressive disorders may be primarily of interest to the psychobiologist, their extent in this condition should be familiar to the internist. Many depressed patients are preoccupied with their loss of energy, libido, and appetite and present first to the internist for a medical evaluation. A thorough assessment of the cardinal symptoms of depressive illness should aid the physician in evaluating the laboratory data and in making the often difficult differential diagnosis between a primary depression and a primary endocrinopathy. Pediatric endocrinologists should be aware that, although major depression is primarily a disorder of adults, it has been found to occur in prepubertal children as well, with some of the same endocrine abnormalities — deficient HGH response to hypoglycemia and hypersecretion of cortisol (Fig. 12–10).

Schizophrenia

Schizophrenia is a psychotic disorder affecting primarily adolescents and young adults. It is characterized by delusions and hallucinations, impaired social functioning, and, frequently, disturbances in thinking and communication, with symptoms lasting at least 6 months and occurring in the absence of signs of organic cognitive impairment. Such patients often have periods of extreme excitement and panic, and these are associated with large increases in corticosteroid and adrenaline excretion. The weight of evidence suggests that such endocrine abnormalities are transient and reflect a stress response rather than an underlying neuroendocrine abnormality, however.

Despite the fact that much circumstantial psychopharmacologic evidence supports the view that the acute psychotic episodes in schizophrenia are associated with hyperactivity of certain brain dopamine pathways, this hyperactivity, if it exists, does not appear to involve the tuberoinfundibular dopamine pathways regulating neuroendocrine function. PRL, for example, is tonically inhibited by dopamine, but baseline levels of PRL and the PRL response to standard doses of neuroleptics (all of which block dopamine transmission) are not abnormal in schizophrenics, nor is the PRL suppression induced by the dopamine precursor L-dopa or by the dopamine agonist apomorphine. Similarly, there is no consistent evidence for abnormal HGH responses to L-dopa or apomorphine, or to insulin-induced hypoglycemia.

As yet there is also no substantial body of evidence suggesting abnormalities in LH or FSH secretion, although these hormones, too, are regulated in part by dopaminergic tracts.

During periods of emotional quiescence, corticosteroid and adrenaline excretion are normal in schizophrenics, and even during periods of emotional arousal, plasma cortisol is generally suppressed by dexamethasone.

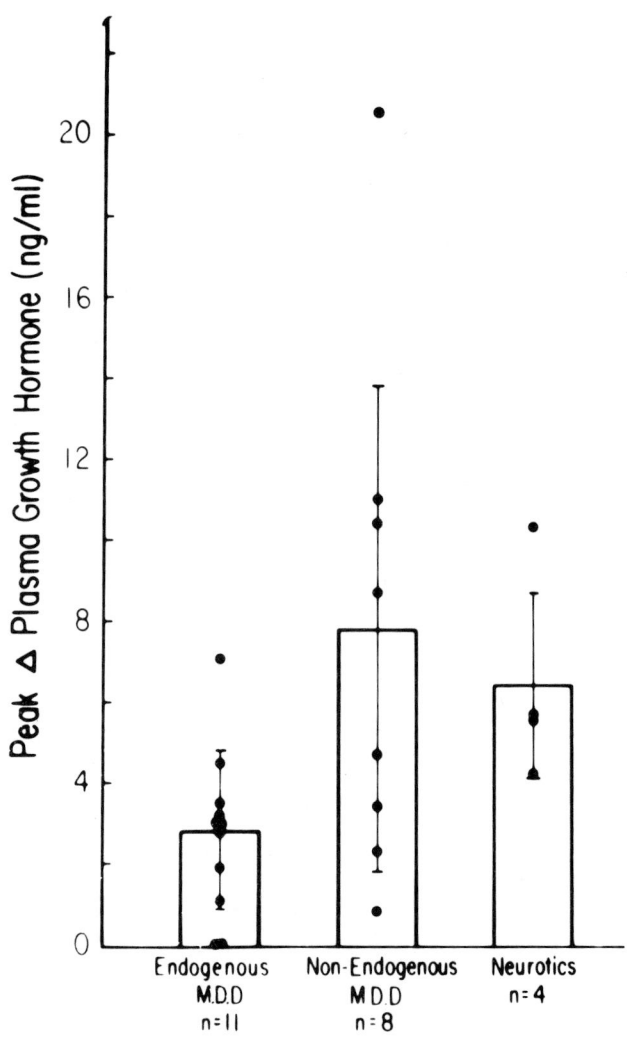

Figure 12–10. Maximal HGH responses to insulin-induced (0.1 U/kg) hypoglycemia in prepubertal children with major depressive and neurotic disorders. All children had adequate and comparable hypoglycemic responses, but the group with endogenous major depressions had deficient HGH responses.

Anorexia Nervosa

This disorder almost exclusively affects adolescent girls and young women. It is stereotyped in its presentation. The patient becomes morbidly afraid of gaining weight and becoming obese and misperceives her bodily image to be fatter than it is. Food is rejected to the point where weight loss falls at least 25% below age-appropriate norms. Amenorrhea is also a cardinal accompanying symptom, generally preceding major weight loss. Sometimes the disorder alternates with bulimia — uncontrollable binge eating, followed by shame and remorse. Mortality from anorexia nervosa ranges from 10 to 25%. The cause of this condition is unknown, nor is there yet compelling evidence for a primarily psychological or a primarily biological etiology.

There are multiple endocrine abnormalities associated with anorexia nervosa. It remains unclear to what extent these changes are secondary to the starvation and loss of body fat (with its role in steroid metabolism) and to what extent they may reflect primary hypothalamic dysfunction manifesting itself in eating disturbances. In general (*but not always*), the hormonal disturbances parallel the weight loss and remit in association with, or soon after, clinical recovery — defined as return to normal weight. Thus, which is cart and which is horse is still uncertain.

Reduced Luteinizing Hormone Secretion

The 24-hour pattern of plasma LH typically reverts to that of early or prepuberty. Prepubertally, LH concentration is normally low and shows no circadian pattern. In early puberty, pulsatile LH surges occur during sleep. In late puberty and after, the adult pattern is established — higher mean levels of LH with pulses throughout the day unlinked to sleep, at least during nonovulatory days (Fig. 12–11).

The regression in LH patterns in anorexia nervosa is associated with the characteristic sign of amenorrhea (Figs. 12–12, 12–13). The response to LRH is often impaired, as is, typically, the response to clomiphene. Atrophy of the gonadotropic cells of the pituitary has been reported in one autopsied case in which special staining methods were used. Normal LH patterns are generally re-established with clinical recovery, although the deficient clomiphene response may persist longer.

Human Growth Hormone Abnormalities

Basal HGH concentration is elevated in about one-third of anorexia nervosa cases and diminished HGH response to hypoglycemia is also frequent. (HGH responses to arginine infusion are generally normal, however.) Again, there is controversy as to whether these disturbances in HGH can be entirely explained by malnutrition.

Cortisol Disturbances

Plasma cortisol concentration is elevated and the circadian curve is flattened. This is only partly due to decreased hepatic metabolism of cortisol, however, since cortisol production is also increased, on a per kg body weight basis. Similar changes are seen in malnutrition from other causes, however.

Thyroid Function

Plasma triiodothyronine (T_3) levels are low, but T_4 is generally normal, suggesting decreased conversion of T_4 to T_3. The TSH response to TRH is not blunted but is slowed.

Differential Diagnosis

The differential diagnosis of anorexia nervosa from panhypopituitarism on the one hand and from depressive illness with anorexia on the other is not difficult. The psychiatric picture, particularly the disturbances in body image and the morbid fear of gaining weight, serves to distinguish it from depressive illness. The laboratory tests, revealing normal or elevated cortisol secretion, generally normal T_4 and generally normal HGH response to arginine, rule out pituitary failure.

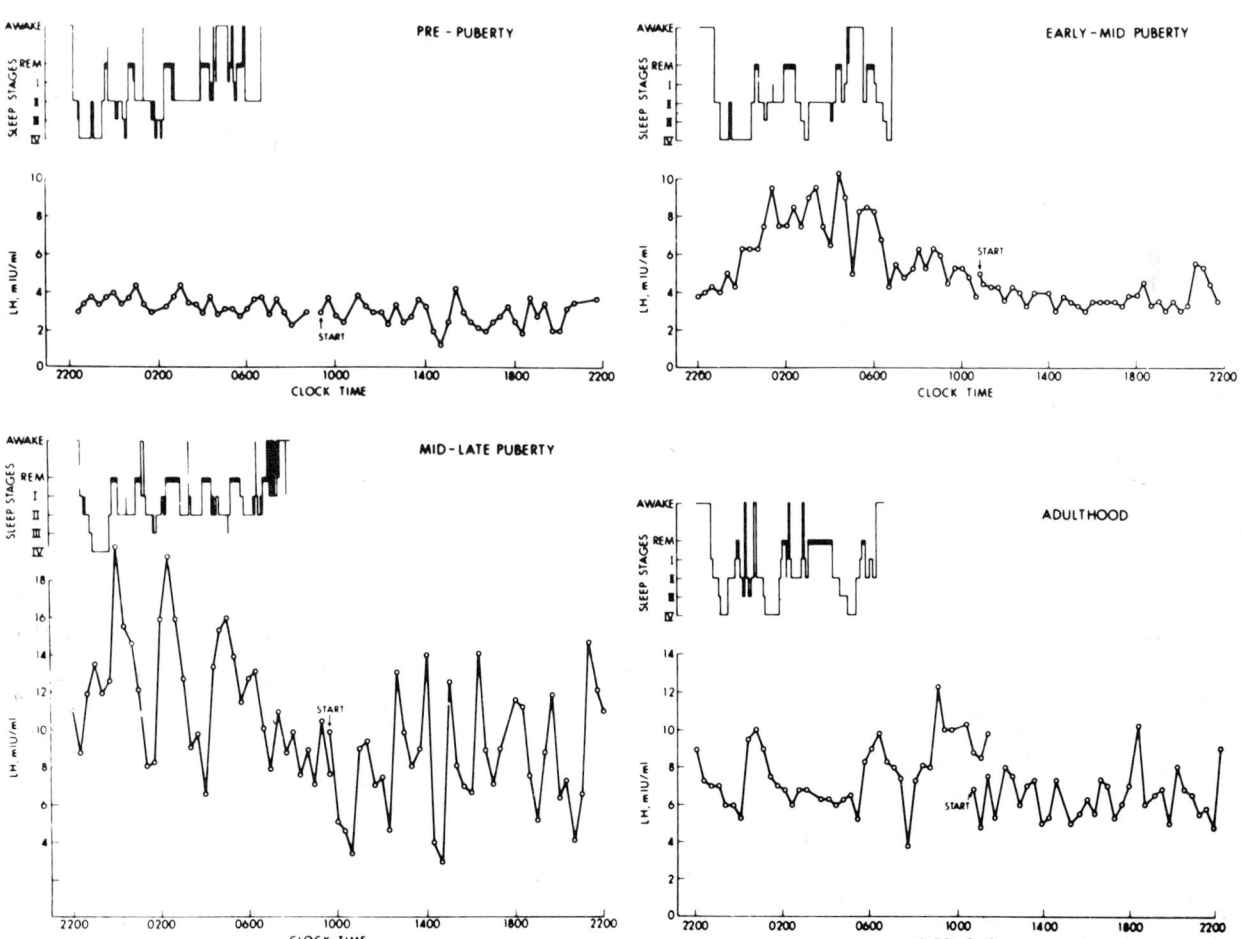

Figure 12–11. Typical 24-hour plasma LH curves and sleep patterns in normal women at different stages of development. (From Katz, J. L., Boyer, R. M., et al.: Toward an elucidation of the psychoendocrinology of anorexia nervosa. In *Hormones, Behavior, and Psychopathology*. Sachar, E. J. (ed.), New York, Raven Press, 1976.)

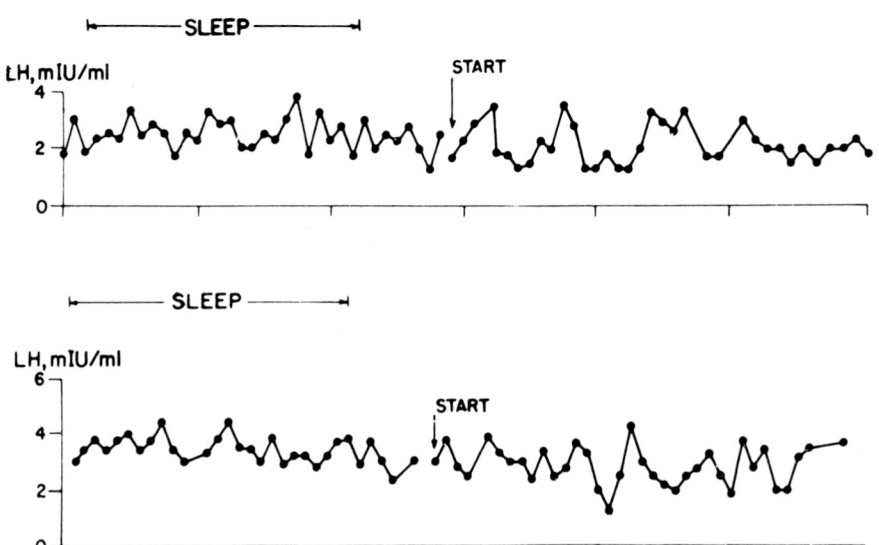

Figure 12–12. Top: Abnormal, prepubertal 24-hour plasma LH curve in a 21-year-old woman with anorexia nervosa. Bottom: Plasma LH pattern in a normal 9-year-old prepubertal girl. (From Katz, J. L., Boyer, R. M., et al.: Toward an elucidation of the psychoendocrinology of anorexia nervosa, In *Hormones, Behavior, and Psychopathology.* Sachar, E. J. (ed.), New York, Raven Press, 1976.)

Treatment

Although many types of pharmacotherapy have been attempted in anorexia nervosa — including neuroleptics, antidepressants, cyproheptadine, and various hormones — none have stood the test of double-blind placebo-controlled trials. The major treatments remain psychological interventions, and behavior modification (focused on specific rates of weight gain) and intensive family therapy (focused partly on power struggles over eating behavior and dependence-independence conflicts) appear to be the most promising current approaches.

"Psychogenic" Amenorrhea

Under conditions of emotional distress, many women will skip one or more periods. Leaving home to go to college or boarding school, life crises, bereavement, and onset of psychiatric disorders such as acute depression or schizophrenia are commonly associated with periods of amenorrhea.

The cause of this situational "stress" amenorrhea is unknown, but it is speculated that stress is associated with a transitory imbalance in hypothalamic neurotransmitters regulating LH.

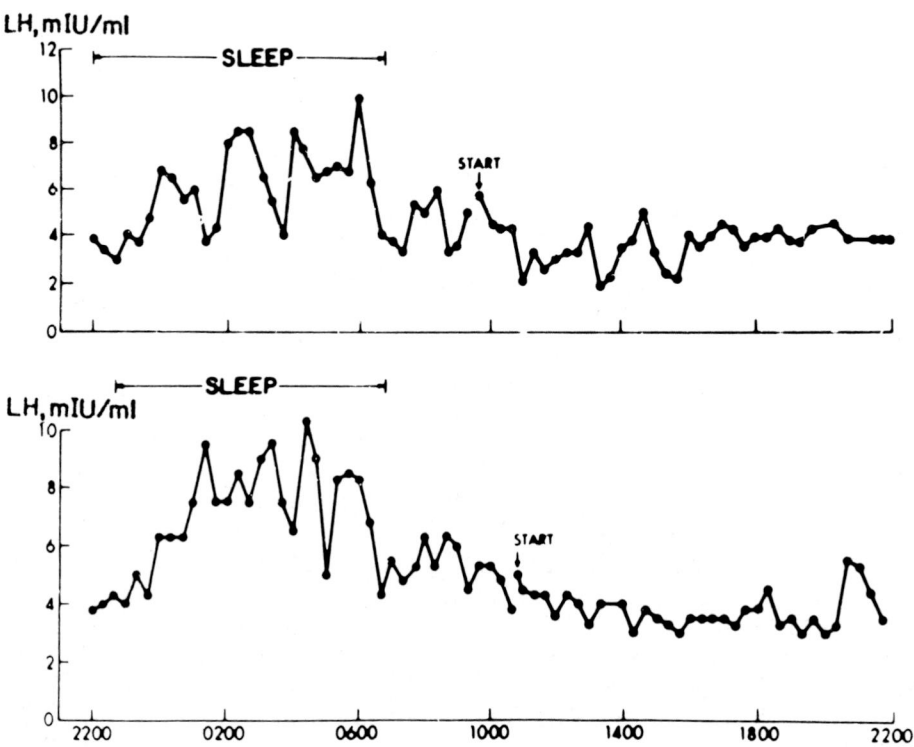

Figure 12–13. Top: Abnormal, early pubertal 24-hour plasma LH pattern in a 17-year-old girl with anorexia nervosa. Bottom: Normal 12-year-old pubertal girl. (From Katz, J. L., Boyer, R. M., et al.: Toward an elucidation of the psychoendocrinology of anorexia nervosa, In *Hormones, Behavior, and Psychopathology* Sachar, E. J. (ed.), New York, Raven Press, 1976.)

On the other hand, many women without obvious endocrine pathology fail to menstruate for many months or years. Some are subsequently revealed to have hyperprolactinemia, or some other disorder, although in many others no cause can be found. The use of the term "psychogenic" for these cases is inappropriate, because there is no evidence from any controlled study that they disproportionately suffer from any particular form of psychopathology or that psychotherapy of any type is efficacious compared to placebo.

Thus, a recent extensive study evaluated 114 patients with amenorrhea without obvious organic cause by clinical interviews, psychological tests, questionnaires, and detailed family histories. These were compared to those gathered from control groups of neurotic outpatients and a random sample of Finnish women. The investigators found that "The amenorrheic group as a whole did not seem to differ from the normal population on social and family background variables. Differences in mental disturbances and personality features were slight on average. Sexual problems were demonstrated, although they were slight. . . . The amenorrheic group appeared very heterogeneous. . . . The average patient did not differ much from an ordinary woman."

It seems, then, that for these cases "idiopathic" amenorrhea would be a better term than "psychogenic," reflecting more accurately our present state of knowledge.

Psychosocial Dwarfism

We are heavily indebted to the workers at Johns Hopkins, particularly Powell and Money and their collaborators, for much of our modern knowledge of this condition. Prepubertal children over the age of 3 with this reversible disorder manifest delayed puberty, markedly reduced stature (average 52% of age norms), and retarded bone age, without evidence of marasmus or other primary medical or endocrine disease. When removed from their family environments into an emotionally supportive hospital setting, however, the children begin to grow again rapidly, tending to catch up with their age norms.

These observations, coupled with the clinical evidence that most, if not all, such children have been grossly neglected, isolated, or abused in their home environments, account for the term "psychosocial dwarfism." In infants and toddlers, there appears to be a similar syndrome, sometimes termed "maternal deprivation with failure to thrive."

Behavioral Manifestations

The children as a group are initially apathetic and withdrawn, avoiding personal contact, emotionally and verbally unresponsive to efforts to engage them, often avoiding even eye contact. Their apathy is occasionally punctuated by brief temper tantrums.

Many of the children also initially appear relatively insensitive to pain, and often self-inflict injuries. Some are encopretic and enuretic. Reports of insomnia and disrupted sleep at home are also common. Many are also described as "roaming" at night, perhaps to find food and drink, and as eating and drinking inappropriate substances. These reports of behavior in the home have to be evaluated cautiously, because the families of such patients often are concealing psychological harassment and physical abuse of the children.

Nearly all these pathologic behaviors rapidly reverse within 48 hours to 2 weeks in a supportive milieu. Indeed, there may even be a transient, evidently compensatory hyperactive period, as the formerly apathetic, withdrawn child hungrily seeks social contact, intensively questions staff, behaves boisterously, and over-reacts emotionally to stimuli. Even the IQ scores of such children typically increase by several points.

Endocrine Manifestations

Growth Hormone

The characteristic endocrine abnormality in virtually all such children on admission is a deficient HGH response to insulin-induced hypoglycemia. The majority also lack an adequate HGH response to arginine infusion and to exercise. In one case in which it was determined, HGH secretion during slow wave sleep was also lacking.

After 4–6 weeks of good nutrition and supportive care, the HGH response is restored in nearly all cases. The previous failure to grow and the subsequent resumption of growth are assumed to be caused by the lack and subsequent return of HGH secretion. One case report, however, suggests that somatomedin may also be suppressed and may return to normal in association with growth resumption.

Adrenal Cortex

Basal corticosteroid excretion is low, as is the response to metyrapone, but the response to ACTH is normal. (This is in contrast to starved patients, who generally have deficient corticosteroid responses to ACTH.) This abnormality also reverts after several weeks of care.

Thyroid

The various indices of thyroid function have been reported as normal in nearly all cases.

Etiology

It has been suggested by some that the immediate cause of the disorder is nutritional, rather than emotional deprivation — that the children have been starved for years by their families. In some infants with the maternal deprivation–failure to grow syndrome, nutritional supplements provided by visiting nurses sufficed to restore normal growth patterns. In the older children with psychosocial dwarfism, however, the crucial role of nutritional deprivation is much less certain. Most of these children are not obviously malnourished for their size, and some are even somewhat obese. The hormonal findings are not congruent with those of starved subjects — basal HGH levels are not elevated and the adrenal response to ACTH is normal. The Hopkins group could not find evidence for nutritional deprivation at home for most of their subjects, although this could have been concealed.

It may be of relevance that in studies of rat pups, maternal separation promptly and specifically suppresses GH secretion. This is true even when nutrition is maintained by an anesthetized mother. On the other hand, contact with an awake mother with ligated nipples immediately restores GH secretion, in the absence of nutrition. Vigorous stroking of separated pups (mimicking the mother's grooming) also restores GH secretion in the absence of nutrition. Thus, at least in the rat, hypothalamic mechanisms exist for nonnutritional suppression of GH secretion by maternal deprivation. It may also be relevant that endogenous depression of adulthood is associated with deficient HGH responses to hypoglycemia, and preliminary data indicate that this abnormality also occurs in prepubertal children with major depressive disorder, endogenous subtype.

PSYCHIATRIC DISTURBANCES ASSOCIATED WITH ENDOCRINOPATHIES AND HORMONE THERAPY

Introduction

Although psychiatric abnormalities associated with endocrine disease have been noted for centuries, and a number of series of clinical reports were published between the 1930s and 1950s, this remains, paradoxically, an underdeveloped area of psychiatric research. In particular, there has been a remarkable lack of work using modern methods of psychiatric diagnosis, comprehensive, quantitative assessments of psychopathology, proper control groups, or any systematic epidemiologic study. Thus, when an endocrine patient is described as hallucinating or delusional, we often have no way of knowing if this reflects an organic brain syndrome or another type of psychosis. Frequently, clinicians assume that all psychoses occurring in medical patients are "schizophrenic" and describe them as such — which is analogous to describing all obese patients as "myxedematous." Schizophrenia is surely the least likely cause of psychosis in a medical patient, with organic mental syndromes the most likely, yet clinicians rarely evaluate cognitive and memory functions in such patients. When a patient is described as "depressed," it is frequently unclear whether he or she is suffering from discouragement and demoralization about his medical condition, is primarily debilitated and fatigued as a nonspecific result of illness, or is actually suffering a syndrome similar in symptom profile to major depression. Surveys of incidence of psychopathology in an endocrine disorder rarely meet standards for unbiased case selection and virtually never include appropriate control groups. All too often important additional relevant medical data are omitted; e.g., electrolyte balance, renal and cardiac function, blood pressure, presence of ketosis, and so on, all of which typically affect mental state. The summaries that follow, therefore, are in most instances clinical impressions, gleaned from case reports, that require further rigorous research by modern methods for firm data.

Hypothyroidism

The severe mental defect associated with untreated cretinism is well known and is related to the essential role of thyroid hormone in brain development. In general, the degree of mental defect is proportional to the length of time before institution of therapy.

Adult onset myxedema is characterized by psychomotor slowing, lethargy, and apathy. Depression, confusion, cognitive impairment, and occasional psychoses ("myxedema madness") have also been reported. Diminution in acuity of taste and smell occurs in most patients.

In a rare example of a thorough, systematic, psychiatric study of an unbiased (albeit small) sample of endocrine patients, Whybrow and associates (1969) examined, consec-

utively, all patients found to have thyroid dysfunction in an endocrine clinic over a 12-month period both before and after treatment. Patients with pre-existing psychiatric or neurologic disorder, mental deficiency, or arteriosclerotic or cardiovascular disease were excluded. Six of the 7 (76%) hypothyroid patients had significant scores for depressive symptoms, as rated by Minnesota Multiphasic Personality Inventory (MMPI) and the Brief Psychiatric Rating Scale (BPRS), and one of these was delusional and suicidal. The symptom profiles in these cases closely resembled those of endogenous depressives. Despair, suicidal thoughts, crying spells, and premonitions of doom were common.

The same patients additionally manifested significant signs of organic cognitive dysfunction, both on clinical mental status examination and on neuropsychological testing. Recent memory, abstraction, and attention were particularly impaired. These findings confirm the impression that the confusion, disorientation, and hallucinations seen in "myxedema madness" are reflections of an organic brain syndrome typically associated with hypothyroidism. In Whybrow's series, after thyroid replacement therapy, the depressive phenomena largely cleared and the cognitive disturbances were ameliorated in all, but some residual intellectual defect was noted in the cases of long-standing myxedema.

There are some clues as to the neurobiologic bases for the depressive and cognitive symptoms of hypothyroidism. As previously noted, a deficit in brain noradrenergic activity is suspected in endogenous depression. There is evidence that thyroid hormone regulates the sensitivity of brain catecholamine receptors. Thus, thyroid hormone–treated rats have augmented responses to brain catecholamine agonists. Hypothyroid rats have increased brain catecholamine turnover, a typical compensatory presynaptic neuronal response to reduced synaptic transmission. Patients with hypothyroidism (who often present with depressive syndromes) respond poorly to tricyclic antidepressants, which are believed to act, in part, by blocking presynaptic neuronal reuptake and catabolism of noradrenalin; after thyroid hormone treatment, such patients generally respond promptly. Furthermore T_3 in small doses (25 μg/d) has been shown to accelerate and potentiate the response of euthyroid depressed patients to antidepressant medication. Thus, a functional noradrenergic deficit caused by receptor insensitivity, induced by thyroid hormone deficiency, may account for the depressive phenomena seen in myxedema.

A similar etiology may underlie the disturbances in memory and attention. In animal behavioral studies, noradrenergic mechanisms have been shown to be critical in mediating short-term memory and attentional processes.

Differential Diagnosis

Because hypothyroidism frequently presents initially as a depressive syndrome very similar to that seen in endogenous depression, it would seem warranted to screen depressed patients seeking psychiatric help for thyroid function as part of a routine evaluation. Similarly, treatment of the recognized hypothyroid patient should include attention to the nearly ubiquitous affective and cognitive disturbances. In Whybrow's series, only one case had been referred for psychiatric consultation, although nearly all cases were suffering marked impairment. Although thyroid hormone is the corrective medication, it is important for the patient and his family to appreciate that the mental difficulties are part of the endocrinopathy and should respond to therapy.

Hyperthyroidism

Anxiety, restlessness, fatigue, and irritability are symptoms experienced by most patients with hyperthyroidism, although apathy, withdrawal, and depression may occasionally be seen, particularly in older patients. The motor restlessness has been aptly described as a great many purposeful movements without any purpose. Clinically, the anxiety is difficult to differentiate from that seen in anxiety neurotics. Although propranolol is helpful in diminishing the cardiac effects of hyperthyroidism, it does not affect the psychic anxiety.

In severely hyperthyroid patients, perceptual disturbances, including visual hallucinations, are frequently noted. Psychotic disorganization with paranoid ideas occasionally occurs.

Cognitive function is impaired, primarily due to difficulties in attention and distractibility.

These various psychological disturbances are replicated by overtreatment with thyroid hormone.

Although there are many anecdotal reports of the onset of hyperthyroidism after severe life stress, there have been no studies to indicate that such antecedent psychosocial stresses are more frequent in hyperthyroid patients than in control subjects.

Hypercortisolism (Cushing's Syndrome)

Psychiatric disturbances are quite common in Cushing's syndrome, whether of adrenal or pituitary origin. Although precise epidemiologic studies have not been conducted, it is estimated that at least one third of cases suffer significant psychiatric morbidity, and the true incidence is probably higher.

Some of the disturbances are caused by the secondary metabolic derangements associated with Cushing's syndrome, such as electrolyte imbalance, diabetes with ketosis, and hypertension with hypertensive encephalopathy. It is not surprising that organic mental syndromes would result from these derangements, leading to confusional episodes, auditory and visual illusions and hallucinations, delusions, and alterations in consciousness.

On the other hand, there is little doubt that cortisol excess *per se* produces profound psychological disturbances. Depression is the most common psychopathological disorder seen, ranging from crying spells and over-responsivity to minor disappointments to full blown syndromes resembling major endogenous depressions. Although the milder forms are hard to differentiate from an understandable reaction to fatigue, debilitation, and physical disfigurement, the severe forms may be associated with depressive delusions and suicidal tendencies. In one series, 10% of cases attempted suicide.

Mild or severe forms of mania are also not infrequent. Typical manifestations are an excessively "pepped-up" feeling, overtalkativeness, overactivity, irritability, decreased sleep, impulsivity, and intrusiveness. In severe forms, elation, grandiose ideas, buying sprees, sexual indiscretions, and even delusions occur. Mixtures of organic and affective syndromes are also seen. Interesting alterations in acuity of taste and smell have been noted in psychophysical testing, although these are rarely complained of by the patients.

The psychiatric disturbances of Cushing's syndrome tend to fluctuate in intensity and in type, perhaps related to fluctuations in hormonal levels and associated metabolic derangements, although such correlational studies have not been done.

Treatment with exogenous corticosteroid preparations are also associated with psychological and psychiatric disturbances, similar to those seen in Cushing's syndrome. The most common response appears to be an amphetamine-like effect: a mild elevation in mood, a "pepped-up" restless feeling, and an increase in irritability, sometimes associated with sleeplessness. It has been reported that some patients become dependent on the mood elevating, energizing effects of steroid therapy, and note anergia and mild depression on steroid withdrawal somewhat analogous to the let-down or "crash" after amphetamine withdrawal.

More severe psychiatric disturbances also occur with corticosteroid therapy: hypomanic or frankly manic syndromes are not uncommon, and mild and severe depressions are also frequent. Although depressions are more common than mania in endogenous Cushing's syndrome, the reverse appears to be the case in corticosteroid therapy. The reason for this interesting, apparent discrepancy in relative incidence is not known.

The precise mechanisms by which the hormonal disturbances exert their mental effects are unknown. Pioneering work by DeWied and his colleagues has established that ACTH itself, independent of its endocrine effects, is psychoactive in animals. ACTH and fragments of the ACTH molecule (ACTH 4–10) influence conditioned learning behavior, as well as memory processes, in rats. There is also extensive literature on animal studies, some of it conflicting, on the effects of ACTH and of corticosteroids on the metabolism of brain neurotransmitters implicated in affective and arousal states and memory processes, including noradrenalin and serotonin.

The possibility is thereby raised that the psychiatric disturbances associated with excess of corticosteroids and decrease of ACTH (e.g., exogenous steroid therapy and primary adrenal Cushing's syndrome) may differ somewhat from those associated with excess of both ACTH and corticosteroids (e.g., pituitary Cushing's syndrome). Thus, anecdotal reports suggest that severe depression was a more common complication during the era of ACTH therapy. No rigorous comparative psychoendocrine analyses have yet been conducted of the various Cushing disorders, however. It is also unknown whether the hypothalamic factor CRF itself is psychoactive.

The psychiatric disturbances associated with Cushing's syndrome remit with correction of the underlying disorder and associated metabolic abnormalities. Interim symptomatic control of the behavioral disturbances may be partially accomplished with supportive care and psychotropic medication. Thus, the confusion associated with organic mental syndromes is alleviated by structuring the environment and keeping it familiar, leaving on a night light, having a clock always visible, and so on. Severe agitation and psychotic episodes can be alleviated with neuroleptics. The depressions are more difficult to treat; the antidepressants act slowly in any case and reportedly are less effective in steroid-induced conditions.

The clinician faces an especially hard dilemma when a patient requiring corticosteroid therapy for medical reasons develops psychiatric disturbances that do not respond to correction of electrolyte, cardiovascular, and other metabolic derangements. Cautious reduction of corticosteroid dose frequently is successful; it is claimed that subsequent reinstitution of a full therapeutic dose can sometimes be achieved without return of the psychiatric disability. Lithium has been reported to prevent the occurrence of psychotic mood disorders during the course of ACTH therapy of multiple sclerosis; in the control group, the incidence was 14%.

One of the most fiendishly difficult clinical problems

occurs when a patient with disseminated lupus erythematosus (LE) receiving steroid therapy develops psychiatric disturbances: Does this reflect CNS LE calling for higher steroid doses or a steroid psychosis calling for lowered dosage? When a careful review of the patient's clinical and medication history fails to provide clues, trial and error adjustment of dose, with serial quantitative assessments of mental function, seems to be the wisest course of action.

Addison's Disease

Apathy, fatigue, somnolence, anorexia, nightmares, and depression are very common psychiatric manifestations of Addison's disease. Confusion and organic psychoses also occur, probably in association with the electrolyte imbalances and hypoglycemia. Hyperacuity of taste and smell is also demonstrable by psychophysical testing, although generally patients are unaware of this.

Adequate corticosteroid replacement therapy reverses the psychopathology, and a recent long-term follow-up study of treated juveniles with Addison's disease revealed no major psychiatric disability. Because steroid requirements sometimes fluctuate, however, the physician should be alert to the reappearance of psychiatric disturbances that may indicate the need for temporary increased dosage.

Hyperparathyroidism

Depression, apathy, confusion, and organic psychoses are quite common in hyperparathyroid states, and not infrequently patients present with the psychiatric disturbance as their initial symptom. The psychologic abnormalities are directly related to the hypercalcemia, rather than to the parathyroid hormone (PTH) *per se*. In general, at serum Ca concentrations between 11 and 16 mg%, symptoms of depression, fatigue, apathy, and inability to concentrate are preponderant, whereas above 16 mg%, organic psychoses and stupor are frequent. The psychiatric disturbances remit promptly after renal dialysis or after successful parathyroid surgery.

Hypoparathyroidism

Idiopathic hypothyroidism, when unrecognized and untreated for a long period of time, is associated with intellectual deterioration in about one third of cases, and after treatment a residual intellectual deficit frequently persists. Organic mental syndromes, including organic psychoses, also occur in about one third of cases, and other patients are reported to suffer from "nervousness," "emotionality," and so on.

Surgical hypoparathyroidism is also associated with organic mental syndromes, including psychoses, but intellectual deficit is rare — probably because the condition is generally recognized and treated quickly. With prompt treatment, the mental symptoms nearly always clear completely.

Hyperinsulinism

With chronic hypoglycemia, cerebral cortical symptoms are prominent and include headaches, faintness, confusion, restlessness, somnolence, irritability, and visual disturbances. More intermittent hypoglycemic states with adrenergic symptoms can closely mimic anxiety states, particularly panic disorder, since both are associated with sudden onset of intense subjective anxiety, tremor, palpitations, perspiration, and dizziness. The reverse error in diagnosis is more commonly made, however: patients with panic disorder (readily treatable with imipramine), are frequently misdiagnosed by internists as hypoglycemic on the basis of clinically insignificant degrees of rebound hypoglycemia after meals.

EFFECTS OF PSYCHOTROPIC AGENTS ON ENDOCRINE FUNCTION

Although it is beyond the scope of this chapter to review exhaustively all the reported effects of every psychoactive agent on all measures of hormonal activity, it is important for the endocrinologist to be aware of the clinically significant endocrine influences of the commonly prescribed drugs, as well as of certain substances of abuse.

Antipsychotic (Neuroleptic) Drugs

The major classes of commonly used antipsychotic drugs include the phenothiazines (e.g., chlorpromazine, thiordiazine, trifluoperazine), the butyrophenones (e.g., haloperidol), thioxanthenes (e.g., thiothixene) dibenzoxazepines (e.g., loxapine), and indolic compounds (e.g., molindone). They are effective in terminating acute psychotic episodes and in preventing recurrence of psychotic episodes in schizophrenics.

Although these medications vary greatly in mg for mg potency in the treatment of psychoses and have major differences in chemical structure, all, without exception, rapidly stimulate PRL secretion.

This is not surprising, because the single neurochemical property all these agents share is that of blocking dopamine transmission across synapses, apparently blocking dopamine receptors. This brain dopamine-blocking property is believed to be an essential feature of the therapeutic action of these drugs in psychoses. The dopamine receptors of the pituitary lactotropic cells are also blocked by antipsychotic drugs, releasing these cells from their tonic inhibition by dopamine from the tuberoinfundibular tract (Fig. 12–14). The relative PRL-stimulating potencies of the various antipsychotic drugs correlate highly with their relative clinical potencies (Fig. 12–15) and with their relative potencies in binding to dopamine receptors. While patients are maintained on neuroleptics, they also sustain elevated PRL lev-

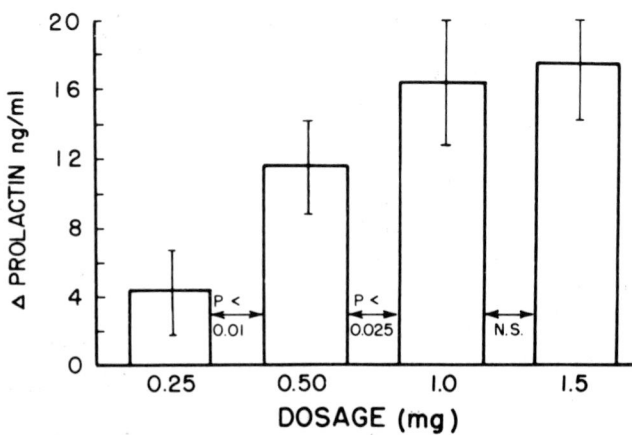

Figure 12–14. Mean maximal PRL increases within 150 min after various intramuscular doses of haloperidol in the same normal young men (n = 7). (From Gruen, P. H., et al.: Prolactin responses to neuroleptics in normal and schizophrenic subjects. *Arch. Gen. Psychiatry* 35:108, 1978.)

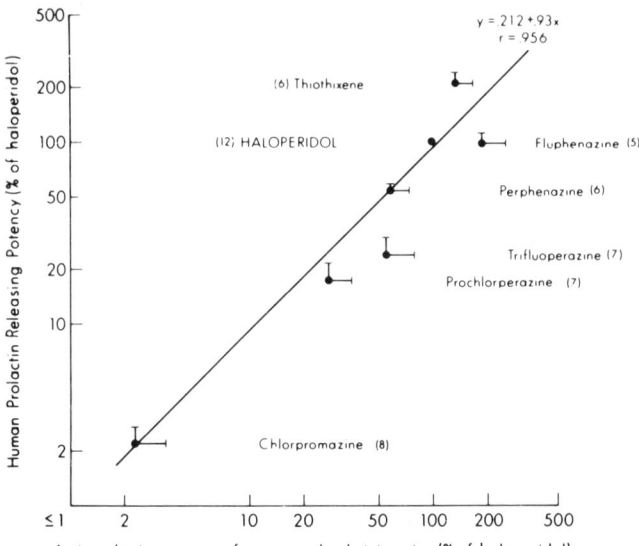

Figure 12–15. Correlation in men between antipsychotic potencies and PRL-stimulating potencies (both expressed relative to haloperidol = 100%) of several neuroleptic drugs. Relative antipsychotic potencies by parenteral administration were gleaned from the literature. PRL = stimulating potencies were determined in groups of normal young men. Example: 1 mg of chlorpromazine has only 2.5% of 1 mg haloperidol's prolactin-stimulating effect in men and also only 2.5% of haloperidol's clinical potency. (From Langer, G., et al.: Human prolactin responses to neuroleptic drugs correlate with antischizophrenic potency. *Nature 266*:639, 1977.)

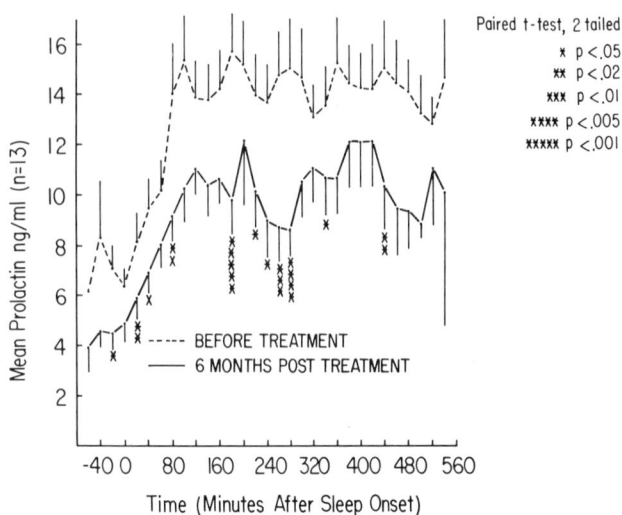

Figure 12–16. Plasma PRL levels during sleep in 13 hyperkinetic boys before beginning dextroamphetamine therapy and in the sixth month of continuous dextroamphetamine therapy. Amphetamine therapy was associated with a reduction in nighttime PRL secretion. Differences between conditions: x = p < .05; xx = p < .02; xxx = p < .01; xxxx = p < .005; xxxxx = p < .001. (From Greenhill, L. et al., *J. Acad. Child Psychiatry*, in press.)

els, at least for many months (although after several years PRL may return to the normal range). Occasionally then, patients maintained on antipsychotic medication will develop galactorrhea. Women have larger PRL responses to neuroleptics than do men, probably because of estrogen potentiation of lactotropic secretion. The PRL response increases with the dose of neuroleptic, up to a point, generally achieving a maximum at dosages equivalent to 500–700 mg of chlorpromazine a day. PRL levels generally return to normal within 3–4 days after discontinuation of antipsychotic medication.

PRL stimulation appears to be the major hormonal effect of neuroleptics. It has not been established that they interfere significantly with physiologic GH or LH secretion in humans, and they appear to have little effect on thyroid function. Although these agents, which also have antianxiety or "tranquilizing" properties, will also diminish the ACTH response to stress, they do not have significant effect on basal or circadian rhythms of ACTH.

Amphetamines

The major clinical use of maintenance dextroamphetamine therapy is in the treatment of children with hyperkinetic syndrome (also called attentional disorder or minimal brain dysfunction). It has recently been shown that chronic treatment with amphetamine suppresses PRL secretion in children, particularly that occurring in association with sleep (Fig. 12–16).

Chronic stimulant therapy of these children is also associated with a slowing of their growth and a reduction in both height and weight velocity. The magnitude of the growth slowing within a group of amphetamine-treated children significantly correlated with the magnitude of the PRL suppression (Fig. 12–17). There is no evidence that PRL itself is a growth factor in humans (though it appears to be in animals), however, so the clinical significance of this correla-

tion is unclear. Secretion of HGH during sleep and in response to insulin-induced hypoglycemia was unaffected by amphetamine therapy, nor was the secretion of cortisol.

Lithium

Lithium carbonate is used mainly in patients with manic-depressive disorders, or with recurrent depressions, since it has been shown that lithium maintenance therapy in such patients significantly reduces both the rate of recurrence and the severity of subsequent affective episodes. The daily dose is usually in the range of 600–1800 mg, adjusted to achieve a predose morning serum concentration of 0.8–1/2 mEq/l. Its mechanism of therapeutic action is still unknown.

Lithium has been found to cause various abnormalities in thyroid function. Lithium concentration in thyroid tissue is about four times the serum concentration. After about 1 month of lithium therapy, there is a generally benign diminution in blood levels of thyroid hormones. Physiologically, lithium inhibits the action of TSH on the thyroid gland, inhibits the uptake of ^{131}I, impairs the conversion of iodotyrosines to idothyronines (e.g., the synthesis of T_4 and T_3), and interferes with release of thyroid hormones. These particular effects of lithium on the thyroid have occasionally resulted in euthyroid goiter, goiter with hypothyroidism, and hypothyroidism with normal-sized thyroid gland. The prevalence of these clinical abnormalities in patients on lithium are reported to range from 3.6% to 15%, whereas changes in the laboratory measures of thyroid function have been found in as many as one third to one half of patients on lithium. Some investigators have found a significantly increased incidence of thyroid autoantibodies in patients who have developed hypothyroidism while on Li^+, suggesting that a subgroup of patients with Li^+-associated hypothyroidism is suffering from autoimmune thyroiditis.

Cases of clinical hypothyroidism associated with lithium treatment are very responsive to the addition of T_4.

Hyperthyroidism has rarely been associated with lithium use (a total of 8 cases in the literature). Some of these cases first manifested hyperthyroidism shortly after lithium withdrawal; this may represent a rebound thyrotoxicity due to

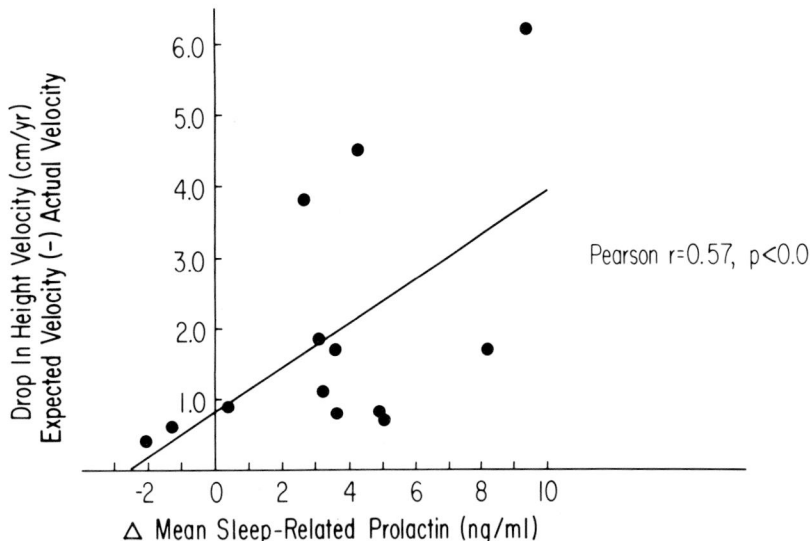

Figure 12–17. Correlation between expected height loss (cm/year) and change from pretreatment levels of mean sleep-related PRL levels (ng/ml) during dextroamphetamine therapy in 13 hyperkinetic boys. In general, the greater the decrease in nighttime PRL levels, the greater was the slowing in height velocity. (From Greenhill, L. et al., *J. Acad. Child Psychiatry* in press.)

the release of the suppressive effect of Li$^+$ on the thyroid. Some cases developed hyperthyroidism during lithium treatment. This may have been a chance occurrence or it may have been due to an increased release of thyroid hormone after an intrathyroid build-up of the iodine stores.

Other hormones do not appear to be affected by lithium therapy in patients who are not experiencing lithium toxicity.

Narcotics and Alcohol

Chronic narcotic administration, either with street drugs or in methadone maintenance, is associated with significant decreases in both LH and testosterone secretion in men. The mechanism is believed to be a primary effect of opiates on the hypothalamic LRH cells, with a secondary fall in circulating LH and testosterone. Administration of the narcotic antagonist, naltrexone, has been reported to increase LH secretion in both abstinent ex-addicts and normal subjects, suggesting a possible role of brain opiates in the regulation of LH in man. Narcotics also reduce cortisol secretion and stimulate PRL.

Alcohol ingestion has been reported to induce a rapid fall in serum testosterone, evidently by competition by alcohol for the testicular reductase enzyme involved in the synthesis of testosterone.

Although plasma LH is low in narcotic addicts, LH is high in alcoholics, evidently as a feedback response to the lowered circulating testosterone levels.

During alcohol withdrawal in chronic alcoholics who develop an abstinence syndrome, elevations of cortisol secretion and blunting of the TSH response to TRH are commonly seen.

BEHAVIORAL EFFECTS OF PEPTIDE HORMONES

The discovery of a variety of peptide hormones in brain tissue, and the growing evidence that many of these peptides act as neurotransmitters or neuromodulators, has led to much recent research to elucidate the behavioral functions of these substances. Most of this research is still in very early stages, nearly all of it focused on animal investigation, and human data are still quite sparse. The summaries presented here, therefore, have to be regarded as highly tentative.

Adrenocorticotropin

As indicated in the section on Cushing's syndrome, animal data indicate an effect of ACTH and its fragments (e.g., ACTH 4–10) on memory, attention, and learning processes in animals. The few human trials have yielded largely negative results, however, ACTH 4–10 does not appear to relieve the transient memory disturbances following electroconvulsive therapy for severe depression or the memory disturbances associated with mild to moderate senility.

Vasopressin

VP has also been shown to have potent behavioral effects in rats, similar to those reported for ACTH 4–10. As yet, however, little data are available from human studies, although studies on patients with mild degrees of senile dementia are in progress.

Thyrotropin-Releasing Hormone

TRH has some psychoactive properties in both animals and man, similar in many but not all respects to a mild dextroamphetamine effect. A brief, mild, alerting arousal and mood-elevating effect has been noted in normal subjects in response to single infusions of 500–100 μ. A similar, mild, lifting of mood lasting up to 24 hours has been noted in some studies of depressed patients, but not in others. In any case, TRH appears to have no role as a clinical treatment for depression.

Cholecystokinin

This peptide hormone has also been found to be present within brain neurons. There is some evidence in monkeys that it may play a role in mediating the satiety response after feeding. There are, as yet, no human data.

Luteinizing Hormone Releasing Hormone

LRH under appropriate conditions can stimulate components of mating behavior in animals. Despite the fact that there are some suggestive, but also conflicting data for a potentiating effect of LRH on libido or potency in men, a recent placebo-controlled trial showed no effect on men with psychogenic impotency.

Somatostatin

Data from one animal study indicated that intraventricular administration of somatostatin was associated with suppression of activity and sedation. There are no human data as yet.

Substance P

Substance P is not only present in intestinal and brain tissue, but also is distributed in substantial concentration along the dorsal horn of the spinal column. Animal studies strongly suggest that it functions as a neurotransmitter mediating pain signals and is antagonistic to opiates in modulating analgesia.

Endorphins and Enkephalins

The explosion of research generated by the discoveries of brain opiate receptors and of endogenous opiate-like peptides produced by brain is still underway. Although much has been learned about the anatomic distribution of the opiate pathways in brain, and some about their function in analgesia, little is known as yet about their other behavioral roles, even in animals, and human data are still miniscule.

The naturally occurring substances are generally unavailable for human studies, and most efforts to infer their functions in man have involved administration of opiate-antagonists such as naloxone. This is a risky strategy, since although naloxone may be a good antagonist for the analgesic effects of the endogenous opiates, it may not be a good antagonist for their other possible behavioral functions.

β-Endorphin

β-endorphin has been found to be present primarily in the anterior and intermediate lobe of the pituitary and in the basal hypothalamus. It appears in peripheral blood together with ACTH. It may therefore play a role in stress-analgesia. In animals it exerts an analgesic effect and, similar to opiates, creates seizure activity on administration and "wet-dog" shakes on withdrawal. In higher doses it produces rigidity and immobility similar to catatonia. These effects are antagonized by naloxone.

In one human study, intraventricular administration of β-endorphin produced several hours of dramatic relief from severe chronic pain. In rats, at least, β-endorphin may play a role in regulation of PRL, LH, and GH secretion, since β-endorphin stimulates secretion of PRL and GH and suppresses LH secretion, and naltrexone administration causes a fall in resting levels of PRL and GH, and a rise in LH.

Enkephalins

The neural pathways in brain and spinal cord containing met-enkephalin and leu-enkephalin have substantially been mapped and in general seem consistent with an important physiological role of these substances in the modulation of pain. Human experiments are somewhat supportive of such a role. Thus, patients with severe, chronic pain who had been implanted with an electrode in the enkephalin-rich central gray area experienced substantial, long-lasting relief after 20–30 min of stimulation. Although there is only a slight effect (if any) of naloxone administration on pain thresholds in normal subjects, pretreatment with narcotic antagonists in pain patients has been reported to block analgesia following acupuncture, and also the analgesic response to placebo.

Of course, exogenous opiates not only affect pain but also have major effects on mood and motivational states. Might endogenous opiates play a similar physiological role in regulating mood, pleasure responses, and motivation? Some of the early animal behavioral studies suggest that enkephalins may play a role in the satisfaction response that reduces drive states. Evidence for a significant psychological role in humans is still lacking, however. Thus, naloxone does not block the pleasure of orgasm, nor can any naltrexone effect be found in batteries of psychological tests administered to normal volunteers. Naloxone and naltrexone also have not had any consistent effect in schizophrenic or manic-depressive patients (although in each study there have been one or two individuals who appeared to have a striking response). Antipsychotic medications have been shown to increase brain levels of enkephalins, so they may play a role in mediating the therapeutic effect of these drugs.

It is worth re-emphasizing that endogenous opiates may exert behavioral actions beyond that of analgesia that are not antagonized by available narcotic antagonists. Synthetic congeners of naturally occurring enkephalins, which are more potent and have longer half-lives, are currently under development and may eventually prove to be powerfully psychoactive.

REFERENCES

Behavioral Influences of Prenatal Hormones

Ehrhardt, A. A.: Prenatal hormone exposure and psychosexual differentiation, In *Topics in Psychoendocrinology.* (Seminars in Psychiatry.) Sachar, E. J. (ed.), New York, Grune and Stratton, 1975.
Ehrhardt, A. A., and Meyer-Bahlburg, H. F. L.: Prenatal sex hormones and the developing brain. Effects on psychosocial differentiation and cognitive function. *Ann. Rev. Med.* 30:417, 1979.
Goy, R. W., and Resko, J. A.: Gonadal hormones and behavior of normal and pseudohermaphroditic nonhuman female primates. *Recent Progr. Horm. Res.* 38:707, 1972.
Money, J., and Schwartz, M.: Dating, romantic and non-romantic friendships and sexuality in 17 early treated andrenogenital females, aged 16 to 25, In *Congenital Adrenal Hyperplasia.* Lee, P. A., et al. (eds.), Baltimore, University Park Press, 1971.

Puberty

Ehrhardt, A. A., and Meyer-Bahlburg, H. S. L.: Psychological correlates of abnormal pubertal development. *Clin. Endocrinol. Metab.* 4:297, 1975.
Hayes, S. E.: Strategies for psychoendocrine studies of puberty. *Psychoneuroendocrinol.* 3:1, 1978.
Rose, R. M., et al.: Androgens and aggressive behavior: a review in recent findings in primates, In *Primate Aggression, Territoriality in Zenophobia.* Holloway, R. L. (ed.), New York, Academic Press Inc., 1974.
Rose, R. M., et al.: Changes in testosterone and behavior during adolescence in the male rhesus monkey. *Psychosom. Med.* 40:60, 1978.
Schmidt, G., and Sigusch, V.: Changes in sexual behavior among young males and females between 1960–1970. *Arch. Sex. Behav.* 2:27, 1972.
Swerdloff, R. S., and Rubin, R. T.: Psychological and endocrine changes in puberty, In *Perspectives in Endocrine Psychobiology.* Branbilla, F., et al. (eds.), New York, Wiley, 1978, p. 287.

Male Sexual Behavior

Comhaire, F., and Verneulen, A.: Plasma testosterone in patients with varicocele and sexual inadequacy. *J. Clin. Endocrinol. Metab.* 40:824, 1975.
Damassa, D. A., Smith, E. R., et al.: The relationship between circulating testosterone levels and sexual behavior. *Horm. Behav.* 8:275, 1977.
Davidson, J. E., Camargo, C. A., et al.: Effects of androgen on sexual behavior in hypogonadal man. *J. Clin. Endocrinol. Metab.* 48:955, 1979.
Davies, T. F., Mountjoy, P. Q., et al.: A double blind cross over trial of gonadotropin releasing hormones (LHRH) in sexually impotent men. *Clin. Endocrinol.* 5:601, 1976.
LaFerle, J., Anderson, D. L., et al.: Psychoendocrine response to sexual arousal in males. *Psychosom. Med.* 40:116, 1978.
Lascattu, L.: Antiandrogens in the treatment of sexual deviation in men. *J. Steroid Biochem.* 6:821, 1975.
Lundberg, P. O., and Wide, L.: Sexual function in males with pituitary tumors. *Fertil. Steril.* 29:175, 1978.

Mauss, J., and Borsch, G.: Effect of long-term testosterone oenanthate administration on male reproductive function: Clinical evaluation, serum FSH, LH, testosterone, and seminal fluid analysis in normal men. *Acta Endocrinol. (KBH)* 78:373, 1975.

Meyer, W. J., Walker, P. A., et al.: Pituitary function in adult males receiving medroxyprogesterone acetate. *Fertil. Steril.* 28:1072, 1977.

Meyer-Bahlburg, H. F. L.: Sex hormones in male sexuality in comparative perspective. *Arch. Sex. Behav.* 6:297, 1977.

Moss, R. L.: Effects of hypothalamic peptides on sex behavior in animal and man, In *Psychopharmacology: A Generation of Progress.* Lipton, M. A., et al. (eds.), New York, Raven Press, 1978.

Rose, R. M.: Neuroendocrine correlates of sexual and aggressive behavior in humans, In *Psychopharmacology: A Generation of Progress.* Lipton, M. A., et al. (eds.), New York, Raven Press, 1978.

Walker, P. A., and Meyer, W. J.: Medroxyprogesterone acetate treatment for paraphiliac sex offenders, In *Violence and the Violent Individual.* Hays, J. R., Roberts, T. K., et al. (eds.), Jamaica, New York, Spectrum Publications Inc., (in press).

Female Sexual Behavior

Abplanalp, J., Donnelly, A. F., et al.: Psychoendocrinology of the menstrual cycle: I. Enjoyment of daily activities and moods. *Psychosom. Med.* 41:587, 1979.

Abplanalp, J., Rose, R. M., et al.: Psychoendocrinology of the menstrual cycle: II. The relationship between enjoyment of activities, moods and reproductive hormones. *Psychosom. Med.* 41:605, 1979.

Adams, D. B., and Gold, A. R.: Rise in female-initiated sexual activity at ovulation and its suppression by oral contraceptives. *N. Engl. J. Med.* 229:1145, 1978.

Baum, M. J., Everitt, B. J., et al.: Hormonal basis of proceptivity and receptivity in female primates. *Arch. Sex. Behav.* 6:173, 1977.

Beach, F. A.: Behavioral endocrinology: An emerging discipline. *Am. Sci.* 63:178, 1975.

Detre, T., Hayashi, T. T., et al.: Management of the menopause. *Ann. Intern. Med.* 88:373, 1978.

Hallstrom, T.: Sexuality in the climacteric. *Clin. Obstet. Gynecol.* 4:227, 1977.

Johansson, B. W., Kaij, L., et al.: On some late effects of bilateral oophorectomy in the age range 15–30 years. *Acta Obstet. Gynecol. Scand.* 54:441, 1975.

Johnson, D. F., and Phoenix, C. H.: Hormonal control of female sexual attractiveness, proceptivity and receptivity in rhesus monkeys. *J. Comp. Physiol. Psychol.* 90:473, 1976.

Meyer-Bahlburg, H. F. L.: Sex hormones and female homosexuality: A critical examination. *Arch. Sex. Behav.* 8:101, 1979.

Michael, R. P., and Zumpe, D.: Effects of androgen administration on sexual invitations by female rhesus monkeys (Macaca Mulatta). *Anim. Behav.* 25:936, 1977.

Rose, R. M.: The psychological effects of androgens and estrogens: A review, In *Psychiatric Complications of Medical Drugs.* Shader, R. I. (ed.), New York, Raven Press, 1972.

Udry, J. R., and Morris, M. N.: Distribution of coitus in the menstrual cycle. *Nature* 220:593, 1968.

Winokur, G.: Depression in the menopause. *Am. J. Psychol.* 130:92, 1973.

Premenstrual Tension Syndrome

Kessel, N., and Coppen, A. A.: The prevalence of common menstrual symptoms. *Lancet* 2:61, 1963.

McCance, R. A., Luff, M. C., et al.: Physical and emotional periodicity in women. *J. Hyg.* 37:571, 1937.

Parlee, M. B.: The premenstrual syndrome. *Psychol. Bull.* 80:454, 1973.

Ruble, D. N.: Premenstrual symptoms: A reinterpretation. *Science* 197:291, 1977.

Smith, S. L.: Mood and the menstrual cycle, In *Topics in Psychoendocrinology.* Sachar, E. J. (ed.), New York, Grune and Stratton, 1975.

Sommer, B.: Stress and menstrual distress. *J. Hum. Stress* 4:5, 1978.

Tonks, C. M.: Premenstrual tension. *Br. J. Psychol.* 9:399, 1975.

Endocrine Responses to Stress

Aakvaag, A., Bentdal, O., et al.: Testosterone and testosterone binding globulin (TeBG) in young men during prolonged stress. *Int. J. Androl.* 1:22, 1978.

Barchas, J. D., Akil, H., et al.: Behavioral neurochemistry: neuroregulators and behavioral states. *Science* 20:965, 1968.

Boyd, A. E., and Reichlin, S.: Neuro control of prolactin secretion in man. *Psychoneuroendocrinol.* 3:113, 1978.

Brown, G. M., Seggie, J. A., et al.: Psychoendocrinology and growth hormone: A review. *Psychoneuroendocrinol.* 3:131, 1978.

Czeisler, C. A., Moore Ede. M. E., et al.: Episodic 24-hour cortisol secretory patterns in patients awaiting elective cardiac surgery. *J. Clin. Endocrinol. Metab.* 42:273, 1976.

Frankenhaueser, M.: Experimental approaches to the study of catecholamines in emotion, In *Emotions — Their Parameters and Measurement.* Levi, L. (ed.), New York, Raven Press, 1975, p. 209.

Greene, W. A., Conron, G., et al.: Psychological correlates of growth hormone and adrenal secretory responses of patients undergoing cardiac catheterization. *Psychosom. Med.* 32:599, 1970.

Guillemin, R., Vargo, T., et al.: Beta-endorphin and adrenocorticotropin are secreted concomitantly by the pituitary gland. *Science* 197:1367, 1977.

Hennessey, J. W., and Levin, S.: Stress, arousal and pituitary-adrenal system (a psychoendocrine hypothesis), In *Progress in Psychobiology and Physiological Psychology.* Sprague, J. M., and Epstein, A. N. (eds.), New York, Academic Press, 1979, p. 133.

Katz, J. L., Weiner, H., et al.: Stress, distress and ego defenses. Psychoendocrine response to impending breast tumor biopsy. *Arch. Gen. Psychol.* 23:131, 1970.

Kreuz, L. E., Rose, R. M., et al.: Suppression of plasma testosterone levels in psychological stress: A longitudinal study of young men in officer candidate school. *Arch. Gen. Psychol.* 26:479, 1972.

Mason, J. W.: A review of psychoendocrine research on the pituitary-adrenal cortical system. *Psychosom. Med.* 30:576, 1968.

Mason, J. W.: Psychological stress and endocrine function, In *Topics in Psychoendocrinology.* Sachar, E. J. (ed.), New York, Grune and Stratton, 1975.

Matsumoto, K., Takeyasu, A., et al.: Plasma testosterone levels following surgical stress in male patients. *Acta Endocrinol.* 65:11, 1970.

Mijulaj, L., Kvetnansky, R., et al.: Catecholamines and corticosteroids in acute and repeated stress, In *Catecholamines and Stress.* Usdin, E. (ed.), New York, Pergamon Press, 1976, p. 445.

Noel, G. L., Suh, H. K., et al.: Human prolactin and growth hormone release during surgery and other conditions of stress. *J. Clin. Endocrinol. Metab.* 35:84, 1972.

Rose, R. M.: Testosterone, aggression and homosexuality: A review of the literature and implications for future research, In *Topics in Psychoendocrinology.* Sachar, E. J. (ed.), New York, Grune and Stratton, 1975.

Rose, R. M., Poe, R. O., et al.: Psychological state and body size as determinants of 17-OHCS excretion. *Arch. Intern. Med.* 121:406, 1968.

Schalch, D. S.: The influence of physical stress and exercise on growth hormone and insulin secretion in man. *J. Lab. Clin. Med.* 69:256, 1967.

Ursin, H., Baade, E., et al.: *Psychobiology of Stress: A Study of Coping Men.* New York, Academic Press, 1978.

Endocrine Disturbances in Psychiatric Disorders

MAJOR DEPRESSIONS

Carroll, B. J.: Neuroendocrine function in psychiatric disorders, In *Psychopharmacology: A Generation of Progress.* Lipton, M. A., DiMascio, A., et al. (eds.), New York, Raven Press, 1978.

Ettigi, P. G., and Brown, G. M.: Psychoendocrine correlates in affective disorder, In *Neuroendocrine Correlates in Neurology and Psychiatry.* Muller, E. E., and Agnoli, A. (eds.), New York, Elsevier-North Holland, 1979.

Puig-Antich, J., Chambers, W., et al.: Cortisol hypersecretion in prepubertal depressive illness: A preliminary report. *Psychoneuroendocrinol.* 4(3):191, 1979.

Sachar, E. J.: Neuroendocrine abnormalities in depressive illness, In *Topics in Psychoendocrinology.* Sachar, E. J. (ed.), New York, Grune & Stratton, 1975.

Sachar, E. J., and Baron, M.: The biology of affective disorders. *Ann. Rev. Neurosci.* 2:505, 1979.

Sachar, E. J., Halbreich, U., et al.: Neurotransmitter regulation of cortisol secretion in depression: Studies of the response to dextroamphetamine, In *Neuroactive Drugs in Endocrinology: Physiologic, Diagnostic and Therapeutic Applications.* Muller, E. E. (ed.), New York, Elsevier-North Holland (in press).

OTHER PSYCHIATRIC DISORDERS

Carroll, B. J.: Neuroendocrine function in psychiatric disorders, In *Psychopharmacology: A Generation of Progress.* Lipton, M. A., DiMascio, A., (eds.), New York, Raven Press, 1978.

Brown, G.: Endocrine aspects of psychosocial dwarfism, In *Hormones, Behavior, and Psychopathology.* Sachar, E. J. (ed.), New York, Raven Press, 1976.

Katz, J. L., Boyer, R. M., et al.: Toward an elucidation of the psychoendocrinology of anorexia nervosa, In *Hormones, Behavior, and Psychopathology.* Sachar, E. J. (ed.), New York, Raven Press, 1976.

Kuhn, C. M., Butler, S. R., et al.: Selective depression of serum growth hormone during maternal deprivation in rat pups. *Science* 201:1034, 1978.

Kuhn, C. M., Evoniuk, G., et al.: Loss of tissue sensitivity to growth hormone during maternal deprivation in rats. *Life Sci.* 25:2089, 1979.

Money, J., Annecillo, C., et al.: Hormonal and behavioral reversals in hyposomatotropic dwarfism, In *Hormones, Behavior, and Psychopathology.* Sachar, E. J. (ed.), New York, Raven Press, 1976.

Psychiatric Disturbances Associated with Endocrinopathies and Hormone Therapy

REVIEWS

Smith, C. K., Barish, J., et al.: Psychiatric disturbance in endocrinologic disease. *Psychosom. Med.* 34:69, 1972.

Sachar, E. J.: Psychiatric disturbances in endocrine diseases: Some issues for research, In *Brain Dysfunction in Metabolic Disorders*. Plum, F. (ed.), New York, Raven Press, (ARNMD Proceedings), 1974.

Whybrow, P. C., and Hurwitz, T.: Psychological disturbances associated with endocrine disease and hormone therapy, In *Hormones, Behavior, and Psychopathology*. Sachar, E. J. (ed.), New York, Raven Press, 1976.

HYPERTHYROIDISM AND HYPOTHYROIDISM

Coppen, A., Whybrow, P. C., et al.: Comparative antidepressant value of 1-tryptophan and imipramine with and without potentiation by liothyronine. *Arch. Gen. Psychiatry 26:*234, 1972.

Lipton, M., Prange, A., et al.: Increased rate of catecholamine synthesis in hypothyroid rats. *Fed. Proc. 27:*399, 1968.

McConnell, R. J., Menendez, C. E., et al.: Defects of taste and smell in patients with hypothyroidism. *Am. J. Med. 59:*354, 1975.

Prange, A., Meek, J., et al.: Catecholamines: Diminished rate of synthesis in rat brain and heart after thyroxine pretreatment. *Life Sci. 9:*901, 1970.

Stein, L.: Reward transmitters: Catecholamines and opioid peptides, In *Psychopharmacology: A Generation of Progress*. Lipton, M. A., DiMascio, A., et al. (eds.), New York, Raven Press, 1978.

Whybrow, P. C., Prange, A. J., et al.: Mental changes accompanying thyroid gland dysfunction. *Arch. Gen. Psychiatry 20:*48, 1969.

HYPERCORTICISM AND HYPOCORTICISM

Carpenter, W. T., Strauss, J., et al.: The psychobiology of cortisol metabolism: Clinical and theoretical implications, In *Psychiatric Complications of Medical Drugs*. Shader, R. I. (ed.), New York, Raven Press, 1972.

Falk, W. E., Mahnke, M. W., et al.: Lithium prophylaxis of corticotropin-induced psychosis. *J.A.M.A. 241:*1011, 1979.

Mattison, B.: Addison's disease and psychoses. *Acta Psychiat. Scand.* [Suppl.] *255:*203, 1974.

Money, J., and Jobaris, R.: Juvenile Addison's disease: Follow-up behavioral studies in 7 cases. *Psychoneuroendocrinol. 2:*149, 1977.

Trethowan, W. H., and Cobb, S.: Neuropsychiatric aspects of Cushing's syndrome. *Arch. Neurol. Psychiatry 67:*283, 1952.

HYPERPARATHYROIDISM AND HYPOPARATHYROIDISM

Denko, J. D., and Kaebling, R.: Psychiatric aspects of hypoparathyroidism. *Acta Psychiat. Scand.* [Suppl.] *38:*7, 1962.

Petersen, P.: Psychiatric disorders in primary hyperparathyroidism. *JCEM 28:*1491, 1968.

Effects of Psychotropic Drugs on Endocrine Function

ANTIPSYCHOTICS

Gruen, P. H., Sachar, E. J., et al.: Prolactin responses to neuroleptics in normal and schizophrenic subjects. *Arch. Gen. Psychiatry 35:*108, 1979.

Meltzer, H. Y., Goode, D. J., et al.: Effect of psychotropic drugs on endocrine function, In *Psychopharmacology: A Generation of Progress*. Lipton, M. A., DiMascio, A., et al. (eds.), New York, Raven Press, 1978.

Sachar, E. J.: Neuroendocrine responses to psychotropic drugs, In *Psychopharmacology: A Generation of Progress*. Lipton, M. A., DiMascio, A., et al. (eds.), New York, Raven Press, 1978.

AMPHETAMINES

Puig-Antich, J., Greenhill, L., et al.: Growth hormone, prolactin and cortisol responses and growth patterns in hyperkinetic children treated with dextroamphetamine. *J. Am. Acad. Child Psychiatry 17:*457, 1978.

LITHIUM

Lazarus, J. H., and Bennie, E. H.: Effect of lithium on thyroid function in man. *Acta Endocrinol. 70:*266, 1972.

Lindstedt, G., Nilsson, L., et al.: On the prevalence, diagnosis, and management of lithium-induced hypothyroidism in psychiatric patients. *Br. J. Psychiatry 130:*452, 1977.

Reisberg, B., and Gershon, S.: Side effects associated with lithium therapy. *Arch. Gen. Psychiatry 36:*879, 1979.

NARCOTICS AND ALCOHOL

Mendelson, J. H., Mello, N. K., et al.: Effects of alcohol on pituitary-gonadal hormones, sexual function, and aggression in human males, In *Psychopharmacology: A Generation of Progress*. Lipton, M. A., DiMascio, A., et al. (eds.), New York, Raven Press, 1978.

Mendelson, J. E., Meyer, R. E., et al.: Effects of heroin and methadone on plasma cortisol and testosterone. *J. Pharm. Exp. Ther. 195:*296, 1975.

Mirin, S. M., Mendelson, J. H., et al.: Acute effects of heroin and naltrexone on testosterone and gonadotropin secretion. *Psychoneuroendocrinol. 1:*359, 1976.

Tolis, G., Hickey, J., et al.: Effects of morphine on serum growth hormone, cortisol, prolactin, and thyroid stimulating hormone in man. *JCEM 41:*797, 1975.

Behavioral Effects of Peptide Hormones

DeWied, D.: Behavioral effects of neuropeptides related to B-LPH, In *Centrally Acting Peptides*. Hughes, J. (ed.), Baltimore, University Park Press, 1978.

Meyerson, B. J.: Hypothalamic hormones and behavior. *Med. Biol. 57:*69, 1979.

Moss, R. L.: Effects of hypothalamic peptides on sex behavior in animal and man, In *Psychopharmacology: A Generation of Progress*. Lipton, M. A., DiMascio, A., et al. (eds.), New York, Raven Press, 1978.

Prange, A. J., Nemeroff, C. B., et al.: Behavioral effects of peptides: Behavioral and clinical studies, In *Psychopharmacology: A Generation of Progress*. Lipton, M. A., DiMascio, A., et al. (eds.), New York, Raven Press, 1978.

Rigter, H., and Van Riezen, H.: Hormones and memory, In *Psychopharmacology: A Generation of Progress*. Lipton, M. A., DiMascio, A., et al. (eds.), New York, Raven Press, 1978.

Usdin, E., Bunney, W. E. (eds.): *Endorphins in Mental Health Research*, New York, Oxford University Press, 1979.

CHAPTER 13

Dysmentation from Metabolic Alterations

by Gilbert S. Omenn

Changes in behavior are often early or significant aspects of the clinical presentation of patients with various endocrine disorders, and these changes may be especially distressing to the patient and the family. It must be admitted that endocrine disorders are not common causes in unselected series of psychiatric patients; on the other hand, the dramatic clinical responses achieved upon effective treatment of many endocrine disorders make proper diagnosis highly rewarding.

Psychobiologic investigations and explanations of normal and abnormal behaviors depend upon a recognition of the fact that the brain is the medium through which behaviors are expressed. Brain functions depend on intrinsic metabolic pathways and cellular connections in the brain and on extrinsic influences mediated by sensory neural inputs and by hormones, metabolites, and other chemicals. The "mind," then, is an artificial construct that gains expression through the functioning of the brain.

Throughout this text, descriptions of the actions of hormones and of the clinical manifestations of endocrine dysfunctions include effects on the brain and behavioral signs and symptoms. Neurotransmitter metabolism, neuroendocrinology, and endocrine relationships of manic-depressive illness and other psychoses are discussed in detail in Chs. 10, 11, and 12. As the late Robert Williams concluded in 1970 in his Presidential Address to the Endocrine Society on "Metabolism and Mentation," there has been surprisingly little systematic analysis of the incidence and types of dysmentation in patients with most types of endocrinopathies.

In this chapter, selected inborn errors of metabolism will be presented in order to explore certain clues to brain functions, to emphasize that certain clinical behavioral features may be related to specific underlying abnormalities, and to introduce an analytic approach to the mechanisms of metabolic effects upon the brain. In addition, behavioral and neurologic consequences of fluid and electrolyte disorders are discussed. Heavy metals, intoxicants, and other chemicals have behavior-modifying effects, but these are outside the scope of this chapter.

The brain seems to have a relatively limited range of clinical responses to hormonal or metabolic disturbances, so that psychiatric consequences are often nonspecific. Emphasis is given here to those disorders with more specific associated behavioral changes.

The metabolic disorders among which we may search for clues to human brain function and dysfunction may be differentiated roughly into those for which the primary lesion is *extrinsic* to the brain and those for which it is *intrinsic* to the brain. Examples are listed in Table 13–1. In phenylketonuria (PKU) and other aminoacidurias, the brain is damaged by normal metabolites in abnormal concentrations, a toxic mechanism, just as the brain may be damaged by lead poisoning from the more external environment. Hypothyroidism differs in representing a deficiency syndrome, in which thyroid hormone, important to brain development and myelination, is lacking. The extrinsic disorders merit considerable attention because they are treatable or preventable by manipulation of the environment by special diets, administration of hormone, or correction of fluid and electrolyte imbalances. Disorders that may be intrinsic to the brain provide clues to metabolic intermediates and metabolic pathways of significance in normal brain functioning, as well as to common patterns of psychiatric and neurologic dysfunction.

METABOLIC DISORDERS EXTRINSIC TO THE BRAIN

Phenylketonuria

Classic PKU results from deficiency in the liver of the enzyme phenylalanine hydroxylase, with resultant defi-

Table 13–1. ORIGIN OF EFFECTS OF METABOLIC DISORDERS

Extrinsic to the brain	Intrinsic to the brain
Phenylketonuria	Lesch-Nyhan syndrome
Urea cycle disorders	Wilson disease
Maple syrup urine disease	Homocystinuria
Galactosemia	Metachromatic leukodystrophy
Hepatic porphyrias	Mucopolysaccharidoses
Hypothyroidism	Wernicke-Korsakoff syndrome
Hypoparathyroidism	
Hyperparathyroidism	
Adrenogenital syndrome	

ciency of production of tyrosine from phenylalanine and with accumulation of phenylalanine itself and phenylpyruvic acid and other metabolites in blood and urine. PKU has been a leading model for study of mental retardation, because it is relatively common and because the dietary management of PKU is one of the most dramatic therapeutic developments in pediatrics and medical genetics. When infants are placed on a diet maintaining optimal levels of phenylalanine in the blood, the chance that nearly normal or normal IQ will result is vastly improved, and normal growth can be achieved. Without treatment, children have a median IQ of about 40, with 95% having IQ less than 50.

Følling identified excess phenylpyruvic acid in the urine of patients with this condition in 1934; thereafter, the ferric chloride test became a simple means of detecting the 1% of patients with PKU among the large population with seemingly similar mental retardation. During the first year of life, there are usually few other clinical clues to the diagnosis. Some 25% have eczema, and those with hyperhidrosis have a musty odor from phenylacetic acid during the first 2 or 3 months. Progressive dilution of skin pigment occurs over the first year because of inhibition of tyrosinase by excess phenylalanine. Nevertheless, the paucity of clinical clues makes biochemic diagnosis via a screening test in the newborn period imperative. Otherwise, the equivalent of an estimated 50 IQ points will be lost if treatment is not initiated until the end of the first year of life. The screening test, developed by Guthrie, utilizes a drop of blood from a heel stick of the infant and measures the extent of growth of phenylalanine-requiring bacteria. Analogous tests have been developed for a series of other rarer inborn errors.

The prevalence of PKU was estimated at 1 case per 20,000 births on the basis of studies of prevalence of PKU among mentally retarded patients. When the screening test was introduced widely and required by law in nearly all states, the apparent incidence nearly doubled. It was recognized only later that many of these additional cases represented hyperphenylalaninemia of heterogeneous origins that would not lead to classic PKU with mental retardation. For this reason, not all children placed on the phenylalanine-restricted diet benefited, and some suffered stunting of growth and even mental retardation. This heterogeneity includes a series of different mutations affecting phenylalanine hydroxylase, causing partial deficiency or altered affinity for the phenylalanine substrate. The former may lead to blood levels of phenylalanine high enough to warrant the special diet. The latter leads to a requirement for higher-than-normal phenylalanine levels in order to make tyrosine, which is essential for protein synthesis, thyroid hormone and catecholamine synthesis, and skin pigmentation.

The detailed enzymology of phenylalanine hydroxylase is quite complicated. Tetrahydrobiopterin is a required co-factor, and the enzyme dihydrofolate reductase is coupled functionally to phenylalanine hydroxylase in order to shuttle the biopterin back and forth between the quinoid and the tetrahydro forms. Deficiency of the dihydrofolate reductase, therefore, can also cause hyperphenylalaninemia. Such a defect was identified in three very unusual patients, who developed feeding difficulties shortly after birth, early evidence of developmental delay, and seizures, with no clinical response to a low-phenylalanine diet that controlled the blood phenylalanine level. By 18 months of age, voluntary movement and social awareness ceased, and the EEG was grossly abnormal. Dihydrofolate reductase deficiency was demonstrated in brain, liver, and culture fibroblasts by Kaufman et al. (1975). Several patients have now been described, with more than one type of abnormality in the reductase enzyme likely. Dihydrofolate reductase deficiency clearly affects intrinsic pathways in the brain, since the same tetrahydrofolate cofactor system is used by tyrosine hydroxylase in the biosynthesis of dopamine and norepinephrine and by tryptophan hydroxylase in the biosynthesis of serotonin (see Ch. 10). Since the neurologic defects are probably due to secondary deficiency of formation of these monoamine neurotransmitters, one patient was treated with dopa, L-5-hydroxytryptophan, and carbidopa and showed progressive improvement during 9 months: myoclonus, uncontrolled movements, tetraplegia, and some skin signs all disappeared.

Behavioral Features

Untreated PKU children were described more than 20 years ago (Wright and Tarjan, 1957) as distinguishable from other mentally deficient children in the same institutions: "... none could be described as friendly, placid, or happy," in striking contrast with Down syndrome children, in particular. The less retarded patients with PKU tend to be restless, jerky, and fearful; destructive and noisy psychotic episodes were observed in 10%. In another series (Paine, 1957), 32% had night terrors or uncontrollable temper tantrums. In fact, hyperactivity, irritability, and uncontrollable temper are often the reasons why these children are admitted to institutions. Even when dietary manipulation sustains development of IQ in the normal range, these children have a higher incidence of restless and hyperactive behavior.

Secondary Metabolic Alterations

The conventional wisdom that heterozygotes are entirely normal and that brain damage starts only after birth in homozygotes with PKU has been challenged. Bessman et al. (1978) deduced that tyrosine deficiency may be an important component of the mental retardation, in addition to the toxic effects of high phenylalanine on glycolytic enzymes, myelination, and various other vulnerable brain processes. Prenatal growth retardation and microcephaly do occur in some PKU newborns, indicating damage during fetal development. The distribution of IQ's within the "normal range" (70–130) of apparently normal siblings of children with PKU has been reported to be bimodal, as would be predicted if the heterozygous sibs (2/3) were more vulnerable than the sibs who did not carry even one gene for PKU (1/3 of sibs). Bessman tested 47 non-PKU offspring of heterozygous mothers and found a significant negative regression coefficient for IQ with the metabolic indicator of dysfunction of phenylalanine hydroxylase (P^2/T ratio, where P is phenylalanine and T is tyrosine).

The higher the P^2/T ratio, the lower the IQ — all well within the normal range (IQ's 86–136). He and his coworkers took the one third of offspring with the lowest P^2/T ratios to be the homozygous normal offspring and the two thirds of the subjects with nonoverlapping higher values to be heterozygotes. Within the normal range, the "heterozygotes" had a statistically significant 10-point lower IQ than the "normals." The hypothesis to explain these findings, and to accommodate the lack of a relationship between IQ and P^2/T in the heterozygous mothers, is that limited prenatal supply of tyrosine due to interaction of heterozygous mother and heterozygous fetus exerts a retarding effect on brain development. The therapeutic recommendation for such a situation is to supplement the diet with tyrosine late in pregnancy, when the brain is growing most rapidly. In mothers with PKU (see later), the appropriate special diet would not only be low in phenylalanine but also be very much supplemented with tyrosine.

Bessman's hypothesis has important implications far beyond the management of pregnancies in families with known cases of PKU. For every homozygote with PKU (1/20,000 births), there are 400 heterozygotes in the general population (2% of the population). Half of these individuals, or 1% of the population, were born to mothers heterozygous for PKU. Thus, the nutritional status of a very large number of pregnancies may be vulnerable to a deficiency of tyrosine. Normally, 95% of ingested phenylalanine is converted to tyrosine, and most dietary proteins have about 3.5% T and 6.5% P. On an 80-gm protein diet, a pregnant woman would ingest 3 gm T and synthesize 5 gm from P, for a total of 8 gm T/day. The heterozygous woman would synthesize half as much, for a total of 5.5 gm/day, reducing the delivery of tyrosine to the maternal-fetal environment by 30%. On a good protein intake, this difference might not matter. Nutritional deficiencies are a leading cause of "non-specific retardation" in both underdeveloped and highly developed countries, however — because of lack of food in the former and chronic nausea or illness-related debilitation in the latter. The most practical means of supplementing the diet with tyrosine is by drinking cow's milk, which is unusually rich (6.2%) in tyrosine.

There are more than 30 enzymes required for the synthesis of the nonessential amino acids. If the phenomenon described here for tyrosine biosynthesis is true, and generalizable, an analogous interaction of maternal and fetal heterozygosity for deficiency of any one of the other enzymes could cause similar genetically predisposed metabolic vulnerability of the brain to nutritional deficiencies.

Maternal Phenylketonuria

The extrinsic origin of brain damage in classic PKU is confirmed by the recognition of effects of maternal PKU on the fetus. These children are far more seriously affected than children with classic PKU, whose mothers are unaffected heterozygous carriers, because the exposure to toxic levels of phenylalanine begins during fetal development of the brain, rather than postnatally. About 25% of children of PKU mothers have had congenital anomalies, and microcephaly, intrauterine growth retardation, and subsequent mental retardation occur in nearly all. The practical implications of this clinical phenomenon are staggering. First, those girls who have been treated successfully with dietary management to age 6 or 8 years will have to be restarted on a special diet during pregnancy, and as early as possible. The diets have generally been considered unpalatable, though more recent formulations are less objectionable. Also, breast feeding is contraindicated, because breast milk has high phenylalanine in these women. Second, without such obstetric management or contraception, the next generation may have as many or more severely retarded children due to PKU as were avoided by successful treatment after mass screening in the parental generation.

Urea Cycle Disorders

The five sequential steps of the urea synthesis cycle involve the amino acids ornithine, citrulline, aspartic acid, and arginine and provide the major pathway for ammonia detoxication. Rare disorders of amino acid metabolism (Table 13–2) are of special interest for two reasons. First, they may provide clues to understanding some of the toxic effects on the brain of liver and kidney failure, particularly those involving excessive circulating concentrations of ammonia. Second, heterozygotes for these rare disorders are not so rare and might account for some of the episodic complaints that bring patients to the endocrinologist or gastroenterologist.

Elevated ammonia levels in blood stimulate overproduction of pyrimidines and their metabolites, including orotic acid. It is claimed (Hindfelt, 1972) that different regions of the brain respond differentially to ammonia intoxication, with the brain stem and cerebellum, then the cerebrum being most sensitive. Decreases in high-energy phosphates may account, at least in part, for proliferation of Alzheimer type II astrocytes in these affected regions. The pathogenesis of mental retardation in these disorders has not been elucidated but probably reflects partial deficiencies of arginine or other essential compounds plus toxic effects of ammonia and of citrulline, which has been shown to inhibit glucose utilization and lactose production in brain *in vitro*.

Complete deficiency of ornithine carbamyl transferase (OCT), determined by an X-linked recessive gene, occurs in males as a lethal condition. Partial deficiency of OCT in heterozygous women has been associated with migraine and cyclic vomiting. Russell (1969) tested blood ammonia and protein tolerance in eight cases of childhood migraine, ophthalmic migraine, or cyclic vomiting; seven had abnormally high ammonia on fasting specimens, and six had abnormal ammonia and protein tolerance tests. Of the four tested, three were proved to be OCT heterozygotes. It is possible that many cases of OCT partial deficiency are not being recognized at present. Even in males, partial OCT deficiency could occur as a result of a different mutation affecting the OCT gene and causing incomplete deficiency of enzyme activity.

The most common lesion in the urea cycle pathway is argininosuccinic aciduria. These patients frequently have distinctively friable, tufted hair (trichorrhexis nodosa). The vast majority have had a late-onset clinical picture of neurologic abnormalities or no symptoms at all, having been detected during family surveys or newborn routine screening. The cases that have had mental retardation almost certainly reflect the bias of ascertainment when similar routine screening is carried out in institutions for the mentally retarded. Symptoms are those of irritability, feeding difficulty, vomiting, and seizures. Protein intakes of greater than 1.5 gm/kg/day are not well tolerated in symptomatic individuals. Because argininosuccinic acid (ASA) is highly polar, it does not diffuse readily from brain to blood, and ASA levels are normally higher in the cerebrospinal fluid (CSF) than in blood.

Table 13–2.   INBORN ERRORS OF AMINO ACID METABOLISM*

Disorder	Enzyme deficient	Behavioral phenotype
A. Phenylalanine Metabolism		
PKU	Phenylalanine hydroxylase	Severe mental retardation (MR); irritable
Hyperphenylalaninemia	Same (? partial deficiency, immaturity of liver development)	Normal IQ or mild MR
"PKU variant"	Dihydropteridine reductase	Dysphagia, convulsions, neurologic signs precede mental deterioration
B. Urea Cycle Disorders		
Hyperammonemia I	Carbamyl phosphate synthetase	Severe MR
Hyperammonemia II	OCT	Lethal X-linked recessive in males Cyclic vomiting, migraine, ataxia in females
Citrullinemia	ASA synthetase	Protein intolerance, neurologic signs
ASA	Argininosuccinic lyase	Seizures, ataxia, severe MR
Hyperargininemia	Arginase	Seizures, diplegia, MR
C. Branched-Chain Amino Acids		
MSUD	Branched-chain ketoacid decarboxylase	Severe MR, ketotic coma
MSUD variant	Same (partial deficiency)	Episodic ataxia, normal IQ
Thiamine-responsive MSUD	Same (altered binding, kinetics)	Developmental retardation, reversed by thiamine
D. Hyperglycinemias		
1. Ketotic		
Propionic acidemia	Propionyl-CoA carboxylase ± responsive to biotin	Attacks of ketoacidosis; early death or MR
Methylmalonic aciduria	Methylmalonyl-CoA mutase ± responsive to vitamin B_{12}	Attacks of severe ketoacidosis
2. Nonketotic	Glycine cleavage system	Severe MR, neurologic signs, seizures
E. Sulfur Amino Acids		
Homocystinuria	Cystathionine synthase (± responsive to B_6)	Moderate MR in only half of cases; ? predisposition to schizophrenic behavior
	Methyltransferase (B_{12} metabolism)	Variable MR, neurologic signs
	Tetrahydrofolate reductase	Schizophrenic syndrome, responsive to folate
Cystathioninuria	Cystathionase	Normal
Sulfite oxidase deficiency	Sulfite oxidase	Congenital neurologic abnormalities, ectopia lentis
F. Miscellaneous		
Histidinemia	Histidase	Mild to moderate MR in some cases (bias of ascertainment); speech impairment in half, probably not causally related
Hyperprolinemia (two types)	Proline oxidase Δ'-pyrroline-5-carboxylate dehydrogenase	Normal; early cases with MR or renal disease due to bias of ascertainment

*See Stanbury et al. (1978), Nyhan (1974), Scriver and Rosenberg (1973).

In evaluating premature newborns with hyperammonemia, it is important to keep in mind that transient hyperammonemia is probably far more common than the inherited disorders of the urea cycle. Most infants treated vigorously for neonatal hyperammonemia have an excellent prognosis. The clinical picture is readily confused with overwhelming sepsis, asphyxia, or central nervous system (CNS) hemorrhage. The cause(s) has not been elucidated, but even moribund neonates have had dramatic responses to respiratory assistance and peritoneal dialysis or exchange transfusion.

Maple Syrup Urine Disease

Maple syrup urine disease (MSUD), due to disorders of branched-chain amino acid metabolism, causes vomiting, muscular hypertonicity, convulsions, coma, and death in the first few weeks of life unless the branched-chain amino acids leucine, isoleucine, and valine are restricted in the diet. A variant of MSUD, in which there is less than complete deficiency of the branched-chain amino acid decarboxylase (Table 13–2), leads to symptoms only episodically, induced by dietary ingestion of the branched-chain amino acids. Initial manifestations have appeared months or years after birth, with attacks of ataxia associated with maple syrup odor and elevations of branched-chain amino acids and ketoacids in urine and blood. Mental and physical development can be normal. It is interesting that the primary symptom is ataxia, since leucine and, to lesser extents, isoleucine and valine are particularly toxic to cerebellum in organ explant systems *in vitro*. Leucine and its ketoacid α-ketoisocaproic acid inhibit myelination and pyruvate and glutamate decarboxylases. There is no information about the susceptibility to neurologic or behavioral impairment in parents who are obligate carriers for the completely deficient infantile-onset form of MSUD. These parents should be investigated after high-protein meals.

Favorable responses to diets low in the branched-chain amino acids suggest that the deleterious effects result from abnormal accumulation of the metabolites proximal to the metabolic block, rather than from insufficiency of metabolites distal. These ataxic attacks are often induced by stress, particularly stress associated with infections, though some acute attacks have no apparent triggering causes. Ingestion of the amino acids simulates the attack clinically.

Yet another variant form of MSUD involves a mutant branched-chain decarboxylase that requires higher than usual concentrations of the cofactor thiamine for its function. These rare patients have been responsive biochemically and clinically to administration of thiamine. They have been asymptomatic in the newborn period. With increased protein intake or intercurrent illness, producing catabolic stress, blood levels of branched-chain ketoacids rise and lethargy, ataxia, and vomiting ensue. A laboratory clue to the diagnosis is the combination of ketones without glucose in the urine.

Vitamin-responsive metabolic disorders may be considered somewhat analogous to vitamin-dependent endocrine disorders. Knowledge of the detailed biochemistry of the metabolic pathway, including the requisite cofactors and the metabolic interconversions of those cofactors, allows effective therapeutic interventions. Other examples are biotin-responsive and B_{12}-responsive ketotic hyperglycinemias (Table 13–2D) and B_6-responsive and folate-responsive homocystinurias (Table 13–2E).

Fluid and Electrolyte Disorders

The major effects of changes in electrolyte concentrations are observed in influences on chemical and electric gradients across cell membranes in excitable tissues. Thus, neurologic and behavioral disturbances are prominent (Table 13–3), as are changes in cardiac function and in skeletal muscle. In general, these changes are entirely reversible with appropriate therapy.

Hypernatremia

The sense of thirst is so strong a defender of the serum sodium concentration that hypernatremia does not occur unless thirst is impaired or rendered ineffective because the person is denied access to water or becomes comatose. Thus, the behavioral status of the patient is closely tied to the mechanisms of hypernatremia. In some cases it is difficult to tell whether the symptoms are due to hypertonicity or to a primary disease process affecting the hypothalamus (intrinsic mechanism). Signs of CNS depression progress from lethargy to coma. In children, signs of irritability and a high-pitched cry are common. Chorea and seizures due to rapid lowering of serum sodium levels occur only occasionally. Deep tendon reflexes are usually unaffected, sometimes increased. Severe cases in childhood can lead to permanent brain damage, with spasticity, seizures, and mental and growth retardation due to subdural effusions, subarachnoid hemorrhages and intracerebral bleeding.

Hyponatremia

The classic description of the subjective manifestations of NaCl deficiency was reported by McCance in 1936. He subjected himself and other volunteers to a salt-free diet and sweating with *ad lib* water intake for 11 days. Serum sodium decreased from 147 to 131 mEq/liter, Cl from 100 to 83 mEq/liter; BUN increased from 15 to 42 mg/dl, and weight loss averaged 2–3 kg total. The very first symptoms of hyponatremia were (and are) strikingly diminished sense of flavor and taste. Nocturnal diuresis, nightmares, cramps in the hands, widespread spasmodic contractions, fatigue, breathlessness, and sense of substernal constriction followed. Then the subjects felt mentally slow, experienced sensations of *déjà vu*, and became apathetic. Recovery was dramatic; in fact, the sense of flavors returned by the end of the first salt-containing meal.

Symptoms of hyponatremia are related to rapid swelling of the brain from overhydration of cells. Outward migration of intracellular sodium and potassium may exacerbate the process. The symptoms are correlated with level of serum sodium and rapidity of its decline, rather than with plasma volume. Thus, either sodium depletion or hyperhydration produces similar effects. When sodium declines very gradually, symptoms and signs may not appear until the serum sodium reaches as low as 110 mEq/liter.

Psychosis may be the dominant feature of hyponatremia, or it may be the cause. In other cases, chronic headache may be the dominant feature. Lightheadedness, headache, and increased CSF pressure with normal CSF protein are common findings. As sodium declines, one notes impaired ability to perform simple tasks, such as mental arithmetic. The patient may fail to recognize relatives or the physician, despite being able to carry on a

Table 13–3. SELECTED SIGNS AND SYMPTOMS OF FLUID AND ELECTROLYTE DERANGEMENTS

Derangement	Psychotic behavior	CNS depression	Neurologic signs	Seizures	Muscular signs	Special features
Hypernatremia	−	++	+	+	−	Impaired thirst
Hyponatremia	++	++	++	+	++	Loss of taste and flavors; nocturia; cramps
Hyperkalemia	−	−	+	−	++	
Hypokalemia	+	++	−	−		
Hypercalcemia	++	++	++	−	++	
Hypocalcemia	++	++	+	−	++	Tetany; dystonic reactions
Hypermagnesemia	−	+	+	−	++	
Hypomagnesemia	+	+	−	−	−	
Acidosis	+	++	+	−	+	
Alkalosis	−	++	+	+	+	Tetany

++ = frequent or prominent feature; + = occasional feature; − = infrequent or rare

reasonable conversation. Many focal signs may occur, including focal seizures. Obviously, serum sodium should be normalized before making judgments on the nature and extent of neurologic deficits. Muscular twitches and tremors may be troublesome. Muscle cramps following hemodialysis may be relieved by raising the serum sodium.

Hyperkalemia

The clinical picture of hyperkalemia includes ascending muscular weakness that can lead to flaccid quadriplegia, but cerebral function is not affected. In the rare inherited disorder hyperkalemic periodic paralysis, stiffness and weakness occur after exercise or during sleep and can be triggered by oral administration of potassium. These individuals appear to have some special susceptibility to levels of serum potassium that are tolerated well by normal persons.

By far the most important effect of hyperkalemia is on the initiation and conduction of the cardiac electric impulse. Arrhythmia or standstill is heralded by characteristic ECG changes. Low serum sodium, low serum calcium, acidosis, and elevated serum magnesium all exaggerate the effects of hyperkalemia. Alterations in serum potassium also influence neuromuscular excitability. The resting membrane potential moves toward the threshold potential with hyperkalemia, thereby inducing a depolarization block with muscular paralysis and slowed ventricular conduction. The threshold potential of -65mv is not altered by changes in serum potassium.

Hypokalemia

Changes in cerebral function are common in hypokalemic patients and include lethargy, apathy, drowsiness, confusion, and irritability. Rarely, coma, delirium, or hallucinations may occur. Potassium depletion has been reported as a cause of acute brain syndrome with confusion, impairment of memory, and disorientation. Cerebral symptoms are not common, however, in patients with familial hypokalemic periodic paralysis, despite profound hypokalemia. This difference may be explained by observations that the potassium balance is markedly negative in other forms of hypokalemia but normal in familial periodic paralysis.

Neuromuscular symptoms are prominent in severe hypokalemia but do not appear until the potassium level declines to about 2.5 mEq/liter. The pattern of weakness is distinctive: the legs are most affected, especially the quadriceps muscles; the upper extremity muscles, cranially innervated muscles, and deep tendon reflexes tend to be normal. With extreme hypokalemia, paralysis of the diaphragm and respiratory muscles can lead to fishmouth breathing and respiratory failure.

Muscle cramps and pain can be so striking as to lead to a diagnosis of rheumatism. The muscles may be tender before weakness occurs. Nocturia, polyuria, and polydipsia are common early signs of potassium depletion due to impaired ability to concentrate the urine. These changes may be accompanied by increase in ammonia in the urine and blood, especially in patients with compromised hepatic function.

The mechanisms of potassium depletion include changes in the resting membrane potential, which is highly sensitive to changes in extracellular potassium concentration, and inhibition of enzymes involved in DNA, RNA, and protein synthesis due to small changes in intracellular potassium concentration.

Hypercalcemia

Patients with hypercalcemia, whether due to vitamin D intoxication, sarcoidosis, or hyperparathyroidism (see Ch. 19), may have a variety of significant psychiatric and neurologic manifestations. In general, symptoms are correlated with serum calcium concentration, but some persons tolerate calcium levels of 16 mg/dl, whereas others have striking symptoms at 12 mg/dl. The variation in symptomatology among individuals with the same calcium level reflects other phenomena that affect behaviors and probably reflects differential susceptibility to the various actions of calcium within cells.

Symptoms commonly include loss of initiative, fatigue, lethargy, weakness, and depression, but some patients are nervous, agitated, and insomniac. Impaired memory, poor calculation, and decreased attention span may progress to confusion, psychomotor retardation, delirium, hallucinations, paranoia, and somnolence. Headache is frequent and CSF protein may be increased.

All of these changes are reversible upon control of the hypercalcemia. The mechanism of effect on the brain is extrinsic in origin, mediated by elevated ionized plasma calcium level; it is possible that hypomagnesemia plays a part. The behavioral symptomatology is similar regardless of the cause. In primary or ectopic hyperparathyroidism, in which plasma parathyroid hormone (PTH) is elevated, symptoms can be reversed with peritoneal dialysis, which lowers the plasma calcium but has little effect on the PTH levels. The effects of calcium are presumably mediated through critical roles in neural and neuromuscular excitability, cell membrane permeability, and certain enzyme functions.

Hypocalcemia

Dysmentation is an underemphasized manifestation of hypocalcemia. Severe emotional and intellectual changes can occur in the absence of other signs or symptoms. Chronic hypocalcemia in childhood, due to idiopathic or pseudohypoparathyroidism, may produce mental retardation. Severe psychoses, sometimes diagnosed as schizophrenia or manic-depressive illness, may develop, usually 3–4 months after neck surgery. In the largest study of its kind (Denko and Kaelbling, 1962), significant behavioral abnormalities were reported in nearly all of 289 patients with hypoparathyroidism. The clinical diagnoses included functional psychoses, pseudoneurosis, organic brain syndrome, and intellectual impairment. Treatment to correct the hypocalcemia brought marked improvement in most patients, but dysmentation was permanent in some, possibly reflecting calcium deposits or structural changes within the brain itself or perhaps owing to coincident behavioral pathology. Calcium deposits occur particularly in the perivascular areas of the caudate nucleus, correlating with occasional occurrence of chorea, athetosis, and parkinsonism. Patients with hypoparathyroidism are unusually susceptible to dystonic reactions to phenothiazines even when normocalcemic; perhaps they have subclinical changes in the basal ganglia. The cardinal manifestation of hypocalcemia, of course, is tetany due to excessive neuromuscular irritability. Hypocalcemia increases the threshold potential E_T, decreasing the difference between E_T and the resting membrane potential. The earliest symptoms usually are not motor, but sensory, with numbness of the fingers and tingling and burning in the extremities and around the lips and tongue.

Hypermagnesemia

Elevated magnesium levels occur almost exclusively in patients wtih renal insufficiency, either with advanced renal failure or from treatment with magnesium-containing salts or antacid mixtures. Excess magnesium blocks neuromuscular transmission by decreasing the amount of acetycholine released at the junction. Peripheral vasodilatation and low blood pressure occur; as magnesium levels rise, nausea and vomiting appear; hypotension can become intractable; lethargy, drowsiness, and dysarthria are noted as signs of CNS depression; deep tendon reflexes are lost (at about 7 mEq/liter); and, finally, paralysis and cardiac arrest may ensue.

Infusion of magnesium into uremic patients (sometimes employed to control uremic convulsions) may cause an accentuation of nausea, lethargy, ataxia, and postural hypotension, all reversed by dialysis. The mild elevation of magnesium in most uremic patients probably contributes negligibly to the symptomatology of renal failure, however.

Hypomagnesemia

Changes in personality attributed to magnesium depletion range from mild depression and nervousness to delirium, hallucinations, and psychosis. Some patients have episodic confusion and irritability. Serum magnesium levels are sometimes low in chronic alcoholism and delirium tremens, but magnesium replacement is not effective as treatment. Hypomagnesemia somehow induces hypocalcemia and hypokalemia, so it is difficult to assess the specific effects of hypomagnesemia. Magnesium deficiency is most common in malabsorption syndromes.

Acidosis

Mild metabolic acidosis, with serum bicarbonate below 20 mEq/liter, is often responsible for lethargy, nausea, anorexia, and headache. With progressive acidosis, disorientation, depressed consciousness, and stupor occur. Seizures are not common. CNS depression is more closely related to pH of the spinal fluid than to pH of the blood. Thus, neurologic signs and dysmentation are much more frequent and severe in respiratory acidosis than in metabolic acidosis, since CO_2 readily diffuses across the blood-brain barrier.

Severe uncompensated respiratory acidosis produces the characteristic syndrome of CO_2 narcosis. Weakness and fatigue, headache, blurred vision, anxiety, and depression progress to irritability, confusion, combative delirium, and somnolence. Asterixis is typical, together with deep sighing respirations of Kussmaul breathing owing to intense stimulation of the respiratory center.

The acidosis and other effects of uremia cause prolonged nerve conduction, peripheral neuropathy, disturbed sleep patterns, asterixis, convulsions, and occasionally psychotic behaviors. The mechanisms of these derangements associated with uremia are very little understood. Retained solutes, deficient substances, hormonal overcompensation, and dialyzable "middle molecules" all have drawn speculation about potential roles in uremic toxicity.

Alkalosis

Severe metabolic alkalosis often occurs in patients with compensated hypercapnea secondary to chronic lung disease when ventilation is suddenly improved. Pco_2 falls rapidly and blood pH rises. Mental confusion and delirium, with focal or generalized seizures, cardiac arrhythmias, and hypotension are likely. The symptoms are reversed if the Pco_2 is allowed to rise. The increase in pH enhances irritability of the peripheral nervous system, as well as the CNS, and causes tetany indistinguishable from that associated with hypocalcemia.

METABOLIC DISORDERS INTRINSIC TO THE BRAIN

Lesch-Nyhan Syndrome

In 1964, a second-year medical student (Lesch) and his professor (Nyhan) reported a most remarkable metabolic/behavioral disorder that now bears their names and that has stimulated a vast array of investigations. Among patients with mental retardation due to inherited metabolic disorders, this syndrome may rank second only to PKU in frequency. The cause is a mutation on the X chromosome affecting the gene for the enzyme hypoxanthine guanine phosphoribosyl transferase (HGPRT), involved in what was previously thought to be a minor pathway of purine metabolism. Boys with this X-linked recessive disorder have virtually complete deficiency of HGPRT in cells throughout the body. The highest activity of HGPRT normally is in the brain, particularly the basal ganglia, where many of the prominent neurologic signs arise in these patients.

Affected males appear normal at birth and for up to 6–8 months postnatally. The earliest symptom is the occurrence of orange sand in the diapers, due to massive excretion of urates (hypoxanthine and uric acid). Screening diagnosis is made most reliably from an elevated uric acid/creatinine ratio. Hematuria or urinary tract stone disease may occur in the early months of life, and later these boys develop any or all of the manifestations of gout: arthritis, tophi, nephropathy, and renal failure. Uric acid stones are radiolucent, so the cause of colicky abdominal pain may be overlooked in early episodes. The manifestations first noted are usually neurologic abnormalities, however. Infants who had been sitting and holding up their heads lose these abilities. After a period of hypotonia, marked hypertonicity develops, with increased deep tendon reflexes and Babinski responses. Spasticity is so severe that bilateral dislocation of the hips often results. Dystonic and athetoid posturing, choreic movements, and athetoid dysarthria and dysphagia are characteristic and are worsened by tension or excitement. Motor disability is so great that none of the patients has walked, and they can sit in a chair only with trunk supports. They appear to have cerebral palsy. Mental development is retarded, with IQ's less than 50, but most learn to speak. In fact, IQ testing in these children is highly suspect. The motor defects make it difficult for them to perform adequately. Writing is impossible, and their behavioral disorder interferes severely. Nevertheless, they usually relate well to people and seem to understand well what is said to them. They have bright, understanding eye contact, and they learn to communicate rather well, considering the dysarthric speech.

Aggressive self-mutilative behavior is an integral and most impressive feature of this syndrome. The behavior begins with the eruption of teeth, though in some patients it was delayed for 3–5 years. Most patients bite their lips or fingers in a stereotyped, highly individualized pattern and with such ferocity that loss of tissue almost always results. The hallmark of the syndrome is a distinct loss of tissue about the upper or lower lip. It is rare to see one of these patients without permanent damage to the lips, unless the primary teeth were removed early. They do not have sensory defect; they scream in pain while they bite themselves. They are really happy only when securely protected from themselves by physical restraints, indicating the insight they, in fact, do have into their propensity to hurt themselves. Sometimes they are engaging children when restrained, with a good sense of humor. When the restraints are removed, however, their personality changes abruptly and they appear terrified. As they get older, they may even call for help. The "switch" in their behavior is more dramatic than the switch described for manic-depressive patients. As they grow older, their behavior becomes more varied, picking with their fingers, scalding in hot water, catching themselves in braces employed for cerebral palsy or in the spokes of a wheelchair. Within their motor limitations, they can constitute a risk to others, including their favorite ward personnel. As they become older, they may become verbally aggressive, with abusive language, but they are remorseful about hurting others. As Nyhan has noted, these children are reminiscent of the principal character of the ballet "Petroushka" with their admixture of good humor and tragedy, unusual posturing, and mitten-like coverings on the hands.

The metabolic disorder has been studied intensively, with many findings, but the link between purine metabolism and the self-mutilative behavior is still a mystery. Uric acid is not formed in the brain. The end-products of purine metabolism in the brain are xanthine and hypoxanthine, and levels of hypoxanthine in the CSF are four times control values. Treatment with allopurinol is indicated to prevent the urinary tract complications, but allopurinol has no effect on the neurologic or behavioral manifestations of the disease.

As little as 5% of normal HGPRT activity is sufficient to prevent development of the neuropsychiatric problems. Patients have been identified with gout due to other mutations affecting HGPRT, leaving 5–15% residual activity. These patients have no neurologic abnormalities or only mild spinocerebellar signs.

Women who carry the Lesch-Nyhan trait in heterozygous form have 100% HGPRT activity in approximately half the cells and no activity in other cells, owing to the process of random inactivation of the X chromosome, as predicted by the Lyon hypothesis. In their bone marrow, however, those cells lacking HGPRT activity are eliminated, so that tests of blood cells from such women show full activity, while tests of skin fibroblasts document the heterozygous state. Whether HGPRT-deficient cells in heterozygous women are also eliminated in the development of the nervous system is unknown. Administration of methylpurines (caffeine, theophylline) in rabbits and rats seems to stimulate excessive self-biting behavior. Methylpurines inhibit phosphodiesterase and raise intracellular concentrations of cAMP. cAMP has emerged as a key intracellular mediator for a great many processes, including the action of hormones in many tissues and of drugs and neurotransmitters in intact and tissue-cultured neuronal systems. Relationships between HGPRT deficiency and cAMP effects are not yet known. The fact that HGPRT activity is normally higher in the brain than in any other tissue and that the activity of amidophosphoribosyltransferase, the likely rate-limiting

step in the *de novo* pathway, is low in the brain, suggests that the brain may be unusually dependent on the salvage pathway for the synthesis of inosinic acid (IMP) and guanylic acid (GMP). In the absence of HGPRT, the brain may be unable to maintain intracellular concentrations of these or the cyclic nucleotides necessary for normal functions. *In vitro*, cultured cells dependent on the salvage pathways for purine nucleotide synthesis grow poorly. Thus, it is possible that impaired cellular proliferation is a feature of the brain dysfunction in Lesch-Nyhan syndrome. Of the six patients whose brains were examined postmortem, four had reduced brain weight, and some mothers of affected boys have remarked on the feebleness of intrauterine contractions. In any case, the purine nucleotide GMP must be synthesized entirely *de novo* in the absence of HGPRT activity, which could lead to depletion of certain critical cofactors, such as ATP or folic acid.

One experimental approach in treating the brain dysfunction has been directed toward replacing the presumed deficiency of either GMP or IMP. Administration of GMP or AMP had no effect, probably because these compounds cross cell membranes very poorly. Adenine has been tried, because it is readily converted to AMP by the enzyme adenine phosphoribosyltransferase and might increase IMP or GMP levels through interconversion or by inhibiting microsomal 5′-nucleotidase. Also, formation of AMP and consumption of phosphoribosylpyrophosphate (PRPP) should reduce the rate of purine synthesis de novo. Studies of cultured fibroblasts with HGPRT deficiency indicated a need for adenine and folic acid. Administration of adenine ± folate to a few patients, even from birth, has had no definitive therapeutic effect, however.

Another possible clue about mechanisms of brain dysfunction involves central adrenergic pathways. Unilateral destruction of a dopamine pathway in the nigrostriatal system with 6-hydroxydopamine occasionally produces self-mutilation in animals, and elevated plasma levels of dopamine β-hydroxylase have been reported in Lesch-Nyhan patients with striking self-mutilation. Patients with other mutations affecting HGPRT but producing only the partial deficiency syndrome without self-mutilation had no such elevation.

There is considerable evidence in studies of rodents that inhibition of serotonin synthesis or lesions in areas rich in serotonin may stimulate aggressive behaviors, whereas treatment with 5-hydroxytryptophan (HTP) can reduce those behaviors. Administration of 5-HTP together with an inhibitor of peripheral decarboxylase activity, such as carbidopa, has been reported by Nyhan to have dramatic effects in reducing mutilative behavior. The effect could be sustained only for 3–4 weeks, owing to tolerance, however. HTP alone is ineffective.

Mintz has devised an ingenious approach to the creation of an animal model for investigation of the pathogenesis of Lesch-Nyhan syndrome. An HGPRT⁻/HGPRT⁺ mosaic mouse has been produced (Dewey et al., 1977) from a normal embryo plus HGPRT⁻ teratocarcinoma cells, combined in the blastocyst stage. Completely HGPRT⁻ progeny will be generated, permitting developmental, physiologic, pharmacologic, and behavioral studies that are impossible with patients. In addition, HGPRT alleles with different residual enzyme activity could be utilized to generate a graded series of HGPRT deficiencies for neurochemical and behavioral correlations.

Attempts at behavior modification with mild aversive techniques of the sort employed with retarded patients with moderate self-mutilative behavior have no effect in these boys, or may even lead to worse behavior. Some have advocated extinction therapy. Perhaps some combinations of pharmacologic and psychologic approaches will be effective.

Wilson Disease: Hepatolenticular Degeneration

Wilson disease, a disorder of copper transport or metabolism, or both, is a rare autosomal recessive disease of young adults, with cirrhosis of the liver and degeneration particularly of the basal ganglia of the brain. Copper deposition can be demonstrated in these organs and in greenish-brown Kayser-Fleischer rings at the limbus of the cornea. The copper-binding serum protein ceruloplasmin is deficient and various tissue proteins are overloaded with loosely bound copper, but the primary lesion in copper metabolism is not yet known. This disorder merits particular emphasis because treatment with the copper-chelating agent D-penicillamine ($\beta\beta$-dimethyl-cysteine) can reverse or prevent copper deposition and clinical signs of the disease. Untreated, this disease is invariably fatal.

Psychiatric and behavioral changes are common but vary in kind and degree. In one series of patients, 60% had significant psychologic manifestations as the first clinical indication of the disease; usually about 20% have such manifestations recognized before the neurologic and hepatic signs emerge. Personality disturbances, hysteria, or schizophrenic behavior may be diagnosed. Intellectual capacities are maintained intact, though observers may be misled by childish personality changes, drooling, difficulties with verbal communication, and eventually a masklike expressionless face. Failure to consider Wilson disease in these patients allows the development of life-threatening complications and needless, ineffective psychiatric therapies.

The neurologic signs vary also. One form of lenticular degeneration is dystonic, with spasticity, rigidity, dysarthria, drooling, and dysphagia, progressing to spasms, contractures, and an unrelenting downhill course with unexplained acute febrile episodes. This form of the disease occurs predominantly in young adults and may lead to death within 1 year, if untreated. Another form of neurologic involvement is pseudosclerosis, with flapping tremors of the wrists and shoulders and with less marked spasticity or rigidity. Occasionally, patients develop seizures or hemiplegia. In undiagnosed patients with cirrhosis, the neurologic complications may incorrectly be thought to be due to hepatic encephalopathy and delay still further the correct diagnosis.

In children, the disease usually begins with chronic active hepatitis, cirrhosis, or an acute hemolytic episode. The Kayser-Fleischer ring has rarely appeared before age 7 years, so diagnosis in children depends upon a high index of suspicion plus laboratory tests.

Since penicillamine can have toxic effects upon the kidney, it is important to recognize that aminoaciduria, glycosuria, proteinuria, and increased renal excretion of uric acid, calcium, and phosphate all occur as part of the disease. The extent of renal abnormality should be characterized before initiating therapy.

It is important to sustain treatment to achieve gradual improvement, even though symptoms and signs may worsen during the first 6–8 weeks of decoppering (Sass-Kortsak and Bearn, 1978). For the relatively few patients who cannot tolerate penicillamine, a new oral decoppering agent, triethylene tetramine dihydrochloride, may prove useful. Finally, in one case, testing the hypothesis that the primary defect in Wilson disease lies in the liver, liver transplantation was carried out. During 4 years of post transplant follow-up while chelation therapy was withheld, the patient improved clinically, his Kayser-Fleischer rings disappeared, and the previously low serum copper and ceruloplasmin levels became normal.

Affected sibs of patients can be diagnosed in the presymptomatic phase of the disease by ceruloplasmin assay and by excessive copper excretion after a standard dose of penicillamine. Treatment should be initiated to prevent the development of the disease in these individuals.

Homocystinuria

Homocystinuria is a fascinating autosomal recessive disorder of the metabolism of sulfur-containing amino acids that illustrates well the matter of genetic heterogeneity (Table 13–2) and provides clues to potentially important aspects of brain metabolism. These patients have skeletal abnormalities approximating the gangling phenotype of Marfan's syndrome, plus displacement of the lens of the eye, blotchy skin, and marked propensity for thromboses of both arteries and veins. Most interesting for this discussion, about half of the patients are described as mentally retarded (IQ below 70). It is not at all clear whether the patients described as having normal IQ reflect heterogeneity of underlying disease mechanisms or whether they also have lost 20 or 30 points in IQ, yet remained in the "normal" range. Some patients have had quite high IQ's (McKusick, 1972). The kind of study that is needed would compare the IQ's of affected individuals with the IQ's of parents and siblings. Psychotic behavior has been noted in some patients and also in their relatives, but no systematic evaluation of these observations is available.

The primary biochemical defect is in the synthesis of the complex amino acid cystathionine from homocysteine and serine by the enzyme cystathionine synthase (CS). In affected persons, the enzyme has less than 5% of normal activity. Although the concentration of cystathionine is similar in the livers of rats and humans, the concentration is very much higher in the brains of humans and monkeys than in the brains of lower animals. Its function is unknown. It is conceivable that cystathionine acts as a neurotransmitter since many amino acids are now suspected of having neurotransmitter roles. In fact, the compounds widely regarded as neurotransmitters (acetylcholine, norepinephrine, dopamine, serotonin, GABA, and epinephrine) may account for only 30% of the synapses in the mammalian brain.

Two forms of CS deficiency can be distinguished by administration of vitamin B_6 (pyridoxine), the cofactor for CS; such treatment leads to prompt metabolic correction in about half the patients. These two forms do not correspond directly with retarded and nonretarded categories, however. Most patients with the B_6-responsive form have normal intelligence, but retarded persons fall into both types. The relative roles of underlying metabolic disorder in the brain and of intracerebral thromboses are hard to assess, especially in the absence of localizing neurologic signs. Nevertheless, it is important to recognize that administration of pyridoxine in the B_6-responsive patients may prevent or even reverse abnormalities in the brain. In several treated children, petit mal seizures ceased and scholastic performance improved as the urine was cleared of homocystine. In another case, severe hyperactive behavior in a child was controlled with pyridoxine. Thus homocystinuria, PKU (described earlier), and Hunter syndrome (discussed later) are all rare causes of the common phenotype of hyperactivity in childhood. Given McKusick's estimate of disease frequency at 1 per 45,000, 1% of the general population would be heterozygous carriers for homocystinuria. Since the biochemical abnormality is present in the brain itself, the detailed behavioral status of carriers is worth investigating.

A previously unrecognized cause of homocystinuria due to deficiency of 5,10-methylenetetrahydrofolate reductase (rather than of CS) presented with a clinical picture of recurrent episodes of mental deterioration and schizophrenic behavior, repeatedly responsive to administration of folic acid (Freeman et al., 1975). The deficient enzyme is necessary to form the folate compound that serves as methyl donor for methylation of homocysteine to methionine and possibly for methylation of some biogenic amines. Such rare metabolic disorders may provide a "handle" on the likely heterogeneity of causes of schizophrenia. The main puzzle in this new disorder is the normal level of methionine, since excess methionine concentrations were presumed to trigger the psychotic behavior observed in some patients with CS-deficient homocystinuria. In fact, the relative roles of elevated levels of methionine and of homocysteine in homocystinuria are not known. Homocysteine appears to be the more important agent in stimulating atherogenesis, however, and the resulting vascular lesions may be the primary causes of the highly variable dysfunction in the central nervous system.

Storage Diseases: Mucopolysaccharidoses

The mucopolysaccharidoses (MPS) have been classified clinically and biochemically into several distinct types. Cell culture experiments have distinguished subtypes that produce degradative enzymes that will correct the excessive storage of the complementary subtype of cells. The present status of this work is summarized briefly in Table 13–4. For the purposes of this discussion, comparison of MPS I, H (Hurler syndrome) with MPS II (Hunter syndrome) will suffice. They are distinguished genetically: MPS I is autosomal recessive; MPS II is X-linked recessive. They are distinguished biochemically by the cross-correction experiments and the different enzymic deficiencies. They can be distinguished clinically, as well. Children with Hurler syndrome tend to have more severe mental retardation, with cortical atrophy and hydrocephalus or ventricular dilatation. Clouding of the cornea is much more common in MPS I, whereas deafness is more common in MPS II. Interestingly, specialists who see these children report that they can easily differentiate boys with these two MPS by examining their behavior and temperament. The children with Hurler syndrome are friendly and affectionate, clumsy, sometimes apathetic. In striking contrast, the boys with Hunter syndrome are characteristically hyperactive and hard to manage. The same mucopolysaccharides accumulate, although the ratio of dermatan to heparan sulfates is usually higher in the Hurler syndrome. The different enzymic activities involved are closely related metabolic steps. Thus it is not at all clear why these children behave so differently, whether it is the amount of MPS, the rate of accumulation, or possibly the sites of accumulation as a function of developmental timing that put the children with Hurler syndrome at greater risk for serious damage. By some standards, however, children with Hunter or Sanfilippo syndrome would be judged even more abnormal in their behavior than would the children with Hurler syndrome.

Storage Diseases: Sphingolipidoses

Very rapid progress has been made in elucidating the enzymic defects and differentiating the clinical pictures of disorders of degradation of complex normal lipids (Table 13–5). Each of these disorders may be considered intrinsic to brain, with the exception of Fabry disease, in which glycolipid deposition affects primarily blood vessels in various organs plus the peripheral and autonomic nervous systems. Considerable clinical heterogeneity has been recognized, with onset of illness in infancy, in childhood, and later in certain of the lipidoses. The detailed biochemical characterization of such clinical heterogeneity is under active investigation, but multiple alleles at the same locus must contribute a good portion of the heterogeneity. When the rate of accumulation is slow or perhaps when an isozyme in brain is not involved, the patient will be spared mental retardation and even later neurologic impairment. Distinctive personality traits or patterns of cognitive defects have not yet been sought among these many newly defined disorders.

The effects on brain function of the stored lipids are not fully explained. Are the effects toxic or mechanical? Do

Table 13–4.   INBORN ERRORS OF MUCOPOLYSACCHARIDE (MSP) DEGRADATION*

Disorder	Eponym	Lysosomal enzyme deficient	Excess urinary MPS	Behavioral phenotype
MPS I, H	Hurler	α-L-Iduronidase	Dermatan and heparan SO$_4$	Severe mental retardation, apathic, friendly, placid
MPS I, S	Scheie	same	same compounds	Normal intelligence
MPS II	Hunter	Iduronate sulfatase	same compounds	Severe mental deterioration, hyperactive behavior
MPS III	Sanfilippo	1. Heparan N-sulfatase 2. N-Ac-α-D-glucosaminidase	Heparan sulfate	Severe mental retardation, hyperactive
MPS IV	Morquio	Hexosamine 6-sulfatase	Keratan sulfate	Normal intelligence
MPS VI	Maroteaux-Lamy	N-Ac-galactosamine-4-sulfatase	Dermatan sulfate	Normal intelligence
MPS VII	—	β-glucuronidase	Dermatan sulfate	Variable mental retardation
MPS VIII	—	Glucosamine-6-sulfate sulfatase	Keratan and heparan SO$_4$	Mental retardation

* After McKusick, V. A., et al.: In *The Metabolic Basis of Inherited Disease*. 4th ed. Stanbury, J. B., et al. (eds.), New York, McGraw-Hill Book Co., 1978.

Table 13–5. INBORN ERRORS OF SPHINGOLIPID METABOLISM*

Syndrome	Enzyme deficient	Behavioral phenotype	Intrinsic to CNS
Generalized gangliosidosis	β-galactosidase	Severe MR	Yes
Sandhoff disease	Hexosaminidase's A and B	Severe MR	Yes
Tay-Sachs disease	Hexosaminidase A	Neurologic signs and mental deterioration	Yes
Fabry disease	Ceramide trihexosidase (α-galactosidase)	Normal. Peripheral neuritis in some cases	No
Metachromatic leukodystrophy			
infantile onset	Arylsulfatase A (cerebroside sulfatase)	Severe MR	Yes
"adult" onset		"Schizophrenia", then neurologic signs and organic dementia	Yes
Krabbe disease (globoid cell leukodystrophy)	Cerebroside β-galactosidase	Severe MR (viscera unaffected)	Yes
Gaucher disease			
chronic non-neuronopathic	Glucocerebrosidase (12–45% activity)	Normal	Probably
acute, neuronopathic	Same (0 activity)	Moderate MR, neurologic signs	Yes
subacute neuronopathic	Same (10–20% activity)	Mild intellectual impairment	Yes
Niemann-Pick disease			
infantile, neuronopathic	Sphingomyelinase (0–9%)	Severe neurologic involvement	Yes
chronic non-neuronopathic	Sphingomyelinase (15–20%) ? different isozyme, less deficient	Normal, but just as severe visceral involvement	??
chronic non-neuronopathic	Sphingomyelinase (less deficient)	Progressive neurologic signs	Yes

*See Stanbury, J. B., et al. (eds.): *The Metabolic Basis of Inherited Disease.* 4th ed. New York, McGraw-Hill Book Co., 1978. Note: there is marked heterogeneity within almost every one of these specific disorders.

deficiencies result from a block in turnover? Are the damaging compounds side-products, since multiple compounds tend to accumulate? In the case of the acute, neuropathic form of Gaucher disease, there is not yet a good correlation of the severity of brain damage with the amount of glucose ceramide found in the brain.

One particularly interesting lipidosis is the adult-onset type of metachromatic leukodystrophy, in which sulfatides are stored because of deficiency and abnormality of arylsulfatase A. Among 19 cases in one review (Austin, 1968), the presenting clinical picture was described as "schizophrenia" in every case. Evidence for an organic dementia was good by the time that distinctive neurologic signs slowly worsened in these patients. This disorder, too, contributes to the iceberg of cases of schizophrenic phenotype. Another lipid storage disorder in which psychotic behavior has been noted is Refsum disease, in which phytanic acid is accumulated, a 20-carbon intermediate of fatty acid degradation. Clinical features are retinitis pigmentosa, peripheral neuropathy, ataxia, sensory disturbances, and changes in skin and bones. Whether some cases with psychosis are due to the phytanic acid storage or simply occur together with Refsum disease in family members remains to be elucidated.

Glycolytic Pathway

The brain, of course, is exquisitely sensitive to lack of oxygen or glucose. My colleagues and I have carried out a number of studies of glycolytic enzymes in brain and other tissues. Most of the 11 enzymes of the glycolytic pathway have tissue-specific isozymes (Table 13–6). Deficiencies of specific enzymes in red blood cells have been recognized as causes of hemolytic anemia. We can predict which patients with hemolytic anemia might also have neurologic impairment. Those with different isozymes in the brain should be spared, whereas those whose enzyme deficiency will be manifest also in brain will be affected. In the cases of tri-

osephosphate isomerase (TPI) and phosphoglycerate kinase (PGK) (see Table 13–6), patients had striking neuropsychiatric symptoms and signs, whereas none of the others were affected. The case of phosphohexose isomerase (PHI) is a reasonable exception, since the hemolytic anemia and enzyme deficiency were mild and the enzyme normally is present in excess activity.

These examples of inferring brain enzyme deficiencies from knowledge of the isozyme patterns of homologous enzymes in blood cells and brain are important for future interpretation of studies of monoamine oxidase (MAO) in platelets and of catechol-O-methyltransferase (COMT) in red blood cells. Low MAO activity was reported in platelets in various groups of psychiatric patients and in patients susceptible to migraine headaches triggered by chocolates, which contain substantial amounts of phenylethylamine, metabolized by MAO. The plasma is a good source of the enzyme dopamine-β-hydroxylase, derived from noradrenergic neurons, from which the enzyme is released together with norepinephrine. Families of individuals with very low dopamine β-hydroxylase activity in serum have been investigated, and an autosomal recessive pattern of inheritance of very low dopamine β-hydroxylase activity was found (Weinshilboum, 1978). No gross clinical differences were noted, but these persons merit detailed behavioral and psychophysiologic investigation. At least some properties of dopamine β-hydroxylase in human brain appear to be the same as dopamine β-hydroxylase in serum. Careful characterization of these peripheral enzymes is essential, utilizing genetic variants to prove or disprove identity between the peripheral enzymes and the corresponding enzyme in brain.

Another valuable peripheral phenomenon for investigation is the platelet active uptake of serotonin, which appears indistinguishable from that of synaptosomes from nerve endings in the brain. Uptake of dopamine into platelets is entirely different from that in brain (Omenn and Smith, 1978), however, showing that detailed pharmacologic and genetic assessment of peripheral models for brain functions is essential.

Table 13–6. CLINICAL CORRELATION OF ISOZYME DATA FOR GLYCOLYTIC ENZYMES

Glycolytic enzymes	Tissue-specific isozymes occur	Deficiency described in red blood cells	
		Hemolytic anemia	Neurologic signs
Hexokinase	+	+	0
Phosphohexose isomerase (PHI)	0	+ (mild)	0
Phosphofructokinase	+	+	0
Aldolase	+	0	
Triosephosphate isomerase (TPI)	0	+	Yes
Glyceraldehyde-3-phosphate dehydrogenase	+	+	0
Phosphoglycerate kinase (PGK)	0	+	Yes
Phosphoglycerate mutase	+	0	
Enolase	+	0	
Pyruvate kinase	+	+	0
Lactate dehydrogenase	+	0	

From Omenn (1976), reprinted from *Behavior Genetics* with permission.

Amino Acid Transport Disorders

Scriver raised the possibility that mental disorders in a few patients with cystinuria might be due to the underlying metabolic disorder. The clinical effects of defective reabsorption of the dibasic amino acids are due to formation of urinary tract stones. Available evidence suggests that amino acid transport systems in the brain might be the same as those in the kidney and intestine, which are abnormal in cystinuric patients. More study of this relationship is indicated.

Another transport disorder is Hartnup disease, in which there are a pellagra-like rash after exposure to sunlight, attacks of cerebellar ataxia, and occasional psychiatric changes ranging from emotional instability to delirium. The condition can be diagnosed by massive urinary excretion of monoamino-monocarboxylic amino acids, but the clinical features are not explained by the aminoaciduria. If the analogy to pellagra is accurate, the episodic neurologic and psychiatric disturbances could be due to nicotinamide deficiency coupled with stress and poor nutrition. Administration of nicotinamide is usually helpful. Whether the disorder is truly intrinsic to brain has not been explored.

The amino acid transport disorder is clearly present in the jejunum, however, where patients retain these specific unabsorbed amino acids for abnormally long periods. Bacterial decomposition produces absorbable compounds, some of which may be toxic. These patients also have a lowered ability to convert tryptophan to kynurenine nicotinamide, which is attributed to the deviation of tryptophan from its normal metabolic route because of the absorptive defect.

Several inherited disorders of the glutathione pathway have been described. Glutathione synthetase deficiency seems to affect red blood cells only, whereas deficiency of γ-glutamylcysteine synthetase in two cases produced both mild hemolytic anemia and spinocerebellar degeneration, peripheral neuropathy, myopathy, and amino aciduria. The γ-glutamyl cycle is known to be important in amino acid transport in the kidney; these observations point to its importance also in the brain. The first of these two patients was a man who was diagnosed at age 29 to have psychotic behavior.

Wernicke-Korsakoff Syndrome

The ophthalmoplegia, ataxia, and lethargy of this syndrome, but probably not the confabulatory psychosis, are known to be due to deficiency of thiamine. Thiamine pyrophosphate is a critical cofactor for transketolase in the pentose-phosphate shunt and for pyruvate and glutamate decarboxylases in the Krebs cycle. Thiamine is normally found in high concentrations in the mammillary bodies and related brain regions. In alcoholics, who are likely to be B-vitamin depleted, thiamine should always be given by injection before intravenous administration of a glucose load.

Blass and Gibson (1977) recently presented evidence to explain why only a few alcoholics with similar thiamine deficiency develop this organ-specific complication. Such individuals have a variant of the thiamine-requiring enzyme transketolase (high Km variant), which makes it need higher concentrations of thiamine in order to have the same enzymic activity. This finding may be considered an example of what must be similar variation in target organ functions for such other organ-specific complications as cirrhosis, pancreatitis, cerebellar degeneration, cardiomyopathy, and fetal alcohol syndrome.

CONCLUSION

Inborn errors of metabolism present valuable experiments of nature for the clinical investigator and important heterogeneity of etiology for the physician planning therapeutic interventions. Just as inborn errors have provided major clues in elucidating the steps of biosynthesis for thyroid and steroid hormones, we may expect that investigations of the brain and other target tissues in patients with specific inborn errors may yield clues to one of our major clinical questions: why are the effects, and especially the behavioral effects, of seemingly similar hormonal or metabolic derangements so different in different patients?

REFERENCES

General

Stanbury, J. B., Wyngaarden, J. B., et al. (eds): *The Metabolic Basis of Inherited Disease*, 4th ed. New York, McGraw-Hill, 1978.

Scriver, C. R., and Rosenberg, L. E.: *Amino Acid Metabolism and Its Disorders*. Philadelphia, W. B. Saunders, 1973.

Nyhan, W. L. (ed.): *Heritable Disorders of Amino Acid Metabolism: Patterns of Clinical Expression and Genetic Variation*. New York, John Wiley and Sons, 1974.

Maxwell, M. H., and Kleeman, C. R. (eds.): *Clinical Disorders of Fluid and Electrolyte Metabolism*. 3rd ed. New York, McGraw-Hill, 1980.

Articles

Austin, J., et al.: Metachromatic leukodystrophy (MLD). VIII. MLD in adults; diagnosis and pathogenesis. *Arch. Neurol.* 18:225, 1968.

Ballard, R. A., et al.: Transient hyperammonemia of the preterm infant. *N. Engl. J. Med.* 299:920, 1978.

Berman, J. L., and Ford, R.: Intelligence quotients and intelligence loss in patients with phenylketonuria and some variant states. *J. Pediatr.* 77:764, 1970.

Bessman, S. P., et al.: Diet, genetics, and mental retardation: interaction between phenylketonuric heterozygous mother and fetus to produce nonspecific diminution of IQ: evidence in support of the justification hypothesis. *Proc. Natl. Acad. Sci. USA* 75:1562, 1978.

Blass, J. P., and Gibson, G. E.: Abnormality of a thiamine-requiring enzyme in patients with Wernicke-Korsakoff syndrome. *N. Engl. J. Med.* 297:1367, 1977.

Cohen, P. T. W., et al.: Restricted variation in the glycolytic enzymes of human brain and erythrocytes. *Nature* 241:229, 1973.

Denko, J. D., and Kaelbling, R.: The psychiatric aspects of hypoparathyroidism. *Acta Psychiatr. Scand.* 38(Suppl. 164):1, 1962.

Dewey, M. J., Martin, D. W., Jr., et al.: Mosaic mice with teratocarcinoma-derived mutant cells deficient in hypoxanthine phosphoribosyltransferase. *Proc. Natl. Acad. Sci. USA* 74:5564, 1977.

Freeman, J. M., et al.: Folate-responsive homocystinuria and "schizophrenia." *N. Engl. J. Med.* 292:491, 1975.

Hindfelt, B.: The effect of sustained hyperammonemia upon the metabolic state of the brain. *Scand. J. Clin. Lab. Invest.* 30:245, 1972.

Kaufman, S., et al.: Phenylketonuria due to a deficiency of dihydropteridine reductase. *N. Engl. J. Med.* 293:785, 1975.

Lesch, M., and Nyhan, W. L.: A familial disorder of uric acid metabolism and central nervous system function. *Am. J. Med.* 36:561, 1964.

McKusick, V. A.: *Heritable Disorders of Connective Tissue*, 4th ed. St. Louis, C. V. Mosby, 1972.

McCance, R. A.: Experimental sodium chloride deficiency in man. *Proc. R. Soc. Med.* 119:245, 1936.

Nyhan, W. L.: Behavior in the Lesch-Nyhan syndrome. *J. Autism Child. Schizo.* 6:235, 1976.

Nyhan, W. L.: The Lesch-Nyan syndrome. *Dev. Med. Child. Neurol.* 20:376, 1978.

Omenn, G. S.: Inborn errors of metabolism: clues to understanding human behavioral disorders. *Behav. Genet.* 6:263, 1976.

Omenn, G. S.: Neurochemistry and behavior in man. *West. J. Med.* 25:434, 1976.

Omenn, G. S., and Smith, L. T.: A common uptake system for serotonin and dopamine in human platelets. *J. Clin. Invest.* 62:235, 1978.

Paine, R. S.: The variability in manifestations of untreated patients with phenylketonuria (phenylpyruvic acid). *Pediatrics* 20:290, 1957.

Petersen, P.: Psychiatric disorders in primary hyperparathyroidism. *J. Clin. Endocrinol.* 28:1491, 1968.

Pueschel, S. M., et al.: Thiamine-responsive intermittent branched chain ketoaciduria. *J Pediatr.* 94:628, 1979.

Richards, F., II, et al.: Familial spinocerebellar degeneration, hemolytic anemia, and glutathione deficiency. *Arch. Intern. Med.* 134:534, 1974.

Russell, A.: A biochemical basis for migraine and cyclical vomiting, In *Enzymopenic Anaemias, Lysosomes and Other Papers.* Allan, J. D., Holt, K. S., et al. (eds.), Baltimore, Williams and Wilkins, 1969, p. 134.

Sandler, M., et al.: A phenylethylamine oxidizing defect in migraine. *Nature* 250:335, 1974.

Sass-Kortsak, A., and Bearn, A. G.: Hereditary disorders of copper metabolism, In Stanbury, J. B., Wyngaarden, J. B., et al. (eds.), *The Metabolic Basis of Inherited Disease.* 4th ed. New York, McGraw-Hill, 1978, p. 1098.

Silberberg, D. H.: Maple syrup urine disease metabolites studied in cerebellum cultures. *J. Neurochem.* 16:1141, 1969.

Smith, I., et al.: New variant of phenylketonuria with progressive neurological illness unresponsive to phenylalanine restriction. *Lancet* 1:1108, 1975.

Walshe, J. M.: Penicillamine, a new oral therapy for Wilson's disease. *Am. J. Med.* 1:487, 1956.

Weinshilboum, R. M.: Human biochemical genetics of plasma dopamine-β-hydroxylase and erythrocyte catechol-O-methyltransferase. *Hum. Genet.* 1(Suppl.):101, 1978.

Williams, R. H.: Metabolism and mentation. Presidential address to the Endocrine Society. *J. Clin. Endocrinol. Metab.* 31:461, 1970.

Wright, S. W., and Tarjan, G.: Phenylketonuria. *A.M.A. J. Dis. Child.* 93:405, 1957.

CHAPTER 14

Gastrointestinal Hormones

By Robert H. Williams*

*This chapter was being written by Dr. Robert H. Williams at the time of his death. It was completed and edited by Drs. John Ensinck and Edwin L. Bierman.

When we consider the large volumes and varieties of food ingested, not uncommonly at a rapid rate, it is clear that the gastrointestinal tract needs a sophisticated "computer system" for optimal digestion, movement, and absorption. A large number of factors are involved in the control of these functions, especially signals provided by the autonomic nervous system and hormones. Many of the latter share origins in the nervous system and are considered neurotransmitters as well as hormones. They include: acetylcholine, ACTH, β-endorphin, bombesin, cholecystokinin, dopamine, enkephalin, enteroglucagon, gastrin, gastroinhibitory polypeptide, histamine, motilin, neurotensin, norepinephrine, pancreatic polypeptide, secretin, serotonin, somatostatin, substance P, and vasoactive intestinal peptide. Whether each of these compounds has been established as a hormone and whether there are others that are not listed that should be considered as gastrointestinal hormones are questions that are considered subsequently.

Several of these substances are released in the gut wall from special endocrine cells and/or nerve terminals (Grube and Forssmann, 1979) (Table 14–1). Most of them are also synthesized in the brain, but are not released into the systemic circulation in sufficient quantities to affect the functions of the gastrointestinal tract. Likewise, most of the hormones in gut cells are synthesized in them and do not become bound to brain cells. There are some that are manufactured in the pancreatic islet and act upon adjacent cells, as well as influencing gastrointestinal function. Directly or indirectly, the brain, gut, and pancreas are interrelated and messages between them are transmitted via special nerves and some hormones. Therefore, it is the intent of this chapter to provide an overview of the hormonal and neural activities of the gastrointestinal tract and their relationships to the brain and pancreas. For more detail, the reader is referred to Chs. 10, 11, 12, and 15. Whereas most of the subsequent discussion is focused on the gastrointestinal tract, it should be recalled that the adenohypophysis, thyroid, parathyroids, and pancreas develop as protrusions from the alimentary canal and are derived from the same cell line as the gut, namely ectoblast (Pearse and Polak, 1978). All of these structures influence the functions of the gastrointestinal tract.

Collectively, the gastrointestinal hormones have major influences on the motility, secretion, digestion, and absorption in the gut. They modify bile flow, the secretion of pancreatic islet hormones, and acinar secretion. They affect the circulation: tonicity of vascular walls, blood pressure, and cardiac output. The mechanisms by which these hormones act differ significantly; hence, some phylogenetic considerations are helpful in understanding the development of their regulatory functions.

Phylogenetic Considerations

The following chronologic sequence in evolution is generally accepted: single cells → multiple cells → specialization in cell function → organs with special functions. With the development of specialty functions, specific cell

Table 14–1. HORMONE RELEASING SITES*
Location of Gut-pancreatic-CNS Hormones in Endocrine Cells and/or Nerve Fibers

	Endocrine Cells†			Nerve Fibers		
	GI	Pancreas	Secretion‡ Granules	CNS	GI	Pancreas
Polypeptide Hormones						
ACTH	G	+	300	+	+	+
Bombesin	P(D₁)	−	120	+	+	−
Cholecystokinin	I	A	250	+	+	+
Endorphin	G?	A	300	+	+	+
Enkephalin	G?	A	300	+	+	+
Enteroglucagon	L(EG)	A	400	+	−	−
Gastrin	G	−	300	+	+	+
GIP	K	A	350	−	−	−
Glucagon	A	A	250	+	−	−
Insulin	−	B	−	+	−	−
Motilin	EC₂	−	350	+	−	−
Neurotensin	N	−	300	+	−	−
Pancreatic Polypeptide	PP(D₂)	PP(D₂)	180	−	+	−
Secretin	S	−	200	−	−	−
Substance P	EC₁	−	300	+	+	+
Somatostatin	D	D	350	+	+	+
TRH	+	+	−	+	−	−
VIP	H	D₁	160	+	+	+
Amines						
Acetylcholine	−	−	−	+	+	+
Dopamine	ECL; G?; S?	−	200	+	+	+
Histamine	ECL; Mast	−	450	+	+	+
Norepinephrine	−	D₁; B; A	−	+	+	+
Serotonin	EC₁; Mast	B₁; A	300	+	+	+

*From Grube, D., and Forssmann, W. G.: Morphology and function of the entero-endocrine cells. *Horm. Metab. Res. 11*:589–606, 1979.
†A = alpha cells; B = beta cells; D= delta cells; G = G cells; H = H cells; I = I cells; K = K cells; L = L cells; N = N cells; P = P cells; S = S cells; EC = enterochromaffin cells; PP = pancreatic polypeptide; TRH = thyrotropin releasing hormone.
‡Size in nm.
CNS = Central nervous system.
GI = Gastrointestinal system.

types have evolved. Compounds are produced which influence the type, speed, and net amount of cell generation, growth, and survival. The actions are diverse: some cause inhibition, others, stimulation. Some exert their action entirely in the cell in which they were synthesized; others leave the cells that generated them, diffuse into intercellular spaces, and influence neighboring cells. With progression of phylogenetic changes, special cells have evolved that produce and release a chemical that transmits a unique message to other cells. These cells are responsive to messages transmitted through high molecular weight protein (most often in the plasma membrane) that can bind this messenger but reject most others. The messenger is considered a *hormone*. When it binds to its specific *receptor* in nearby cells and regulates some of their actions, the hormone is said to have a *paracrine* function.

When the hormone is released by endocrine cells in the gut mucosa, some of it may trickle into the lumen and have significant actions even several centimeters away *(exocrine function)*. When the hormone that is released into the extracellular space is absorbed into the circulation and binds to its receptors at distant sites in sufficient amounts to exert certain actions, it is regarded as having an *endocrine* function.

With the evolution of the larger animal, such as the human, it is necessary to have hormone available to exert appropriate local action on different parts of the gut. Although the total number of hormone-producing cells is considerable, the individual cells are scattered throughout the gut mucosa. Such cells compose the "diffuse endocrine system" of the gut, which collectively is one of the largest endocrine organs in the body (Pearse and Takor, 1979). This diffuseness is probably attributable to their needed paracrine action.

Amine Precursor Uptake and Decarboxylation Cells

The special cells composing the diffuse endocrine system are amine precursor uptake and decarboxylation (APUD) cells. Many of their characteristics are given below.

1. Amine precursor uptake and decarboxylation cells synthesize and secrete most of the hormones in the body, except for the steroids (Pearse and Polak, 1978). They take up amino acids and modify them so that the hormones secreted are amino acid derivations, chiefly amines or peptides (e.g., gut endocrine cells [EC_1]). They can take up 5-hydroxytryptophan and convert it to 5-hydroxytryptamine [serotonin].

2. APUD cells consist of special neurons as well as endocrine cells. These nerve cells and endocrine cells share many characteristics. Pearse and Takor (1979) regarded all of the APUD endocrine cells of the gut as having so many activities like those of nerve cells that they designated them as constituting part of the "diffuse neuroendocrine system." Pearse and associates (1977) consider cell peptide hormones as modified neurotransmitters. Fujita designates APUD endocrine cells as "paraneurons" (Fujita and Kobayashi, 1978).

3. APUD cells are derived from ectoblasts; those in the gut and pancreas originate from the entoderm, but most of the others are of ectodermal origin (Dockray, 1979).

4. APUD endocrine cells are enterochromaffin, argentaffin, or argyrophil clear cells (Pearse and Polak, 1978). They have a fluorogenic amine content.

5. Many of the APUD endocrine cells contain dopamine, serotonin, and histamine as well as a peptide hormone (Owman et al., 1973). These hormones tend to be released together (Fujita and Kobayashi, 1978).

6. APUD hormone binds to its receptor (in most instances in plasma membrane) → acts on its effectors → modifies messenger action → increases or decreases functions such as proteogenesis or glycogenesis.

Whereas some of the endocrine cells secrete enough hormone to enter the plasma to be transported to other tissues of the body in sufficient concentration to produce an *endocrine* action, in other instances little hormone is bound to distant receptors, because the receptors are too few and/or the available hormone too little to bind them so that only a *paracrine* action may result.

Integration of Hormone and Nervous System Actions in the Gut

Integration of actions among different cells is important and this is accomplished through neural and endocrine cells. Both the central nervous system (CNS) and the peripheral nervous system, especially the autonomic nervous system, are essential to these integrative activities. Since the role of the autonomic nervous system is now recognized to be extremely important, a brief review of some of these is now presented.

Nerves of the Gut: Anatomic and Physiologic Considerations

The nerves inside the gut are designated as intrinsic and those outside as extrinsic. The efferent nerve fibers of the gut consist of somatic nerves and the autonomic nervous system. The latter consists of the sympathetic, parasympathetic, and intramural nervous systems of the gut. The somatic nerves are composed of axons of the lower motor neurons, which innervate the pharynx, esophagus, and external anal sphincter. The autonomic component includes axons of preganglionic neurons, cell bodies and axons of the postganglionic neurons, and other intramural neurons and their processes.

The intrinsic nervous system comprises intramural extensions of extrinsic nerves into the gut wall and cell bodies and processes of the intramural neurons (Fig. 14–1). The gut wall has two major nerve plexuses: the myenteric plexus (Auerbach's), located between the longitudinal and circular muscles of the gut, and the submucosal plexus (Meissner's), which is in the submucosal layer. The three smaller plexuses are the subserosal, deep myenteric, and mucosal plexuses. These plexuses, especially Auerbach's and Meissner's, contain the ganglia for the enteric (intramural) nervous system. This enteric nervous system is influenced by intrinsic branches of the sympathetic and parasympathetic nervous systems, but few of its activities are affected by the extrinsic nerves.

The enteric nervous system has been regarded as "the brain of the gut." The efferent intramural neurons are distributed to their effector cells: smooth muscle cells, secretory cells, absorptive cells, or endocrine cells. The axons en route to the target cells branch and rebranch, and as they come in contact with the target cells, have small expansions, designated *varicosities,* that contain vesicles of neurotransmitters and make synaptic contact with effector cells. The vesicles are of two types (Fig. 14–2): (1) agranular vesicles, about 40 nm in diameter and thought to contain acetylcholine; and (2) large granular vesicles, about 125 nm in diameter, with a central dense core approximately 60 nm, that contain aminergic and

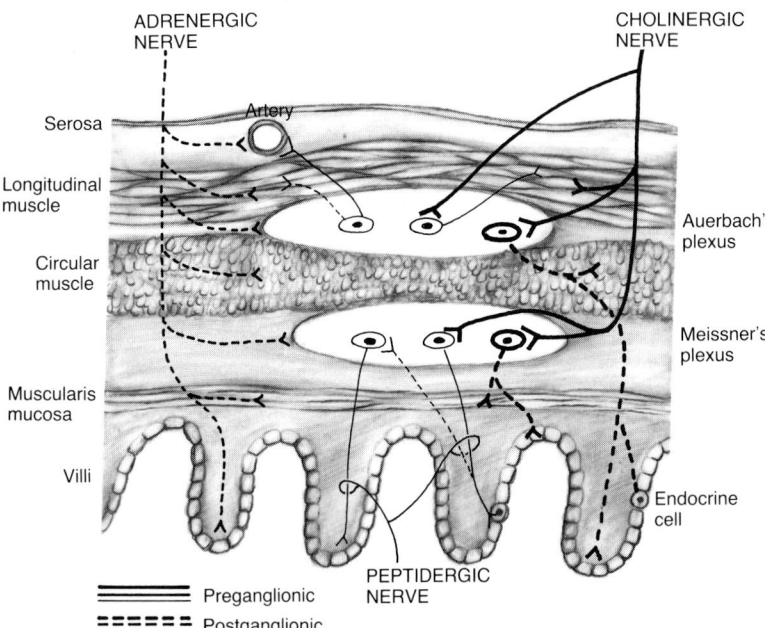

Figure 14–1. The enteric nervous system.

peptidergic transmitters (without cholinergic or adrenergic activity).

Sympathetic Nervous System

The sympathetic nervous system consists of vertebral ganglia, the sympathetic chains, and the prevertebral ganglia, as well as their connections with the central nervous system, and peripheral nerves to the effector cells. The prevertebral ganglia include the celiac, superior mesenteric, and inferior mesenteric ganglia. They provide the postganglionic adrenergic innervation to the gut, liver, gallbladder, and pancreas (Fig. 14–3). The nerves entering the liver and pancreas are "mixed," composed of branches from vagus and sympathetic fibers. These ganglia receive preganglionic cholinergic fibers, which pass through the sympathetic trunk and emerge from them as splanchnic nerves. The prevertebral ganglia contain mostly adrenergic neurons and a few cholinergic neurons, which provide the input from the preganglionic neurons. They also contain incoming signals through the afferent fibers from the gut and from neurons in other ganglia, chromaffin cells, and glial cells. The axons of the prevertebral ganglion cells extend to the effector organs and enter them in company with the blood vessels. The terminal axon from one cell innervates many effector cells, and each is innervated by branches from several adrenergic neurons. The terminal fibers have varicosities that are about 40 nm in diameter, with a dense central core approximately 15 nm in diameter (Fig. 14–2). The adrenergic neurons provide particularly rich innervation to Auerbach's and Meissner's plexuses, but they do not have cell bodies in these ganglia. They also provide a dense plexus in the vasculature of the gut, but do not seem to significantly impinge upon the secretory cells.

Parasympathetic Nervous System

The vagus nerve is the major parasympathetic neural connection to the gut. The vagus is a mixed nerve and carries: (1) parasympathetic preganglionic fibers arising from the visceral (dorsal) motor nucleus of the vagus; (2) somatic efferents with motor neurons in the nucleus ambiguus; and (3) afferent fibers with cell bodies in the jugular and nodose ganglia. About 80% of the fibers in the vagus are afferent. The vagus fibers are not uniformly

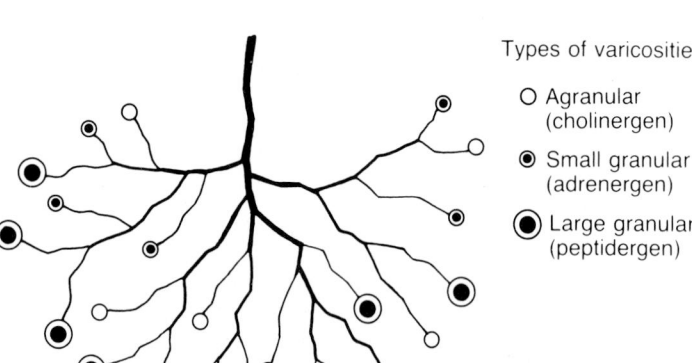

Types of varicosities

O Agranular (cholinergen)

◉ Small granular (adrenergen)

⬤ Large granular (peptidergen)

Figure 14–2. Types of varicosities at axon terminals with their vesicular content of neurotransmitters.

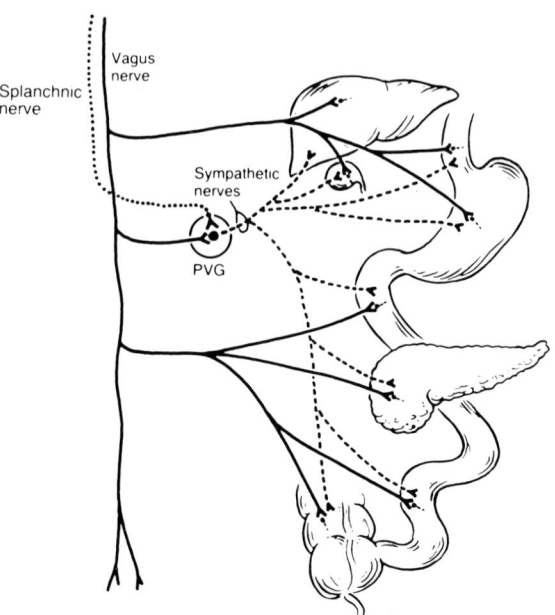

Figure 14–3. Sympathetic innervation of the gastrointestinal tract.

distributed to all the enteric neurons. Most of the preganglionic neurons and several of the postganglionic neurons in the sympathetic and parasympathetic pathways are cholinergic, but some are peptidergic.

The afferent neurons and their processes are widely distributed. Some remain intramural and form a part of the enteric nervous system, whereas others accompany the extrinsic nerves and terminate in the extrinsic autonomic ganglia or the central nervous system.

Connections with the Central Nervous System

The cell bodies of the lower motor neurons of the somatic efferent nerves and those of the preganglionic neurons of both the sympathetic and parasympathetic systems are located in the CNS and receive multiple inputs from other cells there. Afferent fibers in these nerves transmit sensory and other messages from the gut and related organs to the CNS.

AMINERGIC AND PEPTIDERGIC NERVOUS SYSTEM

Traditionally the parasympathetic nervous system has been considered to be composed of cholinergic nerve fibers, and the sympathetic nervous system of adrenergic fibers, but in recent years it has been found that some of the parasympathetic nerves also contain adrenergens and sympathetic fibers contain cholinergens. Morever, an increasing number of aminergic and peptidergic neurotransmitters have been found in the gut, including histamine, serotonin, vasoactive intestinal polypeptide (VIP), substance P, gamma-amino butyric acid (GABA), glycine, L-glutamic acid, and L-aspartic acid (Goyal, 1978; Lundberg et al., 1978; Uvnäs-Wallensten, 1978).

The vagus nerve contains VIP, substance P, enkephalin, somatostatin, gastrin, and serotonin, as well as acetylcholine and a small amount of norepinephrine. Many of the aminergic and peptidergic hormones have been shown to be released by vagal stimulation or by the administration of acetylcholine. The release of some of them is blocked by atropine (Table 14–2).

Table 14–2. NEURAL RELEASE OF GUT HORMONES

Hormone Released	Released By:	
	Acetylcholine	*Vagal Stim.*
Acetylcholine		+ (A+)
Enkephalin		+ (A−)
Epinephrine	+	+
Gastrin	+ (A+)	+ (A−)
GIP	+ (A+)	+ (A+)
Glucagon	+ (A+)	+ (A+)
Histamine	+ (A+)	+ (A+)
Insulin	+ (A+)	+ (A+)
Motilin		+ (A+)
Norepinephrine	+ (A−)	+ (A−)
Pancreatic polypeptide	+ (A+)	+ (A+)
Secretin		+
Serotonin	+ (A+)	+ (A+)
Somatostatin	−	+ (A+)
Substance P		+ (A−)
VIP	+ (A+)	+ (A−)

A+ = blocked by atropine
A− = not blocked by atropine

Innervation of the Pancreas and Liver

Parasympathetic and sympathetic nerve fibers also ramify in the pancreas and liver. Some fibers enter these organs as mixed nerves. Both types of nerves occur in the gallbladder, bile ducts, and liver lobules. Sympathetic nerve fibers richly innervate the blood vessel walls. Both nervous systems are found in the acinar and islet portions of the pancreas as well as the pancreatic ducts. The pancreatic nerves contain acetylcholine, norepinephrine, dopamine, histamine, serotonin, enkephalin, endorphin, ACTH, VIP, somatostatin, substance P, gastrin, and cholecystokinin (CCK).

Patterns of Neurosecretion

The nerve cells communicate with other cells by secretion of neurotransmitters. Many of these cells have characteristics similar to APUD endocrine cells. Different nerve cells may secrete one or more neurotransmitters. The chemical messenger may be synthesized in the body of the cell in accordance with the preprogrammed genetic pattern. The secretory product is packaged into granules in the Golgi apparatus. The granules are then transported by axoplasmic flow (Fig. 11–2) to the nerve endings, where they remain stored until they are released. Whereas many of the neurohormones are synthesized and transported throughout the length of the nerve fiber in this manner, there are others, e.g., acetylcholine, that are synthesized in the nerve terminals and stored there until released. However, in such situations, the nucleus and other portions of the cell body contribute to the synthesis. The hormone is released from the nerve endings, by reverse pinocytosis, in response to propagated action potentials. With membrane polarization Ca^{++} enters the nerve terminal. Ca^{++} exerts several actions, including activating the granule ATPase with the release of plasma membrane ATP. This promotes fusion of the neurosecretory granule membrane and the cell membrane, resulting in extrusion of the hormone-containing granule into the extracellular space. In some instances this space is a synapse, which is a very narrow cleft between the terminals of one neuron and the dendrites of another neuron. The liberated hormone binds to its specific receptor in the second neuron, initiating characteristic neural activity. In this role, the hormone serves as a *neurotransmitter*. One example of many such actions consists of the release of acetylcholine from preganglionic nerve fibers in sympathetic ganglia, where it binds to the sympathetic neurons, promoting changes in the electrical activity resulting in liberation of catecholamine from the nerve terminals of the sympathetic neurons.

Alternatively, the hormones secreted by the nerve cells may become attached to specific receptors in the plasma membranes of non-neuronal cells. Such cells may be endocrine cells, which are then stimulated to secrete another type of hormone. Or such cells may be smooth muscle cells, which are then stimulated to contract, or mucosal cells, which are then stimulated to secrete mucous, water, or electrolytes. This type of nerve action is a *neurocrine* function.

The hormone released from nerve endings may also be secreted into the circulation in sufficient quantities to be transmitted to other organs and to exert actions in them, depending on the cell type to which it becomes specifically bound. This is a *neuroendocrine* action. Whether such actions take place depends on how much is released from the nerves, how much is degraded locally, how much enters the plasma, and how much goes to organs with free specific receptor sites for the hormone.

Hormone Messenger Patterns

Traditionally a hormone has been considered to be a special chemical compound that is synthesized by special cells, secreted into extracellular space, and absorbed into the bloodstream, becomes bound to cells in other parts of the body that have receptor sites for exclusively binding the hormone, and then influences reactions in these cells (Chs. 1 and 2) (Pearse et al., 1977; Grossman, 1979). A standard proof of its hormonal status has been that comparable physiologic responses produced by it could be mimicked by infusing exogenous hormone in an amount sufficient to produce comparable plasma concentrations to what is found with the endogenously released hormone. In the light of accumulated information such a restricted characterization seems unwise. It is preferable to consider designating a chemical compound as a hormone when it manifests one or more of the functional characteristics listed in Table 14–3. Whereas certain hormones may act in only one role, there are others, such as somatostatin, that may serve several functions (Fig. 14–4).

A hormone that exerts a paracrine function can presumably exert an endocrine function provided: (1) a sufficiently large amount is released into extracellular spaces and is absorbed into the bloodstream; (2) there are cells

Table 14–3. MULTIPLE TYPES OF HORMONE FUNCTION

1. Neuroendocrine:	Hormone synthesized in nerve ending; released into extracellular space, absorbed into receptor in cells at some distant site, and affects their function.
	Example: Norepinephrine synthesized in splanchnic nerve ending, released into plasma, and acts on the heart.
2. Endocrine:	Hormone synthesized in one location; released into plasma, binds to its specific receptor in cells at some distant site, and modifies their function.
	Example: Norepinephrine synthesized in enterochromaffin cells in adrenal medulla; released into plasma and acts on heart.
3. Neurocrine:	Hormone synthesized in neurons; released from them into extracellular space, binds to its receptor in nearby cells, and affects their function.
	Example: Norepinephrine synthesized in nerve ending in heart, released there, and acts on muscle cells.
4. Neurotransmission:	Hormone synthesized in neurons, released from the nerve endings, crosses the synapse, binds to its specific receptors in another neuron, and affects its action.
	Example: Acetylcholine is released in sympathetic ganglion from preganglionic nerve fibers, crosses the synapse to bind to its receptor in the postganglionic neurons, and stimulates them to release norepinephrine.
5. Paracrine:	Hormone synthesized in endocrine cells, released from them, binds to its receptor in nearby cells, and affects their function.
	Example: Somatostatin is released from D cells of islet and acts on nearby α and β cells in the same islet.
6. Exocrine:	Hormone synthesized in endocrine cells, released into lumen of gut, and binds to its specific receptor in cells lining the gut at varying distances from the cells that secrete it. It then affects the functions of the cells to which it binds.

some distance away that have a specific receptor for the hormone; and (3) its breakdown in the plasma and in other tissues is not so large as to prevent a sufficient amount of the hormone from arriving at the distantly placed cells bearing its receptors. Moreover, all neurotransmitters are considered as hormones (Fujita and Ko-

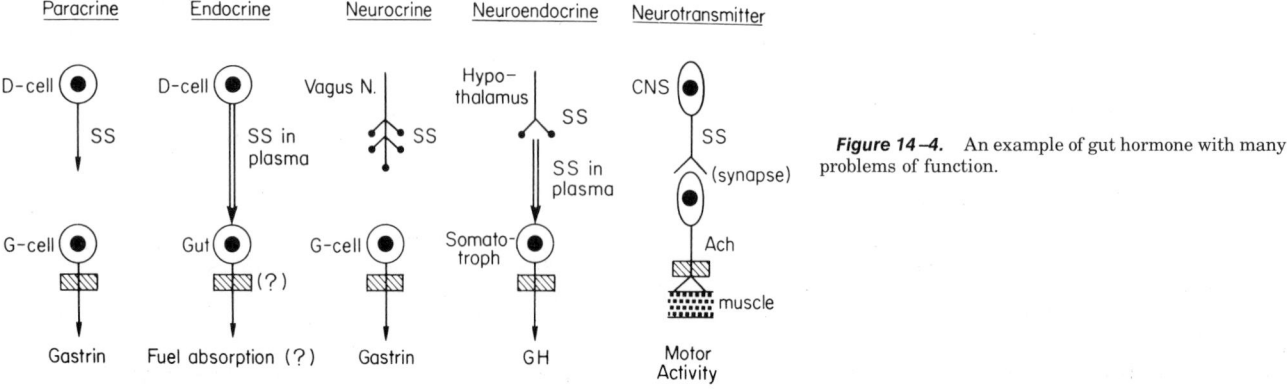

FIVE PATTERNS OF HORMONE FUNCTION FOR SOMATOSTATIN

Figure 14–4. An example of gut hormone with many problems of function.

bayashi, 1978; Pearse and Takor, 1979; Tompkins, 1975), which in most instances are either derivatives of amino acids (e.g., aminergens [Fig. 14–5] and peptidergens [Table 14–1]), or are themselves an amino acid (e.g., glycine).

Certain hormones released by endocrine cells may be taken up by select nerve endings and later released to serve, at least partially, a neurocrine or a neurotransmitter function. Information accumulated thus far suggests that many of the hormones secreted by endocrine cells and/or nerve cells in the gut exert chiefly a paracrine or neurocrine action. One reason, presumably, many of them released in the gut do not exert much action in other tissues is that they are rapidly degraded in the plasma. The half-lives in the plasma of most of them are less than 5 minutes, and in some instances are less than 1 minute.

A number of compounds listed earlier as hormones have not been completely characterized physiologically and chemically. Nevertheless, insulin is considered a hormone, although the mechanism by which it acts has not been established. The compounds listed as gut hormones (Table 14–1) are found in humans to be localized predominantly in specific cell types (Fig. 14–6). Most have been found to have actions which differ from each other.

Traditionally a hormone has been considered to be a compound that transmits a chemical message through the bloodstream, while a neurotransmitter transmits the chemical message through nerves. Since the identical chemical compound can serve either as the blood messenger or the nerve messenger, Grossman (1979) has proposed the word "chemitter" (from *chem*ical transm*itter*) to designate the entire group of APUD hormones. However, in my opinion it is preferable to continue to use the word "hormone" in its broader context with the recognition that it can be transported by different mechanisms and can act in close proximity, or distant, to its site of release.

Correlations of Hormone Functional Patterns with Phylogenetic Changes

As indicated earlier, the phylogenetic transformation from unicellular organisms to the human, with the tremendous increase in the number of cells, resulted in increased specialization of cell functions, and need for coordination of their activities throughout variable distances. The following chronologic, phylogenetic and ontogenic order of sequence of development of the organs and systems apparently resulted: (1) circulation, (2) gut, (3) nervous system, (4) endocrine glands. Presumably, the amine hormones evolved first, followed by peptide hormones and then steroid hormones. Steroids are secreted by organs derived from the mesoderm, which appeared after the ectoderm and endoderm. Steroid hormones are not generated in nerves and they exert relatively little paracrine action. Thus, their main function is endocrine. It seems likely that the following chronologic sequence in the five main functional patterns of nonsteroid hormone actions occurred: (1) paracrine, (2) endocrine, (3) neurocrine, (4) neuroendocrine, (5) neurotransmitter. With each of these five patterns of hormone distribution, different distances are involved, and several methods have been provided for controlling the site, specificity, intensity, duration and other phases of their actions. Some of the major gut hormones are considered in detail in the next sections.

GASTRIN

Gastrin is a linear polypeptide hormone isolated and synthesized by Gregory and associates in the early 1960's (Gregory, 1978).

Chemistry

Multiple molecular species of gastrin have been identified. They comprise: (1) little gastrin (17 amino acids [AA], G_{17}); (2) big gastrin (34 AA, G_{34}); (3) minigastrin (14 AA, G_{14}); (4) big big gastrin (MW $20,000\pm$); (5) component I (C-I), intermediate between G_{34} and big big gastrin; and (6) NH_2-terminal tridecapeptide fragment of G_{17} (NT_{13}). Of these, forms 1, 2, 3, and 6 have been isolated from antral mucosa or gastrinoma tissue and characterized chemically. The others have been recognized immunologically in the circulation, and material resembling them has been found in antral and gastrinoma extracts, but have not been chemically characterized. Besides these six components, there are others in the serum with some characteristics of gastrin; Rehfeld and coworkers (1975) found a total of 20: six component I's, six G_{34}'s, four G_{17}'s, and four G_{14}'s. How many are degraded products and how many exert some biologic actions like gastrin have not been determined. The COOH-terminal end is necessary for the manifestation of gastrin activity, but even a tripeptide consisting of the three last AAs at that end has as full a range of action as larger molecules but is not very potent. Most of the radioimmunoassays for gastrin are

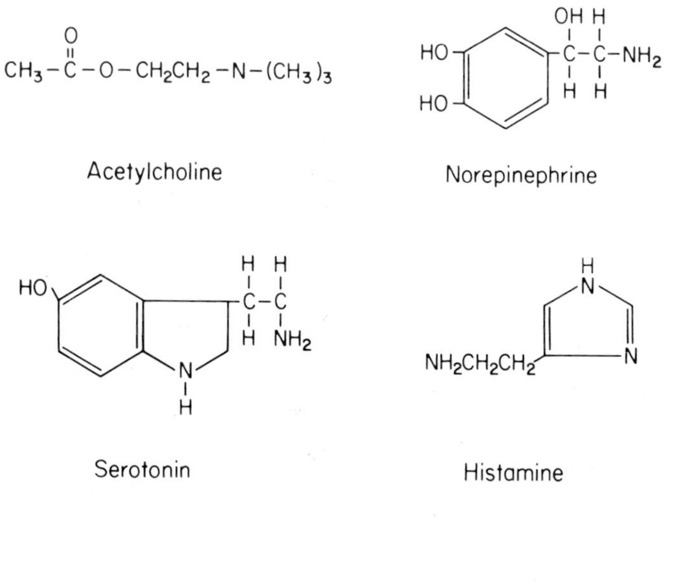

Acetylcholine

Norepinephrine

Figure 14–5. Common APUD amines serving endocrine functions in the gut.

Serotonin

Histamine

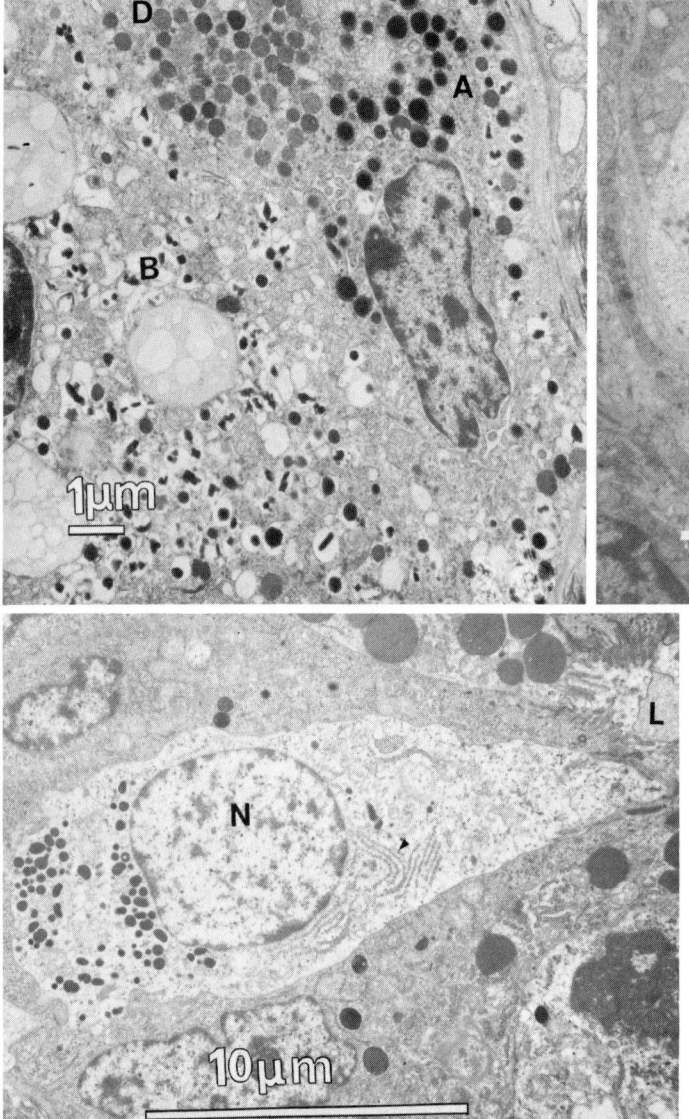

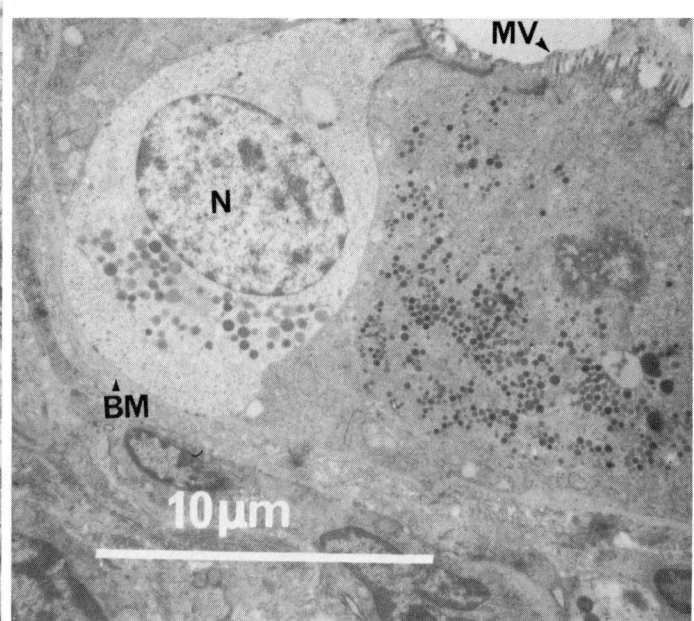

Figure 14-6. (*a*) Section of human pancreas fixed in 3% glutaraldehyde and post fixed in osmium. ×10,000.

  A = glucagon-producing cell
  B = insulin-producing cell
  D = somatostatin-producing cell

(*b*) Section of human duodenum fixed in 3% glutaraldehyde and post fixed in osmium. ×6000.

  N = nucleus
  MV = microvilli
  BM = basement membrane

(*c*) Section of human duodenum fixed in 3% glutaraldehyde and post fixed in osmium. ×6000.

  N = nucleus
  L = lumen

Characteristic intracellular vesicular granules in specific cells of the human pancreas and duodenum producing the same hormone. (Courtesy of Dr. J. M. Polak.)

conducted with antibodies produced by antigenicity induced by the COOH-terminal end. Biologic activity is not influenced by the presence or absence of the sulfate group on tyrosine (AA_{29}). It is not known whether big big gastrin is a circulation form of gastrin or whether it is an artifact. It is not taken up by immunoabsorption columns in which antibodies that bind other forms of gastrin are used.

Component I has a larger molecular weight than G_{34}, and on tryptic digestion, material the size of G_{17} is liberated. The N-terminal tridecapeptide fragment of G_{17} (NT_{13}) was isolated from antral mucosa. It occurs in sulfated and nonsulfated forms and is an inactive gastrin fragment with the N-terminal tridecapeptide sequence of G_{17}. It has also been found in serum. Gregory (1978) has postulated that component I could be the "pre-pro" form of gastrin. From this form G_{34} is presumed to be derived, and from it G_{17} and G_{14}. These reactions probably take place in the G cells.

Gastrin Secretion

Gastrin is released from peptidergic fibers in the vagus nerve. It is also released by endocrine cells in the mucosa (G cells), from which a significant amount passes into the extracellular space. Of this amount, some enters the blood and some flows to surrounding areas and into the lumen.

The factors that influence the secretion of gastrin are listed in Table 14–4. Meal eating is the major physiological stimulus to gastrin release (Fig. 14–7). Paradoxically, acetylcholine and vagal stimulation, as well as vagotomy and atropine, increase the secretion of gastrin. These observations appear valid, but depend upon several factors (Soll and Walsh, 1979). The vagus contains both peptidergic and cholinergic nerve fibers. The former contain several hormones that are released by vagal stimulation and this reaction is not blocked by atropine. Some of the hormones

Table 14–4. FACTORS AFFECTING GASTRIN SECRETION

Increase Gastrin		Decrease Gastrin	No Action
Sham feeding	Acetylcholine	Acid (gut)	Fat
Amino acids (oral)	Atropine	Hyperglycemia	Carbohydrate
Peptides (oral)	Vagal stimulation	Somatostatin	
Calcium (oral)	Vagotomy	Secretin	
Bombesin	β-Adrenergen	Glucagon	
PGE₁		GIP	
Insulin hypo-		VIP	
glycemia		Calcitonin	

Table 14–5. ACTIONS OF GASTRIN

1. Increases secretion of gastric acid and pepsin
2. Increases growth of acid-secreting gastric mucosa
3. Increases pancreatic enzyme secretion
4. Increases water and electrolyte secretion by stomach, pancreas, liver, Brunner's glands
5. Increases water and electrolyte absorption from small intestines
6. Smooth muscle:
   (a) Stimulates contraction of lower esophageal sphincter, stomach, intestine, gallbladder
   (b) Relaxes muscle of pyloric, ileocecal, and Oddi sphincters
7. Decreases absorption of glucose from jejunum
8. Increases secretion of insulin, acetylcholine, somatostatin, and pancreatic polypeptide

released from the vagus inhibit gastrin release (e.g., somatostatin and VIP). Direct electrical stimulation of the vagus releases gastrin, but this is not blocked by atropine. Topical application of acetylcholine to the pyloric mucosa releases gastrin; this reaction is partially blocked by atropine. The gastrin-releasing action of sham feeding or of insulin-induced hypoglycemia is blocked by high doses of atropine but enhanced by low doses (Impicciatore et al., 1977). Vagotomy also increases food-induced gastrin release. In the presence of vagotomy, insulin hypoglycemia increases gastrin release, and in this reaction, catecholamine action is presumed to play some role. Isoproterenol or epinephrine together with phenoxybenzamine increases gastrin, but epinephrine together with propranolol does not (Hayes et al., 1975). The physiologic role of some of these factors that alter gastrin secretion when given in pharmacologic doses is not yet clear.

Distribution and Degradation

Gastrin is found in G cells located chiefly in the midportion of the pyloric glands in the antral part of the stomach. A few G cells are in the crypts of the proximal duodenum. The nerve fibers of the vagus supplying the stomach and duodenum also contain gastrin. Whereas gastrin has been considered to be present in the central nervous system, the question has arisen whether the hormone reacting with the gastrin antibody is gastrin, or CCK, or some other compound. The presence of gastrin in the normal pancreatic islets has not been established conclusively. Little or no gastrin is found in liver, kidney, muscle, or fat.

As discussed earlier, 95% of the gastrin found in extracts of antrum and gastrinoma is in the form of G_{17}. The next most abundant gastrin compound in these tissues is G_{34}. Although a substantially lesser amount is found in tissue, more G_{34} is found in plasma because its half-life is several times longer than that of G_{17}

Actions

Several of the actions of gastrin are listed in Table 14–5. Some resemble those of CCK. For example, the secretion of pancreatic enzymes and contraction of the gallbladder stimulated by gastrin is attributed to the pentapeptide COOH-terminal amino acid identical with CCK. In pharmacologic doses gastrin stimulates insulin secretion. It also increases the secretion of serotonin and calcitonin. Gastrin increases serum Ca^{++}. It may cause hyperplasia of the cells of the oxyntic glands, as well as those of the mucosa of the duodenum and colon, but not those in the antrum (Johnson, 1977).

The primary physiologic actions are to stimulate: (1) gastric acid secretion, (2) growth of acid-secreting gastric mucosa, and (3) secretion of pepsin.

Gastric Acid Secretion

Gastrin is the peptide hormone most clearly identified as a stimulant of gastric acid secretion, and of the different forms of gastrin, G_{17} is the most potent. Gastrin is,

Figure 14–7.   Increase of "little gastrin" (G-17) and "big gastrin" (G-34) after meal ingestion. (From Modigliani, R., Mary, J.-Y., and Bernier, J.-J.: Effects of synthetic human gastrin I on movements of water, electrolytes, and glucose across the human small intestine. *Gastroenterology* 71:971, 1976.)

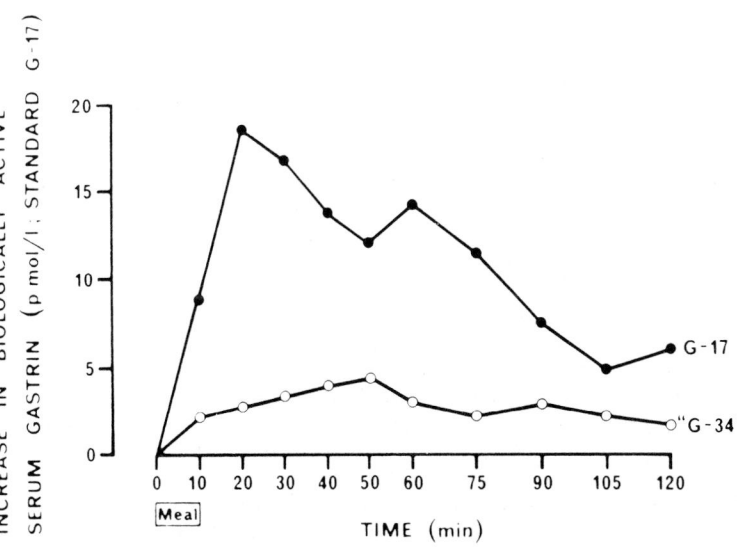

however, one of many factors that contribute to the control of the net amount of acid secreted. For example, the following play some role (Bloom and Polak, 1978): nutrients, pH, VIP, enkephalin, bombesin, neurotensin, somatostatin, histamine, serotonin, prostaglandins, acetylcholine, catecholamine, gastrin, CCK, GIP, and secretin. Gastrin, histamine, and acetylcholine are, however, the major factors ordinarily affecting gastric acid secretion.

Phases of Acid Secretion In Vivo

Some acid is secreted during the fasting state, but the amount is relatively small compared with that resulting from stimulation associated with anticipation or ingestion of food. Three phases have been arbitrarily assigned. They include: cephalic, gastric, and intestinal phases.

Cephalic Phase. This increase in HCl acid release is related to the sight, smell, and taste of food. It seems to be mediated by efferent fibers in the stomach that are in the vagus nerves. With sham feeding, there is direct cholinergic stimulation of the parietal cells as well as increased release of gastrin from the G cells. Apparently one or more substances also are released from the vagus that inhibit acid secretion. The role of the cephalic phase is important; for example, the increased acid response to sham feeding is associated with greater increases in serum gastrin than are found by direct introduction of food into the stomach.

Gastric Phase. When food enters the stomach, acid secretion is stimulated especially by two factors: (1) distention of the stomach, and (2) chemical stimulation of gastrin release. Since distention does not increase gastric concentration, it apparently results from a pyloro-oxyntic reflex. The effects of fundic distention are inhibited by atropine or by vagotomy.

Various food components stimulate gastric acid secretion, especially amino acids and partially digested protein, because they induce increased release of gastrin. Phenylalanine and tryptophan are especially potent.

Intestinal Phase. Food substances entering the intestine may cause either stimulation or inhibition of gastric secretion. Gastrin is present in the proximal duodenum in relatively high concentration, but it has not been established whether gastrin is released from the duodenum by a normal meal. Introduction of fat into the intestines markedly inhibits gastric acid secretion, in part owing to increased release of GIP and CCK. Hypertonic glucose inhibits acid secretion, whether introduced intravenously, orally, or intraduodenally. Acidification of the duodenum inhibits acid secretion. This action may be related in small part to increased release of secretin but has been attributed mostly to the stimulation of an inhibitory neural reflex and possibly to the release of somatostatin which suppresses gastrin secretion.

Role of Histamine in Stimulating Gastric Acid Secretion

Even before gastrin was discovered, histamine was known to be a potent stimulus of acid secretion. Histamine is found in ECL cells in close proximity to the parietal cells. This affords a good opportunity to exert a paracrine action. Although it may have an endocrine function, it is very quickly inactivated both locally, in the plasma, and especially in the liver, therefore making it an unlikely candidate for acting on distant cells. In recent years, it was observed that certain common histamine antagonists

(for example, mepyramine) blocked histamine-induced contraction of the gut but did not block histamine-induced gastric acid secretion. However, three other compounds were discovered (burimamide, metiamide, and cimetidine) that strongly inhibited histamine-stimulated acid release, but did not block the histamine effect on gut contraction. These inhibitors are similar in structure to histamine (Burland and Mills, 1978). Thus they are thought to block histamine action by competition for binding to the H_2 receptors. These and other observations prompted the conclusion that there are two different types of receptors for histamine. The receptor involving acid secretion has been designated as the H_2 receptor and the other type as H_1.

There are certain suggestions that histamine can act through mechanisms additional to those mediated through the H_1 or H_2 receptors. In some instances the action is considered to be muscarinic and hence can be blocked by atropine. In others, it is considered to be beta adrenergic in type and thus can be blocked by propranolol. Stimulation of acid secretion by vagal stimulation or by administration of a cholinergic compound can largely be inhibited by cimetidine. Thus, some investigators (Code, 1977) have suggested that histamine is essential for the acid-secreting action of the parietal cells.

Interrelationships of Major Factors Influencing Acid Secretion

That gastrin secretion is complexly regulated is indicated by blockade by cimetidine, which inhibits chiefly histamine release, and atropine, which suppresses mostly acetylcholine action. The action of acetylcholine is potentiated by histamine and vice versa. Vagotomy decreases the acid secretory response to histamine, gastrin, and vagally mediated stimuli. Two major hypotheses to explain these phenomena have been proposed. It has been postulated that the parietal cell has receptors only for histamine, and both gastrin and acetylcholine promote the release of histamine. Although this model explains the inhibition of gastrin and acetylcholine action by cimetidine, it does not explain the inhibitory action of atropine on gastrin action. Moreover, concentrations of cimetidine that block the response to histamine do not interfere with stimulation by cholinergens and only partially inhibit stimulation by gastrin. Consequently, the other hypothesis states that the parietal cell has specific separate receptors for histamine, gastrin, and cholinergens and that these compounds exert synergistic interactions on these cells. This conjecture is supported by studies of response of isolated parietal cells.

Clinical Disorders Associated with Abnormal Secretion of Gastrin

Excessive secretion of gastrin as a primary event in patients with benign peptic ulcer has not been clearly established. Some patients with duodenal ulcer have an increased number of parietal cells and show inordinate secretion of gastrin in response to a meal in association with a decreased suppressibility of gastrin release by acid (Burland and Milis, 1978). In most of these patients cimetidine is effective in suppressing excessive gastric acid production.

Gastritis may be associated with decreased gastric acid secretion which may lead to secondary hypergastrinemia and hyperplasia of the G cells in the antrum. This condition is especially pronounced in patients with pernicious anemia, in whom the gastrin-producing cells are spared. Impaired gastric emptying can also cause hypergastrinemia that reverts to normal with release of the obstruction. Excessive gastrin levels also result when the antrum is isolated from the flow of acid, as is sometimes found with Billroth II gastric resection.

Hypergastrinemia is most profound with gastrin-producing tumors, with clinical manifestation first described by Zollinger and Ellison — the ZE syndrome (ZES) (McGuigan, 1978). The cardinal features of this syndrome are: (1) excessive gastric acid secretion; (2) severe and recalcitrant upper gastrointestinal ulcerative disease; and (3) pancreatic islet cell tumors. The tumor usually is in the pancreas, but is occasionally in the duodenal wall. Ulcers in the gastrointestines occur in approximately 90% of patients. One or more ulcers may be located in the proximal duodenum, or it may consist of a single ulcer located in the distal duodenum and/or jejunum. There may be several ulcers, in close proximity or scattered in different areas of the duodenum and jejunum. They tend to be very resistant to treatment.

Diarrhea is frequently encountered (30 to 81% of cases) (Bonfils and Bernades, 1974). It may appear as acute bouts with long periods of remission, or there may be massive, persistent watery diarrhea, similar to that experienced by patients with cholera. Steatorrhea commonly occurs. It is due to the excessive acid which cannot be neutralized in the upper small intestine. The low pH causes impairment of lipase activity leading to incomplete hydrolysis of triglyceride. The increased acidification in the duodenum also evokes the release of secretin, which in turn stimulates pancreatic secretion of water and bicarbonate from the pancreatic acinar cells. These cells also may eventually become hyperplastic.

Approximately 60 % of the gastrinomas become malignant. The chronic hypergastrinemia causes hyperplasia of both the parietal and chief cells, with the changes most prominent in the former. Excessive amounts of acid and pepsin are secreted, leading to ulceration.

Although the diagnosis of ZES is very likely when the rates of gastric acid secretion are markedly increased and accompanied by other characteristic features of this syndrome, there are some patients who do not have the typical picture, and further tests are needed. There is an overlap in the rates of basal gastric acid secretion among normals and patients with benign duodenal ulcer or ZES. Frequently they can be distinguished by comparison of the gastric acid secretion in the basal state with that following maximal stimulation produced by either histamine, betazole, or pentagastrin (preferable). These compounds usually do not increase proportionately the rate of acid output in patients with ZES as they do in the other two groups of subjects.

In patients with ZES, the basal gastric acid is usually greater than 60% of what is found after the use of one of the stimulants. A much more satisfactory test is measurement of plasma levels of gastrin. Most of the gastrin extracted from gastrinoma is G_{17}, but the major form in the plasma is G_{34}. Fasting plasma gastrin in normals and patients with ordinary duodenal ulcer average approximately 60 pg/ml (upper limit normal 150 pg/ml). Patients with gastrinoma almost always have >150 pg and not uncommonly >1000 pg/ml. Gastrin level alone will not establish the diagnosis, because patients with pernicious anemia have comparable elevations, but their gastric pH does not drop below 6 even with maximal gastrin stimulation. Similarly, patients with other varieties of gastric atrophy, chronic gastritis, and reduced or absent gastric acid secretion also are likely to have high gastrin levels, provided there are adequate numbers of G cells. Hypergastrinemia occurs also with severe renal disease. Occasionally it is difficult to distinguish patients with gastrinoma from those with antral G cell hyperplasia and common duodenal ulcer. A provocative test is often helpful. Three of these have been used: (1) secretin infusion, (2) a test meal, and (3) a calcium infusion. Of these, the secretin test seems to be the most discriminant. One or two units of secretin (equivalent to 4 to 8 U Boot's secretin) per kilogram is injected intravenously throughout 30 seconds. Serum samples are taken at 5-minute intervals before secretin and for 30 minutes thereafter. In the subjects with ZES, gastrin levels increase usually by >400 pg/ml.

The standard meal test consists of ingestion of one slice of bread, 200 ml of milk, one boiled egg, and 50 g of cheese. Serum samples for gastrin are obtained 15 minutes before and at 15-minute intervals throughout 90 minutes after eating. The highest serum gastrin concentration in ZES subjects usually does not exceed 150% of fasting serum gastrin, whereas those with antral G cell hyperplasia show an increase >150%. Patients with the common duodenal ulcer have intermediate responses.

Treatment of the ZES syndrome usually involves total gastrectomy and removal of tumors where possible. These procedures relieve the symptoms due to gastric hypersecretion. Cimetidine (200 to 300 mg four times daily) has been shown to alleviate the ulcer symptoms by blocking acid secretion. As yet experience is inadequate to determine whether this drug will replace gastrectomy. Streptozotocin treatment of the gastrinoma has been successful in some patients. This drug is usually restricted to patients who have malignant gastrinomas with proven metastases.

ZES Associated with Islet Cell Hyperplasia (Nesidioblastosis)

In a few patients with ZES, general hyperplasia of the pancreatic islets has been found without palpable tumor. It is possible that in these people one or more microadenomata are also present. The hyperplastic islet tissue has not been shown to contain or to release gastrin. The symptoms and complications in these patients are the same as those in patients with ZES associated with adenoma or carcinoma of the islet. Treatment usually involves total gastrectomy; in some instances resection of a large portion of the pancreas causes significant improvement.

Parathyroid Hormone Changes with Peptic Ulcer Disease or with Gastrinoma

There is an increased incidence of peptic ulcers in patients with hyperparathyroidism in whom high levels of plasma gastrin and excess gastric acid have been reported. Following parathyroidectomy some subjects show a substantial decrease in gastric acidity. Patients with hyperparathyroidism who develop peptic ulcer disease may also harbor a gastrinoma, especially if there is an elevation of the fasting serum gastrin concentration. In these persons, it may be helpful to perform a secretin provocative test. Cecchettin and associates (1978) found elevated levels of parathyroid hormone (PTH), calcitonin (CT), and gastrin in 31 patients thought to have gastrinoma. They considered it likely that increased gastrin stimulated increased CT, resulting in decreased serum calcium and a compensatory increase in PTH.

Relationship Between ZES and Multiple Endocrine Adenomatosis

In this group of disorders, hyperplasia and/or tumors of the parathyroids, pancreatic islets, and pituitary are most frequently encountered. In addition, thyroid nodules, carcinoid tumors, and hyperplasia of the adrenal cortices have often been observed in family members. This association has been denoted multiple endocrine adenomatosis (MEA) Type I. Hyperparathyroidism is found in 87% of patients with MEA syndrome, and ZES occurs in approximately 50% of these patients. Fasting serum gastrin levels should be measured and the provocative secretin test should be performed in family members suspected of having this disorder.

CHOLECYSTOKININ

One of the first observed actions of this hormone was its stimulating effect on gallbladder contraction and bile flow; hence the name "cholecystokinin" (CCK) (Ivy and Oldberg, 1928). Subsequently, an intestinal extract was also found to enhance the secretion of pancreatic enzymes and the factor was called "pancreozymin" (Harper and Raper, 1943). Eventually cholecystokinin and pancreozymin were shown to be identical hormone (Jorpes, 1968).

Chemistry

Cholecystokinin is heterogeneous, occurring in different portions of the body in multiple chain lengths of amino acids (Rehfeld, 1978). The predominant form is a 33-AA–containing peptide (CCK_{33}). In addition to the CCK_{33}, the following have been observed: Peptides larger than CCK_{33}, a component presumed to be the COOH-terminal dodecapeptide of CCK_{33} (CCK_{12}), the COOH-terminal octapeptide CCK_{33} (CCK_8), and each half of CCK_8 (Asp-Tyr-$\overset{|}{SO_3H}$

Met-Gly-Trp-Met-Asp-Phe-NH_2). The COOH-terminal end is required for biologic activity, but the full range of actions is manifested by CCK_8. No action is observed if the carboxyterminal amide or the sulfate group attached to the tyrosyl radical is absent. Since the COOH-terminal end of gastrin is also required for its biologic activity, these two hormones share several actions, but vary in their potency. Whether or not they compete for the same binding sites has not been established.

Secretion

Because CCK compounds are rapidly degraded and because immunoassay procedures have not been sufficiently sensitive or specific, evaluation of levels in body fluids and tissues has been difficult. In many of the immunoassays there has been immunologic cross-reactivity between gastrin and CCK, precluding their accurate measurement.

On the basis of bioassay procedures and existing CCK immunoassays, the following factors have been found to increase CCK secretion (Go, 1978; Rayford et al, 1976a): triglyceride, protein, peptides, amino acids (Phe, Met, Val, and Trp have been the most active), Mg^{++}, Ca^{++}, bombesin, and acid. Somatostatin inhibits CCK secretion.

Distribution and Degradation

Rehfeld (1978) found that most of CCK is either in the CNS or in the small intestine. The intestinal wall of the duodenum and jejunum has amounts similar to the high concentrations in the cerebral cortex.

Histochemical studies have demonstrated that CCK cells (I cells) are scattered among mucosal cells of the crypts and villi of the duodenum and jejunum (Buffa et al, 1976; Polak et al, 1975). Virtually no CCK cells were observed in stomach, pancreas, terminal ileum, or colon. Grube and associates (1978) have reported that rat pancreatic α cells contained immunoreactive CCK; others failed to observe this.

CCK is rapidly degraded. The half-life in plasma is less than 3 minutes (Rayford et al., 1976a).

Actions

As indicated in Table 14–6 most of the actions of CCK are in the pancreas, the biliary system, and the gut. It is the most potent hormone in stimulating the pancreas to release digestive enzymes; this action tends to be augmented by both secretin and gastrin. CCK causes strong contractions of the gallbladder and relaxation of the sphincter of Oddi, thereby increasing bile flow into the small intestine; these actions are augmented by gastrin and secretin. CCK mildly stimulates gastric acid release in the basal state, but inhibits gastrin-stimulated secretion of acid and pepsin. It is presumed to have enough similarity in structure to gastrin to have a mild gastrin effect, but by competing with gastrin for binding its receptor, or in some other way, it inhibits gastrin action. It increases the contraction of the antrum (Morgan et al., 1978) and the pyloric sphincter and decreases gastric emptying.

CCK enhances the motility of the small intestine (Stewart and Burks, 1977), which has been attributed to release of acetylcholine. The response of motility to CCK_8 is considered to be mediated by a neurogenic mechanism interacting with non-nicotinic receptors on postganglionic neural elements; this action is blocked by atropine. CCK increases the secretion of Brunner's gland and decreases water and electrolyte absorption from the gut. It also decreases lower esophageal sphincter pressure.

In pharmacologic doses CCK increases insulin secretion (Schatz et al., 1974). We have found that CCK_{33} increases insulin release in dogs comparably to an equimolar amount of CCK_8. Unlike the situation with GIP, CCK releases in-

---

Table 14–6. ACTIONS OF CHOLECYSTOKININ

Pancreas — increases:
    a. Secretion of enzymes, water, and electrolytes into small intestines
    b. Secretion of insulin, glucagon, and pancreatic polypeptide
    c. Acinar growth
    d. cGMP
Biliary system — increases:
    a. Gallbladder contraction and relaxation of sphincter of Oddi, causing increased bile flow to small intestine
    b. Biliary water and bicarbonate
Stomach:
    a. Inhibits gastrin-stimulated secretion of acid and pepsin; increases their basal secretion
    b. Increases contractions of antrum and of pylorus sphincter; decreases gastric emptying
Small intestine:
    a. Increases secretion from Brunner's glands
    b. Decreases water and electrolyte absorption
    c. Increases motility
    d. Increases acetylcholine release
Esophagus:
    a. Decreases lower esophagus sphincter pressure
Appetite and food intake:
    a. Decreases
Increases secretion of GH and calcitonin
Increases blood flow in superior mesenteric artery, and may decrease systemic blood pressure

sulin even with fasting levels of plasma glucose. However, glucose augments CCK_8-induced secretion. The insulin-releasing activity of CCK_8 is brief; for example, despite its continuous infusion in dogs for 30 minutes the plasma insulin levels returned to baseline levels within about 10 minutes (Frame et al., 1976). Its capacity to release glucagon is much slower and weaker than is its insulin-releasing activity. Using an *in vitro* islet culture, we have found that CCK_8 and GIP have about an equal insulin-releasing activity (Fujimoto et al., 1979). *In vitro* the action of CCK_8 in releasing glucagon is also very weak.

In supraphysiologic doses CCK promotes the secretion of growth hormone and calcitonin. Whereas there have been several reports that CCK decreases appetite, the mechanism has not been established. One possibility is that it acts on the appetite center in the CNS. Although the CNS has large concentrations of CCK, whether any normal physiologic effect of CCK on appetite is from hormone that originated in the gut or from CCK stores in the CNS has not been clarified. Little is known of the role of CCK localized in the CNS (Straus et al., 1977).

In pharmacologic amounts CCK has been found to increase the blood flow in the superior mesenteric artery, and it may decrease systemic blood pressure.

Status with Reference to Clinical Disorders

There is not much information on this subject, largely because radioimmunoassays for plasma CCK have not been satisfactory until recently and because the supply of CCK has been limited.

CCK levels rise with acidification of the duodenal contents. This is possibly the reason that CCK levels are high in association with gastrinoma. There are suggestions that there may be abnormalities in the timing of the release of CCK with food ingestion in subjects with duodenal ulcer and in those with "dumping syndrome."

Plasma levels of CCK are increased with plasma exocrine insufficiency (Harvey, 1978) accompanied by hyperplasia of the small intestinal mucosa. CCK may be decreased in patients with severe damage to the upper small intestine, such as is found with nontropical sprue. In celiac disease there is a high basal plasma level of CCK but a diminished rise in CCK in response to food.

SECRETIN

Secretin is a linear peptide released principally from the duodenum when the pH of the duodenal contents is less than 4.5. Its major action is to stimulate the pancreatic acinar cells to release bicarbonate and water, which are transported to the duodenum and change the pH from acid to alkaline, thereby facilitating the action of enzymes.

Chemistry

Secretin has a MW of 3055 and 27 AA. There are a number of similarities in the amino acid sequence among secretin, glucagon, VIP, and GIP (Fig. 14–8). Fourteen of the 27 AA of secretin occupy the same positions as in glucagon, 10 the same as in GIP, and 7 the same as in VIP. The AA between positions 5 and 13 form a helix. Two secretin-type compounds have more than 27 AA, of which conceivably one or more could constitute prosecretin. The secretin molecule must be intact to have full biologic activity; so must the N-terminal histidine. As discussed later, however, fragments of secretin manifest some secretin-type activity.

Secretion

Evaluation of factors that release secretin, the maximal amount of release, and the duration of release has depended more on bioassays than on radioimmunoassays. This is presumably due to the fact that the basal plasma levels and the increment needed to produce an effect are close to the level of sensitivity of the radioimmunoassay for secretin (Boden, 1978; Häcki et al., 1978). Most immunoassays have not shown a rise in secretin with a protein meal, despite a clearly demonstrable increase in pancreatic bicarbonate secretion in association with this meal. Moreover, when secretin is infused a clearly demonstrable increase in pancreatic secretion can be produced, whereas no change in the immunoassayable level of secretin is noted.

There is a consensus that acid in the duodenum promotes secretin secretion. The amount and duration of release are related to the amount of acidification and the length of duodenum and jejunum exposed to the acid. However, a pH of < 4.5 is required for secretin to be released. A decrease of pH to < 3.0 does not augment further the secretion of pancreatic bicarbonate. The secretion of bicarbonate seems to be correlated with the capacity to secrete gastric acid. Some investigators have reported that food increased plasma secretin and fasting decreased it (Schafmayer et al., 1978). Controversy exists as to whether a significant increase in plasma secretin is produced by the administration of fatty acids, amino acids, protein, alchohol, or glucose. Moreover, even when certain of these compounds are associated with an increase in secretin, the implications are that the associated increase in HCL reaching the duodenum is the stimulant rather than the direct effect of the food component.

Distribution and Degradation

Secretin is synthesized and secreted by S cells (Polak et al., 1971), found chiefly in the duodenum. The half-life of secretin in man is approximately 4 minutes (Kolts and McGuigan, 1977). The kidney is the major site of its degradation (40%).

Actions

Pancreas

The principal site of action of secretin is in the pancreatic acinar cells (Table 14–7). These cells have secretin recep-

---

Table 14–7.   ACTIONS OF SECRETIN

Pancreas
   Increase in secretion of H_2O, HCO_3, enzymes
   Increase in secretion of insulin; decreased secretion of glucagon
Biliary system
   Increase in contractions of gallbladder and flow of bile, H_2O, and
      electrolytes
   Increase in level of cAMP in the bile
Stomach
   Decrease in secretion of HCl, but increase in pepsin
   Decrease in gastrin
   Decrease in motility, but increase in pyloric tone
   Inhibition of gastrin-induced parietal cell hyperplasia
   Increase in mucosal thickness
Intestine
   Decrease in muscle tone and duodenal motility
   Increase in absorption of Na^+ and water
   Increase in secretion by Brunner's glands, but not much increase in
      total secretion of water and electrolytes
Other hormones
   Increase in secretion of somatostatin, pancreatic polypeptide, and
      parathyroid hormone

tors in the plasma membrane (Milutinovic et al., 1976). After secretin binds to its receptor on acinar cells, it activates adenyl cyclase, leading to a very significant increase in the secretion by the acinar cells of bicarbonate and water. This action of secretin is augmented by CCK. In turn, secretin augments the action of CCK in stimulating the release of enzymes from the pancreas. Although the intact molecule is needed for full biologic effect, varying size fragments have some activity.

Whereas both *in vitro* (Fujimoto et al., 1979) and *in vivo* secretin increases the release of insulin, the dosages required are in excess of physiologic amounts.

Status with Reference to Clinical Disorders

No secretin-producing tumors have been described. Plasma levels of secretin have been reported to be elevated with uremia, gastrinoma, and untreated diabetes.

The levels of secretin are decreased in celiac disease. In this disorder there is a decrease in the number of S cells and a decrease in the increment of plasma secretin upon duodenal acidification. With ZES there also is a subnormal increment in plasma secretin with duodenal acidification.

Two of the main clinical uses of secretin are: (1) as a test for gastrinoma (see earlier), and (2) as a test for acinar function, in which the amount of bicarbonate and water secreted are noted (Walsh, 1978).

GASTRIC INHIBITORY POLYPEPTIDE

In 1906 Moore and coworkers observed that the duodenum "supplied a chemical excitant for the internal secretion of the pancreas." This unknown factor was designated as "incretin," or "duodenin," which promoted the release of a hormone from the pancreas that would improve carbohydrate tolerance. In 1964 McIntyre and associates reported that glucose given orally stimulated much more insulin secretion and action than the same amount of glucose infused intravenously. Several years later, J. C. Brown and coworkers (1975) discovered that a partially purified extract of CCK contained gastric inhibitory polypeptide (GIP). Its main actions consisted of: (1) inhibition of gastric acid secretion, and (2) stimulation of insulin secretion, when the plasma glucose level is more than 25 mg/dl above fasting. Accumulated data now suggest that GIP seems to fill the role of "incretin," but other gut hormones may also play some role.

Chemistry

GIP is a linear peptide with 43 AA. It has a MW of 5104. As seen in Fig. 14–6, the amino acid sequence of GIP has many similarities to that of VIP, glucagon, and secretin (Bodanszky, 1974). Most of the biologic activity seems to reside between AA 15 and 38. In extracts of human duodenal mucosa and in serum collected after glucose or fat ingestion, chromatographic separation shows two peaks of GIP immunoreactivity, one corresponding to the one with molecular weight of 5104, the other with a significantly higher molecular weight (J. C. Brown and associates, 1978). It is possible that the latter is a proGIP.

Distribution and Degradation

Most GIP is synthesized and released by K cells which are located predominantly in the midzone of the duodenal and jejunal mucosa (Polak et al., 1973; Buffa et al., 1975). In dogs, we found a half-life of GIP in plasma to be approximately 15 minutes. The kidney apparently plays a very important role in the removal and degradation of GIP (O'Dorisio et al., 1977).

Secretion

An increase in plasma GIP is produced by glucose (J. C. Brown et al., 1975; Andersen et al., 1978; Cataland et al., 1974), triglyceride (Falko et al., 1975; Pederson et al., 1975), or by a mixture of AA (Thomas et al., 1977) when administered orally; however, none of these compounds alters GIP levels when given intravenously. A mixed meal or intraduodenally administered HCl increases GIP secretion (Ebert et al., 1979; Creutzfeldt, 1979). Fructose, galactose, and cornstarch cause much less release of GIP than glucose does. The components of corn oil (fatty acids, glycerol) have little or no effect on plasma GIP levels when given orally (Williams and Biesbroeck, 1977). Oral arginine, leucine, phenylalanine, and tryptophan individually administered have no effect on GIP. Many hormones that have been administered intravenously to dogs have not altered fasting GIP levels, but several of them have been found to inhibit somewhat the glucose-induced increase in GIP (Table 14–8). In most instances the effect of the hormone is relatively small. When glucose is given intraduodenally, gastrin and CCK are found to augment the glucose-induced GIP rise (Sirinek et al., 1977).

Analysis of the available data suggests that only those factors that accumulate in the vicinity of the GIP cells exert a physiologic effect on the secretion of GIP. Moreover, accumulated information indicates that for the food components to stimulate GIP release, they must be absorbed by the intestinal mucosa.

Actions

As indicated in Table 14–9, GIP acts on several different tissues. The biologically significant actions are: (1) increase in insulin secretion, and (2) exertion of an enterogastrone action, namely, inhibition of gastric secretion and motility. GIP in physiologic amounts does not stimulate insulin release except in the presence of plasma glucose values > 25 mg/dl above normal fasting levels (Andersen et al., 1978; Pederson and Brown, 1978; Fujimoto et al., 1978) or in the presence of certain amino acid mixtures. Oral glucose in a small dose (0.25 g/kg) does not alter fasting GIP levels despite the fact that a significant increase in insulin is produced (Pederson, et al., 1975). Thus the concentration of glucose necessary to stimulate B cell secretion of insulin is significantly less than that required to release GIP (a high plasma glucose alone will not stimulate GIP release, whereas a relatively small oral dose of glucose constitutes a high concentration in the vicinity of the K cells). Also,

Table 14–8. HORMONES AND DRUGS THAT INHIBIT GLUCOSE-INDUCED GIP RISE

Growth hormone
Diazoxide
Acetylcholine
Isoproterenol
Epinephrine
CCK$_8$
Secretion
Prednisolone
Somatostatin

Table 14-9. ACTIONS OF GIP

Stomach
↓ of gastric acid secretion (stimulated by gastrin, histamine or insulin)
↓ pepsin secretion
↓ gastric motility
↓ gastric emptying
↓ gastric secretion

Small intestines
↑ secretion of H_2O and electrolytes
↓ absorption of H_2O and electrolytes
↓ contraction

Esophagus
↓ contraction of esophageal sphincter

Pancreas
↓ insulin secretion when plasma glucose is > 25 mg/dl above fasting level; oral AA mixture → ↑ plasma GIP and IRI even with basal levels of plasma glucose. Usually no effect on plasma glucagon; increase with certain special stimulants
No effect on acinar cell function

Liver
↑ glucogenesis (physiologic?)
No effect on biliary system

Adipose tissue
↓ in glucagon-induced lipolysis (physiologic?)

certain amino acids that exert a potent effect on insulin release do not release GIP although the relative concentration exposed to the β cells is very small compared with that exposed to the K cells. Since within certain limits the larger the dose of oral glucose, the larger the GIP response and the respective insulin secretion, GIP inhibition of gastric motility and of gastric emptying may be a protective mechanism against the excessive secretion of insulin that might cause hypoglycemia.

Clinical Disorders

No proven cases of tumors producing excess GIP have been reported, but a number of other clinical disorders associated with altered plasma levels of GIP have been observed (Table 14-10). In obesity, excessive levels of GIP occur after ingestion of triglyceride (Ebert and Creutzfeldt, 1978) and glucose (May and Williams, 1978). In patients with severe adult-onset diabetes, glucose-induced GIP rises are exaggerated (J. C. Brown et al., 1975), but this is not found in mild diabetics (May and Williams, 1978). Some juvenile-onset diabetics in ketosis have had elevated basal levels of GIP but a subnormal response to glucose (Ebert and Creutzfeldt, 1978; Reynolds et al., 1979). Insulin adminstration to insulin-dependent diabetics and to nondiabetics does not decrease fasting levels of GIP. With starva-

Table 14-10. CLINICAL DISORDERS WITH ASSOCIATED ABNORMAL GIP RESPONSES

	Basal	Food-induced Glucose	Fat
Obesity	±	↑	↑
Severe diabetes	↑	↑	±
Mild diabetes	±	±	±
Juvenile-onset diabetes (ketosis)	↑	↓	
Starvation	↑	↓	
Uremia	↑	↑	
Truncal vagotomy	↑	↑	
Celiac disease	↓	↓	↓
Pancreatic insufficiency	↑	↓	↓
Cystic fibrosis		↑	↓
Duodenal ulcer	±	↑	
Rapid gastric emptying		↑	↑

tion, baseline levels are increased, but there is often a subnormal response to glucose. The elevated basal and glucose-induced increases in GIP that occur with uremia are presumed to be due to the loss of the marked GIP-degrading activity of the kidneys (O'Dorisio et al, 1977). With celiac disease, there is a decrease in the basal GIP and a subnormal response to glucose and triglyceride (Ebert and Creutzfeldt, 1978), whereas with cystic fibrosis or pancreatitis the response to glucose in appropriately increased and responses to triglyceride are lower than normal. The latter is doubtless due to the deficiency in lipase in the gut, since for triglyceride to stimulate GIP release it is necessary for it to be at least partially hydrolyzed and absorbed by the K cells (Creutzfeldt et al., 1976). With duodenal ulcer, GIP shows an inordinate rise with glucose (Cataland et al., 1977), presumed due to rapid gastric emptying. Indeed, several surgical procedures and other conditions associated with an accelerated rate of transfer of glucose from the stomach into the small intestine tend to produce an excessive initial rise in glucose, GIP, and insulin, leading to hypoglycemia.

VASOACTIVE INTESTINAL POLYPEPTIDE

This linear polypeptide, isolated from hog intestine in 1972 (Said and Mutt, 1972), has 28 AA and a molecular weight of 3326 (Rayford et al., 1976b). There are a number of similarities in structure to secretin, GIP, and glucagon (Fig. 14-8).

Secretion

Little is known about the secretion of vasoactive intestinal peptide (VIP), because it is released locally from nerve endings or from endocrine cells, and relatively small amounts seem to enter the general circulation. The half-time in plasma is ± 1 minute (Domschke et al., 1978). It is released by vagal stimulation or by depolarizing concentrations of K^+ or Ca^{++}. A number of investigators have reported that a mixed meal and other food components do not have any demonstrable effect on VIP secretion.

Distribution

VIP is widely distributed throughout the body but is found in highest concentrations in the nervous system (central, peripheral, autonomic) and the gut (Bryant et al., 1976). Large numbers of VIP-positive nerve cell bodies are found in the hypothalamus in the limbic cortex and neocortex (Fuxe et al., 1977), favoring a neuroendocrine function. VIP is found in the portal hypophyseal blood in concentrations 19 times those in the systemic blood (Said and Porter, 1979) and may lead to the release of some of the pituitary hormones.

VIP is present in all areas of the gastrointestinal tract, in somewhat larger amounts in the colon, ileum, and jejunum, and lesser amounts in the antrum, esophagus, fundus, duodenum, and pancreas. Its concentrations in the gut are many times those of secretin. It is located in the gut in special endocrine cells (H cells) and in nerve fibers. Indeed, it is by far the most abundant of all the peptide hormones found in nerves (Polak et al., 1978). VIP is in the peptidergic nerve fibers, which are especially rich in the vagus nerve and in intrinsic gut nerves (Meissner's and Auerbach's plexuses). In dog pancreas there are many immunoreactive nerve cell bodies that give off axons that heavily

```
                1    2    3    4    5    6    7    8    9   10   11   12   13   14   15   16
GLUCAGON:     HIS- SER- GLN- GLY- THR- PHE- THR- SER- ASP- TYR- SER- LYS- TYR- LEU- ASP- SER-
GIP:          TYR- ALA- GLU- GLY- THR- PHE- ILE- SER- ASP- TYR- SER- ILE- ALA- MET- ASP- LYS-
SECRETIN:     HIS- SER- ASP- GLY- THR- PHE- THR- SER- GLU- LEU- SER- ARG- LEU- ARG- ASP- SER-
VIP:          HIS- SER- ASP- ALA- VAL- PHE- THR- ASP- ASN- TYR- THR- ARG- LEU- ARG- LYS- GLN-

               17   18   19   20   21   22   23   24   25   26   27   28   29 - - - 43
GLUCAGON:     ARG- ARG- ALA- GLN- ASP- PHE- VAL- GLN- TRP- LEU- MET- ASN- THR
GIP:          ILE- ARG- GLN- GLN- ASP- PHE- VAL- ASN- TRP- LEU- LEU- ALA- GLN-  - -GLN
SECRETIN:     ALA- ARG- LEU- GLN- ARG- LEU- LEU- GLN- GLY- LEU- VAL- (NH2)
VIP:          MET- ALA- VAL- LYS- LYS- TYR- LEU- ASN- SER- ILE- LEU- ASN- (NH2)
```

Figure 14–8. Similarities in the primary structure of four peptide gut hormones (porcine) which include some of the same amino acid sequences.

innervate the muscles of the islets and the acini (Larsson et al., 1978). VIP is also found in D1 cells of the islets and nonislets, and binds to acinar cells as well.

VIP is found in significant amounts in the genitourinary organs and lung. It is concentrated particularly in the nerves of the blood vessels and smooth muscle. Degradation of VIP occurs mainly in liver.

Actions

Although a number of actions have been outlined (Table 14–11), the primary physiologic actions may be to: (1) serve as a neurotransmitter, especially in the CNS and in the peripheral autonomic nervous system; (2) relax the smooth muscles of the circulation, especially those in splanchnic, coronary, cerebral, and genitourinary regions; (3) relax the smooth muscles of the gut and genitourinary system; (4) increase the secretion of water and electrolytes from the pancreas and gut; and (5) release hormones from pancreatic islets, gut, and hypothalamus. VIP seems to increase the concentration of cAMP (Schwartz et al., 1974). Most of the actions of VIP tend to be of short duration, because it is rapidly degraded.

Clinical Disorders Involving VIP

The main clinical abnormality involving alterations in VIP secretion and action that has been described so far is that denoted the Verner-Morrison syndrome (VMS). It is characterized by severe watery diarrhea, hypokalemia, and achlorhydria (WDHA syndrome). It has also been called "pancreatic cholera."

Verner-Morrison Syndrome

Pathology. Neoplastic changes in the islets are most frequently found but the tumor may arise in other areas of the body (Said and Faloona, 1975; Bloom, 1978; Modlin et al., 1978). In a few instances there is hyperplasia of the islets and no tumor found anywhere. In about a third of the patients, despite radiographic studies, arteriography, and ultrasonography, no tumor is found.

Pancreatic Islets
Neoplasm. In approximately 60% of the patients there is a β islet cell neoplasm; the exact cell type has not been established; 50% of the neoplasms are malignant.

Islet Cell Hyperplasia, with or without Microadenoma. This is observed in about 10% of the patients.

Extrapancreatic Lesions

Neurotumor. These tumors, composed of endocrine cells and also neural elements, are found in approximately 25% of the patients with this syndrome. The neoplasm may be ganglioneuroma, ganglioblastoma, or pheochromocytoma.

Pulmonary Neoplasm. This WDHA syndrome is a rare

Table 14–11. ACTIONS OF VIP

Esophagus
  Decreases lower esophagus sphincter pressure

Stomach
  Increases adenyl cyclase activity in mucosa
  Decreases food-induced gastrin release
  Decreases gastric acid secretion and pepsin
  Decreases stomach contraction

Small intestine
  Increases adenyl cyclase activity in mucosa
  Increases secretion
  Decreases smooth muscle concentration

Colon
  Increases adenyl cyclase activity
  Increases secretion
  Decreases smooth muscle contraction

Pancreas
  Increases adenyl cyclase activity
  Increases HCO_3 and water secretion; increases enzyme secretion
  Increases secretion of insulin, glucagon, somatostatin

Liver
  Increases adenyl cyclase activity
  Increases glycogenolysis and glucogenesis
  Increases water and electrolyte secretion in biliary system; increases bile flow
  Decreases gallbladder contraction

Circulation
  Vasodilatation, hypotension, tachycardia
  Increases myocardial contraction and cardiac output
  Increases splanchnic and peripheral blood flow

Hypothalamus and pituitary
  Increases the release of growth hormone, prolactin, and LH when injected into 3rd ventricle

Adrenal
  Increases steroidogenesis (1% as potent as ACTH)

Adipose tissue
  Increases adenyl cyclase activity and lipolysis

Miscellaneous
  Decreases platelet aggregation; increases plasma Ca^{++}; decreases plasma K^+; relaxes tracheobronchial smooth muscle

occurrence in patients with primary carcinoma of the lung.

Major Hormone Changes. VIP is the hormone found in excess in most of the patients with VMS.

VIP. In more than 80% of the patients excessive levels of VIP are found in plasma and the tumor tissue; some have also had high levels of VIP in the stool water. The neurotumor tissue has larger concentrations of VIP than the tumor of the pancreatic islets. A number of the patients with islet hyperplasia also have high plasma levels of VIP and higher levels in the tissue than in the normal pancreas. In some instances both plasma and tissue levels have been found to be normal, yet in a significant number of such patients removal of a larger part of the pancreas has caused amelioration of the clinical features of VMS.

VIP has been found to be increased in patients with the short bowel syndrome. This has been attributed to the removal of part of the gut that produced a hormone that tended to inhibit VIP secretion.

Pancreatic Polypeptide (PP). This hormone has been reported to be elevated in the plasma in 70% of the patients with VMS (Modlin et al., 1978). PP has been found in large amounts in pancreatic tumors of patients with VMS, but not in the neural tumors. The PP-producing cells in the pancreas are different from the VIP-producing cells.

Prostaglandins. In 8 of 21 patients with VMS, Jaffe and Condon (1976) found very significant elevations in PGE levels of the plasma.

Pathophysiology

Many of the clinical and laboratory alterations of VMS have been reproduced in normal subjects by the infusion of VIP (Modlin et al., 1978) or of PGE (Jaffe et al., 1977). Three of the major actions of VIP are: (1) vasodilatation, (2) relaxation of the smooth muscle of the gut, and (3) secretion of water and electrolytes into the gut. The last of these changes produces hypovolemia, and with vasodilatation, causes hypotension. The enormous secretion of water and electrolytes into the gut accounts for the very voluminous and watery bowel movement. The achlorhydria or hypochlorhydria is the result of the marked inhibitory actions of VIP on gastric secretion. The hyperglycemia is due to heightened glycogenolysis and increased hepatic glucogenesis.

Jaffe (1978) has given special attention to correlations of prostaglandin levels and diarrhea. PGE_2 and $PGF_2\alpha$ cause diarrhea by increasing contractions of the intestinal smooth muscle and enhancing intestinal secretion of water and electrolytes. These effects are mediated through increases of cyclic nucleotide levels. Since VIP also increases cAMP, an additive effect of these components can be visualized, but PGE changes usually correlate better with the diarrhea than do increments in PGF.

Symptoms and Signs

Plasma. In most patients with VMS the levels of VIP are high and potassium is less than 3 mEq/1. About 25% have hypercalcemia. Bicarbonate tends to be decreased, and acidosis is present. Sodium and chloride are usually normal. Plasma glucose concentrations are elevated in about half the subjects.

Stool. Patients with VMS commonly have numerous voluminous watery bowel movements, tending to several liters each day. In about half this condition persists for many months, whereas in the other half there are periodic partial remissions. The diarrhea tends to persist even with fasting, and occurs without clinically demonstrable lesions in the bowel mucosa. Dehydration is severe and hypokalemia marked, often below 3 mEq/1. Lethargy, weakness, nausea, vomiting, crampy abdominal pain, and weight loss are common. The stools appear somewhat straw-colored, with osmolality similar to that of plasma. Potassium concentration is inversely related whereas the sodium concentration is directly related to stool volume. Acidosis may develop because of bicarbonate loss. During the severe episodes of diarrhea general body flushing may be observed, appearing somewhat like that in carcinoid. In some instances there may be skin pigmentation, psychoneurosis, and hypothermia.

Several other hormonal abnormalities can produce significant diarrhea, with characteristic features listed in Table 14–12.

Kidneys. The concentrating capacity decreases, urea and creatinine increase, and the kidneys may fail from severe hypokalemic nephropathy.

Gut. Radiographic studies do not demonstrate structural abnormalities.

Gastric Contents. Hypochlorhydria or achlorhydria is seen, with little or no gastric secretions observed.

Small Intestine. Intestinal mucosa is usually normal, but sometimes the villi are atrophied.

Pancreas Exocrine Secretion. Basal and secretin-stimulated volume and bicarbonate secretion are normal.

Jaffe et al., 1977 reported a patient with clinical features of WDHA syndrome associated with a tumor in the tail of the pancreas, but assay of the tumor showed low levels of VIP, gastrin, and PGF. Pancreatic polypeptide (PP) content was much less than in the surrounding tissue, but concentrations of PGE were large in the tumor and plasma. Treatment with indomethacin ameliorated the clinical changes and decreased the plasma PGE level, and removal of the tumor abolished the clinical manifestations.

In further studies of prostaglandins in relation to endocrine diarrhea, Jaffe and Condon (1976) found hypernormal levels of PGE in plasma in 8 of 21 patients with pancreatic cholera, 18 of 19 with medullary carcinoma of the thyroid,

Table 14–12. ENDOCRINE DIARRHEAS

	Gastrinoma	Vipoma	Glucagonoma	Carcinoid	Thyroid Medullary Carcinoma
Main tumor site	Islets	Islets	Islets	Gut	Thyroid
Main hormone excess	Gastrin	VIP	Glucagon	Serotonin	Calcitonin
Skin changes	0	++++	++++	++++	0
Blood pressure	N	––	N	––	N
Diarrhea	++	+++++	++	++++	++
Stool volume >liter	+	+++++	rare	+	rare
Watery stools	+++	+++++	+	++++	++
Steatorrhea	++	0	0	+	0
Gastric acidity	+++++	––––	––	N	N
Plasma K+	N	–––	N	N	N
Plasma Ca++	N	+	N	N	
Hyperglycemia	0	++	+++++	+	0
Main drug Rx	Cimetidine	Glucosteroid	Somatostatin	Methysergide	

18 of 22 with carcinoid, and 2 of 29 with ZES. Moreover, as indicated earlier, infusion of prostaglandin in normal subjects has produced several of the features of WDHA. However, even in typical patients with tumors releasing VIP there may be synergistic action of VIP and prostaglandin. In summary, it appears that PGE plays an important role with one or more other hormones in the pathogenesis of diarrhea associated with carcinoid, pancreatic cholera, and medullary carcinoma of the thyroid.

Treatment. Initial attention must be given to replacing the depleted salt and water, and further loss may be inhibited by corticosteroid treatment (e.g., prednisolone, 20 mg or more) daily. In some patients symptoms may be abated by indomethacin. The tumor must be extirpated, if benign. Malignant lesions that are readily removable should be removed, and streptozotocin therapy may be considered (Gagel et al., 1976). When no tumor is found at operation, careful histologic studies should be conducted on frozen sections for the purpose of ascertaining whether there is general hyperplasia of the islets. In this instance, a partial pancreatectomy may be indicated.

SOMATOSTATIN

Somatostatin (SS) is a cyclic tetradecapeptide with a molecular weight of 1639. It was first isolated from hypothalamic tissue by Brazeau and coworkers in 1972. (Brazeau et al., 1978):

$$\text{H Ala Gly Cys Lys Asn Phe Phe Trp Lys Thr Phe Thr Ser Cys COOH}$$
$$1 \quad 2 \quad 3 \quad 4 \quad 5 \quad 6 \quad 7 \quad 8 \quad 9 \quad 10 \quad 11 \quad 12 \quad 13 \quad 14$$

Its designation stems from its action in causing suppression of the release of growth hormone from pituitary cells. Subsequently it has been shown to be widely distributed and to inhibit the secretion of a number of hormones and neurotransmitters.

Distribution and Degradation

In rats the highest concentrations of SS have been found in isolated pancreatic islets and in the stalk median eminence region. It is also distributed in a number of brain regions and such nerves as the vagus, sympathetic ganglia, and intrinsic nerves of several organs. It occurs in very high concentrations in the nerve fibers in the posterior pituitary and is present in nerves in the wall of the gut (Pearse et al., 1977). The vagus, some sympathetic nerves, and intrinsic nerves of the gut also contain SS. It is found in peptidergic or adrenergic nerve fibers rather than in the cholinergic nerves. However, the majority of SS in the gut is in endocrine cells resembling pancreatic D cells. It is also found in the D cells of the pancreas. McIntosh and associates (1978) observed that the concentration of SS in the gastric antrum was more than twice that in the fundus. A significant amount occurs in the proximal duodenum, although much less than in the antrum. The remainder of the gut contains smaller amounts (Yanaihara et al., 1978). Somatostatin also is found in a small number of cells in the parafollicular region of the thyroid gland (Hökfelt et al., 1975).

The D cells and the peptidergic nerve fibers containing SS are found in close proximity to other cell types, the secretion of which is inhibited by SS. Thus, as discussed later, there are indications that most of the actions of SS are of the paracrine or neurocrine nature.

The half-life in plasma in normal subjects is from 1 to 3 minutes (Sheppard et al., 1979).

Secretion

Problems have existed in assaying factors influencing secretion of SS (Schally et al., 1978). The hormone is secreted into the extracellular spaces, and some is presumed to become attached to receptors of nearby cells, the action of which it specifically influences. Within the gut, some goes into the lumen and may spread in the gut secretions to a broader local area. Other portions enter the bloodstream and are distributed throughout the body. However, it is rapidly degraded, especially by the liver. This is evident by the fact that a number of factors increase the concentration of SS in the portal vein but not in the systemic circulation. As yet its function in the circulation is unknown.

The three most important areas of SS actions seem to be in the pituitary, gut, and pancreas. Each of these structures apparently synthesizes its main supply of SS and releases it in accordance with certain needs. Ordinarily, relatively little SS seems to go from one of these sites to the other.

With perifusion of pancreas, an increase in the release of SS is produced by several amino acids, glucose, and a number of neurotransmitters (Ipp et al., 1977).

Electrical stimulation of the vagus causes a release of gastrin and SS into the antral lumen and into the gastric venous blood (Uvnäs-Wallensten et al., 1977). Gastrin also causes SS to be released by the gastric mucosa into the gastric lumen. The higher the pH of the gastric contents, the less the amount of SS released; the reverse also applies.

Intragastric administration of fat, glucose, or casein hydrolysate has been reported to cause a significant increase in the systemic level of plasma SS in the dog. Each of these food substances releases SS from the pancreas, but only glucose and the casein hydrolysate release it from the gastric antrum. Intraduodenal administration of HCl after ligation of the pylorus increases SS release from the pancreas, the antrum, and the fundus. However, when given intragastrically, HCl increased the pancreatic and antral SS but inhibited the release from the fundus (Schusdziarra et al., 1978a). Intragastric glucose increased release of this hormone more than did its introduction intraduodenally. During glucose infusion the peripheral venous levels of SS decreased, whereas after the ingestion of a low-fat, high-protein meal there was increase in SS, but this increase was reduced by the simultaneous administration of intravenous glucose (Schusdziarra et al., 1978b). Perfusion of gastric mucosa with either pentagastrin or with cAMP increases the release of SS (Barden et al., 1979). Intravenous infusion of CCK_8 or secretin increased the release of SS from the stomach and the pancreas, whereas infusion of GIP released it from the pancreas but not from the stomach.

The following seem to be important conclusions about the secretion of SS in species lower than man:

1. Most of the investigations have dealt with the secretion and actions of SS in the areas of the: (a) hypothalamus-hypophysis, (b) stomach and small intestine, and (c) pancreas.

2. It seems likely that most the SS release by any one of these three main areas acts chiefly in the area of its release, although in the case of the gut and pancreas there are many factors that release SS from the gut and from the pancreas.

3. Most of the factors that release SS from the pancreas also release insulin.

4. Whereas perfusion of the pancreas with glucose often releases SS *in vitro*, the *in vivo* infusion of glucose intravenously often decreases the release of SS from pancreas, implicating a role for gastrointestinal factors.

Actions

A large proportion of the activity of SS appears to occur in close proximity to its site of release, irrespective of whether the release is from special endocrine cells (D cells) or from nerve endings. Most of its actions fall into the categories of paracrine or neurocrine, but it also has neurotransmitter, neuroendocrine, and possibly endocrine functions (Luft et al., 1978) (Fig. 14–4). Its most dominant function is to inhibit the release of peptide or amine hormones. It also inhibits a number of actions that do not appear to be dependent on its capacity to release hormone. Since the inhibitory actions that are considered to be nondependent on hormone release seem to involve actions normally augmented by APUD hormones, it is possible that such effect could be associated with its capacity to alter in some way the actions of the APUD hormones, even under basal conditions.

In the pancreas, SS exerts potent inhibitory actions on the release of insulin and glucagon. In addition, it inhibits the secretion of bicarbonate, water, and pancreatic enzymes. It suppresses these acinar functions when stimulated by food, secretin, or CCK, but also under basal conditions. It inhibits the basal release of insulin and glucagon and their release stimulated by glucose, arginine, a standard meal, and other factors.

In the stomach, SS can be released from the nerve fibers and D cells. Numerous D cells are in close proximity to G cells and other cells that release APUD hormones. SS markedly inhibits the release of gastrin, with a consequent decrease in the secretion of gastric juice, acid, and pepsin. However, SS can act directly on the parietal and chief cells to decrease the secretion of acid and pepsin and it also decreases gastric contractions and gastric emptying (Creutzfeldt and Arnold, 1978).

SS decreases the release from the small intestine of numerous hormones: CCK, secretin, GIP, VIP, enteroglucagon, motilin, acetylcholine, catecholamine, neurotensin, substance P, and prostaglandin E_2. It decreases intestinal contractility, decreases gallbladder contraction and bile flow, and delays the absorption of triglyceride, sugar, and other foods (Schusdziarra et al., 1979, 1980), suggesting that SS may be a hormone regulating the absorption of nutrients by the gut.

Additional actions are: the inhibition of the release of renin; inhibition of salivary secretion, basal and stimulated; and a decrease in platelet aggregation. It is not clear yet which of this vast array of actions reflect physiologic control mechanisms, since many require pharmacologic concentrations of SS.

The mechanism by which SS exerts its many actions has not been clearly established. Two aspects that have been given the greatest consideration are its effects on: (1) cAMP concentration and action, and (2) calcium transport. As has been recently reviewed (Hall and Gomez-Pan, 1976; Luft et al., 1978), SS has been shown under certain conditions to decrease the accumulation of cAMP. However, it also affects the net action of cAMP. It tends to decrease the calcium uptake and intracellular calcium transport. Certain of the inhibitory actions of SS have been found to be abolished by increasing calcium concentration in the extracellular fluid (Taminato et al., 1975). On the other hand, there have been observations that seem somewhat in conflict with these generalizations. For example, Wollheim and associates (1977) found that there tends to be a parallel correlation between calcium uptake by islet cells and the release of insulin. Yet SS inhibits insulin secretion but does not affect either calcium influx or efflux. On the other hand, epinephrine inhibits insulin secretion and at the same time inhibits calcium uptake; it does not affect calcium efflux.

Clinical Disorders of Somatostatin Secretion

Diseases of the Gut

With atrophy of the gastric mucosa, the SS concentration in the fundus and antrum is reduced. Chayvialle and coworkers (1978) found a subnormal SS level in the antrum in patients with duodenal ulcer, but Creutzfeldt and Arnold (1978) obtained normal levels. However, they discovered that SS treatment was useful for severely bleeding ulcers. With duodenal ulcers associated with G cell hyperplasia, there is often found a distinctly greater increase in the number of G cells than D cells, thereby presumably upsetting the balance between the amount of gastrin and SS secreted (Pearse et al., 1977). Moreover, the gastric acid and pepsin responses to pentagastrin in these patients are accentuated and the inhibition by somatostatin is subnormal (Konturek, 1978).

Its potential use for treating ulcers acutely remains speculative since the agent has to be administered parenterally and has only a short action.

Somatostatinoma

Larsson and associates (1977) reported a patient with a malignant pancreatic tumor composed of cells indistinguishable from islet D cells. High levels of immunoreactive SS-like material were in the venous drainage from the tumor. Moreover, bioassays of tumor extract strongly inhibited insulin and glucagon secretion from isolated perfused porcine pancreas. The main clinical aspects were hypochlorhydria, steatorrhea, and diabetic glucose tolerance. Peripheral blood samples demonstrated by immunoassay that the insulin, pancreatic polypeptide, and gastrin concentrations were in the range of low to normal, and glucagon was significantly below the normal level. Another patient, reported by Ganda and coworkers (1977), had a benign D-cell tumor that contained large quantities of SS but had only trace amounts of insulin, glucagon, gastrin, VIP, and pancreatic polypeptide. The patient was known to have been diabetic for several years. Upon removal of the tumor, the diabetes disappeared.

Analogs

Experiences accumulated thus far have indicated that the therapeutic usefulness of SS is limited by its multiple effects on many secretory cells and its short duration. With its chronic use, there have been instances observed where it has been associated with increase in blood pressure and decrease in pulse rate, nausea, vomiting, and diarrhea (Lundbaek, 1978). Nonetheless, it has been commonly conceived that by altering the molecule in certain ways so as to increase significantly its duration of action and specificity, while reducing its side effects, it could have benefits in some diseases.

BOMBESIN

Bombesin was first isolated from frog skin (Erspamer and Melchiorri, 1973). It is a tetradecapeptide with a molecular weight of 1620 and this structure (Rayford et al., 1976b):

Glp+-Gln-Arg-Leu-Gly-Asn-Gln-Trp-Ala-Val-Gly-
His-Leu-Met-NH$_2$

It has a wide spectrum of actions, including stimulation of the release of several hormones, pancreatic enzymes, smooth muscle contraction, and hypothermia, as well as changes in cardiovascular and renal functions (Melchiorri, 1978). Little is known of factors governing its secretion. The half-life in the plasma has been estimated to be approximately 5 minutes.

Distribution

Almost all of bombesin is found in nerves and in special endocrine cells in the gut. The stomach has a higher concentration than any other tissue, with the largest quantities being in the antrum and duodenum (Polak et al., 1978.) There also is a relatively large amount throughout the small intestine. Whereas none was found in unextracted rat plasma, significant amounts were demonstrated after its extraction with formic acid (M. Brown et al., 1978a). It was surmised that possibly bombesin was bound to protein in the unextracted plasma, but this is likely to be an artifact of extraction.

Approximately equal amounts of bombesin are found in the wall and in the mucosa of the gut. Bombesin exists in peptidergic nerves in the gut wall and in special endocrine cells, P cells, that are sparsely distributed (Table 14–1) (Solcia et al., 1978; Polak et al., 1976). Nerve fibers containing bombesin are found predominantly in the submucosal region throughout the entire length of the intestine.

Actions

The main actions of bombesin are listed in Table 14–13. Those that are physiologic have not been defined. After its administration intracisternally in rats maintained at 4° C, a marked hypothermia occurs. Whereas the same reaction is produced by neurotensin, bombesin is 10^4 times more potent (M. Brown et al., 1977). The COOH-terminus is needed for it to exert full biologic activity. TRH, PGE, or naloxone blocks bombesin hypothermia. TRH intracisternally increases body temperature. Bombesin inhibits cold-induced increase in TRH and TSH. β-Endorphin has similar actions to bombesin in promoting hypothermia but is much less potent. Its action is blocked by naloxone. No hypothermia is produced by somatostatin, SP, VIP, gastrin, glucagon, LHRH, or bradykinin. Bombesin does not lower the temperature unless the animals are kept in the cold, and it does not lower it even if they are kept at 4° C if it is injected systemically.

Whereas bombesin increases the release of growth hormone and prolactin *in vivo,* it does not do so *in vitro.* It apparently exerts these actions through the hypothalamus. The prolactin-releasing action is not modified by either the histamine antagonist diphenhydramine or by naloxone. However, naloxone blocks the growth hormone–releasing action of bombesin.

Clinical Disorders

McCrossan and associates (1977) have found that with duodenal ulcer there is more than 70% greater than normal number of P cells in the duodenal mucosa. Normally, bombesin is not inhibited by antral acidification. In contrast, other hormones that stimulate gastrin are inhibited by antral acidification.

P cells are increased in number in patients with chronic atrophic gastritis, and also in some with carcinoid, in some with isletoma, and in some with ganglioneuroblastoma (Polak et al., 1978).

MOTILIN

Motilin was accidentally discovered by Brown when he observed that the placing of alkali in the duodenum of dogs causes strong gastric contractions. Subsequently, motilin was isolated and its amino acid sequence determined (J. C. Brown and Dryburgh, 1978). It has 22 AA and a molecular weight of 2698, with the following structure:

Phe-Val-Pro-Ile-Phe-Thr-Tyr-Gly-Glu-Leu-Gln-Arg-
Met-Gln-Glu-Lys-Glu-Arg-Asn-Lys-Gly-Gln

Secretion

As measured by radioimmunoassay, there are considerable variations in the basal circulating levels among individuals. A small increase in plasma motilin is observed after a mixed meal (Christofides et al., 1978). Oral or intravenous fat in man increases plasma motilin, whereas oral or intravenous glucose decreases it (Bloom et al., 1978b). No changes are observed after oral protein. Intraduodenal instillation of alkali decreases plasma motilin in man (Track et al., 1978). Motilin is released at approximately 100-minute intervals during the entire digestive state. Feeding stops the release. The inhibition occurs 1 to 2 hours after the food ingestion when plasma motilin levels are actually decreased. Thus the physiological control of motilin secretion remains to be established.

Table 14–13. ACTIONS OF BOMBESIN

Central nervous system
    Hypothermia (inhibited by SS, TRH, PGE, or naloxone)
    Decreases PGE_2-induced hyperthermia
    Decreases TRH
    Increases epinephrine
    Hyperglycemia
    Analgesia

Gastrointestines
    Increases gastrin and gastric acid secretion
    Increases CCK; decreases VIP
    Contraction of pylorus and ileocecal valve, but decreases motility of remainder of gut

Smooth muscle
    Stimulation of contraction of smooth muscle of uterus, urinary tract, bronchi, gallbladder

Pancreas
    Increases secretion of pancreatic enzymes
    Increases secretion of insulin, glucagon, and pancreatic polypeptide

Pituitary
    Increases secretion of GH and prolactin

Kidney
    Increases renin and erythropoietin
    Constriction of afferent anterioles; decreases blood flow; decreases glomerular filtration; antidiuresis

Circulation
    Tachycardia

Distribution and Degradation

In the gastrointestines motilin-containing cells are found predominantly in the duodenum with a few being in the jejunum and none elsewhere. The pineal gland and the pituitary also contain significant amounts of hormone (Yanaihara et al., 1978). Motilin is inactivated in part by the liver (Itoh et al., 1978).

Actions

Motilin acts on the gastrointestinal tract by altering its motility. It stimulates contraction of the fundus and the antrum and decreases gastric emptying, thereby increasing intragastric pressure. Motilin decreases acid secretion during eating. It also stimulates peristalsis of the small intestine. Significantly, most of its activities do not coincide with food ingestion but are delayed 2 hours or more subsequently. Motilin has been said to be "the housekeeper of the gut." Seemingly, it enhances the movement of various particles in the gut, especially in the small intestine, and clears out the gut in preparation for the next meal. Indeed, motilin is unique in that its actions are restricted to the fasting state (Itoh et al., 1978).

Clinical Studies

Although there are many clinical situations associated with alterations in gut motility, thus far there have been relatively few studies evaluating the status of motilin. There is no difference in the fasting or postprandial motilin in duodenal ulcer patients and normals, even though the ulcer patients have an increase in gastric emptying (Christofides et al., 1978).

PANCREATIC POLYPEPTIDE

Although present almost exclusively in the pancreas, this peptide seems to function largely as an ingestive hormone. Details concerning pancreatic polypeptide (PP) have been presented in a review by Floyd and associates (1977) and discussed in Chapter 15. It has a MW of 4200 and 36 AA, with the following sequence in humans:

Ala-Pro-Leu-Glu-Pro-Val-Tyr-Pro-Gly-Asp-Asp-Ala-Thr-Pro-Glu-Gln-Met-Ala-Gln-Try-Ala-Ala-Asp-Leu-Arg-Arg-Tyr-Ile-Asn-Met-Leu-Thr-Arg-Pro-Arg-Tyr-NH$_2$

PP in man differs from that in ox in the AA in positions 6, 10, 11, and 23, and from that in pig in positions 10, 11, and 23. A tyrosine amide is in the terminal position.

Secretion

By means of specific radioimmunoassay a number of factors have been examined affecting secretion of PP (Table 14–14) (Floyd et al., 1977; Schwartz et al., 1978; Adrian et al., 1978). Floyd and coworkers (1977) have demonstrated a progressive increase in the basal plasma concentration from the third to the seventh decade of life in normal subjects. An increase occurs in plasma PP after a mixed meal or triglyceride or glucose or protein. The rise after glucose or triglyceride is relatively small and of brief duration, whereas that following protein is marked and may last for several hours. An increase in plasma PP occurs after protein ingestion, presumably before much absorption has occurred. Apparently the early response phase is mediated through the vagus (Taylor et al., 1978; Schwartz et al., 1976).

Distribution and Degradation

PP is secreted by special endocrine cells (PP cells). In man, most of these cells are in the peripheral part of pancreatic islets. In dogs many of the cells also occur between acini, being more numerous toward the head of the pancreas; some are in the pancreatic ducts. In dogs a few are also scattered in the stomach and small intestine. In man, the number of PP cells outside the pancreas is so small that after total pancreatectomy essentially no PP can be registered in the radioimmunoassay of plasma.

Actions

Despite the large number of factors that stimulate the release of PP and the relatively high concentrations that are maintained after food intake, thus far relatively few physiologic functions have been ascribed to PP. In pharmacologic doses it stimulates basal acid secretion but inhibits pentagastrin-stimulated acid secretion (Lin et al., 1977). It increases gut motility and increases gastric emptying. It relaxes the pyloric and ileocecal sphincter and the colon. It initially increases pancreas secretion and then inhibits the secretion of pancreatic enzymes, water, and electrolytes from pancreas that is stimulated by secretin together with CCK (Lin and Chance, 1978; Taylor et al., 1979; Greenberg et al., 1978). It relaxes the gallbladder. It does not affect the secretion of insulin or glucagon or the plasma glucose level.

Alterations in Secretion in Various Clinical Disorders

As indicated in Table 14–15, in a number of diseases the secretion of PP is altered significantly (Adrian et al., 1978). Patients with apudomas of different types involving the pancreatic islets have been found to have excessive levels of plasma PP and relatively large amounts of PP in the tumors. Moreover, relatively high PP concentrations were found in the metastatic nodules. Whereas Adrian and associates (1978) found the PP concentration in the surrounding tissue to be similar to that of normal pancreas, Floyd and coworkers (1977) reported that a significant percentage of patients with isletoma had hyperplasia of PP cells in areas of the pancreas not involved by the tumor. Moreover, Floyd and coworkers (1977) found that after removal of the tumor there commonly was not a significant fall of plasma PP; indeed, in some instances it actually rose. Plasma PP levels were not elevated in patient with adenocarcinomas (Adrian et al., 1978).

Table 14–14. SECRETION OF PANCREATIC POLYPEPTIDE

Increased by:	Decreased by:
Mixed meal	Vagotomy
Oral triglyceride	Atropine*
Oral protein	Propantheline*
Amino acids*	Somatostatin*
Oral glucose	
Pentagastrin*	
Vagal stimulation	**No effect:**
Secretin*	Cimetadine*
Sham feeding	Duodenal acidification
Gastric distention (sl)	Catecholamines*
Acetylcholine*	Histamine*
Bethanechol*	Glucagon*
Hypoglycemia (insulin)	PGE$_2$
Fasting (72 hr)	Bombesin
2-Deoxyglucose	
Exercise	
Ca^{++}	
dbcAMP (*in vitro*)	
VIP*	
GIP*	
CCK*	

*Given intravenously.

Table 14–15. CLINICAL DISORDERS ASSOCIATED WITH ABNORMAL AMOUNTS OF PANCREATIC POLYPEPTIDE IN PLASMA AND/OR PANCREAS

Disorders	Increased PP Levels	
	Plasma	Islet Tumor
PP -oma	100%	+
VIP -oma	77%	+
Glucagon-oma	50%	+
Gastrin -oma	26%	+
Insulin -oma	22%	+
		Islets
Juvenile-onset diabetes	+	+
Adult-onset diabetes	+	+
Pancreatic insufficiency	+	+

Bordi and associates (1978) described one patient who was considered to have a tumor producing PP. The person had had longstanding duodenal ulcer and at operation was found to have tumor nodules in the pancreas consisting of PP cells. Plasma and tumor gastrin levels were not elevated. Patients with duodenal ulcers have increased basal levels of PP but show a normal rise with food (Schwartz et al., 1976). Some patients with pancreatic insufficiency have elevated levels of plasma PP, and some patients with chronic pancreatitis have a subnormal increase in PP with insulin hypoglycemia (Sive et al., 1978). Gepts and associates (1978) noted that PP cells tend to become hyperplastic with various pathologic pancreatic changes, for example, mucoviscidosis, pancreatitis, exocrine or endocrine neoplasms, hemochromatosis, and diabetes. Most impressive is the increase found in patients with juvenile-onset diabetes of long duration.

NEUROTENSIN

Neurotensin is a tridecapeptide:
(pyro)Glu-Leu-Try-Glu-Asn-Lys-Pro-Arg-Arg-Pro-
Tyr-Ile-Leu-OH
with a molecular weight of 1692 daltons. It has been isolated from bovine hypothalamus (Carraway and Leeman, 1973), bovine intestine (Carrawy et al., 1978), and human intestine (Hammer et al., 1979). It has been found to have the same structure when isolated from all sources.

Secretion

Some of the immunoreactive hormone in plasma resembles the tridecapeptide, but a large proportion of it is of smaller molecular weight. Since some of these smaller components are more biologically active than the tridecapeptide, it is possible that the latter might be the prohormone, which, after release into the plasma is converted to a more active form.

Distribution and Degradation

Over 95% of the neurotensin in the body is in the gut and brain, with the highest concentrations in the ileum and hypothalamus (Carraway and Leeman, 1976; M. Brown et al., 1978b). The gut has more than nine times as much total neurotensin as the brain. The gut mucosa contains much more neurotensin than the other layers do; it is synthesized and secreted by the N cells (Buchan et al., 1978). Its half-life in the plasma is approximately 1 minute.

Actions

Neurotensin may have endocrine, paracrine, neurotransmitter, neuroendocrine, and neurocrine actions. As listed in Table 14–16, pharmacologic doses of neurotensin promote vasodilatation, increase vascular permeability, decrease plasma volume, increase the hematocrit, produce hypotension, and cause cyanosis. Presumably, neither acetylcholine nor epinephrine plays a signficant role (Bissette et al., 1978) in the actions of the peptide.

Controversy exists with respect to the effect of neurotensin on islet function. We have found in unanesthetized foxhounds that the infusion of neurotensin, 100 ng/kg/min throughout 5-minute intervals, significantly increased insulin secretin without affecting plasma glucose or glucagon. The dosage that we used may approximate physiologic levels. Using far larger doses of neurotensin in anesthetized rats, several investigators (Carraway et al., 1976; Nagai and Frohman, 1978; M. Brown and Vale, 1976) have observed an increased secretion of glucagon, glycogenolysis, and hyperglycemia. The hyperglycemic response apparently results from increased catecholamine and glucagon secretion (Nagai and Frohman, 1978). Upon incubation of neurotensin for short intervals with isolated pancreatic islets plus a low glucose concentration, there was an increase in the release of insulin, glucagon, and-somatostatin; with a high dose of glucose or arginine, neurotensin inhibited the release of these three hormones (Dolais-Kitabgi et al., 1979). Thus at present it is uncertain that neurotensin has any physiologic role in mediating or modulating the secretion of pancreatic glucoregulatory hormones.

Special attention must be given to the possible role of neurotensin as a hypothalamic-releasing factor, particularly since it occurs in the hypothalamus in large concentrations, and because of its releasing action on ACTH, LH, FSH, growth hormone, prolactin, and other hormones.

Neurotensin, when administered intracisternally, produces significant hypothermia (M. Brown et al., 1978b). Neurotensin inserted into the lateral ventricle decreased gastric acid production and mucosal blood flow. Since

Table 14–16. ACTIONS OF NEUROTENSIN

Vascular
    Vasodilatation
    Increases vascular permeability; edema
    Decreases plasma volume; increases hematocrit
    Hypotension
    Cyanosis

Gastrointestinal
    Contraction of fundus and ileum; relaxation of duodenum
    Increases gastrin secretion
    Inhibits pentagastrin-stimulated acid secretion; no decrease in
      histamine effect

Pancreatic islets
    Increases insulin secretion
    Increases glucagon secretion
    (Huge doses in anesthetized animals cause increase in glucagon,
      glycogenolysis, and plasma glucose; they decrease insulin—see text)

Neuroendocrine
    Peptidergic neurotransmitter
    Hypothermia (with intracisternal administration)
    Increases release of ACTH, LH, FSH, GH, and prolactin
    Increases pain

Other actions
    Chemotactic action on neutrophils
    Contraction of uterus

these actions were completely blocked by pretreatment with reserpine or 6-OH-dopamine (Osumi et al., 1978), it is possible that they are mediated through sympathetic neurons.

Abnormalities in Neurotensin Secretion in Disease States

Little is known about neurotensin secretion and action in various clinical disorders. However, patients with the "dumping syndrome" have been found to have increased levels of plasma neurotensin and insulin after oral glucose (Bloom et al., 1978a). Although patients with marked obesity have been observed to have a large increase in the number of N cells in the ileal mucosa, its significance is uncertain.

SUBSTANCE P (SP)

As reviewed by Mroz and Leeman (1977), during the last four decades studies have been conducted on three apparently unrelated biologic activities of this hormone: (1) hypotensive and spasmogenic effects, (2) sialogogic action, and (3) the motor neuron depolarizing action. Von Euler and Gaddum (1931) first designated it as "substance P" in extracts of brain and intestine. Subsequently, Leeman "rediscovered" substance P in hypothalamus and noted that it had a sialogogue action (Leeman and Mroz, 1974). Most of the progress in characterizing this hormone has occurred in the last decade, starting with its purification and chemical characterization by Chang and Leeman (1971), its subsequent synthesis and the provision of a satisfactory immunoassay. It is an undecapeptide amide (molecular weight 1528, bovine). It occurs in the body in several molecular sizes.

Assays

Bioassays have utilized chiefly the following three types of action: (1) sialogogic activity, (2) ileal contraction, and (3) vasodilatation. Relatively little information has accumulated thus far with respect to factors that influence the release of SP. It is released from nerve endings in the brain, spinal cord, and peripheral nerves, and also from specific endocrine cells in the gut (EC$_1$). Vagal stimulation releases SP into the antral lumen (Uvnäs-Wallensten, 1978). SP is rapidly degraded throughout the body.

Distribution

Although SP is located in special endocrine cells in the gut, most is found in nerve cells scattered throughout the body. Nerve cells containing SP are found in the brain, spinal cord, nerve ganglia, peripheral nerves, the autonomic nervous system, and the intrinsic nervous system of the gut. SP is synthesized in the body of nerve cells, transported to nerve endings, and released there. It is widely distributed throughout the brain (Nakata et al., 1978.

Most of the SP in the spinal cord is in dorsal roots and dorsal horns. Membrane-bound dense granules are transported intact through endothelial cells into the blood or are picked up by Schwann cells or fibroblasts. Other granules are broken down locally.

Most smooth muscle-containing organs contain SP. A significant amount of SP is present in the peptidergic fibers of the vagus and is released on stimulation. In the gut, the SP-containing neurons follow VIP fibers as the most numerous of the peptidergic nerve fibers (Hökfeldt et al., 1978). Although SP is found throughout the gastrointestines, the highest concentrations are in the ileum (Yanaihara et al., 1977). SP is concentrated in the intrinsic nervous system of the gut. The SP nerve terminals are expecially numerous in and nearby the myenteric and submucosal plexuses, in muscle layers, and in lamina propria.

Actions

In pharmacologic doses SP affects several systems in the body. Its most important actions are exerted through the nervous system. It seems to be a sensory neurotransmitter involving pain, touch, and temperature. When administered to animals, it also functions as an analgesis (25 times more potent than morphine) (Malick and Goldstein, 1978). In the spinal cord it appears to have an excitatory transmitter role at the synapse between primary afferent neurons and the second-order neurons involved in spinal pain pathways (Powell et al., 1978). In brain, it stimulates a monoaminergic neuron and acts as an excitatory transmitter in nerve terminals that impinge on dopaminergic cell bodies.

Given systemically, it increases the contractions of most of the gastrointestinal smooth muscle (Yau, 1978) and it causes vasodilatation, increased blood flow, hypotension, tachycardia, and flushing. It is one of the most potent vasoactive substances known.

It also causes natriuresis, diuresis, and kaliuresis (Gullner et al., 1979). It tends to decrease renin secretion, increases kallikrein secretion, and increases renal blood flow. It also decreases the sodium and water reabsorption by proximal tubules.

It promotes salivation and increases the secretion by pancreatic acini. Under certain conditions, it has been found to cause increased secretion of growth hormone, prolactin, FSH, LH, and ADH, but to decrease ACTH.

Using anesthetized rats, and very large doses of SP, M. Brown and associates (1976) found that it increased glucagon and plasma glucose but decreased insulin secretion. Some of these changes could be produced by an increased secretion of catecholamine, promoted by the anesthesia and the large dose of SP. Presumably, these hormonal changes result from actions on the hypothalamus.

SP increases the release of histamine from mast cells. Some of the actions attributed to SP could be due at least in part to the release of histamine that it induces.

Mroz and Leeman (1977) stated that there are several thousand-fold differences in the dosages used to produce some of the actions that have been described. It is possible but as yet unproven that SP acts physiologically depending on whether the functions are neuroendocrine, endocrine, paracrine, or neurocrine or neurotransmitter. The amount circulating in the plasma is very small. Effects requiring higher concentrations would necessitate local release on target cells.

Clinical Disorders Associated with Altered Relationships of SP-Containing Cells

In Hirschsprung's disease there is a subnormal amount of SP in the aganglionic segment of the colon. In this disease there is genetic deficiency in the ganglionic cells in the intrinsic nerve plexuses of Auerbach and Meissner. As a result, the colon is severely constricted. The colon proximal to this is dilated and hypertrophied and has elevated concentrations of SP.

In some patients with carcinoid, there are high levels of SP in both the blood and the tumors. The EC_1 cells compose most of the SP-producing argentaffin carcinoids of the ileum. These cells contain both SP and serotonin. It seems reasonable to assume that SP contributes to some of the symptoms and signs of the disease.

LIPOTROPINS, ENDORPHINS, ENKEPHALINS, AND ACTH

These substances are discussed fully in Chs. 3 and 5. The following is a summary of the synthesis, release, distribution, degradation, and action of these substances and their relationship to the gastrointestinal tract.

Presumably all lipotropin is derived from the pituitary. It exerts a mild lipolytic action, but different from some of its constituents, it does not exert a significant opiate action. The endorphins are thought to be derived from lipotropin. They manifest many opiate actions throughout the body, especially in the nervous system and the gut. They complete with morphine and other opiates in the binding of specific receptors. β-Endorphin has many more, and more potent, actions manifested than do γ- and α-endorphins. Its actions on the gastrointestinal tract, pancreas, and biliary system are far more potent than those of morphine. Like morphine, it also has many actions on the nervous system.

Morphine exerts many actions on the gastrointestinal tract, including decreased gastric acid secretion and gastric motility, but increases antral tone. It decreases biliary and pancreatic secretion, causes periodic spasm of the small intestine, decreases the propulsive contractions, decreases peristaltic waves, but increases the tone of the large and small intestines. It increases biliary tract pressure and constriction of the sphincter of Oddi.

Met-enkephalin and leu-enkephalin are found in brain in much higher concentrations than β-LPH. Moreover, there is not a parallelism in the distribution of these two types of compounds; the levels of the enkephalins are not influenced by hypophysectomy. The enkephalins exert potent analgesic and emotional effects as well as other influences on nerve functions. Met-enkephalin, like morphine, increases histamine-induced gastric acid and pepsin secretion and increases the blood flow to the stomach (Konturek et al., 1978). It increases the force of gastric contractility, but decreases the frequency of contraction. It delays gastric emptying. It decreases intestinal contractions but increases intestinal blood flow. It inhibits secretin- and CCK_8-stimualted pancreatic acinar secretion. The enkephalins are degraded within seconds in the plasma and in nerve tissue. Their primary physiologic role seemingly is involved in neurotransmission and neuroregulation. To what extent ACTH directly influences nerve function has not been elucidated.

ACTH-like immunoreactivity has been found in gastrointestinal and pancreatic endocrine cells. In rats this peptide and enkephalin are found in gastrin cells (G cells), but in man the ACTH-like peptide seems to be confined to the duodenum and pancreatic islets (Larsson, 1977). Tumors arising in the gut or pancreatic islets sometimes cause ectopic Cushing's syndrome.

ENTEROGLUCAGON

In the early phases of conducting immunoassays for glucagon, cross-reacting materials were found in extracts of the gut (Unger et al., 1961). These materials were chemically and biologically different from pancreatic glucagon. They have been designated as enteroglucagon, gut glucagon, glucagon-like immunoreactivity (GLI), glycentin, and glucagon immunoreactants. The abbreviation GLI has been most commonly used. Moody and associates (1978) have recently discussed the antigenic sites shared by glucagon and GLI. Most GLIs from the gut have a MW $>10,000$ daltons, but approximately 25 per cent have a MW similar to that of glucagon. One form of GLI has recently been isolated (Sundby et al., 1976). This GLI-I has 100 AA, including all those found in glucagon, and has been specifically denoted "glicentin."

The highest concentration of "glicentin" is detected by specific radioimmunoassay in "L" cells located in the ileum and colon, but there are smaller quantities in the jejunum and duodenum. Essentially none is in the stomach. The pancreas has glicentin-like material. Since glicentin obtained from pancreatic α cells and gut L cells has the full sequence of glucagon, glicentin may really be considered as proglucagon. The L cells presumably do not have the capacity to synthesize glucagon. The presence of a common glicentin-like immunoreactive material in α and L cells suggests that these two cell types are ontogenetically related. The gut GLIs possibly constitute a primitive peptide family which has lost the capacity to synthesize glucagon, VIP, secretin, and GIP, so the L cells may now not have a real significant function (Moody et al., 1978).

GLI has been found in several areas of the dog brain including the hypothalamus, amygdala, and mesencephalon (Conlon et al., 1979). The molecular form of GLI in the brain is seemingly similar to that in the gut. However, in certain brain areas of dogs there also is immunoreactive glucagon with the same molecular weight as pancreatic glucagon.

Plasma GLI increases twofold after duodenal instillation of 20 per cent glucose (2 g/kg). GLI is released from all parts of the small intestine and the colon, but more comes from the ileum and colon than from the upper parts of the small intestine (Frame, 1976). It is also released after: the administration of fat or CCK, and with starvation, insulin hypoglycemia, or a mixed meal (Holst, 1978). It does not affect lipolysis or insulin secretion. Glicentin has no receptors on liver cells, but it increases hepatic glucogenesis. However, to obtain this effect, glicentin presumably must be partially degraded. A large molecular weight basic gut-type glucagon competes with glucagon for binding to liver glucagon receptors, and promotes hepatic glucogenesis and insulin secretion *in vitro* (Holst, 1978).

There are many differences in the plasma response related to glucagon and GLI. Oral glucose or triglyceride increases GLI and decreases glucagon. Hypoglycemia increases glucagon and decreases GLI. Glucagon increases plasma glucose and insulin, but GLI in physiologic amounts has no effect. Thus, a specific physiologic role for GLI remains to be shown.

Possible Relationship of GLI to Pathologic States

A patient with severe colonic and jejunal stasis, malabsorption, and small intestinal villous hypertrophy was found to have a tumor of the kidney. With removal of the tumor, the symptoms and signs and the elevated plasma GLI disappeared. The tumor was found to have a large amount of GLI (Bloom, 1972).

In patients who have rapid transit times associated with surgical procedures, i.e., gastrectomy, pyloroplasty, and/or vagotomy, GLI levels are inordinately increased after oral glucose or mixed meals. Although it has been postulated that

GLI might be involved in hypoglycemia occasionally encountered in these patients, since GLI has not been shown to affect insulin secretion either *in vivo* or *in vitro*, this conjecture has not been substantiated.

ACETYLCHOLINE IN RELATION TO THE GUT, PANCREAS, AND LIVER

Acetylcholine is the principal neurotransmitter in the parasympathetic nervous system. It is synthesized in the nerve terminals. The main enzyme involved in this synthesis, acetyltransferase, is presumed to be synthesized in the neuronal cells and migrates down the axons to the nerve terminals. Choline is taken up by these terminals and is acetylated by acetyl coenzyme A. The acetylcholine is stored in agranular vesicles of the cholinergic nerve terminals until it is released (Fig. 14–2).

This neurotransmitter is concentrated in the following sites: (1) preganglionic nerve terminals of the sympathetic nervous system and of the parasympathetic nervous system, (2) postganglionic nerve fibers of the parasympathetic nervous system, (3) nerve terminals of the postganglionic sympathetic nervous system (in only relatively small amounts), and (4) nerve terminals in the adrenal medulla.

With an increase in action potential in the nerve fibers acetylcholine is released. This is augmented by an increased uptake of calcium. It is also increased by gastrin and CCK. The release is decreased by alpha-adrenergic activity and after vagotomy.

Acetylcholine is probably involved in the propagation of the action potential in many noncholinergic and cholinergic nerve fibers. The actions of acetylcholine at the muscarinic receptors can be blocked by atropine, because atropine competes with acetylcholine in its binding to its receptor. However, the atropine does not block the release of acetylcholine. Nicotinic blockers (e.g., hexamethonium) inhibit acetylcholine action in the autonomic ganglion cells and in neuromuscular junctions.

Acetylcholine increases the tone of the gastrointestinal tract. It increases contraction of the gut, including peristalsis of the stomach and intestines (Brooks, 1977). It increases gut mucosal secretion. In large amounts it can cause nausea, vomiting, diarrhea, abdominal cramps, and defecation. It increases the release of gastrin.

Acetylcholine increases the pancreatic secretion of enzymes, water, and electrolytes. It acts on the pancreatic islets to increase the release of insulin, glucagon, and pancreatic polypeptide, but decreases the secretion of somatostatin.

Acetylcholine increases gallbladder contraction and bile flow. It increases the release of epinephrine, norepinephrine, dopamine, and many other hormones (Table 14–2).

At most of the cholinergic nerve junctions acetylcholinesterase is present. It degrades acetylcholine in fractions of a second, and in this manner limits the intensity and duration of acetylcholine action.

ACTIONS OF THE VAGUS NERVE

The vagus nerve transmits predominantly cholinergen; thus it would be anticipated that vagal stimulation would reproduce the actions of acetylcholine. However, since there are also many peptidergic hormones in the vagus nerve, they may modify the activity of acetylcholine (Table 14–2).

Vagal stimulation increases the swallowing reflex, esophageal peristalsis, relaxation of the esophageal sphincter, and relaxation of the fundus, while increasing the propulsive action of the distal portion of the stomach. Vagal activity results in increased secretion of acid and pepsin; it has both a stimulating and an inhibitory role in gastrin secretion by either stimulating or diminishing its release depending upon the signals from the brain in anticipation of eating or during alimentation.

Pancreas

The vagus is involved in the control of insulin, glucagon, and pancreatic polypeptide secretion, but its precise role has not been defined (Woods and Porte, 1978). Vagal stimulation also increases the secretion by the exocrine pancreas of enzymes, water, and electrolytes.

Vagal activity leads to the contraction of the gallbladder and bile flow. The release of a number of aminergic and peptidergic hormones has been noted but the physiologic significance has yet to be ascertained (Table 14–2).

Peptidergic-Aminergic Nervous System of the Gut and Pancreas

As shown in Table 14–1, there are numerous aminergic and peptidergic hormones in the nerve trunks innervating the gut, and especially in the intramural nervous system. There are also many in the pancreas, but many fewer than in the gut. Since the actions of the various neurotransmitters may be divergent, it is difficult to make generalizations about the specific effects when a given nerve is activated.

The intramural plexuses in the gut wall contain cell bodies and nerve fibers of afferent, efferent, and integrating neurons that are essential for local reactions of the gut. The afferent impulses from mechanoreceptors and chemoreceptors in the mucosa and other parts of the gut go to ganglia and then efferent responses result, such as release of gut hormone. Such reflex arcs are involved in regulating the amount of acid secretion, absorption and secretion into the intestines, esophageal relaxation, peristalsis, relaxation in the proximal stomach and antral peristalsis, propulsive action of the intestine, and defecation reflex. Whereas the cholinergic actions tend to be excitatory, the peptidergic actions are both excitatory and inhibitory.

CATECHOLAMINES

Synthesis and Distribution of Catecholamines

The catecholamines consist of dopamine, norepinephrine, and epinephrine. As discussed in much greater detail in Ch. 10, these are synthesized with tyrosine as the initial substrate (Fig. 10–1). Dopamine and norepinephrine are synthesized in the nerve terminals of postganglionic sympathetic nerve fibers and are stored there until a stimulus is received for their release. Epinephrine is synthesized almost entirely in the adrenal medulla by special endocrine cells.

More than 90% of the total catecholamine in the gut consists of dopamine, much of it in a special type of mast cell. Apparently these cells do not synthesize the hormone but take it up from the extracellular spaces. More than 90% of the catecholamines in the liver and more than 50% in the pancreas consist of dopamine.

The catecholamines are released from adrenergic nerve endings in response to certain action potentials that are transmitted by the axons. Acetylcholine plays a regulating influence, not only by serving as the main transmitter in the synapse between the preganglionic and postganglionic nerves, but also in the terminals of the latter. Also, cholinergic fibers constitute the innervation of the adrenal medullary cells, from which epinephrine and norepinephrine are released. Thus, an increase in acetylcholine promotes a release of all catecholamines. In addition, calcium is involved in the release of all of the catecholamines. Presumably, these same factors influence dopamine release. In Table 14–17 are listed some comparisons of adrenergic and cholinergic actions in the gut, liver, biliary system, and pancreas.

Most of the catecholamine actions in the gastrointestines are on the smooth muscle and the blood vessels. By stimulating contraction of the wall of blood vessels, catecholamines decrease blood flow, which then influences secretion by the gut, but they do not directly affect secretion. They inhibit excitation produced by the intramural neurons and generally inhibit motility of the gut, but stimulate contraction of its sphincters. The effect of the catecholamines in relaxing the smooth muscle of the gut results from an alpha-adrenergic action in decreasing the release of acetylcholine at the presynapse terminal and from inhibition of the excitatory actions of intramural neurons.

Although all three catecholamines are in the pancreas, dopamine is present in largest concentration and presumably exerts the greatest effect. Alpha-adrenergic activity decreases the secretion of insulin and glucagon, but beta-adrenergic activity increases their release (Woods and Porte, 1974). Alpha-adrenergic activity decreases the acinar secretion of the pancreas.

Catecholamines also stimulate glycogenolysis and gluconeogenesis from the liver. They cause relaxation of the gallbladder and bile duct. As discussed in Ch. 11, catecholamines affect the release and action of many hormones within the brain.

The period of action for individual catecholamine molecules is extremely brief. Much of what is released from the nerve endings and not bound to its receptor is taken up again by the nerve endings, and transported into the cytoplasm where monoamine oxidase (MAO) rapidly destroys it. What goes into the bloodstream is either rapidly degraded in the blood or by other organs, especially the liver and kidneys. This degradation is mainly by catechol-O-methyl transferase (COMT). Whereas MAO is in the adrenergic nerve endings, COMT has no selective association with the adrenergic nerves.

The clinical disorders associated with altered catecholamine secretion, action, and metabolism are detailed in Chs. 10, 11, and 12.

Table 14–17. CHOLINERGIC AND ADRENERGIC ACTIONS IN THE STOMACH, INTESTINE, PANCREAS, LIVER, AND BILIARY TRACT

	Receptor	Adrenergic	Cholinergic
Stomach			
Motility	β	Decrease +	Increase +++
Sphincters	α	Contraction +	Relaxation +
Secretion		Decrease (?)	Stimulation +++
Intestine			
Motility	α β	Decrease +	Increase +++
Sphincters	α	Contraction +	Relaxation +
Secretion		Inhibition (?)	Stimulation ++
Liver	β	Glycogenolysis, gluco-neogenesis +++	Glycogenesis +
Gallbladder and ducts		Relaxation +	Contraction +
Pancreas			
Acini	α	Decrease secretion +	Secretion ++
	β	Increase secretion +	

SEROTONIN

Serotonin (5-hydroxytryptamine) is distributed throughout the gastrointestinal tract and the central and peripheral nervous systems. When a large dose is injected into different parts of the body, or when it is released from serotonin-producing tumors (carcinoid), pronounced effects on the neurologic, pulmonary, cardiovascular, endocrine, hematologic, and other systems can be observed. However, only in recent years has very much progress been made in evaluating its role under normal physiological conditions.

Synthesis and Secretion

In the synthesis of serotonin, L-tryptophan is hydroxylated to form 5-hydroxytryptophan and the latter is decarboxylated to form 5-hydroxytryptamine (serotonin). The latter is degraded to form 5-hydroxyindoleacetic acid (5-HIAA). The enzymes catalyzing these reactions are as follows:

$$\text{L-tryptophan} \xrightarrow[\text{hydroxylase}]{\text{tryptophan}} \text{5-hydroxytryptophane}$$

$$\xrightarrow{\text{L-AA decarboxylase}} \text{5-hydroxytryptamine} \xrightarrow{\text{MAO}} \text{5-HIAA}$$

The synthesis of serotonin occurs chiefly in the intestinal enterochromaffin cells or in central or peripheral neurons. What is synthesized outside the brain cannot reach the brain because of the blood-brain barrier, so the brain must synthesize its own supply. The amount synthesized in either location is highly dependent on the amount of nonprotein-bound tryptophan in plasma and the amount of tryptophan hydroxylase. Most of the supply of tryptophan is derived from dietary protein. The protein binding of tryptophan is decreased as the free fatty acid level of the plasma increases, because the latter competes with tryptophan for the binding sites. Consequently, factors that promote lipolysis, with the resulting liberation of free fatty acid, increase the amount of serotonin synthesized (Tagliamonte et al., 1973). The amounts of tryptophan transported into the brain tend to be inversely related to the concentration of neutral amino acids, because of competition for the transport mechanism. These amino acids also interfere with the synthesis of serotonin by the gut cells. Therefore, the intestinal enterochromaffin cells can couple the synthesis and release of serotonin to the quantity and composition of dietary protein, whereas brain neurons respond primarily to the proportion of protein (Colmenares and Wurtman, 1979).

The recent availability of a radioimmunoassay for plasma serotonin has been of great help in evaluating factors influencing the release of this hormone (Jaffe et al., 1978). With a standard meal, the level is found to increase by 30 minutes, reaching a zenith by 60 minutes and falling to basal levels by 2 hours. A strong stimulant for the secretion of serotonin is acid in the duodenum (Fig. 14–9). Glucose causes less rise in blood serotonin than does acid. The source of the serotonin presumably is the enterochromaffin cells of the gut. One should be aware that serotonin is bound to platelets and, despite the fact that both the liver and the lungs have a very rapid serotonin-degrading system, they do not cause degradation as long as the hormone is platelet-bound.

About 90% of the body's supply of serotonin is in the gastrointestinal tract, mainly in the enterochromaffin (EC_1) cells. Most of the remainder is found in platelets and the central nervous system. Some serotonin is found in many types of APUD cells, along with a polypeptide or an amine

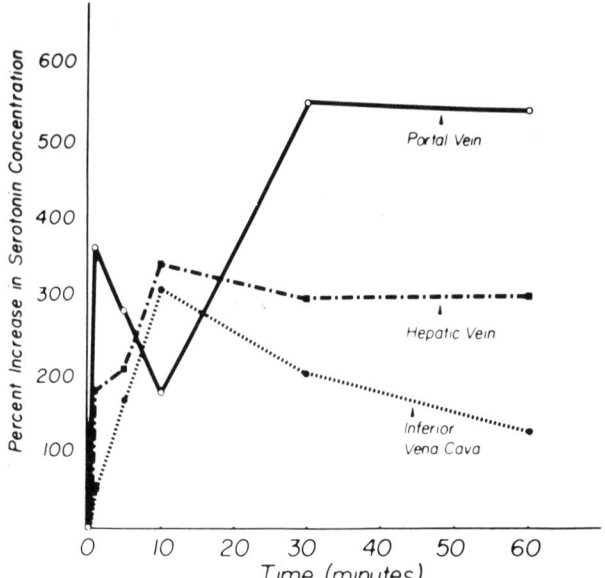

Figure 14–9. The serotonin response of duodenal acidification as measured in the portal, hepatic, and peripheral veins. (From Jaffe, B. M., Kellum, J. M., Jr., et al.: Release and physiologic action of serotonin. In *Gut Hormones.* Bloom, S. R. (ed.), Edinburgh, Churchill Livingstone, 1978.)

hormone (dopamine, histamine). For example, it is found in the α and β cells of the islets, C cells of the thyroid, and substance P neurons in the nervous system (Chan-Palay et al., 1978). It is also located in a number of the other gastrointestinal hormone cells.

The duodenum has a highest concentration of serotonin (Jaffe et al., 1978). Cells of Auerbach's plexus synthesize serotonin and have a high capacity to take up serotonin from the extracellular space. There is also some released from nerve endings of the vagus nerve. There are serotonin receptors in the enteric nervous system, and myenteric neurons synthesize and release serotonin (Vermillion et al., 1979). Recent physiologic observations suggest that serotonin serves as a neurotransmitter within the enteric nervous system.

The turnover time of serotonin in the central nervous system is estimated to be 1 hour, whereas in the gastrointestine it is 17 hours.

Actions

The net actions of serotonin depend very much upon its sites of release and the types and amounts of other hormones released, including many that it may release and also others that are released concomitantly.

Food causes increases in plasma levels of serotonin, but this does not change directly the levels in the brain. Moreover, the serotonin that is synthesized and released in the central nervous system apparently does not influence the function of the rest of the body except indirectly through neurogenic impulses involving it or other components that it has influenced. The impermeability of the blood-brain barrier by serotonin prevents its passage, but does not block the transport of 5-hydroxytryptophan or of tryptophan.

A problem exists in precisely analyzing the actions of serotonin because there are several hormones that affect its release and actions and, conversely, it affects the release and actions of several other hormones. There are many interrelations of serotonin- and catecholamine-releasing actions, both centrally and peripherally. Serotonin can be released

from cells that also contain histamine, dopamine, substance P, and other APUD hormones (Owman, 1973).

Serotonin blocks the release of both insulin and glucagon (Chapter 15). This inhibitive action is counteracted by serotonin antagonists, such as methysergide or cyproheptadine.

Serotonin can cause either gut smooth muscle contraction or relaxation. It can evoke contraction and increase intestinal peristalsis by direct action on the muscle and by exciting certain cells in the intramural ganglia. These stimulative actions can be inhibited by phenoxybenzamine, atropine, or morphine. Serotonin can block muscle contraction by stimulating certain cells in the myenteric plexus that exert inhibitory actions on smooth muscle.

The inhibitory action of serotonin on gastric acid secretion is presumed to result from its release, mostly from the small intestine, its transport through the bloodstream, and then its binding to parietal cells of the stomach where it acts. Therefore, it exerts an endocrine action. This inhibitory action can be demonstrated despite the administration of pentagastrin or after antrectomy or vagotomy. Moreover, this action occurs no matter whether the supply of serotonin is endogenous or exogenous. Serotonin presumably does not exert a significant action by way of the vagus or the antrum.

Considering collectively the many different studies that have been conducted with serotonin, it can act in several ways: as a neurotransmitter, a neuroendocrine, an endocrine, a paracrine, or a neurocrine.

Various studies dealing with the specific mechanism by which serotonin exerts its action indicate that it is dependent upon its capacity to stimulate sodium and calcium intracellular transport, with resulting alterations in membrane permeability.

Clinical Disturbances Associated with Altered Metabolism in Serotonin

These are detailed in Chs. 10 and 12. As discussed in Ch. 10, serotonin usually is the main hormonal component that is secreted by carcinoid tumors. In some patients with such tumors, a large variety of severe changes may occur throughout the body, involving especially mental behavior, gastrointestinal function, and cardiovascular function (Table 10–10). For example, there may be severe diarrhea, abdominal cramps, borborygmi, episodic flushing, telangiectiasia, cyanosis, pellagra-like lesions, bronchial spasmas, wheezing, asthmatic attacks, dyspnea, and valvular lesions of the heart. However, many of these changes and others that occur in this syndrome are only partially caused by serotonin.

HISTAMINE

Histamine is a potent monoaminergic hormone diffusely distributed throughout the body, secreted by endocrine cells and nerve cells. It is designated as histamine because it is an amine found extensively in tissue (*histos*). It is synthesized from histidine with the reaction being catalyzed by histidine decarboxylase.

The largest concentrations of histamine are found in gut mucosa, skin, lungs, and brain. Because histamine is rapidly degraded by body fluids, it is normally not measurable therein. In the gut mucosa, it is found in mast cells and in ECL cells (only a small amount is found in these cells in humans). It has been extracted from peripheral nerve (possibly in mast cells). High concentrations occur in the central nervous system, particularly in the median eminence of the hypothalamus. It is synthesized in the cytoplasm of the nerve endings, stored in synaptic vesicles of the nerve terminals, and released during depolarization with concomitant increase in synthesis (Schwartz, 1975).

With extensive tissue injury, histamine can be released into the circulation with resulting deleterious effects, including death. Histamine is released by stimulation of the vagus or by the ingestion of food.

The actions of histamine are detailed in Chs. 10 and 25. The provision of histamine antagonists has helped to elucidate some of the actions and mechanisms involved. Many of the antagonists act by blocking histamine binding to its receptor, of which there are several, including H_1 receptors and H_2 receptors. Binding to the H_1 receptor is what causes the commonly known features of anaphylaxis. H_1 antagonists include ethanolamines (e.g., diphenhydramine) and ethylenediamines (e.g., pyrilamine). These antagonists inhibit the effects of histamine on capillary permeability and on vascular, bronchial, and many other types of smooth muscle reaction. H_2 antagonists have consisted of burimamide, metiamide, and cimetidine. One of the most important actions involving histamine actions through the H_2 receptor consists of stimulation of gastric acid. In addition to the H_1 and H_2 receptors, there appear to be others which are as yet ill-defined.

Histamine has many different types of actions on the gut, but one of the most important ones is the stimulation of the secretion by the stomach of HCL, pepsin, and other secretions. Acetylcholine and gastrin, as discussed in the section on Gastrin, have a potent stimulating effect on gastric acid secretion, and earlier it was thought that their action was mediated through histamine. Whereas each of these stimulants acts independently, they have synergistic actions. Histamine causes contraction of smooth muscle in various parts of the gastrointestines.

SUMMARY

Clearly the gastrointestinal tract is both a major endocrine organ and a major target for many hormones, released locally and at a distance. The integration of the complex array of chemical signals needed for the smooth functioning of digestion, absorption, and assimilation represents a major challenge for higher organisms which have evolved the "computer system" surveyed in this chapter. It seems not accidental that the first hormone discovered and some of the most recently characterized chemical messengers originated in the gut. Disorders involving gut hormones are playing an ever increasing role in our understanding of endocrine disease.

REFERENCES

Adrian, T. E., Bloom, S. R., et al.: PP — Physiology and pathology, In *Gut Hormones*. Bloom, S. R. (ed.), Edinburgh, Churchill Livingstone, 1978, pp.254–260.

Andersen, D. K., Elahi, D., et al.: Oral glucose augmentation of insulin secretion: interactions of gastric inhibitory polypeptide with ambient glucose and insulin levels. *J. Clin. Invest.* 62:152–161, 1978.

Barden, N., Dupont, A., and Cote, J. -P.: Pentagastrin and adenosine 3',5'-cyclic monophosphate stimulated secretion of somatostatin from perifused rat gastric mucosa. *Life Sci.* 24:739, 1979.

Bissette, G., Manberg, P., et al.: Neurotensin, a biologically active peptide. *Life Sci.* 23:2173–2182, 1978.

Bloom, S. R.: An enteroglucagon tumor *Gut* 13:520–523, 1972.

Bloom, S. R.: VIP and watery diarrhoea VI, In *Gut Hormones*. Bloom, S. R., (ed.), Edinburgh, Churchill Livingstone, 1978, pp. 583–588.

Bloom, S. R., Blackburn, A. M., et al.: Measurement of neurotensin in man: a new circulating peptide hormone affecting insulin release and carbohydrate metabolism. *Diabetologia* 15 Abstract 41, 1978a.

Bloom, S. R., Christofides, N. D., et al.: Release of motilin in man by oral and intravenous nutriments. *Gastroenterology* 74:1010, 1978b.

Bloom, S. R., and Polak, J. M.: Gut hormone overview, In *Gut Hormones*. Bloom, S. R. (ed.), Edinburgh, Churchill Livingstone, 1978, p. 3.

Bodanszky, M.: Gastrointestinal hormones, families of oligoelectrolytes, In *Endocrinology of the Gut*. Chey, W. Y., and Brooks, F. P. (eds.), Thorofare, N.J., Charles B. Slack, 1974.

Boden, G.: The secretin assay, In *Gut Hormones*. Bloom, S. R. (ed.), Edinburgh, Churchill Livingstone, 1978, pp. 169–175.

Bonfils, S., and Bernades, P.: Zollinger-Ellison syndrome: Natural history and diagnosis. *Clin. Gastroenterol.* 3:539, 1974.

Bordi, C., Togni, R., et al.: Human islet cell tumor storing pancreatic polypeptide: a light and electron microscopic study. *J. Clin. Endocrinol. Metab.* 46:215–219, 1978.

Brazeau, P., Epelbaum, J., et al.: Somatostatin: Isolation, characterization, distribution, and blood determination. *Metabolism* 27:1133, 1978.

Brooks, F. P.: Nervous control of gastrointestinal function: neurophysiological considerations, In *Progress in Gastroenterology*. Vol. III. Glass, G. B. J. (ed.), New York, Grune & Stratton, Inc., 1977, pp. 373–393.

Brown, J. C., and Dryburgh, J. R.: Isolation of motilin, In *Gut Hormones*. Bloom, S. R., (ed.), Edinburgh, Churchill Livingstone, 1978, pp. 327–334.

Brown, J. C., Dryburgh, J. R., et al.: Identification and actions of gastric inhibitory polypeptide. *Recent Prog. Horm. Res.* 31:487–532, 1975.

Brown, J. C., Dryburgh, J. R., et al.: Properties and actions of GIP, In *Gut Hormones*. Bloom, S. R. (ed.), Edinburgh, Churchill Livingstone, 1978, pp. 277–282.

Brown, M., Allen, R., et al.: Bombesin-like activity: radioimmunologic assessment in biological tissues. *Life Sci.* 23:2721–2728, 1978a.

Brown, M., Rivier, J., and Vale, W.: Bombesin: potent effects on thermoregulation in the rat. *Science* 196:998–1000, 1977.

Brown, M., Rivier, J., et al.: Neurotensin-like and bombesin-like peptides: CNS distribution and actions. In *Gut Hormones*. Bloom, S. R., (ed.), Edinburgh, Churchill Livingstone, 1978b, pp. 550–558.

Brown, M., and Vale, W.: Effects of neurotensin and substance P on plasma insulin, glucagon and glucose levels. *Endocrinology* 98:819–822, 1976.

Brown, M., Villarreal, J., and Vale, W.: Neurotensin and substance-P: effects on plasma insulin and glucagon levels. *Metabolism* 25:1459–1461, 1976.

Bryant, M. G., Polak, J. M., et al.: Possible dual role for vasoactive intestinal peptide as gastrointestinal hormone and neurotransmitter substance. *Lancet* 1:991–993, 1976.

Buchan, A. M. J., Polak, J. M., et al.: Neurotensin in the gut, In *Gut Hormones*. Bloom, S. R., (ed.), Edinburgh, Churchill Livingstone, 1978, pp. 544–549.

Buffa, R., Polak, J. M., et al.: Identification of the intestinal cells storing gastric inhibitory peptide. *Histochemistry* 43:249–255, 1975.

Buffa, R., Solcia, E., and Go, V. L. W.: Immunohistochemical identification of the cholecystokinin cell in the intestinal mucosa. *Gastroenterology* 70:528, 1976.

Burland, W. L., and Mills, J. G.: Histamine, H_2-receptor blockade and treatment of duodenal ulcer, In *Gut Hormones*. Bloom, S. R. (ed.), Edinburgh, Churchill Livingstone, 1978, p. 638.

Carraway, R. E., Demers, L. M., and Leeman, S. E.: Hyperglycemic effect of neurotensin, a hypothalamic peptide. *Endocrinology* 99:1452–1462, 1976.

Carraway, R., Kitabgi, P., and Leeman, S. E.: The amino acid sequence of radioimmunoassayable neurotensin from bovine intestine. *J. Biol. Chem.* 253:7996–7998, 1978.

Carraway, R., and Leeman, S. E.: The isolation of a new hypotensive peptide, neurotensin, from bovine hypothalami. *J. Biol. Chem.* 218:6854–6861, 1973.

Carraway, R., and Leeman, S. E.: Characterization of radioimmunoassayable neurotensin in the rat. *J. Biol. Chem.* 251:7045–7052, 1976.

Cataland, S., Crockett, S. E., et al.: Gastric inhibitory polypeptide (GIP) stimulation of oral glucose in man. *J. Clin. Endocrinol. Metab.* 39:233–228, 1974.

Cataland, S., O'Dorisio, T. M., et al.: Stimulation of gastric inhibitory polypeptide in normal and duodenal ulcer patients. *Gastroenterology* 73:19–22, 1977.

Cecchettin, M., Albertini, A., et al.: Calcitonin, parathyroid hormone and insulin concentrations in sera from patients with gastrinoma, In *Gastrointestinal Hormones and Pathology of the Digestive System*. Grossman, M., Speranza, V., et al. (eds.), New York, Plenum Press, 1978, p. 117.

Chang, M. M., and Leeman, S. E.: Amino-acid sequence of substance P. *Nature (New Biol.)* 232:86–87, 1971.

Chan-Palay, V., et al.: Serotonin and substance P coexist in neurons of the rat's central nervous system. *Proc. Natl. Acad. Sci. USA* 75:1582, 1978.

Chayvialle, J. A. P., Descos, F., et al.: Somatostatin in mucosa of stomach and duodenum in gastroduodenal disease. *Gastroenterology* 75:13, 1978.

Christofides, N. D., Bloom, S. R., and Besterman, H. S.: Physiology of motilin II, In *Gut Hormones*. Bloom, S. R., (ed.), Edinburgh, Churchill Livingstone, 1978, pp. 343–350.

Code, C. F.: Reflections of histamine, gastric secretion and the H_2 receptor. *Medical Intelligence* 296:1459, 1977.

Colmenares, J. L., and Wurtman, R. J.: The relation between urinary 5-hydroxyindoleacetic acid levels and the ratio of tryptophan to other large neutral amino acids placed in the stomach. *Metabolism* 28:820, 1979.

Conlon, J. M., Samson, W. K., et al.: Glucagon-like polypeptides in canine brain. *Diabetes* 28:700–702, 1979.

Creutzfeldt, W.: The incretin concept today. *Diabetologia* 16:75–85, 1979.

Creutzfeldt, W., and Arnold, R.: Somatostatin and the stomach: Exocrine and endocrine aspects. *Metabolism* 27:1309, 1979.

Creutzfeldt, W., Ebert, R., et al.: Gastric inhibitory polypeptide (GIP), gastrin and insulin: response to test meal in coeliac disease and after duodenopancreatectomy. *Diabetologia* 12:279–286, 1976.

Dockray, G. J.: Evolutionary relationships of the gut hormones. *Fed. Proc.* 38:2295, 1979.

Dolais-Kitabgi, J., Kitabgi, P., et al.: Effect of neurotensin on insulin, glucagon, and somatostatin release from isolated pancreatic islets. *Endocrinology* 105:256–260, 1979.

Domschke, S., Domschke, W., et al.: Pharmacokinetics and pharmacodynamics of VIP in man, In *Gut Hormones*. Bloom, S. R. (ed.), Edinburgh, Churchill Livingstone, 1978, pp. 475–478.

Ebert, R., and Creutzfeldt, W.: Aspects of GIP pathology, In *Gut Hormones*. Bloom, S. R., (ed.), Edinburgh, Churchill Livingstone, 1978, pp. 294–300.

Ebert, R., Illmer, K., and Creutzfeldt, W.: Release of gastric inhibitory polypeptide (GIP) by intraduodenal acidification in rats and humans and abolishment of the incretin effect of acid by GIP-antiserum in rats. *Gastroenterology* 76:515–523, 1979.

Erspamer, V., and Melchiorri, P.: Active polypeptides of the amphibian skin and their synthetic analogues. *Pure Appl. Chem.* 35:463, 1973.

Falko, J. M., Crockett, S. E., et al.: Gastric inhibitory polypeptide (GIP) stimulated by fat ingestion in man. *J. Clin. Endocrinol. Metab.* 41:260–265, 1975.

Floyd, J. C., Jr., Fajans, S. S., et al.: A newly recognized pancreatic polypeptide; plasma levels in health and disease. *Recent Prog. Horm. Res.* 33:519–570, 1977.

Frame, C. M.: The contribution of the distal gastrointestinal tract to glucagonlike immunoreactivity secretion in the rat. *Proc. Soc. Exper. Biol. Med.* 152:667–670, 1976.

Frame, C. M., Davidson, M. B., and Sturdevant, R. A. L.: Effects of the octapeptide of cholecystokinin on insulin and glucagon secretion in the dog. *Endocrinology* 97:549, 1976.

Fujimoto, W. Y., Ensinck, J. W., et al.: Stimulation by gastric inhibitory polypeptide of insulin and glucagon secretion by rat islet cultures (39997). *Proc. Soc. Exper. Biol. Med.* 157:89–93, 1978.

Fujimoto, W. Y., Williams, R. H., and Ensinck, J. W.: Gastric inhibitory polypeptide, cholecystokinin, and secretin effects on insulin and glucagon secretion by islet cultures. *Proc. Soc. Exp. Biol. Med.* 160:349, 1979.

Fujita, T., and Kobayashi, S.: Paraneuronal cells in the GEP endocrine system, In *Gut Hormones*. Bloom, S. R. (ed.), Edinburgh, Churchill Livingstone, 1978, pp. 414–433.

Fuxe, K., Hökfelt, T., et al.: Vasoactive intestinal polypeptide and the nervous system: immunohistochemical evidence for localization in central and peripheral neurons, particularly intracortical neurons of the cerebral cortex. *Neuroscience Letters* 5:241–246, 1977.

Gagel, R. F., Costanza, M. E., et al.: Streptozocin-treated Verner-Morrison syndrome: plasma vasoactive intestinal peptide and tumor responses. *Arch. Intern. Med.* 136:1429–1435, 1976.

Ganda, O. P., Weir, G. C., et al.: "Somatostatinoma": A somatostatin-containing tumor of the endocrine pancreas. *New Eng. J. Med.* 296:963, 1977.

Gepts, W., Baetens, D., and De Mey, J.: The PP cell, In *Gut Hormones*. Bloom, S. R. (ed.), Edinburgh, Churchill Livinstone, 1978, pp. 229–233.

Go, V. L. W.: The physiology of cholecystokinin, In *Gut Hormones*. Bloom, S. R. (ed.), Edinburgh, Churchill Livingstone, 1978, p. 203.

Goyal, R. K.: Neurology of the gut, In *Gastrointestinal Disease*. 2nd ed. Sleisenger, M. H., and Fordtran, J. S. (eds.), Philadelphia, W. B. Saunders Co., 1978, pp. 156–178.

Greenberg, G. R., Adrian, T. E., et al.: Inhibition of pancreas and gallbladder by pancreatic polypeptide. *Lancet* 2:1280–1282, 1978.

Gregory, R. A.: The gastrins: Structure and heterogeneity, In *Gastrointestinal Hormones and Pathology of the Digestive System*. Grossman, M., Speranza, V., et al. (eds.), New York, Plenum Press, 1978, p. 75.

Grossman, M. I.: Neural and hormonal regulation of gastrointestinal function: an overview. *Ann. Rev. Physiol.* 41:27–33, 1979.

Grube, D., and Forssmann, W. G.: Morphology and function of the enteroendocrine cells. *Horm. Metab. Res.* 11:589–606, 1979.

Grube, D., Maier, V., et al.: Immunoreactivity of the endocrine pancreas. Evidence for the presence of cholecystokinin-pancreozymin within the A-cell. *Histochemistry* 56:13, 1978.

Gullner, H-G., Campbell, W. B., and Pettinger, W. A.: Effects of substance P on renin release and renal function in anesthetized dogs. *Life Sci.* 24:237–246, 1979.

Häcki, W. H., Greenberg, G. R., and Bloom, S. R.: Role of secretin in man I, In *Gut Hormones*. Bloom, S. R. (ed.), Edinburgh, Churchill Livingstone, 1978, pp. 182–192.

Hall, R., and Gomez-Pan, A.: The hypothalamic regulatory hormones and their clinical applications, In *Advances in Clinical Chemistry*. Vol. 18. Bodansky, O., and Latner, A. L. (eds.), New York, Academic Press, 1976, p. 189.

Hammer, R. A., Carraway, R., et al.: Isolation of human intestinal neurotensin (NT). *Gastroenterology* 76:1150, 1979.

Harper, A. A., and Raper, H. S.: Pancreozymin, a stimulant of the secretion of pancreatic enzymes in extracts of the small intestine. *J. Physiol.* 102:115–125, 1943.

Harvey, R. F.: Pathology of cholecystokinin in man, In *Gut Hormones*. Bloom, S. R. (ed.), Edinburgh, Churchill Livingstone, 1978, p. 219.

Hayes, J. R., Johnson, D. G., Koerker, D., and Williams, R. H.: Inhibition of gastrin release by somatostatin *in vitro*. *Endocrinology* 96:1374, 1975.

Hökfelt, T., Efendic, S., et al.: Cellular localization of somatostatin in endocrine-like cells and neurons of the rat with special references to the A_1-cells of the pancreatic islets and to the hypothalamus. *Acta Endocrinol.* Suppl. 200, 1975.

Hökfelt, T., Schultzberg, M., et al.: Central and peripheral peptide producing neurons, In *Gut Hormones*. Bloom, S. R. (ed.), Edinburgh, Churchill Livingstone, 1978, pp. 423–433.

Holst, J. J.: Physiology of enteric glucagon-like substances, In *Gut Hormones*. Bloom, S. R. (ed.), Edinburgh, Churchill Livingstone, 1978, pp. 383–386.

Impicciatore, M., Walsh, J. H., and Grossman, M. I.: Low doses of atropine enhance serum gastrin response to food in dogs. *Gastroenterology* 72:995–996, 1977.

Ipp, E., Dobbs, R. E., et al.: The effects of gastrin, gastric inhibitory polypeptide, secretin, and the octapeptide of cholecystokinin upon immunoreactive somatostatin release by the perfused canine pancreas. *J. Clin. Invest.* 60:1216, 1977.

Itoh, Z., Takeuchi, S., et al.: Recent advances in motilin research: its physiological and clinical significance, In *Gastrointestinal Hormones and Pathology of the Digestive System*. Grossman, M., Speranza, V., et al. (eds.), New York, Plenum Press, 1978.

Ivy, A. C., and Oldberg, E.: A hormone mechanism for gall-bladder contraction and evacuation. *Am. J. Physiol.* 86:599–613, 1928.

Jaffe, B. M.: Prostaglandins and serotonin in diarrheogenic syndromes. *Adv. Exp. Med. Biol.* 106:285, 1978.

Jaffe, B. M., and Condon, S.: Prostaglandins E and F in endocrine diarrheagenic syndromes. *Ann. Surg.* 184:516–524, 1976.

Jaffe, B. M., Kellum, J. M., et al.: Release and physiologic action of serotonin, In *Gut Hormones*. Bloom, S. R. (ed.), Edinburgh, Churchill Livingstone, 1978, pp. 515–523.

Jaffe, B. M., Kopen, D. F., et al.: Indomethacin-sensitive pancreatic cholera. *N. Engl. J. Med.* 297:817–821, 1977.

Johnson, L. R.: New aspects of the trophic action of gastrointestinal hormones. *Gastroenterology* 72:788, 1977.

Jorpes, J. E.: Memorial lecture: the isolation and chemistry of secretin and cholecystokinin. *Gastroenterology* 55:157–164, 1968.

Kolts, B. E., and McGuigan, J. E.: Radioimmunoassay measurement of secretin half-life in man. *Gastroenterology* 72:55–60, 1977.

Konturek, S. J.: Somatostatin and gastrointestinal secretion and motility, In *Gastrointestinal Hormones and Pathology of the Digestive System*. Grossman, M., Speranza, V., et al. (eds.), New York, Plenum Press, 1978, p. 227.

Konturek, S. J., Pawlik, W., et al.: Effects of enkephalin on the gastrointestinal tract, In *Gut Hormones*. Bloom, S. R. (ed.), Edinburgh, Churchill Livingstone, 1978, pp. 507–512.

Larsson, L.-I.: Corticotropin-like peptides in central nerves and in endocrine cells of gut and pancreas. *Lancet* 2:1321–1323, 1977.

Larsson, L.-I., Fahrenkrug, J., et al.: Innervation of the pancreas by vasoactive intestinal polypeptide (VIP) immunoreactive nerves. *Life Sci.* 22:773–780, 1978.

Larsson, L.-I., Holst, J. J., et al.: Pancreatic somatostatinoma: Clinical features and physiological implications. *Lancet* 1:666, 1977.

Leeman, S. E., and Mroz, E. A.: Minireview: Substance P. *Life Sci.* 15:2033–2044, 1974.

Lin, T.-M., and Chance, R. E.: Spectrum of gastrointestinal actions of bovine PP, In *Gut Hormones*. Bloom, S. R. (ed.), Edinburgh, Churchill Livingstone, 1978, pp. 242–246.

Lin, T.-M., Evans, D. C., et al.: Bovine pancreatic peptide: action on gastric and pancreatic secretion in dogs. *Am. J. Physiol.* 232:E311–E315, 1977.

Luft, R., Efendic, S., and Hökfelt, T.: Somatostatin — both hormone and neurotransmitter? *Diabetologia* 14:1, 1978.

Lundbaek, K.: Somatostatin: Clinical importance and outlook. *Metabolism* 27:1463, 1978.

Lundberg, J. M., Hökfelt, T., et al.: Peptide neurons in the vagus, splanchnic and sciatic nerves. *Acta Physiol. Scand.* 104:499–501, 1978.

Malick, J. B., and Goldstein, J. M.: Analgesic activity of substance P following intracerebral administration in rats. *Life Sci.* 23:835–844, 1978.

May, J. M., and Williams, R. H.: The effect of endogenous gastric inhibitory polypeptide on glucose-induced insulin secretion in mild diabetes. *Diabetes* 27:849–855, 1978.

McCrossan, M. V., Polak, J. M., et al.: Duodenal bombesin cell pathology. *Gut* 18:A410, 1977.

McGuigan, J. E.: The Zollinger-Ellison syndrome, In *Gastrointestinal Disease.* 2nd ed. Sleisenger, M. H., and Fordtran, J. S. (eds.), Philadelphia, W. B. Saunders Co., 1978, p. 860.

McIntosh, C., Arnold, R., et al.: Gastrointestinal somatostatin in man and dog. *Metabolism* 27:1317, 1978.

McIntyre, N., Holdsworth, C. D., and Turner, D. S.: New interpretation of oral glucose tolerance. *Lancet* 2:20–21, 1964.

Melchiorri, P.: Bombesin and bombesin-like peptides of amphibian skin, In *Gut Hormones.* Bloom, S. R. (ed.), Edinburgh, Churchill Livingstone, 1978, pp. 534–540.

Milutinovic, S., Schulz, I., and Rosselin, G.: The interaction of secretin with pancreatic membranes. *Biochim. Biophys. Acta* 436:113–127, 1976.

Modlin, I. M., Mitchell, S. J., and Bloom, S. R.: The systemic release and pharmacokinetics of VIP, In *Gut Hormones.* Bloom, S. R. (ed.), Edinburgh, Churchill Livingstone, 1978, pp. 470–474.

Moody, A. J., Jacobsen, H., and Sundby, F.: Gastric glucagon and gut glucagon-like immunoreactants, In *Gut Hormones.* Bloom, S. R. (ed.), Edinburgh, Churchill Livingstone, 1978, pp. 369–378.

Moore, B., Edie, E. S., and Abram, J. H.: On the treatment of diabetes mellitus by acid extract of duodenal mucous membrane. *Biochem. J.* 1:28–38, 1906.

Morgan, K. G., Schmalz, P. F., et al.: Electrical and mechanical effects of molecular variants of CCK on antral smooth muscle. *Am. J. Physiol.* 4:E324, 1978.

Mroz, E. A., and Leeman, S. E.: Substance P. *Vitam. Horm.* 35:209–281, 1977.

Nagai, K., and Frohman, L. A.: Neurotensin hyperglycemia: evidence for histamine mediation and the assessment of a possible physiologic role. *Diabetes* 27:577–582, 1978.

Nakata, Y., Kusaka, Y., et al.: Substance P.: regional distribution and specific binding to synaptic membranes in rabbit central nervous system. *Life Sci.* 22:259–268, 1978.

O'Dorisio, T. M., Sirinek, K. R., et al.: Renal effects on serum gastric inhibitory polypeptide (GIP). *Metabolism* 26:651–656, 1977.

Osumi, Y., Nagasaka, Y., et al.: Inhibition of gastric acid secretion and mucosal blood flow induced by intraventricularly applied neurotensin in rats. *Life Sci.* 23:2275–2280, 1978.

Owman, C., Hakanson, R., and Sundler, F.: Occurrence and function of amines in endocrine cells producing polypeptide hormones. *Fed Proc.* 32:1785–1791, 1973.

Pearse, A. G. E., and Polak, J. M.: The diffuse neuroendocrine system and the APUD concept, In *Gut Hormones.* Bloom, S. R. (ed.), Edinburgh, Churchill Livingstone, 1978, pp. 33–39.

Pearse, A. G. E., Polak, J. M., and Bloom, S. R.: The newer gut hormones: cellular sources, physiology, pathology and clinical aspects. *Gastroenterology* 72:746–761, 1977.

Pearse, A. G. E., and Takor, T. T.: Embryology of the diffuse neuroendocrine system and its relationship to the common peptides. *Fed. Proc.* 38:2288–2294, 1979.

Pederson, R. A., and Brown, J. C.: Interaction of gastric inhibitory polypeptide, glucose, and arginine on insulin and glucagon secretion from the perfused rat pancreas. *Endocrinology* 103:610–615, 1978.

Pederson, R. A., Schubert, H. E., and Brown, J. C.: Gastric inhibitory polypeptide: its physiologic release and insulinotropic action in the dog. *Diabetes* 24:1050–1056, 1975.

Polak, J. M., Bishop, A. E., and Bloom, S. R.: Peptidergic neurones as the main autonomic innervation of the gut. *Gastroenterology* 74:1080, 1978.

Polak, J. M., Bloom, S., et al.: Immunofluorescent localization of secretin in the canine duodenum. *Gut* 12:605–610, 1971.

Polak, J. M., Bloom, S. R., et al.: Cellular localization of gastric inhibitory polypeptide in the duodenum and jejunum. *Gut* 14:284–288, 1973.

Polak, J. M., Bloom, S. R., et al.: Identification of cholecystokinin-secreting cells. *Lancet* 2:1016, 1975.

Polak, J. M., Buchan, A. M. J., et al.: Bombesin in the gut, In *Gut Hormones.* Bloom, S. R. (ed.), Edinburgh, Churchill Livingstone, 1978, pp. 541–543.

Polak, J. M., Hobbs, S., et al.: Distribution of a bombesin-like peptide in human gastrointestinal tract. *Lancet* 1:1109–1110, 1976.

Powell, D., Cannon, D., et al.: The pathophysiology of substance P in man, In *Gut Hormones.* Bloom, S. R. (ed.), Edinburgh, Churchill Livingstone, 1978, pp. 524–529.

Rayford, P. L., Miller, T. A., and Thompson, J. C.: Secretin, cholecystokinin and newer gastrointestinal hormones. *New Eng. J. Med.* 294:1093–1101, 1976a.

Rayford, P. L., Miller, T. A., and Thompson, J. C.: Secretin, cholecystokinin, and newer gastrointestinal hormones. *New Eng. J. Med.* 294:1157–1163, 1976b.

Rehfeld, J. F.: Immunochemical studies on cholecystokinin: II. Distribution and molecular heterogeneity in the central nervous system and small intestine of man and hog. *J. Biol. Chem.* 253:4022, 1978.

Rehfeld, J. F., Stadil, F., Malmstrom, J., and Miyata, M.: Gastrin heterogeneity in serum and tissue: A progress report, In *Gastrointestinal Hormones.* Thompson, J. C. (ed.), Austin, University of Texas Press, 1975, p. 43.

Reynolds, C., Tronsgard, N., et al.: Gastric inhibitory polypeptide response to hyper- and hypoglycemia in insulin-dependent diabetics. *J. Clin. Endocrinol. Metab.* 49:255–261, 1979.

Said, S. I., and Faloona, G. R.: Elevated plasma and tissue levels of vasoactive intestinal polypeptide in the watery diarrhea syndrome due to pancreatic, bronchogenic and other tumors. *N. Engl. J. Med.* 294:155–160, 1975.

Said, S. I., and Mutt, V.: Isolation from porcine-intestinal wall of a vasoactive octacosapeptide related to secretin and to glucagon. *Eur. J. Biochem.* 28:199–204, 1972.

Said, S. I., and Porter, J. C.: Vasoactive intestinal polypeptide: release into hypophyseal portal blood. *Life Sci.* 24:227–230, 1979.

Schafmayer, A., Teichmann, R. K., et al.: Physiologic release of secretin measured in peripheral and portal venous blood of dogs. *Digestion* 17:509–515, 1978.

Schally, A. V., Coy, D. H., and Meyers, C. A.: Hypothalamic regulatory hormones: somatostatin. *Ann. Rev. Biochem.* 47:89–128, 1978.

Schatz, H., Otto, J., et al.: Gastrointestinal hormones and function of pancreatic islets: Studies on insulin secretion, ³H-leucine incorporation and intracellular free lucine pool in isolated pancreatic mouse islets. *Endocrinol.* 94:248, 1974.

Schusdziarra, V., Harris, V., et al.: Evidence for a role of splanchnic somatostatin in the homeostasis of ingested nutrients. *Endocrinology* 104:1705, 1979.

Schusdziarra, V., Harris, V., et al.: Pancreatic and gastric somatostatin release in response to intragastric and intraduodenal nutrients and HCl in the dog. *J. Clin. Invest.* 62:509, 1978a.

Schusdziarra, V., Rouiller, D., et al.: The response of plasma somatostatin-like immunoreactivity to nutrients in normal and alloxan diabetic dogs. *Endocrinology* 103:2264, 1978b.

Schusdziarra, V., Zyznar, E., and Rouiller, D.: Splanchnic somatostatin: a hormonal regulator of nutrient homeostasis. *Science* 207:530–532, 1980.

Schwartz, C. J., Kimberg, D. V., et al.: Vasoactive intestinal peptide stimulation of adenylate cyclase and active electrolyte secretion in intestinal mucosa. *J. Clin. Invest.* 54:536–544, 1974.

Schwartz, J.-C.: Histamine as a transmitter in brain. *Life Sci.* 17:503–518, 1975.

Schwartz, T. W., Holst, J. J., et al.: Vagal, cholinergic regulation of pancreatic polypeptide secretion. *J. Clin. Invest.* 61:781–789, 1978.

Schwartz, T. W., Stadil, F., et al.: Pancreatic-polypeptide response to food in duodenal-ulcer patients before and after vagotomy. *Lancet* 1:1102–1105, 1976.

Sheppard, M., Shapiro, B., et al.: Metabolic clearance and plasma half-disappearance time of exogenous somatostatin in man. *J. Clin. Endocrinol. Metab.* 48:50, 1979.

Sirinek, K. R., Cataland, S., et al.: Augmented gastric inhibitory polypeptide response to intraduodenal glucose by exogenous gastrin and cholecystokinin. *Surgery* 82:438–442, 1977.

Sive, A., Vinik, A., et al.: Impaired pancreatic polypeptide secretion in chronic pancreatitis. *J. Clin. Endocrinol. Metab.* 47:556–559, 1978.

Solcia, E., Capella, C., et al.: Endocrine cells of the gut and related growths: recent developments and classification, In *Gut Hormones.* Bloom, S. R. (ed.), Edinburgh, Churchill Livingstone, 1978, pp. 77–81.

Soll, A. H., and Walsh, J. H.: Regulation of gastric acid secretion. *Ann. Rev. Physiol.* 41:35, 1979.

Stewart, J. J., and Burks, T. F.: Actions of cholecystokinin octapeptide on smooth muscle of isolated dog intestine. *Am. J. Physiol.* 232:E306–E310, 1977.

Straus, E., Muller, J. E., et al.: Immunohistochemical localization in rabbit brain of a peptide resembling the COOH-terminal octapeptide of cholecystokinin. *Proc. Natl. Acad. Sci. USA* 74:3033, 1977.

Sundby, F., Jacobsen, H., and Moody, A. J.: Purification and characterization of a protein from porcine gut with glucagon-like immunoreactivity. *Horm. Metab. Res.* 8:366, 1976.

Tagliamonte, A., et al.: Free tryptophan in serum controls brain tryptophan level and serotonin synthesis. *Life Sci.* 12:277, 1973.

Taminato, T., Seino, Y., et al.: Interaction of somatostatin and calcium in regulating insulin release from isolated pancreatic islets of rats. *Biochem. Biophys. Res. Commun.* 66:928, 1975.

Taylor, I. L., Impicciatore, M., et al.: Effect of atropine and vagotomy on pancreatic polypeptide response to a meal in dogs. *Am. J. Physiol.* 235:E443–E447, 1978.

Taylor, I. L., Solomon, T. E., et al.: Pancreatic polypeptide: metabolism and effect on pancreatic secretion in dogs. *Gastroenterology* 76:524–528, 1979.

Thomas, F. B., Shook, D. F., et al.: Localization of gastric inhibitory polypeptide release by intestinal glucose perfusion in man. *Gastroenterology* 72:49–54, 1977.

Tomkins, G. M.: The metabolic code. *Science* 189:760–763, 1975.

Track, N. S., Collins, S., et al.: Motilin release and upper gastrointestinal motility in man, In *Gut Hormones.* Bloom, S. R. (ed.), Edinburgh, Churchill Livingstone, 1978, pp. 351–354.

Unger, R. H., Eisentraut, A. M., et al.: Site of origin of glucagon in dogs and humans. *Clin. Res.* 9:53, 1961.

Uvnäs-Wallensten, K.: Vagal release of antral hormones, In *Gut Hormones*. Bloom, S. R. (ed.), Edinburgh, Churchill Livingstone, 1978, pp. 389–393.

Uvnäs-Wallensten, K., Efendic, S., and Luft, R.: Vagal release of somatostatin into the antral lumen of cats. *Acta Physiol. Scand. 99*:126, 1977.

Vermillion, D. L., et al.: Des 5-hydroxytryptamine influence "purinergic" inhibitory neurons in the intestine? *Am. J. Physiol. 6*:E198, 1979.

Von Euler, U. S., and Gaddum, J. H.: An unidentified depressor substance in certain tissue extracts. *J. Physiol. (Lond.) 72*:74–87, 1931.

Walsh, J. H.: Gastrointestinal peptide hormones and other biologically active peptides, In *Gastrointestinal Disease*. 2nd ed. Sleisenger, M. H., and Fordtran, J. S. (eds.), Philadelphia, W. B. Saunders Co., 1978, pp. 107–155.

Williams, R. H., and Biesbroeck, J.: Effects of single food components on plasma gastric inhibitory polypeptide (GIP), insulin (IRI), and glucose. *Diabetes 26*:374, 1977.

Wollheim, C. B., Kikuchi, M., et al.: Somatostatin- and epinephrine-induced modifications of $^{45}Ca^{++}$ fluxes and insulin release in rat pancreatic islets maintained in tissue culture. *J. Clin. Invest. 60*:1165, 1977.

Woods, S. C., and Porte, D., Jr.: Neural control of the endocrine pancreas. *Physiol. Rev. 54*:596, 1974.

Woods, S. C., and Porte, D., Jr.: The central nervous system, pancreatic hormones, feeding, and obesity. *Adv. Metab. Disord. 9*:283, 1978.

Yanaihara, N., Sakagami, M., et al.: Immunological aspects of secretin, substance P, and VIP. *Gastroenterology 72*:803–810, 1977.

Yanaihara, C., Sato, H., et al.: Motilin-, substance P- and somatostatin-like immunoreactivities in extracts from dog, tupaia and monkey brain and GI tract, in *Gastrointestinal Hormones and Pathology of the Digestive System*. Grossman, M., Speranza, V., et al. (eds.), New York, Plenum Press, 1978, p. 269.

Yau, W. M.: Effect of substance P on intestinal muscle. *Gastroenterology 74*:228–231, 1978.

CHAPTER 15

The Endocrine Pancreas and Diabetes Mellitus

By Daniel Porte, Jr.,
and Jeffrey B. Halter

The exocrine pancreas plays an important role in gastrointestinal function, but it is the endocrine islets which influence metabolism thoughout the body by the actions of insulin and glucagon. The endocrine role of the pancreas was first recognized in 1886 when Minkowski and Von Mering produced diabetes by total pancreatectomy in the dog. This observation occurred 35 years before Banting and Best isolated insulin and 70 years before Sanger demonstrated its amino acid sequence. The chemical synthesis of insulin was reported by Meienhofer in 1963 and Katsoyannis in 1964. In 1967, Steiner discovered that insulin was synthesized as a larger precursor which he called proinsulin. Most recently, Hodgkin reported the three-dimensional structure of insulin.

Diabetes mellitus is the common disease associated with abnormal function of the pancreatic islets; presumably more than 10 million people in the United States are affected. The highest incidence has been reported in Pima Indians; 50% of the group were found by Bennett to have diabetes. This disorder is the fifth leading health-related cause of death in the United States. More than 50% of diabetics die because of coronary heart disease; renal failure is the cause of death of many insulin-dependent diabetics. Diabetes is the second commonest cause of blindness. Its other frequent complications are cerebrovascular disorders, gangrene of the legs, and neuropathy. The total annual costs for the disease in the United States are estimated to be at least 2 billion dollars, including medical care and loss of compensation for work. Much remains to be learned with respect to the etiology and pathogenesis, and there is a great need for improved methods of diagnosis and treatment.

ISLET ANATOMY AND HISTOLOGY

The pancreas develops as dorsal and ventral buds from cells of the duodenal and hepatic diverticulum. From these buds some cells develop mitoses parallel in a plane perpendicular to the axis of the lumen, thereby disrupting tight junction complexes and separating these cells from their neighbors. As the cells further divide, this eventually leads to an accumulation of cells between the basal lamina of the exocrine tissue and the newly forming endocrine mass. Eventually, this mass buds and forms a primitive islet which is distinct from the ductal cells left behind.

The origin of the endocrine cells contained within the primitive pancreatic ducts is still debated. The traditional point of view (Fig. 15–1) suggests derivation from endoderm just as the ductal and acinar cells are derived from the primitive gut. In 1969, Pearse challenged this concept and suggested that the islets originate from neuroectoderm. His evidence focused on a common enzymatic characteristic of polypeptide-secreting endocrine cells to simultaneously synthesize amines from common precursors. Therefore, he classified them as belonging to the APUD (*A*mine *P*recursor *U*ptake and *D*ecarboxylation) series. Pearse has further suggested that all cells having this property arise from the neural crest. While some cells derived from this tissue are known to produce and secrete amines as their primary function (e.g., adrenal medullary cells), he suggests that many endocrine cells secreting peptides still retain the ability to convert specific precursor molecules to their corresponding biogenic amine. Two examples are the conversion of dihydroxyphenylalanine (DOPA) to dopamine and of 5-hydroxytryptophan (5-HTP) to serotonin. In experiments using fetal mouse pancreas, he observed "clear cells"

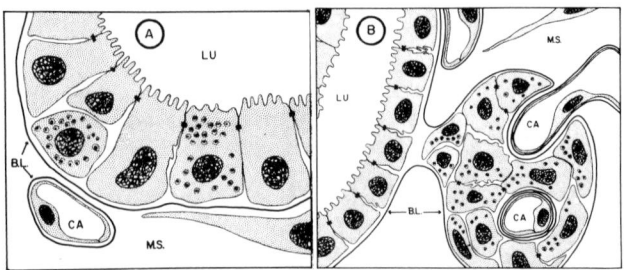

Figure 15–1. Hypothesis for the histiogenesis of the endocrine pancreas. It is suggested that islets are formed by an inversion of the polarity of the axis of cell division. *A*, The axis of division is parallel to the apical-basal cell axis. The consequence of this division is that one of the two daughter cells is no longer joined to its neighbors by junctional complexes. The presence of a few cells containing endocrine gland granules and still facing a lumen indicates that the position is not a regulation in itself. *B*, Repetition of this process leads to an accumulation of endocrine cells between the exocrine cells in the basal lamina. The basal lamina surrounding the newly formed islet can eventually fuse at the origin of the outpocketing, thus separating the intercellular spaces of the endocrine and exocrine cells. At the same time, islets are penetrated by lumen *(LU)*, capillaries *(CA)*, mesenchymal spaces *(M.S.)*, and basal lamina *(B.L.)*. (From Pictet, R. L., and Rutter, W. J.: Development of the embryonic endocrine pancreas. In *Handbook of Physiology*, Section 7: Endocrinology, Vol. 1: *Endocrine Pancreas*. American Physiological Society. Field, J. (ed.), Baltimore, Williams and Wilkins, 1972, p. 41.)

without secretory granules displaying APUD characteristics which later contained typical insulin and glucagon secretory products. He suggests that at a very early stage of development, these cells migrate into the primitive gut and later form the peptide-secreting hormone cells of the gastrointestinal tract and pancreas.

Strong support has been developed for this concept with the discovery of somatostatin as a hormone of both the gut and the endocrine pancreas as well as of hypothalamic and other central nervous system neurons. Since removal of ectoderm from chick and mouse embryos prior to neural crest formation does *not* prevent the development of fully differentiated APUD cells in the gut and pancreatic islets, there is still some question about the hypothesis. However, it is likely that the explanation relates to ectodermal cells populating the endoderm prior to the formation of the neural crest and then migrating with the developing exocrine and ductal cells for the formation of the pancreatic islets in the fashion suggested by Pictet and Rutter. The APUD theory is also supported by the fact that some polypeptide-secreting endocrine cells of known ectodermal origin (e.g., thyroid C-cells) share common cytochemical characteristics with the APUD cells of the endocrine pancreas and gut.

In most species, the glucagon-containing A-cells can be recognized first during embryogenesis, followed by the D-cell and last by the B-cell. In man, A-cells can be recognized at 9 weeks, D-cells at 10 weeks, and B-cells at 11 weeks, but the hormone products themselves can be identified by immunoassay 2–3 weeks earlier. After the third month of gestation, the islets lose their connection with the duct system and remain separated by their own basal lamina from the basal lamina of the interspersed capillaries. Therefore, hormones must cross two basement membranes before they enter the bloodstream. There is an elaborate network of anastomosing capillaries in islets, providing a very rich vascular supply. Electron microscopic studies have shown that the endothelial cells of the capillaries are fenestrated, partly accounting for the rapid appearance of the islet hormones in the circulation after stimulation. Quantitative estimates of the number of islets have been variable. Counts have ranged from 100,000 to 2,500,000 islets in a total pancreas, making up

1–3% of total pancreatic mass. The tail of the pancreas contains more islets than the head. About the thirtieth week of gestation, the density of islets seems to be the greatest with 600–700 per mm², declining to about 130 per mm² at age 5 years. The great bulk of islets are between 100 and 225 μ in diameter, with a range from 50 to 300. After birth, the islets continue to enlarge in size with all cell types participating equally in this growth. In animal studies, the growth rate is proportional to body weight, and there is a linear relationship between the logarithm of body weight and total islet mass. Since the mean islet size increases with age, it would appear that a substantial portion of this growth is the enlargement of already established islets and not the formation of new islets. The source of these new cells is controversial. Replication rates of islet cells are extremely low in postnatal life. Nevertheless, mature cells have been observed to divide and may account for substantial portions of it. Whether the ductal cells or exocrine pancreatic cells can differentiate into islet cells remains a matter of contested conjecture. Polyploid nuclei have been observed in human pancreas, indicating nuclear replication without cell division. The importance of this phenomenon to islet cell mass and function has not been adequately evaluated.

In a normal man, the islets are composed of at least four types of cells: A-, B-, D-, and pancreatic polypeptide (? F-) cells (Figs. 15–2 and 15–3). A-cells secrete glucagon, and B-cells secrete insulin. D-cells contain and secrete so-

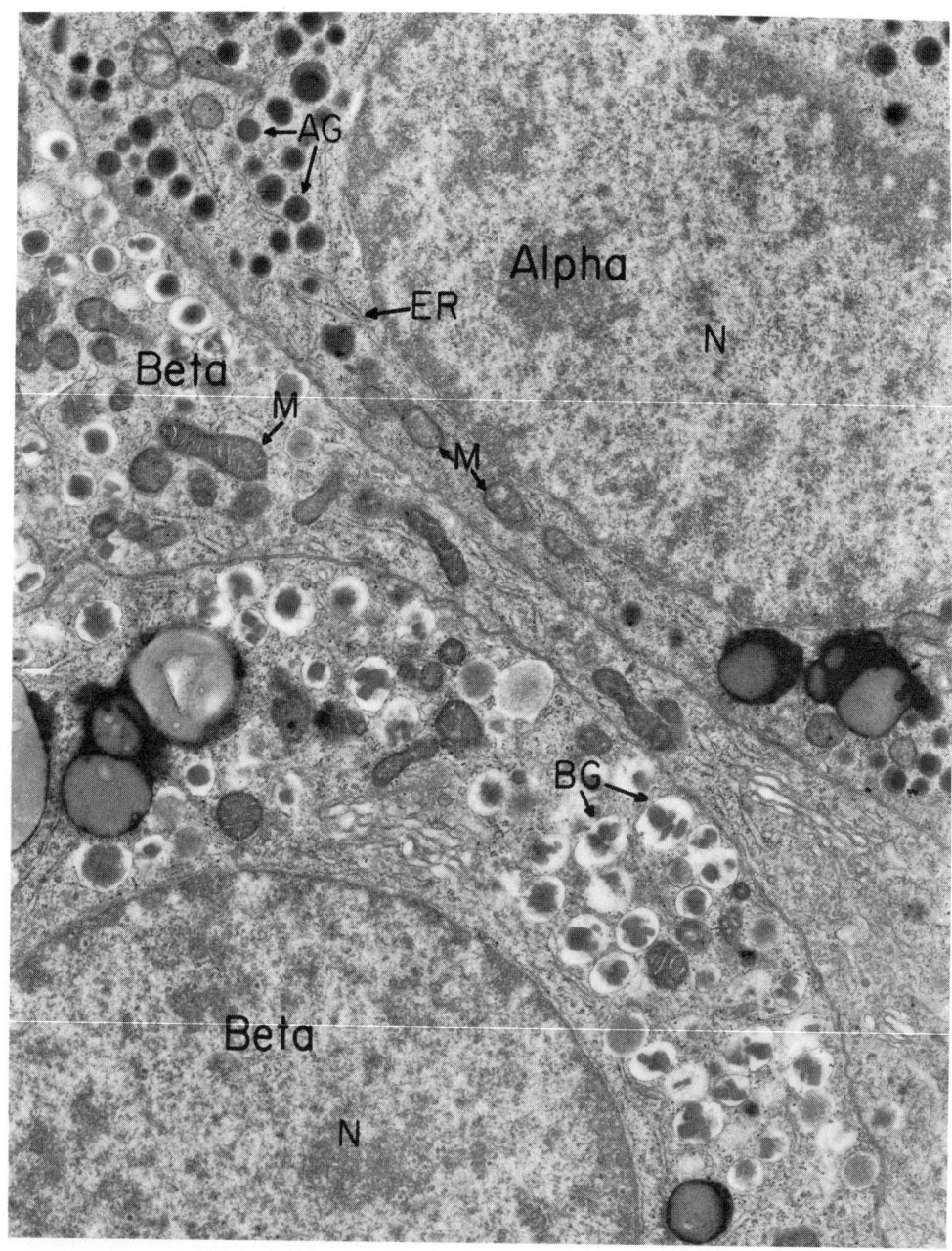

Figure 15–2. Electron micrographs of islets from a man aged 25. Portions of two beta cells are seen, with their characteristic granules *(BG)*, formed by one to four rhomboid crystals enclosed by a limiting membrane. In the alpha cells are round granules *(AG)* with dense center and pale periphery. Nuclei *(N)*, mitochondria *(M)*, and endoplasmic reticulum *(ER)* are noted. (× 17,000.)

matostatin; however, evidence has been presented that, at least in some species, they also contain material which interacts with an antibody for gastrin. There has also been immunoreactive GIP found immunocytochemically in A-cells. The meaning of this dual peptide content is not clear at present. The PP- or "F"-cell contains and secretes pancreatic polypeptide. This cell type is found interspersed in the exocrine pancreas as well. Other cell types have been reported, but they are few in number (less than 2%). In the rat, a reciprocal relation between the A- and F-cell content of individual islets has been found. The composition of islets varies from the head to the tail, with glucagon-rich islets in the tail and pancreatic polypeptide–rich islets in the head. The cytoplasm of all of these cells contains granular endoplasmic reticulum, ribosomes, polysomes, mitochondria, Golgi complex, secretion granules, microtubules, microfilaments, and cytosol.

The detailed fine structure of B-cells varies somewhat

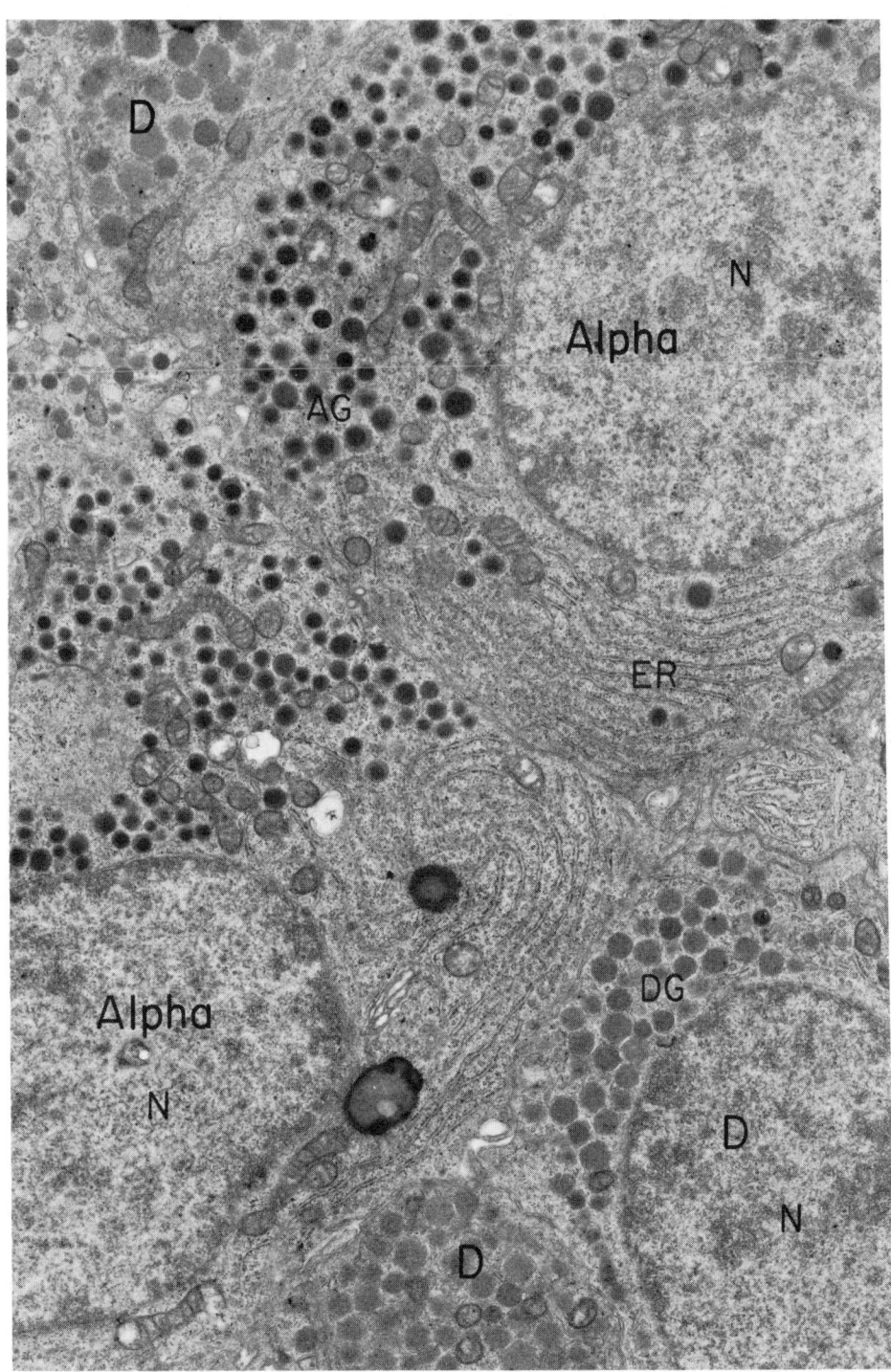

Figure 15–3.   Another part of the same islet shows two alpha cells and part of three D-cells. The D-cells contain numerous closely packed homogeneous granules *(DG)* of less density than the alpha cell granules. A limiting membrane is closely applied to all the granules. (× 14,000.) (Figs. 15–2 and 15–3 were kindly supplied by Dr. Felice Caramia.)

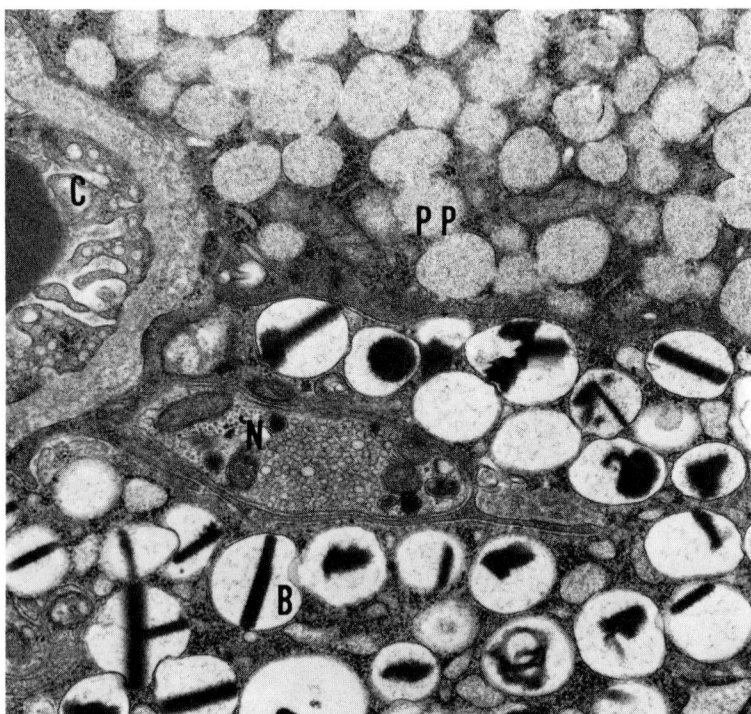

Figure 15–4. Nerve endings *(N)* in a dog pancreatic islet. Note proximity to a B-cell *(B)* and a pancreatic polypeptide cell *(PP)*. A capillary is adjacent *(C)*. (× 24,000.) (Courtesy of Phillip H. Smith, Ph.D.)

in the guinea pig, rabbit, rat, and dog, but the A-cells have a relatively uniform appearance in all of these species. A-cells differ from B-cells in that the concentration and density of the A-granules are greater and the Golgi complex is smaller. The A-cells have smaller granules and a more ovoid nucleus. The granules of the D-cells are less dense and more homogeneous than are the A- and B-granules. The F-cells or PP-cells contain very small granules which are scarce in number. They may be confused with D-cells or degranulated B-cells.

Nerve fibers and their termination on islet cells can be observed by light microscopy. Electron microscopy shows unmyelinated fibers closely applied to plasma membranes of islet cells (Fig. 15–4). Both sympathetic and parasympathetic nerve endings have been identified. These nerve endings are in close association with A-, B-, D-, and F-cells. These nerves function as part of the insulin, glucagon, somatostatin, and pancreatic polypeptide control system.

CHEMISTRY OF INSULIN AND INSULIN PRECURSORS

Proinsulin and Its Precursors

On the basis of physical-chemical principles, it was predicted about a decade ago that the bonds of insulin could form more efficiently by synthesizing disulfide A and B chains as integral parts of one long chain than by synthesizing the chains separately and then combining them. In 1967, Steiner and colleagues showed that insulin was formed from a large molecular weight, single-chain precursor, which they named proinsulin (Fig. 15–5). Subsequently, hormones of the pancreatic alpha cells, parathyroid glands, and pituitary gland have also been found to be formed from larger, biologically less active precursors by limited intracellular proteolysis.

In addition, a larger insulin precursor of about 11,500

daltons has been described. The translation of messenger RNA for insulin in cell-free systems has enabled sufficient synthesis of this material to identify it in the rat and hagfish. The extra amino acids are located exclusively at the amino terminus. There are 24 in the rat sequence. As has been found with other presecretory proteins, there are a large number of amino acids with hydrophobic side chains. It has been hypothesized that these are important for the binding of polysomes to the microsomal membrane in the synthesis of proinsulin. This protein, which has been called pre-proinsulin, is difficult to isolate in the intact cell because it is cleaved to proinsulin almost immediately after synthesis.

The complete structures of porcine and bovine proinsulins are known, and the structure of the nearly intact human connecting peptide segment is known. In these three species, approximately 50% of the connecting peptide (C-peptide) residues are variant (Fig. 15–6), in contrast to the low degree of variance in insulin. The connecting peptide of porcine proinsulin differs from that of bovine and human proinsulin by 12 and 10 residues, respectively. Bovine C-peptide has 26, porcine C-peptide 29, and human C-peptide 31 residues. All three peptides have two glutamic acids very near the amino-terminal region — one glutamic acid located four residues from the carboxyl end and an additional glutamic acid residue located about a third of the way along the peptide chain. This distribution suggests that these residues may interact with specific side chains in the insulin portion of the proinsulin molecule to direct the folding of the peptide chain in a specific manner. Preliminary studies of the monkey C-peptide indicate that it is identical to the human C-peptide except for a single substitution of Pro for Leu at position 5.

Human proinsulin contains four additional basic residues (one Lys, three Arg) not accounted for by the composition of either the insulin or the C-peptide portions of the molecule. It is probable that these residues are arranged in human proinsulin, as they are in bovine and porcine

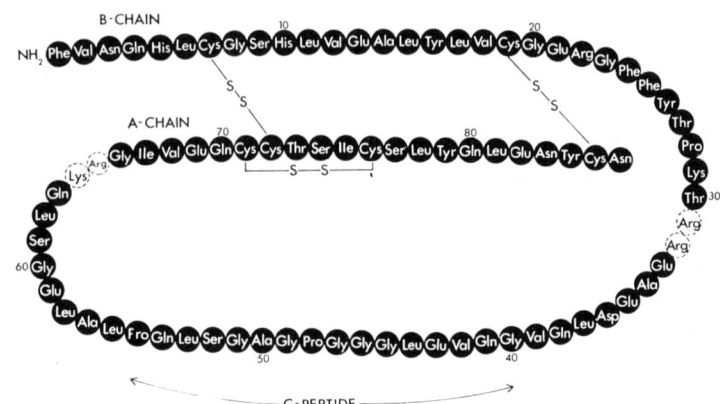

Figure 15–5. Proposed primary structure of human proinsulin. (From Steiner, D. F., et al.: Structural and immunological studies on human proinsulin. In *Diabetes*. Proc. Seventh Cong. Int. Diab. Fed. Rodriguez, R. R., and Vallance-Owen, J. (eds.), Amsterdam, Excerpta Medica Foundation, 1971, p. 281.)

proinsulin, at either end of the C-peptide, linking this peptide to the insulin region. Thus, human proinsulin consists of an 86-residue single-chain polypeptide having the B chain of insulin at its N-terminus linked by two basic residues to the 31-residue C-peptide, which in turn is linked through a second pair of basic residues to the A chain of insulin (see Fig. 15–5). Therefore, this one chain of proinsulin consists of NH₂–B chain–Arg–Arg–C peptide–Lys–Arg–A chain–COOH.

The connecting polypeptide contains acidic residues, proline, lysine, alanine, valine, and leucine but no aromatic residues, histidine, basic amino acids, or sulfur-containing amino acids. Clearly, this must indicate the existence of some specific requirements with regard to the properties of the side-chain groups in this portion of the molecule, perhaps with respect to the maintenance of the appropriate balance between hydrophilic and hydrophobic components in the molecule as a whole. The polar and nonpolar characteristics of the amino acid side chains of C-peptides of different species are preserved when interspecies amino acid substitutions occur. At either end of the C-peptide are regions having a high proportion of polar residues, and just beyond these regions in intact proinsulin there are two additional polar basic residues. These regions of the proinsulin molecule are quite hydrophilic. However, the central portion of the connecting peptide contains a high concentration of glycine residues surrounded by residues that are essentially all nonpolar. This composition indicates that the central part of the

molecule is more flexible and may, in fact, be bent back upon itself through interactions of the nonpolar side chains to produce a hydrophobic micelle, which may interact with some hydrophobic area on the surface of the insulin molecule during peptide folding. This distribution may help to maintain these hydrophilic regions on the outside of the molecule, where they will be readily accessible to the proteolytic cleavage enzymes that convert proinsulin to insulin. A synthetic mini-proinsulin has been synthesized with an artificial reagent to substitute for the C-peptide to cross-link the A and B chains with bismethionyl urea. After its synthesis, the product will reoxidize spontaneously and regain the normal disulfide bond structure with an efficiency and accuracy similar to that of proinsulin.

Some of the immunologic properties of proinsulin are similar to those of insulin. Proinsulin and split proinsulin are about 45% as reactive with insulin antibodies as insulin, on an equimolar basis. Arginine insulins were found to be about 75% as reactive with insulin antibodies as is insulin. Thus, the presence of one or two arginine residues on the COOH-terminus of the B chain may also interfere with antibody binding sites. The antiserum which is used routinely for the immunoassay of insulin cross-reacts with proinsulin to the extent of 25–50% or even more, depending upon what antiserum is used. The lesser reactivity of the proinsulin is most likely due to some of the antibody binding sites on the insulin portion of proinsulin being masked by the connecting peptide. Be-

PROINSULIN C - PEPTIDES

	1	2	3	4	5	6	7	8	9	10	11	12	13	14	15	16
HUMAN:	Glu	Ala	Glu	Asp	Leu	Gln	Val	Gly	Gln	Val	Glu	Leu	Gly	Gly	Gly	Pro
MONKEY:	Glu	Ala	Glu	Asp	Pro	Gln	Val	Gly	Glx	Val	Glx	Leu	Gly	Gly	Gly	Pro
PORCINE:	Glu	Ala	Glu	Asn	Pro	Gln	Ala	Gly	Ala	Val	Glu	Leu	Gly	Gly	Gly	Leu
BOVINE:	Glu	Val	Glu	Gly	Pro	Gln	Val	Gly	Ala	Leu	Glu	Leu	Ala	Gly	Gly	Pro

	17	18	19	20	21	22	23	24	25	26	27	28	29	30	31
HUMAN:	Gly	Ala	Gly	Ser	Leu	Gln	Pro	Leu	Ala	Leu	Glu	Gly	Ser	Leu	Gln
MONKEY:	Gly	Ala	Gly	Ser	Leu	Gln	Pro	Leu	Ala	Leu	Glu	Gly	Ser	Leu	Gln
PORCINE:	Gly	—	Gly	—	Leu	Gln	Ala	Leu	Ala	Leu	Glu	Gly	Pro	Pro	Gln
BOVINE:	Gly	Ala	Gly	—	—	—	—	Gly	Leu	Leu	Glu	Gly	Pro	Pro	Gln

Figure 15–6. Amino acid sequence of C-peptide from four species. (From Steiner, D. F., et al.: Structural and immunological studies on human proinsulin. In *Diabetes*. Proc. Seventh Cong. Int. Diab. Fed. Rodriguez, R. R., and Vallance-Owen, J. (eds.), Amsterdam, Excerpta Medica Foundation, 1971, p. 281.)

cause the amino acid composition of insulin of different species varies relatively little, the antiserum directed against insulin of one species usually cross-reacts with insulin of other species. Moreover, since proinsulin of different species contains the same antigenic determinants in the insulin portion of the molecule, anti-insulin serum generally cross-reacts with heterologous proinsulin. Thus human, bovine, or porcine proinsulin, like insulin of these species, interacts with porcine insulin antiserum. C-peptides have no immunoreactivity against insulin antiserum.

Proinsulin antiserum reacts with both insulin and proinsulin of different species. The cross-reactivity is presumably due to antibodies directed against the antigenic determinants in the insulin portion of the molecule. However, as discussed earlier, there are many species differences in the composition of the C-peptides. Immunoadsorbance with insulin-Sephadex results in a highly specific antiserum which, unlike insulin antiserum, does not cross-react significantly with proinsulin or C-peptide of other species. Proinsulin antiserum which has not been adsorbed by insulin does react with the proinsulin of other species. Since all of the proinsulin-like fragments of the connecting peptides containing sequence B_{33-54} react similarly with porcine proinsulin antiserum, it seems clear that the determinant of reactivity resides in the sequence B_{33-54}, especially B_{41-54}. This sequence is an unusually hydrophobic region and has great variability in the amino acids between species. Leu_{54} is specifically important for immunoreactivity, since removal of this amino acid causes a loss of cross-reactivity.

Human C-peptide coupled to rabbit serum albumin using a water-soluble carbodiimide has been found to produce antibodies sufficient to give sensitivity in immunoassay procedures between 0.05 and 0.1 ng/ml, using a final antiserum dilution 1:1000. However, such an assay probably does not distinguish between intact proinsulin and various partly cleaved intermediate forms that might still have most of the C-peptide portion of the molecule attached to one of the insulin chains. Thus, the plasma proinsulin fraction may be a mixture of both intact proinsulin and various intermediate species. Polyacrylamide gel electrophoresis appears to offer a good approach in separating these immunoreactive substances. C-peptide does not react with insulin antibodies, but it does combine with proinsulin antibodies that are produced by the antigenic determinants in the connecting peptide of proinsulin. Therefore, to measure C-peptide, it is desirable to separate it from proinsulin by means of gel filtration prior to immunoassay.

C-peptide has not been found to have a specific action. Moreover, it does not antagonize or potentiate the effects of insulin, proinsulin, or their intermediates. C-peptide has not been shown to have beneficial effects once it has been removed from proinsulin, although it has been suggested that it aids in the proper reformation of insulin that has been reduced and then reoxidized in the presence of glutathione-insulin-transhydrogenase.

Presumably, many intermediates of proinsulin and insulin could be produced in the body. Among those that have been more commonly found when bovine proinsulin has been subjected to the action of trypsin and carboxypeptidase B are proinsulin without Lys_{59}–Arg_{60} and proinsulin without Arg_{33}–Arg_{32}. Comparable desdipeptides have been derived from porcine proinsulin. Other porcine proinsulin-insulin intermediates produced by trypsin are diarginine insulin and monarginine insulin.

As measured by the mouse convulsion assay, proinsulin and split proinsulin are about 20% as active as insulin, whereas both desdipeptide proinsulin (Lys_{62}–Arg_{63} absent) and desnonapeptide proinsulin (B_{55-63} absent) and both arginine insulins are about 65% as active (Chance). A free NH_2-terminal glycine on the A chain is associated with greater activity, and the same applies to the presence of free COOH-terminal alanine on the B chain. using inhibition of epinephrine-stimulated lipolysis in fat cells for assay, porcine proinsulin, or split proinsulin, has about 3% the activity of insulin, but desnonapeptide proinsulin and arginine insulins are about 75% as active.

Insulin

Crystallization of insulin by Abel (1926) led to studies dealing with its chemical nature. The three-dimensional structure of insulin crystals has been demonstrated by x-ray analysis (Hodgkin). Two atoms of zinc were found to be present with six molecules of insulin in a spheroid unit (Fig. 15–7). The A chain rested in a pocket made by three

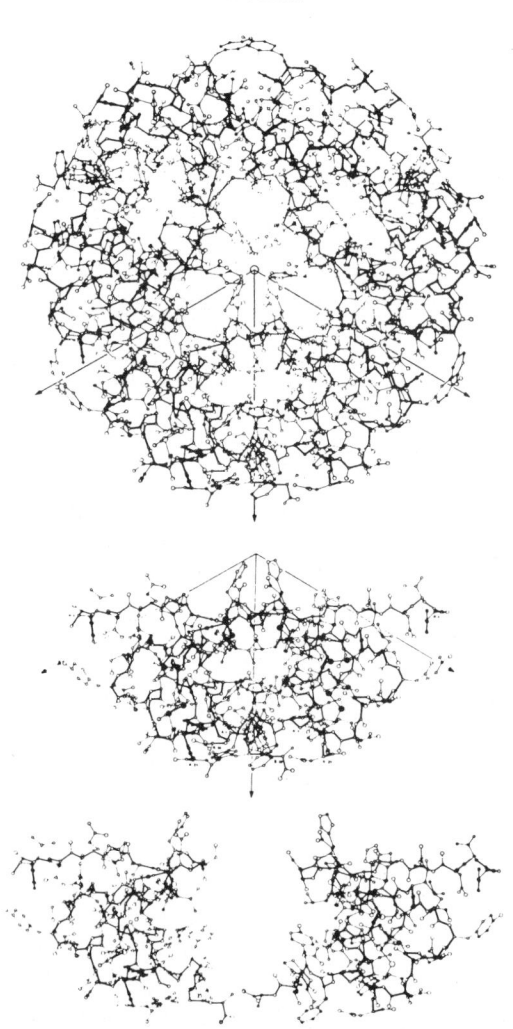

INSULIN

Figure 15–7. Three-dimensional structure of the zinc insulin monomer, dimer, and hexamer. Note the complementary relationships between the insulin molecules as they form a dimer. It is believed that this efficient storage form of insulin with zinc is present in insulin granules. (From Blundell, T., et al.: *Adv. Protein Chem.* 26:279, 1972.)

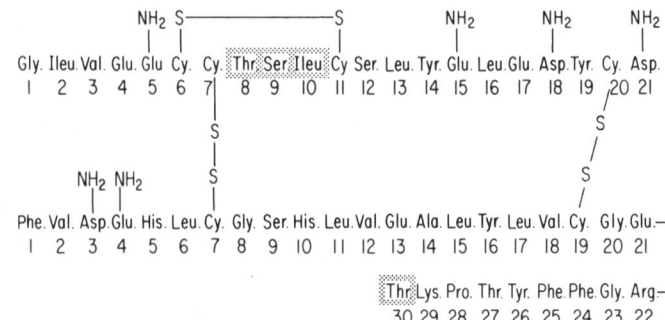

Figure 15–8. Sequence of human insulin. The sequence of insulin from certain animal species differs as follows:

	Chain A			Chain B
	8	9	10	30
Man	Thr	Ser	Ileu	Thr
Pig	Thr	Ser	Ileu	Ala
Rabbit	Thr	Ser	Ileu	Ser
Beef	Ala	Ser	Val	Ala

main sections of the B chain. The covalent bonding of the two chains, through the disulfide residues, were observed to be reinforced by van der Waals interactions between residues belonging to strategically placed nonpolar groups. The surface of the molecule exposed the polar groups, together with a few nonpolar residues. Insulin dimers were found to be compact, cylindrical structures with largely exposed hydrophilic residues and a few hydrophobic residues. The connecting peptide of proinsulin (discussed earlier) directs and holds the A and B chains in a conformation favorable for correct and efficient pairing of cystein residues as proinsulin is released from ribosomal units.

Sanger demonstrated the amino acid sequence of insulin. This was the first protein whose structure was elucidated, and the accomplishment led to the analysis of many other biologically active polypeptides and proteins. The purified molecule has a biologic activity of approximately 25 U/mg. He found insulin to be composed of two long polypeptide chains with a specific amino acid sequence bound together by two disulfide bridges at positions 7 and 20 in the A chain and 7 and 19 in the B chain (Fig. 15–8). The A chain has 21 amino acids and is acidic. The B chain has 30 amino acids and is basic. Also, there is an intrachain disulfide bridge linking positions 6 and 11 in the A chain.

The sequence B_{22-26} is an important part of the molecule for biological activity. Cleavage at B_{22-23} inactivates the hormone, and full biologic activity can be restored in stepwise fashion as the sequence is added back. A very similar sequence is found to be present in nonsuppressible insulin-like activity (NSILA). This molecule is now also called insulin-like growth factor (IGF). This sequence is almost invariant in the insulin molecule among species, compatible with its postulated biologic role. Recent studies show a strikingly similar three-dimensional structure for proinsulin, IGF, and relaxin, despite great disparity of sequence (Fig. 15–9). This three-dimensional view may be important for the biologic similarity of these molecules.

There can be considerable species-specific variations elsewhere in the amino acid sequence; indeed, as many as 29 of the 51 positions can be replaced. The amino acids in the internal ring of the A chain and those immediately adjacent to it on its C-terminal side (positions 12 to 14), as well as the N- and C-terminal parts of the B chain, are most frequently involved in molecular differentiation be-

tween species. These areas exert important antigenic responses in heterologous species. Human insulin differs from porcine insulin by a single amino acid; in the B_{30} position, human insulin has threonine rather than alanine (see Fig. 15–8).

The acid used to extract insulin from the pancreas removes zinc. To crystallize the hormone, it is necessary to add zinc or other metal ions such as nickel, cobalt, or cad-

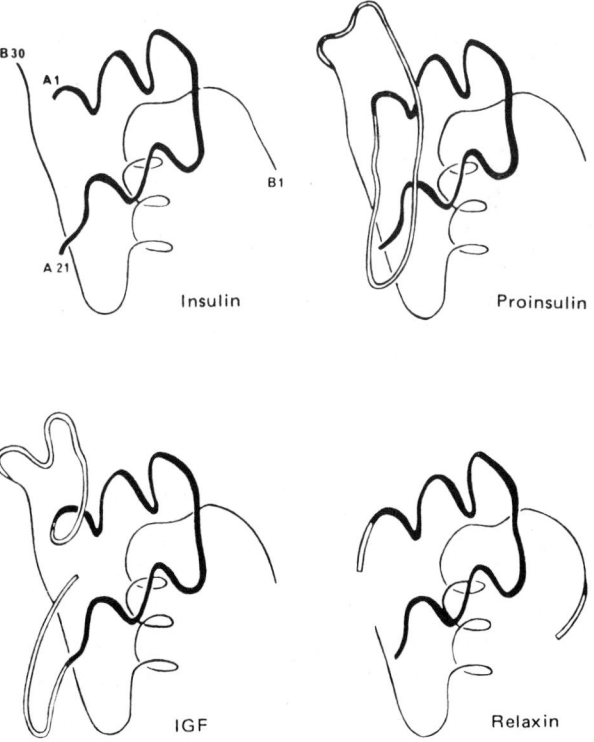

Figure 15–9. Schematic representation of the three-dimensional structure of four metabolic hormones. Despite major sequence differences, these metabolically related peptides show striking similarities which may explain their ability to interact with the same receptors. (From Blundell, T. L., et al.: Insulin-like growth factor: A model for tertiary structure accounting for immunoreactivity and receptor binding. *Proc. Natl. Acad. Sci. USA* 75:180, 1978.)

mium. Crystallin insulin usually contains from 0.3 to 0.6% zinc. Dimers and hexamers are sometimes formed. Insulin is relatively insoluble within the pH range of 4 to 7 (isoelectric point, pH 5.3). Molecular dissociation is favored by extremes of pH and by low ionic strength; concentrated solutions of guanidine hydrochloride also have this effect.

Insulin readily adsorbs loosely to many substances, including cellulose, agar, glassware, and certain serum proteins. When using small amounts of insulin, as in experimental studies, it is important to avoid binding to glassware, paper, and so forth. Many proteins inhibit the adsorption, but albumin and casein are two of the better compounds for preventing this.

For investigative studies, insulin has been labeled in a great variety of ways, but the commonest label used now is ^{125}I. The tyrosyl hydroxyl groups exchange with ^{125}I. More than 75% of the ^{125}I usually is fixed to the A chain, although the B chain also has two tyrosyl groups. Under carefully controlled conditions, it has been possible to label only the A chain, apparently because it is more exposed than the B chain. With heavy radioiodination there is loss of biologic activity as well as alteration in physical-chemical activity of many of the insulin molecules.

INSULIN BIOSYNTHESIS AND STORAGE

The synthesis of insulin begins on ribosomes on the surface of the rough endoplasmic reticulum. It is now believed that the messenger contains a presequence which assists in the association of the polysome with the microsomal membrane. The rat presequence is 24 amino acids long and precedes the B sequence, being attached to the amino terminus of the proinsulin molecule (Fig. 15–10). It has been hypothesized that the single-polypeptide-chain proinsulin, containing from 81 to 86 residues depending on the species, is then directed into the interior of the microsome as a result of the association between the polysome and the microsome. This extra peptide sequence must be rapidly hydrolyzed since pre-proinsulin is not found in extracts of pancreatic islets. After completion of synthesis, the proinsulin molecule spontaneously folds into the appropriate configuration for disulfide bond formation. The conversion of proinsulin to insulin occurs by proteolytic cleavage, which reduces the molecular weight of the protein from 9000 (proinsulin) to one of 6000 (insulin) and one of 3000 (C-peptide). This conversion occurs at the time of, or soon after, the transport of proinsulin to the Golgi complex, where it is packaged into granules. Since the granules contain insulin and C-peptide in equimolar amounts, it seems likely that the packaging occurs first and is followed by cleavage within the granule. Insulin is then complexed with zinc and stored. The B-cell granule also contains lipids and, in some species, monoamines. The complete structure of the B-cell granule is not yet known.

Electron microscopy shows that insulin granules vary considerably in their staining properties. Since there is some evidence that the oldest granules are released first, it appears that these different-staining granules represent stages in the maturing process. However, no more than 2–5% of the total content of the insulin-like materials in pancreas is proinsulin. Therefore, it is unlikely that these changes represent alterations in the relative contents of proinsulin and insulin. The number of B-cell granules is a good indication of the amount of insulin present; however, it does not reflect the synthesis rate or release rate of insulin, but simply the balance between them at any one time. A large quantity of insulin is stored in the pancreas, e.g., about 4 U/g or 200 U in man. In general, when

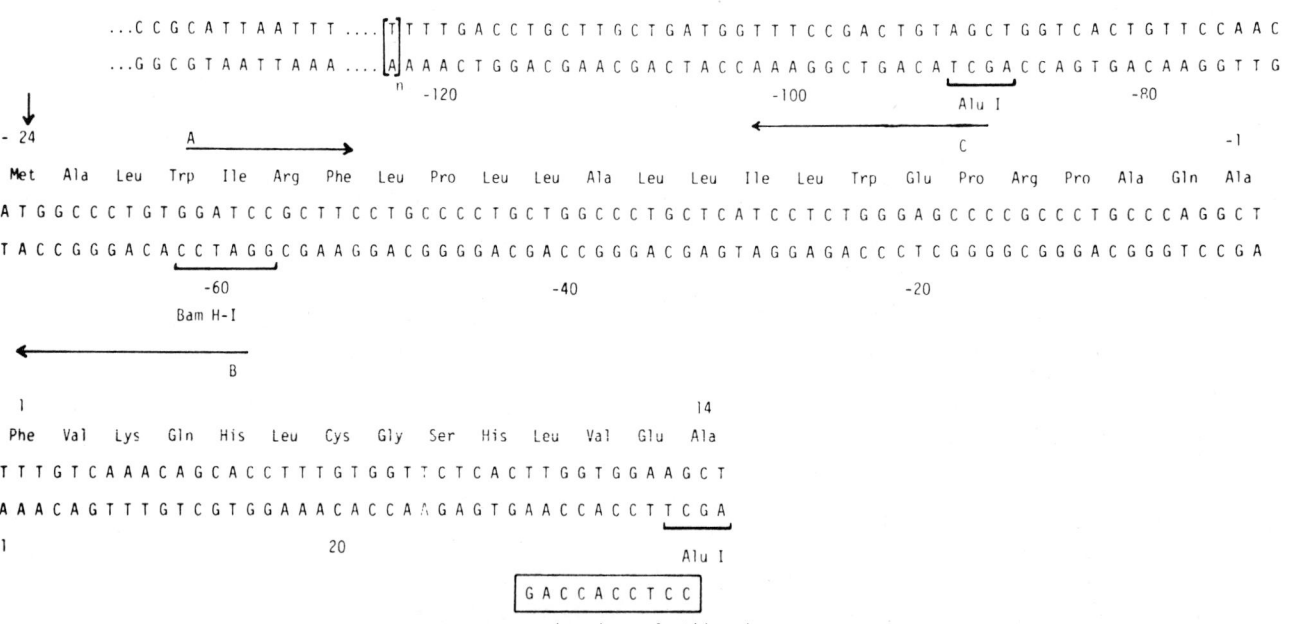

Figure 15–10. Presequence of rat pre-proinsulin shown above (-24-1) and its connection with the first 14 amino acids of the β chain shown below. These are matched with the corresponding primary base and messenger nucleotide sequences. (From Chan, S. J., et al.: Construction and selection of recombinant plasmids containing full-length complementary DNAs corresponding to rat insulins I and II. *Proc. Natl. Acad. Sci.* 76:5036, 1979.)

there is a prolonged decrease in the insulin synthesis and secretion rate, a number of changes in the B-cells are observed, including a decrease in the size of the nuclei, decreased granulation, prominence of the Golgi apparatus, and fewer ribosomes. On the other hand, with an increase in the activity of the B-cells due to continuous glucose stimulation, there is an increase in the size of the nucleus, the granulation tends to diminish, and the Golgi apparatus becomes spread out and more prominent; the RER increases in amount and in the number of prominent ribosome clusters and may become dilated (Fig. 15–11). With continued stimulation of the B-cells by high glucose levels, infiltration with glycogen may be observed. With prolonged marked stimulation, there may be hydropic changes.

Proinsulin synthesis and cleavage and insulin storage are not directly coupled to release; these processes appear to be separately regulated. Insulin synthesis is sensitive to glucose. An increase in synthesis due to glucose can be shown to occur in the absence of insulin secretion — for example, by incubation in a low-calcium medium (Steiner). This effect cannot be reproduced by pyruvate, indicating the specificity of the response and its lack of relationship to the general availability of energy. Sulfonylurea drugs, which are known to cause release of insulin, have not been shown to increase synthesis. The conversion of proinsulin to insulin is known to be an energy-dependent step. A trypsin-like enzyme is believed to be involved but has not been identified with certainty.

INSULIN RELEASE

B-granules are stored until a stimulus for insulin secretion is given. The early change in the release process is a margination of the beta granules to the plasma membrane of the B-cell (Fig. 15–12). The walls of these sacs fuse with the plasma membrane of the cell and rupture, and granules are then liberated into the extracellular space. They then rapidly disappear from the extracellular space, as viewed by electron microscopy, apparently undergoing rapid dissolution. Lacy has called this process of granule ejection into the extracellular fluid *emiocytosis*. With the disappearance of the granule, cytoplasmic projections called microvilli remain. These extend from the surface of the B-cell into the extracellular space. These microvilli have been counted by Lacy and shown to increase in number in proportion to the rate of release of the beta granules by emiocytosis. The additional cell surface produced is eventually taken back up into microvesicles. These are either recycled back to the Golgi complex to be reused or are degraded by lysosomes.

Glucose is the primary regulator of the B-cell; therefore, the mechanism by which glucose regulates insulin secretion has been of intense interest. Both D-mannoheptulose and 2-deoxyglucose inhibit phosphorylation of glucose and inhibit insulin secretion. Xylitol, a sugar alcohol metabolized by the hexose monophosphate shunt pathway, stimulates insulin secretion. Therefore, from two points of view, glucose metabolism has been cor-

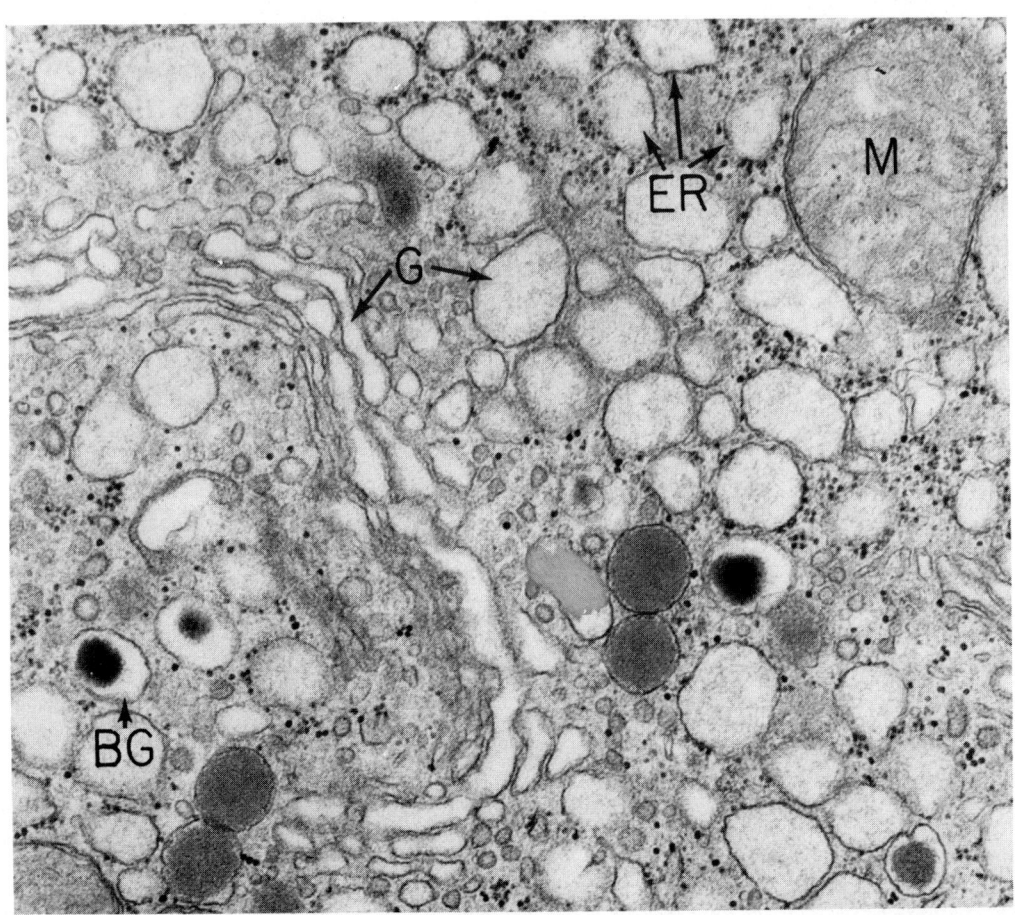

Figure 15–11.   Mouse beta cell stimulated by repeated (21 days) administration of insulin antibody, showing almost total disappearance of B-granules *(BG)*. Endoplasmic reticulum *(ER)*, and Golgi apparatus *(G)* are very prominent. (× 48,000.) (Courtesy of J. Lobothetopoulos.)

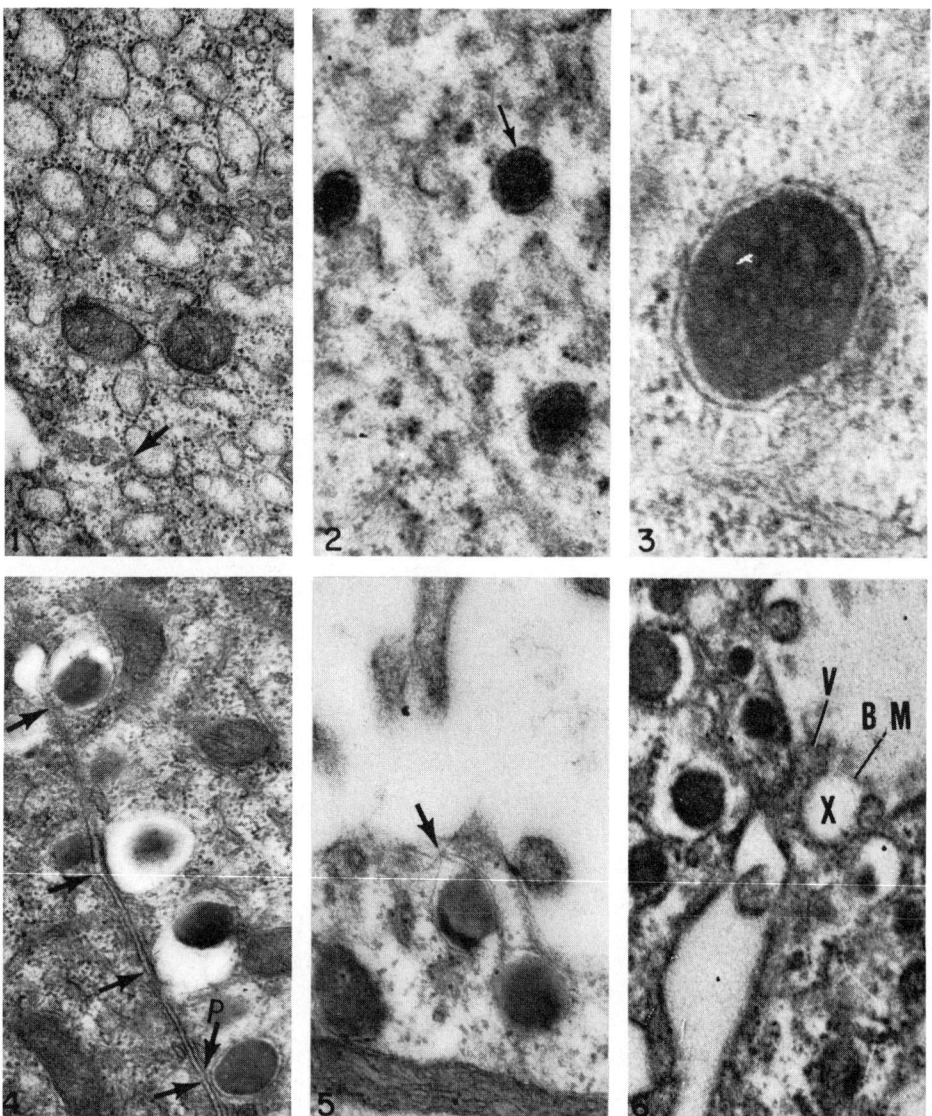

Figure 15–12. Sequential changes in insulin secretion in rats. *1,* Pale, amorphous material in vesicles of RER (↑) (× 34,000). *2,* B-granule with ribonucleoprotein granules attached to the outer surface of its sac (× 45,000). *3,* High magnification of B-granule (× 100,000). *4,* B-granules lining the cell membrane (↑); membranous sac of the granule in the right lower corner is separated from the plasma membrane (× 36,000). *5,* Fusion of the membranous sac of granule with the plasma membrane (P) shown at the arrow (× 55,000). *6,* Space *(X)* previously occupied by a B-granule. Basement membrane *(BM)* overlying the opening of the sac is slightly bulged. The cytoplasm to the left of this protrudes, forming a microvillus *(V)* (× 35,000). (From Williamson, J. R., et al.: Ultrastructural changes in islets of the rat produced by tolbutamide. *Diabetes 10*:460, 1961.)

related with insulin secretion. From this evidence it was concluded that the metabolism of glucose was essential for insulin release.

However, Matchinsky showed that insulin secretion occurs in an intact animal without an increase in the concentration of the metabolic intermediates of glucose in the islet cells. From these studies, he has postulated that early or first-phase insulin secretion is the direct result of the recognition of glucose as a molecule by a "glucoreceptor." Additional support for this idea has been found with studies of alloxan *in vitro.* This compound produces an immediate inhibition of glucose-induced insulin secretion, but has no effect on tolbutamide-induced insulin secretion, indicating that basic secretory mechanisms are intact. Its toxic damage is prevented by glucose, suggesting a competition between them. This protection is stereospe-

cific with better effects of the α-D-glucose anomer than the β-D-glucose anomer. A nonmetabolizable analogue of glucose, 3-*o*-methyl-D-glucose, is also protective, indicating that metabolism is not essential for the protective effect. Since hexose transport remains intact, alloxan does not affect this site of membrane interaction with glucose. Barbituric acid also protects but is known not to be taken up by islet cells. Therefore, a cell membrane site of action is indicated.

The glucoreceptor hypothesis does not eliminate a role for glucose metabolism in insulin release. Rather, it seems likely that glucose initiates release via a membrane-related glucoreceptor mechanism but potentiates the effectiveness of other secretagogues via its intracellular metabolism. This potentiator role appears to be critical, since very few of the other B-cell stimulators will release insulin in the absence of glucose. Glucose also plays a crucial role in insulin synthesis, but the mechanism by which glucose affects insulin synthesis is unknown.

The insulin release process from β-cells has been shown to require extracellular calcium. The rate of insulin release following glucose stimulation is correlated with the rate of calcium uptake by the islet. This has led to the concept that there is a coupling of the stimulus to insulin secretion by calcium in a manner analogous to the stimulus-contraction coupling in muscle. Lacy has also presented evidence for the existence of microtubules in B-cells and for their participation in intracellular transport of the secretory granules to the plasma membrane. His working hypothesis is that calcium triggers a contractile process in which the microtubules facilitate the movement of the granules from the interior of the cell to the cell surface.

Studies with time-lapse cinematography have suggested a simpler role for the microtubular system. Granules have been observed to be in continual motion, an effect which is dependent on glucose. When an inhibitor of microtubular function is present, such as colchicine or vinblastine, granule motion slows or is stopped completely. Under these conditions, insulin secretion is reduced proportionally. At stimulating glucose concentrations (> 100 mg/dl), the rate of motion is not dependent on the amount of glucose, but insulin secretion is. Therefore, motion appears to be necessary for release, but not to control its rate. An analogy can be made with the provision of neurosecretory granules to nerve terminals, which also involves the microtubular system. Provision of granules is a necessary function of the microtubular system in neurons, but release of transmitter is related to sodium-dependent action potentials which increase intracellular calcium.

Another key biochemical regulator of insulin release is intracellular cyclic adenosine monophosphate (cAMP). In the islet, cAMP does not seem to be a direct stimulus of release, as elevation of cAMP levels is not effective in the absence of glucose. Similarly, nonglucose stimuli such as glucagon or β-adrenergic agonists, which are known to activate adenylate cyclase to increase intracellular cAMP, are ineffective in the absence of glucose. Agents such as theophylline or dibutyryl cyclic AMP, which also elevate intracellular cAMP, are effective at extremely low calcium concentrations if glucose is present. Since there is no increase in calcium uptake, but there is an efflux of calcium when theophylline is added to glucose, it has been suggested that cAMP increases intracellular calcium by mobilizing calcium from intracellular stores (mitochondria, granules, or endoplasmic reticulum). Thus, there would be two mechanisms for increasing intracellular calcium to stimulate insulin secretion.

The specific mechanisms mediating an increase in intracellular calcium level by increasing extracellular calcium influx are at present poorly defined. The probable role of other ionic fluxes has been suggested by the description of repetitive islet cell electrical activity which is glucose sensitive. The pattern is complex and most closely resembles that found in smooth muscle cells. It consists of a slow depolarization of the membrane which is glucose sensitive until a "threshold" level of glucose is reached between 100 and 150 mg/dl. At this point, repetitive slow-wave depolarizations begin with superimposed miniature spike action potentials (Fig. 15–13). As glucose concentration increases, the amount of time in which the islet is depolarized at a new plateau potential increases until, at 500 mg/dl, the plateau and its associated spiking activity are constant. A decrease in potassium permeability seems to be the mechanism of the initial glucose-induced depolarization. It has been hypothesized that when the membrane is depolarized to a critical point, a voltage-dependent depolarization to the plateau potential occurs, leading to the spikes which are almost certainly due to a sudden calcium influx. This hypothesis has not been critically tested; nevertheless, there is sufficient evidence to indicate that glucose changes membrane permeability of ions other than calcium as part of the activation process.

A current view of the synthesis, storage, and release of insulin is schematically depicted in Figure 15–14. Although quantitatively *emiocytosis* is probably the most important mechanism of B-granule release, it may not be the only mechanism. For example, it may be that some insulin remains in soluble form and is not incorporated into a recognized granule, that granules dissolve in the cell, releasing insulin to the interior of the cell, or that some granules are released directly from synthetic sites by separate release mechanisms without prolonged storage.

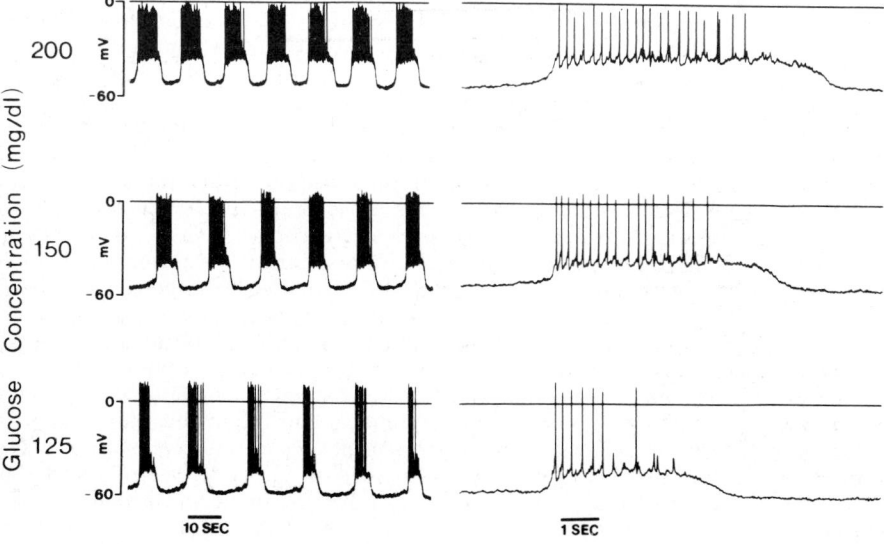

Figure 15–13. Electrical activity from intracellular recording from a single islet cell. Note the increase in duration of the slow-wave depolarization and the greater number of spikes as glucose levels increase. (Courtesy of Daniel L. Cook, M.D., Ph.D.)

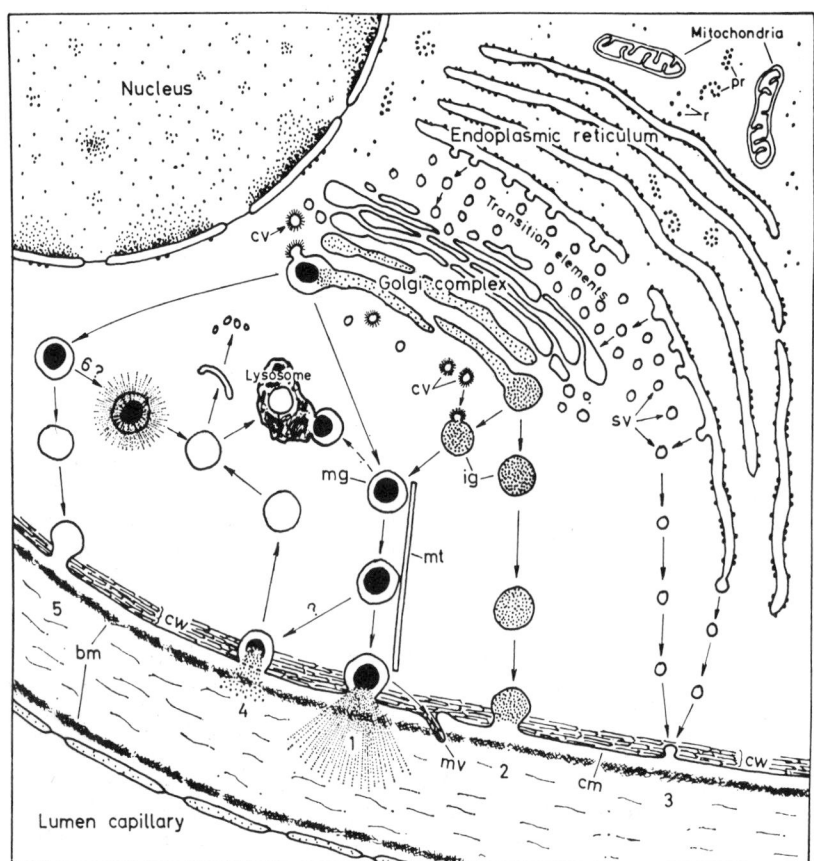

Figure 15–14. Diagrammatic representation of the morphologic events of the secretory process in an insulin-producing cell. Proinsulin is synthesized on the membrane-associated ribosomes of the endoplasmic reticulum and transferred to the Golgi complex by way of transition elements where the granules are formed. (Pro)insulin-containing granules which bud from the Golgi cisternae can be hypothesized to be released by one or more of six possible processes: (1) conventional emiocytosis of mature secretory granules in conjunction with contractile microtubular elements; (2) emiocytosis of immature secretory granules; (3) release of microvesicles independent of the Golgi apparatus; (4) release of insulin from the granule as a result of increased permeability of the granular membrane with retention of the membrane after evacuation of its contents; (5) emiocytosis of granules having previously undergone physical and chemical alteration of granule content; (6) physicochemical change in granule content followed by its passage into the cytoplasm. Although the majority of insulin is probably released by process 1, other methods have not been adequately explored.

Abbreviations: *r* = free ribosome; *pr* = polyribosomes; *sv* = smooth vesicles; *cv* = coated vesicles; *ig* = immature granules; *mg* = mature granules; *mt* = microtubules; *cw* = cell web; *bm* = basement membrane; *mv* = microvillus; *cm* = cell membrane. (From Renold, A.: The beta cell and its responses. Summarizing remarks and some contributions from Geneva. *Diabetes* 21:622, 1971.)

PHYSIOLOGY OF INSULIN SECRETION

Insulin, proinsulin, and C-peptide circulate freely in the plasma. Measurement of insulin is now made by insulin immunoassay. Both proinsulin and insulin interact with the insulin antibody in currently available immunoassays, and therefore both are measured unless plasma is pretreated to separate the two molecules. Gel filtration can be used to separate proinsulin from insulin on the basis of molecular size. Clearly, both peptides contain common immunologic determinants; therefore, it is unlikely that direct immunoassays for insulin will be developed which do not measure some proinsulin. On the other hand, the three-dimensional structure of proinsulin is sufficiently different from that of insulin that proinsulin does not react well with insulin antibodies.

In the basal state (after a 16-hour fast) 5–15 μU/ml of immunoreactive "insulin" (IRI) circulates in plasma of a normal nonobese man; 5–30% of this is proinsulin. Therefore, under these conditions only a small percentage of what is measured as insulin by immunoassay is proinsulin. Turner and Genuth have both estimated posthepatic basal insulin secretory rates of about 0.5 U/hour. Since the methods of estimation were different, these estimates may be reasonably reliable. If the liver extracts about 50% of the insulin delivered to it in a single passage, basal pancreatic insulin output can be estimated to be about 1 U/hour. After intravenous glucose challenge, peak peripheral plasma insulin concentrations occur in 3–5 min. With a maximal 20-g stimulus, this peak is 8–10 times the baseline concentration. After 100 g of oral glucose, the peak peripheral IRI concentration occurs in 30–60 min and is 6–8 times the baseline level. No reliable estimates of true secretion rates after glucose are available, but posthepatic delivery can be estimated by measuring the clearance of insulin and extrapolating from measured peripheral plasma insulin. Maximal rates during first-phase insulin release are estimated to be 10–30 times the basal rate.

Basal Insulin Secretion

The term basal insulin secretion is used to indicate insulin secreted in response to endogenous signals in a sedentary individual after an overnight fast, that is, long enough after the last meal so that absorbed nutrients are no longer having a direct effect upon the pancreatic B-cell. In man, this usually means after an overnight fast of 16 hours. Glucose levels below 100–125 mg/dl are not stimulatory for insulin release in *in vitro* systems. Therefore, insulin secretion in the basal state is probably not a direct function of glucose. On the other hand, none of the other physiologic regulators of insulin secretion are effective *in vitro* in the absence of glucose. Therefore, insulin secretion in the basal state appears to be dependent on the presence of both glucose and nonglucose B-cell modulators. The function of glucose at a concentration below 100 mg/dl is analogous to the permissive ability of steroids to regulate gluconeogenesis by the liver. Since nonglucose stimulators such as amino acids, gut hormones, and autonomic neurotransmitters are variably effective stimulants of the B-cell when glucose is changed between 25 and 100 mg/dl, there is an important interaction between blood glucose levels and nonglucose stimulant levels in the regulation of basal insulin secretion.

Changes in circulating growth hormone, cortisol, thyroxine, somatomammotropin, or estrogens are associated with altered basal insulin secretion. These hormones are, therefore, also believed to be playing a modulatory role in the regulation of basal insulin secretion.

Since basal insulin secretion regulates basal glucose output by the liver as well as peripheral glucose utilization in muscle and adipose tissue, there is a feedback loop between the liver and the pancreas for the regulation of insulin secretion and glucose in the basal state. Although basal glucose levels may not directly affect islet insulin output, these low glucose concentrations are critical to maintenance of basal insulin secretion by regulating the sensitivity of the B-cell to nonglucose stimuli. In this way, the neuroendocrine system sets the gain for islet B-cell function in relation to centrally recognized factors including nutrient history. These interact with the intrinsic glucose-insulin feedback loop between the liver and pancreas. The net sum of all these controllers then determines the endogenous plasma glucose level and endogenous or basal insulin secretion rate. If the net effect of the neuroendocrine factors augments insulin secretion, then basal insulin levels will tend to be higher and basal glucose levels lower. If they tend to inhibit insulin secretion, basal glucose will tend to be higher and basal insulin levels lower. Unfortunately, the relative quantitative importance of all of the neural, hormonal, and substrate influences on basal insulin secretion has not been dissected yet.

Substrate-Induced Insulin Secretion

During meals, substrates are the primary regulators of insulin secretion, and all three major classes — carbohydrates, fats, and proteins — have been shown to influence insulin output.

Carbohydrates. Glucose and fructose are the only important natural sugars in the regulation of insulin secretion. Since fructose is largely converted to glucose during absorption and is a relatively weak stimulus, glucose becomes the dominant carbohydrate regulator. As indicated in the section on insulin release, glucose probably interacts with islet cells in three separate ways — recognition as a molecule, metabolism of glucose specifically, and as a general energy substrate. This is fortunate for the physiologists who model insulin secretion, since almost all the models require more than one controller to explain the complex nonlinear process by which glucose regulates insulin output.

Amino Acids. Leucine was the first amino acid to be shown to stimulate insulin release. This action is exaggerated in pathologic B-cell hyperplasia and tumors and is used as a diagnostic test for patients with suspected B-cell hyperfunction. It now seems that most, if not all, amino acids increase insulin release (Fig. 15–15). Of those tested, arginine is the most potent in man. Different potencies have been suggested for the dog, but this evaluation is complicated by the interaction between the prevailing glucose level and some, but not all, of the amino acids. Thus, leucine can stimulate insulin release *in vitro* in the absence of glucose, but arginine cannot. Responses to both are potentiated by glucose, but arginine more so than leucine. It is of interest that leucine can be oxidized completely by the islet, but arginine poorly, if at all. Therefore, the mechanism of stimulation may vary even among the amino acids. Since nonmetabolizable amino acids can induce insulin release in the presence of glucose, it is clear that some of the stimulation is not due to

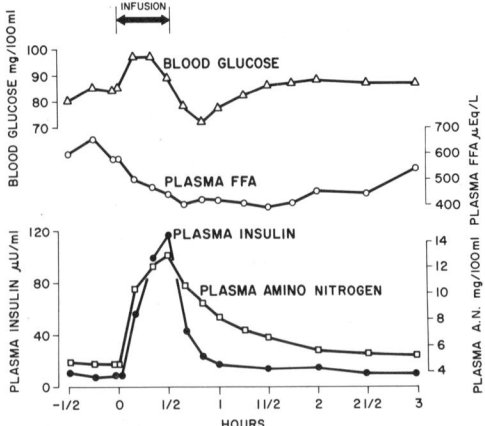

Figure 15–15. With infusion of 30 g of a mixture of 10 essential amino acids in 35 healthy subjects tested 51 times, there is an immediate rise in plasma insulin, correlating with a rise in amino nitrogen. There was only a slight and transient rise in blood glucose but a progressive decline in plasma FFA. (From Floyd, J. C., et al.: Stimulation of insulin secretion by amino acids. *J. Clin. Invest.* 45:1487, 1966.)

metabolism of the amino acid. It seems likely that amino acids have two mechanisms for stimulating insulin secretion. One is related to interaction with a membrane receptor and the other to stimulation of intracellular metabolism. These two functions are not equally present for all the amino acids and, therefore, the glucose dependency of the amino acids varies. Stimulation of insulin release by arginine has been shown to be multiphasic, indicating that the duration of this stimulus is also an important variable. Since experimental administration of protein and glucose together is followed by lower glucose and higher insulin responses than when glucose is given alone, it seems likely that a substantial quantity of insulin secretion following a mixed meal is related to the ingested protein.

Fatty Acids. Oral fat ingestion and intravenous infusion of free fatty acids and ketone bodies have been reported to increase insulin levels. The effect is much greater in dogs than in man. Oral fat ingestion also causes release of gut hormones such as GIP, which can augment insulin secretion. However, since both intravenous and oral administration are effective, it is unlikely that gut hormones are the sole mediators. In any case, some of the insulin secreted during mixed meals can be related to the fat contained in the food. Although fatty acids are weak stimulators of insulin secretion, during starvation they may play a role in ensuring sufficient insulin release to prevent ketoacidosis.

Hormones

Gastrointestinal Hormones. The absorption of foods releases several gastrointestinal hormones — gastrin, secretin, cholecystokinin (CCK), gastric inhibitory polypeptide (GIP), and enteroglucagon. Insulin secretion has been reported to result from stimulation by each of these hormones. Augmentation of the primary response to a substrate has also been found after the simultaneous administration of these hormones and glucose or amino acids. The discovery of this augmentation effect has in large part explained the observation that any substrate given orally produces a larger effect on insulin output than does the same amount of substrate infused intravenously (Fig. 15–16). Physiologically, the release of these augmenting

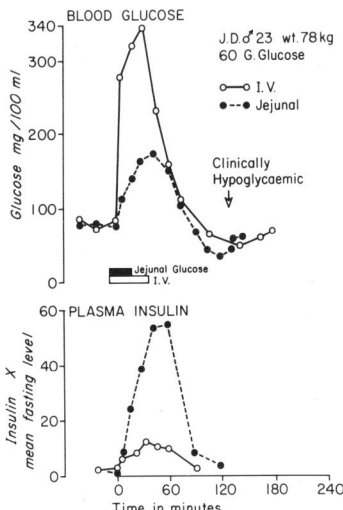

Figure 15–16. Despite the much smaller rise in plasma glucose level following its intrajejunal administration, compared with its intravenous administration, there is a far greater increment in the plasma insulin with the intrajejunal route (>50 × fasting). (From McIntyre, N., et al.: Intestinal factors in the control of insulin secretion. *J. Clin. Endocr.* 25:1317, 1965.)

hormones at the beginning of absorption appears to be useful in that the subsequent nutrient load will be anticipated by the pancreas, resulting in a much larger response. On the other hand, in the absence of simultaneously administered substrates, these hormones have relatively weak effects on islets and predominantly stimulate acute or first-phase insulin release.

The problem has been to identify the physiologic role and the relative importance of these hormones. Studies with secretin, gastrin, and purified CCK suggest these are unlikely to play a physiologic role, as the amounts needed to show a response are unphysiologically high or the hormone is poorly stimulated by exogenous nutrients that are known to produce high plasma insulin levels after oral ingestion. Only GIP now appears to be a good candidate for an important physiologic role. Oral glucose, amino acids, and triglyceride have all been shown independently to stimulate increased levels of immunoreactive GIP. Infusion of the hormone to mimic these physiologic levels results in augmented insulin release when blood sugar is elevated but has very little effect at normal or lower than normal blood glucose levels. Cells containing this hormone have been identified in the gastrointestinal tract, primarily located in the duodenum and to a lesser extent in the jejunum. Increased secretion of this hormone in patients with vagotomy and pyloroplasty may explain some of the postprandial hypoglycemia observed.

The vagus nerve probably also participates in this gastrointestinal augmentation phenomenon either by controlling gastrointestinal hormone release or by its direct stimulating effect on pancreatic B-cells. In rats and dogs, there is good evidence for a vagally mediated "cephalic phase" of insulin secretion which is stimulated by food in the oropharynx and esophagus. This reflex anticipates the absorption of nutrients and improves glucose tolerance.

Glucagon.   Glucagon also increases insulin secretion, even in very small amounts, by a direct B-cell effect. Although glucose regulates insulin and glucagon reciprocally so that as one rises the other tends to fall, amino acids stimulate both simultaneously. Therefore, there are circumstances in which glucagon may be expected to potentiate the insulin-stimulatory properties of amino acids. In addition, glucagon tends to mobilize liver glycogen and prevent the uptake and storage of glucose by the liver during absorption. Presumably, this would allow for the storage of amino acids in peripheral muscles in response to secreted insulin, while at the same time glucagon protects the cerebral cortex from hypoglycemia.

Other Hormones.   A number of other hormones regulate islet function, but not by affecting the release process directly. Their influence can be observed by noting a change in basal insulin secretion and parallel changes in the insulin response to some other stimulants. In this sense, they only regulate the gain of the B-cell. Examples include thyroxine, cortisol (?ACTH), somatomedin (?growth hormone), estrogen, progesterone, and somato-mammotropin. Since most of them antagonize the effects of insulin in peripheral tissues, the net effect of any of these hormones is to produce a new steady state of increased insulin output and B-cell responsiveness with a simultaneous decrease in insulin effectiveness. In this situation it is not clear whether the hormonal effects are primarily on the peripheral tissues with the change in islet function due to a change in circulating substrate or whether there are direct effects of the hormones on the islet B-cell. Most *in vitro* studies have been unable to show effects on islet function; therefore, an indirect mechanism seems likely. Changes in circulating glucose levels seem too small to be playing the feedback role, but there are major changes in stimulatory amino acids during steroid treatment which could be sufficient. Whether other hormonal changes or amino acids might be involved in the adaptation of islet gain by estrogen, progesterone, growth hormone, and so on, needs further study. The beauty of this system is the ability to maintain substrate levels constant over a wide range of hormone concentrations.

Neural Regulation

Ever since Claude Bernard reported hyperglycemia following puncture of the fourth cerebral ventricle, there has been a known relation between blood glucose regulation and the nervous system. In his classic study of the islet, Langerhans recognized the presence of nerves in the pancreatic islets. However, the discovery of pancreatic hyperglycemia and the treatment of diabetes with insulin directed attention away from the central nervous system, and regulation of the islet by substrates was considered to be the sole factor in islet function. This was reinforced by transplantation studies in which the islet functions in the absence of neural signals. While there can be no doubt that the response to nutrients is the result of direct regulation of the islet by substrates, it is now clear that the autonomic nervous system has a major modulating role to play and may be dominant in islet regulation between meals, during periods of starvation, or in response to an environmental change or stress not involving meal ingestion.

The pancreatic islets as well as other endocrine glands are now known to be innervated by both parasympathetic cholinergic neurons and sympathetic adrenergic neurons. As in other organs, they enter along the blood vessels with sympathetic fibers originating in the celiac ganglion and parasympathetic fibers passing through as vagal preganglionic efferents. There is evidence in lower species for purinergic nerves (which use ATP as a transmitter) and peptidergic nerves (which use some polypeptide such as VIP as a transmitter). Afferents are known to be coming from the pancreas, those that convey pain following the splanchnic nerve. It is assumed that some of the afferent vagal fibers

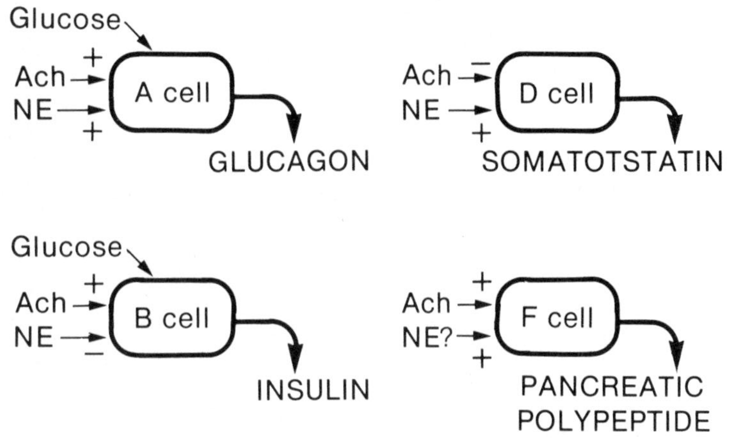

Glucose
Ach + → A cell
NE + →
GLUCAGON

Ach − → D cell
NE + →
SOMATOTSTATIN

Glucose
Ach + → B cell
NE − →
INSULIN

Ach + → F cell
NE? + →
PANCREATIC POLYPEPTIDE

Figure 15–17. A schematic summary of autonomic regulation of islet cells. (From Woods, S. C., et al.: The role of the nervous system in metabolic regulation and its effects on diabetes and obesity. In *Handbook of Diabetes Mellitus.* Brownlee, M. (ed.), New York, Garland Publishing Co., 1981.

also originate from the pancreas, but whether they come from the islet is unknown.

There are no specialized morphologic membrane changes in the islet cells characteristic of neuromuscular synapses. The nerve terminals end blindly within the islet underneath the basal lamina surrounding the islet cells. Nevertheless, individual endings are closely associated with A-, B-, D- and PP cells. This suggests that when neurotransmitters are released, they diffuse through the extracellular space and affect several islet cells simultaneously in a manner analogous to the effects of the autonomic nervous system on smooth muscle groups. Although the nerve terminals may be modest in number, there has recently been demonstrated specialized connections between islet cells which can pass molecules of less than 500 molecular weight. These "gap-junctions" are therefore areas of low electrical resistance. Since islet cells are electrically active during the process of insulin secretion (see Fig. 15–13), it is probable that the neural signals are amplified throughout the islet as a result of this electrical coupling phenomenon. Therefore, this system provides for neural control regardless of direct innervation of each cell. This is similar to what is found in most smooth muscle cells.

Autonomic Transmitters. Both acetylcholine and norepinephrine, the known transmitters of the autonomic nervous system, and the adrenomedullary hormone epinephrine have been shown to influence A-, B-, D-, and PP-cells. Acetylcholine is a direct stimulant of insulin secretion, but its effects are glucose-dependent (Fig. 15–17). Therefore, increased vagal activity will stimulate insulin release only during periods of elevated blood sugar. Atropine blocks this effect, indicating that the receptor is muscarinic in type.

Norepinephrine has complex effects on the islet B-cell. It is perhaps best considered a modulator of insulin secretion since it has both intrinsic stimulation and inhibition properties. When sympathetic nerves are stimulated or when epinephrine or norepinephrine is infused, the predominant effect observed is inhibition of insulin secretion (Figs. 15–17 and 15–18). During continuous infusion, however, there is an apparently paradoxical increase of basal insulin even though there is a continued inhibition of glucose-mediated insulin secretion. This is due to the fact that catecholamines stimulate α-adrenergic receptors to inhibit insulin release while simultaneously stimulating β-adrenergic receptors, which tend to increase insulin secretion. Since phentolamine, an α-adrenergic blocking agent, causes an increase of basal insulin levels when infused, there appears to be tonic α-adrenergically mediated suppression of basal insulin release (Fig. 15–19). On the other hand, the administration of propranolol, a β-adrenergic antagonist, produces a suppression of basal insulin levels. Thus, there appears to be simultaneous tonic β-adrenergically mediated stimulation of insulin secretion (Fig. 15–19).

As blood sugar rises during sympathetic discharge, the ability of catecholamines to suppress islet responses to nonglucose stimuli appears to diminish. The insulin secretory responses to arginine, secretin, and other nonglucose stimuli are often of normal magnitude during catecholamine-induced hyperglycemia. However, these apparently normal insulin responses are a result of the potentiating effect of the induced hyperglycemia. Since this potentiating effect of hyperglycemia does not affect glucose-mediated insulin release, the direct insulin-secreting effect of glucose is still dramatically suppressed. Thus, sympathetic α-

Figure 15–18. Regulation of insulin secretion in man by epinephrine. Note the immediate suppression of insulin secretion and the total block of insulin release to a glucose challenge by the infusion. These are α-adrenergic effects. The slow insulin rise from 120 to 300 minutes is due to β-adrenergic effects which are glucose-dependent.

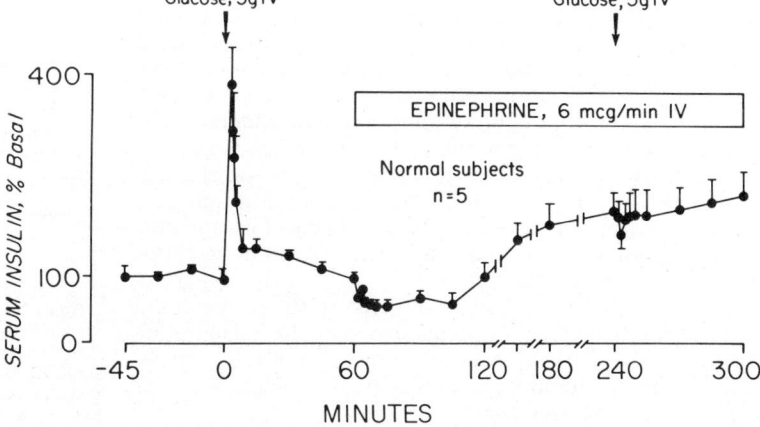

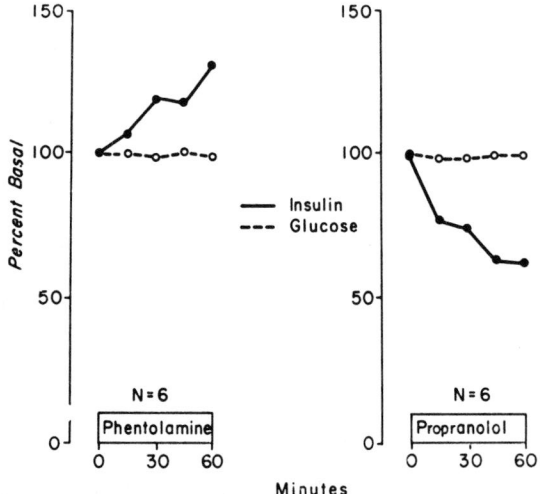

Figure 15-19. A demonstration of tonic adrenergic control of insulin secretion in man. α-Adrenergic blockade with phentolamine and β-adrenergic blockade with propranolol result in either an increase or a decrease in basal insulin secretion (o--o, control; •--•, experimental). (From Robertson, R. P., and Porte, D., Jr.: Adrenergic modulation of basal insulin secretion in man. *Diabetes* 22:1, 1973.)

adrenergic receptors inhibit all stimulatory signals to the B-cell. However, hyperglycemia can compensate for the inhibitory effect on nonglucose stimuli but not for the inhibitory effect on glucose as a direct stimulus. This produces a change in islet function rather than a pure inhibition. The ability of hyperglycemia to compensate for the α-adrenergic block to a nonglucose stimulus appears to be the mechanism by which basal insulin secretion is maintained during the prolonged secretion of epinephrine or norepinephrine.

Somatostatin. Although not a neurotransmitter in the islet, somatostatin is another neural agent which has important inhibitory actions on the secretion of insulin and glucagon. It is present in the D-cell and has been shown to be secreted under the influence of a number of substrates, hormones, and neural modulators. It acts in a directly opposed fashion to acetylcholine. It not only inhibits insulin release but inhibits glucagon release as well as release of a wide variety of nonislet polypeptide hormones. Since it is rapidly inactivated in the circulation, it appears likely that it plays a paracrine role in the endocrine pancreas. Preliminary studies suggest that substrates and gastrointestinal hormones stimulate its release, as does the sympathetic neurotransmitter norepinephrine. Acetylcholine appears to inhibit somatostatin release (see Fig. 15–17). Thus, the effects of the release of neurotransmitters in the islet are relatively complex: acetylcholine directly stimulates insulin and glucagon release, an action amplified by simultaneous inhibition of somatostatin release; on the other hand, norepinephrine stimulates somatostatin release, which should augment catecholamine inhibition of insulin release but inhibit catecholamine stimulation of glucagon release.

Other Islet Monoamines and Prostaglandins. Islet cells are influenced by a number of neurally regulated compounds such as dopamine, serotonin, and the prostaglandins; however, the physiologic significance of these effects is still not entirely clear. Similar to the effects of norepinephrine, both stimulation and inhibition of insulin secretion have been reported. This is probably due to the numerous interactions that are possible. In general, the intracellular monoamines serotonin and dopamine are believed to inhibit insulin release. It has been postulated that they are released with insulin and participate in a feedback system to modulate insulin secretion.

Prostaglandins of the E series are both stimulatory (probably via stimulation of cyclic AMP) and inhibitory. *In vivo* the latter effect predominates. This may be due to the presence of glucose, as the higher of the glucose level *in vitro*, the greater the inhibition found. There is some evidence that α-adrenergic effects are partially mediated by prostaglandin E and some evidence that serotonin mediates the effects of prostaglandin E. Since sympathetic nerve stimulation stimulates the production of prostaglandin E in many tissues, autonomic regulation may involve all of these mediators.

Central Connections. The hypothalamus appears to play the major integrating role in the balance between sympathetic and parasympathetic regulation of the islet. Electrical stimulation of the ventrolateral hypothalamic area elicits an increase of insulin secretion which is blocked by vagotomy. Bilateral destruction of this nucleus results in a marked decrease of insulin levels in rats and lowering of the body weight set point. The ventromedial hypothalamic nucleus when stimulated produces a decrease of insulin and an increase of blood glucose. Bilateral destruction of this nucleus produces hyperinsulinemia, islet hypertrophy, hyperphagia, and obesity. Thus, these centers, which are critical to body weight regulation, have important connections to the endocrine pancreas (Fig. 15–20). The data suggest an important association between the hypothalamus and the endocrine pancreas independent of the regulation of food intake by the hypothalamus. It is presumably this brain area which integrates other environmental influences into the direct control of metabolic hormone secretion. Stress hyperglycemia and the cephalic phase of feeding in which there is direct neural regulation of insulin release are two examples. At the islet level, the integration of substrate, hormonal, and neural influences is via control of the basic insulin secretory process and is schematically summarized in Figure 15–21.

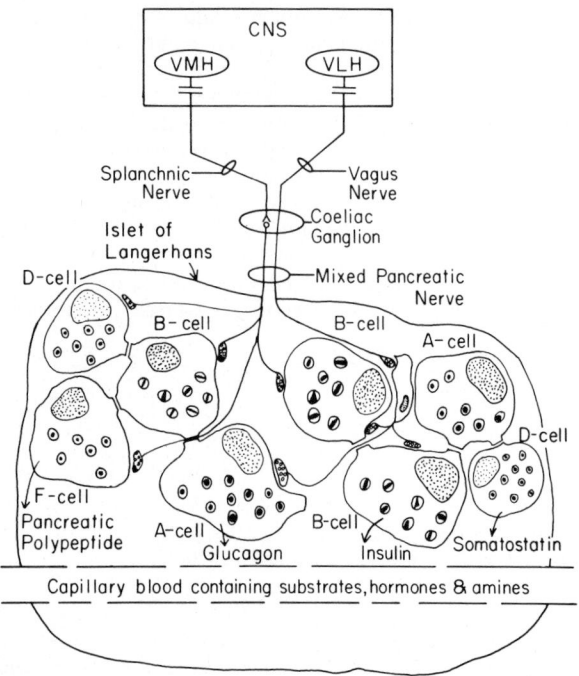

Figure 15-20. Schematic representation of the autonomic innervation of the pancreatic islets (*VMH* = ventromedial hypothalamus; *VLH* = ventrolateral hypothalamus; *CNS* = central nervous system). (From Woods, S. C., et al.: The role of the nervous system in metabolic regulation and its effects on diabetes and obesity. In *Handbook of Diabetes Mellitus.* Brownlee, M. (ed.), New York, Garland Publishing Co., 1981.)

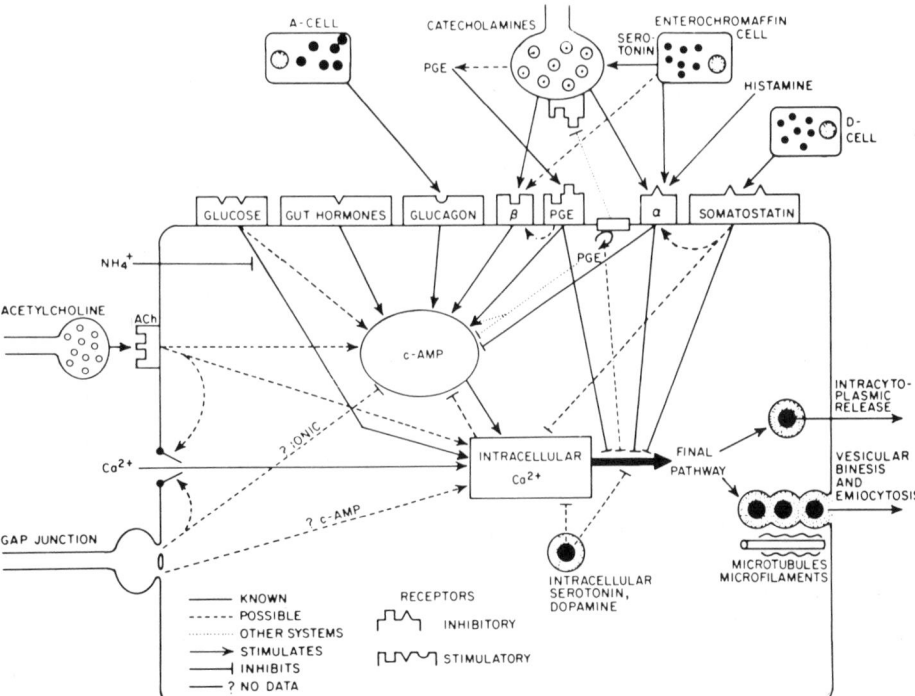

Figure 15–21. Neuroendocrine regulation of the B-cell. A summary description of some of the factors impinging on the basic glucose control of insulin secretion. (From Smith, P. H., and Porte, D., Jr.: Neuropharmacology of the pancreatic islet cells. *Ann. Rev. Pharm. Toxicol. 16*:269, 1976.)

INTERACTING SYSTEMS IN INSULIN SECRETION

Kinetics of Release

Since insulin is the most important storage or anabolic hormone, it is not surprising that its secretion is carefully regulated. As *in vitro* studies show, many substrates and hormones participate in this regulation. The relationship between individual controllers and insulin secretion is a complex function. First, the duration of the stimulus, as well as its strength, determines insulin secretion rate. In addition, a stimulus of fixed duration, but of variable strength, produces a sigmoid dose-response curve of insulin output. To illustrate these effects, we will examine the effects of the primary substrate controllers and the secondary hormonal and neural controllers.

The best studied and probably most important stimulus for insulin secretion is glucose. When glucose is presented to the islet as a sudden increase in concentration and held constant above 100 mg/dl, there is an immediate islet response (30 sec to 1 min) which peaks within a few minutes. Thereafter, the secretion rate falls and then gradually rises to reach another steady level much later (Fig. 15–22). The magnitude of the initial, or first-phase, response depends upon the previous history or gain of the islet, the glucose concentration, and its rate of change. The second phase appears to depend on the metabolism of glucose. This biphasic pattern of insulin secretion has been studied primarily in the rat but is known to occur in man. When a glucose infusion is stopped, insulin secretion quickly returns to control values. The dose-response relationships for both phases of release appear to be sigmoid in nature with a threshold at 100 mg/dl. After the threshold glucose concentration is exceeded, there is a sharp rise in insulin secretory rate with the half-maximal rate at 200 mg/dl and maximal output at above 500 mg/dl.

In order to explain the biphasic pattern of glucose-induced insulin release, mathematical models have been developed which are based upon compartmentation of stored insulin or an interaction between stimulatory and inhibitory signals. Mathematically, these concepts are very similar, and, therefore, the correct approach has not been rigorously defined. The compartmental approach is much easier to understand conceptually. With this system, insulin is described as being in two separate compartments for release. One is small, is available for immediate discharge, and is responsible for the first phase of secretion. The second is much larger. It is responsible for the second, slower phase either by provision to the small compartment or by delayed release directly (Fig. 15–23). Insulin synthesis maintains the size of this larger compartment but may also be responsible for direct release without traversing either storage pool.

This model can be used to describe the response to exogenous glucose *in vitro*. However, in the intact animal, insulin is secreted in the basal state without an exogenous glucose stimulus. Glucose contributes to control of

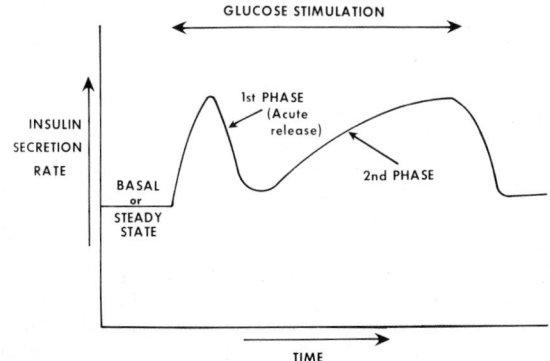

Figure 15–22. The effect of constant glucose stimulation on insulin secretion. Note the two phases of insulin release and their separation from a basal or steady state prior to glucose stimulation.

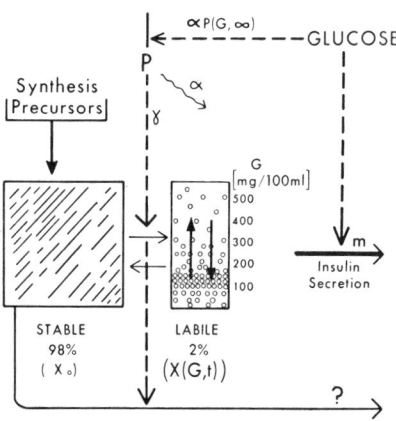

Figure 15–23. A two-compartment model for insulin secretion. This model has been utilized to explain the biphasic insulin release observed in the isolated perfused rat pancreas. Insulin is distributed in units or packets in a labile pool which are released when their glucose threshold is reached. Glucose also controls the provision of insulin to this small compartment through a hypothetical intermediate substance, P. This model can be defined in quantitative terms and has been simulated on a digital computer. (From Grodsky, G. M.: A threshold distribution hypothesis for packet storage of insulin and its mathematical modeling. *J. Clin. Invest.* 51:2050, 1972.)

this type of insulin secretion also, but this control appears to differ from either the first or second phases of exogenous glucose-stimulated insulin release. For this reason, basal insulin secretion has been considered separately from stimulated insulin secretion (see earlier). However, the basal insulin secretion rate can predict insulin responses to challenge. The reason for this predictability is not completely understood but has been interpreted to mean that basal insulin secretion reflects the gain of the islet and that this gain is one of the determinants of the magnitude of the insulin response to an exogenous stimulus. This system of variable gain appears to permit the islet to make long-term adjustments to modulate the response to a sudden challenge to the B-cell. The basal insulin secretion can be used as an index of that gain. It is presumed that many of the substrate and hormonal controllers which have been used to demonstrate stimulated insulin release also participate *in vivo* in the regulation of basal insulin secretion. However, since the basal and stimulated secretory functions are separate, the quantitative interaction between any of these substances and the basal secretory outputs is unknown.

In summary, insulin secretion is considered to be a nonlinear function of substrates and hormonal controller concentrations. It has been subdivided into two broad categories — insulin release in response to an external stimulus and insulin release in the basal state in the absence of an external stimulus. This basal insulin secretion is a reflection of the gain of the islet. The insulin release in response to an external stimulus has been further subdivided into first-phase insulin release and second-phase insulin release, because the duration of the stimulus partly determines the response. First-phase insulin release clearly involves only the release of stored hormone. It has the sigmoid dose-response curve characteristic of a saturable system. Second-phase insulin release stimulated by glucose involves predominantly the release of stored hormone but becomes more and more dependent upon synthesis as its duration persists. Some stimuli, such as glucose, interact with this system by influencing all three types of insulin secretion, but other stimuli interact with only one or two types. With this complexity, it is not surprising that inter-

preting and predicting insulin responses to challenge in the intact animal or man has been difficult.

Clinical Physiology

Clinical tests have been designed using glucose to evaluate insulin secretory responses in man. Most of the early data were confusing because the complex way in which glucose regulates insulin secretion was not appreciated. Therefore, there was no separation of the various phases of insulin release in response to glucose, nor was there separation of basal insulin secretion from insulin secreted in response to a challenge. When the nonlinear nature of the glucose-induced insulin response was defined, it was possible to develop models for man which could be used to interpret the clinical tests. They are very similar to the models that have been developed for the perfused rat pancreas. The model that we have used is shown in Figure 15–24. It consists of two pools (or compartments) — a small pool available for immediate release comparable to that responsible for first-phase insulin secretion, and a much larger pool responsible for second-phase insulin release, which occurs either directly or via the small storage compartment. Insulin synthesis is responsible for refilling the large storage pool and is also a major contributor to insulin secretion in the basal state or after prolonged administration of glucose (several hours).

In clinical testing with oral glucose, the early phases of the test (0–30 min) are dominated by the sensitivity of release of the small storage pool, the size of the small storage pool, and the rate of rise of glucose concentration, i.e., the magnitude of the challenge. The intermediate period (30–90 min) is dominated by the sensitivity of the large storage pool to release insulin and the later phases by the rate of insulin synthesis. When glucose is given rapidly intravenously and there is no further glucose input during the remainder of the test, the two phases of insulin secretion tend to become better separated. The immediate response from the small storage pool is observed for the first 10 min, whereas the second-phase insulin release dominates between 10 and 45 min. Then there is a gradual increase in synthesis-related release after 45 min. The gain of the islet is reflected in insulin secreted in the basal state prior to the stimulus. This output appears to give an index of the size and sensitivity of the storage pools. Thus, in normal subjects, one expects that a greater secretion rate in the basal state will be reflected by greater release from both the small and large storage pools after a challenge. Deviations from this expected response will be discussed in the section on the Pathophysiology of Hyperglycemia.

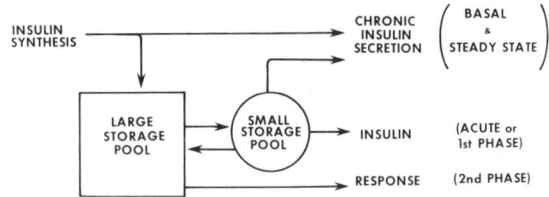

Figure 15–24. Schematic representation of a two-pool model for insulin secretion in man. Glucose is believed to regulate insulin output in three separate ways: (1) as a direct controller of the small storage pool, responding to a rate of change in glucose concentration to produce the rapid or first-phase insulin release; (2) by its metabolism as a controller of the large storage pool to produce a delayed response and a second phase of challenge; and (3) by production of an intermediate which regulates insulin synthesis producing a very delayed response, labeled here "chronic insulin secretion." This delayed response controls insulin secretion in the basal state as well. (From Cook, D.: A systems model study of blood glucose homeostasis. Master's thesis, University of Washington, Seattle, 1969.)

CHEMISTRY OF GLUCAGON

It is difficult to isolate glucagon and insulin from the pancreas separately. Therefore, some commercial insulin preparations still contain glucagon. When the acetone precipitate from pancreas is dissolved in acid and repeatedly dialyzed against dilute sodium acetate and sodium phosphate buffers, glucagon precipitates and is readily crystallized from mild alkaline solution. Traces of zinc and other metals are associated with glucagon, but these metals do not form an integral part of the crystal as they do in insulin. Glucagon is relatively insoluble in water, particularly in the pH range from 3 to 9; its isoelectric point is between pH 7.5 and 8.5. Electrolytes decrease its solubility, but mildly acidic and basic conditions increase it. Alkaline conditions are more favorable than acid since insoluble fibrils form with the latter. Moreover, the alkaline stability of glucagon permits inactivation of trace amounts of insulin.

Glucagon has a molecular weight of 3485. Bromer has shown that the amino acid composition of glucagon is quite different from that of insulin (Fig. 15–25). Glucagon is composed of one long chain. Tryptophan and methionine are constituents of glucagon but not of insulin, while cystine, isoleucine, and proline are components of insulin but not of glucagon. Glucagon is cleaved by carboxypeptidase, trypsin, leucine aminopeptidase, dipeptidyl aminopeptidase I, and chymotrypsin. Since none of the degradation products of glucagon retains hyperglycemic activity, the integrity of most of the molecule seems to be required for physiologic activity.

Although native glucagon contains no metals or prosthetic groups, metal-glucagon complexes are readily prepared; one example is zinc-glucagon. It is less soluble than glucagon and has a prolonged biologic action. In acidic aqueous solutions, glucagon readily forms fibrils and gels that redissolve at pH 11. Glucagon is stable in aqueous solutions for 3 months when kept at 4°C and at pH 2.5–3.0. Molecules of glucagon apparently bind together strongly in solution. Glucagon is capable of conformational alterations, changing from a random coil in aqueous solution to either a beta structure in acidic gels or alpha-helix in the crystal state. Under physiologic conditions, the random coil probably predominates (Bromer).

The gastrointestinal tract has been shown to contain molecules that cross-react immunologically with glucagon. One appears to be immunologically identical and to have the same molecular size as pancreatic glucagon. It has been identified in cells of the stomach which cannot be distinguished from A-cells of the pancreas. Another gut molecule with glucagon-like immunoreactivity (GLI) has now been termed glycentin, since its molecular structure has recently been determined. It is immunologically different and has a larger molecular weight than 3500-dalton pancreatic glucagon. Since it has been shown to contain the structure of glucagon with a C-terminal extension of 1500 daltons, the explanation for the existence of some antibodies which cannot distinguish the two molecules is clear. Glycentin is found in the small intestine in cells similar, but not identical, to the A-cells of the pancreas and stomach. It is known to circulate in plasma. Glycentin concentrations are increased by oral nutrients including glucose, but its regulation is different from that of pancreatic or stomach glucagon.

GLUCAGON STORAGE, SYNTHESIS, AND RELEASE

Although the existence of glucagon has been known almost as long as that of insulin, detailed knowledge of A-cell function is still primitive. A-cell granules show less species variation than do granules of B-cells, presumably because of the great similarity, if not identity, of the primary amino acid sequence among species. A granular endoplasmic reticulum is abundant, as are the typical secretory granules, which are symmetrically round, electron-dense, and surrounded by a limiting membrane. There is a prominent Golgi complex with granules within the complex. Therefore, it is believed that the same synthetic sequence occurs in the A-cell as in the B-cell — that is, synthesis in the endoplasmic reticulum, transport to the Golgi complex, and packaging for export as granules. Glucagon and pancreatic polypeptide are present in a reciprocal relationship in islets. As the islet concentration of one increases, that of the other decreases. Therefore, individual islets can vary greatly in glucagon and pancreatic polypeptide cells.

There is evidence for several larger molecular weight precursors (proglucagon). Details of this biosynthesis are sketchy. In fish islets, a 12,000-dalton immunoreactive glucagon-like molecule is cleaved to a 9000-dalton peptide, then to a 4900 moiety, prior to the final 3500-dalton pancreatic glucagon. A complex scheme has been found in rat islets involving an 18,000-dalton intermediate, followed by cleavage to an 8000- to 10,000-dalton proglucagon which contains glycentin and an N-terminal extension, which is eventually processed to glucagon. A peptide similar to this 9000-weight species circulates in dog and human plasma and is assumed to be a circulating glucagon precursor. Pancreatic glucagon content in most species reported is approximately 5–10 μg/g wet weight. Although some authors, such as Lazarus, have produced evidence that emiocytosis is the method of glucagon secretion, this has not been universally agreed upon (see, for example, Munger). Both calcium and cyclic AMP have been implicated in the regulation of secre-

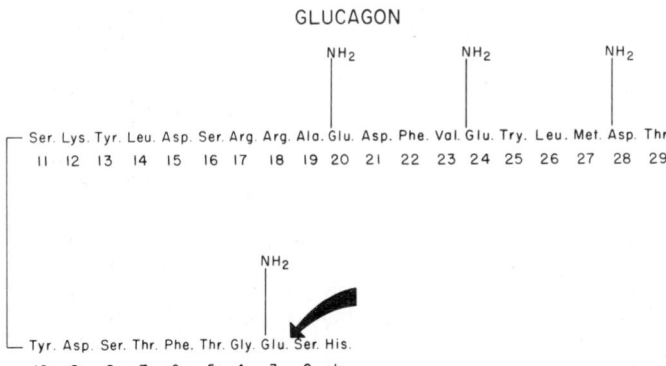

Figure 15–25. Amino acid sequence of glucagon, showing the site of cleavage by dipeptidyl aminopeptidase I.

tion. Increases in cyclic AMP have been associated with an increase in glucagon secretion. The role of calcium has been more controversial, but there appears to be some requirement for calcium during the stimulation by arginine. The recent interest in the physiologic control of glucagon secretion will, it is hoped, stimulate a more complete and penetrating biochemical evaluation of the A-cell.

PHYSIOLOGY OF GLUCAGON SECRETION

The measurement of glucagon in plasma has been considerably more difficult than that of insulin, primarily because of circulating peptides arising from the gastrointestinal tract, with immunologic determinants quite similar to those of pancreatic glucagon. There are cells in the stomach which appear morphologically and immunochemically identical to pancreatic A-cells. These are presumed to release true 3500-dalton glucagon into the plasma. These stomach cells are a major source of this hormone in pancreatectomized animals. They are different from related endocrine gut cells of the small and large intestine which are the source of gut glucagon or glucagon-like immunoreactivity (GLI), recently renamed glicentin. This molecule is of larger molecular weight and different biologic properties but contains the glucagon sequence as part of its primary structure. Therefore, antibodies made to pancreatic glucagon often cross-react with it. Since 1969 several antibodies which are almost specific for pancreatic glucagon have been developed. They apparently do not react with glicentin because of some "protective" effect of the C-terminal extension. These antibodies will react with N-terminally extended molecules, and, therefore, the common gut and pancreatic proglucagons may not be distinguishable in plasma. Although the use of these antibodies has allowed a beginning to be made in understanding the physiology of glucagon secretion, there is still uncertainty about the correctness of the absolute concentrations of glucagon that are reported.

The other major technologic problem has been the finding that plasma contains an enzyme-degrading system which rapidly inactivates glucagon. Presumably, this system exists *in vivo* and contributes to the turnover of the hormone. In addition, glucagon, like insulin, is taken up by the liver and is rapidly removed. The fractional extraction, i.e., the proportion taken out by the liver in a single passage, is unknown but very likely is about 50%. Basal peripheral plasma levels of glucagon are now reported to be less than 50 pg/ml. This is lower than once thought, as investigators have discovered various artifacts in plasma which tend to falsely increase the level. These lower levels are consistent with bioassay experiments concluding that the normal basal concentrations are probably around 50 pg/ml. The kinetics of release have not been evaluated; however, in general terms, it is known that certain substrates, hormones, and the neural system interact to determine the final secretory rate from the pancreas.

The concept has been proposed by Unger that glucagon and insulin form a regulatory couple. Each is controlled by the same factors and both regulate glucose, amino acid, and fatty acid metabolism in the liver. The net effect, then, depends on the relative concentrations of the two hormones. This implies that prediction of the state of activity of the liver depends on the concentration and effects of at least insulin and glucagon. In addition, it may be that the extracellular concentration in the pancreas of each hormone influences the secretion rate of the other. If this concept is correct, it indicates an important role for glucagon as a regulator of metabolism and provides a very sophisticated interactive regulatory system for metabolic processes.

Substrate Controls

Glucose.   There is an inverse relationship between glucagon output and glucose concentration. Thus, hyperglycemia suppresses glucagon secretion (Fig. 15–26) and hypoglycemia augments it. The sensitivity of this response *in vitro* is greater than that to the control of insulin secretion by glucose; thus, *in vitro* the suppression can be observed with as little as 50 mg/dl, a half-maximal effect at 100 mg/dl, and maximal effect at 200 mg/dl. The suppression is monophasic; however, a rapid decrease in glucose concentration may produce a multiphasic glucagon stimulation. The nature of this control has been difficult to study because of the direct effects of insulin to suppress glucagon secretion. Since the effect of glucose occurs at a lower concentration than that at which any insulin secretion occurs and since these effects can be demonstrated in the absence of B-cells, it is clear that glucose has a direct effect independent of its ability to stimulate insulin release. The mechanism for this effect is unknown.

Amino Acids.   Intravenous amino acid and oral protein have been shown to stimulate glucagon secretion (Fig. 15–27). There are major differences in the potency of amino acids to stimulate glucagon release, unrelated to their potency to stimulate insulin secretion. Arginine is the most potent for both, but leucine, another good insulin stimulant, does not increase glucagon secretion. In general, it appears that most glucogenic amino acids increase glucagon output. Some, such as alanine, probably increase only glucagon and not insulin. The physiologic importance of these interactions is presumably to prevent hypoglycemia when protein is ingested and to maximize amino acid storage in peripheral tissues; i.e., if protein stimulated only insulin release, hypoglycemia would tend to develop. Hypoglycemia is pre-

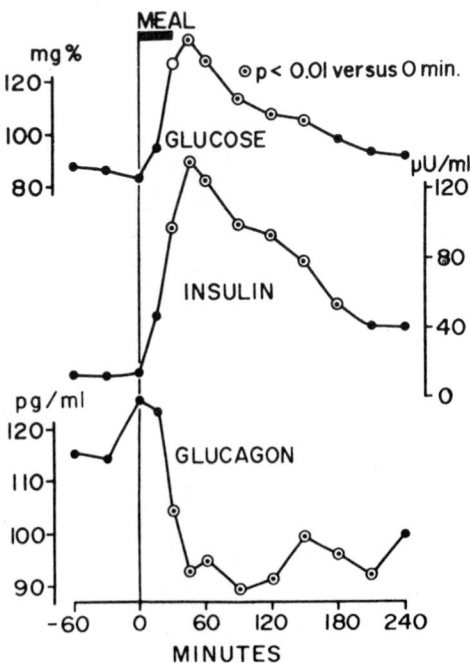

Figure 15–26. Suppression of glucagon by a glucose-containing meal in normal man. (From Unger, R. H.: Glucagon physiology and pathophysiology. *N. Engl. J. Med.* 285:443, 1971.)

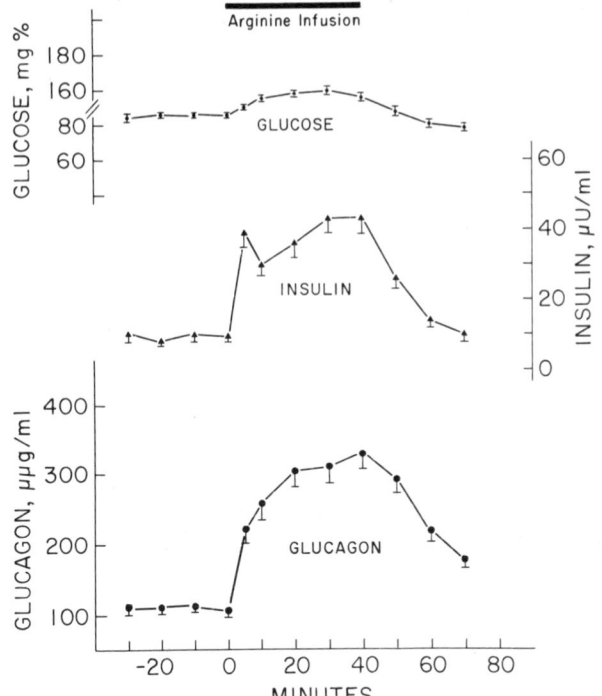

Figure 15–27. Stimulation of glucagon secretion by an arginine infusion in normal man. (From Unger, R. H.: Glucagon physiology and pathophysiology. *N. Engl. J. Med. 285:*443, 1971.)

vented, however, by the simultaneous release of glucagon, which activates liver glycogenolysis. Glucagon also tends to augment insulin secretion, which further accelerates amino acid uptake by muscle.

Fatty Acids. Glucagon is known to activate adipose tissue adenylate cyclase and therefore is a lipolytic hormone. In some species, it is liberated in sufficient quantities to play a role in the acceleration of lipolysis. Therefore, studies have been performed to determine whether fatty acids play a role in the regulation of glucagon secretion. In dogs and in man, elevated fatty acid levels suppress glucagon secretion, whereas lowered fatty acid levels increase glucagon output. Thus all three major substrates regulate both insulin and glucagon secretion.

Endocrine Control

In animals and man, cholecystokinin (CCK) has been found to be a potent stimulator of glucagon secretion. Since this hormone is released during the absorption of protein, the consequent glucagon stimulation is believed to represent an important role for CCK in communicating information from the gastrointestinal tract to the islets. CCK also stimulates insulin release, thus synergizing storage of amino acids with their absorption. Other gut hormones including gastrin and GIP have been shown to have similar effects and may also participate in the regulation of glucagon secretion during meals. Secretin inhibits the aminogenic stimulation of glucagon in the dog, but this finding has not been confirmed in man. While most of these studies have been at pharmacologic levels of gut hormones, they support the concept of an anticipatory mechanism for the regulation of glucagon secretion by gut hormones during meal feeding.

Glucocorticoids have been shown to increase glucagon secretion, possibly by increasing plasma amino acid levels, particularly alanine. Similarly, growth hormone administration has been found to increase glucagon levels, and altered thyroid hormone levels have been associated with changes in glucagon secretion. Since caloric balance plays an important role in glucagon secretion, it is difficult to tell whether these are direct or indirect effects of the hormones. Regardless, it appears that the hormonal control system for glucagon will turn out to be as complex as that for insulin.

Neural Control

An interaction between the sympathetic nervous system and glucagon release had been postulated for a number of years by Sokal. Such an interaction has now been confirmed in many species. Glucagon release is stimulated by epinephrine and in most instances blocked by the β-adrenergic blocking agent propranolol, indicating a β-adrenergic receptor mechanism. Regulation by the adrenergic nervous system has been confirmed by stimulation of pancreatic nerves in the presence of atropine and stimulation of the splanchnic sympathetics or the medial hypothalamus. Under conditions of experimental stress in animals, glucagon secretion tends to be increased. However, studies with adrenergic blocking agents have indicated that the situation is complex, since in some cases the glucagon response is blocked by β-adrenergic blocking agents, but in others only α-adrenergic blocking agents are effective, and in still others, neither works. This apparent paradox has been resolved by demonstrating in the calf both adrenergic and cholinergic control of glucagon secretion during insulin-induced hypoglycemia, thus indicating a redundant neural mechanism to combat life-threatening hypoglycemia. In man glucagon levels are elevated during hypoglycemic stress, but adrenergic blocking agents have relatively little effect on this response. It is not clear whether man is different from other species or whether studies with combinations of blocking agents will be needed in order to uncover the type of neural control mechanism.

The parasympathetic system has been shown to be stimulatory for glucagon secretion. Stimulation of the ventral hypothalamus, the dorsal motor nucleus of the vagus, or the pancreatic branch of the vagus has been shown to increase glucagon secretion. Acetylcholine *in vitro* or in the perfused pancreas is also stimulatory. All of these effects are blocked by atropine, indicating a muscarinic receptor mechanism.

The role of the neurally related intraislet modulators serotonin, dopamine, and the prostaglandins is not yet well defined; however, all have been shown to stimulate glucagon secretion and, therefore, presumably interact with the autonomic nervous system to regulate the A-cell. Finally, peptidergic nerves, particularly those containing vasoactive intestinal polypeptide (VIP), have been described in dogs, cats, and rats. VIP is a potent stimulant of glucagon secretion and may, therefore, be another autonomic nonadrenergic, noncholinergic neuromodulator of the A-cell.

The other potentially important intraislet regulator of glucagon secretion is somatostatin, which would inhibit glucagon release if it is released from the adjacent D-cell. Somatostatin has both substrate and neural controllers as well. Therefore, the autonomic nervous system could regulate insulin and glucagon secretion either directly or indirectly through the modulation of somatostatin release. Functionally, somatostatin appears to be ideally suited to counteract and balance the generally stimulatory actions of acetylcholine. However, it is important to emphasize here that the sympathetic and parasympathetic systems do not always counterbalance each other, since they are both stimulatory to glucagon secretion. A summary of the neuroendocrine regulation of the A-cell is shown in Figure 15–28.

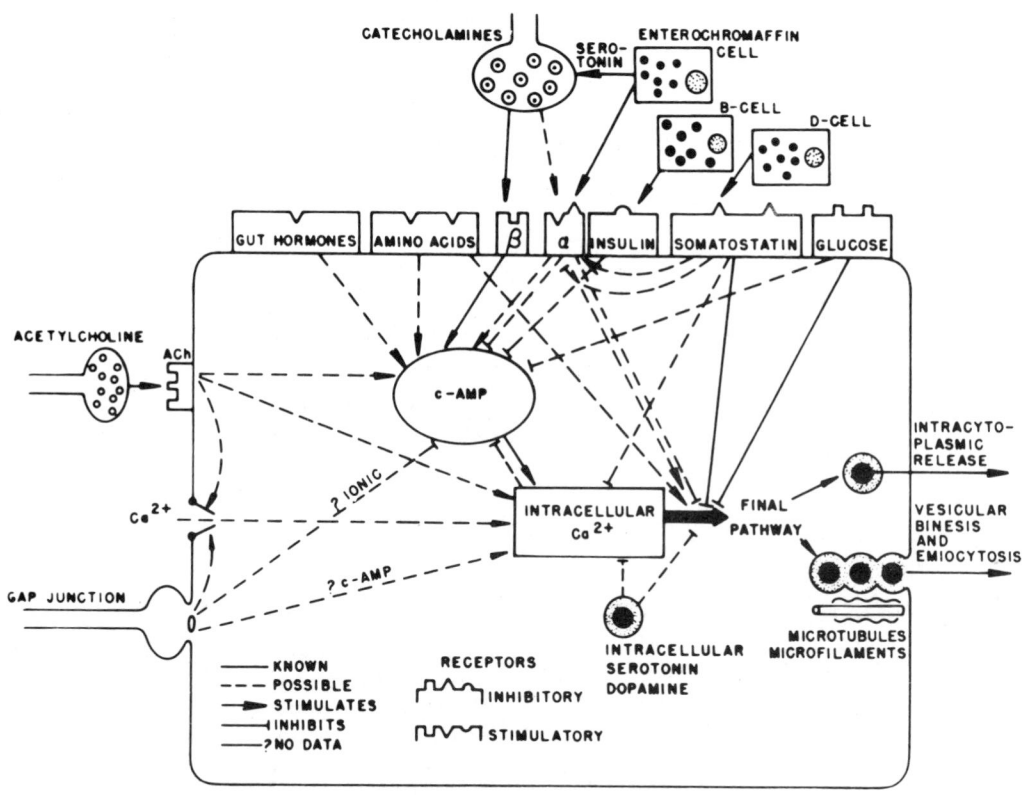

INTERACTING SYSTEMS IN GLUCAGON SECRETION

Figure 15–28. A schematic description of the neuroendocrine regulation of the A-cell. (From Porte, D., Jr., et al.: Neurohumoral regulation of the pancreatic islet A and B cells. *Metabolism 25*:1453, 1976.)

SOMATOSTATIN

Chemistry and Biosynthesis

The third pancreatic hormone, somatostatin, was discovered in 1973 and localized to the pancreas in 1975 after its very surprising effectiveness in suppressing insulin and glucagon secretion was demonstrated in 1974. It was discovered as a side fraction of a hypothalamic extract owing to its ability to suppress release of growth hormone *in vitro*. The 14-amino acid cyclic polypeptide has a 12-membered ring joined by disulfide bonds between two cystine residues (Fig. 15–29). It has been localized in neurons of many areas of the brain including the hypothalamus, midbrain, cortex, pons, cerebellum, and spinal cord, including the afferent spinal ganglia. It is known to inhibit the release of a variety of peptide hormones, but our understanding of its biosyn-

thesis, storage, and release is limited. Since it is contained within the granules of the pancreatic islet D-cell, it is assumed that its biosynthetic sequence is similar to that of other endocrine peptides. Somatostatin-containing D-cells are usually present on the periphery of rat islets but may be scattered throughout the islet in other species. Unlike glucagon and the pancreatic polypeptide, which are usually regionally distributed in a reciprocal relationship, insulin and somatostatin are in a relatively constant ratio throughout all of the islets. Somatostatin content averages 0.35 to 0.4 ng/mg wet weight in rat pancreas or approximately 350 ng for an entire adult pancreas. Islet content is approximately 180 pg/islet. Early biosynthesis studies indicate the likelihood of an initial peptide larger than the native somatostatin. Regulation of this process is not understood at all.

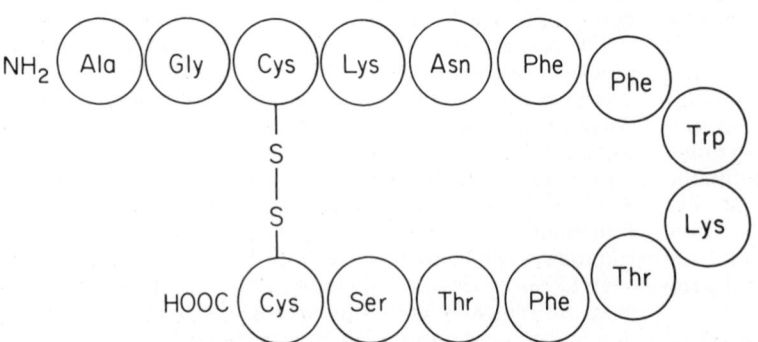

CYCLIC-SOMATOSTATIN

Figure 15–29. Amino acid sequence of hypothalamic somatostatin.

Regulation of Secretion

Studies of somatostatin release are primitive because of difficulties in the radioimmunoassay of plasma levels. There appear to be circulating proteins which either bind in the assay, bind somatostatin, or degrade somatostatin, and interfere with the interaction of the somatostatin with its antibody in a competitive displacement system. Reported plasma levels have ranged all the way from 10 pg/ml to 300 pg/ml. In buffer-perfused organ systems, these artifacts appear to be less important and less of a problem. Most nutrients have been shown to increase somatostatin secretion, including glucose, amino acids, and a fat-protein meal. In addition, hormones such as glucagon and the neurotransmitters of the sympathetic nervous system have been found to stimulate pancreatic somatostatin secretion. Since this latter effect appears to be related to the β-adrenergic receptor, it appears that cyclic AMP is a stimulant to pancreatic somatostatin secretion as it is for insulin and glucagon. Acetylcholine and α-adrenergic stimulation have been shown to inhibit somatostatin release. This response provides for antagonistic effects between the catecholamines and the parasympathetic system (see Fig. 15–17).

The physiologic role of somatostatin as a potential paracrine regulator of insulin and glucagon secretion is not clear. Unger has speculated that its release during nutrient absorption may tend to modulate nutrient entry and the responses of a number of peptide-secreting cells to food ingestion. Another possibility is for somatostatin to participate in the regulation of food intake as a satiety factor analogous to CCK. Studies have shown suppression of single meals by the intraperitoneal injection of somatostatin. Pathophysiologically, somatostatin content of the pancreas can be increased by alloxan diabetes. The number of D-cells also hypertrophies in juvenile-onset diabetes in man. On the other hand, experimental obese hyperglycemic syndromes are characterized by decreased pancreatic somatostatin. Although it has been hypothesized that these changes are related only to the presence or absence of different kinds of diabetes, the possibility that they are due to concomitant changes in body weight and relative adiposity needs to be explored further.

PANCREATIC POLYPEPTIDE

Chemistry

Pancreatic polypeptide was isolated as a contaminant of avian insulin by Kimmell in 1968, but until a similar peptide was identified as a side fraction of commercial insulin preparation in 1975, it was not realized that this peptide existed in mammals. It has a 36-amino acid sequence in all species; however, only about half of the amino acids are the same for birds and mammals. Indeed, there are several sequence differences between various mammalian forms. The human sequence (Ch. 14) differs from bovine in positions 6, 10, 11, and 23 and porcine in positions 10, 11, and 23. The peptide has been identified in special endocrine cells of the endocrine pancreas and in mammals is almost exclusively limited to the pancreas. A similar peptide has been identified in the gastrointestinal tract in some lower species. There has been morphologic evidence for a cell type in the dog different from A, B, and D, which has been called the F-cell. This cell is now known to contain the pancreatic polypeptide. The neutral name given to this peptide is related to the fact that its biologic significance and biologic

activity have not been accurately identified. Nothing is known of its biosynthesis at the present time. The pancreatic polypeptide is found in single cells outside the islets of Langerhans in many species. There is a reciprocal relationship between the concentration of glucagon and pancreatic polypeptide in individual rat islets. There is also a regional separation such that islets in the pancreatic head are particularly high in percentage of pancreatic polypeptide cells and low in the percentage of glucagon-containing A-cells, whereas islets in the tail are relatively rich in glucagon and poor in pancreatic polypeptide.

Pancreatic polypeptide has been shown to deplete liver glycogen and cause lipolysis in the bird, but such effects have not been observed in mammals. The most potent action of the pancreatic polypeptide in the dog is inhibition of pancreatic enzyme secretion and gallbladder contraction. The same effects have been shown in man. It has been reported that the C-terminal hexapeptide has the same biologic actions. No metabolic effects have been described in any mammal which relate directly to the metabolism of glucose, amino acids, or fat.

Regulation of Secretion

Antibodies to pancreatic polypeptide have been relatively easy to raise, and, therefore, there are a number of studies defining the regulation of its secretion in man and in other mammals. Basal levels average about 80 pg/ml and rise 8 to 10 fold after the ingestion of a mixed meal. Protein appears to provide the greatest and most prolonged response. Intravenous administration of glucose or triglyceride produces no effect, but some increase is observed during the intravenous administration of a mixture of amino acids. However, this response is small compared to that observed following a meal. The meal response is blocked by vagotomy or atropine. Metabolic signals such as hypoglycemia which stimulate the vagus will also result in a rapid rise in pancreatic polypeptide. Intravenous administration of a number of gastrointestinal hormones including gastrin, secretin, and cholecystokinin is associated with an increase in pancreatic polypeptide. Therefore, the vagal effects may be direct as well as indirect via gut hormones for the regulation of pancreatic polypeptide secretion (see Fig. 15–17).

Basal levels and responses to challenge are age-dependent, with an increase in both basal and stimulated pancreatic polypeptide responses from the third to the seventh decade of life. Pancreatic polypeptide levels are slightly raised in diabetics of either the maturity-onset, non-insulin-dependent type, or the juvenile-onset, insulin-dependent type. The latter also often have pancreatic polypeptide antibodies owing to the presence of pancreatic polypeptide in the insulin injected in the past. Therefore, true values in many juvenile diabetics are not known. Some patients with pancreatitis also have an elevation of basal pancreatic polypeptide levels, but in those with severe pancreatic disease, greatly reduced pancreatic polypeptide levels may be seen. In those individuals with endocrine pancreatic tumors secreting gastrin, glucagon, insulin, VIP, or somatostatin, there is often a concomitant elevation of pancreatic polypeptide.

In summary, pancreatic polypeptide is a food-related hormone with surprisingly weak metabolic or gastrointestinal effects described to date. Its control seems almost entirely related to the vagus nerve and feeding. Progress has been hampered by limited supplies of the hormone. It seems likely that major effects on gastrointestinal function will be uncovered when this deficit has been remedied.

DISTRIBUTION AND DEGRADATION OF ISLET HORMONES

Insulin Distribution

There are many factors that influence the distribution of insulin, including its rate of degradation in different tissues. When insulin-^{131}I is injected into normal man, less than 15% is present in the plasma after 1 hour. In diabetics and normal men, porcine insulin was found to have a circulating half-life of less than 5 min. Studies with rats showed that almost all tissues accumulate some insulin, but in markedly different concentrations. Brain and red blood cells took up very little hormone, while the greatest concentrations were seen in the kidney and liver. These two organs together with skeletal muscle and plasma accounted for 61% of the insulin-[131]I.

The liver normally removes more insulin than does any other organ, chiefly because insulin secreted by the pancreas must traverse the liver before reaching the peripheral circulation. Several studies indicate that approximately 40–50% of the portal vein insulin is removed by the liver during a single transhepatic passage. Insulin is found in bile with a peak level reached about 45 min after glucose ingestion.

Since the liver normally removes a large amount of secreted insulin, changes in the rate of liver extraction could affect the amount of insulin available to peripheral tissues. Diminished hepatic extraction of insulin has been reported in patients with liver disease, providing a possible explanation for the hyperinsulinemia of these patients. There appears to be little effect of varying physiologic concentrations of insulin *per se* on the hepatic extraction of insulin. However, at pharmacologic insulin levels (200–300 μU/ml), the process seems to saturate. Changes of hepatic extraction of insulin have been reported following administration of glucose or glucagon and during starvation. However, such changes have been rather variable because of technical problems in assessing rates of hepatic extraction during non-steady-state conditions. Thus, although it is clearly established that the liver is a major site of insulin extraction, there is no clear-cut evidence at present that this process is physiologically regulated.

The kidney extracts about 40% of the insulin delivered to it by the systemic circulation in a single passage, a process which does not appear to be saturable. Insulin is filtered through the glomerulus but usually is almost completely reabsorbed from the proximal tubule. The renal medulla extracts very little hormone, whereas the cortex and particularly the proximal convoluted tubules trap large quantities. Glomerular filtration and excretion can account for at most 60% of the insulin removed by the kidney in man. There is now evidence that much of the insulin trapped by tubular cells comes from peritubular capillaries rather than the tubular lumen. In patients with severe renal disease, there is a twofold decrease in the rate of disappearance of ^{125}I-insulin from plasma, presumably due chiefly to an associated decrease in the rate of insulin degradation by the kidney. Small amounts of insulin and proinsulin have been found in human urine.

Once the insulin that has escaped degradation reaches peripheral tissues and crosses the capillary membrane, entering the extracellular fluid, it remains in this lymph fluid much longer than in the blood vascular system. For example, after intravenous glucose administration, lymph insulin was found to peak at about 1 hour, whereas in blood the peak was reached in 5 min. The lymph insulin levels were observed to correlate better with glucose assimilation rates than did serum insulin levels.

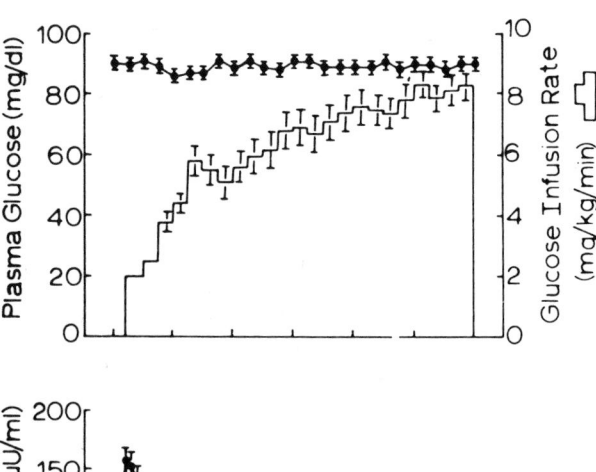

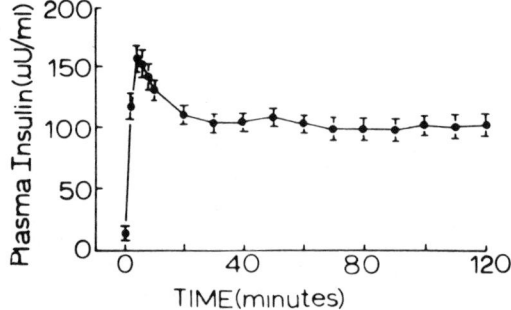

Figure 15–30. Euglycemic glucose clamp study in man. Glucose is infused at a variable rate to maintain euglycemia during infusion of exogenous insulin. Note the increasing glucose infusion rate required over time despite constant hyperinsulinemia. (From DeFronzo, R. A., et al: Glucose clamp technique: a method for quantifying insulin secretion and resistance. *Am. J. Physiol.* 237:E214, 1979.)

The relationship between the time course of distribution of insulin into tissues and the metabolic effects of insulin has been demonstrated in man using the glucose clamp technique. In this procedure, insulin is administered as a bolus followed by a continuous infusion to maintain a constant circulating insulin level. A variable glucose infusion is then given to prevent any change of plasma glucose level. Thus, the rate of glucose infusion at a given time is a measure of total glucose uptake. As illustrated in Figure 15–30, although plasma insulin is constant during 120 min of study, the rate of glucose infusion required to maintain the plasma glucose is continually increasing. It is only toward the end of the study that the maximal effect of insulin is observed. Such studies indicate that there is a considerable lag between the time of appearance of insulin in blood and the time of the maximal effect of the insulin on tissues, presumably representing the time required for distribution of insulin from plasma to tissues. In addition, other studies have demonstrated that insulin action persists after an insulin infusion is stopped and after plasma levels have declined, suggesting that tissue insulin levels fall more slowly.

Proinsulin Distribution

The immunologic half-time of porcine proinsulin has been found to be 20 min in swine and 18 min in baboons. In contrast to insulin, porcine proinsulin and C-peptide are not cleared by isolated perfused rat liver. Dog kidney has been found to extract an amount of proinsulin equivalent to the quantity of insulin extracted. Thus, the kidney is the major organ for the removal of proinsulin.

Since the liver extracts such a large quantity of insulin

and little, if any, proinsulin, this could account for a considerable proportion of the difference in the plasma levels of the two hormonal components following glucose administration. When proinsulin was injected intravenously into rats, no evidence of conversion of proinsulin to insulin was found 1 hour later. Nevertheless, injection of a sufficient amount of proinsulin can produce marked hypoglycemia, suggesting that proinsulin exerts insulin-like effects without being converted to insulin. As discussed earlier, apparently all of the insulin derived from the pancreas results from transformation of proinsulin to insulin induced by a specific enzyme system involving proteolysis. This enzyme system has not been demonstrated in other tissues.

Degradation of Insulin and Proinsulin

Insulin is degraded by essentially all tissues of the body. Little or none is resynthesized from the degraded products. The total degradation by liver and kidney greatly exceeds that of other organs. These two organs appear to remove 80% or more of the total amount secreted. Much of the insulin removed by the kidneys is degraded rather than excreted. The liver, the first organ through which insulin passes after its secretion, has a very active insulin-degrading system. In all tissues studied (except pancreas), proinsulin degradation occurs at less than 10% of the rate of degradation of insulin. Accelerated insulin degradation has been proposed as a mechanism for insulin resistance during pregnancy (placental degradation) and in some patients with diabetes mellitus (fat-tissue degradation of injected insulin).

Tissue Degradation.   Conflicting evidence has been presented regarding the nature of the insulin-degradation system. Some workers have found that 90% of the degradative activity for insulin is located in the supernatant fraction of tissues studied, with liver having the most activity. This degradation is by proteolysis, is relatively specific for insulin (and much less active for proinsulin), and does not depend on the presence of a sulfhydryl reagent such as reduced glutathione. This insulin-specific protease appears to be active at physiologic insulin levels. Comparison of the properties of partially purified insulin-degrading enzyme from liver, muscle, and kidney has suggested that the enzyme preparation from each organ has similar biochemical properties with high specificity for insulin. Advantage has been taken of the relative specificity of the insulin protease to develop an assay method for proinsulin. Plasma is assayed for immunoreactive insulin before and after incubation with an insulin protease preparation. Since almost all of the insulin is degraded and no longer binds to the antibody, the residual immunoreactivity represents proinsulin-like material. This assay method appears to be useful only when the total plasma immunoreactive insulin concentration (before enzymatic degradation) is greater than 30 μU/ml.

Other investigators have reported the existence of insulin-degrading activity in the microsomal fraction of tissues. This enzyme has been called glutathione-insulin transhydrogenase. It catalyzes a reductive cleavage of the insulin disulfide bonds by reduced glutathione with liberation of A and B chains in reduced form. This enzyme is active only in the presence of reduced glutathione. It is also present in a wide variety of tissues, but greatest activity is in the liver. The physiologic role of this enzyme outside the pancreas has been questioned since it appears to be active only at supraphysiologic insulin levels.

Receptor-Mediated Degradation.   A major feature of the interaction between insulin and target cells is the specific binding of insulin to cell surface membrane receptors. This interaction is described in more detail in the next section. There is now clear evidence that degradation of insulin occurs as part of the process of binding to receptors. Ultrastructural and biochemical studies of liver and fat cells have demonstrated that following binding, the insulin-receptor complex is internalized to a limited area at the periphery of the cell. This intracellular material eventually associates with lysosomal structures. Although intracellular bound insulin can be eluted intact from receptors early in this process, with time reversibility is lost and increasing degradation of insulin can be demonstrated. Thus, degradation of insulin appears to be a part of the process of the insulin-receptor interaction. Insulin degradation by insulin-specific protease also can occur independently of receptor binding of insulin. For example, degradation of insulin analogues which do not bind to insulin receptors has been demonstrated. In addition, bacitracin, an inhibitor of proteolysis, prevents non-receptor-mediated insulin degradation but has no effect on intracellular insulin degradation related to receptor binding. The relative importance in terms of overall insulin metabolism of receptor-mediated vs. non-receptor-mediated insulin degradation remains to be established.

Glucagon Distribution and Degradation

Early studies of glucagon distribution and degradation involved the use of glucagon labeled with radioisotope. Although the handling of radiolabeled glucagon may be somewhat different from that of the native hormone, generally similar findings have been reported with either. Essentially all tissues take up ^{131}I-glucagon but at markedly different rates. The relative concentrations of ^{131}I-insulin and glucagon in various tissues have been reported to be similar. Liver degrades a higher percentage of glucagon than insulin. Glucagon injected into the general circulation has been reported to have a half-life of approximately 5 min. The metabolic clearance rate of glucagon in normal man, determined by constant infusion of exogenous unlabeled glucagon, has been reported to be approximately 10 ml/kg/min.

Studies with unlabeled glucagon in human subjects showed that no glucagon was present in urine of normal subjects but that glucagon appeared in the urine after intravenous injection of glucagon in patients with proximal renal tubular disease. Glucagon immunoreactivity has been found in bile and increases after administration of exogenous glucagon. Biologically active glucagon similar to that secreted by pancreatic islet cells has been reported to be present in cells of salivary gland, stomach fundus, and small intestine.

Glucagon has been shown to be degraded by many tissues, especially liver and kidney. Glucagon-degrading activity in liver has been found in the residual supernatant fraction after ultracentrifugation of tissue homogenate. Glucagon degradation by liver preparations has been reported to be inhibited by the addition of insulin, cysteine-inactivated insulin, A or B chain of insulin, ACTH, and growth hormone. One type of glucagon-degrading activity has been attributed to dipeptidyl aminopeptidase I. This enzyme also has been found to degrade a wide variety of other peptides. Chloride and sulfhydryl activators are essential for the degradation of glucagon by this aminopeptidase. The enzyme removes the amino-terminal His–Ser of glucagon, thereby producing a loss of biologic activity of the molecule (see Fig. 15–25). Glucagon degradation by a highly purified insulin-specific protease preparation has also been observed. This finding suggests that both insulin and glucagon may share a common degradative pathway.

The importance of renal metabolism of glucagon is demonstrated by the elevated plasma glucagon levels observed in renal failure in both man and experimental animals. Clearance of exogenously administered glucagon has been reported to be reduced by over 50% in patients with renal failure. Elevated glucagon levels in uremic rats have been shown to consist of both the biologically active 3500-dalton species and a 9000-dalton component, a probable glucagon precursor with little biologic activity.

The role of the liver in glucagon metabolism remains somewhat controversial. Several investigators have reported little difference between portal and peripheral immunoassayable glucagon levels, suggesting that the liver plays a minor role in glucagon removal. However, elevated circulating glucagon levels have been found in patients with liver disease and in hepatectomized animals. Furthermore, when gel filtration was used to quantify the various circulating molecular species of glucagon, a large portal-peripheral gradient was observed for the biologically active 3500-dalton fraction in experimental animals, with a calculated hepatic extraction of over 50% for this molecule. This finding contrasted with the lack of evidence of hepatic extraction of the biologically inactive glucagon species in plasma. Thus, measurement of total immunoassayable glucagon may not accurately reflect the importance of hepatic degradation of biologically active glucagon. Overall, glucagon disposal appears to have many features in common with the disposal of insulin: both kidney and liver degrade biologically active hormone, but the kidney is the major site of degradation of larger precursor molecules. Since both hormones are secreted into the portal system, the liver plays a key role in their metabolism. Whether hepatic extraction of biologically active glucagon is a physiologically regulated process remains undetermined.

Somatostatin Distribution and Degradation

In addition to being present in the D-cells of the pancreatic islets, somatostatin is produced in several other tissues. It is widely distributed in the central nervous system, predominantly in neurons of the median eminence and hypothalamus. Somatostatin is also present in smaller amounts in spinal cord and in cell bodies of sympathetic ganglia. It has been identified in parafollicular cells of the thyroid and in stomach, duodenum, and jejunum of several species. Therefore, the source of somatostatin in blood is unclear.

Somatostatin in blood is rapidly degraded. Exogenously infused somatostatin has been reported to have a disappearance half-time of 1–3 min in normal humans with a metabolic clearance rate of approximately 30 ml/kg/min. Degradation of somatostatin occurs spontaneously in plasma and has been demonstrated in a variety of tissues. Because of the lability of somatostatin, blood samples for its measurement must be collected in the presence of inhibitors of degradative enzymes. Although there is evidence of a portal-peripheral gradient for somatostatin, the metabolic clearance rate has been reported to be normal in patients with liver disease. In contrast, a diminished metabolic clearance rate of somatostatin has been found in patients with renal failure, suggesting an important role for the kidneys in somatostatin metabolism. There is evidence that the kidney is twice as effective as the liver in the clearance of somatostatin from the circulation.

ACTION OF ISLET HORMONES

Insulin Action

Insulin directly or indirectly affects the function of every organ of the body. The effects of insulin depend at least on (1) amount of insulin secreted, (2) insulin distribution, (3) type of tissue, (4) amount of insulin binding to its specific receptor, (5) post-receptor events inside the cell, (6) types and amounts of nutrients inside and outside the cells, (7) ionic composition and concentrations, and (8) amounts and types of other hormones. Some of the tissues in which insulin has been shown to affect glucose uptake and metabolism are listed in Table 15-1; adipose tissue, muscle, and liver have been studied in greatest detail (Fig. 15–31).

Cellular Responses to Insulin

Insulin stimulates metabolic reactions for the synthesis and/or storage of carbohydrates, fats, proteins, and nucleic acids. It regulates membrane transport of many substances and mediates the formation of macromolecules in cells, which then are used in cell structure, energy stores, and regulation of many cell functions. Insulin stimulates the synthesis of protein from amino acids, nucleic acids from mononucleotides, polysaccharides from monosaccharides, and complex lipids from fatty acids (Fig. 15–32).

The following are some of the specific actions of insulin. Insulin increases (1) plasma membrane transport of glucose and certain other monosaccharides, some amino acids, some fatty acids, potassium, and magnesium; (2) magnesium-activated sodium-potassium ATPase activity; (3) glucose oxidation; (4) glycogenesis; (5) lipogenesis; (6) protein synthesis; and (7) formation of ATP, DNA, and RNA. Insulin decreases (1) glycogenolysis, (2) lipolysis, (3) proteolysis, (4) gluconeogenesis, (5) ureogenesis, and (6) ketogenesis. Insulin does not stimulate glucose transport in red blood cells or in most areas of the brain, nor does it promote tubular reabsorption of glucose by the kidney or glucose absorption by the intestinal mucosa.

Insulin Receptor

A series of studies reported by several groups of investigators in the early 1970's demonstrated that insulin binds to specific proteins on the plasma membrane of cells of a variety of tissues. Such studies provided direct evidence that, like other peptide hormones, insulin's mechanism of action is initiated by binding to a cell surface membrane receptor. Such specific insulin receptors have now been demonstrated on fat, liver, and muscle cells in which the insulin binding can be related to the biologic effects of insulin. In addition, insulin binding sites with similar properties have been found in tissues such as brain, placenta, and kidney as well as fibroblasts, platelets, red blood cells, granulocytes, and mononuclear white blood cells. Since blood cells can be easily obtained, they have been used extensively for studies of insulin receptors *in vivo*.

The characteristics of the insulin-receptor interaction are quite similar in all of these cell types and are similar to the general characteristics of hormone-receptor interactions. Specific insulin binding (i.e., that amount of radiolabeled insulin bound to cells that can be displaced by addition of an excess of unlabeled insulin) occurs rapidly (within minutes at 37°C), is rapidly reversible, and is saturable. The insulin receptor has a high degree of specificity for binding biologi-

Liver Cell   Muscle Cell

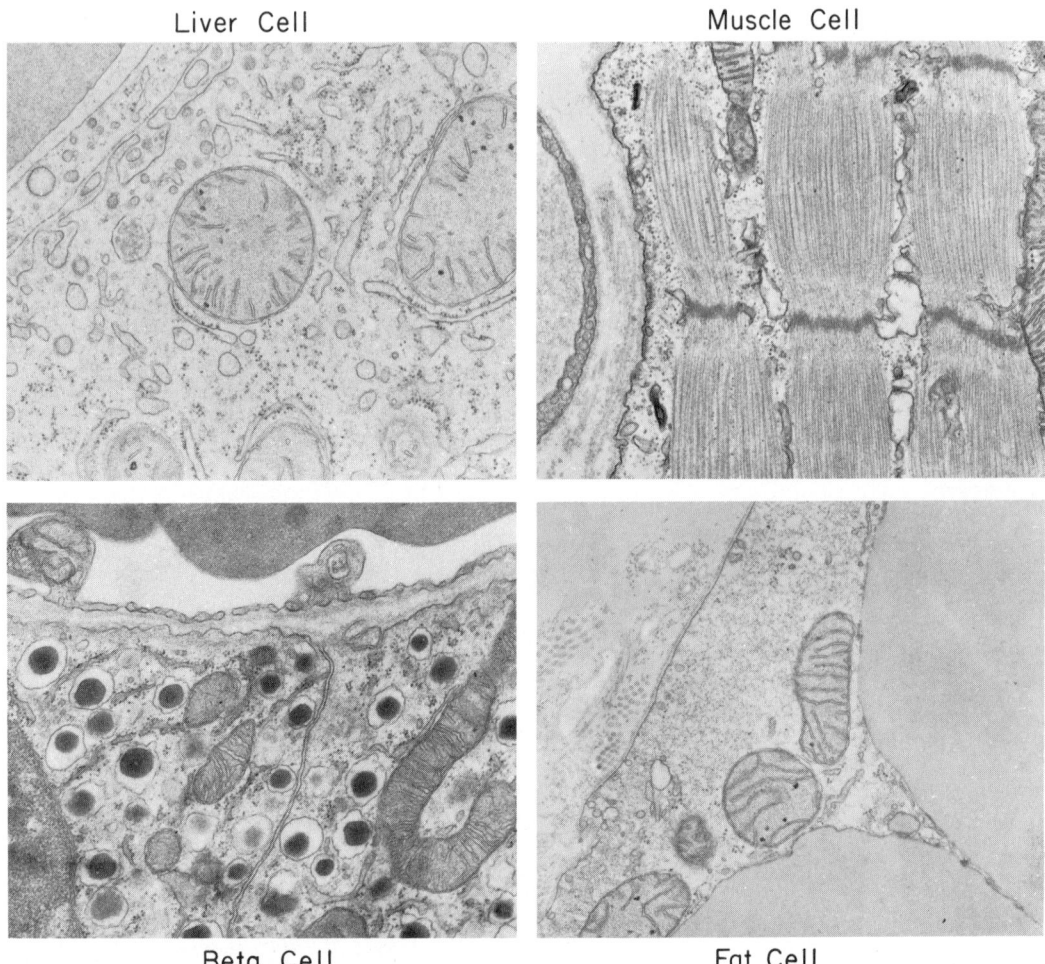

Beta Cell   Fat Cell

Figure 15–31.   Site of synthesis of insulin and the three tissue sites of action that have been studied most extensively. Insulin promotes protein synthesis in each of these tissues. In adipose tissue, its major function consists of synthesis and storage of fat. In muscle, its chief function is to stimulate protein synthesis. It inhibits gluconeogenesis and ketogenesis in the liver. ($\times$ 36,000.) (Photomicrographs kindly supplied by J. Luft and J. Logothetopoulos.)

cally active insulin and insulin derivatives. Furthermore, insulin and its derivatives compete for binding in direct proportion to the degree of insulin-like biologic activity of each molecule (Fig. 15–33). For example, the proinsulin molecule has approximately 5% of the biologic activity of insulin, and displacement of a given amount of insulin from its receptor requires 20 times as much proinsulin. Bound insulin is not displaced by noninsulin peptides such as growth hormone, ACTH, and glucagon even when each hormone is added in very high concentrations. By studying the binding characteristics of a variety of insulin analogues to fat cell insulin receptors, the region of the insulin molecule that binds to the receptor has been identified (Fig. 15–34).

Radiolabeled or fluorescence-labeled insulin preparations have been used as markers to identify and purify the portion of the cell membrane which binds insulin. As a result,

some information about the protein chemistry of the insulin receptor is now available. The insulin receptor appears to be a disulfide-linked glycoprotein complex with a total molecular weight of approximately 300,000. The most simple model for the insulin receptor is illustrated in Figure 15–35. In this hypothetical model, there are two large components, each 125,000 molecular weight, and two smaller components, all linked by disulfide bonds. When the disulfide bonds are broken, insulin binding is associated with a 125,000 molecular weight protein, presumably one or both of the large components of the proposed receptor model. In

Table 15–1.   TISSUES RESPONSIVE TO INSULIN

Muscle (skeletal and heart)	Cartilage and bone
Adipose tissue	Skin
Liver	Lens
Leukocytes	Pituitary
Mammary glands	Peripheral nerve
Seminal vesicles	Aorta
Fibroblasts	Thymocytes
Smooth muscle cells	Brain

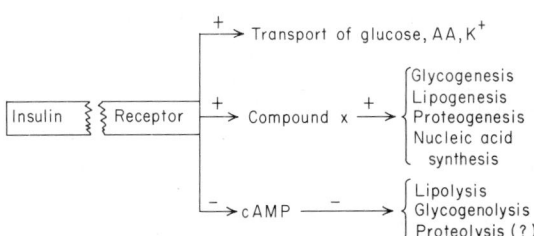

Figure 15–32.   Insulin becomes attached to a specific receptor on the plasma membrane. It then initiates changes in the membrane which affect transportation of specific compounds and affects functions of the nucleus, polysomes, and other subcellular components. (+ signifies increase; − signifies decrease.)

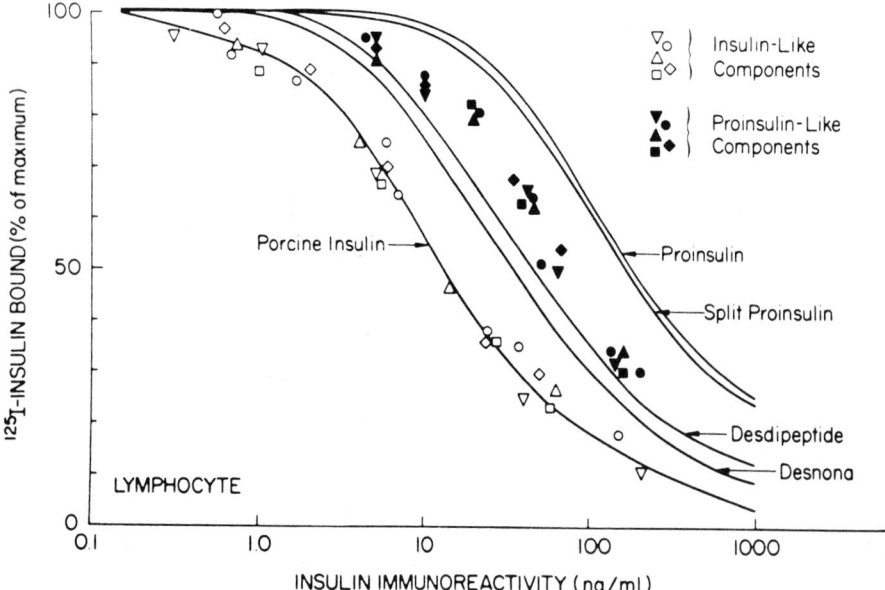

Figure 15–33. Displacement curves for ^{125}I-porcine insulin specifically bound to cultured human lymphocytes. Various concentrations of unlabeled porcine insulin, proinsulin, proinsulin intermediates (split desdipeptide and desnonapeptide proinsulin), and pooled immunoreactive human plasma components are compared. Note that approximately 20 times more proinsulin than porcine insulin is required for equal displacement of bound labeled insulin (From Kahn, R. C., et al.: Receptors for peptide hormones. New insights into the pathophysiology of disease states in man. *Ann. Int. Med. 86*:205, 1977.)

the model the glucose transport system is shown to be adjacent to the insulin receptor. Although a number of studies suggest that the insulin receptor and glucose transport system are closely linked, current evidence indicates that they are separate components of the cell surface membrane.

There has been considerable debate in the past about whether insulin's sole site of interaction with cells is on the cell surface. However, there is now clear ultrastructural evidence from several laboratories that insulin-receptor complexes are internalized. In addition, much of the internalized insulin can be eluted intact, particularly in the

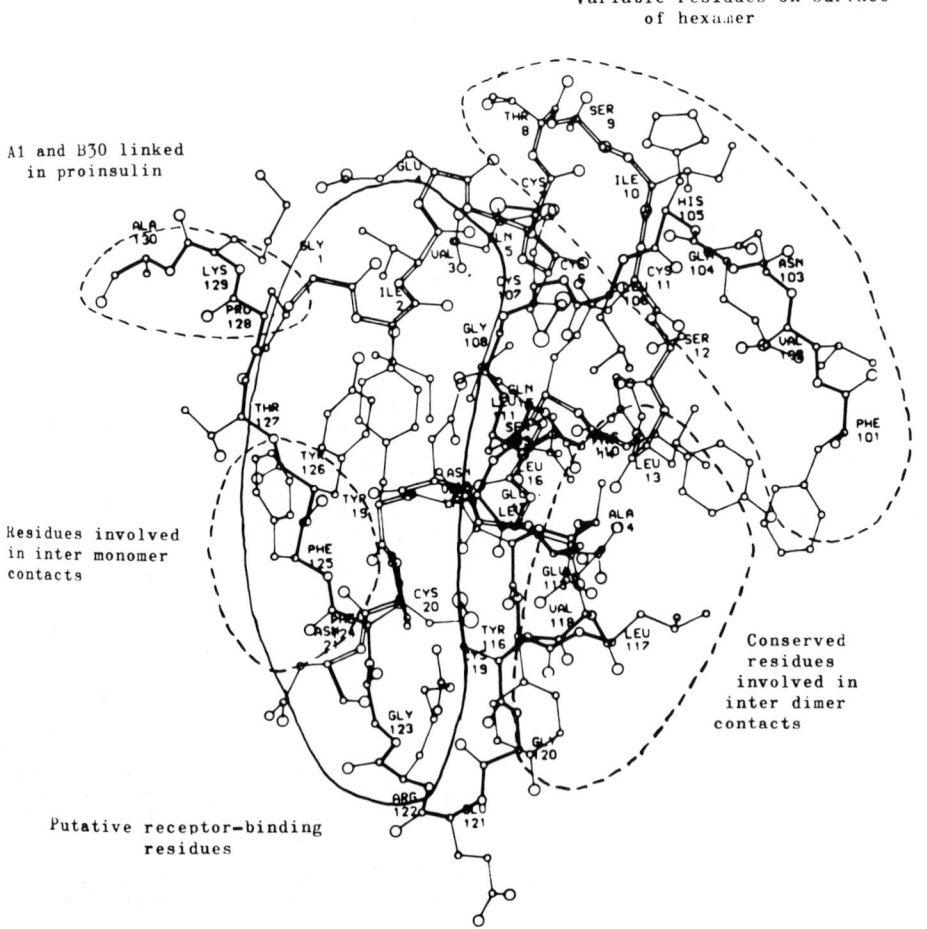

Figure 15–34. View of the insulin monomer indicating how the surface may be described in terms of functions of various regions of the molecule. The residues important for binding to the insulin receptor are enclosed by the solid line. (From Blundell, T. L., and Wood, S. P.: Is the evolution of insulin Darwinian or due to selectively neutral mutation? *Nature 257*:197, 1975.)

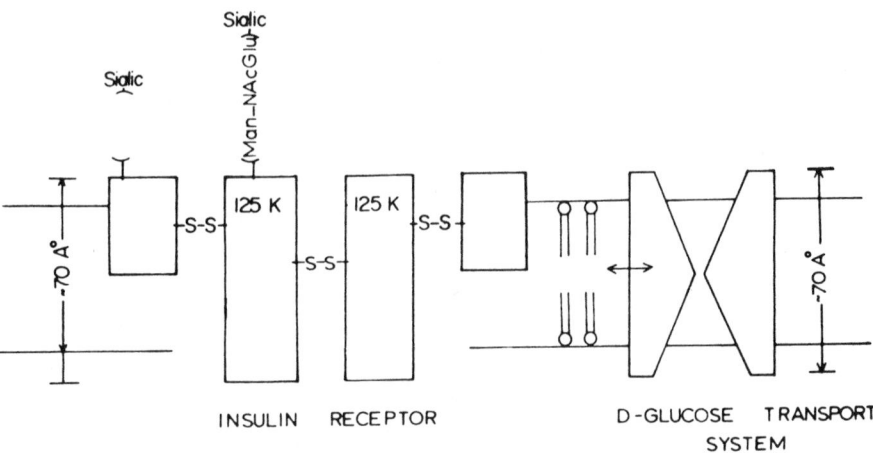

Figure 15–35. A hypothetical model for the insulin receptor. It illustrates some aspects of the protein chemistry of the insulin receptor and D-glucose transport system present in liver and adipocyte plasma membrane. The insulin receptor exists as a disulfide-linked complex with a total molecular weight of approximately 300,000, containing at least one insulin-binding subunit with an apparent molecular weight of approximately 125,000. In this model the D-glucose transport system is shown to be a separate, but closely linked, component of the plasma membrane. (From Czech, M. P.: Insulin action and the regulation of hexose transport. *Diabetes 29*:399, 1980.)

initial few minutes after internalization. As illustrated schematically in Figure 15–36, the internalized insulin-receptor complexes eventually become associated with lysosomal structures where degradation of insulin occurs with time. Presumably, degradation of the insulin receptor also occurs at this site. The penetration of insulin into the cell raises the possibility that insulin or a degradation product of insulin could be a direct intracellular mediator of insulin action. However, at present there is no direct evidence to support this possibility. Insulin receptors have also been identified in the membranous structures of the endoplasmic reticulum and Golgi apparatus. These sites presumably are the location of insulin receptor synthesis and subsequent transport to the cell surface. Although insulin and insulin receptors have also been reported on the nuclear membrane, several laboratories have been unable to confirm this finding.

A number of studies have demonstrated that the binding of insulin to target cells is a complex process that is not readily explained by a simple interaction of insulin with one class of binding sites. One way to express a hormone-receptor binding relationship is to plot the ratio of specifically bound hormone to free hormone as a function of bound hormone as increasing amounts of hormone are added (Scatchard analysis). When there is a single class of binding sites, there is a linear inverse relationship between the bound/free ratio of hormone and the amount of hormone specifically bound to receptors. However, this relationship is curvilinear for the interaction between insulin and its receptors (Fig. 15–37). The observation that there is accelerated dissociation of bound radiolabeled insulin with the addition of unlabeled hormone also indicates that the insulin binding sites are not homogeneous.

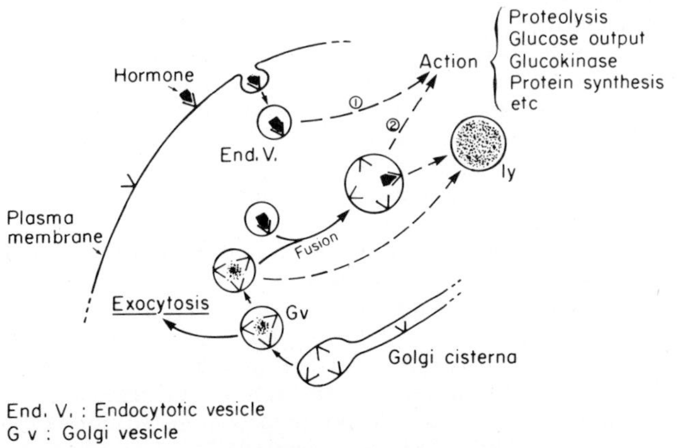

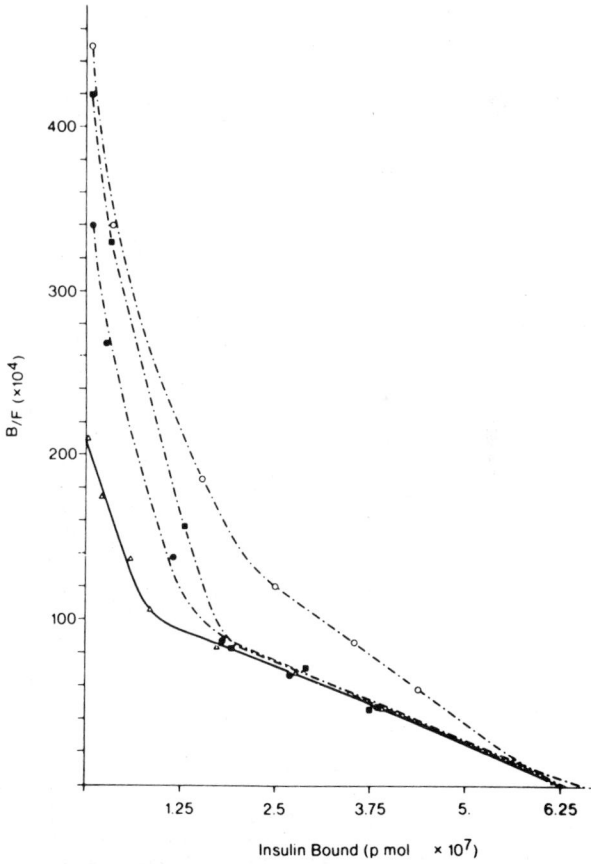

Figure 15–37. Scatchard plot of insulin binding to isolated adipocytes of control rats (△), and of rats fasted for 24 (•), 48 (○), and 72 (■) hours. The ratio of specifically bound to free hormone (B/F) is on the ordinate, and the amount of bound hormone is on the abscissa. The slope has been used as a measure of receptor affinity and the intercept as a measure of receptor number. The steeper slopes of the curves in the cells of the fasted rats have been interpreted to indicate greater binding affinity. (From Olefsky, J. M.: Effects of fasting on insulin binding, glucose transport, and glucose oxidation in isolated rat adipocytes. Relationships between insulin receptors and insulin action. *J. Clin. Invest. 58*:1450, 1976.)

End. V. : Endocytotic vesicle
G v : Golgi vesicle

Figure 15–36. A model illustrating the internalization of insulin-receptor complexes. The association of these complexes with endocytotic vesicles *(End. V.)*, Golgi vesicles *(Gv)*, and lysosomes *(ly)* is shown. Internalization of insulin may be an important mechanism for insulin degradation and/or initiation of insulin action either directly from endocytotic vesicles *(1)* or after processing via Golgi vesicles *(2)*. (From Posner, B. I., et al.: Intracellular insulin and insulin receptors: Nature and significance. In *Proc. 10th Cong. Int. Diab. Fed.* Amsterdam, Excerpta Medica Foundation, 1980.)

One possible explanation for these findings is that there are two or more classes of binding sites, each with a different affinity for insulin. Alternatively, it has been suggested that there is really only one class of binding sites, but that the interaction of insulin molecules with binding sites leads to a change in cell membrane structure. As a result, unoccupied binding sites are transformed into a configuration which has decreased affinity for insulin (negative cooperativity or site-site interactions). Using fluorescence microscopy to visualize the binding of high concentrations of fluorescent analogues of insulin to fibroblasts, aggregation of insulin-receptor complexes into patches has been demonstrated. This aggregation process appears to be an important component of the initiation of insulin action, at least with regard to enhancement of glucose transport (see later), and may be the physical correlate of the proposed negative cooperativity of insulin receptors.

Although the interpretation of the insulin-receptor binding interaction remains controversial, it has been clearly established that only a small percentage of insulin receptors are occupied at concentrations of insulin that have maximal physiologic effects. The presence of a large residual pool of "spare" receptors has provided a theoretical basis for the regulation of biologic sensitivity to insulin as a result of a change of receptor binding alone. Thus, a decrease in receptor binding would not be expected to change the maximal effect of insulin, since there would still be enough "spare" sites available for binding. However, the *concentration* of insulin required to achieve sufficient receptor occupancy for a maximal effect would change considerably. Thus, a reduction of receptor binding would result in a shift of the insulin biologic effect dose-response curve, but with no change of the maximal insulin effect. This concept has spurred considerable investigative effort to determine whether insulin binding to receptors is a regulated process and, if so, whether changes of receptor binding are related to altered biologic sensitivity to insulin.

Regulation of Insulin Receptors

A large number of studies have provided evidence to support the concept that insulin binding to membrane receptors is a regulated process. The most well established regulator of insulin binding is insulin itself. Studies *in vitro* in several different cell types have demonstrated that incubation of cells with insulin results in a decrease (downregulation) of insulin binding by these cells. Subsequent studies of these cell types *in vivo* in experimental animals and in man have all supported the general concept that receptor binding is inversely related to circulating insulin: when insulin levels are high, receptor binding is "downregulated," and when insulin levels are low, receptor binding is "upregulated." Thus, conditions such as obesity and high-carbohydrate diet are associated with elevated insulin levels and low receptor binding. In contrast, fasting and exercise are associated with decreased insulin levels and increased receptor binding. Receptor binding is increased in growth hormone or glucocorticoid deficiency and decreased when growth hormone or glucocorticoid is present in excess. Whether these are direct effects of the hormones or indirect effects due to accompanying alterations of insulin levels is not established.

The changes in receptor binding just described might be expected to cause predictable changes in cell sensitivity to insulin (i.e., increased binding equals increased sensitivity; decreased binding equals decreased sensitivity). However, the cellular response to insulin depends on post-receptor events as well as receptor binding. In fact, there is substantial evidence that regulation of the glucose transport system by insulin (see later) may at times be in the opposite direction of insulin regulation of receptors. Thus, a high-carbohydrate diet results in diminished insulin binding, but the capacity of the glucose transport system increases. The overall result is increased *in vivo* insulin sensitivity despite decreased insulin binding to tissues. The relationship between insulin binding and tissue sensitivity to insulin is even more complex during fasting. Insulin binding has been reported to increase during fasting in a variety of cell types (see Fig. 15–37). However, sensitivity to insulin in fasting man as assessed by the glucose clamp technique is diminished, and there is a marked impairment of insulin-mediated glucose uptake and glucose oxidation in fat cells of fasted rats. In contrast, insulin effectiveness in stimulating glucose transport and metabolism is enhanced in skeletal muscle of mice and rats during starvation.

Thus, regulation of insulin binding to cell membrane receptors has been demonstrated and may contribute to sensitivity of the cell to the actions of insulin. However, one cannot predict overall cell responsiveness to insulin on the basis of receptor binding alone, since post-receptor events are also important and may predominate. The relationship between alterations of receptor binding and insulin resistance in obesity and diabetes is also complex and will be discussed later.

Post-Receptor Events

As indicated in the preceding paragraphs, the initial step of insulin action, binding to specific receptors on the surface membrane of cells, has been well characterized. The ultimate effects of insulin on enzyme activation and the ensuing cellular responses are also relatively well described. However, the intracellular signal or signals that are generated as a result of the binding of insulin to its receptor and that mediate insulin effects are still poorly understood. The effect of insulin to block the lipolytic effect of a number of hormones may be due to inhibition of cyclic AMP production by these hormones. However, this mechanism is not the only one involved in the antilipolytic effects of insulin. In addition, cyclic AMP is clearly not the mediator of the effect of insulin to increase glucose transport. Alterations of calcium flux, changes of cellular pH, physical changes in cell membrane structure as a result of insulin binding, insulin itself or insulin degradation products or some other intracellular peptide, redox reactions in the membrane and alterations of cellular sulfhydryl groups, and membrane components released by proteolysis have all been proposed as mediators of insulin's effects. However, there is no definitive evidence establishing any of these mechanisms.

Glucose Transport System.   The insulin-sensitive glucose transport system has been studied extensively. Glucose transport is an effect of insulin that appears to be very closely related to insulin receptor binding and that can be quantified relatively accurately by using radiolabeled glucose analogues that are transported but not metabolized. There is considerable evidence for the existence of an insulin-sensitive glucose transport system in skeletal muscle, cardiac muscle, and adipose tissue, but glucose transport in the liver does not appear to be affected by insulin. Although insulin has been clearly shown to facilitate the diffusion of glucose into insulin-sensitive cells, the mechanism for this facilitation remains controversial. Some studies have suggested that insulin causes recruitment of new glucose transport protein from the Golgi apparatus and incorporation of this protein into the plasma membrane, thereby increasing the total number of glucose-transporting units.

Other studies have supported the hypothesis that insulin converts inactive transport molecules to active ones.

Some of the key points relative to the specificity of this hexose transport system are as follows:

1. It exhibits stereospecificity, being receptive to sugars such as galactose, D-xylose, and L-arabinose, but not to D-arabinose, rhamnose, gluconate, or glucuronate.

2. It demonstrates saturation kinetics, indicating a limited availability of a specific carrier.

3. The rate of entry of the sugars into the cell interior is relatively slow compared with their diffusion into the extracellular fluid.

4. The insulin-sensitive sugars compete with each other for transport.

5. In rat diaphragm the insulin effect is more temperature-sensitive than would be expected by simple diffusion.

One might expect that enhancing sugar entry in the absence of insulin, as for example by increasing the extracellular glucose concentration, should result in the same metabolic changes as follow addition of insulin in the presence of a lower concentration of glucose. Although for the most part this is true, there are a number of differences. One is that insulin promotes greater usage of glucose for the formation of glycogen than for other pathways. This has been attributed to the capacity of insulin to stimulate glycogen synthetase. Anoxia and certain inhibitors of oxidative phosphorylation greatly augment the entry of glucose into cells, but many of the metabolic consequences differ considerably from those of insulin; for example, the amount of glycogenesis is greatly decreased.

Many agents which have effects on cell membranes can activate the glucose transport system. Of particular interest has been the activation of glucose transport by a variety of agents that have multivalent binding sites for the plasma membrane. These include plant lectins such as concanavalin A and wheat germ agglutinin. Although it is not likely that these agents bind exclusively to the insulin receptor, they do initiate patching on the cell membrane in a manner similar to the aggregation of insulin-receptor complexes (see earlier). These agents also have insulin-like effects on fat-cell lipolysis.

Similar activation of glucose transport has been demonstrated by antibodies to the insulin receptor as well as by antibodies to plasma membrane constituents. These latter antibodies do not interfere with insulin binding and can activate the glucose transport system in trypsinized fat cells which are unable to bind insulin. Monovalent fragments of these same antibodies do not affect glucose transport, but this activity can be restored by the addition of antibodies to the fragments. All of these data indicate that agents capable of binding multivalently to the cell membrane will also have insulin-like effects on the glucose transport system. However, whether such membrane protein cross-linking is an obligatory step in the action of insulin itself has not been established.

The structural relationship between the insulin receptor and the glucose transport system has also been evaluated. Ferritin-insulin has been used to visualize insulin receptors on fat cell membranes. These studies have demonstrated single receptors as well as groups of two to six receptors, independent of the binding of insulin to these receptors. When the plant lectin cytochalasin B was used to disrupt the groups of receptors, glucose transport activity was blocked. Cytochalasin D, a related compound which has similar effects on cell function as cytochalasin B, but does not disaggregate groups of insulin receptors, had no effect on glucose transport activity. These findings have suggested that there is a very close structural relationship between the insulin receptor and the glucose transport system. However, analysis of the glucose transport protein isolated from cell membranes has indicated that it is structurally distinct from the insulin receptor protein (see Fig. 15–35). Cytochalasin B has also been used to estimate the number of glucose-transporting units, since it appears to bind specifically to them.

In addition to responding rapidly to insulin, there is now considerable evidence to suggest that there is a long-term regulation by insulin of the responsiveness of the glucose transport system to insulin. Induction of hyperinsulinemia in rats by daily insulin injections or by high-carbohydrate feeding increases maximal insulin-mediated glucose transport activity in fat cells. Conversely, during hypoinsulinemia induced by starvation or streptozotocin diabetes, responsiveness of the glucose transport system of fat cells to insulin was inhibited. As indicated earlier, these effects may override changes of insulin binding, which occur in the opposite direction in these circumstances.

Response to Insulin by Individual Tissues

Fat. The main function of adipose tissue is to serve as a reservoir of energy. It has the highest concentration of calories of any tissue in the body. The average normal-weight man has about 15 kg of adipose tissue, 90% of which is triglyceride (approximately 120,000 calories). The water content is about 15 μL/100 mg, whereas muscle has five times this level. The concentrations of free fatty acids (FFA), glucose, and single amino acids are relatively low. Adipose tissue does not liberate glucose but can release large quantities of FFA (lipolysis) and some amino acids. Insulin is the principal hormone that promotes storage of nutrients in adipose tissue and prevents lipolysis. Insulin increases glucose uptake and oxidation by fat cells. It markedly increases formation of triglyceride by (1) increasing synthesis of fatty acid in the fat cells, (2) increasing the uptake of glucose, the immediate precursor of α-glycerol phosphate, which is needed for triglyceride synthesis, and (3) maintaining activity of lipoprotein lipase for chylomicron metabolism and uptake.

As indicated in Table 15–2, there are many compounds that affect lipolysis. Glucosteroids and growth hormone (GH) promote induction of lipase. These hormones and thyroid hormone markedly augment the lipolytic effect of catecholamines. Most compounds that increase lipolysis have been demonstrated to increase the level of cAMP, and the reverse applies to those that reduce lipolysis. Presumably, an increase in cAMP causes the regulator protein to release protein kinase (PK), which then stimulates the phosphorylation of lipase, thereby promoting an increase in the rate of hydrolysis of triglyceride to FFA and glycerol.

Table 15–2. COMPOUNDS THAT AFFECT LIPOLYSIS IN ADIPOSE TISSUE

Increase Lipolysis:	
Catecholamines	Chorionic somatomammotropin
Serotonin	ACTH
Thyroid hormones	MSH, α and β
Glucagon	TSH
Secretin	LH
Glucosteroids	Vasopressin (arginine)
GH	Methyl xanthines
Decrease Lipolysis:	
Insulin	Nicotinic acid
Prostaglandin E	β-Adrenergic blockers

In summary: lipolytic hormone → cAMP → unbound PK → lipase → triglyceride hydrolysis → FFA and glycerol. Under some conditions, insulin apparently decreases the level of cAMP and decreases activation of protein kinase. Less insulin is needed to inhibit lipolysis than to affect glucose uptake, glucose oxidation, cAMP level, or the blood glucose level.

FFA are liberated from fat cells when there is insufficient α-glycerol phosphate for reesterification. Conversely, lipolysis decreases when α-glycerol phosphate or β-hydroxybutyrate increases. Lactate inhibits lipase activity and glycolysis. This may partly account for the decrease in ketogenesis as lactic acidosis develops. Compounds that promote lipolysis tend to increase the efflux of K^+ from cells and decrease both glucose oxidation and protein synthesis.

Muscle. After the transport of glucose into the muscle cells, hexokinase catalyzes its phosphorylation. As G-6-P accumulates, it exerts an allosteric effect in its inhibition of hexokinase activity, and in so doing it is competing with one of the substrates, ATP. Thus, the inhibitory effect depends upon the ratio of G-6-P to ATP. The entry of glucose into the cell is the main limiting step as long as insulin is not present, but when it is present, G-6-P is the main limiting factor which adjusts the rate of glucose phosphorylation to that of overall utilization of the hexose monophosphate pool in resting muscle. Adipose tissue is similar in these regards.

Many of insulin's actions on muscle are similar to those on adipose tissue, but in muscle it causes relatively more synthesis of protein, nucleotides, and glycogen, and much less synthesis of triglyceride. Relatively little energy is stored in the form of triglyceride, and the total amount of energy stored in the form of glycogen is not very great despite the large muscle mass. Insulin increases glycolysis and the oxidation of glucose and pyruvate. Muscle is the main source of alanine, glutamine, pyruvate, and lactate, which in turn are used in the liver for gluconeogenesis (discussed later). Insulin increases protein synthesis *in vitro* in the absence of added amino acid or of glucose and stimulates formation of certain amino acids from carbohydrates. It increases the attachment of monoribosomes to mRNA and increases the ratio of polyribosomes to monoribosomes. It also increases the total levels of RNA, mRNA, and DNA.

Insulin also influences the electrical potential of muscle. There is a difference in electrical potential between extracellular fluid and the inside of muscle fibers. Insulin affects the flux of a number of ions. It leads to a net increase in intracellular K^+ and decrease in Na^+. The effect on K^+ is highly sensitive, requiring only minute amounts of insulin; hyperpolarization of the membrane occurs with increased intracellular K^+ and also with increased permeability to Cl^-. These electrolyte shifts appear very important in determining the amount of polarization produced by insulin. It has been suggested that the changes in the membrane potential may play an important role in many of the transport functions of the cell wall.

Liver. The liver is the major endogenous source of plasma glucose and plays an important role in the synthesis of glycogen, lipids, and proteins (Table 15–3). The total amount of glycogen in the liver at any one time is far less than in the muscle, and the total synthesis of fatty acids is considerably less than in the adipose tissue, but the synthesis of protein is relatively large. Liver can also readily degrade glycogen, lipids, and proteins to provide energy in the form of glucose, ketones, and other substances. All of these reactions are significantly influenced by insulin, di-

Table 15–3. ACTIONS OF INSULIN IN LIVER*

Increase	Decrease
Glucose phosphorylation	Glycogenolysis
Glycogenesis	Lipolysis
Glycolysis	Gluconeogenesis
Pentose phosphate shunt	Proteolysis
Proteogenesis	Fatty acid oxidation
Lipogenesis	Ketogenesis
ATP	Ureogenesis
DNA	Uptake of alanine and other
RNA	glucogenic substrates
Mg^{++}, K^+ uptake	cAMP
	Protein kinase activity

*The extent to which these actions are subsidiary is unknown. The activities of numerous enzymes are altered by insulin, most of them presumably by subsidiary reactions. Some of them involved are:

A. *Increased activity:* glucokinase, glycogen synthetase, glycolytic enzymes (phosphofructokinase and pyruvate kinase), TCA cycle enzymes (pyruvate dehydrogenase, citrate synthetase), lipogenic enzymes, proteogenic enzymes, DNA polymerase, RNA polymerase.

B. *Decreased activity:* glycogen phosphorylase, glucose-6-phosphatase, gluconeogenetic enzymes (pyruvate carboxylase, phosphoenolpyruvate carboxykinase, fructose-1,6-diphosphatase), fatty acid oxidizing enzymes, and ketogenesis enzymes.

rectly or indirectly. It should be remembered that the liver is exposed to much higher concentrations of insulin than are the other tissues. Insulin is secreted by the pancreas into the portal system and, therefore, must traverse the liver before reaching the systemic circulation. Because of hepatic extraction of insulin, portal vein insulin levels are approximately 2½ times as high as peripheral levels.

Unlike muscle and adipose tissue, where the activity of a specific glucose transport system is increased by insulin, liver cells are freely permeable to glucose. Within them the initial reaction is phosphorylation with the formation of G-6-P, which is catalyzed by hexokinase and a unique enzyme, glucokinase. The key ways in which glucokinase differs from hexokinase are as follows:

1. Its K_m for glucose is 100 times greater.

2. There is no allosteric inhibition by G-6-P (there is with hexokinase).

3. Phosphorylation of fructose and glucosamine is poor (good with hexokinase).

4. There is strong competitive inhibition by N-acetylglucosamine.

5. The enzyme is unstable *in vitro*.

6. The content in starved animals is markedly decreased (hexokinase is unchanged).

7. It is low or absent in diabetic animals (hexokinase is unchanged).

Both of these enzymes are soluble, require ATP-Mg as phosphoryl donors, yield glucose 6-phosphate as the primary product, and are moderately sensitive to inhibition by ADP-Mg. There is evidence that glucokinase is an inducible enzyme, with insulin rather than glucose serving as the inducer. Insulin exerts long-term control of the amount of enzyme present, but short-term regulation is based on the sensitivity of the enzyme to changes in glucose concentration within the physiologic range.

The amount of glucokinase activity is greatly decreased during starvation. It increases within a few hours after the administration of insulin. However, its reappearance is blocked by inhibitors of protein synthesis or of RNA synthesis. Two other enzymes involved in glycolysis that are stimulated by insulin are phosphofructokinase and pyruvate kinase. Insulin exerts a stimulating effect on glycogen synthetase, which is a key enzyme in the synthesis of glycogen. Insulin increases the activities of glucose-6-

GLYCOGENESIS and GLYCOGENOLYSIS

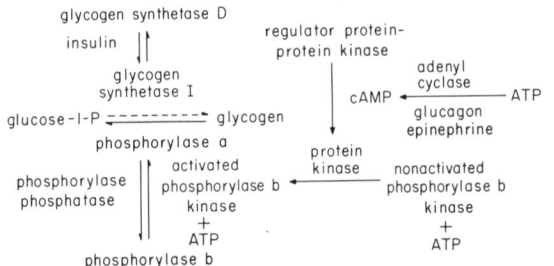

Figure 15–38. Glucagon and epinephrine, by promoting an increase in cAMP, lead to increased glycogenolysis. By decreasing cAMP and increasing glycogen synthetase activity, insulin decreases glycogenolysis and increases glycogenesis.

phosphate dehydrogenase and 6-phosphogluconate dehydrogenase. With increased activities in the hexose monophosphate shunt, TPNH is produced which is utilized in lipid synthesis. Synthesis of fatty acids in the liver in insulin deficiency states may be reduced by more than 90%.

As the blood sugar level rises above approximately 120 mg/100 ml, release of glucose from the liver is normally inhibited, and glucose uptake by the liver increases. These changes are mediated by insulin. As shown in Figure 15–38, under the influence of insulin, glycogen synthetase is activated so that glucose is stored by the liver in the form of glycogen. As the blood sugar level falls, there is correspondingly less output and uptake of glucose by the liver. With decreased insulin effect, increasing amounts of lipolysis and gluconeogenesis are stimulated. These processes are stimulated during diabetes and starvation and by increases of GH, glucosteroids, epinephrine, glucagon, and other lipolytic hormones. Insulin antagonizes the action of these counterregulatory hormones which increase cAMP-stimulated glycogenolysis, gluconeogenesis, potassium loss, and phosphoenolpyruvate carboxykinase activity. However, a number of the effects insulin has on the liver are apparently not activated through its influence on the cAMP concentration.

Insulin also has major effects on hepatic handling of FFA. FFA are taken up by the liver in proportion to their plasma concentration. They are then metabolized completely to CO_2, or partially to ketone bodies, or esterified with glycerol phosphate to form triglyceride (TG). The newly synthesized TG is largely secreted into the plasma as very low density lipoprotein. The balance between oxidation-ketogenesis and TG synthesis appears to be regulated by both insulin and glucagon (see following section on regulation of ketogenesis by glucagon). The amount of fatty acid synthesized by the liver is small compared with that taken up from the plasma. Insulin increases hepatic fatty acid synthesis, partly because of its stimulation of fatty acid synthetase. In the intact animal, increasing the delivery of FFA and amino acids to the liver may result in a decrease rather than an increase in hepatic glucose output. This decrease results from the augmented secretion of endogenous insulin that is stimulated by the elevated levels of FFA and amino acids. However, in states of insulin deficiency, increased delivery of FFA and amino acids to the liver will accelerate hepatic gluconeogenesis.

Glucagon Action

Glucagon is an important regulator of carbohydrate metabolism. Its major site of action is the liver, where it stimulates glycogenolysis and also promotes gluconeogenesis, pro-

teolysis, and ketogenesis. Glucagon in physiologic amounts increases intracellular cyclic AMP in the liver, and in pharmacologic doses can cause similar increases in heart, skeletal muscle, and adipose tissue.

Cellular Mechanism of Action

The first step in glucagon action is binding to a specific cell surface membrane receptor. The characteristics of this interaction have been studied extensively in liver, fat, and myocardial cells. As a result of the binding of glucagon to its receptor, the enzyme adenylate cyclase is activated and cyclic AMP is generated. This coupling of the glucagon-receptor complex to adenylate cyclase is facilitated by GTP (guanine triphosphate), which appears to cause conformational changes of the enzyme and receptor molecules. The cyclic AMP generated acts as an intracellular second messenger by activating protein kinases which in turn phosphorylate other regulatory proteins in the cell. Although glucagon has been shown to increase intracellular cyclic AMP levels in a variety of tissues including fat and muscle, a physiologic role for glucagon to regulate any tissue except the liver has not been established. Since the interaction of hormones with receptors has been demonstrated to be a regulated process for some hormones, a number of studies have been done to determine whether the glucagon-receptor interaction is also regulated. However, such studies have provided conflicting results so that it is unclear whether regulation of glucagon receptors in fact occurs.

Response to Glucagon by Individual Tissues

Liver. The importance of glucagon to the maintenance of the circulating glucose level in the fasting state has been demonstrated by the fall of the glucose level when glucagon secretion is inhibited by somatostatin. This fall of plasma glucose during glucagon deficiency is due to diminished hepatic glucose production (Fig. 15–39). Glucagon increases hepatic glucose production by stimulating both glycogenolysis and gluconeogenesis. Glycogenolysis results from activation of phosphorylase by protein kinases under the influence of cyclic AMP generated by the interaction of the glucagon-receptor complex with adenylate cyclase (see Fig. 15–38). The mechanism by which glucagon increases hepatic gluconeogenesis is less clear but may be related to increased liver uptake of precursors for gluconeogenesis as well as to intrahepatic effects. Glucagon appears to physiologically regulate both glycogenolysis and gluconeogenesis in man, since hepatic glucose production falls when glucagon deficiency is induced either after an overnight fast (when glycogenolysis predominates) or during a more prolonged fast (when gluconeogenesis predominates).

The effect of glucagon on hepatic glucose production has been reported to be transitory, since glucose production returns toward baseline values with time despite continuing glucagon deficiency or glucagon excess. However, this apparent transitory effect is due in part to counterregulatory events. For example, the hyperglycemia and increased insulin secretion that develop during glucagon administration will each tend to inhibit hepatic glucose production. When such counterregulatory processes are prevented, glucagon has been shown to cause a more persistent increase of glucose production and glucagon deficiency results in a more persistent decline of hepatic glucose production.

Glucagon also appears to play a key role in hepatic lipid metabolism. Glucagon can cause lipolysis in the liver, providing a direct source of FFA for oxidation. In addition, there is now evidence that glucagon can regulate ketone production from FFA by liver cells. In a manner analogous to causing cyclic AMP–mediated activation of phosphorylase resulting in glycogenolysis (see earlier), glucagon stimulation of hepatic adenylate cyclase results in inactivation of acetyl-CoA carboxylase, the enzyme which converts acetyl-CoA to malonyl-CoA to initiate triglyceride synthesis. Malonyl-CoA also inhibits activity of carnitine acetyl transferase I, the enzyme which facilitates transport of fatty acids into mitochondria for oxidation (Fig. 15–40). Thus, under the influence of glucagon, malonyl-CoA production drops, carnitine acetyl transferase I activity increases, and FFA are shunted away from triglyceride synthesis and into the mitochondria where ketogenesis occurs. These effects are antagonized by insulin so that glucagon stimulates ketogenesis most effectively in the presence of insulin deficiency. The conversion of the liver from an organ of triglyceride synthesis to one of ketone production is an important physiologic

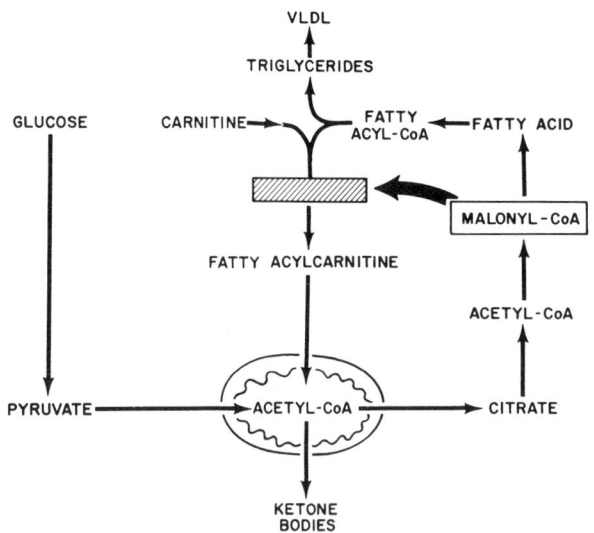

Figure 15–40. Schematic diagram illustrating the critical role of malonyl-CoA in fatty acid utilization. When malonyl-CoA is high, fatty acids will be utilized for triglyceride synthesis in the liver. When malonyl-CoA is low, fatty acids will be diverted into the mitochondria where oxidation occurs. Glucagon inhibits conversion of acetyl-CoA to malonyl-CoA, resulting in use of FFA for oxidation. Insulin can oppose this action of glucagon. (From McGarry, J. D.: New perspectives in the regulation of ketogenesis. *Diabetes* 28:517, 1979.)

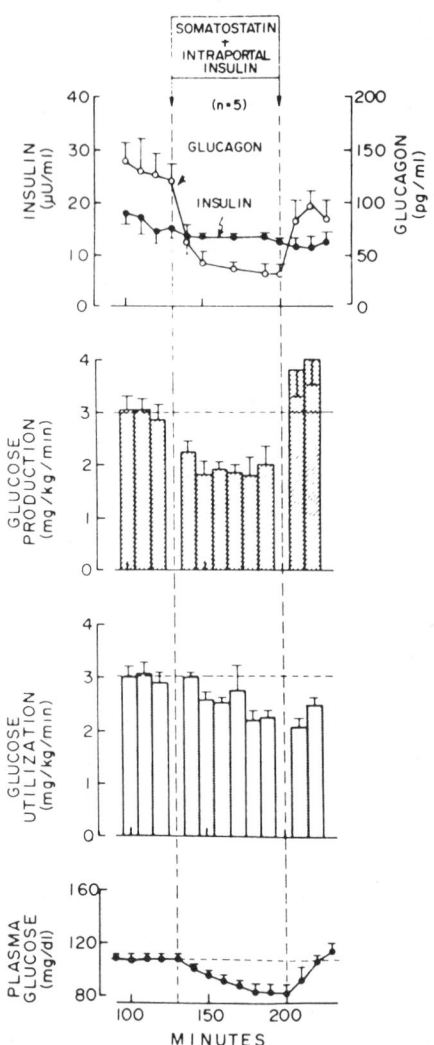

Figure 15–39. A demonstration of the importance of basal glucagon to basal glucose production. A somatostatin infusion (1 μg/kg/min) is combined with intraportal insulin replacement (400 μU/kg/min). Arterial plasma insulin and glucagon and glucose turnover are measured in anesthetized dogs after an overnight fast. Note that selective glucagon deficiency is associated with a fall of glucose production and a fall of plasma glucose. (From Cherrington, A. D., et al.: The role of insulin and glucagon in the regulation of basal glucose production in the postabsorptive dog. *J. Clin. Invest.* 58:1407, 1976.)

adaptation during starvation. However, when there is marked insulin deficiency and glucagon excess, accelerated ketogenesis can result in severe metabolic acidosis (see section on Diabetic Ketoacidosis).

Other Organs. As already indicated, glucagon can stimulate adenylate cyclase activity in a number of tissues. However, whether these effects of glucagon are important physiologically is uncertain. In fat cells glucagon, like a variety of other hormones, can stimulate hormone-sensitive lipase, resulting in lipolysis. FFA released by this potential effect of glucagon would become a source of increased substrate for the liver, providing an indirect mechanism by which glucagon could also augment ketogenesis. Glucagon stimulates cardiac adenylate cyclase, resulting in an increased force of myocardial contraction and increased cardiac output. However, glucagon has not proved useful as a treatment for acute heart failure. In large doses glucagon can also inhibit gastric and intestinal motility and diminish gastric and pancreatic exocrine secretion. This latter effect has been used as a rationale for treatment of acute pancreatitis with glucagon. Glucagon administration has been reported to have a natriuretic effect in man and to antagonize effects of mineralocorticoids. This effect of glucagon has been postulated to be a contributing factor to the natriuresis of fasting.

Somatostatin Action

Somatostatin has profound effects on a variety of tissues. Its physiologic role as a hypothalamic modulator of anterior pituitary function is discussed in Chapter 14. In addition, somatostatin has major effects on gastrointestinal and pancreatic function. However, the physiologic role of somatostatin released from D cells of the endocrine pancreas is not known. Its potent inhibitory effects on insulin and glucagon secretion suggest that somatostatin may be an important regulator of nutrient homeostasis.

Cellular Mechanism of Action

There is preliminary evidence that somatostatin initiates its biologic effects by interaction with cell surface membrane receptors. However, an intracellular binding protein for somatostatin has also been demonstrated, and there is evidence that somatostatin has effects on subcellular components. Thus, somatostatin may act intracellularly as well as on the cell surface. Study of a variety of synthetic analogues of somatostatin has suggested that receptors for somatostatin may be somewhat different in various tissues, since differential inhibition of hormone secretion can be demonstrated. For example, although native somatostatin is a potent inhibitor of both insulin and glucagon release, several somatostatin analogues retain the potent inhibiting effect on insulin secretion but have minimal effects on glucagon secretion (Fig. 15–41).

Because somatostatin is an inhibitor of the secretory function of so many different cell types, it is thought that it inhibits a key step in stimulus-secretion coupling. However, the nature of this inhibitory action is not yet well understood. Somatostatin has been reported to inhibit cyclic AMP production in pancreatic islets. However, it has a number of effects on islet cells that cannot be explained simply by alterations of cyclic AMP. Similarly, it has been suggested that somatostatin interferes with pancreatic islet function

Table 15–4. GASTROINTESTINAL AND PANCREATIC FUNCTIONS INHIBITED BY SOMATOSTATIN ADMINISTRATION

Organ	Effect Inhibited
Stomach	Motility, acid and pepsin secretion
Exocrine pancreas	Bicarbonate and enzyme secretion
Gallbladder	Contraction
Small intestine	Motility, carbohydrate absorption
Splanchnic blood vessels	Blood flow
GI tract endocrine cells	Hormone release: gastrin, CCK, VIP, motilin, GIP, secretin
Endocrine pancreas	Hormone release: glucagon, insulin, pancreatic polypeptide

by altering calcium fluxes. However, somatostatin can inhibit hormone release stimulated by elevated cytosol calcium levels, and physiologic variations of ambient calcium levels do not reverse somatostatin effects. The finding that somatostatin inhibits glucose-induced electrical activity in islet cells suggests that some other alteration of transmembrane ion fluxes in response to secretagogues may underlie somatostatin action.

Somatostatin and Nutrient Absorption and Disposition

The effects of pharmacologic doses of somatostatin on various aspects of nutrient absorption and disposition are listed in Table 15–4. The overall effects of somatostatin administration are to inhibit nutrient absorption from stomach and small intestine both by decreasing motility of these organs and by inhibiting release of factors that contribute to digestion of nutrients. It also is capable of reducing food intake by an effect on satiety mechanisms. The effects of somatostatin to decrease splanchnic blood flow are consistent with its effects to diminish the activity of splanchnic organs. Although these diverse effects on gastrointestinal function can be demonstrated during somatostatin administration, the physiologic role of endogenous somatostatin on gastrointestinal function is not known.

Somatostatin can profoundly inhibit secretion of both insulin and glucagon. This inhibition applies to the basal state as well as to responses to all known secretagogues. A physiologic role for endogenous somatostatin to regulate insulin and glucagon secretion has been suggested by findings that antibodies to somatostatin can increase glucagon and insulin release from islets *in vitro*. Although the acute effect of somatostatin is to cause a fall of blood sugar due to inhibition of glucagon release, infusion of somatostatin for several hours results in hyperglycemia. This presumably is a result of the effects of prolonged insulin deficiency predominating over coexistent effects of glucagon deficiency. Some *in vitro* studies have suggested that somatostatin in high doses may have direct effects on the liver to inhibit glucose production. However, most studies have found no direct effect of somatostatin, and no evidence of somatostatin binding to receptors has been found in liver tissue.

PHYSIOLOGICAL REGULATION OF PLASMA GLUCOSE

Overnight Fast. The basal plasma glucose concentration is carefully regulated through a feedback system involving the liver and the endocrine pancreas. In the absence of meal feeding, the source of plasma glucose is entirely the liver. After an overnight fast, glucose is metabolized largely in the

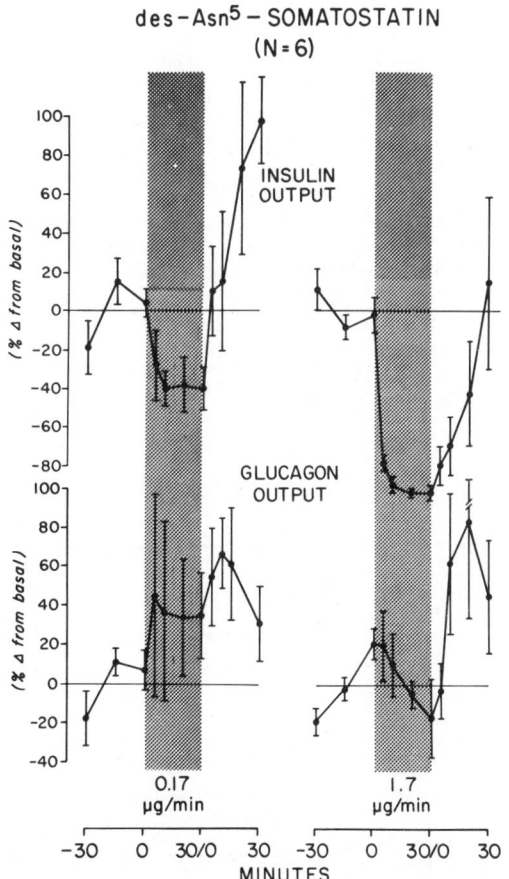

Figure 15–41. Selective inhibition of glucagon secretion by a somatostatin analogue. Although native somatostatin is a potent inhibitor of both insulin and glucagon secretion, this somatostatin analogue clearly inhibits pancreatic insulin output at doses that do not inhibit glucagon output. (From Taborsky, G. J., Jr., et al.: Differential effects of somatostatin analogues on α- and β-cells of the pancreas. *Am. J. Physiol. 236:*E123, 1979.)

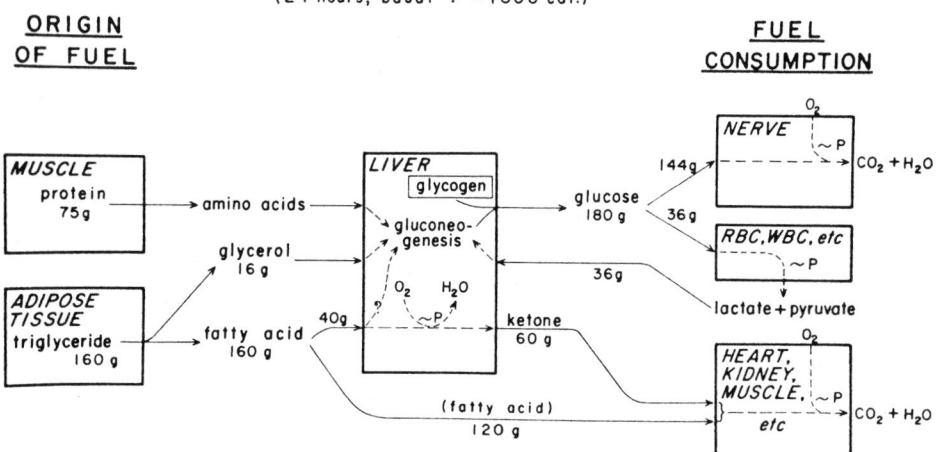

Figure 15–42. Quantitative metabolic turnover in the basal state. (From Cahill, G. F., Jr.: Starvation in man. *N. Engl. J. Med. 282:*668, 1970.)

brain, to a lesser extent in other insulin-insensitive tissues such as the gut and red blood cells, and to a small extent in insulin-sensitive tissues such as muscle and fat. A number of quantitative estimates have been made of the rate of glucose turnover and its relative distribution; however, the rates reported vary widely. A reasonable mean estimate is that approximately 100 mg/kg body weight/hour of glucose is released from the liver after an overnight fast. If this rate of glucose production is maintained for 1 day, it would amount to approximately 180 g for an average man. About 80% of this total would be completely oxidized to carbon dioxide and water by the brain. The rest is metabolized by other tissues largely to lactate which is released back into the circulation for reutilization by liver for gluconeogenesis (the Cori cycle) (Fig. 15–42). The brain, therefore, is the major determinant of glucose turnover rate in the basal state.

The endocrine pancreas plays an important role in this feedback loop between the liver, brain, and peripheral tissues (Fig. 15–43). Regulation of liver glucose production is dependent on the concentration of insulin and glucagon. If there is a selective deficiency of insulin, there is an immediate but slow rise in glucose output by the liver, resulting in hyperglycemia. If there is a decrease in glucagon, there is an immediate decrease in glucose output and glucose concentration in the plasma. Any change in tissue utilization of glucose would also be reflected in a change in basal plasma glucose level. Restoration of the original plasma glucose level will occur owing to the regulation of pancreatic insulin and glucagon secretion by glucose. Thus, if peripheral glucose utilization rises, the glucose level will fall, the insulin level will fall, the glucagon level will rise, and the system will readapt by increasing hepatic glucose output.

This fundamental feedback loop is sensitive to the concentrations of cortisol, thyroxine, epinephrine, norepinephrine, and acetylcholine (Fig. 15–44). Thus, if cortisol levels increase, there will be a tendency to increased glucose output from the liver and decreased glucose utilization in the peripheral tissues. As glucose levels rise, the pancreas will restore the glucose level toward its original value by increasing insulin secretion. Complete adaptation cannot occur, however, as there would be no stimulus for increased insulin secretion. Therefore, a new steady state is reached at some value between that expected for the effects of cortisol on peripheral tissues and liver and that expected for the degree of hyperinsulinemia observed. Thus, the fasting plasma glucose level represents the sum total of the basic liver,

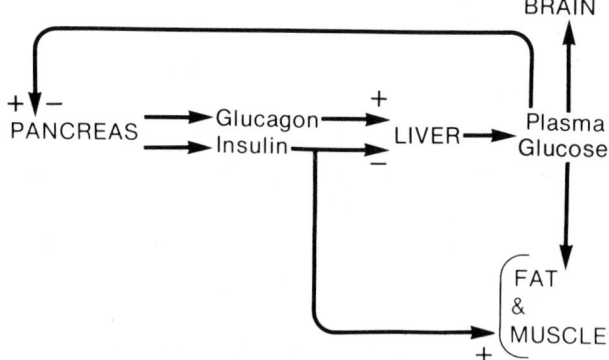

Figure 15–43. Basal feedback loop for the regulation of plasma glucose. Glucose regulates insulin and glucagon secretion, which in turn control hepatic glucose production. This output is matched with insulin-modulated glucose uptake in muscle and fat and insulin-independent glucose uptake in brain to close the loop. (From Woods, S. C., et al.: The role of the nervous system in metabolic regulation and its effects in diabetes and obesity. In *Handbook of Diabetes Mellitus.* Brownlee, M. (ed.), New York, Garland Publishing Co., 1981.)

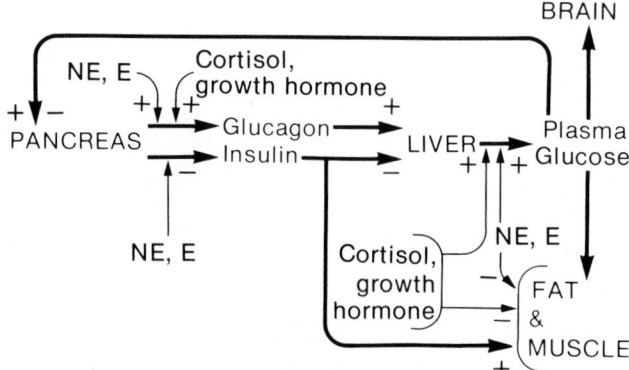

Figure 15–44. Modulation of the basal feedback loop by counterregulatory hormones. The final plasma glucose will be determined by these plus all other factors which can influence the liver, pancreas, or peripheral tissues. (From Woods, S. C., et al.: The role of the nervous system in metabolic regulation and its effects on diabetes and obesity. In *Handbook of Diabetes Mellitus.* Brownlee, M. (ed.), New York, Garland Publishing Co., 1981.)

pancreas, and peripheral tissue feedback system, plus all of the neuroendocrine influences which potentially can regulate glucose utilization and production. It is regulated within a narrow range and tends to remain remarkably constant from day to day, month to month, and year to year.

Response to Meal Feeding. During the process of the ingestion and storage of nutrients, plasma glucose is maintained within relatively narrow limits by the neuroendocrine system despite major changes in glucose turnover rate. The plasma glucose level of healthy subjects rarely rises more than 50 mg/dl after feeding, regardless of the type of nutrient ingested. The response system begins with a cephalic phase involving the endocrine pancreas as well as the salivary glands and gastric acid secretion. Either the sight, smell, or taste of food in the oral pharynx is sufficient to elicit insulin secretion in man in response to the knowledge that food is about to be eaten. In animals it is possible to train an insulin response by repeated injections of either glucose or tolbutamide in the presence of a neural conditioning stimulus. It has also been demonstrated that animals trained to expect meals at certain times will secrete insulin at the time of the expected meal even if the meal is withheld. The importance of this cephalic phase of insulin secretion to the efficiency of carbohydrate metabolism has been demonstrated in rats. Ingestion of a meal via stomach tube by these animals does not elicit an early insulin response and is followed by a higher and more prolonged elevation of plasma glucose than occurs when the same meal is eaten spontaneously through the oral route. It is not known whether the taste of the food is important in this response, but it has been observed that non-nutritive sweeteners such as saccharin can elicit it. Therefore, the cephalic phase of insulin release is not necessarily related to the caloric value of the ingested meal.

The gastric and intestinal phases of absorption are associated with other noncaloric stimuli to the pancreas from the release of the gut hormones gastrin, cholecystokinin (CCK), enteroglucagon (glycentin), and gastrointestinal inhibitory polypeptide (GIP), which augment the insulin and/or glucagon response to food during absorption. These hormones are also involved in the stimulation of gastric juice and intestinal and pancreatic secretions which are critical for the digestive process. It is these cephalic- and gastrointestinal-phase hormones and neural factors which are responsible for the observation that nutrients given orally produce greater insulin responses and better carbohydrate tolerance than the same nutrients given intravenously. Alterations of the liver uptake of glucose have not been described in relationship to this system. However, it seems likely that the liver will also be found to change its metabolism from one of glucose production to glucose uptake not only in direct relationship to the concentrations of insulin and glucagon to which it is exposed, but also in relationship to one or more gut factors and neural signals which are part of meal feeding.

Recently, afferent neurons from the gastrointestinal tract and pancreas which respond directly to glucose and other nutrients have been described. Therefore, it is possible that there may be neural as well as hormone signals for nutrients during the gastrointestinal phase of digestion and absorption. The insulin responses to efferent parasympathetic signals are blocked by atropine in most experimental conditions and are therefore believed to be due to stimulation of cholinergic efferents to the islet. Although glucagon elevations might be expected under meal-feeding conditions because of the increase in vagal activity, it seems likely that the simultaneous increase in plasma glucose occurring as a result of glucose absorption probably masks this neural response.

Many of the same hormones and related neural afferents provide information to the central nervous system regarding ingestion of a meal. Some of them have been shown to be important satiety factors when tested experimentally. Thus, CCK or somatostatin injected shortly before food exposure in hungry rats or baboons suppresses the size of a subsequent meal. Furthermore, the intraduodenal instillation of foods known to stimulate large increases in CCK produce the same suppression of the feeding response in rough proportion to the expected elevation of CCK. It has, therefore, been presumed that the ability of intraduodenal food to suppress spontaneous meal size in proportion to the amount of calories given intraduodenally is due to the metering of the food ingested by the previously described hormonal and neural response systems. This process is probably an important component of a feeding system for the regulation of body weight (Fig. 15–45).

The nutrients, hormones, and neural regulators interact in the islet in a complex way. It is now generally believed that the primary regulators of the islet on a minute to minute basis are the substrates glucose, amino acids, and fatty acids, with glucose playing the key role because it not only regulates the secretion of insulin and glucagon directly, but modulates responses to the other substrates and all of the neural and hormonal factors. However, the set of the islet or its gain prior to the ingestion of the meal is determined by the circulating endogenous signals (i.e., the premeal levels of glucose, amino acids, and fatty acids in circulation plus the hormonal and neuronal milieu due to hormones and transmitters regulated by the central nervous system). The islet hormones then respond to a meal in proportion to the substrates ingested as modulated by the previous meal-feeding pattern of that particular animal which, in turn, is reflected in the neural and hormonal signals present during the intermeal interval. During the meal the hormones and neural factors change, resulting in a continuous adaptation during the meal and a changing gain of the islet to the primary substrate controllers. This system then returns toward basal as the substrates are cleared from the blood. Because of the complexity of this regulatory system, the islet should be viewed as a sophisticated substrate integrator which modulates the response to nutrients by the previous feeding experience of the animal (Fig. 15–46). The outputs from this integration are the release rates of insulin and glucagon (also somatostatin and pancreatic polypeptide?) which act as a regulatory couple for the disposal of ingested nutrients while maintaining plasma glucose within the narrow range necessary for normal brain function.

Since in the basal state 80% of circulating glucose is taken

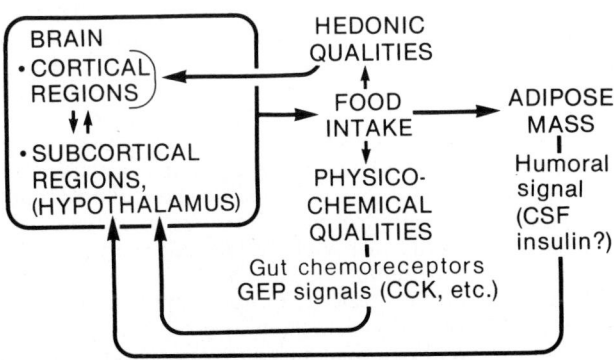

Figure 15–45. A hypothetical system to integrate feeding behavior (food intake) with meal quality and body adiposity. (*GEP* = gastro-entero-pancreatic hormones). (From Porte, D., Jr., and Woods, S. C., In *Proc. 10th Cong. Int. Diab. Fed.* Amsterdam, Excerpta Medica Foundation, 1980.)

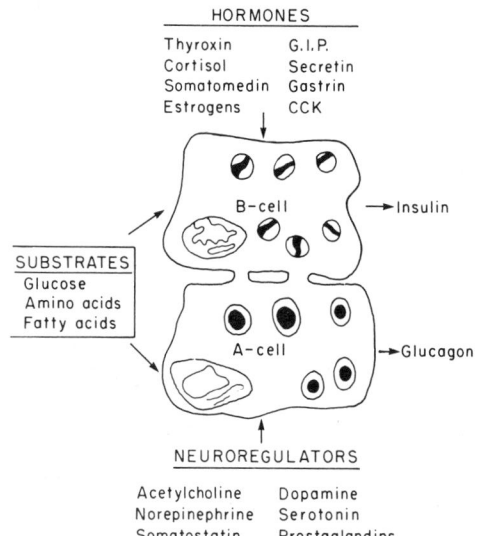

Figure 15–46. The islet as a nutrient integrator. The primary substrate control is modulated by the neuroendocrine system to regulate the output of glucagon and insulin for metabolic processes. (From Woods, S. C., et al.: The role of the nervous system in metabolic regulation and its effects on diabetes and obesity. In *Handbook of Diabetes Mellitus.* Brownlee, M. (ed.), New York, Garland Publishing Co., 1980.)

up by the central nervous system, its need plays a major role in the set and operation of the basal glucose regulatory process. During meals the extra carbohydrate, fat, and protein being absorbed need to be stored in the liver, muscle, and adipose tissue. The major organ concerned with this adaptation and change is the liver, which must decrease its uptake of amino acids, reduce gluconeogenesis, take up rather than produce glucose, and shunt fatty acids into triglycerides for storage in adipose tissue. Again, insulin and glucagon are critical factors for this transformation, although it now appears that glucose itself in the presence of insulin may also play an important role in regulating hepatic glucose uptake. Although quantitative data are scanty, during the absorption of a pure carbohydrate load the liver appears to take up a significant portion of the glucose as it is passed through the portal vein from the gastrointestinal tract prior to entering the systemic circulation. It is a highly efficient process with at least 30%, and perhaps as much as 60%, of a very large load metabolized in this way. The uncertainty is due to debate over the validity of a number of radioisotopic techniques used to measure this uptake. It is a critical question because carbohydrate-tolerance testing for the diagnosis of hyperglycemia may be more dependent upon glucose metabolism in the liver than that in peripheral organs. The possibility that altered hepatic glucose metabolism is a potential cause for poor carbohydrate tolerance in a number of metabolically abnormal states has not been adequately evaluated.

In contrast to glucose uptake by the liver, which is very closely regulated by both insulin and glucagon, regulation of glucose uptake by muscle and adipose tissue is almost solely determined by insulin. However, this insulin action can be modulated by a variety of peripherally acting counterregulatory hormones, including the catecholamines norepinephrine and epinephrine, cortisol, thyroxine, and somatomedin. Since these same hormones may play a role in modulating the action of insulin on the liver, nutrient metabolism during meals is a complex function of the neuroendocrine response to food ingestion.

Response to Exercise. Despite a major change in fuel utilization during exercise, plasma glucose levels remain constant. The mechanism for this adaptation varies with the severity of the exercise and its duration. With any level of exercise there is an increase in glucose utilization by muscle. This increase is not dependent upon an increase in insulin but will not occur in the absence of insulin. It is most likely that a greater blood flow to muscle during exercise increases the number of insulin receptors exposed to insulin, thereby mediating an increase in glucose uptake without an increase in concentration of either glucose or insulin.

Since glucose uptake increases during exercise, glucose production by the liver must also increase if the plasma glucose level is to be maintained. In most studies, mild exercise is accompanied primarily by a decrease in vagal tone, leading to an increase in heart rate, and by a relatively small increase in sympathetic activity associated with small decreases in insulin release. As a consequence of both events, there is also an increase in fatty acid mobilization. The fall of insulin secretion could explain increased glucose production during exercise. However, since hypoglycemia does not occur during mild exercise in pancreatectomized animals or man in whom insulin is constantly infused intraportally or intravenously, it appears that the decrease in insulin is not important to the blood glucose adaptation that occurs. Therefore, either a change in autonomic tone to the liver or direct feedback regulation by glucose is the mechanism by which hepatic glucose release increases in parallel with muscular work. During exercise that is more vigorous and/or longer in duration, there is greater stimulation of the sympathetic nervous system activity, resulting in greater lipolysis, which provides more fatty acids for muscular work. Although there is a continuous parallel increase in muscle glucose uptake as well, during heavy exercise the predominant fuel becomes fatty acids. During very heavy workloads, glucose levels do tend to decline and are associated with a marked increase in epinephrine as well as norepinephrine levels. Prevention of the glucose decline by infusing glucose leads to amelioration of the epinephrine response, indicating that small changes in plasma glucose are centrally perceived after a very modest decline during exercise and lead to counterregulatory autonomic responses.

Glucagon levels also rise during heavy exercise. This increase can be partly reduced by maintaining euglycemia, but this stimulation cannot be blocked by either β-adrenergic or α-adrenergic blocking agents. Therefore, the mechanism for the glucagon response to heavy exercise is not clear. It is possible that insufficient concentrations of blocking agents were used to inhibit neuronally released norepinephrine, or it may be that there are other transmitters involved in the process. Since insulin levels tend to be low, it seems likely that glucagon does play a significant role in the metabolic adaptation of the liver.

Glucose responses to carbohydrate ingestion during exercise can be highly variable, depending upon the level and duration of exercise. If the workload is low, and the predominant adaptation is vagal, carbohydrate tolerance may be normal or increased owing to the accelerated utilization of glucose by muscle and the limited inhibition of insulin secretion by mild exercise. The higher catecholamine levels at greater workloads will markedly inhibit insulin release in response to carbohydrate challenge. Therefore, carbohydrate intolerance will be observed despite the increase in glucose uptake by muscle.

EXPERIMENTAL HYPERGLYCEMIA

Ever since the original demonstration that total pancreatectomy produces hyperglycemia followed by ketoacidosis and death, animal models for diabetes mellitus have played an important role in the understanding of the pathophysiology and etiology of the disease. The replacement of insulin was shown by Banting and Best to restore such pancreatectomized animals to apparent good health. Such models have been particularly useful for understanding the consequences of insulin deficiency and the regulation of fuel physiology. However, interest in the etiology of the disease has not been fully satisfied by either this model or models involving chemical destruction of the islets or the use of anti-insulin serum. It has become clear that such models, while useful for evaluating insulin-dependent-type diabetes, do not appear to be clinically similar to the much more common non-insulin-dependent type.

Thus, more recent attention has been focused on a variety of spontaneous rodent syndromes characterized by hyperglycemia and obesity. For those interested in the potential genetic contribution to this syndrome, such animal models are advantageous because of the short generation time for understanding the mode of inheritance. One major outcome of these studies has been the recognition of the large number of genetic variants associated with hyperglycemia and the importance of the interaction of environmental factors with background genetic stock upon the phenotypic expression of a gene for hyperglycemia and obesity. Thus, there are now a large number of animal models for human diabetes mellitus (Table 15–5). However, it is not clear which of them, if any, are directly relevant to any specific affected human patient. Such diversity suggests that human diabetes is unlikely to represent anything less complex than that already found in these experimental animals. The major disappointing feature of the spontaneously diabetic rodent models described to date is the apparent absence of the chronic vascular lesions which characterize human diabetes. The reasons for this are uncertain but may depend upon inherent differences in the vasculature of these species, the relative crudeness of the measurements that have been made, and/or the relatively short duration of diabetes in most of the animals studied. However, some microvascular and neuropathic changes resembling those in human diabetes have been reported in several spontaneously diabetic rat and mouse strains as well as in some animals made hyperglycemic by pancreatectomy or toxic drug administration.

Pancreatectomy

Total or partial pancreatectomy, while effective in producing insulin-deficiency-type diabetes, also produces a deficiency of pancreatic somatostatin, glucagon, and pancreatic polypeptide. It is of interest, therefore, that so much of the pancreas needs to be removed before clinically evident hyperglycemia occurs. It has been estimated that at least 75% removal is required. One explanation for this phenomenon has been related to the removal of glucagon. However, more recent studies indicate that glucagon, probably arising from the stomach, is present in the circulation after pancreatectomy and prevents a total glucagon deficiency syndrome. It is also possible that there is a great deal of pancreatic reserve, because the partially pancreatectomized animal is known to be more sensitive to other diabetogenic or hyperglycemic agents such as streptozotocin, alloxan, and a variety of hormonal treatments. No careful quantitative comparative studies between animal species has been made in terms of total islet volume or the amount of islet material that must be removed in order to produce severe hyperglycemia. However, all species seem to require almost complete removal. While total pancreatectomy leads to a ketosis-prone state, this is not true of partial pancreatectomy. The difference can be related to the amount of insulin-producing tissue removed.

Just as in severe human chronic pancreatitis or pancreatectomized man, totally pancreatectomized animals are difficult to treat and oscillate between hypoglycemia and hyperglycemia. Subtotal pancreatectomy in rats is followed by an intense islet regeneration, but this decreases as time goes on. After 1–2 months the partially pancreatectomized rat may develop sustained hyperglycemia. This response is not observed in dogs; however, it may depend upon the age of the animal when the pancreatectomy is performed. Of interest is the fact that the regenerative capacity may be increased by steroids, at least in rabbits.

Table 15–5. ANIMAL MODELS FOR DIABETES MELLITUS

Type and Species	Characteristics
Surgical	
Pancreatectomy	Acute pan-islet hormone deficiency.
(Dog, cat, rat)	Brittle, requires > 90% removal. Exocrine insufficiency always present. Ketosis-prone.
Chemical	
Alloxan	Selective B-cell deficiency. Graded abnormality from mild hyperglycemia to ketoacidosis may be seen. Glucose protective.
(Rat, mouse, primate, dog)	
Streptozotocin	Relatively selective B-cell deficiency.
(Rat, mouse)	Reliable dose response with graded effects.
	Nicotinamide protective. Multiple small doses can produce a different form with delayed islitis.
Viral	
EMC-M variant	Only certain strains susceptible.
(Mouse)	
Spontaneous Hyperglycemia	
Ketosis-resistant syndromes:	Most of these animals show beta cell hyperplasia and hyperinsulinemia during their life.
Yellow (A^y) — mouse	obese
Obese (ob) — mouse	obese, severity of hyperglycemia depends on background strain
Adipose (ad) — mouse	obese
Diabetes (db) — mouse	obese, severity of hyperglycemia depends on background strain, often fatal with ketosis
KK (polygenic) — rat	lean, but insulin-resistant
Psammomys obesus — sand rat	obese, may not be hyperglycemic at all
Acomys cahirinus — spiny mouse	related to the gerbil; hyperglycemia depends on diet
Ketosis-prone syndromes:	Generally lean with low insulin levels.
Chinese hamster (polygenic)	variable inheritance; clinical presentation varies from mild hyperglycemia to ketosis-prone syndrome
BB rat (polygenic?)	islitis with sudden onset; selective B-cell loss; die in ketoacidosis

Chemical Hyperglycemia

Alloxan. Alloxan was shown to be toxic to the B-cell after hyperglycemia had been found following its intravenous administration. It has been shown to produce hyperglycemia in most animal species except the guinea pig and chicken. The response to the drug is triphasic, with an initial hyperglycemia, presumably due to a stress response or interference with B-cell function, followed by marked hypoglycemia, presumably due to its destructive B-cell action and release of insulin, and then a permanent hyperglycemia due to B-cell damage. Depending on the dose and the animal, varying degrees of hyperglycemia are observed, from mild to severe with ketoacidosis.

The toxic effect appears to be extracellular since alloxan is not taken up by the islets but remains in the extracellular fluid space. Alloxan blocks glucose-stimulated insulin release both *in vivo* and *in vitro* prior to destruction of the B-cells. Since the destructive effect of alloxan is protected by glucose and glucose analogues, some of which, such as 2-deoxy-D-glucose and 3-o-methyl glucose, are not metabolized, it has been hypothesized that alloxan has a direct toxic effect on a "glucoreceptor." Consistent with this idea, both the alpha anomer of glucose and the alpha anomer of 3-o-methyl glucose are better protectors against the B-cell toxicity of alloxan than the beta anomer. The short half-life of the drug in plasma of 1–2 min is also consistent with this idea.

Histologically, after alloxan administration one observes loss of granules, followed by fragmentation of the cytoplasm, and within a few hours clumping of nuclear chromatin and aggregation of interchromatic material in the nucleus of the B-cells. There is no evidence of an effect on A-cells in any species. The drug is not particularly effective in treating insulin-producing tumors of the pancreas in man, and it is of interest that the same tumors are not well stimulated by glucose. Since the drug can be shown to inhibit insulin release by short-term treatment *in vitro*, it seems likely that the initial hyperglycemic phase is due to the direct inhibition of insulin release. Toxic effects on other organs, particularly the liver, are well known; however, these and some toxic renal effects have not been well described or widely reported. It has been shown that alloxan will induce a reversible decrease in the glucose sensitivity of the tongue. That is, alloxan placed directly on the tongue reduces recorded nerve impulses from taste receptors stimulated by glucose. Similarly, alloxan has been given into the cerebrospinal fluid of rats and a blockade of 2-deoxy-D-glucose-induced eating has been observed. These studies suggest that there are glucose receptor systems outside of the B-cells which are similarly sensitive to alloxan. For these reasons the effects of alloxan treatment on neural and vascular changes in chronically hyperglycemic animals needs to be interpreted with some caution.

Streptozotocin. This compound was discovered as a fermentation product of *Streptomyces achromogenes*. It was shown to inhibit the growth of certain tumors and cultured cells. When used as an antitumor agent, it was found to produce hyperglycemia and low insulin levels. It is now known to be a toxic chemical for the B-cell in a variety of species, including the guinea pig, but not in fish or chicken. The ineffectiveness of streptozotocin in the chicken may not be due to a resistance of B-cells to streptozotocin, since pancreatectomy produces hypoglycemia in birds. In some species the A-cells are damaged as well as B-cells. Therefore, the toxic islet effects of streptozotocin are *not* as specific as those of alloxan. The clinical response to the drug is an initial hyperglycemia followed by hypoglycemia and then permanent hyperglycemia. The initial response is associated with inhibition of insulin release by islets from treated animals studied *in vitro*. Inhibition of insulin release can also be observed by the direct use of the drug with normal islets *in vitro*. The hypoglycemic phase is probably due to a marked increase in the release of insulin during the toxic destruction of B-cells.

Streptozotocin is an analogue of 2-deoxy-D-glucose with an N-nitroso-N methylurea group. In contrast to the effect of alloxan, streptozotocin hyperglycemia is not blocked by glucose or epinephrine. However, streptozotocin effects are blocked by 2-deoxy-D-glucose and 3-o-methyl glucose. The glucose portion of streptozotocin is not an absolute requirement for its hyperglycemic effect since N-nitroso-N methylurea alone can produce B-cell damage. However, the relative ineffectiveness of this latter compound has suggested the hypothesis that the glucose portion of the molecule facilitates its entry into the B-cell and maximizes its toxic effects. Damage is much slower than that caused by alloxan, and the half-life of the drug is much longer *in vivo*. The earliest pathologic changes are observed at 1 hour, but nothing major occurs until about 2 hours after injection, when there is some early margination of nuclear chromatin and compact nuclei. Between 4 and 6 hours the endoplasmic reticulum becomes pronounced, and cellular destruction follows later. Eventually, the B-cells degranulate and become pyknotic. While in many species the A- and D-cells are not significantly affected, some (such as the Chinese hamster) show complete and permanent loss of almost all islet cells.

Protection from streptozotocin is provided by nicotinamide, which may be given as long as 1–2 hours later. Islet cell NAD levels are markedly decreased by streptozotocin, an effect which can also be prevented by the administration of nicotinamide. Pyrazinamide and phenytoin, inhibitors of insulin secretion, have also been shown to be protective, suggesting that the protective effect may be related to inhibition of insulin secretion. Interestingly, the alpha anomer of streptozotocin is more toxic than the beta anomer to rats. Unlike alloxan, streptozotocin is toxic to islet cell tumors and can be used in patients for the treatment of islet cell carcinoma. Toxic effects in other tissues, particularly the kidney, have been reported. These effects may interfere with the use of this agent for antitumor therapy. Of interest is the lack of hyperglycemia in treated patients, suggesting that the normal B-cells are relatively resistant in man (? owing to tumor-induced suppression).

Spontaneous Hyperglycemia in Animals

Spontaneous hyperglycemia in animals can be clinically segregated into two syndromes quite analogous to those found in man. One syndrome is associated with insulin resistance and has a prolonged course without treatment and without ketosis. The other syndrome is associated with severe insulin deficiency, a tendency to ketoacidosis, and very little if any weight gain. Almost all syndromes are a result of a combination of genetic and environmental factors. In the obesity-hyperglycemia syndromes, diet quantity and quality appear to be important, as are the background genetic stock and the specific genetic variant associated with the syndrome. In the lean animals autoimmunity or viruses appear to be important factors, but these are also related to background genetic stock and genetic factors. A large number of animal models are available, and there is considerable variation in the genetics. In some the major effect is related to a single dominant gene, but in others there is a single recessive gene, polygenetic inheritance, or an unknown familial disposition. Listed in Table 15–5 are the common ketosis-prone and resistant syndromes.

Obese Hyperglycemia. A number of rat and mouse

models are characterized by obesity and hyperglycemia. Plasma insulin levels are elevated in proportion to the degree of obesity. However, despite the hyperinsulinemia, these animals are unable to overcome the insulin resistance associated with the obesity. In some animals the insulin resistance appears to be independent of the degree of obesity, but this is not always clear-cut. In these animals beta cell hyperplasia is marked, but if it diminishes with time and insulin levels decrease, hyperglycemia will become severe. It appears as though the islet in some of these syndromes is capable of responding by hypertrophy and hyperplasia, thereby minimizing the effects of peripheral insulin resistance and resulting in minimal hyperglycemia. In contrast, in other syndromes the islet cannot keep up and hyperglycemia develops.

In the ob/ob and db/db syndromes, the genetic background plays an important role in the severity of the hyperglycemia. Thus, if the background is C57/6J, a milder degree of hyperglycemia and more severe hyperinsulinemia is present. If the background is a related C57/KSJ, then the syndrome may consist of more severe hyperglycemia and lesser degrees of obesity. Thus, the ob/ob and db/db genes appear to produce similar effects leading to mild to moderate hyperglycemia and obesity on one background stock, but hyperglycemia and ketosis-prone diabetes on another background stock. However, even on the same background there are differences, indicating that these genes are not the same and not related to the same locus.

In the other animal models for obesity and hyperglycemia there is a great variation in degree of obesity and hyperglycemia ranging from pure obesity and little hyperglycemia to rather severe hyperglycemia with modest amounts of obesity. It is important to emphasize the variability of the clinical syndromes observed in the various models by different workers and at different times. Therefore, there must be important environmental, nutritional, and laboratory influences which play a role in the clinical syndrome observed. Increased food intake is a constant feature of this group of animals. From parabiotic experiments it has been proposed that ob/ob mice fail to produce a circulating satiety factor, whereas db/db mice are unable to respond to such a factor and, therefore, fail to suppress appetite when parabiosed to normal animals. However, the true mechanism for the explanation of the obesity in these syndromes is not yet known. Decreased energy expenditure is a general feature of these conditions and presumably contributes to the caloric retention. Lipogenesis is extremely active and lipolysis is suppressed. However, this appears to be related to the extremely high ambient insulin levels found during the obese stage. Whether the hyperphagia is the explanation for the hyperinsulinemia or whether the hyperinsulinemia is primary has not been determined. However, it is clear that hyperglycemia late in these syndromes is due to a diminished ability to maintain the extremely high insulin levels necessary for normal carbohydrate metabolism.

Ketosis-Prone Syndromes. Lean animals with clear-cut evidence of decreased beta cell function (decreased beta cell content of insulin and decreased insulin levels) can be found in the late stages of the C57 black/KSJ db/db mouse, the Chinese hamster, the EMC-M variant virally induced hyperglycemia, and the BB rat. These all appear to be models for the insulin-dependent type of diabetes mellitus. In most cases, the reason for the poor B-cell replication or B-cell destruction is not known. However, in the db/db mouse model and the Chinese hamster an early phase of hyperphagia, probable insulin resistance, and islet cell hyperplasia seems to be followed by poor islet cell replication and ketosis-prone hyperglycemia. In the Chinese hamster polygenic inheritance with at least four genes has been considered the minimal model for explanation of the observed frequency of hyperglycemia. When any two genes are inherited, the animals become hyperglycemic. There is no late insulin resistance and there are no major abnormalities in B-cells, just a reduced number as time progresses. In the BB rat a rather sudden form of hyperglycemia of great severity appears somewhere between the 50th and 100th days of life. There is no obesity and insulin levels are low. If not treated, these animals rapidly become ketotic and die. In the islets a destructive inflammatory lesion is observed. If insulin treatment is given, the number of islets decreases and the number of B-cells diminishes to almost zero.

The observation that certain mouse strains develop hyperglycemia following exposure to the M variant of the encephalomyocarditis (EMC) virus has provided direct evidence for the ability of viruses to produce islet damage. In susceptible animals high titers of viral antigen can be found within B-cells. The extent and severity of the islet lesion varies greatly from one islet to another and from one animal to another in the same experiment. At the time of hyperglycemia the islet cells are usually degranulated, but there is insulin deficiency in the serum. During the second week of infection, interstitial and peri-insular infiltrates of lymphocytes are found in many islets. In some, degenerating B-cells are observed. The outcome of the infection can be anything from complete recovery to quite severe hyperglycemia and hypoinsulinemia. Susceptibility to the virus is strain- and sex-dependent, with males being more susceptible than females. However, administration of male hormone to females renders them susceptible to the infection, while castration of male mice is protective. Genetic susceptibility is independent of the H-2 histocompatability marker in mice, since animals with the same H-2 group can vary in their susceptibility. Cells of resistant mice are resistant to the EMC virus infection *in vitro*. Thus, either the cells have a reduced number of virus receptors or they fail to support production of virus in some way.

Whether a virus plays any role in the BB rat or Chinese hamster is unknown. The inflammatory response in the BB rat suggests that an infectious process may be involved. However, no clear-cut viral particles have been described. In one strain of guinea pigs in which sporadic hyperglycemia was observed, the hyperglycemia was associated with the presence of a transmitted agent; however, the agent has not been isolated or identified.

Autoimmune Hyperglycemia. The presence of inflammatory cells in virus-induced diabetes and the rather delayed destruction of B-cells has suggested the possibility that immune mechanisms may play a role in B-cell destruction. The observation that multiple small doses of streptozotocin produce a delayed hyperglycemia associated with a mononuclear infiltrate in the presence of more visible murine viral particles in the B-cells has given further impetus to this suggestion. Inflammatory mononuclear cells are observed between 5 and 10 days after the last injection of streptozotocin, and the hyperglycemia progressively increases with time. Numerous C-type virus particles were observed in B-cells but not in A- and D-cells. Interestingly, there is also genetic variation in the susceptibility to multiple doses of streptozotocin so that only some strains are susceptible. The authors suggest that this lesion results from direct beta cell toxicity of streptozotocin followed by virus induction and a later cell-mediated autoimmune reaction which leads to the inflammatory changes, B-cell destruction, and hyperglycemia. Because of the known inflammatory changes in early human insulin-dependent diabetes and the association of the human disease with autoimmune-related HLA factors, this model has been of considerable interest to investigators.

DIABETES MELLITUS

General Principles

Diabetes mellitus is not a disease in the classic sense. It has no distinct and definable pathogenesis, etiology, invariable set of clinical findings, specific laboratory tests, or definitive and curative therapy. Rather, diabetes mellitus should be viewed as a syndrome — a clinical entity which can involve any or all of a long list of symptoms and clinical laboratory findings — which shows a variable response to therapy. The term diabetes mellitus, then, is one of convenience for the physician, rather than one that conveys definite pathologic meaning for the patient. Because abnormalities of glucose metabolism have been easiest to measure and were the first discovered, the major focus has been to define the disease by glucose measurements. Thus, various commissions and committees have periodically attempted to define the normal limits of glucose metabolism. Yet there are no standards of normal limits upon which all agree. This is largely because carbohydrate tolerance is distributed as a continuous function. The lack of a clear separation of normal from abnormal carbohydrate tolerance may be due to the distance of the measurement from the underlying genetic abnormality, to multigenetic regulation of carbohydrate metabolism, or to the variable interaction of hereditary with environmental factors. Therefore, in the absence of a genetic factor which can be measured, the presence or absence of diabetes mellitus can be only imprecisely assigned. Nevertheless, most clinicians can make a pragmatic diagnosis most of the time. In doing so, we consider that four general areas are affected in the complete clinical syndrome and that these should be considered in making a clinical diagnosis.

1. *Hyperglycemia.* There is an abnormality of carbohydrate metabolism resulting in hyperglycemia and often associated with accelerated fat and protein catabolism. This abnormality probably contributes to the other features but seems unlikely to be their sole cause.

2. *Large-vessel disease.* There is accelerated atherosclerosis and medial calcification.

3. *Microvascular disease.* There is an abnormality of capillary basement membranes characterized by thickness and abnormal function. These capillary-related lesions are often termed the microvascular or small-vessel concomitants of diabetes.

4. *Neuropathy.* There are peripheral sensory and motor defects, autonomic nervous system dysfunction, segmental demyelination, and abnormalities of Schwann cells.

None of these findings is specific for diabetes, as each is also found in other diseases and syndromes. It is likely that more than one mechanism can produce each of these four abnormal findings. Since the primary defect in diabetes is unknown, a patient with any one or all of these abnormalities must be considered a possible diabetic. The final decision is based on clinical and laboratory observations and depends largely on the particular frame of reference and concept of the term "diabetes mellitus" for each clinician. Therefore, for purposes of discussions to follow, we shall use the term "diabetes" in reference to the sum total of all clinical and laboratory observations, and such terms as hyperglycemia and thickened basement membrane to describe specific measured or observed findings. Because plasma glucose can be measured simply and accurately, it remains the standard most often used, but better markers for diabetes mellitus are hoped for in the future.

Clinical Classification

For many years clinicians have recognized differences in the presentation and clinical course of patients with diabetes mellitus. In some instances, abnormalities of other endocrine systems were recognized, and these are now considered to be diseases associated with hyperglycemia such as Cushing's syndrome, acromegaly, and chronic pancreatitis. After eliminating these various known causes for hyperglycemia, one is left with a group of patients with varying degrees of hyperglycemia without an obvious explanation and who have an increased likelihood of atherosclerosis, microvascular disease, and neuropathy. Even within this group there are obvious clinical differences. Therefore, terms such as juvenile diabetes and maturity diabetes were used to separate them on the basis of the age of diagnosis.

In the past few years, it has become clear that not only are there clinical differences, but that genetic factor(s) differ between these various clinical types. A summary of the differences in the two most common types is given in Table 15–6. In each case the genetic differences interact with environmental factors to produce the final clinical picture. However, just as the genetic trait varies, so does the nature of the important environmental factor. Thus, season appears to be a factor in the onset of juvenile diabetes, but diet and obesity are important to maturity diabetes. It has also become apparent that the original clinical terms used to segregate these types of patients are inappropriate because many patients who have a disease clinically similar to juve-

Table 15–6. CLINICAL CHARACTERISTICS OF THE TWO MAJOR TYPES OF DIABETES MELLITUS

NIH Diabetes Data Group Terminology*	Insulin-Dependent Diabetes Mellitus (IDDM)	Non-Insulin-Dependent Diabetes Mellitus (NIDDM)
Alternate Clinical Terminology	*Juvenile-Onset Diabetes (JOD)* *Brittle Diabetes*	*Maturity-Onset Diabetes (MOD)* *Adult-Onset Diabetes (AOD)* *Stable Diabetes*
Age at onset	Usually less than 45 years	Usually over 30 years
Genetics	Less than 10% of 1st-degree relatives affected	More than 20% of 1st-degree relatives affected
HLA	Associated with HLA-B-8, BW-15, DW-3, and DW-4	No HLA association
Immunity	Increased incidence of autoimmune phenomena	No increase in autoimmune phenomena
Body weight	Usually lean	Usually obese
Metabolism	Ketosis-prone	Ketosis-resistant
Treatment	Insulin	Weight loss; may need oral agent or insulin

Diabetes 28:1039–1057, 1979.

Table 15–7. CLASSIFICATION OF DIABETES MELLITUS

Traditional Clinical Classification (with Alternate Nomenclature)	NIH Diabetes Data Group Classification*

1. Juvenile-Onset-Type Diabetes (JOD)
   (a) Ketosis-prone diabetes
   (b) Juvenile-onset diabetes
   (c) Severe diabetes
   (d) Brittle diabetes
	1. Insulin-Dependent Diabetes Mellitus, Type I (IDDM)

2. Maturity-Onset-Type Diabetes (MOD)
   (a) Adult-onset diabetes (AOD)
   (b) Ketosis-resistant diabetes
   (c) Mild Diabetes
   (d) Obesity-hyperglycemia
   (e) Maturity-onset diabetes
   (f) Stable diabetes
	2. Non-Insulin-Dependent Diabetes Mellitus, Type II (NIDDM)
	   1. Nonobese NIDDM
	   2. Obese NIDDM

3. Maturity-Onset-Type Diabetes in the Young (MODY)
   (a) Familial maturity diabetes
   (b) Maturity-onset diabetes of youth	

4. Gestational Diabetes	4. Gestational Diabetes
5. Secondary Diabetes	5. Diabetes Mellitus and Impaired Glucose Tolerance Associated with Other Conditions
6. Congenital Insulin Resistance with Acanthosis Nigricans	6. Diabetes Mellitus Secondary to Congenital Insulin Receptor Deficiency
7. Acquired Insulin Resistance with Acanthosis Nigricans	7. Diabetes Mellitus Secondary to Insulin Receptor Antibody
8. Familial Autoimmune Diabetes	8. Diabetes Mellitus Secondary to Familial Autoimmunity

Diabetes 28:1039–1057, 1979.

nile diabetes have its onset after the age of 21 years, and a number of individuals with the clinical type of maturity diabetes have its onset in adolescence. In no case is it known what the genetic factor is and how it interacts with the environment. Therefore, the number of diseases which are covered by the term diabetes mellitus is unclear at the present time. As seen in Table 15–7, a number of different entities have been distinguished to date in which a different abnormal genetic etiology is almost certain.

A major aid in segregating diabetes mellitus into its component parts has been clinical studies in monozygotic twins. Pyke and his colleagues used the British Diabetes Association Registry to identify more than 90 pairs in whom at least one twin had diabetes mellitus (Fig. 15–47). Analysis of the frequency of concordance and discordance revealed a striking age-related phenomenon. In almost all twins diagnosed as diabetic after the age of 45, there was complete concordance for diabetes in the other twin within 3–4 years; in contrast, only 50% of the twins of those diagnosed under the age of 45 ever developed clinical diabetes mellitus (Table 15–8). Further analysis indicated that those diagnosed under the age of 45 were almost always sudden-onset, insulin-treated, juvenile-diabetes-type patients, while those diagnosed over the age of 45 were almost always slow-onset, non-insulin-dependent, maturity-diabetes-type patients.

From these data alone, it is clear that there must be some environmental factor which is important to juvenile-onset-type diabetes, whereas genetic factors alone can be sufficient to result in the development of maturity-onset-type diabetes. However, this does not mean that all maturity-onset-type

diabetics have the same genetic abnormality, nor does it mean that juvenile-onset-type diabetics lack a genetic predisposing factor. In the section to follow we will discuss these various clinical syndromes, attempting to identify features by which they can be distinguished and the potential role of genetic factors in their etiology. This will be followed by discussion of the environmental factors and their interaction with the onset and progression of the disease.

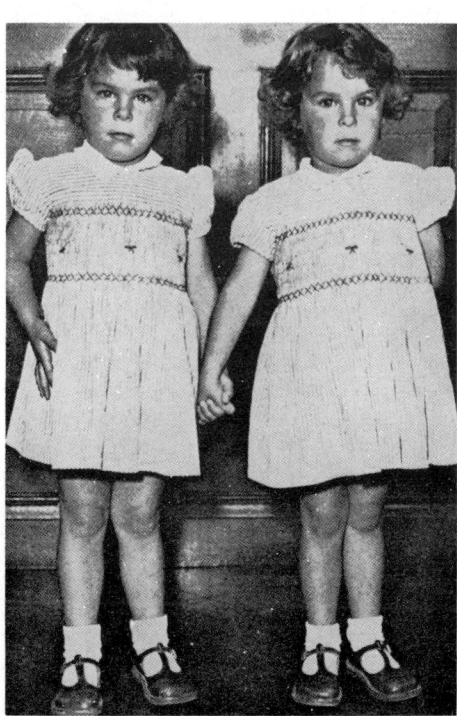

Figure 15–47. Identical twins with acute onset of diabetes appearing simultaneously at age 2½ years. (From Lister, J.: *The Clinical Syndrome of Diabetes Mellitus.* London, H. K. Lewis and Co., 1959.)

Table 15–8. DIABETES MELLITUS IN TWINS*

Age at Diagnosis	Concordant	Discordant
<45	54	52
>45	39	5

*From Pyke, D. A., Workshop on Etiology and Pathogenesis of Insulin Dependent Diabetes Mellitus. September 8–10, 1977, Juvenile Diabetes Foundation.

Juvenile-Onset-Type Diabetes (JOD)

Under proposed new terminology this will be called insulin-dependent diabetes (IDD). Insulin deficiency is the most characteristic finding of this type of diabetes mellitus. It is the classic type that we have known for over 2000 years, with sudden onset, severe hyperglycemia, and rapid progression to ketoacidosis and death unless treated with insulin. About 50% of these patients are diagnosed before the age of 21, with a peak incidence near puberty. Although some cases have been described in children under 1 year of age, this is not considered a congenital disease. Clinically, patients with IDD are lean, and even after treatment there is little tendency to obesity. Diagnosis is usually not a problem as they are almost always grossly hyperglycemic and symptomatic with borderline or overt ketosis in the absence of insulin treatment. They do not respond to oral sulfonylurea agents and at autopsy have gross B-cell failure. There may be a period after diagnosis during which insulin treatment is not essential, the so-called "honeymoon" phase, but this is almost always transient.

While the twin studies indicate that there must be an important environmental influence in the pathogenesis of this syndrome, there is also good evidence of an important genetic factor. It has been clearly shown that juvenile-onset-type diabetes in Caucasians is associated with HLA antigens B8 and Bw15 of the histocompatibility system. This risk increases in persons with HLA antigens Dw3 and Dw4 with which there is a linkage disequilibrium. Linkage disequilibrium applies to genes which are so close together that there is not a random distribution in the population. Since this same association is not found in maturity-onset-type diabetes, it is clear that the syndromes must be genetically different. While the relative increase in risk is small for an individual who has B8 or Bw15 (see Table 15–9), the increased risk of an individual who has Dw3 or Dw4 suggests that another gene (or genes) in linkage disequilibrium with these factors is responsible for the increased susceptibility to juvenile-onset diabetes. This hypothesis is strengthened by the fact that siblings with diabetes almost always have at least one HLA tissue antigen haplotype in common. In siblings completely matched for tissue type (i.e., share both parental gene sets) the frequency of juvenile-onset-type diabetes rivals that of monozygotic twins. This is true whether or not the diabetic subjects have any of the diabetes-related HLA antigens.

Thus, it appears that there is a gene or genes in the HLA region of the sixth chromosome which predispose to juvenile-onset diabetes. At least two such genes seem likely, since the presence of HLA B8/Bw15 and HLA Dw3/Dw4 are additive risks. Thus, someone homozygous for B8 or Dw3 has no different risk than a heterozygote, but a heterozygote B8/Bw15 or Dw3/Dw4 has 2–10 times the risk of those individuals with either HLA type alone. IDD is also associated with an increased risk of having autoantibodies to thyroid tissue and an increased risk of clinical Hashimoto's thyroiditis, another syndrome associated with HLA B8.

This finding has reinforced the concept that the diabetes susceptibility genes are somehow linked to the immune response system and can confer an increased sensitivity to a noxious environmental event leading to B-cell destruction (? viruses; see later). Consistent with this idea is the demonstration of circulating antibodies to human islet cell cytoplasmic antigens at the time of diagnosis of IDD. These autoantibodies are unusual in that they disappear with time after the diagnosis is made. In some series the incidence has been as high as 90% within the first month, dropping to about 50% positive after 1 year and 25% positive after 5 years. Antibodies to surface antigens of rat islet cells have also been reported. The etiology of this immune response is unknown and its clinical significance uncertain. Its absence in maturity-onset-type diabetes is consistent with the separation of these syndromes into two disease types. In patients with recent onset of hyperglycemia, the presence of islet cell antibodies is a good predictor of a future need for insulin treatment.

Unfortunately, at the present time there is no absolute marker for juvenile-onset diabetes. Although insulin treatment may be given, this does not necessarily mean that the patient is ketosis-prone and insulin-dependent. Therefore, in individual cases, particularly in the older age group, it may be very difficult to correctly place a specific patient into the appropriate syndrome category.

Maturity-Onset-Type Diabetes (MOD)

Under new terminology this will be called non-insulin-dependent diabetes (NIDD). The ability to survive without ketoacidosis in the absence of insulin therapy is the distinguishing characteristic of these patients. This disease usually has a slow onset and in the beginning is often asymptomatic, making it difficult to date the onset of the metabolic abnormality. Despite its clear genetic character, the clinical onset of the disease is relatively late and may not appear until the 60's, 70's, or 80's. In fact, there appears to be a continuous increase in the percentage of the population so identified with age. Another major clinical characteristic is obesity. At least 80% of these patients are greater than 15% over ideal body weight at the time of diagnosis. Therefore, it might best be called the obesity-hyperglycemia syndrome. It is also associated with retinopathy, nephropathy, microvascular disease, neuropathy, and atherosclerosis. The most common cause of morbidity and mortality is related to the cardiovascular system. While insulin treatment is not necessary for survival, it is often used therapeutically and is effective. Thus, all insulin-treated patients do not necessarily have insulin-dependent diabetes.

There is no associated HLA antigen type, and the mode of inheritance of the genetic factor or factors is unknown. Socioeconomic factors seem to be important in the age of onset and frequency of this type of diabetes, probably because of the important role of nutrition and body weight in its clinical presentation. There is a higher incidence of non-insulin-dependent diabetes in family members of patients who have this disease than of those with juvenile-onset-type diabetes. For this reason a great deal of effort has been made to identify the disease early by developing diagnostic tests which segregate early maturity diabetics from the normal population. One factor that has made this goal difficult to accomplish is that carbohydrate tolerance deteriorates with age even in normal persons. However, as a result of such testing, stages in the development of overt hypergly-

Table 15–9. HLA AND RELATIVE RISK OF INSULIN-DEPENDENT DIABETES MELLITUS (IDDM) IN WHITE POPULATIONS*

HLA Locus	A	B	C	D	DR
Alleles (relative risk)	1 (1.1)	7 (0.5)	W_3 (1.4)	W_2 (0.4)	W_2 (0.4)
		8 (2.7)		W_3 (2.7)	W_3 (4.8)
		15 (2.0)		W_4 (4.8)	W_4 (2.6)

*From Friedman, J. M., and Fialkow, P. F.: The genetics of diabetes mellitus. In *Progress in Medical Genetics.* Vol. IV. Steinberg, A. G., Bearn, A. G., et al. (eds.), Philadelphia, W. B. Saunders, 1980.

cemia have become evident. Since in many patients there is a variation over time in carbohydrate metabolism, different tests may pick up the abnormality at different stages. Furthermore, the more subtle the abnormality, the more likely there will be overlap with a significant percentage of a normal population group. Thus, the staging is fraught with difficulty as the tests used to place people in the various categories are rather nonspecific and the phenotypic changes are at some distance from the gene or genes that one wishes to identify. Nevertheless, identification of stages of non-insulin-dependent diabetes has usefulness in providing communication between physicians.

Stages of Maturity-Onset-Type Diabetes

Because one or more hereditary factors are believed to be essential parts of the disease and therefore are present at birth, an attempt has been made to separate the syndrome of maturity-onset-type diabetes into the clinical phases as they present themselves to the physician. These classifications are based upon the presence or absence of hyperglycemia or the degree of measurable carbohydrate intolerance. Several such classifications are shown in Table 15–10 and discussed in the following paragraphs, using the newly proposed NIH terminology. This approach ignores the vascular and neuropathic facets of the disease. The separation between categories is arbitrary. Such a classification does not mean to imply that an individual necessarily progresses from one stage of carbohydrate abnormality to the next, or that there is any specific order to the various categories that have been proposed. They are simply definitions which are used for communication between clinicians. Thus, in the natural history of carbohydrate intolerance, progression or regression from one stage to the next (1) may never occur, (2) may occur very slowly over many years, or (3) may be rapid and explosive. Carbohydrate metabolism appears to fluctuate from time to time in many individuals, particularly in persons with maturity-onset-type diabetes mellitus.

Potential Abnormality of Glucose Tolerance. This category is essentially theoretical in that it designates individuals who have the diabetic gene or genes but in whom there is no measurable carbohydrate abnormality. It covers the interval between conception and the time when abnormalities in glucose metabolism can be identified. This diagnosis can be correctly applied with high certainty to the nondiabetic identical twin of a NIDD patient and with less certainty to

the offspring of two NIDD parents. However, since the specific genetic abnormality of the disease has not yet been determined, this diagnosis cannot be made prospectively. The glucose metabolism of groups of individuals with high genetic risk have been studied. In general, subnormal plasma insulin responses to glucose, amino acid, and tolbutamide administration have been found in these genetically high-risk individuals.

Previous Abnormality of Glucose Tolerance. This has also been called subclinical diabetes or latent diabetes. The fasting blood sugar and the glucose tolerance test are normal. Diabetes is suspected because of decreased glucose tolerance after cortisone administration or after certain other types of drug therapy, during pregnancy, or with stressful illnesses such as myocardial infarction or surgery. Since few long-term follow-ups of such patients have been made, the percentage of genetically abnormal persons uncovered by stress hyperglycemia is unknown.

Impaired Glucose Tolerance. This has also been variously described as chemical diabetes, latent diabetes, or asymptomatic diabetes. Since this terminology overlaps with the previous category, there has been quite a bit of confusion. The fasting blood sugar is normal, but the glucose tolerance test is abnormal. Normal performance in a glucose tolerance test usually includes 95% of an age-corrected population as normal. However, this cut-off point has been quite variable and is responsible for most of the controversy in defining this group. Appropriate standards are discussed in the section on Carbohydrate Tolerance Testing.

Overt Diabetes Mellitus. This has also been termed clinical diabetes and is the form of the disease that has been familiar to medical practitioners for many years. Fasting blood sugar is *always* elevated, and the most severely affected patients have classic signs and symptoms of the disease. Patients with similar degrees of hyperglycemia of nongenetic cause (e.g., Cushing's syndrome or pheochromocytoma) are considered by most physicians not to have diabetes, simply because this scheme is based upon the concept that maturity-onset diabetes includes a genetic component by definition.

Maturity-Onset Diabetes of Youth (MODY)

In 1974 Tattersall described a family in which the pattern and presentation of diabetes were distinctly unusual. Clinically, a large number of family members had maturity-

Table 15–10. CRITERIA AND STAGING FOR MATURITY-ONSET-TYPE DIABETES MELLITUS

Terminology Employed by:

Fajans*	Prediabetes	Subclinical diabetes	Latent diabetes	Overt diabetes
American Diabetes Association	Prediabetes	Suspected diabetes	Chemical or latent diabetes	Overt diabetes
British Diabetes Association	Potential diabetes	Latent diabetes	Asymptomatic diabetes (subclinical or chemical)	Clinical diabetes
NIH Diabetes Data Group†	Potential abnormality of glucose tolerance (Pot AGT)	Previous abnormality of glucose tolerance (Pre AGT)	Impaired glucose tolerance (IGT)	Diabetes mellitus (DM)

Findings:

Fasting plasma glucose	Normal	Normal	Normal	Abnormal
Glucose tolerance test	Normal	Normal; abnormal during pregnancy, stress	Abnormal	Abnormal (not necessary for diagnosis)
Cortisone–glucose tolerance test	Normal	Abnormal	—	—

*Fajans, S.: What is diabetes? Definition, diagnosis, and course. *Med. Clin. N. Am.* 55:793, 1971.
†*Diabetes* 28:1039–1057, 1979.

onset-type diabetes; however, many had the diagnosis made during the early teens and twenties, and many remained hyperglycemic for many years with a stable elevation of blood sugar. Analysis of this and two other families indicated inheritance as a Mendelian dominant trait. This was deduced because there was a pattern of three generations of direct inheritance, almost every affected individual had an affected parent, and the ratio of affected to nonaffected in the offspring of affected individuals was approximately 1:1. Since that time a number of similar families have been recorded around the world. The separation of these families from other individuals with maturity-onset-type diabetes may be difficult unless a large number of family members are available for analysis. They appear clinically indistinguishable. In the original family descriptions, the prevalence of neuropathy, retinopathy, and atherosclerosis appeared to be unusually low. However, in some of the later family descriptions, a variety of chronic vascular degenerative changes have been observed. Therefore, it is not clear that all families with a dominant genetic pattern of overt hyperglycemia have the same genetic abnormality. This syndrome is not associated with any characteristic HLA distribution, nor is obesity a particularly prominent feature.

Insulin Receptor Defects

Recent studies have delineated a new clinical syndrome of insulin resistance with maturity-onset-type diabetes of variable degrees of hyperglycemia associated with acanthosis nigricans. Within this group there appear to be two major types. One is clearly familial and occurs in young females who have associated hirsutism, polycystic ovaries, mild virilization, and early accelerated growth. Insulin binding to circulating monocytes in these patients is significantly depressed owing primarily to a decrease in the number of insulin receptor sites per cell. Insulin secretory responses tend to be excessive and basal insulin levels are elevated. There generally tends to be an inverse relationship between the insulin response to challenge and the degree of hyperglycemia. Thus, these patients appear to have a hereditary defect in insulin receptors leading to insulin resistance and compensatory hyperinsulinism. In time, and to a variable degree, the pancreas is unable to continue to secrete insulin in such high amounts, and so carbohydrate intolerance or frank overt maturity-onset-type diabetes occurs. At this point, large amounts of insulin may have to be injected to control hyperglycemia. In some patients thousands of units per day may not be sufficient. In contrast to obese individuals with a similar type of insulin receptor defect, the binding abnormality in these types of patients is not reversed by 72 hours of fasting, indicating that the receptor defect is not secondary to hyperinsulinism but is related to some other metabolic change or to a primary receptor abnormality.

The second group of patients with insulin receptor defects tends to be older but also tends to be female and to have acanthosis nigricans. In addition, they often have other features suggestive of some type of autoimmune disease such as hypergammaglobulinemia, proteinuria, chronic nephritis, leukopenia, arthralgia, or positive antinuclear and anti-DNA antibodies. Studies in these patients have shown the presence of a circulating antibody directed against some portion of the insulin receptor which impairs insulin binding to the patient's cells and can be shown to impair insulin binding to normal cells *in vitro*. When these antibodies are removed from the patient's cells *in vitro*, the insulin binding returns to normal. The titers of these antibodies change during the patient's disease either spontaneously or as a result of treatment, and the insulin resistance changes accordingly. In some cases the antibodies are weak agonists of the insulin receptor. Therefore, when added in the absence of insulin, they have insulin-like activity. This apparent paradox has also been observed clinically, with an occasional patient found to be hypoglycemic. The syndrome is generally not familial and presumably represents a rather unusual manifestation of an autoimmune process in which antibodies to a normal tissue constituent are generated. Because of the general polymorphism of antibodies, it would appear that each patient has a somewhat different antibody type. Generally, however, they all interfere with carbohydrate metabolism by reducing the binding of insulin.

Familial Autoimmune Endocrine Dysfunction with Diabetes

A small number of families have been reported who have familial autoimmune thyroiditis and hypothyroidism, pernicious anemia, Addison's disease and hypocortisolism, hypoparathyroidism, hypopituitarism, and diabetes mellitus. Family members may have one, two, or all of the manifestations of the disease. Associated antibodies to one or more of the endocrine glands almost always appear before the clinical onset of the endocrine hypofunction syndrome, including islet cell antibodies prior to hyperglycemia. The diabetes usually progresses to the insulin-dependent type; however, the age of onset is older than in the usual juvenile-onset type and more consistent with the 40's and 50's age of onset of the usual endocrine autoimmune syndromes. Although juvenile-onset-type diabetes is associated with an increased incidence of thyroid antibodies and thyroiditis, these families clearly have an additional problem. If the diabetes presents first, it is difficult to make this diagnosis without a positive family history. However, the clinician should be alert to the possibility of other endocrine deficiency states. If one family member with this condition is identified, others should be evaluated, as it is relatively common among family members (? a dominant genetic disorder). In contrast to findings in the usual patient with juvenile-onset-type diabetes and islet cell antibodies, these antibodies in patients with the autoimmune syndrome do not disappear with time but seem to persist, perhaps even increasing in titer with time after diagnosis. In common with other autoimmune syndromes, the frequency of diagnosis is greater in females than in males. Therefore, from many points of view this is clinically and probably etiologically a separate form of diabetes mellitus.

Environmental Factors and Diabetes Mellitus

Viruses and Autoimmunity. A viral etiology or association for juvenile-onset diabetes mellitus was proposed more than 50 years ago by Gunderson, who found an association between community outbreaks of mumps and the occurrence of the disease. More recently other common human viruses have been implicated, but to date none have been definitively demonstrated to produce the disease. Many features of juvenile-onset diabetes are consistent with a viral etiology. Thus, the prevalence of new cases has been shown to have seasonal differences, with an increase during the time of high incidence of viral infections. Those studies which have documented an association between certain histocompatibility antigens and juvenile-onset diabetes have suggested that the closely linked immune response system might affect B-cell susceptibility to a virus or another noxious agent. The presence of specific antibodies and cell-mediated immunity against islet cells in patients with juvenile-onset diabetes has been used as evidence to support the viral pathogenesis. Finally, the inflammatory changes often observed in the islets of children dying shortly after the onset of the disease have been interpreted to be a residue of a viral or an immunopathologic event or both. Inflammatory reactions in the pancreas have also been observed in infants dying of disseminated virus infections.

Serologic studies have implicated coxsackie B-4 in the etiology of juvenile-onset-type diabetes; however, the high incidence of positive titers observed in early studies has not been consistent in follow-up evaluation, and in some age groups with diabetes a deficiency of coxsackie B-4 viral titers has been reported. Attempts to use this virus in animal models has been only sporadically successful. Thus, at the present time, the viral etiology of juvenile-onset diabetes remains an unproved but interesting hypothesis. However, all of this conjecture has been greatly strengthened by the observation of EMC-M variant virus–induced hyperglycemia and islitis in certain rodent models.

Autoimmune phenomena are common in patients with juvenile-onset-type diabetes. Cell-mediated immunity to islets was observed first using the migration-inhibition test. Using antigens extracted from the endocrine pancreas, immunity was associated with a delayed-type hypersensitivity reaction in skin testing. The response was not to insulin but could be obtained from whole pancreas homogenates or human insulinoma extracts. More recently, specific cytotoxicity was demonstrated with cultured human insulinoma cells and lymphocytes from insulin-dependent diabetes patients. In some studies use of mitochondrial antigens from other tissues produced the same response, but in others such controls were entirely negative. Tests for cell-mediated immunity are extraordinarily difficult to perform and to control; however, enough positive results have been reported that the phenomenon seems well established.

Evidence of humoral autoantibodies occurring very early in the disease has now been reported from a number of laboratories. These islet cell antibodies require the use of fresh human postmortem pancreas from blood group O donors as the antigen. Since these antibodies produce a rather weak fluorescence, the titers must be relatively low or the pancreatic antigens relatively rare. The percent positive approaches 90% within the first month of diagnosis but then decreases over time rather rapidly. The prevalence of islet cell antibodies (ICA) in the normal control population is very low, with most authors reporting less than 2%. The antibody reacts with all types of islet endocrine cells and is related to cytoplasmic antigens. Recently, another antibody which reacts with surface antigens from rat B-cells has been described. Although many patients have both antibodies, some have only one or the other. Finally, one group of investigators demonstrated serum antibodies reacting with cell surfaces of a viable insulinoma cell in almost 90% of a group of insulin-dependent diabetic patients regardless of duration of disease. This finding has not been confirmed and therefore its validity at the present time is unknown.

Diet and Obesity. The most common associated finding in patients with maturity-onset-type diabetes is obesity. In the diabetic population diagnosed over age 30, about 80–90% are more than 15% over ideal body weight. During periods of food scarcity such as major wars or famine, when there is a decrease in body weight, the incidence of diagnosed maturity-onset-type diabetes mellitus declines. Despite this very evident association, the mechanism and its relationship to specific dietary factors are not totally agreed upon at the present time. This is partly because the degree of obesity does not always correlate directly with the degree of hyper-glycemia, even in relatively standardized population studies. This lack of correlation may be related to the fact that not only the degree but the duration of obesity may play some role in the appearance of clinically recognizable hyperglycemia. In addition, there must be some other factors because populations with similar degrees of obesity vary greatly in the prevalence of diabetes. Thus, in some native populations such as the Pima Indians in the southwestern United States, overt hyperglycemia is very frequently associated with obestiy, whereas Eskimos or Athabascan Indians with similar degrees of obesity have much less frequent hyperglycemia. Such findings have raised the question whether specific dietary nutrients are involved or whether some genetic difference influences the response to obesity. Since dietary restriction or weight loss will reverse the hyperglycemia in almost all such patients and eliminate it in a fair proportion, it is clear that this is not simply a chance association, but a directly related one. Many of the obese hyperglycemic subjects develop other features of the diabetic syndrome, including accelerated atherogenesis, microvascular disease, and neuropathy. Therefore, the presence or absence of vascular degenerative changes does not segregate this syndrome.

The major influence of obesity on carbohydrate metabolism has been demonstrated to be a decreased sensitivity to insulin action in the liver, muscle, and adipose tissue. This decrease in efficacy can be overcome by additional endogenous insulin secretion or exogenous insulin administration. Therefore, more insulin needs to be secreted by the obese individual to maintain carbohydrate homeostasis and to maintain fat and protein metabolism comparable to that of nonobese subjects. This has led to the concept that obesity represents an environmental factor which imposes a continuous stress on the mechanisms for the synthesis and secretion of insulin and the replication of B-cells in the islet. It has been hypothesized that in the genetically susceptible individual there is a deficiency in the ability to respond to this stress which, over time, leads to sustained hyperglycemia. Obesity and hyperglycemia appear to be inherited together in animal studies; therefore, it is possible that the obesity is less environmental than genetic but is dependent upon the ready availability of food calories.

This obesity factor must be taken into account when comparing the prevalence of diabetes in various races, sexes, and socioeconomic groups. Thus, the increasing incidence of diabetes after age 30 (the number of new cases for each age group) is not found in societies in which middle-aged people tend to be lean. The increasing incidence of hyperglycemia with age in Western societies may not be related to aging as much as it is to the greater duration of obesity in the older population. Similarly, it has been reported that females have a greater incidence of maturity-onset diabetes than males. Recently, this difference has been disappearing, a finding perhaps related to the increasing fatness of males between the ages of 30 and 50 in our now sedentary society and partly due to the social pressures for leanness in females in the upper socioeconomic classes. Even the association of parity in females with the incidence of maturity-onset-type diabetes may be related to obesity, since there is a direct correlation between body weight and parity in most societies.

Thus, as more studies are performed, the association between obesity and hyperglycemia becomes more obvious. Some population studies of lean and obese groups over the age of 30 show a direct linear correlation between the degree of hyperglycemia and the relative body weight (Fig. 15–48). Since obesity is also familial, the question is whether obesity alone can cause hyperglycemia if it is severe enough and persists for long enough. Studies of families have sug-

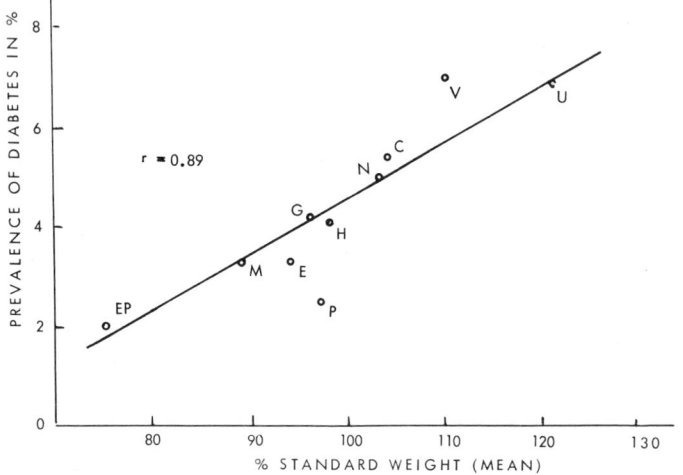

Figure 15–48. Correlation analysis showing the increase in diabetes in populations of increased body weight. (EP = East Pakistan; M = Malaya; E = El Salvador; P = Panama; G = Guatemala; H = Honduras; N = Nicaragua; C = Costa Rica; V = Venezuela; and U = Uruguay.) (From West, K. M., and Kalbfleisch, J. M.: Influence of nutritional factors on prevalence of diabetes. *Diabetes* 20:99, 1971.)

gested that thin relatives of obese maturity-onset-type diabetics do not have a very high risk of maturity-onset-type diabetes. Some obese Indian populations and the Sumo wrestlers of Japan have a high incidence of hyperglycemia even though family histories are relatively unchanged from the general population. There are many factors which tend to hide this association. One is that obese diabetics with marked hyperglycemia will tend to lose weight and therefore may have only a *history* of obesity rather than obesity present at the time of diagnosis. Second, an excessive death rate in this group tends to obscure the relationship when the usual cross-sectional method of analysis is used. Of interest is one prospective study in men aged 40–49 years in which obese men had a 12% incidence of diabetes in one decade, almost 30 times the frequency observed in those of normal body weight.

The evidence for a specific dietary factor in the pathogenesis of maturity onset diabetes is much less convincing. For example, most populations with a high prevalence of maturity-onset diabetes consume high-fat diets, but low rates of diabetes have been observed in some lean populations that consume substantial amounts of fat. However, in animal studies the best way to fatten an ordinarily lean rodent is to use a high-fat diet. Thus, the type of diet may predispose to obesity rather than hyperglycemia directly. In some instances it has been proposed that diets high in carbohydrate might predispose to hyperglycemia; however, most population studies show an inverse correlation between dietary carbohydrate and the frequency of hyperglycemia. Some investigators believe that dietary sucrose is a stress to the endocrine pancreas, and under certain conditions animals have been made hyperglycemic by diets very high in sucrose. However, in almost all cases this has been associated with obesity, and the same degree of carbohydrate intolerance can be produced by induction of obesity with other nutrients such as starch, fat, protein, or alcohol. Thus, although the prevalence of diabetes is higher in populations in which sucrose consumption is high, careful evaluation has not shown a very good association between sucrose intake *per se* and hyperglycemia when the studies are corrected for varying rates of obesity. Finally, there has been a suggestion that dietary fiber may play a role. It is true that populations with diets high in fiber have a lower incidence of hyperglycemia. However, these tend to be lean populations, and it is not clear whether the change is due to the fiber in the diet or the influence of dietary fiber on the relative degrees of obesity.

In summary, obesity is an important factor in the in-

cidence and probably the prevalence of maturity-onset-type diabetes mellitus. Whether this is wholly environmental and cultural or partially genetic in man is unknown at the present time. Although many specific dietary nutrients have been suspected, none have been shown to be operating outside of the influence of these nutrients on body weight and relative adipose mass.

Stress. The metabolic response to stress is associated with a neuroendocrine activation that will tend to elevate the plasma glucose. If the injury is severe, carbohydrate intolerance can be converted to overt hyperglycemia in apparently normal individuals. The hormones involved are norepinephrine, epinephrine, cortisol, growth hormone, and glucagon. Since the plasma glucose level is a simple product of hepatic glucose production and peripheral tissue removal, it is the influence of the hormones on these two processes which is responsible for the hyperglycemia observed (Fig. 15–49). The stress response may also include elevated prolactin and depressed gonadotropin secretion; however, these hormones are not known to play a role in carbohydrate metabolism.

Since the normal response to an increased glucose output by the liver or decreased utilization by peripheral tissues is an adaptive increase in insulin secretion, neuroendocrine factors which tend to inhibit this B-cell response play a critical role in stress hyperglycemia. Therefore, the catecholamines epinephrine and norepinephrine, and perhaps the intrapancreatic islet regulator somatostatin, are probably essential components of the hyperglycemia. For this reason, the original idea that stress hyperglycemia is primarily due to alterations in liver and peripheral tissues, whereas diabetes mellitus is a syndrome of pancreatic insulin deficiency, has broken down, resulting in great confusion regarding the differential diagnosis of hyperglycemia. It now appears that both components play a role in most patients with maturity-onset-type diabetes, and the same is true of stress hyperglycemia. Impaired islet adaptation is probably related to somatostatin or the catecholamines in stressed normal individuals with hyperglycemia, but the mechanism for the poor islet adaptation in nonstressed maturity-onset-type diabetes is unknown.

The situation may be further confused by the possibility that patients with maturity-onset-type diabetes are more sensitive to the hyperglycemic actions of the stress hormones. Furthermore, neuroendocrine counterregulatory hyperglycemic hormones may be elevated in patients with diabetes mellitus without an obvious stress. This has raised the possibility that there is an intrinsic neuroendocrine

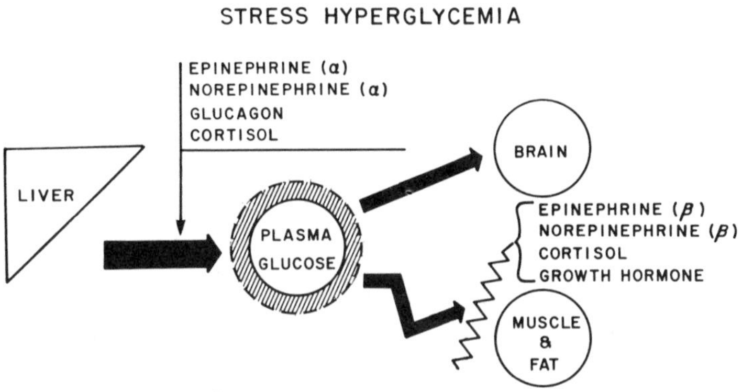

STRESS HYPERGLYCEMIA

Figure 15–49. Neuroendocrine control mechanisms for stress hyperglycemia. Either hepatic glucose output is increased, or insulin-mediated glucose transport is decreased, or both.

abnormality in some individuals with the diabetic syndrome or that the hyperglycemia itself is an activator of the stress hormones. Certainly in the most hyperglycemic, glycosuric, ketotic, volume-depleted patients there is ample evidence that the metabolically abnormal state itself leads to activation of the stress-related hormones and contributes to the vicious circle of hyperglycemia leading to neuroendocrine stress responses leading to further hyperglycemia (see Fig. 15–89 in the section on Diabetic Ketoacidosis).

Thus, a variety of traumatic, metabolic, physiologic, and perhaps even psychic states can be associated with carbohydrate intolerance. When the stress is eliminated, carbohydrate tolerance improves. The question is whether any sudden change in neuroendocrine function can lead to permanent alterations in carbohydrate metabolism. Medical-legal problems may arise when hyperglycemia is first noted following a stressful event (e.g., the trauma of an automobile accident, cerebral trauma, or other trauma related to emotional and neurologic illnesses). While hyperglycemia can obviously be produced in such a circumstance in a normal individual, the authors are inclined to believe that there is not sufficient evidence that stress *per se* can produce a permanent diabetic syndrome in a genetically unaffected person. Similarly, since more than 90% of the pancreas must be removed to produce surgically induced hyperglycemia, it would require massive trauma to lead to a diabetic syndrome on this basis. It is possible, however, that neuroendocrine abnormalities may persist over a longer period of time. In this situation, it is unknown whether they may be responsible for an increased incidence or prevalence of maturity-onset-type diabetes.

Drugs. Other environmental influences that may produce carbohydrate intolerance or overt hyperglycemia include a number of drugs. Among the more common are the benzothiadiazine (thiazide) diuretics, phenytoin (Dilantin), glucocorticoids, and the estrogen component of birth control pills. While the two former drugs inhibit insulin secretion, the latter appear to induce a state of insulin resistance. At reasonable dose levels, most normal people compensate for the insulin resistance by the secretion of additional amounts of insulin. Certain individuals appear unable to maintain this response, and hyperglycemia appears. In most instances when these hormones are withdrawn, carbohydrate tolerance reverts to normal. In some cases ketoacidosis has been precipitated, but this is unusual. However, even in these instances there is a marked improvement in carbohydrate metabolism after the removal of the offending drug. It is not clear whether these are true expressions of the diabetic syndrome precipitated by the drugs (they usually have not been given long enough or to large enough groups for any effect on the vascular or neural components of the diabetic syndrome to have been observed) or manifestations of some unusual sensitivity to the side effects of the drug. Experience

with the cortisone–glucose tolerance test indicates that individuals who react abnormally to this test subsequently have a distinctly higher incidence of overt diabetes than do those with a normal response. Thus, at least some of the individuals who develop drug-induced hyperglycemia may have the genetic abnormality of the diabetic syndrome. Other drugs affecting carbohydrate tolerance testing are discussed later.

Prevalence and Incidence

Because a specific method of identifying the maturity-onset-type diabetic subject is lacking, the prevalence (percentage of population affected) and the incidence (number of new cases per year) have been approximate at best. It is clear, however, that maturity-onset diabetes is one of the most common chronic diseases, affecting 1–5% of the total population. The prevalence appears to increase in populations which are (1) older, (2) obese, (3) female, (4) Jewish, and (5) well supplied with physicians. Approximately 10 times as many cases of diabetes are diagnosed in people over the age of 45 as in those under 45; thus, the juvenile-onset type is much less frequent. The incidence of maturity-onset diabetes in females is approximately 25% higher than in males. A positive family history increases the frequency two to four times. The incidence of diabetes can only be estimated from data of the annual number of newly diagnosed cases because information about the true appearance of new disease is lacking. Even these data are scanty but have been estimated at 5–10% of the total number per year, making about 200,000 new cases per year in the United States.

Genetic Risk

Since the mode of inheritance of diabetes is still in question, accurate genetic counseling is impossible. The best approach would be a simple table to delineate for the clinician the statistics of inheriting a diabetic genotype. Perhaps a more practical approach is the assessment of risk based upon clinical diabetes rather than upon the presence of the diabetic gene or an abnormality of glucose tolerance. Such a practical approach and a discussion of its uses and limitations are given in Chapter 27.

Pathophysiology of Hyperglycemia

Juvenile-Onset-Type Diabetes Mellitus

Insulin. This form of diabetes is clearly associated with a deficiency of insulin secretion. For many years it was believed that complete destruction of the islets had occurred at the time of diagnosis. This belief appeared to be confirmed by the inability of such patients to secrete insulin in response to any islet challenge. However, it has been observed that basal insulin levels are often maintained near normal (but probably only because of the severe hyperglycemia), and ketoacidosis does not always lead to permanent insulin therapy. Furthermore, there is the peculiar phenomenon of the honeymoon period, which is frequently observed during the first year or two of treatment. Marked improvement in carbohydrate tolerance is observed during this period, sometimes to the point where insulin therapy may be stopped for a short period of time. Insulin measurements at this time in patients without antibodies have demonstrated a partial restoration of insulin secretion, indicating that some of the damage to the islet is reversible. Because of circulating antibodies to insulin and their ability to bind endogenous and exogenous insulin, it was for a long time impossible to further assess insulin secretion during insulin therapy. However, with the discovery of the synthetic sequence of insulin via proinsulin, and the ultimate packaging and release of the connecting peptide with the insulin molecule, it became apparent that endogenous insulin secretion could be distinguished from exogenous insulin administration by the measurement of C-peptide.

The development of a practical assay has had to overcome some formidable obstacles. First, because of species differences, only human C-peptide can be used as antigen and radioactive tracer. Second, labeling with ^{125}I can be accomplished only if a tyrosine residue is coupled to the C-peptide. Third, proinsulin will cross-react with the C-peptide assay and if bound to antibody in significant con-

centrations may interfere with the measurement of C-peptide. Therefore, these complexes must be removed prior to assay. Finally, the C-peptide antibodies generated have been shown to interact with some nonspecific substances in plasma leading to different numbers depending upon the antisera used. Nevertheless, it is possible now to obtain qualitative, if not quantitative, results which indicate a significant persistence of endogenous insulin secretion in many juvenile-onset diabetic patients. This residual insulin secretion is a mirror image of the hyperglycemia in the untreated patient, being extremely low during ketoacidosis but then recovering during insulin treatment and finally increasing further as insulin dosage is diminished during spontaneous remission. However, as the disease progresses, C-peptide immunoreactivity disappears from serum and is rarely present 10 years after diagnosis (Fig. 15–50). Comparative studies of stable and unstable diabetics have demonstrated higher levels of C-peptide immunoreactivity in the stable group and very low or nondetectable levels in the unstable group (Fig. 15–51). It is of interest that the unstable group also demonstrates a greater abnormality of glucagon secretion in response to glucose than the stable group. While these findings are important to therapeutic considerations in diabetes mellitus, the clinical value of this assay is in the diagnosis of insulin-producing tumors, discussed in Chapter 16.

Glucagon.   Secretion of this hormone is also abnormal in juvenile-onset diabetes. Basal levels are particularly high during ketoacidosis or in very poorly controlled patients. When tested with arginine, these subjects hyperrespond (Fig. 15–52). When such patients are injected with glucose, there is no suppression of the elevated level. Insulin treatment will usually reverse the abnormality and restore basal glucagon concentrations to the normal range. If glucose is infused after insulin treatment, glucagon will be suppressed but only to about 50% of the normal response. However, if insulin is added to the glucose infusion, glucagon suppression may become normal. This may require very large injections of insulin, giving plasma concentra-

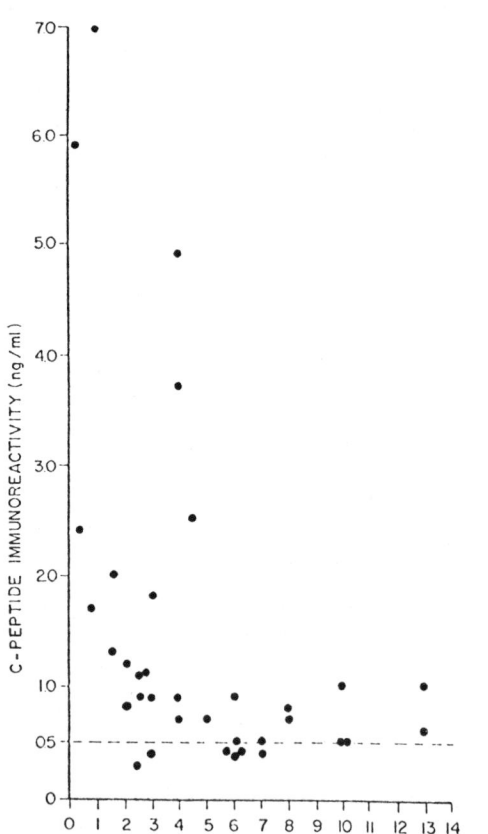

Figure 15–50.   Frequency of residual insulin secretion as estimated from the C-peptide assay vs. years after diagnosis of IDD. Each circle represents an individual subject. (From Grajwer, L. A., et al.: Control of juvenile diabetes mellitus and its relationship to endogenous insulin secretion as measured by C-peptide immunoreactivity. *J. Pediatr. 90*:42, 1977.)

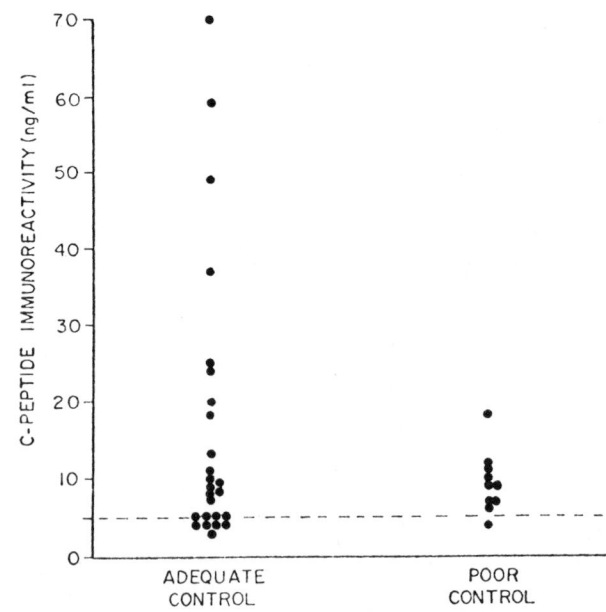

Figure 15–51.   Differences in C-peptide levels in groups of patients in whom control was classified as clinically poor or adequate. (From Grajwer, L. A., et al.: Control of juvenile diabetes mellitus and its relationship to endogenous insulin secretion as measured by C-peptide immunoreactivity. *J. Pediatr. 90*:42, 1977.)

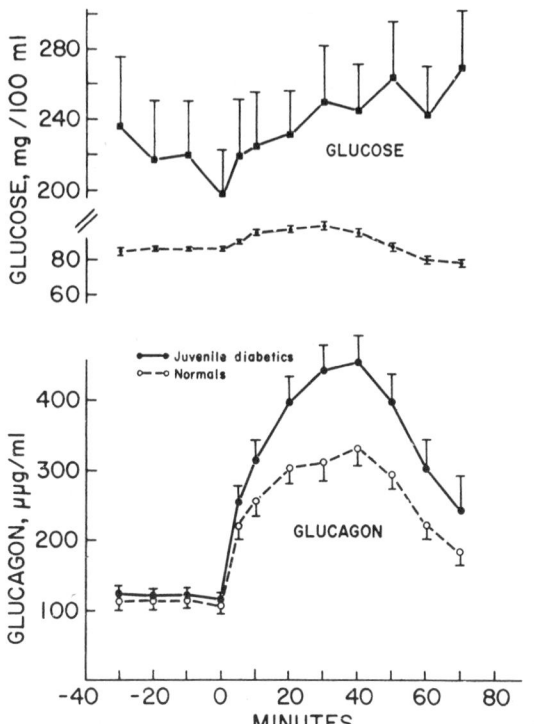

Figure 15-52. Glucagon responses to intravenous arginine in normal and insulin-dependent diabetic subjects. Note the inordinately great and statistically significant higher glucagon response to this intravenous amino acid challenge in the diabetic subjects. (From Unger, R. H., et al.: Studies of pancreatic alpha cell function in normal and diabetic subjects. *J. Clin. Invest.* 49:837, 1970.)

tions higher than those found in normal subjects after a glucose pulse without insulin.

If sufficient insulin is given to produce hypoglycemia, the normal glucagon elevation in response to this hypoglycemic stimulus is not observed. Thus, glucose is perceived poorly when it is elevated or when it is abnormally depressed, while nonglucose stimuli such as arginine produce at least normal and perhaps supernormal glucagon responses. Similarly, fatty acid elevations are capable of suppressing the A-cell normally. During meal feeding the usual balance between stimulatory and inhibitory forces in normal subjects after mixed meals may be converted into a hyperglucagonemic response in the juvenile-onset-type diabetic. While these responses can be normalized by injections of insulin, the amount required is often quite large. Therefore, it seems likely that glucagon levels are often inappropriate for the metabolic state and contribute significantly to hyperglycemia in juvenile-onset-type diabetes. If insulin treatment is stopped experimentally, glucagon levels rise quite rapidly. The prevention of this rise by the infusion of somatostatin has been shown to delay hyperglycemia and ketonemia. However, these studies were complicated by the fact that growth hormone levels were also suppressed. Thus, it is possible that there may be an interaction between these two counterregulatory hormones rather than the effect being due solely to glucagon suppression.

Somatostatin. Little is known about the role of somatostatin in this syndrome; however, increased somatostatin content and increased numbers of D-cells have been reported in the pancreases of juvenile-onset-type diabetics and in experimental models of diabetes produced by alloxan and streptozotocin. If this finding is indicative of increased or inappropriate somatostatin release, its suppressive effects

on the small amounts of residual B-cells could contribute significantly to the state of insulin deficiency in insulin-dependent diabetics.

Other Counterregulatory Hormones and Stress. Elevations of epinephrine, norepinephrine, cortisol, and growth hormone have also been reported in juvenile-onset-type diabetics at the time of diagnosis and during keto-acidosis or periods of poor metabolic control. Since all of these hormones are elevated in stress and are important to stress hyperglycemia, they must be playing a role in the hyperglycemia and metabolic abnormalities found in juvenile-onset-type diabetics. Since uncontrolled diabetes leads to glycosuria, volume depletion, baroreceptor activation, and at least sympathetic autonomic stimulation, if not activation of pituitary ACTH and growth hormone, it seems likely that many of these neuroendocrine hormonal abnormalities are secondary to the insulin deficiency. Through a vicious circle their stimulation continues and maintains the metabolic abnormality. However, even during periods of exceedingly good control, subtle abnormalities of growth hormone and glucagon may remain. Therefore, these hormones probably contribute to the hyperglycemia observed in most patients most of the time. Since the normal response to these hormones is hyperglycemia, which then feeds back to the normal islet to stimulate insulin secretion in a modulatory way, the inability to respond with an increase in insulin also exaggerates the hyperglycemic response to stress in the juvenile-onset-type diabetic.

Thus, modulation of any or all of these hormones can result in lower plasma glucose levels in insulinopenic diabetics. Since it is difficult to control the environment or the individual response to stress, in some rare instances pharmacologic modification of the stress response has been attempted as a therapeutic intervention. While the use of propranolol in juvenile-type diabetics has many potentially hazardous side effects, this treatment did in some instances reduce the frequency of ketoacidosis. The hypophysectomized diabetic animal is also known to become less hyperglycemic during stress testing. Therefore, whether or not the diabetic state itself is associated with an abnormality in the regulation of these hormones, it is clear that they can contribute significantly to the variability of control in severely insulinopenic subjects and must be considered during the treatment of such patients.

Insulin Resistance. In the untreated state most of these patients can be shown to have mild degrees of insulin resistance. This is not surprising in view of the elevations of most of the counterregulatory hormones just discussed. In ketoacidosis it has been shown that the degree of insulin resistance is surprisingly mild considering the gross abnormalities observed in metabolism. Recently, effective treatment for this syndrome has been demonstrated with use of relatively small amounts of insulin (i.e., between 3 and 5 units per hour). Since this dose is twice the estimated endogenous posthepatic secretory rate, some degree of insulin resistance may still be present, but it would be relatively mild. Since during treatment most of these counterregulatory hormone levels fall to or toward normal, this insulin-resistant state would be expected to be ameliorated. However, studies of insulin effectiveness during steady-state glucose infusions in such patients have still demonstrated some degree of insulin resistance, even in the treated patient when the metabolic abnormalities of diabetes are under reasonable control. Whether this is due to residual counterregulatory hormone activity or to an intrinsic feature of the diabetic state in juvenile-onset-type diabetes is not clear. In animal studies of insulin deficiency in the untreated state, an increase in insulin receptor number has been reported. In well treated patients peripheral insulin levels are high, probably because the ordinary exogenous insulin treatment schedules require relatively high insulin levels in order to provide for normal suppression of hepatic glucose release. These high peripheral insulin levels may result in a pathophysiologic suppression of insulin receptors in muscle and adipose tissue and produce resistance to the injected hormone.

Many insulin preparations are still antigenic. Therefore, as treatment progresses, another cause of reduced sensitivity to exogenous insulin emerges. Since the antibodies produced are polymorphic, there is a wide range in their ability to bind, release, and interfere with insulin action. Generally speaking, the binding is reversible so that insulin antibodies serve as a reservoir for circulating free insulin. However, it is clear from the use of injected insulin antibodies in animals that insulin bound to antibody is no longer able to stimulate the insulin receptor. All antibodies that have been made to insulin demonstrate this phenomenon. The development of insulin antibodies may be an important patient variable which partly explains the wide range of insulin dosages that are used to control hyperglycemia in juvenile-onset-type diabetic patients. The clinical development and significance of these antibodies are discussed later.

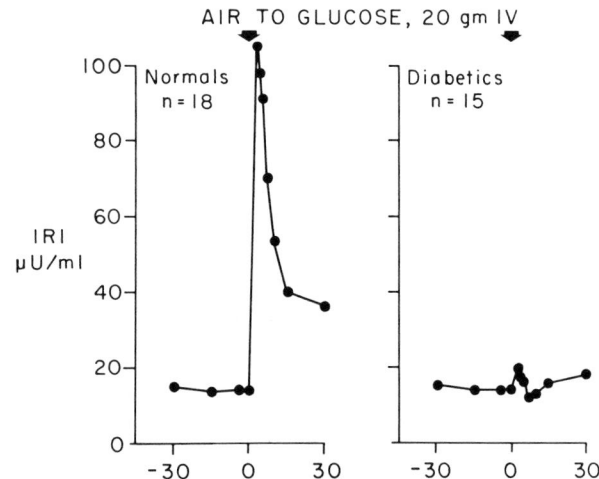

Figure 15–53. Comparison of the acute insulin responses to 20 g glucose in normal and diabetic subjects with fasting plasma glucose greater than 120 mg/dl.

Maturity-Onset-Type Diabetes Mellitus

As will be discussed later in the section on carbohydrate tolerance testing, the diagnosis of maturity-onset-type diabetes is insecure unless fasting hyperglycemia (fasting plasma glucose [FPG] greater than 140 mg/dl on more than one occasion) is present. In such hyperglycemic patients there is a characteristic abnormality of the insulin secretory response to glucose. However, the abnormality may be subtle and will not be detectable in all patients unless the glucose challenge is given intravenously. Despite this islet abnormality, it seems unlikely that the hyperglycemia is related solely to defective insulin secretion; more likely it is due to a complex mix of B-cell deficiency, other abnormal hormonal factors, and insulin resistance. This should lead to heterogeneity in maturity-onset-type diabetes, but aside from maturity-onset diabetes of youth, the rare cases with insulin receptor defects and one genetic abnormality of the insulin molecule, clear-cut heterogeneity within this group has not been defined yet.

Insulin. Insulin secretion in the basal state is normal in patients with modest fasting hyperglycemia (115–200 mg/dl). Basal insulin levels may in fact be elevated owing to the frequent presence of obesity in this group of patients. However, in both normal subjects and maturity-onset diabetics, basal insulin levels are not correlated with basal glucose but instead increase or decrease with changes in relative adiposity. Presumably this is a compensatory change related to the insulin resistance of obesity. This compensation remains nearly intact in patients with mild to moderate fasting hyperglycemia.

After intravenous glucose challenge in normal subjects a maximal increase in insulin occurs within the first 3–5 min and is comparable to the first-phase insulin secretion during square-wave stimulation *in vitro*. In all maturity-onset-type diabetics (FPG > 120 mg/dl) there is no acute or first-phase insulin increase during the intravenous glucose tolerance test (Figs. 15–53 and 15–54). Insulin levels between 10 and 60 min after the glucose pulse are comparable to the second-phase insulin response *in vitro* and are variable. The second-phase response of obese subjects is increased in proportion to body weight when FPG is less than 120 mg/dl, but decreased in subjects with basal hyperglygy-

cemia greater than 120 mg/dl. Second-phase responses to intravenous glucose of lean maturity-onset-type diabetics are reduced in those with FPG greater than 120 mg/dl and particularly so in those with FPG greater than 200 mg/dl.

Since the higher islet gain of obesity is reflected in the increased basal insulin levels and in an increased insulin response to glucose, the effect of obesity can be corrected for by calculating the relative insulin response, that is, the insulin response as a proportion of the basal level. When insulin responses are calculated in this way, obese as well as lean subjects with FPG of up to 120 mg/dl demonstrate a normal second phase of glucose-induced insulin secretion (Fig. 15–55). Using this same method of calculating insulin secretion, there is a 50% mean reduction in the relative first-phase insulin response to glucose in patients with FPG levels between 100 and 115 mg/dl and carbohydrate intolerance. If one calculates the glucose disappearance rate (K glucose or K_g), there will be a good correlation between this measure of glucose tolerance and the relative acute insulin response to glucose challenge. Thus, the first-phase insulin response diminishes in proportion to carbohydrate

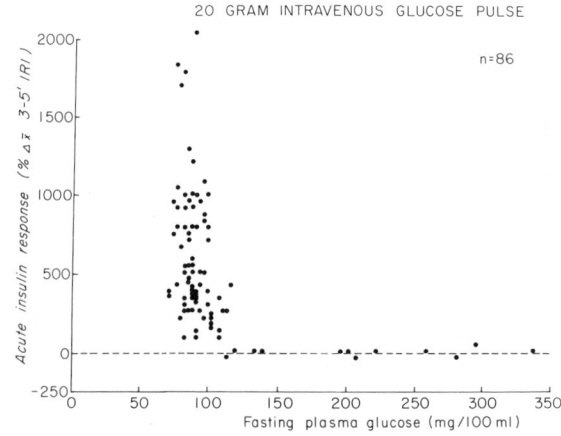

Figure 15–54. The relation of acute or first-phase insulin secretion to a 20-g glucose challenge and fasting plasma glucose. Note the lack of any rapid insulin response when fasting plasma glucose exceeds 120 mg/dl. (From Brunzell, J. D., et al.: Relationships between fasting plasma glucose levels and insulin secretion during intravenous glucose tolerance tests. *J. Clin. Endocrinol. Metab. 42*:182, 1976.)

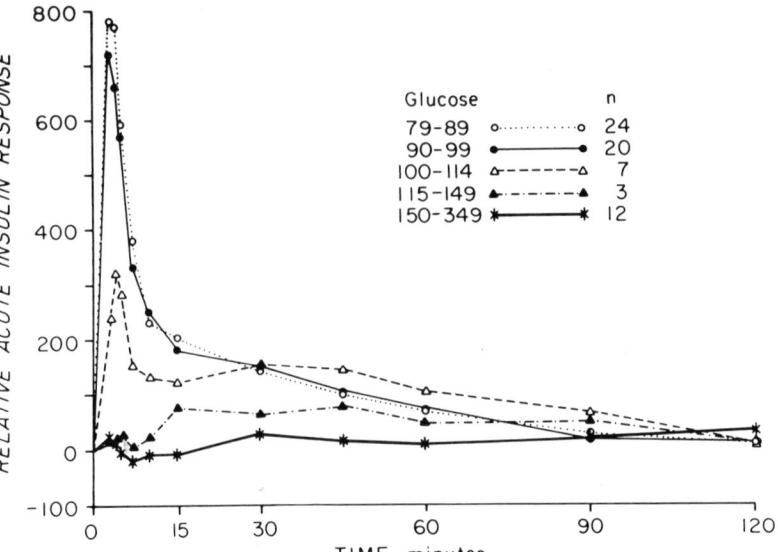

Figure 15–55. The relative insulin response in relation to fasting plasma glucose (FPG). Note the normal responses until FPG exceeds 100 mg/dl, the loss of first phase when FPG is greater than 115 mg/dl, and the presence of a second phase until FPG exceeds 150 mg/dl. (From Brunzell, J. D., et al.: Relationships between fasting plasma glucose levels and insulin secretion during intravenous glucose tolerance tests. *J. Clin. Endocrinol. Metab.* 42:182, 1976.)

intolerance (FPG 100–115) and is lost completely in overt diabetes (FPG > 120). The second-phase response is only gradually reduced until significant glycosuria appears (FPG > 200).

When nonglucose stimulants are used to test B-cell function, the picture is somewhat different. The bolus injection of either the gut hormone secretin, the β-adrenergic agonist isoproterenol, the amino acid arginine, or the drug tolbutamide is followed by acute insulin responses which are normal for body weight in maturity-onset diabetics who have FPG levels up to about 200 mg/dl (Fig. 15–56). Thus, it appears that the defect in the diabetic islet primarily affects glucose. Since the first phase of glucose-induced insulin secretion is completely lost in such patients, we have suggested that a specific glucose receptor defect exists in maturity-onset-type diabetes. As the intracellular mechanisms underlying this response to glucose are unknown, the nature of the defect in molecular terms is not clear. However, early hypotheses that adenylate cyclase or cyclic AMP might be involved seem unlikely because of the persistence of a normal response to the β-adrenergic adenylate cyclase stimulator isoproterenol.

More recently analyses have been directed at an explanation for the normal responses observed to the nonglucose stimulants and to the maintenance of normal basal insulin levels in maturity-onset-type diabetes. We have shown that increases and decreases in steady-state plasma glucose concentrations are important to insulin responses to nonglucose stimulants in normal subjects and maturity-onset-type diabetics. We have used the term potentiation to describe this regulatory effect of glucose. The relationship between the plasma glucose level and the insulin response to a nonglucose stimulant can be expressed as a slope of glucose potentiation. Diabetic subjects have a much flatter slope of potentiation than normals (Fig. 15–57). Therefore, a greater change of glucose level is required to influence insulin responses to the nonglucose stimulants in maturity-onset diabetes. This means that the basal glucose level of both normals and maturity-onset diabetics is critical for maintenance of the response to the nonglucose stimulants. Since nonglucose signals are important for basal insulin secretion as well, it seems likely that the basal glucose level is also a major regulator of this islet function. In this way, the hyperglycemia of maturity-onset diabetes will tend to compensate for the impairment of glucose potentiation. However, when the defect is so severe that it would require

Figure 15–56. A comparison of the acute insulin response (AIR) to the β-adrenergic agonist isoproterenol in normals and diabetic subjects with fasting plasma glucose (FPG) between 115 and 250 mg/dl. The two groups are matched for relative adiposity. This normal response is dependent on the hyperglycemia. Diabetics with FPG greater than 300 mg/dl are decompensated and the response is abnormal.

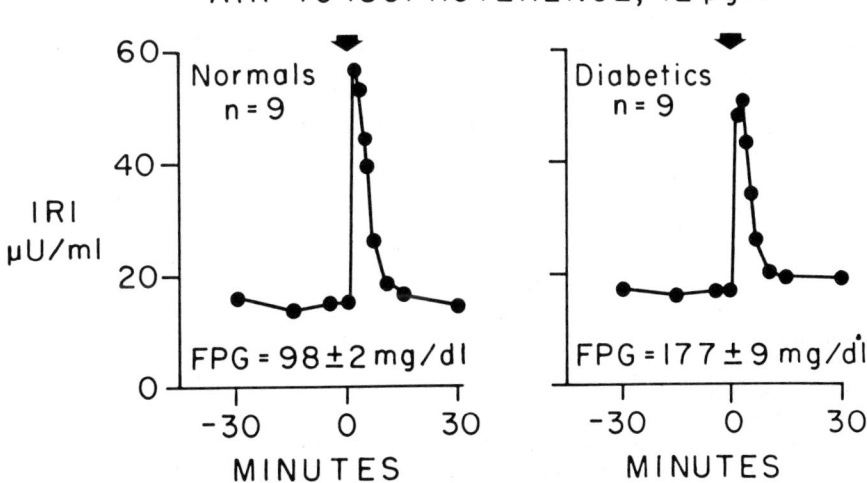

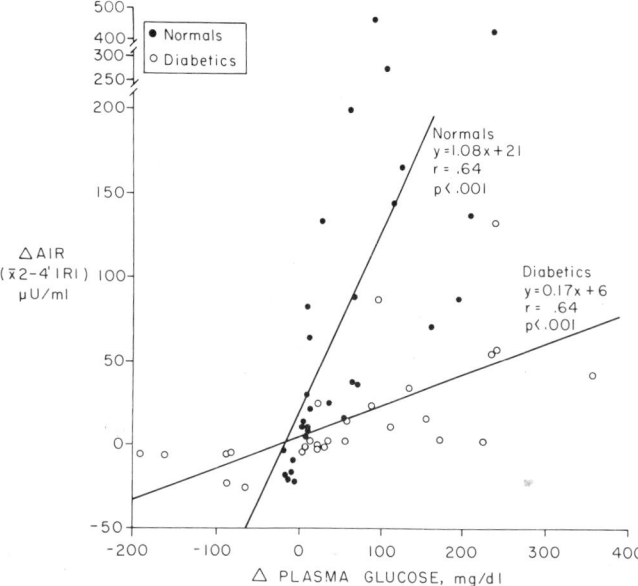

Figure 15–57. Slope of glucose potentiation in normal subjects and non-insulin-dependent diabetics. The acute insulin response at four different glucose levels in 10 diabetics and 18 normal controls are compared. Note the defect in glucose potentiation of the insulin response ($\triangle$ AIR = $\triangle$ acute insulin release) to a maximal dose of isoproterenol (Isuprel) in the diabetics. (From Halter, J. B, et al.: Potentiation of insulin secretory responses by plasma glucose levels in man: evidence that hyperglycemia diabetes compensates for impaired glucose potentiation. *J. Clin. Endocrinol. Metab. 48*:946, 1970.)

glucose levels to be greater than the renal threshold, complete compensation cannot occur. This probably explains the low basal insulin levels observed in patients with FPG levels above 200 mg/dl and the tendency for very hyperglycemic subjects to have poor insulin responses to all nonglucose stimulants. Such patients are unable to maintain glucose levels high enough to compensate for poor glucose potentiation as the kidney excretes glucose.

We have proposed that hyperglycemia is compensatory for the defective B-cell glucose potentiation in maturity-onset-type diabetes, thereby maintaining basal plasma insulin, glucose turnover, and insulin responses to nonglucose stimuli within the normal range until glycosuria prevents this effect. This compensation is so precise that there is a log-linear relation between FPG and the slope of potentiation for the nonglucose stimulants. This finding supports the notion of a feedback loop between the islet, liver, and periphery for the regulation of basal glucose and basal insulin. Such a concept can explain why FPG levels remain as constant as they do in patients with maturity-onset diabetes. Such patients would be regulating around a hyperglycemic set point for basal glucose just as the normal population regulates at a lower plasma glucose level.

Maturity-onset-type diabetes can then be characterized by an early loss of first-phase glucose-induced insulin release and a parallel deficiency in glucose potentiation. However, the latter can be compensated for by a progressive rise of FPG levels so that basal insulin, glucose output by the liver, and uptake by peripheral tissues are near normal (Fig. 15–58). When the renal threshold is exceeded, compensation is no longer possible. At this point, basal insulin levels can no longer be maintained, and there is a progressive increase in basal glucose production by the liver and decreased peripheral glucose utilization. This inability to maintain carbohydrate utilization leads to stimulation of dietary nutrient intake to complete the characteristic triad of polyuria, polydipsia, and polyphagia of the

decompensated diabetic state. Eventually, there may be inadequate suppression of fatty acid mobilization and ketosis.

Oral glucose tolerance tests show the same relation between insulin secretion and impaired tolerance in maturity-onset diabetes; however, many patients with fasting hyperglycemia who do not respond at all to intravenous glucose will still secrete insulin during the oral test. The explanation for this difference is almost certainly related to gut hormone stimulation of insulin release and the potentiation of this response by hyperglycemia. Even in the oral test, however, when either suitably matched control groups with equal degrees of obesity are used or the relative insulin response in relationship to the basal level is calculated, there is a relative deficiency of insulin release in response to challenge with declining glucose tolerance (Fig. 15–59).

Glucagon. Abnormalities of glucagon secretion can also be demonstrated in maturity-onset-type diabetes. The precise nature of the abnormality and whether it is an independent change contributing to hyperglycemia or whether it is secondary to the hypoinsulinemia is still a matter of debate. Part of the reason for this confusion is the fact that A-cell secretion of glucagon is regulated by both the prevailing glucose level and the prevailing insulin level. Although it is thought by some that all of this regulation is by glucose and

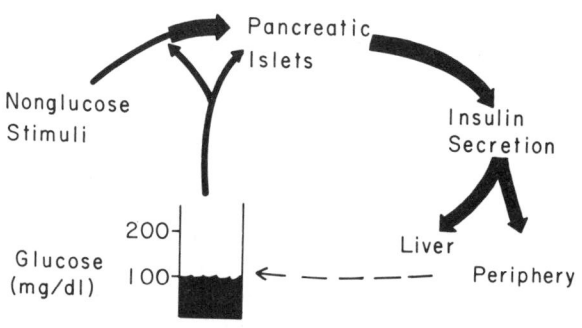

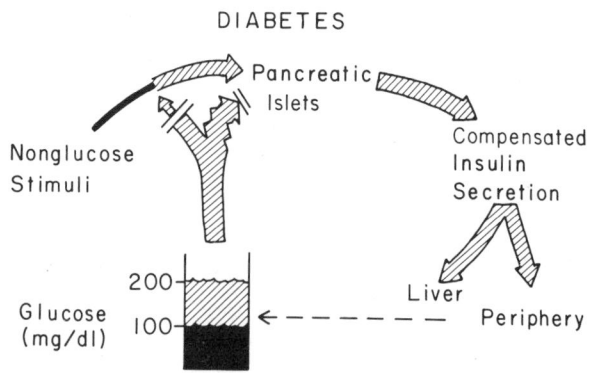

Figure 15–58. Insulin secretion in maturity-onset-type diabetes (non-insulin-dependent diabetes). In the normal subject (above), glucose has dual effects: a direct increase of insulin secretion *and* potentiation of nonglucose stimuli. In diabetes (below), glucose is not able to stimulate the pancreatic B-cell directly, but is still capable of potentiating nonglucose stimuli. Insulin secretion to every stimulus except glucose is compensated, but at the price of hyperglycemia, which reaches a new stable, but elevated, steady state. (From Halter, J. B., and Porte, D., Jr.: Current concepts of insulin secretion in diabetes mellitus. In *Diabetes Mellitus Volume V.* Rifkin, H., and Raskin, P. (eds.), Bowie, Maryland, Robert J. Brady Company, 1981.)

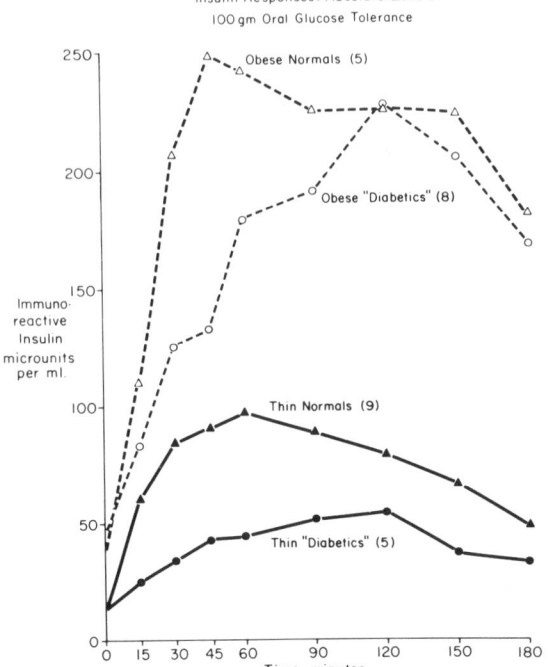

Figure 15–59. The interaction of obesity and diabetes on insulin responses during oral glucose (100 g) tolerance test. Note that obese diabetics secrete more insulin than thin normal subjects, but less insulin than obese normals. Both obese groups and both thin groups start with the same basal insulin levels, despite the difference in carbohydrate tolerance. (From Bagdade, J. D., et al.: The significance of basal insulin levels in the evaluation of the insulin response to glucose in diabetic and nondiabetic subjects. *J. Clin. Invest.* 46:1553, 1967.)

by others that all of this regulation is by insulin, it seems likely that both are independently involved. Since the B-cell is adjacent to the A-cell, the actual concentration of insulin which is regulating A-cell function is not known. Therefore, it is very difficult to know just how representative peripheral insulin levels are for the intraislet concentrations which are presumably affecting glucagon release. In fact, this may differ in different patients if there is a disturbance in cell number or function. This change may or may not be reflected in peripheral insulin levels to the same degree. Furthermore, the basic physiology of this system has not been very well identified and documented. There are no studies in which the levels of glucose and insulin have been varied independently of one another or in which one has been eliminated by clamp and the other varied and the output of glucagon observed except in a few instances *in vitro*. The relevance of these *in vitro* studies to human diabetes is difficult to assess since the various animal models have not been totally consistent.

With these caveats, the following changes have been observed. In subjects with fasting hyperglycemia greater than 200 mg/dl, basal glucagon levels may be elevated and hyperresponsive to infused amino acids. In maturity-onset diabetics with basal plasma glucose levels between 120 and 200 mg/dl, normal basal plasma glucagon levels and normal responses to amino acid stimulation are observed. Unger has argued that the latter are, in fact, still elevated in relationship to the prevailing hyperglycemia. Since in this group some glucose sensitivity has been retained, this is a reasonable argument. The problem is that it is impossible to test the idea by lowering the plasma glucose levels without infusing insulin. Since insulin itself will lower basal glucagon levels, a reduction of glucagon levels by insulin

treatment does not mean that the original values were abnormally high.

In addition, as glucose concentrations fall further and hypoglycemia is achieved, glucagon levels tend to increase. It is clear that glucagon release during hypoglycemia will occur in maturity-onset diabetic patients and that at comparable degrees of hypoglycemia the response is normal. However, the magnitude of this response is partly related to glucose levels and partly related to the counterregulatory neuroglucopenic stimulation by catecholamines, growth hormone, and cortisol. Therefore, it is very difficult to judge the normality of the glucagon response, particularly when it is understood that maturity-onset-type diabetic patients can hyperrespond to such stimuli. Thus, a defective glucagon response to hypoglycemia may be compensated by an increased response to the adrenergic discharge.

When challenged with intravenous glucose, this type of patient (FPG 120–200) has been shown to have a normal suppression. However, the suppression of glucagon by intravenous glucose is a slow phenomenon. Therefore, as the deficient early insulin response is translated into poor glucose disposal rates, there are greater degrees of hyperglycemia. Thus, while there may be less insulin to suppress glucagon, there may be more glucose, causing only an *apparently* normal suppression by glucose. Such a possibility is suggested by the observation that severely hyperglycemic subjects with elevated glucagon levels are usually hyperresponsive to amino acid infusion and have a decreased suppression to intravenous glucose.

In summary, intravenous glucose and insulin tend to produce qualitatively normal responses, but these responses may, in fact, be quantitatively diminished. The problem with precise interpretation is the ability of insulin and glucose to independently regulate glucagon secretion and our inability to test these two stimuli independently of one another or, in fact, to provide comparable stimuli in terms of insulin and glucose concentrations to the islets of maturity-onset diabetics and normal subjects. Since it is clear that an islet glucagon response can occur, the abnormality must be a quantitative and not a qualitative change in maturity-onset-type diabetes.

The situation with oral meal feeding challenges is somewhat more clear-cut. Feeding a carbohydrate meal leads to a gross abnormality in glucagon secretion in maturity-onset diabetes, and after carbohydrate meals there is a paradoxical increase rather than the usual suppression (Fig. 15–60). After protein meals the increase is normal (Fig. 15–61). In contrast to findings in juvenile-onset-type diabetics, the abnormal responses to a carbohydrate meal are not made normal by the administration of insulin, either as a pretreatment or simultaneously with the meal. However, some of the same problems exist in the interpretation of these data. Thus, the administration of insulin alone tends to suppress the response by simultaneously reducing plasma glucose levels which would tend to exaggerate the response. Nevertheless, it seems reasonable to conclude that the abnormal response to a carbohydrate meal is probably not due to simple insulin deficiency and suggests the possibility that glucose recognition by the A-cell is abnormal in such patients.

This may have important implications for the meal-related hyperglycemia observed in such patients, since they will apparently not suppress glucagon normally with mixed meals but, in fact, may have an increase that is due to the protein ingestion which is not adequately balanced by the usual carbohydrate-induced decrease. The pathophysiologic significance of even this point is controversial, since constant infusion of glucagon in normal subjects does not result in significant carbohydrate intolerance. Apparently, this is

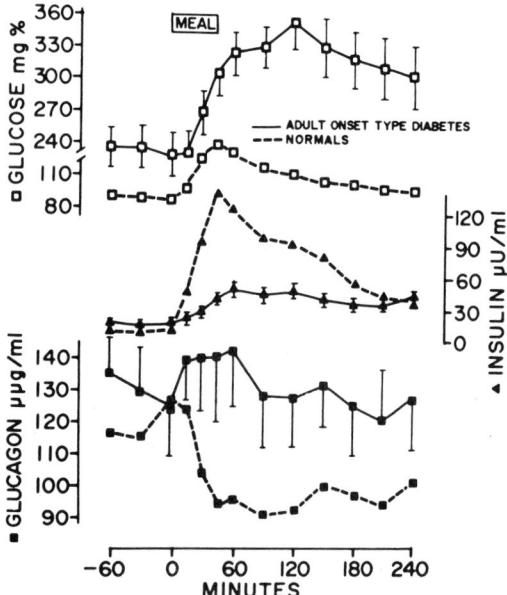

Figure 15–60. The effect of a carbohydrate meal on plasma glucose, insulin, and glucagon. Note the poor insulin response and the lack of glucagon suppression in the diabetic subjects. (From Müller, D., et al.: *New Engl. J. Med.* 283:109, 1970.)

due to the capacity of the islet to adapt to such a stress and ameliorate the consequences of a mild increase in glucagon. Since many of the maturity-onset-type diabetic patients secrete insulin during meal feeding, it is not clear that suppression of glucagon secretion is likely to be as important to postprandial hyperglycemia as it might be in the juvenile-onset patients who have no islet B-cell response. Unfortunately, selective somatostatin analogues which suppress glucagon but not insulin secretion are not available, and therefore this concept has not been tested yet.

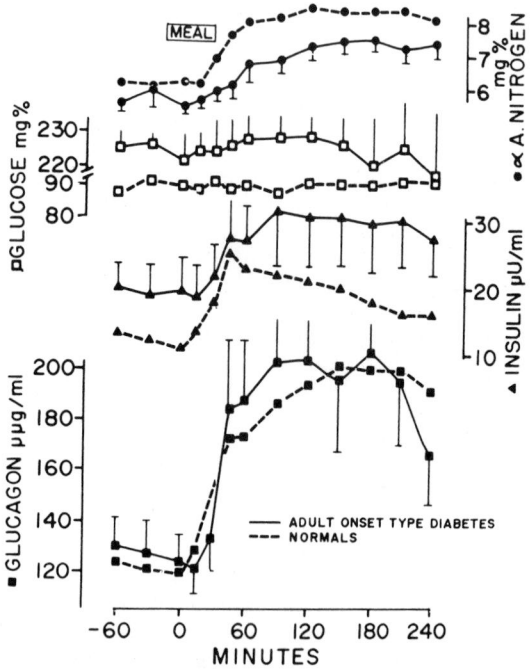

Figure 15–61. The effect of a protein meal on plasma glucose, glucagon, and insulin. Note the prompt rise in glucagon to this mixed amino acid meal. The rise in glucagon in the diabetic subjects has been interpreted to be inappropriate, in view of the severe degree of hyperglycemia. (From Müller, D., et al.: Abnormal alpha-cell function in diabetes. Response to carbohydrate and protein ingestion. *New Engl. J. Med.* 283:109, 1970.)

Somatostatin. D-cells have been found to be decreased in experimental animal models of obesity-hyperglycemia. This decrease may be related to the obesity rather than the diabetes. Unfortunately, no studies are available from human subjects. Somatostatin has been shown to produce hyperglycemia in such patients owing to its suppression of insulin secretion. In experimental animals, infusion of somatostatin produces a diabetic-like state with many similarities to the glucose and insulin findings in maturity-onset-type diabetes. Thus, while there is no evidence that somatostatin abnormalities contribute to the maturity-onset diabetic syndrome, maturity-onset-type diabetes appears to be a state which is pathophysiologically analogous to an increase in somatostatin's effect on the islet B-cells. Further studies of the mechanism of this hormone's effect on the B-cell may therefore provide important clues to the mechanism of the abnormality found in the maturity-onset-diabetic islet.

Other Counterregulatory Hormones and Stress. There are no described abnormalities of ACTH or cortisol secretion; however, studies of these hormones in relationship to carbohydrate tolerance have not been performed. Abnormal growth hormone responses to glucose ingestion have been reported with a paradoxical increase in some maturity-onset-type diabetics rather than the usual decrease. However, there have been relatively few studies, and the patients have not been well characterized. In an interesting study of the children of two diabetic parents, the same paradoxical response was observed in some offspring who had very little, if any, carbohydrate intolerance. Unfortunately, the clinical type of diabetes of the parents was not reported, and, therefore, whether these families had maturity-onset-type diabetes or juvenile-onset-type diabetes is unknown. The problem with growth hormone has been its unpredictable and sporadic release patterns which make careful quantitative analysis of its output difficult. No abnormalities of basal growth hormone levels have been reported except in some very severely hyperglycemic patients. The lack of suppression of growth hormone by glucose ingestion has made the diagnosis of acromegaly in diabetic subjects of the maturity-onset type somewhat difficult. Particularly in women with diabetes, modest growth hormone elevations during glucose tolerance testing must not be ascribed to a pituitary tumor.

The question arises whether the B-cell abnormality in maturity-onset-type diabetes is due to an intrinsic structural or metabolic process within the islet or whether it is caused by some imbalance of neuroendocrine input or due to a change of the sensitivity of the B-cell systems to these stimuli. There is already some evidence in support of the latter point of view. For example, increased insulin release may be observed in maturity-onset-type diabetics during infusion of the α-adrenergic blocking agent phentolamine. In addition, there has also been an increase of insulin release after the administration of the serotonin blocking agent methysergide and during the infusion of the prostaglandin synthesis inhibitor sodium salicylate. Thus, an increase of activity or sensitivity to any one of these inhibitors can be implicated in the impairment of insulin release in maturity-onset-type diabetes. Since pancreatic somatostatin levels have been reported to be increased in experimental diabetes and juvenile-onset-type diabetes, it is even possible that an increase in somatostatin levels or increased sensitivity of somatostatin receptors may play a role in the poor insulin response to glucose. However, all of these changes may be secondary rather than primary effects.

Increased levels of glucagon, cortisol, growth hormone, and the catecholamines have been found in ketotic diabetics, particularly of the juvenile-onset type (Fig. 15–91 in the section on Diabetic Ketoacidosis) but also in some apparently unstressed patients with maturity-onset-type diabetes. These hormone abnormalities could make a significant contribution to the hyperglycemia of such patients. These abnormalities appear to be secondary to the hyperglycemia and metabolic disturbance in many cases, since treatment reduces most of these levels toward or to normal. Hyperglycemia leads to glycosuria, volume depletion, and baroreceptor stimulation. Since this change should be followed by sympathetic nervous system activation, a pathophysiologic explanation is straightforward. Diabetes, in this context, is a form of stress, and there is a vicious circle in which the underlying pancreatic abnormality leads to hyperglycemia, which leads to a neuroendocrine stress response, which leads to more hyperglycemia, and so on.

However, more subtle abnormalities of many of these same hormones have been reported in relatively mild hyperglycemia in which a baroreceptor-mediated stress response seems unlikely. On the basis of these observations, we have postulated that there may be a generalized abnormality of glucose regulation of all of the neuroendocrine cells in maturity-onset diabetes (a defective "glucoreceptor"), of which the islet and the B-cell are simply the most prominent. Thus, it may not be necessary to ascribe all of the hormonal changes to impaired insulin secretion in maturity-onset-type diabetics.

If poor islet adaptation is a common finding in maturity-onset diabetes, then individuals with this lesion would necessarily be expected to be more sensitive to the ordinary influences of environmental stress. Thus, it is not difficult to explain rather wide swings of carbohydrate control when the stressors discussed previously are activated in either asymptomatic or symptomatic patients with diabetes of the maturity-onset type. Some experimental efforts have been directed to the study of stress responses, but only in juvenile-onset patients. It has been found that poorly controlled juvenile-onset-type diabetics develop ketosis during stress interviews, and this response is proportional to the baseline level of carbohydrate control. In another study, the metabolic effects of a stress hormone have been blocked to study its importance to the development of ketosis. In two difficult to manage patients with recurrent ketoacidosis, oral propranolol therapy to inhibit β-adrenergically mediated lipolysis was associated with a marked reduction in the frequency of hospitalization for ketoacidosis. While studies of the sensitivity of maturity-onset diabetic patients to stress hormones have not been performed as yet, it would seem certain that the presence of a glucose-insensitive B-cell would increase the glycemic response to sympathetic arousal and/or increasing levels of glucagon, cortisol, and growth hormone. Such sensitivity may, in fact, explain the well established increase in the incidence of cortisol-induced hyperglycemia in family members of diabetic patients and the need for insulin in maturity-onset diabetes during surgery or infection.

In summary, neuroendocrine abnormalities are common in patients with maturity-onset diabetes mellitus. Even in the apparently unstressed individual, increased sensitivity or increased levels of stress-related hormones and neural inputs may contribute either etiologically or pathophysiologically to the hyperglycemia observed. A pathophysiologic separation of stress hyperglycemia from maturity-onset-type diabetes mellitus can be difficult. Both involve alterations of the regulation of hepatic glucose output and peripheral sensitivity of tissues to insulin, as well as alterations of islet function. Therefore, regardless of etiologic significance, neuroendocrine control systems must be taken into account during the diagnosis, evaluation, and treatment of maturity-onset-type diabetes mellitus in man.

Insulin Resistance. Insulin resistance plays an important role in the hyperglycemia of maturity-onset-type diabetes. Since obesity, increased activity of the counterregulatory hormones, and insulin deficiency are known causes of insulin resistance, the mechanisms involved in an individual patient are complex. Some authors believe that there are additional unknown mechanisms which are important in many patients. However, to evaluate this last possibility, it is necessary to define and characterize known mechanisms to determine whether or not they are sufficient explanation for the insulin resistance found in most maturity-onset-type diabetic patients. It is our present view that the three known mechanisms, i.e., obesity, insulin deficiency, and activation of the counterregulatory hormones, are sufficient, but that their simultaneous presence and interaction in the same patient create confusion in evaluation.

The insulin resistance of obesity has been known for many years. The ability to increase insulin sensitivity with weight loss and decrease it with weight gain indicates that this is a secondary phenomenon related to calorie ingestion. In simple obesity without carbohydrate intolerance, there is a dramatic compensatory hyperinsulinemia. Insulin levels are elevated in the basal state and after challenge with nutrients. Presumably, increased insulin secretion compensates for the insulin resistance to maintain normal glucose, amino acid, and fatty acid levels in such patients. The stimulus for this compensation is unknown. If it is due to a simple feedback loop between plasma glucose and beta cell function, then it is hard to explain what is an apparently perfect compensation. Therefore, it is possible that only small elevations of plasma glucose are necessary in order to provide for increased stimulation of the islet.

Since many other factors influence islet function, it is possible that some of these factors are changed by increases or decreases in body weight and that these signals play a major role in stimulating islet function to overcome insulin resistance. The excellence of the compensation is shown by the linear relationship between basal insulin levels and relative body weight. This compensation persists even in maturity-onset-type diabetic patients, although it requires higher fasting plasma glucose levels, suggesting that plasma glucose may also play an important role in the nondiabetic obese. Since growth hormone levels appear to be suppressed in obese individuals, this seems an unlikely explanation for the resistance observed. Furthermore, although some increase in cortisol production has been found, circulating levels appear to be normal and normally responsive to exogenous steroid suppression. Since glucagon secretion has also been found to be normal, changes in counterregulatory hormones appear to be an unlikely explanation for the insulin resistance of obesity. However, there are little data at present regarding catecholamine levels in obesity.

The question whether the change in insulin sensitivity in obesity is due to reduced effectiveness of insulin which can be completely compensated by an increased insulin concentration versus a decrease in hormone responsiveness which is manifested as a decreased response to a maximal insulin challenge has not been adequately resolved. It is known that there is a proportionate reduction of insulin binding to its receptor as relative adiposity increases. However, the decrease in receptor binding that has been observed should not change the maximal insulin response, since only 10% of insulin receptors need to be stimulated for a maximal physiologic action *in vitro*. The finding that even very large doses of insulin are relatively ineffective in obesity has suggested that there are post-receptor defects as well as decreased receptor binding. In fact, current evidence suggests that the insulin receptor defect may be entirely secondary to the hyperinsulinemia, since the number of insulin receptors has been shown to be regulated by the circulating insulin concentrations to which the cell is exposed.

This simple receptor downregulation has been demonstrated in rodent models of obesity as a reduced sensitivity to insulin stimulation of initial rates of glucose uptake, but with a rightward shift of the maximal dose-response curve such that maximal glucose uptake rates are the same for the obese and lean fat cell. However, in the same obese fat cell preparation there is a marked defect in glucose oxidation, particularly in the activity of the hexose monophosphate shunt and the conversion of glucose to fatty acid. Since this defect is not reversed by large amounts of insulin, it likely represents a post-receptor problem. Therefore, there appear to be two independent mechanisms producing insulin resistance in the rodent models. The relative importance of these two types (receptor vs. post-receptor) to human obesity is not known. While the insulin receptor changes are present in all tissues studied, the intracellular glucose oxidation defect has been found only in adipocytes and may not be present in other cells.

Studies *in vivo* have suggested a relationship between whole-body insulin sensitivity and insulin binding, between insulin binding and basal insulin, and between basal insulin and relative adiposity. If this generally holds true, then most of the insulin resistance in maturity-onset-type diabetes would appear to be due to the associated obesity. However, a number of investigators have reported elevated basal insulin levels and evidence of insulin resistance in maturity-onset-type diabetic subjects who are not obese by anthropometric measurement. Since the fat cell size of these patients has been reported to be increased, they appear to have a form of obesity in which fat cell size is increased but total fat mass is not. However, a more likely explanation is that estimates of body fat mass are not sensitive enough to detect obesity when it is due only to an increase in fat cell size.

Insulin deficiency and hyperglycemia induced in animals with alloxan and/or streptozotocin is also characterized by insulin resistance in adipocytes and skeletal muscle. This abnormality is due to a decrease in the number of cellular transport systems for glucose and is reflected by a decreased insulin responsiveness of the tissues. Similar findings have been reported in overt maturity-onset-type diabetics when adipose tissue metabolism of glucose has been compared with suitably matched, similarly obese, nondiabetic controls. Since treatment reverses these abnormalities, they seem to be due to insulin deficiency.

In summary, insulin resistance is common in maturity-onset-type diabetes. Two known important mechanisms contribute. One, obesity, is an insulin-resistant state associated with hyperinsulinemia, downregulation of insulin receptors, and possible post-receptor defects in glucose metabolism. These abnormalities are proportional to the degree of obesity and are reversed by weight loss. Insulin resistance can also be produced by insulin deficiency. Although insulin deficiency is associated with upregulation of insulin receptors, there is a decrease in the number of glucose transport systems, resulting in resistance to insulin action. These changes can be reversed by insulin treatment if there is careful attention to the prevention of overinsulinization, which can lead to insulin resistance by downregulating insulin receptors.

Obesity alone does not necessarily cause hyperglycemia. The insulin resistance of obesity is often compensated for by an increase in insulin secretion through an adaptive response of the islet due either to a feedback mechanism through plasma glucose levels or to some other response related to the increased ingestion of calories. If only the glucose level is involved, mild degrees of carbohydrate intolerance may be a result of this phenomenon, since a completely compensated system would have no glucose stimulus to maintain the compensation. Overt hyperglycemia appears to be due to insulin deficiency when, for reasons as yet unknown, the islet either fails to adapt or fails to continue to adapt. As a result of this decrease in islet responsiveness, progressive hyperglycemia and the syndrome of maturity-onset-type diabetes develops. Although it has been claimed that patients with maturity-onset-type diabetes can be found who have insulin resistance without obesity and without insulin deficiency, the complexities of analysis to date have not convinced us that such individuals exist.

Stress Hyperglycemia

The neuroendocrine responses to a variety of noxious influences are generally characterized by the stimulation of sympathetic neurons and the release of hormones which tend to elevate plasma glucose. Therefore, hyperglycemia can be either due to the presence of diabetes mellitus or a response to environmental stressors. It was originally believed that this stress response affected neural and hormonal factors which regulated the production of glucose by the liver or the utilization of glucose by the peripheral tissues, whereas maturity-onset diabetes mellitus was due only to a defect in pancreatic insulin secretion. This clear segregation into two different syndromes has not proved true. It is now clear that the mechanisms of hyperglycemia are quite similar. Therefore, it may be very difficult to separate them. For the purposes of this discussion, we wish to characterize the pathophysiology of hyperglycemia which is found in genetically normal individuals in response to environmental stress in relation to pancreatic hormone secretion, other counterregulatory hormone secretion, and insulin resistance. While there is a general tendency for all stress hyperglycemia to be pathophysiologically similar because of the stimulation of the same hormones and neural tracts, there are differences depending on the cause, and these differences may be important, particularly to treatment.

The purpose of the metabolic response system during stress is to maintain glucose flux to the central nervous system whenever there is a threat to oxygenation or flow and to increase glucose flux to damaged tissues in response to trauma or injury for the reparative process. For this purpose, there are two general mechanisms available. One is to increase hepatic gluconeogenesis and glycogenolysis by decreasing insulin and increasing glucagon, epinephrine, norepinephrine, cortisol, and growth hormone. The sensitivity to these factors is dependent on thyroxine, triiodothyronine, somatomammotropin, and the estrogens. The other mechanism is to reduce glucose utilization in peripheral tissues. This is accomplished by decreasing insulin and increasing epinephrine and norepinephrine, cortisol, and growth hormone. In this case, thyroxine, triiodothyronine, and the estrogens regulate the sensitivity to the shorter-term modulators of insulin-sensitive glucose uptake. In stress hyperglycemia either one or both of these mechanisms come into play to a variable degree. Therefore, glucose turnover may not correlate with the plasma glucose level. Glucose turnover can be increased markedly with minimal changes of glucose concentration or reduced in the presence of hyperglycemia. This is due to the relationship between glucose output from the liver and glucose utilization by the periphery. Plasma glucose levels simply reflect the balance between the two processes and not their absolute rate.

The nervous system is the key to stress hyperglycemia because it is absolutely dependent upon a continuous supply of glucose. If brain blood flow or oxygenation is reduced, the only way that adequate substrate delivery and oxidation can be maintained is to increase glucose concentration. The input sensors for this regulatory system include oxygen and pH chemoreceptors in the aortic and carotid bodies, pressure receptors in the carotid sinus and aortic arch, skin temperature receptors, peripheral pain receptors, central glucose receptors, and brain cortex mechanisms which can be activated by the cognitive recognition of an environmental threat.

Physiologically, many of these mechanisms are activated during exercise to increase glucose production and impair insulin-mediated glucose transport. However, the same exercise, by activating the somatic motor system, is responsible for an insulin-dependent, but non-insulin-mediated, increase in glucose removal from the plasma compartment by the exercising muscle. These processes are so precisely balanced during exercise that the plasma glucose level remains constant. However, in pathophysiologic stress, increased sympathetic nervous system activity and increased counterregulatory hormone release usually occur without exercise, and it is these states that are associated with hyperglycemia and carbohydrate intolerance. Common clinical examples include burn, surgery, trauma, hypoxia, hypothermia, and myocardial infarction. Since they all involve sympathetic stimulation and increased secretion of catabolic counterregulatory hormones, there is a similarity in the metabolic response; however, there are also differences, and therefore each must be evaluated independently to develop appropriate treatment recommendations (Fig. 15–62).

Burn. Major burn injury is associated with a hypercatabolic state characterized by elevations of cortisol, growth hormone, and glucagon and increased sympathetic nervous system activity. The initial hyperglycemia is largely due to inhibition of glucose utilization, probably related to impaired insulin release secondary to sympathetic nervous system stimulation of the islet. However, during the convalescent phase there is a marked increase of glucose turnover associated with increased glucose production by the liver, presumably related to gluconeogenesis stimulated by glucagon, cortisol, and growth hormone. This increase occurs despite a rise of insulin levels and in the presence of demonstrable insulin resistance. The net effect is a major increase of glucose flux to the injured peripheral tissues. Depending on the patient, there may be metabolic decom-

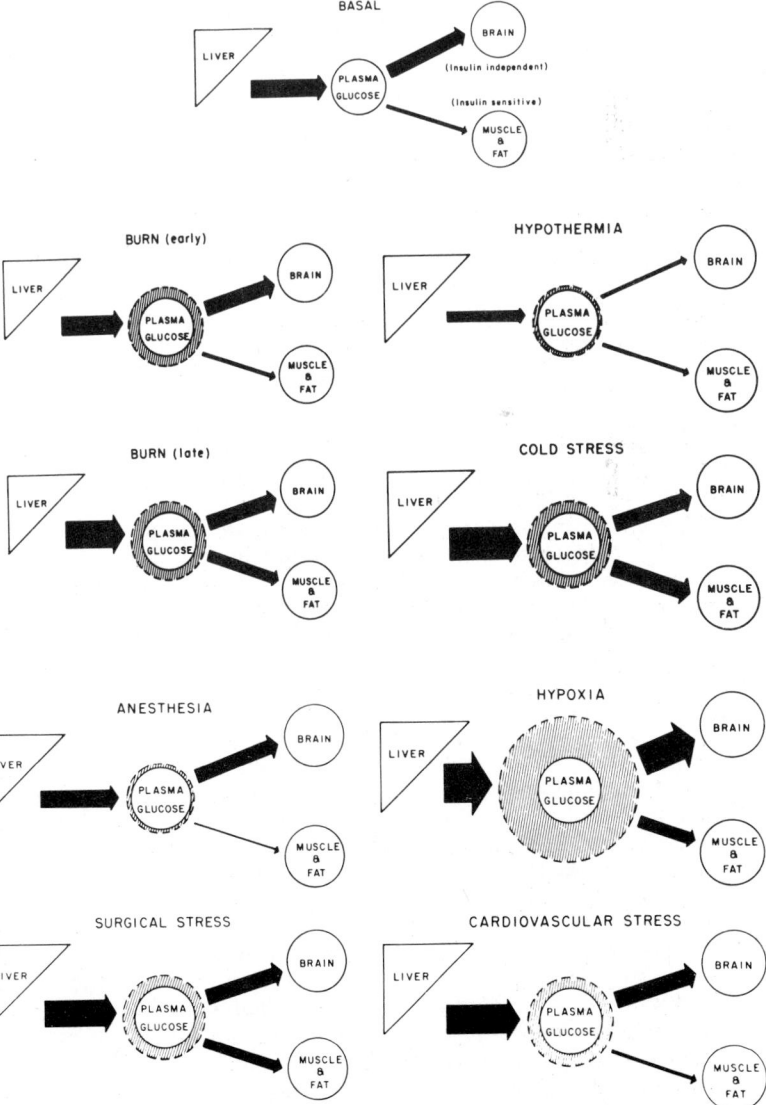

Figure 15–62. A schematic summary of stress hyperglycemia. The overnight-fasted individual is depicted. The relative arrow size represents the magnitude of glucose flux. Input is only from the liver; removal is either to the brain (insulin-dependent) or to muscle and fat (insulin-sensitive). Note the major differences for the various stressors in total flux and relative degrees of hyperglycemia. (From Porte, D., Jr., et al.: Neural control of the pancreatic islet and its relation to stress hyperglycemia. In *Diabetes Mellitus: A Pathophysiological Approach to Clinical Practice.* Marliss, E. B. (ed.), New York, John Wiley & Sons, 1981, in press.)

pensation with hyperglycemia and glycosuria or there may be resolution to a new steady state with completely adaptive hyperinsulinemia and increased glucose turnover at normal glucose levels.

Sepsis. Sepsis may be associated with hyperglycemia and hypoinsulinemia or euglycemia and hyperinsulinemia, depending upon the nature of the organism and the degree of inflammatory response. In gram-negative sepsis with hypotension, increased sympathetic activity and hyperglycemia are common. In the absence of hypotension, leukocyte endogenous mediators (LEM) released from white cells may play a predominant role in the metabolic changes, since these have been shown to increase glucagon secretion, raise blood glucose, and, in the absence of an associated sympathetic response, increase insulin secretion. Thus, increased glucose turnover may occur with little hyperglycemia or even hypoglycemia. Since some of these same mediators from leukocytes may stimulate the central nervous system to produce fever and other toxic signs which tend to increase fuel utilization, the metabolic picture can vary.

Trauma, Surgery, and Anesthesia. Trauma and surgery are invariably associated with hyperglycemia and carbohydrate intolerance. However, the nature of the metabolic response and its degree are clearly influenced by the type and effect of the anesthetic agents. It is now clearly recognized that the pain and stimulation of afferent neural systems play a major role in the metabolic and endocrine responses to surgery and trauma, although psychic factors may have some role. At present there is little evidence of circulating "toxic" factors emanating from the site of injury, since the use of local anesthetics to block peripheral pain impulses appears to prevent both the sympathetic and the catabolic hormone responses observed. Many anesthetic agents in the doses used clinically act primarily at the cortical level and only to a limited extent at the hypothalamus or lower centers. Therefore, afferent pain stimuli may still produce metabolic and endocrine responses in the anesthetized surgical patient. For this reason, the same qualitative increase in sympathetic nervous system activity, glucagon, cortisol, and growth hormone may occur during general anesthesia without analgesia as during trauma in unanesthetized patients. If the anesthetic is also analgesic or the dose is high enough to influence the hypothalamus and brain stem, the anesthetic agents may suppress sympathetic stimulation. Thus, the type and depth of anesthesia are important variables. In addition, there are other stimuli which may modulate these responses. Individuals with shock, hypoxia, or reduced blood pressure will have other non-pain-related stimuli to sympathetic nervous system activity and counterregulatory hormone activation. It is therefore the interplay among these forces which determines the metabolic response.

While pain from afferent nerve fiber plays a major stimulatory role in the increased sympathetic nervous system and counterregulatory neuroendocrine mechanisms, anesthetics tend to depress these responses. The degree of suppression and its type vary with each agent. These responses can be modulated by baroreceptor, chemoreceptor, and psychic stimulatory factors. Cortisol and growth hormone responses tend to parallel those of epinephrine and activation of sympathetic neurons. Hyperglycemia and poor insulin secretory responses to glucose are common, but these effects have a variety of causes.

Hypothermia. Hypothermia is observed when the thermogenic response to cold stress is suppressed by prolonged or accidental exposure or is overwhelmed by deliberate total-body cooling during surgical anesthesia. Since anesthetic agents may produce variable degrees of inhibition of shivering or sympathetic responses, operating room exposure under anesthesia may itself be sufficient to induce hypothermia in subjects undergoing operation. If the sympathetic response to cold stress is impaired, glucose levels may not rise and carbohydrate tolerance may not be very much reduced. If the hypothermia is due to exaggerated cold exposure beyond the body's capacity to generate heat, or if there is only reduction in shivering but not sympathetic stimulation due to the anesthesia, hyperglycemia and rather severe carbohydrate intolerance will be observed. During severe hypothermia both the production and utilization of glucose are reduced but balanced. Therefore, endogenous hyperglycemia may not occur despite very severe carbohydrate intolerance to exogenous glucose administration. This intolerance is partly due to the reduced utilization of glucose by hypothermic tissue plus a direct inhibition of pancreatic insulin release by stimulation of pancreatic α-adrenergic receptors from sympathetic activation. During rewarming a striking insulin response can be obtained, leading to rather rapid shifts of electrolyte balance including severe hypokalemia secondary to suddenly accelerated potassium uptake and glucose utilization. Such alterations may play a critical role in eventual recovery.

Hypoxia. Hypoxia is a well recognized stimulant of sympathetic nervous system activity. Marked hyperglycemia can occur during hypoxia owing to rapid glycogenolysis, and its counterregulation by insulin is blocked. α-Adrenergic blockade produces hypoglycemia by reversing the glycogenolysis and impaired insulin secretion, indicating an important role of α-adrenergic receptor activation in this form of stress hyperglycemia. It is of interest that the β-adrenergic receptor is directly inhibited by hypoxia. Therefore, the lipolytic effects of catecholamines do not occur or are markedly blunted. Reduced β-adrenergic regulation of the islet is also found, thus further magnifying the α-adrenergic-mediated inhibition of insulin release (which is usually modulated by simultaneous β-adrenergic stimulation). Thus, the usual dual receptor control of the islet by catecholamines is changed by hypoxia from mixed α- and β-adrenergic stimulation to almost pure α-adrenergic effects.

Cardiovascular Disease. Patients with recent myocardial infarction often have a type of stress hyperglycemia. At the onset of myocardial infarction, there is an immediate increase in plasma catecholamines, followed later by increases in the other stress hormones glucagon, cortisol, and growth hormone. Impaired insulin secretion is prominent in these patients, and prolonged hyperglycemia is not unusual. Since, as already discussed, the metabolic effects of catecholamines depend upon oxygenation, there are numerous other factors which modulate the degree of hyperglycemia eventually observed. Many patients with diabetes have cardiovascular disease; it may, therefore, be difficult to distinguish between diabetes with stress hyperglycemia and stress hyperglycemia alone in any specific patient. Since the heart may be dependent upon glucose and/or insulin for function, particularly during the stress of injury and local hypoxia, the administration of glucose, insulin, and/or potassium has become an important, although controversial, treatment in the clinical care of such patients.

Clinical Management of Stress Hyperglycemia. Stress responses which occur in normal animals or man may or may not be beneficial for long-term survival. Thus, evaluation of hyperglycemia found under such circumstances must be made prior to a treatment decision. While maladaptive responses may be a significant cause of morbidity and mortality in man during stress, there are many circumstances in which hyperglycemia may be beneficial or even essential for survival. One of the main determinations to be made is whether or not hyperglycemia is in any way associated with reduced glucose flux to the central nervous system. Since the central nervous system is the prime utilizer of glucose between meals and is totally dependent upon maintenance of at least 50% of this flux, cerebral blood flow and oxygenation are critical parameters for evaluation. Thus, in hypovolemic, hypotensive, or hypoxic states, reversal of the hyperglycemia by diverting flux to insulin-sensitive tissues or by reducing hepatic gluconeogenesis with insulin is contraindicated unless the primary condition is corrected or marked hyperglycemia is present. In fact, under some circumstances it may be advisable to increase glucose levels further in an attempt to maintain glucose flux to the central nervous system. In the absence of significant glycosuria and electrolyte loss, hyperglycemia has no known detrimental short-term side effects; therefore, one should err on the side of maintaining an elevated plasma glucose level.

On the other hand, if the stress hyperglycemia can be related to an increased need of peripheral tissues for nutrients, this delivery of glucose can often be accelerated by the use of insulin alone or with additional glucose. Thus, substrate can be provided without the potentially harmful side effects of glycosuria, electrolyte loss, hyperosmolarity, and so forth. In burn and trauma, in which there is increased body metabolism as part of the reparative process, insulin has been shown to be beneficial, probably by diminishing muscle protein wasting and liver gluconeogenesis. This process can obviously be accelerated by the utilization of alternate substrates or additional glucose. It is clear that adequate nutrition should not be withheld in order to maintain normal plasma glucose levels. Rather, insulin treatment should be given along with the nutrients to maintain relative euglycemia during a high caloric intake, which may reach as high as 5000–6000 calories per day. Similar considerations may be present in myocardial infarction, in which ischemic tissue may benefit from increased glucose intake and decreased fatty acid mobilization. In these patients it is likely that the heart remains insulin-sensitive; therefore, glucose uptake will increase even as glucose levels fall. However, cerebral blood flow needs to be assessed to assure an adequate supply of substrate to this insulin-insensitive tissue (at least as far as glucose uptake is concerned). In cases of hypothermia in which total-body metabolism is reduced, hyperglycemia appears not to be useful and can usually be prevented simply by giving less carbohydrate exogenously.

Thus, treatment considerations vary from patient to patient and depend upon the nature of the stress and the specific response to that stress in the individual case. Associated conditions may play an important role in this evaluation. In the final analysis the questions that must be asked are: Is the hyperglycemic state more harmful than helpful, and will the treatment be beneficial and decrease risk? An understanding of the neuroendocrine response to stress and its actions upon substrate-utilizing systems is essential for this decision.

Diagnosis and Detection

Clinical Signs and Symptoms of Diabetes

Signs and symptoms in diabetes may be related solely to the poor metabolism of carbohydrate and overmobilization of fat in this syndrome, or they may result from large- and small-vessel disease or neuropathy. Patients with cardinal clinical signs related to poor carbohydrate metabolism complain of polyuria, polydipsia, polyphagia, weight loss, and loss of strength. Less common are repeated skin infections,

particularly vulvar (with or without pruritus), refractive changes with blurring of vision, anorexia, headache, and drowsiness. Such symptoms may be explosive in their onset and are usually related to a coincident infection or some other stress which may simultaneously increase the need for insulin and decrease the ability to secrete it. Sudden onset of symptomatic hyperglycemia is more common in younger subjects but may occur at any age. Milder forms are more stable, appear to progress more slowly, and are therefore more common in older age groups. However, it has become clear in screening surveys of high-risk families that many young patients have gross abnormalities of carbohydrate metabolism with minimal symptoms and can be relatively stable over many years.

Some patients will come to the physician with symptoms related only to atherosclerotic complications, such as myocardial infarction or peripheral vascular disease, or with chronic renal failure secondary to microvascular disease. In others, neuropathy may be the chief complaint, usually a polyneuropathy with pain and numbness as the initiating symptoms. An acute mononeuritis involving any peripheral nerve may also be a presenting symptom. Loss of motor function is usually the most prominent finding in mononeuritis. Autonomic insufficiency may be manifested as nocturnal diarrhea, incontinence, nausea, orthostatic hypotension, or impotence. However, the frequency of complaints related to large-vessel disease, microangiopathy, and neuropathy generally increase with the duration of known carbohydrate abnormalities. Therefore, such complaints are less likely to be initial symptoms. Their listing here emphasizes the basic problem that early detection of maturity-onset-type diabetes is difficult because often this is an asymptomatic disease for many years. This fact has led to great emphasis on carbohydrate tolerance testing as a method of early case finding. In view of the fact that treatment of carbohydrate intolerance is controversial, except for weight reduction of overweight individuals, the usefulness of carbohydrate tolerance testing remains unproved.

Laboratory Diagnosis

Insulin-dependent juvenile-onset-type diabetes rarely presents a problem in diagnosis. The onset is sudden and the hyperglycemia severe. Maturity-onset-type diabetes is quite different. Onset is slow and hyperglycemia is readily reversible by caloric restriction. It is often asymptomatic for long periods of time. Despite the importance of neuropathy, microangiopathy, and large-vessel disease to the diabetic syndrome, they are rarely useful in the diagnosis of maturity-onset-type diabetes because the diagnosis has been almost wholly based upon hyperglycemia. This is partly because of the lack of quantitative methods for evaluating the degree of abnormality of these other findings and partly because none of these findings is specific for the diabetic syndrome. However, Siperstein measured the basement membrane in biopsy specimens of human muscle and found increased thickness in 97% of overt diabetics. Other investigators have observed these changes less frequently. Furthermore, some consider these abnormalities to be "complications" of the disease in view of the fact that hyperglycemia usually precedes their diagnosis. The degree of hyperglycemia in some individuals with neuropathy or microvascular disease is so slight that it cannot be clearly distinguished from that of the normal aging population. Therefore, controversy persists as to whether or not hyperglycemia causes the "complications," or whether they are separate abnormalities in the same syndrome.

Since the plasma glucose level is regulated by many hormones and neural inputs, hyperglycemia may result from a variety of changes in body metabolism. In carbohydrate tolerance tests of normal populations, therefore, some of the hyperglycemia may be due to physiologically normal responses to stress. In general, tests that are the least sensitive in showing hyperglycemia tend to be the most specific for maturity-onset-type diabetes. To establish a sure diagnosis, it is therefore best to start with the most specific and least sensitive tests and probably to limit the testing to studies which are necessary to make a therapeutic decision. Since at present there is considerable controversy about which level of blood sugar should induce the physician to treat the patient, the number and type of tests will depend on the willingness of any individual physician to treat. The screening tests most generally used are (1) urine glucose plus acetone; (2) fasting plasma glucose; and (3) glucose tolerance test, either oral or intravenous.

Urine Glucose and Ketone Assay. Since the major purpose of all of these tests is to estimate abnormalities in glucose metabolism, it is desirable to use routinely only those methods that measure glucose specifically. The most specific method available involves glucose oxidase, which oxidizes glucose to gluconic acid and liberates hydrogen peroxide, which is measured. This is applied to either the blood or the urine. Strips impregnated with the enzyme are available which can quite easily detect 125 mg/100 ml of glucose in the urine. However, for daily follow-up, the color changes are relatively small, and it may be difficult for a patient to detect accurately the amount of glucose present. Furthermore, some drugs, such as ascorbic acid, may interfere with the detection of glucose by this method. Copper sulfate solutions or Clinitest tablets are the alternative method, but these will also detect other sugars, such as fructose, lactose, galactose, and pentoses; large quantities of drugs, such as salicylates, aminopyrine, para-aminobenzoic acid, chloral hydrate, and ascorbic acid; or normal metabolites, such as uric acid and creatinine. Therefore, there is no ideal urine test. If glucose is present, ketone bodies should also be determined. In general, this is most quickly and conveniently done by use of specifically prepared nitroprusside reagent in tablet, stick, or powder form: Acetest tablet, Ketostix, or Labstix (Ames Company, Elkhart, Indiana); or Denco Acetone Test Powder (Denver Clinical Manufacturing Company, New York, New York). In either case, the reaction color is much more sensitive to acetoacetic acid than to acetone and, therefore, is only a qualitative evaluation of ketone body excretion. Phthalein or the urine preservative 8-hydroxyquinoline may give false-positive results.

Blood or Plasma Glucose Assay. An anticoagulant of some type may be used to prepare specimens — usually oxalate, heparinate, or EDTA. Heparinate is one of the most useful anticoagulants. When measurements of Na^+, K^+, or BUN (urease method) are included, it is desirable to use lithium heparinate rather than the Na^+, K^+, or NH_4^+ derivative. Sodium EDTA (1 mg/ml blood) can be used as an anticoagulant, but it interferes with various enzyme tests on blood. Since many clinical laboratories now used automated devices that perform multiple simultaneous assays, glucose measurements are routinely done in serum or plasma. Blood at room temperature loses ± 7 mg glucose/100 ml per hour owing to glycolysis in red blood cells; at 4°C the loss is ± 2 mg/100 ml. Because of this time-related fall in glucose levels in whole blood, samples should be centrifuged as soon as possible to separate off the red blood cells. Fluoride can be used to preserve glucose in whole blood (1–2 mg NaF/ml blood). This amount of fluoride does not inhibit glucose oxidase activity but prevents significant glycolysis for 8 hours at room temperature and for 48+ hours at 4°C. Fluoride also does not inhibit hexokinase activity, which can be used for glucose assay. Even with the use of fluoride, it is desirable to centrifuge the blood within an hour or so and then to refrigerate the plasma. Instead of heparinate, oxalate may be used (2 mg oxalate powder and 2 mg fluoride/1 ml blood).

Some automated glucose methods use ferricyanide or copper sulfate as a reagent. These reagents are sensitive to certain nonsugar reducing substances, such as creatinine and bilirubin, and will give falsely high readings in patients who have uremia or jaundice. Other automated systems use glucose oxidase or hexokinase methods, which are specific for glucose. Venous plasma glucose has been used for most standard tests, but it is important to remember that arterial or capillary values may be considerably higher, particularly during glucose tolerance testing. The use of plasma or serum rather than whole blood in the determination of glucose eliminates the complicating factor of anemia as a cause of increased blood glucose values. If it is necessary to compare whole blood with plasma, one must remember to make a 15% correction. This is because of the lower glucose concentration of the red cells in relationship to their volume. The correction can be calculated by using the formula: whole blood glucose = plasma glucose $\times [1 - (0.3 \times hct \times 10^{-2})]$. This correction allows one to measure plasma glucose and compare it with whole blood glucose.

Mellituria

Mellituria, sugar in the urine, should under any circumstance make one strongly suspicious of diabetes. However, glycosuria may occur in normal individuals in sufficient amount to cause a positive reaction with one of the more sensitive glucose oxidase tapes. In addition, some rare individuals have a low renal threshold, which leads to glycosuria at normal blood glucose concentrations (renal glycosuria). During pregnancy a lower threshold is common and must be distinguished from pathologic hyperglycemia. Certain hexoses and pentoses may cause a positive copper reduction test, such as Benedict's test or Clinitest, whereas the more specific glucose oxidase tests are negative, indicating nonglucose mellituria. Repeated gross glycosuria without any other underlying cause should be sufficient to make a tentative diagnosis of diabetes mellitus. This *should* be confirmed by a gross abnormality of fasting plasma glucose, since glycosuria does not ordinarily occur unless the plasma glucose level exceeds 180–200 mg/100 ml.

Renal Glycosuria. The maximal renal tubular transport rate for glucose is approximately 300–350 mg/min. Thus, the presence of glucose in the urine will depend not only on the concentration of arterial glucose but also on the dynamics of glomerular perfusion, filtration rate, individual nephron reabsorption rate, and urine flow. Since these vary considerably from person to person, glucose may appear in the urine at varying arterial glucose levels. Most physicians will not consider a diagnosis of nondiabetic renal glycosuria unless there is a significant amount of glucose in the urine after an overnight fast. When this criterion is used, the syndrome is very rare and consists of several related familial genetic defects. In the Joslin Clinic series reported by Marble, only 85 cases of renal mellituria were found among 50,000 patients. The renal threshold for glucose in this syndrome is altered in two ways: either there is a low tubular transport maximum (low Tm for glucose) or there is a change in the relationship between the glucose load and the reabsorbed glucose, such that the maximum is not changed, but the efficiency of reabsorption is reduced for any glucose load (increased glucose splay). Some families have one of these abnormalities, but other families have both of the abnormalities, indicating some degree of genetic heterogeneity. Some families demonstrate an autosomal dominant pattern; others suggest an autosomal recessive. Most of the patients do not have an associated abnormality of the gastrointestinal tract, but a series of patients has been described with both glucose and galactose malabsorption along with renal glycosuria. Aside from this group, the rest of the patients are not ill, absorb and metabolize glucose normally, and are generally asymptomatic.

Fanconi Syndrome. A heterogeneous group of patients with a common defect in tubular reabsorption of a variety of substances can be considered to have the "Fanconi syndrome." Glycosuria is common but is probably one of the least important aspects of the syndrome. This is because of the impairment in the reabsorption of water, PO_4^{3-}, Na^{1+}, HCO_3^{1-}, amino acids, and other organic acids. Although cystinosis is one of the more common causes of this syndrome, a wide variety of conditions in which this syndrome occurs are listed in Table 15–11. Total glucose loss is small and does not contribute in any significant way to the symptomatology but may alert the clinician to the possibility of primary renal disease.

Nonglucose Mellituria. Fructose, galactose, lactose, maltose, mannoheptulose, and L-xylulose have been found in the urine, usually in conjunction with a familial metabolic disorder. All these sugars give a positive copper reduction test but do not react with glucose oxidase. Fructose appears readily in the urine, as there is no tubular reabsorption of this sugar, and it does not compete with glucose or galactose for absorption or reabsorption.

Three separate familial disorders with fructosuria have been described. *Essential fructosuria* is an asymptomatic disorder inherited as an autosomal recessive trait which is due to a defect in the reactivity of fructokinase, the enzyme which phosphorylates fructose in the liver. When fructokinase activity is diminished, fructose appears in the urine after an oral load, as it is metabolized more slowly by the nonspecific phosphorylating hexokinases. Approximately 10–20% of the amount of fructose ingested is excreted. It is a benign asymptomatic condition and requires no treatment. A more serious condition, *hereditary fructose intolerance,* is characterized by hypoglycemia (see Ch. 16), nausea, and vomiting following a fructose load, which leads to hepatomegaly, jaundice, Fanconi syndrome, and fructosuria. It is due to a deficiency of fructose-1-phosphate aldolase. There is complete inhibition of glucose output by the liver after fructose ingestion in this disease by a mechanism not completely understood. Most family studies indicate that an autosomal recessive gene is responsible. A similar syndrome with hypoglycemia and fructosuria, but without liver disease, has been described, called *familial galactose and fructose intolerance* (see Ch. 16), since both sugars produce hypoglycemia. The biochemical and genetic abnormality is completely unknown.

Galactosemia and galactosuria resulting from hereditary defects in the metabolism of galactose have been described as a result of two separate biochemical abnormalities. First, a defect in galactose-1-phosphate uridyltransferase is found in children and results in nutritional failure, liver disease, cataracts, and mental retardation. This *transferase-deficiency galactosemia* is present in a variety of tissues, including the liver and red blood cells, and leads to the accumulation of galactose-1-phosphate, which appears to be toxic. The second syndrome, due to *galactokinase deficiency,* is seen in older subjects and leads primarily to cataracts by accumulation of galactitol via an alternative metabolic pathway in the lens. These are both autosomal recessive disorders in which galactosuria is present only after galactose ingestion.

The presence of L-xylulose in the urine has been termed *chronic essential pentosuria.* In contrast to the other syndromes, the sugar is found in the urine regardless of dietary ingestion. This is because there is a block in the metabolism of glucuronic acid at the step in which xylulose is dehydrogenated to xylitol. It is a benign disorder, again due to an autosomal recessive gene, primarily restricted to Jews and estimated at 1:40,000 to 1:50,000 in the American population.

Lactosuria occurs physiologically during the period of postpartum lactation. Occasionally, lactose may also be found in the urine during the last few days of a normal pregnancy. In the more severe cases of intestinal lactase deficiency, lactose may also appear in the urine, but this is not common in the milder forms of the syndrome.

Fasting Plasma Glucose

The normal fasting glucose level in venous plasma is between 60 and 115 mg/100 ml. Values above 120 mg/100 ml, when confirmed, are usually considered diagnostic of overt diabetes, although the NIH data group suggests 140 mg/dl as a more conservative value to use (see Table 15–13). There is reasonable agreement that persistent fasting hyperglycemia in the absence of complicating illness is sufficient for a diagnosis of diabetes. A substantial number of individuals with apparently abnormal glucose tolerance tests may have normal fasting plasma glucose values. In some clinics, these individuals are considered chemical diabetics, while in others an abnormality of carbohydrate tolerance is recorded, but the term "diabetes" is not used. The NIH data group has recently recommended the term "impaired glucose tolerance" for this group. In the few incomplete long-term studies available, from 1–5% of this group progress to fasting hyperglycemia per year; however, the relationship between development of other neurovascular concomitants of the diabetic syndrome and the blood glucose level is not known. In population studies of large-vessel disease, there is a linear relationship between blood glucose and atherosclerotic complications. Reliance on the fasting glucose for diagnostic purposes has the advantage that most other transient metabolic disorders interfering with carbohydrate metabolism do not usually produce fasting hyperglycemia in otherwise normal individuals.

Table 15–11. CAUSES OF CYSTINOSIS AND THE FANCONI SYNDROME*

I. Metabolic defect with Fanconi syndrome as a major finding
  A. Cystinosis
  B. Idiopathic
  C. Lowe's syndrome
  D. Tyrosinemia
II. Metabolic defect with Fanconi syndrome not a major finding
  A. Galactosemia
  B. Glycogen storage disease (glucose-6-phosphatase deficiency)
  C. Hereditary fructose intolerance
  D. Wilson's disease
III. Other conditions
  A. Human kidney transplantation
  B. Multiple myeloma
IV. Exogenous toxins
  A. Heavy metals
  B. Lysol (cresol) burn
  C. Maleic acid (in rats)
  D. Methyl-c-chromone
  E. Degraded tetracycline

*From Schneider, J. A., and Seegmiller, J. E., In *The Metabolic Basis of Inherited Disease.* 3rd ed. Stanbury, J. B., Wyngaarden, J. B.; et al. (eds.), New York, McGraw-Hill, 1972, p. 1581.

Carbohydrate Tolerance Testing

Carbohydrate tolerance testing has been used extensively in the hope of detecting individuals affected with maturity-onset-type diabetes prior to the development of vascular and neurologic problems. Such testing is by far the most sensitive detection device available but suffers from lack of specificity. It is abnormal in a wide variety of diseases and is influenced by dietary and other variables which are often not controlled. In order to use the test it is essential that it be performed under *standardized* test conditions. Standardized procedures for drawing blood samples must be followed at precise times, and other causes of carbohydrate intolerance should be considered in evaluating the results. Because of the importance of all the variables and the frequency with which one is misled, the authors feel that a random measurement of postprandial blood sugar is unsatisfactory in the diagnosis of carbohydrate intolerance and often is misleading when used as a screening or detection test. Since the concentration of the plasma glucose during glucose tolerance testing depends on (1) the fasting plasma glucose level, i.e., the point of starting, (2) the rate of absorption of glucose, and (3) its uptake by tissues and excretion in urine, it is obvious that the glucose values during the test are only partly related to the utilization of glucose by tissues during the test.

Oral Glucose Tolerance Test (OGTT)

Indications. It should be emphasized that an OGTT adds little diagnostic information in a patient with fasting hyperglycemia and so should not be performed in such individuals. The following may be indications for an OGTT in individuals with a normal fasting plasma glucose: (1) family history of diabetes; (2) a normal fasting plasma glucose and symptoms or signs compatible with diabetes with or without its concomitants (retinopathy, neuropathy, nephropathy, hypercholesterolemia, hypertriglyceridemia, coronary disease, peripheral vascular disease, or cerebrovascular disease, particularly when these are apparent before the age of 50); (3) glucosuria (fasting plasma glucose normal); (4) abnormal postprandial or random plasma glucose level (this applies whether the patient is pregnant, sick, or receiving drug treatment at the time of the test); (5) pregnancy in a woman with a history of spontaneous abortion, premature labor, stillbirth, neonatal death, large baby, hydramnios, or toxemia; and (6) symptoms suggestive of reactive hypoglycemia (see Ch. 16).

Preparation of Subjects for OGTT. It is important to prepare the patient psychologically and physically for the OGTT. The patient is often told that he will have "a test for diabetes." Since there is great fear and distress in the minds of some patients about the possibility of being labeled diabetic, this in itself could lead to a false-positive result. We strongly emphasize the importance of having the proper diet preparation for at least 3 days before the test for each subject who is to receive an OGTT. If the patient has been on a weight-reduction regimen, he should have this dietary preparation for at least 5 days. Each day he should receive a standard diet with maintenance calories, adequate protein, and a minimum of 300 g/day of carbohydrate. Some clinicians state that 150 g/day of carbohydrate is sufficient. However, as emphasized by Seltzer, there are times when this can be inadequate. It is necessary for the subject to fast for 10–12 hours before the test. On the day of the test, he must not have even black coffee or tea and should not smoke. On that day, he should have relatively little exercise and should rest for 30 minutes before the test is started, between 7 and 9 A.M. In every way, he should be put at ease mentally and physically before and during the test. If he has an acute illness, the test should be postponed. It is especially important that he not be receiving drugs that influence the test. Indeed, since there are so many that can affect the procedure, all drugs possible should be omitted for 3 days prior to the test. Table 15–12 lists some of the more common ones that may influence the results of the OGTT.

Test Procedures. Venous blood is preferable to capillary specimens (finger prick or ear prick), but in patients offering difficulties with venipuncture, capillary blood can be used (capillary blood glucose values are closer to arterial than to venous levels). The capillary values are only 2–3 mg higher than the venous after an overnight fast, but after carbohydrate loading in normal subjects, the capillary level may be 20–30 mg/100 ml higher than venous and remain much higher for more than an hour after glucose ingestion. Capillary glucose levels are distinctly more variable than venous; the flow is often less dependable and may be mixed with lymph. Plasma or serum specimens are more satisfactory than whole blood for glucose analysis. Plasma reflects more accurately the absorption, production, and tissue uptake of glucose. Plasma values are independent of the hematocrit level; variations in hematocrit can account for distinct differences in whole blood glucose levels, since glucose levels in plasma are about 15% higher than those in whole blood. Serum glucose values are about the same as plasma values, but if 2–3 hours are allowed for the blood to clot at room temperature, as much as 40 mg glucose/100 ml can disappear from normal blood by means of glycolysis. Therefore, specimens of blood should either be protected from red cell glycolysis or be separated from red cells quickly.

A specified carbohydrate load is *essential* as a challenge. Glucose is preferable and meals should not be used. For example, West reported in middle-aged and older subjects that the 2-hour blood glucose level was 21 mg/100 ml higher after 75 g of oral glucose than after breakfast containing 75 g of carbohydrate. One hour after glucose, it was 49 mg/ml higher than after the test breakfast. We prefer flavored glucose to Glucola, but the latter is more palatable and may be a useful substitute in some instances when nausea and other gastrointestinal symptoms are associated with glucose administration. Glucola consists of corn syrup in carbonated water flavored with cola or cherry; it contains the equivalent of 75 g of glucose.

Glucose, 1.75 g/kg ideal body weight, is given orally as a 25% solution, with up to 5 min permitted for ingestion. Most normal adults can be given a standard 100 g of glucose; however, some groups have used 40 g/m², while others have

Table 15–12. COMMON DRUGS AND HORMONES AFFECTING GLUCOSE TOLERANCE

Associated with Hyperglycemia		Associated with Hypoglycemia
ACTH	Growth hormone	Ethanol
Aldosterone	Haloperidol	
Caffeine	Indomethacin	MAO inhibitors
Catecholamines	Isoniazid	Methimazole
Chlorpromazine	Lithium carbonate	Oxyphenbutazone
Chlorthalidone	Nicotine	PAS
Chorionic somato-mammotropin	Nicotinic acid	Probenecid
	Oral contraceptives	Propranolol
Clonidine	Phenothiazines	Salicylates
Corticosteroids	Phenytoin	Sulfonamide
Diazoxide	Thiazides	
Ethacrynic acid	Tricyclic antidepressants	
Furosemide		
Glucagon		

used 75 g. Within limits, the amount of glucose seems to make only a small difference in the response; however, the true significance of this variable is still unknown. Blood specimens are drawn at 0, 0.5, 1, 1.5, 2, and 3 hours. They are also collected at 4 and 5 hours if reactive hypoglycemia is suspected. The times for the collection of the specimens are related to the beginning of the swallowing of the glucose solution. Undue stasis of the blood should be avoided when collecting the venous specimens. We prefer to use an indwelling scalp vein needle to avoid repeated venipunctures during the test.

Results and Their Interpretation

Ages 15 to 50. As discussed in other parts of this chapter, many factors influence the level of plasma glucose. Thus, one glucose tolerance test may be inadequate for determining whether a given subject has an abnormal carbohydrate tolerance test. When MacDonald assessed variation in the results of OGTT in 400 male volunteers, he found that, in a series of six tests on each individual over a period of 1 year, some had plasma glucose levels that were interpreted as borderline or diagnostic of chemical diabetes on some occasions but normal test results at other times. On the other hand, there were many who consistently had the same range of plasma glucose values all six times during the year. Since we know that during the early stages of diabetes some patients show marked fluctuations in their carbohydrate tolerance, we must be cautious in concluding on the basis of a single negative result that a person is free of diabetes or on the basis of a positive result that he has the disease.

A flat glucose curve is seen occasionally. It may or may not be due to faulty intestinal absorption; a similar curve is observed occasionally after the intravenous administration of glucose. The most characteristic alterations in the glucose tolerance curves are (1) increased apogee, (2) delayed return to normal, and (3) late hypoglycemia (3- to 5-hour interval). The delay in return of plasma glucose to basal is the most helpful factor in the diagnosis of abnormal carbohydrate tolerance. The apogee tends to be found in the ½-hour specimen and is of variable magnitude. Conn and colleagues observed late hypoglycemia accompanied by symptoms during OGTT in 100 diabetics, 44% of whom had a family history of diabetes. This hypoglycemia usually occurs between 2.5 and 5 hours after glucose ingestion.

Table 15–13 gives the upper limit of normal for *plasma* glucose under a variety of circumstances with a variety of proposed criteria. Consideration of all the glucose levels collectively has more value and reliability than consideration of any one individually. As seen by the Fajans-Conn criteria, abnormal tolerance is diagnosed when all three values equal or exceed those given. With the criteria of Wilkerson, abnormal tolerance is indicated if three values exceed or equal the four values given; with the point system, it is diagnosed when the values equal or exceed two points. Some investigators claim that when the sum of the 0-, 1-, 2-, and 3-hour specimens equals or exceeds 600, abnormal tolerance is present. Recently, the NIH has assembled a group of experts who have again attempted to suggest standard criteria for evaluation. The NIH data group considered a fasting plasma glucose value of more than 140 mg/dl diagnostic of diabetes mellitus. Glucose intolerance was considered to be present in subjects with a fasting glucose level less than 140 mg/dl who have a glucose level greater than 200 mg/dl any time in the first 2 hours *plus* a value more than 140 mg/dl at 2 hours during the OGTT.

Children. Normal children have lower glucose levels during OGTT than active young adults. Moreover, the curves are slightly lower in children below the age of 6 years than in those from 6 to 13; 25% of these young children have flat OGTT curves (all values less than 110 mg/100 ml). Thus,

Table 15–13. CRITERIA FOR DIAGNOSIS OF ABNORMAL OR IMPAIRED ORAL GLUCOSE TOLERANCE (ADJUSTED FOR PLASMA GLUCOSE)

	Criteria Based on Plasma Glucose (mg/dl)
Fajans and Conn* 1.75 g/kg of ideal weight	1 hr — >185 1½ hr — >160 2 hr — >140 All three values abnormal for diagnosis
USPHS-Wilkerson†	Fasting — >130 = 1 point 1 hr — >195 = ½ point 2 hr — >140 = ½ point 3 hr — >130 = 1 point Points for abnormal values; 2 points for diagnosis
ADA‡ m² 40 g/m²	Fasting — >115 1 hr — >185 1½ hr — >165 2 hr — >140 Elevated fasting or all three values abnormal for diagnosis
Pregnancy — O'Sullivan§ 100 g to all subjects National Diabetes Data Group (NIH)	Fasting — >105 1 hr — >190 2 hr — > 165 3 hr ← — >145 Two or three values abnormal for diagnosis of gestational diabetes
Children — Seltzer¶ 1.75 g/kg	Capillary whole blood Fasting — >115 1 hr — >175 2 hr — >140 3 hr — >125 Elevated fasting or two of three post-test values abnormal for diagnosis
National Diabetes Data Group (NIH) 75 g to all subjects	0.5, 1.0, or 1.5 hr — >200 *and* 2 hr — >140 Both values abnormal for diagnosis of impaired glucose tolerance Diabetes = Fasting — >140 or 2 hr *and* 0.5, 1.0, or 1.5 hr — >200 Children—2 hr > 140 for diagnosis of impaired glucose tolerance

*Ann. N.Y. Acad. Sci. 82:208, 1959.
†J. Chronic Dis. 13:6, 1961.
‡Diabetes 18:299, 1969.
§Diabetes 13:278, 1964.
　Diabetes 28:1039–1057, 1979.
¶Diabetes Mellitus: Theory and Practice. Ellenberg, M., and Rifkin, H. (eds.), New York, McGraw-Hill, 1970, p. 480.

a test exceeding adult standards in a child indicates a greater loss of physiologic carbohydrate tolerance than does the same finding in adults. A test with at least two values of 1, 2, and 3 hours above 175, 140, and 125 mg/100 ml capillary blood, respectively, was considered abnormal by Seltzer. However, the NIH data group has returned to more conservative criteria (Table 15–13) of 140 mg/dl fasting *and* two postglucose values of more than 200 mg/dl for the diagnosis of diabetes. Impaired tolerance was defined as a fasting value less than 140 mg/dl, but a 2-hour value greater than 140 mg/dl.

The Elderly. It is even more difficult to interpret the OGTT in the elderly. With some standards so many elderly persons are found to have decreased tolerance that most diabetologists regard this as a physiologic change in the aged, rather than a marker for mild diabetes mellitus. However, an important question to be answered is whether this change is contributing to the aging process or simply a result of some aspect of normal aging. Andres has reviewed the problem of changes in glucose responses with aging. According to a National Health Survey using oral glucose (50 g), males showed an increase in the 1-hour blood glucose concentration of 10 mg/dl/decade; the increase in females was 13 mg/dl/decade. The percentage of male subjects with 1-hour values greater than 160 mg/dl was 1% in the 18–24 year group, 15% in the middle-aged group, and 25% in the 75–79 year group; females had values of 5, 25, and 58%, respectively. With a 50-g dose of glucose, there was a greater deviation from normal after 1 hour than after 2 hours, but the reverse was true with 100 g. Jackson found in 144 healthy, active, elderly subjects living in homes for the aged, none of whom had previously been designated as having diabetes, that 48% were hyperglycemic during an OGTT using conventional Fajans and Conn criteria. In order to eliminate the problem of using fixed criteria, Andres constructed a nomogram which ranks 2-hour blood glucose levels with age, based on a series of OGTT's using 1.75 g glucose per kilogram (Fig. 15–63). This nomogram allows one to compare the ranking of an individual test to an age-matched cohort. In this way, the tester does not have to arbitrarily assign an individual to a normal or abnormal group. However, this method leaves the physician with a problem. What percentage of a group is expected to have impaired glucose tolerance? While there is no simple solution, the deterioration of carbohydrate tolerance with age has led to the newer, more conservative criteria for the diagnosis of diabetes mellitus. Thus, although there will be an increasing percentage of the population with age who will have carbohydrate intolerance when the currently recommended criteria by the NIH data group are used, the aging effect will not meet the criteria for a diagnosis of diabetes mellitus.

Seltzer has suggested that some of the decrease in glucose tolerance observed in the aged group is due to their relatively low intake of carbohydrate. When two groups of elderly subjects were given glucose (100 g) before and after high-carbohydrate intake for 3 days, the 2-hour blood sugar level was less in more than 90% of the subjects prepared with extra carbohydrate. Many of those studied without a high-carbohydrate diet had glucose intolerance by standard criteria. These observations could be of great significance; others should pursue similar investigations.

Intravenous Glucose Tolerance Test (IVGTT)

For satisfactory results with the IVGTT, the same precautions that were emphasized in the discussion of the OGTT must be followed. This test is generally used clinically in patients with significant gastrointestinal disturbances (for example, after stomach operations) and whenever there might be unduly rapid or slow absorption of glucose. It has advantages in that it can be performed within 1 hour, and the results are expressed as a single number. The oral test is more physiologic in that the oral route is the usual mechanism for ingress of food. Oral glucose, but not intravenous glucose, stimulates the secretion of several gastrointestinal hormones, which in turn have a highly significant effect on the secretion and action of insulin. In most instances, the dose of glucose selected for IVGTT has been 25 g; more recently, the dose of 50 g/1.73 m^2 body surface area has been employed, or 0.5 g/kg of body weight. As long as more than 20 g is given, the glucose disappearance rate is the same. Glucose is usually administered as a 25 or 50% solution, and the infusion must be completed within 2 min.

The results are expressed by the so-called K value which signifies the decrease in blood glucose in percentage per minute. Between 10 and 30 minutes after glucose administration, the curve forms a straight line on semilogarithmic paper, indicating that the decrease is exponential. When one selects on the abscissa the time interval during which the blood glucose has fallen from a certain value to half that value ("half-time"), the K value can be simply calculated as follows:

$$K_{glucose} = K_g = \frac{0.693}{T_{1/2}} \times 100\%/min$$

Lundbaek found the average figure for nondiabetic patients to be 1.72. This value declines with age to approximately 1.3. A K_g between 0.9 and 1.1 is a borderline result. Overt diabetics always have K_g values below this level. However, a small number of apparently healthy subjects also have low K_g values, indicating that caution should be used in the interpretation of this test. The K_g level is influenced significantly by the effect of insulin on hepatic glucose output and peripheral glucose removal.

Cortisone – Oral Glucose Tolerance Test

The administration of cortisone or other drugs that diminish the peripheral sensitivity to injected insulin may impair performance in a carbohydrate tolerance test in susceptible subjects and, after prolonged administration of large doses, may even lead to the appearance of clinical diabetes mellitus. The long-term follow-up of subjects who demonstrate less than average glucose tolerance after cortisone is unknown. Therefore, at the present time this test serves only a research function. Subjects receive 50–62.5 mg of cortisone acetate, 8.5 and 2 hours before an OGTT. A positive test in a person under age 50 consists of plasma glucose values exceeding 185 at 1 hour, 170 at 1.5 hours, and 160 at 2 hours. The finding that subjects with diabetic family histories perform less well than those without such histories has been the greatest stimulus to its use as a diagnostic test. Fajans and Conn reported that only 3% of a control group performed as poorly as 28% of a group of diabetic relatives, with a substantial portion of these individuals eventually receiving a diag-

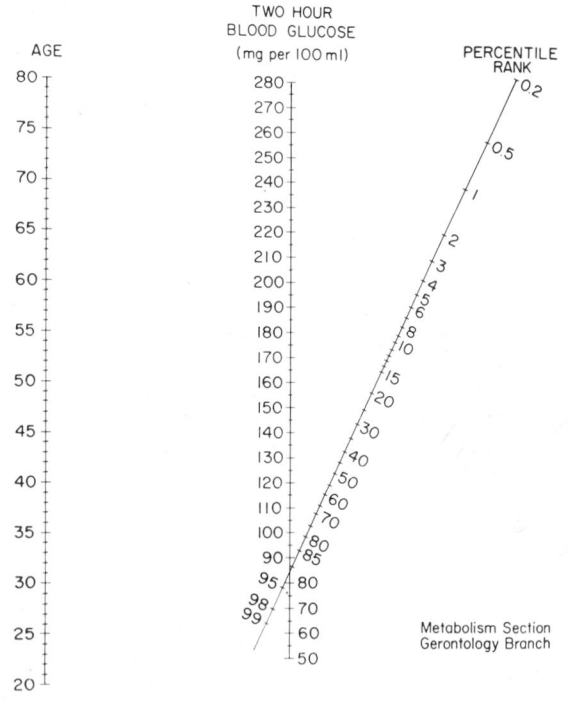

Figure 15–63. A nomogram for the determination of percentile performance 2 hours after an oral glucose load (1.75 g/kg ideal body weight), showing age corrections. This study is based upon free-living adults with no apparent disease eating their usual diet. (From Andres, R.: Aging and diabetes. *Med. Clin. N. Amer.* 55:841, 1971.)

nosis of overt diabetes. Performance on this test is also worse in older subjects; therefore, the age of the subject must be taken into account in interpreting the result of the test. Since glucocorticoid administration is known to be followed by increased insulin output in normal subjects, this test appears to determine the ability of the pancreas to augment its insulin secretion in response to impaired insulin effectiveness.

Pancreatic Pathology in Diabetes

The pathology of the pancreas varies greatly in diabetes. Four types of lesions have been observed: (1) glycogen infiltration of B-cells, (2) hydropic degeneration of the B-cells, (3) hyalinization of the islets, and (4) lymphocytic infiltration of the islets (Fig. 15–64). Since more than 80% of the normal pancreas must be removed for frank and permanent hyperglycemia to be produced, it is difficult to relate the metabolic findings in most patients to the pathology. This degree of destruction is rarely observed in the average case of maturity-onset diabetes mellitus. However, there is an increased incidence of hyperglycemia in chronic pancreatitis, occasional cases are associated with pancreatic carcinoma, and there is a definite association between hyperglycemia and hemochromatosis. A decrease in the number of granules in B-cells is common and is accompanied by a decrease in insulin content. Wrenshall found that in normal individuals the amount of insulin extractable from the pancreas corre-

lates best with the body surface area and is greatest in the most obese individuals. The amount of extractable insulin and the number of B-cells increase with age from early childhood until they reach the adult level at age 12–16 years. In general, diabetic subjects had lesser amounts of pancreatic insulin than nondiabetic controls. This reduction averaged 40%, but most of the difference was in subjects under the age of 20 with insulin-dependent diabetes. It is also important to point out that patients in this study with hypoglycemia rather than hyperglycemia also had very low levels of pancreatic insulin. Thus, low extractable insulin levels did not necessarily correlate with a decreased insulin secretion. In animals low-granulation states have been observed under conditions of very great insulin secretion, which presumably depleted stores, and in conditions in which insulin secretion has been very low for long periods, presumably owing to atrophy of stores.

Among other pancreatic pathologic changes associated with diabetes, the most common is vacuolization of the B-cells. These vacuoles give a positive PAS reaction, suggesting glycogen within them. Such alterations are usually only found at autopsy when there has been consistent untreated hyperglycemia, and they do not occur in the treated diabetic syndrome. Similar findings are observed in untreated experimental diabetes, in which there may also be an increase in glycogen of the ductular epithelium. Occasionally, these vacuoles become complex and contain lipids as well as carbohydrates. Such lesions have been called "hydropic degeneration" and have been considered by some to be precursors to B-cell death.

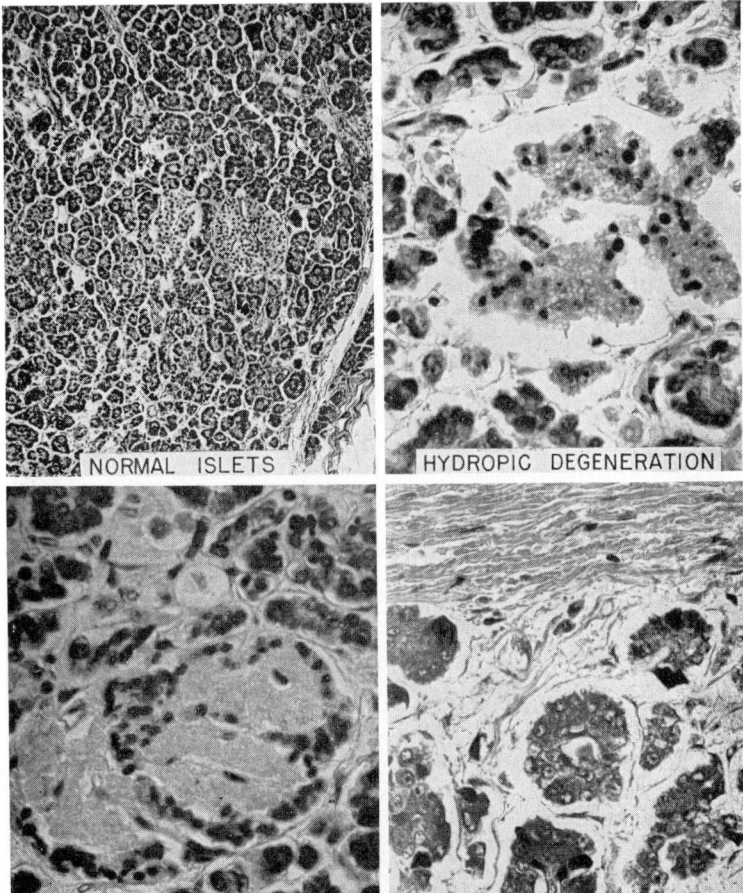

Figure 15–64. Islet changes found in patients with diabetes mellitus.

NORMAL ISLETS

HYDROPIC DEGENERATION

HYALINE DEGENERATION

FIBROSIS

Hyalinization of the islets is relatively common, occurring in approximately 30–40% of diabetics examined. This hyaline material consists of deposits of a homogeneous, subendothelial, acidophilic substance. A similar material may be found in nondiabetic subjects. There is a better correlation between the amount of hyaline and the age of the patient than between the former and the duration or severity of the carbohydrate abnormality. There is considerable evidence that this hyaline material is, or closely resembles, amyloid, which has raised questions regarding autoimmunity in the causation of diabetes mellitus. Such suppositions have been somewhat strengthened by the lymphocytic infiltrations observed in the absence of generalized pancreatic inflammatory disease in insulin-dependent diabetics examined soon after the onset of diabetes. This finding has been termed "insulitis" and is of interest since viral and autoimmune etiologies have been proposed for juvenile-onset-type diabetes.

Clinical Pathology of Diabetic Neurovascular Disease

There are no *specific* pathologic findings associated with diabetes mellitus. However, degenerative changes occur in many organ systems and lead to considerable morbidity and mortality. The following pathophysiologic changes can be thought of as complications of the disease, but are unlikely to be due solely to the direct effects of insulin deficiency (either relative or absolute) or hyperglycemia. Rather, they are concomitants of the disease produced by the *interaction* of other risk factors with hyperglycemia and insulin deficiency in diabetes mellitus in ways which are not well understood.

Macrovascular Disease — Arteriosclerosis

Arteriosclerosis involving the entire vascular system can be present. Findings in the larger arteries and coronary circulation are identical to those in nondiabetic subjects but seem to be more frequent and to occur at an earlier age in the diabetic population. Thus, there appears to be no specific large-vessel morphologic lesion related to diabetes (Strandness). Cardiovascular lesions account for 75–80% of the total mortality in diabetes and have therefore assumed great importance as the cause of premature death in this syndrome. The degree of vascular disease does not appear to be proportional to the alterations in carbohydrate metabolism but correlates best with the duration of the disease and the age of the patient. White, for example, found that there was a 92% incidence of vascular disease in juvenile diabetics who had the disease for more than 20 years. This acceleration of the development of vascular disease greatly reduces the sex differences found in the normal population. Thus, the presence of diabetes in females aged 20–50 years is likely to increase the frequency of macrovascular disease eight- to ten-fold.

Arteriosclerosis consists of two independent but related processes — *atherosclerosis* and *medial calcification.* Atherosclerosis consists of the proliferation of connective tissue cells followed by accumulation of lipids in the subintimal tissues of arteries to form lipid-filled plaques or atheromas. The lipid appears to be deposited or synthesized in smooth muscle cells that proliferate and migrate from the media into the intima and become transformed into foamy cells. These cells eventually rupture, leading to the noncellular deposition of lipid (Fig. 15–65). The fatty plaques then can undergo further changes, such as fibrosis, calcifica-

tion, and ulceration, eventually leading to thrombosis and arterial occlusion (see Chapter 17).

For reasons that are not completely clear, advanced vascular disease in the lower legs is common in diabetics and particularly severe, leading to gangrene or death of the affected extremity. It has been suggested that the concomitant neuropathy and loss of pain and touch sensation may explain the high frequency of lower-leg vascular complications seen in the diabetic population; however, there may be an interaction between capillary microangiopathy and arteriosclerosis which is also important. Diabetics also develop atherosclerotic complications in the cerebral circulation and in the renal and mesenteric circulations, leading to occlusive disease and complications in these organs as well.

Medial calcification or Mönckeberg's calcific medial sclerosis may also lead to an increased firmness in the arterial wall and thus can contribute to arteriosclerosis. The process by which calcium is deposited in the muscular wall is unknown; however, it is independent of atherosclerosis and ordinarily does not lead to vascular occlusion. It may occur in nondiabetic individuals, but in patients below the age of 40 diabetes is almost always present. Since calcification also occurs in the complicated atherosclerotic lesion, it is not possible to determine from an x-ray whether one is dealing with atherosclerosis or medial calcification. It has been reported that there is a tendency for medial calcification and atherosclerosis not to affect simultaneously the same portions of the artery.

Arteriolosclerosis. This appears to be an entirely separate pathologic process which is prominent in diabetics but indistinguishable from that found in essential hypertension. It appears as a concentric hyaline thickening of the arterioles, widening of the endothelium, and eventual encroachment on the vascular lumen by a plaque which stains with PAS. There is some evidence that this material is related to, or resembles, basement membrane, since it is PAS-positive and presumably contains glycoprotein. However, the exact nature of the deposit is unknown. The prevalent site in the diabetic is the kidney, particularly if the individual has had clinical nephropathy, but other organs, including the pancreas, are frequently involved.

Capillary Microangiopathy

The morphologic feature which characterizes diabetic microangiopathy is a thickened capillary basement membrane. This thickening has been reported in practically every capillary bed, including skin, skeletal muscle, adipose tissue, kidney, pancreas, and peripheral nerves; however, it has been best documented and studied in skeletal muscle capillaries and kidney. The involvement is not global, however, and even within the various skeletal muscles some areas may be thicker than others. Although some have suggested that this lesion is specific for diabetes, recent evidence suggests that it occurs in other diseases, although rather rarely, and is then usually associated with some type of inflammatory process.

The cause of this basement membrane thickening is unclear, largely because little is known about the normal composition, origin, and function of the basement membrane. Studies by Spiro have greatly expanded our knowledge of the glycoprotein contained within this structure. His analysis has been based upon the glomerular basement membrane, in which carbohydrates make up about 10% of the glycoprotein as glucose, galactose, mannose, hexosamines, sialic acids, and fucose. It is of interest that this is one of the few glycoproteins that has been shown to contain glucose. There are unusually large amounts of hydroxypro-

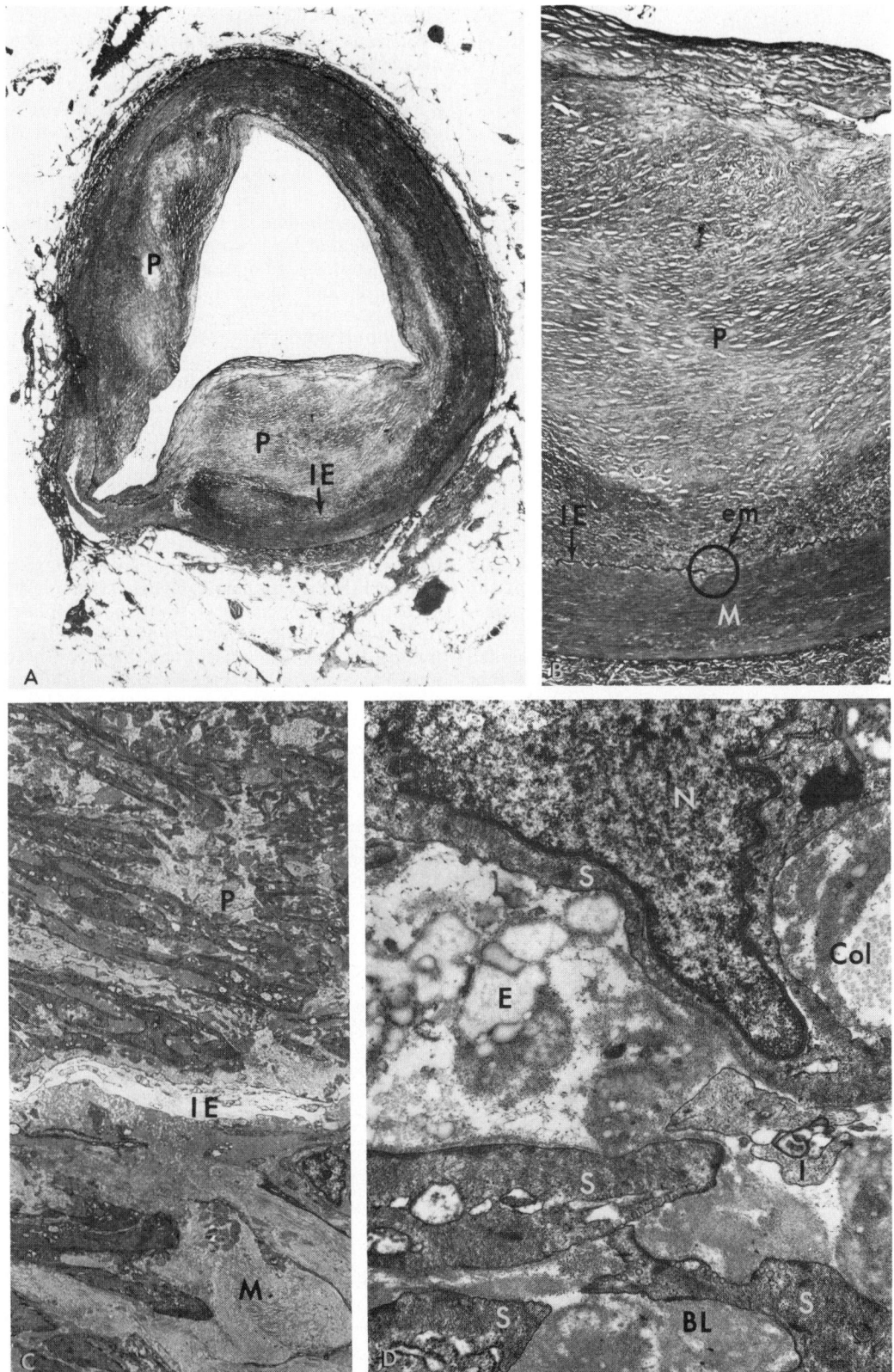

Figure 15–65. Coronary artery obtained 3 hours post mortem from male, aged 52, with atherosclerosis. *A*, Cross section of artery near branch point (× 20). *P* indicates each of two fibrous plaques; *IE* is internal elastic membrane delimiting plaque from arterial media. *B*, Magnification (× 63) of portion of lower plaque seen in *A* compared with media *(M)*. Lighter color of plaque *(P)* shows presence of abundant collagen and basement lamina material surrounding cells. *C*, Electron micrograph (× 1800) of region indicated in *B* at base of plaque. Cells in plaque region *(P)* are somewhat distorted smooth muscle cells. Larger smooth muscle cells in more regular arrays appear under the internal elastic membrane *(IE)* in the media *(M)*. *D*, Electron micrograph (× 14,500) showing portions of four smooth muscle cells *(S)* forming the plaque. *N* is a portion of nucleus of one cell. Collagen *(Col)*, some elastic *(E)*, and much basal lamina *(BL)* type material are irregularly distributed between the cells. Lipid present but not evident is *not* a prominent feature of this plaque, as is frequently the case with other plaques. (Courtesy of Dr. Earl P. Benditt and Dr. Ned Moss.)

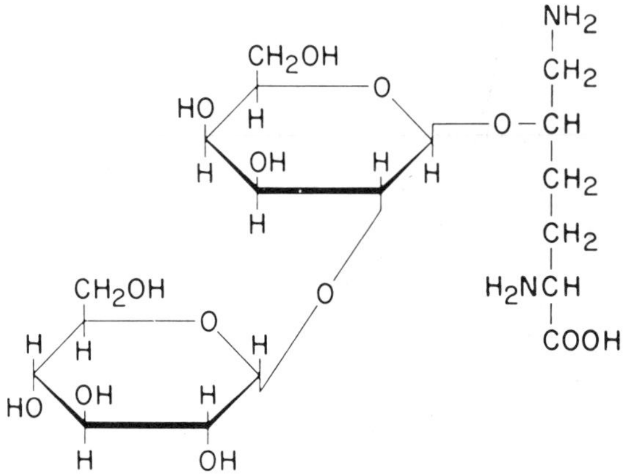

Figure 15–66. Structure and peptide attachment of the disaccharide unit of the glomerular basement membrane (2-*O* α-D-glucopyranosyl-*O*-β-D-galactopyranosylhydroxylysine). (From Spiro, R. G.: The structure of the disaccharide unit of the renal glomerular basement membrane. *J. Biol. Chem.* 242:4813, 1967.)

line and hydroxylysine. The hydroxylysine content is of importance because a large number of these residues are involved in the linkages to a disaccharide unit containing glucose and galactose (Fig. 15–66). In the studies of the diabetic basement membrane, a normal glycoprotein composition was found, except for an increased amount of hydroxylysine residues and an increase in the hydroxylysine-linked disaccharide units. From these findings he postulated that increased availability of glucose for glycoprotein synthesis is in part responsible for the chemical abnormality described.

The finding in experimental diabetes of increased activity of glucosyltransferase, an enzyme responsible for the assembly of the hydroxylysine-linked disaccharide units of the glomerular basement membrane, which is reversed by insulin treatment, has suggested that this enzymatic activity may be involved in the abnormal production of glycoproteins in diabetes mellitus. Spiro's postulate is that the hyperglycemia of diabetes causes excessive basement membrane synthesis because the kidney is an organ which utilizes glucose without insulin being present. However, two other investigators have failed to confirm the findings. Whether this discrepancy is due to different methods of patient selection or to methodologic differences in the isolation of glomerular basement membrane is not clear. The issue has been further confounded by the reports by Siperstein that a similar morphologic lesion of muscle capillaries occurs prior to development of hyperglycemia in a significant number of individuals with two diabetic parents. These observations have led him to hypothesize that these lesions are concomitants of the disease unrelated to the presence of hyperglycemia.

It has been suggested by Vracko that basal lamina provides a microskeleton for cellular regeneration and that its apparent thickening may be related to increased cell turnover. According to this concept, the "thickening" is due to accumulation of abnormally large numbers of normally thick layers of basal lamina, each layer being deposited by a new cell-generation replication. This intriguing idea, which suggests that accumulated layers of basal lamina reflect an accelerated cell turnover in the diabetic population, requires further evaluation. Examples of a normal-appearing basal lamina in skeletal muscle capillary and accumulation of multiple layers as the process occurs with advancing age in a nondiabetic subject and in diabetes mellitus are shown in Figure 15–67.

All investigators agree that long-term diabetics, regardless of treatment, have thickened basement membranes in

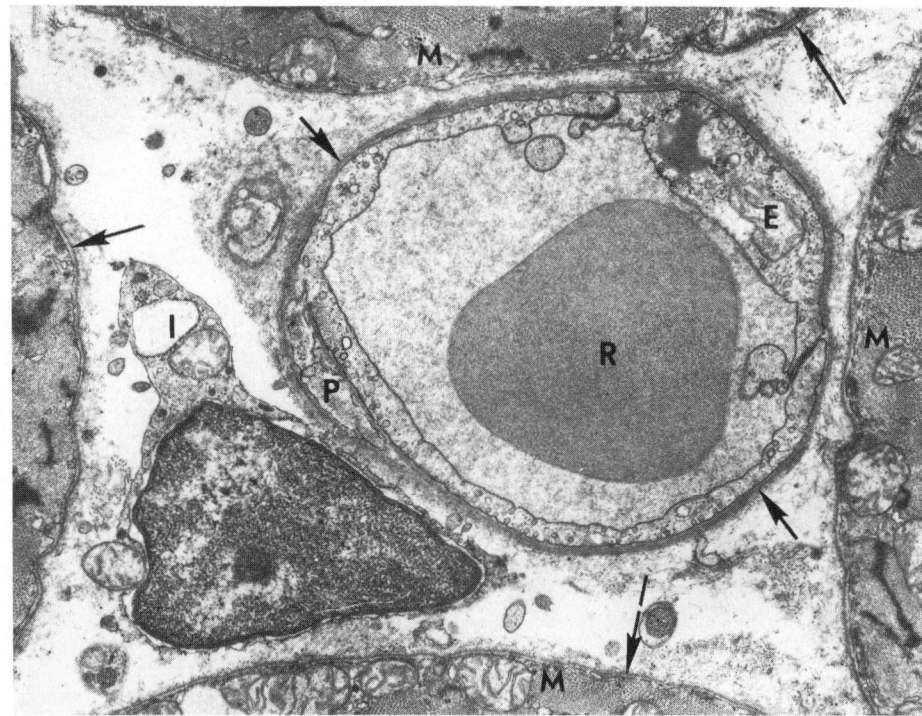

Figure 15–67. Cross sections of tibial skeletal muscle from a 9-year-old nondiabetic boy *(A)*, a 69-year-old nondiabetic man *(B)*, and a 68-year-old diabetic man *(C)*, showing portions of muscle fibers *(M)*, their basal lamina (long arrows), interstitial cells *(I)* and capillaries composed of basal lamina (short arrows), pericytes *(P)*, endothelium *(E)*, endothelial nuclei *(N)*, and red blood cells *(R)*. *A* shows structures as they normally occur in a young individual. In *B* and *C*, the basal lamina investment is "thickened" because of the accumulation of abnormal numbers of basal lamina layers (short arrows).

Illustration continued on opposite page

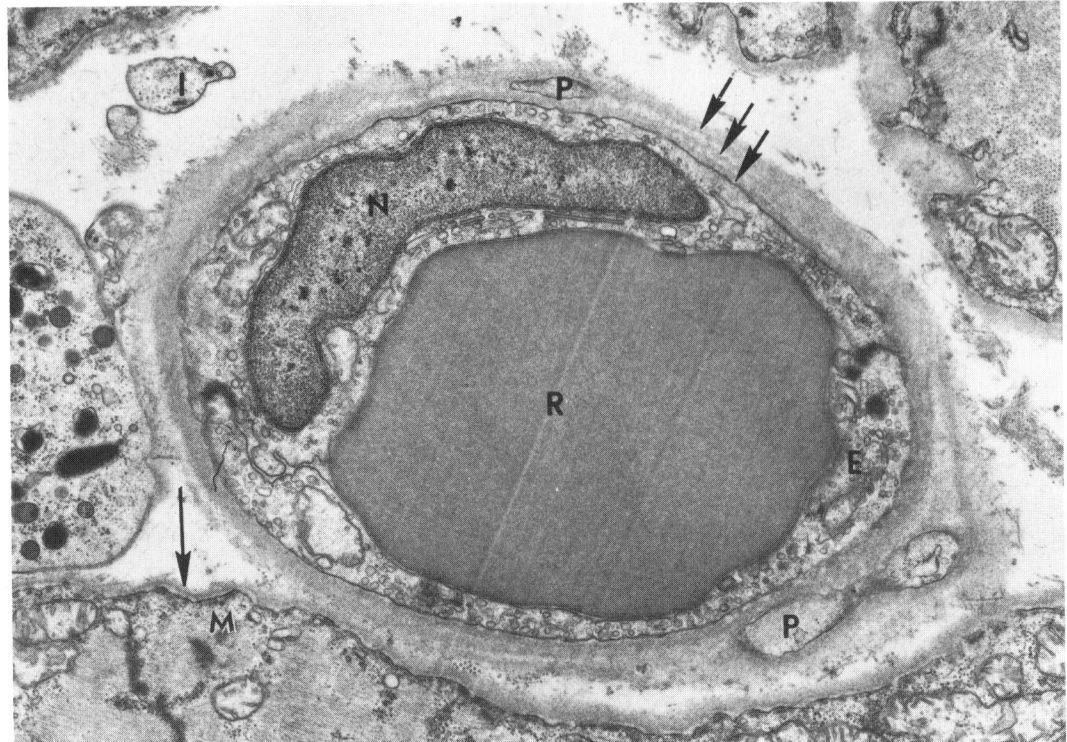

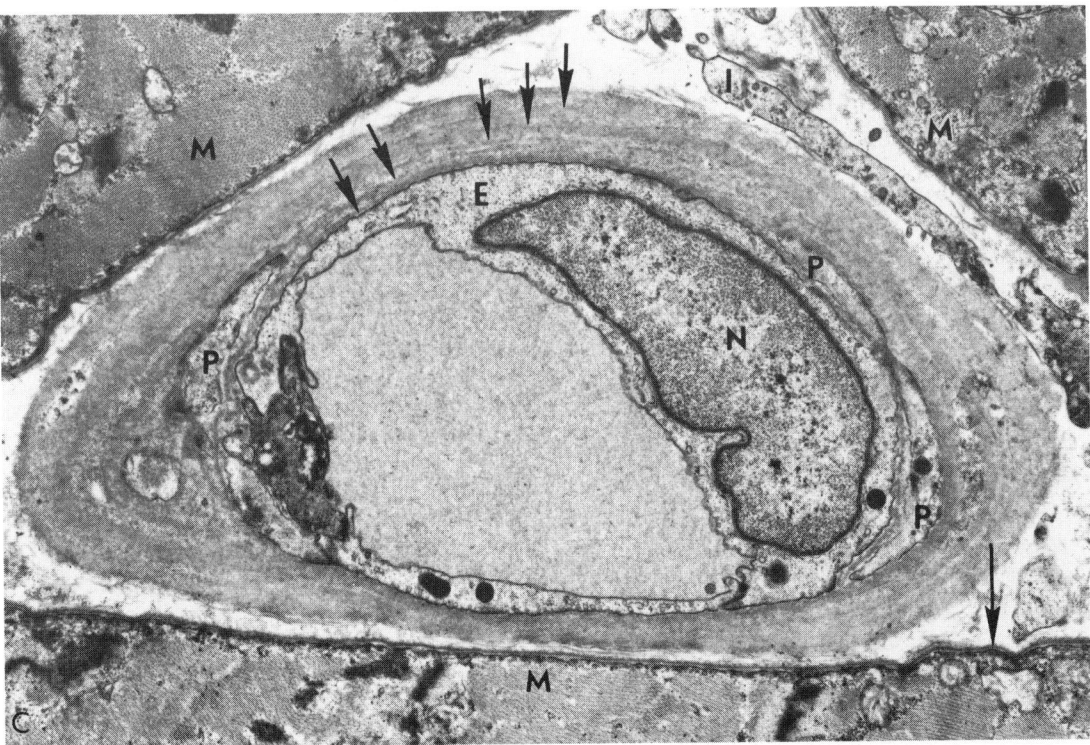

Figure 15–67. Continued. The capillary from the diabetic *(C)* has accumulated at least five layers, while that from the aged nondiabetic has three layers. Cell debris, which is present between the layers of basal lamina in diabetic capillaries, indicates that cell death has occurred. That basal lamina layers have not been produced by the same cell generation is suggested by the presence of a single layer of basal lamina between pericytes and endothelial cells. Layering of basal lamina identical to that seen in *B* and *C* can be produced in nondiabetic animals by alternating cycles of endothelial cell death and regeneration. All electron micrographs are shown at approximately the same magnification (× 14,700). (Electron micrographs and their interpretation provided by Dr. Rudolf Vracko.)

comparison with suitably matched control subjects. However, Williamson found that this is an age-related phenomenon; that is, the basement membrane gets thicker normally with aging, and this age effect is a critical factor in estimating the degree of thickening. Siperstein did not find an age-related effect, nor did he find the duration or degree of carbohydrate intolerance important in its intensity. Further investigations have suggested that both groups of investigators are correct; that is, basement membrane thickening does occur as part of the aging process. However, the major change is related to puberty, and this is exaggerated in diabetes. It may occur prior to, or independently of, the carbohydrate abnormality as an integral part of the diabetic syndrome, but the duration of carbohydrate intolerance increases the chance of finding such a lesion. Despite the use of muscle capillary basement membranes to investigate this lesion, the primary clinical importance of microangiopathy is related to chronic renal disease and blindness due to retinal involvement, the kidney and the eye being the two organs most clearly associated with severe functional deterioration.

The relation between the pathologic finding and the functional changes is very unclear at present. Early on the capillaries appear to leak large protein molecules more readily, despite the morphologic appearance of "thickening."

It is possible that a focal lesion may explain such a phenomenon or that an abnormal protein interferes with function. While the lesion is similar in the various organs, the eventual pathophysiology is quite different and is often different in timing and degree, suggesting that other factors play a major role in each organ affected. A review of these problems and the various studies which relate vascular disease to diabetes has been written by Brownlee and Cahill. While their bias is to relate the changes to hyperglycemia and insulin deficiency, their review indicates that further research will clearly be required.

Symmetric Neuropathy

Dysfunction of the brain, spinal cord, and peripheral nerves appears to be an integral part of the diabetic syndrome. It had been claimed, particularly by Fagerberg from vascular performance studies in diabetes, that there is a vascular cause for the peripheral neuropathy, partly because the two lesions appear to progress simultaneously in many diabetic subjects. However, since both the vascular abnormality and the peripheral neuropathy are dependent upon time and duration of illness, one does not necessarily cause the other. More recent evidence obtained by light microscop-

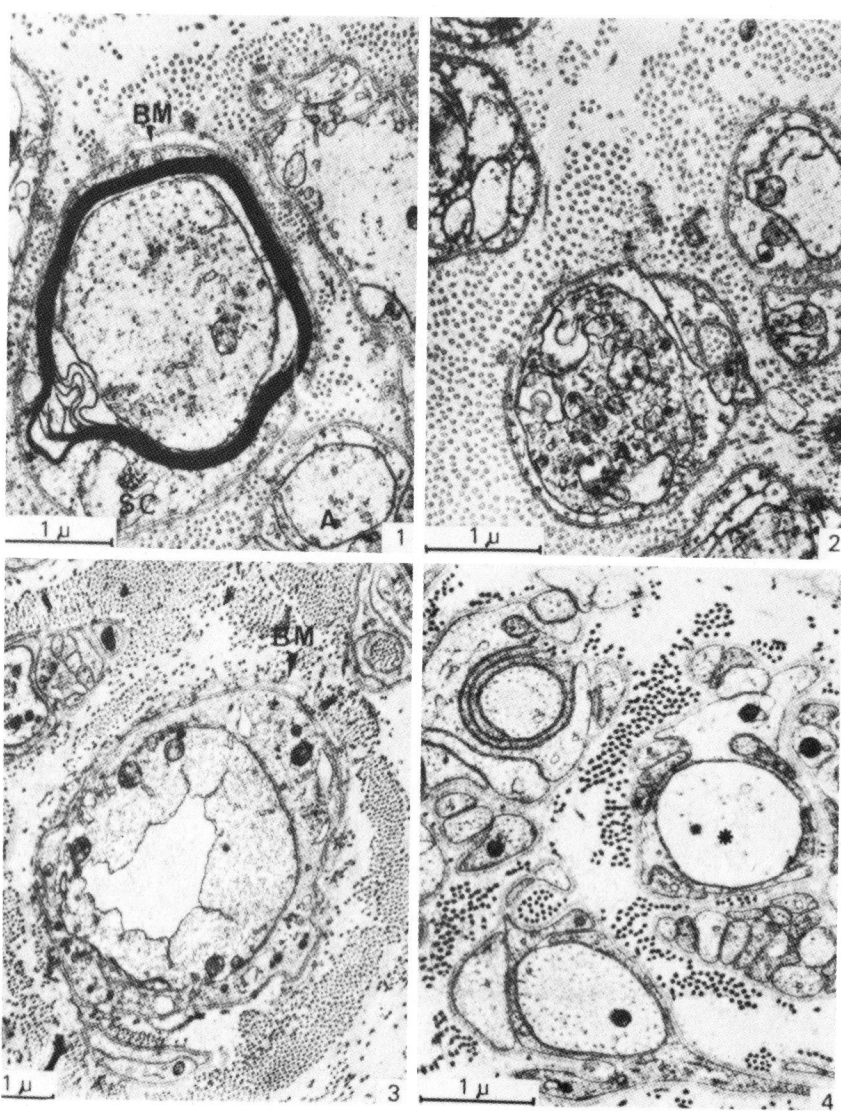

Figure 15–68. Morphology of early neuropathy showing progressive axonal damage in nonmyelinated diabetic nerves. *1,* Transverse section through a thinly myelinated and nonmyelinated nerve fiber *(A).* There is axonal degeneration characterized by disintegration of neural filaments and vesicular proliferation and hyperplasia of the Schwann cell *(SC)* basement membrane *(BM). 2,* Transverse section though several nonmyelinated nerve fibers. There is axonal degeneration characterized by accumulation of organelles in the axoplasm. *3,* Transverse section through several nonmyelinated nerve fibers. There is axonal degeneration characterized by a distended vacuole in the axis cylinder. *4,* Transverse section through several nonmyelinated nerve fibers. One axis cylinder is completely devoid of normal axoplasmic organelles (*). (From Bischoff, A.: Ultrastructural pathology of peripheral nervous system in early diabetes. In *Vascular and Neurological Changes in Early Diabetes.* Camerini-Davalos, A., and Cole, H. S. (eds.), New York, Academic Press, 1973.)

ic examination of myelinated nerves has suggested that the lesion is a thickening of the Schwann cell basement membrane and a segmental demyelinization as described by Thomas and Lascelles. However, examination of nonmyelinated nerves has shown what appears to be a primary axonal loss and shrinkage with perineural edema (Fig. 15–68). Thus, the site of abnormality may be related to the Schwann cell, the axon, or both. It is even possible that this varies with the type of nerve fiber. No morphologic changes were observed in early studies of animal models of diabetes. However, more recently loss of axonal area was found early in experimental diabetes and segmental demyelinization later, again suggesting a primary axonal problem. Eventually, one may find marked degeneration of the dorsal root ganglia and associated axons. These observations of morphologic changes in the nerves have been partly substantiated by biochemical analysis of nerve biopsy specimens, which show changes in the lipid composition. The pathology of changes occasionally found in the spinal cord and central nervous system is obscure.

Reduced motor and sensory nerve conduction velocity (NCV) has been observed in both human diabetes and animal models. Slowed sciatic NCV has been documented 14 days after induction of experimental diabetes with streptozotocin in rats, suggesting that the abnormality of nerve function may be directly related to a metabolic effect of this insulin-deficient state. The degree of impaired NCV has been related to the duration of the disease in patients with juvenile-onset-type diabetes. However, as illustrated in Figure 15–69, the degree of impairment of motor NCV has recently been found to be correlated with the degree of fasting hyperglycemia in untreated patients with maturity-onset diabetes. These patients had diabetes of relatively recent onset and had no clinical findings of neuropathy. Thus, both the duration of diabetes and the degree of metabolic disturbance appear to influence this measurement of nerve function.

Although the autonomic nervous system (ANS) is frequently affected in diabetics, the mechanism by which abnormalities occur has received little attention, except for one investigation which showed dendrite degeneration in the peripheral sympathetic ganglia. An abnormality of afferent input into the autonomic nervous system has also been implicated by Whalen in the gastrointestinal tract, since jejunal dilation is not followed by pain, and in other studies suggesting that postural hypotension can be due to lack of afferent baroreceptor function. Despite the evidence of permanent structural damage to the nerves, clinical neuropathy varies greatly from time to time, suggesting either that these lesions can be repaired or that the function of these nerves is dependent upon metabolic or functional changes that are reversible.

There have been several theories relating to the etiology of the neuropathy. They are: (1) an accumulation of sugar alcohol, leading to swelling and tissue damage; (2) a deficiency of intracellular myoinositol, leading to impaired membrane phospholipid function; (3) a deficiency of myelin synthesis due to hypoinsulinemia, leading to segmental myelin loss; (4) glycosylation of neural membrane proteins with impairment of neural function; and (5) accelerated death and turnover of Schwann cells either secondary to cell injury from any of the above or directly due to diabetes independent of the metabolic abnormality, leading to a thickening and accumulation of abnormal basal lamina and impaired nerve function.

The first of these theories is receiving the most serious attention now because it is based on good evidence that lens cataract formation can be induced by increased activity of the polyol pathway of glucose metabolism. This pathway

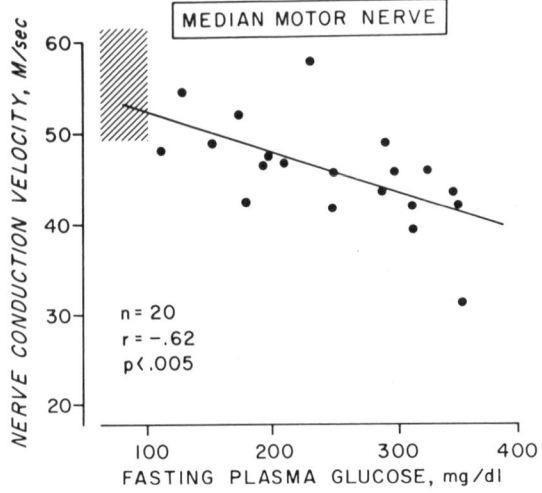

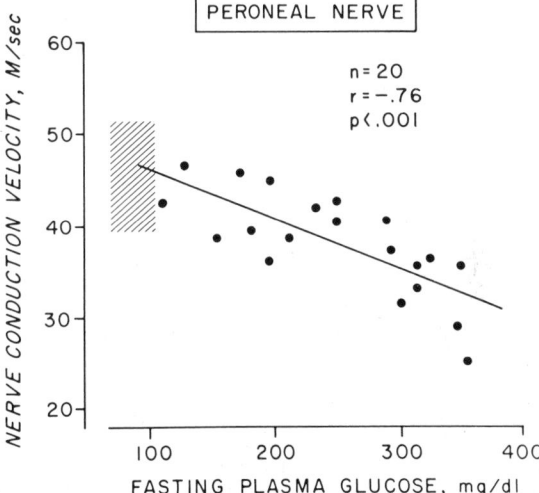

Figure 15–69. Relationship between median and peroneal motor nerve conduction velocity (NCV) and the fasting plasma glucose (FPG) level of untreated, non-insulin-dependent diabetics. The shaded area represents the range of values for age-matched normals. Diabetics with higher FPG levels have proportionately reduced motor NCV. (Adapted from Graf, R. J., Halter, J. B., et al.: Nerve conduction abnormalities in untreated maturity onset diabetes: Relation to levels of fasting plasma glucose and glycosylated hemoglobin. *Ann. Intern. Med. 90:*298, 1979.)

consists of two enzymes (Fig. 15–70) which convert sugars (such as glucose) to their corresponding alcohols (sorbitol) by an enzyme, aldose reductase, which is present in lens, nerve Schwann cells, and other tissues insensitive to the glucose transport acceleration by insulin. The sugar alcohols are relatively impermeable to biologic membranes but osmotically active. They can be further oxidized by another enzyme (sorbitol dehydrogenase) to secondary sugars (fructose) for further metabolism. Since aldose reductase has a high K_m (or low affinity) for glucose, it is active only during hyperglycemia. Because of the limited ability of the dehydrogenase to metabolize the product, intracellular intermediates (sorbitol and fructose) accumulate. This sequence has been demonstrated to play a role in some types of lens cataracts, since inhibitors of the enzyme aldose reductase prevent cataract formation. However, the localization of the enzyme to Schwann cells and not axons makes the jump to diabetic neuropathy a little more tenuous. Furthermore, it has been shown that oral myoinositol supplements improve nerve conduction velocity in diabetic rats without changing aldose reductase. However, it is possible that the loss of myoinositol

$$D-GLUCOSE + TPNH \xrightarrow[\text{Reductase}]{\text{Aldose}} SORBITOL + TPN^+$$

$$SORBITOL + DPN^+ \xrightarrow[\text{Dehydrogenase}]{\text{Sorbitol}} FRUCTOSE + DPNH$$

Figure 15–70. The polyol pathway for the metabolism of glucose.

from diabetic nerve is secondary to accelerated sorbitol pathway activity; therefore, this hypothesis still remains one of the best at present.

Cardiovascular System

Heart

Atherosclerotic coronary heart disease is the commonest cause of death in diabetics (Fig. 15–71). Partamian found that coronary heart disease accounted for 53.3% of the deaths in diabetics. Within 2 months of the initial myocardial infarction, 38% had died; 54.7% of those with a subsequent myocardial infarct died. Only 37.8% of those with a subsequent infarct survived more than 5 years. Other reports indicate that among nondiabetics with myocardial infarctions, 49–83% survive more than 5 years. In diabetic subjects, females show a greater increase in relative risk for myocardial infarction than males. Those with myocardial infarcts frequently had other vascular concomitants, such as retinopathy and glomerulosclerosis or peripheral vascular disease or both. The incidence of coronary disease is dependent to some extent on the duration of the diabetes, the degree of hyperglycemia, the age of the patient, the presence of other complicating illnesses, such as hypertension and obesity, and risk factors such as smoking. The presence of ketoacidosis during acute myocardial infarction worsens the prognosis. Population studies have shown a relationship between atherosclerotic complications and blood sugar. Whether subnormal glucose utilization affects lipid and protein metabolism, or whether some common underlying abnormality leads to both hyperglycemia and atherosclerosis, is not clear at this time.

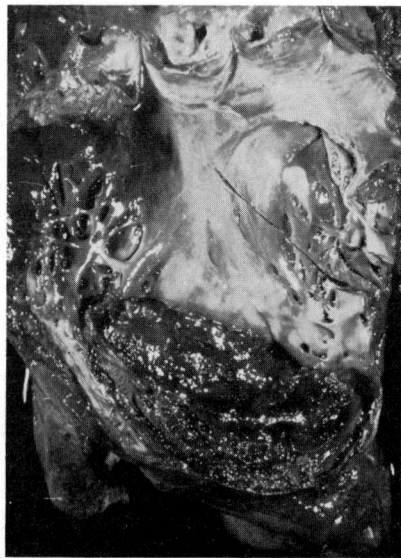

Figure 15–71. Myocardial infarction resulting from coronary atherosclerosis, the commonest cause of death in diabetics.

A large proportion of individuals who previously have not been regarded as having diabetes are noted to have glycosuria and hyperglycemia at the time of an acute myocardial infarction. Thus, the question is raised whether such individuals have diabetes. When the hyperglycemia and glycosuria last 2 weeks or longer, the diagnosis of diabetes is likely. When they last only a few days, the diagnosis is uncertain, but this is likely to represent stress hyperglycemia. Diabetes should be suspected and the patient checked with respect to its possible progression. Treatment during the acute phase depends on the degree of carbohydrate imbalance regardless of the diagnosis.

Cardiomyopathy. Chest pain or signs of congestive heart failure in a diabetic are not necessarily due to coronary artery disease. Several studies using both invasive and noninvasive cardiac diagnostic techniques have documented the presence of myocardial dysfunction in diabetics who do not have significant coronary artery stenosis. Patients with few or no cardiac symptoms have been shown to have evidence of increased ventricular wall stiffness, whereas symptomatic diabetics have diminished myocardial contractility as well. The findings are similar to those observed in nondiabetic patients with cardiomyopathy of other etiologies, such as alcoholism. Postmortem studies of diabetics dying of heart failure have documented widespread accumulation of PAS-positive glycoprotein and increased fibrosis in hearts without evidence of extensive narrowing of either large or small coronary vessels. Recently, microaneurysms similar to those in the retina have also been described in diabetic hearts. Thus, in addition to being at risk for development of coronary atherosclerosis, diabetics may also be subject to a myopathic process in the heart.

Prevention. An effort should be made to reduce risk factors for atherosclerosis. Weight reduction is instituted when there is obesity. Hypertension is lowered when present. Regular exercise of moderate degree is encouraged. Smoking should be omitted. Control of the carbohydrate abnormalities is discussed elsewhere. Hyperlipidemia should be considered and treated as discussed in Chapter 17.

Peripheral Vessels

Peripheral occlusive vascular disease is primarily due to atherosclerosis and is not related to medial calcification, which is also common in diabetes. Although all the larger arteries may be involved to varying degrees with atherosclerosis, it is more common and severe in the arteries of the legs.

Symptoms of peripheral vascular disease are rare before the age of 50. They are most typically those of intermittent claudication, with coldness of the feet, pain, and various paresthesias — burning, tingling, and numbness. The numbness may be due either to vascular narrowing or to an associated neuropathy. On physical examination, the skin of the lower legs and feet appears atrophic, shiny, and cool, with marked redness in the dependent position and a waxy pallor on elevation of the legs. Dependent rubor is a sign of arterial insufficiency when there is no venous stasis. The volume of pulsation of the posterior tibial artery and the dorsalis pedis artery of the foot varies markedly. At times pulsations may be normal, but usually they are reduced.

Although hypertension contributes to atherosclerosis in some instances, one-third of the diabetics with gangrene are found not to have hypertension. Gangrene develops as rapidly in diabetics with mild hyperglycemia as in diabetics with severe hyperglycemia. In some patients with gangrene, a carbohydrate abnormality is not apparent until later. Bartels, for example, studied 100 consecutive patients with peripheral vascular disease of the lower extremities; the patients were unselected except that all those who had a history of diabetes or glycosuria were eliminated. There was some evidence of abnormal glucose tolerance in 59%. Only 23% of the whole group had entirely normal results. Thus, carbohydrate intolerance appears to be unusually common in patients with peripheral vascular disease.

Goldner reported on the natural history of diabetes in 71 patients with amputation of one limb. Other concomitants were common: 8% had retinopathy, 36% nephropathy, and 63% neuropathy. Twenty-nine of the 41 patients studied within 2 years of amputation had lesions of the second leg, and 47 of the 71 studied had involvement of the second leg within 5 years after involvement of the first. Thirty-two of these 47 subsequently had to have the other leg amputated. These observations emphasize the progressive nature of the disease.

Vasodilators are not of much help, possibly because they dilate the more healthy blood vessels and draw blood away from the sclerotic ones. Exercise is good, and walking to the point of claudication should be encouraged. Buerger's exercises or some modifications are also indicated. Tobacco should be avoided. Endarterectomy and bypass operations, although useful, are not often of much long-term help. Alcohol injection into the nerve fibers and sympathectomy rarely prove to be of any significant value.

Gangrene. Complete occlusion of a major vessel may lead to gangrene. An occasional instance of gangrene of the upper extremities has been reported, and the mesenteric arteries may be involved sufficiently to produce abdominal angina and mesenteric infarction. In diabetics the frequency and the degree of involvement of the lower extremities are the same for both sexes; in nondiabetics such gangrene is distinctly more common in males. Bell found that gangrene was 156 times more frequent in diabetics than in nondiabetics in the fifth decade, and 85 times more common in the seventh. An important, but often overlooked, factor is the concomitant peripheral neuropathy which may contribute to this high incidence of gangrene by lack of recognition of leg trauma.

Gangrene may involve small areas or an entire foot or leg (Fig. 15–72). In one study the gangrene extended above the ankle in only 7% of diabetics, compared with 50% of nondiabetics. This is probably because atherosclerosis in the smaller arteries is more common in diabetics than in nondiabetics, possibly because of microangiopathy. When the larger arteries are occluded, the gangrene tends to be massive, whereas it tends to be spotty with occlusions of the smaller arteries and arterioles. Spotty distribution is found in 70% of diabetics. Fifteen to twenty-five per cent of diabetics with gangrene have been reported to have normal or only slightly decreased pulsations in the corresponding dorsalis pedis artery. There is a better opportunity for developing a collateral circulation with atherosclerotic occlusion when only the larger vessels are involved, possibly because the smaller blood vessels that will participate in the collateral circulation are available. Therefore, gangrene results from an occlusion more often in diabetics because of the frequency of small-artery involvement.

The major goal is prevention of gangrene by avoiding trauma and infection and by not restricting blood flow. The patient can accomplish this to some extent by keeping the feet clean, applying lanolin or some other bland ointment to hard, dry areas on the feet, wearing clean footwear, avoiding garters, and wearing only properly fitting shoes. One should also avoid undue exposure to cold and heat, trim the toenails carefully and insert a wedge of cotton under ingrowing

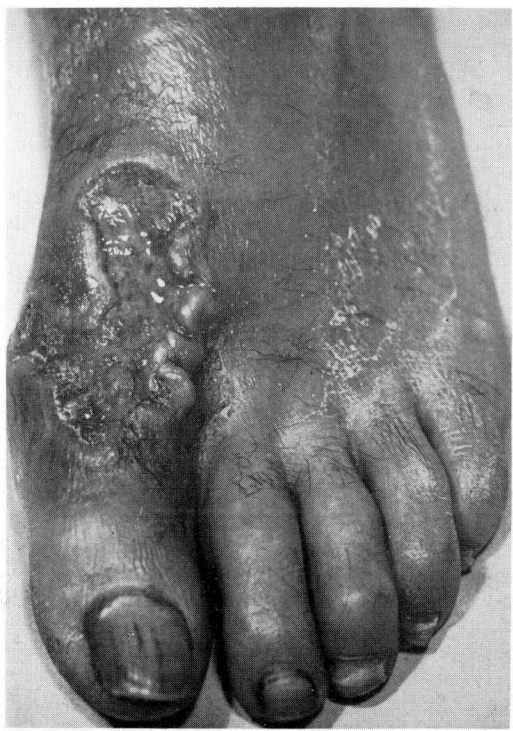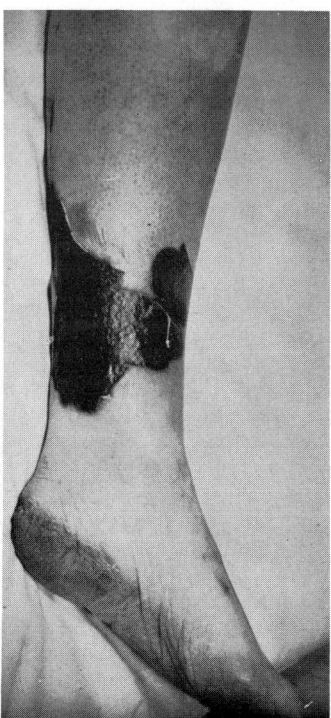

Figure 15–72. Gangrene in diabetics. *Left,* The more common type of gangrene in which only part of the foot is involved. *Right,* Gangrene due to atherosclerosis of the large arteries of the leg, involving the entire lower leg. Gangrene is over 40 times more common in diabetics than nondiabetics.

toenails, remove calluses by soaking in warm water and rubbing off the surplus skin with a coarse towel, avoiding the use of adhesive on the skin, and treating associated dermatophytoses. Despite these measures, gangrene may still occur. When present, it may be wet or dry. Since the pathology and clinical picture of these two types differ, they are discussed separately.

Dry Gangrene. This can be defined as tissue necrosis resulting from arterial occlusion. It often starts in association with trauma of a mechanical, thermal, or chemical type. The swelling induced by the injury further impairs an already poor circulation and, consequently, the tissue dies. Corns and calluses are frequently the sites at which gangrene begins. When dry gangrene appears, the patient should be kept in bed and the gangrenous area exposed to air free of dressings, antiseptics, or ointments. It is advisable to cover the foot with a cradle which will prevent pressure from the covers. The leg should be placed so that pressure to the heel is avoided. Heat should not be used because this increases the oxygen demand and thereby makes the gangrene worse. The head of the bed should be elevated slightly so that the feet are about 8 inches below the level of the heart. Buerger's exercises may be used. Salicylates or phenylbutazone (Butazolidin) is given for pain. Every effort is made to control carbohydrate metabolism. The aim in the treatment of dry gangrene is to promote mummification and a sharp line of demarcation between the dead and viable tissue. This is then followed by a conservative amputation.

Wet Gangrene. This can be defined as tissue death complicated by infection. The outcome depends on whether the trouble is caused predominantly by vascular insufficiency or by infection. Surgical drainage, antibiotics, and intermittent use of wet dressings are often employed for wet gangrene, but amputation is indicated unless the process largely clears in a couple of weeks. Roentgenograms should be taken to determine whether osteomyelitis is present. Either type of gangrene commonly requires amputation.

Kidney and Urinary Tract

Two nephropathies occur almost exclusively in diabetes: nodular glomerulosclerosis and tubular nephrosis. There are, in addition, several other renal lesions that are less specific for diabetes but that occur with increased frequency: diffuse glomerulosclerosis, atherosclerosis, arteriosclerosis, pyelonephritis, necrotizing papillitis, acute tubular necrosis, and toxemia of pregnancy.

Glomerulosclerosis (GS)

On the basis of the differences in the pathologic appearance, there are three types of GS: nodular, diffuse, and exudative.

Nodular Glomerulosclerosis. This lesion is found in about one quarter of diabetic patients dying in hospitals. It is characterized by spherical nodules 20–100 μ in diameter situated at the periphery of the glomerular capillary tufts (Fig. 15–73). They appear laminated and have one or more layers of nuclei embedded around the circumference. There are prominent reticulin fibers and deposition of significant quantities of PAS-positive glycoproteins as well as of other carbohydrates and lipids. This material by electron microscopy appears as nodular accumulations of "basement membrane" in the mesangium. This is the most specific glomerular lesion of diabetes. It has also been called Kimmelstiel-Wilson syndrome or nodular intercapillary GS. Kimmelstiel and Wilson concentrated on the nodular form,

but the more common and less specific diffuse lesion was described by Bell. It is the latter lesion that accounts for uremia in most insulin-dependent diabetes. It is desirable to drop the "intercapillary" terminology in relation to this syndrome because the changes are primarily in the mesangium.

Diffuse Glomerulosclerosis. This condition consists of thickening of the capillary basement membrane. Except in the early stages, all the loops of the glomerular tufts are involved, though not to the same degree. The capillary lumens are reduced in size and eventually become occluded. The thickened basement membrane, which is PAS-positive, then spreads to involve the endothelial cells, leading eventually to extensive diffuse deposits. In contrast to nodular GS, however, reticulin fibers are not demonstrable. This lesion is more common in diabetics than in nondiabetics, but it is less specific for diabetes than is nodular GS. It is believed that the diffuse lesion is the precursor of the nodular lesion in diabetics.

Exudative Glomerulosclerosis. This is the least common of the three lesions and the least specific for diabetes. Its mechanism and pathology appear to be entirely different. Part of the deposit is seen as a clear, intensely eosinophilic substance within Bowman's space but attached to the capsular surface of the glomerular tuft. It shows staining characteristics of fibrinoid. It does not contain collagen but does contain triglyceride, cholesterol, and PAS-positive polysaccharides. A lesion similar to the exudative type has been produced in animals by cortisone administration.

Clinical Considerations. An early diagnosis of diabetic nephropathy can be established in the relatively large proportion of the diabetics who eventually develop it by frequent evaluation of renal function. Renal biopsies of 51 diabetics — half without clinically diagnosed renal disease — were reported by Solomon. He concluded that "all patients with diabetes had some glomerular alterations." The major lesion was diffuse GS due to thickening of the capillary basement membrane and prominence of the intercapillary space or mesangium. The same material accumulated to produce nodules in the more severe cases. He found no correlation between the degree of diabetic nephropathy and the degree of systemic involvement of the cardiovascular or nervous system.

Renal disease may be expected clinically in 50% of all diabetics who survive more than 20 years; it is present pathologically in essentially all insulin-dependent diabetics who survive for 20 years. Consequently, the physician should measure the creatinine clearance every 1–2 years in all diabetics, as well as following the serum creatinine level. The urine characteristically shows proteinuria, white blood cells, and granular casts. These alterations increase in intensity as the process becomes advanced but may be detected early in the course of the disease with use of new sensitive immunoassays for urinary albumin. Eventually, hypoalbuminemia with the nephrotic syndrome, nitrogen retention, and hypertension may be observed. The degree of these changes is an indication, at least in part, of the intensity of the GS. As renal impairment becomes severe, a decrease in glycosuria may be noted. This is due partly to the decrease in glomerular filtration and the relatively greater impairment of glomerular function than of tubular function, permitting reabsorption of a greater proportion of the filtered glucose. This decrease in glycosuria may also be due to the fact that the degradation of insulin, which normally occurs to a significant extent in the kidneys, is reduced so that a given amount of insulin is more effective.

The alterations of renal function occurring with GS are not pathognomonic of this condition; therefore, it is important to be sure that renal disease in patients who have only minimal

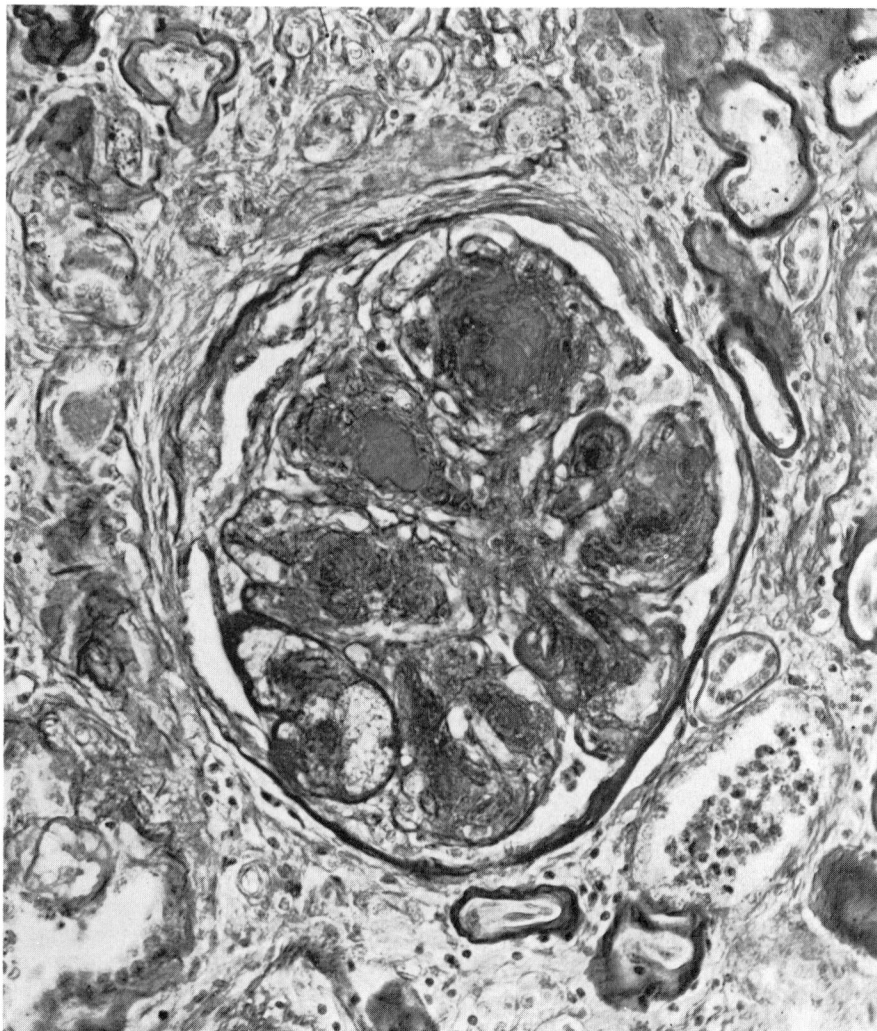

Figure 15–73. Nodular glomerulosclerosis. A considerable amount of PAS-positive material is present. Since the changes involve essentially all glomeruli, it is easy to see how the nephrotic syndrome and uremia are produced. This patient also had chronic and acute pyelonephritis, arteriosclerosis, retinopathy, neuropathy, and a small myocardial infarction. (Alcian blue PAS stain.) (Courtesy of Dr. Karl Mottet.)

hyperglycemia is really due to diabetes rather than some primary renal condition. One should (1) ascertain whether other evidence of microangiopathy is present, and (2) attempt to eliminate other nephropathies that might account for the renal changes under observation. Evidence of renal infection should be sought. It should be emphasized, however, that pyelonephritis is very commonly associated with diabetes and, indeed, often coexists with GS. Occasionally renal biopsy is indicated, since it is usually not difficult to establish the diagnosis when the tissue can be studied.

Some studies have suggested that the more poorly controlled the carbohydrate metabolism, the greater the incidence and severity of GS. However, it may be that the poor control is not due to lack of proper effort or ability on the part of either the patient or the physician; it may simply be that the diabetic process is more intense in these subjects. Moreover, the severity of the GS is not well correlated with the degree of the carbohydrate abnormality. Sometimes GS is observed even before there is evidence of hyperglycemia and glycosuria. At the other extreme, severe alterations in carbohydrate metabolism may exist over many years with no clinical or microscopic evidence of GS. In the absence of a prospective study, the relation between control of carbohydrate metabolism and nephropathy remains unclear.

As the GS progresses, the physician has the problem of dealing with the nephrotic syndrome, uremia, cardiac failure, and other manifestations of microangiopathy, such as retinopathy and blindness. Numerous symptomatic measures may be employed. Nevertheless, the disease process tends to be progressive and irreversible once it has become advanced. In recent years, chronic hemodialysis and renal transplantation have become more readily available. Since a significant number (about 40%) of deaths in juvenile-onset-type diabetes can be related to renal failure after 20–30 years of diabetes, when many of the patients are still young, an increasing number of patients are referred for treatment. However, uremia increases the risk of serious atherosclerosis, even after dialysis or transplantation. Therefore, treatment with either modality has had a high complication rate, particularly in males. Follow-up of the transplanted kidney has demonstrated evidence of asymptomatic vascular lesions within 2–3 years.

Tubular Nephrosis

In tubular nephrosis, tubular epithelial cells show vacuoles containing glycogen. These are especially common in the proximal tubules. Their presence is well correlated with the degree of hyperglycemia and is probably reversible. There does not appear to be an associated tubular functional abnormality. When GS is present, a similar peritubular PAS-positive polysaccharide is often found, possibly related to similar basement membrane thickening.

Arteriosclerosis and Atherosclerosis

Bell found severe atherosclerosis in the small renal arteries examined post mortem in 83% of diabetics over age 50. Hyalinization of the arterioles (arteriosclerosis) was equally common and tended to involve both the efferent and the afferent juxtaglomerular arterioles. The efferent arteriolar involvement is almost pathognomonic for diabetes. The renal involvement from atherosclerosis and hyaline arteriosclerosis does not appear different from this type of vascular disease seen in other organs and tissues.

Infections of the Kidney and Urinary Tract

Frequently infection develops in the kidney or urinary tract or both. It is important to detect such developments promptly and to eliminate them. The infection intensifies the manifestations of the diabetes and may also eventually lead to significant impairment in kidney function. The most important considerations are to look for and correct obstructions, to select the most appropriate antibiotic, and to give it in sufficiently large doses to eliminate the infection completely. Catheterization should be avoided as much as possible. Carefully collected clean-voided specimens can be used both for immediate direct examination and for urine cultures.

Pyelonephritis. As mentioned earlier, pyelonephritis is frequent in diabetics. When glucose is present in the urine, it may be more difficult to eradicate the infection. Under such conditions, improved carbohydrate regulation should be combined with antimicrobial therapy.

Necrotizing Renal Papillitis. This is a very acute, relatively rare form of pyelonephritis associated with severe infection, which produces ischemic necrosis of the renal papillae (Fig. 15–74). It occurs in diabetics much more often than in nondiabetics. It is characterized by fever, hematuria, renal colic, and rapidly advancing azotemia. Characteristic pyelographic changes are observed, and sloughed portions of the renal papillae may be found in the urine. The bacteria involved should be identified and treatment based upon their drug sensitivity.

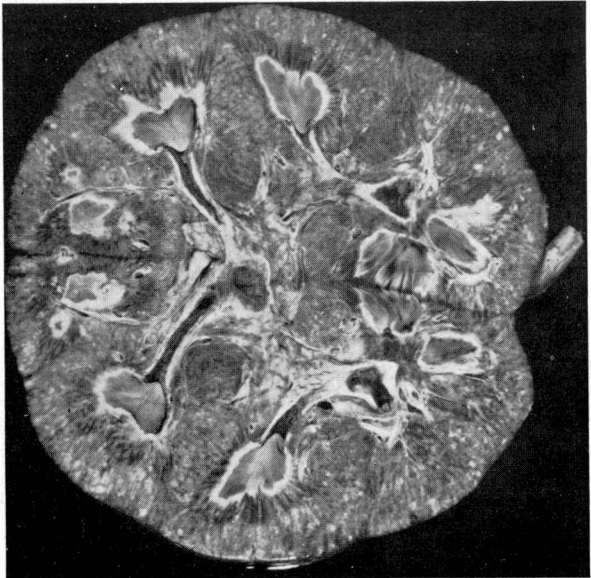

Figure 15–74. Extensive acute necrotizing renal papillitis in a diabetic. Massive infarction involves the renal papillae.

Acute Tubular Necrosis

Acute tubular necrosis occasionally occurs as a complication of diabetic coma, usually when there are prolonged periods of hypotension and shock. Acute renal failure can also be precipitated in diabetic patients with renal disease who receive injections of iodinated contrast material for diagnostic purposes. This problem has been observed following both intravenous pyelography and coronary angiography in diabetics with elevated serum creatinine levels. Thus, these diagnostic procedures should be performed only for clear indications in such patients, and these patients should be followed very carefully after the procedure for evidence of acute renal failure.

Toxemia of Pregnancy

There is an increased incidence of preeclampsia and eclampsia in diabetics. The glomeruli may become enlarged and ischemic. There is swelling of the epithelial cells, basement membrane, and endothelial cells. The major clinical changes are hypertension, proteinuria, and edema, sometimes with intermittent retinal vascular spasm.

Eye

Retina

Changes in the retina in diabetics are common and among the most characteristic findings in the syndrome. Because of the opportunity for direct observation, the changes in the eyes may be followed more easily than those in the kidneys and other tissues.

The earliest change may be a functional abnormality of the blood vessels. The capillary patterns are distorted, and the veins appear distended, tortuous, and sacculated. These changes are now known to be associated with an increased permeability of retinal capillaries. This can be demonstrated as a diffuse leak of fluorescein during angiography which can be quantitated by microfluorophotometry. The presence of severe venous dilatory changes in the retina of a young individual is almost pathognomonic for diabetes. The pathologic retinal alterations may be classified as two types: background or nonproliferative retinopathy and proliferative diabetic retinopathy. Diabetic retinopathy can usually be distinguished from other types of retinal disease (Table 15–14).

Background Retinopathy. This is the most common type of diabetic retinopathy. It is characterized by the presence of microaneurysms, edema, exudates, and small hemorrhages. All of these abnormalities are localized within the retina.

Microaneurysms. Microaneurysms tend to be among the earliest and most specific lesions in the retina (Fig. 15–75). Minute aneurysmal dilation of the capillaries, arterioles, or occasionally the venules occurs. These aneurysms average 30–90 μ in diameter. The exact mechanism for their production is not known. They progress to a thick-walled sac, which stains densely with PAS. Infiltration with lipids may be observed early in their development, and eventually thrombosis, as well as leakage and rupture, may occur. Many hypotheses have been advanced to explain this lesion, including venous stasis, hyaline deposition, capillary basement membrane thickening, a disorder of polysaccharide metabolism, and loss of mural pericytes; none has been established as the sole etiologic mechanism. However, pathologically there are several definitely associated features: (1) increased basement membrane width, (2) loss of mural cells

Table 15-14. CLINICAL PATHOLOGY OF DIABETIC RETINOPATHY

Stage	Pathologic Lesion	Source	Ophthalmoscopic Recognition
I. Diagnostic of diabetes	Central microaneurysms Central waxy exudates	Capillaries (venous), especially at bifurcations	*Punctate* lesions resembling round, dotted hemorrhages and white dots of hyalinized lesions respectively around the macula and the optic disk; a few halo hemorrhages around the microaneurysms
II. Suggestive of diabetes	Patchy hyaline exudates and confluent, round hemorrhages still mostly in the central area	Capillaries	*Confluent* patchy central lesions, including smooth, waxy, lipid exudates and hemorrhages
III. End-stage of a number of conditions other than diabetes	Venous thromboses; widespread, massive exudates; retinal and vitreous hemorrhages; new vessels arising from the disk area; retinitis proliferans; retinal detachment	Capillaries and veins	Diffuse thickening and tortuosity of retinal veins; diffuse yellow to gray exudates and circinate hemorrhages; new vessels and fibrous tissue arising from the optic disk and invading the vitreous humor; gray areas of retinal detachment and vitreous hemorrhages
Mixed stages	All of above or in varying combinations, with Stage I lesions always present	Capillaries and veins	Findings as above singly or in combination with those of Stage I present, unless obscured by subsequent changes
Associated changes: Hypertensive Renal Arteriosclerotic May occur at any time	Exudates and hemorrhages Arteriolosclerosis Arteriosclerosis	Capillaries, veins, arteries	A-V nicking; spasms of vessels; wooly exudates; striate or flame-shaped hemorrhages A-V nicking; widened light reflex

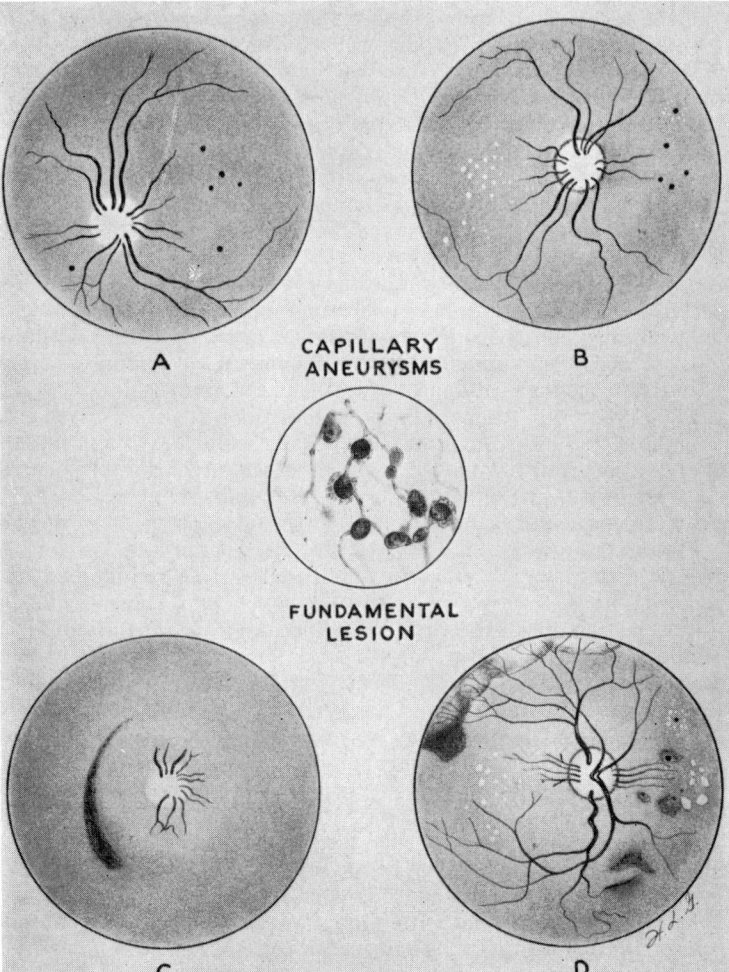

Figure 15-75. Characteristic eyeground changes in diabetic retinopathy as seen by ophthalmoscopic examination. Early punctate hemorrhages, *A* and *B* (right), with waxy, round exudates, *B* (left). *C,* Vitreous hemorrhage obscuring all but the nerve head. *D,* Proliferative retinopathy with fibrosis emanating from the nerve head; retinal detachment (top); flame-shaped hemorrhage and tortuosity of the retinal venules (below the center). The fundamental capillary lesions, the "microaneurysms," are shown in the center as they appear in a high-power microscopic view.

or pericytes, and (3) arteriolosclerosis, which is similar to that found in the kidney and elsewhere. Microaneurysms appear through the ophthalmoscope as small, round, red dots along the course of the capillaries. They tend to be most numerous in the perimacular region. They are usually associated with areas of capillary closure or occlusion. It is possible that local hypoxia stimulates their formation. Such aneurysms may occasionally occur with conditions other than diabetes, such as malignant hypertension, pernicious anemia, obstruction of the central vein, sickle cell anemia, and hypercorticosteroidism (iatrogenic or endogenous). However, they tend to be much more numerous and to occur with much greater frequency in diabetes.

Exudates and Hemorrhages. In time, the microaneurysms become more numerous. After they have been present for several months, they may even seem to be disappearing. This may be due to rupture, hemorrhage, or leakage of plasma proteins. These hemorrhages are small, localized, blot-and-dot-shaped lesions with well defined, relatively deep margins; or they may be larger, more superficial, flame-shaped lesions. Eventually these proteins are organized into deposits which consist chiefly of hyalinized material and lipids that stain heavily with PAS. The exudates are close to the microaneurysms, beginning on the vitreous side of the retina but eventually including all layers. Cotton-wool spots are sometimes visualized as white fluffy exudates even in the absence of hypertension. It has been suggested that these represent accumulation of axoplasmic debris as the result of interruption of axoplasmic transport by ischemia. Edema may be an important associated finding, particularly if the macula is involved. This causes a fuzzy or hazy appearance and is a result of an incompetent endothelial cell barrier.

Particularly in the early stages of the retinopathy, there may be a considerable period of remissions and exacerbations. The course is variable, but hemorrhages and exudates are never permanent lesions. Spontaneous improvement is common; thus, the evaluation of various treatment programs has been particularly difficult.

Maculopathy. This is a condition in which severe edema or a plaque of hard exudate impairs macula function. Usually there are associated microaneurysms and hemorrhage. It is difficult to see with the ophthalmoscope, but can be suspected when a large number of surrounding hard exudates are seen or when a sudden deterioration of vision occurs without an obvious explanation. This lesion is most commonly found in the maturity-onset diabetic, but often after less than 5 years of known diabetes duration. It can be diagnosed by fluorescein angiography and careful slit-lamp examination. Macular edema is the most common cause of decreased visual activity in diabetics, although peripheral vision is unaffected.

Proliferative Diabetic Retinopathy. In approximately 25% of diabetics with retinopathy, a proliferative change occurs. This is observed as small vessels arising from the disk or elsewhere in the retina growing along the surface of the retina and/or into the vitreous. Since background retinopathy precedes the proliferative stage, such patients usually have microaneurysms, hemorrhages, and exudates. However, these findings may seem to improve or even disappear with the development of proliferative retinopathy. Although the proliferative stage has been assumed to begin with retinal hemorrhage into the vitreous, it is now clear that vessel growth precedes such an event. Vessel growth appears to result from release of vasoproliferative factors from ischemic retinal tissue. This leads to an ingrowth of blood vessels and invasion with fibrous tissue. With contraction of the resulting scar tissue, separation of the retina and hemorrhage may occur. The hemorrhages and the neovascularization may occur anywhere in the retina, but tend

to be more numerous in the vicinity of the optic disk. A decrease or total loss of vision may result.

The proliferative changes tend to be more frequent in juvenile-onset diabetics, but this may be related to the length of time required for the changes in the retina to develop. On the average, proliferative retinopathy is found 15 years from the time of the diagnosis in younger diabetics, as opposed to only about 6-10 years in older diabetics. It therefore tends to develop in individuals with diabetes of long duration. The prognosis for vision depends on the site of the new vessels. Eyes with new vessels on the disk have a 40% chance of losing vision in 1 year. Those with peripheral lesions do better, but this complication is a major cause of severe vision loss in diabetes. Although it is particularly likely to be associated with glomerulosclerosis and other chronic manifestations of diabetes, in one-third of the patients albuminuria and hypertension are absent. Proliferative retinopathy is not absolutely specific for diabetes. It is found occasionally with retinal vein occlusion and sickle cell anemia.

Treatment of Retinopathy. The treatment of ocular concomitants of diabetes is a major therapeutic problem. Diabetic retinopathy now stands as the second leading cause of new blindness. Although data on the relationship between carbohydrate regulation and the ocular changes in diabetics are not consistent, there are reports of a significantly higher incidence of retinopathy in patients judged to have been under poor control than in those with better control. Moreover, some have found that patients under poor control have a higher incidence of the more severe forms of diabetic retinopathy. In evaluating these kinds of retrospective data, the problem is that control may have been poorer in some subjects because the disease was more fulminant.

In retrospective studies of 180 blind diabetic patients, Berkow found that the average age at onset of diabetes in the entire group was 14.6 years, and the mean age at onset of severe blindness was 31.4 years. Among 85 diabetics, the average life span after the onset of severe blindness due to diabetic retinopathy was 5.8 years. Thus, the life expectancy of a diabetic is very poor after the onset of blindness due to retinopathy. This, of course, is important in weighing the recommendation of major therapeutic procedures such as pituitary ablation.

Photocoagulation. Photocoagulation has displaced and superseded pituitary ablation in the treatment of diabetic retinopathy. The light energy of xenon, and more recently that of argon lasers, has been used to produce first a burn and then a scar in the retina by absorption of light energy by the retinal pigment epithelium. At first photocoagulation was directed toward specific abnormal areas of neovascularization and suspected bleeding sites, but later it was directed toward microaneurysms, hemorrhages, and exudates. In a symposium on photocoagulation, stabilization of angiopathy was claimed to occur in 65% of the treated eyes. Most recently retinal lesions have not been treated alone, but rather 800-2000 small retinal scars have been made by argon laser throughout the retina. The mechanism by which such scars reduce proliferative retinopathy is currently unknown. Preliminary results have been encouraging from two double-blind trials. They have carefully documented maintenance of vision with a 60% reduction in blindness in patients with new vessels on the disk in the first 2 years. The present recommendations are for treatment if there are (1) moderate or severe new vessels on or within 1 disk diameter of the optic disk, (2) mild new vessels on or within 1 disk diameter of the optic disk if fresh hemorrhage is present, or (3) moderate or severe new vessels elsewhere if fresh hemorrhage is present.

The procedure is not without its hazards, however, as

complex lesions may bleed as a result of the treatment, leading to retinal detachment and vitreous hemorrhage. Nevertheless, it is a relatively simple procedure in expert hands and has excited much enthusiasm. These encouraging results have made it more important to detect and treat such lesions before severe deterioration of vision occurs. Severe retinopathy is unlikely to occur within 5 years of diagnosis in diabetics diagnosed before the age of 25. However, after that time in young patients and in older patients, a yearly examination with pupil dilation is recommended.

Vitrectomy.   This is another promising approach for patients with diabetic retinopathy. It is a procedure requiring special technical skill in which vitreous is removed from the eye and replaced with saline. It has been used to remove blood or fibrous bands in the vitreous following retinal hemorrhage and to cut scar tissue on the retina which has caused retinal detachment. However, vitrectomy has potential serious complications including retinal tears, glaucoma, and additional retinal hemorrhage. Therefore, this procedure has generally been reserved for eyes which have already had persistent major visual loss due to vitreous hemorrhage or in which progressive traction retinal detachment is occurring.

Pituitary Ablation.   The chance observation by Poulsen of significant improvement in diabetic retinopathy of a woman who developed postpartum hypopituitarism led to the introduction of the therapeutic induction of hypopituitarism as the treatment for diabetic retinopathy. The value of this treatment has been highly controversial, but after more than 20 years of experience, certain generalizations seem to hold true. First, retinopathy often progresses after complete pituitary removal; therefore, this form of therapy can be considered only a temporary expedient. Second, there is some alleviation of the retinopathy in a substantial number of individuals in whom the procedure is performed, but this usually means no progression rather than reversal of the process. Third, since there are many complications associated with the induction of hypopituitarism in a diabetic patient, the treatment itself may be very hazardous. Fourth, although there may be improvement of the retinopathy or lack of progression, other areas of microangiopathy, as in the kidney, are not beneficially influenced by hypophysectomy. Therefore, in individuals who have severe atherosclerosis, neuropathy, or nephropathy, operative intervention is contraindicated.

The total explanation for the reported beneficial effects is unknown, but reduction of growth hormone secretion is believed to be the most important factor. The type of procedure used to produce the hypopituitarism appears to be of lesser importance than the operator's skill and experience with a specific technique. Therefore, benefits have been reported with surgical ablation, stalk section, and pituitary irradiation. Unfortunately, control studies of the effectiveness of this procedure are very few. The authors are aware of only one study in which patients were chosen randomly for follow-up or treatment, and this study involved only 12 patients (Lundbaek). Total surgical mortality has been less than 10%, and stabilization or improvement has been reported in 50–80% of subjects so treated, the variability depending primarily on the patients selected for this approach. Since stabilization or improvement in untreated patients approaches 30%, the experience with hypophysectomy has not been very encouraging. Retinal photocoagulation, which appears to be a much simpler procedure, has drastically reduced the indication for pituitary ablation. At present, the only remaining indication *may be* "florid" retinopathy in a young diabetic (Kohner).

Conjunctiva

The dilation of venules in the retinas of diabetic subjects has also been observed in the conjunctival vessels by Ditzel. In contrast to findings in normal subjects, venule diameter may vary in the course of 1 day (Fig. 15–76). Ditzel found that the early conjunctival changes consisted of elongation and distention of the venular end of the capillary. This dilation becomes more fixed as the duration of diabetes increases and tends to become irreversible in most subjects with diabetes of over 15 years' duration. At this time there tends to be sausage-shaped sacculation and actual evidence of exudation. However, the dilation is not specific for diabetes and has been observed in patients with infections of various types.

Iris

In untreated diabetes, an excess of glycogen is deposited in the pigment epithelium of the posterior surface of the iris, leading to depigmentation of that layer. This process can be seen externally and gives the iris a moth-eaten appearance. Sometimes neovascularization of the anterior surface of the iris and the anterior chamber results in a hemorrhagic glaucoma (rubeosis iridis). These changes are usually associated with proliferative retinopathy, but they are sometimes seen with central vein occlusion.

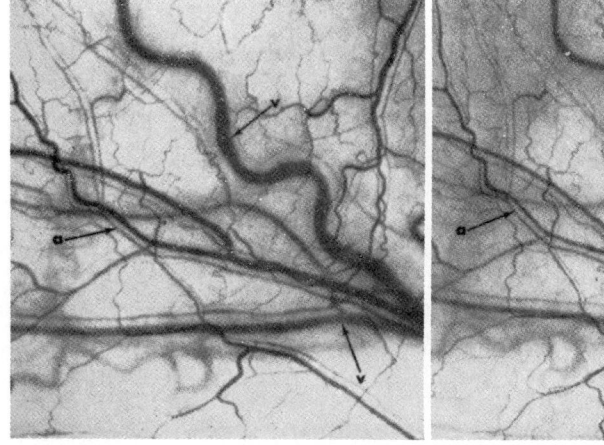

Figure 15–76. Reversibility of venular dilation and congestion between 8:00 A.M. (left) and 4:00 P.M. (right) in an insulin-treated female diabetic aged 22. (× 48.) (From Ditzel, J., et al.: Early vascular changes in diabetes mellitus. *Metabolism* 9:400, 1960.)

Lens

Abnormalities of lens function and structure are very common in diabetics. Two types of cataracts have been described in diabetics, metabolic (or snowflake) and senile. The metabolic type tends to occur particularly in the insulin-treated diabetic and may be related to the degree of glucose control. These cataracts have a snowflake appearance and start in the subcapsular region of the lens. The senile type appears more often in the elderly patient and is similar to the cataracts in nondiabetic elderly subjects. The presence of this type of cataract appears to be no more frequent in the diabetic than in the nondiabetic population, but they are said to mature more rapidly in the diabetic and lead to an increase in cataract extraction rate. Hyperglycemia alone can induce cataracts in experimental animals which are probably similar to the metabolic cataracts of the diabetic. This is one of the few instances in which a pathologic change can apparently be directly related to the carbohydrate abnormality.

The mechanism by which cataracts occur in diabetics has been clarified by studies of lens metabolism. These studies have indicated that the relatively poorly transported sugar alcohol sorbitol is present in high concentrations when cataracts have been induced by high extracellular glucose levels. Aldose reductase is the enzyme responsible for the reduction of glucose to sorbitol and is known to be present in lens tissue. It is apparently the presence of the same enzyme that is responsible for the conversion of galactose to its polyol and which in turn may be responsible for cataract formation in galactosemia. In euglycemic individuals there is no buildup of the polyol because the production of sorbitol is limited, and there is time for its further oxidation to fructose by the enzyme sorbitol dehydrogenase. In contrast, in the hyperglycemic state intracellular glucose levels increase in insulin-independent tissues, thereby increasing the production of sorbitol. This increase in production raises tissue levels markedly, apparently because of the relatively slow further metabolism to fructose. These two factors combined are responsible for the high sorbitol levels. It has been hypothesized that sorbitol increases intracellular osmolarity and subsequent water uptake, which directly or via changes in myoinositol metabolism promotes cataract formation. A similar metabolic pathway (the polyol pathway) in peripheral nerves has been described by Gabbay and may contribute to some of the neural abnormalities found in diabetes.

Alterations in accommodation and in refraction are also often observed, particularly in insulin-treated diabetics. These abnormalities are most likely related to osmotic changes in the lens, but some of them are possibly due to metabolic alterations of the ciliary body. Myopia may suddenly appear, as may other refractive alterations. These changes in accommodation and in refraction tend to be corrected rapidly by an improvement in the carbohydrate abnormality. For this reason, changes in the patient's glasses should not be prescribed until a steady state of regulation of the carbohydrate metabolism has been attained.

Nervous System

The neuropathic disturbances can be classified into five groups: radiculopathy, mononeuropathy, polyneuropathy, amyotrophy, and autonomic neuropathy (Fig. 15–77).

Radiculopathy

Diabetic radiculopathy is an infrequent form of peripheral neuropathy. The disorder is characterized by lancinating pain in the distribution of a single dermatome. When it involves a root of brachial or lumbar distribution, distinction from a herniated nucleus pulposus is sometimes difficult. When nerve roots are affected near the dorsal root ganglion, proximal degeneration may ensue. This results in a loss of

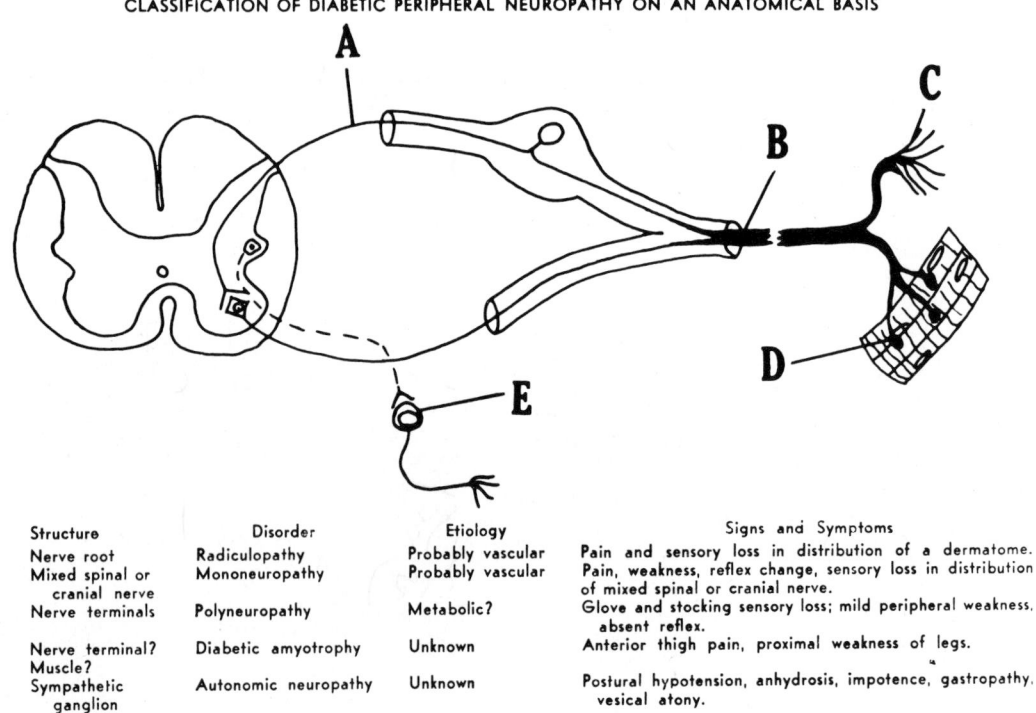

CLASSIFICATION OF DIABETIC PERIPHERAL NEUROPATHY ON AN ANATOMICAL BASIS

	Structure	Disorder	Etiology	Signs and Symptoms
A	Nerve root	Radiculopathy	Probably vascular	Pain and sensory loss in distribution of a dermatome.
B	Mixed spinal or cranial nerve	Mononeuropathy	Probably vascular	Pain, weakness, reflex change, sensory loss in distribution of mixed spinal or cranial nerve.
C	Nerve terminals	Polyneuropathy	Metabolic?	Glove and stocking sensory loss; mild peripheral weakness, absent reflex.
D	Nerve terminal? Muscle?	Diabetic amyotrophy	Unknown	Anterior thigh pain, proximal weakness of legs.
E	Sympathetic ganglion	Autonomic neuropathy	Unknown	Postural hypotension, anhydrosis, impotence, gastropathy, vesical atony.

Figure 15–77. Diabetic peripheral neuropathy. (From Locke, S.: The peripheral nervous system in diabetes mellitus. *Diabetes 13*:307, 1964.)

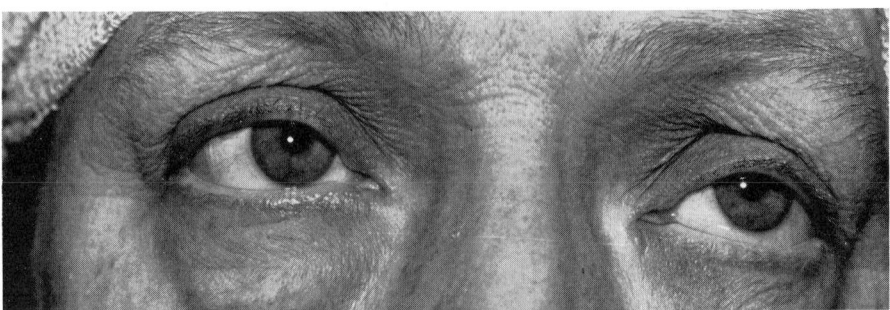

Figure 15–78. Paresis of external rotation of the left eye of a patient, aged 55, with diabetes of 20 years' duration. Function is usually regained within a few months.

myelin and axis cylinders in the posterior columns of the spinal cord and is associated with impairment of position sense, positive Romberg's sign, and loss of deep tendon reflexes. When pupillary abnormalities are noted in association with this disorder, the patient with lancinating pain may be diagnosed as having diabetic pseudotabes.

Mononeuropathy

Mononeuropathy, in contrast to radiculopathy, affects a major nerve trunk. It has often been assumed that the lesion involves a larger blood vessel than in the radicular syndrome, but a vascular basis for this lesion has never been proved. Pain may be prominent; sensory loss, motor weakness, and deprivation of sympathetic innervation in the distribution of a major spinal or cranial nerve contribute to the symptomatology. Clinically, there is acute onset of weakness or sensory loss in an arm or leg. Corresponding to this there is an absence of the appropriate reflex. Palpation of the nerve may disclose striking tenderness. The spinal fluid appears unremarkable. Spontaneous recovery is the rule.

Cranial nerve palsies belong to this group. Involvement of the third, fifth, sixth, seventh, eighth, tenth, and twelfth cranial nerves has been reported, but rarely are any of the nerves affected except those influencing facial contractions and extraocular movements. The third and the sixth nerves are most often involved. Paralysis of the extraocular movements occurs in approximately 1% of the diabetics and is in large part confined to patients over age 50 with longstanding diabetes. Diplopia and ptosis are two common manifestations (Fig. 15–78). The paralysis is associated with retrobulbar pain and pain in the forehead on the affected side. The prognosis is good, with most patients recovering in 2–3 months.

Polyneuropathy

The most frequent form of diabetic neuropathy is the distal, bilateral, comparatively symmetric polyneuropathy, which is clinically predominantly sensory, but electrophysiologically both motor and sensory. The sensory loss and associated motor weakness do not conform to the distribution of a single nerve root or peripheral nerve but involve the distribution of overlapping peripheral terminals of many segmental nerves. Since the longest nerves are most affected, symptoms appear earlier and more severely in the feet. The sensory loss is greatest in the most peripheral portion and less proximally. This produces the so-called *"glove-and-stocking"* loss of sensation which characterizes the disorder. Symptoms may be scarce, and in the early stages many patients are unaware of the sensory disturbance until their attention is called to it by the examiner. Despite the defect in sensory perception, lancinating pain

radiating down the leg or occasionally in the arms, particularly at night, may be a disabling symptom. There is often an associated dysesthesia, particularly on the soles of the feet, with complaints of burning or itching or extreme sensitivity of the skin to touch with an unpleasant feeling. An early finding is loss of deep reflexes of the ankle or knee. There is diminished vibration sense and touch, but these are not well delineated and are difficult to quantify. If available, biothesiometry can be used to quantitate the abnormality of vibration sense. The small muscles of the hands and feet may become weak and atrophy, leading to subtle but rather characteristic functional changes (Fig. 15–79).

Nerve conduction velocity is symmetrically and diffusely reduced in affected patients, but nerve conduction is also often reduced in patients without obvious clinical evidence of neuropathy. Interestingly, motor nerves are often better for study, and the median motor nerve of the upper limb is more reliable than the tibial or peroneal nerve of the lower limb, despite the greater symptomatology of the sensory system of the leg. Trophic changes of the extremities may be associated with a distal polyneuropathy. The feet are often cold and blue with shiny, thin skin and loss of hair. Owing to the associated autonomic neuropathy, there may be anhidrosis. Perforating neurotrophic ulcers and Charcot's joints can be related to the lack of sensation (Fig. 15–80).

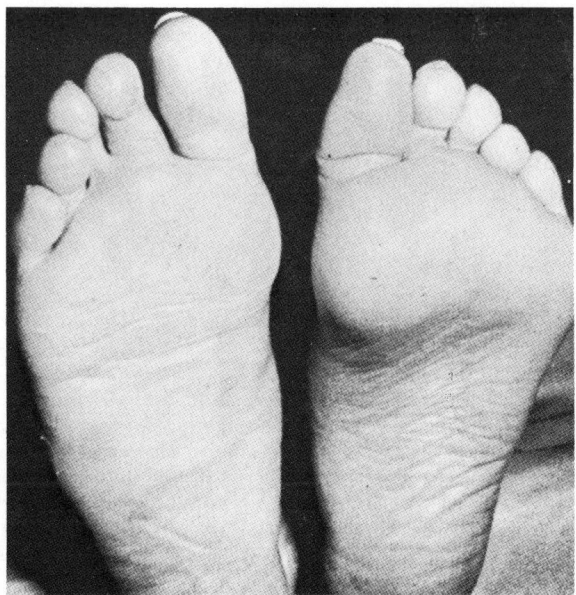

Figure 15–79. The diabetic foot on the left, compared with the normal foot on the right. Note the loss of small muscle function leading to the characteristic flattening of the arch and retraction of the toes. (Courtesy of M. Ellenberg.)

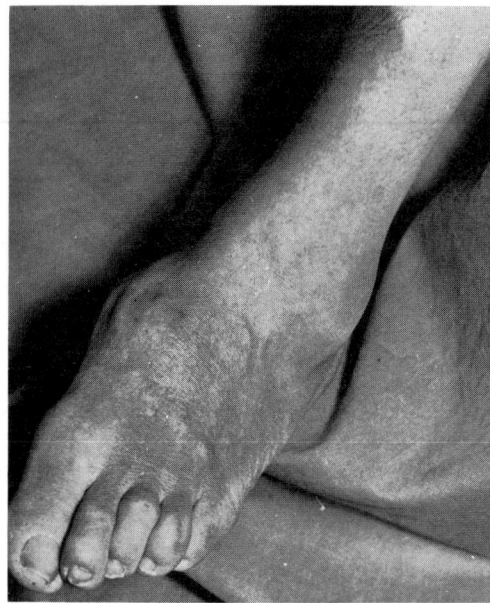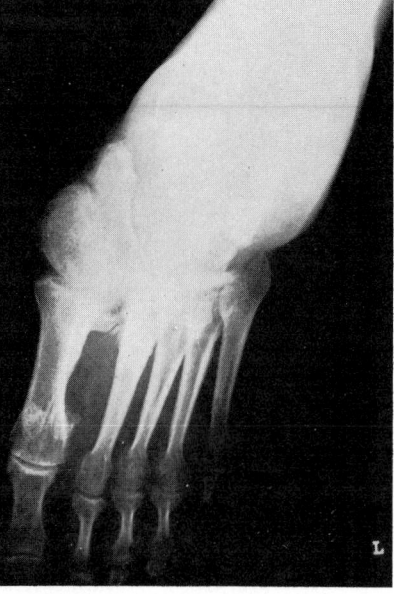

Figure 15–80. Diabetic neuropathy with Charcot type of joints. The patient was 65 years old and had mild diabetes of unknown duration — probably many years. In diabetes, contrary to syphilis, the Charcot type of joint change is much commoner in distal joints than in proximal.

Treatment. Treatment of this diffuse neuropathy is never very satisfactory. Recent evidence suggests that reduction of plasma glucose is associated with an increase of motor nerve conduction velocity, suggesting that better diabetes control may be important to prevention. However, it is sometimes observed that the symptoms get worse after the beginning of treatment. The explanation for the pain and dysesthesia is unknown, and their relation to the diffuse loss of afferent sensory nerve function is not completely clear. Treatment of these complaints is purely symptomatic and may require narcotic analgesics. A number of drugs can be tried, but the course of painful neuropathy is so variable that they are difficult to evaluate. Phenytoin (Dilantin) 300 mg/day can be tried for patients with lancinating leg pains. It is either effective within a week or two or of no value at all. Recently, fluphenazine and amitryptiline alone or in combination have been offered. These are toxic drugs and must be used with caution. The natural history seems to be slow progression of neuropathy with oscillating symptoms of pain, dysesthesia, and weakness. It is critical for the patient to be aware of his sensory loss to minimize injury, particularly to the lower leg and foot. Any minor ulceration should be promptly treated. If it is not infected and not ischemic, reduction of trauma or weight bearing is usually very effective. At times, special shoes to redistribute weight-bearing surfaces may be necessary.

Amyotrophy

The syndrome of diabetic amyotrophy is found characteristically in elderly men with mild abnormalities of glucose metabolism. In this syndrome a prominent weakness of the iliopsoas, quadriceps, gluteal, and hamstring muscles with muscle wasting, fasciculation, weight loss, and myalgia is associated with dysesthesias of the anterior thigh, extensor plantar responses, and an ill defined sensory loss to pin prick. This disease may be difficult to distinguish from a number of other neuropathies and myopathies. The spinal fluid protein may reach levels as high as 200 mg/dl in diabetic amyotrophy. The electromyogram suggests primary muscle disease as well as the neurogenic lesion. Muscle biopsy reveals a characteristic pattern of single-fiber atrophy. Severe weight loss or diabetic cachexia may be a prominent finding. The symptoms often improve within 18–24 months.

Autonomic Neuropathy

It has become apparent that the autonomic nervous system is involved diffusely, and often early, in the course of diabetes, although in general there is a relationship between the duration of the disease and the severity of the autonomic neuropathy. When the viscera are involved, it may be difficult to distinguish this syndrome clinically from an intrinsic lesion of the organ.

Gastrointestinal Tract. Gastroparesis similar to that found after vagotomy has been observed and results in a dilated stomach and slow peristalsis (Fig. 15–81). Gallbladder dysfunction has also been attributed to autonomic neuropathy, but lacking any way of specifically delineating the neurologic lesion, it is difficult to determine whether such a lesion exists in any given patient. Nocturnal diarrhea is another feature associated with autonomic neuropathy. It must be differentiated from steatorrhea from pancreatic insufficiency or celiac sprue, which may both be found in diabetic patients. Occasionally small bowel stasis leads to bacterial overgrowth. The associated diarrhea will respond to broad-spectrum antibiotics, but this is often not the case and one is left with unexplained diarrhea in a diabetic with other signs and symptoms of autonomic neuropathy. Relief of some of these symptoms and improvement of erratic diabetes control has been reported after the drug metoclopramide has been given. Because jejunal biopsy usually reveals normal mucosa, it is assumed that nocturnal diarrhea is related to an associated neurologic abnormality leading to excess water loss in the colon. Although many drugs which suppress intestinal motility have been tried, we find codeine to be superior to the others. Diabetic diarrhea is a distressing problem, and its clinical fluctuations are often hard to explain.

Urogenital System. Urinary retention due to an atonic bladder may contribute to the urinary tract infections found so commonly in the older diabetic. It is often possible to elicit a history of increasing periods between micturition, weakness of stream, a muted sensation of bladder fullness, and incontinence. A voiding urogram demonstrating reten-

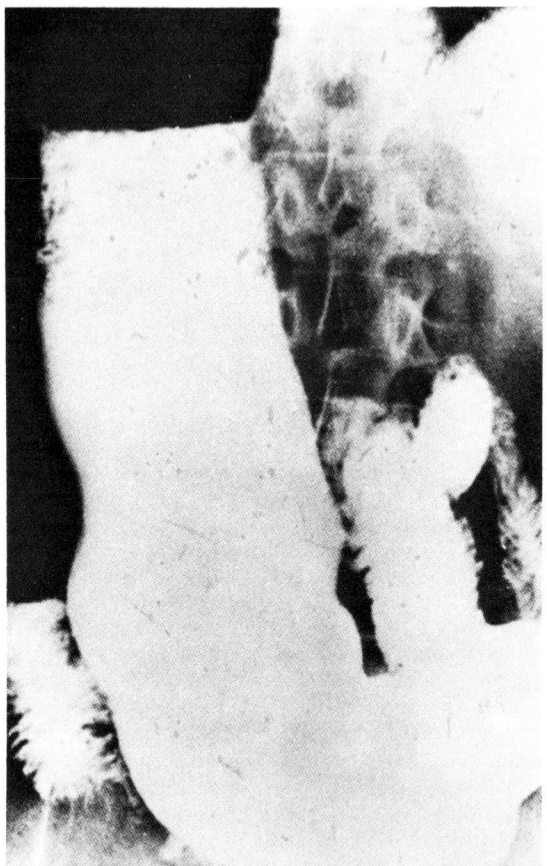

Figure 15–81. Massive distention of the stomach in diabetes mellitus. This has been called gastroparesis and is a consequence of autonomic neuropathy. (Courtesy of M. Ellenberg.)

tion and/or an abnormal cystometrogram may be needed to establish the diagnosis (Fig. 15–82). Drugs which increase bladder tone such as bethanechol (Urecholine) are helpful early on; however, male diabetics who have repeated infections or a large residual volume despite treatment generally require transurethral resection of the prostate. Recent studies suggest that abnormalities of bladder sensation and neural responses to stimulation occur early and commonly in diabetes prior to symptomatic bladder dysfunction. Therefore, the clinician should be aware that decompensation (urinary retention) is probably a late stage of this disorder.

Sexual impotence in the male is now recognized as perhaps the *most common* symptom of autonomic neuropathy in diabetes. It has been partly overlooked in the past, mainly because of poor history taking. Recent studies have reported impotence in as many as 60% of patients within 5 years of diagnosis of diabetes. The major problem is slow loss of erectile function due to diminished parasympathetic function. Orgasm may still be possible early on, but soon is lost because of either secondary failure or later sympathetic nervous system abnormalities. An accurate diagnosis and counseling are important. Psychogenic impotence can usually be distinguished by a careful history. It is typified by its selectivity and periodicity, the presence of morning erections, and the ability to masturbate successfully. Diabetic impotence is a slow and ongoing process. There is usually not a loss of libido. The measurement of overnight penile tumescence by mercury strain gauge can be very helpful in documenting the abnormality (Fig. 15–83). Plasma levels of testosterone, LH, and FSH are usually, but not always, normal. Even if there are some abnormalities of the regulation of these reproductive hormones, testosterone treatment has not often proved useful.

A frank discussion of sexual function is critical for every diabetic patient, as serious marital discord and insecurity

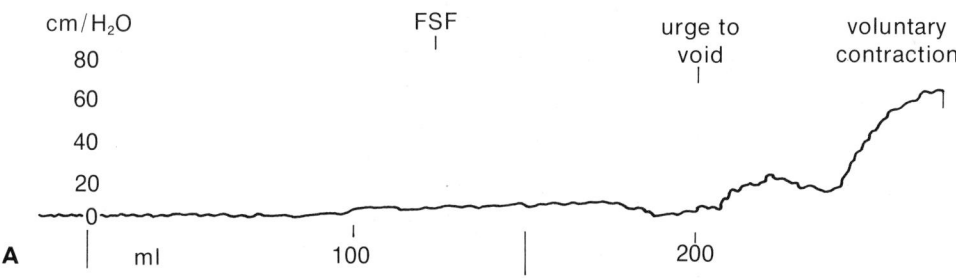

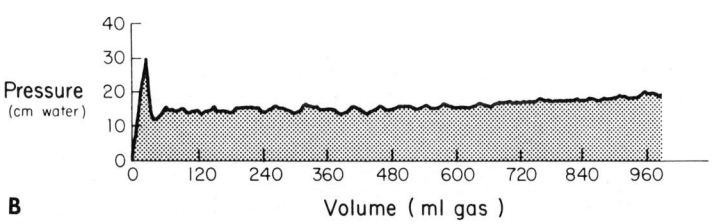

Figure 15–82. *A*, Normal cystomegtrogram. Note bladder contraction and pressure rise after 250 ml. *B*, Cystometrogram from a diabetic patient with severe vesicular dysfunction. Note the minimal change in pressure as the bladder is filled with 1000 ml. (From Blaivas, J. G., et al., In *Clinical Neuro-Urology.* Krane, R. J., and Siroky, M. B. (eds.), Boston, Little, Brown & Co., 1979.)

Typical (condensed) NPT patterns:

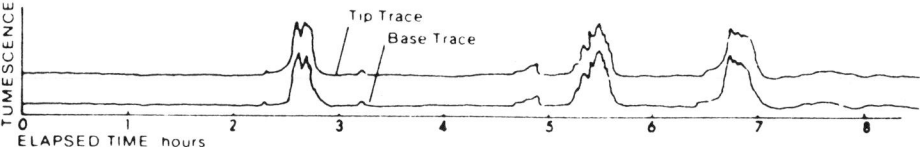

This tracing indicates significant tumescence activity. Organic impotence can be ruled out.

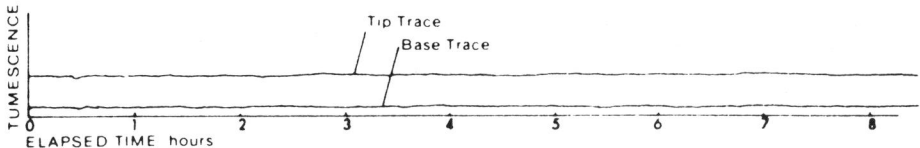

Figure 15–83. Penile tumescence recorded overnight. Normal subject at top, diabetic with impotence at bottom. Note the lack of any tumescence in this clear-cut example of organic impotence. (From Furlow, W. L., et al., In *Clinical Neuro-Urology*. Krane, R. J. and Siroky, M. B. (eds.), Boston, Little, Brown & Co., 1979.)

may result without it. Silicone penile prostheses have been implanted in some patients to allow maintenance of some sexual function. These carry a risk of infection and may be painful, but have often been effective and important to the conjugal pair.

Cardiovascular System. Autonomic control of the heart and resistance vessels is often abnormal in diabetes. Tests of heart rate response to respiration and the Valsalva maneuver suggest an early abnormality of vagal nerve function. The most sensitive index is the measurement of beat-to-beat variation of heart rate during deep breathing. Owing to cyclic vagal tone, the heart rate varies by more than 15 beats per minute in normal persons under age 50. This heart-rate variation is abolished by atropine and is reduced in diabetics (Fig. 15–84). Diminished sympathetic tone is probably also present. Total autonomic denervation of the heart has been reported. As a result of these changes, resting tachycardia is common.

Assumption of upright posture may be followed by hypotension in diabetics with autonomic dysfunction. This is best assessed by measuring blood pressure *2 minutes* after standing. A drop in mean arterial pressure (diastolic pressure + one-third of the pulse pressure) of more than 10 mm Hg is abnormal. Plasma catecholamine responses are highly variable. In some patients with autonomic neuropathy both the basal level and the response are low, while in others the basal level and the response may be normal or even elevated (Cryer). Because the stimulus is greater than normal in such patients (a lower blood pressure), the plasma catecholamine responses alone are probably not a reliable index of the adequacy of vasomotor tone. Heart rate responses may be delayed, but also may appear relatively normal shortly after standing — probably because of the greater fall in blood pressure which provides a greater stimulus. These findings emphasize the difficulty in assessing autonomic function by the use of a reflex in which the clinician is unable to control the strength of stimulation.

Insulin administration has recently been shown to produce direct cardiovascular effects. After injection of a large bolus, there is an increase in heart rate. This response is not

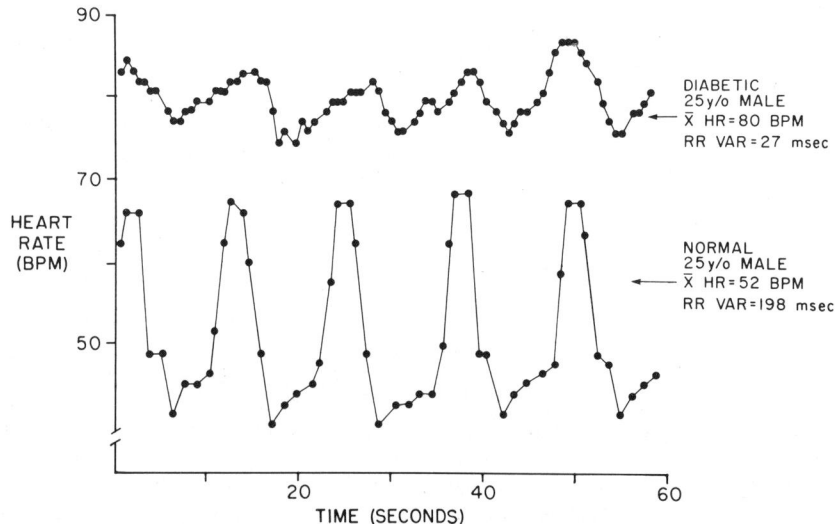

Figure 15–84. Beat-to-beat variation (RR VAR) in heart rate. A 25-year-old man with diabetes of 10 years' duration compared with an aged-matched control. Note the faster rate and reduced variation. Both are characteristic of loss of vagal function. (Courtesy of Michael A. Pfeifer, M.D.)

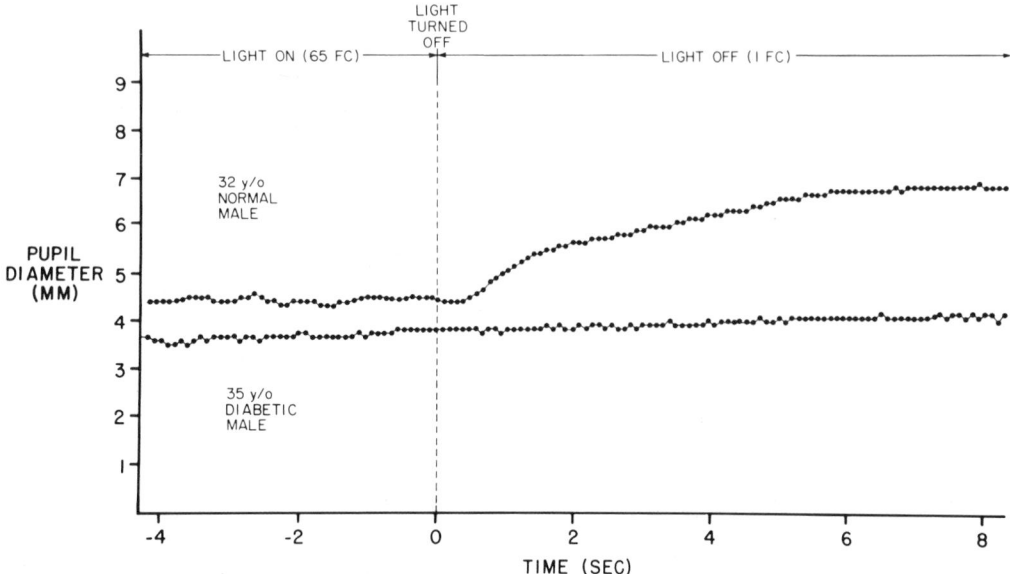

Figure 15–85. Pupil function in diabetic neuropathy. Pupillary dilation during the dark is absent in the diabetic owing to loss of sympathetic pupillary dilator tone. Resting pupil size in the light may also be smaller for the same reason. (Courtesy of Michael A. Pfeifer, M.D.)

due to hypoglycemia, but to arterial vasodilation, a reduction in plasma volume and venous return, or both. In patients with intact cardiovascular reflexes blood pressure is maintained as the heart rate (and probably vasomotor tone) is increased. In diabetics with autonomic neuropathy, the blood pressure may drop as a result of inadequate compensation, and this may lead to fainting in the upright position. This response can simulate hypoglycemia in an insulin-treated patient and cause the patient and his doctor considerable confusion.

In patients with severe autonomic problems cardiorespiratory arrest has occurred, often in association with anesthesia for minor operations. We now recognize that some anesthetics such as barbiturates and halothane suppress autonomic nervous system tone. It is possible that patients with autonomic neuropathy are supersensitive to this effect. There is also evidence of altered respiratory center function during vagal blockade, which may contribute. Sudden unexplained death has been reported in such patients.

Treatment of postural hypotension involves awareness on the part of the patient of the need to change position slowly and of the potential effects of insulin injection. It may be necessary to use elastic stockings to minimize venous pooling, or to add mineralocorticoids such as 9-α-fluorohydrocortisone to the regimen. These patients should avoid autonomic blocking drugs, since intrinsic heart disease is common and heart failure may be precipitated by treatment. Finding the proper balance may be quite difficult.

Sweat Glands. These glands are innervated by *cholinergic* sympathetic fibers. Loss of normal responses to increased environmental temperature is part of the symptomatology of diabetic autonomic neuropathy. The loss is usually bilateral, and more often peripheral in the legs and arms, but may involve the trunk or face. Patients may complain of heat intolerance and loss of sweating, but many complain of *excessive* sweating in uninvolved areas. Gustatory sweating may occur, since food ingestion may increase body heat production. Skin temperature may show abnormal patterns owing to loss of vasomotor tone; therefore, the feet may be unusually warm, but be unable to sweat.

Pupil. The pupil size is totally controlled by autonomic fibers. Light stimulation causes pupillary constriction via parasympathetic pathways. This is balanced by sympathetic α-adrenergic dilator tone related to arousal and mental-emotional state. In diabetics pupil size may be small and irregular, and the reactions to light and to dark may be sluggish because of impaired input from both systems (Fig. 15–85). Infrequently, a true Argyll-Robertson pupil can be found.

Spinal Fluid Changes

Approximately 70% of patients with diabetic neuropathy have an increase in spinal fluid protein (50–100 mg/100 ml). This protein presumably arises from the damage to nerve roots adjacent to the spinal cord.

Spinal Cord Disease

Diabetic myelopathy is rare, but it has been found occasionally. The spinal cord may show segmentally localized degeneration in the posterior columns, and localized necrosis and degenerative changes in the lateral columns as well. Thickening and hyalinization of the arterioles in the involved areas have been observed. The symptomatology is determined by the site and extent of involvement.

Skin

Three types of skin lesions have been found with a high degree of frequency in diabetes mellitus and have at one time or another been considered specific for it; hence the names diabetic dermopathy, necrobiosis lipoidica diabeticorum, and xanthoma diabeticorum. None of these lesions is absolutely specific for diabetes, and at times questions have been raised whether they are even more frequent in the diabetic population. Most studies seem to show that they are, but it is clear that none of these lesions can be considered specific for diabetes mellitus.

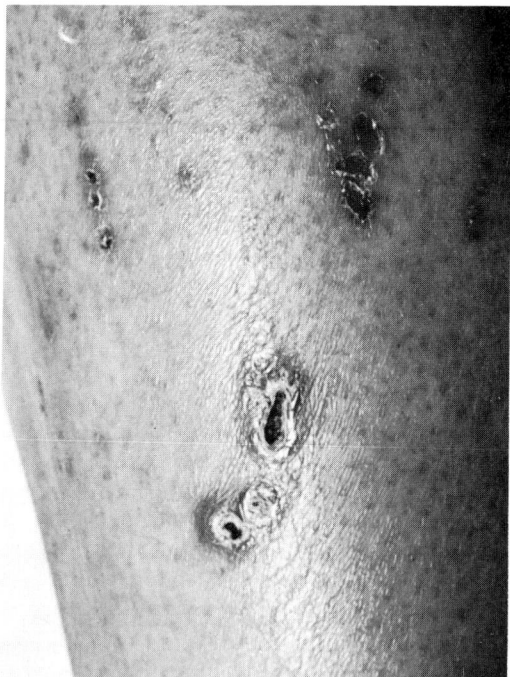

Figure 15–86. Early lesions of dermopathy showing central crusting; in this patient the lesions appear in a somewhat linear arrangement. (From Binkley, G. W.: Dermopathy in the diabetic syndrome. *Arch. Derm., 92*:625, 1965.)

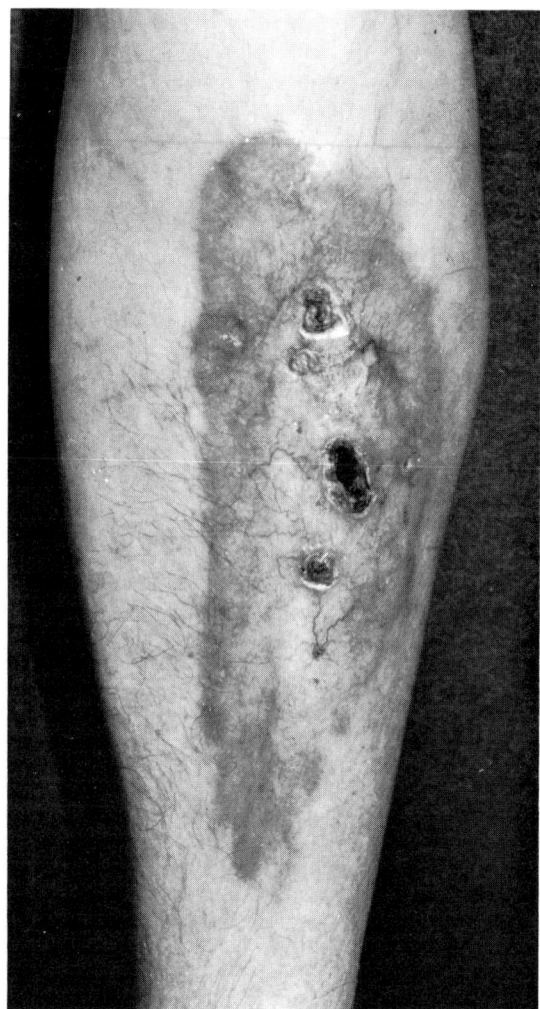

Figure 15–87. Extensive dry ulcerative plaque of necrobiosis lipoidica diabeticorum. (Courtesy of Dr. George Odland.)

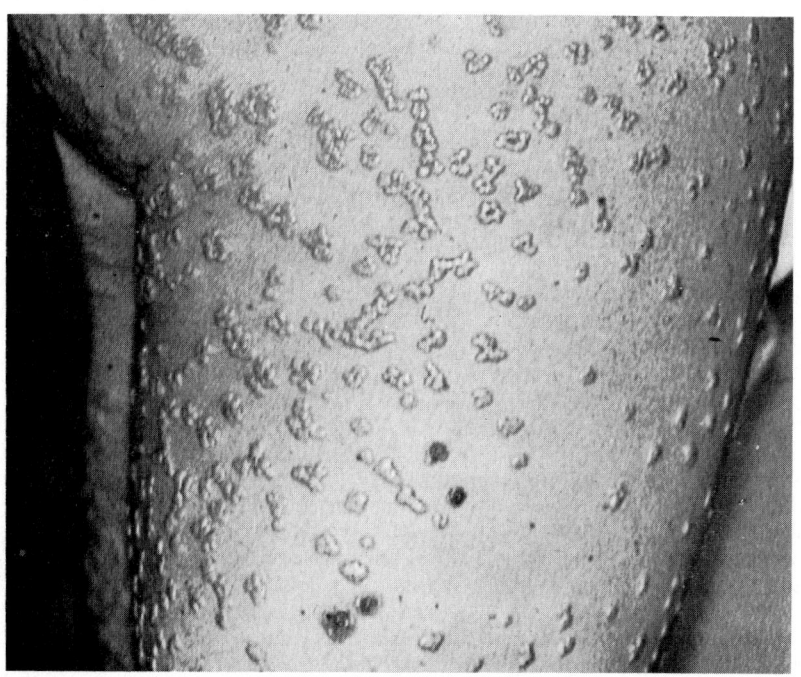

Figure 15–88. Xanthoma diabeticorum. These eruptive xanthomas, composed chiefly of lipid deposits, are not confined to diabetics.

Diabetic Dermopathy

The lesion has been described by Binkley to consist of red or red-brown papules that evolve into sharply circumscribed atrophic patches, usually located in the pretibial area (Fig. 15–86). They are often hyperpigmented and scaly. It was thought the skin lesions were similar to other microangiopathic changes in diabetes mellitus; however, Danowski has been unable to confirm this, and he reports finding similar lesions in a fair number of normal individuals and in subjects with a variety of other endocrine disorders with no abnormality of glucose tolerance.

Necrobiosis Lipoidica Diabeticorum

This lesion occurs in the same location and is described as a sharply bordered, plaquelike lesion, beginning as a red or red-brown lesion, which eventually expands to form a shiny atrophic plaque (Fig. 15–87). Dermal vessels become sclerotic, and an obliterative endarteritis occurs.

Xanthoma Diabeticorum

This term is used to describe typical eruptive xanthomas which arise whenever chylomicronemia occurs in the presence of uncontrolled diabetes mellitus (Fig. 15–88). These lesions are seen in the syndrome of diabetic lipemia and are identical to those found whenever chylomicrons are circulating in very high concentrations from any cause; therefore, these xanthomas are not specific for diabetes mellitus. Physically they are small red-yellow papules that arise in crops and have an erythematous base. They develop primarily on the buttocks, elbows, and backs of the thighs — the extensor surfaces. Chemical analysis has revealed typical chylomicron triglyceride and fatty acids.

Skin Infection

It is not clear whether patients with diabetes mellitus are more likely to have bacterial or mycotic infections, but it is generally agreed that when such infections occur, they are more difficult to control than in nonhyperglycemic individuals. Perineal pruritus in a diabetic is almost always associated with *Candida albicans* and occurs in both the pregnant and nonpregnant female. Glycosuria seems to be an important factor in the maintenance of the lesion; however, Candida infection may occur on other areas of the body, most usually in the intertriginous regions.

The occurrence of a fungal infection of the interdigital areas in the diabetic can be a problem because the epidermal fissures and erosions serve as portals of entry for other organisms which can lead to cellulitis and gangrene. Prophylaxis should be used in all diabetics and prompt treatment started to eradicate the fungus, either with local agents if the infection is minor or with systemic antifungal agents for well entrenched, longstanding problems.

Immune System

Granulocyte function may be impaired in diabetes. This abnormality is corrected by treatment of the hyperglycemia. Chemotaxis, phagocytosis, and intracellular killing are all impaired. These cells are known to have insulin receptors; therefore, it is likely that these abnormalities are a direct consequence of insulin lack. Reticuloendothelial system function has also been reported to be abnormal. T-lymphocyte and B-lymphocyte activity is probably reduced secondary to insulin deficiency, and monocytes have also been shown to have insulin receptors. Despite these abnormalities and the clinical description of increased number and severity of a variety of infections, it has been difficult to prove an increased infection rate in diabetes. Rather, it seems that once the barriers to infection have been breached, diabetics respond less well than normal subjects. At present the evidence suggests that good control with insulin treatment is important during infections in diabetic patients.

Hyperlipoproteinemia

Hypercholesterolemia and/or hypertriglyceridemia is common in diabetes mellitus. This abnormality has many different causes, and it is important to segregate them out. In general, it is assumed that hyperlipidemia is a risk factor for atherosclerosis and participates in the increased incidence of macrovascular disease in diabetes mellitus. Occasionally, hypertriglyceridemia may become so severe (>1500 mg/dl) that there is the additional threat of pancreatitis as a direct result.

Juvenile-Onset-Type Diabetes Mellitus. Hyperlipidemia in patients with juvenile-onset-type, insulin-dependent diabetes seems to be secondary to insulin deficiency. The primary problem is a deficiency of activity of lipoprotein lipase, the enzyme responsible for the hydrolysis of triglyceride from the very low density lipoproteins (VLDL) and chylomicrons. As a result, there is an increase in these lipoproteins until their concentration is high enough to overcome the removal block. At this point, there is a coexistent deficiency of high density lipoproteins (HDL), since they originate in part in VLDL, but a normal turnover rate of triglyceride. It has also been reported that hypercholesterolemia and an increase in low density lipoprotein (LDL) levels are present. The frequency of this finding has been quite variable. This may be due in part to the variable use in the past of high-fat, cholesterol-rich diets for dietary management of some diabetics. In addition, there may be some alteration in the LDL receptor–mediated cholesterol-removal mechanism, which varies either with the degree of insulin deficiency or with the patient type. Regardless, the degree of hypercholesterolemia due to an abnormality of LDL metabolism is small compared with the major effects of insulin deficiency to impair lipoprotein lipase activity and elevate VLDL and chylomicron triglyceride-rich lipoproteins.

During insulin treatment, lipoprotein lipase activity increases and triglyceride levels fall, so that in well treated patients, both VLDL and LDL levels are restored to normal values. The response takes weeks to months and will fluctuate if plasma glucose control varies. Recently, some evidence has been presented to suggest that lipoprotein lipase activity in adipose tissue and HDL levels may become "supernormal" in very tightly controlled patients. This finding suggests that achievement of euglycemia in such very well controlled insulin-treated patients results from maintaining peripheral hyperinsulinemia. Whether this will have adverse side effects is not clear at present.

The presence of defective lipoprotein-removal mechanisms in insulin-deficient patients also makes them more susceptible to any other cause of hyperlipidemia. The most common are alcohol-induced hyperlipidemia, estrogen-induced hyperlipidemia, hyperlipidemia secondary to hypothyroidism, uremia, or the nephrotic syndrome, and the presence of any of the familial hyperlipidemias. These interactions can cause severe hyperlipidemia and are discussed more fully in Chapt r 17.

Maturity-Onset-Type Diabetes Mellitus. The interactions between lipoprotein lipase deficiency and LDL receptor–removal problems due to insulin deficiency are much more complex in maturity-onset-type diabetics. This is largely because of the associated obesity which can markedly aggravate the removal problem by increasing lipoprotein synthesis. Complexity is also greater because of the relatively high frequency of familial hyperlipidemia and maturity-onset-type diabetes in the same family. While the evidence suggests that these are two independently segregating familial syndromes, they often coexist. When this happens, the individual with both disorders is more likely to have severe, symptomatic hyperlipoproteinemia and therefore is more likely to be referred to a physician. In addition, alcohol, estrogen, thyroid deficiency, uremia, and the nephrotic syndrome will all interact with the hyperglycemia in maturity-onset-type diabetes to exacerbate the lipoprotein abnormality. Again, evidence now suggests that persistent reduction of plasma glucose for 2–3 months is required before these other complicating factors can be fully evaluated. It is a general rule of thumb that any diabetic with a plasma triglyceride level greater than 1000 mg/dl has at least one other cause for the hyperlipidemia. A full discussion of hyperlipidemia, its etiology, and treatment is given in Chapter 17.

Diabetic Ketoacidosis (DKA)

DKA is a profound alteration of metabolism resulting from a deficiency of insulin action. This deficiency of insulin action leads to hyperglycemia, increased lipolysis, ketogenesis, systemic acidosis, and depletion of intracellular and extracellular water and electrolytes. Intimately associated with the development of DKA, and contributing to many of the findings, is increased secretion of the stress-related hormones: catecholamines, glucagon, cortisol, and growth hormone. Severe DKA can result in deep coma and, in the period before the discovery of insulin, was uniformly fatal. Although this condition is now treatable, most series continue to report death rates in the range of 5–10%. A patient who has had a clear-cut episode of DKA is generally classified as being an insulin-dependent juvenile-onset-type diabetic.

Pathogenesis

DKA results from a complex interplay among insulin deficiency, increased stress hormone levels, and intravascular volume depletion. As illustrated in Figures 15–89 and 15–90, the manifestations of this interaction include hyperglycemia, hyperosmolality, and ketonemia, the cardinal features of DKA.

Insulin Deficiency

The mechanism by which insulin deficiency occurs in patients with DKA is not always known. Withholding of insulin therapy in a patient with insulin-dependent diabetes can certainly result in severe insulin deficiency. In previously undiagnosed patients it is generally presumed that progressive and/or acute beta cell injury leads to deficient insulin release. Since catecholamines are known to inhibit insulin secretion, the occurrence of an acute stressful illness resulting in release of catecholamines in an untreated, relatively stable diabetic could conceivably precipitate a state of severe insulin deficiency.

Insulin ineffectiveness can also result from factors which interfere with insulin action. Thus the release of stress hormones which can antagonize the actions of insulin provides another mechanism whereby a stressful illness could lead to impaired insulin action in an otherwise stable patient. Insulin resistance can also occur as a result of the development of insulin-binding antibodies or alterations of insulin receptor function or post-receptor events. However, DKA is uncommon in insulin-resistant syndromes such as obesity.

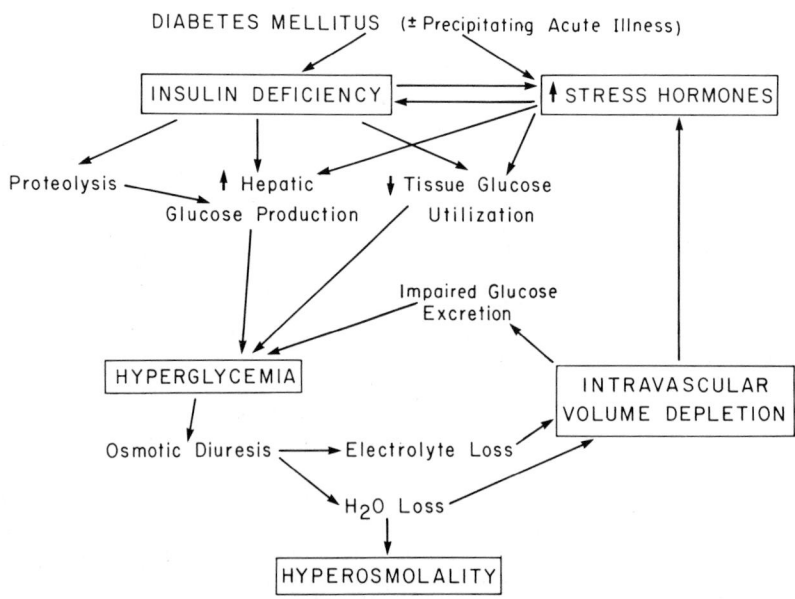

Figure 15–89. Pathogenesis of hyperglycemia during diabetic ketoacidosis (DKA) and other situations of poor diabetes control. The combination of insulin deficiency and increased stress hormones leads to hyperglycemia, osmotic diuresis, hyperosmolality, and volume depletion. Volume depletion completes the cycle by impairing glucose excretion and stimulating further stress hormone release.

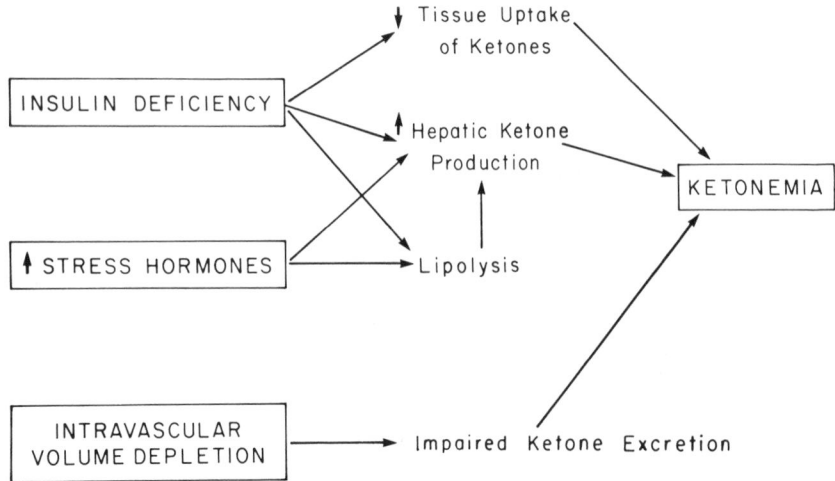

Figure 15–90. Pathogenesis of ketonemia during DKA. The interaction of insulin deficiency, increased stress hormones, and volume depletion (due to uncontrolled hyperglycemia, as shown in Fig. 15–89) leads to increased ketogenesis and impaired ketone removal, resulting in accumulation of ketones in the circulation.

Stress Hormone Release

Elevated circulating levels of catecholamines, glucagon, growth hormone, and cortisol occur during DKA (Fig. 15–91). The factors which can contribute to such elevations are illustrated in Figure 15–62. Acute illnesses, which often accompany or precede DKA, may be associated with a stress hormone response. Such stress responses have been documented during a variety of situations including surgical stress, burn, trauma, and myocardial infarction, or following the administration of bacterial pyrogen. Intravascular volume depletion and systemic acidosis, major features of DKA, are known stimuli of the sympathetic nervous system. Insulin deficiency *per se* has also been postulated to be a cause of increased release of glucagon and growth hormone.

Volume Depletion

Intravascular volume depletion is frequently associated with DKA and is an important factor determining the se-

verity of the metabolic alterations of DKA. When the circulating glucose concentration exceeds the renal tubular reabsorption maximum, glucosuria ensues with an obligate water loss. This osmotic diuresis interferes with the renal mechanisms for reabsorption of solutes, resulting in loss of sodium and an acceleration of extracellular volume depletion. As illustrated in Figure 15–89, a vicious cycle ensues in which volume depletion stimulates release of stress hormones which contribute to increased production and impaired tissue removal of glucose, thereby increasing the load of glucose presented to the kidney and resulting in more osmotic diuresis with further loss of water and sodium. Losses can be so massive that even patients who are feeling well otherwise may be unable to ingest adequate amounts of fluids to keep up. More debilitated patients or those with a concurrent gastrointestinal illness may develop severe volume depletion very rapidly.

Several other factors also contribute to natriuresis during DKA. There is evidence that insulin can enhance sodium reabsorption by the kidney, while glucagon inhibits sodium reabsorption. Thus, during insulin deficiency and glucagon excess as occurs during DKA, renal excretion of sodium is

Figure 15–91. Mean circulating levels of stress hormones, expressed as a percentage of normal concentrations, in patients with DKA. These data have been summarized from several different series of patients. (From Schade, D. S., and Eaton, R. P.: Pathogenesis of diabetic ketoacidosis: A reappraisal. *Diabetes Care* 2:296, 1979.)

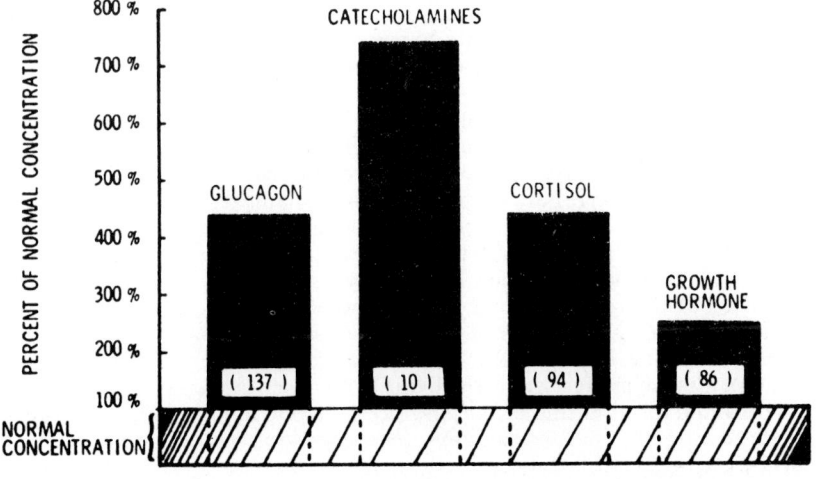

favored. Renal excretion of ketoacids also leads to an obligate increase in the excretion of cations, predominantly sodium.

Hyperglycemia

Hyperglycemia during DKA results from increased hepatic glucose production, decreased tissue glucose utilization, and impaired renal excretion of glucose. The interactions of insulin deficiency, increased stress hormones, and intravascular volume depletion to produce these alterations of glucose homeostasis are illustrated in Figure 15–89.

Renal Glucose Excretion. As will be indicated, a number of factors result in increased glucose production and impaired tissue utilization of glucose during DKA. It is important to emphasize that once the circulating glucose level exceeds the renal threshold for maximal reabsorption (approximately 200 mg/dl), the kidneys become a major site for the removal of glucose. Thus, in the presence of normal kidney function and sufficient renal perfusion to allow adequate clearance of glucose from plasma, the plasma glucose level will not rise appreciably above the threshold concentration for maximal reabsorption.

It is also important to emphasize that large amounts of salt and water are lost during the osmotic diuresis that accompanies renal excretion of glucose. Unless this salt and water is adequately replaced, intravascular volume depletion will occur (see Fig. 15–89). Volume depletion will lead to decreased perfusion of the kidneys, diminished clearance of glucose from plasma, and a further rise of the plasma glucose level. For this reason the degree of hyperglycemia occurring during DKA will depend to a large extent on the degree to which salt and water intake maintains intravascular volume. Some patients with DKA are able to ingest the massive amounts of fluids needed to keep up with urine losses and present with plasma glucose levels of only 200–300 mg/dl. Other patients who are unable to maintain an adequate fluid intake can develop marked hyperglycemia, presenting with plasma glucose levels greater than 1000 mg/dl. Thus, the plasma glucose level at the time of presentation of a patient with DKA should be viewed primarily as an index of renal perfusion and/or function (analogous to the BUN), rather than as a measure of the severity of insulin deficiency.

Glucose Production. The load of glucose which the kidneys must handle during DKA is determined by the relationship between hepatic production and tissue utilization of glucose. Hepatic glucose production has been shown to be increased in ketotic or markedly hyperglycemic diabetics. As discussed earlier in this chapter, insulin and glucagon release by pancreatic islets plays an important role in the regulation of hepatic glucose production. Since insulin secretion is markedly impaired or absent in DKA and glucagon levels are elevated, increased hepatic glucose production is not surprising. Both cortisol and catecholamines are also elevated in DKA and contribute to hepatic glucose production. Furthermore, there is evidence that cortisol, catecholamines, and glucagon have synergistic effects on the liver so that glucose production in the presence of all three is greater than the sum of the effects of each. Thus the hormone milieu during DKA overwhelmingly favors increased glucose production by the liver. Under such circumstances, the rate-limiting factor for glucose production may be the availability of substrates for gluconeogenesis (amino acids, glycerol, and lactate).

The other major organ capable of producing glucose is the kidney. All of the enzymes necessary for gluconeogenesis are found in renal tissue. There is evidence that renal glucose production can increase dramatically in animals during experimental diabetes, an effect that can be reversed with insulin administration. It is certainly possible that stress hormones could have effects on glucose production by the kidney similar to the effects these hormones have on the liver. However, the effects of stress hormones on renal glucose production are not known. A known regulator of renal gluconeogenesis is systemic acidosis. As amino acids are metabolized in order to produce ammonia for acid excretion, the rest of the molecule is converted to glucose. Thus, in addition to being a major site of glucose excretion during DKA, the kidneys may be an important source of increased glucose production.

Glucose Uptake. The other major factor contributing to the increased load of glucose which the kidneys must handle during DKA is diminished tissue utilization of glucose. Glucose uptake by liver, muscle, and fat cells is facilitated by insulin and inhibited by catecholamines, cortisol, and growth hormone. Neural tissue does not require insulin for glucose uptake. However, because of the massive amounts of ketones produced, they may become an important fuel of neural tissue during DKA (analogous to the situation during fasting), thereby further diminishing glucose utilization.

Ketonemia

Ketonemia occurs during DKA primarily as a result of increased hepatic production of ketones, although decreased tissue uptake of ketones and diminished renal excretion of ketones also contribute to the severity of the ketonemia. The interactions of insulin deficiency, increased stress hormones, and intravascular volume depletion to produce these alterations of ketone production and removal are illustrated in Figure 15–90.

Ketone Production. The ketone bodies are acetoacetate, acetone, and betahydroxybutyrate. The mechanism by which their production is regulated has been studied intensively. As a result, the factors regulating hepatic ketogenesis during DKA are now quite well understood. A major controller of ketogenesis is the availability of free fatty acids (FFA), the substrate for this process. FFA become available to the liver as a result of triglyceride catabolism, leading to FFA release from fat cells. This process of lipolysis is regulated by the adipose tissue enzyme hormone-sensitive lipase. Since insulin is the major hormone which inhibits the activity of this lipolytic enzyme, insulin deficiency rapidly leads to lipolysis and increased circulating levels of FFA. Hormone-sensitive lipase activity increases under the influence of a variety of other hormones including catecholamines, cortisol, and growth hormone. Thus, elevated stress hormone levels during DKA can also play a substantial role in increasing availability of FFA.

Since hepatic extraction of FFA is proportional to the FFA level, increased lipolysis leads directly to increased liver uptake of FFA. In hepatocytes FFA either can be reesterified to form triglycerides, a process occurring in the cytosol, or can enter the mitochondria and be oxidized to acetyl CoA, the substrate for ketone production. Thus, the rate at which FFA enter mitochondria of the liver cells is a major determinant of whether FFA are reesterified or become available for ketone production. FFA entry into mitochondria is dependent on the activity of the enzyme carnitine acetyl transferase I (CAT I), located on the outer surface of the inner mitochondrial membrane. When tissue carnitine levels are high, this enzyme is active and FFA entry into mitochondria is facilitated.

There is now substantial evidence that malonyl CoA is a potent inhibitor of CAT I (see Fig. 15–40). Since malonyl CoA is the first intermediate along the pathway of fat synthesis from acetyl CoA, the process controlling its production thereby simultaneously regulates use of FFA for fuel storage or fuel utilization. When an ample supply of acetyl CoA is produced in the cytosol via the glycolytic pathway, malonyl CoA production is enhanced. Increased malonyl CoA levels lead to a fall of CAT I activity and decreased tissue carnitine levels, thereby preventing access of FFA to mitochondria and favoring triglyceride synthesis. Conversely, malonyl CoA production is low during DKA because of inhibition of glycolysis by low insulin and high glucagon levels. In addition, there is inhibition by glucagon of acetyl CoA carboxylase, the enzyme converting acetyl CoA to malonyl CoA. As a result, tissue carnitine levels are high, CAT I activity is increased, and FFA readily enter the mitochondria.

Ketone Removal. In addition to massive increases of ketone production during DKA, ketone removal is impaired. There is evidence that tissue uptake of ketones is insulin-dependent. Thus insulin deficiency may further promote ketonemia by impairing utilization of ketones by tissues. The rate of removal of ketones from blood is also dependent on renal clearance and excretion. As already discussed, diminished renal perfusion due to hypovolemia frequently is present in DKA. Thus impaired renal clearance of ketones may contribute to the degree of ketonemia.

Systemic Acidosis

Ketoacidosis. The marked overproduction of the keto acids, betahydroxybutyric acid and acetoacetic acid, coupled with impaired removal, leads to their accumulation in blood. Since these fatty acids fully dissociate at physiologic pH, hydrogen ions are released which must be buffered by blood constituents. Bicarbonate plays a major role in this regard by forming carbonic acid, which by dissociating to form CO_2 allows respiratory elimination of the product of this reaction. As systemic acidosis develops, respiratory drive is stimulated. The ensuing hyperventilation enhances the efficiency of acid neutralization by accelerating CO_2 elimination. Bicarbonate is also lost in the urine as part of the mechanism for renal excretion of acid during systemic acidosis. As a result of these processes the serum bicarbonate level falls. Tissue uptake and oxidation of ketoacids results in their neutralization and regeneration of bicarbonate. However, ketone production may exceed the capacity of tissues to metabolize them, and, as already indicated, tissue uptake of ketoacids is impaired in the presence of insulin deficiency.

The kidney also plays an important role in the body's compensatory response to systemic acidosis. Ammonia production and subsequent excretion of ammonium ions is a major mechanism for elimination of excess acid. However, as already indicated, the process by which ammonia is produced by the kidney results in gluconeogenesis. Thus, this mechanism of renal compensation for acidosis would tend to contribute to glucose overproduction during DKA. Tubular excretion of hydrogen ions associated with sodium reabsorption is another important mechanism for elimination of excess acid. However, this mechanism is not very effective during an osmotic diuresis such as occurs with severe hyperglycemia. Furthermore, as volume depletion and impaired renal perfusion occur, both renal mechanisms for eliminating acid become impaired.

Lactic Acidosis. An additional factor that can contribute to systemic acidosis in a patient with DKA is the overproduction of lactic acid, superimposing lactic acidosis upon ketoacidosis. In the presence of the enzyme lactic acid dehydrogenase and NADH, large amounts of pyruvate, the end-product of anaerobic glycolysis, can be converted to lactate. However, lactate is readily converted back to pyruvate when there is sufficient tissue oxygenation so that oxidative phosphorylation generates adequate amounts of NAD. During DKA several factors may result in impaired tissue oxygen delivery, thereby providing a setting for excessive accumulation of lactic acid. These factors include hypovolemia, diminished erythrocyte 2,3-DPG levels, and the presence of concurrent vascular disease in some patients. In addition, mitochondrial fatty acid oxidation, which is favored during DKA, generates NADH and acetyl CoA, both of which inhibit pyruvate dehydrogenase, the enzyme complex which converts lactate back to pyruvate.

Coma

Many patients with DKA present with mental obtundation or coma. The precise etiology for the altered mental status of DKA is not established. The degree of alteration of the mental status correlates most closely with the degree of hyperosmolality of body fluids, although other factors may contribute to this finding, including severe acidosis, cellular dehydration, and diminished tissue oxygenation.

Clinical Features

Precipitating Factors

Withdrawal of insulin in a patient with insulin-dependent diabetes mellitus can result in the development of DKA in a matter of hours. However, studies using somatostatin to suppress glucagon release or using adrenergic blocking drugs have demonstrated that both the speed with which DKA develops and its severity are related to the stress hormone responses as well as to the insulin withdrawal itself. Thus, a diabetic patient whose metabolic state is marginally compensated on inadequate therapeutic doses of insulin or by borderline endogenous insulin secretion may be unable to handle the increased metabolic demands associated with stress hormone release during an acute illness, and DKA may result. For this reason it is important to search for a precipitating illness, particularly an infection, in patients with DKA. Low rates of insulin secretion can also be observed in normal subjects (e.g., during a fast), but normal persons will respond to stress hormone–induced hyperglycemia by secreting adequate amounts of insulin to prevent massive ketogenesis and the development of ketoacidosis. Thus, although there is abundant evidence that stress hormones contribute to many of the metabolic alterations during DKA, beta cell function must be severely impaired if DKA is to occur.

History

Patients with no prior history of diabetes mellitus generally present with the classic symptoms of polydipsia, polyuria, polyphagia, and weight loss. These symptoms may be gradually progressive over a period of several weeks or explosive in onset. The polyuria is due to the osmotic diuresis accompanying marked hyperglycemia. Polydipsia represents the normal thirst response to volume depletion and hyperosmolality of body fluids. Polyphagia is apparently the normal response to negative caloric balance and weight

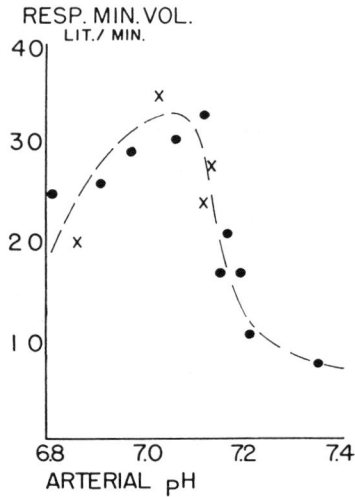

Figure 15–92. With decrease in plasma pH, the pulmonary ventilation increases, reaching a maximum at about pH 7.1; with further decrease in pH, the ventilation decreases. Thus, with decreasing rate of ventilation, the patient may be changing for either the better or the worse. The circles consist of data from patients who ultimately recovered and the crosses from those who succumbed. (From Kety, S. S., et al.: Blood flow and oxygen consumption of human brain in diabetic acidosis and coma. *J. Clin. Invest.* 27:500, 1948.)

loss during the development of DKA. However, the precise mechanism by which appetite stimulation occurs is not established. In some patients anorexia, rather than hyperphagia, may be a prominent symptom. Anorexia may develop as the metabolic state deteriorates or may be a symptom of a concurrent gastrointestinal illness. The mental status may be unaffected or a history of gradual deterioration into coma may be present.

DKA often appears to develop more rapidly in a patient previously known to have insulin-dependent diabetes mellitus. There is frequently a history of a rather abrupt onset of very poor diabetes control in a patient who had been apparently stable on an insulin treatment regimen. This change is usually associated with gastrointestinal symptoms or some other acute illness which results in an inappropriate reduction of insulin dosage by the patient.

Examination

The classic findings on examination of a patient with DKA include hyperventilation, a fruity odor to the breath, and signs of volume depletion. The deep, rapid Kussmaul breathing pattern represents respiratory compensation for the metabolic acidosis. When this sign is present, the pH is generally below 7.20. With profound acidosis (pH less than 7.0) the respiration rate may actually decrease owing to brain stem depressant effects of the acidosis (Fig. 15–92). The fruity breath is caused by acetone elimination via the lungs. Signs of volume depletion may include poor skin turgor, dry mucous membranes, flat neck veins, and a postural blood pressure drop.

The mental status should be carefully assessed because it is an important sign to follow during treatment of DKA. The initial mental status may range from perfectly normal to deep coma. It is also important to evaluate cardiac function. Patients with DKA may have underlying heart disease or may have acute cardiac problems due to acidosis or electrolyte abnormalities. Since patients with DKA often present with a history of gastrointestinal symptoms, evidence of an acute abdominal event such as appendicitis or pancreatitis should be searched for. Finally, there may be

physical signs of other precipitating illness, particularly infection. The presence of fever should never be ascribed to DKA alone. In fact, hypothermia often accompanies DKA, and fever has often been absent even in the presence of well documented infection. Thus, the presence of fever is strongly suggestive of a concurrent infection, but the absence of fever cannot be used as a sign that infection is not present.

Laboratory Findings

Substrates

Glucose. As indicated previously, plasma glucose varies widely in patients presenting in DKA, from levels of 200–300 mg/dl, approaching the normal renal threshold for maximal glucose reabsorption, to levels well over 1000 mg/dl. The degree of hyperglycemia depends to a large extent on the degree of impairment of renal perfusion. However, hyperglycemia is invariably present, and its detection can help to rapidly establish the diagnosis of DKA in a comatose patient. Reagent-impregnated test strips can be used for gross bedside enzymatic measurement of blood glucose. However, current clinical laboratory methodology can allow accurate plasma glucose measurements within minutes. Such methods should be relied upon when readily available, since bedside reagent strip measurements performed by untrained individuals can give misleading results.

Ketones. The diagnosis of DKA is confirmed by the finding of elevated blood ketone levels. The presence of ketonuria can also be established by using reagent strips, but this does not necessarily signify that DKA is present. Ketonemia can be demonstrated at the bedside with nitroprusside (available in pill or powder form), which forms a purple color in the presence of acetoacetate. A strongly positive nitroprusside reaction in undiluted plasma is diagnostic of significant ketonemia.

The nitroprusside test has also been used to semiquantify the amount of ketonemia by performing serial dilutions of plasma. However, this procedure is generally unsatisfactory for quantifying ketonemia for two reasons. First, visual inspection of the color reaction in diluted plasma samples becomes rather subjective and unreproducible. Second, and of major importance, is that nitroprusside does not react with betahydroxybutyrate, the predominant circulating ketone. The ratio of betahydroxybutyrate to acetoacetate in patients with DKA can range from 3:1 to as high as 30:1. The equilibrium point between betahydroxybutyrate and acetoacetate is dependent on the mitochondrial NADH-NAD ratio. When NADH is present in excess, the reaction favors betahydroxybutyrate production. As indicated earlier, fatty acid oxidation and diminished tissue oxygenation both result in NADH accumulation, thereby increasing conversion of acetoacetate to betahydroxybutyrate. Thus, even accurate measurements of acetoacetate with the nitroprusside test may give a misleading estimate of the degree of total ketonemia.

Fortunately, the nitroprusside test is very sensitive, so that qualitatively positive results occur even when there is a marked shift of the betahydroxybutyrate-acetoacetate ratio. It must be remembered, however, that under some conditions this test may be negative in the presence of significant ketonemia. An accurate measurement of betahydroxybutyrate in plasma can be performed by specific enzymatic assay. Such a measurement is helpful in situations in which DKA is suspected but the nitroprusside test is negative or only weakly positive.

Amino Acids. A number of alterations of circulating amino acids during DKA have been described. Concentrations of gluconeogenic precursors such as alanine, glycine, threonine, and serine are decreased, presumably because of augmented uptake by the liver and perhaps the kidneys as well. In contrast, levels of the branched-chain amino acids valine, leucine, and isoleucine are elevated in DKA. Release of these latter amino acids into blood is highly dependent on insulin. Since the branched-chain amino acids are substrates for ketogenesis, their increased release may contribute to ketosis in DKA.

Lactate. As indicated earlier, the metabolic state during DKA favors lactate overproduction, particularly in circumstances in which tissue oxygenation is impaired. Lactate can be used as a substrate for gluconeogenesis. However, blood lactate levels in DKA are generally elevated above the normal upper limit of 1.4 mmol/l and contribute to the degree of metabolic acidosis. A level of greater than 7.0 mmol/l is generally used as an arbitrary criterion for the diagnosis of lactic acidosis. Such a level is exceeded in some cases of DKA. Systemic acidosis out of proportion to the degree of apparent ketonemia should suggest the presence of lactic acidosis. Assay methods for measurement of lactate in plasma are generally available and can confirm such a diagnosis.

Lipids. The alterations of lipid metabolism accompanying DKA may be reflected in marked abnormalities of circulating lipoproteins and products of lipolysis. Plasma levels of both FFA and glycerol are elevated. Although triglyceride synthesis by the liver is inhibited in DKA, tissue removal of triglyceride is grossly abnormal. Activity of lipoprotein lipase, the major enzyme involved in catabolism of triglyceride-rich lipoproteins, is dependent on insulin. Thus, the insulin deficiency of DKA leads to marked inhibition of lipoprotein lipase activity. As a result, large amounts of chylomicrons and very low density lipoproteins may be present in plasma, giving it a lipemic appearance. Chylomicronemia is particularly likely to occur in polyphagic patients who are unable to catabolize absorbed fat because of the lipoprotein lipase deficiency. Chylomicronemia may result in pancreatitis which can precipitate or exacerbate DKA. In addition, chylomicrons in plasma can lead to spuriously low measurements of serum sodium, thereby leading to underestimation of the degree of hyperosmolality during DKA.

Electrolytes and Acid-Base Balance

As DKA develops, large losses of body water and electrolytes occur, primarily owing to the osmotic diuresis which accompanies hyperglycemia. Average deficits in patients with DKA are listed in Table 15–15. However, the magnitude of the specific deficits in a given patient may vary considerably from these averages, depending upon the length of time during which DKA developed and the degree to which the patient was able to maintain fluid and electrolyte intake.

Arterial Blood Gases. Measurement of arterial blood gases establishes the presence and severity of metabolic acidosis and should be performed immediately in patients suspected of having DKA. The pH may be as low as 6.8 and is accompanied by a pCO_2 that may be less than 20 mm Hg. The calculated bicarbonate value is subnormal, and when plasma bicarbonate is assayed, it is frequently less than 10 mEq/l. Hypoxemia is generally not present. If the pO_2 is found to be low, a primary pulmonary condition such as pneumonia or congestive heart failure with pulmonary edema is likely to coexist with DKA.

Osmolality. Elevated serum osmolality is present in DKA except in the rare patient who is able to keep up with the massive water losses accompanying the osmotic diuresis. Serum osmolality can be measured accurately in the clinical laboratory. However, a reasonably accurate estimation can be made from serum glucose and electrolyte measurements, unless chylomicronemia is present. The following formula can be used to estimate effective serum osmolality:

$$\text{Serum osmolality} = 2 \times [Na + K\ (mEq/l)] + \text{serum glucose (mg/dl)} \div 18$$

The measured serum osmolality will also include the contribution of serum urea, which may be elevated in DKA. However, since urea is freely permeable into cells, it does not contribute to the effective osmolality of extracellular fluids.

Sodium. The serum sodium concentration of a patient with DKA may be low, normal, or elevated depending on the relationship between salt and water losses as DKA develops. The osmotic effects of hyperglycemia lead to loss of intracellular water into the extracellular space, tending to lower the serum sodium concentration. However, although large amounts of sodium are lost in the urine during osmotic diuresis, water is lost in excess of sodium, tending to result in an increase in serum sodium. As hyperosmolality develops as a result of the water diuresis, the thirst mechanism is stimulated, leading to water ingestion which will lower the serum sodium. Thus, although the serum sodium concentration may vary depending on these factors, it is important to emphasize that virtually all patients with DKA are sodium-depleted. As already indicated, interpretation of the serum sodium concentration should take into account the possibility that coexistent chylomicronemia during DKA will spuriously lower serum sodium.

Potassium. As with the serum sodium concentration, the serum potassium concentration of patients with DKA does not accurately reflect the status of total body stores. The potassium deficit in DKA may be as high as 10 mEq/kg body weight owing to osmotic diuresis, acidosis, and gastrointestinal losses in some patients. Despite this deficit, the serum potassium is often high at the time of diagnosis of DKA. High serum potassium is due to volume contraction and the shift of potassium from the intracellular to extracellular space which accompanies systemic acidosis. The finding of a normal or low serum potassium in a patient presenting with DKA generally indicates a severe total-body potassium deficit that will require vigorous replacement during therapy to avoid hypokalemia. A reasonable estimate of the total-body potassium deficit can be obtained if the serum potassium and arterial blood pH are known (Fig. 15–93).

Table 15–15. AVERAGE FLUID AND ELECTROLYTE DEFICIT IN DKA*

Substance	Amount of Deficit (per kg body weight)
Water	100 ml
Sodium	7 mEq
Potassium	5 mEq
Chloride	5 mEq
Magnesium	0.5 mEq
Phosphate	1 mEq

*Note: Actual deficits in individual patients may vary widely.

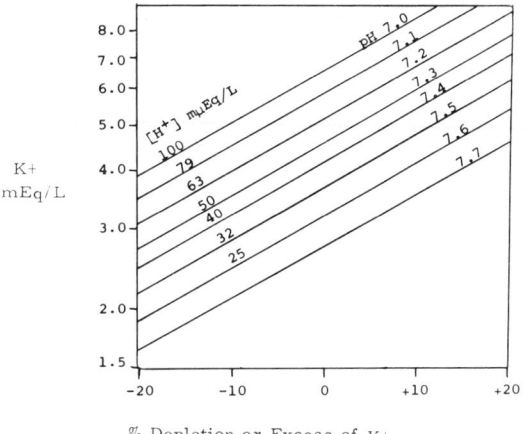

Figure 15–93. To use this nomogram a line parallel to the baseline is drawn from the level of serum K^+. The point at which it crosses the line showing either the pH or carbon dioxide–combining power of the plasma at that time indicates the extent of abnormal deviation of the body K^+. Therefore, this nomogram can be used to signify therapeutic needs in correcting the level of the body K^+. (From the Division of Nephrology, University of Washington, Seattle.)

Phosphate. The relationship between circulating and total-body phosphate levels during DKA is analogous to that for potassium. Total-body phosphate depletion results from osmotic diuresis and acidosis. However, serum phosphate levels are generally normal or elevated initially in DKA. During therapy plasma phosphate may drop precipitously. Intracellular depletion of phosphate results in diminished levels of erythrocyte 2,3-DPG. When the 2,3-DPG concentration is low, hemoglobin affinity for oxygen increases, thereby tending to impair oxygen delivery to tissues. However, since acidosis has the opposite effect on hemoglobin affinity for oxygen, there is little net effect in patients presenting with DKA.

Hormones

Insulin. Although deficient insulin action is clearly present in patients with DKA, circulating insulin levels (measured by radioimmunoassay) of patients with DKA are often similar to insulin levels of normal subjects after an overnight fast. However, such insulin levels clearly represent inadequate insulin secretion in response to the hyperglycemia present during DKA. Normal people develop only mild ketosis during prolonged fasting when insulin levels fall even further. Thus, the grossly abnormal metabolic state of DKA is not solely a result of absolute insulin deficiency, but of the combination of low insulin levels, stress hormone secretion, and volume depletion.

Stress Hormones. The combination of insulin deficiency, hypovolemia, acidosis, and concurrent acute illness results in elevations of circulating levels of stress hormones (see Fig. 15–91). Plasma glucagon, growth hormone, and norepinephrine levels are frequently 10 times normal, while plasma epinephrine may be 50 times normal. Plasma cortisol, aldosterone, and renin activity are generally five times normal levels.

Other Findings

Leukocytosis is common in patients with DKA. Counts in the range of 15,000–30,000 occur in the absence of docu-

mented infection. Thus, neither leukocytosis nor fever is a reliable sign to diagnose or exclude the presence of infection in a patient with DKA. The hemoglobin concentration is generally normal but may be elevated in severely dehydrated patients.

Serum amylase levels and renal clearance of amylase have both been reported to be elevated in patients with DKA who have no other clinical findings of pancreatitis. There is evidence that the source of this amylase is the liver, rather than the pancreas. Since serum lipase levels are not elevated in uncomplicated DKA, this test should be used in a patient with DKA who has clinical findings suggestive of pancreatitis. Serum creatine phosphokinase and transaminase levels are also frequently elevated during DKA. The cause of these findings is not established but may relate to effects of intracellular phosphorus deficiency on muscle membrane stability.

Differential Diagnosis

The diagnosis of DKA is usually not difficult to make once it is considered. Hyperglycemia, ketonemia, and systemic acidosis can generally be documented in a matter of minutes and the diagnosis established. However, there are a number of other causes of coma and/or acidosis which should be kept in mind.

Coma in the Diabetic. Hypoglycemia is the most important diagnosis to rule out in any patient with coma of undetermined etiology. Intravenous glucose is generally easy to administer and is relatively nontoxic, even in a patient who is already hyperglycemic. Therefore, it should be given after blood has been obtained for serum glucose measurement if there is any question about the etiology of the coma. Hyperosmolar coma without ketoacidosis also occurs in diabetics (see later). The findings of both ketonemia and systemic acidosis easily rule out this diagnosis. Intracranial injury or illness (hemorrhage, infarction, infection) should be ruled out in any comatose diabetic, regardless of whether DKA is present. Finally, drug overdosage should also be considered in a comatose diabetic. Although systemic acidosis may be present with ingestion of some drugs (e.g., salicylates, methanol, ethylene glycol), the absence of ketonemia helps to rule out DKA.

Metabolic Acidosis. Lactic acidosis without significant ketonemia can occur in a diabetic, generally as a result of a major acute illness associated with diminished perfusion of tissues. Diabetics treated with the hypoglycemic agent phenformin may also develop lactic acidosis. The coexistence of ketonemia in such patients may be overlooked since the mitochondrial NADH-NAD ratio markedly favors production of betahydroxybutyrate, which does not give a nitroprusside reaction. Treatment of the metabolic state during lactic acidosis in a diabetic is similar to treatment of DKA. However, identification and vigorous treatment of an underlying major illness is essential if the patient is to survive.

Systemic acidosis may also appear in diabetics who develop renal disease. Either renal tubular damage alone or generalized renal parenchymal disease can interfere with excretion of the body's normal acid load. Thus, ketosis-prone diabetics may become even more susceptible to developing DKA if they develop renal disease.

Ketosis. Normal individuals will develop mild ketosis during starvation. Thus, the presence of ketosis in a starving diabetic may not necessarily indicate that DKA is present. Starvation ketosis generally results in only a weakly positive serum nitroprusside test and causes only minor systemic acidosis. However, starvation plus alcohol ingestion can result in a ketoacidosis syndrome without hyperglycemia in nondiabetics. The exact pathogenesis of this condition is not established but appears to be related to inhibition of gluconeogenesis by alcohol, leading to an acceleration of ketogenesis. As a result, hypoglycemia rather than hyperglycemia tends to be present. Because liver metabolism of alcohol increases the mitochondrial NADA-NAD ratio, betahydroxybutyrate production is greatly enhanced compared to that of acetoacetate. Thus, during alcohol ketoacidosis, the nitroprusside test also tends to be negative or only weakly positive. Systemic acidosis, though present in this syndrome, tends to be mild.

Management

DKA is a life-threatening condition which requires aggressive, but careful, management. The dramatic, life-saving effects of insulin administration to patients with DKA following discovery of insulin demonstrated the importance of insulin therapy for this condition. Insulin is now readily available and easy to administer. As a result, it is most unusual for a patient with DKA to receive inadequate insulin therapy. However, the importance of intensive fluid and electrolyte replacement in the treatment of DKA has not been so readily appreciated. Fluid and electrolyte deficits are not easy to quantify accurately, and most physicians are not accustomed to administering the massive amounts required to replace these deficits. Thus, many patients are somewhat undertreated for this aspect of DKA, particularly those with the most severe cases. Identification of underlying or precipitating conditions and their vigorous management are also important to insure a good outcome. A summary of the overall approach to treatment of DKA is presented in Table 15–16. It is important to emphasize that these general guidelines should be modified as needed for each patient, since individual needs may vary considerably.

Insulin

Once a diagnosis of DKA is established, insulin should be administered immediately. The goal of insulin therapy is to rapidly achieve and maintain adequate *tissue* levels of insulin to reverse the processes of lipolysis, ketogenesis, overproduction of glucose, and impaired tissue uptake of glucose which contribute to the pathogenesis of DKA. There is now abundant evidence that in most patients who have DKA, this therapeutic goal can be achieved with relatively modest doses of insulin that result in circulating insulin levels in the physiologic range (Fig. 15–94).

Although high levels of stress hormones and other features of DKA may lead to some resistance to insulin action, severe insulin resistance requiring pharmacologic doses of insulin is unusual. Reversal of DKA can be accomplished in most adult patients in a matter of hours with appropriate fluid therapy (see later) plus 5 to 10 units of regular insulin per hour administered either subcutaneously, intramuscularly, or by constant intravenous infusion (Fig. 15–95). A somewhat more rapid metabolic response is achieved with an immediate priming dose of 10–30 units of regular insulin intravenously. Similar satisfactory control of DKA can be achieved in children with comparably reduced insulin doses.

These doses of insulin result in circulating insulin levels of 50–150 μU/ml. In the absence of insulin resistance, such insulin levels are usually more than adequate to fully inhibit lipolysis and hepatic glucose production. Although

Table 15–16.   TREATMENT PROTOCOL FOR DKA*

	Initial Phase	Recovery Phase
Insulin	1. 10–20 units regular insulin IV bolus + 5–10 units/hour IV (infusion), IM, or subcutaneously; the IV route should be used in any hypotensive patient	1. As acidosis is reversed, ↓ to 5–10 units q 2–4 hours
	2. Increase hourly dose if serum glucose does not fall despite adequate fluid therapy	2. When patient is eating, begin long-acting insulin
Fluids	1. 0.9% NaCl at 1000 ml/hour	1. When BP stable, urine output brisk, and serum glucose falling, ↓ to 0.45% NaCl at 250–500 ml/hour
	2. Replace sodium deficit in 4–6 hours (average = 500 mEq)	2. When serum glucose < 250 mg/dl add 5% glucose to IV fluids
		3. Replace H_2O deficit over 12–24 hours (average = 5–10 l)
Potassium	1. Serum K⁺ high: begin KCl at 20 mEq/hour after urine output established	1. Adjust dose of KCl by serum K⁺ measurements
	2. Serum K⁺ normal or low: begin KCl at 20 mEq/hour immediately; reduce rate by 50% if patient is oliguric	2. Continue oral KCl replacement for 1 week to correct total deficit
	3. Monitor EKG; measure serum K⁺ q 1–2 hours	
Bicarbonate	1. pH < 7.0: give as needed to raise pH to 7.0	1. No bicarbonate
	2. pH 7.0–7.2: ± small amounts (not > 88 mEq)	
	3. pH > 7.2: no bicarbonate	
Phosphorus	1. If patient is not oliguric, may give potassium phosphate 10 mEq/hour (decrease dose of KCl accordingly)	1. No phosphorus
	2. Measure serum phosphorus and calcium frequently	
General measures	1. Comatose patient: nasogastric tube, bladder catheter	1. Remove catheter as soon as possible
	2. Identify and treat any precipitating illness	2. Continue to observe for signs of a precipitating or complicating illness
	3. Consider low-dose heparin	

*Note: These are general guidelines. Since there may be wide variation of individual patient needs, there is no substitute for careful monitoring of each patient, particularly in the early phase of therapy of DKA.

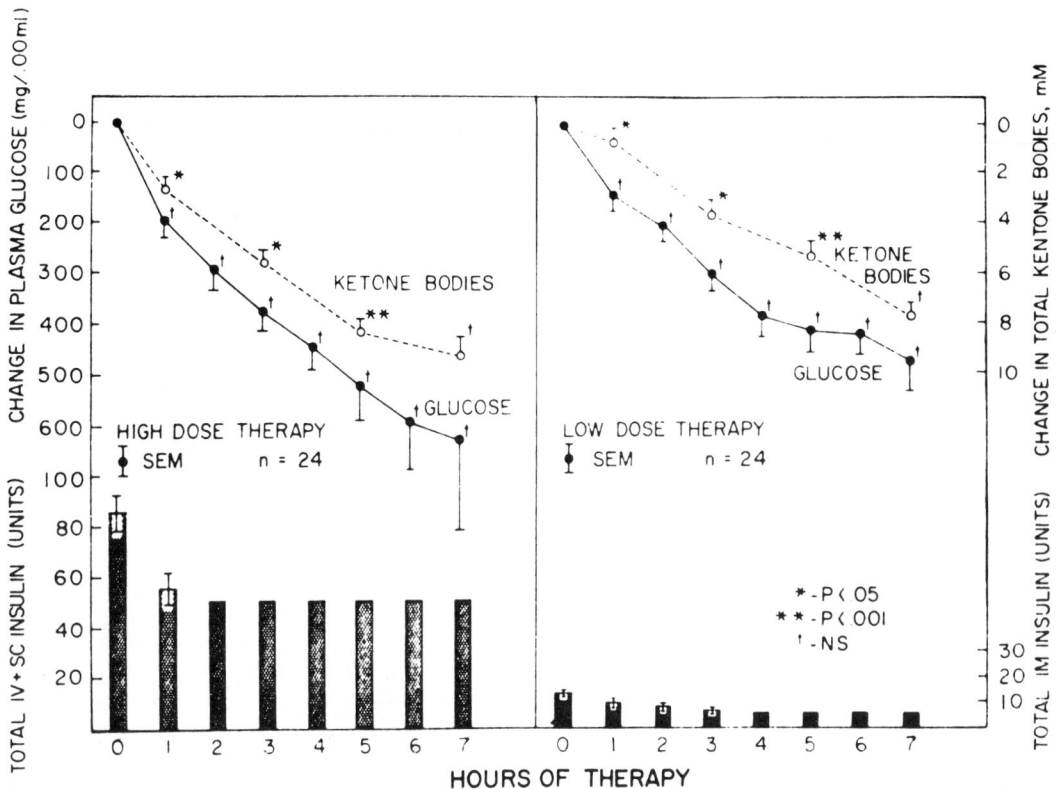

Figure 15–94.   Comparison of the effects of high- and low-dose insulin regimens on the fall of plasma glucose and total ketone bodies in patients with DKA. No significant differences were observed between the two groups in the fall of glucose levels. Ketone body concentrations fell more rapidly initially in the high-dose insulin group, but were not different after 7 hours of treatment. (From Kitabchi, A., et al.: The efficacy of low-dose versus conventional therapy of insulin for treatment of diabetic ketoacidosis. *Ann. Int. Med. 84*:633, 1976.)

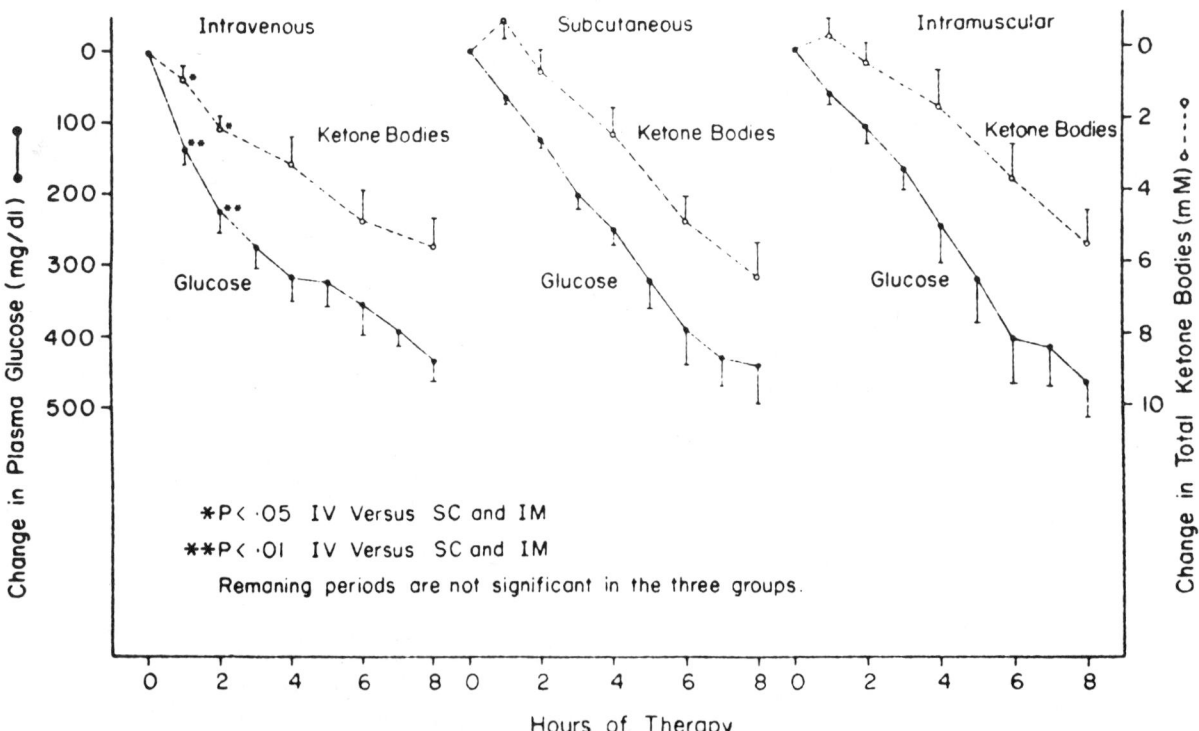

Figure 15–95.   Comparison of the effects of intravenous, subcutaneous, and intramuscular low-dose insulin regimens on changes of plasma glucose and total ketone bodies in patients with DKA (15 patients in each group). Both plasma glucose and ketone bodies fell more rapidly initially in the group receiving intravenous insulin, but no significant differences were present after 3 hours of treatment. (From Fisher, J. N., et al.: Diabetic ketoacidosis: low-dose insulin therapy by various routes. *N. Engl. J. Med. 297*:238, 1977.)

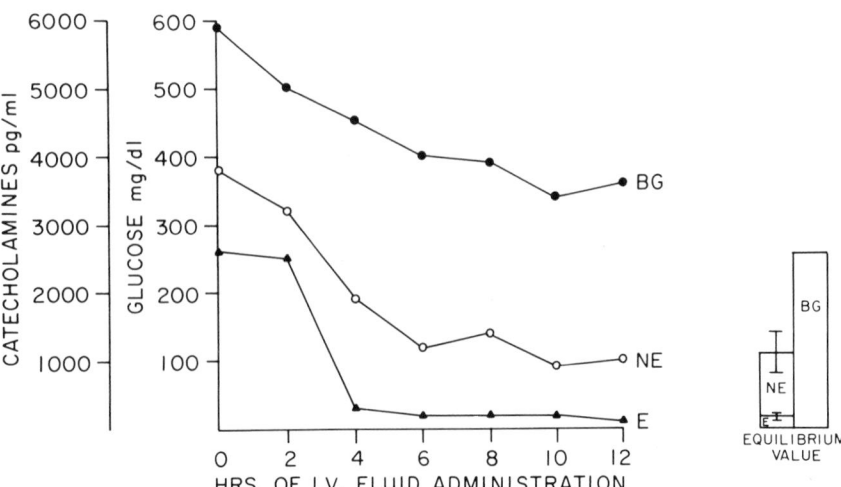

Figure 15–96. Mean levels of plasma norepinephrine *(NE)*, epinephrine *(E)*, and blood glucose *(BG)* during treatment of severe hyperglycemia with fluid therapy alone (no insulin given). The equilibrium values are the levels at the end of the period of treatment with fluids alone, just prior to initiation of insulin therapy. (Modified from Waldhäusl, W., et al.: Severe hyperglycemia: Effects of rehydration on endocrine derangements and blood glucose concentration. *Diabetes* 28:577, 1979.)

tissue uptake of glucose will also be augmented at these levels of insulin, maximal tissue uptake of glucose may require as much as 500 µU/ml insulin. However, it must be remembered that these effects occur only when adequate tissue levels of insulin are achieved. Under normal circumstances equilibration of exogenously administered insulin with peripheral tissues will take 2–3 hours (see Fig. 15–30). The hypovolemia and vasoconstriction present initially in DKA may further retard delivery of insulin to tissues. For these reasons, a considerable lag may exist between the time of initial insulin administration or a change of dose and the time of the maximal metabolic effects of the insulin. Thus, the administration of repeated pharmacologic doses of insulin early in the treatment of DKA tends to cause accelerated tissue uptake of glucose several hours later (when maximal tissue insulin levels have been achieved), a setting which can result in hypoglycemia.

Several randomized studies have indicated that the route of insulin administration does not appreciably affect the rate of recovery from DKA. However, intravenous insulin administration is probably preferable in severely volume-depleted patients in whom systemic delivery of subcutaneous or intramuscular insulin may be delayed by poor absorption. Albumin has often been added to continuous insulin infusions to prevent sticking of insulin to glass and to intravenous tubing. However, simply flushing an intravenous administration system with an insulin solution prior to its use will quickly saturate nonspecific insulin binding sites. A simple dilution of regular insulin in 0.9% saline can then be used for continuous intravenous administration.

When adequate tissue insulinization has been achieved, as indicated by reversal of systemic acidosis and a fall of serum glucose below 300 mg/dl, the frequency of regular insulin administration can be reduced to once every 2–6 hours subcutaneously. As the patient improves so that food is being eaten regularly, long-acting insulin preparations can be reinstituted. In the rare patient whose acidosis does not begin to improve within 2–4 hours, the hourly dose of insulin can be increased.

Glucose

Glucose-containing intravenous fluids should be utilized once the serum glucose falls below 250 mg/dl to increase carbohydrate utilization by tissues and to avoid development of hypoglycemia. Since some patients present with only modestly elevated serum glucose levels, the addition of glucose to intravenous solutions may be necessary early in the course of therapy. It should be remembered that although the plasma half-life of insulin is short, the tissue half-life is much longer and is the physiologically important variable. Thus, the plasma glucose level will continue to fall for some time after discontinuation of insulin or a reduction of insulin dose unless glucose is administered.

Fluids and Electrolytes

The goals of fluid and electrolyte therapy of DKA are restoration of intravascular volume within a few hours by replacing sodium deficits, more gradual replacement of total-body water deficits, and steady replacement of potassium once oliguric renal failure has been ruled out. Restoration of intravascular volume by aggressive fluid therapy is the major factor in reducing serum glucose and osmolality, since fluid replacement will remove a major stimulus for stress hormone secretion and improve renal perfusion, thereby increasing glucose elimination. This has been dramatically demonstrated by Waldhäusl and associates, who delayed treatment of DKA with insulin, and observed a marked decrease of plasma glucose and suppression of elevated stress hormone levels with fluid therapy alone (Fig. 15–96).

Sodium and Water. Initially, 0.9% NaCl should be administered at the rate of 1 l/hr in adults (and comparable rates in children). Hypotensive or severely volume-depleted patients without evidence of heart disease can be given saline at an even more rapid rate. It is virtually impossible to know precisely how sodium-depleted an individual patient is. The average patient has lost approximately 10% of his body weight at the time of presentation with DKA. Half of this is extracellular fluid (which should be replaced with 0.9% NaCl) and the rest intracellular fluid (replaceable with water alone). However, volume deficits will vary widely, depending on the fluid intake of each patient as DKA developed. Therefore, adequacy of sodium replacement should be assessed clinically by monitoring urine output and following the serum glucose level. Failure of the serum glucose to fall after initiation of therapy for DKA is more likely to be a result of inadequate volume replacement than of an insufficient dose of insulin. Once the urine flow has become brisk and the serum glucose begins to fall, the rate of fluid administration can be reduced, and 0.45% NaCl rather than 0.9% NaCl can be used. Although most of the sodium deficit should be replaced in the first 4–6 hours, the total-body water deficit should be more gradually replaced over 12–24 hours.

Potassium. Potassium replacement during DKA is designed to avoid the life-threatening complications of hyperkalemia or hypokalemia. In the majority of patients presenting with an elevated serum potassium, potassium replacement should not be started until urine output is documented. Subsequently, potassium should be given by intravenous infusion at the rate of 20 mEq/hr to avoid severe hypokalemia as potassium shifts back intracellularly with correction of acidosis and increased cellular glucose uptake. Either chloride or phosphate potassium salts can be used (however, note the caution given under the heading Phosphorus). Once oral intake is established, potassium replacement should be continued orally. The average total-body potassium deficit is 5–10 mEq/kg.

Patients presenting with a low or normal serum potassium are at particular risk of developing profound hypokalemia during treatment of DKA. Potassium administration should be started immediately in such patients even if urine output is reduced. The serum potassium should be monitored carefully in all patients during therapy of DKA, but particular care must be taken with patients who are oliguric. The electrocardiogram can be used to evaluate high-risk patients at the bedside for alterations of potassium homeostasis. Hyperkalemia results in tall, peaked T-waves and widening of the QRS complex. Hypokalemia causes prolongation of the Q-T interval, depressed S-T segments, inverted T-waves, and prominent U-waves.

Bicarbonate. The use of sodium bicarbonate to neutralize the acidosis of DKA is somewhat controversial because there are potential adverse effects associated with its use. Since severe acidosis (pH less than 7.0) can cause depression of respiratory and cardiac function, bicarbonate may be used to raise the pH above 7.0. However, acidosis shifts the oxyhemoglobin dissociation curve to the right, making oxygen more available to tissues. As the acidosis is neutralized rapidly, oxygen delivery to tissues may become impaired, since erythrocyte 2,3-DPG levels are generally low in DKA. Thus, rapid correction of acidosis may be potentially hazardous in a diabetic with underlying vascular disease and poor perfusion due to hypovolemia. In addition, bicarbonate administration will correct central nervous system acidosis much more slowly, since it does not penetrate the blood-brain barrier very well. With rapid correction of systemic acidosis, peripheral chemoreceptor-mediated respiratory drive will be diminished and more CO_2 will be retained in the circulation. Since CO_2 diffuses well across the blood-brain barrier, central nervous system acidosis may actually worsen when systemic acidosis is rapidly corrected with bicarbonate. Such central nervous system acidosis may contribute to a transient worsening of mental status during the treatment of some patients with DKA. Finally, acute correction of acidosis with bicarbonate will increase potassium uptake by cells and may precipitously lower the serum potassium level.

Because of these considerations, the goal of bicarbonate therapy should be to only partially correct severe acidosis when present. Patients presenting with a pH greater than 7.2 should not be treated with bicarbonate. Those with pH between 7.0 and 7.2 can receive small amounts (no more than 88 mEq) or none at all. In deciding whether to administer bicarbonate to a patient with DKA, one should also consider that no study has shown that bicarbonate administration alters the course of DKA. For this reason, we rarely use bicarbonate therapy.

Phosphorus. Replacement of phosphorus deficits of patients with DKA has both theoretical advantages and po-

tential hazards, and it has not been shown to alter the course of DKA. The administration of 1 mEq/kg of phosphorus (as phosphate) has been shown to prevent the marked hypophosphatemia that generally accompanies treatment of DKA and to modestly enhance the recovery of erythrocyte levels of 2,3-DPG. Thus, phosphorus therapy might prevent complications of hypophosphatemia such as cardiac dysfunction and enhance delivery of oxygen to tissues. Phosphorus can be administered as a potassium phosphate salt, allowing simultaneous replacement of these two electrolytes. However, overaggressive phosphate therapy, particularly in a patient with poor renal function, can result in severe hypocalcemia owing to precipitation of calcium phosphate in tissues. Thus, adequacy of renal function should be established before phosphate therapy is initiated, and serum calcium should be monitored.

General Measures

Patients presenting in coma should have a nasogastric tube inserted and a bladder catheter placed. Nasogastric fluid and electrolyte losses should, of course, be replaced in addition to the usual fluid and electrolyte therapy. Bladder catheterization should also be performed in awake patients who have had no urine output in the first 4–6 hours to differentiate acute renal failure from bladder dysfunction. Oxygen should be administered to any patient who is hypoxic. Since a thromboembolic event is a potential complication of DKA (see later), low-dose heparin therapy should be considered in comatose, elderly, or severely volume-depleted patients. We do not recommend routine antibiotic coverage in the absence of a specific site of infection in patients with DKA. However, since neither leukocytosis nor fever is a reliable indicator of infection in DKA (see earlier), broad-spectrum antibiotics should be used in hypotensive patients until sepsis can be ruled out by blood and urine cultures.

Assessing Adequacy of Treatment

The most important clinical features to follow during treatment of DKA are the patient's mental status and urine output. Gradual improvement of mental status should occur. A deterioration of mental status is a poor prognostic sign requiring aggressive evaluation for cerebral edema or to diagnose some other brain insult (e.g., cerebrovascular accident). Poor urine output despite intensive fluid administration suggests occurrence of acute renal failure, which will require major readjustments of the usual regimen of fluid and electrolyte therapy. In addition, clinical signs of an underlying precipitating illness may evolve as treatment of DKA proceeds. Such signs should be followed up so that appropriate intervention for such an illness can be made rapidly.

The clinical laboratory should be utilized to provide information about the metabolic state to guide therapy during treatment of DKA. Initially, serum glucose, potassium, and bicarbonate should be measured hourly to determine adequacy of fluid replacement and insulin administration. Once it is clear that improvement is occurring, these measurements should still be made every 2 hours until the serum glucose and potassium have stabilized and acidosis has largely disappeared. Patients with severe acidosis should have the arterial pH repeated hourly until it has increased to 7.20. Serum calcium and phosphate should also be checked in patients receiving phosphate therapy. For reasons outlined previously, repeated semiquantitative serum ketone measurements are not generally helpful and may be misleading. The serum bicarbonate and pH should be relied upon to determine adequacy of reversal of ketoacidosis.

Complications of DKA

The major causes of death in DKA are infection, ischemic vascular disease, shock, and, in children, cerebral edema. A number of factors have been identified that are associated with a poor prognosis. Among these are age of the patient; severe volume depletion associated with hyperosmolality, hypotension, and renal failure; the presence of coma; and the occurrence of a severe precipitating illness such as septicemia or myocardial infarction. When DKA occurs during pregnancy, there is a very high incidence of fetal loss.

Central Nervous System. Hypoglycemia and cerebral edema are the two major central nervous system complications of DKA therapy. Hypoglycemia is uncommon with low-dose insulin regimens including use of glucose in intravenous solutions when the plasma glucose falls below 250 mg/dl. Hypoglycemia occurs more frequently with higher-dose insulin regimens. Frequent monitoring of serum glucose should allow early recognition and treatment of hypoglycemia.

Cerebral edema is a life-threatening complication of DKA. It is rare in adults but still occurs in younger patients with DKA. The pathogenesis is not known but may be related to a number of features of DKA and its therapy. Rapid lowering of serum osmolality during DKA therapy can lead to a dysequilibrium between plasma and cerebrospinal fluid owing to retention of undefined osmotically active molecules (idiogenic osmoles) generated as hyperosmolality develops or as a result of a slower reduction of cerebrospinal fluid glucose compared to peripheral glucose levels. Such a dysequilibrium would result in shifts of water into the central nervous system, leading to cerebral edema. This potential hazard of rapid lowering of hyperosmolality during DKA therapy has been cited as an additional reason for more gradual reduction of hyperglycemia with a low-dose insulin regimen. Other possible, but unsubstantiated, explanations for cerebral edema include diminished central nervous system oxygenation, worsening central nervous system acidosis due to peripheral alkali therapy, and accumulation of sorbitol in brain tissue.

Clinically, cerebral edema should be suspected in a young patient whose level of consciousness deteriorates despite a good metabolic response to DKA therapy. The presence of papilledema supports this diagnosis, and cerebral edema can be confirmed by finding elevated cerebrospinal fluid pressure on lumbar puncture. Aggressive therapy with steroids and mannitol should be instituted and neurosurgical consultation obtained once a diagnosis is made.

Cardiovascular System. Myocardial infarction as a precipitating illness or as a result of hypovolemia and diminished tissue oxygenation is associated with a high mortality rate in patients with DKA. As already mentioned, muscle enzymes may be nonspecifically elevated in serum during DKA. Thus, a diagnosis of myocardial infarction in a patient with DKA should not depend on enzyme measurements alone. Congestive heart failure is a potential complication of severe acidosis, hypophosphatemia, and administration of large amounts of sodium. However, heart failure rarely occurs during DKA in the absence of myocardial infarction, perhaps because of the marked volume depletion generally present. Peripheral edema often occurs for a few days after successful treatment of DKA. The sodium-retaining effects of insulin on the kidney may contribute to

this finding. Cardiac arrhythmia may result from potassium shifts during DKA therapy. However, this complication is preventable by careful monitoring of serum potassium.

Thrombosis or insufficiency of any of a variety of arteries may also occur during DKA. Cerebral or abdominal organ infarction is particularly disastrous. Again, the etiology of these events may be multifactorial. Hypovolemia and impaired tissue oxygenation in the presence of underlying vascular disease can contribute to tissue ischemia. In addition, a number of alterations of platelet function and coagulation factors have been reported in uncontrolled diabetics, all of which could contribute to the formation of intravascular clots. There have been no studies on the efficacy of anticoagulants or antiplatelet drugs in the prevention of ischemic events during DKA. The relatively low general incidence of such events would require that such a study be done on the few patients who may be at highest risk — older subjects presenting with severe hypovolemia.

Infection and Shock. Overwhelming infection continues to be a major cause of death in DKA. Aggressive diagnosis and therapy of infections is of obvious importance. However, neither leukocytosis nor fever is a helpful marker of infection in DKA since leukocytosis is common in noninfected patients and normal or low body temperature is common in infected diabetics. Because of the low overall incidence of bacterial infection in patients with DKA, routine broad-spectrum antibiotic coverage should not be given in the absence of specific evidence of infection. However, such antibiotic coverage should probably be administered to hypotensive patients until sepsis can be ruled out. Profound hypovolemia is the major factor in addition to infection that contributes to shock and acute renal failure during DKA. Aggressive fluid and sodium administration is the approach to be used under these circumstances. Acute renal failure will complicate fluid and electrolyte therapy, and dialysis may be necessary to manage this problem.

Prevention of DKA

Since DKA continues to be a potentially fatal complication of diabetes mellitus, efforts should be made to prevent its occurrence. Insulin-dependent diabetics should be cautioned against large decreases in insulin dose for any reason without consulting a physician. Particular care must be taken by the patient during any acute illness resulting in diminished food intake. Although hypoglycemia can result from continued use of normal doses of insulin, DKA may occur if the insulin dose is cut back too drastically. We suggest that at least half of the usual morning dose of insulin be taken, unless the patient is aglycosuric at the time. The patient should be instructed about appropriate electrolyte-containing fluids to use when a gastrointestinal illness occurs.

Early recognition of the signs of DKA by the patient is important since delay in diagnosis has been associated with increased mortality. Since volume depletion is a major factor in the development of DKA, patients should be advised to contact a physician whenever they are unable to maintain fluid intake in the face of continued heavy glycosuria. Urine testing for ketones can allow early detection of metabolic decompensation. Education of the patient's family may also be helpful in the early detection of DKA and its prevention.

Hyperosmolar Coma

The term hyperosmolar coma has been used to describe a syndrome characterized by marked hyperglycemia, a large total-body water deficit resulting in hyperosmolality of body fluids, the lack of significant ketosis, and the presence of varying degrees of alteration of mental status. In general, this diagnosis is given to a patient in whom the serum glucose is greater than 600 mg/dl, the serum osmolality is greater than 350 mOsm/kg, and undiluted serum does not have a strongly positive nitroprusside test. Patients selected on the basis of these criteria have a relatively characteristic clinical picture which differs markedly from the findings of most patients with DKA. These patients are generally non-insulin-dependent diabetics over age 60, have underlying renal disease, and usually have a major identifiable concomitant acute illness. The mortality rate of such patients is high, reportedly in the range of 30–50%.

It is apparent that the diagnosis of hyperosmolar coma is based on rather arbitrary criteria. Many diabetics have episodes of moderate hyperosmolality unassociated with ketosis but are not given a diagnosis of hyperosmolar coma. Severe hyperosmolality is also a major feature of DKA. The pathogenesis of hyperglycemia and hyperosmolality is probably quite similar in all of these circumstances. Furthermore, it is becoming increasingly clear that a therapeutic approach emphasizing replacement of salt and water deficits as well as adequate tissue insulinization should be used whether the patient has hyperosmolar coma, DKA, or simply poor diabetes control.

Pathogenesis

The mechanisms by which hyperglycemia and hyperosmolality develop in patients with hyperosmolar coma are similar to those that occur in DKA (see Fig. 15–89). Primary beta cell failure and/or inhibition of beta cell function by stress-related adrenergic activation results in inadequate insulin secretion. Under the influence of elevated stress hormone levels and impaired beta cell responsiveness, glucose production increases and glucose uptake by tissues is inhibited. As a result, hyperglycemia develops. The subsequent cycle of hyperglycemia → osmotic diuresis → salt and water depletion → decreased renal perfusion and increased stress hormone release leads to progressively more severe hyperglycemia and hyperosmolality. The presence of underlying renal disease in many of the patients with the syndrome tends to accelerate the development of hyperglycemia by limiting glucose excretion. An underlying major illness also frequently is present, providing an additional stimulus for stress hormone secretion and interfering with the patient's ability to replace salt and water losses.

The major unsolved question about the syndrome of hyperosmolar coma is why these patients with evidence of a severe deficiency of insulin action do not develop significant ketosis. The lack of ketosis could be explained if tissue insulin levels were adequate to prevent lipolysis or ketogenesis but inadequate to maintain glucose homeostasis. Since lipolysis can be inhibited by lower levels of insulin than are required to facilitate tissue glucose uptake or to inhibit hepatic glucose production, such a circumstance is theoretically possible. However, measurements of circulating insulin levels have not supported this hypothesis, since patients with DKA have immunoreactive insulin levels similar to those of patients with the hyperosmolar coma syndrome. Alternatively, it is possible that portal vein insulin levels are higher in hyperosmolar coma or that fat and/or liver cells of patients with this syndrome are more sensitive to the insulin that is present.

If insulin deficiency is comparable in patients with DKA and hyperosmolar coma, one must then postulate that in patients with hyperosmolar coma there is either the existence of another antilipolytic or antiketogenic substance or the lack of substances that promote lipolysis or ketogenesis. Thus far, the emphasis has been on control of lipolysis, since FFA levels in patients with hyperosmolar coma are generally much lower than in those with DKA, although this finding is somewhat variable. Hyperosmolality *per se* has been reported to inhibit lipolysis. Although serum osmolality tends to be higher in hyperosmolar coma than in DKA, many patients with DKA also have a very high serum osmolality. Prostaglandin E_2 is the only known major inhibitor of lipolysis other than insulin. Thus, a marked increase of PGE_2 production could prevent the occurrence of ketosis. No studies to date have tested this hypothesis. A lack of lipolytic hormones would also tend to prevent ketosis; however, studies to date have not documented deficiencies in growth hormone, cortisol, glucagon, or catecholamine release in patients with hyperosmolar coma. The occasional reports of the occurrence of this syndrome in patients with high levels of FFA suggest that some patients may have a defect of hepatic ketogenesis. However, no studies have established a mechanism for such an effect.

Clinical Features

Perhaps the most cogent justification for identifying hyperosmolar coma as a syndrome distinct from other states of poor diabetes control is the characteristic clinical findings manifested by most of the patients. In the largest reported series (Arieff and Carroll), two-thirds of the patients were over age 60 and one-half had no previous diagnosis of diabetes mellitus. Of those patients with a known history of diabetes, none had been treated with insulin. Most of the patients with hyperosmolar coma have underlying renal disease, and most have an identifiable major precipitating illness. This illness is generally either an infection or an acute cerebrovascular event. Other patients have been using a drug which may have contributed to the development of hyperosmolar coma. Such drugs include phenytoin, diuretics, corticosteroids, and some immunosuppressive agents. Hyperosmolar coma has also occurred in patients with acromegaly, thyrotoxicosis, and Cushing's syndrome.

There is generally a history of polyuria, polydipsia, and weight loss preceding a deterioration of mental status which leads to hospitalization. Since many patients have an associated major acute illness, the signs and symptoms of the illness may be predominant. Thus, the symptoms associated with hyperglycemia may be elicited only in retrospect after the diagnosis of hyperosmolar coma is established by laboratory tests. On examination, patients have varying degrees of obtundation, signs of the associated illness (particularly fever), and evidence of marked volume depletion: postural hypotension, flat neck veins, decreased skin turgor, and dry mucous membranes. A variety of neurologic findings may be present with or without a cerebrovascular event. These include focal or general motor seizures, aphasia, hemiplegia, sensory deficits, and hyperreflexia. The explanation for these findings appears to be multifocal brain hemorrhages and infarctions, which have been observed at autopsy in some of these patients. Since ketonemia is minimal, there is no acetone odor to the breath, and Kussmaul respirations are generally not present.

The syndrome of hyperglycemic hyperosmolar coma may also develop in the hospital in severely ill patients receiving hypertonic glucose solutions for nutritional support or in patients with renal failure undergoing peritoneal dialysis with hypertonic glucose solutions. Patients with burns or who are undergoing major surgery in which hypothermia is used as an adjunctive measure are particularly at risk of developing hyperosmolar coma if they are not managed carefully. Such patients are not necessarily diabetic, and they may have normal carbohydrate metabolism after recovery from the acute problem.

Laboratory Findings

By definition, marked hyperglycemia and hyperosmolality are present. Findings are generally similar to those of patients with DKA, but the hyperosmolality may be even more pronounced. The major laboratory finding that differentiates this syndrome from DKA is the lack of significant ketonemia. The nitroprusside test should not be strongly positive in undiluted serum. Since ketonemia is mild or absent, there may be no systemic acidosis. However, because of the marked hypovolemia and resulting diminished tissue perfusion, lactic acidosis may occur. As indicated earlier, the mitochondrial redox state during lactic acidosis may tend to obscure the coexistence of ketoacidosis by favoring the formation of betahydroxybutyrate, which is not measured by the nitroprusside test. Thus, when systemic acidosis is present, a diagnosis of hyperosmolar coma rather than DKA can be established only by measurement of serum betahydroxybutyrate and lactate to determine whether excess amounts of one or both are present. As will be indicated, such measurements may be academic, since the current approach to therapy of both DKA and hyperosmolar coma is the same.

Management

The major emphasis in treatment of hyperosmolar coma has been focused on aggressive replacement of the massive salt and water deficits which characterize the syndrome and on identification and treatment of any associated acute illness. The general approach to fluid and electrolyte therapy should be similar to that previously outlined for DKA (see Table 15–16): initial administration of large amounts of 0.9% NaCl to restore intravascular volume and improve tissue perfusion, then more gradual replacement of the water deficit over 12–48 hours. These patients must be monitored with particular care, since they may have underlying heart disease which will limit their ability to tolerate salt loading, and they often have renal disease which may limit their ability to excrete a solute load.

In contrast to DKA, for which in the past there has been an overemphasis on insulin therapy and an underemphasis on fluid management, the role of insulin in the treatment of hyperosmolar coma has perhaps been underemphasized. As indicated in the discussion of therapy of DKA, aggressive fluid therapy alone can lower the serum glucose dramatically by improving renal perfusion so that glucose can be eliminated by the kidneys and by reducing the levels of stress hormones which augment glucose production. Similar lowering of serum glucose can occur with fluids alone in most patients with hyperosmolar coma. However, fluid therapy may be less efficacious in patients with underlying renal disease, who may not be able to excrete glucose efficiently even when renal perfusion is adequate. Of even more theoretical importance is the potential adverse effect of starving insulin-dependent tissues by reducing levels of glucose without providing insulin. In DKA, insulin-dependent tissues have access to large amounts of ketones for fuel. However, glucose is the only major fuel available (by definition) in hyperosmolar coma. Thus, insulin treatment may be important not only to help reduce hyperglycemia but also to supply fuel to starved insulin-dependent tissues.

It has been observed that most patients with hyperosmolar coma are rather sensitive to insulin, requiring only modest doses to establish metabolic control. However, the current low-dose regimens described earlier for patients with DKA can be applied with equal effectiveness and little risk of hypoglycemia in patients with hyperosmolar coma. It should be re-emphasized, however, that once the serum glucose falls below 250 mg/dl, glucose should be added to intravenous fluids and the frequency of insulin administration reduced to once every 4–6 hours. Insulin therapy does involve the potential risk of development of hypokalemia as potassium shifts into cells under the influence of insulin. Thus, as in DKA, serum potassium should be monitored carefully, and replacement of the total-body potassium deficit should begin as soon as urine output is established.

Complications

The high mortality rate of patients with hyperosmolar coma appears to be related primarily to the associated major illness which accompanies this syndrome. Thus, most deaths have been due to infection or vascular events, and relatively few have been ascribed to the hyperosmolar state *per se*. Infections and vascular events have also appeared to occur as a direct result of the severe debilitation and volume depletion of some patients. These events presumably could be prevented by aggressive fluid management and careful attention to bronchopulmonary toilet and iatrogenic sites where infections could be introduced (intravenous lines and bladder catheters).

Long-Term Management of Diabetes

General Principles

Long-term treatment of diabetes has been generally directed toward control of the glucose level in the hope of preventing or reversing the microvascular, atherosclerotic, and neuropathic changes found in diabetes mellitus. Despite several decades of experience and a great number of retrospective analyses, it is still not clear whether this goal can be achieved. There is general agreement that treatment of overt diabetes should be directed toward control of the measurable metabolic abnormalities in order to normalize fat, protein, and carbohydrate metabolism. One usually sets a series of priorities in relation to the known metabolic effects of relative or absolute insulin deficiency present in overt diabetes: *first*, control of excessive fatty acid mobilization and oxidation (i.e., treatment and prevention of ketoacidosis); *second*, control of excessive protein catabolism and muscle wasting, carbohydrate wastage, and urinary caloric loss (overt diabetes). That these two goals require treatment is universally agreed. However, after these two goals have been reached, the patient is often left with asymptomatic hyperglycemia. Treatment of overt diabetes to the point of eliminating ketosis and glycosuria will restore total daily carbohydrate, protein, and fat turnover to normal. Since these metabolic indices are not quantitatively abnormal in aglycosuric hyperglycemic diabetics, we are left with two unanswered questions: (1) does further control of hyperglycemia *per se* provide any additional benefit to the patient? and (2) is it possible to achieve this degree of control of hyperglycemia with the therapeutic modalities currently available?

The description of a number of insulin-independent pathways, such as those leading to the synthesis of the sugar alcohol sorbitol, glycosylated hemoglobin, and basement membrane glycoproteins, which may be increased in hyperglycemic subjects has raised the possibility that hyperglycemia *per se* is deleterious to health. Unfortunately, it is currently impossible to therapeutically simulate the complexities of normal insulin secretion over a prolonged period of time in order to achieve normal glucose homeostasis. Therefore, an adequate test of the hypothesis that control of hyperglycemia would prevent or improve all of the degenerative neural and vascular changes of the diabetic syndrome has not been possible. The studies that have been done with current therapeutic modalities have not supported the concept that treatment of mild hyperglycemia and glucose intolerance does reduce the mortality rate of mild maturity-onset diabetics. On the other hand, it seems likely that treatment may delay the chronic neural and vascular diseases of the more severely hyperglycemic diabetic. On this hypothetical basis, we would suggest that one should intervene therapeutically to attempt to prevent excessive excursions of blood glucose, particularly those leading to symptomatic glycosuria and hypoglycemia. However, at the present time it is not warranted to institute a regimen that fails to permit the patient to live a reasonably comfortable life.

Dietary Therapy

The inability to restore insulin secretion in a truly physiologic manner requires that diet be an *essential* part of all therapeutic programs. Since the fundamental physiologic abnormality in diabetes is the inability to store calories properly for later use, dietary therapy should stress caloric control and regularity. In general, sufficient calories should be provided to achieve and maintain ideal body weight (in children and adolescents, this includes normal growth and development). Thus, if the patient is malnourished and underweight, he must be provided with additional calories to restore weight. If he is overnourished or obese, caloric restriction must be prescribed. An average nonobese adult uses 30–50 cal/kg/day for weight maintenance, while an obese individual may require only 20–30 cal/kg/day. From many metabolic studies, we have found that weight maintenance in a metabolic ward (i.e., that for sedentary activity in adults) can be calculated from the following formula: cal/kg/day = 52.2 − [15.5 × % ideal weight (kg actual weight/kg ideal weight)]. This formula is valid up to 250% of ideal weight using the Metropolitan Life tables for medium frame. Increased activity increases caloric need; therefore, younger individuals tend to require more calories on a weight basis. This increased need may be as high as 50–60 cal/kg/day in children.

Although major emphasis in the past was placed on the proportion of carbohydrate, fat, and protein calories of the diet, in the last 10 years many studies have suggested that this proportional distribution is of less importance. In fact, clinicians over the years have prescribed diets varying from 10 to 65% carbohydrate, and all have claimed therapeutic successes. As far as glucose control is concerned, the percentage of carbohydrate content of the diet does not usually seem to have much influence on hyperglycemia and glycosuria, provided that calories remain constant and caloric distribution is unchanged. As stated by Albrink and Davidson, perhaps the most that can be concluded is that diabetics tolerate an amazingly wide range of dietary carbohydrate intake, and there is very little firm evidence either for or against any specific percentage of carbohydrate in the diet with respect to its long-range effect on the control of

Table 15–17. DIET THERAPY FOR DIABETES MELLITUS

MOD (NIDDM)	JOD (IDDM)
Key features are:	Key features are:
1. Caloric restriction (diet or behavior modification)	1. Adequate calories for growth and exercise.
2. Low-fat, low-cholesterol intake (high-fiber?)	2. Distribution of food during the day
3. Adequate micronutrient intake (vitamins and minerals)	3. Day-to-day regularity of total calories and meal timing

plasma glucose. For this reason, the American Diabetes Association has recommended a diet that contains roughly normal proportions of calories from carbohydrate, protein, and fat (45–50% carbohydrate and 40% fat) or, more recently, a low-fat, high-carbohydrate diet (50–60% carbohydrate, 30% fat). This freedom to prescribe carbohydrate calories is particularly important in view of the recent desire of many physicians to use low–animal fat and low-cholesterol diets in the hope of preventing atherosclerosis. It is the authors' belief that such a diet, inherently high in carbohydrate content, is in fact desirable for the diabetic population.

Having decided on the total caloric content, distribution, and type of diet to be prescribed, the physician is faced with the necessity of educating the patient to achieve these therapeutic goals. The further the prescribed diet deviates from the average American diet, the greater the need for precise and careful dietary instruction. Therefore, the time spent in education should be proportional to the complexity of the diet. In general, it is best to work closely with a nutritionist or educator who will implement the plan. In recent years, it has become clear that dietary goals and emphasis should be quite different for insulin-treated and non-insulin-treated patients (Table 15–17). Therefore, the treatment program should reflect the metabolic differences in these two types of diabetes.

Juvenile-Onset-Type Diabetes (JOD). This group of insulin-dependent diabetics (IDDM) is generally lean and quite active. Since there is little tendency to obesity, caloric restriction is rarely indicated. The major problem is to match caloric intake to the timing and quantity of exercise, insulin, and food calories. Random food selection and appetite are usually adequate to maintain weight and nutrition; however, a knowledge of caloric values is necessary to maintain the same caloric equivalence of meals taken at the same time each day. Because of the long-acting insulin preparations used, most such patients will require three meals a day *and* an evening snack. In children, the number of meals may be increased to six. Caloric values of foods can be learned by either weighing foods or using the food-exchange system developed by the American Diabetes Association and the American Dietetic Association. The system was devised to simplify dietary prescription by segregating foods into exchange lists, each food group on the list containing about the same amount of carbohydrate, protein, and fat as any other food on the list. It allows for reasonable variety in the meals and yet does not require the accurate weighing of food prior to preparation, although it is still essential for the patient to be aware of the caloric value of foods.

However, random selection will usually lead to a diet containing approximately 45–50% of calories as carbohydrate. Thus, in lean, insulin-dependent diabetics, it has not always been necessary to prescribe a calorie-controlled diet. An example of this approach is the use of the unmeasured diet in diabetic subjects of normal body weight. The patient is instructed to eat food that is balanced in composition, but the quantity ingested is regulated by his appetite rather than by prescription. Such an individual, however, is expected to eat approximately the same amount of food each day at each meal; in the studies performed by Knowles and colleagues, four to six meals per day were prescribed. Follow-up suggested that this type of diet plan is as effective as a more complex prescribed diet for insulin-treated diabetics of normal body weight. Owing to the propensity of such patients to develop accelerated atherosclerosis, we suggest that low-cholesterol, low–saturated fat diets be encouraged for this group.

Maturity-Onset-Type Diabetes (MOD). Although non-insulin-dependent patients (NIDDM) also require a dietary program, the diet requirements are usually quite different. In most subjects with milder degrees of carbohydrate intolerance, obesity is a major problem; therefore, caloric control should be instituted. Again, a balanced diet is explained and provided, but the total number of calories is reduced. Because caloric restriction reduces the ability to respond to sudden nutrient ingestion, it is even more important that dietary regularity be instituted in such patients and that intermittent periods of fasting and feasting are avoided as the obese diabetic attempts to regulate body weight. Since this group of patients may respond to caloric restriction alone with significant improvement in glycosuria and hyperglycemia, insulin and oral therapeutic agents are not given until the effectiveness of dietary control can be evaluated. At the present time, it is our practice to instruct patients in the caloric value of foods, to prescribe total caloric levels to be adhered to by each patient, and to attempt to achieve this without a complex dietary program. In subjects unable to reduce weight satisfactorily, we often use the exchange list as a means to educate the patient about the caloric value of a wide variety of foods. This list is then used to maintain a desired caloric intake until ideal weight is achieved. In our experience, even this type of dietary approach is often unsuccessful and other approaches become necessary. Most recently, we have attempted some form of group therapy or behavior modification in the hope of improving the response rate, but in the long run we are no more successful than others, and only a few of the obese subjects ever attain ideal weight in our clinic. However, even modest weight reduction is often associated with marked improvement in carbohydrate metabolism; therefore, caloric restriction and weight loss should be a major focus for the newly diagnosed patient.

In lean individuals with maturity-onset-type diabetes, diet may have only minimal benefit. However, the size and distribution of individual caloric loads can be a factor. It is quite clear that insulin secretion in response to food stimulation is inadequate in such lean, maturity-onset diabetics and that this defect is most obvious when large caloric loads are given. This probably explains the greater diagnostic discrimination of the 100-g OGTT compared with the 50-g test, and the 20- to 40-g IVGTT compared with the 5- to 10-g test. Thus, even in the lean non-insulin-treated diabetic, large caloric loads should be avoided. Most such patients should eat at least three meals a day. This type of meal spacing also requires caloric regularity from day to day. Although normal individuals can cope with caloric intakes that vary widely from day to day, i.e., 5000 cal one day and 1000 cal the next, the maturity-onset-type diabetic does poorly under such circumstances. It is this inability to handle large caloric loads that is probably responsible for the clinical observation that "cheating" on diabetic diets results in prompt glycosuria. It is the inappropriately large caloric load, rather than the type of foodstuffs eaten, that leads to the immediate hyperglycemia and glycosuria.

Exercise

Exercsie increases glucose utilization by a mechanism which does not depend upon increased secretion of insulin. This increased utilization is balanced by an increased output of glucose by the liver in normal individuals. Therefore, plasma glucose levels are not changed. The mechanism for the compensation is not completely clear, but activation of the sympathetic nervous system to increase hepatic glucose output is believed to be important. Insulin release is suppressed in the normal individual by this activation which allows the increase in hepatic glucose output to occur. In the insulin-treated diabetic, increased blood flow to the subcutaneous tissues during exercise has been shown to increase circulating insulin levels by mobilization of the injected depot. Under these conditions, hepatic glucose production is restrained and muscle glucose uptake accelerates even more, leading to a rather precipitous decline in plasma glucose and potentially resulting in frank hypoglycemia. The risk of hypoglycemia can be minimized by food ingestion immediately before the exercise or by instituting a plan that will include regular amounts of exercise at specified times.

Chronic exercise training has been shown to increase insulin sensitivity. The mechanism appears to be related to an increase in the number and affinity of insulin receptors. Therefore, with regular exercise there is not only an improvement in exercise efficiency but a change in insulin sensitivity. These changes are also associated, as in non-diabetics, with a decrease in VLDL triglyceride concentration and an increase in HDL cholesterol levels, both of which tend to be associated with a decreased risk of macrovascular disease. These effects take some time to be manifested (1–2 weeks) but are lost very quickly (1–2 days) and may explain some of the marked variation in insulin requirement observed in insulin-treated patients who exercise intermittently.

The non-insulin-treated diabetic has no subcutaneous insulin depot to mobilize, and sympathetic suppression of insulin secretion is intact. Therefore, hypoglycemia during exercise does not occur. The same effects of chronic exercise training on insulin sensitivity and plasma lipids may be expected in these patients and should be considered as part of an overall plan for diabetes treatment.

Education

The diabetic must substitute external control of diet and insulin, for which he is responsible, for internal control of insulin which in the normal individual keeps plasma glucose levels relatively constant. Therefore, education in the physiology of normal metabolism and in the external controls that will be prescribed by the physician is an essential part of the treatment program. In general, it is probably best to think of the diabetic as caring for his own disease with the advice and consultation of the physician rather than as a patient for whom all the therapeutic decisions are made by the physician. The diabetic should be aware of the effects of diet and exercise on metabolic control and be cognizant of methods of measuring the degree of metabolic control as reflected in the urine and blood. He also should be able to make adjustments in his treatment program, depending upon his physiologic and pathophysiologic state as it changes from day to day. Much of this information can be imparted through formal classwork, but the physician should use the routine clinic visit for continuing education of the diabetic. In general, it is preferable for the formal education programs to be coordinated in a community or area so that there may be interaction between the patient, other diabetics, and the instructor. There is a growing tendency for this work to be done by paramedical personnel as part of a teaching unit.

The following areas should be part of any teaching program: (1) the clinical signs and symptoms and genetic aspects of the disease and the general nature of the disordered pathophysiology; (2) discussion of diet, including a general discussion of the metabolism of various foodstuffs, the need for regularity in diet, the specific nature of the dietary program recommended for the individual patient, and the importance of interaction between diet, insulin, and exercise on metabolic control; (3) insulin — every patient should be capable of injecting himself with insulin, whether or not the therapeutic program requires this form of therapy at the moment. The nature and source of insulin, types and action of insulin, method of injection, and side effects of insulin therapy should be covered; (4) oral hypoglycemic agents, with a general discussion of the differences between insulin and the oral agents, the nature of the oral agents available, and a frank discussion of their uses and limitations; (5) methodology for urine and blood testing, with specific instruction on glycosuria and ketonuria; and (6) general health care, which needs to be emphasized particularly for the diabetic, such as care of the lower extremities, handling of minor infections and illnesses, diagnosis and therapy of dermatophytoses, and some discussion of the concomitants of diabetes, particularly the microangiopathy, neuropathy, and large-vessel disease.

Insulin Treatment

When the ability to secrete insulin in response to a challenge diminishes sufficiently, the patient with diabetes mellitus begins to lose significant portions of his daily calories as glycosuria. With this caloric loss there is increased gluconeogenesis to maintain carbohydrate metabolism and a reduction of body protein. At this point, a severe complication of insulin deficiency, ketoacidosis, can occur. Such individuals require exogenous insulin in order to maintain weight without caloric excess. Insulin secretion in the normal individual is regulated by the nature and amount of exogenous foodstuffs in order to maintain normal metabolism of ingested carbohydrate, fat, and protein. The patient with insulin-dependent diabetes mellitus differs from a normal individual in that he receives a fixed dose of insulin to which he must match his food intake, as there will not be the normal peaks of insulin in association with food ingestion. Therefore, even with insulin therapy, diabetic patients are unable to store foodstuffs as efficiently as a normal individual who responds to the challenge by suddenly secreting insulin. Since exogenous insulin treatment is an inadequate physiologic replacement, the attainment of reasonable metabolic control requires an understanding of the properties of the various insulin preparations, the nature of the interaction of injected insulin with basic metabolic processes, and the potential complications of insulin therapy.

Insulin Preparations

Data on a variety of insulin preparations are given in Table 15–18. All of these preparations consist of recrystallized extracts of either beef or pork pancreas which have been commercially purified to approximately 95% insulin. The 5% contamination consists of insulin polymers, proinsulin intermediates, and degradation products. There has been continued improvement in purifying the product, with great progress made recently by using Sephadex chromatography to exclude the larger molecular weight aggregates and ion-exchange chromatography to eliminate insulin-sized peptides with different charge characteristics such as VIP, glucagon, somatostatin, and pancreatic polypeptide. At the present time, all commercial insulins are chromatographed on Sephadex and are at least 99% pure. Since beef insulin has different antigenic properties, a number of manufacturers also prepare pure pork insulin. Apparently, because of the closer structural similarity to human insulin, the pork insulins are generally less antigenic. With the elimination of the higher molecular weight forms of insulin and the noninsulin peptides, the only residual cause of insulin antibody formation is in the species difference. Therefore, commercial attempts to synthesize human insulin in bacteria have begun. At present, ion-exchange chromatography is used largely for pure pork insulin preparations. These specially purified insulins are now called "monocomponent," "single-peak," or "single-component" insulin, depending on the manufacturer and the purity. Since contaminating peptides are not always identifiable, it is not clear that these preparations are the same or that different lots from the same manufacturer are always the same. However, in general, only these latter very highly purified insulins have been found to have reduced clinical antigenicity.

Crystalline Zinc Insulin (CZI), Neutral Regular Insulin. Crystalline zinc insulin and neutral regular insulin are the forms that are most rapidly acting and metabolized. Originally, this form of insulin was available only in a solution of pH 2.5–3.5. When injected subcutaneously, it is possible that some was precipitated by the tissue change to pH 7.5, thus altering the clinical pharmacology of the preparation. Neutral regular insulin was therefore introduced and has largely replaced the acid-pH CZI. The other preparations have been modified so as to prolong the effect of injected insulin. Neutral regular insulin, crystalline zinc insulin, and semilente insulin (see later) are the only forms which can be given intravenously. They may also be injected subcutaneously 15–30 minutes before a meal, so that the circulating levels will parallel nutrient influx during and after the meal.

Table 15–18. AMERICAN PREPARATIONS OF INSULIN

Type of Insulin	Buffer	pH	Suspension	Zinc mg/100 U	Interval of Maximal Action (hr)	Total Duration of Action (hr)
Lente series						
Semilente	Acetate	7.1–7.5	Amorphous	0.2 –0.25	4–6	12–16
Lente	Acetate	7.1–7.5	(30% Amor. 70% Cry.)	0.2 –0.25	8–12	18–24
Ultralente	Acetate	7.1–7.5	Crystalline	0.2 –0.25	16–18	30–36
Crystalline zinc	None	2.5–3.5	(Solution)	0.01–0.04	4–6	6–8
NPH (isophane)	Phosphate	7.1–7.4	Crystalline	0.01–0.04	8–12	18–24
Protamine zinc	Phosphate	7.1–7.4	Amorphous	0.2 –0.25	14–20	24–36

Protamine Zinc Insulin (PZI). The initial modification of insulin to prolong its duration of action was made by Hagedorn and coworkers, who found that a properly buffered solution containing the protein protamine would produce a precipitate with poor solubility and slow absorption. Prior to the introduction of PZI as a therapeutic agent in the 1930's, regular insulin alone was insufficient to prevent dwarfism in some patients. The introduction (1936) of the first long-acting insulin prevented this disabling consequence. PZI has a very long duration of action which has limited its use. Another problem with this material is its excess content of protamine, which binds any crystalline insulin put into the same syringe, thereby making it also long-acting. This led to development of neutral protamine Hagedorn (NPH) insulin.

Neutral Protamine Hagedorn (NPH) Insulin. Partly because of the difficulty in mixing crystalline zinc insulin and protamine zinc insulin, and partly because of the very long duration of action of PZI, a near-stoichiometric mixture of protamine and insulin with a shorter duration of action and compatibility with crystalline zinc insulin was rapidly adopted world-wide in the 1930's. Available for subcutaneous injection, NPH insulin has a pattern of action that was more closely related to normal meal-eating patterns than those of the other insulins available at the time. It is still widely used in the United States.

Lente Insulins. In the 1950's, a series of insulins was produced in which zinc insulin crystals were of two different types which in acetate buffer yielded a very long-acting form similar to PZI and a very short-acting form similar to crystalline zinc insulin. The advantage of these different forms was that they permitted the patient to mix the long- and short-acting insulins in any combination desired. The lack of an extra protein, such as protamine or globin, in lente insulins also reduced allergic reactions. A mixture of 70% of the long-acting form (ultralente) and 30% of the short-acting form (semilente) gave a time course of action very similar to that of NPH insulin and is marketed as lente insulin. With this series of insulins, any combination of long- and short-acting insulin can be prescribed in a compatible form, making it very popular. Some idealized curves for the various types of insulin are given in Figure 15–97. At present, ultralente is available only as a beef preparation since it has not been possible to produce a long-acting ultralente-type insulin from pure pork insulin. Thus, purified intermediate-acting lente insulin is by necessity a beef-pork mixture.

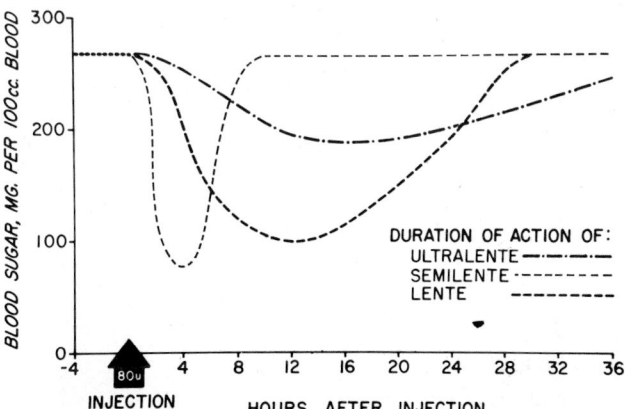

Figure 15–97. The extremes in rates and degrees of hypoglycemic effects are demonstrated by ultralente and semilente insulin preparations after subcutaneous injection. Intermediate types of responses result from mixtures of these solutions, as illustrated by lente insulin, which is composed of 70 parts of ultralente and 30 parts of semilente.

Clinical Pharmacology

Insulin injected subcutaneously must be absorbed into the bloodstream to be effective. Therefore, differences in the rates of absorption from different sites contribute to variations in response. Recent studies have shown that the increased blood flow of exercise markedly increases the absorption of insulin and may totally account for hypoglycemia in insulin-treated diabetics during exercise. This effect is greater when subcutaneous insulin is injected into the exercising limb (usually the leg) than into the abdominal wall. This effect does not seem to occur at all during continuous intravenous infusions, suggesting that either increased delivery of insulin to exercising muscle is not important to the increase in glucose metabolism by muscle or that such an effect is balanced by decreased insulin delivery to the liver during exercise. At rest, the abdominal site provides for the fastest rate of absorption.

In general, all types of commercial insulin are stable, even when stored for moderate intervals at room temperature. Although it is desirable to keep insulin refrigerated to maintain full potency, during periods of traveling there is no appreciable loss of activity at room temperature — even up to a month. Insulin put into intravenous fluids, as is sometimes done during surgery, has caused problems, one of which is the binding of insulin to the intravenous tubing. As much as 50% of the insulin can bind to glass and plastic surfaces when the fluid contains no protein, but this occurs only at very low concentrations. More important, since there is no fixed ratio between insulin and glucose administration in any individual case, hyperglycemia or hypoglycemia may result from simultaneous intravenous administration of glucose and insulin. For this reason, separate infusion rates must be used to control insulin and glucose delivery.

Physicians and patients should be aware of factors that determine responses to insulin. In general, the larger the dose of any insulin, the longer is its duration of action and the later is its maximal effect. Therefore, in an insulin-resistant patient who requires more than 200 U of insulin a day, regular crystalline zinc insulin may be effective for as long as NPH or lente insulin in other diabetics. Important factors that are determinants of the insulin "requirement" are hormones that antagonize insulin action, insulin-resistant states, and the amount of circulating insulin antibodies. The catecholamines, estrogens, growth hormone, chorionic somatomammotropin, and the corticosteroids induce insulin resistance. Therefore with all other factors remaining equal, excess of any of these hormones increases the need for insulin. Certain physiologic and pathophysiologic states will have the same effect. The most important of these, obesity, always induces insulin resistance in proportion to the degree of adiposity and necessitates larger amounts of insulin for maintaining metabolic control. Chronic liver disease and uremia may also produce insulin-resistant states.

Insulin Antibodies. Insulin-binding antibodies of the IgG or IgM type are produced in significant amounts in any diabetic patient treated with nonpurified insulin for more than 30 days. The levels have not been accurately quantified, but in some patients they are high enough to markedly impair insulin action. High levels of insulin antibodies and periodic variations in their amounts may cause difficulty in the regulation of insulin therapy. In many patients who require more than 200 U of insulin per day, a high antibody titer is present. Whenever more than average insulin dosage is required or there is a significant problem in glucose regulation, it is desirable to consider the use of insulin preparations that are less immunogenic or to consider modifying the antibody response in some fashion. Since most commercial insulin is a beef-pork mixture and the antibody titers to beef insulin are higher, switching to highly purified pork insulin may result in a lessening of insulin requirement. There is recent evidence that the immunogenic component of commercial insulin preparations is only in small part due to the single-component (6000 molecular weight) hormone and to a greater extent due to some form of molecular aggregate. It has been found that the use of insulin more purified than the present commercial supply causes less antibody production. The level of antibody itself and its amount of insulin binding may also be reduced by the administration of glucosteroids. Usually, fairly high doses of a potent glucosteroid such as prednisone, 40–60 mg/day, must be given. Although glucosteroids induce peripheral insulin resistance, this effect may be outweighed by reduction in antibody titer in patients with very high insulin antibody levels and may be sufficient to markedly reduce insulin requirement.

Allergic Reactions. Local reactions to the injection of insulin are not unusual, but their true incidence is unknown. The range in published studies has varied from 1–56%. This variability is probably because the majority of reactions are mild and unreported. The presence of such a side effect appears to be unrelated to the development of circulating IgG and IgM insulin antibodies, which neutralize the effects of the injected hormone; that is, there appears to be no tendency for those with high circulating IgG antibody titers to develop allergy more frequently than those with low titers. On the other hand, there is a reasonable correlation with circulating IgE antibodies. The incidence of these allergic reactions appears to be decreasing, perhaps because of the increased purity of insulin preparations, indicating that some of the reactions are due to the contaminants. Some authors have concluded that the added protamine has produced some of these allergic reactions and that the use of non-protamine-containing insulin preparations may be beneficial. Since these local allergic responses are probably related to IgE insulin antibodies, it is not certain they will disappear altogether, even with purified insulin and no IgG antibodies.

The most common local reactions are relatively mild and include stinging or itching at the injection site, which may or may not be followed by heat, induration, erythema, and an urticarial reaction. Fortunately more than 95% of the reactions are local and mild. Usually, the patients can be treated systemically with antihistaminic compounds, and the type of insulin need not be changed. If a change of insulin is needed because of persistence or severity of the allergic response, purified pork insulin should be tried first. If this is not effective, pure beef insulin can be tried. In any case, protamine should be eliminated by using the lente series.

Some patients develop generalized urticaria accompanied by nausea, vomiting, diarrhea, or, in rare instances, angioneurotic edema and serum sickness. Occasionally, reports have been made of anaphylactic shock and, in a few instances, purpura as well. Since insulin is often a necessary treatment regardless of the hypersensitive state, treatment of the allergy is usually necessary. The immediate treatment is epinephrine and/or steroids. The long-term treatment of systemic insulin allergy is desensitization. Kits for this purpose are available from Eli Lilly Company. The usual procedure is intradermal and then subsequent subcutaneous injection of small doses of insulin on ½- to 2-hour schedules until tolerance can be induced. Usually purified pork insulin is used for this purpose. Once desensitized, patients need to be treated with insulin at least twice daily to maintain tolerance.

The most important predisposing cause of insulin allergy and high levels of insulin antibodies is intermittent use of insulin. Individuals who will be treated intermittently during pregnancy or infection or for some other reason should use the most highly purified insulins available to minimize this complication.

Lipodystrophy. The subcutaneous injection of insulin in certain susceptible patients may result in either hypertrophy or atrophy of the local adipose tissue mass (Fig. 15–98). The hypertrophy is easily explainable by insulin's known action on the synthesis of lipids by fat cells. The cause of the atrophy, which occurs mostly in young women and children, is related in some way to the pharmacology of injectable insulin, as it does not occur during the use of purified insulin and can be treated by the local injection of single-component pork insulin into the site. The lipolysis induced by less pure insulin seems to relate to the immune system, as it correlates well with other evidence of local allergy. Once treated by local injection of single-component insulin, the patient should be continued on purified insulin and the site avoided unless a recurrence develops.

Clinical Insulin Use

Research into insulin secretion using the C-peptide assay and the development of a variety of mechanical systems to infuse insulin has radically changed our understanding of the therapeutic use of insulin. The management of the insulin-dependent, juvenile-onset-type patient who has very little residual endogenous insulin secretion is quite different from the insulin treatment of a maturity-onset, non-insulin-dependent diabetic who failed to respond to diet or a sulfonylurea. However, the major goals for the two types of patients are the same: first, to give enough insulin to free the diabetic of symptoms of hyperglycemia and glycosuria; second, to avoid hypoglycemia; and third, to control the hyperglycemia as physiologically as possible in the hope of reduc-

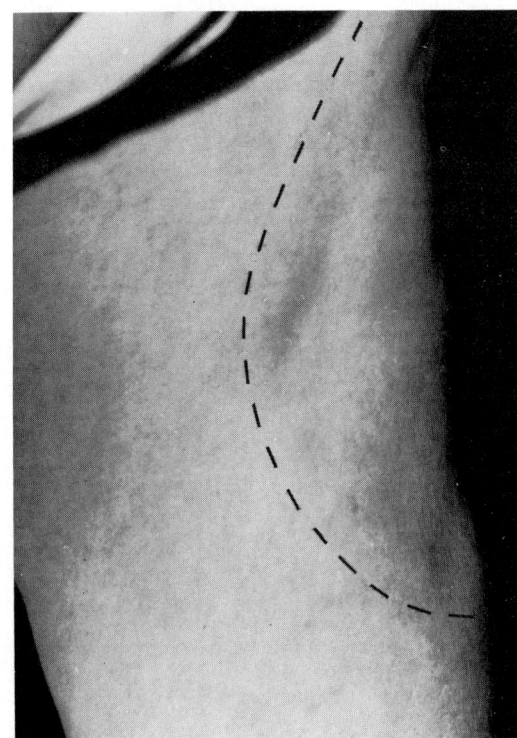

Figure 15–98. Lipoatrophy. Marked disappearance of subcutaneous fat in localized area of thigh (to right of broken line), leaving prominent depression. This was the site of frequent insulin injections. Atrophy sometimes also occurs in areas not injected.

ing the frequency and severity of the neurovascular complications. Conflict arises between these last two goals because as plasma glucose levels become more normal, hypoglycemia often becomes more frequent.

Juvenile-Onset-Type Diabetes (Insulin-Dependent Diabetes). These patients may have a brief period of meaningful insulin secretory return after diagnosis ("honeymoon period"), which some have claimed is prolonged by prompt and effective insulin therapy with nonantigenic insulin. However, this period is usually short regardless of therapy. Sooner or later these patients require replacement of both basal insulin secretion and insulin responses to meal ingestion. Since about half of normal total insulin secretion is basal (i.e., not a response to nutrient stimulation), the use of one injection of insulin a day is rarely very effective in insulin-dependent patients. Therefore, we usually begin with two injections per day. However, a major problem in this group of patients is their marked variability in exercise pattern, leading to irregular mobilization of the depot insulin with any kind of reasonable activity level. To prevent this problem we usually recommend food just prior to exercise to cover the increased insulin absorption. The lack of such a hypoglycemic response to exercise during continuous intravenous insulin infusion suggests that a major problem with present insulin preparations is that they do not release a constant amount of hormone throughout the day and night after one subcutaneous injection. In some patients shortacting regular insulin can be used 30 minutes before a meal. However, this approach is rarely effective without some long-acting insulin given to cover insulin need during the night. It has recently been observed that the insulin requirement rises rather substantially between 6 and 8 A.M. The explanation is not clear (cortisol? catecholamines? arousal?), but this phenomenon may contribute significantly to morning hyperglycemia *without* hypoglycemia during the night. Patients over the age of 8 years should inject themselves. For those with vision problems, a ratchet syringe holder is available which allows the partially sighted to continue to inject themselves accurately.

Unsuspected hypoglycemia is a major concern in insulin-treated patients. Younger diabetics may be overtreated with insulin, leading to rebound hyperglycemia (Somogyi effect) due to stimulation of counterregulatory hormones. Since hypoglycemia occurring during the night is often undetected, the frequency of this complication has been debated. Nocturnal hypoglycemia can be suspected when hyperglycemia and glycosuria are observed only in the morning and do not respond to more insulin. It can also be suspected when there is need for more than 1 unit of insulin per kilogram per day. A test for unsuspected hypoglycemia is to reduce the insulin dosage by half *gradually* over 2–3 days to see if the postulated rebound morning hyperglycemia improves. The past use of carbohydrate-restricted diets may have contributed to this problem; therefore, it may vary in frequency from clinic to clinic. In our experience, it is more often suspected than found.

Another complication of insulin treatment is sudden vasodilation as a result of a direct effect of insulin on the vascular system (Watkins). Since the older insulin-treated patient with autonomic neuropathy may not have a normal reflex vasoconstriction response, blood pressure can decline precipitously, leading to sudden syncope. It is critical to differentiate this hypotensive problem from a hypoglycemic reaction.

Some patients are difficult to manage regardless of attempts by the physician to understand the problem. Experience has focused on a number of potential causes to explain the etiology of "brittle diabetes." The following are some common findings: (1) severe insulin deficiency (total lack of C-peptide secretion); (2) errors in management (a deficiency of patient education or knowledge); (3) intercurrent illness; (4) Somogyi effect (see earlier); (5) important factors influencing the dynamics of insulin action (injection site, exercise, insulin antibodies); and (6) psychosocial factors which interfere with the maintenance of a diabetic regimen such as conflicts with the treatment goal, anxiety about the disease, frustration, parental rebellion, and emotional stress.

Recent efforts to develop a mechanical device capable of measuring plasma glucose and infusing insulin by computer-controlled response have been partially successful (closed-loop artificial pancreas). However, to date the product is unwieldy, inefficient, and unable to be used for more than 1 day at a time. Nevertheless, the experimental results indicate that the timing of insulin delivery is critical to good metabolic control. It is also clear that peripheral administration of insulin (rather than the physiologic intraportal route) probably leads to systemic hyperinsulinemia. It has also become clear that the continuous infusion of a basal level of insulin is very important to diabetes control, particularly overnight, and that some patients will probably not be well controlled without a device which can deliver insulin in this way.

Because of the complexity of this closed-loop system, a number of investigators and the National Institutes of Health have studied the use of a simpler "open-loop" device to infuse insulin without a glucose sensor. The infusions have been given either intravenously, intraperitoneally, or subcutaneously as a preprogrammed pattern of a continuous low basal level plus intermittent bolus injections prior to meals. Surprisingly, preliminary studies show improvement in diabetes control even with open-loop subcutaneous insulin administration. The explanation for the effectiveness of such treatment with minimal reported hypoglycemia is not really understood (or even believed by some!). It may be that the elimination of a subcutaneous depot so that delivery is independent of blood flow and exercise is a major mechanism. If this is the case, the subcutaneously infused patient resembles a non-insulin-dependent diabetic in whom the basal insulin infusion rate is not high enough to cause hypoglycemia between meals, and in whom meals are covered by administration of an insulin bolus.

Maturity-Onset-Type Diabetes (Non-Insulin-Dependent Diabetes). Many of these patients are either lean to begin with or are obese and will not lose weight. The choice between sulfonylurea drugs and insulin for these patients is very arbitrary at the present time. We are more likely to use insulin in patients who are young and lean. In the obese patient and in the older patient, we are more conservative in beginning nondietary treatment and usually do not use drugs in asymptomatic patients. Insulin treatment in these patients is far easier than in the juvenile insulin-dependent type, as they have sufficient residual insulin secretion to prevent ketoacidosis. Therefore, one injection of intermediate-acting insulin is usually sufficient to restore reasonable control of hyperglycemia. Our usual practice is to increase this dose until urine glucose is negative prior to the evening meal. If hyperglycemia occurs in the morning after breakfast, short-acting insulin is added. If hyperglycemia is present on arising, then two insulin doses per day are used, split 70% and 30%. This two-dose type of insulin therapy is rarely necessary in these patients. Since exercise and site of injection are important modifiers of insulin delivery in this group, we either adjust the dose of insulin on exercise days or add calories prior to exercise and advise the use of the abdominal site.

Monitoring Insulin Treatment. Urine glucose has been the key to home monitoring. We like to have the urine glucose measured at least once daily even in relatively stable

$$\beta A \text{---} NH_2 + \quad
\begin{array}{c}
HC=O \\
| \\
HCOH \\
| \\
HOCH \\
| \\
HCOH \\
| \\
HCOH \\
| \\
CH_2OH
\end{array}
\rightleftharpoons
\begin{array}{c}
HC=N\text{---}\beta A \\
| \\
HCOH \\
| \\
HOCH \\
| \\
HCOH \\
| \\
HCOH \\
| \\
CH_2OH
\end{array}
\xrightarrow{\text{Amadori}}
\begin{array}{c}
CH_2\text{---}NH\text{---}\beta A \\
| \\
C=O \\
| \\
HOCH \\
| \\
HCOH \\
| \\
HCOH \\
| \\
CH_2OH
\end{array}$$

glucose aldimine (Schiff base) ketoamine

Hb A ⟶ Hb A$_{1c}$

Figure 15–99. Chemistry of the nonenzymatic formation of HbA$_{1c}$. The aldimine reaction is easily reversible and rapid. The ketoamine formation is slow and essentially nonreversible. N—βA indicates the terminal valine amine of the β chain of HbA.

patients. Plasma glucose should also be measured in patients with reasonable control. Although random glucose estimations provide some information, our experience is that a *fasting plasma glucose* is the single best value for monitoring carbohydrate metabolism. This is particularly true for the adult patients being treated with one injection daily. The development of glucose oxidase sticks and a meter to read them has introduced the possibility of home plasma glucose monitoring. While this is a laborious and difficult task, there appears no doubt that some diabetics can substantially improve metabolic control while monitoring their own plasma glucose at home using conventionally injected insulin. Usually multiple doses of short-acting insulin have been given to such patients with one or two doses of intermediate-acting insulin per day. The major problem has been to evaluate the degree of long-term glucose control. This has been markedly improved by the discovery of hemoglobin A$_{1c}$.

Glycosylated Hemoglobin. Ten years ago Trivelli noted that a fast-migrating fraction of hemoglobin (HbA$_{1c}$) was elevated in diabetic patients. At first there was disappointment when it was found to be elevated in all diabetics but not in the unaffected twin of a diabetic, indicating that this hemoglobin variant was not a genetic marker for diabetes. Later it was shown that HbA$_{1c}$ results from the formation of an irreversible bond between glucose and the N-terminal valine of the Hb β chain (Fig. 15–99). This process of permanent glycosylation is nonenzymatic and occurs slowly *in vivo*. Thus, the percentage of hemoglobin that is glycosylated in a given red blood cell is directly proportional to the amount of time the cell has been exposed to glucose and the glucose concentration. As a result, older red cells have a higher percentage of glycosylated hemoglobin than

younger cells, and the half-life of glycosylated hemoglobin parallels that of the red blood cell. Because of its long half-life, the concentration of glycosylated hemoglobin rises and falls slowly when plasma glucose rises and falls with treatment of diabetes. This nonenzymatic process of glycosylation has been shown to occur in other red cell membrane proteins and elsewhere in the hemoglobin molecule itself. While this form of glycosylation may have implications for the structural changes in proteins important to diabetic neurovascular disease, the immediate practical significance is the ability to assess long-term glucose control by measuring HbA$_{1c}$ or glycosylated hemoglobin.

A number of assay methods have been developed for these compounds, including ion-exchange chromatography, colorimetry, high-pressure liquid chromatography, gel electrofocusing, and immunoassay. At present, none of these methods has been standardized; therefore, while they are internally consistent, there is some probability of difference from laboratory to laboratory and method to method. Nevertheless, it is clear that glycosylated hemoglobin declines slowly with a lag of 3–6 weeks to a new steady level after plasma glucose declines (Fig. 15–100) and rises to a steady elevated level with the same slow half-time of accumulation during periods of poor control. Since there is a long lag between changes of glucose level and the eventual change of glycosylated hemoglobin, use of the glycosylated hemoglobin level alone to assess the response to a change of therapy can be misleading unless sufficient time is allowed. For example, it is possible to have an elevated glycosylated hemoglobin for weeks after plasma glucose has been therapeutically lowered into the normal range.

However, in insulin-dependent patients the level of glycosylated hemoglobin does provide a better index of the integrated glucose level over a period of time than urine or plasma glucose measurements and can be an excellent patient education tool. The glycosylated hemoglobin level of stable maturity-onset-type diabetics relates well to fasting plasma glucose (Fig. 15–101). A discrepancy of the expected relationship between these variables can alert the physician to a change in treatment efficacy, recent instability of control, or the likelihood that the clinic plasma glucose measurement is *not* a good reflection of levels in the home environment for a particular patient.

Patient Instruction. The patient, or in some instances a relative or friend, must be given instruction regarding the use of insulin therapy. The FDA has now phased out all U-40/ml and U-80/ml insulin. Therefore, only 100 U/ml insulin should be used. A syringe should be prescribed with only one set of units on the barrel. This metric system using 100 U/ml of solution is simple and convenient to use. There has been a growing use of disposable syringes and needles for the diabetic population. It has been found that one such syringe and needle may be used for several days with safety, thus markedly reducing the cost. The advantage of disposable needles is their consistently sharp point. Either a 24- or

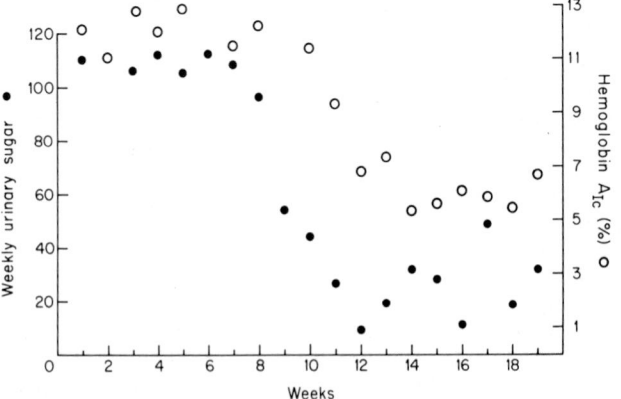

Figure 15–100. Time course of urine glucose and HbA$_{1c}$ during improved glucose control. Urine glucose declines between 6 and 8 weeks. Note the 2- to 4-week lag in the decline in the HbA$_{1c}$. (From Koenig, R. J., et al.: Correlation of glucose regulation and hemoglobin A$_{1c}$ in diabetes mellitus. *N. Engl. J. Med.* 295:417, 1976.)

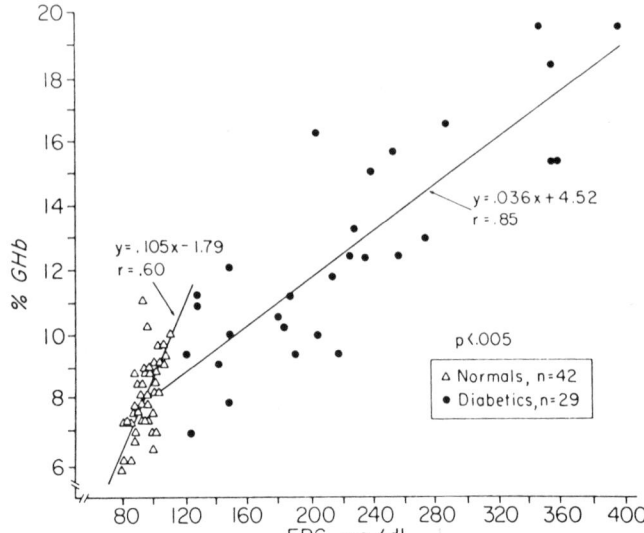

Figure 15–101. Relation between fasting plasma glucose (FPG) and glycosylated hemoglobin (GHb) in normal and treated and untreated stable maturity-onset-type, non-insulin-dependent diabetics. It is likely that there is a continuous curve rather than two straight lines. This relationship can be used to assess the stability of such a patient by a simultaneous measurement of GHb and FPG. (From Graf, R. J., et al.: Glycosylated hemoglobin in normal subjects and maturity onset diabetics; evidence for a saturable system in man. *Diabetes* 27:834, 1978.)

26-gauge needle of ½-inch length is satisfactory. Patients should be instructed in a method of injection which uses a different site each time, preferably moving up one thigh and down the other and then the abdominal wall. The arms may also be used if necessary. It is desirable for the physician to induce a minor hypoglycemic reaction so that the patient will be acquainted with its manifestations and its relief by carbohydrate-containing liquids. The patient should have a card or a Medic-Alert tag to indicate that he is a diabetic and is taking insulin.

Oral Hypoglycemic Agents

There are two groups of oral drugs which effectively lower the blood sugar. In one group, the active portion is a sulfonylurea radical, so that drugs in this group are called sulfonylureas (Fig. 15–102). They are derivatives of sulfur-

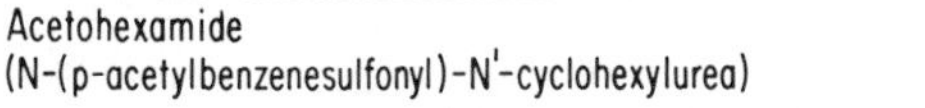

$$CH_3-\langle\bigcirc\rangle-SO_2-NH-CO-NH-CH_2-CH_2-CH_2-CH_3$$
Tolbutamide
(1-butyl-3-p-tolylsulfonylurea)

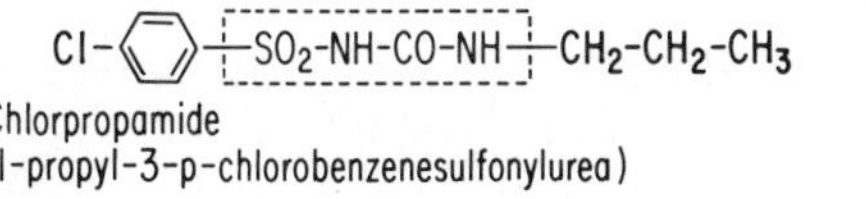

$$CH_3-\langle\bigcirc\rangle-SO_2-NH-CO-NH-N\langle\begin{matrix}CH_2-CH_2-CH_2\\CH_2-CH_2-CH_2\end{matrix}$$
Tolazamide
(1-(hexahydro-1-azepinyl)-3-p-tolylsulfonylurea)

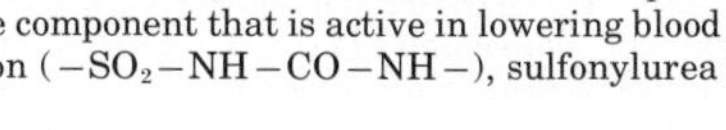

$$CH_3-CO-\langle\bigcirc\rangle-SO_2-NH-CO-NH-\langle\bigcirc\rangle$$
Acetohexamide
(N-(p-acetylbenzenesulfonyl)-N'-cyclohexylurea)

$$Cl-\langle\bigcirc\rangle-SO_2-NH-CO-NH-CH_2-CH_2-CH_3$$
Chlorpropamide
(1-propyl-3-p-chlorobenzenesulfonylurea)

Figure 15–102. Four oral antidiabetic compounds that are most often used. The component that is active in lowering blood glucose is the rectangular portion ($-SO_2-NH-CO-NH-$), sulfonylurea radical.

containing antibiotics which are ineffective as antimicrobial agents. Although their potency, metabolism, and side effects differ, their major mechanism of action is believed to be the same, and therefore they are discussed together. The other class of compounds are biguanides, which have an entirely different mode of action. They depend on the presence of the biguanide radical, which is a complex linear grouping of nitrogen, carbon, and hydrogen. Because of their propensity to increase the frequency of lactic acidosis, they have been removed from the market in the United States.

When these oral agents were first prescribed, there was much hope that their use in chemical or mild, overt diabetic subjects would improve longevity by inhibiting progression of atherosclerosis, microvascular disease, and neuropathy. However, the report of the University Group Diabetes Program (UGDP) in 1971 and 1972 indicated that patients with mild hyperglycemia treated with tolbutamide for 8 years had a higher, rather than lower, incidence of death from cardiovascular disease than did untreated control patients. Subsequently, phenformin (phenethylbiguanide) was also found to be associated with an increased incidence of cardiovascular deaths. While other investigators have reported net benefits from these drugs, their observations have been less carefully controlled and in different types of patients. Therefore, the UGDP report has created a persistent controversy concerning the use not only of tolbutamide, but also of other sulfonylureas. We do not yet know to what extent the long-range advantages of these other sulfonylureas outweigh their disadvantages. Therefore, at the present time, a number of factors must be considered in deciding between insulin and oral hypoglycemic therapy. The patients should share in the decision, if possible, and be aware of the inherent risks of both forms of treatment of altered carbohydrate metabolism.

Insulin therapy requires meticulous attention. Dosage must be adjusted in relation to exercise and meals, and hypoglycemia is a fairly frequent complication in cases of severe diabetes. Effective self-administration of insulin requires more patient education and greater visual acuity than does oral therapy. Oral hypoglycemic agents are rarely associated with hypoglycemia but may interact with other drugs ingested by the patient; occasionally, they may be associated with unwanted side effects or may have their effectiveness altered by changes in hepatic metabolism or renal excretion. Some of these drugs may increase the risk of cardiovascular death. Therefore, no hard and fast rules can be made, and each patient's problem must be approached individually.

Sulfonylureas

Mechanism of Action. In general, it appears that the mechanism of action of each sulfonylurea is similar, but the potency and duration of action differ considerably. The presence of responsive islets is necessary for these compounds to lower plasma glucose. Since they can all be shown to increase the secretion of insulin acutely, it is generally believed that this is the primary mechanism of action. However, under certain circumstances it is possible to demonstrate some increase in the sensitivity of peripheral tissues and liver to the effects of insulin and an increase in insulin receptor number; therefore, it may be that some plasma glucose lowering is related to an interaction of sulfonylurea drugs with organs other than the pancreas. In clinical studies, one can demonstrate increased basal insulin secretion and insulin output in response to challenge for several weeks after starting a sulfonylurea. However, long-term administration of these compounds is generally associated with a sustained blood sugar–lowering action and the return of plasma insulin to pretreatment levels.

Such findings have been interpreted in two ways: either the initial effect is due to increased insulin secretion and the delayed effect is to improve insulin-stimulated peripheral glucose uptake so that no increase in insulin secretion is necessary; or the chronic effects are related to an increased sensitivity of the pancreatic B-cell to the same glucose challenge, so that the same insulin levels are achieved after glucose administration, but with less absolute hyperglycemia needed. The authors are inclined to favor a primary pancreatic mechanism. In fact, the primary effect of the drugs is on the fasting glucose level, with little alteration of plasma glucose increments after a challenge in long-term sulfonylurea-treated patients. Thus, over a period of time, fasting plasma glucose decreases while insulin output, which can be related to this fasting plasma glucose, remains the same, suggesting that in the basal state the sulfonylurea itself is now partly responsible for the insulin secreted. The deficient insulin response after challenge remains about the same, and postchallenge plasma glucose levels are lower only because of the lowered fasting level. Thus, the deficient insulin response to meal challenge and impaired glucose response to the meal in diabetic subjects is not really improved by these agents. Rather, it is the fasting plasma glucose that is lowered and the insulin output in relation to glucose level in the fasting state that is increased by sulfonylurea administration. Physiologically, carbohydrate tolerance usually remains abnormal, even though postchallenge glucose concentrations are lower during treatment with a sulfonylurea agent.

The nature and mechanism of the B-cell response to these compounds is largely unknown. In general, it is believed that there is no increase in B-cell size or number with the most commonly used compounds. However, some authors have suggested that the more recent "second-generation" compounds may actually increase the number of B-cells. The specific details of the mechanism by which sulfonylureas increase insulin release is unknown, but studies *in vitro* suggest that it is not quite the same mechanism of action as that of glucose. In particular, it appears that insulin synthesis, which is definitely stimulated by glucose, is not increased by sulfonylureas.

Metabolism and Excretion.   Although the sulfonylureas probably interact with the B-cell by a common mechanism, there are major differences in their degradation, rates of absorption, and methods of excretion. The compounds with short action are usually metabolized in the liver to inactive forms which are then excreted in the urine. The longer-acting compounds are metabolized poorly, if at all, by the liver and are excreted unchanged in the urine. These drugs or their metabolites may induce hypoglycemia. In the case of a poorly metabolized drug, binding to plasma protein plays an important role in duration of action.

Tolbutamide is carboxylated in the liver to an inactive compound, carboxytolbutamide, which is excreted in the urine. When it is given orally, the biologic half-life is about 3–5 hours. Therefore, the duration of action is short and not dependent upon renal function. *Acetohexamide* is also rapidly metabolized by the liver to form hydroxyhexamide. However, in this case the metabolic product is also a hypoglycemic agent and is believed to be somewhat more potent than the parent compound. Approximately 75% of acetohexamide is excreted in this more active form. Since the liver does not diminish the hypoglycemic potency of the compound, the material has an intermediate duration of action which is dependent upon renal excretion and plasma protein binding, which is relatively weak. *Tolazamide* is also rapidly metabolized to at least six metabolic products, but many of them

induce hypoglycemia. This leads to an intermediate duration of action very similar to that of acetohexamide, but at a somewhat lower dose. *Chlorpropamide,* the longest-acting compound of the group, is very poorly metabolized. It is tightly bound to protein and is therefore active for long periods. Since it is dependent upon renal excretion for the termination of its activity, it is contraindicated for individuals with significantly reduced renal function.

Second-Generation Drugs.   Two new agents of markedly increased potency have been tested extensively in Europe and are planned for release in the United States. They are glibenclamide (Daonil, Euglucon, Diabeta, or Micronase) and glipizide (Fig. 15–103). They are approximately 20–100 times more potent than the older sulfonylurea drugs; however, a maximally effective dose produces approximately the same glucose lowering as a maximally effective dose of the currently available drugs. Side effects seem to be roughly the same as for the currently available drugs, but the flush after alcohol and hyponatremia found in some patients with chlorpropamide have not been observed.

Drug Interactions.   The potency of any sulfonylurea may be altered by other drugs. One of the most common effects reported consists of augmentation of the hypoglycemic potency of the sulfonylureas. This is probably observed more frequently because hypoglycemia is clinically obvious and important, whereas a diminution in the potency of the agent and hyperglycemia may erroneously be attributed to some other factor. Drugs such as sulfaphenazole, phenylbutazone, probenecid, salicylate, bishydroxycoumarin, alcohol, sulfisoxazole, and monoamine oxidase inhibitors have been implicated in severe hypoglycemia associated with sulfonylurea administration. It is likely that these compounds either decrease sulfonylurea excretion or reduce its binding to plasma proteins. Some of the foregoing drugs may produce only subclinical hypoglycemia when given alone, yet significantly augment the hypoglycemic action of sulfonylureas. Because of the prolonged hypoglycemic activity of sulfonylureas in these clinical settings, observation and treatment may be required for more than 24 hours (Seltzer). Bolus injections of glucose given under such circumstances may be expected to produce very large increases in endogenous insulin secretion, which will produce subsequent (and perhaps even greater) hypoglycemia. Therefore, a continuous infusion of glucose should be started and continued until the drug has been clearly metabolized or excreted.

Compounds that may antagonize the hypoglycemic action of sulfonylureas include thiazides, corticosteroids, chloram-

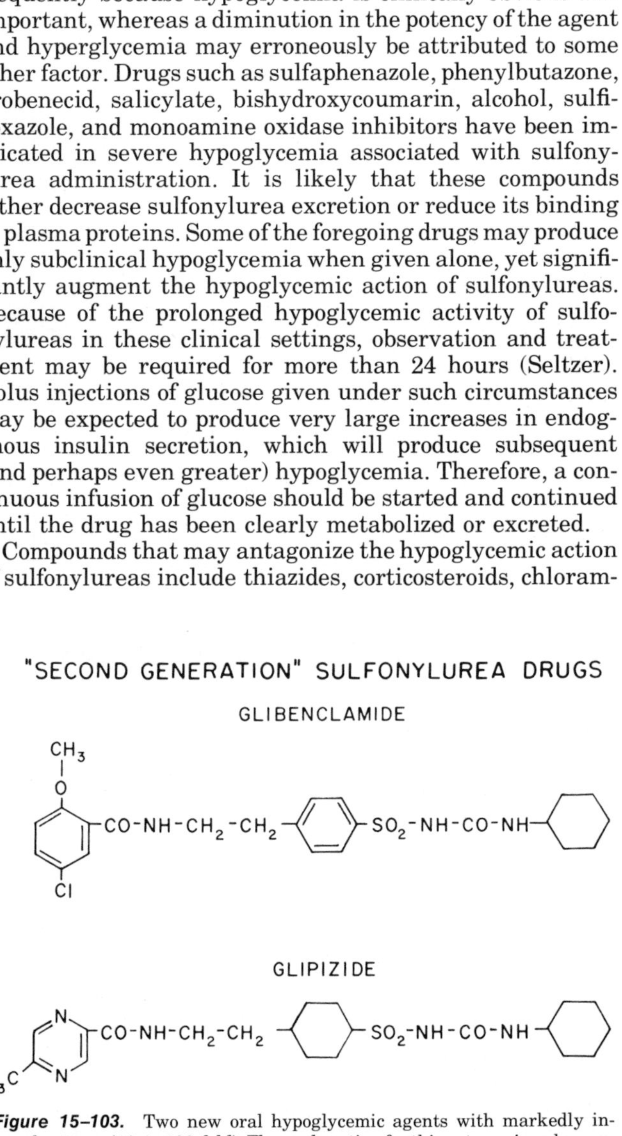

"SECOND GENERATION" SULFONYLUREA DRUGS

GLIBENCLAMIDE

GLIPIZIDE

Figure 15–103.   Two new oral hypoglycemic agents with markedly increased potency (10- to 100-fold). The explanation for this potency is unknown, but is not related to a change in metabolic disposition.

phenicol, furosemide, the oral contraceptives, and propranolol. A change in any of these medications may alter plasma glucose levels. This must be kept in mind for those patients starting *or* stopping them.

Hypoglycemia. Hypoglycemia is rare with moderate doses of sulfonylureas given to patients who are in relatively good health and who do not have significant impairment of renal or liver function. However, sulfonylurea-induced hypoglycemia may occur without any other drug therapy. This is not really a side effect but is either a manifestation of overdosage with sulfonylurea or, more likely, the result of dosages that are clinically inappropriate. Thus more than 90% of reported episodes of severe sulfonylurea-induced hypoglycemia have occurred in acutely or chronically starved patients or in patients who had demonstrable hepatic or renal impairment or both. This is often compounded by the intake of alcohol, which by itself causes hypoglycemia in the starved individual.

Toxic Side Effects. Many of these compounds have effects on metabolism independent of their hypoglycemic properties. The magnitude of the effect may vary considerably depending upon the specific drug, but, in general, differences in their effects are quantitative and not qualitative.

Thyroid Gland. Many reports indicate that sulfonylureas, particularly tolbutamide, decrease ^{131}I uptake. This change appears to be transient and can be reversed by iodide administration. Since only an occasional patient has been reported with goiter and myxedema apparently related to sulfonylurea therapy, it seems likely that some underlying abnormality of thyroid function must be present for the drug to cause hypothyroidism.

Antidiuretic Hormone-like Effect. Some patients treated with chlorpropamide have developed symptomatic hyponatremia and water intoxication. Chlorpropamide appears to have an effect on renal tubules similar to that of antidiuretic hormone (ADH) and has even been used to treat patients with ADH insufficiency. Some ADH seems to be necessary for this effect to occur, and there is also evidence of increased release of the hormone during chlorpropamide therapy. ADH exerts its antidiuretic action by stimulating adenylate cyclase activity; chlorpropamide presumably augments this enzyme reaction in some manner. No other sulfonylurea has been reported to significantly potentiate ADH secretion or action.

Gastrointestinal Tract. Intestinal symptoms such as anorexia, nausea, vomiting, diarrhea, and abdominal pain are observed in about 5% of patients treated with sulfonylureas, but this incidence is not much higher than that associated with placebo ingestion. A reaction to alcohol similar to that seen after disulfiram, with a clinical syndrome of headache, flushing, and tachycardia, may be seen in a number of patients treated with a sulfonylurea, almost exclusively chlorpropamide. The mechanism of this reaction is unknown but is of sufficient importance and magnitude to make patients aware of such a possibility when beginning treatment with a sulfonylurea. It has recently been reported that this response is genetically determined and that there is a subgroup of patients in whom the flushing response can regularly be elicited after chlorpropamide administration. Such data suggest genetic heterogeneity in the non-insulin-dependent group of diabetics. In the families studied to date, there has been a preponderance of cases of maturity-onset-type diabetes of youth (MODY), and the flush and carbohydrate intolerance have segregated together.

Hepatic reactions to these drugs are less frequent, but mild to severe cholestatic jaundice has been reported. The greater the hypoglycemic potency of the drug, the more likely it is to cause liver impairment. This toxic effect is dose-related, especially with chlorpropamide. Hepatocellular damage has been suggested at times, but liver biopsies usually have shown only canalicular bile stasis, similar to that reported for chlorpromazine.

Skin. Maculopapular eruptions have been reported, often with pruritus, and are probably symptoms of allergic hypersensitivity.

Hematopoietic System. Hematologic toxicity has been reported rarely; it includes agranulocytosis and pancytopenia.

Cardiovascular System. The sulfonylurea compounds have been used not only for control of symptomatic hyperglycemia but also in the hope of reducing diabetic concomitants such as microvascular disease, atherosclerosis, and neuropathy. Many of these patients have elevated blood sugar but only minimal to moderate glycosuria. To determine the true efficacy of this therapy, the National Institutes of Health sponsored observations of mild diabetics for 8 years. The patients were divided into five groups and received either (1) placebo administration, (2) tolbutamide, (3) phenformin, (4) a fixed dose of insulin, or (5) a variable dose of insulin. The study was started in 1961, and the results caused a furor in 1970 when it was reported that, compared with placebo or insulin groups, there was an increase in cardiovascular-related deaths in a group of more than 200 patients treated with tolbutamide in a fixed dose. As a result, the Food and Drug Administration recommended that oral hypoglycemic agents be used only when diet alone is ineffective and insulin impractical or unacceptable. The data (Table 15–19) showed an increase in cardiovascular-related deaths for the tolbutamide group (Fig. 15–104) and later an increase in cardiovascular-related deaths for the phenformin-treated group. Although both tolbutamide and phenformin groups had an increase in total mortality, this was not statistically different from that of the other groups. The increasing percentage of deaths related to cardiovascular disease became apparent between the third and fifth years of the study. Because of this increase, the study was discontinued in the eighth year and the recommendations just referred to were made.

Many criticisms of this study are available, perhaps the best of which are summarized by Feinstein and Cornfield. These two authors suggest that a difference in cardiovascular mortality was not established by the study. The study investigators thought this interpretation to be unlikely, but possible. On the other hand, no critic has suggested that a beneficial effect of the drugs was likely to have been overlooked. Therefore, there is no evidence that these oral compounds prevent the vascular abnormalities of diabetes in patients with *mild* hyperglycemia treated with a fixed dose of tolbutamide. Whether this applies to patients with more symptomatic hyperglycemia is not known. It is hoped that these studies will lead to more research into the basic nature of the diabetic defect and to better therapy for all aspects of

Table 15–19. NUMBER OF DEATHS OF DIABETIC PATIENTS TREATED WITH TOLBUTAMIDE, INSULIN, OR PHENFORMIN*

	Tolbutamide	Insulin[†] Standard	Insulin[‡] Variable	Placebo	Phenformin[§]
Total Deaths	30	20	18	21	31
CV-Related Deaths	26	13	12	10	26

*UGDP Study – 823 patients, *Diabetes* 19:747, 1970.
[†]10–16 U, depending on body surface area.
[‡]Dosage varied to lower blood sugar.
[§]Added and reported later.

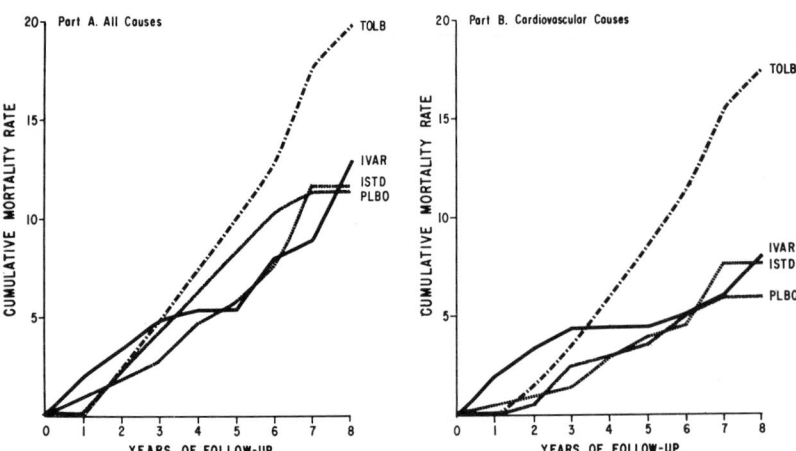

CUMULATIVE MORTALITY RATES
PER 100 POPULATION AT RISK
BY YEAR OF FOLLOW-UP

Figure 15–104. Results of the cumulative mortality statistics for the 8-year University Group Diabetes Program (UGDP) Study. Rates are given per 100 population at risk by year of follow-up. *TOLB* = tolbutamide, 1.5 g/day; *IVAR* = insulin, enough to keep blood sugar normal; *ISTD* = insulin, 10–16 units based on surface area; *PLBO* = placebo. (From Meinert, C. L., et al.: A study of the effects of hypoglycemic agents on vascular complications in patients with adult-onset diabetes. II. Mortality results. *Diabetes* 19:789, 1970.)

the disease. Comparable observations of the results of prolonged use of chlorpropamide, acetohexamide, tolazamide, and other sulfonylureas have not been reported, but there are many similarities in chemical characteristics and biologic activity.

Dosage and Practical Use. The choice of sulfonylurea depends on its potency, biologic half-life, cost, and side effects. Some of the most potent compounds are those most slowly metabolized and therefore the most likely to produce unwanted hypoglycemia. In a diabetic taking insulin, it is not possible to predict with certainty whether a sulfonylurea can be used satisfactorily as a substitute. Since the reports of the University Group Diabetes Program (UGDP) studies, this substitution has become much less frequent. In general, individuals who have had episodes of ketoacidosis or who use more than 40 U of insulin per day, unless there is significant obesity, are unlikely to be responsive to sulfonylureas. The dosage used is that necessary to maintain blood sugar at the desired level up to the maximum indicated for each compound (Table 15–20). The incidence of secondary failures is not established but appears to be about 5% per year. Sulfonylureas are rarely used for pregnant women in the United States, but in some investigations in Scotland and South Africa, no ill-effects were reported. During elective surgery, minor infections, and other minor illnesses, it is not necessary to substitute insulin unless ketosis appears. During emergency surgery or severe infections, it is best to substitute insulin. It is of some interest that 30% of patients who were clearly hyperglycemic prior to oral agent treatment could be maintained without sulfonylurea therapy when pills were withdrawn from all subjects randomly in an outpatient diabetic clinic. This suggests that the disease may fluctuate from time to time and has raised consideration of the desirability of intermittent rather than continuous treatment of symptomatic hyperglycemia and glycosuria.

Recapitulation and Conclusions Concerning Diet, Drug, and Insulin Therapy in Diabetes

Despite major scientific advances in the last 50 years, there is insufficient knowledge of the basic etiology and pathogenesis of diabetes. Therefore, treatment directed toward the vascular and neuropathic concomitants of the disease has been inadequate. Insulin treatment for severe insulin deficiency (insulin-dependent diabetes) is obvious. Treatment for milder carbohydrate abnormalities is more complex. Obese, overt, non-insulin-dependent diabetics with hyperglycemia and glycosuria should begin with caloric restriction; oral drugs or insulin treatment is to be started only when there are indications that diet (caloric control) cannot achieve or is not achieving control of the glycosuria. The choice of therapy between insulin and the oral antidiabetic agents in this group can be made only after the possible problems and benefits from both forms of therapy are considered and discussed with the patient. A long-term program must be developed. The therapy of asymptomatic hyperglycemia (chemical diabetes) remains a very controversial issue. In view of the difficulties with insulin therapy and the potential hazards of the oral antidiabetic agents, many physicians at the present time treat such patients only with diet (caloric restriction). This choice is influenced by the age of the patient. At the present time the authors are not inclined to treat with pills or insulin a patient who has a fasting plasma glucose less than 140 mg/dl. We usually treat anyone with a fasting plasma glucose greater than 200 mg/dl unless there is some specific contraindication. When the fasting plasma glucose is between 140 and 200 mg/dl, we are likely to treat any symptomatic patient and are more aggressive in asymptomatic patients who are younger and do not have significant cardiovascular or renal disease at the time of diagnosis.

Table 15–20. DOSAGE OF ORAL SULFONYLUREA COMPOUNDS

| Generic Names | Trade Names | Total Daily Doses (g) | | Doses Per Day | Approx. Duration of Action (hr) |
		Common	*Range**		
Tolbutamide	Orinase	1.5	0.5 –3.0	2–3	6–10
Acetohexamide	Dymelor	0.75	0.25–1.25	1–2	10–16
Tolazamide	Tolinase	0.25	0.1 –0.75	1	10–16
Chlorpropamide	Diabinese	0.25	0.1 –0.5	1	40–72

*The increase in the antidiabetic effect must be weighed against a possible increase in side effects.

Pregnancy and Diabetes

Pregnancy is an example of the effects of stress on carbohydrate metabolism. In the normal individual, compensation maintains glucose concentrations with only slight changes; however, this occurs at the expense of a total reorganization of many of the factors that impinge upon carbohydrate, fat, and protein metabolism. In a susceptible individual, clinical diabetes may become manifest. Pregnancy not only tends to place stress on carbohydrate metabolism in a diabetic but may also influence adversely the vascular concomitants of the disease. Furthermore, although fertility in the diabetic female is only slightly subnormal, the chance of a diabetic mother producing a live child is decreased, and the number of surviving children is also decreased. The diagnosis of diabetes is more difficult during pregnancy, and treatment of altered carbohydrate metabolism in the pregnant diabetic must be changed as the pregnancy progresses. In contrast to the controversy that surrounds close blood sugar management in other aspects of the diabetic syndrome, this is not the case in the pregnant diabetic, since the outcome of the pregnancy will partly depend upon the degree of carbohydrate control.

Pregnancy and Carbohydrate Tolerance

The predominant effect of pregnancy on carbohydrate metabolism is related to the hormonal changes induced by the pregnancy, and to the presence of the fetus, which depends upon the mother for its entire fuel (mostly glucose) and nutrient supply. All the hormones that are secreted in increased amounts during pregnancy (including estrogen, progesterone, chorionic somatomammotropin, and corticosteroids) antagonize the effects of insulin on carbohydrate uptake and utilization, thus inducing a state of peripheral insulin resistance. At the same time, there is an accelerated utilization of stored nutrients and glucose to feed the fetus overnight and between meals, so that in the morning the normal pregnant woman often has a lower fasting blood glucose level, elevated FFA levels, and mild ketonuria. Furthermore, there is evidence that destruction of insulin occurs in the placenta, thus accelerating the peripheral turnover of this hormone. This requires more insulin secretion to maintain adequate plasma levels. The effect of an uncomplicated pregnancy to produce a minimal change in glucose tolerance but markedly higher insulin levels is shown in the top of Figure 15–105. This insulin-resistant state is reversed immediately after delivery.

Diagnosis of Diabetes. Standards for the diagnosis of diabetes by carbohydrate tolerance testing are clearly altered by the pregnant state. In general, the upper limit of normal for a fasting blood sugar is reduced approximately 10 mg/dl because of the accelerated utilization of glucose during fasting; however, the values after challenge are raised 5–10 mg/dl because of the insulin antagonism (see Table 15–13). The use of urine glucose excretion as an index of diabetes is not advisable, since normal pregnancy reduces the apparent renal threshold for glucose. Thus, a significant number of normal women have glycosuria during pregnancy.

Because of the impact of hyperglycemia on pregnancy outcome, it has now become more important to detect it during pregnancy. A fasting plasma glucose should be measured at least once in the third trimester. A glucose tolerance test should be performed in any pregnant woman with glycosuria or in a woman with a previous history of large babies or a complicated pregnancy. Individuals with carbohydrate intolerance may not always be treated; however, their detection will alert the physician to institute closer monitoring.

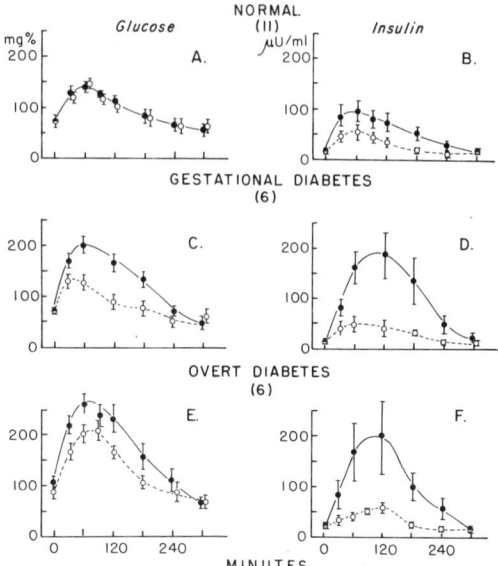

Figure 15–105. The effect of pregnancy on glucose and insulin. Note that with nondiabetic pregnancy (•—•), the glucose tolerance tests were the same as they were post partum (○--○), but much higher levels of plasma immunoassayable insulin were attained than in the postpartum period. The glucose levels in diabetics were higher during pregnancy than following delivery, despite far greater plasma insulin levels. (From Kalkhoff, R., et al.: Diabetogenic factors associated with pregnancy. *Trans. Ass. Amer. Physicians* 77:270, 1964.)

Interaction of Diabetes and Pregnancy

Recognizing that pregnancy is a stress to carbohydrate metabolism, it is logical to expect that the patient with clinical diabetes, whether treated with insulin or oral agents, will experience a change in the need for insulin. Because of the numerous factors influenced by the pregnancy, it is impossible to predict exactly the net effect in every patient; however, in general terms, insulin requirement or the need to begin insulin therapy in an asymptomatic patient will increase during the second half of the pregnancy. Note, for example, the further deterioration in glucose tolerance of subjects with mild prepartum carbohydrate intolerance in Figure 15–105. Most clinics, therefore, will switch patients who are on oral agents to insulin, at least for the duration of the pregnancy. During the first half of the pregnancy, the increased utilization of glucose by the fetus may balance the contrainsulin hormones that have been secreted so that the insulin requirement may not change; in fact, in some cases, it may decrease. This depends in part upon the nutrition of the pregnant woman, as the food intake may fluctuate widely during the first trimester. The greater the food intake, the greater the need for insulin. In the second and third trimesters, insulin requirements will almost always increase because of the insulin-antagonistic hormones.

Ketoacidosis during pregnancy is associated with a marked increase in fetal death rate. Most pregnant diabetics are seen more frequently and managed more closely to prevent this complication, as the fetal death rate may increase to 30% or more. On the other hand, accelerated fasting or starvation ketosis is common in normal pregnancies and must be distinguished from ketoacidosis. In general, this is fairly straightforward, since starvation ketosis alone is not associated with significant hyperglycemia. The use of carbohydrate-restricted diets may accelerate ketogenesis in the diabetic population. Therefore, such diets are definitely contraindicated during pregnancy. It is usually preferable to *increase* the carbohydrate content of the diet in the pregnant diabetic. Should starvation ketosis develop, it can be treated quite easily by the administration of a glucose solution, usually orally. Management of ketoacidosis in the pregnant diabetic is no different from that in the nonpregnant diabetic.

The more challenging problem is to determine whether pregnancy has adverse effects on the vascular pathology of diabetes in addition to its effects on carbohydrate metabolism. There seems to be no doubt that preeclampsia is more common in diabetic patients. In the presence of severe renal disease or rapidly accelerating renal disease, termination of the pregnancy is usually indicated. It is not clear whether the retinopathy, neuropathy, and large-vessel disease are compromised by pregnancy, but it is the general feeling of most clinicians that there is some acceleration of these processes. However, no incontrovertible evidence has been forthcoming. The presence of significant vascular disease considerably reduces the possibility of a live baby, and it is generally felt, therefore, that pregnancy is contraindicated in such a patient.

Infant of the Diabetic Mother

Excessive body weight and size and neonatal hypoglycemia are well recognized fetal complications of a diabetic pregnancy. Fetal hyperinsulinemia has been documented and, since insulin does not pass the placental barrier, it is believed due to the hyperglycemia of the mother. It seems likely that this increased fetal insulin output acts as a growth factor and leads to the increased body fat and visceromegaly. The postpartum hypoglycemia probably results from continued insulin secretion in the absence of glucose supplied by the placenta. There is true hypertrophy and hyperplasia of the pancreas in these infants. Most authors have reported an increase in congenital anomalies in infants of diabetic mothers, but lack of rigidly controlled studies makes this still a controversial point. Fetal loss may be high in the diabetic pregnancy, and intrauterine death tends to increase after the 37th week of pregnancy. This fact has led to the development of criteria for accelerating delivery. On the other hand, premature removal of the fetus leads to an increased incidence of the fetal respiratory distress syndrome, also a major problem. The problem of picking an optimal delivery time is illustrated in Figure 15–106. According to White, 80% of diabetic pregnancies result in a live birth, compared to 90% in the general population;

perinatal mortality occurs in about 10% of deliveries, compared with 3% of deliveries among nondiabetics; however, with close monitoring some clinics have reduced fetal loss in the diabetic group to 3–4%.

Management of the Pregnant Diabetic

There are three major goals in the treatment of the pregnant diabetic. The first is to prevent ketosis and hypoglycemia, the second is to minimize hyperglycemia and glycosuria, and the third is to optimize the length of gestation. Diet in the pregnant diabetic is essentially unchanged, except for an increase in total calories to allow a weight gain of approximately 20–25 pounds per pregnancy and maintenance of at least a normal carbohydrate intake. In the gestational diabetic, this weight gain should be monitored closely, as excessive weight gain may exacerbate the hyperglycemia while caloric temperance will minimize it. Carbohydrates should not be restricted in view of the rapid switch from the fed to the fasting state which takes place during the normal pregnancy. This diet regimen will ordinarily require somewhere between 35 and 40 cal/kg of *ideal* body weight, with at least 45% of calories as carbohydrate. Since this is the same proportion of carbohydrate calories as in an average American diet, it can be approached usually by self-selection. As in other patients with the diabetic syndrome, regularity of diet and total daily caloric intake are probably the most important features, along with intermittent snacks (four to six feedings daily) to minimize wide swings in blood glucose. Glycosuria will occur in many diabetic patients on such a regimen because of the low renal threshold of pregnancy. It may be necessary to determine the renal threshold in each patient in order to assess properly the degree of glucose control that is achievable without risking serious hypoglycemia.

Glucose tolerance testing, particularly in women with glycosuria, should identify a group of patients with carbohydrate intolerance. While treatment with insulin may not be used in this group, it is an important test because it alerts the physician to a high-risk pregnancy and indicates a need for close observation. Thus, women with "gestational diabetes" are treated the same as women with overt diabetes regarding obstetric management and close metabolic observation. If fasting plasma glucose is elevated, treatment with insulin will almost certainly be required.

In the juvenile-onset, insulin-dependent diabetic, two doses of insulin are usually required. The goal is to keep plasma glucose below 170–180 mg/100 ml. Insulin treatment is usually not given in gestational diabetes until the fasting plasma glucose exceeds 105 mg/100 ml. Close monitoring is required throughout, but particularly so after the 32nd week. All authors agree that frequent clinic visits are absolutely essential to maximize fetal salvage rate. Recently, home blood glucose monitoring and multiple doses of insulin have been used to keep plasma glucose as normal as possible (<150 mg/dl).

The major problem in diabetic pregnancy is to determine the optimal time for delivery. The general goal is to allow the pregnancy to go at least 35 weeks and then to check the patient carefully until the 37th or 38th week, if possible. It is probably advisable to hospitalize the patient at the 35th week so that determinations of fetal status and maturity can be made frequently. This is partly related to estimation of uterine size and fetal weight, but more usually is dependent upon endocrine testing. Estriol and pregnanediol measurements can be used to get an estimate of fetal-placental mass. The figures vary widely from patient to patient, and therefore serial measurements in an individual are better.

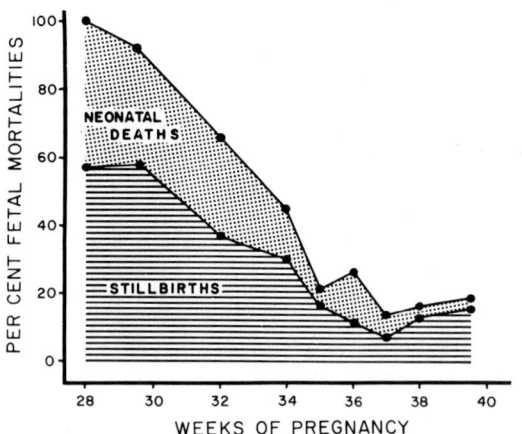

Figure 15–106. Fetal mortality in 705 diabetic pregnancies according to duration. (From Miller, M., In *On the Nature and Treatment of Diabetes*. Leibel, B. S., and Wrenshall, G. A. (eds.), Amsterdam, Excerpta Medica Foundation, 1965.)

Urine estriol excretion of less than 10 mg/24 hr is suspicious, and less than 5 mg/24 hr suggests that fetal death is likely. Plasma somatomammotropin may also be a useful index of placental function, values above 5 μg/ml after the 35th week being rarely associated with fetal distress in labor. Levels below 4 μg/ml suggest a high risk.

Tests of fetal maturity using amniotic fluid have also been recommended. These employ the bilirubin content, creatinine concentration, phospholipid content, and the cytology of the desquamated fetal cells. The evaluation of these procedures has been discussed by Tyson. All are aimed at determining as precisely as possible whether there is sufficient fetal maturity for survival and the probability of the respiratory distress syndrome. The critical factor appears to be the production of sufficient lung surfactant by the fetus. This can be estimated by the lecithin-to-sphingomyelin ratio or the absolute values of lecithin. A ratio of 1.8 within 48 hours of delivery or a content of 3.5 mg/dl is associated with a low incidence of respiratory distress. If delivery is necessary, steroid administration to the mother may induce lecithin synthesis and be a useful adjunct.

Induction of labor is performed when the maximal chance of the fetus living has been realized, and if the induction is unsuccessful, cesarean section is performed. Some clinics perform cesarean section on all such patients, whereas others attempt a vaginal delivery first, usually with 30–50% success. After delivery there is a rapid reduction in insulin resistance, which should be anticipated by decreasing insulin dosage to prepregnancy levels or lower (two-thirds the third-trimester dosage).

Contraception and Sterilization

Both estrogen and progestogen, as already mentioned, clearly promote insulin resistance and may cause frankly abnormal glucose tolerance tests in a significant number of women taking these hormones. Thus, diabetic patients are likely to find similar changes occurring while taking these pills that occur normally during pregnancy. If the patient already has carbohydrate intolerance, the pills may precipitate overt clinical diabetes and are, therefore, clearly contraindicated. In the insulin-treated diabetic, there may be a small increase in insulin requirement, but it is not known whether this increase in any way alters the vascular concomitants of the syndrome. Lacking this information, it has been recommended that the oral contraceptives not be used by diabetic patients; however, the physician must weigh the risks of a possible pregnancy against the risk of unknown effects of oral contraceptives in a patient who is unwilling to be sterilized or to use other methods of contraception. In general, pregnancy is ill advised in the presence of significant large-vessel disease, microvascular disease, or neuropathy, as fetal salvage rate is low, and the likelihood of long-term survival of the mother may be reduced.

Other Diseases and Syndromes with Hyperglycemia (Secondary Diabetes)

A very large number of syndromes and diseases are associated with an inappropriately high plasma glucose level. Some of them are listed in Table 15–21, and some of the

Table 15–21. DISEASES AND SYNDROMES WITH HYPERGLYCEMIA

1. Pancreatic diseases
   (a) Neonatal
       (1) Congenital absence of islets
   (b) Postnatal
       (1) Pancreatitis (calcific, alcoholic, relapsing, infectious, nutritional)
       (2) Pancreatic neoplasia
       (3) Cystic fibrosis
       (4) Toxic destruction—Vacor (rat poison)
       (5) Iron overload (hemochromatosis)
       (6) Trauma
       (7) Pancreatectomy
2. Hormonal
   (a) Counterregulatory hormone excess
       (1) Glucosteroid excess—Cushing's syndrome
       (2) Catecholamine excess—pheochromocytoma
       (3) Growth hormone excess—acromegaly
       (4) Glucagon excess—glucagonoma syndrome
   (b) Other endocrine-metabolic syndromes
       (1) Mineral-corticoid excess (hypokalemia)
       (2) Congenital growth hormone deficiency—Laron dwarf or ateliotic dwarf (growth failure)
       (3) Hypoparathyroidism (hypocalcemia)
       (4) Carcinoid syndrome (hyperserotoninemia)
       (5) Somatostatinoma (hypersomatostatinemia)
       (6) Hyperthyroidism
       (7) Prolactinoma
       (8) Hepatic cirrhosis (hypokalemia?)
3. Genetic syndromes

(1) Acute intermittent porphyria	(11) Klinefelter's syndrome
(2) Alström's syndrome	(12) Laurence-Moon-Biedl syndrome
(3) Ataxia-telangiectasia	(13) Lipoatrophic diabetes
(4) Cockayne's syndrome	(14) Machado's disease
(5) Diabetes insipidus, nerve deafness, and hyperglycemia	(15) Mendenhall's syndrome
(6) Down's syndrome	(16) Myotonic dystrophy
(7) Friedreich's ataxia	(17) Optic atrophy with hyperglycemia
(8) Glycogen storage disease	(18) Prader-Willi syndrome
(9) Herrman's syndrome	(19) Refsum's syndrome
(10) Huntington's chorea	(20) Turner's syndrome
	(21) Werner's syndrome

more common ones are described in the following paragraphs. Since the mechanism of hyperglycemia must involve either impaired islet function or inefficient metabolic utilization of glucose, the ultimate etiology of hyperglycemia in idiopathic diabetes mellitus and in these diseases and syndromes must be the same. Nevertheless, they are separated for discussion purposes because the etiology in these syndromes may be different from that of idiopathic diabetes mellitus. However, as the etiology of insulin-dependent diabetes and non-insulin-dependent diabetes becomes unraveled, we are left with a quandary. If insulin-dependent diabetes should be related to a virus, does this make it secondary diabetes or idiopathic primary diabetes? Thus, it is clear that this artificial separation is beginning to break down rapidly and will in a few years have no meaning at all.

The problem is further complicated by the frequency of non-insulin-dependent diabetes mellitus. Most of the syndromes described in this section are not ketosis-prone, although many such patients are treated with insulin. The frequency of non-insulin-dependent diabetes mellitus is so high that the occurrence of two diseases in the same individual would not be all that unlikely. Therefore, very often the more hyperglycemic individuals with pancreatitis, hemochromatosis, acromegaly, Cushing's syndrome, and so forth may in fact be individuals with idiopathic non-insulin-dependent diabetes mellitus whose disease has become clinically evident by the superimposition of a second illness. The degree of hyperglycemia may vary considerably from patient to patient, and there is often some question whether the disease or syndrome is truly associated with hyperglycemia in the absence of an underlying genetic predisposition to non-insulin-dependent diabetes mellitus. Since there is no marker at present for NIDDM, these two possibilities cannot be distinguished at the present time.

Pancreatic Disease and Hyperglycemia

Pancreatitis

History and Types.   Inflammatory disease of the pancreas is frequently associated with hyperglycemia. This is an extremely heterogeneous group of disorders in which the pathophysiology is not usually understood. The common associated findings are excessive alcohol intake, gallbladder disease, malnutrition, or ingestion of a diet high in tapioca (cassava). Any of these types may be associated with calcification of the pancreas. The disease may be characterized by repeated episodes of acute inflammation and/or a more chronic process leading to pancreatic destruction, pseudocyst formation, and pain. Pain is also a major feature of the acute episode, and since this is often exaggerated by food intake, weight loss is common. In long-term cases, exocrine insufficiency may develop, and therefore malnutrition is often associated with chronic pancreatitis. This variability in food intake may play an important role in the clinical manifestations of hyperglycemia. Jaundice may occur and may be related to the underlying gallbladder disease or an associated independent injury of the liver, or may be secondary to the pancreatitis itself owing to peripancreatic edema, a cyst, or stenosis of an intrapancreatic duct.

Hyperglycemia during an acute episode is common and may be exacerbated by the administration of intravenous glucose. Chronic hyperglycemia is variable and is said to occur in approximately one-third of cases, with approximately another one-third of cases demonstrating glucose intolerance during glucose tolerance tests. Fasting hyperglycemia is usually a sign of advanced disease. In general,

the degree of glucose intolerance can be correlated with the severity of pancreatic exocrine insufficiency. The true frequency of retinopathy, nephropathy, and neuropathy is unknown and is complicated by the associated alcoholism in many of these patients. Nevertheless, there are clearly many patients who develop all of these findings of the idiopathic diabetes syndrome. The clinical impression is that these findings are less frequent and less severe than in idiopathic diabetes mellitus, but data to support this impression are not available.

Incidence.   Although the disease is relatively rare, it has been written about frequently because of its severity. In England, the death rate is approximately 10 per million and the incidence rate is approximately 50 per million, which increases with age. There are no known genetic associations, and therefore it is presumed that the etiology is environmental, with different environmental factors being important in different areas of the world and in individual cases. Persistent hyperglycemia after an acute episode with hyperglycemia is not common. When it does occur, it is often found in patients with a family history of non-insulin-dependent diabetes without pancreatitis.

Pathology.   The pathology is quite variable; however, early on it appears to be focal in nature with an affected lobule often surrounded by normal ones. Protein precipitates are frequent findings in the ducts and often seem to precede the other lesions. It has been suggested that there is a loss of ductular lining epithelium early and encroachment of periductal connective tissue to produce stenosis, which is then followed by the chronic sclerosing fibrosis characteristic of the syndrome. In general, the pancreas tends to diminish in size in proportion to the severity of the clinical disease. Calcification is common and can often be observed by x-ray which usually shows it to be spotty and granular. Most of these calcifications are stones of varying sizes in the ducts. The endocrine pancreas appears to be somewhat resistant to the destructive process, and therefore apparently normal-looking islets by light microscopy are often found in areas of relatively severe fibrosis. Because of the loss of exocrine tissue, the islets may seem to be more prominent, but this is an artifact of tissue loss rather than islet hypertrophy. Eventually there may be islet inflammation and loss of islet cells, possibly related to involvement of blood vessels of the organ. Despite the relatively normal appearance by light microscopy, cyto-histochemistry of the islets in chronic pancreastitis reveals a reduced ratio of B- to A- cells so that A-cells almost equal B-cells in number while the number of D-cells appears to remain unchanged. Pancreatic polypeptide–rich islets are found more frequently; however, it is not known whether this is an artifact of the shrinkage of the pancreas or a true change in the frequency of this islet cell type.

Pathophysiology of Hyperglycemia.   Studies are limited and mostly performed in patients with alcoholic pancreatitis during the chronic phase of the disease. Vinik reported a reduced insulin response to glucose challenge both orally and intravenously. In general, the reduction in insulin secretion paralleled the degree of hyperglycemia. With intense stimulation, a group of pancreatitis patients with normal glucose tolerance still could be distinguished from normal controls by having slightly higher plasma glucose responses and slightly lower insulin secretion. Quantitatively, these responses could not be distinguished from those of non-insulin-dependent diabetics without a history of chronic pancreatitis. It was not possible in these studies to correlate the degree of pancreatic insufficiency with the hormone or glycemic responses; however, the authors point out the difficulty in evaluating exocrine pancreatic function quantitatively.

Intravenous glucose reveals a defect in first-phase insulin secretion. As in non-insulin-dependent diabetes, the insulin responses to arginine are normal unless severe hyperglycemia is present. In contrast to non-insulin-dependent diabetics, insulin responses to tolbutamide are markedly deficient. This has been interpreted to indicate that in pancreatitics there is a quantitative loss of B-cells, whereas in non-insulin-dependent diabetics there is a functional change in which the number of B-cells may be normal but they have specific diminution in their sensitivity to glucose.

The insulin response to combined injections of secretin and cholecystokinin (which may have been contaminated with GIP) was also defective. However, during the infusion of glucose, the CCK-PZ responses were moderately diminished while specific GIP responses were very severely diminished. These same findings were observed in the idiopathic diabetic group. Thus, it would appear that insulin release is abnormal in chronic pancreatitis, but it still can be modulated by glucose. A reduction in B-cell number would explain the findings.

In confirmation of what was observed morphologically, glucagon secretion is either normal or increased. In acute pancreatitis the elevation has been three- to four-fold. In chronic pancreatitis the most hyperglycemic individuals tend to have the highest glucagon levels and the more normally carbohydrate-tolerant the lowest. Glucagon responses to β-adrenergic agonists or CCK-PZ are usually normal or increased. The net result of all these changes is to suggest that in the patients with pancreatitis there is a loss of B-cell mass with maintenance of A-cell function at normal or supernormal levels. The explanation for the change in the ratio of A- to B-cells and the rather selective loss of B-cells remains unknown.

Treatment.   Despite the loss of B-cells as the probable etiology of this syndrome, patients may respond to sulfonylurea drugs early on, although many will eventually require insulin. Management is not particularly difficult unless malabsorption becomes a problem. When present, erratic food absorption may contribute significantly to intermittent episodes of hyperglycemia and hypoglycemia.

Pancreatic Destruction and Infiltration

Pancreatectomy.   Surgical pancreatectomy does not usually result in significant hyperglycemia unless more than three quarters of the pancreas is removed, and insulin-dependent hyperglycemia will not usually occur unless 85–90% of the pancreas is removed. Thus, there is a tremendous functional reserve in normal islets. This raises some serious questions regarding the importance of pancreatic destruction in pancreatitis, cystic fibrosis, neoplasia, and other diseases when they are associated with hyperglycemia. However, it may be that the residual presence and perhaps increase in activity of pancreatic A-cells secreting glucagon may play an important role in the degree of hyperglycemia observed in such circumstances.

The original reports suggesting normal glucagon levels in pancreatectomized man appear to have been related to an artifactual elevation of glucagon levels secondary to a glucagon-like molecule being released from the gut, which is biologically inactive but is measured in the radioimmunoassay. In dogs, stomach glucagon, which is identical to 3500-molecular-weight pancreatic glucagon, can make a considerable contribution to circulating plasma glucagon after pancreatectomy, but this does not seem to be the case in other species, including man. Hyperglycemia after total pancreatectomy is quite labile and frequently difficult to control. Such patients are often quite lean, do not eat well, have malabsorption and fluctuate rapidly between very insulin-sensitive hypoglycemia and severe hyperglycemia. Multiple doses of regular insulin along with long-acting insulin are usually required. Chronic diabetic complications are not often observed, perhaps because of the relatively short life span of patients who require major pancreatic surgery.

Trauma.   Owing to the degree of traumatic loss of endocrine pancreas that must occur, chronic hyperglycemic following trauma which can be directly attributed to the trauma is rare. Certainly, if the hyperglycemia does not occur very shortly after the trauma, it seems very unlikely that it would occur later. During severe trauma, it is common for hyperglycemia to occur as a result of the stress of the traumatic event. This is usually transient and, although it may require insulin treatment, does not necessarily mean that the patient has developed permanent diabetes. Because of the massive destruction required for permanent diabetes, it is likely that trauma sufficient to produce this much damage to the pancreas would usually be fatal, and therefore instances of chronic diabetes due to trauma are quite unusual.

Neoplasia.   Carcinoma of the pancreas is common, and hyperglycemia associated with it occurs in 7–10% of cases. This is more than would be expected, but the low frequency of hyperglycemia appears to be due to the focal nature of the disease and the dispersed nature of the pancreatic islets.

Diseases of Iron Excess

The association between hyperglycemia, diabetes mellitus, and hemochromatosis was described more than 100 years ago. Most of the association is between primary hemochromatosis, a presumed genetic disorder, and hyperglycemia, but there is good evidence for an association between secondary iron overload and hyperglycemia as well.

Primary Hemochromatosis.   The incidence of diabetes has been reported to be quite variable in primary hemochromatosis. However, the percentage is usually quite high and in the range of about 75% of patients. Although cirrhosis of any cause may be associated with glucose intolerance, there seems to be quite a difference between that secondary to hemochromatosis and that associated with cirrhosis of other etiologies. In clinical terms, the association of hyperglycemia is early in patients with primary hemochromatosis, but rather late in patients with alcoholic cirrhosis. Frequently a diagnosis of diabetes is made prior to a diagnosis of hemochromatosis. Hyperglycemia has been reported to be the most common presenting sign in some series.

However, in 1968 Balcerzak challenged the idea that the cause of the hyperglycemia was directly related to the iron overload itself. He found a strong familial tendency for hyperglycemia entirely independent of iron overload in families with hemochromatosis and hyperglycemia. Thus, he raised the question whether the coexistence of hemochromatosis and hyperglycemia represents the chance association of two diseases rather than a cause and effect relationship. Related studies have suggested that patients with hemochromatosis without diabetes tend to have relatives with diabetes less frequently than those patients with hemochromatosis and diabetes. Although the disorder is 10 times more common in males than females, this does not reflect the incidence of the underlying disorder but appears to be partly related to the chronic loss of iron that protects females from the clinical manifestations of the iron-absorptive abnormality. The evidence is that the genetic defect is not X-linked, but the true nature of the genetic disorder has not been determined. Thus, whether one gene or several genes are involved is not clear.

Excessive siderosis is seen in the liver primarily in the periportal parenchyma and later throughout the lobules and ductular epithelium. Periportal fibrosis eventually occurs, leading to a multilobular cirrhosis. Extensive iron deposition is also seen in the pancreas but mostly in the acinar tissue rather than the islets of Langerhans, which often appear histologically normal. Testicular atrophy is frequent, but since there are no hemosiderin deposits in the testes, the failure is probably at the pituitary level. Other findings of clinical hypopituitarism have been described.

Quantification of B-cells has not been made, and therefore the explanation for the hyperglycemia is not totally clear. The hyperglycemia is usually of the non-insulin-dependent type, with a somewhat earlier age of onset. Many patients have been treated with insulin, but ketoacidosis does not appear to be common. In one series reported by Dymock, 27% of the diabetic patients had nephropathy, neuropathy, or peripheral vascular disease and 31% had diabetic retinopathy with the mean duration of diabetes of approximately 8.5 years. Since there is a question whether these individuals have an association of idiopathic diabetes mellitus with hemochromatosis or whether they have iron overload alone causing hyperglycemia, it is not possible to make conclusions regarding the etiology of chronic diabetic complications from such findings. Despite questions regarding the association between the two diseases, a number of careful studies have found that the patients treated with iron removal show improved glucose tolerance and reduction in insulin dosage. Even if these changes do not occur, it appears that progression of the cirrhosis is halted along with progression of the hyperglycemia.

Secondary Iron Overload. This syndrome is found in thalassemia major and in excessive iron ingestion in the Bantu of South Africa. Abnormal glucose tolerance has been found in both syndromes. Again, glucose-intolerant patients were more likely to have glucose-intolerant relatives than non-glucose-intolerant patients. Interestingly, other endocrine dysfunction such as pituitary insufficiency has also been reported in secondary iron overload, suggesting direct toxic effects of iron. Reliable insulin secretory studies in these syndromes have not been reported; therefore, the pathogenesis of the hyperglycemia is not known.

Counterregulatory Hormone Excess and Hyperglycemia

Excess production of any of the counterregulatory hormones including growth hormone, glucosteroids, glucagon, and the catecholamines is associated with increased frequency of hyperglycemia, which may be clinically difficult to differentiate from idiopathic diabetes mellitus. The hyperglycemia in each case is ameliorated or disappears after treatment of the underlying disorder. Therefore, hyperglycemia in these patients is believed to be secondary. However, there is great variability in the degree of hyperglycemia and in the reported frequency of chronic complications associated with these types of secondary diabetes. Therefore, it is still unknown whether this is an association between idiopathic diabetes mellitus which has been exacerbated by counterregulatory hormone excess or whether the hyperglycemia observed is solely related to the excess counterregulatory hormone secretion. Since normal subjects have at least glucose intolerance and often fasting hyperglycemia with an excess of these hormones, this question cannot be answered until a nonmetabolic genetic marker for non-insulin-dependent diabetes is found.

Acromegaly (Excess Growth Hormone Secretion). Acromegaly is caused by excessive autonomous secretion of growth hormone from a pituitary adenoma. The prevalence of glucose intolerance is reported to be at least 60% of patients. One-third of these will have elevated fasting plasma glucose, and of those with overt hyperglycemia, approximately one-third may require insulin treatment. With this wide range of carbohydrate intolerance, it is not clear whether a percentage of patients have inherited a gene related to non-insulin-dependent diabetes mellitus which has been exaggerated by the acromegaly or whether all of the findings are strictly related to excessive growth hormone. Renal, retinal, and neurologic complications are relatively unusual in acromegalic patients with fasting hyperglycemia; however, it has been reported that thickened muscle capillary basement membranes are commonly found in such patients.

Pathologically, a small or large tumor is almost always evident, and after removal of the tumor or reduction of the growth hormone levels by pituitary irradiation, there is a parallel decrease in plasma glucose levels and improvement in indices of insulin resistance. Therefore, although animal studies suggest that permanent hyperglycemia can be induced by giving large amounts of growth hormone to partially pancreatectomized dogs or cats, most of the human findings suggest that the hyperglycemia is largely reversible. High circulating levels of insulin are found in most patients until frank overt diabetes supervenes, when insulin secretion is either normal or subnormal. Glucose and insulin are normal in about 15 or 20% of patients. In almost all of the rest, there is resistance to the action of insulin.

Therefore, it appears that the degree of hyperglycemia is partially related to how effectively the islet is able to overcome insulin resistance, which seems to be the primary effect of growth hormone excess. There is an inverse relationship between the concentration of insulin receptors on circulating monocytes and basal plasma insulin levels in these patients, but the degree of resistance is greater than that found in other insulin-resistant states; i.e., receptor binding is less than that found in obesity. In some cases, receptor affinity is increased, which may explain the variable clinical findings and lack of insulin resistance in some subjects. If treatment is required, it will often mean large doses of insulin if sulfonylureas are not effective. After treatment of the acromegaly, this insulin resistance should be reversed as plasma growth hormone levels fall. While it is assumed that the effects of growth hormone are indirect through somatomedin, this has not as yet been shown to be the case; therefore, the mechanism for this alteration in peripheral metabolism of glucose remains somewhat undefined.

Cushing's Syndrome (Glucosteroid Hormone Excess). Cushing's syndrome is caused by a chronic increase in plasma glucosteroid levels. It may be related to exogenous administration of glucosteroids or ACTH or to endogenous hypersecretion of adrenal steroids or endogenous hypersecretion of ACTH due to a pituitary tumor or an ACTH-secreting neoplasm. Carbohydrate intolerance is very common in Cushing's syndrome and can be found in almost all patients, although probably less than 20% have fasting hyperglycemia. This syndrome is associated with insulin resistance and insulin secretion which is increased but inadequate to prevent the hyperglycemia. Hypoinsulinemia may actually be observed in the most severely hyperglycemic patients. Experimentally, there is often islet cell hyperplasia after steroid treatment, and therefore some of the effects may be related directly to an alteration of islet function by steroids.

The mechanism of the insulin resistance is partially related to a change in affinity of insulin receptors in the liver and adipose membranes. Thus, unlike other forms of insulin resistance, the change of the insulin receptor appears to be a reduction of the affinity of binding and not the number of binding sites. Despite these changes, there is considerable evidence that there are important postreceptor defects induced by steroids. In addition, there is a marked increase in glucose production by the liver due to a direct stimulation of gluconeogenesis by steroids and an indirect effect of glucosteroids to increase glucagon secretion. Basal plasma glucagon and glucagon responses to challenge have both been reported to be elevated. Individual susceptibility must be important to the hyperglycemia, since steroids have been used to detect latent diabetic states in family members of non-insulin-dependent diabetics. Following removal of the steroid or treatment of the Cushing's syndrome, hyperglycemia will ameliorate or disappear. Occasional patients with high doses of steroids may need insulin treatment and can develop ketoacidosis. Yet even in these patients, removal of the excess steroids may allow carbohydrate metabolism to revert to normal.

Pheochromocytoma (Catecholamine Excess). The clinical manifestations of pheochromocytoma result from increased amounts of circulating epinephrine and norepinephrine. Since epinephrine is a far more potent hyperglycemic amine, metabolic effects are usually better correlated with its concentration than with that of norepinephrine. The plasma catecholamines are at least twice and often 10 to 100 times as high as the levels found in normal subjects. Carbohydrate intolerance is common and is probably present in most patients with this syndrome. Nevertheless, fasting hyperglycemia is relatively unusual. In some patients insulin treatment has been required. Regardless of the degree of glucose intolerance, marked amelioration or disappearance of the carbohydrate-intolerant state may occur after tumor removal. Even if diagnosis is delayed, treatment of the tumor almost always leads to complete reversion of the carbohydrate-intolerant state. Pathophysiologically, the syndrome consists of a mixture of inhibition of insulin secretion by α-adrenergic effects, stimulation of hepatic gluconeogenesis and glycogenolysis by both α- and β-adrenergic effects, and β-adrenergic peripheral resistance to insulin action. The relative contribution of these multisystem changes to any one case of hyperglycemia is not clear.

Glucagonoma. A number of islet cell secreting tumors releasing large amounts of glucagon into the circulation have been reported. Histochemically, these tumors are composed of A-cells, and many are malignant. The clinical syndrome is characterized by a severe dermatitis (necrolytic migratory erythema), variable degrees of glucose intolerance, weight loss, malnutrition, and hypoaminoacidemia with markedly elevated levels of plasma glucagon. The most surprising finding has been the mildness of the hyperglycemia considering the severity of the hyperglucagonemia. Insulin levels are often elevated; therefore, presumably the hyperglucagonemia is modulated by feedback stimulation of the beta cell. In some patients, carbohydrate metabolism has apparently been normal. This may be due to the variable nature of the species of glucagon circulating.

While the 3500-dalton glucagon molecule is present in most cases, some are also characterized by high concentrations of a larger molecular weight 10,000-dalton species. Its biologic activity is uncertain, but is certainly less than that of the 3500-molecular-weight material. Most of the patients have been women, and most have been over 45 years of age. Removal of the tumor is usually associated with reversion of the skin lesion and loss of carbohydrate intolerance.

Other Hormonal Syndromes with Hyperglycemia

A number of other hormonally abnormal states are characterized by hyperglycemia secondary to the change in hormone secretion rate. In most instances, the pathophysiology is explainable by the known effects of the syndrome on pancreatic islet function (hypokalemia, hypocalcemia, hyperserotoninemia, hypersomatostinemia). In some instances, it is not clear whether the association is due solely to the hormonal abnormality or whether it is due to the association of idiopathic diabetes mellitus (usually of a non-insulin-dependent type) with an aggravating endocrine-metabolic factor.

The association of hyperglycemia with isolated growth hormone deficiency demonstrates the difficulties in unraveling these relationships. Merimee has reported that *atelio-tic dwarfs* have a high incidence of hyperglycemia as adults, but that this condition is not associated with any of the microvascular complications of diabetes mellitus. Analysis of the *Laron dwarfs*, in whom growth hormone levels are elevated but there is a failure of growth hormone action, reveals the same findings. However, the explanation for hyperglycemia associated with growth hormone deficiency has been confusing, particularly because of the association of growth hormone excess with the same metabolic findings. Studies of the Laron dwarfs have shown *hypoglycemia* and increased sensitivity to insulin during the prepubertal years and the development of carbohydrate intolerance only postpubertally. While extensive studies of the younger ateliotic dwarfs have not been made, it seems likely that a similar course exists — that is, hypoglycemia and marked insulin sensitivity in young children with very low insulin levels, and somewhat higher insulin levels but deficient insulin responses and hyperglycemia as adults.

One potential explanation would be to hypothesize that the normal pubertal growth of islets is dependent upon growth hormone. Patients who develop growth hormone deficiency as children would then be unable to have adequate islet growth as they mature, thereby leaving them relatively deficient in insulin secretory capacity as adults. This hypothesis would also explain why adults who develop isolated growth hormone deficiency or adult hypopituitary patients with growth hormone deficiency do not develop hyperglycemia and are in fact hypoglycemic and extremely insulin-sensitive. It would seem likely that increased insulin sensitivity is always present with growth hormone deficiency, but that the degree of glucose regulation depends upon whether islet B-cell growth has occurred prior to the deficiency or not. The finding that ateliotic dwarfs fail to show significant microvascular disease or retinopathy on careful examination may indicate the multifactorial nature of the chronic microvascular changes found in idiopathic diabetes mellitus.

REFERENCES

General

Bloom, S. R. (eds.): *Gut Hormones.* Edinburgh, Churchill Livingstone, 1978.

Creutzfeldt, W., Kobberling, J., and Neel, J. V. (eds.): *The Genetics of Diabetes Mellitus.* New York, Springer-Verlag, 1976.

Ellenberg, M., and Rifkin, H. (eds.): *Diabetes Mellitus: Theory and Practice.* New York, McGraw-Hill, 1970.

Fajans, S. (ed.): *Diabetes Mellitus.* Bethesda, Md., DHEW Publication No. (NIH) 76–854, 1976.

Fajans, S. S., and Sussman, K. E. (eds.): *Diabetes Mellitus, Diagnosis and Treatment.* Vol. III. New York, American Diabetes Association, 1971.

Knowles, H. C. (ed.): Proc. Fiftieth Anniv. Insulin Symp., Indianapolis. *Diabetes* 21 (Suppl. 2), 1971.

Lefebvre, P. J., and Unger, R. H.: *Glucagon: Molecular Physiology, Clinical and Therapeutic Implications.* New York, Pergamon Press, 1972.

Marble, A., White, P., Bradley, R. F., and Krall, L. P. (eds.): *Joslin's Diabetes Mellitus.* Philadelphia, Lea & Febiger, 1971.

Podolsky, S. (ed.): Symposium on Diabetes Mellitus. *Med. Clin, N. Am.* 62:625–829, 1978.

Podolsky, S., and Viswanatha, M. (eds.): *Secondary Diabetes.* New York, Raven Press, 1980.

Pyke, D. A. (ed.): Diabetes and Related Disorders. *Clin. Endocrinol. Metab.* 1:599, 1972.

Shafrir, E. (ed.): Impact of insulin on metabolic pathways. Intern. Symp. Fiftieth Anniv. Insulin, Jerusalem. *Israel J. Med. Sci.* 8:271, 1972.

Stanbury, J. B., Wyngaarden, J. B., et al. (eds.): *The Metabolic Basic of Inherited Disease.* 3rd Ed. New York, McGraw-Hill, 1972.

Steiner, D. F., and Freinkel, N. (eds.): *Handbook of Physiology,* Section 7: *Endocrinology,* Vol. 1: *Endocrine Pancreas.* American Physiological Society. Baltimore, Williams & Wilkins. 1972.

Sussman, K. E. (ed.): *Juvenile-Type Diabetes and Its Complications: Theoretical and Practical Considerations.* Springfield, Ill., Charles C Thomas, 1971.

Sussman, K. E., and Metz, R. J. S.: *Diabetes Mellitus.* Vol. IV. New York, American Diabetes Association, 1975.

Tattersall, R. B. (ed.): Diabetes. *Clin. Endocrinol. Metab.* 6:283–522, 1977.

Volk, B. W., and Wellman, K. F. (eds.): *The Diabetic Pancreas.* New York, Plenum, 1977.

Waldhäusl, W. K. (ed.): Diabetes, 1979. Proc. Tenth Cong. Internat. Diabetes Fed., Vienna, Austria. Amsterdam, Excerpta Medica Foundation, 1980.

Williams, R. H. (ed.): *Diabetes.* New York, Paul B. Hoeber Co., 1960.

Williams, R. H., and Ensinck, J. W.: Secretion, fates and actions of insulin and related products. *Diabetes* 15:623, 1966.

Islet Anatomy and the Chemistry and Synthesis of Pancreatic Hormones

Brandenburg, D., Gattner, H. G., et al.: The biochemistry of insulin. In *Diabetes.* Proc. Seventh Cong. Internat. Diabetes Fed. Rodriguez, R. R., and Vallance-Owen, J. (eds.), Amsterdam, Excerpta Medica Foundation, 1971.

Bromer, W. W.: Chemistry of glucagon and gastrin. In *Handbook of Physiology,* Section 7: *Endocrinology,* Vol. 1: *Endocrine Pancreas.* Steiner, D. F., and Freinkel, N. (eds.), American Physiological Society. Baltimore, Williams & Wilkins, 1972.

Buffa, R., Capella, C., et al.: Vasoactive intestinal peptide (VIP) cells in the pancreas and gastrointestinal mucosa: An immunohistochemical and ultrastructural study. *Histochemistry* 50:217, 1977.

Chance, R. E.: Chemical, physical, biological, and immunological studies on porcine proinsulin and related polypeptides. In *Diabetes.* Proc. Seventh Cong. Internat. Diabetes Fed. Rodrigues, R. R., and Vallance-Owen, J. (eds.), Amsterdam, Excerpta Medica Foundation, 1971.

Chance, R. E.: Amino acid sequences of proinsulins and intermediates. *Diabetes* 21 (Suppl. 2):461, 1972.

Hodgkin, D. C.: The structure of insulin. *Diabetes* 21:1131, 1972.

Humbel, R. E., Bosshard, H. R., et al.: Chemistry of insulin. In *Handbook of Physiology,* Section 7: *Endocrinology,* Vol. 1: *Endocrine Pancreas.* Steiner, D. F., and Freinkel, N. (eds.), American Physiological Society. Baltimore, Williams & Wilkins, 1972.

Jacobsen, H. A., Demandt, A., et al.: Sequence analysis of porcine gut GLI-I. *Biochim. Biophys. Acta* 493:542, 1977.

Kimmel, J. R., Hayden, L. J., and Pollock, H. G.: Isolation and characterization of a new pancreatic polypeptide hormone. *J. Biol. Chem.* 250:9369, 1975.

Lacy, P., and Greider, M. H.: Ultrastructural organization of mammalian pancreatic islets. In *Handbook of Physiology,* Section 7: *Endocrinology,* Vol. 1: *Endocrine Pancreas.* Steiner, D. F., and Freinkel, N. (eds.), American Physiological Society. Baltimore, Williams & Wilkins, 1972.

Langslow, D. R., Kimmel, J. R., et al.: Studies of the distribution of a new avian pancreatic polypeptide and insulin among birds, reptiles, amphibians, and mammals. *Endocrinology* 93:558, 1973.

Larsson, L. I., Fahrenkrug, J., et al.: Innervation of the pancreas by vasoactive intestinal polypeptide (VIP) immunoreactive nerves. *Life Sci.* 22:773, 1978.

Larsson, L. I., Sundler, F., et al: Immunohistochemical localization of human pancreatic polypeptide. *Cell Tissue Res.* 156:167, 1975.

Like, A., and Orci, L.: Embryogenesis of the human pancreatic islets: a light and electron microscopic study. *Diabetes* 21:511, 1972.

Lin, T. M., and Chance, R. E.: Candidate hormones of the gut. VI. Bovine pancreatic polypeptide (BPP) and avian pancreatic polypeptide (APP). *Gastroenterology* 67:737, 1974.

Munger, B.: The histology, cytochemistry and ultrastructure of pancreatic islet A-cells. In *Glucagon: Molecular Physiology, Clinical and Therapeutic Implications.* Lefebvre, P. J., and Unger, R. H. (eds.), New York, Pergamon Press, 1972.

Orci, L., Baetens, D., et al.: Pancreatic polypeptide and glucagon: Non-random distribution in pancreatic islets. *Life Sci.* 19:1811, 1976.

Oyer, P., Cho, S., et al.: Studies on human proinsulin. Isolation and amino acid sequence of the human pancreatic c-peptide. *J. Biol. Chem.* 246:1375, 1971.

Pearse, A. G. E., and Takor, T. T.: Embryology of the diffuse neuroendocrine system and its relationship to the common peptides. *Fed. Proc.* 38:2288, 1979.

Pictet, R. L., Clark, W. R., et al.: An ultrastructural analysis of the developing embryonic pancreas. *Dev. Biol.* 29:436, 1972.

Pictet, R. L., Rall, L. B., et al.: The neural crest and the origin of the insulin-producing and other gastrointestinal hormone-producing cells. *Science* 191:191, 1976.

Pictet, R., and Rutter, W. J.: Development of the embryonic endocrine pancreas. In *Handbook of Physiology,* Section 7: *Endocrinology,* Vol. I: *Endocrine Pancreas.* Field, J. (ed.), American Physiological Society. Baltimore, Williams & Wilkins, 1972.

Rubenstein, A. H., and Steiner, D. F.: Proinsulin. *Ann. Rev. Med.* 22:1, 1971.

Ruttenberg, M. A.: Human insulin: facile synthesis by modification of porcine insulin. *Science* 177:623, 1972.

Sanger, F.: Chemistry of insulin. *Science* 129:1340, 1959.

Smith, L. F.: Amino acid sequences of insulins. *Diabetes* 21:457, 1972.

Steiner, D. F.: Insulin today. *Diabetes* 26:322, 1977.

Sundby, F.: Species variations in the primary structure of glucagon. *Metabolism* 25:1319, 1976.

Tager, H. S., and Markese, T.: Intestinal and pancreatic glucagon-like peptides. *J. Biol. Chem.* 254:2229, 1979.

Tager, H. S., Patzelt, C., et al.: Biosynthesis of islet hormones. *Ann. N.Y. Acad. Sci.* 343:133, 1980.

Release of Pancreatic Hormones

Adrian, T. E., Besterman, H. S., et al.: Mechanism of pancreatic polypeptide release in man. *Lancet* 1:161, 1977.

Adrian, T. E., Bloom, S. R., et al.: Physiology and pathology. In *Gut Hormones.* Bloom, S. R. (ed.), Edinburgh, Churchill Livingston, 1978.

Adrian, T. E., Bloom, S. R., et al.: Pancreatic polypeptide, glucagon and insulin secretion from the isolated perfused canine pancreas. *Diabetologia* 14:413, 1978.

Anderson, D. K., Elahi, D., et al.: Oral glucose augmentation of insulin secretion. Interaction of gastric inhibitory polypeptide with ambient glucose and insulin levels. *J. Clin. Invest.* 62:152, 1978.

Bagdade, J. D., Bierman, E. L., et al.: The significance of basal insulin levels in the evaluation of the insulin response to glucose in diabetic and nondiabetic subjects. *J. Clin. Invest.* 46:1549, 1967.

Brown, J. C., and Otte, S. C.: Gastrointestinal hormones and the control of insulin secretion. *Diabetes* 27:782, 1978.

Brown, M., Rivier, J., et al.: Somatostatin. Analogs with selected biological activities. *Science* 196:1467, 1977.

Cerasi, E., and Luft, R.: The plasma insulin response to glucose infusion in healthy subjects and in diabetes mellitus. *Acta Endocrinol.* 55:278, 1967.

Dean, P. M., and Matthews, E. K.: Electrical activity in pancreatic islet cells: effect of ions. *J. Physiol. (London)* 210:265, 1970.

Dean, P. M., and Matthews, E. K.: Glucose induced electrical activity in pancreatic islet cells. *J. Physiol. (London)* 210:255, 1970.

Floyd, J. C., Fajans, S. S., et al.: A newly recognized pancreatic polypeptide; plasma levels in health and disease. *Recent Prog. Horm. Res.* 33:519, 1977.

Frohman, L. A., and Bernardis, L. L.: Effect of hypothalamic stimulation on plasma glucose, insulin, and glucagon levels. *Amer. J. Physiol.* 221:1596, 1971.

Ganda, O., Weir, G., et al.: Somatostatinoma: A somatostatin containing tumor of the endocrine pancreas. *N. Engl. J. Med.* 296:963, 1977.

Gerich, J. E., Charles, M. A., et al.: Regulation of pancreatic insulin and glucagon secretion. *Ann. Rev. Physiol.* 38:353, 1976.

Gerich, J., and Lorenzi, M.: The role of the autonomic nervous system and somatostatin in the control of insulin and glucagon secretion. In *Frontiers in Neuroendocrinology,* Vol. 5. Ganong, W., and Martini, L. (eds.), New York, Raven Press, 1977.

Goodner, C. J., and Porte, D., Jr.: Determinants of basal islet secretion in man. In *Handbook of Physiology,* Section 7: *Endocrinology,* Vol. 1: *Endocrine Pancreas.* Steiner, D. F., and Freinkel, N. (eds.). American Physiological Society. Baltimore, Williams & Wilkins, 1972.

Greenberg, C. R., McClog, R. F., et al: Inhibition of pancreas and gall bladder by pancreatic polypeptide. *Lancet* 2:1280, 1978.

Grodsky, G. M.: A threshold distribution hypothesis for packet storage of insulin and its mathematical modeling. *J. Clin. Invest.* 51:2047, 1972.

Guillemin, R., and Gerich, J. E.: Somatostatin: physiological and clinical significance. *Ann. Rev. Med.* 27:379, 1976.

Koerker, D. J., Ruch, W., et al.: Somatostatin: Hypothalamic inhibitor of the endocrine pancreas. *Science* 184:482, 1974.

Lacy, P.: Beta cell secretion — from the standpoint of a pathobiologist. *Diabetes* 19:895, 1970.

Lambert, A. E.: The regulation of insulin secretion. *Rev. Physiol. Biochem. Pharmacol.* 75:98, 1976.

Lazarus, S. S., Shapiro, S., et al.: Secretory granule formation and release in rabbit pancreatic A-cells. *Diabetes* 17:152, 1968.

Luft, R., Efendic, S., et al.: Somatostatin — both hormone and neurotransmitter? *Diabetologia* 14:1, 1978.

Lundbaek, K., and Hansen, A. P.: Diabetes mellitus and somatostatin. *Dan. Med. Bull.* 24:1, 1977.

Matschinsky, F. M., Landgraf, R., et al.: Glucoreceptor mechanisms in islets of Langerhans. *Diabetes* 21:555, 1972.

McIntyre, N., Holdsworth, C. D., et al.: Intestinal factors in the control of insulin secretion. *J. Clin. Endocrinol.* 25:1317, 1965.

Palmer, J. P., and Porte, D., Jr.: Central nervous system control of glucagon secretion. In *Comprehensive Endocrinology, Glucagon.* Unger, R. H. (ed.), New York, Elsevier-North Holland, 1981 (in press).

Porte, D., Jr., and Bagdade, J. D.: Human insulin secretion: an integrated approach. *Ann. Rev. Med.* 21:219, 1970.

Porte, D., Jr., Girardier, L., et al.: Neural regulation of insulin secretion in the dog. *J. Clin. Invest.* 52:210, 1973.

Porte, D., Jr., and Robertson, R. P.: Control of insulin secretion by catecholamines, stress, and the sympathetic nervous system. *Fed. Proc.* 32:1792, 1973.

Robertson, R. P., and Porte, D., Jr.: Adrenergic modulation of basal insulin secretion in man. *Diabetes* 22:1, 1973.

Rocha, D. M., Faloona, G., et al.: Glucagon-stimulating activity of 20 amino acids in dogs. *J. Clin. Invest.* 51:2346, 1972.

Rubenstein, A. H., Block, M. B., et al.: Proinsulin and c-peptide in blood. *Diabetes* 21 (Suppl. 2):661, 1972.

Samols, E., and Weir, G. C.: Adrenergic modulation of pancreatic A, B, and D cells. *J. Clin. Invest.* 63:230, 1979.

Schwartz, T. W., Stadil, F., et al.: Pancreatic polypeptide response to food in duodenal ulcer patients before and after vagotomy. *Lancet* 1:1102, 1976.

Smith, P. H., and Porte, D., Jr.: Neuropharmacology of the pancreatic islets. *Annu. Rev. Pharmacol. Toxicol.* 16:269, 1976.

Smith, P. H., Woods, S. C., et al.: Control of the endocrine pancreas by the autonomic nervous system and related neural factors. In *Integrative Functions of the Autonomic Nervous System.* Brooks, C. McC, Koizuma, K., et al. (eds.), Tokyo and New York, University of Tokyo Press and Elsevier, 1979.

Sokal, J. E.: Glucagon — an essential hormone. *Amer. J. Med.* 41:331, 1966.

Taborsky, G. J., Jr., Smith, P. H., et al.: Differential effects of somatostatin analogues on α- and β-cells of the pancreas. *Amer. J. Physiol.* 236: E123, 1979.

Turner, R. C., Grayburn, J. A., et al.: Measurement of the insulin delivery rate in man. *J. Clin. Endocrinol.* 33:279, 1971.

Unger, R. H., Dobbs, R. E., et al.: Insulin, glucagon, and somatostatin secretion in the regulation of metabolism. *Ann. Rev. Physiol.* 40:307, 1978.

Unger, R. J., and Orci, L.: Physiology and pathophysiology of glucagon. *Physiol. Rev.* 56:778, 1976.

Vale, W., Brazeau, P., et al.: Somatostatin. *Recent Prog. Horm. Res.* 34:365, 1975.

Wollheim, C., Blondel, B., et al.: Somatostatin inhibition of pancreatic glucagon release from monolayer cultures and interactions with calcium. *Endocrinology* 111:911, 1977.

Woods, S. C., and Porte, D., Jr.: Neural control of the endocrine pancreas. *Physiol. Rev.* 54:596, 1974.

Yalow, R. S., and Berson, S. A.: Immunoassay of endogenous plasma insulin in man. *J. Clin. Invest.* 39:1157, 1960.

Distribution and Degradation – Insulin and Proinsulin

Burghen, G. A., Kitabchi, A. E., et al.: Characterization of a rat liver protease with specificity for insulin. *Endocrinology* 91:633, 1972.

Carpentier, J.-L., Gorden, P., et al.: Lysosomal association of internalized ^{125}I-insulin in isolated rat hepatocytes. *J. Clin. Invest.* 63:1249, 1979.

De Fronzo, R. A., Tobin, J. D., et al.: Glucose clamp technique: a method for quantifying insulin secretion and resistance. *Amer. J. Physiol.* 237:E214, 1979.

Duckworth, W. C., Heinemann, M. A., et al.: Purification of insulin-specific protease by affinity chromatography. *Proc. Natl. Acad. Sci. USA* 69:3698, 1972.

Elgee, N. J., Williams, R. H., et al: Distribution and degradation studies with insulin-I^{131}. *J. Clin. Invest.* 33:1252, 1954.

Genuth, S. M.: Metabolic clearance of insulin in man. *Diabetes* 21:1003, 1972.

Horwitz, D. L., Starr, J. I., et al.: Proinsulin, insulin and C-peptide concentrations in human portal and peripheral blood. *J. Clin. Invest.* 55:1278, 1975.

Kahn, C. R., and Baird, K.: The fate of insulin bound to adipocytes. Evidence for compartmentalization and processing. *J. Biol. Chem.* 253:4900, 1978.

Kitabchi, A. E.: Proinsulin and C-peptide: A review. *Metabolism* 26:547, 1977.

Kitabchi, A. E., Duckworth, W. C., et al.: Direct measurement of proinsulin in human plasma by the use of an insulin-degrading enzyme. *J. Clin. Invest.* 50:1792, 1971.

Mirsky, I. A.: The metabolism of insulin. *Diabetes* 13:225, 1964.

Posner, B. I., Josefsberg, Z., et al.: Intracellular polypeptide hormone receptors. Characterization of insulin binding sites in Golgi fractions from the liver of female rats. *J. Biol. Chem.* 253:4067, 1978.

Posner, B. I., Verma, A. K., et al.: intracellular insulin and insulin receptors: Nature and significance. In *Diabetes, 1979.* Proc. Tenth Cong. Internat. Diabetes Fed. Waldhäusl, W. K. (ed.), Amsterdam, Excerpta Medica Foundation, 1980.

Rabkin, R., and Kitabchi, A. E.: Factors influencing the handling of insulin by the isolated rat kidney. *J. Clin. Invest.* 62:169, 1978.

Rödmark, S., Bloom, G., et al.: Hepatic extraction of exogenous insulin and glucagon in the dog. *Endocrinology* 102:806, 1978.

Savage, P. J., Flock, E. V., et al.: C-peptide and insulin secretion in Pima Indians and Caucasians: constant fractional hepatic extraction over a wide range of insulin concentrations and in obesity. *J. Clin. Endocrinol. Metab.* 48:594, 1979.

Distribution and Degradation – Glucagon and Somatostatin

Duckworth, W. C., and Kitabchi, A. E.: Insulin and glucagon degradation by the same enzyme. *Diabetes* 23:536, 1974.

Ensinck, J. W., Shepard, C., et al.: Use of benzamidine as a proteolytic inhibitor in the radioimmunoassay of glucagon in plasma. *J. Clin. Endocrinol.* 35:463, 1972.

Jaspan, J. B., Huen, A. H-J., et al.: The role of the liver in glucagon metabolism. *J. Clin. Invest.* 60:421, 1977.

McDonald, J. K., Callahan, P. X., et al.: Inactivation and degradation of glucagon by dipeptidyl aminopeptidase I (cathepsin C) of rat liver. *J. Biol. Chem.* 244:6199, 1969.

Sheppard, M., Shapiro, B., et al.: Metabolic clearance and plasma half-disappearance time of exogenous somatostatin in man. *J. Clin. Endocrinol. Metab.* 48:50, 1979.

Sherwin, R. S., Bastl, C., et al.: Influence of uremia and hemodialysis on the turnover and metabolic effects of glucagon. *J. Clin. Invest.* 57:722, 1976.

Mechanism of Action of Islet Hormones – Insulin

Blundell, T. L., and Wood, S. P.: Is the evolution of insulin Darwinian or due to selectively neutral mutation? *Nature* 257:197, 1975.

Czech, M. P.: Insulin action and the regulation of hexose transport. *Diabetes* 29:399, 1980.

DeMeyts, P., Bianco, A. F., et al.: Site-site interactions among insulin receptors. Characterization of the negative cooperativity. *J. Biol. Chem.* 251:1877, 1976.

Ensinck, J. W., and Williams, R. H.: Hormonal and nonhormonal factors modifying man's response to insulin. In *Handbook of Physiology,* Section 7: *Endocrinology,* Vol. 1: *Endocrine Pancreas.* Steiner, D. F., and Freinkel, N. (eds.), American Physiological Society. Baltimore, Williams & Wilkins, 1972.

Exton, J. H.: Gluconeogenesis. *Metabolism* 21:945, 1972.

Felig, P.: The glucose-alanine cycle. *Metabolism* 22:179, 1973.

Freychet, P.: The interactions of proinsulin with insulin receptors on the plasma membrane of the liver. *J. Clin. Invest.* 54:1020, 1974.

Freychet, P., Roth, J., et al.: Insulin receptors in the liver: specific binding of (I-125) insulin to the plasma membrane and its relation to insulin bioactivity. *Proc. Natl. Acad. Sci. USA* 68:1833, 1971.

Illiano, G., and Cuatrecasas, P.: Modulation of adenylate cyclase activity in liver and fat cell membranes by insulin. *Science* 175:906, 1972.

Insel, P. A., Liljenquist, J. E., et al.: Insulin control of glucose metabolism in man. A new kinetic analysis. *J. Clin. Invest.* 55:1057, 1975.

Jarett, L., and Smith, R. M.: Effect of cytochalasin B and D on groups of insulin receptors and on insulin action in rat adipocytes. Possible evidence for a structural relationship of the insulin receptor to the glucose transport system. *J. Clin. invest.* 63:571, 1979.

Kahn, C. R., Baird, K., et al.: Effects of autoantibodies to the insulin receptor on isolated adipocytes. Studies of insulin binding and insulin action. *J. Clin. Invest.* 60:1094, 1977.

Kahn, C. R., Megyesi, K., et al.: Receptors for peptide hormones. New insights into the pathophysiology of disease states in man. *Ann. Intern. Med.* 86:205, 1977.

Kolterman, O. G., Greenfield, M., et al.: Effect of a high carbohydrate diet on insulin binding to adipocytes and on insulin action in vivo in man. *Diabetes* 28:731, 1979.

Lakshmanan, M. R., Nepokroeff, C. M., et al.: Control of the synthesis of fatty-acid synthetase in rat liver by insulin, glucagon, and adenosine 3',5' cyclic monophosphate. *Proc. Natl. Acad. Sci. USA* 69:3516, 1972.

Le Marchard-Brustel, Y., and Freychet, P.: Effect of fasting and streptozotocin diabetes on insulin binding and action in the isolated mouse soleus muscle. *J. Clin. Invest.* 64:1505, 1979.

Olefsky, J. M.: Effects of fasting on insulin binding, glucose transport, and glucose oxidation in isolated rat adipocytes. Relationships between insulin receptors and insulin action. *J. Clin. Invest.* 58:1450, 1976.

Pollet, R. J., Standaert, M. L., et al.: Insulin binding to the human lymphocyte receptor. Evaluation of the negative cooperativity model. *J. Biol. Chem.* 252:5828, 1977.

Pullen, R. A., Lindsay, D. G., et al.: Receptor-binding region of insulin. *Nature* 259:369, 1976.

Schlessinger, J., Shechter, Y., et al.: Direct visualization of binding, aggregation, and internalization of insulin and epidermal growth factor on living fibroblastic cells. *Proc. Natl. Acad. Sci. USA* 75:2659, 1978.

Sols, A.: Regulation of liver glucokinase and muscle hexokinase. In *On the Nature and Treatment of Diabetes.* Leibel, B. A., and Wrenshall, G. A. (eds.), Amsterdam, Excerpta Medica Foundation, 1965.

Zierler, K. L: Possible mechanisms of insulin action on membrane potential and ion fluxes. *Amer. J. Med.* 40:735, 1966.

Mechanism of Action of Islet Hormones – Glucagon

Cherrington, A. D., Chiasson, J. L., et al.: The role of insulin and glucagon in the regulation of basal glucose production in the postabsorptive dog. *J. Clin. Invest.* 58:1407, 1976.

Cherrington, A. D., Liljenquist, J. E., et al.: Importance of hypoglycemia-induced glucose production during isolated glucagon deficiency. *Amer. J. Physiol.* 236:E263, 1979.

Lad, P. M., Welton, A. F., et al.: Evidence for distinct guanine nucleotide sites in the regulation of the glucagon receptor and of adenylate cyclase activity. *J. Biol. Chem.* 252:5942, 1977.

Levey, G. S.: The glucagon receptor and adenylate cyclase. *Metabolism* 24:301, 1975.

Liljenquist, J. E., Meuller, G. L., et al.: Evidence for an important role of glucagon in the regulation of hepatic glucose production in normal man. *J. Clin. Invest.* 59:369, 1977.

Mallette, L. E., Exton, J. H., et al.: Effects of glucagon on amino acid transport and utilization in the perfused rat liver. *J. Biol. Chem.* 244:5724, 1969.

McGarry, J. D.: New perspectives in the regulation of ketogenesis. *Diabetes* 28:517, 1979.

Rodbell, M. Birnbaumer, L., et al.: The reaction of glucagon with its receptor: evidence for discrete regions of activity and binding in the glucagon molecule. *Proc. Natl. Acad. Sci. USA* 68:909, 1971.

Spark, R. F., Arky, R. A., et al.: Renin, aldosterone and glucagon in the natriuresis of fasting. *N. Engl. J. Med.* 292:1335, 1975.

Wahren, J. Efendic, S., et al.: Influence of somatostatin on splanchnic glucose metabolism in postabsorptive and 60-hour fasted humans. *J. Clin. Invest.* 59:299, 1977.

Witters, L. A., Kovaloff, E. M., et al.: Glucagon regulation of protein phosphorylation: identification of acetyl coenzyme A carboxylase as a substrate. *J. Biol. Chem.* 254:245, 1979.

Witters, L. A., and Trasko, C. S.: Regulation of hepatic free fatty acid metabolism by glucagon and insulin. *Amer. J. Physiol.* 237:E23, 1979.

Mechanism of Action – Somatostatin

Chideckel, E. W., Palmer, J., et al.: Somatostatin blockade of acute and chronic stimuli of the endocrine pancreas and the consequences of this blockade on glucose homeostasis. *J. Clin. Invest.* 55:754, 1975.

Gerich, J. E.: Somatostatin. In *Diabetes Mellitus: A Pathophysiologic Approach to Clinical Practice.* Assan, R., Girard, J. R., and Marliss, E. B. (ed.) (in press, 1981).

Luft, R., Efendic, S., et al.: Somatostatin — both hormone and neurotransmitter? *Diabetologia* 14:1, 1978.

Pace, C. S., Murphy, M., et al.: Somatostatin inhibition of glucose-induced electrical activity in cultured rat islet cells. *Amer. J. Physiol.* 233:C164, 1977.

Taborsky, G. J., Jr., Smith, P. H., et al.: Differential effects of somatostatin analogues on α- and β-cells of the pancreas. *Amer. J. Physiol.* 236:E123, 1979.

Experimental Hyperglycemia

Bray, G. A.: The Zucker fatty rat: a review. *Fed. Proc.* 36:148, 1977.

Bray, G. A., and York, D. A.: Genetically transmitted obesity in rodents. *Physiol. Rev.* 51:598, 1971.

Bray, G. A., and York, D. A.: Hypothalamic and genetic obesity in experimental animals: An autonomic and endocrine hypothesis. *Physiol. Rev.* 59:719, 1979.

Coleman, D. L.: Obese and diabetes: two mutant genes causing diabetes-obesity syndromes in mice. *Diabetologia* 14:141, 1978.

Craighead, J. E.: The role of viruses in the pathogenesis of pancreatic disease and diabetes mellitus. *Prog. Med. Virol.* 19:161, 1975.

Craighead, J. E.: Viral diabetes. In *The Diabetic Pancreas.* Volk, B. W., and Wellmann, K. F. (eds.) New York, Plenum, 1977, p. 467.

Dulin, W. E., and Soret, M. G.: Chemically and hormonally induced diabetes. In *The Diabetic Pancreas.* Volk, B. W., and Wellmann, K. F. (eds.), New York, Plenum, 1977, p. 425.

Fischer, L. J., and Rickert, D. E.: Pancreatic islet-cell toxicity. *CRC Crit. Rev. Toxicol.* 3:231, 1975.

Herberg, L., and Coleman, D. L.: Laboratory animals exhibiting obesity and diabetes syndromes. *Metabolism* 26:59, 1977.

Like, A. A.: Spontaneous diabetes in animals. In *The Diabetic Pancreas.* Volk, B. W., and Wellmann, K. F. (eds.), New York, Plenum, 1977, p. 381.

Like, A. A., Gerritsen, G. C., et al.: Studies in the diabetic Chinese hamster: electron microscopy of pancreatic islets. *Diabetologia* 10:509, 1974.

Like, A. A., Gerritsen, G. C., et al.: Studies in the diabetic Chinese hamster: light microscopy and autoradiography of pancreatic islets. *Diabetologia* 10:501, 1974.

Like, A. A., and Rossini, A. A.: Streptozotocin-induced pancreatic insulinitis: New model of diabetes mellitus. *Science* 193:415, 1976.

Nakhooda, A. F., Like, A. A., et al.: The spontaneously diabetic Wistar rat. Metabolic and morphologic studies. *Diabetes* 26:100, 1977.

Notkins, A. L.: Virus-induced diabetes mellitus: brief review. *Arch. Virol.* 54:1, 1977.

Renold, A. E., Chang, A. Y., et al.: Third Brook Lodge Workshop on spontaneous diabetes in laboratory animals. *Diabetologia* 10:491, 1974.

Rerup, C. C.: Drugs producing diabetes through damage of the insulin secreting cells. *Pharmacol. Rev.* 22:485, 1970.

Yoon, J. W., Onodera, T., et al.: Passage of encephalomyocarditis virus and severity of diabetes in susceptible and resistant strains in mice. *J. Gen. Virol.* 37:225, 1977.

Yoon, J. W., Onodera, T., et al.: Virus-induced diabetes mellitus. XV. Beta cell damage and insulin-dependent hyperglycemia in mice infected with coxsackie virus B4. *J. Exp. Med.* 148:1068, 1978.

Clinical Diagnosis, Testing, and Definition of Diabetes Mellitus

Andres, R.: Effect of age in interpretation of glucose and tolbutamide tolerance tests. In *Diabetes Mellitus: Diagnosis and Treatment.* Fajans, S. S., and Sussman, K. E. (eds.), New York, American Diabetes Association, 1971.

Bennett, P. H., and Miller, M. (eds.): Epidemiology of diabetes mellitus. *Adv. Metab. Disord.* 9:1, 1978.

Bierman, E. L., Bagdade, J. D., et al.: Obesity and diabetes: the odd couple. *Amer. J. Clin. Nutr.* 21:1434, 1968.

Bottazzo, G. F., Florin-Christensen, A., et al.: Islet cell antibodies in diabetes mellitus with autoimmune polyendocrine deficiencies. *Lancet* 2:1279, 1974.

Caird, F. I., Pirie, A., et al.: *Diabetes and the Aged.* Oxford, Blackwell, 1969.

Dillon, R. S.: Importance of the hematocrit in interpretation of blood sugar. *Diabetes* 14:672, 1965.

Fajans, S. S., and Conn, J. W.: Prediabetes, subclinical diabetes, and latent clinical diabetes: interpretation, diagnosis and treatment. In *On the Nature and Treatment of Diabetes.* Leibel, B. S., and Wrenshall, G. A. (eds.), Amsterdam, Excerpta Medica Foundation, 1965.

Field, R. A., and Skyler, J. S.: Nonglucose mellituria. In *Diabetes Mellitus: Theory and Practice.* Ellenberg, M., and Rifkin, H. (eds.) New York, McGraw-Hill, 1970.

Flier, J. S., Kahn, C. R., et al.: Characterization of antibodies to the insulin receptor. A cause of insulin-resistant diabetes in man. *J. Clin. Invest.* 58:1442, 1976.

Friedman, J. M., and Fialkow, P. J.: The genetics of diabetes mellitus. In *Progress in Medical Genetics.* Vol. IV. Steinberg, A. G., Bearn, A. G., et al. (eds.), Philadelphia, W. B. Saunders, 1980.

Goldstein, S., and Podolsky, S.: The genetics of diabetes mellitus. *Med. Clin. North Am.* 62:639, 1978.

Irvine, W. J., McCallum, C. J., et al.: Pancreatic islet-cell antibodies in diabetes mellitus correlated with the duration and type of diabetes, coexistent autoimmune disease and HLA type. *Diabetes* 26:138, 1977.

Jackson, W. P. U., and Vinik, A. I.: Hyperglycemia and diabetes in the elderly. In *Diabetes Mellitus: Theory and Practice.* Ellenberg, M., and Rifkin, H. (eds.), New York, McGraw-Hill, 1970.

Krane, S.: Renal glycosuria. In *The Metabolic Basis of Inherited Disease.* Stanbury, J. B., Wyngaarden, J. B., et al. (eds.), New York, McGraw-Hill, 1972.

Lundbaek, K.: Intravenous glucose tolerance as a tool in definition and diagnosis of diabetes mellitus. *Brit. Med. J.* 1:1507, 1962.

Marble, A.: Nondiabetic mellituria. In *Joslin's Diabetes Mellitus.* Marble, A., White, P., et al. (eds.), Philadelphia, Lea & Febiger, 1971.

McDonald, G. W., Fisher, G. F., et al.: Reproducibility of the oral glucose tolerance test. *Diabetes* 14:473, 1965.

National Diabetes Data Group: Classification and diagnosis of diabetes mellitus and other categories of glucose intolerance. *Diabetes* 28:1039, 1979.

Nerup, J., Kromann, H., et al.: HLA and insulin-dependent diabetes mellitus. *Postgrad. Med. J.* 55:8, 1979.

Nerup, J., Platz, P., et al.: HLA, autoimmunity and insulin-dependent diabetes mellitus. In *The Genetics of Diabetes Mellitus.* Creutzfeldt, W., Kobberling, J., et al. (eds.), New York, Springer-Verlag, 1976.

Pyke, D. A.: Glucose tolerance and serum insulin in identical twins of diabetics. *Br. Med. J.* 4:649, 1970.

Seltzer, H. S.: Diagnosis of diabetes. In *Diabetes Mellitus: Theory and Practice.* Ellenberg, M., and Rifkin, H. (eds.), New York, McGraw-Hill, 1970.

Seltzer, H. S., Fajans, S. S., et al.: Spontaneous hypoglycemia as an early manifestation of diabetes mellitus. *Diabetes* 5:437, 1956.

Siperstein, M. D.: The glucose tolerance test: a pitfall in the diagnosis of diabetes mellitus. *Adv. Intern. Med.* 20:297, 1975.

Streeten, D. H. P., Gerstein, M. D., et al.: Reduced glucose tolerance in elderly human subjects. *Diabetes* 14:579, 1965.

Tattersall, R. B., and Fajans, S. S.: A difference between the inheritance of classical juvenile-onset and maturity-onset type diabetes of young people. *Diabetes* 24:44, 1975.

White, P.: Childhood diabetes. Its course and influence on the second and third generations. *Diabetes* 9:345, 1960.

Physiology of Plasma Glucose and Pathophysiology of Hyperglycemia

Allison, S. P., Chamberlain, M. J., et al.: Intravenous glucose tolerance, insulin, glucose, and free fatty acid levels after myocardial infarction. *Br. Med. J.* 4:776, 1969.

Baum, D., and Porte, D., Jr.: Stress hyperglycemia and the adrenergic regulation of pancreatic hormones in hypoxia. *Metabolism* 29:1176, 1980.

Cahill, G.: Starvation in man. *N. Engl. J. Med.* 282:668, 1970.

Eff, C., Faber, O., et al.: Persistent insulin secretion, assessed by plasma c-peptide estimation in long term juvenile diabetics with a low insulin requirement. *Diabetologia* 15:169, 1978.

Felig, P.: Amino acid metabolism in man. *Ann. Rev. Biochem.* 44:933, 1975.

Felig, P., Wahren, J., et al.: Insulin, glucagon, and somatostatin in normal physiology and diabetes mellitus. *Diabetes* 25:1091, 1976.

Halter, J. B., Graf, R. J., et al.: Potentiation of insulin secretory response by plasma glucose levels in man: evidence that hyperglycemia in diabetes compensates for impaired glucose potentiation. *J. Clin. Endocrinol. Metab.* 48:946, 1979.

Halter, J. B., and Porte, D., Jr.: Current concepts of insulin secretion in diabetes mellitus. In *Diabetes Mellitus: Diagnosis and Treatment*. Rifkin, H., and Raskin, P. (eds.), New York, American Diabetes Association, 1981.

Horwitz, D. L., Rubenstein, A. H., et al.: Proinsulin and c-peptide in diabetes. *Med. Clin. North Am.* 62:723, 1978.

Lukomsky, P. E., and Oganov, R. G.: Blood plasma catecholamines and their urinary excretion in patients with myocardial infarction. *Amer. Heart J.* 83:182, 1972.

Miller, L. V., Stokes, J. D., et al.: Diabetes mellitus and autonomic dysfunction after Vacor rodenticide ingestion. *Diabetes Care* 1:73, 1978.

Newsholme, E. A.: Carbohydrate metabolism in vivo: Regulation of the blood glucose level. *Clin. Endocrinol. Metab.* 5:543, 1976.

Opie, L. H., and Stubbs, W. A.: Carbohydrate metabolism in cardiovascular disease. *Clin. Endocrinol. Metab.* 5:703, 1976.

Porte, D., Jr.: Sympathetic regulation of insulin secretion and its relation to diabetes mellitus. *Arch. Intern. Med.* 123:252, 1969.

Porte, D., Jr., Woods, S. C., et al.: Neural control of the pancreatic islet and its relation to stress hyperglycemia. In *Diabetes Mellitus: A Pathologic Approach to Clinical Practice*. Assan, R., Girard, G., and Marliss, E. B. (eds.), New York, John Wiley & Sons, 1981 (in press).

Reaven, G. M., and Olefsky, J. M.: The role of insulin resistance in the pathogenesis of diabetes mellitus. *Adv. Metab. Disord.* 9:313, 1978.

Robertson, R. P., Halter, J. B., et al.: A role for alpha-adrenergic receptors in abnormal insulin secretion in diabetes mellitus. *J. Clin. Invest.* 57:791, 1976.

Robertson, R. P., and Porte, D., Jr.: The glucose receptor: a defective mechanism in diabetes mellitus distinct from the β-adrenergic receptor. *J. Clin. Invest.* 52:870, 1973.

Searle, G.: The use of isotope turnover techniques in the study of carbohydrate metabolism in man. *Clin. Endocrinol. Metab.* 5:783, 1976.

Sherwin, R. S., Fisher, M., et al.: Hyperglucagonemia and blood glucose regulation in normal, obese, and diabetic subjects. *N. Engl. J. Med.* 294:455, 1976.

Taylor, S. H., and Majid, P. A.: Insulin and the heart. *J. Mol. Cell. Cardiol.* 2:293, 1971.

Unger, R. H.: Diabetes and the alpha cell. *Diabetes* 25:136, 1975.

Unger, R., and Orci, L.: Possible roles of pancreatic D-cell in normal and diabetic states. *Diabetes* 26:241, 1977.

Vranic, M., Horvath, S., et al. (eds.): Conference on diabetes and exercise. *Diabetes* 28 (Suppl. 1):1, 1979.

West, K. M., and Kalbfleisch, J. M.: Influence of nutritional factors on prevalence of diabetes. *Diabetes* 20:99, 1971.

West, K. M., Oakley, E. L., et al.: Nutritional factors in the etiology of diabetes. In *Epidemiology of Diabetes*. Keen, H. (ed.), London, W. H. D. and International Diabetes Federation, 1978.

Wilmore, D. W.: Carbohydrate metabolism in trauma. *Clin. Endocrinol. Metab.* 5:731, 1976.

Woods, S. C., and Porte, D., Jr.: The central nervous system, pancreatic hormones, feeding and obesity. *Adv. Metab. Disord.* 9:282, 1978.

Woods, S. C., Smith, P. H., et al.: The role of the nervous system in metabolic regulation and its effects on diabetes and obesity. In *Handbook of Diabetes Mellitus*. Brownlee, M. (ed.), New York, Garland Publishing Co., 1980 (in press).

Yoon, J-W., Austin, M., et al.: Virus-induced diabetes mellitus. *N. Engl. J. Med.* 300:1173, 1979.

Pathology of Diabetes Mellitus and Its Complications

Arieff, A. I.: Kidney, water, and electrolyte metabolism in diabetes mellitus. In *The Kidney*. Brenner, B. M., and Rector, F. C., Jr. (eds.), Philadelphia, W. B. Saunders, 1976.

Bagdade, J. D.: Infection in diabetes. *Postgrad. Med.* 59:160, 1976.

Bartels, C. C., and Rullo, F. R.: Unsuspected diabetes mellitus in peripheral vascular disease. *N. Engl. J. Med.* 259:633, 1958.

Beisswenger, P. G., and Spiro, R. G.: Human glomerular basement membrane: chemical alteration in diabetes mellitus. *Science* 168:596, 1970.

Bell, E. T.: *Diabetes Mellitus*. Springield, Ill., Charles C Thomas, 1960.

Binkley, G. W.: Dermopathy in the diabetic syndrome. *Arch. Derm.* 92:625, 1965.

Bischoff, A.: Ultrastructural pathology of peripheral nervous system in early diabetes. In *Vascular and Neurological Changes in Early Diabetes*. Camerini-Davalos, A., and Cole, H. S. (eds.), New York, Academic Press, 1973.

Blankenship, G. W., and Skyler, J. S.: Diabetic retinopathy: a general survey. *Diabetes Care* 1:127, 1978.

Bradley, W. E. (ed.): Aspects of diabetic autonomic neuropathy. *Ann. Intern. Med.* 92:289, 1980.

Brownlee, M., and Cahill, G. F., Jr.: Diabetic control and vascular complications. *Atherosclerosis Rev.* 4:29, 1979.

Clarke, B. F., Ewing, D. J., et al.: Diabetic autonomic neuropathy. *Diabetologia* 17:195, 1979.

Clements, R. S., Jr.: Diabetic neuropathy — new concepts of its etiology. *Diabetes* 28:604, 1979.

Cryer, P. E., Silverberg, A. B., Santiago, J. V., et al.: Plasma catecholamines in diabetes. The syndromes of hypoadrenergic and hyperadrenergic postural hypotension. *Amer. J. Med.* 64:407, 1978.

Danowski, T. S., Sabeh, G., et al.: Skin spots and diabetes mellitus. *Br. J. Derm.* 80:275, 1968.

Ditzel, J., Beaven, D. W., et al.: Early vascular changes in diabetes mellitus. *Metabolism* 9:400, 1960.

Ellenberg, M.: Diabetic neuropathy: clinical aspects. *Metabolism* 25:1627, 1976.

Fagerberg, S. E.: Recent advances in diabetic neuropathy, In *On the Nature and Treatment of Diabetes*. Leibel, B. S., and Wrenshall, G. A. (eds.), Amsterdam, Excerpta Medica Foundation, 1965.

Gabbay, K. H.: The sorbitol pathway and the complications of diabetes. *N. Engl. J. Med.* 288:831, 1973.

Gabbay, K. H., Merola, L. O., et al.: Sorbitol pathway: presence in nerve and cord with substrate accumulation in diabetes. *Science* 151:209, 1966.

Gepts, W.: Pancreatic pathology of juvenile diabetes mellitus. In *Secondary Diabetes*. Podolsky, S. (ed.), New York, Raven Press, 1980.

Goldner, M. G.: The fate of the second leg in the diabetic amputee. *Diabetes* 9:100, 1960.

Graf, R. J., Halter, J. B., et al.: Nerve conduction abnormalities in untreated maturity-onset diabetes: Relation to levels of fasting plasma glucose and glycosylated hemoglobin. *Ann. Intern. Med.* 90:298, 1979.

Hosking, D. J., Bennett, T., et al.: Diabetic autonomic neuropathy. *Diabetes* 27:1043, 1978.

Jarrett, J.: Diabetes and the heart: coronary heart disease. *Clin. Endocrinol. Metab.* 6:389, 1977.

Kalant, N.: Diabetic glomerulosclerosis: current status. *Can. Med. Assoc. J.* 119:146, 1978.

Kohner, E. M.: Diabetic retinopathy. *Clin. Endocrinol. Metab.* 6:345, 1977.

Ledet, T., Newbauer, B., et al.: Diabetic cardiopathy. *Diabetologia* 16:207, 1979.

Liang, J. C., and Goldberg, M. F.: Treatment of diabetic retinopathy. *Diabetes* 29:841, 1980.

Locke, S.: The peripheral nervous system in diabetes mellitus. *Diabetes* 13:307, 1964.

Lundbaek, K., Malmros, R., et al.: Hypophysectomy for diabetic angiopathy. A controlled clinical trial. In *Symposium on Treatment of Diabetic Retinopathy*. Goldberg, M. F., and Fine, S. L. (eds.), Washington, D. C., U.S. Public Health Service Publication, 1968.

Mauer, S. M., Miller, K., et al: Immunopathology of renal extracellular membranes in kidneys transplanted into patients with diabetes mellitus. *Diabetes* 25:709, 1976.

McMillan, D. E., and Ditzel, J. (eds.): Conference on diabetic microangiopathy. *Diabetes* 25 (Suppl. 2):805, 1976.

Mustard, J. F., and Packham, M. A.: Platelets and diabetes mellitus. *N. Engl. J. Med.* 297:1345, 1977.

Partamian, J. O., and Bradley, R. F.: Acute myocardial infarction in 258 cases of diabetes. *N. Engl. J. Med.* 273:455, 1965.

Poulsen, J. F.: Houssay phenomenon in man: recovery from retinopathy in a case of diabetes with Simond's disease. *Diabetes* 2:7, 1953.

Regan, T. J., Lyons, M. M., et al.: Evidence for cardiomyopathy in familial diabetes mellitus. *J. Clin. Invest.* 60:885, 1977.

Robertson, H. D., and Polk, H. C. J.: The mechanism of infection in patients with diabetes mellitus: a review of leukocyte malfunction. *Surgery* 75:123, 1974.

Ross, R., and Glomset, J. A.: The pathogenesis of atherosclerosis. *N. Engl. J. Med.* 295:369, 420, 1976.

Salomon, M. I.: Diabetic nephropathy: clinicopathologic correlation. A study based on renal biopsies. *Metabolism* 12:687, 1963.

Siperstein, M. D., Unger, R. H., et al.: Studies of muscle capillary basement membranes in normal subjects, diabetic, and prediabetic patients. *J. Clin. Invest.* 47:1973, 1968.

Spiro, R. G.: Search for a biochemical basis of diabetic microangiopathy. *Diabetologia* 12:1, 1976.

Strandness, D. E., Jr., Priest, R. E., et al.: Combined clinical and pathologic study of diabetic and nondiabetic peripheral arterial disease. *Diabetes* 12:366, 1964.

Thomas, P. K., and Lascelles, R. G.: The pathology of diabetic neuropathy. *Quart. J. Med.* 35:489, 1966.

Volk, B. W., and Wellmann, K. F.: Pancreatic pathology of maturity-onset diabetes mellitus. In *Secondary Diabetes.* Podolsky, S. (ed.) New York, Raven Press, 1980.

Vracko, R.: Basal lamina layering in diabetes mellitus: evidence for accelerated rate of cell death and cell regeneration. *Diabetes* 23:94, 1974.

Vracko, R., and Benditt, E. P.: Restricted replicative life-span of diabetic fibroblasts in vitro: Its relation to microangiopathy. *Fed. Proc.* 34:68, 1975.

Watkins, P. J., Parson, V., et al.: The prognosis and management of diabetic nephropathy. *Clin. Nephrol.* 7:243, 1977.

Weinrauch, L. A., Healy, R. W., et al.: Coronary angiography and acute renal failure in diabetic azotemic nephropathy. *Ann. Intern. Med.* 86:56, 1977.

Williamson, J. R., Vogler, N. J., et al.: Microvascular disease in diabetes. *Med. Clin. N. Amer.* 55:847, 1971.

Wrenshall, G. A., and Best, C. H.: Extractable insulin of the pancreas and effectiveness of oral hypoglycemic sulfonylureas in the treatment of diabetes in man — a comparison. *Canad. Med. Assoc. J.* 74:968, 1956.

Zincke, H., Woods, J. E., et al.: Renal transplantation in patients with insulin-dependent diabetes mellitus. *J.A.M.A.* 237:1101, 1977.

Ketoacidosis and Hyperosmolar Coma

Alberti, K. G. M. M., and Hockaday, T. D. R.: Diabetic coma: a reappraisal after five years. *Clin. Endocrinol. Metab.* 6:421, 1977.

Arieff, A. I., and Carroll, H. J.: Nonketotic hyperosmolar coma with hyperglycemia: clinical features, pathophysiology, renal function, acid-base balance, plasma cerebrospinal fluid equilibria and the effects of therapy in 37 cases. *Medicine* 51: 73, 1972.

Arieff, A. I., and Kleeman, C. R.: Studies on mechanisms of cerebral edema in diabetic comas. Effects of hyperglycemia and rapid lowering of plasma glucose in normal rabbits. *J. Clin. Invest.* 52:571, 1973.

Biegelman. P. M.: Severe diabetic ketoacidosis (diabetic "coma"). 482 episodes in 257 patients; experience of three years. *Diabetes* 20:490, 1971.

Clements, R. S., Jr., Blumenthal, S. A., et al.: Increased cerebrospinal-fluid pressure during treatment of diabetic ketosis. *Lancet* 1:671, 1971.

Clements, R. S., Jr., and Vourganti, B.: Fatal diabetic ketoacidosis: Major causes and approaches to their prevention. *Diabetes Care* 1:314, 1978.

Felig, P.: Diabetic ketoacidosis. *N. Engl. J. Med.* 290:1360, 1974.

Fisher, J. N., Shahshahani, M. N., et al.: Diabetic ketoacidosis: low-dose insulin therapy by various routes. *N. Engl. J. Med.* 297:238, 1977.

Kitabchi, A. E., Ayyagari, V., et al.: The efficacy of low-dose versus conventional therapy of insulin for treatment of diabetic ketoacidosis. *Ann. Intern. Med.* 84:633, 1976.

Kreisberg, R. A.: Diabetic ketoacidosis: New concepts and trends in pathogenesis and treatment. *Ann. Intern. Med.* 88:681, 1978.

Levy, L. J., Duga, J., et al.: Ketoacidosis associated with alcoholism in nondiabetic subjects. *Ann. Intern. Med.* 78:213, 1973.

Schade, D. S., and Eaton, R. P.: Pathogenesis of diabetic ketoacidosis: A reappraisal. *Diabetes Care* 2:296, 1979.

Schade, D. S., and Eaton, P. R.: The temporal relationship between endogenously secreted stress hormones and metabolic decompensation in diabetic man. *J. Clin. Endocrinol. Metab.* 50:131, 1980.

Turpin, B. P., Duckworth, W. C., et al.: Simulated hyperglycemic hyperosmolar syndrome. Impaired insulin and epinephrine effects upon lipolysis in the isolated rat fat cell. *J. Clin. Invest.* 63:403, 1979.

Vinicor, F., Lehrner, L. M., et al.: Hyperamylasemia in diabetes ketoacidosis: Sources and significance. *Ann. Intern. Med.* 91:200, 1979.

Waldhäusl, W., Kleinberger, G., et al.: Severe hyperglycemia: Effects of rehydration on endocrine derangements and blood glucose concentration. *Diabetes* 28:577, 1979.

Treatment of Diabetes

Albrink, M. J., and Davidson, P. C.: Dietary therapy and prophylaxis of vascular disease in diabetics. *Med. Clin. North Am.* 55:877, 1971.

Brunzell, J. D., Lerner, R. L., et al.: Improved glucose tolerance with high carbohydrate feeding in mild diabetes. *N. Engl. J. Med.* 284:521, 1971.

Brunzell, J. D., Lerner, R. L., et al.: Effect of a fat free, high carbohydrate diet on diabetic subjects with fasting hyperglycemia. *Diabetes* 23:138, 1974.

Bucholtz, H. K.: Insulin allergy: An approach to therapy. *South. Med. J.* 69:1118, 1976.

Bunn, H. F., Gabbay, K. H., et al.: The glycosylation of hemoglobin: relevance to diabetes mellitus. *Science* 200:21, 1978.

Chu, P. C., Conway, M. J., et al.: The pattern of response of plasma insulin and glucose to meals and fasting during chlorpropamide therapy. *Ann. Intern. Med.* 68:757, 1968.

Committee on Nutrition of the American Diabetes Association: Principles of nutrition and dietary recommendations for patients with diabetes mellitus. *Diabetes* 20:633, 1971.

Cornfield, J.: The University Group Diabetes Program. A further statistical analysis of the mortality findings. *J.A.M.A.* 217:1676, 1971.

Crapo, P. A., Reaven, G., et al.: Plasma glucose and insulin responses to orally administered simple and complex carbohydrates. *Diabetes* 25:741, 1976.

Davidson, J. K.: Controlling diabetes mellitus with diet therapy. *Postgrad. Med.* 59:114, 1976.

Dolovich, J., Schnatz, J., et al.: Insulin allergy and insulin resistance. *J. Allergy* 46:127, 1970.

Feinstein, A. R.: Clinical biostatistics. VIII. An analytic appraisal of the University Group Diabetes Program (UGDP) study. *Clin. Pharmacol. Ther.* 12:167, 1971.

Galloway, J. A., and Bresler, R.: Insulin treatment in diabetes. *Med. Clin. N. Am.* 62:663, 1978.

Graf, R. J., Halter, J. B., et al: Glycosylated hemoglobin in normal subjects and maturity onset diabetics; evidence for a saturable system in man. *Diabetes* 27:834, 1978.

Knowles, H. C., Jr., Guest, G. M., et al.: The course of juvenile diabetes treated with unmeasured diet. *Diabetes* 14:239, 1965.

Koenig, R. J., Peterson, C. M., et al.: Correlation of glucose regulation and hemoglobin A_{1c} in diabetes mellitus. *N. Engl. J. Med.* 295:417, 1976.

Koivisto, V., and Felig, P.: Effects of leg exercise on insulin absorption in diabetic patients. *N. Engl. J. Med.* 298:79, 1978.

Krall, L. P., and Chabot, V. A.: Oral hypoglycemia agent update. *Med. Clin. North Am.* 62:681, 1978.

Olefsky, J. H., and Reaven, G. M.: Effects of sulfonylurea therapy on insulin binding to mononuclear leukocytes of diabetic patients. *Amer. J. Med.* 60:89, 1976.

Pecoraro, R. E., Graf, R. J., et al.: Comparison of a colorimetric assay for glycosylated hemoglobin with ion-exchange chromatography. *Diabetes* 28:1120, 1979.

Pfeifer, M. A., Halter, J. B., et al.: Potentiation of insulin secretion to nonglucose stimuli in normal man by tolbutamide. *Diabetes* 29:335, 1980.

Pyke, D. A., and Leslie, R. D. G.: Chlorpropamide alcohol flushing: a definition of its relation to non-insulin dependent diabetes. *Br. Med. J.* 2:1521, 1978.

Schlichtkrull, J., Brange, J. et al.: Clinical aspects of insulin-antigenicity. *Diabetes* 21:649, 1972.

Seltzer, S., and Holbrooke, S.: Drug-induced hypoglycemia. *Diabetes* 21:955, 1972.

Shen, S. W., and Bressler, R.: Clinical pharmacology of oral antidiabetic agents. *N. Engl. J. Med.* 296:493, 787, 1977.

Skyler, J. S., Lasky, I. A., et al.: Home blood glucose monitoring as an aid in diabetes management. *Diabetes Care* 1:150, 1978.

Sönksen, P. H.: The evolution of insulin treatment. *Clin. Endocrinol. Metab.* 6:481, 1977.

Stone, D. B., and Conner, W. E.: The prolonged effects of a low cholesterol, high carbohydrate diet upon the serum lipids in diabetic patients. *Diabetes* 12:127, 1963.

Tamborlane, W. V., Sherwin, R. S., et al.: Reduction to normal of plasma glucose in juvenile diabetes by subcutaneous administration of insulin with a portable infusion pump. *N. Engl. J. Med.* 300:573, 1979.

Trivelli, L. A., Ranney, H. M., et al.: Hemoglobin components in patients with diabetes mellitus. *N. Engl. J. Med.* 284:353, 1971.

University Group Diabetes Program: A study of the effects of hypoglycemic agents on vascular complications of patients with adult-onset diabetes: I. Design. II. Mortality results. *Diabetes* 19 (Suppl. 2):747, 1970.

Weissman, P. N., Shenkman, L., et al.: Chlorpropamide hyponatremia. *N. Engl. J. Med.* 284:65, 1971.

West, K. M.: Diet therapy of diabetes: An analysis of failure. *Ann. Intern. Med.* 79: 425, 1973.

Yue, D. K., and Turtle, J. R.: New forms of insulin and their use in the treatment of diabetes. *Diabetes* 26:341, 1977.

Zinman, B., Murray, F. T., et al.: Glucoregulation during moderate exercise in insulin treated diabetics. *J. Clin. Endocrinol. Metab.* 45:641, 1977.

Pregnancy and Diabetes

Beck, P., Parker, M. L., et al.: Radioimmunologic measurement of human placental lactogen in plasma by a double antibody method during normal and diabetic pregnancies. *J. Clin. Endocrinol. Metab.* 25:1457, 1965.

Beischer, N. A., and Brown, J. B.: Current status of estrogen assays in obstetrics and gynecology. Part 2: Estrogen assays in late pregnancy. *Obstet. Gynecol. Surv.* 27:303, 1972.

Essex, N. L., Pyke, D. A., et al.: Diabetic pregnancy. *Br. Med. J.* 5:89, 1973.

Felig, P.: Body fuel metabolism and diabetes mellitus in pregnancy. *Med. Clin. North Am.* 61:43, 1977.

Freinkel, N., and Metzger, B. E.: Some considerations of fuel economy in the fed state during late human pregnancy. In *Early Diabetes in Early Life*. Camerini-Davalos, R. A., and Cole, H. S. (eds.), New York, Academic Press, 1975.

Gabbe, S. G., Lowensohn, R. I., et al.: Lecithin/sphingomyelin ratio in pregnancies complicated by diabetes mellitus. *Amer. J. Obstet. Gynecol.* 128:757, 1977.

Gabbe, S. G., Mestman, J. H., et al.: Management and outcome of class A diabetes mellitus. *Amer. J. Obstet. Gynecol.* 127:465, 1977.

Gabbe, S. G., Mestman, J. H., et al.: Management and outcome of pregnancy in diabetes mellitus, classes B to R. *Amer. J. Obstet. Gynecol.* 129:723, 1977.

Kalkhoff, R. K.: Effects of oral contraceptive agents on carbohydrate metabolism. *J. Steroid Biochem.* 6:949, 1975.

Knopp, R. H., Childs, M. T., et al.: Dietary management of the pregnant diabetic. In *Current Concepts of Nutrition*, Vol. 6. New York, John Wiley & Sons, 1979.

O'Sullivan, J. B., Charles, D., et al.: Gestational diabetes and perinatal mortality rate. *Amer. J. Obstet. Gynecol.* 116:901, 1973.

Pedersen, J.: Goals and end-points in management of diabetic pregnancy. In *Early Diabetes in Early Life*. Camerini-Davalos, R. A., and Cole, H. S. (eds.), New York, Academic Press, 1975.

Pedersen, J.: *The Pregnant Diabetic and Her Newborn*. Copenhagen, Munksgaard, 1977.

Tyson, J. E.: Obstetrical management of the pregnant diabetic. *Med. Clin. North Am.* 55:961, 1971.

Tyson, J. E., and Hock, R. A.: Gestational and pregestational diabetes: an approach to therapy. *Am. J. Obstet. Gynecol.* 125:1009, 1976.

White, P.: Pregnancy and diabetes. In *Joslin's Diabetes Mellitus*. Marble, A., White, P., et al. (eds.), Philadelphia, Lea & Febiger, 1971.

Other Diseases with Hyperglycemia

Balcerzak, S. P., Mintz, D. H., and Westerman, M. P.: Diabetes mellitus and idiopathic hemochromatosis. *Amer. J. Med. Sci.* 255:53, 1968.

Dymock, I. W., and Williams, R.: Haemochromatosis and diabetes. *Postgrad. Med. J.* Suppl., p. 79, 1971.

Goldstein, S., and Podolsky, S.: The genetics of diabetes mellitus. *Med. Clin. North Am.* 62:639, 1978.

Johnston, D. G., and Alberti, K. G. M. M.: Carbohydrate metabolism in liver disease. *Clin. Endocrinol. Metab.* 5:675, 1976.

Merimee, T. J.: A follow-up study of vascular disease in growth-hormone-deficient dwarfs with diabetes. *N. Eng. J. Med.* 298:1217, 1978.

Podolsky, S., and Viswanatha, M. (eds.): *Secondary Diabetes*. New York, Raven Press, 1980.

Rimoin, D. L.: Genetic syndromes associated with glucose intolerance. In *The Genetics of Diabetes Mellitus*. Creutzfeldt, W., Kobberling, J., et al. (eds.), New York, Springer-Verlag, 1976.

CHAPTER 16

Disorders Causing Hypoglycemia

By John W. Ensinck
and Robert H. Williams

Humans expend energy continuously, yet they feed intermittently; hence they must store nutrients for consumption between meals and as a contingency for the demands of exercise and prolonged fasting. The major endogenous fuel repositories are in the form of triglyceride in adipose tissue, protein in muscle, and glycogen in muscle and liver. Most tissues can meet their energy requirements by using glucose derived from liver glycogen or free fatty acids (FFA) originating from triglyceride, whereas the central nervous system (CNS) and, to a lesser extent, some other specialized organs depend almost exclusively upon glucose as their energy substrate during postprandial phases and short-term fasts. Because the maintenance of plasma glucose concentration within relatively narrow bounds is essential to normal function, a highly integrated system for fuel assimilation and *de novo* generation of glucose has evolved. In normal humans, the circulating plasma glucose levels, ranging from 50–115 mg/dl by 5–6 hours post cibum and after overnight fasting, are the resultant of a complex synchronized interaction between neural and hormonal factors. Hypoglycemia is defined as an abnormal depression of the extracellular glucose concentration reflected in plasma. When plasma glucose levels fall below 50 mg/dl (blood glucose levels < 40 mg/dl), symptoms and signs of adrenergic hyperactivity or nervous system depression, or a combination of the two, usually, but not invariably, result. Since hypoglycemia, *per se,* represents a perturbation of normal glucose homeostasis by diverse causes, the diagnosis and rational treatment of glucopenia require an understanding of the mechanisms of normal glucose regulation. These are detailed in Ch. 15 and recapitulated briefly in the following sections.

GLUCOSE HOMEOSTASIS IN THE FED STATE

The diet of the average adult in the Western world consists of approximately 50% carbohydrate, 35% fat, and 15% protein. After food ingestion, a rise in plasma sugar concentration occurs due to glucose absorbed from the intestinal tract. Typically, of the 300–400 g of nonfibrous carbohydrate eaten daily, 50% is starch, 30% sucrose, 10% glucose, and the remainder is milk lactose. Within the gut lumen and intestinal brush border, the complex carbohydrates are hydrolyzed to monosaccharides — glucose (80%), fructose (15%), and galactose (5%), which, with the exception of fructose, subsequently are actively transported to blood by a carrier-mediated system within the intestinal cells.[42] A variable amount of polysaccharides comprising soluble and insoluble fibers (gums, pectins, celluloses, lignins), mostly derived from plant sources, are not digested in the small intestine and are unavailable as nutrients; however, they play an important role in determining the rate of intestinal transit and absorption of food stuffs.[3] As with carbohydrates, proteins, and fats are cleaved enzymically within the gut and transported as amino acids and mono- and diglycerides, respectively, by energy-requiring carrier systems. It is to be emphasized that the rates of gastrointestinal transit, digestion, and absorption of these various nutrients vary from individual to individual, and from meal to meal. These are determined by food composition, amounts ingested, posture, exercise, and psychogenic factors that alter propulsion, intralumenal mixing, and contents of intestinal juices.[59] In general, after a mixed meal, plasma glucose is usually returned to preprandial levels within 2–3 hours; however, aminoacidemia and lipemia may persist for 8 hours or beyond.[20, 42]

The passage and absorption of fuels from the alimentary tract trigger a number of signals that facilitate the disposition of the transported nutrients into energy stores in various organs (Ch. 14). Concomitantly, the release of insulin, the primary anabolic glucoregulatory hormone, is increased, usually associated with a brief rise or decline in the secretion of hormones governing catabolic processes, dependent upon the composition of the meal. Intracellular glucose is the primary substrate that evokes the release of insulin.[40] Several amino acids, notably arginine, lysine, and leucine, act synergistically with glucose to stimulate insulin secretion. A number of gastrointestinal hormones that influence gut motility, digestion, and absorption of nutrients also enhance the secretion of islet cell hormones, including insulin, glucagon, somatostatin (SRIF), and pancreatic polypeptide (Ch. 14). The term "incretin" denotes one or more gastrointestinal hormones that augment glucose-mediated insulin release (enteroinsular axis). As reviewed by Creutzfeldt,[21] the best characterized of these is gastric inhibitory polypeptide (GIP), which is secreted by the gut cells during absorption of nutrients and by HCL. In addition, increased cholinergic activity occurring during alimentation may enhance the secretion of insulin by direct vagal innervation of B cells.[125] Consequently, following the ingestion of a mixed meal, an array of factors contribute to augment the release of insulin, which has a predominant anabolic action on fuel utilization and storage.

In attempts to mimic the plasma glucose patterns occurring during feeding, glucose solutions (50–100 g) have been traditionally given orally to subjects after an overnight fast, and the alterations in plasma (or blood) glucose levels monitored for the ensuing 5 hours.[37] It is important to be aware that this procedure does not precisely reproduce conditions after ingestion of meals consisting of complex carbohydrates, fats, and proteins, which affect gastric emptying, intestinal motility, and rates of absorption of each other in a manner entirely different from that of a pure glucose solution.[91] Furthermore, the profiles after intake of glucose solutions are not highly reproducible in any given individual. Despite these reservations, because "normal" criteria for the oral glucose tolerance test (OGTT) have been repetitively published, it continues to be the reference test for detecting disturbed glucose homeostasis during alimentation. Within this restricted context, it is appropriate to examine the dynamic events contributing to the rise and decline in plasma glucose following an OGTT, as described by Freinkel (Table 16–1, Fig. 16–1).[37] The rising limb of

Table 16–1. FACTORS INVOLVED IN GLUCOSE DISPOSITION AFTER ORAL CARBOHYDRATE

Ascent of Plasma Glucose
Gastric transit time and rate of intestinal absorption
Release of insulin (glucose, enteric and neural factors)
Inhibition of glucose efflux from liver
Distribution in glucose compartments

Zenith
Outflow equals inflow

Descent of Plasma Glucose
Persistent but diminishing glucose absorption
Decline in insulin release
Resumption of hepatic glucose efflux
Glucopenia with counter-regulation

the plasma glucose level coincides with the delivery of glucose into the circulation from the gastrointestinal tract, at a rate that is determined by gastric emptying and intestinal absorption. Glucose transit through the stomach is intermittent and is determined by waves of gastric motility and pyloric relaxation, which are reflexly governed through complex neural and hormonal pathways mediated by hydrogen ion concentration and osmotic receptors in the stomach and upper intestine.[59] Normally, the stomach empties approximately one third of a 750 ml volume of 10% glucose within 30 min. When gastric emptying time is decreased by operative procedures affecting the gastric outlet, such as gastrectomy or pyloroplasty, the accelerated glucose delivery to the intestine leads to more rapid absorption. In normal persons, the increasing glucose concentrations abetted by cholinergic signals and the release of "incretins" stimulate insulin secretion with elevated insulin levels usually demonstrable in the peripheral blood within 20 min after carbohydrate ingestion (Fig. 16–1). The increased insulin, in conjunction with a decline in glucagon, results in a decrease in hepatic glucose output by inhibition of glycogenolysis and

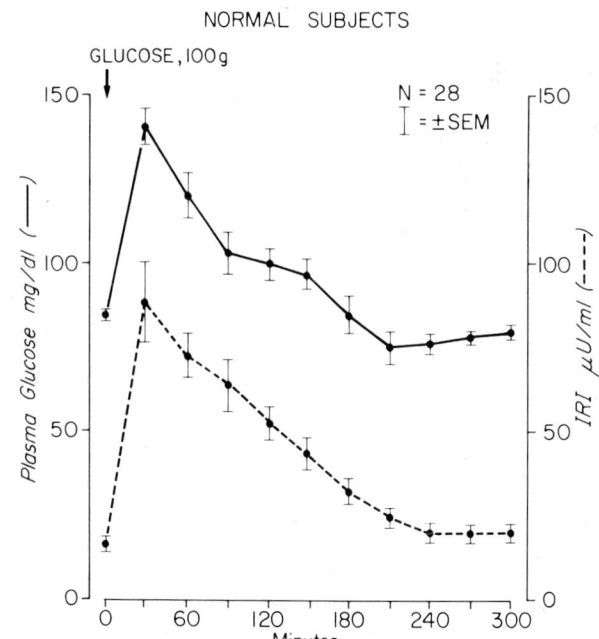

Figure 16–1. Plasma glucose and insulin (IRI) in 28 healthy men and women. (Modified from Hofeldt, F. D., Lufkin, E. G., et al.: Are abnormalities in insulin secretion responsible for reactive hypoglycemia? *Diabetes* 23:589, 1974.

gluconeogenesis.[12, 40] The liver, which is freely permeable to glucose, extracts approximately 50% of the splanchnic glucose load, which is then phosphorylated through the action of glucokinase (type IV hexokinase), a reaction controlled by insulin. Most of the carbohydrate assimilated by the liver is converted to glycogen, catalyzed by a cascade of enzyme reactions, including glycogen synthase, which is regulated by insulin (Fig. 15–38). DeFronzo and coworkers have evidence that an unidentified gastrointestinal factor also enhances insulin-mediated hepatic glucose uptake.[23] Therefore, in the fed state, the liver, in the presence of insulin, constitutes an important reservoir for glucose storage.

Sugar, which is not sequestered in the liver, eventually is distributed within the extracellular space, accounting for the increasing plasma glucose levels. Hyperglycemia stimulates additional release of insulin, thereby promoting the translocation of extracellular glucose, primarily into muscle and fat. In these tissues, insulin also enhances glucose oxidation, glycogen synthesis, amino acid transport, protein synthesis, and potassium and phosphate influx. In addition, insulin inhibits the release of amino acids from muscle; in adipose cells, it also restrains lipolysis and enhances lipogenesis.[12] These anabolic effects on fat are readily demonstrated by a decrease in circulating FFA derived from triglyceride, coinciding with the ascending plasma sugar concentration. Under normal circumstances, the utilization of glucose by insulin-sensitive tissues increases in conjunction with the rising level of insulin, and usually the plasma glucose level peaks within 1 hour, seldom exceeding 160 mg/dl, coinciding with a transitory steady state. Thereafter, plasma sugar levels decline, owing to both increased utilization of glucose and its diminishing delivery from the intestinal lumen. Although plasma sugar levels are most often displayed as smooth curves, more frequent analyses reveal a number of peaks with parallel fluctuations in insulin concentrations.[67] Nonetheless, a direct correlation between glucose and insulin levels has not been shown, and the eventual return to preprandial levels of glucose and FFA cannot be attributed solely to diminishing insulin action as a result of the degradation of this hormone. Complex interaction between hormones and neural signals within the islet also contribute to oscillatory patterns of release of islet cell hormones during the postabsorptive period.[125] Concurrent with the decline in plasma glucose, there is a gradual resumption of hepatic glucose production reflecting a fall in ambient insulin levels, a decrease in insulin receptors, and increased release of hormones that counterregulate the action of insulin on both glucose output from the liver and uptake by peripheral tissue, preventing a continued drop in plasma sugar during the postabsorptive phase. It has been claimed that up to 48% of the normal population have blood glucose levels that fall below 50 mg/dl within 2–5 hours after an OGTT without symptoms.[53] More realistically, however, plasma glucose levels of less than 50 mg/dl occur in less than 10% of the population and are usually associated with symptoms.[91] It is to be emphasized that dietary composition will alter hormonal secretory patterns, as well as tissue responses. Thus, antecedent diets high in carbohydrate and low in fat tend to enhance insulin synthesis and release and augment cellular sensitivity to insulin action. Of interest, affinity of insulin for its receptors increases within 5 hours after an OGTT, possibly accounting for the heightened insulin responsiveness.[87] Paradoxically, decreases in affinity of insulin for its receptors have been reported with short-term, high carbohydrate intake, whereas with protracted periods of high carbohydrate ingestion, the number of receptors declines. Conversely, carbohydrate restriction often results in impaired insulin secretory patterns and carbohydrate intolerance mimicking mild diabetes mellitus. Therefore, interpretation of the OGTT is dependent upon standardization of dietary composition, usually by having the individual ingest food containing 250–300 g of carbohydrate daily for 3 days before testing.[65]

GLUCOSE HOMEOSTASIS DURING FASTING

In the postabsorptive phase, which gradually evolves within 4–6 hours after eating, into protracted periods of fasting (usually not exceeding 24 hours), glucose production is maintained at the expenditure of other fuel sources, as reviewed by Cahill.[13] Thus, homeostasis is preserved by altering a number of metabolic pathways, mediated by an integration of neural and hormonal signals to mobilize stores of glucose to insure proper functioning of the CNS, mainly brain, which oxidizes 100 mg of glucose per min to CO_2 and water. In the average 70-kg man, caloric reserves reside in adipose tissue triglyceride (85%), muscle protein (15%), and muscle and liver glycogen (< 1%). Between meals and during emergent situations induced by stress or exercise, hepatic glycogen is the primary source for maintaining glucose concentrations, with gluconeogenesis contributing 25%. With prolonged fasting, depletion of glycogen necessitates the switching over to gluconeogenesis for almost all glucose produced. The body attempts to conserve protein for mechanical catalytic processes within the cell; consequently, FFA and ketones from the liver are the major fuels used by most tissues. Throughout a 24-hour fast, a normal man who expends 1800 calories uses about 75 g of protein and 160 g of triglyceride to generate about 180 g of glucose (Fig. 16–2). Most of the glucose is diverted to brain and the remainder to skeletal muscle and the cellular elements of the blood, peripheral nerves, and renal medullae, where it is utilized through glycolytic pathways. When food deprivation is extended, muscle becomes almost entirely de-

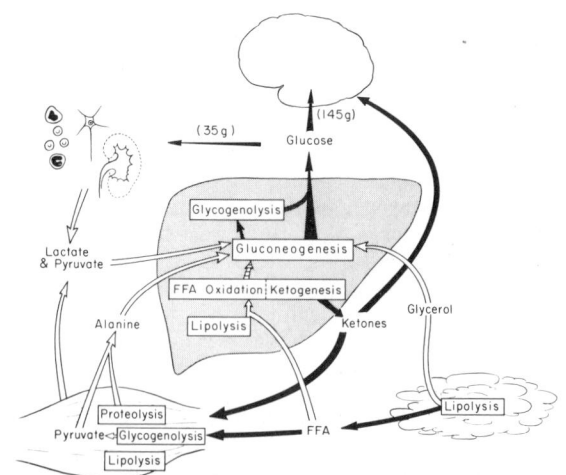

Figure 16–2. Scheme of fuel disposition in normal humans (70 kg), fasted for 24 hr and consuming 1800 cal. Glucose directed primarily for cerebral consumption is released from hepatic glycogen, and new glucose is generated from precursors derived from fat, muscle, blood cells, nerve, and renal medullae. Free fatty acids (FFA) from triglyceride hydrolysis and ketones from hepatic ketogenesis are oxidized in muscle and brain as alternate energy sources.

pendent upon FFA and ketoacids for its energy needs. During fasting, free glucose is virtually confined to the extracellular compartments and intracellular water of the liver, nervous system, and erythron, to which it is freely permeable (equivalent to 50% of body weight). In the average person, the glucose pool in the postabsorptive period comprises 10–20 g at plasma concentrations ranging from 50–70 mg/dl, and the glucose turnover approximates 180 g/day, 80% of which is oxidized internally to CO_2 and water by brain, and the remainder returned as lactate and pyruvate.

When the glucose pool is abruptly depleted, i.e., insulin-induced hypoglycemia, the major source of replacement is hepatic glycogen. Despite the storage of 500 g of carbohydrate as this complex glucose polymer in both muscle and liver, only the latter (and to an insignificant extent, the renal cortex) is capable of rapid conversion of glycogen to free glucose. Normally, hepatic glycogen content is 80–100 g. Through the mediation of a complex cascade of enzymic reactions, glycogen is reduced to glucose-6-phosphate and then to free glucose by the action of glucose-6-phosphatase (Figs. 15–38 and 16–3). Under physiologic conditions, glycogenolysis in the liver is stimulated by glucagon and probably catecholamines, which activate phosphorylase (Fig. 15–38).[30, 47] In the immediate postabsorptive period, 75–85% of net glucose balance is furnished by glycogen, but usually within 24–48 hours glycogen reserves are dissipated with only around 10 g preserved for emergency use, and therefore the glucose pool must be replenished by *de novo* synthesis of glucose from precursors derived from other fuels.

The site of gluconeogenesis and sources of precursors depend upon the duration of the fast. During brief fasting, 90% of total gluconeogenesis occurs in the liver, with the kidney assuming importance as a source of glucose

during protracted starvation.[13] Of the gluconeogenic precursors in humans, glycerol is only a minor contributor. Resynthesis of glucose from pyruvate and lactate represents a major route of disposal of lactate originating from glycolytic processes in blood cells and nervous tissue. With exercise, anaerobic glycolytic catabolism in muscle is increased, with enhanced production of lactate, which is diverted to gluconeogenesis. The most important gluconeogenic substrates are amino acids derived from proteolysis in muscle. All amino acids, except leucine, are potential glucogenic precursors in humans; however, alanine, synthesized from pyruvate, and, to a lesser extent, glutamine have been shown by Felig[33] to be the preferential glucogenic amino acids utilized during the immediate postabsorptive period and during exercise (Ch. 15).

The sequence of major reactions by which substrates are converted to glucose and glycogen in the hepatic cell is shown schematically in Figs. 15–38 and 16–3. The various factors regulating these complex processes have been reviewed by Exton.[30] In brief, they include (a) determinants influencing the provision of substrates. These comprise diet, fasting, obesity, and hormones. (b) Substrate uptake by the liver. Among the potential gluconeogenic precursors, only amino acids are hormonally dependent with regard to hepatic influx. Splanchnic uptake of alanine and other glucogenic amino acids is diminished by insulin and increased by glucagon, cortisol, and growth hormone (GH). (c) Mitochondrial metabolite transport. This is probably carrier-mediated and may be regulated by epinephrine, glucagon, and cortisol. (d) Enzymic control points, as indicated in Figures 15–38 and 16–3. The four rate-limiting enzymes in the gluconeogenic pathway are (1) glucose-6-phosphatase; (2) fructose, 1,6-diphosphatase; (3) phosphoenolpyruvate carboxykinase; (4) pyruvate carboxylase. The diversion of the three-carbon skeleton of pyruvate to oxaloacetate, with ultimate transformation to glucose, involves a number of reactions, one or more of which may be the major sites of regulation by cortisol, glucagon, and insulin. Acetyl CoA is an obligate activator of pyruvate carboxylase and may play a central role in the availability of oxaloacetate in gluconeogenesis. The high Km glucokinase is important in hepatic release because it provides adaptation to glucose delivery to the liver. It is decreased during starvation and insulin deprivation, thereby diminishing glucose influx. Within the period extending from the postabsorptive phase through brief fasting, it is clear that the gradual decline of insulin and the rise in glucagon are the major determinants favoring augmented hepatic glycogenolysis and gluconeogenesis. In addition, the lowered insulin concentration leads to diminished glucose uptake in muscle and adipose tissue with concomitant increased lipolysis and proteolysis, thereby providing a flow of glucogenic precursors (Fig. 16–4).

With prolonged periods of fasting, glucose output gradually falls to about 90 g per day, with a concurrent decline in protein catabolism manifested by a marked decrease in alanine levels. In order to sustain the metabolic requirements of brain and other tissues and to conserve body protein, there is an adaptation to the burning of fat as an energy source. In the immediate postprandial period in an environment of excess glucose, lipogenesis and re-esterification in fat cells are catalyzed by insulin, whereas in the postabsorptive phase and during protracted fasting, lipolysis is augmented as a function of the reduced availability of insulin and coincident increased release of counter-regulatory hormones. From the

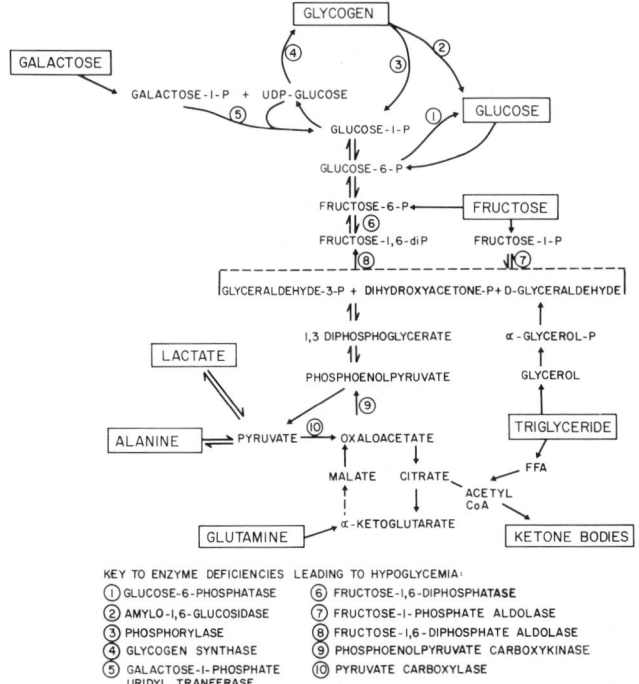

KEY TO ENZYME DEFICIENCIES LEADING TO HYPOGLYCEMIA:

① GLUCOSE-6-PHOSPHATASE
② AMYLO-1,6-GLUCOSIDASE
③ PHOSPHORYLASE
④ GLYCOGEN SYNTHASE
⑤ GALACTOSE-1-PHOSPHATE URIDYL TRANFERASE
⑥ FRUCTOSE-1,6-DIPHOSPHATASE
⑦ FRUCTOSE-1-PHOSPHATE ALDOLASE
⑧ FRUCTOSE-1,6-DIPHOSPHATE ALDOLASE
⑨ PHOSPHOENOLPYRUVATE CARBOXYKINASE
⑩ PYRUVATE CARBOXYLASE

Figure 16–3. Pathways of gluconeogenesis, glucogenesis, and glycogenolysis within the liver.

GLUCOSE CONSUMPTION

(Brain)

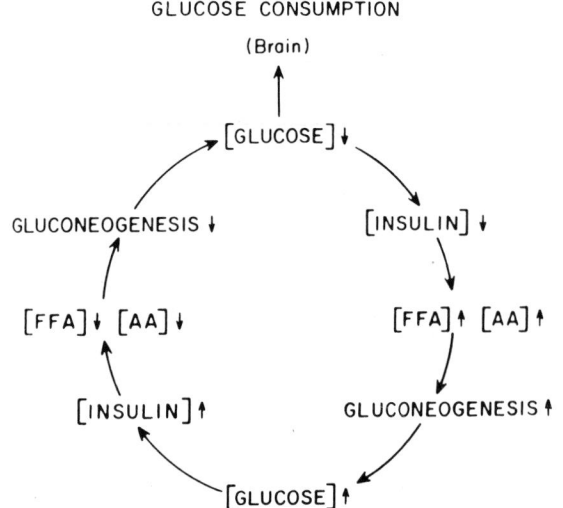

Figure 16–4. Cycle of glucose homeostasis in fasting. Substrates or hormones in brackets refer to plasma concentrations. (From Cahill, G. F., Jr.: Starvation in man. *N. Engl. J. Med. 282*:671, 1970.)

mediated oxidation within hepatic mitochondria. During the postabsorptive period, 40% of FFA (3 g/hr) is taken up by the liver and (1) oxidized via acetyl CoA to ketoacids, (2) metabolized to CO_2 or water, or (3) re-esterified to form triglyceride, which is stored within hepatic cells and subsequently secreted in the form of lipoprotein. Ketoacids are minor metabolic fuels during the early postprandial stage; however, in later phases of fasting, ketogenesis is doubled and ketoacids assume major importance as energy sources. These adaptative processes, whereby fat substitutes for glucose in muscle, are also applicable to the CNS. In the past, the brain was considered to have a chronic obligate requirement for glucose; now, during protracted fasting and in the early neonatal period, ketoacids are recognized as the principal fuels utilized by brain. Hence, during starvation, the adaptation of virtually all tissues to fat as energy sources, concurrent with restriction in gluconeogenesis, may be explained teleologically as a compensatory mechanism to minimize protein breakdown for survival. Plasma glucose concentrations gradually decline within 3–4 days of fasting, accompanied by a decrease in insulin release. Muscle proteolysis and hepatic conversion of amino acid into glucose are augmented in a setting of low ambient insulin levels. In normal and obese healthy males, plasma glucose levels fall by 20–30% within 3–4 days of fasting, but usually not below 50 mg/dl. Merimee and Tyson[86] have recently observed that a number of healthy, nonobese, premenopausal women achieved glucose values below 40 mg/dl by 24 hours and less than 30 mg/dl by 72 hours (Fig. 16–5). Although insulin levels were not distinguished between men and women, glucagon levels were higher (Fig. 16–6) with in-

immediate postabsorptive period into early and late starvation, FFA influx into plasma is doubled.

It has not been established that FFA are converted directly to glucose within the liver; nonetheless, they have been shown to influence gluconeogenic processes indirectly through the provision of energy derived from carnitine-

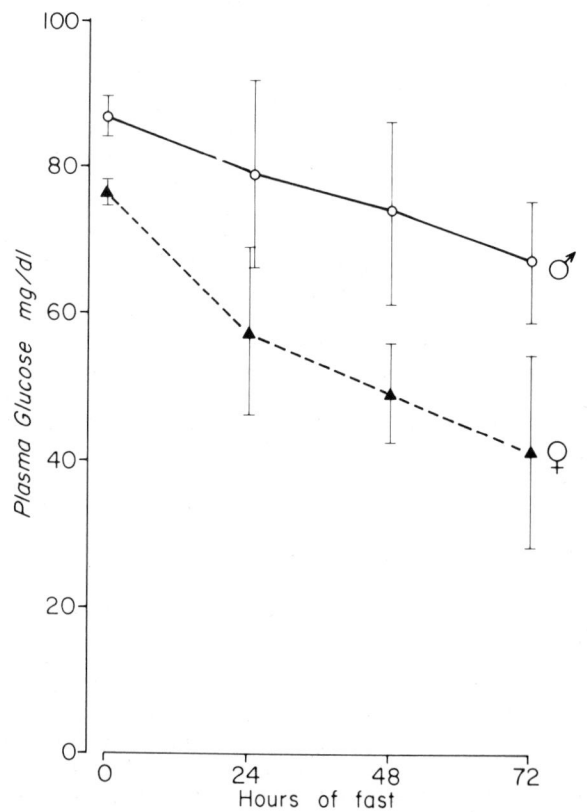

Figure 16–5. Mean plasma glucose concentrations in healthy, nonobese men (N = 12) and women (N = 35) during 3 days of fasting. (Adapted from Merimee, T. J., and Tyson, J. E.: Stabilization of plasma glucose during fasting; normal variations in two separate studies. *N. Engl. J. Med. 291*:1275, 1974.)

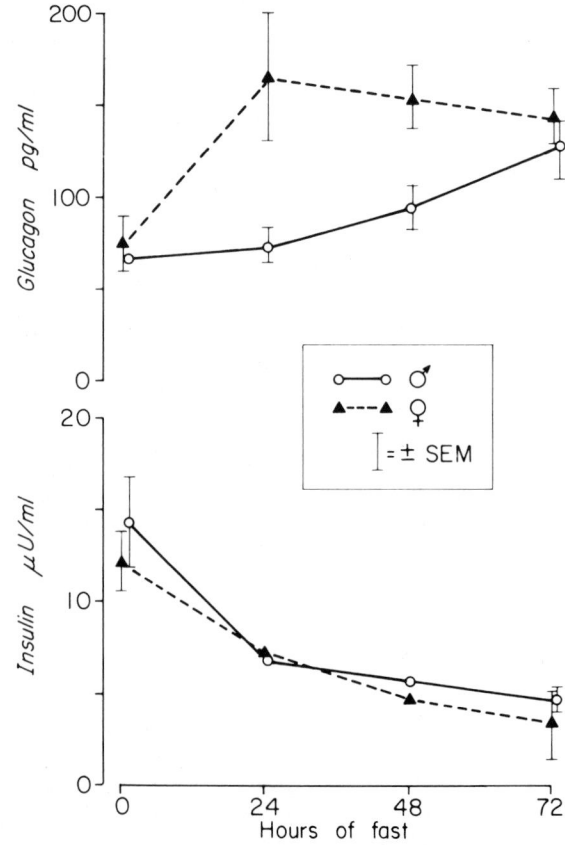

Figure 16–6. Plasma concentrations of glucagon and insulin in healthy, nonobese men (N = 8) and women (N = 7) during fasting. (Adapted from Merimee, T. J., Misben, R. I., et al.: *J. Clin. Endocrinol. Metabol. 46*:414, 1978.)

creased concentrations of FFA, and ketonuria was more prominent and detected earlier in the course of fasting in women than in men.[85] Evidently the rate of gluconeogenesis is slower in females during protracted fasting and has important implications in setting standards for detection of hypoglycemia in the adult.

In contrast to the adult, the newborn infant and young child are particularly vulnerable to disturbances in glucose homeostasis as a result of the dramatic metabolic changes occurring during transition from intrauterine to extrauterine life. The general principles of fuel utilization observed in the adult apply to the infant; however, the glucose requirements in the young child appear to be two- to threefold greater than in the adult. One of the factors that probably contributes to the high glucose needs is the relative increase in the ratio of brain to total body mass. Cornblath and Schwartz[18] and Pagliara and coworkers[88] have summarized several of the distinctive features of metabolism within the fetal-neonatal transition. To defend blood glucose levels during the immediate hours after birth, the infant relies on glycogenolysis and gluconeogenesis. Since most of the gluconeogenic precursors originate from protein stores in the newborn infant and young child in whom protein mass is smaller than in the adult, sustained glucose production may be compromised, accounting for the susceptibility of neonates to develop fasting hypoglycemia.

HORMONES COUNTERACTING INSULIN

To protect the brain against abrupt diversion of glucose to subsidiary organs during insulin excess and to enable mobilization of alternative fuels during fasting, a neuroendocrine control system has been evolved that for the most part opposes the anabolic action of insulin. Hormones known to exert anti-insulin effects at physiologic levels include glucagon, catecholamines, GH, glucocorticoids and thyroid hormones.[29] Relevant aspects of their role in glucose regulation are highlighted here. More detailed descriptions of their other actions and clinical syndromes are found in preceding chapters.

Glucagon

Glucagon-containing cells (A cells) have been found in the upper gastrointestinal tract as well as in the pancreatic islets, reflecting a common embryonic origin of gut and pancreas. Other peptides with some of the immunochemical and biologic properties of glucagon occur in the mammalian intestinal tract ("gut glucagon," glucagon-like immunoreactivity [GLI], glicentin). In humans, circulating glucagon is derived from pancreatic A cells in most physiologic situations. It acts to promote glucose production by stimulating glycogenolysis and gluconeogenesis. As reviewed by Unger and Orci,[121] under basal conditions, glucagon is important in the maintenance of glucose production. In the postprandial phases, when hepatic glucose stores are mobilized, an increase in glucagon secretion is coordinated with a decline in insulin output. In order to meet emergency fuel requirements during strenuous exercise and various clinical conditions of "stress," glucagon release is stimulated, thereby augmenting glycogenolysis. Since hepatic cAMP levels are increased by glucagon and decreased by insulin, the mechanism of the rapid effects of these hormones on glycogen breakdown or storage is explained, at least in part, by the reciprocal actions of these hormones on cAMP-dependent

protein kinase activity that in turn modify phosphorylase and glycogen synthase activities (Fig. 15–38).[47] It has recently been shown that the effects of glucagon on glycogenolysis are evanescent, with a "down regulation" of the glucagon receptor, leading to a drop in enzyme activities involved in glycogenolysis. In contrast, gluconeogenesis stimulated by glucagon persists for long periods in the postabsorptive state. The mechanism by which glucagon induces gluconeogenesis is still unsettled. It has been proposed that glucagon depresses the activities of hepatic pyruvate kinase and phosphofructokinase by changing both the degree of dephosphorylation of the enzymes and the concentration of the allosteric activator, fructose 1-6 diphosphate, allowing complex coordination of the fructose 6-phosphate and phosphoenolpyruvate cycle (Fig. 15–38 and 16–3).[47]

Glucagon, when given in pharmacologic doses, has been shown to promote insulin release; however, a physiologic role for either glucagon or "gut glucagon" in the control of insulin secretion is unresolved. For reasons given by Creutzfeldt,[21] gut glucagon, released during food absorption, is probably not an incretin. To what extent glucagon released locally within the islet plays a physiologic role in insulin secretion during nutrient absorption is conjectural. Glucagon release is inhibited by glucose; therefore, it seems unlikely that it would influence insulin secretion after carbohydrate feeding. Since glucagon secretion is increased by amino acids, it may exert an insulinotropic effect with ingestion of protein in a mixed meal, however.

Recently, a number of stimuli and inhibitors of glucagon secretion have been described in *in vitro* pancreatic systems and subprimate species. Nonetheless, it is uncertain whether all exert physiologic control. Of the various factors so far studied in humans, the most profound increases (five- to tenfold) in plasma glucagon levels are achieved by parenteral amino acids, notably arginine and alanine or following the ingestion of protein.[121] Consequently, it has been implied that circulating amino acids, specifically alanine, may be an important A-cell stimulus, during both fasting and absorption of a protein-containing meal. Glucagon secretion is also stimulated by hypoglycemia, as depicted in Fig. 16–7. Conversely, glucose has been shown to markedly suppress basal plasma glucagon levels. In men, glucagon levels gradually rise to a peak of 150% of basal by the 3rd to 4th day of fasting. In contrast, women tend to have greater increases in plasma glucagon, associated with lower plasma glucose levels during fasting (Fig. 16–6).[85] Unger has proposed that the A cell senses intracellular glucose concentration by an insulin-dependent mechanism that determines the rate of release of glucagon. Recently, it has been shown that SRIF inhibits glucagon release, and its location in the D cell, adjacent to the A cell in the islet, suggests that it may exert a "paracrine" inhibitory influence on glucagon secretion.[121] In addition, it seems likely that the sympathetic nervous system is involved in glucagon release. In situations in which catecholamine secretion is markedly augmented, such as in patients with pheochromocytoma, in severe exercise, infection, trauma, or in diabetic ketoacidosis, elevated glucagon levels have been found. Although considerable evidence indicates a direct glucagonotropic effect of catecholamines in various species, the mechanism is uncertain. In acute hypoglycemia and in protracted starvation, conditions in which activation of the sympathetic nervous system occurs, no consistent inhibition of hyperglucagonemia has been shown by either α- or β-adrenergic blockade; hence, one may infer that the sympathetic nervous system is not the primary determin-

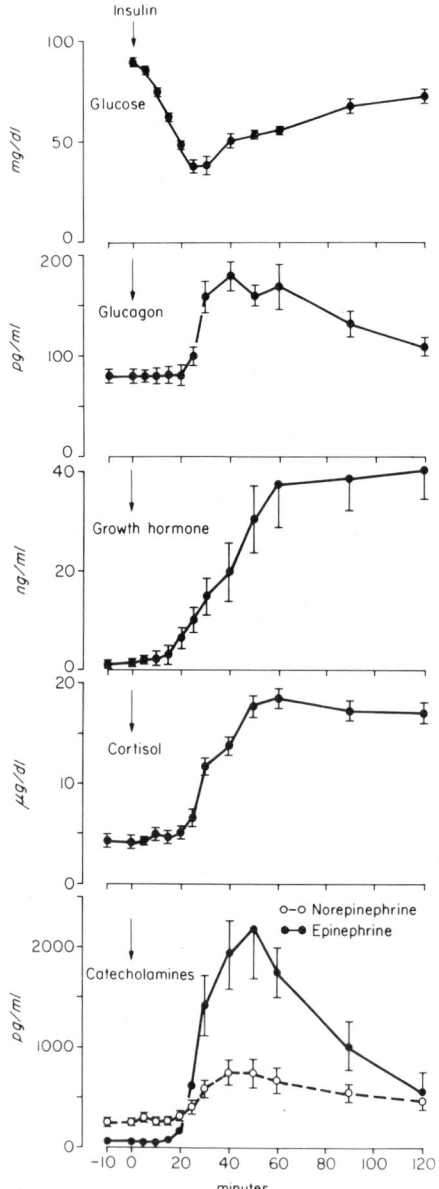

Figure 16-7. Changes in glucoregulatory hormones in six healthy men after administration of insulin (0.15 U/kg IV). (Adapted from Garber, A. J., Cryer, P. E., et al.: The role of adrenergic mechanisms in the substrate and hormonal response to insulin-induced hypoglycemia in man. *J. Clin. Invest.* 58:7, 1976.)

ant of glucagon release in humans under these circumstances. At present, it is uncertain which is the primary stimulus to the A cell during conditions of physiologic need. It is conceivable that during hypoglycemia and exercise, glucagon is released as a consequence of intra-A-cell glucopenia, whereas during fasting, multiple signals, including low blood glucose and insulin and elevated amino acids, act in conjunction to effect a sustained hypersecretion of glucagon to meet gluconeogenic requirements. Of interest, with protracted starvation, glucagon hypersecretion declines concomitant with a drop in the metabolic clearance of this hormone.

It is now established that glucagon has a direct effect on ketogenesis in the liver. In the presence of the lower ambient insulin, glucagon leads to a diversion of glucose to ketones by augmenting hepatic carnitine levels, thereby catalyzing fatty acid oxidation.

When given in supraphysiologic doses *in vivo*, glucagon has several extrahepatic effects on fuel disposition, including elevations of FFA and decreased levels of amino acids, with negative nitrogen balance, indicating a catabolic effect on adipose tissue and muscle. Under physiologic circumstances, a direct effect of glucagon on either skeletal muscle or adipose tissue of humans has not been substantiated, and the major site of action of glucagon would appear to be confined to the liver. Viewed physiologically, the balance between the effects of glucagon and insulin may be the most important factor in influencing hepatic glucose output, and the bihormonal ratio, which is altered during feeding and fasting, has been cited as the crucial control for glucose release by the liver.[121]

Catecholamines

Epinephrine and norepinephrine have major effects on fuel disposition by influencing glucose generation, lipolysis, and release and action of insulin (Ch. 15). Hyperglycemia results from epinephrine infusion, which has been ascribed to the effects of this catecholamine on hepatic glycogenolysis and gluconeogenesis with decreased utilization in muscle.[50] Whether or not epinephrine has a direct effect on glucose output by the liver is controversial, since in isolated liver systems, it does not evoke glycogenolysis at levels achieved in the circulation of humans during stress. It is possible that some of the apparent catecholaminergic effect on hepatic glucose production is mediated through glucagon release. Nonetheless, judging from studies in lower species and recent studies by Garber and coworkers,[39] it seems highly likely that activation of the splanchnic sympathetic nerves may induce hepatic glycogenolysis in humans and that during glucopenia, the increased levels of circulating epinephrine also enhance significantly hepatic glucose output. At physiologic concentrations of epinephrine, glycogen breakdown occurs in muscle with resultant increased plasma lactate, which is a precursor for gluconeogenesis. With supraphysiologic doses, epinephrine inhibits insulin-mediated glucose transport in muscle, possibly by blocking glucose phosphorylation; however, when epinephrine is infused in the human forearm at concentrations achieved during stress, glucose uptake is not diminished, despite increased blood flow and concurrent glycogenolysis. Based upon studies in glucocorticoid-treated, adrenalectomized patients given SRIF to block glucagon secretion, the restoration of glucose following insulin-induced hypoglycemia is impaired, suggesting that catecholamines provide a secondary line of defense against hypoglycemia, particularly when glucagon secretion is deficient. A prominent physiologic effect of catecholamines on fuel metabolism relates to their role in enhancing lipolysis, thereby providing FFA and glycerol for gluconeogenesis.[50] An additional major indirect control on glucose homeostasis exerted by the sympathetic nervous system is through the regulation of insulin release. Both epinephrine and norepinephrine inhibit insulin secretion in humans despite concurrent hyperglycemia. This blockade is mediated through β-adrenergic receptors on the islet B cell (Ch. 15). With insulin-induced hypoglycemia, fasting, profound exercise, and orthostatic changes, secretion of both epinephrine and norepinephrine is enhanced (Fig. 16–7). Thus, during acute hypoglycemia and fasting, the combined effect of activation of the sympathetic nervous system is to decrease insulin release and enhance hepatic glucose output.

Growth Hormone

Growth hormone (GH) serves an anabolic role in promoting protein synthesis, yet exerts a catabolic or antianabolic effect on fat and carbohydrate metabolism.[29, 90] The influence of GH on carbohydrate metabolism is complex. An effect of GH on carbohydrate tolerance in humans is supported by a number of clinical observations, such as the high incidence of diabetes in acromegaly and the exacerbation of hyperglycemia by GH in hypophysectomized, diabetic patients.[76] It is well known that GH exerts a modest and transient blood glucose lowering effect in humans, however. Insulin release is suppressed after GH administration, whereas glucagon secretion is diminished only when the hypoglycemic effects of GH are maximum. Apparently, GH induces simultaneously an inhibition of glucose production by the liver, as well as a decrease in the peripheral glucose utilization. This action is short-lived in contrast to the diabetogenic action of GH. The mechanism of the hypoglycemic effect is obscure and may not be physiologic. This hormone profoundly influences human fat metabolism. After a delay of 30–120 min following GH administration, lipolysis is observed. Before lipolysis is manifested, however, GH increases FFA uptake and oxidation in skeletal muscle and impedes insulin-mediated glucose assimilation. The lipolytic activity of GH is potentiated by glucocorticoids.[29]

Glucose utilization is decreased in acromegalic patients or after injection of pharmacologic amounts of GH. In persons with acromegaly, hyperinsulinemia is frequent, and tissue insensitivity to insulin action has been demonstrated. The magnitude of plasma GH elevation, the severity of hyperinsulinemia, and the degree of insulin resistance are correlated with a decrease in receptor concentration on circulating monocytes, which is considered to reflect similar alterations in tissue receptors. Conversely, in patients with isolated GH deficiency, insulin binding to monocytes is increased and returns to normal after treatment, corresponding to change in *in vivo* sensitivity to insulin.[111] It is uncertain whether these effects on insulin receptors are mediated directly by GH or indirectly through an effect of insulin on its receptors. Since GH does not have these anti-insulin effects on tissue sensitivity or receptor alteration *in vivo*, it has been inferred that this hormone induces the synthesis of an active product. Though one or more of the five related somatomedin-like polypeptides, which are GH-dependent,[16] may be responsible for the effects of GH on fuel utilization, the "insulin-like" activities of these circulating polypeptides are difficult to reconcile with their anti-insulin action.

A primary control of GH secretion is the plasma glucose level, presumably monitored by the hypothalamus, which in turn sends signals to the pituitary (Ch. 3). Despite the fact that GH release is induced by acute hypoglycemia, it is unlikely that it is involved as an anti-insulin substance in acute regulation of glucose levels. In fasting humans, individual levels of GH are variable and do not correlate with circulating fuels. In ateliotic dwarfs lacking GH, however, profound falls in plasma glucose, with high levels of FFA and ketoacids, have been observed, attesting to a glucoregulatory role for GH in the fasting state.

Glucocorticoids

Glucocorticoids, represented mainly by cortisol, have diverse effects on fuel metabolism that, in general, are opposite to those of insulin and tend to elevate plasma sugar concentrations.[6] Thus, chronic excessive glucocorticoid levels increase total body carbohydrate, and fasting plasma glucose concentrations are frequently elevated associated with impaired glucose tolerance. Conversely, adrenalectomized animals have decreased glycogen in liver and muscle; therefore, in patients with glucocorticoid deficiency, the hypoglycemia occurring during fasting and the attenuated posthypoglycemia rebound after insulin are probably due to decreased hepatic glucose output with augmented peripheral glucose uptake.[29] Impairment of peripheral glucose utilization with chronic steroid administration has not been adequately documented in humans. In isolated muscle from adrenalectomized animals, increased insulin sensitivity has been found however. A block in glucose phosphorylation in muscle has been proposed as a site of steroid action. Glucocorticoids also inhibit glucose utilization and esterification in adipose tissue, and after a time lag, lipolysis is enhanced. In addition, chronic steroid excess eventuates in augmented protein catabolism with increased amino acid levels and urinary nitrogen excretion. After adrenalectomy, the main effects on muscle and fat are the depletion of glycogen stores, amino acids, and products of lipolysis. Thus, glucocorticoids affect predominantly the pathways leading to glucose formation by mechanisms that are uncertain and designated as "permissive" since they permit other hormones to produce normal responses.[74] Glucocorticoid treatment is associated with activation of glycogen synthase by glucose-6-phosphate and pyruvate carboxylase by acetyl CoA, accompanied by saturation of gluconeogenic enzymes by precursors and indirect inhibition of glycolysis by FFA, resulting in increased glucogenesis. Adaptation to chronic steroid administration is reflected by *de novo* formation of gluconeogenic enzymes, presumably through actions on nuclear DNA-dependent RNA synthesis. Therefore, a lack of steroids eventually results in deficient gluconeogenesis. Cortisol release is also enhanced with the stress of hypoglycemia (Fig. 16–7) but probably does not play an immediate role in glucose rebound and is unlikely to contribute directly to the moment-to-moment oscillations in glucose levels.

Thyroid Hormones

That thyroid hormones influence fuel regulation is supported by the generalized increased catabolism associated with hyperthyroid states in humans. In excess, thyroid hormones cause increased oxygen consumption, glucose oxidation, glycogen depletion, gluconeogenesis, ketogenesis, lipolysis, and proteolysis.[52] They markedly potentiate the effects of catecholamines on fuel mobilization and are associated with insulin resistance, with a trend to elevated insulin levels. Conversely, their deficiency may lead to glucopenia during fasting.[82] Since the biologic action is measured in hours or days and the concentrations are not altered acutely, thyroid hormones are not involved in moment-to-moment regulation of plasma glucose levels.

Summary of Actions of Anti-Insulin Hormones

In Table 16–2, the major actions of hormones that oppose insulin and tend to replenish the glucose pool during fasting and hypoglycemia are summarized. In general, they act in concert to meet energy demands by one or more of the following: (1) augmentation of hepatic glucose output through direct stimulation of pathways leading to glycogenolysis and gluconeogenesis, (2) provision of glu-

Table 16–2.   PROBABLE PHYSIOLOGIC ACTIONS OF INSULIN-COUNTERACTING HORMONES IN MAN

	Insulin Release	Muscle Glucose Uptake	Hepatic Glucogenesis	Ketogenesis	Lipolysis	Proteolysis
Catecholamines	↓	↓	↑	↑	↑	↑
Glucagon	—	—	↑	↑	—	—
Growth hormone	—	↓	—	↑	↑	↓
Glucocorticoids	—	—	↑	↑	↑	↑
Thyroid hormones	—	—	↑	↑	↑	↑

↑ = increase; ↓ = decrease; — = no significant primary effect

cogenic precursors, (3) hindrance of glucose uptake and assimilation in insulin-sensitive tissues, (4) inhibition of insulin release, and (5) mobilization of alternative fuel sources.

THE NERVOUS SYSTEM IN FUEL HOMEOSTASIS

The brain normally relies constantly on glucose for its energy needs and is uniquely vulnerable to acute depletion of circulating glucose. To protect cerebral function from glucopenia, a highly responsive, integrated nervous system has evolved to analyze ambient glucose levels and rapidly transmit signals to the periphery for the mobilization of appropriate hormones and substrates to replenish the extracellular glucose reservoir. Although not established in humans, evidence in lower species favors the inclusion of the limbic system and hypothalamus as the "visceral brain" that governs autonomic neural responses. The ventromedial hypothalamic (VMH) and lateral hypothalamic (LH) nuclei have been postulated as mutually interacting centers in the neural regulation of carbohydrate and lipid metabolism. A reciprocal relationship exists between VMH and LH. There is mounting evidence in favor of glucoreceptors that "sense" intracellular glucose levels in both VMH and LH regions, with reciprocal firing of the sympathetic parasympathetic nervous systems during fasting and feeding.[125] The mechanism whereby the brain alters the flow of fuel involves (1) the sympathetic nervous fibers ramifying in vascular walls and around parenchymal cells of adipose tissue, muscle, liver, pancreatic islets, and adrenal medulla; (2) the parasympathetic enervation of the pancreas; and (3) a portal system serving as a conduit to the pituitary for transmission of specific peptide releasing and inhibitory hormones, which modulate the secretion of hypophyseal polypeptide hormones.[96] In humans, stimulation of the adrenergic system is related to the rate of decline and degree of reduction of blood glucose attained during hypoglycemia (Fig. 16–7). By extrapolation from studies in animals, centers sensitive to high and low concentrations of glucose probably exist in the human "visceral brain," and it is likely that cells within the VMH nucleus monitor plasma glucose levels and, through tonic activity of the autonomic nervous system, exert a control on fuel mobilization. Indirect evidence in lower mammals also favors the suggestion by Mayer that cells in this region may be dependent upon insulin for glucose transport, and insulin receptors have been demonstrated in cells in various regions of the CNS. In addition, there is a circadian periodicity in hormonal release, as well as substrate mobilization and utilization, that presumably reflects cyclic activity of the nervous system.[69] Thus, in humans who have fasted briefly, plasma glucose and insulin levels peak in the early morning hours and reach an ebb in the late afternoon, whereas the converse temporal relationships apply to FFA and amino acids. Cortisol, which is intermittently released from the adrenal cortex throughout the day, reaches a maximum level between 4 and 8 AM, correlating with increased ACTH secretion. In contrast, GH concentrations are highest with the onset of deep sleep. In recent studies in nonhuman primates, it has been observed that glucose, insulin, and glucagon oscillate in synchrony with a periodicity of less than 10 min, with insulin cycling in, and glucagon out of, phase with glucose. It seems likely, therefore, that superimposed upon the stimuli evoked by feeding or fasting, the rhythmic waxing and waning of the autonomic nervous system regulates substrate flow and hormonal release, which act conjointly to control plasma glucose levels.

CLINICAL AND PATHOLOGIC FEATURES OF HYPOGLYCEMIA

Since cerebral cells have limited stores of glycogen, circulating glucose is the major reservoir for this fuel. Glucose is transported across the blood-brain barrier by a process of facilitated transfusion, which is not dependent upon insulin.[77] It is subsequently phosphorylated. Most of the intracellular glucose is converted to amino acids and the remainder (30%) is oxidized to CO_2 and water by glycolytic processes. In general, glucose oxidation parallels cerebral oxygen uptake; however, the brain cannot tolerate anoxia beyond a few minutes, whereas glucose deprivation is associated with longer survival, presumably because nervous tissue metabolizes additional substrates derived from glycogen, amino acids, ketoacids, and protein. Studies in the rabbit further differentiate hypoglycemia from anoxia in that glucopenia is accompanied by intracellular shifts of electrolytes (Na^+, K^+) and edema, which are not found in hypoxia.[4] As an approximation, the degree to which a given area of the brain is affected by glucose lack depends upon the order of its phylogenetic evolution. In descending order, the areas with the greatest glucose dependence and oxygen consumption are the neocortex and the various anatomic areas of the primitive brain, which regulate cardiorespiratory activities.[51] Despite a reasonable correlation between plasma sugar levels and neuroglucopenic effects, occasionally there is a discrepancy between them. In contrast to the episodic glucose translocation in muscle or fat, glucose extraction by the cerebral cortex is relatively constant, and its uptake does not correlate with plasma glucose levels.

The clinical manifestations of hypoglycemia are usually not apparent until the plasma glucose has fallen below 50 mg/dl (blood glucose of 45 mg/dl). It is to be stressed that no absolute correlation exists between symptomatology and level of circulating glucose, however. As summarized by Permutt,[91] a number of reports have cited the occurrence of asymptomatic individuals with blood glucoses of less than 45 mg/dl, and conversely, in some patients, neuroglucopenic symptoms from prior hypoglycemia may persist after extracellular glucose levels are normal. Furthermore, since the clinical features of hypoglycemia simulate those of hypoxia, symptoms may occur at higher plasma glucose levels in patients with compromised cerebral circulation, exemplified by atherosclerosis in the elderly. Nonetheless, it is important operationally to designate biochemical hypoglycemia arbitrarily as a blood glucose of less than 45 mg/dl, based upon the observation that the majority of asymptomatic, normal persons will have higher values.

In the adult, the clinical picture of neuroglucopenia may be protean; however, two distinct clinical patterns predominate, attributable to (1) activation of the adrenergic nervous system and (2) perturbation in cortical and subcortical function (Table 16–3). Usually, the constellation of symptoms associated with activation of the sympathoadrenomedullary system include one or more of the following: faintness, weakness, tremulousness, nervousness, anxiety, hunger, palpitations, tachycardia, and diaphoresis. In general, activation of the sympathetic nervous system is more likely to occur with a rapid fall in circulating glucose. Although not resolved as yet, it seems likely that it is not solely the rate of fall, but rather a threshold of glucose achieved that determines the triggering of the sympathetic discharge. Activation of the sympathetic nervous system, with concomitant glucopenia, causes inhibition of insulin release and enhanced secretion of glucoregulatory hormones, leading to hepatic glycogenolysis (Fig. 16–7).

Cerebral manifestations of abrupt hypoglycemia may also consist of headache, blurred vision, diplopia, lethargy, confusion, inappropriate affect, and motor incoordination. If counter-regulatory mechanisms are inadequate and the plasma glucose falls to persistently low levels, more primitive parts of the brain are depressed. A wide array of psychiatric and neurologic disorders may be mimicked, including bizarre behavior patterns and depressed sensory and motor function, with paralysis, seizures, and the loss of consciousness.[51] It is particularly noteworthy that patients with hypoglycemia are frequently misdiagnosed as being neurotic or as having nonmetabolic organic brain syndromes. Psychotic

Table 16–3. SYMPTOMS AND SIGNS OF HYPOGLYCEMIA

Adult	
Adrenergic	*Neuroglucopenic*
Tremulousness	Headache
Anxiety	Weakness
Hunger	Diplopia
Sweating	Confusion
Palpitations	Amnesia
Tachycardia	Incoordination
	Seizures
	Coma

Infant
Tremors
Cyanosis
Convulsions
Apnea
Tachypnea, Respiratory Distress
Weak Cry
Limpness
Refusal to Eat
Eye Rolling

behavior and dementia due to chronic hypoglycemia may be difficult to differentiate from other causes. Among the neurologic diseases, various types of epilepsy, particularly in children, must be ruled out. With protracted hypoglycemia, neurologic dysfunction may progress to coma and death from failure of the medullary centers controlling cardiorespiratory function. Although the clinical presentation of hypoglycemia may vary from individual to individual, the sequential manifestations and patterns of recurrence often tend to be repetitive in any one person. Unless glucose levels have been continuously low, resulting in cell death, restoration to euglycemia usually reverses the symptoms and signs of hypoglycemia. In the neonate, the signs and symptoms are manifest in patterns different from those of adults (Table 16–3). They are nonspecific and mimic other diseases of the newborn. Depending upon the duration and degree of glucopenia, recovery may be immediate or prolonged over days. Irreversible damage to neural cells may permanently impair mental function, personality, and motor and sensory nerve functions. Fever (38–39° C) may occur, attributable to cerebral edema. Conversely, profound hypothermia may accompany hypoglycemia. The evolution from coma to death may range from minutes to months. Both electroencephalographic and histologic changes due to severe neuroglucopenia resemble those of anoxia. β and δ waves replace the dominant α waves; these changes may be irreversible. In patients who die from hypoglycemia, the brain shows spotty ischemic necrosis, which is most marked in the cerebral cortex, basal ganglia, hippocampus, and vasomotor centers. Acute alterations include scattered petechiae, congestion, and nerve swelling (Fig. 16–8), with ultimate loss of cells with glial reaction and demyelination.[51] Most of the damage due to hypoglycemia occurs in the brain, but peripheral nerve degeneration is sometimes encountered.

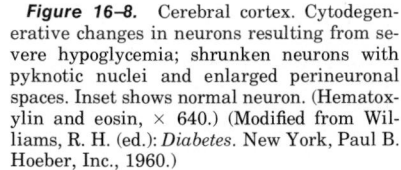

Figure 16–8. Cerebral cortex. Cytodegenerative changes in neurons resulting from severe hypoglycemia; shrunken neurons with pyknotic nuclei and enlarged perineuronal spaces. Inset shows normal neuron. (Hematoxylin and eosin, × 640.) (Modified from Williams, R. H. (ed.): *Diabetes.* New York, Paul B. Hoeber, Inc., 1960.)

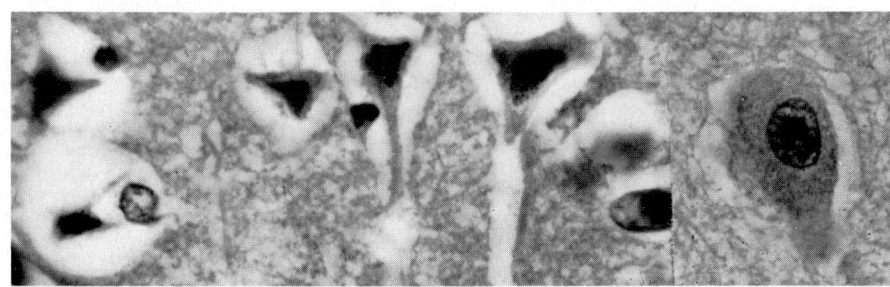

DISORDERS MISATTRIBUTED TO HYPOGLYCEMIA (NONHYPOGLYCEMIA)

The diverse clinical features of hypoglycemia may be imitated by a wide spectrum of other disorders. The most common are psychiatric and neurologic syndromes in which vasomotor and behavioral disturbances are singularly prominent. Patients with ischemic vascular disease involving the brain or heart may have complaints that are difficult to distinguish from those of hypoglycemia and, correspondingly, are at a greater risk for infarction if hypoglycemia should occur. Intoxication from amphetamines, ethanol, barbiturates, or other drugs may simulate the adrenergic actions and cerebral depressive phases of neuroglucopenia. Perhaps the most compelling concern to legitimate physicians has been pointed out by Yager and Young[126] and has been termed nonhypoglycemia. This connotes a number of somatic complaints, such as fatigue, spasms, palpitations, numbness, tingling, pain, severe sweating, and mental dullness, which have led the patient to the self-diagnosis of hypoglycemia. In addition, hypoglycemia has been implicated as the underlying condition for depression, chronic fatigue, allergies, nervous breakdown, alcoholism, juvenile delinquency, childhood behavior problems, drug addiction, and inadequate sexual performance. The lay press has equated energy with blood sugar and exploited hypoglycemia as a universal cause accounting for a welter of aberrant psychosocial behavior. This misguided zeal has been expropriated by a number of professionals who have profited from what has been termed "hypoglycemia quackery." The claim that hypoglycemia underlies a number of diseases stems from the results of a number of uncontrolled OGTT's and reported efficacy of dietary treatments plus chronic glucocorticoid administration. Since raising blood glucose in patients with symptoms purported to be due to reactive hypoglycemia has little impact on alleviating their symptoms, it is difficult to link their complaints to neuroglucopenia. Because of the widespread enthusiasm for hypoglycemia as a cause for a number of ailments, the American Diabetes Association, in collaboration with other societies, has published statements to downplay the prominence of this misattribution.[26] Since hypoglycemia as a valid cause for disease is relatively uncommon, following appropriate examinations and tests necessary to exclude other diseases, it behooves the physician to reassure such patients that hypoglycemia does not underlie their symptoms and to appropriately treat those with potentially remediable personality disorders.

CLASSIFICATION OF DISORDERS CAUSING HYPOGLYCEMIA

Since a low plasma glucose level by itself does not provide a diagnosis, appropriate treatment requires establishment of the etiology of the hypoglycemia. A number of categories have been proposed on the basis of physiologic mechanisms, organic systems involved, and clinical presentations.[17, 18, 31, 78] Each of these classifications has merit; however, we favor the listing in Table 16–4, in which hypoglycemia in the adult is classified by causes related to fed and fasting states and those due to pharmacologic and toxic agents. This format has the advantage of relative simplicity based upon known mechanisms of fuel regulation and thereby facilitates a logical approach to diagnosis and treatment. With the exception of the frequency of hypoglycemic episodes in patients receiving insulin or sulfonylureas, symptomatic hypoglycemic disorders are uncommon. In the infant and child, the incidence and causes of hypoglycemia are

Table 16–4. CLASSIFICATION OF CAUSES OF HYPOGLYCEMIA

I. Nutrient-Induced and Spontaneous Hypoglycemia
  A. Nutrient-induced hypoglycemia
    Postabsorptive ("reactive") hypoglycemia
    1. Induced by glucose
      a. Alimentary
      b. Idiopathic
      c. Diabetes mellitus
      d. Endocrine deficiency
    2. Induced by galactose (galactosemia)
    3. Induced by fructose (hereditary fructose intolerance)
    4. Induced by leucine (leucine hypersensitivity)
  B. Spontaneous hypoglycemia
    Fasting hypoglycemia
    1. Deficient nutrient intake
    2. Deficient glucose production
      a. Inborn errors of glucogenesis
        1. Disorders of glycogen metabolism
        2. Disorders of gluconeogenesis
          a. Deficient gluconeogenesis due to defects in substrate conversion
          b. Deficient gluconeogenesis due to substrate limitation
      b. Acquired liver dysfunction
        —cellular disruption, neoplasia
      c. Deficiencies of counter-insulin glucoregulatory hormones
        —glucocorticoids, thyroid, glucagon, and catecholamines
      d. Extrapancreatic neoplasms (mesotheliomas and carcinomas)
      e. Idiopathic hypoglycemia of infancy and childhood
    3. Overutilization of glucose
      a. Hypersecretion of insulin
        1. Intrinsic abnormalities of pancreatic B cells (insulinoma)
        2. Autoimmune hypoglycemia
        3. Neonatal hypoglycemia (diabetic mothers)
        4. Erythroblastosis fetalis
      b. Increased insulin sensitivity
      c. Miscellaneous syndromes

II. Pharmacogenic and Toxic Causes of Hypoglycemia
  A. Exogenous insulin administration (factitious, inadvertent)
  B. Sulfonylureas
  C. Ethanol
  D. Miscellaneous compounds

markedly different from those encountered in adults. Therefore, for convenience in appraising the most common causes of hypoglycemia in the very young, an alternate classification is given in Table 16–5.

Table 16–5. CAUSES OF NEONATAL AND INFANTILE HYPOGLYCEMIA

I. Transient Hypoglycemia
  A. Small infant for gestational age
  B. Preterm infant
  C. Infant of mother with toxemia
  D. Infant of mother with diabetes
  E. Erythroblastosis
  F. Perinatal asphyxia
  G. Cold stress
  H. Respiratory distress
  I. Polycythemia

II. Persistent Hypoglycemia
  A. Deficient glucose production
    1. Limited substrate
      a. Ketotic hypoglycemia
    2. Deficiency in gluconeogenic enzymes
    3. Disorders of glycogen storage
    4. Deficiencies of counterinsulin glucoregulatory hormones
  B. Galactosemia
  C. Hereditary fructose intolerance·
  D. Leucine hypersensitivity
  E. Intrinsic abnormalities of pancreatic B-cell hyperplasia (insulinoma)

DIAGNOSTIC APPROACHES IN THE EVALUATION OF HYPOGLYCEMIA

The astute clinician may suspect the presence of hypoglycemia from the history and occasional appearance of a unique constellation of physical signs in an infant or adult. More commonly, the symptoms are subtle and intermittent and attributed to psychosomatic disorders. Hypoglycemia is arbitrarily defined as occurring when plasma glucose drops below 50 mg/dl (true blood glucose below 45 mg/dl). In symptomatic individuals, the following issues should be addressed: (1) Is the patient taking parenteral or oral medications that might cause hypoglycemia? (2) Do clinical manifestations occur only within the immediate postabsorptive period (within 5 hours of eating)? (3) Is *symptomatic* hypoglycemia manifested during periods of fasting (in excess of 6 hours postprandially)? Plasma sugar levels obtained sporadically when the patient has symptoms suggesting neuroglucopenia may often be within normal limits or elevated because of counter-regulation. Hence, a systematic approach to the work-up of a patient will depend upon the relationship of the symptom-complex to the fed and fasting conditions. In contrast to adult standards, fasting blood glucose levels of the neonate are normally in the hypoglycemic range for several days after birth. In the premature infant (less than 37 weeks' gestation) and full-term infant (37–42 weeks' gestation), values range from 40 to 50 mg/dl and from 45 to 55 mg/dl, respectively. Between 1 and 5 weeks thereafter, glucose levels reach the normal adult range.[18]

Since carbohydrate restriction followed by a glucose challenge may result in hypoglycemia in normals by altering the secretory reserve of counter-regulatory hormones, in order to permit meaningful interpretation of tests the adult patient should ingest at least 250 g of carbohydrate daily for a minimum of 3 days before testing (Ch. 15). In the infant and child, a diet containing 10 g carbohydrate per kg body weight is recommended.[18] The following procedures are those that may be used in (1) establishing the presence of hypoglycemia and (2) suggesting the underlying cause. The intent of this section is solely to describe the mechanics of the procedures. The appropriate use of the tests, their interpretation, and their reliability are detailed under specific disorders.

Special Tests Aiding in Establishing Diagnosis of Hypoglycemia

Fasting Plasma Glucose Level

Food is restricted after 6 PM the preceding night, and a venous sample for plasma or blood sugar is obtained between 7 AM and 9 AM. Values for fasting plasma sugar in excess of 60 mg/dl *usually* exclude intrinsic causes inhibiting glycogenolysis and gluconeogenesis; in 30–50% of patients with insulin-producing tumors, however, the plasma sugar concentration may not fall to hypoglycemic ranges within 12 hours.

Plasma Levels of Insulin, Proinsulin, and C-Peptide

The quantification of insulin concentration in plasma is of great value in discriminating states of insulin hypersecretion from other causes of hypoglycemia. Insulin, measured by radioimmunoassay, is expressed as immunoreactive insulin (IRI) in μU/ml and is usually available through hospital or commercial laboratories. Determinations should be obtained after overnight or during protracted periods of fasting with corresponding glucose levels and at short intervals after specific provocative or suppression tests. IRI levels are virtually of no assistance in the diagnosis of postprandial ("reactive") hypoglycemia.

Proinsulin, which is a biosynthetic precursor of insulin, is normally released into the circulation in small amounts (between 5 and 22%) and cross-reacts in the insulin radioimmunoassay (Ch. 15). Proinsulin is distinguished from IRI by means of its larger molecular weight (MW) requiring gel filtration and therefore is restricted to research laboratories. Patients with insulinoma frequently have high basal levels of proinsulin.[1, 118]

Normally, insulin is cleaved from proinsulin within the pancreatic B cell, and the peptide bridge, termed the C-peptide, is released in equimolar amounts with insulin (Ch. 15). In states of endogenous hyperinsulinism, C-peptide levels are elevated and are particularly useful in exogenous insulin suppression tests for diagnosis of insulinoma and, specifically, in diabetic patients suspected of having an insulin-producing tumor.[56, 118] In individuals surreptitiously self-administering insulin, low levels of C-peptide virtually exclude the diagnosis of endogenous hyperinsulinism as a cause of this factitious hypoglycemia.[103]

Oral Glucose Tolerance Test

After an overnight fast, the adult patient ingests within 5 min 100 g (60 g/m² body surface) of a standardized glucose solution (i.e., Glucola), and plasma or blood samples are obtained for glucose measurements at 0, 30, 60, 90, 120, 180, 240, and 300 min.[65] In addition, plasma specimens should be obtained when the patient reports symptoms. Although the OGTT is the standard procedure for establishing the presence of postabsorptive ("reactive") hypoglycemia, it is not an ideal test, since it does not simulate the composition of a normal diet and is not highly reproducible in any given individual. The physician should be cautioned in overinterpreting marginal values in a single OGTT and is advised to repeat the test in such instances. In the neonate and child, the glucose is administered orally in dose of 1.75 g/kg as 20% solution. The OGTT in childhood is not often indicated, since glucose-induced "reactive" hypoglycemia is rare and the test is of no use in diagnosis of idiopathic hypoglycemia.

Intravenous Glucose Tolerance Test

If patients develop hypoglycemic symptoms during an OGTT, it may occasionally be helpful to assess plasma glucose responses to glucose by a route independent of its rate of absorption from the gut. Glucose, 0.5 g/kg body weight, is injected within 1 min. Plasma glucose levels are obtained beforehand and at 10-min intervals for 60 min thereafter. The log rate of disappearance of glucose (Kg) is calculated.[114] In contrast to patients with diabetes mellitus, normal values for Kg are found in individuals with early-phase reactive hypoglycemia.

Oral Leucine Test

L-leucine (150–200 mg/kg body weight) in tomato juice is given by mouth or by stomach tube, and plasma concentrations of glucose and insulin measured beforehand at 15-min intervals for 2 hours.[18] Leucine stimulates an acute and marked release of insulin in children with symptomatic hypoglycemia due to leucine hypersensitivity and in 70% of patients with insulin-producing tumors. Between 30 and 45 min after intake of leucine, a plasma sugar value below 50 mg/dl (or 50% of fasting value) is suggestive of one of these disorders.[35, 84]

Prolonged Fast

In order to test the integrity of regulation of glucogenesis during fasting as well as the possibility of sporadic hypersecretion of insulin, subjects may fast up to 72 hours, with periodic moderate exercise. Plasma samples for glucose and insulin are obtained at 6-hour intervals, or when the person has symptoms suggesting hypoglycemia.[32] Close monitoring of the patients within a hospital environment is imperative. Symptoms of neuroglucopenia coupled with plasma glucose levels below 50 mg/dl in men and 35 mg/dl in women are strongly suggestive of an organic cause of hypoglycemia. An inappropriately elevated plasma insulin level in the presence of fasting hypoglycemia is virtually diagnostic of B-cell hyperfunction.[109]

Suppression Tests

Normally, proinsulin, insulin, and C-peptide in the circulation decrease during fasting and hypoglycemia. In patients in whom excessive insulin secretion from autonomously functioning cells is sporadic and difficult to document, despite fasting hypoglycemia, insulin-induced suppression tests may be helpful. Turner introduced the method of infusing fish insulin to cause hypoglycemia with measurement of IRI not cross-reacting with fish insulin and reported excellent discrimination between normal subjects and patients with insulinomas.[120] In the United States, fish insulin is not available. Rubenstein and colleagues used pork or beef insulin infusions (0.1 U/kg/hr) to achieve hypoglycemia, with measurement of C-peptide levels during the infusion.[103] Inappropriately high levels of C-peptide or proinsulin during glucopenia are found in greater than 90% of patients with insulinoma. C-peptide assays are available through commercial laboratories.

Provocative Tests for Insulin Hypersecretion

In patients with hypoglycemia due to abnormal patterns of insulin secretion, the following tests have been devised to accentuate the release of insulin from the abnormal B cell: (1) *Intravenous tolbutamide.* After an overnight fast, tolbutamide (1 g) is infused within 30 sec, and plasma is obtained for glucose and insulin levels at 0, 2, 5, 15, 30, 45, 60, 90, 120, 150, and 180 min.[35] In normal individuals, the peak level of insulin usually occurs within 5 min, whereas the nadir for plasma glucose is within 15–30 min and is normally 50% of basal level. In most instances, insulin and glucose have returned to original levels by 90–120 min. In contrast, profound and protracted hypoglycemia associated with an inordinate release of insulin may occur after tolbutamide administration in patients with hyperfunctioning B cells. An exaggerated insulin response is also found in patients with obesity, acromegaly, or Cushing's syndrome and after anabolic steroid treatment; pronounced hypoglycemia does not accompany these clinical states of insulin resistance, however. Because of the potential to have severe and protracted hypoglycemia after tolbutamide administration, the patient should be under continuous surveillance and parenteral glucose should be given to abort severe neuroglucopenic

symptoms. (2) *Intravenous glucagon.* After an overnight fast, glucagon (1 mg) is infused within 30 sec and samples obtained for glucose and insulin at 0, 2, 5, 10, 15, 30, 45, 60, 90, and 120 min.[79] As glucagon promotes acute insulin release and hepatic glycogenolysis, it has a twofold advantage in assessing patients with hypoglycemia. If excessive insulin responses are found within the first few minutes after parenteral glucagon, islet cell hyperfunction is probable. In contrast, blunted glucose responses with normal insulin rises implicate hepatic or other endocrine organ dysfunction in the genesis of the hypoglycemia. (3) *Calcium infusion.* Intravenous administration of calcium gluconate (4 mg Ca^{++}/kg/hr for 4 hours) has been recommended to evoke inordinate insulin secretion in patients with autonomously functioning B cells, thereby distinguishing them from normal individuals who have little or no rise in insulin levels.[102]

Circulating Insulin Antibodies

Antibodies to insulin usually result from injection of insulin from bovine or pork sources after periods exceeding 1 month and are common in insulin-treated diabetics. In a patient in whom hypoglycemia is suspected to be self-induced, the detection of titers of insulin antibody in the plasma would also justify more intensive efforts to ascertain whether insulin has been administered secretly.[105] Antibodies to human insulin have been reported in a few patients with "autoimmune" hypoglycemia.[41]

NUTRIENT INDUCED AND SPONTANEOUS HYPOGLYCEMIA

Postabsorptive "Reactive" Hypoglycemia

Most nonpharmacogenic causes of symptomatic hypoglycemia are directly related to food ingestion, with symptoms appearing at varying intervals within 5 hours of eating. The syndrome of postabsorptive or "reactive" hypoglycemia reflects abnormalities evoked by one or more of the dietary constituents and can be classified on the basis of their induction by (1) glucose, (2) galactose, (3) fructose, and (4) leucine. In general, the glucopenic syndromes associated with dietary intake of galactose, fructose, and leucine are rare and genetically transmitted, predominating in infancy and childhood. In contrast, the "reactive" hypoglycemia after glucose ingestion occurs most frequently in adults and is by far the most common cause of symptomatic hypoglycemia.

Hypoglycemia Induced by Glucose

With exception of patients with pancreatic B cell tumors, subjects with "reactive" hypoglycemia following ingestion are characterized by either normal or increased fasting plasma glucose levels, and within 5 hours after food intake, they sustain an abrupt decline in circulating glucose, usually followed by a rapid rebound. The hypoglycemic pattern is temporally related to the rate of plasma sugar ascent and the level and duration of the plasma sugar zenith. For the most part, the symptoms reflect activation of the adrenergic nervous system, coinciding with the rapid fall in plasma glucose to a nadir, which triggers catecholamine discharge. They usually subside within 15–20 min. Although disorientation may occur at low blood sugars, loss of consciousness and convulsions are unusual but may go unnoticed by the patient. The glucose-stimulated hypoglycemic disorders are usually attributed to one or more of the following defects: (1) hypersecretion of insulin, (2) hypersensitivity of peripheral tissues to insulin, or (3) deficiency of counter-regulatory hormones. Although it has been claimed that following an OGTT, these syndromes can be distinguished based on the configuration of the plasma glucose profile and time of onset of hypoglycemia, the OGTT in a given person may be quite variable, and, as pointed out by Permutt,[91] there may be difficulties in characterizing mechanisms underlying the hypoglycemia because of the variation in the individual's responses on serial OGTT. Hofeldt and associates[53] and Lefebvre and coworkers,[72] have examined large series of patients with "reactive" hypoglycemia by measuring glucose profiles with coincident evaluation of insulin and counter-regulatory hormones (glucagon and cortisol) and concluded that the patients with reactive hypoglycemia compose a group with multiple etiologies. As part of the spectrum, it is possible to distinguish patients with early-phase reactive hypoglycemia from those with late-phase ("lag") glucopenic manifestations.[63] The majority fall within an ill-defined group designated idiopathic, however.[53, 72] From a practical viewpoint, the physician faced with a patient with "reactive" hypoglycemia will obtain the essential information from the clinical history and measurement of glucose profiles during an OGTT, and the ordering of insulin levels does not add any further diagnostic or therapeutic insights and, because of the expense, should be discouraged.

Alimentary Hypoglycemia

In patients who have undergone gastrointestinal surgery (partial or total gastrectomy, gastrojejunostomy, or pyloroplasty), symptomatic hypoglycemia may occur 90–180 min after meals. The incidence of the symptoms attributable to hypoglycemia in such patients is difficult to ascertain, since they may overlap those associated with the "dumping" syndrome. It has been claimed that 5–10% of patients with gastric outlet surgery have symptoms due either to "dumping" or to hypoglycemia. Chemical hypoglycemia, when tested by OGTT, has been reported as high as 80%, with symptoms in approximately 30% of patients. Symptoms vary from a vague feeling of uneasiness to marked manifestations of hyperepinephrinemia, and in a very few, neuropsychiatric disturbances with seizures and coma have been reported.[46] Typically, patients have a rapid ascending limb of plasma glucose, achieving a peak usually exceeding 200 mg/dl, followed by an abrupt descent to hypoglycemia. Exaggerated insulin responses are usually, but not invariably, found (Fig. 16–9). Since the Kg following intravenous glucose and insulin release after provocative tests are normal, the abnormality is unlikely to reside in the pancreas. The quick rise to high blood glucose levels is due to the increased rate of delivery of hypertonic glucose into the small bowel as a consequence of the elimination of the gastric reservoir or impaired pyloric sphincter ("tachyalimentation").[91] Although not proved, it seems likely that the enteric humoral signal to the B cell, now believed to be GIP, may contribute to the inordinate insulin release concomitant with the hyperglycemic stimulus.[21] The rate of gastric emptying has been reported to stimulate release of other gastrointestinal hormone, such as "gut glucagon"; however, no systematic examination of GIP or "gut glucagon" levels in patients with alimentary hypoglycemia has been undertaken. It is also possible that vasoactive peptides and neural signals augmented during heightened glucose absorption may also abet glucose-mediated insulin secretion.

Within 60 minutes after food ingestion, symptoms of upper gastric discomfort, fullness, nausea, weakness, and palpita-

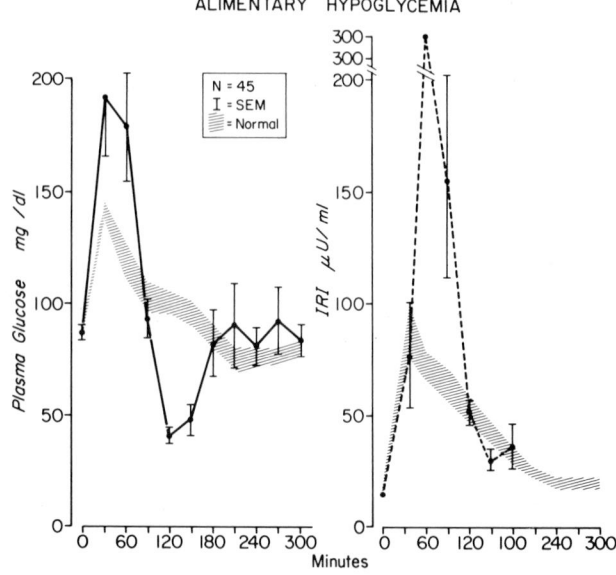

ALIMENTARY HYPOGLYCEMIA

Figure 16–9. Plasma glucose and plasma insulin (IRI) concentrations during an OGTT in patients with alimentary postabsorptive hypoglycemia. Glucose is given at 0. (Modified from Hofeldt, F. D., Lufkin, E. G., et al.: *Diabetes* 23:589, 1974.)

tions occur in patients after surgical procedures that increase gastric emptying and have been designated the "dumping" syndrome. The mechanism has been ascribed to distention of the jejunum due to rapid increase in osmolality within the bowel lumen, resulting in enhanced transfer of food from the blood into the gut. Vasoactive factors, such as gut peptides, serotonin, and kinin-like activities, have also been implicated in the hyperperistalsis and in the vasomotor hyperactivity that characterize this disorder. The "dumping" syndrome and the later manifestations of hypoglycemia, if they occur together, may be difficult to distinguish from each other.

Reactive hypoglycemia with a nadir of blood sugar within 3 hours has been reported in 20–50% of patients with peptic ulcers in whom insulin levels tend to be elevated.[127] It is conceivable that in these tense, apprehensive patients with an ulcer diathesis, the hyperinsulinemia is related to the enhanced gastric motility and accelerated glucose absorption. Since it has been demonstrated that patients with active duodenal ulcer disease release more GIP after mixed meals or glucose, it seems plausible that GIP may contribute to the hyperinsulinemia in these subjects as well as in patients with gastric surgical procedures.[21]

In some individuals with symptomatic early-onset hypoglycemia, with concomitant hyperinsulinemia, neither gastrointestinal surgery nor peptic ulcer disease can be invoked. Some, but not all, have had documented increased gastric emptying. Although the mechanism is unknown, it is possible that some of these patients have an intrinsic abnormality in intestinal absorption of glucose triggering insulin hypersecretion.[91]

Idiopathic Hypoglycemia

A low plasma sugar level 2–4 hours after food intake in apparently healthy young adults has been cited as the most common hypoglycemic syndrome.[17, 63] These individuals tend to be of thin habitus, emotionally unstable, tense, anxious, and compulsive in personality. It is noteworthy that these syndromes may occur in obese and normal weight individuals. The somatic manifestations of a hyperactive autonomic nervous system may be reflected by gastric hypermotility, excessive gastric acid, nausea, vomiting, and an irritable colon. It has been conjectured that the glucopenic manifestations in such patients reflect an altered neuroendocrine "set" that has led to the designation of "functional" or vagotonic hypoglycemia.[17] Measurements of insulin responses in these individuals have failed to reveal any consistent abnormality, either temporally or in the amounts of insulin released (Fig. 16–10). Hofeldt and colleagues[54] and Lefebvre and associates[72] have emphasized the heterogeneity of insulin responses in patients with idiopathic hypoglycemia and concede the possibility that defective counter regulation or excessive sensitivity to insulin may explain the hypoglycemia in these patients. In some patients with renal glycosuria, "reactive" hypoglycemia without apparent hyperinsulinemia has been found.[72] The mechanism remains obscure.

Diabetes Mellitus

Low plasma glucose levels occurring 3–5 hours after meals have been occasionally reported early in the development of diabetes mellitus in adults.[17, 63] It is an uncommon finding in the diabetic population and therefore is an unreliable premonitory clinical clue to impending diabetes mellitus. In patients who do manifest "reactive" hypoglycemia, fasting plasma glucose levels are normal or slightly elevated and the postprandial glucose ascent is slow, with a high zenith (exceeding 150 mg/dl) with a persistence of hyperglycemia, followed by a gradual fall to hypoglycemic levels. These individuals often are obese and have strongly positive family histories of diabetes mellitus.[72] Plasma insulin levels tend to rise in a sluggish fashion, with excessive concentrations achieved by 2–4 hours. The decline in plasma glucose has been considered to be due to inappropriately high insulin levels (Fig. 16–11). Both the glucose and the insulin responses to a variety of intravenous stimuli are usually attenuated in these patients, and the fall in plasma glucose is usually less precipitous and the nadir higher than in other causes of "reactive" hypoglycemia. Correspondingly, symptoms are usually mild and transitory. It has been the experience of some clinicians with time that these patients progress into more advanced stages of diabetes mellitus with the disappearance of the postprandial hypoglycemia. It should be emphasized that carbohydrate restriction in allegedly normal individuals will occasionally mimic the postprandial glucose profile seen in patients with early-onset diabetes, thereby leading to the misattribution of both diabetes and hypoglycemia to healthy persons.[92]

"Reactive" Hypoglycemia Associated with Endocrine Deficiency Syndromes

Postprandial hypoglycemia occurring during the transition from fed to fasting phase may occasionally occur in syndromes of deficiency of counterinsulin glucoregulatory hormones, when glycogenolysis and gluconeogenesis are impaired. Since virtually all such patients who have postprandial hypoglycemia will also have fasting glucopenia, they are described in detail under the section entitled "Fasting Hypoglycemia."

Treatment of Glucose-Induced Postabsorptive Hypoglycemia

With the exception of the syndromes of spontaneous hypoglycemia occurring in both postprandial and fasting conditions, the induction of the hypoglycemic attack in patients with "reactive" hypoglycemia is the direct consequence of ingestion of dietary carbohydrates. Patients who are best characterized as having early- and late-onset "reactive" hypoglycemia tend to share an exaggerated insulin response to ingested glucose. Therefore, the primary strategy in attempting to mitigate symptoms is to manipulate the composition and the frequency of dietary intake. This is coupled with the reinforcement of the benign nature of this disorder and the avoidance of drugs that might tend to aggravate hypoglycemia. Furthermore, since the distinction between true "reactive" hypoglycemia and the syndrome of "nonhypoglycemia" may be difficult to categorically establish without repetitive OGTT, tactful counseling by the physician to avoid misattribution is strongly recommended. Selective use of drugs may also be beneficial.

Diet. Because of the varied dietary preferences in the population, no universally accepted dietary prescription can

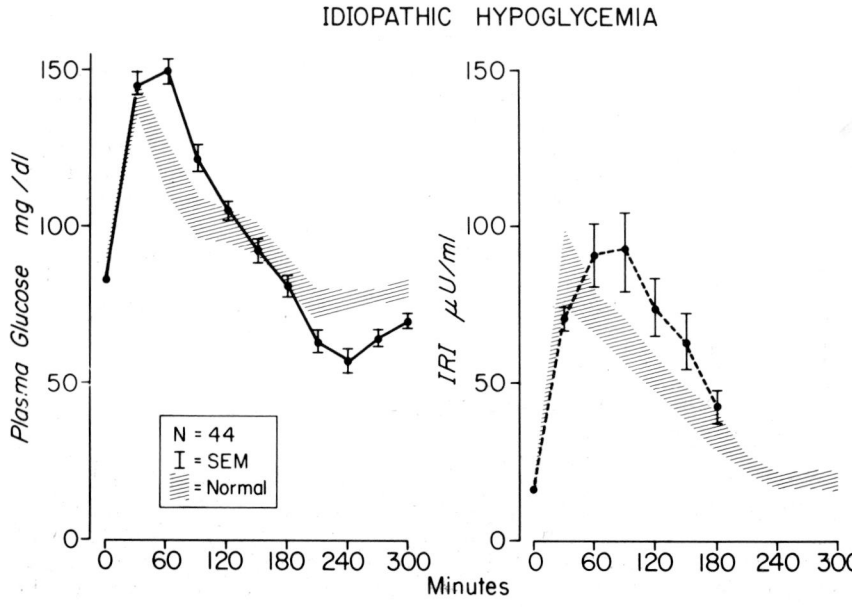

IDIOPATHIC HYPOGLYCEMIA

N = 44
I = SEM
= Normal

Figure 16–10. Plasma glucose and plasma insulin (IRI) concentrations during an OGTT in patients with idiopathic postabsorptive hypoglycemia. Glucose is given at 0. (Modified from Hofeldt, F. D., Lufkin, E. G., et al.: *Diabetes* 23:589, 1974.)

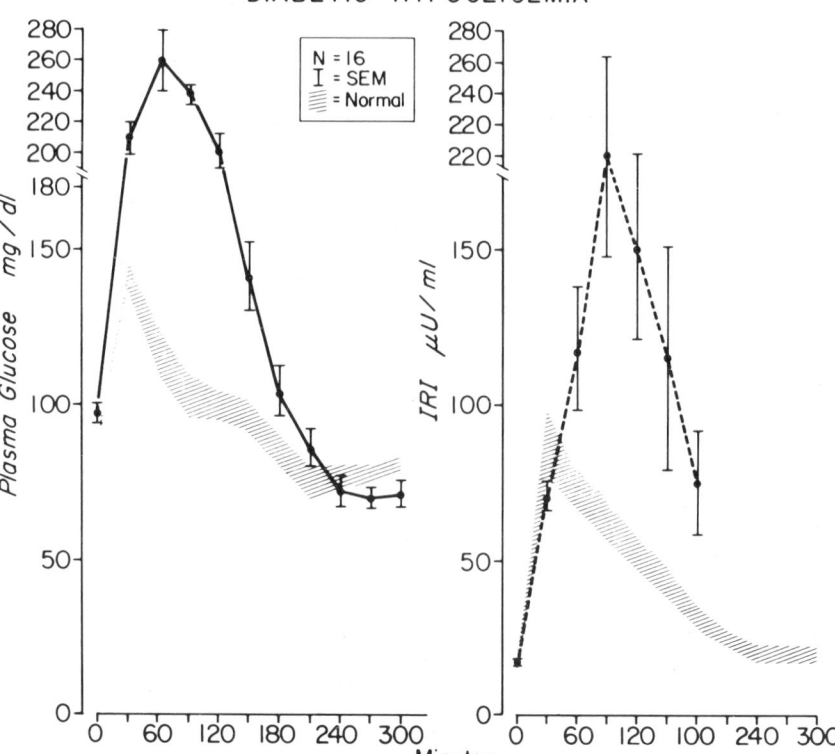

Figure 16–11. Plasma glucose and plasma insulin (IRI) concentrations during OGTT in patients with diabetic postabsorptive hypoglycemia. Glucose is given at 0. (Modified from Hofeldt, F. D., Lufkin, E. G., et al.: *Diabetes* 23:589, 1974.)

be applied to all patients, and thus the recommendations of foods must be tailored to cope with the variations in dietary habits in affected subjects. Moreover, the efficacy of any dietary regimen has not been proved, and of necessity, the physician may have to improvise dietary formulations to alleviate the individual patient's symptoms. With these reservations, the guidelines for dietary maneuvers are based upon the patterns of symptoms and glucose profile after an OGTT.[91] In those persons with alimentary hypoglycemia attributable to rapid transit time, it is advisable to change both the composition of the food and the frequency of eating. Since marked restriction of carbohydrate is neither desirable nor feasible in Western cultures, allocation of carbohydrates should be maintained between 45 and 50% of total calories. Refined sugars, however, which are rapidly absorbed, should be discouraged and substituted by food containing complex carbohydrates that require hydrolysis in the gut. The inclusion of foods high in "crude fiber," which form gels, i.e., 10–20 g of pectin or related polysaccharides, may decrease intestinal transit time and absorption, thereby preventing glucopenic symptoms.[58] High-fat, low-carbohydrate diets are to be discouraged because they are likely to aggravate hypoglycemia, particularly if the patient periodically ingests high-carbohydrate food.[92] High protein intake has been advocated, and in some patients, rapid excursions of blood glucose are dampened by small, high-protein feedings. The frequency of eating may be modified depending upon patients' caloric needs, sense of satiety, and symptoms. Thus, meals normally taken three times daily may be adjusted to divert more calories to snacks every 2–3 hours. Similar dietary maneuvers have been found to be effective in patients with idiopathic "reactive" hypoglycemia and that attributable to mild diabetes mellitus. The obese patient should also be advised to restrict total caloric intake within the framework of the just mentioned dietary prescription until ideal body weight is achieved. Although ethanol potentiates glucose-stimulated insulin secretion under cer-

tain circumstances, it has not been established that when ingested in moderation with meals that it contributes to the reactive hypoglycemia. Practically, modest ethanol intake should not be proscribed but rather the effect on hypoglycemic symptoms should be individually assessed.

Drugs. In patients with accelerated glucose absorption, anticholinergic drugs have been employed to inhibit vagal action, thereby delaying gastric emptying. Propantheline, in doses from 7.5 to 30 mg 30 min before each meal, has been found to alleviate glucopenic symptoms in some patients.[93] In the anxious hyperkinetic person, avoidance of caffeine-containing beverages and cigarettes should be strongly urged, and sedatives, such as phenobarbital (30 mg 2–3 times daily) or diazepam (2.5–5 mg 2 times daily), may be effective in mitigating symptoms. A number of other pharmacologic agents have also been reported to improve hypoglycemic symptoms based upon their potential to inhibit insulin secretion. These include diazoxide, diphenylhydantoin and propranolol. As yet, evaluation of the efficacy of these drugs has been inadequate to justify their use. Propanolol may abate adrenergic symptoms through β blockade; however, it does not affect plasma glucose levels, and in the occasional patient, unconsciousness may occur without any premonitory adrenergic symptoms. In subjects with hypoglycemia associated with early-onset diabetes, a beneficial effect has been reported with the use of sulfonylureas (tolbutamide 0.5–2.0 g in divided doses daily), possibly through partial restoration of the sensitivity of the B cell to respond to normal physiologic signals.[2]

Surgery. Occasionally, in patients with disabling reactive hypoglycemia as a consequence of gastric surgery who do not respond to dietary manipulations or drugs, operations to reverse the distorted gastrointestinal relationships may be beneficial. Fink and colleagues[34] noted a significant improvement in 11 patients in whom the jejunal segment of the bowel was reversed at either the gastric outlet or the ligament of Treitz.

Hypoglycemia Induced by Galactose
(Galactosemia)

The term "galactosemia" describes two rare, hereditary syndromes resulting from the inability to metabolize galactose, which is derived from the hydrolysis of milk lactose in the intestinal mucosa. Both disorders, resulting in galactosemia and galactosuria, are transmitted by autosomal recessive inheritance and are due to specific enzymic defects involved in the conversion of galactose to glucose, leading to toxic accumulation of galactose (Fig. 16–3).[107] Galactokinase deficiency galactosemia has been described in only a few patients ranging from infancy to middle age. Lack of this enzyme limits conversion of galactose-1-phosphate. The patients present with lenticular cataracts, and hypoglycemia is not a feature of this syndrome.

Glucopenia is found within the constellation of nutritional failure, liver disease, cataracts, and mental retardation occurring in infants after lactose ingestion due to a deficiency in galactose-1-phosphate uridyl transferase (transferase deficiency galactosemia). Neonates with transferase deficiency galactosemia fail to thrive and have vomiting or diarrhea or both after milk ingestion. Within a few days, jaundice, hepatomegaly, and cataracts ensue. Growth and development are impaired and mental retardation is often observed after the first few months of life. A few patients, mostly black, who are homozygous for this disorder, may survive into adulthood without striking clinical manifestations.[107] This implies that they are capable of metabolizing galactose by alternate pathways. In affected infants, liver function tests are usually deranged, accompanied by hyperchloremic acidosis, albuminuria, and aminoaciduria. Hypoglycemic attacks usually coincide with hypergalactosemia but are not an invariable consequence of lactose ingestion. Although the relative contribution of the low plasma sugar to the initial symptom complex is uncertain, it seems likely that persistent neuroglucopenia is a major factor in the evolution of the mental deterioration. As a result of transferase enzymic deficiency, galactose-1-phosphate accumulates in many tissues, and the occasional severe hypoglycemic episodes have been attributed to decreased hepatic gluconeogenesis. *In vitro*, it has been shown there is an inhibition of hepatic phosphoglucomutase, which catalyzes the conversion of glucose-1-phosphate to glucose-6-phosphate. In addition, the elevated galactose-1-phosphate may interfere with renal tubular resorption of amino acids, leading to diminished circulating gluconeogenic precursors. Death occurs from inanition and multiorgan injury, possibly as a result of the toxicity of galactitol, which accumulates along with galactose-1-phosphate.

The disease should be suspected on clinical grounds in a setting of mellituria due to galactose. Both galactosemia and galactosuria, however, may be intermittent. A galactose tolerance test is hazardous and should be avoided. The diagnosis is confirmed by direct assay of red cell transferase activity, which is low or absent. Although the occurrence of transferase deficiency galactosemia is uncommon (1/62,000), routine screening in newborn infants for this disorder has been strongly endorsed because it may not be recognized, and death due to sepsis occurs in about 30% of those with untreated classic galactosemia. Management of these patients consists of elimination of dietary galactose, which, if accomplished, results in striking regression of all symptoms and signs. In pregnant women with affected children, restriction of lactose intake is recommended, since the disease probably affects the fetus. Despite apparent improvement in galactose tolerance with age in some patients, suggesting that alternative pathways for galactose metabolism develop in maturity, strict adherence to a galactose-free diet has been advocated indefinitely.

Hypoglycemia Induced by Fructose (Hereditary Fructose Intolerance)

Fructose is an important source of dietary carbohydrate, which is absorbed by the gut by carrier-mediated diffusion and is normally converted to glucose by liver, kidney, and small intestine. The disorder of fructose metabolism denoted "hereditary fructose intolerance" is characterized by protracted vomiting and severe hypoglycemia shortly after the intake of fructose-containing food. The disease, transmitted through an autosomal recessive gene, is the consequence of a deficiency of hepatic fructose-1-phosphate aldolase (Fig. 16–3).[38] This results in the accumulation of fructose-1-phosphate with abnormally high plasma fructose levels and fructosuria after oral or intravenous fructose. Infant and adult patients with this abnormality are healthy and asymptomatic unless they eat fructose-containing food. The clinical picture of chronic fructose poisoning in small children consists of failure to thrive, vomiting, episodic and marked hypoglycemia, jaundice, and hepatomegaly, with albuminuria and aminoaciduria. Typically, the children develop a strong aversion to fructose-containing foods, notably sweets, which probably explains why the characteristic features are usually not found in adults. Clinical manifestations can be evoked by intravenous fructose administration. The smallest dose that always produces hypoglycemic symptoms without causing nausea and vomiting is 0.25 g/kg body weight in adults or 3 g/m^2 body area in children. Levels of plasma glucose and phosphorus fall gradually and remain low for several hours. Hypophosphatemia precedes hypoglycemia and may be the only abnormal finding when a very small amount of fructose is given. Glucopenia, which is frequently profound, is not associated with hyperinsulinism. As detailed by Froesch, the disorder is best explained by the deficiency of hepatic fructose-1-phosphate aldolase, leading to the accumulation of fructose-1-phosphate after fructose ingestion.[38] The latter, in conjunction with depleted inorganic phosphorus inhibits phosphorylase, thereby interfering with glycogenolysis. In addition, gluconeogenesis is impaired, presumably due to deficient ATP. The therapeutic approach to this disorder is the avoidance of fructose in the diet.

Hereditary fructose intolerance should not be confused with essential fructosuria, which is a rare, genetically transmitted, harmless abnormality manifested as fructosemia and fructosuria, reflecting a failure of conversion to fructose-1-phosphate due to a deficiency of hepatic fructokinase. Hypoglycemia has never been found in this benign condition.

Hypoglycemia Induced by Amino
Acids (Familial Leucine Hypersensitivity)

In an evaluation of children with hypoglycemia designated as idiopathic familial hypoglycemia of childhood, Cochrane and associates reported that approximately 60% of infants in this group were distinguished by the association of glucopenia with the ingestion of L-leucine.[18] Subsequent studies suggest that perhaps one third of all infants with idiopathic hypoglycemia may be leucine-sensitive. The clinical syndrome is usually apparent within the first 2 years of life, affecting both sexes equally and manifested by severe fasting glucopenia with profound "reactive" hypoglycemia after the intake of dietary protein with a high leucine content. The nadir of the blood sugar most often occurs within 30–60 min after food ingestion. Seizures may occur with prolonged fasting, and permanent neurologic damage with mental retardation are common sequelae. In most instances, by the time the patient reaches the age of 5–6 years, these amino acid–induced hypoglycemic attacks have spontaneously abated. There is a clustering of this disease in families; the patterns of inheritance are not certain, however. Spontaneous leucine-induced hypoglycemia occurs in adults, but it is extremely rare and is usually elicited postprandially. There are no pathognomonic signs or symptoms of this disorder. It is important to distinguish these patients from individuals with nesidioblastosis and insulin-producing tumors, two thirds of whom release excessive amounts of insulin after intake of foods high in leucine.

Although a number of amino acids are insulinogenic in normal individuals, the provocation of hypoglycemia in affected children is almost exclusively found after L-leucine ingestion. Occasionally, hypoglycemia is induced by L-isoleucine, L-valine, and L-serine, as well as α-ketoisocaproic acid. Leucine administered either orally or intravenously to healthy subjects causes moderate rises in insulin levels, which become more pronounced with concurrent administration of sulfonylureas.[35] Thus, it seems plausible that leucine-induced hypoglycemia in susceptible children represents a marked exaggeration of physiologic responses to this amino acid. The reason for the B cell hypersensitivity to leucine is unclear. Postmortem examination in several of these patients has revealed islet cell hyperplasia in about 50%. Pancreatic insulin content has not been consistently abnormal. The high frequency of fasting hypoglycemia in the face of normal plasma insulin levels also implies that additional factors involved in glucogenesis may be impaired.

The diagnosis is established by demonstrating a decrease in plasma glucose in excess of 20 mg/dl after oral leucine, or 25 mg/dl after its intravenous administration (150–250 mg/kg body weight).[89] This challenge usually results in a two- to threefold rise in plasma insulin levels above basal. Although severe hypoglycemia may be exacerbated by leucine in patients with nesidioblastosis or insulinomas as well as in leucine-sensitive patients, the former conditions are rare in childhood. Insulin responses to tolbutamide in subjects with leucine hypersensitivity tend to be within normal limits. Since it is imperative to differentiate such patients from those harboring insulin-producing tumors, diagnostic maneuvers to exclude a functioning islet cell neoplasm should be undertaken (discussed later).

There is no specific treatment for patients with this disorder. In general, the hypoglycemic episodes are managed by dietary maneuvers, use of drugs, and, occasionally, surgical measures.[89] It has been suggested, but not proved, that restriction of leucine content in the diet is beneficial. L-leucine is essential for normal growth and development, however, and since the minimum daily requirement is approximately 150–230 mg/kg, hypoglycemic episodes may be provoked by food containing obligatory amounts of leucine. Diets high in complex carbohydrates are recommended. Glucocorticoids occasionally cause amelioration of the hypoglycemia, but in general, salutary responses have been disappointing. Adverse effects, particularly growth retardation, may preclude their use. Diazoxide, in oral doses of 10–15 mg/kg, may be effective in control of the hypoglycemic attack.[80] Every effort should be made to control the glucopenic attacks by conservative measures, since the disease is usually self-limited in these children. Occasionally, when such measures fail, a 70% pancreactectomy has been found to relieve hypoglycemic symptoms.[89]

Fasting Hypoglycemia

As detailed in preceding sections, during the transition from the fed to the fasted state, a number of factors operate normally to regulate the provision of fuels for glucose homeostasis. Usually within 5–6 hours after eating, the stabilization of blood glucose levels reflects increased hepatic glucose output, coincident with a rise in circulating gluconeogenic precursors. Hypoglycemia that occurs spontaneously in the fasting state can be conveniently categorized into disorders in which the primary abnormality is either an underproduction of glucose, or alternatively, due to excessive glucose utilization. If glucogenesis is greatly reduced or glucose disposal is markedly accelerated, hypoglycemia may occur by 4–5 hours after eating and be misconstrued as the consequence of ingested nutrients. In such instances, however, the glucopenia is usually profound and persists without appropriate counter-regulation and usually does not present a problem in clinical differentiation from the hypoglycemic syndromes that are related solely to nutrient intake. In some children with both fasting and "reactive" types of hypoglycemia, the mechanisms are multifactorial or uncertain; therefore, they have been classified as "idiopathic." The disorders resulting in spontaneous fasting hypoglycemia are uncommon, representing less than 1% of the glucopenic syndromes. Nonetheless, because patients often have profound hypoglycemia and several of the causes can be cured or managed effectively, establishing the etiology of the hypoglycemia is paramount.

Nutrient Loss

Hypoglycemia resulting from chronic malabsorption of nutrients without marked inanition is a rare occurrence. Lifshitz and coworkers[73] noted symptomatic hypoglycemia in 23 of 403 infants with bacteria-induced diarrhea with monosaccharide intolerance, only after treatment with a carbohydrate-free, high-protein intake. It is likely that the low blood sugars result from depleted protein stores in conjunction with amino acid–induced hyperinsulinism. Spontaneous hypoglycemia has been reported sporadically in individuals who have been chronically deprived of calories during famines and in young women with anorexia nervosa. In such patients with excessive wasting of muscle and adipose tissue, hypoglycemia is attributable to inadequate gluconeogenic precursors. Hypoglycemia associated with kwashiorkor in Africa and Jamaica occurs usually in subjects with marked marasmus. Although it has been claimed that hypoglycemia occurs in persons with massive renal glucosuria, this genetically transmitted abnormality is extremely rare (53 of 18,000 cases in Joslin's series), and none had documented glucopenia.

Deficient Glucose Production

Inborn Errors of Glucogenesis

Disorders of Glycogen Metabolism. Inherited disorders involving glycogen synthesis or degradation in various tissues due to specific enzyme deficiencies have long been recognized, and their clinical features are distinctive. The clinical manifestations, including hypoglycemia, appear early in infancy and childhood, and their severity is related to the degree of enzyme impairment affecting glycogen metabolism and the availability of alternative fuels.

Despite the delineation of specific enzymic defects in several of these entities, there are a few patients with clinical features resembling the classic grouping of the glycogenosis in whom the enzyme abnormalities have not been precisely defined. Nevertheless, a classification of the types of glycogenosis, with major organ involvement and specific enzyme abnormalities that have been identified so far, is given in Table 16–6. With the exceptions of Type IV glycogenosis and the syndrome attributed to a lack of glycogen synthase, patients with each type have in common excessive deposition of glycogen in various organs, and, in most, the enzyme defects are transmitted as autosomal recessive traits. Of the nine inherited diseases of glycogen metabolism, only Types I, III, VI, and O develop hypoglycemia.[57]

Glycogen storage diseases Types I, III, and VI share several clinical features; however, the clinical courses of the latter two are milder than that of Type I, which accounts for 25% of glycogen storage diseases. Children with Type I glycogenosis usually are short in stature, with normal proportions. Hypotonia and a tendency to obesity are also frequent. Massive hepatomegaly, the most striking and characteristic physical finding, persists throughout life, whereas enlargement of the kidneys may require radiographic or ultrasonic confirmation because of the prominence of the liver. Most patients also have xanthomas located typically over the extensor surfaces of the extremities. Fasting hypoglycemia occurs shortly after birth and is variable in severity, with plasma glucose concentrations ranging as low as 10 mg/dl, often without symptoms. Chronic hypoglycemia is associated with hypercholesterolemia, hyperlipoproteinemia, and ketonemia, especially during periods of inadequate carbohydrate intake. High lactic acid levels culminating in metabolic acidosis and the hyperlipidemia with excess lipid deposition in skin and liver are due to the excessive mobilization of gluconeogenic precursors in response to hypoglycemia. Gout may strike affected persons, particularly during early adulthood. Hyperuricemia is the consequence of both increased production of uric acid and competitive inhibition of its renal elimination by the elevated ketoacids.

Individuals with Type I glycogenosis characteristically have minimal or absent hyperglycemic responses to epinephrine, glucagon, galactose, or fructose. Varying degrees of carbohydrate intolerance are found by OGTT, and insulin responses are usually blunted. The extraordinary accumulation of glycogen (greater than 5 g/dl) with normal structure in liver and kidney is due to a lack of the enzyme *glucose-6-phosphatase*, which catalyzes the hydrolysis of glucose-6-phosphate to glucose (Fig. 16–3). Despite this defect in a key enzyme, a number of patients survive into adulthood, and therefore glucose must be derived from glucose-6-phosphate by nonspecific phosphatases. Hepatomas are frequently found in adult patients. The biochemical diagnosis is made by demonstration of increased amounts of normal glycogen by histochemical staining and absence of glucose-6-phosphatase in freshly frozen liver, which is best obtained by open biopsy.

Patients with Type III glycogen storage disease cannot be distinguished by physical examination from those with Type I. In Israel, Type III disease accounts for 73% of the glycogen storage disorders in non-Ashkenazic Jews. The clinical course tends to be less severe, though marked hypoglycemia with convulsions may occur. The hepatomegaly inexplicably tends to diminish at puberty, and renal enlargement is not found. Hyperglycemia after epinephrine and glucagon is variable, and lactose and fructose are readily converted to glucose. Because of the deficiency of *amylo-1,6-glucosidase* or "debrancher enzyme" (Fig. 16–3), abnormal forms of glycogen accumulate in large amounts in the liver. The diagnosis is confirmed by histochemical evidence of abnormally short outer branched chains of glycogen in muscle or liver.

Hers has described a heterogeneous group of patients with clinical features resembling the milder forms of Type I glycogenosis. An abnormality in *phosphorylase kinase* has been shown in some of these patients presenting with features similar to the manifestations of Type V and classified as Type VIII. Others have been found to have reduced activity of hepatic *phosphorylase*, eventuating in impaired generation of glucose-1-phosphate (Fig. 16–3). The former is inherited as an X-linked recessive trait; the latter is transmitted as an autosomal recessive. The two types are clinically indistinguishable. In a few patients a defect in hepatic *glycogen synthase* has been found (Type O). Failure to thrive is the only clinical manifestation other than hypoglycemic attacks. The liver is not enlarged, fasting ketonuria is associated, and, since plasma alanine levels tend to be low, it is possible the hypoglycemia is due to limitation of substrate with impaired gluconeogenesis. Administration of glucagon in the fed state increases blood glucose but has no effect during fasting. The diagnosis is established by appropriate assay of liver for abnormalities in the respective enzymes.

Since there are no specific means of rectifying the enzyme abnormalities in patients with glycogen storage disease, therapy is directed toward ameliorating the hypoglycemic attacks and attempting to reduce hepatic size in the Type I disorder. Frequent feedings high in starch and low in fat have been helpful, and recently the constant nocturnal infusion of high-glucose formula through a nasogastric tube has been reported to reverse many of the metabolic abnormalities.[45] Experience with the use of repository forms of glucagon or infusions of catecholamines has been unsatis-

Table 16–6. DISORDERS OF GLYCOGEN STORAGE

Type	Eponym	Organs	Enzyme Defect	Glycogen Structure	Fasting Hypoglycemia	Clinical Features
I	Von Gierke's disease	Liver, kidney, intestine	Glucose-6-phosphatase	Normal	+++	Early onset, hepatomegaly, xanthomatosis
II	Pompe's disease	Generalized	α-1,4-glucosidase	Normal	0	Hypotonia, cardiomegaly, death from cardiorespiratory failure
III	Cori's disease	Liver, muscle, heart, erythrocytes	Amylo,1,6-glucosidase	Abnormal	++	Similar to type I but less severe
IV	Anderson's disease	Liver, leukocytes	α-1,4-glucan: 1,4-glucan-6-glucosyl transferase	Abnormal	0	Hypotonia, hepatosplenomegaly, death due to progressive cirrhosis
V	McArdle's disease	Muscle	Phosphorylase	Normal	0	Muscle cramping with exercise, myoglobinuria
VI	Her's disease	Liver, leukocytes	Phosphorylase	Normal	+	Similar to type I but less severe
VII	–	Muscle, erythrocytes	Phosphofructokinase	Normal	0	Muscle cramping with exercise, myoglobinuria
VIII	–	Liver, leukocytes	Phosphorylase b kinase	Normal	0	Hepatomegaly
0	–	Liver	Glycogen synthase	Normal	++	Failure to thrive

factory. Diazoxide, acting by several mechanisms, including inhibition of hepatic glucose uptake and glycogenolysis and insulin release, has been beneficial in a few patients in whom it has been used. Portocaval transposition or shunt preceded by long-term parenteral nutrition has been associated with dramatic reduction in hepatomegaly with partial rectification of some of the metabolic abnormalities.[57] Nonetheless, fasting hypoglycemia may continue, necessitating provision of carbohydrate by intranasal or intravenous route. In patients with Type III and Type VI glycogenosis, hypoglycemia can usually be mitigated by frequent feedings or intranasal glucose administration. Since these disorders tend to improve spontaneously with time, surgical procedures are usually not warranted.

Disorders of Gluconeogenesis

Impaired Gluconeogenesis Due to Defects in Substrate Conversion. Disorders in which abnormalities in key enzymes are involved in gluconeogenesis are extremely rare, occur sporadically, or are genetically transmitted. In affected children, circulating gluconeogenic precursors, such as alanine, glycerol, and lactate, are normal.

Nine well-documented cases of a deficiency of *fructose-1,6-diphosphatase* have been reported in children ranging from 5 months to 6 years and in one adult.[115] The patients are chronically ill with metabolic acidosis and hepatomegaly, and lethal hypoglycemia may be precipitated by infection. Since the glycogenolytic system is intact, glucagon administration produces a glycemic response in the immediate postprandial period, but not after a short period of fasting. Infusions of fructose, glycerol, and gluconeogenic amino acids produce glucopenia, leading to the speculation that they cannot be transformed to glucose, with the accumulation of triosephosphates below the level of fructose-1,6-diphosphate. This may inhibit glycogenolysis. The diagnosis is established by demonstrating a lack of the enzyme in an hepatic biopsy specimen. Treatment is directed to replenishing glucose during acute exacerbations and rectifying lactic acidosis by bicarbonate infusion. A diet containing 55% carbohydrate and 12% protein has been found to be effective in minimizing these metabolic abnormalities during nonstressful periods. Folic acid, 15 mg/day, has also been claimed to improve hypoglycemia in two patients with this disorder.

A small number of infants have been described with hepatomegaly and recurrent hypoglycemia, eventuating in death in all subjects. Absolute deficiencies of *phosphoenol pyruvate carboxykinase* were documented.[55] Chronic infantile lactic acidosis with hypoglycemia associated with disturbances in pyruvate oxidation or organic acidemia and Leigh's subacute necrotizing encephalomyopathy have been reported in a few infants. *Pyruvate carboxylase* activity in liver was markedly depressed.[24]

Hypoglycemia is a prominent feature of children with *Reye's syndrome* under 5 years of age. The clinical manifestations include protracted vomiting, hyperpnea, and mental deterioration. Death from apnea is frequent. The symptom complex is often precipitated by upper respiratory infection. Elevations of plasma lactate, pyruvate, alanine, and glutamine coincide with the hypoglycemia, and transient deficiencies in the activity of hepatic *pyruvate carboxylase* and *pyruvate dehydrogenase* are considered to account for the inability to generate new glucose from circulating precursors.

Hypoglycemia has been noted in newborns as one of the metabolic anomalies associated with defects occurring in the degradative steps of the three-branched chain amino acids — leucine, valine and isoleucine. This extremely rare disease is transmitted by an autosomal recessive gene and has been termed "branched-chain ketonuria" or "maple syrup urine disease."[22] The syndrome is due to a block in oxidative decarboxylation of α-ketoisocaproic acid, α-keto-β-methyl-valeric acid, and α-keto-isovaleric acid, resulting in accumulation of their branched-chain amino acid precursors. Affected infants are normal at birth but fail to thrive, vomit, become lethargic, and have muscle hypotonicity and convulsions. Approximately 50% develop symptomatic hypoglycemia. Mental retardation and neurologic deficits are frequent. Few survive beyond 2 years, and death is usually caused by intercurrent infection. The only distinctive feature is the odor of the urine, which resembles that of burnt sugar. The diagnosis is confirmed by measurement of elevated branched-chain ketoacids or amino acids in blood and urine and demonstration of the enzyme defect in peripheral leukocytes. The pathogenesis of the hypoglycemia is uncertain. Despite low plasma alanine levels, the glucopenia would not appear to be substrate-limited, since alanine infusion before and after correction of the hyperaminoacidemia fails to evoke a glycemic response. A diet with reduced amounts of branched-chain amino acids tends to diminish the serious complications of the disease. The severe restrictions in food selection imposed by this dietary regimen are extremely difficult, however, and require sophisticated medical care, with monitoring of amino acids and capabilities of coping with the episodic severe glucopenia by intravenous glucose. Exchange transfusion and peritoneal dialysis have also been advocated but experience is limited.

Impaired Gluconeogenesis Due to Substrate Limitation (Ketotic Hypoglycemia). In 1964, Colle and Ulstrom[16] described the clinical features of "ketotic hypoglycemia," which is the most common form of glucopenia in children. The typical patient is a hyperactive male of short stature and low weight. Hypoglycemia is most frequently encountered between the ages of 18 months and 5 years. Low plasma glucose is episodically found in the morning after carbohydrate deprivation and is accompanied by vomiting and ketonuria. Symptoms are promptly reverted by parenteral glucose, and between attacks the patients are normoglycemic and have no abnormalities in plasma glucose or insulin responses to intravenous glucose, tolbutamide, L-leucine, glucagon or epinephrine. Symptomatic hypoglycemia in these patients is invariably provoked within 24 hours by a hypocaloric, low-carbohydrate diet high in fat content. Ketonuria is not a constant feature. During hypoglycemic episodes provoked by ketogenic diets or after brief caloric restriction, glucagon administration fails to elevate blood glucose levels. Insulin, glucagon, GH, and cortisol levels are appropriate for the degree of glycemia during an attack. A deficiency in gluconeogenic precursors, notably alanine, rather than a defective hepatic gluconeogenic apparatus *per se*, is responsible for the impaired glucose homeostasis.[89] Although decreased circulating epinephrine levels have been reported in several patients,[14] this is not universal and it seems unlikely that hypoepinephrinemia is a major factor in this syndrome.

Treatment of hypoglycemic attacks is empirical and primarily prophylactic. It is desirable to maintain adequate caloric intake with frequent feedings high in carbohydrate content during periods when acetonuria is demonstrable.[18, 89] Hypoglycemia is often aggravated by infections, which should be treated by appropriate measures, and parenteral glucose infusion may be necessary.

Acquired Liver Dysfunction

In view of the central role of the liver in glucogenesis and the evidence that hepatectomy in experimental animals causes sustained glucopenia, hypoglycemia would be expected to be a common complication of severe liver disease. Yet the functional reserve of the liver is such that more than 80% of its mass may be removed without significant disturbance of glucose homeostasis. Hence, fasting hypoglycemia is evident only when there is widespread injury or destruction of the liver parenchyma. Moreover, there is no correlation between the development of hypoglycemia and severity of hepatic disease as measured by conventional liver function tests. Fasting hypoglycemia has been observed with a wide spectrum of hepatic diseases, but the incidence is small in patients with cirrhosis, metastatic carcinoma, and hepatitis.[128] Rarely, patients with fulminant hepatitis have marked hypoglycemia, and deranged glucose metabolism may occasionally be associated with diseases such as ascending cholangitis, hepatic abscesses, and empyema of the gallbladder. Glucopenia is infrequently observed in the terminal phases of Laennec's cirrhosis, yet alcoholics who have impaired liver function varying from massive hepatic fatty infiltration to cirrhosis may also develop hypoglycemia because of the toxic effects of excessive ethanol ingestion, in conjunction with inadequate caloric intake (described later). In some patients with severe congestive heart failure, passive congestion of the liver with damage to hepatic cells may disrupt glucogenesis, resulting in hypoglycemia. Occasionally, in the third trimester of pregnancy, women may develop acute fulminant hepatitis, eventuating in atrophy of the liver, and marked hypoglycemia ensues. A variety of hepatotoxins, notably phosphorus, chloroform, carbon tetrachloride, glycol, and halothane, may cause massive necrosis with attendant hypoglycemia. Hepatic infiltration by metastatic carcinoma is rarely extensive enough to diminish the glucogenic capacity of the liver. Primary tumors of the liver are not infrequently associated with hypoglycemia for reasons other than hepatic cellular destruction.

The hypoglycemia resulting from hepatocellular dysfunction is explained by deficient gluconeogenesis and glycogenolysis causing a reduction in hepatic glucose output. The impaired capability of the liver to form glycogen or release glucose is reflected by the fasting hypoglycemia with elevated postprandial plasma glucose concentrations that gradually decline to low levels, usually by 4–5 hours, when alimentary sources of glucose are depleted. The diagnosis of liver disease is usually evident from other features of hepatocellular failure. Treatment of acute fulminant hepatic disease entails the maintenance of plasma sugar levels with parenteral glucose administration. Restoration of glucose homeostasis usually occurs with liver regeneration. In patients with marginal residual hepatic function, frequent feedings high in carbohydrates may be necessary to minimize glucopenic episodes.

Deficiencies of Counterinsulin Glucoregulatory Hormones

As summarized previously (Table 16–2), glucocorticoids, GH, glucagon, and catecholamines operate in concert to counter the action of insulin during the transition from the fed to the fasting state and provide signals for *de novo* glucose formation. In addition, thyroid hormones are involved in glucose homeostasis. Although each hormone may act by several mechanisms, deficiencies in secretion of glucagon, catecholamines, glucocorticoids, and thyroid hormones result primarily in impaired hepatic glucogenesis. Despite its lipolytic activity leading to glucogenic precursors, GH would appear to exert its major effect on glucose metabolism by impeding insulin action in peripheral tis-

sues; therefore, GH insufficiency is discussed under hypoglycemia due to excessive utilization of glucose.

Glucocorticoid Deficiency. Diseases intrinsic to the adrenal cortex or as a consequence of ACTH lack, resulting in decreased secretion of glucocorticoids, are commonly associated with plasma glucose levels of less than 60 mg/dl, which may fall further to symptomatic ranges with food deprivation.[123] Since cortisol influences glucose homeostasis by mechanisms involving delivery of gluconeogenic precursors, "permissive" actions on hepatic gluconeogenesis, and possibly anti-insulin effects on peripheral tissues, patients with inadequate glucocorticoid production are vulnerable to intermittent fasting hypoglycemia and sensitive to insulin administered exogenously.[6] Spontaneous glucocorticoid insufficiency may be due to (1) primary adrenal failure (Addison's disease), (2) congenital enzymic defects in the pathways of cortisol synthesis (adrenogenital syndrome), and (3) defective ACTH secretion (panhypopituitarism, solitary ACTH deficiency, or diminished CRF release). Glucopenia may also be encountered in patients after bilateral adrenalectomy if steroid replacement is inadequate. In most instances, the symptoms and signs of spontaneous deficiency syndromes of the adrenal or pituitary are striking, so that the diagnosis is suspected on clinical grounds. Since cortisol deficiency with concomitant hypoglycemia can occur secondary to a solitary defect in ACTH secretion, the clinical findings may be atypical. The clinical features and procedures used to establish the diagnosis of these disorders are detailed in Ch. 5. Hypoglycemia due to glucocorticoid lack is rectified completely by administration of one of several naturally occurring or synthetic glucocorticoids (e.g., cortisol, 20–30 mg daily, or prednisone, 5–7.5 mg daily).

Thyroid Insufficiency. Fasting hypoglycemia is uncommon in hypothyroidism. In some hypothyroid patients, plasma glucose levels after an overnight fast may range between the 35 and 45 mg/dl associated with glucopenic symptoms.[82] In these patients, there is a delay in plasma glucose rebound after insulin-induced hypoglycemia. The cause of hypoglycemia in thyroid hormone-deficient subjects is probably multifactorial, involving a reduction in delivery of gluconeogenic precursors, i.e., lactate, and a defect in their conversion to glucose in the liver at the level of action of pyruvate carboxylase. The clinical features of hypothyroidism and the diagnostic approaches are described in Ch. 4. Replacement of the lacking thyroid hormones by administration of oral L-thyroxine, 0.1–0.2 mg daily corrects the hypoglycemic manifestations.

Glucagon Insufficiency. Fasting hypoglycemia has been reported in a few infants and adults who, by histologic evaluation at autopsy, had marked reduction of pancreatic A cells relative to B cells. These findings led to the conjecture that the relative lack of glucagon might explain the hypoglycemia on the basis of impaired hepatic glycogenolysis and gluconeogenesis; however, no measurements of plasma glucagon levels were performed.[43] In 1970, Bleicher described a man believed to have hypoglycemia as a consequence of glucagon deficiency.[7] The patient had recurrent glucopenia both with fasting and after ingestion of protein. Plasma glucose responses to oral glucose resembled those seen in diabetic patients. With extended fasting, insulin and glucagon levels were very low. After arginine infusions, plasma glucagon concentrations remained virtually unmeasurable. Following treatment with a high-carbohydrate diet, glucopenic symptoms were alleviated. Recently, severe hypoglycemia has been described in a neonate that was rectified by parental glucagon.[122] Inappropriately low circulating glucagon levels, unresponsive to amino acid infusion, were documented. A comprehensive search for alternative mechanisms for the hypoglycemia was unrevealing. Thus, spontaneous pancreatic A-cell insufficiency appears to be an exceedingly rare cause of hypoglycemia in both the infant and the adult. A blunted glucagon response to severe glucopenia has been observed in infants of diabetic mothers, and a transitory lack of glucagon has been implicated in this form of neonatal hypoglycemia.

Disorders of Sympathetic Nervous System. Catecholamines antagonize the actions of insulin in glucose homeostasis, yet it is conjectural whether spontaneous hypoglycemia can be ascribed to deficiency states of the sympathetic nervous system. Among children with fasting hypoglycemia of undetermined etiology (idiopathic hypoglycemia of childhood), a subgroup with some of the features of "ketogenic hypoglycemia" has been found to have markedly diminished circulating epinephrine levels or diminished urinary excretion of epinephrine under basal conditions.[14, 16] Moreover, following insulin-induced hypoglycemia, these affected children have little or no increment in epinephrine excretion, whereas normal children respond with a 5- to 20-fold increase. The quantitative defect in adrenal medullary secretion is in keeping with the clinical evidence of lack of catecholamine effects. These patients show an increased sensitivity to insulin with a prolonged fall in plasma glucose levels, yet they have normal hyperglycemic responses to exogenously administered epinephrine. Since norepinephrine metabolism in these children is apparently unaltered, it has been proposed that the pathogenesis is related to the inability to synthesize epinephrine within the adrenal medulla. Tietze has demonstrated that some of these children have impaired release of cortisol as well as catecholamines.[117] Because glucocorticoids promote synthesis of epinephrine by activation of phenylethanolamine-N-methyl transferase, it is possible that adrenocortical dysfunction contributes to decreased epinephrine production. Despite the findings of deficiency of epinephrine in these patients, it seems improbable that hypoglycemia can be attributed solely to a deficiency of circulating catecholamines in view of the well-documented experience that hypoglycemia does not occur in patients following bilateral adrenalectomy when they have received adequate replacement therapy with glucocorticoids. Furthermore, adults with familial dysautonomia or patients with sympathetic denervation virtually never have spontaneous fasting hypoglycemia. Thus it is unlikely that catecholamine deficiency is the primary derangement leading to glucopenia in some patients with neonatal hypoglycemia.

Renal Disease

In diabetic and nondiabetic patients with renal failure, prolonged spontaneous hypoglycemia may occur. Among the 18 reported patients, those with diabetes were not taking insulin.[104] The hypoglycemia is intermittent and often profound. Anorexia often preceded hypoglycemic attacks and varying degrees of metabolic acidosis were present in all. Because several of the patients were under treatment with hemodialysis or peritoneal dialysis and an assortment of drugs, it is difficult to be certain as to a common mechanism for the deranged glucose homeostasis in renal failure. In the few patients so far studied, the evidence points to an abnormality in hepatic gluconeogenesis with decreased circulating levels of gluconeogenic precursors, i.e., alanine. Although the case reports are meager, it is possible that hypoglycemia in a malnourished uremic subject may be more common than hitherto realized. It should be suspected in moribund uremic patients, and, if found, treated promptly with parenteral glucose.

Extrapancreatic Neoplasms

As reviewed by Laurent and colleagues,[71] hypoglycemia accompanies tumors that do not originate from insulin-producing cells in the pancreas. This association is rare (approximately 250 reported cases). Occasionally, it may be difficult to distinguish this syndrome from that associated with insulin-producing tumors, particularly when malignantly transformed islets have metastasized. In most instances, however, the diagnosis can be established by clinical criteria. As indicated in Table 16–7, these nonendocrine neoplasms are heterogeneous in composition and location. The tumors derived from ectodermal and endodermal anlagen originate in a number of different organs, whereas more than 40% evolving from mesoderm are situated within the thoracic and peritoneal cavities, with the highest frequency in the retroperitoneal space. The mesenchymal tumors are diverse histologically, but most are classified as fibrosarcomas, rhabdomyosarcomas, leiomyosarcomas, or fibromas. They are usually of low-grade malignancy, enlarge slowly, and are frequently of extraordinary size (2–4 kg and occasionally > 20 kg). They most commonly occur in older individuals, with equal sex distribution. The initial symptoms are likely to be related to glucopenia, and the patient may be unaware of the large tumor, which is detected by physical signs or radiologic or ultrasonic examination. Fasting plasma glucose levels may be extremely low without activation of the sympathetic nervous system, and the clinical manifestations are primarily those of depressed cerebral function. Extrapancreatic neoplasms originating in a number of organs, accompanied by glucopenia, also tend to be large and generally slow-growing. Among Chinese subjects with hepatocellular carcinoma, McFadzean and Yeung [83] have characterized a group of poorly differentiated tumors with accelerated growth, accompanied by rapid and continuous depletion of the extracellular glucose pool.

The pathogenesis of the hypoglycemia associated with these massive tumors has not been clearly established. Studies of the glucose kinetics in some of these patients suggest the cause is multifactorial. Thus, in any individual, increased glucose utilization, decreased glucose production, defective glycogen synthesis and release, and impaired mobilization of alternate metabolic substrates may coexist, all contributing to the profound hypoglycemia.[68] In only a few instances has there been adequate documentation of increased glucose consumption by the gigantic tumor mass. In these patients, glucose turnover rates have been shown to be elevated, with excessive diversion of blood glucose or utilization by the neoplastic tissue, with conversion to lactic acid through anaerobic glycolysis. Although augmented as-

Table 16–7. DISTRIBUTION OF EXTRAPANCREATIC (NON-BETA CELL) TUMORS ASSOCIATED WITH HYPOGLYCEMIA*

Origin	Distribution (%)
Mesenchymal	45
Hepatoma	23
Adrenocortical carcinoma	10
Gastrointestinal carcinoma	8
Lymphoma	6
Miscellaneous (ovary, lung, kidney)	8
	100

*After Laurent, J., et al.: *Hypoglycaemic Tumours.* New York, American Elsevier, 1971.

similation of glucose may contribute to the glucopenia, considerable data indicate that these neoplasms release a factor influencing glucose homeostasis. There is virtually no compelling evidence that these tumors are able to synthesize and store insulin or its precursors.[110] Circulating levels of immunoreactive insulin are very low, and little or no rise is obtained after various insulinogenic stimuli. Therefore, a causal relationship between insulin and the putative tumor hypoglycemic factor is untenable. Most recent data have pointed to a substance produced by these neoplasms that inhibits hepatic gluconeogenesis. By isotopic techniques, diminished glucose production by the liver has been found in some of these patients, and in one person with mesenchymal tumor, a factor of low MW extracted from the tumor has been reported to inhibit the conversion of lactate to glucose in an isolated liver perfusion system. Since tryptophan has been shown to interfere with gluconeogenesis and has been found in elevated amounts in plasma of a few patients with malignancy, this amino acid or its metabolites have been proposed as the inhibitory substance. Nevertheless, neither tryptophan nor its metabolites have been found to be increased in all patients examined. Recently, renewed interest has been focused on nonsuppressible insulin-like activity (NSILA), one of the growth factors with insulin-like properties, as a potential candidate for the hypoglycemic factor elaborated by some of these tumors. The properties of NSILA-s and NSILA-p have been reviewed by Poffenbarger[94] and are also discussed in Ch. 15. Megyesi and colleagues first reported elevated circulating NSILA-s levels in 8 of 13 patients with hypoglycemia and extrapancreatic neoplasms.[101] This relationship has not been confirmed by others. Recently, elevated serum levels of NSILA-p have been found in 8 of 11 patients with non-B cell tumors. Despite these associations, it is still premature to attribute the hypoglycemia to either one or the other of these substances, and additional studies are necessary to establish whether an antigluconeogenic humoral factor elaborated by the tumors is responsible for the hypoglycemia. A large intrathoracic or intra-abdominal mass, in conjunction with hypoglycemia and low levels of circulating immunoreactive insulin and relative hyporesponsiveness to insulintropic stimuli, distinguishes patients with nonpancreatic neoplasms from those with insulin-producing tumors. Occasionally, remissions can be effected by surgical resection. For the most part, the size and location of the tumors preclude their complete removal, and, in general, they are resistant to radiation or chemotherapy. Hence, treatment is directed primarily to maintenance of tolerable plasma glucose levels by frequent intake of food high in carbohydrates. Glucocorticoids in pharmacologic doses occasionally provide some benefit. Diazoxide has usually been ineffectual.

Idiopathic Hypoglycemia of Infancy and Childhood

A number of hypoglycemic disorders occurring in the newborn and extending into adolescence have been characterized clinically and the pathogenesis explained in part, so that they are no longer classified as idiopathic. In spite of advances in our understanding of the mechanisms underlying several of these hypoglycemic syndromes, there remains a group of children with causes of low plasma sugar that are unresolved, and therefore are retained under this ill-defined category.[89]

The highest incidence of hypoglycemia in humans is during the neonatal period. As many as 10% of all neonates have at least one abnormally low blood glucose reading.

The incidence of symptomatic transient neonatal hypoglycemia approximates 0.3% of all live births.[18] In the newborn with idiopathic transient hypoglycemia, plasma glucose levels of less than 20 mg/dl are frequently seen. The susceptible infants are usually males of low birth weight for the period of gestation, with a tendency to polycythemia, primary nervous system damage or anomalies, and hypocalcemia. Clinical manifestations occur within 72 hours and usually include tremors, jitteriness and twitchiness, cyanosis, convulsions, apnea, respiratory abnormalities, apathy, high-pitched or weak cry, limpness, and refusal to feed. Hypoglycemia in infants who are small for gestational age is probably related to diminished hepatic glycogen storage owing to poor intrauterine nutrition. Additional contributing factors include a high basal metabolic rate and exaggerated insulin response to change in blood glucose, with impaired gluconeogenesis. Premature infants born prior to 37 weeks' gestation are at greater risk for hypoglycemia because of deficient hepatic glycogen stores. Treatment consists of parenteral glucose administration, and usually within a few days, plasma sugar levels return to normal.

Of the cases of hypoglycemia developing in children before the age of 2 years, the majority have been shown to be related to hypersensitivity to leucine, have been induced by a ketogenic diet, or have nesidioblastosis or an islet cell adenoma (discussed later). Nevertheless, a small group remains without a well-defined mechanism for the hypoglycemia. Low blood sugars may be continuous or intermittent, and symptoms are variable in severity. Eventually the hypoglycemia undergoes spontaneous remission over a period of months or years. Although a familial tendency was originally stressed, this has not been invariable. Of possible significance is the fact that five of seven affected children reported by Rosenbloom and Sherman[100] ultimately developed diabetes mellitus, and a high proportion of close relatives of these children had abnormal carbohydrate tolerance. High insulin levels were not found during episodic hypoglycemia in these children, but it is possible that an abnormality in insulin release may have been a factor in the glucopenic phases of this disorder.

Overutilization of Glucose

Hypersecretion of Insulin

Intrinsic Abnormalities of Pancreatic B Cells (Neoplastic Transformation, Insulinoma). A relationship between hypoglycemia and pancreatic B-cell tumors was recognized in 1927, and it is now established that the clinical syndrome is due to excessive insulin production and release by the autonomously functioning B cells. Despite tremendous enthusiasm in correctly diagnosing this disorder because of a high likelihood of curing hypoglycemia, it is an uncommon cause of glucopenia. At routine autopsy, the incidence of islet cell tumors has been reported to vary from 1 in 8,000 to 1 in 63. In a survey at the Mayo Clinic, in 10,314 autopsies, 44 islet cell tumors were found, 8 of which were functional.[75] Probably a realistic estimate of clinically important hyperfunctional tumors is less than 1 to 100,000. The pathologic classification includes (1) nesidioblastosis representing diffuse islet cell proliferation from ductal epithelium, (2) diffuse B-cell hyperplasia, (3) microadenomatosis, (4) B-cell adenoma, and (5) carcinoma. Of these, benign adenomata are found in 90% of cases.[109] They are multiple in less than 8%. The majority measure 10–50 mm (90% < 20 mm) in diameter, with an occasional adenoma under 1 mm. Single adenomata have a comparable frequency distribution in the head, body, and tail of the pancreas. Microadenomatosis scattered among normal sites is uncommon. Approximately 10% of insulin-producing tumors are malignant and metastasize most frequently to the liver and regional lymph nodes. Histologic differentiation between adenoma and carcinoma in pancreatic masses may be difficult, and the diagnosis of malignancy requires evidence of capsular invasion or extrapancreatic extension. Nesidioblastosis and B-cell hyperplasia are extremely rare and, although not exclusively, are most likely to be encountered in infants.[116]

The clinical features of hyperfunctioning B-cell tumors appear most frequently in persons 30–60 years of age, with a slight predilection to affect women in later years in life. Functional adenomas are rare in the newborn (less than 20 reported cases) and in adolescents (less than 60 reported cases).[116] Since the symptoms may mimic a wide variety of neuropsychiatric disorders and may be intermittent and nonspecific, the diagnosis may be unsuspected for many years. Aberrant behavior patterns and disturbances in consciousness are the most common features.[19] Symptoms occur episodically but often appear before breakfast and late in the afternoon and are ameliorated shortly after eating. They are frequently exacerbated by protracted fasting or vigorous physical exercise. Because of the gradual decline in plasma sugar, often achieving levels less than 25 mg/dl, a triggering of catecholamine release may not occur, and confusion, amnesia, and loss of consciousness with the depression of vasomotor function may be the initial or sole manifestations. Hunger is an uncommon symptom, and there is no strong correlation with obesity. Between attacks there are no distinctive physical findings; depending upon the duration and degree of hypoglycemia, insidious intellectual deterioration may occur. Because insulin may be released sporadically by the tumor and symptoms are often misattributed for years, there is no correlation between clinical manifestations and size of adenoma. The clinical picture associated with hyperfunctional carcinoma may be impossible to differentiate from that of the benign cell neoplasm early in the course and will depend upon findings at laparotomy, with histopathologic confirmation. Clues to cancer include increased frequency and severity of the hypoglycemic episodes with metastases indicated by an enlarged nodular liver.[10] Although it has been common experience that functioning islet cell carcinomas usually grow rapidly, with death occurring within 2–3 years of diagnosis, most of the patients are detected when the tumor has spread. It is also possible that they may have been harboring the malignantly transformed tumors for years, and case reports attest to the indolent nature of some of these tumors in a few patients.[62]

Obviously, hypoglycemia in this setting is the direct consequence of the actions of excessive levels of insulin and its precursors released by the neoplastic B cell. The combined actions of insulin, including inhibition of hepatic glucose output and diminished flow of gluconeogenic precursors, with concomitant augmented glucose translocation into peripheral tissues deplete the extracellular glucose pool, often with great rapidity. Despite the release of several counterregulatory hormones, their actions are overwhelmed by the inordinate amounts of circulating insulin. Partial protection against the excess insulin may be afforded by the adaptation of insulin receptors to high levels, leading to a decrease in their number.[101] Insulinomas are composed entirely of islet cells. Frequently, insulin-containing granules in the B cells are immature, implicating abnormalities in synthesis, storage, and release of insulin. This is corroborated by the aberrant control of insulin secretion in these neoplasms, which are usually autonomous. Normally, granular discharge of insulin is linked to the ambient glucose level and also modulated by a number of ancillary signals.

In contrast, in insulinomas, insulin may be released episodically or continuously at inappropriately low blood sugar concentrations. The capricious, unregulated discharge of insulin accounts for the unpredictable temporal relationship to meals and the variable degree of hypoglycemia. A further index of the abnormal secretory apparatus is provided by the reversal of the relative responsiveness of the B cell to physiologic and pharmacologic stimuli. Thus, the normal B cell usually responds to glucose > tolbutamide > glucagon > leucine, whereas the neoplastic B cell hyperresponds to glucagon > tolbutamide > leucine > glucose. This transposition of the order of sensitivity to insulin release provides the basis for the provocative tests of insulin hypersecretion in insulinomas.[35] Furthermore, the relative refractoriness of neoplastic cells to glucose explains the erratic responses to oral glucose. Not infrequently, during an OGTT the patient with a functional adenoma will display a "diabetic" profile.[64] Deranged synthesis and release of insulin has been demonstrated by the excessively high levels of C-peptide, proinsulin, and related insulin precursors in plasma of patients with insulinomas. C-peptide levels are inappropriately elevated in patients with insulinomas. Although tumor content of insulin and related peptides is usually elevated in the adenoma relative to adjacent nonaffected pancreas, there is no relationship between plasma levels and tumor content of insulin precursors at time of surgical resection.

An insulinoma may be suspected in a patient who fulfills the triad described by Whipple (symptomatic, fasting hypoglycemia reversed by glucose).[17] Nonetheless, since these criteria are nonspecific, confirmation of the clinical suspicion of this disorder depends upon (1) documentation of levels of insulin (C-peptide or proinsulin) that are inappropriately elevated for the prevailing plasma glucose levels and (2) identification of the pancreatic tumor.

The diagnosis of inappropriate hyperinsulinism due to B-cell dysfunction is best established during the fasting state.[31] After fasting for 12–14 hours, 80% of patients with islet cell tumors will have abnormally low levels of plasma glucose with inappropriately high insulin concentrations. Since basal insulin and glucose levels normally decline with fasting, establishment of criteria for abnormalcy is essential. Service and coworkers[109] have used the values of IRI levels greater than 6 μU/ml in conjunction with plasma glucose levels below the normal fasting range to improve the accuracy of diagnosis (Fig. 16–12). Occasionally, difficulties may be encountered in interpretation in extremely obese individuals who have elevated basal insulin levels associated with their increased adipose mass. Furthermore, since secretion from insulinomas may be sporadic, it is often necessary to repeat the analysis on several mornings. With more prolonged periods of food deprivation, there is an increased likelihood of demonstrating inappropriate levels of glucose and insulin. Consequently, it may be necessary to hospitalize patients to subject them to fasting for up to 72 hours under close supervision with periodic blood sampling, particularly at times when they become symptomatic. Moderate exercise may be superimposed to precipitate a hypoglycemic episode. In the series reported by Scholz[106], 75% of patients had glucopenic reactions within 24 hours of onset of fast and in only two was it necessary to continue food deprivation beyond 48 hours. Patients with islet cell carcinoma usually develop profound hypoglycemia with markedly elevated immunoreactive insulin levels within 24 hours. In these patients, as well as in the individual with equivocally low insulin levels, the measurement of circulating proinsulin-like substances, if elevated in a setting of hypoglycemia, establishes the diagnosis.[118]

Inhibition of endogenous secretion of insulin, C-peptide,

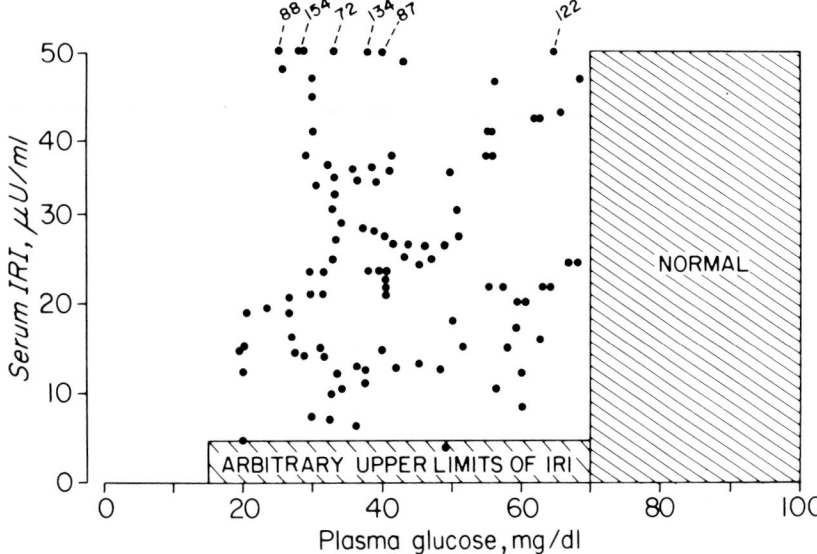

Figure 16–12. Simultaneous, unstimulated, fasting (overnight) plasma glucose and serum insulin (IRI) levels for patients with insulinoma (144 points from 27 patients). Normal fasting state ranges are shown by hatched areas, and arbitary upper limits of IRI of 6 μU/ml at low levels of plasma glucose. (Adapted from Service, F. J., Dale, A. J., et al.: Insulinoma: clinical and diagnostic features of 60 consecutive cases. *Mayo Clin. Proc. 51*:417, 1976.)

and proinsulin by glucopenia, induced by infusing insulin, has been proposed as a useful test in patients suspected of having autonomously functioning B cells and is usually performed in those individuals who have equivocal findings of insulin and glucose levels during fasting. The principle is based upon the normal suppression of insulin C-peptide or proinsulin levels during hypoglycemia, whereas those with hyperfunctioning tissue will not show inhibition. The induction of hypoglycemia with fish insulin and the suppression of endogenous insulin levels provide excellent differentiation between patients with insulinomas and normal subjects[119]; fish insulin is not readily available throughout the world, however. Horowitz and coworkers[56] have employed the measurement of C-peptide levels during hypoglycemia produced by the infusion of porcine or bovine insulin. In normal individuals, the C-peptide level falls to less than 2 ng/ml and glucose levels are less than 50 ml/dl. In 11 of 12 patients with surgically identified islet cell adenomas studied by these investigators, suppression of endogenous C-peptide secretion was impaired. Normal or near-normal suppression of C-peptide secretion has also been reported in patients with proven islet cell adenomas, however; this discrepancy reflects the heterogeneity of the tumors as well as the longer circulating half-life of the C-peptide compared with that of insulin.[118] The measurement of C-peptide levels is of particular usefulness in insulin-treated diabetic patients with circulating insulin antibodies who might be suspected of having an insulinoma, as well as in those individuals surreptitiously self-administering insulin.

Measurement of plasma human proinsulin during insulin-induced hypoglycemia in 15 patients with insulinoma studied by Turner and Heding[118] have shown excellent discrimination; however, the restriction of the measurement of human proinsulin to research laboratories limits its general applicability.

Several techniques that elicit insulin release have been used in an attempt to characterize patients with islet cell neoplasms based on a hypernormal response. It is to be reiterated that after oral glucose loading, plasma sugar levels are frequently difficult to interpret in patients with insulinoma. Typically, the profile of blood glucose responses tends to be considerably lower than normal throughout a 5-hour test period; however, not infrequently, the responses may paradoxically resemble the patterns characteristic of diabetes mellitus. This widely variable response reflects the autonomous nature of the tumor and therefore precludes the OGTT as a useful diagnostic test. Leucine administered orally (or occasionally intravenously) may cause an excessive insulin response in patients with islet cell tumors, as well as in children with leucine hypersensitivity. Leucine testing is associated with a high proportion of falsely negative responses, and generally has fallen into disfavor, however.[64] Pharmacologic tests to evoke excessive release of insulin in attempt to distinguish patients with islet cell neoplasms include (1) intravenous tolbutamide, (2) intravenous glucagon, and (3) intravenous calcium.[35, 79, 102] With islet cell tumors, the tolbutamide response is characterized by an acute decline in plasma glucose with an attenuated rebound during 120–150 min. Plasma insulin usually rises rapidly to very high levels, which are sustained for 40–90 min (Fig. 16–13). In some series, 90% of patients have an abnormal response, yet a number of false-negative and false-positive results have also been reported.[64] Tolbutamide should not be administered to patients with fasting plasma glucose below 45 mg/dl, and the test should be terminated with parenteral glucose if the patient becomes disoriented or unconscious. Similarly, intravenous glucagon causes an inordinate release of insulin in patients with insulinoma, and, because it induces glycogenolysis with hyperglycemia, it is safer than tolbutamide and may be advantageous in evaluation of older subjects. Nonetheless, as with tolbutamide, a number of false-positive and false-negative results have been encountered. In a few patients, calcium infusion significantly increased plasma insulin levels and reduced blood glucose, which was not found in normal volunteers. Its usefulness is yet to be established.

From the accumulated experience, it would appear that no single provocative test or suppression test will categorically establish the diagnosis of endogenous hyperinsulinism in all patients. The best discriminate test for autonomous B cell hyperfunction is the measurement of glucose and insulin levels during fasting, and the tolbutamide test is a useful adjunctive procedure that is readily available. The measurement of proinsulin levels and the insulin suppression test are most likely to be helpful in patients with equivocal results during the fast and tolbutamide test. Tests to foretell malignant transformation in islet cell tumors prior to laparotomy with histopathologic confirmation have not been highly reliable. In general, patients with islet cell carcinoma tend to

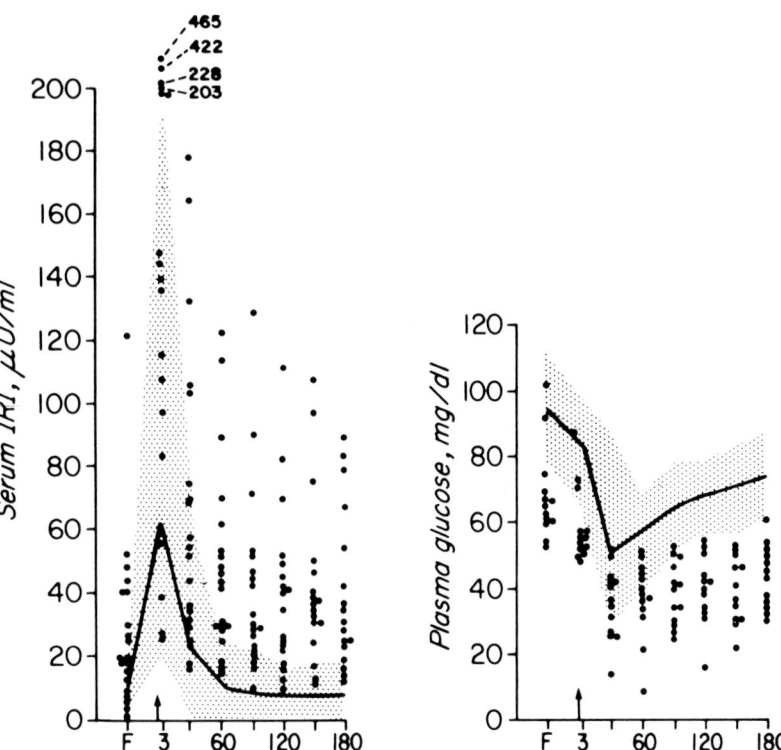

Figure 16–13. Plasma glucose and serum insulin (IRI) in patients with insulinomas given tolbutamide (1.0 g IV). Shaded areas and solid lines represent range and mean for control group. Arrow indicates injection of tolbutamide. (Modified from Service, F. J., Dale, A. J., et al.: Insulinoma: clinical and diagnostic features of 60 consecutive cases. *Mayo Clin. Proc. 51*:417, 1976.)

Minutes after tolbutamide

have higher percentages of circulating proinsulin-like substances. Nevertheless, since there is no correlation between the level of hormonal differentiation and the degree of cellular differentiation, it cannot be used as a predictor of cancer.[10, 49] Kahn and associates[61] have examined plasma levels of hCG and the subunits (hCG-α, hCG-β) as potential tumor markers in 14 patients with proven malignant insulinoma and found that 50% of hCG-α, 21% of hCG-β, and 25% of hCG were elevated. In contrast, in 41 patients with benign insulinomas, none of these markers were high. Therefore, the increased ectopic production of these polypeptides may be helpful in suggesting a malignant neoplasm and also may be used to follow results of therapy.

Once the diagnosis of hyperinsulinism has been confirmed, the localization of an intrapancreatic mass may be aided preoperatively by angiographic techniques using selective catheterization of the celiac and superior mesenteric arteries. The success of positive radiographic identification ranges from 20–80% (mean 63%), and the variation in accuracy probably reflects the dimensions and vascularity of the tumor as well as the advancing technology and experience of the radiologist.[99] Occasional false localization of bonafide insulinomas has occurred. Malignant transformation may be suspected if the tumor exceeds 3 cm in diameter and if the tumor margins are not well circumscribed. Angiography may also provide evidence of liver metastases before they can be appreciated by conventional liver scanning techniques. The use of selective catheterization of splenic and portal veins at laparotomy, with measurement of insulin levels in venous effluents, may occasionally be helpful retrospectively in localizing tumors in regions of the pancreas when surgeons were unable to identify a small lesion.[120] Although these procedures may be of assistance in guiding the surgeon, the localization of the tumor can only be confirmed by palpation at laparotomy or located in serial frozen sections.

Treatment of Patients with Abnormal B-Cell Function. In patients in whom there are no medical contraindications to a laparotomy, surgical resection of the solitary functional benign islet cell tumor will effect a cure. Because of the threat of sporadic, sustained hypoglycemia during the operation, the anesthesiologist should be alerted to the need for supplementary intravenous infusion of glucose. A short trial of diazoxide plus a diuretic, i.e. benzothiadiazine, prior to laparotomy has been recommended to minimize glucopenia during surgery.[31] Preoperative administration of glucose, with or without intramuscular or intravenous glucocorticoids, has also been advocated routinely as prophylaxis against hypoglycemia and occasional high postoperative fever encountered in these patients. Alternatively, the medical consultant may opt not to infuse glucose, since a small adenoma may not be palpated or may be overlooked on pancreatic sections, and serial plasma glucose levels, which rise after resection of the adenoma, may serve as an indication to cease the search. In all cases, low plasma sugar concentrations should be assiduously avoided because of the potential for cerebral damage. If the tumor is not discovered within the pancreas or in the usual sites of ectopic rest formation, progressive sectioning of the pancreas from tail to head is undertaken, with examination of the specimens by the pathologist as well as frequent monitoring of plasma glucose. At the University of Washington, our surgical colleagues usually do not exceed 80% pancreatectomy as a primary procedure. In neonates with persistent hypoglycemia attributable to nesidioblastosis or pancreatic hyperplasia, an 80% pancreatectomy will frequently alleviate the clinical manifestations of hyperinsulinemia. In some series, blind partial pancreatectomy has been reported to remove from 25–34% of insulinomas. Because in approximately 10% of cases more than one tumor is found, it is important to carefully palpate the entire pancreas after localization of a presumed solitary mass. As reviewed by Stefanini,[112] the outcome of operations in 1067 cases of insulinoma was cure in 63%, persistent hypoglycemia in 16%, and long-term hyperglycemia in 10%. Operative mortality was 11%. Complications included pancreatitis, peritonitis, chronic fistulae, and pseudocysts. Failure to find tumors or persistent postoperative hypoglycemia may require reoperation, and in the cases with recurrent hyperinsulinemia from nesidioblastosis or hyperplasia, a total pancreatectomy may be necessary.[116] In patients in whom surgery may be delayed, refused, or deemed inappropriate, dietary and pharmacologic management must be provided with the object of maintaining normal or moderately elevated plasma glucose levels. Dietary manipulations by frequent intake of foods high in complex carbohydrates, which are more slowly absorbed, may minimize severe glucopenic symptoms. During hypoglycemic attacks, fruit juices or candy should be taken. With profound unremitting hypoglycemia, continuous infusion of 10–20% glucose may be needed. In addition, a number of hormones and pharmacologic agents have been used with varying success in attempts to maintain euglycemia. Zinc glucagon (1–5 mg), administered subcutaneously or intramuscularly, may elevate plasma sugar for several hours. Epinephrine also increases plasma glucose, but it requires intravenous administration and may have adverse cardiovascular effects. Glucocorticoids, administered intramuscularly as cortisone acetate (100–200 mg) or intravenously as hydrocortisone hemisuccinate (100 mg) may blunt the glucopenic manifestations. Diphenylhydantoin (100 mg tid) and propranolol (40–60 mg qid) have been reported to diminish insulin secretion in patients with benign or malignant insulinoma, but they are not universally effective. Furthermore, propranolol may attenuate or abolish the premonitory adrenergic symptoms when blood glucose falls. In most instances, all of these hormones or drugs, given singularly or in combination, are temporarily palliative and often have undesirable side effects.

Diazoxide, a nondiuretic benzothiadiazene, has proved to be beneficial in patients with hypoglycemia of diverse etiology, notably those with hyperinsulinism.[80] Diazoxide has also raised plasma glucose levels in a few patients with "idiopathic hypoglycemia of childhood" and occasionally in individuals with Type I glycogen storage disease.[89] Diazoxide acts by inhibiting insulin secretion as well as by enhancing the release of epinephrine, which also impedes insulin output. In addition, this drug directly enhances hepatic glycogenolysis and decreases glucose uptake in muscle in inhibiting phosphodiesterases. Therapeutic oral doses of diazoxide vary between 300 and 800 mg/day in patients with insulinoma. Because diazoxide causes sodium retention, the diuretic trichlormethiazide is used concomitantly to alleviate edema. Other major adverse effects include gastrointestinal irritation, hypertrichosis, and agranulocytosis. Intravenous diazoxide may rarely cause hypotension. Although this drug provides an important adjunct in therapy of patients with intractable hypoglycemia and patients have been managed for several years on oral diazoxide,[31] in some individuals with islet cell carcinoma and in most with hypoglycemia due to extrapancreatic neoplasms, this agent is ineffectual.

The most commonly used drug to treat patients with metastatic islet cell carcinoma is streptozocin, an antibiotic containing the structure N-methyl-nitroso-urea-glucosamine, which has been shown to be cytotoxic to pancreatic B cells and to inhibit DNA-dependent RNA synthesis in tumor cells.[11] Patients treated with this drug experience remission of symptomatic hypoglycemia along with objective evidence of tumor regression lasting for several months and occasionally a few years. Streptozocin has been administered by peripheral vein or into the celiac artery to maximize concentration within the pancreas and liver. Currently rec-

ommended intravenous dosage is 500 mg/m² body surface area daily for 5 days, which is repeated as necessary, dependent on signs of tumor regression and the effects on renal function, since nephrotoxicity, due to renal tubular damage, is the most serious side effect. In addition, nausea and vomiting and reversible hepatitis are invariable sequelae from this drug. 5-Fluorouracil (5-FU), at 500 mg/m² for 5 days may be given concomitantly. A few patients have received mithramycin, Adriamycin, and L-asparaginase with variable remission of hypoglycemic symptoms.[31] The toxicity of these agents usually precludes their repetitive use.

Insulinoma Associated with Other Endocrine Syndromes. Functioning B-cell tumors may coexist with other primary endocrine abnormalities. The syndromes of multiple endocrine adenomatosis (MEA) are characterized by the appearance of several tumors or hyperplasia involving diverse endocrine organs. These constellations are typically familial, and the transformation of specific endocrine cells tends to cluster into two major groups. In "MEA Type I" there is an association of tumors or hyperplasia of the parathyroids, pancreatic islets, and pituitary.[5] The second group, "MEA Type II," is classified into Type IIA— medullary thyroid carcinoma, pheochromocytoma, and hyperparathyroidism — and Type IIB — medullary thyroid carcinoma, pheochromocytoma, rarely parathyroid disorders, with mucosal ganglial neuroromatosis, extending from lips to the rectum.[113, 124] In MEA Type I, clinical manifestations of hyperparathyroidism, hyper- and hypofunction of the pituitary, intractable ulcer disease, and hyperglycemia or glucopenia may appear in various combinations. In one extensive review of MEA Type I, pancreatic islet cell involvement was found in 69 of 85 cases, with hypoglycemia in 36%.[5] In patients with the severe peptic ulcer diathesis (Zollinger-Ellison syndrome), elevated basal acid secretion, the hallmark of this disorder, is due to excessive gastrin production from one or more islet cell tumors. In 260 patients with gastrin-secreting adenomas, Ellison and Wilson[27] found that 10 had coexisting insulinomas.

The common denominator of the diverse endocrine organ involvement in MEA remains speculative. Since many of the endocrine cells that become transformed share certain biochemic features, i.e., amine precursor uptake and decarboxylation (APUD), and are probably embryologically derived from neurally programmed cells of epiblastic origin (Ch. 14), it is possible that the abnormality resides in information coding in all affected tissues. APUDomas presumably represent mutations in germinal cells that may be inherited by an autosomal mechanism leading to a predisposition to hyperplasia, and neoplastic transformation may be imparted from the environment, i.e., virus.[66] Practically, in a setting of hypoglycemia attributable to a pancreatic islet cell tumor, with a family history positive for other endocrine dysfunction, the clinician should be alerted to the possibility of other endocrine abnormalities in the patient, and, conversely, the possibility of an insulin-producing tumor in one or more of the patient's relatives should be kept in mind.

Sporadic reports have appeared describing patients with islet cell tumors in whom insulin, gastrin, glucagon, and pancreatic polypeptide, in combination, have been excessively produced, reflecting autonomous hyperfunction of one or more of the four major islet cell types.[70] In addition, in a few patients with islet cell carcinoma, the ectopic manufacture of polypeptide hormones, including ACTH, MSH, vasopressin, and parathyroid hormone (PTH) in one or more constellations has also been documented. Thus, manifestations of hypoglycemia may coexist with the clinical picture of other endocrine abnormalities because of hormones elaborated by neoplastic pancreatic tissue. The aberrant production of hormones normally manufactured by islet cells has been thought to be due to activation of genetic structural information that is derepressed during neoplastic transformation. in patients with multiple endocrine dysfunction, the diagnostic approaches and treatment of the insulin-secreting pancreatic tumors are similar to those described in the preceding section.

Autoimmune Hypoglycemia. A syndrome of fasting or postprandial hypoglycemic episodes associated with spuriously high values for serum insulin detected by radioimmunoassay has been described in 9 persons ranging in age from 3 days to 77 years.[41] In all patients, antibodies against human and other mammalian insulin were found; no specific antibodies directed to C-peptides of bovine or porcine proinsulins could be detected, however. Conventional causes for hypoglycemia were excluded, and no evidence for surreptitious self-administration of insulin could be obtained. Thus, an autoimmune origin for the insulin antibodies in patients with this syndrome has been postulated. The pathogenesis of the hypoglycemia in patients with this disorder is yet to be clarified. Since several have displayed a diabetic OGTT, it is conceivable that the circulating antibodies may prevent the immediate action of the bound hormone, and under unknown circumstances, the binding activity of hormone to antibody is altered, resulting in excessive release of insulin at inappropriate times. Because of the complex nature of the disorder and difficulty in distinguishing it from factitious hypoglycemia, the diagnosis can only be established by forwarding appropriate samples to selected research laboratories. Treatment would seemingly be directed to the maintenance of adequate carbohydrate in the diet and intravenous glucose emergently.

Neonatal Hypoglycemia In Infants of Diabetic Mothers. During the first 48–72 hours of life, infants born to mothers with overt or gestational diabetes may have sustained hypoglycemia with plasma glucose below 15 mg/dl. They often have cherubic appearance and have a propensity for a variety of malformations, with acute respiratory distress syndrome a prominent clinical feature. The degree of glucopenia has been shown to correlate with maternal carbohydrate tolerance. It is now well established that affected neonates have elevated circulating insulin levels with increased pancreatic insulin content and B-cell hyperplasia.[81] The most plausible explanation for the transitory hyperinsulinemia is that the fetus is exposed to chronic hyperglycemia originating from the maternal circulation, thereby inducing B-cell hyperfunction. At birth, gluconeogenic mechanisms are inhibited by high levels of plasma insulin, leading to hypoglycemia. Paradoxically, increased insulin receptor binding has been reported, which may lead to increased insulin sensitivity. This effect may be aggravated by temporarily suppressed glucagon secretion as a consequence of persistent hyperglycemia in the fetus. Hypoglycemia also occurs in infants of diabetic mothers who have received sulfonylurea compounds, which are transported across the placenta and cause fetal hyperinsulinism. In most patients, frequent feedings suffice to revert plasma glucose to normal within a few days. Occasionally, parenteral glucose is required. Glucagon, 0.1–0.3 mg/kg, intramuscularly, has also been effective. Since the underlying cause of neonatal hypoglycemia is related to maternal hyperglycemia, efforts should be made to more effectively "control" the degree of hyperglycemia in the mother throughout pregnancy.

Erythroblastosis Fetalis. In infants who sustain hemolysis because of Rh immunization (erythroblastosis fetalis), hypoglycemia may occur during the first 3 days of life.[95] The severity of the glucopenia is inversely correlated with the cord blood hemoglobin concentration. Plasma insulin levels in cord blood have been shown to be elevated during the first 24 hours after birth, and pancreatic islet cell hyperplasia with increased insulin content has been documented. During exchange transfusion, plasma insulin levels have been noted to rise markedly. Although the mechanism is uncertain, it has been postulated that insulin in the fetus is rapidly destroyed by the hemolyzed red cells, leading to a compensatory islet cell hyperplasia. Therefore, in the newborn, the increased hyperinsulinemia occurring during the exchange transfusion may be explained by the diminished insulin degradation after replacement with nonhemolyzed cells. Treatment is primarily supportive, with parenteral glucose, and if the child survives the hemolytic crises, glucopenia remits spontaneously.

Miscellaneous Syndromes

Beckwith and Widman initially drew attention to a syndrome in neonates consisting of macroglossia, omphalocele, postnatal gigantism, visceromegaly, and various other defects inherited as an autosomal recessive trait.[98] Between 30 and 50% of affected infants have hypoglycemia. Islet cell hyperplasia has been reported in a few patients without consistent changes in pancreatic insulin content.[89] Insulin levels in patients with Beckwith's syndrome tend to be markedly elevated. The pathogenesis of the pancreatic abnormalities is unresolved.

Donohue first described an infant with elfin-like facial features, hirsutism, and multiple endocrine abnormalities, including hypoglycemia; this syndrome has been called leprechaunism.[98] Glucopenia occurs episodically during fasting, interspersed with hyperglycemia. Islet cell hyperplasia has been noted along with marked hyperinsulinemia and insulin resistance. A defect in insulin action beyond the level of the cell membrane receptor has been suggested.

Hypersensitivity to Insulin

Growth Hormone Deficiency. Symptomatic fasting hypoglycemia is found in approximately 10% of patients with panhypopituitarism maintained on glucocorticoids and is due to lack of GH.[8] That GH modifies the action of insulin has been established in hypophysectomized humans by the marked attenuation of the rebound of plasma glucose after insulin, which is rectified by GH administration. These data indicate that, in the absence of GH, peripheral glucose utilization is increased, owing to the unopposed action of insulin. Increased numbers and affinities of insulin receptor sites on circulating monocytes have been recently shown in patients with isolated GH deficiency, which may contribute to heightened insulin sensitivity.[111] Hypoglycemia may occur both during the fasting and 5–6 hours post cibum in patients with GH deficiency. A variety of lesions may lead to partial or total GH lack (Ch. 5). These include chromophobe adenomas, craniopharyngiomas, and more rarely, granulomatous infiltrations and acute pituitary necrosis due to postpartum hemorrhage, carotid aneurysms, or thrombosis. Hypoglycemia occurs in patients who have had hypophysectomy for carcinoma of the breast or for treatment of retinopathy in insulin-dependent diabetics. In the latter patient, difficulty in their management occurs owing to increased sensitivity to exogenous insulin. Low blood sugar may accompany pituitary dwarfism, which describes forms of short stature from genetically transmitted defects in GH secretion. It is now recognized that absence of GH may occur as an isolated phenomenon or in combination with deficiencies of one or more other tropic hormones. Six distinct forms of hereditary pituitary dwarfism have been reviewed by Rimoin and Schimke.[98] They include congenital absence of the pituitary, familial panhypopituitarism, isolated GH deficiency I, isolated GH deficiency II, Laron-type dwarfism, and pygmies. They share some clinical features, including a normal appearance at birth with a gradual growth retardation. Each of the different categories has characteristic physical findings. Except in dwarfs with isolated GH deficiency II and pygmies, fasting hypoglycemic attacks occur early in life and are more severe in those dwarfs who also have ACTH deficiencies. In patients with isolated GH deficiency I and Laron-type dwarfism, the spontaneous occurrence of hypoglycemia lessens with age. With the exception of dwarfs with isolated GH deficiency II, all groups have diminished insulin secretion and are hypersensitive to exogenous insulin. GH levels measured during fasting and in response to various stimuli are low in all but the Laron-type dwarf and the pygmy. Pygmies have been shown unresponsive to exogenous GH. Because they have normal somatomedin levels, it has been postulated that there is a disturbance in the somatomedin target cell interaction. In the Laron dwarf, somatomedin levels are low, and the most plausible explanation for the syndrome is a defect in GH receptors.[14] The procedures to establish the diagnosis of GH deficiency in states of pituitary hypofunction and dwarfism are detailed in Ch. 5. Because of its scarcity, human GH, which rectifies the abnormalities in glucose homeostasis, is reserved primarily for treatment of short stature in GH-deficient children. In adults, specific therapy of hypoglycemic episodes requires dietary manipulation by frequent feedings high in complex carbohydrates and, when appropriate, by use of maintenance oral glucocorticoids.

PHARMACOGENIC AND TOXIC CAUSES OF HYPOGLYCEMIA

Exogenous Insulin Administration

Self-administration of insulin is the most common cause of hypoglycemia. In almost all instances, the patients are diabetic; occasionally, however, for bizarre psychologic reasons, individuals may inject themselves surreptitiously with insulin to simulate organic disease. This so-called "factitious" cause of hypoglycemia is usually encountered in young women with some exposure to medical practice, i.e., nurse's aides. The clandestine use of insulin results in symptoms mimicking those of organic hyperinsulinism and may lead the physician to embark on an enthusiastic work-up for an insulin-producing tumor. Factitious hypoglycemia should be suspected in a patient with an inconsistent history and numerous hospitalizations, often resulting in laparotomy for a variety of abdominal complaints. Such individuals have been described as having Munchausen's syndrome ("problem peregrinating patients," since they wander from hospital to hospital). The psychopathology of this condition is uncertain and is usually resistant to therapy. In all persons who are suspected of fraudulent hypoglycemia, finding low plasma levels of C-peptide in the face of high insulin levels during periods of hypoglycemia would virtually exclude the presence of endogenous hyperinsulinism.[105] The presence of insulin antibodies also would strengthen the suspicion of a "foreign" source of insulin. An intensive search for an insulin ampule or syringe should be undertaken and addition of ^{131}I hippuran to the discovered ampule with the detection of radioisotope in the patient's urine confirms the diagnosis.

Hypoglycemic episodes among insulin-dependent brittle diabetics are the rule rather than the exception, and the ill consequences are far more common and serious than are generally appreciated. Abnormal EEG's have been found in 50% of diabetics with frequent severe insulin reactions.[44]

These adverse responses to insulin are correlated with the severity and instability of the diabetes. Although the symptoms vary from individual to individual, they tend to have a characteristic pattern for each subject. The rapid decline in plasma sugar usually triggers the sympathetic nervous system with characteristic adrenergic symptoms. This constellation is most frequently seen in patients receiving short-acting insulin. Convulsions are more frequent in children than in adults. Most attacks are reversed spontaneously by endogenous counter-regulation or are aborted by food intake before marked cerebral cortical depression occurs. With intermediate and long-acting insulins, notably protamine zinc insulin, plasma sugar levels may fall more gradually without activating the sympathetic nervous system, resulting in depression of higher cortical centers eventuating in convulsions or coma or both. Because of these untoward effects, many of the long-acting insulins have fallen into disfavor among clinicians. Additional factors that may precipitate hypoglycemia in such patients are (1) decreased or delayed food intake, (2) strenuous or prolonged exercise without additional nutrients, and (3) excessive ethanol ingestion with avoidance of food. A cardinal point to be emphasized in the management of such patients is the early recognition and prompt treatment of the hypoglycemia. In the insulin-dependent diabetic who is first seen in an emergency room in a comatose state, it is essential to distinguish glucopenia from hyperglycemic ketoacidosis. The major clinical and laboratory findings that differentiate these disorders are outlined in Table 16–8. If the physician is uncertain as to which is the cause of the coma, it is wise to administer parenteral glucose promptly after obtaining a sample for glucose analysis, since in this instance, less cerebral damage is likely to ensue from an error of commission than from one of omission.

Sulfonylureas

Seltzer,[108] in a review of the published cases of severe drug-induced hypoglycemia in 1972, found 220 of 473 cases attributable to sulfonylureas, with the greatest number due to chlorpropamide. The incidence of hypoglycemia with sulfonylureas is doubtless greater than is documented in the literature. It has been estimated that about 5% of individuals receiving oral hypoglycemic agents have glucopenic reactions. The mechanisms of actions of sulfonylureas are detailed in Ch. 15. The drugs initially stimulate insulin release but chronically inhibit both its synthesis and secretion. Long-term sulfonylurea therapy alters the plasma membrane of cells, thereby enhancing their responsiveness to insulin action, perhaps by increasing the number of insulin receptors. It is not known how these agents produce sustained hypoglycemia in susceptible subjects. Although the development of hypoglycemia after sulfonylureas may be idiosyncratic, a number of factors predispose to the drug-induced glucopenia: (1) decreased food intake or chronic malnutrition, (2) age, particularly in youths or in elderly, (3) abnormality in hepatic or renal function, and (4) adrenal cortical insufficiency. Thus, the adverse effects are most likely to be encountered in the older diabetic who is undernourished with impaired liver or renal function of both. In addition, sulfonylurea-induced hypoglycemia may be potentiated by ethanol, salicylates, sulfonamides, bishydroxycoumarin, and phenylbutazone. Glucopenic reactions may be profound and last for many hours or days. Since it cannot be predicted in advance who may be sensitive to the sulfonylureas, it is important to avoid large doses in elderly subjects with abnormal liver or kidney function and to discontinue potentiating drugs. Factitious hypoglycemia may also be

Table 16–8. DIFFERENTIAL DIAGNOSIS IN COMA OF KNOWN DIABETIC

	Hypoglycemia	Ketoacidosis
History	Insufficient food, excess insulin, excess exercise.	Insufficient insulin, infection, gastrointestinal upset.
Onset	Following *short-acting insulin:* Suddenly, a few hours after injection. Following *long-acting insulin:* relatively slower, many hours after injection.	Gradual over many hours.
Course	Anxiety, sweating, hunger, headache, diplopia, incoordination, twitching, convulsions, coma. (Headache, nausea, and haziness especially following long-acting insulin.)	Polyuria, polydipsia, anorexia, nausea, vomiting, labored deep breathing, weakness, drowsiness, possible fever and abdominal pain, coma.
Physical findings	Pale moist skin, full rapid pulse, dilated pupils, normal breathing, blood pressure normal or elevated, overactive reflexes, positive Babinski sign.	Florid, dry skin, Kussmaul breathing with acetone odor, decreased blood pressure, weak rapid pulse, soft eyeballs.
Laboratory findings	Second urine specimen sugar- and ketone-free, low blood sugar, normal serum CO_2.	Urine contains sugar and ketone bodies, high blood sugar, low serum CO_2.

induced with sulfonylureas, and because both insulin and C-peptide levels are elevated, it may be virtually impossible to rule out an insulinoma by conventional approaches. It is therefore important to screen blood and urine for sulfonylureas in patients suspected of taking these drugs.[60] Treatment of patients with severe protracted hypoglycemia from these agents requires hospitalization and parenteral glucose administration until the drug has been eliminated.

Ethanol

Disturbances of mental function, disorders of personality, convulsions, and neurologic manifestations are sequelae of the chronic abuse of ethanol. This picture may be seen in alcoholics with normal plasma sugar levels, but hypoglycemia may also accompany ethyl alcohol ingestion and simulate the clinical presentation of acute alcoholic intoxication. The clinical and biochemical characteristics of ethanol-induced hypoglycemia have been extensively investigated by Freinkel.[36] The toxic effects on multiple biologic systems of alcohol are well established.[48] Alcoholic hypoglycemia is most frequently seen in a setting of chronic ethanol intake in an adult; a profound drop in plasma sugar may occur in binge drinkers and also in adolescents during their first encounter with alcohol, however. Typically, the alcoholic who develops hypoglycemia will be malnourished and will have been drinking ethanol without food for several hours prior to the onset of glucopenia. He may be brought to the emergency room either confused or comatose, with physical findings that are difficult to differentiate from those of acute alcoholic stupor. The unsuspecting physician may ascribe these features to intoxication rather than to neuroglucopenia because of the odor of alcohol on the breath. Plasma glucose is usually below 45 mg/dl and may be less than 10 mg/dl. Coincidentally, there is ketonuria with diminished plasma CO_2 content. Hepatic function, measured by conventional laboratory tests, may be marginally abnormal. Glycogenolytic responses to exogenous glucagon are markedly attenuated, and plasma insulin levels are low, with enhanced sensitivity to exogenously administered insulin and tolbutamide. The OGTT in a chronic alcoholic often reveals a diabetic configuration. In animal models as well as in humans who have received sufficient intravenous ethanol to simulate intake to the level of mild intoxication, hypoglycemia is evoked during relatively short periods of fasting, compatible with an interference with gluconeogenesis. In healthy volunteers, the induction of glucopenia by ethanol requires several days of preliminary fasting, whereas in chronic alcoholics, this occurs within a shorter period. In the liver, alcohol is oxidized to acetate with simultaneous reduction of diphosphopyridine nucleotide (NAD to $NADH_2$). The increase in the $NADH_2$:NAD ratio leads to a diversion of NAD from normal substrate oxidation required for gluconeogenesis. Gluconeogenic precursors, such as lactate and glutamate, which normally enter pathways via pyruvate or α-ketoglutarate, accumulate in the unfavorable redox environment. The net effect is to inhibit substrate flow, with eventual suppression of gluconeogenesis. Therefore, in a setting of decreased glycogen reserves, as in fasting, alcohol makes the recipient vulnerable to hypoglycemia. It is to be remembered that glucopenia occurs not only in malnourished chronic alcoholics but also in weekend spree drinkers and may be a potentiating factor in hypoglycemia in insulin-requiring diabetics and patients taking oral sulfonylureas. In most instances, the intravenous administration of glucose results in a prompt and dramatic reversal of all neurologic manifestations of hypoglycemia. Nevertheless, mortality in adults from ingestion of toxic amounts of alcohol is about 10%, and in children, it has been reported as high as 25%. Prophylactically, susceptible alcoholics should be persuaded, if possible, to diminish ethanol intake and to eat more regularly.

Miscellaneous Compounds

Several pharmacologic agents and toxins have been reported to cause glucopenia in humans. In isolated case reports, commonly used drugs such as sulfonamides, chloramphenacol, oxytetracycline, salicylates, phenylbutazone, coumarin derivatives, probenecid, haloperidol, chlorpromazine, propoxyphene, anabolic steroids, and monoamine oxidase inhibitors have been incriminated as causes of profound hypoglycemia. The mechanisms of the drug-induced glucopenia may be through potentiation of the actions of sulfonylureas or insulin in diabetics, and in nondiabetic subjects some of these agents may act by interfering with gluconeogenesis. Hypoglycemia has been noted during perhexalene therapy of coronary artery disease, and it has been suggested that it induces hyperinsulinism. Propranolol, a β-adrenergic blocker, may cause hypoglycemia in individuals who are (1) severely ill and undernourished, (2) diabetics on insulin or receiving sulfonylureas, (3) on a weight reduction program, (4) undergoing vigorous exercise, (5) ingesting excessive amounts of alcohol, or (6) on hemodialysis. The mechanisms are uncertain; they usually occur in situations of food deprivation and are probably related to adrenergic blockade affecting lipolysis and hepatic glucose production, however.[97] The use of these drugs should be either discontinued or carefully monitored in diabetic patients requiring insulin or sulfonylureas.

In Jamaica, profound hypoglycemia in association with protracted vomiting has been observed in undernourished children who have inadvertently eaten the unripened fruit of the tropical plant, *Blighia sapida* (ackee fruit).[9] The amino acid, L-α-amino-β-methylenecyclopropionic acid (hypoglycin) contained in the ackee fruit is converted to its acetic acid derivative in the liver, where it interferes with carnitine-dependent oxidation of long-chained fatty acids, thus limiting energy for generation of new glucose. These drug- or toxin-induced hypoglycemic attacks are treated by parenteral glucose administration and discontinuance of the intake of the offending substance.

REFERENCES

1. Alsever, R. N., Stjernholm, M. R., et al.: Clinical correlations of serum proinsulin-like material in inslet cell tumors. *Diabetologia* 12:527, 1976.
2. Anderson, J. W., and Herman, R. H.: Treatment of reactive hypoglycemia with sulfonylureas. *Am. J. Med. Sci.* 261:16, 1971.
3. Anderson, J. W., and Lin Chen, W. J.: Plant fiber, carbohydrate and lipid metabolism. *Am. J. Clin. Nutr.* 32:346, 1979.
4. Arieff, A. I., Doerner, T., et al.: Mechanisms of seizures in coma in hypoglycemia: evidence for a direct effect of insulin on electrolyte transport in brain. *J. Clin. Invest.* 54:654, 1974.
5. Ballard, H. S., Frame, B., et al.: Familial multiple endocrine adenoma — peptic ulcer complex. *Medicine (Baltimore)* 43:481, 1964.
6. Baxter, J. D., and Forsham, P. H.: Tissue effects of glucocorticoids. *Am. J. Med.* 53:573, 1972.
7. Bleicher, S. J., Levy, L. J., et al.: Glucagon deficiency hypoglycemia — a new syndrome. *Clin. Res.* 18:355, 1970.
8. Brasel, J. A., Wright, J. C., et al.: An evaluation of 75 patients with hypopituitarism beginning in childhood. *Am. J. Med.* 38:484, 1965.
9. Bressler, R., Corredor, C., et al.: Hypoglycin and hypoglycin-like compounds. *Pharmacol. Rev.* 21:105, 1969.
10. Broder, L. E., and Carter, S. K.: Pancreatic islet cell carcinoma. 1. Clinical features of 52 patients. *Ann. Intern. Med.* 79:101, 1973.
11. Broder, L. E., and Carter, S. K.: Pancreatic islet cell carcinoma. II. Results of therapy with streptozotocin in 52 patients. *Ann. Intern. Med.* 79:108, 1973.
12. Cahill, J. F., Jr.: Physiology of insulin in man. *Diabetes* 20:785, 1971.
13. Cahill, J. F., Jr.: Starvation in man. *N. Engl. J. Med.* 282:668, 1970.
14. Chochinov, R. V., and Daughaday, W. H.: Current concepts of somatomedin and other biologically related growth factors. *Diabetes* 25:994, 1976.
15. Christensen, N. J.: Hypoadrenalinemia during insulin hypoglycemia in children with ketotic hypoglycemia. *J. Clin. Endocrinol. Metab.* 38:107, 1974.
16. Colle, E., and Ulstrom, R. A.: Ketotic hypoglycemia. *J. Pediatr.* 64:632, 1964.
17. Conn, J. W., and Seltzer, H. S.: Spontaneous hypoglycemia. *Am. J. Med.* 19:460, 1955.
18. Cornblath, M., and Schwartz, R.: Disorders of Carbohydrate Metabolism in Infancy, 2nd ed. Philadelphia, W. B. Saunders, 1976, p. 345.
19. Crain, E. L., Jr., and Thorn, G. W.: Functional pancreatic islet cell adenomas. *Medicine* 28:427, 1949.
20. Crapo, P. A., Reaven, G., et al.: Plasma glucose and insulin responses to orally administered simple and complex carbohydrates. *Diabetes* 25:741, 1976.
21. Creutzfeldt, W.: The incretin concept today. *Diabetologia* 16:75, 1979.
22. Dancis, J., and Levitz, M.: Abnormalities of branched-chained amino acid metabolism, In *The Metabolic Basis of Inherited Disease*, 4th ed. Stanbury, J. B., Wyngaarden, J. B., et al. (eds), New York McGraw-Hill, 1978, p. 401.
23. DeFronzo, R. A., Ferrannini, E., et al.: Influence of hyperinsulinemia, hyperglycemia, and the route of glucose administration on splanchnic glucose exchange. *Proc. Natl. Acad. Sci. USA* 75:5173, 1978.
24. DeVivo, D. C., Haymond, M. W., et al.: Pyruvate carboxylase deficiency and infantile lactic acidosis. *J. Clin. Endocrinol. Metab.* 45:845, 1977.
25. DeVivo, D. C., and Keating, J. P.: Reye's syndrome. *Adv. Pediatr.* 22:175, 1976.
26. Diabetes, Statement on Hypoglycemia. *Diabetes* 22:137, 1973.
27. Ellison, E. H., and Wilson, S. D.: Ulcerogenic tumor of the pancreas, In *Progress in Clinical Cancer*. Vol 3. Ariel, I. M. (ed.), New York, Grune and Stratton, 1967, p. 225.
28. Ensinck, J. W., and Bierman, E. L.: Dietary management of diabetes mellitus. *Ann. Rev. Med.* 30:155, 1979.
29. Ensinck, J. W., and Williams, R. H.: Hormonal and nonhormonal factors modifying man's response to insulin, In *Handbook of Physiology* Section 7: *Endocrinology (Endocrine Pancreas.* Steiner, D. S., and Freinkel, N. [eds.]) Baltimore, Williams and Wilkins, American Physiological Society 1972, p. 665.
30. Exton, J. H.: Gluconeogenesis. *Metabolism* 21:945, 1972.
31. Fajans, S. S., and Floyd, J. C., Jr.: Diagnosis and medical management of insulinomas. *Ann. Rev. Med.* 30:313, 1979.
32. Fajans, S. S., and Floyd, J. C., Jr.: Fasting hypoglycemia in adults. *N. Engl. J. Med.* 294:766, 1976.
33. Felig, P.: Interaction of insulin in amino acid metabolism in the regulation of gluconeogenesis. *Israel J. Med. Sci.* 8:262, 1972.
34. Fink, W. J., Hucke, S. T., et al.: Treatment of postoperative reactive hypoglycemia by a reversed intestinal segment. *Am. J. Surg.* 131:19, 1976.
35. Floyd, J. C., Jr., Fajans, S. S., et al.: Plasma insulin and organic hyperinsulinism, comparative effects of tolbutamide, leucine and glucose. *J. Clin. Endocrinol.* 24:747, 1964.
36. Freinkel, N., Cohn, A. K., et al.: Alcoholic hypoglycemia: a prototype of the hypoglycemias induced in the fasting state, In *Diabetes*. Ostman, J. (ed.), New York, American Elsevier, 1969, p. 873.
37. Freinkel, N., and Metzger, B. E.: Oral glucose tolerance curve in hypoglycemia in the fed state. *N. Engl. J. Med.* 28:820, 1969.
38. Froesch, E. R.: Essential fructosuria, hereditary fructose intolerance, and fructose-1, 6-diphosphatase deficiency, In *The Metabolic Basis of Inherited Disease*. 4th ed. Stanbury, J. B., Wyngaarden, J. B., et al. (eds.), New York, McGraw-Hill, 1978, p. 121.
39. Garber, A. J., Cryer, P. E., et al.: The role of adrenergic mechanisms in the substrate and hormonal response to insulin-induced hypoglycemia in man. *J. Clin. Invest.* 58:7, 1976.
40. Gerich, J. E., Charles, M. A., et al.: Regulation of pancreatic insulin and glucagon secretion. *Ann. Rev. Physiol.* 38:353, 1976.
41. Goldman, J., Baldwin, D., et al.: Characterization of circulating insulin and proinsulin-binding antibodies in autoimmune hypoglycemia. *J. Clin. Invest.* 63:1050, 1979.
42. Gray, G. M.: Mechanism of digestion and absorption of foods, In *Gastrointestinal Disease, Pathophysiology, Diagnosis and Management*. Sleisenger, M., and Fordtran, J. S. (eds.), Philadelphia, W. B. Saunders, 1978, p. 241.
43. Grollman, A., McCaleb, W. E., et al.: Glucagon deficiency as a cause of hypoglycemia. *Metabolism* 13:686, 1964.
44. Greenblatt, M., Murrary, J., et al.: Electroencephalographic studies in diabetes mellitus. *N. Engl. J. Med.* 234:119, 1946.
45. Greene, H. L., Slonim, A. E., et al.: Continuous nocturnal intragastric feeding for management of type I glycogen storage disease. *N. Engl. J. Med.* 294:423, 1976.
46. Hafken, L., Leichter, S., et al.: Organic brain dysfunction as a possible consequence of postgastrectomy hypoglycemia. *Am. J. Psychiatry* 132:12, 1975.
47. Hansen, R. W., and Mehlman, M. A. (eds.): *Gluconeogenesis, Its Regulation in Mammalian Species*. New York, John Wiley and Sons, 1976.
48. Hawkins, R. D., and Kalant, H.: The metabolism of ethanol and its metabolic effects. *Pharmacol. Rev.* 24:67, 1972.
49. Hayashi, M., Floyd, J. C., Jr., et al.: Insulin, proinsulin, glucagon and gastrin in pancreatic tumors and in plasma of patients with organic hyperinsulinism. *J. Clin. Endocrinol. Metab.* 44:681, 1977.
50. Himms-Hagen, J.: Sympathetic regulation of metabolism. *Pharmacol. Rev.* 19:367, 1967.
51. Himwich, H. E.: *Brain Metabolism in Cerebral Disorders*. Baltimore, Williams and Wilkins, 1951.
52. Hoch, F. L.: Metabolic effects of thyroid hormones, In *Handbook of Physiology*, Section 7: *Endocrinology*. Baltimore, Williams and Wilkins, 1974, American Physiological Society, Greep, R. O., and Cestwood, E. B. (eds.) p. 391.
53. Hofeldt, F. D., Adler, R. A., et al.: Postprandial hypoglycemia, fact or fiction? *J.A.M.A.* 233:1309, 1975.
54. Hofeldt, F. D., Lufkin, E. G., et al.: Are abnormalities in insulin secretion responsible for reactive hypoglycemia? *Diabetes* 23:589, 1974.
55. Hommes, F. A., Bendienk, E., et al.: Two cases of phosphoenolpyruvate carboxykinase deficiency. *Acta Paediatr. Scand.* 65:233, 1976.
56. Horowitz, D. L., Rubenstein, A. H., et al.: Prolonged suppression of insulin release by insulin-induced hypoglycemia demonstrated by C-peptide assay. *Horm. Metab. Res.* 7:449, 1975.
57. Howell, R. R.: The glycogen storage diseases, In *The Metabolic Basis of Inherited Disease*. 4th ed. Stanbury, J. B., Wyngaarden, J. B., et al. (eds.), New York, McGraw-Hill, 1978, p. 137.
58. Jenkins, D. J. A., Gassull, M. A., et al.: Effect of dietary fiber on complications of gastric surgery: prevention of postprandial hypoglycemia by pectin. *Gastroenterology* 72:215, 1977.
59. Johansson, C.: Studies of gastrointestinal interactions, VII characterisi-

tics of the absorption pattern of sugar, fat and protein from composite meals in man, a quantitative study. *Scand. J. Gastroenterol.* 10:33, 1975.

60. Jordan, R. M., Kammer, H., et al.: Sulfonylurea-induced factitious hypoglycemia. *Arch. Intern. Med. 137:*390, 1977.
61. Kahn, C. R., Rosen, S. W., et al.: Ectopic production of chorionic gonadotropin and its subunits by islet cell tumors. *N. Engl. J. Med.* 297:565, 1977.
62. Kernen, J. A., Scofield, G., et al.: Long survival with islet cell carcinoma of the pancreas. *Am. J. Clin. Pathol. 39:*137, 1963.
63. Khurana, R. C., Dhawer, B. P. S., et al.: Glucose, tolbutamide and leucine tolerances in hypoglycemia; reactive hypoglycemia as a variant of normal or chemical diabetes mellitus. *Postgrad. Med.* 53:118, 1973.
64. Khurana, R. C., Nolan, S., et al.: Insulin glucose patterns in control subjects and in proven insulinoma. *Am. J. Med. Sci. 262:*115, 1971.
65. Klimt, E. R., Prout, T. E., et al.: Standardization of the oral glucose tolerance test. Report of the committee on statistics of the American Diabetes Association. *Diabetes 18:*299, 1969.
66. Knudson, A. G., and Strong, L. C.: Mutation cancer, neuroblastoma and pheochromocytoma. *Am. J. Hum. Genet. 24:*514, 1972.
67. Kraegen, E. W., Young, J. D., et al.: Oscillations in blood glucose and insulin after oral glucose. *Horm. Metab. Res. 4:*409, 1972.
68. Kreisberg, R. A., and Pennington, L. F.: Tumor hypoglycemia: A heterogeneous disorder. *Metabolism 19:*445, 1970.
69. Krieger, D. T. (ed.): *Endocrine Rhythms.* New York, Raven Press, 1979.
70. Larsson, L. I., Grimelius, L., et al.: Mixed endocrine pancreatic tumors producing several pepetide hormones. *Am. J. Pathol. 79:*271, 1975.
71. Laurent, J., Debry, G., et al.: *Hypoglycemic Tumors.* New York, American Elsevier, 1971.
72. Lefebvre, P. J., Luyckx, A. S., et al.: Studies in the pathogenesis of reactive hypoglycemia: role of insulin and glucagon in hypoglycemia. Proceedings of European Symposium Supplement Series 6, Hormone and Metabolic Research. Stuttgart, George Thieme, 1976, p. 91
73. Lifshitz, F., Coella-Ramirez, P., et al.: Monosaccharide intolerance and hypoglycemia in infants with diarrhea. *J. Pediatr. 77:*595, 1970.
74. Litwack, G. (ed.): *Biochemical Actions of Hormones.* Vol. 2 New York, Academic Press, 1972.
75. Lopez-Kruger, R., and Dockerty, M. B.: Tumors of the islets of Langerhans. *Surg. Gynecol. Obstet. 85:*495, 1947.
76. Luft, R., and Cerasi, E.: Human growth hormone as a regulator of blood glucose concentrations and as a diabetogenic substance. *Diabetologica 4:*1, 1968.
77. Lund-Anderson, H.: Transport of glucose from blood to brain. *Physiol. Rev. 59:*305, 1979.
78. Marks, V., and Rose, F. C.: *Hypoglycemia.* Oxford, Blackwell, 1965.
79. Marks, V., and Samols, E.: Diagnostic tests for evaluating hypoglycemia, In *Diabetes.* Ostman, J. (ed.), New York, American Elsevier, 1969, p. 864.
80. Marks, V., and Samols, E.: Diazoxide therapy of intractable hypoglycemia. *Ann. N. Y. Acad. Sci. 150:*442, 1968.
81. Martin, F. I. R., Dahlenburg, G. W., et al.: Neonatal hypoglycemia in infants of insulin-dependent diabetic mothers. *Arch. Dis. Child.* 50:472, 1975.
82. McDaniel, H. G., Pittman, C. S., et al.: Carbohydrate metabolism in hypothyroid myopathy. *Metabolism 26:*867, 1977.
83. McFadzean, A. J. S., and Yeung, R. T. T.: Further observations of hypoglycemia in hepato-cellular carcinoma. *Am. J. Med. 47:*220, 1969.
84. McQuarrie, I.: Idiopathic spontaneously occurring hypoglycemia in infants. *Am. J. Dis. Child. 87:*399, 1954.
85. Merimee, T. J., Misbin, R. I., et al.: Sex variations in free fatty acids and ketones during fasting. Evidence for a role of glucagon. *J. Clin. Endocrinol. Metab. 46:*414, 1978.
86. Merimee, T. H., and Tyson, J. E.: Stabilization of plasma glucose during fasting. *N. Engl. J. Med. 291:*1275, 1974.
87. Muggeo, M., Bar, R. S., et al.: Changes in affinity of insulin receptors following oral glucose in normal adults. *J. Clin. Endocrinol. Metab.* 44:1206, 1977.
88. Pagliara, A. S., Karl, I. E., et al.: Hypoglycemia in infancy and childhood. I. *J. Pediatr. 82:*365, 1973.
89. Pagliara, A. S., Karl, I. E., et al.: Hypoglycemia in infancy and childhood. II. *J. Pediatr. 82:*558, 1973.
90. Pecile, A., and Mueller, E. E. (eds.): *Growth and Growth Hormone.* New York, American Elsevier, 1971.
91. Permutt, M. A.: Postprandial hypoglycemia. *Diabetes 25:*719, 1976.
92. Permutt, M. A., Delmez, J., et al.: Effects of carbohydrate restriction on the hypoglycemia phase of the glucose tolerance test. *J. Clin. Endocrinol. Metab. 43:*1088, 1976.
93. Permutt, M. A., Keller, D., et al.: Cholinergic blockade in reactive hypoglycemia. *Diabetes 26:*121, 1977.
94. Poffenberger, P. L.: Non-suppressible insulin-like proteins in health and disease, In *Special Topics in Endocrinology and Metabolism.* Vol. 1. Cohen, M. P., and Foa, P. P. (eds.), New York, R. Liss, 1979, p. 110.

95. Raivio, K. O., and Oesterlund, K.: Hypoglycemia and hyperinsulinemia associated with erythroblastosis fetalis. *Pediatrics 483:*217, 1969.
96. Reichlin, S., Baldessarini, R. J., et al. (eds.): *The Hypothalamus.* Vol. 56. New York, Raven Press, 1978.
97. Reveno, W. E., and Rosenbaum, H.: Propranolol and hypoglycemia. *Lancet 1:*920, 1968.
98. Rimoin, D. L., and Schimke, R. N.: *Genetic Disorders of the Endocrine Glands.* St. Louis, C. V. Mosby, 1971.
99. Robins, J. M., Bookstein, J., et al.: Selective angiography in localizing islet cell tumors of the pancreas. *Radiology 106:*525, 1973.
100. Rosenbloom, A. L., and Sherman, L.: Natural history of idiopathic hypoglycemia of infancy and its relation to diabetes mellitus. *N. Engl. J. Med. 274:*815, 1966.
101. Roth, J., Kahn, C. R., et al.: Receptors for insulin, NSILA-S and growth hormone: applications to disease states in man. *Recent Progr. Horm. Res. 31:*95, 1975.
102. Roy, B. K., Abuid, J., et al.: Insulin release in response to calcium in the diagnosis of insulinoma. *Metabolism 28:*246, 1979.
103. Rubenstein, A. H., Kuzuya, H., et al.: Clinical significance of circulating C-peptide in diabetes mellitus and hypoglycemic disorders. *Arch. Intern. Med. 137:*625, 1977.
104. Rutsky, E. A., McDaniel, H. G., et al.: Spontaneous hypoglycemia in chronic renal failure. *Arch. Intern. Med. 138:*1364, 1978.
105. Scarlett, J. A., Mako, M. E., et al.: Factitious hypoglycemia: diagnosis by measurement of serum C-peptide immunoreactivity and in insulin-binding antibodies. *N. Engl. J. Med. 297:*1029, 1977.
106. Schoz, D. A., ReMine, W. H., et al.: Hyperinsulinism: review of 95 cases of functional pancreatic islet cell tumors. *Mayo Clin. Proc. 35:*545, 1960.
107. Segal, S.: Disorders of galactose metabolism, In The *Metabolic Basis of Inherited Disease.* 4th ed. Stanbury, J. B., Wyngaarden, J. B., et al. (eds.), New York, McGraw-Hill, 1978, p. 160.
108. Seltzer, H. S.: Drug-induced hypoglycemia. *Diabetes 21:*955, 1972.
109. Service, F. J., Dale, A. J., et al.: Insulinoma. Clinical and diagnostic features of 60 consecutive cases. *Mayo Clin. Proc. 51:*417, 1976.
110. Skrabanek, T., and Powell, D.: Ectopic insulin and Occam's razor: reappraisal of the riddle of tumor hypoglycemia. *Clin. Endocrinol.* 9:141, 1978.
111. Soman, B., Tamborlane, W., et al.: Insulin binding and insulin sensitivity in isolated growth hormone deficiency. *N. Engl. J. Med. 299:*1025, 1978.
112. Stefanini, P.: Beta islet cell tumors of the pancreas: results of a study on 1067 cases. *Surgery 75:*597, 1974.
113. Steiner, A. L., Goodman, A. D., et al.: Study of a kindred with pheochromocytoma medullary thyroid carcinoma, hyperparathyroidism, and Cushings disease. Multiple endocrine neoplasia Type II *Medicine (Baltimore) 5:*371, 1968.
114. Streeten, D. H., Gerstein, M. M., et al.: Measurement of glucose disposal rates in normal and diabetic human subjects after repeated intravenous injections of glucose. *J. Clin. Endocrinol. 24:*751, 1964.
115. Taunton, O. D., Greene, H. L., et al.: Fructose-1, 6-diphosphatase deficiency, hypoglycemia and a response to folate therapy in a mother and her daughter. *Biochem. Med. 19:*260, 1978.
116. Thomas, C. G., Jr., Underwood, L. E., et al.: Neonatal and infantile hypoglycemia due to insulin excess: new aspects and diagnosis in surgical management. *Ann. Surg. 185:*505, 1977.
117. Tietze, H. U., Zurbrügg, R. R., et al.: Occurrence of impaired cortisol regulation in children with hypoglycemia associated with adrenal medullary hyporesponsiveness. *J. Clin. Endocrinol. 34:*948, 1972.
118. Turner, R. C., and Heding, L. G.: Plasma proinsulin C-peptide and insulin in diagnostic suppression tests for insulinoma. *Diabetologia* 13:571, 1977.
119. Turner, R. C., and Johnson, P. C.: Suppression of insulin release by fish insulin-induced hypoglycemia with reference to diagnosis of insulinomas. *Lancet 1:*1843, 1973.
120. Turner, R. C., Lee, E. C. G., et al.: Localization of insulinomas. *Lancet* 1:515, 1978.
121. Unger, R. H., and Orci, L.: Physiology and pathophysiology of glucagon. *Physiol. Rev. 56:*779, 1976.
122. Vidnes, J., and Oyasaeter, S.: Glucagon deficiency causing severe neonatal hypoglycemia in a patient with normal insulin secretion. *Pediatr. Res. 11:*943, 1977.
123. Wajchenberg, B. L., Perieira, A. A., et al.: On the mechanism of insulin hypersensitivity in adrenocortical insufficiency. *Diabetes 13:*170, 1964.
124. Wermer, P.: Mutiple endocrineadenomatosis; multiple hormone-producing tumors, a familial syndrome, In *Endocrine Secreting Tumors of the GI Tract.* Bonfils, S. (eds.), Clin. Gastroenterol., Philadelphia, W. B. Saunders, 1974, Ch. 13.
125. Woods, S., and Porte, D., Jr.: The central nervous system, pancreatic hormones, feeding and obesity. *Adv. Metab. Disord. 9:*283, 1978.
126. Yager, J., and Young, R. T.: Non-hypoglycemia is an epidemic condition. *N. Engl. J. Med. 291:*907, 1974.
127. Zieve, L., Jones, D. J., et al.: Functional hypoglycemia in peptic ulcer. *Postgrad. Med. 40:*159, 1966.
128. Zimmerman, H. J., Thomas, L. J., et al.: Fasting blood sugar in hepatic disease with reference to infrequency of hypoglycemia. *Arch. Intern. Med. 91:*577, 1953.

CHAPTER 17

Disorders of Lipid Metabolism

By Edwin L. Bierman
and John A. Glomset

INTRODUCTION

Four interrelated disorders of lipid metabolism, all affected by hormones and diet, account for much of the morbidity and mortality in clinical medicine. These disorders are obesity, hyperlipidemia, atherosclerosis, and cholelithiasis. Although the last two in particular are usually associated with specialties other than endocrinology, i.e., cardiology and surgery, it is likely that physicians interested in endocrinology and metabolism will be increasingly involved in their management. Emphasis in the future will certainly be on prevention, and there is reason to believe that this will require long-term control of triglyceride and cholesterol metabolism, with attention to all four disorders. Although current understanding of lipid metabolism and hormone-lipid interrelationships is far from complete and rational preventive care is not yet possible, enough is known to formulate a tentative framework of pathophysiologic concepts as an aid to following the rapid developments in this area. Furthermore, an understanding of the numerous hormone-lipid interrelationships as discussed in other chapters has become crucial to the student of endocrinology. Particular lipids, especially phospholipids, comprise important structural components of all membranes, and those in plasma membranes are likely to play a central role in the mechanism of action of a variety of hormones. Many hormones are intimately linked to the transport of fat as fuel, and disordered lipid metabolism is often an early sign of an altered endocrine state. Conversely, altered lipid metabolism can profoundly influence hormone production, distribution, and action.

The aim of this chapter is to provide such a pathophysiologic framework of lipid metabolism and hormone-lipid relationships, then a discussion of present knowledge concerning hyperlipidemia, diabetes, atherosclerosis, and cholelithiasis in relation to it. Aspects of lipid metabolism in relation to obesity will be found in Ch. 18. Emphasis in this chapter is on triglyceride, fatty acids, and cholesterol, because of the very close relationship between disordered triglyceride and cholesterol metabolism and these major diseases.

TRIGLYCERIDE METABOLISM: FAT AS FUEL

Aside from its role in insulating the body against heat loss, the major function of triglyceride is to provide an efficient storage form for energy. The importance of triglyceride as a fuel can be appreciated from the fact that enough is usually stored to support many weeks of fasting, whereas carbohydrate is stored in amounts sufficient to last only a few hours (Cahill, 1970). The advantages of triglyceride are that it yields more than twice as many calories per gram as either carbohydrate or protein and that it requires less than half the amount of intracellular water for storage. Both advantages depend upon the long-chain fatty acid components of triglyceride, which yield large amounts of energy when oxidized and are only slightly soluble in water. The same properties, however, necessitate the special mechanisms of transport and metabolic control discussed later.

Digestion and Absorption

Human diets contain highly variable amounts of triglyceride (fat) provided by both plant and animal foods. Typical "western" diets provide as much as 40% of the total calories in the form of triglyceride, but on a world-wide scale, this type of diet is geographically as well as historically unusual. The less affluent most often consume much less triglyceride and much more carbohydrate.

Most dietary triglyceride is absorbed in the duodenum and proximal jejunum after undergoing partial hydrolysis. The water-insoluble triglycerides of food spontaneously aggregate into large oil droplets when mechanically mixed with the aqueous secretions of the gastrointestinal tract. Transfer of triglyceride from these oil droplets across mucosal cell membranes is extremely inefficient, but upon partial hydrolysis, smaller aggregates (micelles) can be formed, greatly increasing the total surface area and facilitating transfer. The events that occur during hydrolysis are schematically illustrated in Fig. 17–1. Conjugated cholic and dihydroxycholanic acids from bile (Table 17–1), secreted into the intestinal lumen in response to dietary fat, act as detergents to disrupt and disperse the oil droplets (Hofmann and Small, 1967). They are able to do this because of their unique configuration. The polar hydroxyl groups all project from the same side of the rela-

Table 17–1. MAJOR ORGANIC COMPONENTS OF HUMAN GALLBLADDER BILE*

	mg/ml Bile
Dihydroxycholanic acids	48.9
Cholic acid	32.2
Phospholipid†	27.3
Protein	5.0
Cholesterol	3.0
Bilirubin	2.8

*From Nakayma and Miyake: *J. Lab. Clin. Med.* 67:78, 1966.
†>95% lecithin (Phillips).

tively flat ring structure (Fig. 17–2), creating a hydrophilic side that spontaneously aligns towards the aqueous phase and a hydrophobic side that associates with the surface of the oil droplets. This association causes the oil droplets to become negatively charged, because of the acidic groups of the bile acids, and promotes their dispersion. Bile acids also promote the action of the triglyceride hydrolase secreted in pancreatic juice. This enzyme attacks the triglyceride of the oil droplets, mainly forming monoglycerides and free fatty acids (FFA). This causes a large increase in the area of the oil-water interface, because bile acids combine with the monoglycerides and FFA to form micelles, i.e., aggregates that are so small (about 5 nm in diameter) that they yield a clear solution in aqueous media.

The surface area of the intestinal mucosa also is enlarged by finger-like villi that project into the lumen and are covered by epithelial cells. These cells themselves have an enlarged surface because of the presence of microvilli (Fig. 17–3). Since the micelles formed by digestion are small enough to enter the spaces between the microvilli, they can come into direct contact with the unstirred aqueous layer immediately adjacent to the cell surface, and rapid transfer of monoglyceride and FFA through this layer and into the cells can occur. Within the cells, the monoglyceride, FFA, and small amount of free glycerol formed during digestion are reconverted into triglyceride (Fig. 17–4), packaged into lipoproteins, and secreted into the lymph. These processes occur rapidly, as can be demonstrated by sequential electron microscopy. Within 20–30 min after the introduction of fat into the intestinal lumen, the Golgi region is crowded with lipid, and within 1 hour, the lipid can be observed in the extracellular

Figure 17–1. Schematic representation of events during the hydrolysis and absorption of triglyceride. ⤙, conjugated bile salt; ←, free fatty acid; ⤚, monoglyceride. (From Senior, J. R.: Intestinal absorption of fats. *J. Lipid Res.* 5:495, 1964.)

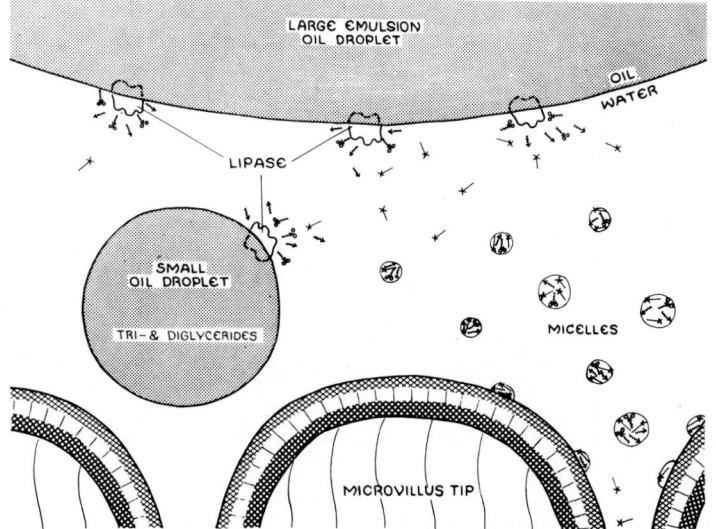

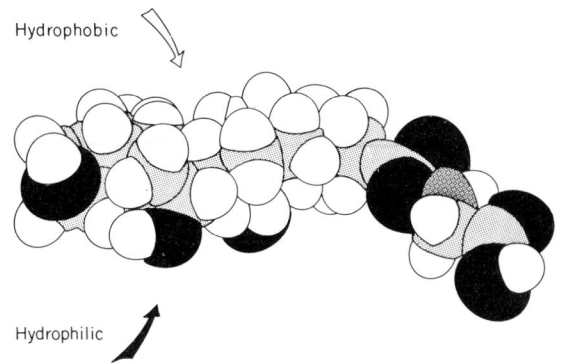

Hydrophobic

Hydrophilic

Figure 17–2.   Model of taurocholic acid. Black areas are oxygen atoms, gray areas carbon atoms, white areas hydrogen atoms.

space at the base of the cell, ready for entrance into the lymphatic system (Fig. 17–3).

The enzymic reactions within the mucosal cells include not only reformation of triglyceride but also formation of phospholipid, unesterified cholesterol, cholesteryl ester, and specific proteins (lipoprotein apoproteins), which have a high capacity to bind lipids. Much of the phospholipid is formed by acylation of lysophosphatidylcholine, absorbed from the intestinal lumen. Unesterified cholesterol also can be absorbed from the intestinal lumen, or it can be biosynthesized from acetyl Coenzyme A (Acetyl CoA) (see p. 885). Some of this cholesterol is esterified by an acyl Coenzyme A:cholesterol acyltransferase (ACAT). The apolipoproteins formed by the mucosal cells include apolipoproteins A-I, A-II, A-IV, and B. Apparently the phospholipid, unesterified cholesterol, and apoproteins form a hydrophilic surface layer surrounding a "core" of more hydrophobic triglycerides and cholesteryl esters (Table 17–2). The finished products of this activity, observed within the Golgi region, are lipid-rich particles of dimensions comparable to those of the chylomicrons and very low density lipoproteins (VLDL) of thoracic duct lymph (75–500 nm) (Table 17–3). The composition of the particles probably differs somewhat from that of lymph particles, however, because rapid changes occur upon mixing

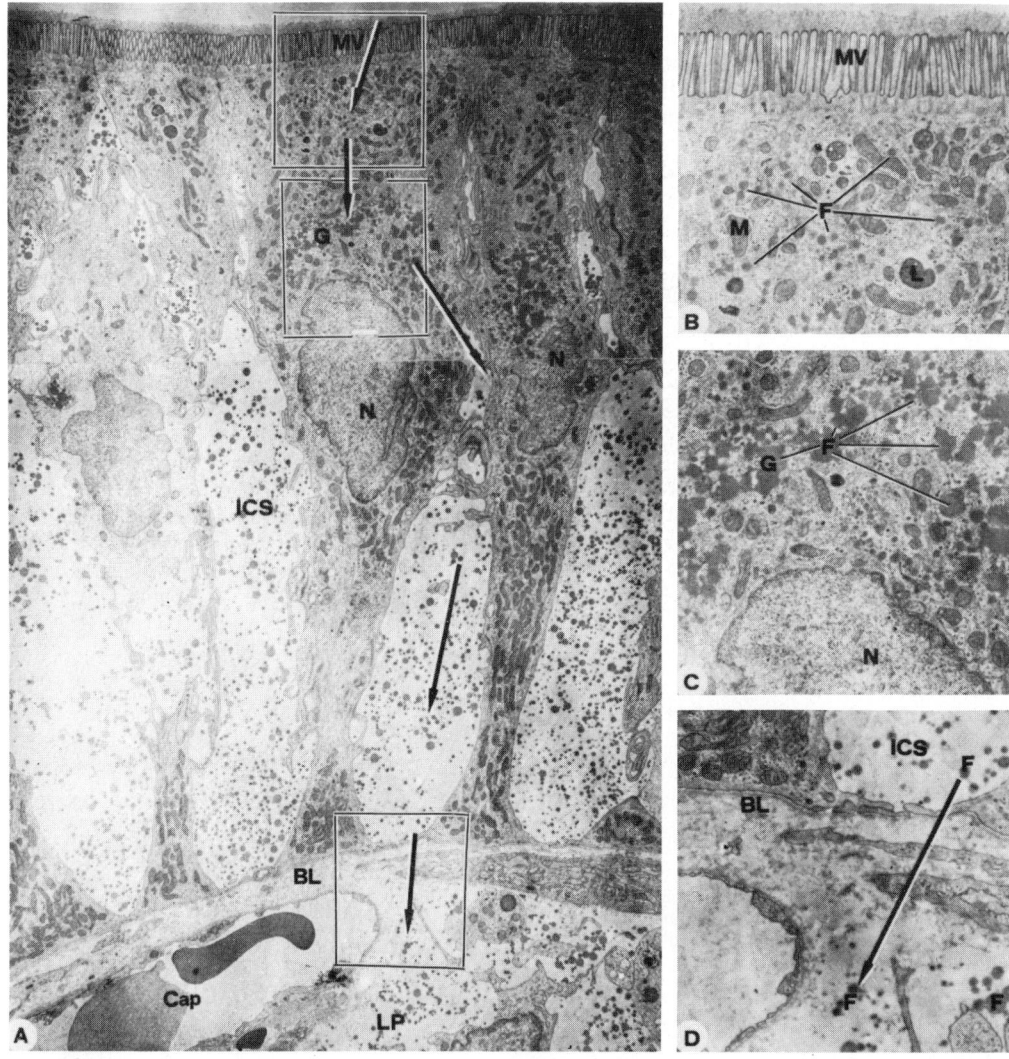

Figure 17–3.   Fat absorption in the jejunum of humans. The large picture on the left (*A*) is a montage of electron micrographs of absorptive cells at the tip of a villus fixed with osmic acid and embedded in epon. (×5,000). The three outlined areas (*B, C, D*) are shown to the right at a greater magnification (×12,000). This biopsy was obtained with a peroral biopsy tube 60 min after a fat meal had been given intragastrically. The large arrows delineate the sequential movement of fat, F, seen as dark grayish globules, from the lumen to the apical area of the cell, then to the Golgi area, G, the intercellular spaces, ICS, and, finally, to the lamina propria, LP, where they will enter lacteals. MV, microvilli; M, mitochondrion; N, nucleus; BL, basal lamina; L, lysosome; Cap, capillary. (Courtesy of Dr. Stanley S. Shimoda, Division of Gastroenterology, University of Washington.)

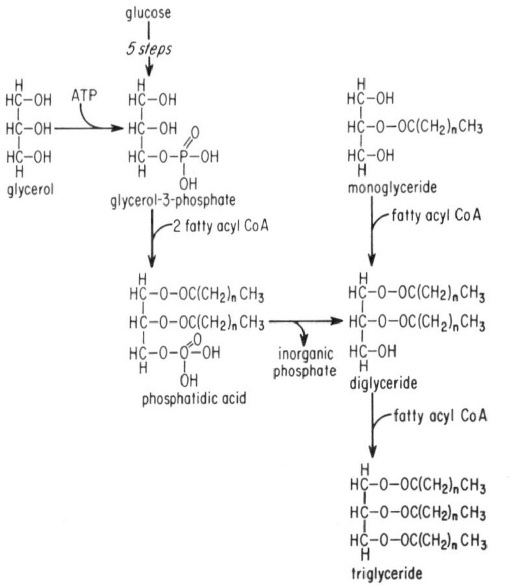

Figure 17–4. Synthesis of triglyceride within the mucosal cell. Note that the major pathway utilizes the monoglyceride formed during digestion. ATP, adenosine triphosphate; CoA, coenzyme A.

Table 17–2. LYMPH CHYLOMICRONS (Obtained by thoracic duct cannulation from human subject fed corn oil.)*

	Protein†	Triglyceride‡	Phospholipid	Cholesterol‡
Chylomicron	0.58%	96.5%	2.9%	0.6%
"Membrane"	11.5%	43.0%	52.8%	4.8%

*From Zilversmit, D. B.: *J. Clin. Invest.* 44:1610, 1965.
†Per cent total weight.
‡Per cent total lipid.

chylomicrons with plasma (Bierman and Strandness, 1966; Minari and Zilversmit, 1963), and similar changes probably begin to occur as soon as the particles are secreted from the mucosal cells into the lymph. These changes include loss of phospholipid and apolipoproteins A-I and A-II and uptake of unesterified cholesterol and apolipoproteins C-I, C-II, C-III, and E. The apolipoproteins acquired by transfer from the plasma appear to be major determinants of the stability and ultimate fate of the particles. In particular, apolipoprotein C-II is known to activate lipoprotein lipase (LPL), an enzyme that catalyzes the first step in the removal of chylomicrons from plasma.

Lipoprotein Lipase

Normally chylomicrons begin to appear in plasma soon after a fatty meal and reach a maximum concentration within 4–5 hours. Because chylomicrons are so large that they scatter light, they frequently cause turbidity of the plasma (postalimentary lipemia). Studies using chylomi-

crons labeled with radioactive triglyceride have demonstrated their rapid removal from the plasma and have shown that the fate of the triglyceride depends on nutritional and hormonal factors. Partial hydrolysis of the chylomicron triglyceride by LPL is believed to occur at the lumenal surface of capillary cells, where tight complexes with infused chylomicrons can be demonstrated by electron microscopy (Fig. 17–5). Evidence from several sources suggests that LPL absorbed on the cell surface initiates the hydrolysis (Robinson, 1970). This enzyme, formerly referred to as "post-heparin lipolytic activity" (PHLA) or "clearing factor" lipase because it is partially released into plasma upon injection of heparin and can sometimes "clear" lipemic plasma, appears initially to form free fatty acids and partial glycerides. Subsequently, the partial glycerides may be further hydrolyzed within pinocytotic vacuoles of the capillary cells (Blanchette-Mackie and Scow, 1971). Finally, FFA are presumably released into the extravascular space, where they become available for uptake by tissue cells or for recirculation into the plasma. The liberated glycerol re-enters the bloodstream and is mainly metabolized by the liver and kidney.

Because LPL appears to be a rate-limiting factor in chylomicron removal that directs the flow of chylomicron fatty acid into tissues, and because it has been implicated in diseases associated with hypertriglyceridemia (see under "Hyperlipidemia"), the factors that influence the distribution and activity of the enzyme are of special interest. LPL activity has been demonstrated in several tissues (Robinson, 1970), but adipose tissue, heart, and mammary gland have received the most attention. The activity in adipose tissue decreases during fasting and in diabetes, is higher in the fed state, and is highest in animals that have been fasted and subsequently refed (Bez-

Table 17–3. COMPOSITION AND PROPERTIES OF MAJOR PLASMA LIPOPROTEINS

Designation; Electrophoretic Mobility	Size, Density	Major "Core" Lipid	Major Apolipo-Proteins*	Source of Nascent Particles	Direct Enzymic Attack By
Chylomicrons	100–500 nm; d<0.940 g/ml	TG	Apo C,E,B	Gut	LPL
VLDL; Pre-β	30–70 nm; d<1.006 g/ml	TG	Apo C,E,B	Liver, gut, remnant of chylos	LPL
IDL; β	20–30 nm; 1.006–1.019 g/ml	CE	Apo E,B	Remnants of VLDL	LPL?
LDL; β	20 nm; 1.019–1.003 g/ml	CE	Apo B	Remnants of VLDL, IDL	
HDL; α₁	10 nm; 1.063–1.21 g/ml	CE	Apo A-I, A-II,C,E	Liver, gut	LCAT

*Major apolipoproteins of circulating particles.

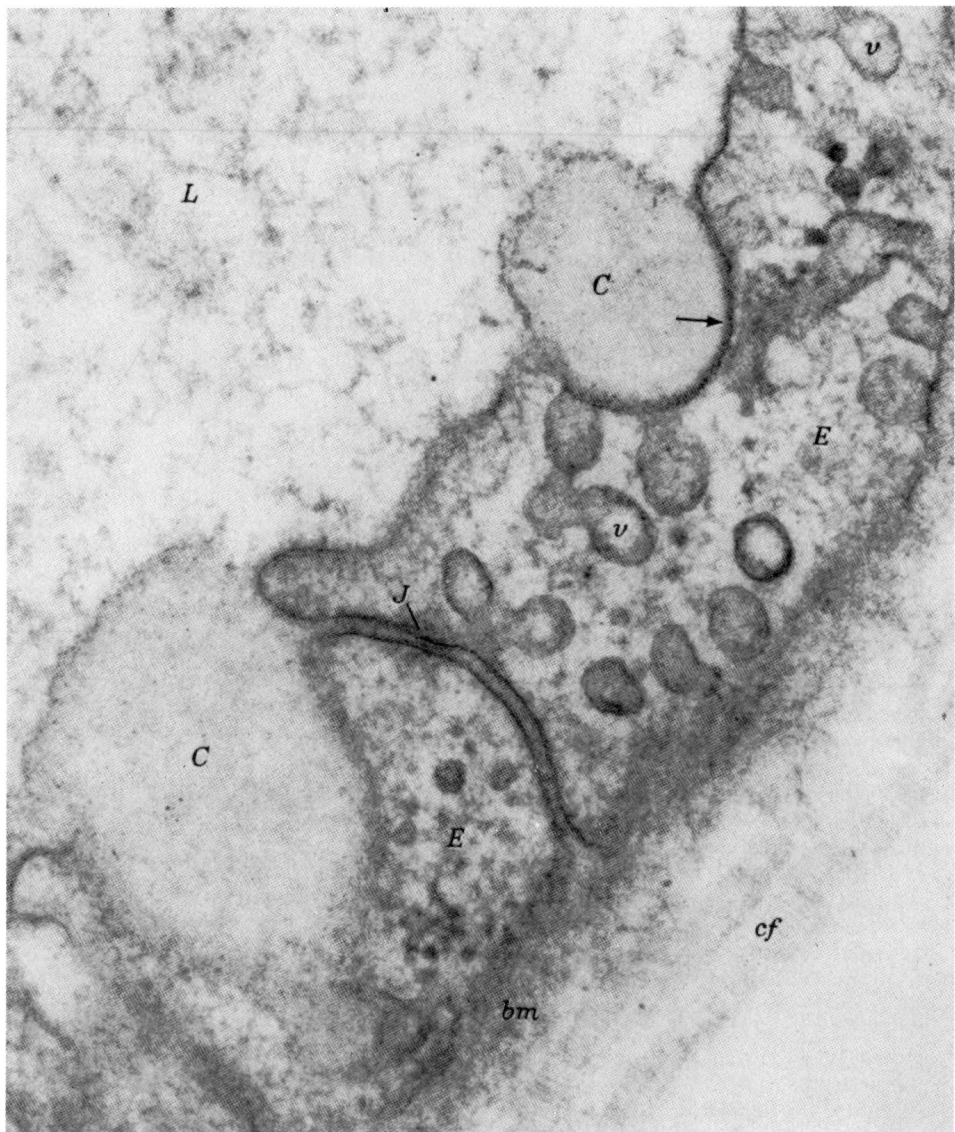

Figure 17–5. Detail of the capillary endothelium of a rat mammary gland 10 min after the intravenous injection of chyle. L, capillary lumen; C, chylomicron; E, endothelium; J, cell junction; v, vesicle; bm, basement membrane; cf, collagen fiber. Lead citrate stain (× 140,000). (From Schoefl, G. I., and French, J. E.: Vascular permeability to particulate fat: morphological observations on vessels of lactating mammary gland and of lung. *Proc. Royal Soc.* [Biol.] *169*:153, 1968.)

man et al., 1962). In contrast, the activity of heart muscle increases during prolonged fasting (Hollenberg, 1960). In mammary tissues, enzyme activity is relatively low until parturition, when it increases as much as 10-fold (McBride and Korn, 1963). The factors responsible for these changes are best understood for adipose tissue. Evidence exists that the LPL of this tissue is synthesized by the fat cells, though only a relatively small proportion of the total tissue activity can be demonstrated within the cells themselves (Cunningham and Robinson, 1969). The fat cells synthesize LPL in the presence of glucose and insulin but not in the presence of agents that increase intracellular free fatty acid levels (Patten, 1970). They also release the enzyme in the presence of glucose and insulin (Stewart and Schotz, 1971). Although subsequent events remain to be clarified, the released enzyme presumably becomes associated with the vasculature. The bound enzyme appears to have a short half-life, and this causes the total activity of the tissue to be highly depend-

ent on glucose and insulin. Studies *in vivo* show multiphasic release into the circulation after heparin administration (Brunzell et al., 1975), consistent with this scheme. Note that glucose and insulin not only increase adipose tissue LPL activity, thereby directing the flow of chylomicron fatty acids into the extracellular space surrounding the adipocyte, but also stimulate intracellular re-esterification of this fatty acid by promoting the formation of glycerol phosphate within the cell (Fig. 17–6).

Production of Triglyceride from Carbohydrate

When dietary fat is replaced by carbohydrate, endogenous synthesis of fatty acid increases in both adipose tissue and liver. This biosynthesis also is dependent upon glucose and insulin. Fatty acids synthesized within fat cells are esterified to glycerol phosphate formed from glucose and converted to triglyceride for storage. Those synthesized in the liver also are converted mainly to triglyc-

PLASMA   ENDOTHELIAL CELL   ADIPOCYTE

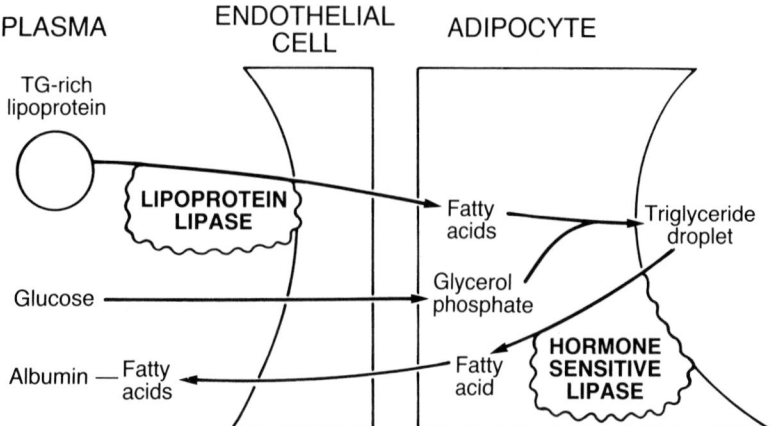

Figure 17-6. The regulatory role of lipoprotein lipase (LPL) and hormone-sensitive lipase in the deposition and mobilization of adipose tissue triglyceride. Insulin promotes triglyceride storage by enhancing LPL activity and fatty acid esterification via glycerol phosphate formation from glucose, while simultaneously limiting fatty acid mobilization by inhibiting hormone-sensitive lipase activity.

eride, but most of the newly formed triglyceride is packaged into VLDL, secreted into the plasma, and removed within minutes to hours by mechanisms probably similar to those involved in removal of chylomicron triglyceride.

The pathways of fatty acid biosynthesis and the mechanisms that control them appear to be similar in adipose tissue and liver. Fatty acids are synthesized from two-carbon units and hydrogen, both of which are mainly derived from glucose. Activated two-carbon units (acetyl CoA) are formed from pyruvate within the mitochondria by the pyruvate dehydrogenase reaction (see Ch. 15). Since fatty acid biosynthesis occurs outside the mitochondria, the two-carbon units must be transferred across the relatively impermeable mitochondrial membrane. The principal pathway of transfer appears to involve condensation of acetyl CoA with oxalacetate to form citrate. The citrate is transferred across the membrane by a membrane carrier protein or permease and reconverted to acetyl CoA and oxalacetate outside the mitochondria by cleavage in the presence of ATP and CoA (Srere, 1959; Spencer and Lowenstein, 1967). Eight acetyl CoA molecules are required for synthesis of one molecule of palmitic acid (16 carbon atoms). One acetyl group appears to be transferred directly to a carrier protein-enzyme complex (fatty acid synthetase). The remaining seven are first carboxylated by a key enzyme, acetyl CoA carboxylase, to form malonyl CoA (Fig. 17-7). Subsequently, the malonyl groups are successively transferred to fatty acid synthetase and condensed to form a long hydrocarbon chain. With each transfer of a malonyl group, one molecule of CoA and one of CO_2 are released. At each step, four atoms of hydrogen, transferred from two molecules of NADPH, are required to convert the elongated chain into a saturated hydrocarbon. The NADPH appears to be derived from two separate pathways, the "pentose shunt" (Ch. 15), which produces two molecules of NADPH during the oxidation of glucose-6-phosphate and 6-phosphogluconate, and the "malic enzyme" pathway. In the latter, the oxalacetate produced by the citrate cleavage reaction is first reduced by NADH to form malate. Then the malate is reoxidized by NADP in the presence of "malic enzyme" (malic dehydrogenase)(Lardy et al., 1965), to form NADPH, pyruvate, and CO_2. Palmitic acid synthesized by this sequence of condensation and reduction steps can be activated to form palmityl CoA and directly esterified to form triglycerides and other lipids, or it can be elongated or dehydrogenated or both to form other fatty acids. Elongation occurs within the mitochondria or in association with the endoplasmic reticulum (mi-

crosomes). Dehydrogenation occurs in the endoplasmic reticulum closely coupled to chain elongation.

The rate of fatty acid biosynthesis is highest on hypercaloric, high-carbohydrate diets, low on fat-rich diets, and lowest during prolonged starvation or diabetes. The factors that cause these differences are not completely understood, but some potential mechanisms of fine and coarse control have been identified. For example, acetyl CoA carboxylase may be subject to allosteric regulation, since high concentrations of citrate cause the enzyme to form an active aggregate, whereas increased concentrations of long-chain fatty acyl CoA rapidly promote disaggregation to a smaller inactive form (Lane and Moss, 1971). There is also evidence for regulation by phosphorylation-dephosphorylation (Lee and Kim, 1977). This mechanism is also involved in the regulation of pyruvate dehydrogenase (Jungas, 1971). In the presence of substances that increase tissue concentrations of cyclic AMP (cAMP) (see Ch. 15), this enzyme is phosphorylated and thereby inactivated, whereas, in the presence of glucose and insulin, the enzyme is rapidly dephosphorylated to its active form. The activation or inactivation of pyruvate dehydrogenase appears at least partly to explain the rapid changes in fatty acid biosynthesis noted in various physiologic conditions, but slower changes in the concentrations of other enzymes also occur, and these appear to explain more long-term physiologic effects. Thus the rates of biosynthesis of glucokinase, the citrate cleavage en-

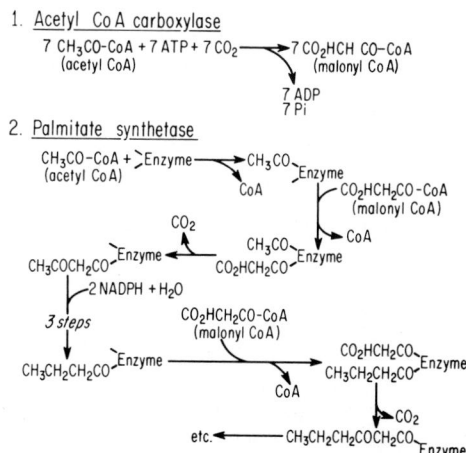

Figure 17-7. Schematic representation of the formation of palmitic acid in the extramitochondrial fluid. ATP, adenosine triphosphate; ADP, adenosine diphosphate; CoA, coenzyme A; Pi, inorganic phosphate.

zyme, acetyl CoA carboxylase, fatty acid synthetase, glucose-6-phosphate dehydrogenase (G6PD), 6-phosphogluconate dehydrogenase, and malic enzyme all are coordinately affected by diet, producing a coarse control of fatty acid biosynthesis.

Whether fatty acids are synthesized slowly or rapidly by liver cells, VLDL are still formed and secreted into the plasma. They can be recognized in the Golgi region of the cell prior to secretion. Like chylomicrons, they contain large amounts of triglyceride, probably surrounded by a layer of protein, phospholipid, and unesterified cholesterol. Although the apoproteins of freshly secreted human or primate VLDL have not yet been studied, human VLDL have been isolated from plasma and contain mainly apoproteins B, C, and E (Kane et al., 1975). The apolipoprotein C-II of VLDL, like that of chylomicrons, facilitates the hydrolysis of VLDL triglyceride by lipoprotein lipase.

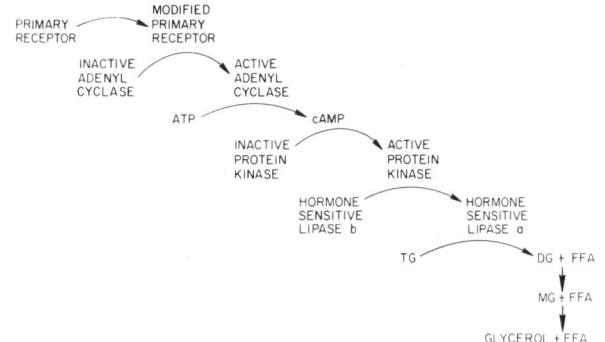

Figure 17–8. Cascade of reactions involved in the activation of hormone-sensitive lipase. (From Steinberg, D., and Huttunen, J. K., In *Advances in Cyclic Nucleotide Research*. Vol. 1. Greengard, P., Paoletti, R., et al. (eds.), New York, Raven Press, 1972, pp. 47–62.)

Release of Fatty Acids from Adipose Tissue Stores

Net release of FFA and glycerol from adipose tissue triglyceride occurs during several physiologic conditions, including exercise, stress, and fasting, as well as in uncontrolled diabetes. Hormones play an important part in this release. Some hormones, and perhaps autonomic nervous stimulation (Table 17–4), increase lipolysis within minutes by promoting formation of cAMP, which stimulates a protein kinase that activates a rate-limiting triglyceride hydrolase, "hormone-sensitive lipase" (Fig. 17–8). Thyroid hormone appears to increase the sensitivity of adipose tissue to these hormones, whereas insulin and prostaglandin PGE₁ inhibit their action, apparently by blocking formation of cAMP (Butcher, 1970). Growth hormone (GH) stimulates lipolysis in a different way. *In vitro*, in the presence of dexamethasone, it increases release of FFA from adipose tissue but only after a time lag of about 2 hours (Fain et al., 1965). This effect can be inhibited by actinomycin and puromycin, which suggests that the biosynthesis of new protein is involved. Once the effect has developed, however, it is insensitive to agents that block protein synthesis but is sensitive to inhibition by insulin. This suggests that the new protein synthesized is the hormone-sensitive triglyceride hydrolase. The synergism between GH and corticosteroids and the relatively long time lag are of interest because both features characterize the action of GH *in vivo*. Why so many hormones activate FFA release is not known; however, the hormones involved in the rapid mobilization of FFA seem to be different from those involved in the slower release of FFA during growth, fasting, or diabetes. Fain and coworkers

(1965) have suggested that the hormones may not be equally sensitive to inhibition by insulin, and that this differential sensitivity may permit a fine control of FFA release during different physiologic conditions.

Fate of Plasma Free Fatty Acids

When glycerol and FFA are released from adipose tissue, they circulate briefly in the plasma. If lipolysis is brisk, the plasma concentrations of these metabolites rise. The rise only partially reflects the rate of lipolysis, however, since uptake by the tissues is proportional to the concentration in the plasma. The glycerol is mainly metabolized in the kidney and the liver, where it is phosphorylated by glycerophosphokinase and either reutilized for triglyceride formation or used for gluconeogenesis (Wagle et al., 1966). The fatty acids circulate as albumin complexes. Their disposal is greatly dependent upon blood flow. During intense exercise, when the flow of blood through the splanchnic bed is reduced, they are largely oxidized in muscle. Those taken up by the liver are activated by reaction with ATP and CoA to form acyl CoA. The activated acyl groups are then either converted to triglyceride or other lipids and secreted as VLDL, oxidized to CO_2, or converted into ketone bodies, depending on nutritional and hormonal conditions. In the presence of glucose and insulin, conversion to VLDL triglyceride predominates. During fasting or in diabetes, when glucose or insulin or both are diminished, most of the acyl groups are oxidized or converted into ketone bodies.

Fatty Acid Oxidation and Ketogenesis

In order for oxidation and ketogenesis to occur, activated fatty acids must be transported into the mitochondria by a specific mechanism. Neither FFA nor their CoA derivatives formed outside the mitochondria readily penetrate mitochondrial membranes, but the soluble fluid of the cell (cytosol) contains an enzyme that reversibly transfers fatty acyl groups from CoA to carnitine, and acylcarnitine derivatives can enter the mitochondria. Once inside, a second enzyme (Kopec and Fritz, 1971) causes essentially irreversible transfer of the acyl groups from acylcarnitine to mitochondrial CoA, thus effectively preventing the fatty acids from returning to the cytosol. The fatty acyl CoA derivatives then enter the β-oxidation pathway and contribute to the formation of reduced coenzymes (NADH and FADH) and acetyl CoA.

Table 17–4. HORMONES THAT AFFECT
LIPOLYSIS *IN VITRO*

Rapid Stimulation
    Catecholamines (β1 agonists)
    ACTH
    Glucagon
    Secretion
    α and β MSH
    VIP
Slow Stimulation
    Growth hormone
    Glucocorticoids
Suppression
    Insulin
    Prostaglandin (PGE₁)
    GIP

When small amounts of fatty acids are oxidized, the reduced coenzymes largely enter the electron transport pathway within the mitochondria and yield ATP and H_2O. The acetyl CoA condenses with oxalacetate to form citrate and is either transported across the mitochondrial membrane by the permease system and reconverted to fatty acid or oxidized to CO_2 by the enzymes of the citric acid cycle. During fasting and in uncontrolled diabetes, however, the flow of FFA into the liver is greatly increased. Under these conditions, production of VLDL triglyceride from these fatty acids is limited, and reduced coenzymes and acetyl CoA within the mitochondria accumulate. The acetyl CoA molecules then condense successively to form acetoacetyl CoA and hydroxymethylglutaryl CoA, whereupon the latter is cleaved to yield acetoacetate and acetyl CoA. This causes the release of CoA, which can then be used in the metabolism of additional fatty acids by the β-oxidation pathway. In addition, the free acetoacetate formed can be reduced by the excess mitochondrial NADH to form β-hydroxybutyrate, thus liberating NAD for use in β-oxidation. Alternatively, it can decompose spontaneously to yield acetone, which accounts for the increased concentrations of all three metabolites in the plasma during ketogenesis.

The fate of the blood ketones, like that of the blood fatty acids, depends on nutritional and hormonal conditions. After a short period of fasting, acetoacetate and β-hydroxybutyrate are mainly metabolized by peripheral tissues such as muscle, but after longer periods, the brain apparently develops the capacity to metabolize these substrates (Cahill, 1970). In muscle, the acetoacetate and β-hydroxybutyrate must be converted into derivatives of mitochondrial CoA before being cleaved to acetyl CoA and oxidized via the citric acid cycle. Since fatty acids taken up from the blood by muscle also must be converted into derivatives of mitochondrial CoA before they can be metabolized, the two substrate types compete with each other. Moreover, both compete for the CoA ordinarily utilized by the pyruvate dehydrogenase reaction in converting pyruvate derived from glucose to acetyl CoA. This competition, along with the conversion of pyruvate dehydrogenase to its less active phosphorylated form in the presence of increased concentrations of FFA (Wieland et al., 1971) may partially account for the decreased utilization of glucose by muscle noted during fasting and diabetes (Randle et al., 1963).

Summary: Hormonal Effects

Adipocyte triglyceride is formed from fatty acids provided by either dietary fat or biosynthesis. Fatty acids from dietary fat are largely transported to adipose tissue as chylomicrons. Those formed by biosynthesis either arise within fat cells or are formed in the liver and transported to adipose tissue as VLDL triglycerides. Formation of triglyceride within adipocytes and liver is dependent upon the availability of glucose and insulin. Both are required for fatty acid biosynthesis and for formation of triglyceride glycerol, both may enhance packaging and secretion of VLDL, and both promote transport of triglyceride to adipose tissue by increasing the activity of adipose tissue LPL.

Glucose and insulin also diminish release of FFA from adipocytes. Insulin blocks activation of a cAMP-dependent, intracellular, hormone-sensitive triglyceride hydrolase by epinephrine, ACTH, and other hormones; glucose and insulin promote re-esterification of hydrolyzed fatty acid.

The availability of glucose and insulin also appears to determine the fate of FFA taken up by the liver. In the absence of one or both, only a small proportion of the FFA is converted to triglyceride and secreted as VLDL (Basso and Havel, 1970). The bulk of the FFA is converted to acylcarnitine, transported into the mitochondria, and either oxidized or used to form ketone bodies. The reaction that forms acylcarnitine (carnitine acyltransferase I) may be a critical control point in this process. It is blocked by malonyl CoA (McGarry et al., 1977), an intermediate in the biosynthesis of fatty acids (Fig. 17–9).

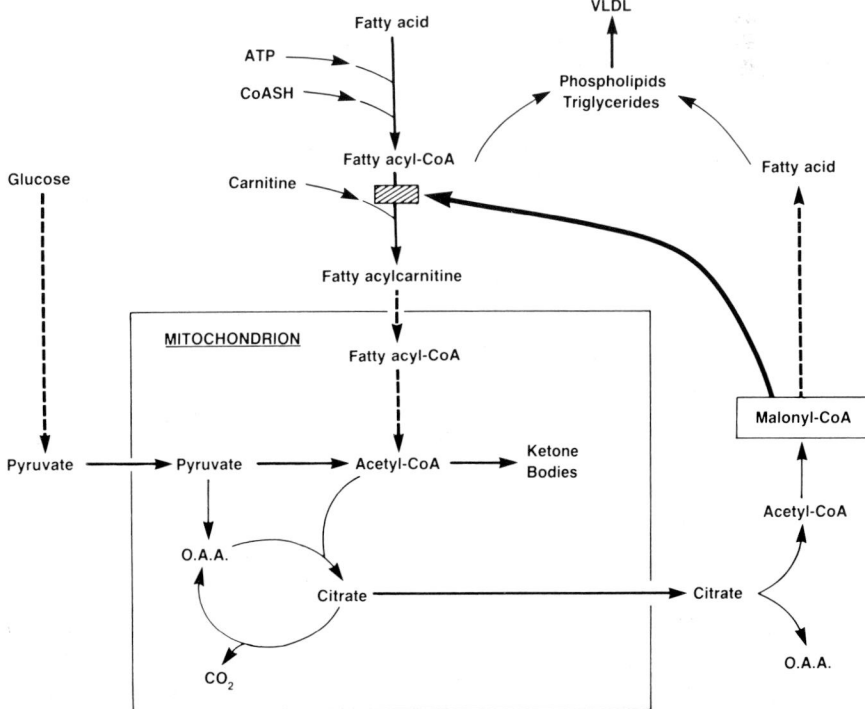

Figure 17–9. Pathways of fatty acid oxidation and synthesis in the hepatocyte. (Adapted from McGarry, J. D., et al.: A possible role for malonyl-CoA in the regulation of hepatic fatty acid oxidation and ketogenesis. *J. Clin. Invest.* 60:265, 1977.)

The transfer of large amounts of acylcarnitine into the mitochondria, coupled with the limited ability of the liver to oxidize the fatty acyl groups to CO_2 accounts at least partially for the greatly increased formation of ketone bodies observed in diabetes. Finally, lack of insulin apparently contributes to the ketosis of diabetes in still another way, by decreasing the utilization of acetoacetate by peripheral tissues (Balasse and Havel, 1971). This effect probably depends on the role of insulin in controlling plasma FFA levels, since fatty acids compete with acetoacetate for mitochondrial CoA.

Insulin lack also affects the concentration of circulating plasma triglyceride. In fasting and diabetes, adipose tissue LPL is diminished, and this increases the concentration of VLDL and especially chylomicron triglyceride in plasma by slowing the rate of their removal.

CHOLESTEROL METABOLISM

Form and Function

Cholesterol is important as a precursor of bile acids and steroid hormones, but particularly as a component (with phospholipids) of plasma membranes and plasma lipoproteins. Its wedgelike shape (Fig. 17–10) and single hydrophilic hydroxyl group apparently adapt it uniquely for intercalation between molecules of phospholipid (Demel et al., 1972). "Mosaics" formed by this intercalation appear to contribute importantly to the structure of outer cell membranes (plasma membranes) and plasma lipoproteins. Apparently, the presence of cholesterol in these mosaics markedly decreases the permeability of membranes to water-soluble compounds (deKruyff et al., 1972) and decreases membrane fluidity. The water insolubility of cholesterol and the inability of most tissues to degrade it presumably contribute to its value as a cell membrane constituent, but, as in the case of triglyceride, its hydrophobic properties complicate the processes of transport and metabolism.

Biosynthesis and Transport of Cholesterol

No dietary requirement for cholesterol exists, since most mammalian cells can synthesize it from acetyl CoA (Dietschy and Wilson, 1970). "Western" diets, rich in eggs, dairy products, and meat (Table 17–5), generally provide 0.5 to 1.0 g of exogenous cholesterol per day, however, and this cholesterol contributes significantly to body pools. A considerable proportion of the cholesterol of food is esterified, and the esters are probably not directly absorbed. Pancreatic juice contains a cholesteryl ester hydrolase that in the presence of trihydroxy bile acids catalyzes the hydrolysis of cholesteryl esters in the intestinal lumen to form FFA and unesterified cholesterol. The latter mixes with the unesterified cholesterol of food, bile, and possibly desquamated mucosal cells, and considerable amounts can be absorbed. The process of absorption is not well understood, but it seems to be passive rather than active, and the following events probably occur. Unesterified cholesterol in the intestinal lumen is taken up by mixed micelles of bile acid and FFA, monoglyceride, or lysolecithin. As a component of these micelles, cholesterol then enters the spaces between the microvilli of the mucosal cells and becomes available for net transfer into the cell. When net transfer occurs, it is probably to replace mucosal unesterified cholesterol that has been incorporated onto the surfaces of newly formed chylomicrons or intestinal VLDL or that has been esterified within the cell and incorporated into the triglyceride-rich "cores" of these lipoproteins (Fig. 17–11). If net transfer does not occur but FFA, monoglycerides, or lysolecithin molecules are taken up, the micelles are disrupted and cholesterol precipitates, no longer capable of being absorbed (Simmonds et al., 1967).

The intracellular mechanism by which cholesterol is transferred from the microvillar membrane to the site of lipoprotein synthesis has not been delineated. It is not even certain that chylomicrons secreted into the intestinal lymph contain enough unesterified cholesterol to form a fully stable surface layer since Minari and Zilversmit (1963) have shown that dog lymph chylomicrons rapidly take up additional unesterified cholesterol immediately upon being mixed with dog plasma. Nevertheless, the amount of chylomicron cholesterol secreted into the intestinal lymph can be estimated by assuming that approximately 100 g of chylomicron triglyceride is secreted each day and that the content of chylomicron unesterified and esterified cholesterol is 1.6% and 1.5%, respectively

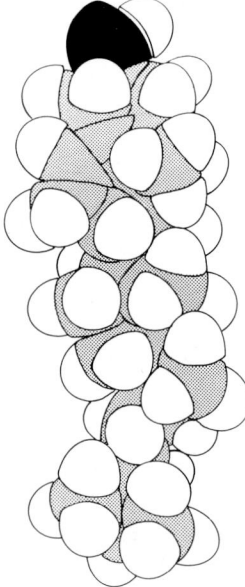

Figure 17–10. Schematic representation of the molecular size and shape of unesterified cholesterol.

Table 17–5.   CHOLESTEROL CONTENT OF SOME COMMON FOODS*

Food	Cholesterol (mg/100 g wet weight)
Eggs	470–650
Butter	280
Lobster, shrimp, oysters, roe	>200
Liver, kidney, brain, tripe, sweetbreads, heart, lung	>150
Cheese	130–160
Cream (35% fat)	124
Meat	70–140
Fish	60–90
Fowl	60–90
Milk (skim)	3
Cottage cheese	1

*From Kritchevsky, D.: *Cholesterol.* New York, John Wiley & Sons, 1958.

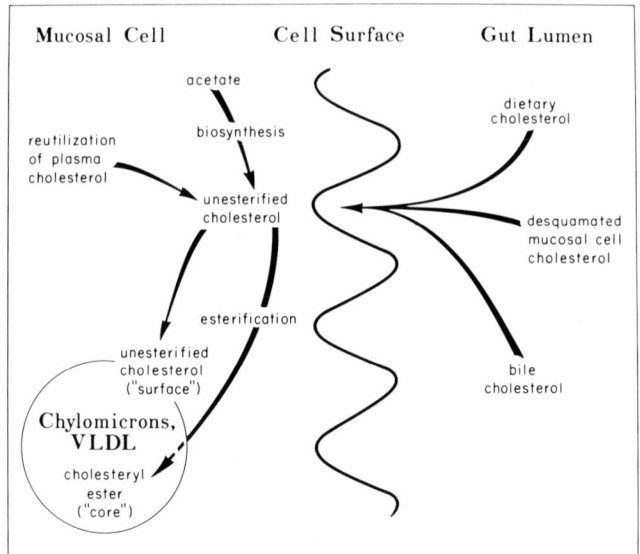

Figure 17–11. Alternate sources of the cholesterol of chylomicrons and VLDL formed by cells of the intestinal mucosa. (From Glomset, J. A., and Norum, K. R.: The metabolic role of lecithin:cholesterol acyltransferase: perspectives from pathology. *Adv. Lipid Res., 11*:1, 1973.)

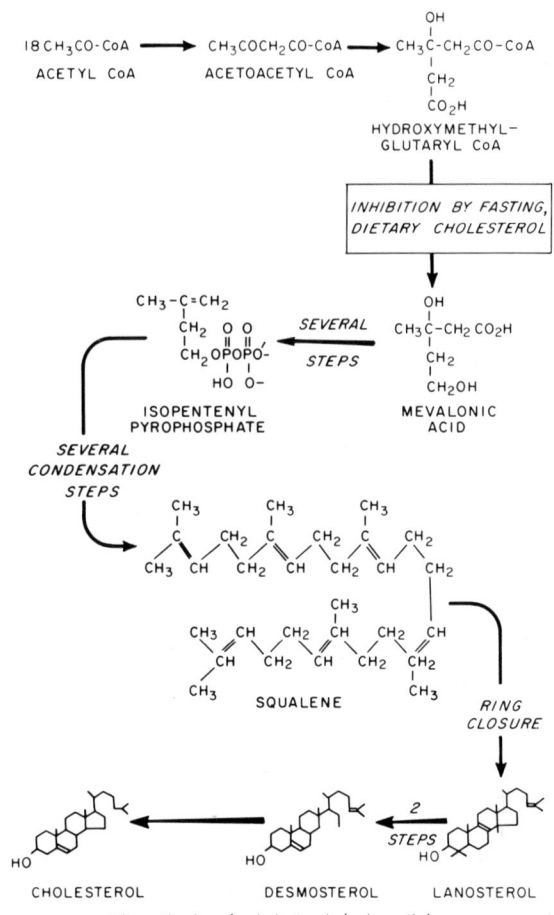

Biosynthesis of cholesterol (schematic)

Figure 17–12. Partial representation of reactions involved in cholesterol biosynthesis.

(Kostner and Holasek, 1972). If these assumptions are valid, then the amounts of cholesterol secreted as chylomicron unesterified cholesterol and cholesteryl ester are about 2 g/day and 1 g/day, respectively (Glomset and Norum, 1973).

Within minutes after chylomicrons and intestinal VLDL enter the plasma, the triglyceride of these lipoproteins begins to be removed by LPL (see p. 879). Removal of the cholesterol of these lipoproteins, however, does not occur by the same mechanism or at the same time. Instead, cholesterol continues to circulate in the plasma, associated with one or more chylomicron remnants (Mjøs et al., 1975). Experiments in rats have shown that the cholesteryl esters of these remnants are removed relatively rapidly and then hydrolyzed by a liver cholesteryl ester hydrolase (Stein et al., 1969). The fate of the unesterified cholesterol, phospholipid, and apoproteins remains to be fully clarified (see later).

Cholesterol enters the plasma not only as a component of chylomicrons and intestinal VLDL, but also as a component of hepatic VLDL. The liver is able to synthesize all of the cholesterol required from acetyl CoA by a multistage series of condensation reactions (Fig. 17–12) similar to that present in most cells. The reaction sequence is at least partially inhibited in most subjects, however, because of feedback inhibition by dietary cholesterol (Siperstein, 1970). Cholesterol biosynthesis in the liver appears to be particularly sensitive to dietary cholesterol, because of the liver's special role in metabolizing the cholesterol of chylomicron remnants. Studies using perfused rat livers (Sherril and Dietschy, 1978) have shown that uptake of these particles leads to decreased activity of an enzyme that acts as an important regulator of cholesterol biosynthesis (Shapiro and Rodwell, 1971). This enzyme, hydroxymethylglutaryl (HMG) CoA reductase, catalyzes the essentially irreversible formation of mevalonic acid, the first committed metabolite in the biosynthesis of cholesterol. Decreased activity of this enzyme diminishes formation of hepatic cholesterol and somewhat limits the effect of diet on increasing hepatic cholesterol levels.

In some species, hepatic VLDL contain both unesterified cholesterol and cholesteryl ester. Human liver, however, appears to contain only small amounts of the ACAT that forms these esters and presumably secretes VLDL that only contain surface unesterified cholesterol. The amount of this cholesterol that enters the plasma each day is difficult to evaluate, but it is probably of the order of 1–3 g (Glomset and Norum, 1973). As mentioned earlier, the triglyceride of hepatic VLDL is hydrolyzed by peripheral LPL, just as in the case of the triglyceride of chylomicrons. Thus the unesterified cholesterol of the hepatic VLDL can be presumed to become associated with "remnants" not unlike those formed from chylomicrons and intestinal VLDL (Mjøs et al., 1975).

"Remnants" of rat VLDL seem largely to be taken up by the liver, whereas human VLDL are mainly converted to intermediate density lipoproteins and low density lipoproteins (LDL) that remain for hours to days in the circulation (see later). The basis for this important species difference has not yet been established. One factor likely to be involved is control of remnant removal by the liver, however. Another is a plasma enzyme, lecithin:cholesterol acyltransferase (LCAT), that appears to modify VLDL and remnants of VLDL in the circulation. Before the action of this enzyme is discussed, it is important to review what is known about its lipoprotein substrates, the high density lipoproteins (HDL).

HDL are lipoproteins, rich in phospholipid and cholesteryl ester, that circulate in the plasma and lymph

(Glomset, 1979). The principal apolipoprotein components of HDL are apolipoproteins A-I and A-II, although smaller amounts of other apolipoproteins such as C apolipoproteins and apolipoprotein E also are present (Table 17–3). The precursors of HDL are largely, if not exclusively, formed in the liver and intestine. HDL secreted by these organs are disc-shaped particles that contain apolipoproteins in association with a bilayer of phospholipid and unesterified cholesterol. Triglyceride-rich lipoproteins, such as chylomicrons, also contribute components to circulating HDL.

In addition to secreting "nascent" HDL, the liver also forms and secretes LCAT. Activated by apolipoprotein A-I, LCAT acts on nascent HDL to form cholesteryl ester. Accumulation of cholesteryl ester in a "core" converts the disc-shaped HDL to globular particles. The metabolic role of the LCAT reaction appears to differ in different species (Glomset, 1979) and may be particularly complex in humans. One of its roles in humans is clearly associated with the metabolism of triglyceride-rich lipoproteins, however.

Attack by LPL on triglyceride-rich lipoproteins removes much of the triglyceride in the interior core. Although some surface phospholipid also may be removed (Chajek and Eisenberg, 1978), more surface lipid remains than is required to cover the core lipid of the remnant lipoproteins. This "excess" surface lipid appears to transfer to HDL, where it is acted upon by LCAT. The cholesteryl esters formed are transferred back to the triglyceride-containing remnant lipoproteins by one or more cholesteryl ester exchange proteins (Pattnaik and Zilversmit, 1979; Chajek and Fielding, 1978). These reactions and others alter the composition and properties of the remnant lipoproteins. Depending on the size and density of these lipoproteins, they are recognized as VLDL, intermediate density lipoproteins (IDL), or LDL.

Removal of these lipoproteins from the plasma presumably is mediated by receptors that are located on cell surfaces. Receptors in many extrahepatic cells appear to bind lipoproteins containing apolipoproteins B and E (Goldstein and Brown, 1977). Most is known about the receptor associated with skin fibroblasts. Upon interacting with this receptor, these lipoproteins such as LDL are taken up into the cells by endocytosis. Fusion of the endocytotic vesicles with lysosomes subsequently leads to degradation of the lipoproteins, and liberated components such as cholesterol can be used for metabolic processes within the cell. Liberated cholesterol appears also to down regulate HMG CoA reductase, so that biosynthesis of cholesterol from acetyl CoA diminishes or ceases, and also down regulates the receptor itself.

In the case of fibroblasts and similar cells, most cholesterol that is either taken up or synthesized is probably utilized for the formation of membranes. Cholesterol taken up by other cells clearly fills additional needs as well, however. Evidence has been obtained in rats, for example, that HDL are recognized and taken up by the adrenal, testis, and ovary (Gwynne et al., 1976; Anderson and Dietschy, 1977). It seems likely that these endocrine glands have cell surface receptors that recognize apolipoprotein A-I and that HDL cholesterol as well as LDL cholesterol is used as a precursor for steroid hormones.

Hepatic Metabolism of Cholesterol

Less is known about receptors for lipoproteins on hepatocyte membranes, though uptake of lipoprotein cholesterol by the liver is likely to play a key role in cholesterol homeostasis. The liver requires cholesterol not only for the formation of membranes but also for the formation of VLDL and HDL

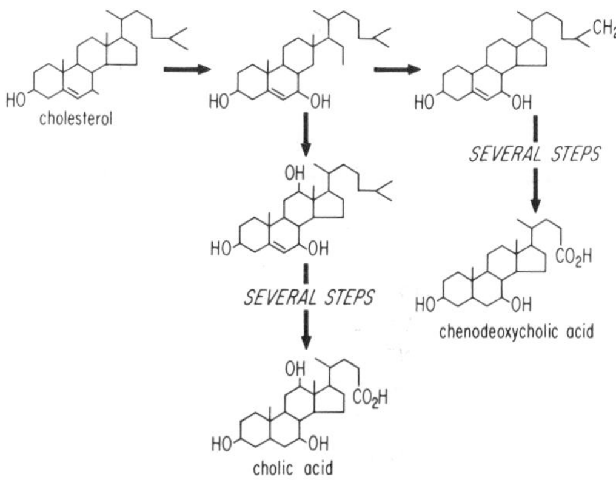

Figure 17–13. Principal steps in the conversion of cholesterol to bile acids.

(discussed earlier) and for the formation of bile. The unesterified cholesterol used for bile formation is either converted into bile acids or secreted directly.

Conversion into bile acids occurs by a series of reactions located in the endoplasmic reticulum, cytosol, and mitochondria (Fig. 17–13). In dogs and rats, this conversion increases several-fold when the animals are fed cholesterol. In humans, however, the response appears to be much more limited, and increased amounts of cholesterol are secreted instead (Quintao et al., 1971). This important species difference may predispose humans to the formation of cholesterol gallstones. Why humans are unable to increase bile acid formation in response to dietary cholesterol is not understood, but it may depend on the 7 α-hydroxylase that catalyzes the first step in bile acid formation. It is generally agreed that this step is an important control point in bile acid biosynthesis (Boyd and Percy-Robb, 1971), and its negative feedback control by bile acids has already been demonstrated.

The mechanisms that promote the direct secretion of cholesterol in bile are not understood, but it has been established that bile acids promote the secretion of biliary lecithin (Entenman et al., 1968) and that bile acids and lecithin together form micelles that can solubilize cholesterol. Bile containing these micelles is stored in the gallbladder and released into the intestine in response to fatty meals. Within the intestinal lumen, the micelles are presumably disrupted as the bile salts participate in the hydrolysis and transport of dietary fat. The lecithin is partially hydrolyzed by a pancreatic lecithinase, and the cholesterol mixes with that of the diet. A substantial recirculation (enterohepatic circulation) of each of these bile components occurs, however, since the bile salts are very efficiently absorbed by an active mechanism in the distal ileum (Dietschy and Wilson, 1970) and return to the liver complexed to the albumin of the portal blood; the lecithin (resynthesized in the mucosa) and cholesterol return to the liver as components of chylomicrons and VLDL. Nevertheless, a small proportion of the bile acids and a considerably larger proportion of the bile cholesterol escape reabsorption during each recirculation of the bile, and since the number of recirculations per day has been estimated to be as great as 10, a substantial amount of cholesterol and bile acid is lost in the feces.

Summary: Hormonal Effects

Adequate amounts of cholesterol for the body's needs are provided by biosynthesis, so that dietary cholesterol is superfluous and increases body pools, particularly in the plasma and bile. There is no evidence that absorption of dietary cholesterol is regulated by hormones. Instead, absorption seems to be a passive process, dependent on the amount of unesterified cholesterol required for "packaging" the triglyceride of chylomicrons and intestinal VLDL and on the amount of cholesterol esterified within mucosal cells and included in the "cores" of these lipoproteins. The amount of dietary cholesterol absorbed probably depends also on the amount of endogenous cholesterol provided by the bile and desquamated mucosal cells and on local biosynthesis within the mucosal cells.

Much of the body's cholesterol, and particularly that of the plasma pool, is formed within the liver, where several controls are operative. Both dietary cholesterol and fasting decrease cholesterol synthesis by the liver, and hypoinsulinism has a similar effect (Lehner et al., 1971). Furthermore, hepatic cholesterol biosynthesis is under circadian control, even in fasted or adrenalectomized animals. Finally, cholesterol biosynthesis is decreased in hypothyroidism and increased in hyperthyroidism.

The concentration of cholesterol in blood plasma depends not only on the amount of cholesterol absorbed and biosynthesized but also on the rates at which chylomicrons, VLDL, LDL, and HDL enter and leave the plasma. These rates appear to be affected by several hormones, including estrogens, androgens, adrenal steroids, glucagon, insulin, and thyroid hormone (Margolis and Capuzzi, 1972). The latter is of particular interest because of its effect on the concentration of LDL, the major carrier of cholesterol in the plasma. In hypothyroidism, both the rate of LDL formation and the rate of LDL clearance from the plasma are slowed, and a new steady state concentration of LDL is reached that is considerably higher than that in euthyroid or hyperthyroid individuals.

Lipoprotein removal from the plasma is mediated by receptors associated with the surface of cells. Most cells appear to have receptors that recognize apolipoproteins B and E, but some cells may have receptors for apolipoprotein A-I and other apolipoproteins. In vitro, hormones such as insulin and thyroid hormones appear to enhance cell surface lipoprotein receptor activity (Chait et al., 1978, 1979a, 1979b; Bierman et al., 1980). Uptake of lipoprotein cholesterol by the liver is likely to be influenced by the mechanisms of secretion of cholesterol and bile acids in bile. Here, too, hormones appear to be important. Thyroid hormones are known to increase bile steroid secretion in both humans (Miettinen, 1968) and experimental animals, and effects of estrogens on bile acid formation (Kritchevsky et al., 1963) and bile flow have been demonstrated in rats and mice. Biliary secretion of cholesterol and bile acids play a major role in regulating body cholesterol pools, because significant amounts of these components escape reabsorption during repeated daily enterohepatic circulations and are excreted in the feces. This is the main means by which cholesterol input through ingestion and biosynthesis is balanced by cholesterol output.

HYPERLIPIDEMIA

Definition and Classification

Hyperlipidemia consists of an excessive accumulation of one or more of the major lipids transported in plasma and is usually a manifestation of an underlying disorder in lipid metabolism. For clinical purposes, hyperlipidemia may manifest as hypercholesterolemia or hypertriglyceridemia, or both. Thus levels of the lipid-carrying molecular aggregates — the lipoproteins (p. 879) — are elevated (hyperlipoproteinemia). The older term "lipemia" or "hyperlipemia" refers to the turbid or lactescent plasma visible when the large, triglyceride-rich particles accumulate (p. 879).

Aside from producing overt signs and symptoms such as xanthoma, lipemia retinalis, and acute abdominal crises (pancreatitis), elevated plasma concentrations of certain lipids and lipoproteins are associated with an increased risk of atherosclerotic disease. It is this risk that is generally used as the guideline for arbitrarily deciding which lipid levels are abnormally high. Although there is a continuous gradient of risk throughout the population (see p. 900), individuals whose triglyceride or cholesterol levels are in the upper 5% for their age and sex are most likely to develop atherosclerotic complications (Goldstein et al., 1973a). Consequently, such persons have been arbitrarily defined as hyperlipidemic (Table 17–6). Thus, as with obesity, the definition of "disease" is somewhat arbitrary, since there are continuous distributions of both plasma levels and morbidity

Table 17–6.   MEAN AND UPPER 95TH PERCENTILE VALUES FOR FASTING PLASMA CHOLESTEROL AND TRIGLYCERIDE LEVELS*

Age (yrs)	Cholesterol		Triglyceride	
	Mean	95th Percentile	Mean	95th Percentile
		(mg/dl)		
MALES				
0–10	160	200	55	100
10–20	155	200	70	140
20–30	175	230	110	225
30–39	195	260	135	290
40–49	210	270	150	320
50–59	215	275	145	305
60–69	215	275	140	280
70+	205	270	130	260
FEMALES				
0–10	160	200	60	110
10–20	160	200	75	130
20–30	165	220	75	140
30–39	180	235	85	160
40–49	200	260	100	200
50–59	225	295	120	250
60–69	230	300	130	240
70+	230	290	130	235

*Adapted from data derived from cross-sectional plasma lipid distributions among 48,431 caucasoid participants in Visit 1 of the Lipid Research Clinics Prevalence Study of 11 North American populations (The Lipid Research Clinics Program Data Book: Selected Variables in 11 North American Populations. Vol. I. Physiologic and Sociodemographic Characteristics, 1979). Ninety-fifth percentile values approximate +2 standard deviations above the mean for cholesterol. Since triglyceride levels are not normally distributed, mean values will be higher than median values. Data for females restricted to those not taking estrogen-containing drugs, since females taking sex hormones have altered plasma lipid levels (Wallace et al., 1977).

risk in the population. Also, since populations vary widely, it is meaningless to select arbitrary limits for normality that can be usefully applied to all populations. Ultimately the level at which preventive treatment can be successfully applied will influence our definition of abnormality.

Excessive lipid accumulation in plasma can result from either defective removal from plasma or excessive endogenous production or both. These abnormalities may be primary or may occur as a secondary result of other diseases, such as endocrine disorders (diabetes or hypothyroidism, for example), or as a result of therapy with certain hormones or drugs.

The primary forms of hyperlipidemia are generally divided into familial, in which clear evidence of a genetic predisposition ("monogenic" or "polygenic") is based on the presence of the disorder in closely related family members, and sporadic, in which neither genetic nor known secondary factors appear to play a role. The primary and secondary hyperlipidemias are generally characterized by similar symptoms and laboratory abnormalities, however, and the metabolic sequelae appear to be comparable.

Differentiation between primary and secondary hyperlipidemia, which is sometimes extremely difficult, is the cornerstone of successful therapy, since the secondary hyperlipidemias may be corrected simply by treatment of the causative disease, when possible, or by withdrawal of the offending medication.

Hyperlipidemia has been classified into six types, based on the specific electrophoretic patterns of the various lipoproteins in plasma (Beaumont et al., 1970). Thus excess chylomicrons have been designated as Type I hyperlipoproteinemia, excess β lipoproteins as Type IIA, excess broad-β lipoproteins (mobility between VLDL and LDL) as Type III, excess pre-β lipoproteins as Type IV, and an excess of both chylomicrons and pre-β lipoproteins as Type V. Increases of both β and pre-β lipoproteins characterize Type IIB.

However, these types of patterns are not specific since the plasma lipoprotein pattern may change with time in any individual, a phenomenon to be expected because of the precursor-product relationships in the metabolism of VLDL and LDL and the profound effects of diet on VLDL transport (Havel, 1977) (see p. 882). Classification solely by this morphologic method, furthermore, does not reflect the pathophysiologic or genetic mechanisms responsible for the disorders. A single mechanism may lead to several different lipoprotein patterns, and conversely, a single pattern may reflect a variety of diseases or mechanisms. Table 17–7 presents a classification of hyperlipoproteinemias based on pathophysiologic characteristics. The common secondary causes of lipid disorders and the types of associated hyperlipoproteinemia are depicted in Table 17–8. Discrete familial hyperlipidemic disorders that have been defined are summarized in Table 17–9 and recently reviewed by Motulsky (1976). These more comprehensive classifications clearly elucidate the disorders for purposes of diagnosis; they also yield a more complete understanding of the rationale for different approaches to therapy.

Excessive Triglyceride Production

"Endogenous" Lipemia

Although a specific defect has not been demonstrated, this disorder appears to result from accelerated hepatic production of pre-β lipoproteins (VLDL) (Reaven et al., 1965; Nikkilä, 1978). In its mildest, most frequent form, endogenous lipemia has a Type IV lipoprotein pattern (increased VLDL) and may be seen in familial forms of hypertriglyceridemia, i.e. familial hypertriglyceridemia and familial combined hyperlipidemia (Table 17–9). When increased lipogenesis is more marked, however, removal mechanisms are saturated

Table 17–7. PATHOPHYSIOLOGIC CLASSIFICATION OF THE HYPERLIPIDEMIAS

Mechanism	Disorders Primary	Disorders Secondary	Lipoprotein Abnormalities	Common Xanthomas	Early Atherosclerosis
1. Increased Triglyceride Input: Postprandial state Increased endogenous VLDL synthesis	Familial hypertriglyceridemia	Hyperinsulinemic states obesity estrogen R_x glucocorticoid R_x uremia growth hormone excess Alcohol Pregnancy	↑ Chylos, VLDL ↑ VLDL ↑ VLDL, chylos	None Eruptive	
2. Decreased Triglyceride Catabolism: Abnormal lipoprotein lipase (LPL) function	Adipose tissue LPL deficiency LPL activator (apo C-II) deficiency	Insulin deficiency (diabetes) Hypothyroidism Uremia Dysglobulinemia (SLE, myeloma, lymphoma, macroglobulinemia)	↑ VLDL, chylos	Eruptive	
3. Abnormal Remnant Catabolism: Core lipid accumulation	Broad-beta disease (Dysbetalipoproteinemia)	Hypothyroidism	↑ remnants, VLDL chylos ↑ apo E (↓ apo E-III)	Planar (palmar); tuberous, tuberoeruptive	Coronary; peripheral vascular disease
Surface lipid accumulation	LCAT deficiency	Liver disease	Discs, LP-X		
4. Abnormal LDL Catabolism	Familial hypercholesterolemia	Hypothyroidism Anorexia nervosa	↑ LDL	Tendon	Coronary
5. Mechanisms Unknown: Combined Hyperlipidemias (multiple lipoprotein phenotypes)	Familial combined hyperlipidemia	Hypothyroidism Nephrotic syndrome	↑ LDL and/or VLDL		Coronary

Table 17–8. SECONDARY HYPERLIPIDEMIA

Cause of Hyperlipidemia	Chylomicrons I	Chylomicrons + VLDL V	VLDL IV	Broad-beta III	LDL IIA	LDL + VLDL IIB
Endocrine						
Diabetes						
Severe	+	+				
Moderate		+	+	+		+
Mild		+	+	+		
Corticosteroid R$_x$						
High dose	+	+				
Low dose or Cushing's syndrome			+		+	+
Hypothyroidism		+	+	+	+	+
Hypopituitarism (ateliotic dwarfism)		+	+			
Acromegaly			+			
Anorexia nervosa					+	
Estrogen or oral contraceptive R$_x$		+	+			
Nonendocrine						
Renal disease						
Nephrotic syndrome		+	+		+	+
Uremia		+	+			
Alcohol		+	+			
Dysglobulinemia	+	+		+	+	
Glycogen storage disease	+	+				
Congenital lipodystrophy (total or partial)		+	+			
Werner's syndrome					+	+
Acute intermittent porphyria					+	
Liver disease				+	LP-X	

and are unable to assimilate all of the additional lipid derived from the diet. In these situations, chylomicrons derived from exogenous fat may accumulate as well, leading to a Type V lipoprotein pattern sometimes referred to as "mixed lipemia" (Havel, 1977). This commonly occurs in endogenous lipemia when two causes producing increased triglyceride production are present simultaneously, e.g. estrogen treatment in a patient with familial hypertriglyceridemia (see p. 893). It also occurs when triglyceride removal defects are associated with factors promoting triglyceride synthesis, such as excess alcohol intake (Ginsberg et al., 1974); it can occur in some diabetics (Bierman et al., 1970).

Endogenous lipemia is not associated with xanthoma unless hyperchylomicronemia supervenes. Familial forms occur quite frequently, however; one form in particular is associated with an increased prevalence of premature coronary atherosclerosis when combined with increased β lipoproteins (see "Combined Hyperlipidemia," p. 891) (Goldstein et al., 1973b; Brunzell et al., 1976). Basal triglyceride levels are characteristically elevated, and since the VLDL that accumulate also contain significant amounts of cholesterol, total plasma cholesterol also may be increased.

Increased production of triglyceride-rich VLDL often occurs during weight gain, during ethanol ingestion, during the last trimester of pregnancy, or during therapy with corticosteroids or estrogenic agents. Estrogen-containing oral contraceptive steroids have been shown to produce uniformly a 50–100% increase in plasma triglyceride levels (Hazzard et al., 1969); in some individuals, gross hypertriglyceridemia has been unmasked (Davidoff et al., 1973) (see "Hyperlipidemia and Estrogens," p. 893). Hypertriglyceridemia also has been observed as a consequence of nonnephrotic chronic renal failure (Bagdade et al., 1968a).

Because of the markedly elevated fasting triglyceride levels observed in these patients following highcarbohydrate, fat-free diets, it was once believed that their metabolic defect was related specifically to carbohydrate, and the disorder was termed "carbohydrate-induced lipemia." It is now clear, however, that "carbohydrate induction" is a normal phenomenon, since healthy subjects not accustomed to eating high-carbohydrate–low-fat diets have been found to transiently double basal triglyceride levels in response to fat-free diets (Bierman and Porte, 1968; Glueck et al., 1969a). The distinguishing feature in patients with "endogenous" lipemia is abnormal triglyceride regulation in

Table 17–9. GENETIC HYPERLIPIDEMIAS

Disorder	Plasma Lipoprotein Pattern*	Genetic Mechanism	Primary Defect	Estimated Population Frequency
Familial hypercholesterolemia (monogenic)	IIA, IIB	Autosomal dominant	LDL receptor	1–2/1,000
Polygenic hypercholesterolemia	IIA, IIB	Polygenic	Unknown	—
Familial hypertriglyceridemia	IV, V	Autosomal dominant	Unknown	2/1,000
Familial combined hyperlipidemia	IIA, IIB, IV, V	Autosomal dominant	Unknown	3–5/1,000
Broad-beta disease (familial dysbetalipoproteinemia)	III, IV, V	Autosomal recessive	Apoprotein E-III	1/10,000
Lipoprotein lipase deficiency	I, V	Autosomal recessive	Lipoprotein lipase	Rare
Apolipoprotein CII deficiency	I, V	Autosomal recessive	Apoprotein C-II	Rare
LCAT deficiency	—	Autosomal recessive	Lecithin cholesterol acyl transferase	Rare

*Electrophoretic classification.

the basal state after ingestion of normal amounts of carbohydrate and fat. Increasing the proportion of carbohydrate in the diet accentuates the hypertriglyceridemia but does not cause it.

Many patients with primary endogenous lipemia share characteristics other than their lipoprotein accumulation, namely obesity, mild glucose intolerance without clinical diabetes, and hyperinsulinism — factors that may contribute to excessive hepatic production of triglyceride. (This phenomenon is described in the section "Hypertriglyceridemia and Diabetes Mellitus.") Hypertriglyceridemia as a clinical problem can be conveniently dissected in terms of some currently held views regarding pathophysiology (Table 17–7).

Triglyceride Removal Defects

Lipoprotein Lipase Deficiency

Since impaired LPL activity leads to defective removal of all triglyceride-rich lipoproteins, it produces either a predominance of chylomicrons derived from dietary fat (Type I lipoprotein pattern) or an accumulation of chylomicrons together with VLDL derived from the liver (Type V). This accumulation may vary in type with age (children have less VLDL) and diet (fat ingestion increases the concentration of chylomicrons).

Although LPL deficiency may occasionally be seen in its congenital form (Table 17–9), it is more frequently acquired, as in severe insulin-dependent diabetes; hypothyroidism; prolonged, high-dose corticosteroid therapy; uremia, dysgammaglobulinemia; and acute pancreatitis (Table 17–8) (Brunzell et al., 1978).

The Type I pattern is more likely to occur in the familial disorder, manifesting itself in childhood with typical episodes of eruptive xanthoma and with the acute abdominal pain of pancreatitis. On the other hand, the Type V pattern is more frequent in adults, largely because they accumulate more endogenous VLDL than do children.

Regardless of underlying cause or age of onset, hyperchylomicronemia can be associated with a syndrome (Chait et al., 1978), including lipemia retinalis, acute pancreatitis, and eruptive xanthoma due to deposits of chylomicrons in the skin (Parker et al., 1970). The xanthomas (Fig. 17–14) are usually located over extensor surfaces of the arms, lower extremities, buttocks, or back and often wax and wane with dietary fat content and the degree or duration of the disorder. Dyspnea and dementia may also be associated with hyperchylomicronemia.

In the laboratory, hyperchylomicronemia may be recognized easily by a characteristic creamlike layer atop fresh plasma after centrifugation or brief refrigeration. Diagnosis of LPL deficiency is suggested by findings of a markedly elevated plasma triglyceride level accompanied by normal or only slightly increased cholesterol concentrations, and it is confirmed by subnormal LPL activity in postheparin plasma or in biopsies of adipose tissue.

Impaired Lipoprotein Lipase Function

Defective function of LPL may occur and produce milder degrees of hypertriglyceridemia, with or without chylomicronemia. Enzyme assay in plasma may be normal. However, studies of triglyceride transport have shown that, in some individuals, LPL can be depleted by prolonged infusions of heparin (Brunzell et al., 1975). In these individuals, an as yet unknown proportion of those with hypertriglyceridemia, the synthesis of LPL appears to be unable to compensate for the reactions that deplete the enzyme.

Most of these hypertriglyceridemic patients are also moderately severe diabetics and the severity of the lipoprotein abnormality seems to be directly related to the height of the fasting blood glucose, which suggests that insulin deficiency is responsible for the impaired LPL activity. (This is described further in the section "Hypertriglyceridemia and Diabetes Mellitus.") The defect appears to be related to low adipose tissue LPL activity (Pykalisto et al., 1975). A rare cause of impaired LPL function is an inherited deficiency of the activator apoprotein C-II (Breckenridge et al., 1978).

Defective Remnant Removal

"Broad-Beta" Disease

In this disorder LPL function is normal, but by-products of its action ("remnants") appear to accumulate. These remnants are spherical particles of low to very low density containing a core rich in cholesterol ester and a surface rich in apoproteins B and E (see p. 886). Remnant lipoproteins separate by density with VLDL and IDL but have the electrophoretic β mobility of LDL, hence the origin of the other descriptive term for the disorder, dysbetalipoproteinemia. Remnant accumulation appears to be due to a defect in remnant removal (Chait et al., 1977). Although it may occasionally be acquired (Hazzard and Bierman, 1971) (Table 17–8), broad-beta disease is predominantly familial, inherited with an autosomal recessive pattern. As with several other inherited lipoprotein disorders, the pateints are extremely prone to develop both coronary and peripheral

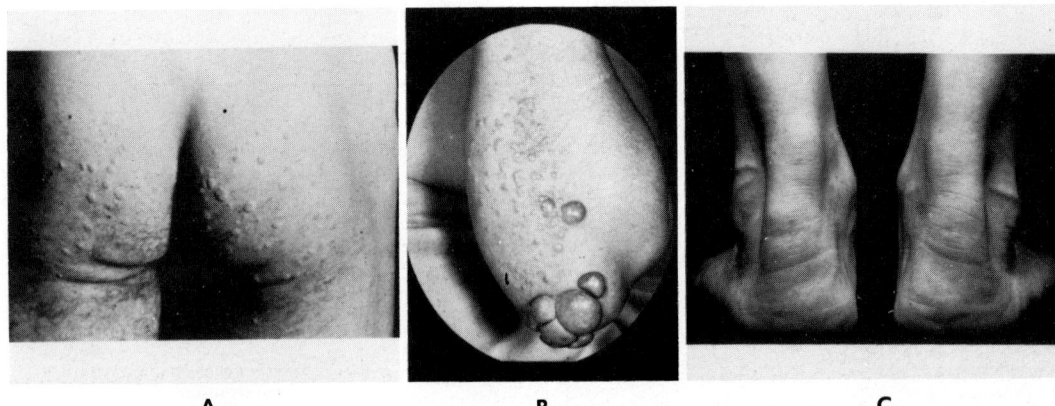

    A   **B**   **C**

Figure 17–14. Various types of xanthomas seen in different hyperlipidemic disorders. *A,* Eruptive xanthomas distributed over the skin of the buttocks. *B,* Tuberous xanthomas on the elbow. Eruptive xanthomas are also present. *C,* Tendinous xanthomas of the Achilles tendons.

vascular atherosclerosis at an early age (Morganroth et al., 1975). The disorder is rare in premenopausal females and is usually not expressed before adulthood.

Diagnosis of the disease is strongly suggested by findings of (1) planar and tuberous xanthomas that are almost pathognomonic when they are present (Fig. 17–14), (2) both plasma triglycerides and cholesterol levels elevated in approximately a 1:1 ratio, and (3) a Type III lipoprotein pattern on paper or agarose electrophoresis (since these "remnants" have a mobility intermediate between pre-β and β lipoproteins, the pattern presents as a broad smear between those two lipoprotein zones). For a definitive diagnosis, however, preparative ultracentrifugation of plasma and electrophoretic and compositional analysis of VLDL are usually required, particularly in asymptomatic patients (Hazzard et al., 1972). The presence of β migrating VLDL and an abnormally cholesterol-rich VLDL fraction confirm the diagnosis. Recently abnormalities in the amount and composition of the apoprotein E fraction have been found to be characteristic of the disease (Havel and Kane, 1973; Kushwaha et al., 1977a; Utermann et al., 1977). The apoprotein E content of VLDL is increased. However, a complete deficiency of one of 4 isoforms of apoprotein E distinguished by isoelectric focusing, apoprotein E-III, inherited as a homozygous trait, is always found. An additional abnormality is necessary for complete expression of the disease, since the heterozygous trait is extremely common (about 15% of the general population) (Utermann et al., 1979). About 1% of unselected asymptomatic normolipidemic individuals are homozygous for the E-III deficiency, yet only about 1 in 50 of these individuals with complete E-III deficiency has the disease.

Familial Lecithin:Cholesterol Acyltransferase Deficiency

This disorder, characterized by absence or near absence of LCAT from the plasma (Gjone et al., 1978), is associated with many plasma lipoprotein abnormalities. The content of cholesteryl ester in all of the lipoproteins is low; abnormal particles, rich in unesterified cholesterol and phospholipid are found in the LDL fraction. Since the concentration of these particles decreases when the patients consume fat-free diets, it has been suggested (Glomset et al., 1975) that the particles may be surface remnants of chylomicrons.

The clinical features of the rare disease usually include moderate anemia and proteinuria, as well as corneal opacities. In middle age, renal dysfunction can progress to the nephrotic syndrome and ultimately renal failure. Laboratory features include β migrating VLDL that contain *low* amounts of cholesteryl ester and absent or barely detectable α lipoproteins. Liver function tests are normal in contrast to biliary obstruction or hepatitis, which yield similar, though less pronounced, plasma lipoprotein abnormalities (Sabesin et al., 1977).

Defective Low Density Lipoprotein Removal

Hyperbetalipoproteinemia

This widespread disorder, whose primary form was recognized early as "essential hypercholesterolemia," is characterized by an accumulation of the cholesterol-rich β lipoproteins (Type II), apparently because of defective catabolism (Langer et al., 1972). Skin fibroblasts and monocytes cultured from persons homozygous for familial hypercholesterolemia have absent or defective LDL receptors (see p. 886), and therefore cannot normally bind, internalize, or catabolize LDL and cannot normally suppress cholesterol

synthesis (Brown and Goldstein, 1976). Heterozygotes are affected to a lesser degree.

Both familial (monogenic and polygenic) and sporadic varieties of hyperbetalipoproteinemia are prevalent and may be associated with obesity. LDL elevation also occurs secondary to hypothyroidism, in which the removal rate appears to be decreased (Walton et al., 1965), and to the nephrotic syndrome, in which production may be increased (Scott et al., 1970). Occasionally, it occurs in patients with acute intermittent porphyria (Lees et al., 1970) or with myeloma (Taylor et al., 1978), in which an abnormal globulin is believed to bind to β lipoprotein and diminish its clearance rate (Savin, 1965). Hypercholesterolemia is also frequently seen in patients with obstructive liver disease in whom an abnormal cholesterol-rich lipoprotein accumulates (LP-X) (Seidel et al., 1969), and it may occur in those who have ingested excessive amounts of dietary cholesterol or saturated fats.

Regardless of the cause of accumulation of these cholesterol-rich lipoproteins, the risk of coronary atherosclerosis is high, and cardiovascular complications are frequent. Familial hypercholesterolemia expresses early in life (Schrott et al., 1972) and has been documented in cord blood samples (Glueck et al., 1971).

Severe hypercholesterolemia is associated with a specific kind of xanthoma, the tendinous xanthoma, which may be nodular or diffuse but usually appears on the extensor forearm tendons, Achilles tendons (Fig. 17–14), or tendons of the hand. Their presence strongly suggests familial hypercholesterolemia; they typically appear during the first decade of life in individuals with the extremely rare homozygous form of this autosomal dominant disorder.

Combined Hyperlipidemia

Frequently associated wtih coronary atherosclerosis, this disorder ("multiple lipoprotein type hyperlipidemia") was only recently recognized as a distinct entity (Goldstein et al., 1973b; Rose et al., 1973; Nikkilä and Aro, 1973); the precise pathophysiologic mechanisms have not yet been established. This familial disease may present with a variety of lipoprotein types (II-B, II, or IV) in affected individuals in the same family. Thus, patients may have hypertriglyceridemia, hypercholesterolemia, or both; phenotypic expression in any individual also may change with time.

In a study by Goldstein and colleagues (1973a; 1973b) of 500 consecutive 3-month survivors of myocardial infarction in Seattle, in which more than 2600 relatives were tested, this disorder was the most frequent genetic type (Fig. 17–15). It was associated with 30% of the cases of myocardial infarction in patients who had hyperlipidemia (one third of all cases), whereas familial hypertriglyceridemia accounted for 14%, and familial hypercholesterolemia only 10%. Among families of patients with hypertriglyceridemia in another study, myocardial infarction was four times more prevalent and occurred at younger ages in affected individuals with familial combined hyperlipidemia compared to controls or to those with familial hypertriglyceridemia (Brunzell et al., 1976). At present, diagnosis can be established only by family studies; both plasma cholesterol and triglycerides are elevated and lipoprotein analysis shows a combined pattern of elevated LDL and VLDL in some, but not all, family members.

Hypertriglyceridemia and Diabetes Mellitus

Alterations in fat transport often resulting in hypertriglyceridemia are well-recognized concomitants of diabetes mel-

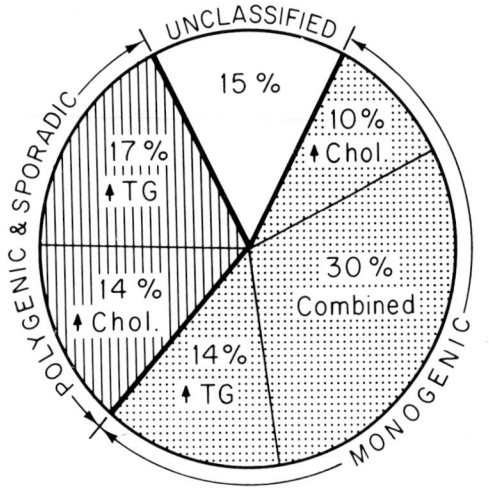

Figure 17–15.   Genetic analysis of hyperlipidemia in 164 M I survivors.

litus. In large groups of diabetics, elevated plasma triglyceride levels coexist in about one third of patients (Bierman and Porte, 1968) and appear to be related to the critical role of insulin in both the removal of triglyceride-rich lipoproteins from plasma and their production. Abnormalities in insulin availability are associated with two distinct pathophysiologic disturbances that affect the production ("endogenous lipemia") and removal ("diabetic lipemia") of triglyceride in acquired hypertriglyceridemia. These more distinct abnormalities appear to be extremes of a spectrum, with varying effects of obesity (high insulin) and diabetes (low insulin) merging between them.

Severe Diabetes: Diabetic Lipemia

Insulin availability appears to be necessary for normal function of LPL (see p. 879); thus, the extreme insulin deficiency associated with severe, uncontrolled diabetes mellitus leads to diabetic lipemia, an acquired form of LPL deficiency.

LPL activity, assessed either indirectly as plasma postheparin lipolytic activity (PHLA) or directly in adipose tissue, is low in patients with the diabetic lipemia syndrome (Bagdade et al., 1967). Although this disorder was recognized in 5% of diabetics before the insulin era, it is now relatively rare. When it occurs, the underlying enzyme deficiency is reversed with appropriate insulin repletion; it promptly restores normal LPL activity, improves triglyceride removal, and reduces plasma triglyceride levels.

Diabetic lipemia can be mimicked by brief withdrawal of insulin from insulin-dependent juvenile diabetics; the enzyme activity decreases and triglyceride levels rise within 48 hours (Bagdade et al., 1968b). The diabetic lipemia syndrome has also been observed as a complication of recurrent alcoholic pancreatitis and during prolonged treatment with high doses of corticosteroids (Bagdade et al., 1969; 1970).

Marked hypertriglyceridemia (plasma triglyceride levels above 2000 mg/dl with chylomicronemia) appears to result from the interaction of two different diseases in the same patient — in this case insulin deficiency superimposed on a separately inherited familial form of hypertriglyceridemia (Brunzell and Schrott, 1973; Brunzell et al., 1975a). Insulin treatment restores triglyceride levels to those seen in nondiabetic hypertriglyceridemic relatives.

Moderate Diabetes: Lipoprotein Lipase Depletion

More subtle insulin deficiency occurs in patients with moderately severe diabetes, those with mild, fasting hyperglycemia in the range of 130–160 mg/dl. Studies by Brunzell and coworkers (1975b) have demonstrated PHLA abnormalities in these individuals despite normal levels of LPL by standard assay. In contrast to normally sustained levels of PHLA during a 5-hour infusion of a large dose of heparin, the PHLA levels of these subjects consistently drop significantly after the 2nd hour. The severity of this "PHLA depletion" appears to be related to the degree of insulin deficiency, judged by fasting glucose levels, and is reflected by low adipose tissue LPL activity (Pykalisto et al., 1975). A comparable phenomenon has been observed in alloxan diabetic rats (Atkin and Meng, 1972).

Most diabetics with hypertriglyceridemia fall into this category, which really represents another acquired form of "removal" lipemia, in which either chylomicrons, VLDL, or both accumulate in plasma. As with severe insulin-deficient diabetics, these persons will respond to replacement therapy. When LPL deficiency occurs in a patient who is being treated for diabetes, it usually indicates that therapy is suboptimal and that treatment requires re-evaluation.

Mild Glucose Intolerance: "Endogenous" Lipemia

By a completely different mechanism, excess insulin associated with the obese patient who frequently has mild glucose intolerance leads to another lipid defect, an acquired form of overproduction hypertriglyceridemia. This disorder also may be seen in individuals with diabetes that has been well-treated. Aside from its effect on LPL activity, insulin (among other substances) appears to act on the liver to promote VLDL production (Topping and Mayes, 1972), presumably by enhancing lipogenesis and lipoprotein packaging and by preventing hepatic triglyceride breakdown (see Figs. 17–9 and 18–11). Several clinical studies have shown that elevated serum immunoreactive insulin (IRI) levels, both in the basal state and after glucose stimulation, are directly related to basal plasma triglyceride levels in normal subjects as well as in those with endogenous lipemia (Olefsky et al., 1974a).

The fact that most patients with endogenous lipemia are also mildly, glucose-intolerant (fasting glucose levels are frequently normal, however) led to the idea that the glucose intolerance was causing the hypertriglyceridemia. It is now apparent that early insulin responses to glucose are similar in patients with hypertriglyceridemia and in subjects with normal triglyceride levels who have comparable degrees of mild glucose intolerance (Bagdade et al., 1971), and correction of glucose intolerance during oral sulfonylurea therapy does not lower triglyceride levels (Belknap et al., 1967). This suggests that glucose intolerance, with its associated abnormality of early insulin release, is not etiologically related to hypertriglyceridemia. Conversely, hypertriglyceridemia does not appear to cause the glucose intolerance (see later).

Obesity is the most prevalent of several secondary factors (see Fig. 18–11) that induce endogenous hypertriglyceridemia by invoking mechanisms that impair the action of insulin on glucose metabolism in peripheral tissue. This reduced responsiveness (insulin "resistance") by some unknown process is "sensed" by the pancreas, which attempts to compensate and secrete additional insulin. The hyperinsulinemia associated with adiposity is well documented (Ch. 18). The basal hyperinsulinemia often observed in persons with endogenous lipemia is fully accounted for by the degree of coexisting adiposity (Bagdade et al., 1971). In one form, familial hypertriglyceridemia, the triglyceride regulatory mechanism appears to be more sensitive to insulin, however, resulting in higher plasma triglyceride levels for a given insulin level (Brunzell and Bierman, 1977). Correlations between adiposity and plasma triglyceride levels have been observed in both sexes, at all ages, using such indices of adiposity as relative weight, skin-fold thickness, and actual measurements of percentage of body fat (reviewed by Bierman et al., 1970).

Most patients with endogenous lipemia and mild glucose intolerance have a long history of obesity. As might be expected, obesity-related hypertriglyceridemia responds dramatically to weight reduction, which reverses basal hyperinsulinemia, hypertriglyceridemia, and glucose intolerance. The other forms of hypertriglyceridemia associated with hyperinsulinemia respond to reduction or removal of the offending hormone or drug or to correction of a causative disorder.

Hyperlipidemia and Hypothyroidism

In addition to the elevated cholesterol-rich β lipoprotein levels (p. 891) frequently observed in hypothyroidism, deficiency of thyroid hormone exerts profound effects on triglyceride transport, often leading to hypertriglyceridemia. The severity of the effect is in large part related to the degree of hormone deficiency, whether primary or secondary to pituitary disorders, and thus the presence or absence of hypertriglyceridemia or hypercholesterolemia offers little diagnostic aid in the differentiation between primary and secondary hypothyroidism.

Availability of adequate thyroid hormone is essential for normal activity of LPL. In hypothyroidism, low LPL appears to be reciprocally related to hypertriglyceridemia, and the abnormalities are reversible with thyroid replacement (Pykalisto et al., 1967). As with insulin deficiency, the degree and type of triglyceride-rich lipoprotein accumulation may vary in severity and type with diet and age. Reversible hypertriglyceridemia associated with low LPL has been reported in a 14-month old cretin (Baum et al., 1973).

The normal removal of chylomicron and VLDL remnants (p. 885) also appears to be affected by hypothyroidism, since a Type III lipoprotein pattern and all the features of "broad-beta" disease can become clinically manifest with thyroid insufficiency and reversible with treatment (Hazzard and Bierman, 1972).

Although fatty acid mobilization from adipose tissue may be decreased in hypothyroidism, thereby reducing fatty acid flux to the liver, diminished hepatic production of triglyceride-rich lipoproteins is presumably insufficient to fully counterbalance impairment of removal.

Thus a wide variety of patterns of hyperlipoproteinemia can be produced by hypothyroidism (Table 17–8). In a large series of patients with primary myxedema reported by Koppers and Palumbo (1972), the majority of patients (53%) were hyperlipidemic, with increased VLDL or LDL levels or both. In addition, the broad-beta pattern and fasting chylomicronemia were not unusual. Although individuals with hypothyroidism appear to be excessively predisposed to atherosclerosis, the role of these varieties of secondary hyperlipidemia in that regard is unknown.

Hyperlipidemia and Estrogens

Estrogens, like insulin, influence both the production and the removal of plasma lipoproteins. In most women receiving estrogen-containing oral contraceptive steroids, some increase in plasma triglyceride and VLDL levels occurs (Hazzard et al., 1969; Wallace et al., 1979). This increase appears to be proportional to the estrogen (but not the progestogen) content of the medication and to the pretreatment triglyceride levels. In population surveys, women below age 25 taking oral contraceptives have plasma triglyceride levels averaging 48% higher than those of women not taking drugs (Wallace et al., 1977). These levels remain in the normal range in most instances, however, and the long-term effect of this increase remains unknown. In a few instances, massive hypertriglyceridemia, chylomicronemia, and life-threatening pancreatitis ensue (Davidoff et al., 1973), usually when estrogen therapy is given to a patient with a previously unrecognized familial form of hypertriglyceridemia (such as familial hypertriglyceridemia or familial combined hyperlipidemia). The mechanism of the estrogen-induced increase in plasma triglyceride levels appears to be related to an enhanced hepatic VLDL triglyceride production rate (Kekki and Nikkilä, 1971: Glueck et al., 1975), perhaps modulated by increased insulin levels (Hazzard et al., 1969). Efficiency of triglyceride removal may also be enhanced by estrogen, but not enough to keep pace with accelerated triglyceride input. Adipose tissue LPL levels remain normal (Applebaum et al., 1977).

In contrast to these effects on triglyceride-rich lipoproteins, estrogens appear to enhance the clearance of cholesterol-rich lipoproteins and thus may be therapeutic in certain familial hyperlipidemias. In broad-beta disease, exogenous estrogens dramatically lower cholesterol and triglyceride levels, normalize the altered VLDL lipid composition and apoprotein concentration (see pp. 890 and 891), and correct the impaired removal of remnants (Kushwaha et al., 1977b; Chait et al., 1977). The inherited apolipoprotein E-III deficiency persists, however. Preliminary results suggest that estrogen may lower LDL cholesterol levels in postmenopausal women with familial hypercholesterolemia (Nikkilä and Tikkanen, 1978), perhaps by enhancing catabolism. Thus, it is essential to measure plasma triglyceride and cholesterol levels prior to starting estrogen or estrogen-containing oral contraceptive therapy, and these drugs should be avoided in patients with pre-existing hypertriglyceridemia, unless it can be shown to be due to broad-beta disease.

Hyperlipidemia and Atherosclerosis

Premature atherosclerosis may be associated with lipoprotein abnormalities. Hyperbetalipoproteinemia is frequently associated with premature atherosclerosis whether genetically determined (Goldstein et al., 1973b), as in familial hypercholesterolemia, familial combined hyperlipidemia, or polygenic hypercholesterolemia, or whether a secondary manifestation of hypothyroidism, nephrotic syndrome, or high cholesterol and saturated fat intake. Endogenous hypertriglyceridemia may be associated with premature atherosclerosis in some specific disorders; this association may not be apparent in studies of whole populations. Patients with elevated VLDL levels who come from families with familial combined hyperlipidemia appear to be at increased risk (Brunzell et al., 1976). Patients with comparably elevated VLDL levels from families with familial hypertriglyceridemia may not have an increased risk. In addition, increased VLDL levels may increase the risk for premature atherosclerosis when associated with other risk factors such as in diabetes (Santen et al., 1972), and in patients who smoke and are hypertensive while on chronic hemodialysis (Haire et al., 1978). Individuals in whom remnants accumulate with resulting hypercholesterolemia and hypertriglyceridemia are also at risk for early development of atherosclerosis (Morganroth et al., 1975).

Recently it has been re-emphasized that HDL seems to confer protection against the development of premature atherosclerosis and therefore might be considered an "anti-risk factor" (Glomset, 1979; Castelli et al., 1977a). That is, individuals with high HDL cholesterol levels have less atherosclerosis, whereas those with low HDL have more. Females characteristically have higher HDL than do males; HDL can be increased by estrogen and reduced by androgen. Rare genetic hyperalphalipoproteinemia syndromes (high HDL) have been associated with increased longevity (Glueck et al., 1977). The role of the interrelationship between HDL and VLDL (which vary in inverse fashion) and the association of HDL with other atherosclerosis-modifying factors such as diabetes (Nikkilä and Hormila, 1978), exercise (Wood et al., 1977), and alcohol (Castelli et al., 1977b) remain speculative.

Laboratory Tests in Differential Diagnosis

The first step in the diagnosis of hyperlipidemia is routine quantitative measurement of both cholesterol and triglyceride levels in fasting serum or plasma. When values are above normal (exceed the 95th percentile matched for age and sex, Table 17–6) and verified at least once more, a combination of personal, dietary, drug, and family histories, a thorough examination, and laboratory tests are necessary to define the specific lipid disorder accurately.

Further studies of plasma obtained after an overnight fast may yield additional information regarding the underlying abnormality. The formation of a cream layer in the cold always indicates the presence of chylomicrons, which often points to a deficiency in triglyceride removal. When a high concentration of triglyceride-rich VLDL is present, the plasma also appears turbid. For practical purposes, completely clear plasma or serum suggests a normal triglyceride level and rules out disorders of chylomicron and VLDL transport.

Because lipoproteins carry varying amounts of triglyceride and cholesterol, the relative degree of elevation of these two lipids in whole plasma is often helpful. In hyperchylomicronemia, the triglyceride-cholesterol ratio is high, 10:1 or higher. In hyperbetalipoproteinemia, the triglyceride-cholesterol ratio may be as low as 1:2 or less, and in broad-beta disease the ratio is about 1:1. On the other hand, in the common combined disorder, since both LDL and VLDL may be increased in varying proportions, ratios of lipids in plasma can be misleading.

Electrophoretic studies, which have been used to define qualitatively abnormal lipoprotein patterns (see p. 888) are usually not necessary (Fredrickson, 1975) and, although formerly emphasized, may now be irrelevant for diagnostic or therapeutic decisions. When serum measurements show only an elevated cholesterol level, there is a very close correlation between serum cholesterol and LDL cholesterol levels. Occasionally, in certain individuals (usually younger females), a mildly increased serum cholesterol may be due to elevated HDL levels. These can be distinguished by precipitation methods. In situations with marked degrees of hypertriglyceridemia, electrophoretic studies are often inadequate for definitive diagnosis. Not infrequently, high levels of triglycerides will produce a smearing effect, so that some of the patterns merge. For example, it is often difficult to distinguish among Types III, IV, and V by paper or agarose electrophoresis alone. Determination of plasma lipoprotein patterns by electrophoresis alone does not define disease (see p. 888) or distinguish discrete genetic disorders, such as familial hypercholesterolemia, from familial combined hyperlipidemia. In some situations, only ultracentrifugation of plasma will provide an answer (as in the definition of broad-beta disease); in others, more detailed family studies, including measurement of fasting cholesterol and triglyceride levels among first-degree relatives, are most helpful. Familial hypercholesterolemia in affected children can be detected in cord blood samples. Aside from that disorder, familial LPL deficiency, and familial LCAT deficiency, other familial forms of hyperlipidemia are not detectable before puberty.

Recently much interest has been generated in the measurement of HDL cholesterol levels since high HDL has been associated with decreased risk of myocardial infarction in population studies (see p. 900). The value of HDL cholesterol measurements for predicting the occurrence of myocardial infarction in the individual patient has not been established, however. Because of the inverse relationship between VLDL and HDL, low HDL cholesterol levels in the patient with hypertriglyceridemia are difficult to interpret.

Estimation of LDL concentration ("β quantification") can now be simply obtained from measurements of serum cholesterol and triglycerides coupled with an independent measurement of HDL cholesterol. This estimate (serum cholesterol minus serum triglycerides/5 minus HDL cholesterol) correlates closely with LDL cholesterol measured directly after ultracentrifugation (Friedewald et al., 1972). It is a reliable approximation in patients with triglyceride levels below about 400 mg/dl but cannot be used in those with broad-beta disease whose VLDL triglyceride:cholesterol ratio is much less than the normal value of about 5:1.

Guidelines for Therapy

Before a therapeutic program for hyperlipidemia is undertaken, the possible underlying secondary causes should be thoroughly investigated since these are very frequent. In general, a thorough history plus laboratory tests for thyroid and liver function, serum glucose, and plasma and urine protein levels will elucidate the secondary forms of hyperlipidemia. These may be simpler to treat, since it is usually only a matter of withdrawal of inciting pharmacologic agents or treatment of the underlying illness.

When underlying causes cannot be elucidated, it must be assumed that the disorder is primary, either familial or sporadic. Although diet and drugs are the treatment mainstays of hyperlipidemia, therapy must be aimed at the pathophysiology associated with the disorder rather than at a particular lipoprotein pattern, which often is nonspecific.

Diet

Provided the patient will cooperate, dietary restriction alone is often very effective in lowering blood lipids in most hyperlipidemias (Olefsky et al., 1974b; Leelarthaepin et al., 1974). The exception is familial hypercholesterolemia, for which optimal diet alone rarely achieves more than a 20% reduction in cholesterol levels (Lees and Wilson, 1971; Evans et al., 1972). In all primary or sporadic disorders, however, dietary therapy should always be attempted initially. Only when the hyperlipidemia proves refractory should pharmacologic agents be considered.

LPL deficiency, in which hypertriglyceridemia is aggravated by dietary fat, is best handled simply by restriction of fat intake and optionally substituting short- or medium-chain triglycerides. The rationale for this substitution depends on the fact that short- and medium chain triglycerides are absorbed directly via the portal vein, bypassing chylomicron formation and transport through intestinal lymphatics (p. 879). When severe insulin deficiency is causing the enzyme deficiency, the patient should be vigorously treated with insulin. In lipemia associated with impaired LPL activity in conjunction with hyperglycemia, either insulin or oral antidiabetic agents are effective in correcting the disorder.

Most other types of hyperlipidemia respond to a basic diet that is low in cholesterol and saturated fat. Since obesity aggravates the hyperlipidemias by promoting production of VLDL, this diet should be hypocaloric until the patient achieves ideal body weight. Such a diet most likely will contain a high proportion of carbohydrate (more than 50% of total calories), but in most instances this is of little concern, even in patients with endogenous lipemia. Although triglyceride levels are reportedly highest on high carbohydrate diets, this only occurs in the postabsorptive state following an overnight fast. Studies of 24-hour patterns of triglyceride levels in patients with hypertriglyceridemia have shown them to be actually lower on higher-carbohydrate diets compared with diets higher in fat than in carbohydrate (Schlierf et al., 1971). If control of hypertriglyceridemia is meant to imply lowering of all-day levels, as in diabetic therapy, evidence suggests that a calorie-restricted, relatively low-fat, high carbohydrate diet would be desirable for the control of the endogenous hypertriglyceridemias. A recent outpatient study (Sommariva et al., 1978) has shown that even for overnight fasting triglyceride levels, a low-fat diet may be more effective than a low-carbohydrate diet for long-term management.

Thus a disproportionate restriction of carbohydrates in the diet of these patients is not usually justified. Alcohol, which may increase triglyceride production by altering the caloric balance and directly stimulating hepatic syntheses (Kudzma and Schonfeld, 1971), should be discouraged in patients with any disorder in the transport of VLDL. In patients with hypercholesterolemia, particular emphasis must be placed on lowering the intake of cholesterol-containing foods. Decreasing the dietary intake from the average American consumption of 500–750 mg/day to less than 250 mg/day is an essential step in therapy, since dietary cholesterol will accumulate beyond the ability of the body to reduce the amount synthesized (Fig. 17–16) and increase the amount secreted (see p. 886). Saturated fat intake should also be curtailed to less than 10% of total calories (American Heart

Association, 1978), since these fatty acids also appear to raise serum cholesterol levels. Cholesterol and saturated fat usually occur in the same foods, however, so that the dietary regimen would probably be similar. Because they have such a high risk of developing premature atherosclerosis, children of patients with familial hypercholesterolemia should be screened in infancy and childhood and appropriate management instituted as early in life as possible, although improvement in outcome has not been proved. Dietary management has been shown to reduce cholesterol levels during the first year of life in infants with familial hypercholesterolemia (Glueck and Tsang, 1971).

The value of substituting unsaturated for saturated fat in diets for patients with hypercholesterolemia is debatable. A diet high in unsaturated fats appears to be less efficient in lowering cholesterol levels than restriction of cholesterol and saturated fats without the substitution. Furthermore, the long-term effects of highly unsaturated fat diets remains unknown, and the mechanism by which unsaturated fat appears to lower cholesterol levels may not necessarily be by increasing cholesterol excretion but could include redistribution of the sterol between plasma and tissues. Thus current recommendations of the American Heart Association limit intake of polyunsaturated fats to no more than 10% of total calories. Increase of the P/S ratio to about 1.0 is thereby achieved mainly by reduction of saturated fat intake. Reduction of the proportion of fat calories to 30–35% of the total would therefore require a reciprocal increase in the proportion of carbohydrate calories to 50% or more.

Thus there is a single basic diet for all the common forms of hyperlipidemia. This low-calorie, low saturated–fat, low-cholesterol diet that is appropriate for patients with hyperlipidemia is a prudent diet for the population at large. In practice, it translates into limitation of animal fats and substitution of vegetable oils and carbohydrates. It carries little known risk in adults and is effective in lowering both cholesterol and triglyceride, not only in the fasting state (i.e., early morning) but throughout the day. It should be individualized to fit the patient: for example, special attention should be paid to dietary cholesterol restriction for patients with familial hypercholesterolemia and to alcohol restriction for those with hypertriglyceridemia and elevated VLDL. The role of increased dietary fiber of various types as an aid to lipid lowering is currently being evaluated.

Pharmacologic Agents

When dietary restrictions or weight reduction or both are ineffective or when the patient fails to cooperate, a number of agents may be added to the therapeutic regimen (reviewed by Yeshurun and Gotto, 1976). Drugs that act by reducing hepatic triglyceride production — clofibrate, nicotinic acid, para-aminosalicylic acid (PAS-C), phenformin — are all effective (Bierman et al., 1970; Carlson, 1969; Stout et al., 1974; Berkowitz, 1971; Goldberg et al., 1978a) in disorders involving that mechanism: endogenous lipemia and broad-beta disease. Patients with broad-beta disease have been found to respond particularly well to combined weight reduction and clofibrate or to estrogen, which despite increasing triglyceride production, has recently been found to uniquely reverse the metabolic abnormalities in this disorder (see p. 890). Estrogen treatment remains experimental, however, and, because of its tendency to provoke atherosclerotic and thrombotic complications, its use should be restricted to selected female patients who fail to respond to clofibrate.

Certain anabolic and progestational agents, such as oxandrolone and norethindrone, have been found to be effective in some patients with primary triglyceride removal disorders

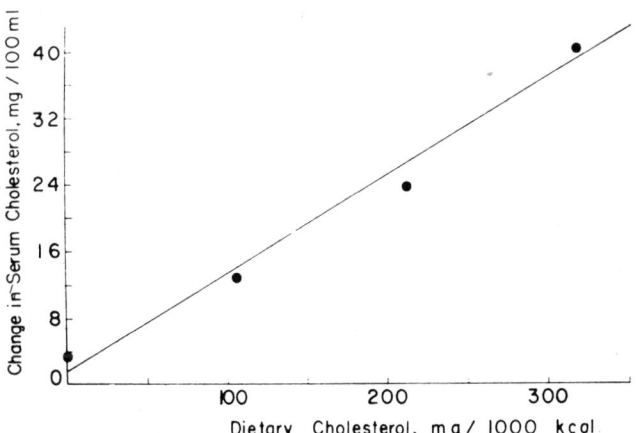

Figure 17–16. Relationship between cholesterol intake and the change in serum cholesterol following 21 days on a cholesterol-free formula diet of constant fatty acid composition. (Adapted from Mattson, F. H., Erickson, B. A., et al.: Effect of dietary cholesterol on serum cholesterol in man. *Am. J. Clin. Nutr.* 25:589, 1972.)

(Glueck et al., 1969b), perhaps by acceleration of the removal rate of triglyceride-rich lipoproteins from plasma (Glueck et al., 1973), apparently independent of enhancement of the effect of LPL (Enholm et al., 1975).

By directly diverting cholesterol and bile acids from the intestine to the feces, bile acid binding agents, such as cholestyramine and colestipol (12–24 g/day for adults), enhance cholesterol excretion and interfere with enterohepatic recycling (see p. 886). Consequently, these agents are useful in lowering plasma cholesterol levels in patients with hypercholesterolemia due to increased LDL levels. Although dextrothyroxine has been shown to reduce both plasma cholesterol and triglyceride levels by 10–15%, presumably by stimulating removal processes more than synthesis, this drug was withdrawn from a large, secondary, drug prevention trial because of a higher mortality and morbidity among patients with coronary heart disease treated with the drug (Stamler, 1972). It is quite likely that the lipid-lowering action of thyroid hormone and its analogues is not separable from the stimulating effect on tissue oxygen consumption. A recently introduced drug, probucol, which lowers LDL levels, is being used in the treatment of hypercholesterolemia; its efficacy remains to be established.

Combinations of drugs are seldom indicated except in the severe familial monogenic form of hypercholesterolemia — when cholesterol levels exceed 400 mg/dl. In these highly resistant patients, a combination of nicotinic acid and bile acid binding agent has been particularly effective in normalizing cholesterol levels (Kane et al., 1978). Perhaps in the future, combined therapy may prove useful in the treatment of familial combined hyperlipidemia.

Side effects of these lipid lowering agents need to be considered particularly since they are needed for long-term use in the primary hyperlipidemias. Clofibrate in usual adult doses (1.5–2.0 gm/day) has been associated with an increased incidence of gallstones (Palmer, 1978; Oliver, 1978) (see p. 903). In patients with impaired ability to metabolize the drug, such as those with uremia or hepatic disease, clofibrate induces an acute myopathy associated with increased serum creatine phosphokinase levels; doses should be drastically reduced to 1.0–1.5 g/week (Goldberg et al., 1977). Nicotinic acid is associated with severe flushing; this can be minimized and tolerated by a gradual increase in dose from 100 mg thrice daily with meals to a total dose of 55–85 mg/kg body weight/day. Bile acid binding agents are constipating, and while lowering serum cholesterol may actually increase VLDL synthesis and aggravate hypertriglyceridemia in some patients; this effect may be transient, however.

Surgery

Surgeons at a number of medical centers are currently performing partial ileal bypass operations on patients with severe, resistant heterozygous familial hypercholesterolemia (Scott, 1972). The procedure results in increased excretion of cholesterol degradation products in the stool. At present, however, the surgical approach should be regarded as experimental, for little is known about the long-term effects of the surgery itself. A remarkable lowering of LDL and cholesterol levels was obtained in several young patients with the very rare and severe homozygous form of familial hypercholesterolemia after portacaval shunt procedures (Starzl et al., 1978). This approach also is now under intensive study. Plasmapheresis as an alternative therapeutic approach to severe familial hypercholesterolemia is also being investigated (Thompson, 1975).

Comment on Therapy

The association between hypertriglyceridemia, hypercholesterolemia, and atherosclerotic disease in persons with and without hyperglycemia has been amply confirmed in a variety of population studies. Although various factors have thus far been implicated, the mechanisms that account for this relationship are yet to be clearly elucidated; they are discussed in more detail in the section "Atherosclerosis."

The rationale for treating symptomatic hyperlipidemia is obvious. Prevention of the potentially fatal complication of acute pancreatitis is an absolute indication for treatment of marked hypertriglyceridemia with chylomicronemia. Treatment of asymptomatic disorders is based on the yet unproven "lipid hypothesis" — that lowering lipid levels will decrease morbidity and mortality from associated atherosclerosis. Recently published results of the large WHO clofibrate trial (Oliver, 1978) have provided the most convincing evidence to date favoring the lipid hypothesis, since cholesterol lowering was associated with a reduced incidence of nonfatal myocardial infarctions. The lack of reduction in total mortality in that study remains unsettling, however. Therefore, the decision as to whom should be treated and when (Ahrens, 1976) is not yet on a rational footing and must await the results of the controlled intervention trials that are currently in progress.

ATHEROSCLEROSIS

Atherosclerosis has been defined as "a variable combination of changes of the intima of arteries . . . consisting of the focal accumulation of lipids, complex carbohydrates, blood and blood products, fibrous tissue and calcium deposits, and associated with medial changes" (WHO Study Group, 1958). Because of its connection with coronary heart disease, cerebrovascular disease, and peripheral vascular disease, atherosclerosis is associated with higher morbidity and mortality than is any other disorder in the western world. Progress toward clarification of its etiology has been slow for several reasons, however. First, it tends to develop insidiously for many years in ostensibly healthy individuals, and no satisfactory method is available for directly studying this important phase of the disease. Second, when clinical symptoms finally develop, atherosclerosis is usually advanced and is only one of a complex group of precipitating factors. This makes evaluation of the course of the primary disease process even more difficult. Finally, because of the difficulty of making satisfactory studies of humans *in vivo*, conclusions with respect to pathogenesis and therapy have had to depend on statistical correlations between the incidence or prevalence of overt vascular disease and plasma lipid concentrations, hypertension, cigarette smoking, obesity, diabetes, and other "risk factors"; the study of specimens obtained at autopsy; and investigations of experimental atherosclerosis in animals. Despite these difficulties, there is strong evidence that lipids play an important role in atherosclerosis, and they have repeatedly been implicated in connection with the pathogenesis, prophylaxis, and treatment of the disease. Consequently, it is important that those involved in the management of diseases of lipid metabolism be acquainted with present knowledge in this area.

Pathogenesis

Structural Factors and Definitions

Normal arteries vary not only in size and degree of branching but also in histologic and chemical composition. This also is true of the arteries most prone to develop atherosclerosis, including the aorta and the coronary and cerebral arteries. Nevertheless, all arteries are composed of three distinguishable layers: the intima, the media, and the adventitia. The *intima* is the primary focus of the developing atherosclerotic process. It is composed of several elements. First, a single layer of endothelial cells, the endothelium, borders on the arterial lumen. Next to this are variable numbers of smooth muscle cells and variable amounts of collagen and other extracellular connective tissue components. Finally, the intima is limited by a layer of elastic tissue, the *internal elastic lamina*. The overall thickness of the intima increases with age because of proliferation of smooth muscle cells and is particularly pronounced at sites of arterial branching. This thickening appears to be correlated with the susceptibility of arteries to atherosclerotic change. The *media* of arteries like the coronaries is mainly composed of smooth muscle cells surrounded by an extracellular matrix of collagen, elastic fibers, and proteoglycans. In the larger arteries, layers of elastic tissue are particularly prominent. The *adventitia* is mainly composed of loose connective tissue.

Fatty Streaks

The earliest macroscopically detectable fatty change in arteries is the so-called fatty streak, regarded by many pathologists as an early stage of atherosclerosis. This is a small yellow-gray area that is characteristically flat and does not compromise the arterial lumen. The yellow-gray color is largely caused by lipid within smooth muscle cells, macrophages, and "foam" cells (Fig. 17–17). The lipid is mainly cholesterol (Table 17–10), most of which is esterified to oleic and palmitic acid. Little phospholipid or triglyceride appears to be present, since the relative content of these lipids in fatty streaks is less than that in lesion-free intima. Despite the presumed relation between fatty streaks and fibrous atherosclerotic plaques, the prevalence and location of fatty streaks are not generally correlated with the prevalence and location of fibrous lesions. Fatty streaks occur in all populations studied, irrespective of the propensity of these populations to develop clinical vascular disease. They begin in childhood (in the aorta) and in late adolescence (in the

coronary and cerebral arteries), increase with age, and do not necessarily "progress" into fibrous lesions. Even in populations susceptible to atherosclerosis, the location of fatty streaks in the aorta and the extent of intimal involvement do not parallel the location and extent of fibrous lesions. Only in the coronary arteries have better correlations been observed (Geer et al., 1968).

Fibrous Plaques

Fibrous plaques differ from fatty streaks not only in prevalence and location but also in appearance, composition, and effects. They are pearly white, considerably larger than fatty streaks, and cause the intimal surface to bulge outward into the lumen. A major part of the lipid is extracellular, often mixed with what appears to be cell debris to form "gruel." Although this lipid, like that of fatty streaks, is mainly cholesteryl ester (Table 17–10), linoleic rather than oleic acid is the principal esterified fatty acid. Consequently, the composition of the cholesteryl ester resembles that of plasma lipoprotein cholesteryl ester rather than fatty streak cholesteryl ester. Another distinctive feature of fibrous plaques is the presence of large numbers of smooth muscle cells and

Table 17–10. LIPID DISTRIBUTION IN DIFFERENT TYPES OF PLAQUE

	Normal Intima†	Fatty Streaks*	Fatty Nodules*	Fibrous Plaques*	Calcified Fibrous Plaques*
Total Lipid (mg./100 mg. dry tissue)	11	28	61	47	50
Percentage Distribution					
Cholesteryl ester	42	60	65	54	56
Unesterified cholesterol	13	12	14	18	22
Triglyceride	15	10	9	11	7
Phospholipid	29	18	14	16	15

†Age group 40–59. (Data from Smith, E. B., Evans, P. H., et al.: *J. Atherosclerosis Res.* 7:177, 1967.)
*Without amorphous lipid. (Reproduced from Smith, E. B.: *J. Atherosclerosis Res.* 5:231, 1965.)

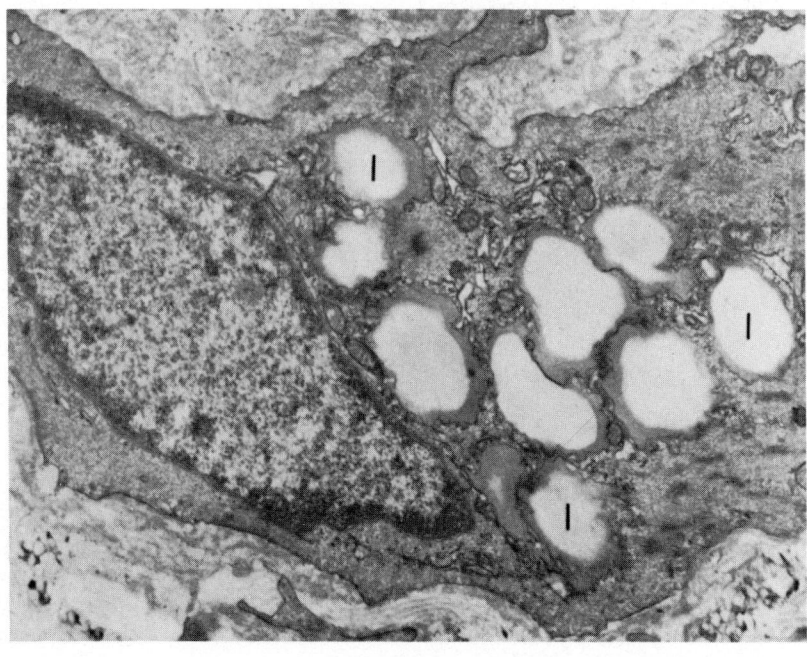

Figure 17–17. Electron micrograph (× 15,000) of smooth muscle cell in fatty streaks in human intima. Lipid inclusions are labeled I. They are irregular in contour and lined by a single membrane. The lipid is moderately electron-dense; the central portion of the inclusions is electron-lucent, probably because of extraction of a portion of the lipid during tissue processing. (From Geer, J.: Fine structure of human aortic intimal thickening and fatty streaks. *Lab. Invest.* 14:1764, 1965.)

Table 17–11. CONNECTIVE TISSUE COMPONENTS AND LIPIDS OF DIFFERENT TYPES OF LESION

	Collagen (Calculated) (mg/100 mg protein)	Mucopoly-saccharide (Calculated) (mg/100 mg protein)	Total Lipid (mg/100 mg protein)
Fatty streaks and nodules	26 (24)*	3.0 (2.6)	31 (9)
Fibrous plaques	41 (25)	2.5 (2.6)	47 (11)
Calcified plaques	61 (24)	1.2 (3.0)	109 (9)

*Controls given in parentheses. (From Smith, E. B.: *J. Atherosclerosis Res.* 5:241, 1965.)

large amounts of collagen (Table 17–11). These usually form a cap between the lumen and the extracellular lipid, and, in older individuals, the collagen is the cap's dominant component. The presumption is that many of the smooth muscle cells have disintegrated and contributed to the lipid-rich extracellular gruel. In older individuals, too, fibrous plaques contain increasing amounts of calcium. These *complicated lesions* are the ones that frequently are associated with clinical symptoms. With increasing cell degeneration and accumulation of gruel, the wall of the artery becomes progressively weaker, and rupture of the intima can occur, causing aneurysm and death by hemorrhage. Alternatively, arterial emboli can form when fragments of diseased intima dislodge into the arterial lumen, or stenosis and impaired organ function can occur as smaller arteries gradually become occluded by widespread atherosclerotic thickening (Fig. 17–18). Stenosis of the coronaries can cause sudden death from ischemic heart disease following what would otherwise be trivial alterations in coronary blood supply and demand. In those who survive an acute ischemic episode,

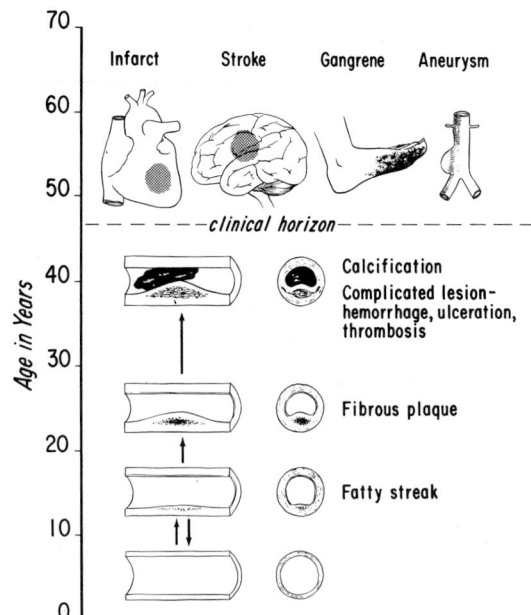

Natural History of Atherosclerosis

Figure 17–19. Diagrammatic concept of the pathogenesis of atherosclerosis. (From McGill, H., et al., In *Atherosclerosis and Its Origin.* Sandler, M., and Bourne, J. (eds.), New York, Academic Press, 1963.)

thrombosis can subsequently lead to complete occlusion. This has been documented in about 50% of the patients who die of acute ischemic heart disease (Crawford, 1961; Roberts and Buja, 1972). A scheme that generally summarizes these concepts is shown in Fig. 17–19.

Etiologic Factors

Injury to the Arterial Endothelium

Since atherosclerosis tends to be focal rather than generalized, its pathogenesis ultimately will have to be explained in terms of local factors that affect the biology of arterial endothelial and smooth muscle cells. Hemodynamic and structural factors probably influence the biochemistry of cells and predispose specific regions of selected arteries to atherosclerosis. One suggested possibility is that turbulent blood flow or shear associated with bending and branching of arteries locally "injures" the endothelium and induces platelet aggregation and the formation of organized microthrombi (French, 1970; Ross and Glomset, 1973). Another is that increased intimal permeability to blood proteins occurs either because of turbulence or because of disruption of the endothelium at arterial sites close to branch points that are more firmly anchored and less able to evenly dissipate stresses caused by pulse waves (French, 1966).

One reason why the arterial endothelium is thought to be so critical is that it presumably influences the ingress of blood proteins like LDL and fibrinogen, which have been identified in arteries and may play an important role in atherosclerosis. A second reason is that endothelial dysfunction may lead to the proliferation of smooth muscle cells associated with the formation of fibrous plaques. Experimental removal of the arterial enodthelium immediately causes aggregation of platelets on the injured surface followed by proliferation of smooth muscle cells and formation of a raised lesion (Stemerman and Ross, 1972). This proliferation of

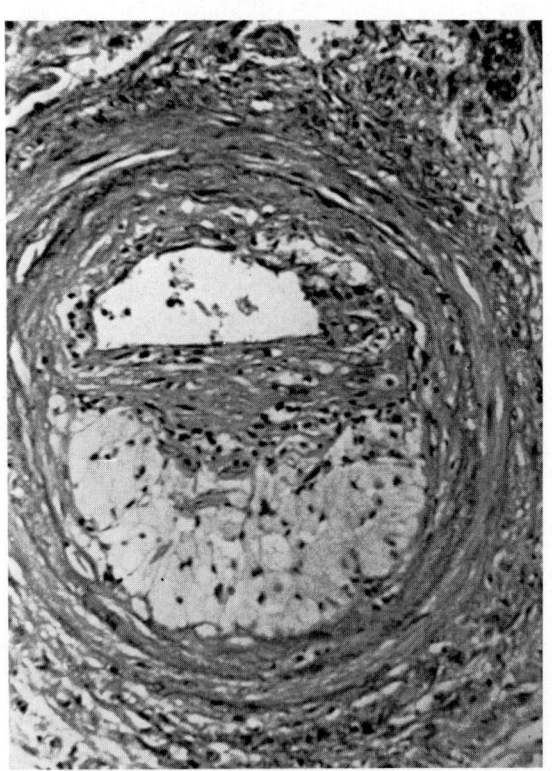

Figure 17–18. A cross section of a small artery with a large, eccentric aggregation of intimal smooth muscle cells loaded with lipid. (Courtesy of S. L. Robbins.)

arterial smooth muscle cells apparently occurs in response to a mitogen released from platelet α-granules (Ross and Glomset, 1976).

Lipids

Many factors probably interact to produce fibrous and complicated lesions, but lipids are clearly of special importance. As shown in Tables 17–10 and 17–11, one third to one half of the calcium-free dry weight of atherosclerotic plaques is lipid, more than 70% of which is cholesterol. In addition, the risk of developing atherosclerotic heart disease is directly correlated with plasma cholesterol concentrations both within (Fig. 17–20) and among populations. Finally, atherosclerosis can be induced in nonhuman primates by dietary measures that increase the concentration of cholesterol in plasma.

The mechanism by which cholesterol and other lipids accumulate in plaques is not yet understood, but three possible sources of the lipid have been proposed: local biosynthesis within the arterial wall, the platelets of encrusted mural thrombi, and plasma lipoproteins that have filtered into the intima. Probably all three are involved to some extent. Nevertheless, most of the extracellular cholesterol is probably derived from the plasma. One reason for believing this has already been mentioned, i.e., the similarity in fatty acid composition between the cholesteryl esters of plaques and those of plasma lipoproteins. A second reason is that isotopic studies of the plaque cholesterol of humans and experimental animals have indicated that biosynthesis by the cells of the arterial wall is too limited to account for more than a small proportion of the total cholesterol present. A third reason is that LDL have been demonstrated in the intima of the arteries (Smith and Slater, 1972) and that the concentration of these lipoproteins is directly related to their concentration in plasma (Fig. 17–21), which in turn is direct-

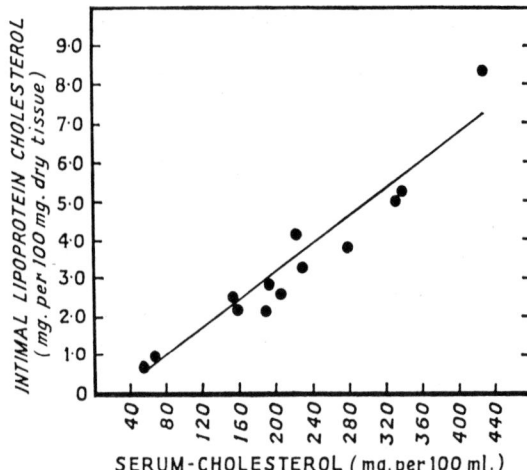

Figure 17–21. Immunologically detectable low-density lipoprotein in the intima of arteries as a function of low-density lipoprotein concentration in plasma. (From Smith, E. B., and Slater, R. S.: Relationship between low-density lipoprotein in aortic intima and serum-lipid levels. *Lancet* 1:463, 1972.)

ly related to the risk of developing atherosclerotic heart disease (Fig. 17–20). A fourth reason is that arterial smooth muscle cells are known (Bierman and Albers, 1976) to contain a receptor that promotes the uptake and degradation of LDL.

If most of the lipid of plaques is derived from plasma lipoproteins, why does it accumulate in arteries, and how does the accumulated lipid affect the biology of the arterial wall? These unanswered questions appear to be of central importance to our understanding of the pathogenesis of atherosclerosis. Smith and her colleagues have already shown that fine droplets of extracellular lipid are present even in arteries that have a normal macroscopic appearance, and that this lipid is rich in cholesteryl ester and increases with age (Fig. 17–22). Since the percentage of linoleic acid present also increases with age and approaches that of the cholesteryl esters of plasma lipoproteins, it is highly likely that this "perifibrous" lipid is derived from plasma lipoproteins. Presumably, all that is required for this lipid to accumulate is some nonenzymic or enzymic mechanism that would alter the lipoproteins in such a way as to render them insoluble and thus incapable of diffusing out of the intima. One possibility is that lipoproteins absorb to the intimal connective tissue matrix. Since both LDL and VLDL readily

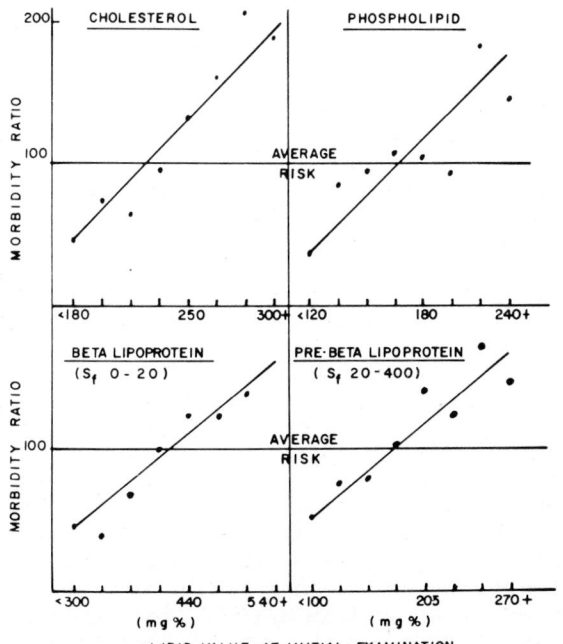

Figure 17–20. Risk of developing overt coronary heart disease (morbidity ratio) as a function of plasma lipid and lipoprotein concentrations. (From Kannel, W. B., Garcia, M. J., et al.: Serum lipid precursors of coronary heart disease. *Hum. Pathol.* 2:129, 1971.)

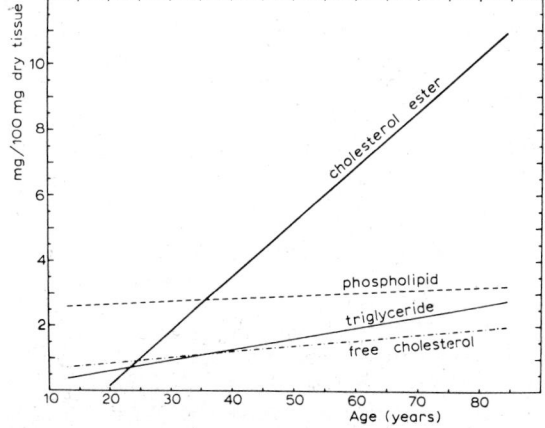

Figure 17–22. Lipids of the normal intima of human arteries as a function of age. (From Smith, E. B., Evans, P. H., et al.: Lipid in the aortic intima. The correlation of morphological and chemical characteristics. *J. Atheroscler. Res.* 7:171, 1967.)

form complexes with sulfated polysaccharides of the type found in the arterial wall, absorption of this type might explain the association between plasma VLDL or triglyceride concentrations (Fig. 17–20), (Carlson and Böttiger, 1972; Goldstein et al., 1973a) and coronary heart disease. Another possibility is that LDL or VLDL trapped within extracellular connective tissue matrices undergo slow, spontaneous denaturation or precipitate after being attacked by extracellular enzymes. Should this be so, the biologic disposal mechanisms of the organism, very poorly understood in the case of the artery, might be inadequate to cope with the problem.

Intracellular lipid probably accumulates primarily through direct uptake of extracellular lipoprotein. Uptake of medium lipoproteins by arterial cells grown in culture has been demonstrated by several investigators, and uptake probably also occurs *in vivo*, since Smith and Slater (1972) found that the concentration of soluble LDL immediately surrounding fatty streaks is considerably lower than that in normal intima. Once taken up by arterial cells, the lipoproteins are degraded by lysosomal esterases and proteases and the cholesterol re-esterified within the cell. The effect of the accumulated cholesteryl ester on the subsequent fate of the cells has not yet been clarified, although the presumption is that cell damage and ultimately cell death occur and that this contributes to the formation of fibrous plaques.

Another question that has arisen in connection with the "atherogenicity" of plasma lipoproteins is whether or not a risk-free concentration of plasma lipoprotein cholesterol exists and whether or not some lipoproteins promote while others prevent atherogenesis. Studies of the comparative geography of atherosclerosis suggest that plasma cholesterol concentrations below approximately 140–150 mg/dl tend to be correlated with relative freedom from atherosclerotic heart disease, but prospective studies in western countries have not yet provided information with regard to this point because of the relatively small proportion of individuals older than 40 who have plasma cholesterol concentrations below 175 mg/dl. They have indicated, however, that individuals who have plasma cholesterol concentrations below 175 mg/dl are at lower risk than are individuals who have plasma cholesterol concentrations of 200 mg/dl. Thus, most individuals who have "normal" plasma cholesterol concentrations by commonly used western standards do not have *optimal* concentrations. Below the arbitrary upper concentration limits used to define "hyperlipidemia" (Table 17–6), a 75 mg/dl increment in the concentration of plasma cholesterol is still associated with an increased risk of developing atherosclerotic heart disease equivalent to that of aging 10 years (Westlund and Nicolaysen, 1966).

Increased concentrations of cholesterol in plasma usually reflect increased concentrations of LDL, and direct measurements have shown that increased concentrations of LDL correlate with increased risk of developing coronary heart disease (Fig. 17–20). However, there are reasons for believing that other lipoproteins, such as VLDL, rich in cholesteryl ester and apo E may be atherogenic (see p. 882). On the other hand, the concentration of HDL appears to show an inverse correlation to the risk of developing coronary heart disease (Castelli et al., 1977) (see p. 886). Although it has been presumed that this correlation depends on the ability of HDL to remove cholesterol from the arterial wall, this remains to be proved. Another possibility (Glomset, 1979) is that the seemingly "protective" effect of HDL simply reflects an inverse correlation between the concentration of HDL and that of chylomicron or VLDL "remnants."

Other Risk Factors

In western populations, several other risk factors, including hypertension, cigarette smoking, obesity, diabetes, male sex, and age, have been correlated with the incidence of atherosclerotic heart disease. These factors appear to exacerbate the effects of high plasma lipid concentrations but apparently do not cause extensive atherosclerosis by themselves, since populations that exhibit a high prevalence of hypertension, obesity, and diabetes but low plasma lipid concentrations do not seem to be at high risk of developing coronary heart disease.

Like the effect of plasma lipids, that of hypertension on atherosclerotic heart disease is almost linear. Presumably, intimal permeability increases progressively with increasing blood pressure and influences the metabolism of arterial cells. Although the response of these cells is only now being studied, evidence is already available that experimental hypertension increases the content of sulfated mucopolysaccharide in the aorta (Hollander et al., 1968).

It is largely because obese individuals tend to be hypertensive and have higher plasma lipid concentrations that they are at increased risk of developing coronary heart disease. If they are compared to thin individuals who have similar degrees of hypertension and similar plasma lipid concentrations, the effect of obesity largely disappears (Keys et al., 1972). Only when sudden death is considered separately from myocardial infarction that occurs at rest (Kannel et al., 1967) does a distinct, independent effect of obesity emerge, presumably because obesity increases the cardiac work load and thereby the burden of physical activity on an already compromised coronary circulation. Whether or not obesity is considered an independent risk factor, its frequent association with hypertension, hyperlipidemia, and hyperglycemia (see later), all potentially reversible with weight reduction, should focus particular attention on this problem.

That diabetics are particularly susceptible to atherosclerotic vascular disease as well as microangiopathy has long been appreciated. Definitive proof that hyperglycemia is a risk factor for coronary heart disease independent of hypercholesterolemia or hypertension, however, was obtained in prospective studies (Ostrander, 1970). It is still not clear that hyperglycemia is a risk factor independent of hypertriglyceridemia, since the two are closely correlated (see under "Hyperlipidemia"). Studies in animals have not yet clarified this question. Indeed, the effect of diabetes has been found to differ in different species. Diabetic rats and monkeys (Lehner et al., 1971) are more susceptible to atherosclerosis. Alloxan diabetes actually protects against the atherosclerosis induced in rabbits by feeding them cholesterol, however (Duff and McMillan, 1949). It has been suggested (Stout, 1977) that high circulating insulin levels, characteristic of both the obese adult diabetic and the insulin-treated diabetic, promote atherogenesis by enhancing arterial smooth muscle cell proliferation and lipid synthesis.

Sex is another factor that influences the incidence of atherosclerosis, at least in Caucasians. Particularly in the coronary arteries but also in the aorta, the prevalence of atherosclerotic plaques is greater in males than in females. In addition, prospective studies such as that done in Framingham (Kannel et al., 1971) have shown that the incidence of coronary heart disease in males is about twice that in females and that an even greater differential exists among males and females below the age of 50. The basis for this sex differential remains to be explained. There is no direct evidence that it is caused by estrogens, since the incidence of coronary heart disease rises almost linearly with age in females and does not appear to be affected by menopause. Furthermore, the sex differential is not universal, since very little if any difference in the incidence of atherosclerosis can be demonstrated among male and female Negroes (Tejada et al., 1968), and even the sex differential in Caucasians is obliterated in diabetics. Nevertheless, sex hormones do affect risk factors associated with coronary heart disease, and this has led some investigators to fear that the sex differential may be reversed in normal females taking oral contraceptives. Thus estrogen-containing oral contraceptives tend to alter lipid and lipoprotein levels (see p. 893), impair carbohydrate tolerance, promote hypertension, and alter blood coagulation (Hazzard et al., 1969; Ygge et al., 1969; Chidell, 1970).

Other risk factors that have been identified include smoking, physical activity, and psychologic behavior pattern. For a discussion of these and other risk factors, the reader is referred to a review by Epstein and Ostrander (1971).

Prevention and Treatment

Obviously a great need exists for a rational therapeutic approach to atherosclerosis, but such an approach is unfortunately not yet at hand. One problem has been that treatment has seldom been attempted until after the onset of clinical symptoms; i.e., after the primary disease process has progressed to the point at which little hope of regression seems justified. Consequently, it is not surprising that attempts at therapy have met with relatively little success. A second problem is that, although most investigators would agree that prevention of atherosclerosis is the only rational approach, this might have to be begun in childhood and would certainly have to be carried out for decades. The paradox is that ultimate proof of the efficacy of a given therapeutic regimen probably will demand this type of long-term approach in a large population, whereas many physicians not unreasonably feel that before such long-term therapy is begun proof of efficacy should already be at hand. Fortunately, a means of circumventing this dilemma may be provided by the series of Lipid Clinics established throughout the United States by the National Institute of Heart and Lung Diseases. These clinics are conducting carefully designed attempts to reduce plasma lipid concentrations in individuals defined as having hyperlipidemia and who are thus at high risk of developing atherosclerotic disease. Although these individuals may not necessarily respond in the same way as individuals who have lower concentrations of plasma lipids, the evidence obtained may provide the necessary impetus for large-scale therapeutic trials in the general population.

In the mean time, what can be done? Apart from surgery to improve the coronary circulation (Baue, 1969), the approach usually advocated is to treat when possible the recognized risk factors. For a general review of the problem, the reader is referred to a review by Dawber and Thomas (1971), and for detailed discussions of obesity and hyperlipidemia to Ch. 18 and to earlier sections of this chapter. The dietary measures recommended to mitigate hyperlipidemia can be applied generally to reduce serum lipid levels in anyone concerned about the risk of developing atherosclerotic vascular disease. Furthermore, more rigorous dietary approaches can be justified for offspring of families with known forms of primary hyperlipidemia (see p. 888) or with a family history of early atherosclerosis. The long-term use of pharmacologic agents is more controversial. As for the therapeutic use of hormones, both thyroid hormones and estrogens have been tried but were later discontinued because of side effects. Justification for hormone therapy exists only when deficiency is to be corrected, as in the case of diabetes and hypothyroidism.

CHOLESTEROL GALLSTONES

Gallstones occur frequently in western countries and appear to be increasing in prevalence in newly "westernized" countries like Japan (Miyake and Johnston, 1968). Some gallstones are mainly composed of bile pigments or insoluble calcium salts but most contain at least 70–80% cholesterol and at times as much as 98% cholesterol. These cholesterol-rich stones are of particular interest because of increasing evidence that they are formed when hepatic cholesterol excretion exceeds the normal solubilizing capacity of the bile. In other words, "cholesterol cholelithiasis" can be considered a "disease" of cholesterol metabolism. In the following presentation, the prevalence of gallstones in various population groups, the factors believed to solubilize cholesterol in bile, and recent studies that directly pertain to gallstone formation in humans will be briefly discussed. For additional details, the reader should consult a recent review by Bennion and Grundy (1978).

Many studies have demonstrated that the prevalence of gallstones increases with age. For example, in a review of a large necropsy series, the overall incidence of gallstones in females was 27.1%, whereas the incidence in females between the ages of 80 and 89 was 38.0%, and a qualitatively similar relation was found in males (Torvik and Hoivik, 1960). The cause of the apparent increase with age is not understood. The tendency to form gallstones may be a simple function of age in all individuals. On the other hand, a process of selection may be operative; i.e., the mechanisms that promote gallstone formation may favor longevity by protecting individuals from premature vascular disease. Studies of Indians from the southwestern United States seem to support this concept (discussed later). Most authors agree that cholesterol gallstones occur more frequently in females than in males. For example, in the study by Torvik and Hoivik (1960), the overall incidence of gallstones in males (12.7%) was less than half that found in females, and a similar sex-related difference was found by Friedman and coworkers (1966) and by Horn (1956) (Fig. 17–23). The studies by Horn and by Hove and Geill (1968) are of interest, since they suggest that the sex differential tends to diminish in aged individuals. The effect of parity may explain part of the sex differential. In Horn's study, the incidence of gallstones in women below the age of 50 increased in proportion

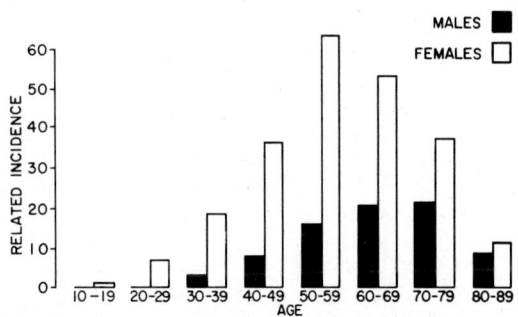

Figure 17–23. Incidence of cholelithiasis in Birmingham males and females as a function of age. "Related incidence" is the ratio of the number of cases in each group to the population (of Great Britain) in the corresponding group (number of cases per million population). (From Horn, G.: Observations on aetiology of cholelithiasis. Br. Med. J. 2:732, 1956.)

to the number of children they had borne, although women with no children still had a higher incidence of gallstones than had men. Another factor that affects the relative incidence of gallstones is body weight. In Horn's study, women below the age of 50 who had gallstones were 25 pounds heavier on the average than were women without gallstones. Furthermore, Van der Linden (1961) found a small but probably significant correlation between subscapular and lateral skin-fold thicknesses and incidence of surgically verified cholelithiasis in women. He found the correlation less obvious, however, than is suggested by the catch phrase "fat, fertile female" found in some textbooks.

It has been suggested that the incidence of cholelithiasis may be affected by various endocrine abnormalities, such as hypothyroidism and diabetes. Both thyroid hormone and insulin are known to affect sterol metabolism, and untreated hypothyroidism and diabetes are characterized by high serum lipid levels (see under "Hyperlipidemia"). So far no evidence that cholelithiasis occurs more frequently in myxedema is available, however, and in fact several cases of coincident cholelithiasis and hyperthyroidism are known (Bockus, 1965). In the case of diabetes, evidence is conflicting, possibly because of the relation between diabetes and obesity. In two large autopsy series, the incidence of gallstones was found to be almost twice as high in diabetics as it was in nondiabetics (Robertson and Dochat, 1944; Lieber, 1952). Nevertheless, Feldman and Feldman (1954) reviewed the findings of 1319 autopsies and found that gallstones were no more prevalent in diabetics than they were in nondiabetics.

Solubilization of Cholesterol in Bile

Although cholesterol is essentially insoluble in water, significant amounts are solubilized in bile (Table 17-1) because of the combined presence of bile acids and lecithin (Isaksson, 1953; Small, 1970). Physical studies of bile acid–lecithin-water mixtures (Small et al., 1969) suggest the presence of mixed micelles of the general composition and shape indicated in Fig. 17-24. Studies in model systems (Carey and Small, 1973) have shown that mixed micelles of bile and lecithin can solubilize up to three times as much cholesterol as can solutions of bile acids alone. Nevertheless, the ability of these mixed micelles to solubilize cholesterol is limited. Moreover, the composition of normal bile can be shown to be compatible with complete solubilization, whereas that of bile containing gallstones is supersaturated with cholesterol. Thus it is apparent that understanding of the pathology of cholesterol stone formation and ultimate treatment or prevention of the disease must be sought in terms of the factors that regulate the proportions of cholesterol, bile salts, and lecithin in the bile.

Bile Secretion

The hepatic mechanisms of bile secretion are not yet understood, although bile acids, secretin, and polyunsaturated fatty acids (Campbell et al., 1972) are recognized choleretics. Furthermore, it is clear that the relative proportions of bile acids, lecithin, cholesterol, and water are not rigidly fixed. Thus, in some American Indian tribes, the prevalence of cholesterol gallstones is unusually high. (It approaches 80% in women.) These Indians consume a diet similar in lipid content to that of caucasoid Americans but have higher concentrations of biliary cholesterol and lower concentrations of plasma cholesterol (Grundy et al., 1972a). Furthermore, their bile acid pools are unusually small (Vlahcevic et al., 1972). Apparently, the increased concentrations of biliary cholesterol relative to bile acid lead to gallstone formation, whereas the low concentrations of plasma cholesterol are associated with relative freedom from cardiovascular disease. Even in the same individual, however, the relative concentrations of biliary components vary. Both increased cholesterol intake (Quintao et al., 1971) and increased cholesterol production in obese individuals (Miettinen, 1971; Grundy et al., 1972a) cause increased excretion of biliary cholesterol without markedly affecting bile acid excretion. Moreover, the secretion of water by bile duct canaliculi, affected by bile acids, secretin, and estrogens (Gumucio and Valdiviesco, 1971), appears to undergo cyclic daily (McSherry et al., 1971) as well as monthly variations. All of these factors may well promote gallstone formation in obese western women.

Treatment and Prevention

Cholesterol crystals form and grow to clinically manifest size in the gallbladder, so rational prevention will have to be directed both toward the supersaturated bile and to the

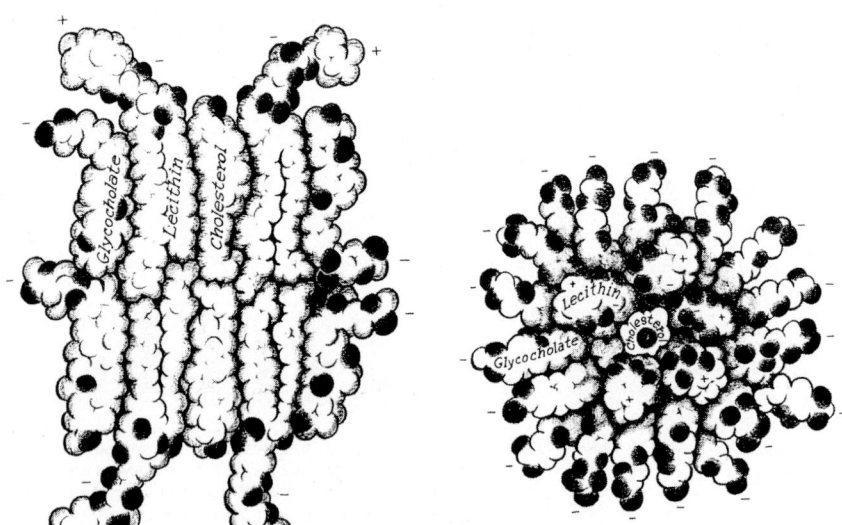

Figure 17–24. Schematic drawing of a bile micelle based on molecular models of unesterified cholesterol, glycocholic acid, and lecithin. Left side = sagittal section through micelle; right side = micelle seen from top; dark areas = oxygen atoms.

factors that initiate precipitation of cholesterol. A basis for this type of preventive management is likely to be provided within the not too distant future, since techniques are now available for determining the effects of diet and drugs on bile secretion in humans (Grundy et al., 1972b). Already it seems likely that restriction of calories and cholesterol will be important, especially since gallstones can be produced experimentally in monkeys simply by feeding them butter and cholesterol (Osuga and Portman, 1972). This should be considered, particularly in patients being treated with polyunsaturated fats or clofibrate to reduce plasma cholesterol concentrations, since both forms of treatment can increase cholesterol excretion (Connor et al., 1969; Grundy, Ahrens et al., 1972) and since treatment with clofibrate has been reported to increase the incidence of cholelithiasis (Cooper et al., 1975). Another approach, introduced by Thistle and Schoenfield (1971), is to dissolve pre-existing gallstones by increasing bile acid concentrations through oral administration of chenodeoxycholic acid. When 0.75–4.5 g of this acid were given daily to seven women with gallstones, the gallstones diminished in four of the women over a period of 6–22 months; liver function and morphology remained normal (Danzinger et al., 1972).

REFERENCES

Ahrens, E. R., Jr.: The management of hyperlipidemia: whether, rather than how. *Ann. Intern. Med.* 85:87, 1976.

American Heart Association: *Diet and Coronary Heart Disease Statement.* 1978.

Andersen, J. M., and Dietschy, J. M.: Regulation of sterol synthesis in 16 tissues of rat. II. Role of rat and human high and low density lipoproteins and of rat chylomicron remnants. *J. Biol. Chem.* 252:3652, 1977.

Applebaum, D. M., et al.: Effect of estrogen on post-heparin lipolytic activity. Selective decline in hepatic triglyceride lipase. *J. Clin. Invest.* 59:601, 1977.

Atkin, E., and Meng, H. C.: Release of clearing factor lipase (lipoprotein lipase) *in vivo* and from isolated perfused hearts of alloxan diabetic rats. *Diabetes* 21:149, 1972.

Bagdade, J. D., et al.: Diabetic lipemia: a form of acquired fat-induced lipemia. *N. Engl. J. Med.* 276:427, 1967.

Bagdade, J. D., et al.: Hypertriglyceridemia; a metabolic consequence of chronic renal failure. *N. Engl. J. Med.* 279:181, 1968a.

Bagdade, J. D., et al.: Acute insulin withdrawal and the regulation of plasma triglyceride removal in diabetic subjects. *Diabetes* 17:127, 1968b.

Bagdade, J. D.: Diabetic lipaemia complicating acute pancreatitis. *Lancet* 2:1041, 1969.

Bagdade, J. D., et al.: Steroid-induced lipemia. *Arch. Intern. Med.* 125:129, 1970.

Bagdade, J. D., et al.: Influence of obesity on the relationship between insulin and triglyceride levels in endogeneous hypertriglyceridemia. *Diabetes* 20:664, 1971.

Balasse, E. O., and Havel, R. J.: Evidence for an effect of insulin on the peripheral utilization of ketone bodies in dogs. *J. Clin. Invest.* 50:801, 1971.

Basso, L. V., and Havel, R. J.: Hepatic metabolism of free fatty acids in normal and diabetic dogs. *J. Clin. Invest.* 48:537, 1970.

Baue, A.: Survey for coronary artery disease. *J.A.M.A.* 208:849, 1969.

Baum, D., et al.: An abnormality of triglyceride metabolism in infantile hypothyroidism. *Am. J. Dis. Child.* 125:612, 1973.

Beaumont, J. L., et al.: Classification of hyperlipidaemias and hyperlipoproteinaemias. *Bull. WHO* 43:891, 1970.

Belknap, B. H., et al.: In *Tolbutamide After Ten Years.* Butterfield, W. J. H., and Van Westering, W. (eds.), Amsterdam, Excerpta Medica, No. 149, 1967.

Bennion, L. J., and Grundy, S. M.: Risk factors for the development of cholelithiasis in man. *N. Engl. J. Med.* 299:1161, 1221, 1978.

Berkowitz, D.: Long-term treatment of hyperlipidemic patients with clofibrate. *J.A.M.A.* 218:1002, 1971.

Bezman, A., et al.: Relation between the incorporation of triglyceride fatty acids and heparin-released lipoprotein lipase from adipose tissue slices. *J. Lipid Res.* 3:427, 1962.

Bierman, E. L.: The role of hormones associated with atherogenesis in modulating cellular metabolism of lipoproteins. In *Atherosclerosis V,* Gotto, A. (ed.) New York, Springer Verlag, 1980.

Bierman, E. L., and Albers, J. J.: Lipoprotein uptake and degradation by human arterial smooth muscle cells in tissue culture. *Ann. NY Acad. Sci.* 275:199, 1976.

Bierman, E. L., et al.: On the mechanism of action of Atromid-S on triglyceride transport in man. *Trans. Assoc. Am. Physicians* 83:211, 1970.

Bierman, E. L., and Porte, D., Jr.: Carbohydrate intolerance and lipemia. *Ann. Intern. Med.* 68:926, 1968.

Bierman, E. L., et al.: Hypertriglyceridemia and glucose intolerance in man, In *Adipose Tissue, Regulation and Metabolic Function.* Jeanrenaud, B., and Hepp, D. (eds.), New York, Academic Press, 1970.

Bierman, E. L., and Strandness, D. E.: Formation of secondary fat particles from lymph chylomicrons in the dog. *Am. J. Physiol.* 210:13, 1966.

Blanchette-Mackie, E. J., and Scow, R. O.: Sites of lipoprotein lipase activity in adipose tissue perfused with chylomicrons. Electron microscope and chemical study. *J. Cell Biol.* 51:1, 1971.

Bockus, H.: Cholelithiasis, In *Gastroenterology.* 3rd ed. Vol. 3. Bockus, H. (ed.), Philadelphia, W. B. Saunders Co., 1965.

Boyd, G. S., and Percy-Robb, I. W.: Enzymatic regulation of bile acid synthesis. *Am. J. Med.* 51:580, 1971.

Breckenridge, W. C., et al.: Hypertriglyceridemia associated with deficiency of apolipoprotein C-II. *N. Engl. J. Med.* 298:1265, 1978.

Brown, M. S., and Goldstein, J. L.: Receptor-mediated control of cholesterol metabolism. *Science* 191:150, 1976.

Brunzell, J. D., and Bierman, E. L.: Plasma triglyceride and insulin levels in familial hypertriglyceridemia. *Ann. Intern. Med.* 87:198, 1977.

Brunzell, J. D., et al.: Pathophysiology of lipoprotein transport. *Metabolism* 27:1109, 1978.

Brunzell, J. D., et al.: Evidence for diabetes mellitus and genetic forms of hypertriglyceridemia as independent entities. *Metabolism* 24:1115, 1975a.

Brunzell, J. D., et al.: Reversible abnormalities in postheparin lipolytic activity during the late phase of release in diabetes mellitus (postheparin lipolytic activity in diabetes). *Metabolism* 24:1123, 1975b.

Brunzell, J. D., and Schrott, H. G.: The interaction of familial and secondary causes of hypertriglyceridemia: role in pancreatitis. *Trans. Assoc. Am. Physicians* 86:245, 1973.

Brunzell, J. D., et al.: Myocardial infarction in the familial forms of hypertriglyceridemia. *Metabolism* 25:313, 1976.

Butcher, R. A.: The role of cyclic AMP in the actions of some lipolytic and anti-lipolytic agents, In *Adipose Tissues, Regulation and Metabolic Functions.* Jeanrenaud, B., and Hepp, D. (eds.), New York, Academic Press, 1970.

Cahill, G. F., Jr.: Starvation in man. *N. Engl. J. Med.* 282:668, 1970.

Campbell, C. B., et al.: Dietary factors affecting biliary lipid secretion in the rhesus monkey. A mechanism for the hypercholesterolaemic action of polyunsaturated fat. *Eur. J. Clin. Invest.* 2:332, 1972.

Carey, M. C., and Small, D. M.: The physical chemistry of cholesterol solubility in bile: evidence that supersaturated bile is frequent in healthy man. *J. Clin. Invest.* 52:1467, 1973.

Carlson, L. A.: The effect of nicotinic acid treatment on the chemical composition of plasma lipoprotein classes in man, In *Advances in Experimental Medicine and Biology.* Vol. 4. Holmes, W. L., Carlson, L. A., and Paoletti, R. (eds.), New York, Plenum Press, 1969.

Carlson, L. A., and Böttiger, L. E.: Ischaemic heart disease in relation to fasting values of plasma triglycerides and cholesterol. *Lancet* 1:865, 1972.

Castelli, W. P., et al.: HDL cholesterol and other lipids in coronary heart disease. The cooperative lipoprotein phenotyping study. *Circulation* 55:767, 1977a.

Castelli, W. P., et al.: Alcohol and blood lipids. The cooperative lipoprotein phenotyping study. *Lancet* 2:153, 1977b.

Chait, A., et al.: Type-III hyperlipoproteinaemia ("remnant removal disease"). Insight into the pathogenetic mechanism. *Lancet* 1:1176, 1977.

Chait, A., et al.: Regulatory role of insulin in the degradation of low density lipoprotein by cultured human skin fibroblasts. *Biochim. Biophys. Acta* 529:292, 1978.

Chait, A., et al.: Regulatory role of triiodothyronine in the degradation of low density lipoprotein by cultured human skin fibroblasts. *J. Clin. Endocrinol. Metab.* 48:887, 1979a.

Chait, A., et al.: Low density lipoprotein receptor activity in cultured human skin fibroblasts. Mechanism of insulin-induced stimulation. J. Clin. Invest. 64:1309, 1979b.

Chait, A., et al.: Chylomicronemia syndrome. *Clin. Res.* 26:127A, 1978.

Chajek, T., and Eisenberg, S.: Very low density lipoprotein. Metabolism of phospholipids, cholesterol, and apolipoprotein C in the isolated perfused rat heart. *J. Clin. Invest.* 61:1654, 1978.

Chajek, T., and Fielding, C. J.: Isolation and characterization of a human serum cholesteryl ester transfer protein. *Proc. Nat. Acad. Sci. USA* 75:3445, 1978.

Chidell, M. P.: Oral contraceptives and blood pressure. *Practitioner* 205:58, 1970.

Connor, W. E., et al.: Cholesterol balance and feral neutral steroid and bile acid excretion in normal men fed dietary fats of different fatty acid composition. *J. Clin. Invest.* 48:1363, 1969.

Cooper, J., et al.: Clofibrate and gallstones. *Lancet* 1:1083, 1975.

Crawford, T.: Morphological aspects in the pathogenesis of atherosclerosis. *J. Atherosclerosis Res.* 1:3, 1961.

Cunningham, V. J., and Robinson, D. S.: Clearing factor lipase in adipose tissue. Distinction of different states of the enzyme and the possible role of the fat cell in the maintenance of tissue activity. *Biochem. J. 112*:203, 1969.

Danzinger, R. G., et al.: Dissolution of cholesterol gallstones by chenodeoxycholic acid. *N. Engl. J. Med. 286*:1, 1972.

Davidoff, F., et al.: Marked hyperlipidemia and pancreatitis associated with oral contraceptive therapy. *N. Engl. J. Med. 289*:552, 1973.

Dawber, T. R., and Thomas, H. E., Jr.: Prevention of myocardial infarction. *Progr. Cardiovasc. Dis. 13*:343, 1971.

deKruyff, B., et al.: The effect of cholesterol and epicholesterol incorporation on the permeability and on the phase transition of intact Acholeplasma laidlawii cell membranes and derived liposomes. *Biochim. Biophys. Acta 225*:331, 1972.

Demel, R. A., et al.: Structural requirements of sterols for the interaction with lecithin at the air-water interfall. *Biochim. Biophys. Acta 255*:304, 1972.

Dietschy, J. M., and Wilson, J. D.: Regulation of cholesterol metabolism. *N. Engl. J. Med. 282*:1128, 1179, 1241, 1970.

Duff, G. L., and McMillan, G. C.: Effect of alloxan diabetes on experimental cholesterol atherosclerosis in the rabbit. *J. Exp. Med. 89*:611, 1949.

Enholm, C., et al.: Effect of oxandrolone treatment on the activity of lipoprotein lipase, hepatic lipase and phospholipase A_1 of human postheparin plasma. *N. Engl. J. Med. 292*:1314, 1975.

Entenman, C., et al.: Bile acids and lipid metabolism. I. Stimulation of bile lipid excretion by various bile acids. *Proc. Soc. Exp. Biol. Med. 127*:1008, 1968.

Epstein, F. H., and Ostrander, L. D., Jr.: Detection of individual susceptibility toward coronary disease. *Progr. Cardiovasc. Dis. 13*:324, 1971.

Evans, D. W., et al.: Feasibility of long-term plasma-cholesterol reduction by diet. *Lancet 1*:172, 1972.

Fain, J., et al.: Effect of growth hormone and dexamethasone on lipolysis and metabolism in isolated fat cells of the rat. *J. Biol. Chem. 240*:3522, 1965.

Feldman, M., and Feldman, M., Jr.: The incidence of cholelithiasis, cholesterosis, and liver disease in diabetes mellitus. *Diabetes 3*:305, 1954.

Fredrickson, D. S.: It's time to be practical (editorial). *Circulation 51*:209, 1975.

French, J. E.: Atherosclerosis in relation to the structure and function of the arterial intima, with special reference to the endothelium. *Int. Rev. Exp. Pathol. 5*:253, 1966.

French, J. E.: Formation and fate of a thrombus, In *Atherosclerosis*. Proceedings of the Second International Symposium on Atherosclerosis. Jones, R. J. (ed.), New York, Springer-Verlag, 1970.

Friedewald, W. T., et al.: Estimation of the concentration of low-density lipoprotein cholesterol in plasma, without use of the preparative ultracentrifuge. *Clin. Chem. 18*:499, 1972.

Friedman, G. D., et al.: The epidemiology of gallbladder disease: observations in the Framingham study. *J. Chronic Dis. 19*:273, 1966.

Geer, J. C., et al.: Histologic characteristics of coronary artery fatty streaks. *Lab. Invest. 18*:565, 1968.

Ginsberg, H., et al.: Moderate ethanol ingestion and plasma triglyceride levels: A study in normal and hypertriglyceridemic persons. *Ann. Intern. Med. 80*:143, 1974.

Gjone, E., et al.: Familial lecithin: cholesterol acyltransferase deficiency, In *Metabolic Basis for Inherited Disease*. 4th ed. Stanbury, J., Wyngaarden, J., et al. (eds.), New York, McGraw-Hill, 1978.

Glomset, J. A.: High density lipoproteins in human health and disease, In *Advances in Internal Medicine*. Vol. 25. Siperstein, M. D., and Stollarman, G. H. (eds.), Chicago, Yearbook Medical Publishers, 1979.

Glomset, J. A., and Norum, K. R.: The metabolic role of lecithin: cholesterol acyltransferase. Perspectives from pathology. *Adv. Lipid Res. 11*:1, 1973.

Glomset, J. A., et al.: Plasma lipoproteins in familial lecithin: cholesterol acyltransferase deficiency: Effects of dietary manipulation. *Scand. J. Clin. Lab. Invest. 35* (Suppl. 142):3, 1975.

Glueck, C. J., et al.: Effects of estrogenic compounds on triglyceride kinetics. *Metabolism 24*:537, 1975.

Glueck, C. J., et al.: Triglyceride removal efficiency and lipoprotein lipases: effects of oxandrolone. *Metabolism 22*:807, 1973.

Glueck, C. J., et al.: Immunoreactive insulin, glucose tolerance, and carbohydrate inducibility in types II, III, IV, and V hyperlipoproteinemia. *Diabetes 18*:739, 1969a.

Glueck, C. J., et al.: Amelioration of hypertriglyceridemia by progestational drugs in familial type-V hyperlipoproteinemia. *Lancet 1*:1290, 1969b.

Glueck, C. J., et al.: Neonatal familial type II hyperlipoproteinemia: cord blood cholesterol in 1800 births. *Metabolism 20*:597, 1971.

Glueck, C. J., and Tsang, R. C.: Pediatric familial type II hyperlipoproteinemia: effects of diet on plasma cholesterol in the first year of life. *Am. J. Clin. Nutr. 25*:224, 1972.

Glueck, C. J., et al.: Hyperalpha- and hypobeta-lipoproteinemia in octogenarian kindreds. *Atherosclerosis 27*:387, 1977.

Goldberg, A. P., et al.: Control of clofibrate toxicity in uremic hypertriglyceridemia. *Clin. Pharmacol. Ther. 21*:317, 1977.

Goldberg, A. P., et al.: Treatment of hypertriglyceridemia with para-aminosalicylic acid-C: A possible mechanism of action. *Metabolism 27*:1648, 1978a.

Goldberg, A. P., et al.: Adipose tissue lipoprotein lipase in chronic hemodia-

lysis: Role in plasma triglyceride metabolism. *J. Clin. Endocrinol. Metab. 47*:1173, 1978b.

Goldstein, J. L., and Brown, M. S.: The low-density lipoprotein pathway and its relation to atherosclerosis. *Ann. Rev. Biochem. 46*:897, 1977.

Goldstein, J. L., et al.: Hyperlipidemia in coronary heart disease. I. Lipid levels in 500 survivors of myocardial infarction. *J. Clin. Invest. 52*:1533, 1973a.

Goldstein, J. L., et al.: Hyperlipidemia in coronary heart disease. II. Genetic analysis of lipid levels in 176 families and delineation of a new inherited disorder, combined hyperlipidemia. *J. Clin. Invest. 52*:1544, 1973b.

Grundy, S. M., Ahrens, E. H., Jr., et al.: Mechanisms of action of clofibrate on cholesterol metabolism in patients with hyperlipidemia. *J. Lipid Res. 13*:531, 1972.

Grundy, S. M., et al.: Mechanisms of lithogenic bile formation in American Indian women with cholesterol gallstones. *J. Clin. Invest. 51*:3026, 1972a.

Grundy, S. M., and Metzger, A. L.: A physiological method for estimation of hepatic secretion of biliary lipids in man. *Gastroenterology 62*:1200, 1972b.

Gumucio, J. J., and Valdiviesco, V. D.: Studies on the mechanism of the ethynylestradiol impairment of bile flow and bile salt excretion in the rat. *Gastroenterology 61*:339, 1971.

Gwynne, J. T., et al.: Adrenal cholesterol uptake from plasma lipoproteins: regulation by corticotrophin. *Proc. Nat. Acad. Sci. USA 73*:4329, 1976.

Haire, H. M., et al.: Smoking, hypertension, and mortality in a maintenance dialysis population. *Cardiovasc. Med. 3*:1163, 1978.

Havel, R. J.: Classification of the hyperlipidemias. *Ann. Rev. Med. 28*:195, 1977.

Havel, R. J., and Kane, J. P.: Primary dysbetalipoproteinemia: Predominance of a specific apoprotein species in triglyceride-rich lipoproteins. *Proc. Nat. Acad. Sci. USA 70*:2015, 1973.

Hazzard, W. R., and Bierman, E. L.: Aggravation of broad-beta disease (type III hyperlipoproteinemia) by hypothyroidism. *Arch. Intern. Med. 130*:22, 1972.

Hazzard, W. R., et al.: Abnormal lipid composition of very low density lipoproteins in the diagnosis of broad-beta disease (type III hyperlipoproteinemia). *Metabolism 21*:1009, 1972.

Hazzard, W. R., et al.: Studies on the mechanism of increased plasma triglyceride levels induced by oral contraceptives. *N. Engl. J. Med. 280*:471, 1969.

Hofmann, A. F., and Small, D. M.: Detergent properties of bile salts: Correlation with physiological function. *Ann. Rev. Med. 18*:333, 1967.

Hollander, W., et al.: Arterial wall metabolism in experimental hypertension of coarctation of the aorta of short duration. *J. Clin. Invest. 47*:1221, 1968.

Hollenberg, C. H.: The effect of fasting on the lipoprotein lipase activity of rat heart and diaphragm. *J. Clin. Invest. 39*:1282, 1960.

Horn, G.: Observations on the aetiology of cholelithiasis. *Br. Med. J. 2*:732, 1956.

Hove, E., and Geill, T.: Serum cholesterol and incidence of gallstones. *Geriatrics 23*:114, 1968.

Isaksson, V.: Dissolving power of LBS for cholesterol. *Acta Soc. Med. Ups. 59*:298, 1953.

Jungas, R. L.: Hormonal regulation of pyruvate dehydrogenase. *Metabolism 20*:43, 1971.

Kane, J. P., et al.: Apolipoprotein composition of very low density lipoproteins of human serum. *J. Clin. Invest. 56*:1622, 1975.

Kane, J. P., et al.: Heterozygous familial hypercholesterolemia: treatment with combined drug regimens. *Clin. Res. 26*:529A, 1978.

Kannel, W. B., et al.: Serum lipid precursors of coronary heart disease. *Hum. Pathol. 2*:129, 1971.

Kannel, W. B., et al.: Relation of body weight to development of coronary heart disease. The Framingham Study. *Circulation 35*:734, 1967.

Kekki, M., and Nikkilä, E. A.: Plasma triglyceride turnover during use of oral contraceptives. *Metabolism 20*:878, 1971.

Keys, A., et al.: Coronary heart disease: overweight and obesity as risk factors. *Ann. Intern. Med. 77*:15, 1972.

Kopec, B., and Fritz, I. B.: Properties of a purified carnitine palmitoyltransferase, and evidence for the existence of other carnitine acyltransferases. *Can. J. Biochem. 49*:941, 1971.

Koppers, L. E., and Palumbo, P. J.: Lipid disturbances in endocrine disorders. *Med. Clin. North Am. 56*:1013, 1972.

Kostner, G., and Holasek, A.: Characterization and quantitation of the apolipoproteins from human chylomicrons. *Biochemistry 11*:1217, 1972.

Kritchevsky, D., et al.: Influence of sex and sex hormones on the oxidation of cholester-26-C^{14} by rat liver mitochondria. *J. Lipid Res. 4*:188, 1963.

Kudzma, D. J., and Schonfeld, G.: Alcoholic hyperlipidemia: induction by alcohol but not by carbohydrate. *J. Lab. Clin. Med. 77*:384, 1971.

Kushwaha, R. S., et al.: Type III hyperlipoproteinemia: diagnosis in whole plasma by apolipoprotein-E immunoassay. *Ann. Intern. Med. 86*:509, 1977a.

Kushwaha, R. S., et al.: Type III hyperlipoproteinemia: paradoxical hypolipidemic response to estrogen. *Ann. Intern. Med. 87*:517, 1977b.

Lane, M. D., and Moss, J.: Regulation of fatty acid synthesis in animal tissues, In *Metabolic Pathways*, 3rd ed. Vol. V. Vogel, H. J. (ed.), New York, Academic Press, 1971.

Langer, T., et al.: The metabolism of low density lipoprotein in familial type II hyperlipoproteinemia. *J. Clin. Invest.* 51:1528, 1972.

Lardy, H. A., et al.: Hormonal control of enzymes participating in glucogenesis and lipogenesis. *J. Cell. Comp. Physiol.* 66:39, 1965.

Lee, K.-H., and Kim, K.-H.: Regulation of rat liver acetyl Coenzyme A carboxylase. Evidence for interconversion between active and inactive forms of enzyme by phosphorylation and dephosphorylation. *J. Biol. Chem.* 252:1748, 1977.

Leelarthaepin, B., et al.: Obesity, diet, and type-II hyperlipidaemia. *Lancet* 2:1217, 1974.

Lees, R. S., et al.: Hyperbeta-lipoproteinemia in acute intermittent porphyria. *N. Engl. J. Med.* 282:432, 1970.

Lees, R. S., and Wilson, D. E.: The treatment of hyperlipidemia. *N. Engl. J. Med.* 284:186, 1971.

Lehner, N. D. M., et al.: The effect of insulin deficiency, hypothyroidism, and hypertension on atherosclerosis in the squirrel monkey. *Exp. Mol. Pathol.* 15:230, 1971.

Lieber, M.: Incidence of gallstones and their correlation with other diseases. *Ann. Surg.* 135:394, 1952.

Margolis, S., and Capuzzi, D.: Serum-lipoprotein synthesis and metabolism, In *Blood Lipids and Lipoproteins: Quantitation, Composition and Metabolism.* Nelson, G. J. (ed.), New York, John Wiley & Sons, 1972.

McBride, O. W., and Korn, E. D.: The lipoprotein lipase of mammary gland and the correlation of its activity to lactation. *J. Lipid Res.* 4:17, 1963.

McGarry, J. D., et al.: A possible role for malonyl-CoA in the regulation of hepatic fatty acid oxidation and ketogenesis. *J. Clin. Invest.* 60:265, 1977.

McSherry, C. K., et al.: Composition of basal and stimulated hepatic bile in baboons, and the formation of cholesterol gallstones. *Proc. Nat. Acad. Sci. USA* 68:1564, 1971.

Miettinen, T. A.: Mechanism of serum cholesterol reduction by thyroid hormones in hypothyrodism. *J. Lab. Clin. Med.* 71:537, 1968.

Miettinen, T. A.: Cholesterol production in obesity. *Circulation* 44:842, 1971.

Minari, O., and Zilversmit, D. B.: Behavior of dog lymph chylomicron lipid constituents during incubation with serum. *J. Lipid Res.* 4:424, 1963.

Miyake, H., and Johnston, C. G.: Gallstones: ethnological studies. *Digestion* 1:219, 1968.

Mjøs, O. D., et al.: Characterization of remnants produced during the metabolism of triglyceride-rich lipoproteins of blood plasma and intestinal lymph in the rat. *J. Clin. Invest.* 56:603, 1975.

Morganroth, J., et al.: The biochemical, clinical, and genetic features of type III hyperlipoproteinemia. *Ann. Intern. Med.* 82:158, 1975.

Motulsky, A. G.: The genetic hyperlipidemias. *N. Engl. J. Med.* 294:823, 1976.

Nikkilä, E. A.: Metabolic and endocrine control of plasma high density lipoprotein concentration. Relation to catabolism of triglyceride-rich lipoproteins, In *High Density Lipoproteins and Atherosclerosis.* Gotto, A. M., Jr., Miller, N. E., et al. (eds.), New York, Elsevier/North-Holland Biomedical Press, 1978.

Nikkilä, E. A., and Aro, A.: Family study of serum lipids and lipoproteins in coronary heart-disease. *Lancet* 1:954, 1973.

Nikkilä, E. A., and Hormila, P.: Serum lipids and lipoproteins in insulin-treated diabetes: demonstration of increased high density lipoprotein concentrations. *Diabetes* 27:1078, 1978.

Nikkilä, E. A., and Tikkanen, M.: Effective treatment of postmenopausal type II hyperlipoproteinemia with natural estrogen. 32nd Annual Meeting, Council on Arteriosclerosis, American Society for the Study of Arteriosclerosis, American Heart Association Monograph No. 61, 1978, p. 31: *Circulation*, 58(Suppl. II): 1978.

Olefsky, J. M., et al.: Reappraisal of the role of insulin in hypertriglyceridemia. *Am. J. Med.* 57:551, 1974a.

Olefsky, J. M., et al.: Effects of weight reduction on obesity: studies of lipid and carbohydrate metabolism in normal and hyperlipoproteinemic subjects. *J. Clin. Invest.* 53:64, 1974b.

Oliver, M. F.: Cholesterol, coronaries, clofibrate, and death. *N. Engl. J. Med.* 299:1360, 1978.

Osuga, T., and Portman, O. W.: Relationship between bile composition and gallstone formation in squirrel monkeys. *Gastroenterology* 63:122, 1972.

Ostrander, L. D., Jr.: Hyperglycemia and vascular disease in Tecumseh, Michigan, In *Early Diabetes.* Camerini-Davalos, D., and Cole, H. S. (eds.), New York, Academic Press, 1970.

Palmer, R. H.: Prevalence of gallstones in hyperlipidemia and incidence during treatment with clofibrate and/or cholestyramine. *Trans. Assoc. Am. Physicians* 91:424, 1978.

Parker, F., et al.: Evidence for the plasma chylomicron origin of lipids accumulating in diabetic eruptive xanthomas: a correlative lipid biochemical, histochemical and electron microscopic study. *J. Clin. Invest.* 49:2172, 1970.

Patten, R. L.: The reciprocal regulation of lipoprotein lipase activity and hormone-sensitive lipase activity in rat adipocytes. *J. Biol. Chem.* 245:557, 1970.

Pattnaik, N. M., and Zilversmit, D. B.: Interaction of cholesteryl ester exchange protein with human plasma lipoproteins and phospholipid vesicles. *J. Biol. Chem.* 254:2782, 1979.

Pykälistö, O., et al.: Reversal of decreased human adipose tissue lipoprotein lipase and hypertriglyceridemia after treatment of hypothyroidism. *J. Clin. Endocrinol. Metab.* 43:591, 1976.

Pykälistö, O. J., et al.: Determinants of human adipose tissue lipoprotein lipase: effect of diabetes and obesity on basal- and diet-induced activity. *J. Clin. Invest.* 56:1108, 1975.

Quintao, E., et al.: Effects of dietary cholesterol on the regulation of total body cholesterol in man. *J. Lipid Res.* 12:233, 1971.

Randle, P., et al.: The glucose fatty acid cycle. Its role in insulin sensitivity and the metabolic disturbance of diabetes mellitus. *Lancet* 1:785, 1963.

Reaven, G. M., et al.: Kinetics of triglyceride turnover of very low density lipoproteins of human plasma. *J. Clin. Invest.* 44:1826, 1965.

Roberts, W. C., and Buja, L. M.: The frequency and significance of coronary arterial thrombi and other observations in fatal acute myocardial infarction. *Am. J. Med.* 52:425, 1972.

Robertson, H., and Dochat, G.: Pregnancy and gallstones: collective review. *Surg. Gynecol. Obstet.* 78:193, 1944.

Robinson, D. S.: The function of the plasma triglycerides in fatty acid transport, In *Comprehensive Biochemistry.* Florkin, M., and Stotz, E. H. (eds.), New York, Elsevier, 1970.

Rose, H. G., et al.: Inheritance of combined hyperlipoproteinemia: evidence for a new lipoprotein phenotype. *Am. J. Med.* 54:148, 1973.

Ross, R., and Glomset, J. A.: Atherosclerosis: a problem in the biology of the arterial smooth muscle cell. *Science* 180:1332, 1973.

Ross, R., and Glomset, J. A.: The pathogenesis of atherosclerosis. *N. Engl. J. Med.* 295:369, 420, 1976.

Sabesin, S. M., et al.: Abnormal plasma lipoproteins and lecithin-cholesterol acyltransferase deficiency in alcoholic liver disease. *Gastroenterology* 72:510, 1977.

Santen, R. J., et al.: Atherosclerosis in diabetes mellitus. *Arch. Intern. Med.* 130:833, 1972.

Savin, R. C.: Hyperglobulinemic purpura terminating in myeloma, hyperlipemia and xanthomatoses. *Arch. Dermatol.* 96:679, 1965.

Schlierf, G., et al.: Diurnal patterns of plasma triglycerides and free fatty acids in normal subjects and in patients with endogenous (type IV) hyperlipoproteinemia. *Nutr. Metab.* 13:80, 1971.

Schrott, H. G., et al.: Familial hypercholesterolemia in a large kindred. *Ann. Intern. Med.* 76:711, 1972.

Scott, H. W., Jr.: Metabolic surgery for hyperlipidemia and atherosclerosis. *Am. J. Surg.* 123:3, 1972.

Scott, P. J., et al.: Low density lipoprotein peptide metabolism in nephrotic syndrome: a comparison with patterns observed in other syndromes characterized by hyperlipoproteinemia. *Aust. Ann. Med.* 1:1, 1974.

Seidel, D., et al.: A lipoprotein characterizing obstructive jaundice. I. Method for quantitative separation and identification of lipoproteins in jaundiced subjects. *J. Clin. Invest.* 48:1211, 1969.

Shapiro, D. J., and Rodwell, V. W.: Regulation of hepatic 3-hydroxy-3-methylglutaryl coenzyme A reductase and cholesterol synthesis. *J. Biol. Chem.* 246:3210, 1971.

Sherril, B. C., and Dietschy, J. M.: Characterization of the sinusoidal transport process responsible for uptake of chylomicrons by the liver. *J. Biol. Chem.* 253:1859, 1978.

Simmonds, W. J., et al.: Absorption of cholesterol from a micellar solution: intestinal perfusion studies in man. *J. Clin. Invest.* 46:874, 1967.

Siperstein, M. D.: Regulation of cholesterol biosynthesis in normal and malignant tissues, In *Current Topics in Cellular Regulation.* Horecker, B. L., and Stadtman, E. R. (eds.), New York, Academic Press, 1970.

Small, D. M.: The formation of gallstones. *Adv. Intern. Med.* 16:243, 1970.

Small, D. M., et al.: Studies on simple and mixed bile salt micelles by nuclear magnetic resonance spectroscopy. *Biochim. Biophys. Acta* 176:178, 1969.

Smith, E. B., and Slater, R. S.: Relationship between low-density lipoprotein in aortic intima and serum-lipid levels. *Lancet* 1:463, 1972.

Sommariva, D., et al.: Low-fat diet versus low-carbohydrate diet in the treatment of type IV hyperlipoproteinaemia. *Atherosclerosis* 29:43, 1978.

Spencer, A. F., and Lowenstein, J. M.: Citrate content of liver and kidney of rat in various metabolic states and in fluoracete poisoning. *Biochem. J.* 103:342, 1967.

Srere, P. A.: The citrate cleavage enzyme. I. Distribution and purification. *J. Biol. Chem.* 234:2544, 1959.

Stamler, J.: The Coronary Drug Project: Findings leading to further modifications of its protocol with respect to dextrothyroxine. *J.A.M.A.* 220:996, 1972.

Starzl, T. E., et al.: Portacaval shunt and hyperlipidemia. *Arch. Surg.* 113:71, 1978.

Stein, O., et al.: The metabolism of chylomicron cholesteryl ester in rat liver. *J. Cell Biol.* 43:410, 1969.

Stemerman, M. B., and Ross, R.: Experimental atherosclerosis. I. Fibrous plaque formation in primates. An electron microscopic study. *J. Exp. Med.* 136:769, 1972.

Stewart, J. E., and Schotz, M. D.: Studies on release of lipoprotein lipase activity from fat cells. *J. Biol. Chem.* 246:5749, 1971.

Stout, R. W.: The relationship of abnormal circulating insulin levels to atherosclerosis. *Atherosclerosis* 27:1, 1977.

Stout, R. W., et al.: Effect of phenformin on lipid transport in hypertrigly-ceridemia. *Metabolism 23*:815, 1974.

Taylor, J. S., et al.: Plane xanthoma and multiple myeloma with lipoprotein-paraprotein complexing. *Arch. Dermatol. 114*:425, 1978.

Tejada, C., et al.: Distribution of coronary and aortic atherosclerosis by geographic location, race, and sex. *Lab. Invest. 18*:509, 1968.

Thistle, J. L., and Schoenfield, L. J.: Lithogenic bile among young Indian women. *N. Engl. J. Med. 284*:177, 1971.

Thompson, G. R., et al.: Plasma exchange in the management of homozygous familial hypercholesterolaemia. *Lancet 1*:1208, 1975.

Topping, D. L., and Mayes, P. A.: The immediate effects of insulin and fructose on the metabolism of the perfused liver: Changes in lipoprotein secretion, fatty acid oxidation and esterification, lipogenesis and car-bohydrate metabolism. *Biochem. J. 126*:295, 1972.

Torvik, A., and Hoivik, B.: Gallstones in an autopsy series. *Acta Chir. Scand. 120*:168, 1960.

Utermann, G., et al.: Studies on the metabolic defect in broad-β disease (hyperlipoproteinaemia type III). *Clin. Genetics 12*:139, 1977.

Utermann, G., et al.: Polymorphism of apolipoprotein E. II. Genetics of hyperlipoproteinemia type III. *Clin. Genetics 15*:37, 1979.

Van der Linden, W.: Some biological traits in female gallstone disease patients. *Acta Chir. Scand.* (suppl.) 269, 1961.

Vlahcevic, Z. R., et al.: Relationship of bile acid pool size to the formation of lithogenic bile in female Indians of the Southwest. *Gastroenterology 62*:73, 1972.

Wagle, S., et al.: Studies on glucose synthesis by rat liver and kidney cortex slices. *Life Sci. 5*:655, 1966.

Wallace, R. B., et al.: Altered plasma lipid and lipoprotein levels associated with oral contraceptive and oestrogen use. Report from the Medications Working Group of the Lipid Research Clinics Program. *Lancet 2*:111, 1979.

Wallace, R. B., et al.: Altered plasma-lipids associated with oral contracep-tive oestrogen consumption. The Lipid Research Clinic Program. *Lancet 2*:11, 1977.

Walton, K. W., et al.: Alterations of metabolism and turnover of I[131] low density lipoprotein in myxedema and thyrotoxicosis. *Clin. Sci. 29*:217, 1965.

Westlund, K., and Nicolaysen, R.: Serum cholesterol and risk of mortality and morbidity. A 3-year follow-up of 6,886 men. *Scand. J. Clin. Lab. Invest. 18* (Suppl. 87):1, 1966.

Wieland, O., et al.: Interconversion of pyruvate dehydrogenase in rat heart muscle upon perfusion with fatty acids or ketone bodies *FEBS Lett. 12*:295, 1971.

Wood, P. D., et al.: Plasma lipoprotein distributions in male and female runners. *Ann. NY Acad. Sci. 301*:748, 1977.

World Health Organization Study Group: Classification of atherosclerotic lesions. Tech. Rep. Ser. No. 143, 1958.

Yeshurun, D., and Gotto, A. M. Jr.: Drug treatment of hyperlipidemia. *Am. J. Med. 60*:379, 1976.

Ygge, J., et al.: Changes in blood coagulation and fibrinolysis in women receiving oral contraceptives. Comparison between treatment and un-treated women in a longitudinal study. *Am. J. Obstet. Gynecol. 104*:87, 1969.

CHAPTER 18

Obesity

By Edwin L. Bierman
and Jules Hirsch

Obesity is the most common disorder of metabolism in humans and is also one of the oldest documented metabolic disturbances in history. A limestone statuette dating from the stone age has been unearthed (Venus of Willendorf, Fig. 18–1) that appears to be the most ancient example of obesity, antedating the development of agriculture by about 10,000 years. Although almost prehistoric, the ancient Venus has the body build of a present-day middle-aged fat woman (Fig. 18–2). Similar historical evidence for obesity is found in Egyptian mummies and Greek sculpture. Despite the prevalence throughout centuries of this abnormality, characterized by markedly different environmental stresses and dietary habits, the dis-

order persists, and we are not much closer to elucidation of its pathogenesis or to elaboration of long-term successful measures for therapy.

DEFINITION AND MEASUREMENT

It is not clear whether obesity represents a "disease" or a common clinical manifestation of a group of disorders. The definition is necessarily arbitrary, since body weight (more accurately, quantity of body fat) is continuously distributed in populations, with no clear division between individuals who are obese and individuals who are thin. A definition of obesity would be made easier if there was a distinct point at which a clear influence of obesity on morbidity and mortality began. This is not the case, however, since there is a continually progressive excess mortality for increasing degrees of overweight beyond about 25%, based on insurance company actuarial standards (Fig. 18–3). Moreover, the metabolic, physiologic, and pathophysiologic consequences (discussed later) appear to increase continuously with the degree of deviation above average weight.

Body weight, although the simplest index of obesity, is not always the best reflection of the relative proportion of adipose tissue in the body or of total adipose mass. The latter needs to be determined or estimated if knowledge of the degree of excess adiposity is desirable. Weight adjusted to body size gives a better indication. For clinical purposes, per cent ideal body weight (relative weight) based on insurance company tables (Table 18–1) usually gives a rough approximation of the degree of adiposity. For common usage, obesity can be defined as that body weight more than 20% above ideal body weight.

A variety of methods for assessment of total body fat, such as body density, x-ray, distribution of fat-soluble

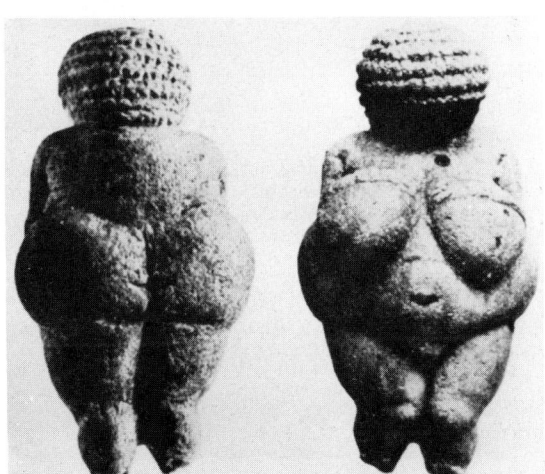

Figure 18–1. Venus of Willendorf. Limestone statuette, circa early Stone Age, 22,000 B.C.

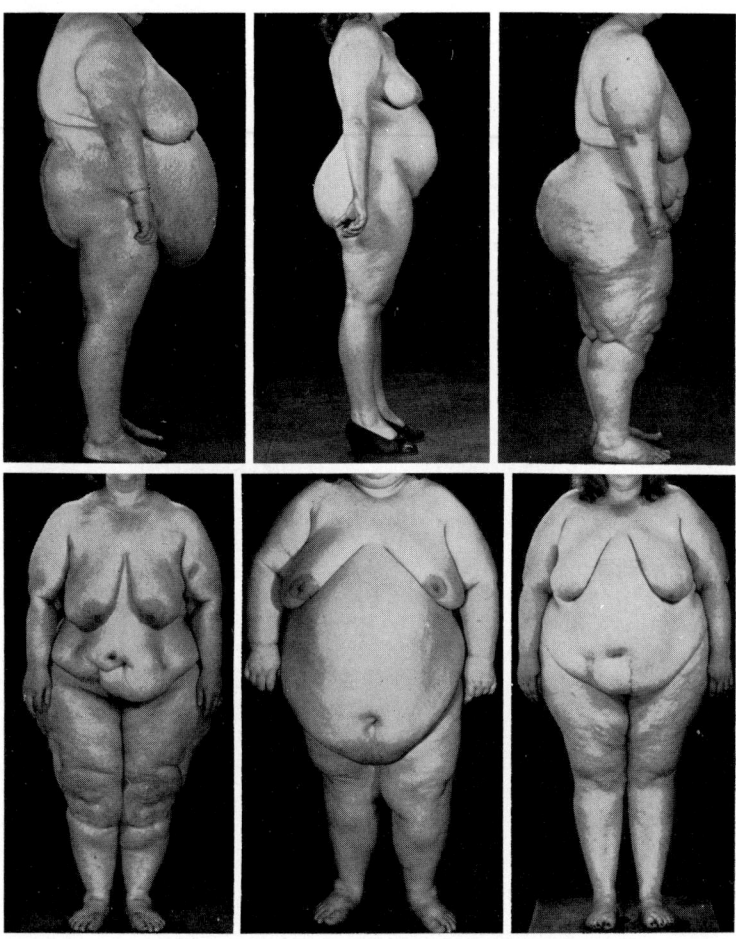

Figure 18–2. Note marked variations in distribution of fat. *Top center,* This patient consulted the Obstetrics Clinic many times for question of pregnancy, which she never had. *Lower center,* Chronic hospitalization was necessary because of incapacitation from obesity. *Lower right,* This patient's hyperphagia began exactly 1 day after she fell from a ladder and injured her head, at age 11. The correlation with possible hypothalamic injury seemed excellent in this patient, but such occurrences are rare.

gases, total body water, and total body potassium-40, have been used for research purposes. In addition, a variety of anthropometric measurements (limb and trunk diameters, circumferences, and skin-fold thicknesses) have been used to derive regression equations that correlate closely with per cent body fat determined by independent means (Steinkamp et al., 1965). The weight/height^2 index (kg/m^2; Body Mass index) is the most useful anthropo-

MORTALITY OF OVERWEIGHT MEN SUBSEQUENT TO WEIGHT REDUCTION AND OF ALL OVERWEIGHT MEN

Cases Accepted for Ordinary Insurance in 1935-53, Traced to Policy Anniversary in 1954

Overweight Group (Per cent Overweight at Issue)	**Mortality Ratio** (Ratio for All Standard Risks = 100 %)

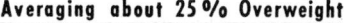

Averaging about 25 % Overweight

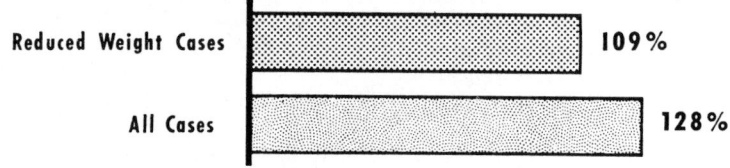

Reduced Weight Cases   109 %

All Cases   128 %

Figure 18–3. The high mortality rate associated with marked obesity falls to a normal level with loss of obesity. (Build and Blood Pressure Study, 1959, published by the Society of Actuaries.)

Averaging 35-40 % Overweight

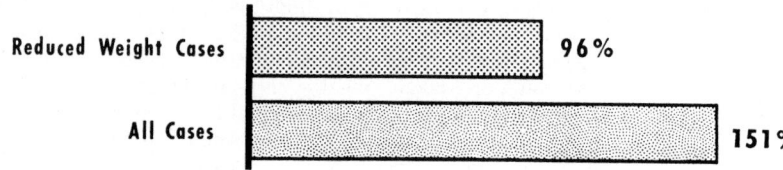

Reduced Weight Cases   96 %

All Cases   151 %

Table 18–1. GUIDELINES FOR BODY WEIGHT*

Metric Height (m)†	Men (Weight in kg) Average	Acceptable Weight Range		Women (Weight in kg) Average	Acceptable Weight Range	
1.45				46.0	42	53
1.48				46.5	42	54
1.50				47.0	43	55
1.52				48.5	44	57
1.54				49.5	44	58
1.56				50.4	45	58
1.58	55.8	51	64	51.3	46	59
1.60	57.6	52	65	52.6	48	61
1.62	58.6	53	66	54.0	49	62
1.64	59.6	54	67	55.4	50	64
1.66	60.0	55	69	56.8	51	65
1.68	61.7	56	71	56.8	52	66
1.70	63.5	58	73	60.0	53	67
1.72	65.0	59	74	61.3	55	69
1.74	66.5	60	75	62.6	56	70
1.76	68.0	62	77	64.0	58	72
1.78	69.4	64	79	65.3	59	74
1.80	71.0	65	80			
1.82	72.6	66	82			
1.84	74.2	67	84			
1.86	75.8	69	86			
1.88	77.6	71	88			
1.90	79.3	73	90			
1.92	81.0	75	93			

Nonmetric Height** Ft In	(Weight in lbs) Average	Acceptable Weight Range		(Weight in lbs) Average	Acceptable Weight Range	
4 10				102	92	119
4 11				104	94	122
5 0				107	96	125
5 1				110	99	128
5 2	123	112	141	113	102	131
5 3	127	115	144	116	105	134
5 4	130	118	148	120	108	138
5 5	133	121	152	123	111	142
5 6	136	124	156	128	114	146
5 7	140	128	161	132	118	150
5 8	145	132	166	136	122	154
5 9	149	136	170	140	126	158
5 10	153	140	174	144	130	163
5 11	158	144	179	148	134	168
6 0	162	148	184		138	173
6 1	166	152	189	152		
6 2	171	156	194			
6 3	176	160	199			
6 4	181	164	204			

*Adapted from the recommendations of the Fogarty Center Conference 1973 (Bray, 1975). Data from the Metropolitan Life Insurance Company tables.

†Height without shoes, weight without clothes

NOMOGRAPH FOR BODY MASS INDEX (KG/M^2)

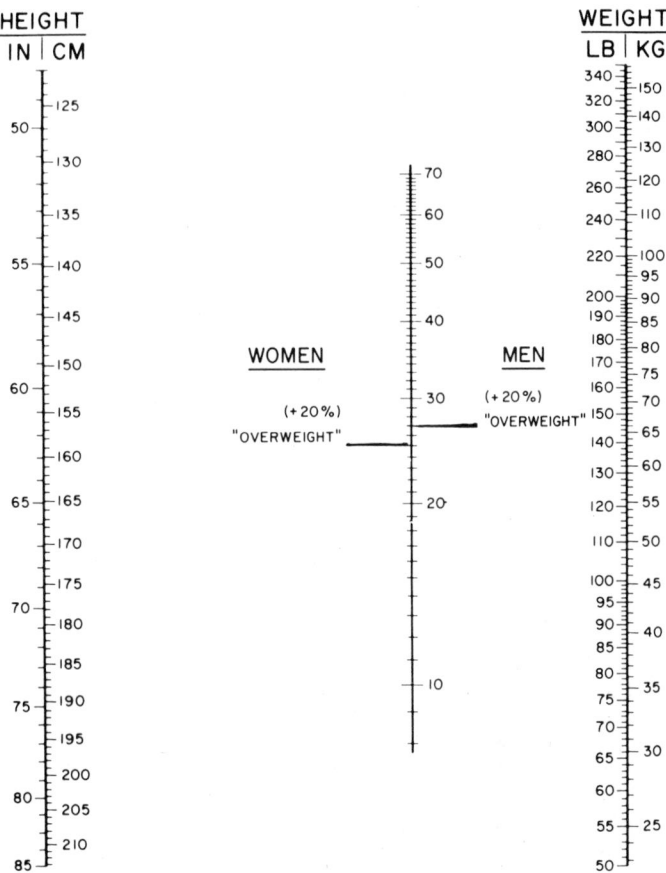

Figure 18–4. The ratio weight/height^2 (metric units) is read from the central scale after a straight edge is placed between height and body weight. "Desirable" body mass index ranges suggested from life insurance data are males: 20–25; females: 19–24. (Adapted from Thomas, A. E., et al.: A nomograph method for assessing body weight. *Am. J. Clin. Nutr. 29:*302, 1976.)

metric measurement and the simplest to obtain; it de-emphasizes the effect of stature on body weight and also correlates closely with adiposity (Edwards and Whyte, 1962). It has been recommended that obesity be defined as a body mass index of greater than 27 for men and greater than 25 for women; these figures closely correspond to a per cent ideal body weight of 120% (Fig. 18–4). Tables for the distribution of subscapular and triceps skin-fold thickness measurements in large populations have been published (Mayer, 1966; Montoye et al., 1965) that also provide an accurate guide. Mayer (1966) suggests that triceps skin-fold thickness greater than 23 mm in men and 30 mm in women should be defined as obesity.

CLINICAL TYPES

Although it has been clear for some time that there are two clinical types of obesity, little metabolic or physiologic evidence has been available until recently to support such a clinical concept. In one type (lifelong obesity), patients give a characteristic history. Although generally of normal birth weight, they tend to have been heavier as children since early grade school, to have had a large spurt in weight gain during puberty, and (in females who have been pregnant) to give a history of irreversibly gaining weight with each successive pregnancy. These individuals usually have tried all available methods and fads promoted for caloric restriction and weight reduction to no permanent avail. After successful weight loss, regardless of the program, they usually return gradually to approximately their prereduction level of overweight. These individuals tend to be grossly obese (more than 150% of ideal body weight) adults.

The other clinical type (adult-onset obesity) is much more common and essentially represents "middle-age spread." These individuals give a history of being thin or of average weight until age 20–40, when weight gain associated with a more sedentary existence and other environmental factors begins. This type of weight gain in

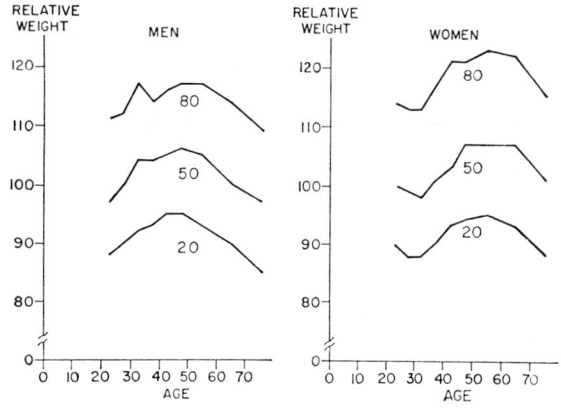

Figure 18-5. Relative weight index for males and females (20th, 50th, and 80th percentiles) throughout adulthood from a cross-sectional study of a total community — Tecumseh, Michigan. (From Montoye, H. J., Epstein, F. H., et al.: The measurement of body fatness: a study in a total community. *Am. J. Clin. Nutr. 16*:417, 1965.)

adult life is extremely common and is seen in most affluent populations as evidenced by a cross-sectional analysis of a total, free-living community (Fig. 18–5). It appears that there is a gradual increase in relative body weight (compared with ideal) until the middle years, after which there is some decline. Since this is not a longitudinal study of the same individuals throughout life, it is possible that the reason for this decline in relative weight in later years reflects the increased morbidity and mortality associated with marked overweight.

A possible explanation for weight gain during adult life that does not appear to be tenable is a decrease in basal energy utilization with aging. Basal oxygen consumption declines only slightly during adult life (Fig. 18–6). Body composition is changing, however, even at constant body weight. There is a larger proportion of body fat and a smaller proportion of lean body mass with age. Thus, basal oxygen consumption in terms of lean body mass, predominantly muscle and bone, may actually be virtually constant with age. Therefore, adult-onset obesity simply may reflect an imbalance between caloric intake and utilization, based on the fact that such individuals do not reduce their caloric intake with age appropriately for their change in body composition. Ahrens (1970) has calculated that the daily caloric requirement for weight maintenance of adults decreases 43 calories/decade/m²

surface area for males and 27 calories/decade/m² surface area for females.

These two broad clinical types of obesity were recognized by Albrink and Meigs (1964), who proposed that adult-onset obesity is mainly central in location (the "middle-aged spread"), whereas lifelong obesity might be peripheral as well as central. For peripheral localization of adiposity, skin-fold thickness of the forearm or the triceps is measured and compared with skin-fold thickness over the tip of the scapula. Weight gain during adult life is significantly correlated with costal, scapular, and, to a lesser extent, triceps skin-fold thickness but not with ulnar skin-fold thickness. Thus forearm fat is minimally influenced by adult-onset obesity, whereas adipose tissue of the trunk is most influenced by weight gain during adult life.

PATHOPHYSIOLOGY

A possible pathophysiologic basis for these clinical observations was first proposed by Bjurulf (1959), who suggested that some forms of obesity might be due to increased numbers of cells. Proof of this hypothesis was provided by the elegant experiments of Hirsch and his coworkers (1966). They demonstrated that grossly obese humans (lifelong) characteristically have an increase in adipose cell number as well as in adipose cell size. After weight reduction, adipose cell size shrinks, but hypercellularity remains fixed (Fig. 18–7).

Adult-onset obesity is usually not as severe and appears to be characterized predominantly by adipose cell hypertrophy, with only minimal increase in cell number. Thus, all human obesity is accompanied by cellular enlargement. Adipocyte hyperplasia is not in clear evidence until body weight is over 170% ideal. At higher weights, hyperplasia becomes increasingly marked (Fig. 18–8).

Adipose cell number appears to be determined very early in life. In studies with rats, animals subjected to overnutrition before weaning maintained greater numbers of adipose cells throughout life than did litter mates subjected to undernutrition prior to weaning (Knittle and Hirsch, 1968). Weight changes during adult life did not influence the cell number of these animals. Studies in humans also have shown that adipose cell number is determined early in life (Knittle et al., 1979; Häger et al., 1977). In the nonobese, two periods of enhanced adipose cell proliferation have been identified: within the

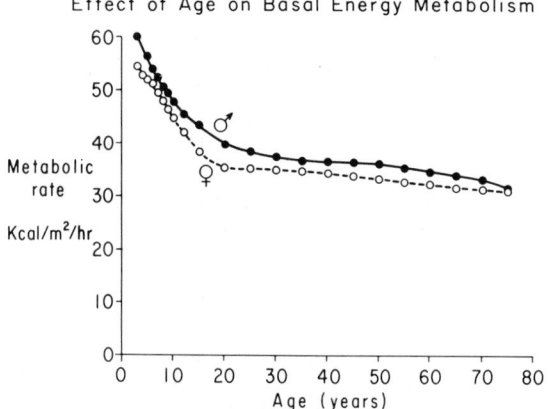

Figure 18-6. Values for basal metabolic rate (kcal/m²/hr) for normal males and females. (From *Handbook of Biological Data,* National Academy of Sciences, National Research Council. Spector, W. S. (ed.), Philadelphia, W. B. Saunders, 1961.)

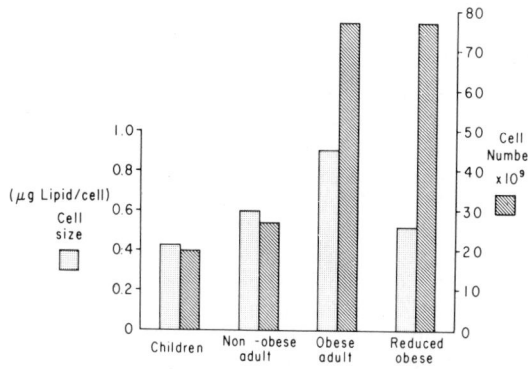

Figure 18-7. A comparison of adipose cell size and adipose cell number in nonobese children and adults and in obese adults before and after weight reduction. (Adapted from the data of Hirsch, J., Knittle, J., et al.: All lipid content and cell number in obese and nonobese human adipose tissue. *J. Clin. Invest. 45*:1023, 1966.)

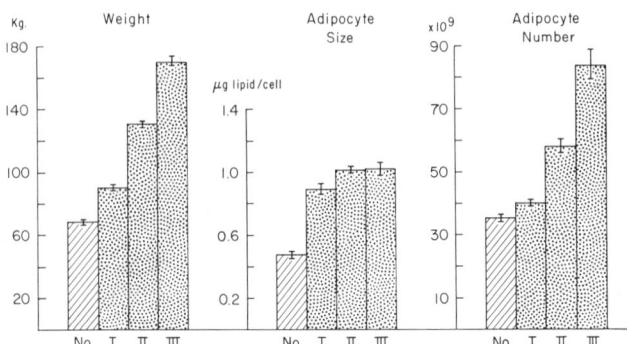

Obese groups vs Non-obese

Figure 18–8. Means ± s.e. mean are shown for nonobese control subjects (No) as well as for each of three groups of obese. Severity of obesity was determined by percentage ideal body weight (IBW). Group I, 115–170% IBW; Group II, 170–240% IBW; Group III, above 240% IBW. (From Hirsch, J., and Batchelor, B.: Adipose tissue cellularity in human obesity. *Clin. Endocrinol. Metabol. 5*:299, 1976.)

first 2 years of life and again prior to puberty. In obese children, adipose cell number is already significantly increased by age 2 and increases rapidly throughout childhood, exceeding the mean cell number found in nonobese adults by age 11.

This may have profound implications with regard to the effect of feeding patterns during infancy and early childhood on the subsequent development of lifelong obesity. It has been shown that excessive weight gain within the first 6 months of life is correlated with overweight at the ages of 6–8 years (Eid, 1970) and at the ages of 20–30 years (Charney et al., 1976). Thus it appears that the rapidity of weight gain in infancy is a better guide to the risk of obesity in later years than is the weight of the parents. Although less than one third of obese adults were overweight children, most overweight children be-

come obese adults. The familial aggregation of obesity (Mayer, 1965),* then, could be explained in part by a familial aggregation of eating patterns, particularly as applied to nutrition in early life. There also appears to be an important genetic influence, since body weights and skin-fold thicknesses of identical twins are correlated more closely than are those of fraternal twins (Newman et al., 1937; Borjeson, 1976).

Experimental Obesity

Support for this concept has been derived from studies of experimental obesity in humans by Sims and coworkers (1973). They force-fed volunteers and with some difficulty produced 20–30% increments in weight (Fig. 18–9) associated with centripetal distribution of excess fat, which was predominantly due to an increase in adipose cell size without a change in adipose cell number. Prompt, spontaneous reversal of adipose increment and cell size was achieved at the termination of the experimental forced feeding.

Studies of experimental obesity in animals also lend some support to these concepts. Genetically transmitted obesity in rodents is characterized by adipose cell hyperplasia as well as by hypertrophy; experimentally induced obesity, such as that which can be obtained by destruction of the ventromedial nucleus of the hypothalamus, is associated with hypertrophy alone (Johnson and Hirsch, 1972). There is evidence that prolonged feeding of highly palatable diets to rats can provoke an increase in cell number even in adult life (Faust et al., 1978). Furthermore, adipose tissue regeneration will occur at some adipose sites of the rat after lipectomy (Faust et al., 1977). It is unknown whether or not such increases in cell number

---

*Fewer than 10% of children are overweight when both parents are thin; 50% are overweight when one parent is obese; 80% are overweight when both parents are obese.

Figure 18–9. Experimental obesity in a human volunteer before (*top*) and after (*bottom*) overfeeding. (Courtesy of E. A. Sims.)

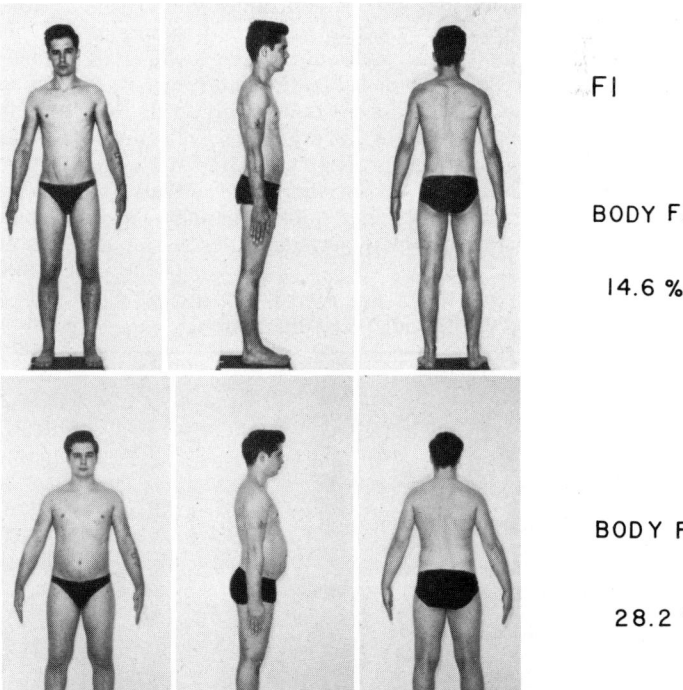

FI

BODY FAT

14.6 %

BODY FAT

28.2 %

Table 18–2. TYPES OF OBESITY

	Hyperplastic	Hypertrophic
Severity	Marked	Moderate
History	Lifelong	Adult-onset
Fat distribution	Peripheral and central	Central ("middle-age spread")
Adipose cellularity	↑ cell number and ↑ cell size	↑ cell size only
Insulin resistance	Related to cell size	Related to cell size
Metabolic consequences	Related to cell size	Related to cell size
Long-term response to R_x	Poor	Fair

can occur in the human adult. It may be that in certain periods of life (e.g., pregnancy), endocrine alterations "permit" a renewal of cellular hyperplasia. In neither animal nor human studies has there been any evidence for a decrease in cell number, however, short of actual surgical removal of tissue. A summary of the two broad general categories of obesity is given in Table 18–2. All obesity is hypertrophic because the adipose cells are enlarged, but only certain individuals have adipose hyperplasia. Massive obesity is usually of the juvenile-onset, lifelong hyperplastic type.

ETIOLOGY

Possible factors in the pathogenesis of adipose cell hypertrophy are listed in Table 18–3. No primary biochemical lesion of adipose tissue has ever been firmly documented as a cause of generalized obesity in humans. Genetic factors play a role, but their mechanism remains unknown. Estrogen-androgen balance also appears to influence the site and amount of adipose tissue deposition, since women and prepubertal children have a proportion of subcutaneous fat higher than that of men. Regulation by insulin in cerebrospinal fluid has also been proposed (Woods and Porte, 1978). Little is known of the etiologic basis for adipose cell hyperplasia.

Only in rare instances of hypothalamic obesity in humans, in which damage to the ventromedial hypothalamic nucleus occurs as a result of tumor or trauma, can an etiology be defined and, with surgical removal of the tumor, obesity cured. This hypothalamic center appears to regulate the deposition of adipose tissue triglyceride. Formerly its role as an appetite or satiety center was emphasized (ventrolateral nucleus = feeding center; ventromedial nucleus = inhibitory or satiety center). Thus this center has been thought by many to be related to obesity in humans via inappropriate hyperphagia derived at the

Table 18–3. POSSIBLE FACTORS IN THE PATHOGENESIS OF OBESITY (ADIPOCYTE HYPERTROPHY)

Excessive Lipid Deposition
  Increased food intake
  Hypothalamic lesions
  Adipose cell hyperplasia
  Hyperlipogenesis
  Increased lipoprotein lipase activity

Diminished Lipid Mobilization
  Decrease in lipolytic hormones
  Defective adipose-cell lipolysis
  Abnormality of autonomic innervation

Diminished Lipid Utilization
  Aging
  Defective lipid oxidation
  Defective thermogenesis
  Inactivity

hypothalamic level. Studies (Frohman et al., 1969; Hustvedt and Løvø, 1972) have shown that experimentally induced hypothalamic lesions alter insulin levels and lipogenesis independent of changes in food intake, however. Neural mediation of the rise in insulin appears to be the primary factor in the development of hypothalamic obesity (Inoue et al., 1978). Anomalous insulin secretion after hypothalamic injury in humans also has been observed and is possibly linked to the development of obesity in these individuals (Bray and Gallagher, 1975). In any event, the relevance to the common types of human obesity of experimental animal models in which obesity is produced by injury to the hypothalamus is open to question. For a thorough description of the various genetic experimental animal models of obesity, the reader is referred to several reviews (Bray and York, 1971; Assimacopoulos-Jeannet and Jeanrenaud, 1976).

Cerebral and emotional influences on eating patterns surely play a role in obesity, but, aside from overt psychiatric disturbances, the general role of altered behavioral patterns in the etiology of obesity has been difficult to define, and a specific type of personality associated with obesity has yet to be distinguished. Cultural influences and socioeconomic status have a strong influence on the prevalence of obesity (Garn et al., 1977). As Stunkard (1977) has pointed out, every social factor studied has been strongly correlated with obesity and thus must be considered a determinant. No less important, habit and environment appear to influence appetite regulation. The experiments of Schachter (1968) have indicated that external cues differentially affect behavior of obese and normal subjects. It appears that obese individuals are stimulated by environmental influences such as ready availability of food, flavor, time of day, and the like. In contrast, thin individuals appear to be stimulated to eat by internal cues presumably related to physiologic appetite regulation. Careful studies of taste sensitivity and susceptibility to external influence in obese and normal-weight subjects failed to substantiate these findings (Grinker et al., 1972). These experiments are of necessity extremely complex and difficult to interpret, however. In theory, a nonobese individual may eat when hungry, an obese person may eat because it's time to eat and the food is appetizing. If food is not readily available or is not appetizing, as shown by the ingenious "black box" feeding experiments of Campbell and coworkers (1971), in which subjects fed themselves through an automatic liquid formula dispensing device without being able to monitor the amount of intake, an obese individual will actually consume far fewer calories than will his or her thin control counterpart. In addition to eating behavior influencing the degree of adiposity, the reverse is also true. Profound adiposity, particularly of the lifelong type, leads to numerous psychologic and psychiatric disturbances which may not be reversible with weight reduction (Bruch, 1957). In fact, in some instances, weight reduction can lead to profound behavioral changes in affective state and perception of self-image. These changes have been shown to be particularly severe after weight loss in those patients who have been obese since childhood. Obesity beginning in adult life may be reversible, with fewer long-term adverse consequences (Grinker et al., 1973; Stunkard and Rush, 1974).

METABOLIC FEATURES

Regardless of the cause or type of obesity, the metabolic consequences are predictable. They appear to relate only to fat cell size, and virtually all metabolic disturbances tested are inducible with weight gain (Sims et al., 1973) and reversible with weight reduction. Thus, although numerous hormonal imbalances have been described in obesity, they are likely to be consequences of the obese state, not causes of it.

The metabolic alteration with the most profound influence on metabolism is the acquired resistance to the action of insulin on glucose utilization by fat and muscle cells that appears to be a direct function of increased fat cell size. Insulin resistance associated with adiposity has been demonstrated both *in vivo*, by the observation that peripheral glucose uptake across the forearm in response to either exogenous or endogenous insulin is less in obesity (Rabinowitz and Zierler, 1962; Butterfield et al., 1965), and *in vitro*, by studies of the metabolism of glucose in isolated fat (Salans et al., 1974; Czech et al., 1977). Since Bjorntorp's studies suggested that physical training decreased hyperinsulinemia in obesity without diminishing adiposity, muscle metabolism presumably plays an important role in the insulin resistance of obesity (Bjorntorp et al., 1977). *In vitro* studies of muscle from obese rats have shown evidence of impaired insulin action (Davidson, 1978; Czech et al., 1978), possibly resulting from decreased numbers of insulin receptors (Olefsky et al., 1976). One of the consequences of this resistance to the action of insulin appears to be a feedback compensatory hyperinsulinism. The beta cells of the pancreatic islets are stimulated by an unknown mechanism to produce more insulin, and beta cell hypertrophy eventually results. The signal is as yet unknown but may be neuronal or hormonal or may involve small changes in glucose, fatty acids, or specific amino acids. In any case, the result is an increase in circulating insulin levels (basal and in response to a variety of stimuli) that is directly related to the degree of adiposity (Fig. 18–10) and is reversible with weight reduction (Bagdade et al., 1967; Kalkhoff et al., 1971). It is not simply a matter of body weight or lean body mass that is associated with hyperinsulinemia, since very muscular individuals who are heavy do not appear to have hyperinsulinism. Insulin resistance and hyperinsulinism can be induced in normal subjects by weight gain and reversed in obese subjects by weight reduction (Horton et al., 1975). Compensatory hyperinsulinism appears to be a common pathway for a multitude of other factors that produce resistance peripherally to the action of insulin (Fig. 18–11).

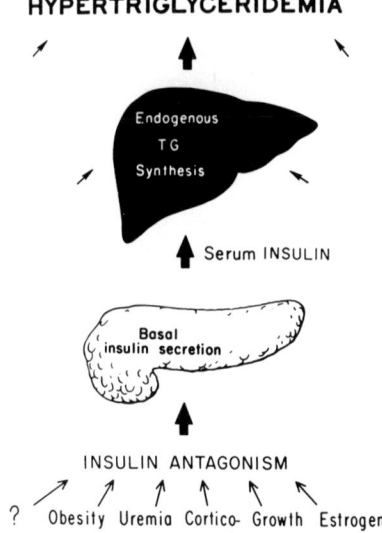

HYPERTRIGLYCERIDEMIA

Figure 18–11.

It has recently been shown that circulating levels of insulin regulate their own receptors on cell surfaces (Bar et al., 1976). Thus obesity has been associated with fewer numbers of insulin receptors on muscle, liver, monocyte, and adipose cell surfaces, thereby further contributing to insulin resistance and impaired glucose utilization by cells. In addition to decreased insulin sensitivity resulting from fewer insulin receptors, decreased insulin responsiveness of adipose tissue contributes to the insulin resistance of obesity. Postreceptor defects in large fat cells involving blunted pentose shunt and fatty acid synthesis activity leading to impaired capacity to utilize glucose have been described (Czech et al., 1977).

The emergence of adult-onset diabetes mellitus in the population may well be profoundly influenced by the degree and duration of obesity (West, 1978) (Ch. 15). One concept is that prolonged hyperinsulinism might lead to beta cell "exhaustion" in those individuals who are genetically susceptible. As is well known, when the pressure is off after successful weight reduction, glucose intolerance is reversed. Thus glucose intolerance in the obese adult may represent "high-output failure," in which the beta cell has failed to compensate fully for the degree of peripheral insulin resistance associated with adiposity. Abnormal growth hormone (GH) regulation has been associated with obesity (lack of a normal rise with starvation, hypoglycemia, or arginine stimulation), but the significance of this finding and its relation to the glucose intolerance of obesity is not understood. These changes in insulin and GH regulation in obesity can be found even in early childhood (Parra et al., 1971).

Fatty acid mobilization appears to be less affected by the insulin resistance associated with adiposity. Impairment of the insulin effect on lipolysis would be expected to lead to enhancement of fat mobilization. In simple obesity (uncomplicated by glucose intolerance), however, lipolysis does not appear to be increased, as reflected by normal to low plasma free fatty acid (FFA) and glycerol levels (Bagdade et al., 1969), unimpaired braking of lipolysis after oral glucose, and apparently normal stimulation after administration of fat-mobilizing hormones. Furthermore, studies *in vivo* of human forearm metabolism (Rabinowitz and Zierler, 1962) have shown no increase in arteriovenous FFA output by subcutaneous tissue in simple obesity. Björntorp and Ostman (1971) have shown

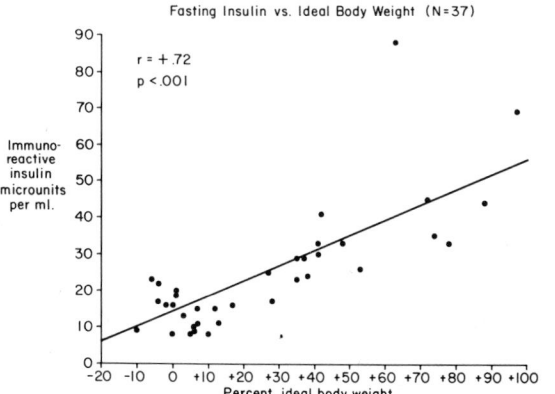

Figure 18–10. Basal serum insulin levels in thin and obese men plotted as a function of % IBW (an index of adiposity). (Adapted from Bagdade, J. D., Bierman, E. L., et al.: The significance of basal insulin levels in the evaluation of the insulin response to glucose in diabetic and nondiabetic subjects. *J. Clin. Invest.* 46:1549, 1967.)

that plasma glycerol levels appear to be correlated with fat cell number but not with fat cell size. Thus it appears likely that in other studies in which elevated FFA and glycerol plasma levels and turnover rates were reported in obese subjects, enhanced lipolysis was a function of the presence of adipose tissue hyperplasia or concomitant glucose intolerance. Furthermore, it is doubtful that enhanced lipolysis, when present, plays a major regulatory role in the hyperinsulinism of obesity. Alternatively, there is little evidence that decreased lipolysis, or resistance to normal fat mobilizing stimuli (hormonal, neuronal), plays an etiologic role in adipose cell hypertrophy (Table 18–3) except in the very rare cases of triglyceride storage disease (Galton et al., 1974).

The peculiar "resistance to ketosis" attributed to obese patients refers to the prolonged interval of fasting (usually more than 2–3 days), in comparison to thin individuals, before ketonuria is observed. This parallels the prolonged decline in elevated insulin levels in obesity observed during total fasting (Bagdade et al., 1972), which suggests that the liver remains well insulinized during fasting in obesity for a longer period of time, resulting in a continuing diversion of fatty acids to nonketogenic pathways (McGarry and Foster, 1976). (There is little evidence that the insulin resistance of adipose tissue and muscle associated with adiposity extends to the liver.) Higher insulin levels would also explain the often observed delay and blunted mobilization of fatty acids when obese patients begin fasting. In addition, the "resistance" of obese individuals to the hypoglycemia induced by ethanol after fasting (Arky and Freinkel, 1967) may reflect expanded hepatic glycogen reserves consequent to hyperinsulinemia.

Lipoprotein lipase (LPL — the enzyme in adipose tissue responsible for assimilation of fatty acids contained in circulating triglyceride-rich lipoproteins) (Ch. 17) appears to be sensitive to the availability of insulin, and its activity is increased in hypertrophic adipose cells (Pykälistö et al., 1975). Increased adipose tissue LPL activity could lead to an enhanced tendency for deposition of dietary and endogenous fat in adipose tissue in obesity. A possible primary role for this enzyme in the etiology of obesity in some individuals is suggested by the report that reduced obese individuals maintain high levels of LPL activity in adipose cells (Schwartz and Brunzell, 1978). If this finding is confirmed, there may be a biochemical basis for the difficulty some obese individuals have in maintaining a reduced state following weight reduction. Observations in the genetically obese rat indicate that LPL activity in adipose cells is increased early in development even before the animals become obese (Gruen et al., 1978). This suggests that early increments in adipose tissue LPL in the "preobese" state may contribute to the development of fat cell hypertrophy during the development of genetic obesity in the rat and is a useful predictor of the onset of obesity. Similar findings have emerged from studies of a cultured mouse preadipocyte cell line (3T3-L1 cells), in which increased LPL activity precedes the accumulation of triglyceride in these cells (Eckel et al., 1977). These findings are consistent with the idea that adipose tissue mass is regulated by as yet unknown neurohumoral factors that may operate by modulating adipose tissue LPL activity.

Other alterations in adipose cell metabolism in obesity have been sought, particularly those involving lipogenesis. Bray (1976) has demonstrated a deficiency of intramitochondrial glycerophosphate dehydrogenase in human obesity that theoretically could have effects on lipogenesis; however, "hyperlipogenesis" has not been demonstrable in humans. The demonstration by Miller and colleagues (1967) that increased thermogenesis can be induced in humans as well as in animals by increased caloric intake raises the intriguing possibility that defects in adaptive thermogenesis might be associated with obesity. In accord with this suggestion, overfed nonobese individuals consume more calories than can be accounted for by the gain in weight, and after weight is gained, it requires many more calories/m² surface area for weight maintenance (Sims et al., 1973). Large individual differences in energy expenditure have been documented (Garrow, 1978), lending support to the observation that some individuals eat much more than others, yet become no fatter.

Another metabolic consequence of obesity is hypertriglyceridemia, which may result in part from the associated hyperinsulinism. Triglyceride levels in populations are correlated with relative body weight, skin-fold thickness, and particularly with weight gain in adult life (Albrink et al., 1962). In a variety of studies (Bierman et al., 1970; Olefsky et al., 1974), circulating insulin levels are significantly associated with triglyceride levels, and since insulin is one of the factors involved in endogenous triglyceride-rich lipoprotein secretion by the liver (Ch. 17), a hypothetic pathway can be devised to explain these results (Fig. 18–11). In hypertriglyceridemic individuals, it is of interest that the hyperinsulinemia is correlated with both relative body weight and fat cell size (Bagdade et al., 1971; Bjorntorp et al., 1971). In such individuals, both hyperinsulinemia and hypertriglyceridemia are reversible with weight reduction (Olefsky et al., 1974). Both hyperinsulinemia and increased endogenous triglyceride production rates have been produced with overfeeding in an experimental animal model for obesity, the desert sand rat (Robertson et al., 1973). The role of obesity in determining the serum lipid levels in populations as a whole is suggested by the superimposibility of age-related curves of relative body weight, plasma triglycerides, and plasma cholesterol in males and females (Fig. 18–12).

Serum cholesterol levels are less closely linked with obesity, but nevertheless a significant relationship exists

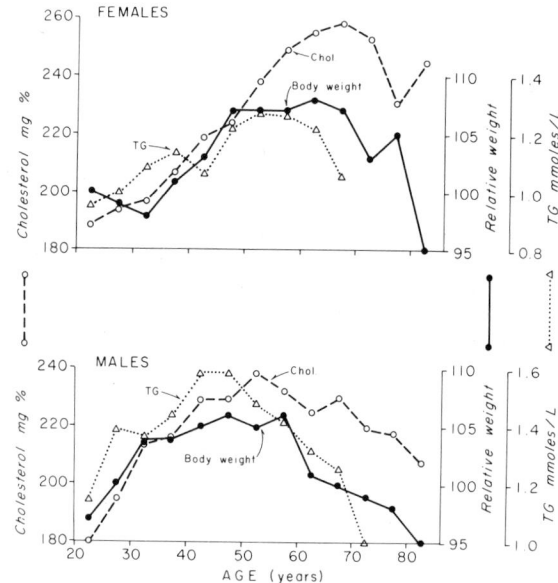

Figure 18–12. Superimposition of values throughout the adult age span for an index of relative body weight, serum cholesterol, and serum triglyceride levels. Weight and cholesterol from the Tecumseh study of a total community (Montoye) and triglycerides from the healthy subgroup studied in Stockholm (Carlson and Lindstedt).

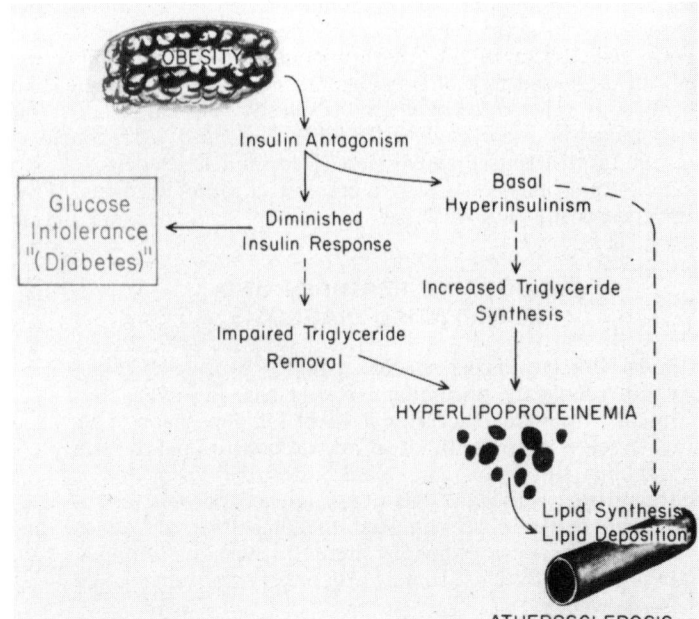

Figure 18–13.

(Montoye et al., 1966). This could be explained in part by the observation that cholesterol production rate appears to be related to the degree of adiposity (Nestel et al., 1973; Smith et al., 1976; Miettinen, 1971). This relationship may be linked to the increased propensity of obese individuals to develop gallstones (Ch. 17).

The influence of obesity on glucose and lipid levels also may be related to the increased tendency for obese individuals to develop all the complications of atherosclerosis (Ch. 17). Possible mechanisms linking obesity, altered carbohydrate and fat metabolism, and atherosclerosis are indicated in Fig. 18–13. The metabolic and endocrine alterations produced as a consequence of human obesity are summarized in Table 18–4. For further discussion of the metabolic aspects of obesity, the reader is referred to recent reviews (Sims et al., 1973; Bray, 1976; Czech and Reaven, 1900). From metabolic considerations alone, it would appear appropriate to define obesity in terms of adipose tissue fat cell size.

PHYSIOLOGIC FEATURES

The physiologic consequences of obesity lead to a variety of clinical manifestations and diseases (Table 18–5) (Mann, 1974). Every organ system appears to be involved. In the respiratory system, alveolar hypoventilation eventually leads to carbon dioxide retention and somnolence (the pickwickian syndrome). In the cardiovascular system, cor pulmonale associated with pulmonary hypertension is common, and nonspecific myocardial lesions have been de-

scribed. Obesity is associated with four major risk factors for atherosclerosis, i.e., hypertension, diabetes, hypercholesterolemia, and hypertriglyceridemia (Ch. 17). Therefore, it is not surprising that obese individuals have more atherosclerotic manifestations, particularly angina pectoris, and are more prone to sudden death. Nonspecific gastrointestinal symptoms (bloating, dyspepsia) are frequent. A fatty liver is common, with mild abnormalities in SGPT and LDH that become normal with weight reduction. With severe caloric restriction, serum bilirubin may rise moderately, but this quickly reverts to normal when adequate calories are given to maintain weight. In addition to the arterial lesions of atherosclerosis, varicose veins are common. Flabby and redundant skin produces moist folds, resulting in a propensity to fungal and yeast skin lesions (particularly in the axillae and perineal region and under the breasts). Gallstones and cholecystitis are more common in obese individuals (Ch. 17). Osteoarthritis is more common and severe, and the prevalence of gout is increased. Women who are obese tend to have irregular menses and increased morbidity associated with pregnancy and again after childbearing ceases. The incidence of toxemia of pregnancy and hypertension is increased. Ob-

Table 18–4. METABOLIC AND ENDOCRINE CONSEQUENCES OF OBESITY

↓ Sensitivity to insulin (muscle, adipose tissue)
Hyperinsulinemia
↓ Glucose tolerance; hyperglycemia
Hyperaminoacidemia
Hypertriglyceridemia
Hypercholesterolemia
↓ Growth hormone responses
"Resistance" to ketosis
↑ 17-Hydroxycorticoid excretion

Table 18–5. PATHOPHYSIOLOGIC CONSEQUENCES OF OBESITY

System	Condition
Respiratory	Alveolar hypoventilation (pickwickian syndrome)
Cardiovascular	Atherosclerosis Hypertension Cor pulmonale Varicose veins and thromboembolism
Gastrointestinal	Fatty liver Gallstones
Musculoskeletal	Osteoarthritis Gout
Genitourinary	Oligomenorrhea Toxemia of pregnancy Endometrial carcinoma

stetric risk is higher due to longer duration of labor, larger babies, more cesarean sections, and higher anesthetic risk. Later in life, there are more uterine fibroids and an increased risk of development of endometrial cancer directly related to the degree of obesity. The large adipose mass is associated with both increased estrogen storage and increased conversion of adrenal androgens to estrone that may result in increased chronic hormonal stimulation of the uterus.

ENDOCRINE FEATURES AND DIFFERENTIAL DIAGNOSIS

Endocrine lesions as specific primary causes of adiposity are relatively uncommon. It is clear, however, that hormones influence the regulation of fat deposition. This may involve a general effect on adipocyte metabolism throughout the body (e.g., insulin, thyroid hormone) or characteristic regional effects (e.g., glucocorticoids, estrogen). Hyperinsulinism can lead to adiposity, as well as vice versa, as exemplified by patients with insulinoma. Individuals with this tumor are only rarely markedly obese, however.

Although much attention has been paid to hypothyroidism and milder degrees of "hypometabolism" as a cause of obesity and vast quantities of thyroid hormone have been administered for treatment, there is no evidence for deficiency of thyroid hormone secretion as a primary cause in most cases. Most of the weight gain associated with the development of myxedema is due to the accumulation of fluid (Ch. 4) rather than to adipose mass. Furthermore, the administration of thyroid hormone to obese patients may result in a loss of lean body mass exceeding the loss of fat (Kyle et al., 1966) and in increased appetite. Circulating thyroid hormone levels, thyroidal ^{131}I uptake, and Achilles reflex times are usually normal.

The fat deposition associated with hyperadrenocorticism (Cushing's syndrome) is characteristic (Ch. 5). Helpful diagnostic clinical features, in addition to fat distribution, that distinguish the much more common obese individual with mild hypertension and glucose intolerance from the individual with obesity secondary to adrenal hypersecretion include thick rather than thin skin, pale rather than purplish striae, absence of plethora, preservation of muscle strength, and absence of osteoporosis. Laboratory tests are also helpful. Polycythemia in obesity (in contrast to Cushing's syndrome) is found rarely and appears to be associated with cor pulmonale when present. Higher than normal urinary excretion rates of hydroxycorticoids and an increase in cortisol turnover may be present (Simkin, 1961), but these changes correlate with the increase in lean body mass associated with obesity. Blood cortisol levels tend to be normal in obesity and are usually suppressible. Although the overnight dexamethasone suppression test (Ch. 5) often distinguishes obesity from Cushing's syndrome, incomplete suppression may be seen in obesity. The diurnal rhythm in adrenal steroid secretion appears to be maintained (Schteingart and Conn, 1965).

Gonadal deficiency certainly is not a common cause of obesity. Although in animals it has been shown that castration is often followed by obesity, this association has been much less prominent in humans. Nevertheless, it has been observed to occur, particularly when the castration is performed after puberty. Moreover, some eunuchoid males are found to be somewhat obese and tend to lose some of the obesity after the administration of testosterone. Gonadal hormones do not constitute a satisfactory therapeutic measure for obesity unless there is definite

evidence of their deficiency. Women with the Stein-Leventhal syndrome tend to be obese (Ch. 7). The obesity may result from the secretion by the ovary of steroids with actions similar to those of some of the adrenal steroids.

With classic hypersomatotropinism (acromegaly), obesity is not a characteristic feature. Furthermore, there is no increase in plasma levels of GH in randomly selected obese patients. In fact, with fasting, hypoglycemia, exercise, and arginine stimulation, the expected rise in circulating growth hormone is much more sluggish in obesity (Rabinowitz, 1968). Therefore, treatment of obesity with various pituitary hormones has little rational basis. Although daily subcutaneous injections of human chorionic gonadotropin (hCG) have been advocated by some to promote weight loss, controlled studies indicate no beneficial effect from this form of therapy.

Hypothalamic syndromes resulting from lesions affecting the ventromedial nucleus are extremely rare causes of obesity in humans. In the case of gross lesions found in the vicinity of the hypothalamus, e.g., craniopharyngioma (Fig. 18–14), or lesions due to trauma, obesity associated with hypogonadotropic hypogonadism and in some instances with diabetes insipidus is part of the syndrome. It is not clear to what extent impairment of the secretion of hypothalamic pituitary releasing factors might contribute to the obesity.

Obesity also rarely may be present in early childhood as part of a variety of congenital syndromes such as adiposogenital dystrophy (Fröhlich's syndrome), Prader-Willi syndrome, Laurence-Moon-Bardet-Biedl syndrome, Alström's syndrome, and pseudohypoparathyroidism. The

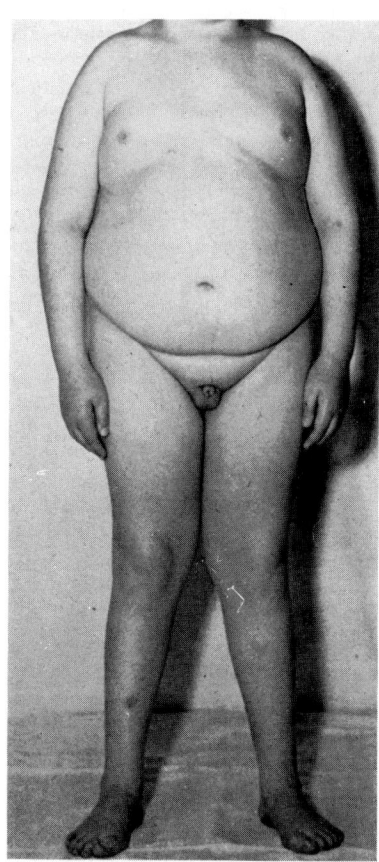

Figure 18–14. Boy aged 19 with craniopharyngioma that was associated with hypogonadotropic hypogonadism and excess fat in hip, abdominal, and pectoral regions. Genu valgum is apparent.

cause of the obesity in these syndromes remains unknown, although structural or functional hypothalamic defects have been postulated (Fiser et al., 1974) in the Prader-Willi syndrome ("HHHO syndrome" or hypotonia, hypomentia, hypogonadism, obesity). Hypothalamic function appears to be normal in the heterogeneous Laurence-Moon-Bardet-Biedl group of syndromes (Toledo et al., 1977).

Unusual distributions of adiposity can occur. Partial lipodystrophy is an unusual variation of congenital lipodystrophy (lipoatrophy), in which subcutaneous fat is totally absent from a portion of the body and hypertrophied in the remainder. In multiple lipomatosis, a frequently familial disorder characterized by localized, discrete, subcutaneous fat deposits throughout the body (Fig. 18–15), stored triglyceride in lipoma cells appears to be unavailable for mobilization even during starvation, despite the morphologic and biochemical resemblance of these cells to the more usual adipose tissue cells.

Thus, less than 1% of obesity can be ascribed to an identifiable cause or aggravating factor. There is no rationale for the use of the popular diagnostic terms "exogenous" and "endogenous" obesity, which have no pathophysiologic meaning.

TREATMENT

The prognosis for treatment of obesity appears to vary with the clinical type. Lifelong obesity is frustrating to treat and leads to much grief on the part of both physician and patient. In view of the poor results after long-term follow-up of a variety of weight reduction schemes (which may be very successful over the short term), this form of obesity may be virtually irreversible. It is a common experience in obesity clinics that less than 5% of the markedly (presumably lifelong) obese patients ever attain

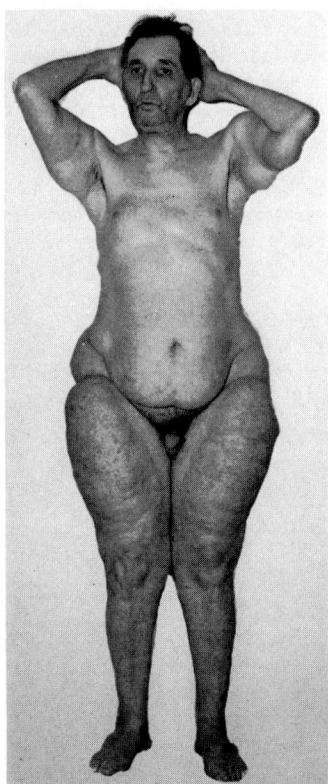

Figure 18–15. Unusual variety of lipomatosis.

normal weight, and few can maintain a short-term weight loss in excess of 40 pounds (Stunkard, 1976; Bray, 1976). On the other hand, adult-onset obesity should be amenable to treatment, so that most of the metabolic and pathophysiologic consequences of enlarged adipose cell mass should be avoidable. Furthermore, excess mortality associated with obesity (Table 18–6) appears to be preventable (Fig. 18–3).

In theory, obesity can be treated by reduction of caloric intake or increase of caloric expenditure or both. In special circumstances, particularly as applied to lifelong obesity, surgical techniques to decrease gastrointestinal absorption of food and to decrease fat storage capacity by resection of large amounts of tissues have been used. Weight loss can be achieved by caloric restriction, regardless of the nature of the diet. The amount of weight loss depends largely on the degree of negative energy balance that is attained. Unfortunately, oxygen consumption declines in parallel with weight loss (Dole, 1959; Bray, 1969), making it more difficult to maintain a steady degree of weight loss over the long term.

Diet

Although there have been many suggestions that the macronutrient composition of the calorically restricted diet is important for successful weight reduction, there is no firm evidence that a calorie is anything more or less than a calorie, regardless of the food source from which it is derived. Despite the popularity of many calorically unbalanced diets, Bortz and coworkers (1967), Kinsell and coworkers (1964), and others have clearly shown that the rate of weight loss on low-calorie diets high in protein is the same as the rate on diets high in fat or high in carbohydrate. Previous observations that indicated less rapid weight loss with high-carbohydrate, low-calorie diets have been attributed to short-term treatment in which changes in salt and water balance obscure changes in weight. It is apparent that an obese individual has a marked propensity to retain sodium during weight reduction and that this tendency is transiently exaggerated by carbohydrate in the diet (Elsbach and Schwartz, 1961; Bortz et al., 1967). Carbohydrate-depleted ("ketogenic") diets increase weight loss solely by affecting water excretion (Van Itallie and Yang, 1977). Long-term ketosis and mild acidosis seen with severely hypocaloric diets or carbohydrate-restricted diets (less than 50 gm/day) may cause decreased bone mineralization and amenorrhea.

Meal frequency may play a role in the degree of success; frequent feedings may be more likely to promote weight loss than less frequent consumption of larger loads, which may lead to abnormal eating patterns, such

Table 18–6. RATIO OF DEATH RATE OF OBESE TO STANDARD RISK INDIVIDUALS ANALYZED AS TO CAUSE OF DEATH (BARR)

Condition	Men	Women
Diabetes	3.83	3.72
Cirrhosis of liver	2.49	1.47
Appendicitis	2.23	1.95
Biliary calculi	2.06	2.84
Chronic nephritis	1.91	2.12
Cerebral hemorrhage	1.59	1.62
Coronary disease	1.42	1.75
Auto accidents	1.31	1.20
Suicides	0.78	0.73
Tuberculosis	0.21	0.35

as the night-eating syndrome described by Stunkard (1955). Fabry and his associates (1964) report that obesity is more common in individuals who eat less frequently; however, Bortz and colleagues (1966) and Young and coworkers (1971) could find no evidence of an effect of feeding frequency on the rate of weight loss in obese subjects. Total starvation has been promoted as a rapid route to achieve or start weight loss (Drenick et al., 1964). The additional metabolic and other consequences of prolonged total starvation, such as unexplained anemia, body potassium depletion, hyperuricemia, gout, ketosis, lactic acidosis, liver function abnormalities, arrhythmias, hypotension, and, rarely, sudden death (Lawlor and Wells, 1969), have limited the utility of this form of treatment, however. Furthermore, it has been shown that the additional weight loss achieved by total starvation over that achieved by a 600–800 calorie diet is achieved by a selective loss in lean body mass rather than by additional loss of fat mass (Ball et al., 1976). The protein-modified fast may reduce nitrogen loss but does not influence the other side effects of starvation. Total fasting supplemented with liquid protein hydrolysates has been associated with increased mortality, in some cases as a result of potassium depletion. Long-term follow-up of more than 200 markedly obese patients (presumably with hyperplastic obesity) who lost up to 100 pounds by total fasting has shown that 50% returned to their starting weight within 3 years and that less than 10% remained reduced 9 years later (Johnson and Drenick, 1977).

Thus a minimal quantity of protein and carbohydrate in weight reduction diets appears necessary, although the body has an unusual capacity to conserve nitrogen. Adequate carbohydrate intake appears to be necessary for utilization of amino acids for protein deposition (Gelfand et al., 1979). In principle, it is clear that the aim of a weight reduction diet should be to keep normal body composition as well as to attain normal weight. There is no evidence to support the superiority of any form of low-calorie diet over that of any other (Hood et al., 1970; Lewis et al., 1977). Thus a practical dietary recommendation for long-term management of obesity would be 15–20 cal/kg ideal body weight, containing 20% protein, 45% carbohydrate, and 35% fat calories. Substitution of one or more meals each day by fixed composition liquid formulas appears to have contributed to successful initiation of weight loss in many individuals. Unbalanced formulations, such as the high protein, "protein sparing" formula,

however, appear to be associated with the same untoward consequences as seen with total starvation and other carbohydrate-deprived regimens. When psychological problems appear prominent, emotional support may be necessary. The success of weight reduction groups for many individuals indicates that support of the "group therapy" type may be a useful adjunct.

Exercise

The most common method for promoting caloric expenditure in obese individuals is increased exercise. Obese patients, particularly adolescent females, are consistently less active than are thin individuals (Stunkard, 1976). In practice, obese individuals on weight reduction diets tend spontaneously to decrease their activity further, perhaps to compensate for decreased caloric intake in an attempt to preserve their fat mass. Exercising animals appear to gain less weight than do free-eating sedentary controls as a result of both an increase in caloric expenditure and a decrease in food intake (Oscai and Holloszy, 1969). Exercise results in a significant decrease in the percentage of body fat, with a proportional increase in lean body mass. Sedentary calorie-restricted animals have a higher fat content than do exercising animals of the same weight. Thus exercise does appear to influence both body composition and food intake and should be part of reducing regimens. Exercise alone, however, does not appear to be an effective means of weight reduction, since the caloric equivalent of most activities is easily nullified by small amounts of food intake (Table 18–7).

Drugs and Hormones

Appetite suppressants (usually amphetamine derivatives) are of limited utility, since their effect is transient and rarely leads to more than a 10% weight reduction (see Bray [1976] or Sullivan and Comai [1978] for recent reviews of the pharmacology of anorexigenic drugs). Since the treatment of obesity is lifelong, such drugs have no demonstrable role in the long-term management of obesity. Since neural regulation of adipose mass appears likely, however, future development of drugs altering such mechanisms holds promise. Thyroid hormone administration has been widely used to increase the oxygen consumption of obese patients regardless of whether or not

Table 18–7. ENERGY EQUIVALENTS OF TYPICAL FOODS EXPRESSED IN TERMS OF VARIOUS ACTIVITIES*

Food	Calories	Minutes of Activity				
		Reclining	Walking	Bicycling	Swimming	Running
Apple (large)	100	78	19	12	9	5
Beer (1 glass)	114	88	22	14	10	6
Bread and butter	78	60	15	10	7	4
Carrot	42	32	8	5	4	2
Cookie (1 plain)	15	12	3	2	1	1
Chicken (½ fried)	232	178	45	28	21	12
Egg (boiled)	77	59	15	9	7	4
Ham (2 slices)	167	128	32	20	15	9
Hamburger	350	269	67	43	31	18
Milk (1 glass)	166	128	32	20	15	9
Orange (medium)	68	52	13	8	6	4
Pie, apple (⅙)	377	290	73	46	34	19
Pork chop (loin)	314	242	60	38	28	16
Spaghetti (1 serving)	400	310	77	49	36	21

*Adapted from Mayer, J.: *Overweight. Causes, Cost and Control.* New Jersey, Prentice-Hall, 1968, pp. 80–81.

they suffer from hypothyroidism or "hypometabolism." Studies of body composition have shown that the accelerated weight loss from superimposition of thyroid hormone treatment on a low-calorie diet is due to a differential loss of lean body mass rather than to loss of fat tissue. Numerous other hormones (e.g., hCG, GH, progesterone) have been promoted for their ability to help achieve weight loss in obese individuals, but none are effective (Rivlin, 1975). Evaluation of drugs becomes a problem, since the routine of frequent physician visits, weight measurement, emotional support, medication, and diet itself promotes weight loss, and it is difficult to ascribe success to a particular medication. Furthermore, weight loss may result predominantly from loss of fluid, as with the widely dispensed diuretics, rather than from loss of adipose mass.

Surgery

Surgical procedures designed to interfere with ingestion of food (gastric exclusion, jaw wiring) or with intestinal absorption (jejunoileal bypass) have caused marked and persistent weight loss. The jejunoileal bypass operation is being used as a radical form of treatment of severe and refractory obesity in an attempt to prevent early morbidity and mortality in such individuals. This surgical procedure was devised to eliminate functionally a sufficient length of jejunum and ileum to produce weight loss and to reduce serum lipids without producing clinical steatorrhea. The distal ileum is essentially bypassed. Unfortunately, as reviewed in a recent symposium (Bray and Benfield, 1977), bypass surgery has been followed in several instances by massive fatty changes in the liver, cholestasis, fibrosis, interstitial inflammation, and fatal hepatic necrosis. Other complications include high operative mortality, severe crippling diarrhea, electrolyte imbalance, arthritis, osteomalacia, and oxalate renal stones. Because of fewer reported complications, it has been suggested that gastric bypass is preferable to intestinal bypass as operative treatment (Mason et al., 1978). At the present time, however, caution in the use of these experimental surgical procedures appears warranted. There is no rationale for adipectomy in the management of lifelong obesity, although the disorder is characterized by adipose cell hyperplasia. Experimental studies in animals lead to little optimism, since lipectomy of large subcutaneous fat depots of rats is followed by compensatory hyperplasia of the remaining subcutaneous adipose tissue (Faust et al., 1977). The main reason for not performing lipectomy in obese humans is probably the technical one of removing sufficient fat without compromising circulation. Efforts at lipectomy done simultaneously with jejunoileal shunt surgery often leads to breakdown of the surgical incision with wound infection and dehiscence.

Behavior Modification

Behavior modification therapy, group psychotherapy, and self-help groups have been relatively successful in management of mild to moderate obesity. Since there are a number of documented differences in the feeding behavior of obese and thin individuals, the newer methods of behavior control have been applied to overeating (Stuart and Davis, 1972). Behavior modification therapy is based on re-educating the patient to manipulate the environment in order to suppress eating stimuli. Techniques used include frequent weighing, keeping diaries of eating and other activities, changes in meal-eating behavior pattern, and analysis of situations leading to deviations from the prescribed diet. Short-term success in small groups of patients have been reported and this approach appears to have promise, particularly as an adjunct to other forms of therapy. Long-term success remains unknown.

CONCLUSIONS

It can no longer be assumed that obesity is simply the result of overeating and that every fat person is simply an overfed normal one. Certainly, most slightly overweight middle-aged individuals are fundamentally normal but have eaten a little too much and exercised much too little. The grossly overweight patient who has had his problem throughout life suffers from a disorder that we do not yet understand and have been unable to cure. Nevertheless, some of the complications or correlates of obesity can be treated, and the obese individual who has experienced multiple failures in weight reduction requires sympathetic attention. "I can't help you unless you lose weight" is a phrase that should rarely be used — if ever. Diabetes mellitus, hypertension, and hyperlipidemia may accompany obesity and can be managed, even though weight loss, were it achievable, would be the most desirable approach.

REFERENCES

Ahrens, E. H., Jr.: The use of liquid formula diets in metabolic studies: 15 years' experience, In *Advances in Metabolic Disorders*. Levine, R., and Luft, R. (eds.), New York, Academic Press, 1970, p. 297.

Albrink, M. J., and Meigs, J. W.: Interrelationship between skinfold thickness, serum lipids and blood sugar in normal men. *Am. J. Clin. Nutr.* 15:255, 1964.

Albrink, M. J., et al.: weight gain and serum triglycerides in normal men. *N. Engl. J. Med.* 266:484, 1962.

Arky, R. A., and Freinkel, N.: Alcohol hypoglycemia. V. Alcohol infusion to test gluconeogenesis in starvation, with special reference to obesity. *N. Engl. J. Med.* 274:426, 1967.

Assimacopoulos-Jeannet, F., and Jeanrenaud, B.: The hormonal and metabolic basis of experimental obesity. *Clin. Endocrinol. Metabol.* 5:337, 1976.

Bagdade, J. D., et al.: Significance of basal insulin levels in the evaluation of the insulin response to glucose in diabetic and nondiabetic subjects. *J. Clin. Invest.* 46:1549, 1967.

Bagdade, J. D., et al.: The interaction of diabetes and obesity on the regulation of fat mobilization in man. *Diabetes* 18:759, 1969.

Bagdade, J. D., et al.: Influence of obesity on the relationship between insulin and triglyceride levels in endogenous hypertriglyceridemia. *Diabetes* 20:664, 1971.

Bagdade, J. D., et al.: Counter-regulation of basal insulin secretion during alcohol hypoglycemia in diabetic and normal subjects. *Diabetes* 21:65, 1972.

Ball, M. F., et al.: Comparative effects of caloric restriction and metabolic acceleration on body composition in obesity. *J. Clin. Endocrinol.* 27:273, 1967.

Bar, R. S., et al.: Fluctuations in the affinity and concentration of insulin receptors on circulating monocytes of obese patients. *J. Clin. Invest.* 58:1123, 1976.

Bierman, E. L., et al.: Hypertriglyceridemia and glucose intolerance in man. In *Adipose Tissue, Regulation and Metabolic Functions*. Jeanrenaud, B., and Hepp, D. (eds.), New York, Academic Press, 1970.

Bjorntorp, P., and Ostman, J.: Human adipose tissue dynamics and regulation. *Adv. Metabol. Dis.* 5:277, 1971.

Bjorntorp, P., et al.: Adipose tissue fat cell size and number in relation to metabolism in endogenous hypertriglyceridemia. *Acta Med. Scand.* 190:363, 1971.

Bjorntorp, P., et al.: Physical training in human hyperplastic obesity. IV. Effects on the hormonal status. *Metabolism* 26:319, 1977.

Bjurulf, P.: Atherosclerosis and body-build with special reference to size and number of subcutaneous fat cells. *Acta Med. Scand.* 166(Suppl. 349):1, 1959.

Borjeson, M.: The aetiology of obesity in children. A study of 101 twin pairs. *Acta Paediatr. Scand.* 65:279, 1976.

Bortz, W. M., et al.: Weight loss and frequency of feeding. *N. Engl. J. Med.* 274:376, 1966.

Bortz, W. M., et al.: Fat, carbohydrate, salt, and weight loss. *Am. J. Clin. Nutr.* 20:1104, 1967.

Bray, G. A.: Effect of caloric restriction on energy expenditure in obese patients. *Lancet* 2:397, 1969.

Bray, G. A.: The obese patient, In *Major Problems in Internal Medicine.* Vol. IX. Smith, L. H., Jr. (ed.), Philadelphia, W. B. Saunders, 1976.

Bray, G. A., and Benfield, J. R.: Intestinal bypass for obesity: a summary and perspective. *Am. J. Clin. Nutr.* 30:121, 1977.

Bray, G. A., and Gallagher, T. F., Jr.: Manifestations of hypothalamic obesity in man. A comprehensive investigation of 8 patients and a review of the literature. *Medicine* 54:301, 1975.

Bray, G. A., and York, D. A.: Genetically transmitted obesity in rodents. *Physiol. Rev.* 51:598, 1971.

Bruch, H.: *The Importance of Overweight.* New York, W. W. Norton & Co., 1957.

Butterfield, W. J. H., et al.: Peripheral metabolism of glucose and free fatty acids during oral glucose tolerance tests. *Metabolism* 14:851, 1965.

Campbell, R. G., et al.: Studies of food-intake regulation in man. Responses to variations in nutritive density in lean and obese subjects. *N. Engl. J. Med.* 285:1042, 1971.

Charney, E., et al.: Childhood antecedents of adult obesity. Do chubby infants become obese adults? *N. Engl. J. Med.* 295:6, 1976.

Czech, M. P., and Reaven, G. M.: Insulin insensitivity. *Metabolism* 27(Suppl. 2): 1829, 1978.

Czech, M. P., et al.: Biochemical basis of fat cell insulin resistance in obese rodents and man. *Metabolism* 26:1057, 1977.

Czech, M. P., et al.: Insulin response in skeletal muscle and fat cells of the genetically obese Zucker rat. *Metabolism* 27(Suppl. 2):1967, 1978.

Davidson, M. B.: Primary insulin antagonism of glucose transport in muscle from the older-obese rat. *Metabolism* 27(Suppl. 2):1994, 1978.

Dole, V. P.: Body fat. *Sci Am.* 201:71, 1959.

Drenick, E. J., et al.: Prolonged starvation as treatment for severe obesity. *J.A.M.A.* 187:100, 1964.

Eckel, R. H., et al.: Development of lipoprotein lipase in cultured 3T3-L1 cells. *Biochem. Biophys. Res. Commun.* 78:288, 1977.

Edwards, K. D. G., and Whyte, H. M.: The simple measurement of obesity. *Clin. Sci.* 22:347, 1962.

Eid, E. E.: Follow-up study of physical growth of children who had excessive weight gain in first six months of life. *Br. Med. J.* 2:74, 1970.

Elsbach, P., and Schwartz, I. L.: Salt and water metabolism during weight reduction. *Metabolism* 10:595, 1961.

Fabry, P., et al.: The frequency of meals: Its relation to overweight, hypercholesterolemia, and decreased glucose-tolerance. *Lancet* 2:614, 1964.

Faust, I. M., et al.: Adipose tissue regeneration following lipectomy. *Science* 197:391, 1977.

Faust, I. M., et al.: Diet-induced adipocyte number increase in adult rats: a new model of obesity. *Am. J. Physiol.* 235:E279, 1978.

Fiser, R. H., Jr., et al.: Evidence for hypothalamic-pituitary dysfunction in the Prader-Willi syndrome. *Ped. Res.* 8:368, 1974.

Frohman, L. A., et al.: Plasma insulin and triglyceride levels after hypothalamic lesions in weanling rats. *Am. J. Physiol.* 216:1496, 1969.

Galton, D. J., et al.: Triglyceride storage disease. A group of inborn errors of triglyceride metabolism. *Q. J. Med.* 43:63, 1974.

Garn, S. M., et al.: Level of education, level of income, and level of fatness in adults. *Am. J. Clin. Nutr.* 30:721, 1977.

Garrow, J. S.: *Energy Balance and Obesity in Man.* New York, Elsevier-North Holland Press, 1978.

Gelfand, R. A., et al.: Dietary carbohydrate and metabolism of ingested protein. *Lancet* 1:65, 1979.

Grinker, J., et al.: Taste sensitivity and susceptibility to external influence in obese and normal weight subjects. *J. Pers. Soc. Psychol.* 22:320, 1972.

Grinker, J., et al.: The affective responses of obese patients to weight reduction: A differentiation based on age at onset of obesity. *Psychosom. Med.* 35:57, 1973.

Gruen, R., et al.: Increased adipose tissue lipoprotein lipase activity during the development of the genetically obese rat (fa/fa). *Metabolism* 27(Suppl. 2):1955, 1978.

Häger, A., et al.: Body fat and adipose tissue cellularity in infants: a longitudinal study. *Metabolism* 26:607, 1977.

Hirsch, J., and Batchelor, B.: Adipose tissue cellularity in human obesity. *Clin. Endocrinol. Metabol.* 5:299, 1976.

Hirsch, J., et al.: Cell lipid content and cell number in obese and nonobese human adipose tissue. *J. Clin. Invest.* 45:1023, 1966.

Hood, C. E. A., et al.: Observations on obese patients eating isocaloric reducing diets with varying proportions of carbohydrate. *Br. J. Nutr.* 24:39, 1970.

Horton, E. S., et al.: Endocrine and metabolic alterations in spontaneous and experimental obesity, In *Obesity in Perspective.* Bray, G. A. (ed.), Fogarty International Series on Preventive Medicine. DHEW Publication No. (NIH) 75-708, Vol. II, Part 2, 1975, p. 323.

Hustvedt, B. E., and Løvø, A.: Correlation between hyperinsulinemia and hyperphagia in rats with ventromedial hypothalamic lesions. *Acta Physiol. Scand.* 84:29, 1972.

Inoue, S., et al.: Transplantation of pancreatic β-cells prevents development of hypothalamic obesity in rats. *Am. J. Physiol.* 235:E266, 1978.

Johnson, D., and Drenick, E. J.: Therapeutic fasting in morbid obesity. *Arch. Intern. Med.* 137:1381, 1977.

Johnson, P. R., and Hirsch, J.: Cellularity of adipose depots in six strains of genetically obese mice. *J. Lipid Res.* 13:2, 1972.

Kalkhoff, R. K., et al.: Metabolic effects of weight loss in obese subjects. Changes in plasma substrate levels, insulin and growth hormone responses. *Diabetes* 20:83, 1971.

Kinsell, L. W., et al.: Calories do count. *Metabolism* 13:195, 1964.

Knittle, J. L., and Hirsch, J.: Effect of early nutrition on the development of rat epididymal fat pads: cellularity and metabolism. *J. Clin. Invest.* 47:2091, 1968.

Knittle, J. L., et al.: The growth of adipose tissue in children and adolescents. Cross-sectional and longitudinal studies of adipose cell number and size. *J. Clin. Invest.* 63:239, 1979.

Kyle, L. H., et al.: Effect of thyroid hormone on body composition in myxedema and obesity. *N. Engl. J. Med.* 275:12, 1966.

Lawlor, T., and Wells, D. G.: Metabolic hazards of fasting. *Am. J. Clin. Nutr.* 22:1142, 1969.

Lewis, S. B., et al.: Effect of diet composition on metabolic adaptations to hypocaloric nutrition: comparison of high carbohydrate and high fat isocaloric diets. *Am. J. Clin. Nutr.* 30:160, 1977.

Mann, G. V.: Influence of obesity on health. *N. Engl. J. Med.* 291:178, 1974.

Mason, E. E., et al.: Gastric bypass for obesity after ten years experience. *Int. J. Obesity* 2:197, 1978.

Mayer, J.: Genetic factors in human obesity. *Ann. N.Y. Acad. Sci.* 131:412, 1916.

Mayer, J.: Some aspects of the problem of regulation of food intake and obesity. *N. Engl. J. Med.* 274:610, 1966.

Mayer, J.: *Overweight Causes, Cost, and Control.* Englewood Cliffs, N.J., Prentice-Hall, 1968.

McGarry, J. D., and Foster, D. W.: Ketogenesis and its regulation. *Am. J. Med.* 61:9, 1976.

Miettinen, T. A.: Cholesterol production in obesity. *Circulation* 44:842, 1971.

Miller, D. S., et al.: Gluttony. 2. Thermogenesis in overeating man. *Am. J. Clin. Nutr.* 20:1223, 1967.

Montoye, H. J., et al.: The measurement of body fatness. A study in a total community. *Am. J. Clin. Nutr.* 16:417, 1965.

Montoye, H. J., et al.: Relationship between serum cholesterol and body fatness, an epidemiologic study. *Am. J. Clin. Nutr.* 18:397, 1966.

Nestel, P. J., et al.: Cholesterol metabolism in human obesity. *J. Clin. Invest.* 52:2389, 1973.

Newman, J., et al.: *Twins, a Study of Heredity and Environment.* Chicago, University of Chicago Press, 1937.

Olefsky, J., et al.: Effects of weight reduction on obesity: studies of lipid and carbohydrate metabolism in normal and hyperlipoproteinemic subjects. *J. Clin. Invest.* 53:64, 1974.

Olefsky, J., et al.: Insulin receptors of skeletal muscle: specific insulin binding sites and demonstration of decreased numbers of sites in obese rats. *Metabolism* 25:179, 1976.

Oscai, L. B., and Holloszy, J. O.: Effects of weight changes produced by exercise, food restriction, or overeating on body composition. *J. Clin. Invest.* 48:2124, 1969.

Parra, A., et al.: Correlative studies in obese children and adolescents concerning body composition and plasma insulin and growth hormone levels. *Pediatr. Res.* 5:605, 1971.

Pykälistö, O. J., et al.: Determinants of human adipose tissue lipoprotein lipase: Effect of diabetes and obesity on basal- and diet-induced activity. *J. Clin. Invest.* 56:1108, 1975.

Rabinowitz, D.: Hormonal profile and forearm metabolism in human obesity. *Am. J. Clin. Nutr.* 21:1438, 1968.

Rabinowitz, D., and Zierler, K. L.: Forearm metabolism in obesity and its response to intrarterial insulin. Characterization of insulin resistance and evidence for adaptive hyperinsulinism. *J. Clin. Invest.* 41:2173, 1962.

Rivlin, R. S.: Drug therapy: therapy of obesity with hormones. *N. Engl. J. Med.* 292:26, 1975.

Robertson, R. P., et al.: Accelerated triglyceride secretion: a metabolic consequence of obesity. *J. Clin. Invest.* 52:1620, 1973.

Salans, L. B., et al.: Glucose metabolism and the response to insulin by human adipose tissue in spontaneous and experimental obesity: effects of dietary composition and adipose cell size. *J. Clin. Invest.* 53:848, 1974.

Schachter, S.: Obesity and eating. Internal and external cues differentially affect the eating behavior of obese and normal subjects. *Science* 161:751, 1968.

Schteingart, D. E., and Conn, J. W.: Characteristics of the increased adrenocortical function observed in many obese patients. *Ann. N.Y. Acad. Sci.* 131:388, 1965.

Schwartz, R. S., and Brunzell, J. D.: Increased adipose-tissue lipoprotein-lipase activity in moderately obese men after weight reduction. *Lancet* 1:1230, 1978.

Simkin, B.: Urinary 17-ketosteroid and 17-ketogenic steroid excretion in obese patients. *N. Engl. J. Med. 264*:974, 1961.

Sims, E. A. H., et al.: Endocrine and metabolic effects of experimental obesity in man. *Rec. Progr. Horm. Res. 29*:457, 1973.

Smith, F. R., et al.: Parameters of the three-pool model of the turnover of plasma cholesterol in normal and hyperlipidemic humans. *J. Clin. Invest. 57*:137, 1976.

Steinkamp, R. C., et al.: Measures of body fat and related factors in normal adults. II. A simple clinical method to estimate body fat and lean body mass. *J. Chronic Dis. 18*:1291, 1965.

Stuart, R. B., and Davis, B.: *Slim Chance in a Fat World: Behavioral Control of Obesity.* Champaign, Research Press Co., 1972.

Stunkard, A. J.: *The Pain of Obesity.* Palo Alto, CA, Bull Publishing Co., 1976.

Stunkard, A. J.: Obesity and the social environment: current status, future prospects, In *Food and Nutrition in Health and Disease.* Moss, N. H., and Mayer, J. (eds.), New York, New York Academy of Sciences, 1977, p. 298.

Stunkard, A. J., and Rush, J.: Dieting and depression reexamined: A critical review of reports of untoward responses during weight reduction for obesity. Ann. Intern. Med. 81:526, 1974.

Stunkard, A. J., et al.: The night-eating syndrome: A pattern of food intake among certain obese patients. *Am. J. Med. 19*:78, 1955.

Sullivan, A. C., and Comai, K.: Pharmacological treatment of obesity. *Int. J. Obesity 2*:167, 1978.

Thomas, A. E., et al.: A nomograph method for assessing body weight. *Am. J. Clin. Nutr. 29*:302, 1976.

Toledo, S. P. A., et al.: Evaluation of the hypothalamic-pituitary-gonadal function in the Bardet-Biedl syndrome. *Metabolism 26*:1277, 1977.

Van Itallie, T. B., and Yang, M. U.: Diet and weight loss. *N. Engl. J. Med. 297*:1158, 1977.

West, K. M.: *Epidemiology of Diabetes and Its Vascular Lesions.* New York, Elsevier-North Holland Press, 1978.

Woods, S. C., and Porte, D., Jr.: The central nervous system, pancreatic hormones, feeding and obesity. *Adv. Metabol. Dis. 9*:283, 1978.

Young, C. M., et al.: Frequency of feeding, weight reduction, and body composition. *J. Am. Diabetic Assoc. 59*:466, 1971.

CHAPTER 19

Parathyroid Hormone, Calcitonin, and the Calciferols

By G. D. Aurbach,

Stephen J. Marx,

and Allen M. Spiegel

INTRODUCTION

In this chapter we present a broad survey of endocrine control of mineral (calcium, magnesium, and phosphorus metabolism and the disturbances of these systems encountered in medical practice. Major recent developments are emphasized, and orientation is provided when knowledge is incomplete or rapidly evolving. Parathyroid hormone (PTH), calcitonin (CT), and the calciferols are the principal calcitropic hormones. Together with extracellular calcium, they synergize with and feed back upon each other to determine their own secretion rates and actions. They regulate processes as diverse as skeletal turnover and availability of cytoplasmic calcium for intracellular signaling. Since the last edition of this text, impressive new facts have been uncovered relating to each of these hormones. Pathways of biosynthesis, secretion, transport, and action have all been studied in detail. Studies of the biosynthesis of PTH have provided new insights into the general mechanisms of polypeptide translation and packaging, and the complete amino acid sequence has been determined for the ribosomal translation product, "pre-proparathyroid hormone" (pre-pro PTH), the precursor of the prohormone, which in turn is converted to the hormonal form that is stored in and secreted from the gland. Each of the calcitropic hormones now can be assayed with great sensitivity and it is possible to diagnose accurately hereditary and acquired disorders in calciferol metabolism. The premalignant phase of C-cell neoplasia has been established as a clinical model for diagnosis and treatment of premalignant processes. Calcitropic drugs such as the diphosphonates are now employed with an increased under-

standing of their mechanisms of action. Basic research has led to development of new therapeutic approaches. Heterologous transplantation of bone marrow has been used to cure congenital osteopetrosis, and newly recognized hormones have been used to treat specific deficiencies (mono- or dihydroxylated cholecalciferols for hereditary or acquired renal 25-hydroxyvitamin D 1-α hydroxylation defects) or metabolic disorders (calcitonin in Paget's disease) of uncertain etiology.

The chapter begins with a review of basic concepts of mineral metabolism and its normal endocrine regulation. The manifestations and treatment of clinical disorders are described next, and the final section represents a summary of laboratory techniques used in diagnosis. The bibliography includes a selection of original reports and detailed reviews that can serve as the starting point in the search for additional information.

CALCIUM, MAGNESIUM, AND PHOSPHORUS METABOLISM

Evolution of Roles for Calcium, Magnesium, and Phosphorus

Complex organic molecules evolved in the primordial atmosphere and oceans, and the development of membranes permitted the compartmentalization of biochemical reactions in a medium of regulated composition. The cytoplasm of animal cells shows a composition radically different from that of present-day oceans and lakes (Table 19–1). To maintain a consistent cytoplasmic ionic compo-

Table 19–1.   MINERAL COMPOSITION OF SOLUTIONS

Solution	Calcium (mM)	Magnesium (mM)	Inorganic Phosphate (mM)
Ocean (Pacific)	10	48	0.001
Lake (Huron)	0.90	0.25	0.003
Cytoplasm—Squid axon			
Total	0.3	6.7	3.0
Ionized	0.0001	3.5	1.5
Plasma			
Hagfish*	5.4	10.4	1.0
Salmon (ocean phase male)	2.3	1.0	4.7
Salmon (freshwater phase male)	2.9	1.8	4.5
Human	2.4	0.9	1.2

*The hagfish is a "primitive" ocean dweller without a skeleton.

sition, cells recognize and respond to changes in plasma membrane permeability. Such changes influence transmembrane fluxes of ions following concentration gradients, and ion fluxes for ions with large transmembrane concentration gradients (sodium, potassium, and calcium) serve as signals for transmission of information into and among cells. The evolutionary pressures that led to selection of magnesium and phosphorus as major cytoplasmic components are poorly understood. Many cellular reactions are dependent upon the availability of organic and inorganic phosphate. Phosphate functions as a major cytoplasmic buffer, the basis for energy exchange, and an essential component of membranes and nucleic acids. Phosphorus is scarce in the earth's crust and must be concentrated by all plant and animal species; its availability in the sea and soil is one limiting factor for population growth of all organisms. Calcium salts are limited in solubility at physiologic pH and could precipitate if in millimolar concentrations in cytosol. Magnesium salts are more soluble; this, and the greater abundance of magnesium than of calcium in ocean water (Table 19–1), may help explain why magnesium evolved as the principal cytoplasmic divalent cation. With the evolution of multicellular life forms, extracellular fluids (ECF) replaced ocean water as the immediate cellular environment. Adaptation to fresh water and then to a terrestrial habitat was accompanied by increasing specialization to regulate the plasma concentrations of important minerals such as calcium, magnesium, and phosphate. In mammals, the majority of the total body calcium, magnesium, and phosphate is in the skeleton (Table 19–2). An endoskeleton composed of hydroxyapatite $[Ca_5(OH)(PO_4)_3]$ provides not only mechanical support but also a reservoir of these important but sparingly soluble minerals.

Extracellular Compartments
External Sources and Nutrition

Large amounts of calcium, magnesium, and phosphate must be regularly supplied to the body. Since these substances are not present in appreciable quantities in the atmosphere, dietary sources must meet metabolic demands. The recommended daily allowances for adults in the United States are 800 mg of calcium, 350 mg of magnesium, and 800 mg of phosphorus. True mineral dietary requirements have not been established. Phosphorus and magnesium are present in adequate amounts in most dietary components, and any but a grossly unbalanced diet will meet the minimal requirements. Symptomatic nutritional deficiency of phosphorus develops in normal subjects only with dietary restriction of phosphorus combined with ingestion of phosphate binders (aluminum hydroxide antacid preparations). Selective and symptomatic nutritional deficiency of magnesium has been observed only with synthetic diets designed for the purpose of inducing this state. Calcium content is high in dairy products (Table 19–3). Dietary calcium intake as nondairy components (200–300 mg/day) is relatively consistent among most human populations, but there are major population differences in intake of dairy products throughout the world, ranging from 100 to more than 1000 mg/day. In the United States, dairy products contribute approximately 800 mg of calcium to the average daily diet. The consequences for humans on a diet critically low in calcium or calcium:phosphorus ratio are not established. In rats, a low-calcium diet retards skeletal growth. The usual calcium:phosphorus ratio (wt:wt) in the diet of most species is approximately 1.0, and large decreases in this ratio by administration of a diet high in phosphorus promote in-

Table 19–2.   DISTRIBUTION OF CALCIUM, MAGNESIUM, AND PHOSPHORUS IN THE BODY OF A 70 KG HUMAN ADULT*

Compartment	Calcium (g)	Magnesium (g)	Phosphorus (g)
Bones and teeth	1300 (99)	14 (54)	600 (86)
Extracellular fluid	1 (0.1)	0.3 (1)	0.2 (0.03)
Cells	7 (1.0)	12 (46)	100 (14)

*Numbers in parentheses indicate percent of total for each element.

Table 19–3. CALCIUM, MAGNESIUM, AND PHOSPHORUS CONTENT OF FOODS
(FROM USDA AGRICULTURE HANDBOOKS 8 [1975] AND 8–1 [1976])*

Food	Calcium	Magnesium	Phosphorus
Vegetables			
Carrots	37	23	36
Peas	26	35	116
Lima beans	52	67	142
Spinach	93	88	51
Tomato	13	14	27
Lettuce	35	11	26
Potato (peeled)	7	22	53
Corn	3	48	111
Fruit			
Apple	7	5	10
Orange	41	11	20
Banana	8	33	26
Meat			
Fish steak (flounder)	54	30	885
Beef steak	10	20	150
Liver (beef)	8	13	352
Chicken	12	20	200
Miscellaneous			
Bread (rye)	75	42	147
Almond (shelled)	234	270	504
Chicken egg (white & yolk)	54	11	205
Salt	253	120	0
Dairy			
Bovine milk	119	13	93
Bovine skim milk	123	11	101
Human milk	33	4	14
Butter	24	2	23
Brick cheese	674	24	451
Cottage cheese	60	5	132

*All entries expressed as mg per 100 g edible portion.

creased parathyroid secretion and increased skeletal resorption rates. In the United States, the recommended dietary calcium:phosphorus ratio is 1.0, but average dietary ratios range from 0.3 to 0.9. The higher values reflect greater consumption of milk with a calcium:phosphorus ratio of 1.3 (Table 19–3).

Plasma and Extracellular Fluid

Less than 2% of the body content of calcium, magnesium, or phosphorus is in the plasma and extracellular fluid (ECF) at any moment (Table 19–2), yet the concentrations of these minerals in ECF are controlled within narrow limits. Plasma calcium participates in multiple processes, including proteolysis (e.g., the clotting and kinin generation cascades), regulation of plasma membrane potential, and exocytosis; its normal concentration in plasma is 4.4–5.2 mEq/l (mean ± 2 standard deviation [SD]), with minor variation dependent on laboratory methods. Calcium introduced into the ECF rapidly equilibrates with an additional calcium pool of even greater calcium content. The anatomic locations of this portion of the miscible or central pool are not well defined but probably include mitochondria and surfaces of bone mineral. Normal plasma concentrations of magnesium (1.5–2.0 mEq/l) and phosphate (1.0–1.7 mM) encompass larger fractional variations from the means.

Plasma is a complex solution, and only the ionized fraction of total plasma calcium participates directly in most biologic reactions (Table 19–4). The focal point of endocrine regulation for mineral metabolism is the concentration of ionized calcium in plasma, but due to major technical problems, this remains difficult to measure accurately. The minute to minute and interindividual variation is very small, however. Change in circulating ionized calcium concentration is a major signal for modification of secre-

tion rates of PTH and CT. Ionized calcium concentration differs among the compartments of the ECF. In the cochlear endolymph of rats, the total calcium concentration is 30 μM, of which most is ionized. It may change in one compartment without changes in others. Ionized calcium concentrations are reduced 20% in the cerebrospinal fluid (CSF) adjacent to cerebellar cells undergoing repetitive stimulation and 90% with severe depression of central nervous system (CNS) function. Albumin accounts for 70% of the protein binding of calcium in serum. Some myeloma globulins can bind enough calcium to increase total serum calcium concentration without affecting the ionized fraction, however. Albumin contains approximately 12 similar calcium-binding regions per molecule. In vivo, only 20% of these sites are occupied at any time. Proportional binding increases with rise in pH such that, within the physiologic range, ionized calcium concentration changes approximately −0.1 mEq/l for each +0.1 unit change in pH. The concentration of albumin in the circulation varies independently of that for ionized calcium and is a major source of intra- and interindividual variations in total concentration of calcium in serum. A simple "correction" for this effect is to adjust total serum calcium concentration +1 mg/dl for each 1 g/dl reduction of albumin concentration below normal and to apply an opposite correction for high serum albumin concentrations. Serum concentrations of albumin are higher in males than in females by 0.2 g/dl, increase with the hemoconcentration of upright posture or use of tourniquets, and decrease in certain chronic illnesses (chronic hepatic disease and nephrotic syndrome in particular).

A small portion of circulating calcium is in the form of complexes, half with bicarbonate and the remainder with phosphate, citrate, and other anions. The ionized plus complexed forms of calcium constitute the free or filterable calcium. The small radii of these complexes allow free diffusion through small pores and inclusion in the

Table 19–4. STATES OF CALCIUM, MAGNESIUM, AND PHOSPHORUS IN HUMAN PLASMA*

State	Calcium (mEq)	Magnesium (mEq)	Phosphate (mM)**
Protein-bound	2.30 (45)	0.55 (31)	0.15 (13)
Filtrable or free†			
Complexed	0.50 (10)	0.15 (9)	0.40 (35)
Ionized	2.15 (44)	1.05 (60)	0.60 (52)

*Numbers in parentheses indicate percentage of total for each mineral.
**Since phosphate circulates as $H_2PO_4^{-2}$ and HPO_4^{-1}, expression as mEq/l would be inappropriate.
†Free = complexed + ionized.

renal glomerular filtrate. The concentration of complexed calcium in serum increases during renal failure due to accumulation of phosphate, sulfate, and other small anions. Infusion of calcium chelators such as edetate (EDTA) or citrate (often a preservative in banked blood) can complex enough calcium to cause symptoms of hypocalcemia.

The proportional distribution of magnesium as ionized, protein-bound, and complexed is similar to that for calcium in serum (Table 19–4). Magnesium competes for the same sites on albumin as does calcium; lower binding affinity of these sites for magnesium than for calcium results in a larger proportion of magnesium in free or diffusible forms. The homeostatic mechanisms regulating magnesium in the ECF are poorly understood. Ionized magnesium elicits responses similar to those from calcium ion with regard to secretion of PTH and CT, though the parathyroid gland shows a greater sensitivity to calcium than to magnesium. Magnesium transport across organs (see later) changes similarly to, but less than, calcium transport in response to PTH, CT, and calciferol.

Seventy percent of the phosphorus in the circulation is covalently bound in phospholipids and phosphoproteins. The remaining 30% is inorganic phosphate in serum and is referred to herein as phosphate or phosphorus. Serum phosphate concentrations are higher in infants than in adults (see Fig. 19–70). Small amounts of phosphate are noncovalently bound to protein (5–15%). The majority circulates as ions or complexes of HPO_4^{-2} and $H_2PO_4^{-1}$, with the usual molar ratio of these anions being 4:1. Changes in total body phosphate stores modulate by unknown mechanisms the activity of the renal 25-OH-D 1 α hydroxylase enzyme and thereby contribute to the determination of circulating concentrations of 1,25-(OH)₂-D. Phosphate depletion leads to increased activity of this enzyme even in the total absence of the parathyroid glands. Phosphate ion does not have direct effects on the secretion rates for PTH or CT; however, each of the major calcitropic hormones, PTH, CT, and vitamin D, affect phosphate fluxes into and out of the plasma compartments.

Calcium, Magnesium, and Phosphate Transport Across Organs

In the steady state, large amounts of calcium, magnesium, and phosphate continuously enter and leave plasma via intestine, kidney, and bone. Each of the three organs contributes to regulation of plasma concentrations of these minerals. Each (1) employs independent mechanisms to regulate ion influx to plasma, others to regulate efflux; (2) contains ion-transporting cells that are polarized with a redundant plasma membrane on the side not exposed to plasma — renal tubular and intestinal mucosal cells possess a brush border, whereas the analogous structure in bone is the ruffled border on the bone face of actively resorbing osteoclasts; and (3) is responsive to one or more of the three major calcitropic hormones.

Intestines

Calcium absorption *in vivo* and *in vitro* is a composite of saturable and nonsaturable processes (Fig. 19–1). The saturable components provide a form of short-term compensation for variation in dietary calcium availability and insure that net calcium absorption varies less than exogenous supply. Within the physiologic range, net absorption of phosphate (and magnesium) varies linearly with dietary supply. Thus the intestine plays a greater role in the adaptation to changes in exogenous availability of calcium than in that of phosphate or magnesium.

Net absorption is the difference between lumen to plasma and plasma to lumen flux (the latter includes the contents of all the digestive juices). The interrelations of absorption of calcium, magnesium, and phosphate are complex. In rats, the net absorption rate for calcium is greatest in the duodenum *in vitro*, although considerable absorption occurs in the jejunum because of the rapid transit time of food through the duodenum *in vivo*. Net lumen to plasma flux for phosphate is greater in the jejunum than it is in the duodenum; in this segment, net movement of phosphate to plasma is far greater than that of calcium. With renal failure, intestinal calcium absorption decreases more than magnesium absorption. The intestinal absorption of calcium, magnesium, and phosphate is depressed in vitamin D deficiency and increased with vitamin D excess; although net calcium absorption varies over a wide range, from 15 to 70% depending on calciferol status, magnesium and phosphate absorption show much smaller deviations from the norm.

Calcium absorption is increased by dietary sugars; lactose stimulates calcium absorption even in vitamin D–deficient animals. The lactose effect occurs whether it is administered before or together with calcium, suggesting

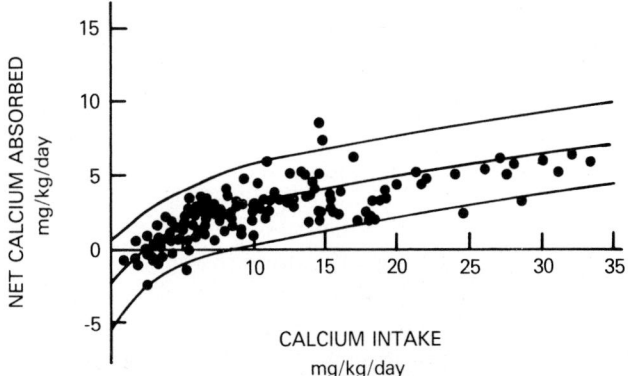

Figure 19–1. Relationship between net absorbed calcium and dietary calcium intake in normal subjects. Data from 212 balance studies on healthy individuals aged 19–83 years. Note the suggestion of a multicomponent process, saturable (decreasing slope) at low dietary calcium intake and nonsaturable (constant slope) at intakes above 10 mg/kg/day. (From Wilkinson, R.: Absorption of calcium, phosphorus, and magnesium. In *Calcium, Phosphate and Magnesium Metabolism.* Nordin, B. E. C. (ed.), New York, Churchill-Livingstone, 1976.

that this represents an effect on mucosal energy metabolism.

Net intestinal absorption of calcium is subject to metabolic regulation. Long-term adaptations are determined by alterations in calciferol metabolism and intestinal responsiveness to the calciferol metabolites. PTH probably has no direct action on the intestinal translocation of minerals, but it affects important control indirectly by regulating 1,25-$(OH)_2$-D synthesis. CT does not significantly influence intestinal calcium fluxes. Deficiency of either calcium or phosphorus leads to increased production of 1,25-$(OH)_2$-D.

Kidneys

Ions and complexes not bound to proteins cross the renal glomerulus. In a 70-k adult with a glomerular filtration rate (GFR) of 120 ml/min and an ECF volume of 12 L, a volume equivalent to the ECF traverses the glomerulus each 100 min. Approximately 65% of the glomerular filtrate is resorbed in the proximal tubule. Phosphate is avidly reabsorbed by the early portion of the proximal convoluted tubule. This is a sodium-dependent process that is under inhibitory regulation of PTH and other factors that decrease fractional sodium resorption by the proximal tubule (sodium loading, volume expansion, and carbonic anhydrase inhibition). Large differences in phosphate delivery from the proximal tubule are not compensated for in the distal segments, though there is uncertainty concerning the possibilities of small contributions from phosphate secretion and resorption in distal segments. Phosphate secretion does occur in the nephrons of nonmammalian species. Phosphate reabsorption by the mammalian kidney can be modeled simply as a high-affinity system operating near saturation. When filtered phosphate rises beyond a threshold concentration, the overflow is virtually completely excreted into the urine. When filtered phosphate load drops below the threshold, it is efficiently resorbed (Fig. 19–2). The urine content is equivalent to 5–20% of the filtered phosphate load, but only 0.5–

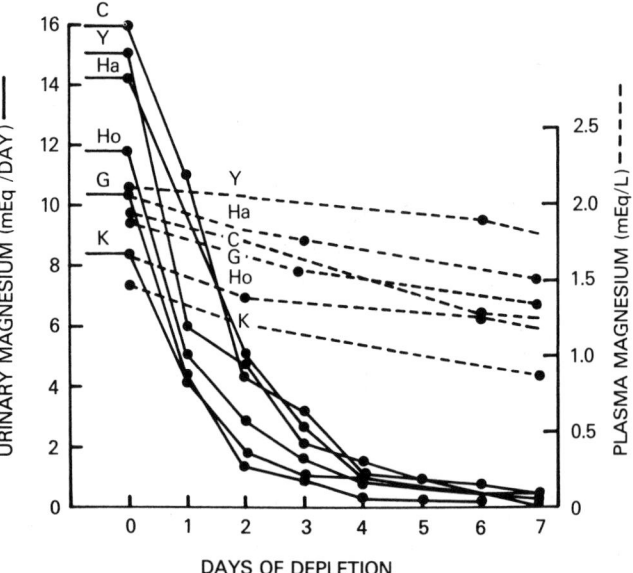

Figure 19–3. Effect of a synethetic magnesium-deficient diet on plasma magnesium concentration and urine magnesium excretion in six patients. (Modified from Shils, M. E.: Experimental human magnesium depletion. *Medicine* 48:61, 1969 p. 65.)

5% for calcium and 2–10% for magnesium. Calcium and magnesium concentrations of late proximal fluid are similar to that in glomerular filtrate (GF). These divalent cations are translocated in the proximal tubules with sodium-driven bulk flow. The major contribution to regulation of divalent cation exchange between plasma and renal filtrate occurs in the distal tubules. Calcium is actively reabsorbed in the thick ascending limb of the distal tubule. Distal calcium transport sites are also capable of translocating magnesium, though there are mechanisms for transporting one or the other divalent cation preferentially. Thiazide diuretics or lithium preferentially decrease the renal clearance of calcium with little effect on renal magnesium clearance. In contrast, restriction of dietary magnesium leads, by unknown mechanisms, to rapid and selective renal conservation of magnesium without large decreases in serum concentration of magnesium (Fig. 19–3). PTH increases distal tubular resorption of calcium and probably magnesium. It is for this reason that the maintenance of normocalcemia in hypoparathyroidism may only be possible with a high rate of calcium flow into the urine (i.e. hypercalciuria). CT increases the renal clearance of sodium, calcium, magnesium, and phosphate; in human adults, these actions may be significant only with pharmacologic concentrations of this agent. Calciferol metabolites probably have only minor effects on the renal handling of calcium, magnesium, and phosphate. Multiple exogenous influences result in direct or indirect changes in renal excretion rate of calcium or magnesium (see "Urinary Calcium Excretion," p. 1021).

Bones

The extracellular pool of calcium, magnesium, and phosphate is in equilibrium with much larger pools of each. A large portion of these pools is in bone, the blood supply of which accounts for 5–25% of the cardiac output. This equilibrium damps the amplitude of concentration changes in plasma that result from hourly variation in exchange across the intestines. In normal adults, ECF calcium efflux to bone (bone apposition) and influx from bone (mineral resorption) are each approximately 8

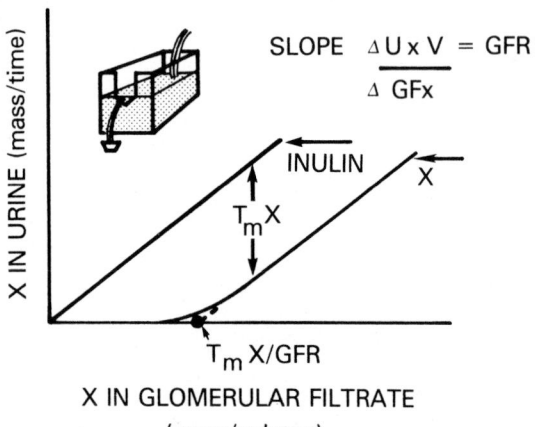

Figure 19–2. Relationship between urinary excretion and filtered load of solutes (X) for which the kidney has a threshold of excretion. For inulin (or creatinine) there is no threshold and excretion is a fixed fraction of load, the fraction being identical to that for renal clearance. For X (calcium, phosphate, or magnesium), clearance is a function of filtered load. Beyond the load at maximal resorption, the slope is identical to GFR. Maximal tubular resorption of X is the vertical distance between the lines or its equivalent, the Y (abscissa) intercept. The X (ordinate) intercept of the extrapolated line is T_mX/GFR or the "theoretical renal threshold" of X. The inset shows how the level of the tank outlet (threshold) influences content of the tank (serum concentration) when there is equilibrium of influx and outflux.

mg/kg/day, a composite of passive exchange with crystal faces and active transport by bone cells. Bone can participate in regulation of ECF mineral concentration by two mechanisms, one a balance between osteoblastic apposition and osteoclastic resorption and the other resulting from osteocytic mineral exchange between ECF and haversian bone. The relative contributions of these two mechanisms are not known. Bidirectional and net fluxes of calcium and phosphate between plasma and bone are determined, in large part, by circulating PTH and vitamin D metabolites. Bone mineral homeostasis and its regulation by hormones are considered in detail in later sections of this chapter.

Steady State and Normal Variation From It

At zero net external mineral exchange (zero mineral balance), skeletal mineral apposition must equal skeletal mineral resorption. Calcium, magnesium, and phosphate content in urine approximates that of net intestinal absorption; losses by perspiration are negligible. Typical daily exchanges of calcium, magnesium, and phosphate in the body are illustrated in Fig. 19–4. Many short-term and long-term deviations from the steady state occur. Some of the common ones are considered here.

There is net entry of calcium across the intestine following oral intake. Total calcium concentration in plasma reaches a peak 2.5–3 hours later; the amplitude of the change in total serum calcium concentration is approximately 0.5 mEq/l after a large oral calcium load (1000 mg). Since magnesium and phosphate are absorbed less preferentially than calcium is in the duodenum, their net intestinal absorption varies less with phasic inputs (meals). Other nutrients interact with mineral homeostasis. For example, carbohydrate loads determine changes in phosphate exchange as phosphate enters cells during glucose uptake. Furthermore, the renal clearances of calcium and magnesium increase after an oral glucose load.

The mediators of these changes are not known. After an oral calcium load in rats, CT secretion blunts the rise in serum calcium concentration. The increase in CT secretion rate may be controlled through hormones released by the intestines, since it occurs with minimal or no change in serum calcium concentration.

Bone mineral mass is responsive to alterations in physical activity. Weightlessness or immobilization leads to net loss of mineral from skeletal stores. Prolonged immobilization, particularly during periods of high bone turnover, leads to loss of skeletal mineral with negative calcium balances of 200 mg/day in adults. It causes hypercalciuria and sometimes nephrocalcinosis or hypercalcemia. The skeletal loss reflects increased mineral resorption rate and variable changes in mineral apposition.

Pregnancy and lactation make demands on maternal mineral homeostasis. The calcium demands of shell formation in fowl represent the extreme case. In domestic chickens the calcium content of the egg shell is 2 g or approximately 10% the calcium mass of the maternal skeleton, yet the process of shell mineralization requires less than 24 hours. In anticipation of shell formation, the chicken develops a specialized form of medullary bone with high mineral turnover rates. In comparison, the human neonate contains 20–30 g of calcium, and most mineralization occurs in the last trimester, thus requiring an average of 250 mg of calcium daily during this period. Daily maternal calcium losses during normal lactation are similar. Maternal skeletal turnover increases by approximately 50% already in the second trimester before fetal mineral accumulation reaches high daily rates.

Changes in mineral mass accompany growth and senescence. During the pubertal growth spurt, net daily positive calcium balance approximates 400 mg/day. Skeletal bone mass reaches a plateau in the third decade and then gradually falls at rates that are sex dependent. After the menopause, annual losses of skeletal mass average 1–2%/year in females, equivalent to 30–60 mg calcium per day (see under "Osteoporosis," p. 1006).

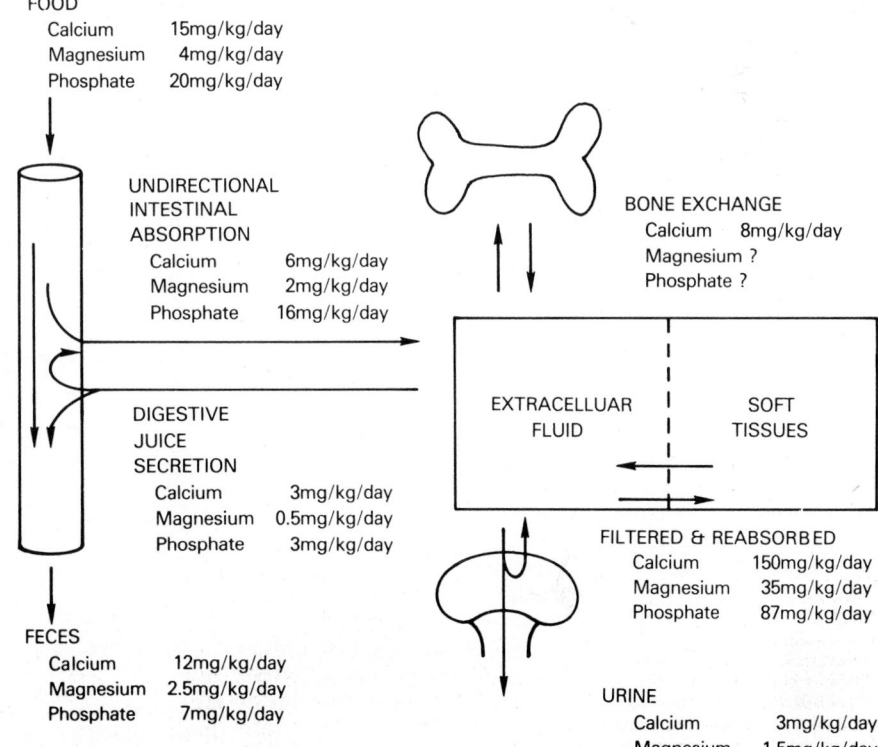

Figure 19–4. Typical daily exchanges of calcium, magnesium, and phosphate among anatomic compartments in adults.

FOOD
Calcium	15mg/kg/day
Magnesium	4mg/kg/day
Phosphate	20mg/kg/day

UNDIRECTIONAL INTESTINAL ABSORPTION
Calcium	6mg/kg/day
Magnesium	2mg/kg/day
Phosphate	16mg/kg/day

BONE EXCHANGE
Calcium	8mg/kg/day
Magnesium	?
Phosphate	?

DIGESTIVE JUICE SECRETION
Calcium	3mg/kg/day
Magnesium	0.5mg/kg/day
Phosphate	3mg/kg/day

EXTRACELLUAR FLUID   SOFT TISSUES

FILTERED & REABSORBED
Calcium	150mg/kg/day
Magnesium	35mg/kg/day
Phosphate	87mg/kg/day

FECES
Calcium	12mg/kg/day
Magnesium	2.5mg/kg/day
Phosphate	7mg/kg/day

URINE
Calcium	3mg/kg/day
Magnesium	1.5mg/kg/day
Phosphate	13mg/kg/day

Calcium, Magnesium, and Phosphate in Cytosol

Each of these three elements is important in the metabolism of all cells, but little is known about regulation of their concentrations in cytosol because technology is not sufficiently advanced for valid or facile measurements. The concentrations of magnesium and phosphate in cytoplasm are within an order of magnitude of those in plasma. Of the magnesium in cytosol, 50–90% is complexed to phosphate, citrate, and other anions such as the adenosine phosphates. In particular, all enzymes utilizing ATP interact with it in the form of $MgATP^{-2}$. Phosphate is covalently incorporated in many proteins, lipids, and nucleic acids. Many enzymes undergo dramatic shifts in activity when modified by phosphorylation or dephosphorylation.

Ionized calcium has been determined in the cytoplasm of a limited number of cell types. Basal concentrations are in the range of 10–100 nM, with dramatic rises upon plasma membrane depolarization or mobilization of sequestered intracellular calcium as during muscle contraction. When small localized fluxes of calcium into the cytosol occur, the change in concentration is restricted to only a small portion of the cytosol volume because of the limited mobility of calcium ions in cytoplasm and the effectiveness of various calcium sequestering systems that restore cytosol–ionized calcium concentration to the baseline. The determinants of ionized calcium concentration in the cytoplasm are largely unknown.

Ionized calcium concentration in cytosol changes with changes in calcium fluxes across membranes. Separate processes determine influx and efflux rates of calcium for cytosol. Two sites at which influx is regulated are the plasma membrane and, in muscle, the sarcoplasmic reticulum. Excitation of striated muscle leads, by unknown mechanisms, to release of calcium into cytosol from stores in the sarcoplasmic reticulum. Excitation of almost all secretory cells leads to increased permeability of the plasma membrane, allowing calcium to move down its concentration gradient into cytosol. For example, in the adrenal medulla, the neurotransmitter acetylcholine promotes calcium influx into the cell. The chromaffin cells contain, in addition to actomyosin, a calcium-dependent protein, synexin, that promotes fusion of chromaffin granule membranes with each other and presumably with the plasma membrane during exocytosis. The parathyroid cell seems to be an exception as PTH secretion is increased with decrease in extracellular calcium concentration (although ionized calcium concentration has not yet been determined in the cytoplasm of parathyroid cells). The interactions of many hormones with plasma membrane receptors lead to changes in transmembrane calcium flux. For example, in the pancreatic acinar cell, cholecystokinin or acetylcholine interacts with distinct receptors, leading to increased calcium efflux from the cell and to increases in cellular cyclic GMP (cGMP) concentration; secretin interacts with receptors presumably on the same cell to increase cellular cyclic AMP (cAMP) without changing plasma membrane calcium fluxes. In analogous ways, PTH and CT may modulate calcium fluxes in their target cells. In suspensions of monkey kidney cells, PTH increases the contents of cellular calcium compartments, increases calcium influx rate, and also increases intercompartmental calcium fluxes. In similar studies, CT also increased renal cellular calcium content but by a completely different mechanism, inhibiting cellular calcium efflux. In hamster renal tubules, PTH causes rises in cellular content of cAMP and cGMP. The PTH-induced changes in cellular cGMP are dependent on the presence of extracellular calcium and can be mimicked by ionophores that induce major shifts in cellular calcium fluxes. Indirect evidence suggests that some actions of PTH on osteoclasts and osteoblasts may be mediated by increases in cell (and perhaps also cytosol) calcium content. Exposure of dispersed bone cells to PTH leads to increased calcium uptake without change in cellular calcium efflux. PTH, vitamin D, and calcium ionophores can all evoke similar responses in bone preparations, suggesting that changes in cytosol-ionized calcium or calcium-binding proteins may be common pathways in the responses to these agents. The rapid PTH-induced changes in target cell calcium content may account for the early (first 60 min) drop in serum calcium concentration after PTH administration prior to mobilization of large amounts of calcium from extracellular pools into plasma (Fig. 19–5).

Maintenance of low concentration of ionized calcium in cytosol is dependent upon active transport. Energy-requiring calcium pumps have been identified in plasma membrane, sarcoplasmic and endoplasmic reticula, and mitochondria. In non-nucleated erythrocytes the plasma membrane calcium pump is the sole mechanism for ejection of calcium from the cytosol. In cardiac muscle cells, the plasma membrane represents only 0.1% of the membrane surface exposed to cytosol; in these cells the sarcoplasmic reticulum and mitochondria have a major role in regulating calcium efflux from cytosol. Relaxation of striated muscle contraction occurs with rapid removal of cytoplasmic calcium into sarcoplasmic reticulum. In many cells small changes in ionized calcium concentration can be buffered by the plasma membrane calcium pump or even by passive binding to calcium-binding proteins in the cytoplasm. In the presence of physiologic concentrations of magnesium, the calcium pumps of mitochondria and sarcoplasmic reticulum have a weaker affinity for calcium. Since these organelles have weak affinity but high capacity for calcium, they are well suited for removal of calcium when ionized calcium concentration rises abruptly, as for example during striated muscle contraction.

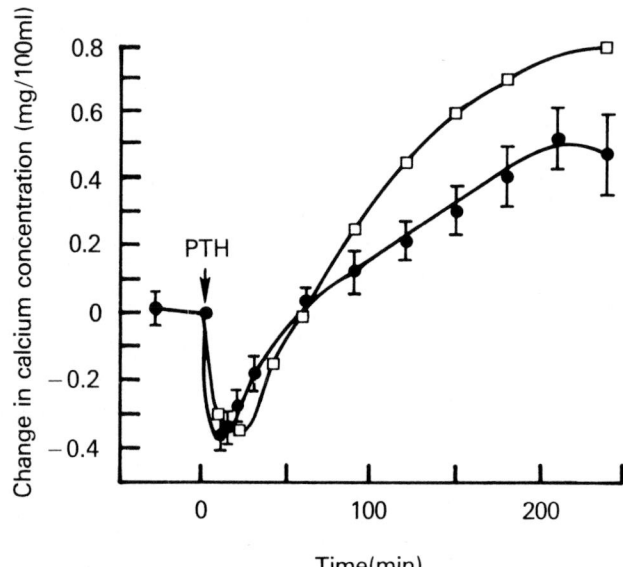

Figure 19–5. Comparison of extracellular calcium concentrations in response to PTH *in vitro* and *in vivo*. Serum calcium concentration change after administration of bovine PTH to dogs (□) and medium calcium concentration change after exposure of mouse calvaria bones to bovine PTH (•). (Modified from Parsons, J. A., et al.: *Endocrinology* 89:735, 1971, and from Robertson, W. G., et al.: *Clin. Sci.* 43:715, 1972.)

Plasma membranes undergo complex interactions with cytosol calcium. Not only do changes in membrane permeability and pump activity regulate calcium fluxes into and out of cytosol, but cytosolic calcium in turn affects several membrane properties. In the erythrocyte, an increased ionized calcium in cytosol increases potassium permeability. In contrast, a local rise in cytosolic calcium to 5×10^{-5} M in blowfly salivary gland cells results in closure of intercellular plasma membrane pores, thereby isolating the cell from direct cytoplasmic contact with neighboring cells.

Generally, mitochondria contain most of the intracellular calcium. Large amounts of amorphous calcium phosphate can be sequestered in mitochondria without forming organized crystals. Mitochondrial calcium accumulation is particularly prominent in dystrophic cells or cells exposed to prolonged hypercalcemia; accumulation is also high in chondrocytes of calcifying cartilage and in osteoclasts of healing bone fractures, however. Mitochondria contain a mechanism for active accumulation of calcium that is extremely effective when cytoplasmic ionized calcium concentration is above normal (10^{-7} M in squid axon), but it is not known whether mitochondria normally discharge large amounts of calcium. Some of the factors that cause calcium discharge from mitochondria include sodium, phosphate, prostaglandins, and an oxidized state of the pyridine nucleotide equilibrium in the matrix or its coupled adenylate nucleotide equilibrium in the cytosol. A slow release of calcium by relatively oxidized mitochondria could activate a series of enzymes (phosphorylase kinase, pyruvate dehydrogenase phosphatase, lipases, and mitochondrial oxidation of β hydroxybutyrate) to restore reducing potential in the cell and its mitochondria.

Intracellular Calcium-Binding Proteins

Many cytoplasmic enzyme activities are sensitive to changes in ionized calcium concentration within the "physiologic" range. These include adenylate cyclase, guanylate cyclase, cAMP phosphodiesterase, actomyosin ATPase, and phosphorylase b kinase. The types of modulation and the relative concentrations of these enzymes determine, in part, the message that changes in cytoplasmic calcium concentration will convey to the remainder of the cell. The calcium sensitivity of many of the just-mentioned enzymes is conveyed by interactions with regulatory proteins that have critical calcium binding sites (Fig. 19-6). Changes in cytoplasmic ionized calcium concentration may regulate a host of processes determined by contractile proteins. These include striated muscle contraction, secretory granule exocytosis, mitotic spindle function, and ciliary beating. The mechanism of calcium regulation has been studied in great detail for striated muscle. Muscle contraction is effected by the sliding of actin and myosin filaments along their long axes, energized by ATP hydrolysis. This activity, actomyosin ATPase, is inhibited by a mixture of several cytosol proteins (tropomyosin, troponin C, troponin I, and troponin T) in the absence of calcium. Increases in ionized calcium concentration to more than 10^{-7} M abolish this inhibition. The actomyosin ATPase inhibitory activity is a property of the tropomyosin-troponin complex, whereas the calcium-dependent release from inhibition is a property of the troponin C. Rabbit striated muscle troponin C is a 17,000 dalton peptide containing four homologous regions (presumably the result of two successive gene duplications) that bind divalent cations. The process of calcium binding in troponin C leads to large conformation changes that modulate the interaction of tropomyosin with actomyosin ATPase. The complete amino acid sequences of C troponins from several species have been determined. They show striking homologies to the sequences of several other major calcium-binding proteins (parvalbumins, myosin light chains, calcium-dependent regulatory proteins [calmodulins], and vitamin D–dependent calcium-binding proteins). The vitamin D–dependent calcium-binding proteins are present in the cytosols of all known vitamin D target tissues. They are considered in more detail in the section on intestinal action of calciferol (p. 956).

BONE

Chemistry and Structure

Skeletal tissue consists primarily of an extracellular matrix containing organic (35% by weight) and inorganic (65%) components. Although cells account for a minor fraction of bone volume, they carry out the dual functions of the skeletal system. By regulating the amount and distribution of inorganic matrix (which contains 95% of total

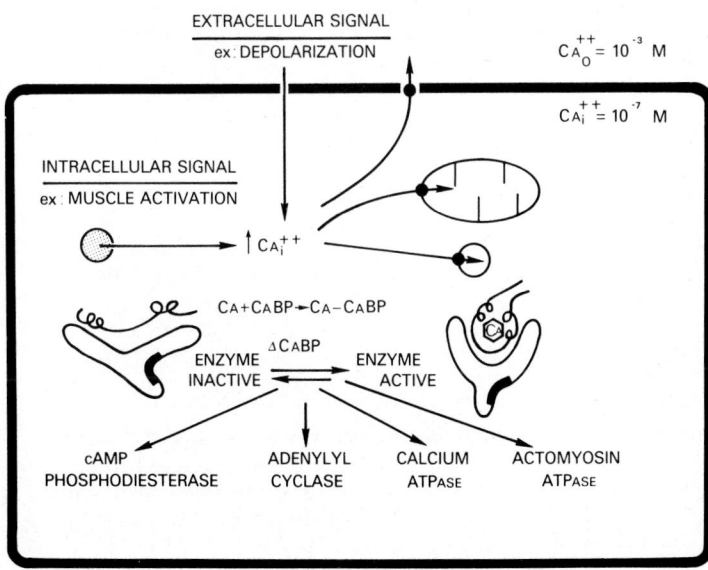

Figure 19–6. Calcium as a cytoplasmic messenger. Extra- or intracellular signals change the ionized calcium concentration in cytosol until active pumps restore the basal concentration. This change in ionic calcium activity causes rapid conformational shifts in calcium-binding proteins (troponin C, vitamin D–dependent calcium binding protein, and calcium dependent regulatory protein), which modulate cytosol enzyme activities. Enzyme active site is schematized as a solid bar on the enzyme protein.

body calcium), bone cells help maintain serum calcium concentration within a narrow range (mineral homeostasis). Bone cells are also responsible for continuous resorption and formation of extracellular matrix (remodeling), allowing response of the skeletal system to the mechanical forces resulting from physical activity (skeletal homeostasis).

Chemistry of Extracellular Matrix

Organic Components

Collagen Structure

Collagen is the major organic component of extracellular matrix. The collagen molecule has a rigid rodlike structure (14 × 300 nm) and is composed of three polypeptide ("α") chains held together in helical fashion by covalent and noncovalent forces. Multiple collagen molecules are assembled together end-to-end to form "fibrils" that are approximately 5–7 molecules thick; the fibrils in turn are arranged in bundles or "fibers" that can be seen by light microscopy in the extracellular bone matrix. Electron microscopy (EM) of collagen fibrils reveals cross striations with a characteristic periodicity (64–70 nm). The striations are due to the staggered arrangement of individual molecules within the fibril (Fig. 19–7). In re-

gions where adjacent molecules overlap ("overlap zone"), an increase in charge density results in the striation noted by EM. Gaps (40 nm) between the end of one molecule and the head of the next result in "hole zones" (visualized on EM by negative staining); these are the major sites of mineral deposition.

The primary amino acid sequences of the chains of collagen from several species have been elucidated. Bone collagen molecules are composed of two identical "α_1" chains and a homologous but distinct "α_2" chain. This so-called type I collagen is also found in skin but differs from collagen found in cartilage (type II — $3\alpha_1$ chains), elastic tissue (type III), and basement membranes (type IV). The primary structure of collagen is distinct and includes glycine at every third amino acid position and high contents of proline and lysine.

Properties unique to bone collagen are conferred by several post-translational modifications. Approximately one fifth of the lysine residues and one half of the proline residues are hydroxylated. Hydroxylysine may be further modified by glycosylation. The rigidity of the imino acid residues (proline and hydroxyproline) and hydrogen bonding of hydroxyproline help stabilize the extended triple helical conformation of the collagen molecule. Intramolecular and intermolecular cross-links (primarily lysine and hydroxylysine residues) help stabilize the collagen fibril structure. Although bone and skin collagen are equivalent in primary structure, they differ significantly in terms of post-translational modification (extent of lysine hydroxylation and glycosylation and number and type of cross-links). These differences probably account for the physical properties specific for bone collagen, which is more densely packed, less hydrated, less soluble, and of greater mechanical strength and thermal stability than is skin collagen.

Collagen Biosynthesis (Fig. 19–8)

Individual α chains are synthesized in a precursor form ("pre α chain") that contains additional N- and C-terminal residues. Separate intracellular enzymes catalyze the hydroxylation of lysine and proline residues; ascorbic acid is a necessary cofactor for these hydroxylations. Triple helix formation may be initiated by noncovalent forces, but interchain disulfide bridges between cysteines located in the C-terminal portions of the α chains help to stabilize the triple helix conformation. Enzymatic glycosylation of hydroxylysines may facilitate extrusion of the procollagen molecule from the cell. Several enzymes, collectively referred to as procollagen peptidases, act extracellularly to cleave N- and C-terminal moieties, leaving a largely triple helical molecule. The copper-requiring enzyme, lysyl oxidase, converts certain of the lysine and hydroxylysine residues to α-aminoadipic acid semialdehyde and 5-hydroxy-α-aminoadipic acid semialdehyde respectively. These modified residues interact with each other and with other amino groups to form intra- and intermolecular cross-links that help to bind collagen molecules into fibrils. Lysyl oxidase is inhibited by the lathyrogen, β-aminoproprionitrile.

Collagen Metabolism

There is evidence for breakdown of both old and recently synthesized collagen molecules. Urinary hydroxyproline excretion has been used as a rough index of collagen metabolism. It should be recognized, however, that uri-

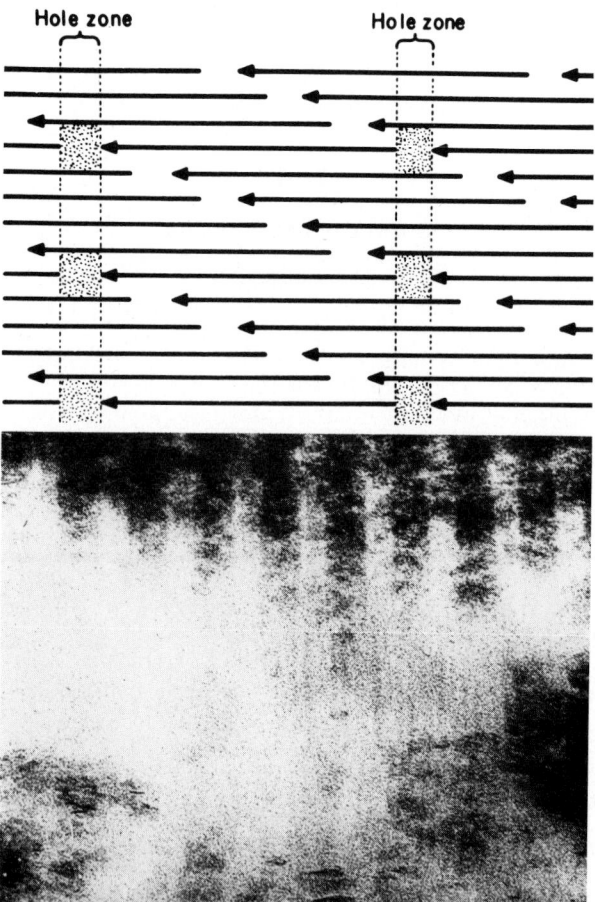

Figure 19–7. The staggered arrangement of individual molecules in collagen fibers results in "hole zones" between the "head" of one molecule and the "tail" of the next. Mineral deposition (bottom panel) begins within the "hole zones." (From Glimcher, M. J., and Krane, S. N.: Treatise on Collagen 2, Part B, New York, Academic Press, 1968.)

SYNTHESIS

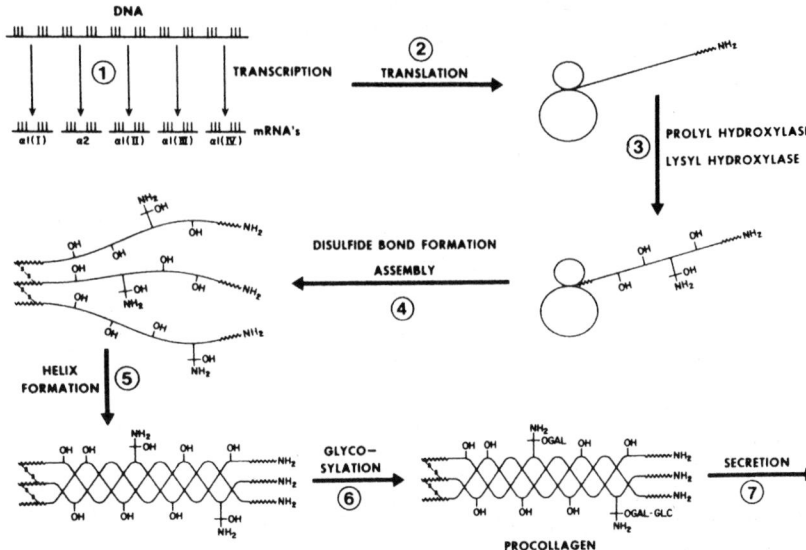

EXTRACELLULAR MATURATION

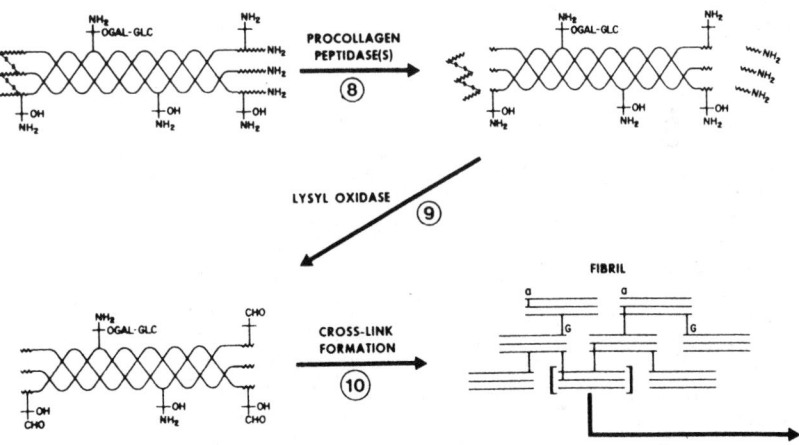

Figure 19–8. A simplified outline of the major steps in collagen synthesis and fibril formation. (From Raisz, L.: In *Metabolic Bone Disease.* Avioli, L., and Krane, S. (eds.), Vol. I. New York, Academic Press, 1977, p. 14.)

nary hydroxyproline represents only a small fraction of total collagen degradation and is not specific for bone, as opposed to skin and other collagen breakdown. Nonetheless, in diseases characterized by increased bone resorption (Paget's, hyperparathyroidism), total urinary hydroxyproline is increased, reflecting matrix breakdown. Ninety per cent of total urinary hydroxyproline consists of dialyzable dipeptides and tripeptides. Approximately 10% consists of nondialyzable components (average molecular weight [MW] = 5000) that appear to reflect exclusively breakdown of recently synthesized collagen. Thus nondialyzable urinary hydroxyproline is increased in clinical states characterized by increased bone formation (healing osteitis fibrosa, Paget's disease).

Noncollagen Organic Matrix Components

A minor fraction (~10%) of the organic matrix consists of noncollagen components, including glycoproteins, acid mucopolysaccharides, and lipids, most of which have not been well characterized. There is some evidence that these components are important in the process of minera-

lization (discussed later). Approximately 20% of noncollagenous matrix protein consists of osteocalcin, a protein containing the unique calcium-binding amino acid, γ-carboxyglutamic acid. Osteocalcin synthesis is vitamin K–dependent, but the bone protein is distinct in structure from the vitamin K–dependent clotting factors synthesized in the liver.

Inorganic Components

The inorganic portion of bone matrix is composed primarily of calcium and phosphate. Initially, calcium and phosphate are deposited as amorphous salts but later undergo rearrangements into a crystalline structure that resembles hydroxyapatite [$Ca_{10}(PO_4)_6(OH)_2$]. Several other ions, including Na, K, Mg, and CO_3 in varying proportions, may be found in the hydration shell of bone hydroxyapatite crystals. Varying amounts of fluoroapatite, depending on fluoride intake, also are formed. The microcrystalline form of bone mineral matrix provides a large surface area for exchange of ions.

Mineralization

Despite intensive research, the mechanism of bone matrix mineralization is not fully understood. Suggestive evidence exists concerning the importance of several factors discussed briefly here. Calcium and phosphate ions in the ECF are thought to be in metastable equilibrium; i.e., their concentrations exceed the solubility product (Ca × P), and they may be kept from forming a solid phase by inhibitors of calcification such as inorganic pyrophosphate. Osteoblasts contain abundant alkaline phosphatase activity and the serum concentration of this enzyme is known to be increased in states of increased bone formation. It is attractive to speculate that alkaline phosphatase activity facilitates mineralization by cleaving phosphate groups and thus either decreasing the effectiveness of inhibitors of calcification or increasing the local phosphate concentration in sites of mineralization. Definitive evidence to prove either hypothesis is lacking. Calcium and phosphate concentration at the site of mineralization may be regulated by the membrane-like action of the osteoblast layer present on the bone-forming surface. Calcium is taken up by various intracellular organelles, in particular mitochondria. There is evidence that calcium- and phosphate-rich membrane-lined vesicles are also extruded into the extracellular matrix; it has been suggested that these calcium- and phosphate-filled "matrix vesicles" help to initiate the process of mineralization but experimental evidence for the role of matrix vesicles has been obtained only in states of rapid matrix formation and mineralization.

Attention has also been directed at the role of the organic matrix components in the process of calcification. Minor glycoprotein components may be important in that their concentration decreases abruptly in sites where bone matrix is being mineralized. Thus glycoproteins might act as inhibitors of calcification that must be degraded before the process can begin.

The major organic component of bone matrix, collagen, undoubtedly plays a vital role in the normal mineralization process. The unique structure of collagen provides spaces ("hole zones," see Fig. 19–7) sufficiently large to accommodate the mineral phase of bone without disruption of the fibrils themselves. EM evidence confirms that the majority of the solid phase calcium and phosphate is located *within* the collagen fibrils and is highly ordered; i.e. the long axes of the crystals run parallel to the collagen fibrils and the mineral has the same (64–70 nm) periodicity as the collagen fibril has. In addition to its passive role as the major site of mineral deposition, there is considerable evidence to suggest that the collagen fibril itself may serve as a heterogeneous nucleation catalyst in the mineralization process. Binding of calcium or phosphate or both to side chain groups on collagen amino acid residues may be the initiating factor in further calcium and phosphate precipitation and ultimate calcification. Such a role for collagen would help to explain the localization of the majority of the mineral phase within the collagen fibrils. Thus, the structure of the collagen molecule dictates its unique physical properties, including the ability to serve as the site of, and possibly also the catalyst for, mineral deposition.

Once mineralization of bone matrix is initiated, it proceeds rapidly, so that within 6–12 hours, 60–70% of the final amount of mineral is deposited ("primary mineralization phase"). Subsequently, mineralization occurs much more slowly and may not be complete until 1–2 months later ("secondary mineralization phase").

Bone Structure

Cortical and Trabecular Bone

Eighty per cent of skeletal mass is made up of cortical (compact) bone and 20% of trabecular (cancellous, spongy) bone. The former is found principally in the shafts of long bones and the latter in vertebrae, most flat bones, and the ends of long bones. Microscopic analysis of cortical bone reveals closely packed osteons (haversian systems), consisting of concentric lamellae of bone surrounding a central (haversian) canal, interstitial lamellae, which represent the remains of remodeled osteons (see "Skeletal Remodeling," p. 934), and circumferential lamellae at the periosteal and endosteal surfaces of the bone. The dense structure of cortical bone is pierced by the osteonal central canals as well as so-called Volkmann canals, which radiate from the central canals to connect neighboring osteons and to form an anastomotic network through which blood and lymph vessels course from the cortex to the periosteum. In trabecular bone, lamellae are arranged in longitudinal bundles. The individual trabeculae anastomose within the marrow cavity, and their arrangement is dictated by the mechanical stresses upon the bone. Although cortical bone makes up the majority of skeletal mass, its surface area (about 3.2 m²) is significantly smaller than that of trabecular bone (about 16 m²).

Woven and Lamellar Bone

The organic extracellular bone matrix may be arranged in woven or lamellar fashion. This distinction is readily made when decalcified bone is examined with the polarizing microscope. In woven bone, coarse collagen bundles are irregularly distributed and osteocytes randomly positioned. In lamellar bone, collagen bundles are highly ordered; when viewed under polarized light, alternating isotropic and anisotropic bands (2–3 μ thick) are visible. Osteocytes are evenly distributed and their lone axes run parallel to those of the lamellae. Woven bone (also termed immature or fibrous) is characteristically seen in embryonic bone and is not normally present after 2 years of age. It appears to be associated with states of rapid bone formation and remodeling and is thus found in fracture callus as well as in Paget's disease and osteitis fibrosa (Fig. 19–9).

Bone Histology

Three main bone cell types, the osteoblast, osteocyte, and osteoclast, are recognized, although their origin and functions are incompletely known. Osteoblasts are located at the bone forming surface and are responsible for elaborating the organic components of the extracellular matrix. The unmineralized matrix forms the *osteoid* seam or zone; approximately 10 days after the osteoid is formed, mineralization begins. During this interval it is believed that collagen is modified (maturation) to facilitate calcification. The junction between mineralized bone and unmineralized osteoid is known as the *calcification front*. This region selectively incorporates tetracyclines and this property has been exploited to calculate the linear rate of mineral deposition (Fig. 19–10). After administering 2 doses of tetracycline at a defined time interval and obtaining a bone biopsy, one can measure the distance between fluorescent bands of incorporated tetracycline. Calculations based on rib biopsy specimens yield values of about 1 μ/day.

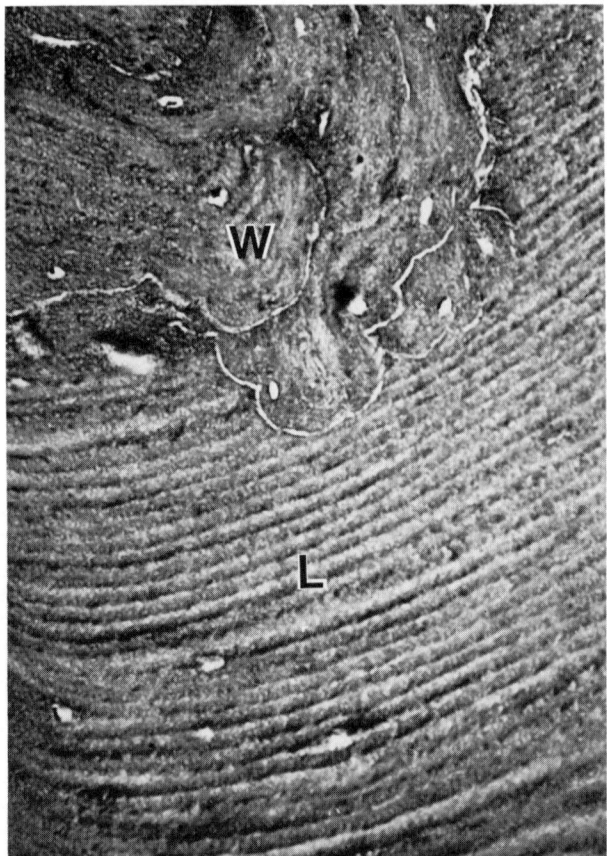

Figure 19–9. Lamellar (L) and woven (W) bone from a patient with Paget's disease. Decalcified, H & E stain, differential contrast optics, magnification × 280. (From Aaron, J.: Histology and microanatomy of bone. In *Calcium, Phosphate and Magnesium Metabolism.* Nordin, B. E. C. (ed.), New York, Churchill-Livingstone, 1976, p. 306.)

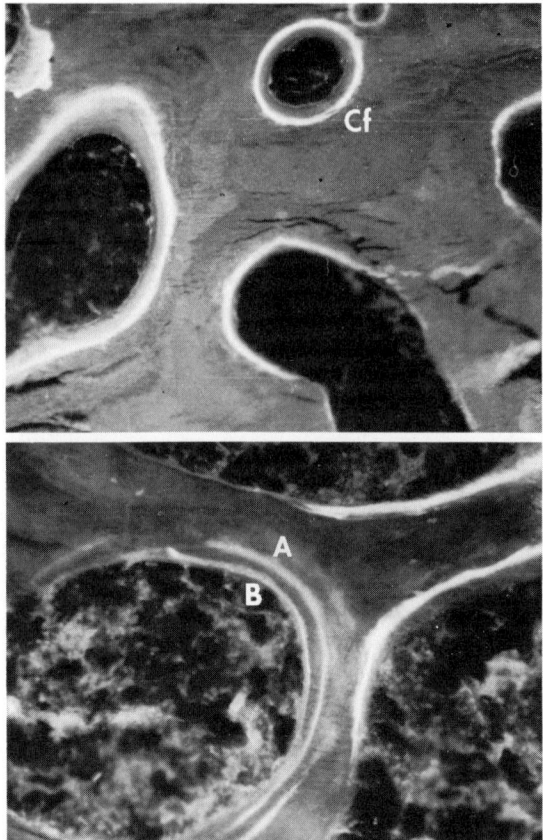

Figure 19–10. Tetracycline labels sites of active mineralization and is deposited at the calcification front (Cf, top panel). Double-label technique can be used to measure rate of mineralization; label A was administered about 10 days before label B (bottom panel). Undecalcified iliac crest, ultraviolet light, magnified × 113. (From Aaron, J.: Histology and microanatomy of bone. In *Calcium, Phosphate and Magnesium Metabolism.* Nordin, B. E. C. (ed.), New York, Churchill-Livingstone, 1976, p. 314.)

Osteoblasts, after forming the organic matrix, eventually become surrounded by it and are then termed osteocytes. This arbitrary distinction obviously does not imply an abrupt alteration in functional properties and indeed ultrastructural evidence (discussed later) indicates that "young" osteocytes show many osteoblastic features. Osteoclasts, like osteoblasts, are present at the bone surface but are localized to regions of active bone resorption.

Bone Cell Origin

Labeling studies with ³H thymidine have been used to identify proliferating osteoprogenitor cells at the bone surface. These cells are indistinguishable from fibroblasts by light microscopy. The preosteoblast is generally thought to derive from primitive mesenchymal cells. A ³H thymidine label can be followed from preosteoblasts to osteoblasts and finally to osteocytes, a process that takes about 5 days in rats. Several authors have postulated a common precursor cell for osteoblasts and osteoclasts, but recent evidence, based on experiments with congenitally osteopetrotic mice, suggests that the osteoclastic precursor may be a circulating monocytic cell. Mice with the grey-lethal mutation lack normal osteoclastic bone resorption but can be "cured" by parabiosis with normal litter mates or by giving them bone marrow or spleen transplants from normal litter mates. Definitive identification of the cell type responsible for res-

toration of normal bone resorption has not yet been achieved.

Bone Cell Ultrastructure

Osteoblasts

Active osteoblasts are cuboidal in shape and approximately 20 μ in diameter. The cytoplasm is basophilic, reflecting the extensive rough endoplasmic reticulum characteristic of cells actively engaged in protein synthesis. A well-developed Golgi apparatus, which may play an important role in collagen processing and extrusion, is also seen with the electron microscope. Abundant alkaline phosphatase activity is demonstrable histochemically. Osteoblastic cell processes may extend within the osteoid zone and communicate with osteocytes (see later). The inactive osteoblast assumes a more flattened fibroblastic appearance; a layer of flattened osteoblasts covering the bone surface may act like a membrane controlling the flow of ions across the bone surface.

Osteocytes

Osteoblasts, once surrounded by matrix, are termed osteocytes. Each cell is surrounded by its own lacuna, but an extensive canalicular system connects osteocytes and surface osteoblasts and probably serves as a channel for the flow of ions and nutrients. The ultrastructure of osteocytes is quite variable; intracellular organelles may be poorly developed, suggesting a metabolically inactive cell, or a well-developed Golgi and endoplasmic reticulum may be seen, reflecting active synthetic function. The presence of numerous mitochondria and cytoplasmic vacuoles in certain osteocytes implies a role in bone resorption. In states characterized by excessive PTH secretion, enlargement of the osteocytic perilacunar space is often observed. This has been interpreted to signify PTH stimulation of "osteocytic osteolysis." The importance of this process in mineral homeostasis is not clear, but several authors have suggested that osteocytic osteolysis may be responsible for rapid movement of calcium from bone into the ECF. As bone ages, there is a progressive decrease in the number of viable osteocytes and a resultant hypermineralization of the osteocytic canaliculi termed "micropetrosis."

Osteoclasts

These are multinucleated cells that may reach 100 μ in diameter. Cinematography has shown that the osteoclast is highly mobile. It moves along the bone surface actively resorbing bone and leaving resorption lacunae in its wake. The cytoplasm contains abundant mitochondria, as well as vacuoles and vesicles that may be involved in the resorption process. Histochemical studies show the presence of significant amounts of lysosomal (e.g., acid phosphatase) and mitochondrial (e.g., succinic dehydrogenase) enzymes. At the resorption surface, the plasma membrane of the osteoclast has a redundant structure referred to as the "ruffled border" (Fig. 19–11). Osteoclasts, under normal circumstances, do not resorb unmineralized osteoid; the precise sequence of resorptive events is still unknown; i.e., does organic matrix removal precede mineral removal or vice versa? Crystals of hydroxyapatite and collagen fibrils have been observed be-

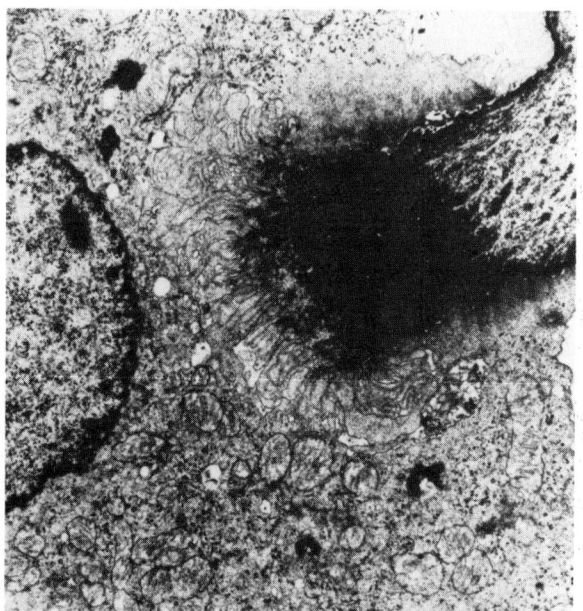

Figure 19–11. Electron micrograph of an osteoclast from fetal rat bone cultured with PTH. "Clear zone" of the osteoclast surrounds a bone spicule. Invaginations of the cell membrane adjacent to the bone spicule constitute the ruffled border responsible for resorbing mineral and matrix. Magnified × 9100. (From Holtrop, M. E., Raisz, L. G., et al.: The effects of parathyroid hormone, colchicine, and calcitonin on the ultrastructure and the activity of osteoclasts in organ culture. *J. Cell Biol. 60*:346, 1974.)

tween the resorbing surface and the ruffled border but have not been identified within the osteoclast itself. Active bone resorption is characterized by an increase in several forms of enzyme activity at the bone surface. Collagenase activity initiates cleavage of collagen fibrils, and other lysosomal enzymes may participate in further breakdown of collagenase cleavage products as well as noncollagen organic matrix components. Osteoclasts stimulated by PTH also form significant amounts of lactic and hyaluronic acid, but the role of these materials in the resorptive process has not been clarified.

Skeletal Homeostasis

Skeletal Growth

With the exception of flat bones such as the skull, bones grow by a process termed endochondral ossification. Early in embryonic development, primitive mesenchymal cells form a cartilage rudiment similar in shape to the bone ultimately to be formed. Along the shaft (diaphysis) newly formed osteoblasts lay down a "collar" of bone. Continued periosteal formation of new lamellae enlarge this collar, and late in fetal life haversian remodeling (discussed later) begins, resulting in the formation of the cortex. Endosteal resorption occurs but does not keep pace with periosteal apposition; as a result the cortex thickens as the marrow cavity is enlarged. At the metaphyseal ends of the bone, trabeculae of calcified cartilage form the "primary spongiosa." These are resorbed and replaced by bony trabeculae in the secondary spongiosa. An epiphyseal ossification center develops at each end; this region is responsible for linear growth of bone. Successive layers of cartilage — resting, proliferating, maturing and calcifying zones — make up the so-called epiphyseal growth plate. With maturity the epiphyseal centers ossify and further linear growth ceases. Cartilage remains only on the articular surface. Bone mass continues to increase through the third and fourth decade primarily through a continued excess of periosteal apposition relative to endosteal resorption, but after the fourth decade there is a gradual loss of bone mass, which becomes more rapid in females following menopause (see "Osteoporosis," p. 1006).

Skeletal Remodeling

Mechanism of Remodeling

Even after growth ceases, bone continues to be a metabolically active tissue. Constant skeletal remodeling occurs in response to both the mineral homeostatic and the structural requirements of the body. Remodeling involves the concerted action of osteoblasts and osteoclasts in the processes of bone formation and resorption. This may occur at endosteal and periosteal surfaces, as well as in the cortex. Intracortical (haversian) remodeling requires resorption of previously deposited bone to make room for new bone formation. This is accomplished by a "cutting cone" of osteoclasts that removes everything in its longitudinal path and is followed by blood vessels and bone-forming cells that line the newly formed cavity with concentric bone lamellae. The newly formed osteons (haversian systems) may be 200 μ in diameter and several mm long; their long axes run parallel to the long bone shaft. The remains of old, partially resorbed osteons form the interstitial lamellae and lack a central canal. A cement line demarcates the border between resorbed bone and newly formed bone. Disturbances in haversian remodeling occur as the individual ages. These include an increase in size of central canal and decreased mineralization and irregularity of the osteons. As a result, cortical bone of elderly individuals may be more porous.

Parameters of Remodeling

The surfaces involved in bone formation and resorption can be quantitated on bone biopsy specimens. The relationship — (number of bone forming or resorptive surfaces) = (osteoclast or osteoblast activation rate) × (period of formative or resorptive activity) — has been used to interpret the static measurements performed on a single biopsy specimen.

Measurements performed on normal trabecular bone from the iliac crest show that about 12% of total surface is being resorbed and 24% represents newly formed bone. Based on the just-mentioned relationship, it has been concluded that in trabecular bone of iliac crest, the rate of resorption is normally twice the rate of formation. Static measurements of bone surfaces may give similar results in several metabolic bone diseases. Thus osteoid borders may be increased in both osteomalacia and hyperthyroidism, but in the former this occurs because bone formation is prolonged (by delay in mineralization) whereas in the latter it reflects a general increase in remodeling and therefore activation rate.

Control of Remodeling

Remodeling is affected by biochemical and physical factors. PTH, CT, and 1,25-$(OH)_2$ vitamin D are the main hormonal influences upon the skeletal system. The major skeletal effect of PTH is to increase bone resorption. Vitamin D plays a permissive role in this effect of PTH. CT, particularly in young animals, inhibits resorption. The detailed skeletal actions of these agents are described elsewhere (see "Actions of PTH on Bone," p. 944; "Calcitonin — Actions on Bone," p. 952; and "Actions of Calciferol — Skeletal Actions," p. 957). Other agents, including thyroid hormones, cortisol, estrogens, GH, prostaglandins, and osteoclast-activating factor, also exert important skeletal effects (see "Miscellaneous Endogenous Calcitropic Factors," p. 961).

Humoral agents affect bone cells through defined biochemical mechanisms (e.g., binding to receptors, increase in intracellular cAMP). Mechanical forces are clearly of great importance in controlling remodeling, but the mechanisms that convert a physical input (mechanical force applied to bone) into a biologic output (remodeled bone resulting from concerted osteoblast and osteoclast action) remain to be elucidated. Applied forces are capable of inducing electrical fields in bone. This so-called piezo electric effect could help modulate the remodeling response to mechanical forces, since it has been shown that bone accumulates preferentially at the negatively charged portion of the field. This has the effect of reducing the compressive stress applied to this area of bone. Mechanical stress on bone *in vitro* also causes increased prostaglandin formation and increased cAMP concentration, which may influence the resorptive phase of bone remodeling. Further work will be necessary to substantiate these mechanisms, since a better understanding of the effects of mechanical stress could have important implications for therapy of fractures and immobilization osteoporosis.

Bone remodeling is characterized by close *coupling* of resorption and formation, virtually independent of extraskeletal regulating factors (Fig. 19–12). This coupling holds

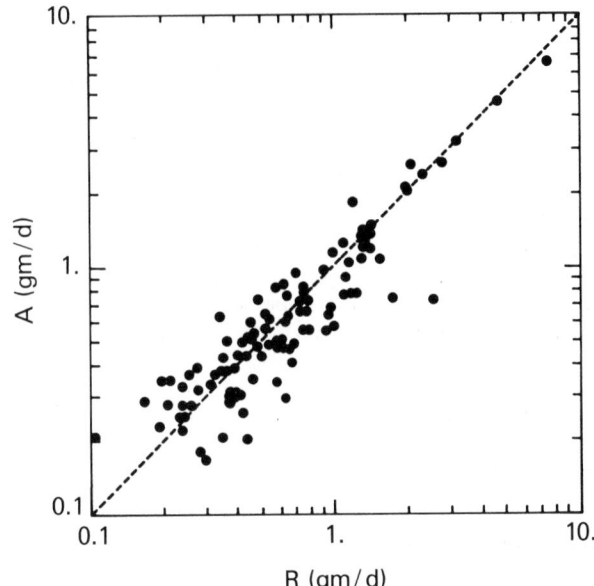

Figure 19–12. Calcium removal (R) from bone plotted as a function of calcium accretion (A) in 108 patients with various disorders of calcium metabolism. (From Harris, W. H., and Heaney, R. P.: Skeletal renewal and metabolic bone disease. *N. Engl. J. Med.* 280:255, 1969.)

at high or low rates of bone turnover. Numerous explanations for the phenomenon of coupling have been proposed but none is entirely satisfactory. Regardless of the mechanism involved, coupling has important therapeutic implications. This is exemplified by the response of osteoporotic subjects to agents that inhibit bone resorption. After several months of therapy to induce an increase in ratio of bone formation to resorption, formation falls, so that the net increase in bone mass may be trivial. A better understanding of the coupling mechanism might permit more effective therapy in metabolic bone disorders.

PARATHYROID GLANDS

Embryology

The parathyroid glands are derived from the endodermal germ layer of the third and fourth pairs of branchial pouches. The lower pair of parathyroids develops (in association with the thymus) from the third branchial pouch. They migrate caudally with the thymus until, at the 18-mm embryo stage, they separate from the thymus and assume their usual position at the lower pole of the thyroid gland. The upper parathyroids derive from the fourth (more caudal) branchial pouch but remain almost stationary during embryologic development, accounting for their final location at the upper pole of the thyroid.

Anatomy

The upper parathyroids are generally located near the junction of the middle thyroid artery and the recurrent laryngeal nerve. They may be flattened against the posterior thyroid capsule or, rarely, actually embedded within the thyroid. Aberrant locations include the tracheoesophageal groove and retroesophageal space. The blood supply is most commonly from the inferior thyroid artery.

The lower parathyroids are more variable in position since they undergo considerable migration. Generally, they are found lateral to the trachea at the lower pole of the thyroid, but they may be located in the anterior mediastinum in association with thymic tissue if separation from the thymus fails to occur during embryologic development. Other aberrant locations include the carotid sheath and, very rarely, the pharyngeal submucosa (possibly related to failure to migrate caudally). The blood supply is usually from the inferior thyroid artery, but aberrant glands in the anterior mediastinum sometimes are supplied by a branch of the internal mammary artery.

At least four parathyroid glands are generally present. More than four glands may occur in as many as 6% of normal individuals. Supernumerary glands have been attributed to division of one or more of the four main glands during development. The parathyroids increase in weight until a plateau is reached in the third or fourth decade of life. Average total weight of the four glands is 120 mg in males and 140 mg in females. The glands are dark tan to yellow in color, depending on fat content. Size and shape vary widely. The most common shape is ellipsoid (average dimension: $6 \times 5 \times 2$ mm), but parathyroids may be flattened or elongated by adjacent structures. Glandular fat cell number begins to increase at puberty and continues to increase until 60–70% of the gland is composed of fat in elderly individuals.

Histology

The chief cell is the major cell type of the parathyroid gland and is responsible for PTH synthesis and secretion. Chief cells are usually arranged in cords and sheets within the gland but follicular and acinar arrangements are sometimes observed. The chief cell is 4–8 μ in diameter with a small central nucleus containing dense chromatin. Chief cells have been segregated into two types on the basis of ultrastructural appearance. The "active" chief cell contains parallel arrays of endoplasmic reticulum in which the precursor protein of PTH is thought to be synthesized. A prominent Golgi region (the probable site of hormone packaging) and membrane-bound granules (presumed to contain PTH) have also been observed. There are generally few secretory granules, and little hormone is stored in the cell. Secretion occurs as granule membranes fuse with the plasma membrane. Microtubules are found in the cell and may be important in movement of secretory granules towards the cell periphery. Secretory mechanisms are discussed on p. 940.

The "inactive" chief cell shows a dispersed endoplasmic reticulum, a smaller Golgi region, abundant glycogen-containing vacuoles, and lipofuscin granules. In the normal gland the ratio of inactive to active chief cells is about 3:1, but in suppressed glands the ratio may approach 10:1. There is a continuous cycle from active to inactive forms of chief cell (including transitional forms).

Oxyphil cells appear after puberty. They are 6–10 μ in diameter and contain a small central pyknotic nucleus, bright eosinophilic cytoplasm, and abundant mitochondria. Oxyphil cells usually show a sparse endoplasmic reticulum and a poorly developed Golgi region and normally may not secrete PTH. It has been speculated that oxyphil cells, which increase in number with age, represent a degenerative form of chief cell.

PARATHYROID HORMONE

Chemistry

PTH was isolated in a highly purified state in 1959, almost 35 years after the first active extract of PTH was prepared by Collip. His method of extraction, it was ultimately proved, leads to production of multiple active polypeptide fragments through mild acid hydrolysis of the native hormone. Although fragmentation of the native polypeptide during extraction was one of the problems hampering purification of the hormone, it ultimately provided the clue that fragments smaller than the native hormone molecule must be biologically active. It is now recognized that the principal form of PTH stored in and released from the parathyroid glands is an 84-amino acid, single-chain polypeptide that is synthesized within the parathyroid gland through precursor forms. After secretion into the circulation, the hormone is metabolized to smaller polypeptide fragments that are inactive.

The total structures of the native 84-amino acid polypeptide hormones from the bovine, porcine, and human species are now known (Fig. 19–13). All three molecules are similar in charge and identical in length and have many amino acid residues in common. The sequence differences between human and bovine or porcine PTH, however, cause distinct immunologic reactivities reflected in incomplete cross-reactivity of human hormone with antibodies developed against porcine or bovine hormone. Generally, results of bioassays indicate that the intact 1–84 human PTH polypeptide is less potent on a molar basis than either bovine or porcine hormone. This reduced biopotency undoubtedly also reflects the significant differences in amino acid sequence. Further, it is possible that the cluster of prolines in the middle region of the human hormone confers unique steric features to the molecule.

Certain other chemical properties are also of significance for interpretation in clinical medicine. (1) The amino terminal third of the molecule is critically important for biologic activity. The sequence 1–27 is the minimum required for detectable biologic activity. Synthetic polypeptides encom-

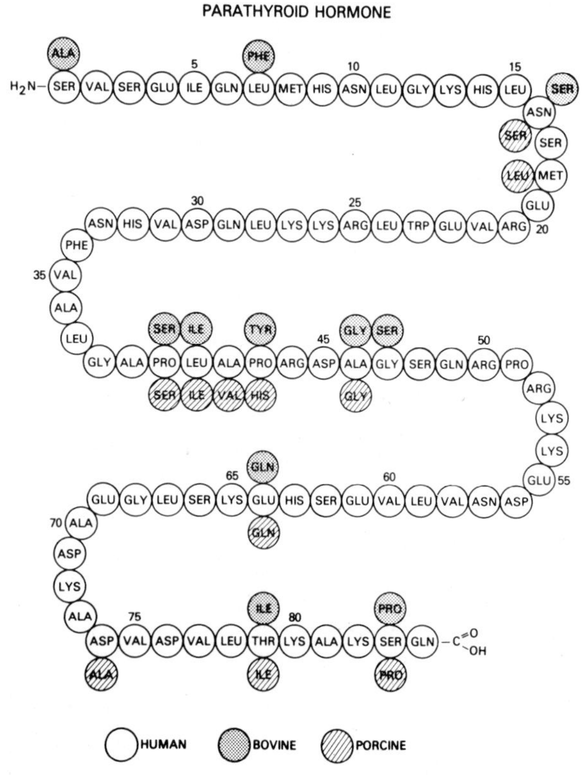

PARATHYROID HORMONE

Figure 19–13. Complete amino acid sequences for bovine, human, and porcine parathyroid hormone. (Courtesy Dr. Henry Keutmann.)

passing the first 34 amino acids generally are fully as active biologically on a molar basis as the entire 1–84 sequence (however, there has not been sufficient pure 1–84 human PTH to allow extensive bioassays to compare with the synthetic fragment). (2) The bovine hormone can be iodinated to the extent of 1 mole/mole of polypeptide on the single tyrosine (postion 43) residue with retention of biologic activity. (3) Oxidation of the methionines in the amino terminus destroys biologic activity; substitution of norleucine for methionine yields synthetic peptides resistant to oxidative inactivation. (4) Most antisera developed against intact human, porcine, or bovine PTH recognize predominantly the C-terminal antigenic sites of the hormone. (5) Removal of the N-terminal amino acid (serine for human or porcine hormone; alanine for bovine) causes greater than 90% loss of biologic potency. (6) These several facts allow for marked discrepancies between biologic and immunologic reactivity of peptide fragments of the hormone identified in gland extracts and in plasma. (7) A synthetic peptide lacking two amino acids (Ala-Ser) at the amino terminus is a competitive inhibitor of PTH action *in vitro*.

Bioassay of Parathyroid Hormone

The original bioassay developed by Collip and Clark was based upon the hormone-induced rise in serum calcium of dogs. This was the method that allowed isolation of the original active extract of parathyroid glands. This assay, still used today in some commercial productions, has been supplanted by development of several much more facile *in vivo* or *in vitro* bioassays for PTH. The *in vivo* assays now used commonly are based on serum calcium measurements in parathyroidectomized rats or in calcium-injected chicks or quail. Perhaps the most commonly used *in vitro* assay depends upon determining activation of renal adenylate cyclase in response to PTH. Crude preparations of renal adenylate cyclase can be obtained and stored indefinitely in liquid nitrogen for use as needed. In this assay the conversion of ^{32}P-labeled ATP to radioactive cAMP is determined *in vitro*. This method appears more precise and more economical of hormone than the *in vivo* assays. This assay as well as the parathyroidectomized rat assay and *in vivo* chick assay have been the major methods utilized in evaluating the biologic activity of synthetic parathyroid-related polypeptides. In general, the biologic potencies of natural as well as synthetic peptides agree closely when tested either *in vitro* or *in vivo*. Interesting differences have been reported, however, in comparing the activity of some synthetic peptides with rat bioassays (either *in vitro* or *in vivo*) and the chick hypercalcemia assay. The chick assay gives relatively more biologic activity for peptides modified at the amino terminus. For this reason, proPTH shows much greater relative biologic activity in the chick hypercalcemia assay than in the *in vitro* adenylate cyclase assay. Similarly, synthetic peptides (representing residues 2–34) devoid of N-terminal alanine show only 50% loss of biologic potency in the chick, but 98%+ loss of activity in the rat adenylate cyclase assay. Conversely, peptides shortened at the C-terminus, e.g., 1–28, show almost full biologic potency with the *in vitro* rat adenylate cyclase assay and virtually complete loss of activity with the *in vivo* chick hypercalcemia assay. These discrepancies undoubtedly are due to differences in distribution or metabolism *in vivo* in the chick, since adenylate cyclase preparations made from chick kidney show a similar biopotency pattern to that found with rat renal adenylate cyclase preparations.

Recent results with isolated bone cells and measurement of cyclic 3',5'-AMP suggest that this system might be developed into a highly sensitive biologic assay. Changes in cAMP content can be observed with PTH at concentrations as low as 10^{-16}M with some cell preparations.

Ultrasensitive Cytochemical Assays

The introduction of highly sensitive techniques for quantitative cytochemistry allows detection of hormones at dilutions 100–1000 times or greater than those utilized even in the best available radioimmunoassay. This approach has led to the development, on an experimental basis, of ultrasensitive assays for PTH in plasma. The method is based on determination of glucose-6-phosphate dehydrogenase (G6PD) activity in the distal convoluted tubules of the guinea pig kidney, which is specifically activated by PTH. It is the G6PD system that has been used as a bioassay for hormone in plasma. Active PTH can be detected at the femtogram level corresponding to 1:1000 dilutions of normal human plasma. This is the most sensitive assay for PTH in plasma and should allow resolution of some of the questions concerning the circulating form of PTH. Unfortunately the assay is cumbersome and time-consuming in performance; thus, unless new modifications allow application on a broader scale, it is not likely to become generally available for clinical use. The implications of this assay are discussed further under "Primary Hyperparathyroidism" and the nature of circulating hormone in that disorder (p. 968). A summary of the nature and characteristics of several bioassays developed for PTH is presented in Table 19–5.

Table 19–5.   BIOASSAYS FOR PARATHYROID HORMONE

Preparation	Parameter	Dose Range, USP units/animal or units/ml
Parathyroidectomized rat	Serum Ca	5–40
Calcium-injected chick or quail	Serum Ca	1–12
Mouse calvaria	Ca release *in vitro*	.01–1.0
Rat long bone	^{45}Ca release *in vitro*	.01–1.0
Mouse calvaria	^{14}CO$_2$ produced *in vitro* from ^{14}C-citrate	.0025–.15
Renal adenylate cyclase	^{32}P-cyclic 3',5'-AMP produced from ^{32}P-ATP	1.4–12
Isolated bone cells	Cyclic 3',5'-AMP	0.1–2
Guinea pig kidney segments	Glucose-6-P-dehydrogenase cytochemical determination	10^{-10}–10^{-6}*

*Fenton, S., Somers, S., et al.: *Clin. Endocrinol.* 9:381, 1978; Chambers, D. J., Dunham, J., et al.: *Clin. Endocrinol.* 9:375, 1978.
References for other methods may be found in Aurbach, G. D., and Chase L. R.: In *Handbook of Physiology;* Section 7: *Endocrinology;* Volume 7: *Parathyroid.* American Physiological Society. Greep, R. O., and Astwood, E. B. (eds.), Baltimore, Williams & Wilkins, 1977, pp. 353–381.

Immunoreactivity and Immunoassay of Parathyroid Hormone

Radioimmunoassays have been developed for PTH from many species, including humans, and for specific peptide sequences within these polypeptide molecules. Since the amino acid sequences vary among hormones from different species, the nature of immunogenic determinants within these peptide molecules differs. Moreover, the sequences that are immunogenic within the polypeptides do not necessarily correspond to the segments that are specifically required for biologic activity. Thus, in radioimmunoassays for any polypeptide hormone, there is opportunity for divergence between biologic reactivity and immunoreactivity of peptide segments within the hormone molecule. There are few hormonal polypeptides wherein divergencies between biologic and immunologic reactivities have been so marked as for PTH. Thus radioimmunoassay, although affording a highly sensitive method for detecting PTH antigen when applied to body fluids, does not afford a valid index for the amount of biologically active PTH in the sample. Indeed, it is now recognized that multiple types of immunoreactive fragments of PTH are found in the circulation. The first observation suggesting heterogeneity of PTH immunoreactive material in the circulation was reported by Berson and Yalow (1966). They had developed two different antisera to bovine PTH. With one antiserum the apparent half-life of the hormone in the circulation was inordinately long. The other antiserum detected a relatively rapid rate of disappearance of the hormone from the plasma after parathyroidectomy (Fig. 19–14). They concluded from these results that there must be more than one form of PTH in the circulation of a human being. Furthermore they found that the half-life of either form of the hormone was prolonged markedly in uremic subjects, and that the hormone extracted from human glands seems different in immunologic reactivity from that in the circulation. These observations were followed by others in several laboratories, with the following general results: (1) Immunologic reactivity in extracts of bovine or human glands differs from that in the general circulation. (2) The discrepancies vary in degree depending upon the antiserum used. (3) In some instances, the immunologic reactivity found in the medium of parathyroid explants differs from that extracted directly from the explant — these discrepancies are seen particularly in long-term (greater than 24 hours) incubations *in vitro*. (4) Gel filtration (a means of separation of molecules by size) of peripheral plasma has indicated that there are immunoreactive PTH-related peptides of varying size in the peripheral circulation. (5) Selective antisera directed specifically at the aminoterminal region of PTH on the one hand versus the carboxyterminal region on the other show discrepant results for PTH concentration in the peripheral circulation when the radioimmunoassay standard is native hormone (i.e., containing a 1:1 ratio of amino and carboxy antigens).

Other Efforts to Improve the Utility of Radioimmunoassays for Clinical Applications

Carboxyterminal- and aminoterminal-"specific" antisera have been developed by adsorbing antisera with aminoterminal or carboxyterminal fragments of the molecule prepared synthetically to yield antisera relatively specific for either segment of the molecule. Antisera have also been developed directly against synthetic polypeptides representing the N-terminal or C-terminal regions. The synthetic fragment representing the C-terminus (residues 53–84) of human PTH is more immunoreactive than "native" (1–84) hormone isolated from human glands. Antisera directed at synthetic peptides representing the aminoterminus (residues 1–34) of human PTH have been developed and applied successfully to assess the hormone in the circulation. Detection of hormone with "aminoterminal" antisera, however, should not be taken to imply that significant quantities of biologically active aminoterminal fragments of the hormone exist in the circulation. Noted earlier was the observation that removal of solely the aminoterminal alanine from PTH destroys greater than 90% of the biologic activity. Moreover, immunoreactivity with the C-terminal-specific antibodies may well represent predominantly large polypeptides, even intact hormone, containing the N-terminal sequences. Further it is important to point out that even "aminoterminal-specific" antisera generally detect concentrations of peptide in the circulation of approximately 200 pg/ml in normal human subjects. The ultrasensitive cytochemical assay results suggest concentrations on the order of only 5–15 pg/ml. This large discrepancy is yet to be clarified. Another problem with PTH radioimmunoas-

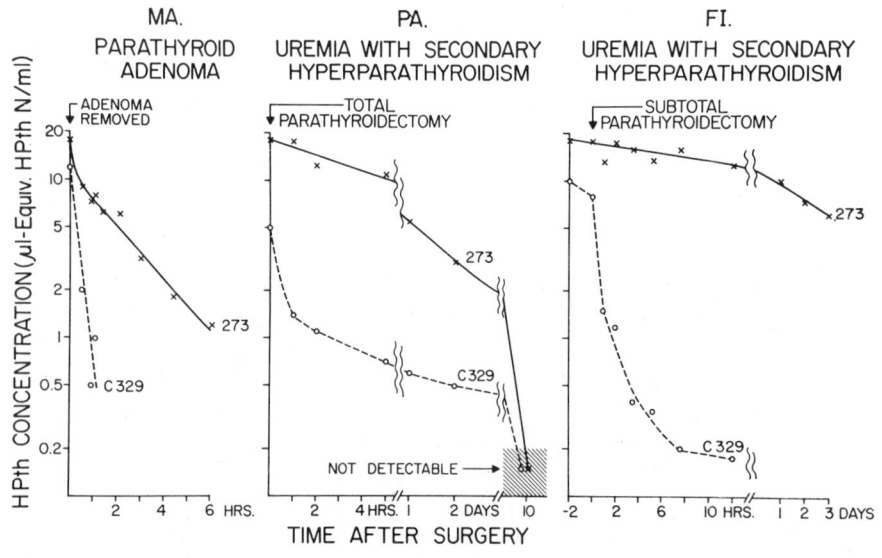

Figure 19–14. Differences in half-life among immunoreactive forms of PTH in the circulation. Results with two different antisera, each sensitive to different immunoreactive regions of the parathyroid hormone molecule, reveal differences in half-lives of parathyroid peptides. Antiserum C-329 recognizes more rapidly disappearing forms of the hormone. Antiserum 273 detects fragments (mostly C-terminal peptides cleaved from PTH) that disappear much more slowly from the circulation. Note that renal impairment causes a reduction in rate of disappearance of each form of the hormone. (From Berson, S. A., and Yalow, R. S.: Immunochemical heterogeneity of parathyroid hormone in plasma. *J. Clin. Endocrinol.* 28:1037, 1968.)

says in general is that they are too insensitive to differentiate between normal and hypoparathyroid states.

Biosynthesis

Recently the base sequences for the entire coding regions of the gene for human and bovine PTH have been determined utilizing cDNA copies of messenger RNA (mRNA). These analyses confirm by an independent method the amino acid sequences for the hormones obtained by classic techniques (Fig. 19–13). PTH is biosynthesized on the ribosome first as a 110-amino acid chain polypeptide called pre-pro PTH. This form of the hormone was first identified in *in vitro* biosynthetic experiments utilizing purified bovine PTH mRNA (mRNA) in a cell-free wheat germ extract capable of carrying out mRNA-directed peptide synthesis. The "pre-pro form" of the hormone is illustrated in Fig. 19–15. In the intact parathyroid cell itself, only biosynthesis of "pro-PTH" and PTH has been observed. It is believed that the amino acids constituting the additional 21-amino acid peptide representing the "pre-prohormone" are rapidly removed as the synthesized polypeptide is elaborated from the cytoplasmic matrix of the rough endoplasmic reticulum. The "pre" sequence is strikingly hydrophobic and probably facilitates movement of the nascent peptides onto or across membranes. Fig. 19–16 depicts the possible intracellular pathway for biosynthesis of PTH. After biosynthesis, proPTH is converted by another proteolytic process to PTH; this conversion occurs in the Golgi region of the cell. Transport from the Golgi may involve microtubular function in that vinblastine and colchicine inhibit the conversion of the proPTH to PTH and may even cause accumulation of the prohormone in the cell.

Initial studies on biosynthesis of PTH utilized incorporation of radioactive amino acids into slices of bovine parathyroid glands. With this experimental approach Cohn, MacGregor, et al. found that a peptide physically different in nature from bovine PTH is synthesized in the gland. It is now known, for example, that this peptide appearing early in the course of amino acid incorporation is distinct from PTH in gel electrophoresis (Fig. 19–17). Later in the course of incubation this labeled peptide is converted to a band migrating with authentic PTH. It is now recognized that the early synthesized material is a prohormone, proPTH, and represents the peptide intermediate through which the major storage and secretory product of the parathyroid

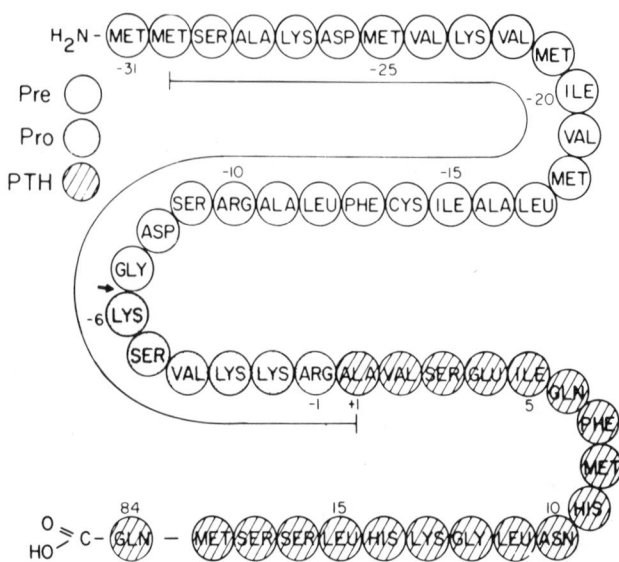

Figure 19–15. Structures for biosynthetic intermediates of parathyroid hormone. "Pre-pro-PTH" is the form in which the molecule is biosynthesized on the ribosomes and includes residues = 31 to 84. The latter is rapidly converted to pro-PTH (= 6 to 84) which is then converted to PTH, the form stored in and elaborated from secretory granules in the gland. See also Figure 19–16. (From Habener, J. F., Kemper, B. W., et al.: Biosynthesis of parathyroid hormone. *Recent Prog. Horm. Res. 33*:249, 1977.)

gland is biosynthesized. The prohormone is a peptide 90 amino acids in length with 6 additional amino acids at the N-terminal portion of the PTH molecule (Fig. 19–15). Presumably there is a specific enzyme in the parathyroid cell that carries out proteolytic cleavage to convert proPTH to PTH. Such an enzyme has not been isolated. It has been shown that trypsin or parathyroid glandular extracts can convert proPTH to PTH, however. ProPTH itself shows very little (less than 0.2% of native hormone) biologic activity when its cleavage is prevented. The additional 6 amino acids at the N-terminus thus strikingly reduce biologic potency of the molecule. This observation is compatible with biologic assays on synthetic parathyroid peptides; in general modification at the N-terminus compromises biologic activity. Conversion of prohormone within the gland to native hormone thus generates a highly potent polypeptide from one that is virtually biologically inactive.

BIOSYNTHETIC PATHWAY FOR PARATHYROID HORMONE
SEQUENTIAL PROTEOLYTIC CLEAVAGES

Figure 19–16. Scheme depicting biosynthesis of precursor and secretory forms of PTH. The "pre-pro PTH" form is biosynthesized on the ribosome and then transported across the membranes of the endoplasmic reticulum with concomitant cleavage to the pre-pro form of the hormone. The "pre-pro" segment may serve a transport function in translocating the biosynthetic precursor across the endoplasmic reticulum membrane. Within the cisterna of the endoplasmic reticulum, the pro-hormone is converted to the 1–84 amino acid PTH for packaging in secretory granules. This PTH molecule is elaborated from secretory granules into the circulation for subsequent interaction with specific PTH receptors in target tissues. The hormone also undergoes degradation to inert forms after secretion from the gland. In addition, some fragments of the molecule may be elaborated directly into the circulation from the parathyroid gland. (From Habener, J. F., Kemper, B. W., et al.: Biosynthesis of parathyroid hormone. *Recent Prog. Horm. Res. 33*:249, 1977.)

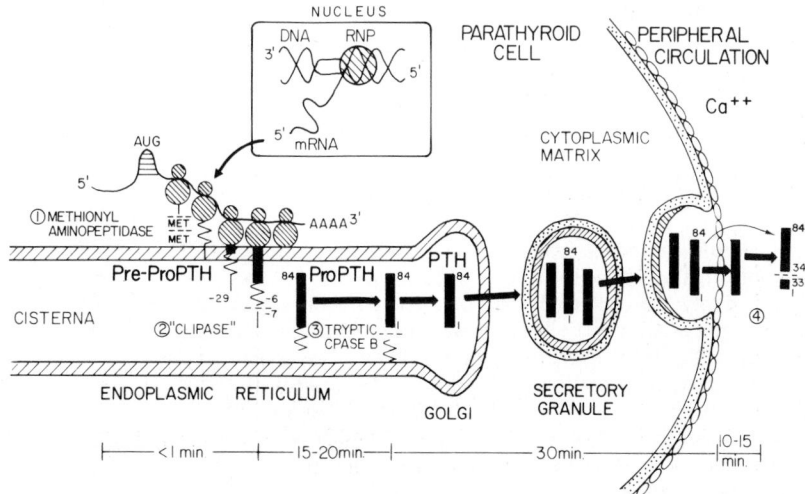

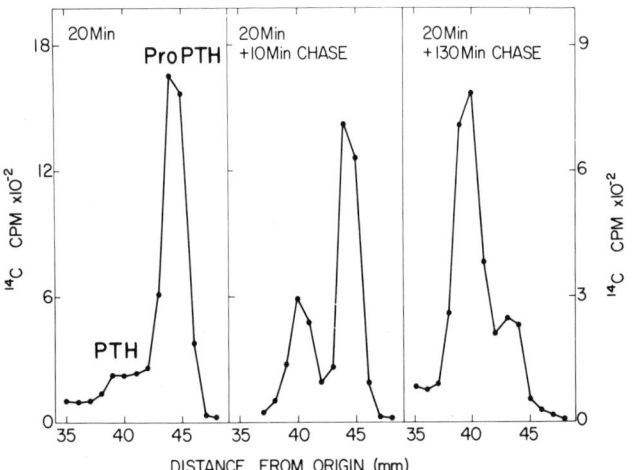

Figure 19–17. Biosynthesis of pro-PTH and conversion to PTH. Analyses by gel electrophoresis were carried out at the intervals shown after adding radioactive amino acids to parathyroid gland slices. This illustrates early production of radioactive pro-PTH and later appearance of radioactivity in PTH molecules. (From Habener, J. F., Kemper, B. W., et al.: Biosynthesis of parathyroid hormone. *Recent Prog. Horm. Res. 33*:249, 1977.)

Secretion of Parathyroid Hormone

It has been recognized for more than a quarter of a century that the concentration of calcium in the circulation is an important controlling factor for PTH secretion. This postulate is based on analyses by bioassay or radioimmunoassay of secreted hormone as well as on determination of radioactive peptides elaborated from glands incubated *in vitro*. It is known from *in vitro* studies, moreover, that a number of factors, e.g., catecholamines, prostaglandins, steroids, as well as several classes of drugs, are capable of influencing PTH secretion.

cAMP represents a major cellular regulator of PTH secretion. β-adrenergic catecholamines, dopamine, secretin, and prostaglandin E_1 each activate adenylate cyclase and cause increased concentrations of cAMP in parathyroid cells or tissue slices *in vitro*. cAMP produced in response to these agonists or in response to cyclic nucleotide phosphodiesterase inhibitors stimulates release of PTH. Conversely certain agents that inhibit PTH release or secretion, for example, calcium, α-adrenergic catecholamines, and prostaglandin $F_2\alpha$, inhibit cAMP accumulation in parathyroid cells. Thus PTH secretion seems to be intimately related to cAMP content of parathyroid cells. It is not known, however, at which stage of secretion cAMP produces its major effect. cAMP, moreover, is not the sole controlling influence on secretion, and the effects of calcium are not solely mediated through controlling cAMP concentration. Changes in calcium concentration affect changes in secretion out of proportion to effects on cAMP concentration.

Effects of Ions on Secretion

Calcium is the classically recognized regulator of PTH secretion and its inhibitory effect on secretion has been extensively documented with *in vivo* as well as *in vitro* experiments. Nevertheless, the precise mechanism whereby calcium regulates secretion has not been established. It is known that in some tissues there is a calcium-binding protein (calmodulin) that regulates either the adenylate cyclase enzyme or cyclic nucleotide phosphodiesterase (or both). Indeed it has been shown that calcium can inhibit adenylate cyclase activity in parathyroid tissue. The effect of

calcium on inhibiting cAMP accumulation is less marked than the effect of calcium on inhibiting PTH release, however. Calcium does not affect acutely the rate of biosynthesis of PTH. It does cause a sharp increase in the rate of intraparathyroid destruction of biosynthesized hormone. It is unknown whether calcium affects transcriptional or translational events within the gland, and there is no evidence that it influences the rate of conversion of proPTH to PTH. It is possible that a major effect of calcium on PTH release is effected at the level of fusion of secretory granules with the cell membrane, a locus apparently influenced in other endocrine tissues by calcium.* In any event, it has yet to be established how calcium exerts its major influence on secretion of PTH from either normal or abnormal parathyroid glands.

Magnesium also can affect PTH secretion. High concentrations of magnesium inhibit in a manner similar to calcium. On the other hand, extremely low concentrations of magnesium *in vitro* or profound hypomagnesemia *in vivo* interfere with PTH secretion.

Effects of Other Agents at the Subcellular Level

Microtubules and microfilaments are important for several types of cellular function, including intracellular transport and release of secretory products. Certain classes of drugs, colchicine, vinblastine, and cytochalasin, cause disruption of microtubular and microfilamentous function. Vinblastine and colchicine have been shown to inhibit secretion of PTH, and the latter was associated with disappearance of microtubules from parathyroid cells. Colchicine and vinblastine interfere with the conversion of proPTH to PTH in the bovine parathyroid cell. Colchicine also is known to cause hypocalcemia *in vivo* and to interfere with the peripheral action of PTH. Recent studies indicate that the predominant effect of colchicine *in vivo* in causing hypocalcemia is mediated peripherally and not through inhibition of secretion of PTH.

Effects of Other Drugs, Hormones and Vitamins

PTH release is dependent upon anion transport across the cell membrane of the parathyroid cell. Release of the hormone is inhibited by reducing external chloride or hydroxyl ion concentration or by interference with transport of these ions. For example, probenecid or disodium 4-acetamido-4'-isothiocyanostilbene-2, 2'-disulfonate (SITS), known anion channel blockers, inhibit release by 90–100%. It is possible that anion transport is part of the mechanism accounting for osmotic swelling of secretory granules with consequent release of hormone into the ECF.

High-affinity binding sites have been found in parathyroid glands for 1,25-dihydroxycholecalciferol (1, 25-[OH]$_2$-D$_3$ and high concentrations of this vitamin D metabolite modulate parathyroid release *in vivo*. 25-Hydroxycholecalciferol as well as 24,25-(OH)$_2$-D and 25,26-(OH)$_2$-D causes acute inhibition of PTH release in the dog. It also is of interest that vitamin D–deficient animals whose serum calcium is corrected by giving 1,25(OH)$_2$-D do not show appropriately suppressed PTH secretion compatible with the treated vi-

---

*In another system (the adrenal medulla) a calcium-binding protein, synexin, has been isolated that is required for fusion of secretory granules. This is but one of many endocrine systems wherein calcium can influence (usually stimulates; the parathyroid is an exception) secretion from endocrine tissue.

tamin D–deficient state. The precise role of vitamin D and its metabolites in regulating secretion is yet to be determined.

Several amines, including TRIS, diethylamine, and lysine amide, can interfere with conversion of proPTH to PTH *in vitro*. It has been proposed that these amines interfere at the level of the Golgi complex. Other factors influencing PTH secretion include vitamin A and cortisol (each are stimulatory). The significance of these observations for general physiology is not known.

Nature of Products Released from Parathyroid Glands

The major form of PTH secreted under normal physiologic conditions represents an active molecule of MW analogous to that of the pure 1–84 polypeptide. There is evidence, however, that under certain circumstances, particularly hypercalcemia, proportionally more fragments of PTH are released into the circulation. Moreover, another secretory product, parathyroid secretory protein (PSP; MW 150,000), has been identified through radioisotope incorporation experiments and is elaborated *in vitro* from gland slices. Its secretion responds to calcium or magnesium in a manner similar to that for PTH. The biologic significance of the PSP is unknown. It might represent a transport protein analogous to the neurophysins, proteins involved in the secretion of oxytocin (OT) and vasopressin (VP).

Metabolism of Parathyroid Hormone

Most of the radioimmunoassayable parathyroid products in the peripheral circulation are smaller than "native" PTH and represent predominantly carboxyterminal fragments of the 84-amino acid polypeptide. There is no general agreement about the biologic or chemical nature of PTH or fragments thereof in the circulation. Cleavage of the molecule carboxyl to residue 27 could conceivably contribute biologically active fragments into the circulation. Identification in plasma of biologically active (thus presumably aminoterminal) peptides shorter than 1–84 has been claimed, and perfusion of the kidney or liver can produce aminoterminal active fragments. On the other hand, there is general agreement that C-terminal peptides (approximately 7000 daltons, representing approximately two thirds of the native molecule at the carboxyterminus) indeed accumulate in the

circulation. Some reports suggest that the peripheral circulation also contains significant amounts of small (approximately 4000 daltons) fragments. Three general approaches have been utilized in attempts to sort out the nature of the circulating hormone: (1) Development of specific (C-reactive vs. N-terminal reactive) antisera; (2) fractionation by size of reactive peptides in plasma — usually gel filtration; and (3) chemical analyses of products after injection of radioactive hormone. Gel filtration studies show that most of the hormone immediately elaborated into the thyroid (parathyroid) veins segregates according to size on gel filtration in a fashion identical to that of native 1–84 polypeptide, whereas material in the peripheral circulation shows very much smaller concentrations of "intact" hormone and high concentrations of C-terminal reactive material approximately 7000 daltons (Fig. 19–18). Similarly gel filtration studies of plasmas containing high concentrations of intact hormone as well as fragments indicate that induction of hypercalcemia causes the intact fraction to disappear rapidly from peripheral circulation without acute change in concentration of fragments (principally C-terminal). The latter fractions also persist for hours (days with renal impairment) after parathyroidectomy when clinical hypoparathyroidism is clearly established. Gel filtration studies similarly show that the material in the peripheral circulation displaying an apparent MW of 7000 daltons show little or no cross-reactivity with antisera developed against the 1–34 synthetic fragment of PTH. Other studies show that after injection of radioiodine-labeled PTH into dogs, there is rapid disappearance of the intact molecule with appearance of carboxyterminal fragments. The micro-sequencing technique has been applied to the radioactive product recovered, and the results support the conclusion that at least one site for cleavage of PTH in the liver is between residues 33 and 34.

Origin of Parathyroid Hormone Fragments in Peripheral Circulation

It is possible that the parathyroid gland itself elaborates directly into the effluent plasma some of the fragments detected in the peripheral circulation. Silverman and Yalow calculated that the half-life and concentration of the fragments in the circulation allowed for the possibility that they were elaborated by the gland directly. More recent experiments analyzing gland effluent *in vivo* or perfusion of glands *in vitro* suggest that significant amounts of C-terminal reactive material may be elaborated directly from the gland.

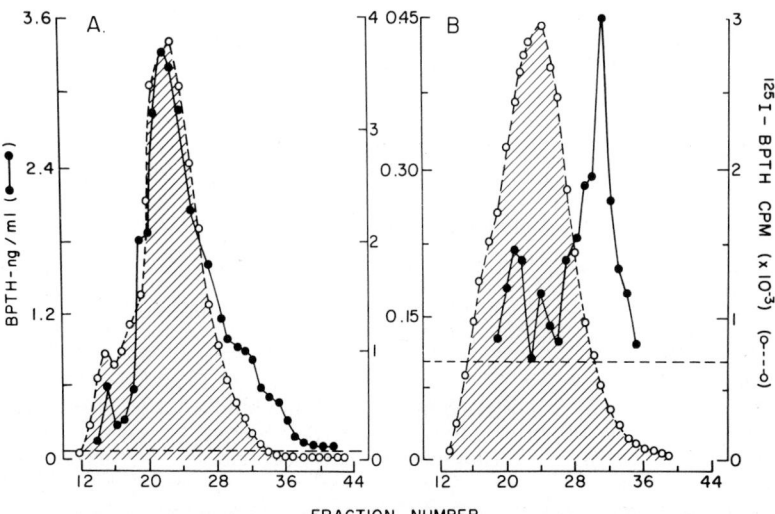

Figure 19–18. Immunoreactive forms of PTH in thyroid veins (A) and peripheral circulation (B) of the cow. The major component as immediately elaborated from the gland into the thyroid vein elutes on gel filtration columns in a position characteristic of the 84-amino acid polypeptide (shaded area). In the peripheral circulation the majority of immunoassayable activity appears in a fraction apparently lower in molecular weight than that immediately elaborated in the gland. (From Aurbach, G. D., and Phang: *Medical Physiology.* Vol. 2, Mountcastle, V. B. (ed.), St. Louis, C. V. Mosby, 1974, p. 1655, with permission.)

Although radioimmunoassay analyses and calculations based on disappearance rates allow for the possibility that parathyroid fragments are produced directly by the parathyroid gland, there is nevertheless clear evidence that part of the fragments in the circulation are generated by peripheral cleavage of intact hormone after it is secreted. Part of the peripheral degradation takes place in the kidney. The perfused dog kidney seems to extract intact PTH and causes degradation of the hormone in the process. The latter studies suggest also that intact PTH is taken up by the kidney (presumably at the plasma front of the tubule cells) independent of glomerular filtration rate (GFR), whereas the clearance of carboxyterminal fragments (via filtration and catabolism in the proximal tubular cells) by the kidney depends upon GFR. The fact that the kidney is an important source of degradation of the hormone as well as a major receptor tissue for action of the hormone has led to the suggestion that degradation of the hormone in the kidney is geared to binding to or release from specific receptors for the hormone. Indeed, it had even been postulated that biologic activity of the hormone was dependent upon cleavage of the 1–84 polypeptide to a smaller (e.g., 1–33) fragment. Available evidence makes the latter unlikely.

Significance of Parathyroid Hormone Fragments

The diverse information on PTH fragments must be evaluated with recognition of the following problems: (1) Neither gel filtration nor immunologic studies with putatively selective antisera necessarily discriminate completely between C-terminal and N-terminal fragments in the circulation; (2) quantitative conversion of endogenously synthesized intact PTH to fragments in the gland or in the periphery has not been documented; (3) there is no precise information on the chemistry of the putative fragments — the crude MW assignments may well be in error and could reflect aberrations in gel filtration characteristics as well as aggregation of smaller peptide fragments; (4) much of the work has been carried out without a standard reference preparation in the immunoassays (indeed there is no general availability of a standard for C-terminal fragments of the molecule); (5) conditions for immunoassay, gel filtration, and *in vitro* or *in vivo* controls for artifactual proteolysis have been lacking or nonuniform.

Summary

The best assessment of the data at this time is as follows: The major substance, if not the sole substance, active at the receptor level under normal physiologic conditions is the 84-amino acid parathyroid polypeptide that is elaborated intact from the glands; there is rapid cleavage of the secreted hormone in the periphery to C-terminal fragments of the molecule, which are biologically inert but immunologically highly reactive; part of the C-terminal material may be derived directly from the gland itself; the C-terminal fragments accumulate to a degree greater than normal in proportion to decrease in renal function. All of these problems compromise simple, direct interpretation of radioimmunoassays for clinical use (see Fig. 19–43).

Physiology

General

Calcium concentration in the ECF is the primary physiologic variable controlled by PTH. The concentration of calcium in the ECF is a function of the rate of transfer of calcium into and out of bone, the glomerular filtrate (GF), and the gastrointestinal tract (see Fig. 19–6). The general aspects of calcium metabolism are reviewed earlier in the chapter. PTH in particular stimulates the rate of reabsorption of calcium from the GF, enhances the rate of calcium resorption from bone, and influences the rate of absorption of calcium from the gastrointestinal tract secondarily through its influence on the renal formation of active vitamin D metabolites. Although the overall results of the influence of PTH on these three tissues, kidney, bone and gut, all lead to an increase in concentration of calcium in the ECF, the effects of the hormone on the different tissues take effect at different rates. The effect on the kidney is the most rapid, and increased clearance of calcium can be observed very rapidly after removal of the parathyroid glands in humans and experimental animals. Changes in resorption of calcium from bone *in vitro* occur in two phases. The earlier phase is manifested by release of calcium into the medium within 2–3 hours in response to the hormone and does not depend upon protein synthesis. The later phase presumably involves activation in biosynthesis of new proteins, particularly lysosomal enzymes, including collagenase and other hydrolytic enzymes, and is blocked by inhibitors of protein synthesis. *In vivo* the hypercalcemic effect attributable to enhanced absorption of calcium from the gut also is relatively slow to develop. This phenomenon depends upon formation of active vitamin D metabolites, which then reach intestinal cells through the circulation. In the intestinal cells the metabolites cause induction of new protein synthesis, in particular synthesis of proteins involved with calcium and phosphate transport across the intestinal wall. This indirect effect of the hormone on calcium absorption from the gut is brought about over a period of 24 hours or longer after administration of hormone.

PTH influences phosphate concentration in the ECF through two mechanisms. A reduction in plasma phosphate is produced by the direct phosphaturic action of PTH on the kidney; this is the predominant effect of the hormone under usual physiologic conditions. A rise in plasma phosphate may follow massive hormone-induced bone resorption with increased release of phosphate as well as other minerals from bone. If renal function is impaired, this effect may predominate. PTH also causes an increase in urinary hydroxyproline excretion, secondary to the hormone's influence on collagen metabolism. The major effects of PTH on kidney, bone, and other organs are discussed in the sections that follow.

Effects of the Parathyroid Hormone on the Kidney

Calcium Reabsorption

Excessive secretion of PTH ultimately is manifested by a rise in urinary calcium excretion. This effect, however, is secondary to the hypercalcemia (and thus high-filtered load of calcium) produced by the hormone. The direct action of the hormone on the kidney causes enhanced fractional reabsorption of calcium from the GF. This renal effect of the hormone is readily apparent in experiments measuring calcium clearance at varying plasma calcium concentrations with or without the influence of PTH. At any given level of calcium load to the kidney, there is decreased calcium clearance under the influence of PTH and increased calcium clearance in the absence of parathyroid secretion. Thus in the few hours after parathyroidectomy in animals or following removal of parathyroid adenomas from human beings, the urinary excretion of calcium increases. It is not until hypocalcemia has developed that urinary calcium excretion decreases. This renal effect of PTH is readily apparent in the golden hamster, which is extremely sensitive to this renal effect of PTH. Parathyroidectomy in this animal causes a marked loss of calcium into the urine, and the hypocalcemia attendant upon parathyroidectomy can be totally accounted for by increased renal loss of calcium during the immediate period following parathyroid ablation. Studies in humans similarly indicate that PTH regulates the reabsorption of calcium from the GF. The determination of renal clearance of calcium as a function of serum calcium can be a useful clinical parameter (Fig. 19–19). Hypoparathyroid or hyperparathyroid subjects show different rates of calcium excretion (expressed as mg/dl GF), which in turn differ significantly from those found in normal subjects.

Although it is clear that PTH influences calcium reabsorption in the nephron, the locus for this effect of the hormone and the mechanism whereby it is brought about have not been clearly established. Calcium clearance is closely linked to sodium clearance in the kidney, and it is possible that calcium and sodium share a common transport mechanism at some locus in the renal tubule. Replacement of sodium by choline or lithium inhibits calcium reabsorption in the proximal tubule, and ouabain, which inhibits sodium-potassium ATPase in the kidney, abolishes active calcium reabsorption in the kidney of the golden hamster. Although the bulk of calcium is reabsorbed in the proximal tubule, the major effect of PTH appears to occur beyond the proximal tubule. Micropuncture studies had suggested that PTH-enhanced calcium reabsorption takes place at some point distal to the ascending thin limb of the loop of Henle. The most recent studies indicate that the thick ascending segment responds to PTH with increased calcium flukes and that cAMP is the intracellular mediator of this effect.

Phosphaturic Effect

The effect of PTH in enhancing phosphate excretion is among the first physiologic effects of PTH discovered and perhaps is the most generally recognized. Nevertheless, the mechanism whereby this effect is brought about is still incompletely understood. This effect of the hormone appears to represent actions at two distinct loci within the nephron, the proximal and distal convoluted tubules. It has variously been proposed that the phosphaturic effect reflects a direct action of PTH on a phosphate transport system or conversely, that the effect is secondary to changes in sodium or bicarbonate (or both) reabsorption. Direct micropuncture

studies have shown that in the dog PTH causes a 30–40% reduction in proximal tubular reabsorption of sodium and phosphate, although this is effected with minimal or undetectable natriuresis. Infusion of dibutyryl cAMP causes a very similar effect on proximal reabsorption of sodium and phosphate. Thus PTH causes a net decrease in proximal reabsorption of phosphate, and this effect is mediated through cAMP generated in response to the hormone. There is recent further evidence that in addition to the proximal effect there is also a distal tubular effect of PTH that similarly produces decreased reabsorption of phosphate. The existence of multiple sites of action of PTH along the course of the nephron is substantiated further by biochemical results on segregated areas of the nephron (see "Mechanism of Action in the Kidney," p. 946).

Since sodium reabsorption is inhibited by PTH in the proximal tubule, it is possible that inhibition of phosphate reabsorption is secondary to effects on sodium. This possibility is made more tenable in that dibutyryl cAMP produces a similar influence on sodium and phosphate in the proximal tubule, and cAMP is known to be capable of regulating sodium transport in a number of tissues. Moreover, it has been shown that catecholamines, another class of hormones also acting through the adenylate cyclase–cAMP system, produce similar effects on sodium transport in the proximal tubule. Another suggestion is that phosphaturia is secondary to changes in intraluminal pH or proximal transport of bicarbonate. A rise in pH and bicarbonate content of the urine was also among the earliest physiologic effects observed for PTH. A rise in pH would change the ratio of $HPO_4^=$ to $H_2PO_4^-$ and consequently decrease the likelihood of reabsorption of phosphate; monovalently charged phosphate presumably is more readily translocated across cell membranes than is the divalently charged ion. Phosphate permeability is much less in the distal nephron than it is in the proximal tubules; thus phosphate rejected by any mechanism in the proximal tubule would likely cause increased elaboration of phosphate into the urine. Another potential factor in the phosphaturic effect is a general increase in proximal tubular cell metabolism caused by the action of PTH. For example, the inotropic action of catecholamines on perfused heart preparations is associated with elaboration of phosphate into the ECF. This presumably is a manifestation of increased cell utilization of ATP, since the rate of elaboration of phosphate into the ECF corresponds stoichiometrically with a decrease in intracellular concentration of creatine phosphate (the intracellular reservoir maintaining ATP concentrations constant).

Effects on Bicarbonate

Alkalinization of urine with increased bicarbonate content was discovered in the earliest tests on biologic responses to extracts of parathyroid glands. Recently, some 50 years after the initial observations, renewed attention has been directed toward the effect of PTH on bicarbonate transport. PTH causes a net inhibition of bicarbonate reabsorption in the proximal renal tubule; this leads to a type of proximal renal tubular acidosis. This is best discerned by studying the Tm for bicarbonate under the conditions of bicarbonate loading. Proximal renal tubular acidosis has been observed in hyperparathyroidism (see under "Primary Hyperparathyroidism"), and marked increases in bicarbonate clearance have been observed after infusion of parathyroid extract into humans. Enhanced delivery of bicarbonate to the distal tubule diminishes calcium reabsorption in the distal tubule, and this is associated with a decrease in calcium-sodium clearance ratio. A number of authors have called attention to the possible interrelationship between bicarbonate and

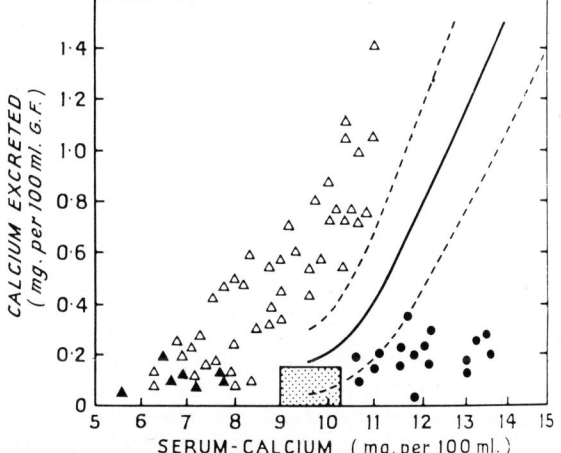

Figure 19–19. The urinary excretion of calcium as a function of serum Ca in normal subjects [solid line ± 2 (SD) — dotted lines] and in patients with hypoparathyroidism (△) and hyperparathyroidism (●). The shaded area represents the normal physiologic situation. (From Nordin, B. E. C., and Peacock, M.: Role of the kidney in regulation of plasma-calcium. *Lancet* 2:1280, 1969.)

phosphate reabsorption in the nephron. The proximal tubule clearly has the potential for bicarbonate transport. (Bicarbonate-induced phosphate excretion was discussed under "Phosphaturic Effect.") Whether the effect of PTH is to inhibit proximal bicarbonate reabsorption or stimulate proximal secretion of bicarbonate is not defined. Phosphate is not the only ion potentially influenced by intraluminal bicarbonate concentration. It has been reported that sodium bicarbonate infusion, even in the absence of PTH, causes increased distal tubular reabsorption of calcium. This suggests that high concentrations of bicarbonate in the distal tubule might facilitate calcium reabsorption.

Other Effects on the Kidney

Micropuncture studies indicate that PTH action mediated by cAMP inhibits isotonic fluid reabsorption in the proximal tubule. The sodium excluded from proximal reabsorption passes to the distal nephron, where presumably significant amounts of it are reabsorbed. The water associated with the sodium is incompletely reabsorbed, giving rise to a net increase in urine flow. This phenomenon may be similar to that observed with catecholamines, another class of hormones influencing ion transport through a cAMP mechanism. There is inhibition of proximal sodium reabsorption, part of which is reabsorbed in the distal tubule, giving rise to an increase in free water clearance. Another manifestation of PTH action on the kidney is an increase in the activity of the 1-α-hydroxylase enzyme leading to an increase in production of 1,25-dihydroxycholecalciferol from the substrate 25-hydroxycholecalciferol (see "Calciferol 1-α Hydroxylation," p. 954). It may be presumed that most or all actions of the hormone on the kidney are affected through the intermediation of cyclic 3',5'-AMP (see "Parathyroid Hormone — Mechanism of Action," p. 946).

Actions of Parathyroid Hormone on Bone

In addition to a direct action on the kidney in maintaining serum calcium, PTH acts directly also on bone, the chief reservoir of calcium within the body. The effect of PTH in mobilizing calcium from bone occurs in two or more phases: an early phase characterized by mobilization of calcium from areas of bone in more rapid equilibrium with the ECF, and a later phase associated with an increased synthesis of bone enzymes, particularly lysosomal enzymes associated with bone resorption. The later phase, but not the early phase, is blocked by inhibitors of protein synthesis. A very rapid (within 1 hour) effect of PTH has been shown *in vitro* as well as *in vivo*. Longer term effects of PTH on bone, release of calcium from bone, may be related to effects on bone remodeling. Bone remodeling, the resorption of older osteons and subsequent replacement with new bone formation, involves the actions of osteoclasts responsible for degradation of bone and subsequent infiltration and function of osteoblasts to synthesize new collagen and allow remineralization of replacement osteons.

PTH stimulates bone formation. Parathyroid tissue grafts to bone cause bone resorption at the surface immediately adjacent to the transplant. At the opposite surface there is increased bone deposition. A number of observers have noted areas of increased bone formation (osteosclerosis) in the bones of some subjects with primary hyperparathyroidism. These effects of PTH on bone formation may be part of an overall effect of PTH on controlling the rate of bone remodeling.

Cell Types Involved

There is an apparent increase in ratio of osteoclasts to osteoblasts in bone upon administration of PTH to experimental animals or in clinical hyperparathyroidism. Such observations led to the concept that osteoclasts represent selectively the target cells for PTH action in bone. It is now clear that PTH influences all three bone cell types — osteoclasts, osteoblasts, and osteocytes. Administration of hormone *in vivo* causes an apparent increase in the extracellular space of bone lacunae, presumptive evidence for resorption of bone immediately surrounding the osteocyte (osteocytic osteolysis). Other physiologic studies indicate that PTH inhibits collagen formation in bone. Since collagen formation in bone is primarily a function of osteoblasts, this is presumptive evidence that PTH can influence this cell type as well. It is now clear from work with separated distinct cell types that PTH affects osteoblastic function as well as osteoclastic function and that there are specific receptors for PTH on each (see discussion later). In general, short-term *in vitro* effects of PTH on osteoblasts are inhibitory, whereas effects on osteoclasts are stimulatory.

The early observations of increased numbers of osteoclasts in bone stimulated by PTH suggested that there was an actual conversion of osteoblasts to osteoclasts or that PTH induced an increased rate of conversion of osteoprogenitor cells to osteoclasts in bone. Neither of these hypotheses is satisfactory in light of recent discoveries about the origin of osteoclast-like cells. Studies on osteopetrotic mice and rats indicate that this disorder can be attributed to abnormal or defective or absent osteoclast function in bone. The defect can be corrected by injection of monocyte cell lines or thymic tissue from normal animals. Resorbing bone is chemotactic for circulating monocytes. Moreover, macrophages have been shown to contain PTH receptors (measured as adenylate cyclase). These several observations suggest strongly that osteoclasts do not find origin in skeletal tissue *per se* but may migrate to bone from thymic or other extraskeletal reticuloendothelial sources. Another interpretation of this set of experiments is that lymphocytes, monocytes, or macrophages may migrate to bone and rather than develop or give rise to osteoclasts directly merely control differentiation of other mesenchymal cells already in bone. This possibility must be considered in at least one of the rat models (IA rat) wherein PTH-activatable adenylate cyclase was detected in the osteoclasts. The osteoclasts, however, were abnormal in that the "ruffled border" response to PTH was lacking.

Scanning EM is another tool that has been acquired recently to study effects of PTH on bone cells. These studies provide further evidence for direct effects of PTH on osteocytes and osteoblasts. PTH brings about a rapid increase in elongation and extension of cellular processes in these cells.

Effects on Bone and Bone Cells In Vitro

Direct resorption of bone incubated or cultured *in vitro* occurs with addition of PTH. This enhanced osteolysis is accompanied by increased activity of osteoclasts and, initially at least, inhibition of osteoblast activity. There are increases in content and release of lysosomal enzymes as well as activation of carbonic anhydrase and an increase in uptake and incorporation of uridine. The increase in total enzyme activity is dependent upon new RNA and protein synthesis. Release of calcium from bone occurs in two phases, the early phase independent of induction of new enzyme synthesis and a later phase dependent upon synthesis of enzymes that lead to hydrolysis of bone collagen, protein, and matrix. Lysosomal enzymes are released rapidly from bone cultured with PTH. β-Glucuronidase is released as early or earlier than detectable release of calcium. Other effects of PTH on bone include enhanced synthesis of hyaluronate determined by incorporation of labeled glucosamine into hyaluronic acid, inhibition of citrate decarboxylation, inhibition of collagen synthesis, and changes in alkaline phosphatase activity. Alkaline phosphatase detected in cytochemical assays increases rapidly (3 min) in bone *in vitro* after exposure to PTH. At later times reduced alkaline phosphatase is observed. The exact mechanisms bringing about these changes are unknown; some or all may be mediated by the clearly defined increases in cell cAMP content in response to PTH (see under "Mechanism of Action," p. 946). Changes in calcium fluxes into and out of bone cells also may represent another intracellular signal initiating or modulating some of these events.

Isolation of Cell Types Sensitive to Parathyroid Hormone

The varied array of multiple effects, some inhibitory, some stimulatory, of PTH on bone *in vitro* is clarified somewhat by recent advances in the separation of bone cells. A technique for liberating cells from fetal calvaria was developed by Peck and his associates over a decade ago. Recent modifications of this technique involve timed release of cells. Cells released early in the course of digestion and cultured for several days are sensitive to both PTH and CT, whereas those released later in the course of digestion and similarly cultured are sensitive only to PTH (Fig. 19–20). The first cell type released is osteoclast-like; the cells released later show osteoblast-like features. These two cell types are distinct in their responses to PTH, 1,25-$(OH)_2$-D_3, and CT. Moreover, the separate cell types differ significantly in the nature of gross changes in mineral and enzyme contents in response to PTH *in vitro* (Table 19–6). Most of the stimulatory influences of PTH are on the osteoclast-like cells and include increases in the lysosomal enzymes. Conversely, the inhibitory influences of PTH on citrate decarboxylation, collagen synthe-

Table 19–6. ACTIONS OF PARATHYROID HORMONE AND CALCITONIN ON ISOLATED BONE CELLS *IN VITRO*

	"CT Cells"	"PT Cells"
Cyclic AMP content	↑ [a]	↑
Hyaluronate synthesis	↑ *	—
Acid phosphatase	↑ *	—
Alkaline phosphatase	—	↓
Prolyl hydroxylase	—	↓
Citrate decarboxylation	—	↓
β-glucuronidase release	↑ *[b]	
Acetylglucosaminidase release	↑ *[b]	

"CT cells" are presumed to represent osteoclasts; "PT cells," osteoblasts. Arrows refer to effect of parathyroid hormone: ↑ = stimulatory, ↓ = inhibitory

a. Calcitonin also increases cAMP content of CT cells.
*Calcitonin inhibits these actions of parathyroid hormone.
b. These effects on lysosomal enzyme release have been described only for whole bone *in vitro* but represent CT cell responses since they are inhibitable by calcitonin. Parathyroid hormone effects also have been described on release of the lysosomal enzymes galactosidase, cathepsin, and acid deoxyribonuclease.

sis, and alkaline phosphatase activity are manifestations of PTH activity primarily on osteoblast-like cells. 1,25-Dihydroxycholecalciferol or high concentrations of calcium affect enzyme activities in a manner similar to PTH or dibutyryl cAMP, suggesting that a change in cell calcium might be a mediator of the effects of increased cell cAMP content.

The new findings concerning action of the hormones on distinct separated cell types provide further evidence that more than one type of bone cell contains receptors for PTH, and the response of a particular cell to the hormone depends upon the nature of the cell and may explain as well the fact that PTH produces anabolic as well as catabolic effects on bone. These observations also are clearly compatible with the possibility that cells bearing PTH receptors are mobilized from distant sites and migrate to bone to mediate osteoclastic resorption. The studies further suggest that the inhibitory effects of PTH on one cell type as well as the stimulatory effects on another are mediated by cAMP.

Effects on the Intestine

Although the intestine represents one of the major organs supplying calcium to the ECF, PTH itself does not directly affect gastrointestinal absorption of calcium. Nevertheless, intestinal absorption of calcium does reflect parathyroid status; absorption is low in hypoparathyroidism and high in hyperparathyroidism and increases after treatment for several days with PTH (Fig. 19–21). The effect of PTH on gastrointestinal absorption of calcium is mediated indirectly through regulation of synthesis of 1,25-dihydroxycholecalciferol in the kidney. It is the latter metabolite of vitamin D that then causes enhanced absorption of calcium from the gastrointestinal tract. This is discussed further in the section on vitamin D metabolism.

Other Effects of Parathyroid Hormone

Intravenous injections of PTH cause an acute transient hypocalcemia that may reflect entry of calcium into cells (see Fig. 19–6). Parathyroid peptide-mediated calcium flux into and out of cells may represent a part of the mechanism of action of PTH and has been observed also with cells *in vitro*. Other effects of PTH observed experimentally include ac-

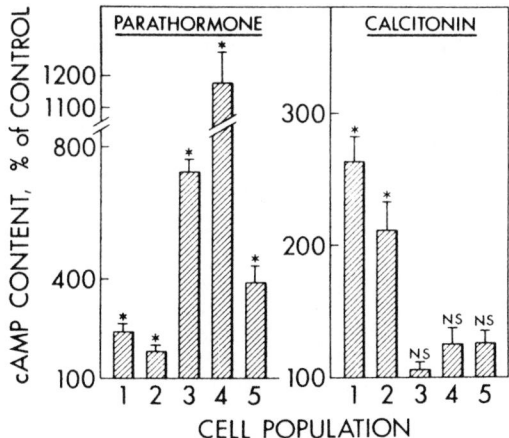

Figure 19–20. Distinct bone cell populations sensitive to PTH and CT, respectively. Cells are released at different rates from bone treated with collagenase *in vitro*. Cells bearing receptors for CT (osteoclast-like) are released early in the course of digestion. Another group of cells (osteoblast-like), released later in the course of digestion, is sensitive to PTH but not to CT. (From Cohn, D. V., and Wong, G. L.: The actions of parathormone, calcitonin, and 1,25-dihydroxycholecalciferol on isolated osteoclast- and osteoblast-like cells in culture. In *Endocrinology of Calcium Metabolism.* Copp, D. H., and Talmage, R. V. (eds.), Amsterdam, Excerpta Medica, 1978, p. 241.)

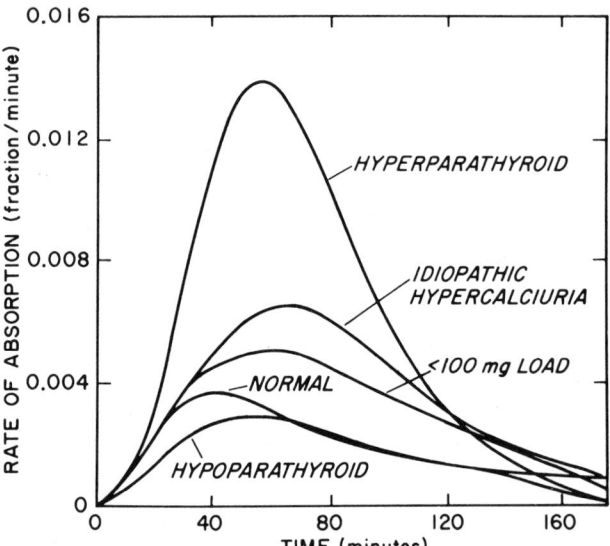

Figure 19–21. Rates of gastrointestinal absorption of calcium as a function of parathyroid status in man. (Modified from Birge, S. J., Peck, W. A., et al.: Study of calcium absorption in man: a kinetic analysis and physiologic model. *J. Clin. Invest. 48*:1705, 1969.)

tions on rates of mitosis of lymphocytes *in vitro*, changes in blood flow through the celiac axis, increased concentrations of calcium in the mammary gland, enhanced lipolysis in isolated fat cells, and increased gluconeogenesis in liver and kidney.

Mechanism of Action of Parathyroid Hormone

Receptors, Cyclic AMP, and Cell Activation

Calcium metabolism is controlled by PTH through interaction with specific receptors on distinct cell types in bone and kidney. Interaction of the hormone with these receptors causes activation of adenylate cyclase and increased generation within the cell of cyclic 3',5'-AMP, which in turn activates systems ultimately leading to increased enzyme and ion transport activities of affected cells. Hormone interaction with cell membranes may also produce other direct consequences such as changes in calcium flux into and out of cells.

Mechanism of Action in the Kidney

The discovery that PTH activates adenylate cyclase in plasma membranes obtained from cells in the kidney makes possible analysis of sites of action of hormones along the course of the nephron. Studies utilizing simple gross anatomic dissection indicated that PTH activates adenylate cyclase predominantly in the renal cortex, whereas vasopressin (VP) stimulates the enzyme in the medulla. These findings fit the physiologic concept that VP acts predominantly on collecting ducts and that calcium and phosphate transport, presumably under the regulation of PTH, occurs in the cortical portions of the nephron. Earlier studies also indicated that areas responsive to CT could be distinguished from the principal loci for either PTH or VP action. Later, elegant microdissection studies and ultrasensitive cytochemical analyses corroborated the earlier studies on gross anatomic dissection and provided much more precise localization of hormone-sensitive loci along the course of the nephron. Several different regions of the nephron from the

glomerulus and proximal cortical tubule through to the thin loop, distal convoluted tubule, and medullary portion of the collecting tubule are identifiable microscopically after microdissection from the kidney. Adenylate cyclase assays on the various segments of the rabbit kidney indicate that PTH receptors are distributed in the cortical regions of both the proximal and the distal tubules. Two areas of the proximal cortical tubule, the early convoluted and the straight portion, respond to PTH. In the distal cortical tubule, parathyroid-sensitive enzyme is found in the granular portion. (In the mouse the cortical ascending limb also responds to PTH.) Distinct sites segregated at least partially from the parathyroid-responsive regions are found for CT (primarily cortical ascending limb), VP (collecting tubule), and catecholamines. The latter acts also in the distal convoluted tubule but at at a site just proximal to the distal site for PTH (Fig. 19–22). The distribution found for PTH-sensitive adenylate cyclase agrees with the physiologic findings that PTH influences phosphate transport at proximal and at distal tubular sites. Information gathered from cytochemical assays for enzymes activated in response to PTH lends further support for two separate regions of the nephron sensitive to PTH. In the proximal convoluted tubule, PTH also causes activation of alkaline phosphatase and carbonic anhydrase. In the distal convoluted tubule, PTH at extremely low concentrations (1–1000 femtograms [fg]/ml) causes activation of G6PD. These findings not only corroborate the previously cited evidence that PTH acts both proximally and distally but also provide further information of theoretical as well as of practical value. The exquisitely sensitive response of G6PD activity in the distal tubule forms the basis for an ultrasensitive biologic assay for PTH (see p. 937).

The studies cited previously on localization of receptors in the kidney obviously provide elegant and precise information on location of receptors but are based upon actions of the hormone at points distal to immediate receptor interaction. The requirement for receptor interaction of PTH for activation of adenylate cyclase is supported further by the studies with a competitive inhibitor of PTH action. The synthetic

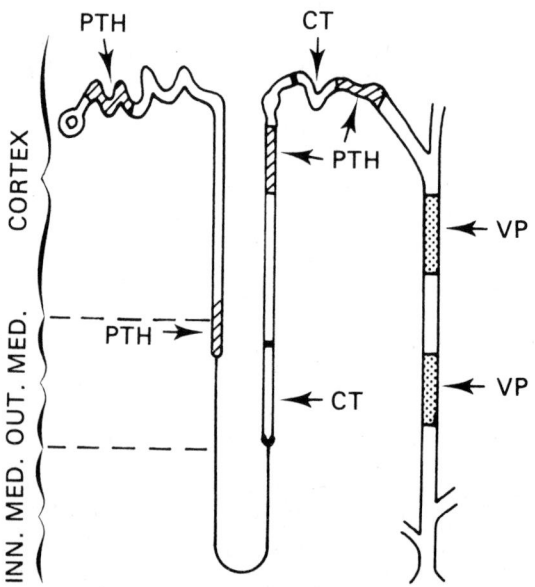

Figure 19–22. Schematic depicting regions of the nephron of the rabbit sensitive to PTH and CT. Discontinuities in hormone response from one region to another are not as abrupt as shown here for illustrative purposes. (Modified from Chabardes, D., Imbert-Teboul, M., et al.: In *Endocrinology of Calcium Metabolism.* Copp, D. H., and Talmage, R. V. (eds.), Amsterdam, Excerpta Medica, 1978, p. 209.)

polypeptide analog of the PTH sequence 3–34 has been shown to competitively inhibit the activation of renal adenylate cyclase by PTH. Some progress has been made toward identifying PTH receptors by direct binding studies, but the technology so far has not advanced to the degree that the interactions determined can be defined as specifically dependent upon biologically relevant PTH molecules. The sensitivity of the competitive binding methods also is insufficient to allow direct determination of hormone receptor interactions on microdissected segments of the nephron. Although several laboratories have provided suggestive evidence that PTH-receptor interactions in the kidney can be identified, the specificity of these interactions has not been definitively established.

Mechanism of Activation of Adenylate Cyclase Enzyme

Studies in several hormone receptor systems indicate that activation of adenylate cyclase by polypeptide or amine hormones is not a function solely dependent upon hormone-receptor interaction. Indeed it is now clear that hormone receptors represent distinct molecules separable from adenylate cyclase itself and that hormonal activation of adenylate cyclase is dependent upon at least three or four interacting proteins or enzymes: (1) hormone receptor, (2) guanine nucleotide and guanine nucleotide binding protein, (3) the adenylate cyclase catalytic unit itself, and (4) GTPase enzyme. The initial interaction of hormone with receptor facilitates binding of an endogenous guanine nucleotide (most likely guanosine triphosphate [GTP]), with a guanine nucleotide-binding protein. The activity of adenylate cyclase is dependent upon interaction with the guanine nucleotide-binding protein and GTP. With GTP bound to it, the regulatory protein–adenylate cyclase complex is active. A guanosine triphosphatase (GTPase) activity is responsible for deactivating adenylate cyclase. Pseudohypoparathyroidism, a disorder apparently representing a defect in renal (and possibly skeletal) receptor–adenylate cyclase complex sensitive to PTH, may be attributable to a defect in the function facilitated by GTP in the adenylate cyclase system (see "Pseudohypoparathyroidism," p. 993). GTP and a nonhydrolyzable guanine nucleotide analog (guanylylimidodiphosphate) are known to facilitate activation of PTH-stimulatable adenylate cyclase. The role of guanine nucleotides in the parathyroid receptor–adenylate cyclase system has not been defined as elegantly as it has been for the catecholamine-activated adenylate cyclase system, however.

Cyclic 3',5'-AMP Accumulation in the Kidney and Effects on Protein Kinase

PTH causes a rapid increase in cAMP concentration in kidney slices or renal tubules incubated *in vitro*. This is largely independent of the vitamin D status of the animal and reflects activation of adenylate cyclase in the plasma membrane of the cells involved. cAMP accumulated in specific receptor-bearing cells causes activation of enzymes and ion transport systems in cells of the nephron that respond physiologically to PTH. Another class of enzymes, protein kinases, responds to cAMP accumulation and catalyzes phosphorylation of cell enzyme and transport systems.

Protein kinases catalyze the transfer of the γ-phosphate of ATP to a hydroxyamino acid (usually serine) in the acceptor protein. Kinase activation by cAMP has been implicated in the inactivation of glycogen synthetase and the activation of phosphorylase, adipocyte lipase, steroidogenesis in the

testis, and ion transport in avian erythrocytes, in toad bladder, and in mammalian kidney. cAMP-sensitive protein kinases are composed of two types of subunits. The regulatory subunit is a protein that specifically binds cAMP. On interaction with cAMP, the regulatory subunit with cAMP bound to it dissociates from the catalytic unit to yield an active kinase enzyme. Of particular interest in the nephron is the apparent polarity of distribution of cAMP-dependent protein kinase. Identification of cAMP by immunofluorescent techniques shows that after injection of PTH there is aggregation of fluorescent granules at the luminal surface of tubular cells. Moreover, separation of luminal brush border membranes from basal lateral membranes of the renal cortical tubule indicates that cAMP-protein kinase is located in the luminal (brush border microvilli) region. Conversely adenylate cyclase sensitive to PTH is located in the basal lateral portion of the cell. These several studies imply that cAMP generated at the plasma membrane in response to PTH-activated adenylate cyclase migrates through the cell, binds to the cAMP receptor kinase complex, and activates the kinase at the luminal surface. The concentration of cAMP at the luminal surface may explain the ready access of cAMP to the luminal fluid and thus the appearance in the urine of large amounts of nephrogenously generated cAMP under the influence of circulating PTH (see discussion on cAMP in the section "Urinary Excretion of 3'5'-cAMP").

Activation of Enzyme and Transport Processes in the Renal Tubule

A number of systems are activated within the renal tubule in response to PTH; alkaline phosphatase, glucose-6-phosphate dehydrogenase, gluconeogenesis, and transport of sodium, phosphate, bicarbonate, and calcium have been documented. Activation of the transport processes and gluconeogenesis seems clearly dependent upon the intermediation of cAMP, in that addition of exogenous dibutyryl cAMP stimulates each of these processes (see discussion under "Parathyroid Hormone — Effects of the Hormone on the Kidney," p. 942). Direct evidence that cAMP is involved in activation of the other enzymes is not available. Since cAMP-dependent protein kinase is concentrated at the luminal brush border of the renal tubular cell, it is possible that the transport phenomena activated thereby also exist in polar distribution along the luminal border of the cell. The fact that cAMP is found in the tubular fluid and that cAMP-dependent kinases are located in the luminal border of cells raises the question of whether cAMP might be a mediator of cell-to-cell communication along the course of the nephron. This phenomenon would allow for the possibility of activation of enzymes within the nephron at a site distant from the cell immediately activated by PTH interaction with specific hormone receptors. There is evidence in *in vitro* systems that cAMP can be a mediator of cell-to-cell communication. Such has not been demonstrated in the nephron, however.

Microtubular Function of Cyclic AMP

Certain functions mediated in receptor tissues by cAMP appear to involve microtubules of cells. Microtubular systems bind colchicine, vinblastine, and cytochalasin, and these agents disrupt microtubular function. Colchicine causes hypocalcemia and interferes with the action of PTH in maintaining calcium concentrations in the ECF. Colchicine and vinblastine also interfere with cell transport processes in the kidney and the action of PTH on bone. These results, the actions of inhibitors on microtubular function and other observations of apparent phosphorylation of microtubular systems by cAMP-regulated protein kinases, allow speculation that microtubules are involved in the cAMP protein kinase–mediated actions of PTH on both bone and kidney.

Mechanism of Parathyroid Hormone Action on Bone

The discussion on physiology of the hormone indicated that there must be PTH receptors on all major types of bone cells, osteoclasts, osteoblasts, and osteocytes. Separation of osteoclast-like from osteoblast-like cells indicates that both types of cells respond to PTH with activation of adenylate cyclase and generation of cyclic 3',5'-AMP. The sequence of events — binding to the hormone receptor, activation of adenylate cyclase, and generation of cAMP — seems clearly implicated in the mechanism of action of PTH on bone cells and consequent mobilization of bone mineral and induction of bone resorption. Incubation of PTH with bone segments *in vitro* causes a rapid and progressive increase in concentration of cAMP in proportion to the amount of PTH added. Hormones not known to induce bone resorption include ACTH, TSH, glucagon, LH, insulin, and GH and cause no change in cAMP content of bone *in vitro*. Conversely, at least one other group of factors, the prostaglandins of the E series, known to produce bone resorption also cause an increase in cAMP content of bone. Further evidence that cAMP is a mediator of bone resorption includes induction by dibutyryl cAMP of lysosomal enzymes in bone and of resorption *in vitro*. Cellular specificity of these responses is not clearly explainable, however. For example, cAMP apparently mediates the stimulatory function of PTH as well as the inhibitory effect of calcitonin on osteoclasts. Perhaps osteoclasts themselves can be subdivided into populations bearing PTH receptors on the one hand and calcitonin receptors on the other. Alternatively, each hormone might influence in distinct ways parallel phenomena (e.g., ion fluxes) that might modulate responses to cAMP. Colchicine *in vitro* disrupts microtubule assemblies in osteoclasts, decreses frequency of ruffled borders on osteoclasts, and prevents hormone-induced resorption of bone.

Cyclic Nucleotides in the Extracellular Fluids

The original novel observations of Sutherland and his collaborators indicated that cyclic nucleotides appear in the ECF and that changes in hormonal status can influence the concentration of cyclic nucleotides therein. They showed that hypophysectomy reduced the urinary excretion of cyclic 3',5'-GMP and that this was restored toward normal by administering thyroxine (T_4) or mixtures of pituitary hormones, or both. In the same set of studies, however, hypophysectomy was without effect on urinary excretion of cyclic 3',5'-AMP even though certain pituitary hormones were known to act through the intermediation of this cyclic nucleotide. It is now clear that part of the cAMP generated extracellularly in response to specific hormones in particular receptor tissues is extruded into the surrounding medium or body fluid. Thus plasma cAMP is derived from diverse tissues and ablation of a single organ does not necessarily cause a major change in concentration of cAMP in plasma. It is likely that the cAMP content of the ECF reflects the sum of contributions of individual tissues, each of which is sensitive to a particular hormone or set of hormones. For example, the cAMP content of the hepatic vein plasma reflects stimulation by endogenous glucagon of hepatic cells; in the adrenal it reflects endogenous ACTH.

Clearance of Cyclic Nucleotides from the Plasma

Half-life for disappearance of cAMP or cyclic 3',5'-GMP from plasma is virtually identical and approximates 30 min. Both cyclic nucleotides appear to distribute in a space exceeding the extracellular volume. Renal clearance of the cyclic nucleotide into the urine accounts for about 20% of the entire clearance of cyclic nucleotides from the miscible pool. In the dog, the kidney accounts for 30% of the total clearance of cAMP from plasma. Only about two thirds of this renal clearance is accounted for by excretion. The remainder appears to represent enzymic destruction within the kidney.

The major sources contributing to plasma cAMP have yet to be defined with certainty. Although PTH, catecholamines, ACTH, and glucagon each in large doses can cause a rise in plasma cAMP, none of the corresponding receptor tissues, liver, kidney, or adrenal, seem to be the major source of plasma cAMP under resting conditions.

Urinary Excretion of 3',5'-cAMP

Although the sources of plasma cAMP are not known in detail, there is considerable knowledge about the origin of cAMP in the urine. Fifty to 60% of cAMP in the urine reflects that cleared from the plasma by glomerular filtration and the remaining 40–50% is contributed directly by the kidney itself (nephrogenous cAMP).

The fact that circulating biologically active PTH is a major influence on urinary cAMP has led to development of this parameter for clinical diagnosis. Injection of PTH causes a striking increase in urinary cAMP excretion; parathyroidectomy either in normal subjects or in those with hyperparathyroidism causes a striking reduction in urinary cAMP excretion. Similarly, infusion of calcium, causing inhibition of parathyroid secretion, leads to decreased urinary cAMP excretion. This effect of PTH is due to the direct activation by the hormone of adenylate cyclase in the renal tubule and consequent release of cAMP (nephrogenous cAMP) from tubular cells into the luminal fluid. Extensive analyses have been carried out on cAMP clearance in normal subjects, in those with hyperparathyroidism, and in those with hypoparathyroidism. Determinations of creatinine and cAMP in the same plasma and urine samples allow calculations of urinary cAMP excretion expressed in a variety of parametric forms: cAMP excretion in nmol/min, in nmol/mg of creatinine, and in nmol/dl of GF; cAMP clearance; clearance ratio for cAMP:creatinine; and nephrogenous cAMP in nmol/dl GF. Presentation of the data as nephrogenous cAMP expressed in nmol/dl of GF gives the sharpest differentiation between hypoparathyroid, normal, and hyperparathyroid groups and the least overlap (see Fig. 19–44). The discrimination between these groups was almost as good when the data were expressed as total urinary cAMP as a function of GFR in nmol of cAMP/dl GF. The latter parameter represents a simple correction of urinary cAMP:creatinine ratio for plasma creatinine ($U_{cAMP}/U_{Cr}) \times P_{Cr}$ without determining plasma cAMP. The parameters expressing cAMP as a function of GF circumvent the disadvantages of expressing urinary cAMP as simply a rate (per unit time or per mg creatinine). Rate *per se* can vary with several other functions, including sex (females excrete less creatinine and thus show a higher basal cAMP:creatinine ratio than do males), debilitating illness, for example hyperthyroidism, or any disturbance causing a decrease in creatinine production.

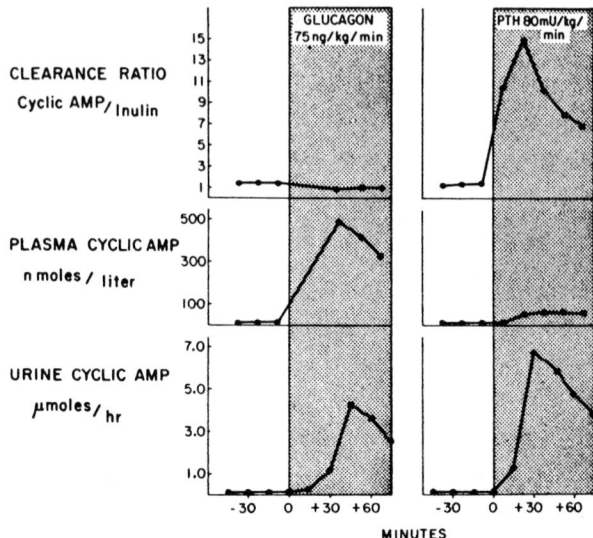

Figure 19–23. Cyclic 3',5'-AMP response patterns to glucagon and PTH in man. Both glucagon and PTH cause an increase in urinary excretion of AMP. PTH causes an increase in nephrogenous cyclic AMP and a marked increase in the clearance ratio of cyclic AMP to creatinine. The increase caused by glucagon reflects AMP cleared from the plasma by GF. (From Kaminsky, N. I., Broadus, A. E., et al.: Effects of parathyroid hormone on plasma and urinary adenosine 3',5'-monophosplate in man. *J. Clin. Invest.* 49:2387, 1970.)

Other Physiologic Influences on Urinary Cyclic AMP Excretion

The injection of glucagon, VP and catecholamines also influences the gross rate of urinary excretion of cAMP. Vasopressin, like PTH, is known to activate adenylate cyclase in specific regions of the nephron. VP, nevertheless, causes only minor changes in excretion of cAMP, and generally the contribution from this action is negligible. Glucagon causes an increase in urinary cAMP, but in this instance the effect reflects the direct action of this hormone on the liver. As a consequence, the concentration of cAMP in plasma (Fig. 19–23) increases markedly and is then cleared by glomerular filtration through the kidney. The effects of glucagon and PTH on urinary excretion of cAMP can be differentiated by the simultaneous measurement of plasma and urine cAMP. Volume expansion also causes an increase in urinary excretion of cAMP, and this effect apparently is mediated at least in part by increased secretion of PTH. Under basal conditions none of these latter factors significantly influence the parameter — cAMP excreted per dl of GF.

CALCITONIN

Parafollicular Cells

Calcitonin in humans is produced by the parafollicular or "C" cells of the thyroid gland. These cells were recognized as being distinct from the iodothyronine-producing follicular cells of the thyroid as early as 1876, but the origin and physiologic role of the parafollicular cells have only recently been elucidated.

Embryology

In submammalian vertebrates, the most caudal (5th) branchial pouch gives rise to a distinct structure, the ultimobranchial body, which has been shown to contain CT-secreting cells. In humans, the ultimobranchial body and the medial portion of the 4th branchial pouch become incor-

porated into the lateral lobes of the thyroid, accounting for the intrathyroidal location of the parafollicular cells. Embryologic studies have shown that the primordial cells that give rise to the parafollicular cells are derived from ectodermal neural crest precursors that migrate ventrally into the branchial pouch rather than from branchial endoderm.

Distribution, Histology and Ultrastructure

Parafollicular cells compose about 0.1% of the epithelial cell mass of the normal adult thyroid and are primarily localized in the central region of the middle third of each lateral lobe. They may occur singly or in clusters; ultrastructural analyses have shown that all C cells are present *within* follicles and are separated from the colloid by the follicular cell cytoplasm and from the interstitium by the follicular basement membrane.

The parafollicular cells are larger than follicular cells and have a large clear nucleus. These morphologic criteria may permit identification of parafollicular cells but definitive identification is provided by a variety of histochemical and immunochemical techniques. Thus, parafollicular cells stain with silver nitrate (argyrophilia) and display masked metachromasia (staining by toluidine blue after mineral acid hydrolysis). Like several other polypeptide-secreting cells (e.g., pancreatic islet cells), parafollicular cells take up and decarboxylate amine precursors such as 5-hydroxytryptophan. The relationship of this property (amine precursor uptake and decarboxylation or APUD) to polypeptide synthesis and secretion has not been clarified.

Immunochemical studies provide direct evidence for the role of parafollicular cells in the synthesis and secretion of CT. Both immunofluorescence and immunoperoxidase techniques have been employed with antibodies directed against CT (Fig. 19–24). These techniques are the most sensitive and specific for identifying parafollicular cells.

Electron microscopy of parafollicular cells shows membrane-bound granules, abundant mitochondria, microtubules, well-developed Golgi region, free ribosomes, and relatively poorly developed rough endoplasmic reticulum. Adrenergic nerve terminals abutting on parafollicular cells have been observed in some studies; this has provoked

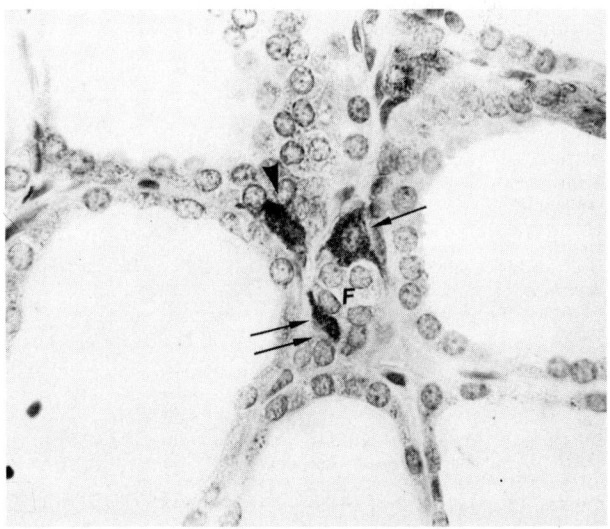

Figure 19–24. Normal adult thyroid gland stained according to the Steinberger peroxidase-antiperoxidase technique, employing a primary antiserum to human CT M and with a methyl green counterstain. The C cell lying in the center (single arrow) has a triangular shape with elongated cytoplasmic processes. Portions of two other C cells (arrow head and double arrows) are also present in this section. Magnification × 640. (Figure kindly provided by Dr. Ronald A. DeLellis.)

speculation regarding sympathetic modulation of CT secretion.

Acute hypercalcemia causes marked degranulation of parafollicular cells. Chronic hypercalcemia leads to hypertrophic changes, including an increase in cell content of free ribosomes, rough endoplasmic reticulum, and Golgi elements.

Chemistry of Calcitonins

Calcitonin polypeptides have been isolated from at least nine different species and uniformly consist of a 32-amino acid polypeptide with an N-terminal 7-membered disulfide ring and a C-terminus of prolineamide. The structures are remarkable in that as many as 19 of the 32 amino acids differ in the most diverse (human versus ovine) forms of the polypeptide. The striking differences in structure of the several forms of CT are apparent in the amino acid sequences shown in Table 19–7. There are, however, a number of features common to the molecules in addition to the aminoterminal disulfide bridge and constant chain length terminated in prolineamide. Six of the seven aminoterminal residues are identical in all CT's, and the sequence variability of the middle region of the molecule (residues 10–27) is more apparent than real. Although no single amino acid in this region is constant in all of the known congeners, they show similar types of side chain function in this region. An acidic residue (aspartic acid or glutamic acid) is found uniformly at position 15, and the only other acid residue is found at position 30. Basic residues are also limited to a few positions. When substitutions for basic residues occur, asparagine or glutamine is the most common replacement. Aromatic residues may exist at positions 12, 13, 16, 19, 22, or 27 but have never been found within the aminoterminal 11 residues. All variants contain at least one aromatic amino acid, but some contain neither tryptophane or tyrosine. The ovine molecule is unique in that it contains three tyrosines.

Certain similarities and differences among the CT congeners are of interest in terms of evolutionary implications. The fish CT's and chicken CT are immunologically similar and represent the most highly biologically potent of the CT molecules. The human and rat hormones are closely related in amino acid sequence and also show a high degree of immunologic cross-reactivity.

Structure-Function Relationships

The availability of natural and synthetic CT congeners has led to development of considerable information concerning structure and activity. The entire 32-amino acid chain appears to be required for significant biologic activity. Even the comparatively long fragments consisting of residues 10–32 or 1–10 joined to residues 20–32 (with omission of the central nonapeptide) are inactive. In fact, shortening the chain by omission of even a few amino acids causes almost complete loss of biologic activity even if the C-terminal prolineamide residue is retained. Methionine, when located at position 8 immediately adjacent to the heptapeptide ring, represents a site of potential inactivation through oxidation. Conversion of the methionine to methionine sulfone at this locus destroys the biologic activity. When methionine is located at position 25, oxidation does not alter biologic activity. An acidic carboxyl function is not essential for activity and indeed substitution of asparagine for the aspartic acid at position 15 in bovine CT enhances biologic potency.

The strikingly enhanced biologic potency of the piscine hormones compared to other CT's is of particular interest. Their amino acid sequences show certain loci (positions 11, 13, 17, 19, 20, and 24) uniquely characteristic to the most active molecules. One possible explanation for enhanced potency of salmon CT I includes an increase in hydrophilicity; however, this property is not seen in salmon CT II or in the eel CT's, which are also highly potent. It is perhaps also important to note that salmon CT shows the highest net positive charge of all the CT's known to date. Deamidation of the carboxylterminal proline (with consequent increase in negative charge in the molecule) leads to reduced biologic activity. Further, substitution of asparagine for aspartic acid at position 15 also enhances activity. Areas of increased positive charge may be of importance in binding to receptors. On the other hand, it is not possible currently to define precisely the structural properties that account for the high biologic potency of the piscine hormone.

Biologic Assay of Calcitonin

Biologic assays for CT generally are based on the hypocalcemic effect on the bone. The simplest bioassays depend upon subcutaneous injection of test material in rats, al-

Table 19–7. AMINO ACID SEQUENCE OF THE CALCITONINS*

Species		2		4	5			8		10		12		14		16
Eel	—	Ser	—	—	—	—	—	Val	—	—	Lys	Leu	Ser	—	Glu	Leu
Salmon I	—	Ser	—	—	—	—	—	Val	—	—	Lys	Leu	Ser	—	Glu	Leu
Salmon II	—	Ser	—	—	—	—	—	Val	—	—	Lys	Leu	Ser	—	—	Leu
Salmon III	—	Ser	—	—	—	—	—	Met	—	—	Lys	Leu	Ser	—	—	Leu
Human	Cys	Gly	Asn	Leu	Ser	Thr	Cys	Met	Leu	Gly	Thr	Tyr	Thr	Gln	Asp	Ph
Rat	—	—	—	—	—	—	—	—	—	—	—	—	—	—	—	Leu
Porcine	—	Ser	—	—	—	—	—	Val	—	Ser	Ala	—	Trp	Arg	Asn	Leu
Bovine	—	Ser	—	—	—	—	—	Val	—	Ser	Ala	—	Trp	Lys	—	Leu
Ovine	—	Ser	—	—	—	—	—	Val	—	Ser	Ala	—	Trp	Lys	—	Leu

Species		18		20		22		24		26		28		30		32
Eel	His	—	Leu	Gln	—	Tyr	—	Arg	—	Asp	Val	—	Ala	—	Thr	—
Salmon I	His	—	Leu	Gln	—	Tyr	—	Arg	—	Asn	Thr	—	Ser	—	Thr	—
Salmon II	His	—	Leu	Gln	—	—	—	Arg	—	Asn	Thr	—	Ala	—	Val	—
Salmon III	His	—	Leu	Gln	—	—	—	Arg	—	Asn	Thr	—	Ala	—	Val	—
Human	Asn	Lys	Phe	His	Thr	Phe	Pro	Gln	Thr	Ala	Ile	Gly	Val	Gly	Ala	Pro-NH$_2$
Rat	—	—	—	—	—	—	—	—	—	Ser	—	—	—	—	—	—
Porcine	—	Asn	—	—	Arg	—	Ser	Gly	Met	Gly	Phe	—	Pro	Glu	Thr	—
Bovine	—	Asn	Tyr	—	Arg	—	Ser	Gly	Met	Gly	Phe	—	Pro	Glu	Thr	—
Ovine	—	Asn	Tyr	—	Arg	Tyr	Ser	Gly	Met	Gly	Phe	—	Pro	Glu	Thr	—

*Table modified from Potts, J. T., Jr., and Aurbach, G. D.: Chemistry of the calcitonins, In *Handbook of Physiology;* Section 7: *Endocrinology;* Volume 7: *Parathyroid.* American Physiological Society. Greep, R. O., and Astwood, E. B. (eds.), Baltimore, Williams & Wilkins, 1977, p. 423.

The entire sequence is shown for human calcitonin. Dashes indicate residues identical to those in human molecule. Residues shown for other calcitonins are only those that differ from human calcitonin. Results for rat calcitonin are those of Raulais et al.: *Eur. J. Biochem.* 64:607, 1976.

though intravenous assays have also been developed. Generally the minimum amount of hormone detected by *in vivo* bioassay is 0.1–1 mU. An *in vitro* assay may be performed with renal membrane adenylate cyclase. This assay has not been generally established but is sensitive to the subnanogram range for salmon CT and should be adaptable for general bioassay use for CT.

Radioimmunoassays

Radioimmunoassays have been established for several species of CT. The first to be developed was for the porcine hormone, the first to be isolated and analyzed for structure. Radioimmunoassays for human CT are based upon antibodies to either synthetic or isolated human CT. In either event, the antigen represents the amino acid sequence found in medullary carcinoma of the thyroid. The structures of porcine, salmon, and human CT differ strikingly (Table 19–7) and, as would be anticipated, there is very poor immunologic cross-reactivity between these hormones. The rat and human hormones are similar, however, and indeed one of the useful radioimmunoassays for rat CT was developed by immunizing rats with human CT. The immunoassays for rat and porcine CT's have been extremely useful for physiologic investigations. The immunoassay for human CT is important in discovery and treatment of medullary carcinoma of the thyroid.

Secretion of Calcitonin

Several secretagogues for CT have been identified. Calcium stimulates secretion of CT in virtually all species tested. In addition, β-adrenergic catecholamines and several peptides, including glucagon (in dogs), cholecystokinin, gastrin, and cerulein, cause release of CT. Cerulein and cholecystokinin share the tetrapeptide C-terminus of pentagastrin. (Pentagastrin and calcium are the principal secretagogues useful in testing for medullary carcinoma [see "Medullary Carcinoma of the Thyroid," p. 1017]). β-Adrenergic catecholamines and glucagon are known to act in receptor tissues by increasing cyclic 3′,5′-AMP content, and indeed theophylline as well as dibutyryl cAMP has also been shown to stimulate CT release. Thus, cAMP is implicated as an intracellular mediator for secretion of CT as well as for secretion of PTH.

The concentration of calcium in the circulation influences the thyroid gland content of CT. Hypocalcemia in parathyroidectomized rats is associated with increased CT content of the thyroid gland, whereas hypercalcemia causes depletion of secretory granules from the C cells of the thyroid and reduced CT content of the thyroid gland. In some species, CT secretion seems critically important for control of blood calcium. Instillation of calcium into the stomach of normal rats causes little or no change in plasma calcium but in thyroidectomized animals causes hypercalcemia. These observations indicate that a gastrointestinal hormone is released in response to calcium or a calcium-containing meal and that this gastrointestinal hormone is a secretagogue for CT. In the pig, instillation of calcium into the stomach causes release of gastrin and also release of CT. Thus it appears that gastrin is one CT secretagogue elaborated in response to alimentary intake of calcium in the pig. Of further interest is the fact that in the pig, PTH at doses insufficient to cause hypercalcemia is capable of stimulating gastrin release. Interrelationships between gastrointestinal and calcitropic hormones appear important in regulation of calcium metabolism in the pig, rat, and other subprimates. Although there is no proven significance for human physiology, such hormone-secretagogue interactions could be relevant in the interpretation of multiple endocrine neoplasia.

Metabolism of Calcitonin

Immunoreactive CT exists in human plasma in multiple forms detected after gel filtration. These immunoreactive peptides in plasma vary in size and quantity with clinical status, renal function, and nature of tissue elaborating CT. High MW species seem to accumulate in chronic renal disease; multiple forms apparently are secreted in medullary thyroid carcinoma as well as in lesions producing CT ectopically. A dimer of CT can be formed from the native hormone. The dimer is inactive but can be converted to the monomer with restoration of biologic activity through reduction with sulfhydryl reagents. The dimer, however, does not appear to represent any of the high MW forms of CT circulating in cases of medullary carcinoma. Of the various forms of immunoreactive CT other than monomer in the circulation, some may represent peptides elaborated from the secretory source. Others represent peripheral conversion of secreted forms. At the present time there is too little known about the metabolism of CT to distinguish the origin of the several high MW forms of immunoreactive CT.

Physiology

General

The effect of CT in lowering serum calcium is the most generally recognized physiologic action of the hormone. Hypophosphatemia accompanies the hypocalcemia, and the concurrence of these two actions suggests that the effects of CT are brought about through the reduction in bone resorption. Studies of radioactive calcium kinetics *in vivo* as well as *in vitro* show changes in specific activity of plasma calcium interpretable as inhibition of release of calcium from a major calcium pool, presumably bone (Fig. 19–25). *In vitro*,

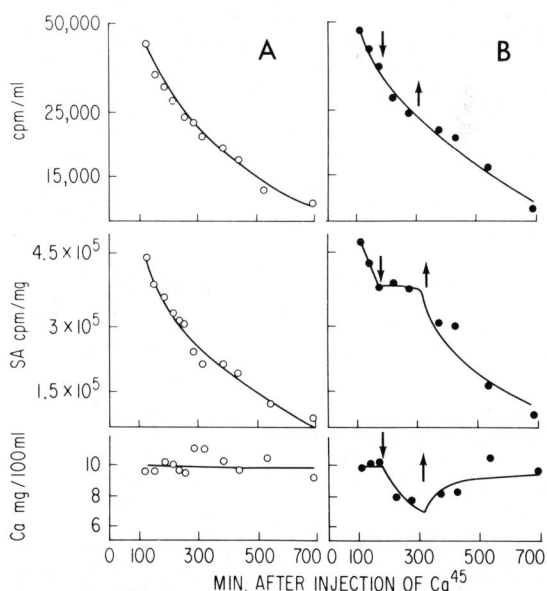

Figure 19–25. Changes in calcium metabolism in the rat in response to CT. Groups of rats were given radioactive calcium intravenously, and serial determinations were made of radioactivity and calcium in blood. Serum calcium remains constant and specific activity changes continuously in plasma of control rats. Rats injected with CT (first arrow) develop acute hypocalcemia and abrupt retardation of decline in specific activity of plasma calcium. Results are interpreted as reflecting inhibition of bone resorption (interruption of supply of stable calcium to the plasma compartment) by CT *in vivo*. (From O'Riordan, J. L., and Aurbach, G. D.: Mode of action of thyrocalcitonin. *Endocrinology* 82:377, 1968.)

CT causes inhibition of the PTH effect on release of radioactive calcium from fetal rat bones. Actions of CT on bone are also evident in the decrease by the hormone of alkaline phosphatase, pyrophosphatase activity, and hydroxyproline production, each accompanying the inhibition of bone resorption. The hypophosphatemic action of CT reflects predominantly inhibition of bone resorption. In addition to this mechanism, however, under certain circumstances CT may by direct action on the kidney cause a modest degree of phosphaturia that also can contribute to hypophosphatemia. Moreover, early in the course of CT action there is also accelerated efflux of phosphate from the ECF.

Actions on Bone

The hypocalcemic activity of CT *in vivo* is effected predominantly by inhibiting calcium resorption from bone and is not dependent on a physiologically functioning kidney, gastrointestinal tract, or parathyroid gland. A direct action on bone is implied also from radioactive calcium kinetic studies in the intact animal. Changes in radioactive calcium specific activity in the plasma compartment in response to CT show that the disappearance rate for radioactive calcium from the ECF (see Fig. 19–25) is not affected by CT. Other evidence that CT directly influences bone includes changes in the morphology, enzyme activity (alkaline phosphatase and pyrophosphatase activity), and collagen metabolism of bone.

Calcitonin inhibits the PTH-induced bone resorption with fetal rat or mouse bone *in vitro*. Bone resorption produced by vitamin A, vitamin D, PTH, dibutyryl cAMP, or prostaglandins, as well as spontaneous bone resorption, is inhibitable by CT *in vitro*. Virtually all resorptive effects, including lysosomal enzyme changes, mineral release, and degradation of collagen, are inhibited upon addition of CT. The magnitude of the inhibitory effect on bone is a function of the rate of bone resorption. At low rates of bone resorption, little effects of CT are observed. At high rates of bone resorption, the inhibitory effects of CT are much greater. After prolonged incubation of skeletal tissue with CT *in vitro*, the effectiveness of the hormone in inhibiting resorption is lost. This effect has been termed "escape phenomenon." This refractoriness to the *in vitro* effects of CT might be directly related to loss of CT receptors ("down regulation of receptors") from the target tissue and consequently decreased production of cAMP in response to the hormone.

Mechanism of Action of Calcitonin

The effects of CT also appear to be mediated, at least in part, by cyclic 3′,5′-AMP. Initial studies with dibutyryl cyclic 3′,5′-AMP indicated that at modest concentrations it caused induction of bone resorption in tissue culture. In the same experiments dibutyryl cAMP added at still higher concentrations caused inhibition of bone resorption and inhibition of the effects of PTH. Thus the effects of high concentrations of dibutyryl cAMP mimic the effects of CT. Later studies indicated that CT itself causes increased accumulation of cAMP in bone and that this is attributable to specific activation of adenylate cyclase by CT *in vitro*. CT also causes activation of renal adenylate cyclase and increased formation of cAMP in the renal tubule. Diverse CT congeners show orders of potency *in vitro* on cAMP production that parallel closely biologic effects *in vivo*. This parallelism in dose-response for physiology and biochemistry (cyclic nucleotide production) supports further the likelihood that cAMP is the mediator of action of CT.

Receptors for Calcitonin and Distribution Among Cell Types

The discussion of the mechanism of action of PTH (p. 946) indicated that adenylate cyclase responses to CT and PTH appear in different regions along the course of the nephron. CT activates adenylate cyclase in the medullary ascending thick limb of the nephron as well as in an area of distal cortical tubule (see Fig. 29–22). Certain CT-sensitive areas respond relatively little to PTH, which activates adenylate cyclase in the proximal convoluted tubule as well as in a more distal region of the distal convoluted tubule of the rabbit. Thus responsive regions for the two hormones differ in distribution along the course of the nephron. There are significant differences in response of bone cells as well (see p. 948). Osteoclastic activity stimulated by PTH is inhibited by CT. Osteoclast-like cells respond to both CT and PTH, whereas osteoblast-like cells respond only to PTH.

Direct Identification of Calcitonin Receptors

Radioiodination with ^{125}I of salmon CT yields an effective ligand for determining direct interaction of CT with specific receptors in target tissues. Specific receptors have been identified on renal plasma membranes and on membranes prepared from fetal rat calvaria (Fig. 19–26). Radioiodinated salmon CT binds with high affinity to membranes in these tissues and dissociates very slowly from the receptor. A series of CT analogs inhibits binding of iodinated CT to the receptor, and the apparent affinities of a series of CT congeners parallel the biologic activity of these compounds (Fig. 19–26). This is the same order of effectiveness of CT analogs in stimulating adenylate cyclase in kidney or bone. Specific receptors for CT have also been identified in certain

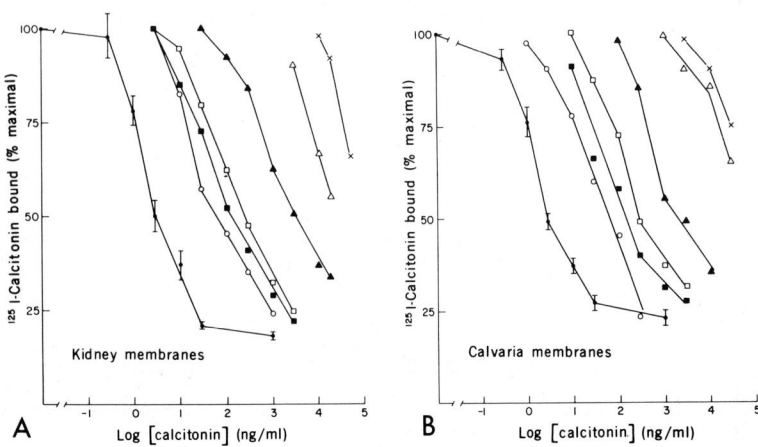

Figure 19–26. Receptor-ligand interactions with CT polypeptides. Renal (A) or skeletal (B) cell membranes were incubated *in vitro* with ^{125}I of salmon CT and indicated amounts of unlabeled congeners. The CT peptides specifically inhibited binding of labeled CT to receptor sites on the membranes. The apparent affinities (taken as concentrations required for half-maximal inhibition) paralleled the biologic effectiveness of the polypeptides. •, salmon CT; ○, porcine CT; ■, ovine CT; □, bovine CT; ▲, human CT; △, human CT fragment amide; X, human CT sulfoxide. (From Marx, S. J., Woodward, C. J., et al.: Calcitonin receptors of kidney and bone. *Science 178*:199, 1972.)

human lymphocyte cell lines. The receptors on these lymphocytes show kinetic characteristics similar to those from rat kidney or bone, and in similar studies human CT shows the lowest apparent affinity for receptors on human lymphocytes as well as on receptors from rat kidney or bone. Thus, in contrast to the marked evolutionary changes in the agonist molecules, there is no evidence suggesting significant genetic modification in the nature of CT receptors. The human hormone shows no greater relative potency when tested against receptors in human tissues than that found with receptors from lower evolutionary forms.

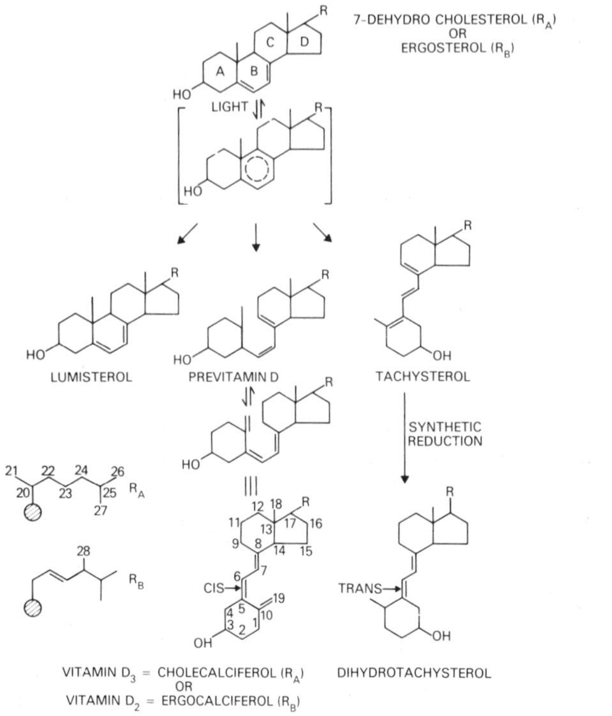

CALCIFEROLS

Vitamin Terminology

Ergocalciferol and cholecalciferol were recognized as essential nutritional factors in the 1920's and 1930's and were labeled as vitamins at that time. In this chapter, the vitamin terminology has been retained for consistency with long-standing usage. The D vitamins are a family of fat-soluble, biologically active, secosteroids. Secosteroids are steroid-related molecules in which one of the four rings has been opened. For the D vitamins, the bond between C9 and C10 of the B ring has been cleaved, giving a conjugated triene structure. The metabolism and mechanism of action of the calciferols are, in many ways, analogous to those of the true steroid hormones.

Metabolic Pathways

Sources of Inactive Precursors — Role of Sunlight

The precursors of vitamin D_2 and vitamin D_3 are produced in plants (ergosterol) and animals (7-dehydrocholesterol). Vitamins D_2 and D_3 differ only with respect to the C17 side chain structure (Fig. 19–27) and are generated nonenzymatically by irradiation of sterol precursors. The precursors are syntheisized *in vivo* by a series of condensations of acetyl coenzyme A analogous to that for the production of other steroid-like compounds. Lanosterol is a precursor for both ergosterol and 7-dehydrocholesterol. The appearance of 7-dehydrocholesterol is the penultimate step in cholesterol biosynthesis, and its conversion to cholesterol is irreversible. 7-Dehydrocholesterol is present in the human dermis and epidermis. Irradiation with near ultraviolet light (230–313 nm wavelength) penetrates as far as the dermis, causing generation of several sterols, including some with antirachitic (vitamin D–like) bioactivity (Fig. 19–27). Skin pigments have been suggested as possible regulators of this process but direct evidence is lacking. At a wavelength of 295 nm there is little generation of products other than previtamin D_3. Previtamin D_3 and vitamin D_3 are isomers that rapidly attain a physicochemical equilibrium that favors vitamin D_3. Exposure of ergosterol to heat and light produces a series of reactions analogous to those seen with 7-dehydrocholesterol (Fig. 19–27). Vitamin D_2 ("irradiated ergosterol") is a synthetic analog of vitamin D_3 used as a dietary supplement in the United States. Ergocalciferol and cholecalciferol appear to have identical biologic properties in humans, and our requirements for the vitamin can be fully satisfied by dietary and endogenous sources. The vitamin D content of an unfortified diet is variable but generally low (see Table 19–16).

Generally, in the temperate zones there is adequate sunlight to allow synthesis and release of sufficient cholecal-

Figure 19–27. Production of cholecalciferol, ergocalciferol, and dihydrotachysterol (DHT_3 or DHT_2) from sterol precursors. DHT is not produced *in vivo*. Note that modification of the 5-6 carbon configuration places the 3-hydroxyl group of DHT in a pseudo-1-hydroxyl configuration.

ciferol by the epidermis to obviate dependence on dietary sources of these sterols. Mean serum concentrations of 25-OH-D reflect season, global latitude, and average hours of solar exposure.

Calciferol 25-Hydroxylation

Ergocalciferol and cholecalciferol are inert when incubated *in vitro* with vitamin D target tissues and, after administration to vitamin D–deficient animals, give responses detectable only after a time lag of 6–12 hours. This time lag reflects the requirement that the calciferols undergo activation by a regulated sequence of hydroxylations (Fig. 19–28)

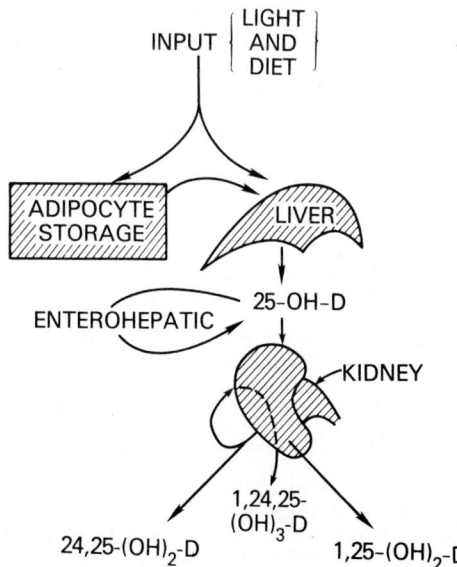

Figure 19–28. Metabolic pathways for production of major biologically active forms of the calciferols.

and then expression by accumulation in the nuclei of target tissues from which they direct changes in cell composition and function. This mechanism of action was uncovered by the use of calciferol radiolabeled to high specific activity. After administration to vitamin D–deficient animals, a series of mono- and dihydroxylated (polar) metabolites were detected (Fig. 19–29). Almost all studies to date have been done with vitamin D–deficient animals in which the conversion to active metabolites is particularly efficient. Less is known of the interconversions of vitamin D in the calciferol replete state, when most metabolism is through storage and degradative pathways.

The initial step in vitamin D activation is introduction of a hydroxyl residue at C25. 25-OH-D$_2$ and 25-OH-D$_3$ act more rapidly *in vivo* than do their precursors, and both show intrinsic activity on intestine and bone *in vitro*, unlike their precursors. Under normal conditions, vitamins D$_2$ and D$_3$ and their 25-hydroxylated forms each constitute approximately 45% of the circulating antirachitic activity. The liver is the principal site of the 25-hydroxylation process, although levels of this activity have been detected in the intestines and kidneys of certain species. There is no detectable conversion of vitamin D$_3$ to 25-OH-D$_3$ *in vivo* in hepatectomized vitamin D–deficient rats. Vitamin D$_3$ 25-hydroxylase activity has been localized to microsomal fractions of the liver. The activity is not stimulated by rachitogenic diets, but there may be a mild degree of product inhibition. In humans and chickens, however, feedback inhibition is not sufficient to prevent the production of toxic amounts of 25-OH-D when intake of vitamin D$_2$ or D$_3$ is high.

Calciferol 1-α Hydroxylation

1α,25-(OH)$_2$-D$_2$ and 1α,25-(OH)$_2$-D$_3$ are the most potent known metabolites of vitamin D, with synthesis rates in normal adults of 0.8–2.4 nM (0.3–1.0 μg) per day. In humans, the normal circulating concentration of 1α,25-(OH)$_2$-D is approximately one thousandth that of 25-OH-D. The 1-α-hydroxylation of 25-OH-D and other vitamin D analogs is the major recognized control point in calciferol metabolism. 25-OH-D 1-α hydroxylase activity has been identified in the kidneys of many species and has not been found in extrarenal sites except bone and the placenta. Nephrectomy, but not ureteral ligation, leads to an abrupt cessation of this activity *in vivo*. The 25-OH-D 1-α hydroxylase activity has been found only in proximal convoluted tubules.

Most studies of the enzyme system have used 25-OH-D$_3$ as a substrate, and it is generally assumed that the same enzyme system can also use as substrates 25-OH-D$_2$, 24,25-(OH)$_2$-D$_3$, 25,26-(OH)$_2$-D$_2$, and probably other 25-hydroxylated metabolites. The enzyme system shares many properties with the steroidogenic mixed function oxidase enzyme systems typified by those of the adrenal cortical mitochondria. Each requires molecular oxygen derived from O$_2$, magnesium, NADPH as a source of electrons, an iron sulfur protein (the chicken kidney protein cross-reacts immunologically with adrenal ferredoxin), and a ferredoxin reductase (thought to be flavoprotein). Cytochrome P-450 serves as the terminal electron donor and oxygenase in the adrenal mitochondrial steroid mono-oxygenase; a similar hemoprotein is involved in the renal system. The renal 25-OH-D 1-α hydroxylase–associated cytochrome binds aminoglutethimide, metyrapone, and carbon monoxide with kinetics similar to those for the adrenal cytochrome P-450.

The hepatic vitamin D 25-hydroxylase activity is not regulated as closely as is the renal 25-OH-D 1-α-hydroxylase system. Regulation of the renal activity may be via modifications of enzyme synthesis, enzyme degradation, or enzyme action (for example, modifications of cofactors). In renal tubules, the activity decays with a half-time of 3.5–4 hours when either protein or RNA synthesis is inhibited, indicating a rapid turnover of both messenger and protein. Even when protein synthesis is inhibited, however, total activity can be increased *in vitro* by incubation with dibutyryl cAMP. Dietary vitamin D deprivation leads to a 5- to 20-fold increase in this activity, and this reverts to normal within several days following acute vitamin D repletion. Administration of excess vitamin D$_3$ to chickens and humans results in accumulation of abnormal amounts of 25-OH vitamin D in serum, whereas the serum concentration of 1α,25-(OH)$_2$-D does not rise outside the normal range. The mechanism whereby the renal tubules respond to vitamin D and calcium depletion under normal circumstances involves an intermediary action of PTH. The renal 25-OH-D 1-α hydroxylase activity decreases to unstimulated levels within 24 hours of parathyroidectomy in vitamin D–depleted chickens. It increases with systemic infusion of PTH, cAMP, or dibutyryl cAMP into thyroparathyroidectomized vitamin D–deficient rats.

Phosphate depletion regulates the renal 25-OH-D 1-α hydroxylase activity by mechanisms independent of PTH (Fig. 19–30), though in chickens the phosphate-associated changes are of a lower magnitude than are those caused by changes in parathyroid status. Phosphate depletion in

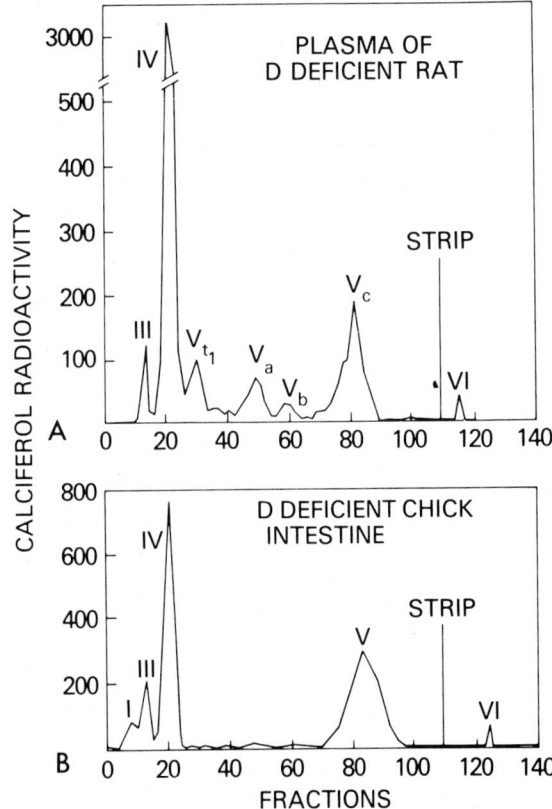

Figure 19–29.   Top: 2.5 μg tritiated cholecalciferol was injected into a calciferol-deficient rat, and plasma was obtained 24 hours later. Lipids were extracted with an organic solvent and chromatographed on a column of sephadex LH-20. The probable major components of the peaks are as follows: III (D$_3$), IV (25-OH-D$_3$), Va (24,25-(OH)$_2$-D$_3$), V$_c$ (25,26-(OH)$_2$-D$_3$), V (1,25-(OH)$_2$-D$_3$). Bottom: Calciferol-deficient chicks were injected with 0.25 μg of tritiated cholecalciferol. Lipids were extracted from the small intestine and chromatographed on a similar column. (Modified from Holick, M. F., and DeLuca, H. F.: *J. Lipid Res.*, 21:460, 1971.)

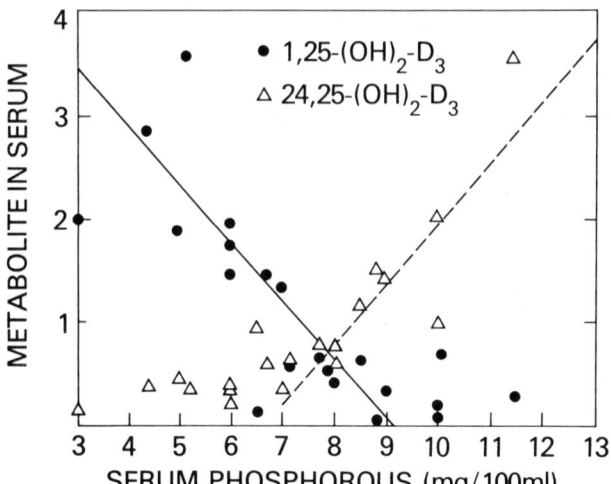

Figure 19–30. Relationship of serum phosphorus concentration to accumulation of dihydroxycholecalciferols in serum. Thyroparathyroidectomized rats received diets of varying amounts of calcium and phosphorus. Tritiated 25-OH-D$_3$ was administered, and serum dihydroxycholecalciferols were chromatographically separated and quantitated by radioactive counting. (From Tanaka, Y., and Deluca, H. F.: The control of 25-hydroxyvitamin D metabolism by inorganic phosphorus. *Arch. Biochem. Biophys. 154*:566, 1973.)

humans, chickens, and rats leads to increased serum concentrations of $1\alpha,25$-(OH)$_2$-D and increased intestinal absorption of calcium and phosphate. It is uncertain whether PTH or calcitonin or both can directly modulate renal tubular 25-OH-D 1-α hydroxylase activity *in vitro*. Since PTH causes major changes in renal phosphate transport, it is possible that some or all of the actions of PTH on this hydroxylase system are mediated by changes in the intracellular or extracellular phosphorus compartment.

Several additional factors have direct or indirect effects on renal 25-OH-D 1-α hydroxylase activity in certain species. For example, in fowl the needs of egg production require sex-dependent controls of mineral metabolism. A kidney from a male Japanese quail produces far less $1\alpha,25$-(OH)$_2$-D than does one from the female. Acute administration of estrogen to the male increases the renal 25-OH-D 1-α hydroxylase activity strikingly within 24 hours. Lactation may also place major stresses on mineral regulation. Serum concentrations of $1\alpha,25$-(OH)$_2$-D are increased during lactation in rats. 1,25-(OH)$_2$D *in vitro* directly leads to rapid inhibition of renal 25-OH-D 1-α hydroxylase activity. Though this enzyme system is sensitive to changing requirements of mineral metabolism, many of the controlling factors remain to be defined.

Calciferol 24-Hydroxylation

Another major metabolite of vitamin D is 24,25-(OH)$_2$-D. Under normal circumstances in humans, its serum concentration is approximately one tenth that of 25-OH-D and 100 times that of $1\alpha,25$-(OH)$_2$-D. The kidney is the principal site of the 24-hydroxylation of 25-OH-D, but anephric animals, including humans, continue to produce this metabolite, although in decreased quantities. Chicken chondrocytes *in vitro* synthesize a polar metabolite from 25-OH-D that is probably 24,25-(OH)$_2$-D$_3$. The rat renal 25-OH-D 24-hydroxylase, like the 1-α hydroxylase, is present in mitochondria. The two renal 25-OH-D hydroxylating systems respond to many of the same modulators but in opposing directions. Variation of dietary phosphorus causes contrasting changes in the two renal activities in the rat (see Fig. 19–30),

though a dependence of the 24-hydroxylase activity on dietary phosphorus has not been observed in the chicken. Administration of $1\alpha,25$-(OH)$_2$-D$_3$ to vitamin D–deficient chicks or rats inhibits metabolism of 25-OH-D to $1\alpha,25$-(OH)$_2$-D within several hours and simultaneously stimulates its metabolism to 24,25-(OH)$_2$-D$_3$. Monkey kidney cells in monolayer culture show decreased 24-hydroxylation of 25-OH-D in the presence of PTH but increased production in response to added $1\alpha,25$-(OH)$_2$-D$_3$ or calcium. In humans, serum concentrations of 24,25-(OH)$_2$-D are in large part determined by availability in serum of the 25-OH-D substrate for the 24-hydroxylase system.

Additional Pathways of Calciferol Metabolism

The list of calciferol metabolites of uncertain role includes 25,26-(OH)$_2$-D, 25-OH-D-26,23-lactone, 1,24,25-(OH)$_3$-D, and C-17 side chain cleavage metabolites. In tissues, vitamin D may be esterified as a palmitate, stearate, oleate, and linoleate. These esters retain antirachitic potency and may be major storage forms of the vitamin. A water-soluble sulfate ester may be the principal form of the vitamin in human and unfortified bovine milk. Numerous unidentified metabolites are excreted in bile. One of the major components is a glucuronide. A water-soluble glycoside of $1\alpha,25$-(OH)$_2$-D$_3$ has been identified in certain plants (see under "Structure-Function Relations," p. 959).

Calciferol Absorption, Transport, Storage, and Excretion

Normally 60–90% of dietary calciferol is absorbed by the small intestine, by mechanisms similar to those that absorb cholesterol and other fat-soluble sterols. Any impairment of fat absorption causes proportional reduction in absorption of vitamins D$_2$ and D$_3$. Absorbed calciferols are initially incorporated into chylomicra; in chylomicron-free blood, vitamins D$_2$ and D$_3$ circulate principally bound to an α globulin, which shows preferential affinity for the 25-hydroxylated forms of the calciferols.

Thirty per cent of tritiated vitamin D$_3$, administered intravenously to vitamin D–deficient rats, is rapidly sequestered within the liver to be released within several hours as tritiated 25-OH-D$_3$. In the vitamin D replete state the percentage of conversion to 25-OH-D is low, and a large portion, perhaps over half, of circulating vitamin D$_2$ or D$_3$ is partitioned into body fat pools. Adipose tissue provides an almost limitless reservoir for vitamin D storage. Consequently, when vitamin D$_2$ or D$_3$ has been ingested in excessive amounts, large amounts are retained in lipid storage, and several months may be required to return the contents of these pools to safe levels. The mechanism for entry of epidermal vitamin D$_3$ into the circulation is probably slow diffusion down a concentration gradient facilitated by binding to carrier proteins in ECF.

Unlike their parent compounds, 25-OH-D$_2$ and 25-OH-D$_3$ possess intrinsic activity *in vitro*. Though more polar than the parent compounds, 25-OH-D is also sparingly soluble in aqueous solutions. 25-OH vitamin D$_2$ and D$_3$ circulate bound to the same α globulin (transcalciferin) that transports the majority of vitamins D$_2$ and D$_3$ in chylomicron-free plasma. This α globulin has a MW of 55,000 and is identical to a protein previously referred to as group-specific component (Gc). There are two major forms with distinct electrophoretic mobility that are the expressions of codominant alleles. Multiple other allelic forms occur in less than 1% of the population but to date no variation in their effectiveness for vitamin D transport has been detected. The 25-OH-D transport globulin is synthesized in the liver, and its concentration rises moderately with estrogenic stimulation, as during pregnancy or treatment with estrogenic contraceptives; under usual conditions males and females have similar serum concentrations, however. It has a single high-affinity vitamin D binding site per molecule, with preferential affinity for the 25-hydroxylated forms. This feature favors partition of the nonhydroxylated forms into adipose tissue while the active 25-hydroxylated forms are retained within the circulation. Normally, less than 5% of its vitamin D binding sites are occupied. Its serum concentration is similar in states of calciferol excess or deficiency. Many species have vitamin D transport proteins that cross-react immunologically with the human protein. Even in the New World monkey, in which 25-OH-D binds to a protein with electrophoretic mobility similar to that of albumin, the binding globulin is immunologically related to the human protein. The 25-OH-D binding globulin of the chicken shows preferential affinity for the vitamin D_3 series over the vitamin D_2 series of analogs, and this accounts for the relative ineffectiveness of ergocalciferol analogs in chickens. The stability and high affinity for 25-hydroxylated forms of the calciferols have allowed use of these transport globulins in competitive binding assays for vitamin D metabolites.

Approximately half of the body pool of 25-OH-D is bound in the circulation to the 25-OH-D binding globulin. This bound form turns over with a half-time of 15 days in normal humans and approximately 45 days in anephric humans (Table 19–8). Most of the remainder of the body's 25-OH-D is inside cells, bound to cytoplasmic proteins. 25-OH-D binding proteins have been identified in the cytosols of all tissues examined, and like the serum 25-OH-D transport globulin they have proved useful as reagents for competitive binding assays of vitamin D metabolites. The majority of cytoplasmic 25-OH-D is bound *in vitro* to a protein that has a different sedimentation coefficient than that of the plasma 25-OH-D binding protein. It shows a spectrum of affinities similar to that of transcalciferin for vitamin D analogs, and the plasma and cytoplasmic proteins are immunologically related. The cytoplasmic 25-OH-D binding protein does not appear when cells are grown in the absence of plasma, and incubation of plasma with cell extracts generates a protein with the sedimentation velocity characteristic of the cytoplasmic 25-OH-D binding protein. It is either a translocated form of the plasma 25-OH-D transport globulin or a contaminating artefact from serum.

One third of tritiated 25-OH-D3 administered intravenously to humans appears in the duodenal lumen within 24 hours and is effectively absorbed in the small intestine, completing an enterohepatic circulation. 25-OH-D is the substrate for further hydroxylations in the 1 α, 24, and 26 positions; all of these occur in the kidney (see sections on hydroxylation) and are subject to varying degrees of metabolic regulation.

The hydroxy metabolites of 25-OH-D, like their precursors, are sparingly soluble in water and also circulate bound to the 25-OH-D transport globulin. Intravenously injected $1\alpha,25$-$(OH)_2$-D_3 has a circulating half-life of approximately 5 hours in the human circulation. During a 6-day period, approximately 15% is excreted as urinary metabolites and 50% as fecal metabolites. The total turnover of $1\alpha,25$-$(OH)_2$-D in adults is 0.3–1.0 mcg/day. Like 25-OH-D, 1,25-$(OH)_2$-D undergoes enterohepatic circulation.

Actions of Calciferols

Intestinal Actions

In the vitamin D–deficient animal, the intestine shows the most dramatic response to vitamin D administration, with large increases in absorption of calcium and lesser increases in absorption of phosphorus and magnesium. Calcium transport along the small and large intestine is regulated by vitamin D; in the rat, however, the basal and stimulated transport rates show a hierarchy with duodenum>jejunum>ileum>colon. Phosphorus absorption by the small intestine in the rat shows a different hierarchy of rates with jejunum>duodenum>ileum. Vitamin D and its active metabolites can determine intestinal calcium and phosphate transport in the total absence of PTH.

In the vitamin D–depleted state, administration of calciferol analogs *in vivo* or *in vitro* produces important alterations in the composition of the intestinal mucosa. The composition changes occur at approximately the same time that the intestinal mucosa increases its mucosal to serosal translocation of calcium. These changes begin approximately 2 hours after addition of $1\alpha,25$-$(OH)_2$-D_3 to intestinal mucosa from vitamin D–deficient animals and will be described in detail as analogous processes occur in other vitamin D target tissues (bone and parathyroid).

The intestinal mucosal epithelium contains a water-soluble calcium-binding protein, the tissue concentration of which mirrors calcium transport rates. Its concentration increases as early as 2 hours after administration *in vivo* or *in vitro* of $1\alpha,25$-$(OH)_2$-D_3 to vitamin D–deficient preparations. It can be detected by calcium-binding properties (competition with a calcium-chelating resin for radioactive calcium) or by immunoassay. Though all tissues contain an array of calcium-binding proteins, few of these proteins cross-react immunologically with the intestinal vitamin D–dependent calcium-binding protein. Small amounts of such cross-reacting material have been identified in bone, parathyroid, kidneys, placenta, pancreas, and brain. The chicken protein has four high-affinity (K_a $2\times(10)^6$M) calcium-binding sites per molecule and a MW of 28,000. The size of the major mammalian intestinal vitamin D–dependent calcium-binding protein is 10,000 daltons, and it contains two calcium-binding sites per molecule. The amino acid sequence of the porcine protein shows major homologies to those of myosin light chains, troponin C, parvalbumin, and calmodulin. The latter are homologous to the intestinal calcium-binding protein and have high affinity for and critical interactions with cytoplasmic calcium (see under "Intracellular Calcium-Binding Proteins," p. 929 and Fig. 19–6). The function of the intestinal vitamin D–dependent calcium-binding protein is not known, although its

Table 19–8. CALCIFEROL POOLS AND TURNOVERS IN HUMAN ADULTS

Metabolite	Body pool (μg)	Circulating half-time (days)	Turnover (μg/day)
Vitamin D*	1000	30	15
25-OH-D	200	15	7
1α, 25-$(OH)_2$-D	0.5	0.2	1

*"D" refers to D_2 plus D_3.

high calcium affinity and evolutionary homologies suggest it would operate at low calcium concentrations such as those anticipated intracellularly.

Skeletal Actions

The antirachitic action of vitamin D has traditionally been measured by an increase in osteoid calcification following vitamin D administration to vitamin D–depleted animals. There are two schools of thought regarding the mechanism of this skeletal effect. According to one view, the only direct action of the calciferols on bone is enhancement of skeletal resorption, the antirachitic effect reflecting provision merely of suitable concentration of calcium and phosphate (reflecting increased intestinal absorption) for mineralization of osteoid (the result primarily of a direct action on the intestine). The alternate view is that, in addition to the just-cited actions, calciferols also have direct anabolic effects on bone.

Most *in vitro* evaluations of the direct skeletal actions of active calciferol analogs have utilized calvaria or long bones of young animals. In these systems the active metabolites mobilize skeletal mineral and matrix. Similar effects occur *in vivo*, in normal or in parathyroidectomized animals. $1\alpha,25\text{-}(OH)_2\text{-}D_3$ is the most potent analog in eliciting these actions. The actions of $1\alpha,25\text{-}(OH)_2\text{-}D_3$ are in many ways similar to the direct actions of PTH on bone. With monolayer cultures of CT-responsive (osteoclast-like) cells from fetal mouse bone, $1\alpha,25\text{-}(OH)_2\text{-}D_3$, like PTH, stimulates the synthesis of hyaluronic acid and increases the activity of acid phosphatase. In monolayers of CT-unresponsive (osteoblast-like) cells, each decreases citrate decarboxylation, collagen synthesis, and alkaline phosphatase activity. Most of the *in vitro* skeletal actions of $1\alpha,25\text{-}(OH)_2\text{-}D_3$ can be elicited with higher concentrations of $24,25\text{-}(OH)_2\text{-}D_3$ or $25\text{-}(OH)\text{-}D_3$, and bone cytosol contains a protein with high selectivity for interaction with $1\alpha,25\text{-}(OH)_2\text{-}D$ similar to the cytosol "receptor" in intestinal mucosa.

Bone is not a homogeneous tissue, however. With rabbit chondrocytes, $24,25\text{-}(OH)_2\text{-}D_3$ stimulates proteoglycan turnover or synthesis at far lower concentrations than does $1\alpha,25\text{-}(OH)_2\text{-}D_3$. This supports the possibility that a response system with specificities different from those with preference for $1\alpha,25\text{-}(OH)_2\text{-}D$ may mediate certain anabolic actions of a spectrum of vitamin D analogs.

Direct Actions Outside Intestine and Skeleton

Several tissues, in addition to intestine and bone, are also calciferol target tissues. Vitamin D and its metabolites act directly on the parathyroid gland although the contribution of these potential feedback loops to normal metabolism is not yet known. *In vitro* $1\alpha,25\text{-}(OH)_2\text{-}D_3$ has shown both stimulatory and inhibitory actions on secretion of PTH. *In vitro* and *in vivo* $24,25\text{-}(OH)_2\text{-}D_3$ and $25,26\text{-}(OH)_2\text{-}D_3$ have shown only inhibitory actions on parathyroid gland size or PTH secretion.

$1\alpha,25\text{-}(OH)_2\text{-}D_3$ also acts directly on the kidney. With monkey kidney monolayer cells it increases the activity of the 25-OH-D 24-hydroxylase. In the thyroparathyroidectomized dog, 25-OH-D decreases the proximal tubular clearance of calcium and phosphorus. In the thyroparathyroidectomized rat, $1\alpha,25\text{-}(OH)_2\text{-}D_3$ decreases the renal calcium clearance, dissociated from changes in sodium clearance, suggestive of a distal tubular site of action.

Biochemical Mechanism of Action

In most systems, active analogs of vitamin D act with time lags of 2 or more hours. This and other evidence has led to a widespread belief that a primary nuclear site of action is involved. Indeed the secosteroidal hormones have many parallels to the classic steroidal hormones in their biochemic mechanisms of action. The most detailed studies have employed intestinal tissues, but there is evidence for analogous mechanisms of action in other tissues (receptors for $1,25\text{-}(OH)_2\text{-}D$ have been identified in many tissues).

Administration of high specific activity radiolabeled vitamin D in physiologic amounts to vitamin D–deficient chickens leads to accumulation of a polar metabolite in the intestine with significant amounts localized to nuclear chromatin. This polar metabolite is $1\alpha,25\text{-}(OH)_2\text{-}D_3$ (Fig. 19–29). The cytosol of chicken intestinal mucosa contains two proteins with high affinity for $1\alpha,25\text{-}(OH)_2\text{-}D_3$. One is presumably the translocated or contaminating serum 25-OH-D transport globulin, the other has the high affinity and specificity for $1\alpha,25\text{-}(OH)_2\text{-}D_3$ characteristic of a target tissue receptor molecule. Thus its specificity for interaction with a series of vitamin D analogs correlates well with their biologic activities *in vitro* and *in vivo*. The initial binding of $1\alpha,25\text{-}(OH)_2\text{-}D_3$ to this molecule is readily dissociable *in vitro* but becomes nondissociable at later times, suggesting a physicochemical modification. This cytosol receptor molecule mediates the translocation of $1\alpha,25\text{-}(OH)_2\text{-}D_3$ to nuclear chromatin, and receptor-bound forms of $1\alpha,25\text{-}(OH)_2\text{-}D_3$ can be extracted from nuclei of the target tissues. At the same early time points that $1\alpha,25\text{-}(OH)_2\text{-}D_3$ becomes associated with target cell nuclear chromatin, an increase occurs in DNA-dependent RNA polymerase II activity. Increased production of an mRNA that codes for the production of immunoreactive intestinal calcium binding protein occurs early after vitamin D treatment of deficient chicks. (Fig. 19–31).

Interactions with Parathyroid Hormone

Since the calciferols and PTH both have striking effects on calcium regulation, it is not surprising that they interact in many ways. The combined actions of the calciferols and PTH allow adaptation to fluctuations in availability of both calcium and phosphorus.

A state of calcium deficiency is sensed by the signal of

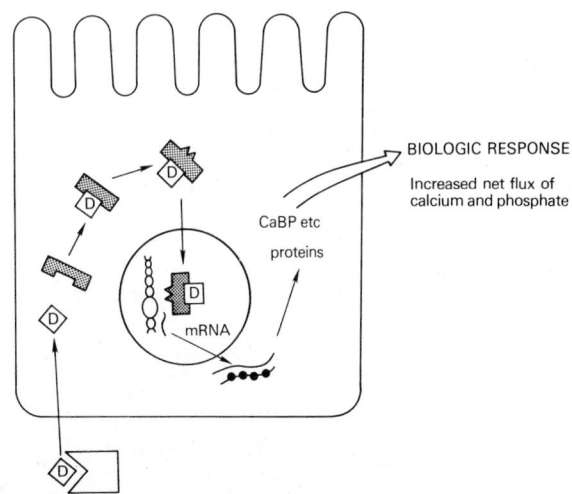

Figure 19–31. Major steps in target cell response to bioactive calciferols.

extracellular hypocalcemia. The release of PTH is increased, causing direct effects on bone and kidney. The skeletal action moves calcium and phosphate into the plasma pool while the renal action facilitates retention of calcium and promotes excretion of phosphate. The skeletal actions are reinforced by increased activity of the renal 25-OH-D 1-α hydroxylase due to increased circulating PTH and hypophosphatemia. Acute hypocalcemia causes a rise in serum concentration of 1α,25-(OH)$_2$-D 12–24 hours later, reflecting increased secretion of PTH (Fig. 19–32). The 1-hydroxylated forms of calciferol act upon bone, kidney, and the intestine to increase both calcium and phosphate content in the circulation. The actions of 1α,25-(OH)$_2$-D$_3$ and PTH on the enzymes of osteoclast-like and osteoblast-like cells in bone are very similar (see section on skeletal actions of calciferols, p. 957), and maximal concentrations of the two hormones do not show additive response, suggesting that both stimulate one final common pathway in bone cells. Increase in an intracellular calcium compartment may be this final pathway. These responses allow for several feedback loops. Increase in serum calcium suppresses PTH release. Calciferol metabolites also have independent effects on the parathyroid gland (see under "Direct Actions Outside Intestine and Skeleton," p. 957). The net response to perceived hypocalcemia is calcium and phosphate mobilization from bone and intestine with balance maintained (or even compromised) by increased renal excretion.

Hypophosphatemia increases the activity of the renal 25-OH-D 1-α hydroxylase system. Hypophosphatemia may have additional effects on metabolism of 1,25-(OH)$_2$-D. An increase in intestinal absorption of calcium and phosphate occurs. Skeletal mineral is also mobilized in response to hypophosphatemia and increased circulating concentration of 1α,25-(OH)$_2$-D$_3$. Increased serum calcium concentration should suppress PTH release. Decrease of the circulating activity of PTH raises the renal threshold for phosphate excretion and simultaneously facilitates the renal excretion of calcium. The net effect is that calcium and phosphate are mobilized from bone and from the intestinal lumen, while calcium balance is maintained (or even compromised) by renal excretion. Mild chronic phosphorus depletion may thus cause absorptive hypercalciuria and nephrolithiasis.

Vitamin D deficiency is a stress simultaneously to supplies of calcium and phosphate. The increase in PTH secretion that occurs, in the absence of adequate 25-OH-D, acts principally on bone and kidney, moving calcium into the circulation at the expense of phosphate that is translocated from bone through the circulation and into urine. There is a relative resistance to the calcemic (presumably bone-mobilizing) action of PTH in this state. PTH-induced tachyphyllaxis at the level of the osteoclast and osteocyte plasma membrane makes little contribution to this resistance. The coating of bone trabeculae by demineralized osteoid may cause resistance to the calcium-mobilizing actions of osteoclasts and osteocytes, however.

This discussion has omitted consideration of potential roles of 24,25-(OH)$_2$-D, CT, and other factors. Undoubtedly the calciferols and PTH interact with many other factors in mineral regulation.

Calciferol Assays

Bioassays

Although *in vivo* bioassays for calciferols are no longer in wide use, some familiarity with them will prevent confusion concerning otherwise puzzling variations in biopotencies. Antirachitic potency has traditionally been assessed by the "line test." Nutritional rickets is induced in test rats. Animals then receive a single dose of standard or unknown, and 7 days later the degree of linear (therefore "line test") calcification in the radial epiphysis is quantitated. One IU (25 ng) of vitamin D$_2$ or D$_3$ per rat will produce a detectable response. In this assay, vitamin D is almost equipotent to 1α,25-(OH)$_2$-D because of the highly efficient conversion of vitamin D to 1,25-(OH)$_2$-D by the vitamin D-deficient animal. In contrast, calciferol analogs of the 5,6 trans series that have low intrinsic target affinity even after 25-hydroxylation are weak (on a molar basis) in this system. Similar antirachitic assays have been developed with chicks. With chicks, vitamin D$_2$ shows only one tenth the potency of vitamin D$_3$, however, because the chicken serum 25-OH-D transport globulin has 10-fold greater affinity for 25-OH vitamin D$_3$ than for D$_2$, with the result that metabolites of the D$_2$ series are cleared more rapidly from serum in the chicken.

In a different type of assay, metabolites are tested for potency in raising the serum calcium concentration in normal or hypoparathyroid animals. Since, in these animals, the renal 25-OH-D 1-α hydroxylation is operating at very low efficiency, the assay is biased toward analogs already possessing a 1-α hydroxy or pseudo 1-α hydroxy configuration. In these "calcemic" assays, the analogs of the 5,6 trans series are approximately equipotent on a molar basis to vitamins D$_2$ and D$_3$, which have a 5,6 cis configuration (see Fig. 19–27).

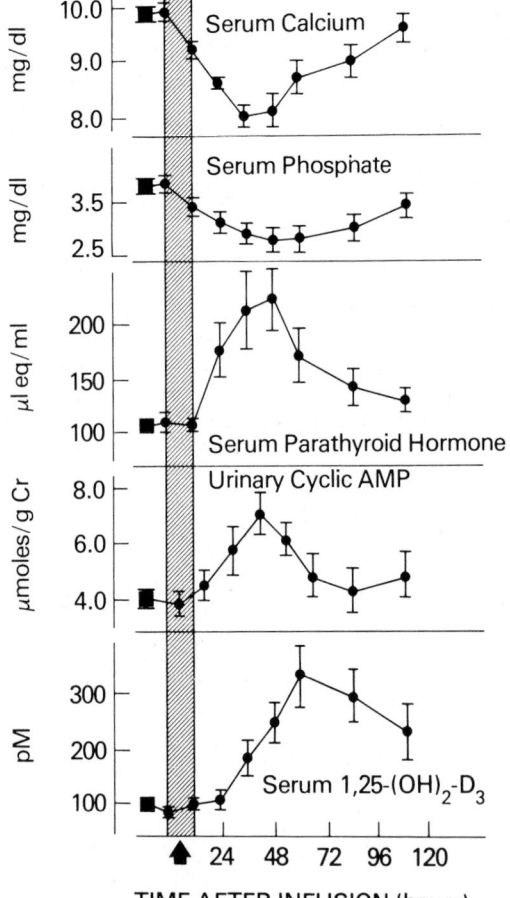

Figure 19–32. Response of the PTH-calciferol axis to hypocalcemia. Eight patients with Paget's disease received mithramycin (25 μg per kg) by infusion (hatched band). Note that the response of serum 1,25-(OH)$_2$-D$_3$ lags 12–24 hours behind the changes in serum PTH and urinary cAMP. (Modified from Bilezikian, J. P., Canfield, R. E., et al.: Response of 1 alpha, 25-dihydroxyvitamin D$_3$ to hypocalcemia in human subjects. *N. Engl. J. Med.* *299*:437, 1978.)

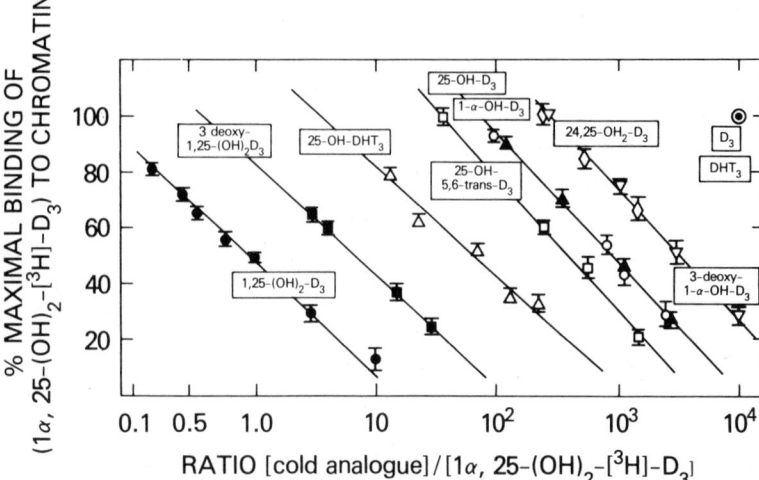

Figure 19–33. Competition of structural analogues of $1,25$-$(OH)_2$-D_3 for its chick intestinal mucosal receptor system. (From Procsal, D. A., Winberry, L., et al.: Dietary regulation of 6-phosphogluconate dehydrogenase synthesis. *J. Biol. Chem.* 250:8382, 1975.)

Some of the most sensitive detection systems in present use take advantage of the high affinities and specificities of target tissues and transport proteins. With fetal rat bones in organ culture, as little as 2 pg of $1,25$-$(OH)_2$-D_3/ml in the medium will cause detectable bone resorption following a 72-hour incubation. Alternatively analogs can be quantitated by competition with high specific activity radiolabeled $1\alpha,25$-$(OH)_2$-D_3 for partially purified receptor proteins from intestinal mucosa (Fig. 19–33). The serum or cytosol 25-OH-D binding proteins have formed the basis for competitive radioligand assays to quantitate 25-hydroxy metabolites of the calciferols (Fig. 19–34). The specificities of the serum transport globulin and cytosol receptor protein are quite different (compare Figs. 19–33 and 19–34). With either system a specific metabolite can be quantitated only after unequivocal separation from other cross-reacting metabolites.

Recently antisera have been raised by immunization with conjugates of calciferol analogs; this shows the feasibility of the radioimmunoassay technique, already proved highly useful in the assessment of other steroidal hormones.

Physicochemical Assays

High concentrations of vitamin D can be quantitated colorimetrically after reaction with antimony trichloride.

The calciferol triene structure has a peak absorbance at 264 nm. Because of its high concentrations in normal plasma, 25-OH-D_2 and 25-OH-D_3 can be isolated and directly quantitated by ultraviolet absorbance. The same method may be applicable to the quantitation of vitamins D_2 and D_3 and $24,25$-$(OH)_2$-D in serum extracts.

All assays in present use must contend with two problems. The first is the need to separate calciferol metabolites from lipids that interfere in a nonspecific manner. This is a particularly difficult problem in assays based solely on ultraviolet absorbance. The second is the need to separate multiple cross-reacting metabolites. The most sensitive and specific assays at present generally require a multistep purification (organic extraction together with radioactive markers for recovery and identification plus a combination of two or three separate chromatographic procedures) prior to measurement by absorbance or by one of the sensitive bioassays.

Structure-Function Relations

The most potent analog to date in most assay systems has been $1\alpha,25$-$(OH)_2$-D. Its biologic effectiveness is attributable to high-affinity interactions with a serum transport globulin and a cytoplasmic receptor protein in target tissues. The

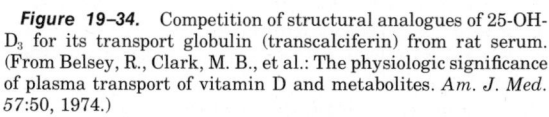

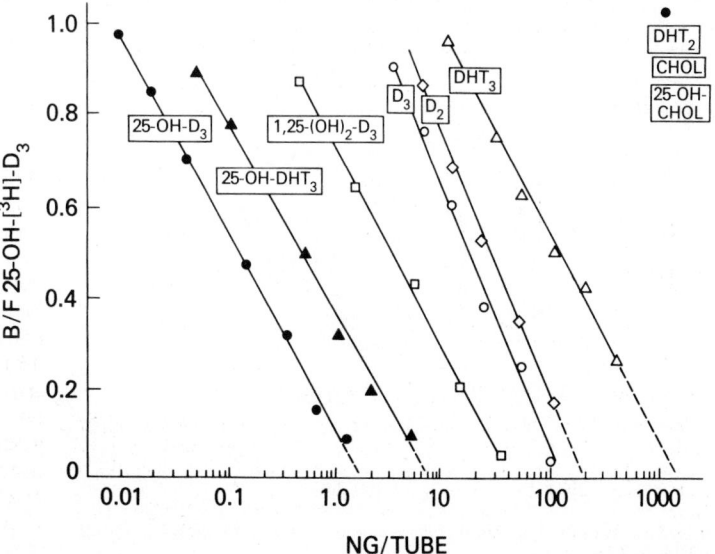

Figure 19–34. Competition of structural analogues of 25-OH-D_3 for its transport globulin (transcalciferin) from rat serum. (From Belsey, R., Clark, M. B., et al.: The physiologic significance of plasma transport of vitamin D and metabolites. *Am. J. Med.* 57:50, 1974.)

mammalian serum vitamin D transport globulins interact preferentially with 25-hydroxy analogs of vitamin D_2 or D_3. Lack of the group favors partition of analogs into adipose stores or excretory pathways when these are administered *in vivo*. 24,25-$(OH)_2$-D has an affinity for the binding globulin similar to that of 25-OH-D; however, A ring modifications such as insertion of the 1-α hydroxyl or deletion of the 3-β hydroxyl result in 10-fold loss of affinity for the serum transport globulin. Side chain lengthening or shortening by one carbon decreases binding affinity to transcalciferin by 10-fold, and greater affinity losses result from progressive modifications in chain length. 24 nor, 25-OH-D_3 was the first synthetic analog shown to block the intestinal calcium transport response to subsequent *in vivo* administration of vitamin D_3. The transport globulin of the chicken interacts only weakly with the C-17 side chain of the vitamin D_2 series, so that in chickens the vitamin D_2 analogs are more rapidly cleared and thus less potent than are comparable analogs of the vitamin D_3 series.

The requirements for direct binding to the intestinal cytoplasmic "receptor" have also been analyzed in detail. Several features of the C-17 side chain are critical. Removal of the 25-hydroxyl group (i.e., 1-α hydroxy D_3) leads to a 900-fold drop in receptor affinity, and insertion of a nearby hydroxyl group, (i.e., 1-α 24R,25-$(OH)_2$-D_3) decreases the affinity twofold to fivefold. Deletion of the 1-α hydroxyl residue causes a 900-fold loss in affinity for the intestinal receptor. Since in humans the circulating concentrations of 25-OH-D are normally approximately 1000 times those of 1α,25-$(OH)_2$D, both metabolites may contribute importantly to mineral regulation in the vitamin D–replete state, however. Synthetic 1-β hydroxy-D_3, in which the 1-hydroxyl is below the plane of the A ring has undetectable activity *in vivo* (less than 1% the antirachitic activity of D_3). The calciferol A ring is flexible in natural solutions with a rapid equilibrium between chair-chair configurations. The consequences of the associated shifts of the 1-α hydroxyl residue from axial to equatorial positions may be important in receptor interaction. The 5,6 cis configuration is not essential, but conversion to a trans configuration results in approximately 100-fold decrease in intrinsic affinity of the 25 hydroxylated forms for the receptor. This rotates the 3-hydroxyl group to a pseudo 1-α configuration (Fig. 19–35), producing a series of synthetic analogs that are active without a need for renal 1-α hydroxylation. From this it can be inferred that neither the 3-β hydroxyl group nor the C-19 methylene group is essential. In most bioassays 24,25-$(OH)_2$-D_3 has actions similar to those of 25-OH-D_3. The unique effects of 24,25-$(OH)_2$-D_3 in other systems (perfused canine parathyroid gland and rat chondrocyte) have raised the possibility of calciferol effector systems with specificities different from those of the major receptor characterized in intestinal mucosal cytosol.

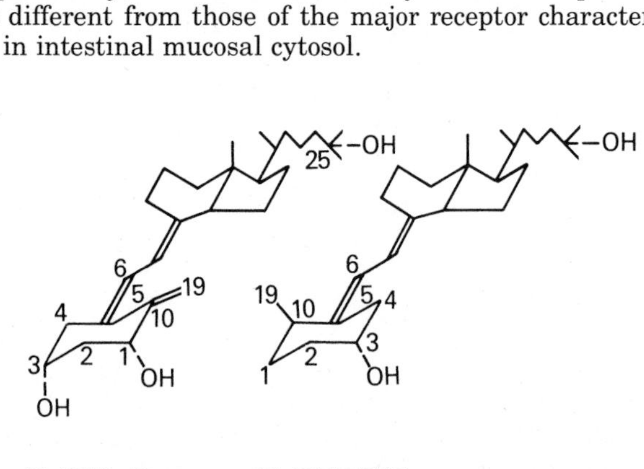

$1\alpha, 25\text{-}(OH)_2\text{-}D_3$ $25\text{-}(OH)\text{-}DHT_3$

Figure 19–35. Possible conformations of 1 alpha, 25-$(OH)_2$-D_3, and 25-OH-dihydrotachysterol$_3$.

Calciferol Pharmacology

A wide range of conditions is responsive to calciferol analogs, including hypoparathyroidism, neonatal hypocalcemia, many forms of rickets and osteomalacia, and uremic secondary hyperparathyroidism. Low circulating concentration of 1α,25-$(OH)_2$-D is a common feature in most of these states, making treatment with calciferol analogs logical. Particular aspects of therapy are discussed in sections dealing with some of the pathologic states; the general pharmacology of calciferol is outlined here.

In most organic solvents these sterols are quite soluble. They can be crystallized from alcohol solutions in the form of long prisms that undergo decomposition at room temperature over two days. Stability is increased by protection from light, oxygen, and heat. Ergocalciferol and cholecalciferol are stable for prolonged periods when dissolved in fats, oils, or propylene glycol. An active water-soluble form of 1α,25-$(OH)_2$-D_3 has been discovered in several species of plants (*Solanum malacoxylon, Cestrum diurnum*, and *Tricetium flavescens*) long known to cause pathologic calcinosis in grazing animals. In these extracts 1α,25-$(OH)_2$-D_3 is linked to one or more glycoside groups at sites that remain to be defined. This indicates the feasibility of development of synthetic water-soluble analogs of the calciferols. Several features that determine the utility of an analog are rate of onset and offset of action and potential to allow endogenous responses to variation in mineral availability. Vitamins D_2 and D_3 show half-times to onset or offset of action of approximately 2 weeks in treatment of hypoparathyroidism. Most of the administered drug accumulates in body fat, and the drug in the circulation must generally be activated by both 25 and 1-α hydroxylation. These features make these drugs particularly useful in patients retaining intact parathyroid-renal axes responsive to variations in mineral availability. If hepatic 25-hydroxylation is intact, vitamins D_2 and D_3 by generating the 25-hydroxylated metabolites also have the potential to be effective even in the anephric patient. Their storage characteristics also make them useful when daily drug administration is not practical or when parenteral therapy is required. Nutritional vitamin D deficiency in adults responds to 5–100 μg/day of vitamin D_2 or D_3; typical requirements are 500–2000 μg/day in most states with clinically evident abnormalities of calciferol metabolism. 25-OH-D_3 differs from vitamin D_3 insofar as a smaller proportion is stored in body fat, and it bypasses hepatic 25-hydroxylation. Thus its onset and offset of action are faster, and it is effective when there is compromise of the hepatic 25-hydroxylation of vitamins D_2 or D_3, as in primary biliary cirrhosis or some cases of neonatal hypocalcemia. Since 25-OH-D has intrinsic agonist activity it retains effectiveness when the renal 25-OH-D 1α hydroxylase system is absent. 1α,25-$(OH)_2$-D_3 is the most potent known natural metabolite of cholecalciferol. Its half-time to onset or offset of action is generally 1–3 days. Thus it is extremely useful when rapid responses are important, as, for example, with symptomatic neonatal hypocalcemia or other forms of tetany. Increases in intestinal calcium absorption occur when normal or vitamin D–deficient adults receive doses in the range of 1 μg daily. This drug bypasses the principal regulatory influence of the parathyroid-renal axis and regulatory controls geared to variations in calcium availability. If PTH or the renal 25-OH-D 1-α hydroxylase response to it is absent, then treatment with any calciferol metabolite will be by a mechanism that provides unregulated circulating metabolite levels sufficient to act on target cells. 1-α hydroxy vitamin D_3 and dihydrotachysterol are synthetic analogs that do not require renal activation to produce a metabolite with an active A ring; each requires 25-hydroxylation by the liver, and 1-α-hydroxy D_3, perhaps because it is more polar, has a more rapid onset and offset of action (3–5 day half-time) than does dihydrotachysterol (7–15 day half-time).

All the calciferol analogs cited previously have similar effects on mineral metabolism in humans. Their initial and major site of action is the intestine, where mucosal to serosal movement of calcium is promoted. Secondary hyperparathyroidism is gradually suppressed by elimination of hypocalcemia and perhaps by direct calciferol metabolite actions on the parathyroid glands. High concentrations of calciferol metabolites may also cause mobilization of calcium and phosphate from skeletal stores. As the serum calcium concentration rises, calcium excretion into the urine increases. In the absence of parathyroid secretion, high renal calcium excretion may occur, even before a normal serum calcium concentration is attained. Hypercalciuria is a potential problem whenever calciferol is used for treatment of hypoparathyroidism. It causes deterioration in renal function even in the absence of hypercalcemia. If uncorrected, this imposes a risk of nephrocalcinosis, nephrolithiasis, and irreversible decrease in glomerular filtration. Decreasing glomerular filtration with continued calcium mobilization from the intestine or skeleton, or both, leads to a vicious cycle of progressive hypercalcemia and worsening renal damage. The nephrotoxic effects of the calciferols are thus indirect, resulting from excesses of calcium in plasma and urine. Vitamin D intoxication occurs whether or not the renal 25-OH-D 1-α hydroxylase regulation is intact. In normal persons, this axis suppresses effectively when high concentrations of calciferol substrate are presented. Thus, excessive intakes of vitamin D_2 are associated with normal serum concentrations of $1\alpha,25$-$(OH)_2$-D_2 but toxic concentrations of 25-$(OH)_2$-D_2 in humans.

Aside from intrinsic potency and underlying disease state, additional considerations will influence dosage requirement. Dietary calcium will determine the quantity of calcium that is available to be mobilized from the intestinal lumen. Major fluctuations in dietary calcium make therapy difficult in states in which the parathyroid-renal regulatory axis is compromised. This problem can be minimized by providing, to all patients, supplemental calcium by mouth, so that dietary variations contribute in only a minor way to a high invariant baseline intake. A supplement equivalent to 15 mg/kg of elemental calcium (for example, 10 grams of calcium lactate for adults) will blunt dietary-associated fluctuations and facilitate abrupt calcium withdrawal if calciferol overdose should occur with a long-acting preparation. Daily flux of calcium out of the central or circulating pool also determines calciferol dosage. At early points in treatment of osteomalacias, large amounts of calcium may be deposited each day in the skeleton. As skeletal pools are repleted, whole body calcium needs, and thus whole body calciferol needs, diminish. Renal excretion of calcium may change abruptly if the patient receives thiazide diuretics (that decrease renal calcium clearance) or loop diuretics (that increase renal calcium clearance). A number of other drugs interact with mineral or calciferol metabolism by mechanisms that are often poorly understood. The reader is referred to "Miscellaneous Endogenous Calcitropic Factors," next, and "Anticonvulsant Osteomalacia," p. 1003 for consideration of interactions with glucocorticoids, estrogens, and anticonvulsants. Lastly, the metabolism of calciferol analogs may change during the course of therapy. Much remains to be learned about changes in metabolite clearance and conversion to active or inactive products during a period of changing mineral status.

Since calciferol therapy is often a long-term commitment, cost and facility of monitoring serum metabolite concentrations should also be considered.

The following principles should serve as general guidelines. (1) Underlying disorders should receive appropriate treatment. (2) In states in which serum concentrations of 25-OH-D are low, treatment should be with analogs that restore normal serum concentrations and allow normal regulation by the parathyroid-renal axis of mineral metabolism. (3) When renal 25-OH-D 1-α hydroxylation is impaired by parathyroid or renal disease, any metabolite that generates target active forms will have similar effects. Selection should be based on considerations of rapidity of action, cost, and facility of monitoring. (4) All analogs have a potential to cause hypercalciuria and irreversible renal damage. (5) Dosage requirements may vary during treatment, especially if the subject receives other drugs concomitantly. Oral calcium supplementation will minimize variations attributable to dietary fluctuation.

Miscellaneous Endogenous Calcitropic Factors

Gonadal Steroids

Lifelong or premature deficiency of the principal estrogens in females or of the principal androgens in males is associated with an increased incidence of osteoporosis. Similarly the endocrine changes occurring about the time of the menopause are associated with acceleration of the rate of loss of bone mass. In addition, among perimenopausal women, the incidence of primary hyperparathyroidism rises, accounting for the female preponderance among patients with this disorder. With loss of normal estrogen secretion, the skeletal actions of PTH seem accentuated, but there has been no unequivocal demonstration of a direct action of estrogens or androgens on bone. In the Japanese quail, estrogen administration *in vivo* to the male or to the ovariectomized female causes a rapid and dramatic increase in the renal 25-OH-D 1-α hydroxylase activity; this action may indicate a direct renal action of gonadal steroids essential for the mineral regulation of an egg-laying species.

The administration of estrogens to menopausal women in "physiologic replacement" amounts leads to the following: slight fall of serum calcium concentration, rise in serum concentration of PTH and 1,25-$(OH)_2$-D, decreased urinary excretion of calcium, and total body calcium retention for at least 6–12 months. All these changes could result from estrogenic interference with net skeletal resorption. Estrogen administration to patients receiving calciferol may increase the calciferol requirement. Occasionally patients with refractory hypercalcemia (bone metastases or parathyroid cancer) will obtain transient decreases in serum calcium concentration when given pharmacologic doses of estrogen.

Glucocorticosteroids

States of glucocorticoid excess are associated with accelerated loss of skeletal mass, particularly from regions of trabecular bone such as the vertebrae. Glucocorticoids antagonize the action of calciferol in states of hypoparathyroidism or calciferol excess. There is an additional therapeutic effect in certain hypercalcemic states, as the consequences of inhibition of tumors that release calcemic factors (myeloma, lymphoma, and some prostaglandin-producing neoplasms). They also inhibit the direct skeletal action of certain osteoclast activating factors (see later).

The histologic appearance of the skeleton with glucocorticoid osteoporosis suggests decreased bone formation and increased bone resorption. The decrease in bone formation has been attributed to inhibition of osteoblast differentiation and function. The increase in bone resorption may be multifactorial in cause. Glucocorticoids lower the serum concentration of calcium and of 1,25-$(OH)_2$-D in humans; this leads to a mild secondary hyperparathyroidism. Furthermore, incubation of rat calvaria bones with physiologic concentrations of glucocorticoids leads to an increase in the tissue cAMP response to PTH; glucocorticoid suppression of skeletal cAMP phosphodiesterase activity accounts in part for this. The hypocalcemic action of glucocorticoids is also multifactorial. It is the inverse of the hypercalcemia that is an expression of glucocorticoid deficiency. Glucocorticoids directly interfere with intestinal calcium absorption, and in addition may interfere with the maintenance of normal plasma concentrations of both 25-OH-D and 1,25-$(OH)_2$-D. Glucocorticosteroids do not compete effectively with the calciferol secosteroids for their high-affinity serum transport proteins or for target issue cytoplasmic receptors.

Thyroid Hormones

Thyrotoxicosis, like immobilization, is associated with hypercalciuria and decrease in bone mass. Careful measurements of plasma ionized calcium in thyrotoxicosis have suggested mild hypercalcemia in many cases. Thyroid hormone *in vitro* leads to a direct stimulation of bone resorption. The histologic features of bone in thyrotoxicosis suggest increased skeletal resorptive and formative activity. An increased quantity of osteoid is the result of an increase in the numbers, not the width, of osteoid borders, reflecting intense osteoblastic activity without any defect in osteoid mineralization. The parathyroid glands are suppressed; the combination of normal to elevated serum concentrations of calcium with decrease of the normal renal action of circulating PTH accounts for a high incidence of hypercalciuria in thyrotoxicosis.

Osteoclast Activating Factors

Factors that activate osteoclasts and stimulate bone resorption *in vitro* have been identified in culture media of activated human leukocytes and cells from patients with multiple myeloma or lymphoma. Osteoclast activating factors (OAF) probably are small proteins and are structurally unrelated to PTH. The resorptive activity of some OAF preparations, unlike that of PTH, is blocked by glucocorticoid concentrations achievable *in vivo*. Mediators such as these or the prostaglandins may account for the bone resorption associated with some skeletal metastases or inflammatory disorders of the skeleton (periodontal disease, arthritis, osteomyelitis).

Prostaglandins

Prostaglandins of the E series, particularly PGE_2, are potent stimulators of bone resorption *in vitro*. The prostaglandin endoperoxides (thromboxanes), prostaglandins of the A, B, and F series, and metabolites of PGE_2 such as 13,14-dihydro-PGE_2 and 15-keto, 13, 14-dihydro-PGE_2 show less potent resorptive activity *in vitro* than does PGE_2. These complex lipids may serve as local mediators of skeletal resorption in the same manner as suggested for the protein OAF. This may be particularly relevant to the bone loss associated with skeletal inflammatory processes such as rheumatoid arthritis or periodontal disease. Hypercalcemia may be a direct result of high circulating concentrations of prostaglandin metabolites in certain patients with

solid tumors (see "Specific Hypercalcemic Disorders — Prostaglandins," p. 987).

PRIMARY HYPERPARATHYROIDISM

Primary hyperparathyroidism can be defined as a state of malregulated hypersecretion of PTH by the parathyroid gland itself. The etiology of the disease has not been established. Genetic factors are involved in some cases since the disease clearly can be hereditary. A number of potential secretagogues for PTH have been identified (see section on secretory control, p. 940). It is conjecture as to whether an endogenous (e.g., antibody as found in hyperthyroidism) or exogenous factor will be identified as causing aberrant parathyroid function through interaction with or regulation of a secretagogue receptor on parathyroid cells. Secondary hyperparathyroidism existing over long periods of time may evolve into primary hyperparathyroidism. Evolution of secondary hyperparathyroidism into primary hyperparathyroidism has sometimes been termed "tertiary hyperparathyroidism." Examples of autonomous primary hyperparathyroidism associated with an adenoma of the parathyroid glands have been reported in long-term osteomalacia as well as in chronic renal disease. Moreover, some cases of adenomatous primary hyperparathyroidism continue to show abnormally high renal clearance of calcium (renal calcium leak) after successful removal of a parathyroid adenoma and correction of hypercalcemia. It has been suggested that chronic loss of calcium through the kidney might represent a stimulus to hyperplasia and ultimate adenomatous growth of the glands and uncontrolled hypersecretion of hormone therefrom. On the other hand, conversion of hyperplastic parathyroid glands to adenomatous glands has never been proved and adenomatous primary hyperparathyroidism itself is not uncommon. Another putative etiologic factor recently advanced is irradiation; three centers have reported histories of prior x-irradiation of the neck in 10–37% of cases of primary hyperparathyroidism.

Prevalence

The apparent prevalence of primary hyperparathyroidism has increased sharply with the advent of more widespread recognition of the disorder and general availability of automated laboratory facilities for routine analysis of serum calcium. In one clinic wherein a consecutive series of 26,000 cases were analyzed for serum calcium, it was concluded that the prevalence of primary hyperparathyroidism is approximately 1:1000. This is a prevalence approximately 10-fold that ascertained in the early original studies on hyperparathyroidism. The high prevalences found in recent surveys are based exclusively on serum calcium measurements and thus do not provide an estimate of numbers of cases requiring treatment. Ascertainment on the basis of hypercalcemia alone thus includes asymptomatic cases of hyperparathyroidism as well as familial hypocalciuric hypercalcemia (FHH) (the exact prevalence of the latter disorder is unknown). Since parathyroidectomy is usually contraindicated in FHH, it is important that such cases be segregated from the population of typical primary hyperparathyroidism.

Pathology

Hypersecretion of PTH with primary hyperparathyroidism may be caused by a single adenoma, primary chief cell or clear cell hyperplasia of all parathyroid glands, or carcinoma.

Histopathology

Adenoma

Parathyroid adenomas may be composed of chief cells, transitional forms between chief and oxyphil cells, and, rarely, solely of oxyphil cells (Figs. 19–36 and 19–37). (Unlike normal oxyphil cells, those found in adenomas contain abundant endoplasmic reticulum and Golgi vesicles.) There may be considerable cellular pleomorphism and atypia. Fat cell fractional content is reduced. Adenomas vary from 500 mg to more than 20 g in weight and may show areas of cystic hemorrhage.

Parathyroid adenoma can be diagnosed only when there is a single enlarged gland and the three remaining glands are grossly and microscopically normal. The distinction between adenomas and hyperplasia cannot be made by examining a single gland. Although the presence of a compressed rim of normal tissue outside the capsule of an enlarged gland has been cited as evidence for the diagnosis of adenoma, a similar appearance occurs in nodular (pseudoadenomatous) chief cell hyperplasia. So-called double or multiple "adenomas" probably represent part of the spectrum of asymmetric chief cell hyperplasia, since removal of "double adenomas" is often followed by recurrence of hyperparathyroidism.

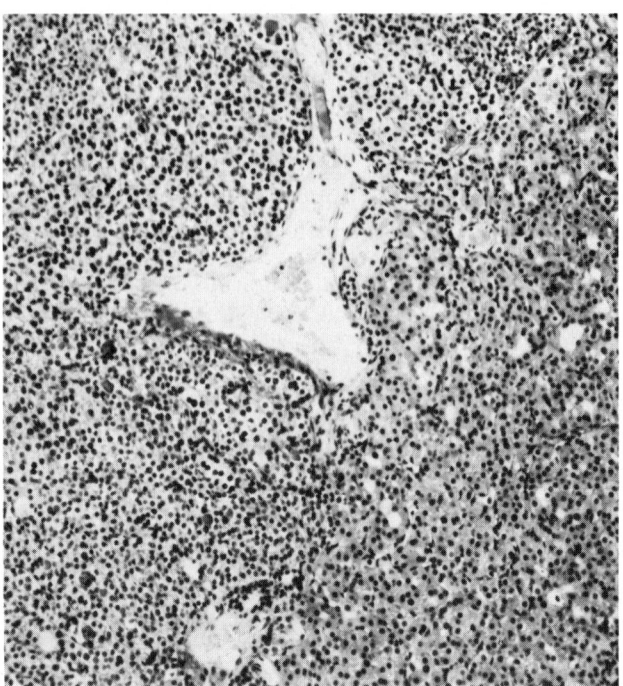

Figure 19–37. Sheets of minimally pleomorphic chief cells with a few intermixed transitional oxyphil cells (upper portion of section) but no stromal fat cells in a patient with primary chief cell hyperplasia. Magnification × 120. (Figure kindly provided by Dr. Benjamin Castleman, reprinted from Tumors of the Parathyroid Glands, *Atlas of Tumor Pathology*, Second Series, Fascicle 14.)

Chief Cell Hyperplasia

Chief cell hyperplasia is diagnosed upon finding more than one parathyroid grossly or microscopically abnormal. Several forms of chief cell hyperplasia have been described. The "classic" variety is the simplest to diagnose, since there is obvious enlargement of several parathyroids. In pseudoadenomatous hyperplasia, a single gland may be grossly enlarged with subtle, if any, enlargement of remaining glands. The minimally enlarged glands, however, have an abnormal histologic appearance with nodularity and an increased chief cell to fat cell ratio. In occult hyperplasia, there is only subtle enlargement of all four glands and a reduction in fat cell content.

Incidence of, and Distinction Between, Adenoma and Chief Cell Hyperplasia

Differentiation between adenoma and chief cell hyperplasia depends on ability to distinguish normal from subtly hyperplastic glands. This may be extremely difficult, particularly in the young; parathyroid glands from subjects less than 30 years old normally contain little fat. No consensus exists on the diagnosis of subtle hyperplasia, and the relative incidence of adenoma versus hyperplasia varies from institution to institution. At one extreme authors argue that virtually *all* cases of primary hyperparathyroidism are due to hyperplasia. At the other extreme are those who claim that adenomas are encountered in about 80% of cases and chief cell hyperplasia in less than 15% of cases. There is general agreement, however, that chief cell hyperplasia is the lesion in essentially all inherited forms of hyperparathyroidism (see "Familial Hypercalcemia," p. 977).

Water-Clear Cell Hyperplasia

The incidence of this lesion has declined to about 1% of all cases of primary hyperparathyroidism, at present. The rea-

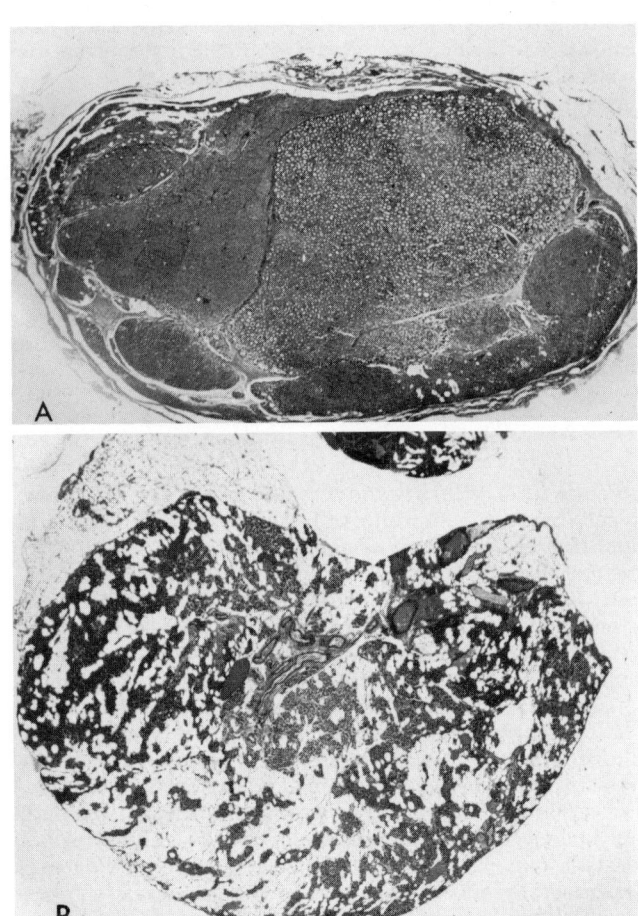

Figure 19–36. (A) Cross-section of an entire hyperplastic gland, showing islands of parathyroid cells in varying patterns. The small solid islands are made up predominantly of oxyphil cells, with the largest island of chief cells in an acinar pattern. Magnification × 11. (B) Cross-section of an entire normal parathyroid gland, demonstrating the usual amount and distribution of stromal fat in a middle-aged person. Magnification × 15. (Figure kindly provided by Dr. Benjamin Castleman, reprinted from Tumors of the Parathyroid Glands, *Atlas of Tumor Pathology*, Second Series, Fascicle 14.)

son for this decline is obscure. Grossly, the superior glands are usually disproportionately enlarged. The empty appearance of water-clear cells is due to the presence of large membrane-lined vacuoles filling the cytoplasm.

Carcinoma

Three to 4% of cases of primary hyperparathyroidism are caused by parathyroid carcinoma. The lesion may be palpable in the neck, and at surgery is often firm and densely adherent to local structures. Characteristic histologic features include capsular and vascular invasion; cells are usually organized into trabeculae separated by thick fibrous bands (Fig. 19–38). Mitotic figures are almost always present. Local invasion, spread to regional lymph nodes, and distant metastases (lung, liver, and bone in order of decreasing frequency) have been described.

Clinical Manifestations

General

Primary hyperparathyroidism is a disease with protean manifestations varying from truly asymptomatic cases to striking systemic symptoms and signs such as weakness, fatigability, headache, weight loss, and depression. The disease tends to segregate into three categories in terms of clinical presentation. In the mildest form there may be no symptoms or signs, and discovery is made only through routine determination of serum calcium. The second form develops insidiously over a period of years and presents predominantly as renal colic. In the third group, the interval between development of symptoms and diagnosis may be much shorter, with marked hypercalcemia, debility, bone pain, and sometimes pathologic fracture. Debility, weight loss, anemia, and elevated sedimentation rate may be prominent enough to suggest systemic malignancy. Symptoms such as polydipsia, polyuria, pruritus, anorexia, nausea and vomiting may develop attendant upon hypercalcemia.

Renal Manifestations

Renal colic is one of the most common symptoms of hyperparathyroidism, occurring in 25–35% of cases. Nephrocal-

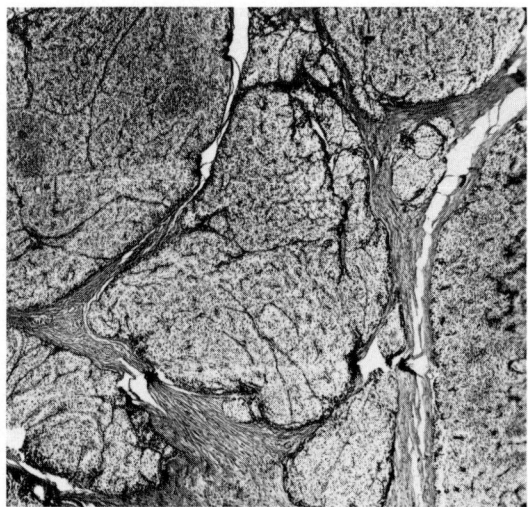

Figure 19–38. Parathyroid carcinoma. Prominent acellular dense fibrous bands separating islands of tumor cells. Magnification × 28. (Figure kindly provided by Dr. Benjamin Castleman, reprinted from Tumors of the Parathyroid Glands, *Atlas of Tumor Pathology*, Second Series, Fascicle 14.)

cinosis and metabolic acidosis (see discussion under "Laboratory Studies," p. 967) are other renal manifestations of primary hyperparathyroidism. Most stones in hyperparathyroidism are calcium oxalate, but calcium phosphate stones also occur and development of either should alert the physician to the possible diagnosis of the underlying disease. Several cases have been reported in association with medullary sponge kidney, but this association may be fortuitous. A recent study shows a high positive correlation between 1,25 $(OH)_2$ vitamin D concentrations in plasma with nephrolithiosis in primary hyperparathyoidism.

Skeletal Manifestations

Bone disease in hyperparathyroidism may present clinically as bone pain, pathologic fracture, bone cysts, or localized swellings of bone encountered as "epulis" of the jaw or "brown tumors" (area of accumulated osteoclasts, osteoblasts, and fibrous tissue) of bones. Histologically the skeletal lesion observed in hyperparathyroidism is osteitis fibrosa cystica (Fig. 19–39), areas of increased bone resorption with large numbers of multinucleated osteoclasts, and fibrous tissue. Occasionally a brown tumor in a small bone such as a phalanx may be the presenting symptom causing the patient to seek medical advice. Bone biopsy in primary hyperparathyroidism may also show areas of decreased mineralization (increased numbers of osteoid seams) as well as areas of osteosclerosis. The roentgenographic signs of bone disease are discussed under "Radiologic Abnormalities in Primary Hyperthyroidism." p. 966.

Several symptoms and signs referable to the joints are recognized in hyperparathyroidism. Gout and pseudogout may be complications of the disease. Chondrocalcinosis and predisposition to attacks of pseudogout occur with greater frequency in primary hyperparathyroidism than they do in the general population. Nonspecific arthralgias involving all of the joints of the hands or sometimes centered in the proximal interphalangeal joints are also reported in primary hyperparathyroidism. The etiology of these nonspecific arthralgias is unknown, but frequently they disappear after correction of the underlying disorder.

Gastrointestinal Manifestations

Peptic ulcer occurs with increased frequency in primary hyperparathyroidism relative to the general clinic population. Hypercalcemia *per se* can cause an increase in serum gastrin as well as an increase in gastric secretion. Moreover, hyperparathyroidism as part of the multiple endocrine neoplasia type I (MEN I) syndrome may be associated with the Zollinger-Ellison syndrome. In the latter instance, pancreatic islet tumors secrete massive amounts of gastrin causing huge increases in acid production by the stomach. The concentrations of gastrin in serum in the Zollinger-Ellison syndrome usually exceed 600 pg/ml. Chronic pancreatitis is another gastrointestinal manifestation that may be associated with primary hyperparathyroidism. The pathophysiology leading to this association is unknown. Pancreatitis may be exacerbated in subjects with worsening hyperparathyroidism as well as in the postoperative phase of parathyroidectomy.

Neurologic Manifestations

Neurologic abnormalities in hyperparathyroidism include emotional lability, slow mentation, poor memory, depression, and neuromuscular abnormalities. Easy fatigabil-

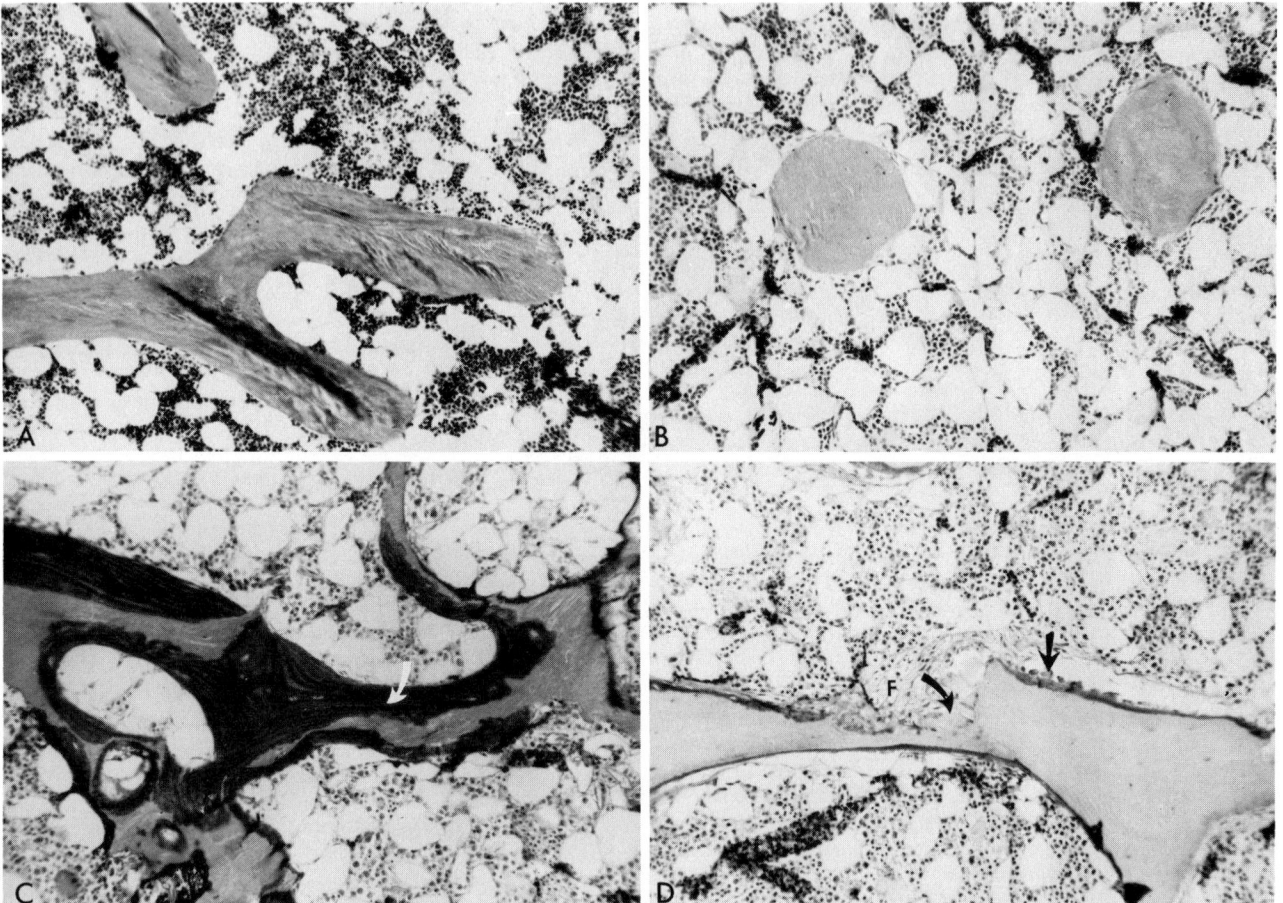

Figure 19–39. Histologic studies of human bone. Sections of undecalcified bone from the iliac crest were stained with Goldner stain and photographed at × 100. (A) Normal trabecular bone. (B) Osteoporosis. The quantity of bone matrix is diminished, but relative proportions of osteoid and cellular elements are normal. (C) Osteomalacia. Bone trabeculae have widened osteoid layers (stained dark). Note normal lamellar structure in the unmineralized osteoid (arrow). (D) Primary hyperparathyroidism. Numerous osteoclasts (curved arrow) are present within a resorption cavity. There is increased quantity of osteoid, much of which is lined by cuboidal osteoblasts (straight arrow). Early peritrabecular marrow fibrosis (osteitis fibrosa) is present (F). (Courtesy of Dr. S. Teitlebaum.)

ity is one of the most prominent symptoms in primary hyperparathyroidism. Muscle weakness, particularly involving the proximal groups of the extremities, can be demonstrated by objective muscle examination in significant numbers of cases. In addition to muscle weakness, fatigability and abnormalities of mental status, occasional patients complain of decreased hearing, dysphasia, anosmia, and dysesthesias. Abnormal tongue movements resembling fasciculations also have been observed in primary hyperparathyroidism. Frequently, neurologic examination will show hyperactive reflexes. Other less frequently encountered neurologic abnormalities include glossal atrophy, decreased vibratory sense in the feet, and glove-and-stocking distribution sensory loss.

Neuromuscular Abnormality in Hyperparathyroidism

Proximal muscle weakness may range in severity from that barely detectable to weakness that obviously limits the subject's activity. The patient may complain of muscle aches and pains and heaviness in the lower extremities with difficulty climbing stairs, getting out of a chair, or getting out of a bathtub. Symptoms in the lower extremities precede those referable to the upper extremities. Loss of muscle strength correlates with changes evident on muscle biopsy. The characteristic finding is muscle atrophy evident most markedly in atrophy of the type II fibers (Fig. 19–40).

Type II fiber atrophy is characteristic of a neuropathic lesion; type II fibers are the first to undergo atrophy upon denervation. Thus it is apparent that the muscle lesion in hyperparathyroidism is a neuropathy and not a myopathy as has occasionally been reported in the literature. The electromyogram in parathyroid neuromuscular disorder shows a polyphasic potential pattern also compatible with denervation. Small-amplitude potentials of short duration on myograms are also observed and again presumably represent neuropathic rather than myopathic changes. Muscle weakness improves significantly upon correction of hyperparathyroidism.

Other Associated Abnormalities

Certain signs and symptoms in hyperparathyroidism may be secondary to hypercalcemia itself. Polyuria and polydipsia (related to associated hypercalciuria) are common, as well as constipation, all complaints possibly relatable to hypercalcemia. In severe hypercalcemia the electrocardiogram may reveal a shortened $Q_{-0}T_C$ interval. Other infrequent abnormalities in hypercalcemia include "band keratopathy," pruritus, subconjunctival deposits of calcium, and ectopic calcifications in lungs, kidneys, arteries, and skin. These forms of ectopic calcification are more likely in association with some degree of renal impairment and phosphate retention. Band keratopathy is recognized as opaque material appearing in parallel lines within the limbus of

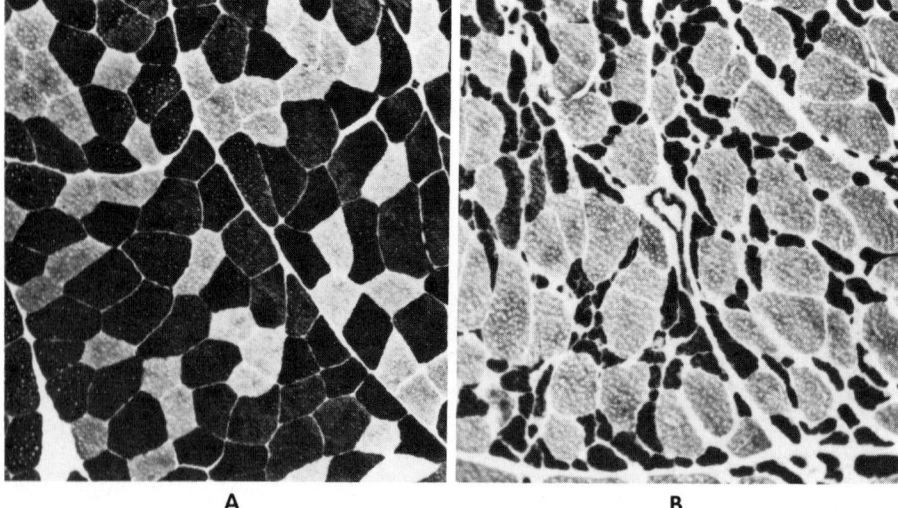

A   B

Figure 19–40. Biopsies of muscle. Section in (A) shows normal quadriceps muscle specimen with slightly larger type II (dark-stained) than type I (light) fibers. (B) Specimen from patient with primary hyperparathyroidism and marked muscle weakness. Note marked atrophy, particularly of type II fibers (ATPase stain). (From Patten, B. M., Bilezikian, J. P., et al.: Neuromuscular disease in primary hyperparathyroidism. *Ann. Int. Med. 80*:182, 1974.)

the eye. Pruritus may be secondary to microscopic deposits of calcium within the skin. Loosening of the teeth and hypermobility of the joints also have been found in hyperparathyroidism, although there is no clear-cut explanation for these phenomena.

Anemia and elevated sedimentation rate are found in significant numbers of patients; indeed anemia was reported in approximately half of the original series from the Massachusetts General Hospital (Albright, Aub, et al., 1934). There is no adequate explanation for the latter abnormalities. Monoclonal gammopathy has been observed as an unrelated coexistent disorder in hyperparathyroidism. These hematologic abnormalities as well as weight loss in some cases heighten concern that hypercalcemia might be due to malignancy. On the other hand, these abnormalities should not deter proper evaluation for hyperparathyroidism nor be taken as definitive criteria diagnostic for hypercalcemia of malignancy.

Hypertension is observed in 20–60% of reported series of primary hyperparathyroidism. There is no single known factor associated with hyperparathyroidism that can be considered the cause of hypertension in the disorder. Moreover, correction of hyperparathyroidism does not regularly lead to cure of the associated hypertension.

Associated Endocrine and Metabolic Disorders

Sporadic occurrence of Hashimoto's disease as well as of Cushing's syndrome in hyperparathyroidism has been reported unrelated to the various types of MEN and in patients whose families are free of endocrine abnormalities. Endocrinopathies associated in familial forms of hyperparathyroidism are discussed separately. Hypokalemia and hypomagnesemia are discussed under other laboratory results.

Radiologic Abnormalities in Primary Hyperparathyroidism

Radiographic evidence of hyperparathyroidism is expressed as subperiosteal resorption (best recognized in the phalanges and distal portions of the clavicles), generalized osteopenia or osteoporosis, demineralization ("salt and pepper pattern") of the skull, bone cysts or brown tumors (evidenced as areas of radiolucency, particularly in the long bones), and occasionally patchy or diffuse areas of increased bone density (osteosclerosis). The symphysis pubis and

sacroiliac joints may appear widened. Nephrocalcinosis as well as nephrolithiasis may be evident on x-rays of the kidney. Tomograms of the kidney may show nephrocalcinosis not detected by routine roentgenograms. Demineralization around the teeth is evidenced as loss of the lamina dura. Chondrocalcinosis is apparent in up to 10% of patients with primary hyperparathyroidism (Fig. 19–41). In severe

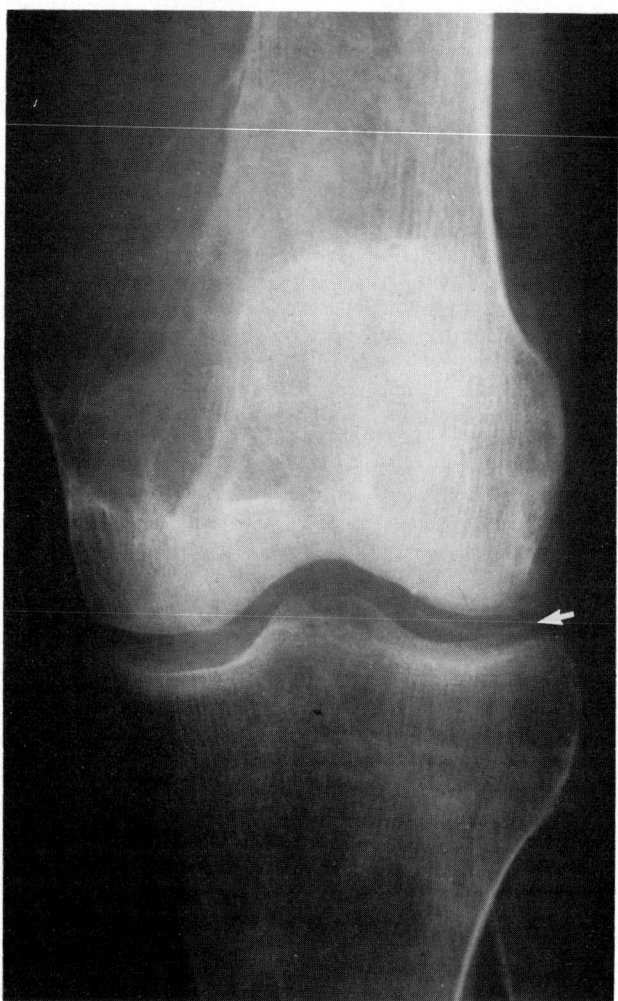

Figure 19–41. Chondrocalcinosis in a patient with osteitis fibrosa cystica. Note intraarticular calcification (arrow).

cases there may also be resorption of the distal phalangeal tufts as well as clubbing of the fingers (Fig. 19–42).

Other occasionally observed roentgenographic features include deviation of the esophagus on esophagogram as a result of impingement by a parathyroid adenoma. Rarely, a mediastinal adenoma is of sufficient size and location to be recognized as an abnormal mass on lateral chest x-ray. Computerized axial tomography (CAT) allows somewhat more frequent recognition of mediastinal lesions.

Other roentgenographic features include signs of ectopic calcification or characteristics of associated diseases. Several cases of extensive pulmonary calcification have been described in hyperparathyroidism. This may occur consequent to intercurrent viral pulmonary infection in subjects with significant hypercalcemia and hyperparathyroidism. Cholelithiasis has been reported in hyperparathyroidism but the incidence does not seem to be significantly greater than that of the general population. Abnormalities found on gastrointestinal x-rays can reflect associated diseases or evidence of MEN. For example, chronic pancreatitis may be evident with calcifications in the pancreas. The increased incidence of peptic ulcer in hyperparathyroidism as well as hypertrophic rugae in the stomach in association with Zollinger-Ellison syndrome may be recognized on upper gastrointestinal series x-rays. Patients who have undergone intravenous phosphate therapy may show evidence of ectopic calcification appearing as calcification of small arteries including the digital arteries.

Laboratory Studies

Hypercalcemia and hypophosphatemia are the classic laboratory hallmarks of primary hyperparathyroidism. Hypercalcemia is almost always found in primary hyperparathyroidism. This reflects the actions of PTH on the kidney and the skeleton to increase reabsorption of calcium from bone and the GF and to stimulate $1,25$-$(OH)_2$-vitamin D production with consequent increased calcium absorption from the gut. Hypophosphatemia is a consequence of the direct action of PTH on the kidney and can be aggravated by hypercalcemia as well. Within the past decade other laboratory parameters for evaluating parathyroid function have become available. These include radioimmunoassay for PTH, urinary cAMP clearance, determination of gastrointestinal absorption of calcium, and determination of vi-

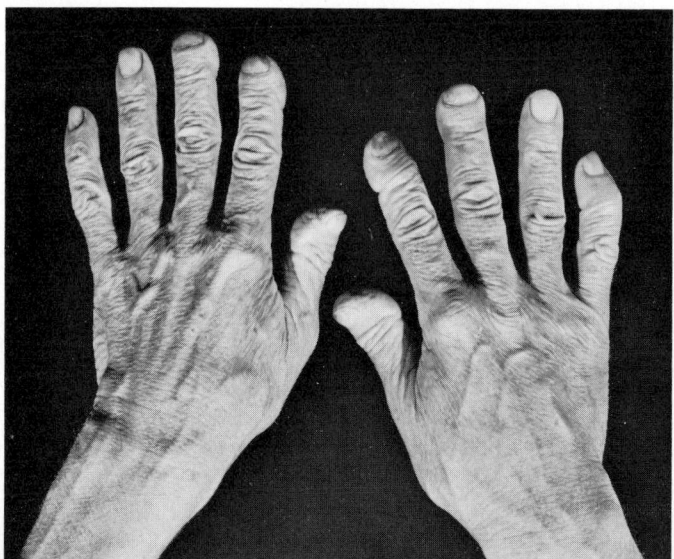

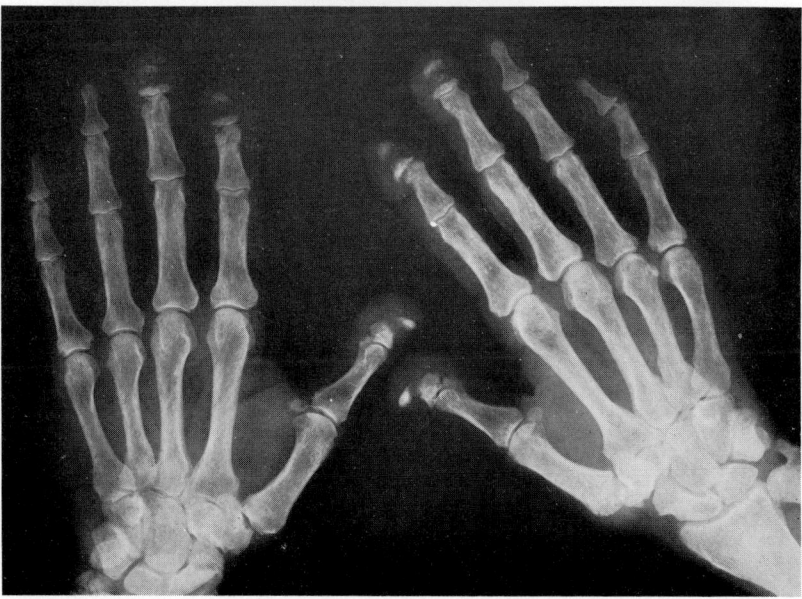

Figure 19–42. Marked periosteal bone erosion in the terminal phalanges of a patient with primary hyperparathyrodism. The erosion has been so extensive that clubbing has resulted.

tamin D metabolites in plasma. These several tests as well as certain ancillary laboratory determinations are discussed later. An outline of laboratory tests for hyperparathyroidism is provided in Table 19–9.

Hypercalcemia

High blood calcium levels are almost always detected in primary hyperparathyroidism. In any one patient, though, particularly in early or mild cases, serial analyses may show fluctuations of serum calcium into and out of the normal range. Some cases of "normocalcemic hyperparathyroidism" represent sampling bias — serum calcium being analyzed near the nadir of such fluctuations in serum calcium. Other causes for apparent normocalcemic hyperparathyroidism or masked hypercalcemia in primary hyperparathyroidism include coexistent vitamin D deficiency, hypoalbuminemia, and acidosis. In the latter two instances ionized calcium will be abnormally high even though total serum calcium concentration is normal. Hypercalcemia that is masked by vitamin D deficiency would become evident upon administration of vitamin D. Hypercalcemia *per se* detected in the general clinic population can be attributed on chance alone to primary hyperparathyroidism in almost half the cases. The differential diagnosis of hypercalcemia is discussed on p. 985.

Plasma Phosphate in Hyperparathyroidism

Generally blood phosphate is low in primary hyperparathyroidism as a consequence of the renal effects of PTH in increasing the clearance of phosphate into urine. Hypophosphatemia, however, is a less reliable parameter for diagnostic purposes. Plasma phosphate varies with phosphate intake, time of sampling, and renal function. True hypophosphatemia is only found in about 50% of cases of primary hyperparathyroidism. Several parameters have been devised in attempts to improve on total serum phosphate concentration as a discriminant in diagnosis. Phosphate clearance, tubular reabsorption of phosphate (TRP), and a phosphate excretion index expressing phosphate excretion per dl of GF and T_m phosphate (tubular maximum for phosphate reabsorption) have all been proposed as better diagnostic indices. None, however, provides highly discriminant diagnostic parameters. In one series of surgically documented hyperparathyroidism, determinations of phosphate clearance or of TRP were abnormal in only 50–60% of cases.

Radioimmunoassay for Parathyroid Hormone

Radioimmunoassays for PTH are discussed extensively under "Parathyroid Hormone," p. 937. The accumulation of inert immunoreactive fragments of the hormone in the circulation, the lack of uniform standards, radioactive tracers, and antisera all make interpretation of results for radioimmunoassays on random samples from peripheral plasma difficult, and sometimes impossible. Problems of interpretation are amplified in proportion to deterioration of renal function. Biologically inert carboxylterminal fragments accumulate to the greatest degree in renal impairment. Even with normal renal function the radioimmunoassays

---

Table 19–9. LABORATORY TESTS IN HYPERPARATHYROIDISM (HPT)

Major Significance	
Total serum calcium	almost always increased; may be intermittent; masked in coexistent vitamin D deficiency; hypoalbuminemia
PTH radioimmunoassay*	nl compatible with HPT; ↑ diagnostic with significant hypercalcemia and no renal impairment
Urinary cAMP	
UcAMP/dl GF**	↑ diagnostic of HPT if malignancy excluded
NcAMP/dl GF†	↓ excludes HPT if renal function nl
Urinary calcium excretion‡	usually ↑; ↓ in FHH; highest in nonparathyroid-related hypercalcemia
Alkaline phosphatase	increased bone fraction indicates significant bone disease (osteitis fibrosis cystica)
Lesser Significance	
Prednisone challenge (30 mg/d × 10)	little or no effect in HPT; Ca falls to nl — suspect vitamin D tox.; sarcoidosis; myeloma (sometimes); "milk-alkali syndrome"
Prot. electrophoresis; bone marrow; B.J. prot.	helps rule out hypercalcemia of malignancy
Bone x-rays	may show signs of HPT — subperiosteal resorption; "salt/pepper skull"; bone cysts helps rule out malignancy
Arteriography (selective)	indicated to localize PT tissue before repeat operation in failed surgery
Venous (selective) catheterization	indicated to localize PT tissue before repeat operation in failed surgery
Ancillary	
Thyroid scan	indicated before arteriography/venography
Serum gastrin	↑ in coexistent Z.E.
TRP/phosphate clearance	abnormal in 50–60% of cases
Calcium absorption test (^{47}Ca)	↑ in HPT
Hematology	↑ sed. rate, anemia in 25% of HPT
Serum chemistry	↑ chloride ↓ CO_2 in some cases; occasionally ↑ K
Kidney x-rays	if suspect nephrolithiasis, nephrocalcinosis
Serum phosphate	usually decreased; nl or ↑ in coexistent renal disease; if high or nl suspect nonparathyroid hypercalcemia
1,25-dihydroxy vitamin D assay	elevated in HPT — not yet generally available
Ionized calcium	elevated in HPT — may be test of choice in future but generally not equal to total Ca determination as diagnostic parameter
Serum magnesium	usually nl or ↓; may be ↑ in FHH

*Normal range (units nonuniform) — varies from one laboratory to another. Some expressed in concentration units for pure standard; others in volume of arbitrary reference plasma.

**Total urinary cAMP expressed as nmol/dl GF, nl range 1.83–4.55 nmol/dl GF.

†Nephrogenous cAMP (NcAMP) = (cAMP/dl GF) — plasma cAMP — nl range 0.29–2.81 nmol/dl GF.

‡May be expressed as mass per 24 hrs or per dl GF, or as Ca/creatinine clearance ratio.

yield higher estimates than bioassays for the concentration of active hormone in the circulation. Recent studies with ultrasensitive histochemical bioassays for PTH indicate that circulating concentrations of biologically active hormone approximate 5–15 pg/ml of plasma. Even the most putatively sophisticated "aminoterminal" immunoassays show concentrations of apparent hormone 10–15 times greater than those determined by the histocytochemical bioassay method. Some examples showing comparative assays using either radioimmunoassay or histocytochemical bioassay for parathyroid in human plasma are presented in Table 19–10 and Fig. 19–43. These data clearly show that most of the immunoreactive PTH in peripheral plasma represents inert metabolites of no physiologic consequence. Also evident are marked discrepancies from one laboratory to another in radioimmunoassay results. Nevertheless, in primary hyperparathyroidism uncomplicated by renal failure, radioimmunoassays usually show abnormally high concentrations of immunoreactive (predominantly inert fragments) hormone in plasma. Hypercalcemia from causes unrelated to PTH and without a renal failure component is appropriately reflected in some assays by undetectable amounts of hormone in plasma. Nonparathyroid-mediated hypercalcemia favors accumulation of fragments (released from the parathyroid gland or formed peripherally) detectable in other assays. High concentrations of PTH in peripheral plasma also have been found in cases of hyperparathyroidism due to ectopic production of the hormone by nonparathyroid tumors. The latter phenomenon can only be established with certainty, however, in cases in which it can be shown that the tumor itself is producing PTH (see "Ectopic Hyperparathyroidism," p. 987). In view of the marked problems in interpreting radioimmunoassay results, it is hazardous to assume that one can differentiate by radioimmunoassay on peripheral plasma ectopically produced PTH and hormone produced by the parathyroid gland itself. Radioimmunoassays for PTH are also useful in the special application of analyzing samples obtained by selective venous catheterization to localize sites of PTH production. This topic is discussed under "Preoperative Localization of Abnormal Parathyroid Glands," p. 973.

Urinary Cyclic 3',5'-AMP

The role of cyclic 3',5'-AMP in the mechanism of action of PTH is discussed extensively under physiology of the hormone (p. 946). Since certain cells in the renal tubule bear specific receptors for PTH, respond to the hormone with an increased concentration of cAMP, and elaborate cAMP directly into the luminal fluid, the rate of excretion of cAMP in the urine reflects the circulating concentration of biologically active PTH. The total amount of cAMP excreted represents cAMP cleared from the plasma by glomerular filtration plus the nephrogenous contribution itself. In primary hyperparathyroidism the total excretion of cAMP in the urine is increased, and parameters of parathyroid secretory

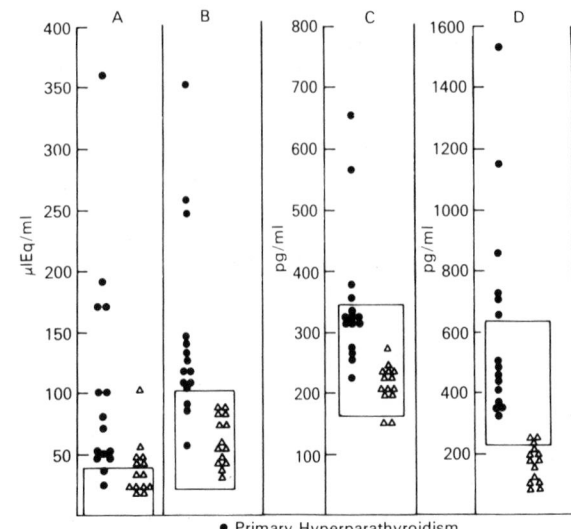

Figure 19–43. Disparate results for radioimmunoassays of PTH. Aliquots of plasma taken from patients with primary hyperparathyroidism (•) or hypercalcemia caused by nonparathyroid malignancy (△) were distributed to four different radioimmunoassay laboratories. The normal range of values for each laboratory is depicted by the rectangle. Note that the overlap between normal and hyperparathyroid subjects varies considerably from one laboratory to another and that in only one laboratory was there adequate discrimination between subjects with primary hyperparathyroidism and those with hypercalcemia due to malignancy. Results indicating normal concentrations of PTH in hypercalcemia of malignancy could be misinterpreted as "parathyroid hormone concentrations too high for the degree of hypercalcemia" and incorrectly suggest the possible diagnosis of hyperparathyroidism, primary or ectopic. (From Raisz, L. G., Yajnik, C. H., et al.: Comparison of commercially available parathyroid hormone immunoassays in the differential diagnosis of hypercalcemia due to primary hyperthyroidism or malignancy. *Ann. Int. Med., 91*:739, 1979.

activity have been based upon this observation. Simultaneous determination of plasma and urine cAMP and creatinine allow calculation of nephrogenous cAMP (Fig. 19–44). Urinary cAMP as a diagnostic parameter has been expressed in several forms. Generally the parameter of greatest discrimination is the expression of nephrogenous cAMP in nmol/dl of GF (see "Urinary Excretion of Cyclic AMP," p. 948). Discrimination almost as great can be obtained by the simple determination of total urinary cAMP/dl of GF (cAMP/mg of creatinine × plasma creatinine). The latter is readily applied to random samples obtained in the general clinic population and is a highly useful screening test for hyperparathyroidism. It should prove valuable in differentiating nonparathyroid-related hypercalcemic states as well as hypoparathyroidism.

Determination of 1,25-Dihydroxycholecalciferol

The influence of PTH on regulating production of 1,25-(OH)-D in the kidney via the 1-hydroxylase enzyme is evi-

Table 19–10. COMPARATIVE RESULTS OF RADIOIMMUNOASSAY AND CYTOCHEMICAL BIOASSAYS FOR PARATHYROID HORMONE IN PLASMA

Subject	n	Serum Calcium (mM)	Bioassay (pg/ml)	RIA (pg/ml)
Normal	(8)	2.42	16.8 ± 3.6	–
Hyperparathyroidism	(8)	2.94	109 ± 35	1920 ± 470
Hypoparathyroidism	(3)	1.84*	0.67 ± .17	–

n = number of subjects
*Two of hypoparathyroid subjects were taking vitamin D.
From Fenton, S., Somers, S., et al.: *Clin. Endocrinol. 9*:381, 1978.

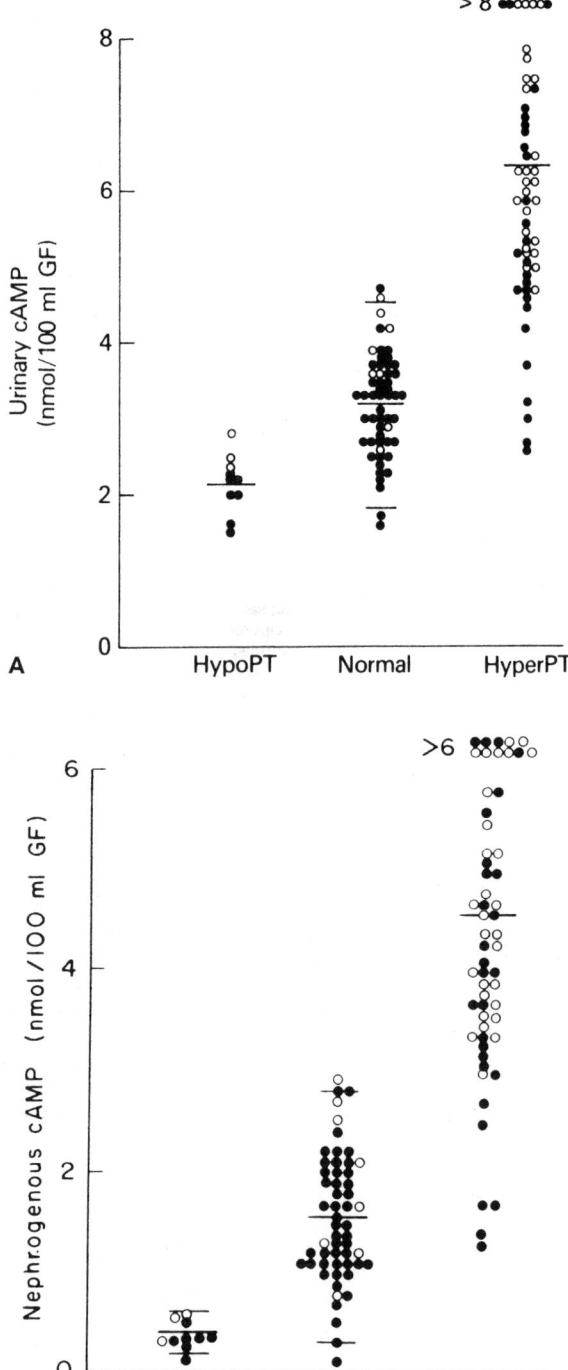

Figure 19–44. Urinary cAMP excretion as a function of parathyroid status. (A) Total urinary cAMP excretion expressed as the parameter cAMP excreted per 100 ml of GF. (B) Nephrogenous cAMP expressed as the parameter nephrogenous cAMP per 100 ml of GF. The parameter shown in (A) is satisfactory for routine clinical testing. Nephrogenous cAMP (B) gives slightly greater discrimination between parathyroid secretory states. Note that each of the parameters affords differentiation of parathyroid hypofunction as well as hyperfunction. Open symbols represent subjects with renal impairment. (From Broadus, A. E., Mahaffey, J. E., et al.: Nephrogenous cyclic adenosine monophosphate as a parathyroid function. *J. Clin. Invest. 60:*771, 1977.)

dent in primary hyperparathyroidism, and increased concentrations of the 1,25 metabolite in plasma have been documented. There is considerable overlap between normal and hyperparathyroid subjects, however. The highly special- ized technology required for these analyses is not generally available. Of interest is the observation that patients with high 1,25-dihydroxyvitamin D concentrations appear more prone to present with renal lithiasis as the expression of primary hyperparathyroidism.

Gastrointestinal Absorption of Calcium in Primary Hyperparathyroidism

Gastrointestinal absorption of calcium is increased in primary hyperparathyroidism as assessed by calcium kinetic studies determining transfer of radioactive calcium from the gastrointestinal tract to blood and bone compartments *in vivo.* Total body retention of radioactive calcium given orally, an index of calcium absorption, is increased in hyperparathyroidism and tends to return toward normal with surgical correction of the disease. Fractional calcium absorption, determined kinetically, is increased in primary hyperparathyroidism and also returns toward normal after parathyroidectomy. The increase in gastrointestinal absorption of calcium in primary hyperparathyroidism presumably reflects enhanced rates of generation of 1,25-dihydroxycholecalciferol by the kidney in response to PTH. The increased circulating concentration of 1,25-dihydroxycholecalciferol (see earlier) is compatible with this view. The difficult techniques for determining gastrointestinal absorption of calcium, the large overlap of results for normal subjects and those with hyperparathyroidism, and the incomplete correlation among other parameters of PTH secretory status all limit the utility of the procedure for routine diagnostic use. It may be of ancillary value in unusual circumstances to determine gastrointestinal absorption of calcium when other parameters, such as PTH radioimmunoassays or cAMP excretion, give equivocal results.

Urinary Calcium and Phosphate Determinations

Urinary phosphate clearance is increased in primary hyperparathyroidism, reflecting the phosphaturic action of PTH as well as the effect of hypercalcemia on renal clearance of phosphate. Parametric expression of urinary phosphate excretion is discussed under "Plasma Phosphate in Hyperparathyroidism" (p. 968). In general, these parameters have not been highly valuable discriminatory indices. Determination of urinary calcium excretion is important in differentiating among several forms of hypercalcemia. Urinary Ca excretion is best expressed as a function of GFR (calcium clearance/creatinine clearance). Such parameters segregate subjects with FHH (see p. 978) and are useful in differentiating parathyroid-related hypercalcemia from those due to nonparathyroid causes. Since PTH causes increased reabsorption of calcium from the GF, there is generally reduced urinary calcium excretion relative to serum calcium in primary hyperparathyroidism. Conversely, in nonparathyroid-related forms of hypercalcemia, parathyroid secretion is inhibited and urinary calcium exceeds normal for any given serum calcium concentration (see Fig. 19–19).

Metabolic Acidosis

Hyperchloremia with reduction of plasma bicarbonate concentration has been described frequently in hyperparathyroidism, whereas metabolic alkalosis with low plasma chloride concentration occurs in nonparathyroid-related hypercalcemias. PTH itself influences the renal tubule causing decreased proximal reabsorption of bicarbonate. This effect of PTH has been described in humans as well as in animals. Patients with hereditary fructose intolerance as

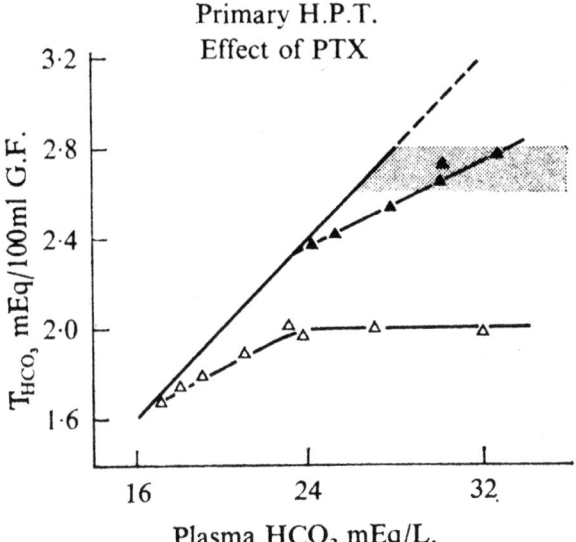

Figure 19–45. Renal capacity for bicarbonate reabsorption in hyperparathyroidism and effect of parathyroidectomy. Bicarbonate reabsorption, expressed as T_m bicarbonate, is reduced under the influence of PTH. This phenomenon can lead to proximal tubular acidosis in hyperparathyroidism and is corrected subsequent to removal of a parathyroid adenoma. (From Muldowney, F. P., Donohoe, J. F., et al.: Parathyroid acidosis in uremia. *Q. J. Med. 41*:321, 1972.)

well as Fanconi syndrome show a type of proximal renal tubular acidosis with bicarbonate loss that resolves with parathyroidectomy. Moreover, it appears likely that at least part of the metabolic acidosis in uremia is attributable to secondary hyperparathyroidism, inducing further proximal tubular rejection of bicarbonate and aggravating thereby the acidosis of renal disease. Muldowney and coworkers showed a defect in proximal reabsorption of bicarbonate in subjects with primary hyperparathyroidism. The defect is revealed particularly well in the test for $TmHCO_3^-$. The test for Tm bicarbonate is carried out by infusing sodium bicarbonate intravenously, attempting to achieve a constant increment in plasma bicarbonate concentration without increasing ECF volume. Results of such tests in primary hyperparathyroidism are illustrated in Fig. 19–45. The abnormality in Tm bicarbonate is corrected after parathyroidectomy.

It seems likely that impaired Tm for bicarbonate under the influence of PTH explains the metabolic acidosis in primary hyperparathyroidism. Occasionally the acidosis becomes even more severe in the first few days following removal of a parathyroid adenoma. This worsening of acidosis may be related to one or more causes: deterioration in renal function after surgery, phosphate depletion, release of hydrogen ion from recalcifying bone, and return of function of residual parathyroid tissue. Phosphate depletion itself has been shown to cause a similar type of proximal tubular bicarbonate wasting.

Parathyroid Secretory Control in Primary Hyperparathyroidism

In the past it has been assumed that PTH secretion in primary hyperparathyroidism is "autonomous" and not suppressible by increasing concentrations of calcium perfusing the glands. Conversely, the glands of secondary hyperparathyroidism have been considered normally suppressible by elevated concentrations of calcium. The concept of strict autonomy has been in doubt since advent of radioimmunoassays for PTH in the circulation. Several early stud-

ies with radioimmunoassays indicate that even certain parathyroid adenomas respond to increments in calcium concentration with reduction in rates of secretion. Recent studies indicate that patterns of response in primary hyperparathyroidism are not absolute. Some glands show no suppressibility *in vivo;* others show suppressed secretion in response to high concentrations of calcium, but the concentrations of calcium required for inhibition are greater than those found with normal glands. Recently an isolated parathyroid cell preparation has been developed that allows study of secretion *in vitro* from normal or abnormal glands removed surgically. Results show the varying characteristics of responsiveness of adenomatous glands. One group is sensitive to inhibition by calcium with apparently normal K_i both *in vivo* and *in vitro* (Fig. 19–46). Another group appears dramatically resistant to suppression by calcium. Again, results *in vitro* compare quite favorably to those *in vivo.* Cells from hyperplastic glands generally show suppression at normal K_i's for calcium. An occasional case of sporadic parathyroid hyperplasia, multiple endocrine neoplasia type II, however, may show nonsuppressibility similar to that found with some adenomas.

Diverse potential secretagogues, including catecholamines and peptides, were discussed in connection with the physiology of PTH. It was noted that β-adrenergic receptors have been identified on parathyroid cells and that β-adrenergic catecholamines stimulate secretion *in vivo* as well as *in vitro* of the hormone from parathyroid cells. Investigation of biogenic amines as potential secretagogues in tissue from primary hyperparathyroidism suggests that β-adrenergic responses vary considerably in abnormal parathyroid cells. Whereas normal bovine parathyroid cells uniformly show β_2-type adrenergic receptors, human parathyroid cells obtained from adenomas or hyperplastic tissue are diverse in receptor class. Preparations obtained from different patients show varying character from β_1- to β_2-type receptors and responses. Moreover, a spectrum of response to β-adrenergic agonists ranges from essentially no increment in cAMP concentration to amounts approaching those found in normal bovine cells. PTH release in response to β-adrenergic agonists as well as to dibutyryl cAMP also varies in pathologic parathyroid tissue and may reflect abnormalities characteristic of tumor cells. Response

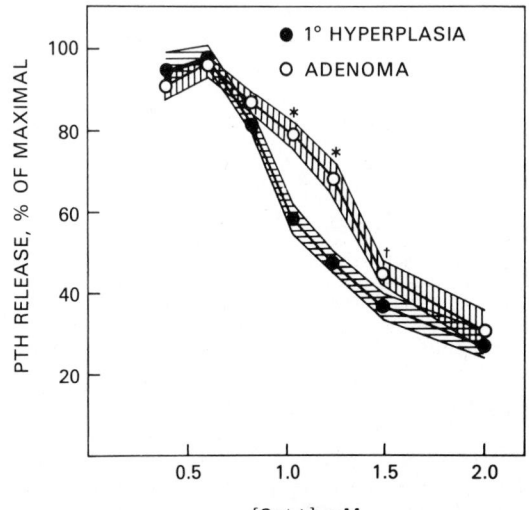

Figure 19–46. Relationship of PTH release to calcium concentration with isolated parathyroid cells *in vitro.* Most hyperplastic cells show calcium inhibition curves that are indistinguishable from normal ones. Adenoma cells show significantly higher K_i's for calcium. (From Brown, E. M., Brennan, M. F., et al.: *J. Clin. Endocrinol. Metab. 46*:267, 1978.)

to unusual secretagogues has also been found with adenomatous tissue. Parathyroid cells obtained from several patients have shown increases in cAMP concentration in response to glucagon. Cells from two other patients responded markedly to histamine. Neither glucagon nor histamine are effective secretagogues with normal bovine tissue. Since it is recognized that tumors may contain "ectopic receptors," it is possible that some of the human parathyroid responses represent pathologic development of receptors that do not normally exist on parathyroid cells.

Other Laboratory Abnormalities

Hypokalemia occurs infrequently in hyperparathyroidism but may become exaggerated in the course of treating patients with phosphate. In other cases hypokalemia may reflect coexistent hyperaldosteronism. There is a general tendency toward hypomagnesemia in primary hyperparathyroidism, and this sometimes is aggravated after surgical correction of the disease. Hypomagnesemia might reflect impaired renal reabsorption of magnesium or long-term bone demineralization (bone is also an important repository for magnesium) in response to hypersecretion of PTH. Low or normal plasma concentrations of magnesium in hyperparathyroidism help differentiate this disorder from FHH (see p. 978), which frequently manifests high normal or elevated concentrations of magnesium in plasma. There also appears to be an increased incidence of hyperuricemia in hyperparathyroidism.

Anemia and elevation of the erythrocyte sedimentation rate are found in primary hyperparathyroidism, particularly in more severe forms of the disease. Recent studies have redirected the attention to the anemia of primary hyperparathyroidism. Anemia correlates with the severity of the disease and signs of hyperparathyroid bone disease on x-ray. There are no specific changes in marrow aspirates or peripheral blood smears, although this form of anemia may represent a type of myelofibrosis.

Summary

Increased total calcium concentration on repeated analysis of plasma remains the hallmark of the disorder. Further tests of parathyroid function permit differentiation between nonparathyroid-related hypercalcemia (functionally suppressed parathyroid glands) and primary hyperparathyroidism. Among the most useful tests are determination of urinary cAMP (expressed as cAMP excretion/dl of GF or nephrogenous cAMP/dl of GF) and radioimmunoassays for PTH. Utilization of these and other tests in the differential diagnosis of hypercalcemia is discussed on p. 985). Tests of primary as well as of ancillary interest in the diagnosis are summarized in Table 19–9.

Differential Diagnosis

The differential diagnosis of primary hyperparathyroidism includes the nonparathyroid causes of hypercalcemia, demineralization of bone, nephrolithiasis, or hypophosphatemia. The differential diagnosis of hypercalcemia, which may be expressed in diverse metabolic, endocrine, or malignant diseases, is discussed separately (p. 985). It is convenient to group those disorders associated with high rates of secretion of PTH, such as primary hyperparathyroidism, ectopic hyperparathyroidism, secondary hyperparathyroidism, or FHH (may show only normal or only modestly ele-

vated parameters of parathyroid function, see p. 978). This group is characterized by laboratory results compatible with the increased rates of parathyroid secretion — high concentrations of PTH in plasma, high rates of excretion of urinary cAMP, and low rates of urinary calcium excretion relative to serum calcium. Virtually all other causes of hypercalcemia are associated with signs of reduced PTH secretion (see p. 985). Significant degrees of renal impairment associated with hypercalcemia of any cause complicate interpretation of PTH radioimmunoassay* as well as cAMP excretion. The latter parameter, however, is severely affected only as GFR drops below 30%.

Other physiologic effects of PTH secretion observed in hyperparathyroidism may serve as differential points. These include hyperchloremic acidosis (reflecting the action of PTH on the rejection of bicarbonate in the proximal tubule of the kidney) and hypophosphatemia, a manifestation of the phosphaturic action of PTH. Conversely, in nonparathyroid-related causes of hypercalcemia there is a tendency to metabolic alkalosis and hyperphosphatemia. The latter two parameters, however, are not uniformly dependable differential points. Moreover, there is a suggestion that in some forms of malignancy and hypercalcemia, hypophosphatemia may exist unrelated to PTH secretion. Certain nonparathyroid-related causes of hypercalcemia are particularly amenable to correction with corticosteroid therapy (see p. 984). The hypercalcemia of hyperparathyroidism, ectopic or primary, almost invariably is resistant to the effects of this treatment with corticosteroids. Laboratory parameters helpful in the differential diagnosis of hyperparathyroidism are presented in Table 19–9.

"Ectopic hyperparathyroidism" in which a nonparathyroid tumor itself produces PTH may be particularly difficult to diagnose because the laboratory findings do not differ from those of hyperparathyroidism caused by parathyroid adenoma or hyperplasia. Diagnosis depends upon suspicion of associated malignancy, localizing the malignancy, and proving that it is the source of ectopic production of PTH. Venous catheterization studies with sampling for PTH radioimmunoassay can be the sole means, other than surgical exploration, to distinguish between ectopic hyperparathyroidism and coexistent primary hyperparathyroidism with unrelated cancer.

Differential Diagnosis of Osteitis Fibrosa Cystica

Although several metabolic diseases of bone may be associated with generalized demineralization of the skeleton, radiolucent areas of bone, or areas of osteosclerosis or increased bone density similar to that found in primary hyperparathyroidism, they frequently can be differentiated on the basis of radiologic appearance as well as of laboratory parameters. Disorders to be considered here include Paget's disease of bone, osteoporosis, osteomalacia, multiple myeloma, malignancy metastatic to bone, polyostotic fibrous dysplasia, secondary hyperparathyroidism, pseudohypoparathyroidism, and solitary bone cysts. Hypercalcemia may be associated with Paget's disease in patients with extensive involvement who are at bed rest. Generally, Paget's disease

---

*Interpretation of radioimmunoassay for PTH is complicated by any degree of renal impairment that causes an increased accumulation in the circulation of biologically inert fragments of the hormone. Not only may the latter accumulate due to decreased clearance in renal impairment, but also hypercalcemia *per se* may favor elaboration of fragments from the gland itself (see discussion concerning secretion and metabolism of PTH, p. 940 and p. 941).

can be differentiated by characteristic lesions found roentgenographically in bone. The laboratory features are distinct from those in primary hyperparathyroidism, and plasma calcium is normal unless the subject becomes immobilized. In osteoporosis serum calcium, phosphate, alkaline phosphatase, and all parameters of parathyroid function are normal. Clinical characteristics of malignant disease as well as roentgenographic appearance should alert the physician to the possibility of malignant metastases in bone. Bone marrow examination also is indicated whenever there is suspicion of underlying skeletal malignancy. Analysis of plasma and urine for myeloma proteins should be routine in suspected cases. Osteomalacia may be caused by hypovitaminosis D, resistance to vitamin D, intestinal malabsorption syndromes, or renal tubular acidosis. In these conditions serum calcium concentration is normal or low, sometimes with tetany. Bone biopsy may be helpful in differentiating various forms of osteomalacia from osteitis fibrosa cystica.

Polyostotic fibrous dysplasia may represent an interesting clinical challenge in that roentgenographic appearance of lesions in bone as well as actual bone biopsy samples resembles strikingly the bone lesions of osteitis fibrosa cystica. In some cases there is associated sexual and somatic precocity in affected females. In general, this disorder can be differentiated from hyperparathyroidism because the bone lesions are not generalized as in primary hyperparathyroidism and all laboratory parameters of parathyroid function are normal. Polyostotic fibrous dysplasia may also be associated with pigmented areas of the skin. There have been occasional case reports of coexistent primary hyperparathyroidism and polyostotic fibrous dysplasia of bone.

Secondary hyperparathyroidism in chronic renal disease may produce the histologic picture of osteitis fibrosa cystica. In general serum phosphate is high, there is a tendency to hypocalcemia, and soft tissue calcification is more severe than it is in primary hyperparathyroidism. Areas of osteomalacia as well as osteitis fibrosa cystica may exist in this condition. Pseudohypoparathyroidism also may be associated with osteitis fibrosa cystica. In these cases the bone appears to be sensitive to the actions of PTH even though the kidney is resistant.

Nephrolithiasis may be associated with a number of metabolic disorders, including idiopathic hypercalciuria, gout, hyperoxaluria or cystinuria, as well as primary hyperparathyroidism. None of these disorders, however, is associated with hypercalcemia, and in virtually all the parameters of parathyroid secretory activity are normal (one form of idiopathic hypercalciuria is associated with increased parathyroid secretory activity). Five to 20% of cases of nephrolithiasis, however, may be attributable to primary hyperparathyroidism. Thus serum calcium should be determined on several occasions in all cases of nephrolithiasis or renal colic.

Nephrocalcinosis

Nephrocalcinosis occurs in several disorders including renal tubular acidosis and pyelonephritis as well as primary hyperparathyroidism. The general laboratory features of primary hyperparathyroidism, however, should establish the correct diagnosis.

Preoperative Localization of Abnormal Parathyroid Glands

Surgical correction of primary hyperparathyroidism is effective in a very high percentage of cases. Since localizing abnormal parathyroid glands during surgery is a problem in 10 to 15% of cases, however, there has been much interest in developing procedures to localize abnormal tissue before surgical intervention. The approaches used include cineesophagography, mediastinography, computerized axial tomography (CAT), arteriography, venography with selective sampling and radioimmunoassay for PTH, radioactive selenomethionine scanning, ultrasonography, and thermography. In addition, there have been attempts to localize abnormal tissue during the course of surgery with intravenous injection of phenothiazine-like dyes. Currently only arteriography and selective venous catheterization with PTH radioimmunoassay represent high yield procedures for preoperative localization of parathyroid lesions. On the other hand, noninvasive procedures such as esophagography and CAT are probably warranted even though the yield with these procedures is low. In rare cases, adenomas are palpable in the neck and mediastinal adenomas occasionally have been detected on simple x-rays of the chest.

Preoperative localization utilizing arteriography and selective venous catheterization should be reserved for and definitely undertaken before further surgery in cases of recurrent hyperparathyroidism or persistent hyperparathyroidism after initial cervical exploration. The relatively high cost of these procedures and the fact that the great majority of cases of primary hyperparathyroidism in the general population can be attributable to a single parathyroid adenoma make it unrealistic to apply these techniques routinely to fresh cases. Moreover, extensive experience in the utilization of these procedures is limited to a small number of research centers. On the other hand, the increased complexity of second or third surgical explorations probably warrants the expense and delay required for angiographic and venous sampling techniques. In these cases, arteriography should be carried out first in an attempt to discover possible lesions as well as potentially to delineate venous anatomy. The nature of lesions can be proved by detecting high concentrations of PTH by radioimmunoassay in plasma of selectively catheterized veins draining the lesion (Fig. 19–47). Arteriography carried out by an experienced angiographer reveals an abnormal mass in approximately 60% of parathyroid adenomas missed at prior surgery. Selective venous sampling with catheterization of the small veins in the neck allows lateralization of parathyroid adenomas in approximately 80% of cases. Arteriographic identification of a mass with subsequent identification of a hormone concentration gradient in a vein draining the lesion is virtually conclusive evidence for the nature of the lesion.

Treatment of Primary Hyperparathyroidism

Asymptomatic Hyperaparathyroidism

The widespread availability of automated reliable analyses for serum calcium has fostered discovery of hypercalcemia in asymptomatic subjects with primary hyperparathyroidism. Indeed, this has led to an apparent 10-fold increase in the prevalence of primary hyperparathyroidism. In early series, cases were discovered primarily through symptoms and signs of the disease. Newer experience with asymptomatic hypercalcemia makes it likely that significant numbers of patients with mild forms of hyperparathyroidism enjoy normal life expectancy without any symptoms or signs of the disease. Some cases previously diagnosed as asymptomatic hyperparathyroidism may in fact be more properly classified as hypocalciuric hypercalcemia (see p. 978).

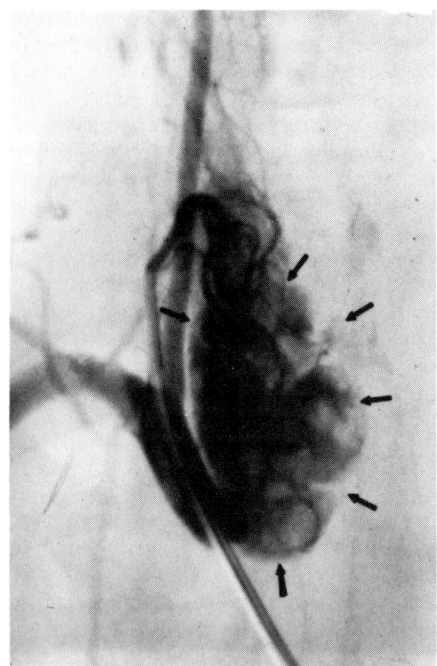
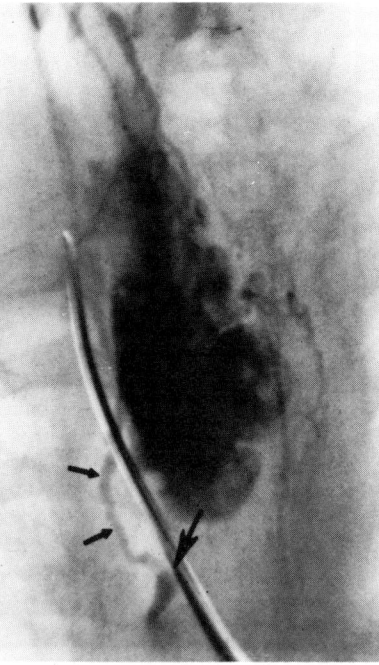

Figure 19–47. Arteriographic localization of large parathyroid adenoma. (A) Arrows outline large parathyroid adenoma filled by radiographic dye injected into right inferior thyroid artery. This phase of the arteriographic study also shows a rich arterial vascular plexus within the gland. (B) Late phase of arteriographic study, showing vein (delineated by arrows) draining the adenoma. Subsequent selective venous sampling showed a very high concentration gradient (sample to peripheral) for PTH at the point marked by the large arrow.

Management of cases of truly asymptomatic hyperparathyroidism is a problem because we do not know the true risk for development of renal and osseous complications in any given patient. A study at the Mayo Clinic of 134 cases of mild or asymptomatic hyperparathyroidism over a 5-year period showed the following results: 20% eventually required surgery (which was unsuccessful in 5 of 29 cases), 58% showed no change in clinical status, 4% died of unrelated causes, and 18% were lost to follow-up. The Mayo Clinic investigators believe that as many as 20% of asymptomatic subjects may develop progression of the disease within 5 years of discovery.

The risk of progression of the disease, the cost of long-term follow-up of such cases, and the psychologic factors (two of the subjects in the Mayo Clinic series underwent surgery strictly on the basis of pressing psychologic factors) must be weighed against the morbidity, cost, and risk of surgical failure in subjects who might otherwise live normal lives without surgical intervention. An approach that is currently useful is as follows: (1) Obtain detailed family history in attempt to exclude FHH, familial hyperparathyroidism, or involvement in multiple endocrine neoplasia type I or type II (see p. 978). Classification into these categories is virtually definitive evidence for multiple gland hyperplasia, which in asymptomatic cases militates against surgical intervention. (2) Test renal function, urinary calcium excretion, and take x-rays of the skeleton. If all these results are normal, surgery probably should be postponed but the patient must be reevaluated for renal, gastrointestinal, and skeletal status at regular periods, e.g., every 6–12 months. Significant evidence for progression of the disease at subsequent examination would be an indication for surgical intervention. (3) Subjects with definite abnormalities in skeletal or renal function even though clinically asymptomatic may be candidates for surgery. (4) Usually the need for developing decisions on these subjects is not urgent. Patients in this "asymptomatic hyperparathyroidism" group followed at the Mayo Clinic and at the National Institutes of Health have so far not developed rapid progressive disease or hypercalcemic crisis requiring emergency surgery. Nevertheless, careful monitoring of this group is still required.

"Normocalcemic primary hyperparathyroidism" was discussed under the diagnosis of hyperparathyroidism. Subjects in this category should be managed in a fashion identical to that outlined for primary hyperparathyroidism in general. Surgery should be considered according to the same criteria outlined previously.

Temporary Treatment

Dehydration and progressive hypercalcemia and deterioration of renal function are the major problems that can be life-threatening in primary hyperparathyroidism. Methods for temporary control of hypercalcemia and dehydration are discussed on p. 982. Some patients with primary hyperparathyroidism have been managed with phosphate administration by mouth for periods of up to 6 months pending clarification of other complications before parathyroidectomy. CT has not proved generally efficacious in controlling hypercalcemia in primary hyperparathyroidism. Mithramycin has been used to reduce hypercalcemia on a short-term basis pending surgery. Repeated use of mithramycin will be detrimental to the blood-forming elements. Corticosteroids, as noted under discussion of diagnosis, are ineffective in controlling the hypercalcemia of primary hyperparathyroidism. Moreover, extensive use of corticosteroids will complicate management before, during, and after surgery.

Emergency Therapy

Occasionally hypercalcemia may become progressive and severe ("hypercalcemic crisis"), leading to marked weakness, mental deterioration, coma, progressive uremia, and death. Aggressive intervention with intravenous fluids, furosemide, and phosphate administration by mouth (see discussion of hypercalcemia, p. 982), as well as administration of mithramycin, may be required. Generally, aggressive use of these measures will allow stabilization of the clinical state pending definitive surgery. Occasionally, hemodialysis against low calcium fluid may be required. Some have advocated emergency surgery; however, it is doubtful that this approach should be entertained until the clinical situation becomes stabilized at least temporarily.

Surgery

The approach taken by the surgeon frequently is influenced by the particular experience with parathyroid pathology at each medical center. Recently reports from a few centers suggest a very high incidence of four-gland parathyroid hyperplasia. The great majority of clinics, however, continue to find that in the general clinic population primary hyperparathyroidism is accounted for in >80% of cases by a single parathyroid adenoma. Particular exceptions are subjects giving a family history for hypercalcemia, hyperparathyroidism, or other manifestations of multiple endocrine neoplasia. The latter groups virtually exclusively show multiple gland hyperplasia as the pathologic basis for primary hyperparathyroidism.

Given that the vast majority of cases represent single parathyroid adenomas, some surgeons favor the following approach: One side of the neck is searched meticulously first. If an adenoma and a normal gland on that side are each proved by biopsy (frozen sections), the adenoma is removed and the wound closed. This leaves the contralateral side undisturbed and suitable for accurate exploration at a future time in the unlikely event that this becomes necessary. If the lesion is not found initially, the surgeon should extend the procedure to the controlateral side and attempt to identify all four parathyroid glands. Biopsy identification of all glands (results of frozen section at surgery should be confirmed by analysis of permanent sections) is then essential for subsequent surgical exploration and also facilitates the diagnosis of hyperplasia. In multiple gland hyperplasia all parathyroid tissue should be removed save for approximately 50 mg of the most normal-appearing gland. If neither hyperplastic nor adenomatous glands are found, dissection should be extended to the retroesophageal and retropharyngeal space as well as retrieving, if possible, the thymic fat pad through the cervical incision. If two normal glands (biopsy identification) have been found on one side of the neck, the surgeon may consider excising the thyroid lobe on the opposite side. Occasional parathyroid adenomas lie entirely within the bed of the thyroid, undetectable by visual inspection. If, after extensive exploration, no abnormal parathyroid tissue is found, a mediastinal exploration should be considered, but only at a later date. Before further surgery is carried out, detailed localization studies should be performed in an attempt to localize the abnormal tissue. The patient's interest is best served by a surgeon having extensive experience in parathyroid surgery.

Reoperative Surgery for Persistent or Recurrent Hyperparathyroidism

Failure at initial neck exploration to find and excise abnormal parathyroid tissue is an indication for temporizing, re-evaluating the diagnosis, and instituting localizing procedures before further surgical intervention. It is best not to proceed with mediastinal exploration at the time of original neck surgery. Most adenomas missed at the time of initial surgical exploration are still to be found within the neck. Moreover, after a prolonged tedious dissection of the neck, neither the surgeon nor the patient is ideally suited to proceed with a further major procedure. It is best to allow a period of several weeks of recovery, if the clinical condition permits, before undertaking localization procedures and considering further surgery. Angiographic and immunoassay sampling procedures are also indicated in subjects who have undergone prior neck surgery unrelated to parathyroid disease. Prior thyroid surgery may sufficiently distort the vascular tree as well as produce sufficient scar tissue to lend additional morbidity to further surgery without localization.

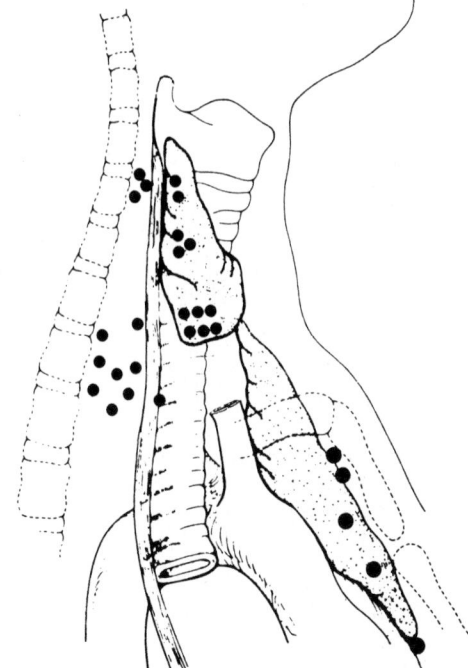

Figure 19–48. Location of parathyroid adenomas missed at initial surgery but found upon subsequent successful surgical exploration. (From Brennan, M. F., Doppman, J. L., et al.: Reoperative parathyroid surgery for persistent hyperparathyroidism. *Surgery 83*:669, 1978.)

Preoperative localization allows the surgeon to plan the type of operation needed and to concentrate on dissecting areas where the pathology is to be found. High mediastinal tumors may be reached through a cervical incision or through a relatively simple "hockey stick" sternum-splitting maneuver. The latter is associated with less morbidity than is a complete sternum-splitting exploration. The locations found for parathyroid lesions in 25 successful reoperative procedures are shown in Fig. 19–48. Note that only five of the lesions represented mediastinal adenomas and of these only three required sternotomy, the remaining two being retrieved from the neck. Note also that a large fraction of the missed glands were found deeply posterior in the neck. Such deep posterior lesions frequently show the "tracheal overlap" sign when detected on arteriography.

Parathyroid Carcinoma

Parathyroid carcinoma is a rare cause of primary hyperparathyroidism and probably accounts for less than 3–4% of cases. It is a relatively slow-growing cancer and is curable in its early stage by adequate local excision. Local spread or dissemination may occur attendant upon rupture of the tumor capsule at the initial operation. Parathyroid carcinoma clearly represents one cause of persistent or recurrent primary hyperparathyroidism. Local recurrences as well as isolated metastases also may be amenable to surgical excision and afford thereby improvement in the hyperparathyroid state.

Postoperative Course

After successful removal of the parathyroid adenoma there is rapid correction of most of the biochemical abnormalities of hyperparathyroidism. Serum calcium begins to fall within hours, may drop through the normal range within 4–12 hours after surgery, and usually reaches a nadir 4–7 days later. Immediately after parathyroidectomy there is a transient increase in urinary calcium; subsequently urinary calcium falls sharply to the undetectable range as hypocalcemia develops. Urinary phosphate excretion falls promptly after parathyroidectomy, but the rapid drop in urinary cAMP is most dramatic and indeed can serve as an intraoperative index of successful parathyroidectomy.

Marked and prolonged hypocalcemia may develop after parathyroidectomy as a result of several possible metabolic perturbations. (1) The most common cause is accelerated skeletal uptake of calcium ("hungry bones") attendant upon abrupt cessation and correction of the excessive bone resorption induced by long-term hyperparathyroidism. The severity and duration of this phenomenon is a function of the degree of bone demineralization previously developed in the course of hyperparathyroidism. This form of bone disease is associated with marked osteoblastic activity in the bone and large amounts of unmineralized osteoid tissue. (2) Hypomagnesemia. Prolonged hyperparathyroidism with marked bone demineralization may lead to total body depletion of magnesium. Following parathyroidectomy with restoration of bone formation, hypomagnesemia may become significant and interfere with secretion or action of PTH from residual normal glands. (3) Permanent or temporary hypoparathyroidism may develop in subjects who have undergone prior parathyroidectomy (the adenoma ultimately excised may represent the sole remaining parathyroid tissue) or in patients undergoing aggressive resection of multiglandular parathyroid hyperplasia. Determination of urinary cAMP in the postoperative period (Fig. 19–49) allows differentiation of hypocalcemia due to hypoparathyroidism, permanent or temporary, from that due to accelerated skeletal remineralization ("hungry bones"). Permanent hypoparathyroidism also is associated with hyperphosphatemia. In one series the achievement of serum phosphate greater than 6 mg/dl heralded permanent hypoparathyroidism. Transient hypocalcemia ("hungry bones") represents a form of osteomalacia and may be preventable by administration of vitamin D metabolites preoperatively. Modest degrees of hypocalcemia in the postoperative period need not be treated beyond ensuring an adequate calcium intake. Significant and symptomatic hypocalcemia may require administration of calcium by vein (5–15 mg/kg of calcium in 500–1500 ml of saline) given slowly over the course of 24 hours. Some patients may require in addition administration of vitamin D or 1,25-dihydroxycholecalciferol. Therapy should be withdrawn as rapidly as clinical progress allows. Definite signs of recovery are usual within 7–10 days postoperatively. It is probably best to allow some degree of hypocalcemia as long as symptoms are controlled because hypercalcemia would tend to inhibit recovery of remaining parathyroid tissue. Excessive calcium or vitamin D should be avoided. Magnesium deficiency should be corrected by intravenous administration (if renal function is satisfactory) of 80–120 mEq of magnesium. Serum magnesium concentration alone does not reflect the severity of total body depletion of magnesium. In magnesium depletion, the urinary magnesium excretion is a useful parameter and will be low so long as significant total depletion of magnesium exists (see Fig. 19–4).

Permanent hypoparathyroidism is usually treated with vitamin D. An experimental program has been developed to correct permanent hypoparathyroidism attendant upon removal of multiple hyperplasic glands or sole remaining adenomatous glands with autotransplantation of part of the tissue to the forearm. One approach is to freeze some of the parathyroid tissue removed at surgery. If hypoparathyroidism develops later, the cryopreserved tissue can then be implanted in the forearm. Transplantation at the time of surgery should probably not be carried out because at that time it is impossible to predict hypoparathyroidism and the necessity for the transplant.

Other complications in the postoperative period include gout, pseudogout, pancreatitis, and worsening of the metabolic acidosis. Arthralgia or arthritis in the postoperative period should alert the physician to the possibility of gout or pseudogout; the latter in particular should be suspected in patients with intra-articular calcification. In some cases, particularly those with compromised renal function, metabolic acidosis may become worsened in the postoperative period. Rarely, bone cysts may be so extensive as to lead to fracture of long bones in patients who return too quickly to vigorous activity. Bone cysts can be differentiated from brown tumors on the basis of remineralization evident on roentgenograms. Brown tumors show dense remineralization within 6–12 months after surgery. Cysts do not remineralize, and if major in extent may require orthopedic intervention and packing with bone chips.

Hyperparathyroidism in Pregnancy

Hyperparathyroidism in pregnancy can pose difficult clinical management problems. In addition to the usual clinical

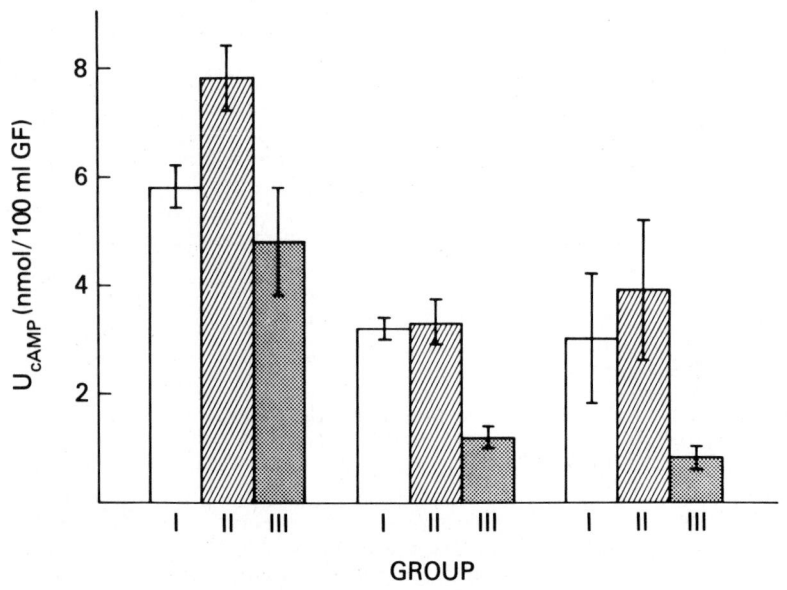

Figure 19–49. Urinary cAMP excretion before parathyroidectomy (set on left), in the early postoperative period (middle set), and 7 to 10 days after parathyroidectomy (set on right). Three types of results were obtained. Group I was normocalcemic postoperatively. Group II required vitamin D transiently for hypocalcemia (due to "hungry bones"). Group III became permanently hypoparathyroid attendant upon removal of sole remaining parathyroid tissue. (From Spiegel, A. M., et al., 1981, in press.)

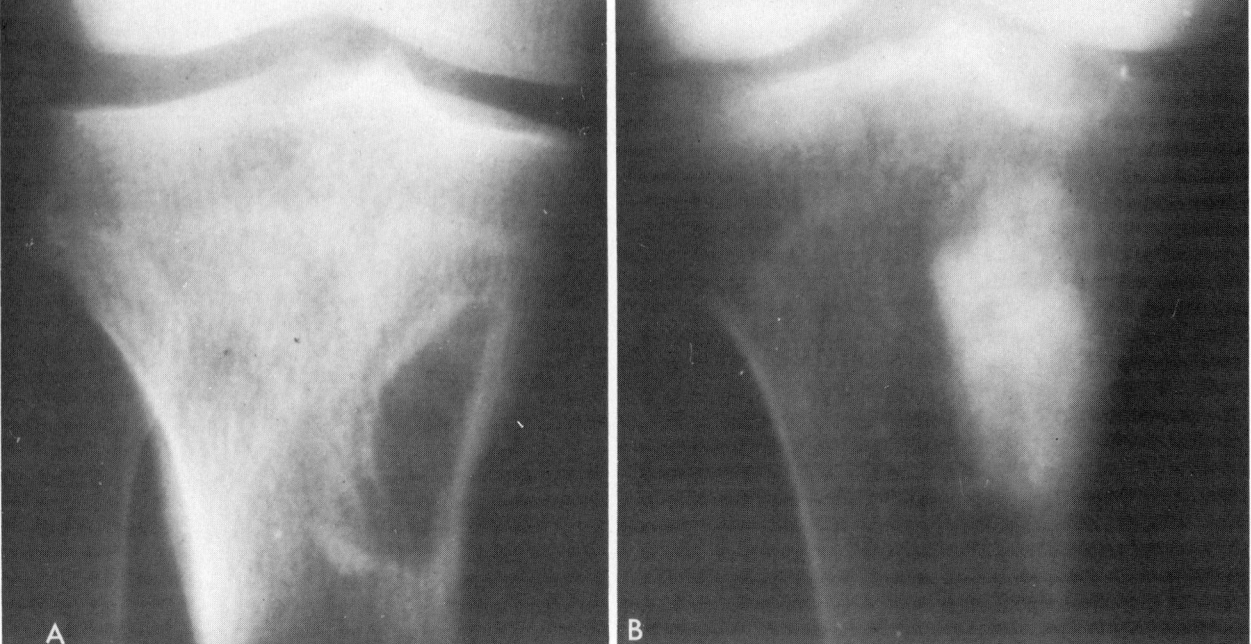

Figure 19–50. Brown tumor of bone before *(A)* and 1 year after *(B)* correction of primary hyperparathyroidism.

expression of the disease — renal, gastrointestinal, and musculoskeletal — for which the mother would be at risk, there is the further challenge of potential risk to the fetus in the event surgery would be required during the first trimester (teratogenicity of anesthetic agents) and neonatal hypocalcemia in the postnatal period. Although hyperparathyroidism is not a rare disease — representing approximately 0.1% of the general clinic population — its prevalence appears to be less in pregnancy. A recent search uncovered only 14 cases reported in a 13-year period. The apparent low incidence might reflect differences in diagnostic screening in prenatal versus medical clinics, a difference in the age of populations surveyed, differences in laboratory methods, or possibly even protection against hyperparathyroidism by the pregnant state. This is a topic clearly in need of further study.

In pregnancy several physiologic mechanisms develop to allow the rapid assimilation of calcium by the fetus. Calcium absorption in the mother increases from approximately 150 mg/day to 400 mg/day at 20 weeks. The placenta develops an efficient calcium transport mechanism that allows the fetal serum calcium to exceed that of the mother. This mechanism may aggravate even further in the fetus the hypercalcemia attendant upon hyperparathyroidism in the mother. The potential detrimental effect of hypercalcemia in hyperparathyroidim thus could be exaggerated in the fetus. The major detrimental influences on the fetus of severe maternal primary hyperparathyroidism are death (as high as 30 per cent, stillbirth, abortion, or neonatal death), failure to thrive in the postnatal period, and delayed neonatal hypocalcemia. Even in the normal fetus PTH secretion apparently is suppressed and is not initiated until approximately 48 hours after birth. The accentuated fetal hypercalcemia attendant upon maternal hyperparathyroidism causes profound and prolonged suppression of PTH secretion until very late in the postnatal period. This late neonatal hypocalcemia occasionally is the first clue to the existence of maternal hyperparathyroidism. Of 11 cases of postnatal hypocalcemia in progeny of 25 mothers with primary hyperparathyroidism, 9 of the babies developed hypocalcemia in the first few weeks of life. One developed hypocalcemia only during weaning at the age of 5 months.

Treatment of Hyperparathyroidism in Pregnancy

Hyperparathyroidism with significant symptoms and signs of the disease should be corrected surgically. The optimum period for surgical intervention is believed to be the second trimester. The possible teratogenic risk of anesthetic agents during the first trimester is considered a relative contraindication to surgery at that time. This risk would necessarily need to be weighed against the risk to the mother should severe hyperparathyroidism develop. There are no available data to evaluate the prognosis of mild primary hyperparathyroidism during pregnancy but it probably has minimal morbidity for mother and fetus.

Neonatal Hyperparathyroidism

Hyperparathyroidism in the neonatal period is rare. The disease is characterized by hypotonia, poor feeding, constipation, and respiratory distress. Marked hypercalcemia, hypophosphatemia, and severe bony demineralization but not nephrocalcinosis have been observed. Histologically the parathyroids have shown hyperplasia of the clear cell or vacuolated chief cell type but never adenoma. There may be generalized bone demineralization and multiple fractures, and a striking feature may be extremely narrow chest. Neonatal hyperparathyroidism has been reported in siblings and also has been described in a family with FHH. Although the disease is rare, recognition and treatment is crucial in that the 1-year survival rate in untreated severe cases is below 50%. The very high incidence of multiple gland hyperplasia in neonatal hyperparthyroidism may require total parathyroidectomy as the surgical approach taken. It is possible that cryopreservation of surgically removed hyperplastic tissue will facilitate reimplantation at a later date of viable parathyroid tissue to the forearm of the patient to correct the expected development of hypoparathyroidism.

Familial Hypercalcemia

Several distinct syndromes of familial hypercalcemia have been delineated. In most, primary hyperparathyroidism has been implicated. A health survey in Sweden indicated a 0.13% prevalence of familial hypercalcemia in a population with a 0.6% prevalence of hypercalcemia. Among cases with primary parathyroid hyperplasia, familial hypercalcemia occurs as frequently as 52%, depending upon the definition of hyperplasia and upon referral bias.

Familial Multiple Endocrine Neoplasia, Type I

This presents with neoplasia, usually benign, of multiple tissues, often with associated hypersecretion of hormones (Table 19–11). It has also been called multiple endocrine adenomatosis (MEA) and Wermer's syndrome. Inheritance is autosomal dominant. Primary hyperparathyroidism is the most common clinical manifestation in the syndrome. Less common features include excessive secretion of gastrin (20–40% of cases), insulin (2–10% of cases), other pancreatic islet peptides (rare glucagon, vasoactive intestinal peptide, etc), and anterior pituitary peptides (rare GH, ACTH, or PRL). The pancreatic cholera syndrome and also nondiarrheogenic pancreatic islet cell tumors are rare causes of a PTH-independent hypercalcemia. Nonsecreting tumor masses may be evident but rarely metastasize. These include lipomas (20%), pituitary chromophobe adenomas, carcinoid tumors, and adrenal and thyroid adenomas. Expression of the trait tends to follow consistent patterns within each kindred. Thus in some kindreds there is a high penetrance for hypergastrinemia whereas in others there is a high penetrance for hyperinsulinemia.

In numerous small kindreds, primary hyperparathyroidism alone has been diagnosed. These might be distinct hereditary syndrome(s) of familial hyperparathyroidism or simply clinical presentations resulting from the statistical likelihood that in many small kindreds FMEN I would present as isolated primary hyperparathyroidism in several members.

The biochemical features of familial multiple endocrine neoplasia (FMEN) type I are those related to excessive secretion by the affected endocrine cells. Since hyperparathyroidism occurs in 95% or more of affected patients, the most simple and useful test for family screening is serum calcium determination. Excessive basal secretion of gastrin may occur in asymptomatic family members, but hypercalcemia is evident in most of them and in 85% or more of those with symptomatic Zollinger-Ellison syndrome.

The cause of the abnormal activation (proliferation and secretion) of endocrine cells in FMEN I is not known. There are interesting similarities between this disorder and the syndrome of neonatal hypoglycemia with nesidioblastosis of the pancreatic islets. Nesidioblastosis is the embryologic process by which pancreatic ductular cells produce buds that differentiate into islets of Langerhans. Neonatal hypoglyce-

mia is one expression of continuation of this process into the postnatal period, with hyperplasia and microadenoma formation in the islets. Islet hormones have multiple actions that could potentially lead to hyperplasia of other endocrine cells, including direct actions on bone, kidney, parathyroid gland, and C (CT-secreting) cells. An equally plausible explanation for FMEN I is a genetic abnormality producing similar growth disturbances in a class of related (mostly endocrine) cell types.

Treatment of FMEN I should be directed at dangerous manifestations; however, several unique features of this disorder should be considered. The primary parathyroid hyperplasia has a greater tendency to recur than sporadic primary parathyroid hyperplasia, sometimes many years after apparently successful subtotal parathyroidectomy. It is thus particularly important to insure that any parathyroid tissue remaining after subtotal parathyroidectomy be in locations easily accessible to later surgery. Hypercalcemia may exacerbate the degree of hypergastrinemia and also the amount of gastric acid secreted at any serum concentration of gastrin. Furthermore, PTH is a secretogogue for gastrin in the dog. Thus, active primary hyperparathyroidism makes evaluation of the gastrin-gastric axis difficult. Family screening should be initiated among the first degree relatives of any patient with MEN I; it is often an hereditary disorder, though it may also arise by new mutation. The syndrome has a high penetrance (for expression of hypercalcemia) after age 30, but generally it cannot be diagnosed by family screening in the first decade of life.

Other Multiple Endocrine Neoplasias

Primary hyperparathyroidism occurs in 20–30% of patients with FMEN type II (Table 19–11) (see under "Hypercalcitoninism," p. 1017). Even more commonly, in a patient without known parathyroid glandular disturbance, diffusely hyperplastic parathyroid glands are discovered at the time of thyroid surgery for familial C cell hyperplasia or C cell cancer. FMEN type IIb or III is a similar but distinct syndrome of hyperfunction of C cells and adrenal chromaffin cells, in which there is a very low incidence of primary hyperparathyroidism. Distinguishing features include mucosal neuromas, ganglioneuromas, and a marfanoid habitus (see section on hypercalcitoninism).

Familial Hypocalciuric Hypercalcemia

FHH, also called familial benign hypercalcemia, is an autosomal dominant trait (Table 19–11) with high penetrance for expression of hypercalcemia at all ages. Its prevalence is similar to that of FMEN I. Most affected persons

Table 19–11. MAJOR FEATURES IN SYNDROMES OF FAMILIAL HYPERCALCEMIA

	Multiple Endocrine Neoplasia Type I	Multiple Endocrine Neoplasia Type II*	Hypocalciuric Hypercalcemia
Inheritance	Autosomal dominant	Autosomal dominant	Autosomal dominant
Penetrance of hypercalcemia, first decade	Low	Low	High
Associated endocrinopathy	Islet cell; anterior pituitary	Medullary thyroid cancer; pheochromocytoma	None
Unique biochemical features	Hypergastrinemia	Hypercalcitoninemia	Low renal clearance of calcium
Subtotal parathyroidectomy	Useful	Useful	Usually no benefit

*MEN type IIB rarely has hypercalcemia or hyperparathyroidism.

have no severe symptoms clearly attributable to the underlying process. Though nephrolithiasis or peptic ulcer disease may occur in 10% of patients, the stone or ulcer diathesis is neither recurrent nor aggressive. Easy fatiguability and muscle weakness are common but generally mild. Subtotal parathyroidectomy almost inevitably is followed by persistence or recurrence of hypercalcemia, and the parathyroid glands are only moderately enlarged.

Hypercalcemia and hypophosphatemia are similar in magnitude to that of typical primary hyperparathyroidism. The biochemical features that differentiate these patients from those with typical primary hyperparathyroidism are higher serum concentrations of magnesium and lower renal clearances of filtered calcium and magnesium (Fig. 19–51). Indices of parathyroid function (immunoreactive PTH, urinary cAMP excretion, and theoretic renal threshold for phosphate excretion) suggest lower circulating PTH activity in FHH than in typical primary hyperparathyroidism.

The etiology of this disorder is not known. It appears to affect divalent cation interactions in both the parathyroid gland and the kidneys. The clinical and biochemical features are distinct from those of MEN syndromes. It shares several clinical and biochemical features with the syndromes of neonatal primary parathyroid hyperplasia. Each causes hypercalcemia in the neonatal period. Neonatal primary parathyroid hyperplasia occurs in either autosomal recessive or autosomal dominant patterns, and mild hypermagnesemia is a common associated feature. Each persists or recurs after subtotal parathyroidectomy, and in each the parathyroid glands show moderate diffuse enlargement. The most useful diagnostic features are the typical familial pattern with onset of hypercalcemia early in the first decade, absence of features of MEN I or MEN II, serum magnesium concentrations that are high or in the upper normal range, and low renal clearances of calcium and magnesium (calcium clearance/creatinine clearance usually below 0.01). Differentiation of this disorder from typical primary hyperparathyroidism may be impossible in the absence of a characteristic family pattern.

The hypercalcemia is not responsive to steroid, natriuretic agents, or subtotal parathyroidectomy. The only measure that has consistently normalized the serum calcium concentration is total parathyroidectomy subsequently treated with calcium or vitamin D or both. This should be undertaken only if clear-cut complications exist. In general these patients have an excellent prognosis and long life expectancy without parathyroidectomy.

Secondary Hyperparathyroidism

Secondary hyperparathyroidism can be defined as a state of compensatory hypersecretion of PTH and may occur in any clinical condition in which there is a tendency towards hypocalcemia. Secondary hyperparathyroidism has been described in chronic renal disease, rickets or osteomalacia, intestinal malabsorption syndromes, Fanconi syndrome, and renal tubular acidosis. Persistent hypersecretion of PTH in these syndromes can produce all of the characteristics of hyperparathyroid bone disease, including osteitis fibrosa and osteosclerosis. A subclass of nephrolithiasis associated with a renal leak for calcium may also represent a type of secondary hyperparathyroidism. This latter condition is associated with a modest degree of hypophosphatemia and increased excretion of urinary cAMP (see "Hypercalciuria and Urolithiasis," p. 1019).

Chronic Renal Failure and Secondary Hyperparathyroidism

Observation of parathyroid hyperplasia and hyperparathyroid bone disease in chronic renal failure as well as classic physiologic observations that experimental animals made uremic were resistant to the effects of PTH led to the recognition of secondary hyperparathyroidism as a consequence of chronic renal disease. The tacit assumption of excessive secretion of PTH in this state was apparently confirmed upon development of the radioimmunoassay for PTH. High concentrations of immunoassayable PTH have been found uniformly in chronic renal failure. Much of the immunoactive hormone that accumulates, however, represents biologically inert C-terminal fragments of the hormonal molecule (see discussion under metabolism and radioimmunoassay of PTH, p. 941). Reports proving high concentrations of circulating biologically active PTH have yet to appear. The gland is capable of releasing biologically active PTH at least in early renal impairment, however, in that the increase in immunoreactive PTH in plasma induced by EDTA infusion is accompanied by a rise in urinary cAMP excretion. Multiple factors are involved in the pathogenesis of this form of secondary hyperparathyroidism. Indeed, the interaction of a complex array of factors is compounded to greater degree in renal failure than it is in any other form of secondary hyperparathyroidism. The factors involved include hypocalcemia, hyperphosphatemia, decreased production of 1,25-dihydroxycholecalciferol, reduced gastrointestinal absorption of calcium, peripheral resistance to the action of PTH, and undoubtedly other factors yet to be recognized. The initial stimulus apparently is a chronic reduction of ionized calcium in the ECF due to renal retention of phosphate; indeed there is a tendency towards frank hypocalcemia due to the hyperphosphatemia in this disorder. Hyperphosphatemia decreases renal production of 1,25-dihydroxy-vitamin D, and reduction in functional renal

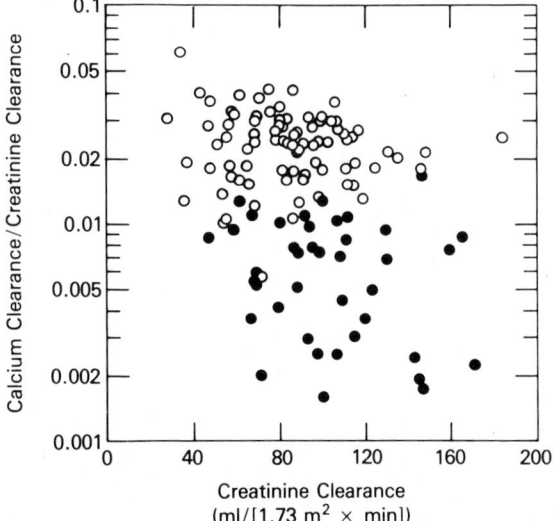

Figure 19–51. Ratio of calcium clearance to creatinine clearance ($[Ca_u \times Cr_p]/[Cr_u \times Ca_p]$) in 90 patients with typical primary hyperparathyroidism ($\circ$) and 40 patients with familial hypocalciuric hypercalcemia ($\bullet$). These data are based on average 24-hour urine excretions and average fasting serum samples (total not filtrable calcium).

mass contributes as well to such reduced production of 1,25-dihydroxy-vitamin D. Hypocalcemia is exaggerated further by decreased gastrointestinal absorption of calcium due to reduced production of the active vitamin D metabolite. A further contributing factor to hypocalcemia is relative skeletal resistance to PTH. The concerted actions of all of the just mentioned factors foster development of hypocalcemia, which is a recognized stimulus to secretion of PTH. Renal impairment, moreover, causes accumulation (decreased renal clearance) of PTH, biologically active hormone, as well as inactive immunoreactive fragments in the circulation. Other hormones including catecholamines also show reduced clearance rate in chronic renal disease. Catecholamines are known secretagogues for PTH, but their contribution to excessive PTH secretion in secondary hyperparathyroidism is unknown. It is possible that other, as yet unknown, secretagogues for PTH contribute still further to hypersecretion of the hormone in chronic renal disease.

✢ Renal Osteodystrophy

The skeletal abnormalities in chronic renal failure reflect osteitis fibrosa cystica, osteomalacia, osteosclerosis, and generalized osteopenia. The degree of involvement of each form of bone disease varies, presumably as a function of the competing effects of resistance to PTH, defective production of vitamin D metabolite, and effects of parathyroid hormone on bone. Any of the classic lesions of primary hyperparathyroidism can occur, although bone cysts apparently are less common. It has been suggested that early in the course of renal impairment the major skeletal pathology reflects osteitis due to the excessive production of PTH. In later stages osteomalacia may be more significant as the effects of impaired formation of 1,25-dihydroxy-vitamin D become evident. Osteosclerosis is noted as discussed under "Primary Hyperparathyroidism" (p. 964). Generalized osteopenia may occur particularly in subjects undergoing chronic hemodialysis.

Clinically, osteodystrophy is expressed most prominently as bone pain. In addition, proximal muscle weakness may develop similar to that observed in primary hyperparathyroidism. The neuropathy associated with muscle weakness was discussed under "Primary Hyperparathyroidism" (p. 964). Osteopenia may lead to development of multiple pathologic fractures.

✢ Management of Renal Osteodystrophy

The general approach is to control plasma phosphate and calcium and to correct osteomalacia. Control of serum phosphate is important to prevent the multiple adverse effects of hyperphosphatemia. Generally this can be effected with the aluminum hydroxide–containing antacids; phosphate depletion should be avoided. Serum calcium can be controlled by giving calcium supplements by mouth and by the use of vitamin D metabolites to increase calcium absorption from the gut. Patients undergoing dialysis can be regulated partially by raising the calcium concentration in the dialysate. This may cause hypercalcemia in the immediate postdialysis period. Persistent hypercalcemia for days to weeks post dialysis requires consideration of possible parathyroid surgery.

The advent of vitamin D metabolites, 1-α-cholecalciferol or 1,25-dihydroxycholecalciferol, makes possible effective correction of poor gastrointestinal absorption of calcium and ostemalacia. These short-acting metabolites as well as dihydrotachysterol previously used for this purpose are advantageous should hypercalcemia develop, requiring prompt reduction in dosage. Use of the vitamin D metabolites requires careful control of blood phosphate, since vitamin D therapy causes an increase not only in calcium absorption but also in phosphate absorption from the gut.

Osteomalacia or rickets due to vitamin D deficiency or "vitamin D dependency" can be associated with hypocalcemia and consequent secondary hyperparathyroidism. In each instance the hypocalcemia is secondary to decreased intestinal transport of calcium, a function dependent on normal action of vitamin D metabolites. These disorders are discussed under "Rickets and Osteomalacia" (p. 998). The secondary hyperparathyroidism in these disorders is readily correctible by appropriate calciferol replacement therapy.

Vitamin D–resistant rickets or phosphate diabetes usually is a sex-linked disorder characterized by a renal reabsorptive defect for phosphate. Chronic phosphate wasting leads to development of an osteomalacia-like skeletal disorder with pseudofractures and stunting of growth. Usually these subjects do not show hypocalcemia and do not express severe secondary hyperparathyroidism unless hypocalcemia develops in the course of treatment with phosphate. The Fanconi syndrome encompasses another type of renal reabsorptive defect involving amino acids, glucose, and phosphate. The renal loss of phosphate (phosphate diabetes) leads to demineralization, rickets, or osteomalacia. Usually serum calcium is normal and severe secondary hyperparathyroidism does not develop unless these is progressive glomerular insufficiency.

HYPERCALCEMIA

Introduction

Hypercalcemia is a common metabolic disturbance that often confronts the practicing physician with formidable diagnostic and therapeutic problems. The clinical spectrum of hypercalcemia ranges from a life-threatening disorder to an asymptomatic biochemical abnormality. Malignancy is probably the leading cause of hypercalcemia in hospitalized patients, but primary hyperparathyroidism may well be the most common diagnosis in hypercalcemia discovered on routine biochemical screening. The pathogenesis, clinical manifestations, diagnosis, and treatment of hypercalcemia in diseases other than primary hyperparathyroidism are discussed in the sections that follow.

Pathogenesis

Hypercalcemia represents an imbalance in calcium flux into and out of the blood compartment (Fig. 19–52A). Increased flux of calcium from bone to blood is the most important cause of hypercalcemia in the majority of patients. The ability of the body to compensate (e.g., increase renal calcium excretion) for increased calcium flux from the large ($\sim$ 1000 g) skeletal calcium reservoir is relatively limited. From the foregoing it is clear that osteolytic factors are of primary pathogenetic importance in most hypercalcemic states. Numerous osteolytic factors have been identified (PTH, prostaglandins, OAF, thyroid hormone, 1,25-(OH_2)-D) and others undoubtedly exist.

Decreased renal calcium excretion and increased intestinal calcium absorption often contribute to increased serum calcium concentration but are rarely the sole cause of hypercalcemia. Reduced renal calcium excretion is most often a consequence of renal failure. A slight reduction in renal function may be sufficient to cause hypercalcemia, if in-

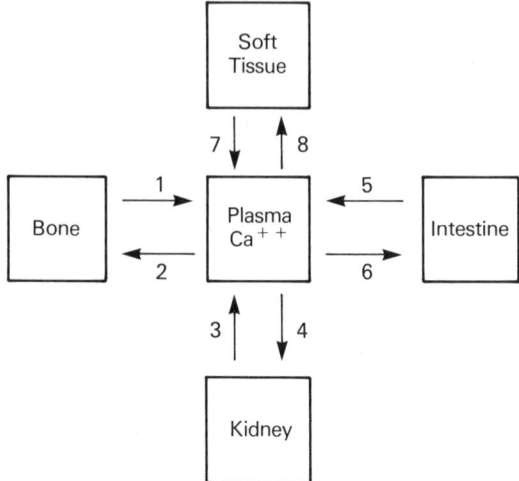

Figure 19–52. Schematic diagram of compartments involved in calcium homeostasis. (A) Hypercalcemia is caused by (1) increased calcium flux from bone to blood produced by osteolytic factors and osteolytic metastases, (4) decreased renal calcium excretion, either functional (e.g., PTH or thiazides) or resulting from impaired renal function, (5) increased intestinal calcium absorption, and (7) increased flux of calcium from soft tissues to blood. (B) Hypocalcemia is caused by (1) decreased calcium flux from bone to blood due to PTH deficiency, (2) increased flux of calcium from blood to bone (e.g., healing osteitis fibrosa, osteoblastic metastases), (3) decreased renal calcium reabsorption due to PTH deficiency, (5) decreased intestinal calcium reabsorption due to 1,25-(OH)₂ D deficiency, (8) increased calcium deposition in soft tissues (e.g., hyperphosphatemia).

creased bone turnover or increased intestinal calcium absorption (or both) is present. PTH and thiazide diuretics reduce renal calcium excretion even when renal function is normal. Increased circulating amounts of vitamin D and increased sensitivity to vitamin D are the major factors leading to increased intestinal calcium absorption. Increased flux of calcium into blood from soft tissue calcium deposits is a theoretic, but unproved, cause of hypercalcemia.

Clinical Manifestations

Hypercalcemia of any etiology can seriously disrupt normal neurologic, gastrointestinal, and renal functions. The severity of symptoms in a given patient is a function of the degree and rapidity of onset of hypercalcemia. Routine determination of serum calcium concentration is important in evaluating patients with a wide variety of complaints, since the symptoms of hypercalcemia are both varied and nonspecific.

Neurologic

CNS manifestations range from lethargy through confusion to coma. The EEG shows slowing and other nonspecific abnormalities that revert to normal (with a variable lag period) after correction of hypercalcemia. In some patients, severe headache is a prominent feature. Depression, paranoia, and a variety of other neuropsychiatric syndromes have been described anecdotally in hypercalcemic patients and in some patients have resolved following correction of hypercalcemia. Generalized muscle weakness and hyporeflexia are characteristic findings in severely hypercalcemic patients. Neuromuscular function may improve dramatically with lowering of serum calcium concentration. CSF protein, in the absence of primary neurologic disease, is almost always normal in hypercalcemic patients.

Gastrointestinal

Constipation, anorexia, nausea, and vomiting are frequently associated with hypercalcemia. Poor fluid intake and fluid loss due to emesis contribute to development of acute hypercalcemic crisis. Hypercalcemia probably increases gastric acid secretion, but the relationship between hypercalcemia, increased gastric acid secretion, and peptic ulcer disease is complex. Hyperparathyroidism, particularly the hereditary form (see "Familial Multiple Endocrine Neoplasia type I," p. 978), is associated with an increased incidence of peptic ulcer disease but there is no clear-cut association between other causes of hypercalcemia and peptic ulcer disease. Acute pancreatitis, although frequently associated with hyperparathyroidism, may occur with other hypercalcemic disorders as well. Reports of pancreatitis in patients with hypercalcemia due to metastatic breast carcinoma or due to calcium infusion suggest that hypercalcemia itself may trigger acute pancreatitis.

Cardiovascular

Hypercalcemia decreases the plateau phase of the cardiac action potential. This is reflected in a shortened S-T segment and consequently a reduced Q-T interval (corrected for heart rate) on the EKG (Fig. 19–53). With hypercalcemia in excess of 16 mg/dl the T wave widens, tending to *increase* the Q-T interval. For this reason, the Q_o-T_c segment (distance from onset of QRS complex to onset of T wave corrected for heart rate) is more reliable indication of hypercalcemia. Arrhythmias are an uncommon manifestation of hypercalcemia; with acute elevation of serum calcium concentration, bradycardia and first degree heart block may occur. Theoretically, hypercalcemia sensitizes the heart to digitalis, but the clinical evidence for this is scant. One should, nonetheless, exercise caution in administering digitalis to hypercalcemic patients.

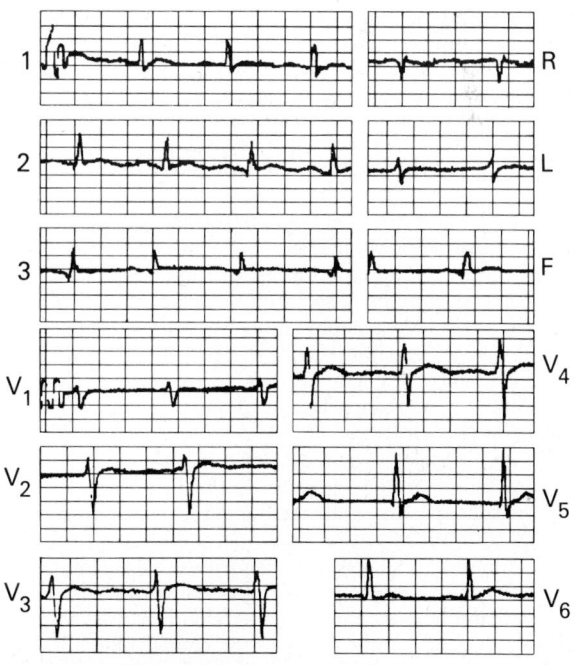

R.M. Age 24 Years

Figure 19–53. Absent S-T segments and short Q-T intervals in hypercalcemia. (From VanderArk, et al.: Electrolytes and the electrocardiogram. Complex electrocardiography. *Cardiovasc. Clin.,* Vol. 5. Philadelphia, F. A. Davis Co., 1973, p. 286.)

Acute elevation of serum calcium concentration may cause a marked rise in blood pressure, possibly through direct vasoconstriction, but the hypertension associated with chronic hypercalcemia may be due to renal damage (see later). Although some reports suggest that hypertension is corrected with cure of hypercalcemia, this is not general and this question needs further study.

Renal

Hypercalcemia impairs renal function in several ways. Hypercalcemia causes polyuria and polydipsia by interfering with the action of ADH on the collecting ducts. Renal blood flow and GFR are reduced. Proximal tubular function may be impaired, causing excessive urinary sodium loss. With persistent hypercalcemia (especially in patients with elevated serum phosphorus concentration), calcium phosphate salts are deposited in the tubules. Focal scarring and inflammation (interstitial nephritis) may develop. In severe cases, nephrocalcinosis will be visible on x-ray, but histologic evidence of renal parenchymal calcification is often present in cases without radiographically detectable nephrocalcinosis. Hypercalciuria and gross urolithiasis may also occur. Superimposed urinary tract infection may aggravate hypercalcemic nephropathy. In the absence of primary glomerular disease, there is generally slight if any proteinuria. Hypercalcemia-induced renal impairment is reversible if the hypercalcemia is of short duration and promptly corrected. Significant improvement in renal function following correction of hypercalcemia cannot be expected in patients with irreversible anatomic damage, including nephrocalcinosis.

Other

Soft-tissue calcification may occur in hypercalcemic patients (see "Extraskeletal Calcification and Ossification," p. 1016). Pruritus may be due to deposits of calcium phosphate in the skin and may improve following correction of hypercalcemia. Calcium activates several of the factors in the clotting system. This may in part account for occasional reports of widespread thrombosis in hypercalcemic patients.

Treatment of Hypercalcemia

Hypercalcemia can be corrected (Fig. 19–52) by (a) inhibiting bone resorption, (b) increasing calcium excretion, and (c) decreasing intestinal calcium absorption. (Soft tissue calcium deposition may be associated with significant reduction in hypercalcemia but is obviously hazardous and should be avoided if at all possible.) Since increased bone resorption is the most important cause of hypercalcemia, agents capable of inhibiting bone resorption are generally most effective in treating hypercalcemia.

Therapy of hypercalcemia often must be instituted without knowledge of the specific diagnosis. Many available forms of therapy are nonspecific. Thus, hydration and increasing calcium excretion by forced sodium diuresis lowers serum calcium concentration regardless of the underlying cause of hypercalcemia. Mithramycin lowers serum calcium concentration by antagonizing the bone resorptive effects of a wide variety of agents. On the other hand, identification of factors causing hypercalcemia allows institution of specific therapy. Destruction of a malignancy (by surgery, radiation, or chemotherapy), correction of thyrotoxicosis, and removal of a parathyroid adenoma are a few examples of specific

treatments that may correct associated hypercalcemia. In addition, several agents often used nonspecifically are considerably more effective in specific disorders. Use of corticosteroids to treat vitamin D intoxication or sarcoidosis is a good example.

Rigid guidelines cannot be set but degree of hypercalcemia, severity of symptoms, and overall status of the patient are factors in deciding whether and how to treat. The mildly hypercalcemic, asymptomatic patient may not require therapy, but a specific diagnosis should be made. Severely symptomatic patients ("hypercalcemia crisis") require emergency measures to correct hypercalcemia. These must be instituted even if the underlying disease is unknown. Sampling blood for PTH and urine for cAMP determinations may be feasible even in acutely ill patients and may assist in subsequent attempts to diagnose the underlying disease. If severe hypercalcemia is corrected, chronic therapy may be necessary to avoid recurrence of hypercalcemic crisis. Unfortunately, chronic therapy of hypercalcemia is generally unsatisfactory, so that whenever feasible, one should treat the underlying disease.

Forms of Therapy

Mobilization

Every effort should be made to avoid immobilization, which tends to accelerate bone resorption and aggravate hypercalcemia. In severely symptomatic patients mobilization may be impossible, but activity should be encouraged as soon as other therapeutic measures have reduced the serum calcium concentration and relieved acute symptoms.

Hydration

Decreased fluid intake (nausea and vomiting) and inability to excrete a concentrated urine cause the dehydration that invariably accompanies severe hypercalcemia. Dehydration lowers GFR and reduces renal calcium excretion; hypercalcemia is in turn aggravated. Rehydration (generally with intravenous saline solution) is an important initial step in treating severely hypercalcemic patients. A rapid fall of 2–3 mg/dl in total serum calcium concentration is typical following rehydration alone. Maintaining adequate hydration is vital in the chronic therapy of hypercalcemia. If adequate oral intake is not feasible, intermittent parenteral hydration may be required to help prevent development of hypercalcemic crisis.

Sodium Diuresis

Since increased sodium excretion leads to increased calcium excretion, sodium diuresis is effective short-term therapy for hypercalcemia of any etiology. Effective therapy requires infusion of large amounts (5–10 l/day) of isotonic saline together with potent diuretics (e.g., furosemide in doses of 100 mg every 2 hours) to insure maximal urinary sodium excretion. With appropriate therapy, urinary calcium excretion of 1–2 g/day can be achieved, and serum calcium concentration may decrease by 2–4 mg/dl in 24 hours. Infusion of sodium sulfate has been reported to be even more effective than saline infusion but in practice sodium sulfate offers little advantage over saline plus diuretics.

Hypokalemia, hypomagnesemia, and congestive heart failure are potential complications of forced sodium diuresis. They can be avoided by careful monitoring of central venous pressure (or pulmonary capillary wedge pressure) and plasma and urine electrolytes and by adequately replacing urinary losses of potassium (which may reach 200 mEq/day) and magnesium. A urinary catheter may be required, especially in obtunded patients. Forced sodium diuresis has been used effectively even in patients with moderately impaired (creatine clearance ~ 20 cc/min) renal function; indeed renal function often improves following correction of hypercalcemia. Severe renal failure, however, precludes use of this form of therapy.

Dialysis

This technique has been used effectively in patients with severe renal failure. Calcium (> 1 g/24 hours) can be removed from the blood either by peritoneal dialysis against calcium-free dialysis fluid or by hemodialysis using distilled water or other calcium-free dialysates. Significant quantities of phosphate may also be dialyzed from the blood; since phosphate depletion would aggravate hypercalcemia, serum phosphorus concentration should be monitored and phosphate supplements given as required.

EDTA

Infused EDTA forms complexes with ionized calcium; the complexes are rapidly excreted by the kidney. Reports of severe renal injury attributed to EDTA infusion have caused this form of therapy for hypercalcemia to be abandoned.

Mithramycin

This cytotoxic substance was initially evaluated as a cancer chemotherapeutic agent. It was moderately effective against a variety of tumors, embryonal cell cancer of the testis being the most responsive, but its use was associated with serious toxicity. The observation that mithramycin frequently caused significant reduction in serum calcium concentration (93% of patients in a large series) prompted evaluation of its efficacy in the treatment of hypercalcemia. It is now clear that mithramycin is a potent inhibitor of bone resorption that probably acts directly on the osteoclast. Reduction in serum calcium concentration produced by mithramycin is accompanied by reduced urinary calcium and hydroxyproline excretion; PTH secretion is not inhibited and may indeed be stimulated by mithramycin-induced hypocalcemia (Fig. 19–54).

Mithramycin can be given in a bolus injection or in an intravenous infusion over several hours. The usual dose is 25 μg/kg body weight. A single dose corrected hypercalcemia within 48 hours in 30 of 41 cases of malignancy. Normocalcemia may persist for a period of days following a single dose but rapid recurrence is also possible depending in part on the underlying illness. Repeat administration is usually effective but cumulative toxicity (see later) limits the frequency with which this agent can be given.

Anorexia and nausea frequently follow mithramycin administration. Hemorrhage and liver and renal damage are the most serious toxic effects. Bleeding is due to thrombocytopenia and inhibition of hepatic clotting factor synthesis. A rise in prothrombin time and release of hepatic enzymes (SGOT, LDH, alkaline phosphatase) indicate liver damage. Proteinuria and azotemia may develop. Toxic effects are most likely after repeated administration of the drug and in patients with pre-existing compromise of bone marrow, liver, and renal function.

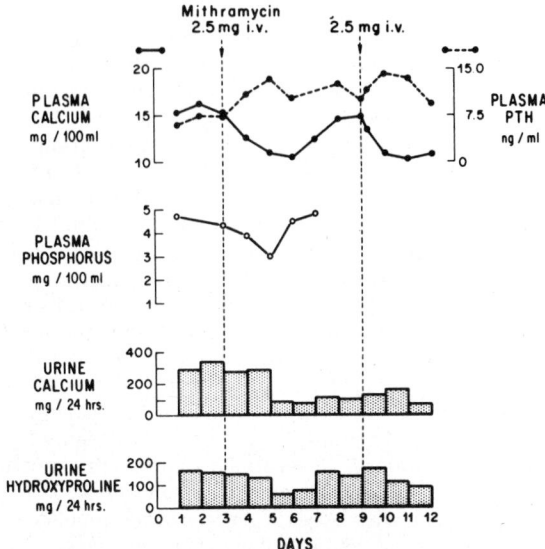

Figure 19–54. Effects of mithramycin on plasma calcium, phosphorus, and PTH and on urine calcium and hydroxyproline in a patient with hypercalcemia caused by parathyroid carcinoma. Note that urine calcium and hydroxyproline decrease, as does plasma calcium, indicating decreased bone resorption. In contrast to these parameters, plasma PTH is *not* reduced. (From Singer, F. R., Neer, R. M., et al.: Mithramycin treatment of intractable hypercalcemia due to parathyroid carcinoma. *N. Engl. J. Med. 283:*635, 1970.)

Calcitonin

CT, effective in inhibiting bone resorption and relatively free of toxicity, might be proposed as the ideal agent but it has not been uniformly effective in lowering serum calcium concentration. Patients with hyperparathyroidism, malignancies, vitamin D intoxication, and other diseases have had good responses, but many "escape" from the effects of CT during continued administration. It has been suggested without good evidence that combining phosphate therapy with CT may prevent "escape." The possibility that combining CT with low doses of other more toxic agents such as mithramycin might reduce toxicity without reducing efficacy has not been adequately evaluated.

Salmon CT is the most potent congener available. Doses used in therapy have been quite variable. The amount given should probably not exceed 8 MRC units/kg body weight given intramuscularly or intravenously every 6 hours, since higher doses are not likely to be more effective. For infusions, dilute gelatin or albumin solution may be used as vehicle. Rarely, nausea and vomiting occur with high doses.

Phosphate

Administration of phosphate intravenously is undoubtedly an effective method for lowering serum calcium concentration. Phosphate has a direct inhibitory effect on bone resorption *in vitro* and this may in part explain its *in vivo* hypocalcemic action. It is also quite likely that acutely raising the serum phosphorus concentration in hypercalcemic subjects leads to the precipitation of calcium phosphate salts. The site of calcium phosphate deposition following phosphate therapy is controversial. **Extensive metastatic calcification** (sometimes associated with *hypocalcemia,* hypotension, renal failure, and death) has been reported to occur in hypercalcemic patients after intravenous phosphate therapy. Other studies suggest that the incidence of soft-tissue calcification with either oral or intravenous phosphate therapy is low and point out that metastatic calcification may be a feature of hypercalcemia itself. The likelihood of developing metastatic calcification following intravenous phosphate may depend on the dose administered, the pretreatment serum phosphorus concentration, and the patient's renal function. A situation analogous to intravenous phosphate infusion occurs in patients undergoing chemotherapy of certain malignancies (Burkitt's lymphoma, lymphoblastic leukemia). Rapid lysis of tumor cells releases a large amount of inorganic phosphate. Hyperphosphatemia, hypocalcemia, renal failure and metastatic calcification have been reported in initially hypercalcemic patients as well as in normocalcemic patients.

Phosphate has generally been administered intravenously in doses up to 50 mmoles (1.5 grams of elemental phosphorus) over 6–8 hours. The decline in serum calcium concentration is directly related to the dose of phosphate given and to the maximal rise in serum phosphorus concentration achieved (Fig. 19–55). Extreme hyperphosphatemia (> 8 mg/dl) may occur with doses in excess of 50 mmoles.

The anorexia that generally accompanies severe hypercalcemia precludes oral administration of phosphates in the acute treatment of hypercalcemia. Once acute symptoms have been relieved by other measures, chronic therapy with phosphates by mouth may be very helpful in preventing recurrence of hypercalcemic crisis. Phosphate by mouth is probably less hazardous than given intravenously since serum phosphorus is increased more gradually. Nonetheless, chronic therapy even orally may cause metastatic calcification, particularly if hyperphosphatemia is produced. Serum phosphorus concentration must be closely monitored (peak concentration may be checked about 2 hours after a dose), particularly in patients with impaired renal function. Therapy is usually initiated with four divided doses to give the equivalent of 2–3 g of elemental phosphorus/day. (Elemental phosphorus constitutes one fifth to one fourth of the weight of most phosphate salt preparations.) The dose may be reduced subsequently, depending on the serum phospho-

rus concentration. Diarrhea and gastrointestinal upset may force reduction in dose in some patients.

Corticosteroids

Corticosteroids are not uniformly effective in lowering serum calcium concentration. In pharmacologic doses, they increase urinary calcium excretion, but this effect is of minor significance. Corticosteroids antagonize the effects of vitamin D by mechanisms that are as yet undefined. In hypercalcemia due to excessive amounts of or excessive sensitivity to (e.g., sarcoidosis) vitamin D, corticosteroids decrease intestinal calcium absorption and bone resorption and lower serum calcium concentration and urinary calcium excretion.

Corticosteroids are also effective in hypercalcemia in several malignancies. Multiple myeloma, leukemias and lymphomas, and some cases of breast carcinoma are the most responsive tumor types. Part or all of the effect may be due to destruction of tumor. Some corticosteroid-responsive tumors (e.g., multiple myeloma, lymphosarcoma) produce osteoclast activating factor (OAF) (see later). The ability of corticosteroids to block the bone resorptive effect of OAF *in vitro* may explain the efficacy of this form of therapy in hypercalcemia due to OAF-producing malignancies. Corticosteroids are ineffective against PTH-mediated bone resorption.

Doses of 40–100 mg/day of prednisone or equivalent have been used to treat hypercalcemia. The side effects of excess corticosteroids are well known. In patients who do not appear to respond (a positive response usually occurs within 1 week), corticosteroids should be immediately withdrawn.

Indomethacin

Indomethacin (25 mg orally every 6 hours) and aspirin (in doses sufficient to reach serum salicylate concentrations of 20–30 mg/dl) are prostaglandin synthetase inhibitors that may correct hypercalcemia caused by production of prostaglandins by tumors (see later). These drugs are ineffective in other forms of hypercalcemia. Prostaglandin determinations are not generally available at present so that a therapeutic trial may be necessary. If the patient is not severely hypercalcemic, this may be appropriate. Even when production of prostaglandins by tumors has been proved, these agents may not be completely effective, particularly in patients with osteolytic metastases.

Summary

Acute treatment of hypercalcemia must be effected on an individual basis. Rehydration and early mobilization are generally applicable. In severely symptomatic patients, additional measures are often required. Forced saline diuresis can be used safely in most patients, if cardiovascular status and serum electrolyte concentrations are carefully monitored. Mithramycin is probably the agent of first choice provided major contraindications (bone marrow, liver, or renal failure) are not present. CT shows low toxicity but is not regularly effective; it should be considered when mithramycin is contraindicated. In our opinion, intravenous phosphate, because of its potential acute toxicity, should be used only in life-threatening hypercalcemia and if CT is ineffective and mithramycin is contraindicated. Several diphosphate analogs, e.g., dichloromethylene diphosphonate, are potent inhibitors of bone resorption and may prove useful in the treatment of hypercalcemia.

There is no entirely satisfactory form of therapy for chronic hypercalcemia. Corticosteroid therapy is useful in

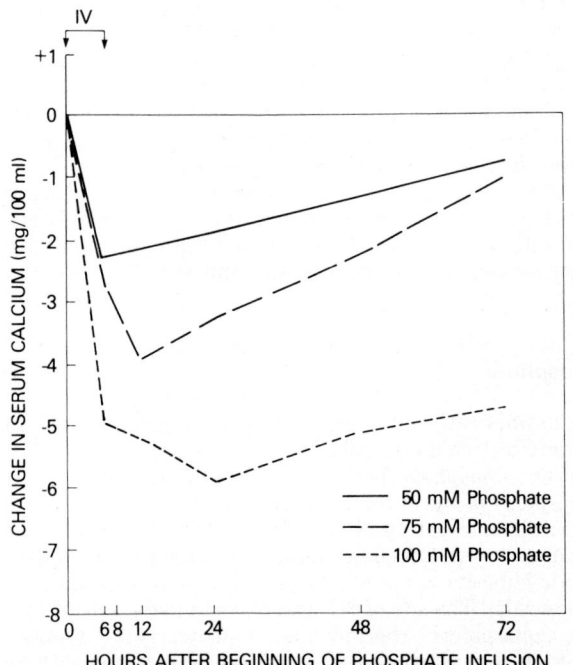

Figure 19–55. Magnitude and duration of decline in serum calcium after intravenous infusion of varying doses (in millimoles) of phosphate. Each line represents the mean response of 4 to 8 hypercalcemic patients. (From Fulmer, D. H., Dimich, A. B., et al.: Treatment of hypercalcemia. Comparison of intravenously administered phosphate, sulfate, and hydrocortisone. *Arch. Int. Med. 129*:927, 1972.)

patients with vitamin D intoxication and sarcoidosis. In patients with hypercalcemia due to malignancy, a therapeutic trial of corticosteroids or indomethacin (or both) may be appropriate. Chronic therapy with oral phosphate can be used in all forms of hypercalcemia. The serum phosphorus concentration and renal function should be monitored closely, and the patient should be examined at frequent intervals for signs of soft-tissue calcification.

Differential Diagnosis of Hypercalcemia

The initial step in evaluating a patient with confirmed hypercalcemia should be assignment to one of two broad categories: PTH-mediated vs. nonPTH-mediated hypercalcemia. This division is of great clinical importance since subsequent diagnostic and therapeutic maneuvers in the two categories are very different (Fig. 19–56). Assessment of circulating PTH activity might in theory readily differentiate hypercalcemic patients into either of these two groups, since hypercalcemia unrelated to parathyroid gland activity should cause suppression of endogenous PTH secretion. In fact, a method for directly measuring circulating amounts of bioactive PTH is not yet generally available, and one must rely on measurements of circulating immunoreactive PTH or of indirect, generally renal, effects of PTH.

The renal effects of PTH are discussed in detail elsewhere (see "Effects of the Hormone on the Kidney," p. 942). Measurement of serum phosphorus, chloride and bicarbonate concentrations, and urinary calcium and phosphorus excretion (normalized for filtered load) sometimes provides suggestive indices for PTH-dependent or independent mechanisms. Results, however, show considerable overlap among these parameters and complicating factors may negate the differential value of these measurements. Thus nausea and vomiting or diuretic therapy render serum chloride and bicarbonate measurement difficult to interpret; hypercalcemia may cause phosphaturia independent of PTH; renal failure may limit the value of urine calcium and phosphorus estimation, even when corrections for reduced creatinine clearance are applied. Several groups have attempted to combine several of these parameters (e.g., serum chloride/phosphate ratio) in an effort to increase diagnostic utility, but the limitations of the individual measurements still apply to the combined indices. Measurement of serum alkaline phosphatase activity has little diagnostic value since it will be normal in the majority of patients with hyperparathyroidism and even if elevated is consistent with some forms of nonPTH-mediated hypercalcemia as well. Radiographic evidence of subperiosteal resorption is quite specific for PTH-mediated hypercalcemia but is rarely present.

Measurements of serum immunoreactive PTH concentration and urinary cAMP excretion are currently the most useful tests for differentiating PTH-mediated from nonPTH-mediated hypercalcemia, but both must be interpreted cautiously, particularly with compromised renal function (see "Primary Hyperparathyroidism — Radioimmunoassay for Parathyroid Hormone," p. 968 and "Urinary Excretion of Cyclic 3',5'-AMP," p. 969). Unequivocal elevations in both U_{cAMP} and serum PTH strongly favor PTH-mediated hypercalcemia but nomograms suggesting that values in the normal range are "inappropriately elevated" in the presence of hypercalcemia cannot be taken at face value. There is a suggestion that a non-PTH hypercalcemic factors(s) secreted by certain malignancies (see later) can cause elevated U_{cAMP} excretion (particularly in the nephrogenous fraction) and such a possibility could limit the utility of this determination. No single parameter provides unequivocal differentiation of PTH-mediated from nonPTH-mediated forms of hypercalcemia; but usually a combination of the previous tests will allow the distinction to be made.

The overwhelming majority of patients with PTH-mediated hypercalcemia suffer from primary hyperparathyroidism. Selective venous catheterization to detect a gradient for PTH in neck veins draining the parathyroids is the only way to exclude a malignancy ectopically secreting PTH; this procedure is usually unnecessary with no evidence suggestive of malignant disease. Patients with nonPTH-mediated hypercalcemia require further diagnostic investigation.

The history may be helpful: (a) chronicity of symptoms argues against malignancy; (b) family history of hypercalcemia or other endocrinopathy suggests MEN I or II or FHH; and (c) clues to other specific disorders, e.g., vitamin D ingestion, should be sought. On physical examination, there may be evidence for specific pathology, e.g., malignancy or sarcoid skin lesions. The presence of soft-tissue calcification (e.g., band keratopathy) argues against uncomplicated hyperparathyroidism. A neck mass generally represents an incidental thyroid nodule but in cases of florid hyperparathyroidism may represent a grossly enlarged (and not necessarily malignant) parathyroid gland. Skeletal radiography and radionuclide scanning should be

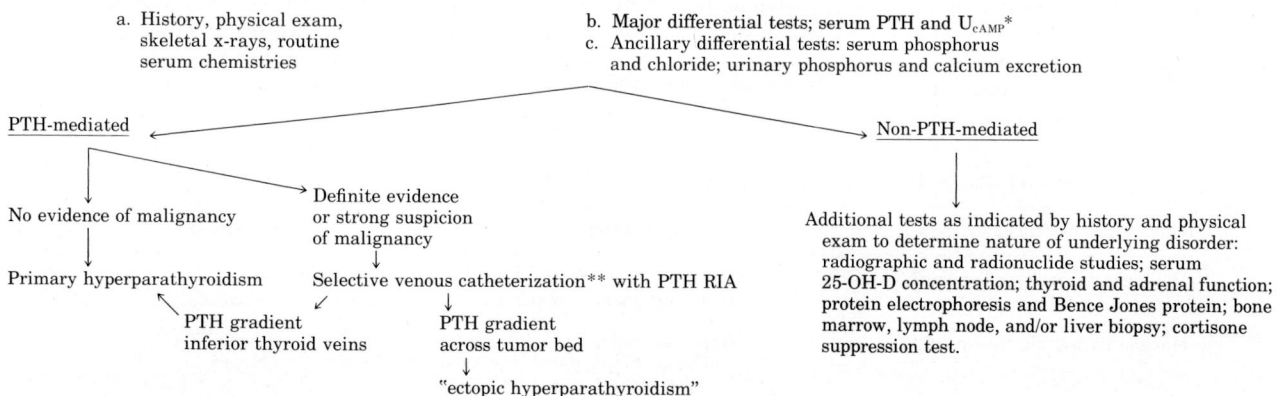

Figure 19–56. Flow diagram for evaluation of hypercalcemia. Hypercalcemia confirmed on multiple determinations; thiazides discontinued; emergency therapy given in severely hypercalcemic patients.

*See "Primary Hyperparathyroidism — Radioimmunoassay for Parathyroid Hormone" (p. 968) and "Parathyroid Hormone — Urinary Excretion of Cyclic 3',5'-AMP" (p. 969) for discussion of pitfalls in interpretation.

**Decision to perform venous catheterization depends on prognosis and status of patient.

performed to detect metastatic lesions or parathyroid bone disease. Additional laboratory studies that may be appropriate, particularly in the nonPTH-mediated group, include (a) liver function tests (e.g., sarcoidosis, malignancy), (b) thyroid and adrenal function tests, (c) protein electrophoresis and urinary Bence Jones protein determination (note that patients with primary hyperparathyroidism may show coincidental benign monoclonal gammopathy), (d) bone marrow aspiration, (e) serum 25-hydroxyvitamin D determination, and (f) additional radiographic or biopsy studies to localize malignancy or evidence of sarcoidosis. Failure to respond to a short course of corticosteroids may help exclude vitamin D intoxication and sarcoidosis; lack of a response supports but does not establish the diagnosis of PTH-mediated hypercalcemia.

In summary, careful clinical and laboratory evaluations permit specific diagnosis in most cases. Neck exploration and parathyroidectomy should not be performed as a diagnostic maneuver but rather as a therapeutic procedure in patients in whom there is a very high likelihood of finding abnormal parathyroid tissue.

Specific Hypercalcemic Disorders

Malignancy

Malignancy is one of the most common causes of hypercalcemia. In patients with disseminated and untreatable malignant disease, the development of hypercalcemia may have little clinical importance, but with the advent of newer and more aggressive forms of treatment, the diagnosis and correction of life-threatening hypercalcemia assumes greater significance. Occasionally, hypercalcemia may be the first manifestation of otherwise occult malignancy; evaluation of hypercalcemia in such cases may permit diagnosis and treatment of the underlying disease.

Increased bone resorption is the final common pathway for tumor-induced hypercalcemia. The role of metastatic bone lesions in this regard has long been appreciated. The observation that some patients with malignancy and hypercalcemia lacked bone metastases raised the possibility of tumor production of a humoral osteolytic factor. Early speculation centered on ectopic production of PTH, and the term "pseudohyperparathyroidism" was applied to this syndrome. Although ectopic production of PTH has now been verified in a few cases of tumor-associated hypercalcemia, recent studies suggest that other osteolytic factors (e.g., prostaglandins) are more often involved. The mechanisms of hypercalcemia associated with malignancy are outlined in Table 19–12. Tumor production of parathyrotropic factors is an additional theoretic possibility for which no conclusive evidence (with the possible exception of pheochromocytoma) has as yet been presented. It should be recognized that classification of tumors with and without bone metastases into separate categories (Table 19–12) is somewhat arbitrary, since humoral factors may play a role in hypercalcemia associated with malignant bone lesions. The section that follows discusses the clinical features and pathogenesis of hypercalcemia associated with specific malignancies.

Malignancy with Bone Metastases

Breast Cancer

Hypercalcemia in patients with breast cancer is almost always associated with bony metastases. The high incidence of breast cancer in the general population and the frequent occurrence (about 65%) of metastatic bone disease in all patients with breast cancer, make this malignancy the leading cause of tumor-associated hypercalcemia, which may occur spontaneously or after administration of estrogens, androgens, and the newer antiestrogens such as tamoxifen. The appropriate management of hypercalcemia after hormone administration is controversial but in most cases therapy with sex steroids should be discontinued and hypercalcemia corrected. A variety of substances (osteolytic plant sterols, prostaglandins) have been incriminated in breast cancer–related hypercalcemia but conclusive evidence for any is lacking. Prostaglandin synthetase inhibitors (see later) have *not* been effective in treating hypercalcemia in patients with breast cancer. A good response to glucocorticoids often but not invariably occurs.

Multiple Myeloma, Lymphoma, Leukemia

Skeletal or bone marrow (or both) involvement are characteristic of these malignancies. In myeloma, skeletal involvement may take the form of focal lytic lesions or diffuse osteoporosis. Recent evidence implicates an OAF in the mechanism of hypercalcemia associated with multiple myeloma and some lymphomas (e.g., Burkitt's). OAF has been isolated from the culture fluid of myeloma cells (but not from peripheral plasma) and has potent bone resorbing activity. OAF production has been correlated with the extent of bone disease in myeloma but not with hypercalcemia (Fig. 19–57). In some hematogenous malignancies (e.g., monocytic leukemia), OAF production is not found but an as yet unidentified (nonPTH and nonprostaglandin) osteolytic factor is produced. The latter, unlike OAF, acts directly, without the mediation of osteoclasts. Glucocorticoids are often quite effective in correcting hypercalcemia due to myeloma, lymphoma, and leukemia. This may in part reflect tumoricidal activity; the ability of glucocorticoids to block OAF-mediated bone resorption *in vitro* suggests an additional therapeutic mechanism.

Table 19–12.   MECHANISMS OF HYPERCALCEMIA ASSOCIATED WITH MALIGNANCY

Hypercalcemia Caused by:	Tumor Type(s)	Mediator(s)
Malignancy metastatic to bone	Myeloma, Burkitt's lymphoma, Breast carcinoma and others	OAF ? others
Malignancy without bone metastases	Hypernephroma Squamous carcinoma of lung, cervix, head and neck, esophagus Pancreatic carcinoma and others	Ectopic PTH, PGE ? others
Coexistent primary hyperparathyroidism (or other nonmalignant disease)	All types	PTH, etc.

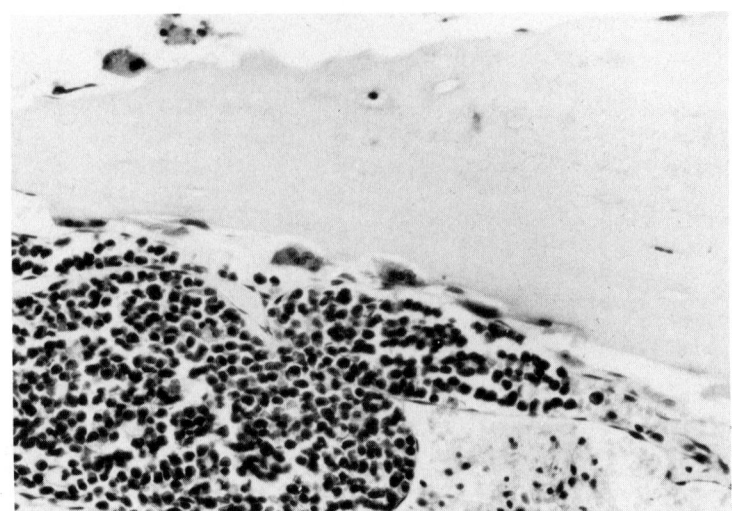

Figure 19–57. Histologic section of an osteolytic lesion in the clavicle of a patient with multiple myeloma, showing increased numbers of osteoclasts in resorption lacunae lying adjacent to myeloma cells. (From Mundy, G. R., Raisz, L. G., et al.: Evidence for the secretion of an osteoclast-stimulating factor in myeloma. *N. Engl. J. Med., 291*:1043, 1974.)

Miscellaneous

Many other tumor types metastasize to bone and may be associated with hypercalcemia. Since the correlation between extent of bony lesions and hypercalcemia is poor, other factors, including production of osteolytic substances (see later), are probably operative in many of these cases.

Malignancy Without Bone Metastases

Tumors may cause hypercalcemia without metastasizing to bone by producing humoral osteolytic factors. Skeletal radiographs do not detect all bone metastases; radionuclide bone scans are more sensitive in detecting skeletal metastases, but in some cases clinically inapparent lesions are observed at autopsy. Correction of hypercalcemia by treatment of the primary tumor (e.g., surgical removal) provides stronger evidence that tumor production of osteolytic substances is involved. Still more direct is demonstration of bone resorbing activity by bioassay in extracts of the tumor. These criteria have been fulfilled in relatively few of the cases reported as examples of hypercalcemia caused by tumor production of osteolytic factors. Nonetheless, there is suggestive evidence that many tumor types, in particular hypernephroma; pancreatic carcinoma; squamous carcinoma of lung, cervix, and esophagus; and other head and neck tumors, cause hypercalcemia by producing osteolytic factors.

Ectopic Hyperparathyroidism

Arteriovenous gradients for PTH across tumor, *in vitro* synthesis of PTH by cultured cells, and correction of hypercalcemia as well as a fall in serum PTH concentration following tumor resection have been demonstrated in a small number of cases of tumor-associated hypercalcemia. These studies support the hypothesis that ectopic production of PTH by tumors may cause hypercalcemia. The overall frequency of ectopic PTH production is controversial. Studies suggesting that this is a common phenomenon are based primarily on radioimmunoassay measurement of elevated or "inappropriately normal" serum PTH concentration in hypercalcemic patients with malignancies. Using different PTH antisera, some laboratories do not detect PTH in the serum of many patients with tumor-associated hypercalcemia, including those lacking bone metastases (see "Primary Hyperparathyroidism — Radioimmunoassay for Parathyroid Hormone," p. 968 and Fig. 19–43). Difficulties in interpretation of radioimmunoassay data as well as failure to exclude coexistent primary hyperparathyroidism in some cases make firm conclusions regarding frequency of ectopic PTH production hazardous. Resolution of this question awaits the availability of sensitive techniques for measuring bioactive PTH.

Prostaglandins

Studies in an animal tumor model prove that tumor production of prostaglandins of the "E" series may cause hypercalcemia. Clinical data supporting this mechanism include the demonstration of elevated urinary excretion of prostaglandin metabolites (PGEM) in some hypercalcemic patients with solid tumors and concommitant lowering of urinary PGEM and serum calcium concentration in the same patient group following administration of prostaglandin synthetase inhibitors such as indomethacin (Fig. 19–58). The source of prostaglandin, i.e., tumor production vs. local production in bone secondary to some other tumor factor, has not been clearly identified in humans. The frequency of prostaglandin-mediated hypercalcemia in cancer patients is also unknown; indiscriminate use of indomethacin to treat tumor-associated hypercalcemia is, therefore, not advisable. Even in patients shown to have elevated urinary PGEM, indomethacin may be ineffective in lowering serum calcium concentration, especially if bony metastases are present.

Other Factors

Some patients with cancer (with or without bone metastases) show hypercalemia, hypercalciuria, elevated nephrogenous UcAMP, and low or undetectable PTH. The factor(s) responsible for this constellation of findings has not yet been identified.

Thyrotoxicosis

Thyrotoxicosis is associated with reduced intestinal calcium absorption, hypercalciuria, and less frequently hypercalcemia; the reported incidence of hypercalcemia in patients with thyroid hormone excess varies widely (2–20%). At least part of this variability may be attributed to failure

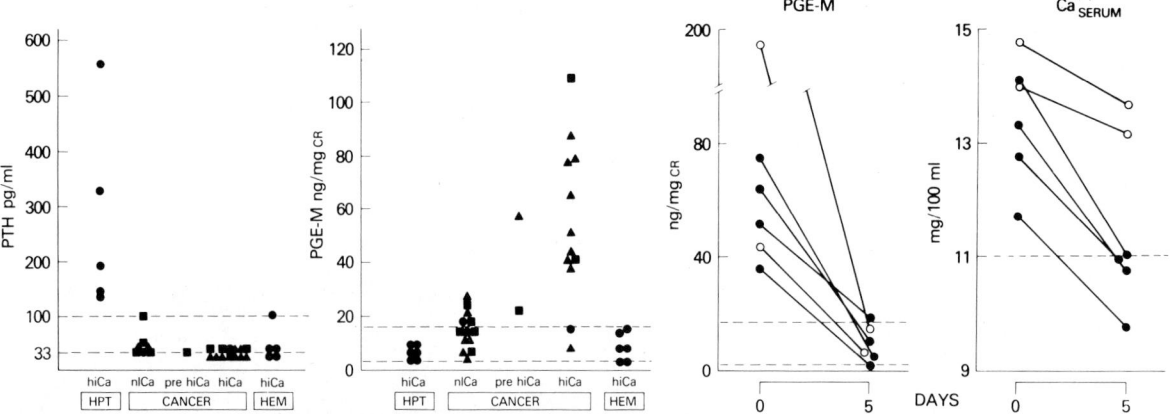

Figure 19–58. Plasma PTH (left) and urinary PGEM (left center) in patients with hyperparathyroidism (HPT), solid tumors (cancer) with varying serum calcium concentrations, and hematogenous malignancies (HEM) with hypercalcemia. Response of urinary PGEM (right center) and serum calcium (right) to indomethacin therapy is shown in hypercalcemic patients with (○) or without (•) bony metastases. (From Seyberth, H. W., Segre, G. V., et al.: Prostaglandins as mediators of hypercalcemia associated with certain types of cancer. *N. Engl. J. Med.*, 293:1278, 1975.)

to exclude coexistent primary hyperparathyroidism. More than 40 patients with coexistent hyperthyroidism and hyperparathyroidism have been reported. Hypercalcemia should not be attributed to hyperthyroidism unless the serum calcium concentration returns to normal and remains normal following specific antithyroid therapy. Radioimmunoassayable serum PTH concentration should be low or "normal" and NcAMP reduced if hypercalcemia is due to thyrotoxicosis. Hypercalcemia caused by thyrotoxicosis is generally mild, but, rarely, severe hypercalcemia occurs and causes symptoms (constipation, mental slowing) that may obscure the diagnosis of hyperthyroidism. Increased bone resorption occurs in thyrotoxicosis and recent evidence suggests that this is a direct effect of thyroid hormone excess. Propranolol (given orally or intravenously) has been reported to correct rapidly hypercalcemia due to thyrotoxicosis in several patients. The ability of propranolol to lower serum calcium concentration in this setting has led to speculation that β-adrenergic catecholamines might play a role in the hypercalcemia of thyrotoxicosis. Further study of the reliability and specificity of propranolol in treating hypercalcemia associated with hyperthyroidism will be needed to verify this hypothesis.

Vitamin D Intoxication

Hypercalcemia due to vitamin D intoxication occurs most commonly in patients being treated for hypoparathyroidism and presents no diagnostic difficulties provided serum calcium concentration is appropriately monitored. Rarely, hypercalcemia is due to surreptitious or inadvertent ingestion of excess vitamin D (as a "health-aid" or as a "remedy" for arthritis); correct diagnosis may be difficult in such cases unless one has a high index of suspicion and takes a careful history (including a check of all medications and vitamins available to the patient). If surreptitious calciferol intake is suspected, serum concentration of 25-OH-D should be determined. Hypercalcemia in hypervitaminosis D causes suppression of PTH secretion, but the frequent occurrence of renal failure in this syndrome may complicate interpretation of radioimmunoassay results for PTH and NcAMP. Soft-tissue calcification (nephrocalcinosis and band keratopathy) is frequently observed because of increased serum calcium *and* phosphorus concentration. The biologic half-life of vitamin D is long, and vitamin D intoxication may persist for months. Vitamin D excess leads to hypercalcemia by increasing both intestinal calcium absorption and

bone resorption. The initial hypercalciuria may dissipate as renal failure progresses. Recent studies suggest that 25-OH D is the principal metabolite responsible for hypercalcemia due to vitamin D intoxication, although 1,25-$(OH)_2$-D, given in excess, is a potent inducer of hypercalcemia. Discontinuation of vitamin D and treatment with glucocorticoids effectively lower serum calcium concentration in most patients (often within 3–4 days). Prolonged therapy as just mentioned may be necessary. CT has also been used successfully but is of secondary importance in treatment of vitamin D intoxication.

Hypervitaminosis A

At least six cases of hypercalcemia attributed to hypervitaminosis A have been reported. Affected patients consumed in excess of 75,000 IU/day, an amount capable of causing increased bone resorption. Since most of the patients also consumed small doses of vitamin D, the hypercalcemia may not be due solely to vitamin A excess but rather to a synergistic action of vitamins A and D. Periosteal calcifications, if present, should suggest vitamin A intoxication, since they are not seen with other causes of hypercalcemia. Discontinuation of vitamin A ingestion corrects the hypercalcemia. There is suggestive but not definite evidence that glucocorticoids will hasten normalization of serum calcium concentration in this condition.

Sarcoidosis with Other Granulomatous Diseases

The incidence of hypercalcemia in sarcoidosis is approximately 17%. Hypercalcemia is more likely in chronic and disseminated disease than in transient or localized disease. Direct bone involvement occurs but is *not* a prerequisite for development of hypercalcemia. Spontaneous fluctuations in serum calcium concentration are common in sarcoidosis; mild hypercalcemia may remit without therapy. Occasional patients, however, show severe hypercalcemia and develop complications that include nephrocalcinosis and uremia. Coexistent primary hyperparathyroidism and sarcoidosis have been reported often, but the neck should be explored only if biochemical evidence for PTH excess is strong and glucocorticoids are ineffective (see later) in correcting hypercalcemia. In sarcoidosis there is increased intestinal absorption of calcium, increased urinary calcium excretion, and hypercalcemia, in decreasing order of frequency. These abnormalities in calcium homeostasis and their correction by glucocorticoids, as well as the observation that many patients with sarcoidosis given small amounts of vitamin D ($\sim$ 10,000 IU/day) become hypercalcemic, have led to the hypothesis of disordered vitamin D metabolism in patients with sarcoidosis. Serum concentrations of vitamin D bioactivity and of 25-OH-D are normal. Recent studies have demonstrated elevated serum 1,25-(OH)$_2$-D in hypercalcemic individuals with sarcoidosis. This would suggest that enhanced formation of 1,25-(OH)$_2$-D may be the lesion causing hypercalcemia in sarcoidosis. Glucocorticoids have been most useful in treating hypercalcemia due to sarcoidosis. Their action may involve both vitamin D antagonism and amelioration of the underlying disorder.

Idiopathic Hypercalcemia in Infancy

This rare syndrome is characterized by hypercalcemia and abnormal growth and development. Clinical features include hypoplastic mandible and low-set ears, giving rise to the characteristic "elfin" facies; cardiac anomalies, most typically supravalvular aortic stenosis; mental retardation; growth retardation; scoliosis; accessory nipples; and abnormal teeth (peglike, widely spaced). The hypercalcemia causes constipation and hypotonia and may lead to nephrocalcinosis and uremia. Affected patients who survive infancy may become normocalcemic. The pathogenesis of the disorder remains unresolved. Abnormal sensitivity to vitamin D has been postulated, but measurements of vitamin D metabolites in affected patients have not as yet been performed. Evidence in favor of a role for vitamin D in the syndrome includes the observation that offspring of rabbits given excessive amounts of vitamin D during pregnancy have facial and aortic anomalies similar to those seen in humans with the disease. Autopsy studies have disclosed normal parathyroids. Therapy consists of reduction in calcium intake and discontinuation of vitamin D ingestion. Glucocorticoids and CT have also been used with some success.

Adrenal Insufficiency

Hypercalcemia may occur as frequently in untreated adrenal insufficiency as do the more familiarly associated electrolyte abnormalities, such as hyponatremia and hyperkalemia. Diagnostic confusion may result from the similarity in symptoms of adrenal insufficiency and severe hypercalcemia. The correct diagnosis has been made in some cases only after a "steroid suppression" test for hypercalcemia. In most cases, it is probably the total, rather than the ionized, serum calcium concentration that is elevated due to hemoconcentration, and possibly increased calcium binding to serum proteins associated with hyponatremia. The hypercalcemia of adrenal insufficiency is readily corrected by appropriate steroid replacement therapy.

Milk-Alkali Syndrome

In 1949, Burnett and coworkers described six patients with hypercalcemia, normal to elevated serum phosphorus concentration, renal insufficiency, and soft-tissue calcification (including band keratopathy and nephrocalcinosis). All of the patients had consumed large amounts of milk and absorbable alkali (generally sodium bicarbonate) for many years as part of treatment for peptic ulcer. Reduced calcium

and alkali intake ameliorated the biochemical abnormalities and symptoms including pruritus. Normal parathyroids were observed at surgery in only one patient but the authors concluded that hyperparathyroidism was not responsible for hypercalcemia in this syndrome. Excessive calcium and alkali intake was postulated to cause soft-tissue calcification, reduction in renal function and urinary calcium excretion, and ultimately hypercalcemia. According to this formulation, PTH secretion should be suppressed, but evidence to support this conclusion has not been presented. At present, the milk-alkali syndrome is rarely encountered, probably because absorbable alkali is no longer in widespread use in the treatment of ulcer disease.

Thiazides

Therapy with thiazide diuretics may lead to hypercalcemia by a variety of mechanisms. In subjects with normal mineral homeostasis, a transient elevation in *total* serum calcium concentration (secondary to hemoconcentration) may occur during the first days of thiazide treatment. Thiazides rarely if ever cause a sustained elevation in serum ionized calcium concentration in normal subjects. Unlike other natriuretic agents, thiazides *increase* renal calcium reabsorption. In patients with high rates of bone resorption and a tendency to hypercalciuria, thiazide diuretics, because of their hypocalciuric effect, may precipitate or aggravate hypercalcemia (Fig. 19–59).

Several lines of evidence suggest that thiazides may also raise serum calcium concentration by extrarenal mechanisms. Thiazide-induced hypercalcemia has been observed in uremic patients on chronic hemodialysis and in vitamin D–treated hypoparathyroid patients. Thiazides did not decrease urinary calcium excretion significantly in either group. Potentiation of PTH action on bone and a direct effect of thiazides on bone appear to be the most likely mechanisms of the effects of thiazides in such patients. Thiazide therapy should be promptly discontinued in patients discovered to be hypercalcemic. Persistent hypercalcemia ($>$ 1 month following discontinuation of thiazide)

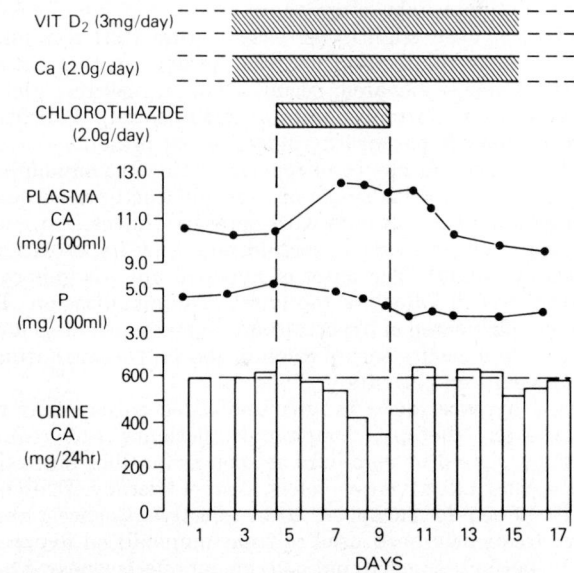

Figure 19–59. Response to chlorothiazide in a patient with idiopathic juvenile osteoporosis also receiving calciferol and supplemental oral calcium. (From Parfitt, A. M.: Chlorothiazide-induced hypercalcemia in juvenile osteoporosis and hyperparathyroidism. *N. Engl. J. Med. 281*:56, 1969.)

indicates that another cause for the hypercalcemia must be sought. In a recent study, 20 of 95 patients discovered on routine screening to be hypercalcemic were receiving thiazides. Hypercalcemia persisted in 14 of 20 following discontinuation of thiazide therapy and primary hyperparathyroidism was proved surgically in each. If hypercalcemia remits after thiazides are stopped, continued follow-up is appropriate. Such patients may have mild primary hyperparathyroidism or other abnormalities and may again develop hypercalcemia.

Immobilization

Immobilization is considered an infrequent cause of hypercalcemia (less than 50 cases have been reported). Since serum calcium determinations are not routinely performed in immobilized patients, the true incidence of immobilization hypercalcemia may be higher. A recent prospective study showed that 6 of 12 patients (ages 4–15 years) immobilized following single limb fractures developed hypercalcemia.

Immobilization causes an increase in the ratio of bone resorption/formation. Patients with high rates of bone turnover (adolescents, Paget's disease) are at greatest risk for developing immobilization hypercalcemia. Excess calcium released from bone is largely excreted by the kidney. Resultant hypercalciuria may lead to renal and bladder stones, urinary obstruction, and impaired renal function. Reduction in renal function leads to reduced calcium excretion and may be sufficient to cause hypercalcemia.

The role of PTH in immobilization hypercalcemia is controversial. Serum PTH concentration has been normal or mildly elevated in most studies. Urinary cAMP excretion (not corrected for GFR) measured in two studies was normal. In theory, one would expect PTH secretion to be suppressed by increased calcium mobilized from bone. The pathogenesis of increased bone resorption following immobilization is unclear, however, and it remains possible that PTH itself plays a role in this process and thus might not be suppressed. Further complicating interpretations are the known difficulties in correlating immunoassayable PTH with bioactive PTH, especially in patients with impaired renal function. Serum PTH measurements should, therefore, be cautiously interpreted in immobilized hypercalcemic patients (who often show mild renal impairment). Normal or even slightly increased serum PTH concentration is *not* an indication for neck surgery in this patient group. Even if elevated, serum PTH and serum calcium concentration normalize after remobilization, indicating that primary hyperparathyroidism is not present.

Hypercalcemia has been reported following immobilization in patients with single or multiple fractures, in quadriplegics, and in patients with extensive burns. Although usually mild, severe hypercalcemia and hypercalcemic crisis may occur. The onset of hypercalcemia is generally several weeks following the onset of immobilization. The nonspecific nature of hypercalcemic symptoms makes it advisable to measure serum calcium concentration routinely in immobilized patients.

Mild hypercalcemia in an immobilized patient may not require any therapy. Symptomatic patients, who require therapy, should be mobilized as soon as feasible, since this is the most effective and safest form of therapy. Exercises while in bed do not appear to be effective. Corticosteroids have frequently been used to treat immobilized hypercalcemic patients but without convincing effectiveness. Phosphate by mouth is useful and has the advantage of reducing urine calcium excretion. CT has also been reported to be effective.

Acute Renal Failure

More than 20 patients with hypercalcemia and acute renal failure have been reported. In virtually every case, renal failure was caused by myoglobinuria secondary to skeletal muscle injury. Hypercalcemia developed most commonly during the diuretic phase and was often severe (> 13 mg/dl) but transient (the longest duration recorded being 5 months). In several cases, soft-tissue calcification (often involving the injured muscles) was seen on x-ray examination. The cause of hypercalcemia in these patients has not been clearly elucidated. Release of calcium from soft-tissue deposits during the diuretic phase has been invoked to explain the hypercalcemia, but this theory remains unproved. (There is evidence that in acute renal failure due to muscle necrosis, hyperphosphatemia is more severe and often leads to calcification of necrotic muscle.) The role of PTH is controversial; difficulties in measuring bioactive PTH in patients with renal failure probably account for the discrepant results obtained in various reports with PTH radioimmunoassay. Subtotal parathyroidectomy was performed in one patient without benefit and is not recommended.

HYPOPARATHYROIDISM

Introduction

Hypoparathyroidism may be defined as a state of decreased secretion or peripheral action of PTH. Secretion may be inadequate, the hormone biologically ineffective, or organ sensitivity to PTH defective (Fig. 19–60). Diminution

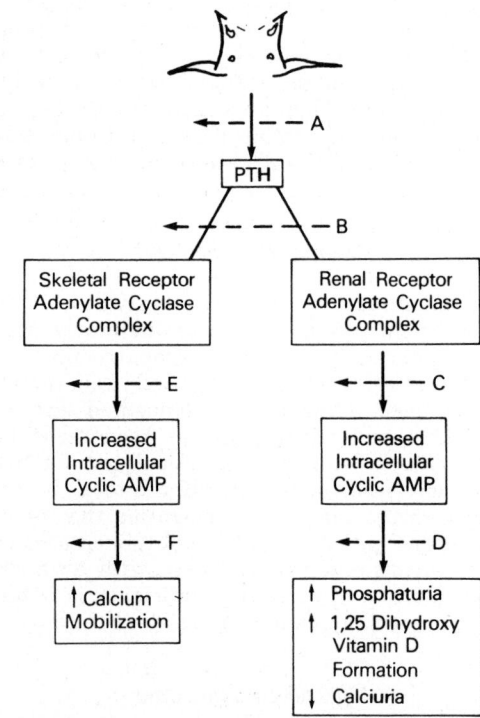

Figure 19–60. Location of defects resulting in hypoparathyroidism. (A) Failure to release PTH (absence or destruction of gland or functional defect, e.g., hypomagnesemia). (B) Biologically ineffective PTH released. (C) Impaired renal cAMP response to PTH (pseudohypoparathyroidism type I). (D) Impaired phosphaturic response to PTH with intact cAMP response (pseudohypoparathyroidism type II). (E) Impaired skeletal cAMP response to PTH (?pseudohypoparathyroidism type I). (F) Impaired skeletal calcium mobilization in response to PTH (pseudohypoparathyroidism, 1,25 vitamin D deficiency).

of PTH action on kidney and bone leads to hypocalcemia and hyperphosphatemia as discussed in the section on hypocalcemia, p. 996.

Clinical Manifestations

Hypocalcemia and hyperphosphatemia lead to an array of signs and symptoms that are independent of the specific cause of hypoparathyroidism. These are discussed in this section; other manifestations are discussed in the sections on individual disorders (see also Table 19–13). Decreased serum ionized calcium concentration increases neuromuscular excitability and may permit the examiner to elicit Chvostek's or Trousseau's sign. (Many normal subjects also show Chvostek's sign so that it should always be sought *before* contemplated neck surgery.) Symptoms may range in severity from mild paresthesias (circumoral tingling and numbness, "needles and pins" feeling in hands and feet) to severe tetany with muscle cramps, carpopedal spasms, laryngeal stridor, and convulsions. Hypocalcemic seizures, unlike the grand mal variety, are usually not associated with loss of consciousness or incontinence and are rarely preceded by an aura. There may be nonspecific abnormalities on EEG, particularly an increase in high voltage slow waves; the EEG reverts to normal with correction of hypocalcemia. A variety of mental changes, including irritability, paranoia, depression, and frank psychosis have been attributed to hypocalcemia. Papilledema, elevated CSF pressure, and neurologic signs mimicking a cerebral tumor may be seen in cases with chronic hypocalcemia.

Intracranial calcifications, particularly in the basal ganglia, are visible on skull x-ray in approximately 20% of patients with chronic hypoparathyroidism. With the more sensitive technique of computerized tomography, intracranial calcifications have been demonstrated in patients with normal standard skull x-rays. A parkinsonian-like syndrome has been associated with hypoparathyroidism in patients with basal ganglia calcification. Increased sensitivity to the dystonic effects of phenothiazines may also be present in hypoparathyroid patients, even in the absence of radiographic evidence of basal ganglia calcification. Calcified basal ganglia may also occur on a familial basis without abnormal parathyroid function.

Calcification of the lens, leading to cataract formation, is an important ocular manifestation of hypoparathyroidism. Correction of hypocalcemia does not lead to regression of cataracts once formed. Development of calcified basal ganglia or cataracts is probably a function of the duration of the hypoparathyroid state and is therefore seen more commonly in pseudohypoparathyroidism and idiopathic hypoparathyroidism than in postsurgical hypoparathyroidism.

Electrocardiographic manifestations of hypocalcemia include prolongation of the Q-T interval (particularly the Q-T corrected for rate) and T-wave changes such as peaking and inversion. The Q-T interval normalizes rapidly after correction of hypocalcemia, but T-wave abnormality may be slower to regress. A prolonged Q-T interval should theoretically predispose to ventricular tachycardia, but this arrhythmia has only rarely been reported in association with hypoparathyroidism. Similarly, hypocalcemia might be expected to cause resistance to the effect of cardiac glycosides and at least one such case has been reported of atrial fibrillation apparently refractory to digitalis. Reversion to normal sinus rhythm occurred only after normocalcemia was restored. Congestive heart failure due to severe hypocalcemia has been reported in neonates, but the role of hypocalcemia in causing congestive heart failure in adults has not been carefully evaluated; reports of improvement in cardiac function after normalization of serum calcium alone are rare.

Abnormalities in dentition occur frequently in children with hypoparathyroidism. Depending on the age of onset of hypoparathyroidism, one may find defective enamel and root formation, dental hypoplasia, or failure of adult teeth to erupt. Untreated hypoparathyroidism during pregnancy may lead to severe skeletal demineralization of the fetus and a state of transient hypoparathyroidism in the neonate.

Differential Diagnosis

Hypocalcemia, hyperphosphatemia, and normal renal function strongly suggest hypoparathyroidism (see also "Hypocalcemic Disorders — Differential Diagnosis," p. 996). The type of hypoparathyroidism may be indicated by the history and physical examination. The patient should be asked about previous neck surgery and about other affected family members. On physical examination there may be a neck scar suggesting postsurgical hypoparathyroidism; features of Albright's hereditary osteodystrophy, suggesting pseudohypoparathyroidism; or vitiligo, alopecia, and moniliasis, suggesting "idiopathic" hypoparathyroidism. Definitive characterization of the form of hypoparathyroidism (Fig. 19–60) requires determination of plasma PTH, urinary cAMP, and the response of urinary cAMP and urinary phosphate to exogenous PTH (Table 19–14). Most patients will show low or undetectable PTH and will respond normally to exogenous PTH, indicating PTH deficiency. These patients may be further subdivided according to the cause of PTH deficiency, e.g., hypomagnesemia, postsurgical, "idiopathic." Elevated concentration in serum PTH coupled with a normal response to exogenous PTH would suggest secretion of a biologically inactive form of PTH. Elevated serum PTH and an abnormal response to exogenous PTH signify resistance to PTH and may be further subdivided according to the site of defect (Fig. 19–60).

Specific Forms of Hypoparathyroidism

Deficient Parathyroid Hormone Secretion

Postsurgical

Tetany following thyroidectomy in humans was first described in 1879. After Erdheim, in 1906, observed that removal of the parathyroids in rats produced tetany, surgeons were more careful to preserve the parathyroid glands during thyroidectomy. The incidence of permanent hypoparathyroidism following thyroidectomy varies widely in surgical series (a range of 0.2–33% has been reported). The extent of thyroid resection, the experience of the surgeon, and the diligence with which hypocalcemia is sought postoperatively all contribute to the apparent variation in incidence. In some patients, postoperative hypocalcemia is transient, suggesting that sufficient viable parathyroid tissue remains to restore normal mineral homeostasis. Such patients, however, may show "decreased parathyroid reserve" and develop hypocalcemia when stressed either experimentally, e.g., by EDTA infusion, or clinically, e.g., during pregnancy and lactation. Occasionally there may be a long latent period before symptoms develop and before hypocalcemia is diagnosed.

Permanent hypoparathyroidism develops in 1% of patients after initial surgery for primary hyperparathyroidism. The risk of permanent hypoparathyroidism increases significantly in subtotal parathyroidectomy for parathyroid hyperplasia or repeated neck surgery for recurrent or persistent disease. In some cases autotransplantation of parathyroid tissue to the forearm is indicated to prevent hypoparathyroidism in these high-risk patients with hyperparathyroidism. Deliberate parathyroidectomy and autotransplantation has also been advocated by some surgeons for patients undergoing thyroid cancer resection. Precise indications for autotransplantation of parathyroids, however, have not been fully established. Complications such as failure of graft function, graft hyperfunction, or unnecessary transplantation make it unwise to perform parathyroid transplants indiscriminately.

Idiopathic Hypoparathyroidism

Deficient PTH secretion without a defined cause (e.g., surgical injury) has been termed "idiopathic hypoparathyroidism." This disease is rare and may occur on a sporadic or familial basis. The mode of inheritance of the familial variety is uncertain, possibly because several forms of the disease exist. Symptoms often begin in childhood but may appear much later, particularly in sporadic cases. The few histologic studies available show parathyroid atrophy with fatty replacement. An autoimmune etiology has been suggested by the presence of antibodies directed against parathyroid tissue in many affected individuals (38% incidence vs. 6% in normal controls). Patients with this disorder may also develop primary adrenal insufficiency and more rarely primary hypothyroidism, primary hypogonadism, diabetes mellitus, and pernicious anemia. Affected individuals should be monitored carefully for these additional endocrine deficiencies. Chronic mucocutaneous moniliasis (due to a defect in cellular immunity), alopecia areata, and vitiligo (with antibodies directed against melanocytes) all occur with increased frequency in patients with idiopathic hypoparathyroidism and bolster the hypothesis that a disordered immune system is responsible for deficient PTH secretion. Monilial lesions may be seen on physical examination and are generally not affected by serum calcium status. Idiopathic hypoparathyroidism is also rarely associated with other syndromes of uncertain etiology, e.g., Kearns-Sayre syndrome (ophthalmoplegia, retinal degeneration, myopathy, and ataxia) and the syndrome of hereditary nephrosis with nerve deafness.

Hypomagnesemia

Hypomagnesemia may result from chronic alcoholism, malabsorption, increased renal clearance in therapy with aminoglycoside antibiotics, prolonged parenteral therapy, or an isolated defect in intestinal absorption of magnesium. Hypocalcemia is frequently associated with hypomagnesemia and can be corrected by magnesium replacement therapy, suggesting a specific role for magnesium depletion in the genesis of the hypocalcemia. Hypomagnesemia-induced peripheral resistance to the effects of PTH has been invoked to explain the development of hypocalcemia, but the results of studies testing the effect of hypomagnesemia on the renal response to PTH (increase in urinary cAMP and phosphaturia) are contradictory. Serum PTH concentrations in patients with hypocalcemia due to hypomagnesemia have been undetectable, normal, or elevated. Recent studies, however, demonstrate an acute rise in serum PTH in patients with hypocalcemia and hypomagnesemia given magnesium intravenously (Fig. 19–61). (In normal subjects, magnesium infusion either suppresses or does not affect PTH secretion). The increase in serum PTH was not accom-

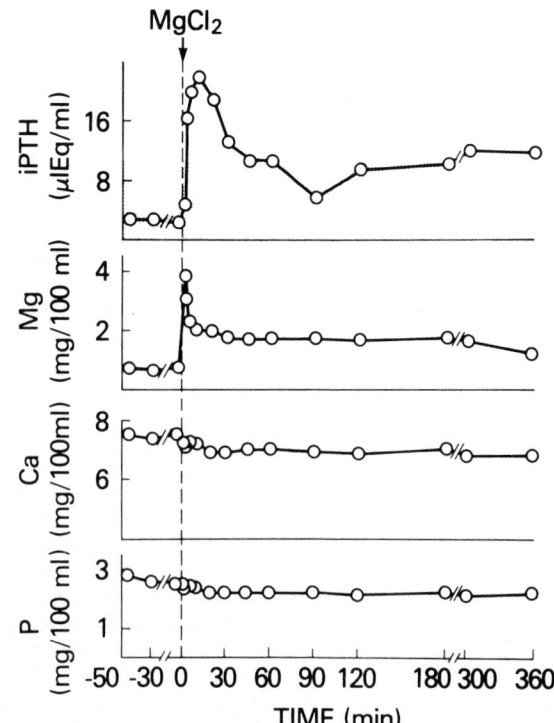

Figure 19–61. Serum PTH, magnesium, calcium, and phosphorus concentrations before and after the intravenous infusion of magnesium chloride (3 mg/magnesium/kg body weight infused over 30 seconds) in a hypomagnesemic, hypocalcemic patient. (From Anast, S., Winnacker, J. L., et al.: Impaired release of parathyroid hormone in magnesium deficiency. *J. Clin. Endocrinol. Metab.* 42:707, 1976.)

panied by acute changes in serum calcium and occurred even in patients with elevated basal serum PTH. It would appear then that the major effect of hypomagnesemia is to impair PTH release (as opposed to synthesis); peripheral resistance to PTH may also contribute to hypocalcemia since, as mentioned, some patients have elevated basal serum PTH. Effects of hypomagnesemia on peripheral metabolism and clearance of PTH have not been carefully studied.

Suppressed PTH Secretion

Elevation of serum calcium by nonparathyroid mechanisms will suppress normal PTH secretion. Acute reduction in serum calcium in this setting (e.g., after administration of mithramycin to a patient with hypercalcemia due to malignancy) may be followed by a brief period of parathyroid suppression leading to hypocalcemia. An analogous situation may occur after removal of a parathyroid adenoma, except that in this case normal parathyroid tissue is suppressed by hypercalcemia due to abnormal parathyroid secretion. Hypocalcemia in the first 2–3 days of life and hypocalcemia in infants of hypercalcemic mothers (see under "Hypocalcemic Disorders," p. 996) are other examples of this mechanism. Unlike the pituitary-adrenal axis, normal parathyroids recover function quickly (generally within 1 week), even after prolonged suppression by hypercalcemia. Hypocalcemia and hypermagnesemia have been reported in women receiving magnesium intravenously for toxemia of pregnancy. Hypermagnesemia could in theory suppress PTH secretion and in one case low serum PTH accompanied hypocalcemia but other etiologies were not definitely excluded.

Miscellaneous Causes of Deficient PTH Secretion

Any process that replaces or destroys sufficient normal parathyroid tissue may cause hypoparathyroidism. Metastases to the parathyroids have been seen at autopsy in 12% of a series of patients dying of malignant disease; breast cancer is the most common primary tumor. Despite the relatively frequent finding of metastases to the parathyroids, hypoparathyroidism caused by tumor replacement is exceedingly rare. Iron storage disease is known to cause gonadal and islet cell failure and has rarely been reported as a cause of hypoparathyroidism. Hypoparathyroidism in patients after radioactive iodine therapy of Graves' disease also is extremely uncommon. Defects in embryogenesis involving the branchial pouches may result in agenesis of the parathyroids, e.g., DiGeorges' syndrome (absent thymus and parathyroids).

Secretion of Biologically Inactive Parathyroid Hormone

Theoretically, hypoparathyroidism could result from secretion by the parathyroids of an abnormal form of PTH, biologically inert but reactive in the radioimmunoassay for PTH. The concentration of defective PTH in serum, moreover, could be elevated if normal feedback regulation of PTH secretion existed. Patients with this putative syndrome would respond normally to exogenous PTH, as do patients with deficient PTH secretion.

To date there have been two reports of patients thought to show hypoparathyroidism due to secretion of ineffective PTH. Both patients were of normal appearance on physical examination, and both showed hypocalcemia, hyperphosphatemia, and elevated serum PTH concentrations in several radioimmunoassays. U_{cAMP} and U_P response to exogenous PTH were said to be normal in both patients. There are problems in interpretation in both cases, however. The first patient was hypomagnesemic (0.7 mg/dl) and the response of serum PTH and calcium to magnesium replacement therapy was not documented. The second patient showed subperiosteal resorption on skeletal x-rays, suggesting that bone response to elevated PTH concentration was intact. Basal U_{cAMP}, moreover, was 11 nmol/mg creatinine, certainly not decreased. Since the phosphaturic response to PTH was rather slight (about 10%), this patient may in fact have pseudohypoparathyroidism type II (see "Hypoparathyroidism — Clinical Features," p. 991).

Hypoparathyroidism Due to Resistance to Parathyroid Hormone

Pseudohypoparathyroidism*

In 1942, Albright and coworkers described three patients with hypocalcemia, hyperphosphatemia, a blunted phosphaturic response to exogenous PTH, and a characteristic physical appearance. They suggested that hypoparathyroidism in these patients was due to target organ unresponsiveness to PTH and termed the syndrome pseudohypoparathyroidism. Subsequent studies have largely confirmed Albright's proposal, but fundamental questions regarding the pathophysiology of this rare disorder remain.

Clinical Features

Affected patients may show a variety of phenotypic features that are not seen in other forms of hypoparathyroidism† (Table 19–13). These include a round face, short stature, obesity, short thick neck, decreased intelligence, and subcutaneous calcification, as well as ossification (Fig. 19–62). Bony anomalies include exostoses and shortening of the metacarpals, metatarsals, and phalanges. Brachydactyly may be asymmetric; the fourth digit is most commonly involved and the second digit least commonly (Fig. 19–63). This constellation of phenotypic features has been termed Albright's hereditary osteodystrophy (AHO) and appears to be expressed independently of the disturbance in calcium metabolism (see later). The disease is clearly hereditary, with the average age at onset of symptoms of hypocalcemia about 8 years. The ratio of involved females to males (2:1) and the family studies are most consistent with an X-linked dominant form of inheritance. Cases of apparent male to male transmission (incompatible with sex linkage) have been reported but not documented with complete laboratory evaluation. Several features of AHO are present in other

---

*Pseudohypoparathyroidism (PHP) — resistance to PTH associated with Albright's hereditary osteodystrophy.

†A single patient with features of AHO and hypoparathyroidism apparently due to deficient PTH secretion has been reported.

Table 19–13. SIGNS AND SYMPTOMS IN TYPES OF HYPOPARATHYROIDISM

	"Classic" Pseudo	Idiopathic	Postsurgical
Increased neuromuscular excitability	+	+	+
Cataracts	+	+	+*
Basal ganglia calcification	+	+	+*
Prolonged Q-T interval on EKG	+	+	+
Papilledema	+	+	+
Dental defects	+	+	+**
Alopecia	−	+	−
Vitiligo	−	+	−
Moniliasis	−	+	−
Hypothyroidism†	+	+	+
Hypoadrenalism	−	+	−
Primary hypogonadism	−	+	−
Albright's hereditary osteodystrophy (brachydactyly, short, obese, round face)	+	−	−
Subcutaneous calcification (and bone formation)	+	−	−

*Uncommon unless long-standing disease present.

**Uncommon since postsurgical hypoparathyroidism rarely seen in children.

†The mechanism of hypothyroidism differs in each of the three forms of hypoparathyroidism.

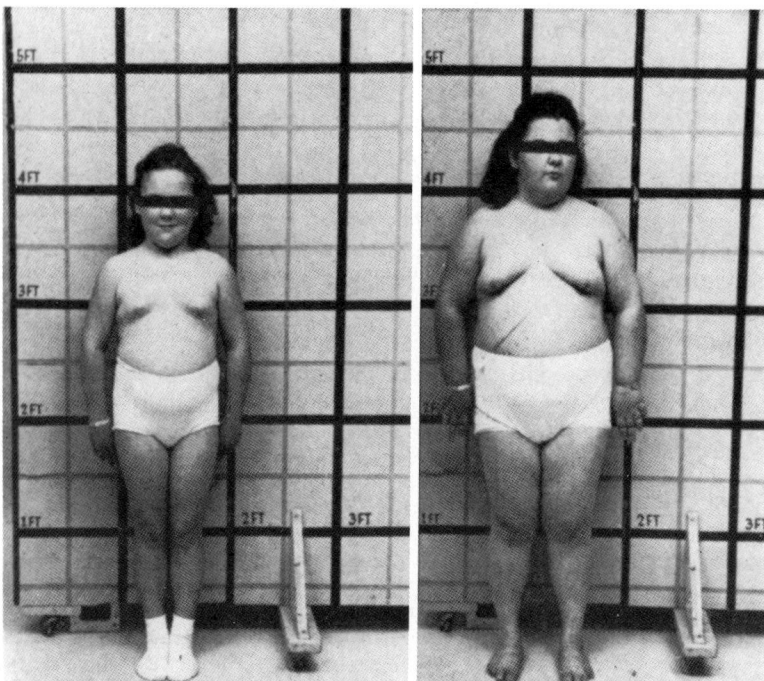

Figure 19–62. Mother and daughter with pseudohypoparathyroidism.

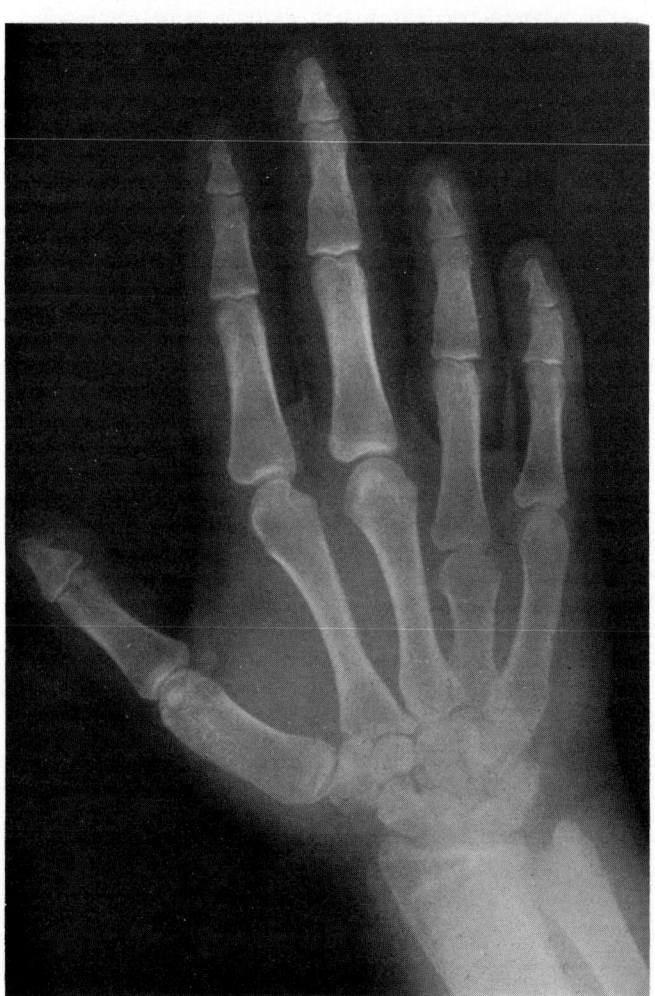

Figure 19–63. Radiograph of hand of patient with pseudohypoparathyroidism. Note shortened fourth metacarpal.

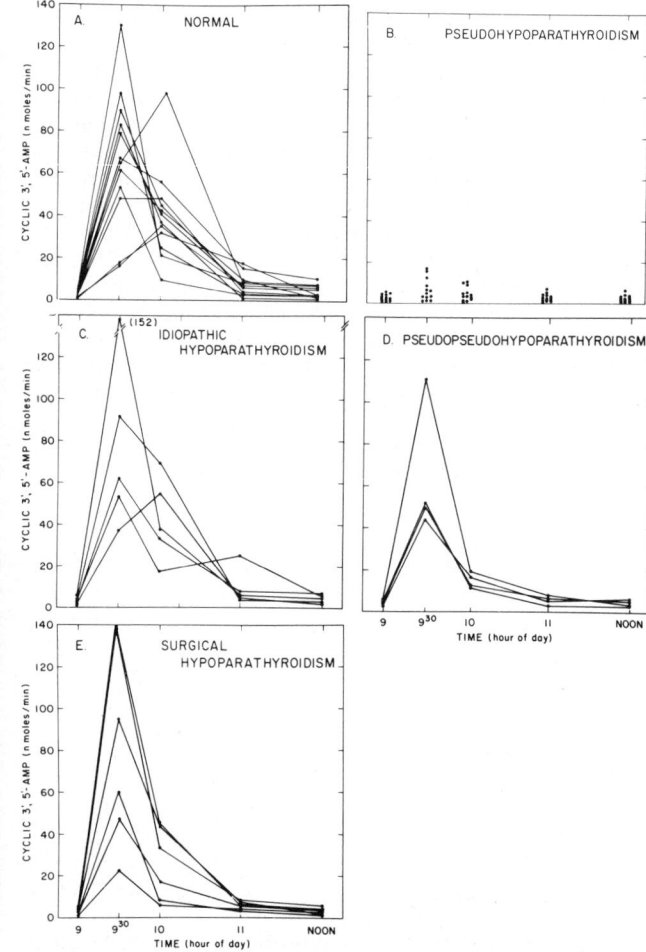

Figure 19–64. Response of U_{cAMP} to PTH infusion (300 units given between 9 A.M. and 9:15 A.M.) in normal subjects and in patients with various forms of hypoparathyroidism. (From Chase, L. R., Melson, G. L., and Aurbach, G. D.: Pseudohypoparathyroidism: defective excretion of 3′,5′-AMP in response to parathyroid hormone. *J. Clin. Invest. 48*:1832, 1969.)

Table 19-14. BIOCHEMICAL CHARACTERISTIC IN TYPES OF HYPOPARATHYROIDISM

	Serum PTH	U_{cAMP}	Exogenous PTH*	
			U_{cAMP} Response	U_P Response
Deficient PTH secretion	low	low	normal	normal
Secretion of ineffective PTH	high**	low	normal	normal
Resistance to PTH—defective receptor-adenylate cyclase complex	high	low	low	low
Resistance to PTH—defect distal to receptor-cyclase complex	high	high	normal	low

*200 units of PTH administered intravenously over 15 min. Urine collected before and after infusion for measurement of cAMP, phosphorus, and creatinine (ref., JCI, Chase et al., 1969).

**High if species secreted cross-reacts with antiserum used in RIA.

disorders, e.g., familial brachydactyly, Turner's syndrome (short stature, brachydactyly), hereditary multiple exostoses, and Gardner's syndrome (exostoses), but response to PTH is normal in all of these. The features of AHO may coexist with normal PTH responsiveness, and this has been termed pseudopseudohypoparathyroidism (PPHP). Within a given family, affected individuals may show AHO with or without abnormal PTH responsiveness. Rarely, transition from PHP to PPHP in a single individual has been reported.

Pathophysiology

As in other forms of hypoparathyroidism, patients with PHP show hypocalcemia and hyperphosphatemia, but serum PTH is elevated in proportion to the degree of hypocalcemia, indicating PTH resistance. Parathyroid hyperplasia has been demonstrated on biopsies obtained from several patients with PHP and biologically active hormone recovered from the glands in one case that was parathyroidectomized. Patients with PHP lack the normal brisk rise in U_{cAMP} after PTH infusion. By contrast, patients with PPHP (as well as idiopathic and surgical hypoparathyroidism) have a normal U_{cAMP} response (Fig. 19-64). Thus a defect in the renal PTH receptor–adenylate cyclase complex seems to account for renal resistance to PTH. Surprisingly, *in vitro* assay of membranes from the kidney of a patient with PHP (obtained at autopsy) showed apparently normal adenylate cyclase activation by PTH. Recently, a study of renal membranes from a single patient with PHP (obtained at renal biopsy) has provided evidence that the guanine nucleotide regulatory component of the adenylate cyclase complex may be defective while both the PTH receptor and catalytic unit of the enzyme are intact. Studies in our laboratory show that red cells from subjects with pseudohypoparathyroidism are deficient in the guanine nucleotide regulatory component (Fig. 19-65). This suggests that a generalized genetic deficiency of the guanine nucleotide regulatory component of adenylate cyclase may be the basis for hormone resistance in pseudohypoparathyroidism.

Skeletal resistance to PTH action in PHP is reflected in the lack of a normal calcemic response to repeated administration of exogenous PTH. This has generally been attributed to a defect in the skeletal adenylate cyclase complex by analogy to the renal lesion. Direct evidence for a defective skeletal adenylate cyclase complex is lacking. Recent studies, moreover, have suggested the possibility that reduced serum 1,25-(OH)$_2$-D (due to hyperphosphatemia or to defective renal response to PTH) contributes to the deficient skeletal response to PTH in PHP (and potentially in other forms of hypoparathyroidism as well). Thus, normal calcemic responses to PTH have been restored by prolonged therapy with vitamin D. In addition, reports of patients with PHP (with AHO) showing radiographic evidence of osteitis fibrosa cystica suggest that bone may be capable of responding to excessive PTH secretion in PHP. Definition of the exact role of 1,25-(OH)$_2$-D deficiency vs. defective skeletal adenylate cyclase in the skeletal resistance (PTH) of patients with PHP awaits development of methods for directly assessing skeletal response to PTH.

Endocrine dysfunction other than parathyroid may occur in PHP. Hypothyroidism (usually primary) has been reported in more than 5 cases; 8 of 10 patients in one study showed an exaggerated TSH response to TRF. PRL response to TRF and other stimuli was recently reported to be defective in six of eight patients with PHP. Elevated gonadotropins in plasma, an exaggerated response to GNRH, oligomenorrhea and hypoestrogenism suggesting gonadal resistance to gonadotropins were described in a single case report. These extra-parathyroidal abnormalities raise the possibility (supported by results discussed before and by Fig. 19-65) that the defect in the adenylate cyclase complex in PHP is more generalized than appreciated heretofore.

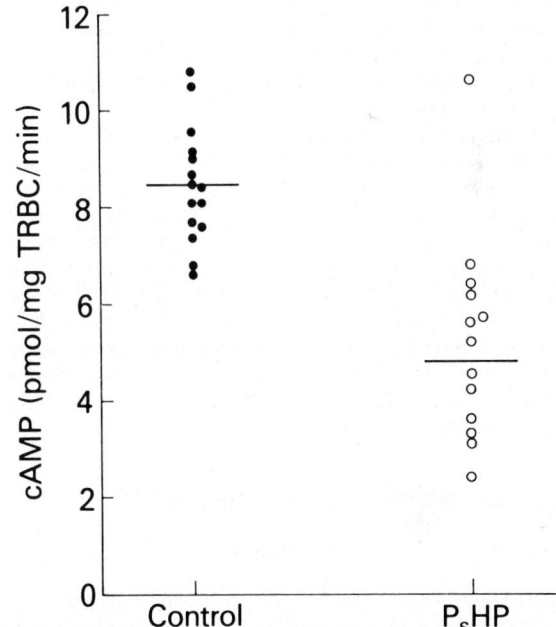

Figure 19-65. Comparison of the guanine nucleotide regulatory component in red cells from control and pseudohypoparathyroid subjects. The component in extracts of human red cell membranes was assayed by mixing with the adenylate cyclase catalytic unit from turkey erythrocyte membranes. Results are expressed as cAMP produced per mg of protein in membrane extract. Human red cells contain the regulatory unit but negligible amounts of the adenylate cyclase catalytic component. Red cells from pseudohypoparathyroidism show significantly (p < .001) reduced content of the regulatory component. (Modified from Levine, et al.: 1980.)

Resistance to Parathyroid Hormone Without Albright's Hereditary Osteodystrophy

Hypoparathyroidism with elevated serum PTH may occur in patients lacking the features of AHO. This constellation of findings appears to be rarer than classic PHP itself. In at least one such case deficient U_{cAMP} response to PTH was reported. More recently, several patients have been described with a normal U_{cAMP} but blunted phosphaturic response to PTH. Such cases have been labeled PHP type II. The nature of the defect in renal response is unknown, but it is presumably localized distal to the generation of cAMP. Normalization of serum calcium may restore the phosphaturic response to PTH in such patients. Lack of a normal calcemic response to PTH may reflect deficiency of 1,25-$(OH)_2$-D rather than an intrinsic skeletal defect.

Therapy

Vitamin D and calcium supplements are the mainstay of therapy of all forms of hypoparathyroidism (with the exception of deficient PTH secretion due to hypomagnesemia, which should be treated by replacing total body magnesium stores). Vitamin D, 50–100,000 units (1–2 mg)/day, together with calcium salts (1–2 g of elemental calcium/day) will correct hypocalcemia in most patients, but the precise dose will vary widely from patient to patient and in a given patient over time. More potent vitamin D metabolites, such as 1-α or 1,25 vitamin D, provide more rapid onset and offset of action but require close monitoring of serum calcium to avoid toxicity (see "Calciferol Pharmacology," p. 000). In the absence of PTH, urinary calcium will be higher than normal at any given serum calcium concentration (Fig. 19–19). To avoid hypercalciuria and nephrolithiasis, serum calcium concentration should generally be maintained in the range of 8–9 mg/dl, assuming the patient can be kept free of neuromuscular symptoms. Patients also receiving glucocorticoids require particularly close monitoring because of antagonistic effects on vitamin D.

Therapy directed at reduction in serum phosphorus, e.g., antacids or acetazolamide, is generally not required since restoration of normocalcemia tends to decrease renal threshold of phosphorus excretion and lower serum phosphorus. A recent report suggests that combined therapy with thiazide diuretics and sodium restriction is capable of maintaining a normal serum calcium concentration in patients wth hypoparathyroidism. Vitamin D was not given to these patients. A potential advantage of this approach is the lack of hypercalciuria, but reduced urinary calcium alone could not account fo the elevation in serum calcium concentration. Further long-term studies are needed to assess the role of this approach in the therapy of hypoparathyroidism.

HYPOCALCEMIC DISORDERS

Introduction

Hyocalcemia occurs in diverse acquired or hereditary diseases. It may be the principal manifestation as in hypoparathyroidism or merely one of a constellation of abnormalities, as in chronic renal failure. Regardless of cause, patients with a low serum ionized calcium concentration often develop symptoms of neuromuscular irritability, including paresthesias, muscle cramps, and seizures. Development of symptoms is not well correlated with the absolute degree of hypocalcemia. The clinical impression that the rate of fall in serum calcium is the critical determinant of whether or not tetany develops has not been substantiated by studies of EDTA-induced hypocalcemia in dogs. Decreased total serum calcium concentration, with a normal ionized fraction can exist with hypoproteinemia or acidosis. These possibilities should be excluded by measuring serum protein concentration and calculating the corrected serum calcium (see section on calcium, plasma, and ECF, p. 000) or by directly measuring ionized calcium. Alkalosis decreases ionized (but not total) serum calcium (a change from pH 7.4 to 7.6 may decrease ionized calcium by 0.5 mEq/l) and may synergize the development of tetany.

Pathophysiology

Hypocalcemia can represent a defect of any of several control points in the homeostatic regulation of calcium concentration (Fig. 19–52B). In most cases the cause is diminished secretion or action of PTH or 1,25-$(OH)_2$-D or both on target organs. As a consequence of deficient PTH concentration, calcium fluxes from bone to ECF and from renal tubular lumen to ECF are reduced; renal clearance of phosphate is decreased, leading to hyperphosphatemia. Deficient PTH action also leads to reduced renal formation of 1,25-$(OH)_2$-D (either directly or secondary to hyperphosphatemia). Low 1,25-$(OH)_2$-D concentration in serum leads to reduced calcium flux from intestinal lumen to blood. Thus diminished calcium entry into the ECF from three anatomic pools (Fig. 19–52B, 1,3, and 5) accounts for hypocalcemia in states of PTH deficiency.

In states of reduced vitamin D effect, calcium flux from intestine to blood will be decreased; in addition, PTH mobilization of calcium from bone to blood is impaired. Both of these factors (Fig. 19–52B, 1 and 5) may produce hypocalcemia. Although reduced intestinal calcium absorption and decreased calcium release from bone are the most frequent causes of hypocalcemia, clinically significant reduction in serum calcium may also result from increased loss of calcium into either soft tissue (Fig. 19–52B, 8), bone (Fig. 19–52B, 2), or other pools (hemodialysis, transplacental). Frank hypocalcemia may develop in such cases if compensatory actions of PTH or 1,25-$(OH)_2$-D are inadequate.

Differential Diagnosis

The clinical and biochemical features in each case will depend on the underlying cause of hypocalcemia. Renal function (serum creatinine, creatinine clearance) and gastrointestinal function (D-xylose tolerance test, serum carotene, quantitation of stool fat) should be evaluated, since renal failure and malabsorption are common causes of hypocalcemia. Skeletal x-rays should be examined for abnormalities, including features suggestive of secondary hyperparathyroidism, osteomalacia, osteoblastic tumor metastases, or bony anomalies suggesting PHP.

History and physical examination may provide diagnostic clues, e.g., cataracts or evidence of neck surgery in the past. Measurement of serum PTH, phosphorus, and 25-OH D and urinary cAMP are essential in defining the category of hypocalcemia (Table 19–15). Serum 1,25-$(OH)_2$-D determination is not generally available at present, but hypocalcemia due to 1,25-$(OH)_2$-D deficiency must be considered with normal serum 25-OH-D and radiographic evidence of rickets, osteomalacia, or secondary hyperparathyroidism.

Table 19–15. BIOCHEMICAL CATEGORIZATION OF HYPOCALCEMIC DISORDERS

Disorder	Serum PTH and U_{cAMP}	Serum P	Alk. P	25-Vitamin D	1,25-Vitamin D
Hypoparathyroidism	low*	high	normal	normal	low
Vitamin D deficiency (e.g., nutritional, malabsorption, liver disease)	high	low	high	low	low normal
Deficient 1,25 vitamin D formation or action (e.g., renal failure, hereditary vitamin D dependency)	high	low	high	normal	low**
Increased bone formation (e.g., healing osteitis fibrosa, osteoblastic metastases)	normal to high	low normal	high	normal	(? high)
Increased soft-tissue calcification (e.g., tumor lysis or phosphate infusion)	normal to high	high	normal	normal	(?)

*PTH-resistant forms have high serum PTH and low (PHP, type I) or high (PHP, type II) U_{cAMP}.
**Elevated in 1,25-$(OH)_2$-D insensitivity.

Specific Causes of Hypocalcemia

Hypoparathyroidism

Disorders in which there is deficient PTH action on kidney and bone are discussed in detail in the preceding section.

Abnormalities in Vitamin D Metabolism

Hypocalcemia may develop in deficiency of vitamin D or its active metabolites 25-vitamin D and 1,25-vitamin D. Both acquired (principally chronic renal failure) and hereditary forms exist and are described fully in the sections on rickets and osteomalacia (p. 998) and on secondary hyperparathyroidism (p. 979).

Disproportionate Net Calcium Influx into Bone

Albright described severe hypocalcemia after removal of a parathyroid adenoma from a patient with osteitis fibrosa cystica. Bone biopsy in the early postoperative period showed increased osteoid formation and osteoblast numbers, with reduction in osteoclasts. Approximately 4 months after surgery, serum calcium became normal, with radiographic and bone biopsy evidence of healing of bone. More recent studies provide direct evidence (serum PTH and U_{cAMP}) for intact parathyroid function in such patients. Hypocalcemia is generally due to PTH resistance associated with greatly increased skeletal demand for calcium ("hungry bones").

A similar mechanism has been invoked to explain hypocalcemia occurring after subtotal thyroidectomy for Graves' disease. In a study of two groups of patients undergoing thyroidectomy (Graves' disease vs. nontoxic goiter), the incidence and timing of postoperative hypocalcemia did not differ. Surgical injury to the parathyroids appears to be the major cause of hypocalcemia after thyroidectomy; "bone hunger" secondary to long-standing Graves' disease may play a minor role in some cases.

Osteoblastic Metastases

Hypocalcemia occurs in association with skeletal metastases, particularly in patients with cancer of prostate and of breast. Twenty-three of 143 patients with bony metastases in one series showed hypocalcemia. When hypoproteinemia and renal failure have been excluded, hypocalcemia has been attributed to increased calcium flux into osteoblastic lesions. Evidence against hypoparathyroidism in such patients includes normal or low concentration of phosphate in serum, but few reported cases show data on PTH concentration. Careful measurement of calcium kinetics is also lacking.

Acute Hyperphosphatemia

An increase in serum phosphate may decrease serum calcium by inhibiting bone resorption or by leading to extraskeletal calcification or by a combination of the two. Exogenous phosphate can be a cause, e.g., intravenous phosphate infusion given to treat hypercalcemia or administration of phosphate enemas to infants. Hypocalcemia due to endogenous phosphate loads also occurs, particularly during chemotherapy of highly responsive tumors such as Burkitt's lymphoma and acute lymphoblastic leukemia. Extensive soft-tissue calcification, renal failure, and death have occurred in several cases.

Pancreatitis

The etiology of hypocalcemia in acute pancreatitis remains obscure despite numerous studies. Calcium soap deposits in areas of fat necrosis have been described in autopsied cases; the amount of calcium deposited in this manner is probably not sufficient in most cases to account for hypocalcemia. More recently humoral mechanisms involving glucagon release from the injured pancreas and secondary increase in CT secretion have been invoked. Elevated serum glucagon and CT concentrations during acute pancreatitis have not been observed in all studies; the relatively weak hypocalcemic effect of these hormones, moreover, makes it unlikely that they account for hypocalcemia of pancreatitis. Inadequate PTH response to hypocalcemia also has been described frequently in acute pancreatitis, but the mechanism for reduced PTH secretion is unknown.

Malabsorption

In certain cases of malabsorption, hypocalcemia may occur even though absorption of vitamin D and magnesium is normal. Fecal fat in excess of 10 g/day may be associated with sufficient calcium malabsorption to cause hypocalcemia.

Calcium Chelators

Substances such as citrate or EDTA reduce ionized (but not total) serum calcium concentration by forming complexes. Clinically this may be encountered during transfusion of citrate anticoagulated blood, e.g., in infants undergoing exchange transfusion or in adults receiving massive amounts of blood (especially with reduced liver function, which delays citrate metabolism). Such patients should be monitored closely, and ionized calcium should be measured if possible to guide treatment with calcium.

Hypercalcitoninemia

Hypercalcitoninemia is generally *not* associated with hypocalcemia because CT is a relatively weak hypocalcemic agent in adult humans. Thus, in patients with medullary carcinoma of the thyroid secreting excess CT, hypocalcemia is distinctly rare. In states of increased bone resorption, e.g., Paget's disease, administration of CT (or other inhibitors of bone resorption, e.g., mithramycin) may lower serum calcium.

Neonatal Hypocalcemia

Hypocalcemia in the first 2–3 days of life occurs with increased frequency in infants who are premature, born to diabetic mothers, or suffer respiratory distress syndrome. High calcium concentration in normal cord blood at term reflects active placental transfer of calcium from mother to fetus and may account for the low serum PTH and high serum CT concentration measured during the first 2–3 days of life. Hypocalcemia occurring later (about 1 week post partum) is often associated with feeding of cow's milk or other high phosphate formula. An inability to excrete sufficient phosphate in the urine at this stage may be involved. Immaturity of the hepatic calciferol 25-hydroxylase system may contribute to rapid depletion of 25-OH-D stores. In cases of maternal hyperparathyroidism, neonatal hypocalcemia may occur after the first week of life, reflecting prolonged but generally transient suppression of parathyroid function in the infant.

Therapy

Whenever possible, any underlying disorder should be treated; resolution of hypocalcemia will generally ensue. When this is not possible, chronic therapy with vitamin D and calcium may be required (see "Calciferol Pharmacology," p. 960 and "Hypoparathyroidism," p. 990). Acute symptomatic hypocalcemia of any cause can be treated by intravenous calcium infusion. Adults requiring urgent treatment can be given 10–20 ml of 10% calcium gluconate (contains about 10 mg elemental calcium/ml) intravenously over 10 min. (In patients taking digitalis, rapid intravenous administration of calcium may be hazardous). In less urgent situations, calcium gluconate may be administered by slow intravenous infusion (20 mg elemental calcium/kg body weight) over 4–8 hours as needed to alleviate symptoms.

RICKETS AND OSTEOMALACIA

Nutritional Vitamin D Deficiency

Prior to 1920, nutritional rickets and osteomalacia were major public health problems, particularly in cities in temperate zones. Recognition of the antirachitic properties of light and of cod liver oil was one of the greatest accomplishments in the field of medical investigation. In the United

States, calciferol needs generally are satisfied through conversion, in the skin, of 7–dehydrocholesterol to cholecalciferol (vitamin D_3) under the influence of ultraviolet radiation. The minimal requirement for vitamin D_2 or vitamin D_3 is approximately 2.5 μg (100 IU)/day in children and adults. Endogenous production of vitamin D_3 normally provides 5–50 times this amount. The recommended dietary allowance of vitamin D is 10 μg (400 IU)/day. In the United States, bovine milk contains added ergocalciferol (or in some regions cholecalciferol), 10 μg/quart, and many dairy and other foods are similarly "fortified." Factors predisposing to nutritional vitamin D deficiency include prematurity, rapid growth with its needs for adequate skeletal calcium and phosphorus, inadequate light exposure, and avoidance of vitamin D–supplemented foods. With deficient solar exposure, a diet unfortified with vitamin D does not normally contain an adequate amount of vitamin D (Table 19–16). In particular, human and bovine milk are probably inadequate sources. Vitamin D sulfate is present in human milk but may not be available for biologic activation. Thus mild rickets can occur during the winter months in otherwise healthy breast-fed infants whose mothers do not provide vitamin D or fortified foods.

Severe nutritional deficiency of vitamin D is now extremely rare in the United States because of the inclusion of supplemental ergocalciferol (vitamin D_2) in most milk and in many other processed foods. Vitamin D deficiency remains a public health problem in many other nations, however. For example, among children of Asian immigrants in Bradford, England, the prevalence of biochemical features of vitamin D deficiency in 1973 was 45%. The clinical and biochemical features of nutritional vitamin D deficiency will be described in detail, as they are relevant to an understanding of many disorders with hereditary or acquired abnormalities of vitamin D metabolism.

Clinical Features

The characteristic skeletal disturbance in vitamin D deficiency, and also in some other metabolic disorders, is osteomalacia, which literally means soft bones. The malacic bone is subject to distortion in shape and to fracture and is particularly prone to develop with vitamin D deficiency in infancy or childhood. The deformities of bone represent the characteristic skeletal appearance seen in rickets. Congenital nutritional rickets occurs only in offspring of mothers with severe vitamin D deficiency. Nutritional rickets may be manifest between the ages of 6 and 24 months, however, and somewhat earlier in premature infants who often have small adipose depots and delayed

Table 19–16. VITAMIN D CONTENT OF UNFORTIFIED FOODS*

Egg Yolk	50
Halibut	44
Herring (fresh or canned)	320
Sardines (canned)	1100–1500
Shrimp	150
Liver (chicken, beef, calf)	0–70
Butter	35
Cheese	12–15
Milk (bovine)	0.3–4
Milk (human)	0–10

*In IU/100 g or /dl. One IU is equivalent to 25 ng of vitamin D2 or D3.

Modified from the International Encyclopedia of Pharmacology and Therapeutics. Vol. 1. Yendt, E. R. (ed.), New York, Pergamon Press, 1970, p. 139.

maturation of the hepatic capacity to utilize 25-hydroxylate calciferols. Deficiencies in bone mineralization are evident particularly in regions of rapid bone growth and turnover. In the first year of life the most rapidly growing bones are in the cranium, wrists, and ribs. Nutritional rickets at this time leads to widened cranial sutures, frontal bossing, posterior flattening of the skull (craniotabes), bulging of costochondral junctions (rachitic rosary), indentation of the ribs at the diaphragmatic insertions (Harrison's groove), and enlargement of the wrists. The rib cage may be so grossly deformed that respiratory failure ensues. Dental eruption is often delayed, and the teeth show irregular pits, grooves, and enamel hypoplasia. There is a severe muscular hypotonia and weakness resulting in a lax, protuberant abdomen. Although linear growth and weight are adequate, the infant may be unable to stand without support until age 3. In older children, proximal muscle weakness may be prominent. Compromised respiratory musculature also undoubtedly contributes to the high incidence of pneumonitis. Signs of other vitamin deficiencies may be present at the same time. Tetany and laryngeal stridor are uncommon, as hypocalcemia is usually mild. After the first year of life the deformities resulting from calciferol deficiency are most severe about the legs because of their rapid growth and weight-bearing function. Most deformities are the result of pressure on weakened growth plates, but in severe rickets bony shafts of the long bones also are deformed and subject to fracture. The ends of the long bones become visibly enlarged. Bowleg (genu varum) or knock-knee (genu valgum) worsens progressively. In long-standing disease there may be coxa vara and rachitic saber shins. Moderate deformities occurring before age 4 may resolve after adequate vitamin D treatment, but those occurring later result in lasting deformity or compromise in adult height or both. When rickets begins later in childhood (age 10) the shafts of the long bones may remain straight while the knee metaphysis becomes angulated. There is an increased susceptibility to pathologic fracture.

The clinical features associated with osteomalacia are subtler than those with rickets. In the mature remodeling skeleton, only 5% or less of calcium is newly laid down each year. Thus, a mineralization defect in adults must be present for several years to produce clinical manifestations. The characteristic symptom, if any, is pain when weight or pressure is applied to the affected bones. Low backache relieved by recumbency is one of the earlier complaints, but the pain may include other portions of the spine, ribs, and feet. A narrowing of the pelvic outlet from inward pressure of the hips may lead to difficulties during childbirth and was once a cause of widespread morbidity. Loss of vertebral height can lead to kyphosis as a late manifestation. The skeletal deformities may be associated with other features of malnutrition. Associated proximal weakness contributes to a waddling gait or severe crippling. Patients with osteomalacia may be referred initially to neurology clinics because of prominent weakness. Often the disease occurs in a series of relapses and remissions, and signs of previous disease activity, such as bowing of the legs, will also be present. The first manifestation may be an acute fracture, the commonest sites being the femoral neck, pubic ramus, spine, or ribs. The previous description is applicable to severe osteomalacia. The incidence and morbidity of mild osteomalacia are presently not known, but with increasing use of bone biopsy and assays for circulating vitamin D metabolites in blood this process will soon be better understood. Sokoloff reported low-grade osteomalacia in 8 femur specimens from an unselected series of 31 Americans with hip fracture, indicating the potential magnitude of this problem. In this study the cause of the histologic lesions was not defined; thus, it would be premature to implicate a deficiency or abnormality in vitamin D metabolism.

Radiographic Features

In children, failure of cartilage calcification results in delayed opacification of the epiphyses and widening of growth plates. In vitamin D deficiency the ends of the growing metaphyses are frayed or irregular, and their usually straight transverse appearance becomes concave or "cupped." They widen owing to the pressure born by a large mass of poorly calcified cartilage (Fig. 19–66). In the di-

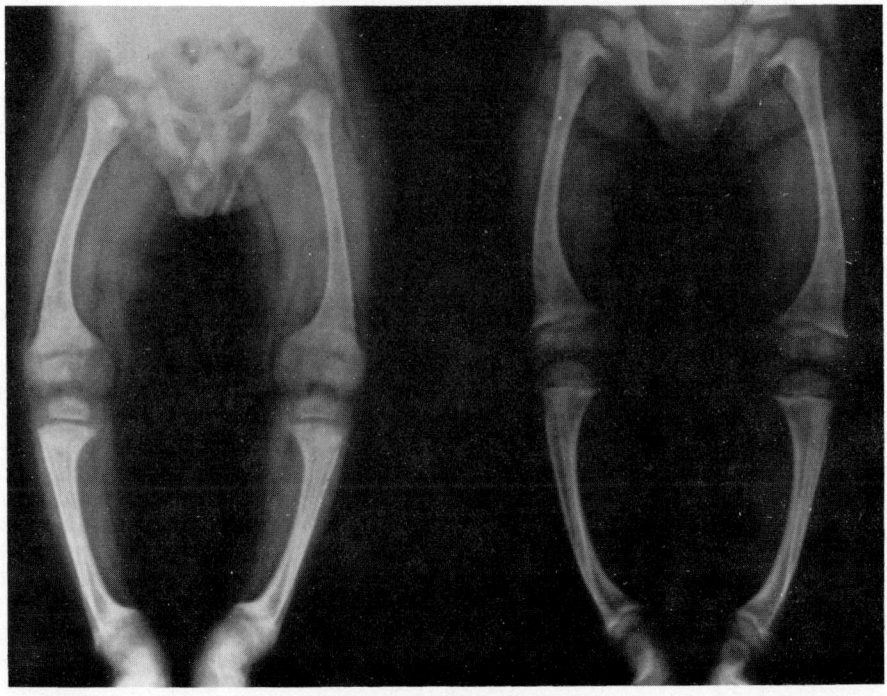

Figure 19–66. Left: Active rickets in a patient with tissue insensitivity to 1,25-(OH)₂-D at age 21 months with genu varum, irregular metaphyses, and widened growth plates. Right: Inactive rickets in the same patient at age 27 months following treatment with massive doses of ergocalciferol (vitamin D₂). (From Marx, S. J., et al.: *J. Clin. Endocrinol.* 47:1303, 1978.)

aphyses, the cortex is thin and the periosteum occasionally fuzzy and bone trabeculae are sparse and coarse. In childhood, the characteristic shaft deformities (genu varum, genu valgum, coxa vara) are present, but pseudofractures are uncommon. There is variable severity of manifestations of secondary hyperparathyroidism. These include irregular lacey subperiosteal erosions especially about the metaphyses of long bones, but the bone cysts and phalangeal lesions present in adults are rarely present in children. Fluctuations in disease severity result in the appearance of thin radiodense growth arrest lines (Harris lines) in the metaphyses parallel to the growth plates. The earliest radiographic feature in healing rickets appears approximately at days 8–30 of treatment as a dense line of calcified cartilage separated from the metaphysis by a small zone of uncalcified cartilage.

Signficant osteomalacia may be present without radiographic manifestations, but there is often a generalized decrease in bone density. Usually there is a decrease in total skeletal mineral content; in certain forms of osteomalacia (for example in approximately half of adults with familial X-linked hypophosphatemia), however, total bone mineral is increased albeit, with excessive quantities of unmineralized osteoid. The most characteristic feature of adult osteomalacia is the pseudofracture, a straight transverse ribbon–like band. Pseudofractures (Looser's zones or Milkman's syndrome) localize, often symmetrically, at the concave sides of the shafts of long bones plus the ribs,

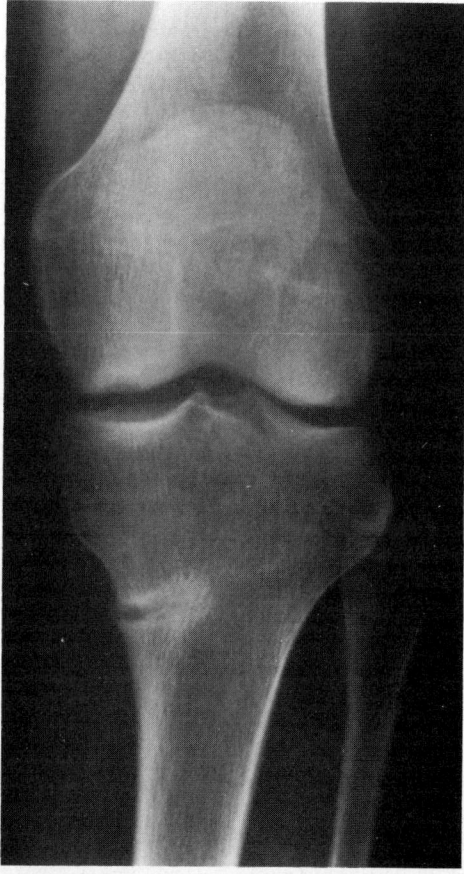

Figure 19–67. Active osteomalacia in a patient with hereditary tissue insensitivity to 1,25-(OH)₂-D (sibling of patient in Fig. 19–66) at age 18 with pseudofracture of the left tibia. (From Marx, S. J., et al.: *J. Clin. Endocrinol.* 47:1303, 1978.)

scapulae, and pubic rami (Fig. 19–67). They probably originate from repeated microfractures with a build-up of uncalcified callus. In some locations they may commence from pressures of pulsating arteries. The medullary cavities are narrowed with trabeculae that are coarse and reduced in numbers. Bone cortex is thinned and, on fine-grain radiographs, contains small intracortical striations of decreased density. Long-standing disease leads to deformities that include bowing of long bones, biconcave vertebrae, and distorted pelvic outlet that has a triangular appearance on standard anteroposterior views. Fractures (sometimes superimposed upon pseudofractures) occur and unite slowly.

Selective malabsorption of calcium leads to secondary hyperparathyroidism with subperiosteal resorption, especially on the medial border of the middle phalanges and erosion of the digital tufts. In severe cases, the associated soft-tissue changes have an outward appearance that resembles clubbing. The long bones may contain sharp-margined cysts, and the symphysis pubis and the sacroiliac joints become widened.

Bone Histology and Biochemistry

The common defect in rickets and osteomalacia is absence or deficiency of regions of osteoid mineralization (mineralization front). The bone mineral density is decreased, and osteoid borders are increased in length, width, and volume. In growing bones the most striking abnormality occurs in regions of endochondral ossification. Systematic histologic studies have been done with rats rendered rachitic by diets deficient in vitamin D and phosphorus. The histologic appearance of the zones of resting and proliferating cartilage are normal. In the zone of maturing cartilage, however, the usually regular columns of chondrocytes are disorganized and greatly increased in length (Fig. 19–68). The zone of hypertrophic cartilage at the diaphyseal end of the columns is sparse. At the diaphyseal end, the calcification front and zone of vascular invasion are distorted or unrecognizable.

Mechanical stress upon the unsupported cellular growth plate leads to the epiphyseal bulging characteristic of rickets. After epiphyseal fusion, these changes can no longer occur. Whenever remodeling occurs there is deficient mineralization, however. The result is osteomalacia, or softening of bones.

Unfortunately the term osteomalacia has been given additional definitions that have led to much confusion. Three widespread definitions of the term are: (1) a decrease in mineralization of osteoid, (2) an increase in osteoid width, and (3) an increase in the proportion of bone surface covered by osteoid independent of width. With vitamin D deficiency all three definitions are acceptable. Prominent osteoid seams reflect an imbalance of osteoid synthesis and osteoid mineralization. For example, in vitamin D–deficient rats, osteoid deposition rate is slowed, but the maturation and mineralization of osteoid are slowed to an even greater extent, with the result that osteoid seams are increased in length and width. Unmineralized osteoid is also prominent in hyperparathyroidism, thyrotoxicosis, Paget's disease, fluorosis, and diphosphonate administration but should not obfuscate proper interpretation of the skeletal abnormalities of these other disorders (see "Causes of Rickets and Osteomalacia — General Considerations in Differential Diagnosis," p. 1002).

In vitamin D deficiency, the mineralization front is absent or decreased in prominence. This is also evident in the periosteocytic lacunae. This latter location may be disproportionally affected in X-linked hypophosphatemia. The

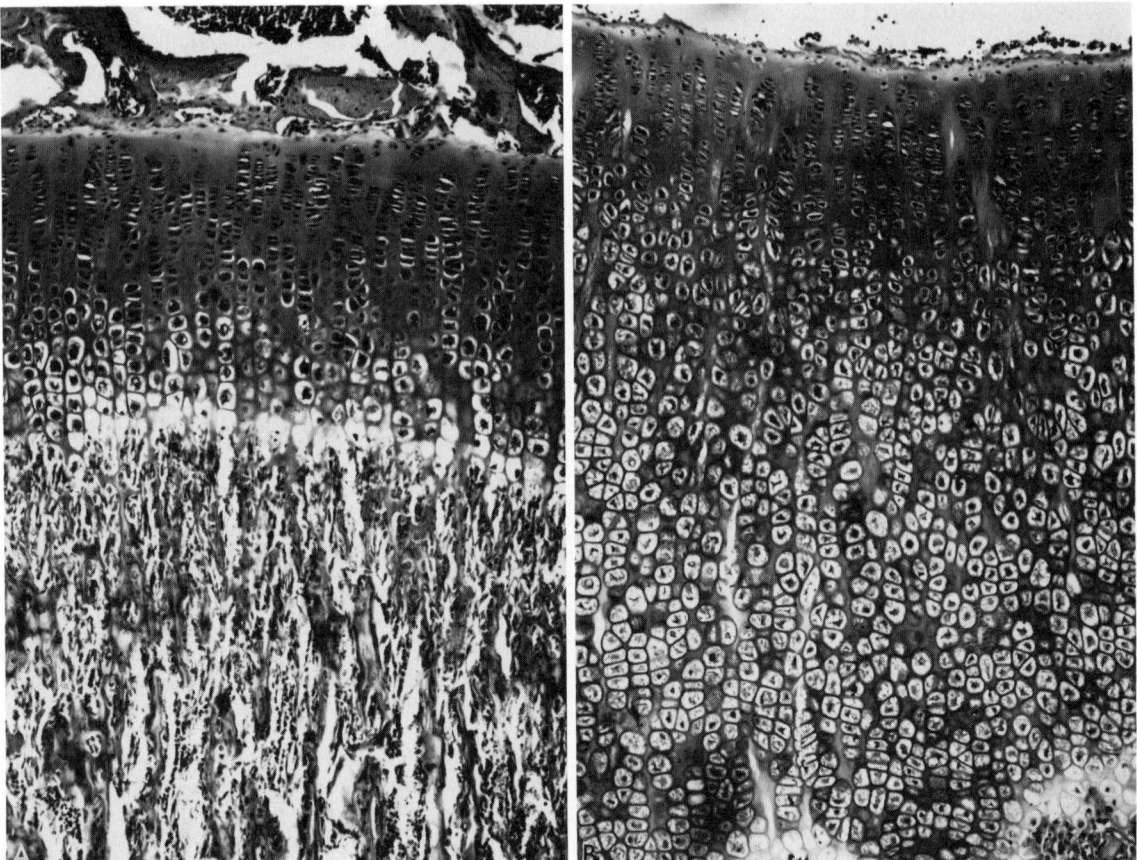

Figure 19–68. (A) Normal epiphyseal plate of immature rat with articular aspect at top. (B) Rat epiphyseal plate after six weeks on a diet deficient in phosphorus and vitamin D. Note increase in axial height of cartilage mass. The normal orderly columns are replaced by increased numbers of cells in irregular rows (× 400). (Courtesy of Dr. H. J. Mankin.)

normal lamellar structure of osteoid is preserved, but with polarized light, the number of lamellae is increased in proportion to the increase in osteoid thickness. Extensive coating of bony surfaces with unmineralized osteoid probably helps account for resistance to the acute skeletal mineral mobilizing effects of PTH. Small zones of unmineralized osteoid may persist deep within mineralized bone even after therapy, and these may contribute to a porotic skeletal appearance. If secondary hyperparathyroidism is present, osteoclast numbers are increased. Regions of reactive tissue with trabeculae of woven (immature) bone correspond to radiographic regions of pseudofracture.

There is disagreement as to whether in vitamin D deficiency the osteoid has a normal mineralization potential. Clearly in vitamin D deficiency the composition of bone and cartilage is abnormal. In addition to the gross deficiency of mineral, there is an increase of lipid within chondrocytes and a decrease in the synthesis rates of RNA, protein, and polysaccharide in the epiphyseal maturation zone. Increased hydroxylation of lysine in vitamin D–deficient bone collagen is similar to that in fetal bone collagen. These changes may all be caused by the structural distortions in the malacic bone, however. In the proliferative zone of the growth plate, DNA synthesis is not abnormal, rachitic cartilage retains a normal quantity and distribution of matrix vesicles, and these retain a normal capacity to accumulate appatite when provided with sufficient mineral substrate *in vitro*. In contrast, when rickets and osteomalacia are induced by administration of diphosphonates to chickens, the matrix vesicles do not accumulate mineral normally *in vitro*.

Laboratory Tests

The principal laboratory features in vitamin D deficiency can be understood by considering only the intestinal actions of vitamin D. Deficient calcium absorption leads to mild hypocalcemia. This promotes secondary hyperparathyroidism. The manifestations of secondary hyperparathyroidism (see "Secondary Hyperparathyroidism," p. 979) include increased plasma PTH concentration, decreased renal threshold for phosphate excretion and hypophosphatemia, and increased circulating concentrations of the skeletal alkaline phosphatase isoenzyme. Often, as a result of secondary hyperparathyroidism, the serum calcium concentration is maintained within the lower portion of the normal range. Urinary calcium is very low, due to the reduced filtered load and the direct renal tubular action of elevated serum concentrations of PTH on renal transport of calcium. In time, skeletal changes become evident first to histologic and later to radiographic evaluations. The circulating concentrations of vitamin D_2 and D_3, 25-hydroxy D_2 and D_3 are all low. Serum 1,25-$(OH)_2$-D_3 and -D_2 may be in the "normal" range, however, though inappropriately low when considered in regard to the degree of secondary hyperparathyroidism. Although net production of 25-OH-D is low in nutritional vitamin D deficiency, the fractional conversion of trace concentrations of radiolabeled vitamin D to 25-OH-D is increased, reflecting contraction of the total vitamin D pool. Assessment of the total serum 25-hydroxy vitamin D concentration, which may include the D_2 and D_3 forms of 25-OH-D, 24,25-$(OH)_2$-D, 25,26-$(OH)_2$-D, 1,25-$(OH)_2$-D, and perhaps other metabolites, is in practice a simple and useful indicator of the state of vitamin D nutrition. A low 25-OH-D concentration alone is not diagnostic of simple dietary deficiency as it also may reflect malabsorption, defective hepatic 25-hydroxylation of vitamin D, or increased clearance of circulating 25-OH-vitamin D. Serum concentrations of 1,25-(OH)$_2$-D may be normal although disproportionally low relative to the degree of secondary hyperparathyroidism.

During the early phases of treatment, because skeletal mineralization may be very rapid, serum calcium concentration may actually decrease and serum activity of alkaline phosphatase may rise. The serum concentration of alkaline phosphatase, after peaking, generally normalizes over several months. The time course of resolution of the secondary hyperparathyroidism is not well delineated, but there seems to be a disproportionate incidence of "primary" hyperparathyroidism among patients with remote histories of treated vitamin D deficiency.

Therapy of Nutritional Vitamin D Deficiency

Treatment and prevention of nutritional vitamin D deficiency has been simple since the discovery of vitamin D in the 1920's. Low doses of ergocalciferol (2–5 μg/day) or even ultraviolet radiation of the skin will effect a satisfactory cure. In practice ergocalciferol is given orally in doses of 125 μg (5000 IU)/day for treatment of nutritional deficiency. Similar amounts are effective in infants and adults. Because of effective storage in body fat, regimens of intermittent high-dose parenteral treatment (stosstherapy) have been employed when day to day cooperation is not optimal. These regimens incur a mild risk of hypercalcemia because of poorly understood differences in individual response, however. The response to vitamin D$_2$ begins within days, and, if a target active metabolite such as 1,25-(OH)$_2$-D$_3$ is given, a change in intestinal calcium absorption is measurable within hours. The early biochemical changes may include decreases in serum and urine concentrations of calcium during early active skeletal mineralization. This can be avoided by supplying extra calcium by mouth (2–3 g of elemental calcium in four divided doses). 1,25-(OH)$_2$-D$_3$ may be useful if there are acute symptoms of tetany, but it is not recommended for maintenance therapy, since it does not replete body calciferol stores or allow regulation of endogenous production of 1–α–hydroxylated calciferol metabolites. Severe symptomatic hypocalcemia should be considered a medical emergency and can be treated with intravenous calcium infusion (15 mg of calcium/kg infused over 6–24 hours). Bone deformities may require orthopedic intervention after the metabolic deficit has been treated.

Causes of Rickets and Osteomalacia

General Considerations in Differential Diagnosis

Rickets and its adult counterpart, osteomalacia, may present in an unmistakable fashion. A large number of conditions can lead to this radiologic or histologic abnormality. Several states associated with active osteoblastic function should be differentiated from the more typical osteomalacic disorders. Very active osteoblastic function is associated with a mild disproportion between osteoid production and calcification, so-called dynamic osteomalacia. During periods of rapid growth severe limitation of dietary calcium can be manifest as rickets, though the more typical lesion in calcium deficiency of animals is osteoporosis. Bone

in the region of a healing fracture will show increased osteoid within 5 days. Disproportionate osteoid may also be present in active Paget's disease, thyrotoxicosis, and primary hyperparathyroidism. In the last case, true vitamin D deficiency may be present simultaneously, even to the point of resulting in normocalcemic or masked primary hyperparathyroidism.

Some generalized skeletal disorders may mimic rickets or osteomalacia. The metaphyseal chondrodystrophies are a spectrum of disorders generally manifested as short-limbed dwarfism. These patients may receive large doses of vitamin D in the belief that they have vitamin D–resistant rickets; the only results are repeated episodes of vitamin D intoxication. In metaphyseal chondrodystrophies metaphyseal growth plates are distorted but not in osteomalacia. The radiographic features mimic rickets but radiographs of the frayed metaphyses show a characteristic sclerotic appearance unlike the undermineralized zone in rickets. Most of the metaphyseal chondrodystrophies are associated with normal serum concentrations of calcium, phosphorus, and alkaline phosphatase, except a severe juvenile form (Jansen type) that often presents with hypercalcemia and its complications. In adults, generalized bony demineralization can reflect one of several disorders, osteoporosis often being a major concern. The diagnosis of osteomalacia is best made by recognizing a precipitating cause and characteristic biochemical abnormalities. An adequate history and several simple laboratory analyses (for example, serum calcium, phosphorus, alkaline phosphatase, creatinine, and 25-OH-vitamin D) (Fig. 19–69) will generally exclude most diagnoses. A bone biopsy may be useful when serum and radiographic features are inconclusive, although experience with the technique is too limited at most centers to be of general value in diagnosis.

Deficiency of 25-OH-Vitamin D

Malabsorption of fat may cause vitamin D deficiency through a combination of malabsorption and increased endogenous loss of 25-OH-vitamin D, representing disruption of the enterohepatic circulation. Often there is also an element of light deprivation or body fat depletion that contributes to compromise of calciferol stores. Rickets or osteomalacia may be early complications of gluten-sensitive enteropathy, pancreatic insufficiency, or intestinal bypass surgery. Children with the combination of malabsorption and vitamin D deficiency may be severely dwarfed. Vitamin D deficiency caused by malabsorption is associated with reduced concentrations of 25-OH-vitamin D in serum.

The serum concentration of 25-OH-vitamin D may be depressed for several reasons in patients with hepatic disorders. Rickets and osteomalacia are common in patients with severe obstructive biliary disease. Malabsorption and disruption of the enterohepatic circulation of calciferol metabolites contribute to this picture. In one study a group of eight patients with primary biliary cirrhosis showed no increase in mean serum concentration of 25-OH-D after a single injection of 2.5 mg ergocalciferol, implicating a decreased hepatic capacity to 25-hydroxylate the vitamin. A similar defect in hepatic production as well as increased metabolism of 25-OH-D contributes to the pathophysiology of certain cases of neonatal hypocalcemia and neonatal rickets. This can be prevented or treated by dietary supplementation with ergocalciferol in doses 4- to 10-fold greater than those recommended for normal neonates. The serum concentration of 25-OH-D drops progressively after birth in premature, but not full-

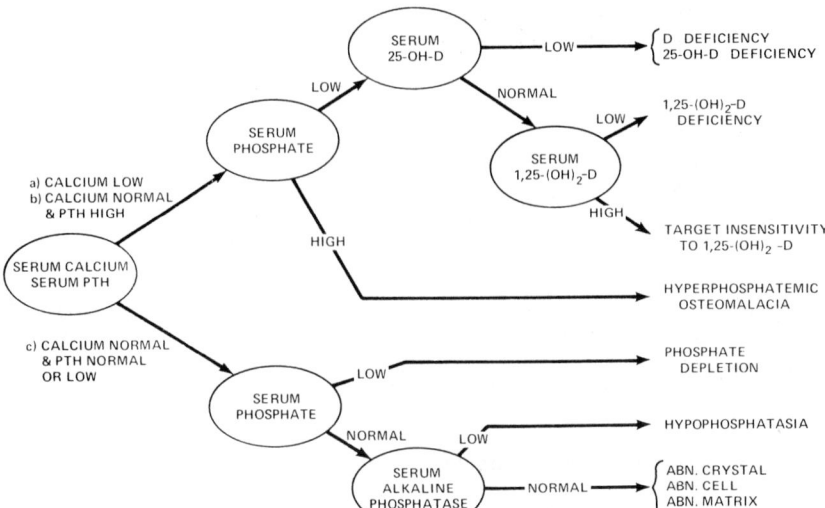

Figure 19–69. Decision tree for evaluation of patients with rickets or osteomalacia. Refer to descriptions of diagnostic categories for further details.

term, infants. Supplementation with ergocalciferol does not prevent this decrease, suggesting immaturity of the hepatic vitamin D 25-hydroxylase system.

The goal of treatment is the restoration of normal serum concentrations of 25-OH vitamin D. The underlying disorder should be corrected if possible. Otherwise, the vitamin D deficiency can be managed with oral or parenteral preparations of ergocalciferol or 25-OH-D, with dosage adjustment to maintain a normal serum concentration of 25-OH-D.

Anticonvulsant-Induced Osteomalacia

With the exception of nutritional and gastrointestinal disorders, many causes of rickets and osteomalacia are not associated with severe reduction of serum concentration of 25-OH-D. Certain drugs interfere with vitamin D metabolism and action by mechanisms that are still poorly understood. Chronic use of anticonvulsants (diphenylhydantoins and barbiturates, particularly when taken in combination) may be associated with florid rickets or osteomalacia with the attendant increase in risk of fracture during seizures. Secondary hyperparathyroidism develops, and serum concentrations of 25-OH-D tend to be mildly diminished but not sufficiently to explain the severity of the skeletal disorder. Reduced serum concentration of 25-OH-D can be due to proliferation of hepatocyte smooth endoplasmic reticulum and shunting of vitamin D metabolism to other unidentified polar metabolites. The serum concentrations of $1,25\text{-(OH)}_2\text{-D}$ were normal or elevated in a series of 25 institutionalized patients receiving diphenylhydantoin or phenobarbital or both. Anticonvulsants affect many tissues and partially inhibit the responses to active calciferol metabolites at both intestine and bone *in vitro*. Whatever the cause(s) of anticonvulsant osteomalacia it can be prevented or treated by supplementation with vitamin D analogs.

Decreased Renal 25-OH-D 1-α-Hydroxylase Activity

Chronic Renal Disease

Low serum concentrations of $1,25\text{-(OH)}_2\text{-D}$ are common to many forms of rickets or osteomalacia. The 25-OH-D 1-α-hydroxylase activity, the most critical and highly regulated step in calciferol metabolism, occurs mainly in the kidney. A number of disease processes impinge directly upon this system. Chronic renal failure leads to widespread disturbances in mineral regulation (see "Secondary Hyperparathyroidism," p. 979), including several distinctive skeletal disturbances.

Under normal circumstances dietary phosphate intake and absorption require that the kidney excrete approximately 10% of the filtered load of phosphate. Phosphate retention, developing early in renal compromise, contributes to most of the components of renal osteodystrophy. In animal models and in humans, restrictions of gastrointestinal absorption of phosphate prevents or delays the early manifestations of renal osteodystrophy. A likely sequence of disease progression is as follows: Renal compromise leads to lower capacity of the 25-OH-D 1-α-hydroxylase system and also to phosphate retention; phosphate retention directly inhibits the renal 25-OH-D 1-α-hydroxylase system further; and azotemia *per se* inhibits the intestinal absorption of calcium. Thus, a complex of factors synergize to lower the serum calcium concentration, and secondary hyperparathyroidism occurs early in this process. Advanced renal failure is associated with low serum concentrations of $1,25\text{-(OH)}_2\text{-D}$ even in the presence of severe secondary hyperparathyroidism. Acidosis occurs both because of damage to the renal acid excretory mechanisms and because of the bicarbonate wasting effect of secondary hyperparathyroidism.

In several other acquired disorders, such as primary renal tubular acidosis, the Fanconi syndromes, the syndrome of tumor osteomalacia, and the syndrome of hyperphosphatemic osteomalacia, decreased production of $1,25\text{-(OH)}_2\text{-D}$ undoubtedly also makes a fundamental contribution (discussed later).

Hereditary

Hereditary vitamin D dependency (pseudo vitamin D deficiency) is a distinct, rare, autosomal recessive disorder. Affected persons manifest typical abnormalities of early onset vitamin D deficiency with hypocalcemia, secondary hyperparathyroidism, and hypophosphatemia. Typically rickets is diagnosed between age 4 and 12 months; it is unresponsive to amounts of ergocalciferol or 25-OH-D that are effective in nutritional rickets, however. Complete cure is attainable but dependent upon continuous treatment with high doses of either of these drugs. Prior to treatment the patients show very low circulating concentrations of

1,25-$(OH)_2$-D. The disorder is responsive to "physiologic" doses of 1,25-$(OH)_2$-D_3, making it highly likely that this represents an abnormality or absence of the renal 25-OH-D 1-α-hydroxylase activity. In some of these cases, serum concentrations of 1,25-$(OH)_2$-D remain low even during effective treatment with ergocalciferol, suggesting a complete absence of the renal 25-OH-D 1-α hydroxylase activity with clinical response dependent upon pharmacologic serum concentrations of 25-OH-D or other weak vitamin D agonists. These patients must be differentiated from those with the more common X-linked familial hypophosphatemia. In the latter biochemically distinct condition, affected patients may remain stable without therapy after adolescence; in vitamin D dependencey, however, manifestations recur whenever therapy is withdrawn.

Decreased Target Sensitivity to 1,25-$(OH)_2$-D

A small number of patients with a disorder resembling vitamin D dependency show high circulating concentrations of 1,25-$(OH)_2$-D. This represents a decrease in target sensitivity to 1,25-$(OH)_2$-D. In some families affected members manifest total alopecia. This disorder will probably prove to be the prototype for a variety of hereditary and acquired interferences with the target tissue responses to the calciferols analogous to the syndromes with decreased target tissue sensitivity to the androgenic steroids.

Hyperphosphatemic Osteomalacia

A few cases of osteomalacia or rickets with hyperphosphatemia have been described. The pathophysiology of the process is diverse, prompting a bewildering array of names. Cases have been found among Asian immigrants to Britain with nutritional vitamin D deficiency and parathyroid failure of unknown etiology, in a patient with idiopathic hypoparathyroidism and normal 25-OH-D stores, and among three siblings in a single family. In the presence of secondary hyperparathyroidism, the deficient phosphaturic response to PTH has led to labels such as pseudohypoparathyroidism type II or hypohyperparathyroidism. The etiology of this process is obscure, but in most cases the serum concentration of 1,25-$(OH)_2$-D has been low or inferred to be low. The hyperphosphatemia may directly inhibit production of 1,25-$(OH)_2$-D_3. A puzzling aspect of this process is the development of osteomalacia, which usually is associated with phosphate depletion.

Phosphate Deficiency Syndromes

The importance of phosphate metabolism in the osteomalacias is underscored by the fact that in rats, where serum phosphate concentration is normally 9.0 mg/dl or double that found in mature humans, only combined restriction of vitamin D and phosphate will foster development of nutritional rickets or osteomalacia. In humans, nutritional deficiency of phosphate is not caused by food faddism because phosphate is widely distributed in all foodstuffs (see Table 19–3). Severe phosphate deficiency can develop with consumption of effective phosphate chelators, however; aluminum hydroxide is the most potent such drug commonly used. Analogous phosphate depletion states may arise during unbalanced alimentation, intravenous feeding, or general dietary restriction in combination with hemodialysis against a low phosphate solution.

Within 5 days of phosphate restriction renal clearance of phosphate becomes nearly undetectable. Continued phosphate depletion leads to hypophosphatemia with increased intestinal absorption of calcium and increased renal excretion of calcium. Both of these effects on calcium flux reflect phosphate-associated changes in vitamin D metabolism. Two effects of phosphate restriction in animals are an increase in renal 25-OH-D 1-α-hydroxylase that is independent of parathyroid function and an increased accumulation of 1,25-$(OH)_2$-D in intestinal target tissues. Even with high serum concentrations of 1,25-$(OH)_2$-D, osteomalacia develops if insufficient phosphate is available in serum to support mineralization of osteoid. If this process continues for several months, patients manifest muscle weakness, anorexia, bone pain, and occasionally elevation of serum alkaline phosphatase activity. Depletion of phosphate may compromise intracellular energy storage mechanisms leading to defective function of muscle cells and of leukocytes, monocytes, and erythrocytes. In dogs, phosphate depletion also leads to intracellular alkalosis and a defect in renal acid excretion.

Rickets and osteomalacia may be caused by conditions with reduced renal threshold for phosphate excretion. This, of course, is an integral feature of secondary hyperparathyroidism and contributes an element of phosphate depletion to all vitamin D deficiency states except those associated with hyperphosphatemia (see "Hyperphosphatemic Osteomalacia"). Decreases in renal threshold for phosphate excretion can also produce severe osteomalacia in the absence of severe secondary hyperparathyroidism.

X-Linked Familial Hypophosphatemia

X-linked familial hypophosphatemia was the first rachitic process recognized to be refractory to vitamin D. It is, by far, the commonest form of hereditary rickets. As with most X-linked processes, the disturbance is most severe in males, who may manifest florid rickets during childhood. Females are more mildly affected, often manifesting only hypophosphatemia. Bone age is retarded and stature is decreased, with the shortening most severe in the legs. Dental caries are increased in frequency. Muscle weakness is less commonly a feature in this disorder than in the hypocalcemic rachitic states. In adults the disease may stabilize without treatment. The radiographic features are basically those of rickets and osteomalacia; in addition, there is a striking propensity to form osteophytes that may limit motion at the elbows, shoulders, and hips or cause spinal ankylosis. Another characteristic radiographic feature is a paradoxically radiopaque skeleton with an increase in total mineral mass. This is a manifestation of mineralization, albeit deficient, of a very large mass of osteoid and may cause confusion with other processes with osteosclerosis. The histologic features resemble those of typical rickets or osteomalacia. The major biochemical features in serum are a normal calcium concentration and a significantly depressed phosphorus concentration. Normal serum calcium concentration and absence of severe secondary hyperparathyroidism are major diagnostic features. Hypophosphatemia is found during fasting and postprandially. It is a manifestation of an abnormally low threshold for renal phosphate excretion and is detectable from age 6 months until old age (Fig. 19–70). Alkaline phosphatase activity in plasma may be high when rickets is most active but is otherwise normal. Intestinal absorption of calcium is mildly decreased and serum calcium is maintained at normal by mild secondary hyperparathyroidism. These features differ from pure phosphate depletion with activation of production of 1,25-$(OH)_2$-D. In fact, defective

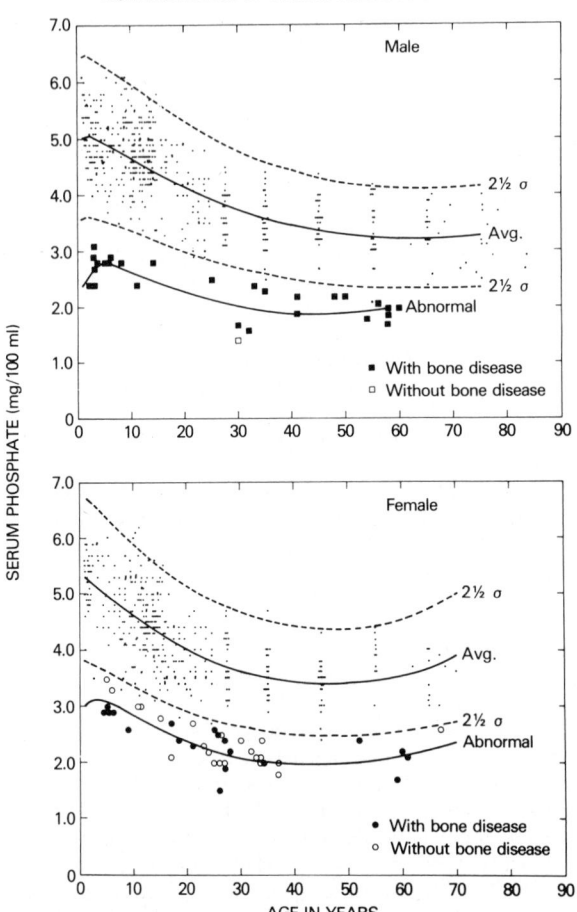

NORMAL RANGE OF SERUM INORGANIC PHOSPHATE

Figure 19–70. Normal serum phosphate concentrations in males and females (dotted curves are computerized fits plus or minus 2.5 standard deviations to estimate range for 99% of normals) compared with concentrations in affected members from five families with x-linked hypophosphatemia. Note that, at all ages, serum phosphate concentrations are outside the 99% confidence limits for normal. (Modified from Greenberg, B. G., Winters, R. W., et al.: The normal range of serum inorganic phosphorus and its utility as a discriminant in the diagnosis of congenital hypophostemia. *J. Clin. Endocrinol. 20*:364, 1960.)

response of the renal 25-OH-D 1-α-hydroxylase is an integral part of this disorder. The cause of hypophosphatemia is the subject of active investigation. There is uncertainty as to whether there is a parallel defect in intestinal phosphate transport. Transport of phosphate by salivary glands and erythrocytes is normal. A promising area of investigation has arisen from the discovery of a strain of mouse with X-linked hypophosphatemic rickets. In these animals, there is a clear abnormality in renal and intestinal transport of phosphate; the skeletal manifestations can be prevented by adding phosphate to the diet but are not improved by treatment with cholecalciferol or 1,25-(OH)₂-D₃. A defect in sodium-dependent phosphate transport occurs in brush border membrane vesicles from kidneys of affected animals.

Although X-linked familial hypophosphatemia varies in intensity, it appears to be a rather homogeneous disorder. A few kindreds show autosomal dominant or autosomal recessive transmission patterns with moderate differences in clinical features. An autosomal recessive variant is associated with increased bone mineral content at early ages, early fusion of the cranial sutures, and nerve deafness. One autosomal dominant variant is associated with glucose intolerance.

There is a large accumulated experience in treatment of these patients with pharmacologic doses of the calciferols. Though skeletal healing may occur, hypophosphatemia persists, suggesting the primacy of the phosphate transport abnormality. Moreover, such therapy incurs a high risk of episodic vitamin D intoxication with irreversible renal damage. Treatment with 25-OH-D₃ or 1,25-(OH)₂-D₃ alone has been similarly unsatisfactory. Better results have been attained by administration of inorganic phosphate at doses equivalent to 1–4 g of elemental phosphorus/day. This must be given by mouth at inconvenient 4-hour intervals in order to maintain a near-normal serum concentration of phosphate. Treatment with 1,25(OH)₂-D₃ improves bone mineralization and allows use of lower doses of phosphate.

Renal Tubular Damage

Several renal tubular disorders may be associated with rickets or osteomalacia disproportionate to the degree of renal failure. Many are disorders affecting the proximal tubule with a stereotyped pattern of renal wastage of phosphate, glucose, bicarbonate, and amino acids (Fanconi syndrome). The major causes include inborn errors of metabolism (cystinosis, galactosemia, glycogen storage disease, hepatorenal form of hereditary tyrosinemia, hereditary fructose intolerance, hepatolenticular degeneraion of Wilson, and the oculocerebrorenal syndrome of Lowe), intoxications (lead, mercury, cadmium, outdated tetracycline, streptozotocin, lysol), immune dysregulations (amyloidosis, Bence Jones proteinuria, Sjögren's syndrome) and idiopathic. At present it is not known to what extent phosphate depletion or deficient production of 1,25-(OH)₂-D contributes to these syndromes. Models for rickets due to proximal tubular disorders have been developed by administering either maleic acid or strontium to rats. Such proximal tubular dysfunction causes decreased production of 1,25-(OH)₂-D, and the skeletal manifestations can be prevented by administration of 1,25-(OH)₂-D₃. A rachitic state also occurs in distal or gradient renal tubular acidosis in association with hypercalciuria, nephrocalcinosis, and secondary hyperparathyroidism; in this disorder, however, the skeletal manifestations can be prevented simply by treatment with sufficient bicarbonate (5–15 mEq/kg/day) to normalize the serum pH. Osteomalacia may also occur with acidosis following ureterosigmoidostomy. Low serum concentrations of 1,25-(OH)₂-D have been directly implicated in this phenomenon. An animal model for these phenomena has been suggested by the observation that ammonium chloride acidosis in vitamin D–deficient rats impairs activity of the renal 25-OH-D 1-α hydroxylase system.

Tumor Osteomalacia

Another syndrome with renal phosphate wastage that resembles X-linked hypophosphatemia or the Fanconi syndrome occurs with a spectrum of neoplastic processes (mostly of mesenchymal origin). Typically, a previously healthy adult develops rapidly progressive hypophosphatemic osteomalacia with normal serum calcium concentration. Removal of a small, usually benign tumor leads to dramatic reversal of the metabolic disturbance. The tumors have included sclerosing or cavernous hemangiomas and ossifying and nonossifying mesenchymal tumors of bone. Analogous disturbances have occurred in prostatic cancer, fibrous dysplasia of bone, the basal cell nevus syndrome, and von Recklinghausen's neurofibromatosis. The identities of the cell of origin and of the presumed humoral mediator(s) remain a fascinating mystery. Low serum concentration of 1,25-(OH)$_2$-D has been documented in a small number of these patients, and it has been suggested that the tumor causes release of factors that perturb the renal 25-OH-D metabolizing enzymes. Whatever the ultimate cause of this syndrome, it should be seriously considered in any normocalcemic adult with a phosphate wasting disorder of unknown etiology. The offending tumor may be small, benign, and extremely difficult to locate.

Rickets and Osteomalacia Due to Bone Cell Disturbance — Familial Hypophosphatasia

Familial hypophosphatasia is generally an autosomal recessive disorder of variable severity. In Toronto the incidence is approximately 1 in 100,000 live births. Its most severe manifestation is infantile rickets with craniostenosis and death around age 1–2 years from complications of hypercalcemia (vomiting, nephrocalcinosis, renal failure). This process has been diagnosed *in utero* by radiography but only in the third trimester. A less severe manifestation in childhood causes premature loss of primary teeth, pseudofractures, and radiolucent zones in long bones with a characteristic notching at the borders of the frayed metaphyses. The skeletal cortices are often thickened with subperiosteal new bone formation and calcification of the paraspinal ligaments. The least severe grade presents in adulthood with premature loss of secondary teeth, fractures, and nephrolithiasis. These persons may give a history of rickets in childhood. The mild adult form has also occurred as an autosomal dominant trait. The characteristic biochemical features are low serum concentrations of alkaline phosphatase due to deficient isoenzyme from bone and a marked increase in serum and urinary phosphorylethanolamine and lesser increases in pyrophosphate. Some affected individuals intermittently show normal circulating total activity of alkaline phosphatase. Urinary hydroxyproline excretion rate is abnormally low. Analysis of bone from affected persons reveals absence or severe deficiency of alkaline phosphatase activity in osteoblasts. This is probably the primary lesion. Increased urinary excretion of phosphorylethanolamine and pyrophosphate reflect the accumulation in plasma of these compounds, which may be natural substrates for osteoblastic alkaline phosphatase. How the accumulation of these phosphoesters relates to the mineralization defect is not known. It is possible that some substrates for the alkaline phosphatase enzyme are mineralization inhibitors that must be cleaved to allow normal mineralization. This explanation is supported by the production of an osteomalacic state by administration of diphosphonates (see later) that are phosphatase-resistant analogs of pyrophosphate. No satisfactory treatment for hypophosphatasia has been developed. Several reports have indicated promising results with phosphate administration, however.

Osteomalacia Due to Bone Matrix Disturbance — Fibrogenesis Imperfecta Ossium and Axial Osteomalacia

Fibrogenesis imperfecta ossium is a rare disorder that has only been diagnosed in patients over the age of 50. It leads to severe skeletal pain, tenderness, and progressive immobilization. Radiographs show a symmetric distribution of coarse, dense trabeculae with periosteal reaction and soft-tissue calcifications. This may resemble Paget's disease

and serum alkaline phosphatase is similarly elevated. The specific diagnostic feature is a loss of usual birefringence of bone collagen fibrils under polarized light. Electron microscopy shows bone collagen fibrils apparently disorganized. In one case collagen solubility was increased in several solvent systems. This disorder may represent an acquired disturbance in matrix structure that will not support normal mineralization. Axial osteomalacia is another rare acquired process seen in several patients age 60–75. Symptoms have been mild and limited to the spine, pelvis, and ribs. Matrix qualities have not been reported in these patients but the disorder has at least a superficial resemblance to fibrogenesis imperfecta ossium.

Rickets and Osteomalacia with Mineralization Inhibitors — Fluorides and Diphosphonates

Diphosphonates are analogs of pyrophosphate with the P-O-P bond replaced by a P-C-P bond. They adsorb to bone mineral and have been useful as bone scanning agents. *In vitro* and *in vivo* they cause diverse effects, including inhibition of apatite crystal deposition and resorption. Certain analogs may selectively block resorption but not deposition. In certain animals, they also directly block the renal 25-OH-D 1-α hydroxylase enzyme.

Inorganic fluoride also accumulates in bone mineral and, like diphosphonate, is used in bone scanning. Chronic ingestion of fluoride (more than 20 mg fluoride ion/day) leads to skeletal fluorosis, a potentially crippling disorder associated with arthralgias, periosteal new bone formation, osteophyte formation, osteosclerosis, and kyphosis. Histologically there is increase in osteoid surface and width. There are also degenerative changes in osteocytes and accumulation of periosteal new bone with a disordered lamellar structure. The etiology of the histologic changes is probably complex. The fluoride content of fluorotic bone is markedly increased and the size of bone crystals is increased. Whether fluorides cause osteomalacia by a direct interaction with bone crystals or by accumulation to cytotoxic concentrations in bone is not known.

METABOLIC BONE DISEASES

Osteoporosis

Osteoporosis is defined as a state of reduced bone mass per unit volume with a normal ratio of mineral to matrix. Since age, race, and sex have important effects on skeletal mass, an individual can be said to show osteoporosis if his skeletal mass is significantly below the normal value for his particular age, race, and sex. This definition may be too restrictive, since loss of bone mass occurs in almost all individuals after age 50; on a longitudinal basis, a high percentage of individuals more than 70 years of age may be said to show osteoporosis.

A reduction in bone mass ultimately must derive from an increase in the ratio of bone resorption to bone formation. An increase in this ratio can occur at several different rates of bone turnover, but in all cases the net result is decreased bone mass.

Bone remodeling is normally regulated by a complex interplay of humoral, metabolic, nutritional, and physical factors, so it is not surprising that many diseases may cause osteoporosis (Table 19–17). Pathogenetic factors are obvious in some diseases states, e.g., excess cortisol in Cushing's disease, but the pathogenesis of the most common form of osteoporosis, variously referred to as primary, senile, or involutional, remains uncertain.

Table 19–17. CAUSES OF OSTEOPOROSIS

1. *Cause unknown*
   Primary (senile, postmenopausal) osteoporosis
   Juvenile osteoporosis

2. *Endocrine abnormalities*
   Glucocorticoid excess
   Thyrotoxicosis
   Hypogonadism

3. *Malignancy*
   Multiple myeloma
   Leukemia
   Lymphoma

4. *Immobilization*

5. *Genetic abnormalities in bone collagen synthesis*
   Homocystinuria
   Ehlers-Danlos syndrome
   Osteogenesis imperfecta

6. *Heparin therapy*
   Systemic mastocytosis (?)

Primary Osteoporosis

Epidemiology and Clinical Significance

Epidemiologic studies show that in approximately 25% of white women over age 60 there is radiographically detectable osteoporosis of the spine. The risk of fracture with minimal trauma is increased in osteoporotic bone, and this risk correlates directly with reduced bone mass (Fig. 19–71). Loss of bone mass in critical weight-bearing areas, e.g., femoral neck and vertebral bodies, compromises structural integrity with potentially disastrous consequences. There are an estimated million fractures per year in American

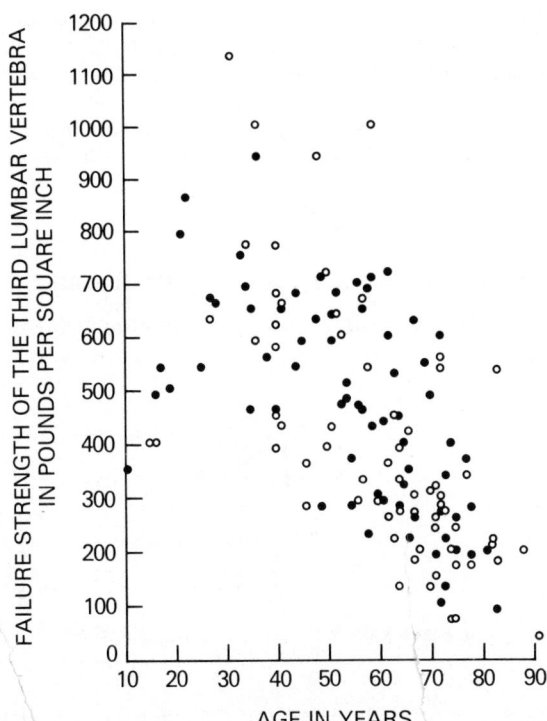

Figure 19–71. Change in vertebral compressive strength with advancing age in 137 cadavers (○ = female; • = male). (From Weaver, J. V., and Chalmers, J.: Cancellous bone: its strength and changes with aging and an evaluation of some methods for measuring its mineral content. *J. Bone Joint Surg.* 48A:289, 1966.)

women over the age of 45 and up to 70% of these fractures are attributed to osteoporosis. The incidence of hip fractures (due to minor trauma) in the U.S. rises from 2/1000/year in women age 50–64 to 10/1000/year in women more than 75, paralleling the rising incidence of osteoporosis. Prevention of bone loss would be expected to reduce the incidence of fractures in the elderly dramatically, but this cannot be accomplished until the factors responsible for bone loss are understood.

Pathogenesis

Methods for Assessing Bone Loss. A brief review of available techniques for studying bone loss in primary osteoporosis will serve to highlight the difficulties encountered in attempting to elucidate the pathogenesis of the disease (see also "Assessments of Bone Metabolism" in the section on utilization of the laboratory, p. 1025). Two major parameters may be quantitated in studying bone loss in osteoporosis. One set of methods (calcium balance studies, radiocalcium kinetics, and skeletal histomorphometry) attempts to measure the ratio of bone resorption to bone formation. There are several limitations to this approach: (1) Significant bone loss may be the result of relatively small changes over long periods of time (a loss of 30 mg of skeletal calcium per day for 30 years will result in about a 30% decrease in skeletal mass). Existing techniques may not be sufficiently accurate and sensitive to detect such changes. (2) Individuals with established osteoporosis (vertebral crush fractures on x-ray) may represent an end-stage of the disease in which increased resorption is no longer present; the "control" population may have higher net resorption since end-stage osteoporosis has not yet been reached. (3) An acute decrease in net resorption after therapeutic intervention does not necessarily lead to increased bone mass, since there may be a compensatory decrease in bone formation. Because of these limitations, the dynamic processes leading to development of osteoporosis have not been elucidated with certainty.

Another approach involves *in vivo* measurement of skeletal mass (or density). Although the trabecular bone of the spinal column is a major region at risk in osteoporosis, vertebral density can only be assessed directly by conventional radiography. Conventional skeletal x-rays are too insensitive to detect subtle changes; more than 30% of skeletal mass must be lost before becoming radiographically detectable. More sensitive techniques for measuring skeletal mass are now available, but these generally assess a localized region of the skeleton that does not necessarily correlate with overall skeletal mass or more importantly with vertebral mass.

Cortical thickness, usually determined on the second metacarpal, allows detection of age-related bone loss, but changes in cortical bone may not adequately reflect trabecular bone loss. The femoral trabecular index is not only a semiquantitative grading system (based on the appearance of the upper femoral trabecular pattern on a pelvic x-ray) but is an index of trabecular bone status. In one study, 97 to 102 patients with vertebral crush fractures scored grade 4 or below while 283 of 316 control subjects scored grade 5 or higher. Other studies utilizing this technique have not confirmed this high degree of discrimination.

Photon absorption densitometry can be used to assess cortical (proximal radius) as well as trabecular (distal radius) bone mineral content. This method is capable of detecting small (<10%) changes in skeletal mass; a weak correlation between measured bone mineral content and likelihood of vertebral crush fracture has been found.

Total body calcium can be determined *in vivo* by the neutron activation technique, which, however, is not widely available. Since 99% of total body calcium is located in the skeleton, this method provides an index of skeletal mass but not the distribution of calcium within the skeleton.

Age-Related Bone Loss. Beginning in the fourth decade of life, there is a progressive fall in skeletal mass (Fig. 19–72). Loss of trabecular bone (characterized by a large resorptive surface) is probably more rapid than loss of cortical bone. (Cortical thinning results from imbalance of endosteal resorption and periosteal apposition).

Loss of bone mass appears to begin earlier in women than in men, precedes the menopause, and is accelerated postmenopausally. Age-related bone loss appears to be a universal phenomenon, but widely varying rates of bone loss have been observed in population studies; genetic and dietary factors, as well as level of physical activity, have been invoked to explain this variation.

Theories Regarding Pathogenesis of Primary Osteoporosis. Two broad formulations have been posed for the pathogenesis of primary osteoporosis. The first is that skeletal mass achieved at maturity is the critical determinant for development of clinical osteoporosis later in life. At maturity skeletal mass is greater in men than in women and in blacks than in whites. Thus elderly white women appear to be the group at highest risk for osteoporosis (Fig. 19–73). An underlying assumption of this theory is that the rate of bone loss is not significantly increased in persons destined to become osteoporotic. Bone loss is merely a "normal" manifestation of the aging process. This theory leaves unanswered the question of why different individuals attain differing amounts of skeletal mass at maturity.

The second theory of pathogenesis is that those destined to become osteoporotic have significantly increased rates of bone loss by comparison with age- and sex-matched normal controls. The factors responsible for increased rates of bone loss in affected individuals may be the same as those operative during the aging process but are exaggerated. These two theories are not mutually exclusive; both require identification of the factor(s) responsible for bone loss.

Many factors are potentially capable of leading to bone loss, but none has been definitely identified as the cause of primary osteoporosis. Albright believed that a primary decrease in bone formation was responsible for bone loss, but most studies assessing bone remodeling suggest that increased resorption is responsible (Fig. 19–74). Increased resorption may be due to increased PTH action on bone. Development of osteoporosis rather than osteitis fibrosa has been attributed to chronic slight elevation in PTH activity. Radioimmunoassay measurements of serum PTH concentration in osteoporotic individuals have in general not shown significant abnormalities, but interpretation is complicated by uncertainty regarding the amount of bioactive hormone being measured in various assays. Several factors have been invoked to account for increased PTH action and bone resorption in osteoporosis.

Estrogen deficiency appears to play an important role in bone loss. Many studies have demonstrated accelerated bone loss after menopause (natural or iatrogenic), independent of age at menopause. It has been suggested that estrogen deficiency may lead to a state of increased sensitivity of bone (but not kidney) to PTH. *In vitro* studies, however, have in general not shown inhibition of PTH-mediated bone resorption by estrogen, except with pharmacologic amounts.

The role of dietary calcium deficiency in osteoporosis is controversial. A clear-cut association between osteoporosis and reduced calcium intake has not been shown. There is a higher incidence of osteoporosis in persons with intestinal

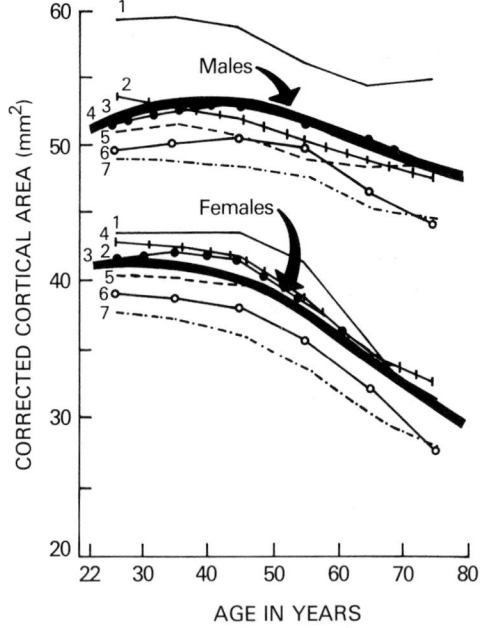

Figure 19–72. Age-related decrease in metacarpal cortical area of males and females from seven different countries. The heavy black lines represent pooled weighted means from all subjects (a total of 5834). (From Garn, S. M., Rohmann, G. G., et al.: Population similarities in the onset and rate of adult endosteal bone loss. *Clin. Orthop. Related Res.* 65:51, 1969.)

lactase deficiency than in subjects with normal lactose absorption, presumably because lactase deficiency leads to avoidance of milk and other calcium-rich milk products. Reduced intestinal calcium absorption and excessive dietary phosphorus intake could lead to secondary hyperparathyroidism and bone loss but definite evidence linking these factors to the development of osteoporosis in humans is lacking.

Additional factors that may play a role in bone loss include relative CT deficiency and reduced physical activity. Decreased basal and stimulated CT secretion in women compared with men has been suggested as a cause for the increased incidence of osteoporosis in women. Epidemiologic studies show a reduced incidence of osteoporosis in ori-

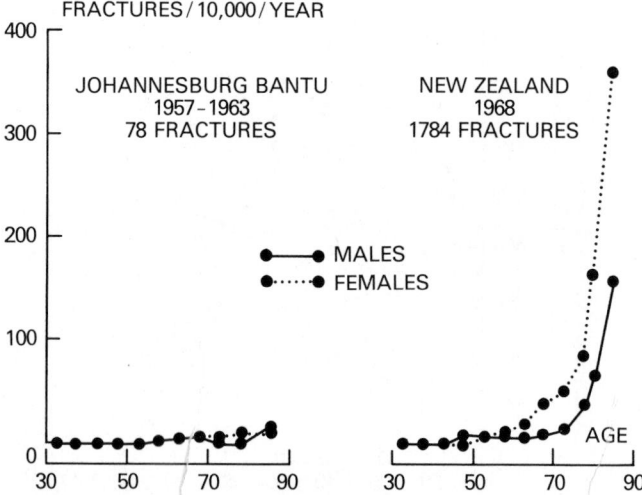

Figure 19–73. Incidence of femoral neck fractures as a function of age in the Johannesburg Bantu population (left) and in New Zealanders (right). (From Cave, W., and Nordin, B. E. C.: International Fracture Survey; First Year Report to the International Health Foundation, 1972 (privately printed. In Nordin, B. E. C. (ed.): *Clinical Physiology and Diagnostic Procedures.* London, Churchill Livingstone, 1976, p. 387.)

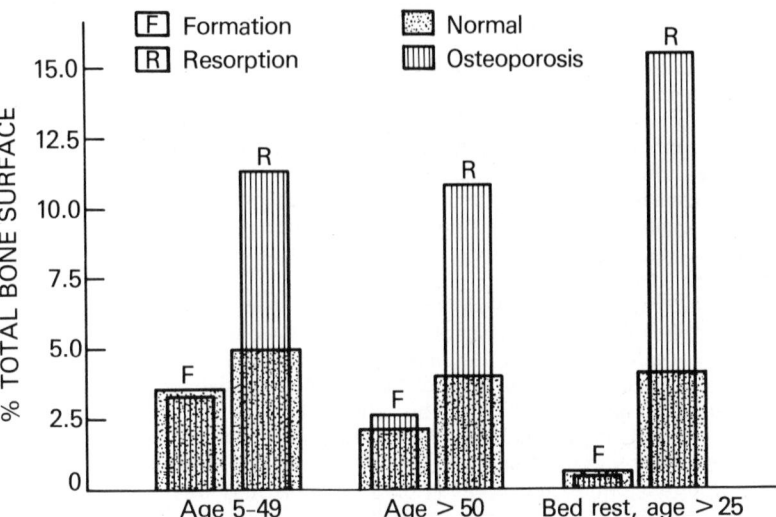

Figure 19–74. Values for bone resorption and formation in patients with juvenile and idiopathic osteoporosis (left), postmenopausal osteoporosis (center), and osteoporotic patients who have been at bed rest (right); each group has age-matched controls. Resorption is greater than normal in all three groups, while formation is not different from normal and is depressed in normal and osteoporotic bed rest groups (right). (From Jowsey, J. O. M., and Offord, K. D.: In *Proceedings, Mechanisms of Localized Bone Loss,* Horton, J. E., Tarphey, T. M., and Davis, W. F. (eds.). Special Supplement to Calcified Tissue Abstracts. Washington, D. C., Information Retrieval, Inc., 1978.)

ental women compared with occidental white women. This difference has been attributed to the more strenuous lifestyle of oriental women.

In summary, the factors reponsible for the bone loss of aging and of primary osteoporosis have not been identified. It is certainly possible that multiple factors combine to cause diminished skeletal mass.

Clinical Features

Radiographic Appearance. Vertebral changes (in order of increasing severity) include loss of horizontal trabeculations (Fig. 19–75), biconcavity due to "ballooning" of the intervertebral discs ("codfish vertebrae"), anterior wedge fractures, and compression fractures. The incidence of vertebral fracture decreases above and below the 12th thoracic vertebra (T-12). Fractures of vertebrae above T-6 are almost never due to primary osteoporosis and should prompt a search for malignancy. Changes in the appendicular skeleton include cortical thinning and loss of trabecular bone in areas such as the femoral neck.

Clinical and Laboratory Evaluation. Many subjects are asymptomatic despite having vertebral crush fractures and are only identified incidentally on x-rays taken for other purposes. When symptoms do occur they may be of two general varieties. Immediately after vertebral crush fracture (usually occurring with minimal trauma or exertion),

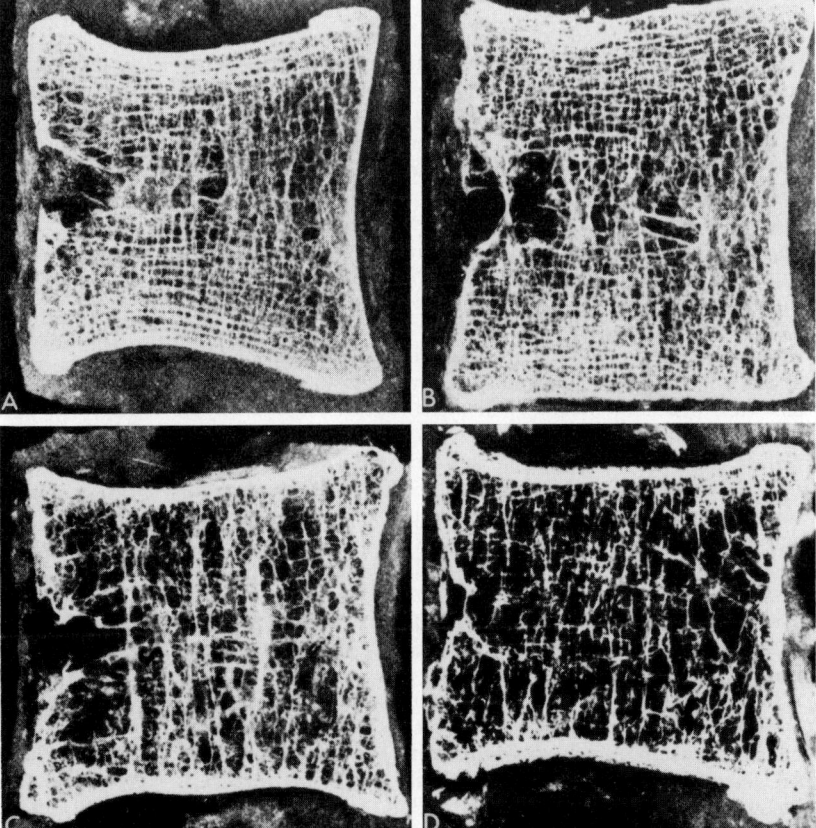

Figure 19–75. Radiographs of sagittal sections taken from second lumbar vertebral body of female subjects of different ages. (A) Age 29, regular trabecular pattern. (B) Age 40, some thinning of transverse trabeculae. (C) Age 84, loss of horizontal trabeculae, thickening of vertical trabeculae. (D) Age 92, further loss of normal trabecular pattern. (From Atkinson, P. J.: Variation in trabecular structure of vertebrae with age. *Calcif. Tissue Res. 1*:24, 1967.)

there may be sharp pain localized over the involved region that will subside within a month regardless of therapy. Analgesics and *temporary* immobilization are appropriate therapy in such cases. Alternatively, chronic, dull, diffuse back pain may be present. Neurologic signs due to nerve root compression are uncommon and if present should lead to a search for other lesions. Progression of vertebral collapse causes loss in height and development of marked dorsal kyphosis ("dowager's hump"). In addition to the spinal column, the femoral neck and distal radius are common fracture sites.

Serum calcium and phosphorus concentrations and alkaline phosphatase activity are generally normal, though serum alkaline phosphatase may rise transiently after a fracture. Osteomalacia may be difficult to distinguish from osteoporosis on skeletal x-rays but should be accompanied by increased serum alkaline phosphatase activity and reduced serum 25-OH-D or or 1,25-(OH)$_2$-D concentration. In certain cases, histologic study of biopsied bone may be necessary to distinguish osteomalacia from osteoporosis. Primary hyperparathyroidism may present with the clinical picture of postmenopausal osteoporosis and should be excluded by measurement of serum calcium, PTH, and urinary cAMP.

Since primary osteoporosis is a diagnosis of exclusion, secondary forms of the disease (Table 19–17) should be excluded. This is particularly true in males, young females, and blacks.

Therapy

Evaluating therapy in osteoporosis is particularly difficult. The ultimate criterion for efficacy is prevention of fracture. Only appropriately controlled long-term longitudinal studies can establish efficacy, and most published studies have either been uncontrolled or short term. There is also a problem inherent in choosing study subjects. If osteoporosis is defined (as it is in the majority of studies) on the basis of radiographically evident vertebral crush fractures, response to therapy may be precluded by the advanced state of disease. Choosing study subjects with "early" disease offers the best chance of observing a therapeutic response, but no definite criteria exist for selecting "pre-osteoporotic" individuals.

Controlled studies suggest that estrogen therapy (25–50 μg ethinyl estradiol/day or equivalent) can prevent the rapid phase of bone loss that occurs in the immediate postmenopausal period (only women undergoing artificial menopause were included in this study). Initiation of estrogen therapy as long as 3–6 years after menopause may lead to slight increases in bone mass. In women maintained on estrogen since menopause, discontinuation of therapy is again followed by rapid bone loss (Fig. 19–76). The implication is that chronic estrogen therapy may be necessary to halt postmenopausal bone loss. Since chronic estrogen use has been linked to an increased incidence of endometrial carcinoma and may cause other serious side effects (thromboembolism, hypertension), it would be advantageous to restrict estrogen therapy to postmenopausal women at greatest risk of developing significant osteoporosis. There is, at present, no definite way to identify this group of patients.

Dietary supplements of calcium (with or without vitamin D) have been reported to cause acute reduction in rates of bone resorption, although results with this form of therapy are less convincing. Dietary calcium intake in the U.S. is below 400 mg/day in many adults. Bone loss might be pre-

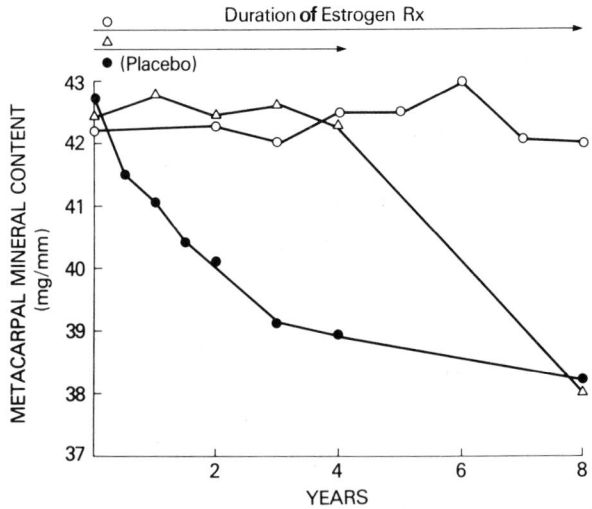

Figure 19–76. Effect of estrogen therapy on postmenopausal bone loss. Metacarpal mineral content (third metacarpal, right hand) was measured by photon absorptiometry over an 8-year period in ovariectomized women maintained with placebo (•), with estrogen (25 μg mestranol/day) for all 8 years (○), or with estrogen for the first 4 years only (△). (From Lindsay, R., Hart, D. M., et al.: Bone response to termination of estrogen treatment. *Lancet* 1:1325, 1978.)

vented by intakes above 1 g/day. Earlier studies suggesting that intravenous infusions of calcium were beneficial have not been confirmed. CT or diphosphonates diminish bone turnover, but increased bone mass has not been observed. Low doses (10 μg/day) of human PTH (1–34 synthetic) appear to increase bone turnover (with a net increase in formation) and increase in trabecular bone mass, but at the expense of cortical bone. A short-term controlled study suggests that exercise delays bone loss but no effect of physical activity was noted in a large cross-sectional study. Therapy with human GH or with oral phosphate supplements has not had any beneficial effects.

Fluoride supplements increase new bone formation but may not increase bone strength. Chronic therapy with high doses of fluoride without calcium supplements may lead to osteomalacia and fluorosis. A controlled study of fluoride (25 mg/day) versus placebo in elderly subjects demonstrated an increase in fracture rate in the fluoride group. Therapy of osteoporosis with the combination of low doses (20 mg/day) of fluoride, vitamin D, and calcium supplements has been advocated. Careful long-term studies will be necessary to evaluate the benefits and potential toxicity of this approach.

In summary, several forms of therapy have been shown to decrease net bone resorption but few have caused a clearcut reduction in bone loss and none has been shown conclusively to prevent fracture. Cyclic therapy with estrogens may be appropriate for carefully selected patients (e.g., young women undergoing surgical menopause), but potentially toxic side effects may limit their usefulness. Increased dietary calcium (1–2 g/day) and increased physical activity may be helpful in preventing bone loss.

Other Causes of Osteoporosis

Glucocorticoid Excess. Osteoporosis is caused by cortisol excess from endogenous (Cushing's disease) and exogenous sources. Children and elderly individuals are at greatest risk of developing significant bone loss. There is positive correlation between duration (but not dose) of steroid therapy and degree of bone loss. Alternate day steroid therapy causes less bone loss in animals than does daily therapy, but data in humans are not available. Osteoporosis may be the principal manifestation of cortisol excess in young adults with micronodular adrenal hyperplasia and in patients with indolent malignancies (medullary carcinoma of the thyroid, carcinoid, thymoma) ectopically secreting ACTH.

Glucocorticoids appear to inhibit bone formation directly and increase bone resorption indirectly. The latter effect may be due to antagonism of vitamin D–mediated intestinal calcium absorption with resultant secondary hyperparathyroidism. The precise mechanism of glucocorticoid interference with vitamin D action (alterations in vitamin D metabolism vs. direct antagonism of 1,25-$(OH)_2$-D effect on the intestine) has not been clarified.

Discontinuation of steroid therapy, if feasible, may allow restoration of bone mass. Prophylactic treatment with vitamin D or one of its active metabolites may be appropriate in high-risk subjects (with careful monitoring of potential toxic effects of vitamin D).

Thyrotoxicosis.   Long-standing thyrotoxicosis may lead to the development of osteoporosis, but significant bone loss is rarely a major feature of the disease. Bone loss is presumably a direct result of thyroid hormone excess since T_4 causes resorption of bone *in vitro*.

Hypogonadism.   Osteoporosis can be associated with hypogonadism either primary or secondary to gonadotropin deficiency. There is an increased incidence of osteoporosis in Klinefelter's syndrome and Turner's syndrome (ovarian dysgenesis). In Turner's syndrome osteoporosis may reflect a more widespread genetic abnormality, since reduced bone mass is evident even before puberty.

Diabetes Mellitus.   Reduced bone mass has been observed in juvenile and adult diabetics. No correlation has been noted between duration of disease and the degree of reduction in bone mass. It has been suggested that insulin deficiency may impair bone formation but the possibility that decreased bone formation is an inherited feature of diabetes has not been excluded.

Disuse Osteoporosis.   Prolonged immobilization leads to negative calcium balance and loss of bone, particularly in weight-bearing sites. Trabecular bone volume may be reduced by one-third after 6 months of bed rest. Space flight (with prolonged weightlessness) may cause similar changes. Studies of skeletal remodeling have shown an initial period of rapid resorption followed by a decrease in net bone turnover.

Juvenile Osteoporosis.   This is a rare disease, usually affecting children 2–3 years before puberty. Complete recovery postpubertally has been described, but in individual cases crippling deformities may result from fractures of long bones and vertebrae. Malignancy (discussed next) must be excluded in such cases. The cause of the disease is unknown.

Malignancy.   Multiple myeloma in adults and lymphoma and leukemia in both adults and children may present with generalized osteoporosis. Bone marrow aspiration is essential in making the diagnosis.

Heparin.   Prolonged treatment with heparin can produce osteoporosis. An association between osteoporosis and systemic mastocytosis has also been attributed to effects of heparin, but a role for other mast cell substances, including histamine, has not been excluded.

Inherited Disorders.   Several inherited disorders are associated with an increased incidence of osteoporosis. These include osteogenesis imperfecta, homocystinuria, Ehlers-Danlos syndrome and Menkes syndrome. Abnormalities in synthesis of mature bone collagen probably lead to impaired bone formation in these disorders.

PAGET'S DISEASE (OSTEITIS DEFORMANS)

Slightly more than 100 years ago, Sir James Paget described a patient with a "rare disease of bones" characterized by deformities of the long bones and skull. Paget's disease is now recognized to be a relatively common disorder, affecting about 3% of the population. Men and women are affected equally. The incidence of the disease rises with age; persons under age 40 are rarely affected.

Pathophysiology

Disordered bone remodeling is the hallmark of Paget's disease. The bone lesions may occur singly or at multiple sites. The initial stage involves excessive bone resorption; at this stage, one may observe a lytic appearance on x-ray ("osteoporosis circumscripta" in the skull). Histologically, there is an abundance of osteoclasts actively resorbing bone. Subsequently, the marrow spaces are occupied by a fibrovascular stroma, and an increase in osteoblast activity leads to excessive bone formation. The combination of disorganized resorption and formation leads to the characteristic "mosaic" pattern, areas of lamellar bone randomly connected by cement lines at the borders of prior resorption (Fig. 19–77). In the final stage, increased cellular activity is not found. Bone in Paget's disease may show increased density on x-ray, but its abnormal structure makes it weaker than normal bone.

Etiology

A genetic basis for Paget's disease is suggested by its familial occurrence (more than 87 families with several involved members have been reported). An autosomal dominant form of inheritance has been postulated but available evidence is inconclusive. An abnormality in collagen extracted from the skin of patients with Paget's disease was observed in a preliminary study, but other studies on bone and skin collagen have not confirmed this finding.

Recently, intranuclear inclusions have been observed in osteoclasts from involved bone. Essentially all patients with Paget's disease studied have shown evidence of these inclusions, but they have not been found in the osteoclasts

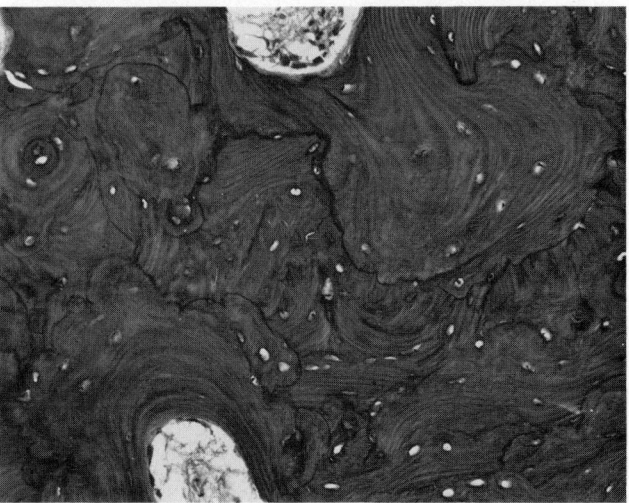

Figure 19–77.   Bone biopsy specimen from a patient with Paget's disease showing the typical mosaic pattern (disorganized lamellar bone and cement lines). Decalcified bone magnified × 80. (From Singer, F. R.: In *Topics in Bone and Mineral Metabolism.* Avioli, L. V. (ed.), New York, Plenum Press, 1977.)

of patients with a variety of other bone disorders, including hyperparathyroidism, osteomalacia, multiple myeloma, and fibrous dysplasia. Similar inclusions have been found only in giant cell tumors of bone. Therapy with CT, which can normalize metabolic parameters (see later), does not lead to disappearance of intranuclear inclusions from osteoclasts. The intranuclear inclusions may be found in 20–40% of osteoclasts in patients with Paget's disease and consist of microfilaments in a paracrystalline array (occasional single microfilaments may also be seen) (Fig. 19–78). The similarity in appearance to the paramyxovirus inclusions found in subacute sclerosing panencephalitis has provoked speculation that Paget's disease may be caused by a slow virus infection. Proof of viral pathogenesis of Paget's disease will require isolation of the virus from bone cells and demonstration that it causes transmission of disease.

Numerous other theories regarding the pathogenesis of Paget's disease have been proposed and discarded. The effectiveness of CT in treatment (see later) prompted speculation unsupported by evidence that CT deficiency is involved in pathogenesis.

Clinical Features

The clinical spectrum of Paget's disease ranges from asymptomatic cases with involvement of a single bone detected on incidental x-ray to crippling deformities and serious neurologic complications. The axial skeleton is more commonly affected than the appendicular. In a large autopsy series, the sites most frequently affected (in decreasing order) were the sacrum, spine, femur, skull, sternum, and pelvis.

Paget's disease may cause pain either because of direct involvement of bone or as a result of complicating degenerative arthritis of joints (usually the hip or knee) adjacent to involved bone. Inadequate tensile strength of involved bone causes bowing of the femur or tibia and may impair walking. Pathologic transverse fractures also occur most commonly in the femur and tibia. The incidence of fracture is approximately 18% in patients with multiple bone involvement. Malignant transformation occurs in less than 1% of patients but portends a poor prognosis. Osteogenic sarcoma is the most frequent malignancy followed by fibrosarcoma. The femur and humerus are the commonest sites of malignant degeneration. Increased pain and rapid soft-tissue swelling are signs of malignant transformation.

Enlargement of affected bone may cause neurologic complications. Overgrowth of the petrous pyramids leads to cochlear dysfunction and a sensorineural type of hearing loss. Vertigo may also occur. Vertebral enlargement can lead to spinal cord compression. Enlargement of the skull may cause basilar impression with compression of the brain stem. Disturbances of speech, swallowing, and gait as well as incontinence and memory loss may develop. Neurosurgical intervention (posterior fossa decompression, laminectomy) is indicated when compressive syndromes occur.

Diagnostic Evaluation

On physical examination there may be signs of deformity in the long bones and the skull may be enlarged. The skin over involved bone may show increased warmth due to increased cutaneous blood flow. Funduscopic examination reveals the presence of angioid streaks in about 15% of patients with polyostotic Paget's disease. These lesions represent cracks just below the retinal vessels in Bruch's membrane.

Elevated serum alkaline phosphatase activity (reflecting increased osteoblastic activity) and increased urinary hydroxyproline excretion (due to increased bone resorption) are characteristic laboratory features of Paget's disease. If only a single site is involved, serum alkaline phosphatase activity may be normal. Serum calcium and phosphorus concentrations are generally normal despite increased bone turnover. Hypercalcemia may occur in patients who are immobilized, but concomitant hyperparathyroidism (and other causes of hypercalcemia) should be excluded. An increased incidence of hyperuricemia has been observed in

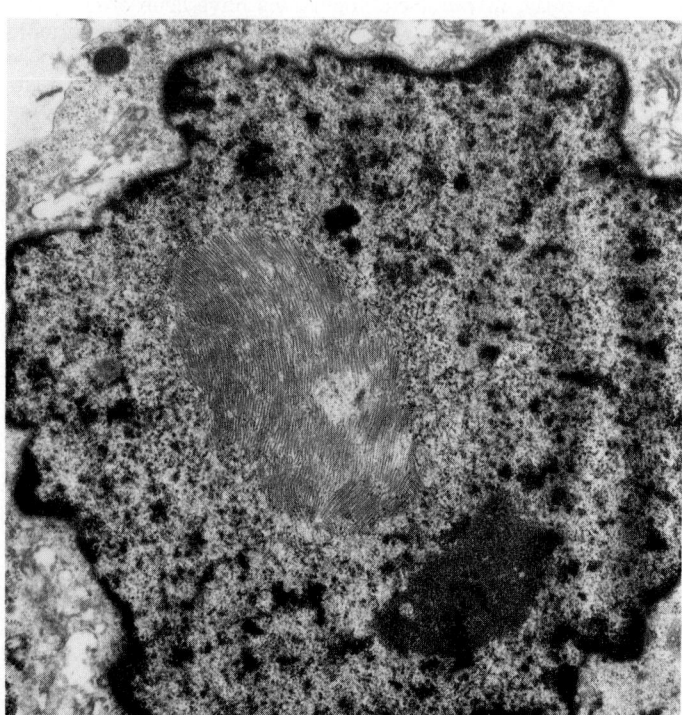

Figure 19–78. Electron micrograph of an osteoclast nucleus from a patient with Paget's disease showing characteristic intranuclear inclusion (consisting of 125° diameter microfilaments). Decalcified bone magnified × 32,400. (Figure kindly supplied by Dr. Barbara G. Mills and Dr. Frederick R. Singer.)

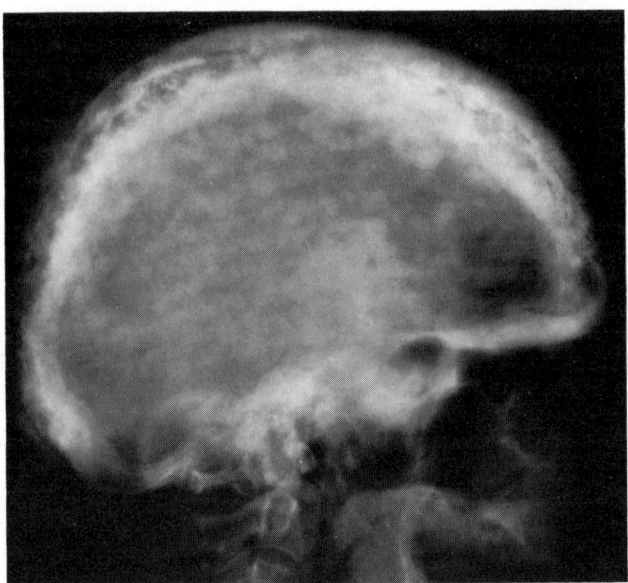

Figure 19–79. Radiograph of skull in a patient with advanced Paget's disease showing thickening, disordered new bone formation ("cottonwool patches") and basilar impression. (From Singer, F. R.: In *Topics in Bone and Mineral Disorders.* Avioli, L. V. (ed.), New York, Plenum Press, 1977.)

Paget's disease; this may be due to increased bone cell turnover.

The bone lesions of Paget's disease show a characteristic radiographic appearance that reflects the disordered bone remodeling observed histologically (Fig. 19–79). Osteoblastic metastases may present a similar appearance, especially pelvic metastases from prostatic carcinoma. Thickening of the pelvic brim and iliopectineal line as well as widening of the pubic and ischial bones are characteristics of Paget's disease in the pelvis and serve to distinguish it from osteoblastic metastases. In rare cases, histologic study of bone biopsies may be necessary to make a definitive diagnosis.

Radiographic evidence of bone involvement does not necessarily reflect continued metabolic activity in osteitis deformans. Scanning with bone-seeking radioactive agents such as technetium diphosphonate allows distinction between active lesions with high uptake and "burned-out" inactive lesions.

Therapy

Several drugs alleviate symptoms, normalize metabolic parameters, and restore normal bone morphology in Paget's disease. Indications for therapy include bone pain, development of neurologic complications, and preparation for surgery on diseased bone. There is no evidence, at present, that prophylactic therapy of the asymptomatic patient is beneficial. Pain due to bone involvement can be relieved by therapy, but patients with degenerative arthritis complicating Paget's disease may not experience relief of pain. Hearing loss is generally not restored by therapy, but case reports have described therapeutic reversal of other neurologic complications. Useful drugs are described in the sections that follow.

Calcitonin

Salmon CT, the most potent form of the hormone, is now generally available for treatment of Paget's disease. The usual starting dose is 20–50 MRC units/day, given subcu-

taneously. Nausea (in less than 10% of patients) appears to be the major side effect. The acute response to the hormone is a transient reduction in serum calcium concentration (by about 25%). Subsequently, urinary hydroxyproline excretion and then serum alkaline phosphatase activity are reduced. This sequence of events suggests that the initial effect of CT is to decrease bone resorption and that bone formation is secondarily reduced. In patients with extreme elevations of urinary hydroxyproline and serum alkaline phosphatase, CT may cause only a 50% reduction, with persistence of abnormal values. Nonetheless x-rays may show apparent normalization of bone, suggesting that persistent elevations of metabolic parameters reflect in part normal bone remodeling. In uncontrolled studies, 88% of patients experienced relief of pain. Discontinuation of treatment after periods as long as a year is often followed by a prolonged therapeutic effect (Fig. 19–80). Available data do not permit a firm conclusion regarding the optimal therapy, i.e., prolonged maintenance vs. intermittent therapy. Resistance to the effects of salmon CT is encountered in some patients; development of a high titer of antibodies accounts for resistance in a minority of cases. Use of human CT may avoid this problem, but this agent is not yet generally available. Continual cycles of relative hypocalcemia after CT might lead to secondary hyperparathyroidism, but patients receiving the drug chronically have not shown evidence of this.

Sodium Etidronate

This drug belongs to the class of diphosphonate compounds that inhibit bone resorption and formation. It has been tested in doses ranging from less than 1–20 mg/kg body weight/day, given orally. Intestinal absorption of the drug may be quite variable. With treatment, urinary hydroxyproline and serum alkaline phosphatase become normal and pain is relieved, as shown in a double-blind controlled study. Diarrhea may occur, particularly at higher doses. Of greater importance is the observation that high doses (10–20 mg/kg) may cause impaired mineralization of osteoid. This may explain the increase in bone pain

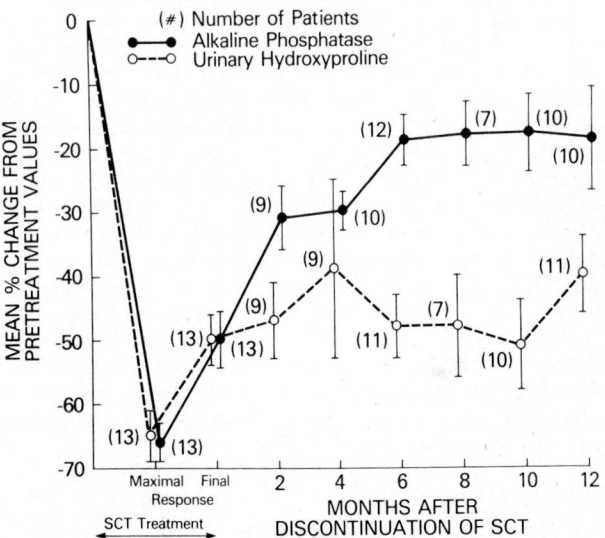

Figure 19–80. Mean (± SEM) % change from pretreatment values in serum alkaline phosphatase and urinary hydroxyproline excretion during and up to 12 months after discontinuation of salmon CT treatment of Paget's disease. (From Avramides, A., Flores, A., et al.: Paget's disease of the bone: observations after cessation of long-term synthetic salmon calcitonin treatment. *J. Clin. Endocrinol. Metab.* 42:461, 1976.)

and incidence of pathologic fractures observed with higher doses in several studies. With a dose of 5 mg/kg, however, metabolic parameters apparently become normal without causing osteomalacia. Maximal therapeutic response to sodium etidronate was achieved by 6 months and, as with CT, discontinuation of therapy was often followed by prolonged "remission."

Mithramycin

This drug inhibits bone resorption directly and causes transient reduction in serum calcium and persistent reduction in urinary hydroxyproline and serum alkaline phosphatase in patients with Paget's disease. Doses of 15–25 μg/kg given intravenously weekly are effective. Nausea and vomiting, renal toxicity, and release of hepatic enzymes are relatively frequent side effects.

In summary, at least three forms of therapy are effective in treating Paget's disease. Salmon CT is expensive and must be given parenterally. Resistant patients may be encountered, but lack of toxicity probably makes it the agent of choice. Diphosphonates appear to be equally effective and can be given orally, but in high doses may cause osteomalacia. The long-term toxicity and effectiveness of lower doses of diphosphonates need to be evaluated. Newer diphosphonate analogs, e.g., dichloromethylene bisphosphonate, may be capable of inhibiting bone resorption without impairing mineralization. Mithramycin should be reserved for failures with other forms of therapy.

Hereditary Bone Dysplasia with Hyperphosphatasia (Juvenile Paget's Disease)

This is a rare hereditary disorder of bone remodeling. More than 15 cases have been reported, with a clustering of cases in Puerto Rican and American Indian families. The mode of inheritance is probably autosomal recessive. The disease begins between 3 and 18 months of age and is generally fatal before adulthood. Characteristically, there is accelerated turnover of membranous bone and a chronic elevation of serum alkaline phosphatase activity and urinary hydroxyproline. Despite superficial resemblances to Paget's disease, this is probably a distinct disorder. Unlike Paget's disease, there is a symmetric involvement of the long bones. Abnormal bone remodeling leads to widened diaphyses and lack of a distinct corticomedullary separation. Bowing of the femur and tibia and increased head size occur. Histopathologic studies demonstrate thickened osteoid seams and a predominance of woven rather than lamellar bone. There are relatively few multinucleated osteoclasts but instead there is evidence of increased osteocytic osteolysis. The cause of the disorder is unknown. CT may be effective in correcting metabolic abnormalities, bone histology, and radiographic appearance. Two children treated for more than 4 months with human CT had decreased pain and increased mobility.

Osteopetrosis

This term has been applied to a clinically and genetically heterogeneous group of skeletal disorders characterized by increased bone density. Three specific subtypes are discussed here.

Early Onset Form

This rare disorder has its onset in infancy and is inherited in an autosomal recessive fashion. Generalized skeletal sclerosis leads to obliteration of the marrow spaces; consequent extramedullary hematopoiesis leads to hepatosplenomegaly. The facial appearance is characterized by frontal bossing, hypertelorism, and exophthalmos. Thickening of the skull causes narrowing of cranial nerve foramina; cranial nerve palsies and hydrocephalus may develop. Pathologic fractures and dental abnormalities are also observed. Some subjects show renal tubular defects causing metabolic acidosis. Death occurs in the first decade, generally from hemorrhage or infection. Skeletal x-rays show increased density, sclerotic foci within bone ("endobones"), and thickened vertebral end plates ("Rugger-jersey spine"). The etiology of the disorder is unknown, but bone biopsies have shown absence of osteoclasts and loss of normal bone resorption. Recent studies in animal models of the human disease (e.g., gray-lethal mice) indicate that the condition can be reversed with bone marrow transplants from normal litter mates. It has been suggested that an osteoclast precursor cell (monocyte?) supplied by the transplanted marrow restores normal bone resorption. This form of therapy has since been attempted in several children. A 3-month-old infant who received bone marrow from an HLA identical sister showed striking clinical and radiographic improvement (Fig. 19–81), but three other children receiving HLA nonidentical marrow have had a less favorable response.

Delayed Onset Form

This disorder is more common and more benign than the early onset form. Inheritance is autosomal dominant. Increased bone density is first observed in childhood. Patients may be asymptomatic and the disease discovered only on incidental x-rays. Mild anemia, cranial nerve palsies, and pathologic fractures are relatively uncommon complications. There may be considerable interfamilial variation in the clinical severity of the disease.

Pycnodysostosis

This disorder is characterized by decreased stature (adult height is < 150 cm) and progressive increase in skeletal density that begins in childhood. Inheritance is autosomal recessive. The skull characteristically shows frontal and occipital bossing and nonclosure of the sutures; the mandibular angle is flattened, giving rise to a receding chin, and the terminal phalanges of the fingers and toes may be shortened. Pathologic fractures may occur. The cause of the disease is unknown. Intermittent elevation in basal serum CT concentration and an exaggerated CT response to calcium and glucagon infusions have been described in a single patient with the disorder. It is unclear whether increased CT secretion is of pathogenetic importance or is merely a secondary feature of the disease.

Several other inherited disorders characterized by increased bone density and dysplasia of bones have been described. These include metaphyseal dysplasia (Pyle's disease), craniometaphyseal dysplasia, endosteal hyperostosis (Van Buchem's disease), and sclero-osteosis. A detailed consideration of these disorders is beyond the scope of this chapter; the interested reader is referred to the review by Beighton and coworkers.

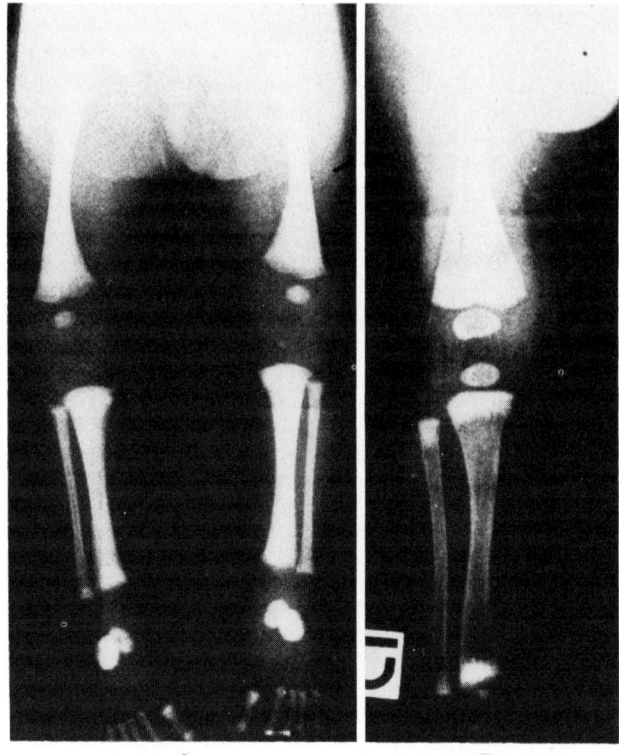

A   **B**

Figure 19–81. (A) Radiographs of lower limb in patient with osteopetrosis at age 2 months before bone marrow transplant and (B) at age 9 months after transplant showing formation of normal medullary bone. (From Ballet, J. J., and Griscelli, C.: Lymphoid cell transplantation in human osteopetrosis. In *Proceedings, Mechanisms of Localized Bone Loss* [Special Supplement to Calcified Tissue Research Abstracts]. Horton, J. E., Tarphey, T. M., and Davis, W. F. (eds.), Washington, D. C., Information Retrieval, Inc., 1978.)

Osteogenesis Imperfecta

The major phenotypic expression of this inherited disorder is a tendency to fracture bones after minimal trauma. The pathogenesis is undefined, and it is possible that there are several genetically distinct entities giving rise to similar clinical expressions. The disease has generally been subdivided into two forms based on the age of onset of fractures, i.e., at birth (congenita) and later in childhood or adulthood (tarda). This classification roughly correlates with the severity of disease, although the clinical course in occasional patients with the congenita form is relatively benign. The pattern of inheritance appears to be autosomal dominant in the tarda form and a positive family history is common; the congenita form may be inherited in autosomal recessive fashion and affected family members are rare.

Several clinical features suggest that the disease may represent a generalized disorder of collagen structure. These include blue sclerae (the choroid pigment is visible beneath abnormally thin sclerae), hyperextensible joints, and "paper" thin skin. In severe cases, frequent fractures may cause crippling deformities and kyphoscoliosis may be present. Abnormal dental development, including failure to form dentin, may be observed. Deafness due to otosclerosis is often associated with osteogenesis imperfecta, but it is not clear if this is an intrinsic feature of the disease.

Increased bone turnover with an excess of resorption has been described in some studies, but this may in part reflect immobilization due to frequent fractures. Other histologic findings in the congenita variety include an increased number of osteocytes and primitive woven bone. Elevations in serum alkaline phosphatase activity and urinary hydroxyproline excretion have been observed but are not the rule. Serum calcium and phosphate concentrations are generally normal. Osteogenesis imperfecta may be confused with juvenile osteoporosis, battered child syndrome, and, in adults, primary osteoporosis. Family history and bone biopsy may be helpful in making the correct diagnosis.

Analysis of bone and skin collagen from patients with osteogenesis imperfecta has yielded conflicting results. Abnormal findings include failure of bone collagen fibrils to form normal fiber bundles, decreased lysine/hydroxylysine ratio, increased synthesis of type III (immature) collagen, and abnormal cross-linking of collagen with an increase in soluble immature forms. An abnormality in mucopolysaccharide metabolism has also been proposed as the primary defect in the disorder. As stated earlier, it is possible that several genetically distinct defects in collagen formation may result in a common phenotype, i.e., abnormal bone matrix with a tendency to fracture.

Therapy with fluoride, androgens, and magnesium oxide has been attempted without much success. CT has been claimed to have a beneficial effect in patients with the tarda form of the disease, but the number of patients treated was small and the objective response (decrease in fracture rate, increase in bone density) was at best slight. Orthopedic surgery (insertion of intramedullary rods) may be appropriate in selected patients to facilitate mobility.

Fibrous Dysplasia

Patients with this rare disease show fibrous replacement of bone in one (monostotic form) or more (polyostotic form) sites. Lesions appear cystic on x-ray, may show sclerotic margins, and may be difficult to distinguish from osteitis fibrosa cystica as well as other cystic bone lesions. The histologic appearance, characterized by a cellular fibroblastic stroma between rare bone spicules, generally permits specific diagnosis. Serum calcium and phosphorus concentrations are normal, but serum alkaline phosphatase activity and urinary hydroxyproline excretion may be increased. The femur, proximal tibia, and skull are the most commonly affected sites. Effective therapy to prevent or halt progression of lesions is not available; orthopedic surgery may be required to correct deformities. The disease generally appears during childhood, but in a minority of patients may develop after age 20.

Pigmented skin lesions (café au lait spots) with irregular borders are frequently observed in patients with fibrous dysplasia. Endocrine and metabolic abnormalities are also associated with fibrous dysplasia (usually the polyostotic form). These include isosexual precocity in affected females, hyperthyroidism, acromegaly and gigantism, glucose intolerance with hyperinsulinism, and adrenal hyperplasia. The triad of polyostotic fibrous dysplasia, pigmented skin lesions, and sexual precocity in girls has been referred to as the McCune-Albright syndrome. The relationship between the bony lesions and the associated sexual precocity (and other endocrine abnormalities) is unexplained. A suggestion that fibrous dysplasia of the base of the skull triggers sexual precocity by interfering with hypothalamic function seems unlikely, since sexual precocity occurs in patients lacking detectable skull involvement.

Acquired hypophosphatemia and osteomalacia have been observed in several patients with fibrous dysplasia. The pathogenesis of hypophosphatemia in these cases is undefined (see p. 1004). Several patients have been reported in whom fibrous dysplasia and primary hyperparathyroidism were said to coexist. This combined diagnosis was based upon persistence of bone lesions after correction of hyperparathyroidism. Other features associated with fibrous dysplasia, e.g., pigmented lesions or sexual precocity, were not present.

Extraskeletal Calcification and Ossification

Deposition of calcium in soft tissues may occur with normal serum calcium and phosphorus concentration in response to injury (dystrophic calcification) or as a result of abnormal serum calcium and phosphorus concentration. Calcium deposits in the skin may cause pruritus and draining ulcers; deposits in muscle and in joint capsules may impair mobility. Parenchymal calcification can cause serious disturbances in renal, pulmonary, and cardiac function. Extraskeletal calcification may be detected on x-rays; some forms of soft-tissue calcification (e.g., tumoral calcinosis, pulmonary parenchymal calcification) may be detected by technetium diphosphonate scanning even before they are detectable radiographically. Calcification of bone matrix in extraskeletal sites is termed ectopic ossification.

Dystrophic Calcification

Soft-tissue calcification is a nonspecific response to many forms of tissue damage. Examples include calcified granulomas following tuberculous infection, pleural calcification in asbestosis and periarticular calcification after joint trauma.

Amorphous calcium phosphate or hydroxyapatite deposits in skin and subcutaneous tissue are often associated with the so-called "collagen-vascular" diseases. This occurs most frequently in scleroderma but may be seen in dermatomyositis and systemic lupus as well. Similar deposits occurring without associated disease have been termed calcinosis universalis.

Dystrophic Ossification

Myositis Ossificans Progressiva

In this rare disorder of unknown etiology, bone is formed in muscle and connective tissue. Males have been said to be affected more frequently than females, but in one large series of 52 patients, two-thirds were females. The disease may be inherited as an autosomal dominant trait with variable penetrance. Eighty per cent of patients display valgus deformity of the great toe. The onset of the disease occurs either immediately after birth or in early childhood. An inflammatory nodule on the back, neck, or head may be the initial lesion; biopsy at this stage may show degenerating muscle fibers, fibroblastic proliferation, and mononuclear cell infiltration. Ectopic cartilage and bone matrix form within the fibrosing muscle and the lesion is successively mineralized and developed into ectopic bone. New lesions may appear spontaneously, after trauma or surgical excision of a previous lesion. Involvement of the trunk generally precedes involvement of the extremities. Ultimately, mobility is severely impaired; thoracic involvement complicated by pneumonia is the usual cause of death. The disease, however, is not invariably fatal and spontaneous fluctuations in the course make it difficult to evaluate the effects of therapy.

Acquired Ectopic Ossification

Ectopic ossification may occur following trauma or neurologic injury (e.g., spinal cord lesions). The most commonly affected sites are adjacent to the hip joint and along the medial side of the thigh. Ankylosis and severely impaired mobility may result.

Therapy of Dystrophic Calcification and Ossification

Many forms of therapy have been tried in calcinosis (associated with scleroderma or dermatomyositis) and in myositis ossificans without much success. Recent reports suggest that sodium etidronate may be of benefit. Favorable responses are attributed to inhibition of calcification, a known effect of diphosphonates, rather than an effect on the primary disease. Although controlled studies have not been performed, regression of lesions has been observed in some patients, and exacerbations appear after discontinuation of therapy in some cases. Not all patients have responded, and toxic effects (osteomalacia, fractures) may be encountered, particularly at higher doses (20 mg/kg).

Calcification Due to Abnormal Serum Calcium and Phosphorus Concentrations

Hypercalcemic Disorders

Soft-tissue calcification may complicate any hypercalcemic disorder (see section on hypercalcemia, p. 980) but occurs most frequently when serum phosphate concentration is concomitantly elevated (e.g., decreased GFR as in vitamin D intoxication) rather than depressed (e.g., uncomplicated primary hyperparathyroidism). Administration of phosphates, particularly intravenously, may cause soft-tissue calcification in hypercalcemic patients. Calcium phosphate precipitates preferentially in sites of localized alkalosis: kidney tubules, lungs, gastric mucosa, and eyes. Other local factors may be of importance in other sites of calcification, e.g., skin and arterial wall.

Hyperphosphatemic Disorders

Extraskeletal calcification can occur with normal or even low serum calcium concentration, if serum phosphate concentration is high. Thus soft-tissue calcification is observed in uremia, in idiopathic hypoparathyroidism, and in PHP (ectopic ossification may occur in the latter). Analysis of calcium deposits from viscera of uremic patients suggests that hypermagnesemia may contribute to soft-tissue mineral deposition.

Tumoral calcinosis is a rare familial disease characterized by massive periarticular calcium phosphate deposition. The disease occurs more frequently in blacks and may be inherited as an autosomal recessive trait. Serum phosphorus concentration is usually elevated, whereas serum calcium concentration is normal. Elevated serum alkaline phosphatase activity and urinary hydroxyproline excretion have been observed in some patients.

Therapy of Ectopic Calcification due to Abnormal Serum Phosphorus and Calcium Concentration

Treatment of the underlying disorders, when feasible, and correction of hypercalcemia (obviously not by administering phosphate) is the appropriate therapy for soft-tissue calcification complicating hypercalcemic illness. Hyperphosphatemic disorders are best treated by reduction in serum phosphate concentration. This may require a combined use of low phosphorus diet and phosphate-binding antacids. Regression of lesions with phosphorus deprivation therapy has been documented in a patient with tumoral calcinosis.

HYPERCALCITONINISM

Medullary Carcinoma of the Thyroid

Calcitonin (or thyrocalcitonin — TCT) was not recognized as a hormone until 1962, and it was not until 1968 that high secretory rates for CT were discovered in a clinical disorder. This is, in part, because in humans CT, unlike many other hormones when secreted at abnormally high rates, does not induce specific metabolic abnormalities. Medullary thyroid cancer, which arises in the parafollicular or C cells, accounts for 10% of thyroid cancers. Its epidemiologic, histologic, and biochemical features differ from those of neoplasms arising from thyroid follicular cells. Unlike the more common thyroid cancers, the male to female ratio is 1:1. The tumor is important also because of frequent hereditary occurrence, association with other endocrine abnormalities, and use as a model for cancerous processes that may be diagnosed on the basis of secretory product markers and treated at early stages.

Clinical Features

The tumor typically presents in patients about 50 years old as one or more palpable thyroid nodules. It grows slowly, spreading via contiguous lymphatics; rapid growth and hematogenous metastases occur infrequently. The sporadic disease may be unicentric in origin, but hereditary occurrences are multicentric, beginning most commonly at the junctions of the middle and upper third of the thyroid lobes, where C cells are present in largest numbers. The tumor may contain or secrete hormones other than CT. These include serotonin, prostaglandins, and ACTH. Immunohistochemical studies have shown that CT and ACTH are synthesized within the same cells. Approximately 20% of affected patients develop diarrhea, variably attributed to intestinal actions of secreted CT, prostaglandins, or serotonin. In FMEN type III, diarrhea may reflect intestinal ganglioneuromatosis (see later). Diarrhea as a manifestation of a humoral tumor product usually indicates the presence of a large tumor bulk and metastases. Other than diarrhea, there have been no clinical features clearly linked to high secretory rates for calcitonin.

Laboratory Analyses

Radioactive thyroid scans are often unremarkable with early stages of the tumor. The tumor may contain large calcifications, unlike the fine, stippled calcifications with papillary thyroid carcinoma (Fig. 19–82); large, calcified, nodular metastases are also highly characteristic. Another characteristic radiographic feature is a fibrotic reaction about metastases in the lungs. Skeletal metastases may assume a lytic or, less commonly, sclerotic appearance. There are distinctive histologic features; the cells are polyhedral or spindle-shaped with variable amounts of stroma and stromal calcification. Almost all contain large amounts of amyloid. The amyloid consists, in part, of aggregates of CT. The tumor cells contain CT and often enzymes relating to the biogenic amine pathways characteristic of neuroectodermal cells. These include dopa decarboxylase and histaminase. Serum calcium and phosphate concentrations are generally normal. In small numbers of patients evaluated by bone biopsy, no uniform abnormalities attributable to CT have been found. Immunoreactive gastrin was moderately decreased in serum in another study, and this was related to a direct inhibitory action of circulating CT on

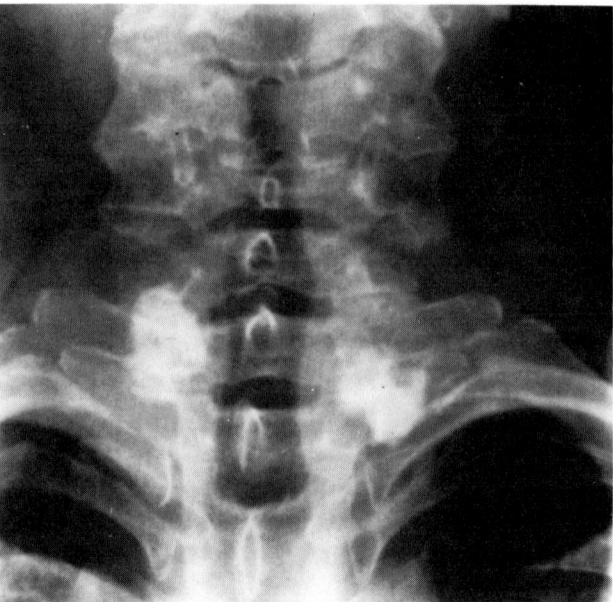

Figure 19–82. Large calcified intrathyroidal masses characteristic of medullary thyroid carcinoma. (Courtesy of Dr. H. Keiser.)

gastrin-secreting cells. The radioimmunoassay of CT in serum is applicable for diagnosis (see later) and follow-up; it has also been used to localize metastases. Serum immunoreactive CT may also be increased in neonates, in azotemia, and in hypercalcemia or hypergastrinemia (both of which may act as secretogogues). Circulating concentrations of other tumor products, such as histaminase and carcinoembryonic antigen, are increased in a large fraction of patients with metastatic medullary thyroid carcinoma.

Therapy

Surgery is considered the treatment of choice, though no studies have yet documented its efficacy in increasing survival. The usual approach is total thyroidectomy with a degree of node removal dependent on evidence of tumor stage. No thyroid tissue should be left because of the malignant potential of residual C cells. The disease presenting as a thyroid mass shows a 10-year postoperative survival of approximately 67%. Family testing allows early diagnosis, and it should be possible to test for potential benefits of treatment in early stages of the disorder. Local radiotherapy or chemotherapy has been used with little success.

Familial Medullary Carcinoma of the Thyroid

Medullary carcinoma of the thyroid occurs in families as an expression of two distinct traits, each with autosomal dominant transmission. The eponym Sipple's syndrome has been applied to both of these hereditary forms, though Sipple's description did not include the multiple neuroma variant. Unlike the sporadic tumor that is often unicentric in origin, familial disease is usually multifocal in the thyroid gland. An early phase of diffuse C-cell hyperplasia can be diagnosed by serial testing (see later).

Familial Multiple Endocrine Neoplasia, Type II (IIA)

For this autosomal dominant trait, there is very high penetrance for medullary thyroid carcinoma in adults. Approximately one third of affected family members also have abnormalities of other endocrine tissues (primary parathyroid hyperplasia or pheochromocytoma or both) (see Table 19–11). All three of the endocrine tissue hyperfunctions have an early stage of hyperplasia that progresses to a nodular phase. In several affected women heterozygous for G6PD, an X chromosome marker, isoenzyme analysis of tumors has suggested that the masses are monoclonal, but each mass may derive from a progenitor cell carrying either X chromosome. Malignant change is rare in the adrenal medulla and has not yet been reported for the parathyroids of these patients. Approximately 10% of affected adults develop hypercalcemia or nephrolithiasis or both. More commonly, the surgeon recognizes diffusely hyperplastic parathyroid glands at the time of surgery directed at the thyroid gland of a normocalcemic patient. It is not known if the parathyroid hyperplasia is a secondary response to a C-cell product; CT, for example, might cause PTH resistance or a direct agonist affect on the parathyroid cell. Moreover, in several affected patients, calcium infusion led to simultaneous increase in secretion of both CT and PTH, in contrast to the anticipated suppression of PTH secretion. On the other hand, some cases do not show calcium stimulation of PTH secretion and parathyroid hyperplasia is not common in patients with sporadic medullary carcinoma of the thyroid or with the multiple neuroma variant of familial medullary carcinoma of the thyroid (see later). Pheochromocytoma may occur, sometimes subtly expressed in members of families with MEN type II or type III. This diagnosis should always be considered prior to administration of general anesthesia. The usual provocative tests for pheochromocytoma are often not helpful for diagnosis in asymptomatic cases of FMEN II, but a biochemically silent adrenal medullary mass may be recognized with standard or computer-assisted tomography of the adrenal beds. In several families, affected persons have manifested a disproportionate increase in urinary excretion of epinephrine versus norepinephrine.

Familial Multiple Endocrine Neoplasia, Type III (IIB)

The C-cell and adrenal medullary abnormalities in these patients are indistinguishable from those of patients with FMEN II (IIA). The major distinguishing feature of this disorder is overgrowth of elements of nerve tissue with the result that the patients develop multiple mucosal neuromas, thickened corneal nerves, and ganglioneuromatosis of the intestine. The mucosal neuromas result in a characteristic facial appearance of buccal and lingual nodules, thick bumpy lips, and thickened tarsal plates (Fig. 19–83). This phenotype can often be diagnosed in the first decade of life. The thickened corneal nerves are best appreciated by slit lamp examination, and an ophthalmologist may be the first to suspect the presence of the underlying disorder. Intestinal ganglioneuromatosis leads to frequent abnormalities of intestinal transit, including diarrhea, constipation, diverticulosis, and megacolon. General muscle development is often poor. Lax joints and the tall, slender body habitus with pectus excavatum or carinatum result in an external appearance resembling that in Marfan's syndrome. No lenticular or vascular abnormalities occur, however.

Early Diagnosis

Recognition of the familial pattern and progression through a premalignant phase make possible diagnosis of hereditary cases long before development of a palpable neck mass. Hopefully, early diagnosis and treatment will improve the life expectancy of these patients. CT radioimmunoassay allows diagnosis of premalignant phases of the disorder in an undefined fraction of cases. High basal concentration of CT in plasma without other conditions known to cause this (pregnancy, uremia, hypergastrinemia, other cancers) is virtually diagnostic of the cancerous phase of the trait. Increased diagnostic sensitivity during the early phases of C-cell hyperfunction is obtained by measuring

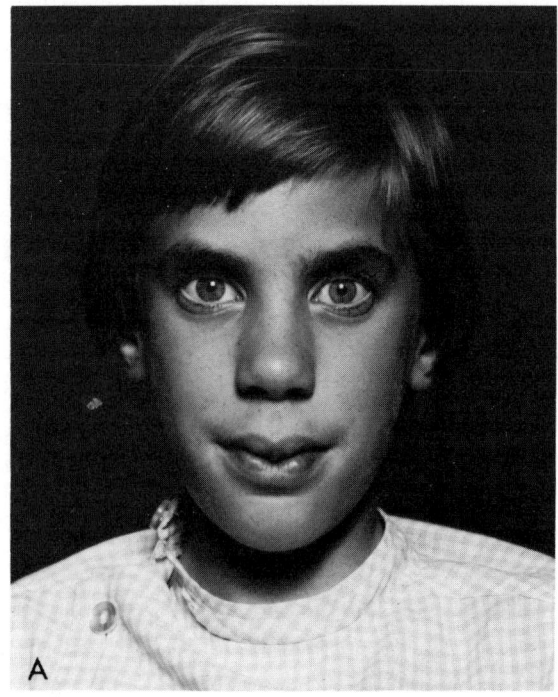

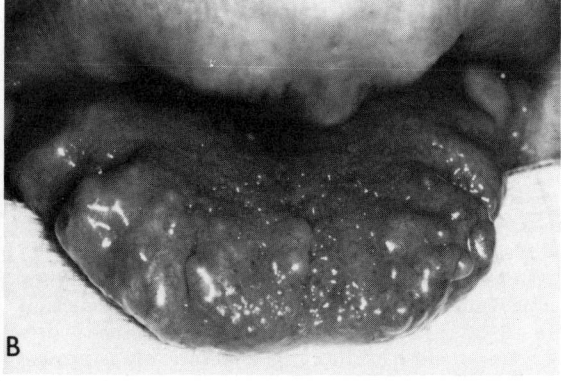

Figure 19–83. *(A)* Characteristic facies of patient with FMEN type III. Note bumpy lips and thickened tarsal plates of eyelids. *(B)* The surface of the tongue is studded with nodular mucosal neuromas. (From Carney, J. A., and Hayles, A. B.: Alimentary tract manifestations of multiple endocrine neoplasia, type 2B. *Mayo Clin. Proc.* 52:543, 1977.)

serum CT concentration after administration of a standardized CT secretagogue. One potent stimulus is an infusion of calcium gluconate (equivalent to 2 mg of elemental calcium/kg) over 1 min followed by pentagastrin (0.5 μg/kg) over 5 sec. This also evokes an unpleasant sensation of retrosternal distress. Serial testing of persons at risk for inheritance of the trait allows diagnosis of the malignant and premalignant phase of C-cell dysfunction in some cases before the age of 10 years.

Other Calcitonin-Producing Tumors

High circulating concentrations of CT may be found in patients with diverse neoplasms and might be caused by CT production by the tumor, decreased clearance of CT by normal catabolic routes, or an increased thyroidal secretion of CT under the influence of subtle hypercalcemia or other tumor-mediated processes. Some tumors that produce and release CT derive from cells of neuroectodermal origin (small cell cancer of the lung, carcinoid tumors, pancreatic islet cell cancer, pheochromocytoma) so that CT secretion by them may not be "ectopic" but an exaggeration of normal secretion. Others, particularly breast cancer, not recognized as neuroectodermal in origin, also have shown CT secretion.

HYPERCALCIURIA AND UROLITHIASIS

In the United States, urolithiasis accounts for approximately 0.1% of all hospitalizations, and 2–4% of all males will experience renal colic at some point in their lives. The precipitation of concretions in the lumina of the urinary tract is one consequence of the kidney's many, often counteracting functions, which include excretion of solutes and conservation of water. The tubules of mammalian and avian kidneys contain long medullary loops that permit elaboration of a concentrated urine. In humans the maximal urinary osmolarity is 1200 mOsm/l, but this can be as high as 5000 in the desert-dwelling kangaroo rat.

The anatomic loci for stones show distinct demographic characteristics. Bladder stones are common among male children in some nutritionally impoverished regions of the world, with a peak incidence at age 2–4 years. The cause is not known but may involve unusual dietary problems such as low protein intake with a diet that is high in oxalates and low in phosphorus. In the U.S. bladder stones occur principally in elderly males or persons with bladder catheters. Stasis with prostatic enlargement or factors associated with indwelling catheters (immobilization hypercalciuria, *Proteus* infection, foreign body, and so on) are important in etiology.

Etiology of Urolithiasis

Three etiologies have been postulated: matrix or anatomic abnormality, deficiency of inhibitor(s) of crystal growth or aggregation, and supersaturation. Urinary stones are predominantly crystalline in composition, but all have an organic component (its matrix) that accounts for 2% or higher of the dry weight. In patients with advanced renal failure and low renal calcium excretion rates, matrix calculi may form with 40–85% matrix by weight. Stone matrix consists of insoluble mucoproteins that often are accumulated in concentric lamellae. There is disagreement as to whether stone surfaces are covered with organic fibrils, and

this could have implications concerning mechanisms of stone growth. Overall amino acid compositions of proteins from stones of calcium oxalate, calcium phosphate, struvite, uric acid, or cystine are similar. Only stones with calcium-containing crystals have high contents of gamma carboxy glutamic acid (gla), however. Clusters of gla residues provide molecular regions with high affinity for calcium and have been identified in a small number of proteins with critical regions for calcium interaction. The biologic properties of the stone matrix proteins are not known.

Stone growth in free suspension is too slow a process to result in a concretion of sufficient size to obstruct a ureter. Anchoring by an anatomic focus increases residence time in the urinary tract. Some stone formers have renal papillary lesions (Randall's plaques), small subepithelial accumulations of hydroxyapatite. Their importance is not known, but 15% of calcium oxalate stones have an eccentric structure or even a smooth indentation suggestive of growth instituted around a papillary focus. Foci of calcification have also been seen within tubules and the interstitium of renal biopsies from patients with calcium oxalate stones. These foci of "intranephronic calculosis" could serve as stone nuclei or might represent merely other manifestations of the stone-forming diathesis.

The second general theory about urinary calculi implicates deficiencies of inhibitors of stone nucleation, growth, or aggregation. Small amounts of normal urine will inhibit these processes when added to solutions that are supersaturated with respect to calcium oxalate or calcium phosphate. Several inhibitory components of normal urine have been identified. These include pyrophosphate, magnesium, citrate, and acidic mucopolysaccharides. The inhibitory properties of these components are related to their adsorption to and interactions with the surfaces of calcium-containing crystals. Heparin-like acidic mucopolysaccharides inhibit crystal aggregation but do not interfere with crystal nucleation or growth.

The third general theory of stone nucleation and growth attributes major importance to urine supersaturation with respect to components of the stone. There is no doubt that this mechanism is important at least for certain types of stone (cystine, uric acid, xanthine). There are at least three distinct phases in crystal development: nucleation, growth, and aggregation. The driving force for nucleation and growth is thermodynamic energy (deltaG) related to the degree of supersaturation of the urine with respect to the crystalline phase:

$$deltaG = RTln(Ai/Ao).$$

R and T are the universal gas constant and temperature, and Ai and Ao are the activity products of the stone salt versus that at saturation equilibrium. As the activity product of an uncharged complex increases, a solution shifts from undersaturation to saturation. In the absence of a nucleating surface the activity product in solution may be increased beyond that at saturation equilibrium without spontaneous precipitation, a condition of metastable supersaturation. Once a critical degree of supersaturation is reached, the solution becomes unstable and spontaneous precipitation proceeds. It is doubtful that this state is ever attained in the urinary tract, where the solution is exposed to particulate debris and other surfaces and undergoes rapid changes in composition. EM of urinary stones often shows spherulic particles that would not occur if the mineral accretion followed idealized assumptions about crystal growth.

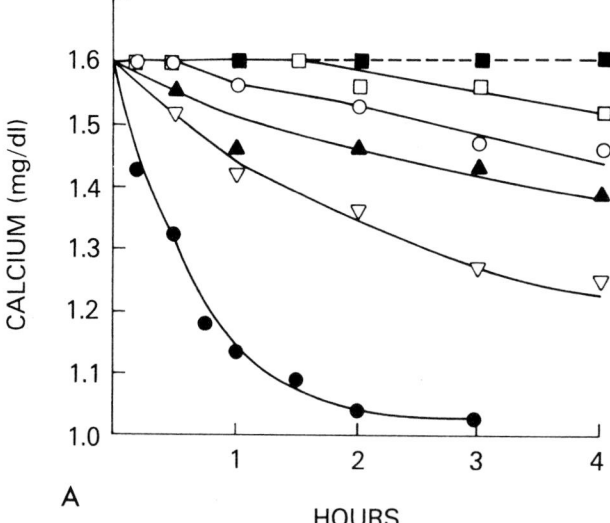

Table 19–18. CRYSTAL COMPONENTS OF KIDNEY STONES FROM AN ANALYSIS OF 10,000 STONES*

Crystal	100%	51–100%	1–50%
Calcium oxalates			
(Monohydrate (whewhellite)	690	3136	4303
Dihydrate (wheddellite)	547	4094	6098
Calcium phosphates			
Carbonate-apatite	20	444	2312
Hydroxyapatite	9	228	3837
Dihydrate (brushite)	17	131	228
Tricalcium phosphate (whitlockite)	3	13	28
Magnesium, ammonium phosphate			
(struvite)	12	912	1570
Other phosphates	1	2	5
Uric acid	350	740	857
Other urates	4	15	87
Cystine	65	88	89
Xanthine	1	1	4

Column heading indicates the % contribution of the identified crystal phase to the total crystal mass of the stone.

Modified from Herring, L. C.: *J. Urol. 88*:545, 1962.

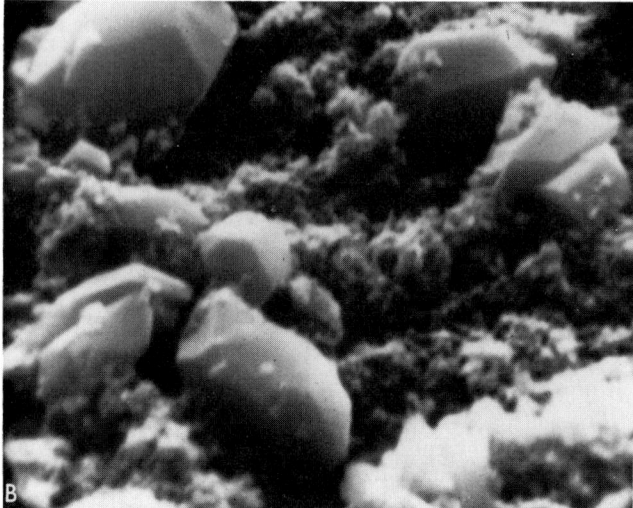

Figure 19–84. *(A)* Effect of surface area of seed on rate of growth of calcium oxalate crystals. To a solution of calcium oxalate with an ionic calcium concentration 2.1 times that at calcium oxalate saturation were added the following seed crystals: none (■), hydroxyapatite 3.7 cm^2 per ml (□), hydroxyapatite 7.7 cm^2 per ml (○), hydroxyapatite 11.5 cm^2 per ml (▲), hydroxyapatite 19.3 cm^2 per ml (△), and calcium oxalate monohydrate 0.8 cm^2 per ml (•). Temperature was maintained at 37°C and pH at 7.4. Calcium remaining in solution was measured at indicated times. *(B)* Scanning electron micrograph (× 9000) of crystals obtained from the solution seeded with hydroxyapatite 3.7 cm^2 per ml 7 hours earlier. Large crystals, in contact with microcrystalline apatite seed, have characteristic morphologic appearance of calcium oxalate monohydrate. (From Meyer, J. L., Begert, J. H., et al.: Epitaxial relationships in urolithiasis: the calcium oxalate monohydrate-hydroxyapatite system. *Clin. Sci. Mol. Med. 49*:369, 1975.)

One component at supersaturating concentrations may accumulate on the surfaces of another component. This process, known as epitaxy, is favored if the crystal lattices of the two components have similar dimensions, as is the case for calcium oxalate mono- and dihydrate, calcium phosphates, uric acid, or sodium urate (Fig. 19–84). Alternatively, nucleation may result from catalytic properties of surface defects in contact with saturated solutions.

Crystal Components of Stone

Analyses of stone composition indicate a high incidence of calcium oxalate stones (whewhellite and wheddellite) and of stones of mixed composition, suggesting the potential importance of epitaxy (Table 19–18). Large stones are generally composed of magnesium ammonium phosphate (struvite) or calcium phosphates (apatite, brushite, octacalcium phosphate), whereas small stones are disproportionately composed of calcium oxalate. When present, calcium phosphates usually occur as minor components (less than 50%); 72.3% ([3136 + 4094]/10,000) of stones have calcium oxalate as the principal (greater than 50%) component. Struvite stones develop in patients with a highly alkaline urine, the result of urinary tract infection with urease-producing organisms (usually *Proteus*) and will not be considered further. Often there is a clear relation between urine and stone composition. To the extent that urine saturation determines the likelihood of stone formation, the important variables are calcium, oxalate, urate, and hydrogen ion concentration and volume. Calcium phosphate shows decreased solubility with increasing pH in the physiologic range; therefore, these stones are found almost exclusively in persistently alkaline urine, as in hyperparathyroidism or other states of hypercalciuric renal tubular acidosis (for example, gradient renal tubular acidosis or carbonic anhydrase inhibitors). In contrast, uric acid solubility rises with increase in pH. The solubility of calcium oxalate is relatively independent of pH within the physiologic range and is influenced more by variation in urinary concentration of oxalate and calcium (Fig. 19–85).

Urinary Excretion of Oxalate

The major known factors determining oxalate content of the urine are dietary intake, intestinal absorption, endogenous production, and urine volume. Accurate quantitation of oxalate in the diet is difficult and estimates of average normal intake vary from 100 to more than 1000 mg/day. Dietary sources of oxalate include rhubarb, spinach, kale, chocolate, cocoa, tea, and fruit juices (20–100 mg oxalate/l). The latter fluids should thus be avoided when seeking increased urine volume to prevent calcium oxalate urolithiasis. Oxalate absorption is a passive diffusional process at all levels of the small and large intestine. Two to 10% of dietary oxalate is normally absorbed and excreted in the urine. Urinary oxalate excretion is normally 10–40 mg/day. It is thought that half is derived from endogenous production. The known causes of a net increase of oxalate absorp-

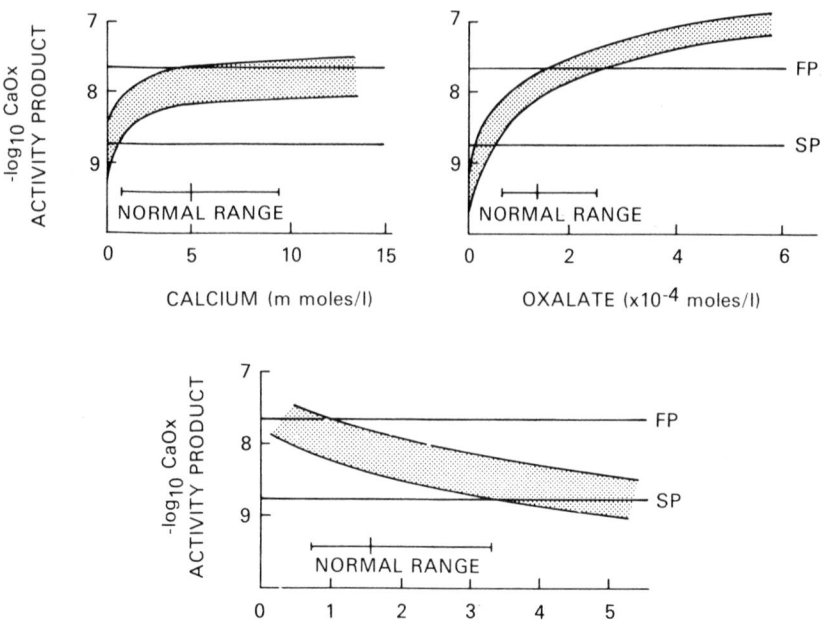

Figure 19–85. The comparative effects of independently changing urinary calcium concentration, urinary oxalate concentration, or urinary volume on the saturation of urine with calcium oxalate. Population normal ranges are shown for each parameter. SP (solubility product) is the calcium oxalate activity product at saturation equilibrium; FP (formation product) is the calcium oxalate activity product leading to spontaneous precipitation of calcium oxalate in vitro. (Courtesy of Dr. W. G. Robertson.)

tion are high oxalate content of the diet and fat malabsorption. Most dietary oxalate precipitates as the insoluble calcium salt in the intestinal lumen and thereby is unavailable for absorption.

Malabsorption of fat causes accumulation of calcium–fatty acid complexes in the intestinal lumen. Oxalate is then associated with sodium and other cations that permit a greater proportion to remain in solution from which it readily enters the circulation and ultimately the urine (enteric hyperoxaluria). Diminished availability of calcium in the intestinal lumen may account for the modest hyperoxaluria occurring in states with increased intestinal absorption of calcium (primary hyperparathyroidism, absorptive hypercalciuria, and dietary calcium restriction). Persons with malabsorptive disorders often develop calcium oxalate urolithiasis. Enteric hyperoxaluria can be decreased by dietary supplementation with calcium but hypercalciuria may then increase the saturation of urine with calcium salts. The optimal treatment is correction of the malabsorption of fat. Alternately improvement can be attained with a low-fat diet supplemented by cholestyramine or other resins capable of binding enteric oxalate.

Increased endogenous production of oxalate occurs with primary hyperoxaluria, types I and II. These are autosomal recessive disorders with similar phenotype. Recurrent passage of calcium oxalate stones begins at an early age; eventually renal damage develops from nephrolithiasis and mineral deposition in the renal parenchyma. Urinary oxalate excretion rate is 100–400 mg/day. The syndromes can be distinguished by the pattern of organic acid excretion. In type I, glycolic acid excretion is abnormally increased. The metabolic defect results in failure of metabolism of glyoxylate to α-hydroxy-β-ketoadipate. Accumulated glyoxalate is metabolized directly to oxalic acid. In the type II syndrome, the excretion rate of L-glyceric acid is high. There is a block in the serine gluconeogenic pathway preventing the conversion of hydroxypyruvate to D-glyceric acid. The mechanism by which this leads to hyperoxaluria is not known, but the conversion of hydroxypyruvate to L-glycerate may be coupled with the conversion of glyoxylate to oxalate. Pyridoxine deficiency causes increased oxalate synthesis and excretion in humans and animals, reflecting

the requirement for this cofactor in conversion of glyoxylate to glycine. The ingestion of oxalate precursors may also result in hyperoxaluria. Ethylene glycol, methoxyflurane, and ascorbic acid each may be converted to oxalate. Ethylene glycol ingestion has led to crystal-associated obstructive uropathy; calcium oxalate deposits are prominent in the renal tubules and parenchyma of the kidney in the small fraction of patients developing renal failure after methoxyflurane anesthesia. Ingestion of large amounts of ascorbic acid (greater than 5 g/day) causes modest increases in urinary oxalate excretion.

Urinary Excretion of Calcium

Calcium ion activity in the urine is determined by filtered load of calcium and multiple factors that modulate the renal handling of filtered calcium, other solutes, and free water. With a 400-mg calcium diet, the 24-hour urine calcium excretion should be less than 250 mg (mean + 2 SD) in adult males and less than 200 mg in females, and these upper limits rise only by 50 mg/day with a 1000-mg calcium diet. Hypercalciuria is associated with an increased incidence of calcium-containing stones. The term hypercalciuria is applied in a statistical sense that need not imply any underlying disorder, however. The only recognized disturbance directly attributable to hypercalciuria is a reversible decrease in the capacity of the kidneys to concentrate urine.

Many agents and disorders are associated with increases in total urinary excretion of calcium. The filtered load of calcium is increased in states with elevated concentrations of ultrafiltrable calcium in plasma; in general, this is equivalent to hypercalcemia. With subnormal PTH secretion caused by hypercalcemia, the renal tubular resorption of calcium decreases producing hypercalciuria. Similarly, with partial parathyroid suppression (serum calcium at the upper normal range), the renal clearance of calcium is high. This occurs with increased influx of calcium to plasma from the intestine (absorptive hypercalciuria: vitamin D excess) or from bone (resorptive hypercalciuria: Paget's disease of bone, thyrotoxicosis, skeletal metastases, immobilization).

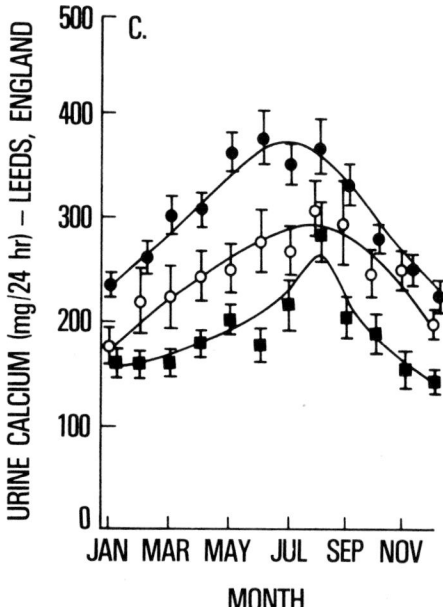

Figure 19–86. Seasonal variation in urine calcium excretion in population of Leeds, England (low annual ultraviolet exposure) — stone formers (closed circles), normal males (open circles), normal women (closed squares). (From Robertson, W. G., Gallagher, J. C., et al.: Seasonal variations in urinary excretion of calcium. *Br. Med. J.* 4:436, 1974.)

In temperate regions there is a seasonal variation in average urinary calcium excretion with a peak in August and a nadir in December (Fig. 19–86). This may reflect variations in solar exposure with consequent fluctuations in endogenous synthesis of cholecalciferol. The relative importance of PTH lack or of CT excess in this process is unknown. Many natriuretic agents decrease distal tubular resorption of calcium. These include dietary salt, certain diuretics (furosemide and ethacrynic acid), mineralocorticoid escape, and CT. The mechanisms by which these four factors cause hypercalciuria may be different. With systemic acidosis, renal calcium clearance increases by unknown mechanisms. Urinary calcium excretion rate doubles after a moderate protein or carbohydrate load, and this may be exaggerated in stone formers. Independent of the dietary calcium content, an increase of dietary protein from a baseline of 80 g up to 700 g/day is associated with a fivefold increase in the rate of urinary calcium excretion. Similar effects occur with ingestion of protein or amino acids.

Calcium-Containing Stones of Uncertain Etiology

In only 50% of cases can a distinct etiology be posed for recurrent urolithiasis (infection, cystinuria, uric acid lithiasis, hyperoxaluria, renal tubular acidosis, primary hyperparathyroidism). Idiopathic urolithiasis (unknown cause) is more common in males than in females (5:1 ratio). In most cases there is mild hypophosphatemia, hypercalciuria, and increased intestinal absorption of calcium. These features constitute the syndrome of idiopathic hypercalciuria. This syndrome is difficult to differentiate from mild primary hyperparathyroidism, but subtotal parathyroidectomy has generally not been beneficial for patients with idiopathic hypercalciuria. Several metabolic patterns have been observed within this large group of patients, and recognition of these patterns might help in understanding etiologic factors and developing appropriate therapy.

Renal Calcium Leak

A subset of patients with "idiopathic hypercalciuria" manifests high concentrations of immunoreactive PTH in plasma. Reduction of urine calcium excretion by administration of thiazide diuretics normalizes urinary calcium excretion, plasma PTH concentration, and low renal phosphate threshold. Some patients with primary hyperparathyroidism show persistent hypercalciuria following surgical cure, suggesting that a calcium leak (and normocalcemic secondary hyperparathyroidism) might have been a long-standing precursor that ultimately led to semiautonomous hyperparathyroidism with normal or high serum calcium concentration. The incidence of renal calcium wastage has varied from 8 to 65% in series of idiopathic calcium urolithiasis.

Other Absorptive Hypercalciurias

The causes of hypophosphatemia in idiopathic hypercalciuria may be diverse (see preceding section). Shen and coworkers evaluated 15 consecutive patients with idiopathic hypercalciuria taking an unrestricted diet. They found a low renal threshold for phosphate excretion, hypophosphatemia, normal or high circulating concentrations of 1α, 25-$(OH)_2$-D, increased intestinal absorption of calcium, and normal or low serum PTH concentration. This may represent a renal phosphate leak. Hypophosphatemia can directly increase the production and effectiveness of 1α, 25-$(OH)_2$-D (see "Calciferol 1-α Hydroxylation," p. 954), leading to increased intestinal absorption of calcium with deleterious consequences. In one study, nine patients thought to have a primary renal phosphate leak and given supplemental phosphate (equivalent of 2g/day of phosphorus) for 8 weeks showed amelioration of all abnormal indices. In another study, 22 of 24 patients with idiopathic hypercalciuria showed absorptive hypercalciuria without hypophosphatemia. An etiologic abnormality of vitamin D metabolism was postulated. The chemical features in patients with renal calcium wastage and in the remaining patients with absorptive hypercalciuria are very similar. Patients with renal calcium wastage should show evidence of secondary hyperparathyroidism (increased serum concentration of PTH and increased urinary excretion rate of cAMP), however, the parathyroids should be suppressed in the other groups. A recent study indicates that in primary hyperparathyroidism high plasma concentrations of 1,25-$(OH)_2$-vitamin D correlate with nephrolithiasis.

Hyperuricosuria with Calcium-Containing Stones

Of 460 stone formers in a large clinic, 14.6% had increased urinary uric acid excretion and 11.7% had increased excretion rates for both uric acid and calcium. Urate concentrations above 300 mg/l at pH above 6.0 indicate that the urine is saturated with respect to sodium urate; although urate may be a minor component of total stone mass, this phase might participate in stone causation. The causes of increased renal excretion of uric acid include high purine content of the diet and high endogenous production rates for purines.

Specialized Tests

Stone Analysis

Evaluation of the patient with urolithiasis begins with analysis of stone composition. Chemical methods are widely available and highly sensitive for detecting even low concentrations of all the major components except oxalate. The mineral composition can also be accurately determined by polarization microscopy; x-ray diffraction analysis provides the most specific crystal identification and is particularly useful when there is a suspicion of an unusual composition. A predominant composition of cystine, uric acid, xanthine, magnesium ammonium phosphate, or even calcium phosphate greatly limits the diagnostic possibilities. Pure calcium phosphate stones are rare and suggest primary hyperparathyroidism or other states with renal tubular acidosis, but these disorders may present with stones of other composition as well.

Urine Composition

Tests of urine composition may give insight into an underlying disorder, particularly if stone analysis is inconclusive or not possible. These tests include the quantitation of the soluble phase, characterization of microcrystalline components, measurement of mineral saturation, and measurement of inhibitors of stone growth.

The urine components most relevant to urolithiasis include cystine, uric acid, calcium, oxalate, and hydrogen ion. Excretion rates of cystine above 40 mg/g creatinine or of uric acid above 1200 mg/g creatinine are grossly abnormal. The reader should consult other sources for discussion of cystine and uric acid stones. There are multiple forms and causes of renal acidification defects; distal renal tubular acidosis, primary hyperparathyroidism, and use of carbonic anhydrase inhibitors are associated with a propensity to form calcium phosphate stones because of limited solubility in alkaline solutions. Hypocitraturia is another feature of classic renal tubular acidosis that contributes to the stone forming diathesis. Stones rarely occur with the Fanconi syndromes or spontaneous proximal renal tubular acidosis probably because of the associated low urinary excretion rate for calcium. If urine pH (tested on the second voiding in the morning) is above 5.5, defects in renal acidification should be tested by administration of an acid load (ammonium chloride 100 mg/kg by mouth) and then by monitoring urine pH hourly for 6 hours. Failure to acidify urine to a pH below 5.3 suggests renal tubular acidosis; validation of the test requires that simultaneous induction of systemic acidosis ("arterialized" venous pH below 7.30 three hours after acid ingestion) be confirmed and urinary tract infection by urease-producing organisms (*B. proteus*) be excluded.

The significance of increased urinary excretion rates for calcium, oxalate, and urate has been discussed previously. High excretion rates of one or more of these occur frequently in patients with recurrent urolithiasis of unknown etiology. There is no consensus concerning the most useful conditions for assessing urinary excretion of these components. Abnormalities of urine composition have been characterized with samples obtained fasting or postprandially or collected for 24 hours. There also is no consensus concerning the merits of taking synthetic, low calcium, or free diets for diagnostic purposes. In the absence of clear advantages for any of these, a 24-hour collection during a free diet would seem most relevant to the conditions leading to stone formation.

Two methods of assessment of urine saturation are under development. One involves chemical quantitation of multiple components of urine and then use of an iterative computer program to derive the theoretic activity product of uncharged complexes for comparison to the activity product at saturation. The other involves chemical quantitation of multiple components in urine before and after incubation to pseudoequilibrium with seed crystals of interest. An empiric activity product ratio (initial versus saturation-equilibrium) is then calculated. For the present these are research tools without proven clinical use. Procedures are also being developed to assay for urine content of inhibitors of crystal growth and aggregation. Quantitation of inhibitory potential is another research tool without proven clinical application.

Other Metabolic Evaluations

Evaluation of parathyroid secretory status, vitamin D metabolism, or intestinal absorption of calcium may help define the causes of urinary tract lithiasis. Certain aspects of these evaluations are discussed in the section on laboratory tests. The ultimate clinical value of these analyses has yet to be established.

In summary, chemical analysis of stones and urine components has value in delineating several metabolic causes of urolithiasis. For the large remainder of cases, etiology is unknown, but perhaps current investigations will lead to the demarcation of additional treatable disorders.

Treatment of Idiopathic Calcium Urolithiasis

After a single episode of urolithiasis, approximately 50% of persons will, if untreated, form additional stones within 10 years. Specific treatment should be initiated for any recognized cause. Treatment for the following conditions will not be discussed in this section: urinary tract infection, primary hyperoxaluria, cystinuria, uric acid urolithiasis, primary hyperparathyroidism, and renal tubular acidosis. Surgical management of urolithiasis also is beyond the scope of this discussion.

Stone disease has been treated by diverse dietary or pharmacologic measures. Hippocrates is generally credited with recognizing the value of hydration in treatment of stone diathesis. Fluid intake should maintain 24-hour urine volume of 3–4 l. In practice such high intake is difficult to maintain, but the thirst mechanisms and the bladder and its sphincters adjust to the increased volume within 4 months. It is most important to maintain a dilute urine at night; thus a glass of water should be taken at bedtime and after urinating in the early morning hours. Tea and fruit juices contain modest amounts of oxalate, and should not be used in large quantities. Excessive intakes of calcium, oxalate, and protein should be avoided but there have been no controlled studies proving efficacy of these dietary restrictions. In particular, severe calcium restriction is not recommended. This may increase the absorption and excretion of oxalate and also carries a risk of long-term negative balance for calcium.

Thiazide Diuretics

Thiazide administration can decrease urinary calcium output by 50% or more in most patients, and, with long-term therapy, urinary oxalate excretion also decreases, perhaps because of decreasing intestinal absorption of calcium and oxalate. Short-acting forms should be taken twice daily, or long-acting forms once daily. Thiazides have been effective in large, unselected groups of patients with idiopathic urolithiasis, including those with normal urine calcium excretion rates. Only patients with medullary sponge kidney have shown resistance to the hypocalciuric action of thiazides.

Inorganic Phosphate

Dietary supplementation with phosphate (equivalent to 30 mg/kg of inorganic phosphorus) as the sodium or potassium salt can decrease urinary calcium output by 50% in many patients. Part of the beneficial result may be attributable to an increased urinary excretion rate of pyrophosphate or other inhibitors of stone growth. In dogs, phosphate infusion into the renal artery causes an ipsilateral increase in renal excretion of pyrophosphate, indicating a direct effect on the kidney. Phosphate treatment for pure calcium phosphate stones may increase the urine supersaturation with respect to calcium phosphate and should not be used in this circumstance. If the hypothesis of a primary renal leak for phosphate in certain patients is confirmed (see "Calcium-Containing Stones of Uncertain Etiology," p. 1022) phosphate would be appropriate treatment for such patients.

Allopurinol

This drug is given if hyperuricosuria may contribute to the stone diathesis. In 48 patients with recurrent calcium oxalate stones and hyperuricosuria as the only known abnormality in urinary composition, treatment with allopurinol was associated with formation of 8 new stones during a period (3.88 years per patient) when 95 new stones might have been predicted from past history.

There are several additional drugs for which there is little accumulated experience.

Cellulose Phosphate

This is a cellulose resin containing esterified phosphate. It adsorbs calcium and magnesium in the intestinal lumen and has been recommended as treatment for intestinal hyperabsorption of calcium. Urinary oxalate excretion increases by 9–50 mg/day during treatment, presumably because of the chelation of enteric calcium. Thus changes in urine saturation with respect to calcium oxalate may be unpredictable. During treatment the mean urinary calcium excretion can be depressed approximately 50%.

Other Drugs

The diphosphonates, pyrophosphate analogs resistant to hydrolysis, are potent inhibitors of crystal growth and aggregation. They are excreted intact in the urine. They cause increased rates of excretion of oxalate, perhaps attributable to chelation of calcium in the intestinal lumen. Furthermore, at the doses of ethane-1-hydroxy-1, 1-diphosphonate (EHDP) required to inhibit crystal growth in urine, EHDP produces osteomalacic changes in bone. Magnesium oxide has been recommended to increase the solubility of oxalate in urine. Pyridoxine has been used because of studies showing that hyperoxaluria occurs with pyridoxine deficiency. Its effectiveness has not been documented.

In summary, there is a need for well-controlled studies on the treatment of idiopathic calcium urolithiasis. The potential for side effects must be considered in committing any patient to a long-term treatment program. Commonly a specific treatable cause cannot be identified, and a high water intake plus thiazides should be recommended. Hyperuricosuria should be treated with appropriate dietary measures or allopurinol.

UTILIZATION OF THE LABORATORY IN ASSESSING CALCITROPIC HORMONES

Standard evaluations of clinical history, radiographs, and mineral concentrations in serum or urine are often inadequate to allow definitive diagnosis and therapy. This section outlines the utility and limitations of specialized tests that are used or discussed most extensively in evaluating patients with disorders relating to the calcitropic hormones and mineral metabolism. Many of these tests require technical expertise and should be undertaken in cooperation with persons experienced in their performance and interpretation.

Assessment of the State of Calcium in Blood

Total calcium concentration in serum can be determined by atomic absorption, colorimetry, or compleximetry (EDTA titration). These methods can provide information that is accurate and precise. It is ionically active calcium that determines membrane excitability and chemical reactivity and regulates the secretion of PTH and CT, however. Total serum calcium does not accurately reflect ionically active calcium when there is variation from normal of the fraction complexed to proteins and other anions.

Calcium ionic activity can be measured directly with electrodes analogous to those used for measuring pH. Serum or plasma are difficult to work with, however, because of change in specimen pH after venipuncture and because of serum protein interference with the operating characteristics of the electrodes. In most clinical laboratories, total calcium is determined with far greater precision than that for determination of calcium ion activity in serum. Current technology does not allow consistent detection of mild abnormalities in calcium ionic activity. The ion-specific electrodes are useful when there are major distortions in the calcium binding activity of serum proteins and also when there are high circulating concentrations of calcium chelators such as citrate, oxalate, EDTA, or unidentified factors.

Filtered load of calcium is of great relevance to urinary excretion of calcium. Filtrable calcium can be assessed *in vitro* by interacting serum or plasma with artificial membranes under conditions that simulate glomerular filtration. Assessment of this fraction removes variation attributable to calcium binding by protein; thus, in theory, it should correlate better with serum ionized calcium concentration than does serum total calcium concentration. Unfortunately, the precision of determinations of ultrafiltrable calcium has generally been even lower than that for ionized calcium. This test will not be clinically useful until more precise methods are developed.

Direct Assays of the Calcitropic Hormones in Blood

Parathyroid Hormone

Most of the immunoreactive PTH in peripheral blood represents inactive metabolites of the hormone. The concentrations are determined by distribution volume, secretion rate, and metabolic clearance. With the most sensitive PTH radioimmunoassays, directed at either amino- or carboxy-terminal antigens, the range of values for documented primary hyperparathyroidism overlaps 10–20% with the normal range. Furthermore, with most assays, immunoreactive PTH concentration is below the lower detection limit of the method in 50–70% of normal subjects. The presence or absence of an increased concentration of immunoreactive PTH, however, is important in assessment of patients with hypocalcemia or hypercalcemia. Determination of serum immunoreactive PTH or PTH bioactivity (see tests of renal clearance of cAMP and phosphate, p. 1026) can document the presence of secondary (hypocalcemia) or primary (hypercalcemia) hyperparathyroidism. The PTH radioimmunoassay is also useful for the localization of PTH-secreting tissues by assessment of superselective samples from the venous beds of the parathyroids or other suspicious tissues.

Calcitonin

The methodologic difficulties for this radioimmunoassay, in general, are similar to those for radioimmunoassay of PTH. Normal basal concentrations are below the lower detection limits of most assays, and, when concentrations are measureable, results with different antisera may not agree as they react with different components of the multiple circulating forms. The difficulty in detecting basal concentrations can, to some extent, be overcome by assessing the concentration after stimulating hormone secretion. Useful stimuli include calcium or pentagastrin or combinations of the two (ethanol and glucagon have been used less). Results with these secretogogues give similar information when performed in a well-standardized manner. The CT radioimmunoassay is useful for the diagnosis of medullary carcinoma of the thyroid, which is virtually always a CT-secreting tumor. When performed with high precision, the CT radioimmunoassay in serum after secretogogue administration may also allow diagnosis of the premalignant phase of this frequently hereditary tumor.

Calciferol Metabolites

Radioligand assays for the calciferol metabolites have the same limitations as those for other steroid-like compounds that circulate at low concentrations. Often serum must be purified by extraction with organic solvents and by one or more column fractionations to eliminate interfering lipids. 25-OH vitamin D can be measured in serum extracts either by ultraviolet absorption or by competitive radioligand assay. The binding proteins used have included serum 25-OH-D transport globulin, cytosol 25-OH-D binding globulin, or antibodies raised against calciferol conjugates. Purification methods resolve 25-OH-D_2 from 25-OH-D_3 but are not usually necessary in clinical application. These assays are sufficiently sensitive to detect concentrations below the normal range and are useful in assessing calciferol excess, calciferol deficiency, or certain abnormalities in calciferol metabolism (malabsorption, decreased hepatic 25-hydroxylation, or increased 25-OH-D clearance). 24,25-$(OH)_2$-vitamin D cross-reacts in most systems that detect 25-OH-D; therefore, these have been adapted to the measurement of 24,25-$(OH)_2$-D. At present, the clinical relevance of this metabolite remains unknown. Normal serum concentrations of 1,25-$(OH)_2$-D are 30 pg/ml or 0.1% of those

of 25-OH-D. Current assays of 1,25-$(OH)_2$-D in serum, therefore, require extensive sample purification and concentration. The binding proteins used have included reconstituted cytosol and chromatin from vitamin D–deficient chick intestine, stabilized cytosol from similar tissue, and antibodies raised against a calciferol conjugate. Though the early assays have been technically demanding, they showed the potential to provide clinically useful information. This assay should find applications in assessment of abnormality of serum calcium concentration, renal osteodystrophy, vitamin D dependency (differentiation of deficiency of renal 25-OH-D 1-α-hydroxylase from target tissue subsensitivity to 1,25-$[(OH)]_2$-D), and abnormal rates of intestinal calcium absorption.

Assessments of Bone Metabolism

Bone Biopsy

Many problems have prevented general use of bone biopsy. Mineral content of the tissue makes it difficult to process. Extraction of the mineral is feasible but eliminates the anatomic relation between the mineral and organic phases. Furthermore, samples from one portion of the skeleton may give information not representative of other portions. Trephine samples are obtained from the anterior superior iliac crest; alternatively, under local or general anesthesia a portion of rib or other tissue can be sampled. Undecalcified sections are imbedded in plastic as preparation for sectioning with a heavy duty microtome. Bone formation and resorption rate are evaluated in static samples by osteoblast and osteoclast counts and by total surface and volume involved in formation or resorption. Other features that can be quantitated include cortical and trabecular bone area and periosteocytic lacunar area. Tetracycline accumulates in the region of the mineralization front, and administration of one or more brief doses of tetracycline at fixed time intervals allows labeling (under fluorescent lighting) of the mineral front at one or more time points. Bone biopsy can give definitive information for diagnosis of osteomalacia, osteogenesis imperfecta, fibrogenesis imperfecta ossium, atypical Paget's disease, and juvenile osteoporosis.

Alkaline Phosphatase in Serum

Alkaline phosphatase activity in serum is a composite of enzymes from multiple sources. In the normal adult most comes from liver and bone with lesser contributions from intestine and other tissues. The osteoblast is considered to be the major skeletal source of circulating alkaline phosphatase activity, but this enzyme is also prominent in chondrocytes and matrix vesicles of bone. The skeletal alkaline phosphatase enzyme differs in electrophoretic mobility from that of the enzyme from the liver; it is also more labile to heat or urea inactivation, two criteria that permit a partial differentiation from the forms released during hepatobiliary disorders. There is no single criterion by which skeletal alkaline phosphatase can be accurately quantitated in serum. The total serum alkaline phosphatase activity is subnormal due to deficiency of the skeletal component in hypophosphatasia. An increase in the skeletal component accounts for the increase in total serum alkaline phosphatase in Paget's disease, hyperparathyroidism, fracture, and growth until puberty. The skeletal contribution may be difficult to quantitate, but alkaline phosphatase is a useful index for disease activity in diffuse Paget's disease.

Hydroxyproline in Urine

Collagen carries virtually all of the body content of hydroxyproline and hydroxylysine. Urinary excretion of hydroxyproline is an index for both rate of bone formation and rate of resorption. It can be greatly elevated in Paget's disease and to a lesser degree in hyperparathyroidism (primary or secondary), thyrotoxicosis, puberty, skeletal metastases, and fracture. The rate of urinary excretion is also determined by dietary intake (patients should consume a low gelatin diet for one day prior to this collection) and turnover of other collagen sources (excretion rates are increased in patients with burns, psoriasis, acromegaly). Of total body collagen, 60% is in bone and 30% in skin. Bone collagen composition differs from that of nonskeletal collagen, and more specific markers of skeletal collagen turnover are being investigated (for example, in the urine a high ratio of glucosyl-galactosyl hydroxylysine/lysine). Approximately 90% of the urine hydroxyproline is peptide-bound; 10% is in the form of large nondialyzable peptides. Excretion of this nondialyzable fraction may be uniquely related to bone formation as it rises following parathyroidectomy at a time when bone resorption and the excretion of total hydroxyproline are decreasing. In each patient urine hydroxyproline excretion rate cannot be directly interpreted as a measure of absolute rate of bone formation or resorption; however, when it is grossly increased, it can be monitored serially as an index of efficacy of therapy.

Calcium Kinetics

Calcium isotopes administered intravenously gradually equilibrate with stable calcium in the body. Serial measurements of isotope in blood, urine, feces, and the whole body or its segments can be analyzed in mathematical terms. Elements of the mathematical solution may correlate with well-defined physiologic processes. In particular, this procedure directly quantitates exchange with slowly equilibrating stores, reflecting bone apposition and bone resorption. Two basic types of equation have been used to fit such data, the multicompartment (linear or branching) and the expanding pool model. With the multicompartment models, three or four separate compartments are required for an optimal fit to the data. The compartment equilibrating most rapidly with injected tracer includes the vascular space but is generally four times as large. Thus there is rapid equilibrium of the tracer with diverse compartments, including ECF and others. The late equilibrating compartments are large and turn over slowly, indicating they must contain principally bone. To assess this slowly equilibrating compartment, sampling must be continued for more than 2 weeks. Expanding pool solutions assume time-dependent alterations of exchange rates of isotope with a single growing central compartment. They lack the attractive feature of constructing compartments with rough anatomic equivalents; they often provide a parsimonious fit for the data, however. With the use of stable calcium isotopes (^{48}Ca) and neutron activation of the sampled specimens, these calculations can be made without giving radioisotopes. Because of expense and the requirement that patients maintain consistent dietary and activity status during a protracted sampling period, calcium kinetic studies of patients are not widely used.

Bone Scanning with Isotopes

Bone-seeking isotopic tracers, particularly polyphosphates and diphosphonates labeled with technetium-99m, adsorb to bone crystal surfaces, allowing imaging of zones of increased turnover or increased vascularity. This technique is particularly valuable in identifying local nonhomogeneities, such as tumor, fracture, Paget's disease, and abscess. It also has the potential to identify diffusely increased rates of skeletal turnover as in hyperparathyroidism and thyrotoxicosis.

Quantitation of Skeletal Mass

Since skeletal strength bears a rough relation to total mineral content, this is a useful indicator of skeletal status. Present definitions of osteoporosis are based on decrease in total or regional skeletal content. In neutron activation analysis, exposure to a neutron flux "activates" a portion of the stable isotope ^{48}Ca to the unstable isotope ^{49}Ca. Gamma emissions from the decay of ^{49}Ca are an index of body calcium content. This method is accurate but used only in a few centers because of the demands in handling the source for the neutron flux. Status of cortical bone can be evaluated by quantitating metacarpal cortical thickness or metacarpal cortical area from standard radiographs. In population studies, these indices show the expected age-related changes with appropriate sex-related differences. There is much interpatient variability; the reproducibility is poor, particularly when separate radiographs are repeated, and there are variations in individual patients attributable to the site analyzed. For photon absorptiometry, a collimated beam of ^{125}I penetrates a bone and radiation attenuation is quantitated. Results with this technique are subject to many of the same limitations as those from quantitative morphometry, though the precision and reproducibility can be better. It has been applied principally to analyses of the radius. This technique may be extended to quantitation of cortical and trabecular bone by simultaneous use of two isotope energies and computerized tomographic analysis (dual channel absorptiometry).

Renal Clearance of Solutes as Indices of Circulating PTH Activity

Cyclic AMP

Normally approximately 50% of urinary cAMP excretion is accounted for by glomerular filtration of cAMP from plasma. The remainder is synthesized and excreted by the kidney under direct influence of circulating PTH and by as yet unidentified factors as well. Correction can be made for variations in serum concentrations of cAMP and in GFR (cAMP to creatinine clearance ratio or nephrogenous urinary cAMP excretion rate corrected for GFR). For example, the cAMP clearance ratio is the ratio between renal clearance of cAMP and clearance of creatinine:

$$\text{cAMP Cl. Ra.} = C_{cAMP}/C_{Cr} = (U_{cAMP} \times S_{Cr})/(S_{cAMP} \times U_{Cr})$$

In hypoparathyroidism it approaches a minimum of 1.0. In hyperparathyroidism it gives data with discriminatory quality stimilar to that from the radioimmunoassay of PTH in serum. cAMP can be quantitated in plasma and urine by radioimmunoassay or by radioligand assays using cytoplasmic cAMP binding proteins. Unlike the PTH radioimmunoassay, this assay includes a working range that extends below the lower limits of the normal range. It is thus particularly useful in assessing degress of hypoparathyroidism. Assessment of renal cAMP excretion after PTH administration is useful in defining states of PTH resistance (see Figure

19–44 and the discussion of pseudohypoparathyroidism types I and II, p. 993).

Phosphate

Another prominent action of PTH is regulation of renal clearance of phosphate. Indices that reflect this action include serum phosphate concentration, the renal tubular reabsorption of phosphate (TRP), and the theoretical renal phosphate threshold (see Fig. 19–2). Tubular reabsorption of phosphate is derived from the following simple relationship:

$$TRP = (Ccr - Cp)/Ccr = 1 - Up \times Scr/Ucr \times Sp.$$

The clearance study is performed in the morning over 2–4 hours with the patient fasting. Because the renal excretion of phosphate is determined by multiple factors other than serum PTH activity, these tests cannot replace the radioimmunoassay of PTH in serum or of cAMP in urine.

Calcium

PTH decreases the renal clearance of calcium. Analysis of the relation between serum calcium concentration and urinary calcium excretion thus provides indirect information about status of the PTH-calciferol axis (see Fig. 19–19). At any serum concentration of calcium, PTH suppression or deficiency is characterized by relative hypercalciuria, whereas PTH excess is characterized by relative hypocalciuria. As factors other than PTH also modulate renal clearance of calcium, these tests complement but do not replace the radioligand assay for PTH in serum or cAMP in urine. Assessment of urine calcium excretion is also relevant for the evaluation of patients with nephrolithiasis (see "Hypercalciuria and Urolithiasis," p. 1019).

Intestinal Interaction with Calcitropic Hormones

Cellular Response to Calciferols

Direct assessment of intestinal cellular responsiveness to calciferols has not yet been developed for clinical use. Assessment of vitamin D receptors and vitamin D-dependent calcium binding proteins in intestinal mucosa may become useful for this purpose.

Mineral Balance

The net balance for any metabolic component is the difference between input and output. Thus the net intestinal balance is the difference between the dietary input and the fecal output. In practice, input and output each are difficult to quantitate. Slow intestinal transit times (a nonabsorbable oral marker such as polyethylene glycol requires 3–6 days to traverse the intestines) and intestinal mixing prevent segregating accurately the fecal output remaining from one meal; thus, balance studies require evaluation periods over several days. Quantitation of input over such a long period requires rigid control of diet and is only possible with a metabolic kitchen and a highly cooperative subject. Optimal equilibration of mineral homeostasis to a constant diet requires a period of several weeks. Since important long-term consequences may derive from balance differences on the order of 50 mg/day, meticulous assessment of total intake and output is demanding but essential. Balance studies are difficult to do outside a research setting.

Isotopic Evaluation of Calcium Absorption

Unidirectional and net (the difference between lumen to plasma and plasma to lumen flux) intestinal absorption can be assessed with calcium isotopes. An isotope (usually ^{47}Ca) is administered orally with a standard meal containing a fixed amount of ^{40}Ca, usually 100 mg. Unidirectional absorption can be estimated from kinetic analysis of the isotope in timed blood samples obtained during the following ½–6 hours. The accuracy of the calculations can be enhanced by solving and correcting for clearance of circulating calcium. This is accomplished by simultaneously administering a different calcium isotope intravenously or by giving the same isotope at a different time and assuming that the patient is in the same metabolic state. Net absorption can also be quantitated by determining the difference between the administered isotope dose and the quantity excreted in feces over the following 7–10 days or by measuring the whole body isotope retention more than 7 days later, when the nonabsorbed tracer (plus that secreted by the intestines) has been eliminated from the intestines. Increased calcium absorption rates occur with calciferol excess, hyperparathyroidism, many cases of calcium nephrolithiasis, and some cases of sarcoidosis. Decreased rates occur with renal failure, hypoparathyroidism, malabsorption, and other calciferol deficiency states.

Response to Oral or Intravenous Calcium

Challenge with oral or intravenous calcium has been advocated in the evaluation of urolithiasis (oral calcium) and parathyroid autonomy (oral or intravenous calcium). These tests are not yet established as clinically useful except for diagnosis of hyperplasia or malignancy of C cells.

REFERENCES

Monographs Concerning Various Aspects of Calcium Metabolism

Aurbach, G. D. (ed.): *Parathyroid Gland. Handbook of Physiology*, Section 7: *Endocrinology*. Vol. VII. American Physiological Society. Greep, R. O., and Astwood, E. B. (eds.), Baltimore, Williams and Wilkins, 1976.

Avioli, L. V., and Krane, S. M.: *Metabolic Bone Disease*. Vol. I. New York, Academic Press, 1977.

Bourne, G. H.: *Biochemistry and Physiology of Bone Calcification and Physiology*. Vol. 4. New York, Academic Press, 1976.

Cheung, W. Y.: *Calcium and Cell Function*. New York, Academic Press, 1980.

Copp, D. H., and Talmage, R. V.: *Endocrinology of Calcium Metabolism*. Proceedings of the Sixth Parathyroid Conference, Vancouver, Canada, June 12–17, 1977. Amsterdam, Excerpta Medica, 1978.

Lawson, D. E. M.: *Vitamin D*. New York, Academic Press, 1978.

Massry, S. G., and Ritz, E.: *Phosphate Metabolism*. New York, Plenum Press, 1976.

Nordin, B. E. C.: *Calcium, Phosphate and Magnesium Metabolism*. New York, Churchill-Livingstone, 1976.

Calcium, Magnesium, and Phosphorus Metabolism

Bell, R. R., Draper, H. H., et al.: Physiological responses of human adults to foods containing phosphate additives. *J. Nutr. 107*:42, 1977.

Borle, A. B., and Uchikawa, T.: Effects of parathyroid hormone on the distribution and transport of calcium in cultured kidney cells. *Endocrinology 102*:1725, 1978.

Goldberg, M., Agus, Z. S., et al.: Renal handling of phosphate, calcium, and magnesium, In *The Kidney*. Vol. I. Brenner, B. M. and Rector, F. C., Sr. (eds.), Philadelphia, W.B. Saunders, 1976, p. 344.

Heaney, R. P.: Calcium kinetics in plasma: As they apply to the measurements of bone formation and resorption rates, In *Biochemistry and*

Physiology of Bone Calcification and Physiology. Vol. 4. Bourne, G. H. (ed.), New York, Academic Press, 1976, p. 105.

Hurwitz, S.: Calcium metabolism in birds, In *Chemical Zoology.* Vol. 10. Florkin, M., and Scheer, B. J. (eds.), New York, Academic Press, 1978, p. 273.

Lennon, E. J., Lemann, J., Jr., et al.: Effect of glucose on urinary cation excretion during extracellular volume expansion in normal man. *J. Clin. Invest.* 53:1424, 1974.

Livingston, D. M., and Wacker, W. E. C.: Magnesium metabolism, In *Handbook of Physiology,* Section 7: *Endocrinology* (Vol VII. *Parathyroid Gland*). American Physiological Society. Greep, R. O., and Astwood, E. B. (eds.), Baltimore, Williams and Wilkins, 1976, p. 215.

Toffaletti, J., Savory, J., et al.: Use of gel filtration to examine the distribution of calcium among serum proteins. *Clin. Chem.* 23:2306, 1977.

Scarpa, A., and Carafoli, E.: *Calcium Transport and Cell Function.* New York, Academic Press, 1978, p. 307.

Urist, M. R.: Biogenesis of bone: calcium and phosphorus in the skeleton and blood in vertebrate evolution, In *Handbook of Physiology,* Section 7: *Endocrinology* (Vol. VII. *Parathyroid Gland*). American Physiological Society. Greep, R. O., and Astwood, E. B. (eds.), Baltimore, Williams and Wilkins, 1976, p. 183.

Walser, M.: Divalent cations: physicochemical state in glomerular filtrate and urine and renal excretion, In *Handbook of Physiology,* American Physiological Society. Orloff, R. O., and Berliner, R. W. (eds.), Baltimore, Williams and Wilkins, 1973, p. 555.

Wasserman, R. H., Corradino, R. A., et al. (eds.): *Calcium-Binding Proteins and Calcium Function.* New York, Elsevier/North-Holland, 1977.

Bone — Chemistry and Structure

Aaron, J.: Histology and microanatomy of bone, In *Calcium, Phosphate and Magnesium Metabolism.* Nordin, B. E. C. (ed.), New York, Churchill-Livingstone, 1976, p. 298.

Aurbach, G. D.: Hormone receptors, cyclic nucleotides and control of cell function, In *The Year in Metabolism 1975–1976.* Freinkel, N. (ed.), New York, Plenum Medical Book Company, 1976, p. 1.

Aurbach, G. D., and Chase, L. R.: Cyclic nucleotides and biochemical actions of parathyroid hormone and calcitonin, In *Handbook of Physiology,* Section 7: *Endocrinology* (Vol. VII. *Parathyroid Gland*). American Physiological Society. Greep, R. O., and Astwood, E. B. (eds.), Baltimore, Williams and Wilkins, 1976, p. 353.

Glimcher, M. J.: Composition, structure and organization of bone and other mineralized tissues and the mechanism of calcification, In *Handbook of Physiology,* Section 7: *Endocrinology* (Vol. VII. *Parathyroid Gland*). American Physiological Society. Greep, R. O., and Astwood, E. B. (eds.), Baltimore, Williams and Wilkins, 1976, p. 25.

Harris, W. H., and Heaney, R. P.: Skeletal renewal and metabolic bone disease. *N. Engl. J. Med.* 280:193, 1969.

Raisz, L. G.: Bone metabolism and calcium regulation, In *Metabolic Bone Disease.* Vol. I. Avioli, L. V., and Krane, S. M. (eds.), New York, Academic Press, 1977, p. 1.

Parathyroid Hormone and Calcitonin

Bank, N.: The effects of changes in tubular pH on renal transport of phosphate. (in press).

Barnicot, N. A.: The local action of the parathyroid and other tissues on bone in intracerebral grafts. *J. Anat.* 82:233, 1948.

Baumann, K., Chan, Y.-L., et al.: Effect of parathyroid hormone and cyclic adenosine 3′,5′-monophosphate on isotonic fluid reabsorption: polarity of proximal tubular cells. *Kidney Intl.* 11:77, 1977.

Belanger, L. F.: Osteolysis: an outlook on its mechanism and causation, In *The Parathyroid Glands: Ultrastructure, Secretion and Function.* Gaillard, P. J., Talmage, R. V., et al. (eds.), Chicago, University of Chicago Press, 1965, p. 137.

Bell, N. H., Avery, S., et al.: Effects of dibutyryl cyclic adenosine 3′,5′-monophosphate and parathyroid extract on calcium and phosphorus metabolism in hypoparathyroidism and pseudohypoparathyroidism. *J. Clin. Invest.* 51:816, 1972.

Berson, S. A., and Yalow, R. S.: Parathyroid hormone in plasma in adenomatous hyperparathyroidism, uremia and bronchiogenic carcinoma. *Science* 154:907, 1966.

Biddulph, D. M., and Wrenn, R. W.: Effects of parathyroid hormone on cyclic AMP, cyclic GMP, and efflux of calcium in isolated renal tubules. *J. Cyclic Nucleotide Res.* 3:129, 1977.

Bourdeau, J. E., and Burg, M. B.: Effect of PTH on calcium transport across the cortical thick ascending limb of Henle's loop. *Am. J. Physiol.* 239:F121, 1980.

Breslau, N., and Moses, A. M.: Renal calcium reabsorption caused by bicarbonate and by chlorothiazide in patients with hormone resistant (pseudo) hypoparathyroidism. *J. Clin. Endocrinol. Metab.* 46:389, 1978.

Broadus, A. E., Kaminsky, N. I., et al.: Kinetic parameters and renal clearances of plasma adenosine 3′,5′-monophosphate and guanosine 3′,5′-monophosphate in man. *J. Clin. Invest.* 49:2222, 1970.

Broadus, A. E., Kaminsky, N. I., et al.: Effects of glucagon on adenosine 3′-5′-monophosphate and guanosine 3′,5′-monophosphate in human plasma and urine. *J. Clin. Invest.* 49:2237, 1970.

Brown, E. M., Carroll, R. J., et al.: Dopaminergic stimulation of cyclic AMP accumulation and parathyroid hormone release from dispersed bovine parathyroid cells. *Proc. Natl. Acad. Sci. USA* 74:4210, 1977.

Brown, E. M., Hurwitz, S., et al.: Beta-adrenergic stimulation of cyclic AMP content and parathyroid hormone release from isolated bovine parathyroid cells. *Endocrinology* 100:1696, 1977.

Brown, E. M., Hurwitz, S., et al.: Direct identification of beta-adrenergic receptors on isolated bovine parathyroid cells. *Endocrinology* 100:1703, 1977.

Brown, E. M., Pazoles, C. J., et al.: Role of anions in parathyroid hormone release from dispersed bovine parathyroid cells. *Proc. Natl. Acad. Sci. USA* 75:876, 1978.

Canterbury, J. M., Lerman, S., et al.: Inhibition of parathyroid hormone secretion by 25-hydroxycholecalciferol and 24,25-dihydroxycholecalciferol in the dog. *J. Clin. Invest.* 61:1375, 1978.

Chabardes, D., Imbert-Teboul, M., et al.: Distribution of adenylate cyclase-linked hormone receptors in the nephron, In *Endocrinology of Metabolism.* Copp, D. H., and Talmage, R. V. (eds.), Amsterdam, Excerpta Medica, 1978, p. 209.

Chambers, D. J., Schäfer, H., et al.: Dose-related activation by PTH of specific enzymes in various regions of the kidney, In *Endocrinology of Calcium Metabolism.* Copp, D. H., and Talmage, R. V. (eds.), Proceedings of the Sixth Parathyroid Conference, Vancouver, Canada, June 12–17, 1977. Amsterdam, Excerpta Medica, 1978, p. 216.

Chang, H. Y.: Grafts of parathyroid and other tissues to bone. *Anat. Rec.* 3:23, 1951.

Cohn, D. V., MacGregor, R. R., et al.: Calcemic fraction-A: biosynthetic peptide precursor of parathyroid hormone. *Proc. Natl. Acad. Sci. USA* 69:1521, 1972.

Cooper, C. W., Bolman, R. M., III, et al.: Interrelationships between calcium, calcemic hormones and gastrointestinal hormones. *Recent Progr. Horm. Res.* 34:259, 1978.

Cooper, C. W., Hirsch, P. F., et al.: Calcitonin — measurement: bioassay, In *Methods in Investigation and Diagnostic Endocrinology.* Vol. 2B. Berson, S. A., and Yalow, R. S. (eds.), New York, Elsevier/North-Holland, 1973, p. 1003.

Dennis, V. W.: Influence of bicarbonate on parathyroid hormone-induced changes in fluid absorption by the proximal tubule. *Kidney Int.* 10:373, 1976.

Dousa, T. P., and Steiner, A. L.: Immunofluorescent localization of cyclic nucleotides in the nephron, In *Endocrinology of Calcium Metabolism.* Copp, D. H., and Talmage, R. V. (eds.), Amsterdam, Excerpta Medica, 1978, p. 221.

Eilon, G., and Raisz, L. G.: Comparison of the effects of stimulators and inhibitors of resorption on the release of lysozomal enzymes and radioactive calcium from fetal bone in organ culture. *Endocrinology* 103:1969, 1978.

Fischer, J. A., Blum, J. W., et al.: Acute parathyroid hormone response to epinephrine in vivo. *J. Clin. Invest.* 52:2434, 1973.

Gill, J. R., Jr., and Casper, A. G. T.: Depression of proximal tubular sodium reabsorption in the dog in response to renal beta-adrenergic stimulation by isoproterenol. *J. Clin. Invest.* 50:112, 1971.

Gold, L. W., Massry, S. G., et al.: Renal bicarbonate wasting during phosphage depletion: a possible cause of altered acid-base homeostasis in hyperparathyroidism. *J. Clin. Invest.* 52:2556, 1973.

Habener, J. F., and Potts, J. T., Jr.: Chemistry, biosynthesis, secretion, and metabolism of parathyroid hormone, In Handbook of Physiology, (Section 7: *Endocrinology* (Vol. VII. *Parathyroid Gland*). American Physiological Society. Greep, R. O., and Astwood, E. B. (eds.), Baltimore, Williams and Wilkins, 1976, p. 313.

Habener, J. F., Powell, D., et al.: Parathyroid hormone: secretion and metabolism in vivo. *Proc. Natl. Acad. Sci. USA* 68:2986, 1971.

Habener, J. F., Rosenblatt, M., et al.: Pre-preparathyroid hormone: amino acid sequence, chemical synthesis, and some biological studies of the precursor region. *Proc. Natl. Acad. Sci. USA* 75:2616, 1978.

Hanley, D. A., Takatsuki, K., et al.: Direct release of parathyroid hormone fragments from functioning bovine parathyroid glands in vitro. *J. Clin. Invest.* 62:1247, 1978.

Heath, D. A., and Aurbach, G. D.: Studies on the binding of ^{125}I-parathyroid hormone to renal cortical membranes. In *Calcium-Regulating Hormones.* Talmage, R. V., Owen, M., et al. (eds.), Proceedings of the Fifth Parathyroid Conference. Amsterdam, Excerpta Medica, 1975, p. 159.

Holtrop, M. E., and King, G. J.: The ultrastructure of the osteoclast and its functional implications. *Clin. Orthop.* 123:177, 1977.

Holtrop, M. E., King, G. J., et al.: Factors influencing osteoclast activity as measured by ultrastructural morphometry, In *Endocrinology of Calcium Metabolism.* Copp, D. H., and Talmage, R. V. (eds.), Amsterdam, Excerpta Medica, 1978, p. 91.

Holtrop, M. E., and Raisz, L. G.: The effects of parathyroid hormone, colchicine, and calcitonin on the ultrastructure and the activity of osteoclasts in organ culture. *J. Cell Biol.* 60:346, 1974.

Hruska, K. A., Martin, K., et al.: Degradation of parathyroid hormone and fragment production by the isolated perfused dog kidney. The effect of glomerular filtration rate and perfusate calcium concentrations. *J. Clin. Invest.* 60:501, 1977.

Insel, P., Balakir, R., et al.: Binding of cyclic AMP to renal brush-border membranes. *J Cyclic Nucleotide Res* 1:107, 1975.

Jones, S. J., and Boyde, A.: Scanning electron microscopy of bone cells in culture, In *Endocrinology of Calcium Metabolism.* Copp, D. H., and Talmage, R. V. (eds.), Amsterdam, Excerpta Medica, 1978, p. 97.

Kemper, B., Habener, J. F., et al.: Parathyroid secretion: discovery of a major calcium-dependent protein. *Science* 187:167, 1974.

Keutmann, H. T.: Chemistry of parathyroid hormone. In DeGroot, L. J., Cahill, G. F., Jr., Martini, L., Nelson, D. H., Odell, W. D., Potts, J. T., Jr., Steinberger, E., and Winegrad, A. I. (eds.), *Endocrinology,* Vol. 2, New York, Grune & Stratton, 1980, pp. 593–597.

Kinne, R., Shlatz, L. J., et al.: Distribution of membrane-bound cyclic AMP-dependent protein kinase in plasma membranes of cells of the kidney cortex. *J. Membr. Biol.* 24:145, 1975.

Kronenberg, H. M., McDevitt, B. E., et al.: Studies of parathyroid hormone biosynthesis using recombinant DNA technology. *Proceedings of the VII International Conference on Calcium Regulating Hormones* (in press).

Marx, S. J., Woodard, C., et al.: Renal receptors for calcitonin: binding and degradation of hormone. *J. Biol. Chem.* 248:4797, 1973.

McKinney, T. D., and Burg, M. B.: Bicarbonate secretion by rabbit cortical collecting tubules in vitro. *J. Clin. Invest.* 61:1421, 1978.

McPartlin, J., Skrabanek, P., et al.: Early effects of parathyroid hormone on rat calvarian bone alkaline phosphatase. *Endocrinology* 103:1573, 1978.

Milhaud, G., Rankin, J. C., et al.: Calcitonin: its hormonal action on the gill. *Proc. Natl. Acad. Sci. USA* 74:4693, 1977.

Minkin, C., Blackman, L., et al.: Effects of parathyroid hormone and calcitonin on adenylate cyclase in murine mononuclear phagocytes. *Biochem. Biophys. Res. Commun.* 76:875, 1977.

Mundy, G. R., Varani, J., et al.: Resorbing bone is chemotactic for monocytes. *Nature* 275:132, 1978.

Munson, P. L.: Studies on the role of the parathyroids in calcium and phosphorus metabolism. *Ann. N.Y. Acad. Sci.* 60:776, 1955.

Munson, P. L.: Physiology and pharmacology of thyrocalcitonin, In *Handbook of Physiology,* Section 7: *Endocrinology* (Vol. VII. *Parathyroid Gland*). American Physiological Society. Greep, R. O., and Astwood, E. B. (eds.), Baltimore, Williams and Wilkins, 1976, p. 443.

Nunez, E. A., and Gershan, M. D.: Cytophysiology of thyroid parafollicular C cells. *Int. Rev. Cytol.* 52:1, 1978.

Pearse, A. G. E.: Morphology and cytochemistry of thyroid and ultimobranchial C cells, In *Handbook of Physiology,* Section 7: *Endocrinology* (Vol. VII. *Parathyroid Gland*). American Physiological Society. Greep, R. O., and Astwood, E. B. (eds.), Baltimore, Williams and Wilkins, 1976, p. 411.

Peck, W. A., Carpenter, J., et al.: Cyclic 3',5'-adenosine monophosphate in isolated bone cells: response to adenosine and parathyroid hormone. *Endocrinology* 94:148, 1974.

Pfeuffer, T.: GTP-binding proteins in membranes and the control of adenylate cyclase activity. *J. Biol. Chem.* 252:7224, 1977.

Potts, J. T., Jr., and Aurbach, G. D.: Chemistry of the calcitonins, In *Handbook of Physiology,* Section 7: *Endocrinology* (Vol. VII. *Parathyroid Gland*). American Physiological Society. Greep, R. O., and Astwood, E. B. (eds.), Baltimore, Williams and Wilkins, 1976, p. 423.

Puschett, J. B.: Renal micropuncture studies of parathyroid hormone action, In *Endocrinology of Calcium Metabolism.* Copp, D. H., and Talmage, R. V. (eds.), Amsterdam, Excerpta Medica, 1978, p. 226.

Raisz, L. G.: Mechanisms of bone resorption, In *Handbook of Physiology,* Section 7: *Endocrinology* (Vol. VII. *Parathyroid Gland*). American Physiological Society. Greep, R. O., and Astwood, E. B. (eds.), Baltimore, Williams and Wilkins, 1976, p. 117.

Raisz, L. G., Brand, J. S., et al.: Interactions of parathyroid hormone and thyrocalcitonin on bone resorption in tissue culture, In *Parathyroid Hormone and Thyrocalcitonin (Calcitonin).* Talmage, R. V., and Belanger, L. F. (eds.), Amsterdam, Excerpta Medica, 1968, p. 370.

Rodan, S. B., and Rodan, G. A.: The effect of parathyroid hormone and thyrocalcitonin on the accumulation of cyclic adenosine 3',5'-monophosphate in freshly isolated bone cells. *J. Biol. Chem.* 249:3068, 1974.

Rodan, G. A., Rodan, S. B., et al.: Parathyroid hormone stimulation of adenylate cyclase activity and lactic acid accumulation in calvaria of osteopetrotic (ia) rats. *Endocrinology* 102:1501, 1978.

Rosenblatt, M., Callahan, E. N., et al.: Parathyroid hormone inhibitors: design, synthesis, and biologic evaluation of hormone and analogues. *J. Biol. Chem.* 252:5847, 1977.

Roth, S. I., and Shiller, A. L.: Comparative anatomy of the parathyroid glands, In *Handbook of Physiology,* Section 7: *Endocrinology* (Vol. VII *Parathyroid Gland*). American Physiological Society. Greep, R. O., and Astwood, E. B. (eds.), Baltimore, Williams and Wilkins, 1976, p. 281.

Shlatz, L. J., Schwarta, I. L., et al.: Distribution of parathyroid hormone-stimulated adenylate cyclase in plasma membranes of cells of the kidney cortex. *J. Membr. Biol.* 24:131, 1975.

Strewler, G. J., and Orloff, J.: Role of cyclic nucleotides in the transport of water and electrolytes, In *Advances in Cyclic Nucleotide Research.* Vol. 8. Greengard, P., and Robisin, G. A. (eds.), New York, Raven Press, 1977, p. 311.

Sutton, R. A. L., and Dirks, J. H.: Renal handling of calcium. *Fed. Proc.* 37:2112, 1978.

Taylor, A. L., Davis, B. B., et al.: Factors influencing the urinary excretion of 3',5'-adenosine monophosphate in humans. *J. Clin. Endocrinol. Metab.* 30:316, 1970.

Vaes, G.: Parathyroid hormone-like action of N^6-2'-O-dibutyryladenosine-3'5' (cyclic)-monophosphate on bone explants in tissue culture. *Nature* 219:939, 1968.

Walker, D. G.: Concentration of splenic lymphocytes with bone resorption-restorative activity (BRRA) by velocity sedimentation at unit gravity, In *Endocrinology of Calcium Metabolism.* Copp, D. H., and Talmage, R. V. (eds.), Amsterdam, Excerpta Medica, 1978, p. 105.

Calciferols

Bell, P. A.: The chemistry of the vitamins D, In *Vitamin D.* Lawson, D. E. M. (ed.), New York, Academic Press, 1978, p. 1.

Corvol, M. T., Dumontier, M. F., et al.: Vitamin D and cartilage. II. Biological activity of 25-hydroxycholecalciferol and 24,25- and 1,25-dihydroxycholecalciferols on cultured growth plate chondrocytes. *Endocrinology* 102:1269, 1978.

Haddad, J. G., Jr., and Walgate, J.: Radioimmunoassay of the binding protein for vitamin D and its metabolites in human serum. *J. Clin. Invest.* 58:1217, 1976.

Holick, M. F., and DeLuca, H. F.: Metabolism of vitamin D, In *Vitamin D.* Lawson, D. E. M. (ed.), New York, Academic Press, 1978, p. 51.

Hughes, M. R., Baylink, D. J., et al.: Radioligand receptor assay for 25-hydroxyvitamin D_2/D_3 and 1-alpha,25-dihydroxyvitamin D_2/D_3. Application to hypervitaminosis D. *J. Clin. Invest.* 58:61, 1976.

Lawson, D. E. M.: Biochemical responses of the intestine to vitamin D, In *Vitamin D.* Lawson, D. E. M. (ed.), New York, Academic Press, 1978, p. 167.

Mawer, E. B., Blackhouse, J., et al.: The distribution and storage of vitamin D and its metabolites in human tissues. *Clin. Sci.* 43:413, 1972.

Norman, A. W.: Calcium and phosphorus absorption, In *Vitamin D.* Lawson, D. E. M. (ed.), New York Academic Press 1978, p. 93.

Tanaka, Y., Castillo, L., et al.: Control of renal vitamin D hydroxylases in birds by sex hormones. *Proc. Natl. Acad. Sci. USA* 73:2701, 1976.

Miscellaneous Endogenous Calcitropic Factors

Aitken, J. M.: Bone metabolism in post-menopausal women, In *The Menopause. A Guide to Current Research and Practice.* Beard, R. J. (ed.), Baltimore, University Press, 1976, p. 95.

Mundy, G. R., Shapiro, J. L., et al.: Direct stimulation of bone resorption by thyroid hormones. *J. Clin. Invest.* 58:529, 1976.

Raisz, L. G., Luben, R. A., et al.: Effect of osteoclast activating factor from human leukocytes on bone metabolism. *J. Clin. Invest.* 56:408, 1975.

Tashjian, A. H., Voelkel, E. F., et al.: Plasma concentrations of 13,14-dihydro-15-keto-prostaglandin E_2 in rabbits bearing the VX₂ carcinoma: effects of hydrocortisone and indomethacin. *Prostaglandins* 14:309, 1977.

Hyperparathyroidism

Albright, F., Aub, J. C., et al.: Hyperparathyroidism. *J.A.M.A. 16*:1276, 1934.

Black, W. C., III, and Utley, J. R.: The differential diagnosis of parathyroid adenoma and chief cell hyperplasia. *Am. J. Clin. Pathol.* 49:761, 1968.

Boonstra, C. E., and Jackson, C. E.: Hyperparathyroidism detected by routine serum calcium analysis. *Ann. Intern. Med.* 63:468, 1965.

Boxer, M., Ellman, L., et al.: Anemia in primary hyperparathyroidism. *Arch. Intern. Med.* 137:588, 1977.

Broadus, A. E., Horst, R. L., et al.: The importance of circulating 1,25-dihydroxyvitamin D in the pathogenesis of hypercalciuria and renal stone formation in primary hyperparathyroidism. *N. Engl. J. Med.* 302:421, 1980.

Capen, C. C., and Roth, S. I.: Ultrastructural and function relationships of normal and pathologic parathyroid cells. *Pathobiol. Annu.* 3:129, 1973.

Castleman, B., Schwartz, A., et al.: Parathyroid hyperplasia in primary hyperparathyroidism. *Cancer* 38:1668, 1976.

Chayen, J., Daly, J. R., et al.: The cytochemical bioassay of hormones. *Recent Progr Horm. Res.* 32:33, 1976.

Cushard, W. G., Creditor, M. A., et al.: Physiologic hyperparathyroidism in pregnancy. *J. Clin. Endocrinol. Metab.* 34:768, 1972.

Delmonico, F. L., et al.: Hyperparathyroidism during pregnancy. *Am. J. Surg.* 131:329, 1976.

Genant, H. K., Baron, J. M., et al.: Osteosclerosis in primary hyperparathyroidism. *Am. J. Med.* 59:104, 1975.

Hanley, D. A., and Sherwood, L. M.: Secondary hypoparathyroidism in chronic renal failure: pathophysiology and treatment. *Med. Clin. North Am.* 62:1319, 1978.

Kaplan, R. A., Haussler, M. R., et al.: The role of 1-alpha,25-dihydroxyvitamin D in the mediation of intestinal hyperabsorption of calcium in primary hyperparathyroidism and absorptive hypercalciuria. *J. Clin. Invest.* 59:756, 1977.

Kaplan, R. O., Snyder, W. H., et al.: Metabolic effects of parathyroidectomy in asymptomatic primary hyperparathyroidism. *J. Clin. Endocrinol. Metab.* 42:415, 1976.

Llach, F., Massry, S. G., et al.: Skeletal resistance to endogenous parathyroid hormone in patients with early renal failure: a possible cause for secondary hyperparathyroidism. *J. Clin. Endocrinol. Metab.* 41:339, 1975.

Mallette, L. E.: Anemia in hypercalcemic hyperparathyroidism. Renewed interest in an old observation. *Arch. Intern. Med.* 137:572, 1977.

Mallette, L. E., Bilezikian, J. P., et al.: Primary hyperparathyroidism: clinical and biochemical features. *Medicine* 53:127, 1974.

Mallette, L. E., Sode, J. E., et al.: Total body retention of orally administered [47]calcium in primary hyperparathyroidism. *J. Clin. Endocrinol. Metab.* 40:582, 1975.

Marx, S. J., Spiegel, A. M., et al.: Familial hypocalciuric hypercalcemia. In *Pediatric Diseases Related to Calcium.* DeLuca, H. F., and Anast, C. S. (eds.), New York, Elsevier/North Holland, 1980, p. 413.

Massry, S. G., Coburn, J. W., et al.: Skeletal resistance to parathyroid hormone in renal failure. *Ann. Intern. Med.* 78:357, 1973.

Morris, R. C., Sebastian, A., et al.: Renal acidosis. *Kidney Int.* 1:322, 1972.

Patten, B. M., Bilezikian, J. P., et al.: Neuromuscular disease in primary hyperparathyroidism. *Ann. Intern. Med.* 80:182, 1974.

Prinz, R. A., Paloyan, E., Lawrence, A. M., et al.: Radiation-associated hyperparathyroidism: A new syndrome? *Surgery* 82:296, 1977.

Purnell, D. C., Scholz, D. A., et al.: Treatment of primary hyperparathyroidism. *Am. J. Med.* 56:800, 1974.

Rao, S. D., Frame, B., et al.: Hyperparathyroidism following head and neck irradiation. *Arch. Intern. Med.* 140:205, 1980.

Schwartz, A., and Castleman, B.: Parathyroid carcinoma: a study of 70 cases. *Cancer* 31:600, 1973.

Shaw, J. W., Oldham, S. B., et al.: Urinary cyclic AMP analyzed as a function of the serum calcium and parathyroid hromone in the differential diagnosis of hypercalcemia. *J. Clin. Invest.* 59:14, 1977.

Silverman, R., and Yalow, R.: Heterogeneity of parathyroid hormone: clinical and physiological implications. *J. Clin. Invest.* 52:1958, 1973.

Spiegel, A. M., Marx, S. J., et al.: Parathyroid function after parathyroidectomy: evaluation by measurement of urinary cAMP and parathyroid hormone in plasma. *Clin. Endocrinol.* (in press).

Wells, S. A., Ellis, G. J., et al.: Parathyroid autotransplantation in primary parathyroid hyperplasia. *N. Engl. J. Med.* 295:57, 1976.

Hypercalcemic Disorders

Benabe, J. E., and Martinez-Maldonads, M.: Hypercalcemic nephropathy. *Arch. Intern. Med.* 138:777, 1978.

Bergstrom, W. H.: Hypercalciuria and hypercalcemia complicating immobilization. *Am. J. Dis. Child.* 132:553, 1978.

Bronsky, D., Dubin, A., et al.: Calcium and the electrocardiogram. II. The electrocardiographic manifestations of hyperparathyroidism and of marked hypercalcemia from various other etiologies. *Am. J. Cardiol.* 7:833, 1961.

Burman, K. D., Monchik, J. M., et al.: Ionized and total serum calcium and parathyroid hormone in hyperthyroidism. *Ann. Intern. Med.* 84:668, 1976.

Burnett, C. H., Commons, R. R., et al.: Hypercalcemia without hypercalciuria of hypophosphatemia, calcinosis and renal insufficiency. A syndrome following prolonged intake of milk and alkali. *N. Engl. J. Med.* 240:787, 1949.

Christensson, T., Hellstrom, K., et al.: Hypercalcemia and primary hyperparathyroidism: prevalence in patients receiving thiazides as detected in a health screen. *Arch. Intern. Med.* 137:1138, 1977.

deTorrente, A., Berl, T., et al.: Hypercalcemia of acute renal failure. *Am. J. Med.* 61:119, 1976.

Frame, B., and Jackson, C. E.: Hypercalcemia and skeletal effects in chronic hypervitaminosis A. *Ann. Intern. Med.* 80:44, 1974.

Hutchins, G. M., Mirvis, S. E., et al.: Supravalvular aortic stenosis with parafollicular cell (C-cell) hyperplasia. *Am. J. Med.* 64:967, 1978.

Neer, R. M., and Potts, J. T., Jr.: Medical management of hypercalcemia and hyperparathyroidism, In DeGroot, L. J., Cahill, G. F., Jr., Martini, J., Nelson, D. H., Odell, W. D., Potts, J. T., Jr., Steinberger, E., and Winegrad, A. I. (ed). *Endocrinology,* Vol. 2, New York, Grune & Stratton, 1980, pp. 725–734.

Raisz, L. B.: New diphosphonates to block bone resorption (Editorial). *N. Engl. J. Med.* 302:347, 1980.

Rodman, J. S., and Sherwood, L. M.: Disorders of mineral metabolism in malignancy, In *Metabolic Bone Disease.* Avioli, L., and Krane, S. (eds.), New York, Academic Press, 1978.

Schneider, A., and Sherwood, L. M.: Calcium homeostasis and the pathogenesis and management of hypercalcemic disorders. *Metabolism* 23:975, 1974.

Stewart, A. F., Horst, R., et al.: Biochemical evaluation of patients with cancer-associated hypercalcemia. *N. Engl. J. Med.* 303:1377, 1980.

Winnacker, J. L., Becker, K. L., et al.: Endocrine aspects of sarcoidosis. *N. Engl. J. Med.* 278:427, 1968.

Hypoparathyroidism and Hypocalcemic Disorders

Avioli, L. V.: The therapeutic approach to hypoparathyroidism. *Am. J. Med.* 57:34, 1974.

Bronsky, D., Kushner, D. S., et al.: Idiopathic hypoparathyroidism and pseudohypoparathyroidism: case reports and review of the literature. *Medicine* 37:317, 1958.

Chase, L. R., Melson, G. L., et al.: Pseudohypoparathyroidism: defective excretion of 3′,5′-AMP in response to parathyroid hormone. *J. Clin. Invest.* 48:1832, 1969.

David, L., and Anast, C.: Calcium metabolism in newborn infants. *J. Clin. Invest.* 54:287, 1974.

Drezner, M. K., and Burch, W. M., Jr.: Altered activity of the nucleotide regulatory site in the PTH sensitive adenylate cyclase from the renal cortex of a patient with pseudohypoparathyroidism. *J. Clin. Invest.* 62:1222, 1978.

Drezner, M., Neelon, F. A., et al.: Pseudohypoparathyroidism type II: a possible defect in the reception of the cyclic AMP signal. *N. Engl. J. Med.* 289:1056, 1973.

Mann, J. B., Alterman, S., et al.: Albright's hereditary osteodystrophy comprising pseudohypoparathyroidism and pseudopseudohypoparathyroidism. *Ann. Intern. Med.* 56:315, 1962.

Nusynowitz, M. L., Frame, B., et al.: The spectrum of the hypoparathyroid states. *Medicine* 55:105, 1976.

Porter, R. H., Cox, B. C., et al.: Treatment of hypoparathyroid patients with chlorthalidane. *N. Engl. J. Med.* 298:578, 1978.

Potts, J. T., Jr.: Pseudohypoparathyroidism, In *Endocrinology,* Vol. 2, DeGroot, L. J., Cahill, G. F., Jr., Martini, L., Potts, J. T., Jr., Nelson, D. H., Steinberger, E., and Winegrad, A. I. (eds.), New York, Grune & Stratton, 1980, pp. 769–776.

Rude, R. K., Oldham, S. B., et al.: PTH secretion in magnesium deficiency. *J. Clin. Endocrinol. Metab.* 47:800, 1978.

Schneider, A. B., and Sherwood, L. M.: Pathogenesis and management of hypoparathyroidism and other hypocalcemic disorders. *Metabolism* 24:871, 1975.

Rickets and Osteomalacia

Dominguez, J. H., Gray, R. W., et al.: Dietary phosphate deprivation in women and men: effects on mineral acid balances, parathyroid hormone and the metabolism of 25-OH-vitamin D. *J. Clin. Endocrinol. Metab.* 43:1056, 1976.

Drezner, M. K., and Feinglos, M. N.: Osteomalacia due to 1-alpha,25-dihydroxycholecalciferol deficiency. Association with a giant cell tumor of bone. *J. Clin. Invest.* 60:1046, 1977.

Hillman, L. S., and Haddad, J. G.: Perinatal vitamin D metabolism. II. Serial 25-hydroxy-vitamin D concentrations in sera of term and premature infants. *J. Pediatr.* 86:928, 1975.

Marx, S. J., Spiegel, A. M., et al.: Familial syndrome of decrease in sensitivity to 1,25-dihydroxyvitamin D. *J. Clin. Endocrinol. Metab.* 47:1303, 1978.

Rasmussen, H., and Anast, C.: Familial hypophosphatemic (vitamin D resistant) rickets and vitamin D-dependent rickets, In *Metabolic Basis of Inherited Disease.* 4th Ed. Stanbury, J. B., Wyngaarden, J. B., et al. (eds.), New York, McGraw-Hill, 1978, p. 1537.

Rasmussen, H., and Bartter, F. C.: Hypophosphatasia, In *Metabolic Basis of Inherited Disease.* 4th Ed. Stanbury, J. B., Wyngaarden, J. B., et al. (eds.), New York, McGraw-Hill, 1978, p. 1340.

Scriver, C. R., Reade, T. M., et al.: Serum 1,25-dihydroxyvitamin D levels in normal subjects and in patients with hereditary rickets or bone disease. *N. Engl. J. Med.* 299:976, 1978.

Sokoloff, L.: Occult osteomalacia in American (USA) patients with fracture of the hip. *Am. J. Surg. Pathol.* 2:21, 1978.

Swan, C. H. J., Shah, K., et al.: Fibrogenesis imperfecta ossium. *Q. J. Med.* 178:233, 1976.

Tenenhouse, H. S., Scriver, C. R., et al.: Renal handling of phosphate in vivo and in vitro by the X-linked hypophosphatemic male mouse: evidence for a defect in the brush border membrane. *Kidney Int.* 14:236, 1978.

Metabolic Bone Disease

Avioli, L. V.: Osteoporosis: pathogenesis and therapy, In *Metabolic Bone Disease.* Vol. I. Avioli, L. V., and Krane, S. M. (eds.), New York, Academic Press, 1977, p. 307.

Ballet, J. J., and Griscelli, C.: Lymphoid cell transplantation in human osteopetrosis, In *Proceedings, Mechanisms of Localized Bone Loss.* (Supplement to Calcified Tissue Abstracts.) Horten, J. E., Tarpley, T. M., et al. (eds.), Washington D.C., Information Retrieval, Inc., 1978, p. 399.

Beighton, P., Horan, F., et al.: A review of the osteopetroses. *Postgrad. Med. J.* 53:507, 1977.

Ehrig, J., and Wilson, D. R.: Fibrous dysplasia of bone and primary hyperparathyroidism. *Ann. Intern. Med.* 77:234, 1972.

Hahn, T. J.: Corticosteroid-induced osteopenia. *Arch Intern. Med. 138*:882, 1978.

Horsman, A.: Bone mass in calcium, phosphate, and magnesium metabolism, In *Clinical Physiology and Diagnostic Procedures.* Nordin, B. E. C. (ed.), London, Churchill-Livingstone, 1976, p. 357.

Jowsey, J., and Offord, K. D.: Osteoporosis: juvenile, idiopathic and postmenopausal, In *Proceedings, Mechanisms of Localized Bone Loss.* (Special Supplement to Calcified Tissue Abstracts.) Horton, J. E., Tarpley, T. M., et al. (eds.), Washington, D.C., Information Retrieval, Inc., 1978.

Rosenberg, E., Lang, R., et al.: Effect of long term calcitonin therapy on the clinical course of osteogenesis imperfecta. *J. Clin. Endocrinol. Metab. 44*:346, 1977.

Singer, F. R.: *Paget's Disease of Bone.* New York, Plenum Press, 1977.

Smith, B., Francis, M. J. O., et al.: Osteogenesis imperfecta — a clinical and biochemical study of a generalized connective tissue disorder. *Q. J. Med. 44*:555, 1975.

Thomson, D. L., and Frame, B.: Involutional osteopenia: current concepts. *Ann. Intern. Med. 85*:789, 1976.

Whalen, J. P., Horwith, M., et al.: Calcitonin treatment in hereditary bone dysplasia with hyperphosphatemia: a radiographic and histologic study of bone. *Am. J. Roentgenol. 129*:29, 1977.

Extraskeletal Calcification and Ossification

Geho, W. B., and Whiteside, J. A.: Experience with disodium etidronate in diseases of ectopic calcification, In *Clinical Aspects of Metabolic Bone Disease.* Frame, B., Parfitt, A. M., and Duncan, H. (eds.), Amsterdam, Excerpta Medica, 1973, p. 506.

Kewalramani, L. S.: Ectopic ossification. *Am. J. Phys. Med. 56*:99, 1977.

Mozaffarion, G., Lafferty, F. W., et al.: Treatment of tumoral calcinosis with phosphorus deprivation. *Ann. Intern. Med. 77*:741, 1972.

Parfitt, A. M.: Soft tissue calcification in uremia. *Arch. Intern. Med. 124*:544, 1969.

Smith, R.: Myositis ossificans progressiva: a review of current problems. *Semin. Arthritis Rheum. 4*:369, 1975.

Hypercalcitonism

Baylin, S. B., Hsu, S. H., et al.: Inherited medullary thyroid carcinoma: a final monoclonal mutation in one of multiple clones of susceptible cells. *Science 199*:429, 1978.

DeLellis, R. A., Nunnemacher, G., et al.: C-cell hyperplasia. An ultrastructural analysis. *Lab. Invest. 36*:237, 1977.

Graze, K., Spiler, I. J., et al.: Natural history of familial medullary thyroid carcinoma. Effect of a program for early diagnosis. *N. Engl. J. Med. 299*:980, 1978.

Khairi, M. R. A., Dexter, R. N., et al.: Pheochromocytoma and medullary thyroid carcinoma: multiple endocrine neoplasia type III. *Medicine 54*:89, 1975.

Wells, S. A., Jr., Baylin, S. B., et al.: Provocative agents and the diagnosis of medullary carcinoma of the thyroid gland. *Ann. Surg. 188*:139, 1978.

Hypercalciuria and Urolithiasis

Coe, F. C.: Treated and untreated recurrent calcium nephrolithiasis in patients with idiopathic hypercalciuria, hyperuricosuria, or no metabolic disorder. *Ann. Intern. 87*:404, 1977.

Coe, F. L.: *Nephrolithiasis. Pathogenesis and Treatment.* Chicago, Year Book Medical Publishers, Inc., 1978.

Pak, C. Y. (ed.): Symposium on urolithiasis. *Kidney Int. 13*:341, 1978.

Pak, C. Y., Hayashi, Y., et al.: Estimation of the state of saturation of brushite and calcium oxalate in urine: a comparison of three methods. *J. Lab. Clin. Med. 89*:891, 1977.

Pak, C. Y., Waters, O., et al.: Mechanism for calcium urolithiasis among patients with hyperuricosuria: supersaturation of urine with respect to monosodium urate. *J. Clin. Invest. 59*:426, 1977.

Robertson, W. G., Peacock, M., et al.: Saturation-inhibition index as a measure of the risk of calcium oxalate stone formation in the urinary tract. *N. Engl. J. Med. 294*:249, 1976.

Shen, F. H., and Baylink, D. J.: Increased serum 1,25-dihydroxyvitamin D in idiopathic hypercalciuria. *J. Lab. Clin. Med. 90*:955, 1977.

van Reen, R. (ed): *Idiopathic Urinary Bladder Stone Disease.* DHEW Pub. No. (NIH) 77-1063, 1977.

Utilization of the Laboratory

Aloia, J. F., Vasrani, A., et al.: Radiographic morphometry and osteopenia in spinal osteoporosis. *J. Nuclear Med. 18*:425, 1977.

Bijvoet, O. L. M.: Kidney function in calcium and phosphate metabolism, In *Metabolic Bone Diseases.* Vol. I. Avioli, L. V., and Krane, S. M. (eds.), New York, Academic Press, 1977, p. 50.

Byers, P. D.: Diagnostic value of bone biopsies, In *Metabolic Bone Diseases.* Vol. I. Avioli, L. V., and Krane, S. M. (eds.), New York, Academic Press, 1977, p. 184.

Eisman, J. A., Shepard, R. M., et al.: Determination of 25-hydroxyvitamin D_2 and 25-hydroxyvitamin D_3 in human plasma using high pressure liquid chromatography. *Anal. Biochem. 80*:298, 1977.

Heath, H., III, and Sizemore, G. W.: Plasma calcitonin in normal man: differences between men and women. *J. Clin. Invest. 60*:1135, 1977.

Krane, S. M., Kantrowitz, F. G., et al.: Urinary excretion of hydroxylysine and its glycosides as an index of collagen degradation. *J. Clin. Invest. 59*:819, 1977.

Posen, S., Cornish, C., et al.: Alkaline phosphatase and metabolic bone disorders, In *Metabolic Bone Diseases.* Vol. I. Avioli, L. V., and Krane, S. M. (eds.), New York, Academic Press, 1977, p. 142.

CHAPTER 20

Effect of Hormones on Water, Sodium, Chloride, and Potassium Metabolism

By Robert W. Schrier
and Alexander Leaf

NORMAL PHYSIOLOGY OF RENAL WATER EXCRETION

The major control of renal water excretion involves a neurohypophyseal-renal reflex mechanism. The humoral component of this mechanism is arginine vasopressin (AVP), the mammalian antidiuretic hormone (ADH). AVP is synthesized from a precursor molecule in the supraoptic and paraventricular nuclei in the hypothalamus. The cells in these nuclei that synthesize AVP appear to be different from those cells that synthesize oxytocin (OT). After synthesis AVP is packaged into neurosecretory granules in the endoplasmic reticulum. The neurosecretory granules containing both AVP and a carrier molecule, neurophysin, are transported along the axons of the synthesizing hypothalamic neurons. The axonal bulbs of these neurons reside in the posterior pituitary gland. The release of the hormone from the posterior pituitary gland into the circulation occurs by the process of exocytosis; both AVP and neurophysins are released into the circulation. The neurophysin that accompanies AVP is immunologically different from that which accompanies OT. Although the neurophysins have not been found to have physiologic properties, they have been used as markers for AVP and OT.

Osmotic and Nonosmotic Regulation of Arginine Vasopressin

The control of synthesis and release the AVP constitutes two pathways, an osmotic and a nonosmotic. The osmotic pathway involves cells in the anterior hypothalamus that were termed "osmoreceptor cells" by Verney; these cells appear to reside outside the blood-brain barrier. With fluid deprivation an increase in extracellular fluid (ECF) osmolality decreases osmoreceptor cell volume, which then triggers an electrical stimulus leading to membrane depolarization, exocytosis, and release of AVP. Conversely, with water ingestion a decrease in ECF osmolality increases osmoreceptor cell volume, which inhibits the electrical discharge and subsequent membrane depolarization of the posterior pituitary membrane. A schematic representation of the sequence of events leading to the synthesis, axonal transport, and AVP release by the osmotic pathway is shown in Fig. 20–1. This osmotic pathway for AVP release is sensitive to 1–2% changes in ECF osmolality.

The nonosmotic pathway for AVP release includes those stimuli that have been shown to alter AVP release in the absence of changes in ECF osmolality. The major nonosmotic stimuli of AVP release are ECF volume depletion and

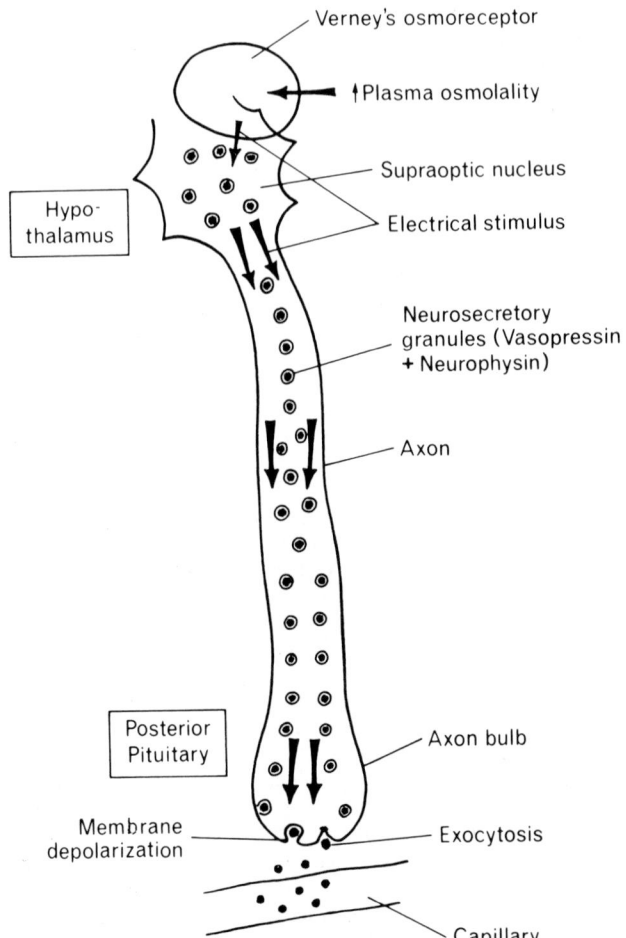

Figure 20–1. Schema of vasopressin release in response to a rise in plasma osmolality. (Published with permission from Schrier, R. W., and Miller, P.: Water metabolism in diabetes insipidus and the syndrome of inappropriate antidiuretic hormone secretion, In, *Pathophysiology of the Kidney.* Kurtzman, N. A., and Martinez-Maldonado, M. (eds.), Springfield, Charles C Thomas, 1977.)

receptors is associated with increased parasympathetic afferent drive and suppression of AVP release. Also, an increase in sympathetic tone that occurs with pain or fright may alter parasympathetic afferent tone and enhance AVP release even in the absence of a detectable fall in pressure at either low or high pressure receptor sites.

The understanding of the interrelationship between the osmotic and nonosmotic pathways for AVP release has recently been advanced by both clinical studies in man and experimental studies in animals. Patients have been studied who present with hypernatremia, adipsia, and maximally concentrated urine in association with a hypothalamic brain lesion. When infused with hypertonic saline to examine the integrity of the osmoreceptor pathway, these patients do not increase their plasma AVP levels as plasma osmolality rises. That is to say, the patients satisfy the criteria for central diabetes insipidus. It was not clear, however, how such patients excreted a concentrated urine in the absence of the osmotic release of AVP. When the nonosmotic baroreceptor pathway for AVP release was tested by lowering blood pressure, however, AVP release was totally normal. These studies therefore explain those patients previously labeled with the diagnosis of "essential hypernatremia" or "reset osmostat." A hypothalamic lesion must destroy the osmoreceptor cells and the adjacent thirst center and leave the baroreceptor pathways that travel from medulla to hypothalamus intact. Presumably, water depletion in these patients occurs and is sufficient to deplete ECF volume and stimulate nonosmotic baroreceptor release of AVP, which then mediates the concentration of urine.

Electrophysiologic studies in the rat suggest that a single cell neuron in the supraoptic nucleus can respond, as judged by changes in electrical activity, to both osmotic and nonosmotic stimuli. This experimental evidence along with aforementioned patient studies suggests the model shown in Fig. 20–2. "Resetting" of the osmoreceptor cells may therefore be interpreted as an interrelationship between osmoreceptor and baroreceptor input into magnocellular hypothalamic neurons in the supraoptic and paraventricular nuclei. Nonosmotic stimulation of AVP release, as may occur with

hypotension. Examples of other stimuli that involve increased adrenergic stimulation and also may cause nonosmotic release of AVP include pain, fright, adrenal insufficiency, cardiac failure, and hypoxia. The phylogenetic evolution of the nonosmotic pathway may have occurred as an integral part of the alarm reaction so that not only is the adrenergic nervous system stimulated but VP is also released in response to stress. Although not as well documented as its antidiuretic properties, AVP does possess vasoconstrictor properties that may be of physiologic and pathophysiologic importance.

The major nonosmotic pathway for AVP release appears to include low pressure receptors in the left atrium and high pressure baroreceptors in the carotid sinus and aortic arch. The parasympathetic afferent pathways from the left atrium and aortic arch travel through the vagus nerve; the parasympathetic afferent pathways from the carotid sinus travel through the glossopharyngeal nerves. The low pressure receptors in the left atrium may perceive early hemodynamic changes, such as a mild decrease in ECF volume, whereas the high pressure arterial baroreceptors may perceive more severe hemodynamic changes as may occur with hypotensive hemorrhage. In any case, it is clear that a fall in left atrial or arterial pressure is associated with diminished parasympathetic afferent drive and release in AVP, whereas a rise in pressure at these low and high pressure

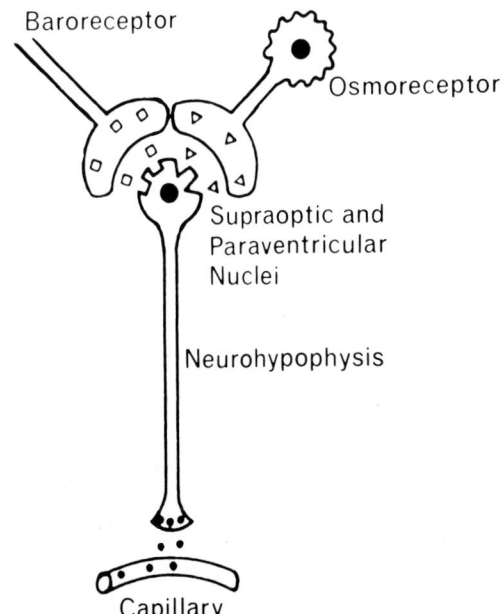

Figure 20–2. Interrelationship between nonosmotic (baroreceptor) and osmotic pathways regulating vasopressin release. (Published with permission from Schrier, R. W., et al.: Osmotic and nonosmotic control of vasopressin release. *Am. J. Physiol. 236*(4):F321, 1979.)

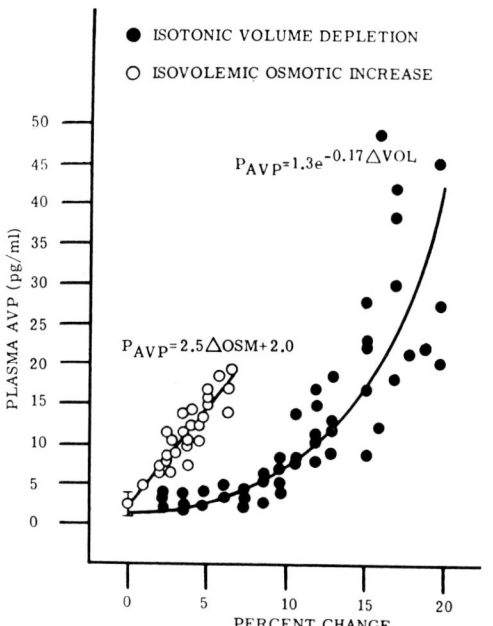

● ISOTONIC VOLUME DEPLETION

○ ISOVOLEMIC OSMOTIC INCREASE

$P_{AVP} = 1.3 e^{-0.17 \Delta VOL}$

$P_{AVP} = 2.5 \Delta OSM + 2.0$

Figure 20–3. Evidence for greater sensitivity for osmotic release of AVP (open circles) and greater potency for nonosmotic release of AVP (solid circles). (Published with permission from Dunn, F. L., et al.: The role of blood osmolality and volume in regulating vasopressin secretion in the rat. *J. Clin. Invest.* 52:3212, 1973.)

volume depletion, may predominate over osmotic suppression of AVP as water retention and hypoosmolality occur. In this regard, it seems clear that although 1–2% change in plasma osmolality alters AVP release, a 5–10% change in blood volume is necessary to stimulate AVP release. Once stimulated, however, the nonosmotic release of AVP occurs in a geometric manner, thus perhaps explaining the potency of this system (Fig. 20–3).

Thirst Mechanism

The existence of a hypothalamic thirst center constitutes a major determinant of fluid intake. The pathways that alter thirst seem to parallel the pathways that regulate AVP release. Specifically, a rise in ECF osmolality stimulates thirst and a fall in ECF osmolality suppresses it, perhaps again by altering cell volume of hypothalamic cells involved in the osmotic regulation of thirst. The stimulation of osmotic thirst in man occurs at a somewhat higher plasma osmolality than the threshold for AVP release (295 vs. 280 mOsm/kg H$_2$O) and thus may constitute a secondary line of defense against water depletion. A nonosmotic pathway for thirst regulation also exists, since ECF volume depletion is known to stimulate thirst in the absence of a change in ECF osmolality. The renin-angiotensin system has been suggested as one mediator of this system, since exogenous angiotensin or renin have been shown to stimulate thirst in animals and nephrectomy has been demonstrated to attenuate the stimulation of thirst by ECF volume depletion. It is not known whether the parasympathetic afferent pathways from low and high pressure baroreceptors are involved in the nonosmotic stimulation of thirst.

Cellular Mechanism of Action of Vasopressin

The primary action of AVP is to increase water permeability of the collecting duct epithelium of the mammalian

nephron. Since during hydropenia the interstitium of the medulla is hypertonic and tubular fluid entering the medullary collecting duct is isotonic, an osmotic gradient is present between the collecting duct lumen and the medullary interstitium. Thus, in the presence of AVP, osmotic water movement occurs across the collecting duct epithelium into the interstitium and vasa recta of the mecullary circulation. The result is concentration of the solute remaining in the urine; in man maximal urinary concentration ranges from 1000 to 1200 mOsm/kg H$_2$O.

The exact mechanism whereby AVP yields the collecting duct epithelium more permeable to water has not been completely defined, but in recent years considerable information has become available about this important process. After release from the posterior pituitary AVP circulates to the kidney and binds the receptors on the contraluminal (plasma) surface of the collecting duct. The AVP receptor binding initiates a sequence of intracellular events that ultimately lead to increased water permeability of the luminal (urine) side of the collecting duct epithelium. Some of the major components of these intracellular events are shown in Fig. 20–4. The AVP-receptor binding activates membrane adenyl cyclase, which catalyzes the conversion of adenine triphosphate (ATP) to 3′,5′-cyclic adenosine monophosphate (cAMP). Cyclic AMP protein kinase then appears to phosphorylate membrane proteins that somehow mediate the enhanced luminal water permeability by increasing either pore size, pore number, or membrane fluidity secondary to particle aggregation. A membrane phosphatase is present that reverses the process. The integrity of microtubules and microfilaments may also be important in mediating the events beyond cAMP generation that lead to increased luminal water permeability. There are also substances or events that may impair cAMP generation and action, including demeclochlortetracycline, lithium, hypokalemia, and prostaglandins. Prostaglandin E$_2$ is present in medullary interstitial and collecting cells, an anatomic location very suitable for modulation of the action of AVP. There is now considerable *in vivo* and *in vitro* evidence that inhibitors of prostaglandin synthetase enhance the tubular action of AVP, and thus enhance urinary concentration.

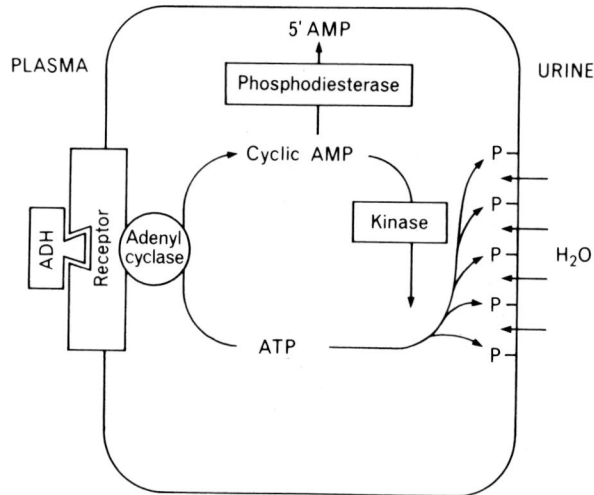

Figure 20–4. Schema of intracellular pathways whereby vasopressin (ADH) increases luminal water permeability of collecting duct cell. (Published with permission from Schrier, R. W., and Miller, P. D.: Water metabolism in diabetes insipidus and the syndrome of inappropriate antidiuretic hormone secretion, In *Pathophysiology of the Kidney.* Kurtzman, N. A., and Martinez-Maldonado, M. (eds.), Springfield, Charles C Thomas, 1977.)

Intrarenal Factors Influencing Renal Water Excretion

The distal portion of the nephron from the loop of Henle and beyond is primarily involved in urinary concentration and dilution. Even so, the volume of fluid delivered to this distal diluting and concentrating segment of the nephron is an important determinant of renal water excretion. The rate of glomerular filtration (GFR) and proximal fluid reabsorption are the primary determinants of fluid delivery to the distal diluting segment. Next, active chloride and passive sodium reabsorption in the water-impermeable thick ascending limb of Henle's loop is an extremely important step in the renal concentrating and diluting mechanism. Specifically, the reabsorption of solute without water (1)

dilutes tubular fluid and (2) constitutes the initiating step in the countercurrent mechanism leading to generation of a hypertonic interstitium. In the presence of AVP the hypotonic distal fluid delivered to the cortical collecting tubule equilibrates with the isotonic cortical interstitium. The resulting isotonic tubular fluid then is delivered to the medullary collecting duct where it equilibrates with the hypertonic medullary interstitium, thus a hypertonic urine results. In the absence of AVP, solute reabsorption continues throughout the water-impermeable distal tubule and collecting duct, thus resulting in a hypotonic urine. These processes of urinary concentration and dilution are depicted schematically in Fig. 20–5A and B.

CLINICAL DISORDERS OF POLYURIA

Polyuria may result from a deficiency of AVP (central diabetes insipidus), a resistance to AVP (nephrogenic diabetes insipidus) or physiologic suppression of AVP (compulsive water drinking).

Central Diabetes Insipidus (Vasopressin-Sensitive)

There are a variety of causes of central diabetes insipidus that are listed in Table 20–1. The severity and duration of the polyuria depend on the location and completeness of the lesion. A lesion below the median eminence will be associated with regeneration of neuronal axons and thus the central diabetes insipidus will be transient. In fact, it can be followed by a period of uncontrolled AVP "leak" from damaged neurons that causes the syndrome of inappropriate secre-

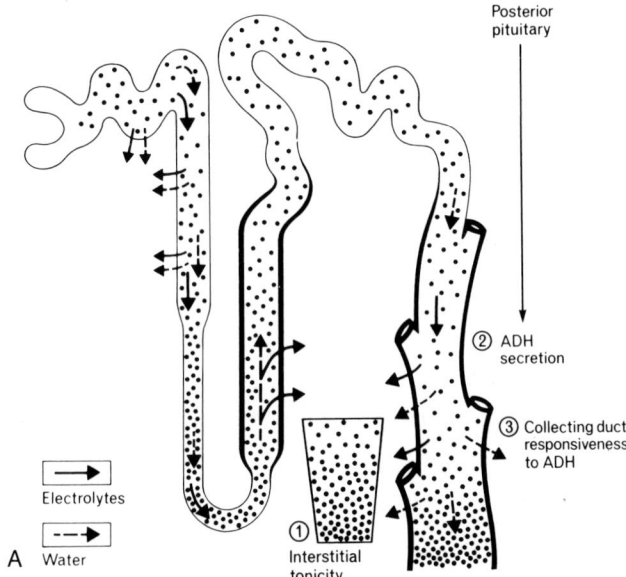

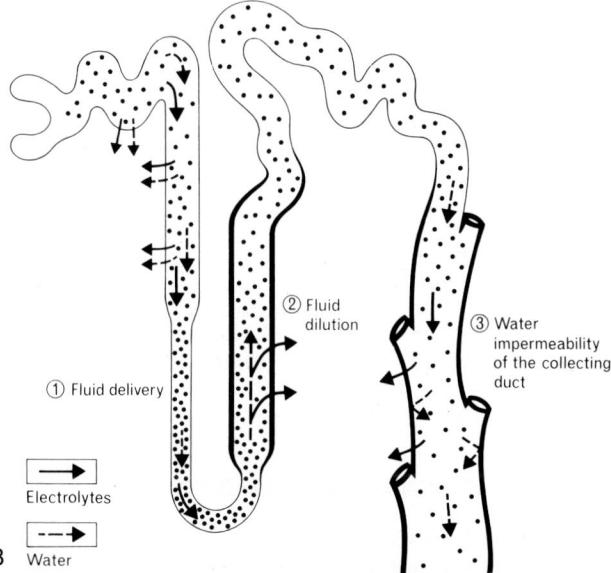

Figure 20–5. *A*, Nephron schema for urinary concentration. *B*, Nephron schema for urinary dilution. (Adapted with permission from Goldberg, M.: Water control and the dysnatremias, In *The Sea Within Us: Clinical Guide in Fluid and Electrolyte Imbalance.* Bricker, N. S. (ed.), Chicago, G. D. Searle, and New York, Science & Medicine Publ. Co., 1975.)

Table 20–1. ETIOLOGIES OF VASOPRESSIN-SENSITIVE DIABETES INSIPIDUS

A. Idiopathic Form
   1. Non-familial form
   2. Familial form

B. Post-Hypophysectomy

C. Trauma
   1. Basilar skull fracture

D. Tumors
   1. Metastatic carcinoma
   2. Craniopharyngioma
   3. Suprasellar cysts
   4. Pinealoma
   5. Leukemia

E. Granuloma
   1. Sarcoid
   2. Tuberculosis
   3. Syphilis

F. Infections
   1. Meningitis
   2. Encephalitis
   3. Landry-Guillain-Barré syndrome

G. Vascular
   1. Cerebral thrombosis or hemorrhage
   2. Cerebral aneurysm
   3. Post-partum necrosis (Sheehan's syndrome)

H. Histiocytosis
   1. Eosinophilic granuloma
   2. Schuller-Christian disease

Published with permission from Berl, T. and Schrier, R. W.: Disorders of serum sodium concentration, In McGaw Fluid and Electrolyte Monograph Series. Irvine, McGaw Laboratories, 1979.

tion of antidiuretic hormone (SIADH). Lesions above the median eminence may cause permanent diabetes insipidus; however, it should be mentioned that only 10% of neurosecretory neurons must remain intact to avoid central diabetes insipidus. Central diabetes insipidus may also be complete or partial. The patient with complete diabetes insipidus has polyuria of at least 10–12 l/day with a urinary osmolality below 100 mOsm/kg H_2O. If an intercedent illness, e.g., viral gastroenteritis, impairs such a patient's capacity to drink, life-threatening hypernatremia will occur rapidly. Also, a hypothalamic lesion may involve the thirst center and cause hypodipsia and hypernatremia. Generally, however, these patients have an intact thirst mechanism so that polydipsia and adequate fluid intake maintain a normal plasma sodium concentration. The patient with partial diabetes insipidus will present with more modest polydipsia and polyuria and, in fact, fluid deprivation may lead to a rise in urinary osmolality above plasma osmolality. Such fluid deprivation should be performed during the daytime and the resulting weight loss should be limited to 3–5% of body weight. After this degree of fluid restriction in the patient with partial diabetes insipidus, urine osmolality will rise further (greater than 10%) in response to exogenous vasopressin (5 U VP subcutaneously), thus confirming a failure to maximally release endogenous AVP. In contrast, the patient with intact baroreceptor pathways and adequate neurosecretory neurons ("essential hypernatremia") should have a maximally concentrated urine after fluid deprivation and indeed may present with a urinary osmolality between 800 and 1200 mOsm/kg H_2O.

There have been various drugs used to treat partial diabetes insipidus, such as chlorpropamide, clofibrate, and carbamazepine, thus avoiding the hypersensitivity reactions and potential vascular consequences of exogenous VP. The new VP analogue, 1-desamino D arginine vasopressin (dDAVP), may now be the drug of choice for treating central diabetes insipidus, however. dDAVP has a long duration of action and is devoid of vascular properties. The analogue can be administered by insufflation (5–20 μg/nostril b i d).

Nephrogenic Diabetes Insipidus (Vasopressin-Resistant)

Nephrogenic diabetes insipidus may be congenital or acquired. The congenital variety was brought to North America by the Ulster clan from Scotland who arrived in Nova Scotia in 1761. The disease has an autosomal dominant pattern of inheritance with male predominance. In infants the diagnosis may become apparent because of hypernatremia, fever, and failure to thrive, in addition to polyuria. Treatment with hydrochlorothiazides or indomethacin has been successful in decreasing the polyuria; both agents probably enhance proximal fluid reabsorption and decrease distal delivery either by a primary action (indomethacin) or secondary to ECF volume depletion (hydrochlorothiazides).

The many causes of acquired nephrogenic diabetes insipidus are listed in Table 20–2. Since most of these causes are associated with some decrease in GFR, the polyuria in acquired nephrogenic diabetes insipidus generally ranges only from 3–6 l/day. Treatment should be focused at the primary disorder, such as cessation of drugs or correction of the hypokalemia, hypercalcemia, or partial urinary tract obstruction. Although the polyuria normally is not of clinical consequence, the patients should be educated about their defect in urinary concentration and thus large daily obligatory urine losses. If such a patient is unable to drink only for 1 day, a 3–6 l negative fluid balance could ensue.

Table 20–2.   ACQUIRED CAUSES OF NEPHROGENIC DIABETES INSIPIDUS

A. Chronic Renal Disease
 1. Polycystic disease
 2. Medullary cystic disease
 3. Pyelonephritis
 4. Ureteral obstruction
 5. Far-advanced renal failure

B. Electrolyte Disorders
 1. Hypokalemia
 2. Hypercalcemia

C. Drugs
 1. Lithium
 2. Demeclocycline
 3. Acetohexamide
 4. Tolazamide
 5. Glycuride
 6. Propoxyphene
 7. Amphotericin
 8. Methoxyflurane
 9. Vinblastine
 10. Colchicine

D. Sickle Cell Disease

E. Dietary Abnormalities
 1. Excessive water intake
 2. Decreased sodium chloride intake
 3. Decreased protein intake

F. Miscellaneous
 1. Multiple myeloma
 2. Amyloidosis
 3. Sjögren's disease
 4. Sarcoidosis

Compulsive (Psychogenic) Water Drinking

Since the normal capacity to excrete water ranges from 15 to 25 l/day, the patient with a habit of compulsive water drinking has symptoms of only polydipsia and polyuria. The polydipsia leads to increased water intake, suppression of endogenous AVP with resultant polyuria. Since chronic water intake diminishes medullary tonicity, the patients develop a resistance to AVP. Thus, with fluid restriction and a 3–5% decrease in body weight, urinary osmolality will increase to hypertonic, but submaximal, levels. In this regard, these patients may respond in a manner similar to patients with polyuria secondary to partial central diabetes insipidus. The difference, however, is that the patient with compulsive water drinking will not respond further to exogenous VP after fluid deprivation, whereas the patient with partial diabetes insipidus will. The responses of patients with central and nephrogenic diabetes insipidus and compulsive water drinking are summarized in Table 20–3. The major danger in a patient with compulsive water drinking is the occurrence of an event, e.g., diuretic treatment, ECF volume depletion, or VP administration, that will impair renal water excretion. Continued ingestion of large volumes of water in this situation can lead to life-threatening acute hyponatremia.

HYPONATREMIC DISORDERS

Patients with polyuria secondary to renal concentrating defects generally are not hypernatremic because thirst stimulation causes a degree of polydipsia necessary to avoid a negative water balance. In contrast, however, patients who are unable to dilute their urine frequently present with some degree of hyponatremia. This is probably because mod-

Table 20–3. RESPONSES TO FLUID DEPRIVATION AND EXOGENOUS VASOPRESSIN

	Number of Cases	Mean U_{osm} with Dehydration	U_{osm} After Vasopressin	% Change (in U_{osm})
Normal subjects	9	1067 ± 68.7	978 ± 79.4	-8.9 ± 3.0
Complete pituitary diabetes insipidus	18	168 ± 13	445 ± 52	180 ± 41.4
Partial pituitary diabetes insipidus	12	437.0 ± 33.6	548.6 ± 28.2	28.5 ± 4.7
Compulsive water-drinking	7	738.2 ± 52.9	779.8 ± 73.1	5 ± 2.2

Data published with permission from Miller, M., et al.: Recognition of partial defects in antidiuretic hormone secretion. *Ann. Intern. Med. 73:*721, 1970.

erate water intake (1–2 l/day) may be primarily owing to habit rather than any dependence on the thirst mechanism. There are several hormonal and nonhormonal disorders that may lead to hyponatremia. A general approach to hyponatremic disorders is based on an evaluation of ECF volume status and urinary sodium concentration; this approach is presented in Fig. 20–6.

Edematous Disorders

Hyponatremia secondary to impaired urinary dilution may occur with the edematous disorders, including congestive heart failure, cirrhosis, and nephrotic syndrome. Two major mechanisms have been proposed as a cause of the hyponatremia with these disorders, namely (1) nonosmotic release of AVP and (2) impaired distal fluid delivery to diluting segment. Most patients with hyponatremia associated with cardiac failure and cirrhosis do have evidence of a diminished GFR and increased proximal tubular reabsorption, events that diminish distal fluid delivery. Infusion of mannitol and plasma have been found to increase free

water excretion in these edematous disorders. Since these agents increase distal fluid delivery in normal subjects, these results have provided evidence for a pathogenetic role of decreased distal delivery in causing the hyponatremia. Alternatively, both mannitol and plasma infusions expand ECF volume and thus provide a nonosmotic stimulus for suppression of AVP. Bioassays have provided conflicting results about the presence of AVP in patients with hyponatremia and cirrhosis or cardiac failure. With the use of a sensitive radioimmunoassay for AVP it is clear that the majority of such patients have detectable levels of AVP even though their level of hypo-osmolality should have normally suppressed AVP to an undetectable level. A decrease in cardiac output with heart failure, and hypoalbuminemia, peripheral vasodilation, and splanchnic venous pooling with cirrhosis seem the most likely factors to decrease "effective" arterial blood volume, thereby stimulating nonosmotic baroreceptor-mediated AVP release. In the absence of an AVP inhibitor it is impossible to quantitate the relative roles of AVP and diminished distal delivery in the hyponatremia. In any case, the standard treatment should be restriction of water intake to less than 750 ml/day.

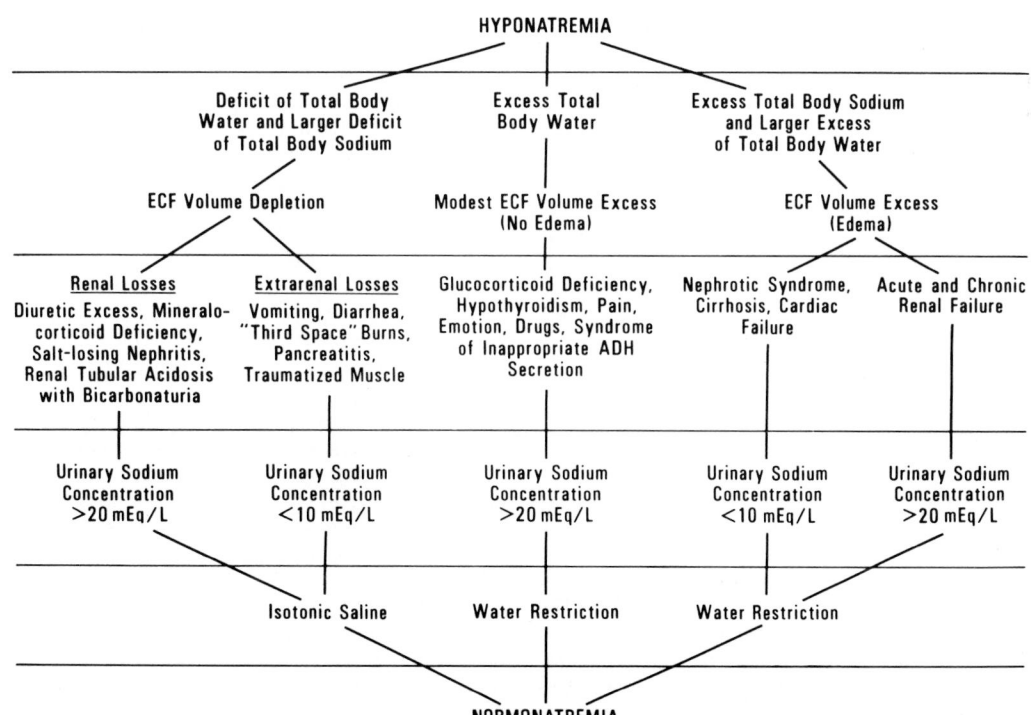

Figure 20–6. Diagnostic approach to hyponatremia with emphasis on ECF volume status and urinary sodium concentration. (Published with permission from Berl, T., et al.: Clinical disorders of water metabolism. *Kidney Int. 10:*117, 1976.)

Adrenal Insufficiency

Hyponatremia secondary to a defect in renal diluting capacity is a frequent occurrence with primary and secondary adrenal insufficiency. In primary adrenal insufficiency (Addison's disease) recent experimental results indicate that the defect in water excretion is due to both glucocorticoid and mineralocorticoid hormone deficiency. The defect with mineralocorticoid deficiency relates primarily to renal sodium wasting and ECF volume depletion. The ECF volume depletion impairs water excretion by stimulating nonosmotic AVP release and diminishing renal hemodynamics and fluid delivery to the distal diluting segments of the nephron. Either chronic mineralocorticoid hormone or sodium chloride replacement will correct this defect in water excretion.

The defect in water excretion associated with glucocorticoid deficiency occurs independent of any evidence of ECF volume depletion. The earliest defect is related to the nonosmotic release of AVP that occurs at a time when impairment in cardiac function is present, thus providing a potential stimulus for baroreceptor-mediated AVP release. More prolonged glucocorticoid deficiency for 2 weeks also will impair renal water excretion by mechanism(s) independent of AVP release. At this time cardiac output and arterial pressure are further diminished. These systemic hemodynamic consequences of prolonged glucocorticoid deficiency are associated with decreased GFR and renal blood flow, increased renal vascular resistance and diminished distal fluid delivery; the latter defect provides the most likely explanation for the AVP-independent defect in water excretion. To date there is no direct evidence that glucocorticoid deficiency renders the collecting duct more permeable to water in the absence of AVP, an earlier proposal to explain the hyponatremia associated with glucocorticoid deficiency. Replacement with physiologic doses of glucocorticoid hormone will correct both the AVP-dependent and AVP-independent defects in water excretion. Both glucocorticoid and mineralocorticoid hormone replacement are necessary to correct the defect in water excretion in the patient with Addison's disease, whereas glucocorticoid hormone alone will correct the defect with secondary (hypopituitarism) adrenal insufficiency, since the renin-angiotensin-aldosterone system is intact. If glucocorticoid replacement does not correct the defect in water excretion in a patient with pituitary disease, it is likely that the patient also has secondary hypothyroidism. In fact, the effects of glucocorticoid or thyroid hormone deficiency to impair water excretion may be so potent as to obscure the presence of partial diabetes insipidus; hormone replacement in such patients therefore may be associated with profound polyuria.

Hypothyroidism

The availability of the radioimmunoassay for AVP has allowed for some clarification of the defect in water excretion associated with the hypothyroid state. In thyroidectomized patients studied after withdrawal of thyroid replacement, a diminution in GFR and distal fluid delivery to the diluting segment is clearly present. The patients are, however, not hyponatremic and AVP levels both before and after a water load are no different as compared to when the same patients have been replaced with thyroid hormone. This AVP-independent defect in water excretion quantitatively impairs the renal capacity to excrete a water load by about 20%. It is clear therefore why such a defect would not lead to hyponatremia, since the renal capacity to excrete water normally ranges from 15 to 25 l/day.

Using a sensitive radioimmunoassay for AVP, the most recent evidence in man, rat, and sheep with advanced hypothyroidism and hyponatremia suggests that the nonosmotic release of AVP is primarily responsible for the defect in water excretion. Whether the known decrease in cardiac output associated with severe hypothyroidism stimulates baroreceptor-mediated release of AVP or some other afferent pathway is involved is not known. There is no evidence that thyroid hormone deficiency enhances the end-organ response to AVP and thereby contributes to the hyponatremia. In fact, both *in vivo* and *in vitro* results indicate that thyroid hormone deficiency impairs the effect of AVP to increase cAMP-mediated water transport. The nonosmotic release of AVP therefore must be sufficient to override this defect in the hyponatremic hypothyroid patient. Chronic replacement of physiologic doses of thyroid hormone corrects both the AVP-dependent and AVP-independent defects in water excretion in the hyponatremic hypothyroid patient.

Syndrome of Inappropriate Antidiuretic Hormone (SIADH)

The diagnosis of SIADH necessitates the exclusion of the causes of hypervolemic (edematous), hypovolemic, and euvolemic hyponatremic disorders, as outlined in Fig. 20–6. It should also be remembered that hyperlipidemic and hyperproteinemic states may cause "pseudohyponatremia." A clue to this diagnosis is that the plasma osmolality will be normal in spite of the presence of hyponatremia. Removal of lipids and proteins reveals a normal plasma sodium concentration when measured on plasma water. The hyperglycemic diabetic patient may also have hyponatremia even though the patient's urinary losses secondary to the glucose-induced osmotic diuresis are hypotonic. This cause of hyponatremia occurs secondary to the osmotic movement of water from cells into the ECF compartment on the basis of the hyperosmotic effect of the elevated blood glucose concentration. During treatment with insulin for every 100 mg/dl fall in blood glucose the plasma sodium concentration will rise approximately 1.6 mEq/l as the osmotic water movement is into cells.

The individual causes of SIADH are listed in Table 20–4. The vast majority of these causes are due to vascular, infectious, and neoplastic processes involving the lungs or central nervous system (CNS). Treatment aimed at the primary disorder is the most appropriate therapeutic approach. If this is not possible, the chronic hyponatremia is best treated by restriction of water intake. Some patients with chronic SIADH, however, will not restrict their water intake and demeclochlortetracycline (600–1200 mg/day) will block the end-organ response to ADH and thereby allow more water intake without the occurrence of hyponatremia. In some patients acute hyponatremia may occur and lead to life-threatening CNS symptoms, including stupor, coma, and convulsions. These symptoms are primarily due to brain edema and may be associated with herniation and death. Acute hyponatremia is much more dangerous than chronic hyponatremia because the cell volume regulatory mechanisms that attenuate cell swelling during chronic hyponatremia are not rapid enough to prevent brain cell swelling during the acute (hours) development of hyponatremia. The cell volume regulatory mechanisms involve extrusion from cells of osmotically active substances (potassium, chloride, and sodium) during hyponatremia, a process that attenuates brain edema. In chronic hypernatremic states idiogenic, osmotically active solute accumulates in brain cells and thus attenuates brain cell dehydration. These idiogenic

Table 20–4. DISORDERS ASSOCIATED WITH THE SYNDROME OF INAPPROPRIATE ANTIDIURETIC HORMONE SECRETION

A. Carcinomas
1. Lung
2. Duodenum
3. Pancreas

B. Pulmonary Disorders
1. Viral pneumonia
2. Bacterial pneumonia
3. Pulmonary abscess
4. Tuberculosis
5. Aspergillosis

C. Central Nervous System Disorders
1. Encephalitis, viral or bacterial
2. Meningitis, viral, bacterial, or tuberculous
3. Acute psychosis
4. Stroke (cerebral thrombosis or hemorrhage)
5. Acute intermittent porphyria
6. Brain tumors
7. Brain abscess
8. Subdural or subarachnoid hematoma or hemorrhage
9. Guillain-Barré syndrome
10. Head trauma

Published with permission from Schrier, R. W., and Berl, T.: Disorders of water metabolism, In *Renal and Electrolyte Disorders.* Schrier, R. W. (ed.), Boston, Little, Brown & Co., 1976.

anions are probably the reason why rapid correction of chronic hypernatremia may lead to brain edema and serious CNS symptoms and sequelae. Acute states of water imbalance, however, should be corrected rapidly, e.g., convulsing patient with development of hyponatremia over a few hours. In such a patient, hypertonic saline or mannitol will rapidly enhance water movement from brain cells to ECF. The renal excretion of this water can be enhanced by use of a loop diuretic, e.g., furosemide (1 mg/kg), thus avoiding excessive volume expansion. The hypertonic saline should be given at a rate that replaces urinary electrolyte losses so that the net effect is a negative water balance.

NORMAL PHYSIOLOGY OF SODIUM, CHLORIDE, AND POTASSIUM EXCRETION

Electrolyte excretion involves both the GFR and tubule reabsorption of solute. The reabsorption of calcium, magnesium and phosphorus will not be discussed here, since Ch. 19 has considered excretion of these ions. Thus, the focus will be primarily on sodium, chloride, and potassium excretion.

Glomerular Filtration

Glomerular filtration is the initial event in urine formation. In normal man, however, approximately 99% of the daily 150 l of filtered water containing 20,000 mEq of sodium and 14,000 mEq of chloride are reabsorbed by the tubules, thus leaving only 1% of glomerular ultrafiltrate to be excreted in urine. Nevertheless, the control of GFR must be considered in any discussion of electrolyte excretion. It is known that GFR remains constant over a wide range of renal perfusion pressures by a process termed renal autoregulation; renal blood flow also participates in this regulatory process. The mechanism responsible for renal autoregulation is not entirely clear, but the transmural pressure gradient across the afferent arteriole appears primarily responsible for the dilatation of this vessel when

renal perfusion pressure falls and the vasoconstriction when renal perfusion pressure rises. There is another important regulatory process involving GFR and the rate of tubular reabsorption that has been termed glomerulotubular balance. With this process, as GFR rises absolute tubular reabsorption increases, and when GFR falls absolute tubular reabsorption falls. This process therefore tends to maintain the fraction of glomerular filtrate (GF) reabsorbed relatively constant, thus buffering against large changes in urinary excretion of water and electrolytes. The exact mechanism responsible for glomerulotubular balance is not known but may involve the rate of substrate delivery to the proximal tubule as well as changes in the peritubular Starling forces.

Several hormones, namely thyroid and glucocorticoids, are known to increase GFR. Several other factors also have been found recently to decrease glomerular capillary permeability, by decreasing either the hydraulic conductivity of the membrane or the membrane's surface area. These factors include angiotensin, VP, several vasodilators and parathyroid hormone (PTH).

Proximal Tubular Reabsorption

The reabsorptive processes in the proximal tubule have been studied intensively both *in vivo* (micropuncture techniques) and *in vitro* (isolated perfused tubules and membrane vesicles) in recent years. The results of these studies have provided considerable understanding about the processes involved in the proximal tubular reabsorption of at least two thirds of filtered sodium, chloride, and water and nearly all of filtered bicarbonate, amino acids, and glucose. The concentration profile of substances reabsorbed along the accessible proximal nephron is shown in Fig. 20–7. Since inulin is not reabsorbed its concentration provides an index of water reabsorption. Since sodium concentration rises very little along the proximal nephron it is clear that this ion is reabsorbed with an isosmotic equivalent of water. The rise in chloride concentration occurs since sodium is reabsorbed secondary to proton secretion and bicarbonate

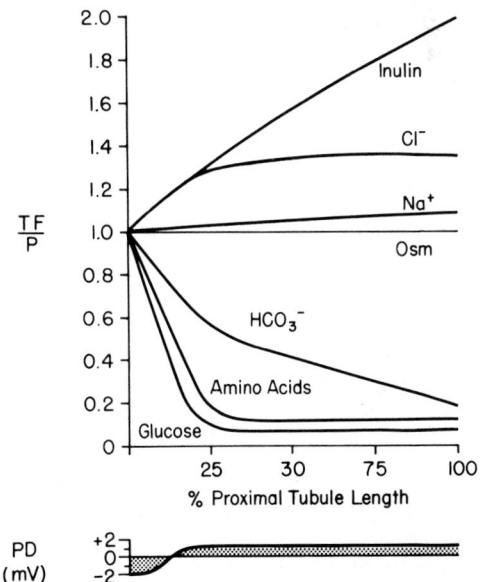

Figure 20–7. Solute profile along proximal tubule. TF/P = tubule fluid concentration/plasma concentration. PD = potential difference. (Published with permission from Schrier, R. W., and Anderson, R. J.: Renal sodium excretion, edematous disorders, and diuretic use, In *Renal and Electrolyte Disorders,* 2nd ed. Schrier, R. W. (ed.), Boston, Little, Brown & Co., in press.)

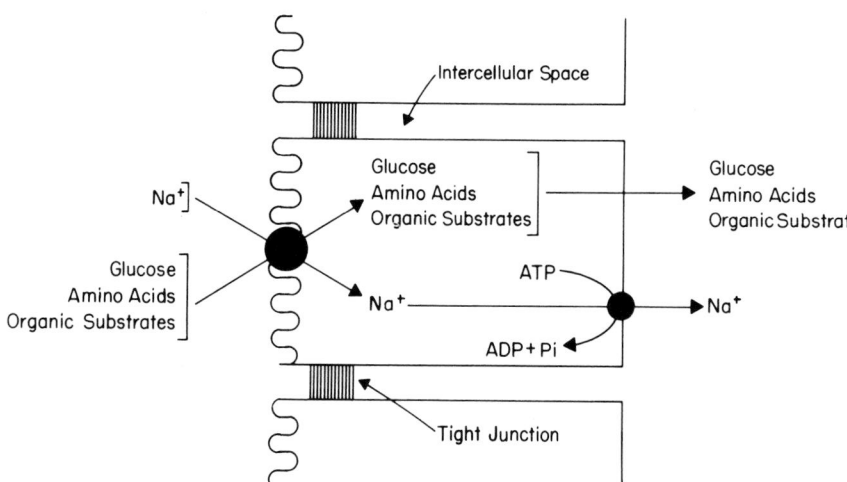

Figure 20–8. Cotransport system in early proximal tubule for glucose, amino acids, and organic substrates with sodium. (Published with permission from Schrier, R. W., and Anderson, R. J.: Renal sodium excretion, edematous disorders, and diuretic use. In *Renal and Electrolyte Disorders.* 2nd ed. Schrier, R. W. (ed.), Boston, Little, Brown & Co., in press.)

reclamation along the early portion of the proximal nephron. Luminal and intracellular carbonic anhydrase are involved in the process of hydrogen ion secretion and bicarbonate reclamation. The increased chloride concentration has been suggested to be a potential driving force for passive sodium chloride reabsorption in the late portion of the proximal tubule. The cotransport system for glucose, amino acids, and organic substrates with sodium in the earlier portion of the proximal tubule is illustrated in Fig. 20–8. Sodium moves along an electrical-chemical gradient into the cell and is transported from the cell by a Na-K-ATPase process on the basal-lateral membrane of the cell. The transport of glucose, amino acids, and organic substrates across the luminal membrane has been shown not to occur in the absence of sodium transport; however, these substances efflux from the cell across the basal-lateral membrane by a process independent of sodium transport but blocked by phloretin.

The reabsorption of potassium in the proximal tubule is nearly complete and is not altered by the ingestion of either a high or low potassium intake. This potassium reabsorption has been found to involve an active process independent of sodium transport. Although there is some evidence for potassium secretion into luminal fluid in the descending limb of Henle's loop, under a variety of experimental conditions only 10% of filtered potassium is present in the early distal convoluted tubule. These results indicate that potassium reabsorptive processes dominate prior to the distal convoluted tubule and that urinary excretion of potassium is primarily regulated by transport processes (reabsorption and secretion) located in the distal segments of the nephron.

There is little direct evidence for hormonal control of proximal tubular reabsorption. A natriuretic hormone has been proposed, but not proved, to mediate the decrease in proximal sodium reabsorption during expansion of ECF volume, however. PTH also has been shown to decrease proximal tubule reabsorption of phosphate, bicarbonate, and sodium. Changes in adrenergic tone also have been found to be a determinant of proximal tubular reabsorption. Further studies, however, will be necessary to delineate totally the intraluminal and peritubular factors that govern proximal tubular reabsorption.

Loop of Henle

Active transport of chloride in the thick ascending limb of Henle's loop has been found to provide the electrical driving force for passive reabsorption of sodium in this segment of the nephron. Since the ascending limb of Henle's loop in this portion of the nephron is always water impermeable, sodium chloride transport dilutes tubular fluid and is the prime mover for generation of a hypertonic medullary interstitium. The ascending limb also has the capacity to increase sodium chloride and water reabsorption in response to enhanced fluid and sodium chloride delivery out of the proximal tubule.

Distal Convoluted Tubule and Collecting Duct

The hypotonic tubular fluid emerging from the loop of Henle does not equilibrate with the isotonic cortical interstitium in the distal convoluted tubule, since this portion of the nephron is not responsive to AVP. Sodium and chloride reabsorption continues in this distal nephron segment, however. The cortical collecting tubule, however, is responsive to AVP; thus the entering hypotonic tubular fluid becomes isotonic along this portion of the nephron. Hydrogen ion and potassium secretion also occurs in this portion of the nephron, a process stimulated by aldosterone. The hydrogen ions secreted are buffered in the tubular lumen by one of the following three processes: (1) Ammonia synthesized in tubular epithelial cells is converted to ammonium in the presence of secreted hydrogen ions; (2) titratable acid, mainly phosphate, buffers hydrogen ion in the tubular lumen; and (3) bicarbonate is converted to carbonic acid in the presence of luminal carbonic anhydrase and hydrogen ion secretion.

There are several factors other than aldosterone that affect potassium excretion. It is clear that high tubular flow rates enhance potassium secretion, probably by rapidly removing secreted potassium and thus re-establishing a more favorable chemical gradient for further potassium secretion. Although this effect of tubular flow may occur independent of distal sodium delivery, it seems likely that at low flow rates increased sodium delivery may enhance potassium secretion by increasing peritubular sodium-potassium exchange and thus intracellular potassium concentration. Such increased peritubular cellular uptake of potassium also may be the mechanism whereby alkalosis increases potassium secretion. Thus, with alkalosis potassium moves into cells as hydrogen ion moves out; the resulting increased intracellular potassium concentration then provides a more favorable chemical gradient for potassium secretion into the tubular lumen. Although the early alterations in potassium secretion and excretion that occur in response to a high or low potassium intake may relate primarily to either stimulation or suppression of aldosterone secretion, changes in cell potassium concentration may be the more importnet chronic determinant of potassium secretion. An increase in peritubular Na-K-ATPase may also be quite important in the improved renal response to chronic as compared to acute potassium loads, probably by enhancing peritubular cellular uptake and increasing potassium secretion.

The outer medullary collecting duct is impermeable to urea, so in the presence of AVP intraluminal urea concentration rises in this nephron segment as water is reabsorbed without urea. Because of this increased urea concentration and the urea permeability of the inner medullary collecting duct, passive urea transport occurs and contributes to the increase in inner medullary tonicity. The urea is also recycled into the ascending limb of Henle's loop, which is urea permeable. Recent findings also suggest that the medullary collecting duct is important in sodium and potassium reabsorption in various circumstances and indeed may be responsible for the fine regulation of urinary excretion of these ions.

Aldosterone

The cortical collecting tubule appears to be the primary site of action of aldosterone. Aldosterone is the most potent known hormonal regulator of electrolyte excretion. The hormone binds to specific protein receptors in collecting duct cells and induces DNA-directed synthesis of RNA with the subsequent formation of a new protein. The role of the new protein is controversial but may either facilitate entry of sodium into the cell or provide a source of increased energy simply for active sodium transport. In either case, the ultimate action of aldosterone is to increase sodium and chloride reabsorption from the tubular lumen and to increase the secretion of hydrogen ion and potassium into the tubular lumen.

The renin-angiotensin system and plasma potassium concentration are the major factors controlling the secretion of aldosterone. Adrenocorticotropin (ACTH) will transiently stimulate aldosterone secretion; however, this effect is not sustained. A rise in plasma potassium concentration stimulates aldosterone secretion even though it suppresses plasma renin activity. Conversely, a fall in plasma potassium concentration suppresses aldosterone secretion even though hypokalemia stimulates renin release. There are three major factors controlling renin release by the juxtaglomerular apparatus. Renin granules have been localized in myoepithelial cells of the afferent arteriole of the glomerular capillary, and alterations in transmural pressure across the afferent arteriole constitute the "baroreceptor" mechanism of renin release. The integrity of the baroreceptor mechanism appears to be dependent on prostacyclines (PGI), which are located in the wall of the afferent arteriole. Specifically, baroreceptor-stimulated release of renin is abolished by pretreatment with inhibitors of prostaglandin synthesis. Renal nerves, primarily by beta receptor stimulation, are the second mechanism modulating renin release; this pathway can be abolished by beta blockade but is independent of inhibition of prostaglandin synthesis. Lastly, the rate of sodium chloride transport across the macula densa cells is another factor regulating renin release. This pathway may also involve the synthesis of prostaglandins, but further studies are necessary to document this possibility. These renin regulatory mechanisms are summarized in Fig. 20–9.

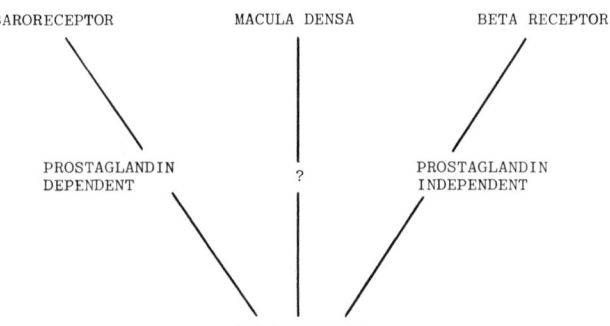

Figure 20–9. Schema for pathways regulating renin release.

Aldosterone Escape

Aldosterone escape, desoxycorticosterone acetate (DOCA) escape, and sodium escape are different terms for the same phenomenon. The exogenous administration of a mineralocorticoid hormone, such as aldosterone or DOCA, causes sodium retention and ECF volume expansion only for a finite period of time, then sodium excretion returns to a level equal to sodium intake. The mechanism for this "escape" from the sodium-retaining effects of a mineralocorticoid hormone is not known. The duration of time necessary for the escape to occur, however, relates to the sodium intake. With a high sodium intake (200 mEq/day) the same ECF volume expansion, e.g., approximately 2 l, occurs earlier, as compared with when the patient is on a low sodium intake (50 mEq/day). The sodium escape also occurs earlier with the high sodium intake, thus suggesting that the degree of ECF volume expansion may be the trigger to the escape phenomenon. Also, it is clear that although there is an escape from the sodium-retaining effect of the mineralocorticoid, the kaliuretic effect of the hormone persists. These findings are therefore compatible with the following hypothesis. No actual "escape" occurs from the sodium-retaining effect of the mineralocorticoid but rather ECF volume expansion with decreased proximal sodium reabsorption and increased distal sodium delivery occurs and obscures the distal sodium-retaining effect of the mineralocorticoid. This would also explain why there is no escape from the kaliuretic effect of the mineralocorticoid, since increased distal flow and sodium delivery enhance potassium secretion.

The most important question in sodium metabolism may be why patients with edematous disorders do not escape from the sodium-retaining effects of aldosterone. The answer to this question is not known. It nevertheless is important to point out several differences between the administration of mineralocorticoid hormone to a normal subject and the secondary hyperaldosteronism associated with edematous disorders. With mineralocorticoid administration the normal subject has an expansion of ECF volume that causes a suppression of the renin-angiotensin system and decreases adrenergic neural tone. In contrast, the patient with nephrotic syndrome, cirrhosis or cardiac failure has an increased aldosterone secretion rate, at least in part, because of activation of the renin-angiotensin system. Thus, the term secondary hyperaldosteronism has been used to describe this situation. These edematous patients not only have increased plasma renin activity but also have evidence of increased adrenergic activity and impaired renal hemodynamics. Taken together, therefore, the renal ischemia, increased renin-angiotensin activity, and enhanced adrenergic tone could be responsible for the failure of these patients to escape from the sodium-retaining effects of mineralocorticoids. Conversely, suppression of the renin-angiotensin system and adrenergic tone and improved renal hemodynamics may be responsible, at least in part, for the "escape" from the sodium-retaining effects of mineralocorticoids in the normal subject or the patient with primary hyperaldosteronism. This hypothesis, although plausible, is in need of investigation. Certainly other explanations are possible to elucidate this difference in the escape phenomenon in primary and secondary hyperaldosteronism. For example, a "natriuretic" hormone may be released in the normal subject secondary to ECF volume expansion and mediate aldosterone escape. In contrast, in the edematous patient, natriuretic hormone is not released because of a persistent decrease in "effective" arterial blood volume secondary to events such as venous sequestration (cirrhosis, cardiac failure), decreased cardiac output (cardiac failure), hypoalbuminemia (nephrotic syndrome and cirrhosis), and peripheral vasodilatation (cirrhosis). These events are probably also responsible for the increased renin-angiotensin and adrenergic activities in edematous patients.

Corticosteroids with Aldosterone-Like Activity

A very large number of corticosteroids, including most compounds with "glucocorticoid activity," share to varying degrees the electrolyte-regulating activity of aldosterone.

11-Desoxycorticosterone (DOC) is an aldosterone-like compound that is of historical importance because it was for many years the principal corticosteroid used in the treatment of Addison's disease. Although DOC is an important intermediate in adrenal biosynthesis of corticosterone and aldosterone, it is not itself released into the blood in biologically significant quantities except under abnormal circumstances. Faulty conversion of DOC to corticosterone is observed in patients with the "hypertensive" variety of congenital adrenal hyperplasia and in individuals treated with a chemical inhibitor of 11-β-hydroxylase such as 2-methyl-1,2-bis(3-pyridyl)-1-propanone (metyrapone). Under such conditions, DOC is secreted in appreciable quantities and acutely causes sodium retention and potassium loss and, over a sufficient period, hypertension.

Corticosterone has electrolyte-regulating activity that is qualitatively similar to that of aldosterone, but it has less than 1 % of the potency of aldosterone. In certain animals, including the rat, corticosterone is the principal glucocorticoid. In man, corticosterone is secreted in quantities on the order of 5 mg/day. Compared with cortisol (hydrocortisone), it is of little importance as a glucocorticoid, and compared with aldosterone, it is of little importance normally as a regulator of electrolyte metabolism.

Aldosterone Antagonists

Aldosterone antagonists are steroids that reverse the effects of aldosterone-like steroids on electrolyte and water excretion. The clearest examples of aldosterone antagonists are the synthetic steroids known as "spirolactones." These compounds have little or no effect upon fluid or electrolyte metabolism when administered in the absence of aldosterone-like steroids, but in the presence of aldosterone-like steroids, the spirolactones cause an increase in excretion of sodium, chloride, and water while diminishing the excretion of potassium, ammonium, and titratable acid. It has been demonstrated that the spirolactones are competitive inhibitors of aldosterone and that they block the attachment of aldosterone-like steroids to a specific receptor substance within cells of the renal tubules. Prog-

esterone is an endogenous aldosterone antagonist. It, and possibly other naturally occurring steroids, also acts by competitively blocking the binding of aldosterone-like steroids to specific receptor proteins within the cytosol and nuclei of responsive cells.

Next, several clinical disorders will be discussed that involve alterations in sodium, chloride, and potassium excretion. Since adrenal disorders are discussed in detail in Ch. 5, the focus in the present chapter will be on the effects of several disorders on electrolyte excretion.

PRIMARY HYPERALDOSTERONISM

Patients with primary hyperaldosteronism have many of the characteristics of a normal subject receiving exogenous mineralocorticoid. For example, ECF volume expansion without edema is characteristic of both circumstances. The major difference is that the normal subject does not become hypertensive before or during the period of aldosterone escape, but perhaps longer periods of exogenous aldosterone excess might cause a rise in blood pressure. In both circumstances, the expansion of ECF volume is associated with an exaggerated response to a saline load. Also, the ECF volume expansion decreases proximal tubular reabsorption and increases distal fluid and sodium delivery. The combination of the increased distal delivery and excess aldosterone activity leads to renal potassium wasting and hypokalemia. If chronic hypokalemia is secondary to extrarenal losses, e.g., gastrointestinal, the urinary potassium concentration should be less than 20 mEq/l, whereas with primary hyperaldosteronism the urinary potassium will be greater than 20 mEq/l. Increased hydrogen ion secretion also occurs and the patients also present with a mild metabolic alkalosis. The chronic hypokalemia is responsible for many of the signs and symptoms of primary hyperaldosteronism, including polydipsia, polyuria, weakness, paresthesias, tetany, and myocardial irritability. The electrocardiogram (ECG) may demonstrate depressed T-waves and the presence of U-waves. It should be pointed out that sodium restriction may diminish distal delivery and ameliorate renal potassium losses in patients with primary hyperaldosteronism. Thus, a low serum potassium (less than 3.5 mEq/l) is a good screening test for primary hyperaldosteronism only if the patient is on a normal sodium intake. The hypokalemic hypertensive patient on a normal sodium intake who is not receiving diuretics therefore should be evaluated for primary hyperaldosteronism. A low plasma renin activity and increased urinary aldosterone excretion support the diagnosis. With saline loading, elevated plasma aldosterone levels are not suppressed but the renal potassium losses are worsened. The adrenal lesion may be an adenoma or adrenal hyperplasia. Since adrenal hyperplasia responds poorly to surgery, this diagnosis is important to establish. A stimulation in plasma renin activity in the upright posture, relatively more DOC than aldosterone, and only a modest degree of hypokalemia provide some clues to the diagnosis of primary aldosteronism secondary to adrenal hyperplasia. Unilateral elevation in adrenal venous aldosterone suggests the presence of an adenoma. Lastly, it should also be remembered that excessive black licorice ingestion may mimic primary hyperaldosteronism.

SECONDARY HYPERALDOSTERONISM

Patients with secondary hyperaldosteronism have associated hyperreninemia, which is in large part responsible for the excess aldosterone. Most of these patients are not hypertensive; however, it should be mentioned that patients with *renal vascular hypertension* and *malignant or accelerated hypertension* have secondary hyperaldosteronism.

Pregnancy also represents a state of secondary hyperaldosteronism since plasma renin activity and concentration also are increased. Estrogen concentrations in blood also are increased during pregnancy and may contribute to the sodium retention that occurs during gestation. As already discussed, patients with *edematous disorders* generally have secondary hyperaldosteronism. The variability in the degree of hyperreninemia and hyperaldosteronism in these edematous disorders may relate to the stage of sodium retention. In the early stages of experimental models of sodium retention, including thoracic vena caval constriction and pulmonary hypertension with right-sided heart failure, plasma renin and aldosterone are quite high and the response to an angiotensin inhibitor is dramatic. The angiotensin inhibitor lowers both blood pressure and plasma aldosterone levels, indicating a dual role of the increased angiotensin activity to increase peripheral vascular resistance and stimulate aldosterone secretion. In the later stages, after considerable sodium retention has occurred, the renin-angiotensin-aldosterone activity returns towards control and no response to the angiotensin antagonist is observed. It thus seems likely that the stage of development of sodium retention is an important determinant of the activity of the renin-angiotensin-aldosterone activity in edematous disorders.

Patients with secondary hyperaldosteronism generally do not present with hypokalemia in the absence of treatment with diuretics. The explanation appears to be that distal fluid and sodium delivery is decreased in edematous disorders as a result of a diminution in GFR and increased reabsorption in the proximal tubule. When diuretics increase fluid and sodium delivery to the potassium secretory site, however, renal potassium losses increase and hypokalemia occurs.

Idiopathic cyclical edema appears to be a variety of secondary hyperaldosteronism that occurs in females and is exacerbated by the upright posture. Body weight increases and calf size enlarges after a day of ambulation, and in some patients the peripheral edema is worse at the time of the menstrual cycle. Recently, a hypothesis explaining the pathogenesis of idiopathic edema in some patients has been proposed. Many such patients commence diuretics for cosmetic reasons such as weight reduction. After prolonged diuretic use a state of hyperreninemia and secondary hyperaldosteronism occurs. With cessation of the diuretics sodium retention, edema, and weight gain occur and the patient or physician usually reinstitutes the diuretic. If diuretics are not restarted, however, the secondary hyperaldosteronism and sodium retention subside over a period of days or weeks and the edema disappears. The largest positive sodium balances and the longest duration necessary for restoration of normal sodium balances appear to occur in those patients with the highest plasma level of renin and aldosterone. Thus, this sequence of events has been described as "diuretic-induced edema." Although this sequence of events may account for some cases of idiopathic edema, it is still possible that a "capillary leak" is the main pathogenetic factor in many cases, particularly in those patients who have not been treated with diuretics.

Bartter's syndrome was described in children with hypokalemic metabolic alkalosis, hypomagnesemia, high plasma renin activity and urinary aldosterone levels, and resistance to the pressor effect of angiotensin. Recently, increased urinary prostaglandin excretion has also been described. The pathogenesis of Bartter's syndrome is not known, but treatment with agents such as indomethacin that inhibit prostaglandin synthesis has had some success. With indomethacin, urinary prostaglandins diminish, sodium retention occurs, plasma renin and aldosterone levels are suppressed, and plasma potassium concentration rises towards normal. It has been suggested recently that a primary defect in chloride transport in the loop of Henle exists that causes renal sodium chloride wasting and increases plasma renin and aldosterone, renal potassium wasting, and the hypokalemia and then stimulates renal prostaglandin synthesis. The prostaglandin inhibition then suppresses renin release and aldosterone activity but the defect in sodium chloride transport persists with increased sodium and fluid delivery to the potassium secretory site. Thus, the hypokalemia of Bartter's syndrome is not totally corrected by indomethacin.

It is important to point out that chronic use of loop diuretics, which inhibit chloride transport, may mimic totally Bartter's syndrome. Moreover, adults may use diuretics surreptitiously and present as though they were patients with Bartter's syndrome. Careful sleuthing and measurement of diuretics in the urine may reveal that the patient's problems actually relate to diuretic abuse; such patients have been termed as having pseudo Bartter's syndrome. Similarly, the patient who is a surreptitious vomiter or who abuses cathartics may present with many of the characteristics of Bartter's syndrome. The urinary chloride concentration will be less than 10 mEq/l in the patient with surreptitious vomiting and will be quite high in the patient who abuses diuretics. The cathartic abuser may present with metabolic acidosis, whereas the patients with diuretic abuse, surreptitious vomiting, or Bartter's syndrome will have metabolic alkalosis. Measurement of phenophthalein in the urine may provide a clue to cathartic abuse, and, if ECF volume depletion is present, the urinary sodium and chloride will be less than 20 mEq/l.

ADRENAL INSUFFICIENCY

The patient with primary adrenal insufficiency presents with symptoms that relate to deficiency of both glucocorticoid and mineralocorticoid deficiency, whereas the patient with pituitary disease and secondary adrenal insufficiency presents with symptoms that relate only to glucocorticoid deficiency. A patient who has been on chronic steroid therapy that is then discontinued also will present primarily with symptoms of glucocorticoid deficiency since the renin-angiotensin-aldosterone system is intact. The glucocorticoid-deficient patient may present with fever, weight loss, lethargy, anorexia, nausea, vomiting, diarrhea, and abdominal pain. Depending on the fluid intake, the patient may or may not be hyponatremic. Excessive pigmentation may or may not be present. Hypotension may be present in the absence of ECF volume depletion since glucocorticoid deficiency is accompanied by a negative inotropic effect on cardiac function and a diminished response of arterioles to norepinephrine. Glucocorticoid deficiency also does not activate the renin-angiotensin system to the degree observed with mineralocorticoid deficiency. This is probably due to the ECF volume depletion with mineralocorticoid deficiency and perhaps diminished renin substrate production with glucocorticoid deficiency. In any case, not only is plasma renin activity higher in mineralocorticoid versus glucocorticoid deficiency but a much more profound fall in blood pressure occurs during the administration of an angiotensin antagonist with mineralocorticoid deficiency.

In the diagnosis of glucocorticoid deficiency it is important to remember that a normal plasma cortisol level does not exclude the diagnosis when obtained during a period of stress. In fact, it supports the diagnosis since a subnormal plasma cortisol level may have become normal in response to very high levels of ACTH. A normal plasma cortisol level obtained during stress therefore should be followed by a 2-hour cosyntropin (Cortrosyn) test. Skull films should be obtained and other endocrine disorders of course should be excluded if secondary adrenal insufficiency or pituitary disease is suspected.

In the patient with Addison's disease, additional adverse effects relating to mineralocorticoid deficiency may be present, since aldosterone increases sodium reabsorption and enhances the secretion of potassium, hydrogen ion, and ammonium in the kidney, salivary glands, and gastrointestinal tract. The patient may have evidence of ECF volume depletion, hyponatremia, hyperkalemia, metabolic acidosis, and prerenal azotemia. The ECF volume depletion occurs secondary to renal sodium losses but may be worsened by poor intake and diarrhea. These patients with mineralocorticoid deficiency therefore tolerate sodium and water loss and potassium or acid loads poorly. Since ACTH has only a transient stimulatory effect on aldosterone, the Addisonian patient during stress may have a normal plasma cortisol but a very low plasma aldosterone level. Although tuberculosis and fungal disease used to be common causes of Addison's disease, an immune disorder may now be the primary cause. The patient with Addison's disease therefore may have other associated, potentially immunologically mediated disorders including pernicious anemia, thyroiditis, hypothyroidism, and diabetes mellitus.

Recently, a state of hyporeninemic hypoaldosteronism has been diagnosed in patients with early diabetic nephropathy or interstitial nephritis. These patients have only mild renal impairment and present with hyperkalemia and hyperchloremic metabolic acidosis. In some patients the hyperkalemia may be severe enough to necessitate treatment with mineralocorticoid replacement. The hyperchloremic acidosis also may be corrected partially by mineralocorticoid replacement. A glucose load in the insulin-deficient diabetic patient with hyporeninemic hypoaldosteronism may precipitate life-threatening hyperkalemia. This is because insulin normally moves potassium and glucose into cells, thus counteracting the osmotic effect of hyperglycemia to increase water movement and potassium movement, perhaps secondary to bulk flow, from the intracellular to ECF compartment. Prostaglandin inhibitors, such as indomethacin, also have been found recently to uncover previous subclinical cases of hyporeninemic hypoaldosteronism. This effect presumably occurs secondary to these agents' capacity to suppress renin release.

Isolated aldosterone deficiency also has been rarely reported in some patients without hyporeninemia. Of course, the Addisonian patient who is replaced only with glucocorticoid hormone may have isolated aldosterone deficiency. This may become apparent only during periods of sodium losses, e.g., diarrhea. Lastly, it should be remembered that restoration of ECF volume depletion in this patient may increase distal fluid delivery to the potassium secretory site and thus correct the hyperkalemia even without mineralocorticoid replacement. Thus, the hyponatremic, hyperkalemic patient whose electrolyte abnormalities correct with saline replacement should still be evaluated for adrenal insufficiency.

HYPERADRENOCORTICISM

Cushing's disease is discussed in Ch. 5. It seems worthy, however, to emphasize that glucocorticoid hormone, particularly in excessive amounts, may affect water and electrolyte excretion. This is probably because glucocorticoid hormone may occupy mineralocorticoid receptors and thus increase tubular sodium reabsorption and enhance potassium and hydrogen ion secretion. This is no doubt the reason that patients with Cushing's syndrome, either spontaneous or iatrogenic, may present with hypokalemic metabolic alkalosis, sodium retention, and hypertension. The Cushing's syndrome secondary to ectopic ACTH produced by tumors may have no other clinical evidence of Cushing's syndrome except severe hypokalemic metabolic alkalosis.

REFERENCES

Water Metabolism

GENERAL

Anderson, B.: Regulation of water intake. *Physiol. Rev. 58*:582, 1978.

Anderson, R. J., et al.: Evidence for an in vivo antagonism between vasopressin and prostaglandin in the mammalian kidney. *J. Clin. Invest. 56*:420, 1975.

Andreoli, T. E., et al.: Questions and replies: Renal mechanisms of urinary concentrating and diluting processes. *Am. J. Physiol. 235*:F1, 1979.

Berl, T., et al.: Clinical disorders of water metabolism. *Kidney Int. 10*:117, 1976.

Berl, T., et al.: Mechanism of suppression of vasopressin during alpha adrenergic stimulation with norepinephrine. *J. Clin. Invest. 53*:219, 1974.

Berl, T., et al.: Mechanism of stimulation of vasopressin release during beta adrenergic stimulation with isoproterenol. *J. Clin. Invest. 53*:857, 1974.

Berl, T., and Schrier, R. W.: Water metabolism and the hypo-osmolar syndromes, In *Sodium and Water Homeostasis* (Contemporary Issues in Nephrology:Vol. 1). Brenner, B. M., and Stein, J. H. (eds.) New York, Churchill Livingstone, 1978.

Berl, T., and Schrier, R. W.: Water metabolism — an overview, In Papper, S., and Whang, R. (eds.), 1978 Symposium Cosponsored by the University of Oklahoma Health Sciences Center and the Veterans Administration. Oklahoma, Veterans Administration, in press.

Dousa, T. P., and Valtin, H.: Cellular actions of vasopressin in the mammalian kidney. *Kidney Int. 10*:46, 1976.

Dunn, F. L., et al.: The role of blood osmolality and volume in regulating vasopressin secretion in the rat. *J. Clin. Invest. 52*:3212, 1973.

Fitzsimons, J. T.: The physiological basis of thirst. *Kidney Int. 10*:3, 1976.

Kokko, J. P., and Rector, F. C., Jr.: Countercurrent multiplication system without active transport in inner medulla. *Kidney Int. 2*:214, 1972.

Kokko, J. P., and Tisher, C. C.: Water movement across nephron segments involved with the countercurrent multiplication system. *Kidney Int. 10*:64, 1976.

Robertson, G. L., et al.: Osmotic control of vasopressin function, In *Disturbances in Body Fluid Osmolality*. American Physiological Society. Andreoli, T. E., Grantham, J. J., et al. (eds.), Baltimore, Williams and Wilkins, 1977.

Robertson, G. L., et al.: The osmoregulation of vasopressin. *Kidney Int. 10*:25, 1976.

Schrier, R. W., and Berl, T.: Mechanism of the antidiuretic effect associated with interruption of parasympathetic pathways. *J. Clin. Invest. 51*:2613, 1972.

Schrier, R. W., and Berl, T.: Mechanism of effect of alpha adrenergic stimulation with norepinephrine on renal water excretion. *J. Clin. Invest. 52*:502, 1973.

Schrier, R. W., et al.: Osmotic and nonosmotic control of vasopressin release. *Am. J. Physiol. 236*:F321, 1979.

Schrier, R. W., et al.: Mechanism of antidiuretic effect of beta adrenergic stimulation. *J. Clin. Invest. 51*:97, 1972.

Schrier, R. W., and Miller, P. D.: Water metabolism in diabetes insipidus and the syndrome of inappropriate antidiuretic hormone secretion, In *Pathophysiology of the Kidney*. Kurtzman, N. A., and Martinez-Maldonado, M. (eds.). Springfield, Charles C Thomas, 1977.

Taylor, A.: Role of microtubules and microfilaments in the action of vasopressin, In *Disturbances in Body Fluid Osmolality*. American Physiological Society. Andreoli, T. E., Grantham, J. J., et al. (eds.), Baltimore, Williams and Wilkins, 1977.

Zimmerman, E. A., and Robinson, A. G.: Hypothalamic neurons secreting vasopressin and neurophysin. *Kidney Int. 10*:12, 1976.

CLINICAL DISORDERS OF POLYURIA

Berl, T., et al.: On the mechanism of polyuria in potassium depletion. The role of polydipsia. *J. Clin. Invest. 60*:620, 1977.

Buckalew, V. M., Jr., and Someren, A.: Renal manifestations of sickle cell disease. *Arch. Intern. Med. 133*:660, 1974.

Carney, S., et al.: A study in vitro of the concentrating defect associated with hypokalemia and hypercalcemia. *Pfleugers Arch. 366*:11, 1976.

Coggins, C. H., and Leaf, A.: Diabetes insipidus. *Am. J. Med. 42*:807, 1967.

Cox, M., and Singh, I.: Lithium and water metabolism. *Am. J. Med. 59*:153, 1975.

Danisi, G., et al.: Effect of chlorpropamide on urinary excretion of water and solute in patients with diabetes insipidus and on water flow across isolated toad bladder. *J. Clin. Endocrinol. Metab. 30*:528, 1970.

Dousa, T. P., and Valtin, H.: Action of antidiuretic hormone in mice with inherited vasopressin-resistant urinary concentration defects. *J. Clin. Invest. 54*:753, 1974.

Fichman, M. P., and Brooker, G.: Deficient renal cyclic adenosine 3′, 5′-monophosphate production in nephrogenic diabetes insipidus. *J. Clin. Endocrinol. Metab. 35*:35, 1972.

Fine, L. G., et al.: Functional profile of isolated uremic nephron. Impaired water permeability and adenylate cyclase responsiveness of the cortical collecting duct to vasopressin. *J. Clin. Invest. 61*:1519, 1978.

Forrest, J. N., Jr., et al.: On the mechanism of lithium-induced diabetes insipidus in man and the rat. *J. Clin. Invest. 53*:1115, 1974.

Forrest, J. N., Jr., et al.: Demeclocycline versus lithium for inappropriate secretion of antidiuretic hormone. *N. Engl. J. Med. 298*:173, 1978.

Halter, J. B., et al.: Selective osmoreceptor dysfunction in the syndrome of chronic hypernatremia. *J. Clin. Endocrinol. Metab. 44*:609, 1977.

Hogan, G. R., et al.: Pathogenesis of seizures occurring during restoration of plasma tonicity to normal in animals previously chronically hypernatremic. *Peidatrics 43*:54, 1969.

Lascelles, P. T., and Lewis, P. D.: Hypodipsia and hypernatremia associated with hypothalamic and suprasellar lesions. *Brain 95*:249, 1972.

Orloff, J., and Burg, M. B.: Vasopressin-resistant diabetes insipidus, In *The Metabolic Basis of Inherited Disease*. 3rd ed. Stanbury, J., Wyngaarden, J. B., et al. (eds.), New York, McGraw-Hill Book Co., Inc., 1972.

Pawlson, L. G., et al.: Effect of vasopressin on renal cyclic AMP generation in potassium-deficiency and patients with sickle hemoglobin. *Metabolism 19*:694, 1970.

Rado, J. P., et al.: Individual differences in antidiuretic response induced by dDAVP in diabetes insipidus. *Horm. Metab. Res. 8*:155, 1976.

Robinson, A. G.: DDAVP in the treatment of central diabetes insipidus. *N. Engl. J. Med. 294*:507, 1976.

Singer, I., and Forrest, J. V.: Drug-induced states of nephrogenic diabetes insipidus. *Kidney Int. 10*:82, 1976.

Sridhar, C. B., et al.: Syndrome of hypernatremia, hypodipsia and partial diabetes insipidus: A new interpretation. *J. Clin. Endocrinol. Metab. 38*:890, 1974.

Tannen, R. L., et al.: Vasopressin-resistant hyposthenuria in advanced chronic renal disease. *N. Engl. J. Med. 280*:1135, 1969.

HYPONATREMIC DISORDERS

Anderson, R. J., et al.: Mechanisms of portal hypertension-induced alterations in renal hemodynamics, renal water excretion, and renin secretion. *J. Clin. Invest. 58*:964, 1976.

Anderson, R. J., et al.: Mechanism of effect of thoracic inferior vena cava constriction on renal water excretion. *J. Clin. Invest. 54*:1473, 1974.

Arieff, A. I., and Guisado, R.: Effects on the central nervous system of hypernatremic and hyponatremic states. *Kidney Int. 10*:104, 1976.

Arieff, A. I., et al.: Neurological manifestations and morbidity of hyponatremia: Correlation with brain water and electrolytes. *Medicine* (Baltimore) *55*:121, 1976.

Bell, N. H., et al.: An explanation for abnormal water retention and hypoosmolality in congestive heart failure. *Am. J. Med. 35*:351, 1964.

Boykin, J., et al.: Role of plasma vasopressin in impaired water excretion of glucocorticoid deficiency. *J. Clin. Invest. 62*:738, 1978.

Boykin, J., et al.: Persistent plasma vasopressin levels in the hypoosmolar state associated with mineralocorticoid deficiency. *Min. Electrolyte Metab. 2*:310, 1979.

DeFronzo, R. A., et al.: Water intoxication in man after cyclophosphamide therapy. *Ann. Intern. Med. 78*:861, 1973.

Dubovsky, S. L., et al.: Syndrome of inappropriate secretion of antidiuretic hormone with exacerbated psychosis. *Ann. Intern. Med. 79*:551, 1973.

Hantman, D., et al.: Rapid correction of hyponatremia in the syndrome of inappropriate secretion of antidiuretic hormone: An alternative treatment to hypertonic saline. *Ann. Intern. Med. 78*:870, 1973.

Kleeman, C. R., et al.: Mechanisms of impaired water excretion in adrenal and pituitary insufficiency. IV. Antidiuretic hormone in primary and secondary adrenal insufficiency. *J. Clin. Invest. 43*:1641, 1964.

Linas, S. L., et al.: Vasopressin in the impaired water excretion of glucocorticoid deficiency. *Kidney Int.* (in press).

Miller, M., and Moses, A. M.: Drug-induced states of impaired water excretion in mammalian kidney. *Kidney Int. 10*:38, 1976.

Nolph, K. D., and Schrier, R. W.: Sodium, potassium and water metabolism in the syndrome of inappropriate antidiuretic hormone secretion. *Am. J. Med. 49*:534, 1970.

Schedl, H. P., and Bartter, F. C.: An explanation for and experimental correction of the abnormal water diuresis in cirrhosis. *J. Clin. Invest. 39*:248, 1960.

Schrier, R. W.: New treatments for hyponatremia. *N. Engl. J. Med. 298*:214, 1978.

Schrier, R. W., and Linas, S. L.: Mechanisms of the defect in water excretion in adrenal insufficiency (editorial). *Mineral Electrolyte Metab.* (in press).

Schrier, R. W., and Szatalowicz, V. L.: Disorders of water metabolism, In *Contributions to Nephrology: Disturbances of Water and Electrolyte Metabolism*. 7th Symposium on Nephrology, Hanover, Germany, (in press).

Seif, S. M.: Neurohypophyseal peptides in hypothyroid rats. Plasma levels and kidney response. *Metabolism 28*:137, 1979.

Skowsky, W. R., and Kikuchi, T. H.: The role of vasopressin in the impaired water excretion of myxedema. *Am. J. Med. 64*:613, 1978.

Ufferman, R. C., and Schrier, R. W.: Importance of sodium intake and mineralocorticoid hormone in the impaired water excretion in adrenal insufficiency. *J. Clin. Invest. 51*:1639, 1972.

Sodium, Chloride, and Potassium Excretion

GENERAL

Anderson, R. J., et al.: Prostaglandins: Effects on blood pressure, renal blood flow, sodium and water excretion. *Kidney Int. 10*:205, 1976.

Bello-Reusse, E., et al.: Effects of acute unilateral renal denervation in the rat. *J. Clin. Invest. 56*:208, 1975.

Bello-Reusse, E., et al.: Effect of renal sympathetic nerve stimulation on proximal water and sodium reabsorption. *J. Clin. Invest. 57*:1104, 1976.

Berl, T., et al.: Prostaglandins in the beta-adrenergic and baroreceptor-mediated secretion of renin. *Am. J. Physiol. 235*:F472, 1979.

Brenner, B. M., and Berliner, R. W.: The transport of potassium, In *Handbook of Physiology (Renal Physiology)*, Section 8, Chapter 16. American Physiological Society. Orloff, J., and Berliner, R. W. (eds.), Baltimore, Williams and Wilkins, 1973, pp. 497–519.

Burg, M. B.: The renal handling of sodium chloride, In *The Kidney*. Brenner, B. M., and Rector, F. C. (eds.), Philadelphia, W. B. Saunders, 1976.

Burg, M. B., and Green, N.: Function of the thick ascending limb of Henle's loop. *Am. J. Physiol. 224*:659, 1973.

Clarkson, E. M., et al.: Two natriuretic substances in extracts of urine from normal man when salt-depleted and salt-loaded. *Kidney Int. 10*:381, 1976.

Davis, J. O.: Control of renin release. *Hosp. Prac. 9*:55, 1974.

de Wardener, H. E.: The control of sodium excretion. *Am. J. Physiol. 235*:F163, 1978.

Dumond, A. E., and Mulholland, J. H.: Hepatic lymph in cirrhosis, In *Progress in Liver Disease* Vol. II. Popper, H., and Shaffner, F. (eds.), New York, Grune and Stratton, 1965.

Giebisch, G.: Renal potassium excretion, In *The Kidney: Morphology, Biochemistry, Physiology*, Vol. III. Rouiller, C., and Muller, A. F. (eds.), New York, Academic Press, 1971.

Good, D. W., and Wright, F. S.: Luminal influences on potassium secretion: Sodium concentration and fluid flow rate. *Am. J. Physiol. 236*:F192, 1979.

Henrich, W. L., et al.: Mechanisms of renin secretion during hemorrhage in the dog. *J. Clin. Invest. 64*:1, 1979.

Kinne, R.: Current concepts of renal proximal tubular function. *Contrib. Nephrol. 14*:14, 1978.

Lameiere, N. H., et al.: Heterogeneity of renal function. *Ann. Rev. Physiol. 39*:159, 1977.

Linas, S. L., et al.: Studies on the mechanism of renal potassium conservation in the rat. *Kidney Int. 15*:601, 1979.

Nizet, A.: The isolated perfused kidney: Possibilities, limitations and results. *Kidney Int. 7*:1, 1975.

Patrick, J.: Assessment of body potassium stores. *Kidney Int. 11*:476, 1977.

Peterson, L. N., and Wright, F. S.: Effect of sodium intake on renal potassium excretion. *Am. J. Physiol. 233*:F225, 1977.

Porter, G. A., and Edelman, I. S.: The action of aldosterone and related corticosteroids on sodium transport across the toad bladder. *J. Clin. Invest. 43*:611, 1964.

Reineck, H. J., et al.: Net potassium addition beyond the superficial distal tubule of the rat. *Am. J. Physiol. 235*:F104, 1978.

Schrier, R. W., and de Wardener, H. E.: Tubular reabsorption of sodium ion: Influence of factors other than aldosterone and glomerular filtration rate. *N. Engl. J. Med. 285*:1231; 1292, 1971.

Sharp, G. W. G., and Leaf, A.: Biological action of aldosterone in vitro. *Nature 202*:1185, 1964.

Sharp, G. W. G., and Leaf, A.: The mechanism of action of aldosterone. *Physiol. Rev. 46*:593, 1966.

Tannen, R. L.: Relationship of renal ammonia production and potassium homeostasis. *Kidney Int. 11*:453, 1977.

Tucker, B. J., and Blantz, R.: Determinants of proximal tubular reabsorption as mechanisms of glomerular tubular balance. *Am. J. Physiol. 235*:F142, 1978.

Wright, F. S.: Potassium transport by the renal tubule, In *Kidney and Urinary Tract Physiology*. (MTP International Review of Science-Physiology Series: Vol. 6.) Thurau, K. (ed.), Baltimore, University Park Press, 1974.

EDEMATOUS STATES AND ADRENOCORTICAL DISORDERS

Ammon, R. A., et al.: Glucose-induced hyperkalemia with normal aldosterone levels. *Ann. Intern. Med.* 89:349, 1978.

Bartter, F., et al.: Hyperplasia of the juxtaglomerular complex with hyperaldosteronism and hypokalemic alkalosis: A new syndrome. *Am. J. Med.* 33:811, 1962.

Bernard, D. B., et al.: Renal sodium retention during volume expansion in experimental nephrotic syndrome. *Kidney Int.* 14:478, 1978.

Better, O. S., and Massry, S. G.: Effect of chronic bile duct obstruction on renal handling of salt and water. *J. Clin. Invest.* 51:402, 1972.

Brunner, F. P., and Frick, P. G.: Hypokalemia, metabolic alkalosis, and hypernatraemia due to "massive" sodium penicillin therapy. *Br. Med. J.* 4:550, 1968.

Cannon, P. J.: The kidney in heart failure. *N. Engl. J. Med.* 296:26, 1977.

Chaimovitz, C., et al.: Mechanism of increased renal tubular sodium reabsorption in cirrhosis. *Am. J. Med.* 52:198, 1972.

Chonko, A. M., et al.: The role of renin and aldosterone in the salt retention of edema. *Am. J. Med.* 63:881, 1977.

Conn, J. W.: Primary aldosteronism, a new clinical syndrome. *J. Lab. Clin. Med.* 45:3, 1955.

Conn, J. W.: Hypertension, the potassium ion and impaired carbohydrate tolerance. *N. Engl. J. Med.* 273:1135, 1965.

Conn, J. W., et al.: Licorice-induced pseudoaldosteronism. *J.A.M.A.* 205:492, 1968.

Coppage, W. S., et al.: Inhibition of aldosterone secretion and modification of electrolyte excretion in man by a chemical inhibitor of 11-beta-hydroxylation. *J. Clin. Invest.* 38:2101, 1959.

Epstein, M., et al.: Determinants of deranged sodium and water homeostasis in decompensated cirrhosis. *J. Lab. Clin. Med.* 87:822, 1976.

Flambaum, C. D., et al.: Serial evaluation of the renin-angiotensin-aldosterone system in caval dogs. *Circ. Res.* 42:778, 1978.

Gaffney, T. E., and Braunwald, E.: Importance of the adrenergic nervous system in the support of circulatory function in patients with congestive heart failure. *Am. J. Med.* 34:320, 1963.

Giebisch, G.: Some reflections on the mechanism of renal tubular potassium transport. *Yale J. Biol. Med.* 8:315, 1975.

Gill, J. R.: Edema. *Ann. Rev. Med.* 21:269, 1970.

Gill, J. R., Jr., et al.: Bartter's syndrome: A disorder characterized by high urinary prostaglandin and a dependence of hyper-reninemia on prostaglandin synthesis. *Am. J. Med.* 61:43, 1976.

Gill, J. R., Jr., and Bartter, F. G.: Evidence for a prostaglandin-independent defect in chloride reabsorption in the loop of Henle as a proximal cause of Bartter's syndrome. *Am. J. Med.* 65:766, 1978.

Grausz, H., et al.: Effect of plasma albumin on sodium reabsorption in patients with nephrotic syndrome. *Kidney Int.* 1:47, 1972.

Gregory, P. B., et al.: Complications of diuresis in the alcoholic patients with ascites: A controlled trial. *Gastroenterology* 73:534, 1977.

Gross, E. G., et al.: Hypokalemic myopathy with myoglobinuria associated with licorice ingestion. *N. Engl. J. Med.* 274:602, 1966.

Hodin, E., and Remington, J. H.: Villous adenoma with severe electrolyte depletion. *Dis. Colon Rectum* 12:36, 1969.

Kassirer, J. P., and Harrington, J. T.: Diuretics and potassium metabolism: A reassessment of the need, effectiveness and safety of potassium therapy. *Kidney Int.* 11:505, 1977.

Knochel, J. P.: Role of glucoregulatory hormones in potassium homeostasis. *Kidney Int.* 11:443, 1977.

Knochel, J. P., and Schlein, E. M.: On the mechanism of rhabdomyolysis in potassium depletion. *J. Clin. Invest.* 51:1750, 1972.

Kuchel, O., et al.: Inappropriate response to upright posture: A precipitating factor in the pathogenesis of idiopathic edema. *Ann. Intern. Med.* 73:245, 1970.

Lancestremere, R. G., et al.: Renal failure in Laennec's cirrhosis. II. Simultaneous determination of cardiac output and renal hemodynamics. *J. Clin. Invest.* 41:1922, 1962.

Landau, R. L., and Lugibihl, K.: Inhibition of the sodium-retaining influence of aldosterone by progesterone. *J. Clin. Endocrinol.* 18:1237, 1958.

Levinsky, N. G.: Refractory ascites in cirrhosis. *Kidney Int.* 14:93, 1978.

Levy, M.: Sodium retention and ascites formation in dogs with experimental portal cirrhosis. *Am. J. Physiol.* 233:F572, 1977.

Levy, M.: Sodium retention in dogs with cirrhosis and ascites: Efferent mechanisms. *Am. J. Physiol.* 233:F586, 1977.

Levy, M., and Allotey, J. B.: Temporal relationships between urinary salt retention and altered systemic hemodynamics in dogs with experimental cirrhosis. *J. Lab. Clin. Med.* 82:560, 1978.

Levy, M., and Wexler, M. J.: Renal sodium retention and ascites formation in dogs with experimental cirrhosis but without portal hypertension or increased splanchnic vascular capacity. *J. Lab. Clin. Med.* 91:520, 1978.

Liddle, G. W.: Aldosterone antagonists. *Arch. Intern. Med.* 102:998, 1958.

Lieberman, F. L., et al.: The relationship of plasma volume, portal hypertension, ascites and renal sodium retention in cirrhosis: The overflow theory of ascites formation. *Ann. N. Y. Acad. Sci.* 170:202, 1970.

Lifschitz, M. D., and Schrier, R. W.: Alterations in cardiac output with chronic constriction of thoracic inferior vena cava. *Am. J. Physiol.* 225:1364, 1973.

Lipner, H. I., et al.: The behavior of carbenicillin as a nonreabsorbable anion. *J. Lab. Clin. Med.* 86:183, 1975.

MacGregor, G. A., et al.: Is idiopathic edema idiopathic? *Lancet* 1:397, 1979.

Oliver, W. J., et al.: Demonstration of increased catecholamine excretion in the nephrotic syndrome. *Proc. Soc. Exp. Biol. Med.* 125:1176, 1967.

Perez, G., et al.: Selective hypoaldosteronism with hyperkalemia. *Ann. Intern. Med.* 76:757, 1972.

Rosoff, L., et al.: Studies of renin and aldosterone in cirrhotic patients with ascites. *Gastroenterology* 69:698, 1975.

Schambelan, M., et al.: Isolated hypoaldosteronism in adults. A renin-deficiency syndrome. *N. Engl. J. Med.* 287:573, 1972.

Schrier, R. W., et al.: Effect of furosemide on free water excretion in edematous patients with hyponatremia. *Kidney Int.* 3:30, 1973.

Shear, L., et al.: Compartmentalization of ascites and edema in patients with hepatic cirrhosis. *N. Engl. J. Med.* 282:1391, 1970.

Streeten, D. H.: Idiopathic edema: Pathogenesis, clinical features, and treatment. *Metabolism* 27:353, 1978.

Wallace, M., et al.: Persistent alkalosis and hypokalemia caused by surreptitious vomiting. *Q. J. Med.* 37:577, 1968.

Watkins, L., et al.: The renin-angiotensin system in congestive failure in conscious dogs. *J. Clin. Invest.* 57:1606, 1977.

Zucker, I. H., et al.: The mechanism of adaptation of left atrial stretch receptors in dogs with chronic congestive heart failure. *J. Clin. Invest.* 60:323, 1977.

CHAPTER 21

The Prostaglandins

By James B. Lee

Since the previous edition published 6 years ago, a truly enormous amount of literature has appeared on the subject of prostaglandins (PG's), to the extent that approximately 2500 articles now appear annually, making this topic one of the most extensively and profoundly studied subjects in biology and medicine. The reason for this exponential growth, from a single article in 1961 to its present rate plateauing in 1976, is that these compounds have perhaps the most diverse and potent biologic activities on virtually every cellular tissue and organ system of any naturally occurring compounds hitherto discovered. This burgeoning literature naturally makes it impossible for a single author to authoritatively and completely review the subject, particularly when much of the published data is conflicting, confusing, and at times irreconcilable. Nevertheless, the author has attempted to define what he personally believes are the salient pieces of essential information for the student and professional uninitiated to this relatively new and rapidly expanding field. References have been held to a minimum, important citations being omitted for clarity and conciseness, and highly controversial and confusing data have been briefly treated. The interested reader who wishes more intimate knowledge of any given area of PG research has been provided with a source of excellent review articles. The entire subject has recently been reviewed in detail (Berti et al., 1977; Samuelsson and Paoletti, 1976; Horrobin, 1978; Lee, 1980).

HISTORICAL ASPECTS

The PGs are a unique group of cyclic fatty acids with vast and potent biologic effects involving almost every organ system in a variety of species including the human. Biologic activity ascribable to these compounds was first discovered in the early 1930s independently by Kurzrok and Lieb, Goldblatt, and von Euler, who observed that extracts of seminal vesicles or human semen caused contraction of the isolated uterus and lowering of blood pressure. Von Euler further characterized the responsible compounds as fatty acids and named them prostaglandins. Some 25 years later in 1960, Bergström and Sjövall isolated and identified two classes of prostaglandins in sheep seminal vesicles — PGE and PGF. Biologic activity ultimately ascribable to a third class, PGA, was discovered in rabbit kidney medulla (Lee et al., 1963). This third class of prostaglandins, originally called medullin, was first isolated in 1965 from rabbit kidney medulla and subsequently identified as PGA_2 (Lee et al., 1965, 1967; Lee, 1967). PGE_2 and $PGF_2\alpha$ were also isolated and identified in rabbit kidney medulla. In addition to these PGs, PGB, C, D, G, H, and I have been more recently described, together with a non-PG structure thromboxane, which is derived from PG precursors. All of these compounds possess varying stimulatory or inhibitory functions on biological processes, actions that form the substance of this chapter.

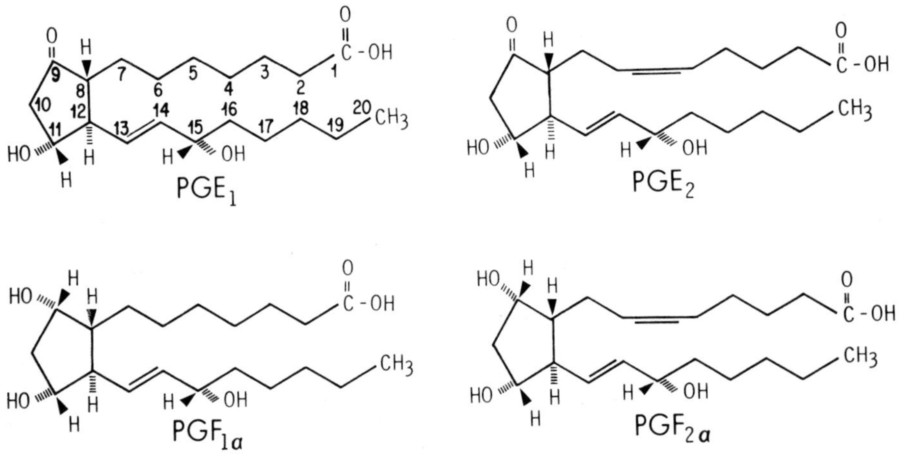

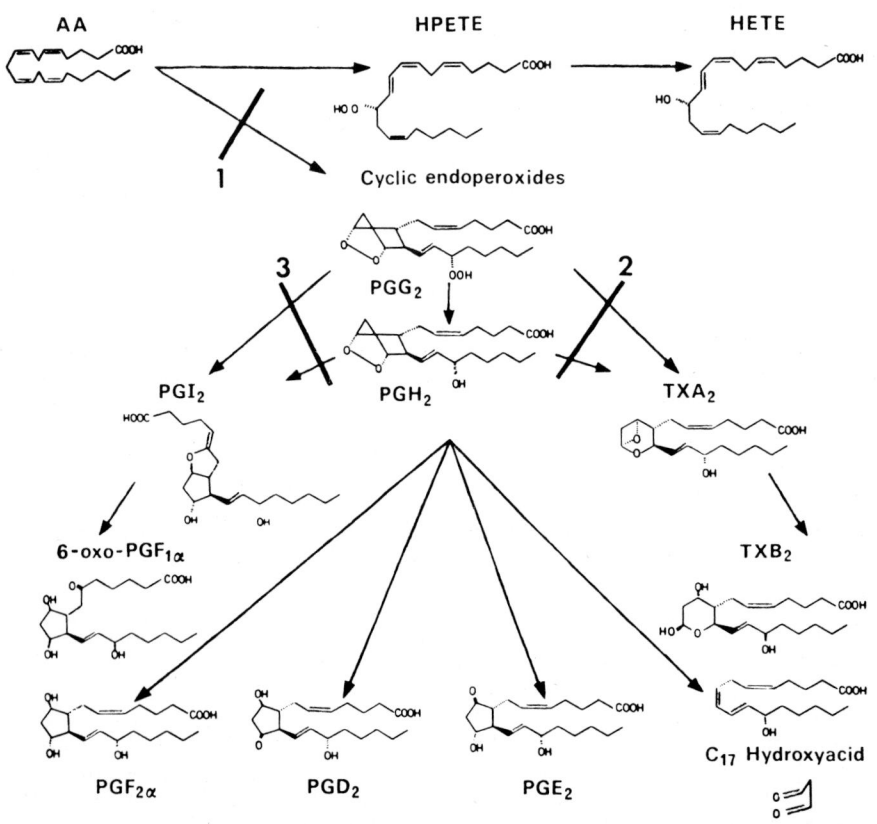

Figure 21–1. Structures of prostaglandins E and F.

STRUCTURAL CONSIDERATIONS

The structures of PGE and PGF are shown in Fig. 21–1 as prototypes for the other PG compounds, the structures of which are shown in Figs. 21–2 and 21–3 in the discussion on synthesis and metabolism. It is evident from Fig. 21–1 that the PGs are composed of a basic 20-carbon fatty acid containing a cyclopentane ring, the so-called hypothetical prostanoic acid. The carbons are numbered 1–20 from the carboxyl to the terminal methyl group. The PGs differ from one another in containing various degrees of substitution or unsaturation in the ring as well as in the aliphatic side chains, which confers upon them varying biological activities in much the same fashion as alterations in the steroid molecule result in marked changes in steroidogenic actions. PGE differs from PGF only in that there is a keto in position 9 in PGE and a hydroxyl in position 9 in PGF, the latter resulting in two stereochemical types of which PGFα is naturally occurring. The designations PGE_1, PGE_2, or PGE_3 refer only to the number of double bonds in the aliphatic side chains. Of all the PGs, the PG_2s are by far the most abundant naturally occurring class.

Figure 21–2. Metabolic pathways of PG biosynthesis from arachidonic acid. The sites where cyclo-oxygenase inhibitors (aspirin-like drugs), thromboxane synthetase inhibitors (imidazole and 1-methyl imidazole), and prostacyclin synthetase inhibitors (15-hydroperoxyarachidonic acid and 13-hydroperoxylinoleic acid) act are indicated by the numerals 1, 2, and 3, respectively. (From Moncada, S., and Vane, J. R.: Unstable metabolites of arachidonic acid and their role in haemostasis and thrombosis. *Brit. Med. Bull. 34*:129–135, 1978. With permission of the publisher.)

Abbreviations:
  AA: arachidonic acid
  HETE: 12-hydroxyarachidonic acid
  HPETE: 12-hydroxyperoxyarachidonic acid
  PGI₂: prostacyclin
  TXA₂: thromboxane A₂
  TXB₂: thromboxane B₂

BIOSYNTHESIS AND METABOLISM

Prostaglandin Formation

The immediate precursors of PG synthesis are essential unsaturated fatty acids esterified to membrane phospholipids, triglycerides, or sterols. It is believed the majority of diet-derived essential fatty acids are incorporated into phospholipid after which, with the appropriate stimulus, phospholipase A is activated, with liberation of the essential fatty acid and subsequent synthesis to PGs. For PGE_1 and $PGF_1\alpha$, the precursor is 8-11-14-eicosatrienoic acid (dihomo-γ-linolenic acid) and for PGE_2 and $PGF_2\alpha$ is 5, 8, 11, 14-eicosatetraenoic acid (arachidonic acid). PGE_3 can be formed from 5, 8, 11, 14, 17-eicosapentaenoic acid. The most ubiquitous pathway in mammalian tissue involves PG_2s derived from arachidonic acid. Fig. 21-2 summarizes the overall synthesis of PG_2s from arachidonic acid.

Following release of arachidonic acid there are two enzymes involved in its subsequent metabolism. The first is a lipoxygenase that forms unstable 12-hydroperoxy arachidonic acid (HPETE) and the stable hydroxy arachidonic acid (HETE). The second and more important enzyme is a cyclo-oxygenase that forms the biologically active endoperoxide PGG_2. This reaction has been shown by Smith and Willis (1971) and Ferreira and coworkers (1971) to be inhibited by aspirin, indomethacin, and other nonsteroidal anti-inflammatory agents, an effect that has been utilized widely in PG research in efforts to determine physiologic roles for endogenously produced PGs. PGG_2 is converted to PGH_2, from which PGE_2, PGD_2, and $PGF_2\alpha$ are formed. The enzymic formation of PGA_2 (PGE_2 dehydrated at position 10 in the ring) is controversial, a topic that will be treated briefly in the discussion on metabolism.

In addition to the classic prostaglandins, it has been shown by Hamberg and coworkers (1975) in platelets that unstable PGG_2 and PGH_2 can be metabolized by thromboxane synthetase to the potent platelet aggregating and vasoconstricting unstable thromboxane A_2, which is in turn converted to the inactive but stable thromboxane B_2, the former reaction being inhibited by imidazole. Lastly, PGG_2 and PGH_2 released from platelets can be converted by prostacyclin synthetase in vascular endothelium to the vasodilating and platelet inhibitory unstable PGI_2 (Bunting et al., 1976), which is metabolized to the stable but inactive 6-keto $PGF_1\alpha$ (Fig. 21-2).

In summary, therefore, PGs are formed ubiquitously throughout the body from PG endoperoxides derived from essential fatty acids, particularly arachidonic acid, in response to a host of variable stimuli. In platelets interacting with vascular endothelium, thromboxanes can also be formed from PG endoperoxides. The details of PG synthesis have recently been reviewed by Maclouf and associates (1977).

Prostaglandin Degradation

Since PGE and PGF are metabolized in a single passage through the lung by 15-PG dehydrogenase (PGDH) to inactive 15-keto PGEs or PGF, they do not function as circulating hormones in the classic sense. On the other hand, PGA and PGI compounds, both of which are vasodilatory, selectively escape metabolism by the lung and thus theoretically could function as circulating compounds. 15-Keto-PGE or PGF is subsequently reduced to 15-keto-13, 14 dihydro PG by PG reductase (13 PGR). 15-Keto-13, 14 dihydro PGs are subsequently transformed into the water-soluble tetranor compounds that appear in the urine by a process of β oxidation of the carboxyl side chain with loss of a 4-carbon fragment and by oxidation of the terminal carbon of the omega chain. 15-Keto-13, 14 dihydro PGs may also be converted to 13, 14 dihydro PGs, which in certain instances possess as much if not more biologic activity as the parent compounds. Fig 21-3 summarizes the metabolism of PGE_2.

The facile dehydration of PGE_2 to PGA_2 can occur enzymically and nonenzymically. Although the existence of PGA_2 has been questioned since it has not been found by G.C./mass spectrometry in renal medulla or human plasma, the existence of definite human plasma immunoreactive PGA material, the presence of a highly specific PGA 15 OH-PGDH in the kidney, the demonstration of enzymic conversion of PGE to PGA in human plasma and the natural occurrence of PGA in certain species of coral have left the precise status of PGA highly controversial. The metabolism of PGI_2 and thromboxane A_2 has been alluded to previously.

Prostaglandin Release

Once synthesized, PGs are released locally, where they may act as local mediators of cellular action leading to a wide variety of functional changes followed by local metabolism or secondary "overflow" release into the venous circulation for eventual metabolism by the lung, or both. The stimuli for PG synthesis and release are diverse, including spontaneous release, neural stimulation, hypoxia, 5-hydroxytryptamine (serotonin), acetylcholine, histamine, norepinephrine, vasopressin (VP), angiotensin II, and bra-

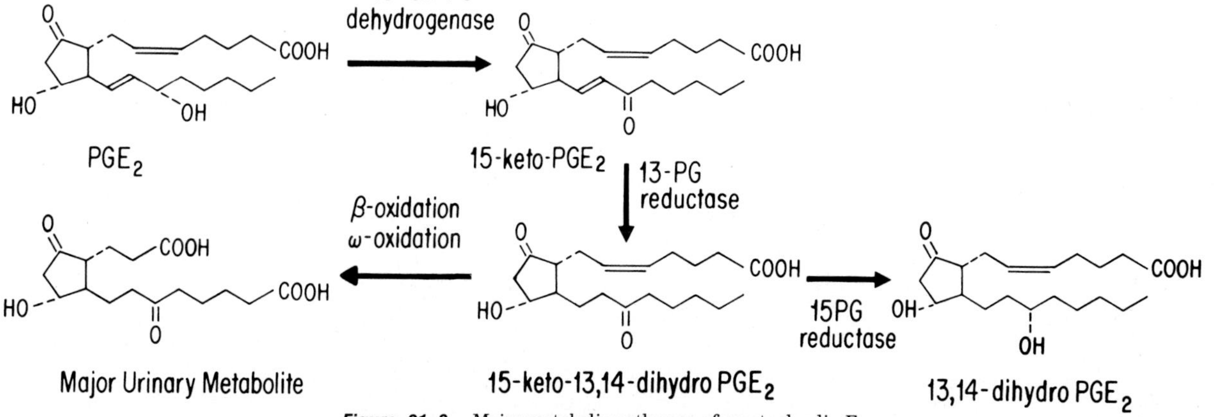

Figure 21-3. Major metabolic pathways of prostaglandin E_2.

dykinin to name a few. It is precisely these apparent conflicting and at times nonspecific stimuli of PG release that have led to so much confusion in the literature regarding possible physiologic roles for these compounds. In this regard it is important to note that the actions of released PGs are nonspecific, the same PG stimulating some target cell actions and inhibiting others. Any specificity of PG action is defived not from the particular PG but from the interaction of PGs with receptors specific for a particular cellular genotype leading to a response characteristic for the function of the cell being stimulated or inhibited by PGs.

BIOLOGIC ACTIONS

3′,5′-Cyclic AMP

The biologic actions of the prostaglandins are the most varied of any naturally occurring compounds. The actions of the prostaglandins are closely linked to changes in 3′,5′-cyclic AMP (cAMP), the same prostaglandin stimulating adenyl cyclase in one tissue and inhibiting it in another. When prostaglandins give rise to an increase in cAMP, target cell action is enhanced (Table 21–1). Conversely, when cell function is depressed by prostaglandins there is a decrease in cAMP (Table 21–2). It is now apparent, however, with the recent discovery of PGI_2 and thromboxane $(TX)A_2$, that these have more potent effects on both cAMP and cGMP than the PGEs. Thus PGI_2 is more potent than PGE_1 in stimulating platelet adenyl cyclase. Since there is a greater sensitivity of the PG receptor to PGI_2, it is quite possible PGI_2 may be the natural ligand that binds to the receptor. Furthermore TXA_2 is a potent inhibitor of PGE_1-stimulated cAMP in human platelets, and inhibition of TXA_2 by imidazole blocks the actions of lipolytic hormones (catecholamines) on both lipolysis and cAMP formation, suggesting that TXA_2 may be required for coupling between receptors and adenyl cyclase.

Fig. 21–4 illustrates a suggested mechanism by which prostaglandins exert a role in the transmission of the mes-

Table 21–2. TISSUES IN WHICH PROSTAGLANDINS* INHIBIT HORMONALLY INDUCED RESPONSES†

Tissue	Hormone	Response
Toad bladder	Vasopressin	Water transport
Rabbit kidney tubules	Vasopressin	Water transport
Rat adipocytes‡	Epinephrine ACTH TSH Glucagon Growth hormone	Lipolysis
Cerebellar Purkinje cells	Norepinephrine	Inhibition of discharge frequency

*PGE_1 most effective at <0.28 μM.
†From Shaw, J. E., Gibson, W., et al.: *Ann. N.Y. Acad. Sci.* 180:241, 1971, with permission.
‡Inhibition associated with decreased cyclic AMP accumulation.

sages of such tropic hormones as luteinizing hormone (LH), thyrotropin (TSH), and adrenocorticotropin (ACTH). The tropic hormone interacts with a membrane receptor, which leads to an increase in prostaglandin synthetase activity and prostaglandin production. The prostaglandins in turn activate membrane adenyl cyclase, possibly through a specific prostaglandin receptor. The resultant increase in cAMP generated from ATP then produces its action on cell function. Prostaglandins would act as a second messenger and cAMP as a third messenger. The most puzzling aspect, however, is the remarkable nonspecificity of prostaglandin action, augmenting cAMP accumulation in some systems and inhibiting it in others. Unlike other stimulators of adenyl cyclase, whose action is restricted to a particular target cell (parathyroid hormone [PTH] increases cAMP in kidney and bone but not in other tissues), prostaglandins have effects on cAMP in almost every cell line. Specificity, therefore, must reside and be inherent in each cell in a manner as yet unclear. Furthermore, as Horton (1972) has suggested, the fact that prostaglandins interact with cAMP does not identify their biochemical mechanisms of action, which still remain to be defined. It is highly likely that the prostaglandins will be found to function as local intracellular mediators responding to regional stimuli with responses

Table 21–1. TISSUES WHERE PROSTAGLANDINS INCREASE ACCUMULATION OF CYCLIC 3′, 5′-AMP*

Tissue	Species	Prostaglandin	(μM) most active
Lung	Rat	PGE_1	2.8
Spleen	Rat	PGE_1	2.8
Diaphragm	Rat	PGE_1	2.8
Adipose	Rat	PGE_1	2.8
Leucocytes	Human	PGE_1	–
Platelets†	Human	PGE_1	0.28
Platelets	Human	PGE_1	0.01
Platelets	Human	PGE_1	0.1
Platelets	Rabbit	PGE_1	0.1
Platelets	Rabbit	PGE_1	0.15
Liver	Rat	PGE_1	–
Anterior pituitary†	Rat	PGE_1	2.8
Aorta	Rat	PGE_1	2.8
Bone	Rat	PGE_1	–
Gastric mucosa†	Guinea pig	PGE_1	–
Kidney	Dog, rat	PGE_1	–
Heart	Guinea pig	PGE_1	0.01
		$PGF_{1\alpha}$	0.01
Corpus luteum†	Cow	PGE_2	28
Thyroid†	Dog	PGE_2	
Erythrocytes†	Rat	PGE_2	0.03

*From Shaw, J. E., Gibson, W., et al.: *Ann. N.Y. Acad. Sci.* 180:241, 1971, with permission.
†Indicates those tissues in which prostaglandins increase adenyl cyclase activity.

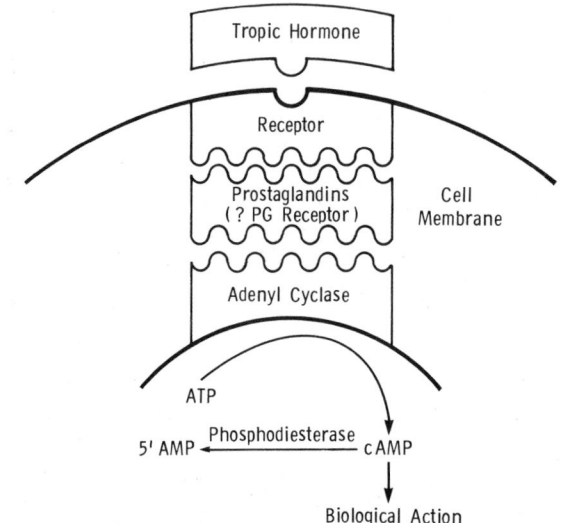

Figure 21–4. Postulated role of the interaction of prostaglandins and cAMP in the transmission of the trophic hormone message. (Reproduced with modification from Speroff, L., et al.: Prostaglandins and reproduction. In *Prostaglandins.* Lee, J. B. [ed.], New York, Medcom, 1973, p. 80, with permission.)

specific to the cells and tissues involved. This subject has been extensively reviewed by Kuehl and associates (1976).

Cardiovascular-Renal System

The original isolation and identification of the renomedullary prostaglandins were the result of a search for renal vasodilators that might account for the so-called antihypertensive function of the kidney. According to this hypothesis, experimental and human hypertension may not solely be the result of an excess activity of vasoconstrictor prohypertensive functions (renin-angiotensin-aldosterone axis and the sympathetic nervous system) but may be the result, at least in part, of a deficiency of vasodilating antihypertensive factors allowing prohypertensive agents to act unopposed, with the ultimate production of hypertension. Although the identification of the renal vasodilatory prostaglandins, PGA_2 and PGE_2, has provided biochemical support for the antihypertensive hypothesis, it soon became evident that these (and other) PGs have many other effects on renal function, such as regulation of renal blood flow, sodium and water excretion, and renin release. Although each of these is interdependent and closely related they will be briefly discussed individually for the sake of clarity. The interested reader is referred to several recent reviews for more detailed discussion of these complex phenomena (Dunn and Hood, 1977; Zins, 1975; Lee, 1978). No attempt will be made to review the cardiac actions of PGs, their effect on the regional and microcirculation and their interaction with the adrenergic nervous system, which are reviewed elsewhere (Nakano, 1973; Hedqvist, 1977; Rose and Kot, 1977; Moncada and Vane, 1978).

Renal Blood Flow and Sodium Excretion

Exogenous administration of PGE_1, PGE_2, PGA_1, PGA_2, PGD_2, PGG_2, PGI_2 and PGH_2 produces renal vasodilation, increase in renal blood flow, and natriuresis. When PG synthesis is increased by administration of arachidonic acid, there is an increase in deep cortical and inner medullary blood flow accompanied by natriuresis, both of which are inhibited by indomethacin. Although these PGs are natriuretic when given exogenously, PG biosynthesis and excretion rise on a low-salt diet and fall on a high-salt diet (Stahl et al., 1979), suggesting that endogenous PGs may actually participate in the antinatriuresis in volume contraction by stimulating the renin-angiotensin-aldosterone axis (vide infra). Loop diuretics such as furosemide, ethacrynic acid, and bumetanide result in increased renal blood flow and natriuresis with enhanced PGE excretion, suggesting that these agents act to release PGs and thereby facilitate sodium excretion. Since indomethacin has not been found by some observers to block diuretic-induced natriuresis, the nature of the interaction of diuretics and PGs remains controversial. It was originally postulated that PGs sustain resting renal blood flow since meclofenamate or indomethacin resulted in a decreased renal blood flow and antinatriuresis in anesthetized animals (Lonigro et al., 1973). This was not observed in the conscious dog (Zins, 1975), however, and it is now believed that intrarenal PG synthesis and release is enhanced to offset any stimulus (anesthesia, surgery, angiotensin II, norepinephrine, renal nerve stimulation, hemorrhage, renal ischemia, etc.) that tends to reduce renal blood flow as a compensatory mechanism to maintain cortical flow. The notable exception to this is the vasodilator bradykinin, which also increases renal PG synthesis. Clinically, this has important connotations, since in pathologic renal states associated with renal vasoconstriction such as acute and chronic renal failure in animals (Mauk et al., 1977) and in humans (Kimberly et al., 1978), PGE synthesis is compensatorily increased and administration of indomethacin results in a marked deterioration of glomerular filtration, renal blood flow, and renal function.

Water Excretion

Original studies (Orloff and Handler, 1965; Grantham and Orloff, 1968) revealed PGE_1 inhibits VP but not cAMP water movement in the toad bladder and isolated collecting duct cell, suggesting an inhibitory effect of PGE_1 on adenyl cyclase. In in vivo studies, inhibition of PG synthesis by aspirin, indomethacin, and meclofenamate results in enhancement of VP-stimulated water reabsorption and maximal urine osmolality. VP in turn stimulates PGE biosynthesis in the renal medulla, an effect associated with a decreased water permeability to VP, suggesting a possible negative feedback system.

Although in hypokalemic dogs there is a rise in urinary PGE (Galvez et al., 1976), and low medium potassium directly stimulates PGE_2 production in the interstitial cell tissue culture (Zusman and Keiser, 1977) and medullary slices (Dusing et al., 1978), recent studies by Attallah et al. have shown that renal PGE_2 synthesis and excretion are markedly diminished in hypokalemic rabbits. This suggests that the hypokalemic polyuria is not mediated by prostaglandins.

Renin Release and Blood Pressure Regulation

Although PGs are natriuretic in animals and PGA_1 has been found to produce a transient, albeit striking, initial rise in renal blood flow in hypertensive man (Lee et al., 1971), volume depletion, whether by sodium restriction (Payakkapan et al., 1975; Davila et al., 1978; Stahl et al., 1979), diuretic administration (Patak et al., 1975; Abe et al., 1977) or following hemodialysis (Juncos et al., 1977), leads to a striking rise in renal prostaglandin production (Fig. 21–5). Since arachidonic acid and PGs all stimulate renin production in vivo and since indomethacin results in a reduction in renin in vivo (Patak et al., 1975; Rumpf et al., 1975) and partially antagonizes the natriuretic and blood pressure lowering effects of furosemide, it has been postulated that volume-depleted renal PG release triggers renin release, leading to angiotensin II generation, an increase in aldosterone, and appropriate sodium retention. Recently, however, with the observation that angiotensin blockade or converting enzyme inhibition leads to a marked decrease in PG synthesis, it has also been postulated that volume depletion leads to a primary rise in renin-angiotensin, which stimulates the release of PGs (Fig. 21–6). Thus a positive feedback system exists between the renin axis and the PG system.

Perhaps the ameliorative effects of low sodium diet, diuretic therapy, and hemodialysis are the result of increased renal, circulating, or local vascular PGs that physiologically may antagonize both adrenergic and angiotensin-mediated vasoconstriction. This is supported by the fact that the decreased vascular reactivity to angiotensin II and norepinephrine in volume-depleted stages is reversed by indomethacin. Clinically this has important considerations in Bartter's syndrome, in which the hyperreninemia, hyperaldosteronism, and hypokalemic alkalosis are associated with elevated plasma and urinary PGs, all of these being reversed by aspirin, indomethacin, and so on (Fichman et al.,

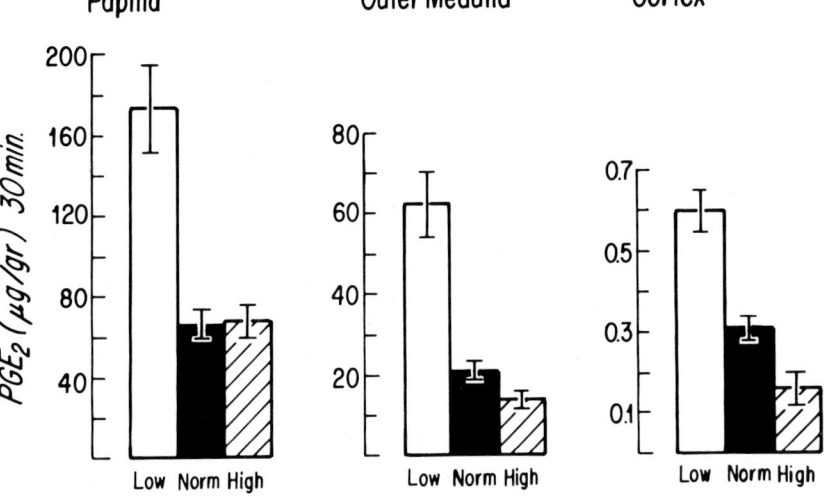

Papilla   **Outer Medulla**   **Cortex**

Figure 21-5. Effect of low-, normal-, and high-salt intakes on *in vitro de novo* PGE$_2$ biosynthesis. Values are means ± SE. PGE$_2$ production is that occurring following incubation in Krebs-Ringer HCO$_3^-$ buffer, 85% N$_2$, 10% O$_2$, 5% CO$_2$, 37° C, 30 min. (Reproduced from Stahl, R. A. K., et al.: Stimulation of rabbit renal PGE$_2$ biosynthesis by dietary sodium restriction. *Am. J. Physiol.* 237:F344, 1979. By permission.)

1976). That excessive PGs in this syndrome are the result of defect in chloride transport and not a primary cause of the syndrome has recently been discussed by Gill and Bartter (1978).

In summary, experimental evidence to date supports an antihypertensive role for the renal or systemic PGs (or both) in the regulation of systemic blood pressure in conformation with the renal antihypertensive endocrine function, a concept that led to the discovery of the renal PGs almost 20 years ago.

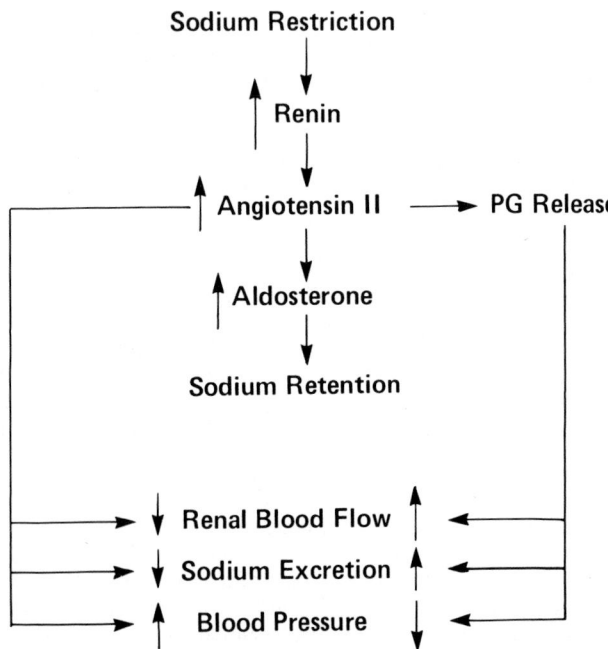

Figure 21-6. Hypothetical schema whereby volume depletion may lead to renin-angiotensin release and physiological antagonism of angiotensin II antinatriuretic and hypertensive actions. (From Lee, J. B.: Prostaglandins and the renin-angiotensin axis. *Clin. Nephrol.* 1980 (in press). With permission.)

Reproductive System

Despite the fact that the PGs were first isolated and are in high concentration in animal and human semen, a role for them in male reproductive physiology has not been established, although effects on seminal fluid transport and sperm motility have been reported. On the other hand, prostaglandins of the E and F classes have marked effects on the female reproductive systems of nonprimates and primates, including the human. Their main actions are to (1) produce luteolysis and decreased progesterone secretion, (2) stimulate gravid and nongravid uterine muscle to contract, (3) mediate LH-induced ovulation, and (4) act at the pituitary-hypothalamic level as mediators of LH releasing factor (LRF) on LH secretion. Most of these actions involve stimulation of adenyl cyclase activity, leading to a rise in intracellular cAMP.

The Estrous Cycle

Ovulation is followed by the development of the corpus luteum and increased progesterone secretion. The most likely series of events that involve PGs leading to luteolysis in the sheep is as follows: During the secretory phase the maturing follicle secretes increased quantities of estradiol that cause a rise in PGF$_2\alpha$ (previously called "uterine luteolysin"). This in turn results in luteolysis and a diminution in progesterone production. The subsequent continuing increase in estradiol then stimulates pituitary LH secretion, which, in a critical concentration relative to follicle stimulating hormone (FSH), initiates ovulation and repetition of the cycle (Fig. 21-7). The mechanism by which PGF$_2\alpha$ acts as a luteolysin is unknown, but its action may be the result of either a reduction in luteal blood flow or a direct inhibition of progesterone synthesis. The latter is most likely the result of inhibition by PGF$_2\alpha$ of luteal cholesterol synthetase, allowing greater esterification of cholesterol esters with concomitant decrease of progesterone precursor and hence of progesterone synthesis (Behrman et al., 1971).

The route by which uterine PGF$_2\alpha$ reaches the ovary in sheep is most likely by a countercurrent mechanism, whereby PGF$_2\alpha$ in the uterine vein is transferred to the ovarian artery, which is anatomically closely interwoven with the vein (McCracken et al., 1971). Since hysterectomy

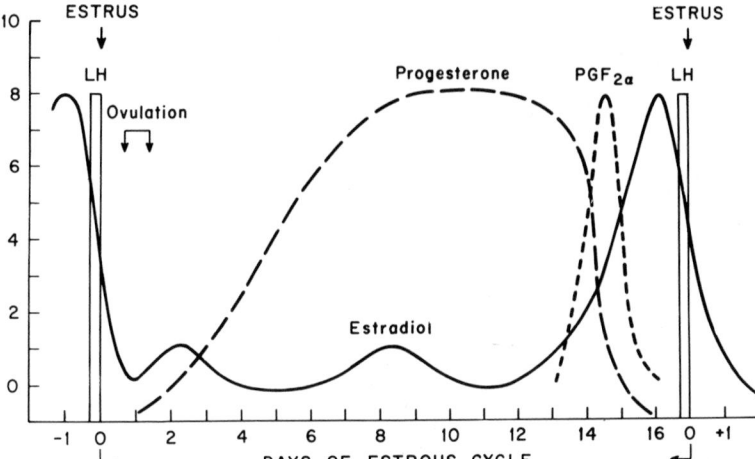

Figure 21–7. A model of the sheep estrous cycle, indicating the key role played by $PGF_{2\alpha}$ in producing the demise of the corpus luteum. (Reproduced from Caldwell, B. V., Tillson, S. A., et al.: The effects of exogenous progesterone and estradiol on prostaglandin F levels in ovariectomized ewes. *Prostaglandins* 1:217, 1972. With permission.)

does not alter the normal ovarian estrous cycle in the human, a uterine-ovarian countercurrent system of this type is unlikely. Human fallopian tube $PGF_2\alpha$ may have a luteolytic role, however, since fallopian tube fluid contains $PGF_2\alpha$, which increases in the immediate preovulatory period under rising estrogen stimulation. The occurrence of a normal estrous cycle after hysterectomy in the human may be explained by the fact that distal fallopian tubes are generally not removed during this procedure. The role of the fallopian tube PGs in the estrous cycle, tubal peristalsis, ciliary activity, and ovum transport has been summarized by Lippes (1975).

The rise in LH in turn stimulates ovarian PG synthesis and ovulation. Evidence of an LH ovulatory surge conditioned by $PGF_2\alpha$-mediated luteolysis and PG-mediated ovulation is supported by the observation that ovulation is inhibited by indomethacin (Armstrong and Griniwick, 1972; Hamada et al., 1977) and aspirin, potent inhibitors of prostaglandin synthesis. Further, PGF levels rise sharply during the preovulatory phase in normal ewes and ewes treated with progesterone plus estrogen but not with progesterone alone (Caldwell et al., 1972).

Evidence that the luteolytic action of $PGF_2\alpha$ may also, at times, be mediated via the pituitary-hypothalamus axis is threefold: (1) Hypothalamic extracts increase pituitary adenyl cyclase and LH release, and $PGF_2\alpha$ increases pituitary cAMP, (2) prostaglandin antagonists block stimulation of LH release by LRF, and (3) estrogen-induced hypothalamic PG production may participate in the preovulatory pulse in LH secretion.

Parturition

Physiologic Considerations

A significant normal role for $PGF_2\alpha$ in the process of parturition has been advanced from experimental work particularly in the rat. The production of $PGF_2\alpha$ by the placenta or uterus is low at the beginning of pregnancy, steadily increasing to very high levels at the onset of labor. Since $PGF_2\alpha$ is known to inhibit progesterone synthesis, it is of interest that there is an initially high activity of tissue PG metabolizing enzyme PGDH, suggesting a protective mechanism during pregnancy to obviate $PGF_2\alpha$-induced abortion by insuring low uterine levels.

Immediately before the onset of labor there is an increase in estrogen leading to an increase in uterine $PGF_2\alpha$ and a decrease in PGDH. The high effective levels of $PGF_2\alpha$ are

believed to decrease progesterone, leading to the onset of labor by an increased uterine sensitivity of oxytocin (OT)-enhanced spontaneous uterine contractions and possibly by a $PGF_2\alpha$-induced decrease in uterine blood flow. This schema is supported by the fact that aspirin and indomethacin result in prolonged parturition in animals and man and induce premature labor in both control and indomethacin-treated pregnancy animals. This subject has been reviewed in detail by Flower (1977)

In addition to a physiologic role in labor, the presence of $PGF_2\alpha$ in menstrual fluid together with its action in contracting gastrointestinal and uterine smooth muscle have suggested a role for $PGF_2\alpha$ in the production of the pain of dysmenorrhea.

Pharmacologic Considerations

$PGF_2\alpha$ and PGE_2 are potent oxytocics whether given orally or parenterally or instilled locally in the gravid uterus (Karim et al., 1968). The intravenous infusion rate necessary to induce labor is 0.5–2.0 μg/min for PGE_2 and 5–10.0 μg/min for $PGF_2\alpha$, and with the exception of hypertonus there are relatively few side effects. The delivery duration ranges from 30 min to almost 20 hours, depending on the state of inducibility. Similar degrees of inducibility with $PGF_2\alpha$ and OT have been noted in difficult and easily inducible patients (Anderson et al., 1972). Although extremely effective oxytocics, PGE and PGF seem to offer little immediate clinical advantage over OT since they are equally effective and act by similar if not interrelated mechanisms. The future clinical use of PGE_2 in labor induction is uncertain, but its highly desirable mechanism of action and its natural occurrence in the female reproductive system may ultimately make it a more attractive agent than OT. This subject has recently been reviewed by Tepperman and coworkers (1977).

Abortion

Karim and Filshei (1970) and Roth-Brandel and associates (1970) first observed the induction of therapeutic abortion in women with high success rates in midtrimester by intravenous injection. Subsequent investigation revealed many side effects, however, particularly nausea and vomiting. The most successful route appears to be a single injection of $PGF_2\alpha$ into the amniotic cavity. Success rates close to 100% have been reported with a mean duration of labor of 22 hours (Anderson et al., 1972). Side effects were few, and the number of incomplete abortions was relatively low (25%). The only current clinical application of prostaglandins is in midtrimester abortion by intra-amniotic injection. Suction curettage still remains preferable to prostaglandin administration during the first trimester. Recently, stimulation of endogenous PGs by drugs inhibiting their metabolism has been reported to be 100% effective in producing abortion (Lerner et al., 1975), possibly leading to a therapeutic use for these agents as antifertility drugs. Although prostaglandins have been suggested as effective "hindsight" oral contraceptive agents, little confirmational evidence has yet been forthcoming.

Hematopoietic System

Platelets

When endothelium is damaged, platelets are known to adhere to subendothelial connective tissue, leading to a release reaction involving secretion of such agents as catecholamines, serotonin, and adenosine diphosphate (ADP), which leads in turn to further platelet aggregation, a phenomenon intricately involved in the intrinsic clotting process. In 1966, Kloeze found that PGE_1 markedly inhibits the aggregation reaction, whereas PGE_2 is a potent stimulator. Subsequent studies revealed that platelets normally contain PGE_2 and $PGF_2\alpha$, that they are released during the clotting process, and that their synthesis and release are inhibited by aspirin, a potent PG synthetase inhibitor. The effect of PGE_2 on platelet aggregation induced by ADP is biphasic; it has little effect during the initial phases of aggregation but produces a prolonged secondary aggregation after exposure to ADP.

If the past 4 years, with the discovery and identification of PGI_2 (prostacyclin) in the vessel wall and thromboxane A_2 (TXA_2) in platelets, there has been widespread interest in the role of these compounds in platelet function, the clotting process, and thrombosis, since these are respectively the most potent platelet inhibitory and platelet aggregating agents hitherto discovered. The mechanism whereby PGs or TXA_2 inhibit or stimulate platelet aggregation appears to involve cAMP, which is itself an inhibitor of platelet aggregation (Table 21–3).

A current model for platelet homeostasis involving the endoperoxide intermediates PGG_2 and PGH_2 and their extremely active products PGI_2 and TXA_2 is shown in Fig. 21–8. Upon initiation of the appropriate stimulus (endothelial injury, plaque formation) platelet arachidonic acid is converted to TXA_2 with promotion of vasoconstriction and platelet aggregation through decreased platelet cAMP production. PGH_2 formed either from endothelial arachidonic acid or from PGH_2 synthesized in the platelet is converted to PGI_2, which results in vasodilation and inhibition of platelet aggregation by cAMP stimulation. It is believed that the action of TXA_2 is through mobilization of calcium

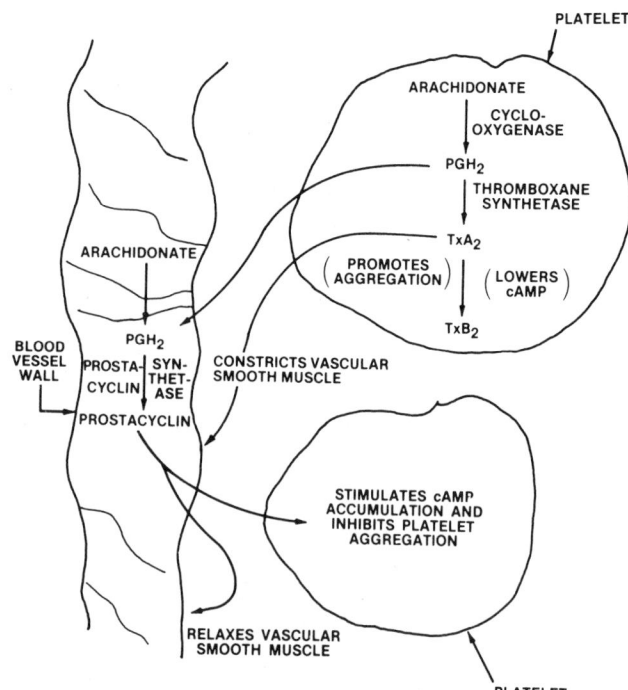

Figure 21–8.   Model of human platelet homeostasis. (From Gorman, R. R.: Modulation of human platelet function by prostacyclin and thromboxane. *Fed. Proc. 38:*83, 1979. With permission.)

from tubular storage sites, the latter being the proximal agent in inhibiting adenyl cyclase and releasing ADP and serotonin from intracellular dense granules. Although aspirin inhibits both PGI_2 and TXA_2 formation, the net effect appears to be prolonged anticlotting effects, since inhibition of TXA_2 synthesis occurs through the entire platelet lifetime and its effects on vascular PGI_2 synthesis are much shorter lasting. The current status of PGI_2 and TXA_2 in the clotting process and the medical implications for future control of deep venous thrombosis, myocardial infarction, stroke, and hypertension have recently been reviewed (Gorman, 1979; Moncada and Vane, 1978).

Erythrocytes

Red cells normally undergo "deformity" as they pass through the capillary system. The degree of deformity may be an important determinant of red cell survival and control of the microcirculation. Furthermore, such deformability is highly dynamic, changing in response to sex, time of day, and a variety of hormones, including prostaglandins. The effect of PGE_1 is to increase deformability, whereas PGE_2 decreases it. $PGF_2\alpha$ is without effect except during certain periods of the menstrual cycle. At low concentrations (10^{-11} M), PGE_1 decreases hemolysis and at higher

Table 21–3.   EFFECT OF PROSTAGLANDINS AND THROMBOXANES ON PLATELET FUNCTION

	Platelet Aggregation*	cAMP	Adenyl Cyclase
PGD_2	↓	↑	↑
PGE_1	↓ ↓	↑ ↑	↑ ↑
PGE_2	↑ ↑	↓ ↓	↓ ↓
PGG_2	↑	↓ **	−
PGH_2	↑	↓ †	↓
PGI_2	↓ ↓ ↓	↑ ↑ ↑	↑ ↑ ↑
TXA_2	↑ ↑ ↑	↓ ↓ ↓	↓ ↓ ↓

*Aggregation induced by ADP; **induced by PGE_1; †induced by PGI_2 ↑ = Augmentation ↓ = Inhibition, PGA and PGF either do not affect or only minimally inhibit platelet aggregation with slight increase in cAMP.

concentrations $(10^{-9}$ M$)$ increases hemolysis (Rasmussen et al., 1977). The reverse is true for PGE$_2$. The significance of these effects, particularly with regard to red cell survival and the state of the microcirculation, remains to be clarified.

PGEs and PGAs also stimulate the production of erythropoietin and may be the principal mediators of erythropoietin produced by the kidney in response to hypoxia, a subject reviewed recently by Fisher and Gross (1977).

The Inflammatory Response

Local Inflammation

The inflammatory response is characterized by increased vascular permeability and vasodilatation with a subsequent migration of leukocytes, leading to the classic signs of redness, heat, pain, and swelling. The induction of the response is multifold and includes burns, trauma, carrageenan administration, infection, and inflammatory diseases of unknown etiology such as rheumatoid arthritis. Bradykinin, serotonin, and histamine released into inflammatory areas by leukocytes have all been proposed as mediators of the response, but the specific agents involved and their interrelationships and mechanisms remain obscure.

Recent evidence has accumulated that prostaglandins may be important mediators of inflammation. In the first place, PGE but not PGF compounds markedly increase histamine-mediated vascular permeability and elicit all the classic signs of inflammation. Secondly, PGEs or PGFs are found in many human skin inflammatory exudates, such as psoriasis, contact dermatitis, burns and ultraviolet injury, as well as in such experimental models as uveitis, carrogeenan inflammation, and rheumatoid arthritis. PGE is leukotactic and prolongs the delayed phase of the inflammatory response when leukocyte invasion occurs. PGF compounds are much weaker and because of their venoconstrictor actions have been suggested as involved in the termination of the inflammatory response. The inflammatory actions of PGE$_2$ are shared to a lesser extent by PGD. Recently, the endoperoxide PGG$_2$ has been suggested as the main PG causing proinflammatory effects (Kuehl et al., 1977). Malondialdehyde (MDA) (a product of endoperoxide fragmentation) and the lysophospholipids are cytotoxic, whereas hydroxy arachidonic acid (HETE), like PGE, is chemotactic for leukocytes during the delayed phase of the inflammatory response.

Lastly, TXA$_2$, as mentioned in the discussion of platelets, is a potent platelet aggregator and may participate in the inflammatory response by this action as well as by its ability to extrude granular serotonin. Fig. 21–9 summarizes the participation of PGs and TX in the inflammatory response. The anti-inflammatory effects of indomethacin and aspirin occur through cyclo-oxygenase inhibition, whereas those of steroids are believed to be through inhibition of release of fatty acids from phospholipids either by phospholipase A$_2$ inhibition or by interfering with release of membrane phospholipids.

The classic clinical example of inflammation is rheumatoid arthritis in which both aspirin and steroids have potent anti-inflammatory effects. Rheumatoid synovium and fluid contain large amounts of PGs, which are believed to promote bone resorption and participate in periarticular bone demineralization characteristic of rheumatoid arthritis.

Despite the fact PGs are proinflammatory, they are also anti-inflammatory, particularly at higher concentrations since they increase cAMP in leukocytes, decrease extrusion of lysozomal enzymes and histamine, and inhibit lymphocyte toxicity, Zurier (1979) has suggested that this retardation of inflammation by pharmacologic amounts of PGs may be a feedback defense mechanism aimed at minimizing injury, particularly the result of an increase in anti-inflammatory PGF that occurs as inflammation decreases.

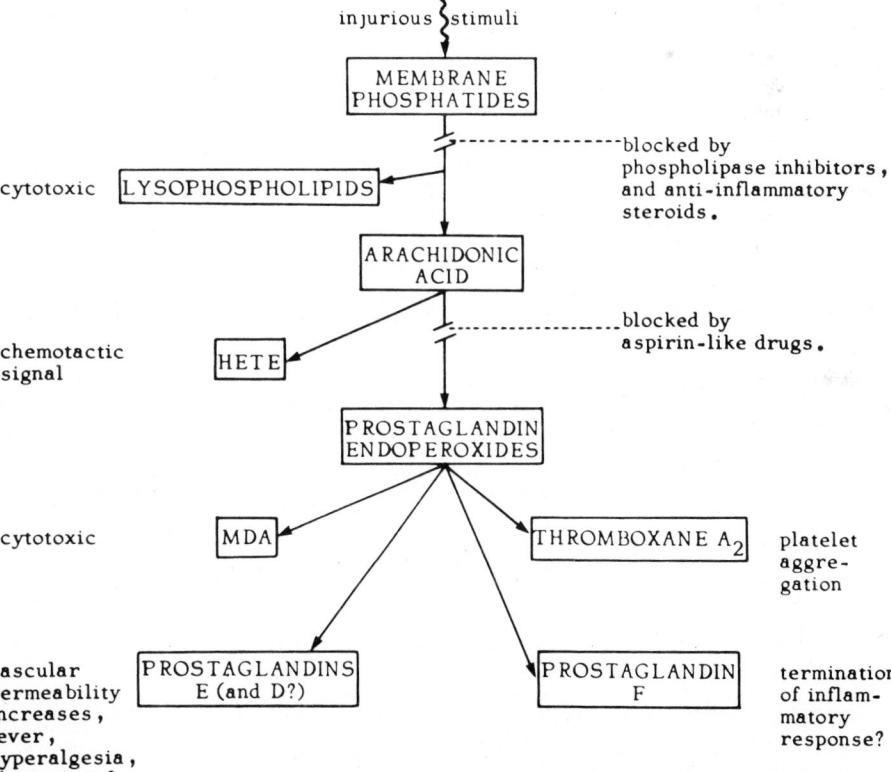

Figure 21–9. Involvement of cellular lipids in the inflammatory process. (From Flower, R. J.: *Prostaglandins and Related Compounds.* Basel, Birkhauser Verlag, 1977. With permission.)

Table 21–4. ASPIRIN AND PROSTAGLANDINS

	Aspirin	PGE
Fever	↓	↑
Headache	↓	↑
Local inflammation	↓	↑
Gastric HCL production	↑	↓
Experimental peptic ulceration	↑	↓
Muscle pain	↓	?

↑ = Augmentation; ↓ = inhibition

Systemic Inflammation

Common systemic manifestations of inflammation are somatic pain and fever, which are classically alleviated by such anti-inflammatory analgesic and antipyretic agents as aspirin, indomethacin, and phenylbutazone, all compounds that markedly inhibit prostaglandin synthesis (Ferreira et al., 1971; Smith and Willis, 1971). There is strong evidence that headache and fever are prostaglandin-mediated since there is a negative correlation between a variety of the effects of aspirin and PGE (Table 21–4). In addition, injection of PGE_1 produces severe headaches when infused into man and pyrogen-induced fever is associated with a rise in hypothalamic $PGF_2\alpha$, both of which are inhibited by indomethacin. Although the evidence is circumstantial, it is likely that most, if not all, of the antiphlogistic actions of the nonsteroidal, anti-inflammatory agents are mediated in large part, by inhibition of PGE synthesis (Vane, 1971). The role of PGs in local and systemic inflammation has recently been reviewed by Zurier (1979) and Flower (1977).

The Immune Response

General Considerations

The immune response can be divided into an afferent and an efferent arm (Parker et al., 1973). In the afferent arm, the antigen localizes in lymphatic tissue and interacts with macrophages and antigen-sensitive lymphocytes of the T (thymus) and B (bone marrow) types, leading to a proliferation of T-memory lymphocytes and antibody-secreting plasma cells, respectively, both with activating antigen specificity. In the effector phase, these sensitized cells and antibodies interact with cellular or soluble antigen to produce immunologic inflammation. In the cellular immune response, the cell may be injured or destroyed by activation of complement with release of lymphokines.

In general, PGEs and PGAs, and to a lesser extent PGFs, inhibit the immune response by inhibiting both T and B-cell activity, in the former instance possibly by inhibition of lymphokine production. The mechanism of action is be-

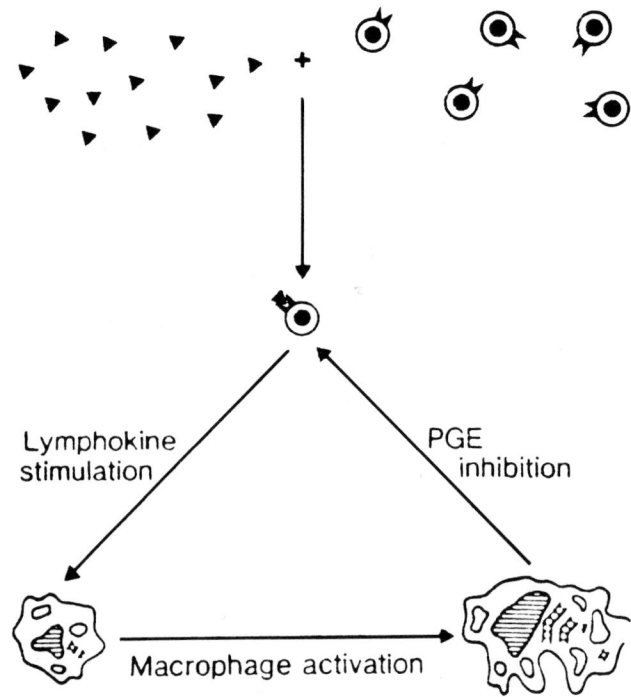

Figure 21–10. Suggested homeostatic mechanism whereby lymphokine-mediated macrophage activation leads to PGE-induced inhibition of lymphocyte activation. (From Meade, C. J., and Mertin, J.: Fatty acids and immunity. *Adv. Lipid Res.* 16:127, 1978. With permission.)

lieved to be mediated by adenyl cyclase activation and increased cAMP (Table 21–5). PGE is believed to be released by lymphokine-activated macrophages inhibiting lymphocyte activation and lymphokine production, a possible homeostatic feedback mechanism (Fig. 21–10). Whereas high concentrations of PGs inhibit the immune response, PG synthetase inhibitors and low PG concentrations enhance it. For recent reviews of this field the interested reader should consult Pelus and Strausser (1977), Meade and Mertin (1978), and Zurier (1979).

Immediate Hypersensitivity

One model of immediate hypersensitivity is antigen-induced histamine release from IgE antibody–sensitized basophils and from the lung, a reaction that is inhibited by catecholamines, cAMP, PGE_1, and PGE_2 but not by $PGF_1\alpha$. The effect of catecholamines is on β-adrenergic receptors, since their inhibition of histamine release can be blocked by

Table 21–5. EFFECT OF PROSTAGLANDINS ON THE IMMUNE RESPONSE

	cAMP Intact Lymphocytes	Immediate Hyper-sensitivity	Leukocyte cAMP*	Delayed Hyper-sensitivity	Lymphocyte Transformation†	Lymphocyte cAMP	Adjuvant Arthritis	Bronchial Smooth Muscle
PGE_1	↑↑↑	↓↓↓	↑↑↑	↓↓↓‡	↓↓↓	↑↑↑	↓↓↓	↓↓↓
PGE_2	↑↑	↓↓↓	↑↑↑	↓↓↓	↓↓↓	↑↑↑	↓↓↓	↓↓↓
$PGF_{1\alpha}$	↑	0	0	0	↓	↑	N.T.	N.T.
$PGF_{2\alpha}$	N.T.	N.T.	↑	N.T.	N.T.	N.T.	0	↑↑↑
PGA_1	↑↑↑	N.T.	↑↑	N.T.	↓↓↓	↑↑↑	N.T.	N.T.
PGA_2	↑↑↑	N.T.	N.T.	N.T.	↓↓	↑↑	0	N.T.

*Values pertain to the immediate hypersensitivity reaction.
†As measured by DNA, RNA, and protein synthesis in phytohemagglutinin-stimulated lymphocyte proliferation.
‡Lymphocyte C-AMP levels elevated.
↑ = Augmentation; ↓ = inhibition; 0 = no effect; N.T. = not tested.

propranolol, whereas no such inhibition occurs with PGE₁. In addition, catecholamine inhibition of histamine release is associated with a rise in leukocyte cAMP, which is blocked by propranolol, whereas the rise in cAMP with prostaglandins is not so inhibited. PGE₁ and PGE₂ are the most potent of all the prostaglandins; the PGA and PGF classes are almost inactive (Table 21–5). The evidence at present suggests that PGE compounds increase cAMP, leading to decreased histamine release using a receptor other than that used by catecholamines.

Delayed Hypersensitivity

cAMP and catecholamines inhibit the delayed hypersensitivity reaction. The most potent inhibitors, however, are prostaglandins PGE₁ and PGE₂; PGF₁α is inactive (Table 21–5). Again, as in acute hypersensitivity, the effect of the catecholamines but not of PGEs is blocked by propranolol. Furthermore, PGE₁ inhibition is associated with a cAMP increase in mononuclear cells. The possible therapeutic implication for such sensitivity reactions as bronchial asthma is noteworthy in that prostaglandins are able to bypass β-adrenergic stimulation of adenyl cyclase and lead to an independent rise in cAMP that, at least theoretically, could act as a second messenger in inhibiting the hypersensitivity reaction.

Lymphocyte Transformation

Catecholamines stimulate adenyl cyclase in human lymphocytes, leading to a rise in cAMP. A simlar rise in cAMP can be elicited by PGE and PGA compounds but to a much lesser degree by the PGF class (Table 21–5). The rise in cAMP is not blocked by propranolol as is that of isoproterenol-induced cAMP, suggesting a non-β-adrenergic mechanism for the prostaglandins. Phytohemagglutinin-induced lymphocyte transformation (measured by protein DNA and RNA synthesis) is inhibited by cAMP as well as by PGA and PGE (Parker, 1972) (Table 21–5); in fact, cell morphology concomitantly returns toward normal under the influence of cAMP.

Bronchial Asthma

Although the cause and mechanisms of human bronchial asthma are unknown, certain important facts are well established. In general, β-adrenergic stimulating agents such as isoproterenol result in bronchodilatation associated with a rise in intracellular cAMP, whereas β-blocking agents of cholinergic stimulation lead to bronchoconstriction associated with a fall in intracellular cAMP. There is increased evidence that asthma is a systemic disorder associated with partial β-adrenergic blockade since (1) asthmatic patients exhibit a reduced generalized metabolic response to epinephrine, (2) the peripheral lymphocytes show a decreased antigenic inactivation by catecholamines and (3) there is a reduction in the rise of lymphocytic cAMP in response to isoproterenol in blood from asthmatics as compared with control (Smith and Parker, 1970).

The possibility of involvement of prostaglandins in asthma stems from the observation that PGE₁ and PGE₂ relax human bronchiolar smooth muscle in vitro, whereas PGF₂α contracts these muscles and inhibits the bronchodilating effect of isoproterenol (Table 21–5). Of great clinical interest is the fact that patients with bronchial asthma respond to cold temperatures with profuse nasal congestion

and bronchiolar constriction and that PGE₁ administration results in nasal vasoconstriction and bronchiolar dilation in such patients (Cuthbert, 1969). There is one group of asthmatic patients whose disease is aggravated by aspirin, suggesting that in this group the bronchiolar constriction may be the result of aspirin inhibition of PGE₂ synthesis. Since both PGE₂ and PGF₂α are present in the lung, it has been suggested that certain forms of asthma may arise in part from a decreased PGE₂/PGF₂α ratio or even from an imbalance of the PG endoperoxides. This subject has recently been reviewed by Gryglewski and Szczeklik (1978).

Adjuvant Arthritis

Intradermal injection of complete Freund's adjuvant produces a severe polyarthritis that is prevented or inhibited by subcutaneous administration of PGE₁ and PGE₂ but not by PGA or PGF compounds (Zurier and Weissman, 1972) (Table 21–5). It has been suggested that one mechanism by which PGE₂ might alleviate experimental arthritis is immunologic, involving inhibition of sensitized lymphocytic migration into the affect joints by increasing lymphocytic cAMP. Drugs that increase the latter compound have been shown to decrease lymphocyte-mediated cytolysis of target cells. Paradoxically, PGE₁ and PGE₂ in smaller doses appear to produce experimental arthritis and are capable of evoking such signs of inflammation as pain, swelling, heat, and redness. In the mouse with experimental lupus erythematosus, PGE₁ treatment prolongs survival and prevents progression of immune complex nephritis, possibly by maintaining an appropriate balance between T and B cells (Zurier et al., 1977a, b). At present, the role of PGEs in inflammation in both experimental and human rheumatoid arthritis is unknown.

Digestive System

Intestinal Motility

PGE₁ and PGE₂, normally present in the gastrointestinal tract, contract longitudinal smooth muscle but inhibit contraction of circular smooth muscle in vitro. PGF₂α, on the other hand, contracts both longitudinal and circular smooth muscle in vitro. PGAs are similar but much weaker than PGF. In the esophagus, in both animals and humans, PGE₁ and PGE₂ relax the cardiac sphincter, whereas PGF₂α increases sphincter tone, suggesting that the former may be useful in the treatment of achalasia and the latter in gastroesophogeal reflex.

In animals, the effect of PGEs and PGF in vivo on intestinal motility is contradictory, with some studies showing intestinal contraction and others relaxation. In the human, admininstration of PGEs results in vomiting, bile reflux, abdominal cramps, and diarrhea, suggesting increased intestinal motility and both pyloric and esophageal sphincter relaxation and reflux. Although the PGE₂ analogue 16,16-dimethyl PGE₂ (16,16-dime-PGE₂) reduces gastric emptying subcutaneously in animals, it accelerates gastric emptying when given orally to humans.

Gastric Secretion

In animals, PGEs, PGAs, and the analogues 15-methyl-PGE₂ (15-me-PGE₂) and 16,16-dime-PGE₂ have marked inhibitory actions on gastric secretion. Both basal secretion (volume, acid, and pepsin) and that following stimulation

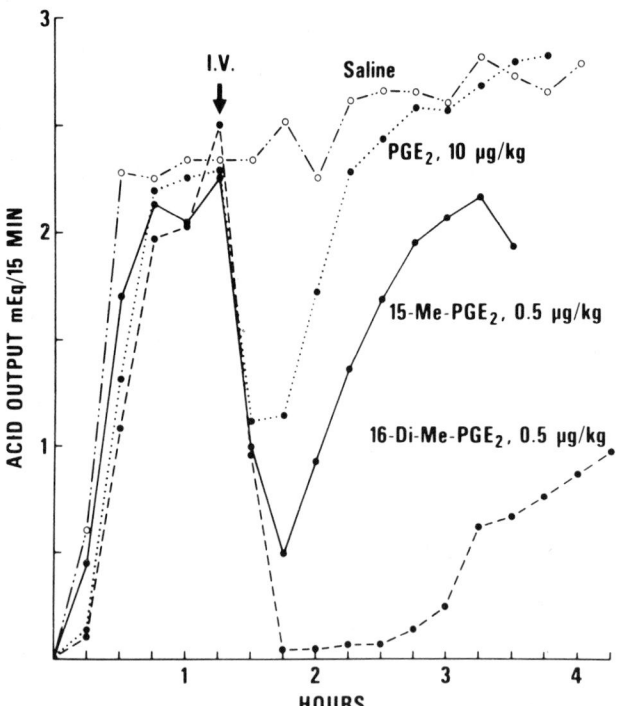

Figure 21–11. Effect of PGEs and their methylated analogues on gastric hydrochloric acid secretion. (From Robert, A.: Prostaglandins and the digestive system. *The Prostaglandins.* Ramwell, P. W. (ed.), New York, Plenum Press, 1977, p. 225.)

with a variety of agents (food, histamine, pentagastrin, insulin, reserpine, and so on) are inhibited *in vitro* and *in vivo*. The most marked antisecretory action was observed following oral, local, or parenteral administration of the analogues 15-me-PGE$_2$, and 16,16-dime-PGE$_2$, their potency being 50–100 times that of the natural PGs with a much longer duration of action (Fig. 21–11).

The mechanism of antisecretory action is unclear, with controversial involvement of cAMP. Clearly the PGs do not appear to act by decreasing gastric blood flow or by an anticholinergic action, since they act in denervated and acetylcholine-blocked preparations. It has been suggested that their antisecretory actions may be a direct local effect on parietal cell secretion, possibly mediated in part by gastrin inhibition.

Peptic Ulceration and Cytoprotection

In animals, gastric ulceration (induced by pyloric ligation, steroids, reserpine, indomethacin, and bile) and duodenal ulceration (induced by histamine and pentagastrin) are prevented by prior oral or parenteral administration of PGE$_1$, PGE$_2$, 15-me-PGE$_2$, and 16,16-dime-PGE$_2$. In 10 humans with proven peptic ulceration, 15-me-PGE$_2$ (150 μg) given orally alleviated epigastric pain and tenderness associated with a rise in gastric pH (Fung et al., 1974) that in a double-blind study was of greater duration than with an antacid and associated with increased gastric epithelial mucous secretion on endoscopy (Fung et al., 1974a). In a double-blind study, Karim and Fung (1976) showed a healing rate with PGE$_2$ (1 mg orally, 4 times a day) of 42% in the treated group and 14% in controls.

Administration of nonsteroidal anti-inflammatory agents in animals produces not only peptic ulceration but also small intestinal ulceration, necrosis, peritonitis, and death that can be obviated by administration of PGA$_2$, PGB$_2$,

PGC$_2$, PGD$_2$, PGF$_2\alpha$ and PGF$_2\beta$, and their methyl analogues, of which the PGEs and PGAs are most potent. This action, termed "cytoprotection" by Robert (1975), suggests that PG-depleted intestinal cells are rendered vulnerable to many noxious intestinal stimuli, particularly bacterial endotoxin (indomethacin is not ulcerogenic in germ-free animals). PG cytoprotection is also evident in the intestinal lesions produced by intestinal toxins and steroids by mechanisms that are unclear but again may involve an antibacterial action of the PGs. Lastly, the antiulcerogenic action of PGs on the stomach and duodenum may not be entirely due to their antisecretory actions but may be in large part the result of their cytoprotective action.

Intestine

PGEs, PGA$_2$, and PGF$_2\alpha$ administered to animals and humans orally, luminally, or parenterally, stimulate sodium, potassium, and chloride accumulation in the small intestine, leading to watery diarrhea, a sequence of events similar to cholera toxin. This fluid accumulation by PGs has been termed enteropooling by Robert (1975). PG-mediated watery diarrhea is believed to occur clinically in syndromes of PG excess, such as medullary carcinoma of the thyroid and amine peptide–secreting tumors.

Miscellaneous Digestive Effects

In the dog salivary gland, PGF$_2\alpha$ and to a much lesser extent PGE$_2$ and PGE$_1$ stimulate salivary flow, an effect inhibited by atropine suggesting the effect is mediated by a cholinergic action. PGA$_2$ and PGE$_2$ have a choleretic action on bile flow stimulated by taurocholate but not secretin. Although PGE$_1$ and 16, 16-dime-PGE$_2$ inhibit pancreatic secretion and stimulated enzyme production in secretin-stimulated dogs, the methyl analogue of PGE$_2$ is essentially without effect in humans.

The actions and roles of prostaglandins on the digestive system with detailed references to the data cited in this section have been reviewed by Wilson (1974) and Robert (1977a,b).

Metabolic and Endocrine Systems

Carbohydrate Metabolism

In *in vitro* studies, PGE compounds increased insulin secretion in isolated pancreatic islet cells (Johnson et al., 1973). On the other hand, in both animal and human studies intravenous PGE$_1$ and PGE$_2$ inhibited both basal and glucose-stimulated insulin release (Robertson et al., 1974; Robertson and Chen, 1977; Sacca et al., 1975). Moreover, PG synthesis inhibition with sodium salicylate administered intravenously resulted in significant improvement in the acute insulin response to glucose stimulation in normal subjects and a restoration of the absent acute insulin response and a fourfold increase in the second phase insulin secretion in adult-onset diabetes (Fig. 21–12). The mechanism of the action of PGEs in inhibiting insulin release is unknown but does not appear to be related to increased somatostatin or serotonin release. Although a role for pancreatic PGE in diabetes mellitus has yet to be established, it is of interest that glucose administration can inhibit PG production (Lambert et al., 1976), an effect enhanced by insulin, suggesting a negative feedback regulatory role of islet cell insulin and PGE on carbohydrate metabolism.

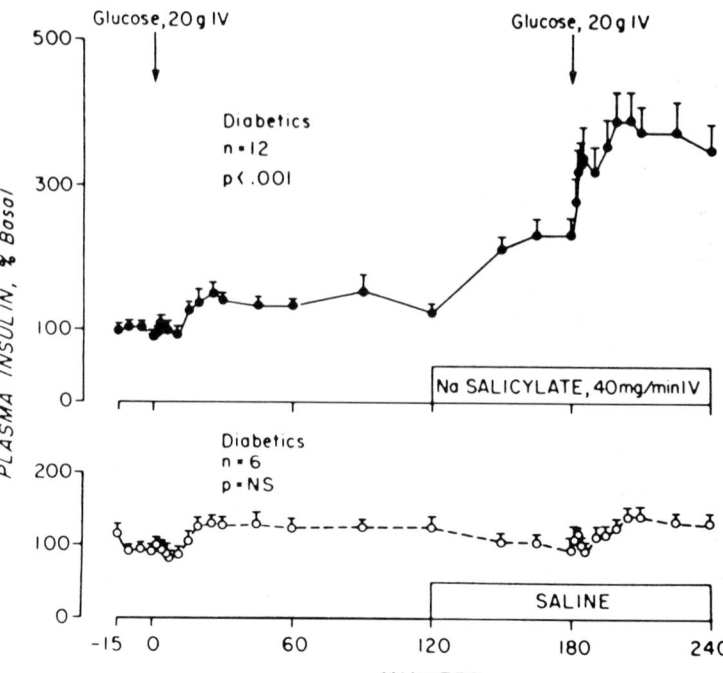

Figure 21–12. Improvement by sodium salicylate of defective insulin secretion in diabetic humans. (From Robertson, R. P., and Chen, M.: A role for prostaglandin E in defective insulin secretion and carbohydrate tolerance in diabetes mellitus. *J. Clin. Invest.* 60:747, 1977. With permission.)

According to this hypothesis, one factor leading to carbohydrate intolerance in diabetes mellitus could be an excessive stimulation of pancreatic PGE (possibly immunologic in nature) leading to blunting of insulin response to glucose loading and carbohydrate intolerance. This subject together with the involvement of TXs in the regulation of oxidative versus glycolytic metabolism has recently been reviewed (Robertson, 1978; Horrobin, 1978).

Fat Metabolism

The lipolytic effects of glucagon, ACTH, and epinephrine are inhibited by PGE$_1$ *in vitro* (Steinberg et al., 1963). The lipolytic agents act by increasing fat-cell adenyl cyclase activity with a subsequent enhanced conversion of ATP to cAMP (Butcher et al., 1967). Theophylline, by inhibiting phosphodiesterase activity, also increases cAMP and lipolysis. Although PGE$_1$ is antilipolytic, it does not inhibit the lipolytic activity cAMP, suggesting that the mechanism of antilipolytic activity of PGE$_1$ is through adenyl cyclase inhibition. The effects of experiments *in vivo* are conflicting, with reports of both lipolytic and antilipolytic effect of PGE$_1$ in dogs and in humans.

The effects of dietary unsaturated fatty acids in lowering blood cholesterol in the human are well known. Since these acids are PG precursors, it is of interest that Ziboh and Hsia (1972) revealed that skin cholesterol esterifying activity, high in essential fatty acid–deficient rats, could be inhibited by PGE$_2$ and that cholesterol hydrolase activity could be activated. A precise physiologic role for PGs in lipid metabolism has yet to be defined, however.

Pituitary Hormone Secretion

Administration of PGE$_2$ and PGF$_2\alpha$ to cattle results in an immediate and striking release of GH and PRL, an observation also observed *in vitro* in cultured pituitary cells (Gautvik and Kris, 1976; Ojeda et al., 1977). Whether the effects of PGF$_2\alpha$ are mediated through the hypothalamus remains

conjectural, however. Although a similar effect has been noted for ACTH release with a subsequent rise in glucocorticoids following PGF$_2\alpha$ administration, the effect of PG's on TSH release is controversial. The effect of PG's on LH and FSH release has been discussed under "Reproductive System," p. 1052.

Thyroid

In contrast to the inhibiting effects on adipose tissue adenyl cyclase, PGE$_1$ stimulates adenyl cyclase in slices of dog thyroid, resulting in an increase in cAMP. Many of the effects of PGE$_1$ mimic those of TSH (Table 21–6), suggesting that TSH may act by elevating thyroid PGE$_1$ concentration. Field and coworkers have presented evidence that dissociates the cAMP effects of other prostaglandins from thyroid hormone production, however, a phenomenon that is largely dose-dependent. This suggests a far more complicated mechanism of action than simple adenyl cyclase activation. Support for TSH stimulation of thyroid prostaglandin production, however, is derived from the fact that it is known that the thyroid contains large amounts of

Table 21–6. COMPARATIVE EFFECTS OF PGE$_1$ (μg per ml.) AND TSH ON VARIOUS PARAMETERS OF THYROID METABOLISM *IN VITRO**

Parameter	PGE$_1$	TSH
Adenyl cyclase	↑ .02	↑
^{3}H-Cyclic AMP	↑ 1	↑
Cyclic AMP	↑ 1	↑
^{14}CO$_2$	↑ 1	↑
^{32}Phospholipid	↑ 100	↑
Colloid droplets	↑ 1	↑

*Adapted from Field, J., Dekker, A., et al.: *Ann. N.Y. Acad. Sci.* 180:278, 1971, with permission. Although PGA$_1$, PGF$_2\alpha$, and PGB$_1$ produce similar effects, the concentrations necessary to elicit a response are generally 100 times greater.

prostaglandin-like compounds (probably PGE_1, PGE_2, and $PGF_2\alpha$) and that TSH stimulates both thyroid prostaglandin production and hormonogenesis. Both hormonogenesis and the accompanying adenyl cyclase rise are inhibited by prostaglandin antagonists. (Thompson et al., 1977).

The only clinical thyroid prostaglandin syndrome so far described is associated with malignant amine peptide–secreting tumors, notably medullary carcinoma of the thyroid. The clinical picture is characterized by profuse watery diarrhea and abdominal cramps that may be the result of excessive PGE_2 or $PGF_2\alpha$ (or both) secretion by the tumor. The syndrome is associated with an increased incidence of pheochromocytoma.

Adrenals

As has been noted, PGs result in increased steroidogenesis through pituitary release of ACTH. PGE_1 and PGE_2 directly stimulate corticosterone and aldosterone production, however, and effect similar to ACTH (Flack et al., 1969; Saruta and Kaplan, 1972). The enhanced steroidogenesis with PGE_2, as with ACTH, appears to be mediated by cAMP. Although these results suggest a mediating role of PG's in the mechanism of action of ACTH, the observation that indomethacin inhibits the PG response but not the steroid response to ACTH (Laychock et al., 1977) leaves the role of PGs in steroid hormonogenesis unresolved.

Calcium and Bone Metabolism

Since the observations of Klein and Raisz (1970) that PGEs stimulate bone resorption *in vitro*, numerous studies have confirmed the potent effects of these PGs on bone metabolism. Although a wide variety of PG's stimulate bone resorption, PGE_1 and PGE_2 are by far the most potent, acting by increasing cAMP in a synergistic fashion with PTH. Morphologically, there is an increase in the size, number, and ruffled borders of the osteoclast. PG's also may inhibit bone formation, since incorporation of proline into collagen by PGs is decreased. Although it is known that PGE is secreted by bone cells, any precise physiologic roles of the PGs in bone metabolism and remodeling, particularly with regard to their interaction with PTH, is unknown.

Clinically, excess PGE has been implicated in the bone resorption of rheumatoid arthritis, periodontal inflammation and the hypercalcemia of neoplasia. Tashjian and associates (1972) first demonstrated that hypercalcemia in experimental animal tumors was the result of tumor-secreting PGE_2, an action that could be prevented by indomethacin. Furthermore, increased concentrations of circulating PGE metabolites have been demonstrated in a variety of experimental neoplasias. In humans, the hypercalcemia of some solid tumors has been shown to (1) be associated with low PTH secretion and excess plasma PGE and (2) be reversed by indomethacin, an action not observed with nonPGE hypercalcemia (hematologic tumors, hyperparathyroidism, and breast tumors). The subject of calcium and bone metabolism has recently been reviewed in detail by Dietrich and Raisz (1975) and Seyberth and coworkers (1978).

The Nervous System

Central

The brain has a high capacity to synthesize PGE_2, $PGF_2\alpha$, and TX, whereas the rate of PG metabolizing enzyme is relatively low, with the exception of high 9-keto-reductase activity. Although PG synthesis is increased by catecholamines, serotonin, and dopamine, the role of PG's in central nervous system (CNS) function remains unresolved.

In the unanesthetized chick and mouse, PGE_1 has sedative, tranquilizing, and anticonvulsive effects. In the mouse, ptosis and ataxia result from PGE_1 administration (Horton, 1964). In the cat, intraventricular administration of PGE_1 produces a loss of spontaneous movements and a catatonic-like state lasting up to 25–48 hours.

Although $PGF_2\alpha$ is without effect on intraventricular administration, intravenous administration of $PGF_2\alpha$ in the chick causes extension of the limbs and dorsiflexion of the neck. Horton and Main (1967) showed that limb extension is the result of an increased gastrocnemius muscle tension secondary to an action of PGF in augmenting central but not peripheral spinal reflexes. Presumably, PGE_1 may have a high inhibitory action of spinal reflexes and a spinal excitatory action. From these considerations as well as the demonstration that PGE (but not PGF) antagonizes norepinephrine inhibition of Purkinje cell discharge (Coceani et al., 1971), it has been suggested that certain prostaglandins may serve as CNS transmitters. The role of PGs in the CNS has been reviewed in detail by Wolfe and associates (1976).

Peripheral

Investigations on peripheral synaptic transmission, reviewed extensively by Hedqvist (1977), reveal that PGE_1 and PGE_2 reversibly inhibit norepinephrine release induced by axonal action potentials. The adrenergic inhibitory actions of the endoperoxides PGG_2, and PGH_2 are believed to result from their conversion to PGE_2 (Hedqvist, 1976). PGAs are less effective than PGE_2, whereas $PGF_2\alpha$, a potent venoconstrictor, enhances the vasoconstrictive response to sympathetic stimulation in the renal and other vascular beds. Since sympathetic stimulation increases synaptic PG release, it is currently believed that there is a negative feedback system whereby sympathetic stimulation leads to an increase in synaptic PGs that reduce the amount of norepinephrine transmitter released.

Ocular Effects

PGE_2, $PGF_2\alpha$, and recently PGI_2 (Kulkarni et al., 1977) have been found to be synthesized in the iris and removed by intraocular transport (Bito, 1974). The main actions of PGs in the eye are to induce miosis and to raise intraocular pressure (Waltzman et al., 1967) by accelerating aqueous humor formation (Eakins, 1976) with little effect on outflow. Both the miotic and glaucoma-like actions of the PGs are antagonized by norepinephrine.

Clinically, the PGs may have a role in inflammatory eye disorders such as uveitis since marked elevation of PGs has been observed in intraocular fluids of animals with mechanical and immunologically induced eye trauma (Eakins, 1976; Podos, 1977). Both the elevated PGs and the inflammation can be inhibited by indomethacin. Although elevated PG levels have been reported in glaucoma, there is no evidence that inflow-promoting PGs play a role in this outflow disorder unless, by accelerating inflow, they aggravate initially an already elevated pressure secondary to diminished outflow. The subject of prostaglandins and the eye has been reviewed by Eakins (1976).

Table 21–7. THERAPEUTIC APPLICATIONS OF THE PROSTAGLANDINS

Current

Prostaglandins	PG Synthesis Inhibition
Midtrimester abortion	Rheumatoid arthritis
	Fever and headache
	Bartter's syndrome

Potential

Hypertension	Patent ductus arteriosus
Congestive Heart Failure	Hypercalcemia of malignancy
Induction of labor	Periodontal inflammation
Infertility	Cholera and certain diarrheal states
Coronary and deep thrombosis	Burns
Peptic ulceration	Lupus erythematosis
Gastric hyperacidity	Glaucoma
Bronchial asthma	
Nasal congestion	

THERAPEUTIC IMPLICATIONS

Although only preliminary human trials with PGs have been undertaken, they hold promise as one of the most revolutionary therapeutic substances ever discovered. The most immediate applications are summarized in Table 21–7. On the basis of their biological effects, certain therapeutic possibilities are obvious, such as their oxytocic, abortive, antacid, and bronchodilator properties in labor, abortion, peptic ulceration, and bronchial asthma, respectively. The inflammatory and bond resorptive actions of the PGs also suggest therapeutic modalities for inhibition of synthesis of these compounds in rheumatoid arthritis, fever, headache, periodontal disease, the human burn syndrome, lupus erythematosus and hypercalcemic states, particularly those associated with malignancy. It is unlikely that the PGE and PGF classes can ultimately be given orally or intravenously because of their side effects, particularly the regard to the gastrointestinal tract. If, as it is postulated, they normally act as local regulators (hormones by definition circulate), new delivery routes will have to be devised to produce a specific therapeutic response in one organ (such as PGE aerosol for bronchial asthma) that would not result in an undesirable effect in a different organ (such as the effect of PGE in stimulating contraction of the uterus). The synthesis of a number of prostaglandin analogues with longer acting and more specific actions offers an alternative in obviating their nonspecific effects.

With regard to a possible therapeutic role in human essential hypertension, it should be remembered that the renal PGs were first discovered during a systematic search for renal vasodilators, deficiency of which had been postulated to underlie the genesis of the hypertensive state. It is of interest in this regard that the PGA and PGI compounds escape degradation by the lungs and could, at least theoretically, function as circulating antihypertensive factors. PGA$_2$, isolated as medullin, was the first PG to be given to a human with essential hypertension (Lee, 1967), in whom it produced a significant fall in blood pressure, acting by causing peripheral vasodilation with a secondary baroreceptor increase in heart rate and cardiac output. Subsequently, intravenous administration of PGA$_1$ in hypertensive patients was found to initially cause a rise in renal blood flow, sodium, and water excretion, all of which returned to preinfusion levels when blood pressure fell to normal levels (Lee et al., 1971). This was associated with a rise in renin activity and a 10% decrease in plasma volume. Thus PGAs (and more recently PGIs) favorably affect renal resistance, sodium and water homeostasis, peripheral resistance, plasma volume, and indirectly the baroreceptor system and cardiac output, all factors intricately woven into the etiologic mosaic of human essential hypertension. The preparation of stable oral analogues of PGAs and for PGIs holds promise for improved specific therapy in essential hypertension, particularly since these compounds possess both vasodilatory and diuretic actions that are the main pharmacologic properties contained in the multiple drug approach to current antihypertensive regimens.

It is now believed that patent ductus arteriosus in the newborn is at least partially PG dependent. In this regard, it is of great interest that PG synthesis inhibition with indomethacin leads to a high incidence of closure, obviating the need for surgery in many instances (Heymann and Rudolph, 1977). Aside from the side effect of renal failure in the immature developing kidney, this treatment has few side effects and may ultimately be the treatment of choice for this relatively common congenital heart disease.

The investigation of PG action holds great promise for revealing as yet undiscovered cellular events. Although there has probably been excessive exuberance for the therapeutic potential of PGs in some areas, it remains likely that further study of these compounds will markedly increase the understanding of many basic biologic processes and provide innovative and possibly revolutionary avenues of medical therapy.

REFERENCES

Anderson, G. G., et al.: Intravenous prostaglandins E$_2$ and F$_2\alpha$ for the induction of term labor. Am. J. Obstet. Gynecol. 112:382, 1972.
Armstrong, D. T., and Grinwich, D. L.: Blockade of spontaneous and LH-induced ovulation in rats by indomethacin, an inhibitor of prostaglandin biosynthesis. Prostaglandins 1:21, 1972.
Attallah, A., et al.: Inhibition of rabbit renal prostaglandin E$_2$ biosynthesis by chronic potassium deficiency. Proc. Endocrine Soc. 1980 (in press).
Behrman, H. R., et al.: Regulation of ovarian cholesterol esters: Evidence for the enzymatic sites of prostaglandin-induced loss of corpora luteum function. Lipids 6:791, 1971.
Bergström, S., and Sjövall, J.: The isolation of prostaglandin F from sheep prostate glands. Acta Chem. Scand. 14:1693, 1960.
Bergström, S., and Sjövall, J.: The isolation of prostaglandin E from sheep prostate glands. Acta Chem. Scand. 14:1701, 1960.
Berti, F., Samuelsson, B., and Velo, G. P. (eds.): Prostaglandins and Thromboxanes (Nato Advanced Study Institutes Series a: Life Sciences, Vol. 13). New York, Plenum Press, 1977.
Bito, L. Z.: The effects of experimental uveitis on anterior uveal prostaglandin transport and aequeous humor composition. Invest. Ophthalmol. 13:959, 1974.
Bunting, S., et al.: Arterial walls generate from prostaglandin endoperoxides a substance (prostaglandin X) which relaxes strips of mesenteric and celiac arteries and inhibits platelet aggregation. Prostaglandins 12:897, 1976.
Butcher, R. W., et al.: The effect of prostaglandin E$_1$ adenosine 3', 5'-monophosphate levels in adipose tissue, In Nobel Symposium – Prostaglandins. Bergström, S., and Samuelsson, B. (eds), New York, John Wiley, 1967, p. 133.
Caldwell, B. V., et al.: The effects of exogenous progesterone and estradiol on prostaglandin F levels in ovariectomized ewes. Prostaglandins 1:217, 1972.
Coceani, F., et al.: Prostaglandins and synaptic activity in spinal cord and cuneate nucleus. Ann. N. Y. Acad. Sci. 80:289, 1971.
Cuthbert, M. F.: Effect on airways resistance to prostaglandin E$_1$ given by aerosol to healthy and asthmatic volunteers. Br. Med. J. 4:723, 1969.
Davila, D., et al: The influence of dietary sodium on urinary prostaglandin excretion. Acta Physiol. Scand. 103:100, 1978.
Dietrich, J. W., and Raisz, L. G.: Prostaglandin in calcium and bone metabolism. Clin. Orthop. Relat. Res. 111:228, 1975.
Düsing, R., et al.: Renal biosynthesis of prostaglandin E$_2$ and F$_2\alpha$: Dependence on extracellular potassium. J. Lab. Clin. Med. 92:669, 1978.
Eakins, K. E.: Prostaglandins and the eye, In Prostaglandins: Physiological, Pharmacological and Pathological Aspects. Karim, S. M. M. (ed), Baltimore, University Park Press, 1976, p. 63.
Ferreira, S. H., et al.: Indomethacin and aspirin abolish prostaglandin release from the spleen. Nature New Biol. 231:237, 1971.
Fichman, M. P., et al.: Role of prostaglandins in the pathogenesis of Bartter's syndrome. Am. J. Med. 60:785, 1976.
Field, J., et al.: In vitro effects of prostaglandins on thyroid gland metabolism. Ann. N. Y. Acad. Sci. 180:278, 1971.

Fisher, J. W., and Gross, D. M.: Effect of prostaglandins on erythropoiesis, In *Prostaglandins in Hematology*. Silver, M. J., Smith, J. B., et al. (eds), New York, Spectrum, 1977, p. 159.

Flack, J. D., et al.: Prostaglandin stimulation of rat corticosteroidogenesis. *Science 163*:691, 1969.

Flower, R. J.: Prostaglandins and related compounds. *Agents Actions* [Suppl.] *(3)*:99, 1977.

Flower, R. J.: The role of prostaglandins in parturition, with special reference to the rat. Ciba Found. Symp. *(47)*:297, 1977.

Fung, W. P., et al.: Double-blind trial of 15(R)-15-methyl prostaglandin E_2 in the relief of peptic ulcer pain. *Ann. Acad. Med. 3*:375, 1974.

Fung, W. P., et al.: Effect of prostaglandin 15(R)-15-methyl-E_2-methyl ester on healing of gastric ulcers: Controlled endoscopic study. *Lancet 2*:10, 1974a.

Galvez, O. G., et al.: Studies of the mechanism of polyuria with hypokalemia. *Kidney Int. 10*:583, 1976.

Gautvik, K. M., and Kris, M.: Effects of prostaglandins on prolactin and growth hormone synthesis and secretion in cultured rat pituitary cells. *Endocrinology 98*:352, 1976.

Gill, J. R., and Bartter, F. C.: Evidence for a prostaglandin-independent defect in chloride reabsorption in the loop of Henle as a proximal cause of Bartter's syndrome. *Am. J. Med. 65*:766, 1978.

Goldblatt, M. W.: Depressor substance in seminal fluid. *Chem Ind. 52*:1056, 1953.

Gorman, R. R.: Modulation of human platelet function by prostacyclin and thromboxane A_2. *Fed. Proc. 38*:83, 1979.

Grantham, J. J., and Orloff, J.: Effect of prostaglandin E_1 on the permeability response of the isolated collecting tubule to vasopressin, adenosine 3', 5'-mono-phosphate and theophylline. *J. Clin. Invest. 47*:1154, 1968.

Gryglewski, R. J., and Szczeklik, A.: Prostaglandins, aspirin, asthma. *Prostaglandins Therap. 4*:1, 1978.

Hamada, Y., et al.: Ovulation in the perfused rabbit ovary: the influence of prostaglandins and prostaglandin inhibitors. *Biol. Reprod. 17*:58, 1977.

Hamberg, M., et al.: Thromboxanes: a new group of biologically active compounds derived from prostaglandin endoperoxides. *Proc. Nat. Acad. Sci. 72*:2994, 1975.

Hedqvist, P.: Prostaglandin action on transmitter release of adrenergic neuroeffector junction. *Adv. Prostaglandin Thromboxane Res. 1*:357, 1976.

Hedqvist, P.: Basic mechanisms of prostaglandin action on autonomic neurotransmission. *Ann. Rev. Pharmacol. Toxicol. 17*:259, 1977.

Heymann, M. A., and Rudolph, A. M.: Ductus arteriosus constriction. *Prostaglandins Therap. 3*:1, 1977.

Horrobin, D. F.: *Prostaglandins. Physiology, Pharmacology and Clinical Significance*. Montreal, Eden Press, 1978.

Horton, E. W.: Action of prostaglandins E_1 and E_3 on the central nervous system. *Br. J. Pharmacol. 22*:189, 1964.

Horton, E. W.: *Prostaglandins*. Berlin, Springer-Verlag, 1972.

Horton, E. W., and Main, I. H. M.: Further observations on the central nervous actions of prostaglandins $F_2\alpha$ and E_1. *Br. J. Pharmacol. 30*:568, 1967.

Johnson, D. G., et al.: Enhanced release of insulin by prostaglandins in isolated pancreatic islets. *Diabetes 22*:658, 1973.

Karim, S. M. M., and Filshei, G. M.: Therapeutic abortion using prostaglandin $F_2\alpha$. *Lancet 1*:157, 1970.

Karim, S. M. M., and Fung, W. P.: Effects of some naturally occurring prostaglandins and synthetic analogues on gastric secretion and ulcer healing in man, In *Advances in Prostaglandin and Thromboxane Research*. Samuelsson, B., and Paoletti, R. (eds.), New York Raven Press, 1976, p. 529.

Karim, S. M. M., et al.: Induction of labor with prostaglandin $F_2\alpha$. *Br. Med. J. 4*:621, 1968.

Kimberly, R. P., et al.: Elevated urinary prostaglandins and the effects of aspirin on renal function in lupus erythematosis. *Ann. Intern. Med. 83*:336, 1978.

Klein, D. C., and Raisz, L. G.: Prostaglandins: stimulation of bone resorption in tissue culture. *Endocrinology 86*:1436, 1970.

Kloeze, J.: Influence of prostaglandins on platelet adhesiveness and platelet aggregation, In *Nobel Symposium – Prostaglandins*. Bergström, S., and Samuelsson, B. (eds.), New York, John Wiley, 1967, p. 241.

Kuehl, F. A., et al.: Prostaglandin-cyclic nucleatide interactions in mammalian tissues, In *Prostaglandins: Chemical and Biochemical Aspects*. Karim, S. M. M. (ed.), Baltimore, University Park Press, 1976, p. 191.

Kuehl, F. A., et al.: Role of prostaglandin endoperoxide PGG_2 in inflammatory processes. *Nature 265*:170, 1977.

Kulkarni, P. S., et al.: Microsomal preparations of normal bovine iris ciliary body generate prostacylin-like but not thromboxane-like activity. *Prostaglandins 12*:465, 1976.

Kurzrok, R., and Lieb, C. C.: Biochemical studies of human semen II. *Proc. Soc. Exp. Biol. Med. 26*:268, 1930.

Lambert, B., et al.: Relationship between prostaglandin biosynthesis and the effect of insulin on hormone stimulated lipolysis in rat adipose tissue. *Biochim. Biophys. Acta 432*:132, 1976.

Laychock, S. G., et al.: Further studies on mechanisms controlling prostaglandin biosynthesis in the cat adrenal cortex. *Endocrinology 100*:74, 1977.

Lee, J. B.: Chemical and physiological properties of renal prostaglandins with emphasis on the cardiovascular effects of medullin in essential human hypertension, In *Nobel Symposium – Prostaglandins*. Bergström, S. and Samuelsson, B. (eds.), New York, John Wiley, 1967, p. 197.

Lee, J. B. (ed.): *The Renal Prostaglandins*, 1977. Montreal, Eden Press, 1978.

Lee, J. B. (ed.) *Comprehensive Endocrinology: The Prostaglandins*. New York, Elsevier-North Holland, 1980 (in press).

Lee, J. B., et al.: Sustained depressor effects of renal medullary extract in the normotensive rat. *Circ. Res. 13*:369, 1963.

Lee, J. B., et al.: Renomedullary depressor substance, medullin: Isolation, chemical characterization and physiological properties. *Circ. Res. 7*:57, 1965.

Lee, J. B., et al.: The identification of prostaglandin E_2, $F_2\alpha$ and A_2 from rabbit kidney medulla. *Biochem. J. 105*:1251, 1967.

Lee, J. B., et al.: Prostaglandin A_1: Antihypertensive and renal effects. *Ann. Intern. Med. 74*:703, 1971.

Lerner, L. J., et al.: Antifertility drugs: novel non-hormonal compounds that inhibit prostaglandin metabolism. *Nature 256*:130, 1975.

Lippes, J.: Applied physiology of the uterine tube, In *Obstetrics and Gynecology Annual*. Wynn, R. M. (ed), New York, Appleton-Century-Crofts, 1975, p. 119.

Lonigro, A. J., et al.: Dependency of renal blood flow on prostaglandin synthesis in the dog. *Circ. Res. 32*:712, 1973.

Maclouf, J., et al.: Recent aspects of prostaglandin biosynthesis: a review. *Biomedicine 26*:362, 1977.

Mauk, R. H., et al.: Effect of prostaglandin E administration in a nephrotoxic and a vasoconstrictor model of acute renal failure. *Kidney Int. 12*:122, 1977.

McCracken, J. A., et al.: Factors affecting the secretion of steroids from the transplanted ovary in the sheep. *Recent Progr. Horm. Res. 27*:537, 1971.

Meade, C. J., and Mertin, J.: Fatty acids and immunity. *Adv. Lipid Res. 16*:27, 1978.

Moncada, S., and Vane, J. R.: Prostacyclin (PGI_2) the vascular wall and vasodilation, In *Mechanism of Vasodilation*. Vanhoutte, P. M., and Leusen, I. (eds.), Basel, S. Karger, 1978, p. 107.

Nakano, J. R.: Cardiovascular actions, In *The Prostaglandins*. Ramwell, P. W. (ed.), New York, Plenum Press, 1973, p.239.

Ojeda, S. R., et al.: Prostaglandin E_2 (PGE_2)-induced growth hormone (GH) release: effect of intrahypothalamic and intrapituitary implants. *Prostaglandins 13*:943, 1977.

Orloff, J., and Handler, J. S.: Effect of prostaglandin E_1 on the permeability response of toad bladder to vasopressin, theophylline and adenosine 3', 5' monophosphate. *Nature 23*:397, 1965.

Parker, C. W.: The role of prostaglandins in the immune response, In *Prostaglandins in Cellular Biology*. Ramwell, P. W., and Pharriss, B. B. (eds.), New York, Plenum Press, 1972, p. 173.

Parker, C. W., et al.: Cyclic AMP and the immune response. *Adv. Cyclic Nucleotide Res. 4*:1, 1973.

Patak, R. V., et al.: Antagonism of the effects of furosemide by indomethacin in normal and hypertensive man. *Prostaglandins 10*:649, 1975.

Payakkapan, W., et al.: Effect of sodium intake on prostaglandin A, renin and aldosterone in normotensive humans. *Kidney Int. 8*:283, 1975.

Pelus, L. M., and Strausser, H. R.: Prostaglandins and the immune response. *Life Sci. 20*:903, 1977.

Podop, S. M.: Prostaglandins, nonsteroidal anti-inflammatory agents and eye disease. *Trans. Am. Opthalmol. Soc. 74*:637, 1977.

Rasmussen, H., and Lake, W.: Prostaglandins and the mammalian erythrocyte, In *Prostaglandins in Hematology*. Silver, M. J., Smith, J. B., et al. (eds.), New York, Spectrum, 1977, p. 187.

Robert, A.: Anti-secretory, anti-ulcer, cytoprotective and diarrheogenic properties of prostaglandins, In *Advances in Prostaglandin and Thromboxane Research*. Samuelsson, B., and Paoletti, R. (eds.), New York, Raven Press, 1975, p. 507.

Robert, A.: Prostaglandins and the digestive system, In *The Prostaglandins*. Ramwell, P. W. (ed.), New York, Plenum, 1977a, p. 225.

Robert, A.: The inhibitory effects of prostaglandins on gastric secretion: their possible role in the treatment of gastric hypersecretion and peptic ulcer, In *Progress in Gastroenterology*. Glass, G. B. J. (ed), New York, Grune and Stratton, 1977b, p. 777.

Robertson, R. P.: PGs and the pathogenesis of diabetes. *Prostaglandins Therap. 4*:1, 1978.

Robertson, R. P., and Chen, M.: A role for prostaglandin E in defective insulin secretion and carbohydrate intolerance in diabetes mellitus. *J. Clin. Invest. 60*:747, 1978.

Robertson, R. P., et al.: Inhibition of *in vivo* insulin secretion by prostaglandin E_1. *J. Clin. Invest. 54*:310, 1974.

Rose, J. C., and Kot, P. A.: Cardiovascular responses to the prostaglandin precursors, In *The Prostaglandins*. Ramwell, P. W. (ed.), New York, Plenum Press, 1977, p. 35.

Roth-Brandel, U., et al: Prostaglandins for induction of therapeutic abortion. *Lancet 1*:191, 1970.

Rumpf, K. W., et al.: The effect of indomethacin on plasma renin activity in man under normal conditions and after stimulation of the renin-angiotensin system. *Prostaglandins 10*:641, 1975.

Sacca, L., et al.: Reduction of circulating insulin levels during the infusion of different prostaglandins in the rat. *Acta Endocrinol. 79*:266, 1975.

Samuelsson, B., and Paoletti, R. (eds.): *Advances in Prostaglandin and Thromboxane Research.* New York, Raven Press, 1976.

Saruta, T., and Kaplan, N. M.: Adrenocortical steroidogenesis: the effects of prostaglandins. *J. Clin. Invest. 51*:2246, 1972.

Seyberth, H. W., et al.: Prostaglandins and hypercalcemic states. *Ann. Rev. Med. 29*:23, 1978.

Smith, J. B., and Willis, A. L.: Aspirin selectively inhibits prostaglandin production in human platelets. *Nature [New Biol.] 231*:235, 1971.

Smith, J. W., and Parker, C. W.: The responsiveness of leukocyte cyclic AMP to adrenergic agents in patients with asthma. *Proc. Cent. Soc. Clin. Res. 43*:76, 1970.

Stahl, R. A. K., et al.: Stimulation of rabbit renal PGE_2 biosynthesis by dietary sodium restriction. *Am. J. Physiol. 237*:F344, 1979.

Steinberg, D., et al.: Effects of prostaglandin E opposing those of catecholamines on blood pressure and on triglyceride breakdown in adipose tissue. *Biochem. Pharmacol. 12*:764, 1963.

Tashjian, A. H., Jr., et al.: Evidence that bone resorption-stimulating factor produced by mouse fibrosarcoma cells is prostaglandin E_2: a new model for the hypercalcemia of cancer. *J. Exp. Med. 136*:1329, 1972.

Tepperman, H. M., et al.: Drugs affecting myometrial contractility in pregnancy. *Clin. Obstet. Gynecol. 20*:423, 1977.

Thompson, M. E., et al.: *In vivo* inhibition of thyroid secretion by indomethacin. *Endocrinology 100*:1060, 1977.

vonEuler, U. S.: Zur Kenntnis der pharmakologischem Wirkungen von nativesekreten und extrakten männlicher accessorischer Geschlectsdrüsen. *Arch. Exp. Path. Pharmakol. 175*:78, 1934.

Vane, J. R.: Inhibition of prostaglandin synthesis as a mechanism of action for aspirin-like drugs. *Nature [New Biol.] 231*:232, 1971.

Waltzman, M. B., and King, C. D.: Prostaglandin influences on intraocular pressure and pupil size. *Am. J. Physiol. 212*:329, 1967.

Wilson, D. E.: Prostaglandins: their actions on the gastrointestinal tract. *Arch. Intern. Med. 133*:112, 1974.

Wolfe, L. S., et al.: The biosynthesis of prostaglandins by brain tissue *in vitro*, In *Advances in Prostaglandin and Thromboxane Research.* Samuelsson, B. and Paoletti, R. (eds.), New York, Raven Press, 1976, p. 345.

Ziboh, V. A., and Hsia, S. L.: Effect of prostaglandin E_2 on rat skin: inhibition of sterol ester biosynthesis and clearing of scaly lesions in essential fatty acid deficiency. *J. Lipid Res. 13*:458, 1972.

Zins, G. R.: Renal prostaglandins. *Am. J. Med. 58*:14, 1975.

Zurier, R. B.: Modulation of inflammation and immune responses by prostaglandins. *Postgrad. Med.* 1980 (in press).

Zurier, R. B., and Weissmann, G.: Effect of prostaglandins upon enzyme release from lysosomes and experimental arthritis, In *Prostaglandins in Cellular Biology*. Ramwell, P. W., and Pharriss, B. B. (eds.), New York, Plenum Press, 1972, p. 151.

Zurier, R. B., et al.: Prostaglandin E_1 treatment of NZB/W mice. I. Prolonged survival of female mice. *Arthritis Rheum. 20*:723, 1977a.

Zurier, R. B., et al.: Prostaglandin E_1 treatment of NZB/W mice. II. Prevention of glomerulonephritis. *Arthritis Rheum. 20*:1449, 1977b.

Zusman, R. M., and Keiser, H. R.: Prostaglandin biosynthesis by rabbit renomedullary interstitial cells in tissue culture. Stimulation by angiotensin II, bradykinin and arginine vasopressin. *J. Clin. Invest. 68*:215, 1977.

CHAPTER 22

The Renin-Aldosterone Axis for Blood Pressure, Electrolyte Homeostasis, and Diagnosis of High Blood Pressure

By John H. Laragh

and Jean E. Sealey

The coherence of a group of hormones, now recognized as the renin-angiotensin-aldosterone system, has only recently been exposed. Angiotensin and aldosterone were studied separately until 1960, when a direct relationship between the activity of these renal and adrenal hormones was established with the discovery by Laragh and associates that angiotensin infusion selectively stimulates aldosterone secretion in normal humans, plus the concurrent exposure of a causal role for both of these hormones in human malignant hypertension. Since then the role of this interaction in electrolyte and blood pressure homeostasis has been increasingly appreciated.

The renin-angiotensin-aldosterone system seems to have been organized primarily for the simultaneous regulation of the interrelated functions of sodium and potassium balance and blood pressure-volume homeostasis. This humoral system is the major, but certainly not the sole, regulator of these vital homeostatic functions, and its activity is coordinated with those of other neurovascular, humoral, and local cellular mechanisms.

THE RENIN SYSTEM DESCRIBED

The renin-angiotensin-aldosterone system regulates sodium balance, fluid volume, and blood pressure as follows (Fig. 22–1): when, as the result of such events as hemorrhage, sodium, depletion, fluid transudation, or alimentary loss, effective blood volume contracts and arterial pressure falls, the kidney's perfusion is reduced, and it secretes renin into the blood stream. Renin, acting enzymatically, hydrolyzes a plasma globulin to release angiotensin I, which is then rapidly hydrolyzed to angiotensin II by pulmonary and plasma-converting enzymes. Angiotensin II, in addition to its pressor action, stimulates aldosterone secretion. Aldosterone acts on the kidney distal tubules to cause sodium retention. This positive sodium balance leads to a secondary retention of water and expansion of the extracellular fluids. Thus angiotensin and aldosterone together act to raise the blood pressure and restore renal perfusion, thereby compensating the system and shutting off the initial signal to renal renin release.

Arterial blood pressure is additionally supported by a coordinated interaction between plasma angiotensin levels and available sodium ions. Since induced sodium retention enhances and sodium depletion diminishes the pressor activity of angiotensin, the product of these two factors determines vascular tone.

Simultaneously, the renin-angiotensin system regulates potassium homeostasis. This activity tends to stabilize plasma potassium levels and so avoids dangerous hyperkalemia which may develop in patients with adrenal insufficiency after a meal of high potassium content. Increases in plasma potassium levels act directly on the adrenal cortex to stimulate aldosterone release. Aldosterone acts on the kidney to promote K^+ loss, at the same time stimulating Na^+ reabsorption by the Na^+-K^+ ion exchange transport system. As the plasma potassium level falls, aldosterone secretion is accordingly reduced. At the same time, increases in plasma potassium act directly on the kidney to inhibit renin release, whereas hypokalemia is a potent stimulus for renin secretion. Thus renal conservation or elimination of potassium ions is closely related to opposite changes in both renin and aldosterone secretion.

The ultimate signal(s) inducing renin release has not yet been identified, but it appears to involve (1) a pressure- or stretch-sensitive receptor in the renal afferent arterioles partially under β-adrenergic-governance, (2) a distal tubular macula densa receptor responsive to changes in sodium supply, (3) changes in autonomic nerve activity, and (4) changes in potassium balance. Additionally, increases in plasma angiotensin levels may "feed

Table 22–1. MECHANISMS GOVERNING RENIN SECRETION

Renal Afferent Detectors:
Arteriolar barostat
Macula densa natriastat or chlorostat

Other Modifiers:
Nervous system and catecholamines
Plasma potassium level
Plasma angiotension II feedback suppression
Other humoral agents:
Vasopressin
Cyclic AMP
Prostaglandins
Renin-stimulating hormone?

back" to retard further renin secretion, and humoral agents may be involved in the mediation of renin release (Table 22–1).

The renin-angiotensin-aldosterone system has two effector hormones: angiotensin II and aldosterone.

Angiotensin II is an octapeptide with three striking physiologic actions: (1) in constricting the arterioles, it is by weight the most potent pressor substance known; (2) it acts directly on the kidney to cause sodium retention with lower dosages and natriuresis with larger amounts; and (3) it acts on the adrenal cortex to evoke a prompt and sustained increase in aldosterone secretion. The concentration of angiotensin II in human venous plasma normally ranges from 10–30 pg/ml.

Aldosterone, the second effector hormone of the system, is an adrenal corticosteroid, unique because of its 18-aldehyde configuration. It acts primarily on the renal tubules to increase the reabsorption of sodium chloride and to promote the elimination of potassium ions. Like angiotensin II, aldosterone is present in relatively minute amounts. In blood, its level is approximately .0001 of that of cortisol. In humans, it ranges from 50–150 pg/ml in venous plasma.

In this system, both the renin substrate and the converting enzymes are ordinarily present in sufficient amounts so that their concentrations are not physiologically rate-limiting for the formation of angiotensin II. Therefore, a relatively small change in the concentration of renin in plasma is usually the major determinant of the final concentration of circulating angiotensin II. By changing the plasma concentrations of the effector components, angiotensin II and aldosterone, this hormonal interaction simultaneously regulates (1) arterial blood pressure, (2) body sodium and water content and thus hydrostatic pressures, and (3) potassium balance.

ABNORMALITIES OF ALDOSTERONE AND RENIN SECRETION IN HUMANS

Major Categories of Disease Involving Oversecretion of Aldosterone

In humans, increased secretion of aldosterone may participate in the pathogenesis of (1) disorders characterized chiefly by potassium wastage, (2) conditions in which there is progressive sodium retention and edema formation, and (3) states characterized mainly by arterial hypertension. The major naturally occurring disorders that involve pathologic oversecretion of aldosterone are summarized in Table 22–2. They are divided into two main groups, primary and secondary aldosteronism (see also Chapter 5).

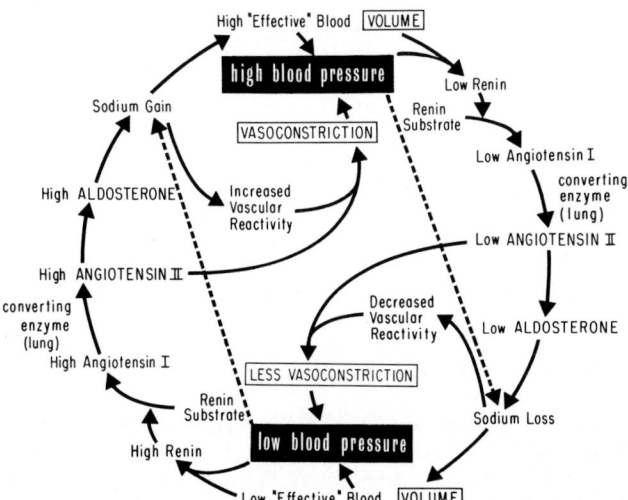

B.P. = VASOCONSTRICTION X VOLUME
(angio)   (aldo)(Na)

Figure 22–1. The renin-angiotensin aldosterone system for blood pressure and for sodium-volume homeostasis.

Table 22–2. OVERSECRETION OF ALDOSTERONE

I. Adrenal in origin
    (a) Primary aldosteronism due to adenoma
    (b) Pseudoprimary aldosteronism (bilateral adrenal
        hyperplasia)
II. Secondary aldosteronism (from extra-adrenal stimulation)
    (a) Edematous states:
        1. Cirrhosis
        2. Nephrosis
        3. Heart failure
    (b) Hypertensive states:
        1. Malignant hypertension
        2. Malignant or severe hypertension due to unilateral
           renal disease
    (c) Alkalotic normotensive states:
        1. Juxtaglomerular cell hyperplasia with potassium
           wastage and retarded growth

Primary Aldosteronism

The term "primary" means that the oversecretion arises from an autonomous aldosterone-secreting adrenal cortical adenoma. The resulting disease is the expression of increased aldosterone secretion in an otherwise healthy patient. The characteristic abnormalities — potassium wastage, polyuria, muscle weakness, hypokalemic alkalosis, and mild arterial hypertension — are entirely corrected by the removal of the offending adenoma.

Pseudoprimary Aldosteronism (Bilateral Adrenal Hyperplasia)

A significant fraction of patients with the clinical syndrome of primary aldosteronism are found at laparotomy to exhibit bilateral adrenal hyperplasia instead of an isolated adenoma. Patients with such hyperplasia appear to have a different pathophysiologic basis for adrenal overactivity, one perhaps involving an extra-adrenal humoral stimulus to both glands. Unlike patients with primary aldosteronism, they are usually not cured of hypertension by adrenal surgery. The condition has therefore been tentatively called pseudoprimary aldosteronism.

Secondary aldosteronism may be defined as increased aldosterone secretion due to stimulation of the adrenal glands from sources extraneous to them. Discrete adrenal tumors are absent, and the oversecretion is the result of bilateral adrenal cortical hyperfunction. In secondary aldosteronism, the oversecretion is usually associated with and seems to be a consequence of other major disturbances, such as nephrosis, cirrhosis, or heart failure. Increased aldosterone secretion also occurs in various forms of hypertensive vascular disease, and for reasons presented below, this too may be considered a form of secondary aldosteronism.

Oversecretion of Aldosterone in Edematous States. Since the report of Deming and Leutscher, it has become generally recognized that patients with nephrosis, cirrhosis, or heart failure excrete increased amounts of urinary aldosterone while becoming edematous.

We have observed marked adrenal cortical hypersecretion of aldosterone in these edematous states, especially in nephrosis and cirrhosis. In general, the values observed in heart failure were considerably lower than those observed in cirrhosis or nephrosis, and in the case of advanced right-sided heart failure, the aldosterone secretion rates were sometimes not significantly increased at all. Furthermore, there was a paradoxical response pattern in heart failure. Sodium administration, which may further embarrass the circulation may induce more,

not less, aldosterone secretion; diuretic therapy, which consistently increases aldosterone secretion in normal subjects, may lower it in those with heart failure, presumably because the sodium diuresis allows cardiac performance to improve. In contrast, hypersecretion of aldosterone in nephrosis and cirrhosis is usually unaffected by changes in dietary salt.

These observations suggest that hemodynamic factors *per se* may be more important than hormonal factors in the edema of congestive heart failure, whereas hormonal factors appear to predominate in the pathogenesis of the edema of nephrosis and cirrhosis. Furthermore, these findings suggest, perhaps, a fundamental difference in the nature of the stimulus for aldosterone secretion under these conditions. All of these disorders are characterized by a tendency for fluid to transude out from the vascular bed, but there are differences in distribution. In heart failure, total blood volume is increased, and there is a generalized increase in venous back pressure. However, in cirrhosis and nephrosis, the effective blood volume and the oncotic pressure may be greatly reduced. Furthermore, central venous pressure is not elevated in cirrhosis or nephrosis. With more study, it may be possible to show how certain of these altered circulatory dynamics are critically involved in eliciting increased renin and aldosterone secretion as part of a homeostatic response.

Aldosterone Secretion in Malignant Hypertension. The physiologic derangements observed in the syndrome of malignant hypertension are of special interest to this discussion because an analysis of this problem revealed the existence of the renin-angiotensin-aldosterone system and its critical involvement in this disorder.

An early study revealed that, unlike other forms of hypertension, aldosterone secretion is consistently and strikingly elevated in malignant hypertension. This syndrome is expressed clinically by neuroretinopathy, severe accelerating hypertension, and evidence of advancing renal disease, and pathologically by necrotizing arteriolitis. The hyperaldosteronism of malignant hypertension is usually accompanied by hypokalemic alkalosis, probably the result of aldosterone excess acting on the kidney. This pattern is still apparent even when renal failure has developed.

The hyperaldosteronism that accompanies malignant hypertension, unlike primary aldosteronism, is not related to the presence of an adrenal tumor, and exploration usually reveals bilateral adrenal hyperplasia. Therefore, it seemed important to identify the extra-adrenal stimulus that might elevate aldosterone secretion in malignant hypertension. Since patients with malignant nephrosclerosis have a tendency to hypokalemic alkalosis, aldosterone stimulation cannot be attributed to increased plasma potassium. In fact, it has been possible to effect further increases in aldosterone secretion by rectifying plasma potassium values. None of the hemodynamic faults, such as those observed in edematous states that might elevate aldosterone, is associated with this disorder. All of these considerations led our group to suspect that in these patients there was another stimulus to the adrenals, probably arising in the kidneys, which are the major site of pathologic change. The studies that defined this vital renal-adrenal relationship linking renin to aldosterone are discussed below.

Renal Juxtaglomerular Cell Hyperplasia (Bartter's Syndrome). Renal juxtaglomerular cell hyperplasia is a very rare disorder described by Bartter and his associates in 1962. It is characterized clinically by chronic renal potassium wastage, hypokalemic alkalosis, and retarded growth and development. Hyperplasia of the renal juxtaglomerular cells occurs but is associated with normotension and the absence of edema. Marked oversecretion of aldosterone occurs in this disorder and is accompanied by marked hypersecretion of renin.

The pathophysiology has been the subject of some debate. Bartter himself proposed that the primary defect might be an unresponsiveness of the arterioles to angiotensin, leading to hypersecretion of renin and aldosterone and chronic kaliuresis. We have suggested as an alternative that the syndrome can be an expression of renal injury or disorder, with a sodium-losing tubular lesion inducing the hyper-reninemia, hyperaldosteronism, and K^+ wastage. It is possible that either one or the other of these mechanisms applies in patients with the syndrome. It is certainly true, too, that other forms of sodium-losing renal diseases can be associated with compensatory increases in renin and aldosterone secretion without elevating the blood pressure (i.e. sodium-losing nephritis).

Physiologic Relationships that Define the Renal-Adrenal Axis

Angiotensin as a Potent Stimulus to Aldosterone Secretion in Humans

The elevated blood pressure and renal involvement that characterize malignant nephrosclerosis led us to suspect a renal pressor substance as the appropriate stimulus for the observed marked increases in aldosterone secretion. This opinion was reinforced by the fact that both the malignant hypertensive state and the aldosteronism of unilateral renal disease could be rectified by removal of the offending kidney. Therefore, we investigated the effects of intravenous infusions of the renal pressor peptide angiotensin and were able to demonstrate that this peptide consistently increases aldosterone secretion in normal subjects. These studies further demonstrated that the stimulation is a specific process that cannot be duplicated by other pressor agents. Furthermore, stimulation occurs without an accompanying increase in adrenal cortisol secretion, and it persists for as long as the angiotensin infusion is applied. Maximum stimulation occurs using doses of angiotensin which are only mildly pressor. Because this stimulation is persistent and selective, angiotensin fulfills the requirements of a tropic hormone for the secretion of aldosterone.

The Renal-Adrenal Hormonal System: Its Relation to Malignant Hypertension and to Other Forms of Primary and Secondary Aldosteronism

Our results permitted proposal of a renal-adrenal interaction for normal control of sodium balance, a derangement of which appears to be involved in the pathogenesis of malignant hypertension. Thus, in malignant hypertension, now also called Laragh's Syndrome, the kidneys appear to have developed a critical degree of damage. When this critical renal damage develops, a sequence is set in motion: renin, secreted into the blood stream in excessive amounts, interacts with the circulating renin substrate to release more angiotensin II; angiotensin II, in addition to raising blood pressure inappropriately by constricting arterioles, also stimulates excessive secretion of aldosterone by the adrenal cortex.

In normal subjects, a feedback loop is closed as aldosterone induces sodium retention and volume expansion and the increased renin secretion ceases. However, in ma-

lignant hypertension, because of kidney damage, a vicious cycle develops. The induced aldosteronism cannot turn off the renin secretion, perhaps partly because it cannot induce appropriate sodium retention in the damaged target organ, kidney. A situation results in which there is too much angiotensin and too much aldosterone in the blood at the same time, leading to more renal and vascular damage. We believe this vicious cycle is crucial to the pathogenesis of the malignant hypertension syndrome.

Indeed, experiments have shown that the simultaneous administration of large doses of angiotensin and aldosterone produces the necrotizing vasculitis so characteristic of malignant hypertension. Neither agent alone has had this effect. Moreover, in humans, total nephrectomy can reverse malignant vasculitis.

Conversely, the benign nature of primary aldosteronism may be attributed to the absence of renin and angiotensin. Thus aldosterone, secreted autonomously in the absence of renal damage, would suppress renal release of renin and prevent the initiation of the vicious cycle that seems to occur in malignant hypertension.

If this is the sequence of events in malignant hypertension, it would seem that oversecretion of aldosterone in this disorder, although not necessarily related to its initiation, is an appropriate consequence of renal damage and contributes to its pathogenesis.

Other studies indicate that the normotensive forms of secondary aldosteronism, in which renin and angiotensin are also presumably increased, are not necessarily accompanied by vascular damage. The secondary aldosteronism in cirrhosis of the liver is a case in point. This disorder is accompanied by the overall abnormal ion distribution usual in edema. Despite the avid renal retention of sodium, cirrhosis is not accompanied by high blood pressure. Patients with cirrhosis also have extremely reduced pressor responses to infusions of angiotensin and, in fact, may rapidly develop tachyphylaxis to pressor effects of drugs. The notable tendency for displacement of sodium and water out of the vascular tree in edematous states may account for the absence of hypertension and of vascular damage in the presence of excess aldosterone and angiotensin. Thus, in these situations a leak renders the central arterial volume chronically deficient in the face of an increased total body sodium.

Human Disorders of Renin Secretion: A Physiologic Classification of Hyperaldosteronism

The studies cited above, indicating that renin, via the generation of angiotensin II, is a potent stimulus for eliciting increased aldosterone secretion, make possible reclassification of most of the naturally occurring disorders or physiologic derangements involving increased aldosterone secretion (Tables 22–3 and 22–4). That practically all of these disorders can be classified by relating them to associated abnormalities in plasma renin activity provides strong additional, albeit circumstantial, evidence in support of the idea that renin and angiotensin do, in fact, constitute the major hormonal control system involved in regulating the secretion of aldosterone. Indeed, there are, to date, very few naturally occurring examples of either physiologic or pathologic hypersecretion of aldosterone that cannot be explained and analyzed in terms of theoretically appropriate abnormalities in plasma renin activity.

This relationship is particularly useful in distinguishing primary from secondary forms of aldosteronism be-

Table 22–3. DISORDERS WITH SUPPRESSED
PLASMA RENIN ACTIVITY

With Adrenal Cortical Disease
  (a) Hypertensive states:
    1. Primary aldosteronism (discrete, usually single, adrenal adenoma)
    2. Pseudoprimary or idiopathic aldosteronism (usually bilateral adrenal cortical hyperplasia)
    3. Glucocorticoid-suppressible aldosteronism
    4. Adrenal carcinoma with mineralocorticoid excess
    5. Adrenal enzyme defects with oversecretion of other mineralocorticoids

Without Adrenal Cortical Disease
  (a) Hypertensive states:
    1. Low-renin essential hypertension
    2. Certain patients with renal parenchymal diseases
    3. Liddle's syndrome
    4. Licorice or mineralocorticoid ingestion
  (b) Normotensive states:
    1. Renal parenchymal diseases
    2. Autonomic disorders with postural hypotension
    3. Uninephrectomized subjects
    4. Drug-induced adrenergic blockers

cause, characteristically, primary aldosteronism due to an oversecreting autonomous adenoma or pseudoprimary aldosteronism due to diffuse adrenal cortical hyperplasia are both associated with suppression of renal renin secretion to subnormal levels. Except for these two conditions and some other even more unusual adrenal cortical disorders listed in Table 22–3 and also discussed in Chapter 5, all other instances of hyperaldosteronism that have been identified in humans can be associated with a prior increase in renal renin secretion, with hyperangiotensinemia appearing to be the direct stimulus to the adrenal for aldosterone oversecretion.

Perhaps surprisingly, practically all observed instances of abnormally suppressed plasma renin activity in humans have been associated with some degree of high blood pressure. The only exceptions to this are certain normotensive patients with chronic bilateral renal disease. Moreover, such suppression of plasma renin levels is not necessarily associated with any demonstrable adrenal cortical dysfunction, as evidenced by the fact that many, perhaps 30%, of all patients with common essential hypertension exhibit suppressed plasma renin levels. Yet

Table 22–4. DISORDERS WITH INCREASED
PLASMA RENIN ACTIVITY

With Consequent Secondary Aldosteronism
  (a) Hypertensive states:
    1. Malignant or severe hypertension
    2. Unilateral renal disease with malignant or severe hypertension
    3. High-renin forms of essential hypertension
    4. Renal parenchymal diseases
    5. Renin-secreting tumors
    6. Oral contraceptive–induced hypertension
  (b) Edematous normotensive states:
    1. Cirrhosis
    2. Nephrosis
    3. Congestive heart failure
  (c) Hypokalemic normotensive states:
    1. Juxtaglomerular cell hyperplasia (Bartter's syndrome)
    2. Other nephropathies with sodium or potassium wastage
    3. Alimentary disorders with electrolyte loss
  (d) Physiologic:
    1. Dietary sodium depletion
    2. Diuretic usage, laxative abuse
    3. Reduced effective blood volume states (hemorrhage, dehydration, upright posture)

Without Consequent Secondary Aldosteronism
  (a) Adrenal cortical insufficiency
  (b) Potassium depletion states (alimentary)

these patients with low-renin essential hypertension do not appear to exhibit oversecretion of a mineralocorticoid.

According to the proposed renin-adrenal hormonal interaction, the lowest plasma renin levels of all would be expected in response to primary excessive adrenal secretion of mineralocorticoid hormones. Similarly, the highest levels of plasma renin might be expected to occur with failure of adrenal cortical function, as in Addison's disease or after total adrenalectomy. In the latter, the feedback loop cannot be closed by an adrenal cortical response, and the initial signal for renin release persists and escalates. The same picture, a high renin and low aldosterone pattern, may result from potassium depletion. Potassium is as effective as angiotensin itself in stimulating aldosterone secretion. Conversely, its deficit has been shown to retard normal adrenal cortical capacity for aldosterone production, and it also affects the kidney in such a way as to stimulate renin secretion.

Table 22–4 shows that, among naturally occurring situations associated with increased plasma renin levels, there are two main types of disorders. The first seems to have as a common mechanism either some compromise of, or deficit in, the so-called "effective" blood volume (total extracellular fluid volume or sodium space), or else this type of disorder is associated with a fall in arterial blood pressure or filling capacity. The second type of stimulus for renin secretion involves certain intrinsic disorders of the kidney. In both mechanisms, the high plasma renin levels can be envisaged as a physiologic response, perceived or misperceived, to volume depletion, which can be induced by internal sequestration of blood, hemorrhage, vomiting, diarrhea, diuretics, or various nephropathies. Following the first line of reasoning, the high plasma renin levels found in cirrhosis with ascites or nephrosis result from the sequestration or transudation of fluid out of the circulation, thereby compromising venous return and the normal filling of the renal arterial bed. In congestive heart failure, poor forward pumping of blood and reduced effective blood volume may signal renin release.

As indicated previously, the increased renin secretion of advanced or malignant hypertensive disease can be related to a critical degree of renal damage. Other renal diseases in which renal tubular dysfunction is reflected in faulty sodium conservation and volume depletion (e.g., renal tubular acidosis, Bartter's syndrome) may also be associated with hyper-reninemia and hyperaldosteronism. In the case of oral contraceptive hypertension, an induced increase in renin substrate levels may be critical to producing too much net renin activity in the face of estrogen-induced sodium retention.

Renin and Aldosterone Secretion in Essential Hypertension

Let us next consider the large problem of patients with benign essential hypertension. In this category, the role of the renal-adrenal axis remains to be fully clarified. A connection between salt metabolism, adrenal cortical activity, and high blood pressure has long been suspected. It has been known, for example, that experimental Goldblatt hypertension can be prevented or corrected by adrenalectomy and that the feeding of salt alone or accompanied by a sodium-retaining steroid can cause hypertension in various species of animal.

The analysis of the relationship of aldosterone and renin secretions to human hypertensive disease poses a particularly difficult problem because patients with essential hypertension may not represent a homogenous etiologic group. Furthermore, the disorder has an insidious onset, and it is often accompanied by occult renal and cardiac complications that, by themselves, might influence the renal-adrenal axis.

Conceptually, it is of fundamental importance to establish whether or not the renal-adrenal axis is abnormal in uncomplicated essential hypertension. Our own earlier measurements indicated that aldosterone secretion and its response to fluctuations in electrolyte balance are most often normal in benign essential hypertension. Other investigators have reported similar findings. In support of these results, it should be noted that these patients are not potassium depleted, a circumstance that may be taken as strong evidence against hyperaldosteronism, because aldosterone excess almost invariably brings about a potassium deficit.

More recently, with the availability of reliable methods for measuring renin and angiotensin, we have investigated the question of whether or not subtle abnormalities in the renin-angiotensin system might be involved in the pathogenesis of essential hypertension. In a study of 219 patients, simultaneous measurements of plasma renin activity and of aldosterone excretion were related to concurrent daily rates of sodium excretion. This is the so-called renin-sodium "profile." The designation of low, normal, or high values for each hormone was made against an index drawn from normal volunteers studied over the same wide and continuous range of sodium balance.

Three major categories of patients with essential hypertension can be identified with respect to plasma renin. Plasma renin activity was subnormal in 27%, normal in 57%, and abnormally increased in 16% of patients. These groups were then further classified with respect to aldosterone excretion to develop a total of eight different categories representing eight different patterns of renin and aldosterone secretion. Thus, with the development of more precise methodology, subtle abnormalities in aldosterone and more flagrant variations in renin have been identified among the population with essential hypertension.

This biochemical "profiling" of hormonal patterns appears to have physiologic relevance. When the observed hormonal patterns were related to the natural history of the disease, it was found that the rate of renin secretion, and also perhaps of aldosterone secretion, was closely related to the risk of heart attack and stroke. Thus none of the 59 patients with low plasma renin suffered a heart attack or stroke, while those with normal or high renin values had significantly greater incidences of these complications. The higher mean age and even greater hypertension of the low-renin group added further weight to the postulate of a protective role for the low-renin condition.

These observations are in harmony with earlier observations on the relationship of excessive renin and aldosterone secretion to the severe vascular disease of malignant hypertension. They suggest that renin and aldosterone secretion may also be involved in a more subtle way in the vascular injury that so often complicates hypertensive disease. Further analysis of these hormonal patterns in essential hypertension promises to define further the nonhomogeneity of this group of patients and has already proven useful in understanding causations, forecasting prognosis, and applying specific therapy.

Renin and Aldosterone Secretion in the Hypertension of Renal Disease

Despite many clinical and experimental studies following the description of Goldblatt hypertension in 1934, it is still difficult to assign a causal role to increased renin secretion in this condition, because many reports have described normal or even low circulating plasma renin levels in significant fractions from experimental animals or patients with this disorder, as well as in hypertensive patients with a whole variety of bilateral parenchymal renal diseases.

This dilemma perhaps may be explained by the existence of two different mechanisms for both experimental or clinical renal hypertension, only one of which involves an increased renin secretion. A recent study by Brunner and associates supports this idea, and provides a rational explanation for the clinical problem posed by patients who appear to have renal hypertension but who, nonetheless, fail to exhibit increases in their plasma renin levels.

In this experimental series, two types of renal hypertension were examined in rats. In each type there was partial occlusion of one renal artery by a clamp, but in one type the opposite kidney was removed, and in the second type the opposite kidney was left in place. In the first type, no beneficial effects were observed from administration of either angiotensin antibody or of a specific peptide inhibitor of angiotensin. However, in the second type, hypertension was completely corrected by either of these procedures. The findings, therefore, describe both renin and non-renin–dependent types of experimental renal hypertension.

The reason for these two different types of renal hypertension, which exhibit different contributions of renin, may be related to differences in their states of sodium balance. Other studies have shown that, with unilateral renal artery constriction, the untouched contralateral kidney appeared to become a sodium-wasting kidney, perhaps from exposure to the systemic arterial hypertension.

Taken altogether, these results suggest that, in experimental renal hypertension, as in other situations, blood pressure is determined by the product of plasma renin activity and the state of sodium balance. Accordingly, in the one-kidney model, hypertension results largely from excessive body sodium content, whereas in the two-kidney model, increased plasma renin activity plays a more predominant role. This concept gains considerable support from reports relating the pressor activity of angiotensin to the state of sodium balance in humans and from experimental studies demonstrating that the activity of angiotensin receptors is directly related to the state of sodium balance.

There are clinical counterparts of these two pressor mechanisms. Indeed, clinical renal hypertension may present the whole spectrum of possible variation between the two extremes illustrated by the experimental models. Accordingly, in chronic bilateral renal disease with hypertension, both volume-dependent and renin-dependent types are well recognized. In the former, reduction of body sodium by diuretics or by ultra-filtration can restore the blood pressure to normal. In the latter group, total nephrectomy, by reducing inappropriately high renin, will correct the hypertension. Undoubtedly, between these two extremes there are patients with renal hypertension in whom more subtle but inappropriate increases in either body sodium relative to renin or in renin relative to body sodium are operating to cause high blood pressure.

Cybernetics of the Hormonal System in Sodium, Potassium, and Blood Pressure Homeostasis

In the light of information from clinical and experimental studies, the renin-angiotensin-aldosterone system appears to play a major role in the normal regulation of electrolyte balance and arterial blood pressure.

It is perhaps appropriate now to consider in more detail just how the hormonal system might operate to accomplish simultaneously the coordinated control of blood pressure and of flow (via sodium and water content), together with the control of potassium balance. In dealing with this question, it is also appropriate to consider to what extent various disorders of electrolyte and fluid balance and of arterial pressure might be explained in terms of disturbance of the hormonal interaction.

In this analysis, it will be assumed for reasons discussed already that (1) angiotensin II is the major tropic hormone for stimulating aldosterone secretion, (2) plasma levels of angiotensin II ordinarily are largely determined by commensurate changes in plasma renin levels, so that, in analyzing the system, changes in plasma renin activity are a reliable index of changes in angiotensin II, and (3) aldosterone secretion, however, is not solely dependent on angiotensin II and also responds to a similar degree to changes in potassium balance.

There appear to be two loci where perturbations in electrolyte and blood pressure homeostasis are detected and transduced. The adrenal cortex perceives changes in potassium balance, and the kidney is responsive to changes in sodium balance or intravascular fluid pressure. Signals so received then induce appropriate changes in the two effector hormones of the system, *angiotensin II* and *aldosterone.* Normally these effectors, in restoring homeostasis, turn off the initial signal.

Sodium-Linked Potassium Homeostasis

The defense of plasma potassium levels within a relatively narrow range, despite wide variations in intake, is one of the most closely guarded homeostatic functions. In this defense, the direct effect of plasma potassium levels on aldosterone secretion can be viewed as part of a system which protects the organism from dangerous hyperkalemia via an aldosterone-induced kaliuresis. Thus, adrenalectomized animals or patients with adrenal insufficiency are prone to hyperkalemia and cardiac arrest after a potassium meal. Conversely, in various states of potassium depletion, the retarding effect of hypokalemia on aldosterone secretion operates to promote renal K^+ conservation. Potassium depletion also simultaneously stimulates renal renin secretion and vice versa. However, there is as yet little information about the role of angiotensin II in potassium homeostasis. Perhaps worthy of further study in this regard are the observations that angiotensin natriuresis in normal subjects only occurs when potassium is given concurrently. The maintenance of potassium balance also invokes coordinated changes in renal sodium transport, as will be discussed.

The Double-Cycle Feedback for Sodium and Potassium Homeostasis

The data discussed in this chapter provide the basis for a cybernetic scheme for coordinated regulation of sodium and potassium homeostasis. Fig. 22–2 in the upper panel describes the "double-cycle feedback" cybernetic system, involving renin (angiotensin) and aldosterone, which simultaneously controls sodium and potassium homeostasis.

The Sodium Cycle. The outer cycle in the figure describes the system for regulation of sodium balance via changes in renin and aldosterone secretion. In this cycle,

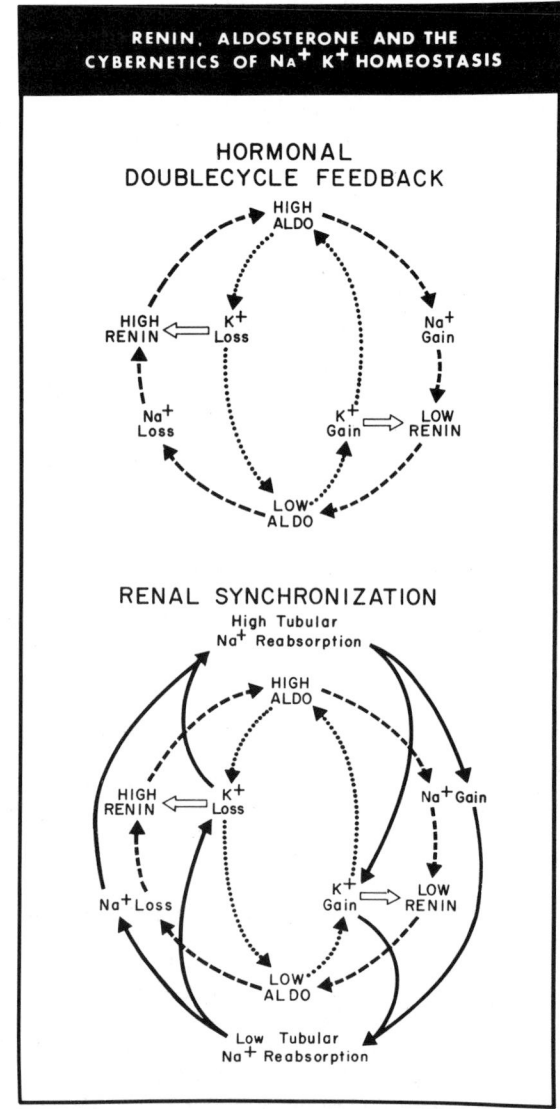

Figure 22–2. *Upper panel,* Hormonal double-cycle feedback system for simultaneous sodium and potassium homeostasis. *Lower panel,* Complementary intrarenal physical factors in renal tubular sodium transport coordinated with dynamic changes in the hormonal system. (From Laragh, J. H., Sealey, J. E., et al.: The control of aldosterone secretion in normal and hypertensive man: abnormal renin-aldosterone patterns in low renin hypertension. *Am. J. Med. 53*:649, 1972.)

any stimulus producing sodium or volume depletion activates renal renin secretion, and this, in turn, stimulates aldosterone secretion. Aldosterone then causes sodium retention with attendant hydremia. This effect, by restoring renal perfusion, operates to turn off the original signal for renin secretion and bring the aldosterone secretory rate back to the null point.

The Potassium Cycle. The inner cycle in the figure describes the system that maintains potassium balance. Ingested potassium ions, by raising plasma potassium, stimulate aldosterone secretion. Aldosterone, in turn, by acting on the renal tubules, restores plasma potassium to normal by promoting renal potassium excretion. As potassium levels in the blood fall, aldosterone secretion is again retarded and restored to the null point. Simultaneously, changes in plasma K^+ also produce direct effects on renal renin secretion, so that a rising plasma potassium suppresses renin secretion and vice versa. It should be noted that the concurrently induced changes in plasma renin activity tend to modulate the effects of potassium on the aldosterone secretory mechanism, so that while potassium stimulates aldosterone secretion, this action is dampened by a concurrently induced fall in plasma renin activity. Accordingly, potassium would exert a much greater stimulatory effect on aldosterone secretion if plasma renin levels remained constant.

Intrarenal hemodynamic adjustments complement and amplify the activity of these hormones in maintaining both sodium and potassium homeostasis. The effect of these changes in intrarenal physical factors on sodium and potassium balance are illustrated in the lower panel of Fig. 22–2. Accordingly, a high sodium intake produces volume expansion, a rise in glomerular filtration rate and in renal blood flow, and changes in intrarenal physical factors, all of which operate to promote renal sodium excretion. These changes also facilitate potassium excretion, because more sodium is delivered to the potassium secretory site in the distal tubule, thereby amplifying the effect of aldosterone and thus increasing potassium excretion. However, potassium wastage is prevented by the high sodium diet–induced fall in aldosterone excretion which concurrently promotes potassium retention and sodium elimination. Completely opposite renal physical effects occur under circumstances of salt and water depletion. This compensatory system is not perfect, since sodium depletion does lead to some potassium retention and very high salt diets might induce K^+ depletion, suggesting that the changes in intrarenal physical factors overcompensate for the hormonal changes.

Deviations in potassium balance can affect renal tubular transport mechanisms either by a direct action or by modifying renal hemodynamic and physical factors. Thus potassium depletion causes increased sodium reabsorption from proximal tubules and resultant decreased sodium delivery to the distal tubule. Clinically, this may cause sodium retention and gross edema even though aldosterone secretion is sharply reduced. Conversely, potassium gain, as can be illustrated by infusing potassium into the renal artery or the peritubular capillaries, can lead to depressed proximal tubular sodium reabsorption, and this may account for the renin-inhibitory action of K^+ as consequent to diverting more Na^+ distally to a macula densa natriastat receptor.

Sodium-Linked Blood Pressure Homeostasis

As indicated already, the maintenance of sodium balance, body fluid volumes, and blood pressure constitutes a closely coordinated homeostatic function. Perturbations of this homeostasis from a whole variety of stimuli are initially perceived by the kidney as a fall in arterial pressure or as a reduction in distal tubular sodium supply, either of which induces renal secretion of renin. This leads to angiotensin II formation and thus to increased aldosterone secretion. The pressor and sodium-retaining effects of these two hormones together operate to restore body fluid volume and renal perfusion, thereby shutting off the initial signal for renin release.

The two effector hormones, angiotensin II and aldosterone, are admirably equipped for these purposes. Thus *angiotensin II* (Fig. 22–1) has three major physiologic actions: (1) it constricts the arterioles to raise arterial pressure, (2) it stimulates adrenal aldosterone secretion, and (3) it acts on the kidney to produce renal sodium retention (not shown in Fig. 22–1). Teleologically, it appears that angiotensin is designed to protect the organism from arterial hypotension or sodium loss or volume contraction. That is to say, it seems to act to defend tissue perfusion, acting immediately to restore pressure and then via aldosterone stimulation to ultimately restore tissue flow. Aldosterone thus works in concert with angiotensin. It acts on the kidney to increase sodium reabsorption, but it has the additional role of maintaining potassium balance by acting on the kidney to promote potassium secretion. Notwithstanding, before accepting this control system as presented, it is appropriate to consider certain seeming paradoxes in its behavior as they occur in physiologic and pathologic situations.

Participation in Physiologic or Secondary Aldosteronism

In view of the fact that angiotensin II is the most potent pressor substance known, the consistent absence of arterial hypertension in many typical examples of secondary aldosteronism (e.g., sodium depletion, cirrhosis, heart failure, and nephrosis) requires an explanation. If angiotensinemia does in fact occur in sodium depletion of normal subjects as well as in the edematous states, why is there no accompanying increase in arterial pressure? The answer to this might possibly reveal a role for angiotensin in essential hypertension and in other hypertensive disorders. Therefore, let us now consider the proposed renin-angiotensin-aldosterone hormonal mechanism in relation to this question.

Dependence of the Vasoactivity of Angiotensin on the State of Sodium Balance

An explanation for the lack of arterial hypertension in states of secondary aldosteronism with presumed angiotensinemia may have been provided by studies of patients with a typical form of secondary hyperaldosteronism, i.e., patients with cirrhosis and ascites, in whom a reduced pressor responsiveness to angiotensin was demonstrated. Such reduced sensitivity was apparent both in acute studies and during infusions lasting several days. The finding seems important because it indicates that increased amounts of angiotensin can circulate and account for hyperaldosteronism without also causing arterial hypertension. This effect could be a nonspecific consequence of a diminished central blood volume because sodium-depleted subjects (and patients forming edema) are less responsive in general to pressor agents. Indeed, a reduced sensitivity to norepinephrine was also observed in these patients.

However, other studies have been able to offer a reasonable explanation for clinical examples of both the *increased* and *decreased* sensitivity to angiotensin. These studies involved the prolonged infusion of angiotensin or of norepinephrine into normal subjects, patients with cirrhosis and ascites, and patients with arterial hypertension. Changing pressor sensitivity to angiotensin could be directly related to concurrently induced changes in the state of sodium balance. In normal subjects, as prolonged angiotensin infusion produced progressive sodium retention, pressor sensitivity increased, so that less and less angiotensin was required to maintain the pressor response. It follows that sodium-depleted normal subjects and cirrhotic subjects exhibited a much reduced sensitivity. Furthermore, in the cirrhotic subjects, in whom it was possible to give even larger doses of angiotensin because of their pressor unresponsiveness, a paradoxical and striking natriuresis occurred, and with this, negative sodium balance pressor sensitivity declined even more. Angiotensin infusions in patients with arterial hypertension also produced natriuresis, and again this negative sodium balance was followed by a declining pressor reactivity to the drug. These studies indicate that angiotensin-induced changes in sodium balance can determine vascular reactivity to the peptide. The experiments further suggest that it was an intravascular accumulation of sodium ions that accounted for the increased sensitivity, because patients with the sodium retention of edema did not exhibit increased sensitivity.

These observations perhaps explain the slowly developing hypertension described in rabbits maintained on initially subpressor infusions of angiotensin, the slowly developing pressor response of rats given renin, the increased pressor response to renin of deoxycorticosterone-treated animals, and the greatly reduced pressor response to angiotensin reported in patients with Addison's disease.

The relationship between angiotensin and available sodium ions may be summarized as follows: (1) in normal subjects, angiotensin causes renal sodium retention and a concomitant *increasing* pressor sensitivity; (2) angiotensin stimulates aldosterone secretion and thus amplifies vascular reactivity by increasing renal sodium retention; (3) however, this sodium-retaining activity of angiotensin appears to have a specific renal feedback component, because with inordinate pressure rises or with larger amounts of exogenous angiotensin, natriuresis (or "escape" from sodium retention) occurs. This natriuresis is greater than that produced by other pressor substances (e.g., norepinephrine), suggesting, in addition, a specific natriuretic action of angiotensin. Taken as a whole, these results suggest an internally controlled system for the regulation of arterial pressure determined by both the blood level of angiotensin and the available sodium ions. The results suggest that, during angiotensin-induced sodium retention, diminishingly small blood levels of angiotensin can act to induce and maintain arterial hypertension, without at the same time being sufficient to increase aldosterone secretion. On the other hand, in normal subjects completely deprived of sodium and in patients forming edema (i.e., transuding), relatively large amounts of angiotensin are unable to raise the blood pressure.

Altered Vascular Receptor Affinity as a Determinant of the Vasoactivity of Angiotensin

Recent research provides more direct evidence for the existence of specific angiotensin II vascular receptors, changes in the activity of which appear to be a determinant of changes in the vasoactivity of angiotensin, with the resultant changes in sodium balance described above. Receptor affinity, as evaluated by determining the amount of angiotensin antibody required to block the blood pressure response to exogenous angiotensin II, was determined in normotensive rats and in various types of hypertensive rats with low, normal, or high salt intakes. Using the immunologic approach, Brunner and his associates found that the binding affinity of angiotensin receptors for exogenous angiotensin was greatly increased by a high-salt diet in normal animals and that it was also greatly increased in animals with various forms of experimental hypertension. These results provide further evidence that there is an important interrelationship between angiotensin pressor responsiveness and sodium balance. They indicate again that angiotensin might, by induction of this mechanism, participate in the pathogenesis of various types of experi-

mental hypertension, even when circulating levels of the hormone itself are not inordinately elevated.

Basis for Participation of the Renal-Adrenal System in Hypertensive Diseases

Quite unlike the states of physiologic and secondary aldosteronism, where hypertension is not ordinarily observed, it is also clear that, in the appropriate settings, high blood pressure can be a cardinal expression of derangements in the renal-adrenal hormonal system. High blood pressure only seems to result when the circulation remains intact, so that any excess fluid retention due to aldosterone excess is reflected in vascular expansion relative to vascular capacity; a steady state results which is characterized by "escape" or a tendency to rapidly excrete any added fluid. This tendency may be viewed as an incipient pressure natriuresis, in which the central circulation is intolerant of any further distention. In the edematous states, on the other hand, fluid increments "leak" rapidly from the central circulation, so that similar vascular-bed filling relative to its capacity does not occur, and the blood pressure remains normal or low. Accordingly, in the edematous states, decompression of the circulation occurs via transudation which precludes a blood-pressure rise, whereas in hypertensive states, the kidney is the run-off site, resisting further increased arterial pressure by natriuresis.

Vasoconstriction-Volume Analysis.   It is apparent from these considerations that hypertension can result either (1) when the vascular bed is overfilled from a fluid surfeit, or (2) when the vascular bed is inappropriately vasoconstricted relative to the available fluid volume. If this reasoning, invoking two interrelated factors, is correct, one might predict that, in extreme situations, there could occur two forms of chronic hypertension, one which would be entirely due to sodium-volume excess, and the other almost entirely related to excessive vasoconstriction (i.e., to excessive pressor activity).

Thus: BP = volume × vasoconstriction

or   BP = (aldosterone) (Na$^+$) × (angiotensin II)

Using this hypothesis, blood pressure is always determined by the product of a volume factor and a vasotonic or pressor factor (both of which are often regulated by the renal-adrenal hormone axis). In this relationship, the vasoconstrictor component is amplified or dampened by concurrent changes in sodium balance, as described above.

For simplicity, in this analysis we shall assume normal cardiac performance, so that the heart has not yet "failed" from any volume or resistance overload. Admittedly, changes in cardiac performance could modify the blood pressure level determined by the other two components. Notwithstanding, let us now consider to what extent various forms of hypertensive disease might be explained in terms of volume and vasoconstriction.

"Volume" Hypertension.   This term describes that extreme of a spectrum in which hypertension seems to be largely due to, or associated with, a maintained excess of sodium and water. In terms of the equation given above, vasoconstrictor activity (i.e., angiotensin II) is minimal or absent in this state. Thus plasma renin activity measurements approach zero. The "volume" factor is maximally excessive because of either (a) excess dietary salt (experimental salt hypertension); (b) excess mineralocorticoid with adequate dietary salt, as in experimental mineralocorticoid hypertension and in primary aldosteronism in humans; or (c) inability to excrete dietary salt, as in certain forms of chronic renal disease and in nephrectomized humans. Physiologically, this type of hypertension would be characterized by minimal vasoconstrictor activity (low plasma renin), relatively dilated (less constricted) arterioles, high plasma and extracellular fluid volumes, and a low blood viscosity and hematocrit. In patients with mineralocorticoid excess, hypokalemia and alkalosis would also be apparent. In all these patients, hypernatriuresis of administered saline would be a prominent feature unless masked by renal dysfunction.

This form of hypertension can be controlled by volume depletion with measures such as a low-salt diet, diuretic therapy, or vigorous ultrafiltration using a hemodialyzer. In patients with mineralocorticoid excess, appropriate adrenal surgery or pharmacologic blockade provides another way for specific correction.

"Vasoconstrictor" Hypertension. This term refers to hypertensive disorders in which arteriolar vasoconstriction is the predominant factor. In terms of the present discussion, it is defined simply as a physiologic excess of renin and therefore angiotensin II. Theoretically, increased autonomic nervous activity or excess norepinephrine should produce an extremely similar picture. In fact, norepinephrine and angiotensin II may synergize or amplify each other, and they may act, at least in part, at similar sites. We are just now beginning to recognize chronic hypertensive states in which there may be sustained increases in α-adrenergic activity instead of angiotensin.

This form of hypertension in its fullest expression is exemplified by human malignant hypertension due to either bilateral or unilateral renal disease and by its experimental counterpart, malignant Goldblatt hypertension. In these states, plasma angiotensin II is markedly elevated. Typically, this is accompanied by secondary aldosteronism and hypokalemia.

Physiologically, this hypertension is characterized by maximal arteriolar vasoconstriction. While one would expect plasma and extracellular fluid volumes to be increased because of the aldosteronism, this volume influence is countered by the vasoconstriction and resultant pressure natriuresis of the severe hypertension, so that the "volume" component in this hypertension may be reduced, especially in the extreme forms. Thus the hematocrit and blood viscosity may be high and the plasma volume reduced. However, as in volume hypertension, hypernatriuresis of administered saline is a prominent feature.

This form of hypertension is controlled by measures that neutralize or eliminate the excessive renin secretion. Thus appropriate unilateral or bilateral nephrectomy can produce dramatic reversal of the hypertension. Short of this, drugs which control renin secretion, such as propranolol or α-methyldopa, can also be of striking benefit. Recently the development of anti-angiotensin (e.g., saralasin) or anti-converting enzyme drugs (e.g., Teprotide or Captopril) have provided highly specific and potent tools for diagnosis and treatment of this renin-induced vasoconstriction. As one might expect, diuretics are of little value here, and they may even produce adverse effects by dehydrating, worsening viscosity and flow, and further stimulating renin secretion. For the same reason, adrenalectomy may not help. Actually, saline infusion may benefit some of these patients by restoring plasma volume, which would suppress renin

and the blood pressure, while improving flow. The saline is best given in conjunction with measures to block the excessive renin-vasoconstriction.

Vasoconstrictor and Volume Factors in Renal Hypertension

Let us then consider to what extent blood pressure elevations in *renal* hypertension might be explained by the product of renin activity and the state of sodium balance, with the latter also acting secondarily to amplify or dampen the activity of angiotensin II, as already described.

In dealing with this problem we have shown that there are two models of experimental renal hypertension which appear to express the two different mechanisms. Two-kidney hypertension (one renal artery maintained partially constricted and the other untouched) is characterized by a high plasma renin level, volume contraction with sodium wastage from the untouched kidney, and a striking drop in blood pressure with administration of either an angiotensin antibody or antagonist. Thus this form seems to fit the requirements of a vasoconstrictor form of hypertension. On the other hand, one-kidney renal hypertension (one renal artery partially constricted, the other kidney removed) in its established form seems to be largely a "volume" hypertension. Accordingly, the latter is characterized by low or normal plasma renin and no effect on blood pressure of angiotensin antibody administration. Here, because of reduced nephron mass, the volume expansion is probably related to a relative inability to excrete sodium.

In clinical renal hypertension may be found the whole spectrum of possible variation between the two extremes illustrated by the experimental models. In chronic bilateral renal diseases with hypertension, both volume-dependent and renin-dependent types are well recognized. In the former, reduction of body sodium by diuretics or by ultrafiltration can restore the blood pressure to normal. In the latter group, total nephrectomy, by reducing inappropriately high renin, will correct the hypertension. Undoubtedly, between these two extremes there are patients with renal hypertension in whom more subtle but inappropriate increases either in volume relative to renin or in renin relative to volume are operating to cause high blood pressure.

Renal-Adrenal Vasoconstriction and Volume Factors in the Spectrum of Essential Hypertension

As indicated above, a variety of abnormal patterns in renin and aldosterone secretion have been described among patients classified as having so-called essential hypertension. In the past this has been taken as evidence that renin is not involved in essential hypertension. However, it is worth considering how these abnormal patterns might emerge, assuming that the hypertension in its established form results from (1) largely vasoconstriction, (2) largely hypervolemia, or (3) an abnormal interaction of the two factors.

Vasoconstriction Essential Hypertension (High-Renin and Medium-Renin Forms)

For this sequence let us assume that the hypertensive process begins as a primary renal disturbance with a subtle increase in renin secretion, angiotensin formation, and then aldosterone secretion. A sequence similar to that observed in the angiotensin infusion studies of normal subjects would ensue. Sodium retention (due to increased aldosterone) and the increased angiotensin would together raise arterial pressure. Increased sodium retention would progressively tend to suppress the excess renin secretion. Thus the amount of angiotensin required to maintain an elevated blood pressure would fall to normal or nearly normal levels because of the increased sodium balance. A point could be reached where angiotensin blood levels would no longer suffice to cause excess aldosterone secretion. This chain of events could produce sustained high blood pressure with no other apparent residual abnormality except for a subtle change in amount or distribution of body sodium ions.

This hypothesis of a mechanism leading to elevated blood pressure in the absence of discernible physiologic fault is in keeping with numerous theories that essential hypertension is a disorder of a regulatory system in which the hypertension has compensated for the system. That is, the initial defect has been masked by a series of readjustments involving feedback mechanisms and changes in the autoregulatory activity by the kidney.

Physiologically, in its established state, this hypertension would exhibit "normal" or slightly high renin and aldosterone secretion. These patterns actually occur in a large number of patients with essential hypertension. In this construction the term "normal-renin" is a misnomer and should be called medium-renin, because in the face of systemic hypertension, renin secretion would not normally be suppressed to very low levels. Hence the kidneys are behaving inappropriately by continuing to secrete renin. This can be proven to be true since when renin-lowering or blocking drugs are given, the blood pressure falls to normal (see below).

Volume Mediated Essential Hypertension (Low-Renin Forms)

Several mechanisms might produce hypertension associated with chronic, albeit subtle, volume expansion. Thus, as in animal models, the chronic ingestion of a very-high-sodium diet theoretically might be a cause. In fact, the amounts required on a weight basis may exceed those usually ingested by humans. Such hypertension would be expected to exhibit a subnormal renin-secretory and a subnormal aldosterone-secretory pattern. Actually, this renin

pattern occurs in about 30% of hypertensive patients who have low plasma renin activity.

A second possible mechanism for chronic volume-expansion hypertension could involve an impaired renal capacity to excrete the amounts of sodium occurring in average diets. Since most hypertensive patients excrete sodium abnormally rapidly, this seems an unlikely causal mechanism unless the hypertension has actually overcompensated for the initial renal defect. Both renin and aldosterone also might be expected to be low in this situation. However, since a renal disturbance is postulated, abnormal renin secretion could be an attendant part.

Another possible mechanism for volume-induced hypertension could result from a primary renal inability to excrete ingested potassium ions. This would lead to elevated plasma potassium levels and thus to increased aldosterone secretion, volume expansion, increased vascular sensitivity, and suppressed plasma renin activity. In the compensated state, potassium balance would be restored to normal, and the established hypertension would be sustained by aldosterone-induced sodium retention with increased vascular sensitivity to angiotensin. This thesis has the attraction of an experimental basis, since potassium gain is known both to stimulate aldosterone and to suppress renin. Moreover, low renin secretion with an inappropriately high aldosterone secretion is a rather common pattern among patients with essential hypertension.

A fourth mechanism for volume-induced essential hypertension involves a primary adrenal disturbance with increased secretion of aldosterone or of another mineralocorticoid. As indicated elsewhere, this leads to volume expansion and suppressed plasma renin levels, but in this situation, unlike the first three, potassium depletion with hypokalemia, the inevitable consequence of mineralocorticoid excess, is almost invariably observed.

While renin-sodium profiling is a powerful tool for subdividing and analyzing essential hypertension, it should be emphasized that the subgroups defined by this technique still may not be homogeneous. Thus, *a priori,* the lowered renin levels suggest overfilling and volume expansion as an important mechanism in low renin hypertension. This in fact often can be easily verified by space measurements and by the fact that blood pressure is normalized simply by administration of a diuretic in two-thirds of these patients. However, something like one-third of low renin patients do not respond to diuretics. Therefore, the profiling technique separates for further research a low renin sub-category in which neither renin nor volume seems to be the pressor factor (Fig. 22–3).

THE VASOCONSTRICTION-VOLUME SPECTRUM IN HYPERTENSION

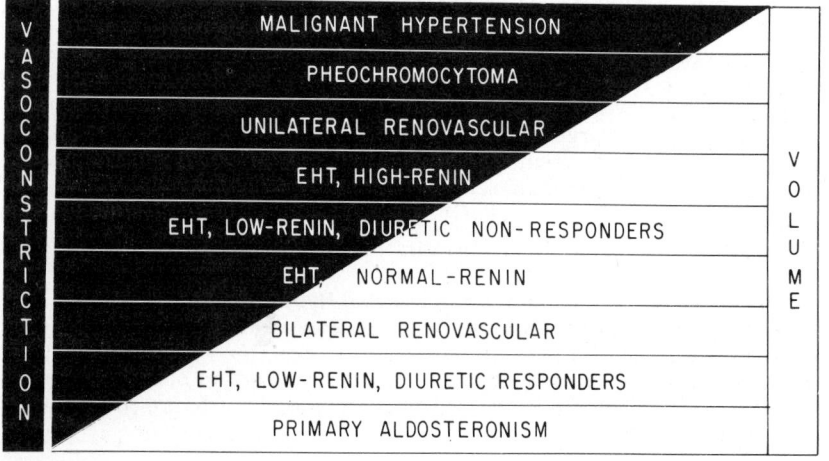

Figure 22–3. Vasoconstriction-volume spectrum in hypertension. Abbreviation EHT indicates essential hypertension. (From Laragh, J. H., et al.: J.A.M.A. *241*:151, 1979.)

Pathophysiologic Implications of "Vasoconstrictor" Hypertension as Contrasted with "Volume" Hypertension

This functional classification of hypertensive states appears to have pathophysiologic correlations both in experimental models and naturally-occurring situations (Fig. 22–3). Thus vasoconstrictor forms of hypertension appear to have more devastating consequences than do volume-expansion forms. In this context, renin-induced forms of hypertension, such as malignant hypertension, are associated with severe vascular injury, and the injection of renin into experimental animals also produces severe vascular injury. Conversely, primary aldosteronism with suppressed renin and a large volume component is usually a benign form of hypertensive disease exhibiting little evidence of vascular injury or target organ damage in the brain, kidneys, and heart. The benign nature of this form of hypertension relative to the vasoconstrictor form may be explained by the more adequate delivery of oxygen and nutrition to the tissues associated with the increased blood volume and relatively dilated arterioles.

While more documentation is required, it now appears that these relationships may also obtain in a more subtle way in various types of essential hypertension. Thus it has been found that patients with low-renin forms of essential hypertension are significantly less prone to the development of heart attacks or strokes than are patients with either normal or high levels of plasma renin activity. If these relationships continue to be observed, they could have important implications for classifying, determining prognosis, and planning treatment.

Meanwhile, from a physiologic standpoint, the data suggest that, given an equal degree of hypertension, arterial-tree distention with hemodilution and low viscosity constitutes, from a biophysical standpoint, a less deleterious situation than does the vasoconstrictor state characterized by a high-resistance arterial tree and a constricted vasculature perfused by a high-viscosity blood.

Pharmacologic Proof of Renin Participation in Most Hypertensive States

Even if the renin system does participate in certain uncommon forms of hypertension, most investigators have doubted a role for it in essential hypertension, probably because of an inability to relate blood pressure levels to renin levels for the group as a whole. However, our research group has long believed that the renin system might participate in certain forms of essential hypertension, since infusion of angiotensin in diminishing amounts, unlike norepinephrine, produces a persistent, partially sodium-dependent hypertension in normal persons.

The effects of various types of antihypertensive drugs on blood pressure and on the renin system provide both theoretical and practical corroboration for the functional characterization of hypertensive disorders in terms of either predominantly vasoconstrictor or volume factors. Moreover, the interactions of these various antihypertensive drugs with the renin system now provide a rational basis for their well-known variations in effectiveness in different patients.

Accordingly, antihypertensive drugs which produce volume depletion — thiazide diuretics and aldosterone antagonists — are especially effective not only in primary aldosteronism but also in most patients with low-renin forms of essential hypertension. Conversely, these drugs are often ineffective or even pressor in high-renin forms of hyperten-

sive disease. Thus, in certain of these latter patients, the induced volume depletion may worsen the situation significantly by exciting more renin secretion, vasoconstriction, and hemoconcentration.

A giant step forward was taken in 1972 when Bühler and associates showed that the antihypertensive action of the β-blocker propranolol hydrochloride is directly related to the preexisting renin level and to the degree that the drug reduces that level. Thus, propranolol was most effective in patients with high renin levels, effective in patients with normal renin levels, and ineffective in patients with low renin levels. To our knowledge, this report provides the first evidence for pressor participation of renin in major fractions of essential hypertension while showing a major mechanism of propranolol's antihypertensive action. It suggested, too, that a normal renin level in a hypertensive patient is in truth abnormal, since the normal response to high blood pressure is a lowered renin secretion (Fig. 22–1).

Studies using experimental drugs to block either angiotensin II action (saralasin acetate) or formation (converting enzyme inhibitor) parallel and extend the propranolol experience. In particular, depressor responses to the converting enzyme inhibitor, which has no intrinsic pressor properties as does saralasin, shows a renin factor supporting some or all of the hypertension in some 70% of patients with essential hypertension, including the patients with high renin levels and most patients with normal renin levels. These parallel results give additional credence to the theory that propranolol's antihypertensive action is largely related to an antirenin effect. In fact, the degree of response to all three antirenin system agents can be predicted from the baseline renin-sodium profile.

All these studies indicate that the plasma renin level is a true reflector of its active vasoconstriction, while the 24-hour urinary sodium measurement gauges the propriety of this vasoconstriction to the fluid-volume status. Moreover, the converse is true. These three antirenin agents are ineffective in the 30% of patients with low-renin essential hypertension who respond instead to diuretics, testifying to their volume dependency.

Considerable research verifies the differing response patterns of hypertensive patients within the renin subgroups to β-blockade as opposed to diuretic therapy. Reciprocal effects reinforce these relationships; not only is propranolol usually ineffective in patients with low renin levels, but, like saralasin, it can be overtly pressor in them. And, diuretics, uniquely effective in patients with low renin levels, can be pressor in the patients with high renin levels. Presumably these already vasoconstricted and hypovolemic patients react to more dehydration with an overshoot renin response. The renin-volume interplay appears as a seesaw. Some patients given diuretics respond with vigorous hyperreninemia, which explains the failure of their blood pressure to fall. Conversely, patients given antirenin agents may not respond because of reactive sodium retention. Altogether, these results are the scientific underpinning for a new era of predictable and selective drug therapy in essential hypertension.

How to Use Renin-Sodium Profiling in Diagnosis and Treatment

Renin-sodium profiling is a new but relatively simple technique which reliably identifies the renin-vasoconstriction factor and its appropriateness to the concurrent volume factor which is estimated from the 24-hour urinary sodium excretion. In practice, in untreated patients or

A FLOW SHEET FOR DIAGNOSIS AND TREATMENT OF HYPERTENSION

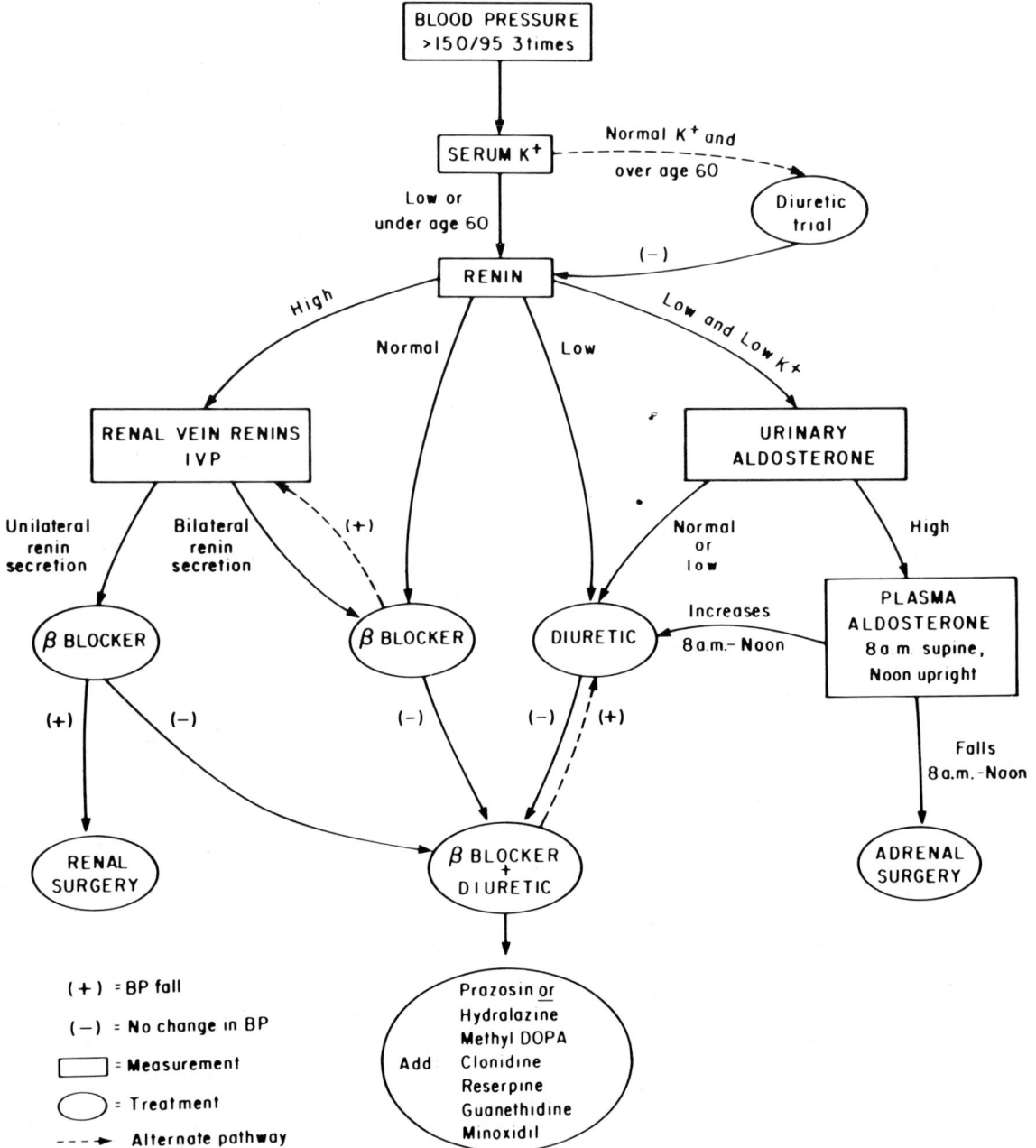

Figure 22–4. Plan for diagnosis and treatment of hypertension. Symbol (+) indicates blood pressure (BP) normalized; (−), BP not normalized; dashed arrow, alternate pathway; K, potassium level.

those withdrawn from therapy for at least three weeks, a 24-hour urine collection is combined with a peripheral plasma renin activity assay from venous blood collected from quietly seated ambulatory patients. The renin value is then plotted against a nomogram derived from normal subjects which allows an evaluation of the normalcy of the renin with respect to the concurrent sodium-volume status.

There are some key technical points to the renin assay which, when overlooked, have led to confusing results. Thus, care should be taken to completely inhibit angiotensinases during the incubation of the plasma sample. This requires the addition of EDTA plus either DFP or PMSF. Secondly, the incubation should be carried out at the acid pH optimum (5.5–6.0) of human renin to achieve maximum sensitivity and stability. Thirdly, chilling of samples should be avoided since this promotes inadvertent activation of inactive renin.

We have recently set forth in detail the methods of a complete, integrated system for diagnosis and for applying simpler, more specific, and more predictable treatment in all hypertension. In it, the renin-sodium profile and a baseline plasma-potassium measurement provide the basis for (1) definitive diagnosis of adrenocortical hypertension, (2) definitive diagnosis of surgically curable renovascular hypertension, (3) the acquisition of baseline data about the relative participation of vasoconstriction and volume factors that enables more specific therapy, and (4) the evaluation of the pace, severity, and outlook of the underlying disorder. The plan also defines an optional procedure for empirical use when a renin profile is not easily available.

Among the advantages of the new system is that for major fractions of all hypertensive patients, it enables, for the long-term commitment, therapy with one drug instead of two, or two instead of three or more, with the attraction that the right type of drug is applied to contain the physiological lesion, i.e., antivolume therapy with a diuretic in patients with low renin levels or anti-renin therapy with a β-blocker in patients with high and normal renin levels (Fig. 22–4). It also reduces the use and aids selection of patients for pyelography and arteriography. In the system (Fig. 22–4), normokalemic patients older than 60 years can first receive diuretics because of the higher prevalence of low-renin hypertension in this age group. Conditions of patients who have low renin levels and hypokalemia (potassium level less than 3.5 mEq/liter) are evaluated for adrenocortical and those of patients with high renin levels for renovascular disease. A mathematical analysis of renal-vein renin levels identifies ipsilateral hypersecretion with ischemia and no secretion contralaterally.

Surgically incurable patients return to the basic treatment program. Patients with normal and high renin levels first receive a β-blocker, and patients with low renin levels receive a diuretic. If either course is only partly corrective, the two are combined. Altogether, this normalizes the conditions of about 85% of patients. Unlike stepped care, drug subtraction and dose reduction are performed whenever blood pressure is normalized to achieve fewest drugs in smallest doses. Only for the small residual resistant group are other less-palatable drugs superimposed in traditional trial-and-error fashion.

Clinical Rewards

Both the clinician and the patient in this new system reap advantages and satisfactions. Especially rewarding is the frequent total long-term control of patients with high renin levels and many patients with normal renin levels

with nothing but a β-blocker, and sometimes with surprisingly small doses. In the traditional stepped-care approach, treatment of this sizable fraction of patients with essential hypertension would begin with a diuretic, and the patient would likely exhibit a poor or no blood pressure response compounded by a new much higher renin level. We suspect that acceleration of this type of hypertension might actually be induced by such therapy. Then drugs such as methyldopa, reserpine, vasodilators, or guanethidine sulfate would be added. The patient would wind up with only partial blood pressure correction, dehydrated and weak, and possibly with impaired mentation, hypokalemia, and impotence.

In our system, this patient group would have about a 75% chance of responding to a β-blocker alone, without side effects and with the possible bonus of protection from ischemic heart disease. Addition of a diuretic would then correct most of the rest. At the low-renin end of the spectrum, too, our method leads to the direct control of the conditions of patients receiving a diuretic alone, again sometimes in surprisingly low doses.

The system enables more precise diagnosis for the entire range of hypertension. Thus, consider the not uncommon younger patient with severe hypertension of recent onset who exhibits a greater than 2:1 renin ratio on renal-vein study and has an abnormal arteriogram. If a preliminary peripheral renin profile is not obtained to establish renin hypersecretion or if an inferior vena caval sample is not collected with the renal-vein samples, the lack of complete suppression of renin secretion in the contralateral kidney can be missed and needless surgery might be performed.

For another example, consider two clinically similar patients, each with a blood pressure of 220/120 mm Hg, one with a low and the other with a high renin-sodium profile. The clinician would probably think differently about these two patients in terms of the pace and severity of their disorder and, therefore, about both direction and urgency of their workup and treatment.

The new framework also prepares clinicians to understand and treat promptly more urgent hypertensive phenomena. A recent study described saralasin withdrawal that triggered notable rebound hyperreninemia and hypertension accompanied by encephalopathy and coma. This description retraces the fulminant vascular events observed with high renin levels in acute or malignant hypertension, in instances of renal injury, following closure of a renal artery graft, or with renin-secreting tumors. In all these, acute hyperreninemia looms as the culprit. Its early identification or exclusion allows better care of the acutely ill patient, especially if one considers that here, too, when antirenin therapy is appropriate, diuretic therapy can be contraindicated, and vice versa.

Altogether, this rational new method ensures both complete diagnosis and more precisely targeted treatments. It entails fewer drugs, lower costs, and fewer disturbances of physical or mental function. This means greater patient compliance and better results.

SUMMARY

A large constellation of clinical and experimental evidence has accumulated which characterizes the renin-angiotensin-aldosterone hormonal concentration. By changing the plasma concentrations of its two effector components, *angiotensin II*, and *aldosterone*, the system works to regulate simultaneously (1) arterial blood pressure, (2) body sodium and water content and thus hydrostatic pressures, and (3) potassium balance.

In this system, the kidney, responding to various stimuli perceived as a fall in arterial pressure or tubular sodium supply, releases renin. Renin liberates angiotensin from a specific circulating plasma globulin. Angiotensin, in turn, stimulates the secretion of aldosterone by the adrenal cortex. Angiotensin and aldosterone together act to restore sodium balance and arterial pressure, thus shutting off the initial signal for renin release.

More specifically, angiotensin II acts immediately to restore blood pressure by causing arteriolar vasoconstriction. The pressor effect is amplified by the sodium-retaining actions of angiotensin, acting directly on the kidneys and via stimulation of aldosterone secretion, to induce renal sodium retention. The increased sodium helps to maintain blood pressure not only by increasing the vasoconstrictor action of angiotensin but also by volume expansion with increased filling of the vascular bed. Thus the renin-angiotensin-aldosterone system maintains blood pressure, first by reducing the capacity of the system (vasoconstriction), and then by increasing the volume of the vascular tree and so restoring precious flow by increasing body sodium content and, therefore, water retention.

At the same time as this sodium-linked blood-pressure homeostasis operates, sodium-linked potassium homeostasis is accomplished by two direct but opposing effects of changes in plasma potassium levels on aldosterone and on renin secretion.

Specific derangements of the renal-adrenal cybernetic system are involved in the pathogenesis of the edematous states of heart failure, cirrhosis, and nephrosis and in certain hypertensive disorders, notably malignant hypertension, primary (adenoma) and pseudoprimary (hyperplasia) adrenal cortical aldosteronism, renovascular hypertension, and oral contraceptive-induced hypertension.

Abnormalities in the renal-adrenal system also occur in the large population of patients with other forms of hypertensive disease, traditionally called essential hypertension. In this problem a cybernetic analysis can be applied in which the hypertension is considered to be the product of two influences, a vasoconstrictor factor and a volume component, each of which may be largely determined by the activity of the renal-adrenal system. This analysis appears to have meaningful pathophysiologic and pharmacologic coordinates.

Accordingly, predominantly vasoconstrictor hypertension is largely renin-sustained, and it is associated with arteriolar vasoconstriction, hemoconcentration, and, with time, evidences of vascular injury. It can be corrected by drugs that reduce renin secretion or which block the formation or action of angiotensin II. This group includes patients with malignant hypertension, more severe forms of renal hypertension, high-renin and most normal-renin essential hypertension.

On the other hand, predominantly volume-factor hypertension is characterized by undue sodium and water retention, a relatively distended or open arterial tree, hemodilation and low blood viscosity, and, with time, less evidence of target organ vascular damage. It can be corrected by volume-depleting natriuretic drugs. This group of patients includes those with primary and pseudoprimary aldosteronism, syndromes of aberrant mineralocorticoid excess, and a large subfraction of patients with essential hypertension in whom renin is suppressed and aldosterone is normal or low.

Areas of uncertainty still exist and should be given special attention. Elucidation of these may finally offer a complete explanation for the genesis of a host of common diseases characterized by hypertension or abnormal sodium or potassium metabolism.

REFERENCES

Ames, R. P., Borkowski, A. J., et al.: Prolonged infusions of angiotensin II and norepinephrine and blood pressure, electrolyte balance, aldosterone and cortisol secretion in normal man and in cirrhosis with ascites. *J. Clin. Invest. 44*:1171, 1965.

Bartter, F. C., Provone, P., et al.: Hyperplasia of the juxtaglomerular complex with hyperaldosteronism and hypokalemic alkalosis. *Amer. J. Med. 33*:811, 1962.

Biglieri, E. G., and Lopez, J. M.: Clinical and laboratory diagnosis of adrenocortical hypertension. *Cardiovasc. Med. 1*:335, 1976.

Brunner, H. R., Baer, J., et al.: The influence of potassium administration and potassium deprivation on plasma renin in normal and hypertensive subjects. *J. Clin. Invest. 49*:2128, 1970.

Brunner, H. R., Kirshman, J. D., et al.: Hypertension of renal origin: evidence for two different mechanisms. *Science 174*:1344, 1971.

Brunner, H. R., Chang, P., et al.: Angiotensin II vascular receptors: their avidity in relationship to sodium balance, the autonomic nervous system, and hypertension. *J. Clin. Invest. 51*:58, 1972.

Brunner, H. R., Laragh, J. H., et al.: Essential hypertension: renin and aldosterone, heart attack and stroke. *New Eng. J. Med. 286*:441, 1972.

Brunner, H. R., Gavras, H., et al.: Hypertension in man. Exposure of the renin and sodium components using angiotensin II blockade. *Circ. Res. 34 & 35: Suppl. I*:I-35, 1974.

Bühler, F. R., Laragh, J. H., et al.: Propranolol inhibition of renin secretion: a specific approach to diagnosis and treatment of renin-dependent hypertensive diseases. *New Eng. J. Med. 287*:1209, 1972.

Bull, M. B., Hillman, R. C., et al.: Renin and aldosterone secretion in man as influenced by changes in electrolyte balance and blood volume. *Circ. Res. 27*:953, 1970.

Cannon, P. J., Leeming, J. M., et al.: Juxtaglomerular cell hyperplasia and secondary hyperaldosteronism (Bartter's syndrome): a reevaluation of the pathophysiology. *Medicine 47*:107, 1968.

Case, D. B., Wallace, J. M., et al.: Estimating renin participation in hypertension. Superiority of converting enzyme inhibitor over saralasin. *Amer. J. Med. 61*:790, 1976.

Case, D. B., Wallace, J. M., et al.: Possible role of renin in hypertension as suggested by renin-sodium profiling and inhibition of converting enzyme. *New Eng. J. Med. 296*:641, 1977.

Case, D. B., Atlas, S. A., et al.: Clinical experience with blockade of the renin-angiotensin-aldosterone system by an oral converting-enzyme inhibitor (SQ 14,225, Captopril) in hypertensive patients. *Prog. in Cardiovasc. Dis.*, Vol. XXI, 1978.

Davis, J. O.: The control of renin release, In *Hypertension Manual*. Laragh, J. H., M.D. (Ed.), New York, Dun-Donnelley Corp., 1974.

Deming, Q. B., and Leutscher, J. A., Jr.: Bioassay of desoxycorticosterone-like material in urine. *Proc. Soc. Exp. Biol. Med. 73*:171, 1950.

Gavras, H., Brunner, H. R., et al.: An angiotensin-converting enzyme inhibitor to identify and treat vasoconstrictor and volume factors in hypertensive patients. *New Engl. J. Med. 291*:817, 1974.

Guyton, A. C., Coleman, T. G., et al.: Arterial pressure regulation. Overriding dominance of the kidneys in long-term regulation and in hypertension. *Amer. J. Med. 52*:584, 1972.

Laragh, J. H., and Stoerk, H. C.: A study of the mechanism of secretion of the sodium-retaining hormone (aldosterone). *J. Clin. Invest. 36*:383, 1957.

Laragh, J. H., Ulick, S., et al.: Aldosterone secretion and primary and malignant hypertension. *J. Clin. Invest. 39*:1091, 1960.

Laragh, J. H., Angers, M., et al.: Hypotensive agents and pressor substances. The effect of epinephrine, norepinephrine, angiotensin II and others on the secretory rate of aldosterone in man. *J.A.M.A. 174*:234, 1960.

Laragh, J. H.: The role of aldosterone in man: Evidence for regulation of electrolyte balance and arterial pressure by renal-adrenal system which may be involved in malignant hypertension. *J.A.M.A. 174*:293, 1960.

Laragh, J. H.: Hormones and pathogenesis of congestive heart failure: Vasopressin, aldosterone and angiotensin II. Further evidence for renal-adrenal interaction from studies in hypertension and cirrhosis. *Circulation 25*:1015, 1962.

Laragh, J. H., Cannon, P. J., et al.: Angiotensin II, norepinephrine and the renal transport of electrolytes and water in normal man and in cirrhosis with ascites. *J. Clin. Invest. 42*:1179, 1963.

Laragh, J. H., Sealey, J. E., et al.: Patterns of adrenal secretion and urinary excretion of aldosterone and plasma renin activity in normal and hypertensive subjects. *Circ. Res. (Suppl. 1) 18 & 19*:158, 1966.

Laragh, J. H., Sealey, J. E., et al.: Oral contraceptives. Renin, aldosterone and high blood pressure. *J.A.M.A. 201*:918, 1967.

Laragh, J. H., Baer, L., et al.: Renin, angiotensin and aldosterone system in pathogenesis and management of hypertensive vascular disease. *Amer. J. Med. 52*:633, 1972.

Laragh, J. H., Sealey, J. E., et al.: The control of aldosterone secretion in normal and hypertensive man: abnormal renin-aldosterone patterns in low renin hypertension. *Amer. J. Med. 53*:649, 1972.

Laragh, J. H.: Vasoconstriction-volume analysis for understanding and treating hypertension: The use of renin and aldosterone profiles. *Amer. J. Med. 55*:261, 1973.

Sealey, J. E., Clark, I., et al.: Potassium balance and the control of renin secretion. *J. Clin. Invest. 49*:2119, 1970.

Sealey, J. E., Gerten-Banes, J., et al.: The renin system: variations in man measured by radioimmunoassay or bioassay. *Kidney International 1*:240, 1972.

Sealey, J. E., Bühler, F. R., et al.: Aldosterone excretion: physiologic variations in man measured by radioimmunoassay or double isotope dilution. *Circ. Res. 31*:367, 1972.

Sealey, J. E., Bühler, F. R., et al.: The physiology of renin secretion in essential hypertension: Estimation of renin secretion rate and renal plasma flow from peripheral and renal vein renin levels. *Amer. J. Med. 55*:391, 1973.

Sealey, J. E., and Laragh, J. H.: A proposed cybernetic system for sodium and potassium homeostasis: Coordination of aldosterone and intrarenal physical factors. *Kidney International 6*:281, 1974.

Sealey, J. E., and Laragh, J. H.: "Prorenin" in human plasma? Methodological and physiological implications. *Circ. Res. 36 & 37 (Suppl I)*:I-10, 1975.

Tobian, L.: A viewpoint concerning the enigma of hypertension. *Amer. J. Med. 52*:595, 1972.

Vaughan, E. D., Jr., Bühler, F. R., et al.: Renin measurements to indicate hypersecretion, and contralateral suppression, estimate renal plasma flow and score for surgical curability. *Amer. J. Med. 55*:402, 1973.

Skin and Hormones

By Frank Parker

The skin is unusually heterogeneous in its cellular composition, comprising, as it does, rapidly proliferating keratinizing epidermal and hair follicle cells, lipid-synthesizing sebaceous glands, pigment-producing melanocytes, and dermal connective tissue cells responsible for the production of fibrous tissue and ground substances. Each cell type has its own unique metabolic pattern, and therefore the integument is capable of a wide variety of biochemical activities.

Many of these metabolic activities are under hormonal regulation. The control of cutaneous pigmentation by melanocyte-stimulating hormone (MSH) is well known, as are the stimulatory effects of androgens on sebaceous glands and certain hair follicles. The regulatory effects of insulin on cutaneous carbohydrate and lipid metabolism are now receiving much attention, and there is a growing awareness that the skin, the largest organ of the body, plays an important role in the total body metabolism of several hormones.

The variety of hormonal effects upon various cellular elements in the skin will be reviewed in this chapter and, when possible, this information will be related to cutaneous clinical findings. In many instances, metabolic aberrations occurring in the skin have helped to explain clinical cutaneous alterations which accompany endocrine diseases.

Expression of hormonal effects at the cellular level depends on the circulating levels of hormones available as well as the ability of specific cellular elements in the skin to react. Excessive amounts of hormone accentuate certain activities of specific cutaneous structures, while deficiencies of a hormone may be expressed either as diminished function in the cutaneous structures or as excessive activity of other hormones, e.g., the interrelationship of corticotropin (ACTH) and cortisol with excess secretion of ACTH in Addisonian patients with decreased cortisol output.

HORMONES AND THE EPIDERMIS AND DERMIS

Glucose and Lipid Metabolism

Qualitatively the skin — in particular, the epidermis — is capable of metabolizing carbohydrate by the same pathways as other tissues to provide both energy (ATP) for the synthetic, energy-requiring processes and various intermediate substances for other metabolic pathways utilized by epidermal cells. Biochemical studies on human and experimental animal epidermis have verified the presence of the anaerobic glycolytic pathway, as well as the oxidative phosphorylative hexose monophosphate shunt and tricarboxylic acid cycle (Fig. 23–1).

Studies on the relative importance of these major pathways in skin have revealed some differences from other tissues of the body. Glycolysis produces ATP at a maximal rate of about 0.1 μM/hr/mg wet weight epidermis, while the respiratory pathways generate the majority of the energy (80% of epidermal ATP) at a rate of about 0.5 μM ATP/hr. Estimates of respiratory activity of human epidermis indicate a CO_2 value of 5.0, higher than the value for smooth muscle or lung tissue. An unusual feature of epidermal metabolism is that most of the glucose assimilated is converted by glycolysis to pyruvate and, particularly, lactic acid (70%) without further degradation to CO_2 by glycolytic or oxidative pathways. Moreover, only 2% of the glucose finds its way through the direct oxidative (hexose monophosphate shunt) pathway, in contrast to glucose metabolism in such organs as liver and muscle. Therefore, although considerable amounts of glucose are assimilated by human epidermis, most of this is not oxidized to CO_2 for energy production through the oxidative pathways. Rather, the primary substrate for epidermal respiration is apparently lipid. This conclusion is supported by the fact that the respiratory quotient (RQ, the ratio of CO_2 formed to oxygen consumed) of epidermis is less than 1.0, a value that results from fatty acid oxidation. β-oxidation of fatty acids generates two-carbon units (acetyl CoA) and reduces nucleotides which in turn form approximately 5 moles of ATP for each mole of acetyl CoA produced (Fig. 23–1).

The epidermis is also an active site of sterol, fatty acid, and polar lipid synthesis, utilizing pyruvate, some amino acids, acetate, and glucose as substrates. Glucose, however, seems to be the major precursor of lipogenesis, being the only compound that stimulates this process in vitro. Glucose also appears to regulate lipogenesis in vivo, since glucose feeding accelerates cutaneous lipid synthesis, while fasting produces the opposite effect. The level of L-glycerol 3-phosphate in the skin fluctuates parallel to lipogenic activity, and the addition of this substance in vitro stimulates lipogenesis, suggesting that this intermediate in the glycolytic pathway (Fig. 23–1) may play a regulatory role in the lipid synthetic processes. Although the hexose monophosphate shunt plays a relatively minor role in epidermal respiration, it does function significantly in lipogenesis, as it supplies about one-half the necessary NADPH for these synthetic reactions.

Cutaneous sterol synthesis proceeds by way of two alternate routes, the Kandutsch-Russell and the Block pathways, which differ in the intermediary steps between lanosterol and cholesterol. One of the Kandutsch-Russell intermediates is 7-dehydrocholesterol, which can be converted by sunlight to vitamin D, providing a teleological basis for the explanation of the operation of this pathway in skin.

Several examples can be cited to demonstate how hormones may affect cutaneous glucose and lipid metabolism, although it is still difficult to relate these metabolic alterations directly to clinical changes in the skin. Hormones have been shown to alter epidermal metabolism in diabetes mellitus. Glucose uptake and utilization and cutaneous lipogenesis are severely impaired in both human and experimental animal diabetics. Insulin reverses these alterations in vivo and even in vitro in skin in contrast to the reported unresponsiveness to insulin of diabetic leukocytes and adipose tissue in vitro. Insulin even stimulates glucose uptake and lipogenesis (via its effect on the hexose monophosphate shunt) in normal skin. How these disturbances in epidermal metabolism contribute, alone or in concert with a variety of other systemic alterations, to the cutaneous complications of diabetics, such as the propensity to bacterial, yeast, and fungal infection, is not yet clear.

A second example of hormonal effects on cutaneous metabolism may be found in the case of thyroxine. Thyrotoxicosis in animals has been shown to stimulate cutaneous respiration as well as to augment glucose assimilation and aerobic metabolism. Whether these changes are brought about directly by the action of thyroxine on the skin or indirectly by altered vascular blood flow or hormone interactions cannot be stated. Nevertheless, the presence of changes in cutaneous metabolism in experimental thyrotoxicosis suggests that these alterations may accompany and underlie clinical abnormalities of the skin in states of thyroid dysfunction.

Another example of hormonal effects on epidermal metabolism is seen in the relationship of cutaneous sterol metabolism to sex hormones. Testosterone and progesterone significantly accelerate sterol ester synthesis via the Kandutsch-Russell pathway. Estrogens inhibit steroidogenesis and concomitantly cause thinning of the epidermis. This decrease in epidermal thickness in relation to alterations in sterol metabolism emphasizes the critical role sterols and their esterification play in the process of epidermal maturation and keratinization. Several drugs, such as nicotinic acid and triparanol, that inhibit cutaneous sterol synthesis induce scaly lesions in the skin reminiscent of ichthyosis. In addition, deficiencies of essential fatty acids which are normally esterified to sterols also lead to abnormal keratinization and scaliness. Last, a

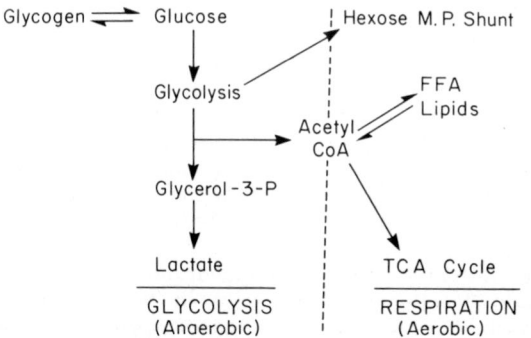

Figure 23–1. A brief résumé of the major pathways of glucose and lipid metabolism demonstrated in the skin.

form of ichthyosis has recently been observed in children born of mothers lacking steroid sulfatase. This X-linked inherited condition was first recognized because women pregnant with affected male fetuses excreted reduced amounts of estriol and had reduced serum estriol concentrations. (The deficient sulfatase is crucial for the formation of estriol.) In addition, these pregnancies did not end in spontaneous labor and delivery, and in every case the affected male children have ichthyosis over the trunk and extremities. It seems likely that the steroid sulfatase plays an important role in maintaining normal keratinization in human epidermis.

Cutaneous Metabolism of Hormones

Sex hormones have long been known to play an important role in the development of secondary sexual characteristics by influencing hair growth and sebaceous gland activity (see discussion under the heading "Hormones and Cutaneous Appendages," below), but the skin has also been noted to participate actively in the metabolism of several hormones including testosterone, progesterone, estrogens, and cortisol. In view of the fact that the skin constitutes 15% of the total body weight, its role in overall body hormone homeostasis and metabolism may be more important than has been assumed.

An unusual feature of normal cutaneous steroid metabolism is that the metabolites of the steroids studied to date all have the 5α configuration in contrast to those of other organs, such as the liver, in which both 5α and 5β isomers are produced. This cutaneous stereospecific reduction at C-5, under the influence of 5α-reductase enzymatic activity, operates upon C-21 steroids (cortisol and progesterone) and C-19 steroids (androgens and estrogens). There is evidence that these steroids compete for the same reductase enzyme, which suggests a complex interplay between the metabolism of one steroid hormone and that of another. For example, progesterone inhibits the 5α reduction of testosterone to the more potent androgen, 5α-dihydrotestosterone. No known direct effect on the skin can at present be attributed to the 5α-pregnane derivatives formed from progesterone, but if these metabolites actively inhibit the reduction of testosterone, they could regulate the formation of potent androgenic substances by the skin. Another comparable situation of steroid competition for the same enzymatic site is seen in the oxidation of the 17β-OL in estradiol and in testosterone by microsomal preparations of human skin. In this instance, an androgen and an estrogen seem to share the same dehydrogenase, which might represent one mechanism by which antagonism between these steroids occurs.

The skin is capable of both activation and inactivation of steroid hormones (Fig 23–2). Several pairs of steroids are known to be reversibly transformed in the skin, including cortisol and cortisone, testosterone and androstenedione, and estradiol and estrone. The equilibrium of these reversible reactions appears to favor oxidative formation of ketones which are less active hormones, i.e., cortisone has less anti-inflammatory activity than cortisol, androstenedione is less androgenic than testosterone, and estrone is less estrogenic than estradiol. In some instances, however, the reverse reductive reactions occur in the skin or mucous membranes, transforming the steroids into more active products. This has been shown, for example, in human vaginal mucosa, where the main product of the interconversion of estrone and estradiol favors the stronger es-

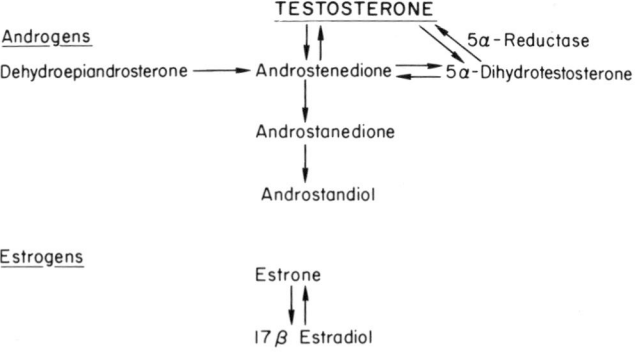

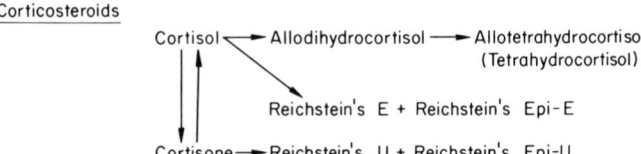

Figure 23–2. The metabolites and interconversions of androgens, estrogens, and corticosteroids by human skin as determined by *in vitro* studies. The formation of allodihydrocortisol and allotetrahydrocortisol is confirmed only in foreskin. Oxidation of 11-β-OH and reduction of 20-one are common to all anatomic sites studied.

trogenic substance, estradiol, but not in human abdominal skin and foreskin, which produce primarily estrone.

Another such example is found in the ability of both male and female skin to form testosterone from the relatively weak androgen, dehydroepiandrosterone, and to further reduce testosterone to the even more potent androgen, 5α-dihydrotestosterone. It would appear that dihydrotestosterone is the most important androgenic metabolite in human skin, and, as in the case of the prostate gland, it may be the active form of androgenic hormone at the tissue receptor site. Those areas of skin that demonstrate the most active conversion rates of testosterone to dihydrotestosterone in both men and women arise from a common anlage in the urogenital ridge (prepuce, clitoris, scrotum, and labium majus), and each of these tissues develops in response to androgenic stimuli. It seems likely that these areas of skin can be likened to accessory sex target organs, and hence steroid metabolism in these specific sites might be particularly sensitive to pathologic aberrations in this metabolic realm.

This point is dramatically demonstrated clinically in the testicular feminization syndrome, in which a basic biochemical defect characteristic of this disorder has been demonstrated in the skin. These patients have a normal male chromosomal pattern, sclerotic but functioning testes, and normal plasma testosterone levels, but they display a phenotypic female physiognomy. Such individuals appear to be suffering from an X-linked recessive inherited defect in the target organ response to testosterone, since skin samples are unable to convert testosterone to 5α-dihydrotestosterone. Although it has been suggested that these patients lack the 5α-reductase enzyme in the skin, they do not respond to dihydrotestosterone therapy either, which implies there is a more basic defect in androgen retention or binding by the target tissues.

The testicular feminization syndrome is only one form of male pseudohermaphroditism in which defects are found in the cutaneous end organ responsiveness to androgens. Two other conditions, familial incomplete male pseudohermaphroditism, Type I and Type II, inherited as X-linked recessive and autosomal recessive traits respectively, have also been found to relate to alterations in target organ response to testosterone. Each of these genetic diseases is characterized by marked ambiguity of external genitalia with partial virilization at puberty. The Type II form has been shown to be due to the deficiency of the 5α-reductase enzyme crucial in converting testosterone to dihydrotestosterone in the urogenital ridge.

Dermal Connective Tissue, Cells, and Hormones

The great bulk of skin is connective tissue stroma consisting of cells (fibroblasts, mast cells, histiocytes), fibrils (collagen and elastic fibers), and interfibrillar amorphous ground substances (glycosaminoglycans). The extracellular components are synthesized by fibroblasts, which are suspended in a three-dimensional network of dense collagen fibers embedded in the nonfibrous, semifluid ground substances.

Glycosaminoglycans are single chain linear macromolecular polymers of disaccharides, whose configuration in solution and moist environs of the dermis assumes random coils which play an important role, along with collagen, in determining the skin's resilience and resistance to compression. Of the half dozen glycosaminoglycans charaterized to date, two occur predominantly in the dermis: hyaluronic acid (repeating units of glucuronic acid and N-acetyl glucosamine) and dermatan sulfate (chondroitin sulfate B, consisting of iduronic acid and N-acetyl galactosamine).

Both the fibrillar and ground substance constituents undergo continuous turnover, and their synthesis and catabolism appear in certain instances to be under hormonal influence. Abnormalities in this balance between the catabolism and anabolism of various dermal components may therefore occur in association with endocrinopathies in the form of changes in cutaneous thickness, compliability and texture.

Effects of Glucocorticoids on the Skin

Excessive quantities of corticosteroid hormones depress proliferation of fibroblasts and inhibit the deposition of both collagen and mucopolysaccharides. Cortisol also accelerates degradation of collagen as evidenced by an increase in soluble collagen.

Cutaneous Signs of Too Much Glucocorticoid.
Endogeneous Glucocorticoids.   Benign and malignant adenomas of the adrenal glands, and bilateral hyperplasia found in association with basophilic pituitary adenomas all result in biosynthesis of cortisol in excessive amounts. The skin in all these conditions appears atrophic, and tissue-paper thin. The clinical impression of atrophic skin has been verified by direct measurement. This loss of collagen and mucopolysaccharides accounts for the increased transparency of the skin, which causes the dermal and subcutaneous vasculature to become apparent as manifested by plethoric facies and broad purple striae on the trunk (abdomen, flanks), upper arms, and thighs. The color fades when the excess synthesis of corticosteroids is arrested, but atrophic white striae remain.

Minor trauma readily produces ecchymosis, presumably because of increased vascular fragility due to the loss of adequate dermal collagen that would otherwise provide support for the vasculature. Decreased vascular tone is also evident as purplish mottling of the lower extremities (cutis marmorata).

Since glucocorticoids have been shown experimentally to inhibit wound healing, it is not surprising that patients with cortisol overproduction also suffer from this problem.

One last striking feature of excess glucocorticoids is the alteration in the body habitus with excessive deposits of fat over the clavicles, back (buffalo hump), abdomen, and cheeks (moon facies), and muscle and fat wasting of the extremities. The cause for this central obesity and peripheral thinning is unknown.

Exogenous Glucocorticoids.   Iatrogenic hypercorticism can cause identical cutaneous changes as endogenous hypercorticism. The severity of the cutaneous signs and symptoms depends on the dose of drug and duration of usage.

Topical potent steroids, applied for long periods of time, can also cause cutaneous atrophy, striae, and telangiectasis. Occasionally, suppression of endogenous steroid production or even hypercorticism (in young individuals) may occur when topical administration of potent steroids is utilized over wide areas of the skin for many weeks. Such effects do not regularly appear in adults when the skin is intact, except with prolonged application to certain sites such as the perianal and scrotal skin where percutaneous absorption is readily obtained. Further, prolonged exposure to as little as 20% of normal skin under occlusion (plastic wraps over topical steroids) results in significant absorption, and therefore care should be taken in treating larger areas of diseased skin with occlusive dressings and potent fluorinated topical steroids.

Cutaneous Signs of Too Little Glucocorticoids.   Deficient formation of adrenal glucocorticoids due to primary adrenal insufficiency (Addison's Disease), secondary adrenal insufficiency (pituitary deficiency), or endogenous blockade of steroidal biosynthetic sequence (adrenogenital syndrome) results in alterations primarily of the pigmentary system or change in hair growth (see discussions under the headings "Hormones, Melanocytes, and Pigmentation," and "Hormones and Cutaneous Appendages," below) rather than changes in the dermal components.

Effects of Somatotropin (Growth Hormone) on the Skin

Excessive quantities of growth hormone (GH) cause fibroblastic proliferation and increased quantities of collagen and mucopolysaccharides to accumulate in the skin. In addition, hyperplasia of the epidermis and dermal appendages such as the pilosebaceous structures is seen.

Cutaneous Signs of Too Much Somatotropin.   Excessive GH elaboration, such as is commonly seen in acromegaly, is recognized clinically by the thickening, coarsening, and edematous leathery consistency of the skin. Over the face, neck and scalp the excessive mass of dermis causes the skin surface to buckle into folds and furrows, imparting a corrugated appearance resembling gyri of the cerebral cortex (cutis verticis gyrata). The cutaneous thickening in these patients has been verified by direct radiologic measurements on the forearm and heel, although the degree of thickening does not correlate closely with the severity of the acromegaly. The eyelids are also thick, as are the lower lip and nose, which are enlarged and protruding. The fingers assume a blunted shape and the overgrowth of fibrous dermal tissue leads to the production of small pedunculated fibromas over the body.

Effects of Thyroid Hormone on the Skin

The thyroid hormones triiodothyronine (T_3) which appears to be the most active thyroid hormone, and thyroxine (T_4) play an important role in the maintenance of normal cutaneous function. Oxygen consumption, mitotic activity, thickness of epidermis, and protein synthesis are increased by thyroid hormone.

Further, thyrotropin and thyroid hormones appear to affect the metabolism of dermal glycosaminoglycans. As is the case for mucopolysaccharides in other organs of the body (e.g., gastrointestinal tract, pericardium, larynx) there is an accumulation of the ground substances in the dermis in individuals deficient in thyroid hormones. It would seem that thyroxine is primarily concerned with the catabolism of dermal hyaluronic acid, its absence leading to a slowing of these degradative processes and the accumulation of ground substance within the skin, while thyrotropin acts directly on connective tissue to stimulate the formation of glycosaminoglycans (increased sulfate-S^{35} incorporation into mucopolysaccharides). This may explain why the accumulation of hyaluronic acid and chondroitin sulfate is so marked in patients with primary myxedema, in whom thyroxine is deficient and thyrotropin levels are increased when compared with secondary myxedematous patients (whose thyrotropin levels are decreased and whose skin amasses smaller quantities of glycoaminoglycans).

Some of the actions of thyroid hormones on skin are mediated by generalized effects on heat production and altered cardiovascular activity. Excessive sweating and increased cutaneous blood flow is seen when increased amounts of thyroid hormones are produced, while the reverse is seen with underproduction of these hormones in myxedema.

Cutaneous Signs of Too Much Thyroid Hormone. Thyrotoxicosis manifests itself in the skin by its warm, moist, soft, and smooth texture related primarily to the peripheral vasodilation and increased blood flow. The changes in the skin have been likened to that of an infant's integument.

Occasionally hyperpigmentation and vitiligo are seen in association with thyrotoxicosis (See the discussion under the heading "Hormones, Melanocytes, and Pigmentation," below.).

Graves' disease, with goiter, thyrotoxicosis, and ophthalmopathy, may also present with pretibial myxedema and acropachy. Accumulation of hyaluronic acid in localized areas on the anteriolateral aspects of one or both legs appears clinically as pink, flesh-colored, or violaceous infiltrated, non-pitting plaques or nodules with prominent, dilated, follicular orifices in the overlying epidermis (peau d'orange) (Fig. 23–3). At times the skin may be verrucous. In extreme cases, the entire lower leg may be involved with thickened skin thrown into folds overhanging the ankle, resembling elephantiasis nostras. The hair over the pretibial lesions is often coarse and very prominent.

Pretibial myxedema may appear while the patient is hypermetabolic, but more often it follows surgical or radioiodine therapy; hence, then, skin alterations cannot be directly related to thyroid function.

The pretibial myxedematous dermal infiltrates frequently occur concomitantly with exophthalmos, and occasionally with clubbing and osteoarthropathy of the digits (acropachy). Exophthalmos, too, results from the accumulation of hyaluronic acid and fluid interposed between the bony socket and the eyeball. The etiology of the mucopolysaccharide accumulation in the skin and eyes is

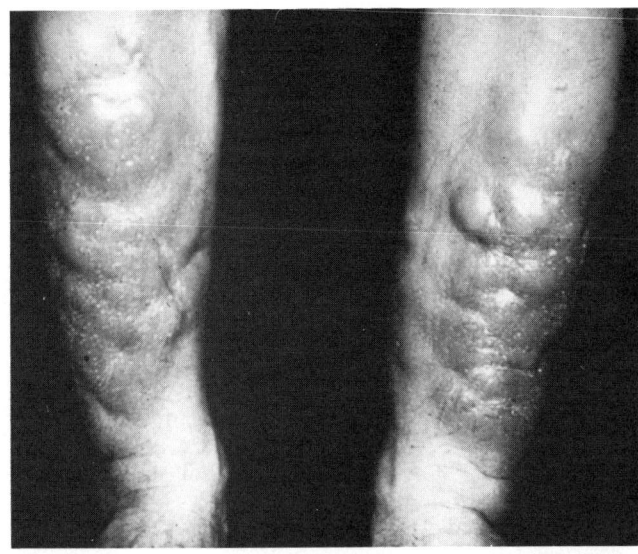

Figure 23–3. Pretibial myxedema is seen as bilateral infiltrated nonpitting nodules with prominent dilated follicular orifices in the overlying epidermis.

unknown, but its occurrence is correlated best with the presence in the blood of long-acting thyroid-stimulating substance (LATS) found in high concentrations in 90% of patients. Whether LATS, an IgG antibody, is directly responsible for initiating the skin lesions is undetermined. Some investigators postulate that this antibody fixes to the skin and elicits a localized antigen-antibody reaction that secondarily stimulates the accumulation of hyaluronic acid. Other workers have failed to demonstrate the presence of LATS in the skin lesions, and several cases have had normal levels of circulating LATS. The cutaneous lesions respond impressively to topically applied fluorinated steroids under occlusive thin plastic wraps.

Cutaneous Signs of Too Little Thyroid Hormone.
The skin in hypothyroidism contains large amounts of hydrophilic hyaluronic acid which is responsible for the puffy, doughy, non-pitting, edematous features of the skin. Recent studies have also identified increased quantities of albumin and other plasma proteins accumulating in the skin of patients with myxedema. The generalized accumulation of albumin in the skin appears to be related to both increased protein extravasation and decreased lymphatic clearance of the serum proteins. The accumulation of mucopolysaccharide and albumin is most striking in the acral parts where the lack of subcutaneous tissue tends to make dermal changes more prominent. Facial changes are particularly characteristic, such as broadened nose, thick lips, puffiness, and lack of facial expressiveness (Fig. 23–4).

There is also dryness of the skin surface with roughness and scaling, particularly over the extensor surfaces of the limbs. In long-standing cases this becomes so marked as to mimic "tree bark" in appearance and texture.

The skin is also cold and pale. The coolness is due to the reduced core temperature and cutaneous vasocontriction. The dryness is due to both decreased sweating as well as a change in the epidermis characterized by thinning and hyperkeratosis.

Further, the skin may take on an ivory-yellow color. The yellow component, most intense on the palms and soles, is related to the accumulation of carotene in the stratum corneum secondary to carotenemia. The pallor is

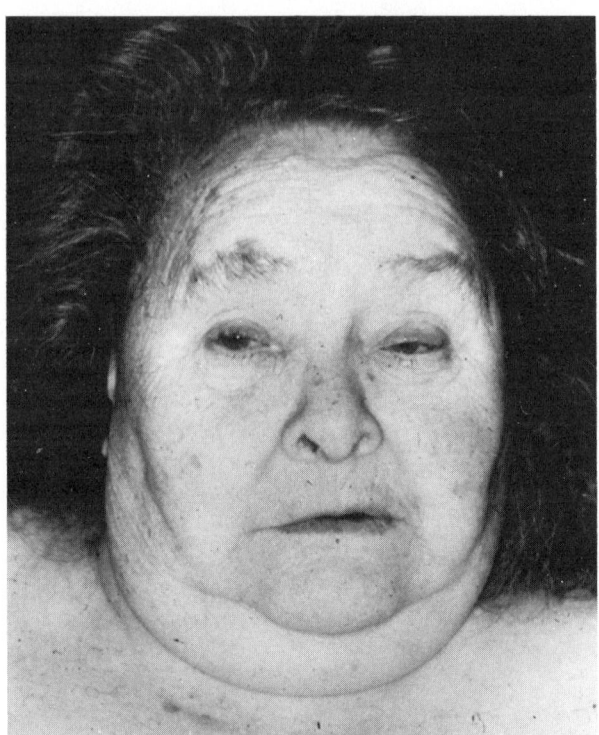

Figure 23-4. Myxedema: Typical features of puffiness and lack of facial expressiveness, along with loss of hair from the lateral margins of the eyebrows.

due to the diffuse accumulation of mucopolysaccharides and water in the dermis as well as the common accompaniment of anemia in myxedema.

Replacement therapy with thyroid hormones mobilizes the dermal glycosaminoglycans with increases in urinary hexosamines.

In addition to the effects hormones have on fibroblasts and the fibrous and amorphous substances they synthesize, the dermal histiocyte also occasionally plays a role in the clinical aberrations of certain endocrine diseases. Patients with diabetes and myxedema and those receiving estrogenic hormones may develop an abnormality in lipoprotein metabolism, leading to large elevations both in β and pre-β lipoproteins and in chylomicrons. These blood lipids infiltrate through dermal capillaries, preferentially in areas subject to stress and pressure, where dermal histiocytes phagocytize the lipids to evolve into foam cells and form xanthomas. Eruptive (small, yellow papules on the extensor surfaces) and tuberous (large, reddish nodules on the elbows and knees) xanthomas are the most common clinical forms found in these patients. The xanthomas resolve concomitant with the decrease in circulating lipoproteins when insulin or thyroid replacement is given for the specific underlying endocrinologic problem.

DERMAL VASCULATURE AND HORMONES

General

Certain cutaneous features of endocrine diseases are related to physiologic or anatomic alterations in the dermal vascular bed. This is not surprising when the extensive arterial and venous microcirculatory networks found in the skin are recalled.

Vascular Alterations in Thyroid Disease

Hyperthyroidism, by virtue of the general effects on increased heat production, heat dissipation, and altered cardiovascular dynamics causes cutaneous vasodilatation and increased cutaneous blood flow (3 to 4 times normal). These changes in turn cause the clinical features so characteristic of the hypermetabolic state such as excessive warmth, softness and smoothness of the skin, and persistent facial flush and palmar erythema.

Vascular Alterations Related to Pheochromocytoma

Paroxysms of blanching and sweating in response to the intermittent release of vasonconstricture catecholamines are often seen in patients with these tumors.

Vascular Alterations in Carcinoid Tumors

Episodes of cyanotic or bright red flushes over the face and upper trunk of patients with ileal or gastric carcinoids are mediated by as yet unidentified substances. Flushing can be provoked pharmacologically by the administration of epinephrine, isoproterenol, and ethanol as well as by physiologic stimuli such as food intake. Some studies have suggested that kinins formed in response to the release of kallikreins synthesized by the tumor are the responsible mediator of these flushes. More recently, however, evidence has been found that gastrin or a related peptide may be one of the flush-producing stimuli. The infusion of somatostatin (a substance shown to block the release and action of gastrin) suppresses flushes in patients with carcinoids. Flushes are also blockaded when a combination of histamine H1 and H2 receptor antagonists is given to patients with carcinoids. Such findings indicate that histamine may be a principal vasodilator eliciting flushing attacks in the carcinoid syndrome.

Estrogens and Vascular Changes

In patients with increased quantities of circulating estrogens angiomas are seen over the face, trunk, and upper extremities as well as palmar erythema. These situations occur in pregnancy and in patients on estrogen therapy or with chronic liver disease.

Diabetes and Vascular Changes

Certain skin alterations associated with diabetes mellitus owe their pathogenesis to alterations in the vasculature. It is likely that abnormalities in lipid, glycolipid and glycoprotein metabolism, prevalent in diabetics, are responsible for the pathologic changes occurring in vessels of all sizes, including large muscular and elastic arteries, arterioles, and capillaries. Premature peripheral large vessel insufficiency secondary to atherosclerotic changes is a frequent occurrence in diabetics, leading initially to loss of hair, and shininess, atrophy, and coolness of the skin over the toes and lower legs, with subsequent ulceration and gangrene. Multiple, sharply demarcated gangrenous ulcerations may occur over the lower extremities in the presence of adequate flow through the large peripheral arteries when arterioles (arteriolosclerosis) and capillaries (microangiopathy) are the major site of vascular damage (Fig. 23-5).

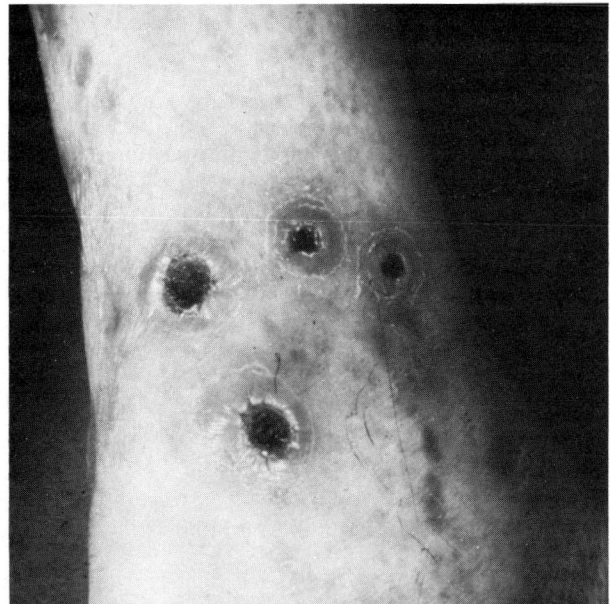

Figure 23–5. Ulcers secondary to microangiopathy. Discrete, punched-out ulcers with eschars over the surface around the ankle region of a diabetic patient with adequate peripheral pulses but severe microangiopathic changes of the skin.

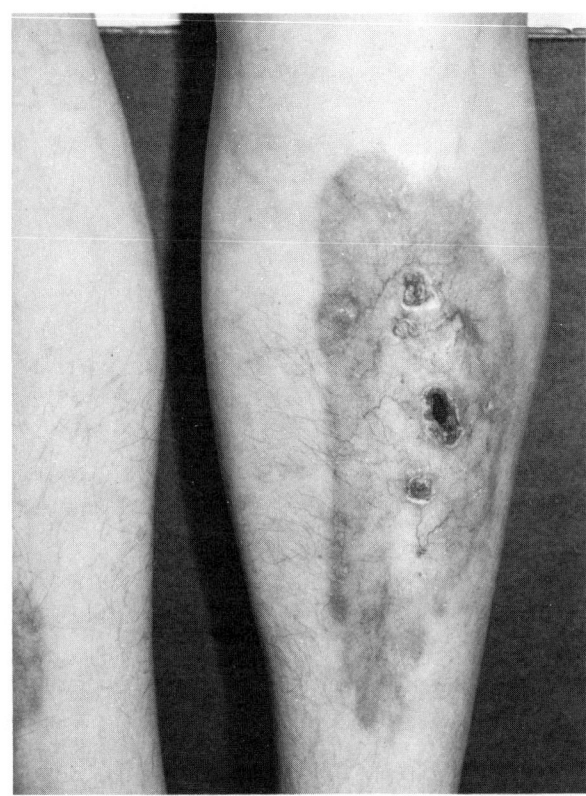

Figure 23–6. Necrobiosis lipoidica diabeticorum: A typical atrophic pretibial plaque, with telangiectatic vessels seen coursing through the center of the lesion. Several ulcers are seen in the plaque.

Several unique cutaneous lesions are seen in diabetics with endarteritic obliterative small vessel disease (intimal proliferation and basement membrane thickening) including necrobiosis lipoidica diabeticorum (NLD), diabetic dermopathy (or shin spots), bullae (bullosis diabeticorum), and erythematous and necrotic cutaneous eruptions. Although these lesions can occur in individuals without diabetes, they are found with sufficient frequency in association with the microangiopathy of this disease that their presence should alert the physician to search for the presence of diabetes. It should be stressed that little is known of how the small-vessel pathologic alterations initiate the clinical features of each of these skin changes.

Necrobiosis Lipoidica Diabeticorum (NLD)

These lesions appear as asymptomatic, sharply circumscribed, shiny, atrophic plaques with an erythematous border and a yellowish central region through which telangiectatic vessels course (Fig. 23–6). In the early stages the lesions appear as papules and nodules that may resemble granuloma annulare or sarcoid. Ulceration may occur in 25–50% of the lesions, often developing after minor degrees of trauma, and with ulceration, pain can become a prominent feature.

The plaques, which vary in size and number, usually occur over the pretibial areas, although they have been found on the trunk, arms, and head. NLD lesions occur in 0.1 to 0.3% of diabetics and the occurrence and course of these lesions are independent of the severity or degree of control of the diabetes.

The lesions precede by two years (range of 1/2 to 14 years) the onset of chemical evidence of diabetes in about 15% of the patients, although many of these patients have a family history of diabetes or other diabetic signs such as large, heavy babies or abnormal cortisone glucose tolerance tests. In 25% of cases, NLD and diabetes (latent, chemical, and overt diabetes) appear concomitant-

ly, while in the remainder the skin lesions are present after the diabetic condition is diagnosed. It should be noted that between 10 and 25% of NLD patients evidence no diabetes. Thus this type of skin lesion, which is characterized histologically by fragmentation and distortion of collagen (necrobiosis), aggregation of epithelioid cells and histiocytes, and thickening of the capillary wall basal lamina, is seen in a certain number of patients without diabetes but is, in every way, identical to the NLD occurring in diabetics.

Spontaneous resolution of small NLD plaques occurs in 13–19% of cases. There is no effective therapy for these skin lesions, and their resolution or progression is unrelated to the severity, the activity, or the adequacy of control of the diabetes. Uncontrolled studies have suggested that NLD lesions may improve with aspirin and dipyridamole therapy. The rationale for this platelet anti-aggregating treatment is the finding of small vessel disease in the lesions as well as defects in platelet behavior in diabetics. Ulcerated NLD lesions may require deep excision which includes diseased underlying perforating vessels, followed by skin grafting.

Diabetic Dermopathy or Shin Spots

These lesions begin as asymptomatic red-brown papules that evolve into sharp circumscribed, atrophic, depressed hyperpigmented patches over the shins and less frequently on the arms (Fig. 23–7). Lesions appear in crops and seldom can be related to antecedent trauma.

Identical skin lesions are observed in 2% of normal individuals and in 20% of patients with a variety of endocrinopathies whose glucose tolerances are normal. The age

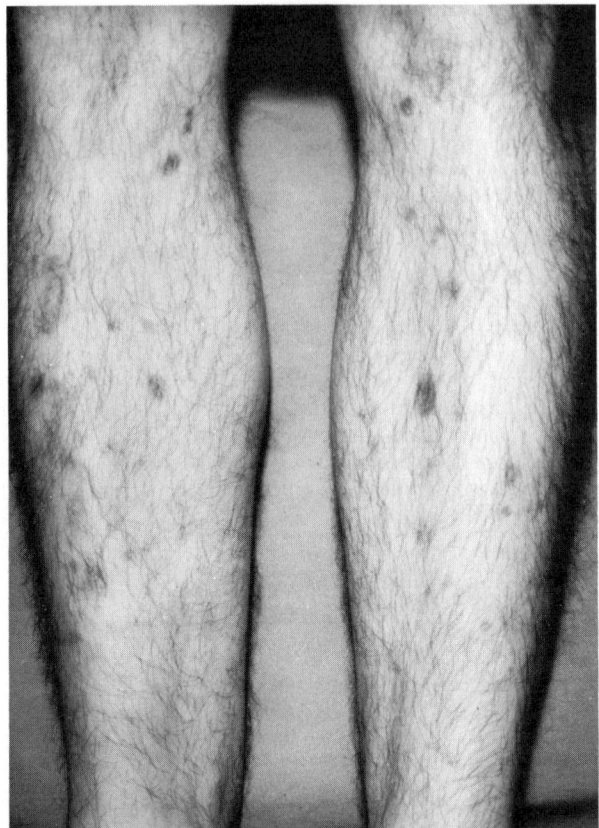

Figure 23–7. Diabetic dermopathy: Circumscribed, atrophic, hyperpigmented shin spots are seen over both pretibial areas.

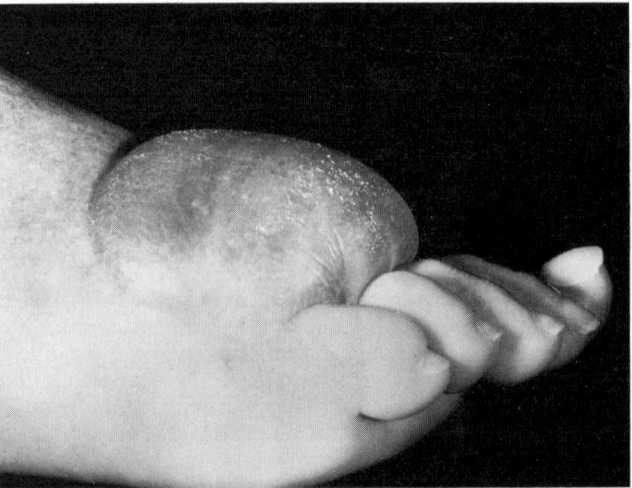

Figure 23–8. Bullosis diabeticorum; A large tense bullous lesion is seen over the dorsum of the foot.

and sex distributions of the occurrence of diabetic shin spots are different from those of NLD. Shin spots occur in 10–30% of female diabetics and 60–65% of male diabetics past the age of 30, while NLD occurs in far fewer diabetics and usually in female diabetics between the second and fourth decades. The incidence of shin spots increases with the longer duration of the diabetic state.

Histologically, the dermal small vessels show intimal thickening and deposition of PAS-positive material in the basement membrane. The shin spots often are seen in association with microangiopathy in other organs; retinal microaneurysms, neuropathy, and nephropathy (50% of patients).

Bullosis Diabeticorum

Such lesions appear as asymptomatic, spontaneously occurring, bacteriologically sterile, tense bullae without surrounding inflammatory reaction over the toes, feet, lower legs, fingers, and forearms. (Fig. 23–8). These blisters vary in size from several millimeters to several centimeters in diameter and usually occur in patients with recognized diabetes, although occasionally they may be the presenting feature leading to the diagnosis of diabetes. The subepidermal bullae usually heal without scarring, but several cases have been reported in which the bullae evolve into circumscribed atrophic patches.

The cause for this rare manifestation of diabetes is unknown, but 75% of affected patients have significant diabetic retinopathy, and a number of diabetic patients with acral bullae have also manifested signs of diabetic neuropathy and even nephropathy.

Erythematous and Necrotic Skin Lesions

Erythemas of the face (rubeosis faciei) and of the extremities have been observed in elderly patients with long-standing diabetes. Erysipelas-like, indurated, painless, swollen areas on the feet and lower legs which may eventuate into painless frank necrosis involving all layers of the skin are seen in elderly diabetics, often following cardiac decompensation, or unilateral edema from venous occlusion and arterial insufficiency. It is likely these cutaneous erythematous and necrotic lesions are manifestations of vascular insufficiency. The patients with cutaneous necrosis may also have destruction of the bones of the foot (metatarsals and phalanges).

The skin lesions are usually reversible. Even necrosis heals in over half of the patients so affected, but characteristically new areas of erythema and necrosis recur in the original site or in other adjacent areas. In most patients the skin of the lower extremities is warm, and good pulses are found.

Certain Cutaneous Diseases More Frequently Associated with Diabetes

1. Scleredema adultorum is an unusual disorder in which there is a painless, scleroderma-like swelling of the skin beginning on the posterior and lateral neck which gradually spreads over a period of several weeks to months to involve the face, shoulders, upper torso, and arms. The onset of this hard, non-pitting edema often begins several weeks after a streptococcal infection. When this is the case, the disease usually resolves spontaneously in several months. However, persistence of the scleredema for many years has been observed in several series of patients in association with diabetes.

2. Glucagonoma Syndrome. Glucagon-secreting tumors of the pancreatic islets cause hyperglycemia and an eczematous or atypical psoriatic-appearing marginated, blistering, and crusting eruption over the lower abdomen, buttocks, perineum, and legs. A beefy red tongue, angular cheilitis, and nail dystrophy may also be present.

Histologically, necrosis and cleft formation in the upper epidermis are seen on skin biopsy. The eruption may precede the diagnosis of the neoplasm by several years and is usually resistant to all forms of topical therapy. Early diagnosis of glucagonoma is difficult because the tumor is clinically silent except for uncomplicated hyperglycemia. Two-thirds of the patients with cutaneous disease have metastatic lesions, usually to the liver, and liver scanning often identifies these metastases. Visceral angiography may also identify the tumor in the pancreas itself, as well as the liver metastases. The diagnosis can also be substantiated when increased levels of plasma glucagon are found. Removal of the primary tumor results in resolution of the skin lesions, but these recur with development of metastases.

3. Acanthosis Nigricans has been described in several patients with glucose intolerance, hyperinsulinemia, and marked resistance to exogenous insulin. Two unique clinical syndromes are found in association with these metabolic and cutaneous alterations. One group of patients includes young females with signs of virilization or accelerated growth in whom cellular insulin receptors are defective. A second group includes older females with signs of immunologic disease (high erythrocyte sedimentation rate, proteinuria, the presence of anti-nuclear and anti-DNA antibodies) in whom circulating antibodies to insulin receptors are found. The acanthosis nigricans is similar to that seen in association with other endocrine diseases (i.e., obesity, pituitary tumors, Cushing's disease) — namely, brown, velvety, hyperkeratotic patches in the body folds.

Cutaneous Complications of Therapy in Diabetes

Oral hypoglycemic agents and parenterally administered insulin have both been found to cause cutaneous alterations.

Sulfonylureas have been associated with a variety of generalized skin eruptions including urticaria, vesiculobullosis eruptions, erythema multiforme, and photosensitivity. Allergic skin reactions due to sulfonylureas usually occur during the first month of treatment. In up to 10% of patients taking sulfonylureas, particularly chlorpropamide, undue sensitivity to even small amounts of alcohol results in severe flushing of the face, throbbing headache, and a feeling of intoxication.

A variety of cutaneous reactions to subcutaneous insulin injections have been observed.

1. Lipodystrophy involving atrophy or hypertrophy of subcutaneous fat at the sites of injections is particularly common in females under 20. The adipose dystrophy which appears as cutaneous depressions seems to be related to contamination of the insulin preparations, since highly purified insulin (single peak and more purified single-component insulin) reverses the lipoatrophy when injected into the atrophic areas. Insulin lipoatrophy, therefore, may be caused by lipolytic substances in commercial preparations.

Localized fat hypertrophy appears as asymptomatic noninflammatory swellings at the sites of insulin injection, most likely due to the local anabolic effects insulin has on adipose tissue.

2. Painful Indurations. Acute, transistory, recurrent, red, and tender indurations that appear about 10 days after insulin injections are begun is one of the commonest complications. Women are more likely to develop such eruptions, the etiology of which is probably related to impurities in insulin preparations.

3. Allergic reactions to insulin. Impurities (consisting of other fractions of islet tissues, insulin precursors, desamidoinsulin, zinc), additives (protamine), preservatives (parabens), and the insulin molecule itself (beef or pork) have all been implicated as allergens. Reactions caused by impurities of insulin preparations are less common now than formerly, since most commercial preparations are "single peak" insulin. Commercial insulin is usually composed of a mixture of beef and pork insulin.

Insulin allergy is common. As many as 56% of patients on insulin may have hypersensitivity reactions ranging from localized pain and swelling, pruritic red papular eruptions, or urticaria, to more generalized urticarial eruptions.

The majority of insulin allergy is due to beef insulin and can be overcome by desensitization and treatment with single-peak pork insulin, which more closely approximates the amino acid sequence of human insulin.

Insulin allergy to zinc recently has been proven in several patients with erythematous, pruritic, papular lesions at the site of insulin injections. Zinc insulin and zinc sulfate–induced transformation and proliferation of peripheral lymphocytes from these patients, and intradermal skin tests to zinc were also positive. With zinc-free insulin the skin eruptions do not recur.

HORMONES, MELANOCYTES, AND PIGMENTATION

Melanin, the major product of the melanocyte, is largely responsible for the coloring of skin. Melanocytes originate in the embryonic neural crest, from which they migrate to form a horizontal network of cells with many cytoplasmic processes or dendrites that intermesh between the basal cells of the epidermis. Melanin is a complex of insoluble, polyquinone, brown or red pigment and protein, formed by the oxidation of tyrosine and 3,4-dihydroxyphenylalanine (DOPA) in the presence of the oxidative enzyme, tyrosinase. Tyrosinase is found within distinctive ultrastructural organelles of the melanocytes, called melanosomes, which are membrane-bound ovoid structures enclosing regularly packed and coiled lamellae upon which melanin is synthesized and deposited. Eventually, when the melanosomes are filled with melanin pigment, all enzymatic activity ceases. They are then referred to as melanin granules, and the granules move out along the melanocytic dendritic processes, where they are transferred to the surrounding epidermal cells (cytocrine activity). Human skin pigmentation, therefore, depends upon not only the amount of melanin synthesized by melanocytes but also the number and dispersion of melanin granules in the adjacent basal cells.

Hormones profoundly influence the melanin pigmentation of man as well as other mammals and amphibia. The precise action of hormones at the cellular level is obscure, although certain parallels exist with a comparable phenomenon in frogs, whereby a number of hormones *in vitro* and *in vivo* rapidly produce hyperpigmentation or lightening of pigmentation by causing dispersion or aggregation of melanin granules throughout the melanocyte's cytoplasm and dendritic processes. This movement of granules in response to hormones can be observed by light microscopy. Table 23–1 lists the effects of certain hormones on both frog and human skin. Note that, in most instances where hormones cause dispersion of melanin granules and thus darkening of amphibian skin, these same hormones causes increased pigmentation in humans, whereas hormones aggregating the granules and thus lightening frog skin have no clinical effect on human pigmentation. "cAMP" has been shown to cause pigment dispersion in frog melanocytes, so that the dispersive effect of MSH and other darkening hormones may be mediated by cAMP. It further appears that microfilaments within the melanocyte's cytoplasm are the transducer between cAMP and pigment granule dispersion. In humans, the

Table 23-1. COMPARATIVE EFFECTS OF VARIOUS HORMONES ON SKIN PIGMENTATION IN FROGS AND MAN

Hormone	Frog Skin		Human Skin	
	Dispersion of Melanin Granules (Darkening Effect)	Aggregation of Melanin Granules (Lightening Effect)	Increased Pigmentation	Decreased Pigmentation
ACTH	+		+ (in large doses)	
α MSH	+		+	
β MSH	+		+	
Estrogens	+		+	
Progesterone	+		+	
Thyroxine		+	+	
Epinephrine		+	No effect	No effect
Norepinephrine		+	No effect	No effect
Hydrocortisone		+	No effect	No effect

increase or decrease in pigmentation initiated by the presence of too much of, or the absence of, certain hormones, such as ACTH, MSH, estrogen, and progesterone, may partially be due to the movement of melanin granules via the same system as in amphibian skin, but it is more likely such changes in pigmentation are the result of alterations in the rate of melanin synthesis and melanin transfer to epidermal cells. MSH increases cAMP in experimental melanomas, and it is possible that the nucleotide is responsible for initiating tyrosinase synthesis and melanin production in human melanocytes. The administration of α MSH to humans results in hyperpigmentation in several days, characterized histologically by increased numbers of melanin granules in the dendrites of melanocytes as well as in epidermal cells.

Marked regional variation exists in the sensitivity of certain melanocytes to specific hormones. For example, during pregnancy estrogens and progesterones stimulate melanogenesis in melanocytes of the areolae and nipples and to a lesser extent in those on the face, midline of the anterior abdominal wall, and genitals.

Table 23-2 summarizes the hormonal imbalances and endocrinologic conditions associated with either hyperpigmentation or hypopigmentation. These changes in pigmentation can be further subdivided, depending upon whether the pigmentary alteration is generalized in nature or localized.

Hyperpigmentation and Endocrinopathies

Generalized Hyperpigmentation

Three pituitary hormones, ACTH, α MSH, and β MSH, are capable of causing generalized hyperpigmentation in humans. A 13 amino-acid polypeptide, α MSH has the same sequence as the first 13 amino acids of ACTH, while human β MSH consists of 22 amino acids whose arrangement is almost identical to the first one-third of the ACTH polypeptide. The skin of humans given injections of MSH begins to darken in 24 hours, and continued daily doses increase the general darkening until the hormone is discontinued, following which normal color returns in 3-5 weeks. The pigmentation in these subjects is most pronounced over the face and mucous membranes and within nevi. Similar pigmentation occurs following ACTH administration, but massive doses (2,400 units/day) must be used.

Normal human pituitary glands contain α MSH and β MSH as identified and quantitated by radioimmunoassay. β MSH accounts for 98% of the MSH activity, while α MSH contributes 2%. In view of the predominance of β MSH in the human pituitary and the somewhat unphysiologic amounts of ACTH required to cause hyperpigmentation, it is generally accepted that β MSH plays the major role in maintaining human pigmentation.

Patients with adrenal cortical insufficiency develop diffuse darkening of the exposed parts, such as face, neck, arms, and dorsum of the hands, as well as the axillae, palmar creases, anogenital region, and buccal mucosa. Nevi darken, new ones may appear, and occasionally darkening of nevi occurs several years before any other pigmentary changes. Scars that develop after the onset of adrenal insufficiency become hyperpigmented as well. Hair becomes darker and longitudinal pigmented bands are observed on the nails. The pigmentary changes are brought on by increased levels of MSH and ACTH in the plasma. Diminution of plasma levels of cortisol provokes a compensatory increased release of pituitary MSH and ACTH, probably mediated through the activation of the respective hypothalamic releasing factor(s).

Table 23-2. HORMONE-INDUCED AND ENDOCRINE-RELATED CHANGES IN CUTANEOUS PIGMENTATION

Increased Pigmentation		Decreased Pigmentation	
Generalized	Localized	Generalized	Localized
Adrenal insufficiency	Pregnancy and anovulatory drugs	Panhypopituitarism	Vitiligo associated with thyroid diseases, adrenal insufficiency, or diabetes
Ectopic ACTH- & MSH-producing neoplasms	Acanthosis nigricans associated with endocrinopathies		
Thyrotoxicosis	Polyostotic fibrous dysplasia (Albright's syndrome)		
	Neurofibromatosis and pheochromocytoma		

Replacement therapy with corticosteroids produces a gradual diminution of the hyperpigmentation. In the treated Addisonian patient, a waxing and waning in the intensity of pigmentary change may be one of the most sensitive indices of changing requirements in the maintenance dose of steroids and so provides an objective criterion for increasing medication.

Vitiligo is associated with primary adrenal failure in as many as 15% of cases and may precede clinical manifestations of adrenal insufficiency.

Generalized hyperpigmentation like that seen in Addison's disease also occurs in some patients with Cushing's disease who undergo bilateral adrenalectomy (with subsequent recognition of enlarging pituitary tumors) and in the ectopic ACTH syndrome caused by various neoplasms, such as carcinomas of the lung, liver, pancreas, and thymus. In each of these instances, plasma ACTH, α MSH, and β MSH have been characteristically elevated. The pigmentary changes are due to β MSH, because the quantity of ACTH and α MSH is too small to account for the amount of melanocyte-stimulating activity. Pituitary tumors emerging after adrenalectomy are associated with marked hyperpigmentation, amenorrhea, and local pressure signs of an expanding pituitary lesion. The hyperpigmentation in this disorder exceeds that found in any other condition and is also associated with the highest blood levels of ACTH and MSH. Radioimmunoassays of tumors taken from hyperpigmented patients with the ectopic ACTH syndrome show large concentrations of β MSH, suggesting that these nonpituitary neoplasms are capable of synthesizing this hormone. Such observations clearly account for the raised plasma levels of this polypeptide and the associated cutaneous pigmentation. In some patients, surgical removal of the tumor has resulted in reversal of cutaneous pigmentation.

The close biologic relationship among α MSH, β MSH, and ACTH can be appreciated from consideration of the fact that all these hormones are found to accompany each other not only in pituitary tissue but also in tumors associated with the ectopic ACTH syndrome, even though the tumors themselves arise from a variety of tissues. One could speculate, therefore, that the synthesis and secretion of these three polypeptides may be controlled by some common mechanism.

Chronic hyperthyroidism can be complicated by generalized hyperpigmentation similar to that seen in Addison's disease. This pigmentation is caused by increased MSH secretion by the pituitary.

Localized Hyperpigmentation

Melasma is a common disorder of large, pale, or sometimes dark brown, irregularly shaped macules over the forehead, upper lips, cheeks, chin, and neck seen in pregnant females. It occurs in association with the hyperpigmentation of the nipples, genitalia, and linea alba universally seen during pregnancy. Existing nevi also darken during pregnancy. Melasma clears several months after delivery, but it is likely to recur with subsequent pregnancies. During pregnancy, increased amounts of MSH and the high levels of estrogens and progesterone augment the pigmentary changes, particularly those over the face.

Melasma is also seen in 23–25% of patients on oral contraceptives. Exposure to ultraviolet light accentuates this facial pigmentation. Unfortunately, in most patients, cessation of the anovulatory pills rarely results in complete resolution of the pigmentation.

Similar facial pigmentation may occur in association with ovarian tumors, diethylstilbestrol treatment of prostatic carcinoma in men, and conjugated estrogens for menopausal women.

Acanthosis nigricans, chiefly recognized for its ominous identification with upper gastrointestinal tract adenocarcinoma in adults, is more commonly seen in a benign setting in children and young adults with several metabolic and endocrinologic diseases. Acanthosis nigricans appears as hyperpigmented, soft, verrucous lesions found symmetrically distributed in the body folds and flexural areas (axillae, neck, groin, and antecubital and popliteal fossae). The lesions can occasionally involve the face, breasts, and inner aspects of the thighs. Perhaps most important in making the diagnosis is the soft, velvety texture imparted to the involved skin, which can be appreciated by gently stroking the skin. Acanthosis is most commonly seen in association with obesity, and if sufficient weight reduction is achieved, the lesions improve. In some instances of acanthosis nigricans, the obesity is related to hypothalamic derangements, as seen in several case reports in children who sustained cranial trauma with concomitant hypothalamic obesity. In other instances, the obesity and acanthosis may be seen in patients with Stein-Leventhal syndrome. Brown and others demonstrated additional links between acanthosis and endocrine disease in a series of 72 patients with these cutaneous lesions, including diabetes mellitus, lipodystrophic diabetes, adrenal insufficiency, hyperthyroidism, myxedema, and testicular carcinoma. In addition, these authors reported upon seven individuals without obesity who had pituitary tumors associated with acromegaly, gigantism, and Cushing's disease, all of whom had marked acanthosis nigricans. The acanthosis improved in only a few patients after their various endocrine disorders were successfully treated. The association of acanthosis with this seemingly large number of unrelated diseases is perplexing and as yet unexplained in the absence of any common denominator in these endocrine diseases which might serve as a pathogenetic mechanism. It is known, however, that diethylstilbestrol and corticosteroids can induce acanthosis in some individuals, so alterations in the levels of circulating hormones may play a direct role.

Two other well-recognized but poorly understood diseases have localized pigmentary changes on the skin and may also be associated with endocrinologic disorders. The first, polyostotic fibrous dysplasia (Albright's syndrome), consists of disseminated osteitis fibrosa bone lesions, often in a segmental distribution; large, circumscribed, irregularly shaped, dark brown, melanotic macules arranged in a linear segmental pattern on one side of the midline of the body and generally overlying the hyperostotic and hypo-ostotic bone lesions; and precocious puberty in females but not males. The coincidence of the cutaneous and bony lesions involving similar segments of the body suggests that a neurologic or embryonic relationship underlies the pathogenesis of this syndrome, but it does not readily explain the association with precocious puberty in the female. The second disease associated with localized cutaneous pigmentation is neurofibromatosis (von Recklinghausen's disease), a dominantly inherited disorder in which a variety of neurogenic tumors are found in conjunction with localized melanin pigmentary macules or so-called café-au-lait spots. The neurogenic tumors involve the cutaneous nerves (neurofibromas), cranial nerves (optic and acoustic neuromas), and even the autonomic nervous system (pheochromocytoma). Approximately 10–15% of patients with neurofibromatosis have pheochromocytomas and associated hypertension. The café-au-lait spots are light brown macules which are usually smaller, more numerous, have less irregular borders, and are more generally distributed over the body than the pigmented macules in Albright's disease. One other useful clinical feature in diagnosing neurofibromatosis is the presence of small, pigmented macules in the axillae (axillary freckling) in a very high percentage of patients. Neural cells and melanocytes both arise from the embryonic neural crest. It appears that proliferation of these neural crest derivatives, including melanocytes, accounts for the clinical findings of neurofibromatosis, suggesting an embryonic defect of neural crest origin.

Hypopigmentation and Endocrinopathies

Generalized Hypopigmentation

Loss of pituitary function results in a decrease in ACTH and MSH, with a resulting generalized hypopigmentation and pallor. Such patients have a decreased ability to tan.

Localized Hypopigmentation

Vitiligo is most commonly seen in patients without endocrine abnormalities, but in some vitiligo patients there appears to be a significant association with such disorders as Addison's disease, thyroid disease, and diabetes. Vitiligo presents as multiple, depigmented, oval or irregularly shaped macules, often symmetrically distributed over the extremities and around the body orifices.

Vitiligo is seen superimposed upon the generalized hyperpigmentation of Addison's disease in 15% of patients. Successful therapy of the adrenal insufficiency not only causes the hyperpigmentation to regress but also may cause the vitiliginous areas to undergo repigmentation.

Vitiligo also appears more frequently in patients with thyroid disease (myxedema, thyroiditis, thyrotoxicosis, non-toxic goiter, and thyroid carcinoma) than would occur by chance alone. Among patients with Graves' disease, 7% have been reported to have vitiligo, but in these instances the clinical pattern of depigmentation is unusual in that it is confined primarily to the extremities, particularly the palms and soles. In some instances, the vitiligo precedes the onset of thyroid dysfunction by several years.

Seven patients with vitiligo have been reported in whom several endocrine diseases were found in each individual, including diabetes, hypothyroidism, and pernicious anemia (another disease in which vitiligo is more frequently found). In these patients, the vitiligo often preceded the development of the multiple diseases by many years; therefore, vitiligo may be an important external manifestation of impending or occult endocrine abnormalities.

The cause for this apparent increased frequency of vitiliginous lesions in association with endocrine disease is unknown, but some studies suggest autoimmune processes might play a role since patients with vitiligo with or without endocrinopathies have various antithyroid, antiadrenal, and antiparietal cell antibodies in their circulation. It has been recognized that melanocytes are absent in vitiliginous skin, and, in like manner, in some patients with diabetes, myxedema, adrenal insufficiency, and pernicious anemia there is a loss of pancreatic islet cells, thyroid acinar cells, adrenal cortical cells, and gastric parietal cells, respectively. There is, of course, no direct evidence that the presence of antibodies directed toward these glands results in this cellular loss, but the analogy of cellular destruction in these endocrine diseases and vitiligo is apparent.

HORMONES AND CUTANEOUS APPENDAGES

Sebaceous Glands

Sebaceous glands on the face, upper back, and chest are dependent upon androgenic stimulation for their development and secretory activity. The glands' holocrine secretion (sebum) is composed of disintegrating sebaceous cells containing large amounts of triglycerides, squalene, and wax esters. The formation of sebum, oiliness of the skin, and occurrence of papulopustular acne result from cellular proliferations and lipid synthesis within the sebaceous glands. Androgens promote cellular turnover and increase the size of the sebaceous gland cells.

The amount of sebum production can be quantitated by collecting and measuring the amount of sebum delivered to a given area of facial skin per unit of time. Sebum production and the histologic size of facial sebaceous glands at various ages reflect the amounts of androgenic hormones produced by the testes, ovaries, and adrenal glands (Fig. 23–3). Before puberty the glands are small and little sebum is secreted. Early in puberty, the glands enlarge, sebum production increases severalfold, and acne may develop in response to the increased production of testicular and ovarian androgens. The administration of low doses of androgen (5 mg methyltestosterone daily) to prepubertal subjects stimulates sebaceous gland size and sebum production within 1-3 weeks. Sebaceous glands, therefore, are exquisitely sensitive to small amounts of androgens in the circulation. Testicular androgens play the predominant role in regulating sebaceous gland activity in the adult male, while androgens synthesized in the ovaries are of prime importance in the female. When testicular or ovarian androgenic stimulation is lost, as occurs after orchiectomy in men being treated for prostatic carcinoma or following menopause in females, there is a diminution in sebum production, but some sebaceous activity is retained in response to the remaining adrenal androgens (mainly dehydroepiandrosterone).

Estrogens administered in large doses to either men or women inhibit sebum production by decreasing the turnover time of the sebaceous cells. This may explain the therapeutic benefits of estrogens and anovulatory drugs in acne patients. It requires large pharmacologic doses of estrogens, however, to overcome the effects of physiologic amounts of androgens.

The apparent central role of androgens in regulating sebaceous gland activity has led to investigations of the metabolism of androgens *in vitro* by sebaceous glands. These studies reveal that the major metabolite of testosterone produced by the glands is dihydrotestosterone. It has, in turn, been suggested that dihydrotestosterone, a very potent androgen, is the primary androgenic stimulus for sebaceous gland activity. Acne-bearing skin produces 2–20 times more dihydrotestosterone than does normal skin, and normal facial skin converts more testosterone to dihydrotestosterone than normal skin from the back. These kinds of studies suggest that there are differences in sebaceous gland androgen metabolism and thus "end-organ" sensitivity to androgens in different regions of the body surface. These regional differences account in part for the distribution of acne, mediated by differential rates of conversion of testosterone to dihydrotestosterone. The individual rates of conversion may also explain the variability in severity of acne seen from patient to patient and the presence of severe acne in some women who have relatively low levels of plasma testosterone as compared to men.

Various endocrinologic disorders are accompanied by changes in sebum production and sometimes acne (Fig. 23–9). Pituitary insufficiency causes decreased sebum production, probably indirectly through its effects on other endocrine glands. Administration of gonadotropin to hypopituitary males results in a rise in sebum secretion. Increased sebum production in patients with acromegaly accounts for their greasy skin. Pituitary ablation decreases sebum excretion, and this decrease is greater in patients with a good therapeutic response to ablation than in those who obtain a poor result. Sebum excretion is said to be a more sensitive indicator of clinical activity in treated acromegaly patients than measurements of serum growth hormone.

Patients with masculinizing androgenic conditions, such as Cushing's disease, adrenal tumors, and adrenogenital syndrome, have significantly elevated rates of sebum production and often concomitant acne. Total or subtotal adrenalectomy in patients with Cushing's disease decreases sebaceous gland activity to normal.

Increased sebum secretion and acne also appear in those ovarian diseases characterized by increased androgen production, such as in certain tumors and polycystic ovaries. When clomiphene is given or wedge resection is performed in patients with polycystic ovaries, the acne disappears.

One additional form of hormonally induced acne should be mentioned — that caused by glucosteroids. Steroid acne is actually a follicular hyperkeratinization, or folliculitis, rather than a stimulation of sebaceous glands. Steroid acne differs from androgen-mediated acne in that the acneform eruption due to steroids consists of numerous small pustules and red papules all in the same stage of development, and no comedones are present. Steroid acne is found mainly on the trunk, shoulders, and upper arms with less involvement of the face, and it may appear as early as 2 weeks after large doses (i.e., greater than 60 mg of prednisone) of steroids are begun.

Hair Growth

Abnormalities in hair growth must be regarded as affecting both hair growth cycle and pattern of distribution of hair types. Hormonal imbalances can alter each of these two aspects of hair growth to cause either increases or decreases in body hair. In assessing clinical problems of hair growth as they may relate to endocrine diseases, it is often of practical value to distinguish between hair pattern abnormalities and growth cycle changes.

Hair Pattern Defined

Hair pattern is determined by the distinctive distribution of two kinds of hair over the body: (1) vellus hairs, which are fine textured and unpigmented and impart a nonhairy appearance to the integument, and (2) terminal hairs, which are coarse, thick, and heavily pigmented and give the impression of hairiness. The proportionate distribution of these two types of hair in various areas of the body is referred to as an individual's hair pattern. Normal hair pattern is determined by the patient's hereditary background as well as hormones, which collectively determine the formation of terminal or vellus hairs in various portions of the skin. An example of this is seen in male pattern baldness, which is genetically determined but requires the presence of androgenic hormones to initiate the transformation of terminal hairs to vellus hairs over the vertex of the scalp in some 60% of Caucasian males by the age of 50 and to a lesser degree in 15% of women past menopause.

Hair Pattern and Hormonal Control

There appear to be three general groupings of hairs, the patterns of which are distinguished by their response to physiologic hormone changes at the time of puberty. These three groups of hair are noted in Table 23–3. They are as follows:

1. Nonsexual hair, which does not depend on hormone stimulation. These hairs are generally of the same type in both pre- and postpubertal individuals (e.g., eyebrows, eyelashes, and hair on forearms and lower legs).

2. Ambosexual hair, which generally changes from vellus to terminal type at puberty in both males and females. These hairs, such as in the axilla and lower pubic triangle, depend upon low levels of circulating androgens from the adrenals and ovaries, as is found in normal females. Ambosexual hair is also found along the frontal hairline, and at puberty these terminal hairs are replaced by vellus hairs with a reshaping and some recession of the facial outline in 80% of girls and nearly 100% of males.

3. Male sexual hairs, such as those found in the beard areas, ears, tip of nose, presternal region, upper pubic triangle, and over certain areas of the temples and vertex of the scalp, occur in follicles which require high levels of circulating androgens for their stimulation. These follicles evolve into terminal hairs in places like the beard area and into vellus hairs over the vertex of the scalp (male baldness) only in the presence of the large amounts of androgens produced in the male.

The pituitary plays a role in determining normal hair

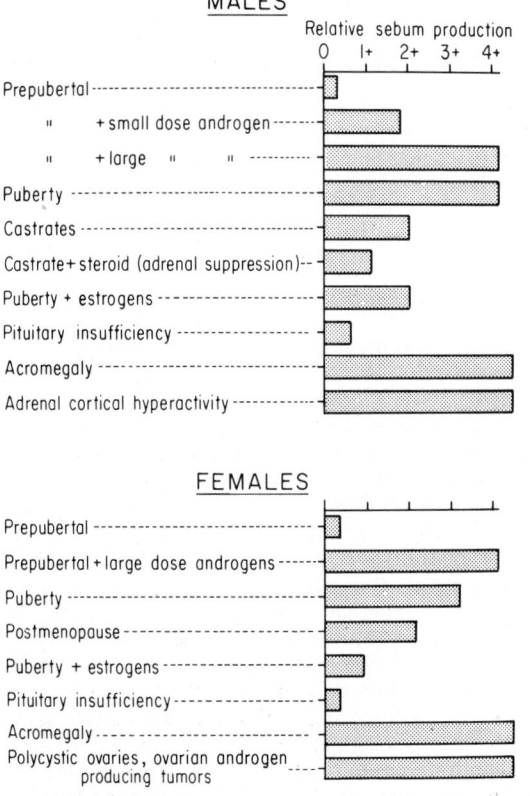

Figure 23–9. Relative amounts of sebum produced in normal males and females in relation to certain endocrinologic disorders.

Table 23–3. HORMONAL CLASSIFICATION OF HAIR PATTERN

Type of Hair Follicle	Hair Regions	Types of Hair Produced		Hormone	
		Prepubertal	Postpubertal	Dependent	Source
Nonsexual hair	Eyebrows and lashes	Terminal	Terminal	Growth hormone	Pituitary
	Forearms and lower legs	Vellus	Terminal		
	Lower parts of scalp	Terminal	Terminal		
Ambosexual hair	Axilla	Vellus	Terminal	Androgen in low concentrations	Adrenal, ovary (females)
	Lower pubic triangle	Vellus	Terminal		Adrenal (males)
	Temporal and vertical parts of scalp	Terminal	Vellus		
Male sexual hair	Beard	Vellus	Terminal	Androgen in high concentrations	Testis
	Ears, nasal tip	Vellus	Terminal		
	Trunk (sternal)	Vellus	Terminal		
	Upper pubic triangle	Vellus	Terminal		
	Temporal and vertical parts of scalp	Terminal	Vellus		

patterns to the extent that it controls androgen production by the ovary, testis, and adrenal. It is likely, however, that pituitary hormones also directly influence hair growth, as in the case of growth hormone, which causes a gradual increase in hair shaft diameter over the limbs and scalp from birth to puberty.

Hormone-Induced Abnormalities in Hair Pattern (Table 23–4)

Clinically it is important to determine if hypertrichosis or alopecia is confined to any one or more of these three groups of hair follicles. If changes occur in nonsexual hair follicles, underlying causative endocrine disturbances are unlikely, whereas cases in which ambosexual or male sexual hair follicles are exclusively affected are usually associated with endocrine disease.

Ambosexual hair is lost in post-pubertal females who develop Addison's disease, and these hairs never grow in females who develop adrenal insufficiency prior to the onset of puberty. Replacement doses of corticosteroids given to females with Addison's disease partly restore axillary hair,

Table 23–4. ABNORMALITIES OF HAIR PATTERN* IN PATIENTS WITH ENDOCRINE DISEASES

Disease	Hair Change		
	Ambosexual Dec.	Male Sexual Inc.	Male Sexual Dec.
Addison's disease	+		
Ovarian agenesis	+		
Polycystic ovaries		+	
Androgen-secreting tumor of ovary or adrenal		+	
Cushing's syndrome		+	
Congenital adrenal hyperplasia		+	
Klinefelter's syndrome			+
Male Turner's syndrome			+
Eunuchism			+
Panhypopituitarism	+		+
Acromegaly	+		
Hypothyroidism	+	+	

*See Table 23–3 for listing of hair types.

and thus some of the effect on the growth of ambosexual hair may be ascribable to the loss of glucocorticoids *per se*. On the other hand, Addison's disease in the adult male is not accompanied by hair loss since the loss of adrenal androgens is overshadowed by the presence of large quantities of testicular androgens. In patients with ovarian agenesis, ambosexual hair is sparse, emphasizing the important role ovarian androgens play in maintaining growth of hair in these follicles. Patients with polycystic ovaries, whose abnormal ovaries synthesize increased amounts of androgens, often have mild to modest amounts of hirsutism of the face, breasts, and upper pubic triangle. Androgen-producing tumors of the ovaries or adrenals cause male sexual hair growth and male pattern baldness in association with other manifestations of masculinization, such as amenorrhea, clitoromegaly, deep voice, and acne. A similar series of events occurs in some patients with Cushing's syndrome and congenital adrenal hyperplasia. In women with virilizing syndromes, the extent of sexual hair growth is influenced in part by the genetic constitution and age of the patient.

Endocrine abnormalities of the testes also affect hair patterns, as exemplified by patients with Klinefelter's syndrome and male Turner's syndrome, in which the hypoandrogenemia accounts for the sparse beard and the axillary and suprapubic male sexual hair. Male eunuchs or males castrated before puberty have similar derangements in male sexual hair patterns, and these patients do not display male pattern baldness unless exogenous testosterone therapy is instituted.

Diseases of the pituitary gland also affect hair growth patterns. Acromegaly with high plasma levels of growth hormone causes an increase in hair shaft diameter, giving the hair over the extremities and scalp a coarse, thick texture. Hypopituitary dwarfs may be totally hairless, and panhypopituitarism in adults results in loss of axillary and pubic hair.

Although diseases of the thyroid gland do not specifically alter ambosexual or male sexual hair, they are associated with changes in hair texture that alter hair pattern. Hyperthyroidism induces a fine, silky textured hair, occasionally associated with diffuse scalp hair loss, while the lack of thyroxine in hypothyroidism causes the hair to be coarse, dry, and brittle. There may also be diffuse and occasionally marked loss of scalp hair as well as loss of hair from the lateral half of the eyebrows. A curious local alteration in hair growth is seen in the pretibial myxedematous plaques of patients with Graves' disease. In these plaques, the hair is coarse and pigmented and grows at an accelerated rate.

Hair Cycle Defined

From the completion of its development in the last month of fetal life, every hair follicle undergoes recurring cycles of active growth, regression, and rest. These stages are known as (1) anagen, the phase of active growth when a new hair shaft is formed by the follicle; (2) catagen, the phase of regression when the hair shaft stops growing and the hair root moves upward within the follicle and becomes club-shaped; and (3) telogen, the resting phase which heralds the ultimate loss of hair from the follicle after a new anagen hair forms in the underlying follicle. When hairs are pulled from the integument, they can be clinically identified. Anagen hairs have elongate roots surrounded by a conspicuous translucent sheath, while catagen and telogen hairs have short, club-shaped roots without a surrounding sheath. If clinical disorders of hair cycle are suspected, it is often useful to examine the roots of a number of hairs under the microscope after forcibly plucking them to determine the relative ratio of anagen to telogen hairs (A/T ratio) in the sampling.

The relative ratio of the number of anagen to telogen hairs in any given region of the body helps to determine the hairiness of that body surface. Regions such as the scalp with large numbers of follicles in anagen phase for long periods of time relative to telogen normally have a high A/T ratio and appear hairy, whereas the generally sparse-appearing general body hair has a low A/T ratio.

Hormone-Induced Abnormalities in Hair Cycle

Hormones influence the hair cycle by either (1) shortening telogen by initiating or prolonging anagen or both in more hair follicles (increase in A/T ratio and increased hairiness), or (2) prolonging telogen while inhibiting the initiation of anagen (decrease in A/T ratio and loss of hair).

Estrogens and probably progesterones stimulate hair growth by initiating anagen. Pregnant females or those on anovulatory drugs may note increasing hairiness over the face, breasts, and extremities. After the estrogenic stimulus is withdrawn, many hairs go into telogen and a telogen effluvium is observed, often involving the scalp with diffuse loss of hair. This occurs 2–3 months after the estrogenic stimulus is withdrawn. Patients concerned about this often impressive loss of scalp hair can be reassured since it is transient and will be replaced in several months. Inexplicably, some women note diffuse balding while on anovulatory drugs. Hair growth commences when the medications are stopped.

Thyroxine stimulates hair growth by initiating anagen, although this does not cause clinical hirsutism in hyperthyroid patients. On the other hand, the diffuse alopecia of the scalp, eyebrow, and other body hair seen in hypothyroidism is partly explained by this loss of anagen stimulus, with a resulting increase in the number of telogen hairs and consequently a decrease in the A/T ratio. Normal anagen-telogen hair relationships are restored during replacement therapy with thyroid hormone.

Hirsutism

Hypertrichosis cannot be defined as a certain amount of hair but rather as more hair than is cosmetically acceptable to a woman living in a given culture. Most cases of hirsutism occur in women with no obvious demonstrable underlying endocrinologic disease. Some of these cases are the expression of a wide variation in hairiness dependent on hereditary factors. In general, dark-haired, pigmented Caucasians of either sex, such as persons of Mediterranean and southern European stock tend to display long coarse hairs on the face, abdomen, and thighs. McKnight reported that in 400 consecutively studied normal women students attending a general medical clinic, 84% had terminal hair on the lower arms and legs; 26 % had hair on the chest and in 35 % pubic hair extended up the linea alba. However, even in patients with apparent ethnic or constitutional hirsutism there is increasing evidence that subtle alterations in androgen metabolism underlie the hypertrichosis.

Hirsutism Associated with Obvious Endocrinologic Disorders or with Virilism.   Endocrinologic disease is more likely to account for hirsutism if features of defeminization or virilism are present, but hirsutism can be a feature of underlying endocrinopathies without associated masculinization such as growth hormone excess due to pituitary tumors, Cushing's syndrome, exogenous usage of glucocorticosteroids and androgens, and the use of certain other drugs such as dilantin and diazoxide. If virilization is present, congenital adrenal hyperplasia, malignant adrenal tumors, and several types of ovarian tumors are more likely to be present. Certain types of endocrine diseases are often associated with virilism:

1. Ovarian Tumors.   Since the gonad is bipotential in early fetal life, tumors of testicular elements may arise in a previously normally functioning ovary. Arrhenoblastomas, hilar cell tumors, and luteomas all have been shown to produce testosterone.

2. Adrenal Tumors.   Malignant tumors may produce virilism, Cushing's syndrome, or a mixture of the two, and frequently hirsutism is the first symptom leading to the detection of these tumors.

3. Congenital Adrenal Hyperplasia often causes precocious growth and virilism and/or hypertension.

4. Polycystic Ovarian Disease is the term applied to a heterogenous group of conditions with a wide clinical spectrum ranging from normal menses and mild hirsutism to complete amenorrhea and virilization. The Stein-Leventhal syndrome (polycystic ovaries, obesity, amenorrhea, and acne) is only one form of polycystic ovarian disease. Other ovarian pathologic processes included in this entity are hyperthecosis and ovarian stromal hyperplasia. In all of these conditions there is excessive secretion of testosterone and androstenedione as evidenced by increased amounts of these hormones in the ovarian venous effluent. Plasma luteinizing hormone (LH) is frequently elevated, while plasma follicle stimulating hormone (FSH) is either low-normal or below normal.

An important feature of polycystic ovarian disease is that it can occur as a dominant inherited disorder. Hypertension, hyperlipidemia, and diabetes mellitus are common in families with ovarian hyperthecosis. The obese, hirsute, hypertensive, diabetic female is frequently considered first to have Cushing's syndrome when first seen by the physician, but such a patient is more likely to have polycystic disease.

Treatment of hyperandrogenism caused by polycystic ovarian disease consists either of suppression of LH by a combination type of oral contraceptive (after one year, a decrease in the rate of hair growth is seen) or wedge resection of ovarian tissue.

Idiopathic Hirsutism.   Patients with normal urinary 17-ketosteroids, normal-sized ovaries, and no evidence of Cushing's disease or adrenal or ovarian tumors, who present with varying degrees of hirsutism are included in this category of hypertrichosis. Some 50 % of hirsute women are in this group. There is a tendency toward obesity and infrequent or anovulatory menses. The excess hair usually appears at puberty and increases into the twenties. Virilism is not present. There may be thick, oily skin and acne.

Excess androgen production by the ovaries or adrenals or both appears to be the basis for the hypertrichosis. In a series of 44 women investigated with unexplained adult onset hirsutism and with elevated testosterone production rates, the ovaries were the predominant source of androgen secretion in 42. Using ovarian and adrenal vein catherizations, testosterone and androstenedione values in the ovarian vein effluents were higher than in the adrenal vein. In half of these individuals dexamethasone suppressed the increased ovarian androgen production.

Patterns of plasma testosterone concentrations in hirsute women are difficult to use for diagnostic purposes, as they are increased to variable degrees in only 35–60 % of cases. Since patterns of sexual hair growth might be more precisely related to free (unbound) plasma androgen levels, measurements have been done on this fraction as well as on the testosterone binding globulin (TeBG) which regulates the amounts of free and bound androgens in the circulation. In one study of Rosenfeld on idiopathic hirsute females, 35 % had elevated total testosterone, while 60 % displayed modest increases in free testosterone. A decreased titer of TeBG was the factor most often found responsible for this altered testosterone binding. However, considerable variation occurs in the levels of total and free androgens in the same patient as shown by additional studies by Rosenfeld. In idiopathic hirsute individuals four distinct plasma androgen patterns are found: 1) total and free plasma androgens are elevated 80 % of the time when frequently studied over a 24-hour period in some patients, 2) free testosterone was constantly elevated while total testosterone was in the high normal range in others, 3) plasma free androgens showed marked fluctuations around the upper limits of normal and 4) plasma free androgens were always normal in certain patients. Because free and total androgen levels fluctuate more widely in hirsute than in normal individuals, a single plasma androgen determination is often not representative nor diagnostic in hirsute women.

The studies of idiopathic hirsutism provide impetus for expanding the spectrum of non-tumorous, androgen-producing ovarian abnormalities that should be included in the group of disorders known as polycystic ovarian disease.

The effectiveness of two oral contraceptives (norethindrone 2 mg mestranol 0.1 mg, and norgestrel 0.5 mg ethinyl estradiol 0.05 mg) in suppressing plasma testosterone, androstenedione, and LH, and in stimulating TeBG, has been shown when these agents are given for six months or longer to idiopathic hirsute individuals. Subjective decrease in the rate of hair growth or a decrease in the amount of facial hair or both are also noted on this therapy.

Approach to Diagnosing Hirsutism. Even though relatively imprecise, one of the few indications for measurement of 24 hour urinary 17-ketosteroids is hirsutism. When the urinary 17-ketosteroids level is above 50 mg/day, an adrenal tumor is likely, especially if dexamethasone does not suppress this high excretion rate. Elevated 17-KS (usually less than 50 mg) also occur with congenital adrenal hyperplasia and a urinary pregnanetriol is useful in distinguishing this entity when there is deficiency in either C21-hydroxylase or 11-β-hydroxylase enzyme activity. Often virilism is seen with adrenal tumors and congenital adrenal hyperplasia with high 17-KS. However, not all androgen secreting adrenal tumors produce urinary 17-KS levels above 30 mg/day, so adrenal vein catherization for measurement of androgen in the effluent plasma may be useful.

Virilizing tumors of the ovaries such as arrhenoblastomas or interstitial cell tumors which produce testosterone usually do not have increased urinary 17-KS.

The majority of hirsute women have normal 17-KS levels and therefore plasma androstenedione (A) and testosterone (T) should be assayed. Plasma TeBG binding capacity should be measured if the plasma A and T levels are normal. A high normal plasma T level with a low TeBG binding capacity is presumptive evidence of hyperandrogenism, since an increase in circulating free T is likely. It may be necessary to obtain several plasma samples at various times in order to get a fair sampling of the plasma A and T levels. High circulating plasma A (exceeding 1000 mg/100 ml) or plasma T (exceeding 250 mg/100ml) suggests an ovarian or adrenal tumor and catherization studies are indicated to localize the tumor site. If plasma A and T are elevated, but not as high as seen with tumors, a three week course of oral combination contraceptive administration is indicated to induce gonadotropin suppression and plasma A and T levels are repeated. If these are reduced to normal, polycystic ovarian disease or idiopathic hirsutism is most likely. If no suppression is seen after a second three week cycle of contraceptive administration, an adrenal or ovarian tumor should be considered.

Hair Follicle Metabolism

Studies on isolated hair follicles have provided information on the metabolic effects hormones have on the follicle cells responsible for hair growth and have further suggested that individual variations in hair growth may reflect differences in hair follicle end-organ response to hormones.

Growing hairs from human integument reveal net shifts in glucose metabolic pathways during the transformation of the resting into the growing anagen stage, which can be summarized as follows: compared with that in resting follicles, glucose utilization in growing follicles increases 200 %, glycolysis 200 %, activity of the pentose cycle 800 %, and metabolism by other pathways 150 %. The most remarkable metabolic change in the transition from telogen to anagen hair, then, is the activation of one of the respiratory pathways, the hexose monophosphate shunt, which also produces large amounts of NADPH. NADPH is apparently important in the metabolism of testosterone by hair follicles. Hair follicles metabolize testosterone to either dihydrotestosterone or androstenedione, but the 5 α-reductase pathway to dihydrotestosterone is dependent upon NADPH. Thus the growing hair follicles, which generate more NADPH, convert larger amounts of testosterone to dihydrotestosterone than resting hairs. Dihydrotestosterone (but not testosterone or androstenedione) in turn has been shown to inhibit adenyl cyclase and reduce intracellular cAMP in scalp hair follicles, while estrone has an opposite effect, increasing follicular cells' AMP.

Follicle Metabolism and Male Pattern Baldness. In the scalp frontal and vertex areas the hair follicles of both male stump-tailed Macaque primates, who routinely display baldness at the time of puberty, and balding human males, an increase of 5 α-reductase activity and accelerated conversion of testosterone to dihydrotestosterone is observed. Thus the limited evidence available to date suggests that those hairs on the scalp that are involved in male pattern baldness do not demonstrate any gross change in the metabolism of testosterone but rather an increased activity of testosterone conversion to dihydrotestosterone.

Table 23–5. GENERAL SUMMARY OF SOME HORMONAL EFFECTS OF VARIOUS COMPONENTS OF THE INTEGUMENT

	Glucose Metabolism	Lipogenesis and Steroidogenesis	Epidermal Hormone Metabolism	Connective Tissue	Vasculature	Melanocytes	Sebaceous Glands	Hair
Insulin	X	X			X			
Testosterone		X	X				X	X
Estrogens		X	X		X	X	X	X
Progesterone		X	X					
Corticosteroids			X	X				
ACTH						X		
MSH						X		
Growth hormone				X			X	X
Thyroxine	X		X	X	X	X		X
TSH			X					

Insulin controls glucose uptake and utilization as well as epidermal lipogenesis. Its relative absence in diabetes is thought to play a role in large and small vessel insufficiency, which leads to gangrene, necrobiosis lipoidica, shin spots, and bullosis diabeticorum.

Testosterone has been shown to accelerate sterol ester synthesis. It is actively metabolized by the epidermis as well as by the sebaceous glands and hair follicles. Indeed, its conversion to dihydrotestosterone correlates with acceleration of sebum production and hair growth, suggesting it is a tissue-active hormone.

Estrogens inhibit sterol metabolism and cause thinning of the epidermis. These hormones are actively metabolized by the epidermis, sebaceous glands, and hair. They suppress sebum production and stimulate hair growth. Excessive amounts cause cutaneous "spiders" and increase pigmentation over the face and nipples.

Progesterone inhibits steroidogenesis in human epidermis and is metabolized by human epidermis.

Corticosteroids are also metabolized by human epidermis. These hormones decrease dermal collagen synthesis, accounting for the thin skin, striae, easy bruising, and poor wound healing seen in Cushing's syndrome.

ACTH in large doses may cause generalized hyperpigmentation.

MSH, particularly β MSH, is the most important hormone in regard to hyperpigmentation. Lack of MSH, as in panhypopituitarism, causes decreased pigmentation.

Growth hormone induces fibroblastic proliferation with increased dermal collagen synthesis, causing thickening of the skin in patients with acromegaly. It also initiates thickening and coarsening of the hair and increased sebum production in patients with acromegaly.

Thyroxine stimulates cutaneous respiration and glucose assimilation in epidermis. It also controls the catabolism of dermal hyaluronic acid, so that in myxedema the catabolism is decreased and hyaluronic acid accumulates in the dermis. High levels of thyroxine, as occur in thyrotoxicosis, increase cutaneous blood flow, giving a soft, smooth texture to the skin. Diffuse pigmentation occasionally occurs in thyrotoxicosis, and thyroxine also stimulates hair growth.

TSH appears to directly stimulate the synthesis of glycosaminoglycans in the dermis.

Follicle Metabolism in Polycystic Ovarian Disease and Idiopathic Hirsutism. *In vitro* observations on pubic hair or skin from the linea alba of hirsute women reveal in several studies that the utilization of testosterone and dehydroisoandrosterone and their conversion to a variety of 5 α-reduced metabolites is significantly greater than that seen in skin from the same locations from normal females. Further, direct estimation of testosterone 5 α-reductase activity in these hairy areas was also elevated, stressing the apparent importance of the 5 α-reductase metabolism in stimulating hair growth in certain hair follicles of the body where hirsutism is observed.

Follicle Metabolism in Testicular Feminization and Male Pseudohermaphroditism. Although no direct studies on hair follicle metabolism in these diseases have been done, studies on fibroblasts and pubic skin have shown there is a defect in the uptake of testosterone, of its conversion to dihydrotestosterone, or a deficiency in the 5 α-reductase enzyme itself. In all of these conditions there is decreased body hair, a scant to absent beard, and no temporal hair line recession, again stressing the crucial role of testosterone conversion to dihydrotestosterone in the growth of ambosexual and sexual hair.

The alterations of androgen metabolism in various hair follicles probably have diverse effects on various pathways of energy metabolism, which in turn inhibit or increase hair growth by affecting the energy supply for keratin synthesis.

CONCLUSION

The wide variety of effects hormones have on the integument clearly marks the skin as an important endocrine end organ (Table 23–5). Although some of the effects can now be directly related to certain clinical cutaneous alterations seen in endocrinologic diseases, for the most part this is not possible, as the hormonal influences on the skin are just now beginning to receive investigative attention. Even so, the cutaneous changes in endocrine disease compel the clinician to examine the skin carefully.

REFERENCES

Hormones and the Epidermis and Dermis

GLUCOSE AND LIPID METABOLISM

Bloch, K.: Biogenesis and transformations of squalene, In *Biosynthesis of Terdenes and Sterols.* Wolstenholme, G. E. W., and O'Connor, M. (eds.), Boston, Little, Brown and Co., 1959.

Crounse, R. G., and Rothberg, S.: Evaluation of the enzymes of the Krebs-Henseleit cycle in human epidermis. *J. Invest. Derm. 36:*287, 1961.

Decker, R. H.: Nature and regulation of energy metabolism in the epidermis. *J. Invest. 57:*351, 1971.

Freinkel, R. K.: Effect of thyroxine administration on the metabolism of guinea pig skin. *J. Invest. Derm. 38:*31, 1962.

Freinkel, R. K.: Metabolism of glucose-C-14 by human skin *in vitro. J. Invest. Derm. 34:*37, 1960.

Gilbert, D.: Demonstration of a respiratory control mechanism in human skin *in vitro. J. Invest. Derm. 43:*45, 1964.

Halprin, K. M., and Ohkawara, A.: Glucose and glycogen metabolism in the human epidermis. *J. Invest. Derm. 46:*43, 1966.

Horlick, L.: Effect of diethylstilbestrol on skin sterols of the male rat. *J. Lipid Res. 9:*773, 1968.

Hsia, S. L.: Potentials in exploring the biochemistry of human skin, In *Essays in Biochemistry.* Vol. 7. Academic Press, 1971.

Hsia, S. L., Dreize, M. A., et al.: Lipid metabolism in human skin. II. A study of lipogenesis in skin of diabetic patients. *J. Invest. Derm. 47:*443, 1966.

Hsia, S. L., Fulton, J. E., et al.: Lipid synthesis from acetate-1-14C by suction blister epidermis and other skin components. *Proc. Soc. Exp. Biol. Med. 135:*285, 1970.

Kalenberg, A., and Kalant, N.: The effect of insulin and diabetes on glucose metabolism in human skin. *Canad. J. Biochem.* 44:801, 1966.

Kandutsch, A. A., and Russell, A. E.: Preputial gland tumor steroids. III. A metabolic pathway from lanosterol to cholesterol. *J. Biol. Chem.* 235:2256, 1960.

Liebsohn, E., Appel, B., et al.: Respiration of human skin: normal values, pathologic changes and effect of certain agents on oxygen uptake. *J. Invest. Derm.* 30:1, 1958.

Menton, D. N.: The effects of essential fatty acid deficiency on the skin of the mouse. *Amer. J. Anat.* 122:337, 1968.

Mier, P. D.: The carbohydrate metabolism of skin. *Brit. J. Derm.* 81 (Suppl. 2):14, 1969.

Nicolaides, N., Reiss, O. K., et al.: Studies of the *in vitro* lipid metabolism of the human skin. I. Biosynthesis in scalp skin. *J. Amer. Chem. Soc.* 77:1535, 1955.

Pomerantz, S. H.: Citric acid cycle in young rat skin. *J. Biol. Chem.* 236:2863, 1961.

Pomerantz, S. H., and Asbornsen, M. T.: Glucose metabolism in young rat skin. *Arch Biochem. Biophys.* 93:147, 1961.

Shapiro, L. J., Weiss, R., et al.: Enzymatic basis of typical x-linked ichthyosis. *Lancet.* Oct. 7, 756, 1978.

Srere, P. A., Chaikoff, J. L., et al.: The extrahepatic synthesis of cholesterol. *J. Biol. Chem.* 182:629, 1950.

Vroman, H. E., Nemecek, R. A., et al.: Synthesis of lipids from acetate by human preputial and abdominal skin *in vitro*. *J. Lipid Res.* 10:507, 1969.

Wheatley, V. R., Hodgins, L. T., et al.: Cutaneous lipogenesis: precursors utilized by guinea pig skin for lipid synthesis. *J. Lipid Res.* 12:347, 1971.

Wilson, J. D.: Studies on the regulation of cholesterol synthesis in the skin and preputial gland of the rat, In *Advances in Biology of Skin.* Vol. IV. *The Sebaceous Glands.* Montagna, W., Ellis, R. A., et al. (eds.), New York, Pergamon Press, 1963.

Yardley, H. J.: Sterol and keratinization. *Brit. J. Derm.* 81 (Suppl. 2):29, 1969.

Yardley, H. J., and Godfrey, G.: Direct evidence for the hexose monophosphate pathway of glucose metabolism in skin. *Biochem. J.* 86:101, 1963.

Yardley, H. J., and Godfrey, G.: Metabolism of phosphate esters and phospholipids in skin maintained *in vitro*. *J. Invest. Derm.* 43:51, 1964.

Ziboh, V. A., and Hsia, S. L.: Lipogenesis in rat skin: a possible regulatory role of glycerol 3-phosphate. *Arch. Biochem. Biophys.* 131:153, 1969.

Ziboh, V. A., Dreize, M. A., et al.: Inhibition of lipid synthesis and glucose-6-phosphate dehydrogenase in rat skin by dehydroepiandrosterone. *J. Lipid Res.* 11:346, 1970.

CUTANEOUS METABOLISM OF HORMONES

Cameron, E. H. D., Baillie, A. H., et al.: Transformation *in vitro* of (7α-³H) dehydroepiandrosterone to (³H) testosterone by skin from men. *J. Endocr.* 35:XIX, 1966.

Frost, P., Gomez, E. C., et al.: Metabolism of progesterone-4-¹⁴C in human skin and vaginal mucosa. *Biochemistry, Easton* 8:948, 1969.

Gomez, E. C., and Hsia, S. L.: Studies on cutaneous metabolism of testosterone-4-¹⁴C and Δ⁴-androstene-3,17-dione-4-¹⁴C in human skin. *Biochemistry, Easton* 7:24, 1968.

Grant, J. K.: The metabolism of steroids by skin in man. *Brit. J. Derm.* 81(Suppl. 2):1969.

Hsia, S. L., and Hao, Y. L.: Metabolic transformations of cortisol-4-¹⁴C in human skin. *Biochemistry, Easton* 5:1469, 1966.

Hsia, S. L., and Hao, Y. L.: Transformation of cortisone to cortisol in human skin. *Steroids* 10:489, 1967.

Kelch, R. P., Lindolm, U. B., et al.: Testosterone metabolism in target tissues. 2. Human fetal and adult reproductive tissues, perianal skin and skeletal muscle. *J. Clin. Endocr.* 32:449, 1971.

Kim, M. H., and Herrmann, W. L.: *In vitro* metabolism of dehydroepiandrosterone sulfate in foreskin, abdominal skin and vagina mucosa. *J. Clin. Endocr.* 28:187, 1968.

Mauvis-Jarvis, P., Bercovici, J. P., et al.: *In vitro* studies on testosterone metabolism by skin of normal males and patients with the syndrome of testicular feminization. *J. Clin. Endocr.* 29:417, 1969.

Mauvis-Jarvis, P., Crepy, O., et al.: Further studies on the pathophysiology of testicular feminization syndrome. *J. Clin. Endocr.* 32:568, 1971.

Northcut, R. C., Island, D., et al.: An explanation for target organ unresponsiveness to testosterone in the testicular feminization syndrome. *J. Clin. Endocr.* 29:422, 1969.

Peterson, R. E., Imperato-McGinley, J. et al.: Male pseudohermaphroditism due to steroid 5α-reductase deficiency. *Am. J. Med.* 62:170, 1977.

Rogone, E. L.: Testosterone metabolism by human male mammary skin. *Steroids* 7:489, 1966.

Rosenfeld, R. L., Lawrence, A. M., et al.: Androgens and androgen responsiveness in the feminizing testicular syndrome. *J. Clin. Endocr.* 32:625, 1971.

Stickland, A. L., and French, F. S.: Absence of response to dihydrotestosterone in the syndrome of testicular feminization. *J. Clin. Endocr.* 29:1284, 1969.

Strauss, J. S., and Pochi, P. E.: Recent advances in androgen metabolism and their relation to the skin. *Arch. Derm.* 100:621, 1969.

Voigt, W., Fernandez, E. P., et al.: Transformation of testosterone into 17β-hydroxy-5α-androstan-3-one by microsomal preparations of human skin. *J. Biol. Chem.* 245:5594, 1970.

Weinstein, G. D., Frost, P., et al.: *In vitro* interconversion of estrone and 17β-estradiol in human skin and vaginal mucosa. *J. Invest. Derm.* 51:4, 1968.

Wilson, J. D., and Walker, J. D.: The conversion of testosterone to 5-α-androstan-17β-ol-3-one (dihydrotestosterone) by skin of man. *J. Clin. Invest.* 48:371, 1969.

Wotiz, H. H., Mescon, H., et al.: The *in vitro* metabolism of testosterone by human skin. *J. Invest. Derm.* 26:113, 1956.

DERMAL CONNECTIVE TISSUE AND HORMONES

Asboe-Hansen, G. Hormonal effects on connective tissue. *Physiol. Rev.* 38:446, 1958.

Asboe-Hansen, G. (ed.): *Hormones and Connective Tissue.* Baltimore, Williams and Wilkins Co., 1966.

Holt, P. J. A., Lazarus, J. et al.: The epidermis in thyroid disease. *Br. J. Derm.* 95:513, 1976.

Kriss, J. P., Pleshakov, V., et al.: Isolation and identification of the long-acting thyroid stimulator and its relation to hyperthyroidism and circumscribed pretibial myxedema. *J. Clin. Endocr.* 27:1005, 1964.

Kriss, J. P., Pleshakov, V., et al.: Therapy with occlusive dressings of pretibial myxedema with fluocinolone acetonide. *J. Clin. Endocr.* 27:595, 1967.

Parker, F., and Short, J. M.: Xanthomatosis associated with hyperlipoproteinemia. *J. Invest. Derm.* 55:71, 1970.

Parving, H., Hansen, J. M., et al.: Mechanisms of edema formation in myxedema-increased protein extravasation and relatively slow lymphatic drainage. *N. Eng. J. Med.* 301:460, 1979.

Schermer, D. R., Roenigk, H. H., et al.: Relationship of long-acting thyroid stimulator to pretibial myxedema. *Arch. Derm.* 102:62, 1970.

Sheppard, R. H., and Meema, H. E.: Skin thickness in endocrine disease. *Ann. Intern. Med.* 66:531, 1967.

Sisson, J. C.: Hyaluronic acid in localized myxedema. *J. Clin. Endocr.* 28:433, 1968.

Szirmai, J. A.: The organization of the dermis, In *Advances in Biology of Skin.* Vol. X. *The Dermis.* Montagna, W., Bentley, J. P., et al. (eds.), New York, Meredith Corp., 1968.

DERMAL VASCULATURE AND HORMONES

Allen, G. E.: Diabetes mellitus and the skin. *Practitioner* 203:189, 1969.

Allen, G. E., and Hadden, D. R.: Bullous lesions of the skin in diabetes (bullosis diabeticorum). *Brit. J. Derm.* 82:216, 1970.

Braverman, I. M.: *Skin Signs of Systemic Disease.* Phiiadelphia, W. B. Saunders Co., 1970.

Danowski, T. S., Sabeh, G., et al.: Shin spots and diabetes mellitus. *Amer. J. Med. Sci.* 251:570, 1966.

Fox, R. H., Goldsmith, R., et al.: Bradykinin as a vasodilator in man. *J. Physiol.* 157:589, 1961.

Frölich, J., Bloomgarden, Z. T., et al.: The carcinoid flush. *N. Eng. J. Med.* 299:1055, 1978.

Jelinek, J. E.: Oral contraceptives and the skin. *Amer. Fam. Physician* 4:68, 1971.

Kahn, C. R., Flier, J. S., et al.: The syndrome of insulin resistance and acanthous nigricans. *N. Eng. J. Med.* 294:739, 1976.

Kontos, H. A., Shapiro, W., et al.: Mechanism of certain abnormalities of the circulation to the limbs in thyrotoxicosis. *J. Clin. Invest.* 44:947, 1965.

Kurwa, A., Roberts, P., et al.: Concurrence of bullous and atrophic skin lesions in diabetes mellitus. *Arch. Derm.* 103:670, 1971.

Levine, R. J., and Sjoerdsma, A.: Pressor amines and the carcinoid flush. *Ann. Intern. Med.* 58:818, 1963.

Mason, D. T., and Melmon, K. L.: Abnormal forearm vascular responses in the carcinoid syndrome: the role of kinins and kinin generating system. *J. Clin. Invest.* 45:1685, 1966.

Melin, H.: An atrophic circumscribed skin lesion in the lower extremities of diabetics. *Acta Med. Scand.* 176(Suppl 423):1, 1964.

Melmon, K. K., Sjoerdsma, A., et al.: Distinctive clinical and therapeutic aspects of the syndrome associated with bronchial carcinoid tumors. *Amer. J. Med.* 39:568, 1965.

Muller, S. A., and Winkelmann, R. K.: Necrobiosis lipoidica diabeticorum. *Arch. Derm.* 93:272, 1966.

Oates, J. A., and Melmon, K. L.: Biochemical and physiologic studies of the kinins in carcinoid syndrome, In *Symposium on Hypotensive Peptides.* Erdos, E. G., Back, N., et al. (eds.), Berlin, Springer Verlag, 1966.

Oates, J. A., and Sjoerdsma, A.: A unique syndrome associated with secretion of 5-hydroxytryptophan by metastatic gastric carcinoids. *Amer. J. Med.* 32:333, 1962.

Roberts, L. J., Marney, S. R., et al.: Blockade of the flush associated with metastatic gastric carcinoid by combined histamine H_1 and H_2 receptor antagonists. *N. Eng. J. Med.* 300:236, 1979.

Hormones, Melanocytes, and Pigmentation

Abe, K., Island, D. P., et al.: Radioimmunologic evidence for α-MSH (melanocyte stimulating hormone) in human pituitary and tumor tissues. *J. Clin. Endocr.* 27:46, 1967.

Abe, K., Nicholson, W. E., et al.: Radioimmunoassay of β-MSH in human plasma and tissues. *J. Clin. Invest.* 46:1609, 1967.

Benedict, P. H., Szabo, G., et al.: Melanotic macules in Albright's syndrome and in neurofibromatosis. *J.A.M.A.* 205:618, 1968.

Bloom, R. E., and Rothman, S.: Juvenile acanthosis nigricans. *Arch. Derm.* 71:413, 1955.

Brostoff, J., Bor, S., et al.: Autoantibodies in patients with vitiligo, *Lancet* 2:177, 1969.

Brown, J., and Winkelmann, R. K.: Acanthosis nigricans. A study of 90 cases. *Medicine* 47:33, 1968.

Brown, J., Winkelmann, R. K., et al.: Acanthosis nigricans and pituitary tumors. J.A.M.A. 198:619, 1966.

Crowe, F. W.: Axillary freckling as a diagnostic aid in neurofibromatosis. *Ann. Intern. Med.* 61:1142, 1964.

Cunliff, W. J., Hall, R., et al.: Vitiligo, thyroid disease and autoimmunity. *Brit. J. Derm.* 80:135, 1968.

Fitzpatrick, T. B., and Mihm, M. C.: Abnormalities of the melanin pigmentary system. In *Dermatology in General Medicine.* Fitzpatrick, T. B., Arndt, K. A., et al. (eds.), New York, McGraw-Hill, 1971.

Katzenellenbogen, I.: Dermatoendocrinological syndrome due to diethylstilbestrol. *J.A.M.A.* 161:1695, 1956.

Kawamura, T., Fitzpatrick, T. B., et al.: *Biology of Normal and Abnormal Melanocytes.* Tokyo, University of Tokyo Press, 1971.

Lee, T. H., and Lee, M. S.: Measurement and electrophoretic study of MSH-like substances in human pregnancy urine. *J. Clin. Endocr.* 29:660, 1969.

Lerner, A. B.: Hormones and skin color. *Sci. Amer.* 205:99, 1061.

Lerner, A. B., and McGuire, J. S.: Melanocyte-stimulating hormone and adrenocorticotrophic hormone. *N. Eng. J. Med.* 270:539, 1964.

Lerner, A. B., Shizume, K., et al.: The mechanism of endocrine control of melanin pigmentation. *J. Clin. Endocr.* 14:1463, 1954.

McGregor, B. C., Katz, H. I., et al.: Vitiligo and multiple glandular insufficiencies. *J.A.M.A.* 219:724, 1972.

McGuire, J., Moellmann, G., et al.: Cytochalasin B and pigment granule translocation. *J. Cell Biol.* 52:754, 1972.

Nelson, D. H., Meakin, J. W., et al.: ACTH-producing tumor of the pituitary gland. *N. Eng. J. Med.* 259:161, 1958.

Ochi, Y., and DeGroot, L. J.: Vitiligo in Graves' disease. *Ann. Intern. Med.* 71:935, 1969.

Quevedo, W. C., Szabo, G., et al.: Biology of the melanin pigmentary system, In *Dermatology in General Medicine.* Fitzpatrick, T. B., Arndt, K. A., et al. (eds.), New York, McGraw-Hill, 1971.

Resnik, C. S.: Melasma induced by oral contraceptive drugs. *J.A.M.A.* 199:601, 1967.

Snell, R. S.: Hormonal control of pigmentation in man and other mammals. In *The Pigmentary System.* Vol. 8. *Advances in Biology of Skin.* Montagna, W., and Hu, F. (eds.), New York, Pergamon Press, 1967.

Snell, R. S., and Bischitz, P. G.: The melanocytes and melanin in human abdominal wall skin: a survey made at different ages in both sexes and during pregnancy. *J. Anat.* 97:361, 1963.

Taleisnik, S., and Orias, R.: A melanocyte-stimulating hormone releasing factor in hypothalamic extracts. *Amer. J. Physiol.* 208:293, 1965.

Taleisnik, S., and Tomatis, M. E.: Melanocyte-stimulating hormone-releasing and inhibiting factors in two hypothalamic extracts. *Endocrinology* 81:819, 1967.

Tucker, W. R., Klink, D., et al.: Insulin resistance and acanthosis nigricans. *Diabetes* 13:395, 1964.

Hormones and Cutaneous Appendages

Sebaceous glands

Burton, J. L., Libman, L. J., et al.: Sebum excretion in acromegaly. *Brit. Med. J.* 139:406, 1972.

Milne, J. A.: The metabolism of androgens by sebaceous glands. *Brit. J. Derm.* 81(Suppl. 2):23, 1969.

Montagna, W., Ellis, R. A., et al.: The sebaceous glands, In *Advances in Biology of Skin IV.* New York, Macmillan Co., 1963.

Pochi, P. E., and Strauss, J. S.: Effect of cyclic administration of conjugated equine estrogens on sebum production. *J. Invest. Derm.* 47:582, 1966.

Pochi, P. E., and Strauss, J. S.: Effect of prednisone on sebaceous gland secretion. *J. Invest. Derm.* 49:456, 1967.

Pochi, P. E., and Strauss, J. S.: Effect of sequential mestranol-chlormadinone on sebum production. *Arch. Derm.* 95:47, 1967.

Pochi, P. E., and Strauss, J. S.: Sebaceous gland response in man to the administration of testosterone. Δ⁴-androstenedione, and dehydroisoandrosterone. *J. Invest. Derm.* 52:32, 1969.

Pochi, P. E., Strauss, J. S., et al.: Plasma testosterone and estrogen levels, urine testosterone excretion, and sebum production in males with acne vulgaris. *J. Clin. Endocr.* 25:1660, 1965.

Sansone, G., and Reisner, R. M.: Differential rates of conversion of testosterone to dihydrotestosterone in acne and in normal human skin — a possible pathogenic factor in acne. *J. Invest. Derm.* 56:366, 1971.

Strauss, J. S.: Diseases of sebaceous glands, In *Dermatology in General Medicine.* Fitzpatrick, T. B., Arndt, K. A., et al. (eds.), New York, McGraw-Hill, 1971.

Strauss, J. S., and Pochi, P. E.: The hormonal control of human sebaceous glands: observations in certain endocrine disorders. *J. Clin. Endocr.* 2:798, 1968.

Strauss, J. S., and Pochi, P. E.: The human sebaceous gland: its regulation by steroidal hormones and its use as an end organ for assaying androgenicity *in vivo.* Recent Progr. Hormone Res. 19:385, 1963.

Summerly, R., and Woodbury, S.: The *in vitro* incorporation of ¹⁴C-acetate into the isolated sebaceous glands and appendage-freed epidermis of human skin. *Brit. J. Derm.* 85:424, 1971.

Sweeney, T. M., Szarnicki, R. J., et al.: The effect of estrogen and androgen on the sebaceous gland turnover time. *J. Invest. Derm.* 53:8, 1969.

Hair growth

Adachi, K., and Kano, M.: Adenyl cyclase in human hair follicles: its inhibition by dihydrotestosterone. *Biochem. Biophys. Res. Commun.* 41:884, 1970.

Adachi, K., Takayasu, S., et al.: Human hair follicles: metabolism and control mechanisms. *J. Soc. Cosmet. Chem.* 21:901, 1970.

Baker, L., Kaye, R., et al.: Diazoxide treatment of idiopathic hypoglycemia of infancy. *J. Pediat.* 71:494, 1967.

Bardin, C. W., and Lipsett, M. B.: Testosterone and androstenedione blood production rates in normal women and women with idiopathic hirsutism or polycystic ovaries. *J. Clin. Invest.* 46:891, 1967.

Bingham, K. D., and Shaw, D. A.: Male pattern baldness and the metabolism of androgens by human scalp skin. *J. Soc. Cosmet. Chem.* 24:523, 1973.

Brooksbank, B. W. L.: Endocrinological aspects of hirsutism. *Physiol. Rev.* 41:623, 1961.

Forbes, A. P.: Hirsutism, In *Dermatology in General Medicine,* Fitzpatrick, T. B., Arndt, K. A., et al. (eds.), New York, McGraw-Hill, 1971.

Freinkel, R. K., and Freinkel, N.: Hair growth and alopecia in hypothyroidism. *Arch. Derm.* 106:349, 1972.

Garn, S. M.: Types and distribution of the hair in man. *Ann. N. Y. Acad. Sci.* 53:498, 1951.

Givens, J. R.: Hirsutism and hyperandrogenism. *Advances in Internal Medicine.* 21:221, 1976. Stollerman, G. H. (ed.)

Givens, J. R., Anderson, R. N., et al.: The effectiveness of two oral contraceptives in suppressing plasma androstenedione, testosterone, LH, and FSH, and in stimulating plasma testosterone-binding capacity in hirsute women. *Am. J. Ob. Gyn.* 124:333, 1976.

Kirschner, M. A., Zucker, I. R., et al.: Idiopathic hirsutism—an ovarian abnormality. *N. Eng. J. Med.* 294:637, 1976.

Kirschner, M. A., and Bardin, C. W.: Androgen production and metabolism in normal and virilized women. *Metabolism* 21:667, 1972.

Kuttenn, F., Mowszowicz, I., et al.: Androgen production and skin metabolism in hirsutism. *J. Endocr.* 75:83, 1977.

Liddle, G. W.: Cushing's syndrome and problems of hirsutism, In *The Hirsute Female.* Greenblatt, R. B. (ed.). Springfield, Illinois, Charles C Thomas, 1963.

Livingston, S., Petersen, D., et al.: Hypertrichosis occurring in association with dilantin therapy. *J. Pediat.* 47:351, 1955.

Lloyd, C. W., Moses, A. M., et al.: Studies of adrenocortical function of women with idiopathic hirsutism: response to 25 units of ACTH. *J. Clin. Endocr.* 23:413, 1963.

Lynfield, Y. L.: Effect of pregnancy on the human hair cycle. *J. Invest. Derm.* 35:323, 1960.

McKnight, E.: The prevalence of "hirsutism" in young women. *Lancet* 1:410, 1964.

Muller, S. A.: Hirsutism. *Amer. J. Med.* 46:803, 1969.

Munroe, D. D.: Disorders of hair, In *Dermatology in General Medicine.* Fitzpatrick, T. B., Arndt, K. A., et al. (eds.), New York, McGraw-Hill, 1971.

Miyazaki, M., Takayasu, S., et al.: Activity of testosterone 5α-reductase in the hair follicles of women with polycystic ovaries. *J. Endocr.* 78:445, 1978.

Perloff, W. H., Channick, B. T., et al.: Clinical management of idiopathic hirsutism (adrenal virilism). *J.A.M.A.* 167:2041, 1958.

Plager, J. E., Cushman, P., et al.: The plasma cortisol response to ACTH in "idiopathic hirsutism." *J. Clin. Invest.* 40:1315, 1961.

Rampini, E., Davis, B. P., et al.: Cyclic changes in the metabolism of estradiol by rat skin during the hair cycle. *J. Invest. Derm.* 57:75, 1971.

Rook, A.: Endocrine influences on hair growth. *Brit. Med. J.* 1:609, 1965.

Rosenfield, R. L.: Plasma free androgen patterns in hirsute women and their diagnostic implications. *Am. J. Med.* 66:417, 1979.

Rosenfeld, R. L.: Plasma testosterone binding — globulin and indexes of the concentration of unbound plasma androgens in normal and hirsute subjects. *J. Clin. Endocr.* 32:717,1971.

Stauss, J. S., and Pochi, P. E.: Recent advances in androgen metabolism and their relation to the skin. *Arch. Derm.* 100:621, 1969.

Thomas, J. P., and Oake, R. J.: Androgen metabolism in the skin of hirsute women. *J. Clin. Endocr.* 38:19, 1974.

Wieland, R. G., Vorys, N., et al.: Studies of female hirsutism. *Amer. J. Med.* 41:927, 1966.

CHAPTER 24

Hormones and the Formed Elements of the Blood

By John W. Adamson, David C. Dale,
and Seymour J. Klebanoff

ERYTHROCYTES

Regulation of Erythropoiesis

The major function of the circulating red cell mass is to provide oxygen to meet tissue metabolic requirements. Under normal circumstances, red cell production is regulated by three factors: the effective red cell mass, which includes both the number of red blood cells as well as the oxygen dissociation characteristics of hemoglobin; the production of erythropoietin; and the proliferative capacity of the erythroid marrow. Disturbances in any one of these regulatory limbs (Fig. 24–1) may result in either an overproduction or an underproduction of red cells.

The hormone primarily responsible for the regulation of erythropoiesis is erythropoietin.[51] This glycoprotein hormone has been isolated from the urine of anemic humans by Miyake.[59] Its specific activity is approximately 8×10^4 IU/mg protein, and its estimated molecular weight (MW) is 47,000 daltons. Although its exact chemical composition is unknown, the molecule contains approximately 70% protein and 30% carbohydrate, of which 11% is sialic acid.[29] The sialic acid moiety prevents the rapid uptake of the hormone by hepatocytes and thus protects the hormone from rapid degradation.

The kidney is the organ primarily responsible for sensing alterations in oxygen availability and for regulating the production of erythropoietin. There are two prevailing concepts of the biogenesis of erythropoietin. The first is that within the kidney there is an enzyme-like factor, erythrogenin, which acts on a plasma substrate to generate the active hormone, erythropoietin.[31] The activating substance is found in the light mitochondrial fraction of centrifuged kidney homogenates. A second concept is that the kidney releases erythropoietin either intact or in the form of a prohormone that is cleaved or modified by a plasma factor, giving rise to active erythropoietin.[66] Regardless of which of these concepts is correct, reduction in oxygen availability to the kidney leads to a rise in both plasma and urinary levels of erythropoietin, whereas states of hyperoxia, e.g., with red cell transfusions, lead to reduced erythropoietin production. Erythropoietin production also may reflect changes in the affinity of hemoglobin for oxygen in blood. Thus, an increase in affinity, indicated by a left shift of the oxygen-hemoglobin dissociation curve, decreases tissue oxygen availability and increases erythropoietin and red cell production.

Erythropoietin acts primarily on morphologically unrecognizable target cells in the bone marrow, inducing terminal differentiation and initiating hemoglobin synthesis. The response involves cell division and the appearance of specific messenger and transfer-RNA's (tRNA's).[28, 58, 69] With increased erythropoietin stimulation, the mitotic interval of marrow normoblasts is moderately shortened and the amount of hemoglobin synthesized per cell is increased.[65] Of clinical significance, the reticulocyte, which normally spends up to 3 days in the marrow, is released prematurely.

Detailed knowledge of erythropoietin metabolism and of the biochemical aspects of its action has been limited by difficulties in hormone measurement and the lack of availability of a sufficient quantity of pure hormone. At present, the most widely used and best standardized technique for measuring erythropoietin is a bioassay employing the poly-

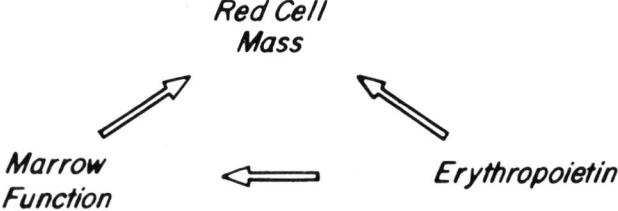

Figure 24–1. Outline of the three major factors participating in the regulation of normal red cell production. (Adapted from Adamson, J. W., and Finch, C. A.: Mechanisms of erythroid marrow activation. *Trans. Assoc. Amer. Physicians* 79:419, 1966.)

Table 24–1. NEOPLASMS ASSOCIATED WITH INCREASED (AUTONOMOUS) ERYTHROPOIETIN PRODUCTION

1. Hypernephroma
2. Hepatoma
3. Cerebellar hemangioblastoma
4. Uterine leiomyoma
5. Pheochromocytoma
6. Bronchogenic carcinoma

cythemic mouse. Endogenous erythropoietin is reduced either by transfusion or by exposing animals to intermittent hypoxic conditions to produce a secondary form of polycythemia and then returning the animals to ambient pressure. In both cases, an absolute functional excess of red cells is achieved, erythropoiesis is suppressed, and the erythropoietic stimulating activity of sera or other biologic materials is more readily detected. Quantitation of erythropoietic stimulating activity in biologic specimens is achieved by comparing the amount of injected radioactive iron appearing in newly-formed red cells in test animals to that appearing in animals injected with known amounts of an International Reference Preparation.* Although assays of serum can be used to detect significant increases in erythropoietin, urinary concentrates must be employed to detect normal or subnormal levels. Unfortunately, the assay techniques are difficult to standardize and their availability is limited. *In vitro* assays, using freshly harvested erythroid cells or immunologic techniques, are being evaluated, but presently available methods are not satisfactory substitutes for *in vivo* assays.[68]

Clinically, increased erythropoietin activity is detected by the reticulocyte count and the presence in the peripheral blood smear of reticulocytes prematurely released from the marrow.[37] These appear in the circulation as large cells containing increased residual cytoplasmic RNA. They have a bluish (polychromatophilic) appearance with Wright's stain. Premature reticulocyte release is confirmed by the marrow radioiron transit time, which reflects primarily the period of reticulocyte maturation in the marrow. This shortens predictably with increases in erythropoietin stimulation. If the proliferative capacity of the bone marrow is normal, its appearance also reflects increased erythropoietin stimulation. Direct examination of the erythropoietin-stimulated marrow reveals erythroid hyperplasia. If erythropoietin stimulation remains high, and there is no reduction in red cell survival, an increased red cell mass will eventually result.

Increased erythropoietin production most frequently occurs in response to a limitation in oxygen availability, as seen with most forms of anemia, in individuals who reside at high altitude or in patients with chronic cardiac or pulmonary disease. It may also be seen in conditions in which hemoglobin affinity for oxygen is modified, as in patients with mutant hemoglobins. Patients with certain solid tumors (Table 24–1) may produce erythropoietin or an erythropoietin-like material.

Most anemias in man are due to a primary impairment in marrow function or to iron deficiency and not to a decrease

in erythropoietin. Hypometabolism and renal disease are two conditions in which impaired production of erythropoietin may contribute to the anemia, however. Although some hormone production persists in these conditions, it is less than expected for the degree of anemia present. Thus, anemia is almost invariably seen with renal disease when the blood creatinine and urea nitrogen exceed 5 and 50 mg/dl, respectively, although there is not a close correlation between renal function and red cell production.[2] The expected shortening of marrow transit time and the appearance of polychromatophilic erythrocytes in the circulation are not seen, however, reflecting the reduced erythropoietin stimulation.

Although erythropoietin is the primary regulator of erythropoiesis, other hormones also influence red cell production. Anemia occasionally accompanies endocrine insufficiency and there are three organs — the thyroid, adrenal, and gonads — whose products influence erythropoiesis and whose dysfunction may result in reduced red cell mass.[82]

Thyroid Hormone

While thyroid hormone is not essential to the production of red cells, it has an important influence on erythropoiesis in experimental animals and man. When thyroid hormone is administered to animals, there is an increase in red cell mass that correlates roughly with oxygen consumption. Hypothyroidism in animals is associated with a decline in the red cell mass that can be restored with thyroid replacement therapy.[30] Mild anemia may accompany hypothyroidism in man; however, the decline in red cell mass may be masked by a reduction in the plasma volume. The incidence of anemia has been reported as high as 30–50% in some series.[53]

The mechanisms leading to anemia in hypothyroidism are complex and may include decreased marrow stimulation as well as deficiencies of iron or vitamins such as B_{12}. The anemia is usually hypoproliferative in nature, with a normal or reduced reticulocyte index. Red cell survival is generally normal. The incidence of iron or vitamin deficiency in hypothyroidism is uncertain, although in the large series reported by Horton, in which anemia was present in 26% of patients, only one fourth of those affected had thyroid hormone deficiency as the single cause of anemia.[38] In the other patients, hematologic recovery required treatment with iron or B_{12} in addition to thyroid hormone replacement.

Iron deficiency complicates hypothyroidism in 5–15% of patients and may result from menorrhagia in females or decreased iron absorption due to achlorhydria. The latter is common in hypothyroidism and is not reversed with thyroid hormone replacement.

Vitamin B_{12} deficiency contributes to the anemia of hypothyroidism in 8–10% of patients. This is of particular interest because of the frequent association of both antiparietal cell and anti-intrinsic factor antibodies with antithyroid antibodies in patients with hypothyroidism and in their

---

*The erythropoietin International Reference Preparation is available from the World Health Organization, International Laboratory for Biological Standards, National Institute of Medical Research, Mill Hill, London, NW7, England.

healthy near-relatives. These associations suggest a general autoimmune disorder involving multiple organs. It is important to follow patients with pernicious anemia for the appearance of hypothyroidism and vice versa since there is not a consistent sequence or time relationship in the development of these two diseases.

The degree of anemia is usually mild; in the group published by Horton, the lowest hemoglobin seen among patients with uncomplicated anemia was 10 g/dl. The peripheral blood findings are nonspecific. The mean corpuscular volume (MCV) may be increased; this macrocytosis does not correlate with B_{12} status and thus may be the result of hypothyroidism alone. Occasional acanthocytes may be seen.

The treatment of the anemia of hypothyroidism is obviously hormone replacement. Iron or vitamin B_{12} levels should be measured and replacement of these factors instituted if deficiencies exist. Although anemia is most prevalent in patients with a low serum iron, iron replacement alone does not completely reverse the anemia in most patients. Because of the reduced plasma volume seen in hypothyroid individuals, the initial response to therapy may be a decline in hematocrit as the plasma volume expands. Complete hematologic recovery may require 6 months of therapy.

Adrenocorticosteroids

Of the blood elements, lymphocytes and eosinophils are the most susceptible to adrenal steroid influences. These hormones also influence erythropoiesis, however, although the exact mechanisms are unknown. In adrenal insufficiency, there is a reduction in erythropoiesis. Anemia is rarely seen, however, as the reduced red cell mass is masked by a concurrent reduction in plasma volume. No specific therapy, other than replacement of adrenocorticosteroids, is required.

When adrenal hormone levels are increased, owing to either Cushing's disease or exogenous administration, the hemoglobin concentration is often 1–2 g/dl above normal.[67] This is due largely to decreased plasma volume and not to a real increase in red cell production. Adrenal glucocorticoids, however, have been used effectively in treating two forms of red cell aplasia: the congenital hypoplastic anemia or Blackfan-Diamond syndrome, and pure red cell aplasia in adults.[50] In the latter instance, the effectiveness of steroids suggests that the anemia is mediated by immune mechanisms directed against the developing normoblast or perhaps against erythropoietin itself.

Androgens

Testosterone and related androgenic derivatives are among the most potent hormones capable of stimulating erythropoiesis. The difference in androgen levels between males and females is probably responsible for the difference in their hemoglobin concentration of 1–2 g/dl. Males with testicular failure have hemoglobin values similar to premenopausal females. A mild anemia accompanying this state is normocytic and normochromic without other distinguishing features. Replacement therapy results in a rise in hemoglobin concentration. The anemia, therefore, may be considered physiologic and does not require independent treatment.

Androgenic hormones have complicated effects on erythropoiesis, but their best-characterized influence is a direct action on the kidney, stimulating erythropoietin production. Administration of androgens to man or experimental animals results in an increase in plasma and urinary levels of erythropoietin and an increase in reticulocyte production, which can be blocked by nephrectomy.[21] Although androgens are frequently used to treat patients with various forms of marrow failure, they are most effective in those instances in which anemia results from decreased marrow stimulation.

Some studies have suggested that, in addition to their stimulation of erythropoietin production, androgens have a direct effect on marrow cells. These studies have generally involved tissue culture techniques, and their relevance to hematopoietic regulation in the intact animal is still speculative.[1] The role of androgenic hormones in hematopoiesis under physiologic conditions can be considered only as a modulating one; hematopoiesis will proceed, despite decreased levels of such hormones.

Pituitary Hormones

A mild to moderate hypoproliferative anemia is commonly seen with hypopituitarism and reflects the combined failure of end organs such as the thyroid, gonads, and adrenals.[13] The anemia results from decreased erythropoietin stimulation associated with the hypometabolic state. In addition to the secondary effects of hormone deficiencies, growth hormone (GH) may be directly required for a full hematologic response. Treatment of pituitary dwarfs with GH increased erythropoietin levels, but it is not clear whether this is a direct effect on erythropoietin production or whether the latter increased in response to increased oxygen consumption or through secondary effects of the hormone on blood volume and growth.[39] Earlier studies suggested the presence of a pituitary factor acting directly and primarily on bone marrow. Current evidence, however, does not convincingly support such a factor.

Estrogens

A mild anemia of 1–3 g/dl may accompany the administration of estrogen or estrogen-like drugs. This is commonly seen in males with prostatic carcinoma treated with diethylstilbestrol. An accompanying fluid retention with expansion of the plasma volume may contribute to the fall in hemoglobin concentration. Estrogens in low doses have been reported to decrease the marrow response to erythropoietin in experimental animals, an effect which was antagonized by the simultaneous administration of 17-α-hydroxyprogesterone or testosterone propionate.[32] At high concentrations, estrogens may suppress erythropoietin formation. There is little direct evidence, however, that the influence of estrogens on red cell formation in man is of major clinical importance.

LEUKOCYTES

Neutrophils, eosinophils, and monocytes are capable of endocytosis, i.e., the uptake of either particulate or nonparticulate material from the extracellular fluid (ECF). In addition, under certain conditions, these cells can release their granule contents into the medium (exocytosis). The phagocytic cells are considered in this section. Other leukocytes, i.e., lymphocytes and basophils, are considered in Ch. 25.

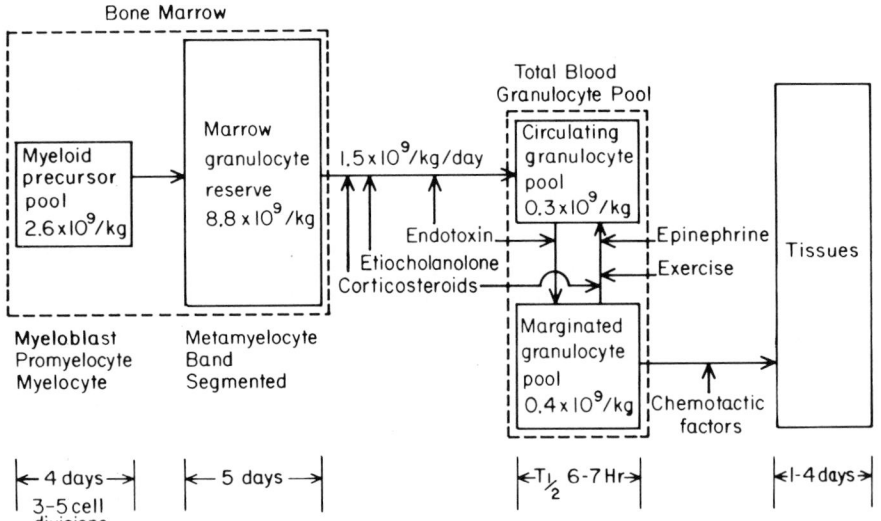

Figure 24–2. Schematic representation of neutrophil kinetics. (Adapted from Klebanoff, S. J., and Clark, R. A.: *The Neutrophil: Function and Clinical Disorders.* New York, Elsevier-North Holland Publishing Co., 1978, p. 74.)

Production

The neutrophil[11, 46, 63] develops in the bone marrow (granulocytopoiesis) beginning with the pluripotential stem cell and continuing through the committed stem cell, myeloblast, promyelocyte, myelocyte, metamyelocyte, and band cell to the mature fully segmented neutrophil (Fig. 24–2). The pluripotential stem cell is a common precursor of the myeloid, erythroid, megakaryocytic, and lymphoid lines, whereas the committed stem cell is recognized by its ability to form a colony of more mature myeloid cells in culture. The myeloblast is a small cell devoid of granules. Azurophil (primary) granules form in the promyelocyte. They bud off from the inner face of the Golgi complex and contain myeloperoxidase, cationic proteins, a number of acid hydrolases, and certain neutral proteases, e.g., elastase and collagenase. Specific (secondary) granules form in the myelocyte. These are smaller and less dense than azurophil granules and develop from the outer face of the Golgi complex. They lack acid hydrolases and myeloperoxidase but contain lactoferrin, most of the cellular lysozyme, and, in some species, alkaline phosphatase. No further cell division occurs beyond the myelocyte stage, although maturation continues.

Eosinophils and monocytes are also bone marrow–derived cells.[8, 11] The eosinophilic promyelocyte and the promonocyte are morphologically very similar to the neutrophilic promyelocyte. The eosinophil can be identified, however, by the development of distinctive membrane-bound cytoplasmic granules. Otherwise its development closely resembles that of the neutrophil. The monocyte, in contrast to the neutrophil and eosinophil, leaves the marrow without undergoing terminal differentiation; it has the capacity both for phagocytosis and for dividing and becoming a long-lived tissue macrophage.

Regulation of Production

It has been presumed for many years that blood leukocyte production is regulated humorally by substances called "leukopoietins." The blood counts for each type of leukocyte are thought to be governed by a separate hormone or group of hormones. Although this concept is widely accepted, no leukopoietic substance has yet been identified as having a specific role in the physiologic regulation of blood leukocytes. Several substances recently have been identified that may have this function, however,[25] and mathematical models for humoral regulation of leukocytes have been constructed as extensions of this basic concept.[71]

"Colony stimulating factor" (CSF) is a substance or group of substances found in serum, urine, and the supernate from *in vitro* cultures of many mammalian cell lines that stimulates granulocytic precursor cells to form colonies in a tissue culture system.[76] The colony-forming cells are hematopoietic stem cells committed to granulocytopoiesis. The colonies that form contain immature and mature neutrophils, monocytes, and macrophages. Human urinary CSF is a sialic acid–containing glycoprotein of MW 45,000–85,000 daltons.[62] It stimulates the growth of human cells as well as cells from several other species. Human serum has colony-stimulating activity, but the stimulating factor has not yet been purified. Human serum also contains inhibitors of colony growth. A fibroblast-derived CSF has been sufficiently purified to permit its measurement in body fluid by radioimmunoassay. Unfortunately, this CSF stimulates mouse, but not human, bone marrow cells, and the antibody to this material does not cross-react with human CSF.[74] Blood and urinary CSF levels, as determined by bioassay, are increased with granulocytopenia in several clinical and experimental settings. Studies to show that CSF administration stimulates *in vivo* granulocytopoiesis or that anti-CSF inhibits granulocyte formation are still needed. The relationship of CSF to other hormones stimulating cell growth, i.e., GH and the somatomedins, is also unclear. Because bacterial endotoxins are so ubiquitous, so difficult to remove from biologic materials and have so many effects on leukocyte formation, distribution, and function, contamination with these substances has caused major problems for the investigation of humoral regulation of leukocyte production.

Lymphocytes and monocytes, but not neutrophils, produce CSF *in vitro* when exposed to certain antigens and mitogens. A selective eosinophil-stimulating CSF is produced by lymphocytes from *Trichinella*-infected animals on re-exposure to *Trichinella in vitro*.[72] This evidence, together with data from *in vivo* studies, strongly suggests that eosinophil production is regulated by humoral factors made by lymphocytes.[8] A serum factor called "eosinophilopoietin" has been detected in animals depleted of eosinophils by repeated administration of antieosinophil serum.[57] This factor increased both blood and bone marrow eosinophils when injected into normal animals, but its physiologic role in regulating eosinophils is not yet known.

Mobilization, Blood Kinetics, and Chemotaxis

Neutrophils and eosinophils are stored in the bone marrow for 1–3 days after they are formed. Cells in this storage pool (marrow granulocyte reserves) can be released into the blood with stress and by administration of endotoxin, glucocorticosteroids, and etiocholanolone[12] (Fig. 24–2). For both endotoxin and etiocholanolone, plasma factors called "leukocytosis inducing factors" have been identified that appear to mediate this effect. These substances are as yet poorly characterized but may be derived from the complement system.

Once released into the blood, the granulocytes are distributed in two pools of approximately equal size. The circulating granulocyte pool consists of those cells that are sampled at venipuncture. The marginated granulocyte pool comprises the cells loosely adherent to blood vessel walls out of the central axial bloodstream. The two pools are in equilibrium. The average half-life of the blood neutrophil is about 6.5 hours; the half-life of the blood eosinophil and monocyte is probably a few hours longer.

Neutrophils are mobilized from the bone marrow in large numbers during infection. Margination and adherence of cells to the blood vessel wall increases, and passage of the adherent neutrophils between the endothelial cells of the small venules occurs. Specific chemotactic factors direct this extravascular migration to sites of microbial invasion. Most microbial species generate relatively low MW ($<$ 3500 daltons) agents that are directly chemotactic for neutrophils. The microorganisms also can initiate chemotactic factor generation through the activation of complement either by the classic or alternative pathways. The predominant chemotactic factor formed is a small MW (about 15,000 daltons) fragment of C5, designated C5a.

Leukocyte Function

Particles recognized by the leukocyte as foreign are taken up and sequestered into intracellular vacuoles. This process of phagocytosis is facilitated by opsonins that bind both to the particle and to specific receptors on the surface of the granulocyte. The predominant complement-derived opsonin, C3b (the large MW fragment of C3), functions primarily to bind the particle to the phagocyte, whereas the ingestion phase is initiated by immunoglobulin that binds to the antigenic sites on the particle and to Fc receptors on the cell surface. Cellular pseudopods, formed as a result of the gelation and contraction of submembranous microfilaments, move around the particle until engulfment is complete. A series of events follow that rapidly leads to the death of the ingested organism. The membrane of the phagocyte vacuole fuses with that of adjacent cytoplasmic granules (both azurophil and specific), and the granule contents are discharged into the vacuolar space. These events are associated with an increase in oxygen consumption and much, if not all, of this extra oxygen consumed is converted to H_2O_2 via a superoxide anion intermediate. The enzyme responsible is believed to be a reduced pyridine nucleotide oxidase. The further reduction of H_2O_2 results in the formation of highly reactive hydroxyl radicals. The respiratory burst is accompanied by the emission of light (chemiluminescence), indicating the formation of electronically excited states. Singlet molecular oxygen is an excited state of oxygen that may be formed by neutrophils during phagocytosis; however, definitive proof of its formation is not yet at hand. Additional aspects of the respiratory burst are increased hexose monophosphate shunt activity and increased nitroblue tetrazolium (NBT) reduction.

The antimicrobial systems of the neutrophil are either oxygen-dependent or oxygen-independent. The oxygen-dependent systems may include H_2O_2 (acting nonenzymatically or in conjunction with myeloperoxidase and a halide), the superoxide anion, hydroxyl radicals, and singlet oxygen. The oxygen-independent antimicrobial systems may include the acid intravacuolar pH, lysozyme, lactoferrin, and cationic proteins. Death of the organisms is followed by their digestion by acid (and possibly neutral) hydrolases. Although the neutrophil is designed for the concentration in the phagocytic vacuole of agents toxic to the ingested organism, leakage or secretion of these agents to the outside of the cell can occur with the potential for damage to adjacent cells.

Adrenocorticosteroids

Leukocyte production, distribution, and function are markedly altered by glucocorticosteroid administration. These effects are the basis for the use of corticosteroids as anti-inflammatory agents. Although there are well-known major quantitative differences in the anti-inflammatory effects of various glucocorticosteroids, there is little factual basis for presuming that any yet available glucocorticosteroid has unique anti-inflammatory properties.[19]

The most easily measured effects of steroids on leukocytes are changes in blood cell counts. In Cushing's syndrome, neutrophilia, eosinopenia, and lymphopenia are observed frequently. In Addison's disease, eosinophilia commonly occurs. Neutrophilia, approximately a doubling of the baseline count, occurs 4 to 6 hours after a single dose of hydrocortisone, prednisone, or dexamethasone; the elevation lasts less than 24 hours. After steroid administration, lymphocytopenia, monocytopenia, and eosinopenia occur within 1 to 2 hours, are maximal within 4 hours, and last less than 24 hours. Tachyphylaxis does not occur even when steroid therapy is prolonged.

The steroid-induced increase in blood neutrophils is attributable to two phenomena: accelerated release of cells from the bone marrow and slower egress of cells from the blood to the tissues. As a result, glucocorticosteroids increase the average sojourn of the blood neutrophil and reduce cell accumulation at sites of inflammation. The precise mechanisms whereby steroids cause these effects are not known, but they may involve changes in cell surface charge or related surface phenomena.[24] The reduction in the adherence of leukocytes from steroid-treated subjects to foreign fibers and endothelial cells may be directly related to a surface effect.[56] The abrupt decrease in blood monocytes and eosinophils with steroid therapy also may be due to a surface effect altering cell distribution. Steroids do not appear to "lyse" these cells, as had been thought previously.

The persisting neutrophilia, monocytopenia, and eosinopenia that occur with prolonged steroid therapy suggest that glucocorticosteroids influence cell production as well as cell distribution and kinetics. In animal studies, it has been demonstrated that glucocorticoids can stimulate neutrophil production.[40] In man this effect has not been clearly demonstrated, but steroids are often included in cancer chemotherapy regimens because of this presumed beneficial effect.

The effects of glucocorticoids on granulocyte chemotaxis, phagocytosis, bactericidal mechanisms, and secretion of enzymes have been intensively investigated. Most investigators have found that these functions are normal for neutrophils from steroid-treated patients,[54] although there is much conflicting data. For monocytes, studies of cells from steroid-treated subjects are more difficult to perform because the steroid-induced monocytopenia limits the number of cells that can be harvested for study. It appears, however,

Table 24–2. GLUCOCORTICOSTEROID EFFECTS ON CELLULAR HOST-DEFENSE MECHANISMS

	Daily Therapy	Alternate-Day Therapy	
		On Day	Off Day
Blood Counts			
Neutrophils	Increased	Increased	Normal
Monocytes	Decreased	Decreased	Normal
Lymphocytes	Decreased	Decreased	Normal
Eosinophils	Decreased	Decreased	Normal
Neutrophil Kinetics			
Blood neutrophil half-life	Increased	Increased	Normal
Neutrophil turnover	Decreased	Decreased	Normal
Inflammatory Responses			
Acute (neutrophils + monocytes)	Decreased	Decreased	Normal
Delayed (monocytes + lymphocytes)	Decreased	Normal	Normal
Cell Function			
Neutrophils	Probably normal	Probably normal	Normal
Monocytes	Decreased	Decreased	Probably normal
Lymphocytes	Decreased	Decreased	Normal

that steroids may suppress monocyte phagocytosis and microbicidal mechanisms.[33, 70] *In vitro* hydrocortisone in very high concentrations will suppress many leukocyte functions,[54] but the relevance of this data to *in vivo* effects is uncertain. The effects of steroids on lymphocytes are presented in Ch. 25.

When patients are treated with alternate-day glucocorticosteroids, several effects of the steroids on leukocytes are noted only on the day the steroids are given. Neutrophil, monocyte, and lymphocyte counts and acute inflammatory responses are normal on the "off" day, whereas they are abnormal on the day steroids are given. It is also noteworthy that delayed hypersensitivity responses, e.g., the tuberculin response, are not suppressed by alternate-day steroid therapy (Table 24–2).

Iodine and Thyroid Hormone Metabolism

Intact phagocytes catalyze both the conversion of iodide to a trichloroacetic acid (TCA)–precipitable form (iodination) and the degradation of the thyroid hormones.

Iodination

When intact neutrophils are incubated with an ingestable particle and radioiodide, a portion of the iodide is converted to a TCA-precipitable form and most of the fixed iodide is located on the ingested particle.[43] Proteolytic digestion reveals labeled monoiodotyrosine, a lesser amount of labeled diiodotyrosine, and a very small amount of labeled thyroxine (T_4).[77] It is not known whether the latter represents *de novo* synthesis or iodine exchange with preformed T_4. Monoiodotyrosine and iodoprotein are detected in the ECF.[78] Iodination is not seen when resting (nonphagocytosing) leukocytes are employed. Iodination by neutrophils results from the interaction of myeloperoxidase, H_2O_2 and iodide.[43] It is very low in leukocytes from patients with chronic granulomatous disease that lack H_2O_2 production and from patients with hereditary myeloperoxidase deficiency.[45] As in the thyroid, iodination is inhibited by goitrogens such as propylthiouracil or methimazole.[48] Iodination also occurs during phagocytosis by monocytes[3] and eosinophils[49] and the mechanism is presumably similar to that which is operative in neutrophils.

Thyroid Hormone Degradation

T_4 and triiodothyronine (T_3) bind to the cell surface of phagocytes and are transferred into the phagocytic vacuole during phagocytosis. Degradation rapidly follows.[47, 85] A small amount of T_3 can be identified as a product of T_4 degradation.[47, 84, 85] Serum inhibits binding and subsequent degradation, presumably due to the competition between serum protein and cellular binding sites for the hormone. Thyroid hormone degradation is dependent on the phagocytosis-induced respiratory burst; it is markedly decreased under hypoxic conditions and in chronic granulomatous disease. Thyroid hormones are degraded by myeloperoxidase and H_2O_2[47]; studies with peroxidase inhibitors and with neutrophils that lack myeloperoxidase have not clearly implicated this enzyme, however.

Role In Vivo

The demonstration of iodination and T_4 degradation by phagocytes raises the question of their occurrence and role *in vivo*. Both are dependent on phagocytosis and therefore would be expected to affect iodine metabolism predominantly during infection. An increased turnover of thyroid hormones during acute infection has been observed in both animals[15] and man[55] Although increased degradation by neutrophils may be partly responsible, other mechanisms may also be involved. There is no evidence that significant *de novo* T_4 synthesis occurs in neutrophils during infection; it is possible that extensive iodination by phagocytes will limit the availability of iodide for T_4 synthesis by the thyroid gland, however. Iodide absorbed as such or released from the thyroid hormones may act as a component of the myeloperoxidase-H_2O_2-halide antimicrobial system of phagocytes.[43]

Insulin

Insulin binds to surface receptors on human granulocytes[22] and, to an even greater degree, monocytes.[9] The monocytes of insulin-resistant patients with obesity,[6] diabetes mellitus,[26] or acanthosis nigricans[41] bind less insulin than do normal cells owing to a decreased concentration of insulin receptors. There is a positive correlation in normal individuals between insulin binding to monocytes and rate of glucose disappearance after glucose or insulin injection.[7] Despite this association, studies of the effect of insulin on glucose metabolism by phagocytes have yielded conflicting results[9, 17] with either a stimulation or no effect reported in different studies. Insulin is degraded by granulocytes, possibly due to the action of glutathione-insulin transhydrogenase.[22] Glucagon also binds to human mononuclear leukocytes.[9, 26]

There have been a number of reports of granulocyte dysfunction in patients with diabetes mellitus. Granulocyte adherence, i.e., the ability of isolated granulocytes to adhere to nylon fiber columns, is impaired in poorly controlled diabetics, with some return of function observed when diabetic control is established.[5] Neutrophil chemotaxis is defective in many, but not all, patients with diabetes.[60] In some instances, the addition of insulin increases the chemotactic responsiveness of diabetic neutrophils. Observations on the phagocytic activity of human diabetic leukocytes have been conflicting, with some reports indicating normal and others depressed phagocytosis.[4] A phagocytic defect in patients with ketoacidosis has been reported[10] and a few reports of a microbicidal defect distinct from that of phagocytosis have appeared.[4, 79]

Estrogens

Estrogen induces a striking influx of eosinophils into the uterus of some experimental animals,[73] and the binding of estrogens by these cells, as well as by human endometrial eosinophils, is observed.[80] This association with uterine eosinophils may be related to the mode of action[81] or tissue degradation[42] of estrogens. Estradiol is oxidized by neutrophils and eosinophils during phagocytosis and is as a result firmly bound, presumably by covalent linkage to cellular components.[44, 49] Oxidation is dependent in part on peroxidase and H_2O_2.[44]

Androgens

In contrast to the male-female differences in erythrocyte levels that are attributed to androgen stimulation of erythropoiesis, there are no sex differences in leukocyte levels and androgen therapy generally does not change the leukocyte count. In patients with aplastic anemia who have granulocytopenia as well as anemia, androgens may elevate both erythrocytes and granulocytes by stimulating cell production in some cases. These effects are currently thought to be mediated by a direct effect of androgens on hematopoietic precursor cells.[75]

Catecholamines

Leukocytes have adrenergic receptors. The interaction of these receptors with circulating catecholamines influences both the destruction and the function of leukocytes. Leukocytosis occurs with stress or administration of either α or β adrenergic agents; the levels of neutrophils, monocytes, and lymphocytes increase.[23] Data are conflicting as to the specificity of this response since α or β blockade may or may not abrogate the response.[16, 20] Epinephrine or isoproterenol administration causes eosinopenia, a response blocked by propranolol.[64]

Phagocytosis and killing of bacteria are not influenced in a major way by catecholamines, although these agents are known to increase hexose monophosphate shunt activity and inhibit iodination.[46] The most important effects of catecholamines on leukocytes may be to elevate intracellular cyclic AMP (cAMP) levels and inhibit the secretion of lysosomal enzymes, an effect that may be particularly important in allergic diseases (see Ch. 25).

Prostaglandin and Thromboxane Synthesis

Arachidonic acid is oxidized by neutrophils[27] and mononuclear phagocytes[14] with the formation of highly reactive products, namely, prostaglandins and thromboxanes. Thromboxane generation by neutrophils and the formation of prostaglandins by mononuclear phagocytes are greatly increased by appropriate cell stimulation. Prostaglandins of the E series inhibit the proliferation of granulocyte-macrophage colony-forming stem cells, raising the possibility that prostaglandin production by mononuclear phagocytes may serve a negative feedback function by limiting stem cell proliferation.[52]

PLATELETS

Regulation of Production

Circulating blood platelets arise from marrow megakaryocytes that are themselves derived from more primitive hematopoietic stem cells. Platelet production is related to both the number of megakaryocytes and their mass. Megakaryocyte mass reflects the extent of nuclear endomitosis that results in the hyperdiploid (4N-64N) mature megakaryocyte. Alterations in platelet count lead to predictable changes in platelet production. With experimentally induced thrombocytopenia, platelet production increases and is associated with an increase in both megakaryocyte number and ploidy.[18, 34] With marrow stimulation, megakaryocyte cytoplasmic maturation is also accelerated and newly released platelets appear larger than normal (increased spreading) on peripheral blood films. With thrombocytosis induced by platelet hypertransfusion, the number and ploidy of megakaryocytes are reduced, and platelet formation falls.[18, 34] An inverse relationship is also normally found between the number of platelets in circulation and the size of marrow megakaryocytes.[36]

Many of these changes are mediated by a humoral factor(s), termed thrombopoietin.[35] Almost nothing is known about thrombopoietin, but clinical studies of disorders of platelet production suggest that more than one regulatory factor may be involved in platelet generation. Thus, in the thrombocytosis accompanying chronic inflammation and iron deficiency, there is a dissociation between the number of megakaryocytes (increased) and their mass (decreased). Although increased in number on smear, circulating platelets appear small.

Hormones and Platelet Number

There are no clearly defined relationships between various hormones and platelet numbers. If changes in the platelet count are observed with endocrine disorders, other causes should be sought. Although estrogens administered to animals in large doses may cause thrombocytopenia,[83] there is little evidence for similar effects in man, and the thrombocytopenia occasionally occurring at or before the time of menses is not known to be hormonally mediated. Glucocorticosteroids are often employed to treat immune-mediated thrombocytopenia, but the effects of these hormones are to interrupt platelet destruction and there appears to be no direct effect on platelet production.

Hormones and Platelet Function

Under normal circumstances, the platelet does not adhere to intact endothelial cells. The biochemistry governing these interactions is slowly becoming known. Cells of the vascular wall produce and release compounds of the prostaglandin series (prostacyclin; PgI$_2$) to prevent platelet adherence.[61] In the platelet itself, arachidonate is converted by the enzyme cyclo-oxygenase to unstable prostaglandin intermediates including PGG$_2$ and thromboxane A$_2$. These unstable factors promote platelet release and aggregation. Thus, it is believed that a delicate balance exists between platelet production of aggregating factors and normal vascular wall to inhibit such adherence. The balance of such reactions is believed to result in thrombus-free microvasculature. Further details of prostaglandin metabolism and the interactions of prostaglandins, platelet function, and endothelial cell interactions are presented in Ch. 21.

REFERENCES

1. Adamson, J. W.: Pharmacological stimulation of marrow function. *Clin. Haematol.* 7:555, 1978.
2. Adamson, J. W., et al.: The kidney and erythropoiesis. *Am. J. Med.* 44:725, 1968.
3. Baehner, R. L., and Johnston, R. B., Jr.: Monocyte function in children with neutropenia and chronic infections. *Blood* 40:31, 1972.
4. Bagdade, J. D.: Phagocytic and microbicidal function in diabetes mellitus. *Acta Endocrinol.* [Suppl.] (Kbh.) 83 (Suppl. 205):27, 1976.
5. Bagdade, J. D., et al.: Impaired granulocyte adherence. A reversible defect in host defense in patients with poorly controlled diabetes. *Diabetes* 27:677, 1978.
6. Bar, R. S., et al.: Fluctuations in the affinity and concentration of insulin receptors on circulating monocytes of obese patients. *J. Clin. Invest.* 58:1123, 1976.
7. Beck-Nielsen, H., and Pedersen, O.: Diurnal variation in insulin binding to human monocytes. *J. Clin. Endocrinol. Metabol.* 47:385, 1978.
8. Beeson, P. B., and Bass, D. A.: *The Eosinophil*. Philadelphia, W. B. Saunders Co., 1977.
9. Blecher, M., and Goldstein, S.: Hormone receptors. VI. On the nature of binding of glucagon and insulin to human circulating mononuclear leukocytes. *Mol. Cell. Endocrinol.* 8:301, 1977.
10. Bybee, J. D., and Rogers, D. E.: The phagocytic activity of polymorphonuclear leukocytes obtained from patients with diabetes mellitus. *J. Lab. Clin. Med.* 64:1, 1964.
11. Cline, M. J.: *The White Cell*. Cambridge, Harvard University Press, 1975.
12. Dale, D. C., et al.: Neutrophil releasing activity in plasma of normal human subjects injected with etiocholanolone. *Proc. Soc. Exp. Biol. Med.* 156:192, 1977.
13. Daughaday, W. H., et al.: Effect of endocrinopathies on blood. *Blood* 3:1342, 1948.
14. Davies, P., et al.: Synthesis and release of oxygenation products of arachidonic acid by mononuclear phagocytes in response to inflammatory stimuli. *Inflammation* 2:335, 1977.
15. DeRubertis, F. R., and Kosch, P. C.: Accelerated host metabolism of L-thyroxine during acute infection: role of the leukocyte and peripheral leukocytosis. *J. Clin. Endocrinol. Metabol.* 40:589, 1975.
16. Ernstrom, U.: Effects of alpha and beta receptor stimulation on the release of lymphocytes and granulocytes from the spleen. *Scand. J. Haematol.* 11:275, 1973.
17. Esmann, V.: The diabetic leukocyte. *Enzyme* 13:32, 1972.
18. Evatt, B. L., and Levin, J.: Measurement of thrombopoiesis in rabbits using ^{75}selenomethionine. *J. Clin. Invest.* 48:1615, 1969.
19. Fauci, A. S., et al.: Glucocorticosteroid therapy: mechanisms of action and clinical considerations. *Ann. Intern. Med.* 84:304, 1976.
20. French, E. B., et al.: Studies on adrenaline induced leukocytosis in normal man. II. The effect of α and β adrenergic blocking agents. *Br. J. Haematol.* 21:423, 1971.
21. Fried, W., et al.: Studies on the erythropoietic stimulating factor in the plasma of mice after receiving testosterone. *J. Lab. Clin. Med.* 68:947, 1966.
22. Fussganger, R. D., et al.: Binding and degradation of insulin by human peripheral granulocytes. Demonstration of specific receptors with high affinity. *J. Biol. Chem.* 251:2761, 1976.
23. Gader, A. M. A., et al.: The effect of adrenaline, noradrenaline, isoprenaline and salbutamol on the resting levels of white blood cells in man. *Scand. J. Haematol.* 14:5, 1975.
24. Gallin, J. I., et al.: Interaction of leukocyte chemotactic factors with the cell surface. *J. Clin. Invest.* 55:967, 1974.
25. Golde, D. W., and Cline, M. J.: Regulation of granulopoiesis. *N. Engl. J. Med.* 291:1388, 1974.
26. Goldstein, S., et al.: Hormone receptors. 5. Binding of glucagon and insulin to human circulating mononuclear cells in diabetes mellitus. *Endocrinol. Res. Commun.* 2:367, 1975.
27. Goldstein, I. M., et al.: Thromboxane generation by human peripheral blood polymorphonuclear leukocytes. *J. Exp. Med.* 148:787, 1978.
28. Goldwasser, E.: Erythropoietin and the differentiation of red blood cells. *Fed. Proc.* 34:2285, 1975.
29. Goldwasser, E., and Kung, C. K. Purification of erythropoietin. *Proc. Natl. Acad. Sci. USA* 68:697, 1971.
30. Gordon, A. S., et al.: Thyroid and blood regeneration in rat. *Am. J. Med. Sci.* 212:385, 1946.
31. Gordon, A. S., et al.: The kidney and erythropoiesis. *Semin. Hematol.* 4:337, 1967.
32. Gordon, A. S., et al.: The renal erythropoietic factor (REF). VII. Relation to sex steroid hormone effects on erythropoiesis. *Proc. Soc. Exp. Biol. Med.* 129:871, 1968.
33. Handin, R. I., et al.: Effect of corticosteroid therapy on the phagocytosis of antibody-coated platelets by human leukocytes. *Blood* 51:711, 1978.
34. Harker, L. A.: Kinetics of thrombopoiesis. *J. Clin. Invest.* 47:458, 1968.
35. Harker, L. A.: Regulation of thrombopoiesis. *Am. J. Physiol.* 218:1376, 1970.
36. Harker, L. A., and Finch, C. A.: Thrombokinetics in man. *J. Clin. Invest.* 48:963, 1969.
37. Hillman, R. S., and Finch, C. A.: *Red Cell Manual*. 4th ed. Philadelphia, F. A. Davis, 1974.
38. Horton, L., et al.: The haematology of hypothyroidism. *Q. J. Med.* 45:101, 1976.
39. Jepson, J. H., et al.: Erythropoietin excretion in a hypopituitary patient. Effects of testosterone and vasopressin. *Arch. Intern. Med.* 122:265, 1968.
40. Joyce, R. A., et al.: Corticosteroid effect on granulopoiesis in mice after cyclophosphamide. *J. Clin. Invest.* 60:277, 1977.
41. Kahn, C. R., et al.: The syndromes of insulin resistance and acanthosis nigricans. Insulin-receptor disorders in man. *N. Engl. J. Med.* 294:739, 1976.
42. Klebanoff, S. J.: Inactivation of estrogen by rat uterine preparations. *Endocrinology* 76:301, 1965.
43. Klebanoff, S. J.: Iodination of bacteria: a bactericidal mechanism. *J. Exp. Med.* 126:1063, 1967.
44. Klebanoff, S. J.: Estrogen binding by leukocytes during phagocytosis. *J. Exp. Med.* 145:983, 1977.
45. Klebanoff, S. J., and Clark, R. A.: Iodination by human polymorphonuclear leukocytes: a re-evaluation. *J. Lab. Clin. Med.* 89:675, 1977.
46. Klebanoff, S. J., and Clark, R. A.: *The Neutrophil: Function and Clinical Disorders*. New York, Elsevier-North Holland Publishing Co., 1978.
47. Klebanoff, S. J., and Green, W. L.: Degradation of thyroid hormones by phagocytosing human leukocytes. *J. Clin. Invest.* 52:60, 1973.
48. Klebanoff, S. J., and Hamon, C. B.: Role of myeloperoxidase-mediated antimicrobial systems in intact leukocytes. *J. Reticuloendothel. Soc.* 12:170, 1972.
49. Klebanoff, S. J., et al.: Functional studies on human peritoneal eosinophils. *Infect. Immun.* 17:167, 1977.
50. Krantz, S. B.: Diagnosis and treatment of pure red cell aplasia. *Med. Clin. North Am.* 60:945, 1976.
51. Krantz, S. B., and Jacobson, L. O.: *Erythropoietin and the Regulation of Erythropoiesis*. Chicago, University of Chicago Press, 1970.
52. Kurland, J. I., et al.: Limitation of excessive myelopoiesis by the intrinsic modulation of macrophage-derived prostaglandin E. *Science* 199:552, 1978.
53. Larsson, S. O.: Anemia and iron metabolism in hypothyroidism. *Acta Med. Scand.* 157:349, 1957.
54. Losito, A., et al.: The effect on polymorphonuclear leukocyte function of prednisolone and azathioprine *in vivo* and prednisolone, azathioprine and 6-mercaptopurine *in vitro*. *Clin. Exp. Immunol.* 32:423, 1978.
55. Lutz, J. H., et al.: Thyroxine binding proteins, free thyroxine and thyroxine turnover interrelationships during acute infectious illness in man. *J. Clin. Endocrinol. Metabol.* 35:230, 1972.
56. MacGregor, R. R.: Granulocyte adherence changes induced by hemodialysis, endotoxin, epinephrine and glucocorticoids. *Ann. Intern. Med.* 86:35, 1977.
57. Mahmoud, A. A. F., et al.: Eosinophilopoietin. *J. Clin. Invest.* 60:675, 1977.
58. Marks, P. A., and Rifkind, R. A.: Protein synthesis: its control in erythropoiesis. *Science* 175:955, 1972.

59. Miyake, T., et al.: Purification of human erythropoietin. *J. Biol. Chem. 252*:5558, 1977.

60. Molenaar, D. M., et al.: Leukocyte chemotaxis in diabetic patients and their nondiabetic first-degree relatives. *Diabetes 25* (Suppl. 2):880, 1976.

61. Moncada, S., et al.: Human arterial and venous tissues generate prostacyclin (prostaglandin X), a potent inhibitor of platelet aggregation. *Lancet 1*:18, 1977.

62. Motoyoshi, K., et al.: Purification and some properties of colony-stimulating factor from normal human urine. *Blood 52*:1012, 1978.

63. Murphy, P.: *The Neutrophil.* New York, Plenum Medical Book Co., 1976.

64. Ohman, J. L., et al.: Effect of propranolol on the eosinopenic responses of cortisol, isoproterenol and aminophylline. *J. Allergy Clin. Immunol. 50*:151, 1972.

65. Papayannopoulou, T., and Finch, C. A.: On the *in vivo* action of erythropoietin: a quantitative analysis. *J. Clin. Invest. 51*:1179, 1972.

66. Peschle, C., and Condorelli, M.: Biogenesis of erythropoietin: evidence for pro-erythropoietin in a subcellular fraction of kidney. *Science 190*:910, 1975.

67. Plotz, C. M., et al.: Natural history of Cushing's syndrome. *Am. J. Med. 13*:597, 1952.

68. Popovic, W. J., and Adamson, J. W.: Erythropoietin assay: present status of methods, pitfalls and results in polycythemic disorders. *CRC Crit. Rev. Clin. Lab. Sci. 10*:57, 1979.

69. Rifkind, R. A., and Marks, P. A.: The regulation of erythropoiesis. *Blood Cells 1*:417, 1975.

70. Rinehart, J. J., et al.: Effects of corticosteroids on human monocyte function. *N. Engl. J. Med. 292*:236, 1975.

71. Rubinow, S. I., and Lebowitz, J. L.: A mathematical model of neutrophil production and control in normal man. *J. Math. Biol. 1*:187, 1975.

72. Ruscetti, F. W., et al.: Specific release of neutrophilic and eosinophilic stimulating factors from sensitized lymphocytes. *Blood 47*:757, 1976.

73. Rytömma, T.: Organ distribution and histochemical properties of eosinophil granulocytes in the rat. *Acta Pathol. Microbiol. Scand. 50*(Suppl. 40):1, 1960.

74. Shattuck, R. K., et al.: Inhibition of diffusion chamber granulocytopoiesis by anti-CSF serum. *Proc. Soc. Exp. Biol. Med. 158*:542, 1978.

75. Singer J. W., et al.: Steroids and hematopoiesis. III. The response of granulocytes and erythroid colony-forming cells to steroids of different classes. *Blood 48*:855, 1976.

76. Stanley, E. R., et al.: Colony stimulating factor and regulation of granulopoiesis and macrophage production. *Fed. Proc. 34*:2272, 1975.

77. Stolc, V.: Stimulation of iodoproteins and thyroxine formation in human leukocytes by phagocytosis. *Biochem. Biophys. Res. Commun. 45*:159, 1971.

78. Stolc, V.: Release of monoiodotyrosine and iodoprotein from human leukocytes. *J. Clin. Endocrinol. Metabol. 37*:397, 1973.

79. Tan, C. V., et al.: Neutrophil dysfunction in diabetes mellitus. *J. Lab. Clin. Med. 85*:26, 1975.

80. Tchernitchin, A., et al.: Radioautographic study of human endometrium superfused with estradiol-17$^\beta$ estrone, estriol and progesterone. *J. Steroid Biochem. 4*:451, 1973.

81. Tchernitchin, A., et al.: Correlation of estrogen-induced uterine eosinophilia with other parameters of estrogen stimulation, produced with estradiol-17$^\beta$ and estriol. *Experientia 31*:993, 1975.

82. Tudhope, G. R.: Endocrine disease. *Clin. Haematol. 1*:475, 1972.

83. Tyslowitz, R., and Dingemanse, E.: Effect of large doses of estrogens on blood picture of dogs. *Endocrinology 29*:817, 1941.

84. Woeber, K. A.: L-Triiodothyronine and L-reverse-triiodothyronine generation in human polymorphonuclear leukocyte. *J. Clin. Invest. 62*:577, 1978.

85. Woeber, K. A., and Ingbar, S. H.: Metabolism of L-thyroxine by phagocytosing human leukocytes. *J. Clin. Invest. 52*:1796, 1973.

CHAPTER 25

Allergy, Immunology, and Hormones

By Paul P. VanArsdel, Jr.

The disciplines of endocrinology and immunology interact, in one way or another, in practically all the organ systems of the body. This chapter will cover only the highlights of this interaction, giving priority to that material not likely to be emphasized elsewhere in this book.

NATURE OF THE IMMUNE RESPONSE

Lymphocyte Classes

Immunologically uncommitted lymphocyte stem cells are produced in large numbers by the bone marrow. There are two major pathways for development of these cells into immunologically competent lymphocytes. One pathway involves obligatory processing by the thymus gland. Most cells that reach the thymus develop into short-lived lymphocytes (thymocytes) that have no known immunologic function. A few, under the influence of antigen, become long-lived, immunologically competent recirculating lymphocytes (T cells) that are responsible for cell-mediated immunity (CMI).

The other pathway involves the development of lymphocytes capable of responding to antigen with the production of humoral antibodies. In fowl, the bursa of Fabricius is the central organ corresponding to the thymus responsible for programming lymphocytes for antibody production. No homologous organ exists in mammals; functionally, a bursal equivalent almost certainly exists, and the processed lymphocytes — precursors of plasma cells in lymphoid germinal centers — are called B cells. T and B cells are differentiated by function rather than by morphology. T cells predominate in peripheral blood, lymph nodes, and thymus; B cells predominate in the bone marrow. The cells are about equal in number in the spleen and tonsils. B cells differentiate into five different classes. Each class, following antigen stimulation, forms a clone of plasma cells in germinal centers that synthesizes antibodies of one immunoglobulin (Ig) class. In descending order of concentration in the circulation, the immunoglobulin classes are IgG, IgA, IgM, IgD, and IgE. The normal concentration of IgG is at least 40,000 times greater than IgE. The most important synthesis of IgA occurs in gut- and respiratory-associated lymphoid tissue, where it is secreted as a dimer into the lumen of the organ rather than into the blood.

The T-cell system also functions to regulate the response of B cells to antigen. One T-cell subpopulation ("helper" cells) must interact with B cells and most antigens before the B cells can develop into specific antibody-producing cells. The only T cell–independent antigens are large polymers with identical repeating units that cause primarily an IgM response. Another T-cell subpopulation inhibits the B-cell response to antigen. These are called "suppressor" cells.

A third class of lymphocytes has neither B nor T markers. Some of these cells have an antibody-dependent cytotoxic function and have been termed K ("killer") cells.

Human lymphocyte classification is becoming steadily more complex as further subpopulations are identified. See reference 3 for a recent review of the subject.

Immunodeficiency States

Much of the knowledge concerning the immune response in man has come from the study of patients in whom the potential for such a response is deficient. Immunodeficiencies fall into three general categories: (1) low immunoglobulin levels and no antibody response to antigen stimulation (B-cell defect); (2) absence of cell-mediated immunity (T-cell defect); and (3) severe combined immunodeficiency (possible stem-cell defect). The first category is heterogeneous and includes congenital X-linked agammaglobulinemia, selective Ig deficiencies, and sporadic or common variable immunodeficiency. The last is also heterogeneous. One subgroup does not appear to have a primary B-cell defect. Instead, antibody synthesis is inhibited by excessive activity of suppressor T cells. Glucocorticoid therapy will cause an increase in immunoglobulin production and antibody formation. The explanation for this paradox is that the suppressor T lymphocytes are much more sensitive to glucocorticoids than the other populations.[33] In the second category is a condition of special interest to the endocrinologist, congenital thymic aplasia (DiGeorge syndrome). Infants with this condition soon succumb to overwhelming bacterial, viral, or fungal infections despite normal antibody responses. The defect is caused by failure of development of the entodermal derivatives of the 3rd and 4th pharyngeal pouches from which the parathyroid glands also develop. Thus hypoparathyroidism is part of the syndrome, and neonatal tetany is the 1st diagnostic clue.[12]

Endocrine Function of the Thymus

Cell-free thymus extracts produce lymphocytopoiesis when injected into animals of the same or different species. In 1964, Osoba and Miller reported that the immunologic capacity of thymectomized animals was partially restored by thymus grafts enclosed in an implanted millipore chamber, suggesting that a secreted humoral factor was responsible.[15] Since then, several factors have been identified and four, each the product of a different group of investigators, have been studied extensively. *Thymic Humoral Factor* (THF), prepared from fresh calf thymus, is a polypeptide with 31 amino acid residues and a molecular weight (MW) of 3220 daltons. It has been reported to activate adenylate cyclase and increase cyclic AMP (cAMP) concentrations in thymocytes and spleen cells.[29]

Thymosin has been partially purified to a group of biologically active peptides (Fraction 5) with the most active (Thymosin α_1) having a MW of 3108. In contrast to THF, Fraction 5 produces an increase in thymocyte cGMP but not cAMP.[9]

Thymopoietin is a somewhat larger polypeptide hormone with a defined amino acid sequence (MW 5562). It is secreted by thymus epithelial cells and induces differentiation of precursor lymphoid cells to thymocytes.[30] Formerly called "Thymin," thymopoietin, in inducing T-cell differentiation also enhances cAMP generation. Thymopoietin is unique among the thymic humoral factors in blocking neuromuscular transmission, but it is doubtful that this action is clinically significant (ie., in the pathogenesis of myasthenia gravis).

In contrast to the others, which are extracted from calf thymus, *Thymic Factor* (TF) is extracted from defibrinated pig blood and has also been identified in the circulation of other species — including man. It also is thought to be secreted by thymus epithelial cells and has a MW of about 1000.[2] This factor appears to stimulate intrathymic differentiation of T cells and the later stages of T-cell maturation.

There is little doubt now that the thymus produces substances that are true hormones, being secreted into the circulation and exerting their effects on remote tissues. Circulating levels of one or more of these substances have been found to decline gradually with age in normals and to be low or absent in severe combined immunodeficiency, the DiGeorge syndrome, post-thymectomy states, systemic

lupus erythematosus, some malignancies, and perhaps bronchial asthma. Active clinical trials are now under way to observe the effect of treatment of immunodeficiency states, autoimmune diseases, malignancies, and even asthama with these substances. The most encouraging clinical results have been in the children with primary thymic deficiency, as in the DiGeorge syndrome. When lymphocyte precursor cells are absent, as in severe combined immunodeficiency, the thymic preparations have had no effect.

Influence of Conventional Hormones on the Immune Response

It is likely that any endocrine system that influences cell growth and metabolism will exert a modest, nonspecific effect on the cell proliferation and protein synthesis involved in CMI and antibody production. Thus, only the more specific and better-known effects will be presented here.

Growth hormone (GH) is required for the normal development of the thymus-dependent immune system in lower mammals. That this represents a specific thymotropic effect is supported by several observations summarized by Pierpaoli and coworkers.[20] Of particular interest is their observation that the pituitaries of neonatally thymectomized mice have enlarged, degranulated acidophilic cells, suggesting a specific interrelationship. GH also stimulates thymocytes *in vitro*.[16] Other studies indicate a possible alteration of immune reactions by hypo- or hyperthyroidism but were not designed to rule out alterations in tissue reaction to the immune response rather than in the response itself.

There is no known human counterpart of the previous observations. Specifically, pituitary or thyroid deficiencies are not associated with any significant deficiency in the immune response.

Sex differences in the occurrence of allergic and immunologic diseases have long been recognized. Asthma occurs in boys about twice as often as in girls, but no immunologic reason has been identified for this difference nor for the reversal in the sex incidence ratio in adult asthmatic patients. Certain autoimmune diseases, such as systemic lupus erythematosus, occur more commonly in women of childbearing age than in others. This association has been reproduced experimentally in the well-known NZB/NZW mouse model for lupus nephritis. Estrogens increase the production of anti-DNA antibodies and the progression of nephritis, whereas androgens have the opposite effect.

Mention should also be made of the effect of androgen, specifically 19-nortestosterone, on the developing chick embryo. This hormone prevents the development of the bursa of Fabricius and, thus, humoral immunity; the thymus is unaffected.[26] This is a well-known model for the study of humoral immunity, but there is no evidence for a comparable, androgenic effect in humans.

Glucocorticosteroids have received by far the greatest amount of attention, clinically and experimentally. Very little of this attention has been devoted to the influence of normal adrenocortical activity on the immune response, although there is some evidence that the development of the lymphoid system is impaired by the absence of the adrenal cortex. On the other hand, an extensive and confusing literature exists regarding the inhibitory effect of pharmacologic doses of glucocorticoids ("steroids") on lymphocytes and the immune response. The confusion is due partly to marked species differences in sensitivity to steroids and partly to the difference in steroid sensitivity of the several stages of lymphocyte development. In sensitive species, such as the mouse, rat, and rabbit, steroids produce marked lysis of the short-lived cells of the thymic cortex and of those B lymphocytes that have not yet been activated by antigen. Humoral antibody response can be inhibited by steroid administration in these species. Once either the T or B cells have been activated by antigen, however, they become steroid-resistant. In other species, including man, steroids have essentially no effect on the immune response at any step. Even though they can produce peripheral lymphopenia in humans and reduction in thymus size in infants, this effect is immunologically insignificant. A possible exception can be found in the immune hematologic reactions. For example, a high glucocorticoid dose does cause a reduction of bone marrow synthesis of IgG antibody during treatment of immune thrombocytopenia, but this is only one of at least three ways by which the drug causes a decrease in cell destruction in this condition (see later). One must look to the inflammatory and other host responses to most allergic events in man to identify significant steroid effects.[25]

MEDIATORS OF IMMUNOLOGIC TISSUE INJURY

When a sensitized individual is exposed to antigen, the resulting reaction develops in one of several characteristic patterns that differ in their immunologic mechanisms. These patterns have been classified by Coombs and Gell[4] into four general types. Although this classification has certain imperfections, it is convenient, widely used, and sufficient for this discussion.

Type I: anaphylactic and atopic reactions. These are initiated by antigen reacting with antibody that has a strong affinity for basophils and tissue mast cells and that generally is of the immunoglobulin E (IgE) class.

Type II: cytotoxic reactions. These occur when IgG or IgM antibody reacts with antigen that is part of, or closely associated with, cells or other tissue elements.

Type III: Arthus-type or immune complex reactions. In these, antigen reacts with antibody (usually IgG) in the fluid phase; the deposition of these complexes leads to tissue injury.

Type IV: tuberculin-type or cell-mediated reactions.

The activity of vasoactive mediators is of paramount importance in the development of Type I reactions, in which the antigen-antibody reaction triggers mediator release from mast cells and basophils; this amplification step permits very minute amounts of antigen and antibody to initiate what may be major clinical reactions.[1] The most two important mediators for producing symptoms in man are histamine and slow-reacting substance of anaphylaxis (SRS-A).*

Histamine

Histamine, the best known and most extensively studied of the autacoids or paracrine hormones, is formed by the enzymic decarboxylation of histidine in mast cells and basophils and is stored within their granules, where it is biologically inert. When antigen and antibody react on the cell surface, a series of calcium-dependent enzymic

steps is activated, leading to the active release of histamine by exocytosis. The released histamine is then metabolized rapidly by oxidative deamination and conjugation and excreted in the urine.[32] The cells are not damaged by the process and proceed to resynthesize their histamine stores. Of course, if damaged by other means, they would also release histamine.

In the short time between release and destruction, histamine causes an increase in vascular permeability associated with constriction of postcapillary venules, vasodilatation, contraction of bronchial and visceral smooth muscle, and stimulation of mucus glands. It can produce the characteristic clinical features of atopic diseases in man, such as urticaria, bronchospasm, rhinitis, and anaphylaxis. These allergic reactions represent the effect of histamine on H_1 receptors, by and large, though some H_2 receptor stimulation may also be involved. H_2 receptors are those involved in the histamine stimulation of gastric acid secretion and cardiac activity. They also are present on human mast cells and basophils — where they apparently aid in self-regulation, because their stimulation by histamine *inhibits* histamine release.

Slow-Reacting Substance of Anaphylaxis

This mediator is an acidic sulfate ester or esters of unknown chemical structure and a MW of about 500 daltons. It is not stored in the mast cell but is synthesized and released from the cell after antigen contact. It is a potent stimulator of bronchial smooth muscle contraction and may have some effect on vascular permeability as well. The response of smooth muscle to this mediator is slower than that to histamine, hence the name. It is not a prostaglandin but is derived from the same precursor, arachidonic acid.[17] The lack of any significant response in most asthmatic patients to antihistaminic drugs lends further support for the concept that SRS-A is the major mediator in asthma.

Eosinophil Chemotactic Factor of Anaphylaxis

Two factors have been identified. They are tetrapeptides with the structure Ala/Val-Gly-Ser-Glu and a MW of about 400 daltons. They exist preformed in human lung mast cells and, after antigen-induced release, are selective chemoattractants for eosinophils. This may be an important homeostatic mechanism, because eosinophils inactivate histamine and SRS-A.

Other Factors in Type I Reactions

A platelet activating factor(s) along with SRS-A is produced from an unknown substrate and secreted in response to antigen. It has a MW of about 1100 daltons. It activates platelets to produce their own mediators, but its clinical significance is unknown. The same statement applies to the release of substances such as kinin-generating and other enzymes, heparin, and a neutrophil chemotactic factor. Complement is not involved in Type I reactions.

Mediators in Other Classes of Reactions

Complement is involved in the genesis of Type II and III reactions. Hormonal mediators are not responsible for cellular injury in Type II reactions, such as autoimmune

---

*Serotonin, a mediator in certain lower animals, has no such function in man.

hemolytic anemia, or thrombocytopenic purpura. The contact of antibody with the antigenic cell surface sets off a complement activation cascade (C1qrs-4-2-3-5-6-7-8-9) that, if it proceeds all the way, causes intravascular cell lysis. This is rare *in vivo*. It is only necessary for the reaction to proceed to the C3 stage for cellular damage to occur. When C3 is activated, one product — C3b — binds to the cell membrane. Macrophages in the reticuloendothelial system have C3b and immunoglobulin receptors and will remove the affected cells by phagocytosis.

In Type III reactions the antigen-antibody complexes fix and activate complement and, if they are soluble, may cause diffuse tissue injury. The activation of complement produces cleavage products C3a and C5a ("anaphylatoxins") that release histamine. In addition, C5a is a chemoattractant for phagocytic cells, which are ultimately responsible for the tissue injury.

Kinins

An extensive literature has accumulated regarding the so-called "kinin hormones." These are specific basic peptides produced by the action of glandular or plasma enzymes (kallikreins) on certain α globulins (kininogens). The major plasma kinin is bradykinin, a nonapeptide with potent physiologic effects: smooth muscle stimulation, vasodilatation, increase in vascular permeability, and pain production.[23] Such effects indicate that the kinins may be important mediators of hypersensitivity reactions; in fact, kinin activation does occur with certain antigen-antibody reactions in experimental animals and, in a few instances, in man. Kinin generation can be produced nonspecifically by any stimulus, however, including tissue injury, that activates Hageman factor. There is still little evidence, other than the recent observation that some kallikrein activity is released from mast cells after exposure to antigen, that kinin generation is anything more than a secondary phenomenon.

Prostaglandins

Prostaglandins (PG's) may play some role in allergic reactions, particularly in the lung, which is a very active metabolic organ in the synthesis and inactivation of these ubiquitous lipids. When a sensitized lung is challenged with specific antigen, PG's are released along with their precursors: thromboxanes and endoperoxides. Prostaglandin $F_{2\alpha}$ (PGF$_{2\alpha}$) and thromboxane A_2 are potent smooth muscle contracting agents.[13] When inhaled by an asthmatic subject, PGF$_{2\alpha}$ produces bronchoconstriction. Since PG synthesis and release can follow several nonspecific stimuli, including the administration of histamine and SRS-A, the PG's are classified with the kinins as secondary mediators; their role in the pathogenesis of allergic reactions, particularly asthma, is questionable. The regulating effect of PG's with a bronchodilating action, PGE, and perhaps PGI$_2$ (prostacyclin) may turn out to be important, however. The following evidence to support this concept is tenuous but intriguing. A small subset of asthmatic patients will develop an asthmatic reaction (that may be life-threatening) after taking aspirin. They react also to indomethacin, which is not a similar drug in an immunochemical sense. The problem also exists with two or three other nonsteroidal anti-inflammatory drugs. These offending drugs have one important property in common: inhibition of cyclooxygenase activity and, thus,

prostaglandin synthesis. Furthermore, the inhibition of PG synthesis may cause a diversion of arachidonic acid metabolism to SRS-A production.[17] There is no explanation as to why only a small proportion of asthmatic patients have this problem, however.

Lymphokines

Type IV reactions involve immunologically committed lymphocytes rather than antibodies. Processes that lead to tissue injury are initiated by substances that are produced by the lymphocytes on exposure to antigen. If one can accept the concept that the lymphoid tissue is an endocrine organ, then these macromolecules can be considered paracrine hormones along with the small MW mediators discussed earlier. Some mediators promote inflammation by (1) macrophage and leukocyte chemotaxis, (2) migration inhibition of macrophages and leukocytes, or (3) direct cell killing. Others include a factor mitogenic for other lymphocytes, an osteoclast stimulating factor, and interferon. Although purification and chemical characterization of lymphokines has not proceeded very far, some information about the main human lymphokines is now available.[5]

	MW
Chemotactic factor	*12,500*
Macrophage migration inhibition factor (MIF)	*25,000*
Neutrophil inhibition factor (LIF)	*68,000*
Lymphotoxin (LT)	*90,000*

INFLUENCE OF THE ENDOCRINE SYSTEM ON THE EXPRESSION OF ALLERGIC AND IMMUNOLOGIC REACTIONS

Acetylcholine and Epinephrine

The autonomic nervous system has a major regulator role in enhancing or antagonizing physiologic changes in the skin, mucous membranes, and bronchi that are characteristic of Type I reactions. For example, acetylcholine can aggravate bronchospasm through psychogenic or nonspecific reflex pathways. It is not a specific mediator of antigen-antibody reactions, however, and thus was not included in the discussion of mediators in the previous section. It probably exerts its effect by stimulating guanylate cyclase, which causes an increase in intracellular cGMP concentration. This change would promote constriction of bronchial smooth muscle directly and also indirectly by enhancing antigen-induced mediator release from mast cells. Epinephrine has the opposite effect on Type I reactions. It is a pharmacologic, or nonspecific, antagonist of histamine and other mediators. By its α-adrenergic action, it is a vasoconstrictor, and by its β-adrenergic action, it is a bronchodilator. It also inhibits antigen-induced release of histamine and SRS-A from sensitized tissues.[31] This inhibition is shared by all agents known to increase the intracellular concentration of cAMP by activation of the enzyme adenylate cyclase. This is a β-adrenergic effect and may be an important part of the therapeutic action of epinephrine in treating reactions such as anaphylaxis. The eosinopenia produced by epinephrine also appears to be a β-adrenergic effect, since it is blocked by a β-adrenergic blocking drug, propranolol.[11] Some patients with asthma and eosinophilia suffer from a relative resistance to endogenous epinephrine, and this may be due to "intrinsic β-adrenergic blockade."[27]

Adrenal Glucocorticoids

In contrast to the lack of substantial effect on antibody production or antigen-antibody interaction, these steroids in pharmacologic doses can reduce substantially the physiologic abnormalities and other signs of tissue injury that are the consequences of hypersensitivity reactions. Extensive clinical observations have established their efficacy in such widely divergent conditions as asthma, serum sickness, and transplant rejection. Fundamental knowledge regarding the mechanisms involved, however, has lagged far behind the accumulation of empirical clinical observations.

The response of Type I reactions to steroid treatment is least well understood. In animals given steroids, the tissue histamine content is diminished, and mast cell synthesis of new histamine following histamine release is inhibited. This is not a significant effect in man, however. During steroid therapy, the typical wheal-and-flare response to an antigen skin test is not altered, indicating in addition that histamine release is not inhibited. When an asthmatic patient inhales an antigen to which he is sensitive, significant bronchospasm develops in a few minutes. After recovery, some individuals develop a second reaction several hours later. Prior steroid administration has been found to inhibit the second reaction —but not the first.[19] The capacity of steroids to produce vasoconstriction and reduce exudation of fluid may play some role in blocking the late asthmatic reaction (as well as having a modest antianaphylactic effect), but this is speculative. In chronic asthma the apparent resistance to β-adrenergic drug action can be diminished by steroid therapy, but the mechanism is not understood.[31] Since blood and tissue eosinophilia is so characteristic of type I hypersensitivity, one might expect some explanation from the eosinopenic effect of steroids. Even this effect is not completely understood, however. It seems to involve decreased marrow release and increased sequestration in some unknown compartment,[10] but such information does not help to explain the therapeutic action of glucocorticoids.

More is known about the action of steroids on other types of hypersensitivity. As mentioned earlier, steroid treatment does cause some reduction in antibody concentration in hematologic reactions, but other actions may be more important therapeutically — namely, elution of antibody off the cell membrane and suppressing the macrophage clearance function.[25]

The inflammation of Type III conditions (serum sickness, systemic lupus erythematosus, certain forms of vasculitis, and other idiopathic diseases collectively referred to as "antigen-antibody complex diseases") can be reduced by steroids via the permeability effect mentioned earlier or, probably more important, by reducing the rate of extrusion of lysosomal contents by neutrophils and macrophages either directly or by reducing their responsiveness to chemotactic factors and, consequently, their accumulation at sites of inflammation.

The inhibitory effect of steroids on Type IV reactions probably involves some of the anti-inflammatory actions mentioned earlier. Also the activity of lymphocyte-derived chemotactic factor and migration inhibition factor is diminished. The reduction in macrophage accumulation means that less antigen is processed to interact with the sensitive lymphocyte, and, either because of this or as a direct steroid action, lymphocyte proliferation is suppressed. The activity of lymphotoxin is also inhibited.[6]

Other Hormones

It has long been known that if a patient with Addison's disease happens to develop asthma, the asthma may be severe and difficult to control. Theoretically, the problem should be greater in those with loss of both the adrenal medulla and the cortex. Bilateral adrenalectomy produces no signs of catecholamine deficiency in nonasthmatic patients, but what would happen in asthmatics is apparently not known. Asthmatic patients, in general, have normal pituitary-adrenal function regardless of the severity of their problem, unless they have been given chronic glucocorticoid therapy.

Thyrotoxicosis also may cause coexisting asthma to be difficult to manage, and restoration of the euthyroid state should ameliorate the asthma problem. There have been several reasons proposed. Increased oxygen demand is one. Depletion of the substrate for cAMP production is another, but cAMP levels are usually high in tissues of hyperthyroid subjects, which should be beneficial. Catecholamine depletion and an increased rate of glucocorticoid degradation have also been raised as possibilities. None provides an adequate explanation, however.[22] Chronic urticaria is also more difficult to control in hyperthyroid patients, and a similar association is suspected between asthma and hyperparathyroidism.

Despite the disease associations with gender mentioned before, there is no evidence that increasing or reducing sex hormone levels has any significant value in treatment of asthma or autoimmune disorders. There is one condition, though, in which hormone treatment has proved valuable. Hereditary angioedema, though not strictly speaking an immunologic disease, has similar manifestations. It is characterized by recurrent episodes of cutaneous or mucous membrane edema and can cause fatal upper airway obstruction. The disease is caused by a deficiency in the activity of a normal inhibitor of the activated first complement component ($\overline{C1}$ or C1 esterase) and is inherited as an autosomal dominant trait. The edema is the result of unregulated activation of later components (C4 and 2) and the generation of vasoactive kinin-like products of these components. In the process, C4 and C2 become depleted, and the reaction subsides. Methyltestosterone treatment had been used for many years with some success in reducing the number of recurrences, but, perhaps because the reason for its use was unclear, it received little attention. Recently this drug and two impeded androgens, oxymethalone and danazol, have been subjected to systematic trials in which serial measurements of the $\overline{C1}$ inhibitor and C4 serum levels were carried out. In addition to unequivocal clinical effectiveness, androgen treatment also causes a return of the low serum levels to normal. It appears, then, that this is a clinically unique example of hormones that seem to act by preventing a genetically determined suppression of normal protein synthesis.[24]

ALLERGIC AND IMMUNOLOGIC REACTIONS TO HORMONES

All the polypeptide hormones can, of themselves, induce an antibody response, and this effect is utilized widely for the preparation of reagents for immunoassay (see later). Protein contaminants of greater size are responsible for most allergic reactions, however, which are usually Type

I, characterized by urticaria and, rarely, anaphylactic shock following hormone injection or by allergic rhinitis and asthma following inhalation of posterior pituitary powder for treatment of diabetes insipidus. Occasionally, sensitivity to posterior pituitary snuff has been manifested by a form of infiltrative lung disease that is associated with precipitating antibodies and thus presumably a Type III reaction.[18] The risk of allergic reactions makes prior skin testing advisable before injecting a hormone such as bovine ACTH. Synthetic corticotropin (Cosyntropin), on the other hand, rarely if ever produces allergic reactions and is now the agent of choice for diagnostic testing. Similarly, synthetic lysine vasopressin (VP) has largely supplanted posterior pituitary powder for nasal administration and has produced very few allergic reactions.

The situation with insulin is considerably more complex. Probably all persons given insulin respond with the production of an insulin-binding antibody, usually of the IgG class. A small proportion of diabetics produce sufficient antibody to be markedly insulin resistant; as the insulin dose is increased, the antibody titer is likely to rise even further.[21] In some instances, antibodies to insulin lack species specificity, reacting not only with bovine insulin but also with all other insulins, including desalinated pork and even human insulin, rendering management extremely difficult. Tissue injury, such as vasculitis or glomerulitis, produced by circulating antibody-insulin complexes is surprisingly rare. Faulk and coworkers[7] have described one insulin-resistant patient with hepatosplenomegaly and a Coombs' test–positive hemolytic anemia due to insulin-antibody complexes, but other stigmata of vasculitis or serum sickness were lacking.

Insulin allergy has little if any relationship to insulin resistance. Except for local erythema and induration, allergy is extremely rare in patients maintained on continuous insulin treatment. Reactions are most likely to occur after a lapse in treatment and are characterized usually by urticaria, occasionally by anaphylactic shock. As expected in Type I reactions, the antibody is of the IgE class. Reactions may occur to protein contaminants or to large MW insulin polymers, but even pure insulin, though only weakly immunogenic, can produce allergic reactions in sensitive patients — a few IgE-mediated reactions have even been reported from human insulin. Pork insulin, having the same structure as human insulin, is less immunogenic than beef insulin. When "single peak" insulins became available, it was hoped that the incidence of allergic reactions would diminish. There is as yet, however, insufficient data on this point.

For patients with systemic or large local reactions to beef-pork insulin one should attempt treatment with single peak pork insulin. If this fails, a trial of highly purified "single component" pork insulin may be successful. This is available from the manufacturer as an investigational new drug.* If that is unsuccessful and alternative treatment is inadequate, then desensitization will be necessary and is usually successful. Desensitization kits with detailed instructions are available from the manufacturer.[8]

Some late-onset local erythema and induration reactions may be IgG-mediated, cell-mediated, or perhaps both. Even insulin-induced lipoatrophy may be allergic. The evidence is that atrophy occurs much less often after single component insulin injections than with the older

products and can be prevented by injecting a small amount (e.g., 0.1 mg) of dexamethasone, which is compatible with insulin in solution.[8]

Allergic reactions to nonpeptide hormones seldom occur. Steroids, for example, are nonimmunogenic in the laboratory unless chemically coupled to carrier protein by reactions that do not occur in vivo. Although at least one convincing case of glucocorticoid-induced anaphylaxis has been reported,[14] practically all reports of steroid allergy are anecdotal and have not been confirmed. The same can be said of the so-called "endogenous steroid allergy" proposed as a cause of cyclic urticaria and other skin reactions in women in scattered reports over half a century.

ANTIBODIES AS HORMONE ASSAY REAGENTS

The development and application of immunoassay for the measurement of hormones in biologic fluids has expanded rapidly over the last decade and is becoming a specialty in itself, quite distinct conceptually from the role of immune mechanisms in disease with which this chapter is primarily concerned. Most of the human peptide hormones will produce specific antibody without special preparation when injected into lower animals. The larger their MW, the greater the antibody response; generally, peptides with a MW less than 5,000 are weak immunogens and may need to be conjugated to a carrier protein to produce a satisfactory antibody response. There are exceptions; satisfactory antisera can be produced to unconjugated vasopressin and gastrin if these are injected with complete adjuvant.

To be immunogenic, all nonpeptide hormones, as well as certain small MW peptides, must be conjugated to an appropriate carrier protein (such as human albumin) and thus act as haptens. Effective conjugation involves the formation of a strong covalent bond. Such a reaction between hormones and protein does not occur naturally.* Conjugation requires synthetic manipulations involving the use of activating chemicals. Agents such as the carbodiimides activate carboxyl groups to form a CO-NH bond. Others, such as the diisocyanates, link two amino groups.

Optimal conditions for antibody production vary widely from one hormone to another relative to species used, mode of administration, and duration of immunization. Within a species, some animals are better antibody producers than others, and a dozen or more may need to be immunized to ensure at least one source of high-titered, high-affinity antibody.

Because of the low concentration and small MW of the hormones, conventional methods of measuring antigen-antibody reactions, such as precipitation of agar, cannot be used for hormone assay. Of numerous methods tried, radioimmunoassay is the most sensitive and can be adapted to assays of all hormones that are available in chemically pure form and that can be labeled with a radioisotope. Standard amounts of antibody and labeled hormone are mixed with the material to be tested. The more unlabeled hormone in the test material, the less labeled hormone is bound to the antibody. This method, then, is a special application of competitive protein-binding assays in which the sensitivity can be very high, because the af-

---

*It was released by the Food and Drug Administration for general use after this chapter was written.

*As mentioned earlier, this fact makes the whole concept of autoimmunity to such hormones as the steroids very tenuous.

finity of specific antibody for a hormone is usually much higher than the affinity of natural hormone-binding serum proteins. A critical step in the procedure is the separation of the radiolabeled hormone bound to antibody from free radiolabeled hormone. In many applications, free hormone can be separated by solid adsorbents such as dextran-treated charcoal. Separation can also be achieved by electrophoresis, by affixing antibody to solids such as agarose beads or the surface of plastic tubes, or by precipitating antigen-antibody complexes with an appropriate anti-immunoglobulin serum (the "double antibody" method).

The lower the concentration of antibody and labeled hormone that can be used in the assay, the greater the sensitivity of the method. Thus the specific activity of the radioisotope label and the binding affinity of the antibody should be as high as possible. Sufficient sensitivity can now be achieved with good reagents to measure hormone concentrations of only a few pg/ml.

Hardly a hormone exists that cannot now be measured by immunoassay. A list of several dozen was presented by Dr. Rosalyn Yalow in her recent Nobel address, and it is by no means complete.[34] The few exceptions are substances such as lymphokines and SRS-A that have not been fully characterized and purified. Detailed methods for assaying hormones and other substances, and clinical applications, can be found in the recent publication by Thorell and Larson.[28]

REFERENCES

1. Austen, K. F.: The chemical mediators of immediate hypersensitivity reactions, In *Immunological Diseases*. 3rd ed. Samter, M. (ed.), Boston, Little, Brown, 1978. Ch. 10.
2. Bach, J-F., and Carnaud, C.: Thymic factors. *Prog. Allergy* 21:342, 1976.
3. Chess, L., and Schlossman, S. F.: Human lymphocyte subpopulations. *Adv. Immunol.* 25:213, 1977.
4. Coombs, R. R. A., and Gell, P. G. H.: Classification of allergic reactions responsible for clinical hypersensitivity and disease. In *Clinical Aspects of Immunology*, 3rd ed. Gell, P. G. H., and Coombs, R. R. A. (eds.), Philadelphia, F. A. Davis Co., 1975, Ch. 25.
5. David, J. R., and Rocklin, R. E.: Lymphocyte mediators: The "lymphokines," In *Immunological Diseases*, 3rd ed. Samter, M. (ed.), Boston, Little Brown, 1978, Ch. 16.
6. Fauci, A. S., Dale, D. C., et al.: Glucocorticosteroid therapy: Mechanisms of action and clinical considerations. *Ann. Intern. Med.* 84:304, 1976.
7. Faulk, W. P., Tomsovic, E. J., et al.: Insulin resistance in juvenile diabetes mellitus. *Am. J. Med.* 49:133, 1970.
8. Galloway, J. A., and Bressler, R.: Insulin treatment in diabetes. *Med. Clin. North Am.* 62:663, 1978.
9. Goldstein, A. L.: Thymosin: Basic properties and clinical potential in the treatment of patients with immunodeficiency diseases and cancer. *Antibiot. Chemother.* 24:47, 1978.
10. Honsinger, R. W., Jr., Silverstein, D., et al.: The eosinophil and allergy: Why? *J. Allergy Clin. Immunol.* 49:142, 1972.
11. Koch-Weser, J.: Beta-adrenergic blockade and circulating eosinophils. *Arch. Intern. Med.* 121:255, 1968.
12. Kretschmer, R., Say B., et al.: Congenital aplasia of the thymus gland (DiGeorge's syndrome). *N. Engl. J. Med.* 279:1295, 1968.
13. Mathé, A. A.: Prostaglandins and the lung. *Prostaglandins* 3:169, 1977.
14. Mendelson, L. M., Meltzer, E. O., et al.: Anaphylaxis-like reactions to corticosteroid therapy. *J. Allergy Clin. Immunol.* 54:125, 1974.
15. Osoba, D., and Miller, J. F. A. P.: The lymphoid tissues and immune responses of neonatally thymectomized mice bearing thymus tissue in millipore diffusion chambers. *J. Exp. Med.* 119:117, 1964.
16. Pandian, M. R., and Talwar, G. P.: Effect of growth hormone on the metabolism of thymus and on the immune response against sheep erythrocytes. *J. Exp. Med.* 134:1095, 1971.
17. Parker, C. A.: Prostaglandins and slow reacting substance. *J. Allergy Clin. Immunol.* 63:1, 1979.
18. Pepys, J.: *Hypersensitivity Diseases of the Lungs Due to Fungi and Organic Dusts*, Basal, S. Karger, 1969, p. 112.
19. Pepys, J.: Clinical and therapeutic significance of patterns of allergic reactions of the lungs to extrinsic agents. *Am. Rev. Respir. Dis.* 116:573, 1977.
20. Pierpaoli, W., Fabris, N., et al.: Developmental hormones and immunological maturation, In *Hormones and the Immune Responses*. Wolstenholme, G. E. W., and Knight, J. (eds.), London, J. & A. Churchill, 1970, p. 126.
21. Pope, C. G.: The immunology of insulin, In *Advances in Immunology*. Vol. 5. Dixon, F. J., Jr., and Humphrey, J. H. (eds.), New York, Academic Press, 1966, p. 209.
22. Reed, C. E., and Townley, R. G.: Asthma: Classification and pathogenesis, In *Allergy, Principles and Practice*. Middleton, E., Jr., Reed, C. E., et al. (eds.), St. Louis, C. V. Mosby Co., 1978, Ch. 36.
23. Rocha e Silva, M.: *Kinin Hormones*. Springfield, Illinois, Charles C Thomas, 1970.
24. Rosen, F. S., and Austen, K. F.: Androgen therapy in hereditary angioneurotic edema. *N. Engl. J. Med.* 295:1476, 1976.
25. Schreiber, A. D.: Clinical immunology of the corticosteroids. *Prog. Clin. Immunol.* 6:103, 1977.
26. Szenberg, A.: Influence of testosterone on the primary lymphoid organs of the chicken, In *Hormones and the Immune Response*. Wolstenholme, G. E. W., and Knight, J. (eds.), London, J. & A. Churchill, 1970, p. 42.
27. Szentivanyi, A.: The beta adrenergic theory of the atopic abnormality in bronchial asthma. *J. Allergy* 42:203, 1968.
28. Thorell, J. I., and Larson, S. M.: *Radioimmunoassay and Related Techniques*. St. Louis, C. V. Mosby Co., 1978.
29. Trainin, N., Small, M., et al.: The role of thymic hormones in regulation of the lymphoid system, In *B and T cells in Immune Recognition*. Loor, F., and Roelants, G. E. (eds.), New York, Wiley, 1977, Ch. 5.
30. Twomey, J. J., Goldstein, G., et al. Bioassay determinations of thymopoietin and thymic hormone levels in human plasma. *Proc. Natl. Acad. Sci. USA* 74:2541, 1977.
31. VanArsdel, P. P., Jr., and Paul, G. H.: Drug therapy in the management of asthma. *Ann. Intern. Med.* 87:68, 1977.
32. VanArsdel, P. P., Jr., and Beall, G. N. The metabolism and functions of histamine. *Arch. Intern. Med.* 106:714, 1960.
33. Waldmann, T. A., and Broder, S.: Suppressor cells in the regulation of the immune response. *Prog. Clin. Immunol.* 3:155, 1977.
34. Yalow, R. S.: Radioimmunoassay: A probe for the fine structure of biologic systems. *Science* 200:1236, 1978.

CHAPTER 26

Autoimmunity and Endocrine Disease

By Robert M. Blizzard

INTRODUCTION AND DEFINITION

Autoimmunity is "self-immunization" and is often associated with "self-destruction." Frequently, the latter is associated with lymphocytic infiltration, with or without formation of lymphoid germinal centers, or fibrosis, or atrophy or a combination of these.

The "autoimmune" diseases are classified as "organ specific" and "nonorgan specific." (Table 26–1).

Autoimmunity is not the only cause of many of these entities, however. For example, probably not all cases of "idiopathic" Addison's disease or all cases of insulin-dependent diabetes mellitus are of autoimmune origin.

Some experts would add a third group, in which polymyositis, active chronic hepatitis, primary biliary cirrhosis, cryptogenic cirrhosis, "autoimmune" diabetes mellitus, and, possibly, myasthenia gravis would be placed. In these entities, only one organ is affected, as in "organ-specific" autoimmunity, but the circulating antibodies cross react with tissues other than the one primarily affected. For example, in active chronic hepatitis, the antibodies are directed against mitochondria of both liver and kidney. The only histopathology is in the liver, however.

Organ- and non-organ-specific autoimmune diseases have the following in common: (1) circulating antibodies that react against normal body constituents, (2) increased immunoglobulins in serum, which may be in any of the classes of immunoglobulins but most frequently are of the IgG or IgM classes, (3) a greater incidence of disease and antibody presence in females than in males, and (4) the measurement of circulating antibodies for purposes of diagnosis.

Ordinarily, in "organ-specific" autoimmune disease the circulating antibodies are directed solely against a cellular component of the affected organ. Exemplary are the antibodies directed against the microsomes of the thyroid follicular cells, which are frequently demonstrable in chronic lymphocytic thyroiditis. In "non-organ-specific" autoimmune diseases the circulating antibodies are directed against a cellular component of multiple organs, and the disease involves multiple tissues. The antinuclear

antibodies found in lupus erythematosus are examples. In the proposed third group of autoimmune diseases, only one organ is affected pathologically, but the antibodies cross react with antigens of multiple tissues, as in the example of hepatitis previously cited.

Certain criteria have been established to unequivocally classify a disease as an autoimmune entity. These include (1) the presence of a circulating antibody or a cellular immune reaction (or both) in patients with the disease, (2) a specific antigen that is demonstrable in the organ or tissue involved in the disease, (3) an antibody or cellular immune reaction that is reproducible in an animal model system by immunization of the animal with an identical or comparable antigen, (4) a disease, similar to that occurring in the human, that is reproducible in the immunized animal, and (5) a disease that can be passively transferred with serum or immunologically competent cells from one animal to another. Not all of these criteria have been met for all of the previously listed diseases, but the majority have been met for most, and the remainder of the diseases are believed to be of similar origin because of frequent association with unequivocal autoimmune dis-

Table 26–1. ORGAN-SPECIFIC AND NON-ORGAN-SPECIFIC AUTOIMMUNE DISEASES

Organ-Specific

Chronic lymphocytic thyroiditis	Insulin dependent diabetes mellitus
Spontaneous myxedema	
Thyrotoxicosis (i.e., Grave's disease)	Premature menopause
Exophthalmos	Pernicious anemia
"Idiopathic" Addison's disease	Atrophic gastritis
"Idiopathic" hypoparathyroidism	Alopecia areata and totalis
Vitiligo	Active chronic hepatitis
Acquired hemolytic anemia	Primary biliary cirrhosis
"Idiopathic" thrombocytopenia purpura	Cryptogenic cirrhosis
Myasthenia gravis	Polymyositis

Non-Organ-Specific

Lupus erythematosus
Rheumatoid arthritis
Dermatomyositis
Periarteritis nodosa

Submitted for publication January 1979.

ease. Alopecia is exemplary of the unproven but presumed autoimmune diseases.

HISTORICAL ASPECTS

Chronic lymphocytic thyroiditis (CLT) is the most completely studied autoimmune endocrinopathy.[1, 19] During the years 1950–1955, laboratory tests that reflected an abnormal production of immunoglobulins, such as the thymol turbidity and cephalin flocculation tests, were frequently found to be abnormal in patients with CLT and in patients with acquired spontaneous myxedema. Roitt and Doniach[31] in 1956 demonstrated circulating antibodies to thyroglobulin in the sera of patients with CLT and in those with spontaneous myxedema. At approximately the same time, Witebsky and Rose[41] were inducing antibody formation to thyroglobulin and other extracts of thyroid tissue in rabbits immunized with these extracts plus Freund's adjuvant. CLT was produced simultaneously in the immunized animals. Most of the postulates for classifying a disease as an autoimmune entity were therefore met for CLT. Passive transfer of the disease process was possible only intermittently, and only then by transferring immunologically competent cells and not circulating antibodies.

In the period from 1960 to 1970, idiopathic hypoparathyroidism, idiopathic Addison's disease, premature menopause, pernicious anemia, active chronic hepatitis, and a few of the other "autoimmune" entities were identified as being associated with circulating antibodies directed against specific antigens of the affected tissue(s). In the mid-1970's some instances of juvenile insulin-dependent diabetes mellitus were found to be associated with circulating antibodies against pancreatic islet cells, and this common endocrinopathy is now believed to be frequently attributable to, or associated with, an autoimmune process. Further historical aspects will be covered in discussions in subsequent sections.

MECHANISMS INVOLVED IN PRODUCING THE AUTOIMMUNE ENDOCRINOPATHIES[1,4]

The various factors that may be involved in the autoimmune processes include
1. Humoral or circulating antibodies, which are not cytotoxic by themselves *in vivo*, although they may be cytotoxic to cells grown in tissue culture.
2. Circulating antibody-antigen complexes, which may be responsible for tissue destruction, as in acquired hemolytic anemia.
3. Antigen-antibody-complement complexes, which may be contributing factors in vitiligo and possibly in other autoimmune entities.
4. "B" or bursa cell production of circulating antibodies of multiple types, i.e., stimulating, blocking, and so on.
5. "T" or thymic cell enhancement or suppression of circulating antibody production by B cells, i.e., the helper or suppressor effect of T cells to stimulate or suppress humoral antibody production by the B cells.
6. "K" or killer cell activity, resulting from an antigen-antibody complex on the target tissue, which invites destruction of the cell.
7. Various combinations and permutations of these events, which may produce a cascading of various mechanisms of self-destruction.

The circulating antibodies are directed against various tissue components, such as those listed in Table 26–2. There are five antinuclear antibodies demonstrable in the indirect Coons' or ultraviolet microscope technique. Circulating antibodies against receptors may be stimulatory, as are the thyroid-stimulating immunoglobulins that substitute for TSH at the TSH receptors, or blocking, as are the antiacetylcholine receptor antibodies in myasthenia gravis. Antibodies against hormones, including cortisol, thyroxine (T_4), growth hormone (GH) and so on, have not been demonstrated as occurring spontaneously, except for anti-insulin antibodies that have been found in a few patients who, allegedly, have not previously received insulin. Antibodies against hormones such as insulin and GH do occur, of course, with exogenous administration, but these are not believed to contribute to an autoimmune disease.

GENETIC AND ENVIRONMENTAL PREDISPOSING FACTORS

Recently, predisposing genetic and environmental factors for autoimmune disease have been suspected. These factors include a genetic predisposition, as indicated by certain human lymphocytic antigen (HLA) haplotypes. The short arm of each chromosome 6 has several subloci

Table 26–2*

Antigen	Antibody	Associated Diseases
Nuclear factors e.g., DNA	Antinuclear factor(s)	Lupus erythematosus, rheumatoid arthritis, active chronic hepatitis, primary biliary cirrhosis, drug toxicity
Microsomal factors e.g., lipoprotein	Antimicrosomal	Addison's insulin-dependent diabetes
Membrane receptors	1. thyroid stimulating immunoglobulins	Thyrotoxicosis
	2. anti-acetylcholine receptors antibodies	Myasthenia gravis
	3. anti-insulin receptors antibodies	Insulin-resistant diabetes mellitus
Mitochondrial factors	Antimitochondrial	Chronic hepatitis
Hormones	Anti-insulin	Hypoglycemia (?)
Thyroglobulin	Antithyroglobulin	Chronic lymphocytic thyroiditis

*These are exemplary antigens, antibodies, and associated diseases and are not meant to be all inclusive.

for HLA types, including HLA-A, HLA-B, HLA-C, and HLA-D. The HLA-B8 haplotype has been associated frequently with thyrotoxicosis, idiopathic Addison's disease, juvenile or insulin-dependent diabetes mellitus, Sjögren's disease, lupus erythematosus, dermatitis herpetiformis, chronic hepatitis, and myasthenia gravis. Surprisingly, no association of HLA-B8 has been confirmed in chronic lymphocytic thyroiditis, although HLA-AW30 has been incriminated. HLA-A1 in combination with HLA-B8 has been found in approximately one half of a group of 16 individuals who have multiple organ–specific autoimmune diseases or polyglandular failure.[13] Further consideration will be given to the HLA haplotypes in the section concerning insulin-dependent diabetes mellitus. Possibly a genetic predisposition may be so dominant that the autoimmune entity, or entities, occur spontaneously without any environmental influence. Such occurs in a strain of obese chickens that are genetically predisposed to develop thyroiditis.

In other individuals with a moderate genetic predisposition, possibly an environmental insult, such as a virus infection, or a chemical insult initiates an autoimmune process. The data to implicate such factors are primarily experimental, but of such quality that the probability that viral or chemical initiating factors play a role in autoimmunity must be mentioned. A diagram to exemplify how genetic and environmental factors may theoretically produce a disease process by themselves, or in combination, is given in Fig. 26–1.

The obscure role of circulating antibodies in contributing to the destructive process of the diseases must be re-emphasized. The presence and demonstration of any of these antibodies reflects a disease process and is therefore often of diagnostic value. These antibodies often disappear soon after being identified, however, and they probably have resulted in some instances from an exogenous insult to the affected organ, with release of antigen and consequent antibody production. The persistence of antibodies may reflect a continuing autoimmune process.

Further aspects concerning the mechanisms involved in the induction and perpetuation of autoimmune endocrinopathies will be covered as each endocrinopathy is discussed.

THYROID AUTOIMMUNE DISEASE

This is the classic example of specific autoimmunity and has been studied in the laboratory more than any other autoimmune entity.[1] This is appropriate as a very large proportion of patients with thyroid disease — particularly in the pediatric age group — has autoimmunity as the basis of disease.

Of 95 pediatric patients seen sequentially in 2 endocrine clinics for goiter (Table 26–3), 33 had CLT and 38 had thyrotoxicosis. Consequently, approximately 75% of children presenting with goiter have autoimmune disease as the cause of that goiter. Acquired hypothyroidism also is usually an autoimmune disease. Therefore, autoimmunity accounts for the majority of thyroid disease seen in children. Similar figures probably apply for adults. The importance of autoimmunity as an etiologic cause for thyroid disease is apparent.

The most readily accepted current thesis explaining the etiology of these thyroid autoimmune diseases is that there is an immunologic defect in the T-cell population that is divided into at least two subtypes — "helper" cells that assist B cells to produce circulating antibodies and "suppressor" cells that inhibit B cells from producing circulating antibodies.[4] With a defect in "normal" suppressor activity, B cells can interact with normal antigens and produce circulating antibodies. The antibodies may vary according to the antigen to which they are exposed; i.e., they may be antibodies directed against thyroglobulin, microsomal components of thyroid cells, or membrane antigens such as the receptors for thyrotropin stimulating hormone (TSH). Antibodies against the latter include the thyroid-stimulating immunoglobulins (TSI) such as long-acting thyroid stimulator (LATS) and LATS-protector (LATS-P). Killer (K) cells, which are probably another subgroup of T cells, may contribute to the lymphocytic infiltration, which is characteristic of CLT, by reacting with an antigen-antibody complex on or in the thyroid cell. These interrelationships are diagrammed in Fig. 26–2. Irvine[19] and Volpe[40] have presented in greater detail variations of this simplified concept.

Since thyrotoxicosis, CLT, and exophthalmos are all autoimmune diseases, they may occur singly or in association (Fig. 26–3). Thyrotoxicosis and exophthalmos particularly occur in association. Occasionally, patients with CLT have associated exophthalmos without any element of thyrotoxicosis. Patients with CLT will occasionally

PRECIPITATING AND PREDISPOSING FACTORS IN AUTOIMMUNITY

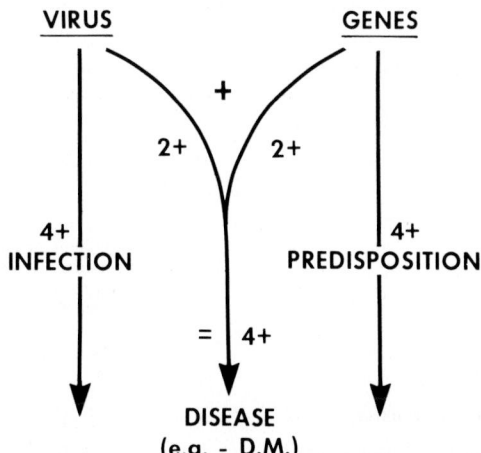

Figure 26–1. Theoretically, precipitating and predisposing factors work together to produce a disease, e.g., insulin-dependent diabetes mellitus. The same disease in theory can occur from an overwhelming viral or chemical insult alone or an overwhelming genetic predisposition. 2+ indicates a mild insult or a moderate predisposition. 4+ indicates an overwhelming insult or predisposition.

Table 26–3. INCIDENCE OF GOITERS IN CHILDREN

Acute suppurative	1
Acute nonsuppurative	5
Lymphocytic thyroiditis	33
Thyrotoxicosis	38
Iodine-induced	2
Carcinoma	1
Colloid (ETIO?)	6
Adenoma	2
Hyperplastic—nontoxic	2
Normal hyperthrophy	5
	95

POSTULATED MECHANISM OF AUTOIMMUNITY IN CLT AND TT

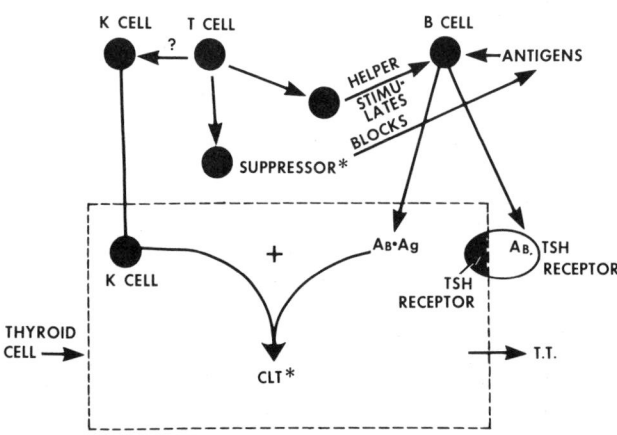

Figure 26–2. K cells may be a type of T cell, as suppressor and helper cells are types of T cells. The basic defect(*) in thyroid autoimmunity is possibly in the activity of suppressor cells. Antibodies are produced in susceptible patients by normal antigens. If antibodies are produced against TSH receptors, thyrotoxicosis results; if against other components, AB·Ag complexes result that theoretically activate K cell activity, and chronic lymphocytic thyroiditis results.

have associated thyrotoxicosis. This probably accounts for most of the patients with "hashitoxicosis." All three entities may occur in the same patient.

The prognosis is variable when a patient has CLT or thyrotoxicosis, or both.[21] The patient may go into temporary or permanent remission. Alternatively, the disease state may stay the same for 25 years without changing, or either disease may progress to hypothyroidism because of progressive destruction of the gland. The latter may occur independent of whether therapy is given or not. The individual also may develop other autoimmune diseases, such as pernicious anemia, alopecia, and so on.

The antibodies used routinely in diagnosing lymphocytic infiltration are those directed against thyroglobulin and against the microsomes of the follicular cells. The usual method of measuring these is to use an agglutination test in which red blood cells are coated with either

THYROID AUTOIMMUNITY AND EXOPHTHALMUS

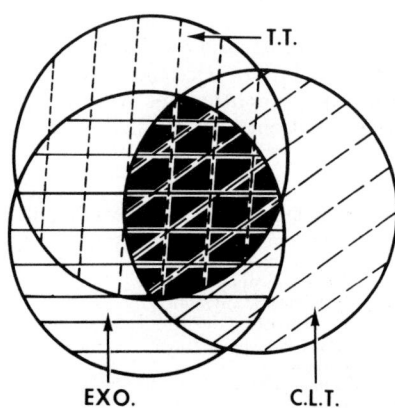

Figure 26–3. Exophthalmos (exo) may occur with or without thyrotoxicosis (T. T.) or with chronic lymphocytic thyroiditis (C.L.T.), or both. When T.T. and C.L.T. occur together, "hashitoxicosis" results. The reason for 1, 2, or 3 of these entities occurring in any single patient remains obscure.

thyroglobulin or microsomal antigen. Therefore, agglutination tests are used to measure the most important antithyroid antibodies. Ninety-five per cent of patients with CLT will have antibodies against the microsomes or thyroglobulin, or both. Children with CLT reportedly have lower titers of antibodies more frequently than do adults with CLT. Titers of 1:8 are significant in children, whereas they are often regarded as being inconsequential in adults. At least one laboratory has found closer correlation between significant disease and the titer of microsomal antibodies than the titer of thyroglobulin antibodies, but further investigation is needed before categorically accepting this as fact.

The TSI's, including LATS and LATS-P, may be measured by bioassay using guinea pigs or mice. TSI's also may be measured by using a TSI receptor assay or by the production of cyclic AMP (cAMP) from thyroid slices in an *in vitro* system. In the receptor assay, TSH is tagged with ^{125}I and is displaced on the receptor with the TSI in serum, if such is present. Since there are several TSI's in serum, it is not suprising that there is not always correlation between the various tests for TSI. For example, Volpe[39, 40] has reported that the stimulating assay is sometimes negative when the receptor assay is positive for TSI. Theoretically, the presence of nonstimulatory TSI blocking antibodies could account for the discrepancy. Measurement of TSI of various types may predict whether a remission of thyrotoxicosis is imminent. Absence of any form of TSI suggests that the patient is in remission and therapy may be unnecessary.

Indications to test for thyroglobulin and microsomal antibodies are given in Table 26–4 and include the investigation of patients who have (1) suspected lymphocytic thyroiditis, to confirm or negate the diagnosis, (2) thyrotoxicosis, to determine if a high titer is present, which might predict imminent thyroid failure from lymphocytic destruction, (3) insulin-dependent diabetes mellitus because of the high coincidence of autoimmune thyroid disease in such patients, (4) Turner's syndrome, (5) Down's syndrome, (6) lupus erythematosus, and (7) juvenile rheumatoid arthritis for the same reason. Patients with these entities should be tested annually for these antibodies, and other methods should be utilized to look for thyroid disease, since a significant percentage of such patients will have associated CLT.

Acute thyroiditis and de Quervain's subacute thyroiditis are probably not autoimmune thyroid diseases. An-

Table 26–4. INDICATIONS TO TEST FOR THYROID ANTIBODIES

Entity	Reason
1. Suspected lymphocytic thyroiditis	1. To confirm or negate the diagnosis
2. Thyrotoxicosis	2. To determine if a high titer is present, which might predict imminent thyroid failure from lymphocytic destruction
3. Insulin-dependent diabetes mellitus	3. Because of the high coincidence of autoimmune disease
4. Turner's syndrome	4. As in #3 above
5. Down's syndrome	5. As in #3 above
6. Lupus erythematosus	6. As in #3 above
7. Juvenile rheumatoid arthritis	7. As in #3 above

tibody production occurs occasionally in these patients but usually is transient, as it sometimes occurs and is transient following surgical removal of the thyroid.

Treatment of autoimmune thyroid disease depends upon the symptoms. T_4 replacement is used for hypothyroidism and for euthyroid patients with CLT. In the latter instance it is recommended to prevent clinical or subclinical hypothyroidism from occurring insidiously. TSH determinations can be performed intermittently to assist in determining the need for T_4 therapy. If the TSH determination becomes elevated, T_4 is unequivocally indicated. Dosage regimens are given elsewhere in this text.

Treatment of thyrotoxicosis remains a choice of surgery, goitrogenic agents, and radioactive iodine. The last is discouraged in children and young adults. Interestingly, TSI has been reported to be present in only 15% of postoperative patients with thyrotoxicosis, in contrast to approximately 50% of patients treated with radioactive iodine or goitrogenic agents. The significance of these differences remains obscure.

For further consideration of the thyroid diseases of autoimmunity the reader is referred to Ch. 4.

EXOPHTHALMOS: A PROBABLE AUTOIMMUNE ENTITY

As diagrammed in Fig. 26–3, exophthalmos occurs alone and with thyrotoxicosis or chronic lymphocytic thyroiditis (or both). When it occurs with thyrotoxicosis, it often correlates poorly with the onset of the thyrotoxic symptoms. The retro-orbital muscles characteristically have lymphocytic infiltration, which is the hallmark of autoimmunity. Edema and mucopolysaccharide deposition also occur.[16]

Utilizing the migration inhibiting factor (MIF) test and testing antigens from retro-orbital muscle and the thyroid, a disturbance of cellular immunity was observed in patients with thyrotoxicosis and exophthalmos and in some patients who had only exophthalmos.[16] The role of thyroglobulin in producing exophthalmos and the affinity of retro-orbital muscle for both thyroglobulin and thyroglobulin-antibody complexes remain obscure. The role of the exophthalmic producing factor (EPF), the IgG of serum, as a factorial agent in causing exophthalmos also is obscure. There appears to be no role of TSH or its fragments. Hypophysectomy has been of little avail. TSH is not antigenic in producing the MIF frequently observed in exophthalmos.

Although the inter-relationship of exophthalmos and autoimmune thyroid disease is still puzzling, it is the consensus that exophthalmos is probably an autoimmune disease itself with a yet unexplained correlation with thyroid autoimmunity. The beneficial response of corticosteroids, if given early in the disease, is in accord with this hypothesis. Cortisol has been effective in alleviating both CLT and the lymphocytic infiltration of the gastric mucosa observed with pernicious anemia.

Of clinical pertinence are the observations of several groups that have studied the incidence of clinical or subclinical thyroid disease (or both) in euthyroid exophthalmic patients whose exophthalmos may be unilateral or bilateral. Hall and coworkers[16] observed that 13 of 26 such patients had 6-hour ^{131}I uptakes that were suppressed following the administration of triiodothyronine (T_3) for 7 days. Solomon and associates[34] found that only 9 of 17 euthyroid patients with exophthalmos had LATS-P. Five euthyroid patients had no detectable LATS-P, thyroid antibodies, or thyroid suppressibility with T_3. Therefore, patients who have exophthalmos and are euthyroid deserve an extensive evaluation of thyroid function. In the absence of any laboratory findings to implicate autoimmune thyroiditis, autoimmune exophthalmos occurring alone should be considered. Gastric antibodies and vitiligo both occur in an increased incidence, as compared with normals, with euthyroid "Grave's" ophthalmopathy.

ISLET CELL AUTOIMMUNE DISEASE

Diabetes mellitus is a disease of hyperglycemia of multiple origins. Type I, as defined by Bottazzo and Doniach,[7, 8] includes all patients who are insulin dependent, although further subcategorization into a juvenile and a polyendocrine type has been proposed. Even the diabetes in patients with insulin dependency is of heterogenous origin, however. For example, Rotter and Rimoin[32] on the basis of recent immunologic and metabolic studies, hypothesize that there are at least two distinct forms of juvenile-onset diabetes, one associated with HLA-B8 and one with HLA-BW15. The former is characterized by autoimmunity, microangiopathy, and a strong association with the HLA-D locus. The HLA-BW15 form is characterized by antibody response to exogenous insulin and a stronger association with the HLA-C locus.

Autoimmunity was postulated as one probable etiology of insulin-dependent diabetes mellitus (IDD) in the early 1960's. This concept developed on the basis of finding lymphocytic infiltration of the islets, which frequently occurred in juvenile patients who died and who had only recently developed IDD, and, particularly, on the basis of the association of IDD in patients and siblings with autoimmune Addison's disease or spontaneous myxedema, or both. Although "Schmidt's syndrome" initially was applied to patients with coincident idiopathic adrenal and thyroid failure, it subsequently was extended to include patients who had IDD plus either or both of these atrophic endocrine diseases. Autoimmunity in IDD could not be proved, however, as islet cell antibodies (ICA) could not be demonstrated in the sera of such patients. Subsequently, Bottazzo and coworkers[7] and MacCuish and associates[27] demonstrated with the use of improved ultraviolet microscopy that some patients with multiple endocrine organ failure (polyglandular autoimmune disease) had ICA, whereas controls did not. Nerup[30] in 1974, utilizing techniques such as production of MIF, implicated an alteration in the cellular immunity of juvenile diabetes.

Currently autoimmune disease is accepted as one etiology of Type I diabetes. Irvine[18] has postulated that some patients may have a marked predisposition to develop autoimmune diabetes mellitus, and others have a moderate predisposition that is activated by an insult to the islets, e.g., a viral infection. In other instances an overwhelming insult may be responsible by itself (see Fig. 26–1). In other instances, an insult such as a viral infection may trigger an autoimmune process. Therefore, Type I or insulin dependent diabetes mellitus will be heterogeneous in origin, even though the characteristics of insulinopenia, insulin dependence, and onset early in life are similar.

Further measurements of ICA since 1974 have been of assistance in subclassifying and further clarifying and disease entities in patients with Type I diabetes. Maclaren and Huang[28] in 1975 demonstrated that 90% of patients with IDD had humoral antibodies against beta cells from an islet-cell adenoma and which were grown in tissue culture. He also demonstrated that lymphocytes from such patients destroyed insulinoma cells grown in culture. Several investigators[2, 7, 18, 27, 30] have now demonstrated that (1) 60–75% of patients with IDD have ICA at the time of diagnosis, (2) the incidence of ICA is greater in females than in males, (3) the incidence of demonstrable ICA decreases with time, so only approximately 5–10% of Type I diabetics have identifiable ICA 5 years post onset, (4) Type I patients with HLA-B8 have persistence of ICA, in contrast to those with HLA-BW15, who have ICA only transiently, (5) the ICA are found more frequently in younger patients, (6) ICA in some instances may appear 7 or 8 years before clinical diabetes is evident, (7) organ-specific autoimmune diseases are frequently associated in patients who have persisting ICA over the years, (8) HLA-B8 is a commonly occurring haplotype in individuals with associated organ-specific autoimmune diseases, and (9) ICA have a common antigen in the cytoplasms of beta, delta, and alpha polypeptide-producing cells and in the vasoactive intestinal peptide–producing cells of the islets, although only the beta cells appear to be destroyed.

Lernmark and coworkers[24] identified circulating antibodies against the islet cell membranes of rat islet cells in 30% of juvenile diabetics, which was independent of the duration of the disease. The importance of finding surface cell antibodies and their relationship to microsomal antibodies is unknown.

The circumstantial evidence that autoimmunity is incriminated as an etiologic factor in at least some patients with Type I diabetes mellitus is substantial, therefore. The HLA-A, B, C, and D loci appear to contribute to the susceptibility of developing IDD. This susceptibility in some instances may be a predisposition to autoimmunity and in other instances to other etiologies. Each of us has two HLA-A genes, two HLA-B genes, etc. Individuals who have HLA-A1, B8, BW15, B18, BW40, CW15, C3, D3, or D4 have a particular predisposition to develop Type I diabetes mellitus. In contrast, individuals having HLA-A11, A32, B5, B7, BW35, C2 or D2 are not prone, and are even possibly resistant, to developing IDD. Individuals with additive "susceptible" HLA types, such as B8 and BW15, are at least twice as susceptible as those with a single "susceptible" gene to developing diabetes of Type I. When HLA-A1 and B8 occur in combination, such individuals are particularly prone to develop polyendocrine gland failure, which often includes diabetes. Recent data suggest that the B8 antigen is in linkage disequilibrium to D3 and that the BW15 antigen is in disequilibrium with C3.

Because of only a transient appearance of antibodies in patients with HLA-BW15, and because of the low incidence of associated autoimmune diseases, some investigators have postulated that this haplotype may indicate a predisposition for an insult, such as a viral infection, to cause the disease. The ICA, which are demonstrable only briefly in individuals with this HLA type, may reflect an insult to the islet, such as the transient appearance of thyroglobulin antibodies that may appear after thyroid surgery or viral thyroiditis in certain individuals. Doniach and Bottazzo[42] have reclassified Type I diabetes into subgroups IA and IB. The latter is thought to have a strong predisposition for autoimmune endocrinopathies with persistence of ICA, in contrast to the findings in Type IA.

Another type of autoimmune disease probably accounts for some cases of insulin resistant diabetes (IRD) mellitus. A syndrome of IRD occurring in association with acanthosis nigricans and the identification of blocking antibodies to insulin receptors have been observed in 10 females and 3 males, 18–65 years of age. Seven of the 13 were black. All had abnormal glucose tolerance tests and severe insulin resistance. Three had spontaneous hypoglycemia at some time in the course of their disease. Eleven of the 13 had acanthosis nigricans. Approximately 30% had an associated overt autoimmune disease, and the others had chemical alterations, such as elevated gamma globulins, suggestive of an immune defect. Insulin and the antibodies to insulin receptors are competitive for binding, and a binding-inhibition assay has been established, as has an immunoprecipitation assay. The monocytes of affected patients do not bind insulin, as occurs in monocytes of unaffected individuals. Not all patients with IRD and acanthosis nigricans have insulin receptor antibodies demonstrable. Kahn and coworkers[20, 14] have described several syndromes that are related but without receptor antibodies. One group has accelerated growth and virilization and a decreased receptor concentration. Another group is similar but has no receptor defect. A third group has lipoatrophic diabetes with insulin resistance and acanthosis nigricans. Some of these patients have a receptor defect and some do not. Further investigation should clarify the role of autoimmunity in these similar, but dissimilar, groups.

Type II diabetes mellitus, which is characterized by hyperinsulinemia, non–insulin dependence, minimal ketonemia, and an onset later in life than that of Type I diabetes, is thought to be not of autoimmune origin, although a strong genetic influence is recognized, as there is almost 100% concordance in identical twins as compared with approximately 50% concordance for IDD.

The implications that autoimmunity can produce or be associated with IDD are many. Therefore, physicians currently should thoroughly interrogate and examine patients with Type I diabetes for coincident autoimmune diseases, such as thyroid autoimmune disease. Screening of the serums of such patients for thyroglobulin and thyroid microsomal antibodies periodically is indicated, as there are numerous studies that describe the increased frequency of thyroid antibodies that reflect thyroid autoimmunity in patients with IDD. Of 85 patients followed in one clinic for juvenile diabetics, 3 became hypothyroid and 2 thyrotoxic. In addition, chemical evidence of primary hypothyroidism was found in 11 other children who had elevated TSH determinations and identifiable thyroid antibodies. The siblings of patients with Type I diabetes should be observed closely for organ-specific autoimmunity.

In the future, determinations for ICA and HLA types may permit predictions that IDD may occur before any clinical or chemical manifestations are present. Further elaboration of the multiple etiologies of Type I diabetes should be possible by correlating these determinations with viral antibody titers or viral infections, or both.

AUTOIMMUNE DISEASE OF THE ADRENAL CORTEX

Addison's disease, i.e., adrenal cortical insufficiency, has been attributed to tuberculosis, histoplasmosis, adrenal hemorrhage, and idiopathic, and other multiple but less common, causes. Adrenal antibodies were initially demonstrated by Anderson and coworkers[3] using a complement fixation method. Blizzard and associates[3] called attention to the high incidence of adrenal antibodies in the sera of patients with idiopathic Addison's disease, using the indirect Coons' technique. The coincidence of many organ-specific autoimmune diseases with adrenal insufficiency produced extensive clinical and genetic investigation that was impressively summarized by Irvine and Barnes. In one series of 114 patients with idiopathic Addison's disease, 27 had autoimmune thyroid disease, 10 had pernicious anemia, 18 had diabetes mellitus, 31 had abnormal gonadal function, and 16 had vitiligo. These associations were rare in patients with tuberculosis as the etiology of adrenal insufficiency.

In addition to these clinical associations, experimental autoimmune adrenalitis has been demonstrated, and the transfer of lymph cells from affected animals has induced adrenalitis in the recipients. Crude adrenal homogenate has been demonstrated to act as an antigen with the lymph cells of affected patients to produce MIF, an indication that "T-cell" hypersensitivity is involved. Volpe[39] failed to find a correlation between MIF and circulating humoral adrenal antibodies, however, and Barnes and Irvine found no abnormal number of T cells or B cells. Regardless, autoimmunity and self-destruction account for the vast majority of cases of idiopathic Addison's disease in the United States and Europe. This destruction is confined to the adrenal cortex. Stimulation of the intact adrenal medulla in these patients with infusions of 2-deoxy-D-glucose (50 mg/kg body weight) increases the urinary output of epinephrine, which assists in differentiating an autoimmune etiology from other causes.

The association of "other" autoimmune diseases often occurs on a genetic basis. Utilizing the personal and family histories and the identification of adrenal antibodies in patients with idiopathic Addison's disease, we were able to classify these patients into four groups, three of which were definitely associated with autoimmunity.[35, 36]

The first group consisted primarily of older adult females with strong personal and family histories of associated autoimmune disease, and the identification of adrenal antibodies in nearly all. Most of these patients had autoimmune thyroid disease or diabetes mellitus with insulin dependency or both. Therefore, many of these patients had *Schmidt's syndrome*. Pernicious anemia, vitiligo, ovarian failure, and alopecia occurred in a few. Hypoparathyroidism and monilia were conspicuously absent. These patients were believed to have a mendelian recessive inheritance pattern with greater penetrance in the females.

The second group also consisted primarily of older adult females but without a personal or family history of associated autoimmune disease. Adrenal antibodies were present in only a few. This group was probably a *heterogeneous population* and may include a few patients who will ultimately develop another autoimmune disease. Autoimmunity could not be implicated in most.

The third group comprised infants, children, and youth who had *polyendocrine glandular failure* consisting of *hypoparathyroidism, Addison's disease* and frequently, *moniliasis* with or without other organ-specific autoimmune disease. Adrenal antibodies were usually present in those with, or in those developing, adrenal insufficiency. There is greater susceptibility for the female with this type of autoimmunity, as compared with the male, to have Addison's disease, in spite of the mendelian recessive pattern of inheritance. In one series 15 of 16 females with monilia and hypoparathyroidism had Addison's disease, but only 5 of 16 males had Addison's disease. No patient who initially had Addison's disease and moniliasis without hypoparathyroidism subsequently developed parathyroid deficiency. Many patients with hypoparathyroidism and moniliasis subsequently developed Addison's disease, however. Further details of these patients are discussed in the section on autoimmune polyglandular endocrine failure.

A fourth group was composed of children who had isolated adrenal insufficiency and a strong sibling history of isolated Addison's disease. Only 27% had demonstrable adrenal antibodies, and those in this 27% were not those with the strong sibling history. Inheritance appeared to be mendelian recessive with a greater male incidence. Autoimmunity is suspect in this minority but could not be incriminated in at least 73% of this group. This also may be a heterogeneous group.

All patients with idiopathic adrenal insufficiency should be tested for adrenal antibodies, and those with adrenal antibodies, or a strong family history for autoimmunity should be tested annually for thyroid and parietal cell antibodies, and, as soon as readily available, islet cell antibodies. Alternatively, very close clinical surveillance for associated diseases is mandatory, as the majority of individuals with these antibodies may develop overt disease of the affected organ(s).

AUTOIMMUNE DISEASE OF THE PARATHYROID GLANDS

Hypoparathyroidism occurs in association with Addison's disease and moniliasis primarily in young patients and is believed to be of autoimmune etiology when associated with these diseases. Not all cases of hypoparathyroidism are of autoimmune origin, and there is little evidence for autoimmunity as the cause of the disease, with the exception of patients with these two associated diseases. Many patients with two or three of these three diseases have other associated atrophic diseases, including pernicious anemia, alopecia, premature ovarian failure, diabetes mellitus, vitiligo, and autoimmune thyroid disease. The inheritance of this syndrome is autosomal recessive. One sibling may have hypoparathyroidism, moniliasis, and adrenal insufficiency, whereas two others may have only one, two, or three of these diseases. Addison's disease frequently follows hypoparathyroidism in such patients, but the reverse seldom, if ever, occurs. The reader may wish to refer to the discussion of polyendocrine autoimmune disease, p. 1123.

Parathyroid antibodies were first demonstrated by Blizzard and coworkers[5] using the indirect Coons test. Others subsequently recognized antibodies in the sera of such patients. The antigen used in our studies was found only in some, but not all, parathyroid adenomas, however. Since normal parathyroid glands are infinitesimally small, inadequate antigen could be obtained from such glands, and the incidence, characteristics, and importance of parathyroid antibodies is less well known than the same parameters for the antibodies against other endocrine tissues.

The role of autoimmunity is well established, however, as Lupulescu produced lymphocytic infiltration, and atrophy of the parathyroid glands of dogs immunized with homogeneous parathyroid extracts and since patients with autoimmune hypoparathyroidism as part of the polyendocrine autoimmune syndrome have abnormalities of T-cell function.[3]

Treatment of hypocalcemia is with dihydrotachysterol or vitamin D. This treatment is discussed further in Ch. 19.

DiGeorge syndrome has similar characteristics in that hypoparathyroidism and moniliasis occur as a result of a developmental defect of the parathyroids and the thymus. The latter is associated with diminished T-cell function, which is circumstantial evidence that the moniliasis results from a T-cell functional abnormality in autoimmune hypoparathyroidism and moniliasis.

Problems associated with this entity were considered under "Autoimmune Disease of the Adrenal Cortex" and will be further considered in the section that follows and under "Polyendocrine and Polyautoimmune Disease."

AUTOIMMUNE DISEASE OF THE GONADS

Premature ovarian failure occurs frequently in young females with the syndrome of hypoparathyroidism, candidiasis, and Addison's disease and in patients with autoimmune Addison's disease with or without other atrophic end organ disease. Twenty-five percent of 157 females with autoimmune Addison's disease had amenorrhea in one series.[3]

Antibodies against steroid-producing cells of the ovary, which cross react with steroid-producing cells of the zona fasciculata, have been demonstrated using the indirect Coons technique.[3, 33] These antibodies, although found in patients with adrenal insufficiency *plus* primary gonadal failure, are not the adrenal antibodies usually found in autoimmune Addison's disease. Premature ovarian failure seldom occurs as an isolated autoimmune entity, i.e., without Addison's disease or hypoparathyroidism, and patients with ovarian failure alone usually have not had ovarian antibodies demonstrated. Ovarian failure has occurred prior to the development of Addison's disease in some females with hypoparathyroidism and Addison's disease, however, and 6 of 13 patients who had only spontaneous premature menopause had antibodies vs. thyroid or parietal cell antigens. This incidence is significantly increased over that in controls.

The histologic alterations of the ovaries in patients whose ovaries were studied were atrophy and lymphocytic and plasma cell infiltration. There were no chromosomal abnormalities in the gonads even when they appeared as "streak" gonads. Cortisone has been effective in re-establishing menstruation in at least one female with this entity. This is not surprising as cortisone reverses the lymphocytic infiltration and function of thyroids with chronic lymphocytic infiltration, providing atrophy has not occurred. Unfortunately, the pharmacologic doses required produce the signs and symptoms of Cushing's syndrome, which are worse than the primary disease.

Two patients with hypoparathyroidism and monilia have had elevated gonadotropins, normal menstruation, and normal estrogen levels.[25] High gonadotropins and apparent gonadal failure in some instances may relate, theoretically, to antibodies against the gonadotropin receptors on the gonad.

Gonadal failure does occur in males with Addison's disease but is much less common than ovarian failure in females. High gonadotropins indicate the gonadal failure.

Observation of females with Addison's disease for primary gonadal failure is important, as 36% of 135 females with Addison's disease had amenorrhea, oligomenorrhea, or menorrhagia.[3] Even if ovarian antibodies are measured, the gonadotropin determinations remain the major diagnostic test to ascertain premature gonadal failure. Treatment, as with most of the autoimmune diseases, is directed toward replacement of the hormones produced by the organ destroyed.

AUTOIMMUNE DISEASE OF THE PITUITARY

A young woman with thyroiditis and adrenal atrophy had extensive lymphocytic infiltration of the pituitary at autopsy. Rarely, patients with organ-specific thyroid and adrenal autoimmune disease have been observed to have GH deficiency, but no pathologic studies of the pituitary have been available. Only a very few patients have had antibodies demonstrable against GH-producing cells.[8] Although autoimmune hypophysitis has been considered as a possible cause of some cases of hypopituitarism, the data to date indicate that autoimmune disease of the pituitary is only a rare cause of pituitary insufficiency. Additional investigation is indicated to ascertain the role that autoimmunity might contribute in some cases of hypopituitarism.

Bottazzo and coworkers[6] identified antibodies to prolactin (PRL)-producing cells in 19 of 287 patients with various types of autoimmune disease. These antibodies were specific for this particular cell and were not against PRL itself. Nine of these patients received thyrotropin releasing hormone (TRH) and seven released PRL secondary to this stimulus. The PRL values were not reported in the other 10. The significance of these antibodies remains obscure.

Fortunately Bottazzo and Doniach[8] have developed an excellent technique to identify the six specific types of pituitary cells, as determined by the hormone they secrete. Utilizing this technique they have identified that most human sera have immunoglobulins that react with ACTH producing cells.

Obviously the role of autoimmunity in relation to pituitary disease requires further investigation. The occasional association of diabetes insipidus with autoimmune entities such as rheumatoid arthritis and the association of optic atrophy, diabetes insipidus, and diabetes mellitus in a common syndrome are suggestive of an autoimmune origin in these syndromes.

NONENDOCRINE AUTOIMMUNE DISEASE

Vitiligo is associated with many organ-specific autoimmune diseases, and the frequent presence of thyroid, adrenal, and gastric-parietal cell antibodies in patients with vitiligo has suggested a common etiology.[26] (See "Polyendocrine and Polyautoimmune Disease.") Anti-*melanocyte* antibodies were found in the sera of two patients with candidiasis, hypoparathyroidism, adrenal insufficiency, and vitiligo.[17] These antibodies appeared to be complement-dependent and bound to intracellular, rather than to cell surface, antigens. This raises the question of whether they are functionally active *in vivo* or represent an epiphenomenon secondary to melanocyte injury.

Myasthenia gravis also is associated with organ-specific autoimmune diseases and is associated with thymic pathology (thymomas or hyperplasia with germinal center formation or both).[10] Many patients with myasthenia, both of the juvenile and adult onset varieties, have antibodies vs. striated muscle, mitochondria, nuclei, and smooth muscle. There are, in addition, however, antibodies vs. the acetylcholine receptors. The latter probably account for the failure of acetylcholine to normally stimulate the neuronal-muscular junction.

Immunization of rabbits with acetylcholine plus Freund's adjuvant has induced a myasthenia-like syndrome. Injection of γ-globulin from myasthenic patients into mice also produces the disease. These experiments add evidence that myasthenia is an autoimmune entity.

The incidence of thyroid antibodies (44% in juvenile and 36.7% in adult onset myasthenia) indicates the strong association of thyroid autoimmunity with myasthenia.[12] The relatives of myasthenic patients also have a high incidence of thyroid antibodies, as both they and the patients have a significant incidence of parietal cell antibodies.

Patients with organ-specific autoimmune diseases often have *alopecia totalis* or *areata* associated with their primary disease. Patients who have alopecia as the only apparent disease have a 10–20% incidence of thyroid antibodies. Alopecia often responds favorably to cortisol treatment. On these bases, alopecia areata and totalis are probably the same disease except for the extent of involvement and are thought to often be attributable to autoimmune phenomenon, although similar lesions have not been produced, as yet, in animals.

Pernicious anemia is associated with parietal cell antibodies in 95% of patients with this disease and with intrinsic antibodies in approximately 50% of these patients. Gastric autoimmunity, as demonstrated by parietal cell antibodies is, next to thyroid autoimmune disease, the most frequently occurring organ-specific autoimmune disease. As is true for CLT, the presence of parietal cell antibodies reflects lymphocytic infiltration (of the gastric mucosa) but does not predict whether pernicious anemia will develop or if the disease will stay subclinical or will regress into remission. The coincidence of autoimmunity of the thyroid gland and the gastric mucosa is discussed further in the next section.

POLYENDOCRINE AND POLYAUTOIMMUNE DISEASE

The concurrence of endocrine and nonendocrine autoimmune diseases is possibly more frequent than the occurrence of one autoimmune disease alone. The coincidence of autoimmune diseases increases significantly with age, although children and adolescents with an autoimmune entity also frequently have coincident diseases.

Many associations have previously been mentioned in this chapter. In early infancy and childhood, the most frequent associations are between candidiasis, hypoparathyroidism, and adrenal insufficiency. This has been termed both *Type I polyendocrine autoimmune disease* and *autoimmune polyendocrine-candidiasis syndrome* (APECS). Pernicious anemia, vitiligo, gonadal failure, alopecia, IDD, and thyroid autoimmune disease also may occur in APECS.[29]

Treatment of moniliasis often is discouraging; treatment of candidiasis recently has been successful in a significant number of patients who have received transfer factor and amphotericin B, however. Kirkpatrick and Greenberg[22] studied 19 patients with chronic mucocutaneous candidiasis, the majority of whom had abnormalities in cell-mediated immunity. All had normal numbers of T and B lymphocytes and normal lymphocyte responses to phytohemagglutinin and concanavalin A, however. Eighteen had negative skin tests and *Candida*. Transfer factor administered over several months with only local treatment with antifungal agents was ineffective. Amphotericin B alone, however, induced remissions in most of the patients. The administration of transfer factor at monthly intervals after remission prolonged the remission times significantly. This treatment may be of significant benefit to those patients who are resistant to antifungal agents.

The association of adrenal insufficiency in association with hypothyroidism or diabetes mellitus with insulin dependency, i.e., *Schmidt's syndrome*, also has been discussed in previous sections. Schmidt's syndrome occurs primarily in adult females, but also occasionally in adult males and in adolescents. This entity has been termed *Type II polyendocrine autoimmune disease*.

The coincidence of insulin-dependent diabetes mellitus with autoimmune thyroid disease was extensively discussed under "Islet Cell Autoimmune Disease." Patients in adolescent and pediatric diabetic clinics should be observed closely for the appearance of thyroid antibodies or symptoms of autoimmune thyroid disease. The latter includes goiter and symptoms of hypo- or hyperthyroidism.

The thyroid autoimmune diseases, i.e., CLT, thyrotoxicosis, and most cases of spontaneous myxedema, are frequently associated with autoimmune disease of the gastric mucosa. Approximately 30% of adults with autoimmune disease of the thyroid will have parietal cell antibodies, and 5–10% of all patients with autoimmune thyroid disease have, or will develop, pernicious anemia. Also, if patients with pernicious anemia are evaluated for thyroid antibodies and overt thyroid disease, the percentages are comparable to those just cited. Therefore, patients with autoimmune thyroid disease should be followed closely for the presence of parietal cell antibodies, if possible, and certainly for any evidence of anemia or decreased vitamin B_{12} levels.

Thyroid autoimmune disease (TAD) also is sometimes associated with vitiligo, myasthenia gravis, alopecia, and IDD. The coincidence of IDD and TAD in children is very significant, as discussed previously. All patients with TAD should be observed closely for symptoms suggestive of diabetes mellitus and, when the measurement of ICA becomes available as a clinical tool, the sera of such patients should be checked annually for these.

The association of vitiligo, particularly with thyrotoxicosis, but also with Addison's disease, alopecia, and diabetes mellitus, has been known for many years. Six instances of vitiligo involving primarily the hands and feet among 90 patients with thyrotoxicosis have been observed. The vitiligo usually preceded the thyrotoxicosis. Since thyroglobulin antibodies, which usually reflect autoimmunity of the thyroid, are significantly increased in patients with vitiligo, patients with vitiligo should be followed closely for subclinical and clinical thyroid disease.

REFERENCES

1. Allison, A. C.: Self tolerance and autoimmunity in the thyroid. *N. Engl. J. Med.* 295:821, 1976.
2. Andersen, O. O., Deckert, T., et al.: *International Symposium. Immunological Aspects of Diabetes Mellitus.* Gentoft, Nordisk Insulanlaboratorium, 1975.
3. Barnes, E. W., and Irvine, W. J.: Addison's disease, ovarian failure, and hypoparathyroidism. *Clin. Endocrinol. Metabol.* 4:379, 1975.
4. Benacerraf, B.: Suppressor T cells and suppressor factor. *Hosp. Pract.* 13:65, 1978.
5. Blizzard, R. M., Chee, D., et al.: The incidence of parathyroid and other antibodies in the serums of patients with eupathic hypoparathyroidism. *Clin. Exp. Immunol.* 1:119, 1966.
6. Bottazzo, G. F., Floren-Christensen, A., et al.: Autoantibodies to prolactin-secreting cells of the human pituitary. *Lancet* 2:97, 1975.
7. Bottazzo, G. F., and Doniach, D.: Pancreatic autoimmunity and HLA antigens. *Lancet* 2:800, 1976.
8. Bottazzo, G. F., and Doniach, D.: The detection of autoantibodies to discrete endocrine cells in anterior pituitary and pancreatic islets. (In press)
9. Brown, J., Solomon, D. H., et al.: Autoimmune thyroid diseases — Graves' and Hashimoto's. *Ann. Intern. Med.* 88:379, 1978.
10. Bundey, S., Doniach, D., et al.: Immunological studies in patients with juvenile-onset myasthenia gravis and in their relatives. *Clin. Exp. Immunol.* 11:321, 1972.
11. Cavalbaro, J. J., Palmer, D. F., et al.: Immunofluorescence detection of autoimmune diseases. Publication of the U.S. Department of Health, Education, and Welfare, Public Health Service Center for Disease Control, Atlanta, Georgia, 30333, January, 1976.
12. Cunlife, W. J., All, R., et al.: Vitiligo, thyroid disease and autoimmunity. *Br. J. Dermatol.* 80:135, 1968.
13. Eisenbarth, G., Wilson, P., et al.: HLA type and occurrence of disease in familial polyglandular failure. *N. Engl. J. Med.* 298:92, 1978.
14. Flier, J. S., Bar, R. S., et al.: The evolving clinical course of patients with insulin receptor autoantibodies: spontaneous remission or receptor proliferation with hypoglycemia. *J. Clin. Endocrinol. Metabol.* 47(5):985, 1978.

15. Galbraith, R. M., and Fudenberg, H. H.: Autoimmunity in chronic active hepatitis and diabetes mellitus. A review. *Clin. Immunol. Immunopathol. 8*:116, 1977.

16. Hall, R., Doniach, D., et al.: Ophthalmic Graves' disease. Diagnoses and pathogeneses. *Lancet 1*:375, 1970.

17. Hertz, K. C., Gazze, L. A., et al.: Autoimmune vitiligo: Detection of antibodies to melanin producing cells. *N. Engl. J. Med. 297*:634, 1977.

18. Irvine, W. J., McCallum, C. J., et al.: Pancreatic islet cell antibodies in diabetes mellitus correlated with the duration and type of diabetes, coexistent autoimmune disease, and HLA type. *Diabetes 26*:138, 1977.

19. Irvine, W. J.: Autoimmunity in endocrine diseases. *Proc. R. Soc. Med. 67*:548, 1974.

20. Kahn, C. R., Flier, J. S., et al.: The syndromes of insulin resistance and acanthosis nigricans: Insulin-receptor disorders in man. *N. Engl. J. Med. 294*:739, 1976.

21. Khangure, M. S., Dingle, P. R., et al.: A long term followup of patients with autoimmune thyroid disease. *Clin. Endocrinol. 6*:41, 1977.

22. Kirkpatrick, C. H., and Greenberg, L. E.: Treatment of mucocutaneous candidiasis with transfer factor, In *Immune Regulators in Transfer Factor.* Khan, A., Kirkpatrick, C. H., et al. (eds.), New York, Academic Press, (in press).

23. Knox, A. J. S., VonWestalp, C., et al.: Thyroid antigen stimulates lymphocytes from patients with Grave's disease to produce thyroid stimulating immunoglobulins. *J. Clin. Endocrinol. Metabol. 43*:3330, 1976.

24. Lernmark, A., Freedman, Z. R., et al.: Islet-cell-surface antibodies in juvenile diabetes mellitus. *N. Engl. J. Med. 299*(8):375, 1978.

25. Lucky, A. W., Rebar, R. W., et al.: Pubertal progression in the presence of elevated serum gonadotropins in girls with multiple endocrine deficiencies. *J. Clin. Endocrinol. Metabol. 45*:57, 1977.

26. Macaron, C., Winter, R. J., et al.: Vitiligo and juvenile diabetes mellitus. *Arch. Dermatol. 113*:15, 1976.

27. MacCuish, A. C., Irvine, W. J., et al.: Antibodies to pancreatic islet cells in insulin-dependent diabetics with coexistent autoimmune disease. *Lancet 2*:1529, 1974.

28. Maclaren, N. K., and Huang, S. W.: Antibody to cultured human insulinoma cells in insulin-dependent diabetes. *Lancet 1*:997, 1975.

29. Myllarniemi, D. D. S., and Perkeentupa, J.: Oral findings in the autoimmune polyendocrine-candidiasis syndrome (APECS) and other forms of hypoparathyroidism. *Oral Surg. 45*:721, 1978.

30. Nerup, J.: In *Immunity and Autoimmunity in Diabetes Mellitus.* Bastenie, P. A., and Gepts, W. (eds.) Amsterdam, 1974.

31. Roitt, I. M., Doniach, D., et al.: Autoantibodies in Hashimoto's disease (lymphadenoid goiter). *Lancet 2*:820, 1956.

32. Rotter, J. I., and Rimoin, D. L.: Heterogeneity in diabetes mellitus-update, 1978. Evidence for further genetic heterogeneity in juvenile-onset insulin-dependent diabetes mellitus. *Diabetes 27*:599, 1978.

33. Ruehsen, M. M., Blizzard, R. M., et al.: Autoimmunity and ovarian failure. *Am. J. Obstet. Gynecol. 112*:693, 1972.

34. Solomon, D. H., Chopra, I. J., et al.: Identification of subgroups of euthyroid Graves' ophthalmopathy. *N. Engl. J. Med. 296*:181, 1977.

35. Spinner, M. W., Blizzard, R. M., et al.: Clinical and genetic heterogeneity in idiopathic Addison's disease and in hypoparathyroidism. *J. Clin. Endocrinol. Metabol. 28*:795, 1968.

36. Spinner, M. W., Blizzard, R. M., et al.: Familial distributions of organ specific antibodies in the blood of patients with Addison's disease and hypoparathyroidism and their relatives. *Clin. Exp. Immunol. 5*:461, 1969.

37. Talai, N.: *Autoimmunity: Genetic, Immunologic, Virologic, and Clinical Aspects. Review.* New York, Academic Press, 1978.

38. Volpe, R.: Thyroiditis: current views of pathogenesis. *Med. Clin. N. Am. 59*:763, 1975.

39. Volpe, R.: The pathogenesis of Graves' disease. An overview. *Clin. Endocrinol. Metabol. 7*:3, 1978.

40. Volpe, R.: The role of autoimmunity in hypoendocrine and hyperendocrine function with special emphasis on autoimmune thyroid disease. *Ann. Intern. Med. 87*:86, 1977.

41. Witebsky, E., and Rose, N. R.: Studies on organ specificity IV. Production of rabbit thyroid antibodies in the rabbit. *J. Immunol. 76*:408, 1956.

42. *Etiology and Pathogenesis of Insulin-Dependent Diabetes Mellitus.* Report of a workshop (Philadelphia, 1977). Co-sponsored by NIAMDD and the Juvenile Diabetes Foundation.

CHAPTER 27

Genetics and Endocrinology

By Joseph L. Goldstein
and Arno G. Motulsky

GENERAL PRINCIPLES OF HEREDITARY DISEASES

As with disease affecting other body systems, genetic factors play a significant role in the pathogenesis of many endocrine and metabolic diseases. In many instances the genetic effects are clearly discernible and easy to analyze. Not infrequently, however, the role of hereditary factors is hard to prove, and the mechanisms involved remain obscure.

In general, "classic" genetic or hereditary diseases transmitted by single-factor inheritance are believed to result from mutations affecting specific parts of the deoxyribonucleic acid (DNA), which carries the genetic information possessed by each cell. These mutations may be of several types, ranging from the substitution of one nucleotide base for another to the addition or deletion of larger segments of DNA. Visible chromosomal aberrations are not found in this type of disease. The principal manifestations of single-gene mutations are usually me-

diated through alterations in the synthesis or structure of proteins. If the mutation affects *structural genes* — genes which control the amino acid sequences of specific proteins — abnormal proteins may be made, or the synthesis of the proteins may be prevented. On the other hand, mutations involving *regulatory genes* possibly exist and may result in the synthesis of abnormal amounts of protein by disturbances in the metabolic and temporal control of their synthesis. At present, the concepts of structural gene mutations have been admirably documented in man, especially for the various abnormal hemoglobins, haptoglobins, and glucose-6-phosphate dehydrogenases.[1] However, understanding of regulatory gene mutations has, so far, been based mainly on work carried out in microorganisms. It is now apparent that the regulation of eukaryotic cells (such as in humans) differs from that of microbial organisms. Nevertheless, recent data regarding the structure of the human hemoglobin gene provide plausible models for the existence of regulatory genes genetically linked to the structural genes.

In some hereditary diseases it is possible to demonstrate directly a genetically determined abnormality or absence of a specific protein or enzyme.[1] In many or even most genetic disorders, only the distal physiologic effects of the mutation are recognizable, and the underlying, or primary, defect is unknown. Nevertheless, it generally seems reasonable to assume that a single primary defect exists whenever a disease is transmitted by a single gene mechanism and that the various manifestations of the disease can all be related to the mutational event by a more or less complicated "pedigree of causes." Whenever the identification of a primary defect is claimed for a disease, it becomes necessary that all clinical and biochemical observations be satisfactorily explained, and that transmission of the proposed defect conform with the observed mode of inheritance.

Recent work in genetic diseases has resulted in the almost constant finding that an entity that appears clinically uniform may represent the end result of different gene mutations (genetic heterogeneity).[2] Considering the complex enzymatic control of metabolism, it is not surprising that interference with different metabolic steps necessary for a given function may lead to a similar end result. In order to demonstrate that a given disease is the result of different mutations, one must ultimately demonstrate biochemical differences between the various forms of the disease. However, such heterogeneity can be strongly suspected if different modes of inheritance (i.e., autosomal recessive or X-linked recessive) are detected in different families with a similar disease. This approach, with careful correlation of detailed genetic, clinical, and biochemical data, has been extremely helpful in the definition of disease entities and for an understanding of the pathophysiology of diseases.

Mechanisms of Genetic Disease

Autosomal Dominant Diseases

Mendelian patterns of inheritance can be categorized as autosomal dominant, autosomal recessive, and X chromosome-linked traits. The distinction between "dominant" and "recessive" must be understood as one of convenience in pedigree analysis rather than as necessarily implying a fundamental difference in genetic mechanisms.[3] The term *dominant* implies that a mutation will be clinically manifest when an individual has a single dose of this mutation (or is heterozygous for it), while *recessive* implies that the double dose (or homozygosity) is required for clinical detection. Genes themselves are never dominant or recessive; their effects, however, are reflected by dominant or recessive inheritance. Individuals who are heterozygous for "recessive" genes often have demonstrable biochemical abnormalities, while those who are homozygous for "dominant" genes may be more severely affected than the heterozygotes.

Autosomal dominant diseases often exhibit considerable clinical variability, both in their penetrance (whether or not they manifest at all) and in their expressivity (the degree to which they manifest). Penetrance is a relative concept, since its assessment varies with the technique used for detection of the trait. In many diseases, penetrance may be rather low if one relies only on history and physical examination but becomes significantly higher when specific laboratory tests are used. Penetrance of less than 100% may be caused by various genetic or environmental modifiers. The genetic modifiers may be genes located on other chromosomes. Not infrequently, the part-

ner gene or allele on the nonmutant homologous chromosome may itself affect clinical expression of the mutant gene. It has been suggested that such modification may be caused by the presence of a series of multiple "normal" allelic forms (isoalleles) that function with different degrees of efficiency.[4] If the normal isoallele works at high capacity, the effect of a mutation might be relatively mild and age of onset delayed. A less efficient isoallele might not produce enough functional gene product, and in that case the mutant allele on the other chromosome would cause more severe disease with an earlier age of onset.

Not infrequently a patient with a dominant disorder is found to have unaffected parents, and a mutation is suspected. A mutation is most likely when the disease under study is highly deleterious and unlikely to lead to reproduction. In less severe disorders, a smaller proportion of cases will be caused by fresh mutations. In general, the frequency of new mutations observed clinically correlates directly with the genetic lethality of the disease. The more lethal the disease, the more common will be cases due to new mutations. For example, some of the rare nonfamilial disorders of sexual development, such as congenital anorchism and congenital absence of the vagina and uterus (Rokitansky-Küstner syndrome), may be the result of a new dominant mutation. Since individuals with these disorders cannot reproduce, the mutation is not transmitted, and the disorder, therefore, appears sporadically. For practical purposes, the presence of several affected sibs rules out mutation since cluster mutations in a gonadal sector are extremely rare.[5] Often when the parents are unaffected, the gene may be carried by one parent in whom the disease was nonpenetrant or of low expressivity. Extramarital paternity is another source of difficulty in interpretation since it is found in about 3% of randomly studied children in the United States and Western Europe.

The basic biochemical defects have been identified in only a few of the approximately 600 autosomal dominant disorders that affect man. These include familial hypercholesterolemia (abnormal cell surface receptor that binds plasma low-density lipoprotein and thereby regulates cholesterol metabolism); heredity methemoglobinemia and several hemolytic anemias due to unstable forms of hemoglobin (abnormal hemoglobin molecule); hereditary angioneurotic edema (abnormal protein inhibitor of an enzyme involved in the serum complement system); dysfibrinogenemias (abnormal subunit aggregation); and acute intermittent porphyria (abnormal enzyme that catalyzes a rate-limiting step in the heme biosynthetic pathway). If these few examples are representative, then mutations causing dominant diseases are likely to involve different types of regulatory molecules, such as membrane receptors, enzymes catalyzing rate-controlling steps in biosynthetic pathways, and molecules that play an inhibitory or activating role in cascade reactions. Abnormal interaction of molecular subunits appears to be another type of mechanism.

Autosomal Recessive Diseases

The clinical picture of autosomal recessive diseases tends to be more uniform than that of dominant diseases, and the age of onset is often early. As a general rule, recessive diseases are more commonly seen in children, while dominant diseases are more frequently encountered in adults. Since with recessive inheritance only one of four children is expected to be affected, multiple cases in a family may not occur, and many isolated or sporadic cases will be found. It can be shown that, in a population in which families with two, three, and four children exist in equal proportions, more than 50% of all cases of a disease due to recessive inheritance will be sporadic, and the genetic etiology will not be apparent from the family history. The presence of autosomal recessive inheritance implies that each clinically normal parent has contributed a single mutant gene to the patient. In the parents, the gene product of the normal allele is sufficient for normal function. With rare recessive diseases, the frequency of consanguineous marriage among the parents is often elevated; the rarer of the gene, the higher the proportion of parental consanguinity.

X-linked Diseases

Mutant genes carried on the X chromosome are characterized by full expression in males (hemizygotes) and variability of expression and penetrance in females (heterozygotes), depending on the particular mutation and on the individual carrying it. Demonstration of genetic linkage to other X-linked traits (such as glucose-6-phosphate dehydrogenase variants, color vision defects, or the blood group Xg[a]) is also of great assistance, as is the observation of cellular mosaicism (see below). X-linked inheritance of rare traits is ruled out by the demonstration of father to son transmission. In common X-linked traits, the mother may be a carrier without clinical manifestation, and spurious father to son transmission may be mimicked.

The understanding of the mechanisms of gene expression for X-linked genes has been greatly advanced by the Lyon hypothesis.[6] According to this hypothesis, only one of the two X chromosomes functions genetically in female cells. Female cells would, therefore, be equivalent in terms of X-chromosome activity to male cells. The nonfunctional X chromosome is heteropyknotic (very condensed in appearance), replicates late in the mitotic cycle ("late-labeling" with tritiated thymidine), and gives rise to the sex chromatin or Barr body.[7] In abnormal states with more than two X chromosomes such as XXX, all but one of the X chromosomes appear to be inactivated. The process of X-chromosome inactivation takes place early in embryonic development and is thought to be random, with inactivation of either the paternally or maternally derived X chromosome in each cell occurring with equal probability. Once inactivation has occurred, the inactivated X chromosome remains nonfunctional, and all progeny of the initial cell will have the same X chromosome inactivated. As a result of the inactivation process, mosaicism of cells in females who are heterozygous for an X-linked mutation will be particularly apparent. One group of cells in a given tissue will be normal; the other will manifest the mutant genotype. Because of the statistical random nature of the inactivation process, about half the cells will, on the average, have the normal X chromosome, while the other half will have the mutant X chromosome. However, chance or selection of one or the other sets of clones of cells may disturb these proportions in any given individual. Depending on the nature of the biochemical defect and on the proportions of mutant and normal X chromosomes in an individual, a genetically heterozygous female may be either virtually undetectable or mildly or severely manifested in the heterozygous state.

Although the Lyon hypothesis assumes complete inactivation of one X chromosome, the phenotype of human sex-chromosome abnormalities and other evidence suggest that this may not be completely true.[7, 8] For example, XO individuals should be identical to XX females and XXY individuals identical to XY males. The existence of considerable differences in these phenotypes suggests that either irreparable damage has been done before the time of inactivation, or that complete inactivation does not occur.

Chromosomal Disorders

Still another category of genetic disease results from chromosomal abnormalities. Chromosomal abnormalities may consist of an increase or a decrease in chromosome number, deletion or inversion of portions of chromosomes, or translocation of bits of chromosomes from one to another. If the sex chromosomes are affected, abnormalities in sexual differentiation may result (e.g., Klinefelter's and Turner's syndromes). Abnormalities of autosomal chromosomes may cause congenital malformations as in Down's syndrome (mongolism). Diseases due to chromosomal aberrations are not usually hereditary or familial but are most frequently caused by an abnormal division of germ cells before fertilization or by mitotic errors in the early cell divisions after fertilization. However, certain chromosome anomalies such as translocations may rarely be carried in a "balanced" state by phenotypically normal carriers and may thus be both hereditary and familial. Since the detection of chromosomal errors is carried out by conventional light microscopy, aberrations involving small chromosomal segments are beyond the resolving power of present methods. A class of genetic diseases with complex malformations which are caused by minute chromosomal defects affecting more than one gene may exist.

Multifactorial Disorders

The genetic element in most common disorders is rarely based on either single-gene (mendelian) or chromosomal abnormalities. Instead, multiple genes are postulated to interact with each other as well as with environmental factors to produce the familial aggregation that is observed in common diseases. The common thyroid diseases, such as thyrotoxicosis, primary hypothyroidism, chronic lymphocytic thyroiditis, and nonendemic goiter, fit into this category, as do, probably, certain forms of diabetes mellitus and coronary heart disease. In multifactorial disorders there is an underlying genetically determined and continuously distributed predisposition, often with a threshold beyond which individuals are at risk to the development of disease.[9, 10] In general, both the first-degree relatives (i.e., parents, sibs, children) and second-degree relatives (i.e., uncles, aunts, nieces, nephews, grandchildren) of a proband with a multifactorial disorder will have an increased absolute risk for the development of the disorder, first-degree relatives being more frequently affected than second-degree relatives. Multifactorial disorders rarely affect more than 5 to 10% of first-degree relatives. The hypothesis of multifactorial inheritance has been made more plausible in recent years by the demonstration of polymorphisms at many gene loci. Thus, at as many as one-third of all gene loci, different forms of a gene (alleles) are present with frequencies that cannot be explained by mutation.[11] Such a large degree of variation in normal genes undoubtedly exerts an important influence on the phenotypic expression of various traits and disease states in man and provides the "genetic background" against which a given gene or genes act. So far, the genetic loci most strikingly associated with predisposition to specific diseases are those that constitute the HLA system.

The HLA System and Disease Susceptibility

The HLA gene complex is located on the short arm of chromosome 6. It consists of four closely linked but distinct loci, which are designated HLA-A, HLA-B, HLA-C, and HLA-D. The products of these genes are proteins that are found on the surface of body cells and that enable an individual's immune system to distinguish its own cells from those of someone else. Each HLA locus in the population consists of multiple alleles, each of which produces an immunologically distinct protein. The specific combination of alleles that occur on one chromosome is termed *haplotype*. Each individual possesses two HLA haplotypes, one inherited from the maternal chromosome and the other from the paternal chromosome. For example, on chromosome 6 inherited from the mother an individual may have allele number 2 at the A locus, allele number 8 at the B locus, allele number 12 at the C locus, and allele number 3 at the D locus, whereas on chromosome 6 inherited from the father he may have allele number 3 at the A locus, allele number 7 at the B locus, allele number 12 at the C locus, and allele number 4 at the D locus.

The HLA system has been shown to be related to a number of diseases, many of which involve a demonstrable type of organ-specific autoimmunity. In order to understand the significance of these relations, it is necessary to understand the genetic term *linkage*. Linkage means that two genetic loci occur in close proximity on one chromosome. Since all of the HLA loci are on chromosome 6, they are all linked with one another. The gene for adrenogenital syndrome due to 21-hydroxylase deficiency is also closely linked to the HLA gene complex (see Adrenogenital Syndromes). All of the genes on any one chromosome are linked to each other, but this linkage may be more or less tight depending on how close the genes are to each other on the chromosome. If they are far apart on the chromosome, there is a good likelihood that a recombination event will take place between them, and they will be transmitted in an independent manner. Such genes are considered to be loosely linked. On the other hand, when genes are very close together on the same chromosome, they will almost always be transmitted to the offspring in the same combination in which they were inherited, and thus they are said to be closely linked. Note that the term *linkage* refers only to the proximity of the genetic loci. It does not say anything about the specific alleles at those loci. The HLA-A and HLA-B loci are linked to each other in every individual, no matter which specific alleles are present at those loci.

Theoretically, the various alleles at the A, B, and C, and D loci should be independently distributed in the population. That is, if an individual has a certain allele at the A locus, this should not affect the allele at the B locus. Such independent assortment should be present since there has been ample time in human evolution for crossing over to occur between all of the HLA loci so that the alleles are randomized. However, in the HLA system, such random assortment of alleles is frequently not observed. For example, if a chromosome happens to have allele number 8 at the B locus (B8), there is a high probability that it will also have a particular allele, namely DW3, at the D locus. The existence of such a nonrandom association between two specific alleles is called *linkage dysequilibrium*.

The reason for the occurrence of linkage dysequilibrium is not known. At least two possibilities exist. First, the mutation that gave rise to the DW3 allele might have occurred on a chromosome that contained the B8 allele, and sufficient time has not elapsed for crossing-over events to have distributed these two alleles randomly in the population. Genetic considerations regarding frequency of crossing over make this unlikely. The second hypothesis is that there is some selective advantage in having these two alleles in combination. It may be that if one has inherited the B8 allele at the B locus, one's survival is enhanced if one has also inherited the DW3 allele at the D locus. This would produce selective pressure to enhance the association between B8 and DW3 in the population.

The clinical importance of the HLA system was first deduced by analogy with a similar system that exists in the mouse. The mouse histocompatibility system is closely linked to genes on the same chromosome that control the immune response. Moreover, certain of the histocompatibility antigens are in linkage dysequilibrium with certain alleles at the immune-response loci. Since the immune-response loci control the ability of an individual to respond to certain types of antigenic challenges, mice that have certain histocompatibility antigens are frequently unable to respond to specific antigenic challenges.

The relevance of the HLA system to the genetics of human endocrine disease stems from the observations that certain alleles at the HLA loci predispose individuals to certain specific diseases. As discussed in more detail later, specific HLA alleles are found with increased frequency in several endocrine diseases, including juvenile-onset diabetes mellitus, thyrotoxicosis, idiopathic Addison's disease, and Schmidt's syndrome.

GENE ACTION IN ENDOCRINE GLANDS

The identification of a gene affecting a specific endocrine function is usually inferred from genetic analysis of family pedigrees showing mendelian inheritance of an endocrine abnormality. The existence of a normal gene can be demonstrated only by the presence and expression of its mutant allele. Since at least 50 phenotypically distinct and simply inherited disorders of the endocrine glands are currently recognized (comprising about 4% of all mendelian disorders now known to exist in man),[12] at least 50 genes exist which affect endocrine function in a major way. Mutation of these genes causes endocrine dysfunction, which is manifested at different physiologic levels, including glandular differentiation and neoplasia; hormone synthesis, secretion, and transport; and hormone action at the target cell level. In most cases, the elucidation of the biochemical nature of these 50 genes (i.e., the isolation and characterization of the normal and abnormal proteins specified by the normal and mutant alleles for each gene) has not been achieved. As more of these endocrine gene products become identified, more "markers" will become available for linkage studies to map the human chromosomes.

Several generalizations can be made regarding the relationship between molecular pathophysiology and mechanism of inheritance in endocrine disorders. The endocrine neoplasia syndromes, such as multiple endocrine adenomatosis, familial hyperparathyroidism without other endocrine gland involvement, and the medullary thyroid carcinoma-pheochromocytoma syndromes, are all inherited as autosomal dominant traits, as is frequently the case for other heritable tumors.[13] As for most enzyme deficiency states in man, the disorders affecting hormone biosynthesis (such as the adrenogenital syndromes and the familial goiters) show an autosomal recessive pattern of inheritance. Finally, it is noteworthy that the best documented examples of hormone resistance in man — e.g., Albright's hereditary osteodystrophy, vitamin D-resistant rickets, nephrogenic diabetes insipidus, and the testicular feminization syndrome (complete type) — result from mutations involving different genes on the X chromosome.

Single-gene–determined endocrine disorders have provided superb investigative models for unraveling the complexities of endocrine physiology and biochemistry. Most impressive has been the use of the various adrenogenital syndromes and of the familial goiters in the delineation of the biosynthesis of adrenocortical hormones and thyroxine, respectively. Since at least 20 mendelian disorders of sexual development are now recognized, it is predictable that the elucidation of the basic defect in each of them will similarly provide the biochemical information necessary to define the basis of sexual differentiation in man.

Many family studies of endocrinologic disease have been published because the operation of genetic factors is striking. Unfortunately, apart from extremely rare disorders, such studies usually are of little value in assessing the *total* role of heredity in the disease under study. In some published reports, genetic factors may be inferred from the data in the family history, but detailed studies on affected family members have not been performed. To

Table 27–1. ENDOCRINE DISORDERS INFLUENCED BY GENETIC FACTORS

Pituitary disorders
  Diabetes insipidus
  Pituitary dwarfism
  Pituitary hypogonadism

Parathyroid disorders
  Hypoparathyroidism
  Albright's hereditary osteodystrophy
  Hyperparathyroidism
  Vitamin D-resistant rickets

Thyroid disorders
  Goiter
  Cretinism
  Myxedema
  Chronic lymphocytic thyroiditis
  Thyrotoxicosis

Pancreatic disorders
  Diabetes mellitus
  Hypoglycemia

Adrenal disorders
  Adrenogenital syndromes
  Adrenal insufficiency
  Bartter's syndrome

Disorders of sexual development
  XX gonadal dysgenesis   XY gonadal dysgenesis
  True hermaphroditism   Testicular feminization
  Reifenstein's syndrome
  Primary male hypogonadism   Pseudovaginal perineoscrotal
  Sertoli-cell-only syndrome   hypospadias
  Stein-Leventhal syndrome   Precocious puberty

Endocrine tumor syndromes
  Multiple endocrine adenomatosis
  Medullary thyroid carcinoma-pheochromocytoma syndromes

Others
  Baldness
  Hirsutism
  Myotonic dystrophy
  Werner's syndrome
  Laurence-Moon-Bardet-Biedl syndrome
  Congenital lipodystrophy

Table 27–2. ENDOCRINE DISORDERS WHICH RARELY OCCUR IN FAMILIAL FORM

Pituitary disorders
  Acromegaly
  Amenorrhea-galactorrhea syndrome
  Hypopituitarism of adult onset
  Inappropriate secretion of ADH
  Anorexia nervosa

Parathyroid disorders
  DiGeorge syndrome

Adrenal disorders
  Cushing's syndrome
  Primary hyperaldosteronism
  Hypoaldosteronism of adult onset

Disorders of sexual development
  Turner's syndrome
  Klinefelter's syndrome
  XYY syndrome
  Mixed gonadal dysgenesis
  Sex-reversed 46/XX male syndrome
  Persistent müllerian duct syndrome (hernia uteri inguinale)
  Congenital anorchia
  Congenital absence of the vagina and uterus (Rokitansky-Küstner syndrome)

Others
  Polyostotic fibrous dysplasia (Albright-McCune-Sternberg syndrome)
  Ectopic hormone-producing tumors

obtain full appreciation of the role of genetic factors in endocrinology, it is imperative that complete individual and family studies be made on nonselected consecutive patients and their family members, using identical criteria in every subject investigated. Although time-consuming and expensive, such studies will be of great help in affording an understanding of the pathophysiology and natural history of these diseases.

Table 27–1 lists those endocrine disorders in which genetic factors have generally been demonstrated to play a significant role. In most of these cases, familial occurrence is frequent enough to warrant a family study. On the other hand, there are a number of endocrine diseases which rarely if ever show familial aggregation (Table 27–2). Although one or two isolated case reports have appeared suggesting familial occurrence of acromegaly, the galactorrhea-amenorrhea syndrome, and primary aldosteronism, most of the available evidence suggests a nongenetic etiology for these as well as the other disorders listed in Table 27–2.

The ectopic polypeptide hormone–producing tumors, although not strictly genetic in the sense that the tumors are heritable, are nevertheless of great genetic interest. Their biologic importance lies not only in that ectopic hormone production can serve as a clue to early diagnosis of cancer, but also in that it provides a model system for the study of the mechanism of genetic derepression of cellular function.[14] These ectopic hormone syndromes are discussed in Chapter 31.

GENETIC COUNSELING IN ENDOCRINOLOGY

When advising parents or potential parents about the risk to subsequent children of having a disorder that has already affected someone in the family, the first step is to be sure of the diagnosis — in particular, to make certain that the problem in question is really of genetic origin.

This is especially important in endocrine disorders with genetic and nongenetic etiologies, such as diabetes insipidus, panhypopituitarism, hypoglycemia, and hyperparathyroidism. Second, if the disease has a hereditary element, there is the problem of genetic heterogeneity.[2] Clinically similar genetic disorders may show different patterns of inheritance. For example, there are two types of familial isolated growth hormone deficiency that resemble each other quite closely, but one shows autosomal recessive and the other autosomal dominant inheritance.[15]

Estimates of recurrence risk are derived in a variety of ways.[16] These will take into account what is known of the genetic mechanism which determines the relevant disorder. When more than one genetic mechanism or when environmental or secondary factors can determine clinically indistinguishable traits, then the *relative* probabilities of the different mechanisms operating in the particular family are considered. For conditions determined by simple mendelian inheritance, there is no particular difficulty in predicting the probability of an offspring being affected, provided that the genotypes of the parents can be recognized. There are, of course, complications associated with failure of penetrance, variability in expression, and new mutations, but in general mendelian principles apply.

The genetic prognosis is usually presented in terms of probability that the couple will produce another affected child. It is important that the counselor make sure that the couple understands the meaning of such absolute risk figures. Although different families initially react in different ways to the same risk (and not always in the way one expects), most couples who ask for genetic advice can be expected to take a responsible course of action on the basis of the information quoted. For genetic diseases in general, when the recurrence risk is high — that is, equal to or greater than 1 in 10 — most parents (66% in Carter's genetic clinic[17]) are deterred from planning further children. When the risks are low — that is, less than 1 in 10 — few (25%) are deterred.

Nearly 100 inherited disorders can now be diagnosed prenatally by amniocentesis.[18] The 21-hydroxylase variety of the adrenogenital syndrome is the only endocrine disorder that has been successfully detected by this technique.[19-21] Elevated levels of pregnanetriol have been found in the amniotic fluid during the *last* trimester of several pregnancies in which the fetus was subsequently proved to be affected with this disorder. Attempts at diagnosis *in utero* earlier in gestation have not been successful[22] but may occasionally be possible on the basis of HLA studies since the gene for the 21-hydroxylase defect is linked to the HLA complex (see Adrenogenital Syndromes). Prenatal knowledge of diagnosis may be lifesaving in the management of male infants known to be at risk for this disease. Affected males often have no genital abnormalities at birth and are thus frequently discharged from the newborn nursery only to return subsequently in adrenal crisis.

Certain inherited endocrine disorders in which expression of the mutant gene is limited to only one sex can be avoided by determining the sex of the fetus and providing the option of selectively aborting fetuses of the appropriate sex. In the diseases listed in Table 27–3, selective abortion is a feasible means of prevention because the disorder is X-linked recessive and affects only males (e.g., diabetes insipidus, vasopressin-resistant type) or because the disorder involves sexual development and is expressed in only one sex (e.g., testicular feminization). In any mendelian disorder for which selective abortion is carried out

Table 27–3. INHERITED ENDOCRINE DISORDERS PREVENTABLE BY SELECTIVE ABORTION

Disorder	Method of Prevention
Diabetes insipidus, vasopressin-resistant type	Selective abortion of XY fetuses
Familial true hermaphroditism	Selective abortion of XX fetuses
Familial XX gonadal dysgenesis	Selective abortion of XX fetuses
Familial XY gonadal dysgenesis	Selective abortion of XY fetuses
Testicular feminization	Selective abortion of XY fetuses
Reifenstein's syndrome	Selective abortion of XY fetuses
5α-Reductase deficiency	Selective abortion of XY fetuses

on the basis of sex alone, one-half of the aborted fetuses will be normal and one-half will be affected. However, many parents prefer abortion on these grounds to prevent the birth of a sick child, particularly if amniocentesis can guarantee a nonaffected infant in a future pregnancy. A more rational approach ultimately will be to make the specific prenatal diagnosis so that only affected fetuses are aborted.

Table 27–4 lists those inherited endocrine disorders in which asymptomatic relatives at risk can be diagnosed by various laboratory tests and then successfully treated by either hormone replacement, prophylactic surgery, or other indicated means. In order that therapy be successful, it must be initiated within the first few months of life for certain of these disorders (e.g., diabetes insipidus, vasopressin-resistant type; vitamin D-resistant rickets; athyreotic cretinism; the adrenogenital syndromes; and familial leucine-sensitive hypoglycemia). In those forms of pituitary dwarfism which respond to treatment (e.g., familial hypopituitarism and isolated growth hormone deficiency), administration of growth hormone must be started in childhood to ensure normal growth. Moreover, in those individuals identified as asymptomatic gene carriers of the familial medullary thyroid carcinoma syndrome, a prophylactic thyroidectomy carried out in adolescence or early adulthood may be lifesaving. Family study to detect and treat affected relatives who are unaware of this disease is, therefore, mandatory in this disorder.

GENETIC DISORDERS OF THE PITUITARY

Diabetes Insipidus

Two hereditary forms of diabetes insipidus are recognized: (1) vasopressin-sensitive diabetes insipidus and (2) vasopressin-resistant, or nephrogenic, diabetes insipidus. Together these two hereditary disorders comprised about one-third of all types of diabetes insipidus seen on the Children's Service of the Massachusetts General Hospital.[23] In this particular series, the familial form of nephrogenic diabetes insipidus was at least 6.5 times more frequent than the familial vasopressin-sensitive type.[23] The most common cause of diabetes insipidus in all series is a nonfamilial form of the vasopressin-sensitive disorder due to brain tumor, such as craniopharyngioma in children[23] and metastatic carcinoma in adults.[24, 25]

Vasopressin-Sensitive Diabetes Insipidus

Hereditary vasopressin-sensitive diabetes insipidus is due to a quantitative reduction in the number of nerve cells in the supraopticohypophysial system,[26] resulting in

Table 27-4. TREATABLE OR PREVENTABLE INHERITED ENDOCRINE DISORDERS FOR WHICH SEARCH IN FAMILY MEMBERS OF AFFECTED PATIENTS IS MANDATORY

Disorder	Mode of Inheritance	Age of Onset	Method of Diagnosis	Treatment	Advantages of Early Diagnosis and Treatment
Diabetes insipidus, vasopressin-resistant type	X-linked recessive	Infancy	Urine concentration tests	Adequate hydration; chlorothiazide	Prevent mental retardation
Familial panhypopituitarism	Autosomal recessive; X-linked recessive	Infancy	Measurement of pituitary, adrenal, gonadal, and thyroid hormones	Replace deficient hormones	Prevent dwarfism, cretinism, adrenal insufficiency, gonadal failure
Isolated growth hormone deficiency	Autosomal recessive; autosomal dominant	Childhood	Measurement of growth hormone responses	Growth hormone	Prevent dwarfism
Pituitary hypogonadism	X-linked recessive; autosomal recessive	Adolescence	Plasma FSH, LH, testosterone	Testosterone	Prevent eunuchoidism
Primary male hypogonadism	X-linked recessive	Adolescence	Plasma FSH, LH, testosterone	Testosterone	Prevent eunuchoidism
Hypoparathyroidism	X-linked recessive; autosomal recessive	Infancy; adolescence	Serum calcium, phosphorus, parathyroid hormone	Calcium lactate; vitamin D	Prevent cataracts and tetany
Hyperparathyroidism	Autosomal dominant	Adulthood	Serum calcium, phosphorus, parathyroid hormone	Parathyroidectomy	Prevent renal damage and other complications of hypercalcemia
Vitamin D-resistant rickets	X-linked dominant	Infancy	Serum calcium, phosphorus, aklaline phosphatase; measurement of urine TRP	Vitamin D (high doses); oral phosphate	Prevent rickets
Familial goiters	Autosomal recessive	Infancy; childhood	PBI; perchlorate test; measurement of iodotyrosines in urine; audiogram	Thyroxine	Prevent cretinism
Hereditary form of athyreotic cretinism	Autosomal recessive	Infancy	PBI	Thyroxine	Prevent cretinism
Adrenogenital syndromes	Autosomal recessive	Infancy	Urinary 17-ketosteroids, pregnanetriol; buccal smear; serum electrolytes	Cortisone acetate	Prevent adrenal crisis and avoid sex identification problems
Adrenal insufficiency	Autosomal recessive; autosomal dominant; X-linked recessive	Infancy; adolescence; adulthood	Serum cortisol, ACTH	Cortisone acetate; DOC	Prevent adrenal crisis
Aldosterone deficiency	Autosomal recessive	Infancy; childhood	Serum electrolytes; measurement of aldosterone secretion	DOC	Prevent hyperkalemia and dehydration
Leucine-sensitive hypoglycemia	Autosomal recessive	Infancy	Blood sugar; measurement of plasma insulin responses	Low protein diet; diazoxide	Prevent convulsions
Multiple endocrine adenomatosis	Autosomal dominant	Adulthood	Serum calcium, phosphorus, blood sugar; gastrointestinal series	Parathyroidectomy; pancreatectomy; ulcer surgery	Prevent complications of hyperparathyroidism, hypoglycemia, peptic ulcer, metastatic cancer
Medullary thyroid carcinoma-pheochromocytoma syndromes	Autosomal dominant	Adulthood	Plasma calcitonin; measurement of blood pressure	Prophylactic thyroidectomy; removal of pheochromocytoma	Prevent thyroid carcinoma and complications of hypertension

a deficiency of circulating plasma vasopressin.[27] A number of families have been reported in which the disease showed the pedigree characteristics of autosomal dominant inheritance. The age of onset is often delayed until adolescence and early adulthood, and there is a wide variability in symptoms in both males and females. Females may be particularly symptomatic during pregnancy, with improvement after menopause.[28] In contrast to nephrogenic diabetes insipidus, hypocaloric dwarfism and mental retardation infrequently occur.[23, 28]

X-linked inheritance of vasopressin-sensitive diabetes insipidus has also been documented in several kindreds.[29] In such families, the males are moderately to severely affected, but female carriers show only mild defects in urine concentration or polyuria, particularly during the last trimester of pregnancy. Such mild effects in heterozygous females are readily understandable on the basis of a partial reduction in hormone-secreting cells, as predicted from the X-inactivation hypothesis. Neither clinical nor laboratory examinations can differentiate between the autosomal and the X-linked varieties of vasopressin-sensitive diabetes insipidus.

Nephrogenic Diabetes Insipidus

In vasopressin-resistant or nephrogenic diabetes insipidus, the renal tubule is completely insensitive to the action of antidiuretic hormone.[30] The biochemical basis for the end-organ unresponsiveness has not been precisely defined. However, physiologic studies suggest the possibility of a deficiency in the renal cyclic AMP receptor system mediated by vasopressin.[31] Almost all cases of nephrogenic diabetes insipidus beginning in childhood are familial, and the genetic pattern is compatible with X-linked recessive inheritance. All males thus far reported exhibit severe clinical signs, while most but not all carrier females manifest a mild form of the disorder, i.e., an abnormal urinary concentration test.[32, 33] One severely affected girl was found to have a deletion of one X chromosome.[34] Bode and Crawford have traced a large number of families to a group of Ulster Scots who settled in Nova Scotia in 1761, and have therefore suggested that most North American Caucasian patients with the disorder descended from these original settlers.[34] At least three Negro families[35-39] and one large Australian aboriginal kindred[38] have been reported with X-linked nephrogenic diabetes insipidus. No close linkage exists between the gene for diabetes insipidus and the Xg[a] blood group.[39]

Pituitary Dwarfism

Pituitary dwarism refers to a heterogeneous group of disorders in which shortness of stature results from a deficiency of growth hormone (GH). At least eight genetically distinct forms of familial dwarfism and GH deficiency have been identified (Table 27–5 and the following paragraphs).[40] Sporadic cases and those forms secondary to birth trauma, cranial irradiation for neoplasia, craniopharyngioma, histiocytosis X, and congenital malformations are also recognized. In Norway, the prevalence of pituitary dwarfism is estimated at 1 case per 100,000 population, with 25% of all cases being hereditary, 60% sporadic, and 15% secondary.[41]

Two of the genetic forms of pituitary dwarfism, congenital absence of the pituitary[42, 43] and abnormal sella turcica syndrome (Ferrier-Stone syndrome),[44, 45] have each been reported in only one family. Both disorders occurred in sibs of both sexes and are therefore presumed to be transmitted as autosomal recessive traits.

Familial Panhypopituitarism

Familial panhypopituitarism (asexual ateliotic dwarfism or multitropic pituitary hormone deficiency) is associated with a deficiency of GH *and* of one or more other pituitary hormones as well. Although the great majority of cases are sporadic, a number of inbred kindreds reported from Switzerland,[46] Yugoslavia,[47] and the Hutterite community of Western Canada[48] provide evidence that the most common familial form of panhypopituitary dwarfism is inherited as an autosomal recessive trait.[40] Recent reports suggest that panhypopituitarism may occasionally occur as an X-linked trait. One of these reports described four male cases in three related sibships connected through females of normal height,[49] and another showed panhypopituitarism in two half-brothers with the same mother.[50] The primary defects causing autosomal recessive and X-linked recessive panhypopituitary dwarfism are unknown.

The clinical features depend on which of the tropic hormones are deficient. There is both interfamilial and intrafamilial variation in the associated hormonal deficiencies. In certain families one individual may lack all of the tropic hormones, whereas another may lack only GH and gonadotropin. However, at least GH and gonadotropin deficiency occur in all affected members; there have been no familial crossovers between familial panhypopituitarism and isolated GH deficiency reported. There are no clinical or endocrine differences between the two genetic forms of familial panhypopituitarism and the more common acquired disease.[51]

Isolated Growth Hormone Deficiency

Analysis of the clinical, genetic, and metabolic features of normally proportioned dwarfs with normal sexual function (midgets or sexual ateliotics) indicates at least two genetically distinct types of isolated GH deficiency.[48] Type I GH deficiency, the more common type, is associated with insulin deficiency, prolonged hypoglycemia following insulin administration, GH responsiveness, wrinkled skin, high-pitched voice, and autosomal recessive inheritance. Type II GH deficiency, characterized by hyperinsulinemia, poor response to administered GH, normal skin, and normal voice, usually occurs as a sporadic disorder, but when it is genetic, it is transmitted as an autosomal dominant trait. The Type II disorder is likely heterogeneous; several families with apparent dominant inheritance who have the metabolic features of the recessive form (i.e., insulin deficiency rather than hyperinsulinemia) have been reported.[51]

Although puberty is frequently delayed to between 16 and 19 years, sexual development, once it occurs, is normal.[48] Cesarean section is required in pregnant affected females since their offspring will be of normal birth weight and length, regardless of whether the child is normal or ateliotic.[40] Pregnancy in these women is followed by normal lactation, suggesting that GH is not essential for normal postpartum lactation.[52]

Autopsies in three cases of the Type I disorder have revealed the presence of typical somatotropic cells in the pituitary and, in one case, the presence of immunoreactive GH, demonstrating the capability of the pituitary to synthesize GH.[53] Thus, the defect in these patients appears to be a deficiency of either GH-releasing factor or a defect in the releasing-hormone receptor of the somatotropic cell.[53]

Laron-Type Dwarfism

Although clinically similar to Type I GH deficiency, this form of familial pituitary dwarfism is distinct metabolically in that it is associated with high fasting levels of immunoreactive GH, low somatomedin (sulfation factor) activity, and metabolic resistant to the action of administered GH.[42] The basic defect appears to involve a defect in the generation of somatomedin, which itself is believed to be due to a generalized deficiency of GH receptors.[53a]

Approximately 40 Laron dwarfs have been identified.[54] Although originally reported in inbred families of Oriental Jewish origin, the disorder has since been described in non-Jewish families from Western Europe and the United States.[40] Consanguinity has been observed in about one-third of all reported cases, strongly suggesting autosomal recessive inheritance.[54]

Pygmies

The African Pygmies vaguely resemble pituitary dwarfs in their size and skeletal proportions but differ in their

Table 27–5. GENETIC FORMS OF PITUITARY DWARFISM*

Disorder	Inheritance
Congenital absence of pituitary	Autosomal recessive
Familial panhypopituitarism	
Type I	Autosomal recessive
Type II	X-linked recessive
Isolated growth hormone deficiency	
Type I	Autosomal recessive
Type II	Autosomal dominant
Laron-type dwarfism	Autosomal recessive
Pygmies	Probably multifactorial (*not* autosomal dominant)
Abnormal sella turcica	Autosomal recessive

*Modified from Rimoin, D. L., and Schimke, R. N.: *Genetic Disorders of the Endocrine Glands.* St. Louis, C. V. Mosby Co., 1971, with permission.

lack of truncal obesity and wrinkled skin.[40] Metabolically, the Pygmies show the unique combination of peripheral unresponsiveness to GH administration in the presence of normal levels of immunoreactive plasma GH and normal serum somatomedin activity.[40] The GH resistance is best explained by an unresponsiveness of peripheral tissues to the actions of somatomedin, suggesting a defect in somatomedin receptors.[51] Pygmy-Bantu hybrids have a normal metabolic response to GH administration and are intermediate in size between the two parental types.[55] No data are available on the inheritance, but a multifactorial mechanism is suggested by the phenotype of the Pygmy-Bantu hybrids.

Pituitary Hypogonadism

Pituitary hypogonadism, resulting from an isolated lack of either one or both of the gonadotropic hormones, FSH and LH, occurs as an accompaniment of organic pituitary impairment and malnutrition and as a primary genetic disorder. Although the heterogeneity of the genetic forms of pituitary hypogonadism has not been well delineated, at least two genetically distinct disorders exist: hypogonadotropic hypogonadism with anosmia (Kallmann's syndrome), inherited as an X-linked trait, and familial isolated gonadotropin deficiency, inherited as an autosomal recessive trait.

Hypogonadotropic Hypogonadism with Anosmia (Kallmann's Syndrome)

The most frequent form of familial hypogonadotropic hypogonadism occurs in males in association with anosmia or hyposmia and is known as Kallmann's syndrome.[56] This disorder has generally been considered to be inherited as an X-linked recessive, the trait being transmitted through females who either are normal or show partial or complete anosmia. However, several families have recently been reported in which dominant inheritance with father to son transmission was documented.[57, 58] The ability to induce fertility in affected males with chorionic gonadotropin should make it possible to determine whether other cases of Kallmann's syndrome, which would otherwise masquerade as an X-linked recessive trait, are the result of autosomal dominant inheritance. Since the anosmia is secondary to an absence of the olfactory lobes of the brain, and since hypoplasia of the hypothalamus has been reported in several autopsied cases,[59] the gonadotropin deficiency may be caused by a developmental anomaly of the brain. Results of LH-releasing hormone stimulation tests suggest that affected men fail to secrete FSH and LH because of a defect at the hypothalamic level.[60] The presence of any one of a number of abnormalities, such as cleft lip and palate, unilateral renal agenesis, ichthyosis, epilepsy, and short metacarpals, has been reported in some families with Kallmann's syndrome,[57, 61-63] but their genetic relationship to the endocrine defect is not well defined. Rarely, hypogonadotropic hypogonadism with anosmia and midline facial anomalies occurs as an autosomal recessive disorder.[64]

Familial Isolated Gonadotropin Deficiency

An isolated deficiency of gonadotropin involving both LH and FSH without anosmia or somatic anomalies has been described as a cause of familial hypogonadism in both males and females in at least four kindreds.[65] Auto-

somal recessive inheritance is suggested by involvement of siblings only and the presence of first-cousin parental consanguinity in one of the families.

Isolated deficiency of LH with normal serum FSH is reported to be the cause of the fertile eunuch syndrome, a disorder of males in which androgen deficiency is seen in combination with near-normal spermatogenesis.[66] This disorder is almost always sporadic, though one sibship with two affected brothers has been reported.[67]

GENETIC DISORDERS OF THE PARATHYROIDS

Hypoparathyroidism

The hereditary forms of hypoparathyroidism are rare disorders and probably comprise no more than one-fourth of all cases of idiopathic hypoparathyroidism.[68, 69] At least three genetically distinct disorders are recognized: (1) familial neonatal hypoparathyroidism; (2) familial hypoparathyroidism without Addison's disease and moniliasis; and (3) familial hypoparathyroidism with Addison's disease and moniliasis.

Familial Neonatal Hypoparathyroidism

Hypoparathyroidism developing in the first weeks of life and manifesting as neonatal tetany is due either to congenital absence of the thymus and parathyroid glands (DiGeorge syndrome), which occurs as a sporadic disorder in both males and females, or to familial neonatal hypoparathyroidism, which is inherited as an X-linked recessive and affects only males.[70, 71] Rarely, unrecognized maternal hyperparathyroidism may lead to suppression of parathyroid function of the newborn causing a clinical picture that transiently resembles neonatal hypoparathyroidism.[72]

Familial Hypoparathyroidism With and Without Addison's Disease and Moniliasis

Idiopathic hypoparathyroidism *without* Addison's disease and moniliasis usually appears after the first 6 months of life and before age 20 years. The distributions of the age of onset do not differ in the familial and nonfamilial cases.[68] Genetic analysis in 13 families suggests autosomal recessive inheritance.[68] Consanguinity has been recorded in several instances.[73]

Hypoparathyroidism developing between the ages of 6 months and 20 years has also been associated with idiopathic Addison's disease and mucocutaneous moniliasis.[74] Most of these cases have been familial, and the inheritance is autosomal recessive.[68] Monoliasis is usually the first manifestation of the disorder, and hypoparathyroidism generally reveals itself before the adrenal insufficiency. In addition, affected siblings may occasionally manifest any combination of pernicious anemia, thyroiditis, ovarian failure, or juvenile cirrhosis. Furthermore, since high titers of anti-endocrine organ antibodies are found in the sera of affected individuals, an inherited autoimmune basis for the disorder has been postulated.[74]

Albright's Hereditary Osteodystrophy

Albright's hereditary osteodystrophy (AHO) is an inherited disorder in which affected family members manifest either pseudohypoparathyroidism (PHP) or pseudo-pseudohypoparathyroidism (PPHP). The population frequency of the disorder is not known, but at least 227 cases had been reported as of 1966.[75] Patients with PHP seek aid at an average age of 8 years with all the clinical and biochemical findings of true idiopathic hypoparathyroidism but do not respond to the administration of parathyroid hormone.[76] In addition, they manifest a variety of skeletal and developmental defects, including shortness of stature, subcutaneous calcifications, ectopic bone formation, shortened metacarpals, roundness of the face, and mental retardation. Not all features are present in all cases, and patients with the skeletal but not the biochemical abnormalities of hypocalcemia and hyperphosphatemia have been designated as having PPHP. It is now generally concluded that PHP and PPHP are part of the same genetic syndrome, since single patients have had both conditions at different ages and many families have been reported in which members with both PHP and PPHP were present.[75]

Aurbach has suggested that the basic defect in AHO may involve a deficient parathyroid hormone receptor–adenyl cyclase system in kidney, bone, and other tissue.[78] Experimental data in support of this hypothesis are based on the observation that little or no cyclic AMP appears in the urine after the administration of parathyroid hormone to subjects with PHP, whereas there is a 10- to 20-fold increase in normal subjects, in patients with true idiopathic hypoparathyroidism, and in patients with a variety of unusual skeletal and developmental defects that resemble AHO, including the basal cell nevus syndrome, familial calcification of the cerebral basal ganglia, Gardner's syndrome, vitamin D-resistant rickets, and Turner's syndrome.[77, 78] The specific component of the parathyroid hormone–sensitive adenyl cyclase receptor system that is deficient is not known, but studies *in vitro* of renal tissue from two patients with PHP showed normal membrane-bound adenyl cyclase activity when tested at saturating concentrations of ATP.[79, 80] However, when detailed kinetic studies were performed, the renal adenyl cyclase showed a threefold lower affinity for ATP, and the *in vitro* response to parathyroid hormone was markedly impaired at subsaturating concentrations of ATP.[79, 80]

On the basis of genetic analysis showing lack of evidence of male to male transmission in families and an affected female to affected male ratio of 2:1, it has been inferred that an X-linked dominant mode of inheritance is operating.[81] On the other hand, the finding that hemizygous males are not more severely affected than are heterozygous females is contrary to what is observed in other X-linked traits. Moreover, the observation that at least 13 unaffected daughters have been born to affected males with AHO[75] is not in keeping with current concepts of X-chromosome inheritance. Finally, while the female to male ratio of all probands with AHO reported as of 1966 is 2.2:1,[75] the sex ratio of their affected sibs is 1.2:1, a value which approaches unity. Taken together, these data suggest either that AHO is in fact inherited as a sex-influenced autosomal dominant rather than an X-linked dominant or that AHO is genetically heterogeneous, comprising both X-linked and autosomal forms. At least one pedigree has been reported in which father to son transmission appears to have occurred.[82]

Hyperparathyroidism

Primary hyperparathyroidism is a common endocrine disorder occurring with a population frequency of 1 in 800.[83] In adults, hereditary forms of primary hyperparathyroidism account for about 20% of all cases and thus occur at a frequency of about 1 in 4000.[83] Three genetic forms are currently recognized, one affecting neonates and two affecting adults. Familial neonatal primary hyperparathyroidism is extremely rare; it affects young infants in the neonatal period and is inherited either as an autosomal recessive[84] or an autosomal dominant trait,[85, 86] Early diagnosis and parathyroidectomy are essential in order to permit survival.[85, 86]

Hyperparathyroidism in adults may occur in families in which there is no other endocrine involvement, or it may be a component of multiple endocrine adenomatosis. Both disorders appear to be inherited as autosomal dominant traits and are probably genetically distinct. In familial hyperparathyroidism, close to half the offspring of affected persons show hypercalcemia in the first two decades, nephrolithiasis and peptic ulcer disease are usual, and concentrations of peptide hormones other than parathyroid hormone are normal.[87]

Jackson has pointed out that male patients with hyperparathyroidism are three times more likely to have a familial disorder than are females. This is because the disorder in general has a male to female ratio of 1:3, while the ratio in hereditary hyperparathyroidism is 1:1. Therefore, if one in five patients with hyperparathyroidism has the hereditary type, then two of every five male patients and two of every 15 female patients should have affected relatives.[83]

Vitamin D-Resistant Rickets with Hypophosphatemia

Familial vitamin D-resistant rickets with hypophosphatemia is a disorder characterized by the development of rickets or osteomalacia, metabolic unresponsiveness to physiologic amounts of vitamin D, and the presence of hypophosphatemia owing to diminished renal tubular reabsorption of phosphate.[88] Current evidence suggests that the basic defect involves a membrane protein that normally mediates the transepithelial transport of phosphate anion.[88] A homologous X-linked mutation in the mouse has been described.[88]

When hypophosphatemia alone is used to identify the presence of the trait, all available genetic data, including sex ratios and segregation analyses, are consistent with a pattern of X-linked dominant inheritance with complete penetrance. Males usually have more severe skeletal disease than do females, as expected from the X-inactivation hypothesis.[88] Diagnosis can be made on the basis of hypophosphaturia in the first weeks of life, and early treatment can prevent the development of phenotypic manifestations in males.[88] Not all cases of vitamin D-resistant rickets are clearly inherited. Of 24 index cases studied by Burnett and Dent, eight (three males, five females) were found to be the only affected member of their respective kindreds.[89] Such sporadic cases could be due to phenocopy, an autosomal recessive trait, illegitimacy, or a new mutation. At least two instances of new mutations in this disorder have been identified.[89]

Vitamin D-resistant rickets needs to be distinguished clinically from a much rarer disorder called vitamin D dependency. This latter disorder has many features in common with vitamin D-resistant rickets, including the fact that all bone lesions heal completely when patients receive pharmacologic doses of vitamin D. The disorder differs from the X-linked vitamin D-resistant rickets by the presence of a myopathy and the autosomal recessive inheritance pattern.[88] Vitamin D dependency appears to be an inborn error of vitamin D hormone biosynthesis, affecting the conversion of 25-hydroxy-vitamin D to 1α,25-di-hydroxy vitamin D. The enzyme defect is presumed to involve the 25-hydroxy-vitamin D-1-hydroxylase in the kidney.[88]

GENETIC DISORDERS OF THE THYROID

Familial Goiter Resulting from Defects in Thyroxine Biosynthesis

This group of diseases is an excellent example of a genetically heterogeneous disorder. Pathophysiologic and biochemical studies have elucidated at least eight different biochemical defects in thyroxine biosynthesis that have the common end result of defective thyroid hormone secretion, hypothyroidism, and goiter formation (Table 27–6).[90] In general, patients affected with the complete defect in these disorders have retarded mental and skeletal development and, if untreated, show the outward appearance of thyroid hormone deficiency. Goiter may be present at birth but more commonly becomes noticeable during childhood. Although these disorders are the only types of thyroid disease in which a marked preponderance of affected females does not occur, females tend to be more severely involved.[91] Most of these defects appear to be inherited as autosomal recessive traits, and, with the exception of the Pendred syndrome, homozygotes are extremely rare, probably occurring no more frequently than 1 in 100,000 for each disorder.

The importance of these rare disorders, however, is out of all proportion to their frequency and relates to the light they throw on the modes of gene action in the causation of thyroid disease in general.[91] In all these defects, heterozygotes, who can be expected to be quite common, show a propensity to goiter formation much in excess of the normal population.[90] Thus, it is likely that the heterozygous states of these disorders contribute to the causation of milder and more common thyroid diseases such as nontoxic goiter (see further).

Pendred's Syndrome (Familial Goiter with Deaf-Mutism)

Pendred's syndrome, characterized by the unique association of goiter and nerve deafness, is the most frequent of the inherited defects in thyroxine biosynthesis. It comprises 7.5% of all individuals with congenital deafness. Moreover, the incidence of the disorder in the general population is estimated at 1 in 50,000.[90, 91] Family studies clearly indicate autosomal recessive inheritance.

Table 27–6. DEFECTS IN THROXINE BIOSYNTHESIS CAUSING FAMILIAL GOITER*

Failure to transport iodide
Failure to form organic iodine
    Complete peroxidase deficiency
    Altered binding of hemin to peroxidase
Pendred's syndrome (goiter with deaf-mutism)
Failure of coupling of iodotyrosines
Failure of iodotyrosine deiodinase activity
Diminished or altered thyroglobulin synthesis
Abnormal iodinated polypeptides in serum

*Modified from Stanbury, J. B., In *The Metabolic Basis of Inherited Diseases.* 4th ed. Stanbury, J. B., Wyngaarden, J. B., et al. (eds.), New York, McGraw-Hill Book Co., 1978.

Studies with ^{131}I have shown that the administration of perchlorate to these patients characteristically causes the thyroid to discharge iodine only partially, a finding which suggests that the basic defect may involve an incomplete failure of organization of iodine.[90] Since direct measurements and characterization of peroxidase activity in thyroid homogenates from patients with Pendred's syndrome have not yet been carried out, its precise biochemical relationship to the several other recognized organification defects listed in Table 27–6 is not known.

In addition to their nerve deafness, patients with Pendred's syndrome can also be distinguished from most other patients with familial goiter by their smaller goiters and euthyroid status. Nerve deafness has been reported, albeit infrequently, in other forms of familial goiter. A single case of cochlear deafness with a partial defect in coupling of iodotyrosines has been reported.[92] Moreover, two brothers with deafness, one of whom was goitrous and had a defect in the coupling of iodotyrosines, have been described.[93] The combination of familial goiter and deaf-mutism has also been reported in a brother and sister who, in addition, had "stippled" epiphyses and end-organ refractoriness to thyroid hormone as determined by elevated plasma thyroxine-bound iodine levels in the presence of euthyroidism. Since the parents of these two siblings were consanguineous, autosomal recessive inheritance is likely.[94]

Nontoxic Goiter

Probably the most frequent cause of simple nontoxic goiter is iodine deficiency, the pathologic changes in the thyroid being due to attempts to compensate for the interference with normal hormone production. The fact that not every person in a hyperendemic area develops goiter, as well as the occasional familial occurrence of simple goiter in nonendemic areas, suggests that genetic factors affect susceptibility to goiter formation.[95] The higher proportion of nontasters of phenylthiocarbamide (PTC tasting is a dominantly inherited genetic polymorphism in which tasters are of the genotypes TT and Tt, while nontasters are tt[96]) among patients in some populations with goiter, and the possibility of genetically determined thyroid autoimmunity in goitrous patients (see later) may explain some of this genetic susceptibility. Moreover, there is further evidence that the mild or incomplete defects in thyroid hormone biosynthesis present in heterozygotes for the various types of familial goiter may sometimes express as euthyroid goiter (discussed earlier). Fraser has estimated that approximately 8% of the general population is heterozygous for one of the genes causing familial goiter.[91] However, heterozygosis of this type alone is clearly not sufficient to cause goiter, since if it were, the family history in cases of nontoxic goiter would be more striking than it is.

Thus it is likely that nontoxic goiter is due to an interaction of the various genetic factors with secondary modifying factors, of which female sex, dietary deficiency of iodine, and dietary excess of goitrogens are the major etiologic factors thus far identified. In this sense, the inheritance of most nontoxic goiters is likely to be polygenic and multifactorial.

At least one form of euthyroid nontoxic goiter is determined by a single gene. Murray and associates described a Scottish family in which 13 members of five generations had nontoxic goiters which appeared in childhood and were characterized by marked intrathyroidal calcification demonstrable roentgenologically. None of the known defects in thyroxine biosynthesis could be implicated. The pedigree was consistent with an autosomal dominant mode of inheritance.[97]

Athyreotic Cretinism

This disorder results from a failure of thyroid development and is probably twice as common a cause of childhood hypothyroidism as are the familial goiters.[98] Most cases are sporadic and occur in females, but a number of families with affected sibs of both sexes have been described, consanguinity having been present in at least three instances.[99]

It is likely that athyreotic cretinism is as heterogeneous as are the familial goiters. One possible mendelian variant of this group is the very rare Kocher-Debre-Semelaigne syndrome, which is characterized by agoitrous cretinism in association with muscular hypertrophy. Cross and associates have identified two affected sibs in an inbred Amish family, thus making autosomal recessive inheritance likely.[100]

Thyroiditis and Adult Hypothyroidism

Thyroid autoantibodies are frequently found in adult patients with both chronic lymphocytic thyroiditis and primary hypothyroidism. Furthermore, a number of family studies have demonstrated an increased occurrence of thyroid autoantibodies in apparently normal relatives of patients with these disorders.[101] Although fathers as well as mothers can transmit the tendency to thyroid autoantibody formation,[102] no firm statement regarding the mode of inheritance can be made yet.[101] In addition to familial clustering of autoantibodies, the familial occurrence of various types of thyroid diseases, including nontoxic goiter and thyrotoxicosis, has been noted among relatives of patients with thyroiditis and primary hypothyroidism.[101] It has been estimated that about one-third of all adult patients with thyroid disease have family members affected with the same or a closely related thyroid disorder.[103]

Thyrotoxicosis

Genetic factors that influence susceptibility to hyperthyroidism have been demonstrated directly in families with thyrotoxicosis. Twin studies strongly suggest the operation of genetic factors, since 47% of identical twins and only 3.1% of nonidentical twins were concordant for thyrotoxicosis.[104]

Several family studies have shown a significant excess of thyrotoxicosis in relatives of those with the disease.[91] Both dominant and recessive modes of inheritance, with relative limitation to women and low penetrance of the gene, have been claimed. Various investigators have found that the incidence of thyroid autoantibodies, as well as of nontoxic goiter, thyroiditis, and primary hypothyroidism, is higher in relatives of thyrotoxic patients than in controls. These findings, coupled with data demonstrating a higher frequency of thyrotoxicosis among relatives of patients with both chronic lymphocytic thyroiditis and thyroid autoantibodies alone, suggest that thyroid autoimmunity may be the most important genetic factor supplying the common etiologic link among thyrotoxicosis, primary hypothyroidism, and thyroiditis. It is not yet clear, however, whether this genetic factor is primarily related to an inherited tendency to form autoantibodies or whether the autoimmune phenomena are secondary to a more fundamental basic lesion. An individual patient with chronic lymphocytic thyroiditis may be clinically hyperthyroid, euthyroid, or hypothyroid at different stages of his disease, thus providing an explanation for the finding of both myxedema and nontoxic goiter in relatives of patients with thyrotoxicosis. Further evidence that a common genetic factor or factors can produce different clinical forms of thyroid disease comes from studies in monozygotic twins, in whom either hypothyroidism with lymphocytic thyroiditis[105] or congenital athyreotic hypothyroidism[106] has been found in one twin and hyperthyroidism in the other.

The most recent focus of attention in unraveling the genetics of thyrotoxicosis has centered on its association with certain HLA antigens. In several large studies, about 40% of patients with thyrotoxicosis were found to have HLA-B8 as compared to only 20% of control subjects.[107] In addition, HLA-DW3 is also found with increased frequency among affected patients; the relative risk in one study for thyrotoxicosis was fivefold in individuals with HLA-DW3. Perhaps the most plausible explanation for this HLA association is that these two HLA antigens are not directly responsible for thyrotoxicosis, but they are marking the presence of another immune-related gene (or genes) which is carried in linkage dysequilibrium in the same haplotype as the HLA DW3 and HLA-B8 alleles (see earlier section, The HLA System and Disease Susceptibility). This other gene is postulated to enhance the development of autoimmunity.

Variants of Serum Thyroxine-Binding Globulin

Several plasma proteins, including prealbumin and thyroxine-binding globulin (TBG), bind thyroxine. Elevation and depression of TBG are associated with high and low protein-bound iodine values, respectively, and occur as familial conditions in euthyroid individuals.[108, 109] Family studies indicate that both TBG deficiency and TBG elevation are inherited as X-linked dominant traits,[109, 110] and both conditions affect the same protein (TBG) with at least two different mutations. The discovery of an XO female with absent TBG is in accord with these genetic data.[111] No linkage of the locus for elevated TBG to the Xg blood group locus could be demonstrated in one family study.[112] Neither condition appears to produce any clinical difficulties, but both must be remembered as causes of falsely low or high PBI values.

GENETIC DISORDERS OF THE ADRENAL

Adrenogenital Syndromes

The disorders of adrenocortical steroid biosynthesis leading to the adrenogenital syndromes and congenital adrenal hyperplasia have been resolved into at least five different specific genetic disorders, each presumably due to a different enzymatic defect.[113] The clinical manifestations vary in each disorder and are dependent on the specific actions of the particular intermediate steroid compound that accumulates (Table 27–7).

All these disorders appear to be inherited as autosomal recessive traits. Most are rare, except for the 21-hydroxylase deficiency, which accounts for more than 90% of all cases currently recognized.[113] The gene frequency for the

Table 27-7. FORMS OF ADRENOGENITAL SYNDROME

Deficiency	Degree of Virilization of Females	Failure of Virilization in Males	Dominant Steroid Secreted	Cortisol	Aldosterone	Comment
21-Hydroxylase Partial	++++	0	17-Hydroxyprogesterone	Normal	Increased	Most common type (95% of total); from 1/3 to 2/3 salt losers
Severe	++++	0	17-Hydroxyprogesterone	Decreased	Decreased	
11β-Hydroxylase	++++	0	11-Deoxycortisol and 11-deoxycorticosterone	Decreased	Decreased	Hypertension
3β-Hydroxysteroid dehydrogenase	+	++++	Δ5-3β-OH compounds (dehydroepiandrosterone)	0	0	Probably second most common; usually salt loss
17α-Hydroxylase	0	++++	Corticosterone and 11-deoxycorticosterone	Decreased	Decreased	No feminization of female; hypertension
20, 22-Desmolase	0	++++	Cholesterol (?)	0	0	Rare; usually salt loss

latter disorder varies among different populations. In the United States, determined in Maryland, the homozygous state is reported at 1 in 67,000,[114] giving a heterozygote frequency of 1 in 125. Figures for Switzerland are 1 in 5000 and 1 in 35, respectively.[115] Southwestern Alaskan Eskimos have the highest frequencies yet reported: 1 in 490 for homozygosity and 1 in 11 for heterozygosity.[116] The reason for these striking population differences in gene frequency is not completely known, but they probably reflect differences in inbreeding in these different areas. While gene frequencies are not affected by inbreeding, a higher frequency of affected homozygotes would be found with high inbreeding levels. If such estimates of homozygote frequency are used for calculations of gene and heterozygote frequencies, as is usually done, misleadingly high gene frequency estimates are obtained.

Recent linkage studies indicate that both the saltwasting and non-salt wasting forms of 21-hydroxylase deficiency are in very close genetic linkage with one of the four HLA loci, namely HLA-B.[117] An important observation in these studies is that no single one of the antigens specified by the HLA-B locus is selectively increased among affected patients, thus indicating a true genetic linkage between the 21-hydroxylase-deficient gene and the HLA-B gene (see earlier section, The HLA System and Disease Susceptibility).

Money and Lewis have reported that among 70 patients with the adrenogenital syndrome, 60% rather than the expected 25% had an IQ of 110 or higher. These data were interpreted to indicate that the higher intelligence in homozygotes is a result of a positive effect of elevated fetal androgen on intellectual development.[118]

Biochemical studies in the rare patients with the desmolase, 3β-hydroxysteroid dehydrogenase, and 17-hydroxylase deficiencies are of particular genetic interest because they indicate that the synthesis of each of these enzymes in both adrenal gland and gonad is under the control of the same gene, since the enzyme deficiency is found in both organs.[113]

Familial Adrenocortical Insufficiency

The familial forms of adrenocortical insufficiency consist of a number of different genetic disorders, each of which is relatively rare. The age of onset of symptoms may provide an initial clue to differential diagnosis. Congenital adrenal hypoplasia, Wolman's disease, and the adrenogenital syndromes (already discussed) become clinically evident in the newborn period; hereditary unresponsiveness to ACTH, uncomplicated Addison's disease, Addison's disease with diffuse cerebral sclerosis, and Addison's disease with hypoparathyroidism and moniliasis usually appear in early childhood, while adrenal insufficiency associated with Schmidt's syndrome develops in late childhood or early adulthood (see the following discussions).

Congenital Adrenal Hypoplasia

On the basis of both histologic and genetic evidence, there are at least two heritable forms of this disorder: (1) an X-linked recessive form involving males and characterized by the persistence of large fetal cells in the adrenal cortex, and (2) an autosomal recessive form involving both sexes in which the histologic abnormality does not appear.[119] The X-linked form has been reported more often than the autosomal recessive form. Both disorders are fatal if not immediately treated with steroids.

Wolman's Disease

This is an abnormality of lipid storage causing adrenal insufficiency, hepatosplenomegaly, and steatorrhea.[120] It is invariably fatal by the age of 6 months despite treatment with steroids. In a newborn with failure to thrive, the presence of bilateral calcification of the adrenals on the abdominal x-ray is highly suggestive of this disorder.

Over 20 patients have been reported, and the inheritance is consistent with that of an autosomal recessive mode. The significant biochemical feature is the accumulation of both cholesterol esters and triglycerides in many organs, because of a total deficiency of lysosomal acid lipase.[121]

Hereditary Unresponsiveness to ACTH

At least 20 patients in 16 families with adrenocortical dysfunction, characterized by deficient hydrocortisone production but normal aldosterone production, have been described.[122] Careful clinical studies have demonstrated ACTH unresponsiveness. Hypoglycemic convulsions and hyperpigmentation have been the two prominent features of this syndrome. Genetic analysis by Franks and Nance revealed an excess of males and a deficiency of consanguineous matings, suggesting the occurrence of both autosomal recessive and X-linked forms of the disorder.[123] ACTH levels in these patients as determined by both immunoassay and bioassay are elevated, thus excluding the possibility of a biologically inactive ACTH molecule.[123] The basic lesion(s) most likely involves a cellular interaction between ACTH and the cortisol biosynthetic system.

Addison's Disease

Idiopathic Addison's disease unassociated with other disorders is frequently familial, especially when it occurs in males below 10 years of age. Spinner and associates found affected relatives in the families of about one-third of all cases of uncomplicated Addison's disease seen at the Endocrine Clinic at Johns Hopkins Hospital.[68] The presence of normal sexual differentiation and the absence of autoantibodies and associated endocrinopathies in these patients separate this entity from other forms of familial adrenal insufficiency (discussed below). Most cases are inherited as a recessive trait, either autosomal or X-linked. The preponderance of males suggests the latter,[68, 124] but no unequivocal X-linked pedigree has yet been reported.

The unique combination of idiopathic Addison's disease and diffuse cerebral sclerosis (Schilder's disease) has been reported in at least 13 families. All fully documented cases have been limited to males, and the pedigrees are characteristic of X-linked recessive inheritance.[125] Close linkage to the Xg^a blood group has been excluded.[126] Clinically, the patients usually first develop adrenal insufficiency during childhood, followed several years later by the onset of spastic paraplegia and mental deterioration. The basic defect is believed to involve the accumulation in the brain and adrenal of cholesteryl esters having an unusually high proportion of fatty acids with a chain length of 24 to 30 carbons rather than the usual length of less than 20.[127]

Addison's disease with hypoparathyroidism and moniliasis is discussed on p. 1133.

The occurrence of Addison's disease of adult onset in association with thyroiditis is called Schmidt's syndrome.[128] An increased incidence of diabetes mellitus, vitiligo, and pernicious anemia, as well as the presence of circulating anti-endocrine tissue antibodies, is also characteristic of this disorder. Patients with Schmidt's syndrome usually have family members who manifest other types of autoimmune diseases. Recent HLA studies suggest that this syndromal association of autoimmune phenomena may be due to unusual genetic susceptibility to immunologic derangement because of the inheritance of a particular immune-response gene in linkage dysequilibrium with the HLA locus on chromosome 6. In a large

family in which three generations were affected with Schmidt's syndrome, Eisenbarth and coworkers found that six of seven affected individuals had the HLA-B8 allele, whereas all 10 unaffected individuals had B alleles other than B8.[129]

Familial Aldosterone Deficiency

Familial aldosterone deficiency results from an abnormality in the conversion of progesterone to aldosterone. Two forms are recognized: one due to a deficiency of 18-hydroxylase[130] and the other due to a deficiency of 18-hydroxydehydrogenase.[131] Both disorders appear to be inherited as autosomal recessive traits. The affected members of one inbred family reported with the 18-hydroxylase defect were severely ill with hyperkalemia, sodium depletion, and intermittent fever. On the other hand, the several families reported with the 18-hydroxydehydrogenase defect manifested only subtle signs, such as mild growth retardation and transient electrolyte disturbances. The 18-hydroxylase disorder is especially frequent in Iranian Jews.[132]

Bartter's Syndrome

Bartter's syndrome is a unique disorder in which juxtaglomerular hyperplasia and hyperaldosteronism are associated with severe hypokalemic alkalosis in the absence of hypertension.[133] Onset is usually in childhood. Dwarfism and chronic renal disease are often present. A disturbance in sodium transport unrelated to elevated levels of aldosterone or renin has been demonstrated *in vitro* in the red blood cells of affected patients, and this may relate to the primary defect of the disorder.[134] Autosomal recessive inheritance seems likely since of 26 cases reported, about half either occurred in sibs, including one pair of monozygotic twins, or resulted from a consanguineous or incestuous mating.[135] More than half of the cases described have occurred in blacks, suggesting a high frequency of the mutant gene in this race.[135]

Variants of Corticosteroid-Binding Globulin

As in the case of thyroxine-binding globulin, inherited variation in the level of serum corticosteroid-binding globulin (CBG) is also known. Both decreases[136] and increases[137] in CBG occur, neither of which has been associated with clinical abnormalities, though both cause abnormalities in the serum cortisol level. The mode of inheritance for CBG decrease appears to be dominant, either autosomal or X-linked, while that of CBG increase presumably involves the same genetic locus, although critical studies are lacking.

DISORDERS OF SEXUAL DEVELOPMENT

Abnormalities in sexual development usually result either from nonfamilial aberrations in sex chromosomes or from inherited single-gene mutations. However, several rare disorders of sexual development have been described in which neither a chromosomal error nor a clear-cut inheritance pattern of the disease can be demonstrated, such as the sex reversed 46/XX male syndrome,[138] the persistent müllerian duct syndrome in the male (hernia uteri inguinale),[139] congenital anorchia,[140] and congenital absence of the vagina and uterus (Rokitansky-Küstner syndrome).[141] It is possible that each of these abnormalities is due to a new dominant single-gene mutation that cannot be transmitted because affected individuals are always sterile. Such cases, therefore, appear as "sporadic" disorders. These "sporadic" abnormalities and the chromosomal errors of sexual development (e.g., Turner's syndrome, Klinefelter's syndrome, and mixed gonadal dysgenesis) are discussed in detail in Chapter 9.

At least 20 different inherited mendelian disorders affecting a variety of steps in sexual development (other than those described for the adrenogenital syndromes) are recognized, and the genetics of the most common of these disorders are discussed in this section. The importance of such rare disorders lies in the fact that the elucidation of the specific biochemical nature of each of these mutations can be expected ultimately to provide the basis of a methodology for carrying out genetic analyses of sexual differentiation in man.[142, 143]

Familial XX and XY Gonadal Dysgenesis

Pure gonadal dysgenesis refers to the occurrence of streak gonads in phenotypic females who lack the somatic anomalies and short stature present in Turner's syndrome. Such women usually have either a 46/XX karyotype (XX gonadal dysgenesis) or a 46/XY karyotype (XY gonadal dysgenesis).[144-146] Familial gonadal dysgenesis should not be confused with Noonan's syndrome, a disorder in which both males and females affected manifest the Turner phenotype but without gonadal abnormalities.[145]

At least 61 individuals with normal female chromosomal complements (46XX) and histologically proven streak gonads have been reported.[145] Nerve deafness has been particularly frequent in this group (incidence of 25%). Although deafness may occur in patients with 45/XO Turner's syndrome, it is usually not due to nerve damage but rather is secondary to middle ear infections.[147]

The occurrence of 16 of these cases in seven sibships is highly suggestive of autosomal recessive inheritance. Moreover, in three of these seven families, and in another family in which a sporadic case appeared, the parents were consanguineous.[148-151] Male sibs in these families appeared to be normal. The autosomal nature of the inheritance of this disorder suggests that genes other than on the X chromosome may be necessary for normal female gonadal development and differentiation.

Of the 62 individuals reported with 46/XY pure gonadal dysgenesis, all have had female phenotypes, and 17 were familial cases.[145, 146] Unlike familial XX gonadal dysgenesis which is inherited as an autosomal recessive trait, familial XY gonadal dysgenesis is not associated with increased parental consanguinity, and affected relatives are not limited to sibs but may also include cousins and aunts. Thus either X-linked recessive or autosomal dominant inheritance with expression only in chromosomal males is the most likely hereditary pattern in this disorder.[145, 151]

Although no family has yet been reported in which pure gonadal dysgenesis was found in both a genetic male and a genetic female, one sibship has been described in which XY gonadal dysgenesis and male pseudohermaphroditism with partial masculinization occurred in two sisters.[152] Patients with XY gonadal dysgenesis, but not XX gonadal dysgenesis, are especially prone to the development of tumors in their streak gonads.[145] It is not known whether the abnormal gene product in this disorder directly suppresses testis-determining loci on the Y chromosome and autosomes or whether it blocks some early stage of testicular morphogenesis.

Familial True Hermaphroditism

True hermaphroditism, defined by the presence of gonadal tissue of both sexes in one individual, is a heterogeneous entity. Sex chromosomal mosaicism, although infrequently demonstrated, is believed to account for the majority of cases.[144] Several examples of true XY/XX hermaphroditism in association with genetic chimeras resulting from the double fertilization of an egg by two sperm have also been reported.[144] Furthermore, a familial form of true hermaphroditism inherited as an autosomal recessive trait represents another mechanism by which this disorder can be produced.[153-155] In the sibship reported by Clayton and associates, all three affected "brothers" had a 46/XX karyotype, hypospadias, and gynecomastia, in addition to both ovarian and testicular tissues.[153]

The mechanism responsible for the gonadal development in true hermaphroditism is unknown. Even if not demonstrable with conventional karyotyping methods, it is assumed that sufficient genetic material derived from the Y chromosome is present (as the result of translocation, nondisjunction, or mutation) to induce the development of testicular tissue. In support of this is the fact that several 46/XX true hermaphrodites with a testis have been shown to be H-Y antigen positive.[143]

Since the familial form of true hermaphroditism in man appears to be inherited as an autosomal recessive, it is possible that many of the sporadic cases of hermaphroditism in which karyotypes fail to show sex-chromosomal mosaicism are, in fact, examples of the inherited form. It is unknown whether homozygosity for this gene, which causes true hermaphroditism in genetic females, has any aberrant effects on the sexual development of genetic males.

Hereditary Male Pseudohermaphroditism

In contrast to the true hermaphrodite who is usually a genetic female with gonadal tissue of both sexes, the male pseudohermaphrodite is a genetic male who has unequivocal male gonadal differentiation (i.e., only testes are present) but has some of the genital appearance of females.[144] In other words, the male pseudohermaphrodite is a genetic and gonadal male who fails to virilize. This failure is due to one of two types of defects that occur during embryonic sexual differentiation: (1) defects in testosterone synthesis, or (2) defects in androgen action (Table 27–8). Those disorders causing defective testosterone synthesis have been described in the earlier section on the adrenogenital syndromes. Those disorders due to defects in androgen action are discussed in the following sections.

Complete Testicular Feminization

The testicular feminization syndrome (complete type) represents the extreme form of male pseudohermaphroditism due to complete failure of virilization. Affected 46/XY individuals are unmistakably feminine in phenotype (i.e., they develop breasts and a typical female body build, with female external genitalia, despite the presence of intra-abdominal testes and the absence of internal female structures such as ovaries, uterus, and fallopian tubes). As a result of the clinical observation that topical and parenteral administration of high doses of methyltestosterone caused no growth of sexual hair in patients with testicular feminization, Wilkins was the first to propose that this disorder was due to end-organ unrespon-

Table 27–8.   CLINICAL AND GENETIC PROFILES OF HEREDITARY MALE PSEUDOHERMAPHRODITISM*

Class	Disorder	Inheritance	Phenotype				
			Müllerian Ducts	*Wolffian Ducts*	*Urogenital Sinus*	*External Genitalia*	*Breast*
Defects in testosterone synthesis	5-Enzyme deficiencies	Autosomal or X-linked recessive	Absent	Variable development	Variable from male to female	Generally female	Usually male
Defects in androgen action	5α-Reductase deficiency	Autosomal recessive	Absent	Male	Female	Clitoro-megaly	Male
	Complete testicular feminization	X-linked recessive	Absent	Absent	Female	Female	Female
	Reifenstein syndrome	X-linked recessive	Absent	Variable development	Variable from male to female	Incomplete male development	Female
	Incomplete testicular feminization	Presumed X-linked recessive	Absent	Male	Female	Clitoro-megaly and posterior fusion	Female

*Modified from Griffin, J. E., and Wilson, J. D.: *Clin. Obstet. Gynec.* 5:457, 1978.

siveness to this male sex hormone.[156] The molecular nature of the androgen resistance has been shown to be due to the absence of a receptor protein specific for the two major androgenic hormones, testosterone and dihydrotestosterone.[157] Fibroblasts cultured from the genital skin of normal men and women express androgen receptors, whereas fibroblasts from affected individuals show undetectable binding activity.

The testicular feminization syndrome (complete type) is the most common form of hereditary male pseudohermaphroditism, the estimated frequency being 1 in 20,000 men in Switzerland[158] and 1 in 62,000 men in Great Britain.[159] Approximately 1 to 2% of females with inguinal hernias prove to have this disorder.[160] Genetic analysis of published pedigree data on this condition is compatible with either X-limited recessive inheritance or autosomal dominant inheritance limited to the male sex. Female carriers can often be recognized by the sparseness of their pubic and axillary hair. Linkage studies in man using the X-linked markers — XG[a] blood group, color blindness, and hemophilia — have failed to show measurable linkage between these genes and that for the testicular feminization syndrome.[161-163] However, tissue culture studies of cloned fibroblasts from mothers of affected patients have provided evidence for mosaicism of the androgen receptor defect, indicating that the mutant gene is X-linked.[164] A homologous mutation in the mouse which is unequivocably X-linked has also been described.[165]

Incomplete Testicular Feminization

Incomplete testicular feminization resembles the complete form of the syndrome in respect to female phenotype, bilateral intra-abdominal testes, and 46/XY karyotype but differs in that ambiguous genitalia are present at birth, and some degree of virilization occurs at puberty. The unique clinical feature of the incomplete syndrome is the finding of breast development and ambiguous genitalia in a phenotypic female.[166] Although the genitalia are primarily female, with clitoromegaly and partially fused labia, the degree of masculinization of the genitalia can be quite variable in different families, suggesting that this disorder is not genetically homogeneous.[166-168]

The frequency of this disorder is uncertain, but in most series it is only about a tenth as common as the complete form. The family history in most cases is uninformative. Since only a few cases have been diagnosed definitively by excluding deficient androgen synthesis as the cause of the pseudohermaphroditism, it is not certain whether the disorder represents new mutations of a dominant disorder or whether the case material is too small to demonstrate autosomal recessive or X-linked recessive inheritance. No convincing pedigree has yet been reported in which complete and incomplete forms of testicular feminization coexist in the same family.[143] Recent studies in cell culture show that affected patients have a partial, but not complete, defect in the androgen receptor protein.[169]

The Reifenstein Syndrome

The Reifenstein syndrome constitutes a spectrum of abnormalities ranging from virtually complete failure of virilization to almost normal masculinization. The most typical phenotype is that of a male with severe hypospadias and gynecomastia. Several other rare clinical syndromes have been described that may ultimately prove to be due to the same mutant gene that gives rise to the Reifenstein defect.[170] For a discussion of the various syndromes by Lubs, Gilbert-Dreyfus, and Rosewater, the reader is referred to reference 171. Each of these disorders was originally assumed to be a distinct nosologic entity, but three extensive pedigrees have recently been described in which affected members of the same family exhibit variable phenotypes that encompass the typical phenotypes of these syndromes as well as the Reifenstein syndrome.[170, 172, 173] Since all three pedigrees are compatible with X-linked inheritance, the simplest interpretation is that the various syndromes of Reifenstein, Lubs, Gilbert-Dreyfus, and Rosewater constitute variable manifestations of a single mutation. For this variably expressed entity, the term "Reifenstein syndrome" or "familial incomplete male pseudohermaphroditism, Type 1" has been suggested.[142]

Studies in cultured fibroblasts have shown that the level of the androgen receptor protein is low in affected patients, ranging from virtually undetectable in some patients to levels intermediate between those seen in complete testicular feminization and the normal range.[169] One interpretation of these biochemical data is that the mutation causing Reifenstein syndrome involves the same genetic locus as the mutation in complete testicular feminization, but that the defect in the former is less severe.

5α-Reductase Deficiency

This disorder, which is also called "familial pseudovaginal perineoscrotal hypospadias" or "familial incomplete male pseudohermaphroditism, Type 2," is characterized by a congenital anomaly of the external genitalia in an otherwise normal male. The defective virilization during embryogenesis is limited to the urogenital sinus and the anlage of the external genitalia. Affected individuals are nearly always raised as females because the genitalia have a severe hypospadias with a perineal urethral opening, cleft scrotum, testes in labioscrotal folds, and a phallus that is mistaken for an enlarged clitoris. At the time of puberty, complete masculinization occurs.[174] Unlike the other forms of male pseudohermaphroditism, there is no breast development.

Genetic studies indicate that the disorder is due to the homozygous expression of an autosomal recessive gene that causes abnormal sexual development only in 46/XY individuals.[174, 175] Consanguinity has been a frequent finding among affected families and is particularly striking in a large pedigree reported from the Dominican Republic.[171]

Inasmuch as testosterone is the fetal androgen responsible for male differentiation of the internal wolffian ducts, whereas dihydrotestosterone is responsible for virilization of the urogenital sinus and the external genitalia, a failure of conversion of testosterone to dihydrotestosterone should result in the precise phenotype observed in these patients. Indeed, studies of intact genital tissues and of cultured genital skin fibroblasts from affected patients have shown that the primary defect is due to a marked deficiency of the 5α-reductase enzyme that normally converts testosterone to dihydrotestosterone.[175]

Familial Male Hypogonadism

A number of families have been described in which hypogonadism unassociated with hermaphroditism, pseudohermaphroditism, and pituitary gonadotropin deficiency occurred in multiple male relatives.[176] Pathogenesis is presumably related to defective androgen production in the testes, though it is unknown whether the mutation(s) involves a biosynthetic enzyme(s) or causes a failure of Leydig cell differentiation. As in most inherited disorders of male sexual development, pedigree analysis cannot distinguish between X-linked recessive and sex-limited autosomal dominant inheritance. This disorder should be distinguished from familial gynecomastia, in which gonadal function is normal and the breast enlargement is thought to be the result of familial sensitivity of the breast to normal circulating levels of androgen and estrogens. Since affected males with familial gynecomastia can reproduce, pedigree analysis can be informative, and it indicates that this trait is transmitted as an autosomal dominant trait limited to males.[177]

Sertoli-Cell-Only Syndrome

In the Sertoli-cell-only syndrome, the seminiferous tubules and germ cells of the testis fail to develop, despite normal Leydig cell development and function.[178] The patients are normally virilized and their only complaint is infertility. The testes are smaller than normal but larger than those of patients with Klinefelter's syndrome. Single-gene inheritance is indicated by the occurrence of two or more affected brothers in several families.[178, 179] The mode of inheritance could either be X-linked or autosomal recessive. The nature of the defect is unknown but may involve a critical step in germ cell differentiation that occurs after formation of the testes from the indifferent gonad.

Stein-Leventhal Syndrome

This disorder is characterized by infertility, secondary amenorrhea, menstrual abnormalities, and hirsutism in women who have enlarged polycystic ovaries. The pathogenesis is not known, though it may involve altered steroid metabolism in the ovary. Detailed genetic analysis in 18 families by Cooper and associates has demonstrated an increased frequency of oligomenorrhea, elevated levels of androgen metabolites in urine and blood, and an increased frequency of polycystic ovaries among the mothers and sisters of index patients. Male relatives were noted to be abnormally hairy. From these data, the inheritance appears to be dominant, probably autosomal.[180]

FAMILIAL PRECOCIOUS PUBERTY

Most cases of isosexual precocious puberty are nonfamilial and are either idiopathic or associated with a central nervous system lesion, a gonadal or adrenal tumor, or polyostotic fibrous dysplasia. These nonfamilial cases occur more often in females than in males.[181] Among the idiopathic forms of precocious puberty, there is a familial variety which predominantly affects males.[182, 183] Since the condition can be transmitted by unaffected females, as well as by affected males, to their sons, X-linked inheritance is excluded, and an autosomal dominant mode of inheritance with male limitation is indicated. Carrier females may either appear normal[184, 185] or show signs of virilization, such as frontal baldness and hirsutism.[183] Certain of the adrenogenital syndromes also cause familial isosexual precocious puberty in males. Familial forms of precocious puberty in females are extremely rare[181] and need to be distinguished from the early onset of sexual development and menarche which may represent the extreme of the normal distribution curve. Since the time of onset of menarche in mothers and daughters, as well as between sisters, shows a significant correlation (r = 0.4), it is likely that multiple genes control this physiologic process.[186]

HIRSUTISM AND BALDNESS

Hair growth patterns show marked variation both qualitatively and quantitatively. That such variation is particularly pronounced when certain racial groups are compared suggests the operation of multiple genetic factors. For example, in African blacks and Orientals, chest and beard growth is greatly diminished.[187]

Probably the best evidence that hair growth is multifactorially determined comes from Lorenzo's detailed family studies of American women with all types of hirsutism (adrenal, ovarian, and idiopathic).[188] For each type of hirsutism, the pattern of hair distribution in female relatives ranged from the normal female distribution to the abnormally hirsute. Correlation coefficients for hair distribution between propositi and their mothers averaged 0.50. No evidence for a major gene effect on hirsutism could be demonstrated in these data.

Pattern baldness, on the other hand, may be controlled by a major gene, whose expression is influenced by both age and hormones.[189, 190] This form of baldness results in the progressive transformation of large stout terminal hairs to short thin vellus hairs and ultimately leads to a reduction in the number of hair follicles of the scalp. Castration before puberty prevents male pattern baldness,[191] while masculinizing tumors will produce pattern baldness in women with bald male relatives.[187, 189] The action of the presumed gene(s) for baldness at the molecular level has not been defined, but its product(s) may interact directly with dihydrotestosterone, the active androgen in male target organs.[192]

FAMILIAL ENDOCRINE TUMOR SYNDROMES

Most endocrine tumors are not heritable, but there are several types of endocrine neoplasia which are determined by a single-gene mechanism. These genetic endocrine tumor syndromes include multiple endocrine adenomatosis and the medullary thyroid carcinoma-pheochromocytoma syndromes. Since the action of the genes causing these tumors has not been identified, very little is known about the pathogenesis of these disorders.

Multiple Endocrine Adenomatosis

More than 50 families have been described in which members have had hyperplasia or tumors (adenomas and, less often, carcinomas) involving one or more of the following endocrine organs: parathyroids, pituitary, pancreatic islets, thyroid, and adrenal cortex.[193-197] The parathyroid and islet-cell tumors are frequently multicentric, and all four parathyroids may be involved. In addition, multiple lipomas of the skin, bronchial adenomas, and intestinal carcinoids may occur. Many of the tumors are functional, and clinical hyperparathyroidism is frequently found. The islet-cell tumors may be either insulin- or gastrin-secreting, giving rise, respectively, to hypoglycemia or the Zollinger-Ellison syndrome of gastric hypersecretion and fulminating peptic ulcerations.[198] In a series of 25 patients with the Zollinger-Ellison syndrome, about 50% had familial multiple endocrine tumors.[198] It is now generally accepted that multiple endocrine adenomatosis and the Zollinger-Ellison syndrome are phenotypic variants of the same mutant gene.[194] Likewise, over half of the families with hereditary hyperparathyroidism actually have multiple endocrine adenomatosis.[83]

The disorder is inherited as an autosomal dominant trait with high penetrance. When 27 asymptomatic adult relatives of five index patients with multiple endocrine tumors were examined, 14 showed evidence of either hypercalcemia, lipomas, or peptic ulcers.[196] Similar to other dominant traits, there is a great deal of phenotypic variability. In the studies of Johnson and associates, the frequency of involvement rose from zero in relatives studied during the first decade of life to more than 50% of those examined during the fifth and sixth decades.[199]

Familial Medullary Thyroid Carcinoma-Pheochromocytoma Syndromes

Schimke has defined a spectrum of six familial syndromes involving medullary thyroid carcinoma and pheochromocytoma[200] (Table 27-9). Medullary thyroid carcinoma comprises less than 10% of all thyroid carcinomas[201] and is characterized histologically by the deposition of amyloid.

Family studies of patients with medullary thyroid carcinoma indicate that the disorder is inherited in an autosomal dominant pattern.[200] While some families show only medullary thyroid carcinoma, others have shown the combination of this tumor with bilateral pheochromocytomas and parathyroid adenomas. The parathyroid tumors are believed to represent a reactive hyperplasia secondary to hypocalcemia that results from excess calcitonin produced by the medullary thyroid tumor.[202] Studies by Melvin and Miller indicate that the first manifestation of this disorder in asymptomatic heterozygotes is an elevated plasma level of calcitonin determined by radioimmunoassay. This assay, therefore, can be used to predict which relatives in an affected family should undergo prophylactic thyroidectomy in order to prevent the onset of thyroid carcinoma.[203]

Patients with medullary thyroid carcinoma and pheochromocytoma may also manifest mucosal neuromas of the tongue, buccal mucosa, and eyelids. These patients also have a characteristic appearance: patulous lips, prognathic jaw, and Marfan-like body habitus.[200] Most cases of this disorder have been sporadic, but several instances of autosomal dominant transmission have been recorded.[200]

In addition to its association with the above syndromes, pheochromocytoma may occur as a familial disorder unassociated with other diseases. As many as 5% of all pheochromocytomas are familial.[204] These familial tumors are often bilateral and multifocal and may be extra-adrenal in location, while the sporadic lesion is usually single. Pheochromocytomas are also rarely seen in association with two mendelian disorders: von Recklinghausen's neurofibromatosis and Lindau-von Hippel disease.[200]

All these various syndromes involving medullary thyroid carcinoma and pheochromocytoma appear to be inherited in an autosomal dominant pattern. Whether they are the result of different gene mutations at the same locus (allelic) or at different loci (nonallelic) or merely reflect variable expression of a single-gene mutation is not known.

Table 27-9. SPECTRUM OF FAMILIAL SYNDROMES INVOLVING MEDULLARY THYROID CARCINOMA AND PHEOCHROMOCYTOMA*

Medullary thyroid carcinoma alone
Medullary thyroid carcinoma with pheochromocytoma and parathyroid adenoma
Medullary thyroid carcinoma, pheochromocytoma, mucosal neuromas and neurofibromas
Pheochromocytoma alone
Pheochromocytoma with neurofibromatosis (von Recklinghausen's disease)
Pheochromocytoma with hemangioblastoma of the retina and cerebellum (Lindau-von Hippel syndrome)

*From Schimke, R. N., In *The Clinical Delineation of Birth Defects X. The Endocrine System.* © 1971 The Williams and Wilkins Company, Baltimore.

DIABETES MELLITUS

While diabetes mellitus has long been considered a hereditary disease and certainly the most common inherited endocrinologic disorder, the mode of inheritance has been the subject of much debate. Rimoin has extensively reviewed the nature of the controversy concerning the genetics of diabetes mellitus.[205-207]

Many studies have demonstrated a higher frequency of diabetes mellitus among relatives of patients than in control populations.[208, 209] Furthermore, studies of twins indicate a higher concordance rate for diabetes between both members of a pair of monozygotic twins compared with dizygotic twins[210-212] (to be discussed later). However, when the precise analysis of the genetic basis of diabetes mellitus has been attempted, the subject has become "in many respects a geneticist's   nightmare . . . [which] . . . presents   almost every impediment to a proper genetic study."[213] Neel has summarized the difficulties involved: (1) frequency of the disease is age-dependent; (2) environmental factors including nutrition influence expression; (3) the nature of the basic defect is unknown; (4) genetic heterogeneity is likely; and (5) precise diagnostic criteria and genetic markers are lacking.[214]

Despite these difficulties, often with investigations in which sources of bias were not or could not be controlled and in which methods of ascertainment and diagnosis were not ideal, many genetic mechanisms have been proposed.[205, 207, 210] Chief among them are autosomal recessive (simple) inheritance and multifactorial (complex) inheritance. Against the autosomal recessive hypothesis for the general American population is the failure to find diabetes in 100% of the children of conjugal diabetics. Even if decreased penetrance is invoked, one still finds no more than 50% of the offspring of two diabetic parents affected, regardless of the criteria used (i.e., clinical diabetes, abnormal oral glucose tolerance, abnormal intravenous glucose tolerance, abnormal cortisone-glucose tolerance, or thickening of muscle capillary basement membranes).[207]

In mice (Mus musculus), inappropriate hyperglycemia may result from at least six distinct mutations, some of which are transmitted as autosomal dominant and others as autosomal recessive traits. Multifactorial forms of hyperglycemia have also been described. If these observations in mice are applicable to the genetics of diabetes in man, then it is quite likely that human diabetes is genetically heterogeneous, and its genetic complexity may, in part, be due to the occurrence in different individuals of various combinations of "diabetes genes," some having a major action and others have minor effects. In support of the idea of genetic heterogeneity in human diabetes is the finding of abnormal carbohydrate tolerance in at least 30 distinct genetic disorders.[207] Both the typical juvenile-onset form (e.g., in the optic-atrophy-diabetes syndrome) and the adult-onset type (e.g., in hemochromatosis) can occur.[207] Although individuals with these syndromes constitute a small fraction of all diabetic patients, they clearly show that distinct mutations at different genetic loci can result in glucose intolerance.

Whatever the exact mode of inheritance, the high frequency of this disease (at least 2% clinically affected in the United States) is of great genetic interest. Since diabetes was commonly a lethal disease until 50 years ago, one would have expected gradual elimination of the gene or genes leading to diabetes. On the contrary, diabetes is a frequently found disease. Since there is no reason to believe that mutations of the genes causing diabetes are more common than other mutations, and since it has not been proved that carriers of the gene(s) for diabetes have an increased number of off-

spring, a yet undetected advantage of the diabetic gene or genes unrelated to the disease itself must be seriously considered. Neel speculated that the ability to mobilize glucose readily may have been of great survival value during times in human evolution in which difficulty in obtaining food was common (the "thrifty genotype" hypothesis).[215]

Genetic Heterogeneity

Twin Studies

In the past few years, direct evidence from several different lines of investigation has emerged supporting the concept that human diabetes mellitus is genetically heterogeneous.[216, 217] Twin studies have provided one line of evidence for the separation of diabetes into at least two genetically distinct forms.[218] In a large group of identical twins with diabetes, Tattersall and Pyke found that of the twin pairs with onset of diabetes at more than 45 years of age, all were concordant, whereas of the pairs with onset at less than 45 years, 50% were discordant and appeared to remain discordant.[218] The finding of 100% concordance for adult-onset diabetic twins implies a stronger genetic component for the adult form of diabetes than had previously been recognized. If adult-onset diabetes is a multifactorial genetic disease, then nearly all of the causal factors must be genetic. The responsible environmental factors, such as obesity, would presumably be those that are common to the vast majority of the population.

The finding of only 50% concordance in juvenile-onset diabetes indicated that this disease has strong environmental as well as genetic components. Since identical twins share all of their genes, the fact that half of them fail to develop diabetes indicates that an environmental challenge is necessary for the development of this disease. Moreover, the environmental challenge must be quite specific since it often affects only one of a pair of identical twins even though both are living in the same household, eating the same food, and so on. That one of a pair of identical twins can be spared any environmental challenge half of the time is in itself quite striking.

An additional practical implication of these twin studies is that if a discordant identical twin of a diabetic child survives childhood without developing diabetes, he will probably never develop diabetes. This finding suggests that one of the environmental factor(s) that triggers juvenile diabetes is a specific event of childhood, such as a viral infection.

HLA Studies

The strongest support for the concept that juvenile-onset and adult-onset diabetes are different genetic entities comes from studies of HLA antigens in diabetic patients (see earlier section, The HLA System and Disease Susceptibility). A definite association between the HLA-B8 and the HLA-BW15 antigens with juvenile-onset diabetes, but not with adult-onset diabetes, has been found in a number of population studies.[217, 219, 220] Individuals with HLA-B8 and HLA-BW15 have 2.4-fold and 5-fold higher risk, respectively, for developing insulin-dependent diabetes than do individuals without these alleles.

Another interesting discovery to emerge from the HLA studies relates to the concept of linkage dysequilibrium. The B8 allele at the B locus is in linkage dysequilibrium with the DW3 allele at the D locus. Thus, most diabetic patients with the B8 allele also have the DW3 allele. Among juvenile

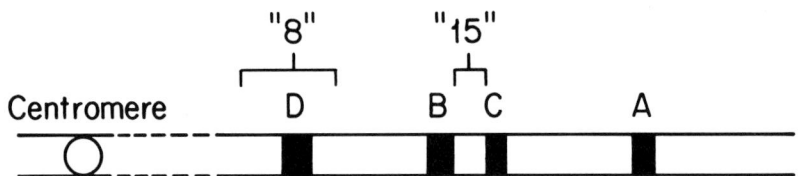

diabetics, the DW3 allele is even more common than the B8 allele, and the apparent association with the B8 allele is probably secondary to the association of the B8 allele with the DW3 allele (58% of juvenile-onset diabetics have the DW3 allele as compared with only 16% of controls[219]). The relative risk for juvenile diabetes if one inherits the DW3 allele is 6.4-fold higher than the risk in the general population.[219] The DW4 allele is also increased in diabetics (42% incidence in juvenile diabetics vs. 16% in the general population). Either the DW3 or the DW4 allele, or both of these alleles, are found in 80% of juvenile diabetic patients as compared with 24% of controls.[219] The simplest interpretation of these data is that there exists a genetic locus whose product can predispose to diabetes mellitus, that this locus is closely linked to the HLA-D locus, and that an allele at this putative locus exists in linkage dysequilibrium with the DW3 allele at the HLA-D locus.[217, 219]

In analogy to the finding that the B8 antigen appears to serve as a marker for a diabetogenic gene close to the HLA-D locus, it has also been shown that the BW15 antigen is in linkage dysequilibrium with the CW3 allele and hence it serves as a marker for a diabetogenic gene close to the C locus. Since the C and D loci are on opposite sides of the B locus, these results suggest that different genes are responsible for the susceptibility to diabetes in B8 and BW15 individuals (Fig. 27–1).[217]

Further support for the concept that the genes causing susceptibility to juvenile-onset diabetes mellitus are located on the 6th chromosome in proximity to the HLA complex comes from studies of the segregation of HLA haplotypes in families in which multiple siblings are affected with juvenile diabetes mellitus, the so-called *diabetes multiplex* families.[221] On the basis of mendelian expectations, there is a 50% chance that a pair of siblings share the same maternal 6th chromosome and hence the same maternal HLA haplotype, a 50% chance that they share the same paternal haplotype, and a 25% chance that they share both of these haplotypes. In a study of 24 families that contained two or more juvenile diabetic siblings, Barbosa found that 55% of the affected siblings shared two HLA haplotypes in common, in contrast to the 25% expected. Forty per cent of the siblings shared one haplotype in common (expected 50%), and only 5% of the siblings shared no HLA haplotypes (25% expected).[221] Stated another way, 95% of the affected pairs of siblings shared at least one HLA haplotype in common, instead of the expected 50%. In only one of the 24 families did a situation exist in which two diabetic siblings did not share one haplotype. The tendency for the affected diabetic siblings to share one or two HLA haplotypes was independent of the particular alleles at the HLA loci on these chromosomes, i.e., the particular alleles at the HLA locus on the diabetogenic 6th chromosome varied from family to family. Yet in each case, one of the 6th chromosomes predisposed to diabetes. These data strongly support the concept that the HLA genes themselves do not predispose to diabetes, but rather there must be a gene or genes on the 6th chromosome located *near* the HLA genes that predispose(s) to diabetes.

Pedigree Analysis

Tattersall and Fajans have identified a genetically distinct group of diabetics called "maturity-onset diabetes of young people."[222] Patients in this group develop diabetes at an early age, but have few symptoms and no ketonuria. Their disease can be controlled without insulin and there is little progression in severity over 20 years. These patients are thus phenotypically different from those with classic juvenile-onset, insulin-dependent diabetes. They also differ from the "garden-variety" adult-onset diabetic in two respects: (1) normal weight, and (2) age of onset below 40 years. Genetic studies provide further evidence for a separate entity. Of the index cases with "maturity-onset diabetes of young people," 85% had a diabetic parent with a similar phenotype, 53% of sibs tested had diabetes, and 46% of the families showed vertical transmission of the trait through three generations, suggesting autosomal dominant inheritance.

The existence of "maturity-onset diabetes of young people" may explain some of the apparent autosomal dominant pedigrees for diabetes that have appeared in the literature. The proportion of diabetic patients who have this disorder and its overall population frequency are important questions that are not yet answered.

Genetic Counseling

Diabetes mellitus is genetically heterogeneous. On the basis of clinical findings (e.g., age of onset and whether or not ketosis is present), studies of HLA antigens, and pedigree analysis, at least three genetically distinct forms of diabetes can now be recognized (Table 27–10). The heterogeneity that

Table 27–10. GENETIC CLASSIFICATION OF DIABETES MELLITUS

Type of Diabetes	Probable Mode of Inheritance	Environmental Factors Promoting Expression
I. Adult-onset, nonketotic	Multifactorial	Obesity

II. Juvenile-onset
  A. Ketotic
     HLA-B8 (DW3) and HLA-BW15 (CW3)
	Multifactorial	? Autoimmunity; ? viral infections; ? autoimmunity precipitated by viral infections

B. Nonketotic Maturity-onset diabetes of young people	Autosomal dominant	None required

has so far been discovered probably represents only the "tip of the iceberg."

In view of this large amount of genetic heterogeneity, it is evident that it would be incorrect to counsel all diabetic patients on the basis of one mode of inheritance. Moreover, the use of empiric risk data compiled without regard to the heterogeneity may be equally misleading. Unfortunately, accurate genetic counseling for the majority of diabetic patients is not possible at the present time. However, the data compiled in Table 27–10 should be useful to the physician as a guideline for explaining the genetic aspects of diabetes to patients.

In addition to discussing genetic aspects, the physician should also make diabetic families aware of the alleged relationship between clinical diabetes or chemical diabetes in the mother and congenital defects in her offspring. The most extensive study found that 44 of 853 infants of diabetic mothers (5.2%) had *major* defects as compared to a 1.2% frequency in control infants of nondiabetic mothers.[223] The most characteristic diabetic embryopathy is the caudal regression syndrome, which consists of agenesis of the sacrum and coccyx, hypoplasia of both femurs, and urogenital abnormalities.[224] Finally, it should be emphasized that, although gestation in the diabetic female is associated with an increased incidence of toxemia and polyhydramnios, the great majority of such pregnancies can be successfully managed with good obstetric care.

FAMILIAL HYPOGLYCEMIAS

The most common form of familial hypoglycemia not associated with other disease affects infants in the first 6 months of life and is characterized by excessive insulin release due to leucine sensitivity. Several families showing autosomal dominant inheritance of this disorder have been reported.[225, 226] Symptoms, including convulsions, may abate with age. Affected family members are often detected only after a challenge with leucine.

Familial hypoglycemia may also be associated with a number of different mendelian disorders including galactosemia, hereditary fructose intolerance, maple syrup urine disease, familial adrenal insufficiency, leprechaunism, various forms of pituitary dwarfism, glycogen storage disease (types I, III, V, and VI), fructose-1-6-diphosphatase deficiency, and multiple endocrine adenomatosis.[227] The hypoglycemias are discussed in detail in Chapter 16.

OBESITY

In man, obesity has been found in association with several rare mendelian disorders, including the Laurence-Moon-Bardet-Biedl syndrome[228] and the Alström syndrome.[229] However, the genetic aspects of the common forms of obesity are less well understood. An association of obesity with both diabetes mellitus[230] and hypertriglyceridemia[231] is unquestioned, and it is possible that a clarification of the genetics of these latter two disorders will provide insight into the genetics of the more common forms of obesity.

Studies of human families show striking aggregation of obesity, and segregation analyses of mating types (stout × stout, stout × normal, normal × normal) suggest a significant genetic contribution.[232] However, because of the problem of assortative matings (i.e., stouts marry stouts and thins marry thins), and because family groups share common eating habits, the genetic significance of these investigations is difficult to interpret. Although studies of twins have been criticized for similar reasons, they do suggest that identical twins are more closely related in weight than are fraternal twins or sibs taken at the same age.

In view of man's variable genetic background, familial obesity is more likely to be multifactorial rather than due to a single factor. Thus the weights of sibs of obese index cases are unimodally distributed with a higher modal weight than the control population, as would be expected with multifactorial inheritance.[233] A variety of physiologic mechanisms leading to obesity, such as the control of the number and size of adipose tissue cells, could be influenced by heredity.

OTHER HEREDITARY SYNDROMES WITH MAJOR ENDOCRINOLOGIC COMPONENTS

Myotonic Dystrophy

The characteristic clinical findings in myotonic dystrophy include myotonia, progressive muscular atrophy, frontal baldness, cataracts, and endocrine symptoms.[234-236] Over 50% of affected males develop testicular atrophy with age, which causes impotence and loss of libido but *not* gynecomastia or loss of male secondary sex characteristics. The frontal baldness does not appear to be directly related to the degree of hypogonadism. Affected females have normal menarche, but about 20% of them have menstrual irregularities, infertility, abortions, or early menopause. A low basal metabolism rate is common, while thyroid function, as assessed by specific tests, is usually normal. Although glucose intolerance and hyperinsulinemia are frequently present,[236] the microangiopathy of "garden-variety" diabetes mellitus does not occur.[236]

The disorder is inherited as an autosomal dominant, usually with delayed onset and marked clinical variability. About 25% of index cases are the result of a new mutation.[237] The most useful clinical methods for identifying subclinical cases in families at risk listed in order of diagnostic success are slit-lamp examination (for lens changes), followed by electromyography (for myotonic discharges), followed by measurement of immunoglobulins (for low IgG).[237] Since the genetic locus for myotonic dystrophy is closely linked to the locus determining the secretor blood group, application of such genetic linkage offers an additional technique for the diagnosis and counseling of family members at risk.[238] The most valuable information can be offered in a family where the affected parent is a secretor married to a nonsecretor, and the coupling phase is known from study of other relatives. If, in such an affected parent, the gene for myotonic dystrophy is on the same chromosome as the gene for secretor, and if the clinically normal offspring is secretornegative, the probability of normality for that offspring is 92%, even when allowance is made for genetic recombination.[238] Since the secretor status can be assessed by amniotic fluid assay, intrauterine diagnosis of myotonic dystrophy and selective abortion may occasionally be possible.

Werner's Syndrome

Werner's syndrome is a condition characterized by autosomal recessive inheritance which simulates premature aging. It is characterized by shortness of stature, a peculiar habitus with thin extremities, cataracts, early graying and loss of hair, a high-pitched voice, atrophy of the skin (especially below the knees), severe vascular disease, and intractable ulcerations of the feet and ankles. Although many endocrinologic defects have been claimed, the only two that are consistently found are a severe testicular atrophy in most males and a mild, relatively insulin-resistant diabetes mellitus affecting about half of all patients.[239] Although patients of both sexes have had children, fertility is markedly reduced. Females often have irregular menses, early menopause, and poor breast development, and the male external genitalia are usually small.

Laurence-Moon-Bardet-Biedl Syndrome

The Laurence-Moon-Bardet-Biedl syndrome is characterized by retinitis pigmentosa, obesity, mental deficiency, polydactylia, and hypogonadotropic hypogonadism.[228, 240, 241] Many other congenital anomalies, such as congenital heart disease, dwarfism, ataxia, nystagmus, and structural defects of the kidney and urogenital tract, have also been reported. There is a high rate of consanguinity among parents (25%), and autosomal recessive inheritance is likely.

In Switzerland, homozygotes occur at a frequency of 1 in 160,000.[241] The syndrome is often seen in an incomplete form, and the basic defect and the reason for the marked clinical variability are not understood. One disorder which superficially resembles the Laurence-Moon-Bardet-Biedl syndrome, but which is probably a separate entity, is the Alström syndrome, an autosomal recessive condition characterized by profound childhood blindness due to retinal degeneration, severe nerve deafness, infantile obesity, chronic nephropathy associated with aminoaciduria and vasopressin-resistant diabetes insipidus, and carbohydrate intolerance. A variety of other metabolic and endocrine abnormalities are present, including baldness, primary hypogonadism in males, hypertriglyceridemia, hyperuricemia, and acanthosis nigricans.[229, 242] The absence of both mental retardation and polydactylia in the Alström syndrome also serves to distinguish this disorder from the Laurence-Moon-Bardet-Biedl syndrome.

Congenital Total Lipodystrophy

Congenital generalized lipodystrophy (Seip-Laurence syndrome) is inherited as an autosomal recessive. It is to be distinguished from noninherited forms of lipodystrophy (partial and total), which usually have an adult onset.[243] Congenital total lipodystrophy has been reported in association with many endocrine and metabolic abnormalities, including hypertriglyceridemia; insulin-resistant nonketotic diabetes mellitus; elevation in basal metabolic rate without other evidence of hyperthyroidism; polycystic ovaries; and acanthosis nigricans. Mental retardation, hepatomegaly, systemic cystic angiomatosis, and acromegaloid facial and acral features have also been described in these patients.[244] The basic defect is not known, and it is also unclear whether congenital lipodystrophy is genetically heterogeneous.

REFERENCES

1. Stanbury, J. B., Wyngaarden, J. B., et al. (eds.): *The Metabolic Basis of Inherited Disease.* 4th ed. New York, McGraw-Hill Book Co., 1978.
2. Childs, B., and DerKaloustian, V. M.: *New Eng. J. Med.* 279:1205–1212, 1267–1274, 1968.
3. Allison, A. C., and Blumberg, B. S.: *Amer. J. Med.* 25:933, 1958.
4. Sutton, H. E. (ed.): *Genetics, Genetic Information, and the Control of Protein Structure and Function.* Transactions of the First Conference. New York, Josiah Macy, Jr., Foundation, 1960.
5. Reed, T. E., and Falls, H. F.: *Amer. J. Hum. Genet.* 7:28, 1959.
6. Lyon, M. F.: *Ann. Rev. Genet.* 2:31, 1968.
7. Epstein, C. J.: *New Eng. J. Med.* 296:318, 1972.
8. Lyon, M. F.: *Biol. Rev.* 47:1, 1972.
9. Cavalli-Sforza, L. L., and Bodmer, W. F.: *The Genetics of Human Populations.* San Francisco, W. H. Freeman and Co., 1971, pp. 508–633.
10. Carter, C. O.: *Brit. Med. Bull.* 25:52, 1969.

11. Harris, H.: *Brit. Med. Bull.* 25:5, 1969.
12. McKusick, V. A.: *Mendelian Inheritance in Man.* 5th ed. Baltimore, Johns Hopkins University Press, 1978.
13. Rimoin, D. L., and Schimke, R. N.: In *The Clinical Delineation of Birth Defects. X. The Endocrine System.* Baltimore, Williams and Wilkins Co., 1971, pp. 5–11.
14. Omenn, G. S.: *Ann. Intern. Med.* 72:136, 1970.
15. Merimee, T. J., Hall, J. G., et al.: *Lancet* 1:963, 1969.
16. Stevenson, A. C., and Davison, B. C. C.: *Genetic Counseling.* Philadelphia, J. B. Lippincott Co., 1970.
17. Carter, C. O., Roberts, J. A. F., et al.: *Lancet* 1:281, 1971.
18. Epstein, C. J., and Golbus, M. S.: *Ann. Rev. Med.* 29:117, 1978.
19. Jeffcoate, T. N. A., Fliegner, J. R. H., et al.: *Lancet* 2:533, 1965.
20. Nichols, J.: *Lancet* 1:1151, 1969.
21. Nichols, J.: *Lancet* 1:83, 1970.
22. Merkatz, I. R., New, M. I., et al.: *J. Pediat.* 75:977, 1969.
23. Crawford, J. D., and Bode, H. H.: In *Endocrine and Genetic Diseases of Childhood.* 2nd ed. Gardner, L. I. (ed.), Philadelphia, W. B. Saunders Co., 1975, pp. 126–158.
24. Blotner, H.: *Metabolism* 7:191, 1958.
25. Thomas, W. C.: *J. Clin. Endocr.* 17:565, 1957.
26. Braverman, L. E., Mancini, J. R., et al.: *Ann. Intern. Med.* 63:503, 1965.
27. Robertson, G. L., Klein, L. A., et al.: *Proc. Natl. Acad. Sci. USA* 66:1298, 1970.
28. Martin, F. I. R.: *Quart. J. Med.* 28:573, 1959.
29. Forssman, H.: *Amer. J. Hum. Genet.* 7:21, 1955.
30. Orloff, J., and Burg, M.: In *The Metabolic Basis of Inherited Disease.* 3rd ed. Stanbury, J. B., Wyngaarden, J. B., and Fredrickson, D. S. (eds.), New York, McGraw-Hill Book Co., 1972, pp. 1567–1580.
31. Verhoeven, G. F. M., and Wilson, J. D.: *Metabolism.* 28:253, 1979.
32. Carter, C., and Simpkiss, M.: *Lancet* 2:1069, 1956.
33. Childs, B., and Sidbury, J. B.: *Pediatrics* 20:177, 1957.
34. Bode, H., and Crawford, J. D.: *New Eng. J. Med.* 280:750, 1969.
35. Kaplan, S. A.: *Amer. J. Dis. Child.* 97:308, 1957.
36. Feigin, R. D., Rimoin, D. L., et al.: *Amer. J. Dis. Child.* 120:64, 1970.
37. Bianchine, J. W., Stambler, A. A., et al.: In *The Clinical Delineation of Birth Defects. X. The Endocrine System.* Baltimore, Williams and Wilkins Co., 1971, pp. 280–281.
38. Schultz, P., and Lines, D. R.: *Humangenetik* 26:79, 1975.
39. Bode, H. E., and Miettinen, O. S.: *Amer. J. Hum. Genet.* 22:221, 1970.
40. Rimoin, D. L., and Schimke, R. N.: *Genetic Disorders of the Endocrine Glands.* St. Louis, C. V. Mosby Co., 1971, pp. 29–42.
41. Seip, M., Trygstad, O., et al.: In *The Clinical Delineation of Birth Defects. X. The Endocrine System.* Baltimore, Williams and Wilkins Co., 1971, p. 33
42. Steiner, M. M., and Boggs, J. D.: *J. Clin. Endocr.* 25:1591, 1965.
43. Sadeghi-Nejad, A., and Senior, B.: *J. Pediat.* 84:79, 1974.
44. Ferrier, P. E., and Stone, E. F.: *Pediatrics* 43:858, 1969.
45. Ozer, F. L.: *Birth Defects: Original Article Series* 10:354, 1974.
46. Hanhart, E.: *Arch. Klaus Stift. Vererbungsforsch.* 1:181, 1925.
47. Zergollern, L.: In *The Clinical Delineation of Birth Defects. X. The Endocrine System.* Baltimore, Williams and Wilkins Co., 1971, pp. 28–32.
48. Rimoin, D. L., Merimee, T. J., et al.: *Recent Prog. Hormone Res.* 24:365, 1968.
49. Phelan, P. D., Connelly, J., et al.: In *The Clinical Delineation of Birth Defects. X. The Endocrine System.* Baltimore, Williams and Wilkins Co., 1971, pp. 24–27.
50. Schimke, R. N., Spaulding, J. J., et al.: In *The Clinical Delineation of Birth Defects. X. The Endocrine System.* Baltimore, Williams and Wilkins Co., 1971, pp. 21–23.
51. Rimoin, D. L., and Horton, W. A.: *J. Pediat.* 92:697, 1978.
52. Rimoin, D. L., Holzman, G. B., et al.: *J. Clin. Endocr.* 28:1183, 1968.
53. Rimoin, D. L.: *Birth Defects: Original Article Series* 12:15, 1976.
53a. Jacobs, L. S., Sneid, D. S., et al.: *J. Clin. Endocr.* 42:403, 1976.
54. Laron, Z.: *Birth Defects: Original Article Series* 10:231, 1974.
55. Merimee, T. J., Rimoin, D. L., et al.: *J. Clin. Invest.* 51:395, 1972.
56. Federman, D. D.: *Abnormal Sexual Development: A Genetic and Endocrine Approach to Differential Diagnosis.* Philadelphia, W. B. Saunders Co., 1967, p. 166.
57. Santen, R. J., and Paulsen, C. A.: *J. Clin. Endocr. Metab.* 36:47, 1973.
58. Merriam, G. R., Beitins, I. Z., et al.: *Amer. J. Dis. Child.* 131:1216, 1977.
59. Gauthier, S.: *Acta Neuroveg.* (Wien) 21:345, 1960.
60. Betend, B., Lebacq, E., Jr., et al.: *Acta Endocr.* 84:246, 1977.
61. Sparkes, R. S., Simpson, R. W., et al.: *Arch. Intern. Med.* (Chicago) 121:534–538, 1968.
62. Barden, C. W.: In *The Clinical Delineation of Birth Defects. X. The Endocrine System.* Baltimore, Williams and Wilkins Co., 1971, pp. 175–178.
63. Christian, J. C., Bixler, D., et al.: In *The Clinical Delineation of Birth Defects. X. The Endocrine System.* Baltimore, Williams and Wilkins Co., 1971, pp. 166–171.

64. Rosen, S. W.: *Proc. 47th Meeting Endocrine Society,* 1965.
65. Ewer, R. W.: *J. Clin. Endocr. 28:*783, 1968.
66. Faiman, C., Hoffman, D. L., et al.: *Mayo Clin. Proc. 43:*661, 1968.
67. McCullagh, E. P., Beck, J. C., et al.: *J. Clin. Endocr. 13:*489, 1953.
68. Spinner, M. W., Blizzard, R. M., et al.: *J. Clin. Endocr. 28:*795, 1968.
69. Aurbach, G. D.: In *The Clinical Delineation of Birth Defects. X. The Endocrine System.* Baltimore, Williams and Wilkins Co., 1971, pp. 48–54.
70. Peden, V. H.: *Amer. J. Hum. Genet. 12:*323, 1960.
71. Bronsky, D., Kiamko, R. T., et al.: *J. Clin. Endocr. 28:*61, 1968.
72. Hutchin, P., and Kessner, D. M.: *Ann. Intern. Med. 61:*1109, 1964.
73. Rimoin, D. L., and Schimke, R. N.: *Genetic Disorders of the Endocrine Glands.* St. Louis, C. V. Mosby Co., 1971, p. 83.
74. Wuepper, K. D., and Fudenberg, H. H.: *Clin. Exp. Immun. 2:*71, 1967.
75. Spranger, J. W.: In *The Clinical Delineation of Birth Defects. IV. Skeletal Dysplasias.* Baltimore, Williams and Wilkins Co., 1969, pp. 122–128.
76. Potts, J. T., Jr.: In *The Metabolic Basis of Inherited Disease.* 4th ed. Stanbury, J. B., Wyngaarden, J. B., et al. (eds.), New York, McGraw-Hill Book Co., 1978, pp. 1350–1365.
77. Chase, L. R., Nelson, G. L., et al.: *J. Clin. Invest. 48:*1832, 1969.
78. Aurbach, G. D., Marcus, R., et al.: *Metabolism 19:*799, 1970.
79. Marcus, R., Wieber, J. F., et al.: *J. Clin. Endocr. 33:*537, 1971.
80. Drezner, M. K., and Burch, W. M.: *Clin. Res. 26:*413A, 1978.
81. Mann, J. B., Alkerman, S., et al.: *Ann. Intern. Med. 56:*315, 1962.
82. Weinberg, A. G., and Stone, R. T.: *J. Pediat. 79:*996, 1971.
83. Jackson, C. E., and Frame, B.: In *The Clinical Delineation of Birth Defects. X. The Endocrine System.* Baltimore, Williams and Wilkins Co., 1971, pp. 66–68.
84. Hillman, D. A., Scriver, C. R., et al.: *New Eng. J. Med. 270:*483, 1964.
85. Spiegel, A. M., Marx, S. J., et al.: *J. Pediat. 90:*269, 1977.
86. Thompson, N. W., Carpenter, L. C., et al.: *Arch. Surg. 113:*100, 1978.
87. Marx, S. J., Spiegel, A. M., et al.: *Amer. J. Med. 62:*698, 1977.
88. Fraser, D., and Scriver, C. R.: *Amer. J. Clin. Nutr. 29:*1315, 1976.
89. Burnett, C. H., Dent, C. E., et al.: *Amer. J. Med. 36:*222, 1964.
90. Stanbury, J. B.: In *The Metabolic Basis of Inherited Disease.* 4th ed. Stanbury, J. B., Wyngaarden, J. B., et al. (eds.), New York, McGraw-Hill Book Co., 1978, pp. 206–239.
91. Fraser, G. R.: In *Progress in Medical Genetics.* Vol. VI. Steinberg, A. G., and Bearn, A. G. (eds.), New York, Grune and Stratton, 1969, pp. 89–116.
92. Hollander, C. S., Prout, T. E., et al.: *Amer. J. Med. 37:*630, 1964.
93. Fontan, A., Rubiana, M., et al.: *Arch. Franc. Pediat. 22:*897, 1965.
94. Refetoff, S., DeWind, L. T., et al.: *J. Clin. Endocr. 27:*279, 1967.
95. Malmos, B., Koutras, D. A., et al.: *J. Clin. Endocr. 26:*688, 1966.
96. Harris, H., Kalmus, H., et al.: *Lancet 2:*1038, 1949.
97. Murray, I. P., Thomson, J. A., et al.: *J. Clin. Endocr. 26:*1039, 1966.
98. Fraser, G. R.: *J. Genet. Hum. 18:*169, 1970.
99. Rimoin, D. L., and Schimke, R. N.: *Genetic Disorders of the Endocrine Glands.* St. Louis, C. V. Mosby Co., 1971, pp. 116–117.
100. Cross, H. E., Hollander, C. S., et al.: *Pediatrics 41:*413, 1968.
101. Fialkow, P. J.: In *Progress in Medical Genetics.* Vol. VI. Steinberg, A. G., and Bearn, A. G. (eds.), New York, Grune and Stratton, 1969, pp. 117–167.
102. Beierwaltes, W. H.: In *The Thyroid.* Hazard, J. B., and Smith, D. E. (eds.), Baltimore, Williams and Wilkins Co., 1964, pp. 58–75.
103. Klein, E.: *Deutsch. Med. Wschr. 85:*314, 1960.
104. Von Verschuer, O.: *Verh. Deutsch. Ges. Inn. Med. 64:*262, 1959.
105. Jayson, M. I. V., Doniach, D., et al.: *Lancet 2:*15, 1967.
106. Townes, P. L., and Bradford, W. L.: *J. Med. Genet. 8:*471, 1971.
107. Friedman, J. M., and Fialkow, P. J.: *Clin. Endocr. Metab. 7:*47, 1978.
108. Beierwaltes, W. H., and Robbins, J.: *J. Clin. Invest. 38:*1683, 1959.
109. Marshall, J. S., Levy, R. P., et al.: *New Eng. J. Med. 274:*469, 1966.
110. Nusynowitz, M. L., Clark, R. F., et al.: *Amer. J. Med. 50:*458, 1971.
111. Refetoff, S., and Selenkow, H.: *New Eng. J. Med. 278:*1081, 1968.
112. Fialkow, P. J., Giblett, E. R., et al.: *J. Clin. Endocr. 30:*66, 1970.
113. Bongiovanni, A. M.: In *The Metabolic Basis of Inherited Disease.* 4th ed. Stanbury, J. B., Wyngaarden, J. B., et al. (eds.), New York, McGraw-Hill Book Co., 1978, pp. 868–893.
114. Childs, B., Grumbach, M. M., et al.: *J. Clin. Invest. 35:*213, 1956.
115. Prader, A.: *Helv. Paediat. Acta 13:*426, 1958.
116. Hirschfeld, A. J., and Fleshman, J. K.: *J. Pediat. 75:*492, 1969.
117. Levine, L. S., Zachmann, M., et al.: *New Eng. J. Med. 299:*911, 1978.
118. Money, J., and Lewis, V.: *Bull. Johns Hopkins Hosp. 118:*365, 1966.
118a. McGuire, L. S., and Omenn, G. S.: *Behav. Genet. 5:*165, 1975.
119. Wein, L., and Mellinger, R. C.: *J. Med. Genet. 7:*27, 1970.
120. Fredrickson, D. S., and Ferrons, V. J.: In *The Metabolic Basis of Inherited Disease.* 4th ed. Stanbury, J. B., Wyngaarden, J. B., et al. (eds.), New York, McGraw-Hill Book Co., 1978, pp. 670–687.
121. Lake, B. D., and Patrick, A. D.: *J. Pediat. 56:*262, 1970.
122. Kelch, R. P., Daniels, G., et al.: *Clin. Res. 19:*202, 1971.
123. Martin, M. M.: In *The Clinical Delineation of Birth Defects. X. The Endocrine System.* Baltimore, Williams and Wilkins Co., 1971, pp. 98–100.

125. Forsyth, C. C., Forbes, M., et al.: *Arch. Dis. Child. 46:*273, 1971.
126. Spira, T. J., Adam, A., et al.: *Lancet 2:*820, 1971.
127. Igarashi, M., Schaumberg, H. H., et al.: *J. Neurochem. 26:*851, 1976.
128. Carpenter, C. C. J., Solomon, N., et al.: *Medicine 43:*153, 1964.
129. Eisenbarth, G., Wilson, P., et al.: *New Eng. J. Med. 298:*92, 1978.
130. Visser, H. K. A., and Cost, W. S.: *Acta Endocr. (Kobenhavn) 47:*589, 1964.
131. David, R., Golan, S., et al.: *Pediatrics 41:*403, 1968.
132. Cohen, T., Theodor, R., et al.: *Clin. Genet. 11:*25, 1977.
133. Bartter, F. C., Pronove, P., et al.: *Amer. J. Med. 33:*811, 1962.
134. Gardner, J., Lapey, A., et al.: *J. Clin. Invest 49:*32a, 1970.
135. Sutherland, L. E., Hartroft, P., et al.: *Acta Pediat. Scand. (Suppl.) 201:*1, 1970.
136. Doe, R. P., Lohrenz, R. N., et al.: *Metabolism 14:*940, 1965.
137. Lohrenz, F., Doe, R. P., et al.: *J. Clin. Endocr. 18:*1073, 1968.
138. de la Chapelle, A.: *Amer. J. Hum. Genet. 24:*71, 1972.
139. Morillo-Cucci, G., and German, J.: In *The Clinical Delineation of Birth Defects. X. The Endocrine System.* Baltimore, Williams and Wilkins Co., 1971, pp. 229–231.
140. Simpson, J. L., Horwith, M., et al.: In *The Clinical Delineation of Birth Defects. X. The Endocrine System.* Baltimore, Williams and Wilkins Co., 1971, pp. 196–200.
141. Leduc, B., Van Campenhout, J., et al.: *Amer. J. Obstet. Gynec. 100:*512, 1968.
142. Wilson, J. D., and Goldstein, J. L.: *Birth Defects: Original Article Series, 11,* 1975.
143. Griffin, J. E., and Wilson, J. D.: *Clin. Obstet. Gynec. 5:*457, 1978.
144. Federman, D. D.: *Abnormal Sexual Development: A Genetic and Endocrine Approach to Differential Diagnosis.* Philadelphia, W. B. Saunders Co., 1967, p. 54.
145. Simpson, J. L.: *Disorders of Sexual Differentiation.* New York, Academic Press, 1977.
146. Summitt, R. L.: In *Progress in Medical Genetics.* Vol. III (new series). Steinberg, A. G., et al. (eds.), Philadelphia, W. B. Saunders Co., 1979, pp. 1–72.
147. Szpunar, J., and Rybak, M.: *Arch. Otolaryng. (Chicago) 87:*34, 1968.
148. Simpson, J. L., and Christakos, A. C.: *Obstet. Gynec. Survey 24:*580, 1969.
149. Perrault, M., Klotz, B., et al.: *Bull. Soc. Med. Paris 67:*79, 1951.
150. Guisti, G., Borghi, A., et al.: *Acta Genet. Med. Gemellol. (Roma) 15:*51, 1966.
151. Sternberg, W. H., Barclay, D. L., et al.: *New Eng. J. Med. 278:*695, 1968.
152. Barr, M. L., Carr, D. H., et al.: *Amer. J. Obstet. Gynec. 99:*1047, 1967.
153. Clayton, G. W., Smith, J. D., et al.: *J. Clin. Endocr. 18:*1349, 1958.
154. Milner, W. A., Garlick, W. B., et al.: *J. Urol. 79:*1003, 1958.
155. Rosenberg, H. S., Clayton, W., et al.: *J. Clin. Endocr. 10:*121, 1963.
156. Wilkins, L. M.: *The Diagnosis and Treatment of Endocrine Disorders in Childhood and Adolescence.* 2nd ed. Springfield, Ill., Charles C Thomas, 1957.
157. Keenan, B. S., Meyer, W. J., III, et al.: *J. Clin. Endocr. 38:*1143, 1974.
158. Hauser, G. A.: In *Intersexuality.* Overdizer, C. (ed.), London, Academic Press, 1963, p. 255.
159. Jagiello, G., and Atwell, J. D.: *Lancet 1:*329, 1962.
160. Kaplan, S. A., Snyder, W. H., et al.: *Amer. J. Dis. Child. 117:*243, 1969.
161. Sanger, R., Tippett, P., et al.: *J. Med. Genet. 6:*26, 1969.
162. Stewart, J. S. S.: *Lancet 2:*592, 1959.
163. Nillson, I. M., Bergman, S., et al.: *Lancet 2:*264, 1959.
164. Meyer, W. J., III, Migeon, B. R., et al.: *Proc. Natl. Acad. Sci. USA 72:*1469, 1975.
165. Lyon, M. F., and Hawkes, S. G.: *Nature (London) 225:*1217, 1970.
166. Park, J. I., and Jones, H. W., Jr.: *Amer. J. Obstet. Gynec. 108:*1197, 1970.
167. Rosenfeld, R. L., Laurence, A. M., et al.: *J. Clin. Endocr. 32:*625, 1971.
168. Saez, J. M., de Peretili, E., et al.: *J. Clin. Endocr. 32:*604, 1971.
169. Griffin, J. E., Punyashthiti, K., et al.: *J. Clin. Invest. 57:*1342, 1976.
170. Wilson, J. D., Harrod, M. J., et al.: *New Eng. J. Med. 290:*1097, 1974.
171. Wilson, J. D., and MacDonald, P. C.: In *The Metabolic Basis of Inherited Disease.* 4th ed. Stanbury, J. B., Wyngaarden, J. B., et al. (eds.), New York, McGraw-Hill Book Co., 1978, pp. 894–913.
172. Gardo, S., and Papp, Z.: *J. Med. Genet. 11:*267, 1974.
173. Walker, A. C., Stack, E. M., et al.: *Med. J. Australia 1:*156, 1970.
174. Simpson, J. L., New, M., et al.: In *The Clinical Delineation of Birth Defects. X. The Endocrine System.* Baltimore, Williams and Wilkins Co., 1971, pp. 140–144.
175. Wilson, J. D.: *J. Biol. Chem. 250:*3498, 1975.
176. Nowakowski, H., and Lenz, W.: *Recent Prog. Hormone Res. 17:*53, 1961.
177. Wallach, E. F., and Garcia, S. R.: *J. Clin. Endocr. 22:*1201, 1962.
178. Howard, R. P., Sniffer, R. C., et al.: *J. Clin. Endocr. 10:*121, 1950.
179. Weyeneth, R.: *Praxis 45:*21, 1956.

180. Cooper, H. E., Spellacy, W. N., et al.: *Amer. J. Obstet. Gynec. 100:*371, 1968.
181. Federman, D. D.: *Abnormal Sexual Development: A Genetic and Endocrine Approach to Differential Diagnosis.* Philadelphia, W. B. Saunders Co., 1967, pp. 159–160, 174–176.
182. Rimoin, D. L., and Schimke, R. N.: *Genetic Disorders of the Endocrine Glands.* St. Louis, C. V. Mosby Co., 1971, pp. 338–340.
183. Beas, F.,Zurbrugg, R. P., et al.: *J. Clin. Endocr. 22:*1095, 1962.
184. Jacobson, A. W., and Macklin, M. T.: *Pediatrics 9:*682, 1952.
185. Jungck, E. C., Brown, N. H., et al.: *Amer. J. Dis. Child. 91:*138, 1956.
186. Zacharias, L., and Wurtman, R. J.: *New Eng. J. Med. 280:*868, 1969.
187. Munro, D. D.: In *Dermatology in General Medicine.* Fitzpatrick, T. B., Arndt, K. A., et al. (eds.), New York, McGraw-Hill Book Co., 1971, pp. 297–330.
188. Lorenzo, E. M.: *J. Clin. Endocr. 31:*556, 1970.
189. Rook, A.: *Brit. Med. J. 1:*609, 1965.
190. Synder, L. H., and Yingling, H. C.: *Hum. Biol. 7:*608, 1935.
191. Hamilton, J. B.: *Amer. J. Anat. 71:*451, 1942.
192. Bruchovksy, N., and Wilson, J. D.: *J. Biol. Chem. 243:*2012, 1968.
193. Wermer, P.: *Amer. J. Med. 35:*205, 1963.
194. Ballard, H. S., Frame, B., et al.: *Medicine 43:*481, 1964.
195. Karback, H. E., and Golindo, D. L.: *Texas Med. 66:*54, 1970.
196. Synder, N., Scurry, M. T., et al.: *Ann. Intern. Med. 76:*53, 1972.
197. Zollinger, R. M., and Craig, T. V.: *Amer. J. Med. 29:*29, 1960.
198. Huizenga, K. A., Goodrick, W. I. M., et al.: *Amer. J. Med. 37:*564, 1964.
199. Johnson, G. J., Summerskill, W. H. J., et al.: *New Eng. J. Med.* 1379, 1967.
200. Schimke, R. N.: In *The Clinical Delineation of Birth Defects. X. The Endocrine System.* Baltimore, Williams and Wilkins Co., 1971, pp. 55–65.
201. Williams, E. D.: *J. Clin. Path. 18:*288, 1965.
202. Melvin, K. E. W., and Tashijian, A. H.: *Proc. Nat. Acad. Sci. USA 59:*1216, 1968.
203. Melvin, K. E. W., Miller, H. H., et al.: *New Eng. J. Med. 285:*1115, 1971.
204. Williams, E. D., and Pollack, D. J.: *J. Path. Bact. 91:*71, 1966.
205. Rimoin, D. L.: *Med. Clin. N. Amer. 55:*807, 1971.
206. Rimoin, D. L.: *Diabetes 16:*346, 1967.
207. Rimoin, D. L., and Schimke, R. N.: *Genetic Disorders of the Endocrine Glands.* St. Louis, C. V. Mosby Co., 1971, pp. 150–216.
208. College of General Practitioners: *Brit. Med. J. 1:*960, 1965.
209. Simpson, N. E.: *Canad. Med. Ass. J. 98:*427, 1968.
210. White, P.: *Med. Clin. N. Amer. 49:*857, 1965.
211. Steiner, F.: *Deutsch. Arch. Klin. Med. 178:*497, 1936.
212. Harvald, B., and Hauge, M.: *Acta Med. Scand. 173:*459, 1963.
213. Neel, J. V., Fajans, S. S., et al.: In *Genetics and the Epidemiology of Chronic Diseases.* Neel, J. V., Shaw, M. W., and Schull, W. J. (eds.), Public Health Service Publication No. 1163, 1965.
214. Neel, J. V.: In *Early Diabetes.* Camerini-Davalos, R., and Cole, H. S. (eds.), New York, Academic Press, 1970, pp. 3–10.
215. Neel, J. V.: *Amer. J. Hum. Genet. 14:*353, 1964.
216. Zonana, J., and Rimoin, D. L.: *New Eng. J. Med. 295:*603, 1976.
217. Rotter, J. I., and Rimoin, D. L.: *Diabetes 27:*599, 1978.
218. Tattersall, R. B., and Pyke, D. A.: *Lancet 2:*1120, 1972.
219. Nerup, J., Platz, P., et al.: In *The Genetics of Diabetes Mellitus.* Creutzfeldt, W., Kobberling, J., et al. (eds.), Berlin, Springer-Verlag, 1976, pp. 106–114.
220. Cudworth, A. G., and Festenstein, H.: *Brit. Med. Bull. 34:*285, 1978.
221. Barbosa, J., King, R., et al.: *J. Clin. Invest. 60:*989, 1977.
222. Tattersall, R. B., and Fajans, S. S.: *Diabetes 24:*44, 1975.
223. Miller, H. C.: *Advances Pediat. 8:*137, 1956.
224. Fields, G. A., Schwarz, R. H., et al.: *Obstet. Gynec. 32:*778, 1968.
225. Ebbin, A. J., Huntley, C., et al.: *Metabolism 16:*926, 1967.
226. Snyder, R. D., and Robinson, A.: *Amer. J. Dis. Child. 113:*566, 1967.
227. Rimoin, D. L., and Schimke, R. N.: *Genetic Disorders of the Endocrine Glands.* St. Louis, C. V. Mosby Co., 1971, pp. 194–200.
228. Blumel, J., and Kniker, W. R.: *Texas Rep. Biol. Med. 17:*391, 1959.
229. Goldstein, J. L., and Fialkow, P. J.: *Medicine 52:*53, 1973.
230. Oakley, W. G., Pyke, D. A., et al.: *Clinical Diabetes and Its Biochemical Basis.* Oxford, Blackwell Scientific Publications Ltd., 1968.
231. Badgade, J. D., Bierman, E. L., et al.: *Diabetes 20:*664, 1971.
232. Mayer, J.: *Bull. N.Y. Acad. Med. 36:*323, 1960.
233. Lenz, W.: *Medizinische Genetik.* 2nd ed. Stuttgart, Georg Thieme Verlag, 1970, pp. 234–238.
234. Caughey, E., and Myrianthopoulos, N. C.: *Dystrophia Myotonia and Related Disorders.* Springfield, Ill., Charles C Thomas, 1963.
235. Drucker, W. D., Rowland, L. P., et al.: *Amer. J. Med. 31:*941, 1961.
236. Huff, T. A., and Lebovitz, H. E.: *J. Clin. Endocr. 28:*992, 1968.
237. Bundey, S., Carter, C. O., et al.: *J. Neurol. Neurosurg. Psychiat. 33:*279, 1970.
238. Renwick, J. H., Bundey, S. E., et al.: *J. Med. Genet. 8:*407, 1971.
239. Epstein, C. J., Martin, G. M., et al.: *Medicine 45:*177, 1966.
240. Cockayne, E. A., Drestin, D., et al.: *Quart. J. Med. 4:*93, 1935.
241. Ammann, F.: *J. Genet. Hum.* (Suppl.) *18:*1, 1970.
242. Alström, C. H., Hallgren, B., et al.: *Acta Psychiat. Neurol. Scand.* (Suppl. 129) *34:*1, 1959.
243. Seip, M., and Trygastad, O.: *Arch. Dis. Child. 38:*447, 1963.
244. Brunzell, J. D., Schankle, S. S., et al.: *Ann. Intern. Med. 69:*501, 1968.

CHAPTER 28

Hormones in Normal and Aberrant Growth

By Louis E. Underwood
and Judson J. Van Wyk

Physical growth includes all of the processes by which a fertilized egg eventually attains the size, form, and function of an adult human. In a more general sense, growth does not cease with the attainment of adulthood since many cells go on replicating throughout life to replace those which are lost through normal attrition or which are destroyed by injury or disease. Although an individual's ultimate capacity for growth and timing of various growth sequences are genetically encoded at the time of conception, we have only limited insight into the complex interactions between hormonal secretion, nutritional status, and specific disease states which influence the expression of these genes.

For many years, knowledge of how hormones affect growth and development was derived by observing the effects of hormonal deficiency or hormonal excess on children and by observing the effect of organ ablation or hormone administration on experimental animals. In recent decades, this information has been amplified vastly by the development of precise, specific methods for measuring the concentrations of nearly every known hormone. We are now progressing to an era in which attention is being focused on the molecular mechanisms by which hormones activate the train of intracellular events which lead either to mitosis or to the production of differentiated cell products. This chapter is addressed to a description of normal human growth and development, of both the entire body and separate tissues; a discussion of the role of hormones and peptide growth factors in these processes; and a discussion of the role of hormones in various disorders of human growth and development.

PATTERNS OF NORMAL GROWTH

Physical Growth

Prenatal Growth

By the end of gestation, the fertilized human ovum will have undergone the equivalent of about 42 successive cell divisions, and if all cells replicated in a uniform manner, only 5 more duplications would be required to reach full adult size.[6] At the end of the embryonic period, which occupies approximately the first 10 postmenstrual weeks, the fetus weighs only 2.8 g and is 3.0 cm in crown-rump length.[7] By this time, however, organogenesis is nearly complete. There then ensues profound acceleration in linear growth, with the peak velocity occurring around the 20th postmenstrual week. At this time, crown-heel length velocity may rise as high as 2.5 cm per week or 130 cm per year (Fig. 28–1). The maximal weight velocity is observed somewhat later, normally around 34 weeks. This weight increment correlates with the acquisition of adipose tissue and results in a doubling of body weight in the last 8 weeks of gestation. As the end of intrauterine life approaches, the rate of growth declines sharply. This normal decline may be, in part, a consequence of uterine filling since it occurs earlier in multiple pregnancies.

Knowledge of fetal age at birth is often of importance in distinguishing prematurely born infants from those who are small as a consequence of intrauterine growth failure (small-for-gestational-age or SGA babies). In assessing gestational age, it should be kept in mind that the convention of equating conception with the last missed menstrual period is misleading since fertilization normally occurs 2 weeks after menstruation; thus the actual duration of gestation is 38 rather than 40 weeks.

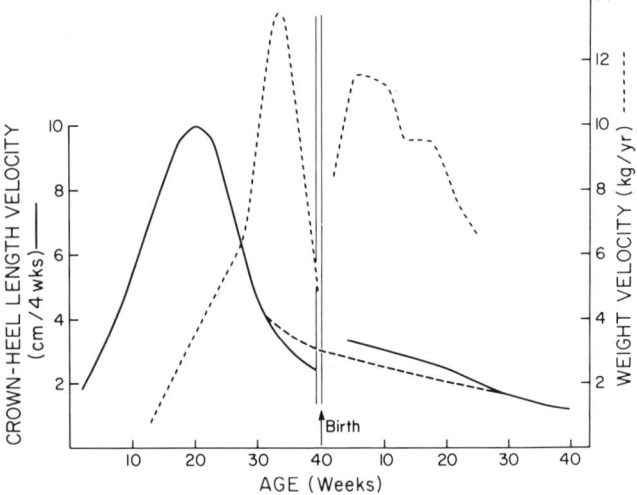

Figure 28–1. Rate of linear growth and weight gain *in utero* and during the first 40 weeks after birth. Note that length velocity is expressed as cm/4 wks. The solid line depicts the actual linear growth rate, and the broken line connecting the prenatal and postnatal length-velocity line depicts the theoretical curve if no uterine restriction took place late in gestation. The lighter dashed line depicts weight velocity. (The figure is redrawn from data compiled and presented by J. M. Tanner.[3])

Errors in determining the age of the fetus at birth are compounded by variations in the interval between menstruation and fertilization and by mistaking early gestational bleeding for menstruation. It is often necessary, therefore, to determine gestational age on the basis of the infant's physical and neuromuscular maturity.[8]

The size of normal infants at birth is determined by a variety of poorly understood genetic and environmental factors. One of these factors is maternal size since the slowing of fetal growth during the last few weeks of gestation is roughly proportional to maternal size and uterine space.[9, 10] There are significant population differences in growth during the prenatal period. For example, American Indians of the Cheyenne tribe have infants with mean birth weights of 3800 g, while infants of the Luni tribe of New Guinea have mean birth weights of 2400 g.[11] Environmental factors such as altitude also may influence intrauterine growth. Infants born in the Andes Mountains of Peru average 1500 g lighter than infants born in Lima, near sea level.[12] Many of the ethnic and environmental variations in birth weight are undoubtedly adaptational responses which improve the chances of the neonate for survival and the mother for further reproductive function. For instance, a mother producing a succession of large infants in a nutritionally insufficient environment would rapidly become malnourished. Similarly, while a large size at birth might be advantageous under optimal circumstances, smaller size at birth is believed to improve fitness for survival under conditions where nutrient supply is limited.

Modest impact on birth weight of infants from normal pregnancies results from: (1) the birth order of the infant — first-born infants being approximately 100 g lighter than later-born infants; (2) sex — male fetuses have higher average birth weights than females, and in mixed, multiple pregnancies, the presence of a male fetus appears to enhance the growth of female fetuses;[13] and (3) advanced maternal age — a striking reduction in birth weight has been observed in first-born infants when maternal age is 38 years or more.[14]

Growth from Birth to Puberty

Growth during the first year of life is extremely rapid, with more than doubling of the birth weight and a 50% increase in the body length. Linear growth velocities, which are as high as 30 cm/yr in the first 2 months of life, decline to one-third of this rate by 10 months and continue to decline sharply until 2 to 3 years.[15-17]

At birth, there is a shift in the factors regulating growth. The dominance of prenatal maternal influences is replaced by the influence of the infant's own genetic, nutritional, and hormone status.[18-21] Whereas at birth, the correlation coefficient between length and adult height is poor (r = 0.31), it improves sharply after birth so that by age 2 years it is 0.8. The latter correlation, which reflects the child's own growth potential, remains constant until the onset of puberty. Smith and colleagues have shown that the linear growth rates of approximately two-thirds of normal infants cross centile channels during the first 12 to 18 months of life, with the number shifting upward on the curve approximately equaling the number shifting downward.[22] Prematurely born infants who are otherwise normal and some infants who are small for gestational age undergo "catch-up" growth. This accelerated rate of growth is most marked during the first 6 months, but in the smallest infants may continue as long as 2 years before a stable growth rate is achieved. As a group, infants who are small for gestational age (SGA) catch up less well than prematurely born infants who are of appropriate size for gestational age (AGA). In one group of SGA babies studied at 4 years of age, 35% remained below the third percentile for both length and head circumference, whereas only 8% of this group had risen above the 50th centile.[23]

At the other end of the spectrum, babies who are exceptionally large at birth, such as those born of multiparous mothers, continue to grow rapidly for several months postnatally and do not begin their deceleration to reach lower centile standings until sometime between the third and seventh months. These children reach their stable childhood growth channel early in their second year of life.

After 2 years of age, the rates of gain in both height and weight show a slow downward trend and reach their nadir just prior to the beginning of the pubertal growth spurt. Before puberty, the mean heights and weights of boys and girls are nearly equal. During this period, most children remain in a remarkably constant centile channel for linear growth, and crossing of several centile channels should be the occasion for investigation.

Pubertal Growth

The impressive acceleration of somatic growth that occurs during puberty is but one component of the spectrum of dramatic changes that transform the child into an adult.[24] Hormonal factors controlling the onset of puberty are discussed in Chapters 6, 7, and 9. The pubertal growth spurt occurs approximately 2 years later in boys than in girls, and this normal delay gives boys, on the average, 2 more years of preadolescent growth than girls. Thus, at the onset of the pubertal growth spurt, boys are on the average 10 cm taller than girls at the corresponding developmental stage. The difference in average stature between men and women is due both to this longer period of preadolescent growth in boys and to their more intense pubertal growth spurt. Furthermore, since extremities grow faster than trunk during the prepubertal period, the leg length in males is generally greater than in females, both in absolute terms and in relation to the trunk.

The pubertal growth spurt is of relatively short duration, normally lasting only about 2 years. The peak height velocity occurs in British boys at a mean age of 14.0 years and averages about 10.3 cm/yr. British girls have their maximal growth velocity at a mean age of 12.14 years and at this time are growing at the average rate of 9.0 cm/yr.[25, 26]

The appearance of secondary sexual characteristics and the hormonal changes of puberty are temporally related to the peak height velocity, regardless of when this occurs.[3, 24] In normal girls, menarche predictably occurs on the descending limb of the height-velocity curve. In girls with sexual precocity, menarche may occur at the same time or slightly before the peak height velocity, whereas in girls with delayed adolescence, menarche occurs later on the descending limb when growth has nearly ceased. Since their growth spurt is late relative to girls', boys' genital and pubic hair development are nearly complete by the time the maximal pubertal growth rate occurs. The relationship between the emergence of other secondary sexual characteristics and the pubertal growth in boys and girls is represented in Figures 28–2 and 28–3.

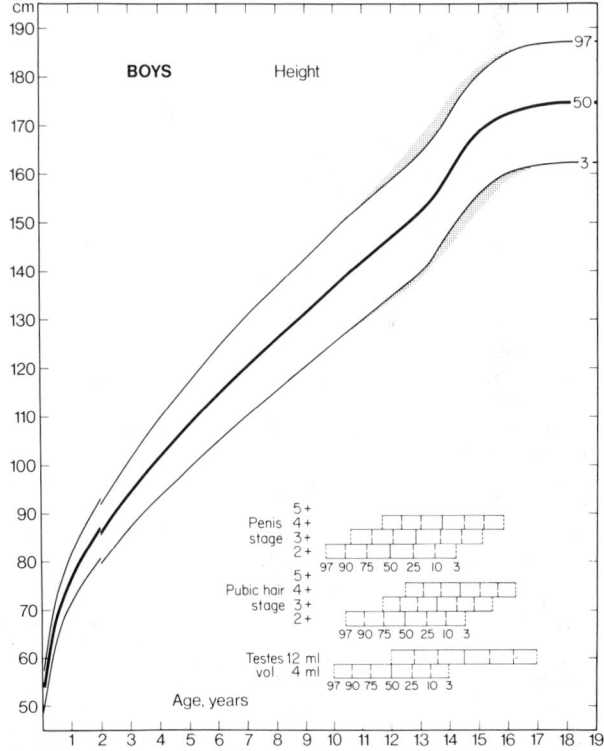

Figure 28–2. Cumulative (height-attained) growth chart for boys. The 97th, 50th, and 3rd centile curves depict the normal growth pattern from data collected by longitudinal as well as cross-sectional observations of British children. The outer (upper and lower) margins of the shaded areas represent the 97th and 3rd centile standards collected only by cross-sectional observations. Ages of attainment of stages of pubertal development (Tanner — see Table 28–4) are plotted by centiles, the 97th centile being the early limit of occurrence of a given pubertal stage and the 3rd centile being the late limit. (The figure is redrawn from charts prepared by J. M. Tanner and R. H. Whitehouse from data published in references 15 and 16. The original charts also contain 10th, 25th, 75th and 90th centile lines. The chart is reproduced here with the kind permission of J. M. Tanner and Castlemead Publications, Hertford, England.)

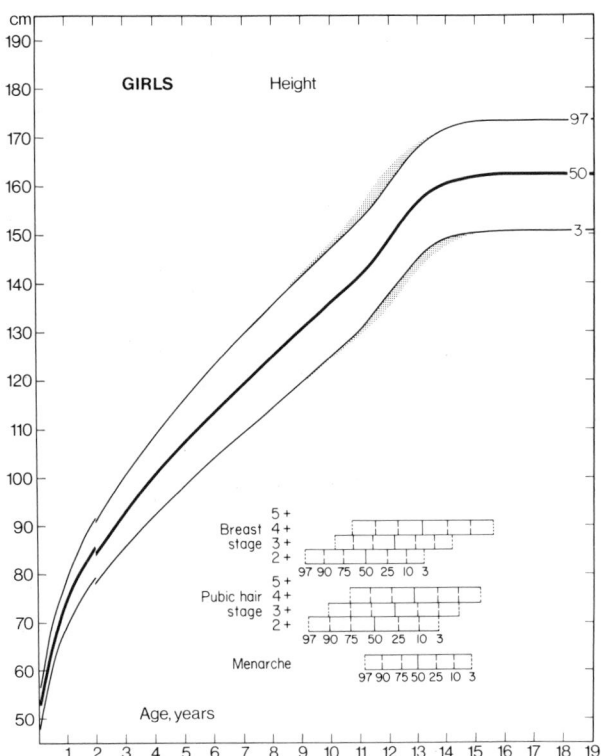

Figure 28–3. Cumulative growth chart for girls. See legend to Figure 28–2. (Redrawn and reproduced with permission of J. M. Tanner and Castlemead Publications, Hertford, England.)

Since linear-growth curves represent a composite of early- and late-maturing children, those curves based on cross-sectional studies of large numbers of children give a misleading picture of an individual child's growth pattern in later childhood. At the onset of their growth spurt, sexually precocious children increase their centile standing in an upward direction and later cross centile channels in a downward direction as their growth rate decelerates and as later-maturing children come into puberty. Similarly, for a time before they begin their own growth spurt, children with delayed adolescence fall into lower centile channels relative to their coevals. Furthermore, the rapidity and duration of adolescent growth reflects hormonal and genetic mechanisms beyond those which control growth during early childhood. Thus, children entering puberty at exactly the same age and weight often show considerably greater scatter in their adult heights than might have been anticipated from their prepubertal growth patterns. While both leg and trunk growth participate in the pubertal growth spurt, trunk growth is relatively greater and is therefore the more important determinant of the amount of growth attained during this period.

The hormonal mechanisms involved in the stimulation of growth at puberty are not well understood[27] (see section on androgens). There are conflicting data concerning growth hormone (GH) secretion during this period. Pubertal GH responses to acute provocative stimuli are greater than those observed before puberty,[28] but integrated concentrations of GH, drawn over 24-hour periods, are not increased in comparison to prepubertal values.[27] A great deal of clinical experience points to the fact that testosterone augments the growth-promoting effect of GH, and there is some evidence in humans that testosterone can stimulate growth in GH-deficient children, albeit at the cost of rapid advancement of skeletal maturation.[27] In females, in whom less impressive elevations of testosterone occur, the stimuli for pubertal growth are even more poorly understood than in males.

Skeletal Age and Physical Maturity

Although in most children, growth and developmental events follow the same orderly pattern, the pace of maturation varies widely. Thus, an individual child's growth performance is better viewed in relationship to his or her stage of physical maturity than in relationship to chronologic age. Since the ossification centers of the bony skeleton mature in an orderly sequence from birth to adulthood, measurement of skeletal maturation provides an objective indicator of overall maturity which is independent of chronologic age, size, and growth rate.

Skeletal maturity, expressed as skeletal age, is best assessed beyond the neonatal period from a single radiograph of the hand and wrist. At minimal radiation dosage, this provides information on 30 bones or about 10% of those in the entire skeleton. Estimation of skeletal maturity traditionally has been made from the *Atlas* of Greulich and Pyle,[29] in which a radiograph of the patient's left hand and wrist is matched with films obtained from "typical children" of various ages. Tanner and associates[30] have devised a more objective method in which a numerical score is assigned to each stage of development of the individual bones of the hand and wrist. This method, although more laborious, has proved to have less variance than the *Atlas* method.[31, 32]

In children with premature or delayed puberty, the skeletal age correlates far better with the onset of the pubertal growth spurt and other events in pubertal development than do either chronologic age or attained height. Using skeletal age, it is possible to predict with some degree of reliability the final adult stature[33-35] and to distinguish between children who will mature early and those in whom sexual development will be delayed.

Organ Growth

Differential Growth of Specific Organs and Tissues

For the most part, growth of individual body parts parallels the pattern described for statural growth. Tissues such as kidney, liver, spleen, and muscle, therefore, experience rapid growth early in life, relative slowing in the prepubertal years, and accelerated growth during puberty. There are several tissues, however, which exhibit marked differences in growth from the general pattern. The brain and eyes are highly developed at birth and attain most of their adult size within the first few years of life. At the opposite end of the growth spectrum are reproductive tissues, which grow very little between the time they are formed *in utero* and the onset of puberty; they then reach adult size in the span of a few years. The lymphoid cell mass progressively increases throughout childhood, reaches its maximum just before puberty, and then slowly declines throughout adulthood.

Growth by Hyperplasia vs. Growth by Hypertrophy: Cell Number vs. Cell Size

The rapid expansion in external dimensions which characterizes childhood growth depends on increases both in the number of cells (hyperplasia) and in the size of the individual cells (hypertrophy).[36] Growth in the early embryo is almost exclusively due to increases in the number of cells, whereas at succeeding stages of development, the balance between hyperplasia and hypertrophy varies markedly among different tissues and at different stages of development. These patterns of growth can be assessed by determining the DNA and protein content of the tissue at different times. DNA content is a good reflection of cell number since the DNA in each diploid nucleus is constant in all cells within a given species and virtually all cellular DNA is chromosomal in origin. The ratio of protein to DNA is commonly used as an index of cell size.

In an effort to bring clarity to the complexities of tissue and organ growth, Goss has proposed a classification of tissues according to the means by which they increase or maintain their mass and by their functional capacity to replace tissue lost by normal attrition or injury.[37, 38] According to his scheme, tissues exhibit growth by: (1) renewal of their cell population, (2) expansion of their cell population, or (3) maintenance of a *static* cell population.

Renewing Tissues. Tissues that renew their cell populations, such as epidermis, gut mucosa, male germ cells, and hemopoietic elements, grow by proliferation from undifferentiated germinal cells and produce cells with highly differentiated functions that have no further mitotic potential. Cells in these tissues have a relatively short life span, and in most instances, the stem cells are compartmentalized in areas separate from the differentiated cells.

Expanding Tissues. The growth of tissues that expand their cell populations differs from that of renewing tissues in that all differentiated, functional cells are capable of mitosis. They exhibit little or no mitotic activity, however, once appropriate organ size is achieved. During adult life, the growth process may be reinitiated in response to tissue injury or loss of tissue mass. Examples of such tissues include the endocrine and exocrine glands, liver, kidney, and lungs.

Mitotically Static Tissues. Tissues such as neurons and skeletal muscle fail to proliferate beyond certain developmental stages. These cells ordinarily are capable of surviving for the life of the entire organism. If they sustain injury, however, they regrow only by cellular hypertrophy or axonal regeneration. This regrowth by multiplication of cytologic organelles is limited by the ultimate size to which the cell is able to enlarge.

In renewing tissues, where growth is primarily the result of cell replication, the processes of growth and tissue repair are nearly identical and change little throughout life. In expanding and static tissues, on the other hand, these processes vary substantially at different ages and stages of growth.

The liver, an expanding tissue, grows by increasing the number and size of cells and has the capacity for spectacular regeneration by cell multiplication throughout most of life. It appears that this regeneration is controlled to a major extent by hormonal factors.[39, 40] In the human brain, a static tissue, most neuronal cell division occurs prenatally, while division of the supporting glial cells is largely a postnatal phenomenon. After the second postnatal year, there is little additional cell replication, and further growth is by hypertrophy. The brain approaches its adult size by the age of 2 years. After injury, individual neurons can undergo hypertrophy, but cell replication does not occur.[41]

There are some cell types and tissues that do not readily fit into Goss's classification. For example, because the skeleton possesses growth zones (epiphyseal plates, perichondrium, and periosteum), it qualifies as a renewing tissue. However, since there is little cell loss and it exhibits growth in adulthood only after injury, it qualifies also as an expanding tissue.

HORMONAL CONTROL OF HUMAN GROWTH

The hormones that are known to exert significant effects on skeletal and somatic growth are growth hormone, thyroxine, cortisol, sex steroids, insulin, and a variety of peptide hormones loosely referred to as growth factors. This section will focus on the relative importance of these substances in controlling growth and the mechanisms by which they act.

Classic Hormones

Growth Hormone

Growth hormone (GH) is by far the most abundant hormone in the human pituitary gland, and the primacy of this hormone in controlling postnatal somatic growth is unquestioned. Nevertheless, perhaps more unresolved questions surround the chemistry and physiology of GH than is the case with any of the other major hormones. Critical questions remain concerning the factors controlling GH secretion, the chemical nature of the active growth principle, and the mechanisms by which GH produces its multiple effects.

In recent years, questions have been raised whether the GH isolated from pituitary glands represents the active growth-promoting peptide or whether this substance is converted to a more active form which is not measured by the usual immunologic techniques. These questions have arisen from several lines of evidence: (1) organ cultures of isolated pituitary glands secrete considerably more bioactive GH than can be accounted for by the quantity of GH that can be measured by radioimmunoassay (RIA); (2) Ellis and Grindeland have presented evidence that jugular vein blood contains much more GH activity as measured in the rat tibial width assay than can be accounted for by RIA;[42, 43] and (3) GH has a variety of metabolic effects that are difficult to explain by a single mechanism (Fig. 28–4).

Whereas the growth-promoting actions of GH on muscle and skeletal tissue are insulin-like, its long-term diabetogenic effects on carbohydrate metabolism and lipolytic effects on fat are opposite to those of insulin. This apparent paradox is further illustrated by the interaction between GH and cortisol in different tissues: in muscle and cartilage, cortisol is catabolic and inhibits the action of GH; on the other hand, cortisol and GH are synergistic in producing the diabetogenic and lipolytic effects.

The work of Lewis and associates[44] suggests one possible mechanism to explain the multiple and seemingly paradoxical actions of GH. These workers found that partial enzymatic digestion of GH with bacterial protease produced three peptides having growth-promoting activity in tibial growth assays. One fraction, however, has more diabetogenic actions than the other two, while another has more growth-promoting effects. Their findings suggest that the active sites coding for the various actions of GH might reside in different parts of the molecule. Using specific radioimmunoassays for their cleaved peptides, they have shown that these substances are not always secreted in concert with the parent hormone.

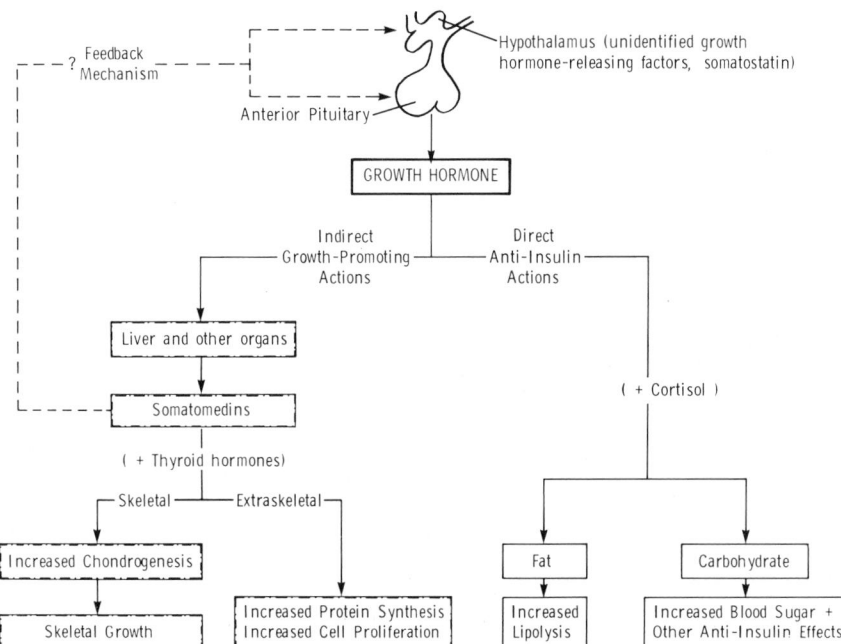

Figure 28-4. Proposed scheme for categorizing the metabolic actions of growth hormone (GH). The direct actions, which are often synergistic with cortisol and antagonistic to insulin, include GH's diabetogenic and lipolytic actions and perhaps its stimulatory action on various hepatic enzymes. The indirect, growth-promoting actions, which are often insulin-like and antagonized by cortisol, are thought to be mediated through the somatomedins.

According to the somatomedin hypothesis of GH action (see section on the somatomedins), the effects of GH on carbohydrate and lipid metabolism are direct, whereas the growth-promoting actions are mediated through the somatomedin family of peptides. This hypothesis has been ably disputed, however, by those who believe that the demonstrated *in vitro* growth-promoting effects of GH are sufficiently convincing that it is unnecessary to invoke the mediation of any secondary hormones.[45] They point out that while the direct *in vitro* effects of GH on cartilage may be small, they are not totally absent, and that too little effort may have been invested in optimizing incubation conditions for the detection of direct GH action.

Thyroid Hormones

Thyroid hormones do not appear to play a significant role in the early growth and development of the human fetus since even those with congenital aplasia of the thyroid gland are of normal size at birth. Pickering and Fisher[46] showed that the major consequences of intrauterine thyroid deficiency in primate fetuses are retardation of osseous and central nervous system development. Human infants suffering from congenital hypothyroidism similarly exhibit obvious immaturity of their skeleton at birth and, although less apparent at this time, neurologic immaturity as well. The critical period of thyroxine-dependent brain growth extends from the last portion of gestation to several months postnatally. Hypothyroidism during this period results in markedly retarded growth of cell bodies, axons, and dendritic connections and delayed myelinization. Although thyroid hormone may act directly on these processes, Walker and coworkers[47] have demonstrated that the administration of thyroxine to mature mice significantly increases the brain concentration of nerve growth factor (NGF). These findings have raised the interesting possibility that the effects of thyroxine on neural maturation may be mediated through NGF.

The importance of thyroid hormones for normal postnatal somatic growth is exemplified by the severe growth failure that regularly accompanies thyroid hormone deficiency. Unlike most other disorders that slow linear growth, severe hypothyroidism causes nearly absolute growth arrest. Following correction of the thyroid hormone deficiency, growth is usually resumed at extraordinarily rapid rates, a period of so-called catch-up growth.

The role of thyroxine on skeletal growth appears to be a permissive one for the action of GH since GH does not stimulate growth in hypothyroid animals. The refractoriness of skeletal tissues to GH in such animals may be due to a defect in the response to somatomedin at the cellular level. Froesch and associates showed that triiodothyronine is necessary to obtain the maximal *in vitro* response of chick cartilage to a purified peptide belonging to the somatomedin family (NSILA).[48]

Thyroid hormone also appears to influence growth at the pituitary level by regulating the synthesis and secretion of GH. Hypothyroid patients frequently have severely blunted GH responses to a variety of provocative stimuli and, perhaps for this reason, their serum somatomedin-C levels are sometimes low.[49] Samuels and coworkers[50] have carried out extensive studies on the effect of thyroid hormone on the induction of the mRNA for GH synthesis in cultured rat pituitary cells. In this system, triiodothyronine causes a 10- to 12-fold increase in GH synthesis after 48 hours in culture.

Insulin

There are a variety of observations which raise the possibility that insulin, in addition to its primary role as the regulator of carbohydrate homeostasis, may function as a stimulator of growth. The contrast between oversized, hyperinsulinemic infants born to diabetic mothers and the poor growth of diabetic newborns with insulin deficiency has given rise to the suggestion that insulin is a primary stimulator of somatic growth in the fetus. Hyperinsulinism is also a constant feature in overgrown infants with the Beckwith-Wiedemann syndrome, and insulinopenia prevails in small newborns with pancreatic agenesis. States of insulin resistance such as leprechaunism have growth failure as a prominent feature.[51, 52] In postnatal life, there are a number of clinical conditions in which insulin deficiency is associated with growth failure and

Table 28–1.   EFFECT OF HORMONES ON GROWTH AND DEVELOPMENT

	Linear Growth	Skeletal Maturation	Effect on Adult Stature (Untreated)
Growth hormone:			
excess	increased*	normal	increased
deficiency	decreased	delayed	decreased
Thyroxine:			
excess	slightly increased	slightly advanced	minimal
deficiency	decreased	delayed*	decreased
Cortisol:			
excess	decreased*	delayed	decreased
Androgen:			
excess	increased	advanced*	decreased
deficiency	increased in extremities	delayed (later childhood)	eunuchoidal
Estrogen:			
excess	increased	advanced*	decreased

*Denotes the effect which usually predominates.

hyperinsulinism is accompanied by overgrowth. Examples of the former include malnutrition, inadequately treated diabetes mellitus, and untreated hypopituitarism. While insulinopenia may be only a compensatory mechanism, the diversity of these conditions raises the question whether, in one or more of them, insulin may be permissive for normal growth. In otherwise normal children with exogenous obesity and in hyperphagic children who have had surgery for craniopharyngioma, insulin levels may be markedly increased, and acceleration of linear growth usually occurs.

In cell-culture systems, insulin, albeit at high concentrations, has been observed to support cell growth,[53] to stimulate DNA synthesis,[54] and to stimulate mitosis in serum-limited medium.[55] It seems unlikely, however, that insulin is a primary growth stimulator under physiologic conditions since high concentrations are required to promote mitosis and tissue growth. Our interpretation is that at physiologic concentrations, insulin is a growth-promoting hormone only to the extent that it is necessary to preserve metabolic homeostasis; only at exceedingly high levels does insulin act as a primary growth stimulant.[88, 156]

Glucocorticoids

Inhibition of growth in the immature animal is one of the cardinal effects of glucocorticoids. Only two to three times the average daily secretion product is required to arrest linear growth.[56] The alert physician, therefore, is presented with an almost foolproof means for differentiating children with states of cortisol excess from those with exogenous obesity (Fig. 28–5). In the former, growth failure is a uniform finding, and even when longitudinal growth data are not available, the patient is nearly always short. In exogenous obesity, however, there is almost always an acceleration of linear growth so that affected children have heights well above the mean for age.

The growth-inhibitory effects of glucocorticoids are not limited to the skeleton since low dosages given to weanling animals inhibit the incorporation of radioactive thymidine into DNA in liver, heart, skeletal muscle, and kid-

ney.[57] Unlike these "nonrenewing" tissues, those tissues which renew and replenish themselves by cell proliferation are relatively resistant to the effects of glucocorticoids. These include gut mucosa, testes, spleen, and the erythropoietic elements of bone marrow.

Glucocorticoids probably do not inhibit growth by suppression of GH secretion. Although in adults large doses of cortisol inhibit GH secretion, in children, excess cortisol has only minimal effects.[58] Furthermore, serum somatomedin-C concentrations determined by radioimmunoassay are not low in patients with glucocorticoid excess, suggesting that suppression of somatomedin generation also can be excluded. Growth hormone administered in conjunction with glucocorticoid will not reverse the growth attenuation caused by the glucocorticoids.[59] These and several other lines of evidence suggest that glucocorticoids inhibit growth by direct action on the target tissue. For example, the addition of micromolar amounts of glucocorticoids to liver cells in a tissue culture result in marked suppression of thymidine incorporation and cell proliferation.[57] Furthermore, high dosages of glucocorticoids have been shown to inhibit directly the synthesis of enzymes concerned with the production of glycosaminoglycans[60] and to induce disruption in the ultrastructure of chondrocytes and extracellular matrix.[61, 62] These changes are not completely reversible. Thus, growth arrest from cortisol excess is not followed by the degree of catch-up growth that characterizes other types of growth failure when the cause is removed.

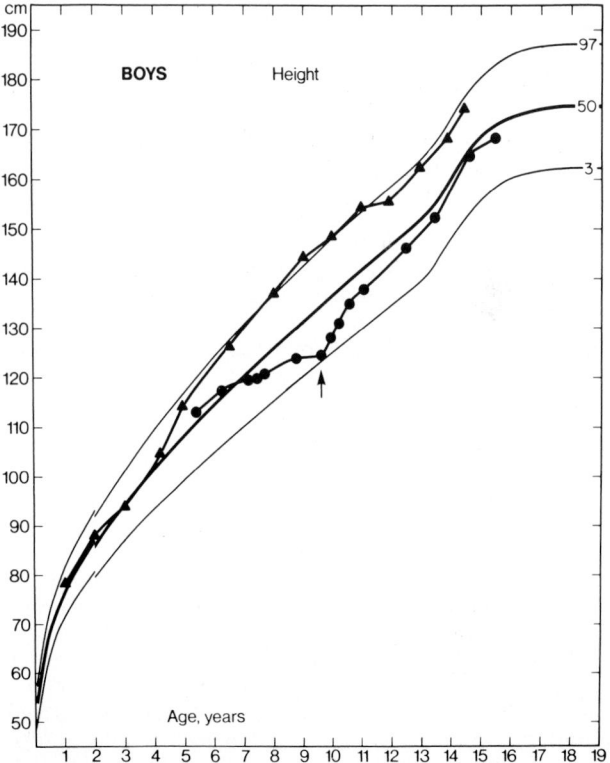

Figure 28–5.   Growth curves of two boys with obesity. The boy depicted by the circles (●—●) had cortisol excess due to Cushing's disease. He experienced the onset of rapid weight gain associated with a decline in linear growth at age 7 years. Diagnosis was made and adrenalectomy was performed at age 9½ years. This was followed by a period of catch-up growth. The boy whose growth is depicted by the triangles (▲—▲) had exogenous obesity. At 9½ years his weight was approximately the same as that of the patient with Cushing's disease but his height was at the 97th centile, reflecting the stimulation of linear growth observed in patients with exogenous obesity.

Androgens

Testosterone and its metabolite dihydrotestosterone are potent anabolic agents that accelerate linear growth and weight gain and increase lean muscle mass when administered to prepubertal children. States of androgen excess, such as androgen-producing tumors, sexual precocity, and virilizing adrenal hyperplasia, are likewise uniformly associated with accelerated linear growth and weight gain.

Studies in humans and animals suggest that the presence of GH is essential for the effective promotion of somatic growth by androgens.[63] Administration of androgens to hypophysectomized rats has no effect on somatic growth,[64] and when androgens are administered along with GH, little, if any, additive effect on growth is observed over that obtained by administering GH alone.[65] In humans with GH deficiency, the growth response to exogenous androgens is markedly diminished;[66] however, following GH replacement, the addition of androgens, in contrast to the acute effects in animals, often causes an impressive augmentation of linear growth over that produced by either hormone given alone.[67, 68]

In addition to the complementary effects with GH, which appear to be the primary mechanism for the stimulation of growth by androgens, there is also evidence that androgens enhance pituitary GH secretion. Administration of testosterone to prepubertal humans enhances peak plasma GH levels after provocative stimuli,[69, 70] without raising basal values.

The disadvantage of using androgenic hormones to stimulate growth in prepubertal children is the propensity of these agents to cause disproportionate stimulation of epiphyseal maturation. The ultimate effect of this discordance is loss of growth potential and diminution of eventual adult stature. By administering graded dosages of methyltestosterone to prepubertal boys with short stature, Sobel found that the effect on epiphyseal maturation was proportional to both the dose and duration of administration, whereas nearly maximal stimulation of growth rate was achieved with the smallest dosage tested.[71] Considerable effort has been expended in the search for synthetic androgens that promote growth without producing virilization and excessive stimulation of epiphyseal maturation. It is unclear whether the growth-promoting effects of the synthetic androgens advertised as growth stimulants have been separated from the androgenic effects or whether these substances are simply weak androgens.

Estrogens

The net effect of estrogens on somatic growth is inhibitory, whereas, as in the case with androgens, the effect on epiphyseal maturation is stimulatory. A number of animal studies show that administration of estrogen decreases linear growth and width of the cartilage growth plate despite increased concentrations of GH in serum.[72-75] In hypophysectomized animals, the widening of the epiphyseal plate induced by exogenous GH is inhibited by simultaneous estrogen treatment.[76] These growth-inhibitory actions may be mediated by the effects of estrogen on somatomedin secretion. Using bioassay methods, it has been shown that estrogens inhibit the GH-induced rise of somatomedin in hypophysectomized rats and in hypopituitary humans[77, 78] and decrease the incorporation of sulfate by cartilage taken from estrogen-treated animals.[79] There is evidence that a direct inhibitory effect of estrogens on somatomedin action is unlikely.[78, 80]

In humans, as in other species, estrogens increase basal plasma GH levels and enhance the GH responses to provocative stimuli. Administration of pharmacologic dosages of estrogens to excessively tall girls leads to attenuation of their growth rates and a decrease in their predicted adult stature.[81-84] Von Puttkamer and associates have found that such treatment lowers the concentration of somatomedin in the girls' sera.[85] Administration of estrogens to patients with acromegaly often produces some clinical improvement with reduction of soft tissue enlargement. This treatment has likewise been associated with increased GH and decreased somatomedin levels.[86]

In spite of overwhelming evidence that estrogens inhibit somatic growth, a paradoxical acceleration of growth often is observed in young children who are exposed to estrogens. It is believed that in children with intact pituitary, gonadal, and adrenal function, there is a concomitant increase in androgens that secondarily causes acceleration of growth. Strengthening this hypothesis are the observations that development of pubic hair and acquisition of other androgen-related secondary sexual characteristics soon follows exposure to estrogens. This mechanism may also account for the acceleration of linear growth seen in estrogen-treated girls with Turner's syndrome.[87]

Peptide Growth Factors

Although the hormones discussed in the preceding section play a pivotal role in the regulation of overall somatic growth and in the growth of sexual organs, it is less clear what role these hormones play in the growth of other specialized tissues. Furthermore, the effect of many hormones on cell division, when they are added in vitro to isolated cell and organ cultures, is often less spectacular than when they are administered in vivo. In recent years, therefore, increasing attention has been directed toward a group of peptide growth factors that are highly active in stimulating cell proliferation in vitro.[88] The production of these growth factors is not confined to the usual "glands of internal secretion." In some instances, however, their secretion may be controlled by the more classic hormones. Since in vivo actions of these substances have been explored only to a limited extent, their position in the hierarchy of growth-regulating mechanisms remains uncertain. Nevertheless, because of their great potency in stimulating cell proliferation, it is apparent that these peptide growth factors are destined to open an entirely new dimension in our understanding of the mechanisms regulating growth at the cellular level.

Among the large number of naturally occurring proteins and peptides that have been described as cell-growth factors are such diverse substances as tripeptides, classic hormones, transferrin, and proteolytic enzymes. Some of these may serve a permissive role in cell maintenance, whereas others may exercise a more dynamic regulatory role. In complex organisms, enormous variations occur between the growth rates of different tissues, and in any given tissue the rate of cell proliferation varies from time to time as a function of age and physiologic circumstance. Thus, in the array of putative growth factors, the most likely candidates for an in vivo regulatory role should be those growth factors which are themselves under strict physiologic regulation and which possess unique specificity for certain cell types. The better characterized peptide growth factors can be divided provisionally into two classes: those whose action is restricted to highly specialized cell types and those that are capable of stimulating the growth of a broader spectrum of tissues.

Tissue-Specific Growth Factors

Erythropoietin. Erythropoiesis is a highly regulated process which under normal circumstances maintains the total red cell mass within narrow limits. The red cell mass is typical of a renewing tissue that is formed from spatially distant precursor cells, the proerythrocytes. Anemia, hemorrhage, or hypoxia stimulates erythropoiesis, whereas artificially produced polycythemia is followed by almost complete cessation of red blood cell formation.

Evidence that a humoral factor regulates erythropoiesis was produced by Reissmann in 1950 who demonstrated that exposure of one parabiotic rat to hypoxia was followed by erythroid hyperplasia in the other rat.[90] It was found subsequently that extracts of blood and urine from hypoxic humans, sheep, and other species are enriched in a peptide growth factor called erythropoietin.[91] Human urinary erythropoietin has been isolated as an acidic sialoprotein with a molecular weight of 39,000 daltons.[92-94]

There is abundant evidence that the kidney is primarily responsible for the production of erythropoietin even though kidney extracts contain only low levels of the active peptide. One theory proposed to explain this paradox is that the renal factor, termed erythrogenin, is in fact an enzyme which acts on a plasma substrate derived from liver to form the biologically active factor.[95] Regardless of the exact mechanism of formation, it is clear that very little erythropoietin is formed in anephric individuals and that the anemia characteristic of renal failure is related to erythropoietin deficiency.[96, 97] Although tissue oxygenation is the major factor in its feedback regulation, erythropoietin production is also under the control of both androgens[98] and GH. Thus, erythropoietin levels are decreased in GH deficiency and increased after GH administration.[99]

A recurrent question that is asked with regard to many growth factors is whether they are primarily cell differentiation factors (which induce protein synthesis and differentiated cell responses in existing cells) or whether they are true mitogens. In many cases, this distinction cannot be made since a single cell division may give rise to daughter cells with new functional properties. In the case of erythropoietin, for example, the proerythrocyte is induced to undergo one wave of mitotic division giving rise to hemoglobin-synthesizing cells which then lack the capacity for further division. Full characterization of the cellular responses to erythropoietin has been difficult, however, since the earliest cells giving rise to proerythrocytes are morphologically undefined. Nevertheless, evidence has been advanced that erythropoietin stimulates several cycles of proliferation in more primitive stem cells before stimulating the terminal wave of mitosis in proerythrocytes.[100, 101]

Colony-Stimulating Factor and Macrophage Growth Factor. The proliferation of white blood cells appears to be controlled by peptide growth factors in a manner analogous to the control of red cell generation by erythropoietin. The term "colony-stimulating factor" (CSF) has been used to describe a class of glycoprotein growth factors which stimulate primitive bone marrow cells to proliferate in soft agar and form colonies of granulocytes and mononuclear phagocytes.[102] The term "macrophage growth factor" (MGF) has been applied to glycoproteins which permit the macrophages harvested from peritoneal exudates to proliferate in liquid-suspension cultures and form colonies consisting solely of mononuclear phagocytes.[103]

The fact that MGF and CSF are defined operationally in terms of different evoked responses does not necessarily mean that they are different substances. Stanley found that MGF activity and CSF activity paralleled each other in such diverse sources as conditioned media from a variety of human and mouse cell lines, mouse serum after the administration of an endotoxin, and ascites fluid after the induction of an inflammatory response.[104, 105] The activity of both is increased in serum and urine after administration of endotoxin, in patients with Hodgkin's disease, and in patients with leukemia. Parallel activity also is found in tissue extracts of salivary gland, kidney, spleen, uterus, lung, and placenta.[106]

Van Zant and Goldwasser found that the addition of CSF to bone marrow cultures caused suppression of erythropoietin-stimulated hemoglobin synthesis, whereas the addition of erythropoietin caused suppression of granulocyte-macrophage colony formation. Both responses were dose-dependent.[108] One possible interpretation of these studies is that erythroid and myeloid stem cells might be identical and that the direction of their subsequent development is dictated by which growth factor

Table 28-2. CHARACTERISTICS OF TISSUE-SPECIFIC GROWTH FACTORS

Name	Site of Origin	Chemical Characteristics	Regulatory Factors	Biologic Effects
Erythropoietin	Kidney (prohormone?) + liver factor; urine from patients with chronic anemia or hypoxia	Glycoprotein MW (human) = 39,000[92]	Anemia, hypoxia; androgens, GH	Proerythrocytes → hemoglobin synthesizing cells; proliferation of earlier precursor cells
Colony-stimulating factor; macrophage growth factor	Conditioned culture media; extracts of kidney, spleen, lung; peritoneal exudates	Glycoproteins MW ≈ 70,000;[107] active subunit = 29,000[104]	Endotoxin, inflammatory agents	WBC precursors → granulocytes and mononuclear phagocytes
Thymic hormones: thymopoietin I and II	Bovine thymus	49-amino acid peptide MW = 5562[111]	TSH? GH?	Proliferation of primitive lymphocytes and differentiation into immunologically competent T cells; restores immunologic competence and growth in neonatally thymectomized mice
α₁ thymosin		28-amino acid peptide MW = 3350[114]		
Nerve growth factor (NGF)	Cobra venom; male mouse submaxillary gland	7S = 130,000; active β subunit = 13,250;[125] homology with proinsulin	Androgens, thyroxine	Differentiation, growth, and survival of sympathetic neurons; growth of embryonic dorsal root ganglia
Ovarian growth factor	Bovine pituitary	Basic peptide MW = 10,000–13,000[131]	?	Physiologic significance unknown; prolongs ovarian cell survival

predominates. Alternatively, these authors suggested that erythroid and myeloid precursor cells are different, but that each possesses receptors with overlapping specificities for both growth factors; occupancy by the "wrong" inducer might then block the action of the growth factor appropriate for that cell type.

Thymic Hormones. The long-disputed role of the thymus as an endocrine organ has been resolved by the isolation of a family of peptides which control the proliferation and maturation of primitive lymphocytes into immunologically competent T cells.[109, 110] Several thymic hormones have been described, each with somewhat different biologic and chemical properties.[111-114]

Thymopoietin is a 49-amino acid, single-chain peptide which induces the differentiation of prothymocytes into immunologically competent T cells with full expression of surface antigens.[115] A synthetic pentapeptide consisting of residues 32 to 36 is able to mimic the action of the native molecule. α_1 Thymosin is a 28-amino acid peptide also purified from bovine thymic extracts.[114, 116, 117] Injections of partially purified thymosin preparations (step 5 material) into athymic dwarf nude mice lead to lymphocyte proliferation, increased rate of somatic growth, and capability of rejecting allografts. Thus, at least some of the thymic hormones are true growth factors as well as differentiating agents. Promising clinical results have been reported following injections of thymosin in children with genetic forms of immunodeficiency disease and in patients with lymphocytopenia secondary to irradiation or drug treatment for cancer.

Although the hormonal dependency of thymic hormones has not been adequately studied, White has suggested that these substances might be under the control of pituitary GH and thyrotropin (TSH). It is also possible that the shrinkage of the thymus gland produced by ACTH and glucocorticoids might involve some interaction with thymic hormones.[117]

Nerve Growth Factor. Bueker observed in 1948 that implantation of a mouse sarcoma into the body walls of chick embryos led to marked enlargement of the dorsal root ganglia innervating that tumor.[118] Levi-Montalcini and Hamburger subsequently showed that sympathetic ganglia also were involved in the growth response to sarcoma implants[119] and that this effect could be exerted across the chorioallantoic membrane. This led them to propose that the sarcoma was producing its effect by secretion of a specific nerve growth factor (NGF).[120-123] The richest sources of NGF are snake venom and submaxillary glands of adult male mice. The latter tissue has served as the primary source of starting material for purification.[124]

In neutral extracts of male mouse submandibular gland, NGF is isolated as a 7S protein possessing a molecular weight of 130,000 daltons. This protein is composed of dimers of three subunits, the bioactive form (β subunit) consisting of a 118-amino acid, 13,250-dalton peptide chain (Fig. 28–6). The precise function of 7S NGF is unknown, but it has been suggested that the active β NGF chains are derived, like insulin, from larger pro-NGF precursor chains through proteolytic cleavage by an esteropeptidase that remains attached as the γ subunit.[125] The active molecule bears substantial homology in both amino acid sequence and three-dimensional structure to proinsulin, suggesting an evolutionary relationship.[126] Nerve growth factor not only acts on highly specific cell types but also exercises its primary function during a portion of embryonic life. NGF stimulates the growth of ganglia in mammals and chicks as the period of neuroblast division approaches its conclusion. In addition, administration of NGF to newborn rats prevents the normal decline in neuronal number which occurs in the first postnatal month. Treatment of newborn or adult mice with NGF causes a marked increase in the adrenergic innervation of salivary glands, blood vessels, intestinal tract, and iris.[120] A number of experimental studies suggest that NGF plays a physiologic role in the maintenance of the sympathetic nervous system in later life.[127] This survival factor role of NGF is perhaps one of its most important functions. Once sympathetic neurons and some sensory neurons have assumed the differentiated status of young, postmitotic neurons, they depend on NGF for survival and, under its influence, progress to mature neurons. Specifically, administration of exogenous NGF prevents death of immature sympathetic neurons whose neurites have been surgically or chemically injured.

While the target cells and morphologic effects of NGF are quite different from those of insulin, the metabolic events which underlie the effects of these hormones are similar. Both hormones stimulate the synthesis of cell-specific enzymes and proteins; both exert positive pleiotypic responses including stimulation of RNA synthesis, polysome formation, glucose utilization, and lipid synthesis; and both promote microtubular polymerization associated with changes in cell shape. This commonality of molecular mechanisms is undoubtedly explained by the structural kinship of the two hormones. Since no direct mitogenic actions of NGF have yet been described, this substance should be regarded as a differentiating factor rather than a true growth factor. This lack of mitogenicity might reflect, however, that its actions are limited to mitotically static tissues which are incapable of division or that an appropriate precursor cell in the early embryo has not yet been identified.

The concentration of NGF in mouse salivary gland is

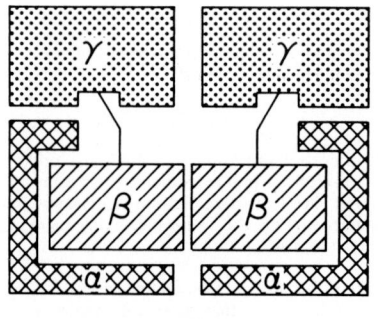

MOUSE 7S NGF

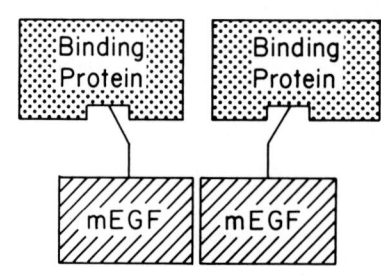

HIGH MOLECULAR WEIGHT
MOUSE EGF

Figure 28–6. Composition of the storage forms of nerve growth factor (NGF) and epidermal growth factor (EGF). The storage form of NGF is 7S NGF (MW 130,000). The biologically active NGF protein (β subunit) exists as a dimer, each chain of which has a molecular weight of 13,250 daltons. This portion of the molecule exhibits biologic activity in the absence of the other components. The γ subunit (MW = 26,000) has arginine esteropeptidase activity and is believed to be involved in cleaving the active (β) form from a pro-NGF molecule. The exact function of the α subunits (MW = 26,500) is unknown but they may serve, along with the γ subunits, to store and protect the active component of the molecule. The high molecular weight storage form of mouse EGF (MW = 74,000) is composed of 2 molecules of active EGF (MW of each = 6045) and 2 molecules

of binding protein (MW of each = 29,300). This binding protein also has arginine esteropeptidase activity that is similar to that of the γ subunit of NGF in its molecular weight, amino acid composition, and immunologic cross-reactivity. They differ, however, in their electrophoretic properties, and the EGF binding protein cannot substitute for the γ NGF subunit in the formation of 7S NGF.

increased markedly by the administration of androgens,[128] and thyroxine increases its concentration in brain.[46] Although it traditionally has been purified from submaxillary glands of adult male mice, salivary glands are not the only source. The prompt fall in the concentration of plasma NGF which follows removal of submaxillary glands is followed by a gradual return to normal levels in spite of failure of these glands to regenerate.[129] This rise in serum concentrations may be accounted for by the finding that the hormone is produced by a variety of tissues including cultures of mouse adrenal medulla, rat skeletal muscle, and chick fibroblast.

Ovarian Growth Factor. During the course of studies designed to elucidate the *in vitro* effect of gonadotropic hormones on cloned ovarian tumor cells, Clark and associates found that crude gonadotropin preparations stimulated these cells to proliferate, whereas more highly purified LH and FSH lacked any ovarian growth-stimulating properties.[130] By fractionating bovine pituitary glands, Gospodarowicz and coworkers were successful in isolating an ovarian growth factor (OGF) which was present as a contaminant in commonly used reference preparations of gonadotropin and TSH.[131] Subsequent studies suggested that OGF functions primarily as a survival factor and its apparent growth-promoting activity is attributable to postponement of cell death.[132] OGF has been partially characterized and found to be a basic carbohydrate-free polypeptide with a molecular weight in the range of 10,000 to 13,000 daltons. Until such time as its physiologic importance becomes more apparent, OGF will be known primarily as the growth factor that brought to light the presence of fibroblastic growth factors in the pituitary and brain (see the following section).

Broad-Spectrum Growth Factors

Fibroblast Growth Factors. During the course of studies with the OGF, Gospodarowicz found that pituitary and brain extracts contain closely related fibroblast growth factors (FGF) which, together with small amounts of serum, are able to stimulate the proliferation of many cell lines of entodermal and mesodermal origin.[88, 133, 134] Pituitary FGF was found to be a basic polypeptide with an apparent molecular weight of 13,400 daltons. Fibroblast growth factor from bovine brain was found to be composed of two peptides, FGF 2 with 107 amino acids and FGF 1 with the same amino acid sequence but an additional 21 residues.[135] Both peptides appear to be components of myelin basic protein (MBP) with the larger FGF corresponding to residues 44 to 166 and the smaller factor corresponding to residues 44 to 153.[136] When injected with adjuvants into guinea pigs and rats, brain-derived FGF preparations induced clinical and histologic signs of autoimmune encephalomyelitis. Whereas brain-derived FGF cross-reacts immunologically with basic myelin, it fails to cross-react with pituitary FGF.

Although FGF was first recognized by its mitogenic effect on Balb/c 3T3 cells, this peptide has been shown to stimulate the division of a wide variety of other cell types. These include bovine adrenal cortex, granulosa and luteal cells, bovine corneal epithelial and endothelial cells, vascular endothelial cells, myoblasts, amniotic fibroblasts, and frog blastemal cells. FGF usually does not provide a complete signal for cell division in these cells, however, unless the medium contains plasma or other hormones such as dexamethasone, insulin, or somatomedin. FGF has no effect on epithelial cells or transformed fibroblasts.[137]

Westall and associates have suggested that FGF may be released *in vivo* by proteolytic digestion of MBP and that such release may have physiologic and pathologic signifi-

cance.[136] For example, in multiple sclerosis, large amounts of acid proteolytic enzymes accumulate in areas of active demyelination and various fragments of MBP are released locally and into cerebrospinal fluid. It is conceivable that FGF released in these situations could trigger the secondary astrocyte proliferation which is characteristic of lesions of multiple sclerosis. More important, since most tissues are innervated by myelinated nerve fibers, release of peptides with FGF activity from injured peripheral myelin may have an important role in initiating wound healing. This may be an efficient, elegant way for an organism to deliver a growth factor which is mitogenic for both fibroblasts and the vascular endothelial cells from which capillaries are formed. In support of this concept was a series of experiments in frogs and other amphibians in which FGF promoted the regeneration of extremities after amputation.[137]

Platelet-Derived Growth Factor and Serum Cationic Growth Factor. Until the observation of Balk in 1971, it was not generally appreciated that plasma is less effective than serum in supporting the proliferation of certain diploid cell lines.[138] Since one obvious difference between plasma and serum is that in the preparation of plasma, formed blood elements are removed before coagulation takes place, Rutherford and Ross combined a platelet extract with plasma and found that the enriched plasma was now equipotent with whole serum in supporting the growth of dermal fibroblasts and aortic smooth muscle cells.[139] Similar observations were made by Kohler and Lipton with mouse 3T3 fibroblasts.[140]

The platelet-derived growth factor now has been purified to apparent homogeneity by Antoniades, Scher, and Stiles from large quantities of outdated human platelets.[141] The purified peptide is highly cationic and, in the reduced state, has an estimated molecular weight of 13,000 to 16,000 daltons.

Several years prior to the isolation of the platelet-derived growth factor, Antoniades and coworkers identified a serum cationic peptide with a similar isoelectric point and a molecular weight estimated at 13,000 daltons.[142] An antibody prepared against this substance cross-reacted with platelet extracts and the concentration of the serum cationic peptide was found to be higher in whole serum than in platelet-poor plasma. Thus, there is reason to believe that the platelet-derived growth factor is not normally found in circulating blood but is released at the site of injury as a consequence of the aggregation and subsequent lysis of platelets. It was long believed that the main function of platelets was to gather at the site of injury and initiate blood coagulation by the release of clotting factors; it has now become apparent that an equally important function is to release a growth factor which initiates the process of wound healing by reprogramming tissue cells to undergo division.

Ross and associates have postulated that the platelet-derived growth factor also may play an important role in the pathogenesis of atherosclerosis.[143] According to his concept, fatty plaques in the walls of blood vessels damage intimal surfaces, thereby attracting platelets to the sites of injury. The release of platelet growth factor at these sites then causes arterial narrowing by stimulating a proliferative response in the arterial walls. If it were possible, therefore, to inhibit the release of platelet growth factor, it might be possible to neutralize the most damaging consequences of atherosclerosis. Harker and coworkers have already demonstrated this possibility by preventing proliferative changes in homocystinemic animals by inhibiting platelet aggregation and lysis.[144]

Epidermal Growth Factor/Urogastrone. Epidermal growth factor (EGF) was discovered by Stanley Cohen in 1962 when he noted that extracts of salivary glands from adult male mice, when injected into newborn mice, greatly accelerated the eruption of their incisor teeth and the open-

Table 28–3. CHARACTERISTICS OF BROAD-SPECTRUM GROWTH FACTORS

Name	Site of Origin	Chemical Characteristics	Factors Stimulating Production	Biologic Actions
Fibroblast growth factors	Pituitary	Polypeptide MW = 13,400 pI = 9.5[134]	?	Stimulates proliferation of cells of entodermal and mesodermal origin in presence of small amounts of serum
	Brain	FGF_1, MW = 13,000 FGF_2, MW = 11,700 (acid- and heat-labile)[135]	Proteolysis of myelin basic protein	Competence factor for fibroblasts
Platelet growth factor (serum cationic peptide)	Platelets	Peptide MW = 38,000 (13,000–16,000 in SDS after reduction); pI = 9.8;[141] acid- and heat-stable	Platelet lysis following aggregation at wound site or during clotting of blood	Similar to FGF where studied; inactive in vascular endothelium; competence factor for fibroblasts
Epidermal growth factor/ urogastrone	Salivary glands	Dimers of 2 subunits = 74,000 MW;[148] active peptide, 6000 MW[146]	Androgen	Stimulates proliferation of cells of ectodermal and mesodermal origin in presence of small amounts of serum; inhibits gastric secretion
Somatomedins	Liver; many other tissues	MW = 6000–8500[156] homologous with proinsulin; SM-C and IGF-I basic (pI = 8.2); IGF_2, SM-A, and MSA more neutral	GH; ?insulin	Sulfate uptake in cartilage; stimulates proliferation of many cell types; insulin-like effects

ing of their eyelids.[145] Indeed, Cohen has been linked with virtually every development connected with EGF.[146-148] Using a difficult *in vivo* assay, he devised an efficient three-step purification procedure from mouse salivary gland, determined the amino acid composition and complete sequence, and clarified many features of the biologic effects of EGF including its interaction with cell membrane receptors.

Mouse EGF is a tightly coiled peptide of 6000 daltons with three disulfide bridges. It occurs natively in salivary gland as a portion of a larger molecule of 74,000 daltons. This prohormone is composed of two molecules of the active peptide and two molecules of a 29,000 molecular weight subunit with arginine esterase activity (Fig. 28–6).

Although EGF, like the NGF, influences differentiation of specialized cells in early life, it is less restricted in its action and stimulates mitogenic activity in fibroblasts, epithelial cells, and mammary cells. It acts primarily on cells of ectodermal origin and a few cell types of mesodermal origin. It is not active on cells of entodermal origin. Like FGF, EGF does not serve as a complete mitogenic signal for most cell types; rather, it is effective only in the presence of small amounts of serum. Topical application of EGF to corneal wounds significantly hastens healing.[149, 150]

Salivary glands from adult male mice contain about 1 μg of EGF per milligram of wet tissue, whereas glands from female or castrated male mice contain less than a tenth of this amount. A rise of immunoreactive EGF in female and castrate male glands following the administration of androgens constitutes one of the most sensitive and specific *in vivo* assays for androgenic activity.[151, 152] It is surprising, therefore, that the levels of EGF in plasma and urine are approximately the same in the adult male, castrate male, and female mice.

The presence of EGF in humans was first described by Ances, who found that blood and urine from pregnant women contained a substance that cross-reacted with mouse EGF in receptor assays.[153] Human EGF subsequently was isolated from urine of pregnant women by using anti-mEGF as an immunoabsorbent. More recently, it has been pointed out that the amino acid sequence of hEGF is very similar, if not

identical, to urogastrone, a peptide which inhibits gastric secretions and protects against peptic ulcers.[154, 155] Completing the linkage are the observations that EGF blocks gastrin secretion and that urogastrone promotes early eye opening in mice.

The Somatomedin Family of Growth Factors. The somatomedins are a family of small peptides ranging in molecular size between 6000 and 8500 daltons. The generic term "somatomedin" implies that the growth-promoting actions of GH (somatotropin) on the skeleton and other tissues are mediated through these substances. Although a substantial body of experimental data is consistent with this hypothesis, rigorous proof based on *in vivo* studies is still lacking.

Four cardinal properties characterize the somatomedin group of peptides: (1) their concentrations in serum are GH-dependent; (2) they stimulate the incorporation of sulfate in proteoglycans of cartilage; (3) they have insulin-like biologic actions; and (4) they stimulate DNA synthesis and cell multiplication in many types of cultured cells.[156-160, 160a] The names applied to the different somatomedins reflect which of these properties were utilized to monitor purification and it is still not clear how many are distinctly different substances.

The Cartilage Sulfation Phenomenon: Somatomedin-A and Somatomedin-C. Salmon and Daughaday observed in 1957 that the incorporation of $^{35}SO_4$ into cartilage explants is stimulated either by normal serum or by serum from GH-treated hypophysectomized rats, but not by serum from untreated hypophysectomized rats.[161] Since the direct addition of GH itself to cartilage explants had no effect, they postulated that the skeletal growth-promoting actions of GH are mediated through a serum "sulfation factor" which is induced *in vivo* by GH action. It was later recognized that the serum "sulfation factor" also stimulates the synthesis in cartilage of RNA, DNA, collagen, and other proteins. Somatomedin-A and somatomedin-C were isolated on the basis of these effects.

Somatomedin-A is a neutral peptide isolated by Hall, Uthne, Fryklund, and Sievertsson using as an assay the incorporation of $^{35}SO_4$ into pelvic rudiments from chick embryos.[162-164] The reported composition of somatomedin-A differs from that of all the other somatomedins by its absence of disulfide bonds.

Somatomedin-C was isolated from acid-ethanol extracts of human plasma by Van Wyk and associates using an assay based on the incorporation of both $^{35}SO_4$ and ^3H-thymidine into costal cartilage segments from young hypophysectomized rats.[165] Somatomedin-C is indistinguishable from insulin-like growth factor I in various radioreceptor assays,[166] and these peptides also exhibit impressive similarities in chemical structure.[167]

Nonsuppressible Insulin-like Activity; Insulin-like Growth Factors. In the years before insulin could be measured directly by RIA, serum concentrations were estimated by biologic assays based on such known effects of insulin as the stimulation of glucose oxidation in rat epididymal fat pads. In such assays, however, less than 10% of the insulin-like activity in serum can be neutralized by insulin-specific antibodies. Froesch and coworkers used the term "nonsuppressible insulin-like activity" (NSILA) to describe those insulin-like substances in serum which do not react with insulin antibodies.[168]

In 1976, Rinderknecht and Humbel isolated two peptides with insulin-like activity which they named NSILA-I and NSILA-II.[169] These substances were found to be GH-dependent and to possess all the growth-promoting properties of the somatomedins. For this reason, they have since been renamed "insulin-like growth factors" (IGF I and IGF II). Both molecules have molecular weights of about 7000 daltons. IGF I, like somatomedin-C, has an isoelectric point of 8.2, whereas IGF II is a more neutral peptide. The complete amino acid sequence of IGF I and IGF II, as determined by Rinderknecht and Humbel, reveals remarkable similarity to that of proinsulin (Fig. 28–7). About 50% of the amino acid residues, the portions of the molecules which correspond with the A and B chains of insulin, are identical to the corresponding residues in proinsulin. The C peptides in the IGFs are shorter and bear no resemblance to the C peptide of proinsulin.[170] In addition, the carboxy terminus of the A chain in IGF is extended by eight amino acids. Blundell and associates have shown that those portions of the IGF I molecule which correspond with the antigenic portions of insulin are folded into the hydrophobic interior of the hydrated molecule, thus explaining the failure to react with insulin antisera.[171] IGF II is more insulin-like than IGF I or somatomedin-C, whereas the serum concentrations of IGF I and somatomedin-C are more GH-dependent than IGF II.[157, 166]

Multiplication-Stimulating Activity. Multiplication-stimulating activity (MSA) is the term coined by Temin to describe the substances in calf serum which stimulate DNA synthesis and cell replication in chick embryo fibroblasts. Pierson and Temin showed that a portion of the mitogenic activity of calf sera is due to a peptide of approximately 6000 daltons.[172] Although not fully purified, their preparation was shown to possess insulin-like activity and to stimulate radiosulfate uptake in cartilage. Cohen and associates demonstrated that the "multiplication-stimulating activity" of rat serum is GH-dependent.[173]

In subsequent work with MSA, several small peptides have been isolated from culture medium in which certain strains of rat hepatocytes have been grown.[174] These cell lines were derived from buffalo rats and were originally cloned on the basis of their ability to proliferate in the absence of serum. Rechler and Nissley have found that media conditioned by the growth of these cells contains several mitogenic substances which possess all of the biologic properties of the somatomedins and cross-react in receptor assays.[175] To identify their origin, these peptides are designated CRL-MSA (conditioned rat liver MSA) and BRL-MSA (buffalo rat liver MSA).

Related Peptides

Nonsuppressible Insulin-like Protein. Using nondenaturing conditions of purification, Poffenbarger has isolated from normal human serum an acid-stable, insulin-like protein of approximately 90,000 daltons.[176, 177] This protein possesses about one-tenth the specific activity of NSILA in epididymal fat pad assays, but is devoid of activity in sulfation factor assays. Although nonsuppressible insulin-like protein (NSILP) may represent a bound form of one of the somatomedins, its apparent lack of activity in cartilage assays fails to support this possibility.

Somatomedin-B. Somatomedin-B is the designation for a serum peptide which induces thymidine incorporation in cultures of human glial cells, but which is inactive in sulfation factor assays[164, 178] and is only partially GH-dependent. This peptide has a molecular weight of 5400 daltons and has been found to be an antiprotease. Somatomedin-B shares few properties with other members of the somatomedin family and the designation is now recognized to be a misnomer.

State of the Somatomedin in Serum. Although all of the somatomedins have been isolated as small peptides with molecular weights ranging between 6000 and 8500 daltons, they circulate in serum as macromolecular complexes.[179] When chromatographed on Sephadex G-200 at neutral pH, approximately 85% of the immunoreactive somatomedin-C is associated with proteins having a molecular weight of

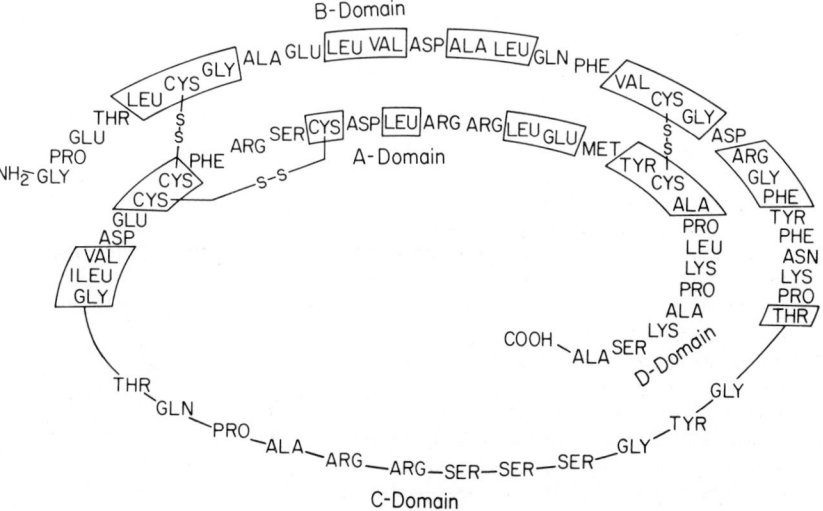

Figure 28–7. Primary structure of insulin-like growth factor I (IGF-I). The residues of the A and B domains of IGF-I that are enclosed in boxes are those which are identical with the insulin-proinsulin molecule. The C domain, which corresponds to the C peptide of proinsulin, has no homology with the latter. The D domain is an 8-residue extension at the carboxy terminus which does not exist in proinsulin. (Structure determined by E. Rinderknecht and R. E. Humbel.[170])

150,000 ± 12,000 daltons and the remainder is associated with smaller proteins, the greatest quantity of which is approximately 38,000 daltons. The 150,000 molecular weight fraction appears to be GH-dependent, since in acromegaly the additional somatomedin is found in this region and in hypopituitarism this fraction is reduced. Acidification of serum separates about 80% of the somatomedin from its binding proteins. The binding proteins undoubtedly prevent rapid fluctuations in serum concentrations, prolong disappearance times, and account for the relatively high concentrations of somatomedin in serum as contrasted with other peptide hormones.

Growth-Promoting Actions of Somatomedin. The limited supply of pure somatomedin peptides has precluded adequate *in vivo* tests of growth promotion. Van den Brande and Van Buul, however, were able to demonstrate an increase of linear growth and weight gain in the genetically hypopituitary Snell dwarf mouse after administrating a plasma extract for 10 days.[180] Although this plasma extract was rich in somatomedin activity, definitive conclusions cannot be made until the experiment is repeated with one of the pure somatomedin preparations. Rothstein and Van Wyk injected pure somatomedin-C into the dorsal lymph sacs of hypophysectomized frogs and were able to demonstrate a proliferative response in the lens epithelium, but the experiment was too short to determine the effect on linear growth.[181]

In cartilage, the somatomedins stimulate a generalized *in vitro* growth response, including cellular proliferation of chondrocytes and synthesis of collagen and noncollagenous proteins. Unlike other peptide growth factors, somatomedin apparently plays a role in the growth of cells derived from all three embryonic origins: entodermal, mesodermal, and ectodermal. These include HeLa cells, chick, mouse, and human fibroblasts, ovarian tumor cells, myoblasts, and pituitary tumor (GH₃) cells, and lens epithelium.[156]

Insulin-like Effects of the Somatomedins. The somatomedins exhibit a full range of *in vitro* insulin-like effects. In fat, they stimulate the conversion of ^{14}C glucose into CO_2, lipids, fatty acids, and glycogen and inhibit epinephrine-stimulated glycerol release. In muscle, they stimulate incorporation of ^{14}C into glycogen and stimulate cellular uptake of amino acids and sugars. Lastly, they inhibit the degradation of insulin in rat kidney cytosol by insulin-specific protease.[156]

Receptor Interactions. All of the insulin-like actions of the somatomedins are consistent with the concept that insulin and the somatomedins have evolved from a common ancestral molecule and hence share some common chemical features. In line with this interpretation was the finding that the somatomedins compete with ^{125}I-insulin for binding to the insulin receptor, although somatomedin is 50 to 100 times less potent than insulin in this regard. A similar potency ratio between the two hormones is found in biologic assays for insulin-like activity. Because of this relatively weak insulin-like activity, it is likely that under ordinary circumstances somatomedin has little or no effect on carbohydrate homeostasis *in vivo*.

The growth-promoting effects of the somatomedins, on the other hand, correlate well with the ability of these peptides to interact with their own specific cell receptors, which are different from the insulin receptor. These receptors are widely distributed in adult tissues and are present in fetal tissues early in gestation. Insulin cross-reacts with these specific somatomedin receptors only at extremely high concentrations.[156]

Origin of the Somatomedins. Analysis of extracts from many different tissues has failed to disclose any single organ where the somatomedin concentration exceeds that in serum. The lack of a readily releasable storage pool is consis-

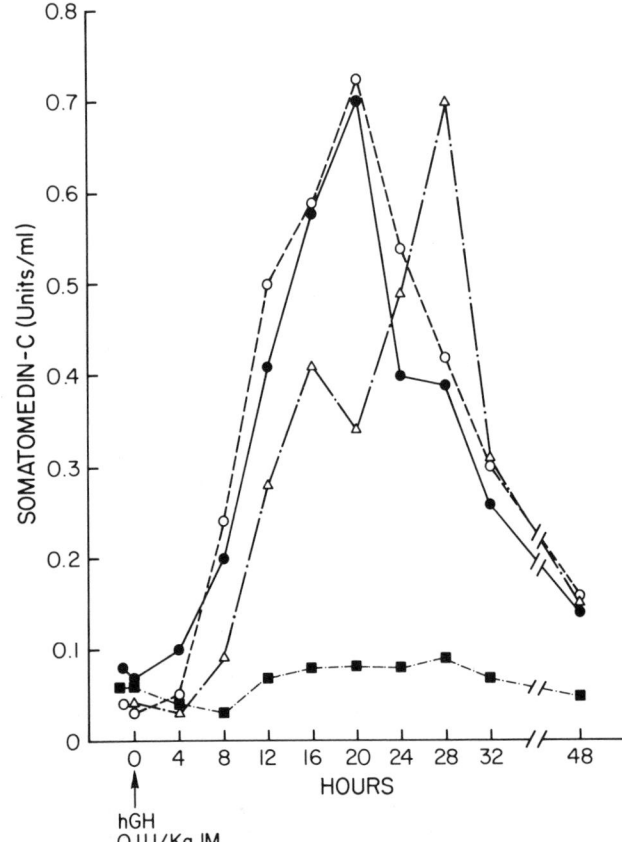

Figure 28–8. Plasma immunoreactive somatomedin-C responses to the intramuscular administration of hGH in four hypopituitary children. Increments in the plasma somatomedin-C level do not occur until 6 to 8 hours after hGH therapy and reach maximal values between 16 and 28 hours. The somatomedin-C level of some patients fails to rise in response to hGH. Although all the factors involved in failure to respond are not known, it appears that a suboptimal nutritional status is one factor which impedes the rise in somatomedin-C. (From Copeland, K. C., et al.: Induction of somatomedin-C in human serum by growth hormone: Dose response relationships and effect on chromatographic profile. *J. Clin. Endocrinol. Metab.* **50**:690–697, 1980.)

tent with the delayed rise in serum somatomedin concentrations following the administration of hGH to hypopituitary children.[182] The first detectable rise occurs at 6 hours, and maximal values are not reached until about 24 hours (Fig. 28–8). Although somatomedin does not appear to be stored in any tissue, it is believed that the liver is a major source since somatomedin is produced by hepatocyte cultures,[183] somatomedin content is higher in hepatic than in portal vein blood, serum concentrations of somatomedin are reduced by hepatectomy or hepatocellular disease,[184] and perfusion of the liver has yielded somatomedin in the effluent. The liver is probably not the only organ involved in somatomedin production, however, since other tissues have been found to produce somatomedin in cell or organ cultures. D'Ercole and associates have shown that somatomedin is produced by explants of a variety of fetal mouse tissues[242] and Weidman and coworkers[185] and Clemmons and Van Wyk[186] have shown production by human fibroblasts.

Physiologic Control of Somatomedin in Serum. For many years, somatomedin in serum could be measured only by bioassays. More recently, results have been based on radioreceptor assays,[189] competitive protein binding assays, or radioimmunoassay.[187, 191] Each of these techniques has somewhat different specificities for each of the somatomedins.

Growth hormone is the single most important regulator of somatomedin in serum. In 58 patients with active acromegaly, Clemmons found that the mean concentration of somatomedin-C was 10 times the mean value in his control population with no overlap between the two groups.[188] In hypopituitarism, serum concentrations are usually less than 20% of normal and rise with hGH administration (Fig. 28–9).

Placental lactogen may be involved in the stimulation of somatomedin production during pregnancy. Ovine placental lactogen is as potent as ovine GH in the induction of somatomedin production by hypophysectomized rats,[243] and serum somatomedin levels tend to rise late in human pregnancy when human placental lactogen levels are also very high.[190] Daughaday found that hypophysectomy of the pregnant rat is not followed by a drop in somatomedin as it is in the normal rat.[244]

Variations in nutritional status may play nearly as important a role as GH in modulating somatomedin concentrations in serum.[192] In rats, levels fall to 40% of basal values after 3 days of fasting. In children with protein-calorie malnutrition, serum somatomedin concentrations are as low as those in hypopituitary patients even though their serum GH levels may be elevated. A similar dissociation between GH and somatomedin is seen in Laron dwarfism where GH levels are high and somatomedin levels are very low. The mechanism of this dissociation appears to be somewhat different, however, since the Laron dwarf appears to have a total inability to respond to GH.

Control of Growth at the Cellular Level

The Mammalian Cell Cycle

The factors which permit certain cells to retain their capacity for repetitive division while impeding this function in other types of cells cannot be resolved until more is known of the mechanism controlling the mammalian cell cycle. While not always directly applicable to *in vivo* growth, observations on growth of eukaryotic cells in culture provide important insights into these mechanisms.[193-196] The cyclic proliferation of cells is segregated into two major nuclear components: a mitotic (M) phase and an intermitotic phase (interphase) (Fig. 28–10). Early observations of the cell cycle were confined to the mitotic phase because its dynamic sequence of events is visible by light microscopy. Mitosis is divided into prophase, in which the nucleus condenses and the chromosomes become shorter and thicker; metaphase, when the chromatids line up on the equatorial plane; anaphase, when the chromatids separate in opposite directions; and telophase, when the chromosomes, in the course of returning to interphase morphology, again lengthen and cytokinesis (cell division) begins.

With the development of chemical and autoradiographic methods for the quantification and timing of DNA replication, three active stages of interphase were recognized. The period of DNA replication, referred to as S (synthesis) phase, is preceded by a gap (G_1) in time between the end of mitosis and the beginning of DNA replication. A second gap (G_2) occurs between the end of DNA replication and the onset of mitosis. During the G_1 and G_2 phases, there is synthesis of structural, catalytic, and regulatory proteins which are unique to each cell type. Fully mature cells may enter a nongrowing, quiescent phase operationally referred to as G_0, in which they are not committed to further cell replication. On the other hand, depending upon cell type and stage of life, they may reenter the cell cycle. It remains to be shown whether resting cells have actually left the cell cycle to enter a distinct G_0 state or are only arrested in a prolonged G_1 phase. While the duration of each stage of the cell cycle is subject to extreme variation, under typical conditions of *in vitro* culture mammalian cells may complete a cycle in 18 to 24 hours. As little as 1 hour of the cycle may be occupied by mitosis, the remainder being taken up by the synthetic processes occupying interphase. The greatest variation is usually found in G_1, and the critical events which regulate proliferation occur primarily in this phase of the cell cycle.

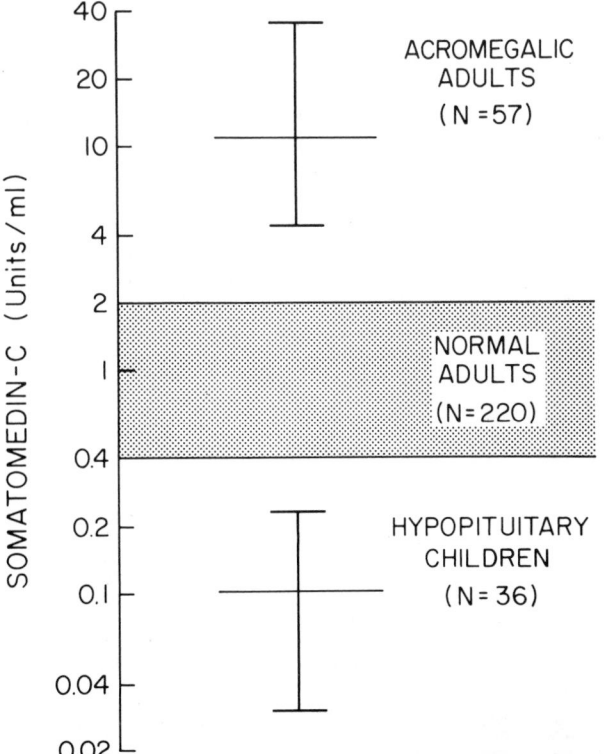

Figure 28–9. Concentration of immunoreactive somatomedin-C in the plasma of normal adults and hypopituitary children and the serum of adults with active acromegaly. The shaded area for normal adults (ages 18 to 64 years) includes 95% of the subjects, whereas the indicators for the hypopituitary and acromegalic patients are means and absolute ranges of values observed. The standard is serum from a large pool of normal adults (Ortho Diagnostics, Raritan, N.J.) and has an assigned potency of 1.66 units/ml.

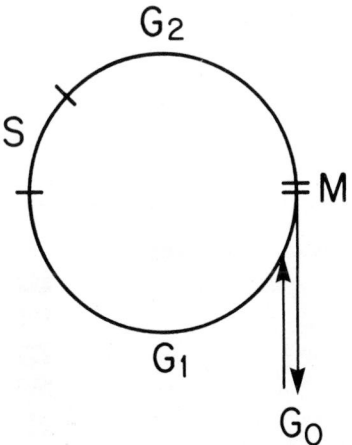

Figure 28–10. The eukaryotic cell cycle (see text).

Effects of Nutrients and Specific Macromolecular Factors on Cell Growth

The responses of cultured cells to growth stimuli are influenced by the source of the cells, their age when plated, and cell density, and by seemingly minor changes in the nutrient media and other culture conditions. Even the responses of well characterized stable cell lines may change from time to time as a consequence of spontaneous transformation or other poorly understood factors. The results obtained in different laboratories, therefore, are frequently contradictory since the experimental conditions are rarely the same. Nevertheless, monolayer cultures of single cell types are capable of providing considerable information on the regulation of cell proliferation and the sequence of biochemical events involved.

The influence of hormones, growth factors, or nutrients on cellular proliferation is commonly evaluated by comparison of the effects produced by serum.[197] The cell types most commonly used for these studies are diploid, nontransformed fibroblasts derived from human skin or from chick or mouse embryos. Although such cells do not replicate in the absence of serum, they can survive and retain their growth potential for long periods of time. The reintroduction of serum into their media is followed by the initiation of DNA synthesis after a lag of about 12 hours, with mitosis beginning several hours later.

It has long been debated whether the function of serum is simply to supply those nutrients which are deficient in most synthetic media or to provide hormones and macromolecular growth factors. It is now clear that this is a false distinction since nutrients and growth factors often act synergistically. McKeehan and Ham, for example, have found that the requirement for macromolecular growth factors is substantially reduced in cells grown in media enriched with optimal concentrations of all the known nutrients.[198]

Although serum contains small amounts of most of the "classic" steroid and peptide hormones, no combination of these hormones is capable of duplicating the effect of serum in the growth of most cell lines. Hayashi and associates have shown, however, that the full effect of serum on the growth of many normal and tumor cell lines can be reproduced with a mixture of peptide growth factors, transferrin, and classic hormones, the exact mixture having been empirically derived for each type of cell[199] (Fig. 28–11).

Action of Peptide Growth Factors on the Cell Cycle

Further understanding of how growth factors and hormones influence the cell cycle has come from the studies of Pledger and associates, who found that an ordered sequence of cellular events ensues when confluent, serum-deprived Balb/c 3T3 mouse fibroblasts are exposed sequentially to various components of serum.[200] In order for such cells to traverse the G_1 phase of the cell cycle and enter S, they must first be rendered "competent." Competence can be achieved by exposure to the platelet-derived growth factor (PDGF) which is released from platelets during the clotting of blood. Once cells are rendered competent, the platelet factor can be removed without impairing the capacity of these cells to subsequently respond to additional mitogenic substances which collectively are called "progression factors." These factors are present in platelet-poor plasma and stimulate competent cells to progress to the S phase of the cell cycle. Neither competence factors nor progression factors can by themselves stimulate stationary fibroblasts to traverse the cell cycle (Fig. 28–12).

Stiles and coworkers showed that the progression factors in platelet-poor plasma can be divided further into those which are GH-dependent and those non GH-dependent factors which are present in plasma from hypopituitary children or hypophysectomized rats.[201] The GH-dependent effect appears to be mediated through the somatomedin family of peptides since full progression factor activity is restored to hypopituitary plasma by the addition of somatomedin-C but not by GH itself. In the absence of somatomedin, competent cells become arrested at a specific restriction point 6 hours prior to the G_1/S boundary.

On the basis of these studies, Stiles and associates have proposed a classification of peptide growth factors which depends on whether they act as "competence factors" or "progression factors." In a systematic survey, they found that FGF and PDGF were interchangeable for inducing competence in Balb/c 3T3 cells and that the somatomedins, insulin, epidermal growth factor and hydrocortisone all, under certain circumstances, possess progression factor activity.

The biochemical responses to the different growth factors and the mechanisms by which one event affects the next is not yet known. Clemmons and associates have shown that

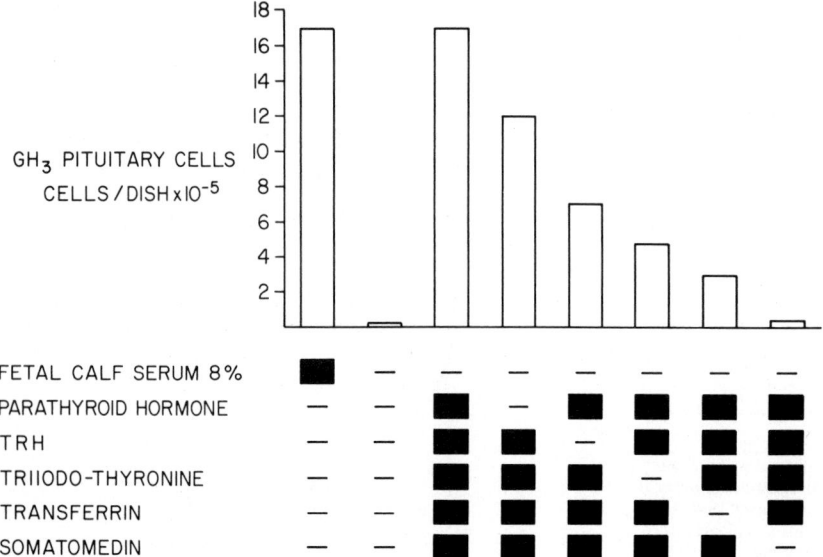

GH₃ PITUITARY CELLS
CELLS/DISH x 10⁻⁵

Figure 28–11. Growth of pituitary GH₃ cells *in vitro*. Addition of parathyroid hormone, thyrotropin-releasing hormone (TRH), triiodothyronine, transferrin, and somatomedin to serum-free cultures produces proliferation of cells equal to that produced by fetal calf serum. Withdrawal in turn of each of the above components results in a progressive decline in cell growth with the most profound effect being exerted by withdrawal of somatomedin. (Adapted from Hayashi, I., and Sato, G. H.: Replacement of serum by hormones permits growth of cells in a defined medium. *Nature* 259:132, 1976.)

ADAPTED FROM HAYASHI AND SATO. NATURE. 259, 132, 1976.

G_0	G_1	S
Competence Formation	Progression (12 hours)	DNA Synthesis

Normal Platelet Poor Plasma

Platelet GF   OR

OR $\begin{bmatrix} \text{hypopit. PPP} \\ \text{(or EGF)} \end{bmatrix}$ + $\begin{bmatrix} \text{somatomedin-C} \\ \text{(or other sms)} \end{bmatrix}$

Fibroblast GF

Figure 28–12. Sequential action of serum factors in stimulating quiescent Balb c/3T3 cells to enter DNA synthesis. The platelet-derived growth factor (or the fibroblast growth factor) renders confluent cells "competent" so that they can respond to "progression factors" in platelet poor plasma (PPP). Hypopituitary PPP (or epidermal growth factor) will advance cells to a point located 6 hours prior to the normal onset of DNA synthesis. Somatomedin-C (or other somatomedins) is required to permit further progression and entry into S.

one effect of rendering cells competent with PDGF or fibroblast growth factor is to increase the binding of ^{125}I-somatomedin-C to cell membrane receptors.[202] Further elucidation of the sequence in which the various growth factors act in the cell cycle may help to delineate the biochemical events leading to cell division.

Cyclic Nucleotides and Cell Growth

Although a number of peptide growth factors have now been shown to interact with cell membrane receptors in the same fashion as classic peptide hormones, the subsequent intracellular events leading to cell division are less well understood than those leading to differentiated cellular responses. Alterations in cyclic nucleotides may be involved in the transmission of pleiotypic signals since transition from G_0 to G_1 often is associated with a fall in intracellular cAMP[203, 204] and cell proliferation is inhibited if cAMP and its dibutyryl analog are added to the culture. On the other hand, cGMP has been shown to promote cell division under certain circumstances, and at least one mitogenic agent has been reported to stimulate a rapid, transient increase in cGMP levels within the cell.[205] Other studies, however, have cast doubt on any role of cGMP as an effector of cell division.[206] Other factors that may be involved in cell division and need further elucidation include calcium,[207] other divalent cations, and intracellular polyamines.[208]

Negative Controls on Cell Proliferation: The Chalone Hypothesis

Bullough has proposed that internal secretions which inhibit cell proliferation play as important a role in regulating mitotic activity as do the humoral factors which stimulate cell proliferation.[209] These substances, for which he has proposed the name chalones, possess four cardinal features: (1) they inhibit cell proliferation in vivo; (2) they are produced by the same tissue on which they act; (3) their actions are reversible; and (4) their action is cell line–specific. The importance of the chalone hypothesis lies in the implicit concept that cells have an inherent tendency to proliferate and that, rather than stimulators, the principal regulators of cell growth are inhibitors which are produced by the organ whose growth they control. More than a dozen chalones have been reported in such diverse tissues as epidermis, fibroblasts, erythrocytes, lymphocytes, melanocytes, kidney, liver, lungs, endometrial tissues, and thyroid. Most have been studied only superficially and reports of their chemical properties often have been contradictory. Those which have been partially characterized have been reported to be peptides with molecular weights varying between 5000 and 40,000 daltons. It has been proposed that chalones act on the

G_1 or G_2 stage of the cell cycle. Opponents of the concept of chalones point out that it has not been possible to unequivocally and consistently demonstrate chalones in tissue culture where the most sensitive techniques are presumably available for their detection.

Evidence for the existence of chalones in active leukemia comes from the finding that the proliferation of normal bone marrow stem cells often is suppressed and their mature progeny may not be detectable in the circulation. Broxmeyer and associates have recovered by extraction and by incubation of leukemic cells a "leukemia-associated inhibitory factor" (LIA) from more than 90% of patients with various types of leukemia.[210] LIA acts in vitro on normal marrow to inhibit growth of cultured granulocytic colony-forming units. It is proposed, therefore, that the LIA "chalone" impairs the production of normal cells, and thereby contributes to the severity of exacerbation of the leukemia process.

Interactions Between Cells

Cultures of single cell types have severe and not always appreciated limitations as a paradigm for interpreting in vivo growth. This is particularly true in embryonic tissues where the direction of differentiation of primordial cells is dependent upon the nature of mesenchyme surrounding them.[211, 212] Ectoderm transplanted from early embryos, for example, maintains the potential for differentiating into a wide spectrum of tissue when exposed to mesenchyme of diverse origins. Pancreatic epithelium will continue its development as pancreas in the presence of any mesenchyme so far tested,[213] whereas salivary gland epithelium undergoes its characteristic morphogenesis only in the presence of its own kind of mesenchyme. There is evidence that such differentiation is under the control of hormone-like signals.[214, 215] Even fully differentiated cells frequently need to be grown in the presence of other cell types to maintain their differentiated state. This is particularly true of epithelial tissues, which tend to dedifferentiate unless grown alone with mesenchymal tissues.

The growth of cells may be influenced by neighboring cells either by direct cellular communication through gap junctions or by modifying the shape of adjacent cells. Gap junctions, described in both vertebrates and invertebrates, are specialized regions of short-range contact between cells.[216, 217] At the site of the gap junction, the intercellular space is narrowed from its normal width of approximately 250 angstroms (Å) to a width of approximately 30 Å. The gap junction particles, made up of protein subunits which are contributed by each abutting cell, form intercellular channels which bridge membranes of adjacent cells and the intercellular space. Studies of cell communications strongly suggest that intercellular junctions facilitate exchange of ions and low molecular weight compounds, such as sugars, amino acids, and nucleotides. There is debate concerning whether large molecules such as RNA and cytoplasmic proteins are transferred.[216, 218, 219] Lawrence and associates[220] cocultured rat granulosa cells with mouse myocardial cells and found that addition of FSH increased the beat frequency in the myocardial cells, whereas addition of norepinephrine caused the secretion of plasminogen activator by the granulosa cells. These responses were found only after gap junctions had been established between the two cell types thus permitting the exchange of cAMP. Such transfer might be important in embryonic growth and differentiation as well as in postnatal growth facilitating the exchange of growth factors between different cell types.

Another mechanism by which cells modify the growth behavior of neighboring cells is by placing restrictions on cellular shape. Gospodarowicz has emphasized the importance of such restrictions in cell shape by comparing the growth characteristics of isolated corneal epithelial cells when plated on various substrata with their growth characteristics in whole-organ cultures or in vivo.[221] When plated on the usual plastic tissue culture dishes, the epithelial cells become flattened and fail to respond to epidermal growth factor, whereas EGF is a powerful mitogen for these cells in vivo or when maintained in organ culture. When these cells were plated on a substratum of collagen or a feeder layer of fibroblasts, the epithelial cells retained their tall columnar configuration and also responded to EGF with a marked increase in cell number. The responses of these corneal epithelial cells to FGF was opposite of that to EGF: when plated on plastic, the flattened cells proliferated in response to FGF, whereas differentiated columnar cells in organ culture were unresponsive to this growth factor. Since the receptors for EGF were not altered by these different culture conditions, Gospodarowicz postulated that cellular shape is one of the major factors which dictates the sensitivity of different cell types to various growth factors. On the basis of more recent studies in which various cell types were grown on a matrix previously laid down by corneal endothelial cells, Gospodarowicz and associates concluded that specific components in the extracellular matrix are among the most important determinants of both in vivo and in vitro cell proliferation.[221a, 221b]

Folkman and Moscona also have emphasized the importance of cell shape by an ingenious series of experiments in which they plated cells in plastic dishes in which the adhesivity had been modified by chemical means. Quantitative changes in adhesivity permitted controlled variation in cell adherence and shape. It was observed that cell adherence and shape varied inversely with DNA synthesis.[222] The limitations of tissue culture for studying cell growth will undoubtedly become increasingly apparent as new mechanisms are discovered to explain the social interactions between different cell types.[223]

Relevance of Growth Factors and Studies of Cellular Growth to Human Physiology and Disease

The discovery of peptide growth factors and their roles in cell differentiation and replication has opened important new frontiers in understanding the regulation not only of linear growth of the skeleton, but also of the growth, functional development, and reparative responses to injury of nearly every system in the body. Much of the rapidly accumulating information on these growth factors has not yet been incorporated into the fabric of classic endocrinology since most of these substances have been isolated in only

trace amounts and sufficient quantities have not been available for administration to living subjects. Further, since rapid, reliable methods have not been available for their quantification, progress has been slow in understanding how the various broad-spectrum growth factors, specialized growth factors, and classic hormones interact in a cooperative or antagonistic fashion in regulating in vivo growth. Nevertheless, several examples can be cited to illustrate how information derived from in vitro cell-growth studies with peptide growth factors might enlarge our understanding of human disease and suggest therapeutic approaches.

The finding that a growth factor, not normally present in circulating blood, is released following the lysis of platelets at the site of vascular injury has refocused attention on the damaging proliferative responses to atherosclerosis.[143] In a similar fashion, following neural injury, FGF might be produced by digestion of myelin basic protein and lead to the focal proliferative changes found in the lesions of multiple sclerosis.[136] The finding that NGF content of the brain is increased by thyroxine suggests a possible mechanism for the attenuated central nervous system development seen in cretins.[46]

If and when sufficient quantities of the peptide growth factors become available for in vivo testing, the therapeutic possibilities so opened could have a major impact on many human diseases. The highly specific growth factors — erythropoietin, macrophage growth factor, and the thymic hormones — all of which act on continuously renewing tissues, would have immediate promise for the treatment of certain forms of anemia, granulocytopenia, and immunodeficiency states; indeed, promising clinical trials have been reported with relatively crude extracts of bovine thymus in both genetic and acquired forms of immunodeficiency. EGF has been found to accelerate the healing of corneal wounds and might find application in the healing of gastric ulcers and other epithelial wounds.[149] The use of somatomedin as a substitute for GH in pituitary dwarfism or in GH-resistant dwarfism, such as Laron dwarfism, might become more than a theoretical possibility if large-scale production were achieved as a result of further advances in recombinant DNA methodology.

Neoplastic diseases must be considered as a fundamental growth disturbance, and evidence is now emerging that certain tumors secrete growth factors, although it remains to be determined whether or not these substances play any role in the undisciplined growth of these cells. Apart from these issues, knowledge of the exact role that peptide growth factors play in the normal cell cycle might make it possible to use growth factors to synchronize the growth of tumor cells in a manner that would make them more vulnerable to mitotic poisons. Whether or not these specific possibilities are realized, these examples serve to illustrate the wide range of clinical applications which could result from further knowledge of peptide growth factors and the mechanisms by which they regulate growth at the cellular level.

DISORDERS OF HUMAN GROWTH

Assessment of Growth and Development

Stature

The assessment of linear growth is one of the most sensitive means for evaluating the overall well-being of the child, since it represents the net expression of genetic make-up, adequacy of nutrition and environment, and the residual effects of past experience with disease. Well kept growth records frequently provide the first clue to endocrine abnor-

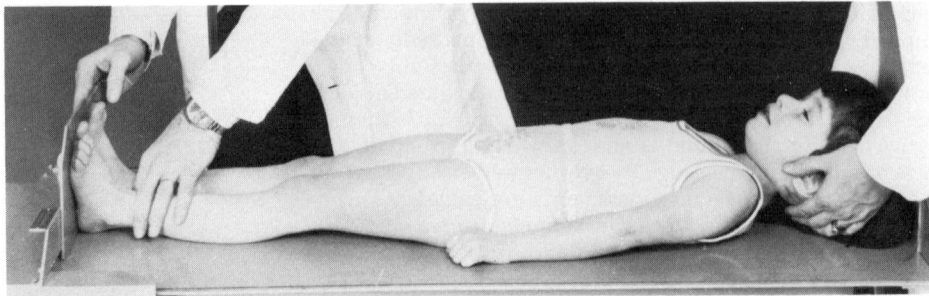

Figure 28–13. Technique for measuring recumbent length. (Courtesy of Noël Cameron, Ph.D., Institute of Child Health, London.)

malities, genetic or chromosomal disorders, malnutrition, or chronic systemic illness. In other instances, growth records may rule against the likelihood of suspected disorders and thus eliminate the need for costly laboratory tests. Despite the simplicity of this noninvasive method for evaluating child health, past growth records frequently are incomplete or grossly inaccurate at the time when concern first surfaces about a child's progress.

Technique of Measurement. Errors of measurement, which may amount to several centimeters, may result from inherent errors in measuring instruments or from improper positioning of the subject.[224] Supine length is generally taken from birth until 24 months of age; thereafter, erect height is used. The best device for measuring the recumbent length of infants is a box with an unyielding horizontal surface and a moving footboard of sufficient size to maintain the soles of the feet on a plane perpendicular to the body axis[3] (Fig. 28–13). The position of the head should be standardized in the Frankfurt plane: i.e., a line running through the outer canthus of the eyes and the external auditory meatus must be perpendicular to the trunk axis. With an uncooperative infant, accurate measurement may require three people to maintain optimal positioning.

It is a commentary on the emphasis most physicians place on accurate longitudinal measurements that most suppliers of medical equipment fail to list precision stadiometers in their catalogs. Instead, the most commonly used device for measuring stature is a weight balance equipped with a moving (and usually flexible) arm. Such devices are nearly worthless for obtaining accurate measurements. A variety of durable stadiometers designed by J. M. Tanner and R. H. Whitehouse for the Harpenden Growth Study in Britain are now available in this country. In the absence of a commercial device, a suitable stadiometer can be made at modest cost by mounting two meter sticks in vertical tandem on any vertical surface at least 12 inches wide and providing a sliding but rigid right-angle device of sufficient size to rest on the crown when the head is held in the Frankfurt plane.

Measurement of height should be made with the patient's feet bare and with the heels, buttocks, and shoulders in contact with the stadiometer. Heels are placed together with medial malleoli touching, if possible, and lordosis is reduced by relaxing the shoulders and applying pressure to the abdomen (Fig. 28–14). Diurnal variations in height are minimized if modest upward pressure is applied to the mastoid processes or the mandibular angles.[225] When a young child is measured, it is often necessary for an assistant to ensure that the plantar surfaces of the heels remain in contact with the floor. The variation between observers of measurement obtained in such fashion should be no more than 0.3 cm. Using these techniques, it is possible to determine a child's growth rate in as little as 3 to 4 months. Because of seasonal variation in growth and other factors, however, it is generally inadvisable to make important decisions about management until growth has been observed for a full year.[226]

Evaluation of Height Measurements. Accurate height measurements are of little value unless interpreted in the light of appropriate norms which have been established for children of the same age and sex and of comparable genetic and environmental background. Since growth is a dynamic process, sequential data from which the current growth rate can be calculated are of far more value than a single measurement. Although many complex formulations have been proposed for the evaluation of linear growth performance, the most useful are simple cumulative growth charts and height-velocity charts. Data on which these charts are based

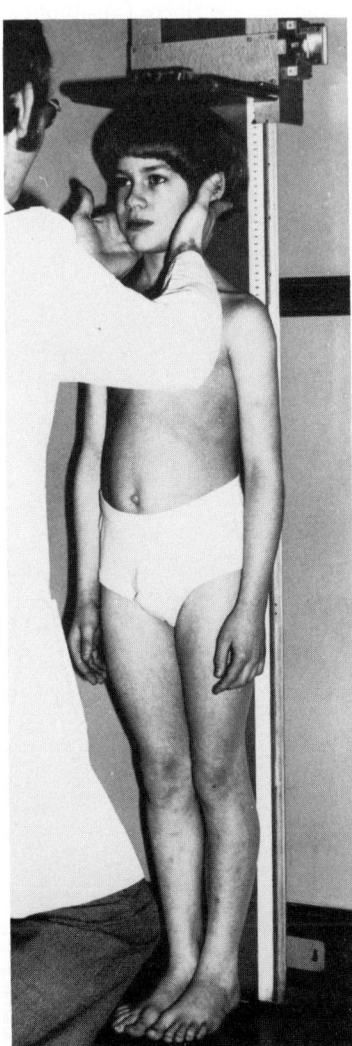

Figure 28–14. Technique for measuring erect height using Harpenden stadiometer with direct digital display of height. (Courtesy of Noël Cameron, Ph.D., Institute of Child Health, London.)

may be derived from cross-sectional studies in which large numbers of individual children, who are supposedly representative of a given population, are measured only once. Group means and population centiles are calculated at each age for the two sexes. Alternatively, growth charts may be derived from longitudinal studies in which a group of subjects are measured periodically over a number of years and the between-measurement increments are calculated.

The cumulative growth charts compiled from a vast data base by the National Center for Health Statistics are cross-sectionally derived and represent the most accurate description of size of children in the United States.[227] Growth charts prepared from cross-sectional data tend to extend and flatten out the growth spurt in a manner that fails to portray the rapid pubertal growth of individual children. The growth charts prepared by Tanner from London children contain longitudinal growth data and more accurately portray growth after the onset of the pubertal growth spurt.[16] Data collected both cross-sectionally and longitudinally are needed to completely define the process of growth. Cross-sectional data are preferable for constructing standards before puberty and for screening patients for growth disorders. Longitudinal data are infinitely better for assessment of pubertal growth and, indeed, are more appropriate for all clinical work which involves reported measurements in a given patient. We have found no serious disadvantage from using these British standards for North Carolina children.

Height-velocity charts (Figs. 28–15 and 28–16) are useful

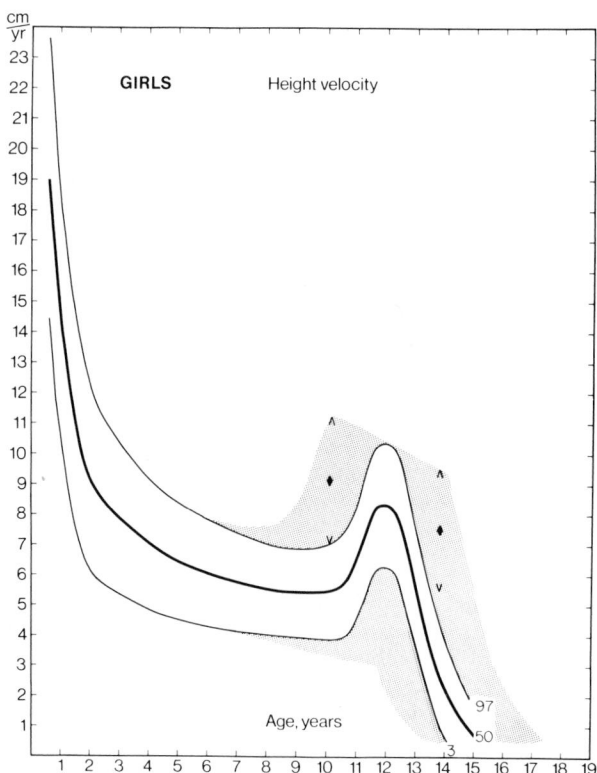

Figure 28–16. Height-velocity chart for girls. See legend to Figure 28–15. (Redrawn and reproduced with the permission of J. M. Tanner and Castlemead Publications, Hertford, England.)

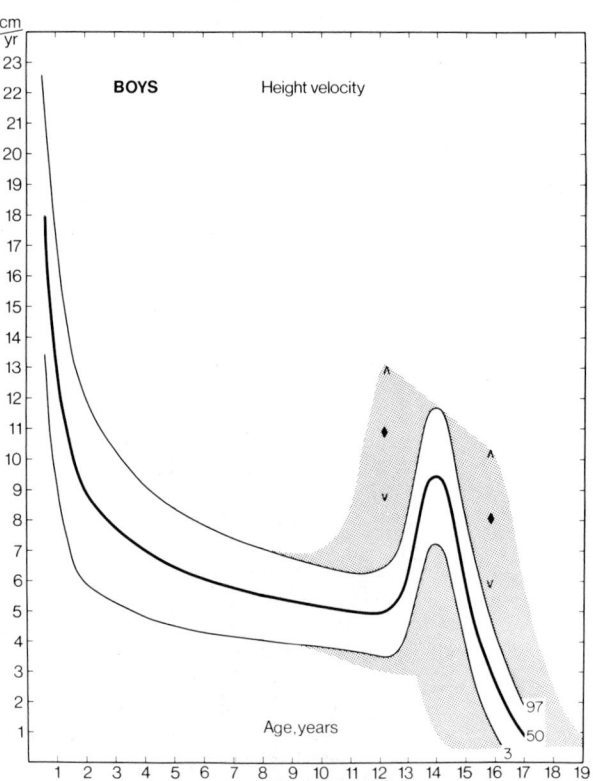

Figure 28–15. Height-velocity chart for boys constructed from longitudinal observations of British children. The 97th, 50th, and 3rd centile curves define the general pattern of growth during puberty. The shaded areas define the velocities of children who have their peak velocities at ages which are up to 2 standard deviations before or after the average age depicted by the centile lines. The arrows and diamonds mark the 97th, 50th, and 3rd centiles of peak velocity when the peak takes place these early or late limits. (The figure is redrawn from charts prepared by J. M. Tanner and R. H. Whitehouse from data published in references 15 and 16. It is reproduced with the permission of J. M. Tanner and Castlemead Publications, Hertford, England.)

in that they accentuate modest changes in growth rate and thereby make it easier to recognize growth-altering processes. They also make it possible to identify the onset of the pubertal growth spurt and the point of maximal height velocity and to anticipate the duration of the growing period. Such data are of great prognostic value in the individual child and are particularly useful in evaluating the acute effects of any therapeutic intervention which might affect the growth process. The height-velocity charts of Tanner have proved eminently satisfactory for these purposes.

"Height age" is a useful means for relating a patient with his peers. Unlike skeletal age, however, it cannot be used as an index of maturity since all adults do not achieve the same height at maturity. The height age of a given child is obtained from the cumulative growth chart by determining the age at which the observed height for the child intersects the 50th centile. The height age of a child is particularly useful in correlating linear growth with skeletal age, weight age, dental age, and other parameters for which age-related norms are available.

Weight

Measurements of weight should be interpreted in relationship to stature rather than to age. In this context, body weight provides primarily an index of nutritional status and adipose deposits, although under special circumstances weight changes reflect alterations in extracellular fluids. Evaluation of the birth weight in relation to the duration of gestation provides important information concerning the adequacy of the intrauterine environment and may provide important clues to the existence of maternal drug or alcohol ingestion, intrauterine infection, various genetic disorders, or, in the case of large babies, diabetes or prediabetes in the mother.

In the older child, severe undernutrition is rarely attributable to a primary endocrine disturbance *per se*, except in long-standing hyperthyroidism. In underweight children, therefore, attention should be more appropriately directed toward the detection of malabsorption syndromes, psychogenic feeding disorders, and systemic illnesses. Similarly, obesity is most commonly due to excessive ingestion of calories and sedentary habits, and a primary endocrine etiology is relatively uncommon. The most common causes of endocrine obesity are primary hypothyroidism and Cushing's syndrome. Both conditions are associated with profound arrest of linear growth, whereas children with exogenous obesity are usually above the 50th centile in stature and are continuing to grow at an accelerated rate. Thus, serial stadiometer measurements in the obese child are usually sufficient to exclude the possibility of either hypothyroidism or Cushing's syndrome and may avert the need for expensive laboratory studies.

Evaluation of Segmental Proportions

Conclusions concerning a child's growth based on total stature can be misleading in disorders selectively affecting the growth of the trunk or extremities. The first suspicion of chondrodystrophies, scoliosis, eunuchoidism, Marfan's syndrome, and similar disorders is often gleaned by finding a disproportion between a child's segmental measurements and those which are normal for age and sex.

The ratio between the upper segment of the body (trunk, neck, and head) and the lower segment (leg length) diminishes from an average value of 1.7 in term babies to slightly less than 1.0 at full maturity. The upper segment can be accurately measured with a child sitting on a stool of fixed height with his back positioned against a stadiometer. The thighs must be horizontal in order to prevent pelvic tilt. The height of the stool is subtracted from the stadiometer reading to obtain the sitting height. The lower segment can be obtained directly by measuring with a steel tape the distance from the floor to the top of the pubic symphysis. Sitting height standards[228, 229] cannot be used for assessment of this measurement, however. In children with deformities affecting only the trunk or legs, a fairly accurate estimate of the true height often can be made after direct measurement of either the normal upper segment or lower segment and calculating the true height from the segmental proportions which are normal for an individual of that age and sex.

Pubertal Development

The simple rating scales proposed by Tanner[24] for grading stages of pubic hair and breast development in girls and pubic hair and genital development in boys have gained wide acceptance as a convenient method for recording pubertal development[230] (Table 28-4).

In girls, development of pubic hair under the stimulus of adrenal androgens is usually, but not always, synchronous with breast development. In a few girls, however, breast development may reach stage III before pubic hair appears; conversely, pubic hair may reach stage III before breast development is apparent. As a rule, growth of axillary hair begins about the time that the breasts reach stage III or IV. The first menstrual period (menarche) is a relatively late pubertal event which must be preceded by sufficient secretion of estrogen to cause uterine growth and proliferation of endometrium. At the time of menarche, the breasts and pubic hair usually have reached stage IV and, almost with-

Table 28-4. STAGES OF DEVELOPMENT OF SECONDARY SEX CHARACTERISTICS*

Boys: Genital (Penis) Development:
Stage 1. Prepubertal: Testes, scrotum, and penis of about the same size and proportion as in early childhood.
Stage 2. Enlargement of scrotum and testes. Skin of scrotum reddens and changes in texture.
Stage 3. Enlargement of penis, which occurs at first mainly in length. Further growth of testes and scrotum.
Stage 4. Increased size of penis with growth in breadth and development of glans. Testes and scrotum larger; scrotal skin darkened.
Stage 5. Genitalia adult in size and shape.

Girls: Breast Development:
Stage 1. Prepubertal: elevation of papilla only.
Stage 2. Breast bud stage: elevation of breast and papilla as small mound. Enlargement of areola diameter.
Stage 3. Further enlargement and elevation of breast and areola, with no separation of their contours.
Stage 4. Projection of areola and papilla to form a secondary mound above the level of the breast.
Stage 5. Mature stage: projection of papilla only, due to recession of the areola to the general contour of the breast.

Both Sexes: Pubic Hair:
Stage 1. Prepubertal: The vellus over the pubes is not further developed than over the abdominal wall.
Stage 2. Sparse growth of long, slightly pigmented downy hair, straight or slightly curled, chiefly at the base of the penis or along labia.
Stage 3. Considerably darker, coarser, and more curled. The hair spreads sparsely over the junction of the pubes.
Stage 4. Hair now adult in type, but area covered is still considerably smaller than in the adult. No spread to the medial surface of the thighs.
Stage 5. Adult in quantity and type with distribution of the horizontal (or classically "feminine") pattern.
Stage 6. Spread up the linea alba (male-type pattern).

*Modified from Tanner, J. M.: *Growth at Adolescence.* 2nd ed. Oxford, Blackwell Scientific Publications, 1962.

out exception, the peak height velocity has been passed and the linear growth rate is slowing.[231] The menarche of early-maturing girls occurs closer to the point of peak height velocity than is normally the case, whereas late-maturing girls undergo menarche at a later point on the velocity curve. On the average, girls grow only 7.3 cm (range: 3 to 11 cm) after menarche.[232]

Although there are no standards for genital development in girls, considerable information concerning pubertal development can be obtained by inspecting the labial membranes for evidence of an estrogen effect. During the prepubertal period, the labial and vulvar membranes are bright red because of the thinness of the epithelial layer. The labia minora have sharp edges and the secretions are watery. An early sign of estrogen stimulation is thickening of the labia minora, the presence of a mucoid vaginal secretion, and change in coloration from bright red to pastel pink. These changes are reflected in the transition from predominantly sparse cuboidal cells with large nuclei to abundant squamous cells with pyknotic nuclei. In addition to vaginal changes, cytologic examination of centrifuged urinary sediment is an exceedingly sensitive method for ascertaining whether or not estrogen secretion has begun. In our hands, examination of urethral cytology has many advantages over the assessment of changes in the vaginal smear. Estrogen secretion can be confirmed by the finding on rectal examination of early uterine enlargement.

In boys, the testes change little in size between birth and the onset of puberty. As puberty begins, however, testicular volume increases as the seminiferous tubules enlarge under gonadotropin stimulation (Fig. 28-17). This testicular enlargement, which can be detected before any other signs of

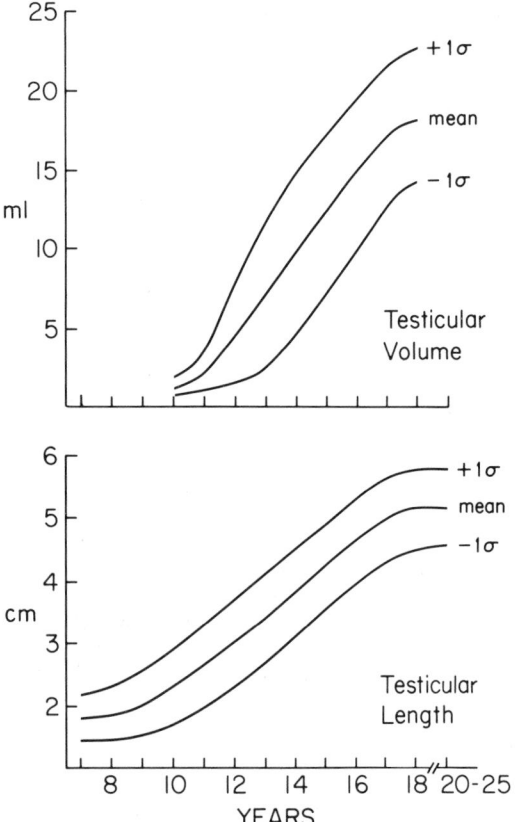

Figure 28–17. Growth of the testis during puberty. Data on mean and 1 standard deviation for the testicular volume are derived from the studies of M. Zachmann and A. Prader.[234] Data on testicular length are taken from Winter, J. S. D., and Faiman, C.: Pituitary-gonadal relations in male children and adolescents. *Pediatr. Res.* 6:126, 1972.

puberty have emerged, is followed by increased vascularity, wrinkling, and enlargement of the scrotal sac and the beginning of pubic hair growth.

The size of the testes may be quantified with a centimeter ruler by direct measurement of the length and width. During the prepubescent period, the testes usually measure less than 2 cm in the long axis.[233] Length exceeding 2.5 cm is excellent evidence for the onset of gonadotropin stimulation. Zachmann and Prader have introduced a set of elliptical models of known volume.[234] By palpating the testis and comparing with these models, it has been found that testicular volumes of 1 to 3 ml are typical for prepubertal boys and that a volume of 4 ml or greater signifies stimulation by gonadotropic hormones. The size of the stretched penis also may be measured with a centimeter ruler.[235]

Growth of pubic hair generally proceeds more slowly than male genital development. Axillary and facial hair do not appear until genital development is well advanced, several years after the appearance of pubic hair. Deepening of the voice is also a relatively late event. Most pubertal males exhibit some enlargement of their areolae and underlying breast tissues and many complain of breast tingling and tenderness during this period. In most instances, this modest adolescent gynecomastia regresses after a period of a few years.[236]

The timing of pubertal events relative to the growth spurt in boys is substantially different from that in girls. Whereas girls usually show acceleration of linear growth at the onset of puberty and reach peak height velocities relatively early in the pubertal process, boys more typically reach their peak height velocities when genital and pubic hair ratings are at stage IV or V.

Prediction of Adult Stature

The impact of retarded or accelerated growth patterns on expectations for eventual adult stature is frequently of more than academic interest, since therapeutic decisions often must be weighed against their ultimate impact on adult height. There is a strong positive correlation between skeletal age and percentage of mature height achieved at any age, and this correlation improves progressively as the child becomes older. Thus, in a group of children of identical stature, those with the least advanced skeletal age in all probability will become taller adults than those whose skeletal development is more mature.

The most widely used tables for height prediction are those published by Bayley and Pinneau,[33] which are reproduced in the Greulich and Pyle *Atlas of Skeletal Development.*[29] Two newer and probably more accurate methods are now available: (1) the method of Tanner and associates[34] utilizes the chronologic age as well as skeletal age and height; and (2) the method of Roche and associates[35] utilizes height, bone age, midparental height, chronologic age, and weight. No matter which method is used, inaccuracies in the height prediction often occur in children with pathologic growth patterns.

Abnormalities of Fetal Growth

There is no good evidence that any hormone of maternal origin occupies a central role in fetal somatic growth.[6, 237-241] Likewise, no hormones of fetal origin have been proven indispensible. Human anencephaly or intrauterine hypophysectomy in experimental animals fails to curtail fetal growth, and even athyrotic fetuses are of normal length at birth. Agonadal infants and infants with virilizing conditions also do not have abnormal birth weights. For reasons stated earlier, the role of insulin in fetal growth is unclear. The possible importance of the placenta as a regulator of fetal growth has emerged only recently. Regarded for many years as an organ through which nutrients reached the fetus and which facilitated disposal of waste products, the placenta is now known to be a major production site for estrogens, peptide hormones, and growth factors. Although the exact role of placental hormones is poorly understood, it is possible that they play a more important role in fetal growth than hormones secreted by fetal endocrine glands.

Since fetal growth results largely from cell proliferation rather than hypertrophy, peptide growth factors may be more important as mitogenic and differentiating factors than classic hormones. Several findings suggest that the somatomedins may play such a role. There are an abundance of cell membrane receptors for somatomedin in fetal tissues, and multiple fetal tissues produce somatomedin *in vitro.*[242] Ovine placental lactogen has been shown to stimulate somatomedin production in hypophysectomized rats,[243] and it has been postulated that one of the functions of placental lactogen in growth is to stimulate somatomedin in the fetus, as well as to increase the levels of somatomedin found in maternal serum. Daughaday and Kapadia showed that following hypophysectomy of the pregnant rat, the maternal serum somatomedin does not fall as it does in the nonpregnant rat.[244] In the human, it has been observed that cord serum somatomedin correlates with birth weight, birth length, and placental weight.[245, 246] The possible importance of epidermal growth factor and nerve growth factor in selected aspects of fetal and neonatal growth has been obvious from the time of their discovery. In addition to its effect on eyelid opening and tooth eruption in neonatal mice, EGF/urogastrone has been shown to be present in human pregnancy urine[153] and to accelerate maturation of fetal sheep lung.[247] Furthermore, EGF receptors are present in placenta and EGF has been shown to stimulate production of hCG.[148]

Low-birth-weight newborns (< 2500 g) may result from pregnancies terminating before the normal period of gestation is completed (premature infants) or from pregnancies in which the rate of intrauterine growth is abnormally slow (small-for-gestational-age or SGA infants). The distinction between the premature and the SGA infant is often crucial since survival rates, perinatal complications, and postnatal growth patterns for the two groups often differ considerably.[248] Since dating the length of gestation by maternal history is often unreliable, a number of methods based on physical, neurologic, and laboratory findings are available to distinguish preterm from SGA infants.[8, 248, 249] Charts for intrauterine growth similar to those for postnatal growth have been developed and greatly facilitate the identification of SGA infants.[250, 251]

The causes of fetal growth retardation include those disorders in which there are intrinsic abnormalities of the fetus, abnormalities of the placenta, and disorders of the mother (Table 28-5). Chromosomal, genetic, and infectious disorders intrinsic to the fetus account for perhaps 10% of all cases. Depending on the precise cause, the growth arrest in infants of this category may be associated with decreased cell number and normal cell size or a decrease in both number and size of cells.[252] In addition to retardation of overall somatic growth, these infants often exhibit dysharmony in the growth of body parts. These variations in rates of growth of specific structures often lead to the development of congenital malformation, asymmetry, and unusual somatic features.

The relationship between maternal nutritional status and fetal growth is a topic of continuing controversy.[253, 254] Most studies show that there is indeed a correlation between maternal weight gain during pregnancy and birth weight. Mild maternal malnutrition or malnutrition occurring late in pregnancy affects only birth weight; more protracted severe nutrient deprivation, however, causes a proportional reduction in the baby's length and head circumference.[255]

In general, the greater the mother's weight gain during pregnancy, the better the infant's growth during the first year of life. Although probably less important, the prepregnancy nutritional status of the mother also is a determinant of fetal growth.

Table 28-5. CLASSIFICATION OF THE CAUSES OF FETAL GROWTH RETARDATION

I. Intrinsic Abnormalities of the Fetus
    Chromosomal and genetic abnormalities
        Autosomal aneuplody—trisomy 21, 13, and 18; deletions of 4p–,
          5p–, etc.
        Sex chromosome aneuplody—XO, Turner syndrome variants
        Primary growth failure syndromes—Silver-Russell syndrome,
          Seckel's syndrome, leprechaunism, chondrodysplasias, etc.
    Congenital infections
        Rubella, cytomegalovirus, toxoplasmosis
    Congenital anomalies
        Bilateral renal agenesis

II. Abnormalities of the Placenta
    Abnormal implantation of placenta
    Vascular malformations
    Hemangiomas
    Progressive vascular disease—infarction, premature aging

III. Maternal Disorders
    Maternal malnutrition
    Vascular disorders—hypertension, toxemia, severe diabetes mellitus
    Uterine malformations—fibroma, bifid uterus
    Drug ingestion—alcohol, narcotics, tobacco

Consumption by a pregnant mother of as little as two alcoholic drinks per day has been found to cause growth retardation in her fetus,[256-258] and infants of alcoholic mothers exhibit more profound growth retardation and morphogenic abnormalities. Fetal growth retardation correlates also with duration of alcohol consumption prior to pregnancy.[259]

Maternal cigarette smoking also causes fetal growth retardation and has an additive effect with ethanol. Growth retardation is proportional to the number of cigarettes smoked,[260] with a decline of 170 to 250 g and as much as 1.5 cm when more than 10 cigarettes per day are smoked.[261]

Between 20 and 45% of infants born to narcotics-addicted mothers are small for gestational age.[262-264] These infants not only are smaller in weight and length, but also have small placentas and reduced brain weight.[265] Raye and associates[266] showed that the fetuses of rabbits given morphine exhibited a dose-related retardation of intrauterine growth. The most dramatic effects were imposed on weight gain, the least on brain growth. These investigators established that growth inhibition is a direct effect of the drug rather than the result of poor caloric intake by the mothers. They showed that fetuses of morphine-treated doe which were pair-fed with control doe showed growth arrest, and fetuses of doe that had caloric restriction equal to that of morphine-treated doe were not growth-retarded.

Abnormalities of Postnatal Growth: Recognition and Diagnostic Assessment

The decision whether or not to embark on diagnostic studies in a short child is made difficult by the lack of any bimodal distribution of height between those normal individuals at the extreme end of the normal distribution curve and those with pathologic causes of growth failure. Approximately 2 million children in this country have statures falling more than 2 standard deviations below the mean for their age, but many of these children have no disease and do not need to be evaluated. On the other hand, a previously normal child who suddenly stops growing may not fall more than 2 standard deviations below the mean for a number of years, but should be investigated long before a subnormal percentile standing calls attention to the problem. Thus, a child's current centile standing must be evaluated in terms of his or her genetic background, gestational and past medical history, physical findings, and, most important, growth trajectory since birth and current growth rate.

In the absence of any universally accepted definition of what constitutes a pathologically short individual, our clinic has adopted a set of pragmatic guidelines which have proved useful in assessing children referred for the evaluation of retarded growth (Table 28-6). In any patient whose stature is more than 3 standard deviations below the mean height for age, an immediate and thorough search is instigated for an etiologic mechanism. In children whose heights are between 2 and 3 standard deviations below the mean, a limited number of screening tests for common causes of growth failure are obtained on the initial clinic visit, and if they are unrevealing, no further studies are undertaken until the current rate of growth is documented over a period usually not less than 6 months. If the growth rate subsequently is found to be subnormal, more extensive testing is undertaken. Children who exhibit a subnormal growth rate for age (less than 3rd percentile on Tanner's incremental charts) are evaluated without regard to whether their absolute height is subnormal. Obviously, these decisions frequently are tempered by historical information and physical findings.

Table 28–6.   GUIDELINES FOR ASSESSMENT OF SHORT STATURE AND RETARDED GROWTH

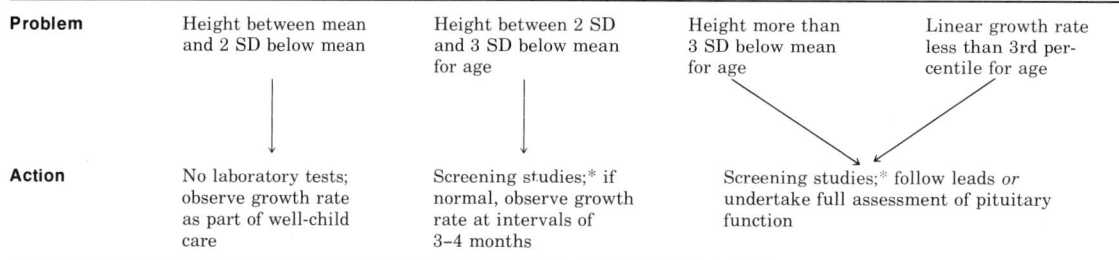

Problem	Height between mean and 2 SD below mean	Height between 2 SD and 3 SD below mean for age	Height more than 3 SD below mean for age	Linear growth rate less than 3rd percentile for age
Action	No laboratory tests; observe growth rate as part of well-child care	Screening studies;* if normal, observe growth rate at intervals of 3–4 months	Screening studies;* follow leads *or* undertake full assessment of pituitary function	

*Screening studies—initial evaluation
 1. Detailed history and physical examination
 2. Analysis of growth trajectory from all available data
 3. Urinalysis—assess ability to acidify and concentrate urine
 4. Blood for urea nitrogen, creatinine, CO_2, electrolytes, calcium, phosphorus, alkaline phosphatase, thyroid hormone, and somatomedin
 5. X-rays of hand and wrist for skeletal maturity; skull films for sella turcica size and abnormalities of sellar area
 6. If patient is female, karyotype for abnormalities of X chromosome

The history should include a complete genetic pedigree to document the stature attained by family members as well as any familial tendency toward delayed or early puberty. The history should take careful note of nutritional adequacy, abnormal fecal patterns, urinary frequency, symptoms of respiratory disease, recurrent or chronic infection and headaches, or other symptoms pointing to an intracranial lesion. The psychosocial environment should not be neglected.

The prenatal and early postnatal status of the patient is particularly crucial. A history of intrauterine growth retardation often suggests some inherent deficiency in the capacity of cells to grow and divide. A history of slow growth in the first few postnatal months may provide clues to malabsorption, congenital heart disease, and various other abnormalities of organ function. If growth failure occurred during a finite period in the distant past and normal growth has intervened since, the history should focus on the interval during which growth failure occurred, and the current evaluation might be restricted to periodic observations of the patient's growth rate.

The physical examination is particularly useful in differentiating non-endocrine-organ-system malfunction from abnormalities of hormone secretion. In states of inadequate food intake, malabsorption, or other organic disease, the failure to gain weight often is more severe than the failure of linear growth. The nutritional status is best evaluated by plotting the child's weight at his height age rather than his chronologic age. Alternatively, skin-fold thickness may be determined. Furthermore, the physical examination may provide clues to skeletal disorders, dysmorphic syndromes, diseases of specific organ systems, and certain endocrine diseases, in particular, hypothyroidism and Cushing's syndrome.

When the history, physical examination, and growth data fail to provide a diagnostic clue, it is essential to screen the patient for some of the more silent causes of growth failure. This screening includes assessment of renal function to rule out unrecognized renal failure and tubular disorders associated with acidosis or hypokalemia, measurement of calcium, phosphorus, and alkaline phosphatase to rule out subtle forms of rickets, thyroid function tests to exclude subclinical hypothyroidism, and measurement of the serum somatomedin concentration to detect GH deficiency. Careful attention should be given to the possibility of a mild, asymptomatic malabsorption syndrome. All female patients with growth retardation of unexplained cause should have a karyotype even though no obvious stigmata of Turner's syndrome are present (see Table 28–6).

Radiologic assessment of skeletal maturation has little value in differential diagnosis since the majority of disorders that retard growth also retard bone age. Determination of the skeletal age is useful, however, in assessing the growth potential of the short child. A normal bone age in a short child may suggest the presence of a previously unrecognized genetic abnormality such as a chondrodysplasia. Sellar x-rays are frequently helpful in disclosing an unsuspected intrasellar tumor or, when the sella is abnormally small, in suggesting hypopituitarism.

Hereditary Short Stature

The wide spectrum of postnatal growth patterns which fall within the range of normality reflects the genetic heterogeneity of the human race, both between and within different ethnic groups. The inheritance of growth potential is polygenic, with genes for stature located on both the sex chromosomes and autosomes. Although stature does not follow strict mendelian laws of inheritance, Tanner and associates have provided charts which take into consideration mean parental height.[267] With these charts, a child whose growth falls more than 2 standard deviations below the population mean will in some instances be found to fall in a more normal range.

The physician should exercise caution in making the diagnosis of familial short stature since applying this designation to the short child tends to preclude further efforts to uncover the cause of the patient's dwarfism. The diagnosis of "familial short stature" frequently has been perpetuated in families in which impaired growth was eventually proved to be the consequence of a defined genetic disorder. Conversely, whereas the short stature of Japanese individuals was formerly thought to have a genetic basis, the improved growth of postwar Japanese children has eloquently demonstrated that "genetic short stature" often may be explained on a nutritional basis. Considering the frequent misuse and abuse of the terms "familial short stature" and "genetic short stature," we believe it would be wise to use these designations only when all the evidence has been weighed and all other causes of growth retardation have been excluded.

The term "constitutional short stature" often is used to describe short children whose height merely reflects their hereditary make-up. Such a term has no precise meaning and should not be used. For the patient who is short but otherwise healthy, has a delayed bone age, is growing at a normal rate, and is destined to have a significant delay in puberty, we prefer the descriptive phrase "constitutional growth delay." These patients are discussed in the section on hypopituitary dwarfism.

Differential Diagnosis of Short Stature and Growth Failure

The causes of short stature and growth failure may be grouped under three broad headings: (1) intrinsic defects of growing tissues, (2) abnormalities in the environment of growing tissues, and (3) hormonal abnormalities.

Intrinsic Defects of Growing Tissues

Generalized intrinsic defects, which include chromosomal abnormalities and some forms of intrauterine growth retardation, may result in slow or abnormal growth of most or all body tissues. On the other hand, the growth defect may be more tissue-limited, as in some chondrodysplasias, where it may be expressed only in the growth of cartilage and bone.

Skeletal Dysplasias. The skeletal dysplasias are a heterogeneous group of disorders, well over 50 in number, which are characterized by short stature and abnormalities in shape and size of the limbs, trunk, and skull. Until 10 to 15 years ago, most affected patients were classified according to gross physical findings, as having either achondroplasia (short limbs) or Morquio's disease (short trunk). The heterogeneous clinical spectrum of these disorders led in turn to a profusion of proposed subclassifications based on Latin and Greek roots and eponyms derived from the observer who first reported specific syndromes.

In 1970, an international classification was proposed for grouping the skeletal dysplasias into two groups.[268, 269] The confusion over classification and the clinical features of these disorders can be expected to persist, however, until the pathophysiologic mechanisms of each subgroup are clearly defined. The reader is referred to references 270 to 274 for information on this group of diseases.

Children with skeletal dysplasias are characterized by abnormal skeletal proportions. Although mild skeletal disorders, such as hypochondroplasia, may not always be apparent on casual examination, their presence may be suggested by measurements of sitting height and span and calculations of the upper/lower segment ratio. If body proportions are abnormal, a detailed family history should be taken and, if possible, other family members should be examined. A radiologic survey of the skeleton also should be carried out. Particular note should be taken of which bones are affected (i.e., vertebral column, long bones, or both) and where within each bone the lesions are localized (i.e., epiphyses, metaphyses, or diaphyses). This information can provide important insight into what adult height can be anticipated, complications that are likely to occur later in life, and the genetic risks in siblings and offspring. In some instances, the diagnosis can be confirmed by microscopic study of the histopathology of the enchondral growth plate. Material for examination may be obtained from the iliac crest or from other growth plates at the time of corrective surgery.

Chromosomal Abnormalities

Abnormalities of Autosomes. Autosomal abnormalities associated with short stature are, with few exceptions, accompanied by significant mental retardation and a variety of readily recognizable physical stigmata. In Down's syndrome, the most common of these autosomal disorders, growth failure is recognizable early in life and is accompanied by substantial delays in bony maturation and epiphyseal fusion.[275-277] The marked reduction in adult stature is attributable primarily to shortness in the lower extremities. Growth in infants and children with Down's syndrome may be delayed further by cretinism or acquired hypothyroidism, both of which occur with increased frequency.

Abnormalities of the X Chromosome. The most significant chromosomal abnormalities causing short stature are those involving absence of or deletion from one of the sex chromosomes. In one clinic, 20% of 255 short girls were proved to have such abnormalities.[278] The phenotypic and genotypic variants of Turner's syndrome have been detailed in Chapter 9.[279] In the context of growth diagnosis, the physician not only should be familiar with the phenotypic features of the classic syndrome but, more important, should be aware that girls with Turner variants may have short stature and slow growth with few or no physical stigmata of the disease (Fig. 28-18). In our experience, the most common variants of Turner's syndrome presenting with few somatic abnormalities other than short stature are isochromosome abnormalities involving the long arm of the X chromosome, deletions of a portion of the X chromosomes, or mosaic patterns of the 45X/46XX or 45X/47XXX variety.

Nuclear chromatin patterns in buccal mucosa are frequently misleading and should be abandoned in favor of a complete karyotype analysis with one or more of the banding techniques. Karyotype analysis of patients suspected of having Turner's syndrome will be necessary no matter what the result of the buccal smear examination. Girls with classic stigmata of Turner's syndrome and a negative buccal smear require karyotype analysis to rule out the presence of a mosaic pattern involving all or part of a Y chromosome (see Chapter 9). Furthermore, buccal smears of girls with isochromosome or mosaic X-chromosomal abnormalities are likely to be chromatin-positive, causing the unwary physician to discard Turner's syndrome as a diagnostic possibility.

A small number of short girls who were later shown to have abnormalities of the X chromosome exhibit normal 46XX karyotypes in their peripheral lymphocytes. In such patients, analysis of skin fibroblasts taken by punch biopsy may reveal a chromosomal abnormality. In several instances we have encountered short girls with normal lymphocyte and skin fibroblast karyotypes who had delayed sexual maturation accompanied by markedly elevated serum LH and FSH concentrations. In these girls, the abnormal cell lines may have been localized to the ovaries and tissues involved in skeletal growth.[280]

Girls with Turner's syndrome fail to undergo the adolescent growth spurt and frequently exhibit progressive slowing of their growth long before their epiphyses approach fusion (Fig. 28-19). The administration of hGH to these girls is without significant effect on their growth rates. Administration of low doses of androgens, usually in the form of a synthetic preparation (e.g., 0.1 mg oxandrolone per kilogram per day) is associated with a twofold to threefold increase in growth rate for a 1- to 2-year period.[281, 282, 285] We do not begin such treatment until after the patient is 10 years of age. Administration of this growth stimulant often provides an important psychologic boost at a critical period and might produce a small increase in adult stature.[283, 284] It has been reported that low dosages of estrogens have a similar stimulatory effect on growth.[87] Although the larger dosages of estrogen required to bring about secondary sexual characteristics should be postponed as long as possible to avoid epiphyseal fusion, psychologic considerations usually make some compromise mandatory. Since autoimmune thyroiditis occurs with increased frequency in girls with Turner's syndrome,[286] the physician should be on the alert for sudden, unexpected deceleration of growth, which may herald the onset of hypothyroidism.

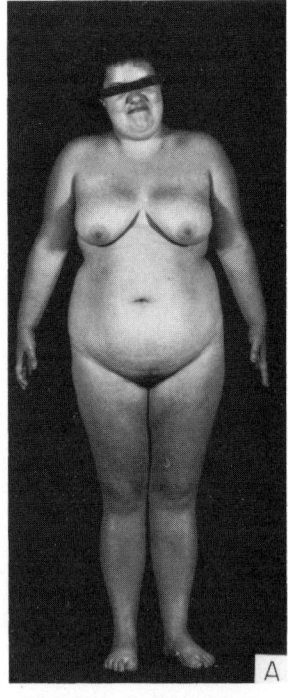
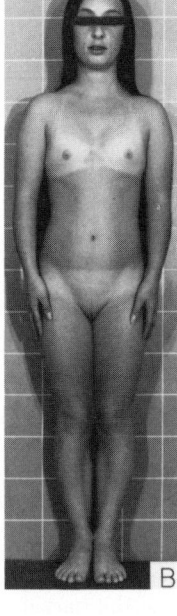
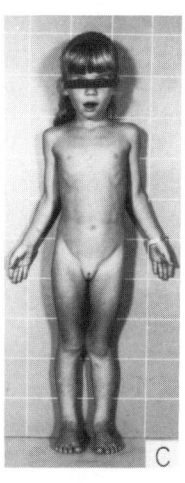

Figure 28–18. Three girls with variants of Turner's syndrome. Patient *A* had no physical signs of Turner's syndrome other than minimal shortening of the fourth metacarpal. She has had regular menses since the age of 10 years. The cell line with 46 XX constitution predominated in peripheral lymphocytes. Patient *B* had no physical stigmata of Turner's syndrome other than short stature and sexual immaturity. She had markedly elevated gonadotropin levels and required cyclic estrogen-progesterone treatment. Patient *C* had cubitus valgus and short stature, but no other stigmata of Turner's syndrome. By the age of 15½ years, she showed incomplete feminization, had a serum FSH level within the normal range, and had no menses.

	45X / 46XX	45X / 46XX qi	45X / 47XXX
Chronological Age (yr.)	15.4	13.2	6.3
Height Age (yr.)	11.4	8.6	3.3

Dysmorphic Dwarfism (Primordial Dwarfism). This group encompasses a variety of distinct disorders of unknown etiology which are characterized by intrauterine growth retardation, postnatal growth failure, and a spectrum of associated abnormalities. These disorders undoubtedly occur as a consequence of single or multiple gene defects or environmental insults during embryogenesis. Typically, blood hormone concentrations are normal and skeletal maturation is normal or only moderately delayed. The older term, primordial dwarfism, is gradually being abandoned as the disorders of these patients are compartmentalized into specific syndrome categories. Some of the more common, better known syndromes in this group are listed in Table 28–7. A more comprehensive description of the features of these syndromes may be found in references 287 to 291.

The categorization of these patients' disorders into specific syndromes serves a useful purpose in alerting the physician to associated abnormalities, and in providing insight into the probable prognosis for physical and intellectual development and life expectancy. Such classification, however, should not lead to cessation of further efforts to understand the etiology and pathophysiology of their problems.

Abnormalities in the Environment of Growing Tissues

Included in this category of disorders are all those systemic diseases which impair growth by adversely affecting the general health and well-being of the growing child. Such growth failure may occur by a variety of mechanisms, including insufficient intake of calories and/or protein, insufficient oxygenation of tissues, electrolyte imbalance, and so forth. In many of these diseases, however, the exact mechanisms of growth retardation are unknown. Although exceptions can be cited, patients with diseases of this type characteristically are poorly nourished and present with weights which are below average for their height. This contrasts with growth failure of endocrine origin in which body weight is often above average for attained height.

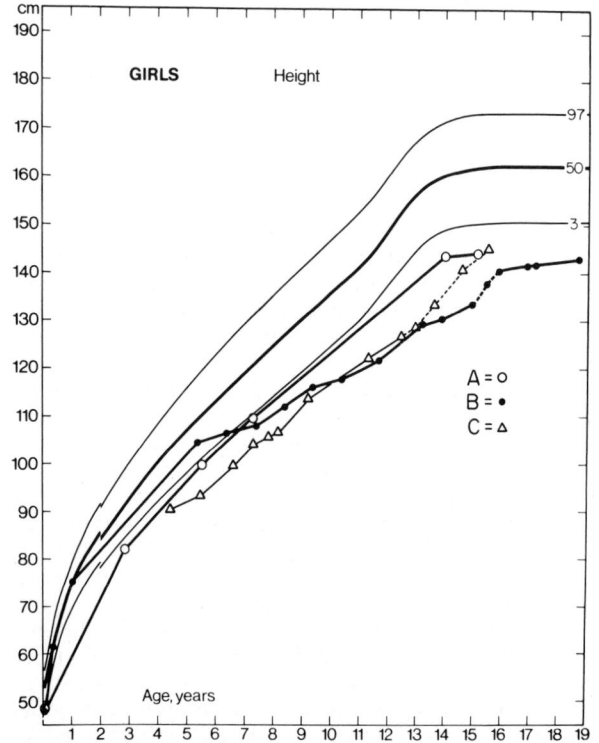

Figure 28–19. Growth curves of the three patients shown in Figure 28–18. The broken lines indicate growth during periods of treatment with oxandrolone.

Table 28-7. DWARFISM ASSOCIATED WITH DYSMORPHIC SYNDROMES OF UNKNOWN CAUSE*

	Principal Features
Prader-Willi syndrome	Intrauterine and postnatal hypotonia; obesity; mental deficiency; hypogonadism; and small hands and feet. Growth retardation may be mild.
Russell-Silver syndrome	Asymmetry; small triangular face; short, incurved fifth finger; renal anomalies; prenatal onset of growth failure.
Noonan syndrome (Turner-like)	Webbing of neck; low posterior hair line; shield chest; pectus excavatum; right-sided congenital heart disease; mental retardation; small penis and cryptorchidism; normal karyotype.
de Lange syndrome	Mental retardation; short nose and anteverted nostrils; abnormal lips and mouth; bushy eyebrows and long curly eyelashes; hypertonicity; abnormal cry.
Bloom syndrome	Facial telangiectatic erythema; malar hypoplasia; microcephaly; prenatal onset of growth failure; predisposition to malignancy.
Seckel syndrome (bird-headed dwarfism)	Microcephaly with premature synostosis; mental retardation; facial hypoplasia with prominent nose; low-set, malformed ears; cryptorchidism; severe growth failure of prenatal onset.
Progeria (Hutchinson-Gilford syndrome)	Premature aging with atherosclerosis; elevated cholesterol; alopecia; thinning of skin; nail hypoplasia; loss of subcutaneous fat; periarticular fibrosis; severe growth failure.
Cockayne syndrome	Mental retardation; deafness; peripheral neuropathy; retinal pigmentation; optic atrophy; microcephaly; photosensitive dermatitis and premature aging.
Leprechaunism	Intrauterine growth failure; prominent eyes; thick lips; large ears; large phallus; breast hyperplasia; hirsutism; islet cell hyperplasia with hyperinsulinism and insulin resistance; severe postnatal growth failure.
Ellis-van Creveld syndrome	Intrauterine growth failure; short extremities; polydactyly; hypoplastic nails; small thorax; short upper lip; congenital cardiac defects.

*The reader is referred to references 272, 273, and 287 to 290 for more complete coverage of these syndromes.

Nutritional Insufficiency. On a global scale, malnutrition is by far the most common cause of growth failure. It is estimated that two-thirds of the world's children are undernourished. Severe growth retardation is associated with the classic clinical pictures of marasmus and kwashiorkor. In the former, in which the intake of both calories and protein are insufficient, there is disappearance of subcutaneous fat, muscle wasting, and shrinkage of internal organs. The chronic diarrhea often seen in this condition results from malnutrition-induced flattening of intestinal mucosa with concomitant deficiencies of intestinal enzymes. These changes, in turn, aggravate the nutritional insufficiency. In kwashiorkor, caloric deprivation usually has been less severe, but the quantity and quality of dietary protein has been inadequate. In its pure form, kwashiorkor may be manifest by persistence of some subcutaneous fat but striking signs of protein deficiency.

In most affected children, the clinical pictures of both marasmus and kwashiorkor are merged. Affected patients typically have elevated serum levels of GH[292] but paradoxically depressed serum somatomedin concentrations.[293] It is

of interest to speculate on the survival value of these relationships: the high GH levels might be expected to increase its direct protein-sparing actions on carbohydrate and fat metabolism while the low somatomedin levels would prevent squandering of protein in growth. With oral feeding and restoration of serum and organ protein, the serum GH falls to normal, and this is followed, after some delay, by an increase in somatomedin and resumption of linear growth.

While full-blown marasmus and kwashiorkor are relatively easy to diagnose, it is much more difficult in the usual clinical setting to recognize children who have growth retardation secondary to modest nutritional deficiency. Not only are accurate dietary histories difficult to document, it is often not clear whether low caloric intake is a cause or a consequence of growth failure. This is so because in normal children a significant portion of the caloric intake is expended in growth; decreased caloric intake, therefore, may be anticipated when growth is arrested. Because of these practical problems, there is often no substitute for hospitalization to observe food intake and short-term weight gain when an adequate diet is available.

Recent studies suggest that growth retardation may be associated not only with inadequate protein and calories, but also with deficiencies of specific dietary components such as zinc and iron. While anemia is the primary manifestation of iron deficiency, reduced appetite and growth failure also may be observed.[294, 295] Zinc deficiency, which results in anorexia and failure to undergo pubertal development, is observed in children with malabsorption syndromes, chronic infection, sickle cell anemia, and liver disease.[296] It remains to be determined how often growth failure results from primary zinc deficiency in the absence of other disease.[297]

Malabsorption Syndromes and Chronic Inflammatory Bowel Disease. In the majority of children with malabsorption syndromes, growth failure is neither the initial presenting complaint nor the primary concern; nevertheless, severe growth failure occasionally may result from clinically mild abnormalities of bowel function. This seems to be particularly true for certain patients with celiac disease (gluten-induced enteropathy) and patients with chronic inflammatory bowel disease. In celiac disease, the onset of symptoms generally occurs in infancy when the patient begins to ingest wheat products containing gluten. In addition to recurrent diarrhea, abdominal distension, and muscular inactivity, these children often exhibit striking apathy and anorexia. Indeed, the anorexia may sometimes contribute more to the growth failure than does fecal wastage due to malabsorption. It is therefore essential when dealing with children with growth failure of unknown cause and evidence of diminished body fat stores not only that a careful history be taken with regard to the quantity and quality of stools, but that quantitative estimates be made of stool fat excretion. In some instances, the diagnosis can be excluded only by a peroral biopsy of the upper intestinal mucosa. Indeed, in patients for whom there is no explanation for growth failure, jejunal biopsy should be considered even though there is no clinical evidence for celiac disease. Regardless of the mechanism of protein-calorie deprivation, children with celiac disease have normal GH responses to provocative stimuli, but low somatomedin activity in serum.[298] The fact that somatomedin does not rise with hGH administration but increases under gluten-free diet suggests that the GH resistance is on the basis of nutritional deficiency.

In Crohn's disease (regional ileitis) or ulcerative colitis, growth failure may have been present for several years before abdominal and bowel complaints bring the child to medical attention. The growth retardation experienced by these children does not appear to be secondary to thyroid or pituitary abnormalities.[299] Careful studies of the diets of children with chronic inflammatory bowel disease show that they consistently have low caloric intake[300] and are in negative nitrogen and caloric balance. It also has been demonstrated that these children can achieve increased growth velocity following improvements in the oral or parenteral supply of nutrients.[300] In the absence of clinical signs of malabsorption, therefore, it is probable that the malabsorptive component of the disease is mild and growth failure is the result of poor caloric intake and modest protein-losing enteropathy.

Chronic Renal Disease. A variety of renal diseases, including chronic renal insufficiency, renal tubular acidosis, and Bartter's syndrome, are associated with profound growth failure.[301] Since in many such patients, clinical signs and symptoms may be minimal or nonexistent, all short patients in whom growth failure is unexplained should have sufficient laboratory tests to rule out these disorders (see earlier section on diagnostic assessment). In general, growth failure from renal disease is most profound in infancy or in the early years of life and is expressed when the glomerular filtration rate falls below 25 ml/min/1.73 m².[304] It seems likely that multiple mechanisms may account for the growth failure of chronic renal disease. It appears that one of the most important is the reduced intake of protein and calories.[302-304]

Many children also have growth failure associated with renal osteodystrophy.[305, 306] This syndrome is characterized by hypocalcemia, hyperphosphatemia, hyperphosphatasia, acidosis, and compensatory elevation of parathyroid hormone levels. Formation of 1,25-dihydroxycholecalciferol (1,25-vitamin D_3) is attenuated because of loss of functional renal parenchyma. As a result of these alterations, formation and remodeling of bone are impaired. In limited studies, the effect of the therapeutic administration of 1,25-vitamin D_3 to these children has been gratifying acceleration of their linear growth.[307]

The availability of somatomedin does not appear to be a rate-limiting factor since serum somatomedin levels are elevated in chronic renal failure.[308, 309] This may possibly be explained by the finding of D'Ercole and associates[310] that, at least in the rat, the kidney is the most active site of somatomedin degradation.

Cardiac Diseases. The growth failure observed in infants and children with severe congenital heart disease undoubtedly reflects tissue hypoxia and the increased energy demands placed on the deformed heart. It frequently correlates with the presence of cyanosis and the severity and chronicity of congestive heart failure, size of the left-to-right shunt, and presence of pulmonary obstructive disease.[311-313] Many patients, however, have low birth weight and extracardiac anomalies and fail to undergo catch-up growth after successful correction of their cardiac defect.[314] The limited growth in these patients may be secondary to intrauterine, noncardiac factors.

Central Nervous System Disease. Many children with mental retardation or other central nervous system disorders are short with no apparent cause.[315] Virtually no effort has been invested in exploring the mechanisms involved in growth failure of these patients. It seems possible that, in many instances, caloric intake is insufficient because of inability to detect hunger, abnormal responses to hunger, and problems related to eating itself. In other instances, growth failure might be secondary to depressed GH secretion, although this does not appear to be a common mechanism.[316]

Diabetes Mellitus. In the preinsulin era, growth failure was one of the prominent features of diabetic children who survived for any length of time. Severe growth failure likewise was observed in the syndrome described by Mauriac, in which poorly controlled diabetic children under treatment with regular, crystalline insulin showed hepatomegaly secondary to increased glycogen deposition and signs of cortisol excess including moon facies and truncal obesity.[317] The blood sugar of such children oscillates recklessly between hypoglycemia and hyperglycemia, and attacks of ketoacidosis occur repeatedly. Growth failure could be a manifestation of recurrent acidosis, chronic cortisol excess,[318] or other factors. Even today, with the use of long-acting insulin preparations, severe growth failure occasionally occurs in children who have had extremely poor diabetic control. Aside from these extreme cases, which occur infrequently, there is evidence that children with diabetes commonly have modest growth failure, even when diabetic control is considered good by other criteria. In one study,[319] a group of over 100 diabetic children were found to be of normal heights at the onset of their disease but to show downward shift in height centile channels within 3 years. The primary effect on growth was a delayed and reduced pubertal growth spurt, and the quality of their diabetic control did not appear to be a determinant of growth rate. Tattersall and Pyke[320] showed a similar decline in growth rate in members of monozygotic twin pairs who developed diabetes before puberty. The group of pubertal diabetics had a mean adult height that was 5.7 cm less than that of unaffected twins in spite of the same general standard of nutrition and what was believed to be adequate diabetic control. The precise cause of such growth failure is not apparent, since GH secretion is not suppressed and caloric intake appears to be sufficient.

The possibility that growth failure in diabetics might result from hypothyroidism secondary to Hashimoto's thyroiditis or to celiac disease should be kept in mind since each of these conditions occurs in diabetics with greater than normal frequency.[321]

Familial Vitamin D-Resistant Rickets. This disorder, which is transmitted as an X-linked trait, is characterized by short stature associated with hypophosphatemia, diminished renal tubular reabsorption of inorganic phosphate, decreased intestinal absorption of calcium, and often rickets or osteomalacia which is unresponsive to physiologic dosages of vitamin D.[322] The growth of the upper segment in this disorder is normal, but the lower segment is shortened, on the average, by 15%.[323] Short stature is due not only to bowing of the legs, since it may occur in patients who exhibit no clinical signs of disease and who have only hypophosphatemia. In patients with more severe disease, the serum alkaline phosphatase also is elevated. In order to achieve as near-normal skeletal growth as possible, it is essential to institute vitamin D and phosphate treatment early and to monitor closely for adequacy of therapy.

Other Metabolic Disorders. A variety of metabolic disorders may be associated with growth delay and short stature and in most instances the exact mechanisms for the effect on growth are unknown. A detailed discussion of each of these disorders is beyond the scope of this chapter. The reader is referred to the comprehensive text of Stanbury and associates.[324]

Hormonal Abnormalities

Growth Hormone Deficiency; Hypopituitarism. In a survey of pituitary disease in Japan,[325] pituitary dwarfism accounted for only 1 of every 80,000 hospital admissions. The incidence of this disorder probably is far greater than this, since in a comprehensive survey of 48,000 Scottish school children, Vimpani and associates[326] found the occurrence rate of severe GH deficiency to be 1 in 4000. More modest growth failure due to less severe GH deficiency probably occurs with even greater frequency.

Patients with pituitary dwarfism can be grouped into three broad categories: those with primary pituitary disease, those with hypothalamic dysfunction, and those who have normal hypothalamic-pituitary function but who are unable to respond to GH (Table 28–8).

Primary Pituitary Failure. A variety of genetic syndromes cause primary GH deficiency. These include pituitary hypoplasia, pituitary aplasia, familial panhypopituitarism, and familial isolated GH deficiency. Primary hypopituitarism also is associated with a variety of developmental defects. In anencephaly, the pituitary is small, deformed, and/or ectopic in location; in holoprosencephaly, absence or malformations of the pituitary gland are associated with impaired midline development of the embryonic forebrain and midline dysplasia of the face.[327] The syndrome of septo-optic dysplasia,[328, 329] is characterized by optic nerve hypoplasia and abnormalities of the septum pellucidum and corpus callosum. Hypopituitarism also occurs with increased frequency in patients with cleft lip and palate.[330] Less common midline central nervous system and cranial defects associated with hypopituitarism have been reviewed by Rimoin and Schimke.[327]

Pituitary destruction also may result from trauma, expanding intrasellar tumors, histiocytosis, granulomata, and therapeutic irradiation of central nervous system and middle ear tumors. Craniopharyngioma, the most common tumor to produce hypopituitarism in children, usually involves primarily the hypothalamus, but may also destroy the pituitary.[331, 332]

Pituitary Dwarfism Secondary to Hypothalamic Dysfunction. Pituitary hypofunction secondary to hypothalamic damage may be caused by a variety of recognized insults. These include: purulent meningitis, granulomata, hydrocephalus, histiocytosis, and hypothalamic tumors such as craniopharyngioma, hamartoma, and neurofibroma. The largest number of patients in this group, however, are those whose disorders are lumped together under the heading of "idiopathic hypopituitarism."

Many cases of idiopathic hypopituitarism may be the result of perinatal insult. Abnormal deliveries and history of perinatal asphyxia have been observed in as many as 50 to 60% of children later shown to be hypopituitary.[325, 333, 334] In a survey of our own patients for abnormalities during the perinatal period (Table 28–9), 65% were found to have at

Table 28–8. CLASSIFICATION OF PITUITARY DWARFISM

Primary Pituitary Disease
Genetic syndromes—aplasia, hypoplasia, familial panhypopituitarism, familial isolated GH deficiency
Intrasellar tumors—adenomas, craniopharyngioma
Nontumorous destruction—trauma, infection, CNS irradiation

Pituitary Deficiency Secondary to Hypothalamic Dysfunction
Idiopathic (many are result of perinatal insult)
  Multiple deficiencies (panhypopituitarism)
  Primarily GH ("isolated")
  Constitutional growth delay (some cases)
Postinfectious
Histiocytosis
Hypothalamic tumor—craniopharyngioma, hamartoma, neurofibroma
Psychosocial dwarfism

States of End-Organ Resistance to Growth Hormone
(high GH, low somatomedin)
  Laron dwarfism
  Biologically inactive GH
  Protein-calorie malnutrition

Table 28–9. COMPLICATIONS OF GESTATION, LABOR AND DELIVERY, AND THE POSTNATAL PERIOD IN CHILDREN WITH "IDIOPATHIC" HYPOPITUITARISM AND IN SIBLING CONTROLS*

	Hypopituitary Patients (N = 46)	Sibling Controls† (N = 54)
Gestation:		
< 37 weeks in duration	7‡	5
Bleeding	13	3§
Toxemia	4	2
Labor and delivery:		
3 hours or less	8	3
24 hours or more	5	3
Breech presentation	11	4§
Difficult forceps	3	0
Cesarean section for fetal indications	2	0
Intrapartum distress and/or asphyxia	10	0
Postnatal complications:		
Seizures	7‖	0
Postnatal infection	2	0
Hyperpyrexia	1	0

*Data from Craft, W. H., et al.: High incidence of perinatal insult in children with idiopathic hypopituitarism. *J. Pediatr.* 96:397–402, 1980.
†Control data were derived from siblings who immediately preceded or followed hypopituitary patients in birth order.
‡Denominator is 42 patients; all others are 46 patients.
§Hypopituitary vs. control; p < 0.005, by chi square method.
‖3 were associated with hypoglycemia.

least one significant perinatal insult and many had two or more insults.[335] Birth weights for these patients are generally normal and the sex ratio is 4:1 in favor of males. The inference that GH deficiency is secondary to hypothalamic dysfunction is based on the observation that most of these children have normal serum TSH and prolactin responses following the administration of thyrotropin-releasing hormone (TRH).[336, 337] Direct confirmation that the pituitary is intact, however, must await testing with a somatotropin-releasing hormone, if and when such becomes available.

Constitutional Growth Delay (Growth Retardation with Delayed Adolescence). Many children are small for age because they are maturing at a slower than normal rate. The syndrome of growth retardation with delayed adolescence, commonly referred to as constitutional growth delay, occurs predominantly in boys and accounts for a high proportion of referrals for growth evaluation.[338] Height and bone age usually are delayed by 2 to 4 years and the onset of pubertal development is delayed by 2 or more years. Often there is a history of delay in growth and pubertal development of the patient's father and other male relatives. Final adult stature, which may not be reached until the age of 20 or more years, is almost always in the low-normal range and sexual development and fertility are normal.

Although most observers look upon this syndrome as a normal, nonendocrine growth variant, we believe that it encompasses a spectrum of clinical severity ranging from the child with normal pituitary function tests who has only minimal delay in growth and pubertal development to the child whose condition many would diagnose as hypopituitary. The gradation between these extremes, both in clinical severity and in GH responses, gives no hint of any clear bimodal distribution. We have found that some of these boys experience significant acceleration of growth with the administration of GH or androgens, and after several months of treatment continue to grow and develop sexually when therapy is withdrawn. Transient, functional hypopituitarism of this type (we use the term "lazy pituitary") has been observed by others.[339-342] Gourmelen and associates[343] found that as many as 20% of 105 adolescent children with growth and pubertal delays had sluggish GH responses to provocative stimuli, but when tested after the onset of puberty, almost all had normal GH secretion. GH responses measured 48 hours after exposure to exogenous androgens also were normal. These patients also responded with an accelerated growth rate following the initiation of hGH therapy, thus supporting the contention that some children with constitutional growth delay may have mild hypopituitarism and that the disease often disappears as puberty progresses.

Slow-growing boys with delayed puberty often have feelings of physical and social inadequacy, and these psychologic factors may affect decisions regarding therapy. For boys with modest growth failure and evidence of early testicular enlargement (>2.5 cm long; >3 ml volume), reassurance that they will mature normally is usually sufficient. For boys with more pronounced delay, a detailed search for causes of growth failure and a thorough assessment of pituitary function are warranted. If no abnormality is found, administration of androgens (50 to 100 mg testosterone enanthate intramuscularly every month; 20 mg methyltestosterone orally each day; or a synthetic anabolic steroid) may be indicated for psychologic reasons even though this may cause some attenuation of final stature. Treatment should be interrupted at frequent intervals, however, to determine whether the patient is progressing spontaneously into puberty.

Psychosocial Dwarfism. It has been recognized for decades that failure to thrive in young children may occur as a result of an inadequate environment.[344-346] In 1967 Powell and associates[347, 348] carefully described a group of emotionally disturbed children coming from hostile environments whose growth patterns resembled those of patients with idiopathic hypopituitarism. These "psychosocial dwarfs" are withdrawn, have retarded speech development, and exhibit bizarre eating habits with polydipsia, tendencies to ingest contaminated food and drink, gorging, and vomiting. When testing is done immediately after admission to the hospital there is evidence of suppressed secretion of GH and ACTH. After a brief period of hospitalization or placement in a foster home, pituitary function, dietary habits, and mental status revert to normal, and linear growth is dramatically accelerated. While these patients may have a component of malabsorption,[347] it appears that the primary defect resides in higher cortical centers and that GH deficiency is mediated by failure of the hypothalamus to stimulate the pituitary.

A clinical picture in infants, similar to the above syndrome, has been referred to as the "maternal deprivation syndrome."[349-351] In these patients, failure to thrive is accompanied by lack of mothering, poor feeding practices, and insufficient caloric intake. Growth hormone secretion, rather than being suppressed, is often normal or even excessive, supporting the contention that caloric deprivation is the major mechanism of growth failure.

We believe that the syndrome of psychosocial dwarfism and the maternal deprivation syndrome represent the extremes of a spectrum: at one end of this spectrum, suppression of pituitary function is the primary mechanism for growth failure, and nutritional deficiency is a relatively minor factor. At the other end of the spectrum, nutritional deprivation predominates and pituitary function is appropriate. We have also observed some children who exhibited transient growth failure concurrent with emotional upheaval within the family. These children resumed normal growth when the emotional environment improved.

Syndromes of Growth Hormone Resistance. The prototype of GH-resistant syndromes is Laron dwarfism,[352] a familial disorder believed to have an autosomal recessive

mode of transmission. Most affected patients are of Middle Eastern extraction and are the products of consanguineous marriages. These children have the physical appearance of severe GH deficiency. Instead of low GH levels, however, they have elevated basal serum GH concentrations and markedly exaggerated GH responses to provocative stimuli, and they fail to muster metabolic and growth responses to the administration of hGH.[353, 354] The somatomedin concentrations in serum are low and do not increase in response to hGH.[355] Although it has been proposed that such children have GH receptor abnormalities, it is possible that they have a postreceptor defect involving the intracellular mechanisms required for responsiveness to GH.

Another GH-resistant variant has been described, in which affected patients also have the physical characteristics of severe GH deficiency, elevated GH concentrations, and low levels of somatomedin in serum.[356] Unlike Laron dwarfs, however, they are able to raise serum somatomedin concentrations and to exhibit linear growth in response to the administration of exogenous hGH. These patients presumably have an abnormal GH molecule, which is immunologically active but biologically inactive.

Clinical Characteristics of Hypopituitary Dwarfism. Children with hypopituitarism are short and exhibit growth curves that deviate progressively away from normal. Growth rates are commonly as slow as 3 cm/yr and almost always less than 4 to 5 cm/yr. In idiopathic cases, growth failure may not be obvious until 2 to 4 years of age. In retrospect, however, it is often possible to establish that growth failure began in the first few months of life (Fig. 28-20). Indeed, when growth failure does not occur until the patient is several years of age, the possibility of pituitary or hypothalamic tumor or another organic cause should be entertained. Affected children have skeletal proportions which are normal for age, tend to be somewhat overweight

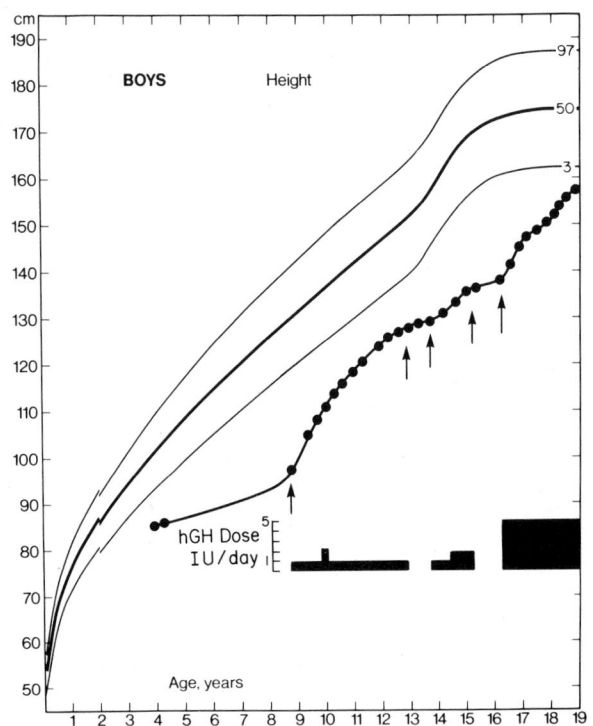

Figure 28-20. Growth curve of a male with idiopathic hypopituitarism (photographs in Figure 28-21) who was treated for several years with hGH. Typical of such patients is the decline in growth response as treatment is continued for long periods of time. At 24 years of age his height is 165 cm (65 inches).

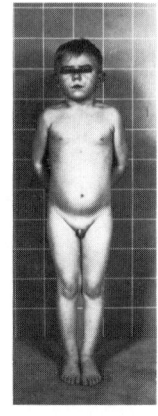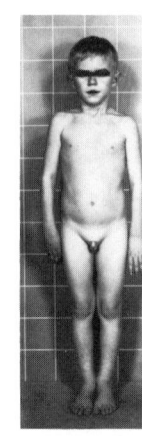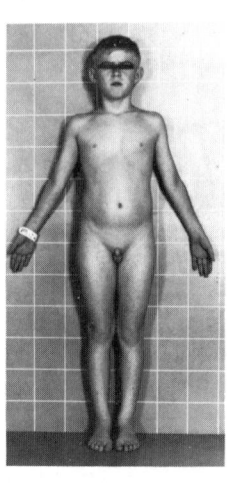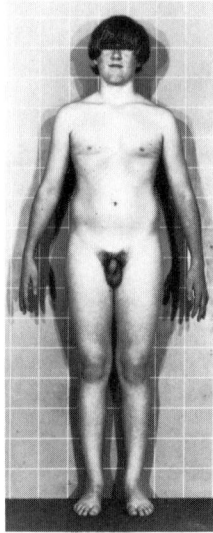

Figure 28–21. Serial photographs of hypopituitary patient whose growth curve is shown in Figure 28–20. Small dosages of oral testosterone propionate were begun at 18.2 years.

Chron. Age	8.8	9.5	12.2	19.3
Height Age	3.0	4.3	8.2	13.8
HGH Rx		9 mo.	41 mo.	9.3 yr.

for height, and may exhibit striking subcutaneous deposits of ripply abdominal fat (Fig. 28–21). Some males who apparently have had prenatal onset of the disorder exhibit micropenis, extremely small testes, and underdeveloped scrotum.[357] Although head circumference is within the normal range for age, the growth of facial bones is retarded, thereby producing a disparity between the size of the face and the calvarium. In the first several years of life, approximately 10% of hypopituitary children have hypoglycemic convulsions. An additional 10% or more are found to have asymptomatic fasting hypoglycemia.[358] Hypoglycemia is usually secondary to combined deficiencies of cortisol and GH and can be corrected only by simultaneous administration of the two hormones.[359] Children with idiopathic hypopituitarism rarely have clinical evidence of hypothyroidism. Serum concentrations of thyroid hormone are frequently below normal or in the low-normal range, however.

Diagnosis of Hypopituitarism. The diagnosis of hypopituitarism is made by careful assessment of the history and physical features of the patient, documentation of the lifelong growth trajectory and current growth rate, and analysis of pituitary function tests. Most of this assessment can be carried out in an ambulatory setting. The skeletal age is invariably delayed and is usually roughly equivalent to height age. This, however, is of little specific diagnostic value. In patients with pituitary tumors or craniopharyngiomas, x-rays may reveal enlargement or ballooning of the sella turcica, erosion of the sphenoid bone, or calcification of a suprasellar mass. On the other hand, the sella turcica is often small in idiopathic hypopituitarism. Sellar volume may be measured from standard skull radiographs and compared to normal standards for age and height.[360, 361] When compared to normal-sized children and children with dwarfism from causes other than hypopituitarism, approximately one-third of our patients with idiopathic hypopituitarism had sellar volumes that were sufficiently small to be diagnostic of the disorder (Fig. 28–22). The finding of a normal sellar volume, however, does not exclude the diagnosis of hypopituitarism.

Measurement of the serum somatomedin-C concentration by RIA is also a useful screening method.[187] Most children with hypopituitarism have somatomedin-C levels below 0.25 unit/ml. Although more information must be collected on the lower limits of the normal range throughout childhood, it

Table 28–10. CLINICAL TESTS OF GROWTH HORMONE SECRETION

	Test Conditions	Time of Growth Hormone Response
Screening Tests:		
Exercise	Patient should be fasting; 15 min moderate exercise, then 5 min vigorous exercise	20–40 min after exercise is begun
Sleep	GH rise occurs with deep sleep (EEG stages 3, 4); with EEG monitoring and frequent sampling, may be used as a more definitive test	Initial peak within 1 hour after onset of deep sleep; awaken patient for sample
Formal Tests:		
Insulin	Regular crystalline insulin 0.05–0.1 U/kg (IV). 50% fall in blood sugar is necessary for adequate test. Nadir blood sugar occurs 20–30 min after insulin is given	45–75 min
Arginine	L-Arginine monohydrochloride, 5–10% solution, 0.5 gm/kg (30 gm for adults), infused over 30 min	60–120 min
L-Dopa	0.5 gm/1.73 m² orally; GH responses are often improved by administering priming doses (0.25 gm/1.73 m² of L-dopa for one or more days prior to the test dose)	45–120 min
Glucagon	0.03 mg/kg IM or SC (maximum of 1 mg)	120–180 min
Propranolol (used to augment responses to primary stimulus)	30–40 mg (children 0.75 mg/kg) orally 30–60 min before glucagon, insulin, arginine, or exercise tests	As with primary stimuli

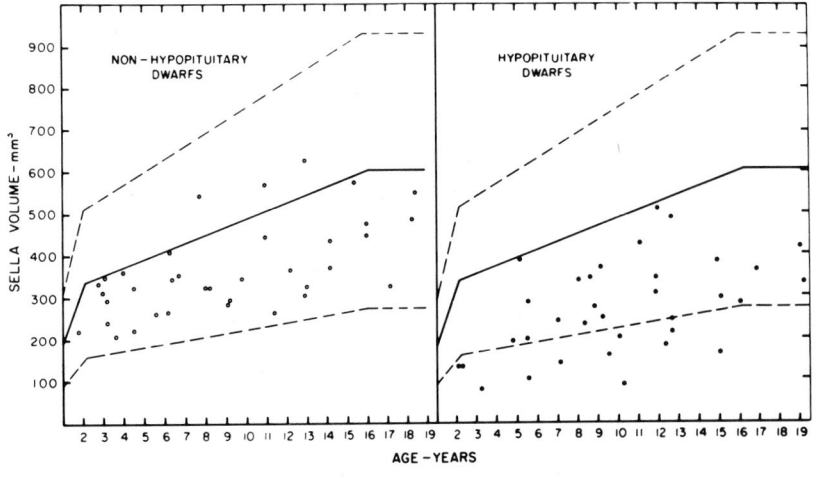

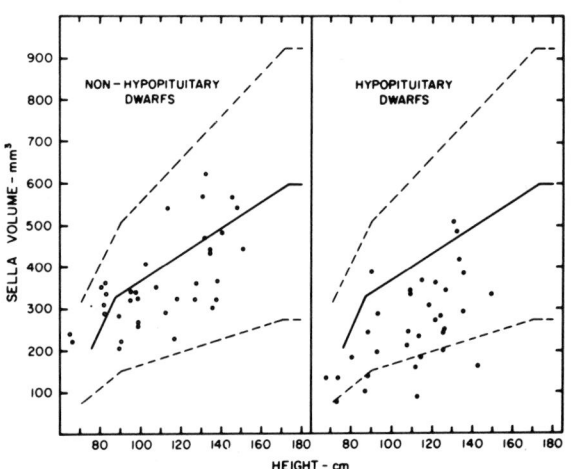

Figure 28–22. Sella turcica volumes as a function of age (top panel) and height (bottom panel) in hypopituitary children (right) and children with dwarfism from causes other than growth hormone deficiency (left). Methods used for derivation of standards are given in reference 361. Sellar volume (V) is calculated using the formula V = ½ (L × D × W). The length (L) represents the longest AP diameter of the sella. The depth (D) is the longest perpendicular dimension between the diaphragmatic line and the sellar floor. The width (W) is taken from the PA projection. (From Underwood, L. E., et al.: New standards for the assessment of sella turcica volume in children. *Radiology* *119*:651, 1976, with permission.)

appears now that after 4 to 5 years of age values below 0.4 unit/ml should be viewed with concern. Since states of insufficient caloric-protein intake also may depress somatomedin-C concentrations, it is important that nutritional status be taken into consideration in interpreting a low value.

Normal serum GH responses to vigorous exercise also may exclude the diagnosis (Table 28–10), but since only 70% of normal children respond to this stimulus, low GH responses are inadequate to confirm the diagnosis. Measurement of GH during deep sleep is also an excellent screening test for GH deficiency. On a single sample taken 1 hour after onset of sleep, 60 to 70% of normal, non-GH-deficient children will have levels greater than 7 ng/ml.[362]

On more definitive testing, subnormal serum GH responses to two or more provocative stimuli are essential components of the diagnosis.[363-365] Although the definition of "subnormal" responses varies considerably from one laboratory to another, most investigators consider responses of less than 7 ng/ml (NIH hGH standards) as indicative of impaired pituitary secretion. The arbitrary nature of such a cutoff value cannot be too strongly emphasized, and it should be recognized that all GH provocative tests occasionally may give misleading results.[366] In our hands, the induction of hypoglycemia with intravenous insulin is the single most reliable method for provoking GH secretion. This test must be done under close monitoring by the physician, however, with an open intravenous line, and with concentrated glucose readily available for treatment of convulsions or unconsciousness. Using these precautions, we have experienced no residual complications in approximately 300 tests. The diagnosis is on firmer footing if, in addition to low GH, deficiencies of other pituitary hormones can be demonstrated. These might include low serum thyroxine, low serum cortisol, impaired cortisol responses to hypoglycemia and ACTH, and impaired serum 11-desoxycortisol or urinary compound S responses to the administration of metyrapone. Our protocol for evaluation of patients with suspected pituitary dwarfism is outlined in Table 28–11. Serum gonadotropin and TSH levels are low in both normal and hypopituitary children; their measurement, therefore, usually is not helpful unless disorders such as Turner's syndrome or primary hypothyroidism have not been excluded.

Treatment of Hypopituitarism. The definitive treatment for GH deficiency in humans is the administration of GH extracted from human pituitary glands obtained at autopsy.[367-369] One gland yields as much as 14 units (7 mg) of purified hGH, enough to treat a 20 to 25-kg child for 2 weeks. The usual therapeutic dosage of hGH is 0.1 unit/kg body weight given intramuscularly every other day or three times weekly. Using this regimen, GH-deficient children almost always have an immediate, spectacular acceleration in linear growth rate. We have observed rates as high as 14 to 15 cm/yr during the first 3 months of treatment. In a group of 42 hypopituitary children treated in our clinic, the mean pre-treatment growth rate was 3.9 ± 1.3 (1 SD) cm/yr, and during the first year of therapy, 8.4 ± 2.0 cm/yr. Young

Table 28–11. A SCHEME FOR EVALUATION OF PITUITARY FUNCTION IN CHILDREN SUSPECTED OF HAVING HYPOPITUITARISM*

Test	Purpose
Skull x-rays	Measurement of sella volume; detect intrasellar or suprasellar mass
Insulin-induced hypoglycemia and L-arginine infusion	GH secretion (see Table 28–10)
Plasma somatomedin-C by RIA	GH secretory status
Serum thyroxine	Detection of chemical hypothyroidism
TSH response to IV TRH	Localization of lesion (hypothalamic vs. pituitary)
Basal A.M. serum cortisol and cortisol level 45 min after administration of 0.25 mg synthetic 1,24-ACTH (Cortrosyn)	Assessment of basal adrenal function. Response to ACTH reflects prior exposure of adrenal to endogenous ACTH
Serum 11-desoxycortisol response to metyrapone (300 mg/m² every 4 hours for 6 doses)	Test of integrity of hypothalamic-pituitary-adrenal axis

*These tests can be completed in less than 72 hours. The day following admission, growth hormone provocative tests are performed in tandem after an overnight fast. TSH responses to TRH may be determined concurrently. The ACTH test is performed the following morning. This ACTH preparation disappears rapidly, so that metyrapone is begun immediately upon the conclusion of the ACTH test. A final blood sample for 11-desoxycortisol is drawn 24 hours later

children respond better than adolescent-age children; obese respond better than thin; and severely GH-deficient children respond better than those with partial deficiencies. As treatment is continued, there is invariably a decline in the growth response, so that after 2 to 4 years the growth velocity may fall below normal. At this point, several months of rest from treatment is advisable, and with resumption of therapy, a renewed growth response is usually obtained.[370] As long as there is a satisfactory growth response, treatment should be continued until a reasonable adult height is reached.

Experimentation with a variety of GH preparations and with different GH dosages has permitted establishment of useful therapeutic guidelines. Larger dosages than those recommended above will produce more rapid growth,[371] but considering the relationship between hGH supply and demand, the routine expenditure of large quantities is prohibitive.[372] Modest dosages of thyroxine should be administered in conjunction with hGH when the pretreatment serum thyroxine level is low or if lowering of thyroxine occurs after hGH treatment has been instituted.[373] In our experience, symptoms of hypoadrenalism are rare and we do not prescribe glucocorticoids unless the patient has symptoms of glucocorticoid deficiency, attacks of hypoglycemia, or laboratory evidence of loss of pituitary-adrenal axis function following removal of a pituitary or hypothalamic tumor. Glucocorticoids should be administered with caution since excessive dosages may attenuate the growth response to hGH. The concurrent administration of androgens and hGH often will augment dramatically the rate of growth of older hypopituitary patients who have been receiving hGH for a long period of time[67] (see section on androgens). In boys, testosterone enanthate in dosages as low as 50 mg/month intramuscularly may more than double the growth rate. Since androgens alone have little or no stimulatory effect on linear growth in GH-deficient patients, they should not be administered without concurrent hGH until after epiphyseal fusion. Once growth has ceased, much larger dosages of androgens can be used, if needed, to bring about full virilization and sexual potency.

Patients who fail to respond or who lose their response to hGH should be assessed for adequacy of dosage and injection technique, thyroid hormone level,[373] and antibodies to hGH.[374, 375] Although development of antibodies to hGH may occur in as many as 30% of treated patients, only rarely have these antibodies been observed to inhibit growth. When large quantities of antibodies are present, a change in hGH preparation may bring about resumption of growth and a decline in antibody concentrations.[376] With the early institution of hGH treatment, hypopituitary patients can experience a normal or near-normal growth pattern and achieve normal adult height.

Primary Hypothyroidism. Growth arrest is perhaps the most constant feature of primary hypothyroidism in infants and children. In newborns with congenital hypothyroidism the disease should be suspected on the basis of poor feeding, unexplained attacks of choking and cyanosis, lethargy, hoarse cry, cutaneous vasomotor instability, and prolonged jaundice. The diagnosis frequently is not made, however, until full-blown signs emerge weeks or months later. Since the early postnatal period constitutes the most critical period of thyroxine-dependent brain maturation, screening programs based on the measurement of thyroxine or TSH on filter-paper blood specimens have been established in many regions.[377]

In older children, acquired hypothyroidism is usually the result of Hashimoto's thyroiditis or decompensation of an ectopic, dysgenetic thyroid gland.[378] In these children clinical signs and symptoms vary in severity and may be so subtle that the physician evaluating a patient for growth failure does not suspect hypothyroidism. The most constant feature is virtually complete growth failure (Fig. 28–23). On the basis of retrospective growth records in our clinic, the aver-

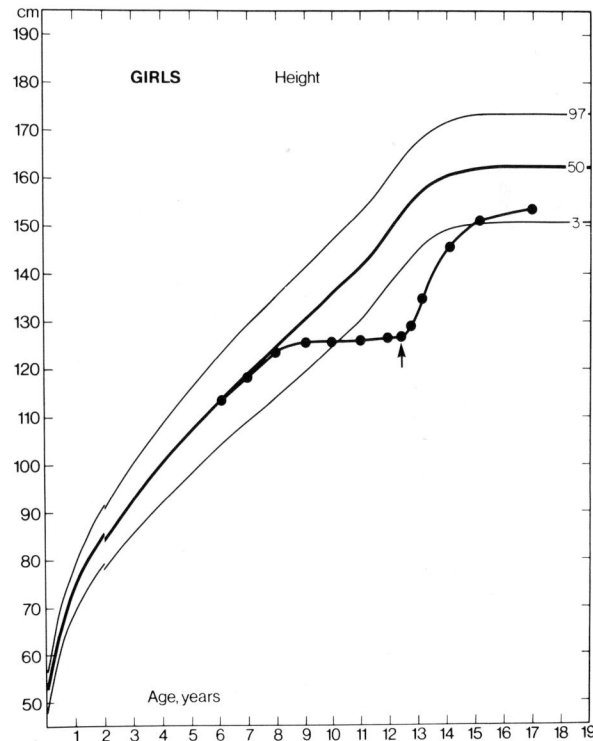

Figure 28–23. Growth chart of girl with primary hypothyroidism diagnosed at 12½ years of age (arrow). The profound growth arrest began at 8 to 9 years and catch-up growth following thyroxine replacement occurred over a 3- to 4-year period.

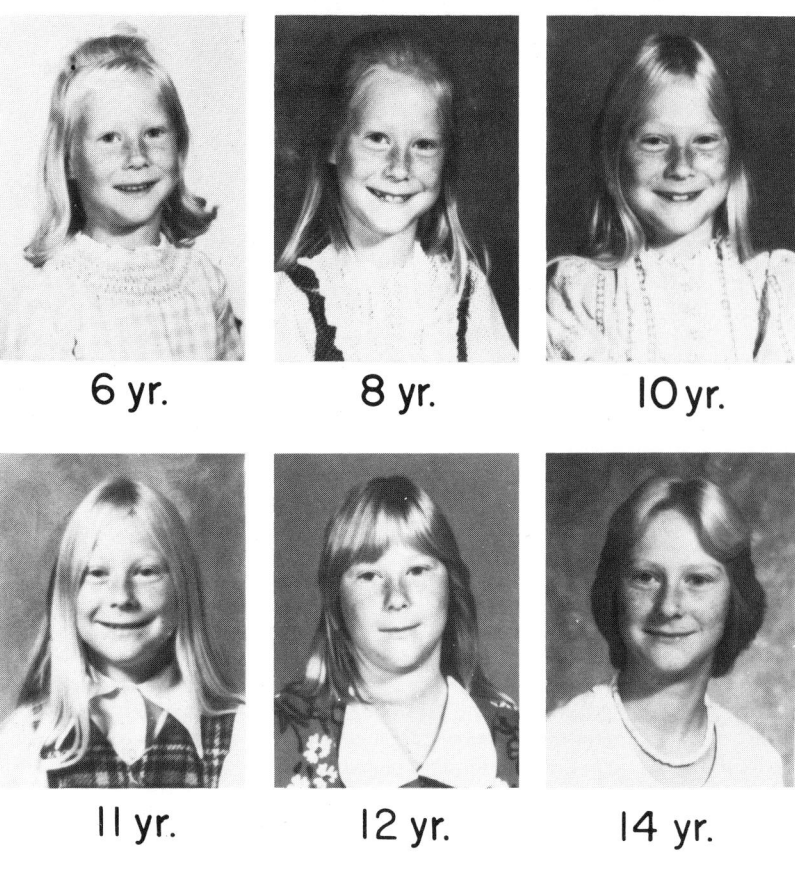

6 yr.   8 yr.   10 yr.

11 yr.   12 yr.   14 yr.

Figure 28–24. Serial photographs of girl with primary hypothyroidism (growth curve shown in Figure 28–23). Facial changes of hypothyroidism are apparent in photograph made at 10 years. Goiter is present at 12 years. The patient had been treated for 1½ years at the time of the last photo.

age duration of acquired hypothyroidism before the disease has been recognized is about 4 years! Inspection of serial photographs in these patients often reveals lack of facial maturation and signs of myxedema concomitant with the onset of growth failure (Fig. 28–24).

The diagnosis is made by demonstrating that the serum thyroxine is low and the TSH is elevated. Skeletal maturation is markedly delayed. In cretins, the diagnosis of athyreosis or thyroid dysgenesis can be made by technetium scanning, and in older children in whom no thyroid can be palpated, scanning for an ectopic gland is indicated. When a gland is palpable the patient's thyroid antibodies should be measured in the search for evidence of Hashimoto's thyroiditis.[379]

Treatment of hypothyroidism is simple and inexpensive and the results are uniformly gratifying. Thyroxine dosages of 100 μg/m² of body surface area are usually sufficient, and adequacy of treatment can be judged from the growth curve and normalization of the serum TSH level. In the first year or so, patients with prolonged growth arrest before treatment will undergo catch-up growth, returning toward the growth channel they occupied before the onset of their disease (see Fig. 28–23).[380, 381] Excessive dosages of thyroxine should be avoided since they will stimulate the disproportionate advancement of skeletal age.

Glucocorticoid Excess. Glucocorticoid excess, whether due to cortisol-secreting adrenal tumors, hypersecretion of ACTH, or pharmacologic therapy, uniformly causes growth arrest[382] (see also section on glucocorticoids). Cortisol-secreting adrenal tumors rarely may be associated with accelerated growth, when androgens are the predominant secretory product. Other signs of glucocorticoid excess include thinning of the skin, vascular fragility, osteoporosis, diminished muscle mass, weakness, obesity, glucose intol-

erance, and occasionally electrolyte disturbances. Truncal obesity may be less prominent than in adults, and some children with Cushing's disease have been observed in whom there were few signs of glucocorticoid excess other than growth failure.[59, 383, 384]

Glucocorticoid excess appears to inhibit growth at the level of the growing tissues since GH secretion is usually normal,[58] serum somatomedin-C concentrations are normal when measured by RIA, and treatment with hGH is ineffective.[59] Although most children with Cushing's syndrome experience some degree of catch-up growth with relief of their condition, the duration and intensity of growth acceleration is often insufficient to return them to normal height centiles. The important determinants of catch-up growth appear to be the duration and intensity of the glucocorticoid exposure and the age of the patient at the time of exposure.[385] Mosier showed that in rats administration of glucocorticoids resulted in permanent, profound biochemical and structural changes in the cartilage of growing animals.[386]

The diagnosis of Cushing's syndrome is often suspected in children and adolescents with exogenous obesity, particularly if they have striae and glucose intolerance. Review of growth charts of patients with exogenous obesity frequently reveals accelerated linear growth, thus making unnecessary a series of costly laboratory tests. In those cases in which the diagnosis remains uncertain, the diagnostic procedures described in Chapter 5 should be followed, with the dosages of dexamethasone and metyrapone reduced in proportion to the surface area of the child.[387]

Growth arrest secondary to the therapeutic administration of supraphysiologic quantities of glucocorticoids can be diminished, along with some of the other side-effects of treatment, by giving single, large doses of medication on alternate days.[388]

Tall Stature

By definition, there are just as many tall children with a stature greater than 2 standard deviations above the mean as there are children with comparable degrees of short stature. There are, however, far fewer pathologic causes of excessive tallness, and concern over this problem surfaces far less frequently. Since, in recent times, normal children have grown faster and reached greater adult stature, it has become more difficult to segregate individuals with pathologic causes of tall stature from those whose tallness reflects optimal growth resulting from excellent health and nutrition. The most useful signs of overgrowth from pathologic causes are the crossing of centile channels upward on the growth chart and the association of abnormalities such as signs of virilization and abnormal body proportions.

Familial Tall Stature: Treatment of Girls with Tall Stature

The vast majority of cases of suspected overgrowth represent variants of the normal growth pattern and reflect the more complete realization of genetic potential. These cases have been variously referred to as "constitutional tall stature" or "familial tall stature." In making the decision of whether a child's tall stature is truly due to hereditary factors, help may be gained by plotting the height and, if possible, the entire growth record of the child's parents. Tall children who do not have tall parents should raise suspicion for a pathologic disorder. If the child is between 2 and 9 years of age, one can relate his height to the height of the parents by using the charts of Tanner and associates.[267] Alternatively, a shorthand method has been proposed for relating the child's height to parental height.[5] In children who have tall parents, diagnostic studies are unnecessary once it has been established that the rate of growth is not accelerated.

In boys, therapy is rarely requested or indicated. In girls, however, tallness more often is regarded as a social handicap, and limitation of growth by the administration of estrogens should be considered. Before undertaking such therapy, it is essential that the adult height be predicted as accurately as possible and the adverse psychologic effects of excessive tallness be weighed against the possible harmful effects of the administration of estrogen. For the latter reasons, we have generally refrained from treating tall girls whose height prediction is less than 183 cm (72 inches). Indeed, some endocrinologists refrain from using this form of treatment at all.[331] Treatment, which has the effect of hastening the onset of puberty, should be instituted well before the first signs of spontaneous puberty are expected to occur and before the bone age is 12 years. Estradiol in doses of 0.15 to 0.30 mg daily have been reported to effect reductions from predicted adult heights of 4.9 to 5.8 cm in girls with initial skeletal ages of 10.5 to 13.0 years, and reductions of 1.8 to 3.6 cm in girls with skeletal ages of 14.0 to 15.5 years.[82, 84] Girls treated with estrogens may experience nausea and excessive weight gain and, unless progestogens are added cyclically, breakthrough bleeding. In view of the recent reports of the long-term adverse effects of estrogen administration, we believe that therapy should be undertaken only in extreme cases and after all known and potential side-effects have been considered.[389]

Excess Production of Pituitary Growth Hormone

Various aspects of excessive GH secretion are reviewed in Chapter 3. Growth hormone hypersecretion in children usually is associated with eosinophilic or chromophobic adenomas. Clinically, this rare disease is characterized by extremely rapid linear growth, overgrowth of soft tissues, and metabolic changes similar to those observed in older acromegalic patients.[390] The physical features of acromegaly such as enlargement of the lower jaw and thickening of the hands and feet usually remain subtle, however, until the disease has been present for many years. If the tumor compresses normal pituitary tissues, there may be signs of TSH, ACTH, and gonadotropin deficiency. Diagnosis can be confirmed by measuring plasma somatomedin levels and by demonstrating that serum GH is elevated and is not suppressed after glucose loading (1.75 g glucose per kilogram of body weight, up to a dosage of 100 g). Abnormalities of the pituitary fossa are usually apparent on sellar tomograms.[332]

Cerebral Gigantism (Sotos Syndrome)

Children with this syndrome are usually above the 90th centile for length and weight at birth and continue to grow rapidly for the first few years of life. After this, some decelerate but remain parallel to the 97th centile. Skeletal maturation is also accelerated, causing puberty to occur early.[391, 392] Children with this syndrome have a large, elongated head, prominent forehead, large ears and jaw, antimongoloid slant to the eyes, elongated chin, and coarse facial features. Most have subnormal intelligence and impaired coordination. Endocrinologically, these children have normal GH secretion and no evidence of thyroid, adrenal, or gonadal dysfunction. The cause of the disorder is not known.

Beckwith-Wiedemann Syndrome

Newborns with this syndrome exhibit marked macrosomia, macroglossia, omphalocele, and hypoglycemia. The

Table 28–12. CAUSES OF STATURAL OVERGROWTH

Prenatal Onset	
Maternal diabetes mellitus	Cushingoid appearance with increased birth weight and length, neonatal hypoglycemia and hypocalcemia, respiratory distress, and jaundice
Beckwith-Wiedemann syndrome	See text
Cerebral gigantism	See text
Postnatal Onset	
Exogenous obesity	Accelerated linear growth accompanying rapid weight gain
Pituitary GH excess	See text
Marfan's syndrome	See text
Sexual precocity and virilizing syndromes	See text
Homocystinuria	Phenotypic characteristics of Marfan's syndrome, mental retardation, excessive homocystine in urine, thromboembolic disease
Total lipodystrophy	Absence of adipose tissue, muscular hypertrophy, enlarged genitalia, diabetes mellitus, enlarged liver, hyperlipidemia; may be associated with acanthosis nigricans and increased GH secretion
Klinefelter's syndrome (47XXY)	Eunuchoid proportions both before and after puberty, small testes, gynecomastia
XYY karyotype	Elevated testosterone in adult; sometimes, impaired intellect and deviant behavior; hairy ears
Hyperthyroidism	Modest acceleration of growth

hypoglycemia, which often is accompanied by islet cell hyperplasia and hyperinsulinism, usually disappears during infancy, but accelerated growth continues postnatally. Skeletal maturation also is advanced, and affected patients exhibit a tendency toward formation of tumors later in life.[393, 394] The mechanism of overgrowth in these patients is unclear, but the hyperinsulinism has been incriminated as a possible cause, and in one patient somatomedin was found to be elevated.[395]

Marfan's Syndrome

Patients with Marfan's syndrome usually are well above average in height but not outside the normal range. They exhibit long limbs with narrow hands and long, slender fingers (arachnodactyly). Their arm span is greater than height and the lower segment is significantly greater than the upper segment. They also exhibit hyperextensible joints, kyphoscoliosis, rib cage deformities, and dislocation of the lens. Death from dissecting aortic aneurysm occurs in early adult life. The nature of the connective tissue defect has not been defined.[396]

Sexual Precocity and Virilizing Disorders

These conditions are the most common endocrine causes of statural overgrowth. In affected children, acceleration of linear growth invariably occurs simultaneously with signs of premature sexual development or inappropriate virilization regardless of whether the disorder is due to congenital adrenal hyperplasia, adrenal tumor, gonadal tumor, or the premature secretion of gonadotropic hormones. Rapid growth is accompanied by accelerated skeletal maturation so that the eventual adult stature is diminished rather than increased. If treatment of the primary disorder is possible, some patients will exhibit "catch-down" growth in an apparent tendency to return to the predisease centile channel (Fig. 28–25). Efforts to curtail the rapid advancement of skeletal age and stature by inhibiting gonadotropin secretion with medroxyprogesterone acetate have proved disappointing. This drug causes suppression of the hypothalamic-pituitary axis[397] and, when given in large dosages, leads to excessive weight gain and other adverse cortisol-like effects.[398] In young girls, smaller dosages of this drug (e.g., 100 mg every 3 to 4 weeks) may prove useful in preventing menstruation and retarding the further development of secondary sexual characteristics.

Two benign conditions which are not associated with accelerated linear growth but may be confused with sexual precocity are premature adrenarche and premature thelarche. In premature adrenarche, pubic hair emerges during the early years of life (before 8 years of age in girls; before 9 years in boys), long before there are any signs of estrogen production or testicular enlargement.[399] Since the normal stimulus which activates adrenal androgen production at puberty is not known, the cause of premature adrenarche is likewise poorly understood. Its frequency is much higher in girls than in boys, and in our experience, it occurs more frequently in black than in white girls. Sometimes, but by no means invariably, it is associated with neurologic defects or mental retardation. Adrenal androgens, in particular, dehydroepiandrosterone sulfate, are elevated and urinary 17 ketosteroid levels may be slightly elevated.[400-402] There also may be a slight advancement of height and bone age. It is important that this condition be differentiated from adrenal hyperplasia and adrenal tumor. In the latter conditions, there are invariably multiple signs of androgen excess including accelerated linear growth, increased muscle mass, clitoral enlargement in girls, voice deepening, and so forth.

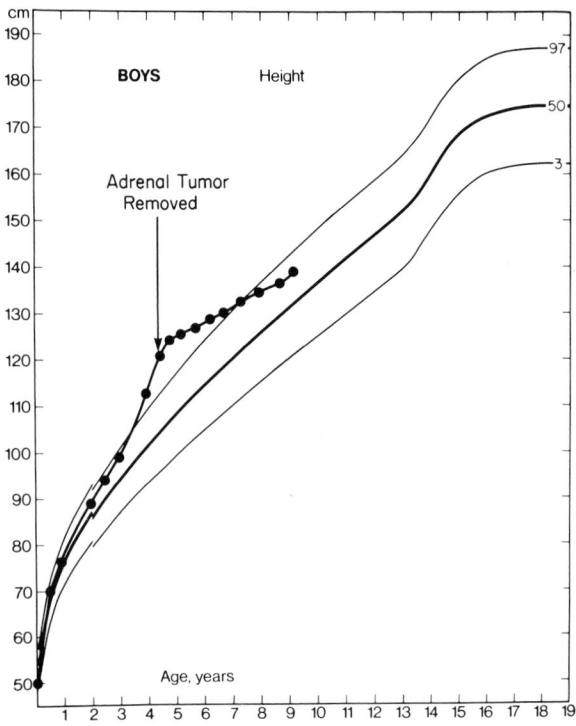

Figure 28–25. Growth curve of boy with virilizing adrenal carcinoma. The patient had a 2-year history of progressive virilization accompanied by acceleration of linear growth. Soon after removal of his tumor, deceleration of growth occurred — so called "catch-down" growth — until his height returned to its original centile channel.

Premature thelarche or benign infantile mammoplasia is an exceedingly frequent finding in young girls, particularly between the first and third years of life. It is characterized by enlargement of the breasts before 8 years of age without other clinical signs of estrogen effect. There is no associated pubic hair, and linear growth usually is not accelerated. Examination of the urinary sediment may reveal a slight degree of epithelial cornification,[403] but serum LH and estradiol levels are not consistently elevated. This benign condition occurs predominantly in well nourished girls. The only requirement for management of this condition is reassurance after the growth rate has been established to be normal and the presence of an ovarian tumor has been excluded by careful physical examination.

Supported by NIH Research Grants AM01022 and HD08299. Judson J. Van Wyk is a recipient of Research Career Award #4K06 AM14115 from the NIH. A Jefferson-Pilot Fellowship in academic medicine provided support for Louis E. Underwood to work in the laboratory of Professor James Tanner and Dr. M. A. Preece (Institute of Child Health, London). Their help in formulating the concepts presented in this chapter and the assistance of Ms. Cindy Sullivan are gratefully acknowledged.

REFERENCES

General Reading

1. Falkner, F., and Tanner, J. M.: *Human Growth*. Vol. I, Principles and Prenatal Growth. Vol. II, Postnatal Growth. New York, Plenum Press, 1978.
2. Falkner, F., and Tanner, J. M.: *Human Growth*. Vol. III, Neurobiology and Nutrition. New York, Plenum Press, 1979.
3. Tanner, J. M.: *Foetus into Man*. Cambridge, Mass., Harvard University Press, 1978.
4. Marshall, W. A.: *Human Growth and Its Disorders*. New York, Academic Press, 1977.
5. Smith, D. W.: *Growth and Its Disorders*. Philadelphia, W. B. Saunders Co., 1977.

Patterns of Human Growth

6. Liggins, G. C.: The drive to fetal growth. In *Fetal Physiology and Medicine: The Basis of Perinatology*. Beard, R. W., and Nathanielsz, P. W. (eds.), Philadelphia, W. B. Saunders Co., 1976, pp. 254–270.

7. Hamilton, W. J., and Mossman, H. W.: *Human Embryology: Prenatal Development of Form and Function*. Baltimore, Williams & Wilkins Co., 1972.

8. Dubowitz, L. M. S., et al.: Clinical assessment of gestational age in the newborn infant. *J. Pediatr.* 77:1–10, 1970.

9. Thomson, A. M., et al.: The assessment of fetal growth. *J Obstet. Gynaecol. Brit. Comm.* 75:903–916, 1968.

10. Bulmer, M. G.: *The Biology of Twinning*. Oxford, Clarendon Press, 1970.

11. Meredith, H. V.: Body weight at birth of viable human infants: a worldwide comparative treatise. *Hum. Biol.* 42:217–264, 1970.

12. Kruger, H., and Arias-Stella, J.: The placenta and the newborn infant at high altitudes. *Am. J. Obstet. Gynecol.* 106:586–591, 1970.

13. Ounsted, C., and Ounsted, M.: Effect of Y chromosome on fetal growth-rate. *Lancet* 2:857–858, 1970.

14. Lobl, M., et al.: Maternal age and intellectual functioning of offspring. *Johns Hopkins Med. J.* 128:347–361, 1971.

15. Tanner, J. M., et al.: Standards from birth to maturity for height, weight, height velocity and weight velocity: British children, 1965. *Arch. Dis. Child.* 41:454–471, 613–635, 1966.

16. Tanner, J. M., and Whitehouse, R. H.: Clinical longitudinal standards for height, weight, height velocity, weight velocity and the stages of puberty. *Arch. Dis. Child.* 51:170–179, 1976.

17. Tanner, J. M., and Whitehouse, R. H.: Height and weight charts from birth to 5 years, allowing for length of gestation. *Arch. Dis. Child.* 48:786–789, 1973.

18. Babson, S. G.: Growth of low-birth-weight infants. *J. Pediatr.* 77:11–18, 1970.

19. Cruise, M. O.: A longitudinal study of the growth of low birth weight infants: velocity and distance growth, birth to 3 years. *Pediatrics* 1:620–628, 1973.

20. Beck, G. J., and van den Berg, B. J.: The relationship of intrauterine growth of low-birth-weight infants to later growth. *J. Pediatr.* 86:504–511, 1975.

21. Falkner, F.: Implications for growth in human twins. In *Human Growth*. Vol. I, Principles and Perinatal Growth. Falkner, F., and Tanner, J. M. (eds), New York, Plenum Press, 1978, pp. 397–413.

22. Smith, D. W., et al.: Shifting linear growth during infancy: illustration of genetic factors in growth from fetal life through infancy. *J. Pediatr.* 89:225–230, 1976.

23. Fitzhardinge, P. M., and Steven, E. M.: The small-for-date infant. I. Later growth patterns. *Pediatrics* 49:671–681, 1972.

24. Tanner, J. M.: *Growth at Adolescence*. 2nd ed. Oxford, Blackwell Scientific Publications, 1962.

25. Marshall, W. A., and Tanner, J. M.: Variations in the pattern of pubertal changes in boys. *Arch. Dis. Child.* 45:13–23, 1970.

26. Marshall, W. A., and Tanner, J. M.: Variations in pattern of pubertal changes in girls. *Arch. Dis. Child.* 44:291–303, 1969.

27. Blizzard, R. M., et al.: The interrelationship of steroids, growth hormone, and other hormones on pubertal growth. In *Control of the Onset of Puberty*. Grumbach, M. M., et al. (eds), New York, John Wiley & Sons, 1974, pp. 342–366.

28. Frasier, S. D., et al.: Effect of adolescence on the serum growth hormone response to hypoglycemia. *J. Pediatr.* 77:465–467, 1970.

29. Greulich, W. W., and Pyle, S. I.: *Radiographic Atlas of Skeletal Development of the Hand and Wrist*. 2nd ed. Stanford, Stanford University Press, 1959.

30. Tanner, J. M., et al.: *Assessment of Skeletal Maturity and Prediction of Adult Height*. London, Academic Press, 1975.

31. Acheson, R. M., et al.: Studies in the reliability of assessing skeletal maturity from x-rays. *Human Biol.* 35:317–349, 1963.

32. Roche, A. F., et al.: A comparison between Greulich-Pyle and Tanner-Whitehouse assessments of skeletal maturity. *Radiology* 98:273–280, 1971.

33. Bayley, N., and Pinneau, S. R.: Tables for predicting adult height from skeletal age: revised for use with the Greulich-Pyle hand standards. *J. Pediatr.* 40:423–441, 1952.

34. Tanner, J. M., et al.: Prediction of adult height from height, bone age and occurrence of menarche at ages 4-16 with allowance for midparent height. *Arch. Dis. Child.* 50:14–26, 1975.

35. Roche, A. F., et al.: The RWT method for the prediction of adult stature. *Pediatrics* 56:1026–1033, 1975.

36. Cheek, D. B.: *Fetal and Postnatal Cellular Growth: Hormones and Nutrition*. New York, John Wiley & Sons, 1975.

37. Goss, R. J.: *Adaptive Growth*. New York, Academic Press, 1964.

38. Goss, R. J.: Adaptive mechanisms of growth control. In *Human Growth*. Vol. I, Principles and Prenatal Growth. Falkner, F., and Tanner, J. M. (eds), New York, Plenum Press, 1978.

39. Leong, G. F., et al.: Effect of partial hepatectomy on DNA synthesis and mitosis in heterotopic partial autografts of rat liver. *Cancer Res.* 24:1496–1501, 1964.

40. Leffert, H. L.: Growth control of differentiated fetal rat hepatocytes in primary monolayer culture. VII. Hormonal control of DNA synthesis and its possible significance to the problem of liver regeneration. *J. Cell Biol.* 62:792–801, 1974.

41. Brasel, J. A., and Gruen, R. K.: Cellular growth: brain, liver, muscle and lung. In *Human Growth*. Vol. 2, Postnatal Growth. Falkner, F., and Tanner, J. M. (eds.), New York, Plenum Press, 1978.

Classic Hormones

42. Ellis, S., and Grindeland, R. E.: Dichotomy between bio and immunoassayable growth hormone. In *Advances in Human Growth Hormone Research*. Raiti, S. (ed.), Washington, D.C., U.S. Govt. Printing office, 1973, pp. 409–433.

43. Ellis, S., et al.: Studies on the bioassayable growth hormone-like activity of plasma. *Recent Prog. Horm. Res.* 34:213–234, 1978.

44. Lewis, U. J., et al.: Enhancement of the hyperglycemic activity of human growth hormone by enzymatic modification. *Endocrinology* 101:1587–1603, 1977.

45. Kostyo, J. L., and Isaksson, O.: Growth hormone and regulation of somatic growth. *Int. Rev. Physiol.* 13:255–274, 1977.

46. Pickering, D. E., and Fisher, D. A.: Therapeutic concepts relating to hypothyroidism in childhood. *J. Chron. Dis.* 7:242–263, 1958.

47. Walker, P. A., et al.: Thyroxine increases nerve growth factor concentration in adult mouse brain. *Science* 204:427–429, 1979.

48. Froesch, E. R., et al.: Non-suppressible insulin-like activity and thyroid hormones: Major pituitary dependent sulfation factors in chick embryo cartilage. *Proc. Natl. Acad. Sci. USA* 73:2904–2908, 1976.

49. Furlanetto, R. W., et al.: The radioimmunoassay for somatomedin-C. In *Somatomedins and Growth*. Giordano, G., Van Wyk, J. J., and Minuto, F. (eds.), New York, Academic Press, 1979.

50. Samuels, H. H., et al.: Control of growth hormone synthesis in cultured GH₁ cells by 3,5,3'-triiodo-L-thyronine and glucocorticoid agonists and antagonists: studies on the independent and synergistic regulation of the growth hormone response. *Biochemistry* 18:715–721, 1979.

51. D'Ercole, A. J., et al.: Leprechaunism: studies of the relationship among hyperinsulinism, insulin resistance and growth retardation. *J. Clin. Endocrinol. Metab.* 48:495–502, 1979.

52. Hill, D. E.: The effect of insulin on fetal growth. *Semin. Perinatol.* 2:319–328, 1978.

53. Gey, G. O., and Thalhimer, W.: Observations of the effects of insulin introduced into the medium of tissue cultures. *J.A.M.A.* 82:1609, 1924.

54. Hollenberg, M. D., and Cuatrecasas, P.: Insulin: interaction with membrane receptors and relationship to cyclic purine nucleotides and cell growth. *Fed. Proc.* 34:1556–1563, 1925.

55. Griffiths, J. B.: Role of serum, insulin and amino acid concentration in contact inhibition of growth of human cells in culture. *Exp. Cell Res.* 75:47–56, 1972.

56. Blodgett, F. M., et al.: Effects of prolonged cortisone therapy on the statural growth, skeletal maturation and metabolic status of children. *New Engl. J. Med.* 254:636–641, 1956.

57. Loeb, J. N.: Corticosteroids and growth. *New Engl. J. Med.* 295:547–552, 1976.

58. Strickland, A. L., et al.: Growth retardation in Cushing's syndrome. *Am. J. Dis. Child.* 123:207–213, 1972.

59. Solomon, I. L., and Schoen, E. J.: Juvenile Cushing's syndrome manifested primarily by growth failure. *Am. J. Dis. Child.* 130:200–202, 1976.

60. Elders, J. M., et al.: Somatomedin and the regulation of skeletal growth. *Ann. Clin. Lab. Sci.* 5:440–451, 1975.

61. Dearden, L. C., and Mosier, H. D., Jr.: Long-term recovery of chondrocytes in the tibial epiphyseal plate in rats after cortisone treatment. *Clin. Orthop.* 87:322–331, 1972.

62. Mosier, H. D., Jr., et al.: Cartilage sulfation and serum somatomedin in rats during and after cortisone-induced growth arrest. *Endocrinology* 99:580–589, 1976.

63. Aynsley-Green, A., et al.: Interrelation of the therapeutic effects of growth hormone and testosterone on growth in hypopituitarism. *J. Pediatr.* 89:992–999, 1976.

64. Simpson, M. E., et al.: Effect of testosterone propionate on the body weight and skeletal system of hypophysectomized rats. Synergism with pituitary growth hormone. *Endocrinology* 35:309–316, 1944.

65. Scow, R. O., and Hagan, S. N.: Effect of testosterone propionate and growth hormone on growth and chemical composition of muscle and other tissues in hypophysectomized male rats. *Endocrinology* 77:852–863, 1965.

66. Zachmann, M., and Prader, A.: Anabolic and androgenic effect of testosterone in sexually immature boys and its dependency on growth hormone. *J. Clin. Endocrinol. Metab.* 30:85–95, 1970.

67. MacGillivray, M., et al.: Enhanced linear growth responses in hypopituitary dwarfs treated with growth hormone plus androgens versus growth hormone alone. *Pediatr. Res. 8*:103–108, 1974.

68. Raiti, S., et al.: Oxandrolone and human growth hormone, comparison of growth-stimulating effects in short children. *Am. J. Dis. Child. 126*:597–600, 1973.

69. Martin, L. G., et al.: Growth hormone secretion enhanced by androgen. *J. Clin. Endocrinol. Metab. 28*:425–428, 1968.

70. Illig, R., and Prader, A.: Effect of testosterone on growth hormone secretion in patients with anorchia and delayed puberty. *J. Clin. Endocrinol. Metab. 30*:615–618, 1970.

71. Sobel, E. H., et al.: The use of methyltestosterone to stimulate growth: relative influence on skeletal maturation and linear growth. *J. Clin. Endocrinol. Metab. 16*:241–248, 1956.

72. Lloyd, H. M., et al.: Effects of stilboestrol on growth hormone secretion and pituitary cell proliferation in the male rat. *J. Endocrinol. 51*:473–478, 1971.

73. Day, H. G., and Follis, R. H., Jr.: Skeletal changes in rats receiving estradiol benzoate as indicated by histological studies and determinations of bone ash, serum calcium and phosphatase. *Endocrinology 28*:83–93, 1941.

74. Geschwind, I. I., and Li, C. H.: *The Hypophyseal Growth Hormone – Nature and Actions.* New York, McGraw-Hill Book Co., 1954.

75. Strickland, A. L., and Sprinz, H.: Studies of the influence of estradiol and growth hormone on the hypophysectomized immature rat epiphyseal cartilage growth plate. *Am. J. Obstet. Gynecol. 115*:471–477, 1973.

76. Josimovich, J. B., et al.: Estrogenic inhibition of growth hormone-induced tibial epiphyseal growth in hypophysectomized rats. *Endocrinology 81*:1428–1430, 1967.

77. Phillips, L. S., et al.: Hormone effects on somatomedin action and somatomedin generation. In *Advances in Human Growth Hormone Research.* Raiti, S. (ed.), DHEW Pub. No. NIH 74–612, Washington, D.C., U.S. Govt. Printing Office, 1974.

78. Wiedemann, E., and Schwartz, E.: Suppression of growth hormone-dependent human serum sulfation factor by estrogen. *J. Clin. Endocrinol. Metab. 34*:51–58, 1972.

79. Herbai, G.: Retardation of body growth and inhibition of sulphate incorporation into costal cartilage of the mouse by various natural and synthetic oestrogens and two oestrogen antagonists. *Acta Soc. Med. Upsal. 75*:209–228, 1970.

80. Phillips, L. S., et al.: Steroid hormone effects on somatomedin. I. Somatomedin action *in vitro. Endocrinology 97*:780–785, 1975.

81. Whitelaw, M. J.: Experiences in treating excessive height in girls with cyclic oestradiol valerate. *Acta Endocrinol. 54*:473–484, 1967.

82. Zachmann, M., et al.: Estrogen treatment of excessively tall girls. *Helv. Paediatr. Acta 30*:11–30, 1975.

83. Frasier, S. D., and Smith, F. G., Jr.: Effect of estrogens on mature height in tall girls: a controlled study. *J. Clin. Endocrinol. Metab. 28*:416–419, 1968.

84. Wettenhall, H. N. B., et al.: Tall girls, a survey of 15 years of management and treatment. *J. Pediatr. 86*:602–610, 1975.

85. Von Puttkamer, K., et al.: Oestrogen treatment of girls with increased growth. *Dtsch. Med. Wochenschr. 102*:983–994, 1977.

86. Schwartz, E., et al.: Mechanism of estrogenic action in acromegaly. *J. Clin. Invest. 48*:260–270, 1969.

87. Alexander, R., et al.: Estrogen treatment of patients with gonadal dysgenesis. (Abstr.) *Pediatr. Res. 12*:364, 1978.

Tissue-Specific Growth Factors

88. Gospodarowicz, D., and Moran, J. S.: Growth factors in mammalian cell culture. *Ann. Rev. Biochem. 45*:531–558, 1976.

89. Goldwasser, E.: Erythropoietin and the differentiation of red blood cells. *Fed. Proc. 34*:2285–2292, 1975.

90. Reissmann, K. R.: Studies on the mechanism of erythropoietic stimulation in parabiotic rats during hypoxia. *Blood 5*:372–380, 1950.

91. Graber, S. E., and Krantz, S. B.: Erythropoietin and the control of red cell production. *Ann. Rev. Med. 29*:51–66, 1978.

92. Miyake, T., et al.: Purification of human erythropoietin. *J. Biol. Chem. 252*:5558–5564, 1977.

93. Goldwasser, E., and Kung, CK-H.: On the mechanism of erythropoietin-induced differentiation. *J. Biol. Chem. 249*:4202–4206, 1974.

94. Dorado, M., et al.: Molecular weight estimation of human erythropoietin by SDS-polyacrylamide gel electrophoresis. *Biochem. Med. 10*:1–7, 1974.

95. Zanjani, E. D., et al.: Biogenesis of erythropoietin: role of the substrate for erythrogenin. *J. Lab. Clin. Med. 77*:751–758, 1971.

96. Jacobson, L. O., et al.: Studies on erythropoiesis. VII. The role of the kidney in the production of erythropoietin. *Trans. Assoc. Am. Physicians 70*:305–317, 1957.

97. Krantz, S B., and Jacobson, L. O.: *Erythropoietin and the Regulation of Erythropoiesis.* Chicago, University of Chicago Press, 1970, pp. 29–31.

98. Alexanian, R.: Erythropoietin and erythropoiesis in anemic man following androgens. *Blood 33*:564–572, 1969.

99. Jepson, J. H., and McGarry, E. E.: Hemopoiesis in pituitary dwarfs treated with human growth hormone and testosterone. *Blood 39*:238–248, 1972.

100. Djaldetti, M., et al.: Erythropoietin effects on fetal mouse erythroid cells. II. Nucleic acid synthesis and the erythropoietin-sensitive cell. *J. Biol. Chem. 247*:731–735, 1972.

101. Glass, J., et al.: Use of cell separation and short term culture techniques to study erythroid cell development. *Blood 46*:705–711, 1975.

102. Bradley, T. R., et al.: Stimulation by leukaemic sera of colony formation in solid agar cultures by proliferation of mouse bone marrow cells. *Nature 213*:926–927, 1967.

103. Virolainen, M., and Defendi, V.: Dependence of macrophage growth *in vitro* upon interaction with other cell types. In *Growth Regulating Substances for Animal Cells in Culture.* Defendi, V., and Stoker, M. (eds.), Philadelphia. The Wistar Institute, 1967.

104. Burgess, A. W., et al.: Purification and properties of colony stimulating factor from mouse lung-conditioned medium. *J. Biol. Chem. 252*:1998–2003, 1977.

105. Stanley, E. R., et al.: Factors regulating macrophage production and growth: Identity of colony-stimulating factor and macrophage growth factor. *J. Exp. Med. 143*:631–647, 1976.

106. Stewart, C. C., and Lin, H.: Macrophage growth factor and its relationship to colony stimulating factor. *J. Reticuloendothel. Soc. 23*:269–285, 1978.

107. Stanley, E. R., and Heard, P. M.: Factors regulating macrophage production and growth. *J. Biol. Chem. 252*:4305–4312, 1977.

108. Van Zant, G., and Goldwasser, E.: Competition between erythropoietin and colony-stimulating factor for target cells in mouse marrow. *Blood 53*:946–965, 1979.

109. Di Sabato, G.: Biochemical aspects of the function of the thymus gland. *Horiz. Biochem. Biophys. 3*:297–325, 1977.

110. Bach, J-F.: Thymic hormones: biochemistry, and biological and clinical activities. *Ann. Rev. Pharmacol. Toxicol. 17*:281–291, 1977.

111. Schlesinger, D. H., and Goldstein, G.: The amino acid sequence of thymopoietin II. *Cell 5*:361–365, 1975.

112. Goldstein, G.: The isolation of thymopoietin (thymin). *Ann. NY Acad. Sci. 249*:177–185, 1975.

113. Low, T. L. K., et al.: The chemistry and biology of thymosin. I. *J. Biol. Chem. 254*:981–986, 1979.

114. Low, T. L. K., and Goldstein, A. L.: The chemistry and biology of thymosin. II. *J. Biol. Chem. 254*:987–995, 1979.

115. Goldstein, G., et al.: A synthetic pentapeptide with biological activity characteristic of the thymic hormone thymopoietin. *Science 204*:1309–1310, 1979.

116. Goldstein, A. L., et al.: Purification and biological activity of thymosin, a hormone of the thymus gland. *Proc. Natl. Acad. Sci. USA 69*:1800–1803, 1972.

117. White, A., and Goldstein, A. L.: The endocrine role of the thymus and its hormone, thymosin, in the regulation of the growth and maturation of host immunological competence. *Adv. Metabol. Disord. 8*:359–374, 1975.

118. Bueker, E. D.: Implantation of tumors in the hind limb field of the embryonic chick and the developmental response of the lumbosacral nervous system. *Anat. Rec. 102*:369–390, 1948.

119. Levi-Montalcini, R., and Hamburger, V.: Selective growth stimulating effects of mouse sarcoma on the sensory and sympathetic nervous system of the chick embryo. *J. Exp. Zool. 116*:321–362, 1951.

120. Mobley, W. C., et al.: Nerve growth factor. *New Engl. J. Med. 297*:1096–1104, 1149–1158, 1211–1218, 1977.

121. Hogue-Angeletti, R. A., et al.: Nerve growth factor: structure and mechanism of action. *Adv. Metabol. Dis. 8*:285–299, 1975.

122. Bradshaw, R. A.: Nerve growth factor. *Ann. Rev. Biochem. 47*:191–216, 1978.

123. Levi-Montalcini, R., and Calissano, P.: The nerve growth factor. *Sci. Am. 240*:44–53, June 1979.

124. Cohen, S.: Purification of a nerve growth promoting protein from the mouse salivary gland and its neuro-cytotoxic antiserum. *Proc. Natl. Acad. Sci. USA 46*:302–311, 1960.

125. Angeletti, R. H., and Bradshaw, R. A.: Nerve growth factor from mouse submaxillary gland: amino acid sequence. *Proc. Natl. Acad. Sci. USA 68*:2417–2420, 1971.

126. Frazier, W. A., et al.: Nerve growth factor and insulin: structural similarities indicate an evolutionary relationship reflected by physiological action. *Science 176*:482–488, 1972.

127. Levi-Montalcini, R., and Angeletti, P. U.: Nerve growth factor. *Physiol. Rev. 48*:534–569, 1968.

128. Hendry, I. A.: Developmental changes in tissue and plasma concentrations of the biologically active species of nerve growth factor in the mouse, by using a two-site radioimmunoassay. *Biochem. J. 128*:1265–1272, 1972.

129. Hendry, I. A., and Iversen, L. L.: Reduction in the concentration of nerve growth factor in mice after sialectomy and castration. *Nature 243*:500–504, 1973.

130. Clark, J. L., et al.: Growth response to hormones by a new rat ovary cell line. *Nature (New Biol.) 236*:180–181, 1972.

131. Gospodarowicz, D., et al.: Purification of a growth factor for ovarian cells from bovine pituitary glands. *Proc. Natl. Acad. Sci. USA* 71:2295–2299, 1974.

132. Nishikawa, K., et al.: Control of ovarian cell growth in culture by serum and pituitary factors. *Proc. Natl. Acad. Sci. USA* 72:483–487, 1975.

Broad-Spectrum Growth Factors

133. Gospodarowicz, D.: Localisation of a fibroblast growth factor and its effect alone and with hydrocortisone on 3T3 cell growth. *Nature* 249:123–127, 1974.

134. Gospodarowicz, D.: Purification of a fibroblast growth factor from bovine pituitary. *J. Biol. Chem.* 250:2515–2520, 1975.

135. Gospodarowicz, D., et al.: Purification of the fibroblast growth factor activity from bovine brain. *J. Biol. Chem.* 253:3736–3743, 1978.

136. Westall, F. C., et al.: Brain-derived fibroblast growth factor: identity with a fragment of the basic protein myelin. *Proc. Natl. Acad. Sci. USA* 75:4675–4678, 1978.

137. Gospodarowicz, D., et al.: Fibroblast growth factor: its localization, purification, mode of action, and physiological significance. *Adv. Metabol Disord.* 8:301–335, 1975.

138. Balk, S. D.: Calcium as a regulator of the proliferation of normal, but not of transformed, chicken fibroblasts in a plasma containing medium. *Proc. Natl. Acad. Sci. USA* 68:271–275, 1971.

139. Rutherford, R. B., and Ross, R.: Platelet factors stimulate fibroblasts and smooth muscle cells quiescent in plasma serum to proliferate. *J. Cell Biol.* 69:196–203, 1976.

140. Kohler, N., and Lipton, A.: Platelets as a source of fibroblast growth-promoting activity. *Exp. Cell Res.* 87:297–301, 1974.

141. Antoniades, H. N., et al.: Purification of human platelet-derived growth factor. *Proc. Natl. Acad. Sci. USA* 76:1809–1813, 1979.

142. Antoniades, H. N., et al.: Isolation of a cationic polypeptide from human serum that stimulates proliferation of 3T3 cells. *Proc. Natl. Acad. Sci. USA* 72:2635–2639, 1975.

143. Ross, R., et al.: A platelet-dependent serum factor that stimulates the proliferation of arterial smooth muscle cells *in vitro*. *Proc. Nat. Acad. Sci. USA* 71:1207–1210, 1974.

144. Harker, L. A., et al.: The role of endothelial cell injury and platelet response in its genesis. *J. Clin. Invest.* 58:731–741, 1976.

145. Cohen, S.: Isolation of a mouse submaxillary gland protein accelerating incisor eruption and eyelid opening in the newborn animal. *J. Biol. Chem.* 237:1555–1562, 1962.

146. Cohen, S., and Taylor, J. M.: Part I. Epidermal growth factor: chemical and biological characterization. *Recent Prog. Horm. Res.* 30:533–550, 1974.

147. Cohen, S., and Savage, C. R.: Part II. Recent studies on the chemistry and biology of epidermal growth factor. *Recent Prog. Horm. Res.* 30:551–574, 1974.

148. Carpenter, G., and Cohen, S.: Epidermal growth factor. *Ann. Rev. Biochem.* 48:193–216, 1979.

149. Savage, C. R., and Cohen, S.: Proliferation of corneal epithelium induced by epidermal growth factor. *Exp. Eye Res.* 15:361–366, 1973.

150. Ho, P. C., et al.: Kinetics of corneal epithelial regeneration and epidermal growth factor. *Invest. Ophthalmol.* 13:804–809, 1974.

151. Byyny, R. L., et al.: Radioimmunoassay of epidermal growth factor. *Endocrinology* 90:1261–1266, 1972.

152. Barthe, P. L., et al.: Submaxillary gland epidermal growth factor. A sensitive index of biologic androgen activity. *Endocrinology* 95:1019–1025, 1974.

153. Ances, I. G.: Serum concentrations of epidermal growth factor in human pregnancy. *Am. J. Obstet. Gynecol.* 115:357–362, 1973.

154. Gregory, H.: Isolation and structure of urogastrone and its relationship to epidermal growth factor. *Nature* 257:325–327, 1975.

155. Gregory, H., et al.: Urogastrone and epidermal growth factor. In *Growth Factors.* Kastrup, K. W., and Nielsen, J. H. (eds.), New York, Pergamon Press, 1977, pp. 75–84.

156. Van Wyk, J. J., and Underwood, L. E.: The somatomedins and their actions. In *Biochemical Actions of Hormones.* Vol. 5. Litwak, G. (ed.), New York, Academic Press, 1978.

157. Zapf, J., et al.: Nonsuppressible insulin-like activity (NSILA) from human serum: recent accomplishments and their physiologic implications. *Metabolism* 27:1803–1828, 1978.

158. Daughaday, W. H.: Hormonal regulation of growth by somatomedin and other tissue growth factors. *Clin. Endocrinol. Metab.* 6:117–135, 1977.

159. Van Wyk, J. J., and Underwood, L. E.: Growth hormone, somatomedins, and growth failure. *Hosp. Prac.* 13:57–67, 1978.

160. Giordano, G., et al.: *Somatomedins and Growth.* New York, Academic Press, 1979.

160a. Phillips, L. S., and Vassilopoulou-Sellin, R.: Somatomedins. *New Engl. J. Med.* 302:371–380, 438–446, 1980.

161. Salmon, W. D., Jr., and Daughaday, W. H.: A hormonally controlled serum factor which stimulates sulfate incorporation by cartilage *in vitro*. *J. Lab. Clin. Med.* 49:825–836, 1957.

162. Hall, K.: Human somatomedin: determination, occurrence, biological activity and purification. *Acta Endocrinol.* Suppl. 163:1–52, 1972.

163. Fryklund, L., et al.: Identification of two somatomedin A active polypeptides and *in vivo* effects of a somatomedin A concentrate. *Biochem. Biophys. Res. Comm.* 61:957–962, 1974.

164. Uthne, K.: Human somatomedins: purification and some studies on their biological actions. *Acta Endocrinol.* Suppl. 175:1–35, 1973.

165. Van Wyk, J. J., et al.: The somatomedins: a family of insulin-like hormones under growth hormone control. *Recent Prog. Horm. Res.* 30:259–318, 1974.

166. Van Wyk, J. J., et al.: Evidence from radioligand assays that somatomedin-C and insulin-like growth factor I are similar to each other and different from other somatomedins. *J. Clin. Endocrinol. Metab.* 50:206–208, 1980.

167. Svoboda, M. E., et al.: Purification of somatomedin-C from human plasma: chemical and biological properties, partial sequence analysis and relationship to other somatomedins. *Biochemistry* 19:790–797, 1980.

168. Froesch, E. R., et al.: Antibody-suppressible and non-suppressible insulin-like activities in human serum and their physiologic significance. *J. Clin. Invest.* 42:1816–1834, 1963.

169. Rinderknecht, E., and Humbel, R. E.: Polypeptides with nonsuppressible insulin-like and cell growth promoting activities in human serum: Isolation, chemical characterization, and some biological properties of forms I and II. *Proc. Natl. Acad. Sci. USA* 73:2365–2369, 1976.

170. Rinderknecht, E., and Humbel, R. E.: The amino acid sequence of human insulin-like growth factor I and its structural homology with pro-insulin. *J. Biol. Chem.* 253:2769–2776, 1978.

171. Blundell, T. L., et al.: Insulin-like growth factor: A model for tertiary structure accounting for immunoreactivity and receptor binding. *Proc. Natl. Acad. Sci. USA* 75:180–184, 1978.

172. Pierson, R. W., Jr., and Temin, H. M.: The partial purification from calf serum of a fraction with multiplication-stimulating activity for chicken fibroblasts in cell culture and with non-suppressible insulin-like activity. *J. Cell. Physiol.* 79:319–329, 1972.

173. Cohen, K. L., et al.: Growth hormone-dependent serum stimulation of DNA synthesis in chick embryo fibroblasts in culture. *Endocrinology* 96:193–198, 1975.

174. Dulak, N. C., and Temin, H. M.: A partially purified polypeptide fraction from rat liver cell conditioned medium with multiplication stimulating activity for embryo fibroblasts. *J. Cell. Physiol.* 81:153–160, 1973.

175. Rechler, M. M., et al.: Purified human somatomedin A and rat multiplication stimulating activity. Mitogens for cultured fibroblasts that cross-react with the same growth peptide receptors. *Eur. J. Biochem.* 82:5–12, 1978.

176. Poffenbarger, P. L.: The purification and partial characterization of an insulin-like protein from human serum. *J. Clin. Invest.* 56:1455–1463, 1975.

177. Poffenbarger, P. L., et al.: Chemistry and physiology of a human serum non-suppressible insulin-like protein (NSILP). In *Somatomedins and Growth.* Giordano, G., Van Wyk, J. J., and Minuto, F. (eds.), New York, Academic Press, 1979.

178. Westermark, B., et al.: Initiation of DNA synthesis of stationary human glia-like cells by a polypeptide fraction from human plasma containing somatomedin activity. *Exp. Cell Res.* 96:58–62, 1975.

179. Hintz, R. L., and Liu, F.: Demonstration of specific plasma protein binding sites for somatomedin. *J. Clin. Endocrinol. Metab.* 45:988–995, 1977.

180. Van Buul-Offers, S., et al.: The Snell dwarf mouse. Interrelationship of growth in length and weight, serum somatomedin activity and sulfate incorporation in costal cartilage during growth hormone, thyroxine and somatomedin treatment. In *Somatomedins and Growth.* Giordano, G., Van Wyk, J. J., and Minuto, F. (eds), New York, Academic Press, 1979, pp. 281–283.

181. Rothstein, H., et al.: Somatomedin-C: restoration of *in vivo* cycle traverse in G₀/G₁ blocked cells of hypophysectomized animals. *Science* 208:410–412, 1980.

182. Copeland, K. C., et al.: Induction of immunoreactive somatomedin-C in human serum by growth hormone: Dose-response relationships and effect on chromatographic profile. *J. Clin. Endocrinol. Metab.* 50:690–697, 1980.

183. Spencer, E. M.: Synthesis by cultured hepatocytes of somatomedin and its binding protein. *FEBS Lett* 99:157–161, 1979.

184. Takano, K., et al.: Somatomedin-A in various clinical conditions in man. In *Somatomedins and Growth.* Giordano, G., Van Wyk, J. J., and Minuto, F. (eds.), New York, Academic Press, 1979.

185. Weidman, E. R., et al.: Production of somatomedin by and mitogenic effects of somatomedin on human fibroblasts. (Abstr.) 61st meeting of the Endocrine Society, 1979.

186. Clemmons, D. R., and Van Wyk, J. J.: Humoral control of somatomedin production by human fibroblasts. Presented to the conference on the Metabolic and Endocrine Aspects of Aging, Bethesda, Md., 1979.

187. Furlanetto, R. W., et al.: Estimation of somatomedin-C levels in normals and patients with pituitary disease by radioimmunoassay. *J. Clin. Invest.* 60:648–657, 1977.

188. Clemmons, D. R., et al.: Evaluation of acromegaly by radioimmunoassay for somatomedin-C. *New Engl. J. Med.* 301:1138–1142, 1979.

189. D'Ercole, A. J., et al.: Serum somatomedin-C in hypopituitarism and in other disorders of growth. *J. Pediatr.* 90:375–381, 1977.

190. Furlanetto, R. W., et al.: Serum immunoreactive somatomedin-C is elevated late in pregnancy. *J. Clin. Endocrinol. Metab.* 47:695–698, 1978.

191. Hall, K., et al.: Immunoreactive somatomedin-A in human serum. *J. Clin. Endocrinol. Metab.* 48:271–278, 1979.

192. Phillips, L. S., and Vassilopoulou-Sellen, R.: Nutritional regulation of somatomedin. *Am. J. Clin. Nutr.* 32:1082–1096, 1979.

Control of Growth at the Cellular Level

193. Holley, R. W. Control of growth of mammalian cells in cell culture. *Nature* 258:487–490, 1975.

194. Pardee, A. B., et al.: Animal cell cycle. *Ann. Rev. Biochem.* 47:715–750, 1978.

195. Rudland, P. S., and Jimenez de Asua, L.: Action of growth factors in the cell cycle. *Biochim. Biophys. Acta* 560:91–133, 1979.

196. Baserga, R.: *Multiplication and Division in Mammalian Cells.* New York, Marcel Dekker, 1976.

197. Temin, H. M., et al.: The role of serum in the control of multiplication of avian and mammalian cells in culture. In *Growth, Nutrition and Metabolism of Cells in Culture.* Cristofalo, V. I., and Rothblat, G. (eds.), New York, Academic Press, 1972, pp. 50–81.

198. McKeehan, W. L., et al.: Improved medium for clonal growth of human diploid fibroblasts at low concentrations of serum protein. *In Vitro* 13:399–416, 1977.

199. Hayashi, I., et al.: Hormonal growth control of cells in culture. *In Vitro* 14:23–30, 1978.

200. Pledger, W. J., et al.: Induction of DNA synthesis in Balb/c 3T3 cells by serum components: re-evaluation of the commitment process. *Proc. Natl. Acad. Sci. USA* 74:4481–4485, 1977.

201. Stiles, C. D., et al.: Dual control of cell growth by somatomedins and platelet-derived growth factor. *Proc. Natl. Acad. Sci. USA* 76:1279–1283, 1979.

202. Clemmons, D. R., et al.: Sequential addition of platelet factor and plasma to fibroblast cultures stimulates somatomedin-C binding early in the cell cycle. *Proc. Natl. Acad. Sci. USA* 1980 (in press).

203. Frank, W.: Cyclic 3',5' AMP and cell proliferation in cultures of embryonic rat cells. *Exp. Cell Res.* 71:238–241, 1972.

204. Otten, J., et al.: Regulation of cell growth by cyclic adenosine 3',5'-monophosphate: Effect of cell density and agents which alter cell growth on cyclic adenosine 3',5'-monophosphate levels in fibroblasts. *J. Biol. Chem.* 247:7082–7087, 1972.

205. Seifert, W. E., and Rudland, P. S.: Possible involvement of cyclic GMP in growth control of cultured mouse cells. *Nature* 248:138–140, 1974.

206. Miller, Z., et al.: Cyclic guanosine monophosphate and cellular growth. *Science* 190:1213–1215, 1975.

207. von Humgen, K., and Roberts, S.: Catecholamine and Ca 2+ activation of adenylate cyclase systems in synaptosomal fractions from rat cerebral cortex. *Nature (New Biol.)* 242:58–60, 1973.

208. Jänne, J., et al.: Polyamines in rapid growth and cancer. *Biochim. Biophys. Acta* 473:241–293, 1978.

209. Bullough, W. S.: Chalone control systems. In *Humoral Control of Growth and Differentiation.* LaBue, J., and Gordon, A. S. (eds.), New York, Academic Press, 1973.

210. Broxmeyer, H. E., et al.: Persistence of inhibitory activity against normal bone marrow cells during remission of acute leukemia. *New Engl. J. Med.* 301:346–351, 1979.

211. Wessell, N. K.: *Tissue Interactions and Development.* Menlo Park, Calif., Benjamin/Cummins, 1977.

212. Grobstein, C.: Mechanisms of organogenetic tissue interaction. *Natl. Cancer Inst. Monogr.* 26:279–294, 1967.

213. Rutter, W. J., et al.: Control of specific synthesis in the developing pancreas. *Natl. Cancer Inst. Monogr.* 13:51–65, 1964.

214. Pictet, R. L., and Rutter, W. J.: The molecular basis of the mesenchymal epithelial interactions in pancreatic development. In *Cellular Interactions in Differentiation.* Karkinen-Jääsheläinen, M., and Saxen, L. (eds.), New York, Academic Press, 1977, pp. 339–350.

215. Karkinen-Jääsheläinen, M., and Saxen, L.: *Cell Interactions in Differentiation.* New York, Academic Press, 1977.

216. DeMello, W. C.: *Intercellular Communications.* New York, Plenum Press, 1977.

217. Staehelin, L. A., and Hull, B. E.: Junctions between living cells. *Sci. Am.* 238:141–152, May 1978.

218. Kolodny, G. M.: Evidence for transfer of macro-molecular RNA between mammalian cells in culture. *Exp. Cell Res.* 65:313–324, 1971.

219. Kolodny, G. M.: Transfer of cytoplasmic and nuclear proteins between cells in culture. *J. Mol. Biol.* 78:197–210, 1973.

220. Lawrence, T. S., et al.: Transmission of hormonal stimulation by cell-to-cell communication. *Nature* 272:501–506, 1978.

221. Gospodarowicz, D., et al.: Determination of cellular shape by the extracellular matrix and its correlation with the control of cellular growth. *Cancer Res.* 38:4155–4171, 1978.

221a. Gospodarowicz, D., Delgado, D., and Vlodavsky, I.: Control of cell proliferation *in vitro* by the extracellular matrix. *Proc. Natl. Acad. Sci. USA* 1980 (in press).

221b. Gospodarowicz, D.: The extracellular matrix and the control of proliferation of vascular endothelial cells. *J. Clin. Invest.* 1980 (in press).

222. Folkman, J., and Moscona, A.: Role of cell shape in growth control. *Nature* 273:345–349, 1978.

223. Folkman, J., and Greenspan, H. P.: Influence of geometry on control of cell growth. *Biochim. Biophys. Acta* 417:211–236, 1975.

Assessment of Growth and Development

224. Cameron, N.: The methods of auxological anthropometry. In *Human Growth.* Vol. II, Postnatal Growth. Falkner, F., and Tanner, J. M. (eds.). New York, Plenum Press, 1978.

225. Whitehouse, R. H., et al.: Diurnal variation in stature and sitting height in 12-14 year old boys. *Ann. Hum. Biol.* 1:103–106, 1974.

226. Marshall, W. A.: Evaluation of growth rate in height over periods of less than one year. *Arch. Dis. Child.* 46:414–420, 1971.

227. National Center for Health Statistics: *NCHS Growth Charts, 1976.* Monthly Vital Statistics Report, Vol. 25, No. 3, Suppl. (HRA) 76-1120. Rockville, Md., Health Resources Administration, 1976.

228. Hamill, P. V. V., et al.: Body weight, stature, and sitting height: white and Negro youths 12–17 years. U.S. DHEW Publication No. (HRA) 74–1608, Series 11, No. 126. Washington, D.C., U.S. Govt. Printing Office, 1973.

229. Tanner, J. M., and Whitehouse, R. H.: *Sitting Height Charts.* Hertford, England, Castlemead Publications, Creaseys of Hertford, Ltd.

230. Marshall, W. A.: Puberty. In *Human Growth.* Vol. II. Postnatal Growth. Falkner, F., and Tanner, J. M. (eds.), New York, Plenum Press, 1978, pp. 141–181.

231. Eveleth, P. B., and Tanner, J. M.: *Worldwide Variation in Human Growth.* London, Cambridge University Press, 1976.

232. Singleton, A., et al.: Croissance de la taille, du segment supérieur et du diamètre biiliaque chez la fille après l'apparition des premières règles. *Arch. Franc. Ped.* 32:859–870, 1975.

233. Laron, Z., and Zilka, E.: Compensatory hypertrophy of testicle in unilateral cryptorchidism. *J. Clin. Endocrinol. Metab.* 29:1409–1413, 1969.

234. Zachmann, M., et al.: Testicular volume during adolescence: cross-sectional and longitudinal studies. *Helv. Paediat. Acta* 29:61–72, 1974.

235. Schonfeld, W. A.: Primary and secondary sexual characteristics: study of their development in males from birth through maturity, with biometric study of penis and testes. *Am. J. Dis. Child.* 65:535–549, 1943.

236. Roche, A. F., et al.: Areolar size during pubescence. *Hum. Biol.* 43:210–223, 1971.

Abnormalities of Fetal Growth

237. Elliott, K., and Knight, J. (eds.): *Size at Birth.* Ciba Foundation Symposium 27. New York, Elsevier Excerpta Medica-North Holland, 1974.

238. Jost, A.: Fetal hormones and fetal growth. *Contrib. Gynecol. Obstet.* 5:1–20, 1979.

239. Naftolin, F.: *Abnormal Fetal Growth: Biological Basis and Consequences.* Berlin, Dahlem Konferenzen, Abakon Verlagsgesellschaft, 1978.

240. Cheek, D. B., et al.: Factors controlling fetal growth. *Clin. Obstet. Gynaecol.* 20:925–942, 1977.

241. Roberts, D. F., and Thomson, A. M.: *The Biology of Human Fetal Growth.* New York, Halstead Press, 1976.

242. D'Ercole, A. J., et al.: Evidence that somatomedin is synthesized by multiple tissues in the fetus. *Develop. Biol.* 75:315–328, 1980.

243. Hurley, T. W., et al.: Ovine placental lactogen induces somatomedin: a possible role in fetal growth. *Endocrinology* 101:1635–1638, 1977.

244. Daughaday, W. H., and Kapadia, M.: Maintenance of serum somatomedin activity in hypophysectomized pregnant rats. *Endocrinology* 102:1317–1320, 1978.

245. Gluckman, P. D., and Brinsmead, M. W.: Somatomedin in cord blood: relationship to gestational age and birth size. *J. Clin. Endocrinol. Metab.* 43:1378–1381, 1976.

246. Underwood, L. E., et al.: Somatomedin and growth: a possible role for somatomedin-C in fetal growth. In *Somatomedins and Growth.* Giordano, G., Van Wyk, J. J., and Minuto, F. (eds.), New York, Academic Press, 1979, pp. 215–222.

247. Catterton, W. Z., et al.: Effect of epidermal growth factors on lung maturation in fetal rabbits. *Pediatr. Res.* 13:104–108, 1979.

248. Battaglia, F. C., and Simmons, M. A.: The low-birth-weight infant. In *Human Growth.* Vol. II, Postnatal Growth. Falkner, F., and Tanner J. M. (eds.), New York, Plenum Press, 1978, pp. 507–555.

249. Lubchenco, L. O.: Assessment of gestational age and development at birth. *Pediatr. Clin. North Am. 17*:125–145, 1970.

250. Lubchenco, L. O., et al.: Intrauterine growth in length and head circumference as estimated from live births at gestational ages from 26–42 weeks. *Pediatrics 37*:403–408, 1966.

251. Tanner, J. M., and Thomson, A. M.: Standards for birth weight at gestation periods from 32–42 weeks allowing for maternal height and weight. *Arch. Dis. Child. 45*:566–569, 1970.

252. Naeye, R. L., and Blanc, W.: Pathogenesis of congenital rubella. *J.A.M.A. 194*:1277–1283, 1965.

253. Bergner, L., and Susser, M. W.: Low birth weight and prenatal nutrition: an interpretive review. *Pediatrics 46*:946–966, 1970.

254. Harding, P. G. R.: Fetal growth and nutrition. In *Perinatal Medicine.* Goodwin, J. W., et al. (eds.), Baltimore, Williams & Wilkins Co., 1976, pp. 255–269.

255. Winick, M.: *Malnutrition and Brain Development.* New York, Oxford University Press, 1976.

256. Jones, K. L., et al.: Pattern of malformation in offspring of chronic alcoholic mothers. *Lancet 1*:1267–1271, 1973.

257. Ouellette, E. M., et al.: Adverse effects on offspring of maternal alcohol abuse during pregnancy. *New Engl. J. Med. 297*:528–530, 1977.

258. Clarren, S. K., and Smith, D. W.: The fetal alcohol syndrome. *New Engl. J. Med. 298*:1063–1067, 1978.

259. Russell, M.: Intrauterine growth in infants born to women with alcohol-related psychiatric diagnoses. *Alcoholism 1*:225–231, 1977.

260. Goldstein, H.: Factors influencing the height of 7-year-old children — results from the national child development study. *Hum. Biol. 43*:92–111, 1972.

261. Hardy, J. B., and Mellits, E. D.: Does maternal smoking during pregnancy have a long-term effect on the child? *Lancet 2*:1332–1336, 1972.

262. Zelson, C., et al.: Neonatal narcotic addiction: 10 year observation. *Pediatrics 48*:178–189, 1971.

263. Zelson, C., et al.: Neonatal narcotic addiction: comparative effects of maternal intake of heroin and methadone. *New Engl. J. Med. 289*:1216–1220, 1973.

264. Reddy, A. M., et al.: Observations on heroin and methadone withdrawal in the newborn. *Pediatrics 48*:353–358, 1971.

265. Naeye, R. L., et al.: Fetal complications of maternal heroin addiction: abnormal growth, infections and episodes of stress. *J. Pediatr. 83*:1055–1061, 1973.

266. Raye, J. R., et al.: Fetal growth retardation following maternal morphine administration: nutritional or drug effect? *Biol. Neonate 32*:222–228, 1977.

Abnormalities of Postnatal Growth

INTRINSIC DEFECTS IN GROWING TISSUES

267. Tanner, J. M., et al.: Standards for children's height at ages 2-9 years allowing for height of parents. *Arch. Dis. Child. 45*:755–762, 1970.

268. Maroteaux, P.: Nomenclature internationale des maladies osseuses constitutionelles. *Ann. Radiol. 13*:455–464, 1970.

269. McKusick, V. A., and Scott, C. I.: A nomenclature for constitutional disorders of bone. *J. Bone Joint Surg. 53A*:978–986, 1971.

270. Rimoin, D. L.: The Chondrodystrophies. *Adv. Hum. Genet. 5*:1–118, 1975.

271. Rimoin, D. L., and Horton, W. A.: Short stature. *J. Pediatr. 92*:523–528, 697–704, 1978.

272. Beighton, P.: *Inherited Disorders of the Skeleton.* Edinburgh, Churchill-Livingstone, 1978.

273. Bailey, J. A.: *Disproportionate Short Stature: Diagnosis and Management.* Philadelphia, W. B. Saunders Co., 1973.

274. Spranger, J. W., et al.: *Bone Dysplasias: An Atlas of Constitutional Disorders of Skeletal Development.* Philadelphia, W. B. Saunders Co., 1974.

275. Smith, D. W., and Wilson, A. C.: *The Child with Down's Syndrome.* Philadelphia, W. B. Saunders Co., 1973.

276. Smith, G. F., and Berg, J. M.: *Down's Anomaly.* Edinburgh, Churchill-Livingstone, 1976.

277. de Grouchy, J., and Turleau, C.: *Clinical Atlas of Human Chromosomes.* New York, John Wiley & Sons, 1977.

278. Brasel, J. A., and Blizzard, R. M.: The influence of the endocrine glands on growth and development. In *Textbook of Endocrinology.* 5th ed. Williams, R. H. (ed.), Philadelphia, W. B. Saunders Co., 1974, pp. 1030–1058.

279. Simpson, J. L.: *Disorders of Sexual Differentiation.* New York, Academic Press, 1976, pp. 259–302.

280. Goldstein, D. E., et al.: Gonadal dysgenesis with 45, XO/46,XX mosaicism demonstrated only in a streak gonad. *J. Pediatr. 90*:604–605, 1977.

281. Johanson, A. J., et al.: Growth in patients with gonadal dysgenesis receiving fluoxymesterone. *J. Pediatr. 75*:1015–1021, 1969.

282. Rosenbloom, A. L., and Frias, J. L.: Oxandrolone for growth promotion in Turner's syndrome. *Am. J. Dis. Child. 125*:385–387, 1973.

283. Urban, M. D., et al.: Oxandrolone therapy in patients with Turner syndrome. *J. Pediatr. 94*:823–827, 1979.

284. Moore, D. C., et al.: Studies of anabolic steroids. VI. Effect of prolonged administration of oxandrolone on growth in children and adolescents with gonadal dysgenesis. *J. Pediatr. 90*:462–466, 1977.

285. Lev-Ran, A.: Androgens, estrogens and the ultimate height in XO gonadal dysgenesis. *Am. J. Dis. Child. 131*:648–649, 1977.

286. Doniach, D., and Polani, P. E.: Thyroid antibodies and sex chromosome anomalies. *Proc. Roy. Soc. Med. 61*:278–280, 1968.

287. Smith, D. W.: *Recognizable Patterns of Human Malformation: Genetic, Embryologic and Clinical Aspects.* Philadelphia, W. B. Saunders Co., 1976.

288. Gorlin, R. J., et al.: *Syndromes of the Head and Neck.* 2nd ed. New York, McGraw-Hill Book Co., 1976.

289. Bergsma, D.: *Birth Defects Atlas and Compendium.* Baltimore, Williams & Wilkins, 1973.

290. Gellis, S. S., and Feingold, M.: *Atlas of Mental Retardation Syndromes.* Washington, D.C., U.S. Govt. Printing Office, 1968.

291. McKusick, V. A.: *Mendelian Inheritance in Man.* 4th ed. Baltimore, Johns Hopkins University Press, 1978.

ABNORMALITIES IN THE ENVIRONMENT OF GROWING TISSUES

292. Pimstone, B., et al.: Growth hormone and protein-calorie malnutrition. Impaired suppression during induced hypoglycemia. *Lancet 2*:1333–1334, 1967.

293. Grant, D. B., et al.: Reduced sulfation factor in undernourished children. *Arch. Dis. Child. 48*:596–600, 1973.

294. Judisch, J. M., et al.: The fallacy of the fat iron-deficient child. *Pediatrics 37*:987–990, 1966.

295. Woodruff, C. W.: Iron deficiency in infancy and childhood. *Pediatr. Clin. North Am. 24*:85–94, 1977.

296. Prasad, A. S.: Zinc: human nutrition and metabolic effects. *Ann. Intern. Med. 73*:631–636, 1970.

297. Hambidge, M. K.: The role of zinc and other trace metals in pediatric nutrition and health. *Pediatr. Clin. North Am. 24*:95–106, 1977.

298. Lecornu, M., et al.: Low serum somatomedin activity in celiac disease. *Helv. Paediatr. Acta 33*:509–516, 1978.

299. Kirschner, B. S., et al.: Growth retardation in inflammatory bowel disease. *Gastroenterology 75*:504–511, 1978.

300. Layden, T., et al.: Reversal of growth arrest in adolescents with Crohn's disease after parenteral alimentation. *Gastroenterology 70*:1017–1026, 1976.

301. Holliday, M. A. (ed.): Symposium on metabolism and growth in children with kidney disease. *Kidney Int. 14*:299–382, 1978.

302. Chantler, C., and Holliday, M. A.: Growth in children with renal disease with particular reference to the effects of calorie malnutrition: a review. *Clin. Nephrol. 1*:228, 1973.

303. Simmons, J. M., et al.: Relation of calorie deficiency to growth failure in children on hemodialysis and the growth response to calorie supplementation. *New Engl. J. Med. 285*:653–656, 1971.

304. Betts, P. R., and Magrath, G.: Growth pattern and dietary intake of children with chronic renal insufficiency. *Brit. Med. J. 2*:189–193, 1974.

305. Avioli, L. V.: Childhood renal osteodystrophy. *Kidney Int. 14*:355–360, 1978.

306. Stickler, G. B., and Bergen, B. J.: A review: short stature in renal disease. *Pediatr. Res. 7*:978–982, 1973.

307. Chesney, R. W.: Increased growth after long-term oral 1α,25-vitamin D₃ in childhood renal osteodystrophy. *New Engl. J. Med. 298*:238–242, 1978.

308. Takano, K., et al.: Serum somatomedin-A in chronic renal failure. *J. Clin. Endocrinol. Metab. 48*:371–376, 1979.

309. Spencer, E. M., et al.: Elevated somatomedin A by radioreceptor assay in children with growth retardation and chronic renal insufficiency. In *Somatomedins and Growth.* Giordano, G., Van Wyk, J. J., and Minuto, F. (eds.), New York, Academic Press, 1979, pp. 341–345.

310. D'Ercole, A. J., et al.: Evidence that somatomedin-C is degraded by the kidney and inhibits insulin degradation. *Endocrinology 101*:577–586, 1977.

311. Mehrizi, A., and Drash, A.: Growth disturbance in congenital heart disease. *J. Pediatr. 61*:418–429, 1962.

312. Feldt, R. H., et al.: Growth of children with congenital heart disease. *Am. J. Dis. Child. 117*:573–579, 1969.

313. Bayer, L., and Robinson, S. J.: Growth history of children with congenital heart defects. *Am. J. Dis. Child. 7*:564–572, 1969.

314. Levy, R. J., et al.: Determinants of growth in patients with ventricular septal defects. *Circulation 57*:793–797, 1978.

315. Mosier, H. D., Jr., et al.: Physical growth in mental defectives. *Pediatrics 36*:465–519, 1965.

316. Frasier, S. D., et al.: Dwarfism and mental retardation: the serum growth hormone response to hypoglycemia. *J. Pediatr. 77*:136–138, 1970.

317. Mandell, F., and Berenberg, W.: The Mauriac syndrome. *Am. J. Dis. Child.* 127:900–902, 1974.
318. McArthur, J. W., et al.: The urinary excretion of corticosteroids in diabetic acidosis. *J. Clin. Endocrinol. Metab.* 10:307–312, 1950.
319. Jivani, S. K. M., and Rayner, P. H. W.: Does control influence the growth of diabetic children? *Arch. Dis. Child.* 48:109–115, 1973.
320. Tattersall, R. B., and Pyke, D. A.: Growth in diabetic children: studies in identical twins. *Lancet* 2:1105–1109, 1973.
321. Thain, M. E., et al.: Coexistence of diabetes mellitus and celiac disease. *J. Pediatr.* 85:527–529, 1974.
322. Williams, T. F., and Winters, R. W.: Familial (hereditary) vitamin D-resistant rickets with hypophosphatemia. In *The Metabolic Basis of Inherited Disease.* 3rd ed. Stanbury, J. B., Wyngaarden, J. B., and Fredrickson, D. S. (eds.), New York, McGraw-Hill Book Co., 1972.
323. McNair, S. L., and Stickler, G. B.: Growth in familial hypophosphatemic vitamin D resistant rickets. *New Engl. J. Med.* 281:511–516, 1969.
324. Stanbury, J. B., et al. (eds.): *The Metabolic Basis of Inherited Disease.* 4th ed. New York, McGraw-Hill Book Co., 1978.

HORMONAL ABNORMALITIES

325. Shizume, K., et al.: Survey studies on pituitary diseases in Japan. *Endocrinol Jpn.* 24:139, 1977.
326. Vimpani, G. V., et al.: Prevalence of severe growth hormone deficiency. *Br. Med. J.* 2:427–430, 1977.
327. Rimoin, D. L., and Schimke, R. N.: *Genetic Disorders of the Endocrine Glands.* St. Louis, C. V. Mosby Co., 1971.
328. Patel, H., et al.: Optic nerve hypoplasia with hypopituitarism. *Am. J. Dis. Child.* 129:175–180, 1975.
329. Kaplan, S. L., et al.: A syndrome of hypopituitary dwarfism, hypoplasia of optic nerves and malformation of the prosencephalon. *Pediatr. Res.* 4:480–481, 1970.
330. Rudman, D., et al.: Prevalence of growth hormone deficiency in children with cleft lip or palate. *J. Pediatr.* 93:378–382, 1978.
331. Frasier, S. D.: Growth disorders in children. *Pediatr. Clin. North Am.* 26:1–14, 1979.
332. Costin, G.: Endocrine disorders associated with tumors of the pituitary and hypothalamus. *Pediatr. Clin. North Am.* 26:15–31, 1979.
333. Bierich, J. R.: On the aetiology of hypopituitary dwarfism. In *Growth and Growth Hormone, Proceedings of the Second International Symposium on Growth Hormone.* Pecile, A., and Muller, E. (eds.), Amsterdam, Excerpta Medica, 1972, p.408.
334. Rona, R. J., and Tanner, J. M.: Aetiology of idiopathic growth hormone deficiency in England and Wales. *Arch. Dis. Child.* 52:197–208, 1977.
335. Craft, W. H., et al.: High incidence of perinatal insult in children with idiopathic hypopituitarism. *J. Pediatr.* 96:397–402, 1980.
336. Costom, B. H., et al.: Effects of thyrotropin-releasing factor on serum TSH: an approach to distinguishing hypothalamic from pituitary forms of idiopathic hypopituitary dwarfism. *J. Clin. Invest.* 50:2219–2225, 1971.
337. Foley, T. P., et al.: Serum thyrotropin responses to synthetic thyrotropin-releasing hormone in normal children and hypopituitary patients: a new test to distinguish primary releasing hormone deficiency from primary pituitary hormone deficiency. *J. Clin. Invest.* 51:431–437, 1972.
338. Prader, A.: Delayed adolescence. *Clin. Endocrinol. Metab.* 4:143–155, 1975.
339. Eastman, C. J., et al.: The effect of puberty on growth hormone secretion in boys with short stature and delayed adolescence. *Aust. N. Z. J. Med.* 1:154–159, 1971.
340. Penny, R., and Blizzard, R. M.: The possible influence of puberty on the release of growth hormone in 3 males with apparent growth hormone deficiency. *J. Clin. Endocrinol. Metab.* 34:82–84, 1972.
341. Illig, R., and Prader, A.: Effect of testosterone on growth hormone secretion in patients with anorchia and delayed puberty. *J. Clin. Endocrinol. Metab.* 30:615–618, 1970.
342. Martin, L. G., et al.: Growth hormone secretion enhanced by androgens. *J. Clin. Endocrinol. Metab.* 28:425–428, 1968.
343. Gourmelen, M., et al.: Transient partial hGH deficiency in prepubertal children with delay of growth. *Pediatr. Res.* 13:221–224, 1979.
344. Widdowson, E. M.: Mental contentment and physical growth. *Lancet* 260:1316–1318, 1951.
345. Patton, R. G., and Gardner, L. I.: Influence of family environment on growth: the syndrome of "maternal deprivation." *Pediatrics* 30:957–962, 1962.
346. Patton, R. G., and Gardner, L. I.: *Growth Failure in Maternal Deprivation.* Springfield, Ill., Charles C Thomas, 1963.
347. Powell, G. F., et al.: Emotional deprivation and growth retardation simulating idiopathic hypopituitarism. I. Clinical evaluation of the syndrome. *New Engl. J. Med.* 276:1271–1278, 1967.
348. Powell, G. F., et al.: Emotional deprivation and growth retardation simulating idiopathic hypopituitarism: II. Endocrinologic evaluation of the syndrome. *New Engl. J. Med.* 276:1279–1283, 1967.
349. Krieger, I., and Mellinger, R. C.: Pituitary function in the deprivation syndrome. *J. Pediatr.* 79:216–225, 1971.
350. Krieger, I., and Chen, Y. C.: Calorie requirements for weight gain in infants with growth failure due to maternal deprivation, undernutrition, and congenital heart disease. A correlation analysis. *Pediatrics* 44:647–654, 1969.
351. Whitten, C. F.: Evidence that growth failure from maternal deprivation is secondary to undereating. *J.A.M.A.* 209:1675–1682, 1969.
352. Laron, Z.: Syndrome of familial dwarfism and high plasma immunoreactive growth hormone. *Isr. J. Med. Sci.* 10:1247–1253, 1974.
353. Laron, Z., et al.: Administration of growth hormone to patients with familial dwarfism with high plasma immunoreactive growth hormone: measurement of sulfation factor, metabolic and linear growth responses. *J. Clin. Endocrinol. Metab.* 33:332–342, 1971.
354. Van den Brande, J. L., et al.: Primary somatomedin deficiency. *Arch. Dis. Child.* 49:297–304, 1974.
355. Daughaday, W. H., et al.: Defective sulfation factor generation: a possible etiologic link in dwarfism. *Trans. Assoc. Am. Physicians* 82:129–138, 1969.
356. Kowarski, A., et al.: Growth failure with normal serum RIA-GH and low somatomedin activity: somatomedin restoration and growth acceleration after exogenous GH. *J. Clin. Endocrinol. Metab.* 47:461–464, 1978.
357. Lovinger, R. D., et al.: Congenital hypopituitarism associated with neonatal hypoglycemia and microphallus: four cases secondary to hypothalamic hormone deficiencies. *J. Pediatr.* 87:1171–1181, 1975.
358. Goodman, H. G., et al.: Growth and growth hormone: VI. A comparison of isolated growth hormone deficiency and multiple pituitary hormone deficiencies in 35 patients with idiopathic hypopituitary dwarfism. *New Engl. J. Med.* 278:57–68, 1968.
359. Underwood, L. E., et al.: Islet cell function and glucose homeostasis in hypopituitary dwarfism: Synergism between growth hormone and cortisone. *J. Pediatr.* 82:28–37, 1973.
360. Underwood, L. E., et al.: Assessment of sella turcica volume in dwarfed children. *J. Clin. Endocrinol. Metab.* 36:734–741, 1973.
361. Underwood, L. E., et al.: New standards for the assessment of sella turcica volume in children. *Radiology* 119:651–654, 1976.
362. Underwood, L. E., et al.: Growth hormone levels during sleep in normal and growth hormone deficient children. *Pediatrics* 48:946–954, 1971.
363. Frasier, S. D.: A review of growth hormone stimulation tests in children. *Pediatrics* 53:929–937, 1974.
364. Joss, E. E.: *Growth Hormone Deficiency in Childhood.* Monographs in Pediatrics, Vol. 5. Basel, S. Karger, 1975.
365. Root, A. W.: *Human Pituitary Growth Hormone.* Springfield, Ill., Charles C Thomas, 1972.
366. Youlton, R., et al.: Growth and growth hormone. IV. Limitations of the growth hormone response to insulin and arginine and of the immunoreactive insulin response to arginine in the assessment of growth hormone deficiency in children. *Pediatrics* 43:989–1004, 1969.
367. Soyka, L. F., et al.: Effectiveness of long-term human growth hormone therapy for short stature in children with growth hormone deficiency. *J. Clin. Endocrinol. Metab.* 30:1–14, 1970.
368. Tanner, J. M., et al.: Effect of human growth hormone treatment for 1 to 7 years on the growth of 100 children, with growth hormone deficiency, low birth weight, inherited smallness, Turner's syndrome and other complaints. *Arch. Dis. Child.* 46:745–782, 1971.
369. Aceto, T., et al.: Collaborative study of the effects of human growth hormone in growth hormone deficiency. I. First year of therapy. *J. Clin. Endocrinol. Metab.* 35:483–496, 1972.
370. Kirkland, R. T., et al.: Results of intermittent human growth hormone (hGH) therapy in hypopituitary dwarfism. *J. Clin. Endocrinol. Metab.* 37:204–211, 1973.
371. Preece, M. A., et al.: Dose dependence of growth response to human growth hormone in growth hormone deficiency. *J. Clin. Endocrinol. Metab.* 42:477–483, 1976.
372. Frasier, S. D., et al.: Collaborative study of the effects of human growth hormone in growth hormone deficiency. IV. Treatment with low doses of human growth hormone based on body weight. *J. Clin. Endocrinol. Metab.* 44:22–31, 1977.
373. Lippe, B. M., et al.: Reversible hypothyroidism in growth hormone-deficient children treated with human growth hormone. *J. Clin. Endocrinol. Metab.* 40:612–618, 1975.
374. Kaplan, S. L., et al.: Antibodies to human growth hormone arising in patients treated with human growth hormone: Incidence characteristics, and effects on growth. In *Advances in Human Growth Hormone Research.* Raiti, S. (ed.), Washington, D.C., U.S. Govt. Printing Office, 1974, p. 725.
375. Frasier, S. D., et al.: Collaborative study of the effects of human

growth hormone in growth hormone deficiency. II. Development and significance of antibodies to human growth hormone during the first year of therapy. *J. Clin. Endocrinol. Metab.* 38:14–18, 1974.

376. Underwood, L. E., et al.: Restoration of growth by human growth hormone (Roos) in hypopituitary dwarfs immunized by other human growth hormone preparations: clinical and immunological studies. *J. Clin. Endocrinol. Metab.* 38:288–297, 1974.

377. Fisher, D. A., et al.: Screening for congenital hypothyroidism: results of screening one million North American infants. *J. Pediatr.* 94:700–705, 1979.

378. Van Wyk, J. J., and Fisher, D. A.: Thyroid. In *Pediatrics.* 16th ed. Rudolph, A. M. (ed.), New York, Appleton-Century-Crofts, 1977, pp. 1663–1693.

379. Hopwood, N. J., et al.: Thyroid antibodies in children and adolescents with thyroid disorders. *J. Pediatr.* 93:57–61, 1978.

380. Prader, A., et al.: Catch-up growth following illness or starvation. *J. Pediatr.* 62:646–659, 1963.

381. Prader, A.: Catch-up growth. In *Paediatrics and Growth.* Barltrop, D. (ed.), London, Fellowship of Postgraduate Medicine, 1978, pp. 133–143.

382. McArthur, R. G., et al.: Cushing's disease in children: findings in 13 cases. *Mayo Clin. Proc.* 47:318–326, 1972.

383. Marie, J., et al.: Les troubles de la croissance staturals dans l'hyper-corticisme spontané acquis de l'enfance. *Ann Pediatr. (Paris)* 13:91, 1966.

384. Lee, P. A., et al.: Short stature as the only clinical sign of Cushing's syndrome. *J. Pediatr.* 86:89–91, 1975.

385. Mosier, H. D., et al.: Failure of catch-up growth after Cushing's syndrome in childhood. *Am. J. Dis. Child.* 124:251–253, 1972.

386. Mosier, H. D., Jr.: Failure of compensatory (catch-up) growth in the rat. *Pediatr. Res.* 5:59–63, 1971.

387. Streeten, D. H. P., et al.: Hypercortisolism in childhood: shortcomings of conventional diagnostic criteria. *Pediatrics* 56:797–803, 1975.

388. Soyka, L. F.: Treatment of nephrotic syndrome in childhood: use of an alternate-day prednisone regimen. *Am. J. Dis. Child.* 113:693–701, 1967.

Tall Stature

389. Report on the conference on estrogen treatment for the young. *Pediatrics* 62(Suppl):1087–1217, 1978.

390. Daughaday, W. H.: Extreme gigantism: analysis of growth velocity and occurrence of severe peripheral neuropathy and neuropathic arthropathy (Charcot joints). *New Engl. J. Med.* 297:1267–1269, 1977.

391. Sotos, J. F., et al.: Cerebral gigantism in childhood: a syndrome of excessively rapid growth with acromegalic features and a non-progressive neurologic disorder. *New Engl. J. Med.* 271:109–116, 1964.

392. Sotos, J. F., et al.: Cerebral gigantism. *Am. J. Dis. Child.* 131:625–627, 1977.

393. Filippi, G., and McKusick, V. A.: The Beckwith-Wiedemann syndrome (the exophthalmos-macroglossia-gigantism syndrome). Report of two cases and review of the literature. *Medicine* 49:279–298, 1970.

394. Sotelo-Avila, C., and Singer, D. B.: Syndrome of hyperplastic fetal visceromegaly and neonatal hypoglycemia — a report of 7 cases. *Pediatrics* 46:240–251, 1970.

395. Schabel, F., and Frisch, H.: Erhohte Somatomedinaktivität beim Beckwith-Wiedemann-Syndrom. *Paediatr. Paedol.* 14:249–257, 1979.

396. McKusick, V. A.: *Heritable Disorders of Connective Tissue.* 4th ed. St. Louis, C.V. Mosby Co., 1972.

397. Sadeghi-Nejad, A., et al.: The effect of medroxyprogesterone acetate on adrenocortical function in children with precocious puberty. *J. Pediatr.* 78:616–624, 1971.

398. Richman, R. A., et al.: Adverse effects of large doses of medroxy-progesterone (MPA) in idiopathic isosexual precocity. *J. Pediatr.* 79:963–971, 1971.

399. Silverman, S. H., et al.: Precocious growth of sexual hair without other secondary sexual development: "Premature pubarche," a constitutional variation of adolescence. *Pediatrics* 10:426–432, 1952.

400. Sizonenko, P. C., and Paunier, L.: Hormonal changes in puberty. III. Correlations of plasma dehydroepiandrosterone, testosterone, FSH, and LH with stages of puberty and bone age in normal boys and girls and in patients with Addison's disease or hypogonadism or with premature or late adrenarche. *J. Clin. Endocrin. Metab.* 41:894–904, 1975.

401. Rappaport, R., et al.: Plasma androgens and LH in scoliotic patients with premature pubarche. *J. Clin. Endocrinol. Metab.* 38:401–406, 1974.

402. Korth-Schutz, S., et al.: Evidence for the adrenal source of androgens in precocious adrenarche. *Acta Endocrinol.* 82:342–352, 1976.

403. Collett-Solbert, P. R., and Grumbach, M. M.: A simplified procedure for evaluating estrogenic effects and the sex chromatin pattern in exfoliated cells in urine: studies in premature thelarche and gynecomastia of adolescence. *J. Pediatr.* 66:883–890, 1965.

CHAPTER 29

Aging and Hormones

By Robert I. Gregerman
and Edwin L. Bierman

In past years, aging was thought by some scientists to be the direct result of deficiency states resulting from age-related failure of the endocrine glands to secrete their hormones. Such thinking now seems naive as the complexities of the processes of aging have become more apparent. Moreover, an overt hormone deficiency state, such as that which occurs at the menopause with ovarian failure and subsequent estrogen lack, is the exception rather than the rule for age-related endocrine changes. In contrast with other hormones, either no deficiency exists in the classic sense, or else the age-related alteration of hormone physiology is subtle. Nonetheless, although mastery of the organs of internal secretion can no longer be viewed as the key to longevity, normal aging does produce a variety of effects on hormone production, secretion, and action. For these reasons, an understanding of age-related changes in endocrine function can make a significant contribution to our concepts of what constitutes "disease," as opposed to time-related physiologic alteration, and to our understanding of the processes of aging.

The practical need for such age-based information has become obvious, and it is now clear that standards of nor-mality in clinical tests of endocrine function must take into account the effects of aging that occur throughout the population. For example, over a number of years, failure to appreciate this phenomenon in connection with age-related changes of glucose tolerance led to probable overestimation of the incidence of diabetes in the adult population and to the frequent initiation of unnecessary therapeutic measures. At the present time, age-related data from normal subjects are beginning to appear earlier and with greater regularity in the evolution of new testing procedures, but the issue of age-based standards from normal subjects for the clinical interpretation of endocrine tests will continue to arise as new tests are developed.

It should be emphasized that useful physiologic and biochemical clinical tests may fail completely to reveal significant age-related events. An unaltered concentration of a hormone in blood, for example, does not mean that age has necessarily been unaccompanied by physiologic changes. The blood level of a hormone is the balance of a number of processes, each of which can be age-influenced. The concentration in blood of a hormone with a relatively constant rate of production results not only from the rate of secretion but also from the concentration in plasma of specific carrier binding proteins, which in turn determine the "free" or metabolically active hormone in plasma and the rate of metabolic destruction or disposal of the hormone, an event which need bear no direct relation to its biologic action. For those hormones whose secretion is episodic or cyclic, the amplitude of the secretory cycles and their frequency are additional age-related variables bearing on the integrated hormonal effect. In addition, concentration in blood is frequently determined by feedback control mechanisms, often in the hypothalamus, the sensitivity of which may be affected by age. Beyond consideration of blood hormone concentration, however, age affects the sensitivity of target-tissue responsiveness through effects on hormone receptors, the plasma membrane–bound adenylate cyclase system, intracellular binding proteins, and other steps related to the expression of hormonal effects. Examples of these age-related phenomena will be pointed out, insofar as they are known, in the discussions of specific hormones, but it should be obvious already that the mere determination of plasma hormone concentration at a given moment or even of the secretion rate of a hormone may give a very incomplete picture of age-related events.

Our attempts to understand endocrine-aging interrelationships in man are, of course, dependent on animal model systems, but the use of animal models is complicated by the fact that it is frequently inappropriate to extrapolate observations made in animals to the situation in man. There are so many qualitative and quantitative differences in the endocrinology of experimental animals and that of the human that such extrapolations, although frequently and sweepingly made, are dangerously deceptive, especially so in connection with age-related events. In our discussion we shall attempt to point out where major differences occur between animals and man and shall mention some occurrences which so far have no counterpart in man, but our major emphasis shall be on what is known about the effects of aging on endocrine gland activity and the metabolism of hormones in the human.

A number of reviews are available which cover general aspects of the biology of aging and the endocrine system (Everitt and Burgess, 1976; Finch and Hayflick, 1977), as well as some of the clinical aspects (Greenblatt, 1978; Schneider, 1978).

ANTERIOR PITUITARY: MORPHOLOGY AND HORMONE CONTENT

A review of the many reports dealing with the weight, histologic appearance, and tropic hormone content of the anterior pituitary during growth and senescence in man and animals can be found elsewhere (Verzár, 1966; Bourne, 1967). Only a summary will be given here. The human data are extremely difficult to interpret, because the gland is of necessity obtained mainly at autopsy, at which time it has usually suffered the effects of one or more disease states, a problem which has been best described in relation to thyroid-stimulating hormone (TSH) (Bakke et al., 1964). With all reservations in mind, it appears that in advanced age the size of the human pituitary decreases minimally, certainly not more than 20% (Calloway et al., 1965; Verzár, 1966). It is not certain whether there is a decrease in ACTH content in old age (Verzár, 1966), but there appears to be no gross decrease in growth hormone (GH) (Gershberg, 1957). Thyrotropin

(TSH) content seems not to be altered (Bakke et al., 1964). Prolactin, although present at a higher concentration in the female than male pituitary, is not altered at advanced age (Yamaji et al., 1976). There is a considerable increase in follicle-stimulating hormone (FSH) in the pituitary of the postmenopausal female, which is in keeping with the increased secretion of FSH that occurs as the result of failure of ovarian estrogen secretion at menopause. Interestingly, the increased plasma FSH and luteinizing hormone (LH) levels of the postmenopausal female are greatly diminished by nonspecific illness (Warren et al., 1977). Comparative data from elderly males also show increased pituitary LH (Ryan, 1962). In contrast, the pituitary of the aged rat of both sexes appears to contain reduced concentrations of FSH and LH (Bruni et al., 1977).

Functionally or physiologically it matters little whether the amount of a pituitary hormone changes with age. The important considerations relate to the release of the hormone in response to appropriate stimuli, which in turn relates to such parameters as age-determined changes in releasing factor secretion, pituitary sensitivity to the releasing factors, and hypothalamic threshold to feedback inhibition, to mention a few. In several instances, limited data that indicate age-related changes are available, and they are discussed below.

POSTERIOR PITUITARY: ANTIDIURETIC HORMONE

Conclusions drawn from a number of extensive studies are that, in the aged rat, neurohypophyseal function and antidiuretic hormone (ADH) secretion are impaired, and that the senescent animal has a modified form of diabetes insipidus (Friedman et al, 1967; see also Dunihue, 1965; Frolkis, 1972). With administration of ADH, a variety of age-related alterations (impaired ability to concentrate urine, increased size of organs, increased muscle sodium, impaired muscle function) are all reversed toward those of the young animal, and life span has been claimed to have been extended. These results have been extrapolated from the rat to account for certain age-related changes in man, but the extrapolation is not justified. The aged human does not exhibit evidence of diabetes insipidus. It is true that the maximal achievable urine osmolality following water deprivation decreases with increasing age, but the defect is apparently a renal one, since the ability of the kidney to respond to exogenous ADH is also decreased. The decrease of maximal urine concentrating ability is in turn related to the decreased glomerular filtration rate that occurs with age rather than to decreased sensitivity to ADH (Lindeman et al., 1966).

Several clinical reports have suggested age-related alterations of the hypothalamic-neurohypophyseal axis in man. For example, development of dilutional hyponatremia following the stress of surgery in the elderly suggested inappropriate secretion of ADH (Deutsch et al., 1966). In addition, a disturbance of the mechanism for ADH release was postulated to account for a syndrome of inappropriate ADH activity in certain elderly diabetics treated with chlorpropamide (Diabinese) (Weissman et al., 1971). Since this drug appears to potentiate ADH rather than to cause its release, it was theorized that the syndrome reflects an inability of some individuals to reduce their output of ADH in response to the stimulus of volume expansion and hypo-osmolality. To date the phenomenon has been seen only in elderly diabetics, suggesting an age-related alteration of hypothalamic–posterior pituitary regulation of ADH secretion. Direct evidence for age-related alteration of ADH release was provided by studies of plasma ADH responses in healthy adult subjects given an osmolar stimulus (hypertonic NaCl) to provoke and ethanol to inhibit ADH release (Helderman et al., 1978). Stimulation with NaCl produced a twofold greater release of ADH in elderly subjects than in the young. Ethanol, a classic inhibitor of ADH release, produced only transient inhibition in the elderly, apparently because in these subjects the osmolar stimulus provided by the ethanol overrides its action to inhibit ADH release. In connection with these observations, two important ADH-synthesizing sites in man, the supraoptic and paraventricular nuclei, show striking age-specific cytologic changes without evidence of cell destruction (Buttlar-Brentano, 1954; Andrew, 1956).

HYPOTHALAMUS: RELEASING HORMONES

The rapidly accumulating information on the hypothalamic regulatory hormones has been recently reviewed (Guillemin, 1978; Schally; 1978). Although there are as yet only a few reports, age has already been shown to affect the physiology of these hormones both during postnatal development and in senescence. A number of different alterations of hypothalamic-pituitary relationships appear to be involved. Responsiveness of the rat pituitary to gonadotropin-releasing hormone (GnRH) reaches a peak during the first weeks of life and then falls off as the animal reaches maturity (Debeljuk et al., 1972). A more extreme change of pituitary sensitivity to a releasing hormone is seen in the senescent rat, the pituitary of which responds only minimally to hypothalamic extracts which have potent GH-releasing activity in young animals (Pecile et al., 1965). Moreover, GHRH appears to be absent from the hypothalamus of the senescent rat. In addition to these alterations of pituitary responsiveness to GnRH and GHRH, the reported reduction in secretion of GnRH in the old female rat may contribute to the loss of reproductive function in this species (Miller and Riegle, 1978a). The decreased secretion of GnRH in the old rat is not, however, due to reduced hypothalamic content of the peptide (Miller and Riegle, 1978b). Comparable information for man is limited, but the impaired response of the pituitary of elderly men to thyrotropin-releasing hormone (TRH) should be recalled in this connection (see Thyrotropin-Releasing Hormone and Thyrotropin).

Other age-related changes of hypothalamic sensitivity have also been proposed (Dilman et al., 1979). These observations as applied to man are open to criticism on numerous grounds, and at this time the conclusions derived from them can only be considered speculative. Nonetheless, there is some evidence that human hypothalamic reactivity is altered during senescence (see Sympathetic Nervous System: Catecholamines). Age-related alteration of feedback in inhibition of gonadotropin secretion by sex steroids has recently been reported (see Gonadotropins under Male Gonadal Function). Age effects on ADH release may also be relevant (see Posterior Pituitary). Moreover, studies in the rat indicate an extremely complex pattern of age-related alterations of hypothalamic function. Evidence has been presented, on the one hand, for increased sensitivity during senescence to direct stimulation by catecholamines and acetylcholine and, on the other, for decreased responses of the hypothalamico-neurohypophyseal system when complex neural pathways are involved (Frolkis and Bezrukov, 1972).

PROLACTIN

Plasma levels of prolactin are both age- and sex-dependent. Until about age 45 years, mean values for men are about two-thirds those of women. In one study levels in women fell considerably with increasing age while those in men increased slightly (Vekemans and Robyn, 1975). In another study age did not appear to influence basal plasma levels (Yamaji et al., 1976). Administration of TRH elevated prolactin to greater levels in women than in men in proportion to the sex difference, with no age effect evident in terms of the magnitude of the peak response. However, the time necessary to reach the peak level after TRH and the rate of decrease was considerably delayed in elderly subjects (Yamaji et al., 1976).

GROWTH HORMONE

The effects of aging on GH levels are complicated by influences of sex and obesity on hormone secretion. In young persons, men have lower basal plasma levels than women, while estrogen given to males raises GH and induces a female pattern of secretion. In the elderly, the influence of sex on basal GH levels is unclear (Laron et al., 1969—F > M; Cartlidge et al., 1970—F = M; Kalk et al., 1973 — M > F). In men no effect of age could be shown on basal levels (Dudl et al., 1973). Nonobese young women (20 to 39 years) had higher GH levels than women of middle age (40 to 59 years). Obese subjects showed no such decrease of GH with age; young obese women had lower levels than their nonobese counterparts. Values for older obese subjects were comparable to those in nonobese women of the same age, a result attributed to a decline with age in the nonobese group and constancy with age in the obese (Vidalon et al., 1973). In yet another study, obese elderly subjects had lower GH levels than lean elderly (Kalk et al., 1973). These divergent results exemplify the complexities of interpreting age effects on hormone levels and the interactions of other variables with aging.

Following stimulation of GH secretion by insulin-induced hypoglycemia, GH increases in young and old subjects. This response has been reported to be considerably diminished in some elderly subjects (Laron et al., 1969). Among the elderly, 20% (all over age 65) were reported to have such grossly decreased responses that, were they younger subjects, a diagnosis of inadequate GH reserve or GH deficiency would have been made. This study is subject to the criticism that in a number of the poor responders the degree of insulin-induced hypoglycemia was inadequate. Furthermore, the degree of obesity was not reported. Others have suggested little influence of age on the response to hypoglycemia, even in very old subjects (Cartlidge et al., 1970; Kalk et al., 1973). In studies of the stimulation of GH secretion by arginine, the expected increase in adiposity with age was reported along with an inverse correlation between GH response and adiposity. Nonetheless, a significant effect of age on arginine-induced GH secretion could not be demonstrated (Dudl et al., 1973).

Despite these reports, impaired secretion of GH appears to accompany physiologic aging. The normal surges of GH secretion which occur during sleep in young adults were entirely abolished in the few middle-aged and elderly subjects studied (Carlson et al., 1972; Finklestein, et al., 1972). Although GH secretory bursts have been thought to be associated with the early stages of deep (slow-wave) sleep, and although this phase of sleep is reduced with aging, no close association could be shown between these two events (Carlson et al., 1972). With regard to GH effects in old age, the limited evidence available indicates that certain metabolic responses are blunted in elderly subjects (Root and Oski, 1969).

THYROID

Attention was drawn many years ago to the influence of age on the thyroid by observations that basal metabolic rate (BMR) decreases with increasing age. Since thyroid hormone (TH) is a major determinant of metabolic rate, a direct relationship between age, TH secretion, and the BMR was suspected. It is now clear that, while BMR and TH secretion rate decrease with age, the two events are not causally related. The decrease of BMR is best explained by an age-related decrease of muscle mass; oxygen consumption per unit of nonmuscle metabolic mass does not decrease with age (Fig. 29–1; Tzankoff and Norris, 1977). The decrease of TH secretion, on the other hand, is currently viewed as a homeostatic adjustment to slowed metabolic disposal of thyroid hormone. These considerations have been reviewed in greater detail elsewhere, together with functional changes related to the neonatal period and age-related data from animal studies (Gregerman and Davis, 1978).

Thyroid Anatomy

With advancing age, the thyroid undergoes fibrosis, cellular infiltrations, and follicular alterations. Microscopic and clinically palpable nodularity also increase with age. There is controversy about whether the overall size of the gland is increased or decreased, but from a functional point of view, the significance of these anatomic changes is minimal, since the thyroid of even very elderly persons functions adequately and maintains its reserve capacity.

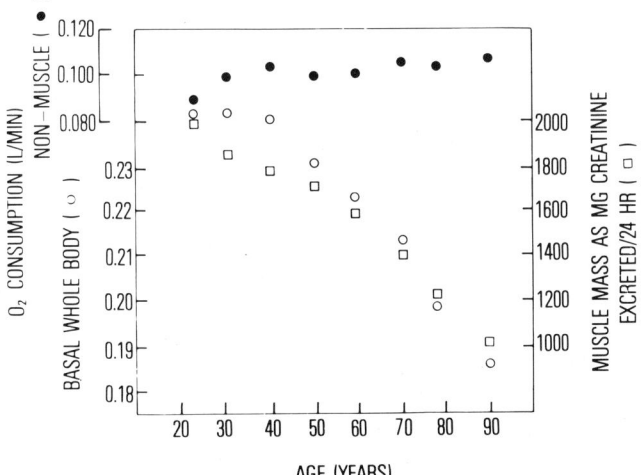

Figure 29–1. Basal oxygen consumption (BMR) and age in male subjects. Note decrease of whole-body oxygen consumption with age (○). Muscle mass, in this study estimated from creatinine excretion (□), also decreases with age. Oxygen consumption calculated per unit nonmuscle metabolic mass (●), however, shows no such decrease. Thus the age-related decrease of BMR is considered to be a function of altered body composition with age rather than a result of diminished thyroid function. Similar age-related decreases of muscle mass can also be shown with measurements of intracellular water or of body potassium. All of these estimates (see also Fig. 29–2) decrease with age. (Modified from Tzankoff, S. P., and Norris, A. H.: Effect of muscle mass decrease on age-related BMR changes. *J. Appl. Physiol.* 43:1001, 1977.)

Thyroid Function Studies

Radioiodide Uptake

While the technical and conceptual limitations of the use of conventional thyroid "function tests" to assess age-related physiologic changes have been reviewed elsewhere (Gregerman and Davis, 1978), the effect of age on the results of the more commonly used tests deserves some mention here. Decreases of radioiodide uptake have been described in elderly subjects, but the magnitude of such changes is small and the statistical variance so large that it serves no useful purpose to establish age-related normal clinical ranges. A partial explanation for the small magnitude of the age-related decrease of uptake is the decrease of renal function in the elderly, which results in alteration of handling of tracer iodide by the thyroid.

The observed decrease of thyroidal radioiodide uptake implies that thyroid function decreases with advancing age. However, the age-related decrease cannot be interpreted without information on plasma inorganic iodide levels during aging. Iodide uptake in absolute terms (AIU) is certainly one measure of hormone formation rate, but must be calculated from the product of thyroid radioiodide clearance and plasma inorganic iodide concentration. Recent data clearly show decreases of AIU in both men and women, despite an increase of plasma iodide in elderly women (Hansen et al., 1975). These data are in agreement with those derived from measurements showing a decline of TH secretion rate (see Thyroxine Disposal).

Plasma Thyroid Hormones and Binding Protein Concentrations

Until recently in most studies of normal healthy adults, plasma thyroxine (T_4) showed no change at advanced age or decreased only slightly. Recent studies of large numbers of subjects do suggest that, despite apparent care to exclude individuals who might be ill, a modest decrease of T_4, not exceeding 15%, may be encountered (Gregerman and Davis, 1978). A recent study reporting elevation of plasma TSH in the elderly did not observe a significant decrease of T_4 in the study population as a whole but did show a decrease in those subjects who had elevated levels of TSH (Sawin et al., 1979). The implications of this observation are discussed separately (see Thyrotropin).

A number of early reports seemed to establish a substantial decrease of plasma triiodothyronine (T_3) with aging (Gregerman and Davis, 1978). Later workers reported only a modest decrease in plasma T_3 (20%) over the adult age span when ill subjects were excluded (Bermudez et al., 1975). However, a careful reexamination of this issue has denied any decrease of T_3 with aging when the elderly subjects were carefully screened for illness (Olsen et al., 1978). The slow resolution of this issue emphasizes again the need for careful clinical screening of subject populations and determination of the influence of illness on plasma hormone levels before attributing changes to aging *per se*.

The concentrations of iodothyronine-binding proteins have been reported to be age-related. Thyroxine-binding globulin (TBG) is said to increase while thyroxine-binding prealbumin (TBPA) falls at advanced age. Despite these changes of binding proteins, neither plasma-free T_4 concentration nor the free T_4 index appears to be affected at advanced age, although one recent report suggests a significant fall of free T_4 (Gregerman and Davis, 1978). In evaluating these reports, one should bear in mind again that the influence of illness may not have been appreciated. For example, in one report elderly healthy subjects were said to have shown a substantial increase of TBG and decreases of T_4 and T_3 (Hesch et al., 1977). The change in T_3 suggests, however, that the population may have included more ill persons than was appreciated; one can only speculate whether the TBG and T_4 results were similarly affected. Acute and chronic illnesses can certainly affect the plasma T_4, the concentrations of both TBG and TBPA, and the free T_4 (Lutz et al., 1972). Since such illnesses are, of course, common in the elderly, changes of these parameters are not readily attributable to age alone (Jefferys et al., 1972).

Studies of these issues in animals are interesting but not readily applicable as model systems for the situation in man. A study of two strains of mice showed plasma T_4 (measured as protein-bound iodine) which decreased 30% and 65% at advanced age, clearly illustrating the importance of genetic determinants (Eleftheriou, 1975). In the rabbit, plasma T_4 is also strain-dependent (Davis et al., 1966). These reports should be kept in mind in interpreting discordant data in widely separated human populations.

Thyrotropin-Releasing Hormone and Thyrotropin

Thyrotropin-Releasing Hormone

The influence of age on the response of the pituitary to TRH has been studied by a number of investigators. The results have varied considerably. Early findings showed a clear and progressive decrease with age in elderly men (Snyder and Utiger, 1972a). The same investigators later were unable to demonstrate an effect of age in elderly women (Snyder and Utiger, 1972b). The decrease with age in men was confirmed by another study from the United States that also failed to observe an age effect in women, although only middle-aged rather than very elderly women were studied (Azizi et al., 1975). In complete contrast, a report on a large number of European subjects showed no age-related decrease of TRH responsiveness in elderly men but did show an unequivocal decrease in elderly females (Wenzel et al., 1974).

These conflicting findings must be compared to a study of a group of Japanese subjects in which TRH responses were unequivocally increased in the elderly (Ohara et al., 1974). Moreover, doses of TRH that produced suboptimal responses in young adults were already maximal in the elderly. Thus, in this population of apparently normal elderly subjects, also characterized by unchanged levels of T_4 but frequently showing elevated levels of basal TSH, aging is accompanied by both increased sensitivity to TRH and hyperresponsiveness with maximal doses. Such results suggest that genetic or subtle environmental factors may strongly influence the endocrine responses during aging in man and call for caution in drawing generalized conclusions from single populations.

Aging in the rat is reported to result in sex-dependent decreased responsiveness to TRH. Maximal response to TRH was decreased by one-half in old animals; no age effect was seen in females. Orchiectomy produced decreased responsiveness to TRH in young but not old animals. Treatment with testosterone reversed the effect of orchiectomy in the young animals and increased TRH response in the old (Chen and Walfish, 1979). Since, in addition, plasma testosterone decreases in the old rat, age-

dependent decrease of testicular function may partially explain the effect of age on TRH responsiveness in this species. The rat, however, may be an inappropriate model for changes in man, since some strains, including the one in which response to TRH was shown to change, show age-related decreases of plasma T_4. Moreover, in man an age-related decrease of testosterone is not a consistent finding (see Male Gonadal Function).

Thyrotropin

Levels of TSH during childhood are similar to those seen in adult life, during which no change occurs until advanced age. Until recently it was believed that plasma TSH concentration does not change with age. Earlier studies in the United States of relatively small numbers of subjects were unable to discern any changes (Azizi et al., 1975; Snyder and Utiger, 1972a), while a number of reports from abroad pointed to an increase of basal TSH at advanced age (Cuttelod et al., 1974; Lauridsen et al., 1974; Lemarchand-Béraud and Vannotti, 1969; Ohara et al., 1974; Wenzel et al., 1974). Recently a study of several hundred elderly men and women in the United States showed that about 3% of elderly men and 8% of elderly women have clearly elevated basal levels of TSH (Sawin et al., 1979). Similar results were reported from a community survey in Great Britain (Turnbridge et al., 1977). In some of the early reports failure to appreciate this finding may have been due to the small numbers of subjects studied. However, the possibility exists that the characteristics of the subject populations account for these differences (see Thyrotropin-Releasing Hormone). Moreover, the finding of elevated basal TSH with aging takes on special significance in view of the possible decrease with age of circulating levels of T_4 and T_3 (see Plasma Thyroid Hormones and Binding Protein Concentrations). Increased basal TSH and hyperresponsiveness to TRH are, of course, features of hypothyroidism, and one might be tempted to interpret these findings as indicative of widespread latent hypothyroidism in the elderly. Such a view is not justified at this time. On the other hand, the identification of a small but significant proportion of the elderly with such subclinical hypothyroidism now seems to be a regular event (see below).

The influence of age on the response of the thyroid to TSH is not resolved. One can infer from the observations that most elderly persons maintain normal plasma T_4 at normal levels of TSH and that no striking age effect exists. An extensive study of thyroidal responsiveness to exogenous heterologous (bovine) TSH in supraphysiologic amounts gave no evidence of diminished responsiveness (Einhorn, 1958), while a decrease was later reported (Lederer and Bataille, 1969; Scazziga et al., 1968). In the one animal species studied (mouse), the thyroidal response to TSH was definitely diminished (Eleftheriou, 1975). During aging in the rat the secretion of a high molecular weight form of TSH has been reported (Klug and Adelman, 1977). The fractional turnover rate of TSH does not appear to be affected by age in the few subjects studied (Cuttelod et al., 1974).

Thyroxine Disposal and Secretion Rate

The decreased thyroidal radioiodide accumulation of adults, together with an unchanging plasma TH concentration with age, led to the conclusion that decreased thyroid activity at advanced age must be due to decreased peripheral disposal of the hormone. Studies with labeled T_4 confirmed this view by demonstrating that the rate of disposal of T_4 decreases with advancing age (Gregerman et al., 1962), an observation which has been repeatedly confirmed (see Gregerman and Davis, 1978). The magnitude of the change is about 50% over the entire adult age span. This is attributed largely to a progressive slowing of the rate of cellular degradation of the hormone. Since the total plasma T_4 is essentially unchanged, and since in the steady state disposal equals secretion, the decrease in the secretion rate of the thyroid is viewed as being homeostatic (see below).

Mechanism of Altered Metabolic Rate of Thyroxine

The mechanism of the age-related slowing of T_4 disposal is not established, but it may relate in part to altered physical activity, since strenuous exercise appears to accelerate the rate of T_4 metabolism in both animals and man. In the available studies of the relationship of age to T_4 disposal rate, the possible importance of exercise was not appreciated and was not controlled. It remains to be shown, however, whether exercise is an important determinant of T_4 disposal rate within the range of normal activities or whether decreased activity such as that seen in the elderly results in decreased disposal rate. The slowed disposal of T_4 with age does provide an explanation for the clinical impression that elderly hypothyroid subjects appear to require less replacement hormone than do young persons to maintain a euthyroid status. These observations are also in keeping with increased sensitivity of the senescent rat to T_4 (Grad, 1969).

In normal man, the rate of metabolism of T_4 and T_3 in the liver is undoubtedly the major determinant of overall TH disposal rate. In animals, disposal is clearly linked to the metabolic pathway for certain drugs and other chemical agents (Oppenheimer et al., 1968) and can be considered an adaptive mechanism; the same is probably true in the human. The age-related slowing of T_4 disposal in normal man and the acceleration of T_4 and T_3 disposal during certain acute illnesses, even in the elderly, is best explained at present by an alteration in this adaptive regulatory mechanism which is clearly influenced by a variety of physiologic and pathophysiologic factors.

Functional State of the Thyroid

For several reasons, the decrease with age of thyroidal secretion of T_4 should not be viewed as gland "failure." First, the thyroid of the elderly person has good reserve, as judged by an unaltered response to stimulation by exogenous TSH. Second, the plasma T_4 does not fall, as is the case when decreased output of hormone is a primary event. Third, the mechanism for activating hormone secretion at a greatly accelerated rate is maintained even in old age, as evidenced by gross acceleration of T_4 turnover during infectious illness in both old and young subjects (Gregerman and Solomon, 1967). Finally, plasma TSH, a sensitive indicator of primary hypothyroidism, is not elevated in most elderly individuals and usually shows an age-related decreased response to TRH stimulation (see Thyrotropin-Releasing Hormone) rather than the increase that is seen in hypothyroidism.

Altered Thyroid Physiology vs. Thyroid Disease in the Elderly

The age-related decrease of T_4 secretion that seems to occur as a continuous process throughout the adult age span (see Thyroxine Disposal) should be conceptually differentiated from altered thyroid function occurring in a small proportion of the elderly population which develops overt or subclinical hypothyroidism. Surveys of hospitalized patients indicate that about 2% of the elderly may be overtly hypothyroid. If the same is true in nonhospitalized populations, at least this number should have elevations of TSH and an additional proportion would be expected to have less fully developed disease with somewhat elevated TSH and moderately decreased T_4. This seems in fact to be the case (Sawin et al., 1979; Turnbridge et al., 1977; see Thyrotropin-Releasing Hormone and Thyrotropin). These recent surveys may also explain other reports of elevations of TSH in "normal" elderly groups along with statistical reduction of T_4. Additional studies are needed to identify thyroid gland failure, i.e., lack of responsiveness to exogenous TSH, in subjects with elevations of endogenous TSH or to identify age-related alterations of thyroidal sensitivity to TSH.

The "Euthyroid Sick Syndrome" vs. Hypothyroidism

Very recently new considerations have arisen in connection with the problem of the diagnosis of hypothyroidism in severely ill and almost invariably elderly patients (Kaptein et al., 1978, 1979). The possibility of hypothyroidism is usually raised by some aspect of the gross appearance of the patient or a finding such as hypothermia. The plasma T_4 and free T_4 index may be well into the hypothyroid range. However, a diagnosis of hypothyroidism cannot be made on the basis of these results alone. The free T_4 will often be found to be normal rather than low; if low, the value will often not be reduced in proportion to the T_4 and free T_4 index. In all such cases the TSH is normal, a finding which rules out primary hypothyroidism but does not exclude the rare possibility of secondary (pituitary) hypothyroidism. The TRH test is said to be normal in these cases, thus excluding secondary hypothyroidism. If clinical recovery ensues, the exception rather than the rule in such cases, the T_4 returns to normal. To date this syndrome has been recognized only in very severely ill patients, but it probably also occurs in chronically ill, nonhospitalized individuals. This phenomenon must be excluded to avoid an incorrect diagnosis of hypothyroidism and inappropriate therapy in these elderly patients.

Hyperthyroidism and Hypothyroidism in the Elderly

The clinical diagnosis of these common diseases is more difficult in the elderly. Many of the features seen in the young may be absent in the elderly, and the old person is much more likely to present with apparent involvement of a single organ system (e.g., heart disease with congestive heart failure). In addition, many aspects of both diseases are nonspecific; in the elderly they are frequently attributed to other disorders. Hyperthyroidism and hypothyroidism in the elderly have been reviewed in detail elsewhere (Davis and Davis, 1974; Zellman, 1968).

The laboratory diagnosis of abnormalities of thyroid function is similarly more difficult in old persons. Elevation of plasma TSH at advanced age and its relationship to hypothyroidism in the elderly population has already been discussed (see Thyrotropin). The occurrence of clinical hyperthyroidism in the face of normal plasma TH concentrations is a major problem. In one group of elderly hyperthyroid patients the most striking finding was the high frequency (35%) of normal concentrations of plasma T_3 (Caplan et al., 1978); elevation of plasma T_3 is almost invariable in younger adults. Similarly, significant proportions of both young and old patients also had normal levels of T_4 and free T_4 index, and a small proportion of both groups had only elevated plasma T_3 and "T_3 toxicosis." The radioiodide uptake was normal in many elderly patients with Graves' disease (30%) and in the majority with toxic nodular goiter (70%) (Caplan et al., 1978), although current lack of diagnostic usefulness of the radioiodide uptake measurement is not unique for the elderly. The limited usefulness of the TRH test in establishing the diagnosis of hyperthyroidism has been implied (see Thyrotropin-Releasing Hormone). An adequate response to TRH serves to exclude a diagnosis of hyperthyroidism in the elderly; inadequate response is not diagnostic, since some normal elderly persons fail to respond to TRH.

The existence, especially in elderly patients, of hyperthyroidism manifested by elevated T_4 but with normal T_3 has been questioned (Gavin et al., 1979). Transient elevations of T_4 do occur in patients with acute nonthyroidal illness; the T_3 is normal or low in such cases. Differentiation of this state from hyperthyroidism may require follow-up observations.

Occult but clinically important thyroid disease can be found in a small proportion of hospitalized patients. A number of surveys are remarkably similar, reporting about 2% occurrence of unsuspected hypothyroidism; hyperthyroidism appears to be much less common in most such surveys (Atkinson et al., 1978).

Effects of Thyroid Hormones in Old Animals

Very little is known about the effects of altered amounts of thyroid hormones on the processes of aging. In mature animals rendered hypothyroid, no effect on longevity was apparent, although excessive amounts of TH produced evidence of accelerated aging of collagen (Everitt and Burgess, 1976).

In terms of TH effects on biochemical parameters, the response of the TH-sensitive mitochondrial α-glycerophosphate dehydrogenase of liver to large amounts of T_3 was markedly reduced during maturation between 1 and 6 months in the rat (Schwartz et al., 1979). On the other hand, in mature and senescent animals age had no effect on the control of α-glycerophosphate dehydrogenase by either reduced or excessive amounts of T_4 (Bulos et al., 1972a). Similarly, control of mitochondrial succinate oxidation was unaffected by age in experimental hypo- and hyperthyroidism (Bulos et al., 1972b). However, the rate of induction of cardiac hypertrophy in mice was slower in old than in adult animals, presumably reflecting the decreased rate of protein synthetic capacity of the hearts of the old animals (Florini et al., 1973). Other studies have reported increased oxygen consumption and protein catabolic responses of old animals given pharmacologic amounts of T_4 (Grad, 1969; Frolkis et al., 1973). In an exception to these reports, resistance of "minimal oxygen consumption" to TH has been reported in aging rats (Denkla, 1974). Thus, old animals show a range of biochemical effects from increased or decreased levels of TH, some being unaffected, others showing delayed or decreased effects, and still others even increased responses, depending on the system involved and the parameter studied.

ADRENALS

Adrenal Anatomy

Age-related changes in adrenal structure and function are highly species-specific. Unique and perhaps the most dramatic are the massive hypertrophy and hyperactivity of the adrenal of the spawning (senescent) Pacific salmon. In other species, however, involutional changes are the rule. Microscopically, one sees accumulation of pigment, connective tissue proliferation, and loss of steroid-containing lipid. Vascular dilation and small hemorrhages are common. Cytologically, the most striking and perhaps functionally most important alteration is the fragmentation and gross alteration of the mitochondrial structure (Bourne, 1967). Size changes in the adrenal may also be seen. In the fowl, for example, the adrenals show an overall decrease in size with age, while in the rat, the zona glomerulosa is selectively and grossly atrophied, with the remainder of the gland relatively little affected. Loss of the zona glomerulosa correlates with decreased juxtaglomerular cell granularity in the kidney and with diminished neurosecretory material in the neurohypophysis. These changes are interpreted as showing diminished activity of the renin-angiotensin-aldosterone system in the aging rat (Dunihue, 1965). Alterations of neurohypophyseal function in the rat are discussed elsewhere (see Antidiuretic Hormone).

The human adrenal shows no major anatomic changes, such as those of decreased gland size or loss of zona glomerulosa, but the microscopic alterations described above are seen, and cortical nodule formation is frequent (Dobbie, 1969). Moreover, a variety of age-related alterations of adrenal secretory activity have been extensively studied and will be discussed below.

Glucocorticoids

For the most important glucocorticoid of man, cortisol, the age-related alterations resemble those of T_4. Plasma cortisol concentrations and diurnal rhythm remain unaltered, even at very advanced age, but secretion rate decreases about 30% over the entire adult age span. This is a consequence of slowed metabolic disposal and undoubtedly the result of an age-related alteration of the enzymatic activities involved in hepatic steroid metabolism (West et al., 1961; Gherondache et al., 1967; Romanoff et al., 1961; Blichert-Toft, 1975). The reduced secretion rate is closely paralleled by an age-related decrease of urinary excretion of the 17-hydroxy and 17-ketogenic steroid metabolites of cortisol. Urinary free cortisol does not change in adults up to age 50; studies of older subjects have not been reported (Juselius and Kenny, 1974). In several species other than man (cattle, goat, rat) plasma glucocorticoid concentrations do not decrease with advancing age (Riegle and Nellor, 1967; Riegle et al., 1968; Hess and Riegle, 1972).

Many investigators have attributed significance to the observation that the excretion of glucocorticoid metabolites and the secretion rate of cortisol, when expressed per unit of creatinine excretion, do not decrease with age (Pincus, 1961; Gherondache et al., 1967). The observation is true, but the physiologic significance of this calculation is nil, since it is total muscle mass that determines creatinine excretion, while the liver, not muscle, is the major site of adrenal steroid metabolism (Moncloa et al., 1963). Thus there is no good physiologic basis for directly relating steroid production to muscle mass or to creatinine excretion. To express glucocorticoid excretion or secretion in terms of any other unrelated measurement that shows an age-correlated decrease would also "abolish" or "correct" the age-related glucocorticoid change and would be equally meaningless. However, expression of excretion of urinary steroid metabolites per unit creatinine remains a clinically useful maneuver.

Although the normal diurnal variation of plasma cortisol is preserved in elderly healthy subjects, in the presence of combinations of common diseases abnormal diurnal patterns are observed (Grad et al., 1971). Such observations emphasize the influence of illness on endocrine function. Careful selection of subjects is essential in studies of human aging to distinguish biologic changes of aging from those secondary to disease states.

Adrenal Androgens

The progressive decrease in men and women of the urinary excretion of 17-ketosteroids with age to mean levels in the elderly that are about one-half those in young adults is a reflection of the decreasing production of the so-called adrenal androgens, secreted chiefly as the sulfate conjugates of dehydroepiandrosterone (DHA) and androsterone. The plasma levels of these specific steroids are closely age-related (Vihko, 1966) and in some individuals practically disappear from the plasma at advanced age (Migeon et al., 1957). Androstenedione of adrenal origin also decreases rather abruptly in women between ages 45 and 55, with little change thereafter (Crilly et al., 1979). Decrease of urinary excretion of DHA is considerably greater than that of total 17-ketosteroids (Gherondache et al., 1967).

The biologic significance of these adrenal secretory products is not known. In the past, attempts have been made to attribute "anabolic" function to the adrenal androgens and to relate them to a "balance" with "catabolic" glucocorticoids and in turn to age-related phenomena, such as osteoporosis and even neoplasia; to date, however, no definite concepts have been established. Unfortunately, the adrenal androgens have not received the study they deserve, although DHA has recently been shown to have some biologic effects, at least in pharmacologic amounts (Schwartz, 1979). Certainly, roles for these steroids in such functions as the maintenance of muscle or of bone have not been excluded (Pincus, 1961). In terms of quantities produced, the adrenal androgens equal or even exceed those of all the other adrenal steroids combined. It would be most remarkable, considering merely the amounts secreted, if they were proved to be devoid of physiologic effects, but until such time as a functional role is demonstrated, we shall remain ignorant of the significance of one of the most striking age-related alterations of hormone secretion.

Aldosterone

Studies of aldosterone metabolism during aging have indicated decreased metabolic clearance rate, decreased secretory rate, and decreased plasma concentration in elderly subjects (Flood et al., 1967; Sambhi et al., 1973; Crane and Harris, 1976). The urinary excretion of aldosterone also falls progressively with age. When sodium intake is unrestricted, the decrease is approximately 40%. The effect of age is more striking when examined under conditions of sodium restriction. Although older persons do augment aldosterone excretion with sodium restriction, a progressive decrease in this adaptive response is seen, so that elderly subjects (age 70) show elevations to levels which are only 30 to 40% of those seen in young adults (Crane and Harris, 1976). In terms of control mechanisms for aldosterone, the secretion of renin shows an age-related decrease which parallels that of aldosterone. In one-third of females over age 70, however, plasma renin levels not only are low but also fail to show the characteristic rise which is usually seen in young subjects during sodium restriction or postural change. These striking age-related alterations of aldosterone and renin secretion have obvious importance for interpreting data from hypertensive populations and, in this context, stress the need for age-related standards.

ACTH and Tests of Adrenocortical Reserve

Adrenal Responses to ACTH

The effect of age on the response of the human adrenal to stimulation by ACTH is controversial. In terms of glucocorticoids, several investigators have reported decreased urinary 17-hydroxysteroid excretion by elderly subjects after ACTH administration, while others have observed no effect of age on urinary excretion or on plasma glucocorticoid response (Gherondache et al., 1967; Moncloa et al., 1963; Blichert-Toft et al., 1970). In regard to the excretion of adrenal androgens after ACTH administration, there is also some disagreement, but definitely decreased responses have been reported (Moncloa et al., 1963). In some species (cow, goat), a striking age effect is seen. Despite the fact that basal levels of plasma corticosteroids are unchanged with age, the old animals show little or no response to ACTH stimulation as measured by plasma concentration of cortisol and corticosterone (Riegle and Nellor, 1967; Riegle et al., 1968). Response to ACTH appears to be grossly intact in the senescent rat, although the steroid output of the old animals is somewhat less after stimulation (Hess and Riegle, 1972). Other studies have indicated that a longer time is required for initiation of ACTH action in the old animals (Rotenberg and Adelman, 1972).

Secretion of dehydroepiandrosterone (DHA) in elderly people has been studied by measurements of plasma DHA following ACTH administration. Basal DHA concentrations were very much lower in the elderly than in the young (see Adrenal Androgens). Although plasma levels increased after ACTH in both groups, responses in the elderly ranged from minimal to delayed, and in no instance did they approach the levels seen in younger subjects (Yamaji and Ibayashi, 1969). This and other observations clearly indicate that age has a greater effect on adrenal androgen production than on the glucocorticoids, and thus age has a highly selective effect on specific pathways of synthesis in the adrenal. The mechanism of this age effect is not known, but recent evidence suggests that adrenal androgen production is regulated by gonadal hormones (Abraham and Maroulis, 1975; Barmach de Niepomniszsze et al., 1973; Maroulis and Abraham, 1976). Since both estrogen and testosterone secretion decrease with age (see Male Gonadal Function and Female Gonadal Function), at least part of the age-related decrease of adrenal androgen secretion may be a consequence of altered gonadal function during aging.

Following administration of ACTH, plasma estrogens increase, presumably owing to increased secretion of androstenedione and its subsequent conversion, principally to estrone. This response to ACTH is well maintained at advanced age, although the increase above basal is somewhat reduced (Murakami et al., 1976; Kley et al., 1975).

ACTH Reserve: Stress and the Metyrapone Test

The effect of age on release of ACTH from the pituitary has been studied indirectly, i.e., as increased plasma cortisol following stress of insulin-induced hypoglycemia or surgery, or as increased plasma desoxycortisol (compound S) following the administration of the 11-hydroxylase inhibitor metyrapone. Recently direct measurements of plasma ACTH have been made during surgery and following metyrapone administration.

Insulin-induced hypoglycemia produces similar effects on plasma cortisol in young and old subjects (Friedman et al., 1969; Cartlidge et al., 1970). Surgical stress also gave no indication of impairment of ACTH release as shown by plasma cortisol responses or radioimmunoassay of plasma ACTH. When metyrapone was given on the fifth postoperative day, plasma ACTH levels were much higher than with surgical stress and no exhaustion of ACTH secretory capacity was evident in the old subjects (Blichert-Toft and Hummer, 1976).

A simple interpretation of the effect of age on the metyrapone test, the most commonly used test of ACTH reserve, is not possible. When metyrapone is given orally, the response, as measured by the excretion of 17-ketogenic steroids, of some elderly subjects is diminished. However, when large doses of the inhibitor are given intravenously and the response is measured in terms of increased plasma compound S (deoxycortisol), the values in the elderly are identical to those in young persons (Jensen and Blichert-Toft, 1970; Blichert-Toft et al., 1970). The explanation for this discrepancy could lie in either the dosage or the route of administration of the drug or both, but could also be related to the measured end point of the response. In view of the slowed rate of steroid disposal in the elderly, it is possible that a moderately diminished adrenal response, owing to impaired ACTH release, could be masked when plasma steroid level rather than urine excretion is used as the index of the response. Thus the available evidence fails to indicate any gross impairment in the elderly of the negative feedback mechanism for the release of ACTH, but some degree of impairment is not excluded.

PANCREATIC AND RELATED HORMONES

Insulin and Age-Related Change of Glucose Tolerance

The gradual decline of glucose tolerance with age has been repeatedly documented (see Chapter 9). Following intravenous or oral glucose loads, glucose levels decrease at a progressively slower rate with advancing age (Andres and Tobin, 1977). Thus, in one representative study, 2 hours after a 100-g oral glucose challenge mean glucose levels were 14 mg/dl higher per decade (O'Sullivan, 1974). This phenomenon requires the use of age-related standards for the diagnosis of diabetes (Davidson, 1979) or a device such as a nomogram (Andres and Tobin, 1977). Fasting glucose has been reported to increase with age, but the effect was small (2 mg/dl decade; Berger et al., 1978) and has not been seen by others (Elahi et al., 1978).

The mechanisms of the age-related decline of glucose tolerance have been extensively investigated in terms of insulin secretion but the results are conflicting. Basal levels of insulin do not appear to change with age (Berger et al., 1978; Elahi et al., 1978). However, it is the early phase of insulin secretion that is an important determinant of glucose tolerance. Some studies have shown impaired early-phase insulin secretion (Andres and Tobin, 1977; Andersen et al., 1976) while others have failed to observe such changes (Dudl and Ensinck, 1977; Palmer and Ensinck, 1975; DeFronzo, 1979).

Another aspect of age-related changes of glucose tolerance relates to possible alterations of insulin sensitivity (or resistance). A critical problem in studies on aging is the confounding effect of adiposity expressed in either absolute or relative terms. The overweight state (obesity) is regularly accompanied by decreased sensitivity to insulin. Since a change of body composition with loss of muscle and increase of fat (relative adiposity) is a regular accompaniment of aging (Dudl and Ensinck, 1973; Novak, 1972; Fig. 29–2), one might expect aging man to show, even at constant body weight, a decline in insulin sensitivity and therefore glucose tolerance. However, effects of aging on glucose tolerance are still apparent even after changes in body composition are taken into account (Davidson, 1979; Dudl and Ensinck, 1973). Theoretical considerations aside, even the experimental data on the issue of insulin sensitivity and age are conflicting. Recent studies have used the same technique of glucose or glucose-insulin infusion ("clamp" technique) but have reported both decreased (DeFronzo, 1979) and unchanged sensitivity to insulin (Andres and Tobin, 1977).

An issue which has never been resolved is that of the nature of the radioimmunologically measured insulin of plasma and the validity of this measurement in aging man. Some data suggest that in older subjects a larger proportion of radioimmunologically reactive hormone is actually proinsulin (Duckworth and Kitabchi, 1976). Since proin-

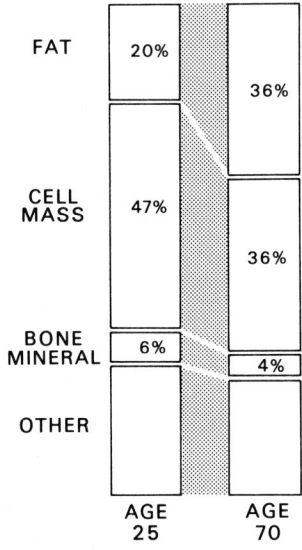

BODY COMPOSITION AND AGE

Figure 29–2. Idealized representation of the age-related change of body composition of male subjects. (Young females [age 25] have nearly twice as much body fat as do males but show a smaller increase of fat [and loss of cell mass] with age than do males.) Since adiposity (increased total body fat) has a major effect on glucose tolerance and insulin secretion (see text), this age-related change of body composition (relative adiposity) may account for some of the effect of age on glucose and insulin metabolism.

sulin is metabolically much less active than insulin, this age-related alteration of secretory pattern may contribute to an explanation of the observed decline in glucose tolerance. Heretofore reported plasma insulin values determined by radioimmunoassay have been based on the assumption that all of the measured material is metabolically active, when in fact in older subjects less than the total amount of the hormone is effective. As recently reviewed, the mechanisms of the effect of aging on glucose metabolism may be heterogeneous and variable among subjects and subject populations (Davidson, 1979).

Studies in animals have not been immediately helpful in explaining the phenomena observed in man. Aging in the rat (also accompanied by increasing adiposity) is associated with increased numbers of β cells and insulin storage in islets but a decrease in glucose-stimulated insulin release (Reaven et al., 1979). Most of these changes in the rat are seen during maturation rather than in senescence. Measurements of insulin receptors in several tissues of the rat suggest a decrease of insulin receptors in liver (Kahn and Roth, 1976) but not in fat (Olefsky and Reaven, 1975).

Studies of insulin binding in human tissues have been limited to circulating monocytes, in which insulin binding was not affected during aging (Helderman, 1978), and cultured fibroblasts, where the data are not consistent, showing increased (Goldstein et al., 1979), unaltered (Hollenberg and Schneider, 1979), and decreased receptors (Ito et al., 1976). The notion that obesity is invariably associated with decreased insulin receptor number has been recently challenged (Misbin et al., 1979), thus further undermining any ready explanation for an effect of adiposity on decreasing glucose tolerance.

Glucagon

Examination of the role of hormones other than insulin has not helped to explain the age-related change of glucose tolerance. Glucagon release is not altered during aging in response to glucose loading (Dudl and Ensinck, 1977). Basal levels of glucagon have been reported to increase with age in one study (Berger et al., 1978) but not in another (Elahi et al., 1978).

Gastrointestinal and Other Hormones

A group of hormones originating in the gastrointestinal tract ("gut hormones") have been shown to play an important role in glucose homeostasis (see Chapter 15). It has long been known that oral glucose causes a much greater release of insulin than does an equal amount of glucose delivered intravenously. This effect is mediated by secretion of an insulinotropic enteric hormone (also known as gastrointestinal inhibitory peptide, GIP) after ingestion of glucose. Studies to date suggest no impairment of GIP secretion in the elderly (Raizes et al., 1976). The plasma concentration of human pancreatic polypeptide, a substance of unknown function, has been found to increase during aging (Berger et al., 1978).

Diabetes Mellitus and Aging

Evidence is accumulating that accelerated aging or senescence characterizes the human diabetic state and its complications (Vracko and Benditt, 1974). Primary abnormalities related to aging may be on a genetic basis, expressed in all cells, and they may be exaggerated by hyperglycemia.

Table 29–1. DIABETES MELLITUS AS ACCELERATED CELLULAR AGING

Cells Showing Premature Death or Impaired Replication Potential	Clinical Abnormality
Beta cells, pancreatic islets	Decreased insulin secretion; hyperglycemia
Alpha cells, pancreatic islets	Increased glucagon secretion; hyperglycemia
Capillary endothelial cells	Basement membrane thickening; microangiopathy
Schwann cells	Neuropathy
Mural cells, retina	Retinopathy
Osteoblasts	Osteoporosis
Arterial endothelial cells	Atherosclerosis
Arterial smooth muscle cells	Atherosclerosis
T cells	Increased autoantibodies
Skin fibroblasts (cell culture)	Unknown

Accelerated aging in tissues may be manifested by decreased replication of β cells of the pancreatic islets in response to injury and accelerated rate of cell death of endothelial cells in capillaries leading to diabetic microangiopathy. Aging of cells can be detected in tissue culture of skin fibroblasts from diabetic patients by decreased replication rates and life span in culture (Vracko and Benditt, 1975; Gleason and Goldstein, 1978; Goldstein et al., 1979; Rowe et al., 1977). The width of muscle capillary basement membrane increases with age in healthy subjects, and this thickening is accelerated in diabetes (Kilo et al., 1972; Jordan and Perley, 1972). The accelerated and premature atherosclerosis found in diabetic patients could in part result from age-related effects on arterial smooth muscle cells and endothelial cells (Bierman and Ross, 1977; Bierman, 1978a). Cultured human arterial smooth muscle cells show decreased replicative life span as a function of donor age (Bierman, 1978b).

Collagen production in cultured fibroblasts from diabetic subjects appears to be abnormal (Kohn and Hensse, 1977). Enzymatic digestion of diaphragm tendon collagen samples allows determination of "chronological ages" in human subjects. In such studies juvenile diabetics appeared to have collagen resembling that of much older subjects (Hamlin et al., 1975). Bone mass, determined by the direct photon absorption method in both juvenile and maturity-onset diabetics, was markedly decreased (Levin et al., 1976; McNair et al., 1978), resembling osteoporosis of aging. It was postulated that generalized osteopenia in diabetes may be due to a decrease in bone formation rather than to an increase in bone loss and may be a manifestation of early aging of all cells as a basic defect of diabetes. A summary is presented in Table 29–1 of the accumulated evidence suggesting that at least some forms of human diabetes mellitus may reflect a cellular abnormality in all tissues related to premature cell death and impaired cellular replication potential associated with accelerated aging.

MALE GONADAL FUNCTION

Sexual Activity in the Male

Although wide individual variation exists, sexual interest, drive, and vigor in the adult male decline with advancing age. Sexual behavior in both elderly men and elderly women appears to be closely related to habits formed during earlier adult life (Pfeiffer and Davis, 1972; Martin, 1977). On the basis of present knowledge, age changes in sexual function cannot be easily related to changes in endocrine status. Recent studies of healthy men clearly show that the age-related decrease of sexual activity is not in the main related to plasma testosterone concentration (Tsitouras et al., 1980). However, in very elderly men sexual activity, though greatly reduced, may yet relate to plasmafree testosterone (see below).

Testosterone

Extensive data indicate that from adolescence to early adulthood plasma testosterone increases greatly, but thereafter no decrease is seen until beyond age 50, after which mean values decrease considerably, according to a number of reports. In those studies which do show age-related decreases of plasma testosterone, the mean for subjects at age 80 to 90 is about 40% of that in the group under age 50. The variability is very great, however. Some subjects in their 80's or even 90's have levels that exceed those in normal young men in their 20's, while in occasional elderly men the values are as low as those found in normal females (Vermeulen et al., 1972). Although most of these investigations purport to give data for healthy elderly subjects, the study groups are often recruited from homes for the elderly. In several reports in which an effort was made to evaluate only the healthiest of elderly subjects, changes of plasma testosterone with age were very small (Pirke and Doerr, 1973; Lewis et al., 1976) or not evident (Harman et al., 1980; Sparrow et al., 1980). In the most recent studies in which no age changes were seen, the data were obtained from several community-dwelling populations, suggesting that health status may indeed have influenced the many earlier reports of decreased plasma testosterone at advanced age. Information on plasma 5α-dihydrotestosterone, most of which arises in the periphery, is less extensive but suggests either a small decrease at advanced age (Pirke and Doerr, 1973; Lewis et al., 1976), — no change (Pirke and Doerr, 1975; Harman and Tsitouras, 1980), or an actual increase (Horton et al., 1975).

Whether the discrepancies between the various studies in man are due to the effects of illness, genetic differences between the populations studied, or as yet unrecognized factors remains to be determined. Some credence must be given to the possible influence of genetic factors, since age-dependent decrease in testosterone production in animals is not only species- but even strain-dependent. Plasma testosterone decreases with age in several strains of rat (Gray, 1978; Tsitouras et al., 1979) and in the rabbit. However, in the mouse such a change is seen in some strains but not in others (Bronson and Desjardins, 1977; Finch et al., 1977).

An additional change with age in plasma testosterone exists, beyond the decrease in total hormone concentration. Some 40 to 45% of the testosterone in plasma is normally associated with a specific testosterone-binding globulin (TeBG). With advancing age the concentration of TeBG increases by up to 50%; the result is an increase in that fraction of hormone that is bound to protein and a decrease in the concentration of free or physiologically active hormone (Vermeulen et al., 1971, 1972; Pirke and Doerr, 1973, 1975). The most recently available study of healthy elderly men, however, reports only a very small increase with age in testosterone binding and no effect at all on free testosterone (Harman and Tsitouras, 1980).

Kinetic studies have directly demonstrated that, when it is observed, decreased plasma testosterone is due to a decrease in rate of hormone production. An age-related decrease in the amount and alteration of the pattern of excretion of testosterone metabolites (androstanediols and androsterone-etiocholanolone ratios) have also been seen (Vermeulen et al., 1972; Zumoff et al., 1976). Although plasma testosterone levels are much lower in females than in males, the available data indicate that no decrease in testosterone occurs during senescence in the female.

Estrogens and Progesterone in the Male

Estrogen production in the male, although always much less than in the female, appears to decrease progressively with age, at least as judged by urinary excretion data, with about 30% less total estrogen being excreted at age 70 than at age 30. However, the biologically more active hormones, estradiol and estrone, together decrease by over 50%, whereas estriol levels are relatively unchanged until late in life, when they decrease slightly, by about 15% (Pincus et al., 1954; Sköldefors et al., 1975). In contrast to the decline of urinary excretion of estrogens, a number of studies have reported increases with age in plasma estradiol and estrone in males. Increased conversion of androstenedione to estrone in peripheral tissues may explain this finding (Hemsell et al., 1974). The physiologic significance of increased estrogens is not apparent, although it may be responsible for the increase of testosterone-binding globulin (TeBG). In any case, the increase in plasma estrogens is not merely secondary to increased TeBG, since free estradiol is increased nearly as much as the total (Pirke and Doerr, 1975). A recent study of healthy elderly men reported no increase in plasma estrogens with age; the same group of subjects showed no decrease in plasma testosterone (Harman and Tsitouras, 1980).

Estrogen in the male arises from both the adrenals and the testes, but the relative contribution of each source to the apparent age-related decrease in estrogen production is not established. The male also produces significant quantities of progesterone, again with both the adrenals and the testes contributing. The production rate in elderly males falls to 40% of that in young subjects. Excretion of urinary pregnanediol, the major metabolite of progesterone, decreases at advanced age to 25% of that seen in young adults (Gherondache et al., 1967).

Gonadotropins in the Male

The very large increase in gonadotropin excretion seen in the postmenopausal or castrate woman has no counterpart in the male, although elderly men show some increase in urinary gonadotropins. The increase in FSH is greater than that in LH (Christiansen, 1972). Plasma LH and FSH also increase and in some very elderly men approach the levels of castrates. Pituitary LH and FSH release can be further increased with GnRH; elderly men show only a slight decrease in responsiveness (Snyder et al., 1975; Harman, 1978). These findings suggest primary gonadal failure as an explanation for the elevation of gonadotropins, as does the report that stimulation of Leydig cell testosterone secretion by hCG is greatly blunted in the elderly (Rubens et al., 1974). The maintained levels of testosterone in the elderly may depend on increased levels of gonadotropins, which would then be viewed as compensatory. Altered regulation of gonadotropin secretion, i.e., decreased sensitivity to feedback inhibition by gonadal hormones, has also been observed recently and may contribute to the finding of elevated gonadotropins in elderly men (Muta et al., 1980).

Studies in animals such as the rat are interesting but do not help explain the phenomena seen in man. The decrease in plasma testosterone in the rat, for example, is accompanied by a decrease in LH and FSH rather than by an increase, as seen in man (Gray, 1978; Simpkins et al., 1977). In this species the decrease in gonadotropins seems to be the primary event leading to decreased testosterone secretion. Decreased gonadotropin secretion may in turn be related to altered hypothalamic neurotransmitter metabolism (Simpkins et al., 1977). A delayed testosterone secretory response to hCG was shown in old animals, while chronic administration abolished the delayed secretory response (Harman et al., 1978). In addition, age effects on Leydig cell function in the rat have been shown *in vitro* as decreased testosterone production in response to hCG. Unlike the results *in vivo,* the testosterone secretory response to hCG could not be restored by prolonged exposure. Gonadotropin receptor numbers were only slightly reduced, and intracellular cAMP formation was unaffected (Tsitouras et al., 1980). Species and strain differences are evident from studies in the mouse. One strain that showed decreased testosterone secretion with age also showed decrease in LH but not FSH (Bronson and Dejardins, 1977), while another strain that showed no change of testosterone had plasma levels of gonadotropins that were unaffected by aging (Finch et al., 1977).

FEMALE GONADAL FUNCTION

Female Reproduction

Cessation of reproductive function in the human female is related to the cessation of ovarian function that occurs at menopause. This event in the human is due primarily not to altered hypothalamic or pituitary function but to changes in the ovary. In contrast, cessation of reproduction in the rat is due not to ovarian or pituitary failure in most of the animals, but to altered hypothalamico-pituitary mechanisms controlling LH release and ovulation. A small proportion of rats show reproductive failure resulting from development of pituitary tumors during senescence (Huang and Meites, 1975). A disturbance of neurotransmitter function has been suspected, since administration of L-dopa restores estrus cycles. Direct injection of dopa into the medial preoptic area is also effective, thus appearing to identify a specific anatomic site of involvement (Cooper et al., 1979).

Estrogens

As an invariable accompaniment to aging in the human female, diminished estrogen production is to be contrasted to the far less predictable decrease of testosterone in the male. Decreased estrogen excretion occurs at the menopause, and mean values for estrogen excretion decline further between ages 50 and 60, but thereafter no additional change is evident. In the elderly female, the ovary ceases completely to secrete either estradiol or estrone. Estradiol blood levels decline by over 90% and those of estrone by about 70% (Longcope, 1971). Nonetheless, the urinary excretion of biologically active estrogen is still about one-fifth of that before the menopause. What estrogen remains is produced from the peripheral conversion of steroid precursors, and, in the case of estrone, continued production originates from androstenedione of adrenal origin.

Kinetic studies have indicated that metabolic clearance rates of both estradiol and estrone decrease by about 25%, a change similar in magnitude to that for testosterone and aldosterone. The newer estimates of decreased production rates of estradiol and estrone are in good agreement with older information obtained from bioassays of urinary estrogens (Pincus et al., 1954).

Menopause

The menopause begins with the termination of menstrual bleeding and is due to cessation of secretion of the ovarian hormones. It is an inevitable result of aging. The age at onset varies widely, with a mean of 50 years, but it may be as early as 42 years or as late as 60. Loss of ovarian follicles, obliteration of ovarian vessels, and fibrosis of ovarian parenchyma are the anatomic correlates. Surgical removal of the ovaries is, of course, followed immediately by menopause.

Menopause is preceded by several years of rising gonadotropin secretion, predominantly FSH. During this period estrogen production, remarkably enough, does not appear to decrease appreciably and ovulation continues (Sherman et al., 1976; Reyes et al., 1977). The explanation of this phenomenon is not at hand. Possibilities include insufficiently sensitive techniques for detecting a premenopausal fall of estrogen production; progressive loss of an ovarian "inhibin"-like substance which may be necessary for suppression of FSH secretion; and age-related alteration of hypothalamico-pituitary sensitivity to feedback inhibition by ovarian hormones. This latter possibility has received some recent support from studies in aging men in whom higher doses of both estrogen and testosterone appear necessary to suppress LH levels (Muta et al., 1980).

Accompanying the hormonal changes are a number of clinical phenomena. Some are simply the result of estrogen deficiency, viz., loss of subcutaneous fat in the vulvar region, leading to atrophic vulvitis and kraurosis vulvae with associated pruritus, and atrophy of vaginal mucosa with loss of rugae and decreased secretion of cervical mucus. These latter changes may lead to dyspareunia in a significant proportion of postmenopausal women but respond readily to local or systemic therapy with estrogens.

The most dramatic symptoms of the menopause are the hot flushes ("flashes") and night sweats that occur in more than half of all women. Typically these episodes are sudden in onset, affect the face and upper thoracic area, and are accompanied by flushing (vasodilatation) and profuse perspiration. Occurring in frequency from every few days to many times daily, these episodes of vasomotor instability are usually thought to disappear within a year or two, but up to 50% of affected women are still symptomatic after 8 years, at least in the case of oophorectomized patients (Aitken et al., 1974). Estrogen therapy is effective in ameliorating or abolishing these episodes. Suggestions that gonadotropin excess rather than estrogen lack is responsible have not been supported by recent work. Although the flush is usually associated with a pulsed release of LH (Tataryn et al., 1979), when estrogen was given over only a few hours, LH release could be abolished without affecting the episodes of flushing (Casper, 1979). Presumably hypothalamic vasomotor function is regulated in feedback fashion by estrogens, but these results show that pulsed gonadotropin release and vasomotor activity can be dissociated.

Other symptoms often associated with the menopause are insomnia, depression, and anxiety. The causal relationship between these phenomena and cessation of estrogen secretion is difficult to assess, as is the effect of replacement therapy. Some evidence suggests that wakefulness may improve with estrogens but effects on psychologic symptoms may not be significant (Thompson and Oswald, 1977).

Estrogen Therapy During Menopause

The place of estrogen therapy for the postmenopausal woman has received considerable attention, most of it more emotional than scientific, and at present no consensus exists. Estrogens have been advocated for preservation of youthful skin, hair, and breasts. No scientific evidence is available to support claims for therapeutic efficacy in these regards. However, there is agreement that estrogens afford prompt relief of vasomotor instability (hot flushes). The only other therapeutic agents used with some success for this purpose are medroxyprogesterone and clonidine. No harmful effects have ever been documented or are likely to occur from short-term, low-dose use of estrogens for the relief of hot flushes. Few would object to the use of estrogens for this purpose or for the treatment of atrophic vaginitis, unless specific contraindication existed.

Little doubt remains that estrogen therapy prevents or greatly slows the age-related loss of bone mineral. Prevention of clinically apparent osteoporosis (fractures) is less well established, although at least retrospective data support this possibility (see Osteoporosis). Before estrogens can be advocated for wide use for the prevention of clinical osteoporosis, questions concerning safety must be resolved. Controversy continues over the issue of whether estrogen increases the risk of endometrial carcinoma, although the current evidence strongly favors such an association. A number of recent studies indicate that the estrogen effect is time-dependent and results in an increased occurrence of endometrial carcinoma after 2 to 6 years of use (Hulka et al., 1980). The possibility of an increased frequency of carcinoma of the breast also continues to be investigated, but a number of studies have failed to show a significant effect in this regard. Estrogen effects on cardiovascular disease and on the coagulation mechanism are also not settled. The data fail to suggest an increase of thromboembolic disease with use of ordinary doses of estrogens in the postmenopausal period, a clear difference from the significant increase seen in premenopausal women treated with estrogen-containing contraceptives. The benefits of therapy in prevention of bone disease, attended by its own morbidity and mortality, will have to be weighed against the risks. This is a judgment which will never be objective. Thus, even if all of these issues are resolved and the risks precisely defined, no firm consensus is likely to emerge. The use of steroids other than estrogens for prevention of bone disease offers promise (see Osteoporosis), but the long-term risks of such therapy also will need assessment.

Practical problems in estrogen therapy also remain. Therapy with orally administered preparations is not defined as regards optimal schedule of administration, the estrogen to be used, or the dose. If the goal of therapy is simulation of the physiologic state that obtains during the years of menstruation, one should probably administer estrogens in cyclic fashion. Cyclic estrogen-progesterone is also feasible. Such therapy does seem to avoid the development of endometrial hyperplasia (Whitehead et al., 1977), a possible precursor of endometrial carcinoma.

The problem of the estrogen to be used and the dose arises because it is difficult to assess an end point of therapy. Physiologic equivalence of the specific estrogens is similarly unresolved. Estradiol, the principal natural estrogen, has been known to be poorly absorbed. Recent preparations of micron-sized particles are better absorbed but even this preparation is rapidly converted to estrone in the gastrointestinal tract (Yen et al., 1975). For this reason and because plasma levels change rapidly, some end point other than hormone concentration in plasma must be used. Plasma gonadotropins are a logical choice, but evidence suggests that hypothalamic sensitivity to feedback suppression may decrease with aging (see Menopause). Thus, greater than physiologic quantities of estrogen may have to be administered after menopause in order to suppress gonadotropins,

and the use of this end point may overestimate the estrogen requirement. This situation is illustrated by the case of the preparation of estrogens (Premarin) that is in widest use in the United States. This material is mainly estrone sulfate. Doses of 0.625 mg daily are thought to be physiologic but fail to suppress gonadotropins to premenopausal values while producing a normal maturation index of vaginal cells and a pharmacologic effect on levels of a number of plasma proteins (e.g., corticosteroid-binding globulin).

Osteoporosis

The progressive decrease of bone density that accompanies aging in both men and women ("involutional osteopenia") is one of the almost inevitable accompaniments of senescence. The rate of bone loss varies between individuals but averages 1% per year after about age 40 in women and somewhat less in men. A clear distinction between this process and that of "osteoporosis" is not possible (Newton-John and Morgan, 1968), but osteoporosis is said to be present when the demineralization is severe and symptomatic and there are fractures, or when the age of onset is unusually early. Methods of assessment of bone mass and remodeling and other aspects of the problem have been reviewed in detail (Thomson and Frame, 1976).

Bone mass in osteoporosis is reduced, but remaining bone is qualitatively intact. Loss of bone is proportionately greater in trabecular bone, comprising 15 to 20% of the total, than in cortical bone. Fractures occur when trabecular bone is reduced by about one-half and are especially common in the vertebrae, the femoral head, and the radius, all of which contain a high proportion of trabecular bone.

The risk of development of clinical osteoporosis is related to a number of factors of which initial bone mass is a major one. Bone mass is greater in men than in women and in blacks as compared to whites; clinical osteoporosis is correspondingly three to five times more frequent in women than in men and is much less frequent in blacks than in whites. Osteoporosis seems to be especially common in whites living in or originating from northern Europe. In Britain, for example, 40% of women over age 60 have osteoporosis; in those over age 70 about 40% have suffered crush fractures of the vertebrae and 10% have had fractures of the wrist. In the United States some 15 million persons have osteoporosis, of which 5 million have had at least one vertebral fracture, including 25% of all women over age 70. Each year an estimated 200,000 hip fractures occur. Many of these are due to underlying osteoporosis.

Diminished gonadal hormone secretion in senescence, especially postmenopausal loss of the protective effect of estrogen in preventing the action of parathyroid hormone (PTH) on bone, was postulated many years ago as a factor in the pathogenesis of this process. The available evidence dealing with PTH levels during aging is discussed elsewhere (see Parathyroid Hormone). Experimentally, estrogen does appear to decrease the sensitivity of bone to PTH (Orimo et al., 1972). A critical review of the relationship of estrogen to the development of osteoporosis is available (Heaney, 1976).

The development of clinical osteoporosis appears better correlated with length of time after menopause and its concomitant estrogen deficiency state than with chronologic age. In addition, surgically induced early menopause is associated with development of osteoporosis in some 80% of cases. Several lines of evidence, however, strongly indicate that the pathogenesis of osteoporosis involves more than a loss of estrogen effect. Not to be forgotten is the fact that bone loss is a phenomenon seen in men as well as women.

Moreover, data exist that show that demineralization begins years before the menopause, the time when estrogen secretion presumably first diminishes. In addition, the effect of estrogen in preventing bone mineral loss diminishes with time. When estrogen replacement was given at menopause, bone density measured at 5 to 10 years was clearly greater than when replacement was not given (Davis et al., 1966; Meema et al., 1975). Thereafter, the difference between those receiving estrogen and those without became progressively less, although a significant difference was still seen after 10 to 15 years of therapy (Davis et al., 1966). By the end of 15 to 20 years, a significant difference was no longer demonstrable. While this retrospective study seemed clearly to establish a delay in demineralization lasting at least 10 to 15 years, even those given estrogen showed progressive demineralization. Other investigations of estrogen treatment of patients with overt osteoporosis showed that, while bone resorption decreased after both short-term and, to a lesser extent, long-term treatment, bone formation, initially unaffected, ultimately decreased (Riggs et al., 1972). Thus, over the longer period (2 to 3 years), the beneficial effect of estrogen was partially negated. Taken together, the data clearly indicate that estrogen therapy is worthwhile for arresting or slowing the progressive bone loss of osteoporosis but that the age-related demineralization process involves other contributing factors. Nonetheless, a major role for estrogen deficiency seems to be receiving additional support. Three prospective, controlled, short-term studies (one of oophorectomized and the others of postmenopausal women) have shown prevention of bone loss by estrogen over 2- to 3-year periods (Aitken et al., 1973; Horsman et al., 1977; Recker et al., 1977). Other prospective observations at 5 years postcastration or after natural menopause have also shown prevention of bone loss by estrogen administration (Lindsay et al., 1976).

Some additional factors that may contribute to postmenopausal bone loss are now under study. Evidence is accumulating that the negative calcium balance of the postmenopausal state is associated with calcium malabsorption in the elderly and that this in turn may be related to an age-related alteration of vitamin D metabolism (Marshall et al., 1977b; Gallagher et al., 1979). Bone loss has been reduced by measures which increase calcium absorption, i.e., by therapy with calcium supplements (Recker et al., 1977; Horsman et al., 1977) and with 1 α-hydroxycholecalciferol (1α-OH D) (Marshall et al., 1977b). This compound is rapidly converted *in vivo* to the active vitamin D_3 metabolite, 1.25 $(OH)_2$ D. The combination of estrogen therapy with an active D_3 metabolite may be even more effective. Results of combined therapy using estrogens with calcium have not yet been reported.

These observations on postmenopausal bone loss have been extended to the therapy of established osteoporosis. Risk factors for these patients, who appear to represent the rapid bone-losers in the postmenopausal population, include low calcium intake, malabsorption of calcium, and low estrogen status (Marshall et al., 1977a). The malabsorption of calcium is resistant to therapy with ordinary vitamin D but responds to 1α-OH D and to 1,25 $(OH)_2$ D (Marshall et al., 1977c; Gallagher et al., 1979).

The plasma levels of 1,25 $(OH)_2$ D appear to decrease in normal elderly subjects and in patients with osteoporosis. Since the levels of the precursor metabolite 25-OH-D are maintained, the suggestion has been made that inadequate metabolic conversion to 1,25 $(OH)_2$ D may contribute to diminished calcium absorption in both the elderly and osteoporotics. Factors that appear to control the degree of metabolic conversion are PTH (low in osteoporotics by the

NH$_2$-terminal assay for PTH) and estrogen (Gallagher et al., 1979). Furthermore, estrogen administration has been reported to correct, at least partially, calcium malabsorption in the elderly (Heaney, 1976).

Steroids other than estrogens are also being investigated for possible use in the prevention of bone loss. It is of interest to note, in connection with the progressive loss of adrenal androgens with age (see Adrenal Androgens), that a synthetic anabolic steroid has short-term and long-term effects similar to those of estrogen (Riggs et al., 1972). A progestogen has also recently been reported to be effective in preventing postmenopausal bone loss, at least for periods up to 1 year (Lindsay et al., 1978). An interesting recent report presents the concept that osteoporosis may be accompanied by a specific type of myopathy and suggests that this process may also respond to therapy with 1α-OH D$_3$ and calcium (Sørensen et al., 1979).

PARATHYROID HORMONE

Diminished gonadal hormone secretion in senescence, especially postmenopausal loss of the protective effect of estrogen in preventing the action of parathyroid hormone (PTH) on bone, was postulated many years ago as a factor in the pathogenesis of osteoporosis. Experimentally, estrogen does appear to decrease the sensitivity of bone to PTH (Orimo et al., 1972).

Several reports on the relationship of age to immunoassayable PTH (iPTH) concentrations unfortunately either do not describe the immunologic specificity of the antibodies used for assay or are known to measure biologically inactive fragments, particularly the C-terminal fragment. Thus, it is difficult to attribute biologic importance to apparent age-related changes of iPTH at this time. Nonetheless, one such study reported findings in a large number of subjects (Roof et al., 1976): iPTH levels showed complicated age-related patterns depending on sex and race. In white males iPTH increased more than two-fold from ages 20 to 30 to ages 50 to 60. Thereafter, iPTH fell progressively to about one-half the peak level at midlife. In contrast, white women showed a fall in iPTH to age 40 to 50 and a subsequent doubling in the group over 80 years. Black men showed a pattern similar to that of whites, but Oriental men showed a steady and striking decrease in iPTH. Black women did not show the midlife nadir of whites and the level did not increase after age 40. Strikingly, the mean levels of iPTH in black women were about one-half those in the whites. In a Japanese population, both men and women showed progressive decrease in iPTH (Fujita et al., 1972). In another study in which it was clear that the iPTH measured represented predominantly the C-terminal (inactive) fragment, a marked increase in iPTH was seen in normal subjects beginning at about age 40 (Wiske et al., 1979). When subjects below and above age 40 were compared, the values were nearly two-fold higher in the older age group, with even higher values being seen in women over age 70. Another smaller study, in which the fragment measured was presumably also the C-terminal fragment, reported even more striking (nine-fold) elevations of iPTH in elderly subjects (Berlyne et al., 1975). In such studies the key question is whether C-terminal fragments are increased because glomerular filtration is the principal mode of disposal of these peptides or whether secondary hyperparathyroidism, presumably due to documented age-related decrease of glomerular filtration rate and possibly contributing to bone mineral loss and osteoporosis, is present in the elderly. The issue may be resolved when age-related measurements of biologically active PTH are available. Preliminary information on this point suggests that NH₂-terminal (1–34) and intact (1–84) PTH remains unchanged with advancing age (Okano et al., 1980) and may actually decrease in osteoporotics relative to their age-matched controls (Gallagher et al., 1979).

The diagnosis of hyperparathyroidism with mild hypercalcemia in the elderly may present some problems. Obviously, assays of PTH may be difficult to interpret, since the C-terminal fragment may be elevated because of age-related phenomena. On the other hand, assays of intact (1–84) hormone may also fail to be helpful, since they are often not elevated even in young patients with parathyroid adenoma. Heightened sensitivity to PTH in the estrogen-lacking postmenopausal woman has also been postulated to account for the relatively high incidence of hyperparathyroidism at this age, previously undetected adenomas being thought to become apparent only after the restraining effect of estrogen is removed. Moreover, occasional postmenopausal women may present with slightly elevated levels of serum calcium and increased calcium excretion, both of which are significantly diminished by treatment with physiologic amounts of estrogen (Gallagher and Nordin, 1972; Riggs et al., 1972; Roof and Gordan, 1978). Some of these cases may be misdiagnosed as being due to parathyroid adenoma and the patients subjected to unnecessary surgical exploration (Roof and Gordan, 1978).

THYROCALCITONIN

The effectiveness of thyrocalcitonin (TCT) is greatly decreased during maturation in the rat. When 1-year-old adult rats are compared with young ones, markedly diminished hypocalcemic and hypophosphatemic effects are seen, even with large doses of hormone (Hirsch and Munson, 1969). Data are not yet available for senescent rats. Diminished hypocalcemic response to TCT may be due to the reduced rate of osseous catabolism that occurs with maturation. The adult rat does appear to secrete a maximally effective amount of TCT in response to the stimulus of hypercalcemia (Orimo and Hirsch, 1973). Other work suggests that in both rats and sheep TCT secretion following hypercalcemic stimulation is decreased during maturation. Comparable measurements are not yet available in the human.

The aged human does respond to exogenous TCT, although no comparison between the responses of old and young has been reported. Since TCT decreases bone resorption, its potential usefulness in the therapy of age-related demineralization and osteoporosis has been explored. Several preliminary studies showed beneficial results, but the most recent data are not encouraging (Jowsey et al., 1971).

SYMPATHETIC NERVOUS SYSTEM: CATECHOLAMINES

Urinary excretion of epinephrine, reflecting basal function of the adrenal medulla, does not change with advancing age in adult man, nor does the excretion of norepinephrine (Kärki, 1956). Nonetheless, elderly subjects differ from young in having diminished adrenal medullary and sympathetico-adrenal responses to certain pharmacologic and psychophysiologic stresses (insulin hypoglycemia, vasomotor conditioning). The response to hypoglycemia is mediated by the hypothalamus, and the effect of age could well be exerted here rather than in the adrenal. Altered hypo-

thalamic reactivity in the aged has, in fact, been inferred from impaired vascular responses to certain drugs (Cohen and Shmavonian, 1967; see also Hypothalamus and Posterior Pituitary: Antidiuretic Hormone). The available observations, however, are in keeping with the clinical impression that elderly diabetics with insulin-induced hypoglycemia are less likely to show the obvious sympathetic symptoms seen in young diabetics, although autonomic dysfunction related to diabetes rather than to age may be responsible.

Progress in this area has been limited by methodologic problems. The difficulties of quantifying catecholamines in plasma limited observations to those derived from measurements of urinary catecholamine or metabolite excretion, rather insensitive indices of sympathetic nervous system activity. Recently, however, reliable assays of plasma norepinephrine have yielded some new information. Plasma norepinephrine does appear to increase significantly with age, although sex and race may be even more important variables (Jones et al., 1978; Brecht and Schoeppe, 1978). Moreover, even the use of plasma norepinephrine as an index of sympathetic nervous activity must at best be an insensitive one, since there is much recycling of the neurotransmitter upon its release.

That alterations of other catecholamine-mediated events in the central nervous system may eventually become apparent is suggested by the finding of decreased levels of norepinephrine and increased monoamine oxidase in human brain with aging (Robinson et al., 1972). On the other hand, altered tissue content need not be related to functional state. For example, the catecholamine content of heart muscle decreases with age in the rat, but this change could not account for the age-related alteration of the mechanical properties of this tissue (Lakatta et al., 1975).

In addition to the age-related changes of the complex sympathetic functions already described, some information suggests altered tissue responsiveness to catecholamines. Examples of such changes include diminished arterial contractile response to norepinephrine in the senescent rat (Tuttle, 1966), decreased lipolytic effect of catecholamines during maturation and senescence in both rat and man, and increased epinephrine-sensitive adenylate cyclase activity in the liver of the senescent rat (Kalish et al., 1977; see Adenylate Cyclase System and Plasma Membrane–Bound Receptors).

HORMONE ACTION

Enzyme Induction

Although the mechanisms of specific enzyme adaptation or induction are complex, hormonal stimuli trigger this phenomenon in many instances. Work in the rat has led to the concept that aging results in a progressive increase in the time required for certain hormone-mediated adaptive enzyme responses. Examples of this age-related time lag include the inductions of hepatic glucokinase by glucose via insulin and of tyrosine aminotransferase by glucocorticoids via ACTH release (Adelman, 1979). In the former, diminished insulin release in response to glucose appears to be the mechanism, while in the latter response the aged rat adrenal requires increased time for the expression of ACTH action, at least in the strain of animal studied (Rotenberg and Adelman, 1972). Induction of the drug-metabolizing enzyme NADPH-cytochrome c reductase by phenobarbital also requires greater time in old animals, suggesting that delayed hormonal responses may be part of a more general age-related change. However, some direct inductions of enzymes, such as hepatic tyrosine aminotransferase and tryptophan pyrrolase by cortisol (Gregerman, 1959; Adelman, 1979) and hepatic α-glycerophosphate dehydrogenase by T_4 (Bulos et al., 1972a), do not appear to be impaired during senescence in the rat, so the time-lag phenomenon is not always observed. Nonetheless, other observations indicate that dose-response effects may be important in demonstrating an effect of age on the rate of enzyme induction (Frolkis, 1970). The complexity of this area is further emphasized by the demonstration that enzyme molecules can undergo alteration during aging (Gershon, 1979).

Adenylate Cyclase System and Plasma Membrane–Bound Receptors

Alterations of membrane structure and function have been thought by many to be of critical importance during aging. Although little definitive information regarding age-related changes of membrane function is available, some changes have been described in relation to hormone-sensitive adenylate cyclase (AC) (see Chapter 16). Most reports in this area deal with maturational rather than postmaturation changes and those of senescence. The available maturational data indicate uniform decreases in hormone-sensitive AC in a variety of animal tissues (Roth, 1979a). No such uniform pattern emerges from the postmaturational studies. In rat brain a number of separate areas (cerebral cortex, cerebellum, hippocampus, and so forth) show decreases in dopamine and norepinephrine-sensitive AC. In the rat adipocyte, no such simple pattern is seen. This cell is responsive to a number of hormones, all of which accelerate lipolysis. When three hormone responses were studied simultaneously, each followed a different pattern. Glucagon-sensitive AC decreased and disappeared during maturation; ACTH responsiveness diminished by about half over the entire life span; and the change of epinephrine-sensitive enzyme was minimal even in the oldest animals (Cooper and Gregerman, 1976). In the liver, little change was seen in the case of glucagon-responsive AC, but the response to epinephrine was markedly increased (Kalish et al., 1977). Thus, even within a single cell type, age-related alterations of hormone-sensitive AC may follow separate patterns for different hormones, and widely different patterns may be seen in various tissues of the same species.

The mechanisms of these changes are only minimally understood. Alterations of hormone-sensitive AC activity could obviously occur via changes of receptor number or affinity or alterations of the catalytic unit of AC or its regulators (calmodulin; GTP-binding proteins), although as yet practically no information is available on these points. In the case of liver, some evidence suggests that age-related alterations of plasma membrane lipid composition may affect the activity of the membrane-bound AC along with other membrane-bound enzymes such as the ATPases (Kalish et al., 1977).

At the cellular level a few age-related changes of hormone responsiveness have been reported in which attempts have been made to define possible alterations of AC-dependent systems. Catecholamine-induced lipolysis, which decreases progressively with aging both in the rat (Jelinková et al., 1972; Masoro et al., 1979) and in man (Berger et al., 1971), is a cAMP-mediated process. A decrease during maturation of cyclase activation in rat fat cells by catecholamines has also been reported (Forn et al., 1970; Cooper and Gregerman, 1976). In this instance an age-related alteration of phosphodiesterase appeared to contribute to the altered hormone response, since phosphodiesterase activity increased as AC decreased (Forn et al., 1970). A recent study also suggested that phosphodiesterase may affect hormone responsiveness of the fat cell in the postmaturation period but that no alterations of β-receptor number or affinity were involved (Dax et al., 1980). The Leydig cell of the senescent rat has been shown to exhibit impaired testosterone secretory response to gonadotropin (hCG) stimulation. A small (20%) reduction of hormone receptors did not account for impaired testosterone formation, since hCG-augmented intracellular cAMP levels were unaffected. The age-related defect in this instance appeared to be distal to the cyclase system (Tsitouras et al., 1979). These reports barely begin to describe this area, but they already clearly indicate that endocrine-related membrane function, i.e., the AC system, is involved in the aging process, and they provide an important clue to the explanation of age-related alterations of hormone sensitivity.

Only a few other studies have examined the relationship of age to membrane-bound receptors; no pattern has yet emerged. Data from human tissues are limited to lymphocytes, in which β-adrenergic receptors decreased with age, and cultured fibroblasts, in which insulin binding has been variously affected, depending, perhaps, on cell-culture conditions (Roth, 1979a, 1979b).

Intracellular Hormone Receptors

The cytosolic hormone receptor proteins that interact with glucocorticoid and sex hormones have been reported to change with age in several species, including man (Table 29–2). In most but not all cases so far examined there has been a decrease in intracellular concentration of the hormone receptor. In only a few of these reports have efforts been made to correlate altered receptor concentrations with age-dependent changes in hormone responsiveness, but several examples in the rat suggest that causal relationships exist. For example, the decrease with age in glucocorticoid receptors of lymphocytes and adipocytes parallels that of the altered glucocorticoid effect on glucose transport. Similar correlations have been made in several cases of androgen and estrogen receptors and the synthesis of specific proteins (Table 29–2). The mechanisms of the apparent alterations of hormone receptor concentrations are not clear. In addition to the obvious possibilities of decreased synthesis or increased degradation, the possibility exists that aging results in synthesis of nonfunctional receptors, as has been seen with certain enzymes. Several studies have noted age-related decreased entry of activated steroid–receptor complexes into nuclei. Both alterations of the nuclei and the existence of age-related cytoplasmic factors which inhibit translocation have been described (Roth, 1979a).

CONCLUSIONS

Aging affects many aspects of endocrine regulation but does not affect all the endocrine glands or all the different hormones secreted by the same gland to the same extent. Although our present knowledge in this area is limited, examples are known of age-related alterations of hormone secretion rates, patterns of secretion, and altered secretory responses to physiologic or pharmacologic stimulation (Fig. 29–3). Diminished secretion is sometimes a primary phenomenon, but age-related decreases in the rate of metabolic

Table 29–2.   CHANGES IN INTRACELLULAR HORMONE RECEPTOR CONCENTRATIONS DURING SENESCENCE*

Hormone Receptor	Receptor Concentration Decrease (D) Increase (I)	Tissue or Cell	Species	Concomitant Biologic Response
Corticosteroid	D	Splenic lymphocytes	Rat	Inhibition of uridine uptake
	D	Cerebral cortex	Rat	
	D	Cortical neurons	Rat	
	D	Skeletal muscle	Rat	
	D	Adipose tissue	Rat	
	D	Adipocytes	Rat	Inhibition of glucose oxidation
	D	Liver	Human	
	D	Lung fibroblasts (WI-38)	Human	Prolongation of *in vitro* life span
Androgen	D	Liver	Rat	Induction of α2u globulin
	D	Ventral prostate	Rat	Maintenance of cell content
	D	Lateral prostate	Rat	
	D	Hypothalamus	Rat	
	D	Pituitary	Rat	
	D	Testes	Rat	
	I	Seminal vesicles	Rat	
Estrogen	D	Uterus	Rat	Induction of phosphofructokinase
	I	Seminal vesicles	Rat	
	D	Uterus	Mouse	
	D	Brain	Rat	Induction of acetylcholinesterase

*Modified from Roth, G. S.: Hormone receptor changes during adulthood and senescence; significance for aging research. *Fed. Proc. 38*:1910, 1979. For references see article.

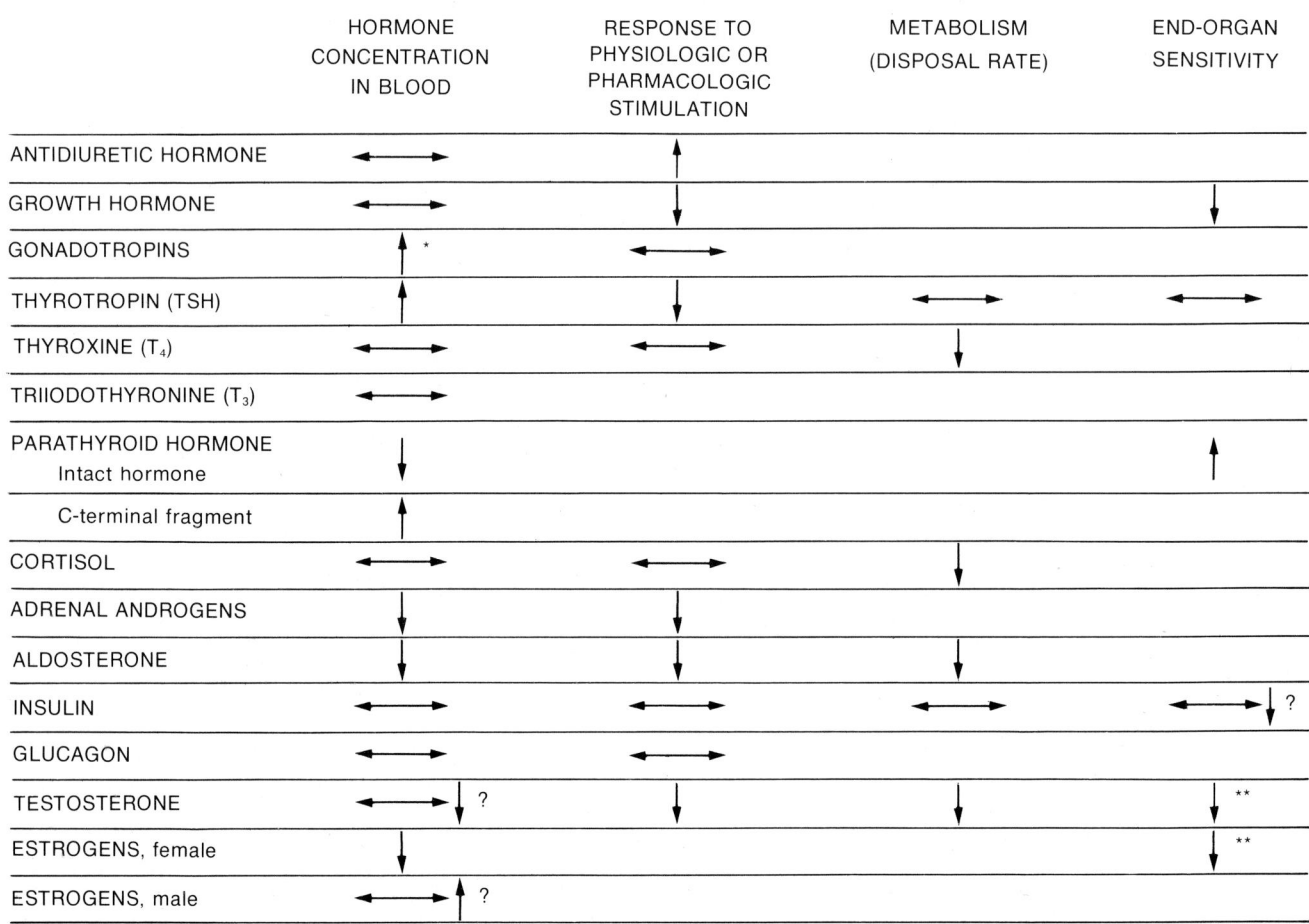

Figure 29–3.   Changes in hormones during aging in man. Symbols: ↑, increase; ↓, decrease; ↔, no change; *, post-menopausal; **, hypothalamic. Blank spaces indicate that no data are currently available.

disposal of some hormones also lead to decreased hormone secretion rates as secondary or homeostatic mechanisms. Age not only can affect the concentration of a specific plasma protein involved in hormone transport but also can influence the concentration of the free or metabolically active portion of that hormone in blood. Target-tissue sensitivity to hormonal effects is sometimes age-related and in certain instances appears to involve alterations of cell surface hormone receptor number, the activity of the adenylate cyclase system, and the concentration of intracellular hormone receptors. From a practical clinical viewpoint, aside from these biochemical and physiologic considerations, age is a variable which must be considered in evaluating normal endocrine function by laboratory methods and in interpreting diagnostic tests.

REFERENCES

Abraham, G. E., and Maroulis, G. B.: Effect of exogenous estrogen on serum pregnenolone, cortisol and androgens in postmenopausal women. *Obstet. Gynecol.* 45:271, 1975.

Adelman, R. C.: Loss of adaptive mechanisms during aging. *Fed. Proc.* 38:1968, 1979.

Aitken, J. M., Davidson, A., et al.: The relationship between menopausal vasomotor symptoms and gonadotropin excretion in urine after oophorectomy. *J. Obstet. Gynaecol. Br. Commonw.* 81:150, 1974.

Aitken, J. M., Hart, D. M., et al.: Oestrogen replacement therapy for prevention of osteoporosis after oophorectomy. *Br. Med. J.* 3:515, 1973.

Andersen, D. K., Elahi, D., et al.: Quantification of biphasic insulin release in three glucose intolerant states: Aging, obesity, and diabetes. *Diabetes* (Suppl. 1) 25:324, 1976 (abstract).

Andres, R., and Tobin, J. D.: Endocrine systems. In *Handbook of the Biology of Aging.* Finch, C. E., and Hayflick, L. (eds.), New York, Van Nostrand Reinhold Co., 1977, pp. 357–378.

Andrew, W.: Structural alterations with aging in the nervous system. *J. Chron Dis.* 3:575, 1956.

Atkinson, R. L., Dahms, W. T., et al.: Occult thyroid disease in an elderly population. *J. Gerontol.* 33:372, 1978.

Azizi, F., Vagenakis, A. G., et al.: Pituitary-thyroid responsiveness to intramuscular thyrotropin-releasing hormone based on analyses of serum thyroxine, tri-iodothyronine and thyrotropin concentrations. *New Eng. J. Med.* 292:273, 1975.

Bakke, J. L., Lawrence, N., et al.: A correlative study of the content of thyroid stimulating hormone (TSH) and cell morphology of the human adenohypophysis. *Am. J. Clin. Path.* 41:576, 1964.

Barmach de Niepomniszsze, A. J., Rosenfeld, R. L., et al.: Adrenal androgen production: dependence on ACTH and gonadal function. *Program 55th Annual Meeting Endocrine Society*, 1973, A-194 (abstract 292).

Berger, D., Crowther, R. C., et al.: Effect of age on fasting plasma levels of pancreatic hormones in man. *J. Clin. Endocr.* 47:1183, 1978.

Berger, M., Preiss, H., et al.: Altersabhängigkeit der Fettzellgrösse und der lipolytischen Aktivität im menschlichen Fettgewebe. *Gerontologia* 17:312, 1971.

Berlyne, G. M., Ben-Ari, J., et al.: The aetiology of senile osteoporosis: Secondary hyperparathyroidism due to renal failure. *Quart. J. Med.* 44:505, 1975.

Bermudez, F., Surks, M. I., et al.: High incidence of decreased serum triiodothyronine concentration in patients with nonthyroid disease. *J. Clin. Endocr.* 41:27, 1975.

Bierman, E. L.: Atherosclerosis and aging. *Fed. Proc.* 37:2832, 1978a.

Bierman, E. L.: The effect of donor age on the *in vitro* lifespan of cultured human arterial smooth-muscle cells. *In Vitro* 14:951, 1978b.

Bierman, E. L., and Ross, R.: Aging and atherosclerosis. In *Atherosclerosis Reviews.* Vol. 2. Paoletti, R., and Gotto, A. M., Jr. (eds.), New York, Raven Press, 1977, p. 79.

Blichert-Toft, M.: Secretion of corticotrophin and somatotrophin by the senescent adenohypophysis in man. *Acta Endocr.* (Kbh.) 78(Suppl. 195) 15, 1975.

Blichert-Toft, M., Blichert-Toft, B., et al.: Pituitary-adrenocortical stimulation in the aged as reflected in levels of plasma cortisol and compound S. *Acta Chir. Scand.* 136:665, 1970.

Blichert-Toft, M., and Hummer, S.: Immunoreactive corticotrophin reserve in old age in man during and after surgical stress. *J. Gerontol.* 31:539, 1976.

Bourne, G. H.: Aging changes in the endocrines, In *Endocrines and Aging.* Gitman, L. (ed.), Springfield, Ill., Charles C Thomas, Publisher, 1967.

Brecht, E. M., and Schoeppe, W.: Relation of plasma noradrenaline to blood pressure, age and sodium balance in patients with stable essential hypertension and in normotensive subjects. *Clin. Sci. Mol. Med.* 55:81s, 1978.

Bronson, F. H., and Desjardins, C.: Reproductive failure in aged CBF1 male mice: Interrelationships between pituitary gonadotropic hormones, testicular function, and mating success. *J. Clin. Endocr.* 101:939, 1977.

Bruni, J. F., Huang, H., et al.: Effects of single and multiple injections of synthetic GnRH on serum LH, FSH and testosterone in young and old male rats. *Biol. Reprod.* 17:309, 1977.

Bulos, B., Shukla, S., et al.: The rate of induction of the mitochondrial α-glycerophosphate dehydrogenase by thyroid hormone in adult and senescent rats. *Mech. Ageing Dev.* 1:227, 1972a.

Bulos, B., Shukla, S., et al.: Effect of thyroid hormone on respiratory control of liver mitochondria from adult and senescent rats. *Arch. Biochem. Biophys.* 151:387, 1972b.

Buttlar-Brentano, K. von: Zur Lebensgeschichte des nucleus basalis, tuberomammillaris, supraopticus und paraventricularis unter normalen und pathogenen Bedingungen. *J. Hirnforsch.* 1:337, 1954.

Calloway, N. O., Foley, C. F., et al.: Uncertainties in geriatric data. II. Organ size. *J. Am. Geriat. Soc.* 13:20, 1965.

Caplan, R. H., Glaser, J. E., et al.: Thyroid function tests in elderly hyperthyroid patients. *J. Am. Geriat. Soc.* 26:116, 1978.

Carlson, H. E., Gillin, J. C., et al.: Absence of sleep-related growth hormone peaks in aged normal subjects and in acromegaly. *J. Clin. Endocr.* 34:1102, 1972.

Cartlidge, N. E. F., Black, M. M., et al.: Pituitary function in the elderly. *Gerontol. Clin.* 12:65, 1970.

Casper, R. F.: Physical, neuroendocrine and neuropharmacologic correlates during menopausal flushes. *Program 61st Annual Meeting Endocrine Society*, 1979, p. 125 (abstract 210).

Chen, H. J., and Walfish, P. G.: Effects of age and testicular function on the pituitary-thyroid system in male rats. *J. Endocr.* 82:53, 1979.

Christiansen, P.: Urinary follicle stimulating hormone and luteinizing hormone in normal adult men. *Acta Endocr.* (Kbh.) 71:1, 1972.

Cohen, S. I., and Shmavonian, B. M.: Catecholamines, vasomotor conditioning and aging, In *Endocrines and Aging.* Gitman, L. (ed.), Springfield, Ill., Charles C Thomas, Publisher, 1967.

Cooper, B., and Gregerman, R. I.: Hormone-sensitive fat cell adenylate cyclase in the rat. Influences of growth, cell size, and aging. *J. Clin. Invest.* 57:161, 1976.

Cooper, R. L., Brandt, S. J., et al.: Induced ovulation in aged female rats by L-dopa implants into the medial preoptic area. *Neuroendocrinology* 28:234, 1979.

Crane, M. G., and Harris, J. J.: Effect of aging on renin activity and aldosterone excretion. *J. Lab. Clin. Med.* 87:947, 1976.

Crilly, R. G., Marshall, D. H., et al.: Effect of age on plasma androstenedione concentration in oophorectomized women. *Clin. Endocr.* 10:199, 1979.

Cuttelod, S., Lemarchand-Béraud, T., et al.: Effect of age and role of kidneys and liver on thyrotropin turnover in man. *Metabolism* 23:101, 1974.

Davidson, M. B.: The effect of aging on carbohydrate metabolism: a review of the English literature and a practical approach to the diagnosis of diabetes mellitus in the elderly. *Metabolism* 28:688, 1979.

Davis, M. E., Lanzl, L. H., et al.: Estrogens and the aging process. The detection, prevention, and retardation of osteoporosis. *J.A.M.A.* 196:219, 1966.

Davis, P. J., and Davis, F. B.: Hyperthyroidism in patients over the age of 60 years: Clinical features in 85 patients. *Medicine* 53:161, 1974.

Dax, E. M., Partilla, J. P., et al.: Epinephrine stimulated lipolysis, β-adrenergic binding, adenylate cyclase, and intracellular cyclic AMP in rat adipocytes during maturation and aging. *Proceedings of the 6th International Congress of Endocrinology*, 1980.

Debeljuk, L., Arimura, A., et al.: Pituitary responsiveness to LH-releasing hormone in intact female rats of different ages. *Endocrinology* 90:1499, 1972.

DeFronzo, R. A.: Glucose intolerance and aging. Evidence for tissue insensitivity to insulin. *Diabetes* 28:1095, 1979.

Denkla, W. D.: Role of the pituitary and thyroid glands in the decline of minimal O_2 consumption with age. *J. Clin. Invest.* 53:572, 1974.

Deutsch, S., Goldberg, M., et al.: Postoperative hyponatremia with the inappropriate release of antidiuretic hormone. *Anesthesia* 27:250, 1966.

Dilman, V. M., Ostroumova, M. N., et al.: Hypothalamic mechanisms of aging and of specific age pathology. II. On the sensitivity threshold of hypothalamo-pituitary complex to homeostatic stimuli in adaptive homeostasis. *Exp. Gerontol.* 14:175, 1979.

Dobbie, J. W.: Adrenocortical nodular hyperplasia: The aging adrenal. *J. Pathol.* 99:1, 1969.

Duckworth, W. C., and Kitabchi, A. E.: The effect of age on plasma proinsulin-like material after oral glucose. *J. Lab. Clin. Med.* 88:359, 1976.

Dudl, R. J., and Ensinck, J. W.: Insulin and glucagon relationships during aging in man. *Metabolism* 26:33, 1977.

Dudl, R. J., Ensinck, J. W., et al.: The effect of age on growth hormone secretion in man. *J. Clin. Endocr.* 37:11, 1973.

Dunihue, F. W.: Reduced juxtaglomerular cell granularity, pituitary neuro-secretary material, and width of the zona glomerulosa in aging rats. *Endocrinology* 77:948, 1965.

Einhorn, J.: Studies on the effect of thyrotropic hormone on thyroid function in man. *Acta Radiol.* Suppl. 160, 1958, 107 pp.

Elahi, D., Muller, D., et al.: Effect of age and obesity on fasting levels of glucose (G), insulin (IRI), glucagon (IRG), and growth hormone (hGH). *31st Annual Scientific Meeting of the Gerontological Society,* 1978, p. 68 (abstract).

Eleftheriou, B. E.: Changes with age in protein-bound iodine (PBI) and body temperature in the mouse. *J. Gerontol.* 30:417, 1975.

Everitt, A. V., and Burgess, J. A. (eds.): *Hypothalamus, Pituitary and Aging.* Springfield, Ill., Charles C Thomas, Publisher, 1976.

Finch, C. E., and Hayflick, L. (eds.): *Handbook of the Biology of Aging.* New York, Van Nostrand Reinhold Co., 1977.

Finch, C. E., Jonec, V., et al.: Hormone production by the pituitary and testes of male C57BL/6J mice during aging. *Endocrinology* 101:1310, 1977.

Finkelstein, J. W., Roffwarg, H. P., et al.: Age-related change in the twenty-four-hour spontaneous secretion of growth hormone. *J. Clin. Endocr.* 35:665, 1972.

Flood, C., Gherondache, C., et al.: The metabolism and secretion of aldosterone in elderly subjects. *J. Clin. Invest.* 46:961, 1967.

Florini, J. R., Saito, Y., et al.: Effect of age on thyroxine induced cardiac hypertrophy in mice. *J. Gerontol.* 28:293, 1973.

Forn, J., Schonhofer, P. S., et al.: The effect of aging on adenyl cyclase and phosphodiesterase activity of isolated fat cells of the rat. *Biochim. Biophys. Acta* 208:304, 1970.

Friedman, M., Green, M. F., et al.: Assessment of hypothalamic-pituitary-adrenal function in the geriatric age group. *J. Gerontol.* 24:292, 1969.

Friedman, S. M., Friedman, C. L., et al.: Adrenal-neurohypophyseal regulation of electrolytes and work performance. Age-related changes in the rat. In *Endocrines and Aging.* Gitman, L. (ed.), Springfield, Ill., Charles C Thomas, Publisher, 1967.

Frolkis, V. V.: On the regulatory mechanism of molecular-genetic alterations during aging. *Exp. Gerontol.* 5:37, 1970.

Frolkis, V. V., and Bezrukov, V. V.: The hypothalamus in aging. *Exp. Gerontol.* 7:169, 1972.

Frolkis, V. V., Verzhikovskaya, N. V., et al.: The thyroid and age. *Exp. Gerontol.* 8:285, 1973.

Fujita, T., Orimo, H., et al.: Radioimmunoassay of serum parathyroid hormone in postmenopausal osteoporosis. *Endocr. Jpn.* 19:571, 1972.

Gallagher, J. C., and Nordin, B. E. C.: Treatment with estrogens of primary hyperparathyroidism in postmenopausal women. *Lancet* 1:503, 1972.

Gallagher, J. C., Riggs, L. H., et al.: Intestinal calcium absorption and serum vitamin D metabolites in normal subjects and osteoporotic patients: Effect of age and dietary calcium. *J. Clin. Invest.* 64:729, 1979.

Gavin, L. A., Rosenthal, M., et al.: The diagnostic dilemma of isolated hyperthyroxinemia in acute illness. *J.A.M.A.* 242:251, 1979.

Gershberg, H.: Growth hormone content and metabolic actions of human pituitary glands. *Endocrinology* 61:160, 1957.

Gershon, D.: Current status of age altered enzymes: alternative mechanisms. *Mech. Ageing Dev.* 9:189, 1979.

Gherondache, C. N., Romanoff, L. P., et al.: Steroid hormones in aging men, In *Endocrines and Aging.* Gitman, L. (ed.), Springfield, Ill., Charles C Thomas, Publisher, 1967.

Gleason, R. E., and Goldstein, S.: Age effect and replicative life-span of fibroblasts of diabetic, prediabetic, and normal donors: Another look at the data. *Science* 202:1217, 1978.

Goldstein, S., Moerman, E. J., et al.: Diabetes mellitus and genetic prediabetes: decreased replicative capacity of cultured skin fibroblasts. *J. Clin. Invest.* 63:358, 1979.

Grad, B.: The metabolic responsiveness of young and old female rats to thyroxine. *J. Gerontol.* 24:5, 1969.

Grad, B., Rosenberg, G. M., et al.: Diurnal variation of the serum cortisol level of geriatric subjects. *J. Gerontol.* 26:351, 1971.

Gray, G. D.: Changes in the levels of luteinizing hormone and testosterone in the circulation of ageing male rats. *J. Endocr.* 76:551, 1978.

Greenblatt, R. B. (ed.): *Geriatric Endocrinology* (Aging, Vol. 5). New York, Raven Press, 1978.

Gregerman, R. I.: Adaptive enzyme responses in the senescent rat: tryptophan peroxidase and tyrosine transaminase. *Am. J. Physiol.* 197:63, 1959.

Gregerman, R. I., and Davis, P. J.: Effects of intrinsic and extrinsic variables on thyroid hormone economy. Intrinsic physiologic variables and nonthyroidal illness. In *The Thyroid.* Werner, S. C., and Ingbar, S. H. (eds.), New York, Harper and Row, 1978, pp. 223–246.

Gregerman, R. I., Gaffney, G. W., et al.: Thyroxine turnover in euthyroid man with special reference to changes with age. *J. Clin. Invest.* 41:2065, 1962.

Gregerman, R. I., and Solomon, N.: Acceleration of thyroxine and triiodothyronine turnover during infections and fever: Implications for the functional state of the thyroid during stress and in senescence. *J. Clin. Endocr.* 27:93, 1967.

Guillemin, R.: Peptides in the brain: The new endocrinology of the neuron. *Science* 202:390, 1978.

Hamlin, C. R., Kohn, R. R., et al.: Apparent accelerated aging of human collagen in diabetes mellitus. *Diabetes* 27:902, 1975.

Hansen, J. M., Skovsted, L., et al.: Age dependent changes in iodine metabolism and thyroid function. *Acta Endocr.* (Kbh.) 79:60, 1975.

Harman, S. M.: Clinical aspects of aging of the male reproductive system. In *The Aging Reproductive System* (Aging, Vol. 4). Schneider, E. L. (ed.), New York, Raven Press, 1978, pp. 29–58.

Harman, S. M., Danner, R. L., et al.: Testosterone secretion in the rat in response to chorionic gonadotrophin: Alterations with age. *Endocrinology* 102:540, 1978.

Harman, S. M., and Tsitouras, P. D.: Reproductive hormones in aging men. I.: Measurement of sex steroids, basal luteinizing hormone, and Leydig cell response to human chorionic gonadotropin. *J. Clin. Endocr.* 1980, in press.

Heaney, R. P.; Estrogens and postmenopausal osteoporosis. *Clin. Obstet. Gynecol.* 19:791, 1976.

Helderman, J. H.: Constancy of pharmacokinetic properties of the lymphocyte insulin receptor in aging man. *31st Annual Scientific Meeting of the Gerontological Society,* 1978, p. 81 (abstract).

Helderman, J. H., Vestal, R. E., et al.: The response of arginine vasopressin to intravenous ethanol and hypertonic saline in man: The impact of aging. *J. Gerontol.* 33:39, 1978.

Hemsell, D. L., Grodin, J. M., et al.: Plasma precursors of estrogen. II. Correlation of extent of conversion of plasma androstenedione to estrone with age. *J. Clin. Endocr.* 38:476, 1974.

Hesch, R. D., Gatz, J., et al.: TBG-dependency of age-related variations of thyroxine and triiodothyronine. *Horm. Metab. Res.* 9:141, 1977.

Hess, G. D., and Riegle, G. D.: Effects of chronic ACTH stimulation on adrenocortical function in young and aged rats. *Am. J. Physiol.* 222:1458, 1972.

Hirsch, P. F., and Munson, P. L.: Thyrocalcitonin. *Physiol. Rev.* 49:548, 1969.

Hollenberg, M. D., and Schneider, E. L.: Receptors for insulin and epidermal growth factor-urogastrone in adult human fibroblasts do not change with donor age. *Mech. Ageing Dev.* 11:37, 1979.

Horsman, A., Gallagher, J. C., et al.: Prospective trial of oestrogen and calcium in postmenopausal women. *Br. Med. J.* 2:789, 1977.

Horton, R., Hsieh, P., et al.: Altered blood androgens in elderly men with prostate hyperplasia. *J. Clin. Endocr.* 41:793, 1975.

Huang, H. H., and Meites, J.: Reproductive capacity of aging female rats. *Neuroendocrinology* 17:289, 1975.

Hulka, B. S., Fowler, W. C., et al.: Estrogen and endometrial cancer: cases in two control groups from North Carolina. *Am. J. Obstet. Gynecol.,* 1980, in press.

Ito, H., Orimo, H., et al.: Reduced insulin action in vitro and the binding of ^{125}I-insulin to the cultured human skin. *Proceedings of the 5th International Congress of Endocrinology,* 1976, p. 261 (abstract).

Jefferys, P. M., Hoffenberg, R., et al.: Thyroid-function tests in the elderly. *Lancet* 1:924, 1972.

Jelinková, M., Stuchlíková, E., et al.: Hormone-sensitive lipolytic activity of the aorta of different age groups of rats. *Exp. Gerontol.* 7:263, 1972.

Jensen, H. K., and Blichert-Toft, M.: Pituitary-adrenal function in old age evaluated by the intravenous metyrapone test. *Acta Endocr.* (Kbh.) 64:431, 1970.

Jones, D. H., Hamilton, C. A., et al.: Plasma noradrenaline, age and blood pressure: a population study. *Clin. Sci. Mol. Med.* 55:73s, 1978.

Jordan, S. W., and Perley, M. J.: Microangiopathy in diabetes mellitus and aging. *Arch. Pathol.* 93:261, 1972.

Jowsey, J., Riggs, B. L., et al.: Effects of prolonged administration of porcine calcitonin in postmenopausal osteoporosis. *J. Clin. Endocr.* 33:752, 1971.

Juselius, R. E., and Kenny, F. M.: Urinary free cortisol excretion during growth and aging; Correlation with cortisol production rate and 17-hydroxycorticosteroid excretion. *Metabolism* 23:847, 1974.

Kahn, C. R., and Roth, J.: Insulin receptors in disease states. In *Hormone Receptor Interaction: Molecular Aspects.* G. S. Levey (ed.), New York, Marcel Dekker, 1976, p. 1.

Kalish, M. I., Katz, M. S., et al.: Epinephrine and glucagon sensitive adenylate cyclases of rat liver during aging. Evidence for membrane instability associated with increased enzymatic activity. *Biochim. Biophys. Acta* 483:452, 1977.

Kalk, W. J., Vinik, A. I., et al.: Growth hormone response to hypoglycemia in the elderly. *J. Gerontol.* 28:431, 1973.

Kaptein, E. M., Kamiel, M. B., et al.: Suppression of thyroid function with severe illness. *Program 60th Annual Meeting of the Endocrine Society,* 1978, p. 111 (abstract).

Kaptein, E. M., Wheeler, W. S., et al.: Thyroid hormone economy in severe illness. *Clin. Res.* 27:21A, 1979 (abstract).

Kärki, N. T.: The urinary excretion of noradrenaline and adrenaline in different age groups, its diurnal variation and the effect of muscular work on it. *Acta Physiol. Scand.* 39(Suppl. 132):7, 1956.

Kilo, C., Vogler, N., et al.: Muscle capillary basement membrane changes related to aging and to diabetes mellitus. *Diabetes* 21:881, 1972.

Kley, H. K., Nieschlag, E., et al.: Age dependence of plasma oestrogen response to HCG and ACTH in men. *Acta Endocr.* (Kbh.) 75:95, 1975.

Klug, T. L., and Adelman, R. C.: Evidence for a large thyrotropin and its accumulation during aging in rats. *Biochem. Biophys. Res. Commun.* 77:1431, 1977.

Kohn, R. R., and Hensse, S.: Abnormal collagen in cultures of fibroblasts from human beings with diabetes mellitus. *Biochem. Biophys. Res. Commun.* 76:765, 1977.

Lakatta, E. G., Gerstenblith, G., et al.: Prolonged contraction duration in aged myocardium. *J. Clin. Invest.* 55:61, 1975.

Laron, Z., Doron, M., et al.: Plasma growth hormone in men and women over 70 years of age, In *Medicine and Sport.* Vol. 4. Brunner, D., and Jokl, E. (eds.), White Plains, New York, Phiebig, 1969.

Lauridsen, U. B., Deckert, T., et al.: Kliniske erfaringer med radioimmunologisk bestemmelse af human tyreotropin (TSH). *Ugeskr. Laeger* 136:1365, 1974.

Lederer, J., and Bataille, J. P.: Senescence et fonction thyroidienne. *Ann. Endocr.* (Paris) 30:598, 1969.

Lemarchand-Béraud, T. H., and Vannotti, A.: Relationship between blood thyrotropin level, protein bound iodine and free thyroxine concentration in man under normal physiological conditions. *Acta Endocr.* (Kbh.) 60:315, 1969.

Levin, M. E., Boisseau, V. C., et al.: Effects of diabetes mellitus on bone mass in juvenile and adult onset diabetes. *New Eng. J. Med.* 294:241, 1976.

Lewis, J. G., Ghanadian, R., et al.: Serum 5α-dihydrotestosterone and testosterone changes with age in men. *Acta Endocr.* (Kbh.) 82:444, 1976.

Lindeman, R. D., Lee, T. D., Jr., et al.: Influence of age, renal disease, hypertension, diuretics, and calcium on the antidiuretic responses to suboptimal infusions of vasopressin. *J. Lab. Clin. Med.* 68:206, 1966.

Lindsay, R., Aitken, J. M., et al.: Long-term prevention of postmenopausal osteoporosis by oestrogen. *Lancet* 1:1038, 1976.

Lindsay, R., Hart, D. M., et al.: Comparative effects of estrogen and a progestogen on bone loss in postmenopausal women. *Clin. Sci. Mol. Med.* 54:193, 1978.

Longcope, C.: Metabolic clearance and blood production rates of estrogens in postmenopausal women. *Am. J. Obstet. Gynec.* 111:778, 1971.

Lutz, J. H., Gregerman, R. I., et al.: Thyroxine binding proteins, free thyroxine and thyroxine turnover interrelationships during acute infectious illness in man. *J. Clin. Endocr.* 35:230, 1972.

Maroulis, G. B., and Abraham, G. E.: Ovarian and adrenal contributions to peripheral steroid levels in postmenopausal women. *Obstet. Gynecol.* 48:151, 1976.

Marshall, D. H., Crilly, R. G., et al.: Plasma androstenedione and oestrone levels in normal and osteoporotic postmenopausal women. *Br. Med. J.* 2:1177, 1977a.

Marshall, D. H., Gallagher, J. C., et al.: The effect of 1 α-hydroxy cholecalciferol and hormone therapy on the calcium balance of post menopausal osteoporosis. *Calcif. Tissue Res.* 22(Suppl.):78, 1977b.

Marshall, D. H., Horsman, A., et al.: The prevention and management of post-menopausal osteoporosis. *Acta Obstet. Gynecol. Scand.* (Suppl. 65):49, 1977c.

Martin, C. E.: Sexual activity in the aging male. In *Handbook of Sexology.* Money, J., and Musaph, H. (eds.), New York, Elsevier-North Holland, 1977.

Masoro, E. J., Bertrand, H., et al.: Analysis and exploration of age-related changes in mammalian structure and function. *Fed. Proc.* 38:1956, 1979.

McNair, P., Madsbad, S., et al.: Osteopenia in insulin treated diabetes mellitus. *Diabetologia* 15:87, 1978.

Meema, S., Bunker, M. L., et al.: Preventive effect of estrogen on postmenopausal bone loss. *Arch. Intern. Med.* 135:1436, 1975.

Migeon, C. J., Keiler, A. R., et al.: Dehydroepiandrosterone and androsterone levels in human plasma. *J. Clin. Endocr.* 17:1051, 1957.

Miller, A. E., and Riegle, G. D.: Serum LH levels following multiple LHRH injections in aging rats. *Proc. Soc. Exp. Biol. Med.* 157:494, 1978a.

Miller, A. E., and Riegle, G. D.: Hypothalamic LH-releasing activity in young and aged intact and gonadectomized rats. *Exp. Aging Res.* 4:145, 1978b.

Misbin, R. I., O'Leary, J. P., et al.: Insulin receptor binding in obesity: A reassessment. *Science* 205:1003, 1979.

Moncloa, F., Gómez, R., et al.: Response to corticotrophin and correlation between excretion of creatinine and urinary steroids and between the clearance of creatinine and urinary steroids in ageing. *Steroids* 1:437, 1963.

Murakami, T., Yamaji, T., et al: The effect of ACTH administration on serum estrogens, LH, and FSH in the aged. *J. Clin. Endocr.* 42:88, 1976.

Muta, K., Kato, K., et al.: Age-related changes in feedback regulation of gonadotropin secretion by sex steroids in men. *Proceedings of the 6th International Congress of Endocrinology*, 1980 (abstract).

Newton-John, H. F., and Morgan, D. B.: Osteoporosis: Disease or senescence? *Lancet* 1:232, 1968.

Novak, L. P.: Aging, total body potassium, fat-free mass, and cell mass in males and females between ages 18 and 85 years. *J. Gerontol.* 27:438, 1972.

Ohara, H., Kobayashi, T., et al.: Thyroid function of the aged as viewed from the pituitary-thyroid system. *Endocr. Jpn.* 21:377, 1974.

Okano, K., Nakai, R., et al.: Effects of age and administration of estrogen on calcium regulating hormones in normal human subjects. *Proceedings of the 6th International Congress of Endocrinology*, 1980 (abstract).

Olefsky, J. M., and Reaven, G. M.: Effects of age and obesity on insulin binding to ioslated adipocytes. *Endocrinology* 96:1486, 1975.

Olsen, T., Laurberg, P., et al.: Low serum triodothyronine and high serum reverse triiodothyronine in old age: An effect of disease not age. *J. Clin. Endocr.* 47:1111, 1978.

Oppenheimer, J. H., Bernstein, G., et al.: Increased thyroxine turnover and thyroidal function after stimulation of hepatocellular binding of thyroxine by phenobarbital. *J. Clin. Invest* 47:1399, 1968.

Orimo, H., Fujita, T., et al.: Increased sensitivity of bone to parathyroid hormone in ovariectomized rats. *Endocrinology* 90:760, 1972.

Orimo, H., and Hirsch, P. F.: Thyrocalcitonin and age. *Endocrinology* 93:1206, 1973.

O'Sullivan, J. B.: Age gradient in blood glucose levels: magnitude and clinical implications. *Diabetes* 23:713, 1974.

Palmer, J. P., and Ensinck, J. W.: Acute-phase insulin secretion and glucose tolerance in young and aged normal men and diabetic patients. *J. Clin. Endocr.* 41:498, 1975.

Pecile, A., Müller, E., et al.: Growth hormone-releasing activity of hypothalamic extracts at different ages. *Endocrinology* 77:241, 1965.

Pfeiffer, E., and Davis, G. C.: Determinants of sexual behavior in middle and old age. *J. Am. Geriat. Soc.* 20:151, 1972.

Pincus, G.: Steroid hormones and aging in man. In *Growth in Living Systems.* Zarrow, M. X. (ed.), New York, Basic Books, 1961.

Pincus, G., Romanoff, L. P., et al.: The excretion of urinary steroids by men and women of various ages. *J. Gerontol.* 9:113, 1954.

Pirke, K. M., and Doerr, P.: Age-related changes and interrelationships between plasma testosterone, oestradiol and testosterone-binding globulin in normal adult males. *Acta Endocr.* (Kbh.) 74:792, 1973.

Pirke, K. M., and Doerr, P.: Plasma DHT in normal adult males and its relation to T. *Acta Endocr.* (Kbh.) 79:357, 1975.

Raizes, G. S., Elahi, D., et al.: Effect of aging on the gastrointestinal mediation of insulin release: The role of gastric inhibitory polypeptide. *29th Annual Scientific Meeting of the Gerontological Society*, 1976, p.50 (abstract).

Reaven, E. P., Gold, G., et al.: Effect of age on glucose-stimulated insulin release by the β-cell of the rat. *J. Clin. Invest.* 64:591, 1979.

Recker, R. R., Saville, P. D., et al.: Effect of estrogens and calcium carbonate on bone loss in postmenopausal women. *Ann. Intern. Med.* 87:649, 1977.

Reyes, F. I., Winter, J. S. D., et al.: Pituitary-ovarian relationships preceding the menopause. I. A cross sectional study of follicle-stimulating hormone, luteinizing hormone, prolactin, estradiol, and progesterone levels. *Am. J. Obstet. Gynecol.* 129:557, 1977.

Riegle, G. D., and Nellor, J. E.: Changes in adrenocortical function during aging in cattle. *J. Gerontol.* 22:83, 1967.

Riegle, G. D., Przekop, F., et al.: Changes in adrenocortical responsiveness to ACTH infusion in aging goats. *J. Gerontol.* 23:187, 1968.

Riggs, B. L., Jowsey, J., et al.: Short- and long-term effects of estrogen and synthetic anabolic hormone in postmenopausal osteoporosis. *J. Clin. Invest.* 51:1659, 1972.

Robinson, D. S., Nies, A., et al.: Ageing, monoamines, and monoamine-oxidase levels. *Lancet* 1:290, 1972.

Romanoff, L. P., Morris, C. W., et al.: The metabolism of cortisol-4-C^{14} in young and elderly men. *J. Clin Endocr.* 21:1413, 1961.

Roof, B. S., and Gordan, G. S.: Hyperparathyroid disease in the aged. In *Geriatric Endocrinology* (Aging Series, Vol. 5). R. B. Greenblatt (ed.), New York, Raven Press, 1978, p. 67.

Roof, B. S., Piel, C. F., et al.: Serum parathyroid hormone levels and serum calcium levels from birth to senescence. *Mech. Ageing Dev.* 5:289, 1976.

Root, A. W., and Oski, F. A.: Effects of human growth hormone in elderly males. *J. Gerontol.* 24:97, 1969.

Rotenberg, S., and Adelman, R. C.: Age-dependent adaptive regulation of adrenocortical function. *Gerontologist* 12:341, 1972.

Roth, G. S.: Hormone action during aging: alterations and mechanisms. *Mech. Ageing Dev.* 9:497, 1979a.

Roth, G. S.: Hormone receptor changes during adulthood and senescence: significance for aging research. *Fed. Proc.* 38:1910, 1979b.

Rowe, D. W., Starman, B. J., et al.: Abnormalities in proliferation and protein synthesis in skin fibroblast cultures from patients with diabetes mellitus. *Diabetes* 26:284, 1977.

Rubens, R., Dhont, M., et al.: Further studies on Leydig cell function in old age. *J. Clin. Endocr.* 39:40, 1974.

Ryan, R. J.: The luteinizing hormone content of human pituitaries. I. Variations with sex and age. *J. Clin. Endocr.* 22:300, 1962.

Sambhi, M. P., Crane, M. G., et al.: Essential hypertension: New concepts about mechanisms. *Ann. Intern. Med.* 79:411, 1973.

Sawin, C. T., Chopra, D., et al.: The aging thyroid. Increased prevalence of elevated serum thyrotropin levels in the elderly. *J.A.M.A.* 242:247, 1979.

Scazzola, B., Lemarchand-Béraud, T., et al.: *Problèmes de Gériatrie.* Paris, Sandoz, 1968, p. 15.

Schally, A. V.: Aspects of hypothalamic regulation of the pituitary gland. *Science* 202:18, 1978.

Schneider, E. L. (ed.): *The Aging Reproductive System* (Aging, Vol. 4). New York, Raven Press, 1978.

Schwartz, A. G.: Inhibition of spontaneous breast cancer formation in female C3H (Avy/a) mice by long-term treatment with dehydroepiandrosterone. *Cancer Res.* 39:1129, 1979.

Schwartz, H. L., Forciea, M. A., et al.: Age-related reduction in response of hepatic enzymes to 3,5,3'-triiodothyronine administration. *Endocrinology 105*:41, 1979.

Sherman, B. M., West, J. H., et al.: The menopausal transition: Analysis of LH, FSH, estradiol and progesterone concentrations during menstrual cycles of older women. *J. Clin. Endocr. 42*:629, 1976.

Simpkins, J. W., Mueller, G. P., et al.: Evidence for depressed catecholamine and enhanced serotonin metabolism in aging male rats: Possible relationship to gonadotropin secretion. *Endocrinology 100*:672, 1977.

Sköldefors, H., Carlstrom, K., et al.: Aging and urinary estrogen excretion in the male. *Acta Obstet. Gynecol. Scand. 54*:89, 1975.

Snyder, P. J., Reitano, P. F., et al.: Serum LH and FSH responses to synthetic gonadotrophin releasing hormone in normal men. *J. Clin. Endocr. 41*:938, 1975.

Snyder, P. J., and Utiger, R. D.: Response to thyrotropin releasing hormone (TRH) in normal man. *J. Clin. Endocr. 34*:380, 1972a.

Snyder, P. J., and Utiger, R. D.: Thyrotropin response to thyrotropin releasing hormone in normal females over forty. *J. Clin. Endocr. 34*:1096, 1972b.

Sørensen, O. H., Lund, B. I., et al.: Myopathy in bone loss of aging: Improvement by treatment with 1α-hydroxycholecalciferol and calcium. *Clin. Sci. 56*:157, 1979.

Sparrow, D., Bosse, R., et al.: The influence of age, alcohol consumption and body build on gonadal function in men. *J. Clin. Endocr.* 1980, in press.

Tataryn, I. V., Meldrum, D. R., et al.: LH, FSH and skin temperature during the menopausal hot flash. *J. Clin. Endocr. 49*:152, 1979.

Thompson, J., and Oswald, I.: Effect of estrogen on the sleep, mood, and anxiety of menopausal women. *Br. Med. J. 2*:1317, 1977.

Thomson, D. L., and Frame, B. Involutional osteopenia: Current concepts. *Ann. Intern. Med. 85*:789, 1976.

Tsitouras, P. D., Kowatch, M. A., et al.: Age-related alterations of isolated rat Leydig cell function: Gonadotropin receptors, adenosine 3',5'-monophosphate response, and testosterone secretion. *Endocrinology 105*:1400, 1979.

Tsitouras, P. D., Martin, C. E., et al.: Relationship of sexual activity to serum testosterone in healthy elderly men. 1980, in press.

Turnbridge, W. M. G., Evered, D. C., et al.: The spectrum of thyroid disease in a community: The Whickham survey. *Clin. Endocr. 7*:481, 1977.

Tuttle, R. S.: Age-related changes in the sensitivity of rat aortic strips to norepinephrine and associated chemical and structural alterations. *J. Gerontol. 21*:510, 1966

Tzankoff, S. P., and Norris, A. H.: Effect of muscle mass decrease on age-related BMR changes. *J. Appl. Physiol. 43*:1001, 1977.

Vekemans, M., and Robyn, C.: Influence of age on serum prolactin levels in women and men. *Br. Med. J. 4*:738, 1975.

Vermeulen, A., Rubens, R., et al.: Testosterone secretion and metabolism in male senescence. *J. Clin. Endocr. 34*:730, 1972.

Vermeulen, A., Stöica, T., et al.: The apparent free testosterone concentration, an index of androgenicity. *J. Clin. Endocr. 33*:759, 1971.

Verzár, F.: Anterior pituitary function in age. In *The Pituitary Gland.* Vol. 2. Donovan, B. T., and Harris, G. W. (eds.), Berkeley, University of California Press, 1966.

Vidalon, C., Khurana, R. C., et al.: Age-related changes in growth hormone in non-diabetic women. *J. Am. Geriat. Soc. 21*:253, 1973.

Vihko, R.: Gas chromatographic-mass spectrometric studies on solvolyzable steroids in human peripheral plasma. *Acta Endocr.* (Kbh.) *52*(Suppl. 109):1, 1966.

Vracko, R., and Benditt, E. P.: Manifestations of diabetes mellitus — their possible relationships to an underlying cell defect. *Am. J. Pathol. 75*:204, 1974.

Vracko, R., and Benditt, E. P.: Restricted replicative life-span of diabetic fibroblasts *in vitro*: its relation to microangiopathy. *Fed. Proc. 34*:68, 1975.

Warren, M. P., Siris, E. S., et al.: The influence of severe illness on gonadotropin secretion in the postmenopausal female. *J. Clin. Endocr. 45*:99, 1977.

Weissman, P. N., Shenkman, L., et al.: Chlorpropamide hyponatremia: Drug-induced inappropriate antidiuretic-hormone activity. *New Eng. J. Med. 284*:65, 1971.

Wenzel, K. W., Meinhold, H., et al.: TRH-stimulationstest mit alters- und geschlectsabhängigem TSH-Anstieg bei Normalpersonen. *Klin. Wochenschr. 52*:721, 1974.

West, C. D., Brown, H., et al.: Adrenocortical function and cortisol metabolism in old age. *J. Clin. Endocr. 21*:1197, 1961.

Whitehead, M. I., McQueen, J., et al.: The effects of cyclical oestrogen therapy and sequential oestrogen/progestogen therapy on the endometrium of post-menopausal women. *Acta Obstet. Gynecol. Scand.* (Suppl. 65):91, 1977.

Wiske, P. S., Epstein, S., et al.: Increases in immunoreactive parathyroid hormone with age. *New Eng. J. Med. 25*:1419, 1979.

Yamaji, T., and Ibayashi, H.: Plasma dehydroepiandrosterone sulfate in normal and pathological conditions. *J. Clin. Endocr. 29*:273, 1969.

Yamaji, T., Shimamoto, K., et al.: Effect of age and sex on circulating and pituitary prolactin levels in human. *Acta Endocr.* (Kbh.) *83*:711, 1976.

Yen, S. S. C., Martin, P. L., et al.: Circulating estradiol, estrone and gonadotropin levels following the administration of orally active 17 β-estradiol in postmenopausal women. *J. Clin. Endocr. 40*:518, 1975.

Zellman, H. E.: Unusual aspects of myxedema. *Geriatrics 23*:140, 1968.

Zumoff, B., Bradlow, H. L., et al.: The influence of age and sex on the metabolism of testosterone. *J. Clin. Endocr. 42*:703, 1976.

CHAPTER 30

Endocrine Responsive Cancers of Man

By Mortimer B. Lipsett
and Marc E. Lippman

INTRODUCTION

Hormones have been implicated in several aspects of cancer genesis and growth. It is likely that hormones "prepare" responsive tissue so that the carcinogenic event can occur (Fig. 30–1). In the absence of this effect, cancer is rare; for example, prostate cancer does not occur in eunuchs, and endometrial cancer occurs in women with Turner's syndrome only when they have been treated with estrogens.[1] Hormones may also be involved in the transformation of latent carcinoma to clinical cancer, as in carcinoma of the prostate (conditional or promoter effect). They have also been postulated to have a role in the carcinogenic process (permissive influence). In none of these cases are the hormones the proximate carcinogens. Additionally, the endocrine milieu is one of the determinants of the rate of growth of such cancers as those of the breast, prostate, and endometrium, and changes in the hormonal environment can alter cancer growth rates.

The current resurgence of interest in the hormone-sensitive cancers derives from increased knowledge of the mechanism of action of hormones. However, the concept underlying many endocrine therapies is essentially simple, namely, that some tumors remain dependent on the hormones that are necessary for growth and maintenance of function of the normal tissue from which the tumor originated. This concept was presaged by the remarkable clinical experiment of Beatson[2] who, in 1896, achieved regression of metastatic breast cancer by oophorectomy. Lacassagne[3] suggested that hormones might be involved in the development of cancer, since he was able to induce mammary carcinoma by estrone in mice with low natural incidence of cancer. Huggins et al.[4] demonstrated that carcinoma of the human prostate regressed after orchiectomy and thereby initiated the modern era of endocrine therapy of cancer. This study was based on his earlier observations that androgen was necessary for function of the prostate, and he then surmised that this dependence survived the process of neoplastic transformation.

In this chapter breast cancer is discussed in depth, first because the principles of endocrine therapy derived from the study of this disease may be applicable generally, and second because the large volume of research in experimental and clinical mammary cancer illuminates the direction of research and therapy to a greater extent than that in other cancers. We shall also discuss lymphoma and carcinomas of the prostate, uterine endometrium, and kidney, with emphasis on the basic endocrinology underlying carcinogenesis and therapy.

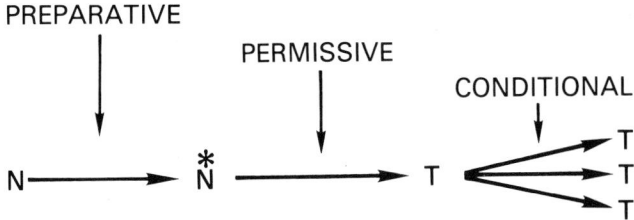

Figure 30–1. Sites of action of steroid hormones on carcinogenesis.

BREAST CANCER

Introduction

Breast cancer is the leading cause of cancer death in women. In 1980, there will be about 100,000 new cases of breast cancer and almost one-half of them will eventually be fatal. To stem this epidemic, high-risk groups must be identified and preventive measures devised. It is in these areas that endocrinologic leads are promising. The large number of women with metastatic disease requires that therapeutic modalities be improved and their selection be made more accurate. Here, too, endocrinology has contributed important new information that has already been shown to be of clinical value. In this section we will briefly review some of the epidemiologic features of breast cancer, particularly as they pertain to the endocrine state, and then discuss more rational approaches to endocrine therapy.

Epidemiology

Epidemiologic studies of breast cancer have provided information concerning such risk factors as genetic potential and chemical, viral, and hormonal factors.[5, 6] These multiple predictors of risk include sex, age, age at menarche and menopause, age at first birth, geographic area of residence, dietary factors, family history of breast cancer (Table 30–1), and a variety of indicators related to steroid hormone concentrations in blood or urine. Many of these risk factors are interdependent; some may be related to endocrine status. Unfortunately, no risk factor, either alone or in combination (with the exception of certain very rare high-risk kindreds), is sufficiently discriminatory at the present time to identify women in whom special therapeutic intervention is warranted. Rather, these epidemiologic factors suggest important and potentially alterable influences in the etiology of breast cancer requiring further study.

Table 30–1. RISK FACTORS

Factor	High Risk	Relative Risk
Religion	Jewish	2
Socioeconomic	Affluent	2
Marital status	Never married	2
Race	Caucasian	2–5
Genetic	Family history	3.5
Diet	Western Europe North America	5
Reproductive history	No lactation	1.5
	Early menarche	1.5
	Nulliparity	2.5
	Late menopause	1.5
	High maternal age at first birth	3
Breast pathology	Prior breast disease	3

The most important risk factors in which endocrine influences may be significant can be grouped under four headings: international variation, reproductive history, familial clustering, and hormonal milieu.

International Variation

A significant epidemiologic finding is the striking variation in rates of breast cancer among various areas of the world. In women at age 50, the incidence of breast cancer is about six times higher in the United States than in Japan or Taiwan.[7] This initially was interpreted as genetic in origin, but the descendants of the Chinese living in Hawaii for several generations have the same rate of breast cancer as do the Caucasians, and first- and second-generation Japanese in Hawaii have rates higher than do women in Japan.[8] It should be noted that the incidence of breast cancer is now increasing in Japan. Therefore, environmental factors must be considered.

The relation of rates to age also has interesting and differential characteristics. In countries with a high incidence of breast cancer, there is a continued increase with age. But in "low-risk" countries, the rate of development of breast cancer decreases after the menopause (Fig. 30–2). DeWaard[9] has suggested that these data imply two different etiologic types of breast cancer. Superimposed on the curve for breast cancer incidence in countries of lower socioeconomic status is an additional type of cancer related to such factors as increased food consumption, increased fat and meat intake, and higher rates of obesity that are generally associated with industrialization.

Reproductive History

Reproductive history has been thoroughly studied. Assigning arbitarily a relative risk of 1 to nulliparous women, it has been claimed that women exhibit nearly a threefold alteration in risk of breast cancer, varying from 0.5 for women having their first child before age 20 to 1.4 for women giving birth after age 37. This protective effect

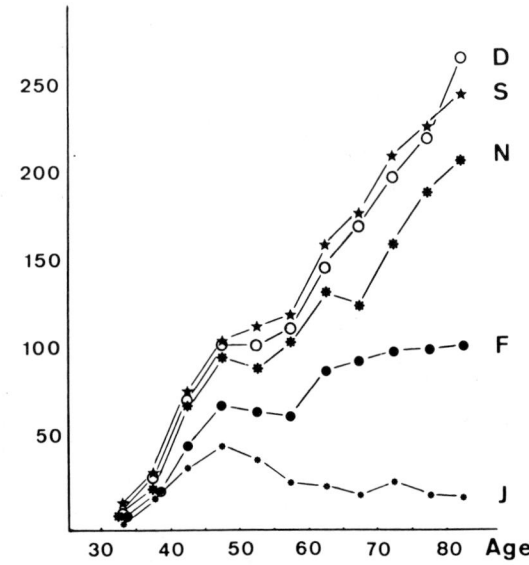

Figure 30–2. Incidence of breast cancer with age in countries with high and low cancer rates. D = Denmark; S = Sweden; N = Norway; F = France; J = Japan. (From DeWaard, F.: *Int. J. Cancer* 4:577, 1969.)

of early age at first birth is maintained throughout life, even among women age 75 and older.[10] In other studies, such effects have not been confirmed.[6]

At the present time, alternative hypotheses suggest that the presumed protective effect of early pregnancy is due either to a permanent pregnancy-induced alteration in the mammary gland or to a chronic postpartum alteration in circulating hormone levels. Study of this issue is critical because identification of the source of this substantial protection against breast cancer risk provided by early first birth might allow prophylactic endocrine manipulations in young women. Generally, it has not appeared likely that this protective effect was due to lactation *per se*,[11, 12] although in one study a protective effect was noted, possibly related to a long duration of lactation.[13] In addition, a recent study in women who nursed their children on only one breast showed a highly significant reduction in breast cancer on that side.[14]

Family History

Family history is an important risk factor in breast cancer. Petrakis[15] has reviewed the evidence supporting genetic components of breast cancer. These include family history of breast cancer, particularly in cases of bilaterality and families with both male and female clustering. Relatively stable incidence rates, as well as stable racial differences, also support the role of genetic factors. Weak associations of breast cancer with HL-A antigens[16] and cerumen type[17] constitute additional evidence. While genetic factors could be expressed at a variety of levels, heritable alteration in the endocrine milieu deserves intensive study. Thus, a comparison of individuals known by family history to be at high risk for breast cancer when compared with an appropriate control group might be expected to yield important insights into hormonal background for development of breast cancer. Two such studies, though well designed, have been relatively disappointing.[18, 19] While the latter study is not yet complete, no statistically significant differences were detected in prolactin, gonadotropin, estrone, estradiol, or estriol concentration. These results are different from those of similar studies of male breast cancer[20] and suggest that genetic effects may be mediated either nonhormonally or via chronic subtle changes in the endocrine milieu that have not been appreciated.

The Hormonal Milieu

It has long been supposed that the hormonal environment may influence the risk of development of breast cancer and the rate of progression of established cancer. This concept has experimental support from studies of induction of mammary cancer in rodents, in which the preparative or conditional role of estrogens can be demonstrated clearly. Investigations of this area in man have been slow for many reasons. Among these were inadequate methods of measurement; rapid fluctuations in the plasma concentrations of some hormones; a variety of characteristics of patients, such as thyroid status, nutrition, age, and liver function, that affect steroid metabolism; and, most important, the real probability that measurement at the time of development of clinical disease has little relevance to the hormonal milieu present during the initial stage of carcinogenesis some 5 to 15 years earlier.

Estrogens. Since the relationship of breast cancer to estrogen seemed obvious, the measurement of urinary estrogens was undertaken by several groups; there were however, no differences between women with breast cancer and those in the normal population. These studies also suffer from the criticism that estrogens should have been measured at the time of carcinogenesis rather than at some stage of clinical disease. Further, the large fluctuations of estrogens during the menstrual cycle and the alterations in route of metabolism with disease or with drugs make interpretation difficult. As noted above, hormonal patterns of presumptively high-risk groups of women did not differ from those of the normal population.

Nevertheless ovarian activity is a clear risk factor in breast cancer. It has long been appreciated that surgical menopause is protective against breast cancer in proportion to the reduction in years of menstrual life.[21] Age at menarche and age at natural menopause are also risk factors in breast cancer, with longer menstrual life associated with a higher risk of breast cancer.[22] This excess risk exists even for very elderly women, an observation which is consistent with a long latent period for some human breast cancers. It seems probable that ovarian estrogen is the causative factor, and it has been shown that the protective effects of early ovariectomy are negated by administration of estrogen.[23] In addition, estrogen treatment of men with prostatic cancer[24] or those undergoing transsexual operations[25] is also associated with an increased risk of breast cancer. In fact, an overwhelming case can be made for disturbances in endogenous estrogen production or metabolism in most cases of male breast cancer.[26]

A popular hypothesis relating estrogens to cancer risk was that a woman with a high urinary excretion of estriol had a decreased risk for breast cancer because estriol was apparently an estrogen antagonist.[27] In support of this hypothesis was the finding that Japanese women (a low-risk group) had higher urinary estriol excretion than did Australian women.[28] However, the hypothesis should be abandoned for the following reasons: First, estriol is an estrogen whose receptor binding characteristics make it act as an antagonist only when it is given intermittently.[29] When it is given continuously, it is a potent estrogen and will act as a promoter of mammary gland carcinogenesis in experimental systems. Second, urinary estriol has no relationship to plasma estriol concentrations or production rates.[30] Further, the ratio of estriol to estrone plus estradiol was not related to differences between estrogen blood levels and production rates in normal women or in women with breast cancer.[30]

Studies of estrogen levels, sources, and production rates have not shown differences between women with early breast cancer and a control population.[31] Similarly, plasma estrogens have not differed between these groups.[32]

Androgens. Bulbrook has summarized early studies as well as his own dealing with discriminant functions based primarily on androgen excretion.[33] Briefly, it was shown that a higher excretion of androgen metabolites was correlated with a greater likelihood of response to adrenalectomy or hypophysectomy. The use of this discriminant function has markedly decreased because of the much higher predictability of estrogen receptors.

Of greater interest was the finding in a prospective trial that urinary etiocholanolone (an androgen metabolite) excretion was lower in women who subsequently developed breast cancer.[34] In a more recent study, the same group showed that women at high risk for breast cancer had the lowest plasma levels of androgens.[34a] Attention has been focused on other androgens; urinary testosterone excretion[35] and plasma testosterone levels[36] were higher in women with early breast cancer. Other conflicting data do not give the endocrinologist confidence that important endocrine abnormalities have been delineated as yet.

Most of the data regarding the hormonal milieu relate to hormones present in plasma or in urine. However, in 1968, Adams and Wong[37, 38] reported that human breast cancer tissue could metabolize dehydroepiandrosterone to androstenedione and possibly to estriol. Cholesterol was converted to C-19 steroids. Dao et al.[39] found that breast cancer tissue could aromatize steroids and isolated estrone and estradiol after incubation with C-19 steroids. Thus the breast cancer cell has the potential to create its own microenvironment and thereby defeat efforts to lower estradiol levels in the surrounding medium. Some breast cancers have the capacity to sulfurylate various steroids, and it has been noted that the absence of the sulfokinase was correlated with a lack of response to adrenalectomy.[39] Recent study of the ability of a metabolite of dehydroepiandrosterone, androstenediol, to compete with estradiol for estrogen receptors[38] suggests a mechanism for relating androgen metabolism to the clinical response to hormonal therapy.

Epidemiology — Exogenous Hormones

Benign Breast Disease

Although most benign breast diseases are not considered to be premalignant, there is strong evidence to suggest that women with benign breast disease have a substantially increased risk (up to four times in one well studied series)[40] of developing breast cancer. While other explanations are possible, it is likely that benign and malignant breast disease share common etiologic factor(s) related to the endocrine milieu. Thus, an examination of the effects of exogenous sex hormones on benign breast disease is of interest. There is now strong evidence from both retrospective analyses[40-44] and prospective studies[45, 46] that oral contraceptive use diminishes risk of benign breast disease. Generally, those studies show a greater protective effect for cystic disease as compared to fibroadenoma. In addition, protection is greater in "long-term users" as compared to "ever users," an important point in favor of a causal relationship. Interestingly, the study conducted by the Royal College of General Practitioners[41] showed the incidence rates for benign breast disease to be inversely related to the amount of progestogen in the preparation. Confirmation of this observation is provided by surveys of women using noncontraceptive estrogen preparations in which no protection against benign breast disease was demonstrated.[42, 47] However, certain forms of benign breast disease such as intraductal papilloma and fibrosing adenosis as well as severe atypia of the ductular lining cells have been associated with a particularly high likelihood of subsequent malignancy.[48, 49] Effects of oral contraceptives on women with these specific histologic features have not been assessed; therefore, it should not be concluded that the effectiveness of oral contraceptives in reducing benign breast disease is equivalent to a protection against breast cancer. It may be that in particular subsets of women with benign breast disease estrogen use increases the risk.

Breast Cancer

There was a small but significant increase in the incidence of breast cancer during the decade 1960 to 1970, a period in which the use of oral contraceptives and postmenopausal estrogens increased sharply.[50] Nevertheless, the many factors that bear on this observation make it difficult to conclude that exogenous estrogens increase breast cancer risk.[50, 51] Multiple retrospective case control studies have failed to reveal a significant overall increase in risk of developing breast cancer among oral contraceptive users.[40, 43, 52-54] However, several observations prevent a totally sanguine view of this conclusion. In general, the time required for tumor promotion in humans is long, and there may not be sufficient experience as yet for firm conclusions. Two studies of younger women showed a relative risk ratio of 1.7 for users of oral contraceptives for more than 8 and 5 years, respectively,[55, 56] although this increase was not statistically significant. Two other studies have failed to show an increase in risk with passage of time.[43, 52] However, in one of these studies[52] oral contraceptives increased the risk of breast cancer in three subsets of patients: nulliparous women, women using the pill prior to the birth of their first child, and women with a history of benign breast disease. Prospective trials of oral contraceptives are negative at this point[45, 52] and, in fact, may suggest a reduction in risk. Longer follow-up studies are required before the risk can be adequately assessed.

There have been many retrospective analyses of women using estrogens after the menopause, and none shows a significant association between use and breast cancer risk.[47, 54-56] In one large retrospective study,[23] a relative risk ratio of 1.3 (of borderline statistical significance) was found for estrogen users. More alarmingly, risk was related to duration of follow-up, with a doubling of this risk ratio after 12 years of use. No follow-up of oral contraceptive users of this duration is available. The risk was greatest in women who took the highest-strength preparation, although it was not related to duration of use. Finally, as with the study of oral contraceptives,[43] risk of cancer was twice as great in women with a history of benign breast disease, and increased sevenfold in women who developed benign breast disease after starting on estrogens.

Hormone Receptors and Endocrine Therapy of Breast Cancer

The fact that some human breast cancers might respond to endocrine manipulations has been appreciated since George Beatson induced tumor regressions in patients following bilateral oophorectomy.[2] Unequivocally, patients who respond to such endocrine therapies have not only palliation of their illness, but substantially longer survival than nonresponders. Despite the clear-cut benefits to responders, only about one-third of unselected patients can be expected to have objective tumor regressions following hormonal therapy. With the advent of effective chemotherapy regimens, a more precise selection of different treatment modalities is necessary.

A variety of empirically derived clinical guidelines (disease-free interval, sites of involvement, and so forth), as well as a few biochemical tests (excretion of androgen metabolites, steroid sulfation), have been suggested as being of value in selecting patients with hormone-responsive tumors. Unfortunately, none of these approaches has proved sufficiently reliable for widespread adoption. However, recent developments in the field of hormone action have brought more accurate means of patient selection.

The first step in steroid hormone action in general, and estrogens in particular, is the binding of the hormone to specific receptor (see Chapter 7). Clearly, functional receptor molecules are a necessary, albeit insufficient, requirement for steroid hormone action. In animal systems, it was shown that regression of mammary cancer in response to hormonal therapy required the presence of estrogen receptors.[57, 58] Subsequently, breast cancer samples were shown to sequester and retain estrogen.[59, 60] Later, Jensen found specific estrogen-binding activity in human breast cancers and showed direct correlations between the presence of estrogen receptor and the likelihood of response to endocrine therapy.[61] In brief, about two-thirds of primary breast cancers contain significant concentrations of estrogen receptor, while a somewhat smaller proportion of metastatic samples are positive for estrogen receptor. Premenopausal patients have tumors that are less frequently estrogen receptor–positive and contain, on average, lower concentrations of receptor than the cancer occurring after the menopause. These observations are only partially explained by the fact that the larger amounts of endogenous estrogen in plasma of premenopausal women mask the binding sites.

Overall, there is a highly significant association between the presence of estrogen receptor and the likelihood of response to endocrine therapy. Predictive accuracy for the test is about 75%. Thus about 75% of the 60% of patients with estrogen receptor–positive tumors respond to endocrine therapy, and 95% of the 40% of patients with estrogen receptor–negative tumors fail to respond. In general, the greater the estrogen receptor content of the tumor, the higher the response rate to endocrine therapy.

While the response rate of tumors apparently lacking estrogen receptors is low, it is not zero. Thus, a single negative assay should be considered as only one component in the selection of appropriate therapy. There are several potential explanations for the observation of an endocrine response in women with purportedly estrogen receptor–negative tumors. First, since steroid receptors are thermolabile proteins, and many methodologic pitfalls may prevent detection of receptor activity. Particularly common problems include incorrect handling and storage of samples. Second, frequently a pathologic diagnosis of metastatic breast cancer may be based on a few tumor cells infiltrating a nonmalignant tissue. Thus, a negative assay may result from an insufficient sampling of malignant cells or even inadvertent biopsy of neighboring nonmalignant tissue. Third, a variety of additive and ablative therapies employed in patients with breast cancer may act via mechanisms mediated by receptors other than estrogen receptors. Thus, even in the absence of estrogen receptor a response to some endocrine manipulations may be observed. Fourth, breast tumors may be heterogeneous with respect to receptor status; thus, a biopsied site which is estrogen receptor–negative may not be representative of other tumor deposits. Fifth, it is possible that some assays are falsely negative since most estrogen receptor analyses are performed on cytoplasmic extracts using conditions which do not permit detection of receptor sites occupied by endogenous hormone. Sixth, it has been shown that even in the absence of endogenous hormone, receptor sites may be localized to the nucleus[62] and therefore missed by standard methodologies. It is in fact somewhat surprising how rarely (about 5%) so-called estrogen receptor–negative tumors respond to endocrine therapy.

It is much more commonly observed that tumors containing estrogen receptor fail to respond to endocrine therapy. The most commonly invoked explanation for this observation is tumor cell heterogeneity. That is, a sufficient number of cells within the tumor sample contain re-

ceptor to give a positive assay result, although the majority are receptor-negative. Were this to be the case, one would anticipate that there might be a quantitative relationship between the concentration of estrogen receptor and the likelihood of observing an endocrine response; this result has been reported.[63] In fact, tumor deposits have been shown to be a heterogeneous mixture of receptor-positive and receptor-negative cells.[64, 65] Second, the presence of estrogen receptor is generally correlated in an apparently nonrational fashion with a variety of endocrine therapies. If, for example, androgen administration induces tumor regressions by a process involving interaction with androgen receptor, then some estrogen receptor–positive, androgen receptor–negative tumors might fail to respond to this endocrine therapy. Third, the presence of receptor may connote hormone-dependent breast cancer but the endocrine therapy may not sufficiently alter the hormonal milieu. For example, pituitary ablation may be incomplete. Additionally, it is well known that about 10 to 15% of patients with metastatic breast cancer who fail to respond to oophorectomy will respond to a subsequent adrenalectomy. Presumably these patients can be assumed to have had hormone-dependent tumors at the time of their oophorectomy and, thus, their tumors would have been estrogen receptor–positive pseudo-hormone-independent. Fourth, any step distal to the initial binding of hormone to receptor may be deranged. Binding of hormone to receptor is only the first step in hormone action. If possible, prediction of hormone dependence could be achieved more certainly if a tumor were assessed for a hormone-inducible function; this would obviously presuppose the presence of receptor. Progesterone receptor,[66] peroxidase,[67-69] and enhanced nucleoside incorporation[70] are being evaluated for their usefulness in this regard. In a model tissue, the uterus, progesterone receptor is induced by estrogen. The presence of progesterone receptor in breast cancer tissue has been assumed to reflect the action of estrogen rather than its binding only. Thus, the presence of progesterone receptor gives some confidence that all the steps of estrogen action are intact.

Despite the many possible explanations for false-positive and false-negative results, steroid receptor studies in breast cancer are extremely valuable. Table 30–2 summarizes the objective response rates to endocrine therapy as a function of estrogen and progesterone receptor status. Thus, for the majority of patients, response to endocrine therapy can be predicted with accuracy.

Recently, two developments have suggested additional ways in which receptor determinations might be of value. Several studies have revealed that patients with estrogen receptor–positive primary breast cancers have a substantially prolonged disease-free interval independent of other

Table 30–2. RESPONSE RATES TO ENDOCRINE THERAPY AS A FUNCTION OF STEROID HORMONE RECEPTOR STATUS IN METASTATIC BREAST CANCER

ER Status	PgR Status	Approximate Objective Response Rate to Endocrine Therapy
Positive	Positive	80%
Positive	Negative	30%
Negative	Positive	Not established
Negative	Negative	5%

ER = Estrogen receptor
PgR = Progesterone receptor

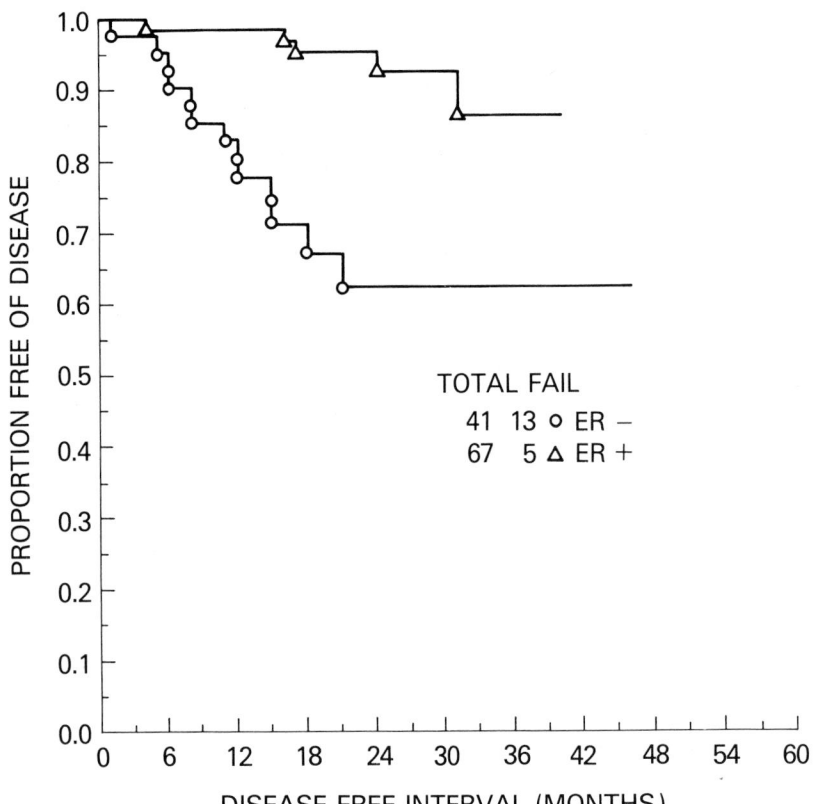

Figure 30–3. Disease-free survival as a function of estrogen receptor status.

Within the figure:

PROPORTION FREE OF DISEASE (y-axis)

DISEASE FREE INTERVAL (MONTHS) (x-axis)

TOTAL FAIL
41 13 ○ ER −
67 5 △ ER +

known prognostic variables including menopausal status, tumor size, histologic grade, and axillary lymph node status.[71-73] In Figure 30–3, the disease-free survival (the time for primary surgery to first recurrence) as a function of estrogen receptor status is shown for a group of women with breast cancer. There is a highly significant prolongation of time from surgery to first recurrence in the estrogen receptor–positive group. Thus, estrogen receptor determinations may aid in selection of patients at higher risk of early recurrence who may benefit from adjuvant therapy. Second, two studies have recently suggested that estrogen receptor–negative tumors have a substantially higher response rate to cytotoxic chemotherapy.[74, 75] This observation is consistent with the findings that less well differentiated tumors, which are more often estrogen receptor–negative, tend to have shorter disease-free intervals and higher thymidine labeling indexes. Since most cytotoxic drugs are far more effective against rapidly dividing cells, one might expect that adjuvant chemotherapy would be more effective in patients with estrogen receptor–negative tumors. Although this hypothesis seems reasonable, a recent study did not confirm the correlation of negative estrogen receptors and a high rate of response to chemotherapy and there is now no agreement on this point.[76]

In rodent mammary carcinoma, prolactin has an important role in the genesis and support of growth of the tumors.[77] Regulation of prolactin receptor content in these tumors is still under investigation, but there does seem to be some relationship between prolactin receptor content and response. As with estrogen receptors, tumors are heterogeneous for prolactin receptor content.[78] Prolactin receptors are present in human breast cancer,[78] but early studies do not suggest a relationship between receptor content and response.[79] The epidemiologic finding that the prolonged use of prolactin-releasing drugs does not increase the incidence of breast cancer[80, 81] is in accord with the few biologic data in humans.

Management of Breast Cancer

Although many aspects of the management of breast cancer fall outside the province of the endocrinologist, it is worthwhile to mention briefly certain aspects of the oncologist's approach to the patient with breast cancer in order to place endocrine manipulations in a proper context.

Basically, it is convenient to divide the management of breast cancer into two phases: The approach to the patient with early-stage disease and the approach to the patient with advanced (metastatic) disease.

Early Breast Cancer

It is important to ensure that all women with early breast cancer have an estrogen receptor assay. In addition to the prognostic significance of the test (Fig. 30–3), there may be other advantages accruing from this assay.

Preliminary data now suggest that the estrogen receptor status of the primary cancer is maintained in the metastases. Thus, knowledge of the receptor status of the primary permits assignment to the appropriate treatment category when metastases develop, even if there is no readily accessible tissue for biopsy. Secondly, a recent unpublished study (Hubay, C., and Pearson, O. H.: NCI Conference on Estrogen Receptors, 1979) shows that receptor-positive patients with positive axillary nodes are benefited by the institution of endocrine adjuvant therapy (tamoxifen) at the time of mastectomy.

MANAGEMENT OF EARLY STAGE BREAST CANCER

All Patients

> 1) Adequate therapy for local control of disease.
> 2) Evaluation of axillary lymph node status.
> 3) ER and PgR* analyses of primary tumor.

Figure 30–4. Approach to therapy for patients with early breast cancer.

Histologic Status of Lymph Nodes	ER Status	Recommended Therapy
Pre menopausal patients		
Involved with tumor	Positive	Combination chemotherapy and/or endocrine therapy
Involved with tumor	Negative	Combination chemotherapy
Negative	Positive	No therapy
Negative	Negative	? Combination chemotherapy
Post menopausal patient		
Involved with tumor	Positive	Endocrine therapy ?
Involved with tumor	Negative	Combination chemotherapy
Negative	Positive	No therapy
Negative	Negative	No therapy

*Role of Progesterone Receptor (PgR) not established.

An approach to patients with early breast cancer is shown in Figure 30–4. The patients require therapy directed at the primary tumor that not only is sufficient for local control of disease but, at the same time, is as attentive to cosmetic outcome as possible. This is an area of active investigation, and therapy is becoming more individualized. In addition, patients require adequate staging, including asesssment of axillary lymph node involvement with tumor and steroid hormone receptor status. On the basis of this evaluation, adjuvant therapy regimens may be considered although their roles remain to be defined.

Metastatic Breast Cancer

While many patients with primary breast cancer will remain free of disease following local therapy (with or without the addition of systemic adjuvant therapy), a substantial number of cancers eventually recur. At this time

endocrine therapy may be attempted. As already mentioned, only about one-third of unselected patients can be expected to achieve a partial response or better. With appropriate consideration of steroid receptor and menopausal status, substantial improvement in response rates can be achieved. One suggested approach is outlined in Figure 30–5. Following appropriate assessment of sites of disease and receptor status, patients may be allocated to differing treatment regimens. Obviously, other factors must be weighed in such decision making, including such prognostic variables as performance status and sites of involvement and issues involving individual patients, such as the relative impact of various treatment modalities on lifestyle. Furthermore, there is substantial latitude in choice of a given endocrine or chemotherapy regimen since the superiority of particular regimens may still be in question. In the next few sections, we will provide some information concerning specific endocrine therapies, with emphasis on the use of antiestrogens and inhibitors of endogenous steroidogenesis.

MANAGEMENT OF METASTATIC BREAST CANCER

All Patients

> 1) Adequate staging of sites of involvement.
> 2a) Biopsy of accessible tumor for ER and PgR status or if not available.
> 2b) Receptor status of primary tumor.

Figure 30–5. Approach to therapy for patients with metastatic breast cancer.

	Pre Menopausal Patients		Post Menopausal Patients	
First therapy	*ER Positive*	*ER Negative*	*ER Positive*	*ER Negative*
	Castration	Combination chemotherapy	Antiestrogens	Combination chemotherapy
	Relapse: Repeat ER Assay		Relapse: Repeat ER Assay	
Second therapy	Endocrine therapy	Chemotherapy	Endocrine therapy	Chemotherapy

Endocrine Therapy of Breast Cancer

Oophorectomy

The removal of the ovaries of premenopausal patients has been known to be an effective treatment for some women with inoperable breast cancer for over 80 years.[2] Using rigid criteria, the regression rate is 25 to 30%,[82, 83] and the median duration of remission is 9 months. In general, surgery is the method of choice, since radiation may require several weeks to be effective, and incomplete destruction of the follicles has been reported.

It is important to be able to evaluate ovarian status accurately. As noted in Chapter 7, a high plasma FSH is a reliable indication of loss of follicles and consequent cessation of estradiol secretion. The low plasma estradiol (< 20 pg/ml) is also characteristic of cessation of ovarian function, but concentrations this low may occur in patients with secondary amenorrhea. The vaginal smear is unreliable for distinguishing between a low secretion rate of estradiol and cessation of ovarian function. In perimenopausal and postmenopausal patients, the regression rate from oophorectomy is well below that of women with ovarian function.[84]

Adrenalectomy and Hypophysectomy

Estrogens persist in blood and urine after ovariectomy. The adrenal cortex secretes a small amount of estrone,[85] but the main source of estrone after castration is the transformation of androstenedione, secreted by the adrenal cortex, to estrone in peripheral tissues.[86] It has been difficult to prove, except inferentially, that the low concentrations of estradiol and estrone characteristic of the menopause are sufficient to support the growth of endocrine-sensitive tumors. However, the demonstration that the absence of an estrogen receptor in tumor tissue predicts that adrenalectomy will fail to be beneficial is additional evidence for this concept. In addition, recent studies of human breast cancer cells maintained in continuous tissue culture have demonstrated that as little as 2 to 3 × 10^{-11} M estradiol is sufficient to stimulate macromolecular synthesis.[87]

The criteria for selection of patients for adrenalectomy or hypophysectomy are several. First, if an estrogen receptor can be identified in metastatic tissue, then the chance of response is about 60%. If the patient has responded to castration, then the likelihood of subsequent response to ablative surgery is above 50%. Whether these two criteria identify the same patients is not known, but it is likely. It is also likely that the longer the free interval, the higher is the remission rate.[88]

The rate of response to adrenalectomy or hypophysectomy has been variously estimated as equal[89] or somewhat in favor of hypophysectomy.[90, 91] The mean duration of remission was also longer after hypophysectomy (15 months versus 8 months).[91] Although these data suggest that hypophysectomy may offer some advantages, the choice of operation must usually be made from more pragmatic considerations, such as the surgical skills available, the sites of metastases, and the age of patient. The management of adrenal and pituitary insufficiency has been discussed elsewhere in this book. It is necessary only to state that the patient can be treated adequately in either case and, when a remission occurs, can often resume full activity.

Androgen Therapy

Lacassagne, who was the first to show that estrogens promoted development of mammary tumors in mice, found that the growth of these tumors could be inhibited by testosterone propionate.[92] Androgen therapy of women with metastatic cancer was initiated 30 years ago. The Cooperative Breast Cancer Group surveyed the response of 521 patients treated with testosterone propionate and reported a remission rate of 21%.[93] The response depended on menopausal status and on sites of metastases. Within 1 year of the menopause, the remission rate was less than 10%, and it was highest 5 years after the menopause. Soft tissue metastases responded most favorably and visceral metastases least. The median period of remission was 8 months. Any androgen, given in large amounts, produces about the same rate of regression. Long-acting preparations should be avoided, since it is then impossible to stop therapy should the disease accelerate, e.g., the sudden development of severe hypercalcemia. The results of trials with many androgens have been summarized.[94]

Attempts have been made to find steroids less androgenic than testosterone, since it may produce virilization that is severe and often distressing. This quest has been generally unsuccessful. A synthetic steroid, Δ'-testololactone, has essentially no androgenic activity and has been reported to produce regression of disease.[95] Although the incidence of remissions was low, their occurrence is evidence that antitumor effect can be independent of androgenicity.

Estrogens

The observation that some patients with breast cancer can respond to estrogen therapy was not predictable, nor was it based on data from animal models. Following the initial observations, however, remission rates of 30 to 37% were reported in two large series[96, 97] when estrogen was used as initial therapy. In a randomized trial of steroid therapy, estrogen produced a 29% remission rate and androgen a 10% remission rate.[98] The duration of response to estrogen has been longer than that to androgen in most series. Estrogen responsiveness increases with years after the menopause. As with androgen and the ablative procedures, the longer the free interval, the higher is the probability of response to estrogen.

When estrogens are used in patients who have relapsed from other therapy, remission rates are low, the chances of response being less than 10%. Also, estrogen is generally ineffective following hypophysectomy or adrenalectomy.

The toxicity from estrogens, even at high doses, is small. Endometrial hyperplasia and breakthrough bleeding are not uncommon and can usually be managed by giving a progestogen, followed by a short period of cessation of hormone therapy to permit sloughing of the endometrium. Salt and water retention, particularly, in the elderly, may occur with any estrogen. Of greatest consequence, however, is hypercalcemia. This can occur abruptly in any patient but is rare in patients 10 or more years after the menopause. Hypercalcemia is managed by withdrawal of estrogen and hydration. Often, on reinstitution of therapy, a regression will be obtained without recurrence of hypercalcemia.

The phenomenon of a response following withdrawal of estrogen or of androgen has been recorded.[99] Thus, new attempts at therapy should generally not be started until at least 2 months after steroids have been stopped. Rapidly advancing disease will, of course, constitute an exception to this suggestion.

Progestogens

A variety of progestogens, both of the C-21-17α-acetoxysteroids, such as medroxyprogesterone, and of the C-19 steroids, such as norethisterone, have been used in patients with breast cancer. In general, remission rates have clustered about 20%,[100, 101] the same as those noted with androgens. The response to progestogens was not influenced by previous response to castration, estrogen, or androgen. Thus progestogens may be given a trial in patients failing to respond to other therapeutic modalities. In general, these agents are without important side-effects. Regression appears to be more common with soft tissue metastases and unusual with bone metastases.

Glucocorticoids

There is little doubt that large doses of any glucocorticoid (equivalent to 200 to 300 mg of cortisol daily) can induce regression of disease at any site. Remissions are short-lived, but the rapid effect of the glucocorticoids makes them useful in rapidly advancing disease. A response to glucocorticoids is not predictive of response to other endocrine modalities. Glucocorticoids are also of value in managing acute difficulties such as hypercalcemia and intracranial metastases.

Antiestrogens

Theoretically, any substance which will antagonize the action of estrogens may be termed an antiestrogen. Many compounds which would fit this definition include a variety of nonspecific inhibitors of protein and RNA synthesis. However, with the possible exception of certain weak, short-acting agonists, such as estriol, all such compounds of clinical relevance developed thus far are derivatives of triphenylethylene. These include nafoxidine and tamoxifen. These compounds compete with estradiol for binding to specific estrogen receptor sites. However, the explanation for their biologic activity is far more complicated and cannot be explained in terms of this effect alone. Detailed information on this subject has been presented recently.[102, 103] It is likely that antiestrogenic compounds after binding to estrogen receptors, translocate these receptors to nuclear sites. A variety of partially conflicting results do not establish with certainty whether these nuclear sites are[104] or are not[105, 106] identical to nuclear sites occupied by estrogen receptor complexes. All such studies are hampered by a failure to either purify or unequivocally identify the specific nuclear "acceptor site" (if it exists at all) that is involved in estrogenic effect.

Nonetheless, antiestrogens have proved extremely useful in the management of postmenopausal breast cancer,[107-109] though their role in premenopausal patients remains to be clarified. Some premenopausal patients may continue to have apparently normal menstrual cycles while exhibiting objective tumor regressions.[110] As already mentioned, antiestrogens have considerable effects which must be termed estrogenic. The vaginal epithelium of postmenopausal women usually shows an estrogenic effect. In addition, some women appear to show a brief "flare" of tumor following the institution of antiestrogen therapy,[111] although very careful attempts to quantify this phenomenon have not been successful.[112]

Antiestrogens are certainly of value in male and female breast cancer,[26, 107-109] since about one-third of patients will benefit from antiestrogen therapy. Thus, these drugs are at least as efficacious as other forms of endocrine manipulation. A particular advantage of the antiestrogens is their almost complete lack of significant toxicity. Tamoxifen administration is not associated with significant myelosuppression or renal, hepatic, or central nervous system toxicity. Particularly encouraging, and of theoretical interest, is that an appreciable response rate has been seen following relapse after successful adrenalectomy.[114] This result is consistent with in vitro studies of human breast cancer which have suggested that antiestrogens are capable of receptor-mediated tumor inhibition, even in the absence of ambient estrogen.[115, 116] Further work is required to delineate the optimal utilization of antiestrogens in breast cancer and other neoplasms.

Pharmacologic Interference with Endogenous Steroidogenesis

Although major ablative endocrine therapies are unquestionably effective for some patients, their substantial hazard has prompted efforts to achieve similar results pharmacologically. It has long been appreciated that transient palliative responses could be seen in some patients with metastatic breast cancer following glucocorticoid administration. Although a direct inhibitory effect of glucocorticoids on human breast cancer cells in long-term tissue culture has been shown,[117] it is likely that partial suppression of adrenal androgen production and subsequent estrogen synthesis played a role. In 1973, Griffiths and colleagues proposed the use of aminoglutethimide combined with dexamethasone to suppress adrenal function.[118] Aminoglutethimide had previously been shown to be a potent inhibitor of the conversion of cholesterol to pregnenolone.[119] While this regimen was effective in some women, subsequent studies by Santen and his colleagues[120] demonstrated that aminoglutethimide substantially shortened the plasma half-life of dexamethasone, and as a result, pituitary ACTH secretion resumed and overrode the adrenal blockade imposed by aminoglutethimide. By substituting hydrocortisone (whose metabolism was not altered by aminoglutethimide) it was possible to derive a fixed-dose regimen which gave adequate adrenal suppression in most patients.[121] Careful measurement of adrenal steroid concentrations in some of these patients suggested that although dehydroepiandrosterone levels declined, there was an initial rise in Δ^4-androstenedione, the immediate precursor of estrone. Since levels of estrone also fell rapidly, it suggested that an important additional activity of aminoglutethimide might be a blockade of peripheral aromatization. This has been substantiated by in vitro measurements in which aminoglutethimide has been shown to inhibit aromatization by human placenta.

Direct comparisons of antisteroidogenic regimens with ablative surgery are under way. Preliminary results have suggested that these nonsurgical modalities may be as effective as surgical means of achieving clinical responses.[121a] It is not unlikely that, if combined with an antiestrogen or antiandrogen, as well as a gonadotropin inhibitor such as danazol or progestin, more widespread use for aminoglutethimide combinations will be found.

ENDOMETRIAL CANCER

Endocrinology

The uterine endometrium is the classic example of a hormone-dependent tissue, its growth and morphology changing cyclically in response to estradiol and progesterone. The identification of the specific uterine cytosol receptor for estradiol in 1960[122] initiated the "receptor" era of endocrinology. The estrogen receptor content of the endometrium is highest in the proliferative phase and is decreased in the luteal phase[123, 124] or by administration of progestins.[125] Progesterone receptor capacity is highest at the time of the estradiol peak[123] and can be induced by estrogens. Estrogen receptor persists in most endometrial carcinomas and the receptor content is inversely correlated with the degree of differentiation,[123] whereas cytosol progesterone receptor capacity[123, 126] and nuclear progesterone receptors[127] are highest in well differentiated cancer.[123] The enzyme, 17β-hydroxysteroid dehydrogenase, that catalyzes the conversion of estradiol to estrone is induced by progesterone content[128] and can serve as an index of progestational effect.

The literature on gynecology is replete with suggestions that the constellation of abnormal estrogen stimulation, disordered anterior pituitary function, diabetes mellitus, obesity, and infertility occur with high frequency in women with endometrial cancer.[129] There is fragmentary evidence for the existence of other factors. Abnormal glucose tolerance tests have been documented in cases of endometrial cancer, and abnormalities of growth hormone secretion were noted in women with endometrial cancer.[130] In biochemical-epidemiologic studies, it was shown that the ratio of estriol to etiocholanolone differed between patients with endometrial cancer and normal controls.[131] A similar study of individual 17-KS and corticoid excretion by patients with endometrial cancer revealed differences between them and several types of matched controls, permitting the construction of a discriminant function.[132] The findings in these last reports do not, of course, distinguish between abnormalities of secretion and of metabolism. These small differences between normal women and those with endometrial carcinoma do not suggest important avenues of research in endometrial cancer.

Epidemiology

There are now clinical, biologic, and epidemiologic data showing that prolonged or unopposed estrogenic stimulation increases the risk of endometrial carcinoma. The biologic evidence is that estrogens probably "prepare" the endometrium for the carcinogenic event. The longer the endometrium is stimulated, the greater the cancer risk, as shown by the association of endometrial carcinoma with the use of estrogens after the menopause[133] and with late menopause. The increase in endometrial cancer among women with estrogen-secreting tumors and the polycystic ovary syndrome[134] emphasizes the role of progesterone-induced endometrial sloughing as a protective mechanism. A higher incidence of endometrial cancer is also seen with several other ovarian abnormalities, such as cortical stromal hyperplasia and persistent stromal thecal cells. In each case, there is reason to believe that estrogen secretion is not excessive. It is, however, continuous, since there are no ovulatory cycles with their accompanying progesterone secretory periods and the subsequent endometrial sloughing. The recent reports of endometrial cancer in women with Turner's syndrome who were treated with estrogens alone is further evidence for this concept. The causal role of continued, unopposed estrogenic stimulus is supported by the high incidence of irregular menses in women with endometrial cancer.[134] The resumption of cyclic ovarian function in response to ovarian wedge resection in the Stein-Leventhal syndrome[135] results in regression of endometrial hyperplasia, and progesterone has also been shown to reverse estrogen-induced endometrial hyperplasia.[136] Since progesterone decreases estradiol receptor (see above), this may be the molecular mechanism underlying these epidemiologic observations.

A risk factor for endometrial carcinoma is obesity. In the premenopausal woman, the association of obesity with anovulatory cycles and amenorrhea may be the physiologic substrate for the association. In the postmenopausal woman, the etiologic pathway has been traced more clearly. After the menopause, the predominant blood estrogen is estrone, derived almost entirely by the conversion in peripheral tissues of androstenedione secreted by the adrenal cortex. The rate of this conversion increases with age[137] and weight,[138] and plasma estrogen concentrations increase with increasing weight.[139] Since fat tissue has the capacity to aromatize androgens, the trail from obesity to greater exposure to estrogens to increased risk for endometrial carcinoma has been opened. Plasma estrone production rates[138] and concentrations[139] are the same in women with endometrial cancer as in weight- and age-matched controls, but the higher incidence of obesity in the women with cancer means that as a group there is greater exposure to estrogen. The mechanism of the factors increasing the risk for endometrial carcinoma are summarized in Figures 30–6 and 30–7.

The association of estrogen use by postmenopausal women and an increased risk of endometrial cancer is impressive and has been reviewed.[129] In essence, relative risk factors for the development of endometrial cancer vary from 4 to 1 to 9 to 1, the risk increasing with the duration of use. This is what might be expected if the endometrium is maintained in a "prepared" state for a longer period, thus allowing more opportunity for the carcinogenic event. It has been claimed that these estimates of excess risk are spurious because of an increased rate of discovery of early endometrial cancer owing to the vaginal bleeding that may accompany estrogen therapy.[141] This argument has been refuted by additional data and theoretical considerations,[133] and it is the consensus that the use of estrogen after the menopause is an important risk factor for endometrial cancer. It should be noted that in all studies of the use of estrogen in postmenopausal women, greater than physiologic doses of estrogen have been used and progestin-induced withdrawal

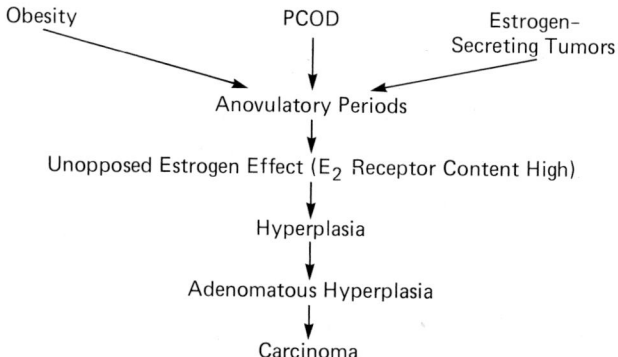

PREMENOPAUSAL WOMEN

Figure 30–6. Mechanisms leading to endometrial carcinoma in premenopausal women. PCOD = Polycystic ovarian disease.

POSTMENOPAUSAL WOMEN

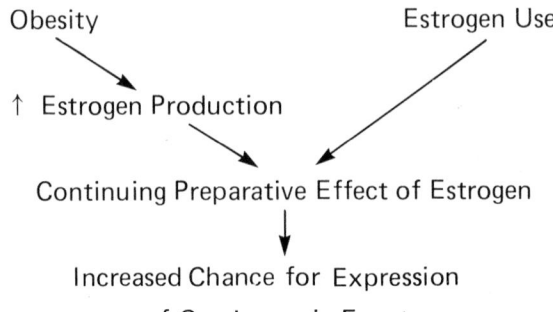

Figure 30–7. Mechanism leading to endometrial carcinoma in postmenopausal women.

bleeding has not generally been part of the regimens. Attention to both these factors would be expected to reduce the risk appreciably.

Therapy

In 1961, Kelley and Baker reported that progestogens could cause regression in about one-third of patients with metastatic endometrial cancer.[140] This has been confirmed with a large series of patients treated at many centers.[142] The response to therapy did not depend on age of patient, site of metastasis, or previous or concurrent therapy. However, women with slowly growing or more differentiated tumors responded better than did those with aggressive cancers. Duration of life after initiation of therapy was 27 months in those who responded and only 7 months in those who did not. These combined data have been duplicated in other reports. It has not mattered which progestogen was used, nor was the dose important,[143] except that large doses seemed to be necessary.

It is the consensus that progestogens should be used in any patient with metastatic disease. It is claimed that the response of pulmonary metastases is better than that of bone metastases, but responses have been noted in all groups. To cite a personal experience, a woman with extensive lytic disease of the pelvis has remained in remission for 15 years, with calcification and remodeling of pelvic bones, on a dose of 100 mg of medroxyprogesterone daily. The remissions seen with progestogens are unique, since they are accomplished with essentially no toxicity. Several studies have clearly demonstrated that quantitative progesterone receptor determinations can be of substantial value in selecting patients suitable for endocrine therapy.

The mechanism behind the effects of progestogen is still only speculation. In the normal estrogen-primed uterus, progesterone causes specific maturational changes, followed by atrophy when a progestogen is continued for long periods. Following administration of progestogens to women with endometrial cancer, mitotic activity ceases, there is increased glandular differentiation, and an increase in cytoplasm-nucleus ratio is seen.[144, 145] Atrophy is also noted.[146] Thus, these changes duplicate those of the normal endometrium during progesterone therapy. The finding that endometrial cancers contain progesterone receptors provides the link to the therapeutic effect. Thus, progesterone decreases estrogen receptors and increases the capacity of the endometrium to metabolize estradiol (see above). As with breast cancer, these tumors may be heterogeneous with respect to cell content of progesterone receptors, thereby accounting for the variability of response.

CARCINOMA OF THE PROSTATE

Epidemiology

Cancer of the prostate is the second most frequent cancer in men in the United States,[147] with more than 60% of the cases occurring in men over 70 years of age The death rate is significantly higher in American blacks than in whites.[148] Of interest was the finding that American black men have an age-standardized incidence rate about six times that of Nigerian black men,[149] although the incidence of latent carcinoma was the same.[150] In this same study, it was reported that the fat intake of patients with carcinoma of the prostate exceeded that of matched controls. It is intriguing to consider that fat intake and possibly testosterone levels act as conditioning factors (see Fig. 30–1) in the transformation of latent to clinical cancer. The role of environmental factors in the etiology of clinical cancer of the prostate has been further supported by the finding that Japanese living in Hawaii have a higher incidence of clinical cancer of the prostate than do Japanese in Japan, although the incidence of latent carcinoma is the same.[151]

Endocrinology

It should be appreciated that studies of the hormone dependency of benign prostatic hypertrophy may not be applicable to the problem of prostate cancer. Benign prostatic hypertrophy, for example, arises from the central zone of the prostate, whereas carcinoma originates in the periphery. It is true, however, that both diseases respond to withdrawal of androgen.

The pioneering work of Huggins[152, 153] established the role of androgen in prostatic function and gave rise to the concept of androgen dependence. The subsequent demonstration that castration caused regression of prostatic cancer in man[4, 154] initiated the era of hormonal management of cancer of the prostate.

In broad outlines, the mechanism of androgen action resembles that of estrogen; i.e., the androgen is bound to a cytosol receptor and transported to the nucleus where it interacts with chromatin.[155] It is almost certain that, in man and many other species, the active intracellular androgen is dihydrotestosterone, a metabolite of testosterone.[156] It has been suggested from studies of prostate in organ culture that a metabolite of dihydrotestosterone, 5α-androstane-3α,17β-diol, specifically stimulates secretion, whereas dihydrotestosterone induces growth.[157] Although both testosterone and androstenedione are precursors of intracellular dihydrotestosterone, apparently high plasma concentrations of testosterone are necessary, since prostate weight is not maintained following castration.

Prolactin plays a role in the prostatic growth of rodents and other species. Hypophysectomy causes a more profound atrophy of the rat prostate than does castration,[158] and endogenous prolactin has been shown to synergize with testosterone in maintaining the male mouse sexual accessory glands.[159] Injection of a prolactin antiserum inhibits prostate growth in rabbits.[160] The prostate has specific prolactin-binding sites and these are androgen-dependent.[161] Thus there may be steroid and peptide hormone interaction in prostate carcinogenesis.

Plasma androgens are the same in men with prostatic cancer as in the normal population.[162-164] The concentrations of androgens in carcinomatous tissue have been variously estimated as higher[165] or lower[166] than in control prostatic tissue (benign prostatic hypertrophy).

In parallel with receptor studies in breast and endometrial cancer, attempts have been made to correlate the content of dihydrotestosterone receptor with response to therapy. In one study, there was a good correlation between receptor content and response to therapy.[167] Sampling errors are only one of the several technical problems that have made these studies difficult.

Therapy

Although the principles of therapy are simple, there is controversy about tactics. If, as proposed by Huggins and those who followed him, it is necessary to decrease plasma androgens to a low level, then orchiectomy should suffice. However, estrogen can inhibit the effect of androgen on prostatic secretion in the absence of the pituitary gland,[168] implying a direct effect of estrogen in addition to its suppression of LH. Thus reasons can be cited for the simultaneous use of orchiectomy and estrogen.

In large, collected series of patients with metastatic disease,[169-171] 3- and 5-year survival rates of treated patients with stage III and IV disease were always better than those of untreated patients. The differences among regimens of castration, estrogen therapy, or combined treatment were not significant at 3 and 5 years. In a more recent study using randomized assignments to therapeutic regimens, no difference was found among the three regimens;[172] however, the use of 5 mg of diethylstilbestrol daily was associated with increased mortality from cardiovascular disease,[172] and these data have been confirmed recently in a study of treatment of patients with coronary artery disease. In a subsequent study, 1 mg of diethylstilbestrol daily was as effective as the 5 mg dose,[173] although the plasma testosterone concentration was not as completely suppressed.[174] The lower dose was not associated with increased cardiovascular mortality. Diethylstilbestrol did not improve the survival curve of stage I and II patients (carcinoma confined to the prostate). There is no evidence that any estrogen is better than another although individual patients may have fewer gastrointestinal reactions to one or another. When patients have responded to either estrogen or orhiectomy, the subsequent use of the other modality has generally proved ineffective.

Remission of disease has usually been defined as a significant lowering of acid phosphatase and relief of pain. Since bone metastases are usually osteoblastic, sufficient remodeling to permit diagnosis of remission may take several years. Nevertheless, regression rates from either orchiectomy or estrogen have been 50 to 80%, varying with grade and stage of disease.[175] The average duration of remission has been 15 months, although remissions lasting over 5 years have been noted.

It has been claimed[176] that in some patients 17-KS excretion rises following orchiectomy, and that this may be associated with reactivation of disease. This idea has persisted without further adequate studies. Recently, it was shown that androstenedione and testosterone plasma concentrations are higher in some patients with prostatic cancer after orchiectomy than has been found generally.[177] Suppression of the adrenal cortex by exogenous glucocorticoids reduced these levels. It seems quite possible that some men, like some postmenopausal women with endometrial hyperplasia, produce higher amounts of androstenedione or its precursor, dehydroepiandrosterone, than does the general population, and that possibly adrenal suppression would be beneficial in this group. Trials of cortisone have been inconclusive, however, although some improvement has been recorded.[178] There is no correlation between clinical relapse and increasing testosterone levels after orchiectomy.[179]

Because of residual androgen production by the adrenal cortex and the possible role of prolactin in maintaining prostate growth and adrenal androgen secretion, adrenalectomy and hypophysectomy have been performed in patients who have relapsed after primary therapy with estrogen or orchiectomy. In general, responses to adrenalectomy have been less satisfactory than to hypophysectomy.[180] In three series, the remission rate for hypophysectomy varies between 40% and 63%.[180-182] The survival of patients classified as having remission was considerably longer than that of the nonresponders.[180]

In none of the series was there a consistent decrease in acid phosphatase accompanying the decrease in pain, as occurs almost invariably after orchiectomy or estrogen therapy. Medical adrenalectomy using aminoglutethimide produced a similar regression rate.[183]

Hypophysectomy often produced clinical remission as defined by decrease in pain and sense of well-being.[184, 185] However, objective evidence of regression of disease occurs much less frequently, as after adrenalectomy. Thus, both procedures may be said to give relatively short-term clinical remissions but to rarely produce objective evidence of regression of disease extending over many months. Although the acid phosphatase has been reported to decrease in responders to hypophysectomy,[180] the data are not convincing. It is thus still premature to recommend any of these procedures routinely for the patient in relapse.

Progestational agents have been used in treatment since they suppress LH and can also act as antiandrogens, competing directly with testosterone for the prostate androgen receptors. In three studies,[186-188] remissions were reported in response to cyproterone acetate, an effective antiandrogen. The agent was given before castration or estrogen therapy and has been ineffective following castration.

A nonsteroidal androgen antagonist, Flutamide, produced substantial regression of disease in untreated patients and had some activity in patients who relapsed following stilbestrol therapy.[189] The drug does not cause a loss of libido, and in the experimental animal its antiandrogenic activity seems to be limited to prostate and germinal vesicles.[190] A "pure" antiandrogen of this type should prove useful both therapeutically and as a probe for androgen dependence.

Testosterone has been given to patients in relapse following orchiectomy. Not all patients show evidence of acceleration of disease, and some have responded symptomatically with relief of pain and increased sense of well-being.[191] There was no objective evidence of regression of disease.

CANCER OF THE KIDNEY

Endocrinology

The kidney is not usually considered an endocrine-responsive tissue, although in the rat, androgen administration causes hypertrophy of the kidney, and an androgen receptor has been identified in mouse kidney.[193] Experimental models of adenocarcinoma of the kidney are rare, the only one being the estrogen-induced renal cell adenoma and adenocarcinoma of the hamster.[194] The histologic pattern of the cancer closely resembles that of the human adenocarcinoma.[195] These tumors can be transplanted to male hamsters only after pretreatment with estrogen,[196] but cannot be induced in females except after ovariectomy, suggesting that ovarian progesterone inhibits induction. An estrogen antagonist decreases the growth rate of a transplantable tumor.[197] The growth of the tumors can be suppressed by cortisone and medroxyprogesterone given concurrrently but not by either agent alone.[198] As in the normal kidney, specific androgen receptors have been demonstrated in the estrogen-dependent hamster carcinoma.[199] Both estrogen and progesterone receptor are present in the primary tumor,[200, 201] the latter presumably the result of estrogen action. Since the first detectable change in the kidney during tumorigenesis was an increase in progesterone receptors,[201] it was of interest to see that there was a further increase with serial passage and increasing autonomy of the tumors.

Evidence that studies of this unique system are relevant to the treatment of human kidney cancer is sparse and depends chiefly on the observation that hormonal therapy, particularly with progestogens, occasionally causes regression of disease. Renal cell cancer occurs twice as commonly in men as in women,[202] thereby minimizing a role for estrogens in tumor induction. In the human renal cell carcinoma, almost two-thirds of the specimens had either estrogen or progesterone receptors.[203] It was suggested that high receptor content was predictive of response to progestational agents.

Therapy

The group of patients treated longest with hormonal therapy has been summarized by Bloom.[204] Of the 80 patients with metastatic disease, 55% underwent remissions (mean duration of 11.5 months). All were treated initially with high doses of medroxyprogesterone and a few secondarily with testosterone. Remissions were rare in the women. The results reported in this series are much better than those given in other series.[204-207] The sex difference among responses recorded by Bloom has not been confirmed because of the limited number of responses noted. An occasional good response to testosterone has also been recorded. There are some data suggesting that treatment with medroxyprogesterone acetate at the time of nephrectomy decreased the rate of recurrence of metastatic disease (Bracci, V., and diSilverio, C., cited in reference 203).

The use of medroxyprogesterone acetate is associated with few side-effects. Although this steroid, in high doses, has a low glucocorticoid potency, neither adrenal atrophy nor Cushing's syndrome has been reported in adults on long-term therapy. The agent causes loss of libido in men via its suppressive effect on LH.[208]

LEUKEMIA AND LYMPHOMA

Glucocorticoids influence the growth, differentiation, and function of virtually every tissue and organ system of the body.[209] Among these diverse effects, inhibitory actions on lymphoid tissue have long been appreciated.[210, 211] Glucocorticoids produce marked lymphocytopenia and thymic atrophy in experimental animals. Thus, these steroids were initially used with great enthusiasm when it was discovered that they could also kill some leukemic lymphoblasts in man.[212, 213] Despite this important observation, there remained several difficulties that prevented their most effective use. First, variable response rates were observed in patients with differing histologic types of acute and chronic leukemia and lymphoma.[214] Thus, the subset of patients likely to benefit from glucocorticoid therapy has not been defined. Second, many patients in whom clinical disease is controlled by glucocorticoid therapy relapse, and inevitably the patient becomes unresponsive to glucocorticoid therapy.[215] Thus, while initial response rates in pediatric acute lymphoblastic leukemia range between 45 and 65%, after primary relapse the rate of subsequent remission induction with glucocorticoids alone falls to 25%.

Furthermore, glucocorticoid administration is associated

with many complications. These include immunosuppression with concomitant nosocomial infections, Cushing's syndrome, diabetes mellitus, poor wound healing, psychosis, and other problems.[209, 216] Since most patients with leukemia die of infectious complications rather than the leukemia *per se,* it is likely that glucocorticoids may be a significant detriment to therapy in some cases. This particular difficulty is amplified by the fact that most patients with leukemia and lymphoma are currently managed by combinations of agents which include glucocorticoids along with cytotoxics. Thus, possibly harmful components in the drug combination, such as the glucocorticoid, may be continued long after they have ceased to be of benefit.

It would therefore be of value to be able to predict in advance when glucocorticoid therapy is indicated. One obvious approach is to measure glucocorticoid sensitivity *in vitro* using some type of cytotoxic or inhibitory end point. Unfortunately, such methods have not proved useful. It is difficult to reliably culture leukemic cell populations and, furthermore, *in vitro* effects of hormones may not be as easily demonstrated as *in vivo* responses.

Studies performed in breast cancer and other malignant diseases supported the notion that quantification of specific steroid receptors for estrogen was useful in predicting response to endocrine therapy.[217] On the basis of this observation, plus a clearer understanding of the mechanism of action of glucocorticoids, several groups sought and found specific glucocorticoid receptors in various populations of human leukemic and lymphoid cells.[218-220]

Glucocorticoid receptors are readily demonstrable in normal peripheral blood lymphocytes as well as in partially purified subpopulations of lymphocytes and monocytes.[221, 222] These receptor proteins are similar to the glucocorticoid receptors more extensively characterized in liver[223] and rat thymocytes.[224] Agents which induce blastic transformation of human lymphoid cells such as liver[223] and rat thymocytes.[224] Agents which induce blastic transformation of human lymphoid cells such as phytohemagglutinin or concanavalin A lead to severalfold increases in intracellular glucocorticoid receptor activity.[221, 225, 226] These lymphoblasts are similar morphologically, and in glucocorticoid receptor content, to human leukemic lymphoblasts.

Early studies in human acute lymphoblastic leukemia suggested that quantitative glucocorticoid receptor analyses would be clinically relevant.[227-230] Glucocorticoid receptors are readily detectable by assay of either cytoplasmic extracts or intact whole cells in most previously untreated patients with acute lymphoblastic leukemia. There is good agreement between concentrations of glucocorticoids which bind to receptor sites and concentrations which inhibit cellular processes. Early data in acute lymphoblastic leukemia suggest that a reasonable correlation may exist between loss of glucocorticoid receptor activity and *in vitro* resistance to glucocorticoids.[228] Furthermore, recent investigations have suggested that there are substantial differences in receptor content of the various types of acute lymphoblastic leukemia of childhood — so-called T-cell leukemias having substantially fewer receptor sites than null cell leukemia.[229] The quantity of receptor in acute lymphoblastic leukemia has recently been shown to correlate with initial complete remission duration.[230] This correlation is independent of known prognostic factors such as cell type, initial white blood cell count, or sex. Thus, at least in acute lymphoblastic leukemia, a role for analyses of glucocorticoid receptors appears established.

Glucocorticoid receptors have also been identified in other leukopathic states including acute myelogenous leukemia,[231, 232] chronic myelogenous leukemia in blast crisis,[232] chronic lymphocytic leukemia,[233-236] and the Sézary syndrome.[223] In none of these illnesses have significant correlations between receptor content and either clinical parameters or prognosis been reliably documented. Clearly "receptorology" as it pertains to glucocorticoid-responsive neoplasia is in an early stage of development and, with the possible exception of acute lymphoblastic leukemia, should be regarded as experimental. Bloomfield and colleagues[236a] have recently shown that quantitative glucocorticoid receptor determinations can accurately distinguish which patients with non-Hodgkin's lymphoma will respond to single agent glucocorticoid therapy.

MISCELLANEOUS

Ovarian Cancer

Ovarian cancer occurs at a higher rate in women with breast cancer[237] and endometrial cancer.[238] Second-generation Japanese women increase their rates of ovarian cancer as they do their rates of breast cancer.[239] The use of estrogen by postmenopausal women has been correlated with a higher risk of ovarian cancer.[240]

Although these data are far from conclusive, they do suggest an association between estrogen and ovarian cancer. Estrogen receptors have been demonstrated in the ovary, but not in the ovarian epithelium, the site of origin of the common ovarian cancers. Nevertheless, progestins have yielded a response rate of 38% in ovarian cancer,[241] and ovarian cancers have been shown to contain both progesterone and estrogen receptors.[242] Thus the tumor behaves as does endometrial cancer, and further biochemical and clinical observation is needed.

Laryngeal Carcinoma

The larynx is a target organ for androgens, as shown by the hypertrophy of the vocal cords at puberty in the male. Androgen receptors have been demonstrated in the human larynx, and similar receptors are present in epithelial cancers of the larynx.[243] Estrogen has been reported to have produced remission in several patients with metastatic disease (Saez, S., Personal communication). These early studies are in accord with the theme of this chapter that cancers derived from a tissue whose growth is stimulated by a hormone may regress following withdrawal of the hormone.

REFERENCES

1. Lipsett, M. B.: *Cancer 43*:1967, 1979.
2. Beatson, G. T.: *Lancet 2*:104, 162, 1896.
3. Lacassagne, A.: *C. R. Soc. Biol.* (Paris) *195*:630, 1932.
4. Huggins, C., et al.: *Arch. Surg. 43*:209, 1941.
5. MacMahon, B., et al.: *J. Natl. Cancer Inst. 50*:21, 1973.
6. Miller, A. B.: *Cancer Res. 38*:3985, 1978.
7. Doll, R., et al.: *Cancer Incidence in Five Continents.* Vol. 2. Berlin, Springer-Verlag, 1966.
8. Haenzel, W., et al.: *J. Natl. Cancer Inst. 40*:43, 1968.
9. DeWaard, F.: *Int. J. Cancer 4*:577, 1969.
10. MacMahon, B., et al.: *Bull. WHO 43*:209, 1970.
11. MacMahon, B., and Feinleib, M.: *J. Natl. Cancer Inst. 24*:733, 1960.
12. Abramson, J. H.: *Isr. J. Med. Sci. 2*:457, 1966.
13. Kamoi, M.: *Tohoku J. Exp. Med. 72*:59, 1960.
14. Ing, R., et al.: *Lancet 2*:124, 1977.
15. Petrakis, N. L.: *Cancer 39*:2709, 1977.
16. Lynch, H. T., et al.: *Cancer 36*:1315, 1975.
17. Petrakis, N. L.: *Science 173*:347, 1971.
18. Pihe, M. C., et al.: *J. Natl. Cancer Inst. 59*:1351, 1977.
19. Fishman, J., et al.: *Cancer Res. 38*:4006, 1978.
20. Everson, R. B., et al.: *Lancet 1*:9, 1976.
21. Feinleib, M.: *J. Natl. Cancer Inst. 41*:315, 1968.
22. Yuasa, S., and MacMahon, B.: *Bull. WHO 42*:192, 1971.
23. Hoover, R., et al.: *N. Engl. J. Med. 295*:401, 1976.
24. Wilson, S. E., and Hutchinson, W. B.: *J. Surg. Oncol. 8*:105, 1976.
25. Symer, W. St. C.: *Br. Med. J. 2*:83, 1968.
26. Everson, R. B., and Lippman, M. E.: In *Breast Cancer: Advances in Research and Treatment.* Vol. III. McGuire, W. (ed.), New York, Plenum Press, 1979, pp. 239–267.
27. Lemon, H. M., et al.: *J.A.M.A. 196*:1128, 1966.
28. MacMahon, B., et al.: *Lancet 2*:900, 1971.
29. Anderson, J. N., et al.: *Endocrinology 96*:160, 1975.
30. Longcope, C., and Pratt, J. H.: *Cancer Res. 38*:4025, 1978.
31. Kirschner, M. A., et al.: *Cancer Res. 38*:4029, 1978.
32. Fishman, J., et al.: *Cancer Res. 38*:4006, 1978.
33. Bullbrook, R. D.: In *Treatment of Breast Cancer.* Atkins, H. (ed.), Baltimore, University Park Press, 1974, p. 177.
34. Bulbrook, R. D., et al.: *Lancet 2*:395, 1971.
34a. Wang, D. Y., et al.: *Europ. J. Cancer 15*:1269, 1979.
35. Grattarola, R., et al.: *Am. J. Obstet. Gynecol. 121*:169, 1975.
36. McFayden, I. J., et al.: *Lancet 1*:1100, 1976.
37. Adams, J. B., and Wong, M. S. F.: *J. Endocrinol. 41*:41, 1968.
38. Adams, J. B., et al.: *Cancer Res. 38*:4036, 1978.
39. Dao, T. L., et al.: In *Estrogen Target Tissues and Neoplasia.* Dao, T. L. (ed.), Chicago, University of Chicago Press, 1972.
40. Kelsey, J. L., et al.: *Am. J. Epidemiol. 107*:236, 1978.
41. Royal College of General Practitioners Oral Contraception Study: *Lancet 1*:624, 1977.
42. Nomura, A., and Comstock, G. W.: *Am. J. Epidemiol. 103*:439, 1976.
43. Paffenbarger, R. S., et al.: *Cancer 39*:1887, 1977.
44. Vessey, M. P., et al.: *Br. Med. J. 3*:719, 1972.
45. Ory, H., et al.: *N. Engl. J. Med. 294*:419, 1976.
46. Vessey, M., et al.: *J. Biosoc. Sci. 8*:373, 1976.
47. Boston Collaborative Drug Surveillance Programme. *N. Engl. J. Med. 290*:15, 1974.
48. Black, M. M., et al.: *Cancer 29*:338, 1972.
49. Kodlin, D., et al.: *Cancer 39*:2603, 1977.
50. Armstrong, B.: *Int. J. Cancer 17*:204, 1976.
51. Vessey, M. P., et al.: *Lancet 1*:941, 1975.
52. Boston Collaborative Drug Surveillance Programme. *Lancet 1*:1399, 1973.
53. Henderson, B. E., et al.: *J. Natl. Cancer Inst. 53*:609, 1974.
54. Sartwell, P. E., et al.: *J. Natl. Cancer Inst. 59*:1589, 1977.
55. Casagrende, J., et al.: *J. Natl. Cancer Inst. 56*:839, 1976.
56. Craig, M. J., et al.: *J. Natl. Cancer Inst. 53*:1577, 1974.
57. McGuire, W. L., and Julian, J. A.: *Endocrinology 89*:969, 1971.
58. Terenius, L.: *Eur. J. Cancer 8*:55, 1972.
59. Folca, P. J., et al.: *Lancet 2*:796, 1961.
60. Korenman, S. G., and Dukes, B. A.: *J. Clin. Endocrinol. 30*:639, 1970.
61. Jensen, E. V., et al.: In *Endogenous Factors Influencing Host-Tumor Balance.* Wissler, R. W., Dao, T. L., and Wood, S., Jr. (eds.), Chicago, University of Chicago Press, 1967.
62. Panko, W. B., and MacLeod, R. M.: *Cancer Res. 38*:1948, 1978.
63. McGuire, W. L.: *Cancer Res. 38*:4289, 1978.
64. Nenci, I.: *Cancer Res. 38*:4204, 1978.
65. Mercer, W. D., et al.: *Proceedings of the American Society of Clinical Pathology,* 1978, abstract 28.
66. McGuire, W. L., Raynaud, J. P., and Baulieu, E. E. (eds.): *Progesterone Receptors in Normal and Neoplastic Tissues.* New York, Raven Press, 1977.
67. Anderson, W. A., et al.: *J. Cell Biol. 64*:668, 1975.
68. DeSombre, E. R., et al.: *Cancer Res. 35*:172, 1975.
69. Duffy, M. J., and Duffy, G.: *Biochem. Soc. Trans. 5*:1738, 1977.
70. Nicole, I., and Saez, S.: *Cancer Res. 38*:4314, 1978.
71. Knight, W. A., et al.: *Cancer Res. 37*:4669, 1977.
72. Maynard, P. V., et al.: *Cancer Res. 38*:4292, 1978.
73. Allegra, J. C., et al.: *Cancer Treat. Rep.* 1271–1277, 1979.
74. Lippman, M. E., et al.: *N. Engl. J. Med. 298*:1223, 1978.
75. Jonat, W., and Maass, H.: *Cancer Res. 38*:4305, 1978.
76. Kiang, D. T., et al.: *N. Engl. J. Med. 229*:1330, 1978.
77. Welsch, C. W., and Meites, J.: *Prog. Cancer Res. Chemother. 9*:71, 1978.
78. Costlow, M. E., and McGuire, W. L.: *Prog. Cancer Res. Chemother. 9*:121, 1978.
79. Pearson, O. H., et al.: *Cancer Res. 28*:4323, 1976.
80. Wagner, S., and Mantel, N.: *Cancer Res. 38*:2703, 1978.
81. Schyse, P. M., et al.: *Arch. Gen. Psychiatry 35*:1291, 1978.
82. Hall, T. C., et al.: *Cancer Chemother. Rep. 31*:47, 1963.
83. Lewison, E. F.: *Cancer 18*:558, 1965.
84. Fracchia, A. A., et al.: *Surg. Gynecol. Obstet. 128*:1221, 1969.
85. Saez, J. M., et al.: *J. Endocrinol. 55*:41, 1972.
86. Grodin, J. M., et al.: *J. Clin. Endocrinol. 36*:207, 1973.
87. Osborne, C. K., and Lippman, M. E.: In *Breast Cancer 2. Experimental Biology.* McGuire, W. (ed.), New York, Plenum Medical Book Co., 1978, p. 103.
88. Wilson, R. E., and Moore, F. D.: In *Prognostic Factors in Breast Cancer.* Forrest, A. P. M., and Kunkler, P. B. (eds.), Edinburgh, Livingstone Press, 1968.
89. Joint Committee on Endocrine Ablative Procedures in Disseminated Mammary Carcinoma. *J.A.M.A., 175*:787, 1961.
90. Hayward, J. L., et al.: In *The Clinical Management of Advanced Breast Cancer.* Second Tenovus Workshop. Joslin, C. A. F., and Gleave, E. N. (eds.), Cardiff, Livingstone, 1970, p. 50.
91. Pearson, O. H., and Ray, B. S.: In *Cancer (Hormone Therapy).* Vol. 6. Raven, R. W. (ed.), London, Butterworth & Co., 1959, Chapter 12.
92. Lacassagne, A.: *C. R. Soc. Biol.* (Paris) *126*:385, 1936.
93. Cooperative Breast Cancer Group: *J.A.M.A. 188*:106, 1964.

94. Cooperative Breat Cancer Group: *Cancer Chemother. Rep. 11*:109, 1961.
95. Goldenberg, J. S.: *Cancer 23*:109, 1969.
96. Kennedy, B. J.: *Cancer 24*:1345, 1969.
97. Stoll, B. A.: *Med. J. Aust. 1*:980, 1964.
98. Kennedy, B. J.: *Surg. Gynecol. Obstet. 120*:1246, 1965.
99. Kaufman, R. J., and Escher, G. C.: *Surg. Gynecol. Obstet. 113*:635, 1961.
100. Kennedy, B. J.: *Cancer 15*:641, 1962.
101. Stoll, B. A.: *Br. Med. J. 2*:338, 1967.
102. McGuire, W. L. (ed.): In *Breast Cancer: Advances in Research and Treatment.* Vol. I. New York, Plenum Medical Book Co., 1977, p. 217.
103. Horwitz, K. B., and McGuire, W. L.: In *Breat Cancer: Advances in Research and Treatment.* Vol. II. McGuire, W. L. (ed.), New York, Plenum Medical Book Co., 1978, p. 155.
104. Katzenellenbogen, B. S., et al.: *Endocrinology 100*:1252, 1977.
105. Roh, T. S., and Baudenstiel, L. J.: *Endocrinology 100*:420, 1977.
106. Rinehart, J. S., et al.: *Acta Endocrinol. 84*:367, 1977.
107. Legha, S., and Muggia, F. M.: *Ann. Intern. Med. 84*:751, 1976.
108. Heuson, J. C.: *Cancer Treat. Rep. 60*:7463, 1976.
109. Bloom, H. J. G., and Boesen, E.: *Br. Med. J. 2*:7, 1974.
110. Manni, A., et al.: *Cancer Treat. Rep. 60*:1445, 1976.
111. McIntosh, I. H., and Thynne, G. S.: *Br. J. Surg. 64*:900, 1977.
112. Tormey, D. C., et al.: *Cancer Treat. Rep. 60*:1451, 1976.
113. Everson, R., and Lippman, M. E.: In *Breast Cancer: Advances in Research and Treatment.* Vol. III. McGuire, W. L. (ed.), New York, Plenum Press, 1979, pp. 239–267.
114. Jain, J., et al.: *Cancer 40*:2063, 1977.
115. Lippman, M. E., et al.: *Cancer Res. 36*:4595, 1976.
116. Lippman, M. E., et al.: *Cancer Treat. Rep. 60*:1421, 1976.
117. Lippman, M. E., et al.: *Cancer Res. 36*:4602, 1976.
118. Griffiths, C. T., et al.: *Cancer 32*:31, 1973.
119. Fishman, L. M., et al.: *J. Clin. Endocrinol. Metab. 27*:481, 1967.
120. Santen, R. J., et al.: *J.A.M.A. 230*:1661, 1974.
121. Santen, R. J., et al.: *Cancer 39*:2948, 1977.
121a. Harvey, H. A.: Cancer *43*:2207, 1979.
122. Jensen, E. V., and Jacobsen, H. I.: *Recent Prog. Horm. Res. 18*:387, 1962.
123. Pollow, K., et al.: *Endocrinology 96*:319, 1975.
124. Bayard, F., et al.: *J. Clin. Endocrinol. Metab. 46*:635, 1978.
125. King, R. J. B., et al.: *Cancer 39*:1094, 1979.
126. Young, P. C. M., et al.: *Am. J. Obstet. Gynecol. 125*:353, 1976.
127. Feil, P. D., et al.: *J. Clin. Endocrinol. Metab. 48*:327, 1979.
128. Gurpide, E., et al.: *J. Steroid Biochem. 7*:891, 1976.
129. Dunn, L. J., and Bradbury, J. T.: *Am. J. Obstet. Gynecol. 97*:465, 1967.
130. Benjamin, F., et al.: *N. Engl. J. Med. 281*:1448, 1969.
131. DeWaard, F., et al.: *Cancer 22*:988, 1968.
132. Sall, S., and Calanog, A.: *Am. J. Obstet. Gynecol. 114*:153, 1972.
133. Antunes, C. M. F., et al.: *N. Engl. J. Med. 300*:9, 1979.
134. Nisker, J. A., et al.: *Am. J. Obstet. Gynecol. 130*:546, 1978.
135. Kaufman, R. H., et al.: *Am. J. Obstet. Gynecol. 77*:1271, 1959.
136. Whitehead, M. I., et al.: *Br. Med. J. 2*:453, 1977.
137. Hensell, D. L., et al.: *J. Clin. Endocrinol. Metab. 38*:476, 1974.
138. MacDonald, P. C., et al.: *Am. J. Obstet. Gynecol. 130*:448, 1978.
139. Judd, H. L., et al.: *J. Clin. Endocrinol. Metab. 43*:272, 1976.
140. Kelley, R. M., and Baker, W. H.: *N. Engl. J. Med. 264*:216, 1961.
141. Feinstein, A. R., and Horowitz, R. I.: *Cancer Res. 38*:4001, 1978.
142. Reifinstein, E. C., Jr.: *Cancer 27*:485, 1971.
143. Malkasian, G. D., Jr., et al.: *Am. J. Obstet. Gynecol. 110*:15, 1971.
144. Sherman, I.: *Obstet. Gynecol. 28*:309, 1966.
145. John, A. H., et al.: *Proceedings St. Thomas Hospital Medical School Symposium,* London, 1971.
146. Bonte, J.: *Proceedings St. Thomas Hospital Medical School Symposium,* London, 1971.
147. Silverberg, E., and Holleb, A. I.: *Cancer 25*:2, 1975.
148. Seidman, H., et al.: *Cancer 26*:2, 1976.
149. Kovi, J., and Heshmat, M. Y.: *Am. J. Epidemiol. 96*:401, 1972.
150. Jackson, M. A., et al.: *Cancer Treat. Rep. 61*:167, 1977.
151. Akazakis, K., and Stennerman, G. N.: *J. Natl. Cancer Inst. 50*:1137, 1973.
152. Huggins, C., and Clark, P. J.: *J. Exp. Med. 72*:547, 1940.
153. Huggins, C., et al.: *J. Exp. Med. 70*:543, 1939.
154. Huggins, C., and Hodges, C. V.: *Cancer Res. 1*:293, 1941.
155. Liao, S., and Fang, S.: *Vitam. Horm. 27*:17, 1969.
156. Wilson, J. D.: *N. Engl. J. Med. 287*:1284, 1972.
157. Baulieu, E. E. et al.: *Nature* (London) *219*:1155, 1968.
158. Grayhack, J. T.: *Natl. Cancer Inst. Monogr. 12*:189, 1963.
159. Peyre, A.: *C. R. Soc. Biol.* (Paris) *162*:1592, 1968.
160. Asano, M., et al.: *J. Urol. 106*:248, 1971.
161. Aragona, C., et al.: *Acta Endocrinol. 84*:402, 1977.
162. Habib, F. K., et al.: *J. Endocrinol. 71*:99, 1976.
163. Sciarra, F., et al.: *J. Steroid Biochem. 2*:313, 1971.
164. Hammond, G. L., et al.: *Clin. Endocrinol. 9*:113, 1978.
165. Geller, J., et al.: *Cancer Res. 38*:4349, 1978.
166. Habib, F. K.: *J. Endocrinol. 71*:99, 1976.
167. Gustafsson, J-A., et al.: *Cancer Res. 38*:4345, 1978.
168. Goodwin, D. A., et al.: *J. Urol. 69*:152, 1961.
169. Nesbit, R. M., and Baum, W. C.: *J.A.M.A. 143*:1317, 1950.
170. Emmett, O. L., et al.: *Br. J. Urol. 83*:471, 1960.
171. Nesbit, R. M., and Plumb, R. T.: *J. Urol. 89*:236, 1963.
172. Veterans Administration Cooperative Urological Research Group: *Surg. Gynecol. Obstet. 124*:1011, 1967.
173. Blackard, C. E.: *Cancer Chemother. Rep. 59*:225, 1975.
174. Shearer, R. J., et al.: *Br. J. Urol. 45*:667, 1973.
175. Schirmer, H. K. A., et al.: *Urol. Digest 4*:15, 1965.
176. Scott, W. W., and Vermeulen, C.: *J. Clin. Endocrinol. 2*:450, 1942.
177. Sciarra, F., et al.: *Clin. Endocrinol. 2*:101, 1973.
178. Mellinger, G. T.: *Surg. Clin. North Am. 45*:1413, 1965.
179. Young, H. H., II, and Kent, J. R.: *J. Urol. 99*:788, 1968.
180. Murphy, P., et al.: *J. Urol. 105*:817, 1971.
181. Scott, W. W., and Schirmer, H. K. A.: In *On Cancer and Hormones: Essays in Experimental Biology.* Boyland, E., et al. (eds.), Chicago, University of Chicago Press, 1962, p. 175.
182. Maddy, J. A., et al.: *Cancer 28*:322, 1971.
183. Sanford E. J., et al.: *J. Urol. 115*:170, 1976.
184. West, C. R., and Murphy, G. P.: *J.A.M.A. 16*:253, 1976.
185. Silverberg, G. D.: *Cancer 39*:1727, 1977.
186. Scott, W. W., and Schirmer, H. K. A.: *Trans. Am. Assoc. Genitourin. Surg. 58*:54, 1966.
187. Giller, J., et al.: *Cancer Chemother. Rep. 51*:51, 1967.
188. Rafla, S., and Johnson, R.: *Curr. Ther. Res. 16*:261, 1974.
189. Aurhart, R. A., et al.: *South. Med. J. 171*:798, 1978.
190. Neri, R., et al.: *Endocrinology 91*:427, 1972.
191. Prout, G. R., and Brewer, W. R.: *Cancer 20*:1871, 1967.
192. Korenchevsky, V., and Ross, M. A.: *Br. Med. J. 1*:645, 1940.
193. Bullock, L. P., et al.: *Biochem. Biophys. Res. Commun. 44*:1537, 1971.
194. Kirkman, H.: *Natle. Cancer Inst. Monogr. 1*:1, 1959.
195. Horning, E. S., and Wittick, J. W.: *Br. J. Cancer 8*:451, 1954.
196. Horning, E. S.: *Br. J. Cancer 10*:678, 1956.
197. Bloom, H. J. G., et al.: *Cancer 20*:2118, 1967.
198. Bloom, H. J.: *Br. J. Cancer 17*:611, 1963.
199. Li, J. J., et al.: *Endocrinology 101*:1006, 1977.
200. Li, J. J., et al.: *Cancer Res. 36*:1127, 1976.
201. Lin, Y. C., et al.: *Cancer Res. 38*:1286, 1978.
202. Wagle, D. G., and Scal, D.: *J. Surg. Oncol. 2*:23, 1970.
203. Concolino, G., et al.: *Cancer Res. 38*:4340, 1978.
204. Bloom, H. J. G.: *Br. J. Cancer 25*:250, 1971.
205. Samuels, M. L., et al.: *Cancer 22*:525, 1968.
206. Talley, R. W., et al.: *J.A.M.A. 207*:322, 1969.
207. Wagle, D. G., and Murphy, G. P.: *Cancer 28*:318, 1971.
208. Gordon, G. G., et al.: *J. Clin. Endocrinol. 30*:449, 1970.
209. Thompson. E. B., and Lippman, M. E.: *Metabolism 23*:159, 1974.
210. Baxter, J. D., and Forsham, P. H.: *Am. J. Med. 53*:573, 1972.
211. Selye, H.: *Endocrinology 21*:169, 1937.
212. Claman, H. N.: *N. Engl. J. Med. 287*:388, 1972.
213. Goldin, A., et al.: *Cancer Chemother. Rep. 55*:309, 1971.
214. Livingston, R. B., and Carter, S. K. (eds.): *Single Agents in Cancer Chemotherapy.* New York, Plenum Press, 1970.
215. Vietti, T. J., et al.: *J. Pediatr. 66*:18, 1965.
216. Kjellstraad, C. M.: *Transplant. Proc. 7*:123, 1975.
217. McGuire, W. L., et al. (eds.): *Estrogen Receptors in Human Breast Cancer.* New York, Raven Press, 1975.
218. Schmidt, T. J., and Thompson, E. B.: In *Endocrine Control in Neoplasia.* Sharma, R. K., and Criss, W. E. (eds.), New York, Raven Press, 1976, p. 263.
219. Lippman, M. E., et al.: *Cancer Res. 38*:4251, 1978.
220. Crabtree, G. R., et al.: *Cancer Res. 38*:4268, 1978.
221. Neifeld, J. P., et al.: *J. Biol. Chem. 254*:2972, 1977.
222. Lippman, M. E., and Barr, R.: *J. Immunol. 118*:1977, 1977.
223. Cake, M. M., and Litwack, G.: In *Biochemical Actions of Hormones.* Vol. 3. Litwack, G. (ed.), New York, Academic Press, 1975, p. 319.
224. Munch, A., and Wira, C.: In *Advances in the Biosciences: Schering Workshop on Steroid Hormone Receptors.* Vol. 7. Raspe, G. (ed.), Oxford, Pergamon Press, 1971, p. 301.
225. Adler, V. V., et al.: *Bull. Exp. Biol. Med. 81*:850, 1976.
226. Smith, K. A., et al.: *Nature 267*:523, 1977.
227. Lippman, M. E., et al.: *Nature* (New Biol.) *242*:157, 1973.
228. Lippman, M. E., et al.: *J. Clin. Invest. 52*:1715, 1973.
229. Konior, G. S., et al.: *Cancer Res. 37*:2688, 1977.
230. Lippman, M. E., et al.: *Cancer Res. 38*:4251, 1978.
231. Lippman, M. E., et al.: *Am. J. Med. 59*:224, 1975.
232. Crabtree, G. R., et al.: *Cancer Res. 38*:4268, 1978.
233. Gailiani, S., et al.: *Cancer Res. 33*:2653, 1978.
234. Homo, F., et al.: *C. R. Acad. Sci.* (D) Paris *280*:1923, 1975.
235. Homo, F., et al.: *Br. J. Haematol. 38*:491, 1978.
236. Terenius, L., et al.: *J. Steroid Biochem. 7*:905, 1976.
236a. Bloomfield, C. D., et al.: Lancet *1*:952, 1980.
237. Schottenfeld, D., and Berg, J.: *J. Natl. Cancer Inst. 46*:161, 1971.
238. Lynch, H. T., et al.: *Am. J. Med. Sci. 252*:381, 1966.
239. Haenszel, W., and Kurihara, M.: *J. Natl. Cancer Inst. 40*:43, 1968.
240. Hoover, R., et al.: *Lancet 2*:533, 1976.
241. Tobias, J. S., and Griffiths, T. C.: *N. Engl. J. Med. 294*:818, 1976.
242. Ehrlich, C. E., et al.: In *Estrogens and Cancer.* Silverberg, S. G., and Major, F. J. (eds.), New York, John Wiley and Sons, 1978, p. 179.
243. Saez, S., and Sakai, F.: *C. R. Acad. Sci.* (D) Paris *280*:935, 1975.

CHAPTER 31

Humoral Manifestations of Cancer

By William D. Odell

INTRODUCTION

In addition to symptoms directly produced by tumor mass or invasion, cancers may produce symptoms by means of production of humoral or hormonal substances. Since this author was first involved in reviewing this subject in 1964,[1] our understanding of the breadth of these syndromes (termed "ectopic hormonal syndromes" by Dr. Grant Liddle[2]) and of their pathogenesis has changed strikingly. Originally humoral production by cancer was considered unusual, and it was postulated that the cause was derepression of genetic information.[1] Now, Odell et al. have postulated that all cancers elaborate proteins or peptides ectopically[3, 4] and that the clinically recognizable syndromes result from elaboration of bioactive proteins. Those cancers not associated with a clinically apparent syndrome produce biologically inactive or only weakly active proteins. Table 31–1 presents the humoral syndromes known to be associated with neoplasms. This table includes several humoral syndromes not related to *hormonal* production.

In this chapter we discuss the endocrine syndromes and hormonal production associated with cancer. Table 31–2 lists the hormones, hormonal fragments, or precursors that have been described to be produced by cancers as part of ectopic syndromes. Note that, with the exception of prostaglandins, all these substances are protein or peptide hormones; none are thyronines (e.g., triiodothyronine or thyroxine) and none are steroids. Thus, with the exception of prostaglandins, ectopic humoral syndromes, where understood, have proved to be produced by cancer elaboration of proteins or peptides. Of course, many syndromes remain poorly understood. As mentioned, early current data indicate that those cancers not associated with any clinically recognizable syndromes

Table 31–1. EXAMPLES OF HUMORAL SUBSTANCES OR SYNDROMES ASSOCIATED WITH NEOPLASMS

1. Hormones
2. Hormone precursors
3. Fetal proteins (e.g., carcinoembryonic antigen, alpha fetal protein)
4. Enzymes (e.g., alkaline phosphatase, thymidine kinase)
5. Central nervous system degenerative conditions
6. Myopathies
7. Myasthenic syndromes
8. Dermatologic syndromes (e.g., dermatomyositis, acanthosis nigricans, pachyderma)
9. Digital clubbing and arthropathies
10. Hematologic diseases (e.g., aplastic anemias, thrombophlebitis)
11. Fever

Table 31–2. HORMONES (ECTOPIC) REPORTED TO BE PRODUCED BY CANCERS

1. ACTH and PROACTH
2. Lipotropin
3. Chorionic gonadotropin
4. Alpha chain
5. Vasopressin
6. Hypoglycemia-producing factor
7. Somatomedins
8. Parathyroid hormone
9. Prostaglandins
10. Osteoclast-activating factor
11. Erythropoietin
12. Hypophosphatemia-producing factor
13. Growth hormone
14. Prolactin
15. Gastrin
16. Secretin
17. Glucagon
18. Corticotropin-releasing hormone
19. Growth hormone–releasing hormone
20. Somatostatin
21. Chorionic somatotropin

PEPTIDE CASCADE

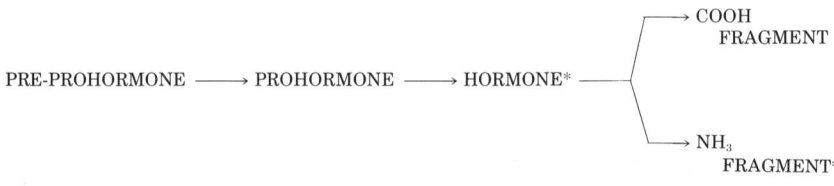

*BIOACTIVE FORMS

Figure 31–1. Schematic representation of the hypothetical peptide cascade through which all protein hormone may evolve during synthesis, storage, secretion, circulation, and degradation.

also produce proteins ectopically, but these proteins are bioinactive. In some instances, at least, they are precursor forms or other metabolic forms of the protein hormones. On the basis of data from many laboratories,[5-18] it is reasonable to hypothesize that all protein hormones evolve during synthesis, storage, secretion, circulation, and degradation through a sort of peptide cascade. Figure 31–1 illustrates this cascade schematically.

THE "PEPTIDE HORMONE CASCADE"

In this scheme protein hormones are synthesized with methionine residues and additional amino acid sequences with poorly understood, if any, purposes. In some instances the precursor protein appears to give rise to several hormones or hormonal substances (e.g., a precursor form of ACTH is metabolized into PROACTH, lipotropin, and the endorphins). Several "PREPRO" and "PRO" forms may exist (we stress that this is a very schematic presentation). With the exception of progastrin, it is likely that these precursor forms of hormones possess little or no biological activity. These forms are metabolized to the biologically active hormones which are the predominant forms normally secreted into the circulation. During circulation or distribution the hormones produce biologic effects and are enzymatically metabolized to various peptide fragments. Commonly the amino terminal fragment may possess bioactivity, while the carboxyl terminal fragments are biologically inert. Various assay systems react differently to each of these hormonal forms. Radioimmunoassay, whose reaction is based on structure, not function, may quantify biologically inactive prohormones or carboxyl fragments (e.g., some ACTH and parathyroid hormone immunoassays). Radioreceptor assays or *in vitro* bioassays may react only with the bioactive forms (e.g., ACTH, chorionic gonadotropin). For the purposes we wish to develop in this chapter, this peptide cascade scheme, while oversimplified from the scientific viewpoint, illustrates how cancers can produce proteins related to hormones, ectopically, and yet not produce clinically recognizable symptoms.

ECTOPIC ACTH PRODUCTION

The association of Cushing's syndrome with carcinoma was first recognized in 1928 and is one of the most common ectopic hormonal syndromes.[19] In the 1960's Liddle et al.[2, 20] published extensive studies using *in vivo* bioassays to characterize the syndrome. These investigators showed that in patients with Cushing's syndrome associated with a cancer, the primary tumor and its metastases contained large amounts of ACTH. Liddle et al.[2] reported findings of

88 patients with this syndrome, and several hundred have been reported in other literature. We summarize from the literature the types of neoplasms that have been associated with Cushing's syndrome and their approximate frequency in Table 31–3.

About 50% of such patients have carcinoma of the lung, predominantly oat cell or small round cell in type. Of all patients with oat cell carcinoma, 2.8% have clinical symptoms or findings of ectopic ACTH syndrome;[21] approximately half of this 2.8% do not have overt clinical Cushing's syndrome but have elevated plasma cortisol which is not suppressed by 8 mg of dexamethasone per day. Considering all patients with clinically recognizable ectopic ACTH syndrome, about 70% have carcinoma of the lung, thymus, or pancreas.

Studies performed by Ratcliffe et al.,[22] Bloomfield et al.,[23] Gewirtz and Yalow,[24] and Wolfsen and Odell[4, 25] have revealed that extracts of all lung carcinomas contain an ACTH-like material measurable by radioimmunoassay. This is independent of histologic type, and in spite of the absence of clinically recognizable manifestations of Cushing's syndrome. The material present in extracts of lung cancers has a molecular weight larger than that of standard ACTH, but little or no activity in *in vitro* ACTH bioassay of dispersed adrenocortical cells[24] or in radioreceptor assays for ACTH.[4, 25] This large molecular form of ACTH is enzymatically converted to bioactive ACTH by incubation with trypsin.[24] It is likely that this substance is one of the precursor molecules of ACTH ("PROACTH").

In further studies of ectopic ACTH, Wolfsen and Odell[4, 25] have shown that if one excludes patients who have a clinically recognizable symptom of excess ACTH production, approximately 72% of patients with lung cancer, independent of histologic type, have elevated immu-

Table 31–3. NEOPLASMS ASSOCIATED WITH ECTOPIC ACTH PRODUCTION

Tumor Type	Approximate Percentage of Cases
Carcinoma of lung	50
Thymic carcinoma	10
Pancreatic carcinoma (including islet cell and carcinoid)	10
Neoplasms from neural crest tissue (pheochromocytoma, neuroblastoma, paraganglioma, ganglioma)	5
Bronchial adenoma (including carcinoid)	2
Medullary carcinoma of the thyroid	5
Miscellaneous*	each < 2

*Carcinoma of ovary, prostate, breast, thyroid, kidney, salivary glands, testes, stomach, colon, gallbladder, esophagus, appendix, etc.

noreactive ACTH; none have elevated receptor-active ACTH.

As indicated in Table 31–3, the clinically apparent ectopic ACTH syndrome is not very common in association with gastrointestinal neoplasms. However, studies of Odell et al.[4] and Wolfsen and Odell[25] demonstrate that extracts of all carcinomas of the colon, stomach, esophagus, and pancreas also contain variable amounts of this large molecular form of ACTH.

Investigation by Eipper and Mains[8, 9] of pituitary ACTH synthesis, using purified messenger RNA from mouse pituitary tumor cell cultures, has revealed that the first messenger RNA product with ACTH immunoactivity has a molecular weight of 31,000. This is converted sequentially to a 23,000, then a 13,000, and finally to the familiar 4500 molecular weight bioactive ACTH. The large molecular weight ACTH material is a glycoprotein and probably is also a precursor of lipotropin (discussed later in this chapter), the endorphins, and possibly calcitonin.

In summary: extracts of virtually all carcinomas contain PROACTH. About three quarters of patients with lung cancer (independent of histologic type) have elevated immunoactive ACTH in blood (PROACTH), which is not biologically active. Those patients having clinically recognizable Cushing's syndrome associated with cancer have increased blood ACTH which is bioactive and measurable by radioimmunoassay, radioreceptor assay, or bioassays.

CANCER PLASMA

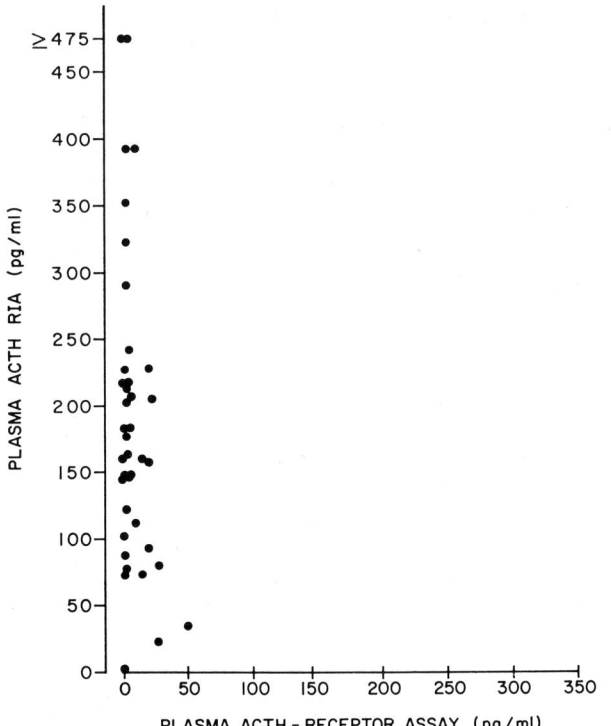

Figure 31–2. Concentration of plasma ACTH quantified by radioimmunoassay (ordinate) plotted against concentration quantified by radioreceptor assay (abscissa). Note that in these patients with carcinoma but no clinical evidence of ectopic ACTH syndrome, radioimmunoassayable ACTH is elevated, yet radioreceptor-assayable ACTH is normal. The material being quantified by RIA is PRO or "BIG" ACTH, which has little reaction in the radioreceptor assay. (From Odell, W. D., et al.: Ectopic peptide synthesis — a universal concomitant of neoplasia. *Trans. Assoc. Am. Physicians* 90:204, 1977.)

Thus, all carcinomas appear to elaborate PROACTH. Those associated with the clinically recognizable ACTH syndrome have cancers that also convert this PROACTH to bioactive ACTH and release this material into blood.

Figure 31–2 shows the ACTH present in blood from patients with various kinds of carcinoma who did not have clinical symptoms of ACTH hypersecretion, as measured by radioimmunoassay and radioreceptor assay.

THE CLINICAL SYNDROME AND ITS DIAGNOSIS

Typical signs of Cushing's syndrome often are absent in patients with ectopic ACTH syndrome, because the carcinomas produce a rapidly fatal course and the typical signs generally take months or years to become evident. However, in patients with slow-growing neoplasms, such as thymoma, bronchial carcinoid, pheochromocytoma, or medullary carcinoma of the thyroid, Cushing's syndrome may be evident months or even years prior to tumor recognition. Any patient with cancer and hypokalemia, muscle weakness, psychosis, increased pigmentation, edema, hypertension, or abnormal glucose tolerance should be suspected of having ectopic ACTH production. In patients without known cancer, but with Cushing's syndrome, the presence of hypokalemia with high plasma cortisol (over 35 μg per 100 ml), high plasma ACTH (over 150 pg/ml), highly elevated 17 ketosteroid excretion, or highly elevated plasma dehydroepiandrosterone sulfate should raise suspicion of ectopic ACTH production. Usually dexamethasone (8 mg/day) will not suppress ACTH or plasma cortisol in the ectopic ACTH syndrome, but will in Cushing's disease. Adrenal cortical adenomas or carcinomas producing Cushing's syndrome are associated with low or undetectable blood ACTH prior to dexamethasone administration. However, some patients with ectopic ACTH production show suppression of both ACTH and cortisol with dexamethasone. This occurs in approximately 50% of patients with bronchial carcinoids[26] and in some patients with thymoma. This phenomenon could be explained by hypothesizing that these tumors produce the hypothalamic peptide corticotropin-releasing hormone (CRH), which produces its effect by stimulating pituitary secretion of ACTH. Glucocorticoids have been shown to suppress CRH activity at the pituitary level. Upton and Amatruda in 1971[27] reported four patients with "ectopic ACTH syndrome" whose tumors contained both ACTH and a CRH-like material.

ECTOPIC LIPOTROPIN PRODUCTION

In 1967 Abe et al.[28] reported that the biologically active material (as tested in melanocyte-stimulating hormone [MSH] bioassays) present in extracts of tumors associated with ectopic ACTH syndromes was predominantly βMSH. Studies by Bloomfield, Scott, and associates[29, 30] and by Bachelot et al.[31] have shown that βMSH *per se* does not exist either in the human pituitary or in blood of normal humans. Neither is it found in blood of patients with Addison's disease, Cushing's disease, or the ectopic ACTH syndrome.* βMSH is an artifact of the extraction-

---

*Subsequent to preparation of this chapter, Abe et al. have confirmed the absence of βMSH in normal subjects and those with Cushing's disease or Addison's disease. However, in ectopic ACTH syndrome, they reported some patients have detectable βMSH *per se*. That is, these neoplasms may enzymatically cleave lipotropin to βMSH, while normally this does not occur. These recent studies have not been confirmed by others.[28]

purification techniques used to prepare it. The molecule giving rise to βMSH in these extraction techniques is probably beta lipotropin, a 91-amino acid protein that contains the entire sequence of βMSH. As discussed earlier, the precursor molecules of ACTH contain the sequence of lipotropin and probably give rise to this protein as well as to ACTH. Thus the material measured by Abe et al.,[28] and which is measured by βMSH radioimmunoassays, is probably lipotropin.

Just as extracts of all carcinomas of the lung (and colon, stomach, esophagus, and so on) contain immunoreactive ACTH, they also contain lipotropin.[4, 32] This material is present in tumor extracts and in blood in amounts that directly correlate with those of PROACTH. Our studies[32] have shown that (as with ACTH) about 60% of patients with carcinoma of the lung, but without clinically recognizable ectopic ACTH secretion, have elevated plasma lipotropin. Lipotropin, as tested in MSH bioassays, has less ability to disperse melanin pigment granules than has MSH and is about equally as potent as ACTH in producing pigmentation. Thus, the hyperpigmentation seen in ectopic ACTH syndrome (and incidentally in Addison's disease, Cushing's disease, and Nelson's syndrome) is poorly understood. It probably relates to a combination of the effects of both ACTH and lipotropin on melanin deposition.

CHORIONIC GONADOTROPIN

Chorionic gonadotropin (CG) is a glycoprotein hormone composed of two peptide chains (alpha and beta) which are not covalently bound.[33-35] Figure 31–3 shows the structure of CG schematically. The alpha chain of CG is very similar in amino acid sequence to the alpha chain of the other human glycoprotein hormones — thyrotropin and luteinizing and follicle-stimulating hormones. The beta chain of CG is very similar in the first 117 amino terminal residues to the beta chain of luteinizing hormone (LH) but in addition possesses a 30-amino acid, carbohydrate-rich tail at the carboxyl terminus. Neither the alpha chain nor the beta chain of any of these glycoproteins possesses bioactivity by itself, but when the beta chain is combined with an alpha chain, a bioactive molecule is formed, the type of bioactivity determined by the beta chain. Several studies have shown that cancers may elaborate intact CG, the free alpha chain, or the beta chain of CG.

Until about 10 years ago it was believed that extrapituitary sources of gonadotropin were relatively rare, for the most part confined to the syncytial and cytotrophoblastic cells of the pregnant primate, the endometrial cusps of the pregnant mare, neoplasms in the human derived from the cytotrophoblast, and teratomas containing such cells.[36] Between 1949 and 1968 about eight isolated case reports of patients with cancer and some evidence of increased gonadotropin production appeared. The forms of cancer included malignant melanoma,[37] adrenal cortical carcinoma,[38] undifferentiated carcinoma,[39] breast carcinoma,[40] renal carcinoma,[41] and carcinoma of the lung.[42-44] The assays used for these studies could not distinguish CG from LH. When the more specific beta chain radioimmunoassay was developed by Vaitukaitis et al.,[45] and large numbers of patients with varying types of neoplasms were studied by Braunstein et al.,[46] it was found that between 6 and 13% of all carcinomas were associated with increased blood CG concentrations.

Subsequently, the story is surprising. Braunstein[47] reported the presence of CG-like material in extracts of normal testes, and Chen et al.[48] reported such a material in the pituitary and urine of a patient with Klinefelter's disease. Studies by Yoshimoto et al. and Odell et al.[4, 49, 50] have revealed that extracts of all *normal* human tissues and of all carcinomas contain a material indistinguishable from CG as studied by beta chain radioimmunoassay and by gonadotropin radioreceptor assay. Figure 31–4 demonstrates dose-response curves of this CG-like material. Since the free beta chain of CG does not react in the radioreceptor assay and LH gives a dose-response line which is not parallel to that of CG in the radioimmunoassay, this material is not the free beta chain of hCG. When this CG-like material was further characterized using the plant lectin* concanavalin A (Con A), it was found that less than 5% bound to Con A columns. In contrast, over 95% of CG obtained from extracts of normal placenta or from blood of pregnant women binds to Con A and is eluted after addition of the carbohydrate competitor alpha methyl glucopyranoside. These Con A studies indicate that the CG material present in extracts of normal tissues possesses either a very different carbohydrate structure from that of placental CG or no carbohydrate. Figure 31–5 shows Con A studies of normal tissue CG. Table 31–4 shows the percentage of binding to Con A of various sources of CG. Van Hall et al.[51] and Tsuruhara et al.[52] have shown that desialated CG is rapidly cleared from the circulation with a half-time of less than 1 minute in the rat; thus it has little biologic potency *in vivo*. However, it has full *in vitro* bioactivity and reacts in radioreceptor assays since degradation or metabolism is not a parameter in *in vitro* assays.

---

*Con A and other plant lectins bind glycoproteins via their carbohydrate moieties. Each lectin has binding sites with carbohydrate specificity. Placental CG binds to Con A because it is rich in carbohydrate moieties of the types that interact with Con A.

Figure 31–3. Chorionic gonadotropin (CG) structure shown schematically: The beta chain of placental CG possesses 147 amino acids. Complex carbohydrate moieties are linked via asparagines at positions 13 and 30 and via serines at positions 117, 131, and 147. The beta chain of CG is identical to that for human LH with the exception that the last 30 amino acids are not present on human LH. The alpha chain of CG contains 92 amino acids and two asparagine-linked complex carbohydrate moieties. The CG alpha differs from human LH alpha by a 2-amino acid inversion and a 3-residue deletion at the amino terminus. The carbohydrate moieties are made up of six different monosaccharides, D-mannose, N-acetylglucosamine, N-acetylgalactosamine, sialic acid, L-fucose, and D-galactose.

Schematic Presentation – hCG Structure

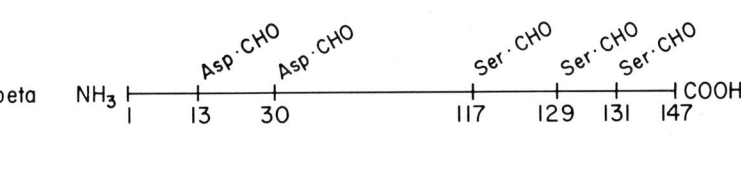

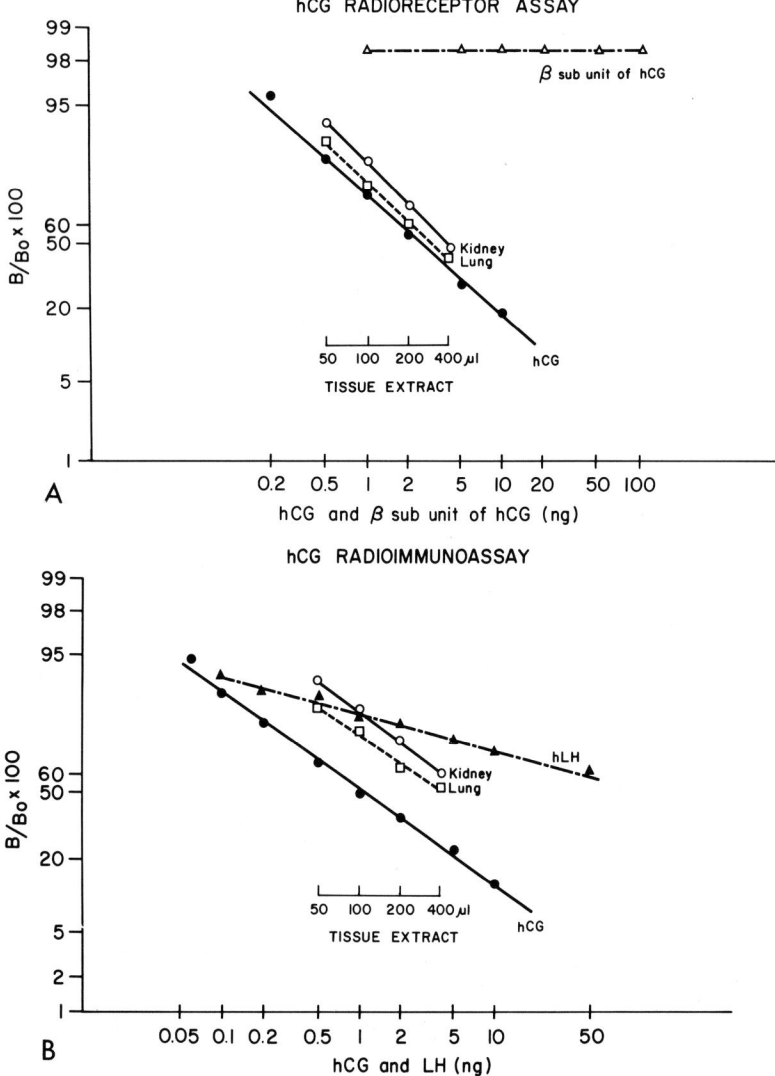

Figure 31–4. *A,* Dose-response curves for extracts of human kidney and lung in the CG (hCG) radioreceptor assay. The free beta subunit of CG does not react in this assay. *B,* Dose-response curves for extracts of human kidney and lung in the CG beta chain radioimmunoassay. Although the beta chain of CG does react in this assay, human luteinizing hormone (hLH) produces a line with a different slope. Taking the data in both figures into consideration, one can conclude that this material is neither hLH nor the free beta chain of CG. Separate studies (not shown) also demonstrate that this is not an enzyme degrading labeled hCG. Such an artifact could produce such results and must be excluded. (From Yoshimoto, Y., et al.: Human chorionic gonadotropin-like material: Presence in normal human tissues. *Am. J. Obstet. Gynecol. 134:*729, 1979.)

We hypothesized from our studies of the CG-like material in normal human tissues that:

1. All normal human tissues synthesize the protein sequence of CG.*

2. The placenta glycosylates this ubiquitous peptide. The added carbohydrate residues protect the protein from rapid degradation, transforming it into a hormone.

On the basis of these studies in normal tissues, it is not

---

*After preparation of this chapter, Morrish, Wolfsen, and Odell demonstrated, using ³⁵S-methionine incorporation, synthesis of this hCG-like material by normal tissues (*Clin. Res. 28:*25A, 1980).

Table 31–4. HCG BINDING TO CONCANAVALIN A

	% Bound ± SEM	**Range**
Normal tissue (10)	6.1 ± 1.6	(0.0–14.6)
Cancer tissue (9)	31.2 ± 9.1	(4.0–86.0)
Placenta (4)	92.5 ± 0.9	(90.1–94.0)
Pregnant serum (3)	100.0	
Cancer serum (8)	54.7 ± 11.9	(3.1–92.5)

surprising that extracts of all carcinomas also contain CG as tested in the beta CG radioimmunoassay and the gonadotropin radioreceptor assay.[53] Figure 31–6 shows the concentrations of CG as measured by radioimmunoassay. Since extracts of all cancers contain CG, and only some 6 to 13% of patients with cancers have detectable blood concentrations of CG, some variable other than production of CG must exist. In contrast to the CG in normal tissues, the CG in cancer extracts has highly variable Con A binding, indicating more variable carbohydrate content (or composition). In further support of our hypothesis that all cancer cells elaborate CG-like material,[53] Acevedo et al.[54] and McManus et al.,[55] using immunofluorescence, have demonstrated CG in most tumor cells.

We conclude from all these studies[53] that:

1. All carcinomas elaborate a CG-like material.

2. The carbohydrate composition of this CG-like material is highly variable.

3. Those carcinomas associated with elevated blood CG either produce increased quantities of CG with altered carbohydrate or glycosylate CG, prolonging its half-time in the circulation.

4. One important variable in using CG as a tumor marker is glycosylation by the tumor cells.

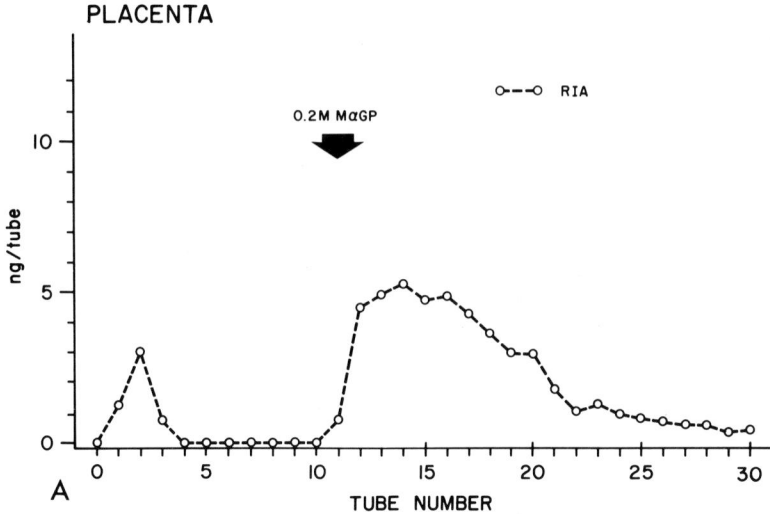

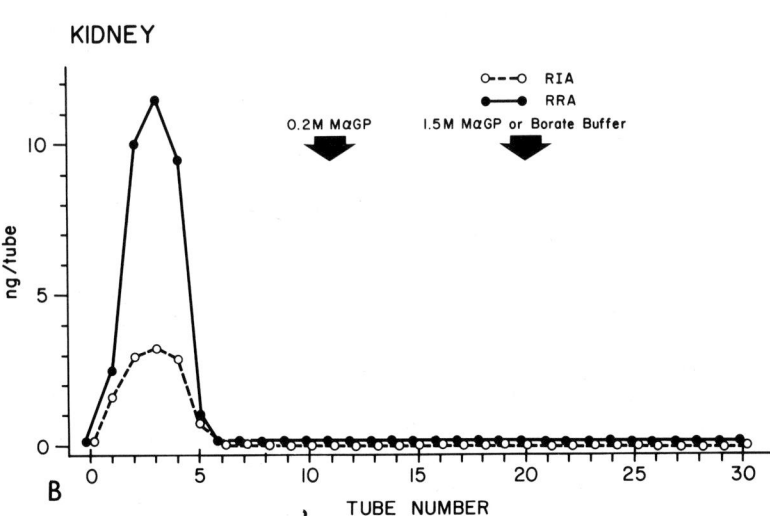

Figure 31–5. These figures show concanavalin A (Con A) column chromatography of CG from placental extracts and from kidney extracts. Over 90% of the CG from placenta (*A*) binds to the Con A column and elutes following addition of 0.2M alpha methyl glucopyranoside (0.2M MαGP). In contrast, over 90% of the kidney CG (*B*) elutes in the void volume; none is detectable following addition of 0.2M MαGP or even more vigorous competitors for carbohydrate binding (1.5M MαGP or borate buffer). (From Yoshimoto, Y., et al.: Human chorionic gonadotropin-like material: Presence in normal human tissue. *Am. J. Obstet. Gynecol. 134*:729, 1979.)

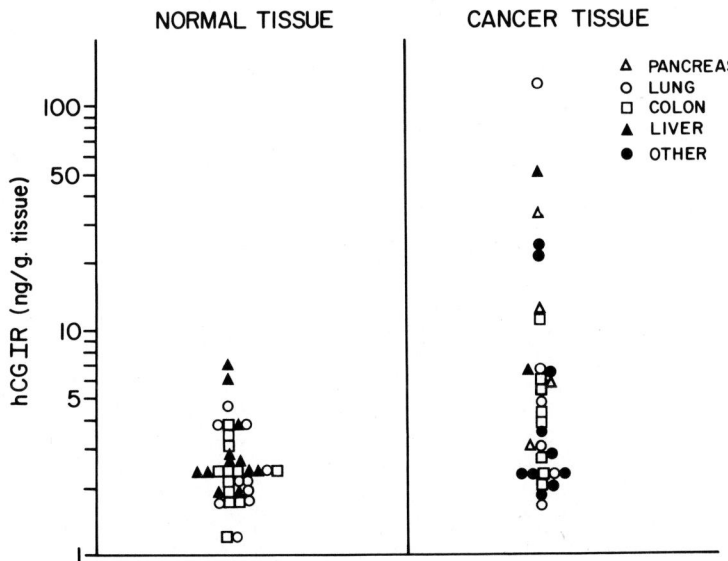

Figure 31–6. Human chorionic gonadotropin immunoreactivity (hCG IR) in acetic acid extracts of various carcinomas and normal tissues. hCG IR is presented on a log scale. (From Yoshimoto, Y., et al.: Glycosylation: A variable in hCG production by cancers. *Am. J. Med. 67*:414, 1979.)

In addition to the production of intact CG-like material, tumors also are able to produce free alpha or beta subunits. In fact, the studies of Odell et al.[4] show that increased blood concentrations of free alpha chain may be more than increased concentrations of CG. Weintraub and Rosen[56] first reported a patient with tumor elaboration of the free beta chain of CG. This patient suffered from anaplastic pancreatic carcinoma. Subsequently, the same authors[57] reported a patient with gastric carcinoid who had large amounts of free alpha chain in serum and tumor extracts. Studies from our laboratory[4, 58] indicated that elevated alpha chain concentrations are found in 30% of men with untreated carcinoma of the lung, 20% of men with untreated gastric carcinoma, and 20% of women with untreated colon carcinoma.. Kahn et al.[59] reported elevated free alpha chain concentrations in blood of 59% of patients with pancreatic islet cell carcinomas, but in no patients with benign islet cell tumors.

HYPOGLYCEMIA AND CANCER

The types of neoplasms producing hypoglycemia as an ectopic humoral syndrome differ from those causing most other humoral syndromes. The largest group, which may be loosely termed mesotheliomas, includes fibrosarcomas, neurofibromas, neurofibrosarcomas, mesenchymomas, and sarcomatous dysembryoplasia. These mesothelial types of neoplasms usually are quite large at the time hypoglycemia is noted; the range of reported size is 800 to 10,000 g and the average is about 2400 g. About two-thirds of these mesotheliomas have occurred in the abdomen, both peritoneal and retroperitoneal. The remaining one-third occur within the thorax. (References of many case reports are given in earlier editions of this textbook.[3, 60] Sex incidence is equal.

Table 31–5 describes the approximate frequency of various types of neoplasms associated with hypoglycemia.

The hypoglycemia associated with hepatic carcinomas does not appear to be caused simply by tumor replacement of normal liver parenchyma and a resultant decrease in hepatic glucose production. Hypoglycemia may occur prior to the diagnosis of a neoplasm, and liver function may be normal or nearly normal. In addition, hypoglycemia is common in association with hepatomas, but rare in association with other metastatic or infiltrative carcinomas involving the liver. As we discuss later, production of hypoglycemia by a hepatoma may not, strictly speaking, be an ectopic humoral syndrome, but an example of a neoplasm retaining sufficient differentiation to produce a substance normally produced by hepatic cells.

Several cases of hypoglycemia associated with malignant diseases of white blood cells have been described.[61-63]

Table 31–5. TYPES OF NEOPLASMS
CAUSING HYPOGLYCEMIA

Tumor Types	Approximate Percentage of Cases
Mesenchymal*	64
Hepatic	21
Adrenal carcinomas	6
Miscellaneous (anaplastic carcinomas, adeno-carcinomas, pseudomyxomas, cholangiomas)	9

*Included in this category are fibrosarcomas, mesotheliomas, neurofibromas, neurofibrosarcomas, spindle cell sarcomas, rhabdomyosarcomas, and leiomyosarcomas.

In some instances such "hypoglycemia" occurs because blood was collected in tubes that permitted continued glucose utilization *in vitro* by the large number of malignant cells.[63] In other cases, a true ectopic humoral syndrome appears to exist.

The etiology of the hypoglycemia remains poorly understood. Extracts of 25 neoplasms were studied in attempts to demonstrate a hypoglycemia-producing factor.[3, 60, 64] By using bioassays (rat diaphragm and epididymal fat pad assays) and studying 10 extracts, insulin-like activity could be demonstrated in all cases. Significantly, acid-alcohol extracts (used for insulin *per se*) contained less bioactivity than saline, water, or buffer extracts. This suggests that the material was not insulin *per se*. Radioimmunoassay (insulin radioimmunoassays) studies of six extracts failed to reveal any insulin activity; three of the same extracts, containing no insulin detectable by radioimmunoassay, did contain activity as measured by bioassay.[64, 65] Thus, on the basis of these earlier studies, the material has biologic activity similar to that of insulin, but fails to react in insulin radioimmunoassays. This suggests that nonsuppressible insulin-like proteins of one or more of the somatomedins might be implicated. As is reviewed in other chapters in this text, the somatomedins are a family of peptides produced by the liver. Somatomedins have biologic properties similar or identical to those of insulin, fail to react in insulin radioimmunoassays (they are structurally different from insulin), but do react in radioreceptor assays for insulin.[66] To further support the postulate that somatomedins produce this syndrome, Megyesi et al.,[67] using a radioreceptor assay for insulin, demonstrated elevated plasma concentrations of nonsuppressible insulin-like activity (NSILA — a somatomedin-like substance) in five of seven patients with cancer and hypoglycemia. Plovnick et al.[68] recently described a woman with intra-abdominal fibrosarcoma and hypoglycemia who had elevated NSIL-P, but low somatomedin activity. It appears possible that the same substance may not be causative in all cases. Several nonsuppressible insulin-like substances and somatomedins have been described. For example, NSIL-P is a 90,000 molecular weight serum glycoprotein with insulin-like biologic properties.[69] The sulfation factor activity of NSIL-P is low, in contrast to that of accepted somatomedins.[70] In contrast, nonsuppressible insulin-like activity soluble (NSILA-S) is a composite of two low molecular weight (5700 to 5900) insulin-like growth factors (IGF-1 and IGF-2).[71] Several somatomedins that are different from either NSIL-P or NSILA-S also exist.[66] On the basis of present knowledge, one or more of the somatomedins, or NSIL-P or NSILA-S, could be elaborated by cancers producing hypoglycemia.

HYPERCALCEMIA

The association of hypercalcemia and cancer was one of the earliest described humoral syndromes. Zondek et al.[72] in 1923 described a man with hypercalcemia and an elevated nonprotein nitrogen of 116 mg per 100 ml. At autopsy, the parathyroids were described as normal, but a carcinoma of the gallbladder was present. In 1936, Gutman et al.[73] described a second patient, a 57-year-old man with hypophosphatemia and hypercalcemia and a bronchogenic carcinoma. The possible cause of this hypercalcemia in some patients with cancer was first suggested by Albright who, in 1941,[74] discussed a patient with renal cell carcinoma and metastases to the ileum who had hypercalcemia and hypophosphatemia. Albright pointed out that hypercalcemia and *hyper*phosphatemia would be expected if bone metastases *per se* caused hypercalcemia. He postulated that the tumor must make a parathyroid hormone–like substance and reviewed the previous two patients described in 1923 and 1936. Albright's patient had no abnormalities in the parathyroid glands at autopsy. In 1964, Tashjian et al.[75] first offered some substantiation of this hypothesis by identifying, using immunochemical techniques, a parathyroid hormone–like material in extracts of carcinomas from patients with hypercalcemia. Subsequently, radioimmunoassay identification was reported by Berson and Yalow[76] and Sherwood et al.[77] Buckle et al.[78] studied in great detail a patient with renal carcinoma and hypercalcemia. An arterial-venous parathyroid hormone (PTH) gradient was demonstrated across the tumor (arterial PTH 0.62 µg/ml). After the tumor was removed, serum PTH fell to normal, and extracts of the renal tumor contained 2200 ng/gm of PTH. Extracts of normal kidney contained no detectable PTH. This patient is the best-documented illustration of ectopic PTH production as a cause of hypercalcemia. A second well studied patient was described by Zidar et al.[79] This patient suffered from acute myeloblastic leukemia and hypercalcemia. On six occasions hypercalcemia recurred, along with relapse of leukemia, and on two of these occasions serum PTH concentrations were elevated. *In vitro* studies showed that the myeloblasts released PTH into the medium, but normal cells did not. These studies led to the belief that hypercalcemia associated with cancer was caused by cancer elaboration of PTH, and in earlier reviews, in 1964 and 1968,[60] this view was expressed.[1]

Some doubts about this viewpoint arose. For example, in 1971 Federman et al.[80] discussed a patient with squamous cell carcinoma, hypercalcemia, and hypophosphatemia who had no detectable plasma PTH. Furthermore, in 1974 Powell et al.[81] carefully studied 11 patients with hypercalcemia, hypophosphatemia, and cancer without bone metastases. In nine, treatment of the tumor by either surgical ablation or chemotherapy restored calcium to normal. PTH was quantified, using several radioimmunoassays designed to react with intact PTH as well as with PTH fragments. With all assays, no PTH was detectable in either tumor extracts or in blood. These same authors indicated that about 50% of other patients with cancer and hypercalcemia whom they had studied had no detectable PTH in tumor extracts. In the tumor extracts from the 11 patients, a substance which caused bone resorption was detectable (using *in vitro* calcium resorption from mouse calvarium). Powell et al.[81] postulated that a substance other than PTH was elaborated by these tumors to produce hypercalcemia.

Certain data from animal studies suggested that prostaglandins might produce hypercalcemia. In 1972 Tashjian et al.[82] studied an animal model of hypercalcemia and cancer, a fibrosarcoma in mice. This tumor elaborated prostaglandin (PG), probably PGE_2. The hypercalcemia in the mouse model was treatable by indomethacin, a potent inhibitor of PG synthesis. These workers also studied a second animal model, the rabbit VX_2 carcinoma, which is associated with hypercalcemia.[83] This tumor also elaborated PG.[13] Prostaglandins had previously been shown to have bone resorption properties *in vitro*.[84] With this background, in 1975, Brereton et al.[85] described a patient with adenocarcinoma of the kidney, without osseous metastases, who had hypercalcemia. Extracts of the neoplasm contained large amounts of prostaglandins, both PGE and PGF. Prostaglandins were not detectable in blood, but this was attributed to lack of assay sensitivity. Modest doses of indomethacin returned blood calcium to normal. Robertson et al.[86] also described a patient with

renal cell carcinoma and hypercalcemia, who had low plasma PTH concentrations and elevated PGE levels by immunoassay. Hepatic metastases contained higher concentrations of PGE than did normal liver and kidney. Ito et al.[87] described a third hypercalcemia patient with renal adenocarcinoma, who had a fall in serum calcium with indomethacin treatment. No measurements of PG were made. In a more extensive study Seyberth et al.[88] evaluated 29 patients with solid tumors. Fourteen of these were hypercalcemic (none had renal carcinoma); 15 had normal blood calcium. Twelve of the 14 hypercalcemic patients had marked increases in urinary PG metabolites; seven of the normocalcemic patients had elevated PG excretion, and the increase was only slight or moderate. In six patients treated with indomethacin or aspirin, urinary PG excretion fell and there was a variable fall in serum calcium. Aspirin is a less potent inhibitor of PG synthesis than is indomethacin. With these data as a background, one might conclude that PG elaboration by cancers is a very common cause of hypercalcemia. However, the story is even more complex, as will be discussed.

For example, Tashjian[89] reported that a number of investigators have found that most patients with hypercalcemia fail to respond to indomethacin therapy. Most intriguing, Benson et al.[90] reported that the metabolism of PTH in normal parathyroid tissue differed from that in carcinomas. Thus the carboxyl fragment of PTH (previously believed to be a peripheral degradation product) is formed intracellularly in parathyroid tissue. This product may be less effectively formed in cancer tissue. Since most PTH assays measure predominantly the carboxyl end of PTH, and "control" or "normal" values are based on measurements in hyperparathyroid patients and normal subjects, the values of such assays in cancer subjects may be difficult to interpret. Thus, "normal" PTH value in a patient with cancer and hypercalcemia could be interpreted as inappropriately low and possibly be implicated in hypercalcemia. With the widespread availability of reliable PTH immunoassays, it is now evident that PTH is very rarely elevated in patients with cancer and hypercalcemia. It is frequently easily detectable, however, when not suppressed to undetectable levels. Whatever the ultimate solution to this problem is, at present it is best to summarize that carcinomas appear to be able to produce hypercalcemia by production of either PTH or prostaglandins or both. The relative frequency of each cause is difficult to state with certainty; estimates vary with types of assays and interpretation of data.

Whatever is the cause, hypercalcemia in cancer is relatively common. Bender and Hansen[91] studied 200 consecutive patients with bronchogenic carcinoma; 12.5% had hypercalcemia. The percentage varied with the histologic type: 23% with epidermoid carcinoma; 12.7% with large cell anaplastic carcinoma; and 2.5% with adenocarcinoma. Fourteen of the 20 patients with hypercalcemia did not have osseous metastases. Table 31–6 shows the approximate frequency of carcinomas associated with hypercalcemia.

A third cause of hypercalcemia associated with malignancy exists — the production of osteoclast-activating factor (OAF). OAF is a protein with molecular weight of about 20,000, normally produced by white blood cells.[92] OAF is about equal to PTH in potency, as tested *in vitro* using bone resorption. Mundy et al.[93] noted that hypercalcemia is common in multiple myeloma, but rare in diseases associated with bone marrow usually packed with diseased cells, e.g., chronic lymphatic leukemia, acute leukemia, or Waldenström's macroglobulinemia. These workers assayed multiple myeloma cells for OAF and

Table 31–6. NEOPLASMS ASSOCIATED WITH HYPERCALCEMIA

Tissue of Origin	Approximate Frequency (Per Cent)
Carcinoma of lung	35
Carcinoma of kidney	24
Carcinoma of ovary	8
Miscellaneous*	each <3

*Carcinoma of breast, uterus, pancreas, urinary bladder, colon, prostate, penis, esophagus, parotid gland, testis (a child), hepatoblastoma (a child), hemangiosarcoma.

found large quantities. PTH was also detectable by radioimmunoassay, but was present in concentrations too low to result in increased bone resorption. Prostaglandins were not detectable. OAF was present in concentrations adequate to explain hypercalcemia. Hypercalcemia also has been reported in association with lymphatic leukemia[94] and acute myeloblastic leukemia;[95] OAF elaboration also could be the cause in these patients. The frequency of hematologic malignant diseases associated with hypercalcemia may be estimated from the study of Laird-Meyers.[96] He reported 430 patients with hypercalcemia and malignancy. Among these were 33 patients with lymphoma and 13 with leukemia.

With the many publications reviewed in this chapter, the reader must bear in mind that standard hyperparathyroidism and cancer may coexist in the same patient. Cystic bone lesions of hyperparathyroidism may mimic metastases. Drezner and Lebovitz[97] attempted to separate such patients by means of excretion of renal cyclic AMP (cAMP). Normal patients excreted 0.05 to 2.40 μMol cAMP/gm creatinine; patients with primary hyperparathyroidism excreted 2.27 to 8.45 μ/Mol; and patients with cancer and nonparathyroid hypercalcemia, 0.5 to 1.30 μ/Mol. In this study of Drezner and Lebovitz, nine patients had hypercalcemia and normal urinary cAMP; six had highly elevated nephrogenic cAMP. Surgical exploration of all patients with elevated cAMP revealed primary hyperparathyroidism in each.

In summary, one may state that primary hyperparathyroidism and cancer may coexist by chance. In solid tumors hypercalcemia may be produced by elaboration of PTH *per se* by the tumor (or by parathyroid glands) or by elaboration of prostaglandins. In hematologic malignant diseases associated with hypercalcemia, the hypercalcemia may be produced by elaboration of another protein, osteoclast-activating factor.

HYPOPHOSPHATEMIA AND NEOPLASMS

A rare syndrome of hypophosphatemia with normal serum calcium has been described in approximately 15 patients with an unusual variety of neoplasms: pleomorphic sarcomas or mesenchymal neoplasms and giant cell tumors of bone. This syndrome is associated with dramatic phosphaturia, normal PTH and calcium concentrations in blood, and rapid reversal upon tumor removal. These patients usually present to the physician with muscle spasms and cramps or symptoms related to severe osteomalacia. In 1977, Drezner and Feinglos[98] reviewed previous reports which described the syndrome and documented the findings presented above and also for the first time studied vitamin D metabolism and response to treatment.

Their patient was a 42-year-old woman with osteomalacia and a giant cell tumor of bone. She had normal plasma PTH measured in several radioimmunoassay systems with both carboxy-terminal specificity and amino-terminal specificity. Serum 20 hydroxycholcalciferol concentrations were normal, while serum 1,25 dihydroxycholecalciferol concentrations were low. Treatment with 3 μg* of 1,25 dihydroxy vitamin D completely abolished hypophosphatemia, which recurred when therapy was stopped. Resection of tumor permanently abolished hypophosphatemia. These workers postulated that these tumors elaborate a substance that inhibits 1-hydroxylation of vitamin D. Additional patients should be studied to further evaluate this possibility, but the findings of Drezner and Feinglos in their well studied patient are very convincing.†

HYPOCALCEMIA AND CANCER

Although, on the basis of present evidence, hypocalcemia associated with cancer may not be produced via ectopic hormone production, it is a most striking and unusual symptom which is poorly understood. We review this subject only briefly to call attention to its occurrence and to indicate that further study is needed. In 1960, Sackner et al.[99] reported a patient with hypocalcemia and lung cancer. Ehrlich et al.[100] and Schwartz and Meiser[101] reported hypocalcemia in response to effective treatment of prostatic carcinoma and chronic leukemia, respectively. Ludwig[102] in 1962 and Hall et al.[103] in 1966 reported hypocalcemia and hypophosphatemia in one and three patients, respectively, with breast cancer and osseous metastases. While vitamin D deficiency and rapid bone formation were considered possible causes, all these reports were published before the relation of magnesium deficiency and PTH secretion and action were known, and hypomagnesemia was not considered or evaluated. Zusman et al.[104] in 1973 reported six children with acute lymphoblastic leukemia receiving various treatment regimens who developed rapid hyperphosphatemia and hypocalcemia. These investigators felt the hyperphosphatemia led to precipitation of calcium phosphate and hypocalcemia. Serum or urinary magnesium was not quantified and magnesium was not administered, but hyperphosphatemia of this degree (5.7 to 9.4 mg per 100 ml) is not expected in hypomagnesemia. The possibility also exists that some of the neoplasms associated with hypocalcemia and normal phosphate levels or hypophosphatemia produce excess calcitonin. This possibility has not yet been evaluated. Hyperphosphatemia, however, would not be expected with excess calcitonin production. Furthermore, it is generally considered that calcitonin is poorly effective in adult humans, and hypocalcemia is not part of the thyroid medullary carcinoma syndrome in which massive levels of circulating calcitonin are often present. More than one cause of the hypocalcemia probably exists — one associated with hyperphosphatemia, perhaps simply a massive phosphate load from dietary sources associated with some decrease in renal function; and a second associated with hypophosphatemia, possibly caused by rapid bone calcification of unknown direct cause.

---

*This is a very high, probably nonphysiologic dose.

†After preparation of this chapter, confirmation of these findings in a second patient appeared (Fukumoto, Y., et al.: Tumor induced vitamin D resistant hypophosphatemic osteomalacia associated with proximal and tubular dysfunction and 1,25 dihydroxyvitamin D deficiency. *J. Clin. Endocrinol. Metab.* 49:873, 1979).

ECTOPIC PRODUCTION OF CALCITONIN

Calcitonin is normally produced by the parafollicular cells of the thyroid and is an excellent marker of tumors developing from these cells — medullary carcinoma. Calcitonin is also elaborated ectopically by a variety of carcinomas. Typically, calcitonin produces no discernible symptoms, but might (certain reservations are expressed later) serve as a tumor marker. The earliest reports were those of Milhaud et al. in 1970,[105] who described a patient with a carcinoid tumor that elaborated calcitonin, and Silva et al. in 1973,[106] who described a man with oat cell carcinoma. In 1974 and 1976 Coombs, Hillyard, et al.[107] and Hillyard, Coombs, et al.[108] described a series of patients with carcinoma of the lung and breast with elevated blood concentrations of calcitonin. Extracts of breast carcinoma contained increased immunoreactive calcitonin. Recently, in studies from our laboratory, Schwartz et al.[109] studied prospectively 240 patients admitted for diagnostic evaluation of possible malignant disease. Of 123 patients subsequently shown to have carcinoma, 35 had highly elevated plasma calcitonin (>150 pg/ml). These included 19 of 49 patients (38%) with carcinoma of the lung, 7 of 29 (24%) with colon cancer, 8 of 21 (38%) with breast cancer, and 6 of 14 (42%) with pancreatic cancer. The association of elevated plasma calcitonin with malignancy is fairly constant from report to report, and ranges from about 45 to 60% for lung carcinoma.[107-109] Interestingly, in some patients, as Silva et al.[110] demonstrated by selective vessel catheterization with assay of calcitonin concentrations, the normal thyroid may be the source of calcitonin and not the tumor itself. This patient was a man with adenocarcinoma of the lung. In this patient, it appears possible that the tumor was producing a substance that stimulated thyroid production of calcitonin. Alternatively, some parameter, only indirectly related to the tumor (e.g., stress or bone vitamin D metabolism), may increase calcitonin production.

Further studies are required to ascertain whether increased thyroidal production is common in cancer.

VASOPRESSIN ELABORATION BY CANCERS

In 1957 Schwartz et al.[111] first described the syndrome of hyponatremia, renal sodium loss, hypervolemia, and inappropriately high urine osmolality in two patients with carcinoma. They attributed this syndrome to sustained elaboration of vasopressin, but the source of vasopressin was uncertain. In a further review of these patients, Bartter and Schwartz[112] commented that in some patients direct vagal stimulation by the lung carcinoma or the presence of brain metastases may cause pituitary hypersecretion of vasopressin; in others the cancer itself could be the source. In 1963, Amatruda et al.,[113] using bioassay, first demonstrated a vasopressin-like material in extracts of tissue from a patient with carcinoma of the lung who suffered from this syndrome. Bower and Mason,[114] using bioassays, also demonstrated the presence of a substance with vasopressin properties in extracts of cancer tissue producing this syndrome. In 1968 Vorherr et al.,[115] using a radioimmunoassay, studied a series of patients with this syndrome; the vasopressin-like material in extracts of cancer tissue reacted identically to arginine vasopressin (AVP). George et al.[116] in 1972 demonstrated direct synthesis of vasopressin by lung cancer by showing incorporation of tritiated amino acids in vitro. In 1976 Hirata et al.[117] studied two patients, using a bioassay, a radioimmunoassay, and gel filtration, and found the material indistinguishable from AVP by these criteria. However, neurophysin also may be elaborated. Hamilton et al.[118] reported the presence of neurophysins in extracts of tumors associated with the syndrome of sustained inappropriate antidiuresis. North et al.[119] studied 26 unselected patients with small cell carcinoma of the lung and found elevated levels of neurophysins in 42% prior to antitumor therapy.

The most common cancer associated with vasopressin production is carcinoma of the lung, predominantly small or oat cell. However, squamous and anaplastic carcinomas also produce this syndrome. It also has been described in patients with prostatic carcinoma,[120] carcinoma of the adrenal cortex,[121] and Hodgkin's disease.[122] Gilby et al.[123] reported that 40% of patients with oat cell carcinoma had sustained inappropriate vasopressin secretion. In 1977 Odell et al.,[4] using an antiserum that reacted with both AVP and the fetal peptide arginine vasotocin (AVT), reported that 41% of 41 patients with lung carcinoma of all histologic types, and 37% of 30 patients with carcinoma of the colon, had inappropriately elevated plasma concentration of AVP/AVT. These concentrations were above the 95% confidence limits of control subjects dehydrated for 18 hours. Many of these patients were not hyponatremic and presumably were susceptible to development of the clinical syndrome if water-loaded. Ginsberg et al.[124] reported that 88% of patients with carcinoma extending outside one hemithorax had abnormal water-load tests, while 4 of 11 (36%) with disease limited to one hemithorax had abnormal tests.

In summary, sustained vasopressin elaboration in patients with cancer appears to be considerably more common than the clinical syndrome of hyponatremia, hypervolemia, renal sodium loss, and inappropriately high urine osmolality. Tumor production of vasopressin probably occurs in about 40% of patients with carcinoma of the lung and colon. Other carcinomas have not been studied adequately for frequency of vasopressin elaboration. Expression of the clinical syndrome is dependent on the patient's being water-loaded. In addition, neurophysins are elaborated by some carcinomas; about 40% of small cell carcinomas of the lung also elaborate this protein.

GROWTH HORMONE AND GROWTH HORMONE–RELEASING HORMONE PRODUCTION BY CANCERS

A small number of patients with acromegaly associated with bronchial carcinoid tumor have been described in recent years.[125-135] Although the association could have been simply fortuitous in some of these patients,[128, 129] in at least five, normal growth hormone (GH) secretion was restored, and/or the clinical syndrome of acromegaly subsided, after removal of the bronchial carcinoid.[125-127] In these cases no therapy was directed to the hypothalamic-pituitary system, suggesting further that the cause was related to the bronchial tumor. Saeed uz Zafar et al.[130] described a well evaluated patient, a 22-year-old female with acromegaly. She had acromegalic features and enlarged sella turcica on x-ray. In 1960 she underwent craniotomy with hypophysectomy; a histologic diagnosis of eosinophilic adenoma was made. The patient also had scoliosis and recurrent episodes of pneumonitis, and after hypophysectomy GH concentrations remained elevated. In 1971, because of the recurrent episodes of pneumonia, she underwent bronchoscopy with discovery of a bronchial adenoma, not visible on chest x-ray. After the surgery which followed, GH concentrations fell to 0.6 ng/ml before and after glucose loading. Extracts of the bronchial carcinoid contained a substance with growth hormone–releasing activity (GHRA) as assessed *in vitro* in a dispersed pituitary cell culture system. The authors concluded that the bronchial carcinoid elaborated a substance with GH-releasing properties. Subsequently Frohman et al.[131] have extracted and partially purified GHRA from tumors from several patients with this syndrome. These data indicate tumor production of GHRA led to development of a pituitary adenoma — an unusual ectopic hormone result.

In addition to the possibility of GHRA production, direct elaboration of GH is feasible. Extracts of lung tumors have been reported to contain immunoreactive GH.[132-136] In the most recent report,[135] a large number of tumor tissue extracts were assayed for GH using radioimmunoassay and radioreceptor assay. In addition, normal tissues (liver, kidney, lungs, spleen, and so forth) were studied. High concentrations (over 10 ng/gm tissue) were rarely found in normal tissues (e.g., one of 76 normal ovaries; none in two livers, four lungs, and four kidneys) but were found in ovarian carcinomas, primary or metastatic. The highest concentrations were found in breast cancer metastases in skin and ovaries, using both radioreceptor and radioimmunoassay techniques. Control studies revealed that these extracts did not degrade the ^{125}I-GH tracer used for assay. Such an enzymatic system can artifactually produce an effect that appears to be GH activity in these assay systems.*

HEMATOLOGIC ABNORMALITIES ASSOCIATED WITH CANCERS

Abnormalities of red cells, white cells, and platelets all have been described to be associated with, and possibly caused by, tumors. The best known syndrome is erythrocytosis, which has been reviewed recently.[137] Over 350 patients have now been described; Table 31–7 lists the frequency of association with various neoplasms.

By using bioassays to quantify erythropoietin, increased blood levels have been found in 96% of patients with cancer and polycythemia. Extracts of tumor or renal cyst fluid contained greater amounts of erythropoietin than normal adjacent tissue in 28 of 44 cases reviewed.[137] One to five per cent of patients with renal neoplasms and 9 to 12% of patients with cerebellar hemangioblastoma have erythrocytosis; elevated plasma erythropoietin may be even more frequent.[138] For example, in 1977 Sulfrin et al.[139] studied 57 patients with renal carcinoma and found increased plasma erythropoietin by bioassay in 63%. Murphy et al.[140, 141] have extensively studied Wilms' tumor, which is associated frequently with polycythemia, and have reported a strong correlation between tumor stage and concentration of plasma erythropoietin. In patients with adrenal cortical tumors and virilizing ovarian tumors erythrocytosis may be related to tumor production of androgens rather than to erythropoietin. Waldman et al.[142] found normal concentrations of erythropoietin in serum and tumor extracts from such patients. Using radiation inactivation of biologic properties to estimate molecular weight, Waldman et al. found that

---

*In all studies of this kind it is imperative to rigorously prove that artifactual assay data will not explain the results. These proofs should include assessment of possible effects on the assay of extract modification of pH, osmolality, and ion content, as well as the presence of enzyme systems which degrade the labeled hormone.

Table 31–7. TUMORS ASSOCIATED WITH ERYTHROCYTOSIS

Neoplasm	Approximate Distribution (Per Cent)
Renal carcinomas	50
Cerebellar hemangioblastomas	20
Benign renal cysts and adenomas	15
Uterine fibroids	6
Miscellaneous*	9

*Hepatomas, adrenal carcinomas, virilizing ovarian neoplasms, lung carcinomas, thymomas, pheochromocytomas.

the molecular weight of tumor erythropoietin was similar to that of erythropoietin produced by the normal kindey.[1, 142]

SYNDROMES OF GASTROINTESTINAL PEPTIDE PRODUCTION

Several clinical syndromes caused by tumor production of peptides normally produced by the gastrointestinal (GI) tract exist. It is debatable whether these represent true ectopic peptide production, for they may represent production by tumors derived from cells that normally produce such substances; in some instances (e.g., alpha cell tumors elaborating glucagon) this is clearly the case.

In 1955, Zollinger and Ellison[143] described the syndrome of severe peptic ulcerations of the stomach, duodenum, and jejunum associated with a pancreatic tumor. This was shown by McGuigan and Trudeau[144] and by Charters et al.[145] to be associated with elevated serum gastrin levels and with the presence in tumor extracts of a material identical to gastrin in radioimmunoassays. Dockray et al.,[146] Gregory,[147] and Walsh and Grossman[148] reported that these tumors contain a mixture of molecular forms — big, big gastrin; big gastrin (34 amino acids); little gastrin (17 amino acids); and minigastrin (13 amino acids) — and that they secrete these multiple forms in response to stimulation by secretin. Big gastrin, little gastrin, and minigastrin are all bioactive in terms of stimulating gastric acid secretion.[148] Immunohistochemical staining has shown more than one peptide-containing cell type in many tumors,[149, 150] and production of both gastrin and vasoactive peptide by such a tumor was reported by Judge et al.[151]

The diagnosis of Zollinger-Ellison (ZE) syndrome may be made by finding elevated basal and calcium-stimulated serum gastrin concentrations and a paradoxical rise in serum gastrin in response to secretin.[152-156] About 40% of patients with the ZE syndrome have gastrinomas that behave as benign tumors. However, in the other 60% the gastrinomas are often multicentric or metastatic when first diagnosed, and total gastrectomy as well as removal of primary and metastatic tumors is desirable.[157-159] Prolonged survival (and, rarely, tumor regression) has been observed following total gastrectomy.[160] When nonresectable malignant gastrinomas are present, treatment with 5-fluorouracil and streptozotocin may decrease tumor size and gastrin production.[161]

Another syndrome of GI hormone production consists of watery diarrhea, hypokalemia, and hypochlorhydria (Verner-Morrison syndrome).[162] This has been described to be produced by pancreatic islet cell carcinomas, bronchogenic cancers, pheochromocytomas, and neuroblastomas.[162-164] This symptom complex has been associated with tumor production of vasoactive intestinal polypeptide,[164-166] of prostaglandin E,[167] of pancreatic polypeptide,[150] of secretin,[168] of serotonin, enteroglucagon, and pancreatic glucagon,[169, 170] and of gastric inhibitory peptide.[171] In addition, over 50% of patients with this syndrome of watery diarrhea, hypokalemia, and hypochlorhydria do have hypercalcemia, which returns to normal if the tumor is resected.[172] Streptozotocin also may decrease symptoms of this tumor if it is unresectable.

Two reports of a renal neoplasm producing enteroglucagon have been made by Gleeson et al.[173] and Bloom.[174] The patient presented with malabsorption with decreased small intestinal motility. In addition, two patients presenting with hyperglycemia associated with a pancreatic tumor elaborating somatostatin have been reported.[175, 176] Since somatostatin is normally produced by the islet cells of the pancreas, this also may not represent true ectopic production.

As indicated, glucagon production by alpha cell tumors is probably not an ectopic humoral syndrome. The clinical presentation of this interesting syndrome consists of bullous eczematoid rash, glossitis, and mild diabetes mellitus.[177]

In 1977 Kahn et al.[59] reported that among patients with functioning islet cell tumors, a malignant tumor was associated with elevations in blood chorionic gonadotropin, or in free alpha or beta peptide chain of chorionic gonadotropin, in 63% of patients. No patient with a benign islet cell tumor had elevations in these peptides. These markers may thus be helpful in preoperative diagnosis of a malignant versus a benign islet cell tumor. Since, as we reviewed earlier in this chapter, many other tumors also produce these peptide markers, the diagnosis of an islet cell tumor must be made on other grounds.

REFERENCES

1. Lipsett, M. B., et al.: Humoral syndromes associated with nonendocrine tumors. Ann. Intern. Med. 61:733, 1964.
2. Liddle, G. W., et al.: Clinical and laboratory studies of ectopic humoral syndromes. Rec. Prog. Horm. Res. 25:283, 1969.
3. Odell, W. D.: Humoral manifestations of nonendocrine neoplasms. In Textbook of Endocrinology. 5th ed. Williams, R. H. (ed.), Philadelphia, W. B. Saunders Co., 1974, p. 1105.
4. Odell, W. D., et al.: Ectopic peptide synthesis — a universal concomitant of neoplasia. Trans. Assoc. Am. Physicians 90:204, 1977.
5. Steiner, D. F., and Oyer, P. E.: The biosynthesis of insulin and a probable precursor of insulin by a human islet cell adenoma. Proc. Nat. Acad. Sci. USA 57:473, 1967.
6. Steiner, D. F.: Insulin today. Diabetes 26:322, 1977.
7. Gewirtz, G., et al.: Big ACTH: Conversion to biologically active ACTH by trypsin. J. Clin. Endocrinol. Metab. 38:227, 1974.
8. Eipper, B. A., et al.: High molecular weight forms of adrenocorticotropic hormone are glycoproteins. J. Biol. Chem. 251:4121, 1976.
9. Mains, R. E., and Eipper, B. A.: Biosynthesis of adrenocorticotropic hormone in mouse pituitary tumor cells. J. Biol. Chem. 251:4115, 1976.
10. Habener, J. F., et al.: Proparathyroid hormone: Biosynthesis by human parathyroid adenomas. Science 178:630, 1972.
11. Habener, J. F., et al.: Pre-proparathyroid hormone identified by cell-free translation of messenger RNA from hyperplastic parathyroid tissue. J. Clin. Invest. 56:1328, 1975.
12. Gregory, R. A., and Tracy, H. J.: Isolation of two "big" gastrins from Zollinger-Ellison tumour tissue. Lancet 2:797, 1972.
13. Noe, B. D., et al.: Glucagon biosynthesis in human pancreatic islets: Preliminary evidence for a biosynthetic intermediate. Horm. Metab. Res. 7:314, 1975.
14. Noe, B. D., and Bauer, G. E.: Evidence for sequential metabolic cleavage of proglucagon to glucagon in glucagon biosynthesis. Endocrinology 97:868, 1975.
15. Stachura, M. E., and Frohman, L. A.: "Large" growth hormone: Ribonucleic acid-associated precursor of other growth hormone forms in rat pituitary. Endocrinology 94:701, 1974.
16. Lingappa, V. R., et al.: Nascent prehormones are intermediates in the biosynthesis of authentic bovine pituitary growth hormone and prolactin. Proc. Nat. Acad. Sci. USA 74:2432, 1977.
17. Bielinska, M., and Boine, I.: MRNA-dependent synthesis of a glyco-

sylated subunit of human chorionic gonadotropin in cell-free extracts derived from ascites tumor cells. Proc. Nat. Acad. Sci. USA 75:1768, 1978.
18. Permutt, M. A., et al.: Cell-free translation of messenger RNA extracted from a human insulinoma. J. Endocrinol. Metab. 46:897, 1977.
19. Brown, V. H.: A case of pluriglandular syndrome: Diabetes of bearded women. Lancet 2:1011, 1928.
20. Meador, C. K., et al.: Cause of Cushing's syndrome arising from "nonendocrine" tissue. J. Clin. Endocrinol. Metab. 22:693, 1962.
21. Kato, Y., et al.: Oat cell carcinoma of the lung. A review of 138 cases. Cancer 23:517, 1969.
22. Ratcliffe, J. G., et al.: Tumour and plasma ACTH syndrome. Clin. Endocrinol. 1:27, 1972.
23. Bloomfield, G. A., et al.: Lung tumors and ACTH production. Clin. Endocrinol. 6:95, 1977.
24. Gewirtz, G., and Yalow, R. S.: Ectopic ACTH production in carcinoma of the lung. J. Clin. Invest. 53:1022, 1974.
25. Wolfsen, A. R., and Odell, W. D.: PROACTH: Use for early detection of lung cancer. Am. J. Med. 66:765, 1979.
26. Mason, A. M. S., et al.: ACTH secretion by bronchial carcinoid tumors. Clin. Endocrinol. 1:3, 1972.
27. Upton, G. V., and Amatruda, T. T., Jr.: Evidence for the presence of tumor peptides with corticotropin-releasing-factor-like activity in the ectopic ACTH syndrome. New Eng. J. Med. 285:419, 1971.
28. Abe, K., et al.: Radioimmunoassay of βMSH in human plasma and tissues. J. Clin. Invsst. 46:1609, 1967.
29. Bloomfield, G. A., and Scott, A. P.: β-Melanocyte stimulating hormone. Proc. R. Soc. Med. 67:748, 1974.
30. Bloomfield, G. A., et al.: A reappraisal of human β-MSH. Nature 252:492, 1974.
31. Bachelot, I., et al.: Pituitary and plasma lipotropins: Demonstration of the artifactual nature of βMSH. J. Clin. Endocrinol. Metab. 44:939, 1977.
32. Odell, W. D., et al.: Ectopic production of lipotropin by cancer. Am. J. Med. 66:631, 1979.
33. Bellisario, E., et al.: Human chorionic gonadotropin. Linear amino acid sequence of the alpha subunit. J. Biol. Chem. 248:6796, 1973.
34. Papkoff, H., et al.: Studies on the structure and function of interstitial cell stimulating hormone. Recent Prog. Horm. Res. 29:563, 1973.
35. Canfield, R. E., et al.: Studies of human chorionic gonadotropin. Recent Prog. Horm. Res. 27:121, 1971.
36. Odell, W. D., et al.: Endocrine aspects of trophoblastic neoplasms. Clin. Obstet. Gynecol. 10:290, 1967.
37. Li, M. C.: Discussion of chemotherapy of choriocarcinoma and related trophoblastic tumors in women. Ann. N.Y. Acad. Sci. 80:280, 1959.
38. Chambers, W. L.: Adrenal cortical carcinoma in a male with excess gonadotropin in the urine. J. Clin. Endocrinol. Metab. 9:451, 1949.
39. Matteini, M.: Su di un caso di ginecomastia associata a tumore retroperitoneale a cellule indifferenziate. Rass. Neurol. Veget. 9:252, 1952.
40. McArthur, J. W.: Para-endocrine phenomena in obstetrics and gynecology. In Progress in Gynecology. Vol. 4. Meigs, J. V., and Sturgis, S. H., (eds.), New York, Grune and Stratton, 1963, p. 146.
41. Case records of Massachusetts General Hospital. Case 13–1972. New Eng. J. Med. 286:713, 1972.
42. Fusco, F. E., and Rosen, S. W.: Gonadotropin-producing anaplastic large-cell carcinomas of the lung. New Eng. J. Med. 284:405, 1966.
43. Faiman, C., et al.: Gonadotropin secretion from a bronchogenic carcinoma. Demonstration by radioimmunoassay. New Eng. J. Med. 277:1395, 1967.
44. Rosen, S. F., et al.: Ectopic gonadotropin production before clinical recognition of bronchogenic carcinoma. New Eng. J. Med. 297:640, 1968.
45. Vaitukaitis, J. L., et al.: A radioimmunoassay which specifically measures human chorionic gonadotropin in the presence of human luteinizing hormone. Am. J. Obstet. Gynecol. 113:751, 1972.
46. Braunstein, G. D., et al.: Ectopic production of human chorionic gonadotropin by neoplasms. Ann. Intern. Med. 78:39, 1973.
47. Braunstein, G. D., et al.: Presence in normal human testes of a chorionic gonadotropin-like substance distinct from human luteinizing hormone. New Eng. J. Med. 293:1339, 1975.
48. Chen, H. C., et al.: Evidence for a gonadotropin from non-pregnant subjects that has physical, immunological and biological similarities to human chorionic gonadotropin. Proc. Nat. Acad. Sci. USA 73:2885, 1976.
49. Yoshimoto, Y., et al.: Human chorionic gonadotropin-like substance in nonendocrine tissues of normal subjects. Science 197:575, 1977.
50. Yoshimoto, Y., et al.: Human chorionic gonadotropin-like material: Presence in normal human tissues. Am. J. Obstet. Gynecol. 134:729, 1979.
51. Van Hall, E. V., et al.: Immunological and biological activity of hCG following progressive desialation. Endocrinology 88:456, 1971.

52. Tsuruhara, T., et al.: Biological properties of hCG after removal of terminal sialic acid and galactose residues. *Endocrinology* 91:296, 1972.

53. Yoshimoto, Y., et al.: Glycosylation: A variable in hCG production by cancers. *Am. J. Med.* 67:414, 1979.

54. Acevedo, H. F., et al.: Choriogonadotropin in cancer cells. III. Further studies *in vitro* and *in vivo* cell systems. *Program of the Endocrine Society Meeting*, 1976, abstract 420.

55. McManus, C. H., et al.: Human chorionic gonadotropin in human neoplastic cells. *Cancer Res.* 36:3476, 1976.

56. Weintraub, B. D., and Rosen, S. W.: Ectopic production of the isolated beta subunit of human chorionic gonadotropin. *J. Clin. Invest.* 52:3135, 1973.

57. Rosen, S. W., and Weintraub, B. D.: Ectopic production of the isolated alpha subunit of the glycoprotein hormones. *New Eng. J. Med.* 290:1441, 1974.

58. Wolfsen, A. R., and Odell, W. D.: Early diagnosis of lung cancer (Ca) using peptide markers. *Clin. Res.* 25:502A, 1977 (abstract).

59. Kahn, R. C., et al.: Ectopic production of chorionic gonadotropin and its subunits by islet cell tumors. *New Engl. J. Med.* 297:565, 1977.

60. Odell, W. D.: Humoral manifestations of nonendocrine neoplasms. In *Textbook of Endocrinology*. 4th ed. Williams, R. H. (ed.), Philadelphia, W. B. Saunders Co., 1968, pp. 1211–1222.

61. Collip, P. J.: Hypoglycemia and leukemia. *Pediatrics* 49:788, 1972.

62. Buffet, C., et al.: Hypoglycemia during lymphosarcoma and reticulosarcoma. *Nouv. Presse Med.* 3:181, 1974.

63. Solomon, J.: Case report: Spurious hypoglycemia and hyperkalemia in myelomonocytic leukemia. *Am. J. Med. Sci.* 267:359, 1974.

64. Field, J. B., et al.: Insulin-like activity of nonpancreatic tumors associated with hypoglycemia. *J. Clin. Endocrinol. Metab.* 23:1229, 1963.

65. Tranquada, R. E., et al.: Hypoglycemia associated with carcinoma of the cecum and syndrome of testicular feminization. *New Eng. J. Med.* 266:1302, 1962.

66. Van Wyk, J. J., et al.: The somatomedins, a family of insulin-like hormones under growth hormone control. *Recent Prog. Horm. Res.* 30:259, 1974.

67. Megyesi, V., et al.: Hypoglycemia in association with extrapancreatic tumors. Demonstration of elevated plasma NSILA-S by a new radioreceptor assay. *J. Clin. Endocrinol. Metab.* 38:931, 1974.

68. Plovnik, H., et al.: Non-β-cell tumor hypoglycemia associated with increased nonsuppressible insulin-like protein (NSILP). *Am. J. Med.* 66:156, 1979.

69. Poffenbarger, P. L.: The purification and partial characterization of an insulin-like protein from human serum. *J. Clin. Invest.* 56:1455, 1975.

70. Poffenbarger, P. L., et al.: Chemistry and physiology of the human serum nonsuppressible insulin-like protein (NSILP). In *Serono Symposia: Somatomedins and Growth.* Giordano, G., and Van Wyle, J. J. (eds.), New York, Academic Press, 1979, pp. 67–83.

71. Rinderknecht, E., and Humbel, R. E.: Two polypeptides with non-suppressible insulin-like and cell growth promoting activities in human serum. Isolation, chemical characterization and some biological properties. *Proc. Nat. Acad. Sci. USA* 73:2365, 1976.

72. Zondek, H., et al.: Die Bedeutung der Kalzium Bestimmung im Blut für diagnose der Niereninsuffizienz. *S. Klin. Med.* 99:129, 1923.

73. Gutman, A. B., et al.: Serum calcium, inorganic phosphorus and phosphatase activity. *Arch. Intern. Med.* 57:379, 1936.

74. Albright, F.: Case records of the Massachusetts General Hospital. No. 27461. *New Eng. J. Med.* 225:789, 1941.

75. Tashjian, A., et al.: Immunochemical identification of parathyroid hormone in non-parathyroid neoplasms associated with hypercalcemia. *J. Exp. Med.* 119:467, 1964.

76. Berson, S. A., and Yalow, R. S.: Parathyroid hormone in plasma in adenomatous hyperparathyroidism, uremia and bronchogenic carcinoma. *Science* 153:907, 1966.

77. Sherwood, L. J.: Production of parathyroid hormone by non-parathyroid tumors. *J. Clin. Endocrinol. Metab.* 27:140, 1967.

78. Buckle, R. M., et al.: Ectopic secretion of parathyroid hormone by a renal adenocarcinoma in a patient with hypercalcemia. *Br. Med. J.* 4:724, 1970.

79. Zider, B. L., et al.: Acute myeloblastic leukemia and hypercalcemia. *New Eng. J. Med.* 295:692, 1976.

80. Federman, D., et al.: Case records of the Massachusetts General Hospital. *New Eng. J. Med.* 284:839, 1971.

81. Powell, D., et al.: Nonparathyroid hypercalcemia in patients with neoplastic diseases. *New Engl. J. Med.* 289:176, 1974.

82. Tashjian, A. H., et al.: Evidence that the bone-resorption-stimulating factor produced by mouse fibrosarcoma cells is prostaglandin E$_2$. A new model for hypercalcemia of cancer. *J. Exp. Med.* 136:1329, 1972.

83. Voelkel, E., et al.: Hypercalcemia and tumor prostaglandins: The VX$_2$ carcinoma model in the rabbit. *Metabolism* 24:973, 1975.

84. Klein, D. C., and Raisz, L. G.: Prostaglandins: Stimulation of bone resorption in tissue culture. *Endocrinology* 86:1436, 1970.

85. Brereton, H., et al.: Indomethacin responsive hypercalcemia in a pa-

tient with renal cell adenocarcinoma. *New Eng. J. Med.* 291:83, 1975.

86. Robertson, R. P., et al.: Elevated prostaglandins and suppressed parathyroid hormone associated with hypercalcemia and renal cell carcinoma. *J. Clin. Endocrinol. Metab.* 41:164, 1975.

87. Ito, H., et al.: Indomethacin responsive hypercalcemia. *New Eng. J. Med.* 293:588, 1975.

88. Seyberth, H. W., et al.: Prostaglandins as mediators of hypercalcemia associated with certain types of cancer. *New Eng. J. Med.* 293:1278, 1975.

89. Tashjian, A. H., Jr.: Prostaglandins, hypercalcemia and cancer. *New Eng. J. Med.* 293:1317, 1975.

90. Benson, R. C., et al.: Immunoreactive forms of circulating parathyroid hormone in primary and ectopic hyperparathyroidism. *J. Clin. Invest.* 54:175, 1974.

91. Bender, R. A., and Hansen, H.: Hypercalcemia in bronchogenic carcinoma. *Ann. Intern. Med.* 80:205, 1974.

92. Luben, R. A., et al.: Partial purification of osteoclast-activating factor from phytohemagglutinin-stimulated human leukocytes. *J. Clin. Invest.* 53:1473, 1974.

93. Mundy, G. R., et al.: Evidence for the secretion of osteoclast stimulating factor in myeloma. *New Eng. J. Med.* 291:1041, 1974.

94. Maudsley, C., and Holman, R. L.: Hypercalcemia in acute leukemia. *Lancet* 1:78, 1957.

95. Kronfield, S. J., and Reynold, T. B.: Leukemia and hypercalcemia. *New Eng. J. Med.* 271:399, 1964.

96. Laird-Meyers, W. P.: Hypercalcemia in neoplastic disease. *Arch. Surg.* 80:308, 1960.

97. Drezner, M. C., and Lebovitz, H. E.: Primary hyperparathyroidism in paraneoplastic hypercalcemia. *Lancet* 1:1004, 1978.

98. Drezner, M. N., and Feinglos, M. N.: Osteomalacia due to 1α,25-dihydroxycholecalciferol deficiency. *J. Clin. Invest.* 60:1046, 1977.

99. Sackner, M. A., et al.: Hypocalcemia in the presence of osteoplastic metastases. *New Eng. J. Med.* 262:173, 1960.

100. Ehrlich, M., et al.: Hypocalcemia, hypoparathyroidism and osteoblastic metastases. *Metabolism* 12:516, 1963.

101. Schwartz, G., and Meiser, J.: Veranderungen des calcium-phosphat Stoffwechsels bei einem Fal von osteoplastichen Metastasen mit Hypocalcemia. *Schweiz. Med. Wochenschr.* 92:1004, 1962.

102. Ludwig, G. R.: Hypocalcemia and hypophosphatemia accompanying osteoblastic osseous metastases: Studies of calcium and phosphate metabolism and parathyroid function. *Ann. Intern. Med.* 56:676, 1962.

103. Hall, T. C., et al.: Hypocalcemia — an unusual metabolic complication of breast cancer. *New Engl. J. Med.* 275:1474, 1966.

104. Zusman, J., et al.: Hyperphosphatemia, hyperphosphaturia and hypocalcemia in acute lymphoblastic leukemia. *New Eng. J. Med.* 289:1335, 1973.

105. Milhaud, G., et al.: Carcinoide sécrétant de la thyrocalcitonine. *C. R. Acad. Sci. (D)* Paris 270:2195, 1970.

106. Silva, O. L., et al.: Ectopic production of calcitonin. *Lancet* 2:317, 1973.

107. Coombes, R. C., et al.: Plasma-immunoreactive-calcitonin in patients with non-thyroid tumours. *Lancet* 1:1080, 1974.

108. Hillyard, C. J., et al.: Calcitonin in breast and lung cancer. *Clin. Endocrinol.* 5:1, 1976.

109. Schwartz, K., et al.: Calcitonin in non-thyroidal cancer. *J. Clin. Endocrinol. Metab.* 49:438, 1979.

110. Silva, O. L., et al.: Hypercalcitonemia in bronchogenic cancer. Evidence for thyroid origin of the hormone. *J.A.M.A.* 234:183, 1975.

111. Schwartz, W. D., et al.: A syndrome of renal sodium loss and hyponatremia probably resulting from inappropriate secretion of antidiuretic hormone. *Am. J. Med.* 23:529, 1957.

112. Bartter, F. C., and Schwartz, W. B.: The syndrome of inappropriate secretion of antidiuretic hormone. *Am. J. Med.* 42:790, 1967.

113. Amatruda, T. T., et al.: Carcinoma of the lung with inappropriate antidiuresis. *New Eng. J. Med.* 269:544, 1963.

114. Bower, B. V., and Mason, D. M.: *Clin Res.* 12:121, 1964 (abstract).

115. Vorherr, H., et al.: Antidiuretic principle in malignant tumor extracts from patients with inappropriate ADH syndrome. *J. Clin. Endocrinol. Metab.* 28:162, 1968.

116. George, J. M., et al.: Bio-synthesis of vasopressin *in vitro* and ultrastructure of a bronchogenic carcinoma. Patient with the syndrome of inappropriate secretion of antidiuretic hormone. *J. Clin. Invest.* 51:141, 1972.

117. Hirata, Y., et al.: Two cases of multiple hormone producing small cell carcinoma of the lung. *Cancer* 38:2575, 1976.

118. Hamilton, B. P. M., et al.: Evidence for the presence of neurophysin in tumours producing the syndrome of inappropriate antidiuresis. *J. Clin. Endocrinol. Metab.* 35:764, 1972.

119. North, W. G., et al.: Human neurophysins as potential tumor markers for small-cell carcinoma. *Clin. Res.* 26:536A, 1978.

120. Sellwood, R. A., et al.: Inappropriate secretion of antidiuretic hormone by carcinoma of the prostate. *Br. J. Surg.* 56:933, 1969.

121. Falchuk, K. R.: Inappropriate antidiuretic hormone-like syndrome as-

sociated with an adrenocortical carcinoma. *Am. J. Med. Sci.* 266:393, 1973.

122. Cassileth, P. A., and Trotman, B. W.: Inappropriate antidiuretic hormone in Hodgkin's disease. *Am. J. Med. Sci.* 265:233, 1973.

123. Gilby, E. D., et al.: Proc. Int. Symp. Biol. Charact. Hum. Tumours, 6th Copenhagen, 1975. In *Advances in Tumour Prevention, Detection and Characterization.* Vol. 3. Davis, W., and Maltoni, C. (eds.): New York, American Elsevier, 1976, p. 132.

124. Ginsberg, S. R., et al.: Syndrome of inappropriate antidiuretic hormone secretion in oat cell carcinoma of the lung. *Clin. Res.* 26:435A, 1978.

125. Dabek, J. T.: Bronchial carcinoid tumor with acromegaly in two patients. *J. Clin. Endocrinol. Metab.* 38:329, 1974.

126. Sonksen, P. H., et al.: Acromegaly caused by bronchial carcinoid tumors. *Clin. Endocrinol.* 5:503, 1976.

127. Leveston, S. A., et al.: Massive GH and ACTH hypersecretion associated with metastatic carcinoid tumor. *Program of the 60th Meeting of the Endocrine Society*, 1978, p. 341.

128. Southern, A. L.: Functioning metastatic bronchial carcinoid with elevated levels of serum and cerebrospinal fluid serotonin and pituitary adenoma. *J. Clin. Endocrinol. Metab.* 20:298, 1960.

129. Weiss, L., and Ingram, M.: Adenomatoid bronchial tumors: A consideration of the carcinoid tumors and the salivary tumors of the bronchial tree. *Cancer* 14:161, 1961.

130. Saeed uz Zafar, M., et al.: Acromegaly associated with bronchial carcinoid tumor: Evidence for ectopic production of growth hormone releasing activity. *J. Clin. Endocrinol. Metab.* 48:66, 1979.

131. Frohman, L. A., Szabo, M., Berelowitz, M., and Stachura, M. E.: Partial purification and characterization of a peptide with growth hormone releasing activity from extrapituitary tumors in patients with acromegaly. *J. Clin. Invest.* 65:43, 1980.

132. Steiner, H., et al.: Ectopic growth hormone production and osteoarthropathy in carcinoma of the bronchus. *Lancet* 1:783, 1968.

133. Cameron, D. P., et al.: On the presence of immunoreactive growth hormone in a bronchogenic carcinoma. *Aust. Ann. Med.* 18:143, 1969.

134. Sparagana, M., et al.: Ectopic growth hormone syndrome associated with lung cancer. *Metabolism* 20:730, 1971.

135. Beck, C., and Burger, H. G.: Evidence for the presence of immunoreactive growth hormone in cancers of the lung and stomach. *Cancer* 30:75, 1972.

136. Kaganowicz, A., et al.: Ectopic human growth hormone in ovaries and breast cancer. *J. Clin. Endocrinol. Metab.* 48:5, 1978.

137. Hammond, D., and Winnick, S.: Paraneoplastic erythrocytosis and ectopic erythropoietins. *Ann. N.Y. Acad. Sci.* 230:219, 1974.

138. Valentine, W. N., et al.: Polycythemia: erythrocytosis and erythremia. *Ann. Intern. Med.* 69:578, 1968.

139. Sulfrin, G., et al.: Hormones in renal cancer. *J. Urol.* 117:433, 1977.

140. Murphy, G. P., et al.: Erythropoietin levels in patients with Wilms' tumor. *N.Y. State J. Med.* 72:487, 1972.

141. Murphy, G. P., et al.: The value of erythropoietin assay in follow-up of Wilms' tumor patients. *Oncology* 33:154, 1976.

142. Waldman, T. A., and Rosse, W. F.: Tumors producing erythropoiesis-stimulating factors. In *Hemoglobin: Its Precursors and Metabolism.* Sunderman, F. W., and Sunderman, F. W., Jr. (eds.), Philadelphia, J. B. Lippincott Co., 1964, p. 276.

143. Zollinger, R. M., and Ellison, E. H.: Primary peptic ulcerations of the jejunum associated with islet cell tumors of the pancreas. *Ann. Surg.* 142:709, 1955.

144. McGuigan, J. E., and Trudeau, W. L.: Immunochemical measurement of elevated levels of gastrin in the serum of patients with pancreatic tumors of the Zollinger-Ellison variety. *New Eng. J. Med.* 278:1308, 1968.

145. Charters, A. C., et al.: Gastrin: Immunochemical properties and measurement by radioimmunoassay. *Surgery* 66:104, 1969.

146. Dockray, G. J., et al.: Relative abundance of big and little gastrins in the tumors of blood of patients with the Zollinger-Ellison syndrome. *Gut* 16:353, 1970.

147. Gregory, R. A.: Heterogeneity of gastrins in blood and tissue. *Ciba Found. Symp.* 41:251, 1975.

148. Walsh, J. H., and Grossman, M. T.: Gastrin. *New Eng. J. Med.* 292:1324, 1975.

149. Larsson, L. I., et al.: Mixed endocrine pancreatic tumors producing several peptide hormones. *Am. J. Pathol.* 79:271, 1975.

150. Larsson, L. I., et al.: Occurrence of human pancreatic polypeptide in pancreatic endocrine tumors. Possible implication in the watery diarrhea syndrome. *Am. J. Pathol.* 85:675, 1976.

151. Judge, D. M., et al.: Vasoactive intestinal polypeptide and gastrin producing islet cell carcinoma. *Arch Pathol. Lab. Med.* 101:262, 1977.

152. Friesen, S. R., et al.: Serum gastrin levels in malignant Zollinger-Ellison syndrome after total gastrectomy and hypophysectomy. *Ann. Surg.* 172:504, 1970.

153. Thompson, J. C., et al.: Clinical role of serum gastrin measurements in the Zollinger-Ellison syndrome. *Am. J. Surg.* 124:250, 1972.

154. Sanzenbacher, L. J., et al.: Prognostic implications of calcium mediated gastrin levels in the ulcerogenic syndrome. *Am. J. Surg.* 125:116, 1973.

155. Morrow, D. J., and Passaro, E., Jr.: Calcium infusion test before and after total gastrectomy in the Zollinger-Ellison syndrome. *Am. J. Surg.* 129:62, 1975.

156. Bradley, E. L., III, and Galambos, J. T.: Diagnosis of gastrinoma by the secretin suppression test. *Surg. Gynecol. Obstet.* 143:784, 1976.

157. Wilson, S. D., and DeCosse, J. J.: Surgical management of the Zollinger-Ellison syndrome. *Surg. Clin. North Am.* 54:395, 1974.

158. Zollinger, R. M., et al.: Observations on the postoperative tumor growth behavior of certain islet cell tumors. *Ann. Surg.* 184:525, 1976.

159. Hofman, J. E., et al.: Duodenal wall tumors and the Zollinger-Ellison syndrome, surgical management. *Arch. Surg.* 107:334, 1973.

160. Friesen, S. R.: Effect of gastrectomy on the Zollinger-Ellison tumor. Observations by second look procedures. *Surgery* 62:609, 1967.

161. Cryer, P. E., and Hill, G. J., II: Pancreatic islet cell carcinoma with hypercalcemia and hypergastrinemia: Response to streptozotocin. *Cancer* 38:2217, 1976.

162. Verner, J. V., and Morrison, A. B.: Islet cell tumor and a syndrome of refractory watery diarrhea and hypokalemia. *Am. J. Med.* 25:374, 1958.

163. Verner, J. V., and Morrison, A. B.: Endocrine pancreatic islet disease with diarrhea. *Arch. Intern. Med.* 133:392, 1974.

164. Said, S. I., and Faloona, G. R.: Elevated plasma and tissue levels of vasoactive intestinal polypeptide in the watery-diarrhea syndrome due to pancreatic, bronchogenic and other tumors. *New Engl. J. Med.* 293:155, 1975.

165. Gagel, R. F., et al.: Streptozotocin-treated Verner-Morrison syndrome: Plasma vasoactive intestinal peptide and tumor responses. *Arch. Intern. Med.* 136:1429, 1976.

166. Said, S. I.: Vasoactive intestinal polypeptide elevated plasma tissue levels in the watery-diarrhea syndrome due to pancreatic and other tumors. *Trans. Assoc. Am. Physicians* 88:87, 1975.

167. Jaffe, B. M., and Condon, S.: Prostaglandins E and F in endocrine diarrheagenic syndromes. *Ann. Surg.* 184:516, 1976.

168. Bradley, E. L., and Galambos, J. T.: Secretin and Zollinger-Ellison syndrome. *Lancet* 1:594, 1972.

169. Burkhardt, A.: The Verner-Morrison syndrome. The clinical picture and pathologic anatomy. *Klin. Wochenschr.* 54:1, 1976.

170. Schmett, M. G., Jr.: Watery diarrhea associated with pancreatic islet cell carcinoma. *Gastroenterology* 69:602, 1975.

171. Elias, E., et al.: Pancreatic cholera due to production of gastric inhibitory polypeptide. *Lancet* 2:791, 1972.

172. Fisher, J. A., et al.: *Clin. Res.* 21:623, 1973 (abstract).

173. Gleeson, M. H., et al.: Endocrine tumor in kidney affecting small bowel structure mobility and absorptive function. *Gut* 12:773, 1971.

174. Bloom, S. R.: An enteroglucagon tumor. *Gut* 13:520, 1972.

175. Ganda, O. T., et al.: Somatostatinoma: A somatostatin containing tumor of the endocrine pancreas. *New Eng. J. Med.* 296:963, 1977.

176. Larsson, L. I., et al.: Pancreatic somatostatinoma: Clinical features and physiological implications. *Lancet* 1:666, 1977.

177. McGavran, W. H., et al.: A glucagon-secreting alpha-cell carcinoma of the pancreas. *New Eng. J. Med.* 274:1408, 1966.

INDEX

Page numbers in *italics* refer to illustrations. Page numbers followed by the letter *t* refer to tables.

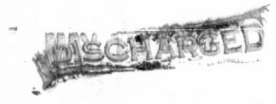

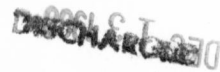